# Environmental & Occupational Medicine

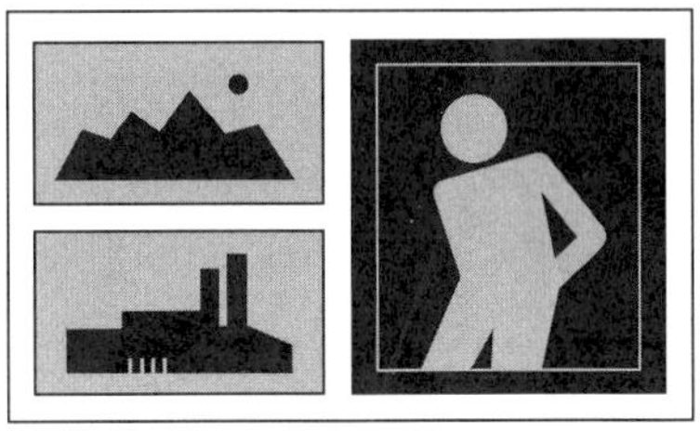

Third Edition

# Environmental & Occupational Medicine

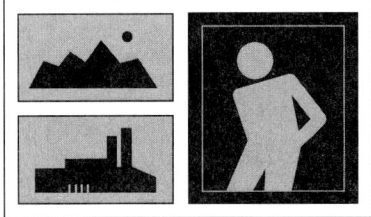

Third Edition

EDITED BY

**WILLIAM N. ROM, M.D., M.P.H.**
*Professor and Chief*
*Division of Pulmonary and Critical Care Medicine*
*Departments of Medicine and Environmental Medicine*
*Director*
*Chest Service*
*Bellevue Hospital Center*
*New York University Medical Center*
*New York, New York*



Lippincott - Raven
PUBLISHERS
Philadelphia • New York

Acquisitions Editor: Joyce-Rachel John
Developmental Editor: Lesa E. Ramsey
Manufacturing Manager: Dennis Teston
Production Manager: Kathleen Bubbeo
Production Editor: Jeffrey Gruenglas
Cover and Logo Design: David Levy
Indexer: Mary Kidd
Compositor: Lippincott–Raven Desktop Division
Printer: Kingsport Press



Printed in the United States of America

9 8 7 6 5 4 3 2 1

**Library of Congress Cataloging-in-Publication Data**

Environmental and occupational medicine / edited by William N. Rom.—
3rd ed.
p. cm.
Includes bibliographical references and index.
ISBN 0-316-75578-8
1. Medicine. Industrial. 2. Environmental toxicology.
3. Environmental health.
[DNLM 1. Occupational Medicine. 2. Environmental Medicine.
3. Occupational Diseases—prevention & control. -WA 400 E61 1998]
RC963.E58 1998
616.9′8--dc21
DNLM/DLC
for Library of Congress 97-42366
CIP

Care has been taken to confirm the accuracy of the information presented and to describe generally accepted practices. However, the authors, editors, and publisher are not responsible for errors or omissions or for any consequences from application of the information in this book and make no warranty, expressed or implied, with respect to the contents of the publication.

The authors, editors, and publisher have exerted every effort to ensure that drug selection and dosage set forth in this text are in accordance with current recommendations and practice at the time of publication. However, in view of ongoing research, changes in government regulations, and the constant flow of information relating to drug therapy and drug reactions, the reader is urged to check the package insert for each drug for any change in indications and dosage and for added warnings and precautions. This is particularly important when the recommended agent is a new or infrequently employed drug.

Some drugs and medical devices presented in this publication have Food and Drug Administration (FDA) clearance for limited use in restricted research settings. It is the responsibility of the health care provider to ascertain the FDA status of each drug or device planned for use in their clinical practice.

*To my wife, Holly, my daughters, Nicole and Meredith,*
*my parents, and the many contributors*
*who make the Earth a greener place*

# Contents

**Other Organ Systems**

## SECTION II: ENVIRONMENTAL AND OCCUPATIONAL EXPOSURES

### Metals



### Organic Chemicals

**Radiation**



**Physical Environment**

**Personal and General Environment**



## SECTION III: CONTROL OF ENVIRONMENTAL AND OCCUPATIONAL DISEASES AND EXPOSURES

# Contributors

**Fred K. Alavi, Ph.D.**
*Assistant Professor*
*Department of Internal Medicine*
*University of South Dakota School of Medicine; and*
*The Royal C. Johnson Veterans Memorial Hospital*
*1400 West 22nd Street*
*Sioux Falls, South Dakota 57105*

**Timothy E. Albertson, M.D.**
*Professor of Medicine and of Medical Pharmacology and Toxicology; and*
*Chief*
*Division of Pulmonary Critical Care Medicine*
*University of California, Davis*
*Davis, California 95616*

**Robert W. Amler, M.D.**
*Clinical Professor*
*Emory University Center School of Medicine*
*Agency for Toxic Substances and Disease Registry*
*U.S. Department of Health and Human Services*
*Atlanta, Georgia 30333*

**W. Kent Anger, M.A., Ph.D.**
*Senior Scientist*
*Center for Research on Occupational and Environmental Toxicology*
*Oregon Health Sciences University*
*3181 Southwest Sam Jackson Park Road, CROET-L606*
*Portland, Oregon 97201-3098*

**Nicholas A. Ashford, Ph.D., J.D.**
*Professor of Technology and Policy*
*School of Engineering*
*Massachusetts Institute of Technology*
*77 Massachusetts Avenue, Room E 40-239*
*Cambridge, Massachusetts 02139*

**Michael D. Attfield, Ph.D.**
*Epidemiologist*
*Epidemiology Investigations Branch*
*National Institute for Occupational Safety and Health*
*Morgantown, West Virginia 26505-2888*

**Dean B. Baker, M.D., M.P.H.**
*Professor and Director*
*Department of Medicine*
*Center for Occupational and Environmental Health*
*University of California, Irvine*
*19722 MacArthur Boulevard*
*Irvine, California 92612*

**Marvin R. Balaan, M.D.**
*Associate Professor of Medicine*
*Section of Pulmonary and Critical Care Medicine*
*Department of Medicine; and*
*Medical Director*
*Respiratory Care and Pulmonary Function Laboratory*
*Robert C. Byrd Health Sciences Center*
*West Virginia University School of Medicine*
*Morgantown, West Virginia 26506-9166*

**Daniel E. Banks, M.D.**
*N. LeRoy Lapp Professor of Medicine, and Chief*
*Section of Pulmonary and Critical Care Medicine*
*Department of Medicine*
*Robert C. Byrd Health Sciences Center*
*West Virginia University School of Medicine*
*Room G280, HSS*
*Morgantown, West Virginia 26506-9166*

**Scott Barnhart, M.D., M.P.H.**
*Associate Professor of Medicine and Environmental Health*
*Department of Medicine*
*University of Washington/Harborview Medical Center*
*325 Ninth Avenue*
*Seattle, Washington 98104*

**William S. Beckett, M.D., M.P.H.**
*Professor*
*Department of Environmental Medicine*
*University of Rochester School of Medicine and Dentistry*
*575 Elmwood Avenue, P.O. Box EHSC*
*Rochester, New York 14642*

**Margaret R. Becklake, M.D., F.R.C.P.**
*Professor Emeritus*
*Department of Medicine and the Joint Departments of Epidemiology and Biostatistics and of Occupational Health*
*McGill University*
*Montréal, Québec H3A 1A3*
*Canada*

**Renate Belville, M.A.**
*Research Assistant Professor*
*Department of Community and Preventive Medicine*
*Mt. Sinai Medical Center*
*One Gustave L. Levy Place*
*New York, New York 10029-6574*

**Paul David Blanc, M.D., M.S.P.H.**
*Associate Professor of Medicine*
*Division of Occupational and Environmental Medicine*
*Department of Medicine*
*University of California, San Francisco*
*350 Parnassus Avenue, Suite 609*
*San Francisco, California 94117*

**Margit L. Bleecker, M.D., Ph.D.**
*Director*
*Center for Occupational and Environmental Neurology*
*Children's Hospital*
*3901 Greenspring Avenue, Suite 101*
*Baltimore, Maryland 21211-1398*

**Jeff Boyd, Ph.D.**
*Associate Attending Biologist*
*Departments of Surgery and Human Genetics*
*Memorial Sloan-Kettering Cancer Center*
*1275 York Avenue*
*New York, New York 10021*

**Paul W. Brandt-Rauf, M.D., Sc.D., Ph.D.**
*Professor*
*Division of Environmental Health Sciences*
*Columbia University School of Public Health*
*60 Haven Avenue B-1*
*New York, New York 10032*

**Arnold R. Brody, Ph.D.**
*Professor*
*Department of Pathology*
*Tulane University Medical Center*
*1430 Tulane Avenue*
*New Orleans, Louisiana 70112*

**Stuart M. Brooks, M.D.**
*Professor of Medicine and Public Health*
*Department of Environmental and Occupational Health*
*College of Public Health*
*University of South Florida*
*13201 Bruce B. Downs Boulevard*
*Tampa, Florida 33612-3805*

**Luz Claudio, Ph.D.**
*Assistant Professor*
*Department of Environmental and Occupational Medicine*
*Mt. Sinai Medical Center*
*One Gustave L. Levy Place*
*New York, New York 10029*

**Beverly S. Cohen, Ph.D.**
*Professor*
*Department of Environmental Medicine*
*New York University Medical Center*
*57 Old Forge Road*
*Tuxedo, New York 10987*

**David E. Cohen, M.D., M.P.H.**
*Assistant Professor*
*Departments of Dermatology and of Occupational and Environmental Dermatology*
*New York University Medical Center*
*550 First Avenue*
*New York, New York 10016*

**Mitchell D. Cohen, M.S., Ph.D.**
*Research Assistant Professor*
*Department of Environmental Medicine*
*New York University Medical Center*
*57 Old Forge Road*
*Tuxedo, New York 10987*

**Theo Colborn, Ph.D.**
*Senior Conservation Scientist*
*Wildlife and Contaminants Program*
*World Wildlife Fund*
*1250 Twenty-Fourth Street Northwest*
*Washington, D.C. 20037-1175*

**Michael J. Colligan, Ph.D.**
*Acting Chief*
*Education and Information Division*
*National Institute for Occupational Safety and Health*
*4676 Columbia Parkway, Mail Stop C-11*
*Cincinnati, Ohio 45226*

**Yvon Cormier, M.D.**
*Professor*
*Department of Medicine*
*Hospital and Université Laval*
*2725 Chemin Ste. Foy*
*Ste. Foy, Québec GIV 4G5*
*Canada*

**Max Costa, Ph.D.**
*Professor and Chairman*
*Department of Environmental Medicine and*
*Professor*
*Department of Pharmacology*
*New York University Medical Center*
*550 First Avenue*
*New York, New York 10016*

**Molly J. Coye, M.D., M.P.H.**
*Vice President*
*The Lewin Group*
*425 Market Street, 16th Floor*
*San Francisco, California 94105*

**Rafael E. de la Hoz, M.D., M.P.H.**
*Attending Physician*
*Chest Service and Occupational Medicine Clinic*
*Bellevue Hospital Center*
*New York University Medical Center*
*462 First Avenue, Room CD349*
*New York, New York 10016*

**Kathleen A. Delaney, M.D.**
*Associate Professor*
*Division of Emergency Medicine*
*University of Texas Southwestern Medical Center*
*5323 Harry Hines Boulevard*
*Dallas, Texas 75235-8579*

**Robert B. Devlin, M.D., Ph.D.**
*Chief*
*Clinical Research Branch*
*National Health and Environmental Effects Research Laboratory*
*U.S. Environmental Protection Agency*
*Maildrop 58D*
*Research Triangle Park, North Carolina 27711*

**Kevin D. Dieckhaus, M.D.**
*Assistant Professor*
*Division of Infectious Diseases*
*Department of Medicine*
*University of Connecticut Health Center*
*263 Farmington Avenue*
*Farmington, Connecticut 06030-3212*

**Douglas W. Dockery, Sc.D.**
*Associate Professor of Environmental Epidemiology*
*Department of Environmental Health*
*Harvard University School of Public Health*
*665 Huntington Avenue*
*Boston, Massachusetts 02115*

**Dana C. Drew, B.S.N.**
*Consultant*
*Occupational Medicine Practice*
*3240 Clifford Circle*
*Pleasanton, California 94588*

**Alan M. Ducatman, M.S., M.D.**
*Professor and Chairman*
*Department of Community Medicine*
*Institute of Occupational and Environmental Health*
*West Virginia University School of Medicine*
*Morgantown, West Virginia 26506-9190*

**David L. Eaton, Ph.D.**
*Professor*
*Department of Environmental Health*
*University of Washington*
*4225 Roosevelt Way Northeast, Suite 100*
*Seattle, Washington 98105-6099*

**Alan L. Engelberg, M.D., M.P.H.**
*Clinical Professor*
*Department of Community and Family Medicine*
*St. Louis University School of Medicine*
*1402 South Grand*
*St. Louis, Missouri 63104*

**Paul R. Epstein, M.D., M.P.H.**
*Associate Director*
*Center for Health and the Global Environment*
*Harvard Medical School*
*Oliver Wendell Holmes Society, Room 263*
*260 Longwood Avenue*
*Boston, Massachusetts 02115*

**Hugh L. Evans, Ph.D.**
*Professor of Environmental Medicine*
*Nelson Institute*
*New York University Medical Center*
*550 First Avenue*
*New York, New York 10016*

**Henry Falk, M.D., M.P.H.**
*Director*
*Division of Environmental Hazards and Health Effects*
*National Center for Environmental Health*
*Centers for Disease Control and Prevention*
*4770 Buford Highway, Northeast*
*Atlanta, Georgia 30341-3724*

**Federico M. Farin, M.D.**
*Research Scientist*
*Department of Environmental Health*
*University of Washington*
*4225 Roosevelt Way Northeast, #100*
*Seattle, Washington 98105-6099*

**Kevin J. Farley, Ph.D.**
*Associate Professor*
*Department of Environmental Engineering*
*Manhattan College*
*Riverdale, New York 10471*

**Jean Spencer Felton, M.D.**
*Clinical Professor*
*Department of Medicine*
*University of California, Irvine;*
*Clinical Professor Emeritus*
*Department of Preventive Medicine*
*University of Southern California*
*Los Angeles; and*
*45150 Cypress Drive, P.O. Box 246*
*Mendocino, California 95460*

**Lawrence J. Fine, M.D., Ph.D.**
*Director*
*Division of Surveillance, Hazard Evaluations, and Field Studies*
*National Institute for Occupational Safety and Health*
*Centers for Disease Control and Prevention*
*4676 Columbia Parkway, Mail Stop R-12*
*Cincinnati, Ohio 45226-1998*

**Alf Fischbein, M.D.**
*Director*
*Department of Life Sciences*
*Division of Environmental and Occupational Health*
*Bar-Ilan University*
*Ramat-Gan 52900; and*
*Department of Research and Development for Occupational and Environmental Health*
*Sanz Medical Center–Laniado Hospital*
*Netanya 42150*
*Israel*

**Mark W. Frampton, M.D.**
*Professor*
*Divisions of Pulmonary/Critical Care and Occupational Medicine*
*Departments of Medicine and Environmental Medicine*
*University of Rochester Medical Center*
*601 Elmwood Avenue, Box 692*
*Rochester, New York 14642*

**George Friedman-Jiménez, M.D.**
*Research Assistant Professor*
*Department of Environmental Medicine and Medicine*
*Bellevue Hospital Center*
*New York University Medical Center*
*462 First Avenue, Room CD349*
*New York, New York 10016*

**Gary D. Gackstetter, D.V.M., M.P.H., Ph.D.**
*Office of the Assistant Secretary of Defense for Health Affairs*
*Department of Defense*
*The Pentagon*
*Defense Drive, Room 3D-366*
*Washington, D.C. 20301-1200*

**Stuart M. Garay, M.D.**
*Clinical Professor of Medicine*
*Division of Pulmonary and Critical Care Medicine*
*New York University Medical Center*
*550 First Avenue*
*New York, New York 10016*

**Richard A. Garibaldi, M.D.**
*Professor*
*Department of Medicine*
*University of Connecticut Health Center*
*263 Farmington Avenue*
*Farmington, Connecticut 06030-3945*

**Seymour J. Garte, Ph.D.**
*Professor*
*Department of Environmental Medicine*
*New York University Medical Center*
*550 First Avenue*
*New York, New York 10016*

**Fredric Gerr, M.D.**
*Associate Professor*
*Division of Environmental and Occupational Health*
*Rollins School of Public Health*
*Emory University*
*1518 Clifton Road*
*Atlanta, Georgia 30322*

**Lewis R. Goldfrank, M.D.**
*Associate Professor*
*Department of Emergency Medicine*
*Bellevue Hospital Center*
*New York University Medical Center; and*
*New York City Poison Center*
*462 First Avenue*
*New York, New York 10016*

**Michael D. Goldstein, M.D., M.P.H.**
*Adjunct Assistant Professor*
*Division of Environmental Health Sciences*
*Columbia University School of Public Health*
*60 Haven Avenue*
*New York, New York 10032*

**Leslie C. Grammer, M.D.**
*Professor*
*Department of Medicine*
*Northwestern University School of Medicine*
*303 East Chicago Avenue*
*Chicago, Illinois 60611*

**Peter D. Griffin, M.D., M.P.H.**
*Corporate Medical Consultant*
*8 Burnham Hill*
*Westport, Connecticut 06880*

**John D. Groopman, Ph.D.**
*Professor*
*Department of Environmental Health Sciences*
*The Johns Hopkins University*
*615 North Wolfe Street*
*Baltimore, Maryland 21205*

**Tee Lamont Guidotti, M.D., M.P.H.**
*Professor of Occupational and Environmental Medicine*
*Department of Public Health Sciences*
*Occupational Health Program*
*University of Alberta*
*13-103 Clinical Science Building*
*Edmonton, Alberta T6G 2G3*
*Canada*

**Janet Guthrie, M.P.A.**
*Program Analyst*
*Office of Policy, Planning, and Evaluation*
*National Institute of Environmental Health Sciences*
*Research Triangle Park, North Carolina 27709-2233*

**William E. Halperin, M.D.**
*Deputy Director*
*Division of Safety Research*
*National Institute for Occupational Safety and Health*
*1095 Willowdale Road*
*Morgantown, West Virginia 26505-2888*

**Manny Halpern, M.A., C.P.E.**
*Adjunct Assistant Professor*
*Occupational and Industrial Orthopaedic Center*
*New York University Medical Center*
*550 First Avenue*
*New York, New York 10016*

**Philip Harber, M.D., M.P.H.**
*Director and Professor*
*Occupational and Environmental Medicine Program*
*Department of Medicine*
*University of California, Los Angeles*
*10911 Weyburn Avenue, #344*
*Los Angeles, California 90095*

**Curtis C. Harris, M.D.**
*Chief*
*Laboratory of Human Carcinogenesis*
*National Cancer Institute*
*National Institutes of Health*
*Building 37, Room 2C01*
*Bethesda, Maryland 20892-4255*

**John G. Hay, M.D.**
*Assistant Professor*
*Departments of Medicine and Pathology*
*New York University Medical Center*
*550 First Avenue, Bellevue 7N-24*
*New York, New York 10016*

**Stephen S. Hecht, Ph.D.**
*Professor of Cancer Prevention*
*University of Minnesota Cancer Center*
*420 Deleware Street Southeast, Box 806 Mayo*
*Minneapolis, Minnesota 55455*

**Clyde Hertzman, M.D., M.Sc.**
*Professor of Medicine*
*Department of Health Care and Epidemiology*
*University of British Columbia*
*5804 Fairview Avenue*
*Vancouver, British Columbia V6T 1Z3*
*Canada*

**Rudi Hiebert, M.A.**
*Epidemiologist*
*Department of Orthopaedics*
*New York University Medical Center; and*
*Acting Director*
*Musculoskeletal Epidemiology Unit*
*Hospital for Joint Diseases*
*301 East 17th Street*
*New York, New York 10016*

**Debie J. Hoivik, Ph.D.**
*Postdoctoral Research Associate*
*Department of Veterinary Physiology and Pharmacology*
*Texas A&M University*
*College Station, Texas 77843-4466*

**John Howard, M.D., J.D.**
*Chief*
*Division of Occupational Safety and Health*
*California Department of Industrial Relations*
*45 Fremont Street, Suite 1200*
*San Francisco, California 94105*

**Hongwei Hsiao, Ph.D.**
*Chief*
*Division of Safety Research*
*National Institute for Occupational Safety and Health*
*1095 Willowdale Road*
*Morgantown, West Virginia 26505-2888*

**Joseph J. Hurrell, Jr., Ph.D.**
*Associate Director for Science*
*Division of Surveillance, Hazard Evaluations, and Field Studies*
*National Institute for Occupational Safety and Health*
*4676 Columbia Parkway*
*Cincinnati, Ohio 45226*

**S. Perwez Hussain, Ph.D.**
*Fellow*
*Laboratory of Human Carcinogenesis*
*National Cancer Institute*
*National Institutes of Health*
*37 Convent Drive*
*Bethesda, Maryland 20892-4255*

**Kenneth C. Hyams, M.D., M.P.H.**
*Head*
*Epidemiology Division*
*Naval Medical Research Institute*
*8901 Wisconsin Avenue*
*Bethesda, Maryland 20889-5607*

**Elizabeth A. Jennison, M.D., M.P.H.**
*Physician, Occupational Medicine*
*Excel Corporate Care Clinic*
*4220 Grand Avenue*
*Middletown, Ohio 45044*

**Stephen C. Joseph, M.D.**
*Deputy Assistant*
*Office of the Assistant Secretary of Defense for Health Affairs*
*Department of Defense*
*The Pentagon*
*360 Pentagon, Mailstop C24*
*Washington, D.C. 20301-1200*

**Agnes B. Kane, M.D., Ph.D.**
*Professor and Chair*
*Department of Pathology and Laboratory Medicine*
*Brown University School of Medicine*
*Biomedical Center, Box G-B529*
*Providence, Rhode Island 02912*

**Shona J. Kelly, M.D.**
*Research Scientist*
*Department of Health Care and Epidemiology*
*University of British Columbia*
*5804 Fairview Avenue*
*Vancouver, British Columbia V6T 1Z3*
*Canada*

**Karl T. Kelsey, M.D., MOH**
*Associate Professor of Occupational Medicine and Radiobiology*
*Department of Cancer Cell Biology; and*
*Occupational Health Program*
*Department of Environmental Health*
*Harvard School of Public Health*
*665 Huntington Avenue*
*Boston, Massachusetts 02115-9957*

**Kaye H. Kilburn, M.D.**
*Ralph Edgington Professor of Medicine*
*Department of Internal Medicine*
*University of Southern California School of Medicine*
*2025 Zonal Avenue*
*Los Angeles, California 90033*

**Joel N. Kline, M.D.**
*Assistant Professor*
*Divisions of Pulmonary and Critical Care and Occupational Medicine*
*Department of Internal Medicine*
*University of Iowa College of Medicine*
*200 Hawkins Drive*
*Iowa City, Iowa 52242*

**Kathleen Kreiss, M.D.**
*Chief*
*Epidemiology Investigations Branch*
*Division of Respiratory Disease Studies*
*National Institute for Occupational Safety and Health*
*1095 Willowdale Road, Mailstop 234*
*Morgantown, West Virginia 26505*

**Bruce P. Krieger, M.D.**
*Professor*
*Division of Pulmonary Medicine*
*University of Miami School of Medicine; and*
*Mt. Sinai Medical Center*
*4300 Alton Road*
*Miami Beach, Florida 33140*

**Joseph LaDou, M.S., M.D.**
*Clinical Professor*
*Division of Occupational and Environmental Medicine*
*Department of Medicine*
*University of California School of Medicine*
*350 Parnassus Avenue, Suite 609*
*San Francisco, California 94143-0924*

**William E. Lambert, Ph.D.**
*Research Associate Professor*
*Epidemiology and Cancer Control Program/ New Mexico Tumor Registry*
*University of New Mexico Health Sciences Center*
*2325 Camino de Salud, Northeast*
*Albuquerque, New Mexico 87131-5306*

**Anthony D. LaMontagne, D.Sc., M.A., M.Ed.**
*Instructor*
*Occupational Health Program*
*Department of Environmental Health*
*Harvard School of Public Health; and*
*Senior Research Scientist*
*New England Research Institutes*
*9 Galen Street*
*Watertown, Massachusetts 02172*

**Philip J. Landrigan, M.D., M.Sc.**
*Ethel H. Wise Professor and Chairman*
*Division of Environmental and Occupational Medicine*
*Department of Community and Preventive Medicine*
*Mt. Sinai School of Medicine*
*One Gustave L. Levy Place, Box 1057*
*New York, New York 10029-6574*

**Robert C. Larsen, M.D., M.P.H.**
*Associate Clinical Professor*
*Department of Psychiatry*
*Center for Occupational Psychiatry*
*University of California, San Francisco*
*690 Market Street, Suite 706*
*San Francisco, California 94104*

**Alexander Leaf, M.D.**
*Jackson Professor Emeritus of Clinical Medicine*
*Department of Medicine*
*Massachusetts General Hospital*
*Harvard Medical School*
*149 Thirteenth Street, Room 4001*
*Charlestown, Massachusetts 02129*

**Grace Kawas Lemasters, Ph.D.**
*Professor*
*Divisions of Environmental Health and Epidemiology*
*Department of Environmental Health*
*University of Cincinnati Medical Center*
*231 Bethesda Avenue*
*Cincinnati, Ohio 45267-0182*

**Richard Letz, Ph.D**
*Associate Professor*
*Department of Behavioral Science and Health Education*
*Rollins School of Public Health*
*Emory University*
*1718 Clifton Road*
*Atlanta, Georgia 30322*

**Stephen M. Levin, M.D.**
*Assistant Professor*
*Department of Community and Preventive Medicine*
*Mt. Sinai Medical Center*
*One Gustave L. Levy Place, Box 1057*
*New York, New York 10029-6574*

**Gene E. Likens, Ph.D.**
*Ecologist*
*Institute of Ecosystem Studies*
*Sharon Turnpike*
*Millbrook, New York 12545*

**Ruth Lilis, M.D.**
*Professor Emeritus, Occupational and Environmental Medicine*
*Department of Community and Preventive Medicine*
*Mt. Sinai Medical Center*
*One Gustave L. Levy Place*
*New York, New York 10029-6574*

**Soo-Yee Lim, Ph.D.**
*Research Psychologist*
*Applied Psychology and Ergonomics Branch*
*National Institute for Occupational Safety and Health*
*4676 Columbia Parkway, MS C-24*
*Cincinnati, Ohio 45226-1998*

**Morton Lippmann, Ph.D.**
*Professor*
*Department of Environmental Medicine*
*New York University Medical Center*
*57 Old Forge Road*
*Tuxedo, New York 10987*

**Dominique F. Lison, M.D., M.I.H., Ph.D.**
*Professor of Toxicology*
*Industrial Toxicology and Occupational Medicine Unit*
*Catholic University of Louvain*
*Clos Chapelle-Aux-Champs, 30.54*
*Brussels 1200*
*Belgium*

**James E. Lockey, M.D., M.S.**
*Professor*
*Department of Environmental Health*
*University of Cincinnati College of Medicine*
*231 Bethesda Avenue (ML 0182)*
*Cincinnati, Ohio 45267-0182*

**Richard F. Lockey, M.D., M.S.**
*Professor*
*Department of Environmental Health*
*University of Cincinnati College of Medicine*
*231 Bethesda Avenue (ML0182)*
*Cincinnati, Ohio 45267-0182*

**Samuel Louie, M.D.**
*Associate Professor of Clinical Internal Medicine*
*Division of Pulmonary and Critical Care Medicine*
*Department of Internal Medicine*
*University of California, Davis*
*Davis, California 95616*

**Emily F. Madden, B.S., M.T.**
*Graduate Research Assistant*
*Department of Toxicology*
*University of Maryland School of Medicine*
*West Redwood Street*
*Baltimore, Maryland 21227*

**David A. Maddox, Ph.D.**
*Professor*
*Department of Internal Medicine*
*University of South Dakota School of Medicine; and*
*The Royal C. Johnson Veterans Memorial Hospital*
*1400 West Twenty-Second Street*
*Sioux Falls, South Dakota 57105*

**Lisa A. Maier, M.D.**
*Instructor/Fellow*
*Department of Medicine*
*Division of Pulmonary and Critical Care Medicine*
*University of Colorado Health Sciences Center; and*
*Division of Environmental and Occupational Health Sciences*
*National Jewish Medical and Research Center*
*1400 Jackson Street, G114*
*Denver, Colorado 80207*

**Douglas W. Mapel, M.D., M.P.H.**
*Assistant Professor*
*Department of Epidemiology and Cancer Control*
*University of New Mexico*
*2325 Camino de Salud, Northeast*
*Albuquerque, New Mexico 87131-5306*

**Martin H. Markowitz, M.D.**
*Assistant Professor*
*Aaron Diamond AIDS Research Center*
*Rockefeller University*
*455 First Avenue, 7th Floor*
*New York, New York 10024*

**Steven B. Markowitz, M.D.**
*Associate Professor*
*Department of Community and Preventive Medicine*
*Mt. Sinai School of Medicine*
*Basic Science Building*
*One Gustave L. Levy Place, Box 1057*
*New York, New York 10029-6574*

**Gary M. Marsh, M.S., Ph.D.**
*Professor*
*Department of Biostatistics*
*Graduate School of Public Health*
*University of Pittsburgh*
*130 DeSoto Street*
*Pittsburgh, Pennsylvania 15261*

**Leonard N. Matheson, Ph.D.**
*Director*
*Work Performance Laboratory*
*Department of Occupational Therapy*
*Washington University School of Medicine*
*4444 Forest Park Avenue*
*St. Louis, Missouri 63108*

**Edward C. Mathews, M.D.**
*Department of Internal Medicine*
*Wilford Hall Medical Center*
*2200 Berquist Drive, Suite 1*
*Lackland Air Force Base, Texas 78236-5300*

**Michael McCann, Ph.D, C.I.H.**
*President*
*Center for Safety in the Arts*
*77 Seventh Avenue, #PHG*
*New York, New York 10011*

**Roger O. McClellan, D.V.M.**
*President and CEO*
*Chemical Industry Institute of Toxicology*
*6 Davis Drive*
*Research Triangle Park, North Carolina 27709*

**Robert J. McCunney, M.D., M.P.H.**
*Director*
*Environmental Medical Services*
*Massachusetts Institute of Technology*
*77 Massachusetts Avenue, 20B-238*
*Cambridge, Massachusetts 02139*

**Ross A. McKinnon, Ph.D.**
*Senior Lecturer*
*School of Pharmacy and Medical Sciences*
*University of South Australia*
*Adelaide, South Australia 5000*
*Australia*

**Louise N. Mehler, M.D.**
*Program Director*
*California Pesticide Illness Surveillance Program*
*University of California, Davis*
*Davis, California 95616*

**Myron A. Mehlman, Ph.D.**
*Adjunct Professor*
*Department of Environmental and Community Medicine*
*University of Medicine and Dentistry of New Jersey–Robert Wood Johnson Medical School*
*681 Frelinghuysen Road*
*Piscataway, New Jersey 08855*

**James M. Melius, M.D., Ph.D.**
*Director*
*New York State Laborer's Health and Safety Trust Fund*
*18 Corporate Woods Boulevard*
*Albany, New York 12211*

**James A. Merchant, M.D., Ph.D.**
*Professor*
*Departments of Preventive Medicine and Internal Medicine; and*
*Department Head*
*Department of Preventive Medicine and Environmental Health*
*Institute for Rural and Environmental Health*
*The University of Iowa College of Medicine*
*100 Oakdale Campus, 126 IREH*
*Iowa City, Iowa 52242-5000*

**John D. Meyer, M.D., M.P.H.**
*Assistant Professor*
*Institute of Occupational and Environmental Health*
*West Virginia University School of Medicine*
*Box 9190*
*Morgantown, West Virginia 26506-9190*

**Jeffrey G. Miller, LL.B.**
*Professor*
*Pace University School of Law*
*Center for Environmental Legal Studies*
*78 North Broadway*
*White Plains, New York 10603*

**Clifford S. Mitchell, M.D., M.S., M.P.H.**
*Assistant Professor of Environmental Health Sciences*
*Department of Environmental Health Sciences*
*The Johns Hopkins University School of Hygiene and Public Health*
*615 North Wolfe Street, Room 7041*
*Baltimore, Maryland 21205*

**Frank L. Mitchell, D.O., M.P.H.**
*Adjunct Associate Professor*
*Department of Environmental and Occupational Health*
*Emory University School of Public Health*
*412 Glencastle Drive Northwest*
*Atlanta, Georgia 30327*

**Luisa T. Molina, Ph.D.**
*Research Scientist*
*Department of Earth, Atmospheric and Planetary Sciences*
*Massachusetts Institute of Technology*
*77 Massachusetts Avenue, Room 54-1812*
*Cambridge, Massachusetts 02139*

**Mario J. Molina, Ph.D. (Nobel laureate)**
*Institute Professor*
*Department of Earth, Atmospheric and Planetary Sciences*
*Massachusetts Institute of Technology*
*77 Massachusetts Avenue, Room 54-1814*
*Cambridge, Massachusetts 02139*

**Gilbert F. Morris, Ph.D.**
*Assistant Professor*
*Department of Pathology and Laboratory Medicine*
*Tulane University Medical Center*
*1430 Tulane Avenue*
*New Orleans, Louisiana 70118*

**Lawrence R. Murphy, Ph.D.**
*Applied Psychology and Ergonomics Branch*
*National Institute for Occupational Safety and Health*
*Centers for Disease Control and Prevention*
*U.S. Public Health Service*
*4676 Columbia Parkway, Mailstop C24*
*Cincinnati, Ohio 45226*

**Piero Mustacchi, M.D., D.Sc. (Honorary)**
*Clinical Professor of Medicine and Epidemiology*
*Department of Epidemiology and Biostatistics and of Medicine*
*School of Medicine*
*University of California, San Francisco*
*San Francisco, California 94143-0560*

**Daniel W. Nebert, M.D.**
*Professor*
*Department of Environmental Health*
*University of Cincinnati Medical Center*
*P.O. Box 670056*
*Cincinnati, Ohio 45267-0056*

**Robert P. Nelson, Jr., M.D.**
*Director*
*Division of Allergy and Clinical Immunology*
*Departments of Medicine and Pediatrics*
*University of South Florida College of Medicine/All Children's Hospital*
*1300 Bruce B. Downs Boulevard (111D)*
*St. Petersburg, Florida 33701*

**Lee S. Newman, M.D.**
*Associate Professor*
*Department of Preventive Medicine and Biometrics*
*University of Colorado Health Sciences Center; and*
*Director, Division of Environmental and Health Sciences*
*National Jewish Medical and Research Center*
*1400 Jackson Street, G010*
*Denver, Colorado 80206*

**Anthony J. Newman-Taylor, M.B., M.Sc.**
*Professor*
*Department of Occupational and Environmental Medicine*
*Royal Brompton Hospital*
*Sydney Street*
*London SW3 6NP*
*England*

**William J. Nicholson, Ph.D.**
*Professor*
*Division of Environmental and Occupational Medicine*
*Department of Community and Preventive Medicine*
*Mt. Sinai School of Medicine*
*One Gustave L. Levy Place*
*New York, New York 10022*

**Margareta Nordin, P.T., D.Sc.**
*Director*
*Occupational and Industrial Orthopaedic Center*
*Hospital for Joint Diseases;*
*Program Director*
*Program of Ergonomics and Biomechanics; and*
*Research Associate Professor*
*Department of Environmental Medicine*
*New York University Medical Center*
*63 Downing Street*
*New York, New York 10014*

**Kenneth Olden, Ph.D.**
*Director*
*National Institute of Environmental Health Sciences and National Toxicology Program*
*National Institutes of Health*
*111 TX Alexander Drive, South Campus*
*Research Triangle Park, North Carolina 27709-2233*

**L. Christine Oliver, M.S., M.D., M.P.H.**
*Assistant Professor of Medicine*
*Department of Medical Services*
*Pulmonary and Critical Care Unit*
*Massachusetts General Hospital; and*
*Harvard Medical School*
*98 North Washington Street, Suite 207*
*Boston, Massachusetts 02114*

**Randall J. Olson, M.D.**
*Professor and Chairman*
*Department of Ophthalmology*
*John A. Moran Eye Center*
*University of Utah Hospital*
*50 North Medical Drive*
*Salt Lake City, Utah 84132*

**Edward B. O'Malley, Ph.D.**
*Adjunct Assistant Professor*
*Division of Pulmonary and Critical Care Medicine*
*New York University Medical Center*
*550 First Avenue*
*New York, New York 10016; and*
*Norwalk Hospital Sleep Disorders Center*
*Norwalk, Connecticut 06856*

**Gilbert S. Omenn, M.D., Ph.D.**
*Executive Vice President for Medical Affairs*
*The University of Michigan*
*1301 Catherine, M7324 Medical Sciences I Building*
*Ann Arbor, Michigan 48109-0624*

**Curtis J. Omiecinski, Ph.D.**
*Professor*
*Department of Environmental Health*
*University of Washington*
*4225 Roosevelt Way Northeast*
*Seattle, Washington 98105-6099*

**Nihat Özkaya, Ph.D. (Deceased)**
*Research Assistant Professor*
*Department of Environmental Medicine*
*New York University Medical Center; and*
*Associate Director*
*Occupational and Industrial Orthopaedic Center*
*Hospital for Joint Diseases*
*63 Downing Street*
*New York, New York 10014*

**George P. Pappas, M.D., M.P.H.**
*Acting Instructor*
*Department of Medicine*
*University of Washington/Harborview Medical Center*
*325 Ninth Avenue*
*Seattle, Washington 98104*

**John E. Parker, M.D.**
*Division of Respiratory Disease Studies*
*National Institute for Occupational Safety and Health*
*Centers for Disease Control and Prevention; and*
*Division of Respiratory Disease Studies*
*Department of Pulmonary and Critical Care Medicine*
*West Virginia University School of Medicine*
*1095 Willowdale Road, Room 240*
*Morgantown, West Virginia 26505-2888*

**Relford E. Patterson, M.D., M.P.H.**
*Adjunct Assistant Professor*
*Department of Preventive Medicine and Biometrics*
*Uniformed Services University of the Health Sciences*
*4301 Jones Bridge Road*
*Bethesda, Maryland 20814*

**Roy Patterson, M.D.**
*Professor*
*Department of Medicine; and*
*Chief, Division of Allergy–Immunology*
*Northwestern University School of Medicine*
*303 East Chicago Avenue*
*Chicago, Illinois 60611*

**Kent W. Peterson, M.D.**
*Clinical Associate Professor*
*Department of Environmental Medicine*
*New York University Medical Center*
*550 First Avenue*
*New York, New York 10016; and*
*Occupational Health Strategies*
*Charlottesville, Virginia 22903-4491*

**Susan H. Pollack, M.D.**
*Department of Pediatrics*
*University of Kentucky College of Medicine*
*740 South Limestone*
*Lexington, Kentucky 40536*

**David M. Rapoport, M.D.**
*Associate Professor and Medical Director*
*Division of Pulmonary and Critical Care Medicine*
*New York University Sleep Disorders Center*
*New York University School of Medicine*
*550 First Avenue*
*New York, New York 10016*

**Joan Reibman, M.D.**
*Associate Professor*
*Division of Pulmonary and Critical Care Medicine*
*Department of Medicine*
*Bellevue Hospital*
*New York University Medical Center*
*550 First Avenue*
*New York, New York 10016*

**Howard E. Rockette, Ph.D.**
*Professor*
*Department of Biostatistics*
*Graduate School of Public Health*
*University of Pittsburgh*
*1600 DeSoto Street*
*Pittsburgh, Pennsylvania 15261*

**Victor L. Roggli, M.D.**
*Professor*
*Department of Pathology*
*Duke University Medical Center*
*508 Fulton Street*
*Durham, North Carolina 27705*

**Timothy J. Rohm, Ph.D.**
*Instructor*
*University of California, Santa Cruz*
*Santa Cruz, California 95192-0100*

**William N. Rom, M.D., M.P.H.**
*Professor and Chief*
*Division of Pulmonary and Critical Care Medicine*
*Departments of Medicine and Environmental Medicine; and*
*Director*
*Chest Service*
*Bellevue Hospital Center*
*New York University Medical Center*
*550 First Avenue*
*New York, New York 10016*

**Roger R. Rosa, Ph.D.**
*Research Psychologist*
*Division of Biomedical and Behavioral Science*
*National Institute for Occupational Safety and Health*
*4676 Columbia Parkway, Mail Stop C-24*
*Cincinnati, Ohio 45226*

**Cecile S. Rose, M.D., M.P.H.**
*Associate Professor*
*Division of Environmental and Occupational Health Sciences*
*Department of Medicine*
*National Jewish Medical and Research Center; and*
*Division of Pulmonary Sciences and Critical Care Medicine*
*Department of Medicine*
*University of Colorado Health Sciences Center*
*1400 Jackson Street*
*Denver, Colorado 80206*

**Herbert S. Rosenkranz, Ph.D.**
*Professor and Chairman*
*Department of Environmental and Occupational Health*
*University of Pittsburgh Graduate School of Public Health*
*RIDC Park, 260 Kappa Drive*
*Pittsburgh, Pennsylvania 15238*

**Kenneth D. Rosenman, M.D.**
*Professor*
*Department of Medicine*
*Michigan State University*
*117 West Fee*
*East Lansing, Michigan 48824-1316*

**Toby G. Rossman, Ph.D.**
*Professor of Environmental Medicine*
*Nelson Institute of Environmental Medicine and*
*Kaplan Comprehensive Cancer Center*
*New York University Medical Center*
*550 First Avenue*
*New York, New York 10016*

**Stephen H. Safe, M.Sc., D. Phil.**
*Sid Kyle Professor of Toxicology*
*Department of Veterinary Physiology and Pharmacology*
*Texas A&M University*
*College Station, Texas 77843-4466*

**John E. Salvaggio, M.D.**
*Henderson Professor of Medicine*
*Department of Medicine*
*Tulane University Medical Center*
*1430 Tulane Avenue*
*New Orleans, Louisiana 70112*

**Jonathan M. Samet, M.D., M.S.**
*Professor and Chairman*
*Department of Epidemiology*
*The Johns Hopkins University School of Hygiene and Public Health*
*615 North Wolfe Street, Suite W6041*
*Baltimore, Maryland 21205*

**Sheldon Wilfred Samuels, A.B.**
*Vice President*
*Ramazzini Institute for Occupational and Environmental Health Research*
*P.O. Box 1570*
*Solomons Island, Maryland 20688*

**Steven L. Sauter, Ph.D.**
*Chief*
*Applied Psychology and Ergonomics Branch*
*National Institute for Occupational Safety and Health*
*4676 Columbia Parkway, MS C-24*
*Cincinnati, Ohio 45226-1998*

**Marc B. Schenker, M.D., M.P.H.**
*Professor and Chair*
*Department of Epidemiology and Preventive Medicine*
*University of California, Davis*
*TB 168*
*Davis, California 95616-8638*

**Richard B. Schlesinger, Ph.D.**
*Professor*
*Department of Environmental Medicine*
*New York University Medical Center*
*550 First Avenue*
*New York, New York 10016*

**Neil W. Schluger, M.D.**
*Assistant Professor of Medicine*
*Division of Pulmonary and Critical Care Medicine*
*Chest Service*
*Bellevue Hospital Center*
*New York University Medical Center*
*550 First Avenue*
*New York, New York 10016*

**James M. Schmitt, M.D., M.S.**
*Medical Director*
*Occupational Medical Service*
*National Institutes of Health*
*10 Center Drive*
*Bethesda, Maryland 20892-1584*

**Teresa M. Schnorr, Ph.D.**
*Assistant Chief*
*Industrywide Studies Branch*
*National Institute for Occupational Safety and Health*
*4676 Columbia Parkway, Mailstop R15*
*Cincinnati, Ohio 45226-1998*

**David A. Schwartz, M.D., M.P.H.**
*Professor*
*Divisions of Pulmonary and Critical Care and Occupational Medicine*
*Department of Internal Medicine*
*University of Iowa College of Medicine*
*200 Hawkins Drive*
*Iowa City, Iowa 52242*

**Jan Schwarz-Miller, M.D., M.P.H., M.P.H.**
*Assistant Clinical Professor*
*Division of Environmental Health Sciences*
*Occupational Medicine Atlantic Health System*
*Columbia University School of Public Health*
*100 Madison Avenue*
*Morristown, New Jersey 07962*

**Kent A. Sepkowitz, M.D., F.A.C.P.**
*Assistant Professor*
*Department of Medicine*
*Memorial Sloan-Kettering Cancer Center*
*Cornell University Medical College*
*1275 York Avenue*
*New York, New York 10021*

**Roy E. Shore, Ph.D.**
*Professor*
*Department of Environmental Medicine*
*New York University Medical Center*
*550 First Avenue*
*New York, New York 10016*

**Ellen K. Silbergeld, Ph.D.**
*Professor*
*Departments of Epidemiology and Preventive Medicine; and*
*Director*
*Program in Human Health and the Environment*
*University of Maryland School of Medicine*
*10 South Pine Street, Mailstop TF9-34*
*Baltimore, Maryland 21201*

**Barbara A. Silverstein, M.D.**
*Research Director*
*Safety and Health Assessment and Research for Prevention*
*Department of Labor and Industries*
*P.O. Box 44330*
*Olympia, Washington 98505*

**O. J. Sizemore**
*Senior Scientist*
*Center for Research on Occupational and Environmental Toxicology*
*Oregon Health Sciences University*
*3181 Southwest Sam Jackson Park Road, CROET-L606*
*Portland, Oregon 97201-3098*

**Mary-Louise Skovron, Ph.D., M.P.H.**
*Genentech, Inc.*
*Medical Affairs/Epidemiology*
*1 DNA Way, MS 88*
*San Francisco, California 94080; and*
*Adjunct Professor*
*New York University Medical Center*
*550 First Avenue*
*New York, New York 10016*

**Donna R. Smith, M.S.W., Ph.D.**
*Senior Vice President*
*Department of Education and Training*
*Substance Abuse Management, Inc.*
*4800 North Federal Highway, Suite 304B*
*Boca Raton, Florida 33431*

**Elizabeth T. Snow, Ph.D.**
*Assistant Professor*
*Department of Environmental Medicine*
*New York University Medical Center*
*57 Old Forge Road*
*Tuxedo, New York 10987*

**John D. Spengler, Ph.D.**
*Professor*
*Department of Environmental Health; and*
*Director*
*Environmental Science and Engineering Program*
*Harvard School of Public Health*
*665 Huntington Avenue, Room 1303*
*Boston, Massachusetts 02115-6021*

**Lynn G. Stansbury, M.D.**
*Staff Physician*
*Occupational Medical Service*
*National Institutes of Health*
*10 Center Drive*
*Bethesda, Maryland 20892-1584*

**N. Kyle Steenland, Ph.D.**
*Senior Epidemiologist*
*National Institute for Occupational Safety and Health*
*4676 Columbia Parkway, Mailstop R13*
*Cincinnati, Ohio 45226*

**Jeanne M. Stellman, Ph.D.**
*Associate Professor of Clinical Public Health*
*Division of Health Policy and Management*
*Columbia University School of Public Health*
*600 West 168th Street*
*New York, New York 10032*

**Steven D. Stellman, Ph.D., M.P.H.**
*Chief*
*Division of Epidemiology*
*American Health Foundation*
*320 East 43rd Street*
*New York, New York 10017*

**Robert F. Stone, M.A.**
*Visiting Research Economist*
*Center for Technology, Policy and Industrial Development*
*Massachusetts Institute of Technology*
*1 Amherst Street, Building E40-238*
*Cambridge, Massachusetts 02139*

**Daniel Storzbach, M.D.**
*Attending Physician*
*Veterans Medical Center*
*Portland, Oregon 97201*

**Karen A. Sullivan, Ph.D.**
*Research Professor and Director*
*Histocompatibility and Immunogenetics Laboratory*
*Department of Medicine*
*Tulane University Medical Center*
*1430 Tulane Avenue, SL-75*
*New Orleans, Louisiana 70112*

**Kay Teschke, Ph.D., M.P.H.**
*Associate Professor*
*Department of Health Care and Epidemiology*
*University of British Columbia*
*5804 Fairview Avenue*
*Vancouver, British Columbia V6T 1Z3*
*Canada*

**Robert V. Thomann, Ph.D.**
*Professor*
*Department of Environmental Engineering*
*Manhattan College*
*Riverdale, New York 10471*

**Valerie M. Thomas, Ph.D.**
*Research Staff*
*Center for Energy and Environmental Studies*
*Princeton University*
*Princeton, New Jersey 08544-5263*

**Arthur C. Upton, M.D.**
*Clinical Professor*
*Department of Environmental and Community Medicine*
*University of Medicine and Dentistry of New Jersey–Robert Wood Johnson Medical School*
*170 Frelinghuysen Road*
*Piscataway, New Jersey 08855-1179*

**Mark J. Utell, M.D.**
*Professor and Director*
*Divisions of Pulmonary/Critical Care and Occupational Medicine*
*Departments of Medicine and Environmental Medicine*
*University of Rochester Medical Center*
*601 Elmwood Avenue—Pulmonary Unit, Box 692*
*Rochester, New York 14642*

**Jan Willem van Doorn, M.D., Ph.D.**
*Director*
*Business Development*
*Occupational and Industrial Orthopaedic and Spine Center*
*Hospital for Joint Diseases*
*301 East 17th Street*
*New York, New York 10016*

**Gregory R. Wagner, M.D.**
*Director*
*Divison of Respiratory Disease Studies*
*National Institute for Occupational Safety and Health*
*1095 Willowdale Road*
*Morgantown, West Virginia 26505-2888*

**John R. Waldman, Ph.D.**
*Research Associate*
*Hudson River Foundation*
*40 West 20th Street*
*New York, New York 10011*

**Joyce A. Walsleben, Ph.D.**
*Assistant Research Professor*
*Division of Pulmonary and Critical Care Medicine; and*
*Director*
*New York University Sleep Disorders Center*
*New York University Medical Center*
*550 First Avenue*
*New York, New York 10016*

**Jia-Sheng Wang, M.D., Ph.D.**
*Assistant Scientist*
*Department of Environmental Health Sciences*
*The Johns Hopkins University*
*615 North Wolfe Street, Room 1102*
*Baltimore, Maryland 21205*

**John H. Ward, M.D.**
*Professor*
*Division of Hematology–Oncology*
*Department of Internal Medicine*
*University of Utah Health Sciences Center*
*50 North Medical Drive*
*Salt Lake City, Utah 84132*

**Donald E. Wasserman, M.S.E.E., M.B.A.**
*Human Vibration and Biomedical Engineering Consultant*
*Biodynamics*
*7910 Mitchell Farm Lane*
*Cincinnati, Ohio 45242-6437*

**Kathleen C. Weathers, Ph.D.**
*Ecologist and Professor*
*Institute of Ecosystem Studies*
*Sharon Turnpike*
*Millbrook, New York 12545*

**Sherri R. Weiser, Ph.D.**
*Adjunct Professor of Ergonomics and Biomechanics*
*Psychological Services*
*Occupational and Industrial Orthopaedic and Spine Center*
*Hospital for Joint Diseases*
*301 East 17th Street*
*New York, New York 10016*

**M. Donald Whorton, M.D.**
*Chief Medical Scientist*
*Environmental Services Health Sciences*
*1135 Atlantic Avenue*
*Alameda, California 94501*

**John K. Wiencke, Ph.D.**
*Associate Professor*
*Department of Epidemiology and Biostatistics*
*School of Medicine*
*University of California, San Francisco*
*500 Parnassus Avenue*
*San Francisco, California 94143-0560*

**Nancy K. Wiese, D.O.**
*Occupational Medicine Consultant*
*Department of Occupational Health Services*
*Cigna Health Care of Arizona*
*Phoenix, Arizona 85006*

**Marc Wilkenfeld, M.D.**
*Research Assistant Professor*
*Department of Environmental Medicine*
*New York University Medical Center*
*550 First Avenue*
*New York, New York 10016*

**Isaac I. Wirgin, M.A., Ph.D.**
*Associate Professor*
*Department of Environmental Medicine*
*New York University Medical Center*
*57 Old Forge Road*
*Tuxedo, New York 10987*

**Norman A. Zabriskie, M.D.**
*Assistant Professor*
*Department of Ophthalmology*
*John A. Moran Eye Center*
*University of Utah Hospital*
*50 North Medical Drive*
*Salt Lake City, Utah 84132*

**Edward T. Zawada, Jr., M.D.**
*Freeman Professor and Chairman*
*Department of Internal Medicine*
*University of South Dakota School of Medicine; and*
*The Royal C. Johnson Veterans Memorial Hospital*
*1400 West 22nd Street*
*Sioux Falls, South Dakota 57105*

**Carl Zetterberg, M.D., Ph.D.**
*Associate Professor*
*Department of Orthopaedics*
*School of Medicine*
*University of Goteborg*
*Sahlgren Hospital*
*S-413, 45 Goteborg*
*Sweden*

**Anatoly Zhitkovich, Ph.D.**
*Assistant Professor*
*Department of Environmental Medicine*
*New York University Medical Center*
*57 Old Forge Road*
*Tuxedo, New York 10987*

# Foreword

Environmental and occupational medicine are specialties that stand at the fascinating interface between clinical medicine and public health. They are specialties that require mastery of all the arts of medicine—history-taking, physical examination, diagnosis, and therapy. In addition, these disciplines also demand knowledge of epidemiology, toxicology, industrial engineering, the behavioral sciences, history, and law.

The specialities of environmental and occupational medicine are heir to several historical traditions (1). They are descendants of Hippocrates, who urged physicians to always consider the interplay between the patient and the environment. These specialties owe much to Ramazzini, Agricola, and Paracelsus, all pioneering physicians who early perceived the relationship between work and disease. More recently, environmental and occupational medicine have been influenced by the sanitary reform movement of the 19th century, by the progressive movement of the 1930s, and by the environmental movement today.

Environmental and occupational medicine are specialties confronting rapid change. Each year hundreds of new synthetic chemical compounds are developed by the chemical industry and are added to the 70,000 chemicals and to the 10,000,000 mixtures, formulations, and blends already in commerce (2). Too frequently, these new chemicals are released in the workplace and in the environment without adequate prior assessment of their potential for toxicity (3). Workers are typically the first to be exposed to these toxicities, and the consequences of careless exposures to untested technologies fall most heavily on workers and on the vulnerable members of our society—infants, children, and the elderly (4). Astute physicians caring for patients exposed to untested chemical toxins repeatedly have had the opportunity to diagnose entirely new disease entities and to recognize emerging epidemics (5–12). Through their identification of these sentinel health events (13), these physicians have made fundamental contributions to the advancement of medicine. These men and women are the heroes of environmental and occupational medicine and the founders of our discipline—Percival Pott, Richard Doll, Alice Hamilton, David Rutstein, and Irving Selikoff.

Prevention of disease is the ultimate goal of environmental and occupational medicine. Prevention is most efficiently accomplished when the cause of disease is identified, the sources and routes of exposure defined, and the exposures eliminated. Such etiologic or "primary" prevention is the holy grail of environmental and occupational medicine. It is far more efficient, cost effective, and humane than "secondary prevention"—the identification and early treatment of persons already exposed to environmental toxins—or than "tertiary prevention"—the treatment of persons already made ill by toxic exposures in order to minimize disability or prevent premature death.

Epidemiology and toxicology are the essential disciplines that provide the scientific basis for prevention of environmental and occupational disease, and they play complementary roles. Epidemiology's great strength is that it permits direct study of the distribution and determinants of disease in human populations. In circumstances where exposures can be quantified, epidemiologists can construct dose-response relationships; the demonstration of such a relationship provides strong evidence for causality (14). Epidemiologists are with increasing frequency incorporating "biological markers" into studies of populations exposed to chemical toxins (15). These biochemical, molecular biological, and physical probes permit precise, individualized assessment of exposures, premorbid effects, and susceptibilities. They permit the early and sensitive detection of environmental and occupational disease, identification of susceptible subpopulations, improved delineation of disease mechanisms (particularly at low dose levels), and better definition of dose-response relationships. Biological markers appear to be powerful tools for both primary and secondary prevention. The inherent limitation of epidemiology is that it can study disease (or the premorbid changes leading to disease) only after human exposure has occurred and only after some degree of damage has already been done.

Toxicology's greatest contribution to disease prevention lies in its ability to identify toxicity prior to human exposure. Premarket toxicologic screening—the evaluation of the toxic potential of new chemical compounds and new technologies before their commercial release—constitutes an extraordinarily effective but too frequently overlooked mechanism for preventing environmental and occupational disease (3). Toxicology also has the potential to provide brilliant insights into the mechanisms by which environmental and occupational toxins cause illness. In recent years a combination of the tools of toxicology with those of molecular biology has enabled identification of the cascade of changes within cells that lead to the development of cancer and to other environmental and occupational diseases of long latency. Also, these tools permit recognition of the acquired and inherited factors that govern susceptibility to environmental and occupational disease. They have begun to enable us to answer such questions as "Why do only approximately 10% of smokers develop lung cancer?" and "Why do only a subset of workers exposed to benzidine develop cancer of the bladder?" (15).

Environmental and occupational medicine are highly interdisciplinary specialties. Successful practice requires the formation of strong partnerships among physicians, nurses, industrial hygienists, safety engineers, trade unionists, industrial managers, and governmental agencies, and additionally requires the building of bridges between health professionals and architects of public policy. Such partnerships enable policymakers to draft laws and regulations founded on good science, which will result in the reduction of toxic exposures and will then accomplish primary prevention of disease. Examples of partnerships between science and policy abound in environmental and occupational medicine, and they have led to bans on dichlorodiphenyltrichloroethane (DDT), stringent reductions in asbestos use, bans on chlorofluorocarbons (CFCs) and the use of polychlorinated biphenyls (PCBs), and an imposition of stringent limits on exposures to benzene, butadiene, silica, and beryllium. More positively, these partnerships have catalyzed development of new closed-system chemical production technologies, promoted the growth of non-polluting industry, and created a sound scientific basis for concepts of sustainable development.

*Environmental and Occupational Medicine*, third edition, is a comprehensive volume that summarizes what we know about occupational and environmental medicine and one that articulates strong principles to guide us as we face the future. It covers the fields of epidemiology, toxicology, clinical medicine, and ethics. It provides guidance for the clinical recognition of environmental and occupational disease and for the identification of sentinel health events (13). It will be an invaluable reference for specialists in the field of environmental and occupational medicine, providing accurate and updated information on a wide range of diseases of toxic origin. *Environmental and Occupational Medicine* will also be a critical reference for the primary care provider who in the course of history-taking may encounter a patient with a new or unexpected disease that may be of toxic origin. It will be the clinician's field guide to toxic chemicals.

Physicians practicing environmental and occupational medicine have a particular responsibility to society. It is our task to inform and warn policymakers and the public about the dangers of uncontrolled release of untested chemicals in the workplace and in the environment. It is our responsibility through sound science to establish links between chemical contamination and its damage to human health (16). It is our duty to give the leaders of our society the advice they need to properly protect our planet and to safeguard human health. This volume, *Environmental and Occupational Medicine*, will guide physicians toward fulfilling these awesome responsibilities.

*Philip J. Landrigan, M.D., M.Sc.*

## REFERENCES


1. Hunter D Sir. *The diseases of occupations.* 6th ed. London: Hodder and Stoughton, 1978.
2. U. S. Environmental Protection Agency, Office of Toxic Substances. *Core activities of the Office of Toxic Substances (Draft Program Plan).* EPA Publication 560/4-76-005. Washington, DC: Environmental Protection Agency (EPA), 1976.
3. National Academy of Sciences. *Toxicity testing: strategies to determine needs and priorities.* Washington, DC: National Academy Press, 1984.
4. National Academy of Sciences. *Pesticides in the diets of infants and children.* Washington, DC: National Academy Press, 1993.
5. Pott P. *Chirurgical observations relative to the cataract, the polypus of the nose, the cancer of the scrotum, the different kinds of ruptures, and the mortification of the toes and feet.* London: Hewes, Clarke and Collins, 1775.
6. Rehn L. Blasengeschwueiste bei Fuchsinarbeitern. *Arch Klin Chir* 1895;50:588–600.

7. Delore P, Borgomano C. Acute leukemia following benzene poisoning. On the toxic origin of certain acute leukemias and their relation to serious anemias. *J Med Lyon* 1928;9:227–233.
8. Doll R, Hill AB. Lung cancer and other causes of death in relation to smoking—a second report on the mortality of British doctors. *Br Med J* 1956;2:1071–1077.
9. Hammond EC, Selikoff IJ, Churg J. Asbestos exposure, smoking and neoplasia. *JAMA* 1968;204(2):106–112.
10. Hammond EC, Selikoff IJ, Seidman H. Asbestos exposure, cigarette smoking and death rates. *Ann NY Acad Sci* 1979;330:473–490.
11. Figueroa WG, Raszowski R, Weiss W. Lung cancer in chloromethyl methyl ether workers. *N Engl J Med* 1973;228:1096–1097.
12. Creech JL Jr, Johnson MN. Angiosarcoma of the liver in the manufacture of polyvinyl chloride. *J Occup Med* 1974;16:150–151.
13. Rutstein DD, Mullan RJ, Frazier TM, Halperin WE, Melius JM, Sestito AP. Sentinel health events (occupational): a basis for physician recognition in public health surveillance. *Am J Public Health* 1983;73:1054–1062.
14. Rinsky RA, Smith AB, Hornung R. Benzene and leukemia: an epidemiologic risk assessment. *New Engl J Med* 1987;316: 1044–1050.
15. Weinstein IB. The scientific basis for carcinogen detection and primary cancer prevention. *Cancer* 1981;47:1133–1141.
16. Chivian E, McCally M, Hu H, Haines A, eds. *Critical condition: human health and the environment.* Cambridge, MA: MIT Press, 1993.

# Preface

*Environmental and Occupational Medicine*, third edition, is riding the crest of a tidal wave of new knowledge and fascination in how the human enterprise affects the workplace and global environment. As glaciers recede and rain becomes increasingly acidic, the science behind these events is critically important for physicians to comprehend. Physician specialties in occupational and environmental medicine and public health are the vanguard teachers of how the environment is affected—whether it is ergonomic design to prevent carpal tunnel syndrome or chlorofluorocarbons causing the destruction of stratospheric ozone.

This third edition has been developed to meet these challenges. It has been planned to aid medical students as they enter the clinical years, for residents and practitioners as a comprehensive resource, and for the public health community as a guide to controlling and preventing disease.

The volume has grown from 125 to 136 chapters and has increased in size to accommodate all of this new knowledge. There are 27 completely new chapters. An additional 42 chapters have been completely rewritten by previous or new authors. Each of the remaining 67 chapters has been closely scrutinized and updated. The contributors in this edition are the leaders in their fields and include Nobel laureates, deans, and bench scientists. There is an expanding coverage of the environmental sciences, particularly the fate of industrial toxicants in the air, water, and/or land. Yet, the same organizational structure remains: an examination of environmental and occupational disease by organ systems, toxicants in the workplace and environment, and control strategies for both diseases and environmental agents.

New issues have arisen in environmental and occupational medicine since the previous edition. Responding to these global challenges are Alexander Leaf and Paul Epstein in "Biological and Medical Implications of Global Warming," Mario and Luisa Molina in "Chlorofluorocarbons and Destruction of the Ozone Layer," Theo Colborn in "Endocrine Disruption from Environmental Toxicants," Kathleen Weathers and Gene Likens in "Acid Rain," and several chapters focusing on chemical permeation of the environment. Noteworthy is a multiauthored chapter devoted to the studies related to Persian Gulf War issues by physicians on the front line in research investigations. The text deals with all types of challenges ranging from multiple chemical sensitivity, low back pain, carpal tunnel syndrome, sick buildings, occupational tuberculosis, ergonomics, biomechanics, human factors, and respirators to managed care and prevention.

*William N. Rom, M.D., M.P.H.*

# Acknowledgments

A volume such as this one owes its existence to the labors and commitment of many contributors. I am indeed grateful to them. Several chapters were edited with significant changes in style, content, and illustrations in order to produce a comprehensive, timely, and accurate volume. I appreciate the patience and cordiality of the contributors as we progressed through the editing process.

I also wish to thank Elena Arvanitopoulos for her excellent assistance as Project Director, and Natalie Little, and Joyce-Rachel John of Lippincott–Raven for helping contributors meet deadlines. I would like to acknowledge the contribution of the many individuals at the Institute of Environmental Medicine at New York University Medical Center.

# SECTION I

## Environmental and Occupational Disease

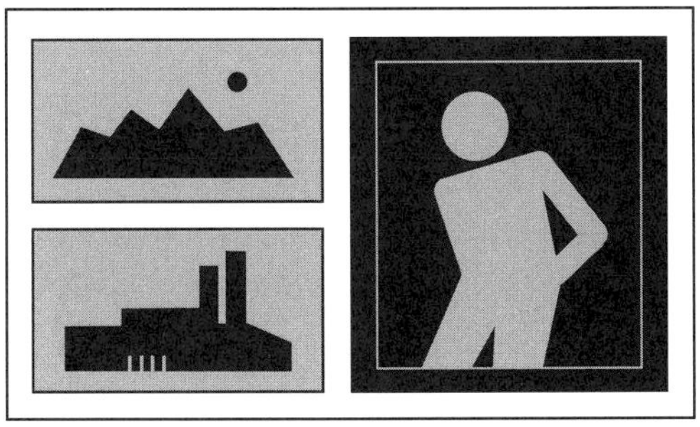

*Environmental and Occupational Medicine, Third Edition,* edited by William N. Rom.
Lippincott–Raven Publishers, Philadelphia © 1998.

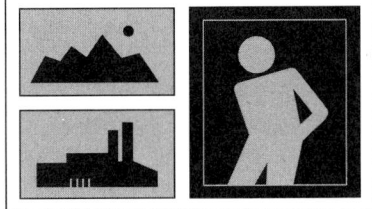

CHAPTER 1

# The Discipline of Environmental and Occupational Medicine

William N. Rom

With roots in the early industrial revolution, industrial medicine has been transformed to corporate practice and to the study of the health effects of environmental and occupational medicine on a global scope. The addition of environmental exposures to the causation of disease or potential for harm has added a profound complexity to the discipline. There is now concern for transnational transport of substances such as mercury from coal combustion or gold mining to lake ecosystems where biotransformation concentrates mercury 225,000-fold greater in fish than in the water. Xenobiotics may act as endocrine hormones in various species and may lead to reproductive disruption. Enhanced ultraviolet radiation from destruction of stratospheric ozone may increase skin cancer in temperate latitudes. The focus in occupational medicine has changed from acute injuries, dermatitis, burns, and lacerations to chronic conditions, especially pneumoconioses, and to issues surrounding airways disease, ergonomics, and the introduction of new solvents that are pertinent to the information and communication age.

## HISTORY

Hippocrates admonished his followers to observe the environment to understand the origins of illnesses in their patients. Agricola observed that miners in Joachimsthal frequently became short of breath and died prematurely (1). In *De Re Metallica* he described dust-aggravated consumption (probably silico-tuberculosis) and remarked that one widow had outlived seven husbands who had mined gold and silver in the Erz Mountains of the Czech-German border. Bernardino Ramazzini (2), recognized worldwide as the father of occupational medicine, dates the birth of the discipline back to 1700 when *De Morbis Artificam Diatriba* was published in Modena, Italy. He discussed diseases of metal diggers, painters, intellectuals, gilders, midwives, glass makers, potters, and sewer workers, noting that their afflictions came from inhaling noxious gases and dusts, or from disorderly motions and improper postures of the body. He described problems of the eye among glassblowers, the symptoms of potters using lead glaze, and the neurologic conditions related to mercurialism. According to Ramazzini, "When a doctor visits a working-class home, he should be content to sit on a three-legged stool if there isn't a gilded chair, and he should take time for his examination; and to the questions recommended by Hippocrates, he should add one more—What is your occupation?" (2). Sir Thomas Legge in 1898 became the first medical inspector of factories in England. He coauthored *Lead Poisoning and Lead Absorption* in 1912 and also investigated anthrax, glassblowers' cataract, industrial skin cancer, toxic jaundice, and poisoning by phosphorus, arsenic, and mercury. An untiring lecturer to medical students in many hospitals, he was knighted in 1925 and continued to stress the importance of including occupational medicine in the medical students' curriculum.

Alice Hamilton was the first American physician to devote her life to the practice of industrial medicine. She wrote *Industrial Poisons in the United States* in 1925 and *Exploring the Dangerous Trades,* her autobiography, in

W. N. Rom: Division of Pulmonary and Critical Care Medicine, Departments of Medicine and Environmental Medicine; and Chest Service, Bellevue Hospital Center, New York University Medical Center, New York, New York 10016.

1943 (3). In studying the lead industries of Illinois, she discovered and ameliorated lead poisoning among bathtub enamelers in Chicago. She wrote about phossy jaw, which occurred among American matchmakers using white or yellow phosphorus. She studied the effects of carbon monoxide among steelworkers, the toxicity of nitroglycerin among munitions makers during World War I, the symptoms of hatters exposed to mercury in Danbury, Connecticut, and the "dead fingers" syndrome of workers utilizing the early jackhammers. She also described the toxic effects to the blood-forming cells from benzene, and the neurologic and physiologic abnormalities of workers exposed to carbon disulfide in the viscose rayon industry. In her autobiography, Dr. Hamilton lamented the status of occupational medicine in the United States (3):

> American medical authorities had never taken industrial diseases seriously, the American Medical Association had never held a meeting on the subject, and while European journals were full of articles on industrial poisonings, the number published in American medical journals up to 1910 could be counted on one's fingers....The employers could, if they wished, shut their eyes to the dangers their workmen faced, for nobody held them responsible, while the workers accepted the risks with fatalistic submissiveness as part of the price one must pay for being poor.

Alice Hamilton was the first woman appointed to the medical faculty at Harvard in 1919.

## SCOPE OF THE OCCUPATIONAL HEALTH AND SAFETY CHALLENGES

In 1994 employers reported 6.3 million work injuries and 515,000 cases of occupational illness in the United States (4). In that same year, occupational injuries alone cost $121 billion in lost wages, productivity, administrative expenses, and health care costs (4). In the United States by the year 2005 there will be 147 million workers; they will be 48% female, 28% minority, and 15% over age 55, representing a strikingly diverse work force. Every 5 seconds a workers in the United States is injured, and every 10 seconds a worker is temporarily or permanently disabled. Manufacturing jobs continue to decline with the service sector now employing 70% of all workers. The 1993 workers' compensation costs of $57 billion reflect only a small portion of the social and economic consequences of occupational injuries and illnesses. Recently, the National Institute for Occupational Safety and Health (NIOSH) and the Occupational Safety and Health Administration (OSHA) celebrated their 25th birthday. In 1970, Congress passed the Occupational Safety and Health Act to assure "so far as possible, every working man and woman in the United States safe and healthful working conditions." The act created NIOSH to identify the causes of work-related diseases and injuries, to evaluate the hazards of new technologies and work practices, to study industrial hygiene and hazard control, and to make recommendations for occupational safety and health standards. NIOSH is an outgrowth of the Office of Industrial Hygiene and Sanitation established in the U.S. Public Health Service in 1914. NIOSH's director reports to the director of the Centers for Disease Control and Prevention, and has research laboratories in Morgantown, West Virginia and Cincinnati, Ohio. OSHA was created to promulgate and enforce standards, with its assistant secretary reporting to the secretary of labor in Washington, D.C.

Priority areas for research have changed over time as disease patterns have been altered by economics and change in work processes (Table 1). Asbestos use has plummeted in developed nations and asbestosis is far less common. Vinyl chloride–induced liver cancers and byssinosis have almost been eliminated. Since 1970, fatal injury rates in coal miners have been reduced by more than 75%, and the prevalence of coal workers' pneumoconiosis has had a general downward trend. However, silicosis persists especially in the foundry industry, and lead poisoning continues to be reported. Occupational lung diseases persist in their prevalence, but asthma, chronic obstructive pulmonary disease (COPD), and irritant-related bronchitis are competing with asbestos exposure for research priority. Allergic and irritant dermatitis (contact dermatitis) is overwhelmingly the most important cause of occupational skin diseases, and they account for 15% to 20% of all reported occupational diseases. From 1983 to 1994 there has been a 26% increase in occupational skin diseases with a rate of 81 cases per $10^5$ workers. Latex in protective gloves causes contact dermatitis or urticaria in 10% of exposed health care workers. Prevention is critically important since 75% of patients with occupational contact dermatitis may develop chronic skin disease. Nearly 30% of COPD and adult asthma may be attributable to occupational exposure, and 9 million workers are occupationally exposed to known sensitizers and irritants associated with asthma (5,6). Research on the effects of various chemicals on reproduction including birth defects, stillbirths, low birth weight, developmental disorders, and impotence remains meager (6). Noise is the most important occupational cause of hearing loss resulting from acute trauma, or more likely, chronic exposure to ototraumatic agents. Factors such as heat and chemicals may interact in causing hearing loss. Health care workers are at risk of tuberculosis, hepatitis B and C, and infection with human immunodeficiency virus. Low back disorders constitute 27% of occupational injuries and are highly preventable with proper work practices. Rapid return to work and focused rehabilitation programs can drastically reduce long-term disability. Over 30% of occupations require some lifting. Workers' compensation for low back disorders average twice the award compared to all other compensable claims. In meat processing plants, for example, working at a fast pace in

**TABLE 1.** *NIOSH occupational research agendas*

| |
|---|
| Disease and injury |
| Acute and chronic airway disease |
| Chronic diseases (selected) |
| Chronic obstructive pulmonary disease |
| Contact dermatitis |
| Depression and anxiety |
| Fertility and pregnancy abnormalities |
| Hearing loss due to noise and nonauditory exposures |
| Low back disorders |
| Molecular correlates of cancer |
| Musculoskeletal disorders of the upper extremities |
| Occupational asthma |
| Occupational cancer |
| Occupational skin diseases |
| Stress |
| Traumatic injuries |
| Work environment and work force |
| Aging populations |
| Behavioral risk |
| Changing economy and work force |
| Construction |
| Emerging technologies |
| Ethics |
| Health care workers |
| Indoor air (environment) |
| Inorganic dusts |
| Interactions (chemical) |
| Latex allergy |
| Mechanical stressors |
| Mineral and synthetic fibers |
| Mixed exposures (includes mixtures of chemicals and/or other agents) |
| Motor vehicles |
| Noise |
| Nonrespiratory routes of exposure |
| Oils and related products |
| Organization of work |
| Pesticides |
| $PM_{10}$ (particulate matter <10 mm) |
| Premature disability |
| Psychosocial factors |
| Sector-focused research |
| Service workers |
| Solvents |
| Small businesses |
| Special populations at risk |
| Violence (assaults) |
| Research tools and approaches |
| Clinical methods research |
| Critical path methods |
| Database linkage |
| Disease surveillance |
| Engineering and technological solutions |
| Exposure assessment methods |
| Hazard surveillance |
| Health services research |
| Injury surveillance |
| Risk assessment methods |
| Social and economic consequences of workplace illness and injury |
| Surveillance research methods |
| Training professionals/impact |

cold environments while using forceful motions in awkward postures places individuals at risk for musculoskeletal disorders of the upper extremities. Musculoskeletal disorders affect the soft tissues of the neck, shoulder, elbow, hand, wrist, and fingers. These include nerves (e.g., carpal tunnel syndrome), tendons (e.g., tenosynovitis, peritendinitis, epicondylitis), and muscles (e.g., tension neck syndrome). In 1994 there were 332,000 musculoskeletal disorders due to repeated trauma reported in U.S. workplaces; this was a 15% increase over 1992 (4). High-risk worker groups for occupational traumatic injuries are construction workers, loggers, miners, farmers, farm workers, adolescents, and older workers. Motor vehicle accidents are the leading cause of injury, but exposure to moving parts on machines, falls, electrocution, and homicide violence are also important. The traditional pneumoconioses, silicosis, and asbestosis are receding in their importance as new technologies redefine the workplace and its exposures.

New emerging technologies include exposures in manufacturing airbags (sodium azide) to new chemicals in oxygenated automotive fuels. More than half the American work force works indoors, and exposures to indoor air pollutants (e.g., formaldehyde) can disrupt the harmony of the workplace. New technologies may improve workplace safety including new respirator filters, new protective clothes for firemen, microsensors to detect environmental contaminants, and substitution of lightweight materials to reduce the risk of low back pain.

Approximately 1.3 million Americans develop cancer each year and 0.5 million die from these diseases. NIOSH estimates that 4% are thought to be related to exposures in the workplace (4). Cancers with well-considered occupational relationships include angiosarcoma of the liver (vinyl chloride), mesothelioma, bladder cancer (21% to 27% occupationally related), and lung (up to 10% occupationally related).

The key to detecting occupational illness is to suspect the diagnosis, and the diagnosis of work-related illness hinges principally on the quality of the occupational and environmental history (5). Asking about a person's occupation is an important routine for every primary care practitioner or specialist and a detailed chronological job history describing what the person did plus relating this to exposures is essential for the occupational medicine practitioner (7). It is important to seek information on whether symptoms abate away from work, and whether any coworkers have similar problems. Often occupational diseases are not correctly diagnosed because they mimic diseases due to other causes (8). The specialist in occupational medicine may wish to conduct a walk-through of the work environment. Public health agencies, including state and county health departments, OSHA, the Mine Safety and Health Administration (MSHA), and NIOSH, may conduct an investigation when a physician reports a sentinel health event. Employees and employers can request an inspection by OSHA, MSHA, or NIOSH, and they can remain anonymous if they so desire. In attempting to confirm the role of current exposure in the patient's illness, the physician can restrict the patient's work temporarily and observe any change in the patient's condition. The physician must determine if the patient needs to change jobs, or whether return to work might exacerbate the condition. Primary care physicians are frequently asked to determine whether a patient has a work-related illness or injury, and whether the condition causes permanent, temporary, or partial impairment (7).

Since there is considerable interest by the public in how the environment may adversely affect health, the environmental and occupational medicine physician needs to understand the health ramifications of environmental problems. The Environmental Protection Agency in 1990 prioritized its leading ecological risks as global climate change, stratospheric ozone depletion, habitat alteration, and species extinction and biodiversity loss. Its leading health risks were criteria air pollutants, toxic air pollutants (e.g., lead, benzene), radon gas, indoor air pollution, drinking water contamination, occupational exposure to chemicals, application of pesticides, and stratospheric ozone depletion. Table 2 lists sources of information to guide postgraduate education and specific inquiries about occupational diseases and exposures. Physicians also need to work constructively with public officials in addressing environmental hazards in the community and in the workplace.

Occupational and environmental medicine seldom achieves the priority status that the discipline deserves (6). For example, in the 1930s a water-diversion project in West Virginia ignored dust controls and wet methods as a tunnel was drilled through a mountain rich in sandstone. The high concentrations of silica at Gauley Bridge resulted in the deaths of hundreds of workers due to acute silicosis. Stanbury and colleagues reevaluated the situation of silicosis in New Jersey in 1995 (9). They identified 329 patients with confirmed silicosis in New Jersey from 1979 to 1992 using a registry in the New Jersey Department of Health. They interviewed 177 of these individuals and only 55 (31%) had filed a workers' compensation claim against their employer. Forty-four claims were settled and 37 (84%) were awarded. Most of the cases had been exposed in manufacturing either in the stone, clay, and glass industries or in foundries. This study suggested that much occupational disease is underappreciated, and that workers do not receive the security from want that the workers' compensation system was supposed to provide. Interestingly, severity of radiologic findings did not affect outcome, whereas more smokers than nonsmokers were awarded payment. Smoking is additive or synergistic with many occupational disorders. Complicating this situation is that workers' compensation administrative judges deny an estimated 60% of occupational disease claims on the initial application. What may make a decision controversial is disagreements among experts on the case definition of occupational asthma, for example, or the competing attributions of asbestos and cigarette smoking for occupational lung disease and cancer.

## PROFESSIONAL EDUCATION

Postgraduate training in occupational medicine spanning 3 years is offered at the residency or fellowship level at more than a dozen medical and public health schools in the United States. The 3 years include a clinical year, a master's in public health or equivalent degree, and a practicum year in supervised corporate medical practice or research. NIOSH funds regional educational resource centers (ERCs), which include occupational medicine residencies as well as graduate programs in industrial hygiene, safety, and nursing. The ERCs encourage multidisciplinary education and research.

Physician specialists in occupational and environmental medicine are in limited supply. Only 60 to 70 board-eligible physicians are produced by residency programs annually. The American Board of Preventive Medicine has certified approximately 1,800 physicians in occupational medicine since certification began 1955. Castorina et al. (10) estimated the supply of these physicians to be 1,200 to 1,500 and the need to be 4,600 to 6,700, with a deficit of 3,100 to 5,500 physicians. These data were based on an optimum utilization with a specialist in environmental and occupational medicine in every medical school, public health department, large group practice, and major corporation. However, funding has lagged in each of these practice modes; medical schools have ceased expanding and are seeking mergers, and corporate occupational medicine departments are downsizing or are being eliminated. The managed care environment is promoting the primary care practitioner with pressure to

**TABLE 2.** *Information sources for environmental and occupational medicine*

| |
|---|
| American College of Occupational and Environmental Medicine (ACOEM), 55 W. Siegers Rd., Arlington Heights, IL 60005-3919; (708) 228-6850. |
| National Institute for Occupational Safety and Health (NIOSH), Robert A. Taft Laboratories, 4676 Columbia Parkway, Cincinnati, OH 45226-1998; (800) 356-4674. |
| Occupational Safety and Health Administration (OSHA), Department of Labor, 200 Constitution Ave., N.W., Washington, DC 20210; (202) 219-8148 (general information), (202) 219-4667 (publications), fax (900) 555-3400. |

minimize specialty consultation. In this context, environmental and occupational medicine can only flourish as part of the medical mainstream.

The American College of Occupational and Environmental Medicine (ACOEM) has grown to approximately 6,000 members. Most of these individuals are not board certified (about three-fourths of the members) and practice part-time. Short-term courses in occupational medicine, including a basic curriculum at the annual ACOEM meeting, meet this growing demand for professional education.

The trainee needs to acquire skills in environmental health, occupational diseases, management and administration, epidemiology, biostatistics, toxicology, health care organizations, dermatology, neurology, pulmonary disease (including classification of the radiographs of the pneumoconioses), ergonomics, safety, and industrial hygiene. An appreciation of the different viewpoints of labor and management is also necessary.

To provide for competence in short-term educational programs for primary care practitioners, Rosenstock and colleagues (11) have recommended that the American Board of Internal Medicine and the American Board of Family Practice offer certificates of added qualifications to diplomates in internal medicine and family practice who have advanced training or experience in occupational and environmental medicine. They envisioned an added year of clinical specialty training, and advocated streamlined dual board certification in internal medicine or family practice. They recapitulated a community-based survey that found that the public identified physicians as one of the most trusted but least informed sources of information about the risks of chemical exposure.

Surveys of environmental and occupational medicine education in medical schools find minimal emphasis of environmental health in the majority of medical schools, and that barriers to more complete representation were lack of environmental and occupational medicine faculty and an overcrowded curriculum (12). Only half of the medical schools specifically teach occupational medicine and 30% require up to 4 hours in the preclinical years (13). Approximately 40% offer a variety of elective courses or clerkships usually in the clinical years. These are taken by only a handful of students. Occupational medicine should be a basic component of the medical school curriculum. Since all doctors will care for workers and work-related illnesses, occupational medicine needs to be integrated into the traditional courses throughout the 4 years. For example, the first year should include the occupational history as part of physical diagnosis, the occupational safety and health laws, workers' compensation, and toxicology (as part of pharmacology). Occupational health and exposures in local and regional industries should be presented. The common occupational diseases should be part of the organ system approach and the internal medicine clerkship. The pulmonary organ system is very important; pneumoconiosis, occupational asthma, lung cancer, hypersensitivity pneumonitis, particle deposition and pulmonary defense mechanisms, and the effects on health of air pollution should all be covered. Occupational dermatology and neurotoxicology are important for course work in dermatology and neurology. Lastly, electives that are available during the summer months and senior year should include preceptorships with unions, industries, or local health agencies. The greatest support for environmental health education comes from the students. Inadequate research funding, lack of faculty, and lack of prestige in environmental and occupational medicine have been cited as potential contributors of the poor showing of environmental and occupational medicine in medical schools' curricula. A separate department of environmental and occupational medicine may maximize research funding and provide a critical mass for teaching in the undergraduate curriculum (14). However, most medical schools have an environmental and occupational medicine program or division as part of a preventive or community medicine department.

In Europe, greater emphasis is placed on occupational medicine, e.g., 24 of 32 medical schools in Italy actually have an institute of occupational medicine (15). A 4-year residency for 60 to 65 physicians per year is offered by 27 of Italy's medical schools, and is funded through the ministry of health. Similar to Italy, the United Kingdom has 85 training posts in occupational medicine, and these individuals enter a 4-year specialty program followed by specialty certification by the faculty of occupational medicine (16). The United Kingdom has over 1,000 occupational medicine specialists who work mainly in a multidisciplinary setting to prevent ill health from workplace factors, and to advise individuals with ill health or disability on fitness for different work activities. The commonest compensable diseases in the United Kingdom are pneumoconiosis, malignant mesothelioma, occupational asthma, occupational deafness, hand-arm vibration syndrome, tendinitis, and dermatitis. Importantly, the journal of the faculty of occupational medicine in the United Kingdom has changed its journal title from the *British Journal of Industrial Medicine* to *Occupational and Environmental Medicine.* Likewise, in the United States the *Journal of Occupational Medicine* has changed its name to the *Journal of Occupational and Environmental Medicine.*

## ENVIRONMENTAL HEALTH: THE CHALLENGE

Environmental medicine focuses on the human health effects from air and water pollution, and in the broader context includes the earth's health, spanning global warming, degradation of the forests and land mass, oceanic pollution, ozone depletion, and loss of biodiversity. Whereas it is important for the environmental and occupational medicine physician to be conversant with occupational medicine, it is the environmental aspect that needs leadership to achieve balance between a healthy people and a healthy planet. Population explosion and its control are critical to ecological balance, e.g., the number of people are increasing from 1 billion in 1800 to 5.3 billion today and 10 billion by 2046. This population pressure will encroach on remaining wild areas, threatening to convert them to agriculture and resource extraction with extraordinary adverse pressures on biodiversity. Only 4,500 areas have been set aside as nature habitats or wilderness areas, equivalent to 3.2% of the planet's land mass. Many of these areas in developing countries are paper parks only, and many others are threatened by overuse by tourists, from multiple use policies including logging and development of private parcels located within the ecosystem, or short-sighted resource extraction policies. A fearful example of the latter is in the United States where the Alaskan plain of the Arctic National Wildlife Refuge is under constant threat from oil development. This narrow corridor north of the Brooks Range experiences an explosion of plant and bird life during the short summer of July and August, and is the calving ground of the porcupine caribou herd. Over 175,000 caribou migrate north through the Brooks Range in the late spring, giving the Arctic plain the distinction of being America's Serengeti. Canada has already preserved the adjacent plain and mountain range as the Yukon National Park and excludes oil development.

As the 20th century comes to a close, there is a resounding alarm from conservation circles about an increasing threat to biodiversity from loss of tropical rain forests and the increasing isolation of island-habitats rather than connected ecological systems where species and their gene pools can flourish and continue to evolve (17). The moist tropics are by far the greatest source of biodiversity, and because all except protected areas will be deforested over the next century, biogeographers predict that one-fourth to one-half of the world's species will disappear. Biodiversity is often equated with species richness including number of species and their biotic and genetic contribution to life. Biotic degradation occurs from population growth, poverty (e.g., deforestation for cooking fuel, trade in rare and endangered species, failure of grass roots support for conservation), the quick economic gain versus long-term benefits from creating and preserving large ecosystems, and cultural imperatives (17). Humanitarian concerns receive more funds and attention than preserving land for water purification and storage and investing in costly air pollution control strategies to obtain clear vistas; however, the preservation of wild areas to enhance discovery of new species for medicine or edible plants for the agricultural industry may hold promise. Because most of the world's people are not only poor but also in a transitional phase from a traditional self-sufficient farm society to a high-impact agricultural society or an industrial-urban one, relatively little value is placed on the protection of nature. New industries in developing countries, such as shipping shrimp north, denude coastlines of their mangrove swamps, and the extraction of coffee, sugarcane, bananas, cacao, mahogany, and other valuable trees, and cattle ranching lead to tremendous pressure on tropical forests in developing countries. Even social redress of the inequities between developing countries and the wealthy nations will not stop their attrition of environmental wealth. Economic necessity continues to press for extraction of old growth timber in the United States where the remaining 15% of virgin climax forests is unlikely to be saved for lack of political will.

Tactics to alter ecosystem degradation are diverse including preservation of wilderness areas, national parks, and wildlife refuges by federal, state, and local governments, and private purchase of valuable land or water areas by groups such as the Nature Conservancy. There is political opposition to this approach, e.g., the difficulty in preserving wild areas in Utah, Montana, etc. where strong antigovernment attitudes predominate, and corporate mergers and takeovers that mandate tremendously accelerated resource extradition to resolve indebtedness, which has adversely affected much of the remaining redwood forest in northern California. Another approach includes legal redress in the judicial system to press for enforcement of environmental laws; on the other hand, building grass roots support in local communities has worked in developing countries. Eco-tourism has contributed to environmental support in countries like Belize and Kenya. In the future, protection of ecosystems will require a pluralistic approach with wild preserves connected by multiple-use corridors. In this regard, biologic and genetic diversity could be preserved for the benefit of mankind. Given a wide appeal, this approach could contribute to reduction of $CO_2$ gases and lessening of global warming and protection of regional water supplies. Desertification in the Sahel, the loss of vast wild areas to hydroelectric projects, and tribal warfare all can lead to habitat destruction and species loss. Importantly, wild areas are necessary for humans to rekindle their spirit, to seek adventure, and to learn to appreciate nature with its intricate laws and delicate balances.

## REFERENCES


1. Hunter D. *The diseases of occupations.* London: Hodder & Stough, 1987.
2. Ramazzini B. Diseases of workers. Translated by Wright WC. In: *De Morbis Artificum Diatriba,* 1713. New York: Hafner, 1964.
3. Hamilton A. *Exploring the dangerous trades.* Boston: Little, Brown, 1943.
4. U.S. Department of Health and Human Services. *National Occupational Research Agenda.* DHHS (NIOSH) Publication No. 96-115. Washington, DC: DHHS.
5. Newman LS. Occupational illness. *N Engl J Med* 1995;333:1128–1134.
6. Cullen MR, Cherniack MG, Rosenstock L. Occupational medicine. *N Engl J Med* 1990;322:594–601, 675–683.
7. Occupational and environmental medicine: the internist's role. *Ann Intern Med* 1990;113:974–982.
8. Landrigan PJ, Baker DB. The recognition and control of occupational disease. *JAMA* 1991;266:676–680.
9. Stanbury M, Joyce P, Kipen H. Silicosis and workers' compensation in New Jersey. *J Occup Environ Med* 1995;37:1342–1347.

10. Castorina JS, Rosenstock L. Physician shortage in occupational and environmental medicine. *Ann Intern Med* 1990;113:983–986.
11. Rosenstock L, Rest KM, Benson JA, et al. Occupational and environmental medicine. Meeting the growing need for clinical services. *N Engl J Med* 1991;325:924–927.
12. Graber DR, Musham C, Bellack JP, Holmes D. Environmental health in medical school curricula: views of academic deans. *J Occup Environ Med* 1995;37:807–811.
13. Levy BS. The teaching of occupational health in American medical schools. *J Med Educ* 1980;55:18–22.
14. Rom WN. Administration of occupational and environmental programs in a medical school: should they be a department? *J Med Educ* 1981;56:914–916.
15. Franco G. The present state of occupational and environmental medicine in Italy. *Int Arch Occup Environ Health* 1995;67:353–358.
16. Harrington JM, Aw TC. Occupational and environmental medicine in the United Kingdom. *Int Arch Occup Environ Health* 1996;68: 69–74.
17. Soulé ME. Conservation: tactics for a constant crisis. *Science* 1991; 253:744–750.

*Environmental and Occupational Medicine, Third Edition,* edited by William N. Rom. Published by Lippincott–Raven Publishers, Philadelphia, 1998.

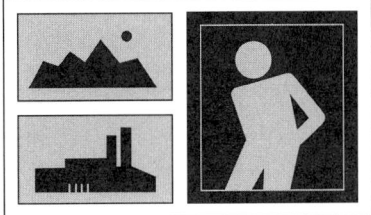

CHAPTER 2

# Recognition and Evaluation of Occupational and Environmental Health Problems

Elizabeth A. Jennison and John E. Parker

Most occupational and environmental diseases present as common medical problems or have nonspecific symptoms. Indeed, it is the etiology, rather than the pathology, that generally distinguishes disorders as occupational or environmental illnesses. It has been estimated that the workplace attribution for over 60% of occupational diseases may be unrecognized (1). Thus, clinicians must maintain a high index of suspicion for disorders that may indeed have an occupational or environmental cause. A brief occupational and environmental history should be part of every medical history. In recognition of this need, the Healthy People 2000 goals for Occupational Safety and Health (2) include the following: "Increase to at least 75% the proportion of primary care providers who routinely elicit occupational health exposures as part of the patient history and provide relevant counsel." The occupational medicine literature contains numerous references to the so-called astute clinicians who first made the connections between occupational exposures and specific disease entities (3). These range from the historical descriptions of scrotal cancer in chimney sweeps to more recent descriptions of angiosarcomas of the liver from vinyl chloride and male infertility associated with dibromochloropropane.

Early diagnosis and proper management can improve outcomes for many occupational and environmental diseases. For example, the duration of exposure after the development of symptoms is a significant predictor of long-term outcome in occupational asthma (4). Recognition of an occupational disease in an individual may serve as a sentinel health event indicating a public health need for intervention to prevent disease in other exposed workers (5). While clinical recognition and evaluation of the contribution of workplace and environmental exposures to morbidity and mortality are mainstays of the specialty of occupational medicine, all physicians should be alert to these conditions in their patients. Extensive knowledge of toxicology is not needed for the evaluation of most occupational and environmental disorders. As in general medicine, the history is the most important aspect of making a diagnosis and is complemented by the findings of the physical examination. Chapter 4 provides a detailed discussion of the occupational and environmental history and physical examination. Laboratory tests and other diagnostic modalities can help confirm suspicions suggested by the history or physical findings.

## DIAGNOSTIC MODALITIES

Levels of many substances or their metabolites are directly measurable in blood or urine. These tests may be used in ongoing biologic monitoring programs, or as part of the diagnostic evaluation in the workup of a single worker or a small group of workers (6). Lead and benzene are the two most common substances for which employers provide ongoing biologic monitoring as part of medical surveillance programs (7). Published references summarize the medical tests recommended by the United States federal government and independent researchers for sub-

E. A. Jennison: Occupational Medicine, Excel Corporate Care Clinic, Middletown, Ohio 45044.

J. E. Parker: Division of Respiratory Disease Studies, National Institute for Occupational Safety and Health, Centers for Disease Control and Prevention; and Department of Pulmonary and Critical Care Medicine, West Virginia University School of Medicine, Morgantown, West Virginia 26505-2888.

stances regulated by the Occupational Safety and Health Administration (OSHA) (8). The sampling time for biologic monitoring may be very critical and must be adhered to, particularly when the levels of the determinant change rapidly or accumulation occurs because of continued exposure to the chemical. If the worker has been unexposed for a significant period of time, the detectable body burden may be low despite the existence of adverse health effects. The physician should keep in mind that results from biologic sampling are reflective of exposure and not direct measures of adverse health effects. There may be considerable variation in the observed effects from a given exposure; persons who have idiosyncratic responses due to sensitization, coexisting conditions, or other intrinsic characteristics may suffer adverse effects from exposures that are generally considered safe.

In medical surveillance settings, audiometric examinations are the most commonly employed testing modality (7). Chest radiographs, preferably classified by the International Labor Organization (ILO) system (9), pulmonary function testing, serial peak flow measurements, and carbon monoxide diffusing capacity are common tools for evaluating pulmonary abnormalities (10). Surveillance end points have been proposed for hepatotoxins (11), nephrotoxins (12), neurologic disorders (13), occupational cancers (14), and infectious diseases (15).

## EVALUATION OF THE WORK SITE

Occupational medicine physicians frequently are asked to participate in work-site evaluations. These evaluations may be performed to determine the work-relatedness of a

**TABLE 1.** *An approach to the collection of health-related data*

Establishing a case definition and confirming cases:

1. Is there a sentinel case or a cluster of reported illnesses?
2. Is there a syndrome-like consistency to the reported symptoms and signs?
3. Have examining physicians confirmed the cases?
4. Are reproductive or "take-home" familial effects recognized or plausible?
5. Once cases are confirmed, can the reported clinical syndrome or case definition be explained by a biologically plausible hypothesis (differential diagnosis), e.g., exposure to chemical, physical, or infectious agents?

Case finding and descriptive epidemiology:

1. Who and how many are ill? (numerator)
2. Who and how many are exposed or at risk? (denominator)
3. Can you estimate the prevalence or attack ratio? (numerator/denominator)
4. Is there evidence of urgency because of the severity, extent, or progression of symptoms?
5. Is there evidence of a unique or high-risk group of affected persons (response by job types, job locations, or tenure at work)?
6. Is there a temporal or spatial pattern to the onset of the problems among individuals or within job categories? Do symptoms vary with process changes, shift changes, weekends, shutdown, or transfer from one job to another?
7. What are the predictive value, sensitivity, and specificity of screening tests available for case identification and case confirmation?
8. Can you characterize the affected or exposed populations by a line listing of name, age, zip code, sex, ethnicity, job classification, date of hire, time in current job, and date and circumstances of onset of symptoms, if any? When available, list previous occupations, smoking history, and other known risk factors.
9. Is there a relevant preemployment medical database? Are routine periodic follow-up examinations performed? Are the compensation, medical, and life insurance records accessible and organized to include information on the employees occupational and medical histories, as well as specific diagnoses?

Analytical epidemiology:

1. Is there an appropriate nearby occupational group available for comparison studies?
2. Does the company, Centers for Disease Control or NIOSH, state health department, federal or state regulatory agency, or a nearby medical center have epidemiologic data on relevant exposures, morbidity, and mortality patterns in the work site and the local community (i.e., the expected values)?
3. If subacute or chronic disease is suspected, can former employees be located and their vital status ascertained? Can the cause of death be ascertained for deceased former employees? Are there historical environmental monitoring records available for former and present employee exposures by job category?
4. Considering the expected distribution and occurrence of similar disease entities that may be attributable to infectious, immune, congenital, vascular, metabolic, neoplastic, degenerative, or psychosocial processes, can you account for any excess of disease by a plausible association with prevalent or historical occupational exposures?
5. Do the size of the population at risk and an available comparison group permit reliable detection of a true excess of disease?

**TABLE 2.** *An approach to the collection of environment-related or work site hazard data*

1. Can you describe the industrial process (or processes) and physical plant, including the nature and adequacy of industrial hygiene control technology (local and general ventilation, etc.)?
2. Are the problems isolated within the workplace by location or job types?
3. Are agents present that are known or suspected to cause the alleged acute, subacute, or chronic health problems?
4. What is the physical form of these agents? By what route or routes of entry are workers exposed?
5. Are there industrial processes for which the composition, exposures, and toxicity of products and by-products are inadequately characterized?
6. Have there recently been changes in the raw materials, maintenance, or operation of industrial processes? Be sure to consider lubricants, additives, solvents, contaminants, products, and by-products, as well as the major industrial agents or processes. Obtain material safety data sheets for suspected agents and the results of bulk analyses for the identification of trace contaminants.
7. If the problems have been chronic, why is the request being made now?
8. What is known about the compliance history and environmental monitoring results of the workplace environment with respect to known agents and established standards?
9. Are labor-management or workers' compensation disputes involved in the request?

single patient's symptoms, to investigate allegations of adverse health effects in a group of workers, to assist in the design of health and safety programs for a facility, or as a work-site "follow-back" study of a sentinel health event (Table 1). These workplace evaluations can range from brief walk-through surveys to more in-depth investigations including medical and environmental testing. The general evaluation format presented here follows that used by National Institute for Occupational Safety and Health (NIOSH) investigators in the Health Hazard Evaluation (HHE) program. The NIOSH teams usually consist of a medical officer and an industrial hygiene professional working together to perform a comprehensive evaluation of occupational hazards in a workplace (Table 2).

Consultants conducting work-site evaluations should gather as much information as possible about the establishment before the site visit. Frequently this begins with a literature search centered around the materials and processes used. The NIOSHTIC database (Table 3) contains citations from the occupational safety and health literature as well as NIOSH reports. It is useful both as a reference source and to determine whether NIOSH has conducted an HHE at this or similar facilities. Other useful electronic databases include MEDLINE (Table 3), a good general medical database, and TOXLINE (Table 3), which is a fairly specific toxicology database. The Registry of Toxic Effects of Chemical Substances (RTECS) (Table 3) is a specialty database, produced by NIOSH, that contains data on toxicity, irritation, mutagenicity, reproductive effects, U.S. government standards for occupational exposure, and other data on more than 100,000 chemical substances. The increasing availability of scientific databases via Internet and World Wide Web technologies makes this information accessible even to occupational health professionals who have limited access to university or government research settings.

All work-site evaluations should begin with an opening conference led by the occupational health consultant. Attendees should include the plant manager, an individual responsible for plant health and safety, and at least one worker representative. This meeting should define the scope and nature of the investigation, address methods of environmental and medical testing, and clarify concerns about trade secret and medical confidentiality issues. All attendees should be given the opportunity to ask questions or express concerns about the investigation process.

Once the opening conference is complete, the consultant team should devote some time to reviewing company health and safety records before actually beginning the walk-through. OSHA 200 logs can provide a good source of information about company injury and illness incidence rates, but company record-keeping practices, including who has responsibility for log maintenance, may result in considerable variability in reporting between firms or from year to year. Logs from a company nurse, physician, or first-aid center may give additional information about injuries and illnesses that were not considered reportable. The company's hazard communication program should be reviewed. A material safety data sheet (MSDS) should be available for each toxic material used in a workplace (16); review of this information can identify many potential occupational hazards. Even a comprehensive set of MSDSs may not reflect all chemical hazards in the workplace since reactive intermediates in the manufacturing process will not be reflected in this information. For example, the 1984 Bhopal disaster in India involved the release of methyl isocyanate, an intermediate in the production process of manufacturing the insecticide carbaryl.

Industrial hygiene data collected by the company or outside consultants should be reviewed. Ideally, personal sampling data are available for a representative number of employees throughout the plant and have been correlated with appropriate medical or biologic monitoring data. In reality, environmental monitoring data may be limited to area samples or to personal samples on a small number of workers. Individual work practices vary enough that two

**TABLE 3.** *Sources of access to the occupational health information*

Most hospitals offer some form of access to the MEDLINE and TOXLINE databases. Hospital librarians usually are quite skilled at searching these databases. They can also assist in locating journal articles and documents identified from literature searches.

For persons who wish to perform their own literature searches and who have basic microcomputer equipment and modem, direct access is available to MEDLINE, TOXLINE, NIOSHTIC, RTECS, and other databases.

Direct access to the MEDLINE and TOXLINE files of the National Library of Medicine can be arranged by contacting:

MEDLARS Management Section
National Library of Medicine
8600 Rockville Pike
Bethesda, MD 20894
Telephone: (800) 272-4787; (301) 496-6193
FAX Number: (301) 496-0822
E-mail: PUBLICINFO@NLM.NIH.GOV

Access the NLM Home Page on the World Wide Web at:
http://nlm.nih.gov

NIOSHTIC and RTECS and other on-line databases are available through private vendors. The list is available from the NIOSH Publications Dissemination office (see address below).

For assistance with obtaining NIOSH publications, contact the following office:

National Institute for Occupational Safety and Health
Publications Dissemination
4676 Columbia Parkway
Cincinnati, OH 45226-1998
Telephone: (800) 356-4674; (513) 533-8287
FAX Number: (513) 533-8573
E-mail: PUBSTAFT

Access the NIOSH Home Page on the World Wide Web at:
http://www.cdc.gov/niosh/homepage.html

To request a NIOSH Health Hazard Evaluation, contact:

Division of Surveillance, Hazard Evaluations, and Field Studies
National Institute for Occupational Safety and Health
Alice Hamilton Laboratory
5555 Ridge Avenue
Cincinnati, OH 45213
Telephone: (800) 356-4674; (513) 841-4428

For assistance with obtaining OSHA publications, contact the following office:

U.S. Department of Labor
Occupational Safety and Health Administration
Publications Office, Room N-3101
200 Constitution Avenue, N.W.
Washington, DC 20210
Telephone: (202) 523-9667

workers doing the same job in nearly identical settings may have quite different exposures. The use of personal protective equipment may also modify individual exposures, although this is difficult to quantify. Workers may be using personal protective equipment without appropriate environmental data to demonstrate a need for it or to assist in appropriate selection. For example, many small firms require hearing protection in areas that are perceived as "noisy," but have never conducted noise surveys. As a result, individuals who should be included in a hearing conservation program may not be, and individuals who work in noisy areas, especially those exposed to impact noise, may be inadequately protected. Similarly, the choice of appropriate respiratory protection also depends on adequate knowledge of the nature and level of air contaminants in the work environment (17).

When permitted, the occupational medical consultant should review any medical surveillance data collected through company programs. This may be difficult to access or look at systematically since a great percentage of occupational medical services are performed by outside clinics rather than in company facilities. Companies may allow consulting physicians to review medical records that their employees have submitted in support of workers' compensation claims. If the consultation is being conducted in response to employee complaints, individuals who have sought medical consultation relating to the occupational conditions under investigation may voluntarily submit copies of their medical records for review.

In addition to the aforementioned medical and environmental information, the database for occupational health and safety consultations should be expanded to include information on company history, the formal statement of company goals, the actual working goals, formal and informal organizational structure, labor-management relations, and regional economic trends (18). For example, one manufacturer noted a sharp upturn in workplace injuries despite continued efforts to improve their safety program. On further review, it was found that the plant had a 50% annual turnover rate, which made it difficult to implement and sustain safety training. The high turnover was attributed to low local unemployment, the plant's requirement of shift rotation while competing employers had fixed shifts, and a wage scale that was on the low end for the area. High worker turnover and high production demands due to product popularity contributed to a high injury rate, despite stated company safety goals.

The walk-through evaluation itself is best accomplished by following the process from the entry of raw materials into the plant until the point where the finished product leaves the facility. This format should allow the consultant to see most job categories and departments and most routine job tasks. Maintenance activities and "rework" of substandard product should be evaluated as well. Tasks that are performed infrequently or are not viewed as an integral part of the production process are often given little attention in company health and safety activities until they are associated with an injury or illness. The use of personal protective equipment in prescribed areas should be observed, as well as employee hygiene practices such as eating, drinking, or smoking in potentially contaminated areas. The physician should keep in mind that exposure may occur through inhalation, ingestion, dermal absorption, or a combination thereof, and should look for evidence of these as the walk-through is conducted.

During the walk-through, it is useful to ask employees about their work. Individual workers can often provide more insight into their specific job task than the plant representative present on the walk-through. Discussions regarding health problems should be brief, informal, and confidential. Initial questions should be open-ended, rather than directed at specific symptoms or complaints. These can be followed with more specific questions about the nature, duration, timing and frequency of symptoms, as well as their association with work activities. It is also helpful to ask workers whether they know of any individuals who left employment with this company for health-related reasons.

If an industrial hygiene consultant is present, the walk-through survey may provide an opportunity for some limited environmental monitoring to help identify workplace contaminants and potential sources or exposure areas in the plant. Direct reading sampling equipment is available to assess airborne chemical contaminants such as carbon monoxide, oxides of nitrogen, acid gases, and combustible hydrocarbons (19). Smoke tubes are a convenient means of observing airflow patterns relating to plant operations or ventilation systems; velocity meters can be used to obtain more exact information on plant ventilation (20).

The findings from the walk-through survey will suggest whether a potential occupational health hazard exists, and whether an in-depth medical or environmental survey, or both, is needed to characterize it. If environmental data demonstrates significant potential exposures, the industrial hygiene consultant may recommend either a thorough one-time survey or an ongoing monitoring program. Ongoing monitoring is particularly useful for exposures to agents whose health effects include long periods with asymptomatic changes and conditions that may benefit from early detection (21). Design of an in-depth medical survey should be based on findings from the walk-through and knowledge about the expected adverse health effects of substances used in the workplace. Outside consultants will usually be limited to conducting cross-sectional studies, with their inherent limitations of measuring disease prevalence rather than incidence and inability to establish a temporal relation between exposure and disease. Other study methodologies, such as cohort and case-control designs may be more appropriate for investigating certain conditions; epidemiologic texts discuss the use and limitations of these study designs (22).

In addition to the technical and scientific skills required for workplace evaluations, health and safety consultants need to develop an understanding of how business and management practices contribute to the occurrence of work-related injury and inhibit adoption and implementation of health and safety recommendations (18). As an example, several employees at a large beverage manufacturer sustained back injuries performing a task known as "repalletization," which involved dismantling finished pallets of product and creating new pallets composed of a mixture of product lines. This task was necessary because the sales force sold the product in case units but the plant had an automated system that produced pallet units. The ergonomics consultant who was asked to reengineer the repalletization task suggested the administrative action of changing sales units to pallets, rather than trying to ergonomically correct an unnecessary task.

When the work-site evaluation is complete, whether after the walk-through or following a more in-depth survey, a report should be issued that summarizes the findings of the investigation and makes appropriate recommendations for continuing health and safety activities within the establishment. For example, the industrial hygienist might recommend appropriate control technology or an ongoing environmental monitoring program. The occupational health physician may recommend, and help the company design, an ongoing medical surveillance program using appropriate screening tests to look for end-organ effects associated with the hazards encountered in the workplace (23). An understanding of the firm's organizational structure is critical to the consultants' ability to bring about change. The consultant must identify and have access to someone with enough authority to facilitate the acceptance and implementation of the final recommendations (18).

## CASE STUDIES

The following cases illustrate the importance of considering an occupational or environmental etiology in evaluating an individual patient, the need for a timely diagnosis, and the concept of an occupational illness in one worker being a sentinel health event suggesting that other workers are at risk.

### Case Study 1

A 41-year-old man with no underlying respiratory problems worked as a maintenance man at a company that used an isocyanate-based polyurethane foam in its products. While working directly with the foaming process, he developed headache, fever, joint pain, dry cough, and shortness of breath. When symptoms worsened, he was taken to the local emergency room, and subsequently admitted to the intensive care unit. No connection was made between his illness and his work; his discharge diagnosis was viral pneumonitis.

He returned to work 2 weeks later, and worked with the polyurethane foam system. Respiratory symptoms developed again, and he was readmitted to the hospital later that day. Discharge diagnoses were bronchitis due to an industrial toxin and pneumonitis due to exposure to industrial toxin.

On returning to work after this second episode, the worker began to note a strong temporal relationship between his proximity to the foaming process and his respiratory symptoms. Three months after his initial illness, he consulted a local pulmonologist who diagnosed his clinical presentation as being consistent with hypersensitivity pneumonitis due to isocyanates. Pulmonary function testing revealed severe restriction with a moderate diffusion defect and mild obstruction. On the advice of the pulmonologist, the worker terminated his employment at that establishment due to inability to avoid exposure to isocyanates.

Two months later this patient was placed on oral steroids. After 2 weeks he developed an acute febrile illness and died. An autopsy revealed bilateral acute bacterial pneumonia and chronic interstitial pneumonitis (24,25).

Delay in recognizing the work-relatedness of the patient's condition resulted in repeated exposure with subsequent morbidity and mortality.

### Case Study 2

A state health department responded to a physician's report of the death of a 55-year-old worker with accelerated silicosis and associated *Mycobacterium kansasii* infection. The man had been a sandblaster for 10 years, most recently in a metal preparation shop.

A work-site evaluation was conducted and revealed that although sandblasters were wearing respiratory protection, it was inadequate to protect them against the very high levels of respirable crystalline silica found in the workplace. Workers reported that coworkers had developed problems while working as sandblasters and that the employer typically hired six to seven new sandblasters each year to replace those who quit. One current worker was identified with severe silicosis, including progressive massive fibrosis, and several workers were found to have simple silicosis. Air sampling outside the blasting room indicated poor containment of the dust, potentially exposing other workers (26).

This case illustrates how a sentinel occupational health event led to investigation of a workplace where an ongoing hazard existed. This also demonstrates the incorporation of medical and environmental testing in a work-site evaluation.

### Case Study 3

A 52-year-old nonsmoking male landscape architect presented to the emergency room with a 6-hour history of dyspnea, fever, headache, and myalgia. Twelve hours prior to presentation he had shoveled composted wood chips and leaves. Examination showed a patient in moderate respiratory distress, with a respiratory rate of 30, heart rate of 120, and an oral temperature of 38.8°C. Lung auscultation revealed fine bibasilar crackles without wheezing. Chest radiographs demonstrated bilateral infiltrates. Arterial $PO_2$ was 53 mm Hg. Systemic steroid therapy and antibiotics were started. A working diagnosis of pneumonia versus hypersensitivity pneumonitis was proposed.

The pulmonary infiltrates and hypoxemia worsened during the next 12 hours, but then improved over the subsequent 3 days. Pulmonary function testing the morning after admission revealed mild restriction (forced vital capacity (FVC) 68% of predicted). The symptoms and infiltrates improved, and the patient was discharged on the third hospital day. One month later he had no respiratory symptoms, and spirometry and diffusing capacity were normal.

Environmental studies revealed that the compost was a suitable substrate for the growth of many fungi and bacteria and measured significant levels of inspirable and respirable dust. These findings supported the clinical diagnosis of organic dust toxic syndrome (ODTS) (27,28).

This case illustrates how nonspecific symptoms may be attributed to common illnesses unless an occupational etiology is sought.

### Case Study 4

A 44-year-old woman developed a severe cough, burning of her eyes and throat, shortness of breath, weakness, wheezing, myalgia, headache, and slurred speech approximately 45 minutes after spraying an aerosolized leather-shoe conditioner on a pair of boots. In the emergency room, she had a temperature of 101.1°F, pulse of 100, and a respiratory rate of 28. She had bilateral rales and an arterial oxygen partial pressure ($PO_2$) of 60 mm Hg on oxygen at 3 L per minute via nasal cannula. A chest x-ray revealed bilateral midzone interstitial infiltrates. Her white blood count was 21,300 cells per $mm^3$, with 90% segmented forms. Liver function tests, electrolytes, urea, and creatinine were normal. Treatment was initiated with antivirals, antibiotics, and a bronchodilator. By the next day, the patient's dyspnea had resolved, she was afebrile, and her pulse and respiratory rate were normal. A repeat chest x-ray showed almost complete clearing of the pulmonary infiltrates.

An 11-year-old boy, who was in an adjacent room when the patient used the leather conditioner, developed a burning throat, shortness of breath, cough, and abdominal pain approximately 45 minutes after exposure. He did not seek medical attention (29).

These cases represent just two of an estimated 500 cases of adverse responses to leather sprays that were reported in 1992 and 1993. Two different leather sprays were implicated; both had been reformulated to comply with the 1990 amendments to the Clean Air Act. Chemical analyses suggested major alterations in the fluorohydrocarbon constituents of the sprays, and laboratory studies also revealed the toxicity of the new products in animals (30).

This case illustrates toxicity associated with an agent in the home environment rather than the workplace. It also demonstrates how changing a product to reduce adverse environmental impact, in this case to comply with the Clean Air Act in an effort to protect the ozone layer, can have unexpected adverse health consequences.

## SUMMARY

The symptoms and physical findings associated with exposure to occupational and environmental hazards are often nonspecific; a suitably high index of suspicion is needed for physicians to detect disease-toxin connections in the workplace. Attention to the occupational history and physical examination, the use of appropriate diagnostic modalities, work-site evaluations, and interactions with other health and safety professionals will enable the clinician to contribute both to the health of the individual patient and to that of the work force as a whole.

## ACKNOWLEDGMENTS

The editor and authors acknowledge Brian A. Boehlecke and Robert S. Bernstein for important contributions to this chapter in earlier editions of this book.

## REFERENCES

1. Brancati FL, Hodgson MJ, Korpf M. Occupational exposures and diseases among medical inpatients. *J Occup Med* 1993;35(2):161–165.
2. Department of Health and Human Services. *Healthy People 2000.* DHHS Publication No. 91-50213 (1991). Washington, DC: DHHS.
3. Fleming LE, Ducatman AM, Shalat SL. Disease clusters: a central and ongoing role in occupational health. *J Occup Med* 1989;33(7): 818–825.
4. Chan-Yeung M. Occupational asthma. *Chest* 1990;98(5):148s–161s.
5. Rutstein D, Mullan J, Frazier TM, Halperin WE, Melius JM, Sestito JP. Sentinel health events (occupational): a basis for physician recognition and public health surveillance. *Am J Public Health* 1983;73: 1054–1062.
6. Rosenberg J, Rempel D. Biological monitoring. In: Rempel D, ed. *Occupational medicine:* state of the art reviews, vol. 5, no. 3, *Medical surveillance in the workplace.* Philadelphia: Hanley & Belfus, 1990; 491–498.
7. Conway H, Simmons J, Talbert T. The Occupational Safety and Health Administration's 1990–1991 Survey of Occupational Medical Surveillance Prevalence and Type of Current Practice. *J Occup Med* 1993; 35(7):659–669.
8. Murthy LI, Halperin WE. Medical screening and biological monitoring. A guide to the literature for physicians. *J Occup Environ Med* 1995;37(2):170–184.
9. ILO. *Guidelines for the use of ILO international classification of radiographs of pneumoconioses.* Occupational Safety and Health Series, No. 22 (rev.). Geneva: International Labor Office, 1980.
10. Balmes JR. Medical surveillance for pulmonary endpoints. In: Rempel D, ed. *Occupational medicine:* state of the art reviews, vol. 5, no. 3, *Medical surveillance in the workplace.* Philadelphia: Hanley & Belfus, 1990;499–514.
11. Harrison R. Medical surveillance for workplace hepatotoxins. In: Rempel D, ed. *Occupational medicine:* state of the art reviews, vol. 5, no. 3, *Medical surveillance in the workplace.* Philadelphia: Hanley & Belfus, 1990;515–530.
12. Kosnett MJ. Medical surveillance for renal endpoints. In: Rempel D, ed. *Occupational medicine:* state of the art reviews, vol. 5, no. 3, *Medical surveillance in the workplace.* Philadelphia: Hanley & Belfus, 1990;531–546.
13. Cone JE, Bowler R, So Y. Medical surveillance for neurologic endpoints. In: Rempel D, ed. *Occupational medicine:* state of the art reviews, vol. 5, no. 3, *Medical surveillance in the workplace.* Philadelphia: Hanley & Belfus, 1990;547–562.
14. Cone JE, Rosenberg J. Medical surveillance and biomonitoring for occupational cancer endpoints. In: Rempel D, ed. *Occupational medicine:* state of the art reviews, vol. 5, no. 3, *Medical surveillance in the workplace.* Philadelphia: Hanley & Belfus, 1990;563–582.
15. Rosenberg J, Clever LH. Medical surveillance of infectious disease endpoints. In: Rempel D, ed. *Occupational medicine:* state of the art reviews, vol. 5, no. 3, *Medical surveillance in the workplace.* Philadelphia: Hanley & Belfus, 1990;583–606.
16. Office of the Federal Register. *CFR:* Code of Federal Regulations. Washington, DC: U.S. Government Printing Office, 1910.1200, hazard communication.
17. NIOSH. *Guide to industrial respiratory protection.* Cincinnati, OH: U.S. Department of Health and Human Services, Public Health Service, Centers for Disease Control, National Institute for Occupational Safety and Health, Division of Safety Research, 1987.

18. Snyder TB, Himmelstein J, Pransky G, Beavers JD. Business analysis in occupational health and safety consultations. *J Occup Med* 1991; 33(10):1040–1045.
19. ACGIH. *Air sampling instruments for evaluation of atmospheric contaminants,* 7th ed. Cincinnati, OH: American Conference of Governmental Industrial Hygienists, 1989.
20. ACGIH. *Industrial ventilation,* 20th ed. Cincinnati, OH: American Conference of Governmental Industrial Hygienists, 1988.
21. Matte TD, Fine L, Meinhardt TJ, Baker EL. Guidelines for medical screening in the workplace. In: Rempel D, ed. *Occupational medicine:* state of the art reviews, vol. 5, no. 3, *Medical surveillance in the workplace.* Philadelphia: Hanley & Belfus, 1990;439–456.
22. Checkoway H, Pearce N, Crawford-Brown DJ. *Research methods in occupational epidemiology.* New York: Oxford University Press, 1989.
23. NIOSH. *Hazard evaluation and technical assistance report:* Asbury Graphite Mills, *Inc., Asbury, NJ.* NIOSH Report No. 93-494. Cincinnati, OH: U.S. Department of Health and Human Services, Public Health Service, Centers for Disease Control and Prevention, National Institute for Occupational Safety and Health, 1994.
24. NIOSH. *Hazard evaluation and technical assistance report:* Distinctive Designs International, *Inc., Russellville, Alabama.* NIOSH Report No. 91-386-2427. Cincinnati, OH: U.S. Department of Health and Human Services, Public Health Service, Centers for Disease Control and Prevention, National Institute for Occupational Safety and Health, 1994.
25. CDC/NIOSH. *Preventing asthma, other respiratory disease, and death due to diisocyanate exposure.* NIOSH Alert, Publication No. 96-111. Cincinnati, OH: U.S. Department of Health and Human Services, Public Health Service, Centers for Disease Control and Prevention, and National Institute for Occupational Safety and Health, March 1996.
26. CDC/NIOSH. *Preventing silicosis and deaths from sandblasting.* NIOSH Alert, Publication No. 92-102. Cincinnati, OH: U.S. Department of Health and Human Services, Public Health Service, Centers for Disease Control and Prevention, and National Institute for Occupational Safety and Health, August 1992.
27. Weber S, Kullman G, Petsonk E, et al. Organic dust exposures from compost handling: case presentation and respiratory exposure assessment. *Am J Ind Med* 1993;24:365–374.
28. CDC/NIOSH. *Preventing organic dust toxic syndrome.* NIOSH Alert, Publication No. 94-102. Cincinnati, OH: U.S. Department of Health and Human Services, Public Health Service, Centers for Disease Control and Prevention, and National Institute for Occupational Safety and Health, April 1994.
29. CDC (Centers for Disease Control and Prevention). Severe acute respiratory illness linked to use of shoe sprays—Colorado, November 1993. *MMWR* 1993;42(46):885–887.
30. Hubbs AF, Castranova V, Ma JYC, et al. Acute lung injury induced by a commercial leather conditioner. *Toxicol Appl Pharmacol* 1997:143; 37–46.

*Environmental and Occupational Medicine, Third Edition,* edited by William N. Rom.
Lippincott–Raven Publishers, Philadelphia © 1998.

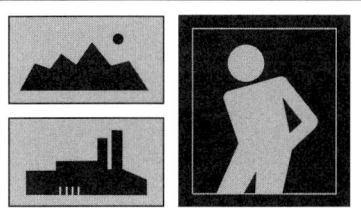

CHAPTER 3

# The Role of Surveillance in Occupational Health

Steven B. Markowitz

Occupational health surveillance entails the systematic monitoring of health events and exposures in working populations in order to prevent and control occupational hazards and their associated diseases and injuries. Occupational health surveillance, like all public health surveillance systems, has four essential components (1,2):

1. to gather information on cases of occupational diseases and injuries and on workplace exposures;
2. to distill and analyze the data;
3. to disseminate organized data to necessary parties, including workers, unions, employers, governmental agencies, and the public; and
4. to intervene on the basis of data to alter the factors that produced these health events and hazards.

Surveillance in occupational health has been more concisely described as counting, evaluating, and acting (3).

The word *surveillance* derives from the French word *surveiller,* "to watch over," which encompasses the twin notions of careful observation and timely intervention. It is important to emphasize that the enumeration and documentation of cases of occupational disease and injury is inseparable from the obligation to attempt to alter the conditions that led to the described occupational health morbidity and mortality (1,4). This obligation to take preventive action on the basis of surveillance data stems from a well-defined series of moral, ethical, and legal responsibilities of employers, governmental agencies, and unions.

Significant gains in occupational health surveillance have been achieved during the past 10 years (5). The National Institute for Occupational Safety and Health (NIOSH) has instituted several new programs including the Sentinel Event Notification Systems for Occupational Risks (SENSOR), the Adult Blood Lead Surveillance and Epidemiology program (ABLES), National Traumatic Occupational Fatalities (NTOF), and the National Occupational Mortality Surveillance (NOMS). The Bureau of Labor Statistics of the Department of Labor redesigned its Annual Survey of Occupational Injuries and Illnesses in 1992 to obtain additional information on selected illness and injuries from employers and has additionally developed a new fatality surveillance initiative, the Census of Fatal Occupational Injuries (CFOI) (5).

Surveillance has at least two meanings in occupational health. Public health surveillance refers to activities undertaken by federal, state, or local governments within their respective jurisdictions to monitor and to follow-up occupational diseases and injuries. This type of surveillance is population-based, i.e., the working public, and the events being studied are suspected or established diagnoses of occupational illness and injury. This chapter describes these activities.

Medical surveillance refers to the ongoing application of medical tests and procedures to individual workers who may be at risk for occupational morbidity to determine whether an occupational disorder may be present. Medical surveillance is generally broad in scope and represents the first step in ascertaining the presence of a work-related problem. If an individual or a population is exposed to a toxin with known effects and the tests and procedures are highly targeted to detect the likely presence of one or more effects in these persons, then this surveillance activity is more aptly described as medical screening (6). A medical surveillance program applies tests and procedures on a group of workers with common

S.B. Markowitz: Department of Community and Preventive Medicine, Mt. Sinai School of Medicine, New York, New York 10029-6574.

exposures for the purpose of identifying individuals who may have occupational illnesses and for the purpose of detecting patterns of illness among the program participants, which may be produced by occupational exposures. Such a program is usually undertaken under the auspices of the individual's employer or union.

In occupational health, there are two kinds of surveillance activities: (a) public health and medical surveillance, as defined above; and (b) hazard surveillance. Hazard surveillance is the monitoring of exposure to chemical agents, physical hazards, or radiation in the workplace. The two types of surveillance data complement each other. This chapter discusses both types of surveillance.

## FUNCTIONS OF OCCUPATIONAL HEALTH SURVEILLANCE

The main purpose of occupational health surveillance is to identify the incidence and prevalence of known occupational diseases and injuries. Gathering descriptive epidemiologic data on the incidence and prevalence of these diseases on an accurate and comprehensive basis is an essential prerequisite for establishing a rational approach to the control of occupational disease and injury. Assessment of the nature, magnitude, and distribution of occupational disease and injury in the United States or in another geographic area requires a sound epidemiologic database. It is only through an epidemiologic assessment of the dimensions of occupational disease that its importance relative to other public health problems, its claim for resources, and the urgency of legal standard setting can be reasonably evaluated. Also, the collection of incidence and prevalence data allows analysis of trends of occupational disease and injury among different groups, at different places, and during different time periods (1). Detecting such trends is useful for determining control and research priorities and strategies and for evaluating the effectiveness of any interventions undertaken (1).

A second broad function of occupational health surveillance is to identify individual cases of occupational disease and injury in order to find and evaluate other individuals from the same workplaces who may be at risk for similar disease and injury. In addition, this process permits the initiation of control activities to ameliorate the hazardous conditions associated with causation of the index case (1,4). A further purpose of case identification may be to assure that the affected individual receives appropriate clinical follow-up, an important consideration in view of the scarcity of clinical occupational medicine specialists (7,8).

Finally, occupational health surveillance is an important means of discovering new associations between occupational agents and accompanying diseases. The potential toxicity of approximately 80% of the chemicals used in the workplace has not been evaluated in humans or in *in vivo* or *in vitro* test systems (9). Discovery of rare diseases, patterns of common diseases, or suspicious exposure-disease associations through surveillance activities in the workplace can provide vital leads for a more conclusive scientific evaluation of the problem and possible verification of new occupational diseases.

## OCCUPATIONAL SENTINEL HEALTH EVENTS

In 1983, Rutstein and investigators from NIOSH (10) adapted the concept of the sentinel health event, which had originally been developed to judge the quality of health care, for use in occupational health surveillance. They defined the occupational sentinel health event as "A disease, disability, or untimely death which is occupationally related and whose occurrence may: 1) provide the impetus for epidemiologic or industrial hygiene studies; or 2) serve as a warning signal that materials substitution, engineering control, personal protection, or medical care may be required."

Rutstein et al. cited 50 diseases and associated occupations and industries in which the weight of available scientific evidence from epidemiologic studies and case reports indicated a causal relationship between occupational exposures and the specified diseases. Several of these diseases are uniquely or almost uniquely caused by occupational agents, such as mesothelioma and the pneumoconioses; most, however, have both occupational and nonoccupational causes, such as asthma, hearing loss, and cancer of the lung and larynx. This list has been updated to include 64 medical conditions (11) and will continue to grow as scientific knowledge about occupational diseases advances.

The occupational sentinel health event concept conveys three important and related notions. First, it is useful as a heuristic device to allow health care providers and public health authorities to sort through health events of individuals and populations to determine a priori which health events and patterns of health events are most likely to be caused by occupational factors, given current knowledge. Second, the sentinel health event concept transforms the actual health problems of individuals into the potential health problems of populations. To recognize the diagnosis of an occupational disease in an individual as a sentinel health event facilitates the identification of others at the workplace who are also ill or who may become ill if exposure continues. Third, the occurrence of a sentinel health event may signify the failure of a system to control known occupational hazards and thereby to prevent cases of unnecessary occupational disease.

Efforts to apply the concept of the sentinel health event to occupational health surveillance have begun. Mortality data from various geographic areas in the United States where occupation is usually coded on the death certificate have been evaluated using the list of occupational sentinel health events and their associated occupations and industries (12–14). Up to 10% to 15% of all deaths may be due to the 50 conditions on the occupational sentinel health event list. However, among these deaths matched to the occupational sentinel health event list, most occurred among individuals who did not work in occupations and/or industries that were cited by Rutstein et al. (10) as being associated with the specified cause of death. Indeed, in only 1% to 2% of all deaths did the death certificate cite as the cause of death an occupation that is associated with an increased risk (10,13,14). Relatively few (<5%) of all deaths that are due to causes on the occupational sentinel health event list are due to diseases that are inherently occupational, e.g., pneumoconioses, extrinsic allergic alveolitis, mesothelioma, and cancer of the scrotum. The list of occupations and industries that were reported to be associated with an increased risk of various occupational diseases may be too restrictive.

These initial studies clearly demonstrate a major limitation of the sentinel health event concept. Except for the limited number of conditions that are uniquely caused by occupational factors, many, if not most, cases of a disease that is considered a potential sentinel health event may not be occupational in origin. The *a priori* likelihood that any individual case of illness or death is an occupational sentinel health event depends on the disease, the nature and intensity of exposures in the occupational setting(s), and the coexistence of other risk factors of disease. Final determination of the work-relatedness of the illness or death in any individual case requires detailed occupational and nonoccupational information. Such detail cannot usually be found in routine data sources. The sentinel health event concept, therefore, may be useful for raising clinical suspicion of occupational disease or for delimiting the universe of disease on which public health authorities must concentrate in their efforts to engage in occupational health surveillance. But the sentinel health concept cannot overcome the ultimate need to link a specific disease with a specific exposure or occupation, which is the sine qua non of accurate and reliable surveillance.

A variation of the sentinel health event model is the sentinel health provider approach to case detection. In this variant, health providers (or facilities) whose practices are likely to include individuals with occupational injuries and illnesses are actively recruited by a public health agency to report a limited number of specified occupational conditions. This approach has been used by NIOSH in the development of its SENSOR program that is described in greater detail below.

## CURRENT OCCUPATIONAL HEALTH SURVEILLANCE ACTIVITIES IN THE UNITED STATES

### Death Certificates

National mortality data have been increasingly used for occupational health surveillance in the United States. This has occurred due to efforts by NIOSH and collaborating state health departments to overcome the historic lack of uniform and accessible information on occupation and industry on the death certificate. Previously, use of national mortality data was limited to diseases that are uniquely caused by occupational agents. Indeed, this application of mortality statistics remains useful.

Evaluation of mortality by occupation was initially accomplished in states where occupational or industrial information was recorded on the death certificate (15–19). In the United States, Milham (15,16) pioneered this approach by examining the occupational distribution of all men who died between 1950 and 1979 in Washington State. In this type of analysis, the proportion of all deaths due to any specific cause for one occupational group is compared with the relevant proportion for all occupations, yielding the proportional mortality ratio (PMR). While this measure of risk has well-known limitations, its advantages in the analysis by mortality include the ability to study occupations that are usually distributed among many workplaces (such as cooks or drycleaner workers), the use of routinely collected data, a large sample size, relatively low expense, and an important health outcome (17–19). Such studies are useful for suggesting new associations between occupations and specific causes of death, but have not been informative about the magnitude and time trends of occupational diseases.

An excellent example of the utility of this approach can be taken from Milham's occupational surveillance of death certificates in Washington State. In 1982, in one of the first studies of the relationship between occupational exposure to electromagnetic radiation and cancer, Milham noted that 10 of 11 occupations with probable exposure to electrical and magnetic fields showed an elevation in PMR for leukemia (20). This clue has led to numerous additional studies, several of which have corroborated the original finding (21–23).

As a result of an intensive cooperative effort between NIOSH, the National Center for Health Statistics, the National Cancer Institute, and the Bureau of the Census, the number of states where occupation and industry is routinely coded on the death certificate increased during the 1980s and early 1990s (5,17). This initiative has been formalized into the National Occupational Mortality Surveillance Program (NOMS). Under NOMS, data from over 500,000 death certificates are collected annually from 23 states (5). These data have been used fruitfully for a number of purposes, especially for tracking deaths due to occupation-specific conditions, such as pneumoconioses. In the *Work-Related Lung Disease Surveillance Report—1996* issued by NIOSH, the numbers, rates, and geographic distribution of deaths are provided for asbestosis, coal workers pneumoconioses, silicosis, byssinosis, and unspecified pneumoconioses (24). These data are derived from the multiple cause of death data files maintained by the National Center for Health Statistics, in which all conditions that are listed on the death certificate, both underlying and contributing, are analyzed. As an example, there were 959 deaths from asbestosis in 1992 in the United States, yielding an age-adjusted mortality rate of 2.9 deaths per 1 million U.S. population, age 15 and over. Breakdowns by age, race, sex, and time trends during the past two decades are also provided (24).

In one of the earliest and the largest mortality surveillance study to date in the United States, Robinson and colleagues (17) analyzed the mortality experience of 880,000 decedents in 14 states by occupation and industry for 1984 and selected other years in the 1980s. More recently, NIOSH investigators have begun to use the NOMS data set to examine the distribution of causes of death among specific occupations and industries. In 1995, Robinson and colleagues at NIOSH (25) published a proportionate mortality experience of construction workers from 19 states. While some of the expected associations, including asbestos-related and silica-related diseases, were found, new findings of cancer and other health outcomes were also observed for specific trades, which would provide useful leads for additional analytical studies. NIOSH investigators have also used the NOMS to examine the proportionate occupational mortality of women in the United States (26).

### Hospital Discharge Data

Diagnoses of hospitalized patients represent a new and potentially excellent source of data for the surveillance of occupational diseases. Studies in several states have shown that hospital discharge data are more sensitive than state workers' compensation records, vital statistics, and Bureau of Labor Statistics surveys in detecting cases of diseases that are specific to occupational settings, such as the pneumoconioses (7,27). In New York State, for example, an annual average of 1,049 people were hospitalized for pneumoconioses in the mid-1980s, compared to 193 newly awarded workers' compensation cases and 95 recorded deaths from these diseases each year during a similar time interval (7).

In addition to providing a more accurate count of the number of people ill with selected serious occupational diseases, hospital discharge data can be usefully followed up to detect and to alter workplace conditions that caused the disease. Thus, Rosenman (27) evaluated workplaces in New Jersey where individuals who were hospitalized for silicosis had previously worked, and found that the majority of these workplaces had never performed air sampling for silica, had never been inspected by OSHA, and did not perform medical surveillance for the detection of silicosis. More recently, Liss and colleagues (28) in Toronto examined the utility of using hospital records for case detection of coal workers' pneumoconiosis, silicosis, and asbestosis.

Advantages of using hospital discharge data for the surveillance of occupational disease are their availability, low cost, relative sensitivity to serious illness, and reasonable accuracy (19,27). Important disadvantages include the lack of information on occupation and industry, the inability to count outpatient cases, and uncertain quality control (19,27). It is likely that hospital discharge data will be increasingly used in occupational health surveillance in future years.

### Physicians' Reports

In an attempt to replicate the strategy successfully utilized for the monitoring and control of infectious diseases, an increasing number of states require physicians to report one or more occupational diseases (29). As of 1988, 32 states required reporting of occupational diseases, though these included ten states where only one occupational disease is reportable, usually lead or pesticide poisoning. In other states, such as Alaska and Maryland, all occupational diseases are reportable (29). In most states, reported cases are used only to count the number of people affected by the disease in the state. In only one-third of the states with reportable disease requirements does a report of a case of occupational disease lead to follow-up activities, such as workplace inspection (30).

Despite the evidence of increased recent interest, physician reporting of occupational diseases to appropriate state governmental authorities is widely acknowledged to be inadequate (31,32). Even in California, where a system for physician reporting has been in place for a number of years (Doctor's First Report of Occupational Illness and Injury) and recorded nearly 50,000 occupational illnesses in 1988 (33), physician compliance with reporting is regarded as incomplete (31).

A promising innovation in occupational health surveillance that was developed by NIOSH in the late 1980s, SENSOR rests on the concept of the sentinel health provider (34). A sentinel provider is a physician or other health care provider (or facility) who, due to their specialty or geographic location, is likely to provide care for workers with occupational disorders. Since sentinel providers represent a small subset of all health care providers, health departments can feasibly organize an active occupational disease reporting system by performing outreach, offering education, and providing timely feedback to sentinel providers. In an early report from three states participating in the SENSOR program (New Jersey, Michigan, and Colorado), physician reports of occupational asthma increased sharply after the state health departments developed concerted educational and outreach programs to identify and recruit sentinel providers (35). Similar results were obtained for reporting of pesticide poisoning due to occupational exposures in Oregon and California.

As part of SENSOR at present, NIOSH provides support to 14 states to develop surveillance systems for 12 occupational conditions, including silicosis, amputations, asthma, burns, cadmium poisoning, carbon monoxide poisoning, carpal tunnel syndrome, childhood injuries, dermatitis, noise-induced hearing loss, pesticide poisoning, and tuberculosis (5). Maizlish and colleagues (36) recently reported on the application of the SENSOR concept to carpal tunnel syndrome in California. They demonstrated the ability of SENSOR methods to identify cases of carpal tunnel syndrome that were not identified by other reporting systems, documented that employers health insurance rather than workers' compensation paid for most of the costs associated with the cases of carpal tunnel syndrome, and identified obstacles to improvement in the workplace conditions that gave rise to the increased risk for developing carpal tunnel syndrome.

**Laboratory Reports**

Reporting of excessive levels of selected toxins in body fluids by clinical laboratories to state health departments is a useful tool for surveillance of poisoning by heavy metals and possibly other workplace agents for which there are reliable and widely used laboratory diagnostic tests. Such reporting allows identification of the workplaces where exposure occurred, categorization of the cases by occupation and industry, estimation of the number of other workers at the index workplace potentially exposed to lead, and assurance of medical follow-up (37). Other metals recorded in the Heavy Metal Registry in New York State include arsenic, mercury, and cadmium.

In the 1990s, NIOSH organized the state-based registries of lead poisoning into the Adult Blood Lead Epidemiology and Surveillance program (ABLES) in order to track elevated blood lead levels among adults in the United States (38). This program has grown since its inception and, as of 1996, obtained reports from 25 states. In 1995, ABLES received 26,459 reports of blood lead levels >25 μg of lead per deciliter of whole blood (%). Through these reports, 12,664 adults with elevated blood lead levels were identified, including nearly 5,000 individuals who represented new cases of elevated blood lead levels (38). NIOSH has continued the ABLES program for several years, allowing analyses of time trends.

Laboratory-based reporting is also performed on selected other exposures, including arsenic, mercury, cadmium, and blood acetyl cholinesterase levels. However, testing and reporting for these results are much less common than for blood lead. In addition, the relative sparsity of agents that can be routinely measured through monitoring bodily fluids provides an inherent limitation to this approach to occupational hazard and disease surveillance.

**Workers' Compensation Reports**

Workers' compensation data provide an intuitively appealing surveillance tool in occupational health, principally because relevant occupational medicine expertise presumably considers combined health and exposure information in the evaluation of the validity of a workers' compensation claim. Unfortunately, the use of workers' compensation records as a credible source for surveillance data is subject to severe limitations, including lack of standardization of eligibility requirements, deficiency of standard case definitions, disincentives to workers and employers to file claims, the lack of physician recognition of chronic occupational diseases with long latency periods, and the usual gap of several years between initial filing and resolution of a claim. The net effect of these limitations is that reliance on workers' compensation data leads to a drastic underreporting of occupational disease.

Thus, in a study by Selikoff (38a) in the early 1980s, less than one-third of insulators who were disabled by asbestos-related disease had even filed for workers' compensation benefits. Similarly, a United States Department of Labor study of workers who reported disability from occupational disease found that less than 5% of these workers received workers' compensation benefits (39). A more recent study in New York State found that the number of people admitted to hospitals for pneumoconioses vastly outnumbered the people who were newly awarded workers' compensation benefits during a similar time period (7). Since workers' compensation systems record simple health events such as dermatitis and musculoskeletal injuries much more readily than complex diseases of long latency, use of such data leads to a skewed picture of the true incidence and distribution of occupational diseases.

The administration of workers compensation on a state by state basis with associated variability has limited its utility as a source for national surveillance purposes. In the early 1990s, the National Council on Compensation Insurance (NCCI) began to collect, analyze, and publish claims data from private workers' compensation insurance providers in 13 states (40). By 1996, NCCI expanded its included number of survey jurisdictions to 41. The use of this data set has been limited so far, but can be expected to grow in the future.

**National Surveys**

The single national occupational health data source that receives the most public attention every year is the Annual Survey of Occupational Injuries and Illnesses conducted by the Bureau of Labor Statistics (BLS) of the United States Department of Labor. The BLS Annual Survey uses a stratified sample of approximately 280,000 workplaces in the private sector, representing nearly 5 million such workplaces. The survey obtains data from the OSHA 200 Log summarized by employers and including information on the numbers of occupational fatalities, injuries, and illnesses, the types of illnesses in broad categories, the nature of the business, the type of industry, and the average employment and total hours worked at the workplace. The OSHA 200 Log is a standardized record of occupational injuries and illnesses that OSHA requires employers to maintain. BLS uses these data to publish annual statistics on the incidence of occupational injuries and illnesses by industry. The great majority of cases of occupational disease now recorded in the BLS Annual Survey are conditions associated with repetitive trauma; this category accounted for 62% of all occupational illnesses in the BLS survey in 1992.

The BLS Annual Survey has been useful in the surveillance of occupational injuries and easily recognized occupational illnesses, especially in the evaluation of alterations in the rates of these conditions over time. However, it has traditionally ignored chronic occupational diseases, such as cancer and chronic neurologic and lung disease, a limitation that reflects the weaknesses of the sources of data from which BLS derives the survey information (31). Also, substantial underrecording of occupational disease on the OSHA 200 Log has been documented and is sometimes based on deliberate falsification of records.

In response to recommendations by the National Academy of Sciences (31), the BLS redesigned its annual survey in the early 1990s. In addition to previous information collected, the new survey includes specific information on workers with occupational illnesses and injuries that are considered serious (i.e., involve 1 or more lost workdays). Newly collected information includes occupation, age, gender, race, length of service, nature of illness/injury, part of body affected, event or exposure, and primary and secondary sources of illness and injury. This redesigned survey was first conducted in 1992.

The redesign of the BLS Annual Survey in 1992 has provided an unprecedented opportunity to examine the extent to which employers record specific chronic diseases as occupational in origin. Categories of disease used in previous BLS surveys were too broad and few to identify diseases of interest such as cancer and heart disease. In the BLS survey in 1992, there were 1,485 cases of coronary heart disease, stroke, cancer and chronic respiratory disease. This number represents 0.8% of all serious occupational illnesses. While the nature of nonserious occupational illnesses recorded in the BLS survey is unknown, they are unlikely to consist of a significant number of cases of coronary heart disease, stroke, cancer, and chronic respiratory disease, given the severity of morbidity that usually accompanies these diseases. Thus, despite the well-demonstrated increase in occupational diseases recorded by the BLS, especially from 1986 to 1992, the four leading causes of death and disease in the United States are still not recorded in large numbers by the occupational disease surveillance system of the BLS.

The National Center for Health Statistics (NCHS), part of the Centers for Disease Control and Prevention, conducts two periodic national health surveys relevant to occupational health surveillance, the National Health Interview Survey (NHIS) and the National Health and Nutrition Examination Survey (NHANES). The NHIS is an annual nationwide survey of approximately 50,000 to 120,000 individuals in the United States designed to collect questionnaire information about morbidity, disability, and medical care (31). The chief advantages of the NHIS are its multistage probability sampling strategy encompassing the entire United States, its availability as public-use data sets, and the large amount of information about demographics and lifestyle factors that it routinely collects (41).

Through a cooperative effort between the NCHS and NIOSH, the NHIS that was conducted in 1988 contained a one-time Occupational Health Supplement (OHS) to gather information on the number and the severity of selected work-related injuries and diseases (41). The OHS interview was administered to 44,233 individuals, a large subset of the overall NHIS survey conducted that year. Tanaka and colleagues at NIOSH (42) recently analyzed OHS results for carpal tunnel syndrome and estimated that 675,000 recently employed workers had prolonged hand discomfort that was considered to be carpal tunnel syndrome by their providers. Occupations showing the highest rates of self-reported carpal tunnel syndrome were in mail service, health care, construction, assembly, and fabrication (42). More recently, Blanc et al. (43) have further analyzed the carpal tunnel syndrome data in the OHS and estimated that 240,578 people in the United States had carpal tunnel syndrome associated with work disability. Other analyses of OHS data have addressed the prevalence of back pain (44,45), dermatitis (45), and occupational injuries (46).

While the analyses have shown that the OHS has important uses, it also has significant limitations. These include its use of self-reports of illness, its lack of inclusion of important chronic occupational diseases such as cancer, and its failure to assess work-related conditions among people who were not employed during the 12 months prior to the interview but who may be disabled as a result of work-related conditions (47).

In contrast to NHIS, NHANES directly assesses the health of a probability sample of 30,000 to 40,000 individuals in the United States by performing physical examinations and laboratory tests in addition to collecting questionnaire information. NHANES was conducted twice in the 1970s and most recently in 1988. NHANES II, which was conducted in the late 1970s, collected limited information on indicators of exposure to lead and selected pesticides (53). Initiated in 1988, NHANES III collected additional data on occupational exposures and disease, especially concerning respiratory and neurologic disease of occupational origin (47).

### Employer Surveillance Programs

Many employers conduct medical surveillance of their work forces and thereby generate a vast amount of medical information that is relevant to the surveillance of occupational diseases. These surveillance programs are undertaken for numerous reasons: to comply with OSHA regulations; to maintain a healthy work force through the detection and treatment of nonoccupational disorders; to ensure that the employee is fit to perform the tasks of the job, including the need to wear a respirator; and to conduct epidemiologic surveillance to uncover patterns of exposure and disease. These activities utilize considerable resources and could potentially make a major contribution to the public health surveillance of occupational diseases. However, since these data are nonuniform, of uncertain quality, and are largely inaccessible outside the companies in which they are collected, their potential use in occupational health surveillance is unrealized (1).

It is an OSHA requirement that employers keep a written record of all occupational injuries and illnesses and basic descriptive data attendant to these events on a standardized instrument (OSHA 200 Log and Summary of Occupational Injuries and Illnesses). OSHA mandates that the employer keep the 200 Log for examination during an OSHA inspection, but does not require that the employer routinely report the log's contents to OSHA. Summaries of the OSHA 200 Log form the basis of the BLS Annual Survey described above.

While few quality-control studies have been undertaken to evaluate the accuracy and completeness of reporting by employers on the 200 Log, it is widely believed that the quality of data on the 200 Log is at best uneven. In a study commissioned by a Panel on Occupational Safety and Health Statistics under the auspices of the U.S. National Research Council, Stanbury et al. (48) identified 66 deaths from occupational injuries in the mid-1980s in New Jersey, using three data sources: OSHA management information system, death certificates, and medical examiners records. They visited 27 employers in whose workplaces occupational injury deaths had occurred in 1983 and who were under the jurisdiction of OSHA. Only 17 of these employers, less than two-thirds, had properly recorded the fatality on the OSHA 200 Log. If obvious work-related deaths are not properly recorded in compliance with OSHA recordkeeping requirements, it is not likely that less serious injuries or illnesses will be recorded with greater accuracy and completeness.

Another OSHA requirement is that employers perform selected medical surveillance tests for workers exposed to a limited number of toxic and infectious agents and noise (49). These are summarized in Table 1. Although not formalized as a standard, OSHA also requires employers to perform regular purified protein derivative (PPD) testing for workers who may be exposed to *Mycobacterium tuberculosis.* Additionally, for 14 well-recognized bladder and lung carcinogens, OSHA requires a physical examination and occupational and medical histories. Unfortunately, the data collected under these OSHA provisions are not routinely reported to OSHA or NIOSH and are not organized into an accessible, uniform, coordinated database, despite the wealth of information collected.

Large employers' associations, especially in the chemical, automobile, and oil industries, have conducted or sponsored epidemiologic studies, especially mortality studies, among their employees. The Chemical Manufacturers' Association has conducted for the past 20 years an ongoing mortality study of more than 10,000 workers employed at 37 U.S. plants that produced vinyl chloride or polyvinyl chloride. In the most recent update of this study, Wong and colleagues (49) found mortality excesses in angiosarcoma, cancer of the liver and biliary tract, cancers of the brain and other central nervous system, and chronic obstructive lung disease. More commonly, employer-sponsored mortality studies are one-time studies that constitute analytic epidemiologic studies designed to address specific hypotheses. Though important, such studies are less useful as surveillance efforts, since they are neither ongoing nor usually timely.

### Occupational Health Clinics

A newly emergent resource for occupational health surveillance has been the development of occupational health clinics that are independent of the workplace and that specialize in the diagnosis and treatment of occupational disease. Several dozen such facilities currently exist in the United States. These clinics can play several roles in enhancing occupational health surveillance (50). First, the clinics can play a primary role in case-finding, i.e., identifying occupational sentinel health events, since they represent a unique organizational source of expertise in clinical occupational medicine. Second, the occupational health clinics can serve as a laboratory for the development and refinement of surveillance case definitions for occupational disease (50). Occupational asthma is an example of such a condition, where several occupational medicine clinics worked jointly with NIOSH to design and evaluate a proposed case definition to be used for surveillance purposes (51). Third, the occupational health clinics can serve as a primary clinical referral resource for the diagnosis and evaluation of workers who are employed at a work site where an index case of occupational disease has been identified.

Occupational health clinics have become organized into a national association (Association of Occupational and Environmental Clinics) to enhance their visibility

**TABLE 1.** *OSHA medical surveillance requirements*

| Exposure | Medical history | Occupational history | Physical examination | Chest radiography | PFTs | Blood tests | Urine tests | Other |
|---|---|---|---|---|---|---|---|---|
| Acrylonitrile | √[a] | √ | √[b] | √ | | | | Fecal occult blood testing |
| Arsenic | √ | √ | √ | √ | | | | Sputum cytology |
| Asbestos | √[b] | √ | √ | √ | √ | | | Respiratory questionnaire |
| Benzene | | | | | | CBC + WBC differential and peripheral blood smear examination | | |
| Blood-borne pathogens | √ | √ | | | | HIV, HBV (postexposure) | | |
| Cadmium | √ | √ | √ | | | Cadmium in blood | $\beta_2$-Microglobulin, cadmium | Standardized questionnaire |
| Coke oven emissions | √ | √ | √ | √ | √ | | Urinalysis, urine cytology | Sputum cytology |
| Cotton dust | √ | | | | √[c] | | | Standardized questionnaire |
| Dibromochloropropane | √[a] | √ | | | | FSH, LH, estrogen (women) | | Sperm count |
| Ethylene oxide | √ | √ | √ | | | CBC | | |
| Formaldehyde | √ | √ | √[d] | √ | √ | | | Standardized questionnaire |
| Hazardous waste | √ | √ | √ | | | | | |
| Lead | √ | √ | √ (including neurologic exam) | | | CBC, BUN, CR, blood lead, ZPP | Urinalysis | |
| Noise | | | | | | | | Baseline and annual audiogram |
| Vinyl chloride | √[a] | | | | | Bilirubin, alkaline phosphatase, SGOT, SGPT, GGTP | | |

[a]Selected topics of interest specified.
[b]Organ system of note is specified for individual chemicals.
[c]Conducted pre- and postexposure.
[d]Contingent on results of questionnaire; see Federal Register part 29 1910.1048 for details.
PFT, pulmonary function tests; SGOT, serum glutamic oxaloacetic transaminase; SGPT, serum glutamic pyruvic transaminase; GGTP, $\gamma$-glutamyl transpeptidase; CBC, complete blood count; BUN, blood urea nitrogen; CR, creatinine; ZPP, zinc protoporphyrin; FSH, follicle-stimulating hormone; LH, luteinizing hormone.
(From U.S. CFR 1910.95, 1910.120, 1910.1001-1910.1101.)

and to collaborate on research and clinical investigations (50). In some states, such as New York, a statewide network of clinical centers has been organized by the State Health Department and receives stable funding from a surcharge on workers' compensation premiums (1,7). The clinical centers in New York State have collaborated in the development of information systems, clinical protocols, and professional education and are beginning to generate substantial data on the numbers of cases of occupational disease in the state.

In a recent example of surveillance activity that can be performed jointly by occupational health clinics, Lax and colleagues (52) recently reported several clusters of lead poisoning among telephone cable strippers from multiple geographic areas in the United States. Although not the first report of lead poisoning in this setting, this study was useful in drawing attention to the continued occurrence of avoidable lead poisoning in a specific group of workers.

## OCCUPATIONAL HAZARD SURVEILLANCE ACTIVITIES IN THE UNITED STATES

Occupational hazard surveillance is the monitoring and analysis of data characterizing workplace exposures. The primary prevention of occupational diseases and injuries depends more directly on hazard surveillance than on health surveillance, since the identification of hazards enables their reduction prior to the onset of ill health effects. Occupational hazard surveillance is less well developed than its health counterpart due to the scarcity of data and data sources and, with the exception of OSHA and NIOSH surveys, the proprietary and inaccessible nature of the hazard data collected by employers.

### OSHA Integrated Management Information System

Nationwide workplace inspections conducted by OSHA are the sole source of uniform and coordinated hazard data involving workplace exposure measurements in the United States. OSHA organizes these data into the Integrated Management Information System (IMIS) and uses them for program operation and evaluation, not for hazard surveillance. OSHA does not publish summary reports characterizing the findings of their inspections.

In the mid-1980s, Froines and colleagues (53–55) and others (7) exploited the OSHA IMIS database to portray the nature, severity, and distribution of occupational exposures by agent and industry. The examples of silica and lead are illustrative. Froines et al. evaluated OSHA inspection results from 1979 to 1982 and found that 46% of the 696 inspections conducted had at least one test sample above the OSHA permissible exposure level (PEL) for silica (54). Similarly for inorganic lead exposure, in the 3,884 inspections conducted by OSHA for inorganic lead exposure between 1979 and 1985, one-third had an air sample above the OSHA PEL, and one-fifth had median air level concentrations of lead above the PEL (55). Such data are very useful, because they facilitate the assessment of the effectiveness of current regulation and enforcement, enable priority setting for workplace intervention, contribute to the estimation of the present and future burden of occupational disease, and, finally, allow for the rational planning of occupational health clinical services (56).

Froines and colleagues emphasize the limitations of using OSHA IMIS data for hazard surveillance. These include the lack of representativeness of the inspection data of all workplaces within given industries, the relatively few agents and industries on which OSHA concentrates its limited inspection resources, and the failure to include some states in the database. It is striking, for example, that 75% of the data in IMIS pertain to only 15 workplace agents (56). Nonetheless, the OSHA IMIS is a unique and underutilized source of national information on occupational hazards.

### NIOSH National Hazard Surveys

In the past two decades, NIOSH has conducted two national surveys to catalog potential workplace exposures. These surveys are the National Occupational Hazard Survey (NOHS) from 1972 to 1974 and the National Occupational Exposure Survey (NOES) from 1981 to 1983. In NOHS, NIOSH industrial hygienists and engineers conducted walk-through surveys and identified possible exposures in a probability sample of 4,636 facilities employing nearly 900,000 employees in more than 600 industries in the United States. Measurements of chemical exposures were not taken and, therefore, NOHS identified only "potential exposures" to the 8,000 hazards and 86,000 unique trade-name products that were found at the workplaces visited. NOHS also collected information on the provision of health services at the workplace, the extent of environmental monitoring conducted at the workplace, and the utilization of personal protective equipment. NOHS has been most widely used to estimate the number and distribution of workers potentially exposed to specific agents (57,58).

In 1981 to 1983, NIOSH conducted NOES to update the information obtained from NOHS and to identify trends in exposures and workplace occupational health activities over the previous decade. In NOES, 4,490 workplaces were visited, and over 10,000 potential hazards and 100,000 trade-name products were identified. Comparison of the results from NOHS and NOES indicate a threefold increase in the proportion of workplaces in which environmental monitoring is conducted, a considerable rise in the availability of health services in plants, and an increase in the coverage provided by worksite–based medical surveillance programs. Characterization of the potential exposures recorded as part of NOES is not yet available, due to the laborious task of identifying the chemical contents of the many trade-name products.

The principal use of NOES has been to estimate the number of employees in the specific industries or occupations who have potential exposures to a large number of individual agents. Burkhart and colleagues (59) used this data set to profile the types of potential exposures that U.S. construction laborers have and the numbers of laborers with these exposures. Others have recently used NOES to characterize the availability of medical services in the private sector by size of firm, union status, and potential exposures at the plant (60).

No national exposure survey comparable to NOES or NOHS has been undertaken by NIOSH in the 1990s.

Other sources of data on workplace hazards include NIOSH health hazard evaluations, the Toxic Release Inventory assembled by the Federal Environmental Protection, and statewide inventories of chemical use gathered by state Departments of Environmental Protection.

Both the OSHA IMIS and the NIOSH national surveys have been used to devise summary hazard ranking schemata as a means of assessing and comparing the overall degree of hazard presented by specific industries. The ranking system based on NOHS data is the Industrial Risk Index (61), while the measure based on OSHA was invented and named the Inspection Based Exposure Ranking by Froines and colleagues (53). These summary measures have been used to rank industries on a regional or national basis by the degree of overall hazard present, to estimate the number of workers employed in the most hazardous industries, and to plan for the provision of necessary occupational health services to serve the workforce in these hazardous industries (7,43).

## CONCLUSION

Occupational health surveillance has made significant gains in the United States during the past decade. The new initiatives undertaken by NIOSH, the Department of Labor, and state health departments are beginning to provide a more complete picture of the nature and extent of the problem of occupational hazards, injuries, and illnesses in the United States.

In 1996, Leigh and colleagues (62) used all available data to construct an estimate of the incidence, mortality, and the direct and indirect costs associated with occupational injuries and illnesses in the United States in 1992. They relied on the national and large regional data sets collected by the NIOSH, the Bureau of Labor Statistics, the National Council on Compensation Insurance, the National Center for Health Statistics, and the Health Care Financing. They combined available data with an attributable risk proportion method to develop the estimates. Approximately 6,500 job-related injury deaths, 13.2 million nonfatal injuries, 60,300 disease deaths, and 862,200 illnesses are estimated to occur annually in the civilian American work force. The total direct ($65 billion) plus indirect ($106 billion) costs were estimated to be $171 billion. Injuries cost $145 billion and illnesses $26 billion. The authors considered that these estimates are likely to be low, especially because they ignore costs associated with pain and suffering as well as those of within-home care provided by family members, and because the number of occupational injuries and illnesses are likely to be undercounted.

These data suggest that occupational health and safety is a costly issue for American workers, employers, and the public at large. Hence, despite recent improvements in occupational health surveillance, much remains to be done. While further improvements can surely be made in the occupational health surveillance systems currently in place, complementary advances in other components of the occupational health system are also needed. Health care providers remain largely uneducated about the risks faced by workers. The numbers of practicing occupational and environmental medicine specialists are still slim. The integration of occupational medicine into primary care is still deficient. Research in occupational health remains woefully underfunded. Since appropriate surveillance depends on the proper functioning of other parts of the health care system, it is not surprising that surveillance efforts in occupational health are seriously impaired. The successes of the past decade to improve occupational health surveillance, however, are cause for optimism. Continued improvement in occupational health surveillance will be an essential component of future efforts to prevent and control occupational diseases.

## REFERENCES

1. Baker EL, Melius JM, Millar JD. Surveillance of occupational illness and injury in the United States: current perspectives and future directions. *J Public Health Policy* 1988:9(2);198–221.
2. Thacker SB, Stroup DF. Future directions for comprehensive public health surveillance and health information systems in the United States. *Am J Epidemiol* 1994;140:383–395.
3. Landrigan PJ. Improving the surveillance of occupational disease. *Am J Public Health* 1989;79:1601–1602.
4. Baker EL, Honchar PA, Fine L. I. Surveillance in occupational illness and injury: concepts and content. *Am J Public Health* 1989;79:9–11.
5. Halperin WE, Ordin DL. Closing the surveillance gap. *Am J Ind Med* 1996;29:223–224.
6. Halperin WE, Frazier TM. Surveillance for the effects of workplace exposure. *Annu Rev Public Health* 1985;6:419–432.
7. Markowitz SB. Fischer E, Fahs MC, Shapiro J, Landrigan P. Occupational disease in New York State. *Am J Ind Med* 1989;16:417–435.
8. Castorino J, Rosenstock L. Physician shortage in occupational and environmental medicine. *Ann Intern Med* 1990;113:983–986.
9. National Research Council. *Toxicity testing strategies to determine needs and priorities.* Washington, DC: National Academic Press, 1984.
10. Rutstein DD, Mullan RJ, Frazier TM, et al. Sentinel health events (occupational): a basis for physician recognition and public health surveillance. *Am J Public Health* 1983;73-1054–1062.
11. Mullan RJ, Murthy LI. Occupational sentinel health events: an updated list for physician recognition and public health surveillance. *Am J Ind Med* 1991;19:775–799.

12. Wagener DK, Buffler PA. Geographic distribution of deaths due to sentinel health event (occupational) causes. *Am J Ind Med* 1989;16: 355–372.
13. Lalich NR, Schuster LI. An application of the sentinel health event (occupational) concept to death certificates. *Am J Public Health* 1987; 77:1310–1314.
14. Feldman JP, Gerber LM. Sentinel health events (occupational): analysis of death certificates among residents of Nassau County, NY between 1980–82 for occupationally related causes of death. *Am J Public Health* 1990;80:158–161.
15. Milham S. *Occupational mortality in Washington State, 1950–1971.* NIOSH publication 76-175. Springfield, VA: National Technical Information Service, 1976.
16. Milham S. *Occupational mortality in Washington State, 1950–1979.* NIOSH publication 83-116. Springfield VA: National Technical Information Service, 1983.
17. Robinson C, Burnett C, Lalich N, et al. *Selected leads from the 1984 Occupational Mortality Surveillance Data.* Springfield, VA: National Technical Information Service, 1990.
18. Dubrow R, Sestito JP, Lalaich NR, et al. Death certificate-based occupational mortality surveillance in the United States. *Am J Ind Med* 1987;11:329–342.
19. Melius JM, Sestito JP, Seligman PJ. IX. Occupational disease surveillance with existing data sources. *Am J Public Health* 1989;79:46–52.
20. Milham S. Mortality from leukemia in workers and exposed to electrical and magnetic fields. *N Engl J Med* 1982;307:2249.
21. Pearce NE, Sheppard RA, Howard JK, Fraser J, Lilley BM. Leukemia in electrical workers in New Zealand. *Lancet* 1985;2:811–812.
22. McDowall ME. Leukemia mortality in electrical workers in England and Wales. *Lancet* 1983;1:246.
23. Linet MS, Malker H, McLaughlin JK, et al. Leukemias and occupation in Sweden: a registry-based analysis. *Am J Ind Med* 1988;14: 319–330.
24. U.S. Department of Health and Human Services. *Work-related lung disease surveillance report 1996.* Washington, DC: Centers for Disease Control, NIOSH, 1996.
25. Robinson C, Stern F, Halperin W, et al. Assessment of mortality in the construction industry in the United States, 1984–1986. *Am J Ind Med* 1995;28:49–70.
26. Burnett CA, Dosemeci M. Using occupational mortality data for surveillance of work-related diseases of women. *J Occup Environ Med* 1994;36:1199–1203.
27. Rosenman KD. Use of hospital discharge data in the surveillance of occupational disease. *Am J Ind Med* 1988;13:281–289.
28. Liss GM, Kuslak RA, Gailitis MM. Hospital records: An underutilized source of information regarding occupational diseases and exposures. *Am J Ind Med* 1997;31:100–106.
29. Freund E, Seligman PJ, Chorba TL, et al. Mandatory reporting of occupational diseases by clinicians. *JAMA* 1989;262:3041–3044.
30. Muldoon JT, Wintermeyer LA, Eure JA, et al. Occupational disease surveillance data sources, 1985. *Am J Public Health* 1987;77: 1006–1008.
31. Pollack, ES, Keimig DG. *Counting injuries and illnesses in the workplace:* proposals for a better system. Washington, DC: National Academy Press, 1987.
32. Wegman DH, Froines JR. Surveillance needs for occupational health. *Am J Public Health* 1985;75:1259–1261.
33. U.S. Department of Labor—Bureau of Labor Statistics. *California: work injuries and illnesses 1989.* Washington, DC: U.S. Department of Labor—Bureau of Labor Statistics, 1989.
34. Baker EL. IV. Sentinel event notification system for occupational risks (SENSOR): the concept. *Am J Public Health* 1989;79:18–20.
35. Matte TD, Hoffman RE, Rosenman KD, et al. Surveillance of occupational asthma under the SENSOR model. *Chest* 1990;98: 173S–178S.
36. Maizlish N, Rudolph L, Dervin K, Sankaranarayan M. Surveillance and prevention of work-related carpal tunnel syndrome: an application of the sentinel events notification system for occupational risks. *Am J Ind Med* 1995;27:715–729.
37. Baser ME, Marion D. A statewide case registry for surveillance of occupational heavy metals absorption. *Am J Public Health* 1990;80: 162–164.
38. Adult blood lead epidemiology and surveillance—United States, first quarter 1996, and annual 1995. *MMWR* 1996;45:628–631.
38a. Selikoff IJ. *Disability compensation for asbestos-associated disease in the United States.* (Private publication.) New York: Mount Sinai School of Medicine, 1982, 440.
39. U.S. Department of labor. *An interim report to Congress on occupational diseases.* Washington, DC: U.S. Government Printing Office, 1980.
40. Murphy PL, Sorock GS, Courtney TK, Webster BS, Leamon TB. Injury and illness in the American workplace: a comparison of data sources. *Am J Ind Med* 1996:30;130–141.
41. Lalich NR, Sestito JP. Occupational health surveillance: contribution from the National Health Interview Survey. *Am J Ind Med* 1997;31: 1–3.
42. Tanaka S, Wild DK, Seligman PJ, Halperin WE, Behrens VJ, Putz-Anderson V. Prevalence and work-relatedness of self-reported carpal tunnel syndrome among U.S. workers: analysis of the occupational health supplement data of 1988 National health Interview survey. *Am J Ind Med* 1995;27:451–470.
43. Blanc PD, Faucett J, Kennedy JJ, Cisternas M, Yelin E. Self-reported carpal tunnel syndrome: predictors of work disability from the National Health Interview Survey occupational health supplement. *Am J Ind Med* 1996;30:262–368.
44. Guo H, Tanaka S, Cameron L, et al. Back pain among workers in the United States: national estimates and workers at high risk. *Am J Ind Med* 1995;28:591–602.
45. Behrens V, Seligman P, Cameron L, Mathias T, Fine L. The prevalence of back pain, hand discomfort, and dermatitis in the U.S. working population. *Am J Public Health* 1994;84:1780–1785.
46. Landen D, Hendricks S. Estimates from the National Health Interview Survey on occupational injury among older workers in the United States. *Scand J Work Environ Health* 1992;18:18–20.
47. Ehrenberg RL. II. Use of direct surveys in the surveillance of occupational illness and injury. *Am J Public Health* 1989;79:12–17.
48. Stanbury M, Goldoft M, O'Leary K. Traumatic occupational fatalities in New Jersey. Appendix C. In: Pollack ES, Keimig DG, eds. *Counting injuries and illnesses in the workplace:* proposals for a better system. Washington, DC: National Academy Press, 1987.
49. Wong O, Whorton MD, Follart DE, Ragland E. An industry-wide epidemiologic study of vinyl chloride Workers, 1942–1982. *Am J Ind Med* 1991;20:317–334.
50. Welch L. XI. The role of occupational health clinics in surveillance of occupational disease. *Am J Public Health* 1989;79:58–60.
51. Klees JE, Rempel D, Barnhart S, et al. Evaluation of a proposed NIOSH surveillance. Case definition for occupational asthma. *Chest* 1990;98:212S–215S.
52. Lax MB, Keough JP, Jeffrey N, et al. Lead poisoning in telephone cable strippers: A new setting for an old problem. *Am J Ind Med* 1996; 351:354.
53. Froines JR, Dellenbaugh CA, Wegman DH. Occupational health surveillance: a means to identify work-related risks. *Am J Public Health* 1986;76:1089–1096.
54. Froines JR, Wegman DH, Dellenbaugh CA. An approach to the characterization of silica exposure in U.S. industry. *Am J Ind Med* 1986; 10:345–361.
55. Froines JR, Bacon S, Segmen DH, et al. Characterization of the airborne concentrations of lead in U.S. industry. *Am J Ind Med* 1990;18: 1–17.
56. Froines J, Wegman D, Eisen E. VI. Hazard surveillance in occupational disease. *Am J Public Health* 1989;79:26–31.
57. Sudin DS, Frazier TM. VII. Hazard surveillance at NIOSH. *Am J Public Health* 1989;79:32–37.
58. Seta JA, Sudin DS. Trends of a decade—a perspective in occupational hazard surveillance, 1970–1983. *MMWR* 1985;34:15SS–24SS.
59. Burkhart G, Schulte PA, Robinson C, Sieber WK, Vossenas P, Ringen K. Job tasks, potential exposures, and health risks of laborers employed in the construction industry. *Am J Ind Med* 1993;24: 413–425.
60. *NOHS-RTECS model for identification of high-risk industrial and occupational groups.* NIOSH publication 83-117. Washington, DC: U.S. Government Printing Office, 1983.
61. Boden LI, Cabral H. Company characteristics and workplace medical testing. *Am J Public Health* 1995;85;1070–1075.
62. Leigh JP, Markowitz SB. Fahs M, Shin C, Landrigan PJ. Occupational injury and illness sin the United States. Estimates of costs, morbidity and mortality. *Arch Intern Med* 1997:157;1557–1568.

*Environmental and Occupational Medicine, Third Edition,* edited by William N. Rom.
Published by Lippincott–Raven Publishers, Philadelphia, 1998.

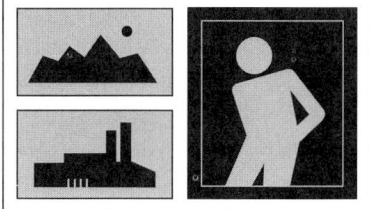

CHAPTER 4

# The Occupational and Environmental History and Examination

Elizabeth A. Jennison and John E. Parker

Bernardino Ramazzini (1), the revered Italian physician who encouraged us all to ask our patients about their occupation, recognized the crucial importance of a good occupational and environmental history. Indeed, a brief occupational and environmental history should be a part of every patient's medical chart. Unfortunately, good occupational histories are often missing. In a recent study of a primary care practice in an academic setting, only 24% of 625 charts reviewed included any mention of the patient's occupation; only 2% included information about toxic exposures, duration of present employment, and former occupations (2).

There are several contexts in which an occupational and environmental history and examination may be performed. The two most common are preplacement physicals and periodic medical screening and surveillance examinations. Less common are return-to-work assessments, exit examinations, and evaluations for specific occupational exposures or diseases. To a greater or lesser extent, all include the same basic components: the occupational/environmental history, the medical history and review of systems, and the physical examination. After these components are discussed, the various examination settings are considered separately as there are unique aspects to each.

E. A. Jennison: Occupational Medicine, Excel Corporate Care Clinic, Middletown, Ohio 45044.

J. E. Parker: Division of Respiratory Disease Studies, National Institute for Occupational Safety and Health, Centers for Disease Control and Prevention; and Department of Pulmonary and Critical Care Medicine, West Virginia University School of Medicine, Morgantown, West Virginia 26505-2888.

## THE OCCUPATIONAL AND ENVIRONMENTAL HISTORY

There are several barriers to obtaining a good occupational and environmental history. Time constraints for both workers and health care providers, coupled with the enormous range of known and potential toxic exposures, make it difficult to obtain a comprehensive history in the general clinical setting. Workers with significant numbers of hazardous exposures may require 30 to 45 minutes to complete a standardized self-administered questionnaire (3). The absence of a widely used, valid, and reliable questionnaire has made it difficult to compare symptom and exposure prevalences gathered in different epidemiologic settings. The Agency for Toxic Substances and Disease Registry (ATSDR) has recommended that the work and exposure survey have three components: an occupational history, an environmental history, and a screening survey to identify occupational exposures (2) (Table 1).

The occupational history should ask the worker to list all jobs held and approximate dates of employment. Significant changes in job duties should be included on this list, even if carried out for the same employer. Workers who have been employed by a large number of firms may fail to recall all jobs; a study of former shipyard workers found that only 50% of those who had worked for a given firm for less than a year recalled working for that firm. Job titles are reported most accurately for jobs with high prestige value (e.g., engineer) or that reflect fairly specific tasks (e.g., electrician, painter). Some tasks may be performed by individuals with different titles; for example, plumbers and sheet-metal workers may perform welding and list their job title as

**TABLE 1.** *Questionnaire structure*

I. Demographics
II. Occupational history
III. Brief review of systems and past medical history
IV. Personal risk factors and environmental history
V. Conditions/symptom-complex modules
  a. Dermatoses
    Irritative contact dermatitis, allergic contact dermatitis, defatting dermatitis, chloracne, and eczema
  b. Mucosal irritations of the eyes, nose, and throat
    Mucosal and upper airway irritation and allergic responses associated with chemical agents and biologic agents
  c. Respiratory disorders
    Chronic bronchitis, emphysema, asthma, chemically induced pulmonary edema, chemical pneumonitis, hypersensitivity pneumonitis, pneumoconiosis (e.g., silicosis, asbestosis, coal workers' pneumoconiosis, byssinosis), metal fume fever, and respiratory tract malignancies
  d. Cardiovascular disorders
  e. Disorders associated with hepatotoxins
    Jaundice and chemical hepatitis
  f. Renal diseases
    Kidney stones, glomerulonephritis, and tubular disorders
  g. Musculoskeletal disorders
    Low back pain syndrome (associated with sprains, strains, disk pathology, arthritis, and degenerative joint disease); repetitive trauma disorders of the hand/wrist (including carpal tunnel syndrome, ulnar nerve compression, De Quervain's disease, degenerative joint disease/arthritis, trigger finger, and tenosynovitis)
  h. Neurotoxic disorders
    Peripheral neuropathy, toxic encephalopathy, and seizure disorders
  i. Noise-induced hearing loss
    Noise-induced hearing loss/deafness and Meniere's syndrome
  j. Psychologic disorders
  k. Infertility and adverse reproductive outcomes
    Diminished fertility, spontaneous abortions, tubal pregnancies, stillbirths, prematurity/low birth weight, birth defects, mental retardation, and childhood cancers
  l. Acute injuries
    Amputations, contusions, fractures/dislocations, lacerations, sprains, electric shocks, and effects of physical agents

"welder."(4). Frequently, neither the job title nor the initial description of job duties provides much insight into potential exposures. Thus, the occupational physician should devote as much or more time to obtaining a good exposure history as is given to listing employers and job titles (Table 2). It is also important to ask patients whether they have supplemental work or if they "moonlight"; many will neglect to list a second job, especially if holding one violates the policies of their primary employer. Ask specifically about farming since many workers who farm part-time fail to list this as a job.

A good starting point in the exposure history is to ask employees, "Have you ever worked with or been exposed to any of the following substances?" Exposures of interest are listed in a simple grid with columns for current or most recent job, any previous job, and activities outside of paid work. Patients find this format easy to complete and it is easily scanned by the physician who should follow-up positive answers with questions about route, dose, duration, and frequency of exposure. In the absence of employer-supplied exposure data, the occupational medicine physician must rely on worker data, despite its limitations. When questioning workers about exposures, it is useful to include both common and chemical terms for substances, as well as any local slang terms. Research has shown that the more general the description of an exposure, the higher the sensitivity and the lower the specificity of worker reporting compared to employer data. Overall, it appears that underreporting of exposures is a greater problem than overreporting (5).

The environmental history should not be ignored. This should include information about the patient's home environment such as water source, heating source, indoor combustion sources, pets, proximity to industry, and proximity to other pollution sources such as dumps or contaminated streams. Information about work performed by family members is included, as "take home" contamination can be significant, especially for asbestos and lead (6). An individual's hobbies are also of interest as these may involve use of toxic substances such as lead (making fishing lures, stained glass work), acquisition of infectious diseases (psittacosis), musculoskeletal risk factors (tennis elbow), or allergic/hypersensitivity phenomena (pigeon fanciers' lung).

**TABLE 2.** *Representative job categories, toxicants, and possible diseases to consider when taking an occupational history*

| Job category | Toxicants | Possible diseases |
|---|---|---|
| Agricultural worker | Pesticides, pathogens, gases, sunlight | Pesticide poisoning, farmer's lung, skin cancer |
| Anesthetist | Anesthetic gases | Reproductive effects, cancer |
| Animal handler | Infectious agents, allergens | Asthma |
| Automobile worker | Asbestos, plastics, lead, solvents | Asbestosis, dermatitis |
| Baker | Flour | Asthma |
| Battery maker | Lead, arsenic | Lead poisoning, cancer |
| Butcher | Vinyl plastic fumes | Meat wrapper's asthma |
| Caisson worker | Pressurized work environments | Caisson disease |
| Carpenter | Wood dust, wood preservatives, adhesives | Nasopharyngeal cancer, dermatitis |
| Cement worker | Cement dust, metals | Dermatitis, bronchitis |
| Ceramic worker | Talc, clays | Pneumoconiosis |
| Demolition worker | Asbestos, wood dust | Asbestosis |
| Drug manufacturer | Hormones, nitroglycerin, etc. | Reproductive effects |
| Dry cleaner | Solvents | Liver disease, dermatitis |
| Dye worker | Dyestuffs, metals, solvents | Bladder cancer, dermatitis |
| Embalmer | Formaldehyde, pathogens | Dermatitis |
| Felt maker | Mercury, polycyclic hydrocarbons | Mercurialism |
| Foundry worker | Silica, molten metals | Silicosis |
| Glass worker | Heat, solvents, metal powders | Cataracts |
| Hospital worker | Infectious agents, cleansers, radiation | Infections, accidents |
| Insulator | Asbestos, fibrous glass | Asbestosis, lung cancer, mesothelioma |
| Jackhammer operator | Vibration | Raynaud's phenomenon |
| Lathe operator | Metal dust, cutting oils | Lung disease, cancers |
| Laundry worker | Bleaches, soaps, alkalis | Dermatitis |
| Lead burner | Lead | Lead poisoning |
| Miner (coal, hard rock, metals, etc.) | Talc, radiation, metals, coal dust, silica | Pneumoconioses, lung cancer |
| Natural gas worker | Polycyclic hydrocarbons | Lung cancer |
| Nuclear worker | Radiation, plutonium | Metal poisoning, cancer |
| Office worker | Poor lighting, poorly designed equipment | Joint problems, eye problems |
| Painter | Paints, solvents, spackling compounds | Neurologic problems |
| Paper maker | Acids, alkalis, solvents, metals | Lung disease, dermatitis |
| Petroleum worker | Polycyclic hydrocarbons, catalysts, zeolites | Cancer, pneumoconiosis |
| Plumber | Lead, solvents, asbestos | Lead poisoning |
| Railroad worker | Creosote, sunlight, oils, solvents, asbestos | Cancer, dermatitis |
| Seaman | Sunlight, asbestos | Cancer, accidents |
| Smelter worker | Metals, heat, sulfur dioxide, arsenic | Cancer |
| Steelworker | Heat, metals, silica | Cataracts, heat stroke |
| Stone cutter | Silica | Silicosis |
| Textile worker | Cotton dust, finishers, dyes, carbon disulfide | Byssinosis, dermatitis, psychosis |
| Varnish maker | Solvents, waxes | Dermatitis |
| Vineyard worker | Arsenic, pesticides | Cancer, dermatitis |
| Welder | Fumes, nonionizing radiation | Lead poisoning, cataracts |

## MEDICAL HISTORY AND REVIEW OF SYMPTOMS

The medical questionnaire should elicit information about previous surgeries, illnesses, hospitalizations, and immunizations. Questions with forced-choice "yes/no" responses seem to have the greatest reliability when evaluated in a test-retest format (7). Patients usually report their medical and drug usage histories accurately when they deal with well-defined chronic conditions such as diabetes. Less well-defined clinical diagnoses, such as arthritis, may be reported with less specificity (8). Smoking history and alcohol use should also be assessed, with the usual caveats about patient underreporting, especially of alcohol intake.

The purpose of an occupational health questionnaire should be specified clearly before the instrument is designed. It would be impractical for questionnaires designed for epidemiologic studies to contain the degree of sensitivity and specificity required to make individual diagnoses. The National Institute for Occupational Safety and Health (NIOSH) has proposed a standardized questionnaire for occupational health research (Table 1), with sections oriented to the NIOSH list of the ten leading work-related diseases and injuries and targeted occupational sentinel health events (9). Examiners should keep in mind that workers may consciously underreport or overreport symptoms for a variety of reasons. Exaggerated reporting of symptoms might be a way of protesting against a hazardous work environment. Underreporting, which is probably more common, may result from lack of awareness of symptoms, denial, or fear of being replaced or dismissed from the workplace (10). Cultural, psychological, and sociologic influences may also impact responses; for example, cigarette smokers may tend not to report minor respiratory symptoms, believing these to be "normal" in a smoker (11). A group of asbestos-exposed workers was observed to have a 50% increase in respiratory symptoms over the course of a year, with no change in pulmonary function or prevalence of radiologic abnormalities. The authors attributed the increase to a change in worker and union attitudes, which lead to greater sensitivity to occupational hazards (12).

The field of respiratory diseases provides examples of the various uses of questionnaires. An early example is the British Medical Research Council (MRC) questionnaire, published in 1960 and revised in 1966 and 1976, and designed to look at the epidemiology of chronic bronchitis and chronic airflow obstruction. Its questions reflect hypotheses about airway obstruction that prevailed in the 1950s, namely that mucus hypersecretion leads to repeated lower respiratory infections and subsequently to airflow obstruction and emphysema. The MRC questionnaire was developed for epidemiologic, not clinical, use; it tends to overdiagnose chronic bronchitis in comparison with physician diagnoses (12). There have been several attempts to develop questionnaires that would be adequate screening tools for asthma, both in occupational and nonoccupational settings. A questionnaire developed by the International Union Against Tuberculosis (IUAT) found that asking "Have you had an attack of asthma in the last 12 months?" had a sensitivity of 50% and a specificity of 96% for discriminating asthmatics from nonasthmatics. Asking, "Have you had any wheezing or whistling in your chest at any time in the last 12 months?" had a sensitivity of 86% and a specificity of 72%. It will continue to be difficult to develop a questionnaire to distinguish asthmatics when strict physiologic criteria defining asthma are lacking (11).

## THE OCCUPATIONAL AND ENVIRONMENTAL PHYSICAL EXAMINATION

The general physical examination, the most common component of occupational and environmental evaluations (13), is no different from examination in any other medical setting. The physician must be alert to the relationship between the workplace and any positive findings; it is estimated that between 60% and 95% of occupational disease goes undiagnosed. A recent study of inpatients on a Veterans Administration general medical service found that 66% of patients had at least one potentially occupational disease, and 68% of these had a relevant occupational exposure that could possibly have contributed to the disease (14). The examination may uncover an occupational disease or a nonoccupational entity that may impact a patient's work capacity.

### Symptoms and Physical Findings

The symptoms associated with exposure to occupational hazards may often be nonspecific, and making the association is difficult unless the physician is knowledgeable and alert. Nonspecific complaints of sleep disturbances, changes in taste or appetite, malaise, headaches, neurologic complaints, or vague abdominal pain may all be related to particular occupational exposures.

Certain findings on physical examination should prompt inquiry about occupational exposure or conditions:

1. General evaluation
   a. Signs of weight loss may be related to a wide variety of toxicants.
   b. Cushingoid facies may be related to work with pharmaceuticals.
   c. Pulse rate and blood pressure may be altered owing to exposure to chemicals such as nitroglycerin.
2. Skin and hair
   a. Skin diseases are the most common occupational health problem.
   b. Skin cancers, dermatitis, and alopecia may be related to a variety of hazards.
   c. White lines in the nail beds may indicate heavy metals exposure.
3. Eye, ear, nose, and throat
   a. Cataracts may develop following exposure to ultraviolet radiation in welding, steel making, or glassblowing, or to microwave or radiofrequency radiation.
   b. Hearing loss often results from workplace noise.
   c. Garlicky breath may result from exposure to metals such as thallium.
4. Chest and respiratory tract
   a. Rales, wheezes, and other unusual sounds may be related to exposure to dusts or allergens in the workplace.
   b. Acute chemically related pulmonary edema can follow exposure to oxides of nitrogen or phosgene.
   c. Cardiac problems may be related to industrial poisons (e.g., arrhythmias following pesticide exposure or premature development of arteriosclerosis following exposure to carbon disulfide.
   d. Carbon monoxide exposure may exacerbate coronary artery disease.
5. Abdomen
   a. Guarding may be due to lead colic.
   b. Evidence of liver disease may follow exposure to a wide range of chemicals, including vinyl chloride, arsenic, and halogenated hydrocarbons.

6. Genitourinary system
   a. Bladder cancer may result from dye exposures.
   b. Renal disease may develop following solvent exposure.
   c. Infertility may be related to chemical exposure such as dibromochloropropane (DBCP).
7. Musculoskeletal system
   a. Back pain, joint pain, missing digits, and other evidence of trauma are often related to work activities.
   b. Raynaud's phenomenon may be secondary to vibration of power tools.
8. Neuropsychiatric
   a. Peripheral neuropathy may result from exposure to chemicals such as n-hexane or methyl butyl ketone, or to lead or mercury.
   b. Psychosis may occur after exposure to mercury or carbon disulfide.
9. Hematologic
   Pallor, bleeding gums, or hematomas may suggest complications resulting from exposure to benzene or ionizing radiation.

Of special note among human illnesses is the increasing evidence of workplace exposure to human carcinogens. Cancers resulting from such toxicants usually do not develop for 20 or more years after the first exposure, and exposure need not continue throughout that period. Unfortunately, even short periods of exposure may cause cancer to develop many years later. Also, our understanding of the multifactorial causation of some cancers is increasing. Examples include the interaction of cigarette smoke with exposure to asbestos or radiation in the development of lung cancer; the damage from the individual exposures is not additive but multiplied.

## LABORATORY STUDIES

Occupational and environmental evaluations frequently include laboratory tests and other diagnostic studies. Many routine laboratory tests have applications in the occupational medicine setting, for example, hematologic profiles to identify adverse effects of benzene exposure. Tests may be specific to the target organ under exposure, such as urinary β2-microglobulin in monitoring cadmium exposure, or to the exposure itself, such as blood lead levels. Which tests are performed, and with what frequency, should be based on knowledge about the condition of interest and the utility of a diagnostic test to detect it. For example, testing for transitory conditions, such as acute infectious diseases, at a single point in time is unlikely to be effective in identifying intercurrent episodes of disease. For occupational diseases with long latency periods, early screening may provide false reassurance that the exposure is not causing adverse effects (15).

## PREPLACEMENT EXAMINATIONS

The preplacement setting is perhaps the most common but least specific application of the occupational and environmental history and examination. Preplacement examinations can assess a candidate's physical suitability for a particular type of employment, provide baseline data useful for measuring early adverse effects of exposure, and identify individuals likely to be vulnerable to certain exposures or having established conditions that could be aggravated by certain types of work (16). Ideally, the employer will provide the physician with a detailed description of the essential functions of the job being offered to the applicant. The physician could then use this information in combination with the history and physical examination findings to assess the candidate's suitability for the job, to identify any accommodations the individual might require, or to recommend against employment in a particular job setting. In reality, the physician often is provided with only the prospective employee's job title.

Under the Americans with Disabilities Act, "otherwise qualified" individuals with disabilities cannot be excluded from employment if they can perform the essential functions of the job, with or without "reasonable accommodation." Individuals who cannot perform the essential functions or who present undue risk to themselves or others may be excluded from employment. The occupational physician often has considerable latitude in defining just what constitutes "undue risk" and inability to perform essential job functions. Thus, there is considerable potential for disagreement among examiners. A recent Dutch study found a notable lack of consensus among experienced occupational physicians with regard to assessing medical fitness for a specific job, even when detailed job requirements were available (17). Physicians who have the opportunity to do so should review the essential job functions with company representatives, including human resources specialists and safety personnel. Lists of essential functions should be limited to tasks that are truly key to job performance. Including unimportant or sporadic tasks increases the probability of rejecting otherwise qualified applicants who could have been employed with minimal accommodations. Once the physician has made his or her recommendations, decisions regarding employability are an administrative function of the hiring organization (18).

## MEDICAL SCREENING AND SURVEILLANCE EXAMINATIONS

Periodic medical screening and surveillance examinations are another frequent service provided by occupational medicine physicians. It is estimated that more than 30% of the United States work force receives periodic occupational health examinations (15). The term *screen-*

*ing* focuses on the individual; screening tests are tools for secondary prevention with the goal of early diagnosis and treatment of disease in exposed workers. True "surveillance" aggregates information about individuals in order to examine patterns within a population. Properly applied, surveillance is a tool for primary prevention through the identification and elimination of the causes of disease.

Screening examinations may be target-organ specific or substance specific, and thus tend to be more focused than preplacement evaluations. Although many are conducted to meet specific OSHA standards, the medical provisions in these standards differ widely in their requirements and degrees of completeness. Requirements for collecting an occupational history range from none (acrylonitrile) to including specific questions (cotton dust). The arsenic standard requires an occupational history, but does not specify what it should include. Most OSHA standards that list medical provisions include a requirement for physical examinations, but the coke oven emissions standard requires only a skin examination, while the cotton dust standard requires pulmonary function testing but has no physical examination requirements.

In many industry groups, 50% of establishments providing medical surveillance do so to satisfy OSHA regulations (19). Thus, a great deal of occupational medical screening data is collected to meet the requirements of various OSHA standards. Unfortunately, most are never used for true surveillance purposes. The OSHA cadmium standard is unique in that any abnormal biologic monitoring result or other lab or clinical finding consistent with toxicity triggers a requirement that the employer reassess employee exposures, work practices, personal hygiene, and engineering controls, and that any identified deficiencies be corrected. Recent calls for a generic OSHA medical surveillance standard suggest that a standardized occupational and medical history be developed and that there be requirements that epidemiologic methods be applied to aggregate clinical data (20).

In addition to satisfying OSHA requirements, employers often conduct medical screening programs for other known occupational hazards, even when full standards do not exist. In both instances the programs can detect early disease and provide intervention at a point when health effects are still minimal. Employers may feel that the purpose of periodic examinations is to demonstrate the absence of adverse health effects in employees exposed to occupational hazards. In a positive light, this may affirm the efficacy of company industrial hygiene practices and employees' use of personal protective equipment. However, there should not be any implication that the lack of adverse health effects means that workers are not exposed to occupational hazards. Screening should not be used to limit disease incidence at a work site by dismissing workers with abnormal findings. Most importantly, medical screening should not be a substitute for hazard control (21).

There are several pitfalls to be avoided by companies who request routine medical examinations and the physicians who perform them (16). Unfortunately, examinations are often performed without consideration of their value. Readers are referred to texts describing the ideal attributes of medical screening examinations. A given test such as a liver enzyme panel may have marginal utility in the evaluation of a given individual, but may be useful for making group comparisons (e.g., exposed versus unexposed cohorts). Periodic examinations may provide a false sense of security to the exposed worker, possibly resulting in a decreased use of personal protective equipment and poor attention to appropriate health and safety practices. Examiners who perform large numbers of routine examinations may perform them by rote and miss subtle clinical findings. Occupational medicine physicians should work with employers to develop appropriate medical screening programs that satisfy applicable regulatory requirements and conscientiously address other occupational hazards.

## RETURN TO WORK ASSESSMENTS

Occupational medicine physicians may be asked to evaluate individuals who are returning to work after a period of absence, be it from occupational or nonoccupational injury or disease. As with preplacement examinations, the physician is charged with determining if employees are fit to perform the jobs to which they are assigned. As in the preplacement setting, the physician needs good information about the job requirements. This can be gathered from company information, worker descriptions, a visit to the job site, or some combination of the three.

The length and format of a return to work examination varies considerably depending on the complexity of the problem at hand. In some instances, the examination may be a simple evaluation to assure that an employee has recovered adequately from an infectious disease to work in a job such as food handling or day care. Occupational medicine physicians may be asked to act as intermediaries between employers and other physicians involved in the employee's care. The occupational medicine physician can assist by making the attending physician more aware of the individual's work requirements and helping to delineate any specific work restrictions. A functional capacity evaluation may be required to resolve any serious discrepancies between the physicians' assessment of the employee's limitations, the employee's self-perceived abilities, and the employer's assessment of the worker's limitations.

For employees returning from an occupational injury or illness, the physician should assess what modifications have been made to the job or workplace to prevent the condition from recurring. Physicians may need to interact with industrial hygienists, safety professionals, engineers, ergonomists, and labor/management teams to help the employee return successfully to the workplace. The occurrence of an occupational injury or illness in a workplace may be considered a "sentinel event" and should be looked upon as an opportunity to improve the working environment to prevent similar conditions in other employees. Finally, the occupational medicine physician should be alert for the possibility that a return to work examination will reveal a previously undetected work-related disease.

## EXIT EXAMINATIONS

The structure and content of exit examinations most closely mirrors that of the periodic medical examination. Exit examinations tend to be either target-organ or substance specific and frequently are used by employers to document that the employee has suffered no adverse health effects from employment or to establish the extent of any such effects. Tests with easily quantifiable results, such as audiograms or pulmonary function tests lend themselves well to determining an individual's status at a given point in time. Some OSHA standards require examinations at termination of employment for individuals who have not had a periodic screening within a certain time frame (asbestos, coke oven emissions). Despite these requirements, exit or termination examinations are the least common occupational and environmental examinations (13). Unless there is good coordination between the personnel and medical or safety functions, employees often leave employment before an exit examination can be scheduled.

## EVALUATIONS FOR SPECIFIC OCCUPATIONAL EXPOSURES OR DISEASES

Evaluation of an individual with a suspected occupational/environmental disease or exposure involves a more targeted history and physical examination than those considered previously. The clinician does not need extensive knowledge of toxicology to evaluate an individual with an apparent occupational disease. The criteria used are the same as those used for the diagnosis of other medical problems. The physician should inquire about the onset and temporal pattern of symptoms in relation to starting new employment, to new or unexpected exposures, and to the workday and workweek. Palliative and provocative factors are also discussed, such as worsening with specific job tasks or improvement on days away from work. A complete physical examination should be performed, with more focused evaluation of the systems involved in an occupational disease or the target organs of a suspected exposure. Appropriate clinical and laboratory tests can provide confirmatory data (2). Some OSHA standards have special provisions for exposure situations; most notable is the benzene standard, which requires that a urinary phenol level be collected at the end of the shift on which the exposure occurred.

## SUMMARY

Occupational and environmental histories and examinations serve two main purposes in occupational health practice. The first is to help place and maintain people in work that is commensurate with their physical and mental capabilities. Preplacement and return-to-work examinations are examples of this application. The second usage is to monitor individuals exposed to environmental hazards associated with work-related diseases. Medical "surveillance" (screening) examinations, exit examinations, and evaluations for specific occupational/environmental exposures or diseases fall into this category. To a greater or lesser extent, all occupational and environmental evaluations contain three basic components: the occupational/environmental history, the medical history and review of systems, and the physical examination.

As our understanding of occupational and environmental medicine becomes more sophisticated, there is an increasing need to relate exposure data and outcomes. Unfortunately, this has become more difficult as increasing amounts of occupational health services are provided by outside clinics rather than corporate medical units. Proposals for a generic OSHA medical surveillance standard suggest that occupational health care providers be required to visit job sites and share information with labor/management safety committees (20). While the history and physical examination are important parts of an occupational health program, physicians can have much greater impact on worker health by participating on interdisciplinary teams with others whose skills relate to environmental assessment and control.

## ACKNOWLEDGMENT

The editor and authors acknowledge Arthur L. Frank for important contributions to this chapter in earlier editions of this book.

## REFERENCES

1. Ramazzini B. Diseases of workers, translated by Wright WC. In: *De Morbis Artificum Diatriba,* 1713. New York: Hafner, 1964.
2. ATSDR. Obtaining an exposure history. *Am Fam Physician* 1993;48(3): 483–491.
3. Rosenstock L, Logerfo J, Heyer NJ, Carter WB. Development and validation of a self-administered occupational health history questionnaire. *J Occup Med* 1984;26(1):50–54.
4. Stewart WF, Tonascia JA, Matanoski G. The validity of questionnaire-reported work history in live respondents. *J Occup Med* 1987;29(10): 795–800.
5. Joffe M. Validity of exposure data derived from a structured questionnaire. *Am J Epidemiol* 1992;135(5):564–570.
6. CDC/NIOSH. Report to Congress on workers' home contamination

study conducted under the Workers' Family Protection Act (29 U.S.C. 671a), September 1995.
7. Gilkison CR, Fenton MV, Lester JW. Getting the story straight: evaluating the test-retest reliability of a university health history questionnaire. *J Am Coll Health* 1992;40(6):247–252.
8. Kehoe R, Wu S-Y, Leske MC, Chylack LT. Comparing self-reported and physician-reported medical history. *Am J Epidemiol* 1994;139(8): 813–818.
9. Ehrenberg RL, Sniezek JE. Development of a standard questionnaire for occupational health research. *Am J Public Health* 1989;79s:15–17.
10. Rodenzo RA, Lundberg I, Escalona E. Development of a questionnaire in Spanish on neurotoxic symptoms. *Am J Ind Med* 1995;28:505–520.
11. Burney P, Chinn S. Developing a new questionnaire for measuring the prevalence and distribution of asthma. *Chest* 1987;91(6):79s–83s.
12. Samet JM. A historical and epidemiologic perspective on respiratory symptoms questionnaires. *Am J Epidemiol* 1978;108:435–456.
13. Conway H, Simmons J, Talbert T. The Occupational Safety and Health Administration's 1990–1991 survey of occupational medical surveillance prevalence and type of current practices. *J Occup Med* 1993; 35(7):659–669.
14. Brancati FL, Hodgson MJ, Karpf M. Occupational exposures and diseases among medical inpatients. *J Occup Med* 1993;35(2):161–165.
15. Halperin WE, Ratcliffe J, Frazier TM, Wilson L, Becker SP, Schulte PA. Medical screening in the workplace: proposed principles. *J Occup Med* 1986;28:547–552.
16. Schilling RSF. The role of medical examination in protecting worker health. *J Occup Med* 1986;28(8):553–557.
17. deKort WL, Uiterweer HW, vanDijk FJ. Agreement on medical fitness for a job. *Scand J Work Environ Health* 1992;18(4):246–251.
18. Hogan JC, Bernacki EJ. Developing job-related preplacement medical examinations. *J Occup Med* 1981;23(7):469–476.
19. Conway H, Simmons J, Talbert T. The purposes of occupational medical surveillance in U.S. industry and related health findings. *J Occup Med* 1993;35(7):670–686.
20. Silverstein M. Analysis of medical screening and surveillance in occupational safety and health administration standards: support for a generic medical surveillance standard. *Am J Ind Med* 1994;26: 283–295.
21. Kennedy SM. Medical screening for occupational disease risk is not a control measure. *Am J Ind Med* 1991;20:271–272.

*Environmental and Occupational Medicine, Third Edition,* edited by William N. Rom.
Lippincott–Raven Publishers, Philadelphia 

CHAPTER 5

# Epidemiology of Occupational Diseases

Gary M. Marsh

Epidemiology is the study of the distribution and determinants of disease in human populations. In contrast to clinical or laboratory research, this study observes large numbers of persons in their everyday home, work, and natural environments, in order to identify and elucidate patterns among various risk factors and the occurrence of disease and injury. A better understanding of these factors affords an opportunity for interventions aimed at reducing or preventing disease.

Occupational epidemiology has evolved during the past several decades as a distinct subdiscipline within the broader fields of epidemiology and occupational medicine. It applies the concepts and methods of these fields to the health determinants of working populations. A major objective of occupational epidemiology is to determine the health consequences of workplace exposures and, when indicated, to make or recommend remedial efforts. Another objective is to provide data useful for setting standards for protection of workers exposed to toxic substances and, more generally, to make projections of risk to members of the population at large who typically experience lower-intensity exposure than those in the workplace. More basic problems, such as elucidating mechanisms of toxicity and dose-response relationships, can also be addressed in occupational epidemiology.

The scope of occupational epidemiologic research is ever increasing. Initially concerned primarily with the study of characteristic occupationally related rare diseases such as lung cancer among gas workers (1), bladder cancer among dyestuff factory workers (2,3), and mesothelioma of the pleura or peritoneum among asbestos workers (4), the field of inquiry has expanded to address a variety of potential occupational disease and injury hazards that workers face today: potential adverse reproductive outcomes among employees of the semiconductor industry, infectious disease risks associated with exposure to genetically modified microorganisms, and cancer risks related to cleanup operations at hazardous waste sites, among others. Fortunately, advances in epidemiologic methods and in the related disciplines of toxicology, industrial hygiene, health physics, and biostatistics can facilitate research into the complex issues that today confront occupational epidemiologists.

## CHARACTERIZATION OF THE OCCUPATIONAL ENVIRONMENT

A primary goal of occupational epidemiology is to determine which specific workplace exposure factors result in disease or injury. This involves the estimation of dose-response relationships that are ultimately used to predict effects in populations other than those studied, forming the bases of occupational and nonoccupational exposure guidelines. The estimability of dose-response relationships depends largely on the quantity and quality of available historical exposure data. In practice, complete and accurate historical exposure data are often nonexistent or unavailable and therefore must be estimated.

Exposure assessment is the scientific process by which historical exposure levels for individual workers are measured or estimated. This is a complex, multidisciplinary process involving the collaborative efforts of occupational epidemiologists, biostatisticians, occupational physicians, industrial hygienists, health physicists, toxicologists, and safety engineers. Several approaches to

G. M. Marsh: Department of Biostatistics, Graduate School of Public Health, University of Pittsburgh, Pittsburgh, Pennsylvania 15261.

qualitative and quantitative exposure assessments have been developed (5–9), although none is yet recognized as an authoritative standard (10). The following section summarizes some basic concepts, techniques, and issues involved in characterizing occupational exposures for epidemiologic studies.

## EXPOSURE VERSUS DOSE

The underlying assumption of dose-response function estimation is that biologic effects arise from damage induced in specific targets, whether organs, tissues, or cells. Predicting the probability or severity of an effect requires estimation of dose, that is, the amount of a substance that reaches the biologic target during some specific time interval. This amount is related to the target burden—the concentration of the substance at or near the target—and to the time interval considered. The rate of delivery is referred to as the dose rate or dose intensity. The concept of biologically active dose is used when only some fraction of the burden can produce an effect.

In most instances, doses and dose rates cannot be measured directly, and surrogate measures must be developed from data on exposures observed in the environment external to the worker. Exposure concentration or intensity is used as a surrogate for dose rate, and cumulative exposure, which combines concentrations with durations, is commonly used as a surrogate for dose. Because dose rate can vary with time, it is often useful in an epidemiologic analysis to consider some summary indicator, such as the average or peak dose rate.

Exposure concentration and cumulative exposure are valid surrogate measures provided that they are directly proportional to dose rates and doses, respectively. Biomathematical (pharmacokinetic) models have been developed for estimating doses of environmental substances when the underlying exposure-dose relationship is nonlinear owing to complex patterns of absorption, retention, and detoxification (8). In general, the choice of a surrogate dose measure depends on the nature of the effect, the affected tissue, the mechanism of occurrence, and the time course of its development and resolution (11).

### Types and Sources of Exposure Data

The first phase in characterizing the workplace environment involves identifying potentially toxic agents and establishing the most relevant routes of exposure. This process can be relatively straightforward for agents of known toxicity (e.g., asbestos in an asbestos textile plant) but extremely complicated in industries where exposures vary greatly by type and intensity and the toxicity of substances, alone or in combination, is often poorly understood (e.g., petrochemical manufacturing) (12). In some situations, workers' reports of symptoms or illness may help to identify at least classes of potentially toxic exposures (e.g., reports of skin rashes or dermatitis indicate the need to identify irritating or sensitizing chemicals).

The types of exposure data needed for an epidemiologic study depend on the health outcomes of interest and the study designs to be used. For example, mortality studies of chronic diseases typically require detailed historical exposure data that span decades of employment, whereas studies of injuries might require data on only current work assignment or job title. Checkoway and coworkers (13) provide a useful exposure classification that indicates how accurate different types of data are for estimating dose. Beginning with the best approximation to dose, these are quantified personal measurements, quantified area or job-specific data, ordinally ranked jobs or tasks, and simple dichotomous categorization of employment (ever/never employed in the industry).

In many respects an investigator's decision about what level to seek within this hierarchy is forced by circumstances (e.g., existence or availability of historical data) rather than choice. For most industry-based studies, the available exposure data fall somewhere in the middle of this range. A notable exception is studies of radiation-exposed workers, which include quantitative personal exposures measured by radiation film badges. Monitoring data obtained from industrial hygiene or health physics surveys may overestimate or otherwise misrepresent true average concentrations when sampling is performed strictly to satisfy compliance testing requirements.

### Exposure Classification Schemes

For industry-based studies that lack personal monitoring data, environmental characterization next involves developing an exposure classification scheme for the various work areas, jobs, and tasks in the industry. Several authors have described approaches to job classification and exposure estimation for epidemiologic study purposes (14–16). This approach can involve the reconstruction of historical exposure profiles (e.g., for studies of chronic diseases with long incubation periods) and/or concurrent prospective exposure estimation (e.g., for surveys of illness or injury or for prospective health surveillance). The classification scheme can be based on quantitative or qualitative occupational exposure categories (ECs), or it may consist simply of groupings of jobs or occupational titles (OTs) that involve relatively similar duties or materials (14). The last scheme requires no explicit assumptions about exposure gradients, although environmental concentration differences may be inferred. A hybrid classification scheme that combines OT and EC approaches was proposed by Marsh (17) as a strategy for pooling work history data in industrywide studies.

An efficient structure for any classification scheme is a matrix of jobs (or work areas) and exposure levels. The matrix can include exposure data of any type for simple or multiple agents, and time or place parameters can be added if exposure concentrations change over time or are available from multiple plant sources.

Classifying jobs and work areas according to exposure levels is a complex task requiring a variety of techniques and data sources. A discussion of some useful data sources is provided by Checkoway and coworkers (13). These include industrial hygiene or health physics sampling data (area or personal), process descriptions and flow charts, plant production records, inspection and accident reports, engineering control and protective equipment, and biologic monitoring results.

Recent studies have shown that industrial hygienists can estimate exposure levels reasonably well for current situations when sufficient information about the operations is available, even if these hygienists have never been in the plant in question or have no monitoring results (18,19). In addition, anecdotal information from employees has been found to be reliable, and reasonably accurate (20).

The final phase of the exposure assessment process for studies lacking personal monitoring data is to link exposure data to individual workers. Work service records (work histories) maintained by company personnel departments usually serve as the primary document in this process. These records typically contain, for each job held, the name of the plant or department, unit or work area, job title, and the associated dates of employment.

Large-scale occupational epidemiologic studies can involve vast amounts of work history data. For example, the ongoing historical cohort mortality study of 40,000 man-made vitreous fiber (MMVF) workers from 17 U.S. plants includes more than 5,500 unique plant or department or job title codes and more than 600,000 individual job entries (21,22). For individual workers in this study, historical exposure profiles are being estimated that include quantitative data on exposure to MMVF and qualitative (ordinal or nominal scale) data on concurrent exposure to five classes of potentially important toxicants: asbestos, arsenic, formaldehyde, phenolics, and polycyclic aromatic hydrocarbon compounds.

In some studies it is necessary to "collapse" work history data into smaller, more manageable numbers of homogeneous categories, to facilitate linkage to the exposure classification scheme.

### Exposure Assessment for Community-Based Studies

Associations of disease risks with occupations can also be examined in studies conducted in the general population, although these generally yield less accurate exposure data than industry-based studies. Sources of exposure data in these studies include personal interviews, hospital records, disease registry records, death certificates, and census data. Perhaps the best use of community-based studies is for screening hypotheses regarding occupational exposures that may warrant more intensive inquiry in subsequent industry-based studies (13).

## MEASUREMENT OF MORBIDITY AND MORTALITY

In addition to an accurate characterization of workplace exposure, the meaningful estimation of exposure-response relationships requires accurate quantification of the presence or occurrence of disease. This section focuses on the "response" side of the exposure-response relationship and summarizes some of the measures of disease frequency and measures of effect that are commonly used in occupational epidemiologic research. Also covered are some basic statistical standardization procedures that are used to facilitate comparison of these measures among groups who differ with respect to age or other factors.

### Measures of Disease Occurrence

The occurrence of disease among working populations is measured using rates and proportions. The choice of a particular measure depends on the study design, the health end point of interest, and whether occurrence is to be measured at a specific point in time or during a specified interval. The measures of disease occurrence described in the following section have specific meaning.

#### *Rates and Risks*

One approach to quantifying the population disease frequency during a specified time interval is to compute the number of newly occurring, or *incident,* cases during the interval of study per number of *person-years of observation.* This quantity is a disease *incidence rate.* The denominator of the incidence rate, person-years, is a quantity that combines the number of persons with their follow-up time. For example, one person followed 1 year and two persons each followed a half year both yield 1 person-year of observation. Other terms for incidence rate are incidence density, instantaneous risk, force of morbidity, and hazard rate. In general, the term *rate* is used to denote the number of new cases per person-time units.

The *mortality rate* is a special form of incidence rate that expresses the incidence of death. For example, if 1,000 workers are followed for 1 year and each of 10 new lung cancer deaths occur at midyear then the mortality rate for lung cancer is $10/(1{,}000 - 0.5(10)) = 0.01005$. For large-scale studies several computer programs are available for performing person-year and rate calculations (23–26).

A second approach to measuring disease occurrence over a specified time interval is to compute the number of incident cases per number of persons at risk at the beginning of the interval. This quantity is a disease risk and represents the probability of developing or dying from a particular disease during the interval of study. Thus, in the above example the 1-year risk of mortality from lung cancer is 10/1000 = 0.01, which is slightly less than the 1-year mortality rate.

Rates are generally more informative measures than risks because they take into account the person-time unit of observation, which in many settings is likely to vary among study members when deaths (or cases) occur at varying points in time. Rates are the central measures of disease occurrence in cohort studies.

*Prevalence* measures denote the number of cases of disease that exist in the population. *Point prevalence* refers to the prevalence at one point in time and is usually expressed as a proportion or percentage. Unlike incidence measures, which focus on events, point prevalence focuses on disease status. For example, if a group of 500 workers is surveyed and 75 report symptoms of respiratory tract disease, while 125 have symptoms of skin disease, the prevalence of respiratory tract disease is 75/500, or 15%, and the prevalence of skin disease is 125/500, or 25%. Note that point prevalence, like risk, does not indicate the rate at which persons develop disease. *Period prevalence* denotes the number of cases that exist during a period of time. Period prevalence is more difficult to interpret, because it combines initial point prevalence with subsequent incidence rates.

Prevalence measures are seldom used in etiologic applications of occupational epidemiologic research because differences in prevalence across time or among groups may be the result of differences in the incidence or duration of disease, or both. This occurs because prevalence ($P$) is approximately equal to the incidence rate ($I$) times average disease duration ($D$), when $P$ is small and $I$ is constant over time, i.e.,

$$P \approx \overline{ID} \qquad [1]$$

Prevalence measures arise primarily in cross-sectional studies and are particularly useful for studying classes of diseases with unmeasurable or uncertain moments of onset (e.g., congenital malformations and nonlethal degenerative diseases) (27).

### Measures of Effect

In occupational epidemiologic research the term *effect* refers to the difference in disease occurrence between two groups of workers that differ with respect to causal exposure characteristics (27). Two types of measures of effect are used in occupational epidemiology, absolute effects and relative effects. The choice of effect measure is guided by the health end point under study and the nature of the inferences to be drawn from the results of the study.

Absolute effect is expressed as the differences in risks, rates, or prevalence between an exposed group and an unexposed but otherwise comparable baseline or reference group. Relative effect is based on the ratio of the absolute effect to a baseline rate. For example, if $I_1$ and $I_0$ are the incidence rates among exposed and unexposed workers, respectively, the absolute effect is $I_1 - I_0$, and the relative effect is $(I_1 - I_0)/I_0 = I_1/I_0 - (0.1)$. Occupational epidemiologists usually refer only to the ratio component $I_1/I_0$, which is known as the *relative risk, relative rate,* or simply *rate ratio.*

The absolute effect measure is often more useful for estimating the magnitude of the occupational health problem presented by the exposure. Also, the absolute effect, unlike the relative effect, is not affected by changes in the baseline incidence rate of disease. On the other hand, the relative effect measure is the preferred one for investigating causation, because it is often a clearer indicator of the strength of an association or, under appropriate circumstances, a causal role (28).

### Summary Measures of Disease Occurrence and Effect

The measures of disease occurrence and effect described above can be expressed as overall summary measures for a group (e.g., crude rates) and as measures for subgroups defined by age, race, sex, or another variable. Crude summary rates have limited usefulness in occupational studies, because they are not mutually comparable across groups that differ with respect to variables associated with the event under study (e.g., age, race, sex). If this occurs, the relationship between exposure and the study event is said to be confounded by the variable. For example, if two groups (say, exposed and unexposed) have different age distributions, age is a confounding variable if disease rates are associated with age. However, while subgroup-specific measures generally provide a more complete and accurate characterization of disease occurrence than do crude summary measures, their utility is limited in studies that contain sparse subgroup-specific data or that involve comparisons of populations that are finely stratified (i.e., subdivided) according to several variables.

Two approaches that can be taken to summarize measures such as rates across subgroups of a confounding variable, while maintaining the unique information contained in subgroup-specific rates, are to compute (a) standardized rates or (b) pooled rates. Following are the summary measures of risk most frequently encountered in occupational studies, such as cohort studies described below, that use rates and person-years. They are described in terms of the crude (unstandardized) data layout in Table 1.

A standardized rate (SR) is simply a weighted average of the subgroup-specific rates. This can be expressed as

**TABLE 1.** *Data layout for a cohort study using rates and person-years*

| | Study (exposed) group | Reference (unexposed) group | Total |
|---|---|---|---|
| Events (cases or deaths) | $a$ | $b$ | $M$ |
| Person-years | $N_1$ | $N_0$ | $T$ |
| Rate | $R_1 = a/N_1$ | $R_0 = b/N_0$ | $R_T = M/T$ |

$$SR = \sum_i W_i R_i \,/\, \sum_i W_i \quad [2]$$

where $i$ represents the subgroups and $W_i$ and $R_i$ are the subgroup-specific weights and incidence (or mortality) rates, respectively. Weights can be derived either internally, from the distribution of the confounder variable (e.g., age) in the study (exposed) group, or externally, from the confounder distribution of a comparison or reference (assumed unexposed) group. The latter approach is known as the direct method of standardization.

Comparison of a study group with a reference group is usually made by taking the ratio of their respective standardized rates. This rate ratio ($RR_s$) is expressed as

$$RR_s = \sum_i W_i R_{1i} \,/\, \sum_i W_i R_{0i} \quad [3]$$

If the $W_i$ are taken from the confounder distribution of the study group (i.e., $W_i = N_{1i}$), the $RR_s$ reduces to the commonly used standardized mortality ratio (SMR), i.e.,

$$SMR = \sum_i a_i \,/\, \sum_i N_{1i} R_{0i} \quad [4]$$

The SMR represents the ratio of the sum of the observed number of events in the study group to the sum of the expected numbers in the study group, where the expected numbers are based on the rates in the reference group.

The SMR is a type of indirectly standardized measure, because its weights are derived internally. The product of the SMR and the crude summary rate in the study group is known as the indirectly standardized rate (ISR):

$$ISR = SMR \cdot R_1 \quad [5]$$

If for $RR_s$ the $W_i$ is taken externally from the confounder distribution of the reference group (i.e., $W_i = N_{0i}$), then $RR_s$ reduces to the standardized rate ratio (SRR) described by Miettinen (29):

$$SRR = \sum_i N_{0i} R_{1i} \,/\, \sum_i b_i \quad [6]$$

The SRR represents the ratio of the number of expected events in the reference group, based on rates in the study group, to the number of observed events in the reference group. The SRR is also referred to as the comparative mortality figure (CMF) (30,31).

Note that, analogous to the expression for ISR, the directly standardized rate (DSR) from above can be expressed as the product of the SRR and the crude summary rate in the reference group:

$$DSR = SRR \cdot R_0 \quad [7]$$

Pooling is an alternative approach to SRR estimation that involves computing a weighted average of the subgroup-specific rate ratios rather than the ratio of weighted averages of subgroup-specific rates as in the $RR_s$. Here, the summary rate ratio is expressed as

$$RR'_s = \sum_i W_i (R_{1i}/R_{0i}) \,/\, \sum_i W_i \quad [8]$$

The Mantel and Haenszel (32) method provides the usual choice of weights for $RR'_s$ where $W_i = b_i N_{1i}/T_i$. With these weights $RR'_s$ becomes

$$RR_{M\text{-}H} = \sum_i a_i (N_{0i}/T_i) \,/\, \sum_i b_i (N_{1i}/T_i) \quad [9]$$

In some occupational studies, such as proportional mortality studies described below, it is not possible to enumerate a population at risk but it is possible to measure the number of events (usually deaths) of interest. In this case, the proportion of deaths from a specific cause (relative to total deaths) can be used in place of death rates to derive summary measures of disease occurrence that resemble and approximate those based on rates.

The following summary measures of proportional mortality are described in terms of the crude data layout in Table 2. For example, if in Table 1 the total person-years of observation in $i$th subgroup of the study and reference groups $N_{1i}$ and $N_{0i}$ are replaced by the corresponding total number of observed deaths, $D_{1i}$ and $D_{0i}$, and the rates in the study and reference groups, $R_{1i}$ and $R_{0i}$, are replaced by the corresponding proportional mortalities, $a/D_{1i}$ and $b/D_{0i}$, the expression for SMR above becomes

$$SPMR = \sum_i a_i \,/\, \sum_i D_{1i} (b_i/D_{0i}) \quad [10]$$

the standardized proportional mortality ratio (SPMR), and the expression for SRR above becomes

$$SePMR = \sum_i D_{0i} \, (a_i/D_{1i}) \,/\, \sum_i b_i \quad [11]$$

the externally standardized proportional mortality ratio (SePMR) described by Zeighami and Morris (33) and Marsh and coworkers (34). The SPMR and SePMR can also be computed within specific disease categories. For example, site-specific cancer mortality can be

**TABLE 2.** *Data layout for proportional mortality studies*

| | Study (exposed) group | Reference (unexposed) group | Total |
|---|---|---|---|
| Cause-specific deaths | $a$ | $b$ | $M$ |
| Total deaths | $D_1$ | $D_0$ | $D$ |
| Proportional mortality | $a/D_1$ | $b/D_0$ | $M/D$ |

expressed as a proportion of all cancer mortality in a proportional cancer mortality ratio (PCMR). The appendix provides a numerical example that illustrates the computation of the summary measures of effect described above.

Several authors have discussed methodologic issues related to the use of these summary measures of effect (35–46). Here are some of the major points:

1. All ratio estimates express disease frequency on a multiplicative scale. Some absolute estimates of effect, expressed on an additive scale, are discussed by Monson (44).
2. When the rate ratio is constant across all subgroups of the confounder, the SMR, SRR, and $RR_{M\text{-}H}$ are equal. Also, for a specific subgroup of the confounder, all three measures provide the same unbiased estimate of the rate ratio.
3. The directly standardized measures (DSR, SRR, and SePMR) are generally more valid than their indirectly standardized counterparts (ISR, SMR, SPMR) for comparing two or more study groups with different confounder distributions. This follows from the fact that the former measures derive their weights externally from a common reference group, whereas the weights of indirect standardization are derived internally from each of the compared study groups.
4. The utility of the directly standardized measures is often limited by the inability to construct stable subgroup-specific rates or proportions within the study groups. This explains the relative popularity of the less valid but more reliable indirect measures, such as the SMR, which are usually based on very stable reference population rates. Thus, the choice between the SMR and SRR as a summary measure of effect involves a trade-off between validity (bias) and reliability (precision).
5. While the proportional mortality-based measures (SPMR and SePMR) are quickly and easily computed, their interpretation (relative to the rate-based measures) is limited, because the number of deaths available for study may not be representative of all deaths occurring in the population, and because of the constraint that proportional mortalities across all causes of death must sum to 1.

Breslow and Day (30) and Checkoway's group (13) provide a more complete discussion of these measures along with related statistical inferential procedures. Computer programs, such as the Occupational Cohort Mortality Analysis Program (OCMAP) for mainframe and microcomputers (23,24,47–49), are also available for the analysis of occupational studies that use these standard measures (25,26). A new program, OCMAP-PLUS, enables a comprehensive analysis of occupational study data in relation to multiple and diverse work history and exposure measures, and provides output files for use by other conventional statistical and epidemiologic data analysis programs (49).

Some other commonly used summary measures of effect are described below in the context of specific occupational epidemiologic study designs.

## CLASSICAL STUDY DESIGNS

The objective of all occupational epidemiologic studies is to examine relationships between possible causal exposures and health risks, where the exposure necessarily precedes the health outcome. In most situations, the limitations imposed by ethics and cost restrict occupational epidemiologic research to nonexperimental, or observational, studies. Because the circumstances of exposure cannot be controlled in observational studies, efforts are directed at identifying naturally occurring exposure conditions that most closely simulate a controlled experiment. This effort is facilitated through the judicious choice of epidemiologic study design and selection of study subjects. For example, follow-up studies of retired employees permit at least some control of exposure to the extent that the study population can be partitioned into a range of homogeneous exposure subgroups (based on employment history at time of retirement) prior to the period of observation, which is presumably exposure free (50).

This section provides an overview of the classical study designs used in occupational epidemiology. The first four designs—the uncontrolled case study, the cross-sectional study, the proportional mortality study, and the ecologic study—usually represent preliminary or pilot investigations used to screen for possible workplace hazards or to generate hypotheses for testing in more complex designs. The last two designs—the cohort study and the case-control study—are the most informative investigations used to test specific etiologic hypotheses and to confirm and quantify degrees of health risk related to causal exposures. This section also describes the basic objectives and components of an occupational epidemiologic surveillance program. Such programs permit continuous monitoring of employee health and provide the exposure and health data resources necessary to conduct specific epidemiologic studies, should the need arise.

### Uncontrolled Case Study

An uncontrolled case study, or case-series report, is not actually a formal epidemiologic investigation but simply the identification and reporting of an unusual occurrence of injury or disease. Typically, no measures of occurrence or effect are computed and exposure estimates, if any, are qualitative. Reports of such occurrences, or "clusters," of disease can be virtually conclusive if they involve very rare illnesses of unknown or poorly understood causes. Classic examples of the uncontrolled case study are the early reports of Pott (45) on scrotal cancer among chimney sweeps, and Creech and Johnson's (51) more recent report on hepatic angiosarcoma among workers exposed to vinyl chloride. These reports, among others, underscore the need for physicians and other health professionals to be alert to the possibility of occupational causes of disease, particularly when the observed health outcome is a very rare disease or an unusual manifestation of a more common condition.

Suspected disease clusters can also be misleading, because they may simply represent a chronic and otherwise unremarkable occurrence within the underlying random distribution of the observed disease (52).

### Cross-Sectional Study

In an occupational cross-sectional study, a survey is conducted to determine and compare the prevalence of disease or health status between groups of workers classified with respect to exposure status. The survey, which often involves random sampling of the target population, can be performed on a one-time basis or on a repetitive basis (health and exposure assessments are made periodically over a period of time). The health assessments may involve clinical examinations, symptom surveys, or direct biologic or physical measurements. Current health status can then be related to either lifetime or current exposures, although in the latter approach the exposure categorization may not be causally relevant to the outcomes under study.

The principal advantage of cross-sectional studies is that they are the best epidemiologic design for studying (a) conditions that are quantitatively measured and that can vary over time (e.g., blood pressure) or (b) relatively frequent nonfatal diseases that have long duration (e.g., chronic bronchitis). The two main limitations of cross-sectional studies are that they measure prevalence rather than incidence and that they are confined to actively employed workers who choose to participate. Workers who have left employment for reasons that might be related to exposure and those who choose not to participate are excluded. Thus these studies are not appropriate for investigating rare diseases or diseases of short duration. Cross-sectional studies also underestimate disease prevalence or severity, particularly for diseases that continue to progress after exposure ceases.

The cross-sectional design was used in a recent study by Schwartz and coworkers (53) to assess the association between blood lead level and hematocrit value in children aged 1 to 5 years living near a primary lead smelter. Marquart and colleagues (54) used the repeated cross-sectional design to assess lung function among welders of zinc-coated steel over five consecutive work shifts. The cross-sectional design was also used to study the independent effects of occupation on lung function in British coal miners (55).

#### *Proportional Mortality Study*

A proportional mortality study is one that includes only observations on deaths when detailed information about the population at risk of dying is not available. This commonly occurs in the occupational setting when death certificates are available for deceased employees from company, union, or insurance company records but it is neither feasible nor desirable to enumerate a complete population at risk from personnel records.

Proportional studies may be viewed as a special type of cross-sectional study (37,42) or as a special type of case-control study (56). In either case, the basic approach in the proportional mortality study is to compare the proportion of total deaths resulting from the disease of interest among different subgroups, as defined by level of exposure (via the SPMR and SePMR summary measures described above). With this approach, therefore, it is possible to test the exposure-response relationship of primary interest only if it can be assumed that exposure is unrelated to the remaining diseases.

Because proportional mortality studies can be performed quickly and inexpensively they serve as an attractive and useful preliminary approach for identifying work-related illnesses. Moreover, the results of a proportional mortality study can be used to approximate those derived from more complex cohort studies if the ascertainment of deaths is complete and is not influenced by differential selection according to cause of death or exposure status. These ideal conditions are generally not met, however, as proportional mortality studies are typically based on death certificates that are readily available rather than those obtained from follow-up of a cohort. John and coworkers (41) provide some general guidelines on the extent to which results of industry-based proportional mortality studies may be biased owing to omission of deaths that were unknown to the company.

Recent examples of the proportional mortality design include studies of garment workers exposed to formaldehyde (57), California agricultural workers (58), corn wet-milling workers (59), and wastewater treatment system workers (60).

### Ecologic Study

Ecologic studies, also called aggregate or descriptive studies, are empiric investigations involving the group rather than the individual as the unit of analysis. The groups may be populations of factories, companies, cities, counties, or nations. The only requirement is that information on the populations studied is available to describe each population with respect to exposure and disease. Ecologic analysis may involve incidence, prevalence, or mortality data, but mortality analysis is most common owing to the widespread availability of such data. For example, U.S. race-, sex-, age-, time period-, and geographic area (state and county)–specific mortality and population data are available for the years 1950 to 1994 from detailed mortality tapes assembled by the National Center for Health Statistics (43).

Exposure is also measured by some overall index. For example, information on socioeconomic status is available for census tracts from the decennial census, and information concerning the percentage of a county population employed in the chemical industry is available from the County and City Data Book (61).

A distinguishing feature of ecologic studies is the lack of information about the joint distribution of the exposure and the disease within each group. The association between exposure and disease is therefore based on measurements averaged over the groups. This can lead to a form of data grouping bias known as aggregation bias (62). Rao and colleagues (63) provide a discussion of this and other biases that arise in the estimation of relative risks from individual and ecologic data.

Ecologic studies are also limited by the use of proxy data for exposure (e.g., cigarette tax data rather than smoking data) and disease (e.g., mortality rather than incidence) and by the unavailability of data necessary to control confounding (27). The general problem of inappropriate inferences from ecologic data has been referred to as the ecologic fallacy (64).

Despite their many limitations, ecologic studies have been useful in providing important clues to occupational and environmental determinants of disease. For example, beginning in the mid-1970s a series of ecologic analyses were published by the epidemiology branch of the National Cancer Institute that implicated industrial factors in the development of various malignant diseases (65). Included among these were reported associations between elevated lung cancer rates and the presence in counties of copper, lead, or zinc smelting or refining plants (66); the petroleum industry and higher rates for cancers of the skin, nasal cavity, and sinuses (67); and the presence of World War II–shipbuilding industry in counties and elevated rates for lung, oropharyngeal, esophageal, and gastric cancers (68).

The findings or hypotheses generated by ecologic studies are often further examined or tested using more informative study designs. For example, in 1992, Day and colleagues (69) reported an excess of hematopoietic and lymphoid neoplasms in an ecologic study of cancer mortality in Kanawha County, West Virginia. In a subsequent case-control study of these neoplasms, Massoudi and coworkers (70) suggested that these neoplasms may be associated with work in the local chemical industry.

### Cohort Study

Among the observational study designs, the cohort study, also called a longitudinal or follow-up study, most closely resembles a controlled experiment and thus provides the most direct approach for evaluating overall patterns of health and disease in a working population. In an occupational cohort study, a presumably disease-free worker population (cohort) is followed over time, and its patterns of disease rates (incidence or mortality) are compared with those of unexposed external reference populations such as a local, state, or national standard population (e.g., via the SMR, SRR, or $RR_{M-H}$ summary measures). Enterline (71) and Gardner (72) provide some guidelines for the choice of appropriate reference populations for cohort studies. Also, if an exposure assessment of the working environment enables classification of workers according to type or level of exposure, disease rate comparisons can be made internally among the subcohorts in an effort to evaluate exposure-response relationships.

Cohort studies can be conducted prospectively (follow-up begins at the time of the study and proceeds into the future), historically (follow-up is conducted for time periods before the initiation of the study), or by combining both approaches. In most cases the historical design is preferred because it affords the most cost-efficient and feasible approach for studying rare diseases or ones that have long induction periods. Historical designs can be limited, however, by the absence or incompleteness of records required to reconstruct a historical cohort and to estimate its associated exposures.

Because rare chronic diseases (e.g., occupationally induced cancers) are often of primary interest, occupational cohort studies must include large numbers of subjects if they are to yield statistically reliable numbers of cases or deaths. In fact, it is not uncommon for a historical cohort study to include as many as 10,000 or more subjects, many of whom were first employed 40 or 50 years before the start of the study. Because of their typically large size, cohort studies are usually costly, time-consuming, and labor intensive, requiring the efforts of a multidisciplinary research team with formidable clerical and computer programming support. Cohort studies are also logistically complex, requiring the coordination of several multiphasic tasks related to exposure assessment, cohort enumeration, cohort follow-up, data processing and analysis, and data quality control. More complete accounts of the operational aspects of cohort studies, including the standard data sources and procedures available for tracing cohorts for disease or death, are provided by Lloyd and Ciocco (73), Redmond and colleagues (74), Monson (75), and Checkoway and coworkers (13).

The occupational epidemiology literature is replete with reports of cohort studies. Recent examples include historical cohort studies of British tin miners (76), U.S. and European MMVF workers (21,22,77), and U.S. workers exposed to formaldehyde (78–80) and chromium pigments (81). Marsh and coworkers (82) recently used the prospective cohort design to study total and cause-specific mortality patterns among chemical workers exposed to β-naphthylamine and other aromatic amines.

Common problems in cohort studies are possible selection bias resulting from incomplete cohort enumeration or follow-up, and possible information bias owing to inconsistent classification of disease influenced by knowledge of exposure. Marsh and Enterline (83) and Marsh (84) describe a method for verifying the completeness of cohorts assembled from industry records that can help to obviate selection bias.

One special form of selection bias that often arises in occupational cohort studies is the so-called healthy worker effect (HWE) (75,85,86). This occurs because an employed population is generally healthier than the unemployed population of the same age, and their death rates from many causes are lower than the corresponding rates in the general population. Also known as the "healthy hire effect" (87), the HWE is attenuated over time as the cohort ages. Cancer death rates appear to suffer less from the HWE than rates for most other causes, and cancer incidence rates probably are less affected than cancer death rates (30). One can adjust for bias due to the HWE by stratification on, or covariate adjustment by, time since hire, or by using internal comparisons.

While the HWE is attributed to the initial selection of healthy people *into* the cohort, workers may also be self-selected to types or to levels of exposures as follow-up progresses and/or workers may cease to be "at risk" for exposure because they have terminated employment. The health worker survivor effect (HWSE) refers to selection of workers *out of* the cohort due to events that evolved since the time of initial employment. The HWSE can occur even in the absence of the HWE. An example of the HWSE given by Robins et al. (88) is the tendency of workers at increased risk of death, such as smokers or workers with emphysema or lung cancer, to terminate early. Because such workers have reduced cumulative levels of occupational exposures relative to their healthier counterparts who do not terminate early, conventional analyses can yield artifactually inverse exposure-response relationships. Further discussion and methods to control for bias due to the HWSE are provided in the Methodological Issues section of this chapter.

Other special forms of selection bias often arise in occupational cohorts. For example, short-term transient workers may have different background disease risks attributable to unfavorable lifestyle factors. On the other hand, their elevated disease risks may reflect the fact that jobs that expose workers to higher levels of toxicants are often assigned to short-term workers.

Cohort studies are also often limited by the unavailability of complete data on certain variables that could potentially confound exposure-response relationships. For example, the results of historical cohort studies of lung cancer can be biased by the confounding effects of cigarette smoking if smoking levels differ between the cohort and the external comparison population or among exposure-specific subgroups of the cohort. Unfortunately, it is generally not feasible to acquire information on cigarette smoking for entire cohorts and adjustments for confounding must be made indirectly (89) or directly (90) in the context of ancillary studies such as a nested case-control study.

The design and statistical analysis aspects of cohort studies are discussed in detail by Breslow and Day (30).

### Case-Control Study

The case-control study, often termed a case-referent or retrospective study, involves the comparison of the exposure profiles of workers who developed the disease of interest (cases) with other workers who were presumably free of the disease at the times when the cases were identified (controls). Ideally, cases and controls should be comparable with respect to the a priori probability of exposure, the method of ascertainment, the method of collection, and the reliability and validity of data on exposure status, potentially confounding variables, and all characteristics (other than exposure) that relate both to the health outcomes and exposure variables under study (i.e., confounding variables). Because, at the outset of a study, it is usually not possible to ascertain the comparability of cases and cohort with respect to potential confounders, efforts are generally made to control for confounding bias either through design (matching cases to one or more confounders on the basis of one or more confounders) or through analysis (stratification by levels of one or more confounders).

Case-control studies can be used to estimate the measures of effect derivable only in cohort studies while reducing the cost and problems of following a cohort (and obtaining data on exposures and confounders on all subjects). Case-control studies do not provide direct measures of disease incidence, but they do yield odds ratios, which estimate relative risks. Consider the crude data layout for a case-control study in Table 3.

The crude odds ratio (OR) is defined as the ratio of the odds of exposure among the cases to the odds of exposure among the controls:

$$OR = (a/b)/(c/d) = ad/bc \qquad [12]$$

The case-control study analysis may be stratified by levels of one or more possible confounding variables (e.g.,

**TABLE 3.** *Data layout for case-control study*

| | Exposed | Unexposed | Total |
|---|---|---|---|
| Cases (events) | $a$ | $b$ | $M_1$ |
| Controls (nonevents) | $c$ | $d$ | $M_0$ |
| Total | $N_1$ | $N_0$ | $T$ |

age or smoking status). If this is done, a pooled summary odds ratio is given by Mantel and Haenszel (32) as

$$OR_{M\text{–}H} = \sum_i a_i(d_i/T_i) \,/\, \sum_i b_i(c_i/T_i) \qquad [13]$$

where summation is taken across all subgroups of the cases and controls. That the odds ratio estimates the relative risk is apparent upon comparing OR and $OR_{M\text{–}H}$ to the expressions for $RR_s$ and $RR_{M\text{–}H}$ presented above.

Two basic types of case-control studies are used in occupational epidemiologic research. A cohort-based study, often called a nested case-control study, is conducted within the framework of an existing occupational cohort, which provides both a basis for complete case ascertainment and a sampling frame for the selection of controls. Nested case-control studies are usually indicated when it is not feasible to obtain data on exposures or potential confounders for all cohort members.

In nested case-control studies, control subjects are usually selected from the cohort by a procedure called incidence density sampling. This involves considering each case in turn and randomly selecting one or more controls from the risk set of persons who were at risk at the age the subject was identified as a case. In some cases the selection of controls is restricted by certain matching variables (i.e., controls are further matched to cases on one or more factors), to either living or dead status (i.e., to avoid differential recall bias), or to diseases (or deaths) that are believed to be unrelated to the exposure under study. The cumulative exposures of the case and the controls, and the status of any confounding variables, are then evaluated as of this age. The relative risk is estimated by forming the ratio of the average exposure of the cases to the average exposure of the controls while adjusting for the confounding variables. Beaumont and coworkers (91) have developed a useful computer program for incidence density sampling. An example of an industry-based nested case-control study is provided by Bond and colleagues (92), who used this design to relate lung cancer mortality to occupational exposures within a chemical production facility. Eisen (93) used the nested case-control design to study larynx cancer in automobile workers exposed to machining fluid.

In another strategy for selecting controls in nested case-control studies, the case-cohort (94), controls are selected at the beginning of the cohort study as a stratified random sample of the entire cohort. This approach eliminates the need to identify cases before selecting controls and can provide controls for several simultaneous case-control studies of various diseases (95). The utility of the case-cohort design is limited by its analytic complexity and the paucity of available statistical methods that allow control for multiple confounders. Enterline and coworkers (96) employed the case-cohort design to control for potential confounding by cigarette smoking in examining the relationship between man-made mineral fiber exposure and respiratory system cancer mortality. The case-cohort design was also used by Baris et al. (97) to study suicide in relation to exposure to electric and magnetic fields among electric utility workers.

The second type of occupational case-control study is the registry-based design. Here, cases are identified from one or more population- or company-based cancer or mortality registries, hospital records, or other community sources, and are compared to controls with respect to occupational factors. Registry-based case-control studies generally are less informative than nested case-control studies with respect to exposure characterization, although they represent the best approach to studying occupational exposures among working groups when cohort enumeration would be difficult or impossible (e.g., agricultural workers or gasoline station attendants).

An example of a comparison-based case-control study is provided by Walrath and coworkers (98), who utilized the E. I. du Pont de Nemours and Company 1956 to 1985 cancer incidence registry (99) to determine whether the risk of developing certain cancers is related to exposure to dimethylformamide. The population-based case-control design is exemplified by the Brender and Suarez (100) examination of the association between paternal occupation and anencephalic births using records of the Texas Department of Health on live births, fetal deaths, and linked live births and fetal deaths.

Case-control studies have numerous other practical and statistical advantages over other designs. They are well suited to testing etiologic hypotheses for specific rare diseases, and they allow investigation of diseases regardless of induction period or duration of expression. They can also evaluate a range of exposures related to the disease. In addition, because the ratio of cases to controls can be fixed by the investigator, for a given sample size and study cost analyses are more statistically efficient than for other designs. In fact, for a given effect size, level of significance, and statistical power, the case-control design requires fewer individuals than the cohort study when the studied health outcome is rarer than the exposure. Compared to a cohort study, the case-control study may also permit a more precise clinical classification of the cases.

A principal limitation of case-control studies is that only one health outcome of interest can be evaluated. Thus, the case-control design may not be as appropriate as a cohort study for exploring the range of health effects resulting from exposure to a certain toxicant. Case-control studies are also inefficient for evaluating the effects of exposures that are rare in the source population for the cases. Their ability to support causal inferences depends on the retrospective of exposure information from records, which may be inaccurate or incomplete, or from human recall, which is subject to differential information bias (recall or amnestic bias) between cases and controls. In general, the greater efficiency of case-control studies is a strength that may compensate for the greater possibility of bias that usually exists.

A thorough review of analytic methods for case-control studies is provided by Breslow and Day (101). Other aspects of case-control studies are discussed in detail by Cole (102) and Schlesselman (103).

### Occupational Epidemiologic Surveillance Programs

Ongoing epidemiologic evaluation of employee health status is becoming an increasingly important component of the corporate occupational health program, because clinical reports and findings of ad hoc morbidity and mortality studies are often insufficient to protect the health of the worker. Unlike traditional medical surveillance systems, which identify and manage individual cases of illness, epidemiologic surveillance involves ongoing systematic analysis and interpretation of the distribution and trends of illness, injury, or mortality in a defined employee population. While they do not have an epidemiologic study design per se, surveillance programs in occupational settings provide the data and an operational framework for the conduct of specific epidemiologic investigations, should the need develop.

Epidemiologic surveillance programs can help employers meet a number of occupational health objectives, such as estimating of baseline rates of illness and mortality, screening for excess risk of illness, providing assistance in the design and interpretation of special studies, and affording prompt response to health-related injuries and participation in health-related programs (e.g., a hypertension screening program).

There are three basic approaches to the development of epidemiologic surveillance programs. The disease registry approach focuses on the enumeration of cases or deaths associated with a health outcome of interest. These data are then linked with appropriate denominator data on persons exposed to different agents to form rates of illness or injury that can be periodically monitored to assess risks in the workplace. In contrast, the exposure-based surveillance approach focuses on subgroups of the employee population that are exposed to particular chemicals of interest or to high concentrations of these chemicals. The exposed persons are then followed over time to monitor possible adverse health outcomes. Medical surveillance, including screening and diagnostic evaluation, may also be included in this exposed persons–based approach. The third approach basically integrates the disease- and exposure-based surveillance systems. This ideal system usually also includes individual employee data on factors (e.g., history of cigarette smoking) that might possibly confound relationships between exposure and disease.

The cancer epidemiologic surveillance program instituted in 1956 by du Pont exemplifies the disease registry approach (99). It uses group health and life insurance records to identify cancer incident cases among active employees and cancer deaths among actives and retirees. Denominator data for incidence and mortality rate computation are provided by company employment and pension records. Examples of the integrated approach to medical and epidemiologic surveillance are the bladder screening programs for chemical workers exposed to β-naphthylamine and other aromatic amines developed by Schulte (104) and Marsh (105) and their coworkers.

## METHODOLOGICAL ISSUES

This section provides a brief overview of some of the most important study design, analysis, and data interpretation issues that arise in occupational epidemiology. A basic understanding of these issues is essential both for persons who wish to design and conduct occupational studies and for those who need to assess the importance and relevance of the published occupational epidemiology literature.

### Precision and Validity

The overall goal of an occupational epidemiology study is to perform accurate measurements of disease occurrence and effect. Sources of error in measurement may be either random or systematic.

Precision in epidemiologic measurements corresponds to the reduction of random error. The primary component of random error is sampling error, which indicates the amount of variation in a measurement that would be obtained if similar studies were repeated a large number of times. Precision is reflected in the variance of a measurement and its associated confidence interval.

Precision can be improved by increasing the size of the study or by modifying its design to increase the efficiency with which information is obtained from a given number of study subjects.

The size of an epidemiologic study is related to the following variables (27):

1. Level of "statistical significance" (alpha level). This is the probability of claiming as a real effect one that is simply a chance occurrence (alpha error).
2. The probability of missing a real effect (beta error). Alternatively, the complement of the beta error, power, can be used. Power is the probability of detecting (as statistically significant) a postulated level of effect.
3. The magnitude of effect.
4. Disease rate in the absence of exposure (or exposure prevalence in the absence of disease).
5. Relative size of the compared groups (i.e., ratio of exposed to unexposed subjects or of cases to controls).

Values of these variables can be used in available "sample size" formulas (106,107) or computer programs (108) to plan or assess the adequacy of the size of a study.

Study efficiency is affected by a variety of design aspects, including the proportion of subjects exposed, the proportion of subjects who have or will develop disease, and the distribution of subjects according to key variables that must be controlled for in the analysis.

Validity in epidemiologic measurements corresponds to the reduction of systematic error. Systematic error, or bias, occurs if there is a difference between what the study is actually estimating and what it is intended to estimate. Systematic error, unlike random error, is not necessarily improved by increasing the size of the study. Validity is usually separated into two components: internal validity, the degree to which the study findings truly represent the phenomena observed among the study sample; and external validity, the degree to which the study findings can be generalized to persons outside the study population. A study must have internal validity before it can be assessed for external validity.

### Selection, Information and Confounding Bias, and Intermediate Variables

As noted throughout this chapter, various types of biases can detract from a study's internal validity. Selection bias is any bias that arises from the manner in which study subjects were selected or the processes by which study participants (or nonparticipants) decided to join (or not join) the study.

Bias related to the instruments and techniques used to collect information on exposure, health outcomes, and other related factors is called information bias. Nondifferential information bias occurs when the likelihood of misclassification is the same for both groups compared. When an effect exists, bias from nondifferential misclassification always is in the direction of the null value (i.e., of no effect) (109). Hence, it is of particular concern in studies that show no association between exposure and disease.

Differential information bias occurs when the likelihood of misclassification is different for each comparison group. This form of bias is potentially more problematic because it can bias the observed effect estimate either toward or away from the null value.

Confounding bias, or confounding, arises from the failure to account for (or control for) the effects of other factors related to the exposure and health outcome. More specifically, if no other bias is present three conditions are necessary for a variable to be a confounder (27):

1. A confounding variable must be a risk factor for the disease.
2. A confounding variable must be associated with the exposure under study in the population from which the cases derive.
3. A confounding variable must not be an intermediate step in the causal pathway between the exposure and the disease.

Cigarette smoking is a classic example of a potential confounding variable in occupational cohort studies of respiratory disease, because it is a known risk factor that can be associated with workplace exposure levels (e.g., working with combustible agents). Also, in studies with time-dependent exposures, employment status (i.e., working or not working) can potentially confound the association between exposure and disease because employment status is necessarily related to exposure (only employed persons can receive workplace exposures), and may be related to the risk of death (either because a change in employment status may signify ill health, or because being unemployed increases the risk of death) (110,111).

Confounding, the most difficult bias to detect and correct, can be controlled in the study design (e.g., by matching), in the statistical analysis (e.g., by stratification), or in both. Sackett (112) provides a useful catalog of biases that can arise in epidemiologic research.

An *intermediate variable* is an independent risk factor for the disease under study that both determines subsequent exposure and is determined by previous exposure to the agent under study. In occupational cohort studies where the HWSE is present, employment status can be an intermediate variable, provided that exposure causes an individual to terminate employment. In this situation, treating employment status as a confounding variable is inappropriate as employment status is on the causal pathway from exposure to disease (i.e., violates condition 3 above).

Methods have been proposed by Robins (113,114) and Robins et al. (88,115) to control bias in cohort studies where the HWSE (and the associated intermediate variable employment status) are present. Stone and Marsh (116) present a review of procedures to control bias from confounding and intermediate variables in occupational cohort studies.

### Criteria Causal Inference in Occupational Epidemiology

Perhaps the most difficult task of the occupational epidemiologist is attempting to determine whether or not an apparent association between an exposure and a health outcome is causal. While epidemiologic studies cannot prove causality, the credibility of a causal connection can be enhanced if several criteria are satisfied. Hill (117) suggested that the following nine criteria be considered in determining whether an association is likely to be causal:

1. Strength: How strong is the association between the suspected risk factor and the observed outcome? Monson (44) offers the following empiric guide to

assessing the strength of association based on the rate ratio:

| Rate ratios | | Strength of association |
|---|---|---|
| 0.9–1.0 | 1.0–1.2 | None |
| 0.7–0.9 | 1.2–1.5 | Weak |
| 0.4–0.7 | 1.5–3.0 | Moderate |
| 0.1–0.4 | 3.0–10.0 | Strong |
| <0.1 | ≥10.0 | Infinite |

2. Consistency: Does the association hold in different settings and among different groups?
3. Specificity: How closely are the specific exposure factor and specific health outcome associated?
4. Temporality: Does the cause (exposure factor) antedate the effect?
5. Biologic gradient: Does a dose-response relationship exist between the exposure and the health outcome?
6. Plausibility: Does the apparent association make sense biologically?
7. Coherence: Is the association consistent with what is known of the natural history and biology of the disease?
8. Experimental evidence: Does any experimental evidence support the hypothesis of an association?
9. Analogy: Are there other examples with similar risk factors and outcomes?

Note that it is not necessary for all of the above criteria to be met in order for a factor to be considered part of the network of causes of a disease. Rather, the weight of the total body of currently available evidence should be used to conclude whether an association is or is not likely to be causal.

Additional or new evidence might support the original conclusion or reverse it at any time, in which case the conclusion should be revised. The tentativeness and subjectiveness of the causal inference process is described eloquently in the words of Hill (117): "All scientific work is incomplete whether it be observational or experimental. All scientific work is liable to be upset or modified by advancing knowledge. That does not confer upon us a freedom to ignore the knowledge we already have, or to postpone the action that it appears to demand at a given time."

## REFERENCES


1. Doll R. The causes of death among gas workers, with special reference to cancer of the lung. *Br J Ind Med* 1952;9:180–185.
2. Case RAM, Hosker ME, McDonald DB, Pearson JT. Tumours of the urinary bladder in workmen engaged in the manufacture and use of certain dyestuff intermediates in the British chemical industry. Part I. *Br J Ind Med* 1954;11:75–104.
3. Mancuso TF, Coulter EJ. Methods of studying the relation of employment and long-term illness in cohort analysis. *Am J Public Health* 1959;49:1525–1536.
4. Wagner JC, Sleggs CA, Marchand P. Diffuse pleural mesothelioma and asbestos exposure in the North Western Cape Province. *Br J Ind Med* 1960;17:260–271.
5. Corn M, Esmen NA. Workplace exposure zones for classification of employee exposures to physical and chemical agents. *Am Ind Hyg Assoc J* 1979;40:47–56.
6. Dosemeci M, Stewart PA, Blair A. Three proposals for retrospective semi-quantitative exposure assessments and their comparison with the other assessment methods. *App Ind Hyg* In press.
7. Esmen NA. Retrospective industrial hygiene surveys. *Am Ind Hyg Assoc* 1979;40:58–65.
8. Smith TJ. Exposure assessment for occupational epidemiology. *Am J Ind Med* 1987;12:249–268.
9. Stewart PA, Blair A, Cubit DA, et al. Estimating historical exposures to formaldehyde in a retrospective mortality study. *Appl Ind Hyg* 1986;1:34–41.
10. Smith T. Introduction. In: Smith TJ, Rappaport SM, eds. *Exposure assessment for epidemiology and hazard control.* Chelsea, MI: Lewis Publishers, 1991;ix–xiv.
11. Smith TJ. Exposure-dose relationships. In: Smith TJ, Rappaport SM, eds. *Exposure assessment for epidemiology and hazard control.* Chelsea, MA: Lewis Publishers 1991;97–114.
12. Ballantyne B. Evaluation of hazards from mixtures of chemicals in the occupational environment. *J Occup Med* 1985;27:85–94.
13. Checkoway H, Pearce NV, Crawford-Brown DJ. *Research methods in occupational epidemiology.* New York: Oxford University Press,1989.
14. Gamble JF, Spirtas R. Job classification and utilization of complete work histories in occupational epidemiology. *J Occup Med* 1976;18: 399–404.
15. Hoar SK, Morrison AS, Cole P, Silverman DT. An occupational and exposure linkage system for the study of occupational carcinogenesis. *J Occup Med* 1980;22:722–726.
16. Socka GE, Langner RR, Olson RD, Storey GL. Computer handling of occupational exposure data. *Am Ind Hyg Assoc J* 1979;40:553–561.
17. Marsh GM. A strategy for merging and analyzing work history data in industry wide occupational epidemiology studies. *Am Ind Hyg Assoc J* 1987;48:414–419.
18. Hawkins N, Evans JS. Subjective estimation of toluene exposures: a calibration study of industrial hygienists. *Appl Ind Hyg* 1989;4:61–68.
19. Krombout H, Costendorp Y, Heederik D, Boleij JSM. Agreement between qualitative exposure estimates and quantitative exposure estimates. *Am J Ind Med* 1987;12:551–562.
20. Hallock MF, Smith TJ, Wegman D. Reconstruction of historical exposures at a transformer manufacturing facility by interview: Analysis of agreement among multiple interviewees. Presented at the American Conference of Industrial Hygiene, St. Louis, 1989.
21. Marsh GM, Enterline PE, Stone RA, Henderson VL. Mortality among a cohort of U.S. man-made mineral fiber workers: 1985 follow-up. *J Occup Med* 1990;32:594–604.
22. Marsh GM, Stone RA, Youk AO, et al. Mortality among United States rock wool and slag wool workers: 1989 update. *J Occup Health Safety Aust NZ* 1996;12:297–312.
23. Marsh GM, Ehland J, Paik M, Preininger M, Caplan R. OCMAP/PC: A user-oriented cohort mortality analysis program for the IBM PC. *Am Stat* 1986;40:308–309.
24. Marsh GM, Preininger ME. OCMAP: a user-oriented occupational cohort mortality analysis program. *Am Stat* 1980;34:245–246.
25. Monson RR. Analysis of relative survival and proportional mortality. *Comput Biomed Res* 1974;7:325–332.
26. Waxweiler RJ, Beaumont JJ, Henry JA, et al. A modified life-table analysis program system for cohort studies. *J Occup Med* 1983;25: 115–124.
27. Rothman KJ. *Modern epidemiology.* Boston: Little, Brown, 1986.
28. Cornfield J, Haenszel W. Some aspects of retrospective studies. *J Chron Dis* 1960;11:523–534.
29. Miettinen OS. Standardization of risk ratios. *Am J Epidemiol* 1972;96: 383–388.
30. Breslow NE, Day NE. *Statistical methods in cancer research.* Lyon: International Agency for Research on Cancer (IARC), 1987;2.
31. Fleiss J. *Statistical methods for rates and proportions,* 2nd ed. New York: Wiley, 1981.
32. Mantel N, Haenszel W. Statistical aspects of the analysis of data from retrospective studies of disease. *J Natl Cancer Inst* 1959;22:719–748.
33. Zeighami E, Morris M. The measurement and interpretation of proportionate mortality. *Am J Epidemiol* 1983;117:90–97.
34. Marsh GM, Winwood J, Rao BR. Prediction of the standardized risk ratio via proportional mortality analysis. *Biometrical* 1987;29: 355–368.

35. Breslow NE, Lubin JH, Marek P, Langholz B. Multiplicative models and cohort analysis. *J Am Stat Assoc* 1983;78:1–12.
36. Chiazze L. Problems of study design and interpretation of industrial mortality experience. *J Occup Med* 1976;18:169–170.
37. Decoufle P, Thomas TI, Pickle LW. Comparison of the proportionate and cause-specific mortality among workers at an energy research laboratory. *Br J Ind Med* 1980;42:525–533.
38. Gaffey WR. A critique of the standardized mortality ratio. *J Occup Med* 1976;18:157–160.
39. Gilbert ES. Some confounding factors in the study of mortality and occupational exposure. *Am J Epidemiol* 1982;116:177–188.
40. Greenland S. Interpretation and estimation of summary ratios under heterogeneity. *Stat Med* 1982;1:217–227.
41. John LR, Marsh GM, Enterline PE. Evaluating occupational hazards using only information known to employers: a comparative study. *Br J Ind Med* 1983;40:346–352.
42. Kupper LL, McMichael AJ, Symons MJ, Most BM. On the utility of proportional mortality analysis. *J Chron Dis* 1978;31:15–22.
43. Marsh GM, Ehland J, Sefcik S. *Mortality and population data system.* Technical report. Pittsburgh: University of Pittsburgh Department of Biostatistics, 1996.
44. Monson RR. *Occupational epidemiology,* 2nd ed. Boca Raton, FL: CRC, 1990.
45. Pott P. *Chirurgical observations.* London: Hawes, Clarke and Collins, 1775.
46. Wong O, Decoufle P. Methodologic issues involving SMR and PMR in occupational studies. *J Occup Med* 1982;24:299–304.
47. Caplan RJ, Marsh GM, Enterline PE. A generalized effective exposure modeling program for assessing dose-response in epidemiologic investigations. *Comput Biomed Res* 1983;16:587–596.
48. Marsh GM, Co-Chien H, Rao BR, Ehland J. OCMAP:Module 6-A new computing algorithm for proportional mortality analysis. *Am Stat* 1989;43:127–128.
49. Marsh GM, Youk AO, Stone RA, Sefcik S, Alcorn C. OCMAP-PLUS: a program for the comprehensive analysis of occupational cohort data. Submitted for publication, 1997.
50. Enterline PE. Pitfalls in epidemiologic research: an examination of the asbestos literature. *J Occup Med* 1976;18:150–156.
51. Creech JL, Johnson MN. Angiosarcoma of liver in the manufacture of polyvinyl chloride. *J Occup Med* 1974;16:150–151.
52. Enterline PE. Evaluating cancer clusters. *Am Ind Hyg Assoc J* 1985; 46:B10–13.
53. Schwartz J, Landrigan PJ, Baker EL, Orenstein WA, Lindern IH. Lead-induced anemia: dose-response relationships and evidence for a threshold. *Am J Public Health* 1990;80:169–172.
54. Marquart H, Smid T, Heederik D, Visschers M. Lung function of welders of zinc-coated mild steel: cross-sectional analysis and changes over five consecutive work shifts. *Am J Ind Med* 1989;16: 289–296.
55. Lewis S, Bennett J, Richards K. A cross sectional study of the independent effect of occupation on lung function in British coal miners. *Occup Environ Med* 1996;53(2);125–128.
56. Miettinen OS, Wang JD. An alternative to the proportionate mortality ratio. *Am J Epidemiol* 1981;114:144–148.
57. Stayner L, Smith AB, Reeve G, et al. Proportionate mortality study of workers in the garment industry exposed to formaldehyde. *Am J Ind Med* 1985;7:229–240.
58. Stubbs HA, Harris J, Spear RC. A proportionate mortality analysis of California agricultural workers 1978-1979. *Am J Ind Med* 1984;6: 305–320.
59. Thomas TI, Krekel S, Hedi M. Proportionate mortality among male corn wet-milling workers. *Int J Epidemiol* 1985;14:432–437.
60. Betemps EJ. Proportional mortality analysis of wastewater treatment system workers by birthplace with comments on amyotrophic lateral sclerosis. *J Occup Med* 1994:36(1):31–35.
61. U.S. Bureau of Census. *County and city data book,* 1995. Washington, DC: U.S. Government Printing Office, 1995.
62. Robinson W. Ecological correlations and the behavior of individuals. *Am Sociol Rev* 1950;15:351–357.
63. Rao BR, Day R, Marsh GM. Estimation of relative risks from individual and ecological correlation studies. In: *Communications in statistics, theory and methods.* 1992;241–268.
64. Morgenstern H. Uses of ecologic analysis in epidemiologic research. *Am J Public Health* 1982;72:1336–l344.
65. Blot W, Fraumeni J, Mason T, Hoover R. Developing clues to environmental cancer: A stepwise approach with the use of cancer mortality data. *Environ Health Perspect* 1979;32:53–58.
66. Blot W, Fraumeni J. Arsenical air pollution and lung cancer. *Lancet* 1975;2:142–144.
67. Blot W, Brinton L, Fraumeni J, Stone B. Cancer mortality in U.S. counties with petroleum industries. *Science* 1977;198:51–53.
68. Blot W, Stone B, Fraumeni J, Morris L. Cancer mortality in U.S. counties with shipyard industries during World War II. *Environ Res* 1979; 18:281–290.
69. Day R, Talbott EO, Marsh GM, Case B. A comparative ecologic study of selected cancers in Kanawha County, WV. *Am J Ind Med* 1992;21: 235–251.
70. Massoudi BL, Talbott EO, Day RD, Swerdlow SH, Marsh GM, Kuller LH. A case- control study of hematopoietic and lymphoid neoplasms: the role of work in the chemical industry. *Am J Ind Med* 1997;31: 21–27.
71. Enterline PE. The estimation of expected rates in occupational disease epidemiology. *Public Health Rep* 1964;79:973–978.
72. Gardner MJ. Considerations in the choice of expected numbers for appropriate comparisons in occupational cohort studies. *Med Lav* 1986;77:23–47.
73. Lloyd JW, Ciocco A. Long-term mortality study of steel-workers. I. Methodology. *J Occup Med* 1969;11:299–310.
74. Redmond CK, Smith ME, Lloyd JW, Rush HW. Long-term mortality study of steelworkers. III. Follow-up. *J Occup Med* 1969;11:513–521.
75. Monson RR. Observations on the healthy worker effect. *J Occup Med* 1986;28:425–433.
76. Hodgson JT, Jones RD. Mortality of a cohort of tin miners 1941-86. *Br J Ind Med* 1990;47:665–676.
77. Simonato L, Fletcher AC, Cherrie JW, et al. The International Agency for Research on Cancer historical cohort study of MMMF-production workers in seven European countries: extension of follow-up. *Ann Occup Hyg* 1987;31:603–624.
78. Blair A, Stewart P, O'Berg M, et al. Mortality among workers exposed to formaldehyde. *J Natl Cancer Inst* 1986;76:1071–1084.
79. Marsh GM, Stone RA, Esmen NA, Henderson VH, Lee KY. Mortality patterns among chemical workers in a factory where formaldehyde was used. *Occup Environ Med* 1996;53:613–617.
80. Marsh GM, Stone RA, Esmen NA, Henderson VL. Mortality among chemical plant workers exposed to formaldehyde and other substances. *J Natl Cancer Inst* 1994;86:384–385.
81. Hayes RB, Sheffet A, Spirtas R. Cancer mortality among a cohort of chromium pigment workers. *Am J Ind Med* 1989;16:127–134.
82. Marsh GM, Leviton LC, Talbott E, et al. The Drake Chemical Workers Health Registry Study: I. Notification and medical of surveillance of a group of workers at high risk of developing bladder cancer. *Am J Ind Med* 1991;19:291–301.
83. Marsh GM, Enterline PE. A method for verifying the completeness of cohorts used in occupational mortality studies. *J Occup Med* 1979;21: 665–670.
84. Marsh GM. Computerized approach to verifying study population data in occupational epidemiology. *J Occup Med* 1982;24:596–601.
85. McMichael AJ. Standardized mortality ratios and the "healthy worker effect": scratching beneath the surface. *J Occup Med* 1976;18: 155–168.
86. Fox AJ, Goldblatt PO. *Longitudinal study:* sociodemographic mortality differentials. London: Her Majesty's Stationery Office, 1982.
87. Arrighi HM, Hertz-Picciotto I. The evolving concept of the healty worker survivor effect. *Epidemiology* 1994;5:189–196.
88. Robins JM, Pambrun M, Chute C, Blevins D. Estimating the effect of formaldehyde exposure on lung cancer and nonmalignant respiratory disease (NMRD) mortality using a new method to control for the healthy worker survivor effect. In: Hogstedt C, Reuterwall C, eds. *Progress in occupational epidemiology.* New York: Elsevier Science Publishers B.V. (Biomedical Division), 1988;75–78.
89. Axelson 0, Steenland K. Indirect methods of assessing the effects of tobacco use in occupational studies. *Am J Ind Med* 1988;13:105–118.
90. Marsh GM, Sachs DPL, Callahan C, Leviton LC, Ricci E, Henderson V. Direct methods of obtaining information on tobacco use in occupational studies. *Am J Ind Med* 1988;13:71–104.
91. Beaumont JJ, Steenland K, Minton A, Meyer S. A computer program for incidence density sampling of controls in case-control studies nested within occupational cohort studies. *Am J Epidemiol* 1989;129:212–219.

92. Bond GG, Flores GH, Shellenberger RJ, Cartmill JB, Fishbeck WA, Cook PR. Nested case-control study of lung cancer among chemical workers. *Am J Epidemiol* 1986;124:53–66.
93. Eisen EA. Mortality studies of machining fluid exposure in the automobile industry. III: A case-control study of larynx cancer. *Am J Ind Med* 1994;26(2):185–202.
94. Prentice RL. A case-cohort design for epidemiologic cohort studies and disease prevention trials. *Biometika* 1986;73:1–11.
95. Kupper LL, McMichael AJ, Spirtas R. A hybrid epidemiologic study design useful in estimating relative risk. *J Am Stat Assoc* 1975;70: 524–528.
96. Enterline PE, Marsh GM, Henderson V, Callahan C. Mortality update of a cohort of U.S. man-made mineral fiber workers. *Ann Occup Hyg* 1987;31:625–656.
97. Baris D, Armstrong BG, Deadman J, Theriault G. A case cohort study of suicide in relation to exposure to electric and magnetic fields among electrical utility workers. *Occup Environ Med* 1996;53(1): 17–24.
98. Walrath J, Fayerweather WE, Gilby PG, Pell S. A case-control study of cancer among du Pont employees with potential for exposure to dimethylformamide. *J Occup Med* 1989;31:432–438.
99. Pell S, O'Berg MT, Karrh BW. Cancer epidemiologic surveillance in the du Pont Company. *J Occup Med* 1978;20:725–740.
100. Brender JD, Suarez L. Paternal occupation and anencephaly. *Am J Epidemiol* 1990;131:517–521.
101. Breslow NE, Day NE. *Statistical methods in cancer research.* Lyon: International Agency for Research on Cancer (IARC), 1980;1.
102. Cole P. The evolving case-control study. *J Chron Dis* 1979;32:15–27.
103. Schlesselman JJ. *Case-control studies:* design, *conduct, analysis.* New York: Oxford University Press, 1982.
104. Schulte P, Ringen K, Altekruse MD, et al. Notification of a cohort of workers at risk of bladder cancer. *J Occup Med* 1985;27:19–28.
105. Marsh GM, Callahan C, Pavlock D, Leviton LC, Talbott EO, Hemstreet G. A protocol for bladder cancer screening and medical surveillance among high-risk groups: the Drake Health Registry experience. *J Occup Med* 1990;32:881–886.
106. Rothman KJ, Boice JD Jr. *Epidemiologic analysis with a programmable calculator.* Chestnut Hill, MA: Epidemiology Resources, 1982;2.
107. Schlesselman JJ. Sample size requirements in cohort and case-control studies of disease. *Am J Epidemiol* 1974;99:381–384.
108. DuPont WD, Plummer WD. Power and sample size calculations. A review and computer program. *Controlled Clin Trials* 1990;11: 116–128.
109. Copeland KT, Checkoway H, McMichael AJ, Holbrook RH. Bias due to misclassification in the estimation of relative risk. *Am J Epidemiol* 1977;105:488–495.
110. Pearce N. Time-related confounders and intermediate variables. *Epidemiology* 1992;3:279–281.
111. Steenland K, Stayner L. The importance of employment status in occupational cohort mortality studies. *Epidemiology* 1991;2:418–423.
112. Sackett DL. Bias in analytic research. *J Chron Dis* 1979;32:51–63.
113. Robins J. A graphical approach to the identification and estimation of causal parameters in mortality studies with sustained exposure periods. *J Chron Dis* 1987;40:139S–161S.
114. Robins J. The control of confounding by intermediate variables. *Stat Med* 1989;8:679–701.
115. Robins JM, Blevins D, Ritter G, Wulfsohn M. G-estimation of the effect of prophylaxis therapy for pneumocystis carinii pneumonia on the survival of AIDS patients. *Epidemiology* 1992;3:319–326.
116. Stone RA, Marsh GM. A review of procedures to control bias in occupational cohort studies. *Am Ind Council Technical Report* 1996 (August).
117. Hill AB. The environment and disease: Association or causation? *Proc R Soc Med* 1965;58:295–300.

## APPENDIX 1. MEASURES OF DISEASE OCCURRENCE AND EFFECT: AN ILLUSTRATION

Table 4 presents data from a hypothetical cohort study in which total death rates and death rates from lung cancer are compared for low-exposure and high-exposure study groups. An external population serves as the common reference group (Table 5). The data layout is presented in Tables 1 and 2.

Table 4 shows that the low- and high-exposure groups have virtually identical crude death rates for lung cancer (0.0084 and 0.0086, respectively). However, the uniformly higher age-specific rates in the high-exposure group suggest that lung cancer mortality may be associated with level of exposure. In this example, age, which is related both to exposure group and to lung cancer rates, is confounding the association between exposure and lung cancer as measured by the crude rates. To control for confounding by age, the techniques of standardization and pooling can be used to compute

**TABLE 4.** *Proportional mortality measures: exposed*

| | Study group 1 (high exposure) | | | | Study group 2 (low exposure) | | | |
|---|---|---|---|---|---|---|---|---|
| | | Deaths | | | | Deaths | | |
| | | All causes | Lung cancer | | | All causes | Lung cancer | |
| Age subgroup $i$ | Person-years ($N_{1i}$) | No. ($D_{1i}$) | No. ($a_i$) | Rate ($R_{1i}$) | Person-years ($N_{1i}$) | No. ($D_{1i}$) | No. ($a_i$) | Rate ($R_{1i}$) |
| 20–44 | 2,500 | 8 | 3 | 0.0012 | 1,000 | 4 | 1 | 0.0010 |
| 45–64 | 1,000 | 14 | 4 | 0.0040 | 1,500 | 18 | 3 | 0.0020 |
| ≥65 | 1,500 | 130 | 36 | 0.0240 | 2,500 | 202 | 38 | 0.0152 |
| Total | 5,000 | 152 | 43 | 0.0086 | 5,000 | 224 | 42 | 0.0084 |

**TABLE 5.** *Proportional mortality measures: reference group*

| Age subgroup *i* | Person-years ($N_{0i}$) | Deaths: All causes ($D_{0i}$) | Lung cancer: Number ($b_i$) | Lung cancer: Rate ($R_{0i}$) |
|---|---|---|---|---|
| 20–44 | 50,000 | 100 | 5 | 0.0001 |
| 45–64 | 35,000 | 400 | 49 | 0.0014 |
| ≥65 | 15,000 | 1,000 | 66 | 0.0044 |
| Total | 100,000 | 1,500 | 120 | 0.0012 |

various summary measures of effect. For example, the lung cancer SMR for the high-exposure group would be computed as follows:

$$SMR_{High} = \frac{(3 + 4 + 36)}{2500\ (0.0001) + 1000\ (0.0014) + 1500\ (0.0044)} = \frac{43}{8.25} = 5.21 \qquad [14]$$

Summary measures expressed as rate ratios ($RR_s$) are usually multiplied by 100, so that deviations from 100 represent percentages of mortality excesses or deficits. Thus,

$$SMR_{High} = 5.21(100) = 521$$

indicating that the high-exposure group had a 421% excess in lung cancer mortality relative to the reference population. Similarly, the SMR for the low-exposure group is found as

$$SMR_{Low} = \frac{(1 + 3 + 38)}{1000\ (0.0001) + 1500\ (0.0014) + 2500\ (0.0044)} * (100) = 318 \qquad [15]$$

indicating a 218% excess in lung cancer mortality. Therefore, because $SMR_{Low}$ is less than $SMR_{High}$, the standardized data suggest an association between exposure and lung cancer.

The directly standardized lung cancer SRR can also be computed for both study groups:

$$SRR_{High} = \frac{(50{,}000)(0.0012) + (35{,}000)(0.0040) + (15{,}000)(0.0240)}{(5 + 49 + 66)} * (100) = 467 \qquad [16]$$

$$SRR_{Low} = \frac{(50{,}000)(0.0010) + (35{,}000)(0.0020) + (15{,}000)(0.0152)}{(5 + 49 + 66)} * (100) = 290 \qquad [17]$$

While the SRR values differ somewhat from the SMR values, the relationship of $SRR_{Low}$ to $SRR_{High}$ holds, again suggesting an association between exposure and lung cancer mortality. Note here that because the age distributions differ in study groups 1 and 2 and age is also related to exposure, the directly standardized SRR is the preferred summary measure.

Using the summary measures computed above, the ISRs for the two study groups are

$$ISR_{High} = (5.21)(0.0086) = 0.0448 \qquad [18]$$

$$ISR_{Low} = (3.18)(0.0084) = 0.0267 \qquad [19]$$

and the DSRs are

$$DSR_{High} = (4.67)(0.0012) = 0.0056 \qquad [20]$$

$$DSR_{Low} = (2.90)(0.0012) = 0.0035 \qquad [21]$$

While the absolute values of ISR and DSR are arbitrary, depending solely on the choice of the reference population, both summary measures again indicate a pattern of greater mortality in the high- than in the low-exposure group.

Pooling can also be used to compute the $RR_{M\text{–}H}$ in both groups:

$$RR_{M\text{–}H_{High}} = \frac{3(50{,}000/52{,}500) + 4(35{,}000/36{,}000) + 36(15{,}000/16{,}500)}{5(2{,}500/52{,}500) + 49(1{,}000/36{,}000) + 66(1{,}500/16{,}500)} * (100) = 519 \qquad [22]$$

$$RR_{M\text{-}H_{Low}} = \frac{1(50{,}000/51{,}000) + 3(35{,}000/36{,}500) + 38(15{,}000/17{,}500)}{5(1{,}000/51{,}000) + 49(1{,}500/36{,}500) + 66(2{,}500/17{,}500)} * (100) = 316 \quad [23]$$

The $RR_{M\text{-}H}$ values are close to the SMR values and reflect the same association between exposure and lung cancer.

Proportional mortality measures could also be computed from Tables 4 and 5 in the situation where the person-years at risk values, $N_{1i}$ and $N_{0i}$, were unknown. These would be

$$SPMR_{High} = \frac{(3 + 4 + 36)}{8(5/100) + 14(49/400) + 130(66/1{,}000)} = 402 \quad [24]$$

$$SPMR_{Low} = \frac{(1 + 3 + 38)}{4(5/100) + 18(49/400) + 202(66/1{,}000)} = 267 \quad [25]$$

Also, the directly standardized SePMRs would be computed as

$$SePMR_{High} = \frac{100(3/8) + 400(4/14) + 1{,}000(36/130)}{(5 + 49 + 66)} = 357 \quad [26]$$

$$SePMR_{Low} = \frac{100(1/4) + 400(3/18) + 1{,}000(38/202)}{(5 + 49 + 66)} = 233 \quad [27]$$

Although the absolute values of the proportional mortality measures differ from their rate-based counterparts, the pattern of both SPMRs and SePMRs again reveals the association between exposure and lung cancer mortality.

These results are summarized in Table 6, which shows that all of the standardized or pooled summary measures of effect reflect the true underlying pattern in age-specific lung cancer rates (i.e., larger in the high-exposure group). This pattern was obscured in the comparison of crude rates between groups 1 and 2 owing to confounding by age.

**TABLE 6.** *Proportional mortality summary measures*

| Summary measure | Study group 1 (high exposure) | Study group 2 (low exposure) |
|---|---|---|
| Crude rate (R) | 0.0086 | 0.0084 |
| SMR | 521 | 318 |
| SRR | 467 | 290 |
| $RR_{M\text{-}H}$ | 519 | 316 |
| ISR | 0.0448 | 0.0267 |
| DSR | 0.0056 | 0.0035 |
| SPMR | 402 | 267 |
| SePMR | 357 | 233 |

*Environmental and Occupational Medicine, Third Edition,* edited by William N. Rom.
Lippincott–Raven Publishers, Philadelphia © 1998.

# CHAPTER 6

# Occupational Biostatistics

Howard E. Rockette

The discipline of statistics is concerned with the description, summarization, and interpretation of data, as well as the development of procedures to accomplish these objectives. Statistical procedures are applicable to a wide variety of research areas. The branch of statistics described in this chapter, occupational biostatistics, is an important tool in the quantitative study of morbidity and mortality in humans, relative to exposure in the workplace. The application of statistical procedures requires an understanding of some fundamental concepts, which are reviewed in this chapter.

## RANDOM SAMPLE

A sample of size *n* selected from a larger population is random if each subgroup of size *n* within the population has equal probability of being selected. When a sample is not random, the occurrence of the characteristic being investigated may be related to the likelihood that an individual was selected for the sample. Therefore, it is necessary to assess bias and selection factors carefully before generalizing from the results of a study based on nonrandom samples.

## RANDOMIZATION

Many studies compare the response in an interest group to the response in a control group. Many statistical procedures require that each individual have equal chances of being in either group. In exposure studies using animal models, this is achieved by "random" assignment of animals to treatment groups. In the occupational environment, however, when we are attempting to relate exposure to response, randomization is seldom possible. The selection procedure may result in an uneven distribution of factors related to response among the exposed and nonexposed groups. An example of this is the phenomenon often referred to as the healthy worker effect (1,2). In a comparison of a mortality index of a working group and a general population group (such as the total male population of the United States), the observed overall mortality rate for the working population often is less than that for the control group. Such a result is hypothesized to be a result of selection into the work force; that is, a person must be reasonably healthy to work. Clearly, the extent of the selection depends on the particular job. The inability to randomize people to exposure categories, and the bias that results, make interpretation of many studies difficult.

## RELATIVE FREQUENCY DISTRIBUTION

The proportion of values that fall within a specified interval is the relative frequency of occurrence of values in that interval. The relative frequency distribution may be displayed graphically in the form of a histogram (Fig. 1). If the selected sample is large and the intervals are sufficiently small, the histogram approximates the relative frequency distribution of the population for the variable of interest. To a great extent the resulting type of distribution determines which statistical tests are applicable. Perhaps the most common distribution is the normal distribution or bell-shaped curve. The term *normal distribution* actually denotes a family of curves in which a specific member of the family is identified by two parameters, usually denoted by $\mu$ and $\sigma$.

H. E. Rockette: Department of Biostatistics, Graduate School of Public Health, University of Pittsburgh, Pittsburgh, Pennsylvania 15261.

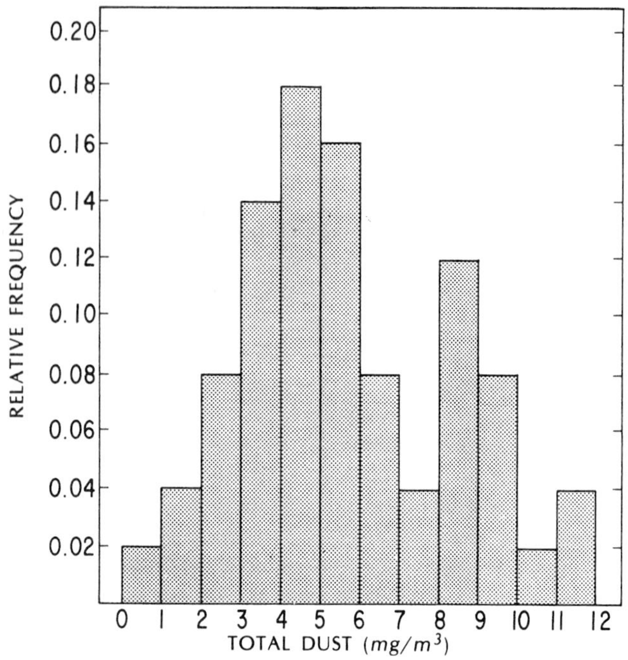


**FIG. 1.** Histogram of exposure to total particulates for a sample job category.

A second distribution common to occupational biostatistics is the *lognormal distribution.* In this distribution, we assume that the logarithm of the variable is normally distributed. For example, the lognormal distribution is frequently used to describe distributions of measurements of particulate air pollutants and particulate sizes.

## STATISTICS

Given a set of observations $x_1, x_2, \ldots, x_n$, it is possible to compute various summary statistics. A statistic serves two roles: it is a useful summary of the data, and, in cases where the data represent a random sample from a population, it is an estimate of a population parameter. Some commonly used statistics are defined in the following paragraphs.

### Arithmetic Mean

Usually denoted as $\bar{x}$, the arithmetic mean is a measure of the central tendency of the data. It is given by the formula

$$\bar{x} = \frac{x_1 + x_2 + \cdots + x_n}{n} \quad [1]$$

If the sample is randomly selected from a larger population, $\bar{x}$ estimates a population mean usually designated as $\mu$.

### Standard Deviation

Usually denoted as $s$, the standard deviation is a measure of the "spread" of the data about $\bar{x}$. It is given by the formula

$$s = \frac{\sqrt{\Sigma(x_i - \bar{x})^2}}{n - 1} \quad [2]$$

The square of the standard deviation, $s^2$, is the variance. If the sample is randomly selected from a larger population, $s$ and $s^2$ estimate the population parameters $\sigma$ and $\sigma^2$.

### Coefficient of Variation

Sometimes used to compare the variability of data with different means, the coefficient of variation is given by the formula

$$CV = (s/\bar{x}) \times 100 \quad [3]$$

### Standard Error

If several samples of a fixed size $n$ are selected and $\bar{x}$ is computed for each sample, a measure of the variability of the arithmetic mean among the samples can be obtained by computing the standard deviation of $\bar{x}$. This is sometimes called the standard error, or $s_{\bar{x}}$, to distinguish it from the standard deviation of $x$. It can be shown that the standard error can be computed by

$$s_{\bar{x}} = s/\sqrt{n} \quad [4]$$

where $s$ is the standard deviation of $x$.

### Geometric Mean

Although $\bar{x}$ is the most commonly used statistic to measure central tendency, there are alternatives. The appropriate choice depends on the type of population from which the sample is selected. For exposure data, the geometric mean is usually a more appropriate choice. The geometric mean can be computed using the formula:

$$\text{Geometric mean} = \sqrt[n]{x_1 \times x_2 \times \cdots \times x_n} \quad [5]$$

Use of this formula is equivalent to transforming the data by taking the logarithm of each observation, computing $\bar{x}$, and then taking the antilogarithm.

*Example 1.* Exposure to polycyclic aromatic hydrocarbon has been associated with an excess of respiratory cancer (3). Time-weighted averages (in milligrams per cubic meter) of benzene solubles were taken for a group of coke oven workers. The measurements are as follows: 0.1, 0.2, 0.05, 0.1, 0.4, 0.2, 0.05. Assuming the data are distributed lognormally, the geometric mean of 0.12 serves as a summary statistic to describe the average measurement.

## CONFIDENCE INTERVAL

In estimating a parameter on the basis of a sample statistic the amount of variability in the estimate can be conveyed by constructing a confidence interval. To construct a confidence interval, the formula $\bar{x} \pm ks/\sqrt{n}$ is used, where $k$ is determined by the specified level of confidence. This specified level of confidence, although arbitrary, is often set at 90% or 95%. For a 95% confidence interval, if the sample is taken from a normal distribution, then $k = 1.96$; 95% of the confidence intervals constructed in this way will contain the unknown parameter.

If the sample is not taken from a population with a normal distribution, then exact confidence intervals may be difficult to compute. One alternative often employed is an asymptotic confidence interval. This is an approximate confidence interval where the approximation improves for large samples. For a wide range of continuous distributions, the confidence intervals used for a normal distribution provide an asymptotic approximation. However, the discrepancy between this approximate interval and an exact confidence interval may be great for small samples.

*Example 2.* Blair and coworkers (4) summarize the mortality patterns of 26,561 workers employed in ten formaldehyde-producing or -using facilities. For white male workers considered to be exposed, they report 201 deaths from lung cancer. The mortality rates from the counties in which the plants were located show that the expected number of deaths is 182. The result of dividing the observed number of deaths by the expected number of deaths and multiplying by 100 is known as the standardized mortality ratio (SMR), in this case 111. Using the method described by Bailor and Ederer (5) to place a confidence interval on an SMR parameter, the 95% confidence interval is 96 to 127. The confidence interval thus provides an interval of values that is likely to contain the unknown parameter. In this case, the confidence interval contains the value of 100 (representing no excess mortality) and thus the observed excess of 111 could be due to chance variation.

## HYPOTHESIS TESTING

A common format used to integrate statistical procedures into a practical application is hypothesis testing. This format follows five steps: (a) specification of a null hypothesis, (b) specification of an alternative hypothesis, (c) selection of an appropriate test statistic, (d) computation of a $P$ value, and (e) rejection or failure to reject the null hypothesis.

### Specification of Hypothesis

The investigator states a hypothesis known as the null hypothesis ($H_0$). This hypothesis is usually stated in such a way that rejection of the hypothesis corresponds to a positive finding. Thus, if one is trying to relate exposure to a health response, the null hypothesis might be that the prevalence of a specified condition is the same for exposed and unexposed groups.

### Specification of an Alternative Hypothesis

The alternative hypothesis represents the statement that is accepted if the null hypothesis is rejected. Thus, if the null hypothesis is that the average exposure in two jobs is the same, the alternative hypothesis may be that the average exposures are different. Sometimes investigators are more specific in their alternative hypothesis. For example, one may specify that $H_1$: $\mu_1 > \mu_2$ (i.e., that a worker in job 1 receives an average exposure greater than the average exposure in job 2). This is called a "one-sided" alternative, as opposed to the alternative $H_1$: $\mu_1 \neq \mu_2$, which is "two-sided" (also known as "two-tailed"). Usually two-sided alternatives are used unless the biologic considerations dictate that only a one-sided alternative is tenable. Before examining the data, the investigator should have selected the form of the alternative hypothesis.

### Selection of an Appropriate Test Statistic

Once the null hypothesis is specified, the test statistic is selected. This statistic is not unique to a particular problem, and the selection of the most appropriate statistic requires some detailed knowledge of the available statistical procedures as well as the biologic aspects of the problem.

### Computation of the *P* Value

The $P$ value indicates the probability that the observed values could be the result of chance. For example, $P = 0.1$ means that if the null hypothesis is true, the result would be expected to occur by chance 10 times out of 100 samples. The computation of the $P$ value follows a general format. The statistic is computed, and then the probability is computed that a value this rare or rarer would be obtained if $H_0$ is true. Thus, a low $P$ value is interpreted as evidence that $H_0$ is false. If a two-sided alternative has been used, we must consider extreme values in either direction. Like the confidence intervals, the $P$ values reported in the literature are sometimes based on large sample approximations and may not be accurate if the sample size is small.

### Decision on Rejection of $H_0$

Note that two errors can be made when the test is actually conducted. A true $H_0$ might be rejected (type I or $\alpha$ error), or a false $H_0$ might be accepted (type II or $\beta$ error). Many times the sample size $n$ and the type I error will be specified, with little concern for type II error. For type I error, the $P$ value is typically set at 0.05 or 0.01 (this is an arbitrary but usual practice). Given the test statistic, the specified type I error, and the form of the alternative hypothesis, those values of the statistic that would lead to rejection can be ascertained. Such a specification requires a knowledge of the distribution of the statistic when $H_0$ is true. Tables of statistical distributions are used to determine those values of the statistic that lead to rejection of $H_0$.

If the $P$ value is less than or equal to the prespecified type I error, $H_0$ is rejected. Often in published studies an asterisk is used to indicate those values rejected at .05 or .01, although a more informative procedure would be to provide the $P$ value.

An alternative method of testing a hypothesis is to construct a 95% $(1 - \alpha)$ confidence interval on the unknown parameter. If the confidence interval does not contain the point specified in the null hypothesis the hypothesis is rejected at $\alpha = 0.05$. In Example 2 we would fail to reject the null hypothesis, $H_0$: SMR = 100, at $\alpha = 0.05$ because the 95% confidence interval includes the value 100. For many statistical procedures, testing hypotheses using confidence intervals produces similar results to those obtained using the formal hypothesis testing procedure outlined in this section.

## SELECTED STATISTICAL PROCEDURES

A common problem is to test the equality of population means given the sample means and variances. The $t$ test, which assumes a normal distribution and equality of population variances, is the most frequently used procedure. The formula used to compute $t$ is

$$t = (\bar{x}_1 - \bar{x}_2)/\sqrt{s^2(1/n_1 + 1/n_2)} \qquad [6]$$

where $s^2$ is a weighted average of the variances of the two samples and $\bar{x}_i$ and $n_i$ are the sample mean and sample size for the $i$th sample. Tables of the $t$ distribution must then be used to determine the $P$ value. If the two samples are paired (i.e., matched controls), the paired $t$ test is more appropriate. For the paired $t$ test, the formula is

$$t = \sqrt{n}\,\bar{x}_d/s_d \qquad [7]$$

where $n$ is the number of pairs, $\bar{x}_d$ is the average difference between pairs, and $s_d$ is the standard deviation of the differences between pairs. Tables of the $t$ distribution are then used to obtain a $P$ value.

The general problem of testing the equality of three or more population means can be resolved using analysis of variance (AOV). Like the $t$ test, which is a special case of this more general procedure, AOV assumes normal distributions and equality of population variances. Although the simplest form of AOV can be viewed as a generalization of the $t$ test, it is also a term used for a wide class of statistical procedures. For example, one may need to test equality of means while adjusting for a second factor that is considered to be a potential confounding variable. Specifically, exposure measurements might be compared for three different jobs where measurements were taken on both the day shift and night shift. Each measurement can be classified into one of the three job categories and one of the two shifts and a 3 × 2 (two factor AOV) could be used to test simultaneously for a difference in population means between shifts or among jobs. If the effect of two factors in a two-way AOV is greater or less than the sum of their individual components, then interaction is present. As long as there are repeated observations in the individual cells (i.e., job-shift categories) it is possible to perform a test for interaction. The concept of interaction is analogous to the epidemiologic concept of effect modification and includes the biologic concepts of synergism and antagonism. Additional AOV procedures include extension of the number of factors beyond two, incorporation of repeated measurements on the same individuals, and specialized designs to increase statistical efficiency. A discussion of the full range of analysis of variance procedures is beyond the scope of this chapter. However, the reader will find a wide diversity of techniques available on the standard statistical packages. These procedures all have the common objective of testing equality of population means for normally distributed data with a specified covariance structure.

Frequently we are interested in testing the hypothesis that the proportion of individuals with a specified characteristic or response is the same in two populations. The problem of testing equality of two proportions is often presented in the format of a 2 × 2 contingency table. The data are placed in a 2 × 2 table as follows:

| | Population I | Population II | |
|---|---|---|---|
| Response | A | B | A + B |
| No response | C | D | C + D |
| | A + C | B + D | |

The sample proportions $\hat{p}_1 = A/(A + C)$ and $\hat{p}_2 = B/(B + D)$ are sample estimates of the proportion of individuals with the specified characteristic in the two populations. The $\chi$-square statistic is used to test the hypothesis:

$$\chi^2 = \frac{(|AD - BC| - (^1\!/_2)N)^2 N}{(A + B)(C + D)(A + C)(B + D)} \qquad [8]$$

The term $(1/2)N$ is a correction for continuity that has been used as an adjustment because a continuous distribution (the $\chi$-square) is being used to approximate a discrete distribution. Simulation studies have shown that the correction tends to be conservative (i.e., rejects the null hypothesis less than the $\alpha$-error would indicate) and, therefore, some statisticians do not recommend its use. To determine the $P$ value for the test based on this statistic, the $\chi$-square distribution with one degree of freedom can be used if we have a reasonable-sized sample. Tables of the distribution are readily available. For small samples or data in which the observations in the two samples have been matched in pairs this test is inappropriate and alternative procedures are used (Fisher's exact test and McNemar's test, respectively).

If one has a 2 × 2 contingency table for each of the several strata and wishes to test across all the strata simultaneously for a difference in proportions in population 1 and population 2, the Mantel-Haenszel $\chi$-square statistic is useful. The test is appropriate if the expected differences in proportions are in the same direction for each of the strata. The Mantel-Haenszel statistic is frequently applied to test simultaneously whether two proportions are equal across various age, race, and sex strata.

Although the previously mentioned uses of the $\chi$-square statistic have been related to testing proportions, other tests utilize this statistical distribution. The $\chi$-square goodness of fit test determines whether an observed distribution closely fits a specified theoretical distribution. Tables of the $\chi$-square distribution are then used to determine a $P$ value. A low $P$ value indicates that the observed distribution is unlikely to have been generated from a population with the specified theoretical distribution.

When a pair of continuous measurements, $x$ and $y$, are obtained on the same individual, it is often useful to investigate the association between $x$ and $y$. If $x$ and $y$ are assumed to obey a bivariate normal distribution, then there are five unknown parameters (i.e., the mean and standard deviation of $x$, the mean and standard deviation of $y$, and the Pearson correlation coefficient $r$, which measures the association of $x$ and $y$). The correlation coefficient ranges between −1 and +1 where +1 indicates $y$ is perfectly related to $x$ by a straight line with positive slope. (−1 if the slope is negative.) If $x$ and $y$ are independent, then the correlation will be zero. A formula for the Pearson correlation coefficient is given by

$$r = (\Sigma(x_i - \overline{x})\ (y_i - \overline{y}))^{1/2}\ /\ s_x s_y \qquad [9]$$

*Example 3.* The average blood lead level of children of 22 workers at a storage battery plant with high risk of exposure to lead oxide were compared to the average blood levels of children in 22 neighborhood control families (6). The implied null hypothesis is that the average blood lead levels in the two populations are the same. The mean blood lead level of employees' children was 31.8 μg/100 ml and the corresponding value for the children of the neighborhood controls was 21.4 μg/100 ml. The computed $t$ value was 3.90 with a corresponding $P < 0.001$. Therefore, the null hypothesis is rejected and the average blood lead levels in the two groups of children are considered different.

*Example 4.* In an investigation of 30 workers exposed to silver nitrate and silver oxide, the complaint of change in ocular color was related to silver particles in the cornea (7). Seventeen of the 19 men who reported a change in eye color had silver particles in the cornea, compared to 4 of the 11 who did not indicate a change in eye color. The implied null hypothesis is that the same proportion of men who complained of a change in eye color and of those who did not would harbor silver particles in their corneas. A statement equivalent to the finding that the two proportions are equal is that complaints relative to a change in eye color are independent of silver particles in the cornea. Fisher's exact test yielded a two-sided $P$ value of 0.004. When the same type of analysis was done to relate change in skin color to silver particles in the conjunctiva, the $P$ value was 0.377. Note that if we would formally test the hypothesis at $\alpha = 0.05$, we would reject the assertion that change in eye color was independent of silver particles in the cornea. We would fail to reject the assertion that skin color was independent of silver particles in the conjunctiva.

*Example 5.* As part of a mortality study in the steel industry, men whose first job in 1953 was in the mason department were compared to other steel industry workers (8). On the assumption of no difference in mortality rates between the masons and the control group, an expected number of deaths was computed. The ratio of the observed and expected number of deaths for white masons was 1.97. A two-sided test of the hypothesis $H_0$: relative risk = 1.0, yields significance at $P < 0.05$. The Mantel-Haenszel $\chi$-square statistic was used, since the data had been analyzed across strata classified by age, calendar year, and plant.

## MULTIPLE COMPARISONS

We will discuss two more concepts related to hypothesis testing, since they are being utilized increasingly in occupational biostatistics. The first concept, related to type I error, we refer to as the multiple comparison problem.

Frequently, a study makes many comparisons each at a specified type I error and one or two tests are rejected. If 20 independent tests are run each at $\alpha = 0.05$, the probability of at least one rejection due to chance is 0.64. Multiple testing of hypotheses in studies may result in more statistically significant findings that are due to chance (sometimes referred to as false positives) than the reader often realizes. Many formal procedures have been developed to address the multiple comparison problem in specific circumstances, but, from a practical standpoint, an adequate solution does not exist to satisfy the needs of most occupational health studies. The investigator must be aware of the risk he runs in placing emphasis on one or two rejections from a large group of tests.

*Example 6.* Eaton and co-workers (9) investigated the prevalence of depression in 104 occupations. Using major depressive disorders as defined by the *Diagnostic and Statistical Manual of Mental Disorders* (DSM-III), third edition, and as measured by the National Institute of Mental Health's Diagnostic Interview Schedule, three occupations had prevalences with a statistically significant elevation when compared with the general employed population. Although the elevations might be related to occupation, given a two-sided $\alpha = 0.05$ test one would expect an average number of 2.6 statistically significant excesses by chance alone. Therefore, although each of the three individual results is significantly elevated, the observation of three statistically significant excesses out of 104 is consistent with the null hypothesis of no association of depressive disorders and occupation.

## STATISTICAL POWER

The second concept relates to type II (or $\beta$) error. The type II error depends on the sample size, the specified type I error, the form of the alternative hypothesis, and the true value in the alternative hypothesis. The probability that the null hypothesis is rejected for a particular value in the alternative is called the power of the test at this point. It is equal to $1 - \beta$. We refer to this concept because of increased awareness among researchers that the failure to reject a test may be due to an insufficient sample size and a corresponding statistical power too low to demonstrate a difference. That is, a negative study may be meaningless if the sample size is inadequate. Ideally, statistical power should be computed before a study is conducted, and it is considered a component of a well-designed study. Methods for determining the sample size required to achieve a given statistical power are well documented in the research literature (10–12).

*Example 7.* Hearne and coworkers (13) report the mortality patterns of a cohort of 1,013 workers exposed to methylene chloride. Hypothesized excesses for this exposure included lung and liver cancer and ischemic heart disease. None of these causes showed a statistically significant excess. To place their negative finding in perspective, the authors report the statistical power for each cause. They estimate 0.90 power of detecting a relative risk of 1.3 for ischemic heart disease, 0.90 power of detecting a 1.7 relative risk for lung cancer, and inadequate power of detecting excesses for liver cancer. Thus the study size was not large enough to adequately test for a liver cancer excess or a 50% lung cancer excess. It should be recognized that most studies have limitations with regard to statistical power. The computation of statistical power quantifies these limitations.

## NONPARAMETRIC PROCEDURES

In closing our discussion of hypothesis testing, it should be noted that many nonparametric test procedures are beginning to replace parametric ones. Parametric procedures such as those based on the normal distribution assume that the statistic is from a particular family of distributions and test whether the unknown parameters are equal to a specified value. Nonparametric procedures do not require that we specify the family of distributions. The test procedure is usually based on ranking the relative magnitude of the observations rather than using the actual measurement. For most of the standard parametric tests there is a corresponding nonparametric procedure that can be used if the form of the underlying distribution is unknown. The Wilcoxon and Wilcoxon matched pairs tests are the nonparametric counterparts of the *t*-test and paired *t*-test. The Kruskal-Wallis test is the nonparametric counterpart of one-way analysis of variance, the Friedman test is the nonparametric counterpart of two-way analysis of variance, and Spearman-rho is a nonparametric alternative to the Pearson correlation coefficient. Many textbooks on nonparametric statistics are available for investigators who feel that their data are not normally distributed and are not willing to make assumptions about the underlying distribution. Since many nonparametric procedures require extensive computations in order to obtain an exact *P* value, historically many applications have relied on approximate procedures. However, improvements in the speed of computers as well as the emergence of software packages that have exact nonparametric procedures have made nonparametric procedures more appealing.

*Example 8.* Stress is believed to cause alterations in the urinary excretion of catecholamines and corticosteroids. To evaluate stress in paramedics and firefighters, Dutton and colleagues (14) acquired 24-hour urine samples from subjects in these two occupations on both working and nonworking days. The primary hypothesis compares the average of the selected urine measurements on a working day to those obtained on a nonworking day. Since each individual provided a sample on both a working and nonworking day, the paired *t*-test could be used to test the null hypothesis. However, the Wilcoxon matched paired test could be used without making the more stringent assumptions of the parametric test. In this case, the investigators applied both tests and found that they reach the same conclusion.

## MODEL

The term *model* is imprecise, but we use it here to refer to those statistical procedures that require a more complex set of mathematical assumptions before the test can be applied. We discuss four different types of models: (a) the simple linear model, (b) multivariate linear models, (c) multiplicative models, and (d) biologic models. The simple linear model assumes a linear relationship of the expected value of a dependent variable $y$ to an independent variable $x$. Since $E(y) = \alpha + \beta x$, the test of the hypothesis $H_0$: $\beta = 0$ could be viewed as a test of whether knowing the value of $x$ contributes information on $E(y)$.

Multivariate linear models assume that the expected value of the dependent variable $y$, is a linear function of a combination of independent variables $x_i$, $i = 1, \ldots, n$. This relationship is described by the equation

$$E(y) = \beta_0 + \beta_1 x_1 + \beta_2 x_2 + \cdots + \beta_n x_n \quad [10]$$

Although not a requirement of the method, it is often assumed that the variable $y$ is normally distributed with a common variance $\sigma^2$, for each possible combination of $x_i$ variables. One advantage of the multivariate model is that it permits characterization of the relationship of a variable $y$ to an independent variable $x_1$, while controlling for a set of other variables $x_2, \ldots, x_n$. Furthermore, interaction terms can be incorporated in the model by defining new variables that are products of the individual variables. Thus, $x_3 = x_1 x_2$ would provide the necessary model to incorporate an interaction term for the variables $x_1$ and $x_2$. The interaction term permits an assessment of whether or not the effect of $x_1$ depends on the value of $x_2$. An important hypothesis when modeling data is the test of whether a particular coefficient is equal to zero. If $\beta_i$ is significantly different from zero, then $x_i$ is significantly associated with the variable $y$. More recently multivariate regression models are being used with distributional assumptions other than normality. In Poisson regression one usually assumes that the log of the expected value of $y$ is given by a linear combination of variables and that probabilities of events can be given by a Poisson distribution. The Poisson distribution is the distribution that characterizes rare events and in the case of occupational biostatistics is often used to indicate the occurrence of death in an occupational cohort.

Multiplicative models are particularly useful for investigating the risk of exposure in occupational studies. If the response variable $y$ is categorical (i.e., dead or alive), then logistic regression can be used to investigate the effect of a set of independent variables on the occurrence of an event. The logistic model assumes that

$$\ln(p/(1-p)) = \beta_0 + \beta_1 x_1 + \cdots + \beta_n x_n \quad [11]$$

The parameter $p$ is the probability that the event of interest occurs, and the quantity $p/(1-p)$ is called the odds ratio. Like multivariate linear regression, logistic regression may be used to investigate the relationship of an outcome to $x_1$ while adjusting for other variables or to include interaction terms. A particularly simple form of the model would define the variable $x_1 = 1$ if the subject is exposed and $x_1 = 0$ if unexposed. Then the test of $\beta_1 = 0$ would determine if outcome is related to exposure, and $e^{\beta_1}$ would be an estimate of the relative odds of an event in the exposed and unexposed groups. Logistic regression models also provide a more general framework in which to analyze contingency tables and so are a useful tool in the analysis of case-control studies, a popular study design in occupational epidemiology.

The continuous counterpart to logistic regression is the proportional hazards model. Instead of using the logarithm of the odds ratio as the dependent variable, the logarithm of the ratio of the hazard functions is used. The hazard function is related to the conditional probability that an event will occur and in an occupational study could represent either a mortality rate or incidence rate. The proportional hazards model assumes that

$$\ln(\lambda_i(t)/\lambda_0(t)) = \beta_1 x_{1i} + \beta_2 x_{2i} + \cdots + \beta_n x_{ni} \quad [12]$$

In this model the ratio of the hazard of the $i$th individual to the baseline hazard rate at any point in time is assumed to be a linear combination of $n$ specified independent variables. The proportional hazards model was the approach used in an analysis of workers at Hanford Works (Richland, WA) to measure low-level radiation (15,16).

We have assumed in our discussion of regression models that the independent variables $x_1, x_2, \ldots, x_n$ are specified in advance and will all be used in the equation characterizing the dependent variable. Because there may be a large number of independent variables it is sometimes useful to select a subset of these variables that contain most of the information regarding the dependent variable. There are several differing model selection approaches including step-up, step-down, and stepwise procedures. Step-up procedures start with the independent variable most highly correlated with the dependent variable and stop when the addition of more variables does not contribute significantly to prediction of the dependent variable.

Step-down procedures start with all independent variables and eliminate ones not contributing significantly to the dependent variable, and stepwise procedures allow variables to both enter and leave the equation during the model building process. These procedures can all be applied to multiple linear regression, logistic regression, and the proportional hazards model. It should be recognized that the model building procedures for different statistical packages may not result in the same set of variables in the final model. The resultant model provides a subset of dependent variables that will explain the variation in the dependent model reasonably well when compared to the result obtained if all variables had been used, but the model is not unique. Thus, these model building techniques serve as a data reduction procedure. Furthermore, it may be difficult to draw biologic conclusions from the final model. A variable may be highly correlated with the dependent variable but excluded from the final model because it is highly correlated to other independent variables already in the model and as a result it does not contribute significant additional information.

Several models that make assumptions about biologic mechanisms have been used in carcinogenic risk assessment. The multistage model (17,18) and its modifications are based on the assumption that a cell becomes malignant only after going through $k$ transitions. As the model has developed, the transition rates between successive stages are not required to be equal, and at least one of the stages is assumed to be linearly related to dose. This model is often criticized for not having a biologic basis, since it has not been demonstrated experimentally that there are more than two transition stages of cancer cells. The two-stage model proposed by Moolgavkar and Knudson (19) is considered to have more biologic basis. It is formulated in terms of cell division, and statistically as a birth–death process. This model views carcinogenesis as the end result of an irreversible two-stage process. It assumes that malignant tumors arise from a single malignant progenitor cell and that malignant transformation of susceptible stem cells is independent of the transformation of other stem cells. The model incorporates mutation rates that summarize the likelihood that during cell division a normal cell will result in an intermediate cell, and a second mutation rate that expresses the likelihood that an intermediate cell will result in a malignant cell during division. A nonmathematical review of various biologic models is given by Chu (20), and Siemiatycki and Thomas (21) provide some examples of how the underlying biologic model is related to the statistical concept of interaction.

Statistical models provide a useful framework in which to test statistical hypotheses, adjust for potential confounders, increase statistical power, and investigate biologic mechanisms. However, analysis based on models can be quite sensitive to deviations from assumptions, and there is a danger of inappropriate use if they are applied casually.

*Example 9.* Foo and co-workers (22) investigated the relationship of postshift toluene levels in blood to the ambient exposure concentrations. Paired samples of toluene were taken from 50 workers and plotted on a graph. The investigators observed a linear relationship of toluene levels in the blood ($y$) and toluene levels in air ($x$). The estimate of the relationship is $y = 0.086 + 0.0130x$, where $y$ is measured in micrograms per milliliter and $x$ is measured in parts per million.

*Example 10.* Claude and associates (23) use a logistic regression model to investigate the effect of lifestyle and occupational risk factors on lower urinary tract cancer. Use of multiple logistic regression enabled them to control for known risk factors. For example, they found a relative risk of 2.6 ($P < 0.05$) for persons who daily drink more than four cups of coffee, after adjustment for cigarette smoking and occupational exposure. The adjustment for cigarette smoking and occupational exposure was accomplished by including these terms in the logistic regression model.

*Example 11.* Marsh and associates (24) apply a proportional hazards model to a cohort of fiberglass, rock wool, and slag wool workers to investigate the effect of exposure on respiratory cancer and nonmalignant respiratory disease. Cumulative respirable fiber (fibers/cc-months) exposure was divided into four categories and a risk ratio of each of the three higher exposure groups was estimated compared to the lowest exposure group. Unadjusted risk ratios for the three higher exposed groups for lung cancer were 0.72, 0.94, and 0.83. The model also was fit including year of hire, plant, and coexposures in order to adjust for potential confounders. After investigating other indices of exposure in a similar manner, the investigators conclude that there is no consistent evidence of an association of cumulative respirable fiber exposure and lung cancer.

*Example 12.* Radecki (25) used multiple stepwise regression to determine a subset of variables associated with prolongation of median and ulnar nerve latency at the wrist. The study population consisted of 1,472 patients with hand or forearm symptoms who were referred for electrodiagnostic evaluation. Factors considered included age, height, weight, body mass index, dominant and average wrist ratios, smoking, alcohol consumption, number of years worked, high-risk occupation, and hand-intensive hobbies. The dependent variable was the difference of the median palmar latency and the ulnar palmar latency. Stepwise regression analysis was done separately for males and females in order to identify a subgroup of variables related to the median minus ulnar/palmar latency. For males the final model included body mass index and wrist ratio, while for females the final model included body mass index, wrist ratio, and age. This does not imply that other independent variables were not related to outcome but that the variable was not important in the model once the variables in the selected model were already included.

## STATISTICAL PACKAGES

The increasing availability of microcomputers and improvements in the development of user-friendly software has increased the range of statistical procedures being applied to many research areas, including occupational and environmental research. Although the relative advantage of one statistical package over another may depend on the specific problem being solved as well as the background and individual preference of the user, there has been considerable progress in making a wide range of statistical procedures available to individuals with a minimal amount of computer and/or statistical skills. The Statistical Package for Social Sciences (SPSS) (26), Statistical Applications Software (SAS) (27), and MINITAB (28) all offer most of the statistical procedures needed for problems encountered in occupational and environmental research. All three packages have a version for Windows. In addition, there are packages that are more specialized and serve to address specific needs that are also very useful. StatXact (29) gives exact procedures for commonly used nonparametric procedures. EGRET (30) is a convenient modeling package that includes logistic regression, Poisson regression, and the proportional hazards model. OCMAP (31) is a package designed to compute standardized mortality ratios for specified subgroups of a cohort; provide age, race, sex, and calendar specific standardized rates for the United States, as well as individual states and counties; and tabulate summary statistics useful when applying the proportional hazards model to occupational cohort data.

## META-ANALYSIS

A common problem of interpreting the research literature is how to synthesize results from different studies of a related hypothesis. These studies may differ in their design, analysis, and conclusions. A wide range of research areas have addressed this problem by applying a body of procedures that are referred to as meta-analysis.

Although there is some disagreement as to what should constitute a meta-analysis, the approach almost always entails a quantitative summary of results across studies investigating a common research question. Its early applications were in the areas of social science, education, and psychology, but it is now frequently employed to combine results across randomized clinical trials evaluating different modes of therapy. More recently, attempts have been made to synthesize results across studies in the area of occupational and environmental epidemiology. These include the evaluation of the effects of passive smoking (32), the relationship of asbestos exposure and gastrointestinal cancer (33), and an evaluation of work-site smoking cessation programs (34).

Advantages of meta-analysis include the potential for greater precision in estimates of risk, a better chance than in the usual reviews of literature of including all relevant studies, and a better indication of the consistency of findings across various studies. The major disadvantages of meta-analysis in occupational epidemiology include the difficulty of combining studies that may differ in design (i.e., case-control versus cohort study), different methods of adjusting for potentially confounding variables, and the likelihood of a wide range of exposure documentation among studies. Meta-analysis is likely to provide a useful tool for synthesizing information from studies in occupational and environmental epidemiology as long as the limitations of the approach are clearly recognized.

*Example 13.* The National Research Council conducted a meta-analysis of lung cancer risk from passive smoking (32). In an analysis based on ten case-control studies and three cohort studies, they estimate that the average risk for a nonsmoking female of a smoking spouse is 1.34, with a corresponding 95% confidence interval of 1.18–1.53.

## APPROPRIATENESS OF STATISTICAL PROCEDURES

The number and diversity of statistical procedures that are used to analyze data in a discipline such as occupational health make it unrealistic to cover all the approaches encountered in the literature. Therefore, the material presented here should be supplemented with reading from standard statistical and epidemiologic texts (see Further Reading). Nevertheless, even with limited statistical knowledge one might pose certain general questions to evaluate whether there has been proper integration of the statistical procedures into the biologic problem:

1. Have the investigators given attention to the assumptions necessary to apply their statistical test?
2. Have the investigators given proper attention to the probability of incorrectly failing to reject the null hypothesis (statistical power)?
3. Have the investigators tested a large number of hypotheses and given undue attention to one or two borderline rejections? The *P* value does not provide accurate information on a chance rejection from a large group of comparisons.
4. If a random sample was not taken and the authors have generalized to a larger population, is such a generalization justified? If they are comparing two nonrandom samples, have they given proper attention to possible selection biases of differences in the two groups in variables related to response?
5. Does the result make sense biologically? Statistical significance does not always result in biologic significance. Are there factors other than those being posed by the investigators that could account for the difference in the summary statistics?

## REFERENCES


1. Fox AJ, Collier PF. Low mortality in industrial cohort studies due to selection for work and survival in the industry. *Br J Prev Soc Med* 1976;30:225–230.
2. Vinni K, Hakama M. Healthy worker effect in the total Finnish population. *Br J Industr Med* 1980;37:180–184.
3. IARC Monographs on the evaluation of the carcinogenic risk of chemicals to humans. Polynuclear aromatic compounds, part 3, industrial exposures in aluminum production, coal gasification, coke production, and iron and steel foundry. Lyon, France: IARC, 1984;34:1–299.
4. Blair A, Stewart P, O'Berg M, et al. Mortality among industrial workers exposed to formaldehyde. *J Natl Cancer Inst* 1986;76:1071–1084.
5. Bailor JC III, Ederer F. Significance factors for the ratio of Poisson variable to its expectation. *Biometrics* 1964;20:639–643.
6. Watson WN, Linden WE, Giguere GC. Increased lead absorption in children of workers in a lead storage battery plant. *J Occup Med* 1978;20:759–761.
7. Rosenman KD, Moss A, Kon, S. Argyria: clinical implications of exposure to silver nitrate and silver oxide. *J Occup Med* 1979;21:430–435.
8. Rockette HE, Redmond CK. Long-term mortality study of steelworkers: X. Mortality patterns among masons. *J Occup Med* 1976;18: 541–545.
9. Eaton WW, Anthony JC, Mandel W, et al. Occupations and the prevalence of major depressive disorder. *J Occup Med* 1990;32:1079–1087.
10. Armstrong B. A simple estimator of minimum detectable relative risk,

sample size or power in cohort studies. *Am J Epidemiol* 1987;126: 356–358.
11. Gordon I. Sample size estimation in occupational mortality studies with the confidence interval theory. *Am J Epidemiol* 1987;125: 158–162.
12. Walter SD. Determination of significant relative risks and optimal sampling procedures in prospective and retrospective comparative studies of various sizes. *Am J Epidemiol* 1977;105:387–397.
13. Hearne TF, Pifer JW, Grose F. Absence of adverse mortality effects in workers exposed to methylene chloride: an update. *J Occup Med* 1990; 32:234–240.
14. Dutton LM, Smolensky MH, Leach CS, et al. Stress levels of ambulance paramedics and firefighters. *J Occup Med* 1978;20:111–115.
15. Mancuso TF, Steward A, Kneale G. Radiation exposures of Hanford workers dying from cancer and other causes. *Health Phys* 1977;33: 369–385.
16. Gilbert ES. The assessment of risks from occupational exposure to ionizing radiation: energy and health. Proceedings of a SIMS conference, Alta, Utah. June 2, 1978;6–30.
17. Armitage P. Multistage models of carcinogenesis. *Environ Health Perspect* 1985;63:195–201.
18. Whittemore A and Keller JB. Quantitative theories of carcinogenesis. *SIAM Rvw* 1978;20(1):1–30.
19. Moolgavkar SH, Knudson AG. Mutation and cancer: a model for human carcinogenesis. *J Natl Cancer Inst* 1981;66:1037–1051.
20. Chu KC. Biomathematical models for cancer: A nonmathematical view of mathematical models for cancer. *J Chron Dis* 1987;40: 1635–1705.
21. Siemiatycki J, Thomas DC. Biological models and statistical interactions: an example from multistage carcinogenesis. *Int J Epidemiol* 1981;10:383–387.
22. Foo SC, Phoon WO, Khoo NY. Toluene in blood after exposure to toluene. *Am Ind Hyg Assoc J* 1988;49:255–258.
23. Claude J, Kunze E, Frentzel-Beyme R, et al. Lifestyle and occupational risk factors in cancer of the lower urinary tract. *Am J Epidemiol* 1986;124:578–589.
24. Marsh G, Stone R, Youk A, et al. Mortality among United States rock wool and slag wool workers: 1989 update. *J Occup Environ Med Aust NZ* 1996;12:297–312.
25. Radecki P. Variability in the median and ulnar nerve latencies: implications for diagnosis entrapment. *J Occup Environ Med* 1995;37: 1293–1299.
26. Noruisis MJ. *SPSS for Windows:* base system user's guide, release 6.0. Chicago, IL: SPSS, 1993.
27. *SAS/STAT user's guide,* version 6. Cary, NC: SAS Institute, 1989.
28. *MINITAB user's guide:* release 11 for Windows. State College: Minitab, 1996.
29. Mehta C, Patel N. StatXact 3 for windows user manual: statistical software for exact nonparametric inference. Cambridge: Cytel, 1995.
30. Mauritsen RH. *EGRET reference manual.* Seattle: Statistics and Epidemiology Research, 1993.
31. Marsh GM, Ehland J, Paik M, Preininger M, Coplin R. OCMAP/PC: a user-oriented occupational cohort mortality analysis program for the IBM PC. *Am Stat* 1986;40:308–309.
32. *Environmental tobacco smoke:* measuring exposures and assessing health effects. Washington, DC: National Academy Press, 1986.
33. Frumkin H, Berlin J. Asbestos exposure and gastrointestinal malignancy review and meta analysis. *Am J Ind Med* 1988;14:79–95.
34. Fisher KJ, Glasgow RE, Terborg JR. Work site smoking cessation: a meta analysis of long-term quit rates from controlled studies. *J Occup Med* 1990;32:429–439.

## FURTHER READING

Brown BW, Hollander M. *Statistics, a biomedical introduction.* New York: Wiley, 1977.

Checkoway H, Pearce NE, Crawford-Brown DJ. *Research methods in occupational epidemiology.* Oxford: Oxford University Press, 1989.

Colton T. *Statistics in medicine.* Boston: Little, Brown, 1974.

Hosmer DW, Lemeshaw S. *Applied logistic regression.* New York: Wiley, 1989.

Hunter JE, Schmidt FL, Jackson GB. *Meta analysis:* cumulating research findings across studies. Beverly Hills: Sage, 1982;4.

Kahn HA, Sempos CT. *Statistical methods in epidemiology.* Oxford: Oxford University Press, 1989.

Kleinbaum DG. *Logistic regression:* a self-learning text. New York: Springer, 1992.

Light RJ, Pillemer DB. *Reviewing research:* the science of summing up. Cambridge: Harvard University Press, 1985.

Monson RR. *Occupational epidemiology,* 2nd ed. Boca Raton, FL: CRC, 1990.

Schlesselman JJ. *Case-control studies:* design, conduct and analysis. Oxford: Oxford University Press, 1982.

*Environmental and Occupational Medicine, Third Edition,* edited by William N. Rom.
Lippincott–Raven Publishers, Philadelphia © 1998.

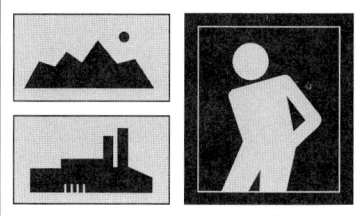

CHAPTER 7

# Impairment, Disability, and Functional Capacity

Alan L. Engelberg and Leonard N. Matheson

The evaluation of permanent impairment and disability, and functional capacity, for the purposes of establishing employability and levels of compensation is an extremely critical function of societies in all industrialized countries. Each year, billions of dollars are paid out because the livelihood of millions of people is altered significantly by injuries and illnesses that affect their ability to carry out economically meaningful activities. Despite the importance of this social function, and despite its basis in the usually sudden alteration of a worker's health status, it is rare to find physicians who have been trained to use their skills in a manner that is helpful to both ill and injured patients and to the administrators or adjudicators who must make the decisions about employability and compensation.

This chapter discusses (1) the distinction between permanent impairment and permanent disability; (2) the distinction between the evaluation and rating of impairment; (3) the role and responsibilities of physicians in the permanent impairment and disability evaluation processes, especially in reporting results of examinations; and (4) the scientific basis for evaluating functional capacity, and how functional capacity relates to one's ability to perform work.

## DISTINCTION BETWEEN PERMANENT IMPAIRMENT AND PERMANENT DISABILITY

Many authors and expert panels have devised definitions of impairment and disability (1–3). The clearest definitions are set forth in the fourth edition of the American Medical Association's *Guides to the Evaluation of Permanent Impairment* (4) (Table 1). The *Guides* define *impairment* as an alteration in health status, which is evaluated by medical means. *Disability* has a broader focus, including not only impairment but how that impairment affects a person's ability to meet demands of life and, in a legal sense, the context in which the impairment is being viewed. For example, for a worker who types frequently at a word processor, complete loss of the use of the fifth finger of the left hand could, in an evaluation for permanent impairment by a physician, be given a rating of, say, 5% of the whole person. But would that constitute permanent disability? First, one would have to ask, Disabled from doing what? If it is from pursuing all aspects of one's occupation, clearly it is not a permanent disability. The mental faculties that allow a person to produce words and concepts on the word processor are intact, and after a few weeks, or perhaps months, one could adapt to make more use of the fourth finger for typing. If, however, one were a concert violinist, then the 5% rating of permanent impairment might well translate into total inability to perform the functions of that livelihood, as it would be impossible for a concert violinist to master the instrument with the use of only four fingers of the left hand. However, even if the violinist were 100% permanently unable to perform the functions of the job, does that mean in a legal context that he or she is disabled? Table 2 shows what standards the violinist's impairment would have to meet for her to be considered disabled in certain legal contexts (5).

It is clear from this example that, since impairment is not a measure of one's ability to perform specific tasks required in a given occupation, there must be something else about a person's health status upon which a measure

A. L. Engelberg: Department of Community and Family Medicine, St. Louis University School of Medicine, St. Louis, Missouri 63104.
L. N. Matheson: Work Performance Laboratory, Department of Occupational Therapy, Washington University School of Medicine, St. Louis, Missouri 63108.

**TABLE 1.** *Definitions of impairment and disability*

| |
|---|
| *Impairment* is the loss of, the loss of use of, or derangement of any body part, system or function. |
| *Permanent impairment* is impairment that has become static or well stabilized with or without medical treatment and is not likely to remit despite medical treatment. |
| *Evaluation of impairment* is acquisition and analysis of information, including clinical evaluation, that is carried out according to the AMA *Guides*. |
| *Rating of impairment* consists of analyzing data accumulated in the course of an impairment evaluation and comparing those data with AMA *Guides* criteria to estimate the extent of the impairment. |
| *Impairment reporting* is explaining the information acquired in the course of evaluating, analyzing, and estimating the extent of an impairment. |
| *Disability* is a decrease in, or the loss or absence of, the capacity of an individual to meet personal, social, or occupational demands, or to meet statutory or regulatory requirements. |
| *Permanent disability* occurs when the degree of capacity becomes static or well stabilized and is not likely to increase despite continuing use of medical or rehabilitative measures. Disability may be caused by medical or by nonmedical factors. |

From ref. 4, pp. 315–317.

of impairment is based. The AMA's *Guides* (4) bases its measures of impairment on activities of daily living (ADL), the life tasks required for self-care and maintenance that all persons learn by the time they reach adulthood, which are taken for granted and do not require special training (Table 3).

Often it is not clear to evaluators of impairment, or to the readers of their reports, how these daily activities are translated into the impairment ratings that are found in books like the AMA's *Guides*. As an illustration, people prefer to position the head so that the eyes easily look straight ahead or slightly down, in order to visualize the space in which the hands work and into which the body steps. Thus a person whose cervical spine is ankylosed in full flexion or full extension would have a considerably greater impairment (40% of the whole person) than a person whose cervical spine is ankylosed in partial flexion or partial extension. A person whose cervical spine is ankylosed in a fully rotated position would have an even greater impairment (50% of the whole person) than one who has ankylosis at full flexion or extension.

## IMPAIRMENT EVALUATION VERSUS IMPAIRMENT RATING

Evaluation and rating of impairment are not synonymous. Unfortunately, because a rating is a single number that purports to reflect a precise measure of a person's health status, evaluators may have a tendency to gear their examinations only toward deriving a rating, and users of evaluation reports may have a tendency merely to use the final number to arrive at a disability rating. In some workers' compensation jurisdictions this is mandated by law. This is an unfortunate consequence of a numerical rating system for impairment. For example, if a statistician reports only a summary statistic, such as a mean, and fails to describe the method by which the mean was obtained (such as sampling strategy or the distribution about the mean), then much useful information is lost.

The most valuable and overlooked part of the AMA's *Guides* is the set of steps for writing an evaluation report (Table 4). The first two steps and their substeps are the most crucial. The first step shows that an evaluation can-

**TABLE 2.** *Legal standards of disability*

| Legal context | Definition |
|---|---|
| Private disability insurance (i.e., contractual) | Disabled for the substantial and material duties of the own occupation (the violinist would have to have purchased a private policy) |
| Workers' compensation | Disability caused by, aggravated by, or arose out of employment (the medical condition must be work related) |
| Family and Medical Leave Act | Disability makes the individual unable to work (i.e., for the sake of taking time off from work) |
| Social Security Disability Insurance | Disabled from substantial gainful employment (i.e., very severely impaired; for example, the violinist could not find a job in the U.S. economy) |
| Americans with Disabilities Act | Worker has an impairment, a history of an impairment, or is regarded as having an impairment that substantially limits major life activities (e.g., inability to engage in broad classes of jobs) |

**TABLE 3.** *Activities of daily living*

| Activity | Example |
|---|---|
| Self-care, personal hygiene | Bathing, grooming, dressing, eating, eliminating |
| Communication | Hearing, speaking, reading, writing, using a keyboard |
| Physical activity | *Intrinsic:* Standing, sitting, reclining, walking, stooping, squatting, kneeling, reaching, bending, twisting, leaning<br>*Functional:* Carrying, lifting, pushing, pulling, climbing, exercising |
| Sensory function | Hearing, seeing, tactile feeling, tasting, smelling |
| Hand functions | Grasping, holding, pinching, percussive movements, sensory discrimination |
| Travel | Riding, driving, traveling by airplane, train, or car |
| Sexual function | Participating in desired sexual activity |
| Sleep | Having restful sleep pattern |
| Social and recreational activities | Participating in individual or group activities, sports, hobbies |

From ref. 4, p. 317.

**TABLE 4.** *Elements of an impairment evaluation report*

Step 1: Medical evaluation

- Medical evaluation includes a narrative history of the medical condition(s) with specific reference to onset and course of the condition, symptoms, findings on previous examination(s), treatments, and responses to treatment, including adverse effects. Information that may be relevant to onset, such as an occupational exposure, should be included.
- Medical evaluation also includes results of the most recent clinical evaluation, including any of the following:
  - Physical examination
  - Laboratory tests
  - Electrocardiogram
  - Radiographic studies
  - Rehabilitation evaluation
  - Character traits mental status examination, including testing of intellectual functioning and
  - Evaluation of other tests or diagnostic procedures
- Current clinical status is assessed, and a statement of plans for future treatment, rehabilitation, and reevaluation is included.
- Diagnoses and clinical impressions are reported.
- The expected date of full or partial recovery is estimated.

Step 2: Analysis of findings

- An explanation of the impact of the medical condition(s) on life activities should be given. The types of activities affected should be listed.
- The medical basis for concluding that the condition and the patient's symptoms have or have not become stable should be explained.
- An explanation should be given of the medical basis for concluding that the individual is or is not likely to suffer sudden, subtle, or other incapacitation as a result of a change in the condition.
- An explanation should be given of the medical basis for concluding that the individual is or is not likely to suffer injury, harm, or further impairment by engaging in activities of daily living or other activities necessary to meet personal, social, and occupational demands.
- Any conclusions that restrictions or accommodations are or are not warranted with respect to daily activities that are required to meet personal, social, and occupational demands should be explained. If restrictions because of risks to the patient or others, or accommodations, are necessary, an explanation of their expected outcome and value should be provided.

Step 3: Comparison of the results of analysis with the impairment criteria

- A description should be given of specific clinical findings related to each impairment, with reference to how the findings relate to and compare with the criteria in the applicable chapter of the AMA *Guides*; references should be made to the absence of, or the examiner's inability to obtain, pertinent data.
- An explanation of each impairment value with reference to the applicable criteria of the AMA *Guides* should be included.
- A summary list of impairment estimates in percent should be included.

From ref. 4.

not be done in a vacuum; the history of the impairing condition, with specific reference to findings on previous examinations, treatments, and responses to treatment, especially if documented in hospital and medical office records, is essential, not only for the evaluator's own understanding of the impairing conditions but also for his or her clear reporting to an administrator or adjudicator. This is especially important when an evaluator's assessment at one point in time differs markedly from what one expected to find given the history of the illness or injury and its treatment to that point.

The second step relies on the definitions of impairment (specifically permanent impairment) and disability and the medical and nonmedical contexts in which the report will be used. Only after carefully collecting information and an analyzing it thoroughly can the evaluator relate the information to a specific set of ratings (step 3). An administrator or adjudicator faced with two widely disparate ratings, one of which is substantiated by complete information and thorough analysis and one of which is not, will rely more heavily on the former report.

## THE SCIENCE OF IMPAIRMENT EVALUATION

A major difficulty of nearly all portions of the AMA's *Guides,* as well as with any other present or past system of evaluating permanent impairment, is the scientific substantiation of the ratings that are given to the clinical parameters that are measured. The human organ system for which the impairment evaluation scheme is most scientifically sound is the respiratory system. The lung responds to endogenous and exogenous insults in only a few ways, and its functions of gas movement and exchange are amenable to a quantifiable physiologic understanding, as measured most easily by spirometry and by the diffusing capacity of carbon monoxide, even in settings outside of hospital-based pulmonary function laboratories (6,7). Thus, for the last 30 years at least, there has never been a question that researchers could test for simple pulmonary functions in populations large enough to develop statistically based normal measurements according to age, sex, and height (8).

Furthermore, the questionnaire on respiratory symptoms that was developed initially by the British Medical Research Council in the 1950s to study the prevalence and causes of chronic bronchitis in Great Britain is an excellent instrument that tests the subjective side of respiratory disease (9). The questionnaire has been validated and modified for use in many countries, including the United States. It provides a standardized format for assessing the symptoms of pulmonary disease, such as cough, wheezing, and dyspnea, and correlating them with results of pulmonary function testing.

The evaluation for impairment of the other organ systems has not been the focus of as much scientific research as the respiratory system. Many of the ratings are not grounded in sound epidemiologic studies of large population groups that would provide normative data to support those ratings. For example, the first edition of the AMA's *Guides* gave impairment ratings for large classes of mental conditions, neuroses, personality disorders, sociopathic personality, psychoses, and organic brain syndrome. A typical statement about rating comes from the section on personality disorders (10): "Evaluation of impairment due to personality disorders is to be made on the basis of lifelong ability of the patient to adapt to the stresses of daily living and could range from zero to 15%. Permanent impairment would rarely exceed 5% on a longitudinal basis."

The *Diagnostic and Statistical Manual,* third edition (11) (DSM-III), eliminated many of these broad categories from the psychiatric lexicon. The DSM-IIIR and DSM-IV continued this approach. In 1984 the American Psychiatric Association assisted the AMA in completely revising the protocols for evaluating mental and behavioral disorders by using "observable" mental status criteria, including intelligence, thinking, perception, judgment, affect, and behavior, plus the ability to handle ADLs and the potential for rehabilitation (12). The AMA altered the criteria for evaluating mental and behavioral impairment in its third and fourth editions of the *Guides* (4), this time following the guidelines of the Social Security Administration (13), which evaluate four very broad parameters: ability to conduct ADL; ability to function socially; ability to concentrate on, persist at, and pace oneself at tasks; and ability to adapt to stress. The AMA (4) also stated, "There is no precise measurement of impairment in mental disorders" (p. 301). Such radical changes among the editions resulted from the lack of a clear scientific basis for any of the schemes that were devised.

Another example of the difficulty in providing scientific substantiation for techniques of impairment evaluation is found in the most recent edition of the AMA's *Guides.* The fourth edition provides two methods of assessing impairment of the spine: the injury, or diagnosis-related estimates (DRE) model, and the range of motion (ROM) model. The former is entirely new, and is based on an ad hoc committee of authorities knowledgeable about the musculoskeletal system, orthopedic surgery, neurosurgery, internal medicine, rehabilitation, impairment evaluation, and medical science. The DRE model is recommended for certain medical conditions of the spine, and the ROM model is recommended for all other medical conditions affecting the spine. That the AMA put forth two models for the clinical evaluation of spine impairment is an indication that the science of such evaluation is progressing, but not to the point that the past tried-and-true method can be abandoned. However, in preparing the users of the *Guides* for the new method while keeping the old method, the AMA provides only one new citation from the scientific literature, and that one pertains to the ROM model (14).

## EXAMPLES OF IMPAIRMENT EVALUATIONS

The following two examples (kindly provided by William R. Shaw, M.D., Denver, Colorado) show how an impairment evaluation scheme such as the AMA's *Guides* is used:

### Case Study 1

Patient B.D., a 37-year-old commercial sprinkler fitter, was seen for an evaluation of impairment resulting from work injuries. While the patient was installing a sprinkler system, he was on a scissors lift about 12 to 14 feet off the ground when the lift toppled, sending him to the concrete floor below. He landed on his right knee and forearm, collapsing forward onto his face. He was hospitalized for 7 weeks with a severely comminuted fracture of the distal femur involving the intracondylar notch, plus a Le Fort II facial fracture. The femoral fracture was treated with traction for approximately 7 weeks, with a fiberglass spica cast for another month, and finally a brace for another month. He was enrolled during the latter period in physical therapy and worked out conscientiously on his own as well as with Nautilus machines. His facial fractures were treated with extensive surgical intervention, including open reduction and internal fixation of facial fractures; exploration of the right orbital floor, with implant reconstruction as well as open reduction and internal fixation of the inferior orbital rim; application of maxillary and mandibular arch bars, and intramaxillary fixation; suspension of the superior orbital rims bilaterally; and bilateral Caldwell-Luc drainage, nasal antral windows, and closed reduction of nasal fractures. The patient had as a residual almost total reduction of the right nasal passage and numbness over the right cheek and upper gum. His jaw popped somewhat, but eating, chewing, and talking were reasonably normal. He had some residual difficulties with speech phonation as a result of the numbness of his lips. He had noted only mild changes in appearance, with a sunken right cheek. Initially he had diplopia, but he felt that this had resolved. Findings at a previous ophthalmologic examination were normal.

The patient's right leg continued to give him moderate discomfort, which was proportionate to activity, particularly climbing stairs and squatting, and which interfered minimally with daily living, causing only occasional inconvenience. He noted no significant effusion of the knee, nor any buckling of the knee for about a year after the injury.

Medical history, social history, and family history were noncontributory. The patient has worked as a sprinkler fitter for the past 16 years. He returned to work just over 6 months after his injury and has worked steadily ever since. Initially, after returning to work he had some difficulty stooping, crawling, and kneeling. He eventually worked without significant disability.

#### *Findings on the Impairment Examination*

Physical examination showed a well-nourished, muscular male in no apparent distress. His head had a mild depression over the right zygomatic arch and inferior orbital rims. The pupils were level on light reflex. No vertical phorias were demonstrated. Corneal reflexes were intact, as were the movements of the extraocular muscles. There was almost complete obstruction of the right nasal passage, with a significantly deviated septum. The neck, chest, heart, and abdomen were entirely normal.

The upper extremities and left lower extremity were normal. Range of motion (ROM) of the right hip and ankle were normal. The right knee showed evidence of placement of surgical traction pins. There was minimal tenderness over the knee, with no effusion. ROM of the right knee was from 3 degrees short of full extension to 133 degrees flexion. ROM of the left knee was from 2 degrees hyperextension to 153 degrees flexion. There was a mild but distinct instability on varus stress of the right knee, although the cruciate ligaments appeared intact. There was a noticeable right pelvic tilt, the right leg measuring between 3/4 and 1/2 inch shorter than the left. There was no atrophy of either lower extremity. The quadriceps were extremely well developed bilaterally.

The neurologic examination was normal except for decreased sensation over the second division of the trigeminal nerve on the right. Corneal reflexes were intact. Radiographs from the time of the injury showed a severely comminuted fracture of the distal femur involving the intracondylar notch, with a fracture of the inferior pole of the patella as well. Follow-up films show exceptionally good alignment following traction and casting; the latest films demonstrated some hypertrophic changes, particularly in the distal femur.

#### *Diagnosis*

The patient suffered severely comminuted facial and distal femur fractures as a result of a fall. He has had unusually good results from treatment, and he has been unusually conscientious in pursuing his own program in addition to monitored physical exercise and reconditioning. His right leg was shortened, and he had minimal residual abnormalities from the facial fractures, including cosmetic changes, minimal speech changes, loss of sensation over the trigeminal distribution, and air passage disruption on the right.

### Case Study 2

Patient R. L. is a 54-year-old male heavy equipment operator with injuries to the right hand and persistent headaches.

While stringing high-tension lines, the patient got caught in an 8-foot-diameter wire reel weighing 17,000 pounds, which turning in its frame trapped his right ankle and pulled his right arm between the reel and the frame. In the process his body was forcibly flexed, so that his right shoulder was pulled to approximately the level of his ankle. The evaluation in the emergency room showed fractures of the right second metacarpal and a sprained ankle. The hand was splinted with the third finger in extreme flexion. Since that time the patient has had persistent symptoms of both headache and hand problems. The headaches were constant and nonpulsatile. No aura or scotoma was present. The headaches gradually built over the day and affected him on a regular, daily basis. He had generally resorted to taking six to eight pills per day of a Canadian over-the-counter medication, each of which contained 8 mg codeine. He developed partial contracture of the hand, which has since resolved, with the exception of a minor contracture at the distal interphalangeal (DIP) joint of the middle finger. He continued to experience loss of sensation in the index finger as well as poor coordination of and manipulation with the right hand. He also experienced mild localized tenderness over the fracture site.

The patient underwent extensive physical therapy, and a variety of medications were prescribed for the headaches. Examinations by many physicians, including neurologists and orthopedists, showed no identifiable lesions of the central nervous system to which the headaches could be attributed.

Before being injured the patient worked with the most sophisticated equipment available, stringing three large wires at a rate of 1,000 feet per minute. With diminished hand coordination he was only able to string a single small wire at a rate of only 500 feet per minute. Demand for his specialized services fell, and his income suffered.

### *Findings at the Impairment Evaluation*

Positive findings were limited to the right upper extremity, which was the patient's dominant extremity. ROMs of the proximal interphalangeal (PIP) and DIP joints of the index finger were normal; flexion of the metacarpophalangeal (MCP) joint of the index finger was limited to 57 degrees; and there was ankylosis of the DIP joint of the middle finger at 20 degrees.

There was a fracture deformity with mild tenderness over the middle of the second metacarpal. There was moderately decreased sensation throughout the right index finger. Radiographs of the right hand showed a healed fracture of the midshaft of the second metacarpal and mild degenerative changes of the wrist. Magnetic resonance imaging of the head was unrevealing.

### *Diagnosis*

Diagnoses included chronic postconcussion headaches and fracture of the second metacarpal of the dominant hand, with residual decreased ROM at the MCP joint, diminished sensation of the index finger, and ankylosis of the DIP of the middle finger.

These case examples show clearly that impairment and disability differ. The patient in case 1 suffered injury to a number of areas of his body. He was working on the job and sustained permanent impairment, so his injuries were deemed compensable by the workers' compensation system. Yet, after 6 months he returned to his job, which he was able to perform without undue difficulty. Thus, he was not disabled to the point that he could not perform his job of many years. The patient in case 2 sustained an injury principally to one part of his body and suffered permanent impairments that were rated at a lower number than the first worker's. He, too, was covered by worker's compensation, but in addition his injury severely limited his ability to perform the tasks of his very specialized job.

## FUNCTIONAL CAPACITY

Functional capacity evaluation (FCE) is a systematic method of measuring a patient's ability to perform meaningful tasks on a safe and dependable basis.

The term *functional* connotes performance of a purposeful, meaningful, or useful task that has a beginning and an end with a result that can be measured. The effect of the patient's impairment on his or her ability to perform meaningful tasks is the focus of functional capacity evaluation (15,16). As such, functional performance is important to measure because it relates to the effect of impairment on disability. Evaluation of disability is based on the measurement of the functional consequences of impairment in tasks that are pertinent to the particular role under consideration (17). Thus, to evaluate the presence or degree of occupational disability, the focus must be on tasks in the worker's role and work environment (18). If the functional consequences are significant and occur in tasks that are critical to the performance of the job, the patient can be described as having an occupational disability (16). The extent and type of occupational disability is dependent on the patient's ability to perform these work-relevant tasks.

The term *capacity* connotes the maximum ability of the patient, beyond the level of tolerance that is measured. Capacity is the patient's immediate potential. The use of this term is somewhat misleading because capacity rarely is measured in a performance task unless the patient is highly trained to perform that particular task.

The term *evaluation* describes a systematic approach to monitoring and reporting performance that requires the evaluator to observe, measure, and interpret the patient's performance in a structured task (19,20). FCE should be distinguished from *functional assessment.* Although the terms sometimes are used interchangeably and some functional assessment instruments are used in FCE, they describe different processes. Generally, FCE is based on performance measurement, while functional assessment is based on expert ratings from observation or on the patient's self-report (21–25).

If the functional consequences of an impairment are sufficiently severe to result in limitation of the patient's ability to work, measurement of the loss of ability in key functional areas of work can be used as an estimate of disability (26,27). Information about the patient's impairment[1] is obtained through a medical examination while information concerning performance in terms of the key functional areas is obtained through an FCE.

The focus of the FCE is on one or more specific components of functional capacity. This occurs as a consequence of selection of those work tasks that are likely to present the greatest challenge to the patient within the context of the presenting impairment.

## OVERVIEW OF MEASUREMENT

Measurement is the basic task performed by the evaluator in a functional capacity evaluation (28–32). The information that is gathered in the FCE is descriptive and, when standards of performance are available, normative (33). Descriptive results are used to compare the patient's current ability with the patient's ability at a previous point in time or with the demands of work. Normative results are used to compare the patient to a reference population. Measurement is dependent on the scale that is used. Functional capacity evaluation uses a wide variety of instruments with various scale attributes. An understanding of these attributes and the limits that they impose on the interpretation and use of the information derived in a FCE is important. The four scales are described in the following sections.

### Nominal

Numbers represent category labels and are used for classification. Examples include diagnostic codes, gender and race classifications, and Waddell's abnormal illness behavior signs (34,35). Nominal data allow the user to distinguish difference between or among members of separately classified groups. No value-based mathematical comparisons are permitted.

### Ordinal

Numbers indicate the rank order of measures. The distance between the ranks is unknown and assumed to vary across the span of the scale. Examples from FCE include scores from activity and depression questionnaires, and scores on functional status questionnaires[2] or manual muscle test ratings. Ordinal data allow the user to distinguish difference from lesser to greater magnitude along one scale. Ordinal data do not allow the magnitude of the difference to be measured with any degree of precision or unambiguous meaning. For example, identical scores in the mid-range on a comprehensive activity questionnaire may be due to an entirely different set of responses from different people. This is a serious limitation in FCE because many of the popular behavior rating scales are ordinal (36). Instruments such as the McGill Pain Questionnaire (37), Dallas Pain Questionnaire (38), and Oswestry Pain Questionnaire (23) are ordinal measures that do not allow scores to be compared or mathematically manipulated with unambiguous meaning.

### Interval

Numbers indicate the rank order of measures with equal intervals between adjacent items at any segment of the scale. However, the interval scale lacks a meaningful zero point. Examples from FCE include scores from quantitated pain questionnaires, visual analog pain scales, and sensory tests. Value-based mathematical comparisons are permitted along the scale but not between scales. Interval data allow the user to distinguish difference from lesser to greater magnitude along one scale and to quantify the difference between scores with precision. Interval data do not allow quantified comparisons between different measures.

### Ratio

Numbers indicate the rank order of measures with equal intervals between adjacent items at any segment of the scale and a zero point that indicates absence of the variable that is being measured. Value-based mathematical comparisons are permitted along the scale and between scales. In FCE, variables such as weight and force are examples of ratio scales. Ratio data allow the user to distinguish difference from lesser to greater magnitude along one scale and to quantify the difference between scales with precision at any point on the scale. Thus, proportional comparisons can be made. In addition, proportional changes across more than one scale can be compared.

The scale of measurement is important because interpretation of performance is restricted by the nature of the scale (39,40). For example, if a scale refers to a patient's

[1]An important assumption for disability rating is that the functional limitations will be a consequence of the impairment. This weak link assumption requires substantial judgment on the part of the physician, assisted by information collected during the evaluation. Without confirmation of the weak link, attribution of measured functional limitations to a particular impairment is difficult to achieve.

[2]Some functional status instruments that are in an ordinal scale can be transformed into an interval scale through the use of Rasch analysis (25). This involves an analysis of the instrument's underlying probability structure of responses in order to develop standardized scores that can be interpreted as scores on an interval scale of measurement. An example is the functional independence measure (20).

strength as "fair-plus" (an ordinal measure), comparison of the patient to others is limited to indicating that he/she is more or less than another patient, without quantifying the magnitude of difference. Generally speaking, the higher the scale of measurement, the more useful it will be (33). For the example of strength, a poor-fair-good rating scale can be used to compare the patient to him- or herself over time as the rehabilitation program progresses. It would be more useful to measure strength using a ratio scale (such as force) because this allows a numerical comparison of the patient over time in addition to comparison of the patient to other people and to the demands of numerous jobs. Because the magnitude of difference is so important in FCE, measures that are based on interval or ratio scales are preferred. If ordinal measures are used, it is preferred that results be converted to standard scores or percentiles and reported as such.

## MODES OF MEASUREMENT

There are several modes of measurement in FCE, each pertinent to a particular type of task. Examples are time-limited and task-limited measurement, each of which is concerned with the patient's speed of performance. In the former mode, the patient is allowed a set period of time to perform a task with the degree of task completion or number of tasks completed as possible performance measures. In the latter mode, the patient is allowed to complete a set task. The time required to complete the task is the performance measure.

A thorough review of the various modes of measurement is beyond the scope of this chapter. Instead, a focus on measurement of strength performance with regard to lifting tasks will be presented. This is useful because these modes of measurement are similar in many ways to other measures of abilities based on strength. Additionally, lifting as a physical ability is arguably the most important physical demand characteristic of work (41–49).

There are three general classes of strength testing in the evaluation of lift capacity, each differentiated in terms of the effect of the test on muscular contraction, considered in terms of both the muscles' force of contraction and the rate of shortening.

### Isometric

Under load, the muscle length is not changed. Force is measured in one biomechanical position. Isometric activity is not as prevalent in daily tasks as muscular contractions to perform tasks that require movement, although the prevalence of isometric tasks is greater for the hand than for any other biomechanical component.

### Isokinetic

Under load, the muscle shortens or (if shortened due to prior concentric contraction) lengthens at a fixed rate as a consequence of external control of the velocity of movement of the biomechanical unit. Force is measured throughout the range of movement.

### Isoinertial

The muscle shortens at a variable rate in response to a constant external resistance. As the biomechanical geometry changes to accomplish movement, changes in muscle length occur at varying velocities. Constant resistance is inferred from the constancy of the mass that is moved because acceleration is assumed to be negligible.

Various technologies have been developed to assess these three general classes of strength tests. The technologies are identified by name in terms of the type of function that each intends to assess. It is important to point out that this leads to confusion in that, due to the complexity of the biomechanical system involved in many tasks, the external system that is used to test the biomechanical system may not be able to sufficiently control the test at the level of the muscle's function so that the intended mode of test is actually achieved. For example, while isokinetic testing intends to evaluate the strength of the biomechanical system at a set velocity, accelerative movement occurs early in the task up to the point at which the desired velocity is achieved. Even after that point, there may be a rebound phenomenon before stabilization at the desired velocity is achieved.

Isometric testing is easiest to achieve in that it ostensibly involves no movement other than the elasticity in the biomechanical units. However, because there are several biomechanical links in the chain that is required if the lifting task is performed while standing, substantial elasticity is present. This elasticity can be controlled through proper instructions and the use of equipment that is sensitive to this phenomenon.

Isoinertial testing is difficult to achieve because lifting and lowering are performed in an environment in which gravity (an accelerative force) controls resistance. Thus, although acceleration is somewhat standardized through control of the vertical range of the task to focus on one biomechanical segment, inertia is not well controlled from person to person because rates of acceleration vary between people. Within the same person across gradually increasing demand levels, acceleration appears to gradually vary inversely to the increasing load.

## LEGAL FRAMEWORK OF FUNCTIONAL CAPACITY EVALUATION

Functional capacity evaluation takes place within the context of professional guidelines as well as numerous state and federal laws. Guidelines for performance testing have been developed and published by the American Psychological Association (50), American Physical Therapy Association (51), and the American Academy of Physical Medicine and Rehabilitation (52). Federal guidelines for testing on which an employment decision is based are found in the Uniform Guidelines for Employee Selection (53). When the testing procedure involves employment of a qualified individual with a disability, the *Americans with Disabilities Act of 1990* (54) is pertinent. Additional standards specific to testing of disabled people have been published (55). There is agreement among the various professional and governmental entities that are concerned with performance testing that selection of a test must be undertaken within the hierarchical context of five standards: safety, reliability, validity, practicality, and utility.

### Safety

Given the known characteristics of the patient, when used properly the test should not be expected to lead to injury. Some functional strength tests have the potential to cause harm to the patient. Well-designed tests provide exclusionary and performance guidelines and procedural rules that must be followed to minimize this likelihood. Safety is a function of the match between the performance demands placed on the patient and the patient's ability to limit performance appropriately (55). Determination of the patient's maximum safe and dependable performance level is a professional judgment made by the evaluator based on the patient's performance during the evaluation. This judgment takes into account the signs, symptoms, and behaviors that indicate that the evaluation has progressed to a point at which the safety of the evaluation cannot be maintained with a reasonable degree of certainty. Thus, the professional evaluator's training and experience to utilize the test's maximum performance indicators is a necessary condition for functional testing.

### Reliability

The test equipment and test protocol should produce a result that is stable within the test trial, and across evaluators, patients, and the date or time of test administration. Reliability can be threatened both externally and internally. External threats are those over which the evaluator has control, such as equipment reliability, protocol reliability, and consistency of protocol application. Internal threats are within the patient and include motivation, fear, and pain avoidance behavior. A functional capacity evaluation requires that the patient put forth maximum voluntary effort in a meaningful task (18,56). The defined task may require full strength, full velocity, endurance, a target number of repetitions, a maximum rate of responding, or some other full effort performance. Characteristics that distinguish performance testing of impaired patients from those who are not impaired are factors such as activity-related pain, fear of reinjury, test anxiety, and the cost-benefit ratio of task performance. While the effect of these factors is difficult to measure with precision, most clinicians agree that they are of significant importance. The functional capacity evaluation must be structured so that it is sensitive to these factors and minimizes their effects.

Intratest reliability (a measure of the patient's consistency of responding) can be assessed through various mathematical means (16,57), using the coefficient of variation statistic as a measure of the consistency of the patient's performance on a repeated-trials task. The coefficient of variation is the population standard deviation, divided by the mean of the scores, expressed as a percentage. Although the specificity of the coefficient of variation statistic appears to be much higher than its sensitivity for the detection of submaximal effort (58), it is widely used and is built in to many FCE test instruments. A more sophisticated indicator of reliability is based on intertest comparisons. In this approach, two or more tests that use a ratio scale of measurement and are biomechanically related are administered, using a protocol that is sensitive to intratest consistency. This approach is especially powerful if the intratest results have demonstrated high consistency (16). Reliability in functional testing has been sparsely studied (59). With a few exceptions, test protocols in which reliability has been scientifically determined have not been agreed upon. In many other instances, tradition has sufficed for scientific rigor. In one example, Caldwell et al. (60) provided guidelines for isometric testing that have been widely referenced and are used as the basis for many strength test protocols. These guidelines were developed for isometric testing of healthy subjects in a laboratory. They were originally presented and have been adopted without any indication that the effect of factors such as the types of instructions were scientifically studied. For example, these guidelines recommend that the evaluator should avoid exhortation of the subject during testing. The avoidance of exhortation is widely practiced with these guidelines cited as the original reference. However, Matheson et al. (61) found that reliability on both an intratest basis and a test-retest (interrater) basis was not dependably achieved without an exhortative instruction set in isokinetic testing of back strength. Also with regard to isokinetic testing, Newton and her colleagues (62) report that test reliability is dependent on factors that currently are not common in clinical practice, such as the opportunity to provide a practice session prior to the test session conducted on a subsequent day.

### Validity

The interpretation of the test score should predict or reflect the patient's performance in a target task. Whereas reliability has to do with the dependability of the measure, validity has to do with the adequacy of the measure (63) to describe or predict performance. A valid measure of functional capacity that can be used with impaired patients must do the following:

1. Allow the clinician to gauge treatment effect by comparing an initial baseline level of performance with performance at the conclusion of the treatment;
2. Make recommendations for return to work by comparing the patient's functional capacity to his or her job demands; and
3. Provide an estimate of disability for rating purposes by comparing the patient's performance to expected values.

The first two purposes are straightforward. The third is problematic because a reference to expected values is not readily available. In certain circumstances, reasonable assumptions can be made about the patient's preimpairment functional capacity. For example, if the patient is a member of an occupational group for which minimum lift capacity standards are known, it can be assumed that the patient has at least the minimum that is required by the standard. This is a rational approach and frequently is used in medicolegal cases. Another standard that is more easily implemented utilizes a normative database. Unfortunately, normative data for functional capacity tests that have been designed for use with impaired patients are rare.

Although there is a long history of validity testing of performance measures to predict productivity in fields such as industrial psychology (64,65), studies of the validity of functional tests to predict injury or disability are rare and often produce conflicting interpretations (66).

### Practicality

The cost of the test should be reasonable. Cost is a function of the capital expenditure for the equipment amortized over the life of the equipment plus wage costs and overhead. Although low-tech approaches to FCE are less expensive initially, if a more expensive high-tech system is able to provide similar results in less time or with lower-wage staff, some of the additional expense for the latter approach may be offset.

### Utility

The usefulness of the procedure is the degree to which it meets the needs of the patient, referrer, and payer. The first four factors in the hierarchy must be adequately addressed for utility to be achieved. Without utility, the test is of no value and will not be supported by the users of the test information.

## BASIC REQUIREMENTS FOR TEST SELECTION

Beyond the legal framework for functional capacity evaluation, the evaluator must use tests that are optimal, given the patient and the evaluation circumstance. There is no single most appropriate test for any one patient or for any one evaluation circumstance. Tests must be selected to meet the unique needs of the patient-role interface that is described above. In addition to these general guidelines, adherence to the following specific guidelines will insure an optimal balance of safety, reliability, and validity:

1. Use only standardized test protocols that have *all* of these characteristics:
   a. Equipment has been demonstrated to be reliable with the level of maintenance that normally will be available;
   b. Test protocol has been demonstrated to be reliable over time on an intrarater basis and interrater basis;
   c. One or more means of intratest confirmation of consistency is available;
   d. One or more means of intertest confirmation of consistency is available; and
   e. Normative data or job demand data are available.
2. Become trained in the use of the test protocols and formally demonstrate skill in the consistent application of the test protocols.
3. Select protocols from those identified in guideline 1 (above) that meet the validity needs and practicality restrictions of the assessment process. Consider each test protocol on a patient basis in response to demands of the target role. These demands should be derived from job analysis data. If these are not available, the *Dictionary of Occupational Titles* can be used, although this information is quite general.
4. After collecting the necessary pretest screening information about the patient to rule out contraindications for testing, administer the test in the standard manner.
5. Evaluate the quality of the data on this basis:
   a. Screen for intratest variability. If more variability exists than is reported to be normal for the protocol, retest;
   b. Screen for intertest variability. If more variability exists than is reported to be normal for the protocol, retest.
6. Interpret the data and report information in terms of the purpose of the functional capacity evaluation.

This approach to FCE will minimize problems with safety, reliability, and validity, thus improving utility. In the field of health care, given the potential for problems in these areas that can harm the patient, practicality must be subordinate to these factors, and should be included only with thoughtful administrative control.

One example of a standardized functional capacity evaluation that was designed to address all of the basic requirements described above is the California Functional Capacity Protocol (Cal-FCP) (67). The Cal-FCP is a 120-minute, 11-part test of functional capacity designed to develop an estimate of lost work capacity to be used in a case management process to address disability rating.

### Case Example

John Smith is a 39-year-old theatrical stage carpenter who suffered a lumbar strain-sprain injury without radiating symptoms on the job. He was excused from work and placed on light self-structured stretching and exercise program for 2 weeks by his physician. Pain was persistent and related to activity. He returned to work on a limited-duty basis after 2 weeks and continued on conservative office-based treatment. However, after 2 additional weeks of treatment, he continued to be symptomatic and requested an orthopedic consultation. Prior to authorizing the consultation, the insurance claims manager requested a Cal-FCP test battery. Test results demonstrated a 39% loss of lift capacity and an attendant 25% loss of work capacity. Additional difficulties were found with Mr. Smith's perception of his functional limitations in that he perceived himself to be much more functionally limited than expected. After reviewing the results, his physician requested 3 weeks of work conditioning in physical therapy, which the claims manager authorized. A follow-up Cal-FCP at the conclusion of the work conditioning program demonstrated lift capacity that was 31% in excess of same-age males based on normative data, with perceived physical capacity consistent with his job duties. Mr. Smith was released to return to full duty work and did so successfully. He did not receive a disability rating.

## REFERENCES

1. Social Security Administration. *Disability evaluations under Social Security.* SSA Publication 05-10089. Washington, DC: USGPO, 1986.
2. American Thoracic Society Ad Hoc Committee on Impairment/disability Criteria. Evaluation of impairment/disability secondary to respiratory disorders. *Am Rev Respir Dis* 1986;134:1205–1209.
3. Kessler HH. *Disability, determination and evaluation.* Philadelphia: Lea & Febiger; 1970;25.
4. American Medical Association. *Guides to the Evaluation of Permanent Impairment,* 4th ed. Chicago: AMA, 1994.
5. Demeter SL, Smith GM, Andersson GBJ. Approach to disability evaluation. In: Demeter SL, Smith GM, Andersson GBJ, eds. *Disability evaluation.* Chicago: American Medical Association, 1996;3.
6. American Thoracic Society Committee on Proficiency Standards for Pulmonary Function Laboratories. Standardization of spirometry—1994 update. *Am J Respir Crit Care Med* 1995;152(3):1107–1136.
7. American Thoracic Society DCO Standardization Conference Single-breath carbon monoxide-diffusing capacity (transfer factor): recommendations for a standard technique. *Am J Respir Crit Care Med* 1995;152(6 part 1):2185–2198.
8. American Thoracic Society: Lung function testing: selection of reference values and interpretive strategies. *Am Rev Respir Dis* 1991;144: 1202–1218.
9. Samet JM. A historical and epidemiologic perspective on respiratory symptoms questionnaires. *Am J Epidemiol* 1978;108:435–446.
10. American Medical Association Committee on the Rating of Mental and Physical Impairments. *Guides to the evaluation of permanent impairment.* Chicago: American Medical Association, 1971;151.
11. American Psychiatric Association. *Diagnostic and statistical manual of mental disorders* (DSM-III), 3rd edition. Washington, DC: APA, 1980.
12. AMA Council on Scientific Affairs. *Guides to the evaluation of permanent impairment,* 2nd ed. Chicago: American Medical Association, 1984;220.
13. Social Security Administration Federal old-age, survivors and disability insurance: listing of impairments. Mental disorders; final rule. (20 CFR 404). *Federal Register* 1985;50:35038–35070.
14. Waddell G. Somerville D, Henderson I, Newton M. Objective clinical evaluation of physical impairment in chronic low back pain. *Spine* 1992;17:617–628.
15. American Occupational Therapy Association. *Uniform terminology for occupational therapy,* 3rd ed. Rockville, MD: American Occupational Therapy Association, 1994.
16. Matheson LN. *Work capacity evaluation for occupational therapists.* Canyon, CA: Rehabilitation Institute of Southern California, 1982.
17. National Advisory Board on Medical Rehabilitation Research. *Report and plan for medical rehabilitation research.* Bethesda, MD: National Institutes of Health, 1992.
18. Velozo CA. Work evaluations: critique of the state of the of the art of functional assessment of work. *Am J Occup Ther* 1993;47(3):203–209.
19. Hart DL. Test and measurements in returning injured workers to work. In: Isernhagen SJ, ed. *Work injury management:* the comprehensive spectrum. Rockville, MD: Aspen, 1994.
20. Isernhagen SJ. Functional capacity evaluation and work hardening perspectives. In: Mayer TG, Mooney JV, Gatchel R, eds. *Contemporary conservative care for painful spinal disorders.* Philadelphia: Lea & Febiger, 1991;328–345.
21. Deyo RA, Centor RM. Assessing the responsiveness of functional scales to clinical change: an analogy to diagnostic test performance. *J Chron Dis* 1986;39(11):891–906.
22. Dodds TA, Martin DP, Stolov WC, Deyo RA. A validation of the functional independence measure and its performance among rehabilitation inpatients. *Arch Phys Med Rehabil* 1993;74:531–536.
23. Fairbank JC, Cooper J, Davies JB, O'Brien JP. The Oswestry low back pain disability questionnaire. *Physiotherapy* 1980;66(8):271–273.
24. Granger CV, Wright BD. Looking ahead to the use of the functional status questionnaire in ambulatory physiatric and primary care: the functional assessment screening questionnaire. In: Granger CV, Gresham GE, eds. *Physical medicine and rehabilitation clinics of North America:* new developments in functional assessment. Philadelphia: WB Saunders, 1993, 104–175.
25. Matheson L, Matheson M, Grant J. Development of a measure of perceived functional ability. *J Occup Rehab* 1993;3(1):15–30.
26. Kirkpatrick JE. Evaluation of grip loss. *Calif Med* 1956;85(5):314–320.
27. Luck JV Jr, Florence DW. A brief history and comparative analysis of disability systems and impairment rating guides. *Orthop Clin North Am* 1988;19(4):839–844.
28. Messick S. The standard problem: meaning and values in measurement and evaluation. *Am Psychol* 1975;30:955–966.
29. Mitchell J. Measurement scales and statistics: a clash of paradigms. *Psychol Bull* 1986;100(3):398–407.
30. Ottenbacher KJ, Tomchek SD. Measurement in rehabilitation research: consistency versus consensus. In: Granger CV, Gresham GE, eds. *Physical medicine and rehabilitation clinics of North America:* new developments in functional assessment. Philadelphia: WB Saunders, 1993, 214–227.
31. Rothstein JM, ed. *Measurement in physical therapy.* New York: Churchill Livingstone, 1985.
32. Wright BD, Linacre JM, Heineman AW. Measuring functional status in rehabilitation. In: Granger CV, Gresham GE, eds. *Physical medicine and rehabilitation clinics of North America:* new developments in functional assessment. Philadelphia: WB Saunders, 1993, 1–22.
33. Portney LG, Watkins MP, eds. *Foundations of clinical research:* applications to practice. Norwalk, CT: Appleton and Lange, 1993.

34. Chan CW. The pain drawing and Waddell's nonorganic physical signs in chronic low-back pain. *Spine* 1993;18(13):1717–1722.
35. Waddell G, Bircher M, Finlayson D, Main CJ. Symptoms and signs: physical disease or illness behavior? *Br Med J* 1984;289:739–741.
36. Fisher WP Jr. Objectivity in measurement: a philosophical history of Rasch's separability theorem. In: Wilson M, ed. *Objective measurement:* theory into practice. Norwood, NJ: Ablex, 1992:29–55.
37. Melzack R. The McGill Pain Questionnaire: major properties and scoring methods. *Pain* 1975;1:277–299.
38. Lawlis GF, Cuencus R, Selby D, McCoy GE. The development of the Dalias pain questionnaire: an assessment of the impact of spinal pain on behavior. *Spine* 1989;14(5):511–515.
39. Angoff WH. *Scales, norms, and equivalent scores.* Princeton, NJ: Educational Testing Service, 1984.
40. Wright BD, Linacre JM, Heineman AW. Measuring functional status in rehabilitation. In: Granger CV, Gresham GE, eds. *Physical medicine and rehabilitation clinics of North America:* new developments in functional assessment. Philadelphia: WB Saunders, 1993, 1–22.
41. Alpert J. The reliability and validity of two new tests of maximum lifting capacity. *J Occup Rehabil* 1991;1(1):13–29.
42. Ayoub MA. Control of manual lifting hazards. I. Training in safe handling. *J Occup Med* 1982;24(8):573–577.
43. Chaffin DB, Andersson GBJ. *Occupational biomechanics.* New York: Wiley, 1984.
44. Garg A, Ayoub MM. What criteria exist for determining how much load can be lifted safely? *Hum Factors* 1980;22(4):475–486.
45. Mital A. Psychophysical capacity of industrial workers for lifting symmetrical and asymmetrical loads symmetrically and asymmetrically for 8-hour work shifts. *Ergonomics* 1992;35(7/8):745–754.
46. Mundt DJ, Kelsey JL, Golden AL. An epidemiologic study of non-occupational lifting as a risk factor for herniated lumbar intervertebral disc. *Spine* 1993;18(5):595–602.
47. National Institute for Occupational Safety and Health. *Work practices guide for manual lifting* [Technical Report 81-122]. Cincinnati, OH: Division of Biomedical and Behavioral Science, NIOSH, 1981.
48. Snook SH, Irvine CH. Maximum acceptable weight of lift. *Am Ind Hyg Assoc J* 1967;28:322–329.
49. Waters TR, Putz-Anderson V. Gaig A, Fine LJ. Revised NIOSH equation for the design and evaluation of manual lifting tasks. *Ergonomics* 1993;36(7):749–776.
50. American Educational Research Association, American Psychological Association, National Council on Measurement in Education. *Standards for educational and psychological testing.* Washington, DC: American Psychological Association, 1986.
51. Task Force on Standards for Measurement in Physical Therapy. Standards for tests and measurements in physical therapy practice. *Phys Ther* 1991;71:589–622.
52. Johnston MV, Keith RD, Hinderer SR. Measurement standards for multidisciplinary medical rehabilitation. *Arch Phys Med Rehabil* 1992; 73:S3–S23.
53. Equal Employment Opportunity Commission. Uniform Guidelines of Employee Selection Procedures. *Federal Register* 1978;43(166): 38290.
54. Equal Employment Opportunity Commission. ADA rules and regulations. *Federal Register* 1991;56(144):35726–35756.
55. Hart DL, Isernhagen SJ, Matheson LN. Guidelines for functional capacity evaluation of people with medical conditions. *J Occup Sports Phys Ther* 1993;18(6):682–686.
56. Ogden-Niemeyer L, Jacobs K. *Work hardening:* state of the art. Thorofare, NJ: Slack, 1989.
57. Hazard RG, Reid S, Fenwick J, Reeves V. Isokinetic trunk and lifting strength measurements: variability as an indicator of effort. *Spine* 1988; 13(1):54–57.
58. Chengalur SN, Smith GA, Nelson RC, Sadoff AM. Assessing sincerity of effort in maximal grip strength tests. *Am J Phys Med Rehab* 1990; 69(3):148–153.
59. Newton M, Waddell G. Trunk strength testing with iso-machines. Part 1. Review of a decade of scientific evidence. *Spine* 1993;18(7): 801–811.
60. Caldwell LS, Chaffior DB, Dukes-Dobos FN. A proposed standard procedure for static muscle strength testing. *Am Ind Hyg Assoc J* 1974; 35:201–206.
61. Matheson L, et al. Effect of instructions on isokinetic trunk strength testing variability, reliability, absolute value, and predictive validity. *Spine* 1992;177(8):914–921.
62. Newton M, Thow M, Sumerville D, Henderson J, Waddell G. Trunk strength testing with iso-machines. Part 2. Experimental evaluation of the Cybex II back testing system in normal subjects and patients with chronic low back pain. *Spine* 1993;18(7):812–824.
63. De Vellis R. *Scale development:* theory and applications. Newbury Park, CA: Sage, 1991.
64. Cronbach LJ. *Dependability of behavioral measurements:* theory of generalizability for scores and profiles. New York: Wiley, 1972.
65. Fleishman EA. On the relation between abilities, learning, and human performance. *Am Psychol* 1972;Nov:1017–1032.
66. Matheson LN, Mooney V, Grant J, Leggett S, Kenny K. Standardized evaluation of work capacity. *J Back Musculoskel Rehabil* 1996;6: 249–264.

*Environmental and Occupational Medicine, Third Edition,* edited by William N. Rom.
Lippincott–Raven Publishers, Philadelphia © 1998.

CHAPTER 8

# Occupational Health and Managed Care into the 21st Century

Dana C. Drew and Molly J. Coye

The focus on health care reform in the United States in 1994 seems like a long time ago. The furious debates and cries of a concerned citizenry have quieted and gone away. What happened? Where are we today? What was, and what will be, the impact on occupational health?

While a national health care plan was not developed, the consciousness of the nation was raised. New language and new ideas, such as managed care, health maintenance organization (HMO), preferred provider organization (PPO), protocols, outcomes, and 24-hour care, became part of everyday life in lay and medical communities. In some states, particularly California and Minnesota, these ideas were old and well established. Other areas found these concepts radical and representative of frightening changes from the status quo. As we head into the next century, the application of managed care is becoming a national reality and it will affect how occupational health care is delivered.

## WHAT IS MANAGED CARE AND HOW DOES IT WORK?

The term *managed care* implies that an entity (a payer or provider) is overseeing the delivery of health care services to a predetermined (or enrolled) group of people. The management of care includes determining what type and level of services are needed, and which provider will deliver the services. This is a far cry from traditional insurance plans where individuals chose their provider and accessed specialty care at will. In managed care individuals are assigned a specific primary care provider who generally acts as the "gatekeeper" in determining access and level of service. The requirement that individuals often provide a copayment at the time of service is meant to decrease utilization as well.

The primary intended difference between managed care and traditional insurance is cost. The goal of managed care is to reduce the cost of health care without reducing the quality of care. In managed care the provider agrees to deliver all required services for a predetermined amount, often a specified reimbursement amount per enrollee (or member), per month of coverage (capitation). This contract is negotiated prior to and regardless of utilization. The provider therefore is at some financial risk. By putting the provider at risk financially, more cost-effective utilization of ancillary and specialty services is encouraged. It then becomes prudent to encourage preventive medicine (wellness) in order to reduce expensive (acute illness, chronic disease state) demand. Quality of care is measured by the appropriateness of the outcomes and degree of utilization.

Managed care vehicles vary in their configuration and administration. HMOs are either of a closed or open model and most strictly direct care and provider choice. PPOs are looser organizations of many providers that tend to allow more provider choice by the individual and have fewer utilization restrictions. The pricing structures vary and employers choose the plans that best meet their needs. Managed care principles have also been applied to state and federal health insurance programs with the iden-

D. C. Drew: Occupational Medicine Practice, Pleasanton, California 94588.
M. J. Coye: The Lewin Group, San Francisco, California 94105.

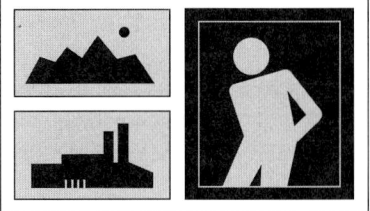

tical intent—reduce cost and maintain, or improve, quality of care.

In group health the focus on prevention is centered in the areas of immunizations, health screenings, and the encouragement of healthy lifestyle choices (such as smoking cessation, exercise, and weight control). Each of these proactive behaviors is intended to reduce the need for curative treatments or for the long-term support of chronic disease states. The managed care focus for those individuals with chronic disease states is the reduction of long-term effects of either the disease or the treatment. In both instances the goal is to increase the quality and quantity of life while managing the cost of care. The problem with managed care and group health is one of compliance. Individuals are not under any obligation to make the best choice for their health and often do not. This can result in excessive utilization and cost, which is counter to the intent of managed care.

The influence of managed care is evident in all health care arenas. The measures of inpatient utilization (length of stay, intensity of service) have dropped as managed care techniques and concepts have been implemented (1). The most notable examples are maternity stays and the use of outpatient, or ambulatory, surgery. Maternity stays currently average 48 hours postpartum as opposed to the 3- or 4-day average stays of just a few years ago. The number and complexity of procedures that are done in an ambulatory, or short stay, setting have risen dramatically. Improved technology and technique, coupled with financial focus, have reduced inpatient utilization to the point that the number of hospital beds required by a community can be reduced by 33% to 50%. Home health care is heavily utilized in geriatrics, maternity, pediatric, and surgical cases. This allows people to return home earlier and still continue to receive services that historically were provided in the inpatient setting. These changes have generally been accomplished while still maintaining quality care.

## IS MANAGED CARE APPLICABLE TO OCCUPATIONAL HEALTH?

What will the influence of managed care be on the practice of occupational medicine? One must first acknowledge the different components of occupational health. Treatment of workers' compensation injuries and illnesses and maintaining medical surveillance compliance with the Occupational Safety and Health Administration (OSHA) (or other occupational safety agency) standards are areas that are well defined. Corporate culture is highly variable and often determines what constitutes occupational health. This may include preplacement examinations, drug screening, health risk appraisals, and wellness programs. These services are delivered either at an on-site service (within the plant or office), at a freestanding clinic, or at some combination thereof.

There are some critical differences between group health and occupational health. The most significant is that the two largest components of occupational health, workers' compensation and medical surveillance, are required by law. Employers do not have a choice as to whether or not they are going to provide this benefit, or at what level. This requirement makes these occupational health services an entitlement or statutory benefit. Other corporate medicine services (preplacement examinations, drug screening, health risk appraisals, etc.) are provided based on corporate culture and prudent business choices. These optional services are dispensable when economic issues arise, but workers' compensation and medical surveillance are not.

There is also a difference as to how injuries and illnesses are treated. A basic premise in managed care is to defer specialty utilization and maintain treatment at the most primary level possible. Conversely, workers' compensation care is much closer to the intensified sports medicine model, where the interventions are early, aggressive, and often provided by a specialist (2). Because wage replacement is part of the expense of workers' compensation, every day an employee is out of work has a direct impact on the cost of care.

Next is the issue of eligibility and level of benefit. Occupational health services are provided from the moment of employment, are completely at the expense of the employer, and are restricted to the employee. On the other hand, group health benefits are often subject to a waiting or eligibility period, generally require some financial contribution from the employee, and are available to family members.

Another difference is the issue of indemnity and ongoing liability. Workers' compensation has an indemnity component that is not present in group health. This indemnity portion includes wage replacement (temporary or permanent), vocational rehabilitation, litigation expense, and temporary and/or permanent disability. Group health liability is restricted to the policy period, while workers' compensation liability can extend over an injured worker's life span, regardless of the policy period.

The last contrast offered for discussion is the type of carrier and financing mechanisms that support group health and occupational health. Group health is provided by health care insurers, while workers' compensation is provided, or administered, by property and casualty insurers or state insurance funds. While these are all insurance entities, they have different focuses, priorities, and incentives. Additionally, workers' compensation premiums are directly related to an employer's experience rating and state laws, while group health premiums are more often based on national, or regional, actuarial information for the population at large.

Table 1 demonstrates the differences between group and occupational health.

**TABLE 1.** *Differences between group health and occupational health*

| Group health | Occupational health |
|---|---|
| Predetermined contracts, subject to employer design, option | Regulated, entitlement, statutory benefit |
| Primary care medicine, deferred specialty utilization | Aggressive, early intervention; high specialty utilization |
| Cost sharing, as much as 50% | First dollar coverage, no employee contribution |
| Defined liability period | Liability period unknown |
| Health care services only | Vocational rehabilitation, litigation expense included |
| No wage replacement | Temporary or permanent disability payments (partial or total) |
| Not often litigated | Litigation rates much higher |

Is there any crossover for managed care from group health to occupational health? This was a topic of discussion during the health care reform debates and generally referred to as 24-hour care. The concept behind 24-hour care was that a single payer would administer care, regardless of causation (occupational versus nonoccupational), theoretically reducing cost and duplicate efforts. However, the government failed to recognize that the solution is not so simple, as the basis for each system is different.

## MANAGED CARE AND WORKERS' COMPENSATION

Workers' compensation has traditionally lagged behind group health by 10 to 15 years in terms of implementing alternative financing mechanisms. In many parts of the country workers' compensation is the last bastion of fee-for-service medicine. However, the trend toward managed care is clear and the economic crises will not tolerate a lengthy lag time in order to achieve cost control.

Twenty-four-hour pilots have been attempted and generally met with dismal results. The recently disbanded program in Oregon highlighted the difficulties, most of which were related to the issue of indemnity (3). However, this is not to say there is no place for managed care in workers' compensation. On the contrary, the spiraling workers' compensation cost increases experienced nationwide, which rose 183% between 1982 and 1991, have instigated multiple reform acts in states across the country (4,5).

Today, it is the workers' compensation component of occupational health that is most visibly affected by managed care. Twenty states have created legislation that define how managed care organizations can provide for the resolution of workers' compensation injuries and illnesses. The variances in legislation, and approaches to cost containment, are significant across the country, yet are designed to address the basic problems, which are universal. The language of these changing laws, and the tenor of discussions by payers, employers, and providers alike, is recognizing that managed care in workers' compensation comes only with managing the entire claim, not just episodes of care.

### Cost Containment Techniques

The most prevalent form of controlling medical costs is a state-mandated fee schedule. Currently 40 of the 51 jurisdictions utilize a fee schedule, most often based on relative value studies (RVS) (California RVS, RBRVS, Blue Cross/Blue Shield (BC/BS) RVS). Fee schedules are sometimes combined with other cost containment vehicles in hopes of managing the medical component of a claim (6).

Preferred provider organizations are often utilized in managing workers' compensation costs. Physician services are provided, sometimes at a discount from the regulated fee schedule, often in exchange for volume (numbers of patients). These organizations can be large and are generally made up of physicians from all specialties (primary and secondary care), many of whom are untrained in occupational medicine, and who rarely understand the unique nuances of the system. The concepts of outcomes and protocols has not been widely implemented as measurement tools.

Bill review is a technique frequently used with a state fee schedule. Bill-review enterprises develop computer programs to compare services billed at usual and customary fee-for-service rates to regulated fee schedules. Bills are then reduced to meet the regulated fee schedule, resulting in an adjusted (lower) payment to the physician.

In addition to utilization review, many payers assign case managers (generally registered nurses) to difficult cases. It is not unusual in the 1990s to have a nurse case manager present with an injured worker for examinations and tests. The nurse case manager represents the employer's and payer's interests in interactions with the physician.

Moves toward capitation, in any form, are slow. The inherent differences between workers' compensation and group health make this a complicated task. Initial discussions have explored carving out just the medical costs for capitation. However, models to determine risk for a population defined by job title, rather than by age or gender, have not evolved to the point where they can be introduced into the marketplace with any degree of confidence.

Analysis indicates that the efforts listed above have had varying degrees of success in the reduction of overall costs. The development of treatment protocols and outcomes, while still embryonic in occupational medicine, appears to hold more promise in managing all the factors in a claim. By the early 1990s new models began to evolve, known as case rates (based on treatment guidelines and outcome goals), that focus on multiple areas of concern. Case rates are constructed with the emphasis, and financial incentive, being on appropriate, yet rapid, resolution of the injury while reducing, or eliminating, time lost from the workplace. In effect, this approach manages both the medical (treatment) and indemnity (lost time) sides of a claim. The introduction of treatment protocols or guidelines, while difficult for some physicians to accept, has the benefit of putting the treatment plan into an objective arena.

### Discussion Points

One of the largest inhibitors to managing an entire claim, rather than elements of it, is the historically adversarial positions held by the various constituents. The payers (and employers), providers, attorneys, and claimants have staked out self-serving positions that do not promote the goal of quality care or appropriate outcomes. The lack of trust between the participants, perhaps influenced by current financing and delivery systems, must be addressed in any new program design.

The question "Isn't the primary care physician the provider of choice?" is often raised.

Primary care training and practices are founded on the concept of delivering care to a patient over a period of years. Primary care physicians are often hesitant to enforce return-to-work guidelines, or suggest transitional duty, for fear that it will alienate their primary care patient (the employee). When these patients (employees) present with work-related discomforts (physical or mental), the tendency often is to take the employee off work, which is counterproductive in an environment where managing the time lost from work is as crucial as managing the medical care.

An advantage of workers' compensation is the ability to influence compliance. Many jurisdictions eliminate benefits when an injured worker ceases being compliant with the treatment regimen. This variant from group health, and any subsequent impact on outcomes, will be an interesting source of study in the future.

It is clear that the momentum is toward managed care. The question is, Will the various entities continue to recognize and address the differences between workers' compensation and group health? Undoubtedly there will be many models proposed and implemented with the intent of containing cost. The challenge will be to manage the indemnity costs as well as the medical costs.

## MANAGED CARE AND MEDICAL SURVEILLANCE

Medical surveillance parallels group health in that both are focused on prevention. Routine biologic monitoring, based on exposure, is intended to detect changes at the earliest possible date in order to intervene as optimally as possible. This is similar to regularly scheduled examinations and screening tests in group health. It seems feasible to develop a managed care product, similar to those in group health, that covers this segment of occupational health. This has not been done primarily because the costs incurred in medical surveillance are not as large as those in group health or workers' compensation, and therefore receive less attention.

Medical surveillance lends itself well to managed care models as it has an epidemiologic basis and its areas of concern are well documented and observed. There are existing guidelines for the monitoring of most occupational exposures and databases established for predictive and trend analysis. The information could be assembled to develop capitation rates based on length of exposure, gender, age, etc.

An important element of medical surveillance is the tracking and retention of historical data. The development of any managed care solution will have to incorporate a long-term data repository, as many exposures require medical records be maintained for the length of employment plus 30 years. This extended requirement is a significant challenge in terms of who will provide this service and how will it be funded.

The question of whether or not medical surveillance can be combined with routine medical care is often asked. The answer is generally negative, as few adults access routine medical care with the same frequency required by medical surveillance. Of additional concern is who should provide medical surveillance care. Primary care physicians are not as well trained as occupational medicine physicians with regard to potential hazardous exposures, their detection, or their consequences. These issues again illustrate some of the significant differences between group health and occupational health, and support the development of unique solutions.

## MANAGED CARE AND CORPORATE MEDICINE

The optional components of occupational health—preplacement examinations, drug screening, executive physicals, health risk appraisals, influenza vaccine programs, wellness programs—or corporate medicine, often fall into the gray area between group health and occupational health. These services are more closely aligned with traditional group health and are often rendered in primary care settings. The relevant issues that exist in medical surveillance apply to corporate medicine as well. While the similarities are strong, and the inclination to combine these services with routine group health care is great, the differences must be understood and addressed.

Preplacement examinations and drug screening are excellent illustrations of these differences. Even though preplacement examinations are relatively straightforward, the provider must be well educated on the Americans with Disability Act in order to determine if an individual can perform the job's "essential functions." Therefore, to best serve all parties, the provider must have in-depth knowledge of the job being filled, its essential functions, and the dynamics and culture of the workplace. Additionally, when a disability exists, the provider must know how and to whom any restrictions must be communicated. As a rule, primary care physicians are not knowledgeable enough about work sites and job descriptions to adequately provide this service.

Drug screening interpretation, whether or not it is regulated by the Department of Transportation, has the potential for litigation and should be provided by an individual who has successfully certified as a medical review officer. Again, these activities require different skills than those generally found in a primary care practice. In both preplacement examinations and drug screening, a lack of education, focus, or desire can contribute to an inappropriate outcome.

In contrast, annual or biannual executive physicals were often offered as a perk by the private sector, municipalities, and governmental agencies. These were generally complex physical assessments, with ancillary testing (lab work, ECG, mammogram, stress treadmill, flexible sigmoidoscopy, etc.), the cost of which easily approached $400 to $500 per person. With the evolution of managed care, and its focus on prevention, many of these programs have been disbanded, because these services are duplicated on the group health side and can be obtained at a much lower cost (already included in the health care premium). In other words, the cost-benefit analysis showed that companies were spending duplicate dollars with little, if any, return on their investment.

To some extent, wellness programs and health screenings have followed the same path as executive physicals. As group health programs offer more programs based on prevention, it is considerably more cost-effective for employers to promote utilization on the group health side rather than pay for a duplicate program within occupational health.

## MANAGED CARE AND ON-SITE PROGRAMS

Large employers often have on-site programs located within a plant or office. Occasionally these programs are staffed by physicians and nurses who are employees of the company, but more often are operated by an organization that has contracted to provide these services. The services delivered include nonoccupationally and occupationally related encounters. The ratio of nonoccupational to occupational visits often approaches 4:1. Contracting organizations use this ratio as a selling point for their programs, the persuasive argument being that employees who receive treatment for minor ailments on-site create less down time by using less sick time or paid time off (7). This is advantageous for both the employer and the contractor, who must have a busy facility to be profitable. The cost savings achieved by an on-site program are often calculated using the local usual and customary fees. This means that the on-site provider can demonstrate that their monthly, or annual, contracted rate is less than if the same services were rendered outside the plant or office.

Managed care also has an effect on that argument. When an employer chooses a managed care plan, the cost of care is not subject to local pricing influence. Managed care plans contract with local primary care physicians for group health (or nonoccupational) services and generally do not have a contract with the on-site provider. The result again is a duplicative expense. The employer is paying the managed care premium to cover all nonoccupational services with local providers, and paying the on-site provider a monthly or annual fee for the availability to render these same services.

## THE CHALLENGES

Occupational health services are delivered in assorted settings and by a variety of providers. Depending on size, a plant or office might have a fully staffed clinic, running 24 hours a day. There are free-standing facilities dedicated to occupational medicine, or those that offer a continuum of urgent care (group health and occupational health) services. Large employers often employ certified occupational health nurses to provide first aid, screening tests, and counseling. Occupational medicine programs frequently supply per diem staff to perform annual examinations, influenza vaccine programs, and other corporate medicine services on-site. Primary care physicians often provide occupational health services to primary care patients.

Nationwide there are fewer than 2,500 board-certified occupational medicine physicians.

The evolution of occupational medicine as an independent field of medicine has been slow. As managed care for group health spreads across the country, the income of many primary and specialty care physicians has been adversely affected. This has influenced many nonoccupational medicine physicians to offer their services to the occupational medicine market. Many of these providers, whether they provide occupational medicine services full or part time, do not understand the unique requirements of occupational health. The utilization of other than dedicated occupational medicine providers contributes to poor outcomes. In short, the delivery system for occupational health is highly fragmented and variable.

Managed care succeeds when large numbers of lives (or enrollees) can be aggregated and directed toward contracted providers. This ensures an adequate revenue stream and patient volume to maintain a practice. Aggregating occupational health within a managed care framework yields a population that is significantly smaller than those in group health as it is composed of employees only, rather than employees and dependents. Likewise, the demand for occupational health services is restricted to workplace concerns rather than general health issues. This lower demand and smaller population make it difficult to establish large enough groups to support a practice. Additionally, many states require that injured workers retain the choice of treating physician, which further dilutes the patient stream.

Compounding the fragmentation, dedicated provider and aggregation issues are the inherent differences between group health and occupational health. The inclusion of non–health care benefits and potential responsibility for permanent or partial disability and wage replacement within a managed care approach are issues that payers and legislators have struggled with during the last several years. A few occupational health elements cross easily into managed care group health programs (executive physicals, wellness programs, health screenings), but the majority (workers' compensation, medical surveillance, preplacement examinations, drug screening) are most appropriately served by a dedicated occupational medicine physician.

Some traditional managed care techniques have been applied in occupational health and have affected the delivery of occupational health services. The concern is will these managed care techniques, which often substitute duration of treatment for intensity of treatment, have a negative impact in an environment where rapid resolution is critical. Can these techniques truly address the long-term, prospective needs of the medical surveillance community?

The primary challenge at hand is the development and application of managed care techniques that recognize and support the unique requirements of occupational health, without providing services that are duplicated in group health. The opportunity lies in modifying group health managed care concepts and coupling them with providers who are dedicated to the practice of occupational medicine. This creates an approach that coordinates all the components, from preplacement examinations that match people with the right skills to the right jobs through 30 years of record retention, and appropriately manages the treatment of workers' compensation injuries as well. Such a coordinated approach will reduce the incidence of occupational injuries and illnesses, thereby reducing the dollars spent on medical care and indemnity. This integration of managed care into occupational health over the next 5 to 10 years will further establish occupational medicine as a unique specialty, as well as better serve employers and employees.

## GLOSSARY

**Bill review**—a cost containment method that compares fees billed to the contracted, or mandated, pricing structure and adjusts them accordingly.

**Capitation**—a managed care strategy that pays a provider a predetermined amount of money per insured individual for each time period covered (i.e., dollars per member/per month).

**Case rate**—the total allowance that will be paid to a provider to manage a specific injury from beginning to end; for example all sprained ankles would pay $x$ dollars and all sprained backs would pay $2x$ dollars.

**Cost containment**—strategies and methodologies designed to control and analyze health care costs.

**Credentialing**—a process by which managed care organizations determine which physicians meet established criteria to provide service.

**Discount**—a negotiated reduction of fees charged against an established pricing structure.

**Eligibility periods**—preestablished waiting periods before a covered member is eligible to receive services and benefits.

**Employer contributions**—payments made by an employer for workers' compensation coverage, generally based on payroll.

**Experience rating**—historical and/or actuarial rating of an employer's accident rate, in terms of frequency and severity.

**Gatekeeper**—the role played by a primary care physician or case manager that determines when, how, and what level of service an individual receives.

**Health Maintenance Organization (HMO)**—a managed care organization that offers specific services for a fixed fee or premium. A closed HMO, such as Kaiser, employs its own physicians and uses its own hospitals and clinics. An open HMO contracts with private physicians to provide services in their own offices.

**Indemnity**—payments on a workers' compensation claim that are not for medical treatment; includes temporary/permanent partial/total disability, legal fees, and nonmedical ancillary costs.

**Internal dispute resolution**—a formal process for employers, insurers, providers, and employees to resolve disagreements outside the judicial system (i.e., arbitration).

**Lost time management**—programs that monitor and manage an employee's rapid, but safe, return to the workplace following an occupational injury or illness.

**Managed Care Organization (MCO)**—an organization that administers health care benefits to enrolled members by monitoring and determining access to benefits and levels of service.

**Managed care**—the administrative philosophy that applies cost containment techniques to a health care delivery system for a designated group of individuals for a contracted period of time.

**Outcomes**—the objective, measurable results of medical intervention in disease and injury management.

**Preferred Provider Organization (PPO)**—a loose association of providers, held together with similar contracts, and credentialed to the same standard, but not necessarily providing service within the same building, city, county, or state.

**Return to work**—the philosophy and programs that encourage rapid return to the workplace, either in a transitional role or at the original job, following an occupational injury or illness.

**Self-insured**—employers who have met established criteria, and have the financial resources, to pay for all claims made by employees for group health or workers' compensation benefits.

**Transitional duty**—alternative tasks, or essential functions of a job that are modified or adapted, which allow an injured worker to return to the workplace before achieving maximum improvement, either on a full- or part-time basis.

**Treatment protocols/guidelines**—a prescribed or suggested treatment pattern, determined by diagnosis, designed to achieve the most favorable outcome in the least amount of time.

**Utilization review**—an independent review of treatment plans and choices designed to monitor quality of care, appropriateness of care, and cost.

**Vocational rehabilitation**—a course of assessment and retraining for individuals who can no longer perform their original job duties as the result of an occupational injury or illness.

**24-hour care**—an insurance concept that integrates group health and workers' compensation coverage to provide health care benefits and coverage 24 hours a day, regardless of causation or place of occurrence.

## REFERENCES


1. The Governance Committee. *Capitation strategy.* Washington, DC: Advisory Board Committee, 1994.
2. Parry T. *Medical benefit delivery, group medical versus workers' compensation in California. Research notes.* San Francisco: California Workers Compensation Institute, 1994 (August).
3. Molmen WP. *Oregon 24-hour coverage pilot experience.* San Francisco: Integrated Benefits Institute, 1997 (February 28).
4. *Fiscal data for state workers' compensation system, 1982–1991. Research bulletin.* Washington, DC: National Foundation for Unemployment and Workers Compensation, 1993 (December 9).
5. Burton JF Jr, Schmidle TP. Workers' compensation insurance rates, national averages up, interstate differences widen. *John Burton's Workers' Compensation Monitor* 1993;5 (January/February).
6. Eccelston SM. *Managed care and medical cost containment in workers compensation, a national inventory, 1995–1996.* Cambridge, MA: 1995 (December);13:15.
7. Pachman JS, Stempien DE, Milles, SS, O'Neill, FN. The hidden savings of an on-site corporate medical center. *J Occup Environ Med* 1996; 38(10):1047–1048.

*Environmental and Occupational Medicine,*
*Third Edition,* edited by William N. Rom.
Lippincott–Raven Publishers, Philadelphia © 1998.

CHAPTER 9

# The Immune System and the Environment

John E. Salvaggio and Karen A. Sullivan

## ENVIRONMENTAL CHEMICALS AND THE IMMUNE SYSTEM

### The Immune System

A brief discussion of the components, development, and function of the immune system is appropriate to provide a background for analysis of disturbances and function of the immune system associated with exposure to environmental agents. The immune system consists of a variety of immunocompetent cells and their products that reside principally in lymphoreticular tissues and interact with virtually all organs of the human body. Subpopulations of these cells with specialized functions act to prevent invasion of tissues by microbial agents and growth of neoplastic cells. They also provide host defense mechanisms against foreign tissues, parasites, aeroallergens, drugs, and environmental chemicals. Overall, immunity is conveyed by the actions and products of these cells.

The immune system is capable of generating a diversity of genetically distinct T- and B-cell clonal populations with multiple specificities. Other immune cells are not endowed with such specificity but depend on T and B cells to orchestrate their immune responsiveness. All cells of the immune system arise from stem cells (1). T and B cells mature and differentiate at separate anatomic sites. By the 8th week of gestation and through early adolescence, lymphoid stem cells enter the thymus. There, they differentiate and divide under the influence of growth and maturational factors released by local epithelial cells. It is during this process that T cells acquire a unique series of membrane-bound glycoproteins or differentiation antigens, which divide them into various sets and subsets. The subsets are defined by surface markers that react with monoclonal antibodies (MAb). Some of the surface antigens are retained by T cells upon leaving the thymus and entering the circulation (Table 1) (2). T cells are referred to as belonging to different clusters of differentiation (CD) groupings (Table 2, since they are defined by their reactions with clusters of MAb. The numbers of CD designations have rapidly expanded and continue to do so. The CDs enumerated in Table 2 were defined by six international workshops (3). The CD3 marker, for example, is present on a very small percentage of mature thymocytes but on all peripheral blood T cells. In contrast, the CD4 and CD8 antigens are coexpressed on approximately 70% of thymocytes and are individually expressed on the subpopulation of exportable mature cells that enter the circulation and harbor the CD3 glycoprotein. T cells carry out multiple functions that are, to some extent, associated with their various subsets.

#### *T Cells*

Circulating T cells can be separated into two major antigenically and functionally distinct subpopulations: (a) the 55% to 70% of peripheral T cells that express the CD3 and CD4 surface differentiation antigens and provide helper-inducer stimuli for all T-T and T-B interactions, and (b) the 25% to 40% of the remaining T cells that express CD3 and CD8 surface molecules and actively suppress both T- and B-cell immune reactivity.

There are other multiple subsets of T cells, which are also subdivided into effector and regulator T cells. A group of effector cytotoxic T cells recognized by MAb

J. E. Salvaggio: Department of Medicine, Tulane University Medical Center, New Orleans, Louisiana 70112.
K. A. Sullivan: Histocompatibility and Immunogenetics Laboratory, Department of Medicine, Tulane University Medical Center, New Orleans, Louisiana 70112.

**TABLE 1.** *The clusters of differentiation phenotype of thymocytes and peripheral T cells*

| | | | |
|---|---|---|---|
| | Bone marrow stem cell | | |
| Thymic capsule | CD2$^-$ CD3$^-$ | CD4$^-$ CD8$^-$ | Stem cells enter capsule at the periphery, then migrate toward capsule interior; we are not considering the fates of several cell types arising at this point, including double-negative, TCR-positive ($\alpha$, $\beta$ or $\gamma\delta$) cells |
| Thymic cortex | CD2$^-$ CD3$^-$<br>CD2$^+$ CD3$^+$<br>CD2$^+$ CD3$^+$ | CD4$^-$ CD8$^-$<br>CD4$^-$<br>CD4$^+$ | TCR-$\beta$-H and $\alpha$-chain genes are rearranged; if successfully expressed, cell moves to the next stage; if not, cell dies |
| Thymic medulla | CD2$^+$CD3$^+$CD4$^+$ | CD2$^+$CD3$^+$CD8$^+$ | If TCR recognizes antigen plus MHC on thymic dendritic cells, cell dies; if not, then cell proceeds to next step |
| Peripheral lymphoid | CD2$^+$CD3$^+$CD4$^+$ (65% of peripheral blood T cells) | CD2$^+$CD3$^+$CD8$^+$ (35% of peripheral blood T cells) | If TCR is restricted to class I or class MHC on thymic epithelium, cell matures to single-positive thymocyte; if not, then cell dies<br>Single-positive thymocytes are restricted to self (thymic) MHC and are depleted or self-reactive cells |

against the CD8 surface marker and carrying the CD8 designation (the same marker borne by suppressor T cells) are perhaps most studied (4). These cells recognize antigens in the context of the class I major histocompatibility complex (MHC) products on chromosome 6, namely human leukocyte antigen loci A, B, and C (HLA-A, HLA-B, HLA-C) (5). When activated, they can kill a target cell of the particular HLA specificity bearing the involved antigen. Thus, persons who are immune to a particular virus, such as mumps or measles virus, have cytotoxic T cells that are able to kill the virus-infected cells of the same HLA haplotype.

T cells that carry out delayed, or so-called type IV hypersensitivity, reactions recognize antigen in the context of the class II components of the MHC (HLA-DR). These effector T cells are recognized by MAb against the CD4 antigen and are referred to as CD4 cells. Their inflammatory reactions are facilitated through production of cytokines, such as the family of interleukins, interferons, and lymphokines.

Regulator or helper T cells that influence the development of effector T cells and B cells are divided into two types. Helper T cells are required for B cells to produce antibody and are recognized by MAb against the CD4 type. These cells also recognize antigen in the context of MHC class II molecules and produce interleukins and lymphokines when activated. A second type of regulator T cell, the suppressor T cell, is recognized by MAb against the CD8 marker. These cells negatively regulate immune responses and probably downregulate helper T cell activity (6). The specific receptors on which they act have not been well studied. They do, however, secrete soluble suppressor lymphokines, and they may be important in developing acquired immune tolerance.

Subclasses of T helper lymphocytes have been identified among antigen-specific T cells depending on the profile of cytokines that they produce (7) as illustrated in Table 3.

In humans, type 1 T-helper cells (Th$_1$) primarily produce interferon-$\gamma$ (IFN-$\gamma$), tumor necrosis factor-$\beta$ (TNF-$\beta$), and interleukin-2 (IL-2). They preferentially develop during infections by intracellular bacteria and trigger phagocyte-mediated host defense with activation of macrophages and induction of delayed hypersensitivity responses. Th$_2$ cells produce primarily IL-4, which stimulates immunoglobulin (Ig)E and IgG$_1$ antibody production, and IL-5, which activates eosinophils. Other T-cell subsets designated Th$_0$ have a less differentiated cytokine profile than Th$_1$ and Th$_2$ cells and may dominate the early stages of some immune responses. IL-10 and IL-13 in conjunction with IL-4 inhibit macrophage functions. Th$_2$ responses are associated with production of mast cells, eosinophils, IgG$_1$, and IgE. They are also thought to exert suppressive effects against the cell-mediated or Th$_1$ response. Because the respective cytokines act antagonistically, these T-cell populations (Th$_1$ and Th$_2$) appear to mutually regulate each other's function (8). In essence, Th$_1$ cells trigger a phagocyte-mediated host defense and tend to be induced by infections with intracellular microorganisms. Th$_2$ type responses are mainly responsible for phagocyte-independent host defense, such as that noted against parasites or allergens mediated by IgE and eosinophils. The main phagocyte-mediated and non-phagocyte-mediated host defense pathways are illustrated in Fig. 1.

There are several caveats concerning Th$_1$ versus Th$_2$ responses. For example, there are few differentiation markers for Th$_1$ and Th$_2$ cells (Th$_1$ cells have IL-12 receptor B2 and P-selectin and E-selectin, whereas Th$_2$ cells do not). Thus, functional characterization of increased cytokine production may not represent a clear state of differentiation but merely the functional consequences of the environment in which the cell is being stimulated. There are also circumstances in which the analogy of the cytokine profile between human and murine Th$_1$ and Th$_2$ lymphocytes is different. For example, in humans Th$_1$ and

**TABLE 2.** *Definition of monoclonal antibody cell surface markers*

| CD | Cell distribution/function | Antibody clusters |
|---|---|---|
| 1a,b,c | Thymocytes, Langerhans cells, B-cell subset, dendritic cells | T cell biased |
| 2 | Thymocytes, T cells, NK cells/LFA-2, E rosette receptor | |
| 2R | Activated T cells, NK cells | |
| 3 | Thymocytes, T cells/T-cell receptor associated | |
| 4 | T helper cells/MHC class II receptor, HIV antigen receptor | |
| 5 | T cells, B-cell subset, B-cell chronic lymphocytic leukemia | |
| 6 | Pan T cells | |
| 7 | Pan T cells/FcR (IgM receptor?) | |
| 8 | T cytotoxic/suppressor cells/MHC class I receptor | |
| 27 | Thymocyte subset, T cells, transformed B cells | |
| 28 | T-cell subset, activated B cells | |
| 45 | Pan leukocyte | |
| 45RA | T-cell subset, B cells, monocytes/ naive T cells | |
| 45RB | T-cell subset, B cells, monocytes, macrophages, granulocytes (weak) | |
| 45RO | T cells, B-cell subset, monocytes, macrophages/memory T cells | |
| w60 | T-cell subset, platelets | |
| 98 | T cells, B cells (weak), NK cells, granulocytes, cell lines | |
| 99 | Thymocytes, Peripheral blood lymphocytes | |
| 99R | T cells, B cells, some leukemias | |
| 9 | Pre-B cells, monocytes, platelets | B cell biased |
| 10 | Lymphoid progenitor cells/CALLA (common ALL antigen) | |
| 19 | B cells | |
| 20 | B cells | |
| 21 | B cells, follicular dendritic cells/C3d/EBV receptor; CR2 | |
| 22 | B cells, hairy cell leukemia | |
| 23 | Activated B cells, activated macrophages, eosinophils, platelets/low-affinity Fc-IgE receptor | |
| 24 | B cells, granulocytes | |
| 37 | B cells, T cells, myeloid cells (weak) | |
| 39 | B cells, monocytes, macrophages, vascular endothelium | |
| 40 | B cells, B-cell leukemias and lymphomas, some carcinomas, monocytes (weak)/receptor for costimulatory signal for B cell proliferation | |
| 72 | B cells | |
| 73 | B-cell subset, T-cell subsets | |
| 74 | B cells, macrophages, monocytes/Ii, invariant chain of HLA class II | |
| w75 | B cells, T-cell subset (weak) | |
| w76 | B cells, T-cell subset | |
| 77 | Activated B cells, follicular center B cells, endothelial cells | |
| w78 | B cells, macrophage subset | |
| 79a,b | B cells/B-cell antigen receptor associated; cell surface expression and signal transduction | |
| 80 | B-cell subset *in vivo*, activated B cells *in vitro*/B7, BB1; ligand for CTLA-4 & CD28 | |
| 81 | B cells, lymphocytes | |
| 11a | Leukocytes/leukocyte function antigen (LFA-1) | Myeloid biased |
| 11b | Granulocytes, monocytes, NK cells/C3bi receptor | |
| 11c | Granulocytes, monocytes, NK cells, B-cell subset, T-cell subset, hairy cell leukemia | |
| w12 | Granulocytes, monocytes, platelets | |
| 13 | Monocytes, granulocytes/MY7 | |
| 14 | Monocytes, granulocytes, macrophages | |
| 15 | Granulocytes, monocytes | |
| 15s | Neutrophils | |
| 16a | Macrophages, NK cells/FcRIII IgG receptor | |
| 16b | Granulocytes | |
| w17 | Granulocytes, monocytes, platelets/lactosyl ceramide | |
| 32 | Granulocytes, monocytes, B cells/FcRII IgG receptor | |
| 33 | Myeloid progenitor cells, monocytes, myeloid leukemias | |
| 35 | Granulocytes except basophils, monocytes, B cells, some NK cells/CR1; C3b receptor | |
| 64 | Monocytes/FcRI IgG receptor | |
| 65 | Granulocytes, monocytes | |
| 66a | Neutrophils | |
| 66b | Granulocytes/previously CD67 | |
| 66c | Neutrophils, Colon carcinoma | |
| 66d | Neutrophils | |

**TABLE 2.** *Continued.*

| CD | Cell distribution/function | Antibody clusters |
|---|---|---|
| 66e | Colon carcinoma, Colon epithelial cells/CEA | Myeloid biased |
| 66f | PMG-1 | |
| 68 | Monocytes, macrophages | |
| 87 | Granulocytes, monocytes, macrophages, activated T cells/urokinase plasminogen activator receptor, UPA-R | |
| 88 | Polymorphonuclear leukocytes, mast cells, macrophages, smooth muscle/C5a receptor | |
| 89 | Neutrophils, monocytes, macrophages, T-cell and B-cell subsets /Fc$\alpha$R, IgA receptor | |
| 91 | Monocytes, some non-hemopoietic cell lines/$\alpha$2 macroglobulin receptor | |
| w92 | Neutrophils, monocytes, endothelial cells, platelets | |
| 93 | Neutrophils, monocytes, endothelial cells | |
| 101 | Granulocytes, macrophages | |
| 114 | G-CSFR | |
| 56 | NK cells | NK cell biased |
| 57 | NK cells, T-cell and B-cell subsets | |
| 94 | NK cells, T-cell subsets | |
| 31 | Platelets, monocytes, macrophages, granulocytes, B cells/gpIIa′ | Platelet biased |
| 36 | Platelets, monocytes, macrophages, B cells (weak)/gpIV or IIIb | |
| 41 | Platelets, megakaryocytes/gpIIb/IIIa | |
| 42a,b,c,d | Platelets, megakaryocytes/gpIX, gpIb, GPIB, gpV | |
| 51 | Platelets (weak)/vitronectin receptor | |
| 61 | Platelets, megakaryocytes/gpIIIa | |
| 63 | Activated platelets, monocytes, macrophages, weakly on T cells, B cells and granulocytes | |
| 107a,b | Activated Platelets/LAMP-1, LAMP-2 | |
| 18 | Leukocytes | Adhesion biased |
| 29 | Ubiquitous (erythrocytes are negative), T helper subset | |
| 43 | Leukocytes (not peripheral B cells), brain cells/binds ICAM-1 | |
| 44 | Leukocytes, erythrocytes, brain cells/mediates leukocyte adhesion | |
| 49a | Activated T cells, monocytes/VLA-1; binds collagen and laminin | |
| 49b | B cells, monocytes, platelets/VLA-2;binds collagen and laminin | |
| 49c | B cells/VLA-3; binds laminin and fibronectin | |
| 49d | Thymocytes, B cells/VLA-4; binds fibronectin, Peyer's patch HEV and VCAM-1 | |
| 49e | T cells, monocytes, platelets/VLA-5; binds fibronectin | |
| 49f | Thymocytes, T cells, monocytes/VLA-6; binds laminin | |
| 50 | Leukocytes (not plasma cells)/ICAM-3 | |
| 54 | PHA blasts, endothelial cells, follicular dendritic cells/ICAM-1 | |
| 55 | Hematopoietic and nonhematopoietic cells/binds C3b | |
| 58 | Hematopoietic and nonhematopoietic cells/LFA-3; binds CD2 | |
| 59 | Hematopoietic and nonhematopoietic cells/binds complement components C8 and C9 | |
| 62E | Endothelial cells | |
| 62L | T cells, B cells, monocytes, NK cells | |
| 62P | Platelets, endothelial cells, megakaryocytes | |
| 102 | Vascular endothelial cells, lymphocytes, monocytes/ICAM-2 | |
| 103 | Intraepithelial lymphocytes, 2–6% peripheral blood lymphocytes | |
| 104 | Epithelial cells, Schwann cells, some tumor cells | |
| 26 | Activated T cells and B cells, macrophages/cofactor for HIV infection | Activation biased |
| 30 | Activated T cells and B cells, Reed-Sternberg cells, embryonal carcinoma, Hodgkin's lymphoma | |
| 40L | Activated $CD4^+$ cells/ligand for CD40 | |
| 69 | Activated T cells, B cells and macrophages, NK cells | |
| 70 | Activated T cells and B cells, Reed-Sternberg cells, macrophages (weakly) | |
| 71 | Activated T cells and B cells, macrophages, proliferating cells/transferrin receptor | |
| 95 | Myeloid and T lymphoblastoid cell lines/FAS; causes apoptosis | |
| 96 | Activated T cells | |
| 97 | Activated cells | |

**TABLE 2.** *Continued.*

| CD | Cell distribution/function | Antibody clusters |
|---|---|---|
| 25 | Activated T cells, B cells and macrophages/TAC; IL-2 receptor | Cytokine biased |
| 115 | Monocytes, macrophages, placenta/M-CSFR; macrophage colony stimulating factor receptor | |
| 116 | Monocytes, neutrophils, eosinophils, fibroblasts, endothelial cells/GM-CSF R; granulocyte, macrophage colony stimulating factor receptor | |
| 117 | Bone marrow progenitor cells/SCF R; stem cell factor receptor | |
| 118 | Broad cellular distribution/IFNα, receptor | |
| 119 | Macrophages, monocytes, B cells, epithelial cells/IFN receptor | |
| 120a,b | Most cell types/TNFR; tumor necrosis factor receptor | |
| 121a | T cells, thymocytes, fibroblasts, endothelial cells/IL-1 receptor | |
| w121b | B cells, macrophages, monocytes/IL-1 receptor | |
| 122 | NK cells, T-cell subset, some B cell lines/IL-2 receptor chain | |
| 123 | Bone marrow stem cells, granulocytes, monocytes, megakaryocytes/IL-3 receptor | |
| 124 | T cells, B cells, hemopoietic precursor cells/IL-4 receptor | |
| w125 | Eosinophils, basophils/IL-5 receptor | |
| 126 | Activated B cells, plasma cells, leukocytes (weakly)/IL-6 receptor | |
| 127 | Bone marrow lymphoid precursors, Pro-B cells, T cells, monocytes/IL-7 receptor | |
| w128 | Neutrophils, basophils, T-cell subset/IL-8 receptor | |
| 130 | Activated B cells, plasma cells, endothelial cells, leukocytes/common subunit of IL-6, IL-11, oncostatin M and leukemia hibitory factor receptors | |
| 34 | Hematopoietic progenitor cells, endothelial cells | Miscellaneous |
| 38 | Plasma cells, pre-B cells, immature T cells, activated T cells | |
| 46 | Hematopoietic cells, nonhematopoietic cells | |
| 47 | All cell types | |
| 48 | Leukocytes | |
| 52 | Leukocytes | |
| 53 | Leukocytes | |
| 82 | Leukocytes | |
| 83 | Activated T cells and B cells, germinal center cells, dendritic cells | |
| 84 | Platelets, monocytes, B cells (weak) | |
| 85 | Monocytes, B cells (weak) | |
| 86 | Monocytes, germinal center cells, activated B cells | |
| 90 | $CD34^+$ prothymocytes, bone marrow cells, cord blood, fetal liver | |
| 100 | Hematopoietic cells | |
| 105 | Endothelial cells, bone marrow cell subset, *in vitro* activated macrophages | |
| 106 | Endothelial cells/VCAM-1 | |
| w108 | Activated spleen T cells, some stromal cells | |
| 109 | Activated T cells, platelets, endothelial cells | |
| 114 | G-CSFR; granulocyte colony stimulating factor receptor | |
| 131 | Common β | |
| 132 | Common γ | |
| 134 | OX40 | |
| 135 | Flt3,Flk4 | |
| w136 | MSP-R; macrophage stimulating protein receptor | |
| w137 | 4-IBB | |
| 138 | Syndecan-1 | |
| 139 | B cell | |
| 140a,b | PDGFRα, β; platelet-derived growth factor receptors | |
| 141 | Thrombomodulin | |
| 142 | Tissue factor | |
| 143 | Angiotensin converting enzyme | |
| 144 | Vascular endothelial cadherin | |
| w145 | Endothelial | |
| 146 | MUC18, S-endo | |
| 147 | Neurothelin, Basigin | |
| 148 | HPTP-eta, p260 phosphatase | |
| w149 | MEM-133 | |
| w150 | SLAM, IPO-3 | |
| 151 | PETA-3 | |
| 152 | CTLA-4 | |

**TABLE 2.** *Continued.*

| CD | Cell distribution/function | Antibody clusters |
|---|---|---|
| 153 | CD30L | Miscellaneous |
| 154 | CD40L, T-BAM | |
| 155 | Polio virus receptor | |
| 156 | ADAM8, MS2 | |
| 157 | BST-1, MO-5 | |
| 158a,b | NK receptors specific for MHC class I | |
| 161 | NKRP-1; NK receptor P1 | |
| 162 | P selectin glycoprotein ligand 1 | |
| 163 | M130 | |
| 164 | MGC-24 | |
| 165 | GP37/AD2 | |
| 166 | Activated leukocyte cell adhesion molecule | |

From ref. 129, p. 52; ref. 130, pp. 53–61; and ref. 131, p. 101.

$Th_2$ subsets both produce IL-2, IL-10, and IL-13 plus granulocyte-macrophage colony-stimulating factor (GM-CSF) and IL-3, as illustrated in Table 3.

In spite of the importance of Th lineage commitment in diseases, the mechanisms that determine whether an immune response will be dominated by a $Th_1$- or $Th_2$-type cell response are not well understood. Among these factors are genetic predisposition, the nature of the offending antigen, various modes of antigen presentation, processing pathways, and genetic factors. The dominant factors that control differentiation of $Th_1$ and $Th_2$ cells from Th precursor cells are likely the cytokine and cytokine-derived mediators in which the T lymphocyte is activated.

Human $Th_1$ and $Th_2$ cells differ not only in their cytokine secretion profiles, but also in their responsiveness to cytokines. For example, both cell types proliferate in response to IL-2, but $Th_2$ cells are considerably more responsive to IL-4 (7). $Th_1$ and $Th_2$ cells also differ in their cytolysis potential and in their mode of help for B-cell antibody synthesis. $Th_1$ and $Th_2$ cells also differ in their degree of activity on monocytes. The primary functional properties of human $Th_1$ and $Th_2$ clones are summarized in Table 4.

Knowledge of mechanisms determining the development and function of $Th_1$ and $Th_2$ cells is essential to our understanding of immunoregulation. The general belief is that in the mouse $Th_1$ and $Th_2$ subsets are derived from a common precursor cell that secretes high levels of IL-2, but little IL-4 or interferon-γ, through a process of antigen-driven extrathymic maturation (9). Other factors that may play a role in driving naive CD4 cells toward differentiation into $Th_1$ or $Th_2$ types are the type of antigen-presenting cells, the nature of the antigen involved, and microenvironmental factors, such as cytokines and hormones, which are thought to regulate $Th_1$ and $Th_2$ balance (10,11). Certain cytokines, such as IL-12, that are powerful interferon-γ inducers, strongly promote $Th_1$ differentiation, whereas IL-4 is by far the most important cytokine

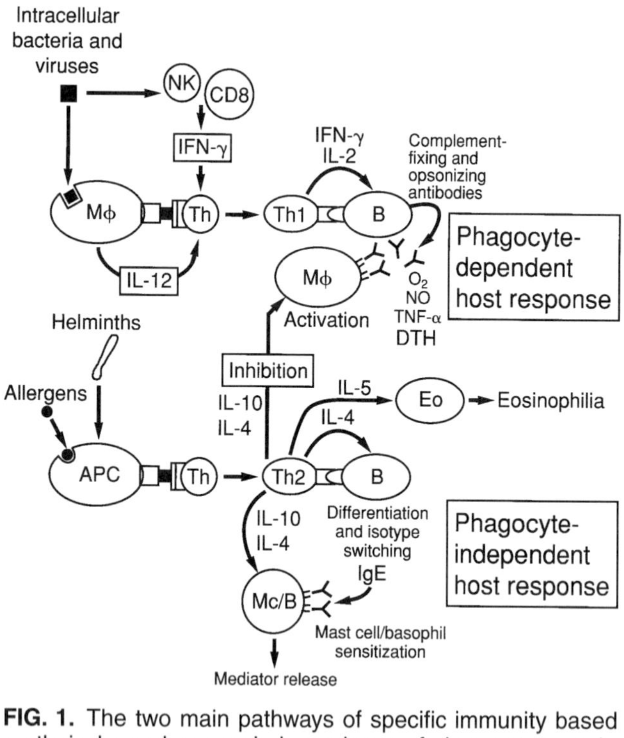


**FIG. 1.** The two main pathways of specific immunity based on their dependence or independence of phagocyte recruitment in the effector response. Th, $CD4^+$ helper T lymphocyte; CD8, $CD8^+$ T lymphocyte; NK, natural killer cell; B, B lymphocyte; DTH, delayed type hypersensitivity; Eo, eosinophilia; APC, antigen preventing cell; Mc/B, cell of the mast cell/basophil lineage; ?, the nature of the cell(s) providing IL-4 at the triad (APC/Ag/Th) recognition level is still unclear. (From ref. 7.)

**TABLE 3.** *Subclasses of T-helper cells*

| T-helper subtypes | $Th_1$ | $Th_2$ | Both |
|---|---|---|---|
| Human | IFN-γ, TNF-β | IL-4, IL-5, IL-9 | GM-CSF, IL-2, IL-3, IL-10, IL-13 |
| Murine | IFN-γ, TNF-β, IL-2 | IL-4, IL-5, IL-6, IL-9, IL-10, IL-13 | GM-CSF, IL-3 |

**TABLE 4.** *Main properties of Th1 and Th2 human CD4⁺ T-cell clones*

| Properties | $Th_1$ | $Th_2$ |
|---|---|---|
| Cytokine secretion | | |
| IFN-γ | +++ | – |
| TNF-β | +++ | – |
| IL-2 | +++ | + |
| TNF-α | +++ | ++ |
| GM-CSF | ++ | ++ |
| IL-3 | ++ | ++ |
| IL-6 | + | +++ |
| IL-10 | + | +++ |
| IL-13 | + | +++ |
| IL-4 | — | +++ |
| IL-5 | — | +++ |
| CD30 expression | + | +++ |
| Regulation by cytokines | | |
| IL-2 | Up | Up |
| IL-4 | | Up |
| IFN-γ | Down | Down |
| IL-10 | +++ | — |
| Cytolysis potential | | |
| B-cell help for Ig synthesis | | |
| IgE | — | +++ |
| IgM, IgG, IgA | | |
| At low T:B cell ratios | +++ | ++ |
| At high T:B cell ratios | — | +++ |
| Macrophage activation | | |
| Induction of PCA | +++ | — |
| TF production | +++ | — |

From ref. 7, p. 123.
+, increased secretion or production; –, decreased secretion or production.

in determining the maturation of naive CD4 cells into $Th_2$ cells.

The discovery of $Th_1$ and $Th_2$ forms of immune responsiveness is very important in our knowledge of the pathogenesis of different diseases of man. Several diseases and other pathophysiologic conditions that are associated with predominant $Th_1$ or $Th_2$ responses are listed in Table 5.

**TABLE 5.** *Pathophysiologic conditions associated with predominant Th1- or Th2-effector responses*

| Th cell subset | Condition |
|---|---|
| $Th_1$ | Autoimmune thyroid diseases |
| | Multiple sclerosis |
| | Type 1 diabetes mellitus |
| | Crohn's disease |
| | Lyme arthritis |
| | Reactive (*Yersinia*-induced) arthritis |
| | Contact dermatitis |
| | Acute allograft refection |
| $Th_2$ | Essential hypereosinophilic syndromes |
| | Vernal conjunctivitis |
| | Atopic disorders (extrinsic asthma allergic rhinitis, atopic eczema) |
| | Reduced protection to many infections |
| | Systemic lupus erythematosus |
| | Progression to AIDS in HIV infection |

Modified from ref. 7, p. 126.

$Th_1$ inflammatory responses may be beneficial when directed against certain pathogenic microorganisms. However, such responses to self antigens are often deleterious, based on animal models of a variety of inflammatory and autoimmune diseases (12,13). It would appear that activation of $Th_1$ responses is central to the pathogenesis of these diseases. Thus, it is possible that inhibition of such autoantigen-specific $Th_1$ responses or administration of $Th_1$-inhibiting cytokines such as IL-10 may be beneficial in the prevention or treatment of these disorders. In other systemic autoimmune diseases, such as systemic lupus erythematosus (SLE), a $Th_2$-type immune response may be involved, particularly in experimental forms of SLE induced by chemicals (14). Atopic diseases, including allergic rhinitis, bronchitis, and atopic dermatitis, are also clearly associated with $Th_2$ responses to common environmental allergens (15–18). IL-4 production by $Th_2$ cells from atopic patients is markedly reduced by specific immunotherapy in the process of clinical improvement (19). Thus, various immunotherapy strategies that downregulate $Th_2$ responses or shift them to $Th_1$ responses are being considered in several disease states (20).

## B Cells

B-cell development begins in the fetal liver and bone marrow between the 8th and 9th week of gestation and continues throughout the lifetime of the host. Early B-cell precursors have immunoglobulin M (IgM) μ chains in their cytoplasm. Development into mature B cells is achieved subsequent to the expression of cytoplasmic and membrane-associated IgM. Mature B cells lose most of their cytoplasmic IgM and acquire surface IgD in addition to IgM. All these changes occur in the absence of antigen (21). Maturation among B lymphocytes continues once they leave the bone marrow environment. Within the peripheral lymphoid organs, certain members of each clone switch from expressing IgM to one of the other major immunoglobulin isotypes (22). Ultimately, the interaction of B cells with antigen and activated helper T cells induces the cells to enter their final stage of development. Terminal differentiation into antibody secreting plasma cells requires additional non–antigen-specific T-cell factors. The ability of the host to mount an antibody response upon repeat exposure to antigen is ensured by B lymphocytes, which have long-lived memory.

### *Third-Population Cells*

Third-population cells (TPCs) are large granular lymphocytes that have a lower nuclear-cytoplasmic ratio and azurophilic cytoplasmic granules (23). They account for as many as 20% of blood lymphocytes. These cells lack the surface antigen receptors of T and B cells, T-cell receptors, and surface immunoglobulin, but their surface phenotype has been delineated with the help of several other monoclonal antibodies to various cytokine and related receptors. A reagent commonly used to identify TPCs is the MAb CD16. The CD16 marker is also expressed by a small number of T cells, by granulocytes, and by some macrophages. Other major surface markers are also present on human TPCs, as is the α chain of the IL-2 receptor. Direct stimulation with IL-2 results in activation of TPCs. TPCs have the ability to kill certain neoplastic cells, virus-infected cells, and other target cells coated with IgG antibodies. Collectively, these activities are referred to as the natural killer (NK) function (24) and antibody-dependent cellular cytotoxicity (ADCC). TPCs also release interferon-γ and other cytokines that are important in facilitating immune and inflammatory responses.

The NK cell activity appears to be regulated by MHC class I molecules as described by the missing self model in which the lack of expression, or masking, of self MHC class I molecules on target cells renders them sensitive to lysis by NK cells (25,26). Recently, cell surface NK cell receptors (NKR) have been identified that are specific for HLA-A, HLA-B, or HLA-C class I molecules and that belong to either the Ig superfamily or the C-type lectin superfamily (27). When NKRs bind to their appropriate MHC molecules, inhibition or activation of NK cell lytic function occurs. Inhibition of NK cell function is the dominant and normal state.

### *Mononuclear Phagocytic and Antigen-Processing Cells*

Cells of the mononuclear phagocyte system derived from the bone marrow consist of two different cell categories that perform different functions. One type of classic phagocytic macrophage has the predominant role of removing particulate antigens. Phagocytic tissue macrophages form a network, the reticuloendothelial system (RES), which is established in many organs. Such monocyte-macrophage cells actively phagocytize organisms *in vitro* and adhere strongly to plastic and glass surfaces. They possess a well-developed Golgi complex and many intracytoplasmic lysosomes, which contain a variety of hydrolases and peroxidases. These are in turn important in killing microorganisms. Human monocyte-macrophages also display multiple surface receptors, many of which are designated or identified by CD markers and have different functions, including triggering of extracellular killing, phagocytosis, and opsonization.

The second group of antigen-processing or antigen-presenting cells (APCs) presents antigen to specific lymphocytes (28). APCs consist of a heterogeneous cell population possessing immunostimulatory capacity. APCs are found primarily in lymph nodes, skin, spleen, and thymus. Some of these cells play a crucial role in the functioning of helper T cells, and others communicate with other leukocytes (29). Among the classic APCs are Langerhans cells of the skin, which migrate via lymphatics into the paracortical areas of draining lymph nodes. Other specialized APCs are the follicular dendritic cells. Still other APC types interdigitate with T cells, providing an efficient mechanism to present antigen carried from other areas, such as the skin, to the draining lymph nodes. Most but not all APC cells have MHC class II surface molecules and other surface markers such as CR1 (CD35).

### *Lymphocyte Activation*

#### *Role of T-Cell Receptor*

T cells possess a definitive surface marker, the T cell-antigen receptor (TCR), of which there are two types: TCR1 and TCR2; both are heterodimers, consisting of two disulfide-length polypeptide chains having some similarity to immunoglobulin molecule chains. Thus, a T cell is defined either by a TCR1 or TCR2, which is associated with the CD3 or pan–T-cell marker (30). The TCR/CD3 complex and other membrane-bound glycoproteins are involved in activating T cells when they are recognized by an appropriate ligand. The TCR recognizes antigen when it is presented on the surface of an APC in the context of some component of the MHC (31). As previously mentioned, helper T cells recognize antigen in the context of class II MHC molecules (HLA-DR), whereas cytotoxic T cells recognize antigen in the context of class I MHC molecules (HLA-A, HLA-B, and HLA-C). When activated by the proper signals, T cells can carry out many functions, including differentiation, proliferation, lymphokine production, and development of effector function. T cells can be specifically activated by an antigen in the context of the proper MHC component and nonspecifically activated by polyclonal activators, such as the plant lectins concanavalin A (ConA) or phytohemagglutinin (PHA). These plant lectins are mitogens interacting with T-cell surface receptors that are different from the antigen-specific TCR. Thus, the response to this type of activation is polyclonal. APCs are also necessary to present these mitogens to T cells. The cellular proliferative response to such a mitogen provides an approximate measure of a person's T-cell functional capacity, although no special antigen-specific clone can be tested by this method. T cell-nonspecific responsiveness is markedly diminished in persons with T-cell defects and in immunosuppressed patients.

When antigen is presented to a T cell by an APC in the context of an MHC that has a specific receptor for that particular antigen-MHC complex, the T cell is activated. Another auxiliary or maturational signal, namely IL-1, is also delivered to the T cell by the APC.

#### *Lymphocyte Stimulation with Mitogens*

Several plant lectins have been used to assess human lymphocyte function. These are generally referred to as

**TABLE 6.** *Nonspecific human lymphocyte mitogens that activate human lymphocytes*

| Mitogen | Abbreviation | Source | Relative specificity |
|---|---|---|---|
| Phytohemagglutinin | PHA | *Phaseolus vulgaris* (kidney bean) | T cells |
| Concanavalin A | ConA | *Canavalia ensiformis* (jack bean) | T cell (different subset from those stimulated by PHA) |
| *Staphylococcus* protein A | SpA,SAC | *Staphylococcus aureus* (Cowan I strain) | B cells, T cell-independent response |
| Pokeweed mitogen | PWM | *Phytolacca americana* | B cells, T cell-dependent |

nonspecific lymphocyte activators or polyclonal mitogens. The substances usually employed, together with their biologic source and relative specificity, are listed in Table 6. There is no evidence that B or T cells can be selectively activated by these mitogens in humans (as they are in rodents), although PHA and ConA are largely mitogenic for T cells, and pokeweed mitogen (PWM) is predominately mitogenic for B cells. Other agents, such as staphylococcal protein A derived from the organism's cell wall, are thought to stimulate human B cells via the IgG Fc receptor. Multiple confounding variables can influence the results of lymphocyte mitogen stimulation assays: possible contamination of cultures with nonlymphoid cells, dose of agent employed, time of incubation, cell-harvesting techniques, cell concentration, and cellular regulatory influences in the culture. Occasionally, mitogens such as ConA can activate suppressor T cells, which may markedly reduce proliferative responses in these particular cultures. Dose-response kinetics are also especially important in lymphocyte activation by mitogens. Altered lymphocyte function can lead to shifts in either dose- or time-response curves to the right or left. Such shifts determine the optimal dose and time of the lymphocyte response. Lymphocyte transformation or responsiveness can also be suppressed or enhanced by multiple nonspecific factors in human serum, and it is important to differentiate this type of humoral modulation of responsiveness to mitogens or antigens from intrinsic suppression of cellular reactivity. Some examples of known lymphocyte-suppressive factors in serum are illustrated in Table 7. The fact that such substances demonstrate suppressive or enhancing effects *in vitro* does not necessarily mean that they act similarly *in vivo*.

Antigens are also used to stimulate smaller numbers of lymphocytes specifically sensitized to the particular antigen under study. Many antigens have been employed in tests for specific lymphocyte activation (Table 8). Most of these antigens are also commonly used to induce delayed hypersensitivity skin test responses. Normal subjects usually demonstrate a good correlation between results obtained with antigen-induced lymphocyte activation and delayed skin test responses.

### *Cytokine and Lymphokine Production*

Following activation, the T cell expands clonally and begins to produce lymphokines or cytokines. A partial list of some lymphokines and related cytokines, including interleukins, interferons, and colony-stimulating factors produced by macrophages, monocytes, and related cell types, together with a list of their targets and activities, is given in Table 9. This collective group of mediators released from antigen-activated T cells represents a group of glycosylated or nonglycosylated polypeptides. Similar cytokines derived from macrophages or other cells are produced under the influence of lymphocyte-derived lymphokines. This large, diverse group of cell-derived mediators can have wide-ranging effects on most organ systems of the body. Studying the biologic role of lymphokines has been difficult, and conflicting results have often been obtained. Three general types of lymphokine-mediated effects have, however, been recognized: (a) costimulant effects—more than one lymphokine is neces-

**TABLE 7.** *Examples of lymphocyte suppressive factors in serum*

| |
|---|
| Serum proteins |
| Albumin (high concentration) |
| Specific antibodies to stimulating antigens |
| Immunoregulatory globulin |
| $\alpha_1$-Acid glycoprotein |
| Pregnancy-associated serum globulins |
| C-reactive protein (CRP) |
| Serum $\alpha$-globulin of amyloid (SAA) |
| $\alpha$-Globulins in cancer, chronic infection, inflammatory diseases |
| $\alpha$-Fetoprotein (AFP) |
| Low-density lipoprotein |
| Antigen-antibody complexes |
| HLA antibodies |
| T cell antibodies |
| Normal serum inhibitors (poorly characterized) |
| Hormones |
| Glucocorticoids |
| Progesterone |
| Estrogens |
| Androgens |
| Prostaglandins |
| Drugs |
| Aspirin |
| Cannabis |
| Chloroquine |
| Ouabain |
| Others |
| Interferon |
| Cyclic nucleotides |
| Chalones |

From ref. 131, vol. 18, p. 294.

**TABLE 8.** *Antigens commonly used to assess human cellular immunity in vitro and in vivo*

| Antigen | Trade name | *In vitro* used | *In vivo* used |
|---|---|---|---|
| Purified protein derivative (PPD) | PPD (Stabilized solution) | X | X |
| *Candida* | Dermatophyton O | X | X |
| Streptokinase/streptodornase | | | X |
| Coccidioidin | Coccidiodin | X | X |
| Tetanus toxoid | Tetanus toxoid | X | X |
| Tumor antigens | | | X |
| Histoincompatible mixed-lymphocyte culture cells | | | X |
| Trichophyton | Dermatophyton | X | |
| Viruses | | | X |

sary to produce an effect; (b) quantitative or dose-dependent effects—a signal from one lymphokine enhances the effect or secretion of another; and (c) a cascading type of activation mediated by a single lymphokine released from an activated cell, which can in turn have a further enhancing effect on the same cell and on other potentially responsive cells.

### *The Interleukins*

The complexity of this system is illustrated by a study of the family of interleukin molecules that mediate many of the effects of T cells on B cells. At least 18 interleukins have been described and their number continues to increase. The best characterized of these is interleukin-1 (IL-1), which is produced by many cell types in response to damage by environmmental agents, pathogens, or antigens.

#### *Interleukin-1 (IL-1)*

The IL-1 family consist of three peptides, IL-1α, IL-1β, and the IL-1 receptor antagonist (IL-1rα or IL-1γ) (32). IL-1α and IL-1β have similar biologic activity and all three proteins interact with similar affinities to the two IL-1 receptors (33). Type I receptors are present on T cells and many other cell types including fibroblasts, endothelial cells, and hepatocytes. On the other hand, type II receptors have been identified on B cells, neutrophils, and bone marrow cells. Type II receptors likely function as the precursor for the soluble IL-1–binding factors (34). IL-1 production may be stimulated by a variety of agents including endotoxins, other cytokines, and microorganisms *(Mycobacterium tuberculosis)* through NF–IL6 (nuclear factor IL-6) and NF-κA binding sites on the promoter (35). One of the most important biologic activities of IL-1 is its function as a lymphocyte activating factor. This includes activation of T cells, B cells, NK cells, and macrophages either directly or indirectly, in order to increase their activity or potentiate their response to other lymphocytes. In the absence of IL-1 no immune response or a state of tolerance develops. IL-1 also enhances B-cell proliferation and increases immunoglobulin synthesis. Administration of IL-1, in addition, produces a bone marrow–derived neutrophilia. IL-1 plays an important role in interacting with the central nervous system (probable astrocytes), subsequently producing fever, lethargy, anorexia, and release of corticotropin-releasing factor. This interleukin also interacts with hepatocytes stimulating synthesis of acute phase response proteins, such as amyloid peptide, C-reactive protein, and complement components. In providing amino acids for this protein synthesis, IL-1 stimulates muscle catabolism, synovial cell proliferation, and bone resorption. These effects of IL-1 on muscles and joints contribute to the arthralgias and myalgias associated with illness. Much of IL-1 proinflammatory activity is due to its induction of arachidonate metabolism with production of many eicosanoids, which function as secondary messengers. IL-1 also induces synthesis of other cytokines, especially TNF, IL-6, and GM-CSF (35). Indeed, it shares many biologic activities with TNF. During the inflammatory process a natural IL-1 receptor antagonist is secreted and upregulated by various cytokines, such as IL-4 and IL-1 itself. Production of IL-1 receptor antagonist modulates the deleterious effects of IL-1 in the natural course of inflammation.

#### *Interleukin-2 (IL-2)*

Interleukin-2, ordinally referred to as T-cell growth factor, has an activating and proliferating effect on T cells and other cell populations (36,37). When T cells are stimulated by antigens in the presence of IL-1, simultaneous secretion of IL-2 occurs together with the expression of high-affinity IL-2 receptors (38,39). The binding of secreted IL-2 to these IL-2r–positive T cells induces T-cell proliferation. IL-2rα (or Tac antigen and CD25) is a glycoprotein (40). IL-2rβ is also glycoprotein with a large intracytoplasmic component (41). The third chain that appears to be essential for high-affinity binding, namely IL-2rγ, has also been identified. Other interleukins, including IL-4, IL-7, IL-9, IL-13, and IL-15, all make use of the γ chain as part of their receptor complexes. IL-2

**TABLE 9.** *Targets and activities of lymphokines and related cytokines*

| Cytokine | Immune system source | Other cells | Principal targets | Principal effects |
|---|---|---|---|---|
| IL-1α<br>IL-1β | Macrophages, large granulocytes, leukocytes, B Cells | Endothelium, fibroblasts, astrocytes, etc. | T cells, B cells, macrophages, endothelium | Lymphocyte activation macrophage stimulation, increased leukocyte and endothelial adhesion, pyrexia, acute-phase proteins |
| IL-2 | T cells | | T cells | T-cell growth factor |
| IL-3 | T cells | | Stem cells | Multilineage colony-stimulating factor |
| IL-4 | T cells | | B cells, T cells | B-cell growth factor |
| IL-5 | T cells | | B cells | B-cell growth and differentiation |
| IL-6 | T cells, B cells, macrophages | Fibroblasts | B cells, hepatocytes | B-cell growth and differentiation, acute-phase response |
| IL-7 | Mononuclear phagocytes | Activated platelets | T cells, B cells | T cell activation |
| IL-8 | Mononuclear phagocytes | Eosinophils, T cells, hepatocytes, epithelial cells, fibroblasts, neutrophils, keratinocytes | Neutrophils, endothelial cells | Neutrophil chemotaxis and endothelial cell adherence, neutrophil degranulation and activation |
| IL-10 | $Th_2$ cells | Mast cells, cytotoxic T cells, B cells | Mononuclear cells, NK cells, $Th_2$ cells, B cells, eosinophils | Inhibits $Th_1$, IFN-γ, and IL-2 production, inhibits eosinophil survival, inhibits IL-4–induced IgE synthesis, inhibits monocyte MHC class II expression, activates (stimulates) B cells and Ig secretion |
| IL-12 | Monocytes, phagocytes | B cells, mast cells | NK cells | Stimulates NK cells and NK cytotoxicity, stimulates IFN-γ and TNF secretion, decreases IL-4 concentration |
| IL-13 | T cells | Mast cells, basophils | B cells, mononuclear cells | Inhibits proinflammatory cytokine production, inhibits allergic responses, inhibits isotope switch to IgE, inhibits expression of low affinity IgE receptors |
| IL-15 | Epithelial cells | Mononuclear cells, muscle, placenta | NK cells, B cells, T cells | T cell growth factor, differentiates NK to LAK cells, stimulates B-cell growth |
| TNF-α | Macrophages, lymphocytes | | Macrophages, granulocytes, tissue cells | Activation of macrophage granulocytes and cytotoxic cells, increased leukocyte and endothelial cell adhesion, cachexia, etc. |
| TNF(LT)-β | T cells | | | |
| IFN-α | Leukocytes | Epithelial fibroblasts | Tissue cells | MHC class I induction, antiviral effect |
| IFN-β | | Epithelial fibroblasts | Tissue cells | MHC class I induction, antiviral effect |
| IFN-γ | T cells, NK cells | Epithelium fibroblasts | Leukocytes, tissue cells | MHC class I induction, macrophage activation, increased endothelial cell and lymphocyte adhesion |
| M-CSF | Monocytes | Endothelium, fibroblasts | Stem cells | Stimulation of division and differentiation |
| Granulocyte-CSF | Macrophages | Fibroblasts | Stem cells | Stimulation of division and differentiation |
| Granulocyte-macriphage CSF | T cells, macrophages | Endothelium, fibroblasts | Stem cells | Stimulation of division and differentiation |
| Macrophage-inhibiting factor | T cells | | Macrophages | Migration inhibition |

From ref. 1, p. 9.9.

receptors are also found on NK cells through which IL-2 causes a more potent cytotoxic response with the differentiation of NK cells into lymphokine-activated killer (LAK) cells (42,43).

Interleukin-2 production has been measured in a variety of immunodeficiencies and autoimmune and related diseases. A marked increase of IL-2, for example, has been noted in certain autoimmune, inflammatory diseases, and production is impaired in a variety of immune deficiency diseases (44–47). Plasma and urine IL-2 receptor levels are also increased during renal allograft rejection and in a variety of inflammatory and infectious diseases.

The IL-2 receptor has also been closely studied using monoclonal antibodies. After cell activation, β chains are actively produced and expressed and receptors are then referred to as being of the high-affinity variety. The β-chain component (Tac peptides) of the IL-2 receptor, often referred to as the soluble IL-2 receptor or as sIL-2r, is released by activated T-cells during many immune-mediated inflammatory responses, including autoimmune diseases, graft versus host reactions, infectious and parasitic diseases, lymphoreticular disorders, multiple sclerosis, and acquired immune deficiency syndrome (AIDS), among others. In some autoimmune diseases, such as SLE and rheumatoid arthritis, high serum levels of IL-2 and IL-2r have been correlated with disease activity.

### *Interleukin-3 (IL-3)*

Interleukin-3 is a potent regulator of growth and differentiation of many hematopoietic and lymphoid progenitor cells (48). It has not been well studied in human diseases, but may play an important role in certain allergic and hematologic diseases.

### *Interleukin-4 (IL-4)*

Interleukin-4 was originally termed B-cell growth factor (49). It is produced by T helper cells, as well as cytotoxic T cells, mast cells, and basophils. It also plays an important role in stimulating MHC class II antigens and low-affinity IgE receptor expression by B cells, resulting in increased antigen-presenting ability of these cells (50). In addition, it induces the immunoglobulin isotope switch from IgM to IgE (51,52). IL-4 synergizes with other interleukins including IL-2, IL-5, and IL-6 to increase secretion of IgE, and IL-4 is absolutely essential for IgE production (53). For example, so called IL-4 knockout mice that are genetically engineered to lack the IL-4 gene are completely unable to synthesize IgE (54), whereas mice that have been engineered to secrete large amounts of IL-4 demonstrate markedly increased IgE levels (55). IL-4 also acts as a growth factor for T-cell function in certain kinds of allergic inflammation. It increases production of cytotoxic T cells and activates NK and LAK cells. Conversely, it has inhibitory effects on ADCC, and down-regulates production of IL-1, IL-6, and TNF-α (56). Finally, IL-4 induces increased adhesiveness of endothelium for T cells, basophils, and other cells by inducing expression of vascular cell adhesion molecule-1 on endothelial cells.

### *Interleukin-5 (IL-5)*

Interleukin-5 was also identified earlier as a B-cell stimulating factor. It is produced by T-helper cells, eosinophils, and mast cells. It interacts with specific receptors composed of α and β chains. IL-5 is now known to be the most important stimulator of eosinophils, inducing maturation of these cells when it interacts with bone marrow precursor cells (57). IL-5 is also chemotactic for eosinophils and it activates mature cells. In addition, it prolongs the survival of these cells and limits apoptosis of eosinophils. IL-5 levels are increased in the hypereosinophilic syndrome, eosinophilia-myalgia syndrome (58), and after bronchial challenge testing. Certain colony-stimulating factors, including IL-3, GM-CSF (59,60), and certain members of the chemokine family, also contribute to the activity of eosinophils and allergic inflammation.

### *Interleukin-6 (IL-6)*

Interleukin-6 plays a very important role in stimulating the final stages of B-lymphocyte maturation into mature plasma cells that secrete immunoglobulins. It is a costimulus for ConA activation of T cells. It also mediates T-cell differentiation, growth, and activation, and like IL-1 induces febrile and acute-phase responses (35). It also stimulates mononuclear phagocytic cells to differentiate and hematopoietic cells to proliferate. Among its other activities are those of neutrophil activation, destruction of tumor cells, and possession of antiviral activity. IL-6 is produced by mononuclear phagocytic cells as well as T cells, B cells, fibrinogen keratinocytes, hepatocytes, neuroglial cells, and bone marrow stromal cells (61,62).

### *Interleukin-7 (IL-7)*

Like IL-6, IL-7 is a costimulus for ConA activation of T cells (63). It is also a growth stimulus for pre–B cells. Its effect in human diseases is not well studied.

### *Interleukin-8 (IL-8) and the Chemokine Family*

Interleukin-8 is the most completely studied member of the so-called chemokine superfamily (64). It is derived from mononuclear phagocytes, eosinophils, T cells, hepatocytes, fibroblasts, keratinocytes, neutrophils, epithelial cells, and chondrocytes. IL-8 is one of the most powerful neutrophil chemotactic cytokines. It also stimulates degranulation of these cells and adherence to endothelial cells.

The chemokines taken as a whole are a family of proteins structurally and functionally related. They include at least 13 members in addition to IL-8 (64). These consist of small proinflammatory cytokines exhibiting up to 50% of homology in amino acid sequence. Some members of the chemokine family including platelet factor-4, macrophage inflammatory protein (MIP), 1α, and neutrophil-activating protein 2, and all share the ability to activate neutrophils. Other members of this family including RANTES, MIP, and monocyte chemotactic peptides (MCP-1) and (MCP-3) contribute uniquely to allergic inflammation by acting as histamine-releasing agents from basophils and mast cells. RANTES is also very effective as a basophil chemoattractant. Conversely, IL-8 inhibits cytokine-mediated histamine release by basophils.

*Interleukin-10 (IL-10)*

Interleukin-10 is a $Th_2$ lymphocyte product that inhibits $Th_1$ IFN-γ and IL-2 production. It can also be produced by other cells including $Th_1$ cells, mast cells, cytotoxic T cells, and B cells. IL-10 inhibits production of IL-1β, IL-6, IL-8, IL-12, and TNF-α by mononuclear cells (65–67), IL-4 and IL-5 by $Th_2$ cells (68), and IFN-γ and TNF-α by NK cells (69). IL-10 also inhibits MHC class II expression by monocytes as well as accessory cell function. Since it inhibits survival of eosinophils and IL-4–induced IgE synthesis, it may play an important modulator role in allergic diseases of man. Conversely, with regard to B lymphocytes, IL-10 functions as an activating factor, stimulating cell production and immunoglobulin secretion (70). Overall, IL-10 inhibits cytokines associated with allergic inflammation and cellular immunity (71). On the other hand, it stimulates humoral and cytotoxic immune responses. The appearance of IL-10 correlates with and may contribute to the downregulation of proinflammatory cytokines. TNF-α is a potent stimulus for IL-10 secretion. These studies suggest a type of feedback mechanism in which an inflammatory stimulus induces TNF-α, which in turn stimulates IL-10 secretion with ultimate feedback into the system to dampen TNF-α synthesis.

*Interleukin-12 (IL-12)*

Interleukin-12 was first described as the stimulatory factor for NK cells (72,73). It is derived from monocytes and phagocytes as well as from B cells and mast cells. It not only stimulates production of NK cells, but it enhances their cytotoxicity and causes secretion of IFN-γ and TNF-α. IL-12 induces increasing concentrations of IFN-γ and decreasing concentrations of IL-4 in responding antigen-specific lymphocytes (74). IL-12–mediated IFN-γ production is likely required for the full expression of the $Th_1$ phenotype (75).

Since mononuclear phagocytes are the major source of IL-12 production, it is probable that antigens processed by macrophages such as intracellular obligate and facultative microorganisms (e.g., mycobacteria, viruses, and other intracellular pathogens) produce predominant $Th_1$ responses.

*Interleukin-13 (IL-13)*

Interleukin-13 shares many of the biologic activities of IL-4 on B cells and mononuclear cells. IL-13 inhibits proinflammatory cytokine production and it induces the IgE isotype switch (76,77). Its receptor is a heterotrimer containing the IL-4r, IL-2rγ, and a unique IL-13–binding component. IFN-γ is also very important in regulation of IgE synthesis. It acts as an inhibitor of allergic responses through its ability to inhibit IL-4–mediated expression of low affinity IgE receptors and the isotype switch to IgE. Thus IgE production appears to be facilitated by a combination of excess IL-4 and IL-13 occurring in the absence of IFN-γ.

*Interleukin-15 (IL-15)*

Interleukin-15 competes for binding sites with IL-2 and has a similar activity to IL-2. IL-15 is produced by epithelium, fibroblasts, mononuclear phagocytic cells, muscle, and placenta (78). Like IL-2, IL-15 is a T-cell growth factor. It differentiates NK into LAK cells, is chemotactic for T-lymphocytes, and stimulates B-cell growth and differentiation.

***Interferon-γ (IFN-γ)***

This is the most important cytokine involved in macrophage activation and cell-mediated immunity (79). It is produced in large quantities by Th lymphocytes, but also to some extent by NK and cytotoxic T cells. It increases class I and II MHC expression stimulating antigen presentation and cytokine production by monocytes. It also stimulates adherence, phagocytosis, and tumoricidal activity of those cells. Overall, it results in accumulation of activated macrophages at the sites of inflammatory cellular immune responses. Like IL-1 and TNF, IFN-γ also induces intercellular adhesion molecule (ICAM-1), thus further stimulating granulocyte adherence to endothelial cells (80). In addition it is an important inhibitor of viral replication and is thought to be an inhibitor of allergic responses via its ability to inhibit IL-4's immediate effects on B cells with a subsequent decrease in IgE secretion.

### *Transforming Growth Factor-β (TGF-β)*

This is a family of peptides that regulate cell growth either via stimulation or inhibition (81). Mesenchymal cells are the main source of TGF-β. TGF-β receptors are present on all cells and TGF-β mediates multiple biologic activities including stimulation of fibrosis and formation of extracellular matrix. It is also inhibitory for B-cell immunoglobulin secretion and cytotoxicity of natural killer cells. The expression of TGF-β during the process of allergic inflammation is often associated with fibrosis, such as that seen in subendocardial hypereosinophilic syndrome.

### *Tumor Necrosis Factor (TNF)*

Tumor necrosis factor consists of two homologous proteins (TNF-α and TNF-β). These proteins were organically described as possessing antitumor effects, and they are directly cytotoxic to neoplastic cells, stimulating antitumor responses by immune cells and inducing hemorrhagic necrosis of neoplasms (82,83). They also induce ICAM-1 expression, permitting the movement of granulocytes into inflammatory areas (80). In addition, they stimulate cartilage degradation, bone resorption, and monocyte and B-cell activation, and they increase the ability of other monocytes to produce inflammatory mediators, such as IL-6 and IL-8. TNF possesses antiviral activity that activates neutrophils and stimulates MHC class I and II expression (84). The severe cachexia and wasting that occurs in cancer and neoplasms in chronic infections is likely caused by TNF due to its capacity to inhibit the enzyme lipoprotein lipase (82). TNF-α and TNF-β are produced by mononuclear phagocytes. TNF-α is also synthesized by neutrophils, lymphocytes, natural killer cells, smooth muscle, and endothelial cells.

## *B-Cell Activation*

A variety of stimuli trigger B-cell activation (83). At least two cytokines contribute to B-lymphocyte maturation in the bone marrow: the lymphoid stem cell growth factors IL-7 and IL-11. IL-6 is essential for the final differentiation of B cells into immunoglobulin-secreting plasma cells (84). The cytokines IL-4 and IL-13 induce isotype switching to the IgE isotype, and TGF-β triggers the IgA isotype switch. IL-10 contributes to generation of IgG isotypes. Many of the cytokines influence B-cell maturation, but are not directly involved in isotype switching.

Specific activation of B cells involves antigen that is complementary to the particular immunoglobulin on the cell surface. B cells can recognize antigen in its free state, unlike T cells. Nonspecific B-cell activation also occurs and involves B-cell mitogens. When activated in the resting state B cells can enlarge, divide, mature, and differentiate into antibody secreting plasma cells.

In the case of so-called T-cell–dependent triggering by certain complex protein antigens, antigen processing cells (APCs) present antigen to a cell that becomes activated and secretes cytokines in contact with specific antigens. Cytokines enable the B cells to transform into antibody-secreting plasma cells that produce antibodies of the classic Ig specific classes (IgG, A, M, D, or E). In other cases, especially when certain polysaccharide antigens are involved, B cells can be triggered directly in a T-cell–independent manner. These antigens are referred to as T-cell–independent antigens. In general, such antigens induce primarily weak IgM responses and poor immune system memory.

## *Immune Response Regulation*

The intensity of an immune response results from a net balance of factors that tend to either amplify or depress the response. Virtually all immune responses are so regulated, and aberrations of immunoregulation are thought to be important in the expression of such variable as autoimmunity, tolerance, hypersensitivity, and perhaps even aging. Immune responses can also be self-regulated. According to the network theory of Jerne (85), all antigen receptors (idiotypes) on T and B cells are capable of inducing complementary anti-idiotypic T or B cells, which by themselves or through their self-products can down-regulate production of the original idiotope. For example, a certain antigen provokes the production of antibody, and this antibody and the B cell that manufactures it bear an antigen receptor, or idiotope, capable of stimulating another clone of B cells to make anti-idiotypic antibodies directed against this antigen receptor.

The host's genetic composition also plays a role in determining immune responsiveness. When an organism fails to respond to certain antigens, in almost all cases the genetic defect can be mapped to part of the MHC. In some cases, immune system unresponsiveness may be associated with inability to manufacture a receptor on T or B cells for a particular antigen. In other cases, an overwhelming stimulation of suppressor rather than helper T cells may occur, leading to tolerance rather than immunity. In humans the linkage between certain autoimmune diseases and haplotypes of the MHC serves as an example of genetic aspects of immunoregulation. This occurs in such diseases as Reiter's syndrome, ankylosing spondylitis, myasthenia gravis, celiac disease, Addison's disease, and insulin-dependent diabetes mellitus, among others (86). The basis for the specific responsiveness of patients with common atopic or IgE-mediated allergic respiratory tract disease is also ill defined but definitely genetic; it predisposes them to overproduce IgE.

## ENVIRONMENTAL AGENTS AND THE IMMUNE SYSTEM

### Environmental Agents and Immunoresponsiveness

In addition to acting as antigens and inducing specific immunity or hypersensitivity states, environmental agents can potentially inhibit or enhance immune responsiveness in a nonspecific immunomodulatory manner at multiple levels. An environmental agent may, for example, exert selective toxicity for one cell type and affect principally only one detectable effector activity, such as TPC (e.g., NK cell) activity or immunoglobulin production by B cells. Conversely, it may affect the development of a bone marrow–derived lymphocyte progenitor cell, resulting in pan immune system suppression. In addition, in the adult host, inhibition or stimulation by an environmental agent of IL-1 secretion, IL-2 synthesis, or the function of other interleukins or their receptors might also result in T-cell, B-cell, or TPC dysfunction.

Discussion of the large number of chemicals, metals, and related inorganic environmental agents alleged to affect the immune system is beyond the scope of this brief review. A few of these agents that affect the immune system in experimental animals, including pesticides, herbicides, solvents, combustion products, and metals, are listed in Table 10. Here we discuss only a few of these substance that have widely recognized environmental significance, to illustrate their potential effects on the immune system.

**TABLE 10.** *Environmental chemicals and related substances reported to affect the immune system in experimental animals*

| Substance (source) | Alteration of immune function |
|---|---|
| Benzo[a]pyrene (incomplete combustion of coal and other fossil fuels) | Decreased antibody production by pulmonary lymph node cells |
| 7,12-Demethylbenz[a]anthracene (incomplete fossil fuel combustion) | Decreased splenic antibody production, decreased resistance to bacterial infection and tumor challenge |
| 3,3′,4,4′-Tetrachloroazoxybenzene (manufacture and degradation of herbicides) | Decreased thymic weight, decreased splenic antibody production, inhibition of macrophage function, depression of bone marrow cellularity |
| Toxaphene (insecticide) | Decreased antibody production, suppressed delayed hypersensitivity responses, reduced macrophage phagocytosis |
| Trichloroethylene (chemical solvent) | Decreased antibody- and cell-mediated immune responses, inhibition of bone marrow stem cell colonization |
| Carbofuran, diazinon (pesticides) | Alteration of serum immunoglobulin levels |
| Chlordane (insecticide) | Depressed contact (T-cell) hypersensitivity |
| Pentachlorophenol (PCP) (pesticide) | Increased tumor susceptibility, reduced susceptibility to viral challenge, suppression of T-cell cytotoxicity, increased macrophage phagocytosis |
| Formaldehyde (cigarette smoke, auto exhaust, smog, incinerators, biomedical research, insulation, industrial processes) | Enhanced resistance to bacterial challenge |
| Nitrogen dioxide (oxidant air pollutant, tobacco smoke) | Alteration of antibody in lung-associated lymph node cells |
| Sulfur dioxide (oxidant air pollutant) | Depressed resistance to bacterial infection |
| Cigarette smoke | Depressed mitogen responses, increased IgE level |
| Fly ash (coal combustion) | Decreased splenic antibody responses |
| Diesel exhaust | Alterations of alveolar macrophages and polymorphonuclear leukocytes, depressed interferon production |
| Organic and inorganic mercurials (natural and industrial contaminant-pesticides, food, etc.) | Induction of autoimmune disease |
| Tin (canning processed food) | Decreased splenic antibody responses |
| Titanium dioxide (paints, cigars) | Abnormalities of macrophage morphology and enzyme production |
| Lead (paints, welding, battery production, smelting, gasoline combustion) | Depressed serum immunoglobulins and complement levels, decreased salivary IgA, depressed antibody-dependent cellular cytotoxicity |
| Silica (sandblasting, glass industry, mining) | Altered T- and B-cell function, antinuclear antibody formation and autoimmune-like disease |
| Cadmium (electroplating, paint and battery manufacture, smelting) | Altered T- and B-cell function, antinuclear antibody formation, immunosuppression, antiglomerular basement membrane antibody |
| Mercury compounds (paints, pharmaceuticals, fungicides, jewelry) | Autoantibody formation, decreased neutrophil chemotaxis, hypergammaglobulinemia |
| Beryllium salts (alloy production; aerospace, electronics, nuclear industries) | Delayed (cell-mediated) hypersensitivity, lymphocyte transformation, lymphokine production |

Studies of experimental animal models have demonstrated the extent and specificity with which some environmental toxins, chemicals, and drugs affect various biologic targets in general and the immune system in particular. It is well known that treatment of certain experimental animals with comparatively high concentrations of environmental toxins (such as those listed in Table 10), can result in bacterial and fungal infections, raising the possibility of environmentally induced immunosuppression. A variety of environmental agents, chemicals, and immunnodepressive drugs are also known to act, collectively or individually, on cellular components of the immune system. Such agents have been used to suppress or dampen hypersensitivity and inflammatory responses in humans. Some immunosuppressive agents such as corticosteroids have multiple actions, among which are the ability to affect lymphocyte trafficking, to inhibit the release of cytokines, and to decrease the formation of inflammatory arachidonic acid metabolites such as prostaglandins and leukotrienes (87). Others, such as the alkylating agent cyclophosphamide, inhibit the division of sensitized lymphocytes and affect CD8 suppressor cells. The agent cyclosporine inhibits helper T-cell function and IL-2 production (88). Certain elements present in trace amounts also have profound effects on the immune system. Beryllium sulfate, for example, can both stimulate and inhibit lymphocyte metabolism and has induced delayed hypersensitivity skin test reactivity and lymphokine production by appropriately sensitized T cells (89,90). Calcium is required during the proliferative stage of the antibody response, but it inhibits the differentiation of spleen cells into immunoglobulin-secreting cells (91). Other metallic salts and fumes, such as nickel, chromium, and platinum compounds, can induce immediate IgE-mediated hypersensitivity reactions (92). Certain metals and related alloys are also well-known causative agents of hypersensitivity conditions such as asthma in humans. These include zinc, vanadium, cobalt, and stainless steel welding fumes among others (93–96).

### Concept of Immunotoxicology

Because of the continued introduction of natural and man-made contaminants into the environment, considerable attention has been focused on various aspects of "immunotoxicology." This field might be defined as the study of the immune system and its cellular components as target organs for detection of general or selective chemically induced toxicity. In spite of the perceived magnitude of this problem, there is a paucity of sound data on the effects on the human immune system of trace amounts of environmental chemicals.

In addition to simple chemicals, other toxic pollutants of aquatic or atmospheric origin, including pesticides, agricultural runoff from fertilizers, acid rain, sludge, garbage, and oil dumping into our oceans, have the potential of posing public health hazards (97). Many of these pollutants can be encountered outdoors as well as in workplaces and homes. Exposure to "immunotoxicants" at dose levels below those that induce severe organ toxicity have the potential to affect the immune system as a primary large target system or to injure the immune system as a secondary target system when the primary target is another organ or system such as lungs, skin, nervous system, or thyroid. When the immune system is a primary target, the immunotoxicant may act simultaneously as a toxin and an antigen, sensitizing the host to future exposure. This is the case with simple elements, such as beryllium, and with many other simple chemicals, such as toluene diisocyanate (TDI) and trimellitie anhydride (TMA), which are known to cause immunologically specific hypersensitivity states but also have profound toxic effects in higher doses. Immunotoxicants may also act as immune response modifiers by inhibiting or enhancing immune reactivity. There is, for example, some evidence for increase in IgE antibody production against common inhalant allergens in association with increasing industrialization and with cigarette smoking (98). Exposure to high levels of ozone has also been reported to augment allergic responses (99), and both diesel exhaust particulates and cigarette smoke have been reported to enhance serum IgE levels and specific IgE antibody production (100,101). The great need to establish diagnostic criteria for alleged affects of "immunotoxins" is emphasized by the increased litigation of cases involving workplace or environmental exposure.

### Environmental Agents and Autoimmunity

Experimental autoimmune diseases, hypergammaglobulinemia, and autoantibody formation have been induced by elemental salts such as mercuric chloride, cadmium, and gold thiomalate. Cadmium, for example, has been reported to induce antinuclear antibody formation in approximately 90% of rodents exposed to this simple element in low concentration (102). Cadmium also has a known immunosuppressive effect in experimental animals. Mercuric chloride is known to induce autoimmune disease in rats and mice with production of autoantibody to the nuclear antigen fibrillen and hypergammaglobulinemia, particularly of the IgE isotype (103). It has been postulated that mercury compounds may cause polyclonal B-cell activation. Gold thiomalate has also been reported to induce antinuclear antibody formation in experimental animals (104).

The mechanism by which these agents induce autoantibody formation currently is unknown. Preliminary evidence suggests, however, that certain nonhistone acid nuclear protein antigens, distinct from DNA and collectively referred to as small nuclear ribonucleoproteins (snRNPs), are capable of being altered by environmental agents such as toxins or infectious agents and rendered immunogenic. SnRNPs represent subcellular intranuclear protein–nucleic acid assemblies or particles that regulate important intracellular events such as pre–messenger RNA (mRNA) splicing. Other nucleoprotein autoantigens are also proving to be of interest in studying potential mechanisms of DNA synthesis and replication. The immune specificity of autoantibodies to these antigens and their relationship to certain autoimmune connective tissue diseases has been thoroughly reviewed (105–107), and it is reasonable to postulate that the immune response to these autoantigens may be driven or directed principally by external environmental agents such as viruses, environmental chemicals, and drugs (108,109). Indeed, some clinical clues to our understanding of how chemicals and other environmental agents may "drive" an immune response to these autoantigens might be provided from continued studies of the autoantibody formation induced by mercuric chloride, cadmium, and gold thiomalate, and from a study of the antihistone antibodies of drug-induced lupus.

In addition to chemicals binding with autoantigens and changing their conformational structure or exposing hidden determinants, it is also possible that chemically induced tissue damage may release autoantigens that were sequestered, resulting in an immune response to the previously sequestered unrecognized determinants. Cross-reactivity between antigenic determinants on chemical agents that are shared with tissue autoantigens has also been postulated. Such cross-reactivity is known to occur with bacteria, but nothing is known about similar cross-reactivity with chemicals. In other cases, chemicals may cause immunoregulatory aberrations. Methyldopa, which has been shown to have effects on suppressor T cells; silica, which can induce autoimmune phenomena and autoantibody formation in humans; and asbestos fibers, which are known to act simultaneously as polyclonal B-cell stimulants and as suppressors of certain T-cell functions, are illustrative examples of such agents (110).

Although little is known about the relationship between environmental chemicals and possible autoimmune disease, there is growing suspicion of a possible association between the two. As an example, numerous autoimmune-like responses have been noted in patients treated with penicillamine. Among the responses to penicillamine have been syndromes resembling systemic lupus erythematosus with autoantibodies to native double-stranded DNA, autoantibodies to thyroid and chronic thyroiditis, bullous pemphigoid with anti-skin basement membrane antibodies, and pemphigus vulgaris with autoantibodies to skin intracellular substance.

## Environmental Agents, the Immune System, and Carcinogenesis

### *The Immune Surveillance Theory of Carcinogenesis*

In this section we review the potential modulatory and carcinogenic properties of certain organic chemicals as they relate to (a) their possible effect on the immune system and (b) the use of certain immunologic tests as diagnostic aids to detect immune system damage.

Advances in biotechnology and molecular biology are contributing to our understanding of the immunology of cancer in general. New diagnostic procedures have improved the sensitivity and specificity of diagnostic techniques for detecting neoplasms, and aided in their classification. The immune surveillance theory of carcinogenesis, which originally derived from our earlier observations that MHC-restricted cytotoxic T cells were involved in graft rejection and that certain types of neoplasms occurred in increased incidence in immunosuppressed persons, has remained a controversial subject. Against this theory is the known observation that thymectomized or athymic mice, which lack functioning T cells, do not have an abnormally high incidence of neoplasms. Furthermore, most spontaneous or non–virus-induced neoplastic cells do not appear to manifest strong tumor-associated antigens on their surface and may not be detected by a specific cellular immune response. It may be that the immune system is important in virus-induced neoplasms or other neoplasms that display some type of strong tissue-specific antigens on their surface rather than neoplasms induced in experimental animals by environmental toxicants. On the other hand, other lymphoid cells of the immune system, such as NK cells and LAK cells, do not necessarily require the presence of MHC antigens to recognize foreign or neoplastic cells as cytotoxic T cells do (111,112).

Contrary to T-cell activation, NK-cell function is reportedly inhibited by recognition of MHC class I and becomes functional in the absence of or, with reduced expression of one or more MHC class I molecules (25,26,113). It is possible that interfering with their numbers or function may increase tumorigenesis. For example, depressed macrophage function has been reported to increase the incidence of tumors. The accumulation of NK cells and tumor-infiltrating lymphocytes (TILs) has been shown to reduce growth and metastatic potential (114,115). In addition, some chemical carcinogens have been shown to reduce NK-cell function. TILs, a heterogeneous group of cells that are isolated directly from tissue neoplasms, NK, and LAK cells are capable of interacting with a variety of neoplastic cell types that are refractive to cytotoxic lymphocytes. The immune system, considered in this broad context, may be capable of serving as a surveillance system for the expression of spontaneous or environmentally induced neoplasms. One might predict that the depression of such relevant effector mechanisms by some carcinogenic environmental chemicals would increase the incidence of neoplasms or metastasis. Likewise, enhancement of the activities of these cell types might theoretically result in a decreased incidence of neoplasms or metastasis. Nonetheless, most human neoplasms are weakly immunogenic and induce little or no rejection potential in any given patient, in spite of their capability of inducing immunoresponsiveness, including antibody formation.

### *Polycyclic Aromatic Hydrocarbons*

Polycyclic aromatic hydrocarbons (PAH) are the result of forest fires, decay of organic matter, burning refuse, and burning fossil fuels (petroleum products and coal), and therefore are widespread in the environment. Exposure to PAHs occurs from daily living, e.g., breathing, eating or drinking contaminated food and water, and smoking. Many of the PAHs, beginning with benzo-[$\alpha$]-pyrene (BAP) found in coal tar (116), have been shown to be carcinogenic. As with most environmental pollutants, few data are available on the immunotoxic effects of these compounds in humans. In general, the carcinogenic PAHs have toxic effects on the immune system in experimental animals. PAHs suppress cell-mediated and humoral immunity and may also have suppressive affects on macrophages and other cellular components of the immune system. The ability to suppress and the degree to which PAHs induce immunosuppression depend on their route of administration, dose, duration of exposure, and, in mice, the strain used.

The PAH most extensively studied in experimental animals for its affects on cell-mediated immunity is 7,12-dimethylbenz-[d]-anthracene (DMBA). DMBA is a potent carcinogen. Following *in vivo* exposure of mice, DMBA has been shown to suppress T-cell mitogen ConA and PHA responses, the mixed lymphocyte reaction (MLR), cytotoxic T lymphocyte generation and activity, cutaneous delayed-type hypersensitivity reactions (DTH), allograft rejection of skin and hearts, NK-cell activity, and production of all forms of interferon (IFN). DMBA also has profound suppressive effects on humoral immunity as measured by serum antibody titers, plaque-forming cell assays (PFC), antibody-dependent cellular cytotoxicity, and resistance to bacterial infections. The suppressive effects of DMBA can be immediate and persist for weeks to months. Following injection into neonates DMBA has been reported to suppress the humoral response permanently. Both T-cell–dependent and T-cell–independent antibody responses are affected. Studies by various investigators have suggested that B cells and B-cell precursors, antigen-presenting cells (APC), or T-helper cells are the primary targets.

3-Methylcholanthrene (MCA) and BAP (strong and moderate carcinogens, respectively) have also been shown to exert suppressive effects on the immune system and can be selective for a particular arm of the immune response. While MCA affects cell-mediated and humoral immunity similarly to DMBA, BAP has less effect on cell-mediated immunity than on humoral immunity. An increased tumor susceptibility following subchronic exposure of mice to BAP was reported at the same time that susceptibility to *Listeria* monocytogenes was unal- •14•
tered. Additionally, exposure to BAP resulted in suppression to TNP-ficoll (a T-independent antigen that stimulates mature B cells) but not to TNP-LPS (a T-independent antigen that stimulates immature B cells), suggesting that BAP acts on mature B cells. DMBA exposure resulted in a persistent suppression to both conjugates, implicating a B-cell precursor effect. The ability of PAHs to suppress humoral immunity is not limited to direct exposure. The PFC response to sheep red blood cells (SRBCs) in mice exposed to BAP in utero (i.e., maternal exposure) was suppressed into adulthood (117).

There is some evidence that the immunosuppressive effects of PAHs are due to cytochrome P-450–dependent metabolic breakdown products similar to those involved in their carcinogenic effect, and binding to Ah receptors inducing Ah gene complex activation (118).

#### *Antibodies*

Monoclonal antibodies (MAbs) have been of help in the serologic classification of tumor-associated antigens. Antibodies have been demonstrated in the serum of humans in association with a variety of neoplasms; their presence has not correlated with host resistance to specific neoplasms. Antibodies are known to mediate antitumor activity via opsonization, complement-dependent cell lysis, enhanced cytotoxicity, phagocytosis, and other mechanisms. There is, however, no strong evidence that these mechanisms are significant in reducing tumor burden of common neoplasms.

#### *T Cells*

Probably the most important immune response to neoplasms has been the T-cell response, which reflects the function of helper-inducer CD4 cells and suppressor cytotoxic CD8 cells. Most neoplasms in humans appear to be poorly immunogenic, and special tests are needed to detect specific cytolytic T-cell activity.

#### *Natural Killer Cells*

Although these cells can bind to and destroy tumor cells *in vitro* via the mechanism of antibody-dependent cellular cytotoxicity (ADCC) or engagement of the activating type of NK-cell receptors, little is known about their role *in vivo* in humans. Data are also insufficient to determine whether ADCC plays a role in tumor resistance in humans. NK cells, however, appear to play an important role in preventing metastasis. Although abnormalities of activity or numbers of NK cells have been reported in cancer and other diseases such as viral infections, autoimmunity, AIDS, and chronic fatigue syndrome, measurement of NK numbers or function cannot be considered to be of diagnostic utility at this time.

*Macrophages*

Macrophages are known to kill neoplastic cells directly through a form of ADCC and through release of cytocidal lysosomal enzymes. They may also indirectly help control growth of neoplasms by producing toxic arachidonic acid metabolites and cytokines. They accumulate in areas of spontaneous tumor regression in humans, but their exact role in controlling human neoplasms is unknown.

*Tumor Infiltrating Lymphocytes*

Tumor infiltrating lymphocytes (TILs) are lymphoid cells of diverse types that actually infiltrate solid neoplasms. Following intravenous inoculation they can survive several months in the circulation or at the tumor site. Retrovirus-mediated gene transfection can provide marker genes to detect and trace those cells.

Therapy with autologous TIL and IL-2 used to treat patients with malignant melanoma has achieved a 38% remission rate (115). Attempts are under way to optimize TIL therapeutic efficacy by employing retrovirus-mediated gene transfection with vectors that express cytokines such as tumor necrosis factor (TNF). In this manner, the lymphocyte may, in essence, serve as a drug delivery agent for transporting potent toxic agents such as TNF directly to tumor sites, augmenting therapeutic efficiency, and reducing systemic toxicity.

Thus, in many experimental animal models, a wide range of antigen-specific and -nonspecific factors can decrease growth of neoplasms, but data are insufficient to allow conclusions about humans. Some investigators have postulated that synthetic chemicals that are known carcinogens in rodents pose little or no risk of inducing human neoplasms. This view is based on, among other things, the premise that the very large doses employed in studies of rodent carcinogenesis cause tumors principally by inducing cytotoxicity, with resulting compensatory cell proliferation that, in turn, converts DNA damage into mutations. These facts notwithstanding, evidence is still inadequate to understand the mechanisms (including immunosurveillance) by which carcinogens exert their effects, and no safe exposure levels or thresholds for diverse human populations are identifiable. It is likely that, in the final analysis, further studies of the molecular biology of carcinogenesis will discover a far more complex combination of mechanisms of tumor induction than those dominated simply by mitogenesis, immunosurveillance, or any other single pathogenic mechanism (119).

**Potential Forms of Immunotoxin- and Lymphokine Receptor-Directed Immunotherapy**

The development of recombinant DNA technology has facilitated production and characterization of cytokines that regulate immune responses in general. Development of MAb technology has allowed identification and selective targeting of specific inflammation-inducing cell subsets and surface molecules to dampen or decrease inflammatory responses caused by environmental poisons, autoantigens, viruses, and related agents. The MHC-associated APC-T cell interaction results in the production of immunoregulatory cytokines such as interleukins and IFN-γ, which modulate the inflammatory response. All of the interleukins appear to play central roles in the regulation and growth of various lymphoid cell populations (120). IL-2 is important in regulating T-cell growth, and the IL-2 receptor is a potential therapeutic target for interfering with IL-2's function. MAb and radiolabeled IL-2 have been used in attempts to chemically characterize several high-affinity and low-affinity subunits or subtypes of the IL-2 receptor. For example, it has been determined that resting or normal monocytes, B cells, and T cells do not express the β chain of the IL-2 receptor. This receptor peptide is expressed by certain abnormal cells and released into the serum in certain autoimmune diseases, lymphomas, allograft rejections, and B-cell, T-cell, and monocytic leukemias. Anti-TAC antibodies can be used as a diagnostic aid to determine the expression of IL-2 receptors on T cells from patients with these diseases. This has provided a basis for therapeutic strategies that could potentially eliminate IL-2 receptor-expressing cells. A better understanding of IL-2 and its receptor system is opening the door for possible immune intervention in several of the above-mentioned diseases, and MAbs that might inhibit or enhance the activity of regulatory cytokines are being used experimentally as potential therapeutic agents. Similar agents, including "blocking" or "inhibiting" peptides that might inhibit the interaction between APCs and T cells by interfering with or inactivating T-cell receptor sites, are also being used experimentally in animal models to prevent or slow the development of autoimmune disease.

Anti–T-cell MAbs are also being used to alter immune function for prevention and reversal of organ allograft rejection. In murine models of certain autoimmune diseases such as systemic lupus erythematosus, rheumatoid arthritis, diabetes mellitus, and myasthenia gravis, administration of these agents is known to suppress autoreactive T-cell activity and the development of autoimmune disease.

Toxin-interleukin therapy is undergoing therapeutic trials. In these cases, a toxin is bound to IL-2 or IL-2 receptor and the fusion protein taken into the cell has an immunotoxic or immunosuppressive effect. These "immunotoxins" may offer new therapeutic perspectives for treating certain autoimmune and neoplastic diseases. They consist of growth factors, antibodies, or hormone coupled to toxins of bacterial or plant origin. The coupled products are specifically designed to target selected neoplastic cells, virus-infected cells, or subsets of normal cells, in order to induce cell damage or death (121). Studies in recent years have demonstrated that their efficacy *in vivo* is usually rather poor because of problems related to instability, inaccessibility of the target cell populations, nonspecific binding, or the development of immunoresponsiveness directed against the immunotoxin after repeated therapy. Nonetheless, several clinical trials have shown some success with either first-generation or improved second-generation immunotoxins (122,123), particularly with cells that are accessible to the circulation such as circulating lymphocytes or macrophages. Problems with allergic reactions and other untoward effects have been noted, but cloning genes for relevant receptor toxins, MAbs, soluble receptors, growth factors, and other ligands has raised the possibility that they could be generated by recombinant DNA technology (124) with subsequent production of the immunotoxins in large quantity. It is to be hoped that functional and structural relationships will be studied to redesign immunotoxins into more clinically effective reagents for use in humans.

Development of MAb to leukocyte "adhesion molecules" might block their access to tissues and prevent inflammation. In order to be recruited into specific tissues, leukocytes must initially bind to endothelial cells that line blood vessels. They then pass through the endothelial cells and basement membranes into tissues to liberate mediators and induce inflammatory tissue responses. For example, T cells migrating through tissues transiently adhere to several types of surrounding cells, enabling them to assess the possible presence of foreign antigen on these cells. A number of adhesion molecules are necessary for proper functioning of T cell–APC interactions. Thus, interference with the function of adhesion molecules may have beneficial effects in retarding inflammatory responses. Recent studies have demonstrated that MAb blocking the function of a certain LFA-1 family (three surface proteins referred to as integrins) of adhesion molecules markedly decreased the intensity of granulocyte-induced inflammatory response in animal models of meningitis.

MAbs have also been used for other purposes, including purging autologous bone marrow of neoplastic cells and eliminating neoplastic cells *in vivo*. Likewise, anti-idiotypic antibodies directed against the TCR itself have been used experimentally to treat T-cell chronic lymphocytic leukemia.

The proliferation of activated B cells that produce IgE is stimulated by IL-4, which also increases the expression of the FC ε receptor on B cells and stimulates mast cell growth. Experiments are under way to develop agents that can interfere with the activity of IL-4 and protect against production of allergic disease. Similar studies are under way to develop agents that can block the IgE receptor sites on mast cells and thus prevent sensitization with IgE molecules.

## CELLULAR ASSAYS FOR DETECTION *IN VITRO* OF CHEMICALLY INDUCED IMMUNE SYSTEM INJURY

### Quantitation of Lymphoid Cells

Studies *in vitro* of quantity and function of cellular components of the immune system may be performed as a means of detecting immunotoxicity in cases of alleged immune system injury by simple chemicals that are not known to sensitize in any immunologically specific manner. These assays use automated methods and are expensive. They depend on the production of MAb against a variety of CD antigens on surfaces of T, B, and NK cells and various T-cell phenotypic subsets, and on flow cytometry using a fluorescence-activated cell sorter (FACS).

By this means, rapid identification and sorting of lymphoid cells reacted with fluorochrome-conjugated antibodies against these surface determinants can be accomplished. When used in this clinical context, such assays are often difficult to interpret because of multiple confounding variables—a wide range of normal values, different normal values in different laboratories, and age- and time-related differences. Other variables such as intercurrent viral infection, cigarette smoking, use of several drugs, and associated disease states can all affect the quantity and function of lymphoid cell populations. It is difficult to base clinical evaluations on results of isolated assessment *in vitro* of quantity and function of immune system cellular components without considering these variables and without knowing the complete case history and physical examination. This is especially difficult when, as is often the case, the subject with alleged environmental injury has no symptoms characteristic of immunodeficiency and no abnormal signs on physical examination. Some conditions have been misdiagnosed as various forms of "immune dysregulation," "immune dysfunction," or even "chemical AIDS" in the absence of evidence of overt clinical disease by history or physical examination on the basis of cellular, immunologic, quantitative, and functional assays using MAbs against CD marker surface antigens. If the confounding variables enumerated above are not considered, and if minor deviations from the norm are interpreted as evidence of clinical "disease" without tempering by sound clinical judgment, misdiagnoses will be made on the basis of abnormal laboratory test results alone.

In the case of alleged environmental injury to humans, it would be prudent to order tests only in the presence of a clinical indication, physical signs or symptoms suggestive of severe immunodeficiency disease, or other abnormal test results. This is particularly true because there is no sound experimental evidence from humans to show that abnormal quantities or function of any particular lymphocyte- or T-cell–phenotypic subset characterizes patients who claim environmental illness following exposure to trace elements of chemicals in the environment. There is today no sound evidence that environmental agents can selectively damage suppressor cells, helper T cells, or any other specific cellular component of the human immune system.

### Diagnostic Evaluation of Alleged Environmental Disease

It would seem prudent to employ the approach described here to evaluate a patient who may have environmentally induced immune disease that allegedly is the result of exposure to small amounts of chemicals or related environmental toxicants.

#### *History and Physical Examination*

The history and physical examination should include a comprehensive environmental exposure history as well as comprehensive investigation of any possible relationship between exposure to environmental or workplace chemicals and development of symptoms. Choice of laboratory tests and the physical examination should be guided by the clinical presentation. For example, if immunodeficiency disease is suspected, simple quantitation of serum immunoglobulins G, A, M, and E, plus IgG subclasses should be performed, plus qualitative assessment of immune system function by specific antibody assays to rule out immunodeficiency.

If the patient has not been told by another person or physician that he or she has some form of immune dysregulation or immune system damage, and if findings of complete history, physical examination, and routine laboratory tests such as complete blood count are normal and there are no symptoms or signs of severe immunodeficiency disease, the physician can reassure the person and proceed no further.

#### *Laboratory Assessment*

If signs and symptoms detected by history and physical examination suggest immunodeficiency disease or if the person has been told that tests in other laboratories have indicated immune system dysfunction or dysregulation, as is sometimes the case, further diagnostic evaluation is in order—evaluation of the humoral and cellular components of the immune system by repeating the relevant assays that were allegedly abnormal, such as immunoglobulin, IgG subclass quantitation, complement component and selected autoantibody assays, and simple B-cell, T-cell, and phenotypic T-cell subset analysis by flow cytometry. These tests are necessary in such a setting to confirm or dispute previously obtained laboratory results, especially when the diagnosis is in dispute and litigation is pending. They should be performed with full consideration for the necessity of proper controls and assessment of the many variables that influence test results.

As noted by the American Academy of Allergy and Immunology Training Program Directors (125), clinical evaluation should never be based on results of isolated *in vitro* assessment of quantity and function of immune system cellular components without consideration of all variables that apply to all of the previously discussed assays and without knowing the complete case history and physical examination in any person tested. The Academy further emphasizes that this is especially true when a test subject with any type of alleged environmental injury has no symptoms characteristic of any immune deficiency or no abnormal signs on physical examination. The training program directors and the Subcommittee on Immunotoxicology, of the Committee on Biologic Markers of the National Research Council, have proposed a tier testing system that may be used to assess patients with known or suspected exposure to an immunotoxicant (126). This system should only be used with knowledge of the case history and evidence that the environmental injury is at least associated with symptoms characteristic of immune deficiency, autoimmunity, or hypersensitivity or with some abnormal signs that suggest a disease state on physical examination. In this testing system, tier-1 procedures may be applied to all persons exposed to immunotoxicants. These include routine assessment of humoral immunity and quantitation of total numbers of T and B cells with surface analysis for CD3, CD4, CD8, and CD20 markers, and routine tests of delayed-type skin hypersensitivity, plus selected autoantibody titers to nuclear antigens. If any of these test results are abnormal, a more extensive second tier procedure may be applied, with the recognition that if a population of exposed persons is involved, only a very small fraction might receive tier-2 testing. This would include testing for induction of a primary antibody response to protein and polysaccharide antigens and induction of a primary delayed skin test type reaction, together with assessment of the proliferative response to both mitogens and special antigens. Quantitation of other lymphoid subtypes could also be performed, including monocytes, NK cells, T cells, and B cells bearing the CD5 marker, CD11, CD16, CD19, CD23, CD64, and the class II major histocompatibility complex on T cells. Levels of cytokines in serum plus secreted activation markers and receptors are also included among the tier-2 tests. Finally, tier-3 tests may be applied to individuals with abnormalities appearing in the tier-2 battery. An example of these tier-3 tests would be performance of nonspecific killing of tumor cell lines to test for NK-cell function. Groups of environmentally exposed persons would also have to be followed sequentially in order to conform to the initial abnormalities and to show evidence of a persistent immune system dysfunction.

The American Academy of Allergy and Immunology Committee also emphasizes that application of these tests, or any portion of them to persons who allege environmental injury can lead to their misuse when slight departures from the norm are considered evidence of injury. When used in a clinical context, these assays are difficult to interpret because of many confounding variables, among which are the wide range of normal values, the varying normal ranges among different laboratories, age- and time-related differences, and other variables including the presence of concurrent viral infections, cigarette smoking, and the influence of drugs, stress, and associated disease states. All can affect the quantity and function of lymphocyte cell populations. For example, the number of CD4 helper T cells can vary by 50% or more (according to some studies, by 100%), depending on the time of day that a blood sample is drawn (127). In addition, lymphocyte composition of the blood differs from that of most body organs and tissues, and peripheral lymphocyte numbers do not necessarily reflect the pathologic changes occurring in specific organs. Furthermore, the peripheral blood contains only approximately 2% of the $500 \times 10^9$ lymphocytes that migrate through the vascular system each day (128). Very small alterations in lymphocyte numbers within the lymph organs can cause major alterations in peripheral blood numbers. Thus, it seems obvious that one cannot make clinical evaluations based on results of isolated *in vitro* assessment, or quantity and function of immune system cellular components, without considering all of these variables and without knowledge of the complete case history and physical examination. Also to be considered in performing these tests is the lack of standardization of flow cytometry, which is only now under consideration, and the experimental nature of several of the monoclonal antibodies.

### *Consultative Advice*

In some cases, particularly of alleged "environmental illness" characterized by multisystem complaints in the absence of positive findings on physical examination and abnormal laboratory test results, it may be wise to obtain psychologic or psychiatric consultation, as these patients are thought by some to have somatoform disorders or related neuropsychiatric problems.

## SUMMARY

Many challenging clinical problems involve suspected immune system damage due to environmental or workplace exposure to a wide range of simple chemicals often encountered in trace or moderate amounts. Some patients present with associated multisystem symptoms, including behavioral and neuropsychiatric manifestations, but no abnormal findings on physical examination and little or no identifiable disorder on gross or microscopic examination of tissues or by laboratory data. Unfortunately, such persons are occasionally declared totally disabled and seek or receive personal injury compensation. Some may be treated with multiple unproven therapeutic modalities. With the increasing industrialization in our environment, it is likely that the number of patients who present for evaluation of these problems will increase.

With these facts in mind, several generalizations can be made concerning the immunosuppressive, immunotoxic, or sensitizing potential of such agent humans. First, environmental chemicals and toxic pollutants of aquatic or atmospheric origin have generally produced immune system defects only when experimental animals were exposed to very high concentrations. Second, there is a paucity of information on the possible immunotoxic or immunoregulatory effects of simple environmental chemicals on humans, although many organic and inorganic chemicals have been demonstrated to induce various forms of hypersensitivity in man. Third, selected B-cell– and T-cell–mediated abnormalities have been produced by such agents in experimental animals independent of their mutagenic or teratogenic effects. There have, however, been no large-scale human cohort or case control epidemiologic studies to show that persons exposed for long periods to low-levels of environmental toxicants demonstrate symptoms directly attributable to immune system compromise.

## REFERENCES


1. Roitt I, Brostoff J, Male D. *Immunology.* London: Gower, 1989.
2. Jackson A, Warner H. Preparation stainings and analysis by flow cytometry of peripheral blood leukocytes. In: Rose N, Friedman H, Fahey J, eds. *Manual of clinical laboratory immunology.* Washington, DC: American Society of Microbiology, 1986;226–235.
3. Organizing Committee for the 6th International Workshop on Human Leukocyte Differentiation Antigens. CD Antigens 1996. *Immunology Today* 1997;18:100–101.
4. Reinherz EL, Schlossman S. The differentiation and function of human T lymphocytes. *Cell* 1980;19:821–827.
5. Zinkernagel RM, Doherty PC. MHC-restricted cytotoxic T cells: studies on the biologic role of polymorphic major transplantation antigens determining T cell restriction—specificity, function, and responsiveness. *Adv Immunol* 1979;27:51–177.
6. Dorf M, Benacerraf B. Suppressor cells and immunoregulation. *Annu Rev Immunol* 1984;2:127–158.
7. Romagnani S. Biology of human $T_H1$ and $T_H2$ cells. *J Clin Immunol* 1995;15:120–130.
8. Seder RA, Seipelt E, Sieper J. Acquisition of lymphokine-producing phenotype by $CD4^+$ T cells. *Annu Rev Immunol* 1994;12:635–673.
9. Swain SL. IL-4 dictates T-cell differentiation. *Res Immunol* 1993;144:616–620.
10. Seder RA, Paul WE, Davis MM, Fazekas de St Groth B. The presence of interleukin 4 during *in vitro* priming determines the lymphocyte-producing potential of $CD4^+$ T cells from T-cell receptor transgenic mice. *J Exp Med* 1992;176:1091–1098.
11. Hsieh CS, Heimberger AB, Gold JS, et al. Differential regulation of T helper phenotype development by IL-4 and IL-10 in an $\alpha\beta$-transgenic system. *Proc Natl Acad Sci USA* 1992;89:6065–6069.
12. Khoury SJ, Hancock WW, Weiner HL. Oral tolerance to myelic basic protein and natural recovery from experimental autoimmune encephalomyelitis are associated with downregulation of inflammatory cytokines and differential upregulation of transforming growth

factor B, interleukin 4, and prostaglandin E expression in the brain. *J Exp Med* 1992;176:1355–1365.
13. Campbell I, Kay TW, Oxbrow L, Harrison LC. Essential role for Interferon- and interleukin-6 in autoimmune insulin-dependent diabetes in NOD/Wehi mice. *J Clin Invest* 1991;87:739–745.
14. Goldman M, Druet P, Gleichmann E. $T_H2$ cells in systemic autoimmunity: insights from allogeneic diseases and chemically-induced autoimmunity. *Immunol Today* 1991;12:223–227.
15. Maggi E, Biswas P, Del Prete GF, et al. Accumulation of $T_H2$-like helper T-cells in the conjunctiva of patients with vernal conjunctivitis. *J Immunol* 1991;146:1169–1174.
16. Del Prete GF, Del Carli M, D'Elois MM, et. al. Allergen exposure induces the activation of allergin-specific $T_H2$ cells in the airway mucosa of patients with allergic respiratory disorders. *Eur J Immunol* 1993;23:1445–1449.
17. van der Heijden FL, Wierenga EA, Bos JD, Kapsenberg ML. High frequency of IL-4 producing $CD4^+$ allergen-specific T lymphocytes in atopic dermatitis lesional skin. *J Invest Dermatol* 1991;97:389–394.
18. Robinson DS, Hamid Q, Ying S, et al. Predominant $T_H2$-like bronchoalveolar T-lymphocyte population in atopic asthma. *N Engl J Med* 1992;326:295–304.
19. Secrist H, Chelen CJ, Wen Y, et al. Allergen immunotherapy decreases interleukin 4 production in $CD4^+$ T-cells from allergic individuals. *J Exp Med* 1993;178:2123–2130.
20. Romagnani S. Regulation of $T_H2$ development in allergy. *Curr Opin Immunol* 1994;6:838–846.
21. Kincade PW. Formation of B lymphocytes in fetal and adult life. *Adv Immunol* 1981;31:177–245.
22. Kuritani T, Cooper MD. Human B-cell differentiation. I. Analysis of immunoglobulin heavy chain switching using monoclonal anti-immunoglobulin M, G, and A antibodies and pokeweed mitogen-induced plasma cell differentiation. *J Exp Med* 1982;155:839–851.
23. Ritz J, Schmidt RE, Michon J, et al. Characterization of functional surface structures on natural killer cells. *Adv Immunol* 1988;42: 181–211.
24. Herberman R, Reynolds C, Ortaldo J. Mechanism of cytotoxicity by natural killer (NK) cells. *Annu Rev Immunol* 1986;4:651–680.
25. Kärre K. How to recognize a foreign submarine. *Immunol Rev* 1997; 155:5–9.
26. Reyburn H, Mandelboim O, Valés-Goméz M, et al. Human NK cells: their ligands, receptors and functions. *Immunol Rev* 1997;155: 119–125.
27. Moretta A, Biassoni R, Bottoin C, et al. Major histocompatibility complex class I-specific receptors on human natural killer and T lymphocytes. *Immunol Rev* 1997;155:105–117.
28. Roitt I, Brostoff J, Male D. *Immunology.* London: Gower, 1989; 2.13–2.14.
29. Unanue ER, Allen PM. The basis for the immunoregulatory role of macrophages and other accessory cells. *Science* 1987;236:551–557.
30. Allison J, Lanier L. Structure function and serology of T-cell antigen receptor complex. *Annu Rev Immunol* 1987;5:503–540.
31. Claman HN. The biology of the immune response. JAMA primer on allergic and immunological diseases. *JAMA* 1987;258:2834–2840.
32. Oppenheim JJ, Kovacs EJ, Matsushima K, Durum K. There is more than one interleukin 1. *Immunol Today* 1986;7:45–56.
33. Dinarello CA. Interleukin-1 and interleukin-1 antagonism. *Blood* 1991;77:1627–1652.
34. Sims JE, Gayle MA, Slack JL, et al. Interleukin 1 signaling occurs exclusively via the type I receptor. *Proc Natl Acad Sci USA* 1994;90:6155–6159.
35. Zhang Y, Rom WN. Regulation of the interleukin-1β (IL-1β) gene by mycobacterial components and lipopolysaccharide is mediated by two nuclear factor-IL6 motifs. *Mol Cell Biol* 1993;13:3831–3837
36. Malkovsky M, Loveland B, North M, et al. Recombinant interleukin-2 directly augments the cytotoxicity of human monocytes. *Nature* 1987;325:262–265.
37. Malkovsky M, Sondel PM, Strober W, Dalgleish AG. The interleukins in acquired disease. *Clin Exp Immunol* 1988;74:151–161.
38. Taniguchi T, Fujita H, Takaoka C, et. al. Structure and expression of a cloned cDNA for human interleukin-2. *Nature* 1983;302:305–310.
39. Smith KA. Interleukin 2. *Annu Rev Immunol* 1984;2:319–333.
40. Leonard WJ, Depper JM, Crabtree GR, et al. Molecular cloning and expression of cDNAs for the human interleukin-2 receptor. *Nature* 1984;311:626–631.
41. Hatekeyama M, Kono T, Kobayashi N, et al. Interaction of the IL-2 receptor with the src- family kinase $p56^{lck}$: identification of novel intermolecular association. *Science* 1991;252:1523–1528.
42. Henney CS, Kuribayashi K, Kern DE, Gillis S. Interleukin-2 augments natural killer cell activity. *Nature* 1981;291:335–338.
43. Siegel JP, Sharon M, Smith PL, Leonard WJ. The IL-2 receptor β chain: role in mediating signals for LAK, NK, and proliferative activities. *Science* 1987;238:75–78.
44. Campen DH, Horwitz DA, Quismorio FP, et al. Serum levels of interleukin 2 receptor and activity of rheumatic disease characterized by immune system activation. *Arthritis Rheum* 1988;31:1358–1364.
45. Josimovic-Alasevic O, Feldmeier HJ, Zwingenberger K, et al. Interleukin 2 receptor in patients with localized and systemic parasitic disease. *Clin Exp Immunol* 1988;72:249–254.
46. Sethi KK, Naher H. Elevated titers of cell-free interleukin 2 receptor in serum and cerebrospinal fluid specimens of patients with acquired immunodeficiency syndrome. *Immunol Lett* 1986;13:179–184.
47. Manoussakis MN, Papdopulos GK, Drosos AA, Moutsopoulos HM. Soluble interleukin 2 receptor molecules in the serum of patients with autoimmune diseases. *Clin Immunol Immunopathol* 1989;50: 321–332.
48. Schrader JW. The panspecific hemopoietin of activated lymphocytes (interleukin 3). *Annu Rev Immunol* 1986;4:205–230.
49. Paul WE, Ohara J. B cell stimulatory factor 1/interleukin 4. *Annu Rev Immunol* 1987;5:429–459.
50. Paul WE. Interleukin-4: a prototypic immunoregulatory lymphokine. *Blood* 1991;77:1859–1870.
51. Romagnani S. Regulation and deregulation of human IgE synthesis. *Immunol Today* 1990;11:316–321.
52. Coffman RL, Ohara J, Bond MW, et al. B cell factor-1 enhances the IgE response of lipopolysaccharide-activated B cells. *J Immunol* 1986;136:4538–4541.
53. Urban J, Katona IM, Paul WE, Finkelman FD. Interleukin 4 is important in protective immunity to a gastrointestinal nematode infection in mice. *Proc Natl Acad Sci USA* 1991;88:5513–5517.
54. Kuhn R, Rajewsky K, Muller W. Generation and analysis of interleukin-4 deficient mice. *Science* 1991;254:707–710.
55. Tepper RI, Levison DA, Stanger BZ, et al. IL-4 induces allergic-like inflammatory disease and alters T cell development in transgenic mice. *Cell* 1990;62:457–467.
56. Fenton MJ, Buras JA, Donnely RP. IL-4 reciprocally regulates IL-1 and IL-1 receptor antagonist expression in human monocytes. *J Immunol* 1992;149:1283–1288.
57. Clutterbuck EJ, Hirst EMA, Sanderson CJ. Human interleukin 5 (IL-5) regulates the production of eosinophils in human bone marrow cultures: comparison and interaction with IL-1, IL-3, IL-6, and GMCSF. *Blood* 1989;73:1504–1512.
58. Owen WF Jr, Petersen J, Sheff DM, et al. Hypodense eosinophils and interleukin 5 activity in the blood of patients with the eosinophilia-myalgia syndrome. *Proc Natl Acad Sci USA* 1990;87:8647–8651.
59. Rothenberg ME, Owen WF, Siberstein DS, et al. Human eosinophils have prolonged survival, enhanced functional properties, and become hypodense when exposed to human interleukin 3. *J Clin Invest* 1988;81:1986–1992.
60. Owen WF Jr, Rothenberg ME, Siberstein DS, et al. Regulation of human eosinophil viability, density, and function by granulocyte/macrophage colony-stimulating factor in the presence of 3T3 fibroblasts. *J Exp Med* 1987;166:129–141.
61. Van Snick J. Interleukin 6: an overview. *Annu Rev Immunol* 1990;8: 253–278.
62. Akina S, Taga T, Kishimoto T. Interleukin-6 in biology and medicine. *Adv Immunol* 1993;54:1–78.
63. Morrissey, PJ, Goodwin RG, Nordan RP, et al. Recombinant interleukin 7, pre-B cell growth factor, has costimulatory activity on purified mature T cells. *J Exp Med* 1989;169:707–716.
64. Oppenheim JJ, Zachariae COC, Mukaida N, Matsushima K. Properties of the novel proinflammatory supergene "intercrine" cytokine family. *Annu Rev Immunol* 1991;9:617–648.
65. Fiorentino DF, Zlotnik A, Mosmann TR, et al. IL-10 inhibits cytokine production by activated macrophages. *J Immunol* 1991;147: 3815–3822.
66. Ralph P, Nakoinz I, Sampson-Johannes A, et al. IL-10, T lymphocyte inhibitor of human blood cell production of IL-1 and tumor necrosis factor. *J Immunol* 1992;148:808–814.

67. D'Andrea A, Aste-Amezaga M, Vaiante NM, et al. Interleukin 10 (IL-10) inhibits human lymphocyte interferon- production by suppressing natural killer cell stimulatory factor/IL-12 synthesis in accessory cells. *J Exp Med* 1993;178:1041–1048.
68. Del Prete G, DeCarli M, Almerigogna F, et al. Human IL-10 is produced by both type 1 helper (Th1) and type 2 helper (Th2) T cell clones and inhibits their antigen-specific proliferation and cytokine production. *J Immunol* 1993;150:353–360.
69. Hsu D-H, Moore KW, Spits H. Differential effects of interleukin-4 and -10 on interleukin-2 induced interferon-γ synthesis and lymphokine-activated killer activity. *Int Immunol* 1992;4:563–569.
70. Rousset F, Garcia E, Defrance T, et al. Human and viral IL-10 are potent growth and differentiation factors for activated human B lymphocytes. *Proc Natl Acad Sci USA* 1992;89:1890–1893.
71. Punnonen J, de Waal Malefyt R, van Vlasselaer P, Gauchat J-F, de Vries JE. IL-10 and viral IL-10 prevent IL-4 induced IgE synthesis by inhibiting the accessory cell function of monocytes. *J Immunol* 1993; 151:1280–1289.
72. Merberg DM, Wolf SF, Clark SC. Sequence similarity between NKSF and the-6/G-CSF family. *Immunol Today* 1992;13:77–78.
73. Brunda MJ. Interleukin-12. *J Leukoc Biol* 1994;55:280–288.
74. Manetti R, Parronchi GP, Giudfizi MG, et al. Natural killer cell stimulatory factor interleukin 12 (IL-12) induces T helper type 1 (Th1)-specific immune responses and inhibits the development of IL-4 producing Th cells. *J Exp Med* 1993;177:1199–1204.
75. Schmitt E, Hoehn P, Huels C, et al. T helper type 1 development of naive $CD4^+$ T cells requires the coordinate action of interleukin-12 and interferon-γ and is inhibited by transforming growth factor-β. *Eur J Immunol* 1994;24:793–798.
76. McKenzie ANJ, Culpeper JA, de Waal Malefyt R, et al. Interleukin-13, a novel T cell-derived cytokine that regulates human monocyte and B cell function. *Proc Natl Acad Sci USA* 1992;90:3735–3739.
77. Zurawski G, de Vries JE. Interleukin 13, an interleukin 4-like cytokine that acts on monocytes and B cells, but not on T cells. *Immunol Today* 1994;15:19–26.
78. Grabstein K, Eisenmann J, Shanebeck K, et al. Cloning of a T cell growth factor that interacts with the β chain of the interleukin-2 receptor. *Science* 1994;264:965–968.
79. Farrar MA, Schreiber RD. The molecular cell biology of interferon- and its receptor. *Annu Rev Immunol* 1993;11:571–611.
80. Weigner CD, Gundel RH, Reilly P, et al. Intercellular adhesion molecule-1 (ICAM-1) in pathogenesis of asthma. *Science* 1990;247: 456–459.
81. Sporn MB, Roberts AB. Transforming growth factor-β: recent progress and new challenges. *J Cell Biol* 1993;119:1017–1021.
82. Beutler B, Cerami A. The biology of cachectin/TNF: a primary mediator of the host response. *Annu Rev Immunol* 1989;7:625–655.
83. Vilcek J, Lee TH. Tumor necrosis factor: new insights into the molecular mechanisms of its multiple actions. *J Biol Chem* 1991;266: 7317–7326.
84. Zhang Y, Broser M, Rom WN. Activation of the interleukin 6 gene by *Mycobacterium tuberculosis* or lipopolysaccharide is mediated by nuclear factors NF-IL6 and NF-κB. *Proc Natl Acad Sci USA* 1994;91: 2225–2229.
85. Jerne NK. Idiotypic networks and other preconceived ideas. *Immunol Rev* 1983;79:5–24.
86. Svejgaard A, Plotz P, Ryder L. HLA and disease-1982: a survey. *Immunol Rev* 1983;70:193–218.
87. Claman H. Glucocorticosteroids I: anti-inflammatory mechanisms. *Hosp Prac* 1983;18:123–134.
88. Bellanti JA. *Immunology,* vol 2. Philadelphia: WB Saunders, 1978; 740.
89. Williams WR, Williams WJ. Development of beryllium lymphocyte transformation tests in chronic beryllium disease. *Int Arch Allergy Appl Immunol* 1982;67:175–180.
90. Newman LS, Bobka C, Schumacher B, et al. Compartmentalized immune response reflects clinical severity of disease. *Am J Respir Crit Care Med* 1994;150:135–142.
91. Diamantstein T, Odenwald MV. Control of the immune response *in vitro* by calcium ions. *Immunology* 1974;27:531–541.
92. Pepys J. Occupational allergy due to platinum complex salts. *Clin Immunol Allergy* 1984;4:131–157.
93. Joules H. Asthma from sensitization to chromium. *Lancet* 1932;223: 182–183.
94. Dolvich J, Evans SL, Nieboer E. Occupational asthma from nickel sensitivity I. Human serum albumin in the antigenic determinant. *Br J Ind Med* 1984;41:51–55.
95. Malo J-L, Cartier A. Occupational asthma due to fumes of galvanized metal. *Chest* 1987;92:375–377.
96. Simonsson BG, Sjoberg A, Rolf C, et al. Acute and long-term airway hyperreactivity in aluminum salt-exposed workers with nocturnal asthma. *Eur J Respir Dis* 1985;66:105–118.
97. Salvaggio JE. Impact of allergy and immunology on our expanding environment. *J Allergy Clin Immunol* 1990;85:689–699.
98. Zetterstrom O, Nordvall SL, Bjorksten B, et al. Increased IgE antibody responses in rats exposed to tobacco smoke. *J Allergy Clin Immunol* 1985;75:594–598.
99. Matsumura Y. The effects of ozone, nitrogen dioxide and sulfur dioxide on the experimentally induced allergic respiratory disorder in guinea pigs. Parts I, II, and III. *Am Rev Respir Dis* 1970;102:430–437, 438–443, 444–447.
100. Muranaka M, Suzoki S, Koizumi K, et al. Adjuvant activity of diesel exhaust particulates for the production of IgE antibody in mice. *J Allergy Clin Immunol* 1986;77:616–623.
101. Kjellman N-IM. Effect of parental smoking on IgE levels in children. *Lancet* 1981;1:993–994.
102. Ohsawa M, Takahashi K, Otsuka F. Induction of anti-nuclear antibodies in mice orally exposed to cadmium at low concentrations. *Clin Exp Immunol* 1988;73:98–102.
103. Pelletliera L, Passquier R, Rossert J, et al. Autoreactive T cells in mercury-induced autoimmunity: ability to induce the autoimmune disease. *J Immunol* 1988;140:750–754.
104. Robinson C, Egorov I, Balazo T. Strain differences in the induction of antinuclear antibodies by mercuric chloride, gold sodium thiomalate, and D-penicillamine in inbred mice. *Fed Proc* 1983;42:1213.
105. Tan EM. Autoantibodies to nuclear antigens (ANA): their immunobiology and medicine. *Adv Immunol* 1982;33:167–240.
106. Harmon CE. Antinuclear antibodies in autoimmune disease. *Med Clin North Am* 1985;69:547–563.
107. Tan EM. Interactions between autoimmunity and molecular and cell biology: bridges between clinical and basic sciences. *J Clin Invest* 1989;84:1–6.
108. Hirsch F, Couderc J, Sapin C, et al. Polyclonal effect of $HgCl_2$ in the rat, its possible role in an experimental autoimmune disease. *Eur J Immunol* 1982;12:620–625.
109. Bigazzi PE. Mechanisms of chemical-induced autoimmunity. In: Dean JH, Luster MI, Munson AE, Amos H, eds. *Immunotoxicity and immunopharmacology.* New York: Raven Press, 1989;277.
110. Bozelka BE, Salvaggio JE. Immunomodulation by environmental contaminants: asbestos, cadmium, and halogenated biphenyls: a review. *Environ Carcinogenesis Revs (J Environ Sci Health)* 1985;3: 1–62.
111. Rosenberg SA, Spiess P, Lafreniere R. New approach to the adoptive immunotherapy of cancer with tumor-infiltrating lymphocytes. *Science* 1986;233:1318–1321.
112. Herberman RB. *NK cells and other natural effector cells.* New York: Academic Press, 1982.
113. Höglund P, Sundbäck J, Olsson-Alheim MY, et al. Host MHC class I gene control of NK-cell specificity in the mouse. *Immunol Rev* 1997; 155:11–28.
114. Topalain S, Soloman D, Rosenberg S. Tumor-specific cytolysis by lymphocytes infiltrating human melanomas. *Immunology* 1989;142: 3714–3725.
115. Rosenberg S, Packard B, Aebersold P, et al. Use of tumor-infiltrating lymphocytes and interleukin-2 in the immunotherapy of patients with metastatic melanoma: A preliminary report. *N Engl J Med* 1988;319: 1676–1680.
116. Woo Y-t, Arcos JC. Environmental Chemicals. In: Sontag JM ed. *Carcinogens in industry and the environment.* New York: Dekker, 1981;168.
117. Urso P, Gengozian N. Depressed humoral immunity and increased tumor incidence in mice following in utero exposure to benzo-[a]-pyrene. *J Toxicol Environ Health* 1980;6:569–576.
118. Ladics GS, Kawabata TT, White KL. Suppression of the *in vitro* humoral immune response of mouse splenocytes by 7, 12-dimethylbenz[a]anthracene metabolites and inhibition of immunosuppression by α-naphthoflavone. *Toxicol Appl Pharmacol* 1991;110:31–44.
119. Perera FA. Carcinogens and human health: Part 1. *Science* 1990;250: 1644–1646.
120. Dinarello CA, Meir JW. Interleukins. *Annu Rev Immunol* 1986;37:173–178.

121. Waldmann TA, Grant A, Tendler C, et al. Lymphokine receptor-directed therapy: a model of immune intervention. *J Clin Immunol* 1990;10:19S–20S.
122. Vitetta ES. Immunotoxins: New therapeutic reagents for autoimmunity, cancer and AIDS. *J Clin Immunol* 1990;10:15S–18S.
123. Byers VS, Baldwin RW. Therapeutic strategies with monoclonal antibodies and immunoconjugates. *Immunology* 1988;65:329–335.
124. Chang MS, Russell DW, Uhr JW, Vitetta ES. Cloning and expression of recombinant, functional ricin B chain. *Proc Natl Acad Sci USA* 1987;84:5640–5644.
125. Salvaggio JE and Controversial Practices Committee (1995). The role of training programs in dealing with controversial practices. *J Clin Immunol* 1994;93:955–966.
126. Subcommittee on Immunotoxicology, Committee on Biologic Markers. *Biologic markers in immunotoxicology.* Washington, DC: National Academy Press, 1992.
127. Giorgi JV. Lymphocytes subset measurements: significance in clinical medicine. In: Rose N, Friedman H, Fahey J, eds. *Manual of clinical laboratory immunology,* 3rd ed. Washington, DC: American Society of Microbiology, 1986;236–246.
128. Westermann J, Reinhard P. Lymphocyte subsets in the blood: a diagnostic window on the lymphoid system? *Immunol Today* 1990;11:406–410.
129. Peter JB. *The use and interpretation of tests in clinical immunology,* 6th ed. Omaha: Interstate Press, 1989.
130. Cruse J, Lewis RE. *Illustrated dictionary of immunology*. Boca Raton, FL: CRC Press, 1995.
131. Stites DP, Stobo JD, Wells JV. *Basic and clinical immunology,* 6th ed. Norwalk, CT: Appleton and Lange, 1987.

*Environmental and Occupational Medicine, Third Edition,* edited by William N. Rom.
Lippincott–Raven Publishers, Philadelphia © 1998.

# CHAPTER 10

# Molecular Biology

John G. Hay

This chapter introduces current concepts in molecular biology and gives an overview of the different techniques used to identify genes and study their expression. The material has been arranged starting from the fundamental, that is, DNA and the genetic code, and progresses through organization of genes, gene polymorphisms and positional cloning, evaluation of gene structure, transcription, cloning of genes, control of gene expression, signal transduction, translation, and protein processing.

## DNA AND THE DOUBLE HELIX

Studies performed in 1928 by Fred Griffith, an English microbiologist, demonstrated that when heat-killed bacteria are mixed with live bacteria the characteristics of the living organisms could change. The pathogenicity of *Diplococcus pneumoniae* is dependent on the possession of a polysaccharide capsule, and the ability to synthesize a capsule can be transferred to nonpathogenic strains by a substance present in pathogenic strains that have been killed by heat. That a nucleic acid, deoxyribonucleic acid (DNA), was this "genetic transforming factor" was demonstrated by the studies of Avery and colleagues (1), reported in 1944.

A nucleic acid is composed of a pentose sugar linked to a phosphate group and a nitrogenous base. The pentose sugar in DNA is 2-deoxyribose, whereas the pentose in RNA is ribose (Fig. 1). One of four different bases—thymine, adenine, cytosine, and guanine—can be linked to the carbon at ring position 1 of deoxyribose. Uracil is found in place of thymine attached to ribose. Adenine and guanine are purines with a double-ring structure, whereas cytosine, uracil, and thymine are pyrimidines and have a single-ring structure (Fig. 2). Nucleosides (pentose plus a base) can be phosphorylated by the addition of a phosphate group on the 3′ or 5′ carbon to become a nucleotide.

J. G. Hay: Departments of Medicine and Pathology, New York University Medical Center, New York, New York 10016.

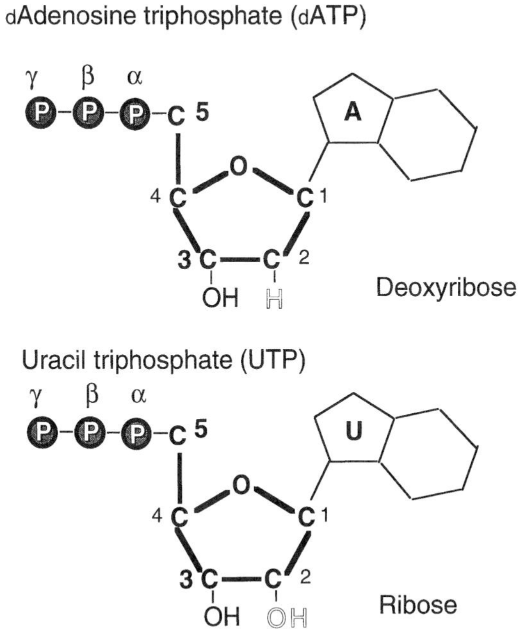


**FIG. 1.** Molecular structure of deoxyribose adenosine triphosphate (dATP) and ribose uracil triphosphate (UTP). The five carbon ring positions of ribose and deoxyribose are numbered. Ribose differs from deoxyribose by the possession of an hydroxyl group at ring position 2. The α, β, and γ-phosphate position on carbon 5 are labeled. dATP has the base adenine bonded to the carbon at position 1 of deoxyribose, and UTP has uracil bonded to the carbon 1 position of ribose.

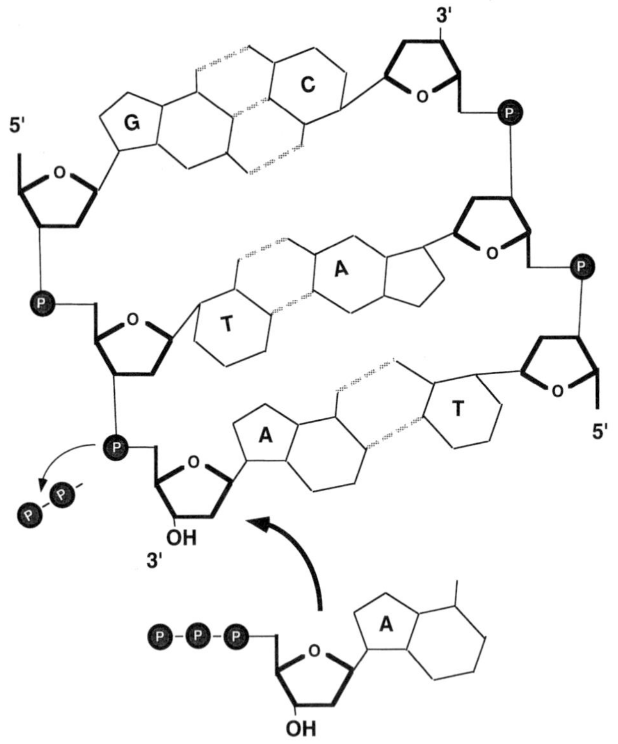


**FIG. 2.** Two DNA strands are bonded together by complementary base pairing, adenine with thymine and cytosine with guanine. Adenine and thymine bond with two hydrogen bonds, and cytosine to guanine with three. The sugar phosphate backbone is composed of deoxyribose sugar moieties linked one to another by a phosphate group through a 5′-3′ phosphodiester linkage. The strands are antiparallel in orientation, one running 5′ to 3′ and the other 3′ to 5′. A new strand is always synthesized in the 5′ to 3′ direction, the next nucleotide aligned with its complementary base and then added by DNA polymerase, with the formation of the phosphodiester bond and the release of pyrophosphate.

Adenosine 5′-triphosphate, a very important molecule in metabolism and energy transfer, has three phosphate groups added to the carbon at position 5 (Fig. 1).

A sugar-phosphate chain is formed by the linking of the pentose sugars together by a phosphate group, the 5′ carbon of one sugar linked to the 3′ carbon of the adjacent sugar by a phosphodiester bond (Fig. 2).

DNA forms a double helix, with two chains or strands intertwined in an antiparallel direction, that is, one strand running in the 5′ to 3′ direction and the other strand in the opposite direction (Fig. 2). The sugar-phosphate backbone is on the outside of the helix, and the base groups are directed toward the inside of the helix. The base groups of one strand associate by hydrogen bonding in a specific manner with the base groups of the other strand. Adenine always bonds to thymine, and guanine always bonds to cytosine; this association is termed complementary base pairing. A purine (two rings) also always bonds to a pyrimidine (one ring), keeping the diameter of the double helix constant.

The association between the two strands of DNA is not permanent. When DNA is replicated, the strands are unwound and separated region by region by an enzyme called a topoisomerase. A new daughter strand is synthesized alongside each of the original single parent strands by assembly of nucleotides by complementary base pairing. The formation of phosphodiester bonds links the nucleotides together into a complementary chain by the action of an enzyme called DNA polymerase, which always synthesizes the new chain in the 5′ to 3′ direction. This form of replication is called semiconservative, in that each of the new double-stranded molecules contains both an old and a new single strand (Fig. 3). As the unwound region of DNA moves along the strand forming a replication fork, the daughter DNA must be synthesized on one strand in segments (DNA polymerase synthesizes always in the 5′ to 3′ direction). These fragments, which are then covalently bonded together, are called "Okazaki fragments."

The two strands of the double helix can also be dissociated or denatured by physical forces including heat and strong alkali. Importantly, when these forces are reversed (cooling or neutralization) the strands will reassociate and realign according to their complementary base pairing. This property of DNA is very valuable in the study of gene structure and expression.

All the genetic hereditary information, from simple organisms such as viruses and bacteria to complex ani-

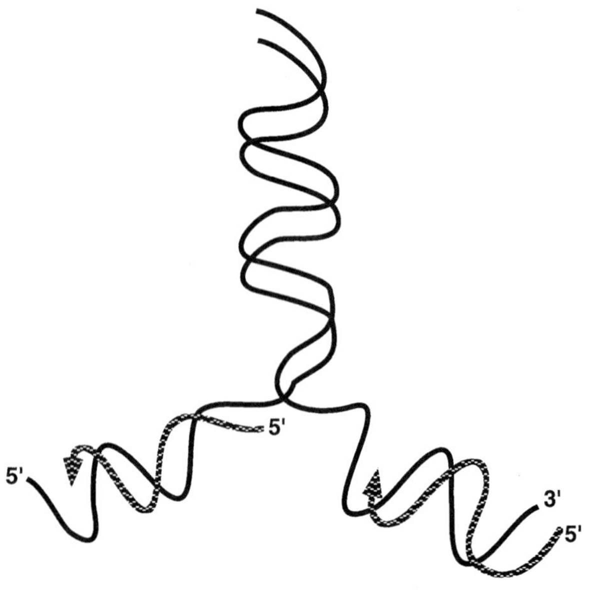


**FIG. 3.** The DNA strands are unwound by a topoisomerase and the daughter strands synthesized on both of the parent strands. Replication is semiconservative; each new copy possesses an old and a new strand.

mals such as humans, are encoded in the sequences of four bases—thymine, adenine, cytosine, and guanine—in strands of DNA (RNA viruses excepted), and this information can be replicated by the formation of daughter strands through complementary base pairing: A-T, T-A, G-C, C-G.

## THE GENETIC CODE AND THE STRUCTURE OF GENES

The inherited genetic information is contained within the linear sequence of bases in DNA, and the gene that is the unit of inheritance contains a sequence of bases that determine the amino acid sequence of a protein. That is, there is a one gene–one protein relationship and the gene is the unit of inheritance.

The genetic code was fully deciphered in 1966 building on data generated by Marshall Nirenberg and Heinrich Matthaei (2). It was discovered that the sequence of bases in DNA determined the amino acid sequence of a protein in a triplet code. That is, a sequence of three bases or a "codon" determined the code for one amino acid. There is considerable redundancy in the system, as the random assortment of four bases at the three positions in the codon could code for 64 amino acids, yet only 20 amino acids are encoded. Most amino acids are therefore encoded by more that one codon, although, in general, of the different possible codons for each amino acid, the first two base positions are the same with redundancy at the third base position. Three codons do not code for an amino acid, and they are the "stop codons" TAA, TAG, and TGA, which terminate protein synthesis.

The human genome contains $3.3 \times 10^9$ base pairs (bp); however, only a small portion of this total amount of DNA actually codes for proteins. The genes themselves are separated from one another by long spans of DNA whose function remains unknown. Even within a gene, not all of the base pairs within the DNA encode amino acids. The protein coding sequence is split up into segments called exons that are separated from one another by long stretches of DNA called introns, whose function again remains largely unknown.

Within the regions of DNA that do not encode proteins, certain sequences can be seen repeated many times. An example of one of these frequently repeated sequences is called an "Alu repeat," which is approximately 300 bp long. There are approximately 500,000 Alu repeats within the human genome.

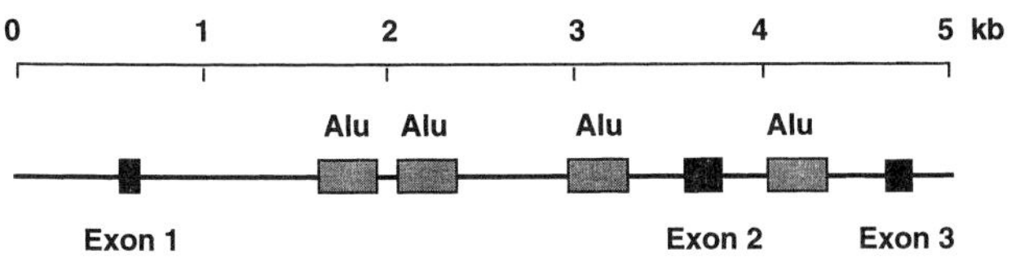


**FIG. 4.** Genomic structure of the human Clara cell 10-kd gene. The three exons and the four Alu repetitive DNA elements within the two introns of the gene are shown (3).

To illustrate the characteristics of genes as just described, the structure of the Clara cell 10-kd protein (CC10) gene is shown in Fig. 4 (3). The CC10 gene spans almost 4 kb of genomic DNA, yet the protein coding sequence is only approximately 400 bp in length and is separated into three short exons. There are also four Alu repeats within the two introns of the CC10 gene.

## IDENTIFICATION OF GENES

Each human cell (diploid) possesses two complete copies ($2N$) of this genetic information, which is split into 22 pairs of chromosomes and the two sex-determining chromosomes. In order for cells to divide, this material has to be duplicated by a process called mitosis. In contrast, meiosis separates one chromosome (at random) from each chromosome pair into two different cells, thereby reducing the number of chromosomes by half ($N$) and forming cells destined to become oocytes or spermatozoa. During the process of meiosis some crossing over of the genetic material occurs from one of each chromosome pair to the other. That is, for each individual chromosome, the gamete will receive chromosome fragments originating from both the grandmother and the grandfather and not directly inherit a whole chromosome from either through the parent.

Alterations can occur in the DNA sequence during meiosis as a result of imperfect crossing over of the pair of chromosomes, which may cause a segment of DNA to be inserted or deleted. Mistakes may also occur during the replication of DNA for mitosis, and DNA can be damaged by a variety of agents. These sequence changes may affect large chromosomal fragments, or perhaps change just one base position (point mutation). Viruses are also able to insert segments of their DNA into the genome. The most frequent variations in the DNA sequence, however, are short repeated sequences often just 2 or 3 bp, repeated up to several hundred times. These repeats, which are called "short tandem repeated sequences," are often highly variable.

All of the changes just described lead to polymorphisms in the genome of an individual, and if they occur in the germ cells they will be inherited in a mendelian manner. A polymorphism may cause an inherited disease by disrupting the function of a gene, but most polymorphisms do not lead to disease. They can, however, be of great value in the evaluation of the inheritance of various segments of DNA that may be close to an abnormal gene that is responsible for a disease. The more variable any polymorphism is in the population (heterozygous), the more valuable it is likely to be.

The evaluation of polymorphisms is of great importance in the technique called "positional cloning," which has had recent success in the identification of genes responsible for human disease including cystic fibrosis (4) and breast cancer susceptibility (mutations in the gene BRCA1) (5). Positional cloning identifies the gene on the bases of inherited polymorphisms. The inheritance of a disease phenotype is studied in relation to the inheritance of various polymorphic markers. The closer the disease-causing gene to the polymorphism being followed, the tighter the linkage with the disease phenotype will be. The further apart the polymorphic marker and the abnormal gene, the more likely a crossover event will have occurred at meiosis, and the marker and the abnormal gene will then not be linked on the same chromosome. It is clear that the closer a marker is to the genetic abnormality, the more closely it will be linked to the disease phenotype. A statistical method called a "lod score" (logarithm of the odds score) is used to evaluate the degree of linkage between a marker and a disease phenotype (6).

### Restriction Fragment Length Polymorphisms

Restriction enzymes are bacterial enzymes that cut up DNA. These enzymes are very specific as to which sequences they cleave, and recognize short nucleotide sequences usually between 4 and 8 bp in length. Between normal individuals there are variations in the DNA sequence, although this is not usually within essential protein coding regions, as this may lead to disease. These changes may include the exchange of one base pair for another, and the addition or deletion of one or several base pairs. If these changes occur within the recognition sequence for a restriction enzyme, that enzyme will no longer be able to cut the DNA strand at that position.

For example, the sequence recognized by the restriction enzyme called RsaI is GTAC. In the following sequence, digestion with RsaI will produce two DNA fragments (n represents any nucleotide:

GTACnnnnnnnnnnnnnnnnGTACnnnnnnnnnnnnnnnGTAC
CATGnnnnnnnnnnnnnnnnCATGnnnnnnnnnnnnnnnCATG
+RsaI
↓
ACnnnnnnnnnnnnnnnnGT    ACnnnnnnnnnnnnnnnGT
TGnnnnnnnnnnnnnnnnCA    TGnnnnnnnnnnnnnnnCA

If one of the bases in the middle sequence is changed, for example A to T, the enzyme RsaI will no longer recognize this site, and will therefore not cleave the DNA at this position. Only one fragment of DNA will therefore be produced following restriction digestion.

GTACnnnnnnnnnnnnnnnnGAACnnnnnnnnnnnnnnnGTAC
CATGnnnnnnnnnnnnnnnnCTTGnnnnnnnnnnnnnnnCATG
+RsaI
↓
ACnnnnnnnnnnnnnnnnGAACnnnnnnnnnnnnnnnGT
TGnnnnnnnnnnnnnnnnCTTGnnnnnnnnnnnnnnnCA

The production of different-sized fragments by a restriction enzyme from the same region of DNA from different individual chromosomes is called a restriction fragment length polymorphism (RFLP). In addition to one base pair changes or "point mutations" as shown above, certain longer sequences can be inserted into the genome. Retroviruses in particular are adept at inserting their viral sequences into the host DNA. Like the point mutations described above, if these changes occur in host DNA sequences that are not part of a protein coding or regulatory region, no effect on the host may be evident, although the change may as described above lead to the development of an RFLP. If the change occurs in the DNA sequence of a germ cell, the mutation will be inherited. Like viral sequences, repetitive sequences including "Alu" repeats can also become inserted into the genome, and these are called transposable elements or transposons.

An example of an RFLP will be illustrated by reference to the CC10 gene (Fig. 5) (3). There is a restriction site for the enzyme RsaI in the middle of the first intron, and a second site just 3′ to the third exon. If this segment of the gene is cleaved with RsaI, a fragment of DNA 1.9 kb in length is generated. If, however, one of the restriction sites contains a point mutation, the enzyme will not cut the DNA at this position and a longer fragment will be generated. In the example shown of a polymorphism in the CC10 gene, rather than a point mutation, there is an insertion of an extra Alu repeat in intron 2 of the polymorphic gene. This insertion results in a longer DNA fragment (2.2 kb) between the two RsaI restriction sites.

To identify RFLPs generated by the digestion of genomic DNA by restriction enzymes, it is necessary to separate fragments of DNA according to their length, and then to identify the same region of DNA from different individuals. The various techniques to do this will now be described.

## TECHNIQUES TO EVALUATE GENE STRUCTURE

### Gel Electrophoresis and Southern Blots

DNA fragments can be separated according to their length by gel electrophoresis. Two types of gel matrix are used, agarose or polyacrylamide. The principles for both are the same; the DNA sample is loaded in a well in the gel, which is submerged in a salt buffer solution. An electrical potential is then applied across the gel (Fig. 6). DNA, being a basic molecule, moves toward the positively charged electrode. The gel matrix acts like a sieve with small DNA fragments moving faster than large fragments. Using the Southern blotting technique, the DNA fragments can be transferred from agarose gels to nylon or nitrocellulose membranes (Fig. 7), and

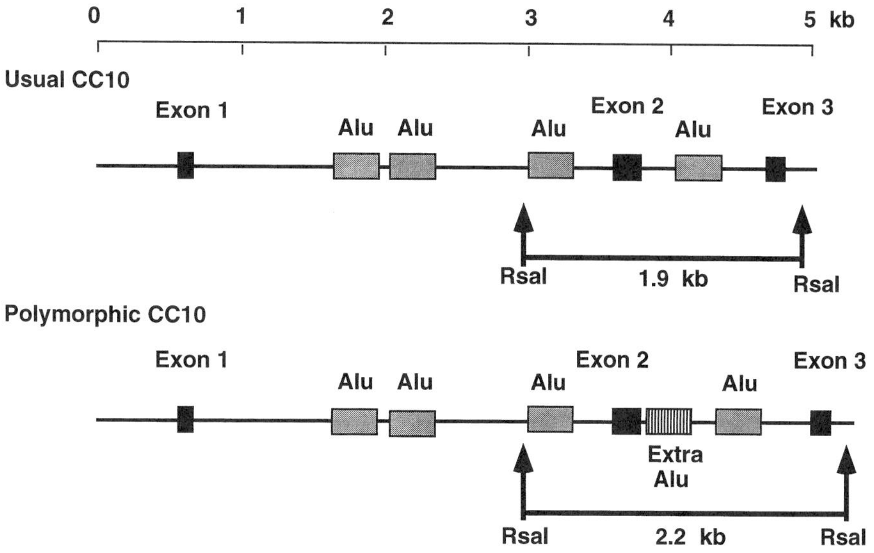


**FIG. 5.** A polymorphic form of the human CC10 gene. An extra Alu repeat is inserted into the second intron of the gene in some chromosomes (about 3%). This leads to a restriction fragment length polymorphism if the gene is digested with several restriction enzymes including RsaI as shown.

the DNA fragment of interest can then be identified by hybridization with a labeled probe (Fig. 8). The analysis of an RFLP in a three-generation family will now be described as an example of how these techniques may be used.

As shown in Fig. 5, the CC10 gene is polymorphic; some individuals have an extra Alu repeat inserted in the second intron. A blood sample has been taken from all the family members of a three-generation family. Genomic DNA is extracted from the white blood cells, and then digested with the restriction enzyme RsaI. The digested DNA is loaded onto an agarose gel and a current applied to separate the DNA fragments (Fig. 6). This procedure will have generated DNA fragments of varying sizes, all separated on the basis of their length. RsaI cuts DNA on an average at 200- to 300-bp intervals; many thousands of fragments will therefore have been generated for each individual.

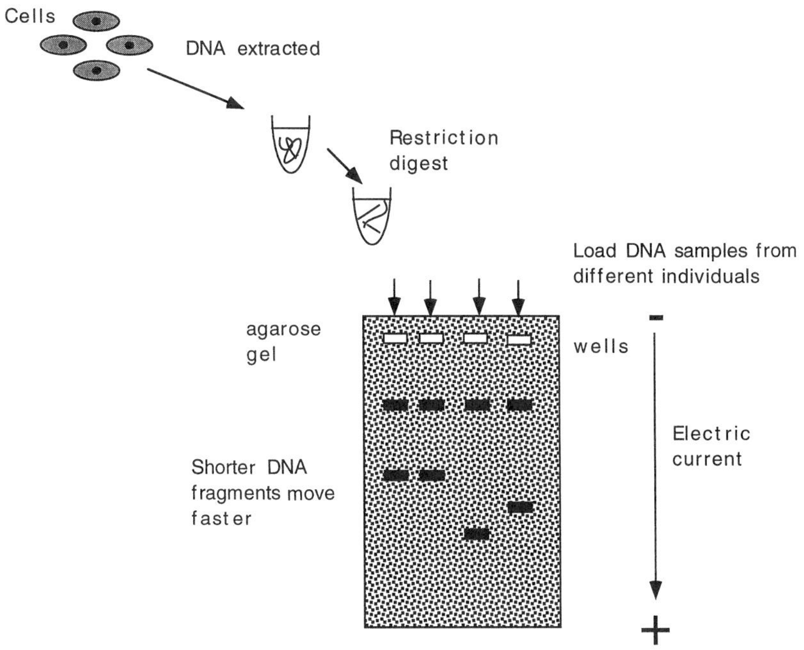


**FIG. 6.** Gel electrophoresis to detect a restriction fragment length polymorphism. Genomic DNA is extracted from cells from different individuals, usually leukocytes. The DNA is digested with a restriction enzyme and then loaded onto an agarose gel. A current is applied to separate the fragments on account of their mobility in the gel, which is dependent on their length.

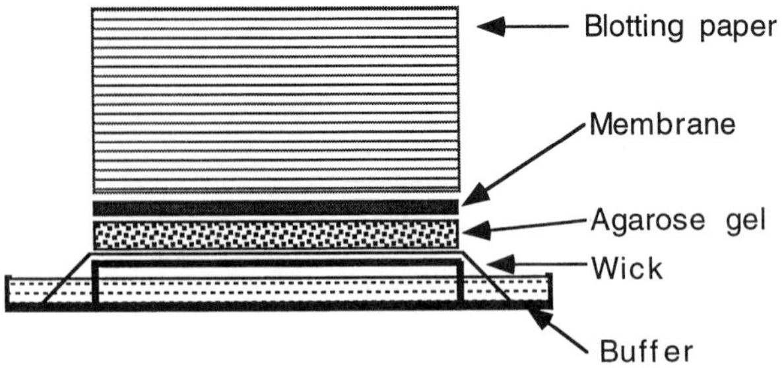


**FIG. 7.** Southern blotting. An agarose gel (from Fig. 6) is placed on top of a wick bathed in a salt buffer. A membrane and several layers of blotting paper are placed on top on the gel. The DNA transfers to the membrane as a result of buffer flow under capillary action.

The DNA fragments are then transferred from the gel to a nylon or nitrocellulose membrane by the technique of Southern blotting (Fig. 7). The agarose gel is placed on top of a wick that is bathed in salt buffer. The membrane is placed on top of the gel, and many layers of absorbent blotting paper on top of the membrane. Over several hours the buffer flows through both the gel and the membrane into the blotting paper by capillary action. The DNA moves with the buffer out of the gel but remains trapped on the undersurface of the membrane. The DNA can then be fixed to the membrane by heat or ultraviolet light.

Visualization of the CC10 gene fragment from all the other thousands of fragments on the membrane is achieved by hybridization with a probe (Fig. 8). The CC10 gene exon 2 sequence, if used as a probe (Fig. 5), will hybridize with the same sequence in genomic DNA by complementary base pairing. If this is the usual CC10 gene that has been digested with RsaI, a 1.9-kb fragment will be identified between the flanking RsaI sites, but if it is the polymorphic CC10 gene, a 2.2-kb fragment will be identified (Fig. 5). These fragments can be visualized by autoradiography if the probe used is radioactive, although there are also other labeling techniques that require different methods of detection.

The results of this analysis are shown in Fig. 9 along with the family tree. The maternal grandmother of the nine children in the family (lane 1) has one polymorphic (2.2 kb) and one usual copy (1.9 kb) of the CC10 gene. None of the other grandparents (lanes 2, 13, and 14) have the polymorphic gene, and they therefore only show one band on the autoradiogram (a similar-sized band from both their maternally and paternally inherited chromosome superimposed). The mother of the children (lane 3), however, does have the extra band that she must have inherited from her mother, and in turn this is inherited by five of the eight children (lanes 4, 5, 8, 9, and 10).

This simple example demonstrates how this technique may resolve the identity of a specific gene associated with a genetic illness. If the polymorphic CC10 gene was

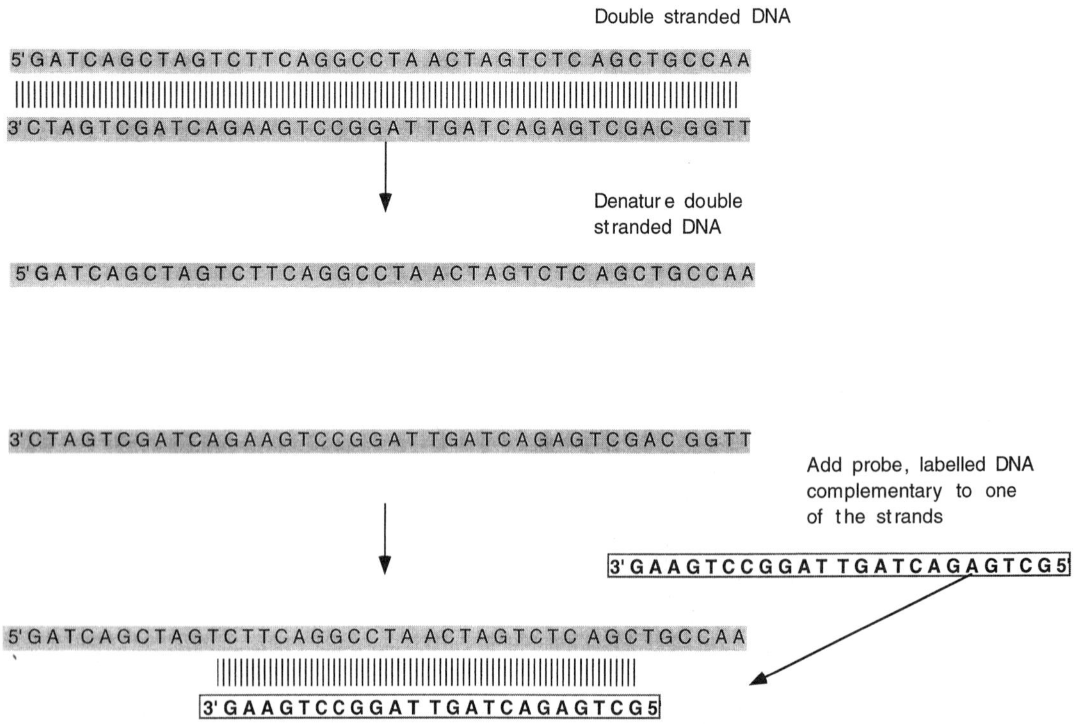


**FIG. 8.** Hybridization with a labeled probe. A length of nucleic acid that is labeled, usually with a radioactive phosphate group, will hybridize by complementary base pairing with a complementary sequence.

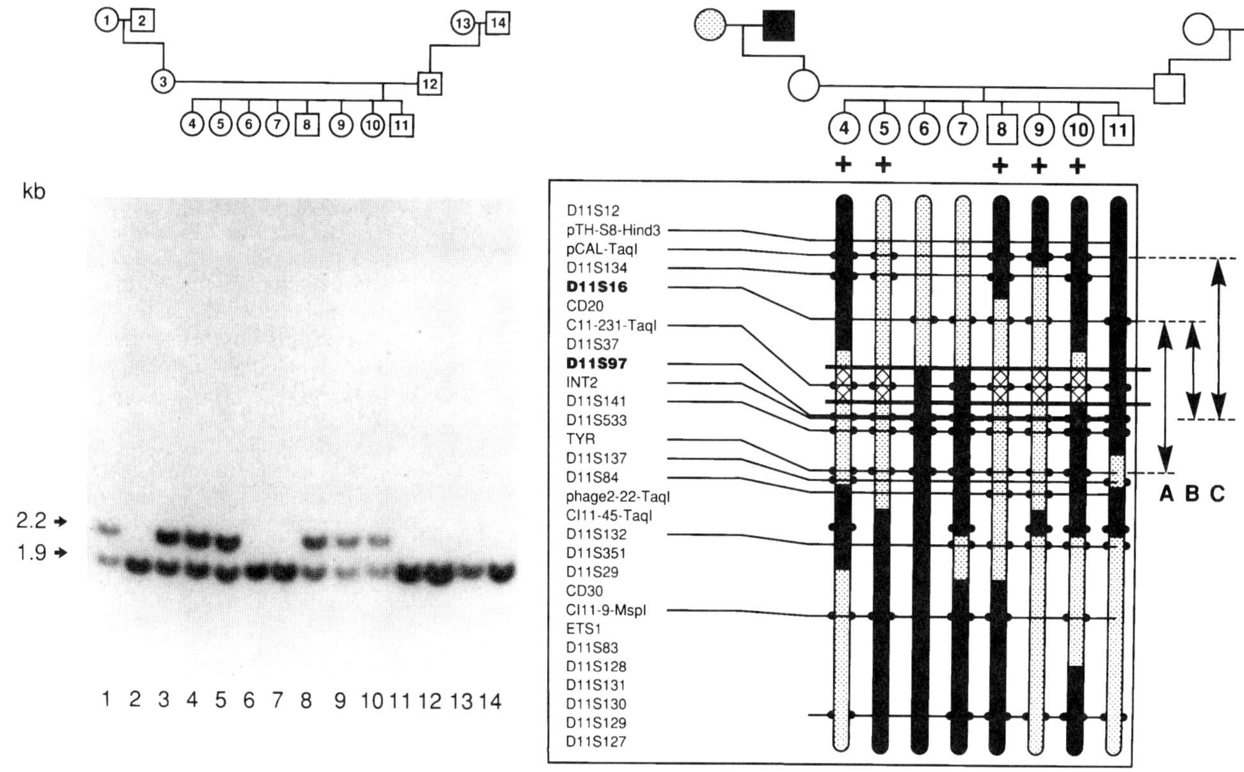


**FIG. 9.** Autoradiogram of a Southern blot hybridized with a $^{32}$P-labeled CC10 cDNA probe 3. Genomic DNA was obtained from the individuals in a three-generation family, digested with the restriction enzyme RsaI, and subjected to gel electrophoresis and Southern blotting. The family tree is shown above the autoradiogram, and the normal length (1.9 kb) and polymorphic (2.2 kb) fragments are marked. (From ref. 3 with permission.)

the cause of asthma, it would be expected that, in the family shown in Fig. 9, the maternal grandmother would have asthma and that this would be inherited by the mother and five of the eight children (lanes 4, 5, 8, 9, and 10) in association with the inheritance of the longer RFLP band and the polymorphic gene. If, however, asthma was not caused by a defect in the CC10 gene but a defect in a gene close by, the maternal grandmother may again have the asthma phenotype and an Alu insertion into the CC10 gene, but her disease is caused by a defect in a gene that is close by. The daughter and most of the children of the family would still inherit asthma (an abnormal IgE receptor gene) along with the longer RFLP because the two genes are close together (linked), but it would be possible to inherit asthma without the longer RFLP band if a crossover event occurred between the CC10 gene and the other gene in some of the children.

The RFLP in the CC10 gene just described is only present in 3% of chromosomes and is either present or absent; this therefore limits the value of such a marker. RFLPs are not the only means of tracking the inheritance of segments of DNA. Within the genome there are frequent "runs" of repeated sequences, perhaps 2 or 3 bp, repeated up to 100 or more times. These repeated sequences, called short tandem repeated sequences or microsatellites, are very variable in length between individuals and thus very useful in the determination of inheritance of a fragment of DNA. That is, for any given microsatellite at one position within the genome, each individual is likely to have a different number of repeats on each of their two copies of DNA at that site. Similarly, two parents are also likely to have a different number of repeats on their two copies, which are likely to be different from each other. The inheritance of a segment of DNA can therefore be identified with considerable precision, and the variability of a microsatellite between individuals is called its heterozygosity. Incidentally, a panel of such microsatellites can be very powerful in linking an individual to blood samples and other biologic material; this technique is called DNA finger printing and is used in forensics.

### DNA Sequencing

Although DNA can be sequenced by chemical methods devised by Maxam and Gilbert (7), Sanger et al. (8) developed an enzymatic reaction that is most frequently used. DNA replicates by the formation of a daughter strand alongside its template by complementary base pairing and the action of DNA polymerase, as described

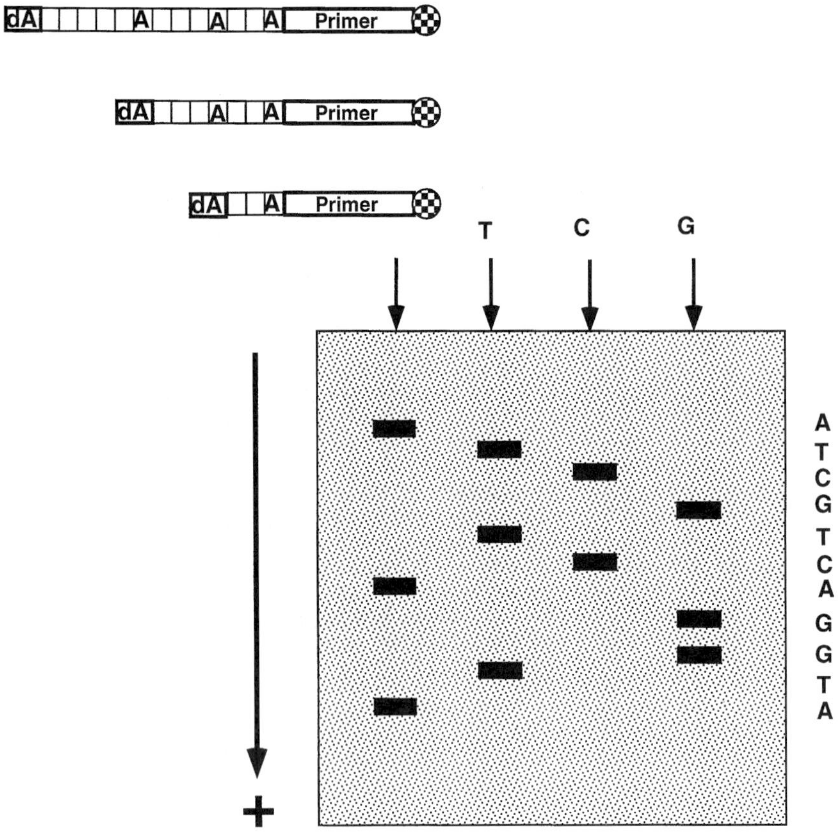


**FIG. 10.** Sequencing reaction using dideoxynucleotides. The reactions are set up containing the DNA strand to be sequenced with the sequencing primer annealed and the four nucleotides dATP, dCTP, dGTP, and dTTP. The daughter strand is then synthesized by complementary base pairing and the incorporation of nucleotides by DNA polymerase. Four reactions are performed in parallel that contain small quantities of either ddCTP, ddGTP, ddTTP, or, as in the figure, ddATP. When the dideoxynucleotide is incorporated, chain elongation is terminated. As only a small proportion of the nucleotide is in the dideoxy form, only a small percentage of the strands will be terminated at any given base position. The products of the four different sequencing reactions (each performed with a different dideoxynucleotide) are run on an acrylamide gel. The primer has been labeled, and the ddATP reaction products are shown as an example. The products from all four reactions are loaded on the gel in the order A, T, C, and G, and can be read from the ladder obtained as shown.

previously and shown in Fig. 2. The new DNA strand is synthesized in the 5′ to 3′ direction by the incorporation of the nucleotides dATP, dCTP, dGTP, and dTTP into the elongating strand of DNA. Sanger et al. discovered that a dideoxyribose would inhibit chain elongation; a dideoxy-sugar incorporated into the elongating strand does not have an hydroxyl group in the 3′ position to form a phosphodiester bond with the next incoming nucleotide. The dideoxy-sugar thus acts as a "chain elongation terminator."

To sequence a length of DNA, first the two stands must be separated or denatured either by heat or alkali. Next a short length of single-stranded DNA approximately 15 or more bp long (an oligonucleotide) is annealed to the strand to be sequenced by reducing the temperature, to allow complementary base pairing to a known sequence within the DNA fragment. This oligonucleotide then acts as a "primer" for DNA polymerase to synthesize the daughter strand by incorporation of the respective complementary bases moving along the parent strand and synthesizing the new strand in the 5′ to 3′ direction. Four reactions are performed, and each is "spiked" at a low concentration with a different dideoxynucleotide to cause some of the elongating chains to be terminated. Each separate reaction is then run on a polyacrylamide gel to separate the different bands and allow the sequence to be read (Fig. 10).

The daughter strands need to be labeled to be visualized, and this is achieved either with a radioactive label or nonradioactive label. A radioactive label can be incorporated into the elongating strands by using a labeled nucleotide, e.g., dATP that has the $\alpha$-phosphate labeled with $^{33}$P. The end-labeling method using the enzyme polynucleotide kinase to transfer a labeled phosphate group from the $\gamma$-position of dATP to the 5′ position of the DNA oligonucleotide primer can also be used.

Automated sequencers follow the same principles, except the primers used in the four different termination reactions have a different fluorescent group attached. The four reactions are then pooled and run on a gel, and the sequential fluorescence detected from the different primers corresponding to the different termination reactions.

### Polymerase Chain Reaction

The polymerase chain reaction (PCR), a technique that enables a segment of DNA to be copied many times over, has revolutionized the practice of molecular biology and has numerous applications.

The technique depends on (a) the ability of double-stranded DNA to separate into single strands at high temperatures, and then reassociate at low temperatures determined by complementary base pairing; and (b) the discovery of DNA polymerase enzymes that are stable at high temperatures; the first was isolated from *thermus aquaticus* (Taq polymerase).

The reaction requires the following ingredients: the template DNA to be amplified, Taq polymerase enzyme, nucleotides to be incorporated into the daughter strands, a pair of oligonucleotide primers complementary to known sequences that flank the DNA segment to be amplified, and an enzyme buffer.

The first step in the reaction is to "denature" the dsDNA by increasing the temperature of the reaction to

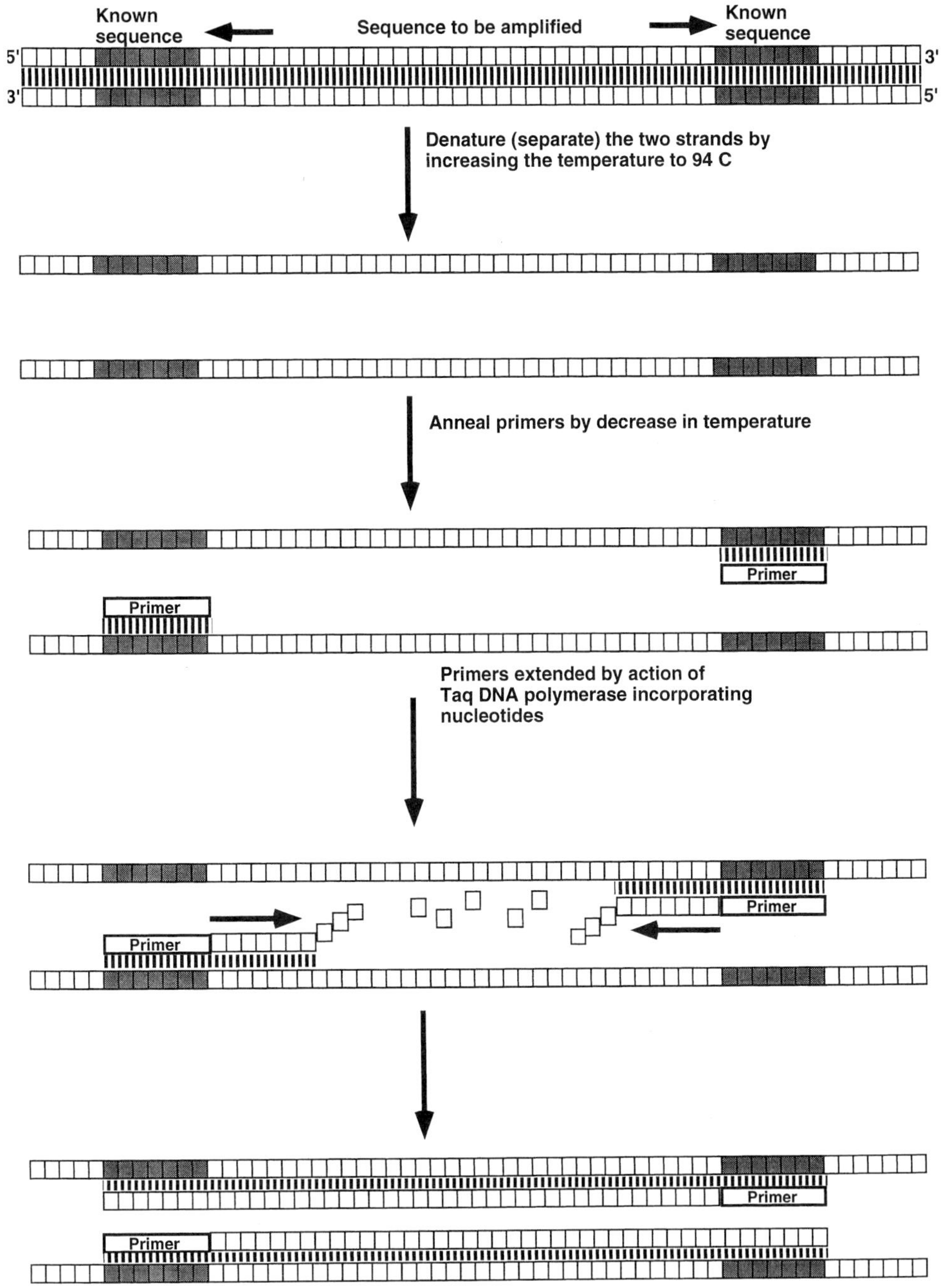


**FIG. 11.** The polymerase chain reaction. It is necessary to know the sequence of flanking nucleotides. The double-stranded segment of template DNA is first denatured (strands separated) by heat, the temperature is then reduced, and the primers annealed to their complementary sequence. The temperature is next increased to 72°C to allow primer extension by the activity of Taq DNA polymerase. The second cycle then commences with strand denaturation by increasing the temperature to 94°C again, and repeated cycles of denaturing, annealing, and extension.

94°C (Fig. 11). Next the temperature is decreased to enable the primers to bind or "anneal" to their complementary sequence. The temperature is then held for a minute or two at 72°C to allow the daughter strands to be synthesized by the action of Taq DNA polymerase that incorporates nucleotides and "extends" the primers, making a new strand in the 5′ to 3′ direction. At the end of this step, two daughter strands will have been synthesized. The cycle is then repeated again with denaturation, primer annealing, and extension. At the end of the second cycle, however, the target sequence will be amplified to four copies, and at the end of the third cycle to eight copies, etc. It is usual to perform 20 or more cycles that will yield millions of copies.

The accuracy of primer binding can be influenced by the temperature set for the annealing step in the reaction. As mentioned previously, G binds to C with greater strength (three H bonds) than A binds to T (two H bonds). For short lengths of DNA, the temperature of annealing can be calculated approximately by allowing 2°C for every A-T bond and 4°C for every G-C bond. Thus, the sequence CACCATGGCATTGCAAGGC will anneal to its exact sister strand at a temperature of 60°(C $((11 \times 4) + (8 \times 2))$. If the annealing temperature for the PCR reaction is set for 64°C, the primer will not anneal and the reaction will not work. If the temperature is set for 45°C, the primer will anneal to the target sequence, but also to other sequences within the genome that do not have an exact match. Performing the PCR reaction with an annealing temperature close to 60°C is likely to give the most specific amplification.

## TRANSCRIPTION AND RNA PROCESSING

Genetic information is stored in the ordered sequence of bases in the strands of DNA that constitute the chromosomes. The unit of inheritance is the gene, and each gene by the sequence of bases it contains encodes the amino acid sequence of a protein. The protein coding sequence within the gene is usually split into short stretches of DNA or exons that are separated by noncoding stretches of DNA or introns.

The chromosomes and thus genes are stored in the nucleus, yet the protein production machinery is within the cytoplasm. Messenger RNA (mRNA) is the courier of information from the gene in the nucleus to the protein production machinery in the cytoplasm. The production of mRNA from a DNA template is called transcription. During the process of RNA production or transcription, the enzyme RNA polymerase synthesizes a daughter strand of RNA by complementary base pairing with the DNA template (Fig. 12). The RNA polymerase is directed to and binds specific sequences (see below) upstream of the coding sequence of the gene. mRNA is synthesized and extended in the 5′ to 3′ direction by reading the sequence from the template DNA gene in the 3′ to 5′ direction. Sequential ribonucleotides rather than deoxyribonucleotides are added; the process is otherwise similar to DNA replication except in transcription the nucleotide uridine triphosphate is used in place of thymidine triphosphate.

RNA polymerase does not distinguish the exons from the introns and makes a complete copy of the gene. Only

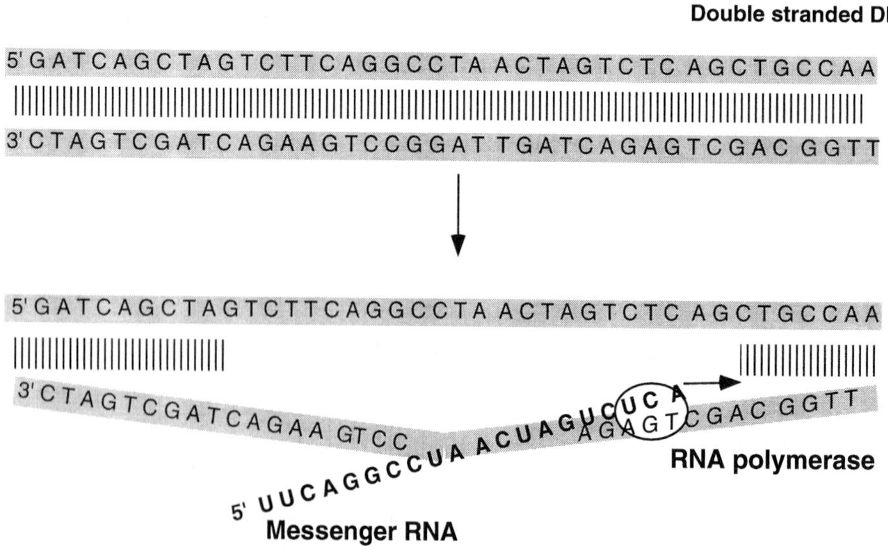


**FIG. 12.** The process of transcription. mRNA is synthesized by RNA polymerase from the noncoding DNA template. The mRNA is synthesized in the 5′ to 3′ direction on the DNA strand that is read in the 3′ to 5′ direction.

one DNA strand is transcribed; the strand that codes for the protein product is called the "sense" strand or coding strand. The mRNA sequence is also a sense sequence and must therefore be synthesized by pairing with the complementary "anti-sense" strand.

### RNA Processing

RNA polymerase does not distinguish sequences that are from the coding exons of a gene from the intron sequences. The initial unprocessed pre-mRNA, which is also called heterogeneous RNA, has to be processed to mRNA. The process of excising the intron sequences from between the exons is called splicing. An enzyme complex called the spliceosome is responsible for performing this task. This enzyme complex recognizes three specific sequences: GT denotes the start and AG the end of an intron, and 18 to 40 bases upstream of the 3′ end of the intron is a branch point motif conforming to the sequence PyNPyPyPu**A**Py(Py = pyrimidine, C or T; Pu = purine, A or G; N = any nucleotide).

After splicing is complete and the final mRNA formed, the protein coding sequence runs uninterrupted from the translation start codon (AUG) to the translation stop codon (UAG). The protein coding sequence is flanked by untranslated sequences, called the 5′ untranslated region (5′ UTR) and the 3′ untranslated region (3′ UTR) upstream and downstream of the protein coding sequence respectively. These flanking regions are also modified by the addition of a "cap" structure that is a modified GTP nucleotide at the 5′ end, and the 3′ end is trimmed by a nuclease and a string of adenines added after the "polyadenylation signal," which is the sequence AAUAAA (Fig. 13).

### Alternative Splicing

In some instances, by a process called "alternative splicing," the same gene may be spliced differently in different tissues, and this may result in the production of two different proteins. The calcitonin/calcitonin-gene regulated peptide gene is an example of a gene that is alternatively spliced; in the thyroid the mRNA comprises exons 1, 2, 3, and 4, and the protein product is calcitonin, yet in the brain the mRNA comprises exons 1, 2, 3, 5, and 6, and the protein product is the calcitonin-gene regulated peptide.

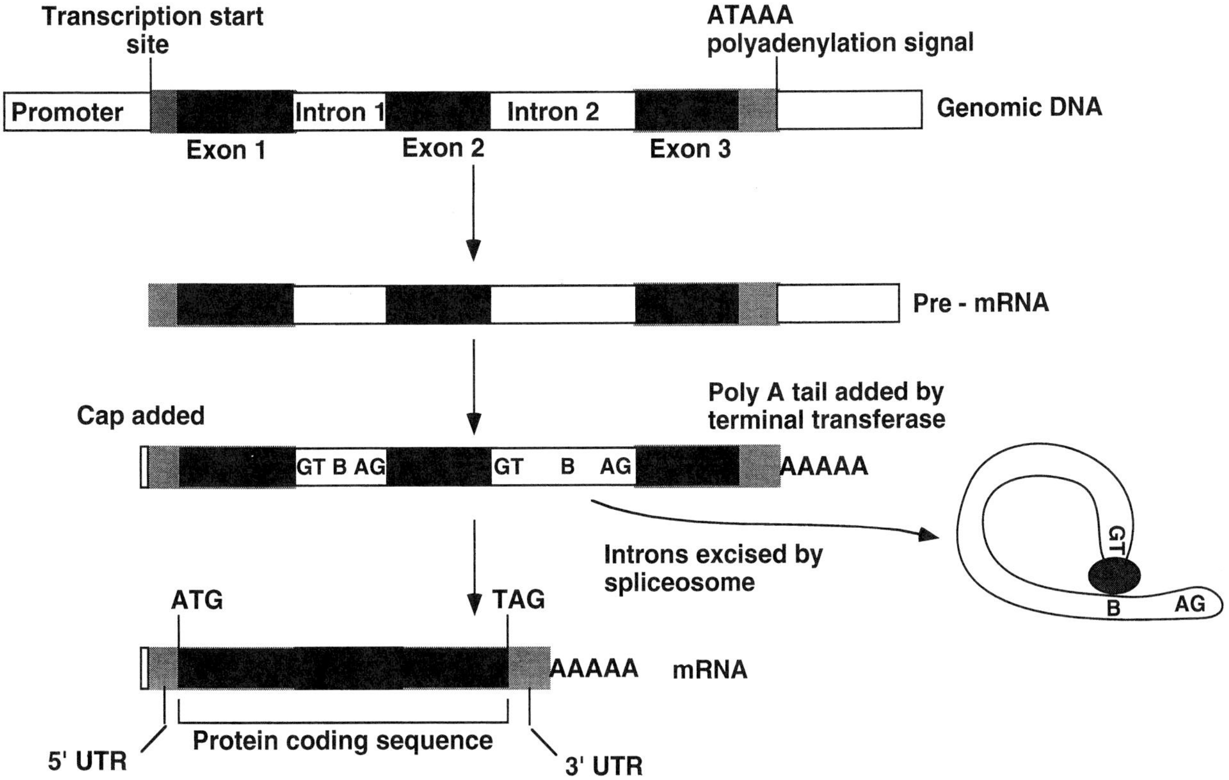


**FIG. 13.** RNA processing. The pre-mRNA is capped by the addition of a modified GTP at the 5′ end, and the 3′ end is trimmed by a nuclease, and a poly A tail is added at the polyadenylation signal. The introns are also spliced out by the spliceosome enzyme complex. The intron has a consensus GT sequence at its 5′ end and a consensus AG at its 3′ end with a conserved branch point sequence (B) in between.

It can also be understood that if an intron fails to be spliced out of the pre-RNA due to a mutation in one of the conserved splicing sequences, an extra section of RNA will remain in the mRNA and be translated and included in the protein. This may totally disrupt the function of the protein, and if the insertion is not in frame, that is, divisible by 3, the remainder of the protein coding sequence will be out of frame and thus encode different amino acids.

In addition to the insertion of an intron sequence into the protein, exons can also be aberrantly excised. Such splicing abnormalities can lead to human disease including neurofibromatosis and cystic fibrosis.

### Evaluation of Exon/Intron Structure

Gene structure can be evaluated by the use of an enzyme called S1 nuclease. In brief, this technique utilizes the property of S1 nuclease to digest single-stranded DNA, but not DNA-RNA hybrids. If a segment of genomic DNA whose gene structure is unknown is taken, denatured (strands separated), and hybridized with mRNA (which will hybridize by complementary base pairing to the exons, but not introns), and then digested with S1 nuclease, only segments of DNA representing the exons will remain intact. These segments can then be evaluated by gel electrophoreses, Southern blotting, and hybridization.

The transcription start site, that is, the position where RNA polymerase starts to synthesize the RNA strand, can also be evaluated in the same manner by S1 nuclease. Additional techniques to evaluate the transcription start include extension of a primer hybridized to the first exon by reverse transcriptase and the use of RNase protection assays.

## CLONING OF GENES

The ability to produce many copies of a gene, that is, to produce recombinant DNA, is a very powerful tool in molecular biology. Segments of DNA can be introduced into bacteria and replicated many thousandfold and thus become available for detailed study in numerous applications.

The isolation of the human cPLA2 gene and the promoter region of this gene will be used to demonstrate the use of recombinant DNA and the principles of screening a DNA library. The human cPLA2 protein is the rate-limiting enzyme in the production of arachidonic acid, an important mediator of inflammation. The structure of the protein and mechanisms regulating expression of the gene in various tissues and in response to various mediators may therefore be of importance in understanding inflammatory pathways, and in the development of therapeutic agents to inhibit inflammatory processes.

The first step is to develop an oligonucleotide probe to hybridize with $cPLA_2$ gene sequences. The cPLA2 protein was isolated from inflammatory exudates and the sequence of a short segment of this protein determined by chemical methods (9,10). The amino acid sequence can be translated into a nucleotide sequence, remembering that a codon of three nucleotides specifies an individual amino acid. The redundancy in the genetic code (more than one code for most amino acids) prevents the exact determination of nucleotide sequence, but the first and the second base for each amino acid can usually be predicted. A "degenerate" oligonucleotide probe is therefore synthesized that conserves the nucleotides that are known to be present and has random nucleotides at the other positions.

The hybridization conditions will have to be "nonstringent" to allow this imperfect probe to bind to its complementary sequence. As previously discussed, the strength with which two complementary strands of DNA bind to each other depends on the relative GC (three bonds) and AT (two bonds) composition. It also depends on the length of the sequence, the buffer composition, and the temperature. The conditions can therefore be adjusted to favor the binding of imperfect sequences (compare with the discussion of conditions for PCR).

The next step is to produce a library of DNA sequences that will contain the sought after cPLA2 gene sequences. A cDNA library is usually screened before a genomic library. Genomic DNA is the form of DNA that is present in the chromosomes, and contains exons, introns, and intervening sequences, whereas cDNA or complementary DNA is a DNA copy of the mRNA and thus contains only gene sequences. To make a cDNA library, a tissue that expresses the cPLA2 gene must be selected, for example, monocytic cells. mRNA is first extracted from the monocytic cells, and converted to cDNA by the use of an enzyme called reverse transcriptase (Fig. 14).

Reverse transcriptase is an enzyme present in retroviruses that is able to synthesize a DNA strand on an RNA template. A poly T primer (oligo dT) can be used to prime the reverse transcriptase based on the knowledge that mRNA has a poly A tail that will be complementary to the poly T primer. A first cDNA strand is thus synthesized on the mRNA template. The second DNA strand is then synthesized by the addition of DNA polymerase, which is self-primed by a hairpin bend that invariably occurs at the end of the DNA (the end of the DNA folds back on itself). cDNA has thus been synthesized.

The next step is to ligate onto both ends of the cDNA strands a short chemically synthesized length of double-stranded DNA or an "adapter" that contains a restriction site. This cDNA library is then digested with the restriction enzyme corresponding to the restriction site in the adapter and ligated into a vector to propagate the library.

Depending on the size of the DNA fragments to be propagated, several different vectors are available, including plasmids, cosmids, and yeast. Phages, which are viral particles that infect bacteria, are the vectors usually chosen. All the essential information for phage replication is avail-

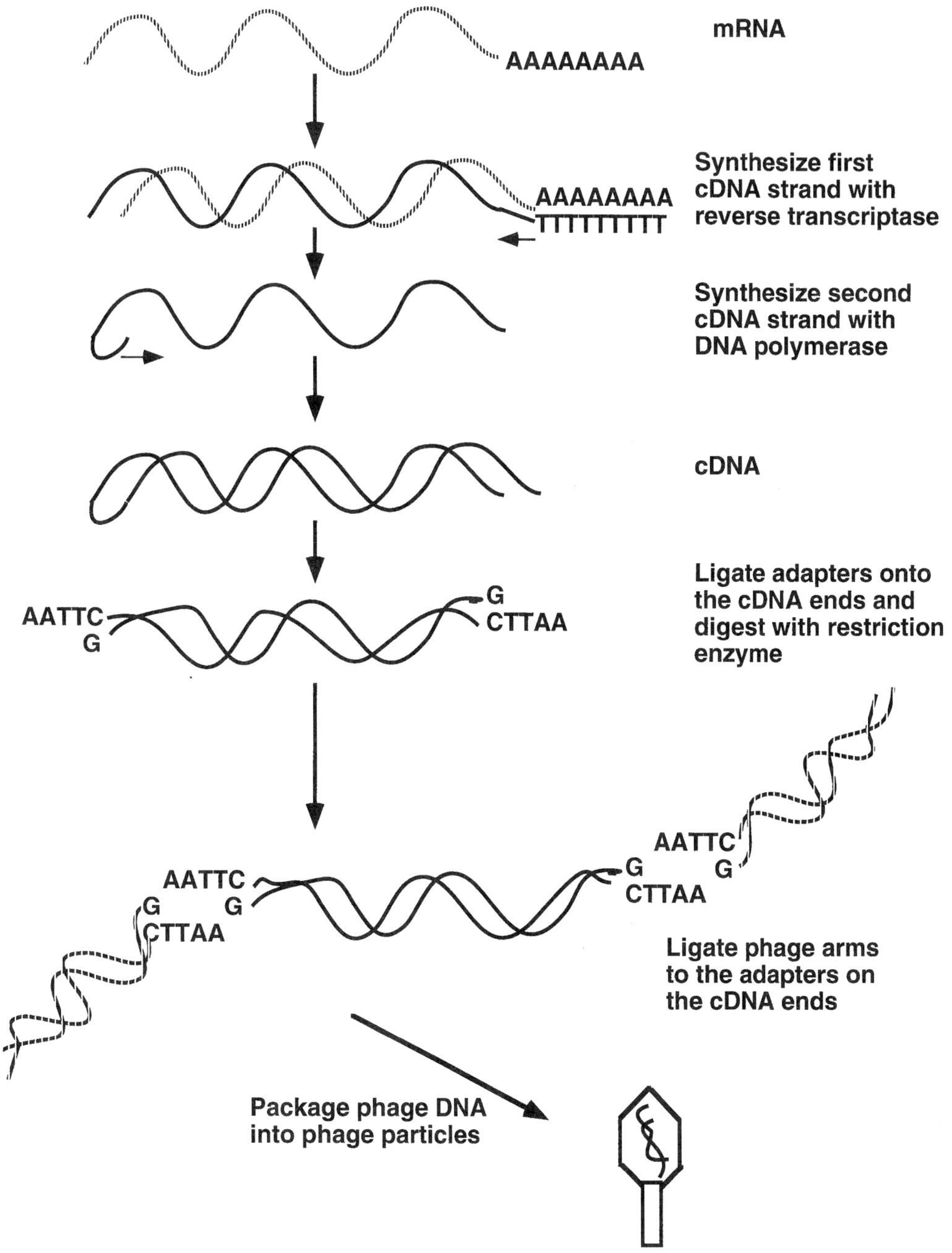


**FIG. 14.** Creation of a cDNA library in a bacteriophage vector. First strand cDNA is synthesized on the mRNA template using reverse transcriptase and a oligo-dT primer. The synthesized 3′ cDNA end forms a hairpin loop to self-prime the second cDNA strand synthesis when DNA polymerase is added. Adapters are ligated onto the cDNA ends, digested with a restriction enzyme, and ligated to phage arms with compatible digested ends. The phage DNA is then packaged into phage particles.

able in the ends of the phage DNA, and these ends can thus be digested from the phages with an appropriate enzyme and ligated onto the cDNA library. The phages can then infect a "lawn" of bacteria on agar plates (Fig. 15).

The phage infectious cycle will cause the bacteria to lyse, and this will be detected as a clear spot on the cloudy bacterial plate. Each clear spot will be the result of an individual phage particle infecting an individual bacterium and replicating and infecting adjacent bacteria to produce a clone of phage particles. These clear areas of lysis are called plaques, and it is possible to have 50,000 discrete plaques on one 15-cm plate of bacteria.

The next step is to lay a nylon membrane on the plaques to absorb some of the DNA. The membrane is

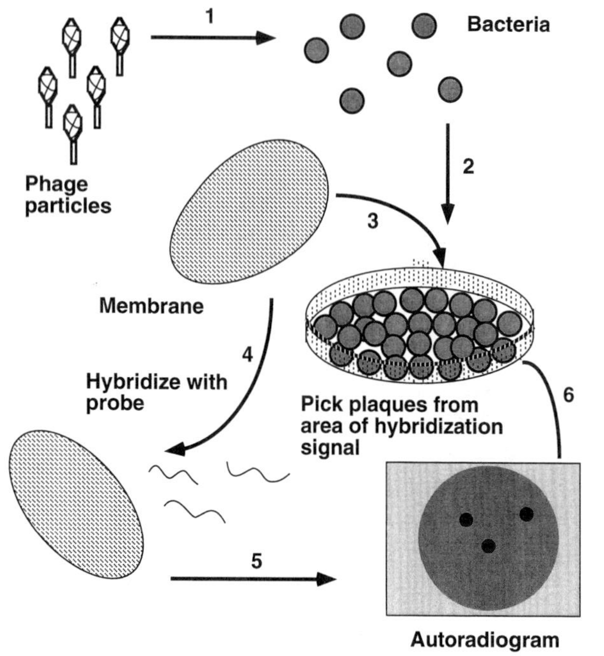


**FIG. 15.** Screening a phage library. A bacterial culture is infected with the phage library and spread onto agar plates. The phage particles replicate within the bacteria and infect surrounding bacteria until each clone derived from one original phage particle infects and causes the lysis of a cluster of bacteria. This is seen as a clear area on the cloudy bacterial lawn, or a plaque. A membrane is then laid on the bacterial lawn allowing some DNA from each of the plaques to transfer to the membrane. The membrane is then hybridized with a probe to the gene being sought, and an autoradiogram obtained. The positive signals on the autoradiogram are aligned with the appropriate region on the bacterial plate, and each positive region picked for a second round of screening.

then hybridized with the labeled probe previously constructed. Any clones that have a DNA sequence homologous to the probe will hybridize to the probe and a positive signal will be seen. If the plate is then reexamined by alignment to the membrane, the region from which the positive signal was obtained can be picked. Phages from this region are isolated and reinfected onto bacterial plates at a low density such that individual clones can be picked and evaluated.

The individual clones that hybridize with the probe are selected, and the DNA between the arms of the phage that should be the cDNA being sought after is digested and extracted from the phage and subcloned into a plasmid and sequenced. Plasmids are small circles of DNA that are able to replicate within bacteria.

Once the cDNA sequence has been cloned, it can be placed in an expression plasmid that will direct the synthesis of the protein in bacteria. The recombinant protein will thus be available for study in large quantities.

If an antibody for the protein product of the gene to be cloned is available, another strategy is to screen an expression library. An expression library contains all the cDNA sequences from a cell type prepared as previously described, but the cDNA sequences are preceded by the necessary sequences in the phage that allow the cDNA to be transcribed and expressed as a protein. The plaques can then be screened with an antibody against the protein product rather than a DNA probe.

The cloned cDNA itself can now be used as a probe to screen a genomic library to isolate the gene in a similar manner. Genomic libraries are constructed by cutting up the genome with a specific restriction enzyme, and then ligating phage arms onto these fragments and continuing as previously described for a cDNA library. It is sometimes necessary to screen up to 1 million plaques (20- × 15-cm plates with 50,000 plaques on each) to isolate the genomic fragment being sought. The promoter region and other regions of the gene can then be futher evaluated.

## CONTROL OF GENE EXPRESSION

### DNase Hypersensitive Sites

The huge amount of DNA within each cell nucleus does not exist in a disorganized tangle, but is neatly arranged in coils around proteins. These proteins that are very positive in charge are called histones (11), and 200 bp of DNA is coiled around an octamer of four pairs of proteins to form a cylinder. This DNA–protein complex is called a nucleosome, and nucleosomes are closely packed adjacent to one another. An additional histone protein is loosely attached between adjacent nucleosomes.

DNase is an enzyme that degrades DNA, and although all the DNA in the chromosomes exists as nucleosomes, different regions are more susceptible than others to DNase degradation. The least susceptible regions of DNA are stretches that do not contain genes. The most susceptible regions of DNA are those within genes that are transcribed in that particular cell, and even within these regions, lengths of DNA within the promoter region appear to be particularly sensitive to DNase degradation; these regions are called DNase-hypersensitive sites. DNase-hypersensitive sites are the lengths of DNA within the promoter of a gene that are likely to bind proteins that regulate the transcriptional machinery.

### Basal Transcription Machinery

As appropriately named, mRNA is the messenger that carries the genetic information from the nucleus to the protein production machinery in the cytosol. Although each nucleated cell in the human body has all the genetic information to make every protein, cell differentiation into specialized cells to form tissues and organs require that certain cell types make some proteins but not others. For example, the hepatocyte is

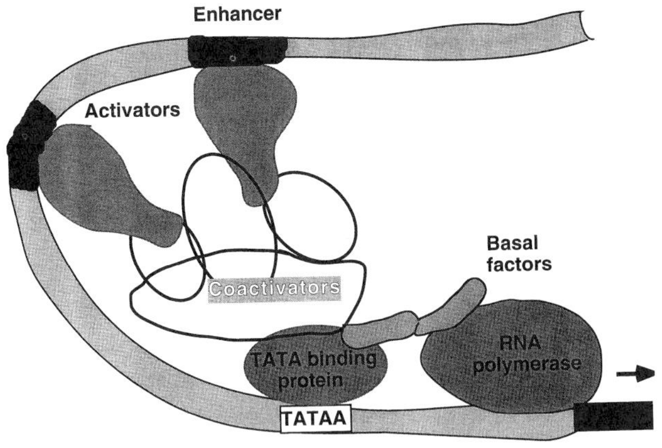


**FIG. 16.** Transcription factors or activators bind to sequence motifs or enhancers within the promoter region. These activating factors bind coactivating proteins that interact and stimulate transcription from the basal transcription machinery.

responsible for the production of albumin, $a_1$-antitrypsin, and various other circulating proteins. The pulmonary type II cell produces the surfactant proteins. It would clearly be inappropriate for the hepatocyte to produce surfactant, or the type II cell clotting factors. As already discussed, the organization of the genome into more or less accessible regions (DNase-hypersensitive regions) may confer some degree of control of gene expression, but the predominant control of gene expression is the control of transcription.

The enzyme RNA polymerase synthesizes the RNA molecule by the sequential addition of ribonucleotides complementary to the DNA sequence. RNA polymerase has to be positioned at the promoter region of the gene to commence synthesis of RNA. Most regulated eukaryotic genes have a conserved sequence approximately 28 bp upstream of the start of transcription. This sequence motif

**TABLE 1.** *Examples of transcription factors and the DNA motifs they recognize*

| Transcription factor/ activation site | Synonym | Inducer | Binding sequence | Domains | Comments |
|---|---|---|---|---|---|
| Activating protein 1 | AP-1 | TPA | TGA$^{G}/_{C}$T$^{C}/_{A}$A | Leucine zipper | Homodimer or heterodimer of Jun and Fos |
| CAAT/enhancer binding protein | C/EBPα | | GTGG$^{T}/_{A}$$^{T}/_{A}$$^{T}/_{A}$G | Leucine zipper | Important for liver and adipose tissue expression; also binds to CAAT box |
| cAMP response element binding protein | CREB | PKA | TGACG$^{C}/_{T}$$^{C}/_{A}$$^{G}/_{A}$ | Leucine zipper | Phosphorylated by PKA |
| CAAT box | CTF/NF-1 | GGCCAATCT | | | Binds to CAAT box |
| Glucocorticoid response element binding protein | GRE | Glucocorticoid | AGAACAN$_3$TGTTCT | Zinc finger | Cytosolic receptor moves to nucleus following glucocorticoid binding |
| Hepatocyte nuclear factor 1 | HNF-1 | | GTTAATNATTAAC | | Important in liver-specific transcription |
| Hepatocyte nuclear factor 3 | HNF-3 | | TATTGA$^{C}/_{T}$TT$^{A}/_{T}$G | Helix turn helix | A family of factors important in liver- and lung-specific transcription |
| Interferon stimulated response element | ISRE | Interferon-α | ACTTTCAGTTTCAT | | Activated by STAT proteins |
| Interferon γ activation site | GAS | Interferon-γ | GTTTCATATTACTCTA | | Activated by STAT proteins |
| Nuclear factor kB | NFkB | TNF | GGGA$^{A}/_{C}$TN$^{T}/_{C}$CC | | Family of factors involved in inflammatory response |
| Nuclear factor IL-6 | NF-IL6 | IL-1, IL-6 | T$^{T}/_{G}$NNGNAA$^{T}/_{G}$ | | |
| | SP-1 | | G/TG/AGGCG/TG/AG/AG/T | Zinc finger | |
| TATA binding protein | TBP | | TATAAA | | Part of basal transcription machinery |
| Thyroid transcription factor 1 | TTF-1 | | GTNNAG | Homeodomain | Important in thyroid and lung-specific transcription |

closely conforms to TATAA, and is called the TATA box. A protein called the TATA binding protein binds to this TATA box, and recruits several other basal factors that form a complex to bind RNA polymerase at the appropriate position to commence transcription.

*Activating factors* or transcription factors are proteins important in stimulating transcription (12–14). These transcription factors bind to specific DNA sequences or "enhancers" in the promoter region of the gene. They are then able to bind a complex of coactivating proteins that in turn interact with the basal transcription proteins and stimulate transcription (Fig. 16). Transcription factors are thus of great importance in the regulation of transcription, both in determining the tissue specificity of gene expression and the cell's response to various signals to modulate the transcription of specific genes.

Transcription factors fall into four major classes based on their protein structure, and these are called helix-turn-helix, zinc finger, leucine zipper, and helix-loop-helix factors. These four classes of protein differ in their structural motifs that interact with DNA.

Jun and fos are transcription factors of the leucine zipper variety, they are able to homodimerize and heterodimerize to form a factor called AP-1 that binds to DNA elements with the sequence TGACTCA, and are thus able to modulate transcription. The factor NFκB is a dimer of two subunits, p65 and p50, which normally resides in the cytoplasm bound to an inhibitory factor IB. In response to various cell signals, often that mediate inflammatory responses, IκB is degraded and NFκB is thus released and able to reach the nucleus where it binds to the sequence motif GGGA(A/C)TN(T/C)CC in the upstream region of several genes, and is then able to modulate transcription of these genes.

The DNA sequence motifs that are recognized by a variety of transcription factors are shown in Table 1.

Transcription factors from several different families, some with widespread expression and others with more limited expression, interact to determine tissue specificity of gene expression. For example, the CCAAT/enhancer binding protein α (C/EBPα), a transcription factor of the leucine zipper family, is abundant in liver and adipose tissues, and stimulates transcription from a number of liver-specific genes. Another group of trans-activating factors that interact with liver-specific genes are homologous to the *Drosophila* homoeotic gene fork head, and are called HNF-3a, HNF-3b, and HNF-3g (15).

### Regulated Genes and Housekeeping Genes

Genes loosely fall into two main groups: those that are responsive to a variety of signals, for instance genes encoding inflammatory mediators, and those that encode products that are required constitutively, for example genes for cellular structural proteins. This latter group of genes that are not subject to substantial regulation are often called housekeeping genes, and usually have a different promoter structure.

Whereas regulated genes typically have a TATA box and a variety of other sequence motifs for transcription factors such as a CAAT box for factor NF1/CTF, or adenosine 3′,5′-cyclic monophosphate (cAMP) response elements (CRE) that might bind the cAMP response element binding protein (CREB). Housekeeping genes typically do not have a TATA box but an "initiator element" that directs transcription, and the reporter region is typically GC rich with multiple SP1 binding sites (GGGGCGGGG).

## SIGNAL TRANSDUCTION

Signal transduction is the mechanism by which an extracellular stimulus is transmitted from the cell's external membrane to elicit a response within the cell, that often results in modification of gene transcription. These pathways are often complex signaling cascades that enable signal amplification and specificity. It is possible to define several different pathways, but as further data accumulate, cooperation between the different pathways becomes more evident.

The activity of protein kinases is an important aspect of the signaling pathways. These enzymes can be grouped into those kinases that phosphorylate threonine or serine on the target molecules, or those that phosphorylate tyrosine. The protein tyrosine kinases can also been grouped into the receptor protein tyrosine kinases where the kinase forms an integral part of a receptor, and the non-receptor protein tyrosine kinases that usually associate with receptors, although they are not themselves an integral part of the receptor.

Families of pathways can also be distinguished based on the second messenger mediating the signaling event, such as cAMP, guanosine 3′,5′-cyclic monophosphate (cGMP), calcium, and diacylglycerol.

cAMP is released from activated adenylyl cyclase and mediates many intracellular pathways, mainly by activating protein kinase A (PKA). cGMP activates a cGMP-dependent protein kinase (PKG) located predominantly in smooth muscle and the brain. Calcium ions bind to the protein calmodulin, the resulting conformational changes activating a number of protein kinases, or calmodulin-dependent protein kinases.

In response to receptor stimulation phospholipase C breaks down phosphatidylinositol 4,5-biphosphate to inositol triphosphate and diacylglycerol (DAG). Phospholipase D is also able to form DAG from phosphatidylcholine. DAG in turn activates protein kinase C (PKC), which has multiple functions within the cell.

## G Proteins

Heterotrimeric guanine nucleotide binding proteins or "G proteins" form the link between a large family of membrane-bound receptors and their effectors or second messengers (16). The α- and β-adrenergic receptors are typical examples of membrane receptors that are linked to their effectors by G proteins. All G protein interacting receptors have seven membrane spanning helices, and are linked to an effector, which is often adenylyl cyclase or phospholipase C. The G proteins themselves are trimeric, composed of α, β, and γ subunits.

The interaction of a hormone with its receptor leads to a guanosine diphosphate (GDP) to guanosine triphosphate (GTP) exchange in the α subunit of the G protein. The α subunit then dissociates from the trimer, diffuses through the membrane, and activates an effector, for example, adenylyl cyclase. The activated adenylyl cyclase releases cAMP, which is thus able to activate cAMP-dependent protein kinase (PKA), which phosphorylates the target molecules. The cAMP response element binding protein (CREB) is one such protein that is phosphorylated, and in its phosphorylated state is able to enter the nucleus and induce transcription from genes with a cAMP response element (CRE) in their promoter.

After a short period of time, the α subunit of the G protein converts GTP to GDP, thereby deactivating itself. The α subunit then reassociates with the β and γ subunits to reform the trimer.

## Receptor Protein Tyrosine Kinases

Receptor protein tyrosine kinases respond to the binding of ligand by dimerization and autophosphorylation on tyrosine This enables the phosphorylated receptor to bind proteins containing "SH2 domains" with subsequent activation of protein serine/threonine kinases. The SH2 domain is a region of the protein that has homology with the noncatalytic region of the c-*src* proto-oncogene and recognizes regions around a phosphorylated tyrosine residue. Many of the receptor protein tyrosine kinases mediate their response through mitogen activated protein (MAP) kinase.

### *Mitogen Activated Protein Kinase Signaling*

Growth factor stimulation is often signaled through a MAP kinase pathway (17), as is illustrated in Fig. 17. An extracellular ligand, for example epidermal growth factor (EGF), binds to its receptor on the cell surface, which results in receptor dimerization and autophosphorylation on tyrosine residues. The phosphorylated receptor then activates Ras, a monomeric or small G protein that itself hydrolyses GTP into GDP. The activation of Ras is mediated through an adapter molecule GRB2, which contains SH2 and SH3 domains and associates with the receptor and a guanine nucleotide exchange factor called SOS. SOS then converts the inactive Ras-GDP to activated Ras-GTP.

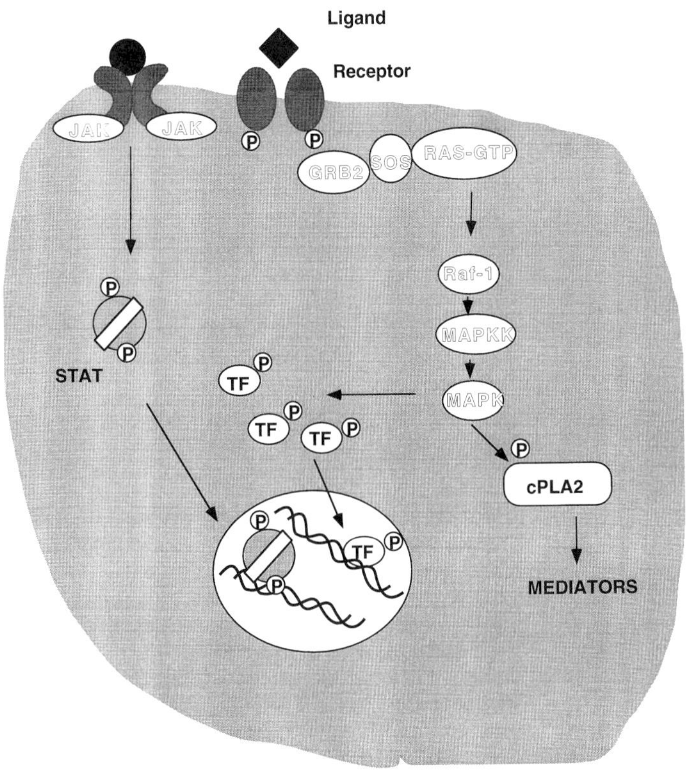


**FIG. 17.** Signal transduction by receptor and nonreceptor protein tyrosine kinases. A receptor protein tyrosine kinase is shown signaling through the MAP kinase pathway to result in activation of transcription factors and cPLA2. A nonreceptor protein tyrosine kinase, JAK, is shown signaling through STAT proteins after activation by a receptor.

This activation of Ras is followed by the sequential activation of several protein kinases; Raf is a threonine/serine kinase that activates MAP kinase kinase (also called MEK), and MAP kinase kinase activates MAP kinase by threonine/tyrosine phosphorylation. Map kinase is then able to phosphorylate transcription factors, for example NF-IL6, c-*fos,* or c-*jun* to modulate transcription to perhaps induce cell proliferation, or phosphorylate cellular enzymes like cPLA2, which results in the liberation of arachidonic acid, a substrate for prostaglandin synthesis.

### Nonreceptor Protein Tyrosine Kinases

Cytokine receptors fall into several family types. Type I receptors include those responsive to most of the interleukin cytokines, type II receptors respond to the interferons and IL-10, type III receptors to tumor necrosis factor, and type IV receptors to IL-1. They do not possess intrinsic protein tyrosine kinase activity, but following receptor activation protein tyrosine kinase activity is rapidly invoked. This kinase activity is mediated by two major families of nonreceptor protein tyrosine kinases, the Src family and the Jak family (18).

#### *The Src Family*

v-*src* was first discovered as an oncogene carried by the Rous sarcoma virus. v-*src* was subsequently shown to be homologous to c-*src*, and both function as protein tyrosine kinases. c-*src* contains two motifs that are found in many cytoplasmic proteins involved in signal transduction, and they are called SH2 and SH3 domains.

The IL-2 receptor binds a member of the src family, Lck, which becomes rapidly activated following receptor occupation.

#### *Jaks and STATs Signaling*

A group of cell surface receptors including a superfamily of cytokine receptors (type 1), examples being IL-2, IL-3, IL-4, and IL-6, and the interferon's (type II) signal through the Jak-STAT pathway (18). Following the binding of ligand, the receptors dimerize, and cytoplasmic protein tyrosine kinases or Jaks associated with the receptors become activated by phosphorylation on tyrosine residues. The activated Jaks then phosphorylate tyrosine residues on the cytoplasmic portion of the receptor, which enables STAT proteins (signal transducers and activators of transcription) to bind to the receptor and become activated by tyrosine phosphorylation. The activated STATs then dimerize and move to the nucleus and activate transcription of various genes.

Interferon-γ, for example, after binding to its receptor, enables activation of Jak1 and Jak2. A STAT protein is then phosphorylated, moves to the nucleus, and activates transcription of genes containing γ-activation sequences (GAS).

#### *NFkB/IkB Pathway*

NFκB is a transcription factor that activates a number of cytokine genes, and is activated in response to tumor necrosis factor as well as other inflammatory stimuli. NFκB is kept in the cytoplasm by association with an inhibitory protein IκB (Fig. 18). However, following TNF

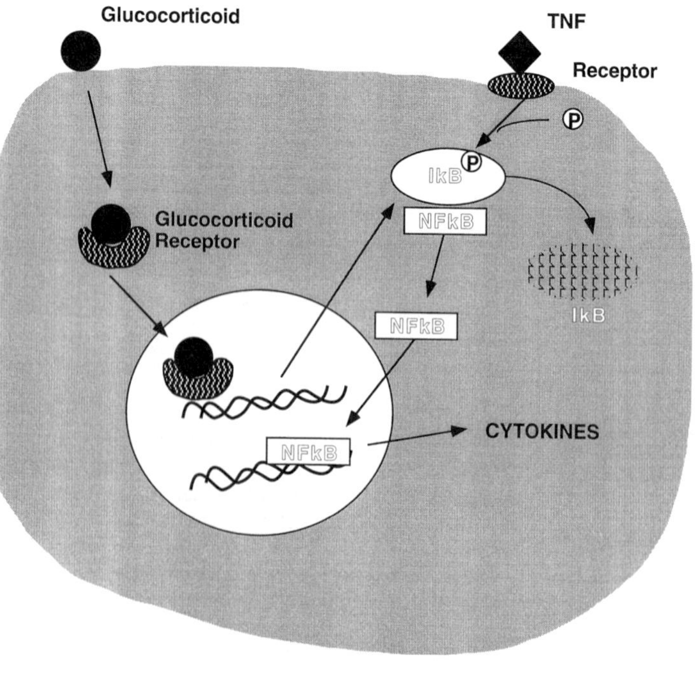


**FIG. 18.** Signal transduction by the transcription factor NFκB and its inhibition by glucocorticoids. TNF signaling is shown as an example; TNF binding to its receptor leads to the phosphorylation of IκB, which causes IκB to degrade. NFκB without IκB bound is able to move to the nucleus and stimulate transcription. Glucocorticoids bind to a cytosolic receptor that then translocates to the nucleus and induces transcription from steroid responsive genes. The IκB gene is an example of a steroid responsive gene, which when overexpressed is able to inhibit the TNF pathway.

binding to its receptor, IκB is phosphorylated by an IκB kinase and subsequently is degraded, thereby allowing NFκB to translocate to the nucleus and activate genes containing a consensus sequence motif for NFκB in their promoter region. Interestingly, glucocorticoids upregulate the IκB gene, and thereby prevent NFκB translocation to the nucleus in response to inflammatory stimuli (19–21).

### *Glucocorticoid Receptor*

The glucocorticoid receptor is part of a family of cytosolic hormone receptors. These receptors are normally inactive in the cytosol in a complex with heat shock proteins (22). Following hormone binding, they translocate to the nucleus and modulate transcription by binding to a specific sequence within the promoters of various genes (Fig. 18).

## EVALUATION OF GENE EXPRESSION

### Northern Blotting

Northern blots are used to evaluate steady-state levels of mRNA expression. RNA is isolated from cells or tissues by a variety of methods, and run on an agarose gel to separate the fragments. The RNA is then transferred from the gel to a nylon membrane in a manner similar to that described for Southern blots. The blots can then be hybridized with specific probes based on the cDNA sequence of the gene being evaluated (23). An example of a Northern blot is shown in Fig. 19.

On some occasions, to detect very low level gene expression, mRNA can be specifically separated from the much larger quantities of ribosomal RNA. This technique takes advantage of the poly A tail that mRNA possesses and uses a T column to bind the mRNA poly A tail.

### Nuclear Run-On Assays

Northern blots are only able to detect steady-state levels of gene expression. This steady-state level is dependent on rate of RNA production and rate of degradation. Nuclear run-on assays are able to detect rates of RNA production. Nuclei are extracted from cells and are quickly chilled to "freeze" ongoing transcription. A radioactively labeled ribonucleotide is then added and transcription in the isolated nuclei allowed to continue. The RNA is then extracted and hybridized with the target gene sequence fixed on a membrane. The gene sequence can be either the cDNA or the genomic sequence (the RNA may not be spliced) cloned in a plasmid. The target DNA bound to the membrane is kept in excess; the strength of the hybridization signal therefore reflects the rate of transcription.

### Posttranscriptional Regulation

Regulation of transcription by a multitude of transcription factors is important in gene regulation, but the stability or the half-life of the mRNA product may also be important. UAA sequences in the 3′ untranslated end of the mRNA transcripts are able to affect the stability of transcripts. For example, tumor necrosis factor-α (TNF-α) inhibits surfactant protein B (SP-B) mRNA expression *in vitro* by decreased SP-B mRNA stability rather than by decreased gene transcription (24). This effect is mediated by an element located in the 3′-UTR region of SP-B mRNA. Further, experimental addition of the 837-bp human SP-B 3′-UTR to a reporter gene mediates a 50% reduction in reporter gene expression induced by TNF-α.

mRNA stability can be evaluated *in vitro* using actinomycin D, which inhibits transcription. The rate of decline of specific mRNA species with time detected by North-

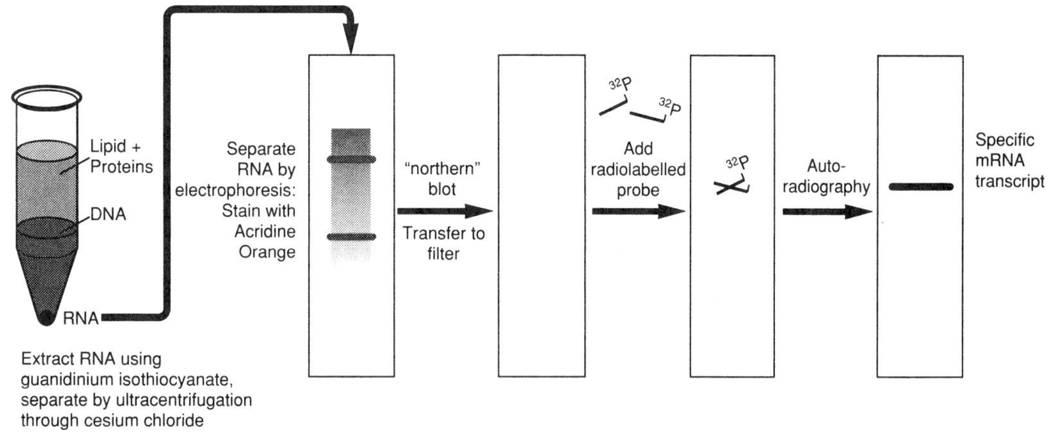


**FIG. 19.** Schematic diagram of the procedures for Northern blot analysis of RNA. Total RNA is isolated and separated by size, using denaturing agarose gel electrophoresis. After transfer of RNA to a solid matrix, specific mRNA is detected by hybridization with radiolabeled gene probes and autoradiography.

ern blotting and hybridization with a specific probe to the gene being evaluated will thus enable the mRNA half-life or stability to be determined.

### *In Situ* Hybridization

Northern blotting of RNA derived from a tissue is able to estimate total amounts of mRNA expressed, but is of little value in determining which cell types within a tissue or population of cells are expressing a particular gene. In situ hybridization is a technique that has this potential. In this technique the cells or tissue are hybridized directly with a labeled RNA probe. This probe is synthesized by *in vitro* transcription from a plasmid. The desired probe sequence is cloned into the plasmid behind a promoter sequence for a bacterial DNA directed RNA polymerase. The RNA polymerase is added to the plasmid in addition to the four ribonucleotides, one of which is labeled, and RNA is synthesized *in vitro*. The transcript is terminated at the end of the probe sequence by previously cutting the plasmid at the end of the sequence so the RNA polymerase will stop and not transcribe other plasmid sequences. Since mRNA conveys the "sense" sequence, the probe to detect expression of RNA within the cell will have to be complementary, that is anti-sense. A sense probe is often used as a control to detect background radioactivity.

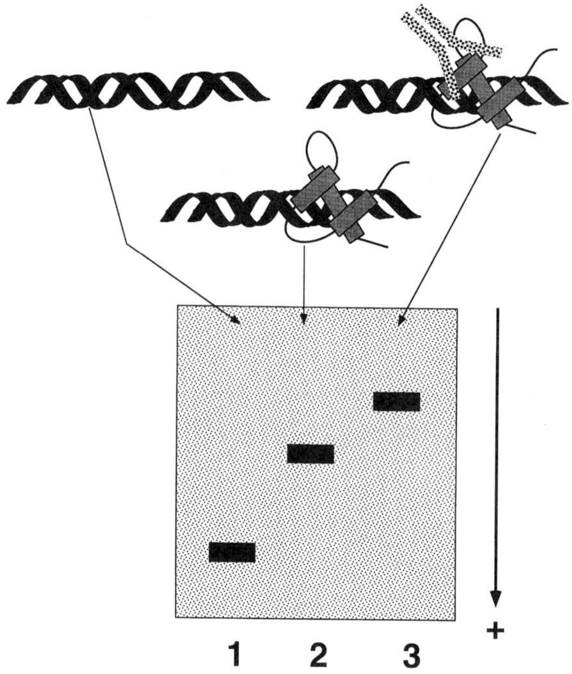


**FIG. 20.** Gel shift assay. The DNA segment presumed to interact with nuclear proteins is run on a polyacrylamide gel (lane 1). After incubation with a protein transcription factor that binds to the DNA segment, the progress of the DNA fragment in the gel is retarded (lane 2); this is called a gel shift. A specific antibody that binds to the protein will retard migration even further (lane 3); this is called a supershift.

## EVALUATION OF DNA PROTEIN INTERACTIONS

### Gel Shift Assay

This is a technique to evaluate the interactions of transcription factors with the promoter element of a gene. It is necessary to have a clone of the promoter element of the gene being evaluated. This DNA fragment is labeled and run on a polyacrylamide gel and then visualized by autoradiography. The fragment will migrate in the gel a distance that is a function of its length (Fig. 20). If, before electrophoresis, the DNA promoter fragment is hybridized with a transcription factor that binds to the promoter region, the DNA will run more slowly as a consequence of the bound protein. This retardation of the mobility of the DNA fragment by the bound protein is called a gel shift.

The transcription factor used to bind to the promoter fragment can be a pure recombinant protein, or can simply be an extract (usually nuclear) from the cell type being studied. To determine the specificity of binding, it is usual to try and inhibit or compete the interaction between the promoter element and the transcription factor by the addition of an excess of oligonucleotides homologous to the sequence it is presumed the transcription factor is binding to. The identity of the transcription factor can also be confirmed by adding to the hybridization mixture a specific antibody against the presumed transcription factor. The bound antibody will again delay the passage of the DNA fragment through the gel, and this is called a supershift (25).

### DNA Footprints

DNA footprinting is another technique to evaluate DNA protein interactions. The concept of this technique is that when a protein is bound to a strand of DNA, it will be more resistant to degradation by the enzyme DNase (compare with discussion on hypersensitive sites). If cloned DNA is taken and mixed with DNase at a concentration that will cleave the strand randomly such that fragments are present in 1-bp increments, the protein-protected region will appear as a footprint in this ladder when the DNA fragments are run on a polyacrylamide gel (Fig. 21).

### Reporter Gene Assays

The use of reporter genes is another method used to evaluate promoter function. Several different reporters are used, including (a) the gene for luciferase that encodes an enzyme isolated from fireflies; luciferase catalyzes the emission of light when mixed with adenosine triphosphate (ATP) and its substrate luciferin; (b) the

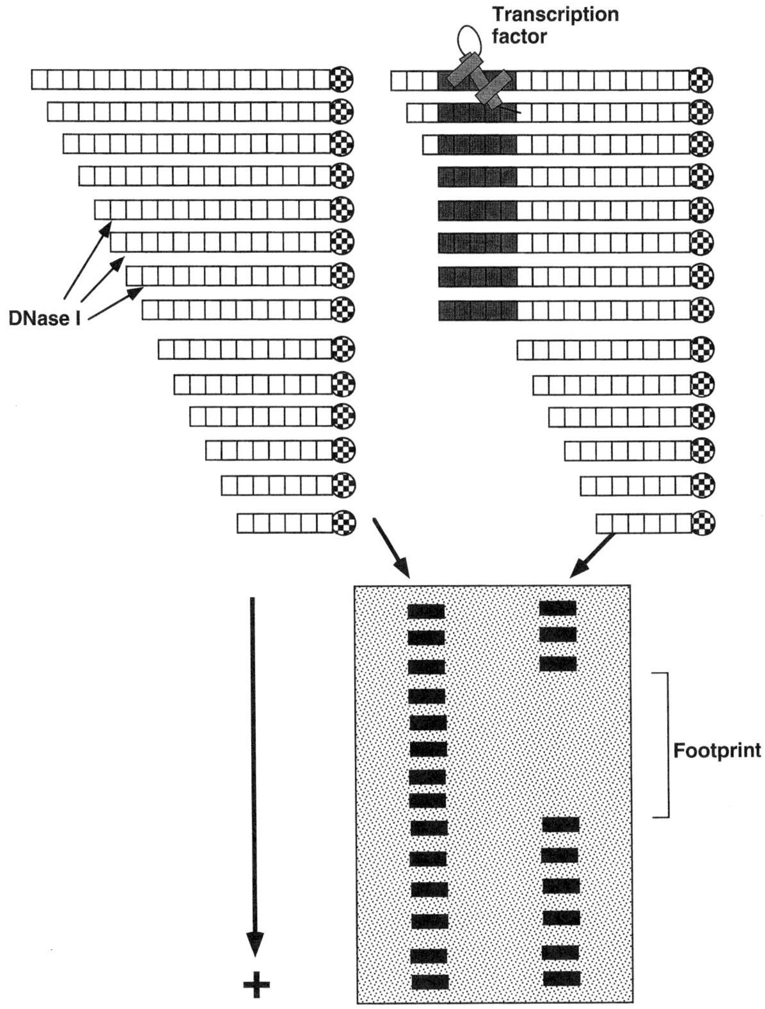


**FIG. 21.** DNA footprinting. Reaction conditions can be adjusted so that DNase I will digest a DNA sequence to yield fragments increasing in size in 1-bp increments. If a transcription factor is bound to part of the sequence, this region will be more resistant to digestion and appear as a footprint when the DNA segments are run on a polyacrylamide gel. The DNA fragments are end labeled so they can be visualized on an autoradiogram.

chloramphenicol acetyl transferase gene (CAT), which catalyzes the acetylation of chloramphenicol; and (c) the β-galactosidase gene, which encodes a protein β-galactosidase that forms a colored product when mixed with its substrate.

The essence of this technique is that the promoter of interest is cloned and inserted into a plasmid in front of a reporter gene. This promoter reporter gene hybrid plasmid can then be transfected into the cell lines being evaluated. Quantification of the activity of the protein derived from the reporter gene in cell lysates will thus indicate the activity of the promoter fragment being evaluated in the cell lines of interest. Subjecting the cell lines to various stimuli, for instance cytokines, which might be expected to modulate promoter activity, and deleting or mutating various segments of the promoter to determine the important regions for promoter activity, will alter the magnitude of reporter gene expression.

An example of the results of a reporter gene assay is shown in Fig. 22. As described in the section on gel shifts and shown in Fig. 22, the human $cPLA_2$ gene promoter contains a polypyrimidine tract (CTCCCTCTTCCCCTTT) that binds a nuclear protein. A 541-bp segment of the $cPLA_2$ promoter drives the luciferase reporter gene with approximately 40% of the efficacy of the positive control promoter from the SV40 virus. When the polypyrimidine tract is deleted from the promoter, the promoter activity decreases to just 10% of the positive control promoter, confirming the importance of this region.

## TRANSLATION AND PROTEIN PROCESSING

Messenger RNA moves from the nucleus to the cytosol where protein synthesis occurs. Ribosomes are protein-RNA complexes that provide the environment for the RNA sequence to be read and catalyze the peptide chain synthesis. Eukaryotic ribosomes are composed of two major subunits, termed 40S and 60S based on their sedimentation rates, and together they form an 80S complex. Within the large 60S particle is a single large rRNA strand 28S in size, and within the smaller ribosome particle an 18S rRNA strand.

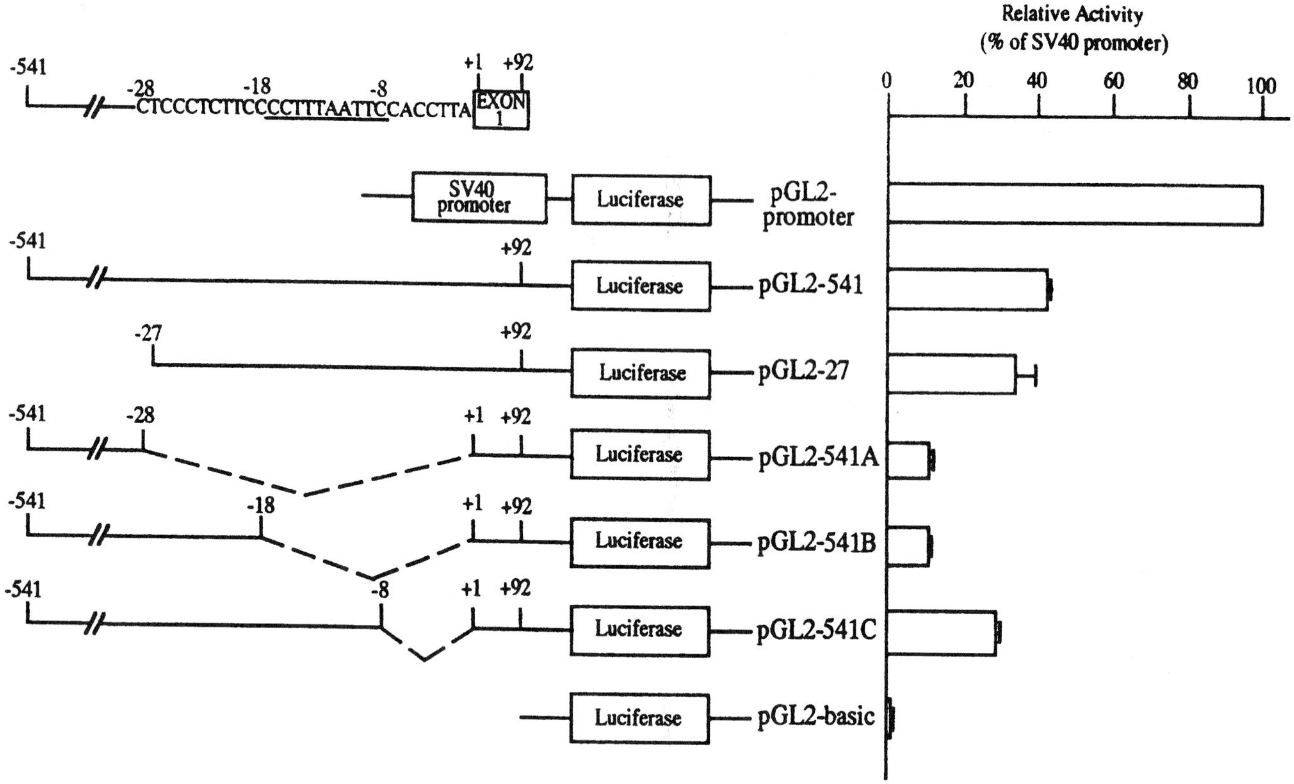


**FIG. 22.** Promoter activity of a 541-bp fragment of the human cPLA2 gene. A 541-bp fragment of the cPLA2 gene promoter has been cloned in front of the luciferase reporter gene. Various segments of the promoter have been deleted as shown; the sequence is shown at the top of the figure. The various constructs have been transfected into HEp-2 laryngeal carcinoma cells, and luciferase activity determined and expressed as percentage of the SV40 promoter that has been used as positive control. It is seen that a 27-bp fragment has as much activity as the 531 bp fragment, and deleting the region between –28 and –8 markedly decreases promoter activity. (From ref. 23 with permission.)

The ribosomes have two sites, an A site and a P site. Amino acids are recruited to the ribosome by another RNA species called transfer RNA (tRNA). The tRNA molecule contains a sequence of three nucleotides or an anti-codon complementary to a codon on the mRNA molecule that encodes a specific amino acid. Each specific tRNA is only able to bind one specific amino acid that is encoded by the anticodon. However, most amino acids can bind to more than one tRNA, that is, for most amino acids there is more than one triplet code. The amino acid is linked to the tRNA by an ester bond and forms an aminoacyl-tRNA.

Protein synthesis thus proceeds through three steps: initiation, elongation, and termination. For the process to be initiated, a specific aminoacyl tRNA must be bound, and in eukaryotes this is Met-tRNAi. This tRNA carries the amino acid methionine, which is always the first amino acid in the peptide chain and binds to the triplet AUG on the mRNA molecule. A different tRNA carries methionine, which is introduced into a elongating peptide chain. Protein synthesis continues until a stop codon is reached corresponding to the triplets UAG, UAA, or UGA.

The sequence of the elongating peptide chain determines the eventual location of the protein. Proteins that are to remain in the cytosol are synthesized in the cytosol, the ribosomes remaining attached to the mRNA but unattached to other organelles. Proteins that are to be located within organelles, within the cell membrane, or secreted from the cell, however, have specific sequences to direct their transfer. For such proteins, preceding the mature protein is a stretch of amino acids called a leader sequence or signal peptide. This sequence binds to a signal recognition particle within the cytosol that temporarily stops translation. The complex then moves to the endoplasmic reticulum (ER), where the signal recognition particle binds to the signal receptor. Protein synthesis then again resumes and the elongating peptide becomes inserted through the membrane of the ER into the lumen, and the signal peptide is cleaved. Ribosomes synthesizing proteins of this type therefore become attached to the endoplasmic reticulum, which gives the ER a granular appearance that is called the rough ER.

Within the ER the protein takes up its folded conformation and is modified by glycosylation, that is, the addition of sugar moieties. There are two main forms of glycosylation: N-linked glycosylation adds a sugar to an asparagine amino acid, and O-linked glycosylation to a serine or threonine.

A protein called Bip, a member of the heat shock family of proteins, assists in the folding of proteins. Proteins that do not fold properly are degraded. Proteins are further modified by passage from the ER through the Golgi apparatus. This occurs by membrane budding with the protein enclosed in an envelope of membrane that buds from the ER and moves to the Golgi and then across the Golgi stacks. Within the Golgi the protein becomes further modified by the addition and removal of sugar moieties.

From the description of transcription, splicing, and translation it is clear that abnormalities in protein structure and function can occur in a number of ways. Large mutations can delete whole genes or large parts of a gene. Single base pair changes may also have devastating effects. A single base pair change may introduce a premature stop codon so that the protein is truncated. The different amino acid encoded by a changed base may affect the folding of a protein so that it cannot be processed in the ER, or may alter the active site or phosphorylation domain of an enzyme or change the susceptibility to glycosylation.

## GENE THERAPY

The understanding of some diseases at the genetic level and the ability to clone and express human genes have led to the possibilities of replacing defective genes as a therapeutic option (26). Gene therapy is the application of genetic principles to treat disease, and thus usually involves the transfer to an individual of a normal copy of a gene to replace one that is defective. Several different options of gene transfer are available depending on the nature of the genetic defect to be corrected.

*Naked DNA* is not well taken up into cells, and the possible applications are therefore limited. However, it has been found that muscle cells are able to take up naked DNA, and although at a low level, the possibilities of using this technique to generate vaccines is being actively pursued. That is, the transferred gene may express sufficient protein to induce an immune response.

*Liposomes* are generating considerable interest in gene therapy studies. Liposomes are charged lipids of two main types, cationic or anionic, that either bind to or engulf DNA. When applied to cells they are endocytosed, and a small fraction is able to break out of the endosome and reach the nucleus where the transferred gene can be expressed. This strategy has been used in preliminary trials for the local transfer of genes to treat cancer or cystic fibrosis.

*Viruses* of several types are efficient gene transfer vectors. **Retroviruses** have been most extensively used to date, and they have the advantage of stable integration into the recipients genome. This ability of retroviruses to integrate means that gene expression should be permanent, although this also has the drawback of random integration, which could disrupt the function of another vital gene. Retroviruses are being evaluated in the treatment of several diseases including cancer, and the first gene therapy protocol involved the use of a retrovirus to transfer a normal copy of the adenosine deaminase gene to children with severe combined immune deficiency (27).

*Adenoviruses* have the advantage of efficient infection of a wide variety of cells including nondividing cells. The transferred gene does not, however, become integrated and expression therefore wanes, and the immune response may limit further administration. Most experience of the use of adenovirus vectors has been obtained in the treatment of cystic fibrosis (28).

*Adeno-associated viruses* and *herpes viruses* are also currently being evaluated as gene therapy vectors.

## REFERENCES


1. Avery OT, MacLeod CM, MacCarty M. Studies on the chemical nature of the substance inducing transformation of pneumococcal types. *J Exp Med* 1944;79:137–158.
2. Nirenberg MW, Matthaei JH. The dependence of cell-free protein synthesis in *E. coli* upon naturally occurring or synthetic polyribonucleotides. *Proc Natl Acad Sci USA* 1961;47:1588–1602.
3. Hay JG, Danel C, Chu CS, Crystal RG. Human CC10 gene expression in airway epithelium and subchromosomal locus suggest linkage to airway disease. *Am J Physiol* 1995;268:L565–575.
4. Rommens JM, Iannuzzi MC, Kerem B, et al. Identification of the cystic fibrosis gene: chromosome walking and jumping. *Science* 1989; 245:1059–1065.
5. Neuhausen SL, Swensen J, Miki Y, et al. A P1-based physical map of the region from D17S776 to D17S78 containing the breast cancer susceptibility gene BRCA1. *Hum Mol Genet* 1994;3:1919–1926.
6. Ott J. *Analysis of human genetic linkage.* Baltimore & London: Johns Hopkins University Press, 1991.
7. Maxam AM, Gilbert W. A new method for sequencing DNA. *Proc Natl Acad Sci USA* 1977;74:560–564.
8. Sanger F, Nicklen S, Coulson AR. DNA sequencing with chain-terminating inhibitors. *Proc Natl Acad Sci USA* 1977;74:5463–5467.
9. Clark JD, Lin LL, Kriz RW, et al. A novel arachidonic acid-selective cytosolic PLA2 contains a Ca(2+)-dependent translocation domain with homology to PKC and GAP. *Cell* 1991;65:1043–1051.
10. Sharp JD, White DL, Chiou XG, et al. Molecular cloning and expression of human Ca(2+)-sensitive cytosolic phospholipase A2. *J Biol Chem* 1991;266:14850–14853.
11. Grunstein M. Histones as regulators of genes. *Sci Am* 1992;267:68–74.
12. Tjian R. Molecular machines that control genes. *Sci Am* 1995;272:54–61.
13. Tjian R, Maniatis T. Transcriptional activation: a complex puzzle with few easy pieces. *Cell* 1994;77:5–8.
14. Latchman DS. Transcription factors: an overview. *Int J Exp Pathol* 1993;74:417–422.
15. Clevidence DE, Overdier DG, Tao W, et al. Identification of nine tissue-specific transcription factors of the hepatocyte nuclear factor 3/forkhead DNA-binding-domain family. *Proc Natl Acad Sci USA* 1993;90:3948–52.
16. Linder ME, Gilman AG. G proteins. *Sci Am* 1992;267:56–65.
17. Seger R, Krebs EG. The MAPK signaling cascade. *FASEB J* 1995;9: 726–735.
18. Ihle JN, Kerr IM. Jaks and Stats in signaling by the cytokine receptor superfamily. *Trends Genet* 1995;11:69–74.
19. Marx J. How the glucocorticoids suppress immunity. *Science* 1995;270: 232–233.
20. Auphan N, DiDonato JA, Rosette C, Helmberg A, Karin M. Immunosuppression by glucocorticoids: inhibition of NFκB activity through induction of IκB synthesis. *Science* 1995;270:286–290.

21. Scheinman RI, Cogswell PC, Lofquist AK, Baldwin AS. Role of transcriptional activation of IκB in mediation of immunosuppression by glucocorticoids. *Science* 1995;270:283–286.
22. Pratt WB, Welsh MJ. Chaperone functions of the heat shock proteins associated with steroid receptors. *Semin Cell Biol* 1994;5:83–93.
23. Miyashita A, Crystal RG, Hay JG. Identification of a 27 bp 5′-flanking region element responsible for the low level constitutive expression of the human cytosolic phospholipase A2 gene. *Nucleic Acids Res* 1995; 23:293–301.
24. Whitsett JA, Clark JC, Wispe JR, Pryhuber GS. Effects of TNF-alpha and phorbol ester on human surfactant protein and MnSOD gene transcription *in vitro*. *Am J Physiol* 1992;262:L688–693.
25. Rosenthal N. Molecular medicine. Recognizing DNA. *N Engl J Med* 1995;333:925–927.
26. Anderson WF. Gene therapy. *Sci Am* 1995;273:124–128.
27. Blaese RM, Culver KW, Miller AD, et al. T lymphocyte-directed gene therapy for ADA SCID: initial trial results after 4 years. *Science* 1995; 270:475–480.
28. Crystal RG. Transfer of gene to humans: early lessons and obstacles to success. *Science* 1995;270:404–410.

*Environmental and Occupational Medicine, Third Edition,* edited by William N. Rom.
Lippincott–Raven Publishers, Philadelphia © 1998.

# CHAPTER 11

# Environmental Carcinogenesis

Seymour J. Garte

At the beginning of the 20th century, when the germ theory of disease causation had become universally accepted, Peyton Rous discovered that a form of cancer in chickens could be transmitted by tumor extracts. According to the recently established criteria of Koch, Rous had discovered a cancer-causing virus, the Rous sarcoma virus, and had proved that cancer, like most of the other killer diseases of the day, could be caused by infectious microorganisms. However, the extension of this result to the idea that all cancers are of viral etiology has proven to be false. Cancers induced solely by viruses are very rare, particularly in humans. In fact, research has shown that certain chemicals, radiation, metals, and fibers can cause cancer in the absence of any virus or biologic agent. More importantly, there is now overwhelming evidence that the preponderance of human cancers owe their origin to such agents present in the human environment. It should be made clear at the outset that the term *environmental* as applied to origins of human cancer is not restricted to such global references as air and water pollution (1) or industrial processes, but also includes more individual interactions such as smoking, diet, specific occupational exposures, and personal habits (2–4). An individual's environment may be quite different from "the environment" in quality and in carcinogenic potency.

The origin of understanding that environmental agents can cause cancer is surprisingly old (5). In the late 18th century, an English surgeon, Percival Pott, determined that the unusually high incidence of cancer of the scrotum in chimney sweeps was due to their occupational exposure to soots and tars (6). Considering the paucity of knowledge of cancer or medicine in general at the time, Pott's contribution is remarkable. It is also the first definitive epidemiologic study on human cancer. Subsequent research into environmental carcinogenesis is primarily a much more recent endeavor. The idea that chemical exposure to chemicals or radiation may be carcinogenic required controlled experiments in animals to be proven.

Although a few reports during the 19th century showed linkage between certain human cancers and occupational exposure to agents such as arsenic, shale oil, and snuff, the first demonstration that a nonbiologic substance could directly cause cancer in a controlled laboratory experiment was done in 1918 by two Japanese scientists who applied coal tar (which had already become suspect in human carcinogenesis) to the skin of rabbit ears and produced carcinomas.

Other scientists investigating a chemical hypothesis for carcinogenesis, devoted years of effort to the tedious task of purifying, testing, and characterizing the chemicals in coal tar that were carcinogenic in pure form. In 1932, a pure chemical, the hydrocarbon dibenzanthracene, was shown for the first time to cause tumors on skin of mice. The following year, benzopyrene, a potent mouse skin carcinogen, was purified from coal tar. In the decades that followed, many other chemicals were discovered to have carcinogenic activity (6).

The identification of radiation as a carcinogen took longer. After the Second World War, a number of human populations that had been exposed to high levels of ionizing radiation (x-rays, alpha rays, etc.) were found to exhibit high frequencies of cancer. These groups included Japanese survivors of the atomic bomb attack at Hiroshima (7), uranium miners, and radium dial painters (8). The latter group was composed of workers who painted watch faces using radium-containing paint, and

S. J. Garte: Department of Environmental Medicine, New York University Medical Center, New York, New York 10016.

who habitually moistened the tips of their fine brushes in their mouths. Women who received radiation as a treatment for mastitis and children who were irradiated as a cure for ringworm have also shown increased cancer rates (8). The ultraviolet nonionizing radiation of sunlight has been clearly implicated in skin cancer (9). This is especially true among fair-colored people, such as those of Irish or English descent who migrated to tropical areas such as Australia or New Zealand. Radiation-induced cancer in experimental laboratory animals has confirmed and extended our knowledge of radiation as a significant environmental carcinogen (10).

The understanding that chemicals and radiation can produce cancer in humans and experimental animals does not directly answer the question of whether such agents are in fact responsible for a significant proportion of human neoplastic disease. Epidemiologic evidence to support the view that a majority (perhaps as high as 80–90%) of human cancer is of environmental origin falls into two main categories. First, there are specific examples of high occupational exposures to agents such as asbestos (11,12) or bis(chloromethyl)ether (13,14) that have been clearly linked to specific types of cancer. Tobacco use (which may account for 30% of all human cancer) is well established as an important etiologic agent by itself and in combination with other environmental agents (see below).

A more general epidemiologic approach to the question is the examination of cancer incidence in various populations. Cancer incidences vary widely among nations and are often more correlated with socioeconomic factors than with ethnic or racial differences. Especially useful is the experience of migratory groups. For example, throughout Japan the rate of stomach cancer in men is five to six times higher than the incidence among Caucasians living in Hawaii (15). The colon cancer rate among Japanese men is four to five times lower than that found among white Hawaiian males. When one examines the cancer pattern in Japanese who moved to Hawaii, the rate of stomach cancer drops to the level seen in white Hawaiians, while the colon cancer rate rises by a similarly dramatic degree. This striking change in the cancer incidence patterns in Japanese who migrated to Hawaii is also seen for cancer of the esophagus, rectum, and prostate among men, and for cancer of the breast, ovary, and uterus among women. A similar analysis was done comparing cancer patterns in American blacks to American whites and African blacks. As an example, American blacks, like American whites, have a tenfold higher incidence of colon cancer and a five- to tenfold lower incidence of liver cancer than African blacks (15).

A sufficiently large number of such migratory populations have been studied to conclude that the large differences seen in cancer incidence patterns in different parts of the world are not due to genetic or heritable factors, but to local environmental or cultural effects. In certain cases such as liver cancer in Africa, viruses such as hepatitis B may have a potentiating or contributing role but clearly cannot be the sufficient cause since a very high proportion of the population is infected that never develops liver cancer. In this case, the ingestion of aflatoxin, a chemical carcinogen found in contaminated grain, is a likely cofactor in the etiology of the disease.

The conclusion from these studies, as well as from the specific epidemiologic evidence on occupational exposure and smoking, is that cancer is an environmental disease. In their classic paper, Doll and Peto (15) estimate that 30% of cancer deaths are attributable to tobacco use, 35% to diet, and less than 5% each to alcohol, occupational exposure, pollution, radiation, and sexual behavior. These authors estimate that 15% to 20% of cancers arise from “unknown” factors such as virus infection and genetic susceptibility.

The major implication of the conclusion that human cancer is largely caused by environmental agents is that it is a preventable disease. While there is a strong consensus that human carcinogenesis is preventable in theory, it is also generally agreed that effective efforts at such prevention requires extensive knowledge of two major areas: the identification and removal of human carcinogens from the environment, and the understanding of basic biologic mechanisms by which chemical and physical agents cause cells to become transformed to malignancy (16). As will be demonstrated, progress in the first area is in fact dependent on the second.

The first area involves issues of risk assessment, dose-response relationships, short-term and animal testing of suspect agents, and epidemiologic and theoretical modeling of carcinogenesis. The second area involves basic research into the mechanisms of carcinogenesis and the ways in which carcinogens interact with cells to trigger a neoplastic response. Historically, these research areas have often remained sheltered from the influences of each other. However, in recent years important progress has been made in understanding the carcinogenic process, and evidence is appearing of collaboration between efforts at cancer risk assessment and cancer molecular biology, such as the emergence of the new field of molecular epidemiology (see below). Since many of the scientific issues behind the problems of carcinogen identification are ultimately related to the basic biology of environmentally induced carcinogenesis, the latter area will be discussed first. Due to the enormous scope of this subject and the volume of research literature that has been generated, the following discussion can do no more than present a brief introductory survey. The reader is referred to the excellent reviews cited in the reference list. Discussions of the molecular biology of carcinogenesis in general and of the role of the p53 tumor suppressor gene in particular can be found in other chapters of this volume.

## MECHANISMS OF CARCINOGENESIS

### Stages of Carcinogenesis

Research into mechanisms of carcinogenesis has moved in the past three to four decades from chemistry to biochemistry to molecular biology. The clear lesson from the mass of data generated from all this work is that the process is enormously complex and may occur via a multitude of pathways (17,18). At the same time, research of the past decade has shed new light on the possibility that cancer induction by disparate agents, including chemicals of astonishingly varied structure, radiation, viruses, and genetic defects, might proceed by a set of related mechanisms involving a large but finite number of specific genes (19,20).

Evidence from animal tumor models, as well as epidemiologic data (21), has established the fact that carcinogenesis involves multiple stages with distinct biologic features. The first stage, called initiation, almost definitely results from an irreversible genetic alteration in a single or small number of cells. The initiated cell, which may be phenotypically normal, must then undergo a clonal expansion to form a benign lesion. This process is called promotion. Conversion of such benign tumors to malignancy occurs through processes collectively known as progression. The degree of malignancy may continue to increase at this stage, with the tumor acquiring properties such as metastatic activity, drug or radiation resistance, and angiogenesis. Although the process of carcinogenesis is operationally divided into stages termed initiation, promotion, and progression, it is important to note that this represents a minimal degree of staging at the biologic level. The number of events or "hits" required to induce a malignant tumor is not known.

Since the first stage of carcinogenesis (initiation) is probably triggered by mutational events produced by direct interaction of carcinogens with DNA, this stage may be thought of as irreversible. In fact, results from experimental animals have shown this to be true (22,23). Initiated cells may remain dormant for many cell cycles, passing the initiating mutations to successive generations of daughter cells. The expansion of a single initiated cell into a clone of transformed cells (promotion) probably occurs through epigenetic mechanisms. Evidence for this comes from studies in the mouse skin carcinogenesis model system (23,24). Tumor promotion in this model, produced by regular repeated applications of promoting compounds such as the phorbol esters or benzoyl peroxide, is a reversible process. The promoting agents themselves do not bind to DNA, although their interaction with the cell indirectly produces alterations in gene expression.

Mouse skin papillomas, liver nodules, and other benign lesions such as adenomas result from promotion of initiated cells by environmental or endogenous compounds such as components in cigarette smoke or estrogen hormones. In the final stages of carcinogenesis the progression of these benign clones to highly malignant, lethal cancers is a complex process that probably involves a series of genetic alterations. The originally monoclonal lesion becomes heterogeneous, with cellular subpopulations characterized by increased genetic instability evolving by selection into more malignant phenotypes at an accelerating rate. The concept of carcinogenesis as a multistage process has been strengthened by observations of several models of human carcinogenesis, where either etiologic factors or molecular events have been associated with different stages. For example, human gastric carcinogenesis proceeds according to the following stages: chronic gastritis, atrophy, intestinal metaplasia, and dysplasia (21). The initial stages of gastritis and atrophy have been associated with excessive salt intake and infection with *Helicobacter pylori.* The intermediate stage of intestinal metaplasia has been linked to ingestion of ascorbic acid and nitrate, and the final stage of dysplasia has been linked with excessive salt intake (21). In another well known model, Vogelstein and his colleagues (25) have demonstrated that in human colon carcinogenesis, each stage of progression from benign polyps through malignant invasive carcinoma is accompanied by specific molecular alterations in oncogenes and tumor suppressor genes.

### Initiation

The idea that the origin of carcinogenesis involves the genetic material was originally called the "somatic mutation hypothesis" and dates back to the 1920s. The long latent period required between exposure to a carcinogen and the onset of cellular transformation requires heritable transmission of the initial effect. This finding, along with an early observation of Boveri (26) that cancer cells often exhibit visible distortions in their chromosomes, makes the DNA a likely target for the initiating stage of carcinogenesis. This idea has been strengthened to the point of general consensus by two additional discoveries that will be discussed further below. First, several groups demonstrated that the great majority of chemical carcinogens interact chemically with DNA (27) and in fact produce mutations by a variety of direct and indirect mechanisms (28). Second, specific genes such as oncogenes or tumor-suppressor genes have been implicated in experimental and human carcinogenesis (20,29).

A large number of chemicals have been shown to be carcinogenic in animals by experiment, and, in far fewer instances, in humans by epidemiologic evidence. The list of known or suspected chemical carcinogens includes agents from a wide variety of chemical classes. Aromatic amines found in dyes, metals such as beryllium and nickel, nitrosamines, chlorinated compounds such as carbon tetrachloride and vinyl chloride, ethionine (an amino acid derivative) fibers such as asbestos, and alkylating agents such as bis(chloro)methylether, methylmethane sulfonate, and methyl nitrosourea are representative of some of the well-known chemical carcinogens. Many of these agents have little in common with each other in terms of their chemistry or biologic action. The polycyclic aromatic hydrocarbons, for example, are large, inert, insoluble, and nonreactive molecules, while certain alkylating agents (like nitrogen mustards, lactones, nitrosamines) are small, soluble, and reactive. On the other hand, not all compounds of a particular class are carcinogenic. Subtle structural changes such as alteration of the stereochemistry or replacement of a substituent functional group can dramatically change the carcinogenic potency of a compound. Research into structure-activity relationships has yielded some general principles but has not been successful at predicting the carcinogenicity of a new chemical compound based solely on structure.

### *Carcinogen Metabolism*

The first step in chemical carcinogenesis actually occurs before interaction of the chemical with the DNA. Many environmental carcinogens including the aromatic hydrocarbons such as benzopyrene and others found in smoke and tar, are not very reactive, and in fact are harmlessly inert. However, most cells of most vertebrate species contain complex detoxification enzyme systems that convert such molecules into highly reactive water-soluble electrophiles (30–32). The purpose of these cytochrome P-450 enzyme systems is to aid in the removal of toxic agents (33). By providing a nonpolar inert molecule with a reactive functional group such as an epoxide or hydroxyl moiety, these enzymes allow for the conjugation of the xenobiotic agent with endogenous compounds such as glutathione or glucose (34), or sulfate (35) derivatives. Such conjugates are then easily excreted from cells and tissues. However, in certain cases the reactive intermediates produced during the reactions catalyzed by P-450 enzymes are able to form complexes with DNA. The DNA-chemical adducts, if not quickly repaired, can lead to mutations and the initiation of neoplasia.

It is ironic that a system designed by evolution to defend the organism from harm caused by toxic chemicals is in fact often directly responsible for the creation of active carcinogens. One might ask how such a phenomenon could arise in the face of natural selection. However, since cancer is a disease whose long latent period results in illness and death generally well past the reproductive age, the processes of natural selection are not fully operative in this case, and therefore the production of carcinogenic intermediates by the cytochrome P-450 system, although harmful to the individual organism, has much less bearing on the evolutionary fitness of the population.

When carcinogens require metabolic activation for activity, the parent compound is called the proximate carcinogen, while the active metabolite that actually reacts with the DNA is called the ultimate carcinogen. The metabolic activation of carcinogens is often species and/or tissue specific and may account for a number of species- or tissue-specific patterns of chemical carcinogen potency (36,37). It has been known for some time that there is chemical specificity in the induction and activity of cytochrome P-450 metabolizing enzymes (38,39). For example, aromatic hydrocarbons such as benzo[*a*]pyrene induce the activity of an enzyme in liver that catalyzes the first step in a metabolic pathway, which leads eventually to the formation of the carcinogenic diol-epoxide derivative (40–42). Treatment with phenobarbital or testosterone or any of a number of other drugs induces different forms of cytochrome P-450 that do not recognize the hydrocarbons as substrates. This specificity implies a multigene family with different regulatory controls and diverse gene products. In fact, many of the genes that compose the P-450 multigene family have been cloned, and although the final number of such genes is not known, it is probably quite large (38,43).

In the case of aromatic hydrocarbons, the mechanism of induction has been intensively investigated. A cytosolic receptor, called the Ah receptor, that binds to toxicants such as dioxin (TCDD) or benzo[*a*]pyrene has been isolated (44,45). The receptor-toxicant complex then moves into the nucleus where it forms a ternary complex with another transcription factor protein, and then interacts with a specific recognition sequence in an enhancer region of several metabolic genes including CYP1A1 (cytochrome P-4501A1) (46). These genes code for enzymes such as aromatic hydrocarbon hydroxylase that are responsible for the first steps in metabolic activation of the toxic compounds.

Metabolism of polycyclic aromatic hydrocarbons such as benzo[*a*]pyrene can occur at many sites on the three to five fused benzene rings that compose these molecules. In fact, cytochrome P-450 catalyzed oxidation does occur at several sites to produce epoxides. Such multiring hydrocarbons contain regions of homologous electron density such as the K-region, and structurally homologous regions such as the bay region (47). Bay region metabolites tend to be more important in carcinogenesis than other sites on typical polycyclic molecules (41,48). As show in Fig. 1 in the case of benzo[*a*]pyrene, it is the 7,8-oxide that is critical for carcinogenic activity, even though epoxides are also formed between carbons 4 and 5, and 9 and 10. The next step is hydration of the epoxide (catalyzed by epoxide hydrase) to form a dihydrodiol. A second oxidation step at the 9,10 positions yields the 7,8-dihydrodiol 9,10-epoxide. Only one of the four possible diastereomeric forms of this compound is responsible for DNA binding and mutagenesis. Of course, the active diol epoxide represents a small fraction of the total metabolic

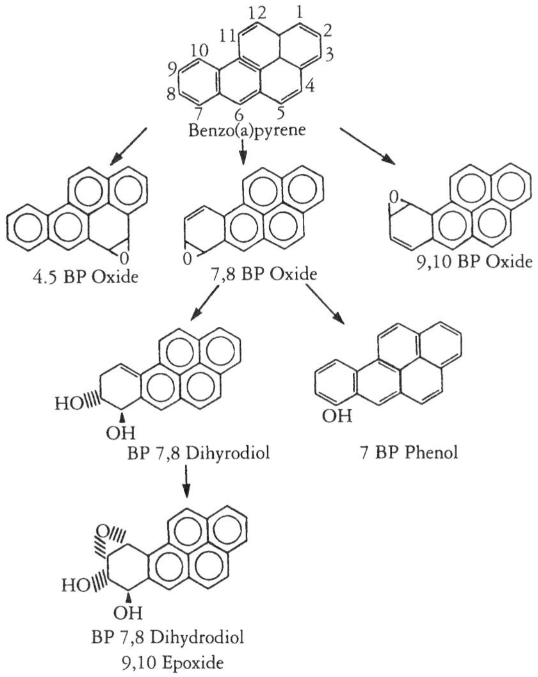


**FIG. 1.** Outline of metabolism of benzo[*a*]pyrene.

profile of benzo[*a*]pyrene. Phenols, quinones, tetrols, and other metabolites are also formed, which eventually participate in conjugation reactions before elimination.

The bay region hypothesis has been confirmed by analysis of the metabolism of many other polycyclic aromatic hydrocarbons such as dibenzanthrancene, 3-methycholanthrene, chrysene, and 7,12-dimethylbenzanthracene. The stereospecificity of carcinogenic activity among chemicals is well established. The enantiomer (mirror image) of benzo[*a*]pyrene-benzo[*e*]pyrene is not active. This principle, which has been found to hold true in numerous examples from several chemical classes, implies a very specific interaction between the carcinogen and a target molecule.

Aromatic hydrocarbons are the best studied, but are not the only class of chemical carcinogens to undergo metabolic activation. The nitrosamines are potent carcinogens that also require a metabolic reaction for activity (49). The parent compound nitrosamines can themselves be synthesized in the gastrointestinal tract from endogenous amines such as amino acids and nitrates used as food additives. This reaction is especially favored in the acidic environment of the human stomach. Ascorbic acid has been shown to block the synthesis of nitrosamines from nitrite (50). Nitrosamines are also important carcinogenic components of cigarette smoke (see below).

Not all chemical carcinogens require metabolic activation. Direct-acting carcinogens also produce adducts on DNA. Alkylating agents such as mustards, methylating agents, and other electrophiles are well-known direct-acting carcinogens (51,52). While carcinogens that require metabolic activation usually exhibit tissue-specific effects related to different enzyme profiles, direct-acting agents often produce tumors in diverse organs depending on route and site of administration, and/or the presence of promoting or cocarcinogenic factors.

Both direct-acting and indirect-acting carcinogens share the feature of chemical interaction with DNA. The ultimate carcinogens are in fact indistinguishable from direct-acting electrophiles in this regard. The chemistry of DNA-carcinogen interactions is complex and involves reactions at diverse sites on the DNA molecule. Covalent adducts to exocyclic and endocyclic oxygens and nitrogens of each of the four bases are the most commonly studied product; however, phosphotriesters, cross-links, and reactions with deoxyribose also occur (30,53–55). The results of the initial reaction between a carcinogen and a target site on the DNA may include formation of a stable covalent adduct (56,57) and/or may rapidly lead to deamination or hydration of the base, DNA strand breaks, or loss of the base (58,59). Lesions such as apurinic sites (loss of a guanine or adenine from the DNA backbone), strand breaks, inter- or intrastrand cross-links, intercalated chemical adducts, and covalent adducts may have one of three consequences for the cell: they may be repaired by repair enzymes (60–63), they may prove lethal to the cell, or they may result in a mutation. Mutations may also occur as a result of faulty or error-prone repair. Depending on the site and nature of the mutation, this consequence may lead to the onset of neoplasia.

### *DNA Adducts*

The metabolism of a carcinogenic compound generally produces a myriad of metabolic products, only one of which (and not necessarily the most abundant) is actually the ultimate carcinogenic agent. Analogously, the interaction of a carcinogenic electrophile such as benzopyrene diol epoxide with DNA may produce a myriad of adducts, only one of which may be responsible for the carcinogenic effect. The formation of DNA adducts by carcinogens, with or without prior metabolic activation, is, with several exceptions, a critical feature of chemicals that can initiate carcinogenesis. Certain adducts, by interfering with the hydrogen bonds that are responsible for normal base pairing (A-T and G-C) may cause mispairing such as G with T (64,65). This will also lead to a permanent mutation after the next cycle of cell division. The connection between certain adducts and the types of mutations they cause has been the subject of extensive research (30,66–69).

The consequences of formation of a DNA adduct depend on the location of the adduct on the DNA, and the nature of the adduct. For example, the normal G-C base pair involves hydrogen bonding between the N1 of guanine and the N2 of cytosine. If an adduct is placed on the $O^6$ position of guanine, this results in a keto-enol type charge distribution, such that the N2 of guanine becomes deprotonated and can no longer form a hydrogen bond with cytosine, but does form a hydrogen bond with the protonated N1 of thymine. Therefore, adducts on $O^6$ of guanine result in a mispairing during cell replication of G with T. Since T normally pairs with A, the end result is a G-C > A-T transition. A similar result is produced by adducts at the $O^4$ position of thymidine. Other adducts such as N-7 of guanine do not interfere with base pairing. However, such adducts may lead to a net positive charge on the base and may cause depurination. Adducts at the N1 and N3 positions of adenine may also lead to depurination (66,70). Loss of a base can lead to mutations, for example, if an A is inserted opposite an apurinic site that has originally contained a G, then a G-C > T-A transversion will result.

It is important to understand that the theoretical implications of the chemical reactivity of carcinogen-DNA adducts are not sufficient alone to predict relative carcinogenic potencies of the different adduct sites. Experiments to empirically determine the mutation frequency as a function of specific adducts have in fact shown that the number of $O^6$ guanine adducts correlates well with mutagenicity (67,71). Correlation with N7 adducts was poor. There is now a general consensus that $O^6$ guanine adducts are important in the carcinogenic mechanisms of certain carcinogens such as direct-acting methylating agents in specific systems (72). However, a role for other DNA lesions cannot be ruled out in general (73,74).

More complex interactions are found between bulky planar hydrocarbons and DNA (75). These molecules may cause base substitution or deletions. The hydrocarbon AAF binds to the C-8 of guanine and can distort the structure of the DNA sufficiently to cause excision repair enzymes to operate. Deamination of cytosine or 5-methyl cytosine produces deoxyuracil or thymidine, respectively. If not repaired, this produces a mutation from C-G to T-A.

The wealth of research on DNA adducts has demonstrated the fundamental importance of DNA effects in carcinogenesis (72,76). Of course, the fact that a carcinogen may cause a mutation in the DNA of a target cell is only of relevance if the mutation occurs at a critical site. Therefore, knowing the type of mutation formed is only a part of the mechanistic story behind the actions of chemical carcinogens. At least as important is the question of precisely where in the genome (in other words which genes) are the critical target(s).

### *DNA Repair*

As stated above, interactions of a chemical carcinogen with DNA usually triggers a repair mechanism. Once an adduct is formed, it may be quickly repaired by mechanisms such as removal of the damaged base by a glycosylase (77,78), or excision of a stretch of bases surrounding the chemical lesion (60,61). Such removal is followed by DNA polymerase catalyzed synthesis of the correct sequence. If the repair is done correctly and rapidly, then no biologic consequences of the original damage will be seen. However, if the repair system itself does not function properly, as is the case with some inherited genetic syndromes (79,80), or if the repair is faulty, then a mutational event becomes possible. If a lesion in the DNA is not repaired because the lesion is not recognized by any repair system, or because the level of damage is so high as to saturate the repair capacity, then there is also a strong possibility for mutagenic consequences. The mechanisms associated with DNA repair are highly complex, and involve several enzyme systems such as methyl transferases (81), glycosylases, and damage-specific repair enzymes of various types (82,83). Any further detailed discussion of this topic is beyond the scope of this general review, and the interested reader should consult the numerous books and reviews (84–-86) dealing with the many facets of this research area.

## Promotion

The phenomenon of tumor promotion was first discovered and has been most actively investigated in mouse skin carcinogenesis (23,24). A fairly low dose of an initiating carcinogen such as the aromatic hydrocarbon dimethylbenzanthracene (DMBA) applied once to the backs of mice will produce few or no tumors. However, if the single initiating dose of carcinogen is followed by repeated frequent administration of the irritating oil from the croton tiglium plant, or its pure active ingredient tetradecanoyl phorbol acetate (TPA) (also known as phorbol myristate acetate [PMA]), then multiple benign papillomas will begin to appear on each mouse within 3 to 6 months. By 1 year, conversion of a papilloma to a malignant squamous cell carcinoma will have occurred in most of the mice. Tumor promoters such as TPA cannot produce cancer without prior initiation. On the other hand, most initiators are whole carcinogens; that is, they can produce tumorigenesis without additional promoting agents, as long as the dose is sufficiently high. It was discovered early on that for the promoting agent to work, there must be only a minimum separation of time (2 to 3 days at most) between promoter applications. An interruption in treatment will result in no tumors. Therefore, tumor promotion, unlike initiation, is a reversible process. Consistent with this is a series of studies showing that unlike complete carcinogens, tumor promoters do not interact with DNA, do not produce mutations, and do exhibit dose thresholds for their effects (87). The mechanism of action of the phorbol ester type of tumor promoter does not therefore involve genotoxicity but is instead an epigenetic phenomenon.

Treatment of mouse skin with TPA produces a pleiotropic effect, at both the cellular and biochemical level. Among the many responses are hyperplasia and inflammation; increased DNA and protein synthesis; increased synthesis of phospholipids, prostaglandins, and ornithine decarboxylase; uncoupling of the β-adrenergic response; and a host of other changes in gene expression and cellular morphology (88). In the early 1980s, it was discovered that a specific receptor exists for TPA, and this receptor is in fact part of the signal transduction enzyme system known as protein kinase C (PKC) (89–91). The tumor-promoting activity of TPA is mediated through its binding and stimulation of PKC. This enzyme is also involved in complex metabolic pathways controlling phosphoinositol and diacylglcyerol turnover as well as $Ca^{2+}$ flux (92).

The phorbol esters are not the only potent tumor promoters in mouse skin. Other agents have varying degrees of activity (88,93–95). These include benzoyl peroxide, teleocidin and its derivatives, mezerein, aplysiotoxin, anthralin, and tobacco smoke condensate. Not all of these agents act by stimulating PKC; thus, there must be alternative mechanisms for tumor promotion in skin. Stimulation of the production of oxygen radicals is one example of proposed alternative mechanisms (96,97). Furthermore, the phenomenon of promotion is not limited to the mouse skin. Compounds such as phenobarbital, DDT, and dioxin are promoters in rat liver (95), high-salt and high-fat diets are promoters for human and animal stomach and colon carcinogenesis (98), saccharin is probably a human bladder tumor promoter, and cigarette smoke is a promoter for cancer of the lung, pancreas, esophagus, and other organs in several species (99).

Endogenous substances such as estrogen hormones have promoting activity in breast carcinogenesis, and testosterone can function as a promoter in a rat prostate carcinogenesis model (100). Tumor promotion is probably therefore a widespread if not universal phenomenon during the pathogenesis of cancer. In mouse skin, it turns out that promotion can itself be separated into at least two stages (101). Whether this is true in other systems is not clear. The expansion of a single initiated cell into a clonal benign lesion (which is the biologic consequence of promotion) very likely can proceed by a number of cellular biochemical mechanisms, but none of these involve genetic damage or alteration.

### Progression

If carcinogenesis were simply a two-stage process—initiation followed by promotion—cancer would not be a lethal disease. The benign lesions (papillomas, nodules, adenomas) that result from promotion are not lethal. However, there is a high probability once the benign clonal tumor is formed that the tumor will be converted to a malignant carcinoma or sarcoma, and that later steps in progression such as invasion and metastases, will occur. There is strong evidence that progression to malignancy, like initiation, is triggered by genetic events (102,103).

Malignant tumors exhibit genetic instability, including a tendency toward aneuploidy, chromosomal aberrations, gene amplification and rearrangements, and increased mutation rate (104,105). Once a tumor passes into the later stages of progression, it becomes heterogeneous and a strong selective pressure begins to favor rapid evolution of the tumor cells to the most malignant phenotype. At this stage tumor cells acquire quite astonishing characteristics such as the ability to dissolve or cross basement membranes, to survive in the bloodstream, to counteract the immune system, to become resistant to the toxic effects of a myriad of drugs or radiation, to stimulate angiogenesis, and generally to survive at the ultimate expense of the host organism.

Genotoxic carcinogens have been shown to increase the rate of conversion of papillomas to carcinomas (106–108). The detailed mechanisms of tumor progression remain less understood than those of initiation or promotion, but certainly increased understanding of this aspect of environmental carcinogenesis is of no less importance.

## CARCINOGEN IDENTIFICATION

The prevention of a large proportion of human cancers should theoretically be possible by the identification and elimination of all carcinogenic agents in the environment. This goal is in fact the implicit basis for several regulatory and legislative initiatives of the United States federal government such as the Delaney Clause and provisions of the Toxic Substance Control Act. The first step in this goal, the identification of environmental carcinogens, is the overall purpose of carcinogen risk assessment. Carcinogen risk assessment can be divided into qualitative and quantitative risk assessment. Qualitative risk assessment simply asks the question of whether an agent is or isn't carcinogenic. This information is not as useful for either research or regulatory purposes as quantitative risk assessment, which addresses the question of how potent an agent is in carcinogenic activity. Different chemicals have been shown to vary in their carcinogenic potency in animals over 6 to 10 orders of magnitude (109–111).

The goal of cancer prevention may be extremely difficult. The difficulties lie largely in the sphere of identification, although in certain instances, even when carcinogens are known, it may be difficult to eliminate them from the environment. The best example of this is tobacco, whose removal from the human environment is more related to issues of politics and economics than science.

### Examples of Environmental Carcinogens

#### *Tobacco*

Smoke from combustion of vegetable matter contains a mixture of gases and particulates. These extremely fine particles consist of various hydrocarbons, mineral ash, and carbon. The hydrocarbons of smoke are similar to the hydrocarbons of coal tar. It was natural, therefore, for early cancer researchers to investigate whether the carcinogenicity of tar and soot might also apply to smoke. Epidemiologic evidence strongly supports the connection between cigarette smoking and lung cancer. Since the early 1950s a large number of studies have shown correlations between smoking history and cancer of the lung as well as other organs (99,112,113). Smoking is also highly synergistic with other environmental carcinogens. For example, the incidence of lung cancer among uranium miners who also smoked was extremely high (8). The same pattern has been seen for asbestos workers and many other groups of people exposed occupationally to chemical carcinogens. One of the most informative studies relates to the incidence of lung cancer as a function of gender. Historically this has been a predominantly male disease. However, after World War II women began to smoke with equal frequency to men. The curve of lung cancer in women began a steep upward trend just 20 years later, paralleling the curve of smoking incidence. This trend is still rising, and lung cancer has begun to outrank breast cancer as the leading cause of cancer mortality among women.

Cigarette smoke contains an amazing variety and number of carcinogens; in fact, it would be hard to deliberately formulate a more carcinogenic mixture than cigarette smoke. In the gas phase are found several nitrosamines such as dimethylnitrosamine, urethane, formaldehyde, and vinyl chloride, all complete carcinogens. In the particulate phase are found the carcinogens benzopyrene, beta-naphthylamine, methylchrysene, benzofluoranthene, benzanthracene, and more than two dozen other aromatic hydrocarbons. Tumor promoters and cocarcinogens such as pyrene, naphthalene, catechol, phenols, methylindoles, methylcarbazoles, and others are also found in smoke. Besides these hydrocarbons, cigarette smoke contains carcinogenic metals such as nickel and cadmium and the radioactive element polonium 210 (114). A large number of the constituents of smoke have proven positive in carcinogenic bioassays. An important class of chemical carcinogens, the nitrosamines, is produced in cigarette smoke from nicotine, the addictive agent (115).

Because tobacco smoke contains so many potent carcinogens of so many types, it is difficult to attribute the carcinogenicity of tobacco to any particular compound. The most likely situation is that various different combinations of initiators, cocarcinogens, and promoters act to produce malignant transformation. Recently, considerable attention has been paid to two lesser known tobacco carcinogens, the nitrosamines and radioactive polonium. The active narcotic agent in tobacco and other related alkaloids is chemically converted during curing, processing, and burning into *N*-nitrosononicotine (NNN), 4-(methylnitrosamino)- 1-(3-pyridye)-1-butanone or nicotine-derived nitrosaminoketone (NNK), 4-(methylnitrosamino)-4-(3-pyridyl)-butanal (NNA), and other carcinogenic nitrosamines. These agents are tobacco specific; they are found in snuff and chewing tobacco as well as in cigarette mainstream and sidestream smoke (115). The nitrosamines NNN and NNK produce tumors in rats, mice, and hamsters in the lung, nasal cavity, esophagus, and trachea. These agents require metabolic activation for their carcinogenic action (116). Human trachea, lung, and other respiratory tissues have been shown to metabolically activate NNN and NNK.

The presence of radioactive elements in cigarette smoke has been known since the 1960s. These elements include radium 226, radon 228, thorium 228, traces of other elements, and polonium 210. Polonium 210 is the most abundant of these in smoke. It is an alpha emitter and is volatile at the temperature of a burning cigarette. Alpha radiation is an intense form of radioactivity known to be carcinogenic in animals and humans. Due to very low solubility, polonium 210 is retained and concentrated in lung tissue longer than other tobacco smoke constituents (114). Research is now being conducted on several biochemical and molecular parameters, such as detection of nitrosamines in urine of smokers, analysis of DNA adducts in lung tissue of smokers who died of lung cancer, and activation of oncogenes in lung tumors, which may further elucidate the precise mechanisms by which inhalation of cigarette smoke causes cancer.

### *Chloromethylethers*

The chloromethylethers—chloromethly methyl ether (CMME or CME) and bis chloromethyl ether (BCME)—are chemicals used in a number of industrial processes. These compounds represent one of the most interesting cases of environmental carcinogen identification, because both epidemiologic (117–124) and animal experimental studies (125–127) as well as structure activity studies (14,128) were done at roughly the same time and all these data were combined in a regulatory decision to prevent any exposure of workers to these agents. The immediate stimulus for the epidemiologic study was the finding of a cluster of lung cancer cases among chemical workers at a CME plant. An industrywide epidemiologic study found an increased risk of lung cancer in CME-exposed workers at one plant where workers were known to have been highly exposed. A clear dose-response relationship with risk ratios exceeding 10 for the longest duration and greatest exposure subgroups was found for this plant (117). Meanwhile several experimental studies using BCME in animal models also showed unequivocal evidence for carcinogenicity of these chemicals. When a single dose of BCME was applied to mouse skin, followed by promotion with TPA, skin tumors were observed (127). In a more relevant inhalation carcinogenesis experiment, rats and hamsters were exposed to BCME 6 hours per day, 5 days per week throughout their lifetime. Forty respiratory tract cancers were found in the 200 exposed rats including 14 cancers of the lung and 26 cancers of the nasal cavity. A clear dose-response relationship was seen (125).

In subsequent years, several groups have done follow-up epidemiologic studies to determine if the initial results on the carcinogenicity of BCME would be confirmed with longer observation time (129,130). In fact, all studies have confirmed the original findings. An industry-wide retrospective epidemiologic study was performed on over 6,000 chemical workers, of whom 2,460 had been exposed to chloromethyl ethers at seven American plants between 1948 and 1980. This study found an average fourfold increased risk of respiratory cancer in one plant, and a sixfold increase in another plant. Significant dose-response relationships were observed with respect to cumulative time-weighted exposures (130). The latent period for the development of lung cancer was found to be from 10 to 19 years after exposure to chloromethyl ethers. This was true for all doses, although some cases were observed with shorter periods of exposure (131). The results from one study suggested that chloromethyl ether exposure affects both early and late stages of the carcinogenic process (130).

The results of the cumulative research on chloromethyl ethers led to a finding by the International Agency for Research in Cancer (IARC) that these compounds are class 1 human carcinogens (Table 1), and also led to industrywide changes in the engineering design of plants to eliminate all human exposure to CME and BCME. As of 1987, the majority of exposed workers had passed through the latent period, and the number of cases seen in recent years are declining toward the control population level (131). Clearly, the case of BCME represents an example of a victory for the research community in that many lives of potentially exposed workers were saved, due to the work of several disciplines. Unfortunately, for many other chemicals, results from different disciplines, as well as laboratories, are not always as clear cut, and therefore regulatory decisions, such as those that prevented further exposure to BCME, are not usually made in such an atmosphere of general consensus (see below).

**TABLE 1.** *Examples of environmental human carcinogens*

| |
|---|
| Acrylonitrile |
| Aflatoxin |
| 4-Amino biphenyl |
| Arsenic |
| Asbestos |
| Benzene |
| Benzidine |
| Beryllium |
| β-Naphthylamine |
| bis(chloro)methylether |
| Chromium compounds |
| Coal tar (aromatic hydrocarbons) |
| Cyclophosphamide |
| Diethylstibesterol (hormone analog) |
| Leather and wood dust |
| Mustard gas (alkylating agents) |
| Neoprene |
| Nickel compounds |
| Nitrosamines |
| Radiation (ionizing and ultraviolet) |
| Tobacco smoke |
| Vinyl chloride |

### *Diet*

The human diet contains numerous carcinogens including naturally occurring chemical carcinogens, synthetic compounds, and compounds produced by cooking (132,133). In the first category are toxins from fungi and plants such as aflatoxin. The second group includes food additives and pesticides. A very important group, the chemicals produced by cooking (pyrolysis), includes polycyclic aromatic hydrocarbons and heterocyclic amines. The latter are produced from creatinine and amino acids in meat and fish, and include such potent carcinogens as 2-amino-1-methyl-6-phenylimidazo [4,5-b]pyridine (PhIP), 2-amino-3,8-dimethylimidazo[4,5-f] quinoxaline (MeIQx), and 2-amino-3-methylimidazo [4,5-f]quinoline (IQ) (134). Other components of diet that have been implicated in human carcinogenesis (either causative or protective) include total calories, fat, choline, methionine, vitamin A, selenium, calcium, zinc, fiber, ethanol, and many nonnutrient components of foods (133).

The idea that diet must play some role in carcinogenesis is not new, and a large body of literature on the effects of fat and caloric restriction on cancer induction in animals has been produced (135,136). Several U.S. and Japanese groups have shown that probable carcinogens can be found in certain foods, especially when prepared in certain ways (137,138). Some of the best known carcinogens in the human diet are aflatoxin, a product of a fungus that grows on grain and peanuts; safrole, contained in many plants such as black pepper; and hydrazenes, found in mushrooms. Other compounds found in celery, potatoes, coffee, and various other plants have been shown to possess carcinogenic and/or mutagenic activity in laboratory tests. Other candidates for human dietary carcinogens are excess animal fat, alcohol, charcoal-broiled meat, nitrates, and nitrites (139,140).

On the other hand, a number of dietary factors probably have anticarcinogenic activity (139,141). These include vitamin E, beta carotene, selenium, fiber (133), ascorbic acid (50), protease inhibitors (142), and certain food additives such as butylated hydroxyanisole (BHA). Consumption of naturally occurring vitamins and minerals, as well as fiber, may explain the consistent epidemiologic demonstrations of reduction of tumor risk with increased consumption of fruits and vegetables.

### *Radiation*

Ionizing and nonionizing radiations are among the most widely known and carefully studied environmental hazards to humans. Among the many cytotoxic effects of radiation exposure are a number of types of DNA damage (143–145). These include single- and double-strand breaks, base substitutions and hydroxylations (for ionizing radiation such as x or gamma radiation), and dimer formation (for nonionizing radiation such as ultraviolet light). The first step in the production of such genotoxic effects is not known for certainty, but considerable evidence points to the involvement of oxygen free radicals such as hydroxyl radicals that are produced by the ionization of water in the cell. The effects of such free radicals in genotoxicity and various stages of carcinogenesis is the subject of considerable research (146). The clastogenic effects of radiation on cells such as chromosomal aberrations have been known for many years. Mutations, gene rearrangements, amplification, and large deletions result from the effects of radiation on the genome. It might be expected, therefore, that in analogy with genotoxic chemical carcinogens, cellular oncogenes should play a role in radiation-induced carcinogenesis. This has been found to be the case in several model tumor systems. Both *ras*, activated by point mutation, and *myc*, activated by amplification and/or rearrangement, have been found in radiation-induced cancers (147–149).

Because of the relative simplicity of dosimetry for radiation compared to chemicals, it has been possible to proceed further in the development of carcinogenic risk assessment models for radiation than for chemicals. This effort has also been aided by the existence of numerous human populations with well-documented radiation exposures. Based on such experimental and empirical data, as well as on theoretical grounds, the cancer incidence has been found to be a function of dose, dose rate, and the linear energy transfer (LET) of the radiation. For high-LET radiation such a neutrons, the dose-response curve is linear at low doses, whereas for low-LET radiation (x-rays, electrons) the incidence is a more complex linear and quadratic function of the dose (150). Fractionated doses, which allow for repair, decrease the tumor yields of low-LET but not of high-LET radiation. Correlation of the physical effects of radiation with biologic observations on cancer incidence and other end points, and with molecular mechanisms including changes in the structure and function of specific oncogenes and/or tumor suppressor genes, represents the major current challenge for elucidation of the mechanisms of radiation carcinogenesis (151).

## Methods for Carcinogen Identification

Chemicals represent the most important class of environmental carcinogens. A critical question for regulatory policy makers, medical practitioners, and research scientists is how can we predict which specific chemical compounds pose a cancer risk to human beings (152). The identification of carcinogens, whether components of foodstuffs or of factory emissions, is a formidable task. There are three broad categories of accepted methods for carcinogen risk assessment: epidemiologic studies on humans, animal bioassays, and short-term tests.

### *Epidemiology*

Sound epidemiologic studies showing that an agent causes cancer in human populations, as has been done for smoking, asbestos, BCME, and ionizing radiation, are the strongest evidence for carcinogenicity. Such evidence is sufficient for strong regulatory action, and is rarely refuted or contradicted. Unfortunately, such epidemiologic data are not usually available, and to date only a relatively small list of chemicals or processes have been implicated as human carcinogens by this criterion (Table 1). For the majority of environmental agents, it is difficult to identify clearly defined exposed populations of sufficient size that can be matched with nonexposed control groups. Furthermore, an agent must be fairly potent to be detected in an epidemiologic study. Finally, since human cancer requires 15 to 30 years to develop after exposure to an agent, it is difficult to use this approach for evaluating new chemicals or for identifying carcinogens before they have caused human disease. Despite these major drawbacks, epidemiologic studies are critically important in the assessment of cancer risks to human beings (153). This is especially true for agents that act via different mechanistic pathways in different species, or for chemicals that produce different quantitative and/or qualitative clinical outcomes in different species. In some cases, cohorts of highly exposed people are available for study because of an industrial accident, or because of an unusually high industrial exposure (154). An example is the case of TCDD or dioxin. This compound is extremely toxic to guinea pigs, but is much less so for mice or humans. It is a tumor promoter in mice, but its carcinogenic potency in humans is still under investigation. Several cohorts of highly exposed people, such as a population living in the vicinity of an industrial accident at Seveso Italy, are being studied to clarify this issue (155). This type of epidemiologic investigation, termed a cohort or prospective study, is extremely informative and valuable, since an exposed (along with the suitable control) population can be followed to determine precisely the magnitude of risk associated with exposure. The overriding disadvantage of this study design is the long period of time (on the order of decades) necessary to complete such studies. An alternative approach is called the case control design, in which people with and without cancer are questioned as to their exposure history (156). These studies are much more common, but may present problems of interpretation due to a number of uncertainties.

*Molecular Epidemiology*

One of the most difficult problems facing epidemiologists who study environmental carcinogenesis is the issue of accurate and objective assessment of exposure. In recent years a new field sometimes called molecular epidemiology, or biomarker research, has had an important impact in providing several possible solutions to this problem (157–160). Biomarker research combines epidemiology with laboratory assays in studies that have been termed transitional epidemiology. The goal of such studies is to better define carcinogen exposure and to more accurately determine individual risk for cancer development based on a more precise understanding of an individual's exposure.

Biomarkers can be used to measure internal dose, biologically effective dose, early disease end points, and prognosis (160). The techniques used in biomarker research include the measurement of DNA and protein adducts (161–163), levels of gene expression (164,165), analysis of mutational spectra (166), immunologic methods, detection of DNA and chromosomal damage, and many others.

Because molecular epidemiologic research involves the relationship between exposure to carcinogenic agents and subsequent cancer induction, this research can have an important impact on cancer risk assessments. Furthermore, biomarker research can be used to design preventive strategies (167).

*Individual Susceptibility*

It has always been clear that individual human beings differ widely in their susceptibility to the carcinogenic effects of environmental agents. For example, although tobacco smoke contains many potent carcinogens, and is responsible for a large number of cancer deaths each year, it remains a fact that not all heavy smokers develop lung cancer, even at late ages. Unlike laboratory animals, which are often inbred strains, human beings are genetically very diverse, and it isn't surprising that such a high level of variability is always observed in human studies, not only for disease end points (168), but also for biochemical and physiologic end points as well (169). This variability is one of the major hurdles facing molecular epidemiologists, who often find that the interindividual variability of an assay result is so high as to mask differences between exposed and control groups of people.

Several types of cancer susceptibility genes are known. One category includes tumor suppressor genes such as p53, Rb, BRCA1, and other genes involved in inherited cancer susceptibility syndromes such as Li-Fraumeni syndrome, retinoblastoma, or familiar breast cancer (29, 170). Another category of genes that is important in human carcinogenesis has an influence on carcinogenic events such as DNA repair or carcinogen metabolism (171–173). A new field of pharmacogenetics (174) has developed to study the role of genes involved in the metabolism of drugs, toxicants, and carcinogens in genetic sensitivity (175,176). Some of the important genes involved in conferring individual differences in metabolism on environmental carcinogens are illustrated in Table 2. Phenotypic and genotypic (sequence) polymorphisms have been found in these genes that directly affect the function of their gene products (177,178). These polymorphisms generally occur at different frequencies in different ethnic populations (179–182), and the human genetics of these polymorphisms can be quite complex (183). Case control studies have shown several such polymorphisms to be associated with increased risk of various cancer types in specific human populations (184–190).

In many cases the biochemical mechanisms by which polymorphisms in such genes exert their effects is fairly straightforward, and is related to the actual dose of the active carcinogenic metabolite that reaches the genome in the target cell. Increased metabolism of a carcinogenic precursor to the ultimate carcinogen, and loss of function of a conjugation mechanism for elimination of the active metabolite, are examples of how alterations in the activity of certain gene products can affect the biologically relevant dose in different individuals, even when exposures are equivalent. These genes function in the context of interaction with the environment (191), since the substrates of their gene products are xenobiotic chemicals or their metabolites. Further study of the genetic basis for individual differences in sensitivity to environmental car-

**TABLE 2.** *Cancer susceptibility genes*

| Gene | Metabolic pathway | Cancer sites |
|---|---|---|
| GSTM1 | Conjugation of organic epoxides with reduced glutathione | Lung, bladder, colon, stomach, breast, liver |
| CYP2D6 | Hydroxylation of lipophilic xenobiotics, possibly NNK | Lung, bladder, breast |
| NAT2 | *N*-Acetylation of arylamines and *N*-hydroxylated heterocyclicaryl amines | Bladder, lung, colorectal, breast |
| CYP1A1 | Metabolism of polycyclic aromatic hydrocarbons, TCDD, and estrogens | Lung, stomach, colon, breast |
| CYP2E1 | Oxidation of *N*-nitrosamines, alcohol | Lung, bladder, colon |

cinogens is a critical requirement for the complete understanding of cancer risk on an individual basis.

### *Animal Bioassays*

When epidemiologic data is unobtainable, the most reliable determination of carcinogenic activity of a chemical is testing in animals. After years of study, the National Toxicology Program has promulgated standardized protocols for such testing to assure consistency in the use of animal species, strains and sexes, dose levels, and methods of analysis and data collection. Without such standardization, it was not uncommon for different laboratories to reach dramatically different conclusions regarding the carcinogenic activity of a particular agent.

Data from animal carcinogenicity assays are generally collected using groups of 20 to 50 animals. Larger groups would be prohibitively expensive. To detect a significant carcinogenic response in this number of chemically exposed animals compared to a similar number of control animals, it is necessary to produce a cancer incidence of at least 10%. To detect any dose response, the incidence must be even higher and is often reported as high as 80% to 100% at the highest dose level. These are extremely high incidence levels compared with those with which regulators are concerned with respect to human carcinogenesis. For example, even a cancer response of 0.01% is quite high for a human population when one realizes that 1 cancer in 10,000 translates to 100 excess cancer cases in 1 million exposed people. Agents released into the environment that cause this level of cancer incidence would be a public health concern if a significant fraction of the national population were exposed.

Therefore, for most agents, the doses that must be administered to test animals in order to detect any response needs to be far higher than the dose expected to be present in the human environment. The only alternative, which is not economically feasible, would be to use 10,000 to 100,000 animals in each test group. Therefore it is generally recommended that the highest dose used in an animal carcinogenicity bioassay be the maximum tolerated dose (MTD). While there may be different precise definitions of the MTD, it is usually determined by the dose that produces the first sign of toxicity, such as minor weight loss. Because of cost, the number of dose groups must be kept low, and three to four doses including a no exposure control are usually used. These doses are often a fraction of the MTD such as $^1/_2$, $^1/_4$, etc. The purpose of using multiple doses is to try to gather information on the shape of the dose-response curve. Such information is critical for reliable risk assessment.

The use of the MTD has come under fire based on the argument that at such high doses, the mutagenic activity of a chemical may be an artifact related to cell proliferation following cell death (192). However, since no alternative has been proposed, or is likely to be available, use of the MTD is the only viable means to choose dose levels for carcinogenicity assays. The use of very high doses does not preclude assessment of quantitative carcinogenic risk at realistically low doses, as long as one assumes that the shape of the dose-response function is linear over the whole dose range. For example, if a dose of 10 mg/kg produces an observed 10% tumor incidence in 50 mice, than a dose of 0.01 mg/kg would be calculated to produce a tumor incidence of 0.01%. Unfortunately, the assumption of linearity for carcinogenesis dose response is often not valid. Some agents such as formaldehyde show very steep dose-response curves with cancer incidence being proportional to the 4th or 5th power of dose. For ionizing radiation, the power of the dose-response curve is a function of the energy content of the radiation. For nonlinear functions of cancer incidence with dose, extrapolation of experimental data produced using high doses to low doses may be very difficult. A number of mathematical models have been devised for the purpose of quantitative risk assessment at low doses (193,194). Some of these models are purely mathematical, while others, such as the multistage model are based partially on knowledge of carcinogenic mechanisms. Pharmacokinetic modeling (195) has also contributed to mechanism-based risk assessment. Use of different models can provide quite different answers when applied to determine the quantitative potency of a carcinogen at low dose. Certain models, which approximate the linear dose-response curve most closely, are termed conservative since they yield relatively high risks at low doses. Decisions concerning which extrapolation formula to use are often difficult, especially in the absence of experimental dose-response data or mechanistic understanding.

A related issue to low-dose risk assessment is the question of thresholds (196). Almost all toxic agents have threshold doses—levels of exposure that are too low to cause a toxic response in any number of target organisms. The question of thresholds can be approached either empirically or theoretically, but will probably never be resolved unequivocally. In a long-term "mega-mouse" experiment using a 10,000 mice/dose group, experimental evidence was obtained to support the idea that for certain carcinogens in certain organs, no threshold exists for carcinogenic response (197,198). The theoretical explanation for a lack of thresholds for carcinogenesis is the low but finite probability that a critical mutation could be caused in a transforming oncogene even by a few molecules of a carcinogen. As the dose increases, the probability of critical damage and cancer incidence increases.

Counterarguments have been raised, specifically in relation to carcinogens such as formaldehyde that have unusually steep dose-response curves, and for carcinogens that are highly cytotoxic. If cytotoxicity is a critical step in the carcinogenic process, then a threshold can be postulated, since cytotoxicity is subject to a threshold effect. Furthermore, if the carcinogen acts as a promoting agent rather than as an initiator, again a threshold may be postulated, since pure tumor promoters have thresholds for effective dose. There is some concern, therefore, that genotoxic (no-threshold, initiating, mutagenic, DNA damaging) agents be regulated differently than nongenotoxic (threshold, promoting, nonmutagenic, non–DNA damaging) agents (87,199).

Although there is validity to the argument that nongenotoxic carcinogens might exhibit truly safe "no effect" levels, such agents must be proven to have only promoting activity and no genotoxicity. Many compounds are both cytotoxic and genotoxic, and may act as both promoters and mutagenic initiators. With the demonstration of any evidence of effects on the DNA, such chemicals must be assumed to be potentially genotoxic, and therefore no totally safe (threshold) level can be postulated.

Animal bioassays have been questioned on other grounds. First, in addition to extrapolation to lower doses, it is also necessary to extrapolate from the test species to humans (200–202). Despite the problems associated with cross-species comparison of carcinogenic activity (203), the majority of known human carcinogens are carcinogenic in rodents, and many chemicals first found to be carcinogenic in animal tests, such as vinyl chloride and bis(chloromethyl)ether, were later confirmed to be carcinogenic in humans by epidemiologic criteria. Arguments have been raised that certain strains of mice commonly used by the National Toxicology Program to test the carcinogenicity of chemicals, such as the C3B6F1 mouse, are unusually sensitive to liver carcinogenesis, possibly by promoting rather than initiating activity, and therefore are not appropriate models for assessing human cancer risk. The carcinogenic potency of some chemicals is specific to certain rodent species or strains (200–202). This specificity may often be a function of different metabolic enzyme profiles. The use of transgenic mice (and more recently rats) represents a new application of molecular biology to toxicology testing. Such strains allow for *in vivo* determination of end points on specific genes, that previously could only be done *in vitro* (204).

### Short-Term Tests

Because of the problems associated with species and strain comparison (205), low-dose extrapolation, and genotoxic or promoting mechanisms, the identification of carcinogens by animal bioassay is clearly not a simple endeavor. To make matters worse, animal bioassays require 2 to 3 years, and are very expensive. Therefore, the number of suspect agents that can be tested by animal bioassay each year is usually less than the number of new chemicals developed or released during the same year. This backlog has led to the development of shorter, cheaper tests that examine the activity of an agent in a surrogate assay that is predictive of its carcinogenic potential. The development and validation of such tests requires sufficient knowledge of carcinogenic mechanisms to render the assays relevant. For example, one of the first and most widespread such assays is the *Salmonella* mutagenesis assay developed by Ames and his colleagues (206,207). This test is based on a measurement of mutations in bacteria. The rationale for use of an assay in organisms that are not relevant to cancer is the mechanistic hypothesis that mutagenic activity is closely associated with carcinogenic activity. In fact, the majority of carcinogens are mutagenic, though many examples are known of nonmutagenic chemicals that cause cancer, as well as mutagenic agents that have not produced tumors in experimental models.

The Ames assay uses specific tester strains of *Salmonella* bacteria that have undergone base substitution or frame-shift mutations in the histidine locus. These bacteria require histidine for growth. However, if a reversion mutation occurs so that the wild-type genotype is restored, colonies of such mutants can be seen growing in histidine-depleted media.

Other mutagenesis assays have been developed both for bacteria and in mammalian cells. The best known of the latter are systems designed to detect mutations in target genes such as the hypoxanthine guanine phosphoribosyl transferase (HGPRT) gene (208). Chinese hamster ovary (CHO) and lung (V79) are the most commonly used cell types for the HGPRT mutation assay. Human lymphocytes have been employed with this assay as a method to detect exposure or sensitivity to mutagenic agents. Mutations in the HGPRT locus are detected by resistance to 6-thioguanine. Unlike the *Salmonella* assay, the HGPRT assay measures forward mutations.

Other short-term tests are generally designed to detect some genotoxic end point. For example, DNA damage can be indirectly measured by analysis of DNA repair rates. This is accomplished by determination of non–replication-associated DNA synthesis or unscheduled DNA synthesis (UDS) (209). Another example is the measurement of damage to chromosomes. A widely used test measures the frequency of sister chromatid exchanges (SCE) (210). This test detects a form of chromosomal rearrangements that are often the end result of DNA strand breaks. Such breaks, either single or double strand, can also be directly measured using techniques such as alkaline elution or alkaline unwinding assays. The micronucleus test (211, 212) and the determination of chromosomal aberrations (213) are also standard assays for determination of genotoxic effects.

There are many other short-term assays for genotoxic effects, and other markers of potential carcinogenic activity. New assays for the detection of nongenotoxic carcinogens have also been developed and utilized (214). Each of these assays, in order to be useful, must possess some degree of mechanistic relevance to carcinogenesis *in vivo* (215,216), must give positive results when known carcinogens are used, but must also exhibit a minimum level of false positives when tested with control substances (217,218). Furthermore, the tests should be rapid, reproducible, and inexpensive.

General consensus among scientists and regulators holds that no single short-term test will ever be devised to unequivocally determine the carcinogenicity of a chemical agent. Instead, batteries of four to six such tests measuring two to three end points in bacterial and mammalian systems may be used as a prescreen to determine the most important agents for further testing in animal bioassays (219,220).

### Cancer Risk Communication

The uncertainties of scientific cancer risk assessment as transmitted by the media have occasionally had an adverse effect on public trust and confidence in the regulatory agencies, and in the pronouncements of health professionals working in environmental carcinogenesis. Improvements in the current public climate regarding carcinogenic risks will probably require new methods for the systematic and consistent communication of comparative cancer risk in a quantitative manner (221). The field of risk communication is devoted to addressing these problems.

## CONCLUSION

Because of the suffering associated with human cancer, as well as increased attention to environmental issues, the subject of environmental carcinogenesis is often shadowed by emotional and political issues in addition to the difficult scientific questions that remain to be answered. Fortunately, the rapid advance in our understanding of the underlying molecular mechanisms of chemical and radiation carcinogenesis promises to provide major dividends in their application to risk assessment, carcinogen identification, and cancer prevention. The application of the tools and concepts of molecular biology to human cancer prevention and epidemiology represents a step forward in translational research with great potential benefits. In the near future it should be possible to use these approaches for identification of highly susceptible individuals, for assessment of carcinogen exposure, for early diagnosis, and for the development of new assays for carcinogen identification. The prevention of human cancer, caused largely by agents in the human environment, is the goal for continued research.

## REFERENCES

1. Lewtas J. Airborne carcinogens. *Pharmacol Toxicol* 1993;72(suppl 1): 55–63.
2. Ames BN. What are the major carcinogens in the etiology of human cancer? Environmental pollution, natural carcinogens, and the causes of human cancer: six errors. *Important Adv Oncol* 1989;1:237–247.
3. Higginson J. Importance of environmental and occupational factors in cancer. *J Toxicol Environ Health* 1980;6:941–952.
4. Nesnow S, Argus M, Bergman H, et al. Chemical carcinogens. A review and analysis of the literature of selected chemicals and the establishment of the Gene-Tox Carcinogen Data Base. A report of the U.S. Environmental Protection Agency Gene-Tox Program. *Mutat Res* 1987;185:1–195.
5. Lawley PD. Historical origins of current concepts of carcinogenesis. *Adv Cancer Res* 1994;65:17–111.
6. Weisburger JH, Williams GM. Chemical carcinogenesis. In: Doull J, Klaassen CD, Amdur MO, eds. *Toxicology:* the basic science of poisons. New York: Macmillian, 1980;84–138.
7. Schull WJ. Atomic bomb survivors: patterns of cancer risk. In: Boice, JD, Fraumeni, JF, eds. *Radiation epidemiology and biological significance.* New York: Raven Press, 1984;21–36.
8. Upton AC, Shore RE, Harley NH The health effects of low-level ionizing radiation. *Annu Rev Public Health* 1992;13:127–150.
9. Emmett E. Ultraviolet radiation as a cause of skin tumors. *CRC Crit Rev Toxicol* 1973;2:211–255.
10. Burns FJ, Albert RE, Garte SJ. Multiple stages in radiation carcinogenesis of rat skin. *Environ Health Perspect* 1989;81:67–72.
11. Barrett JC, Lamb PW, Wiseman RW. Multiple mechanisms for the carcinogenic effects of asbestos and other mineral fibers. *Environ Health Perspect* 1989;81:81–89.
12. Mossman BT, Craighead JE. Mechanisms of asbestos carcinogenesis. *Environ Res* 1981;25:269–280.
13. Pastorino U, Berrino F, Gervasio A, Pesenti V, Riboli E, Crosignani P. Proportion of lung cancers due to occupational exposure. *Int J Cancer* 1984;33:231–237.
14. Van Duuren BL. Comparison of potency of human carcinogens: vinyl chloride, chloromethylmethyl ether and bis(chloromethyl)ether. *Environ Res* 1989;49:143–151.
15. Doll R, Peto R. The causes of cancer: quantitative estimates of avoidable risks of cancer in the United States today. *J Natl Cancer Inst* 1981;66:1191–1308.
16. Higginson J. Environmental carcinogenesis. *Cancer* 1993;72(3 suppl): 971–977.
17. Sugimura T, Terada M, Yokota J, Hirohashi S, Wakabayashi K. Multiple genetic alterations in human carcinogenesis. *Environ Health Perspect* 1992;98:5–12.
18. Garte SJ. Activation of multiple oncogene pathways: a model for experimental carcinogenesis. *J Theor Biol* 1987;129:177–188.
19. Balmain A, Brown K. Oncogene activation in chemical carcinogenesis. *Adv Cancer Res* 1988;51:147–182.
20. Weinberg RA. Oncogenes, antioncogenes, and the molecular bases of multistep carcinogenesis. *Cancer Res* 1989;49:3713–3721.
21. Correa P. Human gastric carcinogenesis: a multistep and multifactorial process. *Cancer Res* 1992;52(24):6735–6740.
22. Pitot HC, Campbell HA, Maronpot R, et al. Critical parameters in the quantitation of the stages of initiation, promotion, and progression in one model of hepatocarcinogenesis in the rat. *Toxicol Pathol* 1989;17: 594–611.
23. Slaga TJ. Overview of tumor promotion in animals. *Environ Health Perspect* 1983;50:3–14.
24. Yuspa SH, Kilkenny A, Roop DR. Aberrant differentiation in mouse skin carcinogenesis. *IARC Sci Publ* 1988;92:3–10.
25. Vogelstein B, Fearon ER, Hamilton SR, et al. Genetic alterations during colorectal-tumor development. *N Engl J Med* 1988;319:525–532.
26. Boveri T. *The origin of malignant tumors.* Baltimore: Williams and Wilkins, 1929.
27. Miller EC, Miller JA. Searches for ultimate chemical carcinogens and their reactions with cellular macromolecules. *Cancer* 1981;10: 2327–2345.
28. Loeb LA. Endogenous carcinogenesis: molecular oncology into the twenty-first century. *Cancer Res* 1989;49:5489–5496.
29. Friend SH, Dryja TP, Weinberg RA. Oncogenes and tumor-suppressing genes. *N Engl J Med* 1988;318:618–622.
30. Conney AH. Induction of microsomal enzymes by foreign chemicals and carcinogenesis by polycyclic aromatic hydrocarbons. *Cancer Res* 1982;42:4875–4917.
31. Garte SJ, Kneip TJ. Metabolism. In: Kneip TJ, Crable JV, eds. *Methods for biological monitoring.* Washington, DC: American Public Health Association, 1988;15–26.
32. Guengerich FP. Metabolic activation of carcinogens. *Pharmacol Ther* 1992;54:17–61.
33. Gonzalez FJ, Jaiswal AK, Nebert DW. P-450 genes: evolution, regula-

tion, and relationship to human cancer and pharmacogenetics. *Cold Spring Harb Symp Quant Biol* 1986;51:879–890.
34. Cmarik JL, Inskeep PB, Meredith MJ, Meyer DJ, Ketterer B, Guengerich FP. Selectivity of rat and human glutathione S-transferases in activation of ethylene dibromide by glutathione conjugation and DNA binding and induction of unscheduled DNA synthesis in human hepatocytes. *Cancer Res* 1990;50:2747–2752.
35. Michejda CJ.Kroeger Koepke MB.. Carcinogen activation by sulfate conjugate formation. *Adv Pharmacol* 1994;27:331–63, 1994.
36. Harris C, Trump BF, Grafstrom R, Autrup H. Differences in metabolism of chemical carcinogens in cultured human epithelial tissue and cells. In: Harris C, Cerutti P, Fox CF, eds. *Mechanisms of chemical carcinogenesis.* New York: Liss, 1982;289–292.
37. Kimura S, Gonzalez FJ, Nebert DW. Tissue-specific expression of the mouse dioxin-inducible P(1)450 and P(3)450 genes: differential transcriptional activation and mRNA stability in liver and extrahepatic tissues. *Mol Cell Biol* 1986;6:1471–1477.
38. Nebert DW, Jones JE, Owens J, Puga A. Evolution of the P-450 gene superfamily. *Prog Clin Biol Res* 1988;274:557–576.
39. Shimada T, Guengerich FP. Inactivation of 1,3-, 1,6-, and 1,8-dinitropyrene by cytochrome P-450 enzymes in human and rat liver microsomes. *Cancer Res* 1990;50:2036–2043.
40. Jeffrey AM, Kinoshita T, Santella RM, Grunberger D, Katz L, Weinstein IB. The chemistry of polycyclic aromatic hydrocarbon-DNA adducts. In: Pullman B, Ts'o POB, Gelboin H, eds. *Carcinogens: fundamental mechanisms and environmental effects.* Amsterdam: Reidel, 1980;565–579.
41. Thakker DR, Levin W, Buening M, et al. Species-specific enhancement by 7,8-benzoflavone of hepatic microsomal metabolism of benzo[*e*]pyrene 9,10-dihydrodiol to bay-region diol epoxides. *Cancer Res* 1981;41:1389–1396.
42. Yang SK, McCourt DW, Roller PP, Gelboin HV. Enzymatic conversion of benzo[*a*]pyrene leading predominantly to the diol-epoxide r-7,t-8-dihydroxy-t-9, 10-oxy-7,8,9,10 -tetrahydrobenzo[*a*]pyrene through a single enantiomer of r-7,t-8-dihydroxy -7,8-dihydrobenzo[*a*]pyrene. *Proc Natl Acad Sci USA* 1976;73:2594–2598.
43. Nebert DW, Nelson DR, Adesnik M, et al. The P-450 superfamily: updated listing of all genes and recommended nomenclature for the chromosomal loci. *DNA* 1989;8:1–13.
44. Hankinson O. The aryl hydrocarbon receptor complex. *Annu Rev Pharmacol Toxicol* 35:307–40, 1995.
45. Burbach KM, Poland A, Bradfield CA. Cloning of the Ah-receptor cDNA reveals a distinctive ligand-activated transcription factor. *Proc Natl Acad Sci USA* 1992;89:8185–8189.
46. Whitelaw ML, Gustafsson JA, Poellinger L. Identification of transactivation and repression functions of the dioxin receptor and its basic helix-loop-helix/PAS partner factor Arnt: inducible versus constitutive modes of regulation. *Mol Cell Biol* 1994;14(12):8343–8355.
47. Phillips DH, Grover PL Polycyclic hydrocarbon activation: bay regions and beyond. *Drug Metab Rev* 1994;26(1-2):443–467.
48. Hemminki K, Cooper CS, Ribeiro O, Grover PL, Sims P. Reactions of "bay-region" and non-"bay-region" diol epoxides of benz[a]anthracene with DNA: Evidence indicating that the major products are hydrocarbon-$N^2$-guanine adducts. *Carcinogenesis* 1980;1:177–286.
49. Montesano R. Alkylation of DNA and tissue specificity in nitrosamine carcinogenesis. *J Supramol Struct Cell Biochem* 1981; 17:259–273.
50. Mirvish SS. Experimental evidence for inhibition of N-nitroso compound formation as a factor in the negative correlation between vitamin C consumption and the incidence of certain cancers. *Cancer Res* 1994;54:1948s–1951s.
51. Den Engelse L, Menkveld GJ, De Brij RJ, Tates AD. Formation and stability of alkylated pyrimidines and purines (including imidazole ring-opened 7-alkylguanine) and alkylphosphoriester in liver DNA of adult rats treated with ethylnitrosourea or dimethylnitrosamine. *Carcinogenesis* 1986;7:393–403.
52. Essigmann JM, Green CL, Croy RG, Fowler KW, Buchi GH, Wogan GN. Interactions of aflatoxin $B_1$ and alkylating agents with DNA: Structural and functional studies. *Cold Spring Harbor Symp Quant Biol* 1983;47:327–337.
53. Eastman A, Mossman BT, Bresnick E. Formation and removal of benzo[*a*]pyrene adducts of DNA in hamster tracheal epithelial cells. *Cancer Res* 1981;41:2605–2610.
54. Geacintov NE, Lee MS, Ibanez V, Amin S, Hecht SS. Differences in conformations of covalent adducts derived from the binding of 5- and 6-methylchrysene diol epoxide stereoisomers to DNA. *Carcinogenesis* 1990;11:985–989.
55. Grunberger D, Santella RM. Alternative conformations of DNA modified by N-2-acetylaminofluorene. *J Supramol Structure Cell Biochem* 1981;17:231–244.
56. Dipple A. DNA adducts of chemical carcinogens. *Carcinogenesis* 1995;16:437–441.
57. Kadlubar FF. DNA adducts of carcinogenic aromatic amines. *IARC Sci Publ* 1994;125:199–216.
58. Huff AC, Topal MD. DNA damage at thymine N-3 abolishes base-pairing capacity during DNA synthesis. *J Biol Chem* 1987;262: 12843–12850.
59. Wogan GN. Detection of DNA damage in studies on cancer etiology and prevention. *IARC Sci Publ* 1988;89:32–51.
60. Bohr VA, Evans MK, Fornace AJ. Biology of disease: DNA repair and its pathogenetic implications. *Lab Invest* 1989;61:143–161.
61. Poirier MC, Beland FA, Deal FH, Swenberg JA. DNA adduct formation and removal in specific liver cell populations during chronic dietary administration of 2-acetylaminofluorene. *Carcinogenesis* 1989; 10:1143–1145.
62. Van Houten B. Nucleotide excision repair in *E. coli. Microbiol Rev* 1990;54:18–51.
63. Williams GM, Bordet C, Cerutti PA, et al. DNA damage and repair in mammalian cells. *IARC Monogr Eval Carcinog Risk* 1980;suppl 2: 201–226.
64. Toorchen D, Lindamood C 3d, Swenberg JA, Topal MD. $O^6$-Methylguanine-DNA transmethylase converts O-methylguanine thymine base pairs to guanine thymine base pairs in DNA. *Carcinogenesis* 1984;5:1733–1735.
65. Williams LD, Shaw BR. Protonated base pairs explain the ambiguous pairing properties of $O^6$-methylguanine. *Proc Natl Acad Sci USA* 1987;84:1779–1783.
66. Drinkwater NR, Miller EC, Miller JA. Estimation of apurinic/apyrimidinic sites and phosphotriesters in deoxyribonucleic acid treated with electrophilic carcinogens and mutagens. *Biochemistry* 1980;19: 5087–5092.
67. Richardson FC, Boucheron JA, Skopek TR, Swenberg JA. Formation of $O^6$-methyldeoxyguanosine at specific sites in a synthetic oligonucleotide designed to resemble a known mutagenic hotspot. *J Biol Chem* 1989;264:838–841.
68. Singer B. The chemical effects of nucleic acid alkylation and their relation to mutagenesis and carcinogenesis. *Prog Nucleic Acid Res Mol Biol* 1975;15:219–284, 330–332.
69. Grollman AP.Shibutani S. Mutagenic specificity of chemical carcinogens as determined by studies of single DNA adducts. *IARC Sci Publ* 1994;125:385–397.
70. Loeb LA, Preston BP. Mutagenesis by apurinic/apyrimidinic sites. *Annu Rev Genet* 1986;20:201–230.
71. Eadie JS, Conrad M, Toorchen D, Topal MD. Mechanism of mutagenesis by $O^6$-methylguanine. *Nature* 1984;308:201–203.
72. Poirier MC. Human exposure monitoring, dosimetry, and cancer risk assessment: the use of antisera specific for carcinogen-DNA adducts and carcinogen-modified DNA. *Drug Metab Rev* 1994;26:87–109.
73. Singer B. Alkylation of the $O^6$ of guanine is only one of many chemical events that may initiate carcinogenesis. *Cancer Invest* 1984;2: 233–238.
74. Swenberg JA, Dyroff MC, Bedell MA, et al. $O^4$-Ethyldeoxythymidine, but not $O^6$-ethyldeoxyguanosine, accumulates in hepatocyte DNA of rats exposed continuously to diethylnitrosamine. *Proc Natl Acad Sci USA* 1984;81:1692–1695.
75. Drinkwater NR, Miller JA, Miller EC, Yang N-C. Covalent intercalative binding to DNA in relation to the mutagenicity of hydrocarbon epoxides and N-acetoxy-acetyl-aminofluorene. *Cancer Res* 1978;38: 3247–3255.
76. Poirier MC, Beland FA. DNA adduct measurements and tumor incidence during chronic carcinogen exposure in animal models: implications for DNA adduct-based human cancer risk assessment. *Chem Res Toxicol* 1992;5:749–755.
77. Singer B, Brent TP. Human lymphoblasts contain DNA glycosylase activity excising N-3 and N-7 methyl and ethyl purines but not $O^6$-alkylguanines or 1-alkyladenines. *Proc Natl Acad Sci USA* 1981;78: 856–860.
78. Sirover MA. Induction of the DNA repair enzyme uracil-DNA glyco-

sylase in stimulated human lymphocytes. *Cancer Res* 1979;39: 2090–2095.
79. Kraemer KH, Levy DD, Parris CN, et al. Xeroderma pigmentosum and related disorders: examining the linkage between defective DNA repair and cancer. *J Invest Dermatol* 1994;103:96S–101S.
80. Savitsky K, Bar-Shira A, Gilad S, et al. A single ataxia telangiectasia gene with a product similar to PI-3kinase. *Science* 1995;268: 1749–1753.
81. Pegg AE, Dolan ME, Moschel RC. Structure, function and inhibition of O6-alkylguanine-DNA alkyltransferase. *Prog Nucleic Acid Res Mol Biol* 1995;51:167–223.
82. Grossman L. Damage recognition by UvrABC. A study of vectorial movement. *Ann NY Acad Sci* 1994;726:252–265.
83. Grollman AP, Johnson F, Tchou J, Eisenberg M. Recognition and repair of 8-oxoguanine and formamidopyrimidine lesions in DNA. *Ann NY Acad Sci* 1994;726:208–213.
84. Bohr VA. DNA repair fine structure and its relation to genomic instability. *Carcinogenesis* 1995;16:2885–2892.
85. Hanawalt PC. Transcription-coupled repair and human disease. *Science* 1994;266:1957–1958.
86. Stewart BW. Role of DNA repair in carcinogenesis. *IARC Sci Publ* 1992;116):307–320.
87. Weisburger JH, Williams GA. Carcinogen testing: current problems and new approaches. *Science* 1981;214:877–880.
88. Colburn NH, Farber E, Weinstein EB, Diamond L, Slaga TJ. American Cancer Society workshop on tumor promotion and antipromotion. *Cancer Res* 1987;47:5509–5513.
89. Castagna M, Takai Y, Kaibuchi K, Sano K, Kikkawa U, Nishizuka Y. Direct activation of calcium-activated phospholipid-dependent protein kinase by tumor-promoting phobol esters. *J Biol Chem* 1982;257: 7847–7851.
90. Dunphy WG, Delclos KB, Blumberg PM. Characterization of specific binding of [$^3$H]phorbol 12,13-dibutyrate and [$^3$H]phorbol 12-myristate 13-acetate to mouse brain. *Cancer Res* 1980;40:3635–3641.
91. Marks F. Gschwendt M. Protein kinase C and skin tumor promotion. *Mutat Res* 1995;333(1-2):161–172.
92. Yuspa SH. Hennings H. Dlugosz A. Tennenbaum T. Glick A. The role of growth factors in mouse skin tumor promotion and premalignant progression. *Prog Clin Biol Res* 1995;391:39–48.
93. Sharkey NA, Hennings H, Yuspa SH, Blumberg PM. Comparison of octahydromezerein and mezerein as protein kinase C activators and as mouse skin tumor promoters. *Carcinogenesis* 1989;10:1937–1941.
94. Slaga TJ, Klein-Szanto ASP, Triplett LL, Yotti LP, Trosko JE. Skin tumor-promoting activity of benzoyl peroxide, a widely used free radical-generating compound. *Science* 1981;213:1023–1025.
95. Solt E, Farber E. New principle for the analysis of chemical carcinogens. *Nature* 1976;263:701–703.
96. Frenkel K. Carcinogen-mediated oxidant formation and oxidative DNA damage. *Pharmacol Ther* 1992;53(1):127–166.
97. Marnett LJ, Ji C, Hancock AB Jr. Modulation of oxidant formation in mouse skin *in vivo* by tumor-promoting phorbol esters. *Cancer Res* 1994;54:1886s–1889s.
98. Birt DF. The influence of dietary fat on carcinogenesis: lessons from experimental models. *Nutr Rev* 1990;48:1–5.
99. Wynder E, Hoffmann D. Tobacco and health. *N Engl J Med* 1985;300: 885–902.
100. Bosland MC, Prinsen MK. Induction of dorsolateral prostate adenocarcinomas and other accessory sex gland lesions in male Wistar rats by a single administration of N-methyl-N-nitrosourea, 7,12-dimethylbenz[a]anthracene, and 3,2′-dimethyl-4-aminobiphenyl after sequential treatment with cyproterone acetate and testosterone propionate. *Cancer Res* 1990;50:691–699.
101. Slaga TJ. Cellular and molecular mechanisms involved in multistage skin carcinogenesis. *Carcinog Compr Surv* 1989;11:1–18.
102. Liu E, Dollbaum C, Scott G, Rochlitz C, Benz C, Smith HS. Molecular lesions involved in the progression of a human breast cancer. *Oncogene* 1988;3:323–327.
103. Pitot HC. Progression: the terminal stage in carcinogenesis. *Jpn J Cancer Res* 1989;80:599–607.
104. Nicolson GL. Tumor cell instability, diversification, and progression to the metastatic phenotype: from oncogene to oncofetal expression. *Cancer Res* 1987;47:1473–1487.
105. Nowell PC. The clonal evolution of tumor cell populations. *Science* 1976;194:23–28.
106. Dotto, GP, O'Connell JO, Patskan G, Conti C, Ariza A, Slaga TJ. Malignant progression of papilloma-derived keratinocytes: differential effects of the ras, neu, and p53 oncogenes. *Mol Carcinogen* 1988; 1:171–179.
107. Harper JR, Roop DR, Yuspa SH. Transfection of the EJ rasHa gene into keratinocytes derived from carcinogen-induced mouse papillomas causes malignant progression. *Mol Cell Biol* 1986;6:3144–3149.
108. Hennings H, Shores R, Balaschak M, Yuspa SH. Sensitivity of subpopulations of mouse skin papillomas to malignant conversion by urethane or 4-nitroquinoline N-oxide. *Cancer Res* 1990;50:653–657.
109. Crouch E, Wilson R. Interspecies comparison of carcinogenic potency. *J Toxicol Environ Health* 1978;5:1095–1118.
110. Gold LS, Slone TH, Backman GM, et al. Third chronological supplement to the carcinogenic potency database: standardized results of animal bioassays published through December 1986 and by the National Toxicology Program through June 1987. *Environ Health Perspect* 1990;84:215–216.
111. Peto R, Pike MC, Bernstein L, Gold LS, Ames BN. The TD50: a proposed general convention for the numerical description of the carcinogenic potency of chemicals in chronic-exposure animal experiments. *Environ Health Perspect* 1984;58:1–8.
112. Upton AC. On the costs of smoking. *Cancer Invest* 1989;7:517–518.
113. Samet JM. The epidemiology of lung cancer. *Chest* 1993;103: 20S–29S.
114. Cohen BS, Eisenbud M, Harley NH. Alpha radioactivity in cigarette smoke. *Radiat Res* 1980;83:190–196.
115. Hecht SS, Hoffmann D. The relevance of tobacco-specific nitrosamines to human cancer. *Cancer Surv* 1989;8:273–294.
116. Hecht SS, Carmella SG, Foiles PG, Murphy SE. Biomarkers for human uptake and metabolic activation of tobacco-specific nitrosamines. *Cancer Res* 1994;54:1912s–1917s.
117. Pasternack BS, Shore RE, Albert RE. Occupational exposure to chloromethyl ethers. A retrospective cohort mortality study (1948–1972). *J Occup Med* 1977;19(11):741–746.
118. Nelson N. The chloroethers—occupational carcinogens: a summary of laboratory and epidemiology studies. *Ann NY Acad Sci* 1876;271: 81–90.
119. Lemen RA, Johnson WM, Wagoner JK, Archer VE. Saccomanno G. Cytologic observations and cancer incidence following exposure to BCME. *Ann NY Acad Sci* 1976;271:71–80.
120. Weiss W, Figueroa WG. The characteristics of lung cancer due to chloromethyl ethers. *J Occup Med* 1976;18(9):623–627.
121. DeFonso LR, Kelton SC Jr. Lung cancer following exposure to chloromethyl methyl ether. An epidemiological study. *Arch Environ Health* 1976;31(3):125–130.
122. Albert RE, Pasternack BS, Shore RE, Nelson N. Identification of occupational settings with very high risks of lung cancer. *J Natl Cancer Inst* 1979;63:1289–1290.
123. Weiss W, Moser RL, Auerbach O. Lung cancer in chloromethyl ether workers. *Am Rev Respir Dis* 1979;120(5):1031–1037.
124. Reznik G, Wagner HH, Atay Z. Lung cancer following exposure to bis(chloromethyl)ether: a case report. *J Environ Pathol Toxicol* 1978; 1(1):105–111.
125. Kuschner M, Laskin S, Drew RT, Cappiello V, Nelson N. Inhalation carcinogenicity of alpha halo ethers. III. Lifetime and limited period inhalation studies with bis(chloromethyl)ether at 0.1 ppm. *Arch Environ Health* 1975;30:73–77.
126. Van Duuren BL, Goldschmidt BM, Seidman I. Carcinogenic activity of di- and trifunctional alpha-chloro ethers and of 1,4-dichlorobutene-2 in ICR/HA swiss mice. *Cancer Res* 1975;35(9):2553–2557.
127. Zajdela F, Croisy A, Barbin A, Malaveille C, Tomatis L. Bartsch H. Carcinogenicity of chloroethylene oxide, an ultimate reactive metabolite of vinyl chloride, and bis(chloromethyl)ether after subcutaneous administration and in initiation-promotion experiments in mice. *Cancer Res* 1980;40(2):352–356.
128. Van Duuren BL. Direct-acting alkylating and acylating agents. DNA adduct formation, structure-activity, and carcinogenesis. *Ann NY Acad Sci* 1988;534:620–634.
129. Gowers DS, DeFonso LR, Schaffer P, et al. Incidence of respiratory cancer among workers exposed to chloromethyl-ethers. *Am J Epidemiol* 1993;137(1):31–42.
130. Collingwood KW, Pasternack BS, Shore RE. An industry-wide study of respiratory cancer in chemical workers exposed to chloromethyl ethers. *J Natl Cancer Inst* 1987;78(6):1127–1136.

131. Maher KV, DeFonso LR. Respiratory cancer among chloromethyl ether workers. *J Natl Cancer Inst* 1987;78(5):839–843.
132. Nagao M, Sugimura T. Carcinogenic factors in food with relevance to colon cancer development. *Mutat Res* 1993;290(1):43–51.
133. Rogers AE, Zeisel SH, Groopman J. Diet and carcinogenesis. *Carcinogenesis* 1993;14(11):2205–2217.
134. Layton DW, Bogen KT, Knize MG, Hatch FT, Johnson VM. Felton JS. Cancer risk of heterocyclic amines in cooked foods: an analysis and implications for research. *Carcinogenesis* 1995;16(1):39–52.
135. Birt DF, Kris ES, Choe M, Pelling JC. Dietary energy and fat effects on tumor promotion. *Cancer Res* 1992;52:2035s–2039s.
136. Ip C. Controversial issues of dietary fat and experimental mammary carcinogenesis. *Prev Med* 1993;22(5):728–737.
137. Sugimura T. Mutagens, carcinogens and tumor promoters in our daily food. *Cancer* 1982;49:1970–1984.
138. Wynder EL. The dietary environment and cancer. *J Am Diet Assoc* 1977;71:385–392.
139. Ames BN. Dietary carcinogens and anti-carcinogens. *J Toxicol Clin Toxicol* 1984;22:291–301.
140. Archer MC. Mechanisms of action of N-nitroso compounds. *Cancer Surv* 1989;8:241–250.
141. Boutwell RK. An overview of the role of diet and nutrition in carcinogenesis. *Prog Clin Biol Res* 1988;259:81–104.
142. Kennedy AR. Prevention of carcinogenesis by protease inhibitors. *Cancer Res* 1994;54:1999s–2005s.
143. Burns FJ, Upton AC, Silini G, eds. *Radiation carcinogenesis and DNA alterations.* New York: Plenum Press, 1986.
144. Grosovsky AJ, de Boer JG, de Jong PJ, Drobetsky EA, Glickman BW. Base substitutions, frameshifts, and small deletions constitute ionizing radiation-induced point mutations in mammalian cells. *Proc Natl Acad Sci USA* 1988;85:185–188.
145. Lloyd DC, Edwards AA, Leonard A, et al. Frequencies of chromosomal aberrations induced in human blood lymphocytes by low doses of X-rays. *Int J Radiat Biol* 1988;53:49–55.
146. Zimmerman R, Cerutti P. Active oxygen acts as a promoter of transformation in mouse embryo C3H/10T1/2/C18 fibroblasts. *Proc Natl Acad Sci USA* 1984;81:2085–2087.
147. Garte SJ, Burns FJ, Ashkenazi-Kimmel T, Felber M, Sawey MJ. Amplification of the c-*myc* oncogene during progression of radiation-induced rat skin tumors. *Cancer Res* 1990;50:3073–3977.
148. Guerrero I, Calzada P, Mayer A, Pellicer A. A molecular approach to leukemogenesis: mouse lymphomas contain an activated c-*ras* oncogene. *Proc Natl Acad Sci* USA 1984;81:202–205.
149. Gumerlock PH, Meyers FJ, Foster BA, Kawakami TG, deVere White RW. Activated c-N-*ras* in radiation-induced acute nonlymphocytic leukemia: twelfth codon aspartic acid. *Radiat Res* 1989;117:198–206.
150. Committee on the Biological Effects of Ionizing Radiation. *Health effects of exposure to ionizing radiation BEIR V.* Washington, DC: National Academy Press, 1990.
151. Upton AC. Biological basis for assessing carcinogenic risks of low-level radiation. *Carcinog Compr Surv* 1985;10:381–401.
152. Shubik P. Chemical carcinogens and human cancer. *Cancer Lett* 1995;93(1):3–7.
153. Moller H. Occurrence of carcinogens in the external environment: epidemiological investigations. *Pharmacol Toxicol* 1993;72(suppl 1): 39–45.
154. Vineis P. Epidemiology of cancer from exposure to arylamines. *Environ Health Perspect* 1994;102(suppl 6):7–10.
155. Bertazzi P, diDomenico A. Chemical, environmental, and health aspects of the Seveso Italy accident. In: Schecter A, ed. *Dioxins and health.* New York: Plenum Press, 1994;587–632.
156. Breslow NE, Day NE. *Statistical methods in cancer research, vol 1. The analysis of case control studies.* Lyon, France: IARC Scientific, 1980.
157. Vineis P. The use of biomarkers in epidemiology: the example of bladder cancer. *Toxicol Lett* 1992;64-65:Spec No. 463-7.
158. Perera F. Biomarkers and molecular epidemiology of occupationally related cancer. *J Toxicol Environ Health* 1993;40(2-3):203–215.
159. Strickland PT, Groopman JD. Biomarkers for assessing environmental exposure to carcinogens in the diet. *Am J Clin Nutr* 1995;61: 710S–720S, 1995
160. Hulka BS. Epidemiological studies using biological markers: issues for Epidemiologists. *Cancer Epidemiol Biomark Prevent* 1991;1: 13–19.
161. Hemminki K. DNA adducts, mutations and cancer. *Carcinogenesis* 1993;14(10):2007–2012.
162. Skipper PL, Peng X, Soohoo CK, Tannenbaum SR. Protein adducts as biomarkers of human carcinogen exposure. *Drug Metab Rev* 1994; 26(1-2):111–124.
163. Strickland PT, Routledge MN, Dipple A. Methodologies for measuring carcinogen adducts in humans. *Cancer Epidemiol Biomarkers Prevent* 1993;2:607–619.
164. Whyatt RM, Garte SJ, Cosma GN, et al. CYP1A1 mRNA levels in placental tissue as a biomarker of environmental exposure. *Cancer Epidemiol Biomarkers Prevent* 1995;4:147–153.
165. Ganguly S, Taioli E, Baranski B, Cohen B, Toniolo P, Garte SJ. Human metallothionein gene expression determined by quantitative RT-PCR as a biomarker of cadmium exposure. Cancer Epid. *Biomark Prevent* 1996;5:297–301.
166. O'Neill JP, Albertini RJ, Nicklas JA. Molecular analysis of mutations induced *in vivo* in humans In: Garte S, ed. *Molecular environmental biology.* Boca Raton, FL: Lewis, 1994;225–246.
167. Groopman JD, Wogan GN, Roebuck BD, Kensler TW. Molecular biomarkers for aflatoxins and their application to human cancer prevention. *Cancer Res* 1994;54:1907s–1911s.
168. Vineis P, Ronco R. Interindividual variation in carcinogen metabolism and bladder cancer risk. *Environ Health Perspect* 1992;98:95–99.
169. Harris CC. Interindividual variation among humans in carcinogen metabolism, DNA adduct formation and DNA repair. *Carcinogenesis* 1989;10:1563–1566.
170. Frebourg T, Friend SH. 1992 Cancer risks from germline p53 mutations. *J Clin Invest* 1992;90(5):1637–1641.
171. Shields PG. Inherited factors and environmental exposures in cancer risk. *J Occup Med* 1993;35(1):34–41.
172. Pelkonen O. Carcinogen metabolism and individual susceptibility. *Scand J Work Environ Health* 1992;18(suppl 1):17–21.
173. Hayes RB. Genetic susceptibility and occupational cancer. *Med Lav* 1995;86(3):206–213.
174. Idle JR, Armstrong M, Boddy AV, et al. The pharmacogenetics of chemical carcinogenesis. *Pharmacogenetics* 1992;2(6):246–258.
175. Hirvonen A. Genetic factors in individual responses to environmental exposures. *J Occup Environ Med* 1995;37(1):37–43.
176. Rothman N. Genetic susceptibility biomarkers in studies of occupational and environmental cancer: methodologic issues. *Toxicol Lett* 1995;77(1-3):221–225.
177. Ikawa S, Uematsu F, Watanabe K, et al. Assessment of cancer susceptibility in humans by use of genetic polymorphisms in carcinogen metabolism. *Pharmacogenetics* 1995;5:Spec No. S154–60.
178. Kaderlik KR, Kadlubar FF. Metabolic polymorphisms and carcinogen-DNA adduct formation in human populations. *Pharmacogenetics* 1995;5:Spec No. S108-17.
179. Cosma G, Crofts F, Currie D, Wirgin I, Toniolo P, Garte SJ. Racial differences in restriction fragment length polymorphisms and messenger RNA inducibility of the human CYP1A1 gene. *Cancer Epidemiol Biomarkers Prevent* 1993;2:53–57.
180. Shields PG, Caporaso NE, Falk RT, et al. Lung cancer, race, and a CYP1A1 genetic polymorphism. *Cancer Epidemiol Biomarkers Prevent* 1993;2:481–485.
181. Stephens EA, Taylor JA, Kaplan N, et al. Ethnic variation in the CYP2E1 gene: polymorphism analysis of 695 African-Americans, European-Americans and Taiwanese. *Pharmacogenetics* 1994;4: 185–192.
182. Crofts F, Cosma GN, Taioli E, Currie DC, Toniolo PT, Garte SJ. A novel CYP1A1 gene polymorphism in African-Americans. *Carcinogenesis* 1993;14:1729–1731.
183. Garte SJ, Trachman J, Crofts F, et al. Distribution of composite CYP1A1 genotypes in Africans, African-Americans and Caucasians. *Hum Hered* 1996;46:121–127.
184. Taioli E, Trachman J, Chen X, Toniolo P, Garte SJ. CYP1A1 RFLP is associated with breast cancer in African American women. *Cancer Res* 1995;55:3757–3758.
185. Taioli E, Crofts F, Demopoulos R, Trachman J, Toniolo P, Garte SJ. An African American specific CYP1A1 polymorphism is associated with adenocarcinoma of the lung. *Cancer Res* 1995;55:472–473.
186. Kato S, Shields PG, Caporaso NE, et al. Analysis of cytochrome P-4502E1 genetic polymorphisms in relation to human lung cancer. *Cancer Epidemiol Biomarkers Prevent* 1994;3:515–518.
187. Hirvonen A, Husgafvel-Pursianen K, Anttila S, Vainio H. The GSTM1

null genotype as a potential risk modifier for squamous cell carcinoma of the lung. *Carcinogenesis* 1993;14:1479–1481.

188. Nakajima T, Elovaara E, Anttila S, et al. Expression and polymorphism of glutathione S-transferase in human lungs: risk factors in smoking-related lung cancer. *Carcinogenesis* 1995;16:707–711.
189. Nakachi K, Imai K, Hayashi S. Kawajiri, K. Polymorphisms of the CYP1A1 and glutathione S-transferase genes associated with susceptibility to lung cancer in relation to cigarette dose in a Japanese population. *Cancer Res* 1993;53:2994–2999.
190. Kihara M, Kihara M, Noda K. Lung cancer risk of GSTM1 null genotype is dependent on the extent of tobacco smoke exposure. *Carcinogen* 1994;15:415–418.
191. Garte SJ, Zocchetti C, Taioli E. Gene-environment interactions in the application of biomarkers of cancer susceptibility in epidemiology.In: Toniolo P, Boffetta P, Shuker D, Hulka B, Pearce N, Rothman N, eds. *Applications of biomarkers in cancer epidemiology.* IARC Scientific Publication No. 142. Lyon, France, 1977, 251–264.
192. Ames BN, Gold LS. Too many rodent carcinogens: mitogenesis increases mutagenesis. *Science* 1990;249:970–971.
193. Brown CC, Chu KC. Additive and multiplicative models and multistage carcinogenesis theory. *Risk Anal* 1989;9:99–105.
194. Moolgavkar SH, Day NE, Stevens RG. Two stage model for carcinogenesis: epidemiology of breast cancer in females. *J Natl Cancer Inst* 1980;65:559–569.
195. Andersen ME, Krewski D, Withey JR. Physiological pharmacokinetics and cancer risk assessment. *Cancer Lett* 1993;69(1):1–14.
196. Upton AC. The question of thresholds for radiation and chemical carcinogenesis. *Cancer Invest* 1989;7:267–276.
197. Cohen SM, Ellwein LB. Proliferative and genotoxic cellular effects in 2-acetylaminofluorene bladder and liver carcinogenesis: biological modeling of the ED01 study. *Toxicol Appl Pharmacol* 1990;104:79–93.
198. Hughes DH, Bruce RD, Hart RW, et al. A report on the workshop on biological and statistical implications of the ED01 study and related data bases. *Fundam Appl Toxicol* 1983;3:129–136.
199. Williams GM. Classification of genotoxic and epigenetic carcinogens using liver culture assays. *Ann NY Acad Sci* 1979;23:60–66.
200. Ashby J. The unique role of rodents in the detection of possible human carcinogens and mutagens. *Mutat Res* 1983;115:177–213.
201. Krewski D, Goddard MJ, Withey JR. Carcinogenic potency and interspecies extrapolation. *Prog Clin Biol Res* 1990;340:323–334.
202. Rall DP. Relevance of animal experiments to humans. *Environ Health Perspect* 1979;32:297–230.
203. Bernstein L, Gold LS, Ames BN, Pike MC, Hoel DG. Some tautologous aspects of the comparison of carcinogenic potency in rats and mice. *Fundam Appl Toxicol* 1985;5:79–86.
204. Gorelick NJ. Overview of mutation assays in transgenic mice for routine testing. *Environ Mol Mutagen* 1995;25(3):218–20.
205. Lijinsky W. Species differences in carcinogenesis. *In Vivo* 1993;7(1): 65–72.
206. Ames BN, Durston WE, Yamasaki E, Lee FD. Carcinogens are mutagens: a simple test system combining liver homogenates for activation and bacteria for detection. *Proc Natl Acad Sci USA* 1973;70: 2281–2285.
207. Maron DM, Ames BN. Revised methods for the Salmonella mutagenicity test. *Mutat Res* 1983;113:173–215.
208. Hsie AW, Casciano DA, Couch DB, Krahn DF, O'Neill JP, Whitfield BL. The use of Chinese hamster ovary cells to quantify specific locus mutation and to determine mutagenicity of chemicals. A report of the Gene-Tox Program. *Mutat Res* 1981;86:193–214.
209. Burlinson B. An *in vivo* unscheduled DNA synthesis (UDS) assay in the rat gastric mucosa: preliminary development. *Carcinogenesis* 1989;10(8):1425–1428.
210. Latt SA, Allen J, Bloom SE, et al. Sister-chromatid exchanges; a report of the Gene-Tox Program. *Mutat Res* 1981;87:17–62.
211. Gocke E. The micronucleus test: its value as a predictor of rodent carcinogens versus its value in risk assessment. *Mutat Res* 1996;352(1-2):189–190.
212. Fritzenschaf H, Kohlpoth M, Rusche B, Schiffmann D. Testing of known carcinogens and noncarcinogens in the Syrian hamster embryo (SHE) micronucleus test *in vitro*;correlations with *in vivo* micronucleus formation and cell transformation. *Mutat Res* 1993;319(1): 47–53.
213. Galloway SM. Chromosome aberrations induced *in vitro*: mechanisms, delayed expression, and intriguing questions. *Environ Mol Mutagen* 1994;23(suppl 24):44–53.
214. Yamasaki H, Ashby J, Bignami M, et al. Nongenotoxic carcinogens: development of detection methods based on mechanisms: a European project. *Mutat Res* 1996;353(1-2):47–63.
215. Travis CC, Wang LA, Waehner MJ. Quantitative correlation of carcinogenic potency with four different classes of short-term test data. *Mutagenesis* 1991;6(5):353–360.
216. Kier LD. Comments and perspective on the EPA workshop on "The relationship between short-term test information and carcinogenicity." *Environ Mol Mutagen* 1988;11(1):147–157.
217. Lovell DP. Screening for possible human carcinogens and mutagens. False positives, false negatives: statistical implications. *Mutat Res* 1989;213(1):43–60.
218. Ashby J. No. 22. Prevalence of carcinogens and short-term test performance—a dangerous statistical illusion? *Mutat Res* 1990;242(3): 261–263.
219. Heinze JH, Poulsen NK. The optimal design of batteries of short-term tests for detecting carcinogens. *Mutat Res* 1983;117:259–269.
220. Ennever FK. Rosenkranz HS. Application of the carcinogenicity prediction and battery selection method to recent National Toxicology Program short-term test data. *Environ Mol Mutagen* 1989;13(4): 332–338.
221. Garte SJ. Communication of relative carcinogenic risks: a quantitative approach. *Risk Anal* 1990;10:467—468.

*Environmental and Occupational Medicine, Third Edition,* edited by William N. Rom.
Lippincott–Raven Publishers, Philadelphia © 1998.

# CHAPTER 12

# Molecular Carcinogenesis

Jeff Boyd

The question of how cancer arises remains one of the most fundamental and complex problems in all of human biology. Understanding cancer will ultimately require an understanding of "what makes a cell a cell" (1). Historically, many theoretical models have received temporary favor in efforts to empirically address the problem of cancer etiology, including those founded upon the action of environmental agents, chemical carcinogens, viruses, somatic chromosomal abnormalities, and congenital predisposition. We now know that all of these paradigms are in fact correct by virtue of their convergence into the genetic paradigm: cancer is the result of an accumulation of mutations in genes that govern the tumor phenotype (2).

There is unlikely to exist, now or ever, a more robust biologic paradigm than the genetic basis of human cancer development. The genetic foundation of carcinogenesis was implied by some of the earliest practitioners of cancer cell biology and cytogenetics. In the mid-19th century, Rudolph Virchow recognized that metastatic cancer cells resemble those of the primary tumor and that all cells of a tumor may arise from a single progenitor cell. Thus, the neoplastic phenotype is heritable from one tumor cell generation to the next, leading to the aphorism *onmis cellulae cellula.* In the early 1900s, Theodor Boveri (3) extended this concept to the cytogenetic level, suggesting that gains and losses of specific chromosomes from abnormal segregation might lead to abnormal cell division and other aspects of the cancer phenotype. Not until the discovery of DNA and elucidation of the genetic code, however, was it possible to begin defining the molecular basis of tumorigenesis in terms of specific mutations in specific genes. In the two decades since Bishop and Varmus described the first vertebrate oncogene (4), the genetic paradigm has been defined in sufficient detail such as to allow an unprecedented optimism regarding our understanding of cancer and thus our ability to diagnose it, provide more accurate prognoses, and, ultimately, to more effectively treat it.

Since genetic mutations are the central etiologic factor in tumorigenesis, a chapter on molecular carcinogenesis must include the basic principles of cancer molecular genetics, including evidence for the multistep, multigenic basis of tumorigenesis, and a summary of our current state of knowledge regarding the genes involved in this process. Molecular carcinogenesis is intimately linked to perturbations in cell cycle regulation, and an overview of the enormous progress recently made in this area is also presented. Related topics with direct clinical implications to be covered include angiogenesis and gene therapy. This chapter complements others in this volume focusing on environmental carcinogenesis and the P53 tumor suppressor gene.

## PRINCIPLES OF CANCER MOLECULAR GENETICS

All cancers are genetic in origin, in the sense that the driving force of tumor development is genetic mutation. A given tumor may arise through the accumulation of mutations that are exclusively somatic in origin, or through the inheritance of a mutation(s) through the germline, followed by the acquisition of additional somatic mutations. These two genetic scenarios distinguish what are colloquially referred to as sporadic and hereditary cancers, respectively (Fig. 1). While the neoplastic phenotype is partially derived from epigenetic alterations in gene expression, the sequential mutation of

J. Boyd: Departments of Surgery and Human Genetics, Memorial Sloan-Kettering Cancer Center, New York, New York 10021.

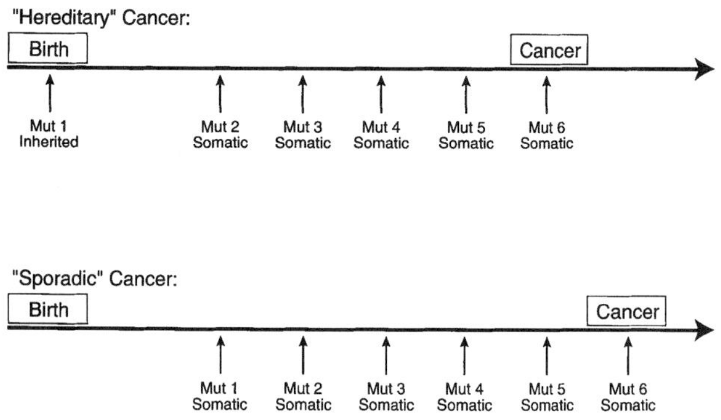


**FIG. 1.** All cancers are genetic. Hereditary cancers differ from sporadic cancers by virtue of association with a predisposing mutation inherited through the germline. In contrast, all of the mutations associated with sporadic tumorigenesis are acquired somatically.

cancer-related genes, with their subsequent selection and accumulation in a clonal population of cells, are the determinant factors in regard to whether a tumor develops and the time required for its development and progression. The data to support this multistep, multigenic paradigm are extensive (5–8), but perhaps the most compelling evidence is that the age-specific incidence rates for most human epithelial tumors increase at roughly the fourth to eighth power of elapsed time, suggesting that a series of four to eight genetic alterations are rate limiting for cancer development (9).

Genetic alterations in cancer cells have thus far been described in two major families of genes, oncogenes (10) and tumor suppressor genes (11). Proteins encoded by oncogenes may generally be viewed as stimulatory and those encoded by tumor suppressor genes as inhibitory to the neoplastic phenotype; mutational activation of proto-oncogenes to oncogenes and mutational inactivation of tumor suppressor genes must both occur for cancer development to take place. Proto-oncogene mutations are nearly always somatic; two known exceptions involve the *RET* and *MET* proto-oncogenes, mutations of which may be inherited through the germline, predisposing to multiple endocrine neoplasia type 2 (12), and papillary renal carcinoma (13), respectively. Tumor suppressor gene mutations may be inherited or acquired somatically. Other than the above-noted exceptions, all hereditary cancer syndromes for which predisposing genes have been identified are linked to tumor suppressor genes.

## Oncogenes

Oncogenes result from gain-of-function mutations in their normal cellular counterpart proto-oncogenes, the normal function of which is to drive cell proliferation in the appropriate contexts. Activated oncogenes behave in a dominant fashion at the cellular level, that is, cell proliferation or development of the neoplastic phenotype is stimulated following the mutation of only one allele. This class of genes was originally discovered through studies of the mechanism of retroviral tumorigenesis (14), which involves viral transduction of the vertebrate proto-oncogene and reintegration into the host genome under the transcriptional control of viral promoters, such that expression is constitutive and thus oncogenic. The most common mechanisms for mutational activation of human proto-oncogenes are gene amplification, typically resulting in overexpression of an otherwise normal protein product, point mutation, generally leading to constitutive activation of a mutant form of the protein product, and chromosomal translocation, which usually results in juxtaposition of the oncogene with the promoter region of a constitutively expressed gene, thus resulting in overexpression of the oncogene-encoded protein. This latter mechanism is most common in hematopoietic malignancies, while the first two are more common in solid cancers. The oncogenes most relevant to human solid malig-

**TABLE 1.** *Summary of representative oncogenes mutated in human solid cancers*

| Gene | Chromosomal location | Function | Mutation | Tumor[a] |
|---|---|---|---|---|
| *RAS (K-, H-, N-)* | 12p12, 11p15, 1p13 | Membrane-associated GTPase; signal transduction | Point mutation (codons 12, 13, or 61) | Many |
| *ERBB-2* | 17q12-q21 | Transmembrane tyrosine kinase receptor | Gene amplification | Breast, ovary, endometrium |
| *MYC (C-, N-, L-)* | 8q24, 2p24, 1p34 | Transcription factor | Gene amplification | C: many; N: neuroblastoma; L: lung |
| *MDM2* | 12q14-q15 | p53-binding protein | Gene amplification | Sarcomas |
| *RET* | 10q11 | Transmembrane tyrosine kinase receptor | Point mutation | Endocrine |
| *MET* | 7q31 | Transmembrane tyrosine kinase receptor | Point mutation | Renal |
| *CCND1 (cyclin D1)* | 11q13 | Cell cycle regulator | Gene amplification | Many |

[a]Carcinoma, unless otherwise specified.

nancies, their mechanism of activation, biochemical function, and the tumor types most often affected by each are summarized in Table 1.

## Tumor Suppressor Genes

The protein products of tumor suppressor genes normally function to inhibit cell proliferation and are inactivated through loss-of-function mutations. Knudson's (15) two-hit model established the paradigm for tumor suppressor gene recessivity at the cellular level, wherein both alleles must typically be inactivated in order for a phenotypic effect to be observed. The most common mutations observed in tumor suppressor genes are point mutations, either missense or nonsense, microdeletions or insertions of one or several nucleotides causing frame shifts, large deletions, and, rarely, translocations. A mutation in one allele, whether germline or somatic, is then revealed following somatic inactivation of the homologous wild-type allele. In theory, the same spectrum of mutational events could contribute to inactivation of the second allele, but what is typically observed in tumors is homozygosity or hemizygosity for the first mutation, indicating loss of the wild-type allele. As originally demonstrated for the retinoblastoma susceptibility gene (16), loss of the second allele may occur through mitotic nondisjunction or recombination mechanisms, or large deletions. This so-called loss of heterozygosity (LOH) has become recognized as the hallmark of tumor suppressor gene inactivation at particular genomic locus. Table 2 summarizes the known tumor suppressor genes, their chromosomal locations, suspected biochemical functions, and the hereditary and sporadic tumors with which they are most commonly associated.

## Genotype to Phenotype

A human cancer represents the end point of a long and complex process involving multiple changes in genotype and phenotype. Human solid tumors are monoclonal in nature; every cell in a given malignancy may be shown to have arisen from a single progenitor cell. As proposed by Nowell (17), the process through which a cell and its offspring sustain and accumulate multiple mutations, with the stepwise selection of variant sublines, is known as clonal evolution or clonal expansion (Fig. 2). A long-term goal in studying the molecular genetics of a particular tumor type is to catalogue the specific genes that are affected by mutations, the relative order in which they are affected (if any), and, ultimately, to use this molecular blueprint to improve methods of diagnosis, prognostication, and treatment. This task will undoubtedly prove difficult, however, as a defining characteristic of cancer is genetic instability (18). There are multiple types of such instability, operative at both the chromosomal and molecular levels. Distinguishing the genetic mutations that are simply the by-product of genetic instability from those are critical to the neoplastic phenotype or, indeed, responsible for increasing genetic instability of one form or another is among the greatest challenges to be faced in cancer research.

The greatest progress in this context has clearly been achieved for colorectal cancer, and a model has been proposed that applies molecular detail for this particular can-

**TABLE 2.** *Summary of representative tumor suppressor genes mutated in human solid cancers*

| Gene | Chromosomal location | Function | Tumors[a] | |
|---|---|---|---|---|
| | | | Hereditary | Sporadic |
| *RB1* | 13q14 | Cell cycle regulator | Retinoblastoma, osteosarcoma | Retinoblastoma, sarcomas, bladder, breast, lung |
| *WT1* | 11p13 | Transcription factor | Wilms' tumor | Wilms' tumor |
| *P53* | 17p13 | Transcription factor; regulator of cell cycle, apoptosis | Li-Fraumeni syndrome | Many |
| *APC* | 5q21-q22 | Signal transduction | Familial adenomatous polyposis | Colorectal, gastric |
| *VHL* | 3p26-p25 | Transcriptional elongation | von Hippel-Lindau syndrome | Renal |
| *hMSH2, hMLH1, hPMS2* | 2p16, 3p21, 7p22 | DNA mismatch repair | Hereditary nonpolyposis colorectal cancer syndrome | Colorectal, endometrial |
| *BRCA1* | 17q12-21 | Transcription factor; DNA repair | Breast, ovary, prostate | Ovary (rare) |
| *BRCA2* | 13q12 | DNA repair | Breast, ovary, others | Ovary (rare) |
| *NF1* | 17q11 | Negative regulator of Ras | Neurofibromatosis | None |
| *DPC4* | 18q21 | TGF-β signaling pathway | None | Pancreatic |
| *CDKN2A (p16)* | 9p21 | Negative regulator of cyclin D | Melanoma | Many |

[a]Carcinoma, unless otherwise specified.

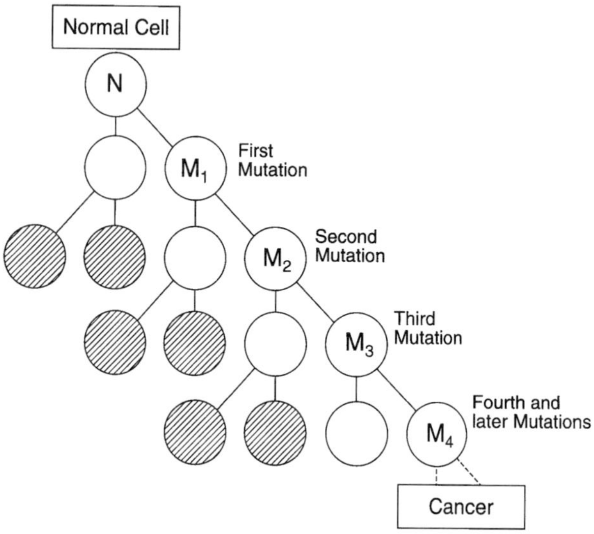


**FIG. 2.** Model of clonal evolution in neoplasia. Following the initiating mutation in a normal cell, stepwise genetic mutations and selective pressures result in a cancer consisting of a clonal population of cells all derived from the original progenitor cell. Each critical mutation in the evolving tumor may be viewed as having provided a selective advantage leading to clonal expansion.

cer type to the general paradigm of multistep tumorigenesis and clonal evolution. In addition to the recent demonstration that most colon cancer cell lines are affected by one of two types of genetic instability (19), specific molecular genetic alterations have been shown to occur at discrete stages of neoplastic progression in the colon, for example, mutation of the *APC* tumor suppressor gene at a very early stage of hyperproliferation, mutation of the *K-RAS* oncogene in the progression of early to intermediate adenoma, and mutation of the *P53* tumor suppressor gene in the progression of late adenoma to carcinoma (20). Several features of colorectal cancer facilitate this type of characterization, including the well-defined histopathologic progression of normal colonic epithelium to cancer and the accessibility of the various premalignant lesions for molecular analyses, as well as the occurrence of some of these genetic mutations in unusually large fractions of all colorectal tumors. The model is limited in applicability to other cancer types, however, as nonmalignant precursor lesions for many solid tumor types (e.g., ovarian cancer) are not readily detectable, and few molecular genetic changes have been described that occur in major fractions of other cancer types.

## THE CELL CYCLE

Although cancer cells possess many abnormal properties, deregulation of the normal constraints on cell proliferation lies at the heart of malignant transformation. A tumor may increase in size through any one of three mechanisms involving alterations pertaining to the cell cycle: shortening of the time of transit of cells through the cycle, a decrease in the rate of cell death, or the reentry of quiescent cells into the cycle. In most human cancers, all three mechanisms appear to be important in regulating tumor growth rate, a critical parameter in determining the biologic aggressiveness of a tumor (21). The classical cell cycle model, consisting of a DNA synthesis (S) phase, a mitosis (M) phase, and two gap ($G_1$ and $G_2$) phases, has now been elucidated in molecular detail (Fig. 3). Critical components of the cycle include the cyclins, cyclin-dependent kinases, inhibitors of cyclin-dependent kinases, and the Rb, p53, and E2F proteins. Many of the protein products of oncogenes and tumor suppressor genes are directly linked to biochemical pathways involving growth factor signaling and control of progression through the cell cycle.

The current model of cell cycle control holds that the transitions between different cell cycle states are regulated at checkpoints (22). A first crucial step in the cell cycle occurs late in the $G_1$ phase at the so-called restriction point, when a cell commits to completing the cycle (23). To pass through this point and enter S phase, growth-promoting signals transduced from the cell surface to the nucleus cause a rapid and transient elevation in the levels of D-type cyclins (in early $G_1$) and cyclin E (in late $G_1$). There are three forms of cyclin D, which are in part cell-type specific; most cells express D3 and either D1 or D2 (24). These cyclins combine with and activate enzymes known as cyclin-dependent kinases (CDKs), primarily CDK4 with the D-type cyclins and CDK2 with cyclin E. CDK4 transfers phosphate groups from adenosine triphosphate (ATP) to the Rb tumor suppressor protein. Rb is hypophosphorylated throughout the $G_1$ phase, phosphorylated just before S phase, and remains hyperphosphorylated until late M phase (25). The Rb protein binds to and sequesters transcription factors critical for the $G_1$ to S transition, notably E2F, and their release following Rb phosphorylation leads to the expression of

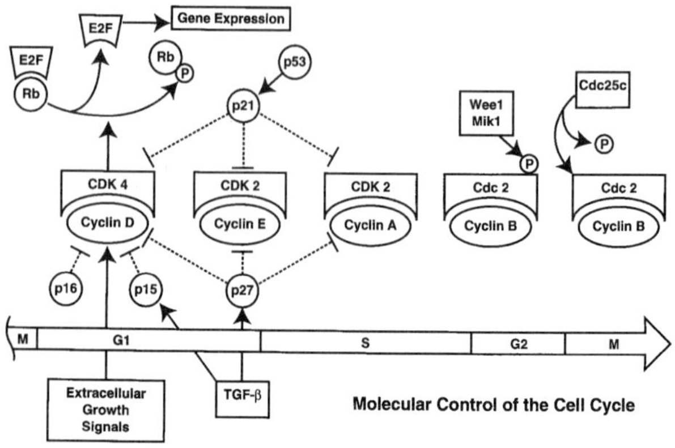


**FIG. 3.** Molecular control of cell cycle progression. A linear version of the various stages of the cell cycle is shown with the various cyclin/cyclin-dependent kinase complexes corresponding to the stages that they control.

genes responsible for further cell cycle progression (26). It is postulated that the cyclin D-CDK4 complex regulates progression through $G_1$, while the cyclin E-CDK2 complex regulates the $G_1$-S transition (27).

Various CDK inhibitor (CDKI) proteins also play a crucial role in the process of $G_1$ progression (27,28). Among these are proteins known as p15 (INK4B or MTS2), p16 (INK4 or MTS1), p21 (SDI1 or WAF1), and p27 (Kip1). The CDKIs act through the formation of stable complexes with cyclin-CDK dimers, disrupting the catalytic function of CDKs. All four of these CDKIs bind to the cyclin D-CDK4/6 dimers, while p21 and p27 also associate with the cyclin E-CDK2 dimer. Several factors are known to regulate expression of the CDKI proteins. Transforming growth factor-β (TGF-β) causes a rapid increase in levels of p15 and p27 messenger RNA (mRNA) and protein, indicating that these CDKIs are responsible for arresting cells in $G_1$ in response to this antimitogenic cytokine. The E2F transcription factor upregulates p16 expression, suggesting the presence of a feedback loop wherein repression of p16 expression by Rb hypophosphorylation leads to increased activity of CDK4 and phosphorylation of Rb. Transcriptional regulation of p21 is accomplished primarily by the p53 tumor suppressor protein, but may be affected by various activated growth factor receptors as well.

The cyclin E-CDK2 complex mediates progression out of $G_1$, and cyclin A expression increases dramatically with the onset of S phase. Cyclin A-CDK2 function then appears to be required for ongoing DNA replication, and again for the $G_2$/M transition. Available evidence suggests that the cyclin A-CDK2 complex participates in the assembly, activation, or regulation of DNA replication structures (29). An additional function of cyclin A may be in programmed cell death (28). The activity of cyclin A–dependent protein kinases is increased in cells undergoing apoptosis, and overexpression of cyclin A induces apoptosis in low serum.

Passage through $G_2$ and traversal of the $G_2$/M checkpoint are mediated by cyclins B1 and B2 in complexes with the Cdc2 kinase (30). Cyclin B-Cdc2 complexes accumulate in an inactive state during S and $G_2$ phases. The Cdc2 kinase component is kept inactive through phosphorylation by Wee1/Mik1-related protein kinases. At the end of $G_2$, a phosphatase known as Cdc25C dephosphorylates and activates Cdc2, allowing the transition into mitosis. In normal cells, DNA damaged by radiation or alkylating agents prevents dephosphorylation of Cdc2, resulting in a $G_2$ arrest. Several ubiquitin-dependent proteolysis events, including the destruction of B-type cyclins, allow the cell to progress completely through mitosis and complete the cell cycle.

Clearly, there are many points in this cell cycle where mutational activation or hyperactivity of cyclins and their associated kinases, or mutational inactivation or hypoactivity of CDKIs, would be expected to exert an oncogenic stimulus. Both cyclins and CDKIs are represented on the list of genes mutated in human cancers, and aberrant expression or activity of these proteins are common in tumors of many types. The gene encoding cyclin D1, *CCND1,* is located on chromosome 11q13 in a region that is amplified in several cancers. Amplification and overexpression are observed most commonly in carcinomas of the breast, lung, stomach, and esophagus, while overexpression alone is seen in a much larger number of cancers (27,31). This oncogene has also been designated *PRAD1* because of its overexpression resulting from a translocation in benign parathyroid adenomas, and as *BCL1* because of a different translocation leading to its overexpression in certain B-cell lymphomas.

The gene encoding p16, *CDKN2A,* is located on chromosome 9p21 in a region that is deleted in many solid tumor types. This tumor suppressor gene is most often disrupted by large homozygous deletions, but may also be inactivated through point mutations (27,32). Germline mutations of *CDKN2A* are also responsible for the majority of the familial melanoma kindreds that show genetic linkage to chromosome 9p21 (33,34). In humans, the genes encoding p16 and p15 lie in tandem on chromosome 9p, and homozygous deletions that include both genes have been observed in several tumor types (27).

Two prototypical human tumor suppressor genes, *RB1* and *P53,* encode proteins that play pivotal roles in $G_1$/S cell cycle progression. Both molecules participate in biochemical pathways that eventually converge on regulation of the E2F transcription factor. Inactivating mutations of *P53* are the most common molecular genetic alterations known in human cancers. Loss of p53 function leads to reduced levels of p21 and hyperactivity of both cyclin D-CDK and cyclin E-CDK complexes, hyperphosphorylation of Rb, and elevated levels of E2F. Mutational inactivation of the *RB1* gene itself, which is seen in several tumor types, would have the same end result; in addition to retinoblastomas and osteosarcomas that are seen in patients with inherited *RB1* mutations, sporadic retinoblastomas, and sarcomas, most if not all small cell lung carcinomas, and a portion of non–small cell lung, bladder, and breast carcinomas exhibit somatic *RB1* mutations (11). The molecular targets of E2F and its related transcription factors are becoming known in increasingly greater detail (35,36), providing a coherent view of the pathway through which Rb and p53 converge in negative control of the cell cycle progression. Binding sites for E2F are present in genes implicated in the induction of S phase, including those encoding thymidine kinase, the proto-oncogenes *MYC* and *MYB,* dihydrofolate reductase, and DNA polymerase-α (37).

## ANGIOGENESIS

The proliferation of new capillaries, termed angiogenesis or neovascularization, is now recognized as a critical pathogenic step in the process of cancer growth, tissue invasion, and metastasis. Although the mechanism through which tumors switch to the angiogenic phenotype remains unknown, it is clear that, like carcinogenesis itself, the process is complex, involves multiple steps and pathways, and depends on a local balance of positive and negative regulatory factors. Since 1971, when Judah Folkman (38) first proposed that solid tumors are unable to grow beyond a finite, limited size in the absence of neovascularization, research has evolved from validating this hypothesis and defining the molecular basis of angiogenesis to, most recently, a focus on the therapeutic potential of insights into mechanisms of angiogenesis. This section summarizes the basic principles of the angiogenesis process, the endogenous factors known to be most centrally involved, and the pharmacologic agents currently in use as potential antineoplastic agents.

Most cancers appear to arise in the absence of observable angiogenesis, expanding to a size of 2 to 3 $mm^3$ before requiring a switch to the angiogenic phenotype for further tumor expansion (39). Prior to this switch, tumors are not quiescent but exhibit an apoptosis rate that equals the rate of cell proliferation (40,41). The genetic mutations that lead to the angiogenesis phenotype are not known, but presumably occur as a late event in tumor evolution and progression. A limited body of data suggests that in some cases, mutational inactivation of the *P53* tumor suppressor gene may contribute to the acquisition of angiogenesis through the decreased production of potent inhibitors of angiogenesis that are positively regulated by p53, such as thrombospondin-1 (39) and glioma-derived angiogenesis inhibitory factor (42). Similarly, inherited and somatic mutations of the *VHL* tumor suppressor gene have been implicated in renal carcinogenesis, and several lines of experimentation suggest that one normal function of the *VHL* gene product may be to suppress the production of vascular endothelial growth factor (VEGF), an important angiogenic protein (43,44). These types of studies will eventually lead to an integration of the molecular pathways controlling the angiogenesis switch with the multistep genetic mutation pathways governing carcinogenesis.

For the present, however, the great majority of angiogenesis research data pertain to a description of those proteins that when aberrantly expressed are involved in the angiogenesis phenotype. This phenotype is not one event, but a cascade of events involving the degradation of endothelial basement membrane, migration of endothelial cells into the perivascular stroma, and initiation of a new capillary sprout; thus, many of the known angiogenic factors (Table 3) possess the ability to stimulate endothelial proteolysis, motility, and growth (45). The process begins with the release of positive angiogenic factors from the primary tumor, among the most well characterized of which are VEGF, the acidic and basic fibroblast growth factors, and angiogenin (46). These factors may also be released from the extracellular matrix or produced by macrophages attracted to the tumor. Negative regulators of angiogenesis must also be decreased; in addition to those discussed earlier, angiostatin is a recently discovered endogenous protein that appears in the circulation in the presence of a growing primary tumor, and disappears when the tumor is removed (47). A large body of indirect data, based on the expression of these proteins and their receptors during tumorigenesis and their effects on endothelial cells, support this model (39). Direct evidence implicating neovascularization in tumor growth and metastasis is derived from studies using immunoneutralizing monoclonal antibodies and pharmacologic agents that specifically inhibit angiogenic factors (48).

**TABLE 3.** *Endogenous angiogenesis factors*

| |
|---|
| Vascular endothelial growth factor (VEGF) |
| Basic fibroblast growth factor (bFGF) |
| Acidic fibroblast growth factor (aFGF) |
| Angiogenin |
| Transforming growth factor-α (TGF-α) |
| Transforming growth factor-β (TGF-β) |
| Tumor necrosis factor-α (TNF-α) |
| Platelet-derived endothelial cell growth factor (PD-ECGF) |
| Granulocyte colony-stimulating factor (G-CSF) |
| Placental growth factor (PGF) |
| Interleukin-8 (IL-8) |
| Hepatocyte growth factor (HGF) |
| Pleiotrophin (PTN) |
| Proliferin |

The process of metastasis is also intimately related with and dependent on angiogenesis. The local migration of tumor cells into the circulation occurs only after neovascularization of the tumor, and new, proliferating capillaries are relatively more porous and contain fragmented basement membranes, thereby facilitating the entry of tumor cells into the circulation (49,50). Migration of tumor and endothelial cells through tissue extracellular matrix is required for both processes, and a class of matrix-degrading metalloenzymes and their endogenous inhibitors, known as matrix metalloproteases (MMPs) and tissue inhibitors of metalloproteases (TIMPs), respectively, are essential in this respect (51,52). These enzymes are secreted by the same cells that produce angiogenic factors and are responsible for degradation of tissue matrix components (e.g., type IV collagen). Most are secreted in an inactive proenzyme form and require activation through a proteolytic cleavage cascade, mediated by molecules such as the urokinase plasminogen activator and receptor (uPA/uPAR) (52–54). Finally, the physical interaction of MMPs, uPAR, and endothelial cell surface integrins has been documented to play a role in cell adhesion, migration, and controlled matrix degradation during endothelial and tumor cell invasion (48).

To translate knowledge of the molecular biology of angiogenesis into clinically useful end points, many attempts have been made to evaluate the presence of angiogenic factors in bodily fluids as they may correlate with clinicopathologic parameters. Specifically, increased serum or urine levels of bFGF and VEGF correlate with the presence or extent of disease in patients with several types of malignancies (55–59). The quantitative assessment of angiogenesis in primary tumor biopsies has also been linked to the risk of developing metastatic disease and to duration of disease-free and overall survival (48,60). Studied most thoroughly in breast cancer, the degree of primary tumor neovascularization as measured by the angiogenic index (number of vessels per microscopic field) was first shown to correlate well with the development of metastatic disease (61). This index was subsequently reported to be responsible for the association between tumor size and grade, the presence of lymph node metastases, and early death in patients with breast cancer (62), and survival in patients presenting with lymph node–negative breast cancers (63,64). Methods to quantitate angiogenesis based on the measurement of blood flow *in vivo* have also been developed, and include color Doppler ultrasound in ovarian and cervical cancers (65,66), and positron emission tomography (PET) scanning in glioma (67).

A number of human clinical trials are currently under way designed to test the clinical utility of inhibitors of angiogenesis in the treatment of malignancy (48,60). Many of these trials utilize Kaposi sarcomas in AIDS patients because the lesions are visible and accessible for biopsy and direct drug injection. The wide range of pharmacologic agents that have shown antiangiogenic activity in laboratory experiments consist of protease inhibitors, cytokines and their modulators, heparin-like molecules, and inhibitors of vascular growth factors (Table 4). Representative compounds from these categories that have entered clinical trials include the matrix metalloprotease inhibitor batimastat (BB-94), the cytokine interleukin-12 (IL-12), the sulfated polysaccharide pentosan polysulfate, and platelet factor-4, which inhibits the interaction of basic fibroblast growth factor with its receptor. One particularly well-studied compound that does not fall into any of these categories is TNP-470, a less toxic synthetic analog of the fungal antibiotic fumagillin (68) that appears to act by specific inhibition of endothelial cell growth through modulation of the G1 cell cycle checkpoint (69). The available data suggest that these compounds may have limited utility in a clinical setting when used alone; greater therapeutic effect may be observed when antiangiogenics are employed in an adjuvant context. Used in combination or between courses of chemotherapy, angiogenesis inhibitors have shown significant promise in the laboratory (70,71).

**TABLE 4.** *Inhibitors of angiogenesis*

| |
|---|
| TNP-470 (AGM-1470) |
| Batimastat (BB-94) |
| Marimastat (BB-2516) |
| Interleukin-12 (IL-12) |
| Pentosan polysulfate |
| Platelet factor 4 (PF4) |
| Thalidomide |
| Tecogalan (SP-PG, DS-4152) |
| Angiostatin |
| CM101 |
| CT2584 |
| Vitaxin |
| Metastat (Col 3) |
| AG3340 |
| GM6001 |

## GENE THERAPY

A logical extension of the significant advances recently achieved in the molecular biology of cancer would seem to lie in the application of this knowledge to the gene-based therapy of cancer. Of the four categories of approaches to cancer gene therapy that have developed, however, only one is based on the principle of correcting a defective gene product in cancer cells. The other three approaches involve (a) the transfer of genes encoding enzymes that convert inactive prodrugs into cytotoxic metabolites; (b) the transfer of genes encoding cytokines and related molecules that enhance immunogenicity against tumors; and (c) the transfer of drug resistance genes into hematopoietic stem cells to increase their resistance to myelosuppressive chemotherapeutic agents (Table 5). This section provides illustrative examples of clinical trials that are under way in each of these three

**TABLE 5.** *Molecular tools for gene therapy*

| |
|---|
| Tumor suppressor genes |
| p53 |
| RB |
| BCL-$x_S$ |
| Suicide genes |
| Thymidine kinase |
| Cytochrome P-450 |
| Deoxycytidine kinase (dCK) |
| Immune modulators |
| Interleukin-2 (IL-2) |
| Macrophage colony-stimulating factor (M-CSF) |
| Granulocyte-macrophage colony-stimulating factor (GM-CSF) |
| Tumor necrosis factor-$\alpha$ (TNF-$\alpha$) |
| Interferon-$\gamma$ (IFN-$\gamma$) |
| B7-1 |
| Drug resistance genes |
| Multidrug resistance gene (MDR)-1 |
| Dihydrofolate reductase (DHFR) |
| $O^6$-methylguanine-DNA-methyltransferase (MGMT) |
| Glutathione-S-transferase (GST) |

categories plus the category based on the principle of correcting a defective gene product, as well as an overview of the technology currently available for accomplishing cancer gene therapy. It should be emphasized that gene therapy is not currently viewed as an approach to the curative therapy of cancers, but rather as an alternative or adjuvant therapy for advanced, recurrent, or otherwise resistant malignancies with the aim of prolonging survival beyond that available with traditional therapeutic modalities.

Gene delivery systems for the transfer of double-stranded DNA to the nucleus of a mammalian target cell are based on the use of plasmids or several types of recombinant viruses, primarily retroviruses and adenoviruses (72). Each of these systems has strengths and weaknesses regarding the accuracy of gene delivery to target cells, the efficiency of gene transfer and expression, and the stability of the foreign molecule in the host cell over time. Plasmid DNA is relatively easy to manipulate and can accept large gene fragments, can be produced stably and cheaply to a high level of purity, and poses none of the risks associated with viral incorporation or replication. Multiple administrations to immunocompetent subjects can be performed as plasmid DNA is poorly immunogenic. The greatest drawback to plasmid-based gene therapy is the low efficiency of gene transfer, but high levels of gene expression can be achieved in a small number of target cells (73,74), and efficiency may be increased greatly through the use of cationic liposomes (75).

The majority of human gene therapy protocols utilize viral vectors, recombinant retrovirues being the first developed for this purpose (76). Integration of proviral DNA into the host genome occurs if cell division proceeds shortly after infection, which is generally an advantage in terms of efficiency of transfer, long-term expression, and selective infection of proliferating tumor cells (77). Slow-growing human tumors would not be as effectively treated, however. The remote possibility of insertional mutagenesis poses a modest safety concern. Other disadvantages of the retroviral vector are the relatively low titers achievable, making this system most appropriate for small, rapidly dividing tumors in confined spaces, such as glioma (78,79). In contrast, adenoviruses may be produced in extremely high titers and can transfer genes to a wide range of nondividing cells with high efficiency (80). They infect host cells as episomes rather that by genomic integration, and are relatively benign human pathogens. Disadvantages of the adenoviral vectors are the absence of stable integration and transfer to daughter cells, and immunogenicity of the viral material. Rapid developments in vector technology have produced less immunogenic vectors (81), and will be expected to improve upon all of the currently available resources for cancer gene therapy.

Cancer gene therapy aimed at correcting genetic defects in tumor cells has focused mainly on the restoration of tumor suppressor gene function (82,83). Although it is frequently assumed that multiple genetic defects would necessarily have to be corrected in a given cancer cell to reverse malignancy, this is an inaccurate interpretation of the multistage genetic paradigm, which predicts that correction of a single critical genetic alteration would in fact be sufficient to render the a tumor cell nonmalignant. This concept is supported experimentally in studies showing that human cancer cell lines may be rendered nontumorigenic by the transfer of a single human chromosome (84,85). Many human cancer cell types have been shown susceptible to the viral-mediated transfer of p53, which generally suppresses growth and/or induces apoptosis (82,83), but has also been found to increase chemosensitivity in transduced cells (86). Predictably, the downstream target of p53, p21, exerts similar effects in experimental gene therapy protocols (87,88). Other genes that have proven efficacious in laboratory studies include the RB tumor suppressor (89) and BCL-$x_S$, a dominant-negative inhibitor of the BCL2 oncogene product (90). Human clinical trials have been reported in which the retroviral-mediated transfer of p53 to lung cancers results in a clinical response (91), and in which the adenoviral-mediated transfer of p53 to lung cancers enhances the response to cisplatin (92).

Perhaps the most common cancer gene therapy protocol tested to date utilizes a form of suicide gene transfer, in which the thymidine kinase gene from herpes simplex virus (HSV-tk) is transferred to recipient tumor cells followed by treatment with the prodrug ganciclovir (93). HSV-tk phosphorylates the otherwise nontoxic ganciclovir more efficiently than mammalian thymidine kinase; the ganciclovir monophosphate is then metabolized by the mammalian enzyme to ganciclovir triphosphate which is incorporated into DNA as a purine analog causing cell death. This method benefits from a "bystander effect," in which neighboring noninfected cells are also killed, through gap junctional transfer of the activated drug *in vitro* (94), or through recruitment of host immune cells and cytokine release *in vivo* (95). In laboratory studies, this protocol is effective in eradicating many types of solid malignancies in animal models, including mesothelioma (96), glioma (97), hepatocellular carcinoma (98), and ovarian carcinoma (99). Clinical trials to test the feasibility of this system in glioma (100) and ovarian cancer (101) have been reported.

The potential for gene therapy to generate systemic tumor immunity has also been explored. This type of response is generally achieved by immunization with transduced irradiated autologous tumor cells or by gene delivery in situ into an established tumor mass, using genes encoding many of the interleukins, especially IL-2, macrophage and granulocyte-macrophage colony-stimulating factors, tumor necrosis factor-$\alpha$, interferon-$\gamma$, and the B7 costimulatory molecule. Interleukin-2 is naturally produced by T cells, and stimulates the activation of T cells, B cells, NK cells, and monocytes. Rejection of tumor challenge may be shown following the injection of irradiated IL-2–transduced tumor cells of many types, including melanoma (102), colorectal carcinoma (103), prostate carcinoma (104), and breast and ovarian carcinoma (105). Transduction of genes encoding granulocyte-macrophage colony-stimulating factor (106), tumor necrosis factor-α (107), and interferon-γ (108) causes tumoricidal activity in several experimental cancer systems. The B7 costimulatory molecule, normally expressed on macrophages and B cells, activates T cells through its interaction with CD28. Vaccination with B7-infected tumor cells, alone or in combination with other immune modulators, generates an antitumor response against tumor challenge and eliminates established tumors of several types (109–111). Recent efforts to apply these approaches in human clinical trials suggest significant potential in cancer treatment (112).

Finally, the transduction of drug resistance genes into hematopoietic cells has been tested as mechanism for allowing higher doses of traditional chemotherapeutic drugs that would otherwise cause severe myelosuppression. The multidrug resistance gene (MDR)-1 gene product is a transmembrane p-glycoprotein that can eliminate a wide range of toxic substances from the cell, including many commonly used cancer cytotoxic agents. Proof of the principle has been demonstrated in several experimental systems, and human clinical trials are now under way (113,114). Other genes tested in this context include those encoding dihydrofolate reductase (DHFR), $O^6$-methylguanine-DNA-methyltransferase (MGMT), and glutathione-S-transferase (GST) (112–114). Attempts to improve the efficacy of current protocols are aimed at the use of two or more drug-resistance genes in combination, and the design of mutant forms of these proteins that offer improved resistance to cytotoxic compounds.

## REFERENCES


1. Watson JD. In: Angier N, ed. *Natural obsessions:* the search for the oncogene. Boston: Houghton Mifflin, 1988;12.
2. Bishop JM. Cancer: the rise of the genetic paradigm. *Genes Dev* 1995;9:1309–1315.
3. Boveri T. *Zur Frage der Erstehung Maligner Tumoren.* Jena: Fischer, 1914.
4. Spector D, Varmus HE, Bishop JM. Nucleotide sequences related to the transforming gene of avian sarcoma virus are present in DNA of uninfected vertebrates. *Proc Natl Acad Sci USA* 1978;75:4102–4106.
5. Weinberg RA. Oncogenes, antioncogenes, and the molecular basis of multistep carcinogenesis. *Cancer Res* 1989;49:3713–3721.
6. Boyd J, Barrett JC. Genetic and cellular basis of multistep carcinogenesis. *Pharmacol Ther* 1990;46:469–486.
7. Bishop JM. Molecular themes in oncogenesis. *Cell* 1991;64:235–248.
8. Vogelstein B, Kinzler KW. The multistep nature of cancer. *Trends Genet* 1993;9:138–141.
9. Renan MJ. How many mutations are required for tumorigenesis? Implications from human cancer data. *Mol Carcinog* 1993;7:139–146.
10. Hunter T. Cooperation between oncogenes. *Cell* 1991;64:249–270.
11. Weinberg RA. Tumor suppressor genes. *Science* 1991;254: 1138–1146.
12. Hofstra RMW, Landsvater RM, Ceccherini I, et al. A mutation in the RET proto-oncogene associated with multiple endocrine neoplasia type 2B and sporadic medullary thyroid carcinoma. *Nature* 1994;367: 375–378.
13. Schmidt L, Duh F.-M, Chen F, et al. Germline and somatic mutations in the tyrosine kinase domain of the MET proto-oncogene in papillary renal carcinomas. *Nature Genet* 1997;16:68–73.
14. Bishop JM. Cellular oncogenes and retroviruses. *Annu Rev Biochem* 1983;52:301–354..
15. Knudson AG. Hereditary cancer, oncogenes, and antioncogenes. *Cancer Res* 1985;45:1437–1443.
16. Cavenee WK, Dryja TP, Phillips RA, et al. Expression of recessive alleles by chromosomal mechanisms in retinoblastoma. *Nature* 1983;305:779–784.
17. Nowell P. The clonal evolution of tumor cell populations. *Science* 1976;194:23–28.
18. Loeb LA. Mutator phenotype may be required for multistage carcinogenesis. *Cancer Res* 1991;51:3075–3079.
19. Lengauer C, Kinzler KW, Vogelstein B. Genetic instability in colorectal cancers. *Nature* 1997;386:623–627.
20. Fearon ER, Vogelstein B. A genetic model for colorectal tumorigenesis. *Cell* 1990;61:759–767.
21. Baserga R. *The biology of cell reproduction.* Cambridge: Harvard University Press, 1985.
22. Nurse P. Ordering S phase and M phase in the cell cycle. *Cell* 1994;79:547–550.
23. Sherr CJ. G1 phase progression: cycling on cue. *Cell* 1994;79: 551–555.
24. Sherr CJ. Mammalian G1 cyclins. *Cell* 1993;73:1059–1065.
25. Hinds PW, Weinberg RA. Tumor suppressor genes. *Curr Opin Genet Dev* 1994;4:135–141.
26. Nevins JR. E2F: A link between the Rb tumor suppressor protein and viral oncoproteins. *Science* 1992;258:424–429.
27. Cordon-Cardo C. Mutation of cell cycle regulators: biological and clinical implications for human neoplasia. *Am J Pathol* 1995;147: 545–560.
28. Hunter T, Pines J. Cyclins and cancer II: cyclin D and CDK inhibitors come of age. *Cell* 1994;79:573–582.
29. Heichman KA, Roberts JM. Rules to replicate by. *Cell* 1994;79: 557–562.
30. Dunphy WG. The decision to enter mitosis. *Trends Cell Biol* 1994;4:202–207.
31. Arnold A. The cyclin D1/PRAD1 oncogene in human neoplasia. *J Invest Med* 1995;43:543–549.
32. Pollock PM, Pearson JV, Hayward NK. Compilation of somatic mutations of the CDKN2 gene in human cancers: non-random distribution of base substitutions. *Genes Chromosomes Cancer* 1996;15:77–88.
33. Hussussian CJ, Struewing JP, Goldstein AM, et al. Germline p16 mutations in familial melanoma. *Nature Genet* 1994;8:15–21.
34. Kamb A, Shattuck-Eidens D, Eeles R, et al. Analysis of the p16 gene (CDKN2) as a candidate for the chromosome 9p melanoma susceptibility locus. *Nature Genet* 1994;8:22–26.
35. La Thangue NB. E2F and the molecular mechanisms of early cell-cycle control. *Biochem Soc Trans* 1996;24:54–59.
36. Sanchez I, Dynlacht BD. Transcriptional control of the cell cycle. *Curr Opin Cell Biol* 1996;8:318–324.
37. Johnson DJ, Schwarz JK, Cress WD, Nevins JR. Expression of transcription factor E2F1 induces quiescent cells to enter S phase. *Nature* 1993;365:349–352.
38. Folkman J. Tumor angiogenesis: therapeutic implications. *N Engl J Med* 1971;285:1182–1186.
39. Folkman J. What is the evidence that tumors are angiogenesis dependent? *J Natl Cancer Inst* 1990;82:4–6.
40. Holmgren L, O'Reilly MS, Folkman J. Dormancy of micrometastases: Balanced proliferation and apoptosis in the presence of angiogenesis suppression. *Nature Med* 1995;1:149–153.
41. O'Reilly MS, Holmgren L, Chen C, Folkman J. Angiostatin induces and sustains dormancy of human primary tumors in mice. *Nature Med* 1996;2:689–692.
42. Van Meir EG, Polverini PJ, Chazin VR, Su Huang H-J, de Tribolet N, Cavenee WK. Release of an inhibitor of angiogenesis upon induction of wild type p53 expression in glioblastoma cells. *Nature Genet* 1994;8:171–176.
43. Wizigmann-Voos S, Breier G, Risau W, Plate KH. Up-regulation of vascular endothelial growth factor and its receptors in von Hippel-Lindau disease-associated and sporadic hemangioblastomas. *Cancer Res* 1995;55:1358–1364.

44. Siemeister G, Weindel K, Mohrs K, Barleon B, Martiny-Baron G, Marme D. Reversion of deregulated expression of vascular endothelial growth factor in human renal carcinoma cells by von Hippel-Lindau tumor suppressor protein. *Cancer Res* 1996;56:2299–2301.
45. Folkman J, Klagsburn M. Angiogenic factors. *Science* 1987;235: 442–447.
46. Folkman J. Angiogenesis in cancer, vascular, rheumatoid and other disease. *Nature Med* 1995;1:27–31.
47. O'Reilly MS, Holmgren L, Shing Y, et al. Angiostatin: a novel angiogenesis inhibitor that mediates the suppression of metastases by a Lewis lung carcinoma. *Cell* 1994;79:315–328.
48. Pluda JM. Tumor-associated angiogenesis: mechanisms, clinical implications, and therapeutic strategies. *Semin Oncol* 1997;24: 203–218.
49. Liotta LA, Kleinerman J, Saidel GM. Quantitative relationships of intravascular tumor cells, tumor vessels, and pulmonary metastases following tumor implantation. *Cancer Res* 1974;34:997–100.
50. Dvorak HF, Nagy JA, Dvorak JT, Dvorak AM. Identification and characterization of the blood vessels of solid tumors that are leaky to circulating macromolecules. *Am J Pathol* 1988;133:95–109.
51. Liotta LA, Steeg PS, Stetler-Stevenson WG. Cancer metastasis and angiogenesis: an imbalance of positive and negative regulation. *Cell* 1991;64:327–336.
52. Ray JM, Stetler-Stevenson WG. The role of matrix metalloproteases and their inhibitors in tumour invasion, metastasis, and angiogenesis. *Eur Respir J* 1994;7:2062–2072.
53. Moscatelli D, Rifkin DB. Membrane and matrix localization of proteinases: a common theme in tumor cell invasion and angiogenesis. *Biochem Biophys Acta* 1988;948:67–85.
54. Saksela O, Rifkin DB. Cell-associated plasminogen activation: regulation and physiological functions. *Annu Rev Cell Biol* 1988;4: 93–126.
55. Fujimoto K, Ichimori Y, Kakizoe T, et al. Increased serum levels of basic fibroblast growth factor in patients with renal cell carcinoma. *Biochem Biophys Res Commun* 1991;180:386–392.
56. Nguyen M, Watanabe H, Budson AE, Richie JP, Hayes DF, Folkman J. Elevated levels of the angiogenic peptide, basic fibroblast growth factor, in the urine of patients with a wide spectrum of cancers. *J Natl Cancer Inst* 1994;86:356–361.
57. Meyer GE, Yu E, Siegal JA, Petteway JC, Blumenstein BA, Brawer MK. Serum basic fibroblast growth factor in men with and without prostate cancer. *Cancer* 1995;76:2304–2311.
58. Kondo S, Asano M, Matsuo K, Ohmori I, Suzuki H. Vascular endothelial growth factor/vascular permeability factor is detectable in the sera of tumor-bearing mice and cancer patients. *Biochem Biophys Acta* 1994;1221:211–214.
59. Yamamoto Y, Toi M, Kondo S. Concentrations of vascular endothelial growth factor in the sera of normal controls and cancer patients. *Clin Cancer Res* 1996;2:821–826.
60. Bicknell R, Harris, AL. Mechanisms and therapeutic implications of angiogenesis. *Curr Opin Oncol* 1996;8:60–65.
61. Weidner N, Semple JP, Welch WR, Folkman J. Tumor angiogenesis and metastasis—correlation in invasive breast carcinoma. *N Engl J Med* 1991;324:1–8.
62. Horak ER, Leek R, Klenk N, et al. Angiogenesis, assessed by platelet-endothelial cell adhesion antibodies, as indicator of node metastases and survival in breast cancer. Lancet 1992;340:1120–1124.
63. Weidner N, Folkman J, Pozza F, et al. Tumor angiogenesis: a new significant and independent prognostic indicator in early-stage breast carcinoma. *J Natl Cancer Inst* 1992;84:1875–1887.
64. Bosari S, Lee AKC, DeLellis RA, Wiley BD, Heatley GJ, Silverman KL. Microvessel quantitation and prognosis in invasive breast cancer. *Hum Pathol* 1992;23:755–761.
65. Wu CC, Lee CN, Chen TM, et al. Incremental angiogenesis assessed by color Doppler ultrasound in the tumorigenesis of ovarian neoplasms. *Cancer* 1994;73:1251–1256.
66. Hsieh CY, Wu CC, Chen TM, et al. Clinical significance of intratumoral blood flow in cervical carcinoma assessed by color Doppler ultrasound. *Cancer* 1995;75:2518–2522.
67. Sasajima T, Mineura K, Sasaki J, et al. Positron emission tomographic assessment of cerebral hemocirculation and glucose metabolism in malignant glioma following treatment with intracarotid recombinant human tumor necrosis factor-alpha. *J Neurol Oncol* 1995;23:67–73.
68. Ingber D, Fujita T, Kishimoto S, et al. Synthetic analogues of fumagillin that inhibit angiogenesis and suppress tumour growth. *Nature* 1990;348:555–557.
69. Antoine N, Greimers R, De-Roanne C, et al. AGM-1470, a potent angiogenesis inhibitor, prevents the entry of normal but not transformed endothelial cells into the G1 phase of the cell cycle. *Cancer Res* 1994;54:2073–2076.
70. Kato T, Sato K, Kakinuma H, Matsuda Y. Enhanced suppression of tumor growth by combination of angiogenesis inhibitor O-(chloroacetyl-carbamoyl) fumagillol (TNP-470) and cytotoxic agents in mice. *Cancer Res* 1994;54:5143–5147.
71. Teicher BA, Holden SA, Ara G, et al. Potentiation of cytotoxic cancer therapies by TNP-470 alone and with other antiangiogenic agents. *Int J Cancer* 1994;57:920–925.
72. Vile R, Russell, SJ. Gene transfer technologies for the gene therapy of cancer. *Gene Ther* 1994;1:88–98.
73. Plautz GE, Yang ZY, Wu B.-Y, Gao X, Huang L, Nabel GJ. Immunotherapy of malignancy by *in vivo* gene therapy into tumors. *Proc Natl Acad Sci USA* 1993;90:4645–4649.
74. Vile RG, Hart IR. *in vitro* and *in vivo* targeting of gene expression to melanoma cells. *Cancer Res* 1993;53:962–967.
75. Zhu N, Liggitt D, Liu Y, Debs R. Systemic gene expression after intravenous DNA delivery into adult mice. *Science* 1993;261:209–211.
76. Miller AD. Human gene therapy comes of age. *Nature* 1992;357: 455–460.
77. Miller AD. Retroviral vectors. *Curr Top Microbiol Immunol* 1992; 158:1–242.
78. Culver KW, Ram Z, Wallbridge S, Ishii H, Oldfield EH, Blaese RM. *in vivo* transfer with retroviral vector-producer cells for treatment of experimental brain tumors. *Science* 1992;256:1550–1552.
79. Ram Z, Culver KW, Walbridge S, Blaese RM, Oldfield EH. In situ retroviral mediated gene transfer for the treatment of brain tumors in rats. *Cancer Res* 1993;53:83–88.
80. Kozarsky KF, Wilson JM. Gene therapy: adenovirus vectors. *Curr Opin Genet Dev* 1993;3:499–503.
81. Yang Y, Nunes FA, Berencsi K, Gonczol E, Englehardt JF, Wilson JM. Inactivation of E2a in recombinant adenoviruses improves the prospect for gene therapy in cystic fibrosis. *Nature Genet* 1994;7: 362–369.
82. Davis BM, Koc ON, Lee K, Gerson SL. Current progress in the gene therapy of cancer. *Curr Opin Oncol* 1996;8:499–508.
83. Roth JA, Cristiano RJ. Gene therapy for cancer: what have we done and where are we going? *J Natl Cancer Inst* 1997;89:21–39.
84. Stanbridge EJ. Human tumor suppressor genes. *Annu Rev Genet* 1990;24:615–657.
85. Goyette MC, Cho K, Fasching CL, et al. Progression of colorectal cancer is associated with multiple tumor suppressor gene defects but inhibition of tumorigenicity is accomplished by correction of any single defect via chromosome transfer. *Mol Cell Biol* 1992;12:1387–1395.
86. Fujiwara T, Grimm EA, Mukhopadhyay T, Zhang W.-W, Owen-Schaub LB, Roth JA. Induction of chemosensitivity in human lung cancer cells *in vivo* by adenovirus-mediated transfer of the wild-type p53 gene. *Cancer Res* 1994;54:2287–2291.
87. Eastham JA, Hall SJ, Sehgal I, et al. *in vivo* gene therapy with p53 or p21 adenovirus for prostate cancer. *Cancer Res* 1995;55:5151–5155.
88. Yang, Z.-Y, Perkins ND, Ohno T, Nabel EG, Nabel GJ. The p21 cyclin-dependent kinase inhibitor suppresses tumorigenicity *in vivo*. *Nature Med* 1995;1:1052–1056.
89. Xu H.-J, Zhou Y, Seigne J, et al. Enhanced tumor suppressor gene therapy via replication-deficient adenovirus vectors expressing an N-terminal truncated protein. *Cancer Res* 1996;56:2245–2249.
90. Ealovega MW, McGinnis PK, Sumantran VN, Clarke MF, Wicha MS. bcl-$x_s$ gene therapy induces apoptosis of human mammary tumors in nude mice. *Cancer Res* 1996;56:1965–1969.
91. Roth JA, Nguyen D, Lawrence DD, et al. Retrovirus-mediated wild-type p53 gene transfer to tumors of patients with lung cancer. *Nature Med* 1996;2:985–991.
92. Nguyen DM, Spitz FR, Yen N, Cristiano RJ, Roth JA. Gene therapy for lung cancer:enhancement of tumor suppression by a combination of sequential systemic cisplatin and adenovirus-mediated p53 gene transfer. *J Thorac Cardiovasc Surg* 1996;112:1372–1376.
93. Moolten FL. Tumor chemosensitivity conferred by inserted herpes thymidine kinase genes: paradigm for a prospective cancer control strategy. *Cancer Res* 1986;46:5276–5281.
94. Bi WL, Parysek LM, Warnick R, Stambrook PJ. *in vitro* evidence

that metabolic cooperation is responsible for the bystander effect observed with HSV tk retroviral gene therapy. *Hum Gene Ther* 1993; 4:725–731.
95. Ramesh R, Marrogi AJ, Munshi A, Abboud CN, Freeman SM. *in vivo* analysis of the "bystander effect": a cytokine cascade. *Exp Hematol* 1996;24:829–838.
96. Smythe WR, Hwang HC, Elshami AA, et al. Treatment of experimental human mesothelioma using adenovirus transfer of the herpes simplex thymidine kinase genes. Ann Surg 1995;222:78–86.
97. Perez-Cruet MJ, Trask TW, Chen SH, Goodman JC, Woo SL, Grossman RG. Adenovirus-mediated gene therapy of experimental gliomas. *J Neurosci Res* 1994;39:506–511.
98. Qian C, Bilbao R, Bruna O, and Prieto J. Induction to sensitivity to ganciclovir in human hepatocellular carcinoma cells by adenovirus-mediated gene transfer of herpes simplex virus thymidine kinase gene. *Hepatology* 1995;22:118–123.
99. Behbakht K, Benjamin I, Chiu H.-C, et al. Adenovirus-mediated gene therapy of ovarian cancer in a mouse model. *Am J Obstet Gynecol* 1996;175:1260–1265.
100. Eck SL, Alavi JB, Alavi A, et al. Treatment of advanced CNS malignancies with the recombinant adenovirus H5.010RSVTK: a phase I trial. *Hum Gene Ther* 1996;7:1465–1482.
101. Link CJ, Moorman D, Seregina T, Levy JP, Schabold KJ. A phase I trial of *in vivo* gene therapy with the herpes simplex thymidine kinase/ganciclovir system for the treatment of refractory or recurrent ovarian cancer. *Hum Gene Ther* 1996;7:1161–1179.
102. Maass G, Schmidt W, Schilcher F, et al. Priming of tumor specific T cells in the draining lymph nodes after immunization with interleukin 2 secreting tumor cells: three consecutive stages may be required for successful tumor vaccination. *Proc Natl Acad Sci USA* 1995;52: 5540–5544.
103. Fakhrai H, Shawler DL, Gjerset R, et al. Cytokine gene therapy with interleukin-2-transduced fibroblasts. *Hum Gene Ther* 1995;6: 591–601.
104. Vieweg J, Boczkowski D, Roberson KM, et al. Efficient gene transfer with adeno-associated virus based plasmids complexed to cationic liposomes for gene therapy of human prostate cancer. *Cancer Res* 1995;55:2366–2372.
105. Philip R, Clary B, Brunette E, et al. Gene modification of primary tumor cells for active immunotherapy of human breast and ovarian cancer. *Clin Cancer Res* 1996;2:59–68.
106. Armstrong CA, Botella R, Galloway TH, et al. Antitumor effects of granulocyte-macrophage colony stimulating factor production by melanoma cells. *Cancer Res* 1996;56:2191–2198.
107. Tos AG, Cignetti A, Rovera G, Foa R. Retroviral vector mediated transfer of the tumor necrosis factor alpha gene into human cancer cells restores an apoptotic cell death program and induces a bystander-killing effect. *Blood* 1996;87:2486–2495.
108. Abe J, Wakimoto H, Tsunoda R, et al. *in vivo* antitumor effect of cytotoxic T lymphocytes engineered to produce interferon-gamma by adenovirus mediated genetic transduction. *Biochem Biophys Res Commun* 1996;218:164–170.
109. Fujii H, Inobe M, Kimura F, et al. Vaccination of tumor cells transfected with the B7-1 (CD80) gene induces the anti-metastatic effect and tumor immunity in mice. *Int J Cancer* 1996;66:219–224.
110. Cayeux S, Beck C, Aicher A, Dorken B, Blankenstein T. Tumor cells co-transfected with interleukin 7 and B7-1 genes induce CD25 and CD28 on tumor infiltrating T lymphocytes and strong vaccines. *Eur J Immunol* 1995;25:2325–2331.
111. Baskar S, Glimcher L, Nabavi N, Jones RT, Ostrand-Rosenberg S. Major histocompatibility complex class II$^{+}$B7-1$^{+}$ tumor cells are potent vaccines for stimulating tumor rejection in tumor bearing mice. *J Exp Med* 1995;181:619–629.
112. Hanania EG, Kavanagh J, Hortobagyi G, Giles RE, Champlin R, Deisseroth AB. Recent advances in the application of gene therapy to human disease. *Am J Med* 1995;99:537–552.
113. Koc ON, Allay JA, Lee K, Davis BM, Reese JS, Gerson SL. Transfer of drug resistance genes into hematopoietic progenitors to improve chemotherapy tolerance. *Semin Oncol* 1996;23:46–65.
114. Rafferty JA, Hickson I, Chinnasamy N, et al. Chemoprotection of normal tissues by transfer of drug resistance genes. *Cancer Metastasis Rev* 1996;15:365–383.

*Environmental and Occupational Medicine, Third Edition,* edited by William N. Rom.
Published by Lippincott–Raven Publishers,
Philadelphia, 1998.

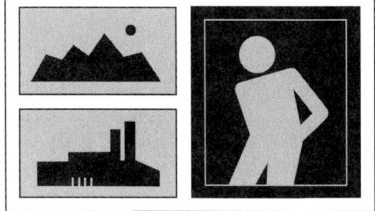

CHAPTER 13

# p53 Tumor Suppressor Gene: At the Crossroads of Molecular Carcinogenesis and Molecular Epidemiology of Human Cancer

S. Perwez Hussain and Curtis C. Harris

## MOLECULAR EPIDEMIOLOGY

Classical epidemiologic studies have identified populations and families at increased cancer risk. Molecular epidemiology has a more ambitious goal, i.e., the identification of individuals at high cancer risk in the general population. Achieving this goal is challenging both current molecular technologies and epidemiologic designs, and exposing bioethical dilemmas.

The two facets of molecular epidemiology of human cancer risk are assessment of carcinogen exposure and inherited or acquired host cancer susceptibility factors (reviewed in refs. 1 and 2). The interaction between these two facets determines an individual's cancer risk. This paradigm can also improve cancer risk assessment (Fig. 1). When combined with carcinogen bioassays in laboratory animals and classical epidemiology, molecular epidemiology can contribute to the four traditional aspects of cancer risk assessment: hazard identification, dose-response assessment, exposure assessment, and risk characterization. Improved cancer risk assessment has broad public health and economic implications (3).

Weighty bioethical consequences follow the identification of high-risk individuals (4). The bioethical issues include autonomy, privacy, justice, and equity (Fig. 1). One can argue that the knowledge of one's risk can be beneficial. However, more encompassing bioethical issues arise such as an individual's responsibility to family members and psychosocial concerns regarding the genetic testing of children (4). Therefore, the uncertainty of the current individual risk assessments and the limited availability of genetic counseling services dictate caution and, many argue, the restriction of genetic testing to those conditions amenable to preventative or therapeutic intervention.

Inherited gene mutations that increase the risk of cancer can be divided into two general categories (Table 1). Predetermining genes increase the risk of cancer with little modulation by environmental factors. Predisposing genes have marked interactive effects with environmental and lifestyle risk factors. For example, inheritance of a defective gene involved in nucleotide excision repair (xeroderma pigmentosum) increases the risk of skin cancer only in individuals exposed to ultraviolet light, so that protection from sunlight is an obvious preventive strategy. Whereas in individuals inheriting a defective predetermining gene, e.g., Li-Fraumeni syndrome with a germline mutation in the p53 tumor suppressor gene, modification of the environment may be a less effective strategy.

## p53 TUMOR SUPPRESSOR GENE

The 18-year history of p53 investigations is a paradigm in cancer research, illustrating the convergence of previously parallel lines of basic, clinical, and epidemiologic

S. P. Hussain and C. C. Harris: Laboratory of Human Carcinogenesis, National Cancer Institute, National Institutes of Health, Bethesda, Maryland 20892-4255.

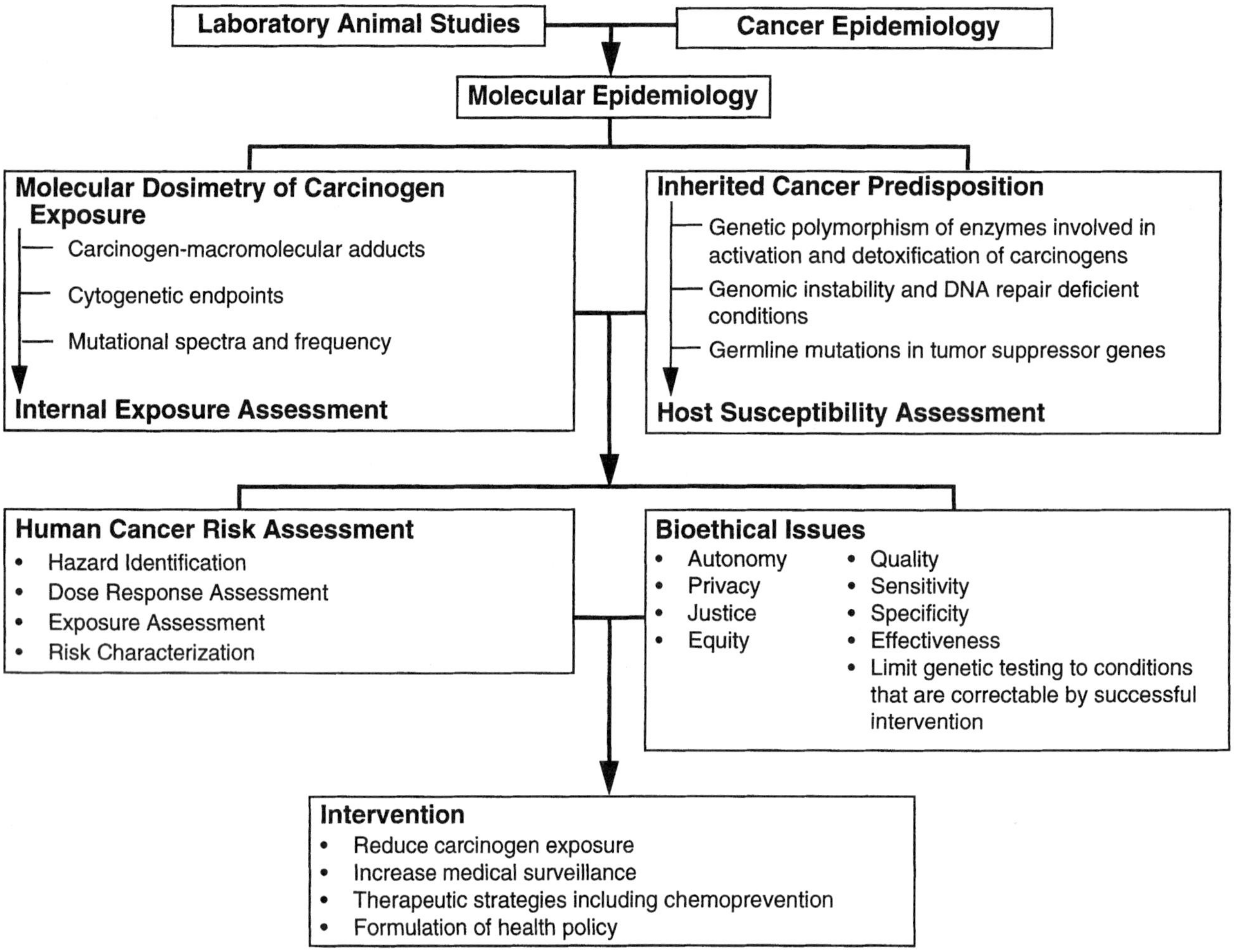


**FIG. 1.** Human cancer risk assessment and bioethical issues associated with molecular epidemiology and human cancer.

investigation and the rapid transfer of research findings from the laboratory to the clinic.

The knowledge acquired during this brief history of scientific advancement indicates that the p53 protein is involved in several central cellular processes including gene transcription, DNA repair, cell cycling, genomic stability, chromosomal segregation, senescence, and apoptosis (programmed cell death) (reviewed in 5–13). Since these complex biochemical processes in themselves are performed by multicomponent protein machines, it is not surprising that the p53 protein is included in these molecular machines and that the multiple effects of oncogenic DNA viruses are mediated in part by their targeting the p53 protein for binding and perturbing its functions (reviewed in 6,8,13) (Fig. 2). Since the number of p53 molecules per cell is limited, i.e., about $10^3$ to $10^4$ per cell, the physiologic state of the cell and the posttranslational modification of p53 must dictate where, when, and how efficiently p53 plays its role as the "guardian of the genome" in response to endogenous and exogenous carcinogens (14,15).

**TABLE 1.** *Familial versus sporadic cancers*

| | Familial (e.g., Li-Fraumeni syndrome) | Sporadic (e.g., smoking-related lung cancer) |
|---|---|---|
| Frequency | Rare | Common |
| Inherited susceptibility | Single | Multiple |
| Etiology | Primarily genetic | Multifactorial |
| Familial pattern | Segregates | Aggregates |
| Environmental effect | Constrained | Critical |
| Genetics | Predetermining | Predisposing |

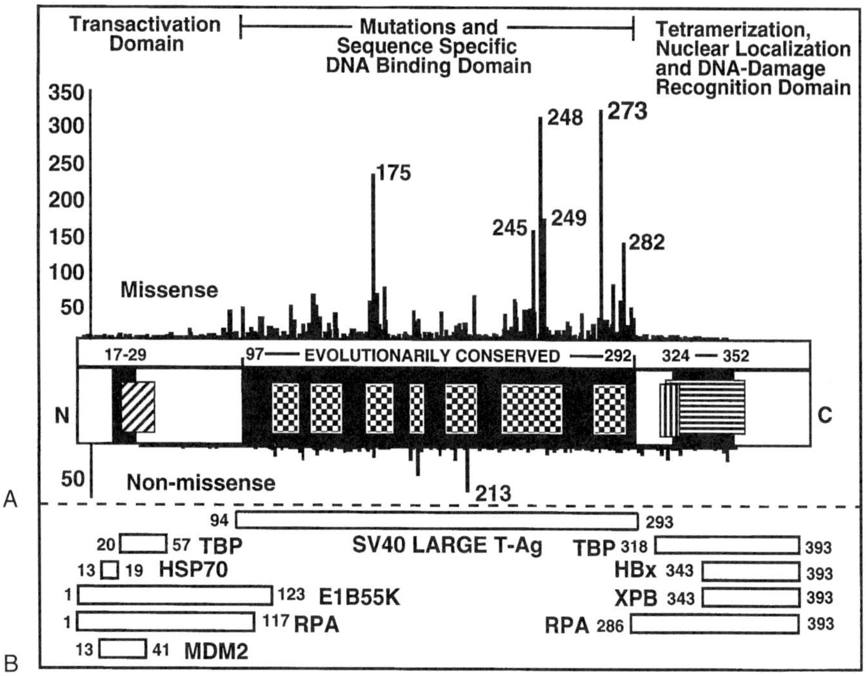


**FIG. 2.** Schematic representation of p53 molecule. The human p53 protein consists of 393 amino acids with functional domains, evolutionarily conserved domains, and regions designated as mutational hot spots (reviewed in 8). **A:** Missense or nonsense mutation. Functional domains include the transactivation region (*diagonally striped block*), sequence-specific DNA binding region (amino acids 100–293), nuclear localization sequence (amino acids 316–325; *vertical-striped block*), and oligomerization region (amino acids 319–360, *horizontal-striped block*). Evolutionarily conserved domains (amino acids 17–29, 97–292, and 324–352; *black areas)* were determined using the multiple alignment construction and analysis workbench program (MACAW) program. Seven mutational hot spot and evolutionarily conserved regions within the large conserved domain are also identified (amino acids 130–142, 151–164, 171–181, 193–200, 213–223, 234–258, and 270–286; *checkered blocks*). *Vertical lines* above the schematic, missense mutations; *lines below schematic,* nonmissense mutations. The majority of missense mutations are in the conserved hydrophobic midregion of the protein that is required for the sequence-specific binding to DNA, the nonmissense (nonsense, frame shift, splicing, and silent mutations) are distributed throughout the protein, determined primarily by sequence context. **B:** Protein-protein interactions: Cellular (e.g., TBP, TATA-binding protein; hsp70, heat shock 70 protein; RPA, replicating protein antigen; mdm2, multiple double minute; XPB, xeroderma pigmentosum) or viral oncoproteins (e.g., E1B55K, adenovirus protein E1B55K; SV40 large T ag, SV40 viral large T antigen; HBx, hepatitis B viral X protein) bind to specific areas of the p53 protein. Functional domains and protein-binding sites (*white bars* underneath) were compiled from references (reviewed in 8).

## DNA DAMAGE AND APOPTOTIC RESPONSE PATHWAYS

The p53 protein is clearly a component of one of the pathways activated in response to DNA damage (Fig. 3) (16–21). Cell cycle arrest at the $G_1$ and $G_2$ checkpoints prior to DNA replication and mitosis, respectively, aids the DNA repair processes and prevents mutations and aneuploidy, whereas apoptosis can be considered a fail-safe mechanism to rid the organism of cells either with severely damaged DNA or cells with a low apoptotic threshold. Double-stranded DNA breaks are especially efficient in causing p53 protein accumulation, possibly by reducing its degradation through the ubiquitin-dependent proteolytic pathway (16–18,21–25). The molecular pathway between DNA damage and p53 protein accumulation is not understood. p53 protein may be involved as one of the sensors of DNA damage. The carboxyl-terminus of p53 can bind nonspecifically to the ends of DNA molecules and catalyze DNA renaturation and strand transfer (26–30). This region of the protein can also bind to extrahelical regions of DNA damage involved in forming insertion/deletion mismatches (31). It will be interesting to determine if p53 recognizes other types of DNA damage including carcinogen-DNA adducts.

Wild-type p53 protein can transcriptionally transactivate genes involved in cell cycle arrest [e.g., $p21^{waf1}$, a potent inhibitor of most cyclin-dependent kinases (32–34)] and interact either with the DNA repair and synthetic machinery [e.g., proliferating cellular nuclear anti-

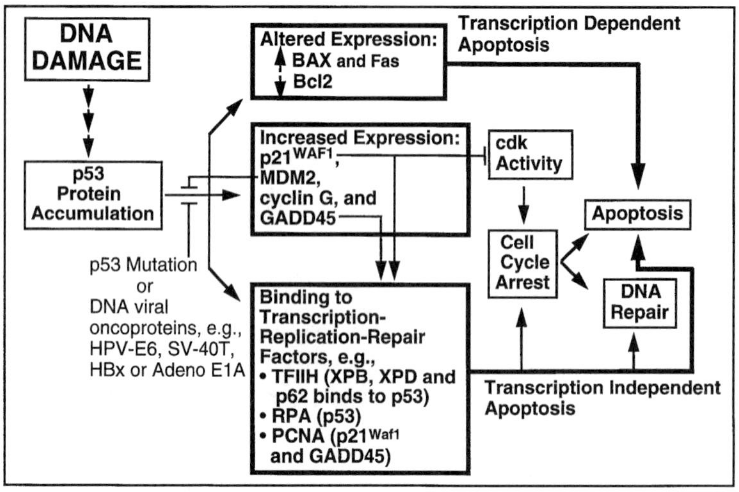


**FIG. 3.** p53 is a component of a DNA damage response pathway. This simplified model does not consider qualitative or quantitative differences due to either cell type or microenvironment. p53 accumulation leads the regulation of cellular genes involved in apoptosis (e.g., BAX, Fas, and Bcl2), cell cycle arrest [e.g., $p21^{Waf1}$, an inhibitor of cyclin dependent kinases (cdk)] and DNA synthesis and repair [e.g., $p21^{Waf1}$ and GADD45 binding to proliferating cell nuclear antigen (PCNA)]. mdm2 protein can bind to p53 protein and inhibit its functions in a negative feedback loop. p53 can also bind directly to proteins involved in DNA synthesis [e.g., replicating protein antigen (RPA)] and transcription, nucleotide excision, and apoptosis [e.g., xeroderma pigmentosum group D (XPD), xeroderma pigmentosum group B (XPB), and p62 of the TFIIH, transcription factor complex IIH]. Therefore, p53 may mediate apoptosis by two inactive pathways, one dependent on p53 function as a transcription transactivator and transrepressor and a second pathway independent of its transcriptional activities and dependent on p53 protein-protein interactions.

gen (PCNA), GADD45, and $p21^{waf1}$ (35,36)] or proteins modulating apoptosis [e.g., Bax and Fas (37,38)]. Certain other genes containing TATA boxes in their promoter regions, e.g., bcl-2 (39), can be transrepressed perhaps by p53 binding to the TATA-binding protein (TBP) and inhibiting its function as a basal transcription factor (40–43). p53 can also inhibit DNA synthesis by a transcription-independent mechanism binding to putative origins of DNA replication and prevent either initiation or early replication fork unwinding (44,45). p53 forms protein-protein complexes with cellular proteins involved in DNA synthesis [e.g., replicating protein antigen (RPA) (46)], DNA repair [e.g., RPA, xeroderma pigmentosum groups B and D (XPB, XPD), p62, topoisomerase I, and Cockayne syndrome group B (CSB) (46–51)], and apoptosis [e.g., XPB and XPD (52)]. Cellular context determines whether p53 can induce apoptosis independent or dependent of its transcription transactivation function and in the absence of RNA and protein synthesis (52–57). Interestingly, cycloheximide, an inhibitor of protein synthesis can induce apoptosis (58–60), and a temperature-sensitive mutant of a basal transcription factor, GG1/$TAF_{II}250$, when inactivated at a nonpermissive temperature, induces apoptosis (61). Cells from patients with CSB, which are deficient in transcribed strand-specific repair, have increased sensitivity to ultraviolet (UV) light–induced apoptosis (62). Since the induction of apoptosis was positively correlated with p53 accumulation and inhibition of transcription, Ljungman and Zhang (62) have speculated that blockage of RNA polymerase by UV damage in the transcribing DNA strand initiates the apoptosis response to UV. All of these results are consistent with the hypothesis that the apoptotic protein machinery is constitutively present in a latent state and does not require the synthesis of additional proteins. Nevertheless, p53 regulation of genes, whose products (e.g., Bax, Bcl2, and $p21^{Waf1}$) may be involved in apoptosis, could modulate a cell's sensitivity to inducers of apoptosis. p53 initiated $G_1$/S cell cycle arrest is primarily mediated by upregulation of $p21^{Waf1}$ (32–34), but $p21^{Waf1}$ is not an inducer of apoptosis in that ionizing radiation induces a p53-dependent apoptosis in $p21^{-/-}$ cells from $p21^{Waf1}$ gene knockout mice (63,64). Therefore, p53 may function by transcription transactivator-dependent and -independent mechanisms in interactive yet distinct pathways of cell cycle arrest and apoptosis.

Normal tissue homeostasis is maintained by balancing positive and negative cell growth regulation. Both external and internal signals can initiate or inhibit cell proliferation. Negative regulation also includes entry of cells into a terminally differentiated, senescent, or apoptotic state. During carcinogenesis, genetic and epigenetic lesions that lead to an imbalance between these growth regulator pathways accumulate in dysplastic and neoplastic cells leading to clonal selection and expansion, thus giving rise to clinical tumors (65). In this scenario of tumor progression, p53 mutations would occur after the initiating events of carcinogenesis. For example, hypoxia may select mutant p53 cells that are resistant to hypoxia-induced apoptosis (66). Deregulation and overexpression of certain cellular and viral oncogenes, e.g., myc, E2F, adenovirus E1a, or human papilloma virus E7, both stimulate proliferation and sensitize cells containing normal p53 and Rb tumor suppressor genes to apoptosis and, again, select for p53 mutant cells (67–70) (Fig. 4). Recent evidence from studies of mice with either a homozygous deletion of Rb or a human papilloma virus E7 transgene indicate that the absence of Rb promotes apoptosis (71,72). When Rb is inactivated, the resultant apoptotic response may be dependent on a normally functioning p53 (reviewed in (70)). Therefore, it is not surprising that (a) oncogenic DNA viruses target both Rb and p53 for inactivation; (b) retinoblastoma, in which Rb is deleted and p53 is normal, is generally sensitive to radiotherapy (73); and (c) p53 is frequently mutated in some human cancer types, e.g., small cell lung carcinoma and Burkitt's lymphoma, which exhibit deregulated myc expression, a p53-dependent apoptosis inducer (reviewed in 74–76). In other cancer types, the Rb pathway is often deregulated either by cyclin $D_1$ overexpression, cyclin-dependent kinase-4 overexpression or activating mutation, or functional inactivation of $p16^{INK4}$ by various mechanisms (reviewed in (77,78)). Cancer cells harboring cellular or viral oncogenes also may be intrinsically sensitive to the apoptotic response mediated by restored wild-type p53 function. Whereas loss of Rb and many other inducers of apoptosis are dependent on p53, physiologic activators of apoptosis such as glucocorticoids and the Fas ligand are independent of p53 and can activate apoptosis in p53 mutant cells.

## STRUCTURE–FUNCTION RELATIONSHIP OF p53

The mutation spectrum can also provide clues to the critical functional regions of the gene that, when mutated, contribute to the carcinogenic process. Since about 80% of the missense mutations are in the sequence-specific DNA-binding midregion of the protein (6–8), investigators have focused on the transcription transactivator function of p53. However, these missense mutations and the resultant amino acid substitutions can cause aberrant protein conformations (79) that also may alter other functional domains including those in the carboxyl terminus of the p53 protein. This positively charged region contains the putative major nuclear localization signal (amino acids 316 to 325), the oligomerization domain (amino acids 319 to 360), and a DNA damage-binding domain (amino acids 318 to 393) (27,80–82). p53 sequence-specific DNA binding and transcriptional transactivation can also be modulated by posttranslational mechanisms including serine phosphorylation (80,83) and the redox regulation of the cysteine residues responsible for binding zinc to p53 (84–86). The func-

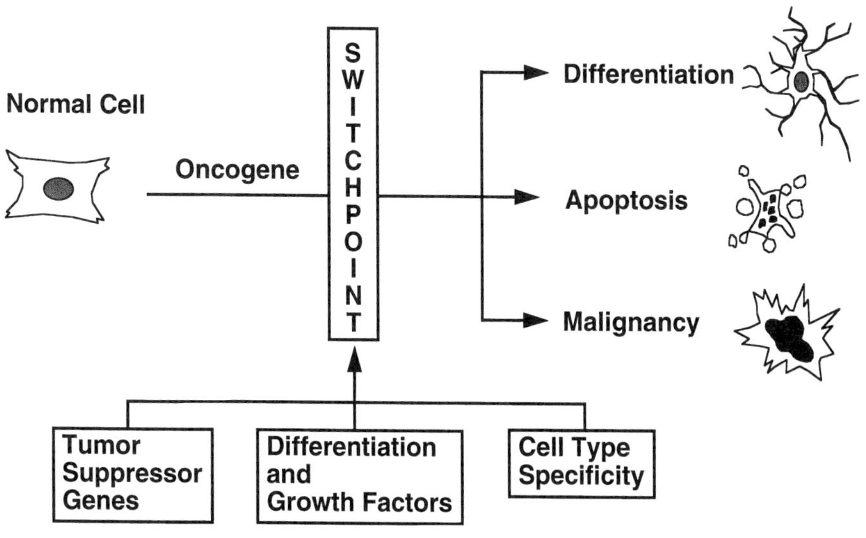


**FIG. 4.** Cellular switch point in response to cellular oncogenes. An inappropriately activated proto-oncogene can lead to differentiation (e.g., Ha-ras in rat PC12 cells), apoptosis (e.g., myc in rodent cells), or neoplastic transformation (e.g., Ha-ras in murine 3T3 cells).

tion-structure relationship revealed by the analysis of the p53 mutation spectrum (7,8), its nuclear magnetic resonance (NMR) and crystallographic three-dimensional structure (87–89), and functional studies of wild-type versus mutant p53 activity (reviewed in (90) have generated both hypotheses for further study and strategies for the development of rational cancer therapy.

## MOLECULAR ARCHAEOLOGY OF p53 MUTATIONS

Mutations can arise by either endogenous mutagenic mechanisms or exogenous mutagenic agents, and are archived in the spectrum of p53 mutations found in human cancer (6–8,10,91,92). Errors introduced during DNA replication, RNA splicing, DNA repair, and DNA deamination are examples of endogenous mutagenic mechanisms. The DNA sequence context is an important factor determining these events. Almost all short deletions and insertions occur at monotonic runs of two or more identical bases or at repeats of 2– to 8–base pair DNA motifs, either in tandem or separated by a short intervening sequence (93). The mechanism that has been most studied is called slipped mispairing, a misalignment of the template DNA strands during replication that leads to either deletion, if the nucleotides excluded from pairing are on the template strand, or insertion, if they are on the primer strand. When direct repeat sequences mispair with a complementary motif nearby, the intervening oligonucleotide sequence may form a loop between the two repeat motifs and be deleted (94,95). More lengthy runs and sequence repeats are more likely to generate frame-shift mutations. The deletions and insertions in the p53 gene found in human tumors also may be biologically selected from the broad array of such mutations occurring in human cells. When compared to the distribution of missense mutations, these types of mutations occur more frequently in exons 2 to 4 (54%) and 9 to 11 (77%) than in exons 5 to 8 (20%). The N-terminus of the p53 protein (encoded by exons 2 to 4) (reviewed in 41,90,96,97) has an abundance of acidic amino acids that are involved in transcriptional function of p53 (98,99) and binds to transcription factors such as TBP in TFIID (40–42,100,101), and experimental studies have shown that multiple point mutations are required to inactivate its transcriptional transactivation function (102). The carboxy-terminus (encoded by exons 9 to 11) of the p53 protein is enriched in basic amino acids that are important in the oligomerization and nuclear localization of the p53 protein (reviewed in 88,89,103,104), recognition of DNA damage (26,105), and induction of apoptosis (52). Multiple point mutations are infrequently found in the p53 gene, which is consistent with the target theory, i.e., exogenous mutagens target the p53 gene within the context of the entire human genome. Therefore, deletions and insertions would be a more efficient mutagenic mechanism than single point mutations in disrupting these N-terminal and C-terminal functional domains.

The p53 mutational spectrum of hepatocellular carcinoma is an example of a molecular linkage between carcinogen exposure and cancer. In liver tumors from persons living in geographic areas in which aflatoxin $B_1$ and hepatitis B virus (HBV) are cancer risk factors, most p53 mutations are at the third nucleotide pair of codon 249 (106–109). A dose-dependent relationship between dietary aflatoxin $B_1$ intake and codon $249^{ser}$ p53 mutations is observed in hepatocellular carcinoma from Asia, Africa, and North America (reviewed in 110). The mutation load of $249^{ser}$ mutant cells in nontumorous liver also is positively correlated with dietary aflatoxin $B_1$ exposure (111). Exposure of aflatoxin B1 to human liver cells *in vitro* produces $249^{ser}$ (AGG → AGT) p53 mutants (112; Mace, Aguilar, Harris, and Pfeifer, unpublished results). These results indicate that expression of the $249^{ser}$ mutant p53 protein provides a specific growth and/or survival advantage to liver cells and are consistent with the hypothesis that p53 mutations can occur early in liver carcinogenesis.

Since cellular context may influence the pathobiologic effects of specific mutants of p53, the $249^{ser}$ mutant may be especially potent in hepatocytes. The enhanced growth rate of p53-null HEP-3B cells by transfected $249^{ser}$ mutant p53 indicates a gain of oncogenic function and is consistent with this hypothesis (113). The $249^{ser}$ mutant p53 also is more effective than other p53 mutants ($143^{ala}$, $175^{his}$, $248^{trp}$, and $282^{his}$) in inhibiting wild-type p53 transcriptional transactivation activity in human liver cells (114). One hypothesis concerning generation of liver cancers with $249^{ser}$ mutation is (a) aflatoxin $B_1$ is metabolically activated to form the promutagenic N7dG adduct, and (b) enhanced cell proliferation due to chronic active viral hepatitis allows both fixation of the G:C to T:A transversion in codon 249 of the p53 gene and selective clonal expansion of the cells containing this mutant p53 gene.

In addition to producing chronic active hepatitis, HBV also has other important pathobiologic effects. For example, hepatitis B viral gene products may form complexes with cellular transcription factors, e.g., ATF2 (115), upregulate transcription of cellular and viral genes (116–120), or activate the ras-raf–mitogen activated protein (MAP) kinase signaling cascade (121). Inactivation of p53 tumor suppressor gene functions including DNA repair and apoptosis may be another consequence of cellular protein-HBV oncoprotein complex formation. Since the HBVX gene is frequently integrated and expressed in human hepatocellular carcinomas from high-risk geographic areas (122,123), the X protein has been found to bind p53 (48,124,125) and to inhibit its sequence specific DNA binding and transcriptional activity (48). HBVX protein also inhibits p53-dependent apoptosis (52). Based on the above results, we have speculated that HBVX protein may modulate p53 function in nucleotide excision DNA repair (47), including repair of $AFB_1$-DNA adducts, and are currently testing this hypothesis. HBV integration also could increase genomic instability, including abnormal chromosomal segregation, and increase rates of DNA recombination (126,127). Therefore, a second hypothesis of liver carcinogenesis emerges in which integration of HBVX gene is the initial event in these high cancer risk geographic areas, and $AFB_1$-mediated $249^{ser}$ p53 mutation is the second genetic lesion that leads to further genomic instability.

Absolute proof of causation cannot be obtained by epidemiologic studies. However, one can invoke the "weight of the evidence" principle. Using this principle, Bradford-Hill (128) proposed criteria in the assessment of cancer causation, including strength of the association (consistency, specificity, and temporality) and biologic plausibility. These criteria can also be utilized in the analysis and extrapolation of results from molecular epidemiology studies. For example, considerable amount of evidence is now consistent with the hypotheses that dietary aflatoxin $B_1$ exposure can produce codon $249^{ser}$ (AGG → AGT) p53 mutations during human liver carcinogenesis (Table 2) and chemical carcinogens, e.g., benzo[*a*]pyrene, in tobacco smoke cause p53 hot-spot mutations in human lung carcinogenesis (Table 3). Such assessments of causation have important implications in the understanding of molecular carcinogenesis and the utilization of evidence from molecular epidemiology studies to formulate both public health policy and medical-legal decisions.

**TABLE 2.** *Assessment of causation by the Bradford-Hill criteria*

- Hypothesis: Dietary aflatoxin $B_1$ exposure can produce $249^{ser}$ (AGG→AGT) p53 mutations during human liver carcinogenesis.
- Strength of association
  - Consistency
    - Positive correlation between estimated dietary aflatoxin $B_1$ exposure and frequency of $249^{ser}$ p53 mutations in 3 different ethnic populations on 3 continents (106,107,129)
  - Specificity
    - $249^{ser}$ p53 mutant are uncommon in other cancer types (8)
  - Temporality
    - $249^{ser}$ p53 mutant cells observed in nontumorous liver in high HCC incidence geographic areas (111)
- Biologic plausibility
  - $AFB_1$ is enzymatically activated by human hepatocytes (130,131) and the 8,9-$AFB_1$ oxide binds to the 3rd base (G) in codon 249 (132)
  - $AFB_1$ exposure to human liver cells (133) *in vitro* produces codon $249^{ser}$ p53 mutations
  - $249^{ser}$ p53 expression inhibits apoptosis (133), p53-mediated transcription (114) and enhances liver cell growth *in vitro* (113)

**TABLE 3.** *Assessment of causation by the Bradford-Hill criteria*

- Hypothesis: Chemical carcinogens, e.g., benzo[*a*]pyrene (BP), in tobacco smoke cause p53 hot-spot mutations at codons 157, 248, and 273 in human lung carcinogenesis
- Strength of association
  - Consistency
    - Cigarette smoking is associated with a dose-response increase in p53 mutations (G to T transversions) in human lung cancer (134)
  - Specificity
    - Codon 157 (GTC->TTC) mutations are uncommon in other types of cancer and have not been found in lung cancer from never smokers (8)
  - Temporality
    - p53 mutations can be found in bronchial dysplasia (135)
- Biologic plausibility
  - BP is metabolically activated and forms BP diol epoxide-DNA adducts in human bronchus *in vitro* (75-fold interindividual variation) (136–138)
  - BP diol epoxide binds to Gs in codons 157, 248, and 273, which are p53 mutational hot spots (139)
  - BP exposure to human cells *in vitro* produces codon 248 (CGG->CTG) p53 mutations (140)
  - Cigarette smoke condensates or BP can neoplastically transform human bronchial epithelial cells in the laboratory (141,142)

## ACKNOWLEDGMENT

We appreciate the editorial and graphic assistance of Dorothea Dudek.

## REFERENCES

1. Harris CC. Chemical and physical carcinogenesis: advances and perspectives. *Cancer Res* 1991;51:5023s–5044s.
2. Perera FP. Molecular epidemiology: Insights into cancer susceptibility, risk assessment, and prevention. *J Natl Cancer Inst* 1996;88: 496–509.
3. National Research Council. Assessment of Toxicology. In: National Academy of Sciences, ed. *Science and judgement in risk assessment.* Washington, DC: National Academy Press, 1994;56–67.
4. Li FP, Garber JE, Friend SH, et al. Recommendations on predictive testing for germ line p53 mutations among cancer-prone individuals. *J Natl Cancer Inst* 1992;84:1156–1160.
5. Harris CC. p53 Tumor suppressor gene: from the basic research laboratory to the clinic—an abridged historical perspective. *Carcinogenesis* 1996;17:1187–1198.
6. Levine AJ, Momand J, Finlay CA. The p53 tumour suppressor gene. *Nature* 1991;351:453–456.
7. Hollstein M, Sidransky D, Vogelstein B, Harris CC. p53 mutations in human cancers. *Science* 1991;253:49–53.
8. Greenblatt MS, Bennett WP, Hollstein M, Harris CC. Mutations in the p53 tumor suppressor gene: clues to cancer etiology and molecular pathogenesis. *Cancer Res* 1994;54:4855–4878.
9. Lane DP. A death in the life of p53. Nature 1993;362:786.
10. Gottlieb TM, Oren M. p53 in growth control and neoplasia. *Biochim Biophys Acta* 1996;1287:77–102.
11. Harris CC. Structure and function of the p53 tumor suppressor gene: clues for rational cancer therapeutic strategies. *J Natl Cancer Inst* 1996;88:1442–1455.
12. Fukasawa K, Choi T, Kuriyama R, Rulong S, Vande Woude GF. Abnormal centrosome amplification in the absence of p53. *Science* 1996;271:1744–1747.

13. Ko LJ, Prives C. p53: puzzle and paradigm. *Genes Dev* 1996;10: 1054–1072.
14. Forrester K, Ambs S, Lupold SE, et al. Nitric oxide-induced p53 accumulation and regulation of inducible nitric oxide synthase (NOS2) expression by wild-type p53. *Proc Natl Acad Sci USA* 1996;93: 2442–2447.
15. Lane DP. Cancer. p53, guardian of the genome [news; comment]. *Nature* 1992;358:15–16.
16. Maltzman W, Czyzyk L. UV irradiation stimulates levels of p53 cellular tumor antigen in nontransformed mouse cells. *Mol Cell Biol* 1984;4:1689–1694.
17. Kastan MB, Radin AI, Kuerbitz SJ, et al. Levels of p53 protein increase with maturation in human hematopoietic cells. *Cancer Res* 1991;51:4279–4286.
18. Kastan MB, Zhan Q, El-Deiry WS, et al. A mammalian cell cycle checkpoint pathway utilizing p53 and GADD45 is defective in ataxia-telangiectasia. *Cell* 1992;71:587–597.
19. Guillouf C, Rosselli F, Krishnaraju K, Moustacchi E, Hoffman B, Liebermann DA. p53 involvement in control of G2 exit of the cell cycle: role in DNA damage-induced apoptosis. *Oncogene* 1995;10: 2263–2270.
20. Powell SN, DeFrank JS, Connell P, et al. Differential sensitivity of p53(-) and p53(+) cells to caffeine-induced radiosensitization and override of G2 delay. *Cancer Res* 1995;55:1643–1648.
21. Nelson WG, Kastan MB. DNA strand breaks: the DNA template alterations that trigger p53-dependent DNA damage response pathways. *Mol Cell Biol* 1994;14:1815–1823.
22. Scheffner M, Werness BA, Huibregtse JM, Levine AJ, Howley PM. The E6 oncoprotein encoded by human papillomavirus types 16 and 18 promotes the degradation of p53. *Cell* 1990;63:1129–1136.
23. Lu X, Lane DP. Differential induction of transcriptionally active p53 following UV or ionizing radiation: defects in chromosome instability syndromes? *Cell* 1993;75:765–778.
24. Di Leonardo A, Linke SP, Clarkin K, Wahl GM. DNA damage triggers a prolonged p53-dependent G1 arrest and long-term induction of Cip1 in normal human fibroblasts. *Genes Dev* 1994;8:2540–2551.
25. Huang LC, Clarkin KC, Wahl GM. Sensitivity and selectivity of the DNA damage sensor responsible for activating p53-dependent G1 arrest. *Proc Natl Acad Sci USA* 1996;93:4827–4832.
26. Jayaraman L, Prives C. Activation of p53 sequence-specific DNA binding by short single strands of DNA requires the p53 C-terminus. *Cell* 1995;81:1021–1029.
27. Brain R, Jenkins JR. Human p53 directs DNA strand reassociation and is photolabelled by 8-azido ATP. *Oncogene* 1994;9:1775–1780.
28. Oberosler P, Hloch P, Ramsperger U, Stahl H. p53-catalyzed annealing of complementary single-stranded nucleic acids. *EMBO J* 1993; 12:2389–2396.
29. Foord OS, Bhattacharya P, Reich Z, Rotter V. A DNA binding domain is contained in the C-terminus of wild type p53 protein. *Nucleic Acids Res* 1991;19:5191–5198.
30. Reed M, Woelker B, Wang P, Wang Y, Anderson ME, Tegtmeyer P. The C-terminal domain of p53 recognizes DNA damaged by ionizing radiation. *Proc Natl Acad Sci USA* 1995;92:9455–9459.
31. Lee S, Elenbase B, Levine A, Griffith J. p53 and its 14kDa C-terminal domain recognize primary DNA damage in the form of insertion/deletion mismatches. *Cell* 1995;81:1013–1020.
32. Harper JW, Adami GR, Wei N, Keyomarsi K, Elledge SJ. The p21 cdk-interacting protein Cip1 is a potent inhibitor of G1 cyclin-dependent kinases. *Cell* 1993;75:805–816.
33. El-Deiry WS, Tokino T, Velculescu VE, et al. WAF1, a potential mediator of p53 tumor suppression. *Cell* 1993;75:817–825.
34. Xiong Y, Hannon GJ, Zhang H, Casso D, Kobayashi R, Beach D. p21 is a universal inhibitor of cyclin kinases [see comments]. *Nature* 1993; 366:701–704.
35. Smith ML, Chen IT, Zhan Q, et al. Interaction of the p53-regulated protein Gadd45 with proliferating cell nuclear antigen. *Science* 1994; 266:1376–1380.
36. Li R, Waga S, Hannon GJ, Beach D, Stillman B. Differential effects by the p21 CDK inhibitor on PCNA-dependent DNA replication and repair. *Nature* 1994;371:534–537.
37. Selvakumaran M, Lin HK, Miyashita T, et al. Immediate early up-regulation of bax expression by p53 but not TGF beta 1: a paradigm for distinct apoptotic pathways. *Oncogene* 1994;9:1791–1798.
38. Miyashita T, Reed JC. Tumor suppressor p53 is a direct transcriptional activator of the human bax gene. *Cell* 1995;80:293–299.
39. Miyashita T, Krajewski S, Krajewska M, et al. Tumor suppressor p53 is a regulator of bcl-2 and bax gene expression *in vitro* and *in vivo*. *Oncogene* 1994;9:1799–1805.
40. Seto E, Usheva A, Zambetti GP, et al. Wild-type p53 binds to the TATA-binding protein and represses transcription. *Proc Natl Acad Sci USA* 1992;89:12028–12032.
41. Liu X, Miller CW, Koeffler PH, Berk AJ. The p53 activation domain binds the TATA box-binding polypeptide in Holo-TFIID, and a neighboring p53 domain inhibits transcription. *Mol Cell Biol* 1993;13: 3291–3300.
42. Truant R, Xiao H, Ingles CJ, Greenblatt J. Direct interaction between the transcriptional activation domain of human p53 and the TATA box-binding protein. *J Biol Chem* 1993;268:2284–2287.
43. Chen X, Farmer G, Zhu H, Prywes R, Prives C. Cooperative DNA binding of p53 with TFIID (TBP): a possible mechanism for transcriptional activation [published erratum appears in *Genes Dev* 1993 Dec;7(12B):2652]. *Genes Dev* 1993;7:1837–1849.
44. Miller SD, Farmer G, Prives C. p53 inhibits DNA replication *in vitro* and in a DNA-binding-dependent manner. *Mol Cell Biol* 1995;15: 6554–6560.
45. Cox LS, Hupp T, Midgley CA, Lane DP. A direct effect of activated human p53 on nuclear DNA replication. *EMBO J* 1995;14: 2099–2105.
46. Dutta A, Ruppert JM, Aster JC, Winchester E. Inhibition of DNA replication factor RPA by p53. *Nature* 1993;365:79–82.
47. Wang XW, Yeh H, Schaeffer L, et al. p53 Modulation of TFIIH-associated nucleotide excision repair activity. *Nature Genet* 1995;10: 188–195.
48. Wang XW, Forrester K, Yeh H, Feitelson MA, Gu JR, Harris CC. Hepatitis B virus X protein inhibits p53 sequence-specific DNA binding, transcriptional activity, and association with transcription factor ERCC3. *Proc Natl Acad Sci USA* 1994;91:2230–2234.
49. Xiao H, Pearson A, Coulombe B, et al. Binding of basal transcription factor TFIIH to the acidic activation domains of VP16 and p53. *Mol Cell Biol* 1994;14:7013–7024.
50. Leveillard T, Andera L, Bissonnette N, et al. Functional interactions between p53 and the TFIIH complex are affected by tumour-associated mutations. *EMBO J* 1996;15:1615–1624.
51. Gobert C, Bracco L, Rossi F, et al. Modulation of DNA topoisomerase I activity by p53. *Biochemistry* 1996;35:5778–5786.
52. Wang XW, Vermeulen W, Coursen JD, et al. The XPB and XPD helicases are components of the p53-mediated apoptosis pathway. *Genes Dev* 1996;10:1219–1232.
53. Caelles C, Helmberg A, Karin M. p53-dependent apoptosis in the absence of transcriptional activation of p53-target genes [see comments]. *Nature* 1994;370:220–223.
54. Haupt Y, Rowan S, Shaulian E, Vousden KH, Oren M. Induction of apoptosis in HeLa cells by trans-activation-deficient p53. *Genes Dev* 1995;9:2170–2183.
55. Wagner AJ, Kokontis JM, Hay N. Myc-mediated apoptosis requires wild-type p53 in a manner independent of cell cycle arrest and the ability of p53 to induce p21waf1/cip1. *Genes Dev* 1994;8:2817–2830.
56. Del Sal G, Ruaro EM, Utrera R, Cole CN, Levine AJ, Schneider C. Gas1-induced growth suppression requires a transactivation-independent p53 function. *Mol Cell Biol* 1995;15:7152–7160.
57. Sakamuro D, Eviner V, Elliott KJ, Showe L, White E, Prendergast GC. c-Myc induces apoptosis in epithelial cells by both p53-dependent and p53-independent mechanisms. *Oncogene* 1995;11:2411–2418.
58. Harris CC, Grady H, Svoboda D. Alterations in pancreatic and hepatic ultrastructure following acute cycloheximide intoxication. *J Ultrastruct Res* 1968;22:240–251.
59. Martin SJ. Protein or RNA synthesis inhibition induces apoptosis of mature human CD4+ T cell blasts. *Immunol Lett* 1993;35:125–134.
60. Bazar LS, Deeg HJ. Ultraviolet B-induced DNA fragmentation (apoptosis) in activated T-lymphocytes and Jurkat cells is augmented by inhibition of RNA and protein synthesis. *Exp Hematol* 1992;20: 80–86.
61. Sekiguchi T, Nakashima T, Hayashida T, et al. Apoptosis is induced in BHK cells by the tsBN462/13 mutation in the CCG1/TAFII250 subunit of the TFIID basal transcription factor. *Exp Cell Res* 1995;218: 490–498.
62. Ljungman M, Zhang F. Blockage of RNA polymerase as a possible trigger for UV light-induced apoptosis. *Oncogene* 1996;13:823–831.

63. Brugarolas J, Chandrasekaran C, Gordon JI, Beach D, Jacks T, Hannon GJ. Radiation-induced cell cycle arrest compromised by p21 deficiency. *Nature* 1995;377:552–557.
64. Deng C, Zhang P, Harper JW, Elledge SJ, Leder P. Mice lacking p21CIP1/WAF1 undergo normal development, but are defective in G1 checkpoint control. *Cell* 1995;82:675–684.
65. Tomlinson IP, Bodmer WF. Failure of programmed cell death and differentiation as causes of tumors: some simple mathematical models. *Proc Natl Acad Sci USA* 1995;92:11130–11134.
66. Graeber TG, Osmanian C, Jacks T, Housman DE, Koch CJ, Lowe SW, et al. Hypoxia-mediated selection of cells with diminished apoptotic potential in solid tumours. *Nature* 1996;379:88–91.
67. Askew DS, Ashmun RA, Simmons BC, Cleveland JL. Constitutive c-myc expression in an IL-3-dependent myeloid cell line suppresses cell cycle arrest and accelerates apoptosis. *Oncogene* 1991;6: 1915–1922.
68. Rao L, Debbas M, Sabbatini P, Hockenbery D, Korsmeyer S, White E. The adenovirus E1A proteins induce apoptosis, which is inhibited by the E1B 19-kDa and Bcl-2 proteins [published erratum appears in *Proc Natl Acad Sci USA* 1992 Oct 15;89(20):9974]. *Proc Natl Acad Sci USA* 1992;89:7742–7746.
69. Evan GI, Wyllie AH, Gilbert CS, et al. Induction of apoptosis in fibroblasts by c-myc protein. *Cell* 1992;69:119–128.
70. White E. Tumour biology. p53, guardian of Rb. *Nature* 1994;371: 21–22.
71. Pan H, Griep AE. Altered cell cycle regulation in the lens of HPV-16 E6 or E7 transgenic mice: implications for tumor suppressor gene function in development. *Genes Dev* 1994;8:1285–1299.
72. Morgenbesser SD, Williams BO, Jacks T, DePinho RA. p53-dependent apoptosis produced by Rb-deficiency in the developing mouse lens [see comments]. *Nature* 1994;371:72–74.
73. Pizzo PA, Horowitz ME, Poplack DG, Hays DM, Kun LE. Solid tumors of childhood. In: DeVita VT Jr, Hellman S, Rosenberg SA, eds. *Cancer:* principles and practice of oncology, 4th ed. Philadelphia: JB Lippincott, 1993;1738–1791.
74. Milner AE, Grand RJ, Waters CM, Gregory CD. Apoptosis in Burkitt lymphoma cells is driven by c-myc. *Oncogene* 1993;8:3385–3391.
75. Carbone DP, Minna JD. The molecular genetics of lung cancer. *Adv Intern Med* 1992;37:153–171.
76. Greenblatt MS, Harris CC. Molecular genetics of lung cancer. *Cancer Surv* 1995;25:293–313.
77. Hunter T. Braking the cycle. *Cell* 1993;75:839–841.
78. Weinberg RA. The retinoblastoma protein and cell cycle control. *Cell* 1995;81:323–330.
79. Milner J, Medcalf EA, Cook AC. Tumor suppressor p53: analysis of wild-type and mutant p53 complexes. *Mol Cell Biol* 1991;11:12–19.
80. Wang Y, Prives C. Increased and altered DNA binding of human p53 by S and G2/M but not G1 cyclin-dependent kinases. *Nature* 1995; 376:88–91.
81. Wu L, Bayle JH, Elenbaas B, Pavletich NP, Levine AJ. Alternatively spliced forms in the carboxy-terminal domain of the p53 protein regulate its ability to promote annealing of complementary single strands of nucleic acids. *Mol Cell Biol* 1995;15:497–504.
82. Bakalkin G, Selivanova G, Yakovleva T, et al. p53 binds single-stranded DNA ends through the C-terminal domain and internal DNA segments via the middle domain. *Nucleic Acids Res* 1995;23:362–369.
83. Mayr GA, Reed M, Wang P, Wang Y, Schwedes JF, Tegtmeyer P. Serine phosphorylation in the NH2 terminus of p53 facilitates transactivation. *Cancer Res* 1995;55:2410–2417.
84. Hainaut P, Milner J. Redox modulation of p53 conformation and sequence-specific DNA binding *in vitro*. *Cancer Res* 1993;53: 4469–4473.
85. Hupp TR, Meek DW, Midgley CA, Lane DP. Activation of the cryptic DNA binding function of mutant forms of p53. *Nucleic Acids Res* 1993;21:3167–3174.
86. Rainwater R, Parks D, Anderson ME, Tegtmeyer P, Mann K. Role of cysteine residues in regulation of p53 function. *Mol Cell Biol* 1995; 15:3892–3903.
87. Cho Y, Gorina S, Jeffrey P, Pavletich NP. Crystal structure of a p53 tumor suppressor-DNA complex: a framework for understanding how mutations inactivate p53. *Science* 1994;265:346–355.
88. Clore GM, Omichinski JG, Sakaguchi K, et al. High-resolution solution structure of the oligomerization domain of p53 by multi-dimensional NMR. *Science* 1994;265:386–391.
89. Jeffrey PD, Gorina S, Pavletich NP. Crystal structure of the tetramerization domain of the p53 tumor suppressor at 1.7 angstroms. *Science* 1995;267:1498–1502.
90. Vogelstein B, Kinzler KW. p53 function and dysfunction. *Cell* 1992; 70:523–526.
91. Harris CC. p53: at the crossroads of molecular carcinogenesis and cancer risk assessment. *Science* 1993;262:1980–1981.
92. Soussi T, Legros Y, Lubin R, Ory K, Schlichtholz B. Multifactorial analysis of p53 alteration in human cancer: a review. *Int J Cancer* 1994;57:1–9.
93. Greenblatt MS, Grollman AP, Harris CC. Deletions and insertions in the p53 tumor suppressor gene in human cancers: confirmation of the DNA polymerase slippage/misalignment model. *Cancer Res* 1996;56: 2130–2136.
94. Jego N, Thomas G, Hamelin R. Short direct repeats flanking deletions, and duplicating insertions in p53 gene in human cancers. *Oncogene* 1993;8:209–213.
95. Krawczak M, Cooper DN. Gene deletions causing human genetic disease: mechanisms of mutagenesis and the role of the local DNA sequence environment. *Hum Genet* 1991;86:425–441.
96. Thut CJ, Chen J-L, Klemm R, Tjian R. p53 transcriptional activation mediated by coactivators TAFii40 and TAFii60. *Science* 1995;267: 100–104.
97. Lu H, Levine AJ. Human TAFII31 protein is a transcriptional coactivator of the p53 protein. *Proc Natl Acad Sci USA* 1995;92: 5154–5158.
98. Raycroft L, Wu H, Lozano G. Transcriptional activation by wild-type but not transforming mutants of the p53 anti-oncogene. *Science* 1990; 249:1049–1051.
99. Fields S, Jang SK. Presence of a potent transcription activating sequence in the p53 protein. *Science* 1990;249:1046–1048.
100. Martin DW, Munoz RM, Subler MA, Deb S. p53 binds to the TATA-binding protein-TATA complex. *J Biol Chem* 1993;268: 13062–13067.
101. Mack DH, Vartikar J, Pipas JM, Laimins LA. Specific repression of TATA-mediated but not initiator-mediated transcription by wild-type p53. *Nature* 1993;363:281–283.
102. Lin J, Chen J, Elenbaas B, Levine AJ. Several hydrophobic amino acids in the p53 amino-terminal domain are required for transcriptional activation, binding to mdm-2 and the adenovirus 5 E1B 55-kD protein. *Genes Dev* 1994;8:1235–1246.
103. Hupp TR, Lane DP. Allosteric activation of latent p53 tetramers. *Curr Biol* 1995;4:865–875.
104. Lee W, Harvey TS, Yin Y, Yau P, Litchfield D, Arrowsmith CH. Solution structure of the tetrameric minimum transforming domain of p53. *Nature Struct Biol* 1994;1:877–890.
105. Bakalkin G, Yakovleva T, Selivanova G, et al. p53 binds single-stranded DNA ends and catalyzes DNA renaturation and strand transfer. *Proc Natl Acad Sci USA* 1994;91:413–417.
106. Hsu IC, Metcalf RA, Sun T, Welsh JA, Wang NJ, Harris CC. Mutational hotspot in the p53 gene in human hepatocellular carcinomas. *Nature* 1991;350:427–428.
107. Bressac B, Kew M, Wands J, Ozturk M. Selective G to T mutations of p53 gene in hepatocellular carcinoma from southern Africa. *Nature* 1991;350:429–431.
108. Scorsone KA, Zhou YZ, Butel JS, Slagle BL. p53 mutations cluster at codon 249 in hepatitis B virus-positive hepatocellular carcinomas from China. *Cancer Res* 1992;52:1635–1638.
109. Li D, Cao Y, He L, Wang NJ, Gu J. Aberrations of p53 gene in human hepatocellular carcinoma from China. *Carcinogenesis* 1993;14: 169–173.
110. Harris CC. The 1995 Walter Hubert Lecture—Molecular epidemiology of human cancer: insights from the mutational analysis of the p53 tumor suppressor gene. *Br J Cancer* 1996;73:261–269.
111. Aguilar F, Harris CC, Sun T, Hollstein M, Cerutti P. Geographic variation of p53 mutational profile in nonmalignant human liver. *Science* 1994;264:1317–1319.
112. Aguilar F, Hussain SP, Cerutti P. Aflatoxin B1 induces the transversion of G→T in codon 249 of the p53 tumor suppressor gene in human hepatocytes. *Proc Natl Acad Sci USA* 1993;90:8586–8590.
113. Ponchel F, Puisieux A, Tabone E, et al. Hepatocarcinoma-specific mutant p53-249ser induces mitotic activity but has no effect on transforming growth factor beta 1-mediated apoptosis. *Cancer Res* 1994; 54:2064–2068.

114. Forrester K, Lupold SE, Ott VL, et al. Effects of p53 mutants on wild-type p53-mediated transactivation are cell type dependent. *Oncogene* 1995;10:2103–2111.
115. Maguire HF, Hoeffler JP, Siddiqui A. HBV X protein alters the DNA binding specificity of CREB and ATF-2 by protein-protein interactions. *Science* 1991;252:842–844.
116. Shirakata Y, Kawada M, Fujiki Y, et al. The X gene of hepatitis B virus induced growth stimulation and tumorigenic transformation of mouse NIH3T3 cells. *Jpn J Cancer Res* 1989;80:617–621.
117. Kekulë AS, Lauer U, Meyer M, Caselmann WH, Hofschneider PH, Koshy R. The preS2/S region of integrated hepatitis B virus DNA encodes a transcriptional transactivator. *Nature* 1990;343:457–461.
118. Twu JS, Schloemer RH. Transcriptional trans-activating function of hepatitis B virus. *J Virol* 1987;61:3448–3453.
119. Spandau DF, Lee CH. trans-activation of viral enhancers by the hepatitis B virus X protein. *J Virol* 1988;62:427–434.
120. Caselmann WH, Meyer M, Kekulë AS, Lauer U, Hofschneider PH, Koshy R. A trans-activator function is generated by integration of hepatitis B virus preS/S sequences in human hepatocellular carcinoma DNA. *Proc Natl Acad Sci USA* 1990;87:2970–2974.
121. Benn J, Schneider RJ. Hepatitis B virus HBx protein activates Ras-GTP complex formation and establishes a Ras, Raf, MAP kinase signaling cascade. *Proc Natl Acad Sci USA* 1994;91:10350–10354.
122. Unsal H, Yakicier C, Marcais C, et al. Genetic heterogeneity of hepatocellular carcinoma. *Proc Natl Acad Sci USA* 1994;91:822–826.
123. Paterlini P, Poussin K, Kew M, Franco D, Brechot C. Selective accumulation of the X transcript of hepatitis B virus in patients negative for hepatitis B surface antigen with hepatocellular carcinoma. *Hepatology* 1995;21:313–321.
124. Feitelson MA, Zhu M, Duan LX, London WT. Hepatitis B x antigen and p53 are associated *in vitro* and in liver tissues from patients with primary hepatocellular carcinoma. *Oncogene* 1993;8:1109–1117.
125. Ueda H, Ullrich SJ, Gangemi JD, et al. Functional inactivation but not structural mutation of p53 causes liver cancer. *Nature Genet* 1995;9:41–47.
126. Hino O, Nomura K, Ohtake K, Kawaguchi T, Sugano H, Kitagawa T. Instability of integrated hepatitis B virus DNA with inverted repeat structure in a transgenic mouse. *Cancer Genet Cytogenet* 1989;37:273–278.
127. Hino O, Tabata S, Hotta Y. Evidence for increased *in vitro* recombination with insertion of human hepatitis B virus DNA. *Proc Natl Acad Sci USA* 1991;88:9248–9252.
128. Hill AB. The environment and disease: association or causation. *Proc R Soc Med* 1965;58:295–300.
129. Soini Y, Chia SC, Bennett WP, et al. An aflatoxin-associated mutational hotspot at codon 249 in the p53 tumor suppressor gene occurs in hepatocellular carcinomas from Mexico. *Carcinogenesis* 1996;17:1007–1012.
130. Autrup H, Harris CC, Wu SM, et al. Activation of chemical carcinogens by cultured human fetal liver, esophagus and stomach. *Chem Biol Interact* 1984;50:15–25.
131. Pfeifer AMA, Cole KE, Smoot DT, et al. SV40 T-antigen immortalized normal human liver epithelial cells express hepatocyte characteristics and metabolize chemical carcinogens. *Proc Natl Acad Sci USA* 1993;90:5123–5127.
132. Puisieux A, Lim S, Groopman J, Ozturk M. Selective targeting of p53 gene mutational hotspots in human cancers by etiologically defined carcinogens. *Cancer Res* 1991;51:6185–6189.
133. Wang XW, Gibson MK, Vermeulen W, et al. Abrogation of p53-induced apoptosis by the hepatitis B virus X gene. *Cancer Res* 1995;55:6012–6016.
134. Takeshima Y, Seyama T, Bennett WP, et al. p53 mutations in lung cancers from non-smoking atomic-bomb survivors. *Lancet* 1993;342:1520–1521.
135. Vahakangas KH, Samet JM, Metcalf RA, et al. Mutations of p53 and ras genes in radon-associated lung cancer from uranium miners. *Lancet* 1992;339:576–580.
136. Harris CC, Genta VM, Frank AL, et al. Carcinogenic polynuclear hydrocarbons bind to macromolecules in cultured human bronchi. *Nature* 1974;252:68–69.
137. Harris CC, Autrup H, Connor RD, Barrett LA, McDowell EM, Trump BF. Interindividual variation in binding of benzo[*a*]pyrene to DNA in cultured human bronchi. *Science* 1976;194:1067–1069.
138. Jeffrey AM, Weinstein IB, Jennette KW, et al. Structures of benzo[*a*]pyrene—nucleic acid adducts formed in human and bovine bronchial explants. *Nature* 1977;269:348–350.
139. Denissenko MF, Pao A, Tang M, Pfeifer GP. Preferential formation of benzo[*a*]pyrene adducts at lung cancer mutational hotspots in P53. *Science* 1996;274:430–432.
140. Cherpillod P, Amstad PA. Benzo[*a*]pyrene-induced mutagenesis of p53 hot-spot codons 248 and 249 in human hepatocytes. *Mol Carcinog* 1995;13:15–20.
141. Klein-Szanto AJ, Iizasa T, Momiki S, et al. A tobacco-specific N-nitrosamine or cigarette smoke condensate causes neoplastic transformation of xenotransplanted human bronchial epithelial cells. *Proc Natl Acad Sci USA* 1992;89:6693–6697.
142. Iizasa T, Momiki S, Bauer B, et al. Invasive tumors derived from xenotransplanted, immortalized human cells after *in vivo* exposure to chemical carcinogens. *Carcinogenesis* 1993;14:1789–1794.

*Environmental and Occupational Medicine,*
*Third Edition,* edited by William N. Rom.
Lippincott–Raven Publishers, Philadelphia © 1998.

# CHAPTER 14

# Biologic Markers

Anatoly Zhitkovich and Max Costa

## RATIONALE FOR THE DEVELOPMENT AND USE OF BIOMARKERS

Much of the knowledge about health effects of exposures to toxic agents has been derived from epidemiologic studies of highly exposed workers and from experimental studies on laboratory animals. In the past, disease risk was easier to detect since workers were exposed to much higher concentrations of toxic agents than in modern industrial settings or compared to the general population. In most current situations potential adverse factors are expected to increase health risk only modestly. Weak associations are difficult to detect in standard epidemiologic studies because they require very large numbers of participants and long waiting periods. Due to the demands by the general public to evaluate exposures now, development of short-term methods to estimate health effects of environmental exposure and efficacy of remediating efforts would be of great value. Apart from being an obstacle in assessing health risks of current exposure, extended waiting intervals in the traditional epidemiologic studies can lead to additional confounding exposures. The majority of diseases can be caused by a large number of different toxic exposures, and the chances of exposure to another causative agent during a 20- to 30-year latency period for cancer induction, for example, becomes very significant.

A need for better risk assessment strategies of toxic exposures is also dictated by the fact that there are subpopulations of exposed individuals who are particularly sensitive to a specific agent. Traditional methods of risk assessment based on environmental measurements obviously cannot identify susceptible subjects. Tobacco smoking can serve as an illustration to this problem. Cigarette smoking is believed to be responsible for almost 80% of 170,000 lung cancer cases occurring in the United States every year (1). Consistent epidemiologic data and isolation of a large number of potent carcinogens from tobacco smoke provided strong evidence that smoking causes lung cancer. Nevertheless, the majority of smokers do not develop lung cancer. In fact, estimates suggest that only about 17% of people who smoke develop any type of cancer. There should be significant differences in individual capabilities to metabolize carcinogens and cope with induced DNA damage leading to this variable susceptibility to the induction of lung cancer by smoking.

Exposure to toxic chemicals has long been monitored through environmental measurements such as analysis of airborne or water concentrations. In many situations environmental measurements are not very reliable since environmental levels are prone to large fluctuations over time. In addition, in many environmental and occupational settings exposures can vary dramatically at different sites and depend on individual hygienic behavior. Additional problems arise when there are multiple routes of exposure to a chemical such as through inhalation, various dietary sources, drinking water, and soil. The heterogeneous distribution of xenobiotics, temporal fluctuations, and individual dietary habits may affect levels of exposure so profoundly that control and case groups become indistinguishable. The questionnaire data can be sometimes quite useful when, for example, exposure to cigarette smoke is analyzed since subjects can rather accu-

A. Zhitkovich: Department of Environmental Medicine, New York University Medical Center, Tuxedo, New York 10987.
M. Costa: Department of Environmental Medicine and Department of Pharmacology, New York University Medical Center, New York, New York 10016.

rately estimate the number of cigarettes they smoked per day. However, this approach is very imprecise when it is applied to assessment of exposures occurring through diet. Polycyclic aromatic hydrocarbons (PAH) are potent human carcinogens and typical examples of xenobiotic exposure to which may occur through many different routes and sources. The general population can be exposed to PAH through smoking, ambient pollution, and consumption of charbroiled food (2). In industrial settings many workers take in PAH via inhalation and dermal uptake (3). All this complexity and extensive variation makes it very difficult to extrapolate environmental measurements of toxicants to an individual human exposure. Consequently, risk assessment can be greatly improved through the development of biologically based measurements that can account for multiple routes of entry, variable exposures, and biologic effects resulting from a specific exposure. A good biomarker can also be helpful in the identification of individuals who may be particularly susceptible to toxic effects of a specific exposure.

## DEFINITION AND CLASSIFICATION

Biologic markers are measurements conducted in biologic samples that evaluate an exposure or biologic effect of that exposure. In 1987, the Committee on Biological Markers of the National Research Council (4) proposed a general concept for biomarkers that became widely accepted by the scientific community. The conceptual framework for biomarkers described the sequence of events occurring between exposure to a toxic agent and the development of disease (Fig. 1). Biomarkers are generally classified into three groups: biomarkers of exposure, biomarkers of effect, and biomarkers of susceptibility. Typical biomarkers of exposure include measurements of the toxin (e.g., cadmium in blood) or its specific metabolite (e.g., S-phenylmercapturic acid for benzene exposure). Detection of a product of interaction between a xenobiotic and an endogenous component also represents an exposure biomarker. The most frequently measured biomarkers of this type are DNA and protein adducts. A biomarker of effect is the biologic response that is mechanistically involved in the pathway leading to injury and disease. Gene mutations or chromosomal rearrangements induced by a carcinogen exposure are examples of biomarkers of effect. It should be noted that there is no sharp division between biomarkers of exposure and effect, and some biomarkers lie at the interface. Most DNA adducts are biomarkers that assess both exposure and effect. A specific DNA adduct is an exposure biomarker since it is the product of the interaction of a particular chemical with DNA, and therefore it provides the measure of a biologically active dose. At the same time, by being directly linked to mutagenic events, DNA adducts give an estimate of the biologic response (mutations). Another example of biomarkers falling at the boundaries of exposure and effect classification are measurements of cholinergic muscarinic receptors and acetylcholinesterase activity as indicators of exposure to organophosphorus insecticides. Decreases in the number of cholinergic muscarinic receptors and acetylcholinesterase activity reflect exposure levels (markers of exposure), but these biologic changes are also believed to be mechanistically involved in the observed neurotoxic effects of exposure to organophosphorus insecticides (markers of biologic effect) (5). Biomarkers of susceptibility can be defined as indicators signaling unusually high sensitivity to a toxic exposure. Biomarkers of susceptibility include measurements of activity of the enzymes involved in the metabolism of an exogenous compound or the cell's ability to efficiently repair DNA damage. Major steps in a continuum of biologic events occurring after exposure can be characterized by biomarkers of the initial exposure, internal dose (e.g., urinary or blood levels of a specific metabolite), biologically active dose (dose at the target site such as DNA or a receptor), early biologic effect (somatic mutations for carcinogens), and altered structure or function (abnormal cell growth) (Fig. 1).

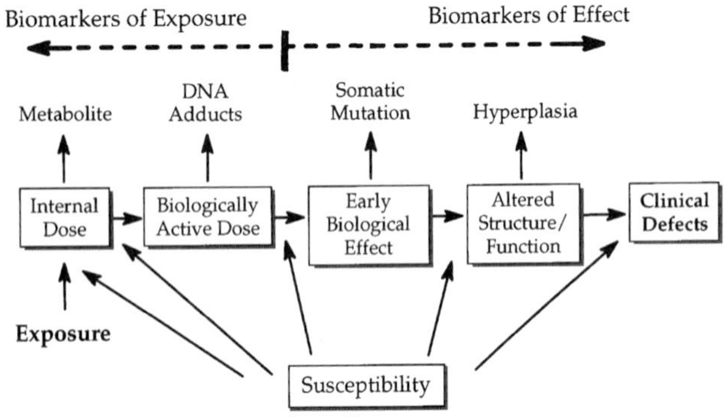


**FIG. 1.** Relationship between exposure and disease. (Adapted from ref. 4.)

The usefulness and limitations of exposure biomarkers reflecting different steps on the exposure-disease pathway can be illustrated by the example of biomonitoring human exposure to carcinogenic chromium (Cr) compounds. Humans are exposed to two major oxidative forms of Cr, Cr(III), and Cr(VI), with only Cr(VI) being toxic and carcinogenic. Toxicity of the Cr(VI) form results from its active accumulation in cells, while Cr(III) has a very low ability to enter cells. Inside the cells all of the Cr(VI) is reduced to Cr(III), and this reduction process is responsible for the induction of DNA damage. Biomonitoring of occupational exposure to Cr (VI) compounds is usually based on measurements of Cr in urine and serum. However, Cr(III) is an essential element, and its dietary levels in these biologic fluids can be high, masking low-level Cr(VI) exposures and leading to a large day-to-day variability. In addition, Cr is readily excreted or redistributed from serum, and therefore Cr measurements in the human serum or urine reflect relatively recent exposure and are useful primarily for heavy industrial exposures. Analysis of Cr in erythrocytes may be more informative by being indicative of exposure to carcinogenic Cr(VI) compounds. Unlike inorganic forms of Cr(III), Cr(VI) can readily enter erythrocytes where it is reduced, and it binds to hemoglobin (6,7). Cr-hemoglobin complexes are quite persistent, and therefore a single determination can potentially estimate cumulative Cr(VI) exposure going back in time. Internal dose measurements based on Cr levels in erythrocytes can provide rather good evidence of exposure to carcinogenic Cr(VI) compounds; however, they do not prove that toxicologic damage has occurred. It is known that Cr(III) can form very stable complexes with many cytoplasmic molecules precluding damage to DNA (8,9). In addition, intracellular metabolism of Cr(VI) and subsequently Cr accumulation kinetics in erythrocytes and nucleated cells were reported to be quite different since ascorbate plays a dominant role in Cr(VI) reduction in lymphocytes and tissue targets (10–12), whereas in erythrocytes glutathione is the most abundant reductant (13,14). Measurements of Cr-DNA adducts would be of significant importance, because they are direct products of damage to a critical genetic target and they are not influenced by dietary Cr(III). Determinations of Cr(VI)-induced DNA-protein cross-links, which are biomarkers of biologically active dose of Cr(VI), provided evidence of significant genetic damage occurring in human populations with what was previously thought to be low exposures to carcinogenic Cr(VI) (15–17).

## BIOMARKERS OF SUSCEPTIBILITY

The majority of carcinogenic chemicals require metabolic activation for the induction of biologic effects. Many organic chemicals can be converted into reactive electrophilic metabolites by the oxidative (phase I) enzymes, which are predominantly cytochrome P-450 (CYPs) enzymes. Phase-II conjugating enzymes such as glutathione-S-transferases (GST), uracil diphosphate (UDP)-glucuronosyltransferases, and N-acetyltransferases (NAT) are considered detoxifying enzymes. A large number of genes encoding phase I and II enzymes have been cloned (18). Development of relatively simple polymerase chain reaction (PCR)-based assays has enabled identification of the allelic variants or genetic defects for a variety of metabolic polymorphisms.

Differences in human susceptibility to lung and urinary bladder cancer have frequently been ascribed to genetic polymorphism in enzymes responsible for metabolizing such potent carcinogens as aromatic amines and polycyclic aromatic hydrocarbons. Cytochrome P-450–dependent oxidation of PAHs leads to the formation of very reactive intermediates that interact with DNA, producing promutagenic adducts. The acetyltransferases, NAT1 and NAT2, participate in the metabolism of aromatic amines by catalyzing detoxification (N-acetylation) or activation (O-acetylation) reactions. Polymorphisms in both NAT1 and NAT2 genes have been shown to be associated with higher risk for bladder cancer. Several epidemiologic studies indicate that NAT2-dependent slow N-acetylation increases bladder cancer risk among workers exposed to aromatic amines (19,20). Slow acetylators exposed to aromatic amines had also higher levels of 4-aminobiphenyl adducts (21,22). The presence of the NAT1*10 genotype and phenotype has also been found to correlate significantly with higher levels of bladder DNA adducts attributable to reactions with aromatic amines (20). Many studies have also observed a significantly increased risk of bladder cancer associated with the lack of the GSTM1 gene (23–25). In agreement with these findings, smokers with the GSTM1 null genotype were found to have several times more mutagenic urine than smokers with the functional gene (26). A significant association has also been found between cigarette smoke–induced lung cancer, levels of DNA adducts in human lung tissue and genetic polymorphism in CYP1A1, CYP2D6, and GSTM1 genes (27–29).

Despite quite interesting findings reported over recent years concerning associations of specific genotypes in phase I and II enzymes and cancer risk, given the number of carcinogen-metabolizing enzymes already identified and the degree of variability in their expression and polymorphism, assessment of a single enzyme or genotype may not be sufficient. Several studies were conducted in an attempt to correlate cancer risk and polymorphism in both CYP1A1 and GSTM1 genes. In one such study on Japanese individuals with squamous cell lung carcinoma, subjects with the CYP1A1 Msp genotype combined with deficient GSTM1 were at a remarkably high cancer risk with an odds ratio of 16 (30). The risk of developing the carcinoma was even higher in individuals who had other susceptible genotype CYP1A1 (Val/Val) combined with GSTM1 null genotype (odds ratio 41.0).

In addition to the importance of carcinogen-metabolizing enzymes, cellular repair capabilities can also play a significant role in predisposition to cancer development. Wei et al. (31) reported that patients with reduced DNA repair capacities and overexposure to sunlight had approximately fivefold elevated risk of basal cell carcinoma than the control group. This risk was even greater (tenfold) in female subjects. In a case-control study on lung cancer, individuals with reduced DNA repair activity were also found to be at an increased risk of developing cancer (32). Considering a large variety of physiologic factors (activating and detoxifying enzymes, DNA repair, etc.) capable of influencing genotoxic outcome in response to carcinogen exposures, a new approach has been taken in several studies aiming at integrating all these variables in one assay. This approach is often termed mutagen sensitivity or mutagen susceptibility assay. For most carcinogens, carcinogenic activity results from adduction of DNA, chromosomal damage, and, subsequently, induction of mutations. Based on mechanistic connection between DNA damage and cancer induction, several investigators sought to compare cancer risk and DNA damage measurements in lymphocytes following *in vitro* exposure to a carcinogen of interest. The two most common genotoxic end points in this type of studies are DNA adducts and chromosomal aberrations. The *in vitro* mutagen sensitivity based on measurements of chromosomal damage was found to be a good biomarker of genetic susceptibility to head and neck squamous cell carcinoma (33), oral cancer (34,35), lung cancer (36,37), and medullary thyroid carcinomas (38). Enhanced formation of DNA adducts in blood lymphocytes following *in vitro* exposure to a tobacco smoke carcinogen benzo[a]-pyrene was also reported to be associated with higher risk for lung cancer (39–41).

## CHARACTERIZATION OF BIOMARKERS

Prior to its application to study human exposure to toxic agents, a number of technical characteristics of a biomarker must be known. The sensitivity and specificity of a biomarker assay, as well as periods of a past exposure integrated in the biomarker response are the primary parameters that must be considered. Practical applications of a biomarker depend significantly on whether the biomarker assay reflects a very recent exposure or integrates exposures over a prolonged period of time. Toxicant-induced adverse health effects usually develop following chronic exposures over years, and therefore biomarkers that provide an estimate of cumulative dose over extended periods of time are the most useful. The ability of a biomarker assay to integrate past exposures can be tested in chronic exposures and by analyzing biomarker levels following cessation of exposure. To have practical utility, a biomarker assay should be sensitive enough to detect low levels of exposures typically experienced by human populations. The applicability of a biologic test is dependent on its signal-to-noise ratio. A biomarker assay with a high signal-to-noise ratio is considered a good assay. Sensitivity and accuracy of a biomarker assay can be determined in laboratory experiments with spiked samples or cells exposed to known amounts of a chemical of interest. Additionally, animal exposures can be performed to determine detection limits and a linear range of response in *in vivo* situations. In cases when a chemical has more than one metabolizing pathway, responsiveness of individual metabolites at different levels of exposure should also be clarified. Relative yields of different metabolites can vary significantly as a function of dose.

The specificity of a biomarker is a very important characteristic, particularly for biomarkers of exposure. The specificity of a biomarker assay can be defined as the ability to detect exposure only to a single agent. Some examples of biomarkers of different specificity are given in Table 1. Not all biomarkers can be expected to be chemically specific. Typically, biomarkers of exposure are the most specific, while biomarkers of effect are the least specific. Effect biomarkers usually measure biologic responses that occur at some time after exposure and in most cases a given response can be affected by many different agents whose pathogenic pathways converge at this end point. Chromosomal aberrations repre-

**TABLE 1.** *Examples of biomarkers with different agent-specificity*

| Specificity | Biomarkers | Exposure |
|---|---|---|
| Low | Sister chromatid exchanges and chromosomal aberrations in peripheral lymphocytes | Clastogens |
| | Micronuclei in buccal cells | Clastogens |
| | 8-oxo dG in urine or lymphocytic DNA | Radiation and many chemicals |
| | *N*-acetyl-β-D-glucosaminidase in urine | Nephrotoxic agents |
| | Mutagenesis at HPRT locus in lymphocytes or glycophoryn A in erythrocytes | Mutagens |
| | Urinary malondialdehyde | Agents causing lipid peroxidation |
| Intermediate | Serum or urinary chromium | Toxic and dietary forms of chromium |
| | Urinary nitrosoproline | Nitrosamines |
| | Immunoassay for PAH-DNA adducts 1-hydroxypyrene in urine | PAH compounds |
| | Cholinergic muscarinic receptors or acetylcholinesterase activity | Organophosphorus insecticides |
| High | Original substance in biologic specimens | For example, cadmium |
| | Substance-specific metabolite | For example, S-phenylmercapturic acid for benzene |
| | Chemical-specific DNA or protein adducts | For example, styrene-hemoglobin for styrene exposure |
| | Biologic response characteristic of specific exposure | δ-Aminolevulinic acid in urine (lead exposure)<br>Urinary porphyrins profiles (mercury exposure) |

sent a widely used biomarker of genotoxic exposures that has a low level of agent specificity. Chromosomal damage can be induced by many industrial and environmental pollutants, radiation, drugs, and lifestyle factors. As a disease biomarker, however, chromosomal aberrations are quite good, having a significant predictive value as the cancer risk factor (42).

Another factor in practical use of biomarkers is a low and consistent background level of the biomarker response in nonexposed population. The consistency of measurements remains an important consideration since thus far biomarkers are typically used to assess populations rather than individuals. A low interindividual variability in biomarker values allows detection of exposure using a small group of individuals. Tight variance in biomarker measurements among control unexposed subjects may also suggest that the biomarker is not strongly affected by some unknown factors associated with, for example, diet or lifestyle. To properly design human studies, a minimal sample size required to detect meaningful increases in the biomarker response should be known. Sensitivity and low interindividual variability are the most important parameters influencing the statistical power of a biomarker. A biomarker assay that requires either a very large number of samples or a highly exposed population cannot have practical utility in assessing human exposures. A recent article by Taioli et al. (43) provides a general strategy and useful examples as to how variability of biomarkers can be estimated, and offers an equation to calculate the minimal sample size. It appears that DNA adduct–based assays require manageable sample sizes, while gene expression biomarkers exhibit very large variability among unexposed individuals and require much larger populations.

Interindividual variability in biomarker measurements among subjects with similar levels of exposure should not be viewed only as a limitation in assessing toxicant's exposures. This person-to-person variation, however, may provide a valuable opportunity to reveal subgroups with higher risk for a specific disease. Biomarkers of genetic damage such as DNA adducts integrate absorbed dose, metabolism, and DNA repair capabilities, and therefore levels of these markers should be expected to better reflect individual risks than the assessment of external exposure. In the instance of DNA adducts, even detection of carcinogen-specific DNA adducts in human populations per se may have important public health implications since formation of premutagenic DNA lesions is generally accepted to be a critical step in the initiation of cancer.

The majority of biomarkers exhibit certain background levels even among persons with no documented exposure to a specific chemical. Baseline measurements among unexposed individuals of some biomarker assays simply reflect nonspecific background noise for a particular methodology. Immunoassays are typical examples of biomarkers of this type. For other assays, biomarker values among unexposed subjects represent true measurements of an agent-specific exposure, as evidenced, for example, by a distinct and characteristic spot on thin-layer chromatography (TLC) plates. Ambient exposure to low levels of toxic chemicals is believed to be responsible for induction of background values for these specific biomarkers. Biomarkers of effect are usually biologic assays, and their background responses can be influenced by endogenous factors. For example, the frequency of mutagenic events in the hypoxanthine phosphoribosyltransferase (HPRT) assay or the number of chromosomal aberrations can be affected by levels of endogenously produced active oxygen species and individual characteristics of DNA repair.

## VALIDATION OF BIOMARKERS

Validation of exposure biomarkers typically involves assessment of their ability to correctly measure a specific exposure. Validation studies of this type must prove that there is a quantitative relationship between a dose and a biomarker level under *in vivo* exposure conditions. Biomarker responses must be observed at exposure levels experienced by humans in environmental or industrial settings. Initial validation can be performed in experimental animals followed by confirmative studies in human populations exposed to different levels of a chemical of interest. Examples of validation studies of exposure biomarkers in animals are the food carcinogens 2-amino-1-methyl-6-phenylimidazol[4,5-b]pyridine (44) and aflatoxins (45,46). In the first study, a linear dose-response relationship was observed for urinary excretion of unmetabolized 2-amino-1-methyl-6-phenylimidazol[4,5-b]pyridine across the entire range of doses, including a dose comparable with known human dietary exposure (44). The excellent dose-response relationship and relevance of doses to human exposures provided validation of the urinary measurements as exposure biomarker. Groopman et al. (46) performed validation of urinary aflatoxin biomarkers in rats exposed to aflatoxin B1. The linear relationship between aflatoxin B1 dose and the excretion of the major DNA adduct, aflatoxin-$N^7$-guanine, was observed. Other oxidative metabolites of aflatoxin B1 did not exhibit linear excretion characteristics. Validity of aflatoxin-albumin adducts as exposure biomarkers was examined by Anwar et al. (45), who found a linear correlation between dose and the levels of aflatoxin-albumin in rats. Interestingly, unlike rats, mice are known to be resistant to hepatocarcinogenic effects of aflatoxins, and aflatoxin-exposed mice showed very low levels of albumin adducts. The usefulness of aflatoxin-$N^7$-guanine measurements in human biomonitoring was confirmed in studies on urinary metabolites in residents of China with a high intake of aflatoxins (47). An immunoaffinity–high-performance liquid chromatography (HPLC) analysis of 24-hour urine samples detected aflatoxin-$N^7$-guanine and aflatoxins M1, P1, and B1. Only aflatoxin-$N^7$-guanine and aflatoxin M1 showed a good correlation with aflatoxin intake. It is noteworthy that the kinetics of formation and urinary excretion of aflatoxin-$N^7$-guanine was very similar in rats and humans (46,47). Pharmacokinetics and metabolism of many other xenobiotics in experimental animals, however, are not always that close to humans.

Development of biologic markers of exposure to benzene based on measurements of blood protein adducts exemplifies the importance of validation studies in exposed human populations. Results of animal experiments on metabolism of benzene revealed formation of a reactive intermediate that binds to cysteine in hemoglobin producing the S-phenylcysteine adduct (48,49). This suggested that S-phenylcysteine adducts of hemoglobin might be applied to human biomonitoring of benzene exposure. However, in occupational studies with levels of exposure as high as 28 ppm benzene, the presence of S-phenylcysteine adducts in human hemoglobin was not detected (49). In contrast, analysis of benzene-albumin adducts in exposed workers revealed a linear dose-response curve (50). Significant differences between rodents and humans were also observed in the metabolism of butadiene based on measurements of urinary metabolites (51). It should be noted that in many situations even for a very good valid biomarker, there may not be a strong correlation of biomarker levels to external exposure data. Exposures from different sources and routes (known and unknown), temporal variability of ambient measurements, and individual characteristics are likely to make external exposure assessments not very accurate.

Effect biomarkers are usually validated by their ability to predict human disease. This can be accomplished in prospective epidemiologic studies by determining biomarkers among an exposed population and comparing these measurements with subsequent disease risk. The major problem with this approach is that it will require a very large population size and a long time to register subsequent health outcome (20 to 30 years for exposures to carcinogens). Until now, only one study of this type has been performed in which chromosomal damage in peripheral lymphocytes was evaluated as a predictor of human cancer risk (42). In this prospective Nordic cohort study, frequency of chromosomal aberrations, sister chromatid exchanges, and micronuclei were determined in lymphocytes of adults with known histories of exposures and were compared to the subsequent cancer outcome. There was no significant association between cancer risk and frequency of sister chromatid exchanges or micronuclei. In contrast, chromosomal aberrations exhibited a statistically significant linear correlation with subsequent cancer risk. A less rigorous approach to the evaluation of biomarkers as a predictor of adverse health effects might be conducted by comparing levels of a biomarker among healthy individuals and those who developed a specific disease. A strong association was found, for example, between levels of DNA adducts and colorectal (52) and lung cancers (53). A major concern with this validation approach is the possibility that disease itself may somehow affect a biomarker of interest.

Adverse health effects caused by exposure to toxic substances can sometimes be modified via chemopreventive interventions. Applying a chemopreventive agent to attenuate health risk and measuring a specific biomarker provide a useful experimental approach to evaluate the relationship between a biomarker and health outcome in animals. Oltipraz is a potent inhibitor of aflatoxin-induced tumorigenesis in rats (54). Studies were performed to examine the impact of oltipraz on levels of serum aflatoxin-albumin, aflatoxin-$N^7$-guanine in urine, and DNA adducts in liver (55,56). Administration of the chemopreventive compound oltipraz reduced total levels of hepatic aflatoxin–DNA adducts and the urinary excretion of aflatoxin-$N^7$-guanine by 76% and 62%, respectively. The intervention with oltipraz in aflatoxin-fed animals produced a similar decrease in binding of aflatoxin to albumin (57). Thus, results of these intervention studies strongly indicated usefulness (validity) of measurements of the excreted aflatoxin–DNA adduct and the aflatoxin-albumin levels since these biomarkers accurately reflected the extent of genotoxic damage in the target tissue (liver) and were directly related to the cancer risk. The administration of *N*-acetylcysteine, a cancer chemopreventive agent, was also reported to considerably reduce several biomarker responses induced by a polycyclic aromatic hydrocarbon fraction obtained from urban particulates (58). As an indirect approach to assess a predictive value of a new biomarker, an examination of its relationship with another valid biomarker can be applied. With carcinogenic compounds, comparative studies can be conducted correlating a biomarker with chromosomal aberrations (DNA damage end points) to assess cancer risk (42). Several biomarkers of exposure to carcinogens were evaluated using this approach (45,59–64).

## BIOLOGIC SAMPLES

Table 2 lists common biologic specimens that are currently used for measurements of biologic markers. Biologic materials collected by invasive techniques are not suitable for routine biologic monitoring, but analysis of chemical-specific responses in internal organs provides valuable information in relationship to biomarker measurements in easily available surrogate tissues. The extent and frequency of use of different specimens varies substantially and is influenced by such factors as the amount of material obtained, relevance to route or targets of exposure, ability to provide an estimate of internal dose, and availability of critical macromolecular targets in the sample. For example, tooth tissue does not react with organic chemicals and it is not a good source of DNA or protein,

**TABLE 2.** *Biologic materials that are used to measure biomarkers*

| | |
|---|---|
| Noninvasive sampling | |
| | Expired air |
| | Breast milk |
| | Semen |
| | Urine |
| | Fingernails |
| | Nasal lavage |
| | Saliva |
| | Hair |
| | Deciduous teeth |
| | Sputum |
| Minimally invasive sampling | |
| | Blood |
| | Nasal epithelium |
| | Buccal cells |
| | Bronchoalveolar lavage |
| Invasive sampling | |
| | Amniotic fluid |
| | Lung tissue |
| | Bone marrow |
| | Adipose tissue |
| | Liver tissue |
| | Bone |

but because of their mineralous nature, teeth are used to measure biomarkers related to metal exposures and microelement intake. Measurements of lead levels in deciduous teeth can estimate a cumulative dose of this toxic metal over extended periods of time (65,66). Determinations of biomarkers in nasal lavage can only provide a short-term measure of exposures to reactive chemicals via inhalation. Exposure to reactive $SO_2$ can be estimated by quantitation of S-sulfonates in nasal lavage, but this biomarker was found to measure exposure occurring only within 24 hours (67). Overall, among all biomaterials blood and urine are the most frequently collected for the purpose of biomarker determinations. The major advantage of these two types of biologic specimens is the ability of urinary and blood biomarkers to reflect internal dose for most chemicals.

Blood biomarkers are a heterogeneous group of biologic measurements that includes detection of an unmodified original chemical, a chemical-specific metabolite, modifications of proteins and DNA, and serum and intracellular measurements. Blood contains large quantities of hemoglobin and albumin, and these proteins can be easily isolated in pure form. Carboxyl, amino, and sulfhydryl groups are the typical sites of adduction by electrophilic compounds. Many protein adducts are stable under physiologic conditions, and this provides an opportunity to assess cumulative exposure over extended time since the life span of human hemoglobin is approximately 120 days. Biologic half-life of albumin adducts is shorter than that of hemoglobin due to a faster metabolic turnover of albumin (68). Measurements of aflatoxin-albumin adducts are reported to give an estimate of aflatoxin exposure over the past 2 to 3 months (62). Protein adducts are surrogate biomarkers that are not mechanistically involved in the pathway leading to disease, but they can be useful as predictive tools as long as the relationship between surrogate and mechanistic biomarkers is known. It is assumed that detection of agent-specific protein adducts can signal occurrence of reactive electrophilic substances that are capable of inflicting damage to target tissues and molecules such as DNA. Liu et al. (69) conducted exposure assessment of trinitrotoluene-exposed workers comparing external levels, hemoglobin adducts, and the prevalence of cataract. They found that levels of trinitrotoluene-hemoglobin adducts significantly correlated not only with the external concentrations but also with the incidence of cataract and the degree of lenticular damage. Meier and Warshawsky (70) analyzed the relationship between hemoglobin and DNA adducts in mice exposed to 7H-dibenzo[*c,g*] carbazole. Liver DNA had the highest level of adducts among all tissues studied, and the extent of liver DNA adduction was proportional to 7H-dibenzo[*c,g*] carbazole-hemoglobin adduct formation. Studies on albumin adducts of hepatocarcinogen aflatoxin B1 demonstrated usefulness of these measurements as evidenced by strong correlation with cytogenetic damage and sensitivity to the hepatocarcinogenic action of aflatoxin B1 (44).

Peripheral blood lymphocytes are the most frequently used cells to assess biomarkers related to potential genotoxic exposures. Certain important characteristics of lymphocytes make them useful to serve as the surrogate tissue for measurements of biologic effects in target tissue. Lymphocytes contain DNA and circulate throughout the human body, and therefore they are exposed to any circulating genotoxic agent or its metabolites. These cells can integrate exposure over extended time intervals since they are long-lived (up to several years) (71) and do not divide *in vivo*. Many *in vitro* studies found that unstimulated lymphocytes have inefficient DNA repair capabilities (72,73), permitting these cells to accumulate detectable DNA damage even from very low exposures. Lymphocytes are also capable of metabolizing many important xenobiotics such as PAHs to DNA-reactive species (74). In addition, lymphocytes are easy to obtain in large quantities from a blood sample. Total leukocyte population of cells can also be used to estimate DNA markers; however, the relatively short-lived granulocytes that constitute 60% to 70% of total leukocytes might not always accumulate detectable levels of DNA damage (75). While lymphocytes may be appropriate tissue to assess risk of hematopoietic cancers, they represent surrogate cells for the assessment of most exposures, and it is very important to determine that quantitative relationships exist between the levels of markers in lymphocytes and tissue targets.

Many studies compared levels of DNA adducts in lymphocytes and tissue targets. In several cases a good correlation between lymphocytic and target tissue adducts was indeed found. For example, Bianchini and Wild (76) performed a comparative analysis of dose-response relationships between exposure to four methylating carcinogens and levels of 7-methylguanine in white blood cells and in cancer target organs. Strong correlation was found between the presence of the DNA adducts in white blood cells and liver for all carcinogens studied. Animal studies on DNA adduct levels of benzo[*a*]pyrene, a typical representative of carcinogenic PAH, also revealed a very good correlation between leukocytic adducts and those in internal organs (77). Significant support for usefulness of adduct measurements in white blood cells to estimate adducts in target tissues was found in human studies comparing DNA damage in lymphocytes and tumors or tissues surrounding the tumor. Several such studies were carried out on cancers related to tobacco smoking. Szyfter and colleagues (78) analyzed smoking-originating aromatic DNA adducts in leukocytes, larynx tumor, and adjacent normal tissues by means of $^{32}$P-labeling assay. The presence of aromatic DNA adducts was detected in all tissue samples obtained after surgery of larynx tumors. The highest number of DNA adducts was observed in larynx tumor samples, and the levels of DNA adducts in larynx (tumor and nontumor) tissues correlated very strongly with those in leukocytes. In another study DNA adducts originated from interactions with hydrophobic aromatic hydrocarbons were examined in lung tissues and lymphocytes obtained from lung cancer patients (79). Total levels of lymphocytic adducts were found to exhibit a linear correlation with total lung adducts. In addition, adduct levels in both tissues decayed at similar rates following smoking cessation. Strong correlation between aromatic DNA adducts in leukocytes and adducts in lung tumor and nontumor tissues was also found by other investigators (53). Usefulness of DNA damage measurements in lymphocytes for other classes of chemicals might not be as good as in the abovementioned examples.

Measurements of biomarkers in urine samples generally reflect recent exposures and are useful largely for assessing accidental overexposures or highly exposed industrial workers. Analysis of spot urinary samples is performed to estimate exposures in populations, whereas individual exposures are more reliably assessed in 24-hour collections. Urinary biomarker measurements are always corrected for a dilution factor by normalizing all determinations for a creatinine content. Typical analysis of urine samples for detection of chemical exposure involves measurement of an original substance or its metabolite. Examples of such determinations are numerous, and these biomarkers can be successfully employed to assess recent exposures by providing measures of internal dose. A substantially smaller group of urinary bioassays can also estimate a biologically effective dose. Exposure to a majority of carcinogens results in the formation of DNA adducts that later can be excised by cell repair systems. For some chemicals, excised adducts are then excreted in urine, and determinations of these adducts can provide a measure of biologically effective doses. There are two well-characterized biomarkers based on measurements of urinary DNA adducts. Urinary excretion of aflatoxin-N$^7$-guanine has been shown to be a good biomarker of aflatoxin exposure in humans and experimental animals as evidenced by strong correlations with aflatoxin intake, DNA adducts in liver, and hepatocarcinogenesis (47,55,56). Exposure to many chemicals is also known to lead to chemical-nonspecific oxidative DNA damage. Among numerous oxidative DNA lesions, premutagenic 8-oxodeoxyguanosine (8-oxodG) is formed in relatively large amounts and this adduct can be measured with high sensitivity by HPLC with electrochemical detection. Many studies were performed utilizing measurements of the urinary excretion of 8-oxodG as a noninvasive biomarker of oxidative DNA damage in humans (80).

Some urinary determinations can be considered biomarkers of altered tissue function. Measurements of urinary excretion of kidney-specific proteins is a standard approach to assess possible nephrotoxic effects of chemical exposures. Examples of such urinary analyses include determinations of *N*-acetyl-β-D-glucosaminidase, β-glucuronidase, and retinol-binding protein. Biologic markers of this type are typically agent-nonspecific. In case of mercury exposure, however, there seems to be a very specific metabolic response in the kidney, resulting in a characteristic pattern of urinary porphyrin excretion (81). Mercury selectively changes porphyrin metabolism in kidney proximal tubule cells, leading to elevated excretion of 4- and 5-carboxyl porphyrins and the appearance of an atypical precoproporphyrin. Using analysis of urinary porphyrin profiles among dentists, a strong correlation was found between the porphyrin assay and the internal dose of mercury (81).

Exposure to many chemical carcinogens leads to elevated incidence of bladder cancer. One of the very promising approaches to estimate biologically active doses of bladder carcinogens is to analyze DNA damage in exfoliated bladder cells, which can be obtained from urine. The life span of urinary bladder cells is estimated to be about 100 days (82), and there are sufficient numbers of recoverable cells to conduct analysis of DNA adducts and chromosomal damage. The most frequently applied genotoxicity test performed on exfoliated urinary bladder cells is the micronuclei assay. Micronuclei observed in exfoliated cells reflect DNA damage inflicted on basal epithelium cells by mutagens. For example, a positive correlation was found between increased micronuclei and ingestion of arsenic, a known bladder carcinogen (83,84). Measurements of tobacco-related DNA adducts in exfoliated urothelial cells was shown to be related to smoking history, urinary mutagenicity, and levels of 4-aminobiphenyl-hemoglobin adducts (85).

Detection of DNA adducts in exfoliated urothelial cells was also successfully applied to assess human exposures to the bladder carcinogen benzidine (86).

## REFERENCES


1. Samet JM, Lerchen ML. Proportion of lung cancer caused by occupation: a critical review. In: Gee L, Morgan KC, Brooks SM, eds. *Occupational lung disease.* New York: Raven Press, 1984;55–65.
2. Rothman N, Correa-Villasenour A, Ford DP, et al. Contribution of occupation and diet to white blood cell polycyclic aromatic hydrocarbon-DNA adducts in wildland firefighters. *Cancer Epidemiol Biomarkers Prevent* 1993;2:341–348.
3. Elovaara E, Heikkila P, Pyy L, Mutanen P, Riihimaki V. Significance of dermal respiratory uptake in creosote workers: exposure to polycyclic aromatic hydrocarbons and urinary excretion of 1-hydroxypyrene. *Occup Environ Med* 1995;52:196–203.
4. National Research Council Committee on Biological Markers. Biological markers in environmental health research. *Environ Health Perspect* 1987;74:3–9.
5. Fitzgerald BB, Costa LG. Modulation of muscarinic receptors and acetylcholinesterase activity in lymphocytes and in brain areas following repeated organophosphate exposure in rats. *Fundam Appl Toxicol* 1993;20:210–216.
6. Lewalter J, Korallus U, Weidemann H. Chromium bond detection in isolated erythrocytes: a new principle of biological monitoring of exposure to hexavalent chromium. *Int Arch Occup Environ Health* 1985;55:305–318.
7. Merritt K, Brown SA. Release of hexavalent chromium from corrosion of stainless steel and cobalt-chromium alloys. *J Biomed Mater Res* 1995;29:627–633.
8. Denniston ML, Uyeki EM. Distribution and HPLC study of chromium-51 binding sites in Chinese hamster ovary cells. *J Toxicol Environ Health* 1987;21:375–386.
9. Hneihen A, Standeven AM, Wetterhahn, KE. Differential binding of chromium (VI) and chromium (III) complexes to salmon sperm nuclei and nuclear DNA and isolated calf thymus DNA. *Carcinogenesis* 1993; 14:1795–1803.
10. Bergsten P, Amitai G, Kehrl J, Dhariwal KR, Klein HG, Leveine M. Millimolar concentrations of ascorbic acid in purified human mononuclear leucocytes. *J Biol Chem* 1989;265:25–84.
11. Suzuki Y, Fukuda K. Reduction of hexavalent chromium by ascorbic acid and glutathione with special reference to the rat lung. *Arch Toxicol* 1990;64:169–176.
12. Standeven AM, Wetterhahn KE. Ascorbate is a principal reductant of Cr(VI) in rat liver and kidney ultrafiltrates. *Carcinogenesis* 1991;12: 1733–1737.
13. Aaseth J, Alexander J Norseth T. Uptake of $^{51}$Cr-chromate by human erythrocytes—a role of glutathione. *Acta Pharmacol Toxicol* 1982;50: 310–315.
14. Vinson, JA, Staretz, ME, Bose, P, Kassm, HM, Basalyga ME. *in vitro* and *in vivo* reduction of erythrocyte sorbitol by ascorbic acid. *Diabetes* 1989;38:1036–1041.
15. Costa M, Zhitkovich A, Toniolo P. DNA-protein crosslinks in welders: molecular implications. *Cancer Res* 1993;53:460–463.
16. Taioli E, Zhitkovich A, Kinney P, Udasin I, Toniolo P, Costa M. Increased DNA-protein crosslinks in lymphocytes of residents living in chromium contaminated areas. *Biol Trace Element Res* 1995;50:175–180.
17. Zhitkovich A, Lukanova A, Popov T, Taioli E, Cohen H, Costa M, Toniolo P. DNA-protein crosslinks in peripheral lymphocytes of individuals exposed to hexavalent chromium compounds. *Biomarkers* 1996;1:86–93.
18. Nelson DR, Kamataki T, Waxman DJ, et al. The P450 superfamily: update on new sequences, gene mapping, accession Nos., early trivial names of enzymes, and nomenclature. *DNA Cell Biol* 1993;12:1–51.
19. Risch A, Wallace DM, Bathers S, Sim E. Slow N-acetylation is a susceptibility factor in occupational and smoking related bladder cancer. *Hum Mol Genet* 1995; 4:231–236.
20. Kadlubar FF, Badawi AF. Genetic susceptibility and carcinogen-DNA adduct formation in human urinary bladder carcinogenesis. *Toxicol Lett* 1995;82–83:627–632.
21. Vineis P, Caporaso N, Tannenbaum SR, et al. Acetylation phenotype, carcinogen-hemoglobin adducts and cigarette smoking. Cancer Res 1990;50:3002–3004.
22. Yu MC, Skipper PL, Taghizadeh K, et al. Acetylator phenotype, aminobiphenyl-hemoglobin adduct levels, and bladder cancer risk in white, black, and Asian men in Los Angeles, California. *J Natl Cancer Inst* 1994;86:712–716.
23. Bell DA, Taylor JA, Paulson D, Robertson CN, Mohler JL, Lucier GW. Genetic risk and carcinogen exposure: a common inherited defect of the carcinogen metabolism gene glutathione transferase (GSTM1) increases susceptibility to bladder cancer. *J Natl Cancer Inst* 1993;85: 1159–1164.
24. Daly AK, Thomas DJ, Cooper J, Pearson WR, Neal DE, Idle JR. Homozygous deletion of gene for glutathione S-transferase M1 in bladder cancer. *Br Med J* 1993;307:481–482.
25. Katoh T, Inatomi H, Nagaoka A, Sugita A. Cytochrome P4501A1 gene polymorphism and homozygous deletion of the glutathione S-transferase M1 gene in urothelial cancer patients. *Carcinogenesis* 1995;16: 655–657.
26. Hirvonen A, Nylund L, Kociba P, Husgafvel-Pursiainen K, Vainio H. Modulation of urinary mutagenicity by genetically determined carcinogen metabolism in smokers. *Carcinogenesis* 1994;15:813–815.
27. Hirvonen A. Genetic factors in individual responses to environmental exposures. *J Occup Environ Med* 1995;37:37–43.
28. Kato S, Bowman ED, Harrington AM, Blomeke B, Schields PG. Human lung carcinogen-DNA adduct levels mediated by genetic polymorphisms *in vivo*. *J Natl Cancer Inst* 1995;87:902–907.
29. Nebert DW, McKinnon RA, Puga A. Human drug-metabolizing enzyme polymorphisms: effect on risk of toxicity and cancer. *DNA Cell Biol* 1996;15: 273–280.
30. Nakachi K, Imai K, Hayashi S, Kawajiri K. Polymorphisms of the CYP1A1 and glutathione S-transferase genes associated with susceptibility to lung cancer in relation to cigarette dose in a Japanese population. *Cancer Res* 1993;53:2994–2999.
31. Wei Q, Matanoski GM, Farmer ER, Hedayati MA, Grossman L. DNA repair and aging in basal cell carcinoma: a molecular epidemiology study. *Proc Natl Acad Sci USA* 1993;90:1614–1618.
32. Wei Q, Cheng L, Hong WK, Spitz MR. Reduced DNA repair capacity in lung cancer patients. *Cancer Res* 1996; 56:4103–4107.
33. Cloos J, Spitz MR, Scantz SP, et al. Genetic susceptibility to head and neck squamous cell carcinoma. *J Natl Cancer Inst* 1996;88:530–535.
34. Ankathil R, Bhattathiri NV, Francis JV, et al. Mutagen sensitivity as a predisposing factor in familial oral cancer. *Int J Cancer* 1996;69:265–267.
35. Trivedi AH, Bakshi SR, Jaju RJ, et al. Elevated mutagen susceptibility in cultured lymphocytes of oral cancer patients. *Anticancer Res* 1995; 15:2589–2592.
36. Wei Q, Gu J, Cheng L, et al. Benzo[*a*]pyrene diol epoxide-induced chromosomal aberrations and risk of lung cancer. *Cancer Res* 1996;56: 3975–3979.
37. Spitz MR, Hsu TC, Wu X, Fueger JJ, Amos CI, Roth JA. Mutagen sensitivity as a biological marker of lung cancer risk in African Americans. *Cancer Epidemiol Biomarkers Prevent* 1995;4:99–103.
38. Hsu TC, Cherry LM, Samaan NA. Differential mutagen susceptibility in cultured lymphocytes of normal individuals and cancer patients. *Cancer Genet Cytogen* 1985;17:307–313.
39. Rudiger HW, Nowak D, Hartmann K, Cerutti P. Enhanced formation of benzo[a]pyrene:DNA adducts in monocytes of patients with a presumed predisposition to lung cancer. *Cancer Res* 1985;45:5890–5894.
40. Li D, Wang M, Cheng L, Spitz MR, Hittelman WH, Wei Q. *in vitro* induction of benzo[a]pyrene diol epoxide-DNA adducts in peripheral lymphocytes as a susceptibility marker for human lung cancer. *Cancer Res* 1996;56:3638–3641.
41. Nowak D, Meyer A, Schmidt-Preuss U, Gatzemeir U, Magnussen H, Rudiger HW. Formation of benzo[a]pyrene-DNA adducts in blood monocytes from lung cancer patients with a familial history of lung cancer. *J Cancer Res Clin Oncol* 1992;118:67–71.
42. Hagmar L, Brogger A, Hansteen IL, et al. Cancer risk in humans predicted by increased levels of chromosomal aberrations in lymphocytes: Nordic study group on the health risk of chromosome damage. *Cancer Res* 1994;54:2919–2922.
43. Taioli E, Kinney P, Zhitkovich A, et al. Application of reliability models to studies of biomarker validation. *Environ Health Perspect* 1994; 102:306–309.
44. Friesen MD, Cummings DA, Garren L, Butler R, Bartsch H, Schut HAJ. Validation in rats of two biomarkers of exposure to the food-

borne carcinogen 2-amino-1-methyl-6-phenylimidazol[4,5-b]pyridine (PhIP): PhIP-DNA adducts and urinary PhIP. *Carcinogenesis* 1996;17:67–72.
45. Anwar WA, Khali MM, Wild CP. Micronuclei, chromosomal aberrations and aflatoxin-albumin adducts in experimental animals after exposure to aflatoxin B1. *Mutat Res* 1994;322:61–67.
46. Groopman JD, Hasler J, Trudel L, Pikul A, Donahue PR, Wogan GN. Molecular dosimetry in rat urine of aflatoxin-N7-guanine and other aflatoxin metabolites by multiple monoclonal antibody affinity chromatography and HPLC. *Cancer Res* 1992;52:267–274.
47. Groopman JD, Zhu J, Donahue PR, et al. Molecular dosimetry of urinary aflatoxin DNA adducts in people living in Guangxi Autonomous Region, People's Republic of China. *Cancer Res* 1992;52:45–51.
48. Sun JD, Medinsky MA, Birnbaum LS, Lucier G, Henderson RF. Benzene hemoglobin adducts in mice and rats: characterization of formation and physiological modeling. *Fundam Appl Toxicol* 1990;15: 468–475.
49. Bechtold WE, Sun JD, Birnbaum LS, et al. S-phenylcysteine formation in hemoglobin as a biological exposure index to benzene. *Arch Toxicol* 1992;66:303–309.
50. Bechtold WE, Willis JK, Sun JD, Griffith WC, Reddy TV. Biological markers of exposure to benzene: S-phenylcysteine in albumin. *Carcinogenesis* 1992;13:1217–1220.
51. Bechtold WE, Strunk MR, Chang IY, Ward JB Jr, Henderson RF. Species differences in urinary butadiene metabolites: comparisons of metabolite ratios between mice, rats, and humans. *Toxicol Appl Pharmacol* 1994;127:44–49.
52. Pfohl-Leszkowitz A, Grosse Y, Carriere V, et al. High levels of DNA adducts in human colon are associated with colorectal cancer. *Cancer Res* 1995;55:5611–5616.
53. Tang D, Santella RM, Blackwood AM, et al. A molecular epidemiological case-control study of lung cancer. *Cancer Epidemiol Biomarkers Prevent* 1995;4:341–346.
54. Roebuck BD, Liu Y-L, Rogers AE, Groopman JD, Kensler TW. Protection against aflatoxin B1-induced hepatocarcinogenesis in F344 rats by 5-(2-pyrazinyl)-4-methyl 1,2-dithiole-3-thione (oltipraz): predictive role for short-term molecular dosimetry. *Cancer Res* 1991;51: 5501–5506.
55. Kensler TW, Groopman JD, Eaton DL, Curphey TJ, Roebuck BD. Potent inhibition of aflatoxin-induced hepatic tumorigenesis by the monofunctional enzyme inducer 1,2-dithiole-3-thione. *Carcinogenesis* 1992;12:95–100.
56. Groopman JD, Egner P, Love-Hunt A, DeMatos P, Kensler TW. Molecular dosimetry of aflatoxin DNA and serum albumin adducts in chemoprotection studies using 1,2-dithiole-3-thione in rats. *Carcinogenesis* 1992;13:101–106.
57. Egner PA, Gange SJ, Dolan PM, Groopman JD, Munoz A, Kensler TW. Levels of aflatoxin-albumin biomarkers in rat plasma are modulated by both long-term and transient interventions with oltipraz. *Carcinogenesis* 1995;16:1769–1773.
58. Izzotti A, Camoirano A, D'Agostini F, et al. Biomarker alterations produced in rat lung by intratracheal instillations of air particulate extracts and chemoprevention with oral N-acetylcysteine. *Cancer Res* 1996;56: 1533–1538.
59. Anwar WA, Shamy MY. Chromosomal aberrations and micronuclei in reinforced plastics workers exposed to styrene. *Mutat Res* 1995;327: 41–47.
60. Sessink PJ, Cerna M, Rossner P, et al. Urinary cyclophosphamide excretion and chromosomal aberrations in peripheral blood lymphocytes after occupational exposure to antineoplastic agents. *Mutat Res* 1994;309:193–199.
61. Jelmert, O, Hansteen, I-L, Langard S. Chromosome damage in lymphocytes of stainless steel welders related to past and current exposure to manual arc welding fumes. *Mutat Res* 1994;320:223–233.
62. Miele M, Donato F, Hall AJ, et al. Aflatoxin exposure and cytogenetic alterations in individuals from the Gambia, West Africa. *Mutat Res* 1996;349:209–217.
63. Sorsa M, Peltonen K, Anderson D, Demopoulos NA, Neumann HG, Osterman-Golkar S. Assessment of environmental and occupational exposures to butadiene as a model for risk estimation of petrochemical emissions. *Mutagenesis* 1996;11:9–17.
64. Van Hammelen P, Severi W, Roosels D, Veulemans H, Kirsch-Volders M. Cytogenetic analysis of lymphocytes from fiberglass-reinforced plastics workers occupationally exposed to styrene. *Mutat Res* 1994;310:157–165.
65. Begerow J, Freier I, Turfeld M, Kramer U, Dunemann L. Internal lead and cadmium exposure in 6-year-old children from western and eastern Germany. *Int Arch Occup Environ Health* 1994;66:243–248.
66. McMichael AJ, Baghurst PA, Vimpani GV, Wigg NR, Robertson EF, Tong S. Tooth lead levels and IQ in school-age children: the Port Pirie Cohort Study. *Am J Epidemiol* 1994;140:489–499.
67. Bechtold WE, Weide JJ, Sandstrom T, et al. Biological markers of exposure to $SO_2$: S-sulfonates in nasal lavage. *J Expos Anal Environ Epidemiol* 1993;3:371–382.
68. DeBord DG, Swearengin TF, Cheever KL, Booth-Jones AD, Wissinger LA. Binding characteristics of ortho-toluidine to rat hemoglobin and albumin. *Arch Toxicol* 1992;66:231–236.
69. Liu YY, Yao M, Fang JL, Wang YW. Monitoring human risk and exposure to trinitrotoluene (TNT) using hemoglobin adducts as biomarkers. *Toxicol Lett* 1995;77:281–287.
70. Meier JR, Warshawsky D. Comparison of blood protein and target organ DNA and protein binding following topical application of benzo[*a*]pyrene and 7H-dibenzo[*c,g*] carbazole to mice. *Carcinogenesis* 1994;15:2233–2240.
71. Brazelmann H, Schmid E, Bauchinger M. Chromosome aberrations in nuclear power plant workers: the influence of dose accumulation and lymphocyte life-time. *Mutat Res* 1994;306:197–202.
72. Barret J-M, Calsou P, Salles. B. Deficient nucleotide excision repair activity in protein extracts from normal human lymphocytes. *Carcinogenesis* 1995;16:1611–1616.
73. Freeman SE, Ryan SL. Excision repair of pyrimidine dimers in human peripheral blood lymphocytes: comparison between mitogen stimulated and unstimulated cells. *Exp Cell Res* 1988;194:143–150.
74. Gupta RC, Early K, Sharma S. Use of human lymphocytes to measure DNA binding capacity of chemical carcinogens. *Proc Natl Acad Sci USA* 1988;85:3513–3517.
75. Savela K, Hemminki K. DNA adducts in leukocytes and granulocytes of smokers and nonsmokers detected by the $^{32}P$-postlabeling assay. *Carcinogenesis* 1991;12:503–508.
76. Bianchini F, Wild CP. Effect of route of administration of environmental methylating agents on 7-methylguanine formation in white blood cells and internal organs: implications for molecular epidemiology. *Cancer Lett* 1994;87:131–137.
77. Reddy MV, Randerath KA. A comparison of DNA adduct formation in white blood cells and internal organs of mice exposed to benzo[a]pyrene, dibenzo[*c,g*]carbazole, safrole and cigarette smoke condensate. *Mutat Res* 1990;24:37–48.
78. Szyfter K, Hemminki K, Szyfter W, Szmeja Z, Banaszewski J, Yang K. Aromatic DNA adducts in larynx biopsies and leukocytes. *Carcinogenesis* 1994; 15: 2195–2199.
79. Wiencke JK, Kelsey KT, Varkonyi A, et al. Correlation of DNA adducts in blood mononuclear cells with tobacco carcinogen-induced damage in human lung. *Cancer Res* 1995;55:4910–4914.
80. Loft S, Fisher-Nielsen A, Jeding IB, Vistisen K, Poulsen HE. 8-hydroxydeoxyguanosine as a urinary biomarker of oxidative DNA damage. *J Toxicol Environ Health* 1993;40:391–404.
81. Woods JS, Martin MD, Naleway CA, Echeverria D. Urinary porphyrin profiles as a biomarker of mercury exposure: studies on dentists with occupational exposure to mercury vapor. *J Toxicol Environ Health* 1993;40:235–246.
82. Clayson DB, Lawson TA. Mechanisms of bladder carcinogenesis. In: Connoly JG, ed. *Carcinoma of the bladder.* New York: Raven Press, 1987;91–100.
83. Warner ML, Moore LE, Smith MT, Kalman DA, Fanning E, Smith AH. Increased micronuclei in exfoliated bladder cells of persons who chronically ingest arsenic-contaminated water in Nevada. *Cancer Epidemiol Biomarkers Prevent* 1994;3:583–590.
84. Moore LE, Smith AH, Hopenhayn-Rich C, Biggs ML, Kalman DA, Smith MT. Micronuclei in exfoliated bladder cells among individuals chronically exposed to arsenic in drinking water. *Cancer Epidemiol Biomarkers Prevent* 1997;6:31–36.
85. Talaska G, Scsamer M, Skipper P, et al. Detection of carcinogen-DNA adducts in exfoliated urothelial cells of cigarette smokers: correlation with smoking, hemoglobin adducts, and urinary mutagenicity. *Cancer Epidemiol Biomarkers Prevent* 1991;1:61–66.
86. Rothman N, Bhatnagar VK, Hayes RB, et al. The impact of interindividual variations in NAT2 activity on benzidine urinary metabolites and urothelial DNA adducts in exposed workers. *Proc Natl Acad Sci USA* 1996;93:5084–5089.

*Environmental and Occupational Medicine, Third Edition,* edited by William N. Rom.
Lippincott–Raven Publishers, Philadelphia © 1998.

# CHAPTER 15

# Environmental Mutagenesis

Ross A. McKinnon and Daniel W. Nebert

The field of environmental mutagenesis is concerned with perturbations in the natural genetic structure of plants, animals, and humans induced by environmentally derived agents of diverse types. These include physical agents such as ionizing radiation, biologic agents, including viruses, and a broad range of chemicals. While having its origins in early observations of mutations secondary to x-rays (1), or mustard gases (2), it was with the founding of the Environmental Mutagenesis Society in 1969 that the biologic significance of mutagenesis became a priority research focus (3). Recent decades have witnessed exciting changes in the field of environmental mutagenesis. A primary stimulus for these developments has been the explosion of molecular biology and recombinant DNA technology that began in the 1970s and continues unabated today. Among the many advances secondary to the introduction of these technologies is a clearer insight into the role of mutation in the etiology of human disease, particularly cancer, and the development of sensitive mutation *in vivo* detection systems utilizing transgenic mice. In addition, the past decade has seen remarkable progress in our understanding of the genetic basis of differential response to chemicals including many environmental pollutants. While a consensus strategy on mutagen avoidance remains elusive, it is clear that recent advances have significantly augmented our capacity to gauge risk and recommend strategies for its minimization.

In this chapter, we first discuss the biologic principles underlying mutagenesis including the types of lesions induced by environmental mutagens. We then provide a brief introduction into the variety of environmental mutagens that humans encounter on a daily basis. Because the field of environmental mutagenesis has its roots firmly grounded in prevention, the bulk of the chapter is devoted to a discussion on the assessment of human exposure and susceptibility to environmental mutagens. Finally, we focus on interindividual differences in genetic toxicity assessment, and particularly on the impact of transgenic mouse models on this field.

## BIOLOGIC PRINCIPLES UNDERLYING MUTAGENESIS

The inherent focus of environmental mutagenesis studies is DNA. DNA is a polymer molecule comprising a linear assembly of monomer units termed nucleotides. Genetic information is expressed by the linear order of approximately three billion base pairs (adenine, guanine, cytosine, and thymine). Several properties of DNA render it unique among cellular macromolecules. First, DNA is self-replicating. Second, it is mutable by a variety of endogenous and exogenous stimuli. Finally, DNA is transmissible. The DNA of higher organisms is ordered into tightly condensed protein-associated structures, termed chromosomes. Chromosomes are the primary means by which genes are segregated and recombined in successive generations. In humans, 46 chromosomes are present, comprising 23 derived from each parent. Each of the 23 chromosome pairs may be distinguished from all others based on their size, shape, and characteristic banding patterns. The study of chromosomal structure is termed cytogenetics, and is of critical importance in assessing the mutagenic impact of environmental agents.

R. A. McKinnon: School of Pharmacy and Medical Sciences, University of South Australia, Adelaide, South Australia 5000, Australia.
D. W. Nebert: Department of Environmental Health, University of Cincinnati Medical Center, Cincinnati, Ohio 45267-0056.

Although the focus of this chapter is environmental mutagenesis, the chemical nature of mutagenesis is consistent for both exogenous and endogenous agents. Mutagenic lesions may be defined as those that inhibit DNA replication or those that allow replication to proceed with diminished fidelity. This results in a heritable alteration in genetic information. When such mutations arise in critical regions, they have the capacity to produce genotoxic disease, primarily cancer and congenital abnormalities. Environmentally induced cellular lesions may be manifest at any level of genetic organization, namely chromosomes, genes, or primary DNA sequence. Whereas chromosomal aberrations are generally identified by classical cytogenetic studies, primary DNA lesions are detected by a broad range of methods utilizing molecular biology techniques.

Although some environmental chemicals are capable of reacting with DNA directly, most require metabolic conversion to electrophilic intermediates, such as epoxides or carbonium ions. Such intermediates are capable of interacting with DNA at multiple nucleophilic sites, within the four possible nucleotide bases and also in the phosphate backbone of DNA. Because any particular mutagen is capable of interacting with DNA at multiple sites to produce a range of adducts, it is difficult to define accurately which type of adducts result in which mutations, and why. In general, compounds with a single electrophilic moiety tend to form simple DNA adducts, while those with multiple loci favor inter- and intramolecular cross-links. Such cross-links may be DNA-DNA or, alternatively, DNA-protein. Other possible modifications include breaks in the phosphodiester backbone and the loss of bases (abasic sites). Clearly, all these modifications have the capacity to impede efficient DNA replication by DNA polymerase. In general, smaller lesions such as mono-adducts are likely to result in base-pair substitutions or frame-shift mutations, whereas bulky adducts and cross-links may result in the gain or loss of large chromosomal fragments. Once fixed, the impact of any of these mutations on human health is dependent on the genetic environment in which it occurs.

## SOURCES OF HUMAN MUTAGENS

Environmental mutagens can be broadly classified into three categories: biologic, physical, and chemical. The primary source of biologic agents is viral pathogens, which are capable of infecting cells and disrupting their genetic blueprint. Physical agents include ionizing radiation, ultraviolet light, and hyperthermia. Among adverse physiologic sequelae resulting from radiation exposure, mutagenic aberrations are the most extensively documented. The genetic effects of ionizing radiation have been extensively studied in a wide spectrum of biologic systems. This includes a number of large studies assessing radiation-induced genetic injury in Japanese atomic bomb survivors (reviewed in refs. 4–6). These studies have been of particular value due to the availability of various cohorts, including survivors of direct high- or low-level exposure as well as two classes of offspring: those in utero at the time of the bombings, and those conceived subsequently.

Chemical agents represent the largest source of environmental mutagens, with humans being constantly exposed to a barrage of natural and synthetic chemicals. Examples of this bombardment include more than 400 chemicals isolated from red wine, while at least 1,000 chemicals are estimated to be produced by a lighted cigarette. Further rich sources of chemicals include cosmetics, diet, drugs, and agriculture. In the United States alone, farmlands annually receive more than 75,000 chemicals in the form of pesticides, herbicides, and fertilizing agents; after uptake by plants and grazing animals, as well as fish in nearby waterways, humans (at the end of the food chain) ingest these chemicals.

Many classes of toxic chemical pollutants have been described. These include aromatic hydrocarbons, halogenated aromatics, nitrosamines, polychlorinated biphenyls (PCBs), and polycyclic aromatic hydrocarbons. Within each of these broad categories exist numerous examples of compounds for which biologic activity (mutagenicity, teratogenicity, carcinogenicity) has been demonstrated (7). While a review of all chemicals documented as genotoxic is beyond the scope of this chapter, extensively studied examples include the industrial solvent benzene (8), various cytostatic drugs employed in cancer chemotherapy (8), heterocyclic amine compounds formed during high temperature cooking of meat products (9,10), the food contaminant aflatoxin B1 (11,12), and combustion products of cigarettes (13,14).

Human contact with the above mutagen-causing agents occurs via three primary routes: inhalation via the respiratory tract, ingestion via the gastrointestinal tract, and absorption through the skin. The fate and time course of mutagens in the body is then dependent on the toxicokinetics of the individual chemicals and the metabolic fingerprint of the exposed individual (discussed below).

### Evaluating Human Genetic and Cancer Risk from Environmental Mutagens

Recognition of the precise risk that chemical, biologic, and physical exposures represent to individuals provides an enormous challenge for biomedical research. The probability that a given chemical exposure will cause mutation is dependent on many variables, including the level of exposure, toxicokinetics and metabolic fate of the chemical, and the inherent reactivity of the chemical intermediate. The current approach to predicting human response to chemical exposure combines two fundamental approaches (Fig. 1): first, monitoring the extent of human exposure through environmental monitoring and the use of biologic markers (biomarkers); and second, predicting the likely response of an individual to a given

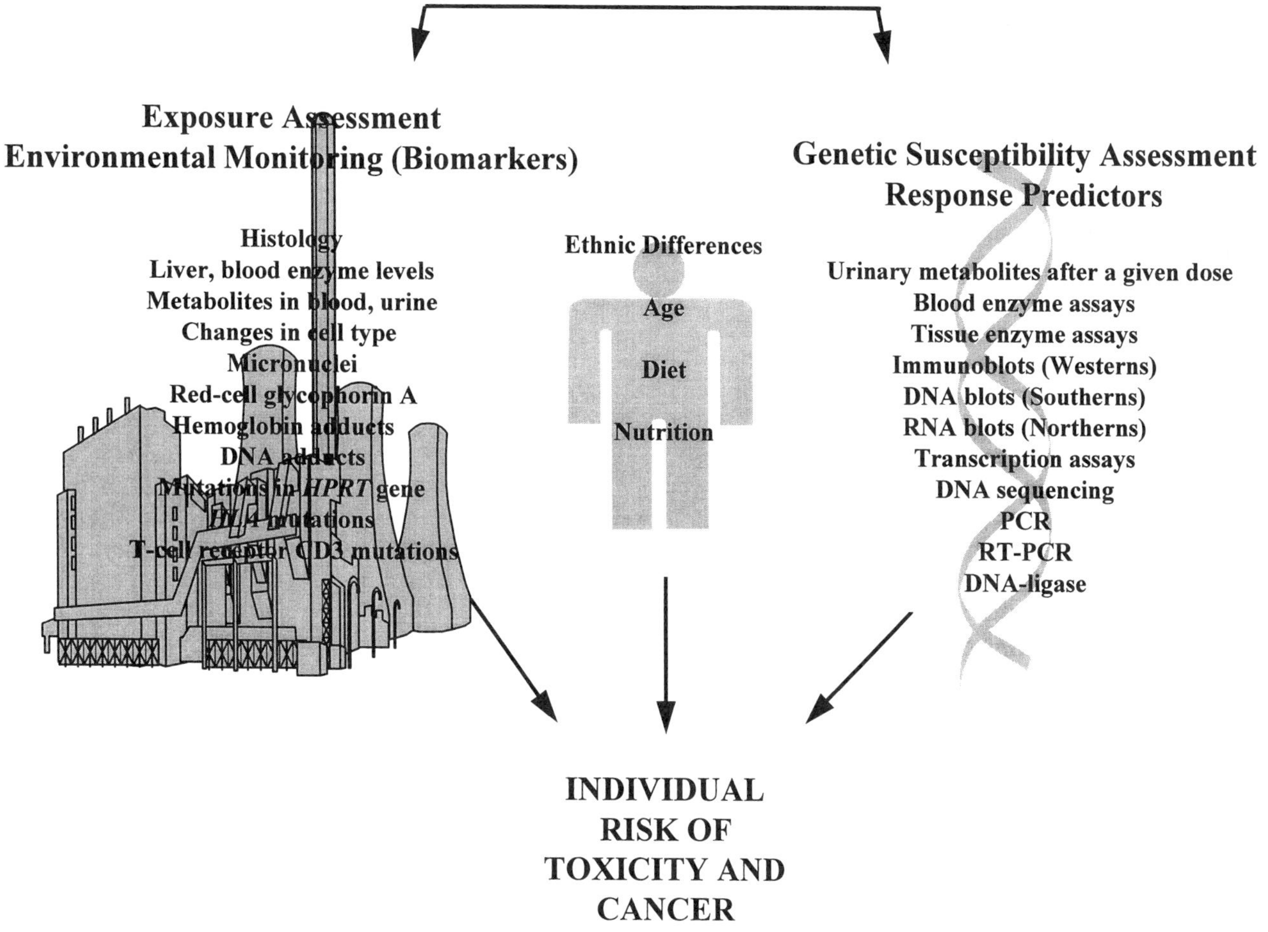


**FIG. 1.** Interrelationships among exposure assessment, ethnic differences, age, diet, nutrition, and genetic susceptibility assessment—all of which contribute to the individual risk of toxicity and cancer.

level of exposure. Environmental monitoring utilizes sampling devices or personal monitoring instruments designed to measure hazardous exposure accurately within a given environment. This type of monitoring is of particular importance for assessing occupational exposures. Biologic monitoring utilizes physiologic fluids, tissues, cells, molecules, or expired air to estimate current or recent exposures to a hazardous agent. It should be noted that although both exposure monitoring and toxic risk prediction are intrinsically important in the overall assessment of risk, the two are distinctly different from one another.

### *Biomarkers of Human Exposure to Environmental Mutagens*

A number of approaches have been developed in an attempt to monitor human populations accurately for exposure to environmental mutagens. These range from epidemiologic studies of exposed human populations to molecular detection of single-base mutations. The various methods developed utilize a variety of chemical and biologic end points. Some of the more widespread methods include cytogenetic analysis of chromosomal aberrations, detection of sister-chromatid exchanges, micronucleus assays, macromolecular adducts detection, and direct measurements of chemical metabolites. The nonepidemiologic methods can be broadly divided into two categories: cytogenetic methods, which are a sensitive monitor of mutagenic effects on the whole genome; and detection of single-gene mutations, which reflect the impact of mutagens on specific targets. The majority of well-established methods utilize peripheral blood lymphocytes due to several features, including their accessibility, ease of culture, and life span.

### *Chromosomal Aberrations*

Many environmental mutagens are capable of inducing chromosomal disruption, causing breakage or rearrangement to occur within or between chromosomes. Such aberrations are generally detected using standard cytogenetic methodology. Two types of chromosomal aberrations are recognized, structural and numerical. Both types of aberration have been associated with adverse effects on human health, especially the development of cancer and congenital malformations. Structural chromosomal aberrations may be further subclassified as chromosome- or chromatid-type aberrations based on the unit of breakage or exchange. Numerical chromosomal aberrations result in deviations from the normal human diploid number of 46, a condition termed aneuploidy (Fig. 2). The hypoploid and hyperploid states refer to a loss and gain of chromosomes, respectively. Mechanisms involved in the generation of aneuploidy include anaphase lag, in which chromosomes separate normally during mitosis or meiosis but one fails to reach the pole, and chromosomal nondisjunction during cell division. Concern over environmental mutagens causing aneuploidy (Fig. 3) is particularly prudent given its implication in an increasing spectrum of human genetic illness, including infertility, spontaneous abortion, and physical and mental handicaps.

Both structural and numerical chromosomal aberrations can be easily studied and quantified in human peripheral lymphocytes. In recent years, the detection of chromosomal abnormalities has been improved significantly with the development and subsequent refinements of the fluorescent in situ hybridization (FISH) technique (reviewed in 15). This sensitive technique involves the hybridization of specific DNA probes to chromosomal specimens and can be used to detect structural or numerical aberrations. Among potential applications of the technique are the characterization of micronuclei (discussed below) and an ability to estimate absorbed radiation dose from past exposures.

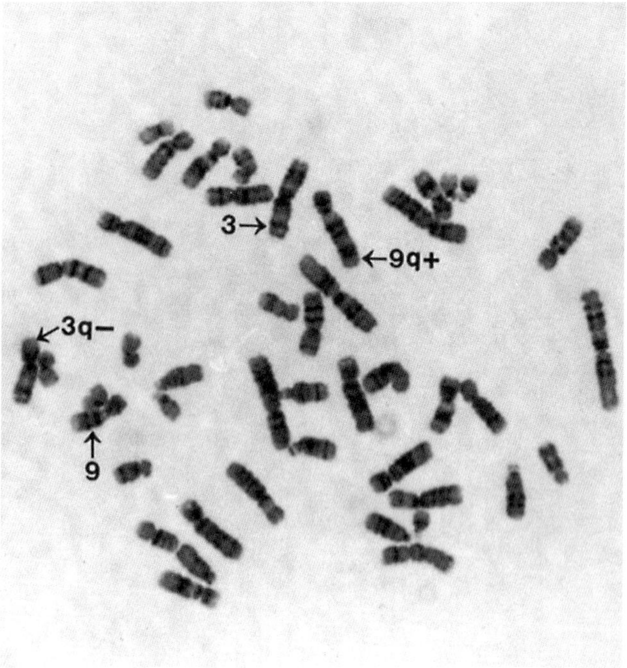


**FIG. 3.** Lymphocyte chromosomal aberrations in a woman with a history of infertility: A balanced reciprocal translocation involving the long arm of chromosomes 3 and 9 occurs in every G-banded metaphase cell. The structurally abnormal chromosomes involved in the exchange, 3 and 9, are identified by the notation 3q- and 9q+, respectively. The normal chromosome of each pair is identified by the numbers 3 and 9.

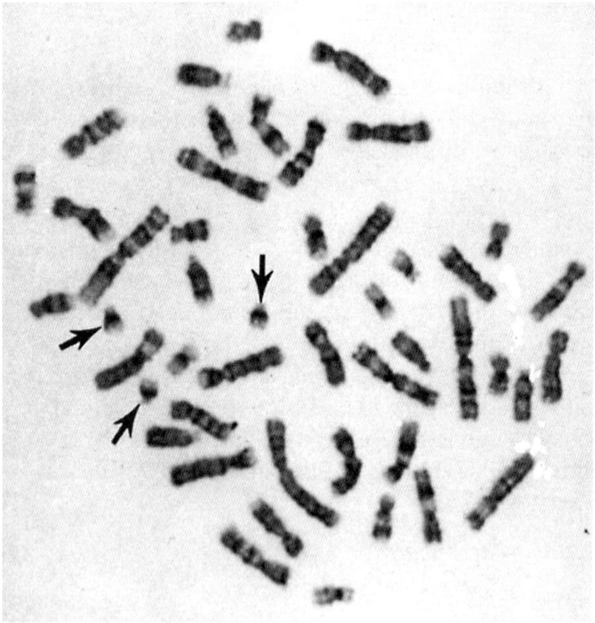

**FIG. 2.** Lymphocyte metaphase spread showing the most frequent numerical human chromosome abnormality, which is due to the presence of an extra chromosome 21 (note three *arrows*). This karyotype (47, XX, +21) represents trisomy 21.

*Sister-Chromatid Exchange*

Unlike the chromosomal aberrations discussed above, sister-chromatid exchange (SCE) does not result in altered chromosomal morphology (Fig. 4). SCEs result from an equal (symmetrical) exchange at a single locus between sister chromatids. They are known to be formed during S-phase replication and involve complete exchange between sister DNA duplexes. Their existence was first demonstrated experimentally by Taylor (16) using tritiated thymidine and autoradiography. In contrast to many chromosomal aberrations, SCEs are compatible with cell survival and occur more frequently. SCEs may be induced by a variety of environmental mutagens, particularly chemicals capable of forming covalent DNA adducts. While the impact of SCEs on human health is not clearly defined, studies have demonstrated their elevation in human populations exposed to several known environmental mutagens (17).

*Micronuclei*

Recent years have seen the widespread use of the micronucleus assay as a rapid, sensitive, quantitative, and

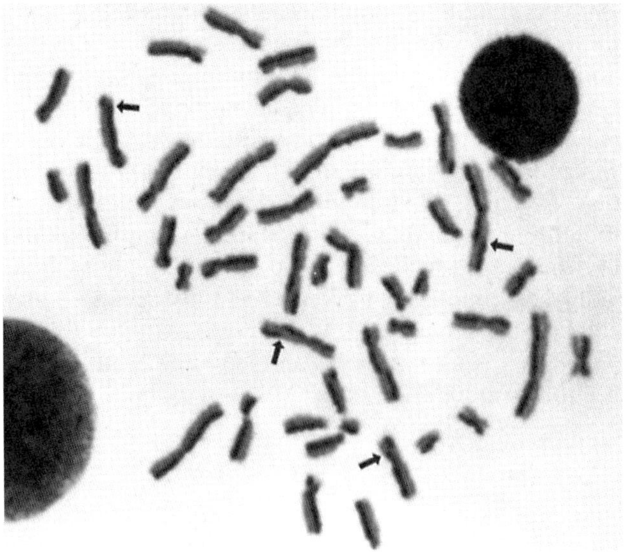

**FIG. 4.** Human lymphocyte at metaphase illustrates differential staining of sister chromatids for each of the 46 chromosomes. A total of 16 sister-chromatid exchanges occur between the dark- and lightly stained chromatids *(arrows)*.

cost-effective assay for assessing genetic damage induced by environmental agents (18,19). Micronuclei are small, round- to oval-shaped DNA-containing structures found in the cytoplasm of a cell (Fig. 5). Micronuclei originate from either whole chromosomes or acentric chromosome fragments that lag behind at anaphase during nuclear division. Consequently, the responsiveness of the micronucleus assay is rapid as it is mainly limited by the time taken for cells to divide following or during intervention. In addition to use as a biomarker of human exposure to environmental mutagens, the rodent micronucleus assays have gained widespread use as screening assays for potential human mutagens (20,21).

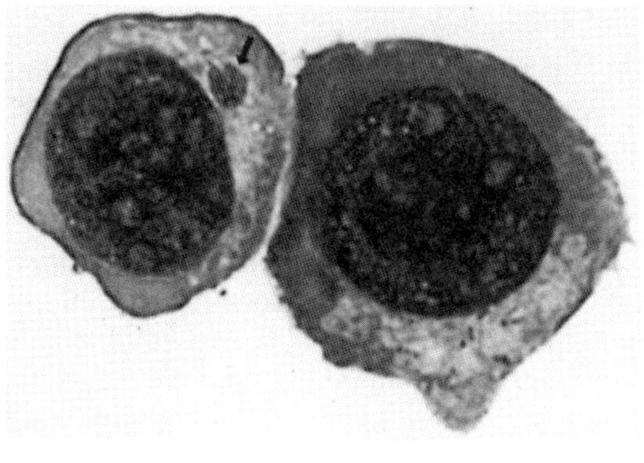

**FIG. 5.** Two interphase lymphocytes prepared by cytocentrifugation following culture and stained with Wright's Giemsa. The left cell shows a micronucleus *(arrow)*; the other cell has normal nuclear structure.

*Macromolecular Adducts*

Steady-state exposure to environmental mutagens is frequently assessed by measuring macromolecular adducts, particularly DNA adducts (22,23). DNA adducts are generally favored, as they provide a clear insight into the penetration of mutagenic species to the molecule of primary concern. The use of DNA adducts as *in vivo* dosimeters of mutagen exposure is complicated, however, by the ability of DNA to repair genotoxic damage. To date, adduct measurements have been essentially restricted to comparisons of exposed populations to unexposed ones, with only limited quantitative risk assessment. DNA adducts are detected by several means, with immunologic assays being the most sensitive and specific (24,25). In addition to direct detection of DNA adducts, urinary measurements of adduct metabolites have also been used as a biomonitor of exposure (26).

Investigations into the utility of detection and quantitation of protein adducts have yielded several important findings relevant to environmental mutagenesis, particularly related to passive smoke inhalation (27). Hemoglobin is generally the preferred protein for adduct studies due to its abundance in blood samples (28). In addition, the 120-day life span of red blood cells and stability of hemoglobin adducts enable cumulative doses of genotoxicants to be determined (29).

***Biomarkers of Individual Susceptibility to Environmental Mutagens***

Biomarkers of susceptibility are measurements designed to highlight individual differences in response to genotoxic influences. Factors likely to be critical in determining individual susceptibility to genotoxicity include metabolic phenotype, immune function, nutritional status, and the efficiency of DNA repair.

*DNA Repair*

The role of DNA repair in determining individual susceptibility to mutagenic agents is inherently obvious. There are well-documented genetically determined interindividual differences in the ability to repair DNA (30–33). Individuals with impaired DNA repair capacity have an increase in irreversible genetic damage secondary to processing of DNA lesions such as adducts. It is now also known that such individuals have an increased susceptibility to cancer. Indeed, many heritable cancer syndromes are related to defects in genes encoding DNA repair enzymes (34,35).

*Metabolic Genotype/Phenotype*

Since most mutagens require metabolic conversion before interacting with DNA, many of the recent advances in determining individual susceptibility to environmental mutagenesis and other chemical-mediated toxicities have evolved from a greater appreciation of the processes by which humans and other mammals detoxify chemicals, and the remarkable complexity of the enzyme systems involved. Collectively, these enzymes are frequently referred to as drug-metabolizing enzymes or xenobiotic-metabolizing enzymes. Both terms are inappropriate, however, given that in addition to drugs and other xenobiotics, these enzymes also have many physiologic substrates; indeed, none of these enzymes metabolizes only foreign chemicals. As we learn more about the biologic and chemical processes leading to human health aberrations, it has become increasingly evident that drug-metabolizing enzymes function in an ambivalent manner. In the majority of cases, lipid-soluble chemicals are converted to more readily excreted water-soluble metabolites. However, it is clear that on many occasions the same enzymes are capable of activating various inert chemicals to highly reactive molecules capable of inducing mutation. These intermediates can then interact with cellular macromolecules such as proteins and DNA. Thus, for each chemical to which humans are exposed, there exists the potential for the competing pathways of metabolic activation and detoxification.

Human genetic differences in the metabolism of various drugs and environmental chemicals have been known for more than four decades (36,37). These differences are frequently referred to as pharmacogenetic or, more broadly, ecogenetic polymorphisms. These polymorphisms represent variant alleles that occur at a relatively high frequency in the population and are generally associated with aberrations in enzyme expression or function. Historically, polymorphisms have usually been identified following unexpected responses to therapeutic agents. More recently, however, the advent of recombinant DNA technology has enabled scientists to identify the precise alterations in genes that are responsible for some of these polymorphisms. Polymorphisms have now been characterized in many drug-metabolizing enzymes, including both phase I and phase II enzymes. As more and more polymorphisms are identified, it is becoming increasingly apparent that each individual possesses a distinct complement of drug-metabolizing enzymes. This diversity might be described as a metabolic fingerprint. It is the complex interplay of the various drug-metabolizing enzyme superfamilies within any individual that will ultimately determine his/her particular response to a given chemical and potential for toxicity (reviewed in 38–41).

The future will no doubt see an explosion in the identification of further polymorphisms (two or more phenotypes in any population) involving drug-metabolizing enzymes. This information will be accompanied by improved, minimally invasive DNA-based tests to identify the genotype associated with the trait, or phenotype, in human populations. Such studies should be particularly informative in evaluating the role of chemicals in the many environmental diseases of presently unclear origin. The consideration of multiple drug-metabolizing enzyme polymorphisms, in combination, is also likely to represent a particularly fertile research area. Such studies will probably clarify the role of chemicals in the causation of many cancers. Collectively, this information should enable the formulation of increasingly individualized advice on avoidance of chemicals likely to be of individual concern. This is the field of preventive toxicology. Such advice will no doubt greatly assist all individuals in coping with the ever-increasing chemical burden to which we are exposed.

## GENETIC TOXICITY ASSESSMENT

The capacity to detect chemically induced mutations is critical to our ability to identify potential human mutagens carcinogens. Genetic toxicity assessment involves the evaluation of chemicals for their capacity to induce mutation at any level of DNA organization. Since 1927 when Herman Müller developed the first assay for detection of mutagenic agents, more than 200 assays have been developed for this purpose. These methods can be grouped into several broad categories: epidemiologic studies, long-term *in vivo* bioassays, mid-term *in vivo* bioassays, short-term *in vivo* bioassays, *in vitro* bioassays, structure-activity relationships, and mechanism-based inference. The exact type, and the number of such assays used, varies from country to country and is constantly evolving.

Epidemiologic studies are potentially very useful, because they utilize humans as the ultimate indicators of disease. Disadvantages include the cost and duration of studies and difficulty in obtaining accurate exposure data, particularly in the case of multiple chemical exposures. An inaccurate exposure (error in phenotype) will wreak havoc on trying to relate this trait to any genotype. Data from long-term *in vivo* bioassays (e.g., 2-year rodent carcinogenesis bioassay) provide excellent correlations with human carcinogens. This is to be expected, given that such systems represent interactive and integrative biologic systems closely related to humans. They are, however, labor- and resource-intensive and generally difficult to replicate. In addition, it is frequently difficult to mimic human exposure conditions, which usually involve multiple chemicals. Short-term *in vivo* and *in vitro* bioassays provide a low-cost alternative to longer-term assays and are frequently used as initial screening assays to select compounds suitable for long-term studies. Short-term tests include a variety of bacterial and mammalian cell bioassays. The primary bacterial system used is the Ames *Salmonella* test. In recent years, several additional bacterial strains have been introduced for this assay, significantly improving its predictive capacity. Structure-activity relationships are relatively simple methods that can be developed from existing chemical and biologic databases. These have proven very reliable for certain classes of compounds, although exceptions to formulated rules are not uncommon. Similar observations and limitations are seen with mechanism-based approaches.

As in other fields, recent advances in recombinant DNA technology have provided many new initiatives in the field of genetic toxicity assessment. Such initiatives have been given added impetus by limitations on the existing assays, including the inability to measure mutations in multiple tissues, large animal numbers required, and difficulties in accurately assessing the mutagenicity of large numbers of chemicals. Recent developments include the use of transgenic rodents for mutation detection and improved metabolic activation models such as stably transformed cell lines expressing human xenobiotic-metabolizing enzymes.

The use of transgenic models has been a revolutionary development in genetic toxicity testing. Transgenic animals are those that have been genetically altered by introduction of foreign DNA sequences into the genome of zygotes or embryos. They may be generated by microinjection of DNA into a zygote pronucleus, infection of embryos with modified retroviruses, or introduction of genetically altered embryonic stem (ES) cells into developing embryos. Whereas these methodologies are generally applied to mice, they are applicable to other species, as evident with the recent development of a transgenic rat mutation detection system. Some of the various transgenic mouse models relevant to environmental mutagenesis are discussed below.

### Mutation Detection Systems

Transgenic rodent models for *in vivo* mutation detection have provided a major advance in our ability to assess tissue-specific mutations following chemical treatment (42,43). Such models are based on the stable insertion into the genome of target genes that can be easily recovered from selected tissues and analyzed for mutations. In these systems animals are exposed to the environmental chemical in question, and after sufficient time to allow fixation of DNA adducts as mutations, genomic DNA is isolated. The target gene is then captured, utilizing either λ-phage packaging or magnetic affinity methods, and assessed for mutations.

The commercially available transgenic rodent systems developed for mutation detection (e.g., Muta Mouse, Big Blue mouse and rat, Xenomouse) generally utilize genes from the *lac* operon of *Escherichia coli.* The *lac* operon is a well-characterized set of coordinately regulated genes involved in lactose uptake and metabolism. The *lacI* gene encodes a repressor protein that, in the absence of inducer (e.g., lactose) binds to the *lacO* operator sequence. When bound, the repressor prevents the transcription of three structural genes, *lacZ* (β-galactosidase), *lacY* (permease), and *lacA* (transacetylase). In the presence of inducer, removal of the repressor protein from *lacO* leads to transcription of the three structural genes. β-galactosidase activity may be measured in *E. coli* by plating on medium containing a chromogenic substrate such as X-gal. Under such conditions, the presence of β-galactosidase activity results in the production of an insoluble blue dye, seen as a blue plaque. Scoring the ratio of blue mutant plaques to colorless nonmutant plaques allows for a quantitative index of mutation frequency in any selected tissue. The *lacZ* gene of the operon acts as the target gene in the Muta Mouse and Xenomouse systems, while the Big Blue systems utilize *lacI* as the target gene. More recently, the number of available mutation detection systems has expanded, providing researchers with an improved capacity to detect and differentiate different types of mutations (44).

### Mice with Increased Cancer Susceptibility

Transgenic mice, with a genetic alteration critical to the development of tumors, but insufficient by itself to produce cancer, are proving valuable models for rapid cancer bioassays. Such genetically altered mice succumb to chemically induced cancer in a fraction of their life span. It is hoped that such mice will greatly reduce the time it currently takes for prospective identification of potential carcinogens. Examples include mice heterozygous for an inactivated tumor suppressor genes such as *p53* (45,46) and those carrying inducible proto-oncogenes (47). Interbreeding of different mouse lines will undoubtedly continue to improve transgenic mouse models relevant to environmental mutagenesis. This is lucidly demonstrated by the commercial availability of a new mouse line combining the mutation detection capability of the Big Blue system with the cancer susceptibility of *p53* inactivation (TSG-p53).

### Xenobiotic-Metabolizing Enzyme Knockout Mice

Another area of transgenesis impacting on the field of environmental mutagenesis is the development of mouse lines lacking individual cytochrome P-450 genes. It has long been recognized, since the pioneering work of James and Elizabeth Miller, that the majority of environmental mutagens require metabolic activation prior to exerting their mutagenic effects. This metabolism generally involves the highly versatile cytochrome P-450 family of enzymes. Mice deficient in individual cytochrome P-450 genes (knockout mice) provide unique *in vivo* systems suitable for accurately defining the role of the targeted enzyme in metabolism. Such mouse lines should enable researchers to define more accurately the metabolic profile of mutagens and carcinogens. As we go to press, two cytochrome P-450 genes have been successfully targeted, *Cyp1a2* (48,49) and *Cyp2e1* (50), and many more are expected to be developed soon. Both Cyp1a2 and Cyp2e1 catalyze the metabolic activation of many mutagens of environmental origin. For example, Cyp1a2 is the principal enzyme involved in the activation of the food-derived heterocyclic amine mutagens to their active form (51,52). It is conceivable that the near future will see human alleles introduced into these mice to replace the target murine alleles. The resultant humanized mice will provide a valuable metabolic activation source for a range of mutagenicity tests.

## CONCLUSION

Protection of our environment and the maintenance of quality of life continue to be public issues of paramount importance. Crucial to both of these goals is an awareness of the presence and magnitude of all toxic risks. Awareness of these risks, when combined with an understanding of individual susceptibility to them, will enable the widespread practice of preventive toxicology. The underlying rationale of environmental mutagenesis is thus the prevention of ill health and injury among exposed populations. There is no doubt that the last few decades have seen remarkable technical advances in biomonitoring related to environmental mutagens and in our ability to identify potential mutagens. Many of these advances have been tempered, however, by methodologic difficulties, particularly with respect to quantitative aspects and extrapolation of laboratory animal data to the human. The existing biomarkers clearly provide sensitivity in detecting low biologically active doses of environmental mutants; however, their precise role in etiologic research relating to environmental mutagens awaits further clarification. With further developments and refinements in molecular biology, it is certain that new, improved markers will be identified to assess environmental exposure. Similar advances can be expected in understanding genetic susceptibility to environmental exposures. These two approaches, when intertwined, should ensure continual improvements in the practice of preventive toxicology.

## REFERENCES


1. Muller HJ. Artificial transmutation of the gene. *Science* 1927;64: 84–87.
2. Auerbach C, Robson JM, Carr JG. The chemical production of mutations. *Science* 1947;105:243–247.
3. Wassom JS. Origins of genetic toxicology and the Environmental Mutagen Society. *Environ Mol Mutagen* 1989;14(suppl 16):1–6.
4. National Research Council. *The effects on populations of exposure to low levels of ionizing radiation.* (BEIR III). Washington, DC: National Academy Press, 1980.
5. National Research Council. *Health effects of exposure to low levels of ionizing radiation.* (BEIR V). Washington, DC: National Academy Press, 1990.
6. Awa AA, Honda T, Neriishi S, et al. Cytogenetic study of atomic bomb survivors, Hiroshima and Nagasaki. In: Obe G, Basler A, eds.*Cytogenetics:* basic and applied aspects. New York: Springer-Verlag, 1987; 345–360.
7. Ames BN. Identifying environmental chemicals causing mutations and cancer. *Science* 1979;204:587–593.
8. Sorsa M, Yager JW. Cytogenic surveillance of occupational exposures. In: Obe G, Basler A, eds. *Cytogenetics:* basic and applied aspects. New York: Springer-Verlag, 1987;345–360.
9. Sugimura T. Studies on environmental chemical carcinogens in Japan. *Science* 1986;233:312–318.
10. Felton J S, Knize MG, Shen NH, Andresen BD, Bjeldanes LF, Hatch FT. Identification of mutagens in cooked beef. *Environ Health Perspect* 1986;67:17–24.
11. Mclean M, Dutton MF. Cellular interactions and metabolism of aflatoxin—an update. *Pharmacol Ther* 1995;65:163–192.
12. Massey TE, Stewart RK, Daniels JM, Liu L. Biochemical and molecular aspects of mammalian susceptibility to aflatoxin. *Proc Soc Exp Biol Med* 1995;208:213–227.
13. Littlefield LG, Joiner EE. Analysis of chromosomal aberrations in lymphocytes of long-term heavy smokers. *Mutat Res* 1986;170: 145–150.
14. Livingston GK, Fineman RM. Correlation of human lymphocyte SCE frequency with smoking history. *Mutat Res* 1983;119:59–64.
15. Natarajan AT, Boei JJWA, Darroudi F, et al. Current cytogenetic methods for detecting exposure and effects of mutagens and carcinogens. *Environ Health Perspect* 1996;104:445–447.
16. Taylor JH. Sister chromatid exchanges in tritium-labeled chromosomes. *Genetics* 1958;43:515–529.
17. Carrano AV. Natarajan AT. Considerations for population monitoring using cytogenetic techniques.*Mutat Res* 1988;204:379–406.
18. Sorsa M, Yager JW. Cytogenetic surveillance of occupational exposures. In: Obe G, Basler A, eds. *Cytogenetics:* basic and applied aspects. New York: Springer-Verlag, 1987;345–360.
19. Livingston GK, Reed RN, Olson BL, Lockey JE. Induction of nuclear aberrations by smokeless tobacco in epithelial cells of human oral mucosa. *Environ Mol Mutagen* 1990;15:136–144.
20. Morita T. Evaluation of the mouse micronucleus assay to screen carcinogens, Mammalian Mutagen Study Group Communications. *Japanese Environmental Mutagen Society* 1993;1:1–32.
21. Ashby J. Evaluation of the rodent micronucleus assay in the screening of IARC carcinogens (Groups 1,2A and 2B)—the summary report of the 6th collaborative study by CSGMT/JEMS. *Mutat Res* 1997;389:1
22. Dipple A. DNA adducts of chemical carcinogens. *Carcinogenesis* 1995;16:437–441.
23. Burkhart JG. Perspectives on molecular assays for measuring mutations in humans and rodents. *Environ Mol Mutagen* 1995;25(suppl 26): 88–101.
24. Keith G, Dirheimer G,. Postlabeling: a sensitive method for studying DNA adducts and their role in carcinogenesis. *Curr Opin Biotechnol* 1996;6:3–11.
25. Yin BY, Whyatt RM, Perera FP, Randall MC, Cooper TB, Santella RM. Determination of 8-hydroxydeoxyguanosine by an immunoaffinity chromatography-monoclonal antibody based ELISA. *Free Radical Biol Med* 1995;18:1023–1132.
26. Groopman JD, Donahue JPR, Zhu J, Chen J, Wogan GN. Aflatoxin metabolism in humans: detection of metabolites and nucleic acid adducts in urine by affinity chromatography. *Proc Natl Acad Sci USA* 1985;82:6492–6496.
27. Wogan GN. Molecular epidemiology in cancer risk assessment and prevention: recent progress and avenues for future research. *Environ Health Perspect* 1992;98:167–178.
28. Neumann HG. Analysis of hemoglobin as a dose monitor for alkylating and arylating agents. *Arch Toxicol* 1984;56:1–6.
29. Osterman-Golkar S, Christakoppoulos A, Zorcec V, Svensson K. Dosimetry of styrene 7,8-oxide in styrene- and styrene oxide-exposed mice and rats by quantification of hemoglobin adducts. *Chem Biol Interact* 1995;95:75–87.
30. Lehmann AR. Xeroderma pigmentosum, Cockayne syndrome and ataxia-telangiectasia: disorders relating DNA repair to carcinogenesis. *Cancer Surv* 1982;1:93–118.
31. Malkin D, Li FP, Strong LC, et al. Germ line p53 mutations in a familial syndrome of breast cancer, sarcoma, and other neoplasms. *Science* 1990;250:1233–1238.
32. Savitsky K, Bar-Shira A, Gilad S, et al. A single ataxia-telangiectasia gene with a product similar to PI-3. *Science* 1995;268;1749–1753.
33. Nicotera TM. Molecular and biochemical aspects of Bloom's syndrome. *Cancer Genet Cytogenet* 1991;53:1–13.
34. Lee W-H, Bookstein R, Hong F, Young L-J, Shew J-Y, Lee Ey-HP. Human retinoblastoma gene: cloning, identification, and sequence. *Science* 1987;235:1394–1399.

35. Nicolaides NC, Papadopoulos N, Liu B, et al. Mutations of two PMS homologues in nonpolyposis colon cancer. *Nature* 1994;371:75–80.
36. Kalow W. *Pharmacogenetics:* heredity and the response to drugs. Philadelphia: WB Saunders, 1962.
37. Kalow W, ed. *Pharmacogenetics of drug metabolism.* New York: Pergamon Press, 1992.
38. Nebert DW, Genes encoding drug-metabolizing enzymes: possible role in human disease. In: Woodhead AD, Bender MA, Leonard RC, eds. *Phenotypic variation in populations.* New York: Plenum, 1988;45–64.
39. Gonzalez FJ, Nebert DW, Evolution of the P-450 gene superfamily: Animal-plant "warfare," molecular drive, and human genetic differences in drug oxidation. *Trends Genet* 1990;6:182–186.
40. Nebert DW, Weber WW, Pharmacogenetics. In: Pratt WB, Taylor PW, eds. *Principles of drug action. The basis of pharmacology,* 3rd ed. New York: Churchill-Livingstone, 1990;469–531.
41. Nebert, DW, McKinnon RA, Puga A. Human drug-metabolizing enzyme polymorphisms: effects on risk of toxicity and cancer. *DNA Cell Biol* 1996;15:273–280.
42. Provost GS, Kretx PL, Hamner RT, et al. Transgenic systems for *in vivo* mutation analysis. *Mutat Res* 1993;288:133–149.
43. Mirsalis JC, Monforte JA, Winegar RA. Transgenic animal models for detection of mutations. *Annu Rev Pharmacol Toxicol* 1995;35:145–164.
44. Nohmi T, Katoh M, Suzuki H, et al. A new transgenic mouse mutagenesis test system using Spi- and 6-thioguanine selections. *Environ Mol Mutagen* 1996;28:465–470.
45. Donehower LA, Harvey M, Slagle BL, et al. Mice deficient for p53 are developmentally normal but susceptible to spontaneous tumors. *Nature* 1992;356:215–221.
46. Harvey M, McArthur MJ, Montgomery CA Jr, Butel JS, Bradley A, Donehower LA. Spontaneous and carcinogen-induced tumorigenesis in p53-deficient mice. *Nature Genet* 1993;5:225–229.
47. Breuer M, Slebos R, Verbeek S, van Lohuizen M, Wientjens E, Berns A. Very high frequency of lymphoma induction by a chemical carcinogen in pim-1 transgenic mice. *Nature* 1989;340:61–63.
48. Pineau T, Fernandez-Salguero P, Lee STT, McPhail T, Ward JM, Gonzalez FJ. Neonatal lethality associated with respiratory distress in mice lacking cytochrome P-450 CYP1A2. *Proc Natl Acad Sci USA* 1995;92: 5134–5138.
49. Liang H-C, Li H, McKinnon RA, Potter SS, Duffy JJ, Puga A, Nebert DW. Cyp1a2(-/-) mice develop normally but display abnormal drug metabolism. *Proc Natl Acad Sci USA* 1996;93:1671–1676.
50. Lee SST, Buters JTM, Pineau T, Fernandez-Salguero P, Gonzalez FJ. Role of Cyp2e1 in the hepatotoxicity of acetaminophen. *J Biol Chem* 1996;271:12063–12067.
51. McManus ME, Burgess WM, Veronese ME, Huggett A, Quattrochi LC, Tukey RH. Metabolism of 2-acetylaminofluorene, benzo[a]pyrene and the activation of food derived heterocyclic amine mutagens by human cytochromes P-450. *Cancer Res* 1990;50:3367–3376.
52. Hammons GJ, Milton D, Stepps K, Guengerich FP, Tukey RH, Kadlubar FF. Metabolism of carcinogenic heterocyclic and aromatic amines by recombinant human cytochrome P-450 enzymes. *Carcinogenesis* 1997;18:851–854.

*Environmental and Occupational Medicine, Third Edition*, edited by William N. Rom.
Lippincott–Raven Publishers, Philadelphia © 1998.

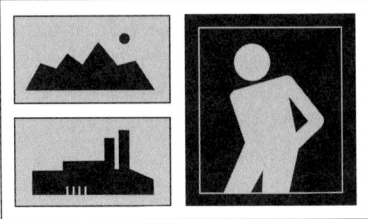

CHAPTER 16

# Experimental and Computational Strategies for the Rapid Identification of Environmental Carcinogens

Herbert S. Rosenkranz

Given the cost and time required to conduct rodent cancer bioassays (3 years, approximately $2 million), a variety of attempts have been made to develop short-term tests and models based on structure-activity relationships (SAR) that predict the carcinogenic effect. Indeed, the discipline of genetic toxicology is concerned with the identification of potential carcinogens based on the results of short-term tests. If short-term tests are to be predictive of carcinogenicity, they should have a mechanistic foundation. Indeed, most such short-term assays are based on the assumption that cancer results from a somatic mutation (1) and that, therefore, assays that can identify agents that affect the genetic material [mutations, chromosome alterations, deoxyribonucleic acid (DNA) damage or alterations (2)] might be expected to identify cancer-causing chemicals. A variety of tests have been based on this hypothesis. At last count, there were approximately 180 of them (3). In fact, the search for more relevant and more predictive short-term assays continues to this day.

Among the latest tests undergoing evaluation is the single-cell microgel electrophoresis (Comet) assay for DNA damage (4) and the *in vitro* micronucleus assay (5). Moreover, the availability of genetically engineered cell lines with widely different cytochrome P-450 isozyme levels is introducing both added sensitivity and complexity to the situation, as these cells—lacking detoxifying enzymes—will result in the generation of additional positive responses that may widen the dichotomy between *in vitro* and *in vivo* assays (6). Indeed, during the early years of genetic toxicology there was a significant concordance between the mutagenicity and carcinogenicity of chemicals, and we accepted the assumption that carcinogens are mutagens (7). Even as our understanding of the mutagenic activation of oncogenes (8,9) and inactivation of suppressor genes (10) appeared to substantiate the somatic mutation theory and the use of short-term genetic toxicity tests to identify carcinogens, however, analysis of the carcinogenicity and short-term test results sponsored by the U.S. National Toxicology Program (NTP) seemed to deny an overall concordance between mutagenicity and carcinogenicity (11–13). To understand the current state of affairs and to use short-term tests wisely, it may be instructive to analyze the events that led from the carcinogens are mutagens hypothesis to its apparent reversal. Such a survey may clarify the current situation and inform the further development of strategies for identifying cancer-causing agents.

The excellent concordance that was obtained originally between measures of DNA damage as by short-term tests and rodent carcinogenesis (7,14,15) derived from the fact that the chemicals originally tested in rodents were alkylating agents, nitrosamines, and polycyclic aromatic hydrocarbons, all potent electrophiles that were carcinogenic as well as DNA reactive (16,17). In fact, during the early phases of the rodent cancer test program very few noncarcinogens were tested. When the first short-term tests were

H. S. Rosenkranz: Department of Environmental and Occupational Health, University of Pittsburgh Graduate School of Public Health, Pittsburgh, Pennsylvania 15238.

developed (2), most of the assays were "validated" against these potent agents, and indeed a prophecy was fulfilled. In fact, so pervasive was the acceptance of the principle that carcinogens are mutagens that when a proven or presumed rodent carcinogen tested negative in a standard short-term test assay such as *Salmonella* (7) or the pol $A^+$/pol $A^-$ DNA repair assay (18), the assay was either modified or discarded in favor of new ones developed to demonstrate the activity of that particular chemical; thus the existence of more than 180 such short-term tests (3). Many of these short-term tests were validated with the potent agents then known to be carcinogens. In parallel with this, the chemicals included in organized cancer bioassay programs were principally structural analogs of chemicals that already had tested positive in the cancer bioassay, i.e., they looked like carcinogens (16). Although this latter fact established a relationship between electrophilic or potentially electrophilic moieties and carcinogenicity (19) and resulted in the identification of structural alerts (20,21), it also produced a carcinogenicity database that contained limited information on the structural features associated with carcinogenicity (22).

When the more rigorous National Cancer Institute/National Toxicology Program (NCI/NTP) rodent bioassay was adopted (23,24), which included two sexes and two species plus greater discrimination with respect to chemicals chosen for inclusion in the bioassay (i.e., with relevance to potential human exposure and use), there was (a) a reasonable assurance that chemicals that tested negative in this protocol could be considered not carcinogenic (25,26), and (b) a gradual shift in the nature of the chemicals recognized as carcinogenic. This derived also from the inclusion of the maximum tolerated dose (MTD) as well as the use of two species, as it has been observed that whereas mutagenic carcinogens cause cancer principally in mice and rats, nonmutagenic carcinogens appear to be restricted to causing cancer in only one species (21,27). Additionally, as a group, nonmutagens appear to be less potent carcinogens than mutagens (28,29) and so would produce a response only at or close to the MTD. Finally, cellular toxicity and the related phenomenon of cell proliferation could well be involved in causing cancer (30–32). These mechanisms would not necessarily involve DNA damage and might be expected to occur when larger doses are administered (33–35), although this is not always the case (36).

These factors would, of course, lead to apparent deterioration of the predictive performance of short-term tests when chemicals of a different nature are included (17). Indeed, an analysis of the results of the NTP bioassay show a number of interesting features. Approximately 350 chemicals have been tested for carcinogenicity in rodents (21,37). Of these, 55% are carcinogens. We do not expect the prevalence of carcinogens in the environment to be so high. The current wisdom suggests that the prevalence is about 10% and in any case does not exceed 20% (38—41). Thus, the chemicals selected for the NTP bioassay represent a biased sample. Additionally, while 42% of all chemicals tested are mutagens, 55% of the carcinogens are mutagens (21). This is significantly different from the 90% to 95% concordance between mutagens and carcinogens that had been suggested earlier (7). This led to the concept of genotoxic as well as nongenotoxic carcinogens (21,42,43).

In parallel with rodent cancer bioassays and *Salmonella* mutagenicity assays, the NTP also tested many of these chemicals for their ability to induce chromosomal aberrations and sister chromatid exchanges in cultured Chinese hamster cells and gene mutations in cultured mouse lymphoma cells. Analysis of the results of these studies led the NTP to conclude that none of these mammalian assays was better than the *Salmonella* assay alone in predicting the carcinogenicity of chemicals in rodents (11,12), although analysis by others suggested that a battery of these tests performed better than the *Salmonella* assay alone, especially in correctly predicting noncarcinogens (44,45). Moreover, the recent application of newer computational techniques (e.g., learning machines) led to the identification of a combination of short-term assays and physical chemical parameters that demonstrated a high predictivity for carcinogens and noncarcinogens that are not mutagenic in *Salmonella* (46). Certainly, the results of these analyses raised many questions regarding the predictive value of these short-term tests and how to proceed practically in identifying safe chemicals to be included in consumer products or used in commerce and industry (13,40,43,47–57). For its part, the NTP, in view of the above results, suggested that perhaps a combination of the *Salmonella* mutagenicity assay *in vitro* with the rodent micronucleus assay *in vivo* (12) would be sufficient to identify potential carcinogens, and the NTP then embarked on a program to test chemicals in the micronucleus test. The evaluation of the results of that exercise is ongoing (58–61). However, even while the applicability of the standard *in vivo* micronucleus assay is being debated, new insight about its mechanism of action is leading to a better understanding of its response to chemical agents. Moreover, the ongoing development of *in vivo* transgenic mouse mutational assays (62,63) might lead to the eventual replacement of the *in vivo* micronucleus assay.

## GENOTOXIC AND NONGENOTOXIC CARCINOGENS

Most investigators agree that owing to the NTP's quality control criteria the rodent cancer data it generated constitute the most authoritative body of carcinogenicity data. It has, therefore, been the subject of detailed analysis by investigators associated with the NTP as well as by outsiders. Based on the many correlations regarding the carcinogenic spectrum of chemicals that have been made, a number of generalizations have been reached. Chemicals that are carcinogenic in only one species generally are not mutagenic, whereas chemicals that are carcinogenic to both mice and rats are also mutagenic in *Salmonella* (21,27). Thus, if we were to use transspecies effect as a measure of "potency," we could conclude that mutagenic carcinogens are more likely to cause cancer in more than one species, and intuitively we could conclude that such chemicals would also be likely to cause cancer in humans. Additionally, although nongenotoxic carcinogens (reserpine, 2,3,7,8-tetrachlorodibenzo-*p*-dioxin) are among the most potent rodent carcinogens known, as a group the mutagenic carcinogens are more potent, on a dose per kilogram basis, than nonmutagenic carcinogens (28,29).

Simultaneously with these analyses, other studies revealed that chemicals recognized as human carcinogens by the International Agency for Research on Cancer are predominantly mutagenic or genotoxic (51,64–66), in contrast to presumed human noncarcinogens, which even though they might be rodent carcinogens are neither mutagens nor genotoxicants (51).

These trends, taken together, have led some to suggest that mutagenic carcinogens pose a greater risk to humans than nonmutagenic ones (13,66—69). At present this issue is far from resolved, but added to the controversy of the role of cellular toxicity in cell proliferation and the validity of using the MTD in the cancer bioassay (31–36), it has resulted in a situation that is very much in flux with respect to the use of short-term tests, and even of the standard NTP rodent bioassay. This unsettled situation is likely to persist until the pathogenic and molecular basis of nonmutagenic (nongenotoxic) carcinogens is elucidated further.

Still, there seems to be consensus that mutagenic or genotoxic carcinogens represent a greater risk to humans, possibly because of the fact that a similar mechanism of cancer induction may be operative in both rodents and humans (e.g., induction of the K-*ras* oncogene or inactivation of the p53 suppressor gene). This analysis identifies genotoxic and nongenotoxic carcinogens by their structural features. This is based on the assumption that at present, nongenotoxic carcinogens cannot be identified by "validated" short-term tests (42,70), although some tests may be in the process of development (e.g., inhibition of cell-to-cell communication, chemical induction of cell proliferation) (30). Moreover, as mentioned earlier, some combinations of validated short-term assays and physical chemical properties can be used to predict the carcinogenicity of *Salmonella* nonmutagens (e.g., nongenotoxic carcinogens) (46). Additionally, using knowledge-based structure-activity approaches (see below), evidence for common structural features of nongenotoxic carcinogens has been presented (71,72).

Although the NTP findings suggested that the *Salmonella* mutagenicity test in isolation is as predictive of carcinogenicity as the other tests (11,12), regulatory guidelines in the United States and elsewhere still call for the use of combinations of tests (73—77). Unfortunately, however, no clear guidance is offered as to which tests are to be included in such batteries or how the results are to be interpreted (78,79). Thus, since as a society we are risk averse and since mutagens and genotoxicants are seen by some as representing increased risk for humans (66), the problem seems to be how to identify reliably mutagenic and genotoxic agents using short-term tests (80). This, then, brings us to the development, validation, deployment, and interpretation of such assays, a crucial point given that we can, presumably, choose from among 180 such short-term tests.

It is fairly well agreed that before a test is accepted, a strict validation process must be completed (81). Unfortunately, all too often this is not done, and tests are used that are neither reliable nor validated. Still, it must be emphasized that no single test, even a validated one, is perfect, but knowledge of its predictive characteristics, as described by sensitivity and specificity, with respect to false-positive and false-negative predictions, will allow its inclusion in a testing program (80,82,83).

Currently, the following steps are recognized in the validation process of short-term tests (81): (a) Intra- and interlaboratory reproducibility of the assay must be established. Ideally, this should be accomplished using coded samples. (b) The database must be established. The nature of the chemicals represented in the database is probably the most difficult parameter to address. Thus, the database should contain representatives of various chemical classes, as well as chemicals that cover the spectrum of mechanisms that are hypothesized to induce carcinogenicity in rodents. To satisfy such requirements, it might seem redundant to say that a variety of chemical classes must be represented in the database; however, this is more easily said than done. Looking at the problem from a chemical point of view, using, for example, the experience of the Gene-Tox Program, initially more than 60 chemical classes were defined (84). As a result, there were very few representatives in each chemical class, so no structural correlations were feasible. Subsequently, the number of chemical classes was reduced to 30 (85). Still, this left many chemical classes underrepresented for the purpose of analyzing the relationship between the performance of the assay and structural features. The newer, knowledge-based structure-activity relational (SAR) methods can bypass this problem (see below). (c) The predictive reliability of short-term tests can be determined and expressed in various ways, including concordance, sensitivity, specificity, and predictivity (86). The latter measure of performance can be expressed formally in a comparative fashion using Bayes' theorem (87). These analyses of the characteristics of a test are based on their performance vis-à-vis certified carcinogens and noncarcinogens. This presents a problem, as the "gold standard" (i.e., rodent cancer bioassay) is usually based on a single bioassay, the reproducibility of which is unknown. Finally, as will be shown below, the database may not be representative of the chemical universe, and a particular test may not have been validated against a particular chemical class if chemicals of that family were not included in the validation set.

Thus, although we can characterize the predictive performance of a short-term test, we know that no single test is perfect; each gives a certain proportion of false-positive as well as false-negative results (80,82,83). The question then facing us is, How can this information be used to advantage to interpret the results of short-term tests? A number of generalizations can be made a priori; thus, a test with high sensitivity and high specificity will have good predictive value for both carcinogens and noncarcinogens, whereas a test with high sensitivity but low specificity will be a good predictor of noncarcinogenicity, and conversely an assay with high specificity but low sensitivity will be a good predictor of carcinogens (87).

## DEPLOYMENT OF COMBINATIONS OF TESTS

Because of a desire to be risk averse, as well as in response to a variety of regulatory requirements, very often we are not satisfied with the results of a single test such as the *Salmonella* mutagenicity assay, even though that assay by itself has been suggested to be a good predictor of carcinogenesis (11,12). This has led to the evolution of the concept of batteries or tiers of tests (6,87–93). These tests may be looked upon in two ways that may be mutually exclusive. Batteries may be constructed to cast as wide a net as possible, to identify most potential carcinogens. Under these conditions, the tests would be mechanistically based to include assays that detect the different mechanisms that have been associated with carcinogenicity—DNA damage, gene mutations, chromosomal rearrangements, loss of heterozygosity, cell transformation, and tumor promotion. In addition, it seems reasonable to include *in vitro* and *in vivo* tests and a combination of tests designed to detect different classes of chemicals. On the other hand, batteries could be constructed to confirm one another. In the latter situation, it might be considered that the two tests, even though they may be different, actually reflect the same mechanism. In the former situation, the tests should be independent of one another, whereas in the latter they would be expected to be dependent and overlapping (94).

Another way to identify the greatest spectrum of chemicals is to match the test performance of assays. Thus, as mentioned above, tests that have high levels of both sensitivity and specificity are good predictors of carcinogens and of noncarcinogens. Tests with high sensitivity but low specificity are good at predicting noncarcinogens, while tests with low sensitivity and high specificity are good predictors of carcinogens. Thus, an ideal battery could consist of tests of high sensitivity and high specificity and equal numbers of tests with high sensitivity but low specificity and high specificity and low sensitivity (87). Owing to the fact that very few tests are both highly sensitive and highly specific (80,82), we might have to settle for less than ideal batteries, which might consist of two assays with high sensitivity but low specificity and two with high specificity but low sensitivity. Indeed, it has been shown that such a semi-ideal battery can be highly predictive as well as cost-effective (82).

Using such an approach it is possible to construct batteries that satisfy not only scientific and regulatory criteria but also statistical ones, including tests for independence (82,95). In addition, such batteries can be made to be risk averse (i.e., to minimize the possibility of false-negative results by including a majority of tests that are very sensitive but not necessarily very specific) (82). In addition, cost and time can also be incorporated as determinants. Thus, if two tests exhibit equal performance characteristics as measured by sensitivity and specificity but different costs, the less expensive one should be adopted, since both would contribute equally to the probabilistic outcome (82).

Methods for modeling these situations have been described (46,80,82). Still, with combinations of tests it is probable that results will be mixed (e.g., combinations of positive and negative results), and we must be prepared to take the appropriate action. A battery consisting of three tests may give rise to eight possible results (82), and unless one is prepared to act on each of the possibilities, the tests should not be performed in the first place. A number of decision rules have been used to assess test results:

1. A single positive result outweighs two or more negatives.
2. A majority rules.
3. A hierarchic approach is used; results of testing in a phylogenetically more advanced system outweigh those from a less advanced one (e.g., a negative result of micronucleus *in vivo* outweighs a positive result on the *Salmonella* test *in vitro*).
4. A weight-of-evidence approach takes into consideration the performance characteristics (sensitivity versus specificity, rates of false-positive and false-negative results). This approach can be coupled to the Bayesian analysis mentioned earlier (80).

The latter approach can be exemplified by the battery consisting of mutagenicity in *Salmonella,* the induction of sister chromatid exchanges (SCE), and chromosomal aberrations (ChA) in cultured Chinese hamster ovary cells. The predictive characteristics of these and other tests for carcinogenicity in rodents are shown in Table 1. Thus, we have one test with fairly good sensitivity and specificity *(Salmonella)*, one assay with acceptable sensitivity but low specificity (SCE), and one assay with low

**TABLE 1.** *Sensitivity and specificity of some short-term tests for carcinogenicity*

| Assay | Sensitivity | Specificity |
|---|---|---|
| Mutagenicity in *Salmonella* | 0.767 | 0.730 |
| Chromosomal aberrations | 0.492 | 0.685 |
| Sister chromatid exchanges | 0.727 | 0.427 |
| Mouse lymphoma mutations | 0.680 | 0.329 |
| Micronuclei *in vivo* | 0.545 | 0.617 |
| Structural alerts for DNA reactivity | 0.703 | 0.693 |

sensitivity but acceptable specificity (ChA). By the considerations listed earlier, this can be considered a balanced battery. Applying Bayes theorem (87) to the sensitivities and specificities of these assays, we can calculate the probability of carcinogenicity of each of the eight possible combinations of results. Thus, it must be realized that because none of the tests is perfect, even if all results are positive or if they are all negative (combinations 1 and 5), these will not yield 100% and 0% probabilities of carcinogenicity, respectively. Rather, the predicted probabilities are 85% and 13%, respectively (Table 2). Moreover, as a consequence of the differences in specificities and sensitivities of individual tests, different combinations of test results will give different predictions. Thus, combinations of two positives and one negative may give a probability of 74% (combination 2), which indicates probable carcinogenicity or 39% (combination 8), which is a marginal prediction of carcinogenicity.

Also illustrated in Table 2 is the effect of the inclusion of an assay [induction of mutations at the thymidine kinase locus of mouse lymphoma cells (MLA)] that is problematic. Although MLA has an unacceptably low specificity and a borderline sensitivity (Table 1) and has been shown not to be predictive of carcinogenicity in rodents (11,12), some regulatory jurisdictions require or recommend the MLA as part of a battery of tests (96,97). However, as clearly shown in Table 2, inclusion of MLA has no effect on the outcome irrespective of whether the results of the assays are positive or negative.

In view of the superiority of the *Salmonella* mutagenicity assay over other short-term assays (11,12), the suggestion has been made that a positive response in *Salmonella* should be followed by an *in vivo* micronucleus assay (MNT) to determine whether the mutagenic/genotoxic potential demonstrated *in vitro* is translated into an *in vivo* response (60,66,98). However, a consideration of the predictive performance of MNT (Table 1) suggests that such a strategy is fraught with problems, some of which have been recognized earlier (60,61,79). This is presumably due to the fact that while genotoxicants undoubtedly can induce MNT, such a biologic response is also induced by nongenotoxicants by a mechanism not directly related to the induction of cancers, e.g., inhibition of tubulin polymerization or the induction of aneuploidy (99).

The problem is one of defining genotoxicity (80) and of gaining an understanding of the potential carcinogenicity of a chemical. It must be stressed, however, that the short-term test approach described herein is only part of the initial process of risk assessment (i.e., hazard identification) and determines the probability of causing cancer in rodents as a result of a genotoxic mechanism. The realization of this risk depends on many additional factors, including route, level, and duration of exposure; physiologic and genetic characteristics of the exposed subject; and other possible concurrent exposures or lifestyle.

## STRUCTURE-ACTIVITY APPROACHES

In view of the recognized shortcomings of short-term assays, and given the fact that they cannot yet be used to

**TABLE 2.** *Predictivity of carcinogenicity of combinations of results obtained with a battery consisting of three assays*

| | Salm | ChA | SCE | Probability* | If MLA⁺ | If MLA⁻ |
|---|---|---|---|---|---|---|
| 1 | + | + | + | 0.85 | 0.85 | 0.85 |
| 2 | + | + | − | 0.74 | 0.74 | 0.73 |
| 3 | + | − | + | 0.73 | 0.73 | 0.72 |
| 4 | + | − | − | 0.57 | 0.58 | 0.57 |
| 5 | − | − | − | 0.13 | 0.13 | 0.13 |
| 6 | − | − | + | 0.23 | 0.23 | 0.23 |
| 7 | − | + | − | 0.24 | 0.24 | 0.24 |
| 8 | − | + | + | 0.39 | 0.39 | 0.38 |

*Based on Bayes theorem, applying a prior value of 0.50.

Salm, mutagenicity in *Salmonella;* ChA, induction of chromosomal aberrations in cultured CHO cells; SCE, induction of sister-chromatid exchanges in cultured CHO cells; MLA, induction of mutations at the thymidine kinase locus of cultured mouse lymphoma cells.

identify nongenotoxic carcinogens, efforts to identify structural features associated with carcinogenicity have proceeded.

There are two ways to approach the elucidation of the structural basis of the carcinogenicity of chemicals: (a) hypothesis-driven and (b) knowledge- or information-based approaches. These two approaches can complement each other.

The hypothesis-driven approach to structure-carcinogenicity elucidation is best illustrated by the structural alerts espoused by Ashby and associates (20,21) (Fig. 1). Thus, based primarily on the pioneering studies of Miller and Miller (19), structural alerts recognize electrophiles or potential electrophiles that may be capable of altering the genetic material. Since the *Salmonella* mutagenicity assay, the most widely used short-term test for predicting carcinogenicity, is not endowed with all of the metabolic machinery of the mammal, structural alerts must be able to recognize potential electrophilic moieties that are not mutagenic in *Salmonella* organisms. These include Michael-type chemicals such as acrylamides, which can be biotransformed to DNA-reactive species by mammals (100). The concept of structural alerts is based on the hypothesis that carcinogenic initiation or progression, or both, depends on an alteration of the cellular DNA. As currently practiced, the identification of structural alerts depends on the human expert's knowledge or intuitive understanding of the carcinogenic process. Unlike current knowledge-based systems, the definition of structural alerts is not based on strict statistical criteria; that is, the recognition of a new structural alert may rest on the experimental results for only two chemicals. One of the chief advantages of the hypothesis-driven approach exemplified by structural alerts is that the human expert is able to call on all of the knowledge accumulated over a lifetime of expertise in chemical carcinogenesis, while strictly information-based approaches are restricted to the data that have been included in a "learning set."

As used by Ashby, Tennant, and their associates (20,21), the structural alerts concept has been extremely useful in conjunction with the results of *Salmonella* mutagenicity assays for classifying carcinogens as genotoxic or nongenotoxic. Indeed, the predictive performance for carcinogenicity in rodents based on the presence of structural alerts for DNA reactivity is close to that demonstrated by the *Salmonella* mutagenicity assay (Table 1). The concept of structural alerts has been especially attractive, as it is in harmony with our understanding of oncogene activation and suppressor gene inactivation, and with the generalization that most recognized human carcinogens are genotoxic (51,64,65), as are rodent carcinogens that affect both mice and rats (21,27). Indeed, the current concept of genotoxic carcinogens has led some to suggest that nongenotoxic rodent carcinogens present less of a human hazard than genotoxic ones (13,66–69). Of course, the success of the structural alerts approach derives in part from a tautology: the majority of the chemicals tested during the initial phase of the organized cancer bioassay program consisted of carcinogens, chemicals that looked like carcinogens, mutagens, and other DNA-reactive agents (16). The practitioners of this approach do not deny that there may be a structural basis for the activity of nongenotoxic carcinogens, but they believe that it is as yet unrecognized and therefore that it is not yet ready for exploration by this approach (101).

The knowledge-based approach is not dependent a priori on a mechanistic hypothesis. Rather, it is based on the

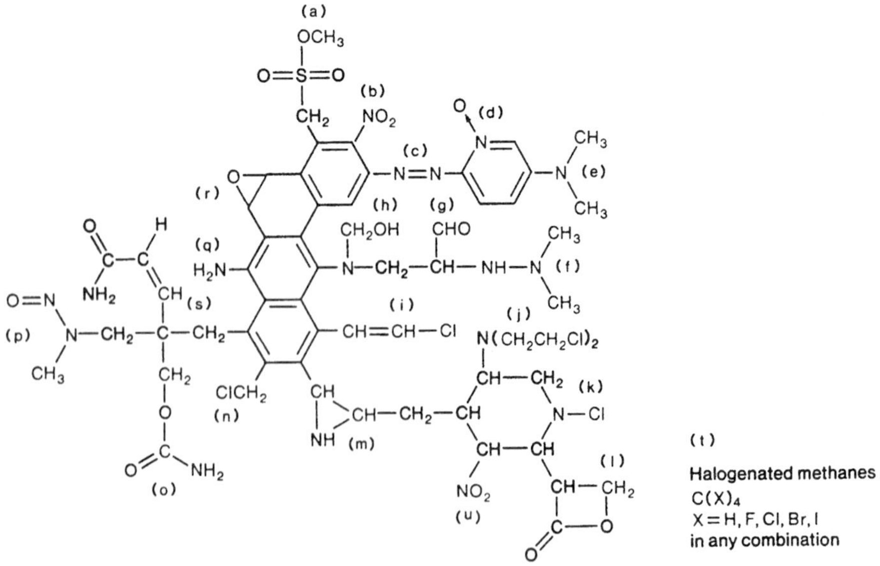


**FIG. 1.** Schematic diagram of composite molecule details the structural alerts. (From ref. 21.)

presumption that there may be a structural basis for cancer causation, including nongenotoxic carcinogenesis, and that its recognition may subsequently lead to the generation of mechanistically based hypotheses. Thus, recent refinements of SAR methods capable of handling noncongeneric databases has resulted in their acceptance as part of the scheme to identify carcinogens (102,103). However, just as with the development of short-term surrogate assays, rigorous procedures relating to the nature of the database, determination of predictive performance, and validation of the resulting SAR models had to be implemented. The development of these diagnostic procedures has lagged behind the implementation of the SAR paradigms. Thus it is generally agreed that the criteria for acceptance of data for model building must be defined rigorously. However, in the case of modeling of the carcinogenic phenomena, the computational toxicologist is hampered by the fact that administration of the chemical may be by the oral, dermal, or inhalation routes. The inclusion of data from these different protocols may make the resulting SAR model noninformative.

To develop a better model, SAR models have been restricted to those agents that have been administered orally. However, retaining a number of chemicals sufficient for model building required pooling of results from bioassays in which test chemicals were administered by gavage, in the food, or in water. This has impact on the nature of the model. Moreover, in developing SAR models of carcinogenesis, we are faced with the unique situation that most chemicals have been tested only once, and thus the reproducibility of the "gold standard" against which the predictive performance of the SAR is judged is not known. The predictive performance of the model cannot be better than that of the assay that is being modeled. Because we lack information regarding the reproducibility of the cancer bioassay, it may be of interest to indicate that the interlaboratory reproducibility of the NTP *Salmonella* mutagenicity assays is approximately 85% (104).

Moreover, only now are criteria dealing with the effect of the size of the database and the nature of the chemical structures contained therein on the performance of the SAR model being evaluated (105,106). Similarly the procedures for validating the SAR models and determining their predictive performances are being addressed currently (107), as is the possibility of combining the predictive features of different SAR models describing the same biologic phenomena, e.g., carcinogenicity (108).

However, in view of the fact that SAR models are being incorporated into regulatory and risk assessment approaches (102,103) and because of their rapidity and cost-effectiveness [in fact a candidate chemical need not be physically available to project its toxicologic profile (109,110)], there is no doubt that the rigorous diagnostics required to determine the general applicability of an SAR model and its predictivity as well as the development of strategies to combine SAR models based on different algorithms will be forthcoming. Finally, advances in programming and personal computer technology are making the SAR methodology widely available to investigators, regulators, and decision makers.

This information-based SAR approach is exemplified by the MULTICASE SAR approach (111,112) (Figs. 2 and 3). Basically, a learning set, consisting of chemical structures and the associated results of the cancer bioassay, is assembled and the expert system is then asked to identify structural determinants associated with biologic activity (Table 3). Typically, MULTICASE recognizes functionalities that resemble the structural alerts described by Ashby [e.g., nitro and amino aromatics (biophore 2; Table 3), bay region, and so on], but additionally the program identifies distance descriptors (e.g., biophore 1; Fig. 3) and functionalities (e.g., biophore 3) not included among the structural alerts. These may be nongenotoxic moieties involved in the carcinogenicity of chemicals that act by mechanisms that do not directly modify the cellular DNA [e.g., receptor-mediated, mitogenesis, toxicity (72,113)]. Still, in view of the fact that the recognized biophore and biophobes achieve good discrimination and correctly identify chemicals as rodent carcinogens or noncarcinogens, we have to accept that they indicate that there is a structural basis for carcinogenicity, including that of chemicals that have a nongenotoxic mechanism (71).

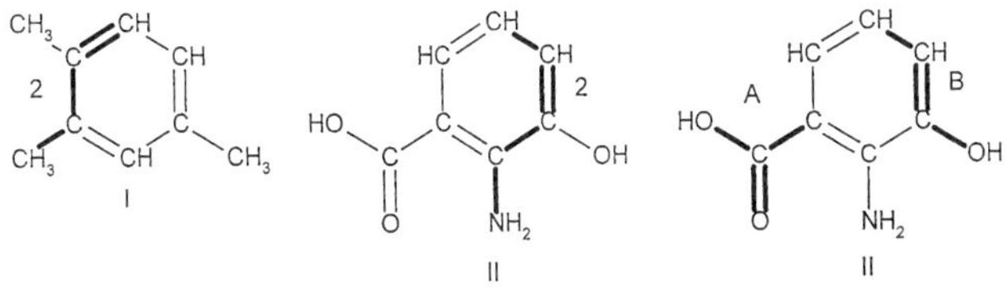


**FIG. 2.** Prediction of the carcinogenicity in mice of 2,5-xylidene (I) and the lack of carcinogenicity of 3-hydroxyanthranilic (II). Both molecules contain biophore 2 (Table 3), which is present in 20 molecules, 16 of which are mouse carcinogens (i.e., 80% probability of carcinogenicity $p$ <.001). The presence of biophore 2 is associated with +44 units of activity. On the other hand, 3-hydroxyanthranilic acid also contains the inactivating modulators -COOH (A) and OH-C=CH-CH= (B), both of which are associated with molecules that contain biophore 2 but are noncarcinogenic. Modulators A and B are associated with -34 and -28 units of activity. Thus 3-hydroxyanthranilic acid, even though it contains biophore 2, which is associated with an 80% probability of carcinogenicity, is predicted to be noncarcinogenic (i.e., 44-34-28 = -18 units). On the other hand, 2,5-xylidene is projected to have an 80% probability of being a mouse carcinogen. Moreover, a projected activity of 44 units of activity corresponds to a potential to cause cancer at a single site in both male and female mice (121). Even though the modulators shown above are structural determinants, they may involve log P (as for biophore 6), highest occupied molecular orbital (HOMO) energy, molecular weight, water solubility and lowest unoccupied molecular orbital (LUMO) energy.

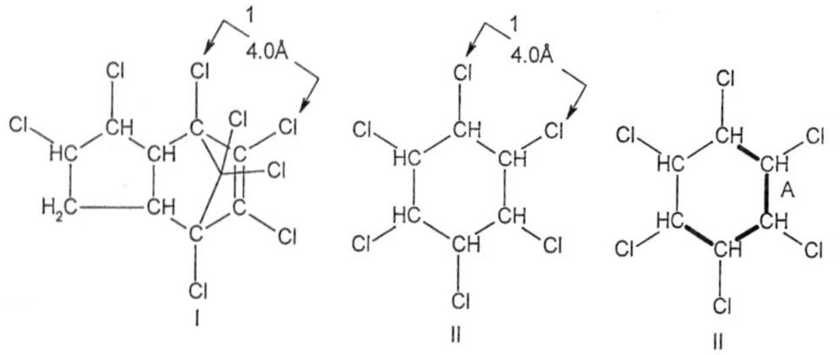

**FIG. 3.** Prediction of the carcinogenicity in mice of chlordane (I) and the lack of carcinogenicity of lindane (II). Both molecules contain biophore 1 (Table 3), which is a lipid anchored distance descriptor (115). In the learning set, this biophore is present in 21 molecules, 17 of which are mouse carcinogens (81% probability of carcinogenicity, $p < .001$). The presence of this biophore is associated with 44 units of activity (see below). However, lindane also contains the inactivating biophore CH-CH-CH-CH-CH- (A), which has been identified in molecules (e.g., endrin, dieldrin) that contain biophore 1 but are devoid of carcinogenicity in mice. Accordingly, in spite of the presence of biophore 1, the carcinogenic potential of lindane is not realized, and it is predicted to be a noncarcinogen. On the other hand, the projected activity of chlordane (44 units) is taken to indicate a potential to cause cancer in male and female mice at a single site (121).

Following the recognition of the carcinogenic biophore, it is up to the expert to interpret its significance, and this in turn may be hypothesis driven. Thus, when investigating the biophores based on an SAR model derived from the Carcinogenic Potency Database of Gold and associates (114), a 6Å distance descriptor that spanned a p-hydroxy-substituted phenyl moiety anchored in a lipophilic center was identified. Further investigation revealed (72) that this biophore was derived from estrogenic carcinogens (e.g., diethylstilbestrol, β-estradiol; Fig. 4). The biophore was present in some antiestrogens but absent in others, and it was absent from phytoestrogens (such as genistein) (115). Our analyses led us to conclude that the lipophilic moiety represented an estrogen receptor recognition ligand, and that the hydroxyl moiety allowed for hydrogen binding to the receptor site (116). Based on these findings we suggested that the 6Å biophore could be used to differentiate between carcinogenic and noncarcinogenic estrogens [e.g., diethylstilbestrol (DES) vs. coumestrol] and to be used in the design of noncarcinogenic antiestrogens (116).

Still, much about the mechanistic significance of the structural moieties associated with nongenotoxic carcinogens remains to be elucidated. However, since it has been recognized that an understanding of the mechanistic basis is essential for identifying the carcinogenic risk represented by exposure to a chemical (102,103,117), it may well be that the nongenotoxic biophore will lead to the recognition that a specific chemical possesses a biophore that is associated with cancer causation that is species and even gender specific and possibly not relevant to humans.

The acceptance of either of the above two SAR approaches (i.e., hypothesis-driven vs. knowledge-based) to the exclusion of the other has important ramifications for the strategy for selecting chemicals for future testing. Thus, as mentioned, currently the rodent carcinogenicity databases are dominated by carcinogens and mutagens (i.e., genotoxic carcinogens). To a large extent this is due to the initial decision to include in the bioassay chemicals that look like carcinogens (16), which in turn leads to tautologies. The net effect, however, is that the informational content of the database is not expanded (22).

If, however, we were to use for the selection of chemicals for further testing an approach that is not primarily hypothesis driven (i.e., DNA reactivity), we would be testing a completely different class of chemicals—chemicals that do not necessarily resemble known carcinogens. In fact, based on the analyses of Ashby, Tennant, and their associates, we have insufficient information on chemicals with known structural alerts to make reliable predictions. On the other hand, if the approach were knowledge based, we would be selecting chemicals characterized by func-

**TABLE 3.** *Major MULTICASE biophores associated with carcinogenicity in mice*

| Fragment | | No. of fragments | Inactives | Marginal | Active | Nr | *p*-value |
|---|---|---|---|---|---|---|---|
| [Cl -] ← 4 Å → [Cl -] | | 21 | 3 | 1 | 17 | 1 | 0.000 |
| $NH_2$–C =C –CH =CH – | | 20 | 4 | 0 | 16 | 2 | 0.004 |
| Cl –C =C –C =CH – | | 4 | 0 | 0 | 4 | 3 | 0.06 |
| O –CH2-CH –CH2– | | 6 | 0 | 0 | 6 | 4 | 0.02 |
| [C –] ← 9.1A → [Cl –] | | 4 | 0 | 0 | 4 | 5 | 0.06 |
| Cl –CH = | | 4 | 0 | 0 | 4 | 6 | 0.06 |
| CH =C. –CO –C. = | | 4 | 0 | 0 | 4 | 7 | 0.06 |
| CH =CH –C =C –CH = | <3-O > | 9 | 1 | 0 | 8 | 8 | 0.01 |
| C1 –C =CH –CH =C –NH2 | | 4 | 0 | 0 | 4 | 9 | 0.06 |

The database was generated under the aegis of the U.S. National Toxicology Program (21,37). Biophores 1 and 2 are shown in Figs. 3 and 2, respectively. Each biophore may be associated with a constellation of specific modulators that either increase or decrease the potential carcinogenicity associated with the biophore (see Figs. 2 and 3). Cl←4Å→Cl indicates a distance descriptor. $NH_2$-C=C-CH=C- indicates that the second carbon atom from the left must be substituted by an atom other than hydrogen. C. indicates a carbon atom shared by 2 ring systems as in anthraquinone. <3-O > indicates that the third atom from the left contains an oxygen substituent.

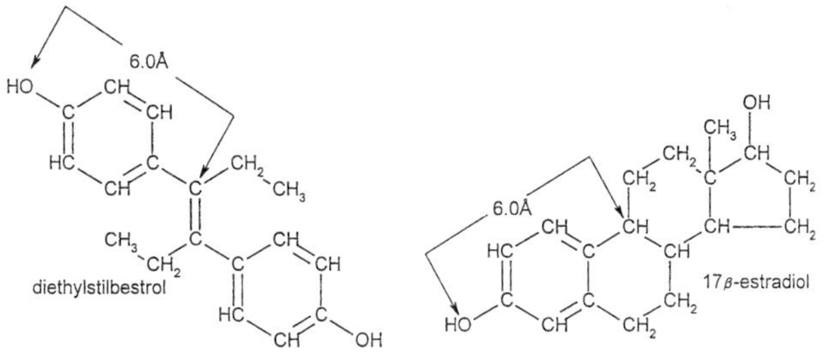


**FIG. 4.** Identification of a 6Å biophore that is anchored in a lipophilic region. This biophore has been identified in carcinogenic estrogens.

tionalities that are as yet unknown with respect to their role in carcinogenicity. Thus, in an analysis of several thousand chemicals representing the universe of chemicals, a number of functionalities were recognized that were not represented among the chemicals tested thus far for carcinogenicity in rodents (22). Some of these were present in a large number of as yet untested chemicals. When using a knowledge-based approach we would want to include chemicals with such unknown functionalities in the bioassay, so as to increase the informational content of the carcinogenicity database and at the same time perhaps recognize additional mechanisms of cancer induction.

## CONCLUSIONS

It would appear that short-term tests to detect mutagenic (genotoxic) carcinogens are available, although relying solely on such assays may yield a number of false-positive results, as noncarcinogenic mutagens do exist. Still, since genotoxic rodent carcinogens may represent a greater risk to humans than nongenotoxic ones, and since we have a societal goal to be risk averse but don't have the resources to carry out extensive cancer bioassays on all chemicals currently used in commerce and industry (92), it appears that judicious selection of a battery of short-term tests may be satisfactory for screening purposes, especially as use of the cancer bioassay as a regulatory tool has been questioned (33–35,92). With respect to nongenotoxic carcinogens, as yet we do not have validated predictive tests, but a consensus is emerging about their mechanisms of action [e.g., dioxins (118), d-limonene(119)], which appear to differ from those of genotoxic carcinogens and may in fact be species and gender specific (119). In parallel with these developments, a number of promising structural approaches have been refined. Additionally, the MULTICASE SAR method, which is a priori information based, does not depend on the results of surrogate tests or on mechanistic hypotheses, and has been shown to be capable of predicting biologic activity with a concordance approaching that of the interlaboratory reproducibility (120). With respect to the prediction of carcinogenicity in rodents, since the experimental reproducibility is not known, the reliability of the predictions must await the results of the cancer bioassays. Still, although the significance of short-term tests and chronic cancer bioassays is currently uncertain, the situation is far from static, and a number of fundamental advances toward determining the causes of cancer will undoubtedly continue to inform the development of methods for identifying cancer-causing chemicals in the workplace and the environment.

## REFERENCES


1. Burdette WS. The significance of mutation in relation to the origin of tumors: a review. *Cancer Res* 1955;15:201–226.
2. Rosenkranz HS. Aspects of microbiology in cancer research. *Annu Rev Microbiol* 1973;27:383–401.
3. IARC. *IARC monographs on the evaluation of the carcinogenic risk of chemicals to humans,* suppl. 6.Lyon, France: International Agency for Research on Cancer, 1988.
4. Singh NP, Tice RR, Stephens RE, Schneider EL. A microgel electrophoresis technique for the direct quantitation of DNA damage and repair in individual fibroblasts cultured on microscope slides. *Mutat Res* 1991;252:289–296.
5. Fenech M, Morley AA. Measurement of micronuclei in lymphocytes. *Mutat Res* 1985;147:29–36.
6. Ashby J. Precedents or possibilities: which should guide the harmonization of mutagenicity test protocols and carcinogen prediction strategies? *Mutat Res* 1993;298:291–295.
7. Ames BN, Durston WE, Yamasaki E, Lee FD. Carcinogens are mutagens: a simple test system combining liver homogenates for activation and bacteria for detection. *Proc Natl Acad Sci USA* 1973;70: 2281–2285.
8. Reynolds SH, Stowers SJ, Patterson RM, Maronpot RR, Aaronson SA, Anderson MW. Activated oncogenes in B6C3F1 mouse liver tumors: Implications for risk assessment. *Science* 1987;237:1309–1316.
9. Stowers SJ, Maronpot RR, Reynolds SH, Anderson MW. The role of oncogenes in chemical carcinogenesis. *Environ Health Perspect* 1987; 75:81–86.
10. Harris CC. p53: at the crossroad of molecular carcinogenesis and risk assessment. *Science* 1993;262:1980–1981.
11. Tennant RW, Margolin BH, Shelby MD, et al. Prediction of chemical carcinogenicity in rodents from *in vitro* genotoxicity assays. *Science* 1987;236:933–941.
12. Zeiger E, Haseman JK, Shelby MD, Margolin BH, Tennant RW. Evaluation of four *in vitro* genetic toxicity tests for predicting rodent carcinogenicity: confirmation of earlier results with 41 additional chemicals. *Environ Mol Mutagen* 1990;16:1–14.
13. Ashby J, Purchase IFH. Reflections on the declining ability of the Salmonella assay to detect rodent carcinogens as positive. *Mutat Res* 1987;205:51–58.
14. Sugimura T, Sato S, Nagao M, et al. Overlapping of carcinogens and mutagens. In: Magee PN, Takayama S, Sugimura T, et al., eds. *Fundamentals in cancer prevention.* Tokyo: University of Tokyo Press, 1976;191–215.
15. Rosenkranz HS, Poirier LA. An evaluation of the mutagenicity and DNA modifying activity of microbial systems of carcinogens and noncarcinogens. *J Natl Cancer Inst* 1979;62:873–892.
16. Clayson DB, Arnold DL. The classification of carcinogens identified in the rodent bioassay as potential risks to humans: What type of substance should be tested next? *Mutat Res* 1991;257:91–106.
17. Rosenkranz HS, Ennever FR. Recent developments in the use of short-term tests to identify carcinogens and noncarcinogens. *ISI Atlas of Science:* Pharmacology 1988;2:211–214.
18. Slater EE, Anderson MD, Rosenkranz HS. Rapid detection of mutagens and carcinogens. *Cancer Res* 1971;31:970–973.
19. Miller JA, Miller EC. Ultimate chemical carcinogens as reactive mutagenic electrophiles. In: Hiatt HH, Watson JD, Winsten JA, eds. *Origins of human cancer.* Cold Spring Harbor, NY: Cold Spring Harbor Laboratory, 1977;605–627.

20. Ashby J. Fundamental structural alerts to potential carcinogenicity or noncarcinogenicity. *Environ Mol Mutagen* 1985;7:919–921.
21. Ashby J, Tennant RW. Definitive relationships among chemical structure, carcinogenicity and mutagenicity for 301 chemicals tested by the U.S. NTP. *Mutat Res* 1991;257:229–306.
22. Takihi N, Rosenkranz HS, Klopman G. Identification of chemicals for testing in the rodent cancer bioassay. *Quality Assurance: Good Practice, Regulation, and Law* 1993;2:232–243.
23. Sontag JM, Page NP, Saffiotti U. *Guidelines for carcinogenicity bioassay in small rodents.* DHEW publication NIH 76-801. Washington, DC: Department of Health, Education and Welfare, 1976.
24. Haseman JK, Huff JE, Zeiger E, McConnell EE. Comparative results of 327 chemical carcinogenicity studies. *Environ Health Perspect* 1987;74:229–235.
25. Shelby MD, Stasiewicz S. Chemicals showing no evidence of carcinogenicity in long-term, two-species rodent studies: the need for short-term test data. *Environ Mutagen* 1984;6:871–878.
26. Clayson DB, Krewski D. The concept of negativity in experimental carcinogenesis. *Mutat Res* 1986;167:233–240.
27. Gold LS, Bernstein L, Magaw R, Slone TH. Interspecies extrapolation in carcinogenesis: Prediction between rats and mice. *Environ Health Perspect* 1989;81:211–219.
28. Rosenkranz HS, Ennever FK. An association between mutagenicity and carcinogenic potency. *Mutat Res* 1990;244:61–65.
29. Parodi S, Malacarne D, Romano P, Taningher M. Are genotoxic carcinogens more potent than nongenotoxic carcinogens? *Environ Health Perspect* 1991;95:199–204.
30. Butterworth BE. Consideration of both genotoxic and nongenotoxic mechanisms in predicting carcinogenic potential. *Mutat Res* 1990;239:117–132.
31. Cohen SM, Ellwein LB. Cell proliferation in carcinogenesis. *Science* 1990;249:1007–1011.
32. Preston-Martin S, Pike MC, Ross RK, Jones PA, Henderson BE. Increased cell division as a cause of human cancer. *Cancer Res* 1990;50:7415–7421.
33. Ames BN, Gold LS. Too many rodent carcinogens: mitogenesis increases mutagenesis. *Science* 1990;249:970–971.
34. Ames BN, Gold LS. Chemical carcinogenesis: Too many rodent carcinogens. *Proc Natl Acad Sci USA* 1990;87:7772–7776.
35. Swenberg JA. Bioassay design and MTD setting: Old methods and new approaches. *Regul Toxicol Pharmacol* 1995;21:44–51.
36. Weinstein IB. Mitogenesis is only one factor in carcinogenesis. *Science* 1991;251:387–388.
37. Ashby J, Tennant RW, Prediction of rodent carcinogenicity for 44 chemicals: results. *Mutagenesis* 1990;9:7–15.
38. Rulis AM. De Minimis and the threshold of regulation. In: Felix CW, ed. *Food production technology.* Chelsea, MI: Lewis, 1986;29–37.
39. Scheuplin R. Perspectives on toxicological risk—an example: Food-borne carcinogenic risk. In: Clayson DB, Munro IC, Swenberg JA, et al., eds. *Programs in predictive toxicology.* New York: Elsevier, 1990; 351–372.
40. Heddle JA. Prediction of chemical carcinogenicity from *in vitro* genetic toxicity. *Mutagenesis* 1988;3:287–291.
41. Huff JG, McConnell EG, Haseman JK. On the proportion of positive results in carcinogenicity studies in animals [letter]. *Environ Mutagen 1985;*7:427.
42. Clayson DB. Can a mechanistic rationale be provided for nongenotoxic carcinogens identified in rodent bioassays? *Mutat Res* 1989;221:53–67.
43. Douglas GR, Blakey DH, Clayson DB. Genotoxicity tests as predictors of carcinogens: an analysis. *Mutat Res* 1988;196:83–93.
44. Ennever FK, Rosenkranz HS. Short-term test results for NTP noncarcinogenesis: An alternate, more predictive battery. *Environ Mutagen* 1986;8:849–865.
45. Ennever FK, Rosenkranz HS. Application of the carcinogenicity prediction and battery selection (CPBS) method to recent National Toxicology Program short-term test data. *Environ Mol Mutagen* 1989;13:332–338.
46. Lee Y, Rosenkranz HS, Buchanan BG, Mattison DR, Klopman G. Learning rules to predict rodent carcinogenicity of non-genotoxic chemicals. *Mutat Res* 1995;328:127–149.
47. Ashby J. Computer-assisted short-term test battery design: Some questions. *Environ Mol Mutagen* 1988;11:443–448.
48. Ashby J. The separate identities of genotoxic and nongenotoxic carcinogens. *Mutagenesis* 1988;3:365–366.
49. Benigni R. Mutagenicity testing: New National Toxicology Program (NTP) data confirm old data but question old interpretations. *Mutagenesis* 1987;2:239–240.
50. Bridges BA. Genetic toxicology at the crossroads—a personal view on the deployment of short-term tests for predicting carcinogenicity. *Mutat Res* 1988;205:25–31.
51. Ennever FK, Noonan TJ, Rosenkranz HS. The predictivity of animal bioassays and short-term genotoxicity tests for carcinogenicity and noncarcinogenicity to humans. *Mutagenesis* 1987;2:73–78.
52. Ennever FK, Rosenkranz HS. Computer-assisted short-term test battery design: Some answers. *Environ Mol Mutagen* 1988;12:349–352.
53. Haseman JK, Margolin BH, Shelby MD, Zeiger E, Tennant RW. Do short-term tests predict rodent carcinogenicity? *Science* 1988;241: 1232–1233.
54. ICPEMC. Testing for mutagens and carcinogens: The role of short-term genotoxicity assays. *Mutat Res* 1988;205:3–12.
55. Kier LD. Comments and perspective on the EPA workshop on The relationship between short-term test information and carcinogenicity. *Environ Mol Mutagen* 1988;11:147–157.
56. Ramel C. Short-term testing—are we looking at wrong end points? *Mutat Res* 1988;205:13–24.
57. Yander G, Lin GHY, Mermelstein R. Selection of batteries in an industrial setting. *Environ Mutagen* 1987;9:357–358.
58. Galloway SM. The micronucleus test and NTP rodent carcinogens: not so many false negatives. *Mutat Res* 1996;352:185–188.
59. Shelby MD, Erexson GL, Hook GJ, Tice RR. Evaluation of a three-exposure mouse bone marrow micronucleus protocol: results with 49 chemicals. *Environ Mol Mutagen* 1993;21:160–179.
60. Tinwell H, Ashby J. Comparative activity of human carcinogens and NTP rodent carcinogens in the mouse bone marrow micronucleus assay. *Environ Health Perspect* 1994;102:758–762.
61. Zeiger E. Strategies and philosophies of genotoxicity testing: what is the question? *Mutat Res* 1994;304:309–314.
62. Morrison V, Ashby J. A preliminary evaluation of the performance of the Muta Mouse and Big Blue (lacl) transgenic mouse mutation assays. *Mutagenesis* 1994;9:367–375.
63. Mirsalis JC, Monforte JA, Winegar RA. Transgenic animal models for measuring mutations *in vivo*. *Crit Rev Toxicol* 1994;24:255–280.
64. Bartsch H, Malaveille C. Prevalence of genotoxic chemicals among animal and human carcinogens evaluated in the IARC Monograph Series. *Cell Biol Toxicol* 1989;5:115–127.
65. Shelby MD. The genetic toxicity of human carcinogens and its implications. *Mutat Res* 1988;204:3–15.
66. Ashby J, Morrod RS. Detection of human carcinogens. *Nature* 1991; 352:185–186.
67. Anderson MF, Higginson J, Krewski D, et al. Safety assessment procedures for indirect food additives. An overview. *Regul Toxicol Pharmacol* 1990;12:2–12.
68. Williams GM. Definition of a human cancer hazard. In: Butterworth BE, Slaga TJ, eds. *Nongenotoxic mechanisms in carcinogenesis.* Cold Spring Harbor, NY: Cold Spring Harbor Laboratory, 1987; 367–380.
69. Ashby J, Purchase IFH. Will all chemicals be carcinogenic to rodents when adequately evaluated? *Mutagenesis* 1993;8:489–493.
70. Upton AC, Clayson DG, Jansen JD, Rosenkranz HS, Williams GM. Report of the International Commission for Protection against Environmental Mutagens and Carcinogens Task Group on the Differentiation between Genotoxic and Nongenotoxic Carcinogens. *Mutat Res* 1984;133:1–49.
71. Rosenkranz HS, Klopman G. Structural basis of carcinogenicity in rodents of genotoxicants and nongenotoxicants. *Mutat Res* 1990;228: 105–124.
72. Rosenkranz HS, Cunningham A, Klopman G. Identification of a 2-D geometric descriptor associated with non-genotoxic carcinogens and some estrogens and antiestrogens. *Mutagenesis* 1996;11:95–100.
73. Loprieno N. Control of commercial chemicals: the sixth amendment to the directive on dangerous chemical substances (79/831/EEC) adopted by the Council of the European Communities. *Chem Mutagens* 1983;8:343–366.
74. ICPEMC. Regulatory approaches to the control of environmental mutagens and carcinogens. *Mutat Res* 1983;114:179–216.
75. Shirasu Y. The Japanese mutagenicity studies' guidelines for pesticide registration. *Mutat Res* 1988;205:393–395.
76. Parry JM. The equivalence of assays within individual guidelines for

the testing of the potential mutagenicity of chemicals: problems associated with battery selection. *Mutat Res* 1988;205:385–392.
77. Auletta AE, Dearfield KL, Cimino MC. Mutagenicity test schemes and guidelines: U.S. EPA Office of Pollution Prevention and Toxics and Office of Pesticide Programs. *Environ Mol Mutagen* 1993;21: 38–45.
78. Kirkland DJ. Genetic toxicology testing requirements: Official and unofficial views from Europe. *Environ Mol Mutagen* 1993;21:8–14.
79. Madle S. Problem of the harmonization of philosophies for genotoxicity testing. *Mutat Res* 1993;300:73–76.
80. Rosenkranz HS, Ennever FK. Quantifying genotoxicity and nongenotoxicity. *Mutat Res* 1988;205:59–67.
81. Balls M, Blaauboer B, Brusick D, et al. Report and recommendations of the CAAT/ERGATT Workshop on the Validation of Toxicity Test Procedures. *ATLA* 1990;18:313–337.
82. Rosenkranz HS, Ennever FK. New approaches to battery selection and interpretation. In: Jolles G, Cordier A, eds. *New trends in genetic risk assessment.* New York: Academic Press, 1989;401–425.
83. Ennever FK, Rosenkranz HS. Methodologies for interpretation of short-term test results which may allow reduction in the use of animals in carcinogenicity testing. *Toxicol Ind Health* 1988;4:137–149.
84. Ray VA, Kier LD, Kannan KL, et al. An approach to identifying specialized batteries of bioassays for specific classes of chemicals: class analysis using mutagenicity and carcinogenicity relationships and phylogenetic concordance and discordance patterns. *Mutat Res* 1987; 185:197–241.
85. Nesnow S, Argus M, Bergman H, et al. Chemical carcinogens: a review and analysis of the literature of selected chemicals and the establishment of the Gene-Tox Carcinogen Database. *Mutat Res* 1987; 185:1–195.
86. Purchase IFH. An appraisal of predictive tests for carcinogenicity. *Mutat Res* 1982;99:53–71.
87. Chankong V, Haimes YY, Rosenkranz HS, Pet-Edwards J. The Carcinogenicity Prediction and Battery Selection (CPBS) method: a Bayesian approach. *Mutat Res* 1985;153:135–166.
88. Bridges BA. Short-term screening for carcinogens. *Nature* 1976;261: 195–200.
89. Brusick D. Principles of genetic toxicology. New York: Plenum Press, 1980;199–202.
90. Flamm WG. A tier system approach to mutagen testing. *Mutat Res* 1974;26:329–333.
91. ICPEMC. Mutagenesis testing as an approach to carcinogenesis. *Mutat Res* 1982;99:73–91.
92. Lave LB, Omenn GS, Heffernan KD, Dranoff G. A model for selecting short-term tests of carcinogenicity. *J Am Coll Toxicol* 1983;2: 125–130.
93. Dean BJ, ed. *Report of the UKEMS Sub-Committee on Guidelines for Mutagenicity Testing. Part I:* Basic test battery; *minimal criteria; professional standards; interpretation; selection of supplementary assays.* Swansen, Wales: United Kingdom Environmental Mutagen Society, 1983.
94. Rosenkranz HS. Demythifiers: short-term tests and intelligence (human or otherwise). *Mutagenesis* 1990;5:299–300.
95. Kim BS, Margolin BH. Predicting carcinogenicity by using batteries of dependent short-term tests. *Environ Health Perspect* 1994;102 (suppl 1):127–130.
96. Combes RD, Stopper H, Caspary WJ. The use of L5178Y mouse lymphoma cells to assess the mutagenic, clastogenic and aneugenic properties of chemicals. *Mutagenesis* 1995;10:403–408.
97. Garriot ML, Casciano DA, Schechtman LM, Probst GS. International Workshop on Mouse Lymphoma Assay Testing Practices and Data Interpretations: Portland, Oregon, May 7, 1994. *Environ Mol Mutagen* 1995;25:162–164.
98. Ashby J, Tinwell H. A sequential approach to testing with the rodent bone marrow micronucleus assay—obviation of the need for statistical analyses of data. *Mutat Res* 1995;327:49–55.
99. ter Haar E, Day BW, Rosenkranz HS. Direct tubulin polymerization perturbation contributes significantly to the induction of micronuclei *in vivo*. *Mutat Res* 1996;350:331–337.
100. Warr TJ, Parry JM, Callander RD, Ashby J. Methyl vinyl sulphone: a new class of Michael-type genotoxin. *Mutat Res* 1990;245: 191–199.
101. Ashby J. Use of short-term tests in determining the genotoxicity or non-genotoxicity of chemicals. In: Vainio H, Magee P, McGregor D, McMichael AJ, eds. *Mechanisms of carcinogenesis in risk identification,* No. 116. Lyon, France: International Agency for Research on Cancer, 1992;135–164.
102. National Research Council. *Science and judgment in risk assessment.* Washington, DC: National Academy Press, 1994.
103. Environmental Protection Agency (EPA). *Proposed guidelines for carcinogen risk assessment.* Washington, DC: EPA, Office of Research and Development, 1996.
104. Piegorsch WW, Zeiger E. Measuring intra-assay agreement for the Ames *Salmonella* assay. In: Rienhoff O, Linberg DAB, eds. *Lecture notes in medical information (statistical methods in toxicology).* Berlin: Springer, 1991;35–41.
105. Liu M, Sussman N, Klopman G, Rosenkranz HS. Estimation of the optimal database size for structure-activity analyses: the *Salmonella* mutagenicity database. *Mutat Res* 1996;358:63–72.
106. Liu M, Sussman N, Klopman G, Rosenkranz HS. Structure-activity and mechanistic relationships: The effects of chemical overlap on structural overlap in databases of varying size and composition. *Mutat Res* 1996;372:79–85.
107. Zhang YP, Sussman N, Klopman G, Rosenkranz HS. Development of methods to ascertain the predictivity and consistency of SAR models: application to the National Toxicology Program rodent carcinogenicity bioassays. *Quant Struct-Act Rehab* 1997;16:290–295.
108. Macina OT, Zhang YP, Rosenkranz HS. Improved predictivity of carcinogens: The use of a battery of SAR Models. In: Kitchin KT, ed. *Testing, predicting and interpreting carcinogenicity.* 1997;9:237.
109. Zhang YP, Macina OT, Rosenkranz HS, Karol MH, Mattison DR, Klopman G. Prediction of the metabolism and toxicological profiles of oxygenates added to gasoline. *Inhalation Toxicol* 1997;9:237–254.
110. Rosenkranz HS, Klopman G. Structure-activity relationships as alternatives in the study of carcinogenesis. In: Goldberg AM, Van Zutphon LFM, eds. *Alternative methods in toxicology and the life sciences,* vol 11. New York: Mary Ann Liebert, 1994;379–390.
111. Klopman G, Rosenkranz HS. Prediction of carcinogenicity/ mutagenicity using Multicase. *Mutat Res* 1994;305:33–46.
112. Klopman G. Multicase 1. A hierarchical computer automated structure evaluation program. *Quant Struct Act Rel* 1992;11:176–184.
113. Rosenkranz HS, Klopman G. Structural evidence for a dichotomy in rodent carcinogenesis: involvement of genetic and cellular toxicity. *Mutat Res* 1993;303:83–89.
114. Gold LS, Manley NB, Slone TH, Garfinkel GB, Rohrbach L, Ames BN. The fifth plot of the Carcinogenic Potency Database: results of animal bioassays published in the general literature through 1988 and by the National Toxicology Program through 1989. *Environ Health Perspect* 1993;100:65–135.
115. Cunningham AR, Rosenkranz HS, Klopman G. Structural analysis of a group of phytoestrogens for the presence of a 2-D geometric descriptor associated with non-genotoxic carcinogens and some estrogens. *Proc Soc Exp Biol Med* 1997;9:237–254.
116. Cunningham AR, Klopman G, Rosenkranz HS. A dichotomy in the lipophilicity of natural estrogens/xenoestrogens and phytoestrogens. *Environ Health Perspect* 1997;105(suppl3):665–668.
117. Vainio H, Magee P, McGregor D, McMichael AJ, eds. *Mechanisms of carcinogenesis in risk identification.* IARC Scientific Publication No. 116. Lyon, France: International Agency for Research on Cancer, 1992.
118. Roberts L. Dioxin risks revisited. *Science* 1991;251:624–626.
119. Hard GC, Whysner J. Risk assessment of d-limonene: an example of male rat-specific renal tumorigens. *Crit Rev Toxicol* 1994;24: 231–254.
120. Zeiger E, Ashby J, Bakale G, Enslein K, Klopman G, Rosenkranz HS. Prediction of Salmonella mutagenicity. *Mutagenesis* 1996;11: 471–484.
121. Rosenkranz HS, Zhang YP, Klopman G. Risk identification using structural concepts: the potential carcinogenicity of praziquantel. *Regul Toxicol Pharmacol* 1995;22:152–161.

*Environmental and Occupational Medicine, Third Edition,* edited by William N. Rom.
Lippincott–Raven Publishers, Philadelphia © 1998.

# CHAPTER 17

# Genetic Susceptibility

David L. Eaton, Federico M. Farin, Curtis J. Omiecinski, and Gilbert S. Omenn

Variation in susceptibility to chemical, infectious, and physical agents encountered in the workplace or in other environments increasingly is being recognized as an important variable in environmental and occupational medicine. There are clinical, policy, and scientific reasons for such attention.

First, workers often ask, "Why me, Doc?" when informed that a particular workplace exposure may account for their medical complaints. "I'm no more exposed and no less careful than the next person." Such clinical encounters put an ethical imperative on learning whether some workers are more susceptible than others to similar exposures and through what mechanisms. The same applies for individuals, families, and population subgroups in the broader community.

Second, key laws require informed analysis about variation in susceptibility. The Occupational Safety and Health Act requires that health standards be such that no worker, even if exposed at the "safe level" (the standard) for a full working lifetime, shall suffer any adverse effects (with allowance for technical feasibility in meeting the standard). The Clean Air Act requires that National Ambient Air Quality Standards protect even the most susceptible subgroups in the population, and do so with an adequate margin of safety. As we reduce harmful exposures in the workplace and the environment more generally, genetic variations could account for a larger proportion of the remaining risk of adverse health effects from chemical and other exposures. Nongenetic factors, including nutritional differences, coexisting exposures, protective practices, and other behavioral and physiologic determinants (smoking, drinking habits, body weight) also need to be considered as part of "host variation." Table 1 shows the place of host variation in the characterization of risks and in regulatory decision-making.

Third, dramatic advances in human genetics and in the technology to test for genetic differences offer promise of practical means for an individualized practice of preventive medicine through risk profiling and through understanding how to modify the effects or end results of various genetic predisposition. Susceptibility genes, unlike major genes associated with colon or breast cancer, for example, are neither necessary nor sufficient to cause disease, but modify the risk; they often have high prevalence in the population, so that even modestly increased absolute risk can lead to a rather high population-attributable risk when there is appropriate exposure (3).

No longer should we think of "nature versus nurture"; rather, we should focus on the interaction of genetic and environmental factors. We call that field "eco-genetics" (4–6). The concept was beautifully articulated early in the 20th century by the discoverer of several inborn errors of metabolism, Sir Archibald Garrod: "In every case of every malady there are two sets of factors at work in the formation of the morbid picture, namely internal or constitutional factors, inherent in the sufferer and usually inherited from his forebearers, and external ones which fire the train" (3).

Nevertheless, as this chapter will document, we are still in the earliest phases of developing eco-genetics into a practical role in occupational and environmental medicine. We have focused on the genetics of key biotransformation enzymes, about which a veritable avalanche of

D. L. Eaton, F. M. Farin, and C. J. Omiecinski: Department of Environmental Health, University of Washington, Seattle, Washington 98105-6099.
G. S. Omenn: Executive Vice President for Medical Affairs, The University of Michigan, Ann Arbor, Michigan 48109-0624.

**TABLE 1.** *Framework for risk assessment and risk management*

| | |
|---|---|
| Identification of hazard | Epidemiology |
| | Toxicology |
| | *in vitro* tests |
| | Structure-activity analyses |
| Characterization of risks | Dose-response (potency) |
| | Exposures |
| | Susceptibility |
| Control/reduction of risks | Information |
| | Personal protection |
| | Regulation |
| | Substitution |

Adapted from refs. 1 and 2.

clinical and scientific studies is occurring. We provide a critical review of the literature, often noting conflicting results (not surprising with small numbers of persons studied in most studies) or lack of knowledge about functional and clinical consequences of the genetic variation discovered. As more is learned, we can confidently predict that profiles of such variation (some protective, some more vulnerable) will need to be studied and eventually tested, not just variation in one gene, one enzyme, or one cell receptor at a time.

This recommendation for combined analysis is analogous to the thrust of the new Risk Management Framework proposed by the presidential/congressional Commission on Risk Assessment and Risk Management: put each environmental problem into public health (or ecological) context (7), analyzing all sources of an ambient exposure and estimating risks of health end points attributable to each agent and each category of sources. Like the commission, we also emphasize the crucial importance of worker and other stakeholder participation in decisions about whether and how to test, what to test for, how to interpret test results, and how to ensure that privacy, confidentiality, access to health insurance and life insurance, and employment status are protected.

## BIOTRANSFORMATION ENZYME POLYMORPHISMS

Most potentially toxic chemicals encountered in the workplace and general environment undergo chemical changes soon after entering the body (Fig. 1). This process of biotransformation occurs predominantly in the liver, although all tissues have some capacity to biotransform most chemicals. Biotransformation of a chemical to its final metabolite(s), which are usually eliminated in urine or bile, is often a multistep process whereby the chemical is first oxidized to a more polar form, then conjugated with an endogenous ligand such as glutathione, sulfate, acetate, or glucuronic acid. Oxidation of most chemicals occurs by the multigene family of enzymes collectively referred to as the cytochromes P-450 (CYP) (Fig. 1). Common variant forms of numerous individual CYP genes have been identified; these "polymorphisms" often confer differences in catalytic activity or level of gene expression, which may result in varying rates and/or extent of oxidation of xenobiotics among individuals.

Analogous multigene families of conjugating enzymes have been identified, including the glutathione S-transferases (GST) and the *N*-acetyltransferases (NAT). Common polymorphisms in these enzymes have been identified in the human population. Most, but not all, conjugation reactions are detoxification reactions, and thus "poor metabolizers" for these enzymes are potentially at increased risk for chemical-related diseases. A large number of molecular epidemiology studies have been completed in the past decade to identify the relative etiologic significance of numerous biotransformation enzyme polymorphisms. The following section summarizes the results of the major studies, and attempts to identify diseases of relevance to the occupational environment where genetic susceptibilities have been substantiated.

### Cytochrome P-450 1A1

Polycyclic aromatic hydrocarbons (PAHs) such as benzo[*a*]pyrene, and other aromatic compounds are oxidized by CYP1A1 to mutagenic and/or carcinogenic metabolites (8). Two common polymorphisms in the CYP1A1 gene have been described, the *Msp*I and *Ile-Val* variants (9); their prevalence varies with ethnic background (Table 2). A third variant allele present in 8% of African-Americans has not been detected in Caucasian or Asians (10,11).

The functional significance of the CYP1A1 variants is unclear. The CYP1A1 *Ile-Val* polymorphism may be associated with increased inducibility (10,29,30), or elevated constitutive expression of the enzyme (31).

In Japanese (9,32–34) and some Caucasians (12,14) CYP1A1 genotypes have been associated with increased risk of smoking-associated lung cancer, but not in others (13,35,36). Smokers with the *Msp*I/*Msp*I or the Val/Val genotype have a significantly higher risk of possessing a mutant p53, a key control gene in cell division (37). One of two studies of the third variant in African-Americans showed an association with adenocarcinoma of the lung (38,39). CYP1A1 polymorphisms also have been associated with increased risk for breast cancer, especially in those who smoked up to 29 pack-years (40), but not for bladder cancer (41).

### Cytochrome P-450 2D6 (Debrisoquine Hydroxylase)

CYP2D6 polymorphisms affect the metabolism and drug/drug interactions of >30 widely used cardiac and antidepressant medications (42). From 7% to 10% of Caucasians have a "poor metabolizer" phenotype, while

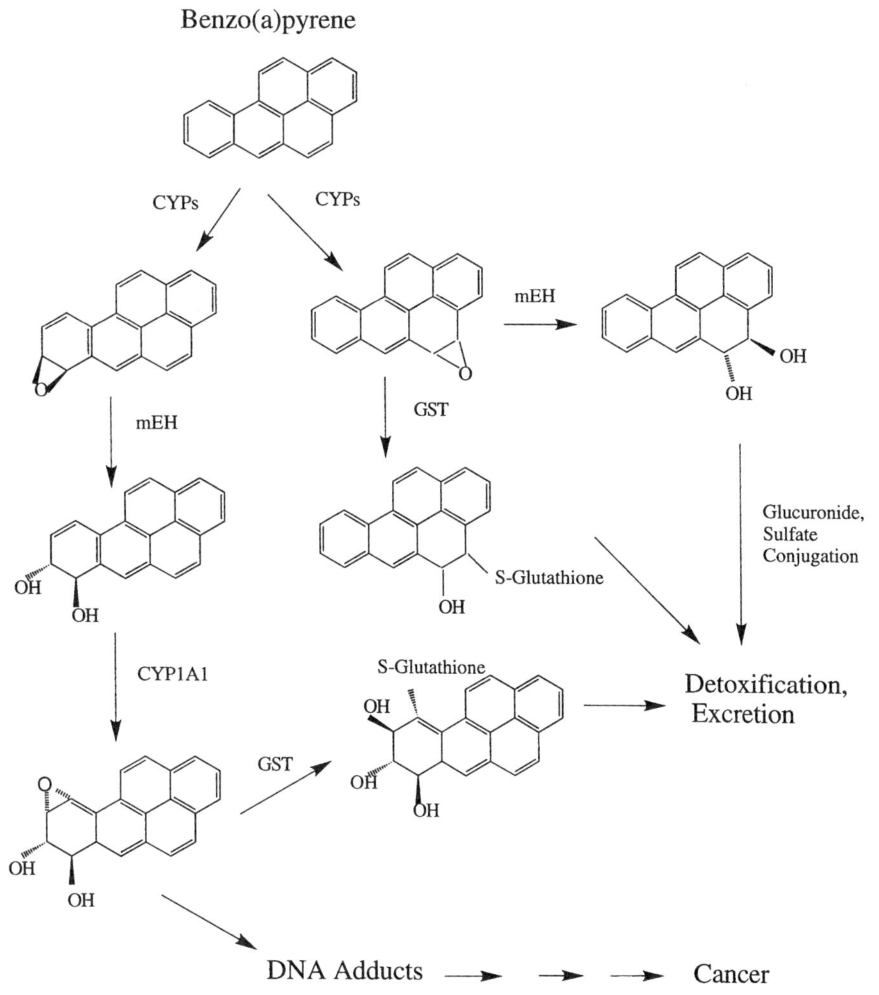


**FIG. 1.** Pathways of benzo[*a*]pyrene activation and detoxification, showing roles of cytochrome P-450, epoxide hydrolase, and glutathione S-transferase enzymes.

**TABLE 2.** *Ethnic variation in the allele frequency of different biotransformation enzyme polymorphisms*

| Polymorphism | Caucasian | Asian | African-American | Reference |
|---|---|---|---|---|
| CYP1A1-MspI | 7–14% | 33% | 23% | 12–14 |
| CYP1A1-Ile-Val | 3% | 20% | 2% | 12,15,16 |
| CYP1A1-MspI (intron 7) | <1% | <1% | 9% | 11 |
| CYP2D6[a] | 7–10% | 1% | NA | 17,18 |
| CYP2E1-DraI | 9% | 31% | 9% | 20 |
| CYP2E1-PstI | 2% | 24% | 5% | 19,20 |
| CYP2E1-RsaI | 2% | 27% | 2% | 19 |
| mEH-113 H/H | 8% | NA | NA | 21 |
| mEH-139 R/R | 5% | NA | NA | 21 |
| GSTM1[b] | 43–52% | 48–60% | 22–35% | 22,23 |
| GSTT1[b] | 15–20% | 60% | 22% | 23–25 |
| NAT2[c] | 40–70% | 32–60% | 68% | 26 |
| Paraoxonase | 50% | variable | variable | 27,28 |

[a]Represents frequency of multiple variant alleles that result in poor metabolizer phenotype.
[b]Represents frequency of individuals who are homozygous for the null (deleted) alleles.
[c]Represents frequency of slow acetylator alleles.
NA, not available.

the rest, the "extensive metabolizers," represent a broad range of activity (17,42–44).

It was hypothesized that extensive metabolizers would activate procarcinogens much more actively than poor metabolizers. Despite numerous reports of associations of CYP2D6 with various disease states, follow-up studies have led to conflicting results. For example, CYP2D6 poor metabolizer phenotype and genotypes were associated with lower risk of lung (45–47) and bladder cancer (48–50), but the strength of any association remains controversial (3). Similarly, early reports of association of CYP2D6 variants with Parkinson's disease (51–54) and schizophrenia (55,56) are now contradicted.

### Cytochrome P-450 1A2

CYP1A2 is a key enzyme in the oxidation of many carcinogens, such as dietary heterocyclic aromatic amines (e.g., MeIQ), aromatic arylamines (e.g., 4-aminobiphenyl), tobacco-specific nitrosamines (e.g., NNK), and aflatoxins, found in the diet, tobacco smoke, and the workplace (57). This enzyme is expressed only in liver, and as much as a 70-fold variation in activity has been described among humans (57, 58). Even though the distribution is polymodal, no genetic basis for these large interindividual differences have been identified (57). Phenotypic differences in activity can be assessed conveniently by determining the ratio of specific metabolites of caffeine in the urine (57). There are currently no molecular epidemiology studies that have assessed the importance of phenotypic variation in CYP1A2 in relation to cancers, but based on *in vitro* studies the rapid metabolizer CYP1A2 phenotype would be expected to be at increased risk for aflatoxin-related liver cancer and perhaps other diet and smoking-related cancers (57).

### Cytochrome P-450 2E1

This cytochrome P-450 metabolizes benzene, trichloroethylene, alcohols, and nitrosamines found in the diet and cigarette smoke (58,59). CYP2E1 is highly expressed in liver and also active in extrahepatic tissues (60); levels vary widely between individuals (61). Allelic frequencies of three CYP2E1 polymorphisms according to ethnic group are listed in Table 2.

The CYP2E1 *Dra* I polymorphism has been associated with susceptibility to cancer of the lung in Japanese (62–64), but not in Scandinavian populations (65,66). Both the *Pst*I polymorphism and the 5′ flanking *Rsa*I polymorphism have shown no increased risk for lung cancer in numerous studies (19,20,65,67,68).

CYP2E1 metabolizes ethanol to acetaldehyde and the hydroxyethyl radical, and is also inducible by alcohol. The *Rsa*I allele has greater transcriptional and enzyme activity, compared to the wild-type allele (69), and has been associated with higher risk of developing alcoholic liver disease among Caucasians with alcohol abuse (70).

### Epoxide Hydrolase

Microsomal epoxide hydrolase (EH) is the key epoxide hydrolase enzyme in biotransformation of drugs and foreign compounds (71), and epoxide derivatives of certain steroids, e.g., estroxide (72). Other forms of EH act on cholesterol epoxides (73), leukotriene A4 (74), *trans*-stilbene oxide, and endogenous arachidonate and prostaglandin-derived epoxide intermediates (75).

Two polymorphisms in microsomal EH have been characterized, coding a Tyr to His substitution at position 113 and a His to Arg substitution at position 139 of the enzyme. In Caucasians Tyr is the predominant amino acid at position 113, while His predominates at position 139 (21). *In vitro* the Tyr113/Arg139 combination has approximately 65% higher activity than the His113/His139 combination (21). Complex regulation of microsomal EH gene expression *in vivo* makes interpretation of the available data quite challenging.

Microsomal EH detoxifies anticonvulsant medications such as phenobarbital, phenytoin, and carbamazepine; phenytoin is a known cause of birth defects (76–78). Data on a direct genetic association between microsomal EH polymorphism and incidence of adverse effects of the drugs are inconclusive (79–81).

Although microsomal EH actually contributes to the bioactivation of certain carcinogenic polycyclic aromatic hydrocarbons, it generally detoxifies most xenobiotic epoxides (Fig. 1). Only a few cancer epidemiology studies have been reported with the EH variants. McGlynn et al. (82) reported an odds ratio of 3.3 for hepatocellular carcinoma (HCC) incidence in a Chinese population possessing at least one low-activity His113 allele, when considered independent of glutathione transferase M1 genotype or hepatitis B virus (HBV) exposure. Individuals with both HBV infection and the high-risk (low-activity) EH genotype exhibited >77 times the risk of HCC compared with individuals with neither factor (82). In contrast, Lancaster et al. (83) found a 2.6-fold increased risk for ovarian cancer with the higher activity Tyr113 EH allele. A bladder cancer study showed no association (41).

### Glutathione S-Transferases

The glutathione S-transferases (GST) are a multigene family of dimeric enzymes that detoxify a variety of xenobiotics by conjugation with glutathione and excretion of the conjugates. There are four major classes of GST enzymes: alpha (GSTA), mu (GSTM), pi (GSTP), and theta (GSTT) (23). GSTM1 and GSTT1 are polymorphic in the human population.

#### *GSTM1 Polymorphism*

Approximately 45% to 55% of the Caucasian population is homozygous for a deletion of the GSTM1 gene (84,85). Ethnic differences in gene frequency are shown in Table 2. In Micronesia, >90% of Polynesians have the null genotype.

GSTM1 detoxifies several carcinogenic epoxides found in cigarette smoke, such as benzo[*a*]pyrene and tobacco-specific nitrosamines. Deletion of the GSTM1 gene and loss of GSTM1 activity places individuals, especially smokers, at increased risk for lung cancer (16,36,37,86–100). Even studies without a statistically significant association between the GSTM1 null genotype and increased risk for lung cancer (88,89,96,97), show a trend in that direction. Two separate meta-analyses of studies completed prior to 1995 found composite odds ratios of 1.41 [95% CI, 1.23–1.60 (100)) and 1.6 (95% CI, 1.26–2.04 (101)] for an association between the GSTM1 null genotype and lung cancer risk. To put these findings in perspective, because of the ~50% frequency for this deletion phenotype and the high incidence of lung cancer in smokers, an increased risk of 60% associated with the GST null genotype in smokers gives an excess number of cancer deaths due to this one gene greater than cancer deaths attributed to breast cancer (e.g. BRCA1 and BRCA2) gene and the human nonpolyposis colon carcinoma (HNPCC) gene combined (3)!

Of the dozen studies of the relationship between the GSTM1 null genotype and bladder cancer, most have demonstrated a significant association (26,41,102–113). A meta-analysis of six studies in Caucasians completed prior to 1995 found an aggregate odds ratio of 1.54 (101). The proportion of total risk for bladder cancers attributable to the GSTM1 polymorphism has been estimated to be 17% to 25% (109,113).

Because smoking is associated with bladder cancer, it is not surprising that the strongest association has been identified in smokers, although several studies have also found increased risk among nonsmokers. Other studies have demonstrated that urine from smokers with the GSTM1 null genotype is more mutagenic than urine from GST-positive smokers (114); both smokers and nonsmokers with the null GSTM1 genotype have a higher level of 3- and 4-aminobiphenyl hemoglobin adducts (115), lending biologic plausibility to such an association. It has been suggested that the GSTM1 null genotype may be related to survival of bladder cancer patients (105).

No association was found between the GST null genotype and bladder cancer among workers with exposure to benzidine (102). There is little reason to expect such an association because GSTM1 is not involved in the detoxification of benzidine.

Several studies have suggested that the GST null genotype is associated with increased risk to stomach cancer (24,116,117), but not all (118). Two studies on GSTM1 genotype and colon cancer suggested an approximate increase in risk of 60% to 70% for the null genotype (106,116), but more recent studies (118–120) have not. Case-control studies of GSTM1 null genotype and breast (24,40,106), brain (121,122), skin (123–126), ovarian (127), cervical (128), anal (129), oral (118,130), and liver (131,132) cancers have been largely negative; in a few instances a trend was noticed or subclassification resulted in marginally significant associations.

Although several studies have implicated human GSTM1 in the detoxification of the potent liver carcinogen, aflatoxin $B_1$ (a fungal toxin contaminant of peanuts and corn) (82,133,134), definitive studies in rodents have found that it is an alpha class GST with high catalytic activity toward AFB-epoxide (135–137). Relative to these rodent alpha class GSTs, human GSTM1 has very low activity toward AFB-epoxide (134–137), and there was no correlation with GSTM1 genotype and phenotype with ability of human liver to conjugate AFB-epoxide *in vitro* (138). Based on the only molecular epidemiology study on GSTM1 and AFB-related liver cancer, GST null individuals exposed to aflatoxin $B_1$ in the diet may be at slightly increased risk of hepatocellular carcinoma relative to GST-positive individuals (82,139). Thus, in the absence of an alpha class GST with high activity toward AFB-epoxide in human liver, the low activity present in GSTM1 could be important in protection against AFB-induced liver cancer in humans.

Although the vast majority of studies of the GSTM1 polymorphism have focused on cancer susceptibility, several other disease end points have also been examined. The GSTM1 null genotype occurred more frequently among solvent-exposed workers with a diagnosis of chronic toxic encephalopathy (CTE) when compared to non-CTE patients referred to a clinic for some degree of psychiatric or neurologic symptoms (140). GSTM1 null individuals were also found to be significantly more likely to have radiographic evidence of nonmalignant asbestos-related disease, compared to the GST-positive individuals (141). Weak associations of the GSTM1 null genotype with endometriosis (142), alcoholic liver disease (142,143), chronic bronchitis (142), and a subset of cystic fibrosis patients (142) have been reported.

### *GSTT1 Polymorphism*

A polymorphism for the theta class GST enzyme in humans was first described in 1994 (144). Like the GSTM1 polymorphism, the T1 polymorphism reflects deletion of a substantial part of the gene. Thus homozygous-deleted individuals lack GSTT1 activity in all tissues. The frequency of the GSTT1 deletion ranges from about 15% in Caucasians to over 60% in certain Asian populations (23). This enzyme has considerable functional significance, because it either activates or detoxifies a variety of oxidative metabolites of important industrial chemicals, including methylene chloride, ethylene dichloride, methyl bromide, ethylene oxide, and 1,3-butadiene (23,145). The gene deletion could decrease risk to some exposures (e.g., ethylene dichloride, which GSTT1 activates to a genotoxic metabolite) while increasing risk to other chemicals (e.g., butadiene, for which GSTT1 detoxifies the butadiene epoxides). GSTT1*0/0 (null genotype) individuals occupationally exposed to butadiene demonstrated a 16-fold increase in sister-chromatid exchange compared to GSTT1-positive individuals with similar exposures (146); chromosomal aberrations were also significantly higher (147).

Several molecular epidemiology studies have been completed already on the relationship between the GSTT1 deletion and cancer. Chen et al. (148) found a 4.3-fold increased risk for myelodysplastic diseases among individuals that were homozygous for the theta deletion. The GSTT1 deletion polymorphism has also been associated with increased risk for astrocytoma and meningioma, although the sample size was small (121). An association with colon cancer was found in one study (118) but not another (120). A third study found GSTT1 null homozygotes were more common in patients who were diagnosed before age 70 (119).

No association between GSTT1 null genotype and skin cancer was found in one study (124), but in a longitudinal study basal cell carcinomas appeared at a significantly greater rate in GSTT1 null individuals [rate ratio 2.15, $p$ <.001 (125)]. GSTT1 deletion was associated with increased risk for bladder cancer in nonsmokers (OR 2.6, 95% CI, 1.1–6.0), but not in intermediate or heavy smokers (41). Other studies on lung (118), oral (118), or gastric (118,120) cancers failed to find any statistically significant association with the GSTT1 null genotype. The significance of this polymorphism will require further study.

### Arylamine *N*-Acetyltransferase

Arylamine *N*-acetyltransferase (NAT) acetylates numerous drugs containing primary aromatic amine or hydrazine groups, including isoniazid, sulfamethazine and other sulfonamides, procainamide, hydrazine, dapsone, and caffeine, as well as the well-known carcinogens β-naphthylamine, 4-aminobiphenyl, benzidine, and 2-aminofluorene (149).

In humans two distinct genes code for *N*-acetyltransferase 1 (NAT1) and *N*-acetyltransferase 2 (NAT2) (150). NAT2 is polymorphic as a result of various point mutations in the coding region (151), making individuals phenotypically slow or rapid acetylators (152). Of Caucasians in Europe and North America, 40% to 70% have the slow acetylator phenotype, making them less efficient than rapid acetylators in the metabolism of certain drugs and chemicals (Table 2). Rapid acetylators are either heterozygous or homozygous for the wild-type alleles; slow acetylators' enzymes are poorly expressed, unstable, or partially reduced in catalytic activity (153).

Combined data from 12 studies of bladder cancer found a 1.5-fold increase in risk for bladder cancer in slow versus rapid acetylators, which increased to 2.2-fold in patients with documented exposure to arylamines (154). Exposures were not the same across all studies, as workers in some studies were exposed to both benzidine and β-napthylamine, whereas others were exposed only to benzidine. It is likely that acetylator phenotype is a risk factor only in association with certain types of exposure.

Separation between acetylator phenotypes was not initially recognized for NAT1; however, recent studies have demonstrated that NAT1 is also "polymorphic" (155,156). NAT1 and NAT2 are both involved in the metabolism of arylamines, but at different points in the pathway. *N*-acetylation of the amine by NAT2 is a detoxification pathway, whereas *O*-acetylation of the P-450–activated hydroxylamine by NAT1 results in further activation to a carcinogenic intermediate. Thus, it has been suggested that individuals with exposure to carcinogenic aromatic amines who possess a combined rapid NAT1–slow NAT2 phenotype/genotype will be at highest risk for the development of urinary bladder cancer (157).

Studies of breast cancer and NAT2 phenotype, as a single variable, generated inconclusive results (158–160). However, in postmenopausal women who smoked more than one pack a day, NAT2 slow acetylator status strongly increased the slight association of smoking with breast cancer risk (161).

Many studies have addressed the association between lung cancer and the NAT2 phenotype, but most have not found a significant association (162–164). Rapid acetylators appear to be more susceptible to develop colorectal cancer than slow acetylators (165–167), although not all studies have found this association (168). Roberts-Thomson et al. (169) investigated both acetylator phenotype and meat intake in 110 patients with colorectal cancer, 89 patients with adenomatous polyps, and 110 controls; rapid acetylator phenotype was associated with an odds ratio of 1.1 for polyps and 1.8 for cancer (2.5 and 8.9 among those less than 64 years of age); the effect was strongly associated with medium and high meat intake, but showed no association with fat, fiber, calcium, or ethanol. Slow acetylators showed no pattern of increased risk with increasing meat intake.

### Combined Genotypes and Cancer Susceptibility

Because biotransformation of xenobiotics is usually a multistep pathway involving both activation and detoxification steps, one might expect that certain combinations of genotypes could be especially predisposing to chemical-induced disease (Table 3). Indeed, in a study of Japanese smokers, the relative risk of individuals with a combination of the Val/*Val* genotype of the CYP1A1 *Ile-Val* polymorphism and the GSTM1 null genotype was 5.8 for lung cancer and 9.1 for squamous cell carcinoma, compared with other combinations of genotypes (16). Another case-control study found that the Japanese who were homozygous for the 3′ noncoding region *Msp*I poly-

**TABLE 3.** *Summary of relationship between various biotransformation polymorphisms and cancer susceptibility*

| Polymorphism[a] | Lung cancer | Bladder cancer | Colon cancer | Breast cancer |
|---|---|---|---|---|
| CYP1A1-any | + | | | + |
| MspI-3′ | + | | | |
| Val/Val | ± | | | |
| MspI, intron 7 | ± | | | ++ |
| CYP2D6 | ± | ± | | |
| CYP2E1 | | | ± | |
| DraI | ± | | | |
| PstI | − | | | |
| RsaI | − | | | |
| NAT1 | | ± | | |
| NAT2 | − | + | + (decrease) | ± |
| GSTM1 | + | + | ± | − |
| GSTT1 | − | + | ± | |
| Combination: | | | | |
| GSTM1 + CYP1A1 | +++ | | | |
| NAT1 + NAT2 | | +++ | | |

[a]Compares the variant genotype (homozygous null for GSTM1 and T1, "slow" metabolizer genotypes for NAT1, NAT2 and CYP2D6) to the wild type genotype. This table represents a crude approximation of effects; many of the "positive" studies are reflective of special at-risk populations (e.g., smokers, occupationally exposed), and are not necessarily reflective of the general population risk.

morphism or individuals with the *Val/Val* genotype of the *Ile-Val* polymorphism in CYP1A1, combined with the GSTM1 null genotype, had odds ratios of 16 and 41 respectively, for lung cancer (170). In contrast, Swedish lung cancer patients showed no association between CYP1A1 allelic variants and an increased susceptibility to lung cancer, but there was an increased risk (OR = 3.0) for squamous cell carcinoma diagnosed before age 66 among patients who carried both the GSTM1 null genotype and one of the rare alleles of the CYP1A1 *Msp*I polymorphism (36).

## GENETIC VARIATION IN SUSCEPTIBILITY TO NONCANCER EFFECTS OF CHEMICALS

### Neurotoxicity

#### *Polymorphic Biotransformation of Pesticides by Plasma Paraoxonase*

In general, health effects other than cancer have received much less attention than predisposition to cancers. However, that is changing, with explicit test protocols and risk assessment guidance for reproductive, developmental, neurobehavioral, immunologic, and various organ-specific toxicities. An important example of a polymorphic biotransformation enzyme affecting neurotoxicity risk is the enzyme paraoxonase. This plasma enzyme inactivates the toxic metabolite of the common organophosphorus pesticide parathion, widely used in agriculture and in the home and garden. Parathion is activated by P-450 enzymes to paraoxon, which both kills insects and damages human nerves by attacking acetylcholinesterase, an enzyme essential for normal cholinergic function. Paraoxonase degrades paraoxon into harmless p-nitrophenol and diethylphosphate products. Different racial and ethnic groups show significant variations in paraoxonase activity, affecting a broad array of OP and carbamate pesticides; Caucasians have a bimodal distribution in activity (Table 2), with 50% low and 50% high activity (a difference of up to threefold), related to a Gln/Arg polymorphism at position 191 in the protein (27,28). In contrast, African, Chinese, Japanese, and Malaysian populations show a wide range of activity with no clear separation between high- and low-activity groups; further genetic dissection of the variation is needed. Low activity is almost unknown among Inuit Alaskans, Zambians, and Australian aborigines tested (171). Although the role of this phosphotriesterase in normal metabolism is unknown, a role in lipid metabolism and cardiovascular disease is suspected, based on the fact that the enzyme is a component of circulating high-density lipoprotein (HDL) (27,28,172).

## PULMONARY DISEASE RELATED TO POLYMORPHIC GENETIC VARIATION

Alpha$_1$-antitrypsin, the most abundant proteinase inhibitor in human plasma, is important in protecting tissues from endogenous proteolytic damage. Persons with deficiencies of this protein are predisposed to damage in the lung, liver, joints, kidneys, and vasculature. Those who are smokers are particularly vulnerable in the lungs, leading to emphysema at an early age, due to the action of neutrophil elastase on lung elastin. More than 75 variants have been discovered; one common deficiency allele (S, with Glu/Val substitution at position 264) occurs in 7% of Caucasians. Individuals homozygous for this allele have 50% to 60% of normal alpha$_1$-antitrypsin activity.

The less common Z allele (Lys/Glu substitution at position 342) reduces activity to 10% to 15% in homozygotes; 3% of the population in Britain carries this allele, which is not found in Africans or Asians (173).

Smoking is the critical factor in these predisposed individuals. The rate of pulmonary deterioration of the elastic matrix of alveolar walls was four times more rapid in deficient smokers as in deficient nonsmokers (174). In MZ heterozygotes (2–5% of Caucasian), the loss of elastic recoil in smokers is about equal to that in ZZ nonsmokers.

There is marked interindividual variation in susceptibility to beryllium oxide–induced lung disease from exposures to power plant emissions as dusts and fumes. Occupational chronic beryllium exposure also occurs in ceramics, electronics, dental alloy, metal extraction, and aerospace workplaces. The polymorphic genetic marker HLA-DP $\beta_1$-Glu69 has been associated in cultured blood lymphocytes from sensitive persons with exaggerated proliferation *in vitro* in the presence of beryllium salts (175). HLA-DR and HLA-DQ alleles may also be associated with acid anhydride–induced asthma (176) and isocyanate-induced asthma (177).

## DIFFERENCES IN SUSCEPTIBILITY TO INFECTIOUS AGENTS

Classic examples of variation in susceptibility include the complete resistance of Duffy-negative red blood cells to infection by vivax malaria plasmodia; the advantage in survival of carriers of glucose-6-phosphate dehydrogenase (G6PD) deficiency, hemoglobin S, and beta-thalassemia genes in infections with falciparum malaria plasmodia; and greater association of likelihood of infection and sites of complications in monozygotic versus dizygotic twins.

Currently of great potential importance in occupational medicine is the exciting evidence from American and Belgian investigators that an identical 32 base pair deletion mutation in the chemokine receptor (CKR-5/CCR-5) that is a cofactor for entry of the HIV virus into $CD4^+$ cells makes such individuals highly resistant to HIV infection and probably to cell-cell transfer of the virus. The truncated protein that results from this deletion mutation loses the third transmembrane loop of this receptor protein in the cell membrane, and thereby loses its biologic activity. Evidence of resistance comes from the extensive histories without apparent infection and the *in vitro* resistance of white blood cells from such individuals to HIV-1 strains (178). These observations from alert clinicians and now epidemiologic and virologic investigators herald a whole new way to interfere with HIV infection. Probably there are other mutations that interfere with HIV infection, since this mutation has been found in only a small fraction of “clinically resistant” individuals.

## HEMOCHROMATOSIS

Hereditary hemochromatosis occurs with a frequency of the homozygote of 1 in 200 to 1 in 2,000 persons in the general Caucasian population. There is a very long presymptomatic period, of 40 years or more, before clinical features become manifest. Practitioners of occupational medicine need to be aware of this disorder. The symptoms are nonspecific fatigue, asthenia, joint pains, loss of libido, impotence, increased skin pigmentation, and liver enlargement. Cirrhosis of the liver, diabetes mellitus, and impairment of cardiac function are major complications of iron storage in the respective organs. If the condition is recognized, treatment is straightforward: periodic phlebotomies. Even cardiac disease may respond to iron depletion; it can definitely be prevented (179). Screening can be performed by testing iron saturation, or now by testing for mutations of an HLA-H gene and protein (His63/Asp and Cys282/Tyr substitutions); this protein is homologous with major histocompatibility complex (MHC) class I molecules (180). Women are less likely to manifest this autosomal dominant condition than men, since they dispose of much of the excess iron through menstruation.

## TESTING PRINCIPLES

As genetic variation is recognized and probes are developed to test for numerous common (polymorphic) variants in genes important to biotransformation and to sites of action of exogenous chemicals, many issues will have to be resolved in order to make ethical and effective use of such technology in preventive, occupational, and environmental medicine (1,181). Tests must have well-characterized sensitivity, specificity, and predictive values in population groups for which they are proposed to be used. Only then can test results be interpreted. The purposes of testing must be agreed upon by all stakeholders before testing is undertaken, even research on testing. It must be agreed who controls the information and who decides who controls the information, so that discrimination in employment and in insurance—based on test results, or even on misinterpretation of test—can be avoided. Since genetic variation is different in different ethnic and racial groups (Table 2), special care must be taken to have appropriate controls and to avoid racial discrimination. Finally, we must use these new tools to identify and control harmful exposures, rather than to exclude the predisposed.

## CONCLUSION

Genetic variation in susceptibility is an essential element of the characterization of risk in diverse human populations. Knowledge is mounting rapidly about genes important in human responses to harmful agents and variation in those genes. Nevertheless, it is a huge leap to define epidemiologically and toxicologically the significance of such variation and to find appropriate applications in the practice of occupational and environmental medicine.

## REFERENCES


1. Omenn GS, Faustman EM. Risk assessment, risk communication, and risk management. In: Detels R, Holland WW, McEwen J, Omenn GS, eds. *Oxford textbook of public health.* New York: Oxford University Press, 1997;969–986.
2. Faustman EM, Omenn GS. Risk assessment. In: Klaassen CD, ed. *Casarett and Doull's toxicology:* the basic science of poisons, 5th ed. New York: McGraw-Hill, 1996;75–88.
3. Caporaso N. Commentary: genetic susceptibility and the common cancers. *Biomarkers* 1996;1:174–177.
4. Omenn GS, Motulsky AG. Ecogenetics: genetic variation in susceptibility to environmental agents. In: Cohen BH, Lilienfeld AM, Huang PC, eds. *Genetic issues in public health and medicine.* Springfield, IL: C. C. Thomas, 1978;83–111.
5. Omenn GS, Gelboin HV. *Genetic variability in responses to chemical exposure.* Banbury Report. Cold Spring Harbor, NY: Cold Spring Harbor Laboratory, 1984.
6. Omenn GS, Omiecinski CJ, Eaton DL. Eco-genetics of chemical carcinogens. In: Cantor C, Caskey T, Hood L, Kamely D, Omenn G, eds. *Biotechnology and human genetic predisposition.* New York: Alan R. Liss, 1990;81–93.
7. Commission on Risk Assessment and Risk Management. *A new framework for environmental health risk management.* Washington, DC: Risk Commission, 1996.
8. Shimada T, Yun CH, Yamazaki H, Gautier JC, Beaune PH, Guengerich FP. Characterization of human lung microsomal cytochrome P-450 1A1 and its role in oxidation of chemical carcinogens. *Mol Pharmacol* 1992;41:856–864.
9. Hayashi S, Watanabe J, Nakachi K, Kawajiri K. Genetic linkage of lung cancer-associated MspI polymorphisms with amino acid replacement in the heme binding region of the human cytochrome P-4501A1 gene. *J Biochem* 1991;110:407–411.
10. Taioli E, Crofts F, Trachman J, Bayo S, Toniolo P, Garte SJ. Radical differences in CYP1A1 genotype and function. *Toxicol Lett* 1995;77:357–362.
11. Crofts F, Cosma G, Currie D, Taioli E, Toniolo P, Garte JS. A novel CYP1A1 gene polymorphism in African-Americans. *Carcinogenesis* 1993;9:1729–1731.
12. Drakoulis N, Cascorbi I, Brockmoller J, Gross CR, Roots I. Polymorphisms in the human CYP1A1 gene as susceptibility factors for lung cancer: exon-7 mutation (4889 A to G), and a T to C mutation in the 3′-flanking region. *Clin Invest* 1994;72:240–248.
13. Tefre T, Ryberg D, Haugen A, et al. Human CYP1A1 (cytochrome P1450) gene: lack of association between the MspI restriction fragment length polymorphism and incidence of lung cancer in a Norwegian population. *Pharmacogenetics* 1991;1:20–25.
14. Xu X, Kelsey KT, Wiencke JK, Wain JC, Christiani DC. Cytochrome P-450 CYP1A1 MspI polymorphisms and lung cancer susceptibility. *Cancer Epidemiol Biomark Prevent* 1996;5:687–692.
15. Taioli E, Trachman J, Chen X, Toniolo P, Garte SJ. A CYP1A1 restriction fragment length polymorphism is associated with breast cancer in African-American women. *Cancer Res* 1995;55:3757–3758.
16. Hayashi S, Watanabe J, Kawajiri K. High susceptibility to lung cancer analyzed in terms of combined genotypes of P-450IA1 and Mu-class glutathione S-transferase genes. *Jpn J Cancer Res* 1992;83:866–870.
17. Daly AK, Brockmoller J, Broly F, et al. Nomenclature for human CYP2D6 alleles. *Pharmacogenetics* 1996;6:193–201.
18. Johansson I, Oscarson M, Yue Q, Bertilsson L, Sjoqvist F, Ingelman-Sundberg M. Genetic analysis of the Chinese cytochrome P-4502D locus: characterization of variant CYP2D6 genes present in subjects with diminished capacity for debrisoquine hydroxylation. *Mol Pharmacol* 1994;46:452–459.
19. Kato S, Shields PG, Caporaso NE, et al. Cytochrome P-450IIE1 genetic polymorphisms, racial variation, and lung cancer risk. *Cancer Res* 1992;52:6712–6715.
20. Kato S, Shields PG, Caporaso NE, et al. Analysis of cytochrome P450 2E1 genetic polymorphisms in relation to human lung cancer. *Cancer Epidemiol Biomark Prevent* 1994;6:515–518.
21. Hassett C, Aicher L, Sidhu JS, Omiecinski CJ. Human microsomal epoxide hydrolase: genetic polymorphism and functional expression *in vitro* of amino acid variants [published erratum appears *in Hum Mol Genet* 1994;3(7):1214]. *Hum Mol Genet* 1994;3:421–428.
22. Chen CL, Liu Q, Relling MV. Simultaneous characterization of glutathione S-transfersase M1 and T1 polymorphisms by polymerase chain reaction in American whites and blacks. *Pharmacogenetics* 1996;6:187–191.
23. Hayes JD, Pulford DJ. The glutathione S-Transferase supergene family: regulation of GST and the contribution of the isoenzymes to cancer chemoprotection and drug resistance. *Crit Rev Biochem Mol Biol* 1995;30:445–600.
24. Harada S, Misawa S, Nakamura T, Tanaka N, Ueno E, Mutzumi N. Detection of GST1 gene deletion by polymerase chain reaction and its possible correlation with stomach cancer in Japanese. *Hum Genet* 1992;90:62–64.
25. Nelson HH, Wiencke JK, Christiani DC, et al. Ethnic differences in the prevalence of the homozygous deleted genotype of glutathione S-transferase theta. *Carcinogenesis* 1995;16:1243–1245.
26. Lin HJ, Han CY, Lin BK, Hardy S. Ethnic distribution of slow acetylator mutations in the polymorphic N-acetyltransferase (NAT2) gene. *Pharmacogenetics* 1994;4:125–134.
27. Adkins S, Gan KN, Mody M, La Du BN. Molecular basis for the polymorphic forms of human serum paraoxonase/arylesterase: glutamine or arginine at position 191, for the respective A or B allozymes. *Am J Hum Genet* 1993;52:598–608.
28. Humbert R, Adler DA, Disteche CM, Hassett C, Omiecinski CJ, Furlong CE. The molecular basis of the human serum paraoxonase activity polymorphism. *Nature Genet* 1993;3:73–76.
29. Cosma G, Crofts F, Currie D, Wirgin I, Toniolo P, Garte SJ. Racial differences in restriction fragment length polymorphisms and messenger RNA inducibility of the human CYP1A1 gene. *Cancer Epidemiol Biomark Prevent* 1993;2:53–57.
30. Crofts F, Taioli E, Trachman J, et al. Functional significance of different human CYP1A1 genotypes. *Carcinogenesis* 1994;15:2961–2963.
31. Kiyohara C, Hirohata T, Inutsuka S. The relationship between aryl hydrocarbon hydroxylase and polymorphisms of the CYP1A1 gene. *Jpn J Cancer Res* 1996;87:18–24.
32. Kawajiri K, Nakachi K, ImaiK, Yoshii A, Shinoda N, Watanabe J. Identification of genetically high risk individuals to lung cancer by DNA polymorphisms of the cytochrome P-4501A1 gene. *FEBS Lett* 1990;263:131–133.
33. Kawajiri K, Nakachi K, Imai K, Watanabe J, Hayashi S. The CYP1A1 gene and cancer susceptibility. *Crit Rev Oncol Hematol* 1993;14: 77–87.
34. Okada T, Kawashima K, Fukushi S, Minakuchi T, Nishimura S. Association between a cytochrome P-450 CYP1A1 genotype and incidence of lung cancer. *Pharmacogenetics* 1994;4:333–340.
35. Hirvonen A, Pursianen KH, Karjalainen A, Antilla S, Vainio H. Point mutational MspI and Ile-Val polymorphism closely linked in the CYP1A1 gene: lack of association with susceptibility to lung cancer in a Finnish study population. *Cancer Epidemiol Biomark Prevent* 1992;1:465–489.
36. Alexandrie AK, Sundberg MI, Seidegard J, Tornling G, Rannug A. Genetic susceptibility to lung cancer with special emphasis on CYP1A1 and GSTM1: a study on host factors in relation to age at onset, gender and histological cancer types. *Carcinogenesis* 1994;15: 1785–1790.
37. Kawajiri K, Eguchi H, Nakachi K, Sekiya T, Yamamoto M. Association of CYP1A1 germ line polymorphisms with mutations of the p53 gene in lung cancer. *Cancer Res* 1996;56:72–76.
38. Taioli ECF, Trachman J, Demopoulos R, Toniolo P, Garte SJ. A specific African-American CYP1A1 polymorphism is associated with adenocarcinoma of the lung. *Cancer Res* 1995;55:472–473.
39. London SJ, Daly AK, Fairbrother KS, et al. Lung cancer risk in African-Americans in relation to a race-specific CYP1A1 polymorphism. *Cancer Res* 1995;55:6035–6037.
40. Ambrosone CB, Freudenheim JL, Graham S, et al. Cytochrome P-4501A1 and glutathione S-transferase (M1) genetic polymorphisms and postmenopausal breast cancer risk. *Cancer Res* 1995;55: 3483–3485.

41. Brockmoller J, Cascorbi I, Kerb R, Roots I. Combined analysis of inherited polymorphisms in arylamine N-acetyltransferase 2, glutathione S-transferases M1 and T1, microsomal epoxide hydrolase, and cytochrome P-450 enzymes as modulators of bladder cancer risk. *Cancer Res* 1996;56:3915–3925.
42. Kroemer HK, Eichelbaum M. "It's the genes, stupid." Molecular bases and clinical consequences of genetic cytochrome P-450 2D6 polymorphism. *Life Sci* 1995;56:2285–2298.
43. Nebert DW, McKinnon RA, Puga A. Human drug-metabolizing enzyme polymorphisms: Effects on risk of toxicity and cancer. *DNA Cell Biol* 1996;15:273–280.
44. Meyer UA, Amrein R, Balant LP, et al. Antidepressants and drug-metabolizing enzymes—expert group report. *Acta Psychiatr Scand* 1996;93:71–79.
45. Shaw GL, Falk RT, Deslauriers J, et al. Debrisoquine metabolism and lung cancer risk. *Cancer Epidemiol Biomark Prevent* 1995;4:41–48.
46. Lennard MS. Genetically determined adverse drug reactions involving metabolism. *Drug Safety* 1993;9:60–77.
47. Caporaso N, DeBaun MR, Rothman N. Lung cancer and CYP2D6 (the debrisoquine polymorphism): sources of heterogeneity in the proposed association. *Pharmacogenetics* 1995;5:S129–134.
48. Chinegwundoh FI, Kaisary AV. Polymorphism and smoking in bladder carcinogenesis. *Br J Urol* 1996;77:672–675.
49. Spurr NK, Gough AC, Chinegwundoh FI, Smith CA. Polymorphisms in drug-metabolizing enzymes as modifiers of cancer risk. *Clin Chem* 1995;41:21864–21869.
50. Caporaso N, Landi MT, Vineis P. Relevance of metabolic polymorphisms to human carcinogenesis: evaluation of epidemiologic evidence. *Pharmacogenetics* 1991;1:4–19.
51. Barbeau A, Cloutier T, Roy M, Plasse L, Paris S, Poirier J. Ecogenetics of Parkinson's disease: 4-hydroxylation of debrisoquine. *Lancet* 1985;2:1213–1216.
52. Agundez JA, Jimenez JeFJ, Luengo A, et al. Association between the oxidative polymorphism and early onset of Parkinson's disease. *Clin Pharmacol Ther* 1995;57:291–298.
53. Landi MT, Ceroni M, Martignoni E, Bertazzi PA, Caporaso NE, Nappi G. Gene-environment interaction in Parkinson's disease. The case of CYP2D6 gene polymorphism. *Adv Neurol* 1996;72:61–72.
54. Bordet R, Broly F, Destee A, Libersa C, Lafitte JJ. Lack of relation between genetic polymorphism of cytochrome P-450IID6 and sporadic idiopathic Parkinson's disease. *Clin Neuropharmacol* 1996;19:213–221.
55. Daniels J, Williams J, Asherson P, McGuffin P, Owen M. No association between schizophrenia and polymorphisms within the genes for debrisoquine 4-hydroxylase (CYP2D6) and the dopamine transporter (DAT). *Am J Med Genet* 1995;60:85–87.
56. Dawson E, Powell JF, Nothen MM, et al. An association study of debrisoquine hydroxylase (CYP2D6) polymorphisms in schizophrenia. *Psychiatr Genet* 1994;4:215–218.
57. Eaton DL, Gallagher EP, Bammler T, Kunze KL. Role of cytochrome P-4501A2 in chemical carcinogenesis: Implications for human variability in expression and enzyme activity. *Pharmacogenetics* 1995;5:259–274.
58. Guengerich FP, Shimada T. Oxidation of toxic and carcinogenic chemicals by human cytochrome P-450 enzymes. *Chem Res Toxicol* 1991;4:391–407.
59. Guengerich FP, Kim DH, Iwasaki M. Role of human cytochrome P-450 IIE1 in the oxidation of many low molecular weight cancer suspects. *Chem Res Toxicol* 1991;4:168–179.
60. deWaziers I, Cugnenc PH, Yang CS, Leroux JP, Beaune PH. Cytochrome P 450 isoenzymes, epoxide hydrolase and glutathione transferases in rat and human hepatic and extrahepatic tissues. *J Pharmacol Exp Ther* 1990;253:387–394.
61. Guengerich FP, Turvy CG. Comparison of levels of several human microsomal cytochrome P-450 enzymes and epoxide hydrolase in normal and disease states using immunochemical analysis of surgical liver samples. *J Pharmacol Exp Ther* 1991;256:1189–1194.
62. Uematsu F, Kikuchi H, Abe T, et al. Msp I polymorphism of the human CYP2E gene. *Nucleic Acids Res* 1991;19:5797.
63. Uematsu F, Kikuchi H, Motomiya M, et al. Human cytochrome P-450IIE1 gene: Dra I polymorphism and susceptibility to cancer. *Tohoku J Exp Med* 1992;168:113–117.
64. Uematsu F, Ikawa S, Kikuchi H, et al. Restriction fragment length polymorphism of the human CYP2E1 (cytochrome P-450IIE1) gene and susceptibility to lung cancer: possible relevance to low smoking exposure. *Pharmacogenetics* 1994;4:58–63.
65. Hirvonen A, Husgafvel-Pursiainen K, Anttila S, Karjalainen A, Vainio H. The human CYP2E1 gene and lung cancer: Dra I and Rsa I restriction fragment length polymorphisms in a Finnish study population. *Carcinogenesis* 1993;14:85–88.
66. Persson I, Johansson I, Bergling H, et al. Genetic polymorphism of cytochrome P-4502E1 in a Swedish population. Relationship to incidence of lung cancer. *FEBS Lett* 1993;319:207–211.
67. Watanabe J, Yang JP, Eguchi H, et al. An Rsa I polymorphism in the CYP2E1 gene does not affect lung cancer risk in a Japanese population. *Jpn J Cancer Res* 1995;86:245–248.
68. Hamada GS, Sugimura H, Suzuki I, et al. The heme-binding region polymorphism of cytochrome P-4501A1 (CYP1A1), rather than the Rsa I polymorphism of IIE1 (CYPIIE1) is associated with lung cancer in Rio De Janeiro. *Cancer Epidemiol Biomark Prevent* 1995;4:63–67.
69. Watanabe J, Hayashi S, Kawajiri K. Different regulation and expression of the human CYP2E1 gene due to Rsa I polymorphism in the 5′-flanking region. *J Biochem* 1994;116:321–326.
70. Pirmohamed M, Kitteringham NR, Quest LJ, et al. Genetic polymorphism of cytochrome P-4502E1 and risk of alcoholic liver disease in Caucasians. *Pharmacogenetics* 1995;5:351–357.
71. Guengerich FP. Epoxide hydrolase: properties and metabolic roles. *Rev Biochem Toxicol* 1982;4:5–30.
72. Fandrich F, Degiuli B, Vogel BU, Arand M, Oesch F. Induction of rat liver microsomal epoxide hydrolase by its endogenous substrate 16 alpha, 17 alpha-epoxyestra-1,3,5-trien-3-ol. *Xenobiotica* 1995;25:239–244.
73. Nashed NT, Michaud DP, Levin W, Jerina DM. Properties of liver microsomal cholesterol 5,6-oxide hydrolase. *Arch Biochem Biophys* 1985;241:149–162.
74. Haeggstrom JZ, Wetterholm A, Medina JF, Samuelsson B. Novel structural and functional properties of leukotriene A4 hydrolase. Implications for the development of enzyme inhibitors. *Adv Prostaglandin Thromboxane Leukotriene Res* 1994;12:3–12.
75. Meijer J, DePierre JW. Cytosolic epoxide hydrolase. *Chem Biol Interact* 1988;64:207–249.
76. Omiecinski CJ, Aicher L, Swenson L. Developmental expression of human microsomal epoxide hydrolase. *J Pharmacol Exp Ther* 1994;269:417–423.
77. Buehler BA, Rao V, Finnell RH. Biochemical and molecular teratology of fetal hydantoin syndrome. *Neurol Clin* 1994;12:741–748.
78. Lindhout D. Pharmacogenetics and drug interactions: role in antiepileptic-drug-induced teratogenesis. *Neurology* 1992;42:43–47.
79. Gaedigk A, Spielberg SP, Grant DM. Characterization of the microsomal epoxide hydrolase gene in patients with anticonvulsant adverse drug reactions. *Pharmacogenetics* 1994;4:142–153.
80. Green VJ, Pirmohamed M, Kitteringham NR, et al. Genetic analysis of microsomal epoxide hydrolase in patients with carbamazepine hypersensitivity. *Biochem Pharmacol* 1995;50:1353–1359.
81. Kerr BM, Rettie AE, Eddy AC, et al. Inhibition of human liver microsomal epoxide hydrolase by valproate and valpromide: *in vitro/in vivo* correlation [published erratum appears in *Clin Pharmacol Ther* 1989;46(3):343]. *Clin Pharmacol Ther* 1989;46:82–93.
82. McGlynn KA, Rosvold EA, Lustbader ED, et al. Susceptibility to hepatocellular carcinoma is associated with genetic variation in enzymatic detoxification of aflatoxin B1. *Proc Natl Acad Sci USA* 1995;92:2384–2387.
83. Lancaster JM, Brownlee HA, Bell DA, et al. Microsomal epoxide hydrolase polymorphism as a risk factor for ovarian cancer. *Mol Carcinog* 1996;17:160–162.
84. Seidegard J, Vorachek WR, Pero RW, Pearson WR. Hereditary differences in the expression of the human glutathione transferase active on trans-stilbene oxide are due to a gene deletion. *Proc Natl Acad Sci USA* 1988;85:7293–7297.
85. Seidegard J, Pero RW, Stille B. Identification of the trans-stilbene oxide-active glutathione transferase in human mononuclear leukocytes and in liver as GST1. *Biochem Genet* 1989;27:253–261.
86. Anttila S, Luostarinen L, Hirvonen A, et al. Pulmonary expression of glutathione S-transferase M3 in lung cancer patients: association with GSTM1 polymorphism, smoking, and asbestos exposure. *Cancer Res* 1995;55:3305–3309.
87. Bell DA, Thompson CL, Taylor J, et al. Genetic monitoring of human

polymorphic cancer susceptibility genes by polymerase chain reaction: application to glutathione transferase mu. *Environ Health Perspect* 1992;98:113–117.
88. Brockmoller J, Kerb R, Drakoulis N, Nitz M, Roots I. Genotype and phenotype of glutathione S-transferase class isoenzymes mu and psi in lung cancer patients and controls. *Cancer Res* 1993;53:1004–1011.
89. Heckbert SR, Weiss NS, Hornung SK, Eaton DL, Motulsky AG. Glutathione S-transferase and epoxide hydrolase activity in human leukocytes in relation to risk of lung cancer and other smoking-related cancers. *J Natl Cancer Inst* 1992;84:414–422.
90. Kawajiri K, Watanabe J, Eguchi H, Hayashi S. Genetic polymorphisms of drug-metabolizing enzymes and lung cancer susceptibility. *Pharmacogenetics* 1995;S70–73.
91. Kihara M, Kihara M, Noda K. Risk of smoking for squamous and small cell carcinomas of the lung modulated by combinations of CYP1A1 and GSTM1 gene polymorphisms in a Japanese population. *Carcinogenesis* 1995;16:2331–2336.
92. Kihara M, Noda K, Kihara M. Distribution of GSTM1 null genotype in relation to gender, age and smoking status in Japanese lung cancer patients. *Pharmacogenetics* 1995;5S74–79.
93. Liu L, Wang LH. Correlation between lung cancer prevalence and activities of aryl hydrocarbon hydroxylase and glutathione S-transferase in human lung tissues. *Biomed Environ Sci* 1988;1:277–282.
94. Hirvonen A, Husgafvel P-K, Anttila S, Vainio H. The GSTM1 null genotype as a potential risk modifier for squamous cell carcinoma of the lung. *Carcinogenesis* 1993;14:1479–1481.
95. Seidegard J, Pero RW, Miller DG, Beattie EJ. A glutathione transferase in human leukocytes as a marker for the susceptibility to lung cancer. *Carcinogenesis* 1986;7:751–753.
96. London SJ, Daly AK, Cooper J, Navidi WC, Carpenter CL, Idle JR. Polymorphism of glutathione S-transferase M1 and lung cancer risk among African-Americans and Caucasians in Los Angeles County, California. *J Natl Cancer Inst* 1995;87:1246–1253.
97. Zhong S, Howie AF, Ketterer B, et al. Glutathione S-transferase mu locus: use of genotyping and phenotyping assays to assess association with lung cancer susceptibility. *Carcinogenesis* 1991;12:1533–1537.
98. ToFigueras J, Gene M, GomezCatalan J, et al. Glutathione-S-transferase M1 and codon 72 p53 polymorphisms in a Northwestern mediterranean population and their relation to lung cancer susceptibility. *Cancer Epidemiol Biomark Prevent* 1996;5:337–342.
99. Nazar S-V, Motulsky AG, Eaton DL, et al. The glutathione S-transferase mu polymorphism as a marker for susceptibility to lung carcinoma. *Cancer Res* 1993;53:2313–2318.
100. McWilliams JE, Sanderson BJ, Harris EL, Richert B-KE, Henner WD. Glutathione S-transferase M1 (GSTM1) deficiency and lung cancer risk. *Cancer Epidemiol Biomark Prevent* 1995;4:589–594.
101. dErrico A, Taioli E, Chen X, Vineis P. Genetic metabolic polymorphisms and the risk of cancer: A review of the literature. *Biomarkers* 1996;1:149–173.
102. Rothman N, Hayes RB, Zenser TV, et al. The glutathione S-transferase M1 (GSTM1) null genotype and benzidine-associated bladder cancer, urine mutagenicity, and exfoliated urothelial cell DNA adducts. *Cancer Epidemiol Biomark Prevent* 1996;5:979–983.
103. Anwar WA, AbdelRahman SZ, ElZein RA, Mostafa HM, Au WW. Genetic polymorphism of GSTM1, CYP2E1 and CYP2D6 in Egyptian bladder cancer patients. *Carcinogenesis* 1996;17:1923–1929.
104. Lafuente A, Zakahary MM, ElAziz MAA, et al. Influence of smoking in the glutathione-S-transferase M1 deficiency-associated risk for squamous cell carcinoma of the bladder in schistosomiasis patients in Egypt. *Br J Cancer* 1996;74:836–838.
105. Okkels H, Sigsgaard T, Wolf H, Autrup H. Glutathione S-transferase mu as a risk factor in bladder tumours. *Pharmacogenetics* 1996;6: 251–256.
106. Zhong S, Wyllie AH, Barnes D, Wolf CR, Spurr NK. Relationship between the GSTM1 genetic polymorphism and susceptibility to bladder, breast and colon cancer. *Carcinogenesis* 1993;14:1821–1824.
107. Lafuente A, Pujol F, Carretero P, Villa JP, Cuchi A. Human glutathione S-transferase mu (GST mu) deficiency as a marker for the susceptibility to bladder and larynx cancer among smokers. *Cancer Lett* 1993; 68:49–54.
108. Lafuente A, Giralt M, Cervello I, Pujol F, Mallol J. Glutathione-S-transferase activity in human superficial transitional cell carcinoma of the bladder. Comparison with healthy controls. *Cancer* 1990;65: 2064–2068.
109. Bell DA, Taylor JA, Paulson DF, Robertson CN, Mohler JL, Lucier GW. Genetic risk and carcinogen exposure: a common inherited defect of the carcinogen-metabolism gene glutathione-S-transferase M1 (GSTM1) that increases susceptibility to bladder cancer. *J Natl Cancer Inst* 1993;85:1159–1164.
110. Daly AK, Thomas DJ, Cooper J, Pearson WR, Neal WR, Idle JR. Homozygous deletion of gene for glutathione S-transferase M1 in bladder cancer. *Br Med J* 1993;307:481–482.
111. Katoh T, Inatomi H, Nagaoka A, Sugita A. Cytochrome P-4501A1 gene polymorphism and homozygous deletion of the glutathione S-transferase M1 gene in urothelial cancer patients. *Carcinogenesis* 1995;16:655–657.
112. Lin HJ, Han CY, Bernstein DA, Hsiao W, Lin BK, Hardy S. Ethnic distribution of the glutathione S-transferase M1-1 (GSTM1) null genotype in 1473 individuals and application to bladder cancer. *Carcinogenesis* 1993;15:1077–1081.
113. Brockmoller J, Kerb R, Drakoulis N, Staffeldt B, Roots I. Glutathione S-transferase M1 and its variants A and B as host factors of bladder cancer susceptibility: a case control study. *Cancer Res* 1994;53: 1004–1011.
114. Hirvonen A, Nylund L, Kociba P, Husgafvel P-K, Vainio H. Modulation of urinary mutagenicity by genetically determined carcinogen metabolism in smokers. *Carcinogenesis* 1994;15:813–815.
115. Yu MC, Ross RK, Chan KK, et al. Glutathione S-transferase M1 genotype affects aminobiphenyl-hemoglobin adduct levels in white, black and Asian smokers and nonsmokers. *Cancer Epidemiol Biomark Prevent* 1995;4:861–864.
116. Strange RC, Matharoo B, Faulder GC, et al. The human glutathione S-transferase: a case control study of the incidence of the GST 1 0 phenotype in patients with adenocarcinoma. *Carcinogenesis* 1991;12:25–28.
117. Kato S, Onda M, Matsukura N, et al. Genetic polymorphisms of the cancer related gene and Helicobacter pylori infection in Japanese gastric cancer patients. An age and gender matched case-control study. *Cancer* 1996;77:1654–1661.
118. Deakin M, Elder J, Hendrickse C, et al. Glutathione S-transferase GSTT1 genotypes and susceptibility to cancer: studies of interactions with GSTM1 in lung, oral, gastric and colorectal cancers. *Carcinogenesis* 1996;17:881–884.
119. Chenevix T-G, Young J, Coggan M, Board P. Glutathione S-transferase M1 and T1 polymorphisms: susceptibility to colon cancer and age of onset. *Carcinogenesis* 1995;16:1655–1657.
120. Katoh T, Nagata N, Kuroda Y, et al. Glutathione S-transferase M1 (GSTM1) and T1 (GSTT1) genetic polymorphism and susceptibility to gastric and colorectal adenocarcinoma. *Carcinogenesis* 1996;17: 1855–1859.
121. Elexpuru C-J, Buxton N, Kandula V, et al. Susceptibility to astrocytoma and meningioma: influence of allelism at glutathione S-transferase (GSTT1 and GSTM1) and cytochrome P-450 (CYP2D6) loci. *Cancer Res* 1995;55:4237–4239.
122. Hand PA, Inskip A, Gilford J, et al. Allelism at the glutathione S-transferase GSTM3 locus: interactions with GSTM1 and GSTT1 as risk factors for astrocytoma. *Carcinogenesis* 1996;17:1919–1922.
123. Heagerty A, Fitzgerald D, Smith A, et al. Glutathione S-transferase GSTM1 phenotypes and protection against cutaneous tumours. *Lancet* 1994;343:266–268.
124. Heagerty A, Smith A, English J, et al. Susceptibility to multiple cutaneous basal cell carcinomas: Significant interactions between glutathione S-transferase GSTM1 genotypes, skin type and male gender. *Br J Cancer* 1996;73:44–48.
125. Lear JT, Heagerty AHM, Smith A, et al. Multiple cutaneous basal cell carcinomas: Glutathione S-transferase (GSTM1, GSTT1) and cytochrome P-450 (CYP2D6, CYP1A1) polymorphisms influence tumour numbers and accrual. *Carcinogenesis* 1996;17:1891–1896.
126. Yengi L, Inskip A, Gilford J, et al. Polymorphism at the glutathione S-transferase locus GSTM3: interactions with cytochrome P-450 and glutathione S-transferase genotypes as risk factors for multiple cutaneous basal cell carcinoma. *Cancer Res* 1996;56:1974–1977.
127. Sarhanis P, Redman C, Perrett C, et al. Epithelial ovarian cancer: Influence of polymorphism at the glutathione S-transferase GSTM1 and GSTT1 loci on p53 expression. *Br J Cancer* 1996;74:1757–1761.
128. Warwick AP, Redman CW, Jones PW, et al. Progression of cervical intraepithelial neoplasia to cervical cancer: interactions of cytochrome P-450 CYP2D6 EM and glutathione s-transferase GSTM1 null genotypes and cigarette smoking. *Br J Cancer* 1994;70:704–708.

129. Chen C, Madeleine MM, Lubinski C, Weiss NS, Tickman EW, Daling JR. Glutathione S-transferase M1 genotypes and the risk of anal cancer: a population-based case-control study. *Cancer Epidemiol Biomark Prevent* 1996;5:985–991.
130. Katoh T. Application of molecular biology to occupational health field–the frequency of gene polymorphism of cytochrome P-450 1A1 and glutathione S-transferase M1 in patients with lung, oral and urothelial cancer. *Sangyo Ika Daigaku Zasshi* 1995;17:271–278.
131. Yu MW, Gladek-Yarborough A, Chiamprasert S, Santella RM, Liaw YF, Chen CJ. Cytochrome P-450 2E1 and glutathione S-transferase M1 polymorphisms and susceptibility to hepatocellular carcinoma. *Gastroenterology* 1995;109:1266–1273.
132. Hsieh LL, Huang RC, Yu MW, Chen CJ, Liaw YF. L-myc, GST M1 genetic polymorphism and hepatocellular carcinoma risk among chronic hepatitis B carriers. *Cancer Lett* 1996;103:171–176.
133. Liu YH, Taylor J, Linko P, Lucier GW, Thompson CL. Glutathione S-transferase mu in human lymphocyte and liver: role in modulating formation of carcinogen-derived DNA adducts. *Carcinogenesis* 1991;12: 2269–2275.
134. Raney KD, Meyer DJ, Ketterer B, Harris TM, Guengerich FP. Glutathione conjugation of aflatoxin $B_1$ *exo-* and *endo*-epoxides by rat and human glutathione S-transferases. *Chem Res Toxicol* 1992;5: 470–478.
135. Buetler TM, Slone D, Eaton DL. Comparison of the aflatoxin $B_1$-8,9-epoxide conjugating activities of two bacterially expressed *alpha* class glutathione S-transferase isozymes from mouse and rat. *Biochem Biophys Res Commun* 1992;188:597–603.
136. Eaton DL, Ramsdell H, Monroe DH. Biotransformation as a determinant of species susceptibility to aflatoxin $B_1$: *in vitro* studies in rats, mouse, monkey, and human liver. In: Pohland AE, Vulus RDJ, Richard JL,eds. *Microbial toxins in foods and feeds:* cellular and molecular modes of action. New York and London: Plenum Press, 1990; 275–290.
137. Eaton DL, Gallagher EP. Mechanisms of aflatoxin carcinogenesis. *Annu Rev Pharmacol Toxicol* 1994;34:135–172.
138. Slone DH, Gallagher EP, Ramsdell HS, et al. Human variability in hepatic glutathione S-transferase mediated conjugation of aflatoxin $B_1$-epoxide and other substrates. *Pharmacogenetics* 1995;5:224–233.
139. Chen CJ, Yu MW, Liaw YF, et al. Chronic hepatitis B carriers with null genotypes of glutathione S-transferase M1 and T1 polymorphisms who are exposed to aflatoxin are at increased risk of hepatocellular carcinoma. *Am J Human Genet* 1996;59:128–134.
140. Soderkvist P, Ahmadi A, Akerback A, Axelson O, Flodin U. Glutathione S-transferase M1 null genotype as a risk modifier for solvent-induced chronic toxic encephalopathy. *Scand J Work Environ Health* 1996;22:360–363.
141. Smith CM, Kelsey KT, Wiencke JK, Leyden K, Levin S, Christiani DC. Inherited glutathione-S-transferase deficiency is a risk factor for pulmonary asbestosis. *Cancer Epidemiol Biomark Prevent* 1994;3: 471–7.
142. Baranov VS, Ivaschenko T, Bakay B, et al. Proportion of the GSTM1 0/0 genotype in some Slavic populations and its correlation with cystic fibrosis and some multifactorial diseases. *Hum Genet* 1996;97:516–520.
143. Savolainen VT, Pajarinen J, Perola M, Penttila A, Karhunen PJ. Glutathione-S-transferase GST M1 "null" genotype and the risk of alcoholic liver disease. *Alcohol Clin Exp Res* 1996;20:1340–1345.
144. Pemble S, Schroeder KR, Spencer SR, et al. Human glutathione S-transferase theta (GSTT1): cDNA cloning and the characterization of a genetic polymorphism. *Biochem J* 1994;300:271–276.
145. Guengerich FP, Thier R, Persmark M, Taylor JB, Pemble SE, Ketterer B. Conjugation of carcinogens by theta class glutathione s-transferases: mechanisms and relevance to variations in human risk. *Pharmacogenetics* 1995;S103–107.
146. Wiencke JK, Pemble S, Ketterer B, Kelsey KT. Gene deletion of glutathione S-transferase theta: correlation with induced genetic damage and potential role in endogenous mutagenesis. *Cancer Epidemiol Biomark Prevent* 1995;4:253–259.
147. Sorsa M, Osterman Golkar S, Peltonen K, Saarikoski ST, Sram R. Assessment of exposure to butadiene in the process industry. *Toxicology* 1996;113:77–83.
148. Chen H, Sandler D, Taylor J, et al. Increased risk for myelodysplastic syndromes in individuals with glutathione transferase theta 1 (GSTT1) gene defect. *Lancet* 1996;347:295–297.
149. Weber WW. *Pharmacogenetics.* New York: Oxford University Press, 1997.
150. Grant DM. Molecular genetics of the N-acetyltransferases. *Pharmacogenetics* 1993;3:45–50.
151. Vatsis KP, Weber WW, Bell DA, et al. Nomenclature for N-acetyltransferases. *Pharmacogenetics* 1995;5:1–17.
152. Kadlubar FF. Biochemical individuality and its implications for drug and carcinogen metabolism: recent insights from acetyltransferase and cytochrome P-4501A2 phenotyping and genotyping in humans. *Drug Metab Rev* 1994;26:37–46.
153. Blum M, Demierre A, Grant DM, Heim M, Meyer UA. Molecular mechanism of slow acetylation of drugs and carcinogens. *Proc Natl Acad Sci USA* 1991;88:5237–5241.
154. Hein DW. Acetylator genotype and arylamine-induced carcinogenesis. *Biochim Biophys Acta* 1988;948:37–66.
155. Weber WW, Vatsis KP. Individual variability in p-aminobenzoic acid N-acetylation by human N-acetyltransferase (NAT1) of peripheral blood. *Pharmacogenetics* 1993;3:209–212.
156. Vatsis KP, Weber WW. Structural heterogeneity of Caucasian N-acetyltransferase at the NAT1 gene locus. *Arch Biochem Biophys* 1993;301:71–76.
157. Badawi AF, Hirvonen A, Bell DA, Lang NP, Kadlubar FF. Role of aromatic amine acetyltransferases, NAT1 and NAT2, in carcinogen-DNA adduct formation in the human urinary bladder. *Cancer Res* 1995;55: 5230–5237.
158. Ladero JM, Fernandez MJ, Palmeiro R, et al. Hepatic acetylator polymorphism in breast cancer patients. *Oncology* 1987;44:341–344.
159. Philip PA, Rogers HJ, Millis RR, Rubens RD, Cartwright RA. Acetylation status and its relationship to breast cancer and other diseases of the breast. *Eur J Cancer Clin Oncol* 1987;23:1701–1706.
160. Webster DJT, Flook D, Jenkins J, Hutchings A, Routledge PA. Drug acetylation in breast cancer. *Br J Cancer* 1989;60:236–237.
161. Ambrosone CB, Freudenheim JL, Graham S, et al. Cigarette smoking, N-acetyltransferase 2 genetic polymorphisms, and breast cancer risk. *JAMA* 1996;276:1494–1501.
162. Martinez C, Agundez JAG, Olivera M, Martin R, Ladero JM, Benitez J. Lung cancer and mutations at the polymorphic NAT2 gene locus. *Pharmacogenetics* 1995;5:207–214.
163. Philip PA, Fitzgerald DL, Cartwright RA, Peake MD, Rogers HJ. Polymorphic N-acetylation capacity in lung cancer. *Carcinogenesis* 1988;9:491–493.
164. Roots I, Drakoulis N, Ploch M, et al. Debrisoquine hydroxylation phenotype, acetylation phenotype, and ABO blood groups as genetic host factors of lung cancer risk. *Klin Wochenschr* 1988;66:87–97.
165. Ilett KF, David BM, Detchon P, Castleden WM, Kwa R. Acetylator phenotype in colorectal carcinoma. *Cancer Res* 1987;47:1466–1469.
166. Lang NP, Chu DZJ, Hunter CF, Kendall DC, Flammang TJ, Kadlubar FF. Role of aromatic amine N-acetyltransferase in human colorectal cancer. *Arch Surg* 1986;121:1259–1261.
167. Wohlleb JC, Hunter CF, Blass B, Kadlubar FF, Chu DZJ, Lang NP. Aromatic amine acetyltransferase as a marker for colorectal cancer: environmental and demographic associations. *Int J Cancer* 1990;46:22–30.
168. Ladero JM, Gonzalez JF, Benitez J, et al. Acetylator polymorphism in human colorectal carcinoma. *Cancer Res* 1991;51:2098–2100.
169. Roberts-Thomson IC, Ryan P, Khoo KK, Hart WJ, McMichael AJ, Butler RN. Diet, acetylator phenotype, and risk of colorectal neoplasia. *Lancet* 1996;347:1372–1374.
170. Nakachi K, Imai K, Hayashi S, Kawajiri K. Polymorphisms of the CYP1A1 and glutathione S-transferase genes associated with susceptibility to lung cancer in relation to cigarette dose in a Japanese population. *Cancer Res* 1993;53:2994–2999.
171. Costa L, Omiecinski CJ, Faustman EM, Omenn GS. Eco-genetics: determining susceptibility to chemical-induced diseases. *Washington Public Health* 1993;11:8–11.
172. Davies HG, Richter RJ, Keifer M, Broomfield C, Sowalla J, Furlong CE. The effect of the human serum paraoxonase polymorphism is reversed with diazoxon, soman and sarin. *Nature Genet* 1996;14:334–336.
173. Cox DW. Alpha-1 antitrypsin deficiency. In: Scriver CR, Beaudet AL, Sly WS, Valle D,eds. *The metabolic and molecular bases of inherited disease.* New York: McGraw-Hill, 1995:2407–2437.
174. Janus ED, Phillips NT, Carrel WT. Smoking, lung function, and alpha-1antitrypsin deficiency. *Lancet* 1985;1:152–154.
175. Richeldi L, Sorrentino R, Saltini C. HLA-DBP beta-1 glutamate 69: agenetic marker of beryllium disease. *Science* 1993;262:242–244.
176. Young RP, Barker R, Cookson W, Newman Taylor AJ. HLA-DR and DP antigen frequencies and the anhydride sensitization. *Am Rev Respir Dis* 1993;147:A113.

177. Bignon JS, Aron Y, Ju LY, al. e. HLA class II alleles in isocyanate-induced asthma. *Am J Respir Crit Care Med* 1994;149:71–75.
178. Hill CM, Littman DR. Natural resistance to HIV? *Nature* 1996;382: 668–669.
179. Cox T. Haemochromatosis: strike while the iron is hot. *Nature Genet* 1996;13:386–388.
180. Feder JN, Gnirke AWT, al. e. A novel MHC class I-like gene is mutated in patients with hereditary haemochromatosis. *Nature Genet* 1996;13:399–408.
181. Khoury M, Group GW. From genes to public health: The application of genetic technology in disease prevention. *Am J Public Health* 1997;86:1717–1722.

*Environmental and Occupational Medicine, Third Edition*, edited by William N. Rom.
Lippincott–Raven Publishers, Philadelphia © 1998.

# CHAPTER 18

# Occupational Exposures and Effects on Male and Female Reproduction

Grace Kawas Lemasters

The past two decades have seen growing concern that environmental and occupational chemicals pose threats to male and female reproductive health, particularly as increasing numbers of women enter the work force. In 1960 the percentages of women and men in the United States civilian labor force under the age of 35 were 33% and 37%; today, these values have risen to 43% and 45%, respectively. The percent of married men in the labor force has decreased since 1960 from 89% to 77% while almost doubling for women, from 32% to 61%. Predictably, the percentage of women under the age of 44 having a child while working also escalated from 38% to 54% during the 1980 to 1992 period. Simultaneously, the fetal loss rate per 1,000 women increased one percentage point from 14.1 to 15.1, and the percent of low birth weight (LBW) (<2,500 g) infants also increased from 6.8% to 7.2%. In the late 1970s, after workplace exposures rendered men infertile, interest was further spawned (1). Today, questions exist as to whether or not the fertility potential of men is declining. These questions were sparked by findings that testicular cancer has increased, and the average human sperm count has been reported to be on the decline—half of that reported in the 1930s. Others disagree, however, citing differences over time in methods and/or technical procedures.

A couple's reproductive success depends on a delicate physiochemical balance within and between the paternal, maternal, and fetal systems. Any disruption in this balance can result in a broad range of adverse effects. Reproductive toxicity is defined as a condition causing deleterious responses in the postpubertal male or female manifested by interference with normal physiologic processes or regulatory mechanisms, organ functioning, and/or the genetic integrity of the sperm or egg cells. Developmental toxicity is defined as a condition producing adverse effects on the developing organism reflected in prenatal or early postnatal death, altered growth, structural abnormalities, and functional deficits. Chances that a couple will experience some form of reproductive impairment are high. Approximately 15% to 20% of all couples report periods of infertility, and a large proportion of all pregnancies end adversely—with preterm delivery (7%), LBW (7%), major malformations (2.2%), infant death (1.3%), or fetal loss (15% to 20%) (2). The cause is usually unknown. To determine whether or not a work force is at enhanced reproductive risk due to chemical exposure, both biologic and epidemiologic parameters must be considered. This chapter reviews the methods applicable in industry to assess these effects. The reproductive abnormalities discussed consist of changes in semen parameters, subfecundity, menstrual abnormalities, fetal loss, LBW, preterm delivery, and congenital anomalies.

G. K. Lemasters: Divisions of Environmental Health and Epidemiology, Department of Environmental Health, University of Cincinnati Medical Center, Cincinnati, Ohio 45267-0182.

## MALE REPRODUCTION

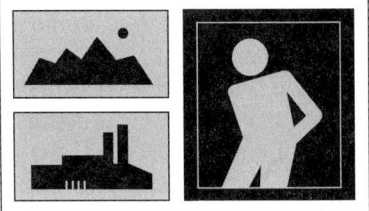

An intact hypothalamic-pituitary-testicular axis as measured by hormonal levels may provide a measure of the successful integration of the male reproductive system. To summarize the male neuroendocrine system, the hypothalamus integrates signals from the central nervous system regulating gonadotropin secretion by the anterior pituitary gland. The Leydig, Sertoli, and germ cells are acted upon by the hormonal secretions of the anterior pituitary gland to regulate spermatogenesis and hormone production by the testes. The gonadotropin-releasing hormone (GnRH) stimulates the anterior pituitary to release luteinizing hormone (LH), follicle-stimulating hormone (FSH), and prolactin. Synthesis and release of testosterone is controlled by LH acting on the Leydig cells, while FSH stimulates biosynthesis of testosterone to estradiol in the Sertoli cells. Spermatogenesis is a time-locked, synchronous process wherein the germ cell proceeds through a series of (a) mitotic divisions for cell proliferation, (b) meiotic divisions generating genetic diversity and decreasing the chromosome number by half, and (c) differentiation steps antecedent to the release of immature spermatozoa from the testes. As sperm are transported through the epididymis, maturational changes occur and full motility and fertilization ability is acquired. The process of spermatogenesis requires approximately 70 days in the human testis; transport time through the epididymis averages 6 days. Any one of the developing cell types, from testicular spermatogonia, spermatocytes, and spermatids, to immature and mature epididymal spermatozoa, may be susceptible to toxic exposures. Sperm assays, therefore, provide both a direct measure of male reproductive impairment and a possible indirect measure of transmission of genetic damage to progeny. This measure of genetic damage may be suggested by changes in DNA content, induced changes in sperm morphology, or a damaged conceptus.

Given the site and timing of insult, varying effects will be observed. The absence of sperm (azoospermia), sperm count less than 20 million per milliliter semen (oligospermia), and sperm with low motility are associated with reduced fertility. For nonmutagenic events the most likely outcome associated with insult to the spermatogonia (stem cell) may be cell death and phagocytosis. Although cell death also may occur in later stages (i.e., the mature forms, spermatids and spermatozoa), the rapidity and efficiency of phagocytic processes are uncertain. The most sensitive end point is speculative. A likely scenario is that perturbing of the biochemical milieu in which the mature cells are maintained may be reflected initially as alterations in motility, followed by decreases in viability, leading to cellular degeneration and eventually decline in concentration (3).

Sperm with abnormal forms (teratosperm) or degenerative forms may be associated with basic interferences of cellular processes necessary for maintaining the integrity and viability of the cell. These abnormal forms are likely to be associated with infertility or early fetal loss. Mutations may be transmitted at conception, resulting in an adverse pregnancy outcome.

Based on a meta-analysis of 60 historical studies and analysis from data available in sperm banks, there may be valid concern about male reproduction. In a study of 1,351 healthy men volunteering for sperm donation, a decrease of 2.1% in sperm concentrations per year was noted, a decrease in sperm motility, and an increase in abnormal spermatozoa. What associations, if any, the above findings have with workplace exposures is unknown. In one example of exposure to a nematocide, 1,2-dibromo-3-chloropropane (DBCP), not only did workers experience sterility, but their exposure was associated with an increased incidence of spontaneous abortions among the wives (1,4).

### Study Design Issues

Methodologic approaches used in studies of fecundity requiring either collection of semen samples or reproductive histories are herein reviewed. In semen assay studies, there are two basic designs, cross-sectional and longitudinal. The cross-sectional study examines the differences between exposed and unexposed men, generally at one point in time, and is probably most appropriate when exposure has occurred over a long period. Chronic exposure to a toxicant may be associated either with damage attributed to bioaccumulation of the toxicant or with repeated cellular insult resulting in the accumulation of injury consistent with physiologic or biochemical disruptions and histopathologic alterations (5,6). This is true if exposure has extended beyond several full cycles of spermatogenesis, the agent is maintained at a steady state during the cycle, and gonadal damage has reached some level of steady state (3,7). The concept of steady-state damage implies that the lesion produces a constant level of effect at a given cell stage. The experience of workers exposed long term to DBCP showed an inverse relationship between sperm count and years of employment (1). Histologic examination of testicular biopsy specimens exhibited a loss of spermatogenic cells and a decrease in the amount of cellularity in the seminiferous tubules (8).

In contrast, in a longitudinal or prospective study men are followed and interval biologic samples are collected. Several stages of sperm development are examined. For men experiencing an acute exposure, such as after an accidental spill, an ideal study is to obtain several semen samples timed to characterize damage at various stages of sperm development. To characterize an insult to spermatogonia, a semen sample should be taken approximately 10 to 13 weeks after exposure, whereas for spermatids and spermatocytes the sampling time frame is 3 to 8 weeks, and for spermatozoa, 1 to 3 weeks.

The most common measures in semen studies are sperm count, sperm velocity, and percentages of motile, viable, and morphologically normal sperm. Several reviews describe basic field methods and methods for obtaining automated semen analysis (9–11). In brief, sperm count is measured as the number of sperm per milliliter of ejaculate or the total number of sperm ejaculated. Sperm velocity (in micrometers per second) is either the swimming speed of sperm along its swimming path or the distance traveled in a straight line from one point in time to another. The percentage of motile sperm measures the proportion of sperm that fulfill at least minimum movement criteria. Computer instruments have been developed to evaluate swimming speed and patterns (10). The percentage of viable sperm is expressed as the portion of living sperm measured by a stain exclusion test or hypo-osmotic swelling. The stain exclusion assays measure structural integrity; functional integrity of sperm membranes (i.e., maintenance of ionic gradients) is assessed by placing sperm in a hypo-osmotic solution to measure cell swelling. Sperm morphology is an assessment of the shape of the sperm head, but it may also incorporate the midpiece and tail. Alterations in sperm morphology may be associated with decreases in fertility, fetal loss, and heritable genetic abnormalities (12). Sperm motility and morphology are considered two sensitive indicators of fertility potential (13,14).

A longitudinal study of semen quality of 45 unexposed men was conducted to obtain data on the statistical variation of these parameters (15). From that study and another (9) the mean sperm concentration, sperm count (millions per ejaculate), semen volume, sperm velocity, percentage of motile sperm, and percentage with normal morphology are summarized in Table 1. From these studies it was concluded that, although sperm count is the most frequently measured variable in occupational field studies, it lacks precision for detecting population differences; the average coefficient of variation among one subject's successive sperm counts is high—44%. Sperm velocity, on the other hand, had low overall inter- and intrasubject coefficients of variations, but the intrasubject variation was greater; overall, fluctuations in one subject's rates were almost as great as those between subjects. This finding suggests that examining multiple samples from any individual may be optimal. Both parameters of morphology and viability have relatively good intraclass correlations and low coefficients of variations, allowing detection of trends and population differences.

**TABLE 1.** *Sperm parameters for an unexposed population*

| Primary outcome | Mean | (1 SD) |
|---|---|---|
| Semen assays | | |
| Sperm concentration (millions/ml) | 47.43 | (22.9) |
| Sperm count (millions/ejaculate) | 204.80 | (199.2) |
| Semen volume (ml) | 2.78 | (0.75) |
| Motile sperm (%) | 59.76 | (20.87) |
| Viable sperm | | |
| 1. By stain exclusion (%) | 71.41 | (7.38) |
| 2. By hypoosmotic stress (%) | 64.08 | (9.04) |
| Sperm morphology | | |
| % Normal | 80.16 | (9.52) |
| % Macro | 1.69 | (2.54) |
| % Micro | 1.10 | (0.99) |
| % Tapered | 2.49 | (3.17) |
| % Double | 0.83 | (1.47) |
| % Absent | 1.43 | (1.29) |
| % Abnormal | 5.71 | (4.45) |
| % Immature | 5.64 | (4.71) |
| % Amorphous | 0.61 | (0.60) |

From ref. 9.

The ultimate question that these tests must address is whether an individual's reproductive potential has been compromised. In classic fertility studies originally conducted by Hammen (16) in 1944 and in follow-up studies (17–20), the predictive utility of four tests were measured: sperm count, sperm motility, abnormal morphology, and sperm viability. Originally, 1,639 men were examined for possible infertility and 783 were reexamined 20 years later. The findings demonstrated a significant correlation of sperm count and sperm motility with the number of living children and interval to first pregnancy. There was no relationship between either count and motility with spontaneous abortions. A sperm count of 5 million per milliliter or fewer was found to have borderline significance for male infertility. Additionally, there was a significant correlation between semen volume and interval to first pregnancy, but no relationship between semen volume and number of living children or spontaneous abortions. In one study, a relationship of low sperm count and abnormal morphology was associated with spontaneous abortions (21) but not in others (22–24).

### *Traditional Semen Assays*

In a typical occupational study involving semen collection, the worker is asked to abstain from ejaculating for 48 hours prior to sample collection. On the appointed day, the participant obtains a sample via masturbation without using lubricants or condoms. The sample is collected either at home or in the clinical setting. If the sample is collected at home, the participant is asked to place the specimen container directly in a vacuum bottle and deliver it to the laboratory within 60 minutes. A video prepared by the National Institute for Occupational Safety and Health (NIOSH) is available that describes procedures to be followed. Guidelines for field studies have been published (25,26).

In addition to semen sample collection, occupational studies require the administration of questionnaires to determine whether other risk factors are operating that might explain the observed effect (rather than the specific exposure of interest). Such factors could be medical conditions such as varicocele, parotitic orchitis, cryptorchidism, febrile or viral disease, diabetes, epilepsy, genitourinary infection, sexually transmitted disease, hypertension, cancer, leprosy, malaria, renal transplantation, sickle cell anemia, testicular biopsy, urogenital tuberculosis, vesiculitis, epididymitis, prostatitis, a history of mumps, convulsions, severe allergic response, genital injuries, diethylstilbestrol use by the mother, history of infertility, or some medications such as estrogens, chlorambucil, cyclophosphamide, and nitrofurantoin.

Use of tobacco, alcohol, or illicit drugs also has been associated with changes in semen parameters (27,28). The components of a field study questionnaire have been outlined and include reproductive history, health questions, lifestyle factors, and exposure to chemical and physical agents (29).

Because of the limited thermoregulatory capacity of the scrotum, elevated scrotal temperature is also a risk factor for lowered sperm count. Activities that contribute include using a hot tub, sauna, hot baths or showers, long-distance running, and tight-fitting underwear. Sperm concentration may change with the season of the year. In a study of 131 outdoor workers in Texas, significantly lower sperm concentrations, total sperm counts per ejaculate, and concentrations of motile sperm were observed during the summer months, as compared to winter (30). After adjustment for other factors, the mean decreases in sperm concentration, count, and number of motile sperm in summer were 32%, 28%, and 24%, respectively. Particularly interesting was the finding that the group at greatest risk for the seasonal effect were the men with the lowest sperm count—those who had the least compensatory ability.

The challenge in occupational studies involving the collection of biologic samples is achieving a high rate of participation. In four NIOSH studies the average rate of participation was approximately 57% (31). A number of measures can be used to enhance participation—incentive payments, maintenance of complete confidentiality and privacy, enlisting the support of both labor and management, on-site recruitment of workers, providing descriptive literature about the study, immediate follow-up, and agreeing to provide results and interpretation of all tests to the participant.

### *Subfecundity*

Another approach for estimating effects of exposure on male reproduction is the collection of reproductive histories from the worker or his mate. Interviewing the worker's wife is preferred; it has been shown that women better recall dates for certain events such as miscarriage (32). Methods described in this section also are applicable to evaluating subfecundity in women.

The terminology of fertility can be confusing. Fertility statistics are based on the ability to deliver a viable child, whereas fecundity impairments are more inclusive and involve the physiologic capacity to conceive. A woman is considered subfecund if she has difficulty becoming pregnant or sustaining a pregnancy over a specified period. Population statistics indicate that approximately 16% of married women between ages 15 and 44 years have fecundity impairments that cannot be surgically repaired (33). This rate is considerably higher in African-Americans than in Caucasian, 23% versus 15%, respectively. Other risk factors for subfecundity are age, marital status, socioeconomic status, gravidity, history of adverse pregnancy outcome, birth control methods, interval since previous pregnancy, body mass, certain infectious or chronic diseases, cigarette smoking, alcohol use, and irradiation. Use of xenobiotics in the home or for hobbies, such as lead, heat, glycol ethers, and carbon disulfide, among others, must be evaluated (34).

Three study approaches may be useful in assessing subfecundity. The first asks specific questions to determine whether the subject has identified a period of time during which the couple was trying to conceive. Dates are obtained for the total period(s) when the couple was trying. The rate and length of time, in days, weeks, or months, when the couple was subfecund are compared for exposed and unexposed. Often a minimum of a full year of unprotected intercourse is the criterion. This interval encompasses about five sperm cycles and may be inappropriate for exposures that are acute or intermittent (35).

A study design used to assess subfecundity of workers exposed to ethylene dibromide compared the observed number of births for exposed person-years to an expected number estimated from birth rates specific to the mother's age, parity, race, and year of birth, and may examine the fertility experience, comparing exposure intervals (36–39). The disadvantages of this approach are that important covariates such as contraceptive history and functional infertility are not considered, expected rates are missing for some ages, cohorts, or parities, and marital status of the study group may not be comparable to that on which national statistics are based. Standardized fertility ratios consider only live births. Thus, other important reproductive events are ignored. Determining the number of contraceptive-free cycles that is required for a couple to conceive after complete termination of birth control is another approach for analyzing subfecundity (34). This time-to-pregnancy or time-to-delivery approach incorporates a larger sample of reproductive experience, as cycles accumulate ending in pregnancy, induced abortion, fetal loss, ectopic pregnancy, or a live birth. Data are collected that may include information on menstrual periods, contraception, and frequency of sexual intercourse. This analysis adjusts for covariates such as cycle length, abstinence, and sporadic use of birth control.

A broad range of rates may be observed, depending on the method of assessment (40). Using a life-event calendar approach that tracks all pregnancies, an overall age-adjusted prevalence of infertility of 20.6% was observed for couples who had not conceived after 24 months of unprotected intercourse. When specific questions were asked about a couple's awareness of dates when they were unable to conceive after trying for 2 years, the overall rate dropped to 12.5%.

The choice of approach for analyzing infertility depends on the study design. If a referent population is unavailable, the standardized fertility analysis is used. If a referent group is available and if considerable details are known on potential confounders, the time-to-pregnancy approach may be preferred. It is prudent to include more than one approach, such as responses to specific questions about the couple's concern or recognition of an infertility problem, the life- event calendar approaches inherent in the standardized fertility rate (SFR), and time-to-pregnancy analyses. Discrepancies may then be revealed and comparisons made.

### Occupational Exposure and Male Reproduction

This section reviews occupational studies on the effects of exposure and male reproduction that were selected either because of their historic importance or because of general interest in research methods. Included are examples of direct effects on semen quality or male-mediated effects expressed as a couple's infertility or as adverse pregnancy outcome (Table 2). Human studies on occupational hazards to male reproduction are reviewed elsewhere (41,42). The first specific reports on reproductive effects of an industrial chemical appeared in the late 1800s and concerned lead toxicity. Unusually high rates of infertility, spontaneous abortion, stillbirth, neonatal death, macrocephaly, and convulsions in offspring were recorded in European lead-working communities (43). Findings in an occupational lead exposure study by Lancranjan et al. (44) indicated that absorption of moderately increased amounts of lead resulted in asthenospermia, hypospermia, and tetraspermia. More recent studies indicate that lead battery workers still experience elevated levels of lead in blood, urine, and semen associated with a decrease in sperm count that is not associated with a change in gonadotropins, prolactin, or testosterone (45). These findings suggest that the effects are not mediated via the hypothalamic-pituitary axis. It was not until the late 1970s, after worker exposure to DBCP had a striking effect on reproduction, that male occupational reproductive effects became a serious concern.

In 1981, shortly after the DBCP study, the Occupational Safety and Health Administration (OSHA) proposed a revision of the existing allowable exposure standard for workers exposed to ethylene dibromide (EDB). This revision, which was based on information that included data from animal studies reporting adverse male reproductive effects (46–50), was designed to protect against cancer and other health effects. EDB was widely used as an active component of pesticides and as a scavenger in leaded gasoline. The manufacturers of EDB objected to this proposed standard because the accumulated epidemiologic evidence was largely negative (51). James Dobbins (52) wrote a thoughtful review concluding that the negative results of these human studies had low power, so that absence of a statistically significant effect did not constitute evidence of safety. [For a detailed discussion of the issue of evidence of safety, see Millard (53).] Dobbins asserted that these studies did not represent evidence that EDB was harmless, for several reasons: the calculated expected levels of fertility were too low, few study subjects were used, one study found important differences between the exposed and unexposed groups, and another lacked a concurrently unexposed group.

Human studies performed subsequent to Dobbins's analysis lend support to the suspicion of the reproductive

**TABLE 2.** *Types of male reproductive effects by occupational exposure*

| | Observed effects | | | |
|---|---|---|---|---|
| Type of exposure | Lowered number of sperm | Abnormal sperm shape | Altered sperm transfer | Altered hormones/ sexual performance |
| Lead | x | x | x | x |
| Dibromochloropropane | x | | | |
| Carbaryl (Sevin) | | x | | |
| Toluenediamine and dinitrotoluene | x | | | |
| Ethylene dibromide | x | x | x | |
| Plastic production (styrene and acetone) | | x | | |
| Ethylene glycol monoethyl ether | x | | | |
| Welding | | x | x | |
| Perchloroethylene | | x | x | |
| Mercury vapor | | | | x |
| Heat | x | | x | |
| Military radar | x | | | |
| Kepone[a] | | | x | |
| Bromine vapor[a] dichlorophenoxy | x | x | x | |
| Radiation[a] (Chernobyl) | x | x | x | x |
| Carbon disulfide | | | | x |
| 2,4 acetic acid (2,4-D) | | x | x | |

Adapted from ref. 245.
[a]Work place accident causes high level exposure.

toxic effects of EDB. A longitudinal study of timber fumigators with short-term exposure to EDB demonstrated that sperm velocity was decreased when pre- and postexposure samples were compared (54). Additionally, a cross-sectional study of 46 men employed in the papaya fumigation industry with an average employment duration of 5 years and an 88 parts per billion (ppb) [8-hour time-weighted average (TWA)] EDB demonstrated a significant decrease in sperm count, viability and motility, and morphologic abnormalities (55,56). No differences were observed, however, in chromosome aberrations or sister-chromatid exchanges (57). These two studies also suggest that short-term acute exposures may slow sperm velocity, but chronic exposure is more likely associated with sperm immobility and cell death.

Workers exposed to trichloroethylene, another hydrocarbon, also were evaluated for a relationship between somatic cell mutations and spermatotoxic effects (58). Numbers and morphology of sperm of 15 metal workers who used trichloroethylene as a degreasing agent were not significantly different from those of unexposed persons. There was a significant correlation, however, in structural chromosome aberrations in cultured lymphocytes, including breaks, gaps, translocations, deletions, inversions, and hyperdiploid cells. Although it has been suggested that changes in sperm morphology may be associated with genetic damage, neither of the above studies on EDB and trichloroethylene confirms a correlation with somatic cell gene damage or spermatogenic changes. That does not preclude the possibility that other germ cell tests (59–61) might have been more sensitive. For example, Martin and coworkers (62) found that the sperm of men exposed to therapeutic ionizing radiation showed a significant increase in chromosome aberrations 36 months after treatment. In contrast, neither radiotherapy nor chemotherapy appears to increase the rates of malformation in offspring of men and women treated with these agents. It is uncertain, however, if specific genetic defects preferentially involve the paternal chromosomes, especially the sex chromosomes, e.g., XYY, XXY, and XO.

Although there are numerous studies on paternal exposures and adverse pregnancy outcomes, the mechanisms of action remain unclear. Little is understood about occupational exposures and the relationship of male-mediated effects on offspring, such as spontaneous abortions, developmental disorders, and childhood cancer. Guidelines for the applications of these genetic end points to studies of human paternal exposure have been developed (63,64). Studies of anesthetists were some of the first to suggest evidence of male-mediated inheritance of mutations due to occupational exposure. Paternal exposure did not appear to influence the overall abortion rate in two studies of male anesthetists (65), but both studies reported a 25% increase in risk of congenital abnormalities in offspring of exposed men. A study of sperm count and morphologic abnormalities suggested no significant differences in semen parameters related to anesthetic gas exposure, but this study was undertaken in operating rooms that had modern gas-scavenging devices (66). A possible link between paternal occupational exposure and germ cell mutations was found with radiation exposure of male workers at the Sellafield nuclear plant in England (67). The relative risks to offspring for leukemia and non-Hodgkin's lymphoma were 6.4 [95% confidence interval (CI) = 1.5–26.3] when fathers received a total ionizing radiation dose of 100 millisieverts (mSv) or more before the children were conceived. Other risk factors, including exposure to x-rays, maternal age, employment elsewhere, eating seafood, and playing on a possibly contaminated beach, did not explain these findings. One proposed mechanism is internal contamination by a radionuclide localized in spermatogonia, and amplified during spermatogenesis, causing a higher incidence of genetic lesions in the offspring (68,69). A provocative finding in a recent study is that decreases in birth weight, gestational age, and fetal growth were related to preconception diagnostic x-rays of fathers (70).

Markers of genome alterations in male gene cells include DNA-adduct detection and a sperm chromatin stability assay. Although the primary action of DBCP is testicular toxicity, it has been shown to also cause massive DNA damage *in vivo* and *in vitro* (71).

Because of their ubiquity, solvents are an increasing concern. Glycol ethers are suspected of having male reproductive effects based on results of animal experiments that indicate that 2-methoxyethanol (2ME) and 2-ethoxyethanol (2EE) and their acetates are toxic to the male reproductive system. Studies of rats, mice, rabbits, and dogs demonstrate an association of 2EE with a variety of adverse outcomes, including testicular atrophy, degeneration of seminiferous tubules, severe oligospermia, abnormal sperm morphology, and reduced sperm motility. Two studies indicate a marginally significant effect of exposure of workers to 2EE and decreased sperm count at both a metal castings company and in painters (72,73), but no other semen parameters were significant. In the study of painters, a stratified analysis by smoking and exposure status was undertaken of those with lower sperm count (not more than 100 million). In smokers the prevalence of lower sperm count was similar regardless of whether they were exposed to 2EE. In nonsmokers, however, 36% of exposed workers had lower sperm count, compared to 16% for the unexposed group. This finding suggests that if occupational exposure is a much weaker risk factor than another, such as smoking, the effects of the weaker factor may be masked owing to the overriding influence that a highly predictive factor has on the outcome (74).

Perchloroethylene is another hydrocarbon that is widely used, particularly in dry cleaning. A study comparing 34 dry cleaners with 48 laundry workers identified no significant differences in sperm concentrations or overall percentage of abnormal forms, but significant dose-related changes were found in sperm shape and lateral head displacement (75). Another study of mixed solvent exposure found a decrease in follicle-stimulating hormone (FSH) after toluene exposure (76).

The advantages and limitations of semen measurements for detecting occupational causes of reproductive impairment are reviewed elsewhere (77,78). The advantages are that a large number of sperm cells can be collected, effects can be detected in workers who are not attempting to conceive (e.g., single men), and early detection may be possible when no alteration in fertility is apparent. The limitations include difficulty in obtaining a high participation rate, and there is much biologic and measurement variability in these tests.

Linking the exposure with the time of conception can be crucial, as the interval between exposure and expression of an event may be brief (e.g., 74 days for a spermatogenic cycle). Obtaining precise identification of the specific exposure period that initiated the event is important to minimize misclassification errors. When the outcomes of pregnancy for the partner of an exposed worker are assessed, the period of exposure just prior to the conception (perhaps the preceding 4 to 6 months) or at conception often is used. Hence, it may not be a worker's total person-years of exposure that are important but the exposure that occurred relative to a critical period of reproductive development (5).

In a survey of pregnancy outcomes among wives of employees exposed to chlorinated dioxins, there was no increase in spontaneous abortions, stillbirths, or infant deaths (79). In this study, however, a worker was considered exposed if during his total employment he had been assigned to a chlorophenol process for at least 1 month. As this study did not link exposures with pregnancies, misclassifications may have resulted. In another study of dioxin exposure in Vietnam veterans, a similar problem prevailed (80). Several years after the exposure, investigators studied the reproductive experience: pregnancy history of the wives of 7,924 Vietnam veterans and 7,364 veterans who did not serve in Vietnam, and semen analysis of 324 Vietnam veterans and 247 other veterans. Although the Vietnam veterans reported a significant excess of birth defects and fetal loss among their partners, the increased prevalence of birth defects was not substantiated with medical records. Reporting or a selection bias was considered a possible explanation. Evaluating birth defects from pregnancies that occur many months to years after the exposure assumes that the mechanism of action is premeiotic damage to the genes or chromosomes of spermatogonial stem cells rather than teratogenesis. This hypothesis has little support in the literature (81). However, there was a lower mean sperm concentration among the Vietnam veterans (64.8 million per milliliter) than among other veterans (79.8 million per milliliter) (82). Compared to referents, the Vietnam veterans were twice as likely to have sperm concentrations less than 20 million per ml, 15.9% and 8.1%, respectively [odds ratio (OR) = 2.7; 95% CI = 1.3–5.7]. There was no significant difference between the two groups in mean percentages of motile and morphologically normal cells. These differences, however, were not sufficient to decrease the fecundity of the veterans but could indicate possible stem cell damage.

Although workplace exposures to mixtures are more the rule than the exception, few studies have attempted to examine these combined effects. Savitz and coworkers (83) investigated exposure to a complex mixture of halogenated hydrocarbons in a survey of male oil, chemical, and atomic workers. This report indicated a significant elevation of infant mortality among their offspring. Infertility, fetal loss, and malformation effects, however, proved undetectable in this instance, and response rate was low. Exposure to mixtures of solvents have been linked to male-mediated effects. McDonald and coworkers (84) reported an increase in spontaneous abortion among the spouses of motor vehicle mechanics, and spontaneous abortions and congenital malformations were observed among the wives of men exposed to 1,1,1-trichloromethane, toluene, and xylene (85). Sewage sludge and waste water are complex mixtures containing heavy metals, persistent pesticides, chlorinated hydrocarbons, and other organic compounds. Individually, many of these compounds have been shown in laboratory studies to affect male reproduction. Morgan and coworkers (86) investigated pregnancy outcomes in 101 wives of workers employed at a petrochemical waste water treatment plant. This study indicated that the risk of fetal loss doubled when the father was exposed to industrial waste water at time of conception. Others suggested, however, that this finding may be artificial, owing to a maternal age factor or recall bias (87,88). A follow-up cross-sectional study of these workers showed no significant effects related to sperm count or morphology (89). In another study of employees of a metropolitan treatment plant who were exposed to industrial wastes, no differences between exposed and unexposed workers were observed in either fetal loss or infertility, but there was a significant difference in their mean sperm counts as well as more subtle changes in morphology (35,90,91).

In summary, workers may experience a range of physical or chemical exposure, from brief but extremely high to continuous low-level exposure. The biologic response may depend on the type of exposure. Therefore, the choice of study design and the decision to collect biologic semen samples or use survey methods will vary, depending on the type, timing, and duration of exposure and the population to be studied. The survey approach may be better equipped to examine historical exposures unless these have been constant over time. Although survey approaches were shown to be as sensitive as use of biologic samples when exposures were very potent (e.g., with DBCP) (77), these methods are probably not sufficiently sensitive for detecting more subtle effects of subfecundity. Semen analysis has been shown to be superior, in some instances, for the detection of the effects of both physical and chemical exposures on male fecundity (90,92).

## FEMALE REPRODUCTION STUDIES

Studies of the reproductive effects of toxicant exposure on female worker populations are unique because two persons may be at risk—the woman, and, if she is pregnant, her developing offspring. Maternal exposure to a toxicant may cause infertility, menstrual disorders, illness during pregnancy, chromosome aberrations, breast milk alteration, early onset of menopause, and suppressed libido. Adverse fetal outcomes include preterm delivery, fetal loss, perinatal death, low birth weight (LBW), altered sex ratio, congenital malformations, childhood malignancies, infant or childhood illness, chromosome aberrations, and developmental disabilities. This section discusses the potential effects of toxic exposure on menstrual cycle variability and adverse pregnancy outcomes.

### Menstrual Cycle Variability

Although women compose about half of the work force, research on the impact of exposures on menses has been limited. Toxic exposures can alter the pattern of menstruation by several means, including inhibition or damage to the follicles, effects on the central nervous system leading to endocrine alterations, damage to the hormone-secreting organs, or disruption of the delicate hormone balance that regulates ovulation and the menstrual cycle. For example, in an experimental study exposing rhesus monkeys to lead in their drinking water, significant changes occurred in progesterone peaks (93).

At birth infant girls' ovaries have between 3 and 4 million follicles each. By puberty the number is fewer than 400,000. During each ovarian cycle a number of follicles start to mature, but most fail. After menopause, few if any follicles are present in the ovaries. Reproductive senescence can occur if xenobiotic agents block oogenesis in the fetus or destroy oocytes, causing premature ovarian failure (94). The sensitive and complex process of ovulation affords several potential targets for damage by industrial chemicals. Damage to the ovulatory process may be expressed in disorders of menstruation, which in turn may be a surrogate of other events such as a decrease in fertility potential or very early pregnancy loss (95).

Although the characteristics of a normal cycle vary between women, variations in individual women are slight. The average age of menarche is 12.5 years (range 9 to 16 years) (96) and the average duration is 2 to 7 days, and the interval between menses ranges from 23 to 35 days (mean 28.1 days) (97,98). Variation in the interval between menses for an individual should not exceed 5 days (99). During each menses the average blood loss is 30 to 100 ml (98). The estimated mean age at natural menopause is 50.5 years. Women whose median cycle length between ages 20 and 35 years was less than 26 days reached menopause 1.4 years earlier than those with cycles between 26 and 32 days, and 2.2 years earlier than those with cycles of 33 days or longer (100).

Menstrual abnormalities can be broadly divided into three categories: (1) cycle length or rhythm, (2) characteristics of bleeding patterns, and (3) the presence of pain. The most dramatic disruption of cycle rhythm is complete absence of menses. There are two types of amenorrhea: primary, the failure to menstruate by age 16 years; and secondary, cessation of menses for 3 months or longer before age 40. Polymenorrhea is the occurrence of menstrual cycles at intervals of less than 18 days (101). Polyhypermenorrhea is periods of heavy flow that occur more frequently than normal. Oligomenorrhea is defined as infrequent menstrual periods, the interval between periods being 40 to 45 days. Metrorrhagia, or intermenstrual bleeding, is uterine bleeding at any time other than during the menstrual period. Irregular cycles may be defined as variations of more than 5 days in an individual woman's cycle length. Women older than 40 generally have shorter cycles, and 7 years before menopause the incidence of abnormally short or long cycles increases. In a study of 1,560 nurses Shortridge (102) found that the proportion of subjects reporting cycles of fewer than 25 days was 4.4% for women aged 30 to 34 years but 8.2% at 40 to 45 years.

For category 2, one characteristic bleeding pattern is excessive flow, referred to as menorrhagia or hypermenorrhea. To quantify the amount of flow, the number of menstrual pads or tampons used may be counted. A menstrual pad and a tampon are considered saturated when they contain 30 to 50 ml and 20 to 30 ml of blood, respectively (103). The number of pads used per day can be a measure of hypermenorrhea, although because of variability in women's hygiene practices this measure can be fairly inaccurate. During the first 2 days of her period, a woman usually uses three to six pads or tampons per day (104). If more than six pads or tampons are used or if clots are present, the flow is abnormally heavy (105).

As noted in category 3, pain also is used to characterize the menstrual cycle. Dysmenorrhea, or painful menstruation, is recognized as symptoms that are severe enough to cause loss of time from work or school. These symptoms may include lower abdominal cramping, backache, aching thighs, nausea, diarrhea, headache, anorexia, irritability, and poor concentration. Primary dysmenorrhea is unrelated to an obvious physical cause while secondary dysmenorrhea is linked to pelvic disease. In a population of 293 workers, it was found that the baseline prevalences of secondary amenorrhea, dysmenorrhea, secondary amenorrhea, intermenstrual bleeding, and hypermenorrhea were 7.9%, 14.0%, 16.4%, and 28.3%, respectively (106).

Studies of the effects of exposure on menstruation must account for the myriad risk factors associated with these conditions. Age is a well-established influence on menstruation. Immediately after menarche and near menopause, the risk for irregular cycles is great. Younger women are more likely to suffer from dysmenorrhea (107). Both underweight and overweight women are at risk for disturbances of menses. The association of anorexia nervosa and amenorrhea is well known (108,109). The relationship between weight loss, anorexia nervosa, and amenorrhea appears to entail a decrease in the ratio of body fat to lean body mass. Vigorous exercise, such as long-distance running, dancing, gymnastics, tennis, skiing, rowing, or fencing, is associated with amenorrhea or oligomenorrhea. Again, this condition is related to the theory of decreased body fat associated with anorexia nervosa. Women who have not borne children are at greater risk for dysmenorrhea and amenorrhea (110). Breast-feeding mothers may not have a period for as long as 6 months postpartum. Female genital tract disease and systemic illnesses also may cause menstrual disturbances. Uremic and dialysis patients are prone to menstrual disturbances; after renal transplantation menstrual function usually returns to normal (111). Virtually all menstrual disturbances secondary to thyroid disease return to normal with treatment. Various medications may influence the menstrual cycle.

Contraceptive methods also influence the cycle. Amenorrhea, irregular bleeding, or intermenstrual flow may occur when a woman begins to take oral contraceptives. Continued use may diminish dysmenorrhea. Most women who stop using birth control pills menstruate within 2 months; however, 2.2% have true postpill amenorrhea, a failure to resume menstruation after a 6-month hiatus in oral contraception (112). After intrauterine contraceptive device (IUD) insertion, the great majority of women experience a 50% to 100% increase in menstrual blood loss, and 54% experience dysmenorrhea (113,114). The effect of tubal ligation remains controversial. One study showed a 7.1% increase in menorrhagia and a 6.0% increase in dysmenorrhea with tubal ligation (115).

Socioeconomic and psychological factors have been reported to influence the menstrual cycle. The effect of stress remains controversial but may be related to amenorrhea, oligomenorrhea, hypermenorrhea, or dysmenorrhea (112,116–118). Amenorrhea and dysmenorrhea do occur more frequently in women who experience stress (102,116). Smokers are at risk for both amenorrhea and dysmenorrhea (107,110). Amenorrhea is also associated with alcoholism. When women stop drinking their menses return (119).

**Occupational Studies**

The attempts to assess menstrual cycle alterations that are related to occupational exposures have been few. Workers exposed to formaldehyde in occupations such as biology, ink making, and embalming report menstrual disorders more frequently than unexposed workers (47.5% versus 9.2%) (120). Studies of women exposed to solvents such as benzene, toluene, and xylene have shown menstrual disturbances, principally associated with abnormal bleeding (121–124). Styrene was reported to be associated with irregular cycles and hypermenorrhea in one study (125), but these findings were not confirmed in a larger study (106). Women working in dry cleaning plants who were exposed to perchloroethylene and other solvents were compared to laundry workers. Exposure in dry cleaning work was associated with a significant excess of menstrual disorders, including cycle length, menorrhagia, dysmenorrhea, and premenstrual syndrome (126). Among petrol workers (also exposed to hydrocarbons) 50% of women older than 40 years reported some type of menstrual disorder, compared to 18.7% of aged-matched controls. Twenty-one percent of these workers experience menorrhagia, versus 8.3% of control subjects (127). Eighty-three percent of workers exposed to trinitrotoluene (TNT) in explosive manufacturing experienced changes in their menstrual cycle; symptoms diminished to 65% and 20% after 1 and 2 years postexposure, respectively (128).

Manufacturing or handling certain drugs may place the female worker at risk. Forty percent of all estrogen plant workers reported intermenstrual bleeding, and the prevalence increased to 50% for the most exposed workers (129). The prevalence of menstrual irregularity and amenorrhea was shown to be higher among nurses who handled cytotoxic drugs than among controls and was most pronounced in those older than 30 years (102). A study of female pharmacists did not, however, support these findings (130). Table 3 summarizes the possible causes of menstrual disorders associated with environmental exposures and other known risk factors.

Exposure to physical hazards has been linked to abnormal menses. Women who experience vibration in occupations such as textile manufacturing are three times more likely (50.7% versus 16.4%) to develop hyperpolymenorrhea and severe dysmenorrhea (131). A few studies have examined the effect of shift work on the menses. The results have been conflicting: two reported irregular menses (132,133), and another no effect on cycle length, duration, or flow (134). Women who work as airline flight attendants experience a variety of menstrual disorders, probably owing to multiple factors—vibration, disruption of circadian rhythms, altitude changes, and solar radiation (135,136); menstrual function, however, has been shown to revert to the preflight status with longer jet flight experience (137).

**TABLE 3.** *A summary of risk factors associated with menstrual disorders*

| Risk factors | Amenorrhea, oligomenorrhea | Hypermenorrhea, polymenorrhea | Irregular cycles/ metrorrhagia | Dysmenorrhea | Type unspecified |
|---|---|---|---|---|---|
| General | | | | | |
| Age | | | x | x | |
| Anorexia nervosa, underweight | x | | | | |
| Obesity | x | | | x | |
| Pregnancy | x | x | x | | |
| Lactation | x | | | | |
| Nulliparity | x | | | x | |
| Female genital tract disorder | | | | | |
| Anatomic abnormality | | | | x | |
| Endometriosis | | | | x | |
| Polyps, fibroids | | x | x | x | |
| Infections | x | x | x | | |
| Chronic pelvic inflammatory disease (PID) | | | | x | |
| Cancer of ovary, uterus, vagina | x | x | x | | |
| Asherman's syndrome | x | x | | x | |
| Systemic illness | | | | | |
| Hemorrhagic disorders | | x | x | | |
| Iron deficiency | | x | | | |
| Systemic lupus erythematosus | | x | | | |
| Diabetes | x | | | | |
| Crohn's disease | x | | | | |
| Hypopituitarism | x | | | | |
| Cushing's syndrome | x | | | | |
| Stroke | x | | | | |
| Sarcoidosis | x | | | | |
| Pituitary lesions | x | | | | |
| Acute febrile illness | x | | | | |
| Renal disease | x | x | x | | |
| Liver disease | x | x | x | | |
| Hypothyroidism | | x | x | | |
| Hyperthroidism | x | | | | |
| Multiple sclerosis | x | | | | |
| Tuberculosis | x | | | | |
| Medications | | | | | |
| Anticoagulants | | x | | | |
| Excessive use of aspirin | | x | | | |
| Tranquilizers, sedatives | x | | | | |
| Steroids | x | | | | |

Few studies have related physical or chemical hazards to determinants of age at menopause. A recent investigation demonstrated the group with earliest natural senescence were African-Americans who reported being very stressed during the prior 6 months (138). Median age at menopause for African-American women reporting stress was 48.4 compared to 49.9 for those without stress and 51.6 for Caucasian women regardless of stress. Other factors significantly related to earlier onset of menopause were irregular cycles, being a current smoker, and being on a weight-reduction diet.

There are many challenges to undertaking investigations of menstrual disorders in working populations. Levels of effort can extend from collecting a one-time questionnaire, to using daily logs, including various hormonal measurements such as salivary and urinary progesterone, urine, human chorionic gonadotropin (hCG), LH, FSH, estrone 3-glucuronide ($E_13G$), and pregnanediol 3-glucuronide (Pd3G) (139). When menstrual history information is collected using questionnaire data, some studies have shown poor reliability (140,141). In a survey of nurses, however, some menstrual related variables were found to have high reliability, including age at menarche and menopause, history of severe irregularity, uterine fibroids, ovarian cysts, endometriosis, pelvic inflammatory disease (PID), and use of oral contraceptives and IUDs (102). The variables that have fair to poor reliability are dysmenorrhea, hypermenorrhea, clotting, and spotting. Methods to improve data collection include restricting the history to a very recent time frame (say, the previous 3 months) or having the patient keep a daily log. A study of nurses, however, has shown that compliance with log keeping can be poor (134). Urine hormone measures could be used as an objective measurement of dysfunction or as a validity measurement, at least in a subpopulation keeping the daily diaries. Decisions must be

**TABLE 3.** *Continued.*

| Risk factors | Amenorrhea, oligomenorrhea | Hypermenorrhea, polymenorrhea | Irregular cycles/ metrorrhagia | Dysmenorrhea | Type unspecified |
|---|---|---|---|---|---|
| Phenothiazines | x | | | | |
| Long-term tetracycline | x | | | | |
| Spironolactone | x | | | | |
| Injectable triamcinolone | | | | | x |
| Methaqualone | | | | | x |
| Contraceptive methods | | | | | |
| IUDs | | x | x | x | |
| Oral contraceptives | x | | x | | |
| Tubal ligation | | x | | x | |
| Socioeconomic and psychological factors | | | | | |
| Stress | x | x | | x | |
| Dissatisfaction with work | | | | x | |
| Unmarried, separated, divorced status | x | | | x | |
| City dwellers | x | | | | |
| Smoking | x | | | x | |
| Alcohol abuse | x | | | x | |
| Vigorous exercise | x | | | | |
| Occuaptional toxicants exposure | | | | | |
| Antineoplastics | x | | x | | |
| Tobacco | | | | | x |
| Fluorine | | | | | x |
| Weaving-industry compounds | | | x | | |
| Cotton/textiles-industry compounds | | x | | | x |
| Formaldehyde | | | | x | x |
| Hormones | x | | x | | x |
| Carbon disulfide | | x | | | |
| Benzol (benzene) | | | | | x |
| Vibration | | x | | x | |
| Croton aldehyde | | x | | x | |
| Petrol | | x | | | x |
| Jet air travel | x | x | x | x | |
| Trinitrotoluene | x | x | x | | |
| Solvents | x | x | x | x | |
| Chloroprene | | | | | x |
| Cadmium | | | | | x |
| Shift work | | | x | x | |
| Superphosphates | | | x | | |
| Perchloroethylene | | | x | x | |

made about the appropriateness of including or excluding persons who have risk factors that are known to strongly influence menses: use of oral contraceptives or an IUD, recent pregnancy, hysterectomy, primary amenorrhea, history of cancer of the reproductive organs, and age over 40 years. One study of 1,525 women found that 49% of the work force had one or more of these conditions; in another, 70% were excluded for similar reasons (106,126).

Although menstrual disorders generally are frequently viewed as less serious than many health end points, the financial impact is high. National cost estimates for work days missed due to menstrual illness for women under age 44 range from $94 to $308 million per day missed (142). Furthermore, menstrual or hormonal disorders may reflect or predict other disorders including subfecundity, early miscarriage, breast cancer, osteoporosis, or cardiovascular disease.

**Adverse Pregnancy Outcomes**

Exposure of the conceptus to a toxicant can result in different effects depending on the phase of embryofetal development—early or late embryogenesis—or the fetal period of development. Adverse responses include fetal death, metabolic or physiologic disorders, structural malformations, growth retardation, functional disorders in the offspring, preterm delivery, and low birth weight (LBW) (143).

Transport time of a fertilized ovum before implantation is between 2 and 6 days. During this early stage the embryo may be exposed to chemical compounds that penetrate into the uterine fluids. Absorption of xenobiotic compounds may be accompanied by degenerative changes, alteration in the blastocytic protein profile, or failure to implant (144–146). Insult during this period is seldom recognized. It is well established experimentally that the embryo is fairly resistant to teratogenic insult at this early stage since cells have not initiated the complex sequence of differentiation (147). Menstrual irregularities may be the only recognized outcome.

The period of late embryogenesis is characterized by differentiation, mobilization, and organization of cells into tissue and organ rudiments. Embryogenesis is the period of greatest sensitivity to teratogens. Wilson (143) outlined many of the possible mechanisms in structural malformations: mutation, chromosome damage, mitotic interference, altered nucleic acid integrity, lack of precursors, altered energy sources, enzyme inhibition, and alteration in membranes. Mediating susceptibility factors include route and level of exposure, pattern of exposure, and genotype. Extrinsic factors such as nutritional deficiencies, or the additive, synergistic, or antagonistic effects associated with multiple exposures may further impact response (143,148,149). Untoward responses during embryogenesis can culminate in spontaneous abortion, gross structural defects, fetal loss, growth retardation, or developmental abnormalities.

The fetal period extends from embryogenesis to birth and is characterized developmentally by growth, histogenesis, and functional maturation. Toxicity may be manifested by a reduction in cell size and number. The brain remains sensitive to injury; myelination is incomplete until after birth. Growth retardation, functional defects, disruption in the pregnancy, behavioral effects, transplacental carcinogenesis, or death may result from toxicity during the fetal period.

The following discussion reviews the biologic, sociologic, and epidemiologic issues concerning the process of evaluating occupational exposures and fetal loss, congenital anomalies, preterm delivery, and LBW. Definitions, estimated incidence rates, and risk factors associated with the specific outcome are described.

### *Fetal Loss*

The developmental stages of the zygote, defined in days from the last menstrual period (LMP) and days from ovulation (DOV), proceed from the blastocyst stage at days 15 to 20 (1 to 6 DOV), with implantation occurring on day 20 or 21 (6 or 7 DOV), to the embryonic period from days 21 to 62 (7 to 48 DOV), and the fetal period from day 63 (49+ DOV) until the designated period of viability, which in reports ranges from 140 to 195 days. Estimates of the probability of pregnancy termination at one of these stages depends on both the definition of fetal loss and the method used to measure the event.

The definition of early versus late fetal loss ranges from the end of week 20 to the end of week 27. The definitions of fetal and infant death recommended by the World Health Organization (WHO) (150) are listed in Table 4. Because the majority of early spontaneously aborted fetuses have chromosome anomalies, Källén

**TABLE 4.** *Definitions of fetal loss and infant death*

| |
|---|
| Spontaneous abortion: ≤500 g *or* 20–22 weeks or 25 cm length |
| Stillbirth: >500 g (>1000 g international) nonviable |
| Early neonatal death: death of a live-born infant at ≤7 days (168 hours) |
| Late neonatal death: death between 7 and 28 days |

(151) suggested that for research purposes a finer distinction should be made between early fetal loss, before 12 weeks' gestation, and later fetal loss. In examining late fetal losses it may be appropriate to include early neonatal deaths, as the causes may be similar. The WHO defines early neonatal death as the death of an infant aged 7 days or younger and late neonatal death as demise between 7 and 29 days. For studies conducted in developing countries, it may be important to distinguish between prepartum and intrapartum deaths. In less developed countries, intrapartum deaths account for a large portion of stillbirths because the process of delivery is the problem. Owing to burial practices or religious customs, however, these data may not be accurately recorded.

Kline and coworkers (152) reviewed nine retrospective or cross-sectional studies. The fetal loss rates before 20 weeks' gestation ranged from 5.5% to 12.6%. When the definition was expanded to include losses up to 28 weeks' gestation, the fetal loss rate varied between 6.2% and 19.6%. The incidence rates of fetal loss among clinically recognized pregnancies in four prospective studies, however, had a relatively narrow range of 11.7% to 14.6% for the gestational period up to 28 weeks (95,153–155). This lower rate, seen in prospective versus retrospective or cross-sectional designs, may be attributable to differences in underlying definitions, misreporting of induced abortions as spontaneous, or misclassification of a delayed or heavy menses as fetal loss.

When early, subclinical pregnancy loss is evaluated using sensitive hormonal assays, e.g., hCG, the total spontaneous abortion rate jumps dramatically. It has been estimated that approximately 15% of fertilized eggs are lost prior to implantation; thus, 85% are available for implantation (154,156–159). In a study using hCG methods (95), the incidence postimplantation of subclinical loss of fertilized ova was 22%, which translates into 19% of the remaining conceptions ($0.85 \times 0.22$); 9% of terminations were recognized—8% of the total available ova ($0.85 \times 0.09$) (160). Thus, the true potential rate of spontaneous abortions among fertilized ova is high, approximately 42% ($0.15 + 0.19 + 0.08$) for fetal losses up to 28 weeks' gestation. Five epidemiologic studies that have used hormonal monitoring in different scenarios have been recently reviewed (139).

Occupational studies have also used records or questionnaire data to identify spontaneous abortions. Recorded data sources include vital statistics and hospital, private practitioner, and outpatient clinic records. Questionnaire data are collected with mailed instruments or in personal or telephone interviews. Use of record systems identifies only a subset of all fetal losses, principally those that occur after the start of prenatal care, typically after two or three missed periods. By interviewing women to obtain reproductive histories, more complete documentation of all recognized losses is possible. Questions that are usually included in reproductive histories include all pregnancy outcomes, prenatal care, family history of adverse pregnancy outcomes, marital history, nutritional status, prepregnancy weight, height, weight gain, use of cigarettes or alcohol, prescription and nonprescription drugs, health status of the mother during and prior to a pregnancy, and exposures at home and in the workplace to physical and chemical agents such as vibration, radiation, metals, solvents, and pesticides (139).

The validity of self-reported pregnancy histories as reported in six studies was verified in hospital or physician records at a rate between 57.5% and 91.8% (median 86.2%) (7). Wilcox and Horney (161) reported that fetal losses before 7 weeks' gestation are confirmed in records at a low rate, 54%. As gestational age advances, so does the likelihood that fetal loss will be recorded; by 9 to 12 weeks' gestation 82% are recorded, and at 13 weeks' gestation 93%. Gestational age ($r$ = .86) followed by information on reproductive histories and various medical procedures was retrieved from medical records (162). Likewise, the interval between the fetal loss and time of interview may be associated with memory errors and a reduction in validity. It has been shown that if the interview occurs within 10 years of the event, recall appears to be good, as it was with 82% of the spontaneous abortions recorded (163). Interview data on spontaneous abortions can be a valid source of information, particularly if the analysis includes those of 9 weeks' gestation or later and those that occurred during the last 10 years. Correlations between medical records and maternal interviews are highest for birth weight ($r$ = .98).

The principal physical, genetic, social, and environmental factors associated with spontaneous abortion are summarized in Table 5. Infections associated with fetal loss include syphilis, rubella, genital *Mycoplasma* infections, herpes simplex, uterine infections, and general hyperpyrexia. One of the most important risk factors for clinically recognized spontaneous abortion is a history of pregnancy ending in fetal loss. Higher gravidity is associated with increased risk, but this may not be independent of a history of spontaneous abortion. Interpretations of gravidity as a risk factor conflict because of its association with maternal age, reproductive history, and heterogeneity of women at different gravidity ranks. Rates of spontaneous abortion are higher for women younger than 16 and older than 36 years. After adjusting for gravidity and a history of pregnancy loss, women older than 40 were shown to have twice the risk of fetal loss of younger women (164). The increased risk for older women is associated with an increase in chromosome anomalies, particularly trisomy (165).

**TABLE 5.** *Factors associated with spontaneous abortions*

| Physical-genetic | Environmental-social |
|---|---|
| Increasing gravidity | Socioeconomic status |
| Maternal age | Smoking history |
| Birth order | Prescribed and recreational drugs |
| Race | Alcohol use |
| Repeat spontaneous abortion | Poor nutrition |
| Insulin-dependent diabetes | Infections |
| Uterine disorders | Spermicides |
| Twinning | Employment |
| | Chemical exposure |

Employment status may be a risk factor regardless of a physical or chemical hazard and may act as a confounder in assessment of occupational exposure and spontaneous abortion. Some investigators suggest that women who stay in the work force are more likely to have had an adverse pregnancy history (163,166); others believe this group is an inherently more fit subpopulation (167,168). In a recent report of 3,315 pregnancies, it was found that employed women had a significantly higher rate of spontaneous abortion (14.5%) than those unemployed [11.7%; risk ratio (RR) = 1.23; 95% CI = 1.02–1.49] (74). Another study of 3,712 employed and 2,215 unemployed women indicated that working women had more favorable demographic and behavior characteristics, such as higher income and better prenatal care, but a less favorable reproductive history (169).

### *Congenital Anomalies*

During the first 60 days after conception, the developing infant may be more sensitive to xenobiotic toxicants than at other stages in the life cycle (143). There are numerous reviews on the causes, mechanisms, and types of malformations (143,170–172). This section highlights data on incidence rates, risk factors for birth defects, and epidemiologic considerations in the assessment of congenital anomalies.

Historically, the terms *terata* and *congenital malformations* refer to structural defects present at birth that may be gross or microscopic, internal or external, hereditary or nonhereditary, single or multiple. *Congenital anomaly* is more broadly defined and includes abnormal behavior, function, and chemistry with malformations as one type of anomaly. Malformations may be single or multiple. Chromosome defects generally produce multiple defects, whereas single-gene changes or exposure to environmental agents may cause either single defects or a syndrome (170). A major malformation can be defined as one that results in death, requires surgery or medical treatment, or constitutes a substantial physical or psychological handicap.

The incidence of malformations depends on the status of the conceptus—live birth, spontaneous abortus, or stillbirth. Miller and Poland (173) found 88% of 28-day-old abortuses were abnormal (73 of 83). By 20 weeks' gestation the overall incidence was 45% (223 of 498). In the early age group, multiple-system defects and severe growth disorganization were found; these anomalies became less frequent with each developmental stage. Another study found a 32% rate of anomalies among 172 stillborn fetuses that weighed more than 500 g ($N$ = 5,964) (174). Birth defect incidence figures for live births depend on the age at diagnosis and varies with the information source—birth certificates, hospital records, physician records, and parental reports—which also reflect the age of the child at diagnosis. Many congenital malformations go undetected at birth and only become evident months to years later. The frequency of major congenital defects was 1.02% when reported shortly after birth, and it more than tripled when the same infants were reexamined at 9 months of age (175). Bierman and coworkers (176) estimated that by age 2, 10% of the surviving infants had anomalies requiring special medical or educational services; an additional 10% sustained minor defects. Overall, the prevalence of major defects fluctuates between 1% and 3%, with a frequency of about 2.24% (177). The prevalence of minor defects ranges between 3% and 15% (average about 10%) (2,170,174, 178,179). The great variation in reported rates for major and minor defects is the result of differences in study populations, definitions, the specialty of the examining physician, and data sources.

Malformation rates are approximately 41% higher for boys than for girls (180). The overall sex differential is explained by the significantly higher rate of anomalies for male genital organs. Frequent anomalies in both sexes include syndactyly, oral clefts, reduction deformities, clubfoot, cardiac anomalies, polydactyly, congenital hydrocephalus, and Down syndrome. Polydactyly is the most common anomaly among African-Americans, accounting for 39% of the total. There is some variability in birth defects by region of the United States (181). For example, the incidence rate for clubfoot is 0.20% in the South, as compared to 0.31% in the North Central region; the rate of ventricular septal defect is 0.13% in the South and 0.23% in the Northeast.

Birth anomalies of known causes are due to genetic factors (27.7%), multifactorial inheritance (23%), uterine factors (2.5%), twinning (0.4%), or teratogens (3.2%) (177). The causes of the remaining 43.2% are unknown and likely multifactorial.

A number of environmental toxicants have been associated with congenital anomalies in offspring. One of the strongest was consumption of food contaminated with methylmercury during gestation in the countries of Japan and Iraq; this causes morphologic, central nervous system, and neurobehavioral abnormalities (182,183). In Japan, the cluster of cases was linked to consumption of fish and shellfish contaminated with mercury derived from the effluent of a chemical factory. The most severely affected offspring were children with cerebral palsy. Further, in 1968 maternal ingestion of polychlorinated biphenyls (PCBs) from contaminated rice oil gave rise to babies with several disorders, including growth retardation, dark brown skin pigmentation, early eruption of teeth, gingival hyperplasia, wide sagittal suture, facial edema, and exophthalmos (184).

One challenge in studying malformations is deciding how to group for analysis (151,152). Often, all malformations are combined or the combination is based on major and minor categories. The rationale for grouping all together is that the majority arise during organogenesis. The advantage of this approach is that the total number of cases is increased, and therefore the statistical power is increased. If, however, the exposure effect is specific to a particular type of malformation (e.g., central nervous system), such grouping could mask an effect. Alternatively, malformations may be grouped by organ system. Though this method may be an improvement, certain defects may dominate the class, such as varus deformities of the feet in the musculoskeletal system. Given a sufficiently large sample, the optimal approach is to divide the defects into pathogenetically homogeneous groups (151). Considerations should be given as well to the exclusion or inclusion of certain malformations, such as those that are likely caused by chromosome defects, autosomal dominant conditions, or malposition in utero. In analyzing congenital anomalies in particular, a balance has to be maintained between maintaining precision and compromising statistical power.

### *Low Birth Weight and Preterm Delivery*

Among the many factors linked to infant survival, physical underdevelopment associated with early delivery, LBW, or both, presents the greatest risk in the U.S. Every year, more than 250,000 infants are born prior to term. If respiratory distress is included as one of the complications of preterm delivery, preterm labor and LBW are directly or indirectly responsible for more neonatal deaths, mental retardation, and neurologic and ophthalmic disorders than any other single cause. Significant fetal weight gain does not begin until the second trimester. The conceptus weighs 1 g at 8 weeks, 141 g at 12 weeks, and 1.1 kg at 28 weeks. An additional 1.1 kg is gained every 6 weeks until term (185). The normal newborn weighs approximately 3,200 g at term.

Several terms often are used interchangeably, and sometimes incorrectly, to describe an infant delivered prior to the expected date of confinement. In 1948, the First World Health Assembly of the WHO (186) defined an immature infant as a live-born infant with a birth weight of 5½ pounds or less. If weight was not specified, gestation less than 37 weeks was used to define an immature infant (187). In 1950, the WHO Expert Group on Prematurity recommended the term *prematurity,* rather than *immaturity,* to denote birth weight of 2,500 g or less (186). This latter definition did not differentiate growth-retarded and small-for-gestational age infants from those delivered early whose weight was appropriate to gestational age. By 1961, the WHO attempted to rectify this problem by defining birth weight of 2,500 g or less as LBW and birth before 37 complete weeks' gestation as prematurity (188). New confusions resulted as some clinicians chose to define prematurity in terms of birth weight while others defined it in terms of gestational age. Finally, the term *prematurity* was discarded. Currently, the WHO (150) recommends the definition of *preterm* as delivery before 37 completed weeks, less than 259 completed days from the first day of the LMP. The American Academy of Fetus and Newborn defined *preterm* as delivery before gestational day 266 (189). LBW was defined as less than 2,500 g, and very low birth weight as less than 1,500 g (190).

It is important to distinguish between symmetric and asymmetric growth retardation. Asymmetric growth retardation (i.e., weight is affected more than skeletal structure) is associated principally with a risk factor operating late in pregnancy; symmetric growth retardation may more likely be associated with a cause operating over the entire length of gestation, such as malnourishment (152). The difference in rates of asymmetric and symmetric growth retardation is especially apparent when developing and developed countries are compared (152). The rate of growth retardation in developing countries is 10% to 43%, and most cases are symmetric, primarily due to poor nourishment. In developed countries the rate of fetal growth retardation is between 3% and 8%, asymmetric, and the result of several factors. In developing countries, more than 60% of LBW infants are small for gestational age (191).

Gestational age is generally measured from the onset of the LMP to the date of delivery. Ovulation occurs approximately 2 weeks after onset of the LMP. There may be an error in estimation of 1 to 4 weeks, depending on the variability of the menstrual cycle. Accuracy of gestational age also depends on the woman's recall of the LMP or the physician's calculation of the expected delivery date. The accuracy of vital statistics records depends not only on this information but on accurate recording in the hospital records and transferral to birth certificates. Thus, the opportunities for error are many.

The risk factors associated with preterm delivery and LBW are summarized in Table 6 (152,152,192,193). Social class, as measured by income or education, persists as a risk factor in situations in which there are no ethnic differences. Other factors that may be associated with social class or race are cigarette smoking, physical work, prenatal care, and nutrition. African-American women deliver twice the number of preterm infants as Caucasian women, and on average a few days earlier. Women between ages 25 and 29 years are least likely to deliver a preterm or a LBW infant. Heavy maternal smoking increases the risk of a preterm or LBW offspring by about 200%. Hyperpyrexia, malaria, hepatitis, measles, and urinary and genital infections have been associated with shortened gestation. More controversy exists about the relevance of vaginitis, cervicitis, and bacteremia. Some maternal medical conditions associated with preterm delivery include multiple birth, incompetence of the cervical os, bicornuate or arcuate uterus, uterine tumors or fibroids, alterations in the estrogen-progesterone ratio, imbalance in oxytocin level, hypertension, and history of adverse pregnancy (194–196). Maternal medical conditions associated with LBW include placental abnormalities, heart disease, viral pneumonia, liver disease, preeclampsia, eclampsia, chronic hypertension, weight gain, and hyperemesis. An adverse pregnancy history of fetal loss, preterm delivery, or LBW infant increases the current risk of having a preterm or LBW infant by a factor of two to four. An interval between births of less than a year triples the risk of LBW. Chromosome anomalies associated with abnormal growth include Down syndrome, trisomy 18, and most malformation syndromes.

Although cigarette smoking has been associated with preterm delivery (197–201), it is also one of the principal exogenous agents most directly linked with lower birth weight (202–209). Smoking during pregnancy has been

**TABLE 6.** *Factors associated with low birth weight and shortened gestation*

| Physical-genetic | Environmental-social |
|---|---|
| Multiple births | Malnutrition |
| Malformed fetus | Low income/poor education |
| Hypertension | Maternal smoking |
| Placental or cord anomaly | Maternal alcohol consumption |
| Maternal medical history | Occupational exposure |
| History of adverse pregnancy outcome | Psychosocial stress |
| Race | |
| [a]Chromosone anomalies | [a]Altitude |
| [a]Sex | [a]History of infections |
| [a]Maternal height, weight, weight gain | |
| [a]Paternal height | |
| [a]Parity | |
| [a]Length of gestation | |
| [a]Shorter interval between pregnancies | |
| [b]*In vitro* fertilization | |
| [b]Hormone imbalance | |

[a]affects birth weight; [b]associated with preterm delivery.

shown to increase the risk of a LBW two to three times and to cause an overall weight deficit of 150 to 400 g (202,208,209). A study by Murphy and colleagues (207) demonstrated that after 21 weeks' gestation the average biparietal diameters of smokers' fetuses were significantly smaller than those of nonsmokers' fetuses—2.65 ± 0.03 and 2.60 ± 0.03, respectively.

Explanations for these reductions in fetal weight and growth vary. Nicotine and carbon monoxide are considered the most likely agents, since both are transferred rapidly and preferentially across the placenta (210,211). Nicotine is a powerful vasoconstrictor. Asmussen and Kjeldsen (212) found significant differences in the size of umbilical vessels of smoking mothers. Carbon monoxide levels in cigarette smoke range from 20,000 to 60,000 parts per million (ppm); carbon monoxide has a 210-times greater affinity for hemoglobin than oxygen (209,213). Thus, the oxygen-carrying capacity of maternal, and especially fetal, blood is reduced, diminishing the amount of oxygen available to fetal tissues. Others have suggested that these effects are not due to smoking but are attributable to characteristics of smokers. Yerushalmy (203), however, found that infants born before their mothers started smoking (i.e., to future smokers) had the same rate of LBW as infants born to mothers who had never smoked. Butler and coworkers (214) studied women who changed their smoking habits during pregnancy; the infant's weight was lower if the mother started to smoke and higher if she stopped.

Probably the most widely used and researched agent associated with fetal growth retardation (as well as congenital anomalies) is ethanol. A case-control study by Ulleland (215) was the first to demonstrate an association between maternal alcohol consumption and LBW. In a prospective study of 9,236 births, Kaminski and associates (216) characterized the alcoholic mother as older, unmarried, high-parity, low socioeconomic level, and a smoker, who experienced early-pregnancy bleeding. After adjusting separately for each of these risk factors, Kaminski found that consumption of more than 1.6 ounces alcohol per day was associated with an increased rate of stillbirth, lower birth weight, and intrauterine growth retardation. Ambient environmental exposure to DDT or lead has been linked to preterm delivery. Historically, both ambient and occupational gestational exposure to lead has been associated with early delivery (217–220). Fifty-six pregnancies of 13 workers exposed to lead in a printing shop had the following outcomes: 26 spontaneous abortions, 9 preterm deliveries, 1 stillbirth, 17 neonatal deaths, and 3 normal infants (218). The reproductive history of 182 women exposed to lead in printing, painting, polishing, or processing of artificial flowers indicated that, of 82 reported pregnancies, 10 ended in spontaneous abortion, 48 in preterm delivery, and 8 in stillbirth; 20 infants died shortly after birth (outcomes were not mutually exclusive) (219). Thirty of these 182 women had been exposed to very toxic levels of lead. A small case-control study of Missouri residents demonstrated that the level of DDT in the blood of preterm infants was more than three times that of full-term infants, 19.5 ppb compared to 5.8 ppb (23 of 67 infants) (220).

In evaluating the possible effects of exposure on birth weight and gestational age, some problematic issues must be considered. Before the effects of exposure on LBW are evaluated, preterm delivery should be analyzed as a possible mediating outcome. The duration of a pregnancy is directly correlated with weight of the offspring.

Duration of exposure can also be correlated with gestational length. Longer pregnancies afford more opportunity for exposure of workers. If enough women work late in pregnancy, the longest cumulative exposure may be associated with the oldest gestational ages and heaviest babies purely as an artifact (221). A number of procedures can be used to overcome this problem, including a variant of survival analyses handling time-dependent covariants. Preterm delivery and LBW can be defined as either dichotomous or continuous variables. The problem with defining birth weight as dichotomous is that valuable information—the specific weight—is lost. Xenobiotics must have a very powerful effect in order to demonstrate a drastic drop in the infant's weight. In a study of more than 1,000 pregnancies, when birth weight was defined as a continuous variable and analyzed in a multiple regression model, the log of birth weight performed best. For this data set, not only was a linear term needed for gestational age but also quadratic and cubic terms (222,223). The paucity of significant findings in the literature in relation to exposures and these outcomes may in part be caused by inadequacies in design and analyses.

### *Occupational Studies of Adverse Pregnancy Outcomes*

There have been a number of reviews on occupational studies associated with adverse pregnancy outcomes (224–226). This discussion focuses on studies of health personnel, laboratory workers, and industries where solvents and other mixtures are used including the microelectronics industry. These specific occupations were chosen because of historic and/or current interest, employment of a large number of women, and exposures potentially representing high risk to pregnant employees.

Health care personnel are exposed to a variety of hazardous agents including infectious agents, radiation, anesthetic gases, and mercury, and a host of hazardous chemicals such as antineoplastics drugs, formaldehyde, and ethylene oxide. One of the first studies associating occupational exposures with congenital anomalies involved operating room personnel exposed to anesthetic gases (227). This investigation included 49,585 exposed and 23,911 unexposed individuals. There was a significant difference in the rate of congenital anomalies for both exposed female workers and wives of exposed male workers. A British study of the offspring of female anesthesiologists (228) also found a threefold increase in anomalies associated with the heart and vessels and significantly lower birth weights (3,347 ± 525 g) than in the controls (3,380 ± 503 g). Veterinarians represent a unique group of health care personnel, exposed not only to anesthetic gases but to radiation, trauma from animal kicks, insecticides, and zoonotic diseases. No difference was found in the rate of spontaneous abortions or in birth weight between female veterinarians and female lawyers (229), but there was a significant excess of birth defects among veterinarians. Exposure of medical personnel to potent medications such as antineoplastics may occur during mixing or administration of the cytotoxic drugs, disposing of syringes, cleaning up spills from tubing and vials, or touching contaminated linens and excreta of patients. Following the publication of the Occupational Safety and Health Administration's (230) recommendations for the handling of antineoplastics, a study found that more than 40% of hospital-based female pharmacists had skin contact with these drugs at least once a month; more than 13% did not have a special preparation area dedicated to antineoplastics, and 12% still did not wear protective gloves when mixing (231). The adverse effects of chemotherapy on gonadal function in both sexes, including azoospermia and ovarian failure, have been reviewed (232). Occupational studies of nurses identified an association between mixing or administering these agents and a significant excess of chromosome anomalies, menstrual dysfunction, malformations, and fetal loss in the offspring (233–236).

Laboratory and other work involving exposures to mixtures have been linked to adverse outcomes. Female laboratory workers in Sweden were shown to have offspring with almost three times the risk of major malformations (237). The offspring of women working in the pulp and paper industry, in either laboratory work or jobs involving refinement, also had increased risk of central nervous system (CNS), heart, and oral cleft defects (238). Women working in industrial or construction work with unspecified exposures had a 50% increase in CNS defects, and women working in transportation and communication had two times the risk of having a child with an oral cleft (239). Toxicants in the semiconductor industry also are complex mixtures and include such reproductive toxins as glycol ethers, xylene, toluene, trichloroethylene, trichloroethane phenols, isopropyl alcohol, arsine gas, boric acid, thallium, lead, cadmium, and radiofrequency and ionizing radiation. Considerable research has been undertaken evaluating the reproductive health of employment in this industry. Initial findings from Pastides et al. (240) reported that 18 pregnant workers working in the diffusion process area had a significant increase in the rate of spontaneous abortion (RR = 2.18, 95% CI = 1.8–4.04), and there was an excess of spontaneous abortions among both photolithography (31.3%) and diffusion (38.9%) workers. Shortly thereafter, another study of a limited subsample of former female workers (144 of 3,371) detected a significant excess of spontaneous abortions among microelectronics assembly workers (241). The low participation rate, however, raised serious concern about selection bias. Three additional studies representing 17 companies reported an excess (although nonsignificant) of spontaneous abortions in semiconductor fabrication workers, with an RR of 1.6 (242) and 1.4 (243,244). For the latter two studies, after jobs were characterized by high exposure to etyleneglycol ethers (EGE), the relative risks more than doubled (244). Work-related stress in this industry also correlated with spontaneous abortions (242,244).

## CHALLENGE TO HEALTH PROFESSIONALS

In this chapter the biologic and epidemiologic issues associated with evaluating reproductive hazards in the workplace were reviewed. The male and female reproductive system and developing conceptus may be relatively sensitive targets for toxicants. It is the health professional's responsibility to understand the potential hazards. One way to achieve this is to have access to a complete and regularly updated inventory of chemicals in a computerized database. Contained in this data system should be all chemicals that are known and suspected to be mutagenic, teratogenic, or spermatotoxic, plus compounds that may act indirectly on the reproductive system, as through the CNS or endocrine system. Several commercial reproductive toxicologic databases are available that can assist this effort. Too often the potential nature, stresses, and physical and chemical hazards in the workplace are not understood.

Ideally, the health professional team, nurse, physician, industrial hygienist, and/or safety officer will be proactive in the recognition and prevention of reproductive hazards. The mission of this team includes informing both management and labor of the nature of workplace hazards. Most convincing to these groups is objective information obtained from a literature review on a particular hazard or on health data collected through a surveillance program. Certainly, there is no reason to repeat the DBCP experience of failing to prevent a potential hazard that should have been suspected years earlier. Maintaining a health surveillance program for exposed workers is another baseline objective. Often, when there is an occupational surveillance program, it is offered only for perceived high-risk jobs. In some instances, however, the jobs that are thought intuitively to carry high risk are not as risky as others because of safety controls that have been put in place. Workers in other locations, such as in maintenance or laboratory, may have varied and hazardous exposures.

Some industries have undertaken pregnancy or fertility surveillance programs. These programs also may include education programs for women who are pregnant or may be planning a pregnancy. The March of Dimes is an excellent resource for educational materials, including brochures, videos, speakers, and generally high-quality teaching programs. All industries should have a maternity policy and provide new mothers assistance in returning to the workplace. There are work-hardening programs for injured employees, but generally no planned program for women who have undergone major physiologic and psychological changes after giving birth. Management and labor need to work closely to ensure that the workplace is a safe environment for men and women and their unborn children.

## REFERENCES


1. Whorton D, Krauss RM, Marshall S, et al. Infertility in male pesticide workers. *Lancet* 1977;2:1259–1261.
2. Bloom AD. *Guidelines for studies of human populations exposed to mutagenic and reproductive hazards.* White Plains, NY: March of Dimes Birth Defects Foundation, 1981.
3. Schrader SM, Kesner JS. Male reproductive toxicology. In: Paul M, ed. *Occupational and environmental reproductive hazards.* Baltimore, MD: Williams & Wilkins, 3–17.
4. Kharrazi M, Potashnik G, Goldsmith JR. Reproductive effects of dibromochloropropane. *Isr J Med Sci* 1980;16:403–406.
5. Lemasters GK, Selevan SG. Use of exposure data in occupational reproductive studies. *Scand J Work Environ Health* 1984;10:1–6.
6. Smyth HF. Industrial toxicology. In: Casarett LJ, Doull J, eds. *Toxicology:* the basic science of poisons. New York: Macmillan, 1975; 683–700.
7. Selevan SG. Methods for environmental quantitative risk assessment. Presented at the Symposium on Environmental Epidemiology, April, 1989, Pittsburgh, PA.
8. Whorton MD. Male occupational reproductive hazards. *West J Med* 1982;137:521–524.
9. Schrader SM, Ratcliffe JM, Turner TW, Hornung RW. The use of new field methods of semen analysis in the study of occupational hazards to reproduction: the example of ethylene dibromide. *J Occup Med* 1987;29:963–966.
10. Moruzzi JF, Wyrobek AJ, Moyall BH, Gledhill BL. Quantification and classification of human sperm morphology by computer-assisted image analysis. *Fertil Steril* 1988;50:142–152.
11. Boyers SP, Davis RO, Katz DF. Automated semen analysis. In: Barbieri RL, ed. *Current problems in obstetrics, gynecology and fertility.* Chicago: Year Book Medical Publishers, 1989;12:173–200.
12. Wyrobek AJ, Watchmaker G, Gordon L. An evaluation of sperm test as indicators of germ-cell damage in men exposed to chemical or physical agents. *Teratogenesis Carcinog Mutagen* 1984;4:83–107.
13. Jouannet P, Ducot B, Fenleux D, Spira A. Male factors and the likelihood of pregnancy in infertile couples. I. Study of sperm characteristics. *Int J Androl* 1988;11:379–394.
14. Grunert JH, deGeyter C, Bordt J, Schneider HPG, Nieschlag E. Does computerized image analysis of sperm movement enhance the predictive value of semen analysis for *in vitro* fertilization results? *Int J Androl* 1989;12:329–338.
15. Schrader SM, Turner TW, Breitenstein MJ, and Simon SD. Longitudinal study of semen quality of unexposed workers. I. Study overview. *Reprod Toxicol* 1988;2:183–190.
16. Hammen R. *Studies of impaired fertility in man with special reference to the male.* Copenhagen: Munksgaard and Milford, 1944.
17. Bostofte E, Serup J, Rebbe H. Hammen semen quality classification and pregnancies obtained during a 20-year follow-up period. *Fertil Steril* 1981;36:84–87.
18. Bostofte E, Serup J, Rebbe H. Relationship between sperm count and semen volume, and pregnancies obtained during a 20-year follow-up period. *Int J Androl* 1982;5:267–275.
19. Bostofte E, Serup J, Rebbe H. Relation between spermatozoa motility and pregnancies obtained during a 20-year follow-up period. Spermatozoa motility and fertility. *Andrologia* 1983;15:682–686.
20. Bostofte E, Serup J, Rebbe H. Relation between number of immobile, spermatozoa and pregnancies obtained during a 20-year follow-up period. Immobile spermatozoa on fertility. *Andrologia* 1984;16: 136–140.
21. Furuhjelm M, Jonson B, Lagergren CG. Quality of human semen in spontaneous abortion. *Int J Fertil* 1962;7:17–21.
22. Kneer M. The habitual aborter. *Dtsch Med Wochenschr* 1957;82: 1059–1061.
23. MacLeod J, Gold RZ. The male factor in fertility and infertility. *Fertil Steril* 1957;8:36–49.
24. Homonnai ZT, Paz GF, Weiss JN, David MP. Relation between semen quality and fate of pregnancy: retrospective study of 534 pregnancies. *Int J Androl* 1980;3:574–584.
25. Wyrobeck, AJ, Schrader SM, Perreault SD, et al. Assessment of reproductive disorders and birth defects in communities near hazardous chemical sites: No. 3 Guidelines for fields studies of male reproductive disorders. *Reprod Toxicol* 1997;11:243–259.
26. Schrader SM, Turner TW, Breitenstein MJ, et al. Measuring male reproductive hormones for occupational field studies. *J Occup Med* 1993;35(6):574–576.
27. Evans HJ, Fletcher J, Torrance M, Hargreave TB. Sperm abnormalities and cigarette smoking. *Lancet* 1981;1:627–629.
28. Wyrobek AJ, Gordon LA, Burkhart JG, et al. An evaluation of human sperm as indicators of chemically induced alterations of spermatogenic function. A report of the U.S. Environmental Protection Agency Gene-Tox Program. *Mutat Res* 1983;115:73–148.
29. Terracciano GJ, Lemasters GK, Amber RW. *Standardized assessment of birth defects and reproductive disorders in environmental health field studies.* HHS PB96-199609. Washington, DC: U.S. Department of Health and Human Services, 1996;79.
30. Levine RJ, Matthew RM, Chenault CB, et al. Differences in the quality of semen in indoor workers during summer and winter. *N Engl J Med* 1990;323:12–16.
31. Grajewski B. Participation rate and nonparticipant characterization. Presented at the EPA/NIOSH Workshop on Methods for Semen Studies in Humans, Alexandria, Va, October 18, 1989.
32. Selevan SG. *Evaluation of data sources for occupational pregnancy outcome studies* [Dissertation]. Cincinnati, OH: University of Cincinnati, 1980.
33. Mosher WD, Pratt WF. *Reproductive impairments among married couples,* United States. DHHS Publication PHS 83-1987. Hyattsville, MD: National Center for Health Statistics, 1982.
34. Baird DD, Wilcox AJ, Weinberg CR. Use of time to pregnancy to study environmental exposure. *Am J Epidemiol* 1986;124:470–480.
35. Lemasters GK, Zenick H, Hertzberg V, Hansen K, Clark S. Fertility of workers chronically exposed to chemically contaminated sewer wastes. *Reprod Toxicol* 1991;5:31–37.
36. Wong O, Utidjian HMD, Karten VS. Retrospective evaluation of reproductive performance of workers exposed to ethylene dibromide (EDB). *J Occup Med* 1979;21:98–102.
37. Levine RJ, Symons MJ, Balogh SA, Arndt DM, Kaswandik NT, Gentile JW. A method for monitoring the fertility of workers. I. Method and pilot studies. *J Occup Med* 1980;22:781–791.
38. Levine RJ, Symons MJ, Balogh SA, Milby TH, Whorton MD. A method for monitoring the fertility of workers. II. Validation of the method among workers exposed to dibromochloropropane. *J Occup Med* 1981;23:183–188.
39. Starr TB, Levine RJ. Assessing effects of occupational exposure on fertility with indirect standardization. *Am J Epidemiol* 1983;118: 897–904.
40. Marchbanks PA, Petersen HB, Rubin GL, Wingo PA, the Cancer and Steroid Hormone Study Group. Research on infertility: definition makes a difference. *Am J Epidemiol* 1989;130:259–267.
41. Schrader SM, Kanitz MH. Occupational hazards to male reproduction. *Occup Environ Med State Art Rev* 1994;9(3):405–414.
42. Lahdetie J. Occupation- and exposure-related studies on human sperm. *J Occup Environ Med* 1995;37(8):922–930.
43. Rom WN. Effects of lead on reproduction. In: Infante PF, Legator MS, eds. *Proceedings of a workshop on methodology for assessing repro-*

*ductive hazards in the work place.* Washington, DC: USGPO, 1980; 33–42.
44. Lancranjan I, Popescu HI, Gavanescu O, Klepsch I, Serbanescu M. Reproductive ability of workmen occupationally exposed to lead. *Arch Environ Health* 1975;30:396–401.
45. Assennato G, Paci C, Baser ME, et al. Sperm count suppression without endocrine dysfunction in lead-exposed men. *Arch Environ Health* 1987;42:124–127.
46. Amir D, Volcani R. Effects of dietary ethylene dibromide in bull semen. *Nature* 1965;206:99–100.
47. Amir D. The sites of spermicidal action of ethylene dibromide in bulls. *J Reprod Fertil* 1973;35:519–525.
48. Amir D. Individual and age differences in the spermicidal effect of ethylene dibromide in bulls. *J Reprod Fertil* 1975;44:561–565.
49. Amir D, Lavon U. Changes in total nitrogen, liproproteins, and amino acids in epididymal and ejaculated spermatozoa of bulls treated orally with ethylene dibromide. *J Reprod Fertil* 1976;47:73–76.
50. Amir D, Esnault C, Nicolle JC, Courot M. DNA and protein changes in the spermatozoa of bulls treated orally with ethylene dibromide. *J Reprod Fertil* 1977;51:453–456.
51. Chemical Manufacturers Association. Comments on OSHA's proposed rule making on occupational exposure to ethylene dibromide. OSHA Docket H-111, Exhibit 19-7. Cited in Dobbins JG. Regulation and the use of negative results from human reproductive studies: the case of ethylene dibromide. *Am J Ind Med* 1987;12:33–45.
52. Dobbins JG. Regulation and the use of negative results from human reproductive studies: the case of ethylene dibromide. *Am J Ind Med* 1987;12:33–45.
53. Millard SP. Proof of safety versus proof of hazard. *Biometrics* 1987;43:719–725.
54. Ratcliffe JM, Schrader SM, Meinhardt TJ, Steenland K, Clapp DE, Turner T. *Semen evaluation of timber fumigators exposed to ethylene dibromide.* NIOSH report TA 83-244. Cincinnati, OH: NIOSH, 1984.
55. Ratcliffe JM, Schrader SM, Steenland K, Clapp DE, Turner T, Hornung RW. Semen quality in papaya workers with long-term exposure to ethylene dibromide. *Br J Ind Med* 1987;44:317–326.
56. Schrader SM, Turner TW, Ratcliffe JM. The effects of ethylene dibromide on semen quality: a comparison of short-term and chronic exposure. *Reprod Toxicol* 1988;2:191–198.
57. Steenland K, Carrano A, Ratcliffe J, Clapp D, Ashworth L, Meinhardt TJ. A cytogenetic study of papaya workers exposed to ethylene dibromide. *Mutat Res* 1986;170:151–160.
58. Rasmussen K, Sabroe S, Wohlert M, Ingerslev HJ, Kappel B, Nielsen J. A genotoxic study of metal workers exposed to trichloroethylene, sperm parameters, and chromosome aberrations in lymphocytes. *Int Arch Occup Environ Health* 1988;60:419–423.
59. Martin RH, Balkan W, Burns K, Rademaker AW, Lin CC, Rudd NL. The chromosome constitution of 1000 human spermatozoa. *Hum Genet* 1983;63:305–309.
60. Brandiff B, Gordon L, Ashworth L, et al. Chromosomes of human sperm: viability among normal individuals. *Hum Genet* 1985;70:18–24.
61. Evenson D, Jost L, Baer R, Turner T, Schrader S. Longitudinal study of sperm chromatin structure of 45 men. *J Androl* 1990;57:35(abstr).
62. Martin RH, Hildebrand K, Yamamoto J, et al. An increased frequency of human sperm chromosomal abnormalities after radiotherapy. *Mutat Res* 1986;174:219–225.
63. Association of Schools of Public Health. *Proposed national strategy for the prevention of leading work related diseases and injury. Part II. Disorders of reproduction.* Washington, DC: National Institute of Mental Health, 1988;1–29.
64. Environmental Protection Agency proposed guidelines for assessing male reproductive risk and request for comments. Part III. *Federal Register* 1988(June 30).
65. Cohen EN, Brown BW, Bruce DL, et al. A survey of anesthetic health hazards among dentists. *J Am Dent Assoc* 1975;90:1291–1296.
66. Wyrobek AJ, Brodsky J, Gordon L, Moore DH, Watchmaker G, Cohen EN. Sperm studies in anesthesiologists. *Anesthesiology* 1981;55:527–532.
67. Gardner MJ, Snee MP, Hall AJ, Powell CA, Downes S, Terrell JD. Results of case-control study of leukemia and lymphoma among young people near Sellafield nuclear plant in West Cumbria. *Br Med J* 1990;30:423–429.
68. Beral V. Leukemia and nuclear installations. *Br Med J* 1990;30:411–412.
69. Riley PA. Leukemia and lymphoma among young people near Sellafield. *Br Med J* 1990;300:676.
70. Shea KM, Little RE, and The ALSPAC Study Team. Is there an association between preconception, paternal x-ray exposure and birth outcome? *Am J Epidemiol* 1997;145(6):546–551.
71. Sœdireund EJ, Brunborg G, Holme JN, Hongses JK, Neeson SD, Dybing E. Cocullate systems for assessing the stability and genotoxicity of reasete DBCT metabolites. *Mutagenesis* 1991;6:25–30.
72. Ratcliffe JM, Schrader SM, Clapp DE, Halperin WE, Turner TW, Hornung RW. Semen quality in workers exposed to 2-ethoxyethanol. *Br J Ind Med* 1989;46:399–406.
73. Welch LS, Schrader SM, Turner TW, Cullen MR. Effects of exposure to ethylene glycol ethers on shipyard painters: II. Male reproduction. *Am J Ind Med* 1988;14:509–526.
74. Lemasters GK, Pinney SM. Employment status as a confounder when affecting occupational exposures and spontaneous abortion. *J Clin Epidemiol* 1989;42:975–981.
75. Eskenazi B, Wyrobek AJ, Fenster L, et al. I. A study of the effects of perchloroethylene exposure on semen quality in dry cleaning workers. *Am J Ind Med* 1991;20:575–591.
76. Morck HI, Winkel P, Gyntelberg F. Health effects of toluene exposure. *Dan Med Bull* 1988;35:196–200.
77. Levine RJ, Blunden PB, DalCorso DR, Starr TB, Ross CE. Superiority of reproductive histories to sperm counts in detecting infertility at a dibromochloropropane manufacturing plant. *J Occup Med* 1983;25:591–597.
78. Schenker MB, Samuels SJ, Perkins C, Lewis EL, Katz DF, Overstreet JW. Prospective surveillance of semen quality in the work place. *J Occup Med* 1988;30:336–344.
79. Townsend JC, Bodner KM, Van Peenen PFD, Olson RD, Cook RR. Survey of reproductive events of wives of employees exposed to chlorinated dioxins. *Am J Epidemiol* 1982;115:695–713.
80. Centers for Disease Control. Health status of Vietnam veterans. II. Physical health. *JAMA* 1988;259:2708–2714.
81. Hatch MC, Stein ZA. Agent orange and risk to reproduction: the limits of epidemiology. *Teratogenesis Carcinog Mutagen* 1986;6:185–202.
82. DeStefano F, Annest JL, Kresnow M, Schrader SM, Katz D. Semen characteristics of Vietnam veterans. *Reprod Toxicol* 1989;3:165–173.
83. Savitz DA, Harley B, Krekel S, Marshall J, Bondy J, Orleans M. Survey of reproductive hazards among oil, chemical and atomic workers exposed to halogenated hydrocarbons. *Am J Ind Med* 1984;6:253–264.
84. McDonald AD, McDonald JC, Armstrong B, Cherry NM, Nolin AD, Robert D. Fathers' occupation and pregnancy outcome. *Br J Ind Med* 1989;46:329–333.
85. Taskinen H, Anttila A, Lindbohm ML, Sallmen M, Hemminki K. Spontaneous abortions and congenital malformations among the wives of men occupationally exposed to organic solvents. *Scand J Work Environ Health* 1989;15:345–352.
86. Morgan R, Kheifets L, Obrinsky D, Whorton M, Foliart D. Fetal loss and work in a wastewater treatment plant. *Am J Public Health* 1984;74:499–501.
87. Goldsmith JR, Burack J. Two comments on fetal loss and wastewater workers. I. Maternal age a factor. *Am J Public Health* 1985;75:98.
88. Rosenberg MJ, Wyrobeck AJ. Two comments on fetal loss in wastewater workers. I. Recall bias in interpretation. *Am J Public Health* 1985;75:98.
89. Rosenberg M, Wyrobeck A, Ratcliffe J, et al. Sperm as an indicator of reproductive risk among petroleum refinery workers. *Br J Ind Med* 1985;42:123–127.
90. Lemasters G, Hansen K, Hertzberg V, Zenick H, Meyer C, Clark S. A fertility evaluation of workers exposed to industrial wastes. *Am J Epidemiol* 1988;128:924.
91. Hertzberg VS, Lemasters GK, Hansen K, Zenick H. Statistical issues in risk assessment of reproductive outcomes with chemical mixtures. *Environ Health Perspect* 1991;90:171–175.
92. Rachootin P, Olsen J. The risk of infertility and delayed conception associated with exposures in the Danish workplace. *J Occup Med* 1983;25:394–402.
93. Morse PA, Molfese D, Laughlin NK. Categorical perception for voicing contrasts in normal and lead-treated Rhesus monkeys: electrophysiological indices. *Brain Lang* 1987;30:63–80.
94. Mattison DR. *Reproductive toxicology.* New York: Alan R. Liss, 1983.

95. Wilcox AJ, Weinberg CR, O'Connor JF, et al. Incidence of early loss of pregnancy. *N Engl J Med* 1988;319:189–194.
96. McFarland KF. Amenorrhea. *Am Fam Physician* 1980;22:95–101.
97. Chiazze L, Brayer FT, Macisco JJ, Parker MP, Duffy BJ. The length and variability of the human menstrual cycle. *JAMA* 1968;203: 377–380.
98. Goldsmith L, Weiss G. Puberty, adolescence and the clinical aspects of normal menstruation. In: Danforth DN, Scott J, eds. *Obstetrics and gynecology.* Philadelphia: JB Lippincott, 1986.
99. Fogel C, Woods N. *Health care of women.* St. Louis: CV Mosby; 1981.
100. Whelen EA, Sandler DP, McConnaughey R, Weinberg CR. Menstrual and reproductive characteristics and age at natural menopause. *Am J Epidemiol* 1990;131:625–632.
101. Tyler S, Woodall G. *Female health and gynecology:* across the life span. Bowie, MD: Brady, 1982.
102. Shortridge LA. Assessment of menstrual variability in working populations. *Reprod Toxicol* 1988;2:171–176.
103. DeGowen EL, DeGowen RL. *Bedside diagnostic examination.* New York: Macmillan, 1976;603–604.
104. Romney S, Gray M, Little A, Merrill J, Quilligan E, Stander R. *Gynecology and obstetrics, the health care of women.* New York: McGraw-Hill, 1975.
105. Hibbard L, Judd H, Lamb E, Nelson R, Ulene A. *The menstrual history.* Atlanta: National Medical Audiovisual Center, 1973 [revised 1977).
106. Lemasters GK, Hagen A, Samuels SJ. Reproductive outcomes in women exposed to solvents in 36 reinforced plastics companies. I. Menstrual dysfunction. *J Occup Med* 1985;27:490–494.
107. Wood C, Larsen L, Williams R. Social and psychological factors in relation to premenstrual tension and menstrual pain. *Aust NZ J Obstet Gynaecol* 1979;19:111–115.
108. Little AB. Gynecologic endocrine disorders. In: Danforth DN, ed. *Obstetrics and gynecology,* 3rd ed. Hagerstown, MD: Harper & Row, 1977;792–811.
109. Baker ER. Menstrual dysfunction and hormonal status in athletic women: a review. *Fertil Steril* 1981;36:691–696.
110. Pettersson F, Fries H, Nillius SJ. Epidemiology of secondary amenorrhea. I. Incidence and prevalence rates. *Am J Obstet Gynecol* 1973;117:80–86.
111. Morley JE, Distiller LA, Epstein S, et al. Menstrual disturbances in chronic renal failure. *Horm Metab Res* 1979;11:68–72.
112. Singh KB. Menstrual disorders in college students. *Am J Obstet Gynecol* 1981;140:299–302.
113. Dawood MY. *Dysmenorrhea.* Baltimore: Williams & Wilkins, 1981; 157–159.
114. Klein SM, Garcia CR. Asherman's syndrome: a critique and current review. *Fertil Steril* 1973;24:722–735.
115. Buytaert PH, Viaene P. Laparoscopic tubal sterilization: postoperative follow-up and late gynecological complaints. *Eur J Obstet Gynecol Reprod Biol* 1980;10:119–124.
116. Fries H, Nillius SJ, Pettersson F. Epidemiology of secondary amenorrhea. II. A retrospective evaluation of etiology with special regard to psychogenic factors and weight loss. *Am J Obstet Gynecol* 1974;118:473–479.
117. Skandhan KP, Pandya AK, Skandhan S, Mehta YB. Academic examination stress versus menstrual cycle. *Panminerva Med* 1981;23: 47–49.
118. Pepitone-Arreola-Rockwell F, Sommer B, Sassenrath EN, Rozee-Koker P, Stringer-Moore D. Job stress and health in working women. *J Hum Stress* 1981;19–26.
119. Ryback RS. Chronic alcohol consumption and menstruation. *JAMA* 1977;238:2143.
120. Griesemer RA, Ulsamer AG, Arcos JC, et al. Report of the federal panel on formaldehyde. *Environ Health Perspect* 1982;43:139–168.
121. Beskrovnaja NJ. Gynecological morbidity in women workers in the rubber industry [translation]. *Gig Tr Prof Zabol* 1979;8:36–38.
122. Michon S. Connection between aromatic hydrocarbons and menstrual disorders analyzed [translation]. *Pol Tyg Lek* 1965;20:1648–1649.
123. Butarewicz L, Gosk S, Gluszczopma M. Examination of the health of female workers in the leather industry, especially from the gynecological viewpoint. *Med Pr* 1969;20:137–140.
124. Syrovadko ON, Skormin VF, Pron'kova EN. Effect of working conditions on the health and some specific functions in female workers exposed to white spirit [translation]. *Gig Tr Prof Zabol* 1973;16:5–8.
125. Zlobina NS, Izyumora AS, Ragulie NY. The effect of low styrene concentrations on the specific functions of the female organism. *Gig Tr Prof Zabol* 1975;18:21–25.
126. Zielhuis GA, Gijsen R, van der Gulden JWJ. Menstrual disorders among dry cleaning workers. *Scand J Work Environ Health* 1989;15:238.
127. Panova Z. Menstrual and reproductive functions and gynaecological morbidity in women occupationally exposed to petrol [translation]. *Letopisi Na Higienno-Epidemiologicnata Sluzba* 1976;20:;RO53–56.
128. Gesher G. *Changes in the menstrual cycle of women occupationally exposed to trinitrotoluene* [translation]. *Parva Nacionalna Koferenciza Na Aspirantite.* Sofia: Medicina I Fizkultura, 1967(April); 159–262.
129. Harrington JM, Stein GF, Rivera RO, deMorales AV. The occupational hazards of formulating oral contraceptives–a survey of plant employees. *Arch Environ Health* 1978;33:12–15.
130. Christensen CJ. *Characterization of exposure to antineoplastic agents and report of symptoms and menstrual function of hospital-based female pharmacists* [Dissertation]. Cincinnati: University of Cincinnati, 1988.
131. Lotis VM, Solovieva IP, Tartakovskya LY. The effect of general vibrations on the female sexual apparatus. *Vopr Okhrany Materinstva Detstva* 1962;10:62–66.
132. Tasto KL, Colligan MJ, Skjei EW, Polly SJ. *Health consequences of shift work.* DHEW [NIOSH) publication 78-154. Washington, DC: USGPO, 1978.
133. Uehata T, Sasakawa N. The fatigue and maternity disturbances of night work on women. *J Hum Ergol* 1982;suppl II:465–474.
134. Kuchinski BB. *The effect of shift work on the menstrual characteristics of nurses* [Dissertation]. Baltimore: Johns Hopkins University, 1989.
135. Iglesias R, Terres A, Chavarria A. Disorders of the menstrual cycle in airline stewardesses. *Aviat Space Environ Med* 1980;51:518–520.
136. Prill HJ, Maar H. Changes in the menstrual cycle caused by altitude. *Med Klin* 1971;66:986–989.
137. Cameron RG. Effect of flying on the menstrual function of air hostesses. *Clin Aviat Aerospace Med* 1969;40:1020–1023.
138. Bromberger JT, Matthews KA, Kuller LH, Wing RR, Meilahn EN, Plantinga P. Prospective study of the determinants of age at menopause. *Am J Epidemiol* 1997;145:124–133.
139. Scialli AR, Swann SH, Amler RW, et al. Assessment of reproductive disorders and birth defects in communities near hazardous chemical sites. II. Female reproductive disorders. *Reprod Toxicol* 1997;11(2/3): 231–242.
140. Matsumoto S, Nogami Y, Ohkuri S. Statistical studies on menstruation: a criticism on the definition of normal menstruation. *Gunma J Med Sci* 1962;11:294–318.
141. Bean JA, Leeper JD, Wallace RB, Sherman BM, Jagger H. Variations in the reporting of menstrual histories. *Am J Epidemiol* 1979;109: 181–185.
142. U.S. Department of Commerce, Bureau of the Census. *Statistical abstract of the United States, 1990,* 110th ed. Washington, DC: U.S. Government Printing Office, 1990;384.
143. Wilson JG. *Environment and birth defects.* New York: Academic Press, 1973.
144. Chang MC. Effects of certain antifertility agents on the development of rabbit ova. *Fertil Steril* 1964;15:97–106.
145. Lutwak-Mann C, Hay MF. Effect on the early embryo of agents administered to the mother. *Br Med J* 1962;2:944.
146. McLachlan JA, Dames NM, Fabro S. Abnormal protein profile in rabbit embryos after maternal exposure to some common environmental chemicals. *Fed Proc* 1970;29:348.
147. Hendrickx AG. Disorders of fertilization, transport, and implantation. In: Lockey J, Lemasters GK, Keye WR, eds. *Reproduction:* the new frontier in occupational and environmental health research. New York: Alan R. Liss, 1984;211–227.
148. Goodwin J, Godden J, Chance G. *Perinatal medicine.* Baltimore: Williams & Wilkins, 1976.
149. Kurzel RB, Cetrulo CL. The effect of environmental pollutants on human reproduction including birth defects. *Environ Sci Technol* 1981;15:626–639.
150. WHO. Recommended definitions, terminology and format for statistical tables related to the perinatal period and use of a new certificate for cause of perinatal deaths. *Acta Obstet Gynaecol Scand* 1977; 56:247–253.

151. Källén B. *Epidemiology of human reproduction.* Boca Raton, FL: CRC Press, 1988.
152. Kline J, Stein Z, Susser M. Conception to birth–epidemiology of prenatal development. Monograph. In: MacMahon B, ed. *Epidemiology and Biostatistics,* vol 14. New York: Oxford University Press, 1989.
153. Miller JF, Williamson E, Glue J, Gordon YB, Grudzinhas JG, Sykes A. Fetal loss after implantation. *Lancet* 1980;2:554–556.
154. Edmonds DK, Lindsay KS, Miller JF, Williamson E, Wood PJ. Early embryonic mortality in women. *Fertil Steril* 1982;38:447–453.
155. Whittaker PG, Taylor A, Lind T. Unsuspected pregnancy loss in healthy women. *Lancet* 1983;1:1126–1127.
156. Leridon H. *Human fertility:* the basic components. Chicago: University of Chicago Press, 1977.
157. Schlesselman JJ. How does one assess the risk of abnormalities from human *in vitro* infertilization? *Am J Obstet Gynecol* 1979;135: 135–148.
158. Jones, Jr. HW, Acosta AA, Andrews MC, et al. What is a pregnancy? A question for programs of *in vitro* fertilization. *Fertil Steril* 1983; 40:728–733.
159. Little AB. There's many a slip 'twixt implantation and the crib. *N Engl J Med* 1988;319:241–242.
160. Hertz-Picciotto I, Samuels SJ. The incidence of early loss of pregnancy. *N Engl J Med* 1988;319:1483–1484.
161. Wilcox AJ, Horney LF. Accuracy of spontaneous abortion recall. *Am J Epidemiol* 1984;120:727–733.
162. Olson JE, Shu XO, Ross JA, Pendergrass T and Robison LL. Medical record validation of maternally reported birth characteristics and pregnancy-related events: a report from the Children's Cancer Group. *Am J Epidemiol* 1997;145:58-67.
163. Axelsson G, Rylander R. Validation of questionnaire reported miscarriage, malformation and birth weight. *Int J Epidemiol* 1984;13:94–98.
164. Risch HA, Weiss NS, Clarke EA, Miller AB. Risk factors for spontaneous abortion and its recurrence. *Am J Epidemiol* 1988;128: 420–430.
165. Hassold T, Quillen SD, Yamane JA. Sex ratio in spontaneous abortions. *Ann Hum Genet* 1983;47:39–47.
166. Marbury MC, Linn S, Monson R, et al. Work and pregnancy. *J Occup Med* 1984;26:415.
167. Joffe M. Biases in research on reproduction and women's work. *Int J Epidemiol* 1985;14:118–123.
168. Murphy JF, Dauncey M, Newcombe R, Garcia J, Elbourne D. Employment in pregnancy: prevalence, maternal characteristics, perinatal outcome. *Lancet* 1984;1:1163–1166.
169. Savitz DA, Whelan EA, Rowland AS, Klackner RC. Maternal employment and reproductive risk factors. *Am J Epidemiol* 1990; 132:933–945.
170. Warkany J. *Congenital malformations:* notes and comments. Chicago: Year Book, 1971.
171. Schardein JL. *Drugs as teratogens.* Cleveland: CRC Press, 1976.
172. Wilson JT, Fraser FC. *Handbook of teratology. mechanisms and pathogenesis.* New York: Plenum Press, 1976.
173. Miller JR, Poland BJ. The value of human abortuses in the surveillance of developmental anomalies: general overview. *Can Med Assoc J* 1970;103:501–502.
174. Nelson MM, Forfar JO. Congenital abnormalities at birth: their association in the same birth. *Dev Med Child Neurol* 1969;11:3–10.
175. Neel JV. A study of major congenital defects in Japanese infants. *Am J Hum Genet* 1958;10:398.
176. Bierman JM, Siegel E, French FE, Simonian K. Analysis of the outcome of all pregnancies in a community. *Am J Obstet Gynecol* 1965; 91:37–45.
177. Nelson K, Holmes LB. Malformations due to presumed spontaneous mutations in newborn infants. *N Engl J Med* 1989;320:19–23.
178. Ekelund H, Kullawder S, Källén B. Major and minor malformations in newborns and infants up to one year of age. *Acta Paediatr Scand* 1970;59:297.
179. Lilenfeld AM. Population differences in frequency of malformations at birth. In: Fraser FC, McKwick VA, Robinson R, eds. *Congenital malformations.* New York: Excerpta Medica, 1970.
180. Congenital anomalies and birth injuries among live births. In: *United States Vital and Health Statistics,* 1978. PHS Series 21 Publication 79-1909. Washington, DC: US DHEW. 1979.
181. Centers for Disease Control. *Congenital malformations surveillance.* Atlanta: CDC, 1988;11–18.
182. Bakir F, Damluji SF, Amin-Zaki L, et al. Methylmercury poisoning in Iraq. *Science* 1973;181:230–241.
183. Amin-Zaki L, Elhassani S, Majeed MA, Clarkson TW, Doherty RA, Greenwood M. Intrauterine methylmercury poisoning in Iraq. *Pediatrics* 1974;54:587–595.
184. Kuratsune M, Yoshimura T, Matsuzaka J, et al. Epidemiologic study of Yusho, a poisoning caused by ingestion of rice oil contaminated with a commercial brand of polychlorinated biphenyls. *Environ Health Perspect* 1972;1:119–128.
185. O'Shaughnessy RW. Uterine blood flow and fetal growth. In: Van Assche FA, Robertson WB, eds. *Fetal growth retardation.* New York: Churchill Livingstone, 1981;101–116.
186. *WHO report on the second session of the Expert Committee on Health Statistics.* Geneva: World Health Organization, 1950.
187. *Manual of the International Statistical Classification of Diseases, Injuries, and Causes of Death,* 6th revision. Geneva: World Health Organization, 1957.
188. *Public health aspects of low birth weight.* Third report of the Expert Committee on Maternal and Child Health. Geneva: World Health Organization, 1961.
189. Keirse MJNC. Epidemiology of preterm labour. In: Keirse MJNC, Anderson ABM, Gravenhorst JB, eds. *Human parturition.* Leiden: Leiden University Press, 1979;219–234.
190. *Prevention of perinatal morbidity and mortality.* Geneva: World Health Organization, 1969.
191. Villar J, Belizan JM. The relative contribution of prematurity and fetal growth retardation to low birth weight in developing and developed societies. *Am J Obstet Gynecol* 1982;143:793–798.
192. Fedrick J, Adelstein P. Factors associated with low birth weight of infants delivered at term. *Br J Obstet Gynaecol* 1978;85:1–7.
193. Kaltreider DF, Kohl S. Epidemiology of preterm delivery. *Clin Obstet Gynecol* 1980;23:17–31.
194. Tamby Raja RL, Anderson ABM, Turnbull AC. Endocrine changes in premature labour. *Br Med J* 1974;4:67–75.
195. Johnson JWC, Dubin NH. Prevention of preterm labor. *Clin Obstet Gynecol* 1980;23:51–73.
196. Vasicka A, Kumaresan P, Han GS, Kumaresan M. Plasma oxytocin in initiation of labor. *Am J Obstet Gynecol* 1978;130:263–273.
197. Buncher CR. Cigarette smoking and duration of pregnancy. *Am J Obstet Gynecol* 1969;46:38–52.
198. Berkowitz GS. An epidemiologic study of preterm delivery. *Am J Epidemiol* 1981;113:81–92.
199. Fedrick J, Anderson ABM. Factors associated with spontaneous preterm birth. *Br J Obstet Gynaecol* 1976;83:342–350.
200. Simpson WJ. A preliminary report on cigarette smoking and the incidence of prematurity. *Am J Obstet Gynecol* 1957;73:808–815.
201. Yerushalmy J. Mother's cigarette smoking and survival of infant. *Am J Obstet Gynecol* 1964;88:505–518.
202. Yerushalmy J. The relationship of parents' cigarette smoking to outcome of pregnancy–implications as to the problems of inferring causation from observed association. *Am J Epidemiol* 1971;93: 443–456.
203. Yerushalmy J. Infants with low birth weight born before their mothers started to smoke cigarettes. *Am J Obstet Gynecol* 1972;112:227–284.
204. Comstock GW, Lundin FE. Parental smoking and perinatal mortality. *Am J Obstet Gynecol* 1967;98:708–718.
205. Comstock GW, Shah FK, Meyer MB, Abbey H. Low birth weight and neonatal mortality rate related to maternal smoking and socioeconomic status. *Am J Obstet Gynecol* 1971;111:53–59.
206. Rush D, Kass EM. Maternal smoking: a reassessment of the association with perinatal mortality. *Am J Epidemiol* 1972;96:183–196.
207. Murphy JF, Drumm JE, Mulcahy R. The effect of maternal cigarette smoking on fetal birth weight and on growth of the fetal biparietal diameter. *Br J Obstet Gynaecol* 1980;87:462–466.
208. Mulcahy R, Murphy JF, Martin F. Placental changes and maternal weight in smoking and non-smoking mothers. *Am J Obstet Gynecol* 1970;106:703–704.
209. Longo LD. The biological effects of carbon monoxide on the pregnant woman, fetus, and newborn infant. *Am J Obstet Gynecol* 1977; 129:69–103.
210. Suzuki K, Horiguchi T, Comas-Urrutia AC, Mueller-Heubach E, Morishima H, Adamsons K. Placental transfer and distribution of nicotine in the pregnant Rhesus monkey. *Am J Obstet Gynecol* 1974;119: 253–256.
211. Cole TV, Hawkins LH, Roberts D. Smoking during pregnancy and its

effect on the fetus. *J Obstet Gynaecol Br Commonwealth* 1972;79: 782–785.
212. Asmussen I, Kjeldsen K. Intimal ultrastructure of human umbilical arteries. Observations on arteries from newborn children of smoking and nonsmoking mothers. *Circ Res* 1975;36:579–589.
213. Pirani BBK. Smoking during pregnancy. *Obstet Gynecol Surv* 1978; 33:1–13.
214. Butler NR, Goldstein H, Ross EM. Cigarette smoking in pregnancy: its influence on birth weight and perinatal mortality. *Br Med J* 1972; 2:127–130.
215. Ulleland CN. The offspring of alcoholic mothers. *Ann NY Acad Sci* 1972;197:167–169.
216. Kaminski M, Rumeau C, Schwartz D. Alcohol consumption in pregnant women and the outcome of pregnancy. *Alcohol Clin Exp Res* 1978;2:155–163.
217. O'Leary JA, Davies JE, Edmundsen W, Feldman M. Correlation of prematurity and DDE levels in fetal whole blood. In: Davies JF, Edmundsen WF, eds. *Epidemiology of DDT.* New York: Futura, 1972; 55–56.
218. Balland C. Gazette Hebdomadaire de Medecine et de Chirurgie. 1896;1141. Cited in Lund C. The effect of chronic lead poisoning on reproductive capacity. *Nord Hyg Tidsskrift* 1936;18:12–20.
219. Lund C. The effect of chronic lead poisoning on reproductive capacity. *Nord Hyg Tidsskrift* 1936;18:12–20.
220. Fahim MS, Fahim Z, Hale DG. Effects of subtoxic lead levels on pregnant women in the state of Missouri. *Res Commun Chem Pathol Pharmacol* 1976;13:309–331.
221. Samuels SJ, Lemasters GK. A statistical problem in relating exposures during pregnancy and length of gestation. *Am J Epidemiol* 1983;118: 435.
222. Lemasters GK, Samuels SJ, Morrison JE, Brooks SM. Reproductive outcomes in pregnant workers employed at 36 reinforced plastics companies. II. Lowered birth weight. *J Occup Med* 1989;31:115–120.
223. Samuels SJ. The statistics of reproductive research. In: *Reproduction:* the new frontier in occupational and environmental health research. New York: Alan R. Liss, 1984.
224. Barlow SM, Sullivan FM. *Reproductive harzards of industrial chemicals.* New York: Academic Press, 1982.
225. Eskenazi B, Brody D, Maurer K. *Reproductive hazards of chemical exposures in the work place.* Washington, DC: Office of Technology Assessment, Congress of the United States, 1984.
226. Rosenberg MJ, Feldblum PJ, Marshall EG. Occupational influences on reproduction: a review of recent literature. *J Occup Med* 1987;29: 584–591.
227. American Society of Anesthesiologists. Occupational disease among operating room personnel. *Anesthesiology* 1974;41:321–340.
228. Pharoah POD, Doyle P, Alberman E. Outcome of pregnancy among women in anaesthetic practice. *Lancet* 1977;1:34–36.
229. Schenker MB, Samuels SJ, Green RS, Wiggins P. Adverse reproductive outcomes among female veterinarians. *Am J Epidemiol* 1990;132: 96–106.
230. Yodaiken RE, Bennett D, eds. OSHA work-practice guidelines for personnel dealing with cytotoxic drugs. *Am J Hosp Pharm* 1986;43: 1193–1204.
231. Christensen CJ, Lemasters GK, Wakeman MJA. Work practices and policies of hospital pharmacists preparing antineoplastic agents. *J Occup Med* 1990;32:508–512.
232. Averette HE, Borke GM, Jarrell MA. Effects of cancer chemotherapy on gonadal function and reproductive capacity. *CA* 1990;40:199–209.
233. Waksvik H, Klepp O, Brogger A. Chromosome analysis of nurses handling cytosatic agents. *Cancer Treat Rep* 1981;65:607–610.
234. Valanis B, Shortridge L, Hertzberg V. Health hazards associated with work exposure to antineoplastic drugs. *Am J Epidemiol* 1984;120:494.
235. Selevan S, Lindbohm M, Hornung RW, Hemminki K. A study of occupational exposure to antineoplastic drugs and fetal loss in nurses. *N Engl J Med* 1985;313:1173–1178.
236. Hemminki K, Kyyronen P, Lindbohm M. Spontaneous abortions and malformations in the offspring of nurses exposed to anesthetic gases, cytostatic drugs, and other potential hazards in hospitals based on registered information of outcome. *J Epidemiol Community Health* 1985; 39:141–147.
237. Meirik O, Källén B, Gauffin U, Ericson A. Major malformations in infants born of women who worked in laboratories while pregnant. *Lancet* 1979;2:91.
238. Blomqvist U, Ericson A, Källén B, Westerholm P. Delivery outcome for women working in the pulp and paper industry. *Scand J Work Environ Health* 1981;7:114–118.
239. Hemminki K, Franssila E, Vainio H. Spontaneous abortion among female chemical workers in Finland. *Int Arch Occup Environ Health* 1980;45:123–126.
240. Pastides H, Calabrese EJ, Hosmer DW, Harris DR. Spontaneous abortion and general illness symptoms among semiconductor manufacturers. *J Occup Med* 1988;30:543–551.
241. Huel G, Mergles D, Bowles R. Evidence for adverse reproductive outcomes among women microelectronic assembly workers. *Br J Ind Med* 1990;47:400–404.
242. Pinney SM and Lemasters GK. Spontaneous abortions and stillbirths in semiconductor employees. *Occup Hyg* 1996;2:387–401.
243. Gray RH, Corn M, Cohen R, et al. *Final report:* The Johns Hopkins University retrospective and prospective studies of reproductive health among IMB employees in semiconductor manufacturing. Baltimore, MD: Johns Hopkins University, 1993.
244. Swan SH, Beaumont JJ, Hammond SK, et al. Historical cohort study of spontaneous abortion among fabrication workers in the semiconductor health study: agent-level analysis. *Am J Ind Med* 1995;28(6):751–769.
245. NIOSH. *The effects of work place hazards on male reproductive health.* 549-180/40015, Publ. No. 96-132. Washington, DC: U.S. Government Printing Office: 1996.

*Environmental and Occupational Medicine,*
*Third Edition,* edited by William N. Rom.
Lippincott–Raven Publishers, Philadelphia © 1998.

CHAPTER 19

# Particle Deposition and Pulmonary Defense Mechanisms

Morton Lippmann

Living organisms must maintain their unique internal biochemical makeup while extracting the substances necessary for survival from a complex, often hazardous external environment. Within the respiratory tract, an elaborate multistaged defense system has evolved to cope with the extraneous substances inevitably taken in along with the required oxygen. Because humans can survive only minutes without oxygen, there is almost continuous intake of air and exposure to the contaminant gases and particles it contains. The average adult male inhales 15 kg of air each day, while he consumes only 1.5 kg of food and 2.0 kg of water; very little selectivity can be exercised over the materials inhaled, compared with the control one has over what is ingested.

Inhaled particles can accumulate at or near their initial deposition sites within lung airways or at other sites along translocation pathways. Particle movement along translocation pathways depends on factors such as the specific deposition site's location in relation to major clearance pathways; the amounts deposited; the nature and depth of surface fluids at the deposition site; the stimulatory or inhibiting effects of the particles on surface fluids, phagocytic cells, and secretory cells and glands; and the presence of preexisting abnormalities contributing to altered particle transport. Unfortunately, our knowledge of the nature and extent of the influence of these critical factors, and perhaps others of comparable influence, remains limited. The nature of the information that is needed for the kinds of analytical dosimetry and pathophysiology that can facilitate a fuller understanding of the mechanisms leading to some chronic lung diseases and the options available for disease prevention are discussed at the end of this chapter.

Depending on where they are deposited, inhaled particles can remain for long periods. They can slowly release toxic substances, and microbial particles can proliferate until irreversible tissue damage has occurred or serious disease has developed. Moreover, the large surface area of the parenchyma (about 70 $m^2$ in an adult male) and short diffusing length necessary for rapid gas exchange between the alveoli and the blood in the surrounding capillaries allow for only a very thin tissue barrier (as little as 0.2 μm) to the entry of microbes and toxic substances into the blood. Because they collect in high local concentrations, the effects from toxic particles can be greater than those from acute exposure to toxic gases, which are often more rapidly dispersed in respiratory tract fluids and diluted by the continuous exchange of air.

## OVERVIEW

The respiratory system's defenses against inhalable particles can be grouped into three lines of defense successively encountered by particles that enter the airways.

The first line of defense for the sensitive deep-lung airways is the progressive mechanical filtration of inspired air through the upper respiratory tract airways: nose, nasopharynx, pharynx, and larynx (during mouth breathing: mouth, oropharynx, and larynx) and the conducting airways of the lower respiratory tract, i.e., the tracheobronchial tree. The deposition of particles along the air passages reduces their penetration into the more vulnera-

M. Lippmann: Department of Environmental Medicine, New York University Medical Center, Tuxedo, New York 10987.

ble gas-exchanging structures—the respiratory bronchioles, alveolar ducts, and alveoli in the periphery of the lung. Receptors in the airways can initiate constriction of bronchial smooth muscle in response to mechanical or chemical irritation, further decreasing the penetration of particles and noxious gases and, in extreme cases, triggering a sneeze or cough, which can actually expel foreign substances from the upper airways or large bronchi of the tracheobronchial tree.

The second line of defense is provided by the fluids that line the airways and gas-exchange structures, and by the clearance mechanisms that physically remove particles from their surfaces. The respiratory tract fluids constitute a physical barrier to the contact of particles on airway surfaces with the bronchial and alveolar epithelia; these fluids may also represent a chemical buffer when they contain substances that give them detoxifying and bactericidal capabilities. In addition, the secretions that coat the ciliated epithelia of the conducting air passages of the upper and lower airways form the viscoelastic fluid. The cilia beat within the less viscous sol layer, propelling particles remaining on the more viscous gel layer along a mucociliary "escalator" to the larynx, where they are swallowed and eliminated via the gastrointestinal tract. In the periphery of the lung, the slow but continuous exudation of fluid and its drainage via the airways and the lymphatic system cleanse the respiratory bronchioles and the alveoli. Finally, resident alveolar macrophages scavenge particles from the surfaces of the alveoli, digesting them and/or removing them via the mucociliary escalator.

The specific immune defenses of the lung, which are brought into play against biochemically active particles that are deposited in the lung, are the last line of defense. These defenses are divided into two major effector systems—antibody production (humoral immunity) and lymphocyte-mediated antigen elimination.

These lines of defense are interdependent and coordinated as well. The aerodynamic size of the particles, the geometry of the airways, and the depth and pattern of respiration determines the pattern of particle deposition and, hence, the mechanisms available for either neutralizing or removing them. Respiratory tract fluids contribute to the mechanical clearance of particles, have nonspecific bactericidal and detoxifying capabilities, and, in immunized hosts, contain antibodies. The alveolar macrophage carries bactericidal enzymes and antimicrobial antibodies for nonspecific and specific defenses in situ, respectively, in addition to its more primitive function of sequestering or physically removing particles. Finally, the specific immune defenses increase the efficiency of the nonspecific defenses by contributing antibodies to the respiratory tract fluids and by facilitating adherence of organisms to alveolar macrophages and increasing their activity.

## PARTICLES

### Definition

Inhalable particles are small droplets or pieces of material—organic or inorganic, viable or nonviable—that can become airborne and penetrate into the oral or nasal airways. They range in size from individual molecules smaller than 0.001 μm in diameter through 1-μm bacteria to visible dust particles of 100 μm diameter or larger. They can be spherical, irregularly shaped, or fibrous (by convention, fibers are particles whose lengths are greater than three times their diameters); for example, an asbestos fiber that penetrates into the lungs may measure from 0.05 μm to a few micrometers in diameter and up to several hundred micrometers in length. Particles can occur naturally or be anthropogenic. They can be formed by the condensation of vapors, the aggregation of smaller particles, or the abrasion or disintegration of bulk material or larger particles. They can be innocuous or harmful, either intrinsically or because toxic or radioactive substances are dissolved in them or have been adsorbed onto them. A collection of airborne particles is called an aerosol.

### Particles of Concern

The viable particles of major concern for health effects are pollens and various microorganisms, including bacteria, viruses, algae, molds, yeasts, fungi, rusts, and spores. Inhalation of these particles is related to a broad range of allergic and infectious diseases. Nonviable particles of concern are those that consist of or contain toxic metals, toxic chemical compounds, or radioactive elements. In addition, lung disease has been associated with the inhalation of naturally occurring crystalline materials such as silica and asbestos. Finally, plant and insect debris contain biochemically active substances that can have harmful effects when inhaled.

### Physical Characterization

Because the diameter, density, and concentration of the particles in an aerosol affect its stability (i.e., the rate at which particles coagulate and how long they remain airborne) as well as its ability to be inhaled and to penetrate through the upper respiratory tract into lung airways, particle diameter, density, and shape are primary determinants of exposure. Particle density is defined by composition and state of aggregation. Particle diameter is more complicated, since most solid particles are irregularly shaped and not amenable to the direct measurement of diameter. Consequently, an operational definition of particle diameter based on the particle's inertial and gravitational motion in air, called the aerodynamic diameter (or aerodynamic resistance diameter if slip correction is included), is commonly used to characterize the effective sizes of particles in an aerosol.

A particle falling through the air under the force of gravity (gravitational sedimentation) accelerates until it reaches a velocity at which the force of gravity is just balanced by the viscous resistive force exerted by the air (Stokes' law). This velocity is known as the terminal settling velocity. Thus the aerodynamic diameter of a particle, however shaped, is taken as the diameter of a unit density sphere that would have the identical terminal settling (Stokes) velocity. Although it is possible to determine effective aerodynamic diameters for fibers in the same way as for more compact particles, the extreme length of fibers affects their deposition in the narrow branching passages of the lung and must be taken into account: fibers tumble and physically intercept the walls of the airways. As a general rule, fibers with length-to-diameter ratios greater than 10 have an aerodynamic diameter three times their actual diameter, but for critical analyses the size of fibers must be specified by both length and diameter.

Since even an aerosol of the most homogeneous particles has a distribution of diameters, the width of that distribution must also be specified. Naturally occurring and mechanically generated aerosols are usually log-normally distributed, so geometric standard deviation ($\sigma g$) is used to describe their distribution. An aerosol can be called monodisperse if $\sigma g < 1.2$, or if, in a given situation, the size range is narrow enough that the particles can be treated as if they all have the median diameter.

Half the particles of an aerosol have diameters smaller than the median physical diameter (count median diameter, CMD) but, because particle mass is proportional to the cube of the diameter, the collective mass of the particles smaller than the CMD may constitute only a small fraction of the aerosol's total mass. Since the amount of toxic material a particle contains is proportional to its mass rather than its diameter, mass median diameter (MMD) is often specified. This is the particle diameter for a particle whose mass falls at the median of the particle mass distribution of the aerosol. Atmospheric aerosols found over urban regions tend to be distributed bimodally: a fine mode centered at about 0.3 μm (MMD) and a coarse mode centered at about 7 μm (MMD) or larger. Mass median aerodynamic diameter (MMAD) corresponds to the unit density equivalent aerodynamic diameter.

For hygroscopic aerosols, particle size as a function of humidity must also be specified. This is an especially important consideration for particle deposition in the respiratory tract, where the warm air is saturated with water. Aqueous particles containing solutes absorb water as they penetrate the airways, continuously growing and changing their deposition characteristics. Although the deposition mechanisms described in the next section are valid for any particle, hygroscopic or not, an estimation of the deposition of a hygroscopic aerosol would need to take particle growth into account by integrating over the particle size-versus-humidity function.

## THE FIRST LINE OF DEFENSE: PARTICLE FILTRATION BY THE AIR PASSAGES

Most inhaled particles with an aerodynamic diameter greater than 3 μm are deposited along the conductive air passages of the upper and lower respiratory tract; i.e., they are mechanically filtered from the air before they can reach the delicate gas-exchanging membranes within the alveolar region. Because the secondary defenses (especially the clearance mechanisms) are very different for the two regions, the anatomic distribution of this deposit, as well as its total mass and chemistry, must be considered before any health effects can be estimated.

Although a particle is physically characterized by its density, diameter, and shape, this is not enough to predict its deposition in the lung airways. The dimensions of the air passages and the pattern of air flow must also be taken into account. The intricacies of mathematical models of particle deposition are beyond the scope of this chapter, but we can briefly describe the lung and try to convey an understanding of the interaction between physical deposition mechanisms and general features of lung structure.

### Lung Morphology

In general, lung morphology is determined by two major constraints: (1) limited access for protection from the environment, and (2) a large surface area interface for air-blood oxygen and carbon dioxide exchange. The evolutionary solution to both constraints is the rapidly branching network of cartilage and smooth muscle lined tubes that constitutes the tracheobronchial tree.

The human tracheobronchial tree has what is known as an asymmetric dichotomous branching pattern, i.e., each segment (the "parent") gives rise to two daughter branches) (1). The major daughter is typically larger (about 30%) and forms a smaller (about 20%) angle with the parent than the minor daughter. Because of this asymmetry, the number of branchings (generations) along different paths from the trachea to the alveoli varies from 7 to 24. Through each successive generation, the airways become smaller, but, because of the exponential growth in the number of airways, the total cross section for airflow and surface area increase rapidly. The gas-exchange region beyond the termination of the tracheobronchial tree of an average adult contains approximately 300 million alveolar air sacs, with a total gas-exchange surface area the size of a tennis court.

To avoid the computational complexity that is introduced by tracheobronchial tree asymmetry, most calculations of particle deposition have used the simpler, symmetric morphometric model of the lung defined by

Weibel (2), which represents an average path. In this model, the airways and their generations (g) are as follows: trachea (g = 0), main bronchi (g = 1), lobar bronchi (g = 2 to 3), segmental bronchi (g = 4), bronchi with cartilage in their walls (g = 5 to 10), terminal bronchi (g = 11), bronchioles with smooth muscle walls (g = 12 to 15), terminal bronchioles (g = 16), respiratory bronchioles (g = 17 to 19), and alveolar ducts (g = 20 to 23), with 21 alveoli (g = 24) per duct.

Weibel tabulated the numbers of airways in each generation and their mean diameters and lengths. He also computed the total cross-sectional area, the total volume, and the cumulative volume for each generation. For a given respiratory pattern, Weibel's tabulated dimensions can be used to compute the approximate air velocity in the airways of any given generation and, with deposition models, to estimate particle deposition in each airway generation.

### Particle Deposition in the Lung

There are five major mechanisms by which particles are deposited in the respiratory tract: impaction, gravitational sedimentation, Brownian diffusion, electrostatic deposition, and interception. Deposition by impaction occurs at airway bifurcations when a particle, owing to its momentum and the aerodynamic forces exerted on it by the stream of air in which it is carried, fails to make the turn into either of the daughter branches and impacts on the bifurcation. Gravitational sedimentation, as discussed earlier, is the settling of particles onto airway surfaces under the force of gravity. For particles smaller than 0.5 μm diameter, the gravitational and inertial effects that cause sedimentation and impaction are no longer influential on deposition. As particles become smaller than 0.5 μm, they are more affected by the random thermal kinetic buffeting (Brownian motion) of the gas molecules in the air around them, and they diffuse to the walls of the air passages—hence, deposition by Brownian diffusion. The relative importance of these three mechanisms—gravitational sedimentation, impaction, and diffusion—for deposition in a given airway depends on the size of the particle, its density, and the velocity of the air moving through that airway. In reality, air turbulence tends to blur the influence of the three mechanisms and to exert a major influence on deposition patterns and efficiencies. If the particles are freshly generated by mechanical disintegration or are sprayed as liquid droplets, they may be highly charged and be deposited by electrostatic image forces that they induce on the airway surfaces. Finally, if the length of a fibrous particle approaches the order of the dimensions of the airway, it may be deposited by physical interception with the airway walls. This is not an important deposition mechanism for particles other than fibers.

Sedimentation and impaction are the most important deposition mechanisms for particles larger than 1 μm. Both increase in proportion to particle density and the square of particle diameter. With increasing air velocity, however, deposition from impaction increases while sedimentation decreases. For this reason, deposition in the large airways (where air velocities are high) is due predominantly to impaction, then shifts to a dominance of sedimentation in the smaller conductive airways, as total airway cross section increases and air velocity drops. The two mechanisms are also distinguishable for their respective dependency on airway length and branching angle. Sedimentation increases with airway length and is independent of branching angle; deposition from impaction increases with the branching angle and is independent of airway length.

It follows that slow, deep breathing enhances sedimentation and leads to relatively uniform deposition of particles throughout the respiratory tract, whereas rapid, shallow breathing increases impaction in the large airways, producing a centralized particle deposition pattern. Though rapid, shallow breathing may protect the gas-exchange regions, it favors high local particle concentrations, or "hot spots," around the bifurcation carinas of the large airways, where the particles impact. Significantly, it has been observed that bronchial carcinomas tend to occur in these same airways (3).

Deposition of particles through Brownian diffusion starts to become significant for particles with diameters smaller than 0.5 μm. A unit density sphere of 1 μm has a terminal sedimentation velocity of 33 μm per second and a diffusion displacement rate of about 13 μm per second, whereas a 0.5-μm unit density sphere has sedimentation and diffusion rates of 9.5 and 20 μm per second, respectively. Like deposition by sedimentation, deposition by diffusion increases with increasing airway length and decreases when air velocity or airway diameter increases. It is greatest in the gas-exchanging structures, where velocities are very low, giving particles time to diffuse to the surrounding surfaces.

Interception is important only for fibers, since their length can be an appreciable fraction of the diameter of the air passages. Because of the large cross section they present for lateral movements, fibers tend to align themselves with airstream lines, effectively resisting impaction and sedimentation, and allowing them to penetrate to the peripheral gas-exchanging structures. Though usually aligned with the stream lines, turbulence can disrupt airflow and causes the fibers to flip end over end. In the periphery of the lung, where fiber lengths are significant in relation to airway dimensions, this flipping results in the interception of a fiber end with a wall, leading to its collection at that point.

While it is possible to estimate total and regional deposition by calculating deposition in each generation and making the appropriate summations, the result is subject to great uncertainty and error. Air turbulence caused by airway branching, surface irregularities, and the flow reversal between inspiration and expiration introduce indeterminate factors, which make exact calculations of air flow and particle deposition impossible. In addition, individual variability in tracheobronchial tree dimensions introduces further uncertainty in the application of such results to any living subject, because the specific airway morphometry is unknown.

An alternative approach to determining the extent of *in vivo* deposition within broad regions of the respiratory tract involves the controlled inhalation of well-defined inert particles that are tagged with nonleaching radioisotopes, followed by a series of external *in vivo* measurements of particle retention as a function of time after the brief inhalation period (4,5). A mass balance can be made using: (a) measurements of the inhaled particles that are exhaled and captured on a filter; (b) the initial measurements of retention of inhaled particles within the head and thorax (as indications of the amounts deposited in the upper and lower respiratory tracts, respectively); and (c) thoracic retention at 1 day after inhalation. The particles that were deposited along ciliated airways within the thorax can be assumed to have moved to the larynx by mucociliary transport within the first 24 hours and be swallowed, whereas those deposited in nonciliated lung airways can be assumed to have cleared to a negligible extent within the first day. The thoracic retention of tagged particles, corrected for radiologic decay, is credited with being deposited initially in the region known variously as the alveolar, pulmonary, or gas-exchange region, and the difference between the initial thoracic retention and the 24-hour retention is credited to deposition in the tracheobronchial region.

The accuracy and applicability of regional deposition estimates based on *in vivo* retention measurements are uncertain, since some of the simplifying assumptions may be invalid. There is evidence that some of the particles deposited within the tracheobronchial region are not cleared from the thorax within the first day. Experiments by Scheuch and Stahlhofen (6), using small boli of tagged particles inhaled near the end of a tidal inspiration, showed prolonged retention of a major fraction. Their a priori assumption that there is a low probability of airborne particle penetration beyond the tracheobronchial region of the particles within the bolus was confirmed by Fang et al. (7) in experiments in which a 40-ml bolus of radioaerosol was drawn into freshly excised human and canine lungs at end inspiration. Autoradiographic examination of fixed slices of these lungs showed negligible penetration beyond about ten generations of airways.

Despite these concerns, data obtained from experimental studies of human volunteers provide the most accurate estimates of regional and total deposition. Figures 1

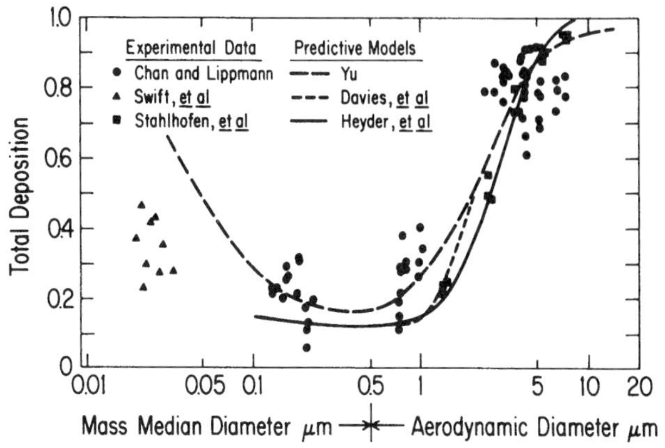


**FIG. 1.** Total deposition (fraction inhaled) as a function of particle size (MMD, d <0.5 μm; MMAD, d >0.5 μm). (From ref. 8.)

through 3 show, respectively, total, tracheobronchial, and alveolar deposition data compiled from several such studies, along with curves generated from empirical and theoretical predictive models (8). The variability of deposition among individuals is apparent from the scatter of the data points.

Using available data on regional particle deposition and measurements of airway sizes as a function of age, Martonen (9) developed a model for tracheobronchial deposition as a function of age, for both iron oxide ($Fe_2O_3$), a nonhygroscopic aerosol, and sulfuric acid ($H_2SO_4$), a very hygroscopic aerosol. The efficiency of tracheobronchial deposition decreases with increasing age (Fig. 4). For a hygroscopic aerosol such as $H_2SO_4$, hygroscopic growth within the airways occurs as the droplets approach equilibrium with the higher-than-ambient air temperature and humidity. When the original droplet size is larger than 0.7 μm, hygroscopic growth increases tracheobronchial deposition; for droplets smaller than 0.5 μm, hygroscopic growth can reduce tracheobronchial deposition.

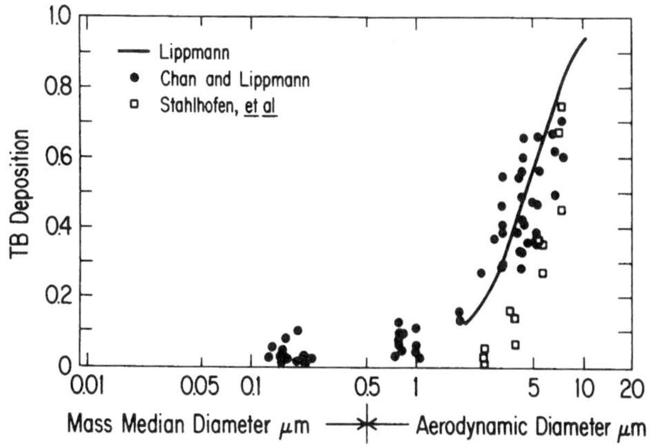


**FIG. 2.** Tracheobronchial (TB) deposition, fraction of aerosol entering the trachea, as a function of particle size (MMD, d <0.5 μm; MMAD, d >0.5 μm). (From ref. 8.)

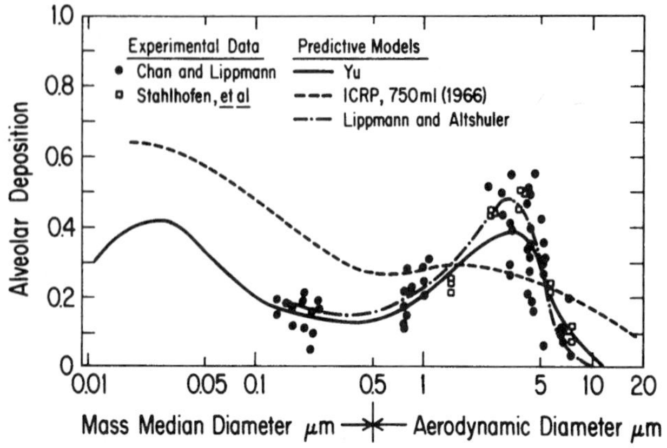


**FIG. 3.** Alveolar (gas-exchanging region) deposition, fraction inhaled, as a function of particle size (MMD, d <0.5 μm; MMAD, d >0.5 μm). (From ref. 8.)

During mouth breathing, particles that deposit in the gas-exchange region represent approximately 15% of the particles inhaled when the size of the particles ranges from 0.1 μm (MMD) to about 1.0 μm (MMAD). As particle size increases, the fraction deposited in the deep lung airways rises to a maximum of approximately 50% for a particle diameter of 3 μm (MMAD). It then falls to zero by 10 μm (MMAD). Particles with MMAD larger than 10 μm are filtered from the inspired air by the upper and lower airways, and do not reach the gas-exchange structures.

Although most experimental studies have used mouth breathing, deposition for nose breathing can also be generally described. For inhaled particles smaller than 1.0 μm diameter, the fraction that is deposited in the gas-exchange region is similar to that for mouth breathing. As particle diameter increases above 1.0 μm (MMAD), however, the deposition fraction for nose breathing, unlike that for mouth breathing, increases only a little, reaching a peak of about 25% at 2.5 μm (MMAD) and then falling to zero by about 8 μm (MMAD). Clearly, nose breathing provides significantly greater protection than mouth breathing against particles of 1 μm diameter or larger.

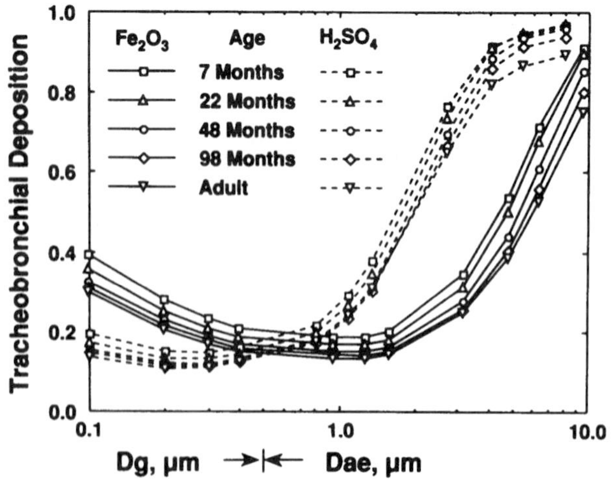


**FIG. 4.** Tracheobronchial deposition of dry $Fe_2O_3$ particles and hygroscopic sulfuric acid droplets in the human lung at various ages. (From ref. 9.)

In actuality, the situation is more complicated. Although some 15% of the population are habitual mouth breathers, most people breathe predominantly through their noses until the ventilation rate reaches about 40 L per minute. At higher flow rates, the amount of inhaled air is split almost evenly between mouth and nose. Miller and coinvestigators (10) called such people "normal augmenters." Using an empiric deposition model based on available regional deposition data, they calculated tracheobronchial deposition at various flow rates for both normal augmenters, and habitual mouth breathers. Tracheobronchial deposition declines with flow rate in normal augmenters up to 30 L per minute, and then, owing to increased impaction in the upstream nasal airways, jumps abruptly as part of the inhaled air bypasses the more efficient filtration of the nasal passages (Fig. 5).

### Localized Retention of Inhaled Particles

Very detailed information on particle deposition and the initial stages of translocation has been obtained in studies in which laboratory animals are briefly exposed to airborne particles shortly before they are sacrificed. Microscopic evaluation of airway sections collected by microdissection provides quantitative information about the distribution of particles on the surfaces of the fluid layers above the epithelial cells as well as the distribution of particles on, within, and beyond the epithelial cells at the time of sacrifice. With serial sacrifice of laboratory animals at various times after the end of inhalation, one can characterize the distribution of retained particles at various anatomic sites as a function of time after end of exposure. This can provide estimates of the kinetics of particle migration into and through the epithelium and along translocation pathways. Studies of deposition and retention within the first day after particle inhalation have been performed at the respiratory acinus (11,12) and within the trachea (13). Examination of particle distribution in lung and lymphatic tissues at later times can provide information on the nature and extent of movement of particles to more distant sites of accumulation and/or any pathologic consequences. Systematic studies can be performed on laboratory animals that are sacrificed at specific times following acute or chronic exposure regimens. Valuable information can also be obtained from human lungs obtained at autopsy, especially when a reliable history of occupational or environmental exposure to the airborne particles of interest is available (14).

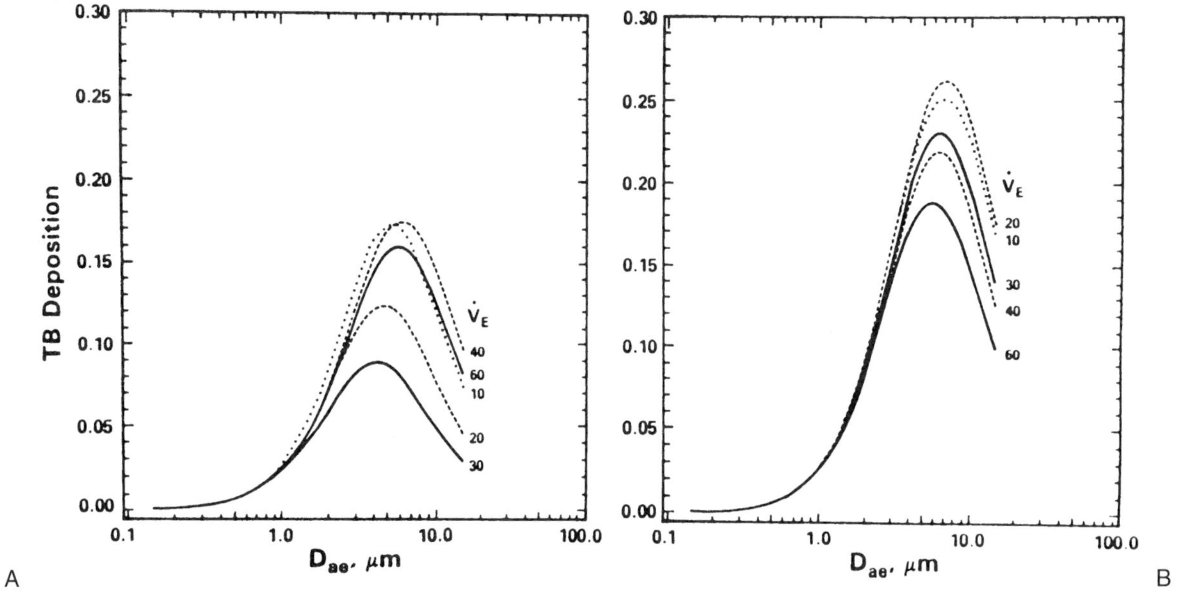


**FIG. 5.** Tracheobronchial deposition of particles for normal augmenters **(A)** and mouth breathers **(B)** as a function of aerodynamic particulate diameter for minute ventilation, Ve, ranging from a resting level (10 L $min^{-1}$) to heavy exercise (60 L $min^{-1}$). (From ref. 10.)

### *Factors Affecting Local Particle Deposition within Lung Airways*

One major misconception in respiratory tract dosimetry is that particle deposition is considered to be relatively uniform in small airways where the dominant deposition mechanisms are sedimentation and diffusion. By contrast, it has long been recognized that in large airways, where inertial impaction is important, there are prominent deposition hot spots at airway bifurcations and other surfaces directly downstream of high-velocity flow streams. The observations by Brody and colleagues (11,12) of hot spots of particle deposition at alveolar duct bifurcations in the rat necessitated a reexamination of the nature of convective flow in small airways of the lung, and some of the studies addressing these phenomena have provided new insights on the aerodynamics and dosimetry of inhaled particles.

### *Airway Geometry and Flow Fields*

Mammalian lungs consist of an array of bifurcating conducting airways of ever smaller size leading to alveolar sacs surrounded by capillaries, where inhaled oxygen ($O_2$) is exchanged for exhaled carbon dioxide ($CO_2$). During each flow cycle the small airways and alveolar sacs expand during inhalation and contract during exhalation. Human lungs differ from other mammalian lungs in that the branching pattern of the approximately 16 generations of conductive airways is nearly symmetric, with each parent airway splitting into two smaller daughter airways of nearly equal size and branching angle. By contrast, four-legged animals of all sizes have highly asymmetric branching wherein the major daughter airway is almost as large and has a small angular change of direction, while the smaller daughter airway is much smaller and extends at a more acute angle from the parent airway (15).

The velocity of the air in the larger airways can be high enough for turbulent flow, whereas in the smaller conductive airways and beyond it is so low that the flow is laminar and viscous. Furthermore, the airway cross section expands during inhalation, with the greatest expansion in the smallest airways. In the turbulent flow regime, the flow profile across a long conduit tends to be relatively flat, with the center-line velocity being only about 10% greater than the average velocity and the flow resistance relatively high because of turbulence and wall resistance. There are also departures from symmetry in the flow profile, since the entry length for flow stabilization is greater than the physical length of each airway segment and there are major directional changes and secondary swirling currents at each bifurcation.

By contrast, the small airways have very short entry lengths and the flow is laminar. During inhalation, the cross section is increasingly divergent as the lungs expand, allowing the development of lubrication flow (16) in which the center-line velocity can be many times greater than the average, with a large proportion of the inspiratory flow in the axial core of each airway. When the flow direction reverses, the cross section for flow decreases and the flow becomes convergent. Under these conditions, the flow, while laminar, has a relatively flat profile, with a greater fraction of the exhalation flow in the annular space around the axial core. For particles of low intrinsic mobility, the net result of each cycle, in terms of convective flow, is a movement of recently inhaled airborne particles along the axial core toward the lung periphery balanced by an equivalent volume of particle-free residual air from the lung periphery. The smaller the tidal volume, the greater the influence of the axial core flow on the depth of penetration of inhaled particles. There is, simultaneously, axial-core flow induced by the beating heart, which causes rapid compressions and expansions of the surrounding airways. The heartbeat creates convective exchange the same way an external high-frequency ventilator used in cardiac surgery does when the heartbeat is temporarily suspended, except that the high-frequency ventilator creates tidal volumes large enough to maintain normal $O_2$-$CO_2$ exchange without creating significant chest motions (16,17).

There are important implications of axial-core flow to localized particle deposition patterns and dosimetry. For normal tidal breathing, the inspiration brings the tidal front into respiratory bronchioles and alveolar ducts, with the inhaled particles being concentrated in the axial core and the air nearer the walls enriched in particle-free residual air. The particles are much closer to the airway bifurcations than to any of the other airway surfaces, and relatively small displacements by sedimentation, diffusion, and image forces can lead to relatively high deposition densities on the surfaces at and near the bifurcation. For quiescent rats, as in the inhalation studies of Brody and Roe (12), this proposed mechanism for particle penetration is highly consistent with the observations that nearly all detectable particles were at or near bifurcations and that deposition density fell rapidly with increasing airway generation. Molecular diffusion allows gas exchange from these vestibular regions, but inhaled particles in the size range from ~0.1 to 2 μm have too little airborne mobility to reach most of the gas exchange surface.

## THE SECOND LINE OF DEFENSE: LUNG FLUIDS AND CLEARANCE

### Upper and Lower Airways

#### *Fluid Lining*

The fluid that lines the upper and lower airways is a mixture of tissue transudates and the secretions of submucosal cells and goblet cells, which are interspersed with the ciliated cells of the surface epithelium. Its major macromolecular components—and the ones responsible for the characteristic viscoelastic properties necessary for mucociliary clearance—are the long-chain glycoprotein molecules, or mucins. These molecules constitute 2% to 3% of normal tracheobronchial secretions (95% is water) and consist of polysaccharide units linked to a polypeptide core. The relative amounts of additional attached groups of fucose, N-acetylneuraminic acid, and sulfates distinguish the different mucins and probably contribute to their buffering capacity, as well as providing a source of sulfhydryls for oxidant neutralization. The physical entanglement of these long glycoprotein molecules is probably the main source of the rheologic (i.e., viscoelastic) properties of mucus.

The submucosal mucous glands, the major source of airway mucus, consist of mucous and serous cells lining a common secretory duct leading to the epithelial surface. Both the quantity and composition of the secretions are influenced by the autonomic nervous system. The same mechanical or chemical irritations that stimulate the contraction of airway smooth muscle cause a discharge of airway secretions. Once secreted, this "mucocolloid" separates into two phases. The continuous beating of the cilia takes place within a low-viscosity sol underlying a discontinuous viscoelastic gel phase in which the long-chain mucopolysaccharide molecules are concentrated.

The goblet cells, cells distended with mucus and so named because of their shape, are found in the epithelia of both upper and lower airways but are most numerous in the large proximal airways of the tracheobronchial tree. Although they produce mucus, their collective secretory output is not nearly as copious as that of the submucosal mucous glands, and they do not respond to autonomic stimulation. They probably serve as local repositories of mucus and help to maintain a baseline level of secretory output, responding only to local stimuli. Clara cells (nonciliated bronchiolar epithelial cells), found mainly in the terminal bronchioles, also contribute to respiratory tract fluids; however, their secretion has yet to be fully characterized.

Other components of the fluid lining the upper and lower airways are the immunoglobulins IgA and IgG, lysozyme, albumin, lactoferrin, transferrin, $\alpha_1$-antitrypsin, haptoglobin, $\alpha_1$-antichymotrypsin, the salivary $\alpha_1$- and $\beta_1$-C-globulins, and $\gamma_1$-acid glycoprotein. IgA, the predominant species of immunoglobulin, is extremely important in mucosal defense against antigens. It is secreted locally as well as being provided by serum transudate along with IgG and albumin. Lysozyme is also produced locally, but the specific sources of the rest are uncertain.

### Mucociliary Clearance

Except for the anterior nares and the posterior nasopharynx, most of the nasal and bronchial epithelia are ciliated; there are about 200 cilia per cell, each approximately 5 μm long (Fig. 6). Coating the epithelia and just covering the cilia is the sol phase of the respiratory tract fluid. Within this sol, the cilia beat about 1,000 times per minute in a metachronous or wavelike pattern, drawing their energy from the dephosphorylation of adenosine triphosphate (ATP). Overlying mucous gel is propelled by means of a fluid coupling between it and the sol underneath as well as by contact with the tips of the beating cilia. Patches of the mucous gel, along with any

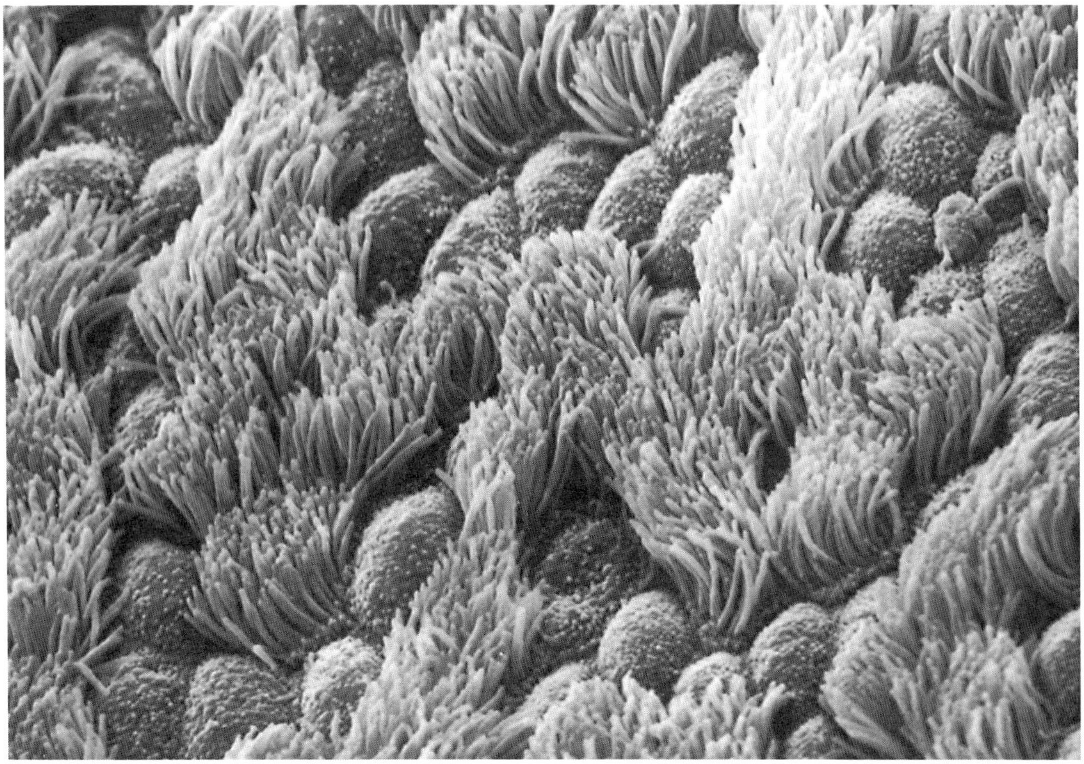

**FIG. 6.** Ciliated tracheal epithelium from adult Fisher 344 rat (×4,700). (Courtesy George Schidlovsky, Brookhaven National Laboratory.)

intermingled particles and other debris, are carried out of the airways on this mucociliary escalator. Particles deposited in the anterior nasopharynx are swept forward to the unciliated nares to be removed mechanically or by nose blowing, whereas those deposited elsewhere in the nose (and virtually all of the particles deposited on the ciliated epithelium of the tracheobronchial tree) are swept toward the pharynx and swallowed.

Local transport velocities in both the nasopharyngeal region and the tracheobronchial tree vary widely; values of less than 1 mm per minute to more than 20 mm per minute have been reported. Although most measurements of mucous transport in the tracheobronchial tree have been confined to the trachea, measurements in smaller bronchi and estimates based on mucus thickness and tracheobronchial tree surface area indicate a velocity gradient from the 5 to 10 mm per minute or so observed in the trachea to an estimated 10 μm per minute in the smallest ciliated airways. The mucus, however, covers only part of the tracheobronchial tree, with discrete mucous plaques in the smaller airways and a consolidated mucous sheet that covers parts of the larger airways. Particles that deposit on serous fluid not covered by mucus remain on the surface for a limited number of hours, during which they can be swept up by mucus moving up the airways on the serous layer. Alternatively, the particles can be wetted with surfactant, drawn into the serous layer, and brought down to the epithelial cell surface to be phagocytosed.

There appears to be a particle size dependence, and possibly a particle composition dependence, on the probabilities of clearance via mucus versus via the epithelial cells (18). Particles larger than 9 μm in diameter are much less likely than smaller ones to be drawn into the serous fluid, and plastic particles are less likely to be displaced through the serous fluid surface than are metal oxide particles. The size dependence may reflect a time dependence for the coating of the particles by an osmiophilic film at the air-mucus surface. The osmiophilic bilayer observed by Gehr et al. (13) at the gel-sol interface could also play a role in the displacement of a particle toward the epithelium. Thus, if mucociliary transport of uncoated particles on the surface of the gel layer is slow, or delayed, the likelihood of migration toward and phagocytosis by the epithelial cells increases.

In general, the transport velocity observed in any given location depends on the arrangement of cilia and on the viscoelastic properties and thickness of both sol and gel phases of the respiratory tract fluid. Too much or too little fluid, or fluid with suboptimal viscoelastic properties, would affect the coupling between the cilia and the mucous gel and impair mucociliary transport. (Patients with bronchitis, for example, have an excess of bronchial secretions and defective mucociliary clearance.) There are also areas where the arrangement of cilia is such that wave patterns conflict and transport is impaired (e.g., in the nasal passages and at the carinas of airway bifurcations).

Impaired transport, combined with the tendency of particles to become impacted in these locations, could make airway bifurcations especially vulnerable (3). Fortunately, both nasal passages and the bifurcations of the large bronchi are the areas where irritant receptors are concentrated and the areas most effectively cleared by sneezes and coughs, respectively.

Measurements of overall nasopharyngeal or tracheobronchial clearance provide more consistent indicators of mucociliary function than local transport rates, because they represent a composite of regional rates, averaging out local variations. Such measurements are provided by experimental studies in which a test aerosol tagged with a γ-ray–emitting isotope is inhaled and its clearance is monitored by external detectors. Data from a study in which tracheobronchial clearance was measured are plotted in Fig. 7A (19). The percentage of particles retained is plotted as a function of time after inhalation. Tracheobronchial clearance is shown by the fall in retention during the first few hours, and its completion by the relatively constant retention level after an average of 6 to 8 hours. Although retention curves can be evaluated in many ways, the time to clearance completion has proved the most reliable parameter because it is the least dependent on the distribution of the deposited particles.

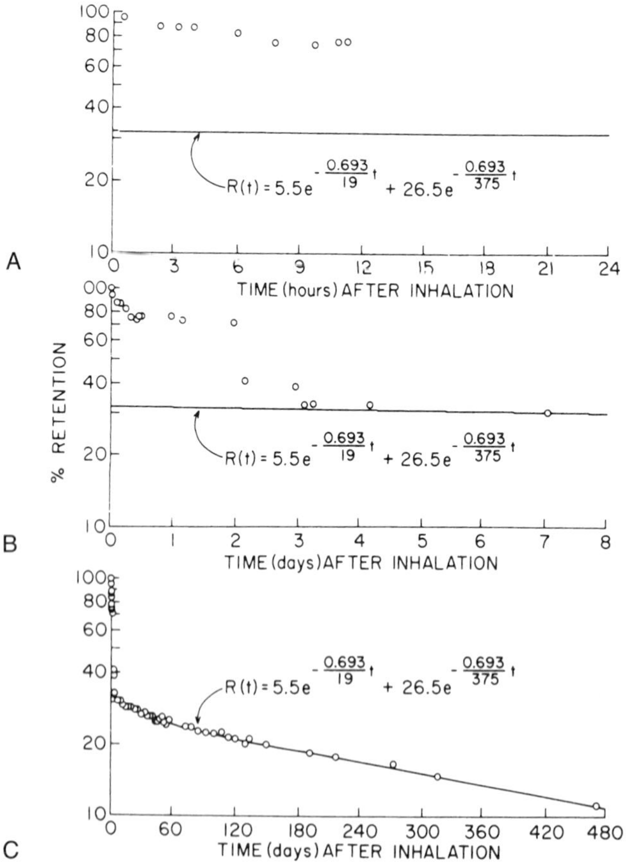


**FIG. 7.** Long-term retention of 4.0 μm (MMAD) polystyrene particles as a function of time after inhalation plotted on three different time scales to show tracheobronchial clearance **(A)**, gastrointestinal elimination **(B)**, and alveolar clearance **(C)**.

Overall, clearance of the ciliated nasopharyngeal region is completed within about 4 hours, and clearance of the ciliated epithelium of the tracheobronchial tree can take as little as 2 or as many as 20 hours (4). Clearance times for the tracheobronchial tree especially, but also nasopharyngeal region clearance times and tracheal transport velocities, appear to be characteristic of an individual. This might be expected, since both local transport velocities and overall clearance rates depend on the quantity and rheologic properties of the respiratory tract secretions as well as respiratory tract morphology and ciliary function. All of these should be fairly constant and, to some extent, unique to an individual. Because the quantity and quality of respiratory tract secretions are influenced by the autonomic nervous system, mucociliary function can also change dramatically. For example, depending on individual clearance characteristics and sensitivity, acute exposure to an irritant like cigarette smoke usually causes a temporary increase in the tracheobronchial clearance rate. Even as mild a stimulant as tea can speed mucociliary clearance, and the administration of an adrenergic agent like isoproterenol can cause clearance to be completed in less than an hour, whereas atropine essentially halts it. More important than these transient changes, however, is the impairment of tracheobronchial clearance associated with lung disease that is often seen in cigarette smokers (20). Although this impairment may be secondary to disease-induced changes in respiratory tract secretions or lung morphology, it will certainly exacerbate any disease condition because it constitutes the breakdown of an important defense mechanism.

## Gas-Exchanging Structures

### *Alveolar Fluid*

The fluid lining the alveoli, like that lining the conducting passages, is a combination of local secretions and plasma transudates. Its most important components are the lipid secretions (surfactants) associated with the type II alveolar cells, which give it its surface tension-reducing properties. These lipids have been identified as the saturated lecithins, principally dipalmitoyl lecithin, together with the unsaturated lecithins and cholesterol. If the surface tension of the fluid film in the alveoli were not reduced, much greater pressures would be required to inflate small alveoli than large alveoli. The smaller alveoli would collapse (atelectasis), the larger ones would overinflate, and uniform ventilation could not be maintained. The fluid plays an important role in lung defense as well. Particles deposited in the alveoli are rapidly coated (opsonized) by the surface-active lipid materials and serum proteins found there, enhancing particle phagocytosis by alveolar macrophages, and even causing direct lysis of some particles.

Alveolar fluid also contains other phospholipids, neutral lipids, carbohydrates, and a number of serum proteins, including albumin, IgA, IgG (an important opsonin), transferrin, $\alpha_1$-antitrypsin, free IgA secretory component, and complement, the last being a system of serum proteins formed through enzymatic cascade that enhances antibody response by promoting phagocytosis, producing lysis of sensitized red blood cells and bacteria, and participating in the inflammatory response to injury.

### *Alveolar Macrophage*

Alveolar macrophages are large (10 to 12 μm) mononuclear phagocytic cells, generally believed to be descendants of bone marrow monocytes, that enter the lung interstitium as monocytes from circulating blood. In the interstitium, the monocytes divide and mature into interstitial macrophages. Many of these cells move out onto the alveolar surface, adapting to the highly aerobic environment to become alveolar macrophages, where they maintain the sterility of the lung by engulfing, neutralizing or digesting, and physically removing pathogenic particles (Fig. 8).

The macrophages reach sites of particle deposition by chance or through chemical attraction to chemotactic substances released by the particles or to particle coatings (opsonins) containing antibodies (especially IgG), antibody-antigen complexes, or complement formed from alveolar fluid. They can also be drawn by chemotactic substances released by lymphocytes and other macrophages as they interact with the particles, amplifying macrophage response. Once in contact with a particle, the macrophage, often stimulated by the opsonins, rapidly engulfs it. Lysosomes (packets of hydrolytic enzymes) then attach themselves to the phagosomal membrane surrounding the ingested pathogen, the lysosomal membranes become continuous with the phagosomal membrane, and the lytic enzymes kill and digest the pathogen.

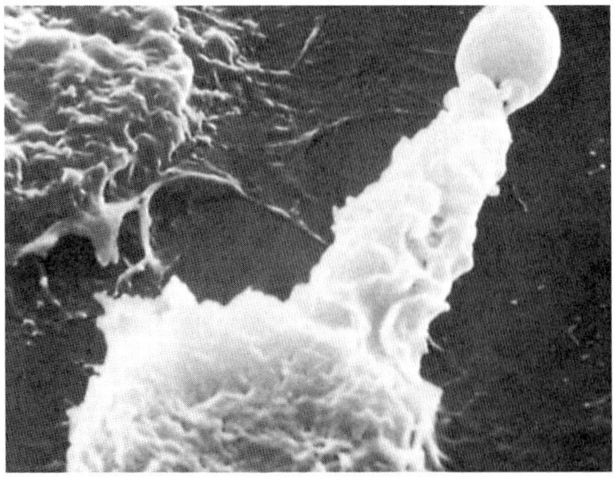

**FIG. 8.** Rabbit alveolar macrophage attaching itself to yeast particle. (Courtesy of John G. Hadley, Owens-Corning Fiberglass, and John Adee, Battelle Northwest.)

Indigestible material remains sequestered in the macrophages and is gradually removed as macrophages migrate from the gas-exchange structures to ciliated airways for clearance via the mucociliary escalator. Often, this material includes antigens, pathogenic particles, or other toxic substances the macrophages are incapable of digesting. Within the interstitium, the interstitial macrophages provide bactericidal and immune-mediated protection against particles that escape alveolar macrophages and penetrate the alveolar epithelium, as well as sequestering them and removing them via the lymphatics.

### *Pulmonary Lymphatics*

The pulmonary lymphatic system is a network of vessels connecting aggregates of immunocompetent lymphoid tissue that drains excess fluids, proteins, and even cells and particles from the pulmonary interstitium. It backs up respiratory tract surface defenses against foreign cells and antigenic particles with both cell-mediated and humoral immune defenses and ties in the lung to the body's systemic immune system. This network is composed of two major plexuses—peribronchovascular and pleural plexus. The peribronchovascular plexus consists of intercommunicating networks located in the connective tissue surrounding the airways, pulmonary arteries, and pulmonary veins, which merge imperceptibly at the level of the bronchioles and arterioles. The pleural plexus is a dense network of small lymphatic vessels localized within the connective tissue of the visceral pleura. The two plexuses are linked by means of small vessels in the interlobular septa as well as by pleural lymphatics that run over the surface of the lung toward the hilus, where they join with the peribronchovascular lymphatics. In the lumen of the vessels, funnel-shaped one-way valves work with vascular and respiratory pressures to maintain slow but steady unidirectional flow of lymph from the periphery of the lung to the larger lymphatic collecting vessels, and finally to the bloodstream via the right lymphatic and thoracic ducts.

Lymphatic "capillaries," arising as blind pouches within lymphoid aggregates at the level of the terminal and respiratory bronchioles and in connective tissue adjacent to alveoli, absorb fluids and particles from the interstitium of the peripheral lung. These vessels are distinguished by their extremely thin walls, interrupted basement membrane, and loose intercellular junctions, which account for the permeability of the lymphatic vessels to serum proteins, cells, and particles. Moving out of the periphery of the lung, the lymphatic vessels feed through more and more highly organized lymphatic tissue. In the walls of the respiratory bronchioles, lymphoepithelial organs bring respiratory epithelium, lymphatic tissue, and blood vessels into proximity. They may serve as functional pathways for the removal of alveolar fluids and particulates from airways to lymphatics. Lymphoid nodules in the walls of medium-sized and large bronchi (bronchus-associated lymphoid tissue, BALT) also provide pathways for the potential interchange of particles and lymphoid cells between air passages and lymphatics for activation of immune defenses. Finally, hilar and tracheobronchial lymph nodes receive the lymphatic drainage for most of the respiratory tract before it reenters the blood.

### *Alveolar Clearance*

The respiratory bronchioles, alveolar ducts, and alveoli, unlike the conducting airways, do not have ciliated epithelia. While the mechanisms responsible for the translocation and retention of particles depositing on the nonciliated epithelium of the gas-exchange region are still poorly understood, it is well known that alveolar macrophages ingest a large proportion of these particles within about 4 to 6 hours, and that particle-laden macrophages find their way onto the mucociliary escalator at the terminal bronchioles, accounting for a phase of particle clearance from the lungs that lasts several weeks.

A mechanism for alveolar clearance via the bronchial airways has been suggested by Patrick and Stirling (21). They propose that particles on the surface of the alveolar lining fluid are drawn onto the mucociliary escalator as the high-surface-tension fluid layer is drawn from the alveolar ducts and respiratory bronchioles. Those particles not cleared to the tracheobronchial tree can be ingested by epithelial cells at their favored deposition sites at alveolar duct bifurcations. There is also speculation that bare particles can migrate to interstitial spaces without being ingested and can contribute to translocation via lymphatic drainage to pleural nodes. The evidence for such translocation is strongest for ultrafine-sized particles (~0.02 μm diameter), as has been noted by Ferin et al. (22). This "membrane" filtration concept may also apply to mineral fibers. Mesothelial tumors are most closely associated with very thin fibers (<0.15 μm diameter), as discussed by Lippmann and Timbrell (14), and one can speculate that the fibers that penetrate the epithelium and migrate most effectively to the pleural surfaces are more likely to cause pleural disease than are those that remain at or near their sites of deposition.

Figure 7 shows particle retention data from a long-term clearance study. The data are plotted on three different time scales so that the difference between tracheobronchial and alveolar clearance rates can be appreciated (19). The particles were 4.0-μm (MMAD) polystyrene microspheres, and the retention is expressed as a percentage of initial deposition. Tracheobronchial clearance (Fig. 7A) is typically completed in about 6 to 8 hours. The elimination of this material from the gastrointestinal tract can be seen in Fig. 7B from the abrupt drop in retention on the second and third days after inhalation. By the fourth day, although particles are passing through the tracheobronchial tree and gastrointestinal tract as they clear, only the gas-exchange region of the lung contains a significant fraction of the particles initially inhaled. Finally, Fig. 7C shows the characteristic two-phase pattern of alveolar clearance observed in healthy persons. Here, the fast phase has a half-time of 19 days, and the slow phase a half-time of 375 days.

Most of the particles that are deposited in the gas-exchange structures, depending on their size and composition, are engulfed by alveolar macrophages. These particle-laden macrophages, as well as the "naked" particles that remain, can then follow one of two major clearance routes: the mucociliary escalator or the alveolar epithelium into the interstitium for clearance via the lymphatics (Fig. 9). There are opposing views, but the particle-laden macrophages probably are cleared principally via the airways and naked particles via both routes. It is not known how the macrophages and particles find their way to the mucociliary escalator, but surface tension and viscosity gradients, respiratory movements, and a slow movement of fluid transudate from the alveoli to the airways have all been suggested. The fast alveolar clearance phase is commonly associated with macrophage activity, and it is

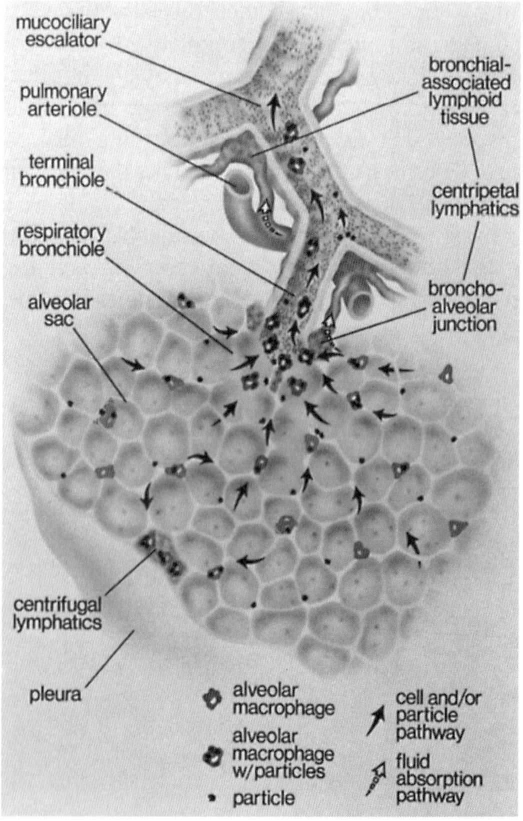


FIG. 9. Alveolar-bronchiolar particle clearance route. (From ref. 36.)

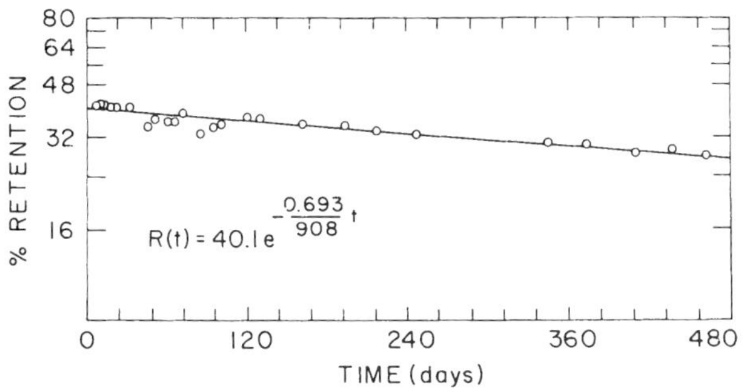


**FIG. 10.** Long-term retention of 4.0-μm (MMAD) polystyrene particle as a function of time for persons with chronic obstructive lung disease. (From ref. 19.)

assumed that particles entering the interstitium clear more slowly; however, no direct correspondence has yet been drawn between the two temporal clearance phases and either clearance route.

Particles that enter the interstitium can also become sequestered there, within macrophages or bound in connective tissue to remain indefinitely. Relatively inert particles such as soot cause the diffuse pigmentation seen at autopsy in lungs of city dwellers, while toxic materials such as silica and asbestos lead to the lung diseases known as silicosis and asbestosis.

Although the role of impaired alveolar clearance in the pathogenesis of lung disease is not yet clear, persons with lung disease have defective alveolar clearance. Figure 10 shows alveolar clearance in a person with chronic obstructive lung disease. The fast clearance phase has disappeared, and the half-time of the slow phase is significantly increased. Cigarette smokers show a similar long-term clearance pattern: no fast phase and slow phase half-times increased in proportion to pack-years of smoking. Since the effects of inhaled particles are often directly related to their retention time, such alterations in alveolar clearance may have consequences that are probably more serious than those resulting from changes in tracheobronchial clearance.

### *Particle Accumulation and Overload*

Cytotoxic particles can kill macrophages in transit to the mucociliary escalator, releasing both the internalized particles and the digestive enzymes that attack epithelial cells. The regenerating epithelial cells can phagocytose the particles and lead to the commonly observed peribronchiolar focal accumulations of particles in the lungs of workers in the dusty trades. Dusts can also accumulate when the normal physiologic capacity is exceeded.

Accumulation of fibers in distal lung airways may slow the clearance of fibers and other particles from the lung as shown by Ferin and Leach (23) and Bolton et al. (24). They found strong evidence for an overload of clearance at high lung burdens of asbestos, especially for the intermediate-rate clearance mechanisms. Their hypothesis is consistent with the results of other inhalation studies in rats with asbestos (25), quartz (26), and diesel soot (27). Vincent et al. (28) modified the overload hypothesis on the basis of rat inhalation studies extending for up to 1 year. They found the lung burden to increase in proportion to the exposure concentration. Because, the general pattern for asbestos in rats is so similar to that for rats inhaling diesel fumes, such accumulations are not specific to fibrous dust. The particular sequestration model favored by Vincent et al. is one in which the longer a particle remains in the lung without being cleared, the more likely it will be sequestrated (and therefore less likely to be cleared).

Morrow (29) developed a general hypothesis that dust overloading, which is typified by a progressive reduction of particle clearance from the deep lung, reflects a breakdown in alveolar macrophage (AM)-mediated dust removal as a result of the loss of AM mobility. The inability of the dust-laden AM to translocate to the mucociliary escalator is correlated with the average composite particle volume per AM in the lung. When the volume of relatively nontoxic particles exceeds approximately 60 $\mu m^3$/AM, the overload effect appears to be initiated. When the distributed particulate volume exceeds ~600 $\mu m^3$ per cell, the AM-mediated particle clearance virtually ceases, and agglomerated particle-laden macrophages remain in the alveolar region. For cytotoxic particles, these effects occur at lower loadings.

Ferin et al. (22) performed additional lung instillation and inhalation studies to further explore the Morrow hypothesis and the respective roles of both AM and polymorphonuclear leukocytes (PMN), whose influx is indicative of a cellular inflammatory response. On the basis of their studies, they concluded that:

- the delivered dose rate of particles to the lung is a determinant of the acute inflammatory PMN response;
- the process of phagocytosis of "nuisance" particles by AMs, rather than the interstitial access of the particles, appears to initiate the influx of PMN into the alveolar space;
- the surface area of the retained particles correlates best with inflammatory parameters rather than the phagocytosed particle numbers, mass, or volume;
- interstitialization of particles appears to be important for inducing interstitial inflammatory responses including the induction of fibrotic reactions; and
- if the interstitialized particle fraction exceeds the particle fraction remaining in the alveolar space, the influx of PMN into the alveolar lumen decreases, conceivably reflecting a reversal of chemotactic gradients from alveolar space toward the interstitial space.

Inhalation studies were performed by Jones et al. (30) in which rats inhaled Union Internationale Contre le Cancer (UICC) amosite asbestos at an approximately constant concentration of 0.1 mg/m$^3$ or, equivalently, 20 fibers/ml for 7 hours/day, 5 days/week, for up to 18 months. The lung burdens were compared with the previous results of higher-exposure concentrations of 1 and 10 mg/m$^3$. Taken together, these results showed lung burdens rising in proportion to exposure concentration and exposure time. This accumulation of lung burden fits a kinetic model that takes account of the sequestration of material at locations in the lung from where it cannot be cleared. A mathematical model that accounts for the effects of both particle concentration and toxicity on rat lung particle retention has been described by Gradon et al. (31). The most direct evidence for the effect of altered dust clearance rates on the retention of inhaled fibers in humans comes from studies of the fiber content of the lungs of asbestos workers in various countries. Timbrell (32) developed a model for fiber deposition and clearance in human lungs based on his analysis of the bivariate diameter and length distributions found in air and lung samples. He observed that the workers with the highest exposure had the most severe lung fibrosis.

## THE THIRD LINE OF DEFENSE: THE IMMUNE SYSTEM

Most antigenic particles that deposit in the respiratory tract do not penetrate the fluid barriers and do not elicit a systemic immune response. As discussed previously, they are enzymatically degraded, neutralized by antibodies already present, and cleared. In addition, the particles that penetrate to the gas-exchange regions are engulfed and deactivated or removed by alveolar macrophages, or by interstitial macrophages if they reach the interstitium.

Sometimes, however, these defenses are not sufficient, and the antigens gain access to lymphoid tissue. In the upper and lower airways, they may move to the lymphoid nodules in the walls of the bronchi or directly through the mucosa. In the gas-exchanging structures, they may be taken up by the lymphoepithelial organs in the walls of the respiratory bronchioles or move into the interstitium to lymphatic capillaries for transport to local lymphoid nodules, and, subsequently, to the hilar and tracheobronchial lymph nodes.

Once sensitized by interaction with antigen, T cells evolve into subsets of effector cells: (a) soluble mediator (lymphokine)-secreting cells, (b) cytotoxic cells, (c) helper cells, and (d) memory cells. Probably most important in the defense of the respiratory tract are the lymphokine-secreting cells. The lymphokines help coordinate the immune response, especially macrophage function. The cytotoxic cells are sensitized T cells that directly kill foreign cells and cells bearing antigens. For example, a heterogeneous population of so-called natural killer (NK) cells is important in resistance against neoplastic cells and cells that harbor viruses.

B cells are bone marrow–derived lymphocytes that congregate in lymphoid tissues, such as the follicles of lymph nodes, and serve as precursors for the antibody-forming cells that effect humoral immunity. There are five major structural types or classes of immunoglobulins, the molecules that function as antibodies: IgA, IgG, IgM, IgD, and IgE. IgA is the predominant immunoglobulin species in the upper and lower airways; most is synthesized locally. It neutralizes viruses and toxins, inhibits microbial growth, agglutinates particles, and, possibly most important, blocks mucosal penetration of antigens. IgG, although present throughout the respiratory tract in local secretions, occurs in relatively high concentrations in the gas-exchange structures, provided mostly by serum transudate. The respiratory tract's major bacterial opsonin, IgG, agglutinates particles, activates complement, neutralizes bacterial exotoxins and viruses, and lyses gram-negative bacteria.

## RESEARCH NEEDS

Research in recent years has created an expanded knowledge base and improved technology that is capable of addressing many unresolved questions. These are divided into specific areas that need further study.

### Flow Profiles in Large Airways

The complications are (a) transition flow regime with partial turbulence, (b) entry lengths as long as or longer than the tube length, (c) varying cross-section for flow from entry to end of airway and during each respiratory cycle, (d) secondary swirling flows created at bifurcations and changing planes of successive bifurcations, (e) ribbed walls and mucous coatings, and (f) temperature and humidity differences between axial air and air at the walls.

### Flow Profiles in Small Airways

Since the flow is laminar in small airways, some of the complications associated with flow patterns in the large airway flow are absent. Some complications are unique to airways in mammalian lungs, such as variable cross-sections from end to end and during the flow cycle, mucous and serous coatings on the walls, and flow resistance that is greater on exhalation than inhalation. Another complication is the sudden increase in cross section at the entry of the alveolar duct, and the corresponding radial expansion of flow during inspiration and contraction during expiration.

### Penetration Depth for Tidal Flow

Tidal air is usually a small fraction of total lung capacity, and respirable particles have very limited intrinsic mobility. Thus, most of the alveolar epithelium receives little or no particle deposition. Most of the deposition in the gas-exchange region occurs at the respiratory acinus on the small airway bifurcations. More quantitation is needed of the surface density of particle deposition in the respiratory acinus, how it varies with tidal volume, and whether there are major interspecies differences in dosimetry at this level of the lung.

### Extent of Hot Spots of Deposition

Impaction accounts for deposition hot spots at large airway bifurcations, at and below the larynx, and at the nares. More data are needed on the influence of turbulence, upstream flow profiles, airway curvature, and branching angles. Research is also needed to define the roles of particle diffusion, sedimentation, interception, and image forces in the migration of respirable particles to surfaces at and adjacent to airway bifurcations.

### Influence of Airway Narrowing on Particle Deposition

Airborne particles are often inhaled along with irritants that cause acute bronchoconstriction and/or persistent airway narrowing. Such agents include cigarette smoke, sulfur dioxide, and ozone. However, the extent and uniformity of airway narrowing produced by these agents and their effects on total and hot spot deposition need further study.

### Spatial Variability in Mucus Coverage and Efficacy

Particles deposited in large airways during normal tidal breathing are more completely cleared within 1 day than are particles deposited from a bolus of aerosol during breath holding. This raises the question of whether mucous coverage is more complete, or mucus velocities are greater at sites that normally receive the highest deposition density in comparison to sites that normally receive little deposition. Perhaps particles deposited on the uncovered sol layer are more readily retained than are particles that deposit on mucus plaques that travel on the sol layer.

### Effects of Particle Size and Composition

Small particles depositing on the sol layer of large airways are more readily wetted and removed from the surface to the epithelial cells than are larger particles. Composition may also affect the rate at which particles are coated with a lipophilic layer.

### Variations in Mucus Secretions

Agents that stimulate mucous secretion can greatly accelerate the rate of mucociliary particle clearance in humans without increasing the amount cleared within the first day. These agents include cigarette smoke (33) and sulfuric acid aerosol (34). On the other hand, a bronchoconstrictive agent such as sulfur dioxide, when given before the tagged particle aerosol, can increase both the amount cleared and the rate of clearance (35), presumably owing to a proximal shift of particle deposition. Chronic cigarette smokers have a greater fraction cleared by mucociliary clearance than do nonsmokers inhaling the same particles at the same rates, which was attributed to increased tracheobronchial deposition within the chronically narrowed airways. Perhaps another reason for more mucociliary clearance in smokers is that their conductive airways are more completely covered by mucus and a greater fraction of particles depositing in the tracheobronchial airways are cleared by mucociliary clearance.

Virtually nothing is known about the clearance pathways and transport rates for those particles deposited in tracheobronchial airways that descend to the epithelial cells.

### Extent of Uptake by Epithelial Cells

As previously discussed, Brody and colleagues (11,12) have shown that some of the particles and fibers deposited at the bifurcations of alveolar ducts in rodents are taken in by type I epithelial cells. Important issues that remain are the fraction of clearance by this route and the pathways taken by the particles beyond the epithelial cells.

### Mechanisms for Epithelial Penetration by Ultrafine Particles

Ultrafine particles and ultrathin fibers (diameter 0.1 μm) penetrate the epithelial lining of the airways more rapidly than do larger particles. The mechanisms and translocation pathways for such particles need to be investigated and described.

### Role of Fibrosis in Limiting Clearance

Cytotoxic particles such as quartz and asbestos can cause lung fibrosis at relatively low dust burdens, whereas almost all insoluble dusts can cause fibrosis when overload conditions are reached. As fibrosis progresses, clearance is retarded. Lesions are detected earlier and are most pronounced in centrilobular foci, perhaps because a bottleneck effect results from the collection of dust-laden macrophages at these sites.

### Validation of an Assay for Determining Critical Dissolution Rates in Relation to Pathogenic Potential

This requires standardization of test cell design, fluid composition and pH, and flow rate through the cell.

**Determination of Critical Dissolution Rates for Pathogenic Potential in Both Laboratory Animals and Humans**

These rates are needed so that assays in animals can be extrapolated to disease risks in humans.

## ACKNOWLEDGMENTS

This chapter retains major text sections prepared for the first edition and modified in the second edition by Dr. Daryl E. Bohning. It also incorporates material originally prepared for a paper by the author entitled Particle Deposition and Accumulation in Human Lungs, which appeared in *Toxic and Carcinogenic Effects of Solid Particles in the Respiratory Tract,* edited by D. L. Dungworth, J. L. Mauderly, and G. Oberdörster (Washington, DC: ILSI Press, 1994). This review was supported as part of a Center program by the National Institute of Environmental Health Sciences, grant ES 00260.

## REFERENCES

1. Horsfield K, Cumming G. Morphology of the bronchial tree in man. *J Appl Physiol* 1968;24:373–383.
2. Weibel ER. *Morphometry of the human lung.* New York: Academic, 1963.
3. Schlesinger RB, Lippmann M. Selective particle deposition and bronchogenic carcinoma. *Environ Res* 1978;15:424–431.
4. Lippmann M, Albert RE. The effect of particle size on the regional deposition of inhaled particles in the human respiratory tract. *Am Ind Hyg Assoc J* 1969;30:257–275.
5. Morsy SM, Werner E, Stahlhofen W, Pohlit W. A detector of adjustable response for the study of lung clearance. *Health Phys* 1977;32: 243–251.
6. Scheuch G, Stahlhofen W. Deposition and dispersion of aerosols in the airways of the human respiratory tract: the effect of particle size. *Exp Lung Res* 1992;18:343–358.
7. Fang CP, Wilson JE, Spektor DM, Lippmann M. Effect of lung airway branching pattern and gas composition on particle deposition in bronchial airways. III. Experimental studies with radioactively tagged aerosol in human and canine lungs. *Exp Lung Res* 1993;19:377–396.
8. Chan TL, Lippmann M. Experimental measurements and empirical modeling of the regional deposition of inhaled particles in humans. *Am Ind Hyg Assoc J* 1980;41:399–409.
9. Martonen TB. Acid aerosol deposition in the developing human lung. In: Masuda S, Takahashi K, eds. *Aerosols: science, industry, health, and environment.* Oxford: Pergamon, 1990;1289–1291.
10. Miller FJ, Martonen TB, Menache MG, et al. Influence of breathing mode and activity level on the regional deposition of inhaled particles and implications for regulatory standards. *Ann Occup Hyg* 1988; 32(suppl 1):3–10.
11. Brody AR, Hill LH, Adkins B Jr, O'Connor RW. Chrysotile asbestos inhalation in rats: deposition pattern and reaction of alveolar epithelium and pulmonary macrophages. *Am Rev Respir Dis* 1981;123: 670–679.
12. Brody AR, Roe MW. Deposition pattern of inorganic particles at the alveolar level in the lungs of rats and mice. *Am Rev Respir Dis* 1983; 128:724–729.
13. Gehr P, Schürch S, Im Hof V, Geiser M. Inhaled particles deposited in the airways are displaced towards the epithelium. *Ann Occup Hyg* 1994;38(suppl 1):197–202.
14. Lippmann M, Timbrell V. Particle loading in the human lung-human experience and implications for exposure limits. *J Aerosol Med* 1990;3: S155–S168.
15. Lippmann M, Schlesinger RB. Interspecies comparisons of particle deposition and mucociliary clearance in tracheobronchial airways. *J Toxicol Environ Health* 1984;13:441–469.
16. Briant JK, Lippmann M. Particle transport through a hollow canine airway cast by high-frequency oscillatory ventilation. *Exp Lung Res* 1992; 18:385–407.
17. Scheuch G, Stahlhofen W. Effect of heart rate on aerosol recovery and dispersion in human conducting airways after periods of breathholding. *Exp Lung Res* 1991;17:763–787.
18. Im Hof V, Geiser M, Schürch S, Gehr P. Clearance of particles deposited on tracheal surfaces in hamsters. *Ann Occup Hyg* 1994; 38(suppl 1):203–209.
19. Bohning DE, Atkins HL, Cohn SH. Long-term particle clearance in man: normal and impaired. *Ann Occup Hyg* 1982;26:259–271.
20. Albert RE, Lippmann M, Briscoe W. The characteristics of bronchial clearance in humans and the effects of cigarette smoking. *Arch Environ Health* 1969;18:738–755.
21. Patrick G, Stirling C. The redistribution of colloidal gold particles in rat lung following local deposition by alveolar micro-injection. *Ann Occup Hyg* 1994;38(suppl 1):225–234.
22. Ferin J, Oberdörster G, Penney DP. Pulmonary retention of ultrafine and fine particles in rats. *Am J Respir Cell Mol Biol* 1992;6:535–542.
23. Ferin J, Leach LJ. The effect of amosite and chrysotile asbestos on the clearance of $TiO_2$ particles from the lung. *Environ Res* 1976;12: 250–254.
24. Bolton RE, Vincent JH, Jones AD, et al. An overload hypothesis for pulmonary clearance of UICC amosite fibers inhaled by rats. *Br J Ind Med* 1983;40:264–272.
25. Wagner JC, Skidmore JW. Asbestos dust deposition and retention in rats. *Ann NY Acad Sci* 1965;132:77–86.
26. Ferin J. Observations concerning alveolar dust clearance. *Ann NY Acad Sci* 1972;200:66–72.
27. Chan TL, Lee PS, Hering WS. Pulmonary retention of inhaled diesel particles after prolonged exposures to diesel exhaust. *Fundam Appl Toxicol* 1984;4:624–631.
28. Vincent JH, Johnston AM, Jones AD, et al. Kinetics of deposition and clearance of inhaled mineral dusts during chronic exposure. *Br J Ind Med* 1985;42:707–715.
29. Morrow PE. Possible mechanisms to explain dust overloading of the lungs. *Fundam Appl Toxicol* 1988;10:369–384.
30. Jones AD, McMillan CH, Johnston AM, et al. Pulmonary clearance of UICC amosite fibers inhaled by rats during chronic exposure at low concentration. *Br J Ind Med* 1988;45:300–304.
31. Gradon L, Pratsinis SE, Podgorski A, Scott SJ, Panda S. Modelling retention of inhaled particles in rat lungs including toxic and overloading effects. *J Aerosol Sci* 1996;27:487–503.
32. Timbrell V. Deposition and retention of fibers in the human lung. *Ann Occup Hyg* 1982;26:347–369.
33. Albert RE, Peterson HT Jr, Bohning DE, Lippmann M. Short-term effects of cigarette smoking on bronchial clearance in humans. *Arch Environ Health* 1975;30:361–367.
34. Leikauf G, Yeates DB, Wales KA, et al. Effects of sulfuric acid aerosol on respiratory mechanics and mucociliary clearance in healthy nonsmoking adults. *Am Ind Hyg Assoc J* 1981;42:273–282.
35. Lippmann M, Altshuler B. Regional deposition of aerosols. In Aharonson EF, Ben-David A, Klingberg MA, eds. *Air pollution and the lung.* Jerusalem: Wiley, 1976;25–48.
36. Green GM, Jakab GJ, Low RB, et al. Defense mechanisms of the respiratory membrane. *Am Rev Respir Dis* 1977;115:479.

*Environmental and Occupational Medicine, Third Edition,* edited by William N. Rom.
Lippincott–Raven Publishers, Philadelphia © 1998.

# CHAPTER 20

# Pulmonary Function Testing

Stuart M. Garay

Pulmonary function testing attempts to detect and quantitate abnormal lung function. Pulmonary function studies usually do not indicate a precise, specific anatomic or pathologic diagnosis. The detection of abnormal lung function by such studies helps assess the severity and progression of a disease process as well as response to therapy. This chapter provides fundamental information on the performance and interpretation of pulmonary function tests used in occupational and environmental medicine.

## HISTORY

In 1831 C.T. Thackrah described a device, known as a pulmometer, which was an inverted bell jar in water that allowed entry of air via a tap at the bottom (1). Thackrah used this device to measure lung function on the basis of occupations in his classic book *The Effects of the Principal Arts, Trades, and Professions on Health and Longevity* (2). Thus, “Nineteen individuals from the 14th Light Dragoons gave an average of 4280 ml a man.” He also concluded that tailors, despite their tendency to curvature of the spine, phthisis, and anal fistula, did not have reduced ventilation: the average exhaled volume was 4,360 ml. It was not until 1846, however, that John Hutchinson designed his water-sealed spirometer and published his systematic assessment of lung volumes in more than 4,000 subjects, classifying them as paupers, First Battalion Grenadier Guards, pugilists and wrestlers, giants and dwarfs, girls, gentlemen, and diseased cases (3,4). Hutchinson’s interest in establishing normal values for vital capacity related to his work with insurance companies, from which he received much of his income. Hutchinson defined vital capacity as the number of cubic inches given by a full expiration following the deepest inspiration. He also described other lung volumes as “complemental air” (inspiratory reserve volume), “breathing air” (tidal volume), “reserve air” (expiratory reserve volume), and “residual air” (residual volume). Hutchinson established the linear relationship between vital capacity and height and firmly established that pulmonary diseases, specifically tuberculosis, resulted in reduced vital capacity. Despite Hutchinson’s major contributions, his spirometer was not frequently utilized; an account in the 1890s contained this comment (1): “At the Brompton Hospital his spirometer was not much used, because patients require education in doing so. ... The instrument was useful in obscure cases.”

In the first quarter of this century spirometers were utilized intensively by physiologists but little by clinicians. By 1930, however, clinicians such as Alvin Barach (5) began exploring the importance of ventilatory measurements for assessing diseases such as asthma and emphysema. Concurrently, in the 1930s and 1940s preoperative assessment in the newly developing field of thoracic surgery spurned the use of quantitative assessment before and after lung resection (6). The deleterious effects of various abdominal operations on lung function was also being recognized (7,8). The establishment by Baldwin and coworkers (9) in 1948 of predictive values for vital capacity based on age, sex, and height led to routine use of this parameter, especially for preoperative evaluation. Finally, the work of Tiffeneau and Pinelli (10) in France during the 1940s and of Gaensler (11,12) in the United States during the late 1940s and early 1950s established the timed vital capacity maneuver, specifically the measurement of that portion of the vital capacity exhaled in

S. M. Garay: Division of Pulmonary and Critical Care Medicine, New York University Medical Center, New York, New York 10016.

the first second, as an accurate method of assessing air flow limitation. In 1933, Hermannsen in Germany described the maximum voluntary ventilation test; Cournand and Richards (13) described this test in the English literature in 1941. They believed this test to be a better assessment of ventilatory function than vital capacity but recognized that it was nonspecific.

The addition of motorized chart recorders to spirometers such as the water-sealed Stead-Wells spirometer allowed graphic analysis of the spirogram in terms of volume versus time (14). Various spirometric indices were proposed in addition to the forced expiratory volume in 1 second ($FEV_1$) and forced vital capacity (FVC). One measurement that gained wide acceptance was the maximal midexpiratory flow ($FEF_2$) introduced by Leuallen and Fowler (15) in 1955, because measurement of the slope of the volume-time curve estimated flow. In the late 1960s, through the early 1970s, direct assessment of air flow limitation was achieved by measuring inspiratory and expiratory flow and plotting these rates against exhaled volume (vital capacity) (16). The forced expiratory maneuver generated the data for both the flow-volume and volume-time curves.

During the past 50 years spirometer designs have proliferated. Today spirometers are either volume-displacement devices such as the water-seal, dry rolling-seal, and bellows-volume spirometers, or flow types such as Fleisch, wire mesh, hot-wire, and turbine pneumotachograph. Volume-displacement spirometers measure exhaled volume directly, whereas flow spirometers measure air flow rate in liters per second and multiply (by seconds) to obtain volume indirectly. Pneumotachographs contain a flow transducer that converts flow into a signal that is integrated electronically to obtain volume.

While computerized spirometers can quickly display both curves and analyze data quickly, studies have demonstrated that some spirometers have errors as great as 1.5 L in the forced vital capacity measurement, or almost 25% (17). Nelson and coworkers (18) demonstrated that only 53% of 57 contemporary commercially available spirometers could meet American Thoracic Society (ATS) performance criteria. Software errors were found in 27% of computerized systems (18). Thus, recommendations for spirometer performance and validation have been published by the ATS (17).

## LUNG VOLUMES

### Measurement of Lung Volumes

Measurement of lung volumes provides fundamental information that makes possible categorization and staging of lung diseases. However, lung volumes provide a static picture and do not measure dynamic performance. The four subdivisions of maximum lung volume described by Hutchinson include the following (Figs. 1 and 2):

1. Tidal volume ($V_T$), the volume of air inspired and expired with each breath
2. Inspiratory reserve volume (IRV), the maximum volume of air that may be inhaled beyond a normal tidal breath
3. Residual volume (RV), the volume of air that remains in the lungs after maximal expiration
4. Expiratory reserve volume (ERV), the maximum volume that may be exhaled between the resting end-tidal position and residual volume.

On the basis of these four volumes, four capacities can be described (Figs. 1 and 2):

1. Total lung capacity (TLC), the amount of air in the chest after a maximum inspiration, equal to the sum of all four lung volumes ($TLC = RV + ERV + V_T + IRV$)
2. Vital capacity (VC), the maximum amount of air expired after a maximum inspiration (i.e., the total amount of air that can be moved in and out of the lungs ($VC = ERV + V_T + IRV = TLC\text{-}RV$)
3. Functional residual capacity (FRC), the amount of air remaining in the lungs at the end-tidal position ($FRC = RV + ERV$)
4. Inspiratory capacity (IC), the maximum volume of air inspired from end-tidal position ($IC = V_T + IRV$).

Spirometric volumes are relatively simple to obtain. The subject is instructed to breathe normally with a resting tidal pattern as the volume is being recorded. Next the subject inspires maximally, then exhales as completely as possible with a slow, continuous, smooth exhalation and returns to tidal breathing. The result is the slow vital capacity (SVC). The forced vital capacity (FVC) is mea-

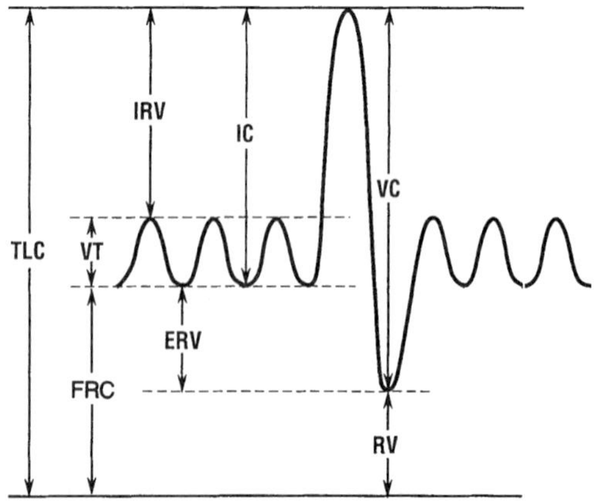


**FIG. 1.** Lung volumes and capacities. TLC, total lung capacity; VC, vital capacity; RV, residual volume; FRC, functional residual capacity; IC, inspiratory capacity; IRV, inspiratory reserve volume; Vt, tidal volume; ERV, expiratory reserve volume.

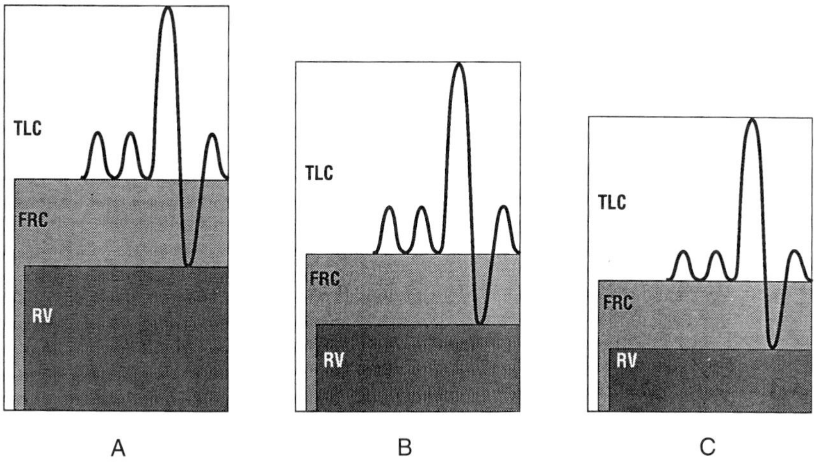


**FIG. 2.** Lung volume patterns in patients with **(A)** obstructive lung disease, **(B)** normal patients, and **(C)** patients with restrictive lung disease. Patients with obstructive lung disease (A) are hyperinflated, resulting in an increased TLC. In addition, air trapping results in a decreased VC as a result of increased RV and FRC. Patients with restrictive lung disease (C) have reduced TLC, FRC, VC, and RV.

sured with virtually the same maneuver, but the patient is instructed to exert maximal forced expiratory effort (17). This maneuver is used to assess air flow. In normal persons the SVC and FVC are virtually equivalent, the difference being no more than 0.2 L. In some individuals who suffer airflow obstruction, forceful exhalation causes airways to close prematurely because of the increased intrathoracic pressure produced. This phenomenon of "air trapping" results from dynamic compression due to increased resistance of intrathoracic airways and loss of elastic recoil. When it is marked, it suggests emphysema (secondary to loss of elastic recoil), but it may be associated with asthma or chronic bronchitis (secondary to bronchospasm). A minimum of three acceptable FVC maneuvers should be attempted, and up to eight maneuvers, to ensure reproducibility (17).

Vital capacity and its subdivisions (ERV, TV, IRC, IC) can be measured by spirometry. Because spirometry does not provide a measure of RV, determination of TLC (TLC = RV + VC) is precluded. Spirometry also cannot provide the end-tidal volume (the FRC). Any one of these three "absolute" volumes can be used to derive the other two by utilizing the appropriate subdivisions of the spirometric vital capacity (Fig. 1). Three different techniques may be used to measure FRC or RV: two multiple-breath, steady-state gas-dilution methods (closed-circuit helium dilution and open-circuit nitrogen washout) and body plethysmography. These methods yield the FRC measurement, from which the spirometrically determined ERV is subtracted to yield RV (RV = FRC − ERV). RV is added to VC to yield TLC (TLC = VC + RV). The single-breath gas-dilution technique, used principally to determine diffusing capacity (see below), measures alveolar volume (VA), which should equal the TLC derived by other methods. While it is not often used to determine TLC, it can provide an "internal check" on the accuracy of TLC as determined by other methods and on the validity of the diffusing capacity ($D_LCO$) measurement. Details of the actual performance of these techniques can be found elsewhere, though a brief overview follows (19–26). Radiographic techniques utilizing planimetry or the ellipsoid method measure TLC, but their accuracy is highly variable, and so they will not be discussed further (27–29).

During multiple-breath steady-state gas-dilution techniques, the patient breathes continuously while a tracer gas is either equilibrated in the lungs (closed-circuit helium dilution) or eliminated (open-circuit nitrogen washout) from the lungs. In the "wash-in" method, the patient breathes helium from a reservoir of known volume and size, thereby diluting its concentration in the lungs. Since the total amount of helium (volume × concentration) does not change, the initial volume and concentration are known, and the final concentration is measured. The final unknown volume (FRC) can be calculated:

$$\text{FRC} = \frac{(\text{Initial helium conc} - \text{Final helium conc})}{\text{Final helium conc}} \times V_S \qquad [1]$$

where $V_S$ = volume in the spirometer.

During the open-circuit nitrogen washout method, the patient breathes 100% oxygen to wash out the nitrogen to a negligible plateau concentration (1% to 2%). This test assumes that the gas within the lungs is 79% nitrogen and then nitrogen concentration in the lungs and atmosphere are in equilibrium. Thus, if the nitrogen is washed out of the lungs and measured, this measurement represents 79% of an unknown volume. As the nitrogen washes out of the lungs, the volume and nitrogen percentage of the exhaled gas are measured. The test is stopped when the nitrogen concentration levels off at a negligible value (1% to 2%):

$$(\text{FRC} \times \text{initial } N_2\%) = (\text{Exhaled vol}) \times (\text{Final } N_2\%) \qquad [2]$$

$$FRC = \frac{(\text{Exhaled vol}) \times (\text{Final } N_2\%)}{(\text{Initial } N_2\%)} \quad [3]$$

Body plethysmography applies Boyle's law, which states that in a closed system the product of pressure and volume within the system remains constant. Consequently, the volume of gas varies inversely with the pressure to which it is subjected. Pfluger is credited with first applying Boyle's law to measure residual volume (30). In 1882 he built a metal cylinder, or *Menschendose* (literally, *man can)*, in which a subject was placed who was instructed to exhale completely to residual volume. Pfluger decompressed the cylinder, causing the alveolar gas to expand; this expansion-derived gas was collected in a spirometer into which the subject breathed. Pfluger calculated the original volume of the lungs, since he already knew the initial alveolar pressure, the new lower pressure, and the volume of the gas leaving the lungs during decompression. He reported values of 400 to 800 ml for RV in normal adult men. The modern body plethysmograph consists of an airtight chamber, a pneumotachograph to measure flow at the mouth, pressure transducers to measure mouth and box pressure, and a solenoid-operated shutter in the mouthpiece. The patient sits in the box, breathing through the mouthpiece. After the door to the box is closed, the mouthpiece shutter is closed at end-tidal position and the patient takes shallow panting breaths with an open glottis at a rate of 1 to 2 per second. The panting maneuver alternatively compresses and decompresses the thorax, resulting in small changes in mouth and box pressures. Since there is no flow, changes in mouth pressure are assumed to be equal to changes in alveolar pressure, and changes in box pressure can be used to calculate thoracic volume by applying Boyle's law:

$$P_1V_1 = P_2V_2 \quad [4]$$

$$P_{FRC} \times V_{FRC} = (P_{FRC} - \Delta P) \times (V_{FRC} - \Delta V) \quad [5]$$

$P_{FRC}$ is alveolar pressure, which equals atmospheric pressure when there is no flow (shutter occluded) at end-tidal position or FRC; $V_{FRC}$ is lung volume at FRC; $\Delta P$ is the small decrease in alveolar pressure that occurs with each inspiratory pant; and AV is the small increase in volume that occurs with each inspiratory pant.

The volume at FRC can then be calculated by rearranging this equation:

$$V_{FRC} = \frac{\Delta V}{\Delta P}(P_{FRC} - \Delta P) \quad [6]$$

The value of $\Delta P$ is very small and therefore can be ignored.

### *Comparison of Techniques: Pitfalls in Measurements of Lung Volume*

Various studies have demonstrated good correlation between the different techniques in normal subjects. Significant differences may occur in disease states. Gas-dilution techniques measure communicating gas volume within the airways. Thus, in patients with bullous disease or severe obstructive airway disease, noncommunicating or poorly communicating airways may result in underestimation of lung volumes by gas-dilution techniques (31). In both the open- and closed-circuit techniques, the RV is measured indirectly as a subdivision of FRC. In practice, the resting end-tidal level is more reproducible than the volume at the extreme of complete inspiration (TLC) or complete expiration (RV). FRC is the lung volume at which the respiratory muscles are at rest and lung and chest wall elastic recoil are counterbalanced. The resting end-tidal volume, as well as the ERV, must be accurately determined. If the subject's pattern of tidal breathing is irregular, the end-tidal position, and therefore the ERV, may be falsely elevated, resulting in a reduced RV (RV = FRC − ERV). Subsequent calculation of the TLC (TLC= VC + RV) will yield an erroneously diminished TLC, misdiagnosing a restrictive process. Finally, with gas techniques, gas analyzer malfunction as well as circuit leaks may produce an FRC value that is disproportionate to other lung function measures. Gas leaks in the system can cause overestimation with the helium-dilution method, resulting in falsely high values.

Plethysmography measures the total intrathoracic volume that is compressed during the panting maneuver. The FRC measurement is subject to error if the study is begun at an inappropriate starting volume (i.e., not at end-tidal position). The measured volume reflects the actual volume in the thorax at the start and end of the study. Plethysmography may overestimate true lung volumes by compressing compliant airways that narrow during the panting procedure, resulting in failure of mouth and alveolar equalization (32,33). A major disadvantage of plethysmography is that the body box is large and expensive. Claustrophobia and physical handicaps prevent certain patients from sitting in the box. Finally, some patients are unable to perform the requisite panting maneuver.

## Application of Lung Volume Measurements

Lung volumes may be altered by disease processes that affect respiratory muscles, chest wall, parenchyma, and airways. FRC represents the point of dynamic equilibrium, when the opposing forces of lung and chest wall recoil are counterbalanced. TLC is determined by inspiratory muscle strength, lung elastic recoil, and, to a lesser extent, chest wall elastic recoil. Finally, expiratory muscle strength, chest wall recoil, and (to a lesser extent) elastic recoil at low lung volumes affect RV.

Determination of all lung volumes (VC, TLC, FRC, and RV) is crucial for assessing the presence of a truly restrictive process. The isolated reduction in vital capacity, as may be detected by simple spirometry, does not imply a restrictive process. Thus, epidemiologic field studies or individual clinical examinations that measure only VC by spirometry can be misleading. Diseases that cause airflow limitation, such as asthma, chronic bronchitis, and emphysema, also result in a diminished vital capacity, usually in conjunction with reduced expiratory flow rate. These "obstructive" diseases usually result in an increase in RV and FRC, whereas with true restrictive processes most or all volumes are reduced. In patients with reduced VC due to chronic obstructive pulmonary disease (COPD), RV and FRC are elevated in proportion to the degree of air flow limitation. TLC variably is affected, being elevated with emphysema, to a lesser degree with chronic bronchitis, and sometimes with asthma [being elevated only during a deteriorating state (34)]. Although an isolated RV elevation is unusual, Vulterini and co-workers (35) observed a significant elevation of RV in 14 patients who had normal VC, $FEV_1$, $FEF_{50\%}$, and airway resistance values. These persons, predominantly cigarette smokers, had decreased measured lung elastic recoil, which led the authors to conclude that they had airway disease. The term *air trapping* is sometimes used to denote an increase in RV, whereas *hyperinflation* refers to an absolute increase in TLC. Yip and coworkers (36) demonstrated that in stable COPD patients FRC is a useful guide to static recoil properties of the lung. An increase in FRC is a useful index of emphysema and the degree of hyperinflation, even in the presence of chronic airway disease.

Restrictive lung disease is often defined physiologically as a decrease in lung volumes, specifically VC and TLC, but the term *restrictive lung disease* is a misnomer. Many different disease processes result in diminished lung volumes. It is more appropriate to modify the "restrictive" by adding an anatomic correlate, for example, restrictive interstitial or parenchymal disease (idiopathic fibrosis, asbestosis, allergic alveolitis), restrictive neuromuscular lung disease (myotonic dystrophy, amyotrophic lateral sclerosis, Guillain-Barré syndrome, diaphragmatic paralysis), restrictive pleural disease (fibrothorax, mesothelioma), restrictive chest wall disease (kyphoscoliosis, ankylosing spondylitis).

A restrictive process may be suggested by reduced VC and normal $FEV_1$/FVC ratio on spirometry. Reduced lung volumes, especially TLC, confirm the presence of a restrictive process. VC and TLC usually fall in parallel, though concurrent reduction in FRC and RV is variable. Restrictive parenchymal processes and chest wall abnormalities such as kyphoscoliosis result in diminished FRC and variable diminution in RV. In contrast, ankylosing spondylitis, a chest wall disorder, results in diminished VC and TLC while FRC and RV are elevated. Finally, neuromuscular disorders usually do not affect FRC; inspiratory muscle weakness results in normal RV, whereas expiratory muscle weakness results in elevated RV. An isolated reduction in FRC is most often associated with obesity or another process (ascites, pregnancy) that increases abdominal girth and contents and reduces ERV. It should be noted that the same mechanism may result in an isolated reduction in VC, which may be measured spirometrically Finally, an isolated reduction in RV often reflects inadequacies in the measurement or the predicted normal value, as opposed to true disease, though it can also reflect parenchymal or chest wall abnormalities, as reported by Owens and coworkers (37), who found 69 patients with isolated reductions in RV with normal VC and the diffusing capacity for CO ($D_LCO$). In 91% (63 patients) definite or probable clinical disease accounted for radiographically apparent parenchymal disease in 38 (congestive heart failure, 12; sarcoidosis, 6; infection, 1; drug toxicity, 1; rheumatoid arthritis, 1) and radiographically apparent chest wall disease in 25 (skeletal deformity, 10; fibrothorax, 7; myasthenia, 2; other, 2).

It should be emphasized that, when it is possible, serial testing is often useful in establishing a diagnosis of restrictive or obstructive disease in patients whose values are borderline or slightly elevated. The range of normal values is often great, as is intersubject variability (see Normal Values, below). Thus, sequentially diminishing lung volumes within the normal range may suggest early restrictive disease, especially if other deficits, such as reduced diffusing capacity (in interstitial disease) or reduced maximum inspiratory and expiratory pressures (in neuromuscular disease), are observed. Indeed, in conjunction with reduced expiratory flow rates, serial lung volume measurements may detect the occasional patient with asthma who has airflow limitation associated with reduced lung volume (38,39). In such cases restrictive lung disease is often misdiagnosed on the basis of one isolated set of pulmonary function test results.

The subject of normal values and predictive equations is discussed in a subsequent section. With respect to lung volumes, considerable differences in normal predictive values have been published (40–44). There may be as much as a 1-L difference between predicted values for the same individual. Traditionally, many laboratories have used 80% to 120% of the predicted value as the outer limits of normal. More recently, the 95th confidence interval (CI) has been advocated to define the lower limit of normal. Viljanen and coauthors (45) defined 95% confidence limits for TLC in men and women as 80% to 125% of the predicted value, and limits for RV of 60% to 160% for men and 65% to 155% for women. However, Crapo and co-workers (46) have stated that a single value for the 95% CI was most appropriate, suggesting that normal values, defined by single values expressed as a percentage predicted (e.g., ±20% for TLC) were not valid. Nonetheless, many clinical laboratories continue to use percentages predicted to grade severity (Table 1). Finally, several studies have found that blacks have lower lung volumes than Caucasians (47). This has been attributed to blacks having shorter trunks and longer legs. As a result,

**TABLE 1.** *Various investigators' results of grading degrees of abnormality for lung volumes[a]*

| | Miller (216) | | Ries/Clausen (81) | | Morris (62) | |
|---|---|---|---|---|---|---|
| | RV | TLC | RV | FRC | TLC | RV |
| Increase | | | | | | |
| Normal | 80–134 | 80–120 | | | | 81–120 |
| Mild | 135–159 | | 135–150 | 135–150 | 120–130 | |
| Moderate | 150–199 | >121 | 150–250 | 150–200 | 130–150 | >121 |
| Severe | 200–249 | | >250 | >200 | >150 | |
| Decrease | | | | | | |
| Mild | 70–79 | | 55–65 | 55–65 | 70–80 | |
| Moderate | 60–69 | ≤79 | 45–55 | 45–55 | 60–70 | |
| Severe | 50–59 | | <45 | <45 | <60 | |

[a]Upper and lower limits of predicted percentage.

some laboratories reduce Caucasian predicted values by 15%.

## STATIC LUNG MECHANICS

### Lung Compliance

Lung compliance measures the distensibility of the lungs. Compliance (C) is defined as the volume change per unit of pressure (P) change (i.e., $C = \Delta V/\Delta P$). Elastic recoil pressure ($P_{EL}$) is the pressure generated by the lungs at a particular lung volume, usually total lung capacity. Compliance of the lungs ($C_L$), of the chest wall ($C_{cw}$), and of the total lung chest wall system ($C_T$) may be measured. Determination of lung compliance ($C_L$) requires measuring intrapleural pressure when there is no flow of air in and out of the lungs at various lung volumes to generate a pressure-volume curve (48) (Fig. 3). An esophageal balloon is passed into the esophagus; esophageal pressure approximates intrapleural pressure in the upright position (49). The subject inspires to TLC and begins slowly exhaling. Inspiratory flow at the mouth is repeatedly interrupted at small volume intervals. Since airway pressure during the occlusion is equal to alveolar pressure, the transpulmonary pressure is determined as the difference between airway and esophageal pressure. The volumes and corresponding pressures are plotted to generate a pressure-volume curve (Fig. 3). Static lung compliance ($C_{LST}$) is the slope of the curve

$$C_{LST} = \frac{\Delta V(\text{liters})}{\Delta P(\text{cm } H_2O)} \quad [7]$$

and is normally recorded in the tidal breathing range (approximately 500 to 1000 ml above FRC).

The static lung compliance is usually related to the absolute lung volume at which the measurement was made, since compliance is directly related to lung volume. The specific compliance is $C_{LST}/V_L$, the volume usually being FRC. The maximum pressure generated at TLC divided by the TLC is known as the coefficient of retraction. Schlueter and coworkers (50) demonstrated that the coefficient of retraction is reduced with emphysema and increased with interstitial disease.

Measurement of lung compliance is not a routine test and is performed selectively or for research purposes. Lung compliance can be measured with a spirometer but more often body plethysmography is used, because the mouth shutter, the pneumotachograph that measures flow, and the pressure transducer are all available in the body box. In a normal adult both $C_L$ and $C_{CW}$ are 0.2 L/cm $H_2O$ each. They can be added in a series to yield $C_T$ of the lungs-chest wall system:

$$\frac{1}{C_L} + \frac{1}{C_{CW}} = \frac{1}{C_T}, \quad [8]$$

thus

$$\frac{1}{0.2} + \frac{1}{0.2} = 10 \quad [9]$$

where the reciprocal of 10 is the total compliance, $C_T = 0.1$ L/cm $H_2O$. The total compliance is less than either of its components, since the chest wall and lungs counterbalance each other.

Lung compliance reflects the elasticity of the parenchyma. With advancing age, changes in connective

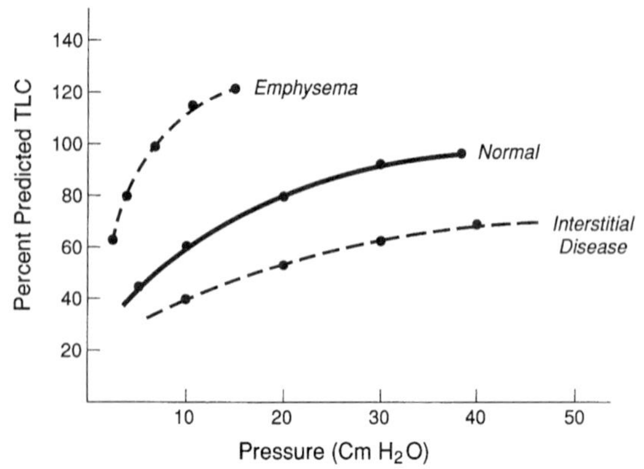


**FIG. 3.** Pressure–volume curve. Representative curves for normal subjects and for patients with emphysema and interstitial lung disease.

tissue alter the elastic fibers in the lungs, increasing the static lung compliance (51–53). Emphysema is the principal disease that results in increased compliance, owing to destruction of elastic tissue in alveolar septa (50,54). Because there is decreased lung elastic recoil, the balance of forces between the lungs and chest wall is altered, resulting in higher lung volumes at end-expiration (FRC). In the acute stage of asthma, patients may also have increased lung compliance, but this reverses following therapy (55). In contrast, lung compliance is decreased with disease processes that result in alveolar filling or interstitial abnormalities (47). Pulmonary edema, atelectasis, and pneumonia account for the former, whereas idiopathic pulmonary fibrosis, asbestosis, radiation, various drug-induced interstitial diseases, and sarcoidosis are some of the diseases that account for the latter (56,57). Fibrotic interstitial disease may result in decreased lung compliance owing to increased connective tissue in the alveolar septa or to a uniform mixture of normal and obliterated alveoli. Finally, chest wall compliance ($C_W$) may also be reduced by kyphoscoliosis or obesity.

The pathophysiologic mechanisms of interstitial disease range from diffuse impairment of all alveoli to a more selective process resulting in a "shrunken lung," in which functioning and nonfunctioning alveoli intermix. Gibson and Pride (57) predicted that the relationship between lung compliance and disease-induced volume loss could not distinguish between the two processes. They, as well as Sharp and colleagues (56), emphasized that altered lung compliance can result from either process. Furthermore, the reduction in lung compliance was disproportionate to the loss of lung volume. More recently, Kanengiser and associates (58) confirmed these findings and found that volume adjustment of compliance resulted in both low and "normal" ratios in patients with severe disease and thus was not helpful for distinguishing the mechanisms or the severity of disease.

## MAXIMAL INSPIRATORY AND EXPIRATORY PRESSURE

The measurement of maximal inspiratory pressure (MIP or $P_{IMAX}$) and maximal expiratory pressure (MEP or $P_{EMAX}$) is used to assess respiratory muscle strength. Maximal respiratory pressure is simple to measure but requires the patient's cooperation and effort. The $P_{IMAX}$ is measured by having the patient rapidly exhale from TLC and occluding the airway at RV. A maximal inspiratory effort is performed against an occluded valve for at least 2 seconds. $P_{EMAX}$ is measured by having the patient inhale from RV; the airway is occluded at TLC and the patient subsequently exhales. The greatest value of three determinations is recorded for both TLC and $P_{EMAX}$. Normal predicted values for maximal respiratory pressures have been reported by Black and Hyatt (59) and by Rochester and Arora (60). $P_{IMAX}$ measures inspiratory muscle strength and normally is not less than –60 cm $H_2O$. A decreased $P_{IMAX}$ is associated with neuromuscular disease and with diaphragmatic dysfunction. Patients with COPD whose lungs are hyperinflated or who have chest wall disorders may also have a decreased $P_{IMAX}$. $P_{EMAX}$ measures the function of accessory muscles of respiration, abdominal muscles, and elastic recoil. Normally, $P_{EMAX}$ is more than 80 to 100 cm $H_2O$. This value is decreased in neuromuscular disorders.

## DYNAMIC LUNG FUNCTION

### Spirometry

Analysis of volume-time or flow-volume relationships provides an assessment of the ventilatory apparatus "in action" (Figs. 4 and 5). Spirometry is the measurement of volume change achieved by various breathing maneuvers. Volume-time analysis utilizes the "simple" or "classic" spirogram, whereas the flow-volume relationships are described by the maximum expiratory flow-volume curve (also referred to as the F-V loop). The same basic maneuver, the FVC maneuver, generates data for both analyses.

### Technical Aspects of Spirometry

The FVC maneuver requires the patient to inhale maximally to TLC and then exhale as rapidly and forcefully as possible. The exhaled volume is plotted on an *x-y* recorder, the *y* axis being volume and *x* axis time. The ATS spirometry recommendations suggest a minimum exhalation time of 6 seconds unless an obvious plateau (at least 2 seconds) has been achieved (17). Often, a longer exhalation (up to 10 seconds) is necessary, especially with advanced COPD. The ATS guidelines recommend three to eight consecutive FVC attempts (see

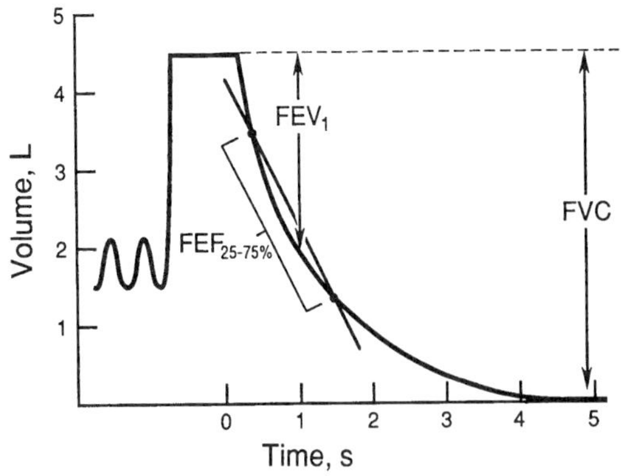


**FIG. 4.** Typical spirogram plotting volume against time. The $FEV_1$ (forced expiratory volume in 1 second) as well as the $FEF_{25–75\%}$ can be determined from the graph. The former can be easily read from the graph. The latter is found by marking the points at which 25% and 75% of the FVC have been expired. The slope of this line can be determined by dividing half of the FVC by the interval between the two points.

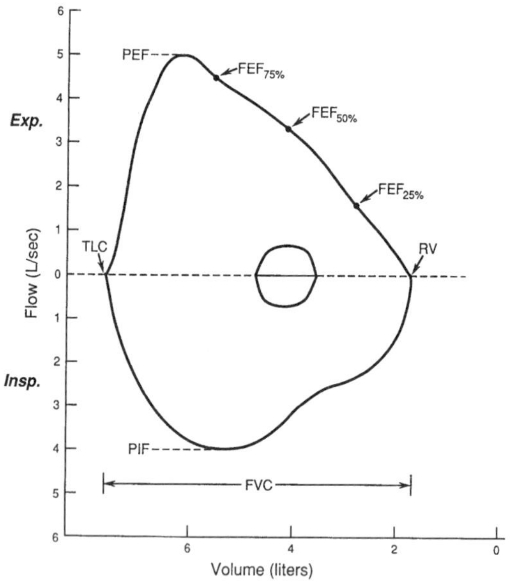


**FIG. 5.** A typical F-V loop demonstrating inspiratory and expiratory limbs. Inspiratory flow rates are measured at 75% ($FEF_{75\%}$), 50% ($FEF_{50\%}$), and 25% ($FEF_{25\%}$) of the FVC. PEF and PIF can also be determined. The end-expiration point occurs at RV; end inspiration at TLC. A smaller tidal loop is sometimes depicted. The end-tidal volume (not depicted) is FRC.

below). The pulmonary function technician must confirm that the patient understood the instructions, and achieved a maximal inspiration with a proper start, a continuous smooth exhalation, and a maximal effort. Gardner et al. (61) summarized complications that render an FVC maneuver unacceptable: coughing during the first second of the maneuver, glottic closure (Valsalva's maneuver), a leak in the system, obstruction of the mouthpiece (by dentures or tongue), and unsatisfactory start of expiration owing to excessive hesitation or a false start. The back-extrapolation method (Fig. 6) is used to determine the start of the FVC. It assumes that the FVC maneuver is initiated at peak flow (which occurs at TLC). A tangent drawn from the steepest part of the slope on the volume-time curve intersects the time axis at 0, or the true start of the FVC maneuver. The extrapolated volume is the volume of air exhaled before time 0. It should be less than 5% of the FVC or 0.100 L, whichever value is greater, for an acceptable maneuver (17,61).

It is desirable to have a minimum of three acceptable FVC maneuvers to ensure maximal effort and provide an accurate reflection of the patient's pulmonary function (17,61,62). The ATS further recommends reproducibility criteria, suggesting that the largest and next to largest FVC from acceptable curves should not vary by more than 5% or 0.100 L, whichever is greater (17). The same criteria are applied to the largest and next to largest $FEV_1$. The largest FVC and the largest $FEV_1$ should be recorded, even if the two values do not come from the same curve. Thus, the "best test" curve is defined (17) as the test that meets acceptability criteria and gives the largest sum of FVC and $FEV_1$. The acceptability criteria are used to determine whether more than three FVC maneuvers should be performed before the reproducibility criteria are applied. The only criterion for unacceptable performance that would eliminate the subject from evaluation is fewer than two acceptable curves. The reproducibility criteria are a guide to whether more than three FVC maneuvers is needed. Poor reproducibility should not be cause for rejecting the curves provided three acceptable maneuvers were obtained. The ATS (17) further states, "Use of data from maneuvers with poor reproducibility is left to the discretion of the interpreter." The ATS committee cautions that if acceptability criteria are not applied before the reproducibility criteria, a passive exhalation maneuver will be labeled as "best" maneuver, because it may give the largest sum of FVC plus $FEV_1$ (17).

Recently, it was suggested that eliminating some patients' data from epidemiologic surveys because of poor reproducibility may eliminate patients inappropriately and result in a population bias (63,64). Patients with airways obstruction have greater coefficients of variation than normal healthy persons (65); some may not fulfill ATS reproducibility criteria. Glindmeyer and coworkers (66) examined potential sources of error in spirometry despite application of ATS acceptability criteria and stressed the need for visual inspection of the curves. Furthermore, the technician who collects the data and the physician who interprets the results must be knowledgeable of technical artifacts and potential effects on each parameter. Indeed, even though FVC maneuvers met ATS quantitative criteria, visual inspection of the tracings revealed visible defects, which were more evident when subjects were followed longitudinally (66). Hankinson

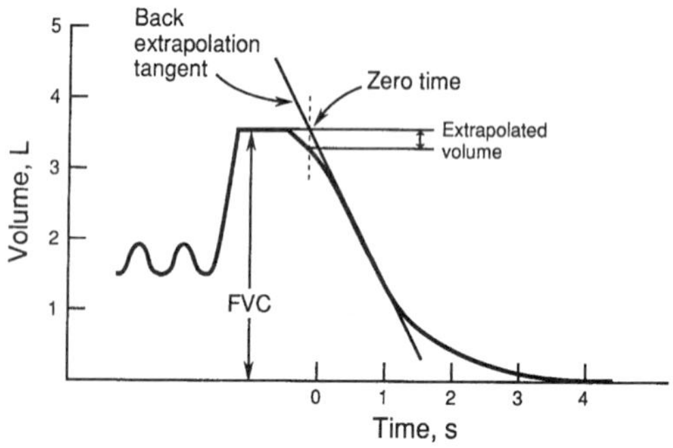


**FIG. 6.** The back-extrapolation method is used to determine the start of test. A straight line is drawn through the steepest portion of the curve, extending to cross the volume baseline. The point of intersection is back-extrapolated to time 0. The $FEV_1$ is measured from this starting point. The *dashed line* from time 0 to the curve is the back-extrapolated volume, which should be less than 5% of the FVC or 100 ml, whichever is greater (see text).

and Bang (67) analyzed 6,486 subjects aged 8 to 90 years from the general population to determine the ability of normal subjects to satisfy the ATS acceptability and reproducibility criteria. They found that subjects younger than age 18 and older than 55 years had more difficulty meeting the ATS reproducibility criteria. In lieu of the ATS criterion, a constant 200-ml reproducibility criterion for FVC and $FEV_1$ was used; the failure rate was similar for all heights, suggesting that basing the ATS criterion on a percentage of FVC and FEV may be inappropriate, especially for younger patients with smaller heights and lung volumes. In addition, there was uniform intrasubject variability for FVC and $FEV_1$, in terms of the mean difference between the largest and next to largest values.

## SPIROMETRIC INTERPRETATION

Interpretation of spirometry requires the determination of whether the patient's test results are less than the lower limits of normal. Many laboratories have classified values of FVC and $FEV_1$ less than 80% of predicted as abnormal. However, this has no statistical basis (68). While some studies have demonstrated that use of 80% of predicted FVC and $FEV_1$ is close to the 5th percentile in adults of average age and height, use of this fixed value (80%) will result in shorter, older subjects being classified as "abnormal," whereas taller younger adults are more likely to be classified as "normal." Similarly, defining a fixed $FEV_1$/FVC ratio as a lower limit of normal is also not recommended in adults because $FEV_1$/FVC is inversely related to age and height. Use of a fixed ratio may result in an increase in impairment associated with aging. Furthermore, some athletes as well as some workers in physically demanding occupations such as mining and deep sea diving may have FVC values relatively larger than $FEV_1$ values, resulting in a lower $FEV_1$/FVC ratio.

One statistically acceptable approach for establishing the lower limits of normal for spirometric measurements is to define the lowest 5% of the reference population as below the lower limit of normal. If individual observations have a Gaussian distribution, the value of the 5th percentile can be calculated as follows: lower limit of normal = predicted value − 1.645 × SEE (where SEE is standard error of the estimate). Finally, lower limits of normal are variable and should not be considered as arbitrary limits that correctly classify all patients. Patient values that are close to the lower limits of normal should be interpreted with caution.

### Flow Rates

Several measurements can be obtained from a volume-time recording of a forced expiration VC maneuver. The maximum volume exhaled in the first second of the FVC maneuver is the $FEV_1$. Although $FEV_1$ is a measure of volume, it is also a measure of mean flow during the first second. Because flow is a function of lung volume, a more sensitive evaluation of flow is derived by relating $FEV_1$ to FVC (i.e., the $FEV_1$/FVC ratio). Normally, humans can exhale 70% to 80% of their FVC in 1 second.

The maximal midexpiratory flow rate ($FEF_{25-75\%}$) is the average flow between 25% and 75% of VC. It is the average rate of flow during the middle half of the FVC maneuver (15). It is determined from the slope of the line connecting the points on the volume-time curve that correspond to 25% and 75% of the FVC (Fig. 4). Previously utilized flow rates $FEF_{200-1200}$ as well as $FEF_{75\%-85\%}$ have not proven useful because of the wide range for 95% confidence limits for normal values. The $FEF_{25-75\%}$ is determined by the later, effort-independent part of forced expiratory maneuver, which does not increase with further effort. Abnormalities in $FEF_{25-75\%}$ may occur in the setting of normal $FEV_1$ and $FEV_1$/FVC, suggesting medium-sized or small airways obstruction. The $FEF_{25-75\%}$ varies significantly in normal subjects. As noted above with respect to $FEV_1$ and FVC measurement, the practice of using 80% of predicted as the lower limit of normal for $FEF_{25-75\%}$ or the instantaneous flow rates generated by the flow-volume loop will also cause some serious errors. For these flow rates, the lower limit of normal is closer to 50% of predicted. Thus its usefulness is limited despite its popularity. The test result also depends in part on subject effort. There is no evidence that the $FEF_{25-75\%}$ is a more reliable measure of flow than others (69). Knudson and Lebowitz (69) have presented data for the percent predicted value of $FEF_{25-75\%}$ above which 95% of asymptomatic nonsmokers fall: for men older than 36 years, 56.2%; for women over 36 years, 57.2% predicted.

The maximum expiratory flow-volume curve (F-V loop) records flow versus volume (16,70) (Fig. 5). The FEF depicts instantaneous flow at variously reported volumes: $FEF_{max}$ or peak expiratory flow rate (PEFR), which occurs at 90% TLC, $FEF_{50\%}$ (FEF at 50% FVC), $FEF_{25\%}$ (FEF at 25% FVC, also reported as $FEF_{75\%}$, i.e., flow after 75% of FVC is exhaled). Normally, on maximal exhalation there is a rapid peak flow (at 90% of the TLC) and a linear decline in instantaneous flow rate as volume (i.e., VC) decreases. The initial portion of the F-V loop (from peak flow to $FEF_{50\%}$) is effort dependent and so can vary. The flow from $FEF_{50\%}$ downward is relatively effort independent; further effort cannot increase flow rates as flow is determined by lung elastic recoil and the flow-resistive properties of the smaller airways (71). Maximal expiratory flow (MEF) at a given volume can be achieved only if the patient generates maximum effort to raise intrathoracic pressure to reach flow limitation. Both inspiratory and expiratory flow rates can be measured. Preferential reductions in the flow rates, as depicted by the inspiratory or expiratory limb or both, may suggest upper airway obstruction (Fig. 7), though poor effort or inspiratory muscle weakness may also reduce inspiratory flow (72,73). As air flow limitation pro-

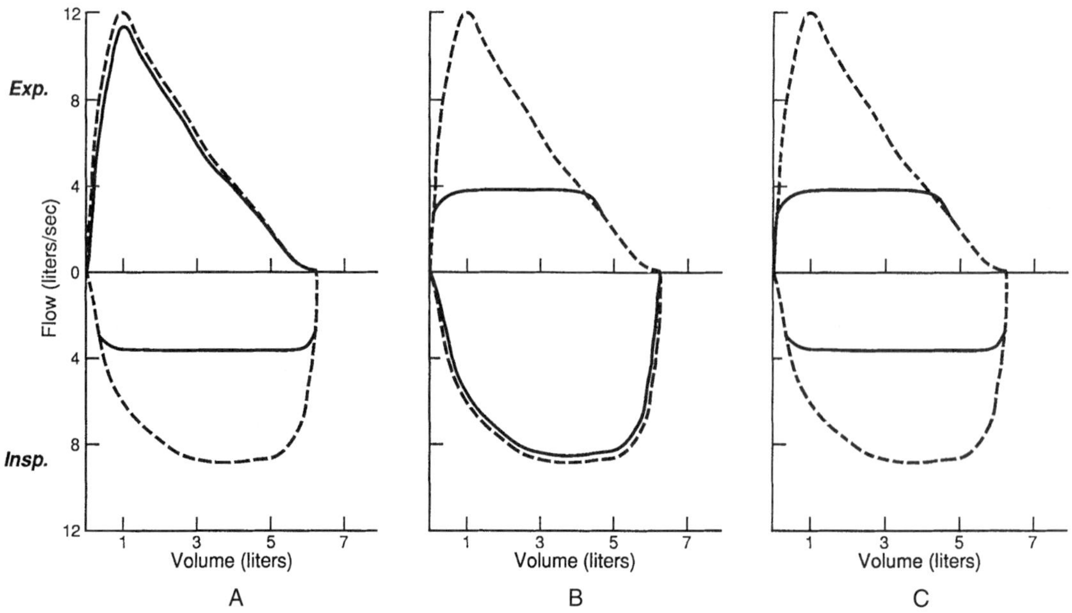


**FIG. 7.** Upper airway obstruction. Variable extrathoracic obstruction **(A)** results in a plateau of the inspiratory limb, while variable extrathoracic obstruction **(B)** results in an expiratory plateau. Fixed upper airway obstruction **(C)** results in a plateau of both inspiratory and expiratory limbs. *Dashed line* represents normal F-V loop; *solid line* represents abnormality.

gresses, reduction in flow rates will start at small lung volumes (71). Eventually, flow rates decrease at greater lung volumes (50% FVC and more). Note, spirometric measurements, including those obtained by the F-V loop, should take into account that flow is a function of lung volume. Thus, the $FEF_{50\%}$ and $FEF_{25\%}$ can be reported as $FEF_{50\%}$/FVC and $FEF_{25\%}$/FVC. Just as flow is reduced proportionately to lung volume in patients with restrictive lung diseases, yielding a normal $FEV_1$/FVC, flow rates generated by the F-V loop can be reduced, but proportionately to the decreased volumes. Indeed, Jayamanne and coworkers (74) have reported "supernormal" F-V ratios in patients with interstitial lung disease, suggesting increased recoil pressure. The shape of the F-V loop allows rapid and easy assessment of flow rates. Following the generation of peak flow ($FEF_{max}$), the expiratory limb of the F-V loop appears as a straight line (Fig. 5). Airflow limitation in the "small airways" initially appears as a scooped-out indentation at the terminal end of the flow-volume loop (between $FEF_{25\%}$ and RV). As airway disease progresses, $FEF_{50\%}$ diminishes as does $FEF_{25–75\%}$. The configuration of the F-V loop reveals a more significant concavity in the expiratory limb (Fig. 8). Dynamic compression due to loss of elastic recoil (as in emphysema) can be suggested by the shape of the loop (see below).

### Clinical Implications of Airflow Limitation

Diseases that cause airflow limitation, such as asthma, chronic bronchitis, and emphysema, cause lower-airway obstruction. For conceptual purposes, the lower airways have been divided into large (central) and small (peripheral) ones. Large airways have internal diameters greater than 2 mm; they usually extend to the ninth generation. Approximately 75% to 80% of total airway resistance occurs in these larger airways. Distal to the ninth generation, airway diameter decreases but cross-sectional area increases. Thus, only about 20% to 25% of total airway resistance occurs in the smaller, peripheral airways. Measuring $FEV_1$ and $FEV_1$/FVC does not detect increased resistance in these smaller airways, but more sensitive tests, such as measuring frequency dependence of compliance does. In addition, the graphic display of flow versus volume may demonstrate such abnormalities as a reduction in $FEF_{25\%}$ when remaining flow rates are normal. Such "small airways obstruction" is found early in asymptomatic cigarette smokers who have otherwise normal pulmonary function (75). The use of a helium-oxygen mixture during measurement of MEF demonstrates that small airways dysfunction exists among smokers, the most sensitive test being the volume of isoflow. Small airways obstruction has been found in various interstitial diseases, presumably secondary to the effect of interstitial fibrosis on the tethering qualities of the small airways (76).

As airway disease becomes more severe in patients with asthma, chronic bronchitis, or emphysema, the diminution in expiratory flow rate becomes more obvious: $FEV_1$, $FEV_1$/FVC ratio, and $FEF_{25–75\%}$ are reduced, as well as all flow rates generated by the F-V loop. Con-

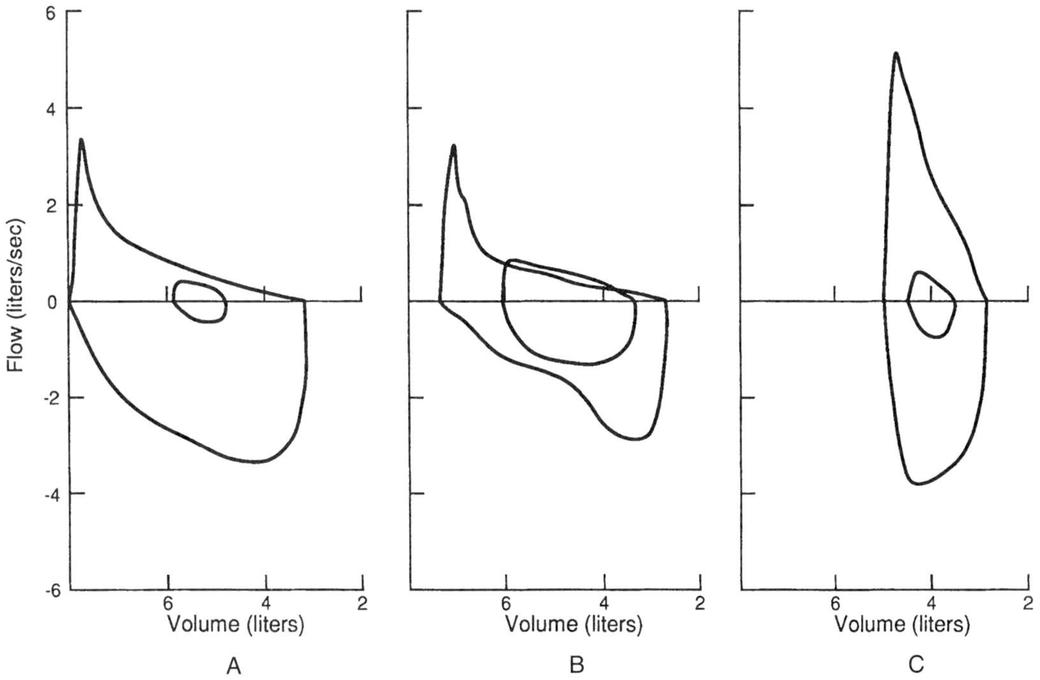


**FIG. 8.** F-V loop configurations. **A:** Airflow limitation in patients with asthma or chronic bronchitis. Flow is decreased at middle and low lung volumes (50% and 25% of FVC). F-V loops A and B are seen in patients with COPD. **B:** Loop is characteristic of patients with emphysema (see text). **C:** Loop is typical of patients with restrictive lung disease with normal or supernormal flow rates (see text).

current abnormalities in lung volume in patients with airflow limitation were discussed above. Jayamanne and coworkers (77) have shown that graphic analysis of the F-V loop can delineate dynamic compression in the large airways in some patients who have lost elastic recoil (i.e., those who have emphysema). The F-V loop contour demonstrates a characteristic abrupt reduction in flow from an already reduced peak flow, with an inflection point within the first 25% of the FVC. The remainder of the expiratory limb is flat, signifying a markedly reduced flow rate (Fig.8).

## Maximum Voluntary Ventilation

The maximum voluntary ventilation (MVV) is the largest volume that can be exhaled over a 10- to 15-second interval; the value is then extrapolated to 1 minute and expressed in liters per minute (13). MVV tests the overall functioning of the respiratory system—the respiratory muscles, airway resistance, and compliance of lungs and chest wall (78). The MVV maneuver exaggerates air trapping and respiratory muscle exertion. The value is decreased with moderately severe airways obstruction (79). In contrast, it may be normal with restrictive disease. Furthermore, a severe reduction in MVV with restrictive interstitial disease suggests an intercurrent problem such as airways obstruction (as in complicated pneumoconiosis) or muscle dysfunction (as in dermatomyositis). With advanced interstitial disease, the MVV may be significantly reduced, but less so than lung volumes (79). Because the maneuver is largely effort dependent and normal values vary much, only a large reduction in MVV is clinically significant. MVV may be calculated indirectly by multiplying the FEV by a factor of 35 to 40. If the measured MVV is significantly less than the calculated MVV, poor effort should be suspected.

### *Airway Resistance*

Airway resistance ($R_{AW}$) is the pressure difference developed per unit of flow (cm $H_2O$/L/sec) ($R_{AW} = P/V$). Clinical measurement of $R_{AW}$ includes the resistance provided by the entire pathway for air flow from mouth, nasopharynx, larynx, central airways, down to the peripheral airways. Thus, the pressure difference is measured between the mouth (atmospheric pressure) and the alveoli. Air flow at the mouth is measured by a pneumotachograph, and alveolar pressure in a body plethysmograph. Detailed guidelines for measuring airway resistance can be found elsewhere (80,81). The inverse of $R_{AW}$, airway conductance ($G_{AW}$), is recorded in L/sec/cm $H_2O$. Specific conductance ($SG_{AW}$) relates the airway conductance to lung volume. Airway conductance is nearly linear with respect to lung volume. $SG_{AW}$ is independent of lung volume.

Airway resistance is elevated with asthma, emphysema, or chronic bronchitis. It is a value more often used in research than in routine clinical evaluation. It is extremely objective, since the patient cannot influence it by lack of effort. Measurement of $R_{AW}$ may be useful in an occasional case when borderline spirometric findings suggest obstructive lung disease. It has also been used in bronchial challenge testing. Some persons lack the coordination required for the panting maneuvers in plethysmography. Voluntary glottic narrowing or panting at lung volumes below FRC may result in a falsely elevated $R_{AW}$.

**Bronchodilator Responsiveness**

Reversibility of airflow limitation is assessed by measuring the response to administration of a bronchodilating drug. Many factors affect the bronchodilator response: cause, chronicity, and severity of air flow limitation, as well as the "bronchomotor state" of the airways at the time of testing (i.e., the degree of abstinence from bronchodilator medication). For example, an asthmatic patient usually demonstrates a greater degree of bronchodilation than a patient with COPD. On the other hand, if that asthmatic patient has taken his bronchodilator medications one half hour before testing, his response may not demonstrate reversibility. In addition, certain technical factors affect whether a bronchodilator response is observed. These include the specific bronchodilator drug used to test the bronchodilator response as well as its route of administration (oral versus inhaled); the dose and method of administration of the bronchodilator drug (metered dose inhaler, spacer, or nebulizer); and the interval between administration of the drug and performance of the test (which may depend on the specific bronchodilator drug). Finally, which test is performed may affect the degree of response. Several detailed reviews of this problem have been published, so the following discussion will be limited (82,83).

Traditionally, flow rates such as $FEV_1$, PEFR, $FEF_{25-75\%}$, and $FEF_{50\%}$ are measured to test bronchodilator response; however, lung volume may increase without a demonstrable increase in flow rate (84,85). Ramsdell and Tisi (84) retrospectively analyzed the bronchodilator response in 241 patients, 129 of whom demonstrated a significant decrease in $R_{AW}$ following bronchodilator administration. Of these 129 patients, 46 exhibited a significant increase in vital capacity (mean increase 465±43 ml) and a decrease in FRC as measured blethysmography (mean decrease of 763±78 ml) with no change in the $FEV_1$/FVC or the $FEF_{25-75\%}$. Ayres and associates (85) found that, following bronchodilator administration, COPD patients may demonstrate decreased $R_{AW}$ without a change in flow rate. When FVC improves without a change in $FEV_1$, it is important to distinguish whether the increase is secondary to a more prolonged expiratory effort or whether there is true bronchodilation, as suggested by measures of expiratory volumes over longer intervals (3 or 6 seconds) (86).

Light and coworkers (87) evaluated various tests and the response to bronchodilators in an effort to determine which is the one best test for evaluating effects of bronchodilator therapy. $FEV_1$, FVC, $FEV_1$/FVC%, $FEF_{25-75\%}$, $SG_{AW}$, and $R_{AW}$ were evaluated. $SG_{AW}$ responded with the greatest improvement, followed by $FEF_{25-75}$%, $FEV_1$, $R_{AW}$, and PVC. Analysis of variance revealed that $FEV_1$ had the greatest discriminatory power, followed by PVC, $SG_{AW}$, and $FEF_{25\%}$. Berger and Smith (88) observed similar results in COPD patients: measurement of $FEV_1$ following bronchodilator administration most often demonstrated acute improvement. In 7% of patients FVC was the only test that demonstrated bronchodilatory response.

Finally, quantification of the bronchodilator response needs to be determined (i.e., what critical percentage of increase above baseline confirms the presence of a bronchodilator response). Pennock and coworkers (89) suggested that this depends on the variability of the results of the test in question. They found that normal subjects demonstrated variability in flow rates that was significant at the 95% confidence limit (see Normal Values, below): 5% in FVC, 5% in $FEV_1$, and 13% in $FEF_{25-75\%}$. Furthermore, patients with obstructive lung disease had even more variable results—almost twice that of normal healthy subjects: 11% in FVC, 13% in $FEV_1$, and 23% in $FEF_{25-75\%}$. Thus, on a given day a truly significant bronchodilator response should be greater than the intrasubject variability. Pennock's group also found that COPD patients may exhibit even greater week-to-week variability: 21% in FVC, 23% in $FEV_1$, and 30% in $FEF_{25-75\%}$. Sourk and Nugent (90) measured the bronchodilator response in normal subjects and calculated 95% confidence intervals: 5.2% for PVC, 10.5% for $FEV_1$, and 49% for $FEF_{25-75\%}$. Following administration of inhaled placebo, confidence intervals for patients were 15% for FVC, 12% for $FEV_1$, and 45% for $FEF_{25-75\%}$.

As a measure of bronchodilator response, percentage of change may be misleading. In patients with severe obstruction, who have very low baseline flow rates, small absolute increases in $FEV_1$ may produce large percentage increases. In addition, in patients who have relatively high (though reduced) flow rates, a significant percentage increase in $FEV_1$ may not occur. Tweeddale and associates (91) studied 150 patients with COPD in an effort to establish criteria for a bronchodilator response. They found that the increments in $FEV_1$ and FVC should be at least 160 and 330 ml, respectively, to achieve the 95% confidence interval that is statistically significant. Anthonisen and coworkers (92) reviewed the bronchodilator response of 985 COPD patients. They found that the absolute increase in $FEV_1$ was directly related to the baseline $FEV_1$; this was in contrast to Tweeddale's group's finding that patients who responded to bronchodilator therapy had similar absolute increases in $FEV_1$, regardless of the degree of obstruction.

Finally, the importance of volume adjustment of postbronchodilator flow rates has been demonstrated by several investigators (93–95). Cockcroft and Bersheid (93) found that if the PVC increases after bronchodilator administration, the $FEF_{25-75\%}$ will not be calculated over the same absolute lung volume as the prebronchodilator $FEF_{25-75\%}$. The postbronchodilator $FEF_{25-75\%}$ underestimates the response, since the increased PVC is secondary to decreased EV. Isovolumetric measurement of the $FEF_{25-75\%}$, that is, measuring the $FEF_{25-75\%}$ at the same pre- and postbronchodilator volume, corrects this problem. This effect has also been demonstrated for flow rates generated by the F-V loop (94,95). Thus, the pre- and postbronchodilator $FEF_{50}\%$ should be measured at the same lung volume exhaled from TLC.

Based on the preceding discussion, ATS criteria that indicate bronchodilator response are as follows: at least 12% increase in $FEV_1$ or FVC with a minimum increase in $FEV_1$ of at least 200 ml. Other criteria include at least 30% increase in $FEF_{50}\%$ or $FEF_{25-75\%}$ isovolume, and at least 20% increase in $FEF_{25}\%$ or $FEF_{25-75\%}$ (83,87).

## DIFFUSING CAPACITY

Diffusing capacity measures factors that affect the transfer of a diffusion-limited gas across the alveolocapillary membrane. The measurement is affected by the physicochemical properties of the test gas, alveolar-capillary membrane thickness, resistance to diffusion by the red cell membrane, and the reaction rates of the test gas and hemoglobin. For clinical purposes carbon monoxide (CO) is used to measure the diffusing capacity. CO combines with hemoglobin 210 times more readily than $O_2$ does but otherwise behaves likewise. Small amounts of CO in the inspired gas produce measurable changes in the concentration of inspired versus expired gas. The diffusing capacity for CO ($D_LCO$) is defined as the amount of carbon monoxide transferred per minute per millimeter mercury of driving pressure:

$$D_LCO = \frac{\dot{V}_{CO}}{\bar{P}_{ACO}} - \bar{P}_{CCO}, \qquad [10]$$

where

$\dot{V}_{CO}$ = amount of CO transferred (ml/min),
$\bar{P}_{ACO}$ = mean alveolar partial pressure of CO (mm Hg), and
$\bar{P}_{CCO}$ = mean pulmonary capillary partial pressure of CO (mm Hg).

Because hemoglobin has such a strong affinity for CO, the partial pressure of CO in blood in nonsmokers is negligible, and the value of $P_{CCO}$ can be ignored. Therefore, the $D_LCO$ can be determined by calculating the $\dot{V}_{CO}$ as the difference between the inspired and expired samples and estimating the mean alveolar $P_{ACO}$. The most widely used technique for calculating $D_LCO$ is the single-breath method, first described in 1914 by Marie Krogh. The development of the single-breath CO diffusion test by August and Marie Krogh was a by-product of their efforts to disprove the oxygen secretion hypothesis advanced by Haldane and Bohr. From his experimental work Haldane had concluded that the $PO_2$ was higher in arterial blood than in the lungs, and thus that absorption of oxygen by the lungs could not be explained by diffusion alone (96). In contrast, the Kroghs measured CO-diffusing capacity in 22 subjects (including some patients who had pneumonia, tuberculosis, asthma, emphysema, or bronchitis). They concluded (97), "The absorption of oxygen and elimination of carbon dioxide in the lungs takes place by diffusion and by diffusion alone." The actual measurement of diffusing capacity was described by Marie Krogh as part of her doctoral thesis (98). In the early 1950s the work of the Kroghs was applied clinically and modified by Ogilvie and Forster and their colleagues (99).

Standards for performing and calculating the $D_LCO$ have been established by the ATS (100). The patient inspires rapidly to TLC a gas mixture of 0.3% CO, 10% helium, and the remainder air (20.9% O2, balance nitrogen) and holds this single breath 10 seconds. The patient exhales: the initial portion (usually 1,000 ml) containing dead space gas is discarded. The remainder is collected and the concentrations of CO and He are analyzed [see the ATS 1995 update (100) for a detailed discussion of the calculation of the CO and He concentrations]. Various factors affect the diffusing capacity: body size, age, hemoglobin concentration, carboxyhemoglobin (COHb) concentration, smoking, lung volume, and ventilation-perfusion abnormalities. Because taller persons have greater lung volume and greater surface area for gas exchange, they have greater diffusing capacity. $D_LCO$ decreases with age; thus, a man aged 70 years has one-third the diffusing capacity he had at age 20. Anemia results in a reduced $D_LCO$, approximately 6% to 7% per gram of hemoglobin reduction, so all measured values should be corrected for the hemoglobin value (101,102). Conversely, polycythemia increases $D_LCO$. Elevations in COHb levels decrease the measured $D_LCO$. This occurs principally in cigarette smokers (103,104). The median COHb level in smokers is 5.0% and the value can be as high as 12%; for nonsmokers it is 1.2%. Because smoking also decreases $D_LCO$ independent of COHb, patients should be asked to refrain from smoking for 24 hours before the test. Some occupations predispose to CO exposure; firefighters, garage attendants, and tunnel workers may have elevated levels of COHb. $D_LCO$ decreases by 1% for each 1% increase in COHb (104). This is due to both a "back-pressure" effect of CO and an "anemia effect." Several proposals have been made to adjust for the back.pressure effect, though this has not been mandated by the ATS (100,105). (The ATS committee considered the cost and inconvenience of doing CO measurements and did not make this correction mandatory.) Failure to make such an adjustment may introduce small but systematic errors in $D_LCO$.

Methodologic issues are addressed fully in the ATS recommendations and so will not be discussed in detail here (100). Several points, however, should be reiterated. Standardization of technique is crucial in light of Clausen et al.'s (106) findings of an interlaboratory coefficient of variation by 12.7% for $D_LCO$, compared to 3.4% for PVC. Saunders (107) found even greater differences in six London laboratories. Sources of variability are (a) test technique, (b) errors in gas analysis, and (c) computation algorithms (108). In addition, the selection of reference equations alters the predicted value, leading to differences in interpretation (109).

The ATS recommendations state that an adequate test is marked by rapid inspiration, inspired volume ($V_I$) greater than 90% of the largest VC, a breath-holding time of 9 to 11 seconds, an adequate washout volume, and an appropriate sample size (100). Since $V_I$ should equal at least 90% of the vital capacity, alveolar volume ($V_A$) should be equivalent to an alternatively measured TLC. At the end of the breath holding a volume of gas must be exhaled, clearing the dead space before the alveolar sample is collected. This washout volume should be 0.75 to 1 L, but 0.5 L is acceptable if the patient's VC is less than 2 L. Furthermore, a sample of 0.5 to 1 L should be collected in less than 4 seconds. Inspiratory time should be less than 2.5 seconds for healthy subjects and less than 4.0 seconds for patients with moderate to severe air flow obstruction. If the inspiratory time is increased to half the breath-holding time (approximately 5 seconds), the $D_LCO$ is reduced by 13% (100). There should be a minimum of two acceptable tests, and the mean of two or more test results should be reported. Duplicate measurements of $D_LCO$ should be within 10%, or 3 ml CO (STPD) $min^{-1}.mm\ Hg^{-1}$, whichever is larger.

If the inspired volume is less than 90% of the VC, the subject failed to hold the breath at TLC or to exhale to RV, or both. Underestimation of $V_A$ results in reduced $D_LCO$ values. Cotes (110) has suggested use of an alternatively derived measurement of alveolar volume (TLC) using the value obtained from rebreathing gas dilution methods or plethysmography and calling that the "maximum $D_LCO$." The ATS statement avoided definitively addressing the issue, but stated that other measurements of $V_A$ could be used for interpretive purposes. Another source of error involves measurement obtained during breath holding (i.e., the time when diffusion occurs). Rapid inspiration and expiration to the alveolar sampling phase reduces the differences that can result from different timing methods. Furthermore, the volume of gas discarded before the alveolar sample is collected may affect the $D_LCO$ measurement. When the washout volume is reduced in a subject with a VC less than 2.0 L, an increase in dead space volume may be added to the alveolar sample, which lowers the CO. When the alveolar sample volume is also reduced in subjects with reduced vital capacity, true alveolar mixing of CO and He may not occur, in which case the $D_LCO$ will be reduced. Finally, if the alveolar volume is collected for longer than 3 seconds, as may occur with severe airways obstruction, $D_LCO$ will be increased. Graham and coworkers (111) have demonstrated that the single-breath $D_LCO$ may be overestimated in patients with air flow obstruction.

There are many published prediction equations for $D_LCO$. Given the current state of the art it is not possible to select a best equation (112). The differences may be due to interlaboratory variation in technique. Possible racial and ethnic differences have not been studied; most study subjects are whites. In a small pilot study, Weissman and Zeballos (113) compared $D_LCO$ in 32 healthy black subjects and 38 healthy whites. They found that blacks had lower $D_LCO$ values but identical $DL/V_A$ values, suggesting that the reduced $D_LCO$ of blacks may be due to smaller lung volume. At the present time the ATS recommends that each laboratory test a limited number of healthy subjects (15 to 20 of each gender), compare the results with published prediction equations, and select the prediction equations that most closely match the measured $D_LCO$ values (100,112).

### Clinical Application of $D_LCO$ Values

$D_LCO$ is a marker of the integrity of the surface area available for gas exchange, which in turn is a function of the alveolar-capillary interface. Disruption of this interface by parenchymal (e.g., emphysema, interstitial lung disease) or vascular (e.g., recurrent pulmonary emboli) processes, as well as absolute loss of surface volume (e.g., pneumonectomy) or decreased hemoglobin oxygen-carrying capacity (anemia), affects the measured $D_LCO$ (Table 2).

**TABLE 2.** *Abnormalities of diffusing capacity*

| |
|---|
| Increased |
| Polycythemia |
| Left-to-right intracardiac shunt |
| Pulmonary hemorrhage (e.g., Goodpasture's syndrome) |
| Asthma (?) |
| Decreased |
| Obstructive lung disease: emphysema, cystic fibrosis |
| Parenchymal interstitial disease: asbestos, drugs (bleomycin, amiodarone), sarcoidosis, allergic alveolitis, collagen vascular disease, Wegener's granulomatosis |
| Cardiovascular disease: acute myocardial infarction (pulmonary edema), mitral stenosis, pulmonary thromboembolism |

Diffuse interstitial lung disease may diminish $D_LCO$ even when the chest radiograph is normal. In a retrospective study of 44 patients with normal chest radiographs and biopsy-proven interstitial disease of various causes, Epler and colleagues (114) found reduced $D_LCO$ in 71% of patients, compared to reduced VC in 57% and reduced TLC in 16%. Diminution in $D_LCO$ has been observed as an early marker of interstitial disease of various causes, including infectious processes. Thus, in a patient who has human immunodeficiency virus (HIV) infection and is not an intravenous drug abuser, and who presents with fever, cough, and dyspnea (with or without hypoxemia), an isolated reduction in $D_LCO$ is very suggestive of *Pneumocystis carinii* pneumonia regardless of radiographic findings (115). Unfortunately, an isolated reduction in $D_LCO$ in a HIV-infected patient is nonspecific; previously, it was described in intravenous drug abusers, and more recently in asymptomatic "HIV-positive" persons as well as those with nonspecific interstitial pneumonitis (116,117).

Miller and co-workers (118) have reported a correlation between $D_LCO$ and progression of radiographic abnormalities in sarcoidosis. Significant hypoxemia occurs only in patients with low diffusing capacity (119). Furthermore, markers of inflammatory activity such as gallium-67 uptake and percentages of T lymphocytes/total lymphocytes in bronchoalveolar lavage fluid of patients with active sarcoidosis correlate with abnormalities in diffusing capacity (120).

In idiopathic pulmonary fibrosis the diffusing capacity is almost always diminished. Tukiainen and coworkers (121) reported on 100 consecutive patients: 97 had reduced $D_LCO$; in contrast, only 70 had reduced FVC. The reduction in $D_LCO$ does not correlate directly with the degree of inflammation or fibrosis found on pathologic examination (122). Risk and colleagues (123) demonstrated a correlation between reduced $D_LCO$ and diminishing gas exchange as determined by an increase in the alveolar-arterial $O_2$ gradient. In 168 patients with a variety of interstitial disorders, including 18 cases of asbestosis, $D_LCO$ below 70% of the predicted value was a good predictor of gas exchange abnormalities. Keogh and co-workers (124) have found that the reduction in $D_LCO$ cannot completely determine the magnitude of gas exchange abnormalities in patients with interstitial lung disease. For example, when patients with idiopathic pulmonary fibrosis were exercised at a $VO_2$ of 1/L per minute, reduced $D_LCO$ accounted for less than 30% of the reduction in $PO_2$. The ATS Committee on Evaluating Respiratory Disability and Impairment considers a $D_LCO$ no higher than 50% of predicted value as a criterion for disability in patients with interstitial lung disease (125).

With asbestosis the diffusing capacity is usually reduced (126). Some investigators have found that reduced diffusing capacity may be an early marker, but others have not (127–133). As with idiopathic pulmonary fibrosis, the extent of asbestosis does not correlate with the magnitude of $D_LCO$ reduction, though this also has been debated. Sue and associates (132) attempted to correlate $D_LCO$ values with gas exchange abnormalities during exercise in shipyard workers exposed to asbestos. They found at least one abnormality of gas exchange during exercise in 14 of 16 workers whose $D_LCO$ was less than 70% of the predicted value. Only 14 of 96 workers with abnormal exercise test results had reduced $D_LCO$. Garcia and colleagues (133) studied a cohort of 286 patients who were exposed at work to asbestos; 53 had an isolated reduction in diffusing capacity. These findings differed from those of Sue's group in that, with the exception of a mild reduction in $VO_2$ percent predicted in asbestos-exposed patients with low $D_LCO$ who were cigarette smokers, all patients had normal gas exchange during exercise. These results should be interpreted cautiously, as the number of patients who were exercised was small in contrast to Sue's study. It is significant, however, that Garcia and coworkers found that the reduced $D_LCO$ correlated with increased inflammatory cells in bronchoalveolar lavage specimens.

Since $D_LCO$ is directly related to alveolar volume, volume adjustment of the absolute $D_LCO$ measurement ($DL/V_A$) has been advocated as a means of differentiating various processes that result in a decreased diffusing capacity (i.e., disease processes that cause reduced lung volume as opposed to diffuse V/Q mismatch) (134). Kanengiser and coinvestigators (58) demonstrated that such an assessment for interstitial diseases does not correlate with the pathophysiology or clinical spectrum of disease. When the predicted $D_LCO$ is divided by the predicted $V_A$, the "normal" $D_L/V_A$ is approximately 4 or 5. Kanengiser's group found both low and "normal" $D_L/V_A$ values in patients with severe disease. Thus, adjusting the measured $D_LCO$ to alveolar volume ($D_L/V_A$) is a way to normalize differences in body size and lung volume when predicting values in normal persons. An absolute reduction in $D_LCO$ concomitant with a reduction in $D_L/V_A$ denotes an abnormality. However, reduced $D_LCO$ in association with reduced lung volume (i.e., $D_L/V_A = 4$ to 5) should not be dismissed as normal in patients with interstitial or alveolar processes. This is in distinction to persons whose measured $D_LCO$ is truly diminished because of a reduction in lung volume (i.e., patients with pneumonectomy, chest wall abnormalities, or neuromuscular disorders) who may have reduced $D_LCO$ (almost 50% in the former case but much less in the latter two conditions) but normal $D_L/V_A$ (134,135).

Patients with emphysema also have a diminished $D_LCO$ with a normal $V_A$, yielding a reduced $D_L/V_A$ ratio. Indeed, a reduction in $D_LCO$ has been used to differentiate emphysema from chronic bronchitis and asthma (136). Asthmatic patients have normal or increased DLCO values (137,138). Gelb and coworkers (139) correlated pathologic evidence of emphysema in lobectomy specimens with reduced diffusing capacity. In some of these patients, emphysema was not suspected because of normal flow rates and lung volumes; thus, isolated reductions in diffusing capacity indicated significant disease. Berend and coworkers (140) found that $D_LCO$ correlated with degree of emphysema, while Burrows and associates (141) and Vandenbergh and co-workers did not (142). Owens and colleagues (143) found that in 19 of 28 patients a $D_LCO$ value below 55% predicted desaturation on exercise. The degree of desaturation correlated with the magnitude of $D_LCO$ reduction.

Because the diffusing capacity is a measure of alveolar capillary membrane integrity, pulmonary vascular abnormalities may also affect the $D_LCO$ value. Recurrent pulmonary emboli, primary and secondary pulmonary hypertension, pulmonary vasculitis, and scleroderma have resulted in diminished $D_LCO$ (144–148). Cardiovascular diseases may also affect the $D_LCO$. Patients with chronic congestive heart failure or severe chronic mitral stenosis may have reduced $D_LCO$, presumably secondary to chronic vascular changes or decreased cardiac output (149–152). Siegel and coworkers (152) found that the reduction in diffusing capacity correlated strongly with a reduced ejection fraction (less than 40%), but only in patients who had inspiratory crackles: 10 of 11 patients with crackles had reduced $D_LCO$ values, but only 2 of 23 patients without crackles. On the other hand, cardiac diseases that cause left-to-right shunting increase pulmonary blood volume, especially in the upper lung zone; the result is increased diffusion and an elevated $D_LCO$ measurement, though it varies (153). Intraalveolar hemorrhage, as observed in Goodpasture's syndrome, may also result in increased $D_LCO$. The additional red blood cells in the alveoli increase CO binding (154).

## ARTERIAL BLOOD GAS ANALYSIS

Technologic advances have made blood gas analysis a routine procedure. The arterial pH, $Paco_2$, and $Po_2$ are measured by specially designed electrodes, and the oxygen saturation and bicarbonate are calculated from these data. Arterial blood gases reflect both the gas exchange efficiency of the lung and the acid-base status of the patient (the latter is not discussed here). Assessment of oxygenation is achieved by determining the $Pao_2$ and the alveolar-arterial $O_2$ gradient [$P(A - a)O_2$]; adequacy of alveolar ventilation is assessed by measuring the $Paco_2$.

The degree of oxygenation of arterial blood is expressed as the partial pressure of oxygen ($Po_2$) or oxygen saturation ($O_2$ Sat). These measurements are related to each other by the sigmoidal oxyhemoglobin (Hb $O_2$) dissociation curve. If one value is known, the other can be derived. The $O_2$ Sat is a determining factor in calculating the $O_2$ content, provided the hemoglobin concentration is adequate. $PaO_2$ values of 40, 50, and 60 mm Hg, respectively, correspond roughly to $O_2$ Sat values of 70, 80, and 90%. When $Po_2$ is greater than 60 mm Hg, disturbances in gas exchange may cause discernible changes in the $Po_2$ and little change in the $O_2$ Sat level because the $O_2$ dissociation curve is flat in the 60- to 100-mm Hg range. Thus, changes in the $Po_2$ level below 60 mm Hg are critical. In the latter circumstance, the $O_2$ Sat level has decreased to less than 90%, and small changes in the $Po_2$ level on the steep part of the $O_2$ dissociation curve ($Po_2$ less than 60 mm Hg) imply great changes in $O_2$ Sat, which is the critical value in the calculation of arterial $O_2$ content. In most clinical situations (except CO poisoning) the $Pao_2$ level is measured; the $O_2$ Sat level can then be calculated. When CO poisoning is suspected, a cooximeter must be used to measure CO concentration and $O_2$ Sat directly, because the $Po_2$ level will not be affected by the CO. If the $O_2$ Sat level is calculated from the misleading $Po_2$ level, it will also be incorrect.

A $Pao_2$ level greater than 90 mm Hg is considered normal if it is not achieved by hyperventilation; however, arterial oxygen tension is a function of altitude, age, and inspired $O_2$ concentration. At a given altitude the $Po_2$ should be multiplied by the fraction local PB/760 (where PB is the barometric pressure). The precise reduction in $Po_2$ level with aging is not fully known, but $Po_2$ values as low as 75 mm Hg may be normal after age 70 years. Empirically derived formulas for calculating predicted arterial $O_2$ tension are as follows (155,156):

$$\text{Seated: } Pao_2 = 104.2 - (0.27 \times \text{age}) \pm 6 \qquad [11]$$

$$\text{Supine: } Pao_2 = 109 - (0.43 \times \text{age}) \pm 4 \qquad [12]$$

(These figures are corrected from the original paper for 760 mm Hg.)

Assessment of gas exchange requires evaluation of both the $Pao_2$ and the $Paco_2$. While a $Pao_2$ less than 80 mm Hg usually indicates significant hypoxemia, the cause is unknown. Patients may suffer this degree of hypoxemia and have a $Pco_2$ value less than 40 mm Hg while hyperventilating (owing to severe asbestosis, acute pulmonary embolus, or acute asthma attack), or they may suffer this degree of hypoxemia and have an increased $Pco_2$ due to severe V/Q mismatch (chronic bronchitis) or hypoventilation (drug overdose, neurologic dysfunction, primary alveolar hypoventilation). One can differentiate between these two groups of disorders by calculating the alveolar-arterial oxygen difference, $P(A - a)O_2$, which assesses the intrinsic gas-exchange properties of the lungs and suggests the cause of the hypoxemia (Table 3).

At sea level [where the fraction of inspired oxygen ($FIo_2$) is 0.21], the important mechanisms for arterial hypoxemia include alveolar hypoventilation, V/Q mismatch (low V/Q), and shunt (V/Q = 0). Calculating the $P(A - a)O_2$ distinguishes these mechanisms; only with alveolar hypoventilation is a normal gradient maintained. An increased $P(A - a)O_2$ suggests V/Q shunt or diffusion abnormalities. Furthermore, response to 100% $O_2$ (for a

**TABLE 3.** *Mechanisms of hypoxemia*

| Cause of hypoxemia | $P_{AO_2}$ | $Pa_{O_2}$ | $P(A-a)O_2$ (RA) | $P(A-a)O_2$ on 100% $O_2$ | $Pa_{CO_2}$ | Examples |
|---|---|---|---|---|---|---|
| Decreased $F_{IO_2}$ | ↓ | ↓ | N | N | ↓ | High altitude |
| Hypoventilation | N | ↓ | N | N | ↑ | Drug overdose |
| Diffusion abnormalities | N | ↓ | ↑ | N | N or ↓ | Interstitial lung disease |
| V/Q mismatch | N | ↓ | ↑ | N | ↓, N, or ↑ | Interstitial lung disease, obstructive lung disease |
| Right-to-left shunt | N | ↓ | ↑ | ↑ | N | Intrapulmonary shunt (ARDS), ASD, VSD |

N, normal; ↑, increased; ↓, decreased; RA, room air; ARDS, adult respiratory distress syndrome; ASD, atrial septal defect; VSD, ventricular septal defect.

minimum of 20 minutes) distinguishes shunt from V/Q mismatch; the latter condition responds by normalizing the calculated gradient. In calculating the $P(A-a)O_2$, the alveolar gas equation reveals that the $P_{AO_2}$ is equal to the partial pressure of the inspired $O_2$ concentration ($P_{IO_2}$) minus the arterial $P_{CO_2}$ ($Pa_{CO_2}$) divided by 0.8 (the respiratory exchange ratio in a steady state). $Pa_{CO_2}$ approximates $P_{ACO_2}$ and is substituted for it. Thus

$$P_{AO_2} = P_{IO_2} - \frac{Pa_{CO_2}}{R} \qquad [13]$$

Because $P_{IO_2} = F_{IO_2}(P_B - P_{H_2O})$, these values can be substituted in the equation for $P_{IO_2}$:

$$P_{AO_2} = F_{IO_2}(P_B - P_{H_2O}) - \frac{Pa_{CO_2}}{R} \qquad [14]$$

In these equations $F_{IO_2}$ is inspired $O_2$ fraction; PB, barometric pressure; and $P_{H_2O}$, water vapor pressure. In room air, $F_{IO_2}$ is 0.21, and in a steady state, R is 0.8; PB, 760 mm Hg; and $P_{H_2O}$, 47 mm Hg. Therefore,

$$P_{AO_2} = 0.21(760 - 47) - \frac{Pa_{CO_2}}{0.8} \qquad [15]$$

$$= 150 - 1.25 \times P_{CO_2}.$$

To summarize,

$$P(A-a)O_2 = 150 - (1.25 \times Pa_{CO_2}) - Pa_{O_2}. \qquad [16]$$

The normal $P(A-a)O_2$ gradient is 10 to 15 mm Hg, but because the arterial $O_2$ value varies with age, the gradient increases likewise (155,156). A quick approximation of the normal $P(A-a)O_2$ gradient is one-third of the patient's age or (age/4) – 5.

Normally, $Pa_{O_2}$ and $P(A-a)O_2$ do not change with mild or moderate exercise. The $O_2$ Sat changes no more than 2% from rest to maximal exercise, which makes it less sensitive to subtle gas-exchange abnormalities. During heavy exercise, the alveolar-arterial oxygen gradient increases but rarely above 30 mm Hg. During maximum work in normal persons the gradient should be no more than 35 mm Hg and $Pa_{O_2}$ at least 75 mm Hg. Hansen and co-workers (157) demonstrated that, in 77 normal "older men" (aged 34 to 74 years), the mean alveolar-arterial $O_2$ gradient was 12.8 ± 7.4 mm Hg at rest and 19.0 ± 88 mm Hg with maximal exercise (157). Only 3 of 77 subjects had a gradient of at least 35 mm Hg. In younger persons the $P(A-a)O_2$ at maximal exercise was no more than 21 mm Hg. Widening of the gradient during exercise suggests a diffusion or V/Q mismatch abnormality.

Administering 100% $O_2$ differentiates between V/Q and shunt mechanisms of hypoxemia. If the problem is V/Q mismatch, the 100% $O_2$ will raise the $Pa_{O_2}$ above 550 mm Hg and the alveolar-arterial gradient will be reduced to normal (i.e., following the administration of 100% $O_2$ the gradient is 100 mm Hg). If a shunt mechanism causes hypoxemia, administration of 100% $O_2$ does not produce a $Pa_{O_2}$ in the 550 mm Hg range. If the problem is shunting, the shunt fraction can be determined by using one of several shunt nomograms (158,159). If cardiac output is normal (arteriovenous difference of 5 ml/100 ml blood), $P(A-a)O_2$ can be used to estimate shunt: each 20-mm Hg increment in the gradient corresponds to a 1% shunt. This is valid only when the $Pa_{O_2}$ is greater than 150 mm Hg.

$Pa_{CO_2}$ values normally range between 37 and 43 mm Hg. The $Pa_{CO_2}$ measures the adequacy of the lung in removing $CO_2$ from the blood coming to it. Altitude below 8,000 feet and age have minimal effects on this value. $Pa_{CO_2}$ can be used as an accurate estimate of alveolar ventilation, because the concentrations of $CO_2$ in alveolar gas and pulmonary capillary blood rapidly equalize (in contrast to arterial and alveolar oxygen). If $CO_2$ production remains constant, arterial $P_{CO_2}$ is inversely related to alveolar ventilation:

$$Pa_{CO_2} \propto \frac{1}{\dot{V}_A}, \dot{V}_A = \text{alveolar ventilation} \qquad [17]$$

Thus, an increased $Pa_{CO_2}$ indicates alveolar hypoventilation; conversely, reduced $Pa_{CO_2}$ indicates alveolar hyperventilation. When the $Pa_{CO_2}$ is abnormal, it is necessary to determine whether the condition is a primary ventilatory abnormality (intrinsic or extrinsic to the lung) or whether the value merely represents compensation for a primary metabolic disturbance (an attempt to achieve acid-base balance). $Pa_{CO_2}$ values are determined in part by acid-base homeostasis, because the $Paco_2$ value is directly proportional to the bicarbonate concentration, the body's primary buffer system.

Measurement of minute ventilation ($\dot{V}E$) can be very helpful in identifying the mechanism of arterial hypercapnia. Minute ventilation is the product of tidal volume and respiratory rate. During each tidal breath, some of the air reaches the alveoli and participates in gas exchange (alveolar ventilation, $\dot{V}A$), while some air remains in the conducting airways (dead space ventilation, $\dot{V}D$). Thus, over a 60-second interval, $\dot{V}E$ is the sum of $\dot{V}A$ and $\dot{V}D$ ($\dot{V}E = \dot{V}A + \dot{V}D$). Minute ventilation ranges from 5 to 8 L per minute, while $\dot{V}A$ is roughly two-thirds of $\dot{V}E$. If a patient develops hypercapnia, $\dot{V}A$ must be reduced. A mathematical solution of the equation governing $\dot{V}E$ reveals that $\dot{V}A = \dot{V}E - \dot{V}D$. Thus, when hypercapnia results in reduced $\dot{V}A$, the mechanism must be either reduced $\dot{V}E$ or increased $\dot{V}D$.

In patients with increased $Paco_2$ and reduced $\dot{V}E$, the mechanism of hypercapnia is alveolar hypoventilation (when $\dot{V}E$ is reduced, $\dot{V}A$ must be reduced). As $Paco_2$ increases, $PAO_2$ decreases, because $PAO_2 = 150 - PCO_2/R$ (see alveolar gas equation above). If the alveolarterial $O_2$ gradient remains normal, this decrease in $PAO_2$ must produce arterial hypoxemia. Causes that should be considered are those that result in decreased ventilatory drive (e.g., sedative drugs, anesthesia, head injury, medullary infarct) or in decreased chest bellows output (e.g., neuromuscular disease, thoracic cage abnormalities).

If arterial hypercapnia is present and measured $\dot{V}E$ is increased, then diseases (such as recurrent pulmonary emboli) that result in increased dead space (anatomic and physiologic) are responsible for the patient's hypercapnia. In this instance the increased $\dot{V}E$ is not adequate to compensate for the increased $\dot{V}D$. Ventilation of nonperfused area also results in increased $\dot{V}D$. The total $\dot{V}E$ value is often increased, but $\dot{V}D$ is increased owing to increased airway resistance (as in the case of asthma or bronchitis) or increased lung compliance (as in the case of emphysema). The local alterations in resistance and compliance produce underventilation of local lung units and so increase the regional $Paco_2$. When lung disease is extensive, compensation by hyperventilating normal lung units cannot prevent systemic arterial hypercapnia.

Arterial hypocapnia indicates hyperventilation, which can also be verified by measuring $\dot{V}E$. The causes for reduced $Paco_2$ include pulmonary (interstitial, airways, or vascular processes) and extrapulmonary ones (anxiety, drugs, meningitis, fever, pain).

### Clinical Application of Blood Gas Analysis

The concept of an alveolar-arterial pressure gradient is central to understanding gas exchange. As noted earlier, calculation of this gradient provides an understanding of the mechanism of hypoxemia in individual patients. Normally, at rest the gradient is 10 to 15 mm Hg, which is attributed to V/Q mismatch and small venous shunts. The value increases with age. During exercise the gradient may decrease, increase, or remain unchanged. Initially, during moderate exercise, more efficient ventilation and perfusion matching result in a decreased gradient. Subsequently, as exercise increases in intensity, increased venous shunting results in an increased gradient.

Risk and coworkers (123) studied 168 patients with various interstitial diseases [sarcoidosis, asbestosis, berylliosis, idiopathic pulmonary fibrosis (IPF)]; they have emphasized that abnormal gas exchange is best evaluated by examining the alveolar-arterial $O_2$ gradient during exercise. The increase in the gradient with exercise correlated best with the severity of the reduction in single-breath diffusing capacity, although the magnitude of the increase could not be predicted from the resting gradient value. Indeed, patients may have a relatively normal resting $P(A - a)O_2$ in the presence of severe disease as evidenced by reduced diffusing capacity and radiographic abnormalities. The increase in gradient occurred with IPF and sarcoidosis, if the $D_LCO$ was no more than 50% and with other disease processes if the $D_LCO$ was 70% or less. It should be noted that the number of patients with other diseases was small in this series (e.g., asbestosis, 10 patients). Risk and coworkers attempted to stratify all measurements of alveolar-arterial $O_2$ gradient during exercise with severity of disease as assessed by $D_LCO$, to see if one measure could be substituted for the other. Approximately 40% of the studies were discordant, and therefore diffusing capacity and alveolar–arterial $O_2$ gradient for exercise complemented each other.

Smith and Agostoni (160) co-workers attempted to measure the sensitivity and specificity of these gradients during exercise and the resting state in asbestos-exposed workers who were predominantly smokers. Ninety-two asbestos-exposed patients were divided into five groups, based on their chest radiograph and pulmonary function status: normal, chronic airflow obstruction (CAO), CAO and pleural disease, pleural disease alone, and asbestosis with or without CAO. As noted previously, smoking increases the alveolar-arterial $O_2$ gradient, especially in the setting of CAO (161–163). Almost half of the asbestos-exposed patients had CAO. Values for $P(A - a)O_2$ at rest did not discriminate between the groups, and at maximum exercise they were higher in asbestosis sufferers. The $P(A - a)O_2/VO_2$ correlated best with asbestosis. Both CAO and asbestosis were associated with increased alveolar-arterial $O_2$ gradient during exercise, but Smith and Agostoni suggested that asbestosis is also present if $P(A - a)O_2/VO_2$ is more than 35 (160). This association was very specific—only 2 of 65 patients without asbestosis had values that would be considered abnormal—but not sensitive; only 9 of 27 patients with presumed asbestosis had incriminating values.

Finally, caution must be exercised when analyzing arterial blood gas values, especially if they are used to determine impairment and disability. Neither "resting" nor "exercise" values can provide helpful independent information on impairment (164–167). Morgan and Zaldivar (168) examined arterial blood gases in 41 coal miners who were applying for disability due to coal worker's pneumoconiosis. They found concurrent diseases, such as cardiac disease, obesity, and COPD, in many patients who had resting hypoxemia, confirming the lack of specificity. More important, variability in $Pa_{CO_2}$ could be attributed to poor quality control, as others have documented (169,170). Furthermore, arterial blood gas analyses did not include information on work load during exercise, oxygen consumption, or heart rate. Finally, position and body weight affect the measurement of $Pa_{O_2}$. Obesity leads to ventilation-perfusion mismatch. When a subject lies supine the diaphragm is pushed upward, further reducing basilar ventilation and increasing mismatch. The $Pa_{O_2}$ of obese patients decreases by 10 to 15 mm Hg in the supine position (171).

## CARDIOPULMONARY EXERCISE TESTING

Exercise testing has achieved clinical importance in evaluation of pulmonary disease. While not without risks, it is a relatively safe test: the reported mortality rate is about 0.01% and morbidity about 0.02% (172). It is, however, both time-consuming and expensive. Although exercise testing is more useful for assessing extent and severity of disease than for establishing specific diagnoses, it can confirm that there is a physiologic basis for dyspnea of unknown cause. Various patterns of response are observed in different disease states: cardiac, ventilatory, and pulmonary vascular limitations can be detected. In addition, exercise testing can help evaluate patients who complain of dyspnea but have few or no objective findings and normal pulmonary function studies. Dyspnea may be due to poor physical fitness or even malingering. In patients with combined cardiopulmonary disease, either or both may be responsible for dyspnea; exercise testing may reveal a distinctive cardiac or pulmonary limitation. Finally, certain persons experience symptoms only with exertion: those with exercise-induced asthma who have normal results on resting pulmonary function studies fall into this category. A detailed review of pulmonary exercise resting is beyond the scope of this chapter but is available elsewhere (173–175).

### Exercise Physiology

During exercise, mechanical energy for muscle work is derived from the conversion of biochemical energy from stored fuel sources—carbohydrates stored as glycogen, fat stored as triglycerides, and protein stored as muscle tissue. A complex series of biochemical reactions within cells produces adenosine triphosphate (ATP), providing the chemical energy to perform work. The mitochondria are the principal site of oxygen consumption and $CO_2$ production.

The normal response to exercise involves a variety of changes designed to accommodate increasing $O_2$ consumption and $CO_2$ production. The normal minute ventilation ($\dot{V}_E$) in a resting adult is 5 to 8 L per minute. During exercise $\dot{V}_E$ may exceed 100 L per minute in untrained subjects and 200 L in conditioned athletes. Most of the initial increase in ventilation is due to increased tidal volume; during maximal exercise tidal volume can approach 50% to 60% of VC. During exercise, alveolar ventilation increases with improved V/Q matching. Total dead space ventilation is unchanged, while the $V_D/V_T$ ratio decreases since tidal volume increases.

Ventilation increases linearly with increasing workload ($\dot{V}_{O_2}$, or oxygen consumption) at low and moderate levels of exercise, following the increase in $\dot{V}_{CO_2}$ ($CO_2$ production; Fig. 9). The maintenance of aerobic metabolism during exercise is critically dependent on continued avail-

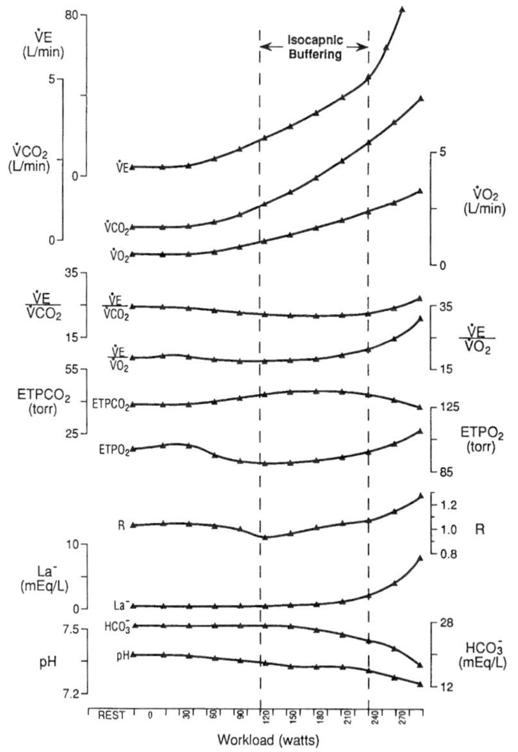


**FIG. 9.** Incremental exercise testing. Breath-by-breath analysis with monitoring of various parameters during incremental exercise (see text). Isocapnic buffering occurs when $\dot{V}_E$ and $\dot{V}_{CO_2}$ increase at the same rate without an increase in $\dot{V}_E/\dot{V}_{CO_2}$, resulting in a constant $ETP_{CO_2}$. After this period $ETP_{CO_2}$ decreases reflecting respiratory compensation for exercise-related metabolic acidosis. The anaerobic threshold can be identified by locating the nadirs of the $\dot{V}_E/\dot{V}_{O_2}$, $ETP_{CO_2}$, and R simultaneous with a plateau of the $\dot{V}_E/\dot{V}_{CO_2}$ and $ETP_{CO_2}$.

ability of $O_2$ at the mitochondrial level. As work load increases, $O_2$ uptake ($\dot{V}O_2$) must rise in compensation or anaerobic metabolism will increase to provide the necessary ATP for muscle utilization. Because of the close correlation between work load and $O_2$ uptake, energy requirements can be expressed in terms of $\dot{V}O_2$. As work load increases, $\dot{V}O_2$ eventually reaches a plateau. The maximum $O_2$ uptake ($\dot{V}O_{2MAX}$) provides a quantifiable assessment of the maximum amount of exercise that a person is capable of. Most normal subjects achieve a $\dot{V}O_{2MAX}$ of about 85% of the predicted value. $\dot{V}O_{2MAX}$ is a function of age. The minute ventilation during exercise may be related to the work (the $\dot{V}O_2$) performed, resulting in the "ventilatory equivalent for oxygen ($\dot{V}E/\dot{V}O_2$)." This value measures "efficiency" of the ventilatory apparatus with the normal range, 20 to 30 L/L $\dot{V}O_2$. The ventilatory equivalent for $CO_2$ ($\dot{V}E/\dot{V}CO_2$) ranges from 25 to 35 L/L $\dot{V}CO_2$ and is a measure of the maximum tolerable work for patients with ventilatory impairment.

At approximately 60% of $\dot{V}O_{2MAX}$, metabolic demand exceeds the capacity for aerobic energy production and must be supplemented by anaerobic oxidation, resulting in the conversion of intracellular pyruvate to lactic acid, with an associated increase in arterial lactate. The production of hydrogen ions is buffered by bicarbonate, with a consequent release of $CO_2$, increasing total $CO_2$ production ($\dot{V}CO_2$). The work level at which this process occurs is known as the anaerobic threshold (AT). Increased work above AT produces increased lactate. The anaerobic threshold work rate (i.e., the level of $\dot{V}O_2$ at which AT occurs), is influenced by fitness, training, hemoglobin concentration, and $FIO_2$. Below AT, the respiratory exchange ratio, R ($R = \dot{V}CO_2/\dot{V}O_2$) ranges from 0.7 to 0.9. Above AT, R rises dramatically, from a nadir at the onset of the anaerobic threshold, achieving values of 1 or greater. The increased hydrogen ion concentration caused by the reduction in serum bicarbonate levels stimulates the carotid bodies to increase ventilation further, lowering the $PaCO_2$ and compensating for the metabolic acidosis. Thus, both the $O_2$ ventilatory equivalent ($\dot{V}E/\dot{V}O_2$) and the end-tidal $PO_2$ ($ETPO_2$) increase from their lowest values, while $\dot{V}E/\dot{V}CO_2$ and ($ETPCO_2$) remain constant, resulting in "isocapnic buffering" for approximately 2 minutes (Fig. 9). The $\dot{V}E$ and $\dot{V}CO_2$ increase linearly up to AT; thereafter they are nonlinear to $\dot{V}CO_2$ as they rise more steadily. The $\dot{V}E/\dot{V}O_2$ is felt to be the most reliable indicator of AT. These parameters provide a noninvasive determination of AT, obviating measurement of lactate.

Recognition of AT is useful; its detection confirms that adequate effort was exerted during testing. AT is a function of physical fitness, normally occurring at 55% to 65% of $\dot{V}O_{2MAX}$. It falls in persons with cardiovascular disease, but patients with severe cardiac disease or severe COPD may be incapable of performing enough aerobic exercise to reach an anaerobic threshold. Ventilatory limitations of COPD allow aerobic exercise only. Below AT, the $\dot{V}E$ may be disproportionately high when $VD/VT$ is increased in severe COPD or pulmonary vascular disease.

The ratio of physiologic dead space to tidal volume measures wasted ventilation and can be calculated using a modification of the Bohr equation:

$$VD/VT = PaCO_2 - P_ECO_2/PaCO_2 \qquad [18]$$

where $P_ECO_2$ is mixed expired $CO_2$. The normal resting $VD/VT = 0.3 \pm 0.035$; the value falls dramatically with the onset of exercise, to 0.20 to 0.25 by the time $\dot{V}O_2$ reaches 1 L and may continue to decline more slowly thereafter. This reduction in $VD/VT$ reflects an increased tidal volume being distributed to well-perfused areas of the lungs. Increased $VD/VT$ often suggests pulmonary vascular disease, especially recurrent pulmonary emboli, but it can occur with parenchymal diseases such as severe emphysema or interstitial lung disease.

At the initiation of exercise in the upright position, cardiac output increases due to increased stroke volume and heart rate (HR). Maximum stroke volume is achieved early in exercise; further increases in cardiac output are due to increasing HR (stroke volume being fixed). Exercise in the supine position has similar effects, but stroke volume is already at maximum at rest. Increased cardiac output allows delivery of more $O_2$ to the exercising muscles. The linear increase in HR parallels $\dot{V}O_2$ and reaches a maximum of 190 to 220 beats per minute in young subjects. The maximum achievable HR is age related: 220 – (patient's age).

$O_2$/pulse ($\dot{V}O_2$/HR), the $O_2$ extraction per heartbeat, is a measure of stroke volume ($\dot{V}O_2/HR = SV = (A - V)\ O_2$ difference). A reduced $O_2$/pulse suggests heart disease, since a higher HR is necessary to maintain cardiac output, to compensate for low stroke volume. However, poor motivation, musculoskeletal limitation, ventilatory limitation, and anemia can also cause a low $O_2$/pulse. High $O_2$/pulse values are associated with beta-blocker therapy, conduction disease, or poor effort, but are also observed in well-trained subjects. During exercise, systolic and diastolic blood pressures increase as a result of improved myocardial contractility and reduced ventricular ejection time; however, the increase is principally in systolic pressure, usually about 100 mm Hg, raising the pressure some 200 to 250 mm Hg. The diastolic pressure usually does not increase more than 20 mm Hg. The rate of increase of systolic and pulse pressure as work increases is a function of age. If the systolic pressure does not rise or the diastolic pressure falls, cardiac output is inappropriate.

Various algorithms have been suggested for assessing cardiopulmonary responses to exercise (Fig. 10) (173–176). Regardless of whether such approaches are used for interpreting exercise studies, the major questions to be answered are these: (a) Was the exercise maximal or submaximal? (b) What was the subject's work capacity (i.e., was 85% to 100% of the predicted $\dot{V}O_{2MAX}$ achieved)? (c) What was the anaerobic threshold? (d) Was there a

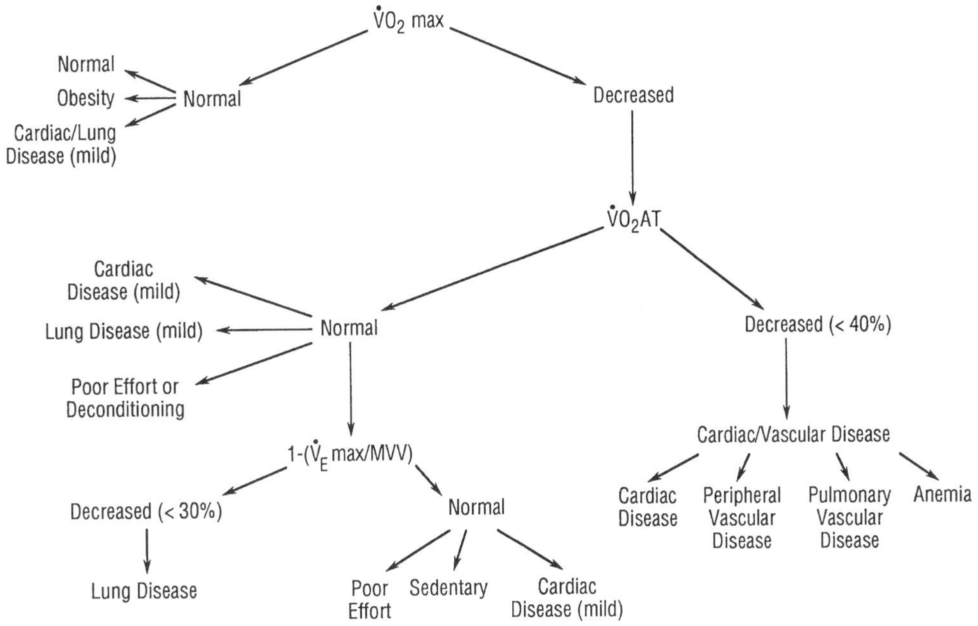


**FIG. 10.** Algorithm for cardiopulmonary stress testing. (Modified from refs. 173 and 174.)

ventilatory limitation? (e) Was gas exchange impaired with respect to abnormal $V_D/V_T$ or $P(A-a)O_2$? Table 4 lists the major differences in exercise parameters among the common disease states.

When the patient's $\dot{V}O_{2MAX}$ is normal, the anaerobic threshold is normal. Normal results are observed in normal or obese subjects and those with mild lung or heart disease. More important, if the $\dot{V}O_{2MAX}$ is less than 85% of the predicted value, determination of AT is pivotal for determining the cause of dyspnea. The $\dot{V}O_2$ at AT and its percentage of the $\dot{V}O_{2MAX}$ are critical numbers. Normal $\dot{V}O_2$ AT/predicted $\dot{V}O_2$ is at least 40%. Decreased $\dot{V}O_2$ at AT indicates cardiac, pulmonary, or peripheral vascular disease. In addition, anemia and chronic metabolic acidosis must be considered. A normal $\dot{V}O_2$ AT in the presence of low work capacity suggests poor effort or deconditioning, or mild cardiac or lung (obstructive or restrictive) disease.

Ventilatory impairment occurs when the breathing reserve ($BR = 1 - \dot{V}E_{MAX}/MVV$) is less than 30% or MVV $- \dot{V}E \geq 15$ L. Normally, at $\dot{V}O_{2MAX}$ the respiratory frequency does not exceed 50 to 60 breaths per minute and the $\dot{V}T$ does not exceed the inspiratory capacity (i.e., $\dot{V}T/FVC = 55–60\%$). Peak tidal volume during exercise varies considerably among patients, and the $\dot{V}T/FVC$ ratio has been suggested as a means of differentiating limitations due to cardiac and pulmonary disease (the latter demonstrate a ratio greater than 50%) (177). Jones and Rebuck (178), as well as Spiro and co-workers (179) have found normal $\dot{V}T/FVC$ ratios in patients with restrictive lung diseases. Similar results have been observed in COPD patients (180).

Recently, Gowda and associates (181) demonstrated no significant difference in $\dot{V}T/FVC$ ratios in COPD, asthma, restrictive lung disease (six cases of IPF, three of sarcoidosis), and heart disease (five cases of mitral valve disease, one of coronary artery disease). The ratios ranged from 44% ± 15% to 54% ± 12%.

Cardiac limitation can be assessed by reviewing the rhythm and rate of the electrocardiogram (ECG) and by determining $O_2$/pulse, heart rate reserve (HRR), and BP response to exercise. The $O_2$/pulse ($\dot{V}O_2/HR$) is a function of stroke volume. Normally it is at least 8.0 ml per heartbeat in females and 12.0 ml per heartbeat in males. A more precise calculation of predicted $O_2$/pulse uses this equation:

$$O_2/\text{pulse} = \frac{\text{predicted}\,\dot{V}O_{2MAX}}{\text{predicted HR}_{max}} \quad [19]$$

Heart rate reserve represents the unused percentage of HR at maximal work: $HRR = 1 - HR_{max}/HR_{pred\ max}$. A low HRR (rapid pulse) may be seen with cardiac disease. A high HRR (slow pulse) may be due to poor effort, conduction disease, blockade, or athletic conditioning. It can also be seen in patients with severe ventilatory impairment that limits exercise and thus reduces HR.

### Technical Aspects of Exercise Testing

Exercise studies are performed on a treadmill or a bicycle ergometer. Each instrument has its advocates. There is little difference between the two, except that the value of $\dot{V}O_2$ achieved on a bicycle is usually 89% to 95% of that obtained on a treadmill. Both incremental and

**TABLE 4.** *Patterns of response to exercise*

| Measurement | Normal value | Cardiac | COPD | ILD | Pulmonary emboli | Pyschogenic malinger | Deconditioning |
|---|---|---|---|---|---|---|---|
| Work capacity $\dot{V}O_{2max}$/pred $\dot{V}O_{2max}$ | >85% | Plateaus at low WR or occurs early | Decreased | Decreased | Decreased | Decreased | Normal or decreased |
| Anaerobic threshold $\dot{V}O_2AT$/pred $\dot{V}O_{2max}$ | >40% | <40% | Normal or indeterminate at close to $\dot{V}O_{2max}$ | Normal or occurs early | Decreased | Normal or not achieved | Normal |
| Breathing reserve $1-(\dot{V})E_{max}/MVV)$ | >30% | Normal | Decreased | Decreased | Normal or decreased | Normal | Normal |
| MVV–$\dot{V}E_{max}$ | >15 L | Normal | Decreased | Decreased | Normal or decreased | Normal | Normal |
| Resp. frequency rest→$WR_{max}$ | 8→50/min | Normal | Increased | >60/min at $WR_{max}$ | Normal or increased | Irregular, rapid | Normal |
| VT/FVC rest→$WR_{max}$ | 0.15→0.6 | Normal | Decreased | Normal but VT/IC=1 | Decreased | Not applicable | Not reliable |
| Gas exchange $P(A–a)O_2$ rest→$WR_{max}$ | 20→<30 | Normal | Abrupt increase as a single step at low WR | Stepwise increase | Increased | Normal | Normal |
| $ET_{CO_2}$ rest→$WR_{max}$ | ±2→<0 | Normal | Increased at $WR_{max}$ | Increased at $WR_{max}$ | Increased | Normal | Normal |
| VD/VT rest→$WR_{max}$ | 0.35→<0.25 | Normal | Increased | Increased | Increased | Normal | Normal |
| HR reserve | <15 beats | $HR_{max}$ reached at low exercise | Normal | Normal | Normal or increased | Normal | Normal |
| $O_2$/pulse ($\dot{V}O_2$/HR) | Females ≥8 ml/beat; males ≥12 ml/beat | Decreased | Decreased but slope normal | Normal | Normal or decreased | Normal or decreased | Normal or decreased |
| Blood pressure at $WR_{max}$ | Systolic <220; diastolic <110 | Systolic >240; diastolic >130; no systolic increase with exercise | Normal | Normal | Normal or decreased diastolic hypertension | Normal | Normal |

steady-state exercise studies can be performed. Most clinical laboratories perform progressive incremental studies, increasing work rates approximately 10 to 25 watts per minute, depending on the subject. The "ramp" method of increasing power continuously at a fixed rate or an electronically controlled cycle ergometer is utilized. Detailed discussion of the technical aspects can be found elsewhere (173–175). To avoid muscle fatigue, a protocol should be chosen that will cause the patient to be symptom limited within 8 to 10 minutes.

Jones developed a four-stage testing procedure. Stage I is progressively incremental, while stages II to IV are steady state (175).

Stage I: Workload, ECG, HR, $\dot{V}_E$, respiratory rate, $\dot{V}O_2$, $\dot{V}CO_2$, and $O_2$ Sat are monitored; R, $O_2$/pulse, $\dot{V}_T$, and $\dot{V}_E/\dot{V}CO_2$ and $\dot{V}_E/\dot{V}O_2$ are derived.

Stage II: Arterial blood gases are added to calculate $V_D/V_T$.

Stage III: Mixed venous partial pressure of $CO_2$, $\overline{P}vCO_2$, in addition to $\overline{P}aCO_2$ and $\dot{V}CO_2$ are measured to calculate cardiac output.

Stage IV: A Swan-Ganz catheter is inserted for hemodynamic measurements.

### Exercise Interpretation

There are four basic patterns of abnormal response to exercise: cardiac, ventilatory, pulmonary vascular, and deconditioning (Table 4). Although a single pattern may be observed, often the pattern is mixed, so it may be extremely difficult to determine if a patient's dyspnea is due to coronary insufficiency, COPD, or both. Likewise, in asbestos workers who have smoked, ventilatory impairment may be due to COPD, asbestos exposure, or intercurrent cardiac disease. Exercise testing has been used to evaluate the cause of respiratory complaints in patients with various pneumoconioses (182). The prevalence of abnormal exercise studies in asbestos-exposed workers varies greatly (183–187). Indeed, the results have been surprising. Several recent large series by Pearle, Agostoni, Sue, and Oren and their respective coinvestigators have concluded that most impairment in much-exposed workers was not pulmonary (183–186). Furthermore, many asbestos workers who complained of dyspnea had significant cardiac disease; those with ventilatory impairment were often cigarette smokers who had chronic air flow obstruction.

### Exercise-Induced Asthma

Exercise-induced asthma (EIA) produces a characteristic response after exercise at maximal or near maximal levels (188–190). Treadmill walking has been suggested as the preferred mode of exercise, since cycling occasionally fails to induce air flow limitation. A constant work rate should be selected, usually 80% of $\dot{V}O_{2MAX}$ or HR to be sustained for 6 to 8 minutes. Spirometry is performed immediately alter exercise and 5, 10, and 20 minutes later. Typically, the $FEV_1$ or $FEF_{25-75\%}$ decreases by 15% compared to preexercise flow rates. The F-V loop reveals decreased flow rates (PEFR, $FEF_{50}$%, $FEF_{25\%}$).

## BRONCHIAL PROVOCATION TESTS

In 1921 Alexander and Paddock (191) induced "asthmalike" attacks in asthma patients by injecting pilocarpine subcutaneously. In the late 1940s Curry (192) demonstrated the ability of inhaled histamine and acetyl-β-methyl choline to provoke bronchospasm in certain susceptible persons (those who had hay fever as well as asthma). Since that time many different methods of inducing bronchoconstriction have been developed and advocated for both research and clinical purposes (193–195). Bronchoprovocation testing can be divided into specific and nonspecific challenges. In recent years attempts to standardize methods have been made in the United States and in Europe (196–198).

Most challenge testing with nonspecific agents such as methacholine chloride can be performed in an outpatient setting, though specific challenges such as aspirin, metabisulfite, and specific antigens that may produce severe or delayed reactions must be done where emergency hospital facilities are available nearby. Many different techniques have been described that differ in the method of inhalation and of aerosol generation. While use of the Rosenthal-French dosimeter in conjunction with a jet nebulizer has been recommended by the National Academy of Allergy and Immunology (196), various other investigators have validated a simple jet nebulizer utilizing tidal breathing for 2 minutes (199, 200). The dosimeter is breath actuated, delivering a predetermined amount of aerosol liquid (usually 0.02 ml) during inspiration. The duration of aerosol delivery is 0.6 seconds. The dosimeter attaches to the DeVilbiss no. 42 or no. 646 nebulizer. When the two methods were compared, there was no difference in response, despite differences in aerosol output by the two methods (200). The dosimeter gave a more central disposition. A greater absolute dose of irritant (histamine) had to be given by the continuous tidal breathing method, since much of the aerosol produced was not inhaled, whereas the dosimeter produced aerosol only during inhalation.

The constrictor response to bronchoprovocation challenges has been measured by various tests for assessing air flow: $FEV_1$, $FEF_{25-75\%}$, $FEF_{50\%}$, PEFR, and specific airway conductance ($SG_{AW}$). A positive response is suggested by a decrement in the following measurements: $FEV_1$ (20%); $FEF_{25-75\%}$ (25%); $FEF_{50\%}$ (30%); PEFR (20%); and $SG_{AW}$ (35%). Measurement of $FEV_1$ is the most widely used measure clinically and epidemiologically because of its high reproducibility and ease of measurement by routine spirometry. Measurement of $SG_{AW}$ requires a body plethysmograph.

Most often the five-dose sequence of methacholine dilutions (with increasing concentration) is used. Baseline spirometry is performed, followed by five inhalations of a buffered saline solution (preserved with 0.04% phenol). Spirometry is repeated to obtain a "saline control." Patients are given five inhalations of increasing concentrations of methacholine (0.025, 0.25, 2.5, 10.0, and 25 mg/ml) if that goal has not been achieved. At each of five inhalations of the incremental concentrations the subject begins at FRC and slowly inhales the dose to TLC. Spirometry is repeated within 5 minutes of each dose until the target decrement is achieved or exceeded. Doses are quantitated in terms of "cumulated units," defined as the inhalation of 1 mg/ml methacholine (Table 5). The challenge test ends if there is at least a 20% reduction in $FEV_1$ (positive response) at any dose or if 188.88 cumulative units are administered and the $FEV_1$ has been reduced by 14% or less (i.e., a negative response). If $FEV_1$ drops 15% to 19% from baseline, the challenge test may be repeated at that concentration or a higher concentration, provided the total dose has not exceeded 188.88 cumulative units. A dose-response curve is constructed, which relates $FEV_1$ in terms of percent saline control value to the cumulative breath units of methacholine administered. This can be plotted on four-cycle semilogarithm arithmetic paper (Fig. 11). One interpolates the dose necessary to produce a 20% decrease in $FEV_1$ ($PD_{20}FEV_1$), which provides a measure of methacholine sensitivity. Note, when other measurements are used, such as $SG_{AW}$, the appropriate percentage reduction is assessed [i.e., 35% reduction in $SG_{AW}$ ($PD_{35}$)]. If the $FEV_1$ decreases by at least 20% following a specific dose unit, $FEV_1$ is measured again 3 minutes later to ensure that it is sustained. Subsequently, the patient inhales a β-adrenergic agonist to reverse the bronchoconstriction.

Alternative methods have been described that do not require a dosimeter; also fewer challenge doses are administered (201). The rebreathing technique of Hargreave and coworkers (202,203) requires 2 minutes of tidal breathing with each concentration. A screening challenge test has also been advocated that uses two concentrations—5 and 25 mg/ml (204). If no reduction in $FEV_1$ has occurred, measurements are made following the inhalation of a saline control—four breaths of 5 mg/ml and four of 25 mml. Braman and Corraro (205) have designed an abbreviated protocol: two breaths of a 25-mg/ml concentration alter the one breath of a 25-mg/ml concentration prior to administering four breaths of 25 mg/ml. The total cumulative dose of methacholine is 200 dose units.

**TABLE 5.** *Classification of response to methacholine-histamine challenge*

| | Response-eliciting dose | |
|---|---|---|
| Response | Cumulative inhaled volume (units) | Drug concentration (mg/ml) |
| None | >250 | >25 |
| Mild | >50–250 | >5–25 |
| Moderate | ≥10–50 | ≥1–5 |
| Marked | <10 | <1.0 |

Modified from ref. 224.

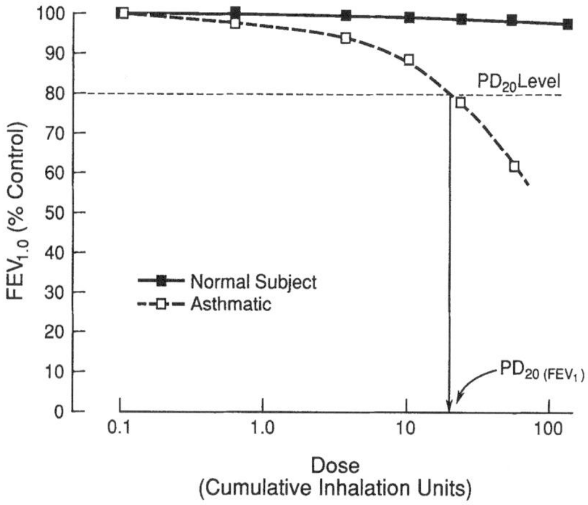


**FIG. 11.** Bronchoprovocation dose-response curve. The $PD_{20}$ is measured in cumulative inhalation units; in this case the challenge agent was methacholine.

While challenge testing most often uses methacholine, histamine, and less often acetylcholine or carbachol, has been used. Studies comparing methacholine and histamine have demonstrated equal reactivity, though side effects such as headaches, throat irritation, and flushing are more common with the latter.

The procedure for antigen challenge is similar to that for methacholine testing (193–195,199,206–208). Following a diluent control measurement, the patient inhales five breaths of the antigen concentration required to elicit a 2+ intradermal response. $FEV_1$ is measured 10 minutes after inhalation. If a reduction less than 15% occurs, the next concentration is administered. As in the methacholine test, the end point for a positive response is a 20% reduction in $FEV_1$. Following antigen challenge, the patient should be observed closely for 24 hours for possible severe late bronchospastic reactions. The results, like those of the previously described tests, are plotted on semilogarithmic paper; one antigen unit equals one inhalation of a 1/5,000 dilution of antigen. The dose of the antigen multiplied by the number of breaths equals the cumulative dose. It should be stressed that antigen testing is potentially far more dangerous than nonspecific challenge testing with methacholine or histamine because of the varied earlier and late reactions. The early responses may be reversed with β-adrenergic agonists, while late reactions, which develop slowly and usually peak 6 to 8 hours later, but can be observed up to 24 hours later, respond poorly to bronchodilators but are ameliorated by corticosteroids if they are given early.

Various reactions can be elicited by antigen testing. Most common are the immediate and late bronchoconstrictive (asthmatic) response. Less frequently there is an immediate bronchoconstrictive response followed by repeated bronchoconstrictive responses. This pattern is seen in workers who are sensitized to western red cedar. Patients with hypersensitivity pneumonitis may demonstrate several different patterns: a late "restrictive" pattern, or an immediate or late reaction. Late reactions are more common in persons exposed long-term or atopic patients. It should be noted that for most tests the standard $FEV_1$ measurement suffices for identifying a positive response. More sophisticated measurements such as F-V loops, lung volumes, airway resistance, and compliance are not necessary. Some patients with hypersensitivity pneumonitis due to long-term low-level exposure may have only a low diffusing capacity and hypoxemia following antigen challenge.

Other types of bronchoprovocation testing can be performed. These include cold-air isocapnic hyperventilation challenge, as well as osmotic challenge utilizing nebulized hypertonic saline (3.6%). Details of these tests are published elsewhere (209,210).

### Challenge Testing Indications

Most patients with asthma (occupationally related or not) do not need challenge testing. Symptoms coupled with demonstration of air flow limitation, as described previously, are sufficient to make the diagnosis. Indeed, provocation testing of confirmed asthma patients can be dangerous. Provocation testing can be used, however, to confirm a diagnosis of asthma in persons whose pulmonary function repeatedly "tests normal" or who have atypical symptoms such as persistent cough without wheezing or dyspnea. Bronchial hyperreactivity can occur in a variety of conditions in addition to asthma: COPD, bronchiolitis, recent viral airway respiratory tract infection, atopy, allergic rhinitis, hay fever, smoke inhalation, cystic fibrosis, post–adult respiratory distress syndrome, sarcoidosis (up to 50% of patients), cigarette smoking, after vaccination, and following chemical irritant exposure. The latter, also known as reactive airways syndrome (RAS), has been described in persons who experienced a single exposure to a high concentration of a noxious irritant such as paint, floor sealant, welding fume, or smoke (211). Patients develop an asthmalike illness but often have normal spirometries; results of methacholine challenge are positive.

### Normal Values

With the publication in 1846 of Hutchinson's *On the Capacity of the Lungs and on the Respiratory Functions with the View of Establishing a Precise and Easy Method of Detecting Disease by the Spirometer* (4), it was recognized that spirometric measurements could be interpreted only by comparing them to values derived from a "normal" population. Now, over 150 years later, we realize that the definition of "normal" depends on the context in which it is applied. Becklake (212) has reviewed in great detail the complex subject of normality as it relates to lung function. Her application of informational theory, which distinguishes "signal" (the information a test is designed to measure) from "noise" (measurement error) attempts to define "normality."

The definition of normal respiratory function depends on the sources of variation in lung function measurements that are of interest (signal) and those that are not (noise). Normal respiratory function may be defined differently by clinicians, physiologists, and epidemiologists. Clinicians are concerned principally with variation due to disease; physiologists in sources of variation other than disease. Epidemiologists, on the other hand, define normal according to specific objectives of a particular study. Measurement errors due to technical factors such as instrumentation variability, procedure variability, differences in administration and interpretation of tests, subject comprehension and cooperation, as well as subject–observer and observer–instrument interaction all contribute to variations in different published reference values. Equally important to the problem of identifying "normal" pulmonary function is the recognition of biologic variation, that is, intrasubject, intersubject, or interpopulation. Intrasubject variation may be due to measurement error noted previously, or to diurnal, seasonal, or endocrine effects. Intersubject variability results from all of the intrasubject factors cited above as well as from age, height, position (standing, sitting), gender, race, physical activity and muscularity, environmental exposures (cigarettes, occupation, urban air pollution, home or office pollution), residence (urban or rural), and socioeconomic position. Finally, interpopulation variability may result from all of these as well as from selection factors that determine inclusion or exclusion from the study population.

Unfortunately, published normal reference values and prediction regression formulae vary considerably, owing to the above considerations (213). Glindmeyer (214) has described the problem as "predictable confusion." He used published predicted regression equations to demonstrate gross differences for predicted normal FVC, $FEV_1$, and $FEF_{25-75\%}$ measurements. Thus, a 25-year-old man whose height is 1,173 cm (68 inches) has a predicted FVC range from 4.45 to 5.48 L, an $FEV_1$ in the range of 3.61 to 4.47 L, and $FEF_{25-75\%}$ in the range of 4.49 to 5.66 L. Similarly, a 55-year-old, 173-cm man has a predicted FVC range of 3.67 to 4.82 L, a predicted $FEV_1$ range of 2.72 to 3.44 L, and a predicted $FEF_{25-75\%}$ range of 2.99 to 4.55 L. Predicted $FEV_1$ and FVC measurements vary by 20% to 30%, and predicted $FEF_{25-75\%}$ by as much as 40%. Finally, the $FEV_1$/FVC ratio ranges from 80% to 91% in subjects aged 25 years and decreases to 70% to 83% at 55 years, yielding an average decline of 2.5% per decade (214).

The problem with prediction equations extends to other testing, including the single-breath diffusing capacity. Clausen (215) has reported testing the single-breath diffusing capacity of one healthy individual in 28 different teaching hospital laboratories. The $D_LCO$ ranged from 28 to 40 ml CO per minute per millimeter mercury. The percent predicted ranged from 84% to 131%. Thus, Clausen concluded, "The unavoidable conclusion . . . is that . . . there is no one recommended set of prediction equations applicable to all labs and patient populations."

Nevertheless, in clinical practice as well as epidemiologic surveys, choices must be made and certain guidelines should be used (213). Prediction equations should be chosen with attention to the technical and biologic factors discussed previously. Attempts should be made to adhere to published recommendations on equipment and standardization of procedures (17,100). Reference values should be selected that are derived from a study population that closely parallels the population served by the laboratory. Equations for similar tests should be taken from the same reference (i.e., $FEV_1$ and FVC predicted values should be obtained from the same reference). Finally, it has been suggested that verification of the "adequacy" and "best fit" of the predicted regression equations should be obtained by individual laboratories testing a cross section of their local normal healthy subjects. A sample size of 20 to 40 subjects is recommended. The equations with the smallest average differences and smallest range of difference should be chosen. If many tested subjects fall outside the limits of normal, three possibilities exist: the "normal" subjects are not normal, there is a problem with the testing methods or equipment, or the predicted equations selected are not suitable for the population being tested by the laboratory in question.

The above discussion notwithstanding, it remains to define the lower limits of normal for a given individual, in an effort to determine dysfunction or actual disease. Three methods have been advocated: percentage of predicted with a normal range of 80% to 120%, the normal 95th percentile, and the 95% CI.

Traditionally, the range of normal has been defined as 20% of the predicted value. Thus, 80% of predicted has been the standard for defining the lower limit of normal for PVC, $FEV_1$, TLC, RV, and MVV, the upper limit of normal being 120% of the predicted values for TLC and RV. Many laboratories have used 75% of predicted value for $FEF_{25-75\%}$ and $D_LCO$ as the lower cutoff point. Miller and coworkers (216,217) have demonstrated that using 80% of the predicted value as a lower limit underestimates the prevalence of abnormalities in a young working population and overestimates the prevalence of abnormalities in an older working population.

While using 80% of the predicted value as the lower limit of normal is simple and may be correct in most clinical situations, there is no statistical basis for its use. Sobol (218) has commented:

> Applying the 80% rule to those functions defined by a regression equation adds another dimension of error ... Percent predicted will deviate from the regression line less for small values than it will for large values. Therefore, small predicted values, as occur in the short and aged, will result in a higher incidence of abnormal findings.

To avoid some of the problems related to size and height, various volume-adjusted ratios have been used, including $FEV_1$/FVC, RV/TLC, and $G_{AW}$/FRC or $SG_{AW}$. The $FEV_1$/FVC ratio is used most widely, dating back to studies in the early 1950s, initially using 0.75 as the cutoff value but more recently using 0.70. However, the $FEV_1$/FVC ratio decreases with age, so a single value cannot be used. Furthermore, in persons older than 70 years the rate of $FEV_1$ decline is less than that of PVC, yielding an increase in the $FEV_1$/FVC ratio. Similarly, the $FEF_{25-75\%}$ and flow rates generated by the F-V loop have been "adjusted" for lung volumes. With respect to the former, the lower limit of $FEF_{25-75\%}$/FVC has been suggested as 0.65. Instantaneous flow rate ratios generated by the F-V loop have been suggested: $FEF_{50}/PVC = 0.98$ and $FEF_{25}/PVC = 0.48$ (219,220). Size compensation (i.e., volume adjustment) has disadvantages when size has different effects on the numerator and denominator, as it does in restrictive disorders. The problem of volume adjustment for $D_LCO$ and mechanics measurements was discussed previously.

A more precise statistical approach for defining the lower limit of normal is based on the predicted value and its variabilities (221,222). Assuming that pulmonary function tests vary in a bell-shaped or gaussian distribution, lower and upper limits of normal can be calculated: the predicted value is $\pm 1.96 \times$ SEE (standard error of the estimates) for a two-tailed *t*-test or the predicted value is $1.65 \times$ SEE for a one-tailed *t*-test. The latter is more often used to define those tests that can only be too low (spirometry), while the former is used for parameters that can be too high or low (lung volumes). Thus, if a value falls above or below the 95th percentile, there is less than a 5% chance that it will be normal. The lower limit of normal is defined as the value above which 95% of a normal population lies.

Recently, the 95% CI has been advocated as the most sophisticated approach for separating normal from abnormal. The difference between the predicted value and the subject's measured value is divided by the value of 1 CI:

$$\frac{\text{Predicted} - \text{Measured}}{\text{CI}} \qquad [20]$$

Both the Cl and the 95th percentile approaches yield the same lower limit of normal provided the measured parameters are distributed in normal gaussian fashion. The lower 95% CI can be estimated by subtracting 1.645 × SEE from the predicted value. Lower 95% CIs have been published for routine spirometry, maximum expiratory flow rates, diffusing capacity, and lung volume measurements. It should be noted that, because of greater SEE values for flow rates generated by the flow-volume curve, the lower 95% confidence limits may be extremely low or zero, and this analysis may not be useful. Finally, Clausen (223) has reminded us that although "the 95% confidence interval has achieved almost sacrosanct status, . . . it is frequently used without thoughtful reflection about its 'clinical significance.' By itself, the lower limit of normal cannot be used to predict the probability of lung disease."

## REFERENCES


1. Spriggs EA. The history of spirometry. *Br J Dis Chest* 1978;72:165–180.
2. Thackrah CT. *The effects of the principal arts, trades, and professions on health and longevity.* London: Longman, Rees, Ornie, Brown and Green, 1831;16–22.
3. Hutchinson J. Lecture on vital statistics, embracing an account of a new instrument for detecting the presence of disease in the system. Part 1. *Lancet* 1844;1:567–570, 594–597.
4. Hutchinson J. On the capacity of the lungs and on the respiratory functions with the view of establishing a precise and easy method of detecting disease by the spirometer. *Trans Med Chir Soc Lond* 1846; 29:137–252.
5. Barach AL. Physiological methods in the diagnosis and treatment of asthma and emphysema. *Ann Intern Med* 1938:12:454–481.
6. Moncrief A. Tests for respiratory efficiency. *Spec Rep Sec Med Res Coun* 1934;198.
7. Churchill ED, McNeil D. The reduction in vital capacity following operation. *Surg Gynecol Obstet* 1927:44:483–488.
8. Beecher HK. Effect of laparotomy on lung volume. Demonstration of a new type of pulmonary collapse. *J Clin* Invest 1933;12:651–658.
9. Baldwin ED, Cournand A, Richards DW. Pulmonary insufficiency. I. Physiological classification, clinical methods of analysis, standard values in normal subjects. *Medicine* 1948:27:243–278.
10. Tiffeneau R, Pinelli A. Air circulant et air captif dans l'exploration de la function ventilatrice pulmonaire. *Paris Med* 1947:133:624–628.
11. Gaensler EA. Analysis of the ventilatory defect by timed vital capacity measurements. *Am Rev Tuberc* 1951:64:256–278.
12. Gaensler EA. An instrument for dynamic vital capacity measurement. *Science* 1951:114:444–446.
13. Cournand A, Richards DW. Pulmonary insufficiency 1. Discussion of a physiological classification and presentation of clinical tests. *Am Rev Tuberc* 1941;44:26–4l.
14. Wells H, Stead WW, Rossing TD, Oghanovich J. Accuracy of an improved spirometer for recording fast breathing. *J Appl Physiol* 1959:14:451–454.
15. Leuallen EC, Fowler WS. Maximal midexpiratory flow. *Am Rev Tuberc* 1955;72:783–800.
16. Hyatt RE, Black LF. The flow-volume curve: a current perspective. *Am Rev Respir Dis* 1973;108:475–481.
17. American Thoracic Society. Standardization of spirometry—1994 update. *Am J Respir Crit Care Med* 1995;152:1107–1136.
18. Nelson SB, Gardner RM, Crapo RD, Jensen RL. Performance evaluation of contemporary spirometers. *Chest* 1990;97:288–297.
19. Meneely GR, Ball CO, Kory RC, et al. A simplified closed-circuit helium-dilution method for the determination of the residual volume of the lungs. *Am J Med* 1960;28:824–831.
20. Darling RC, Cournand A, Richards DW. Studies on the intrapulmonary mixing of gases. II. An open-circuit method for measuring residual air. *J Clin Invest* 1940;19:609–618.
21. Burns CB, Scheinhort DJ. Evaluation of single-breath helium-dilution total lung capacity in obstructive lung disease. *Am Rev Respir Dis* 1984;130:580–583.
22. Dubois AB, Botelho SY, Bedell GN, Marshall R, Comroe JH. A rapid plethysmographic method for measuring thoracic gas volume: a comparison with a nitrogen washout method for measuring functional residual capacity in normal subjects. *J Clin Invest* 1956;35:322–326.
23. Mitchell MM, Renzetti AD Jr. Evaluations of a single-breath method of measuring total lung capacity. *Am Rev Respir Dis* 1968;97:571–58O.
24. Jalowayski AA, Dawson A. Measurement of lung volume: the multiple-breath nitrogen method. In: Clausen JL, ed. *Pulmonary function testing: guidelines and controversies.* New York: Academic Press, 1982;115–127.
25. Zarins LP. Closed-circuit helium-dilution method of lung volume measurement. In: Clausen JL, Zarins LP, eds. *Pulmonary function testing:* guidelines and controversies. New York: Academic Press, 1982;129–140.
26. Zarins LP, Clausen JL. Body plethysmography In: Clausen JL, Zarins LP, eds. *Pulmonary function testing:* guidelines and controversies. New York: Academic Press, 1982;141–153.
27. Harris TR, Pratt PC, Kilburn KH. Total lung capacity measured by roentgenograms. *Am J Med* 1971;50:756–763.
28. Barnhard HJ, Pierce JA, Joyce JW, Bates JH. Roentgenographic determination of total lung capacity. *Am J Med* 1960;28:51–60.
29. Clausen LL, Zarins LP. Estimation of lung volumes from chest radiographs. In: Clausen JL, Zarins LP, eds. *Pulmonary function testing:* guidelines and controversies. New York: Academic Press, 1982; 155–163.
30. Comroe JH. Man-cans. *Am Rev Respir Dis* 1977;1 16:945–950.
31. Burns CB, Scheinhorn DJ. Evaluation of single-breath helium-dilution total lung capacity in obstructive lung disease. *Am Rev Respir Dis* 1984;130:580–583.
32. Shore S, Milic-Emili J, Martin JG. Reassessment of body plethysmographic techniques for the measurement of thoracic gas volume in asthmatics. *Am Rev Respir Dis* 1982;126:515–520.
33. Rodenstein DO, Stanescu DC. Frequency dependence of plethysmographic volume in healthy and asthmatic subjects. *J Appl Physiol* 1983;54:159–165.
34. Woolcock AJ, Read J. Lung volumes in exacerbations of asthma. *Am J Med* 1966;41:259–273.
35. Vulterini S, Bianco MR, Pellicciotti L, Sidoti AM. Lung mechanics in subjects showing increased residual volume without bronchial obstruction. *Thorax* 1980;35:461–466.
36. Yip CK, Epstein H, Goldring RM. Relationship of functional residual capacity to static mechanics in chronic obstructive pulmonary disease. *Am J Med Sci* 1984; 287:3–6.
37. Owens MW, Kinasewitz AT, Anderson MW. Clinical significance of an isolated reduction in residual volume. *Am Rev Respir Dis* 1987; 136:1377–1380.
38. Colp C, Williams MH Jr. Total occlusion of airways producing a restrictive pattern of ventilatory impairment. *Am Rev Respir Dis* 1973; 108:118–122.
39. Hudgel DW, Cooper D, Soubrada J. Reversible restrictive lung disease simulation asthma. *Ann Intern Med* 1976;85:328–332.
40. Goldman HJ, Becklake MR. Respiratory function tests: normal values at median altitudes and the prediction of normal results. *Am Rev Tuberc* 1959;79:457–467.
41. Black LF, Oxfford K, Hyatt RE. Variability in the maximal expiratory flow-volume curve in asymptomatic smokers and nonsmokers. *Am Rev Respir Dis* 1974;110:282–292.
42. Boren HG, Kory RC, Syner JC. The terans Administration-Army cooperative study of pulmonary function. II. The lung volume and its subdivisions in normal men. *Am J Med* 1966;41:96–114.
43. Needham CD, Rogan MC, McDonald I. Normal standards for lung volumes, intrapulmonary gas mixing, and maximum breathing capacity. *Thorax* 1954;9:313–325.
44. Grimby G, Soderholm B. Spirometric studies in normal subjects. III. Static lung volumes and maximum voluntary ventilation in adults, with a note on physical fitness. *Acta Med Scand* 1963;173:199–206.
45. Viljanen AA, Viljanen BC, Halttunen K, Kreus K-E. Body plethys-

mographic studies in nonsmoking, healthy adults. *Scand J Clin Lab Invest* 1982;4(suppl 159):35–50.
46. Crapo RO, Morris AH, Clayton PD, et al. Lung volumes in healthy nonsmoking adults. *Bull Eur Physiopathol Respir* i982;18:419–425.
47. Stinson JM, McPherson GL, Hicks K, et al. Spirometric standards for health black adults. *J Natl Med Assoc* 1981;73:729–733.
48. Dawson A. Elastic recoil and compliance. In: Clausen JL, Zarins LP, eds. *Pulmonary function testing:* guidelines and controversies. New York: Academic Press, 1982, 194–204.
49. Milic-Emili J, Mead J, Turner JM, Glauser EM. Improved technique for estimating pleural pressure from esophageal balloons. *J Appl Physiol* 1964;19:207–211.
50. Schlueter D, Immekus J, Stead W. Relationship between maximal inspiratory pressure and total lung capacity (coefficient of retraction) in normal subjects and in patients with emphysema, asthma, and diffuse pulmonary infiltration. *Am Rev Respir Dis* 1967;96:656–665.
51. Knudson RJ, Clark DF, Kennedy TC, Knudson DE. Effect of aging alone on mechanical properties of the normal adult human lung. *J Appl Physiol* 1977;43:1054–1062.
52. Turner JM, Mead J, Wohl ME. Elasticity of human lungs in relation to age. *J Appl Physiol* 1968;25:664–671.
53. Yernault JC, Baran D, Englert M. Effect of growth and aging on the static mechanical lung properties. *Bull Eur Physiopathol Respir* 1977; 13:777–788.
54. Ebert RV. Elasticity of the lung in pulmonary emphysema. *Ann Intern Med* 1968;69:903–908.
55. Gold WM, Kaufman HS, Nadel JA. Elastic recoil of the lungs in chronic asthmatic patients before and after therapy. *J Appl Physiol* 1967;23:433–438.
56. Sharp J, Sweany S, van Lith P. Physiologic observations in diffuse pulmonary fibrosis and granulomatosis. *Am Rev Respir Dis* 1966;94: 316–331.
57. Gibson GJ, Pride NB. Pulmonary mechanics in fibrosing alveolitis. *Am Rev Respir Dis* 1977;116:637–647.
58. Kanengiser LC, Rapoport DM, Epstein H, Goldring RM. Volume adjustment of mechanics and diffusion in interstitial lung disease: lack of clinical relevance. *Chest* 1989;96:1036–1042.
59. Black LF, Hyatt RE. Maximal respiratory pressures: normal values and relationship to age and sex. *Am Rev Respir Dis* 1969;99:696–702.
60. Rochester DF, Arora NS. Respiratory muscle failure. *Med Clin North Am* 1983;67:573–597.
61. Gardner RM, Crapo RO, Nelson SB. Spirometry and flow-volume curves. *Clin Chest Med* 1989;10:145–154.
62. Morris AH, Kanner RE, Crapo RO, Gardner RM. *Clinical pulmonary function testing:* a manual of uniform laboratory procedure, 2nd ed. Salt Lake City: Inter-mountain Thoracic Society, 1984.
63. Eisen EA, Robins JM, Greaves IA, Wegman DH. Selection effects of repeatability criteria to lung spirometry. *Am J Epidemiol* 1984;120: 734–742.
64. Eisen EA, Oliver LC, Christiani DC, Robins JM, Wegman DH. Effects of spirometry standards in two occupational cohorts. *Am Rev Respir Dis* 1985;132:120–124.
65. Pennock BE, Rogers RM, McCaffree DR. Changes in measured spirometric indices—What is significant? *Chest* 1981;80:97–99.
66. Glindmeyer HW, Jones RN, Barlmian HW, Weill H. Spirometry: quantitative test criteria and test acceptability. *Am Rev Respir Dis* 1987;136:449–452.
67. Hankinson JL, Bang KM. Acceptability and reproducibility criteria of the American Thoracic Society as observed in a sample of the general population. *Am Rev Respir Dis* 1991;143:516–521.
68. American Thoracic Society. Lung function testing: selection of reference values and interpretative strategies. *Am Rev Respir Dis* 1991; 144:1202–1218.
69. Knudson RS, Lebowitz MD. Maximal midexpiratory flow (FEF 25–75%): normal limits and assessment of sensitivity. *Am Rev Respir Dis* 1978;117:609–610.
70. Knudson RJ, Burrows B, Lebowitz MD. The maximal expiratory flow-volume curve: its use in detection of ventilatory abnormalities in a population study. *Am Rev Respir Dis* 1976;114:871–89O.
71. Hyatt RE, Schilder DP, Fry DL. Relationship between maximum expiratory flow and degree of lung inflation. *J Appl Physiol* 1958;13: 331–336.
72. Miller R, Hyatt R. Evaluation of obstructing lesions of the trachea and larynx by flow-volume loops. *Am Rev Respir Dis* 1973;108:475–481.
73. Kryger M, Bode F, Antic R, Anthonisen N. Diagnosis of obstruction of the upper and central airways. *Am J Med* 196;611:85–93.
74. Jayamanne DS, Epstein H, Goldring RM. The influence of lung volume on expiratory flow rates in diffuse interstitial lung disease. *Am J Med Sci* 1978;275:329–336.
75. Dosman J, Bode F, Urbanetti J, Martin R, Macklem PT. The use of a helium-oxygen mixture during maximum expiratory flow to demonstrate obstruction in small airways in smokers. *J Clin Invest* 1975;55: 1090–1099.
76. Fulmer JD, Roberts WC, Von Gral ER, Crystal RG. Small airways in idiopathic pulmonary fibrosis. *J Clin Invest* 1977;60:595–610.
77. Jayamanne DS, Epstein H, Goldring RM. Flow-volume curve contour in COPD: correlation with pulmonary mechanics. *Chest* 1980;77: 749–757.
78. Gaensler EA, Wright GW. Evaluation of respiratory impairment. *Arch Environ Health* 1966;12:146–189.
79. Aldrich TK, Arora NS, Rochester DF. The influence of airway obstruction and respiratory muscle strength on maximal voluntary ventilation in lung disease. *Am Rev Respir Dis* 1982;126:195–199.
80. Dubois AB, Botelbo S, Comroe JH Jr. A new method for measuring airway resistance in man using a body plethysmograph. Values in normal subjects and in patients with respiratory disease. *J Clin Invest* 1956;35:327–335.
81. Ries AL, Clausen JL. Airway resistance. In: Wilson AF, ed. *Pulmonary function testing:* indications and testing. Orlando, FL: Grune & Stratton, 1985, 95–118.
82. Shim C. Response to bronchodilators. *Clin Chest Med* 1989;10: 155–164.
83. Ries A. Response to bronchodilators. In: Clausen JL, Zarins LP eds. *Pulmonary function testing:* guidelines and controversies. New York: Academic Press, 1982;215–221.
84. Ramsdell JW, Tisi GM. Determination of bronchodilation in the clinical pulmonary function laboratory. Role of changes in static lung volumes. *Chest* 1979;76:622–628.
85. Ayres SM, Griesbach SJ, Reimold F, et al. Bronchial component in chronic obstructive lung disease. *Am J Med* 1974;57:183–191.
86. Girard WM, Light RW. Should the PVC be considered in evaluating response to bronchodilator? *Chest* 1983;84:87–89.
87. Light RW, Conrad SH, George RB. The one best test for evaluating effects of bronchodilator therapy. *Chest* 1977;72:512–516.
88. Berger R, Smith D. Acute postbronchodilator changes in pulmonary function parameters in patients with chronic airways obstruction. *Chest* 1988;93:541–546.
89. Pennock BE, Rogers RM, McCaffree DR. Changes in measured spirometric indices: What is significant? *Chest* 1981;80:97–99.
90. Sourk RL, Nugent KM. Bronchodilator testing: confidence intervals derived from placebo inhalations. *Am Rev Respir Dis* 1983;128: 153–157.
91. Tweeddale PM, Alexander F, McHardy GJR. Short-term variability in $FEV_1$ and bronchodilator responsiveness in obstructive ventilatory defects. *Thorax* 1987;42:487–490.
92. Anthonisen NR, Wright EC, IPPB Trial Group. Bronchodilator response in chronic obstructive pulmonary disease. *Am Rev Respir Dis* 1986;133:814–819.
93. Cockcroft DW, Bersheid BA. Volume adjustment of maximal midexpiratory flow: importance of change in total lung capacity. *Chest* 1980;78:595–600.
94. Sherter CB, Connolly JJ, Schilder DP. The significance of volume adjusting the maximum midexpiratory flow in assessing the response to a bronchodilator drug. *Chest* 1978;73:568–571.
95. Lorber DB, Kaltenborn W, Burrows B. Responses to isoproterenol in a general population sample. *Am Rev Respir Dis* 1978;118:856–861.
96. Haldane J, Smith JL. The absorption of oxygen by the lungs. *J Physiol* 1897;22:231–258.
97. Krogh A. On the mechanism of the gas exchange in the lungs. *Scand Arch Physiol* 1910;23:248–278.
98. Krogh M. The diffusion of gases through the lungs of man. *J Physiol (Lond)* 1914;49:271300.
99. Ogilvie CM, Forster RE, Blakemore WS, Morton JW. A standardized breathholding technique for the clinical measurement of the diffusing capacity of the lung for carbon monoxide. *J Clin Invest* 1957;36:1–17.
100. American Thoracic Society. Single-breath carbon monoxide diffusing capacity. Recommendations for a standard technique— 1995 Update. *Am J Respir Crit Care Med* 1995;152:2185–2198.

101. Dinakara P, Blumenthal WS, Johnston RF, Kauffman LA, Solnick PB. The effect of anemia on pulmonary diffusing capacity with derivation of a correction equation. *Am Rev Respir Dis* 1970;102:965–969.
102. Cotes JE, Dabbs JM, Elwood PC, Hall AM, McDonald A, Saunders MJ. Iron-deficiency anemia: its effect on transfer factor for the lung (diffusing capacity) and ventilation and cardiac frequency during submaximal exercise. *Clin Sci* 1972;42:325–335.
103. Frans A, Stanescu DC, Veriter CV, Clerbaux T, Brasseur L. Smoking and diffusing capacity. *Scand Respir Dis* 1975;56:165–183.
104. Mohsenifar Z, Tashkin DP. Effect of carboxyhemoglobin on the single-breath diffusing capacity: derivation of an empirical correction factor. *Respiration* 1979;37:185–191.
105. Leech JA, Martz L, Liben A, Becklake MR. Diffusing capacity for carbon monoxide. *Am Rev Respir* Dis 1985;132:1127–1129.
106. Clausen J, Crapo R, Gardner RM. Interlaboratory comparisons of pulmonary function testing. *Am Rev Respir Dis* 1984;129(suppl A37). Abstract.
107. Saunders RB. Current practice in six London lung function laboratories. *Proc R Soc Med* 1977;70:162–163.
108. Morris AH, Crapo R. Standardization of computation of single-breath transfer factor. *Bull Eur Physiopathol Respir* 1985;21:183–189.
109. Make B, Miller A, Epler G, Gee JBL. Single-breath diffusing capacity in the industrial setting. *Chest* 1982;82:351–356.
110. Cotes JE. *Lung function:* assessment and application in medicine, 4th ed. Oxford: Blackwell Scientific, 1979;235–236.
111. Graham BL, Mink JT, Cotton DJ. Overestimation of the single-breath carbon monoxide diffusing capacity in patients with air-flow obstruction. *Am Rev Respir Dis* 1984;129:403–408.
112. Crapo RO, Forster RE II. Carbon monoxide diffusing capacity. Clin Chest Med 1989;10:187–198.
113. Weissman IM, Zeballos RJ. Lower single-breath carbon monoxide diffusing capacity (DLCO) in black subjects compared to Caucasians. *Chest* 1987;92(suppl):142S.
114. Epler GR, McCloud TC, Gaensler EA, Mikus JP, Carrington CB. Normal chest roentgenograms in chronic diffuse infiltrative lung disease. *N Engl J Med* 1978;298:934–939.
115. Coleman DL, Dodek PM, Golden JA, et al. Correlation between serial pulmonary function tests and fiberoptic bronchoscopy in patients with *Pneumocystis carinii* pneumonia and the acquired immune deficiency syndrome. *Am Rev Respir Dis* 1984;129:491–493.
116. Overland ES, Nolan AJ, Hopewell PC. Alteration of pulmonary function in intravenous drug abusers, prevalence, severity and characterization of gas exchange abnormalities. *Am J Med* 1980;68:231–237.
117. Ognibene FP, Masur H, Rogers P, et al. Nonspecific interstitial pneumonitis without evidence of *Pneumocystis carinii* pneumonia in asymptomatic patients infected with human immunodeficiency virus. *Ann Intern Med* 1988;109:874–879.
118. Miller A, Teirstein AS, Chuang MT. The sequence of physiologic changes in pulmonary sarcoidosis: correlation with radiographic stages and response to therapy. *Mt Sinai J Med* 1977;44:852–865.
119. Matthews JI, Hooper RG. Exercise testing in pulmonary sarcoidosis. *Chest* 1983;83:75–81.
120. Line RB, Hunninghake GW, Keogh BA, Jones AE, Johnston GS, Crystal RG. Gallium-67 scanning to stage the alveolitis of sarcoidosis: correlation with clinical studies, pulmonary function studies and bronchoalveolar lavage. *Am Rev Respir Dis* 1981;123:440–446.
121. Tukiainen P, Taskinen E, Holsti P, Korhola O, Valle M. Prognosis of cryptogenic fibrosing alveolitis. *Thorax* 1983;38:828–833.
122. Fulmer JD, Roberts WC, Von Gal ER, Crystal IG. Morphologic-physiologic correlates of the severity of fibrosis and degree of cellularity in idiopathic pulmonary fibrosis. *J Clin Invest* 1979;63:665–676.
123. Risk T, Epler GR, Gaensler EA. Exercise alveolar-arterial oxygen pressure difference in interstitial lung disease. *Chest* 1984;85:69–74.
124. Keogh BA, Lakatos E, Price D, Crystal RG. Importance of the lower respiratory tract in oxygen transfer: exercise testing in patients with interstitial and destructive lung disease. *Am Rev Respir Dis* 1984; 129(suppl):570–580
125. American Thoracic Society. Evaluation of impairment/disability secondary to respiratory disease. *Am Rev Respir Dis* 1982;126:945–951.
126. Murphy RL, Becklake MR, Broolts SM, et al. Diagnosis of nonmalignant diseases related to asbestos: official statement of the American Thoracic Society. *Am Rev Respir Dis* 1986;134:363–368.
127. Regan GM, Tagg B, Walford J, Thomson ML. The relative importance of clinical, radiological and pulmonary function variables in evaluating asbestosis and chronic obstructive airway disease in asbestos workers. *Clin Sci* 1971;41:569–582.
128. Epler GR, Samet JM, Gaensler EA. Diffusing capacity in the diagnosis of asbestosis. *Chest* 1978;74:336.
129. Britton MG, Hughes DTD, Wener AMJ. Serial pulmonary function tests in patients with asbestosis. *Thorax* 1977;32:45–52.
130. Zedda S, Aresini G, Ghezz I, Sartorelli E. Lung function in relation to radiographic changes in asbestos workers. *Respiration* 1973;30: 132–140.
131. Becklake MR, Fournier-Massey G, McDonald JC, Siemiatycki J, Rossiter CE. Lung function in relation to chest radiographic changes in Quebec asbestos workers. I. Methods, results and conclusions. *Bull Physiopathol Respir* 1970;6:687–699.
132. Sue DY, Oren A, Hansen JE, Wasserman K. Diffusing capacity for carbon monoxide as a predictor of gas exchange during exercise. *N Engl J Med* 1987;316:1301–1306.
133. Garcia JGN, Griffith DE, Williams JS, Blevins WJ, Kronenberg RS. Reduced diffusing capacity as an isolated finding in asbestos- and silica-exposed workers. *Chest* 1990;98:105–111.
134. Ayres LN, Ginsberg ML, Fein J, Wasserman K. Diffusing capacity, specific diffusing capacity and interpretation of diffusion defects. *West J Med* 1975;123:255–264.
135. McIlroy MB, Bates DV. Respiratory function after pneumonectomy. *Thorax* 1957;11:303–311.
136. Gonaalez E, Weil H, Ziskind M, George R. The value of the single-breath diffusing capacity in separating chronic bronchitis from pulmonary emphysema. *Dis Chest* 1968;53:229–236.
137. Ohman JL, Schmidt-Nowara W, Lawrence M, Kazemi H, Lowell FC. The diffusing capacity in asthma. Effect of air-flow obstruction. *Am Rev Respir Dis* 1973;107:932–973.
138. Weitaman RH, Wilson AF. Diffusing capacity and overall ventilation perfusion pressure in asthma. *Am J Med* 1976;57:767–774.
139. Gelb AF, Gold WM, Wright RR, Bruch HR, Nadel JA. Physiologic diagnosis of subclinical emphysema. *Am Rev Respir Dis* 1973; 107:50–65.
140. Berend N, Woolcock AJ, Martin GE. Correlation between the function and the structure of the lung in smokers. *Am Rev Respir Dis* 1979; 119:695–705.
141. Burrows B, Strauss RH, Nider AH. Chronic obstructive lung disease. III. Interrelationships of pulmonary function data. *Am Rev Respir Dis* 1965;91:861–868.
142. Vandenbergh E, Billiet L, Van de Woestijne KP, Gyselen A. Relation between single-breath diffusing capacity and arterial blood gases in chronic obstructive lung disease. *Scand J Respir Dis* 1968;49:92–101.
143. Owens GR, Rogers RM, Pennock BF, Levin D. The diffusing capacity as a predictor of arterial oxygen desaturation during exercise in patients with chronic obstructive pulmonary disease. *N Engl J Med* 1984;310:1218–1221.
144. Nadel JA, Gold WM, Burgess JH. Early diagnosis of chronic pulmonary vascular obstruction: value of pulmonary function tests. *Am J Med* 1968;44:16–25.
145. D'Alonzo GE, Bower JS, Dantaker DR. Differentiation of patients with primary and thromboembolic pulmonary hypertension. *Chest* 1984;85:457–461.
146. Young RH, Mark GJ. Pulmonary vascular changes in scleroderma. *Am J Med* 1978;64:998–1004.
147. Ungerer RG, Tashkin DP, Furst D, et al. Pulmonary hypertension in progressive systemic sclerosis. *Am J Med* 1983;75:65–74.
148. Peters-Golden M, Wise RA, Hochberg MC, Stevens MS, Wigley FM. Carbon monoxide diffusing capacity as predictor of outcome in systemic sclerosis. *Am J Med* 1984;77:1027–1034.
149. Burgess JH. Pulmonary diffusing capacity in disorders of the pulmonary circulation. *Circulation* 1974;49:541–550.
150. Rhodes KM, Evemy K, Nariman S, Gibson GJ. Relation between severity of mitral valve disease and results of routine lung function tests in nonsmokers. *Thorax* 1982;37:751–755.
151. Hales CA, Kazemi H. Pulmonary function after uncomplicated myocardial infarction. *Chest* 1977;72:350–358.
152. Siegel JL, Miller A, Brown LK, DeLuca A, Teirstein A. Pulmonary diffusing capacity in left ventricular dysfunction. *Chest* 1990;98: 550–553.
153. De Troyer A, Yernault JC, Englert M. Mechanics of breathing in patients with atrial septal defect. *Am Rev Respir Dis* 1977;115: 413–421.

154. Ewan PW, Jones HA, Rhodes C, Hughes JMB. Detection of intrapulmonary hemorrhage with carbon monoxide uptake: application of Goodpasture's syndrome. *N Engl J Med* 1976;295:1391–1396.
155. Mellengasrd K. The alveolar-arterial oxygen difference: its size and components in normal man. *Acta Physiol Scand* 1966;67:10–26.
156. Sorbini CA, Grassi V, Solinas E, Muisan G. Arterial oxygen tension in relation to age in healthy subjects. *Respiration* 1968;25:3–13.
157. Hansen JE, Sue DY, Wasserman K. Predicted values for clinical exercise testing. *Am Rev Respir Dis* 1984;129(suppl):S49–S55.
158. Benatar SR, Hewlett AM, Nunn JF. The use of isoshunt lines for control of oxygen therapy. *Br J Anaesth* 1973;45:711–718.
159. Shapiro AR, Peters PM. A nomogram for planning respiratory therapy. *Chest* 1977;72:197–200.
160. Smith DD, Agostoni PG. The discriminatory value of the P(A - a)$O_2$ during exercise in the detection of asbestosis in asbestos exposed workers. *Chest* 1989;95:52–55.
161. Stewart RI, Lewis CM. Arterial oxygenation and oxygen transport during exercise in patients with chronic obstructive pulmonary disease. *Respiration* 1986;49:161–169.
162. Jones NL. Pulmonary gas exchange during exercise in patients with chronic airway obstruction. *Clin Sci* 1966;31:39–50.
163. Kurihara N, Fujimoto S, Terakawa K, Yamamoto M, Takeda T. Prediction of $PaO_2$ during treadmill walking in patients with COPD. *Chest* 1987;91:328–332.
164. Gimenez M, Salinas W, Candina R, et al. Blood gases at rest and exercise for assessment of respiratory impairment in pneumoconioses. *Eur J Respir Dis* 1981;62(suppl):30–31.
165. Refsum HE. Pulmonary gas exchange during and after exercise of short duration in silicosis. *Scand J Clin Lab Invest* 1972;121(suppl): 1–48.
166. Morgan WKC, Lapp NL, Seaton A. Respiratory disability in coal miners. *JAMA* 1980;243:2401–2404.
167. Epler GR, Sober EA, Gavosler EA. Determination of impairment (disability) in interstitial lung disease. *Am Rev Respir Dis* 1980;121: 647–657.
168. Morgan WKC, Zaldivar GL. Blood gas analysis as a determinant of occupationally related disability. *J Occup Med* 1990;32:440–443.
169. Eichorn JH, Cormier AD, Moran A. Accuracy and comparisons in blood gas measurements. *Chest* 1988;94:1–3.
170. Man Kessel AL, Eichorn JH, Clausen J, et al. Interinstrument comparison of blood gas analyzers and the assessment of tonometry using fresh heparinized whole human blood. *Chest* 1987;92:418–422.
171. Said S. Abnormalities of pulmonary gas exchange in obesity. *Ann Intern Med* 1960;94:49–54.
172. Rochmis P, Blackburn H. Exercise tests: a survey of procedures, safety and litigation experience in approximately 170,000 tests. *JAMA* 1971;217:1065–1066.
173. Wasserman K, Hansen JE, Sue DY, Whipp BJ. *Principles of exercise testing and interpretation.* Philadelphia: Lea & Febiger, 1987.
174. Zavala DC. *Manual on exercise testing. A training handbook,* 2nd ed. Iowa City: University of Iowa Press, 1987.
175. Jones NL. *Clinical exercise testing,* 3rd ed. Philadelphia: WB Saunders, 1988.
176. Eschenbacher WL, Mannina A. An algorithm for the interpretation of cardiopulmonary exercise tests. *Chest* 1990;97:263–267.
177. Weber KT, Janicki JS, Likoff MJ. Exercise testing in the evaluation of cardiopulmonary disease. *Clin Chest Med* 1984;5:173–180.
178. Jones NL, Rebuck AS. Tidal volume response to exercise in patients with diffuse fibrosing alveolitis. *Bull Eur Physiopathol Respir* 1979; 15:321–327.
179. Spiro SG, Dowdeswell IRG, Clark TJH. An analysis of submaximal exercise responses in patients with sarcoidosis and fibrosing alveolitis. *Br J Dis Chest* 1981;75:169–180.
180. Spiro SG, Hahn HL, Edwards RHT, Pride NB. An analysis of the physiological strain of submaximal exercise in patients with chronic obstructive bronchitis. *Thorax* 1975;30:415–425.
181. Gowda K, Zintel T, McParland C, Orchard R, Gallagher CG. Diagnostic value of maximal exercise tidal volume. *Chest* 1990;98: 1351–1354.
182. Cotes JE, Zeida J, King B. Lung function impairment as a guide to exercise limitation in work-related lung disorders. *Am Rev Respir Dis* 1988;137:1089–1093.
183. Pearle J. Exercise performance and functional impairment in asbestos-exposed workers. *Chest* 1981;80:701–705.
184. Agostoni P, Smith DD, Schoene RB, Robertson HT, Butler J. Evaluation of breathlessness in asbestos workers. *Am Rev Respir Dis* 1987;135:812–816.
185. Sue DY, Hansen JE, Wasserman K. Lung function and exercise performance in smoking and nonsmoking asbestos-exposed workers. *Am Rev Respir Dis* 1985;132:612–618.
186. Oren A, Sue DY, Hansen JE, Torrance DJ, Wasserman K. The role of exercise testing in impairment evaluation. *Am Rev Respir Dis* 1987; 135:230–235.
187. Howard J, Mohsenifar Z, Brown HV, Koerner SK. Roles of exercise testing in assessing functional respiratory impairment due to asbestos exposure. *J Occup Med* 1982;24:685–689.
188. Anderson SD. Exercise-induced asthma: the state of the art. *Chest* 1985;87:191S–195S.
189. Bleeker ER. Exercise-induced asthma: physiological and clinical considerations. *Clin Chest Med* 1984;5:109–119.
190. Eggleston PA. Pathophysiology of exercise-induced asthma. *Med Sci Sports Exerc* 1986;18:318–321.
191. Alexander HL, Paddock R. Bronchial asthma: response to pilocarpine and epinephrine. *Arch Intern Med* 1921;27:184–191.
192. Curry JJ. Comparative action of acetyl-β-methacholine and histamine on the respiratory tract in normals, patients with hay fever, and subjects with bronchial asthma. *J Clin Invest* 1947;26:430–438.
193. Eiser NM. Bronchial provocation testing. In: Nadel JA, Pauwels R, Snashall PD, eds. *Bronchial hyperresponsiveness.* Oxford: Blackwell Scientific Publications, 1987, 173–256.
194. Braman SS, Corrao WM. Bronchoprovocation testing. *Clin Chest Med* 1989;10:165–176.
195. Spector SL, ed. *Provocative challenge procedures. Background and methodology.* Mount Kisco, NY: Futura, 1989.
196. Chai H, Farr RS, Froehlich LA, et al. Standardization of bronchial inhalation procedures. *J Allergy Clin Immunol* 1975;56:323–327.
197. Eiser NM, Kerrebijn KF, Quanjer PH. Guidelines for standardization of bronchial challenge with (nonspecific) bronchoconstricting agents. Working group. Bronchial hyperreactivity. SEPCR. *Bull Eur Physiopathol Respir* 1983;19:495–514.
198. Guidelines for bronchial inhalation challenges with pharmacologic and antigen agents. *Am Thorac Soc News* 1980;6:11–19.
199. Hargreave FE, Dolovich J, Boulet L-P. Inhalation provocation tests. *Semin Respir Med* 1983;4:224–235.
200. Ryan G, Dolovich MB, Roberts RS, et al. Standardization of inhalation provocation tests: two techniques of aerosol generation and inhalation compared. *Am Rev Respir Dis* 1981;123:195–199.
201. Cockcroft DW. Bronchial inhalation tests II. Measurement of allergic (and occupational) bronchial responsiveness. *Ann Allergy* 1987;59: 89–98.
202. Cockcroft DW, Killian DN, Mellon JJA, Hargreave FE. Bronchial reactivity to histamine: a method and clinical survey. *Clin Allergy* 1977;7:35–43.
203. Hargreave FE, Ryan G, Thomson NC, et al. Bronchial responsiveness to histamine or methacholine in asthma: measurement and clinical significance. *J Allergy Clin Immunol* 1981;68:347–355.
204. Chatharn M, Bleecker ER, Norman P, et al. A screening test for airways reactivity. *Chest* 1982;82:15–18.
205. Myers JR, Corrao WM, Braman SS. Clinical applicability of a methacholine inhalational challenge. *JAMA* 1981;246:225–229.
206. Pepys J, Hutchcroft BJ. Bronchial provocation tests in the etiologic diagnosis and analysis of asthma. *Am Rev Respir Dis* 1975;112:829–859.
207. Burge PS. Aerosol challenge in lung disease. In: Clarke SW, Pavia D, eds. *Aerosols and the lung.* London: Butterworth, 1984, 225–250.
208. Salvaggio JE, Hendrick DJ. The use of bronchial inhalation challenge in the investigation of occupational diseases. In: Spector S, ed. *Provocative challenge procedures. Background and methodology.* Mount Kisco, NY: Futura, 1989, 417–450.
209. Assoufi SK, Dally MD, Newman-Taylor AJ, et al. Cold air test: a simplified standard method for airway reactivity. *Bull Eur Physiopathol Respir* 1986;22:399–402.
210. Anderson SD, Schoeffel RE, Finny M. Evaluation of ultrasonically nebulized solutions for provocation testing in patients with asthma. *Thorax* 1983;38:284–291.
211. Brooks SM, Weiss MA, Bernstein IL. Reactive airways dysfunction syndrome (LADS). *Chest* 1985;88:376–384.
212. Becklake MR. Concepts of normality applied to the measurement of lung function. *Am J Med* 1986;80:1158–1164.

213. Crapo RO. Reference values for lung function tests. *Respir Care* 1989;34:626–634.
214. Glindmeyer HW. Predictable confusion. *J Occup Med* 1981;23: 845–849.
215. Clausen JL. Prediction of normal values. In: Clausen JL, Zarins LP, eds. *Pulmonary function testing:* guidelines and controversies. New York: Academic Press, 1982, 51–61.
216. Miller A, Thornton JC, Smith H, et al. Spirometric abnormality in a normal male reference population: further analysis of the 1971 Oregon survey. *Am J Ind Med* 1980;1:55–68.
217. Miller A, Thornton JC. The interpretation of spirometric measurements in epidemiologic surveys. *Environ Res* 1980;23:444–468.
218. Sobol BJ. The early detection of airway obstruction: another perspective. *Am J Med* 1976;60:619–624.
219. Lapp NL, Hyatt RE. Some factors affecting the relationship of maximal expiratory flow to lung volume in health and disease. *Dis Chest* 1967;59:475–481.
220. Kuperman AS, Riker JB. The predicted normal maximal midexpiratory flow rate. *Am Rev Respir Dis* 1973;107:231–238.
221. Buist AS. Evaluation of lung function: concepts of normality. In: Simmons DH, ed. *Current pulmonology.* New York: John Wiley, 1982;4:141–165.
222. Pennock BE, Cottrell JJ, Rogers RM. Pulmonary function testing. What is normal? *Arch Intern Med* 1983;143:2123–2127.
223. Clausen JL. Prediction of normal values in pulmonary function testing. *Clin Chest Med* 1989;10:135–143.
224. Cropp GJA. Pulmonary function and bronchial challenge testing in office and hospital practice. *Ann Allergy* 1983;51:19.

*Environmental and Occupational Medicine, Third Edition,* edited by William N. Rom.
Lippincott–Raven Publishers, Philadelphia © 1998.

CHAPTER 21

# Chest Radiography for Assessment of the Pneumoconioses

James A. Merchant and David A. Schwartz

Chest radiography was first performed widely to detect pulmonary tuberculosis. Because of the susceptibility of silicosis patients to tuberculosis, miners and other silica-exposed workers were the subject of chest radiographic studies in the 1920s. The classic study of coal trimmers published by Collis and Gilchrist (1) in 1928 clearly demonstrated that pneumoconiosis among coal trimmers arose from coal dust exposure and not, as was previously thought, only from silica exposure. The need for standardization and classification of radiographs for the pneumoconioses was recognized as early as 1930, at the International Conference on Silicosis held in Johannesburg, South Africa. Since then, an international classification has evolved under the auspices of the International Labour Office (ILO) in Geneva, Switzerland. The ILO 1980 International Classification of Radiographs of the Pneumoconioses is now accepted as the standard against which chest radiographs are measured in epidemiologic studies, for medical surveillance, and for clinical evaluation (2).

While the chest radiograph, together with a good occupational history, usually allow the physician to make a presumptive diagnosis of pneumoconiosis, an exposed worker might have one of many other diseases common to the general population. Lesions and conditions that mimic the rounded opacities of silicosis or coal worker's pneumoconiosis include sarcoidosis, histoplasmosis, tuberculosis, bronchial and alveolar carcinoma, and lymphangitic and hematologic metastases (3,4). The many mimics of the linear opacities of asbestosis include scleroderma, idiopathic pulmonary hemosiderosis, amyloidosis, parenchymal Hodgkin's disease, and pulmonary edema (3). The early radiographic changes of asbestosis are also simulated by lung markings commonly found in aged smokers, which often result from centrilobular emphysema (3). As a result, the interpreter of the worker's radiograph must be careful in making a medical assessment, especially to avoid missing treatable conditions. This caution, together with technical care in obtaining high-quality chest radiographs, are both vital in chest radiography for the assessment of pulmonary disease among persons exposed at work. Now added to this well-standardized approach of chest radiography is computed tomography (CT) of the chest, which promises to enhance detection and characterization of pneumoconiotic opacities.

## TECHNICAL ASPECTS

The principal reasons for producing an unacceptable or unreadable chest radiograph are unfamiliarity with the technique and careless technique. Through the rigorous application of basic radiographic technique, the preparation of technically unreadable radiographs can be reduced below 2% in large surveillance programs. This has been achieved in the National Institute of Occupational Safety and Health (NIOSH) National Coal Workers' Health Surveillance Program through adoption of recommendations made by the American College of Radiology Task Force

J. A. Merchant: Departments of Preventive Medicine and Internal Medicine; and Department of Preventive Medicine and Environmental Health, Institute for Rural and Environmental Health, University of Iowa College of Medicine, Iowa City, Iowa 52242-5000.

D. A. Schwartz: Divisions of Pulmonary and Critical Care and Occupational Medicine, Department of Internal Medicine, University of Iowa College of Medicine, Iowa City, Iowa 52242.

**TABLE 1.** *Physical criteria for excellence of technical quality in chest radiographs*

A. Optical density
  1. Hilar regions should exhibit a minimum of 0.2 units of optical density above fog
  2. Parenchymal regions should exhibit a maximum of 1.8 units of optical density above fog

B. Gross image contrast[a]; should fall within the range of 1.0 and 1.4 units of optical density

C. X-rays tube potentials and use of grids
  1. Potentials of 70 to 100 kVp; use grids for all subjects whose posteroanterior dimension exceeds 220 mm
  2. Potentials over 100 kVp; use grid for all subjects

D. Exposure time: not greater than 0.1 second, and preferably 0.05 second or less

E. Film-screen combination: use medium-speed films and screens to assure adequate image detail; good screen-film contact is essential with periodic testing mandatory

F. Processing: maintain strength and temperature of processing chemicals within limits recommended by manufacturer

G. Assumptions
  1. Cleanliness of films and screens and of processing fluid and equipment is maintained
  2. Care in subject positioning is taken
  3. Subject movement is prevented

[a]The difference in optical density between the darkest segment of the lung parenchyma and the lightest portions of the hilar regions. (Reprinted with the kind permission of the International Labour Office, Geneva, Switzerland.)

on Pneumoconiosis (5). Similar recommendations were adopted by the ILO (2) (Table 1).

Many different types of x-ray film and image-intensifying screens are available. Experience has shown that medium-speed film-screen combinations are well suited for recording the small opacities that characterize the pneumoconioses. Combinations of class A and B films are often favored because of their wide variety and because darkroom fogging is less frequently encountered (6).

Image quality describes the clarity with which the radiograph transmits the image recorded on the film to the reader, and, as such, is highly subjective. It has been found to be inversely related to the difficulty the physician encounters in interpreting the radiograph. In addition to this subjective aspect, image quality is strongly affected by the contrast and detail of the image. Detail is often lost because of patient movement, poor film-screen contact, or darkroom fogging, all problems amenable to correction through proper technique. Image contrast is the most common problem in producing a quality chest radiographic image (6). As a useful guide to obtaining suitable contrast, measurement of optical density (in a range between 1.0 and 1.4 units) in the fourth rib interspace may be used by the technologist. Experience has shown that demand for radiographic excellence by the interpreter and training of the technologist are both important in reducing the proportion of unreadable radiographs. A technically unsatisfactory radiograph will result from underexposure, which suggests a greater profusion of pneumoconiotic opacities, or overexposure, which often "burns out" small opacities and so tends to reduce the profusion category. Overexposure is a common problem with high-speed films and must be guarded against.

### Standards for Radiographic Classification of Pneumoconioses

The ILO has been instrumental in promoting and revising classifications since 1950 (previous editions appeared in 1950, 1958, 1968, and 1971). The ILO 1980 International Classification of Radiographs of the Pneumoconioses retained the principles of earlier revisions, maintained the assessment of profusion without change, clarified ambiguities in the 1971 classification, extended the classification of pleural abnormalities, and provided improved standard radiographs based on extensive international reading trials. Updated standard radiographs using new radiographic photocopying methods have been produced by the American College of Radiology (2). Serious students of pneumoconiosis radiography are advised to obtain a copy of the complete classification and the standard radiographs. The classification may be obtained by writing the International Labour Office, 1750 New York Avenue, N.W., Washington, DC 20006.

The classification was initially intended for use only in epidemiologic studies, but it has evolved to serve as a useful evaluation scheme for government and nongovernment surveillance programs, for clinical evaluation, and to assist in evaluating workers for compensation. However, the classification is intended only to codify radiographic opacities and not to define pathologic changes, imply level of impairment, or provide a legal definition of the pneumoconioses for compensation purposes. The classification consists of two compatible written parts—the short classification, more suitable for clinical use, and the complete classification, intended for use in epidemiologic studies—and a set of standard radiographs to illustrate, and sometimes define, specific abnormalities. Its recommendations are intended for use in the classification of only standard posteroanterior chest radiographs.

### Film Quality

Interpretation of a chest radiograph by the ILO 1980 Classifications consists of a series of decisions based on viewing of a two-dimensional image of a very complex three-dimensional structure. The initial decision concerns film quality. This is an important judgment, as it may well determine whether the film is to be read at all. Film quality is graded as follows:

Grade 1. Good
Grade 2. Acceptable for classification for pneumoconiosis

Grade 3. Poor, with technical defect but still acceptable for classification (this grade was added in 1980 in order to allow more historical films or radiographs on deceased workers to be assessed)
Grade 4. Unacceptable

### Consistency with Pneumoconiosis

Given a readable radiograph, the reader must decide whether the radiograph is consistent with pneumoconiosis. If the radiographic changes (parenchymal or pleural) might be due to pneumoconiosis, the next step is classification. If all the appearances are judged to have other causes, the radiographic changes are recorded under Symbols and Comments. Many radiographs are completely normal, requiring only that the reader so indicate by checking that box in the reading form.

### Classification of Small Opacities

If radiographic findings are or might be consistent with pneumoconiosis, three judgments must be made about small opacities: shape and size, extent, and profusion.

#### *Shape and Size*

Classification by shape and size involves identifying primary and secondary types of small opacities on the radiograph.

| PRIMARY | | SECONDARY | |
|---|---|---|---|
| *p* | *s* | *p* | *s* |
| *q* | *t* | *q* | *t* |
| *r* | *u* | *r* | *u* |

Rounded opacities, as defined by diameter or width, are designated by the letters *p, q,* and *r,* and irregular opacities by *s, t,* and *u.*

Type *p.* Diameter 1.5 mm or smaller
Type *q.* Diameter larger than 1.5 mm but not larger than 3.0 mm
Type *r.* Diameter larger than 3.0 mm but not larger than 10.0 mm
Type *s.* Width 1.5 mm or smaller
Type *t.* Width larger than 1.5 mm but not larger than 3.0 mm
Type *u.* Width larger than 3.0 mm but not larger than 10.0 mm

For example, shape and size may be recorded *p/s* or *p/p,* to indicate primary over secondary shape and size opacity. This modification was made in 1980 in recognition of the fact that mixed opacity patterns are very common and that their interpretation should be facilitated.

#### *Extent*

The extent of profusion is judged by recording the lung zone in which small opacities are observed. The six zones correspond to the upper, middle, and lower thirds of the right and left lungs, respectively, not to the anatomic lobes of the lungs.

#### *Profusion*

Profusion is an assessment of the concentration of opacities as compared with that on the standard radiographs. Profusion is graded on a 12-point scale of four major categories, each with three subcategories:

| MAJOR CATEGORY | SUBCATEGORIES | | |
|---|---|---|---|
| Category 0 | 0/– | 0/0 | 0/1 |
| Category 1 | 1/0 | 1/1 | 1/2 |
| Category 2 | 2/1 | 2/2 | 2/3 |
| Category 3 | 3/2 | 3/3 | 3/+ |

Category 0 is defined as no opacities or a concentration of opacities less than the lowest subcategory of category 1 (Fig. 1). Categories 1, 2, and 3 and their subcategories are intended to model a continuum of increasing concentration of opacities (Figs. 2 to 4). Thus, a radiograph that most closely resembles the category 1 standard, but in which consideration was given to category 0, would be classified 1/0: 1 being the primary profusion, and 0 the secondary profusion. Barn door normal radiographs are categorized as 0/–; snowstorm radiographs 3/+. It is helpful to carefully consider the pulmonary vasculature in assessing the degree of profusion. If the interstitial markings are present and the pulmonary vasculature is distinct, the film should be rated as a category 1 profusion. Alternatively, if interstitial markings are pre-

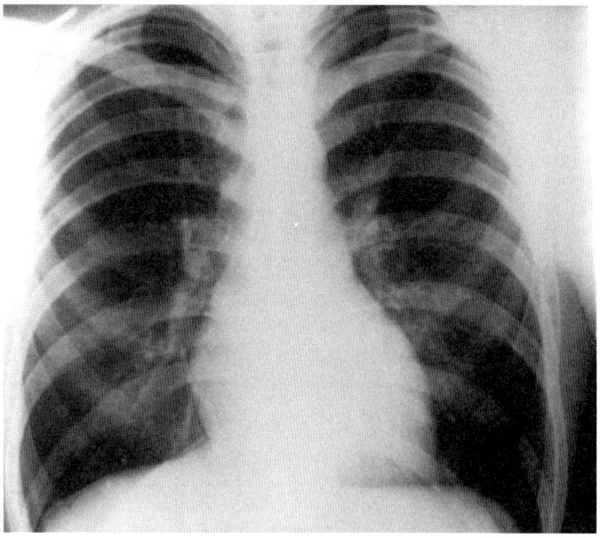

**FIG. 1.** ILO standard radiograph—profusion 0/0.

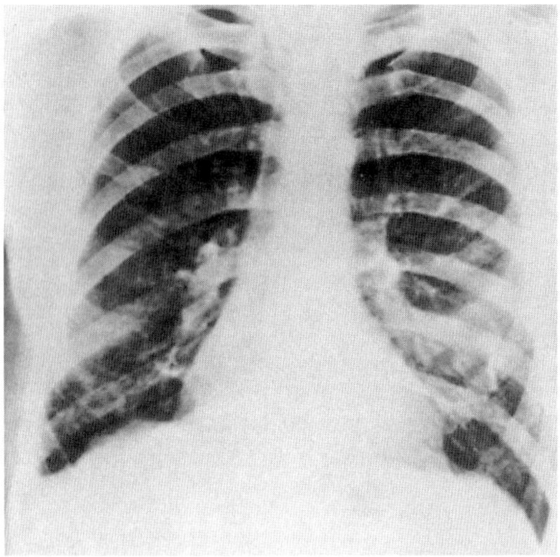

**FIG. 2.** ILO standard radiograph—profusion 1/1 *t/t*.

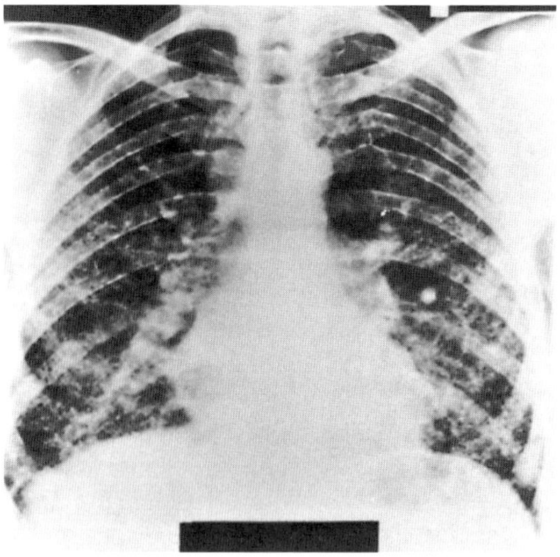

**FIG. 4.** ILO standard radiograph—profusion 3/3 *t/t*.

sent and the pulmonary vasculature is obscured, the film should be rated as a category 3 profusion. Profusion is rated by considering profusion over all affected zones and comparing this integrated profusion with the standard radiographs (Figs. 2 and 4). Where there is a marked difference in profusion between zones (three minor categories or more), the zone or zones with the lowest profusion are ignored.

### Classification of Large Opacities

Large opacities may represent progressive massive fibrosis, a granuloma, a neoplasm, or another medical entity. Because by definition a large opacity is larger than 10 mm diameter, they might be expected to be easy to identify and classify. Experience has shown this is not the case. Experience and judgment are required to determine if the large opacity is consistent with pneumoconiosis, as a background of small opacities frequently suggests. If so, the picture is placed in one of the following categories:

A. An opacity, or several opacities, having a diameter larger than 10 mm but not having a total diameter (sum of all opacities) exceeding 50 mm (Fig. 5)
B. An opacity, or several opacities, larger than 10 mm diameter but with a combined area not larger than the right upper zone
C. One or more large opacities, the combined area of which exceeds the area of the right upper zone

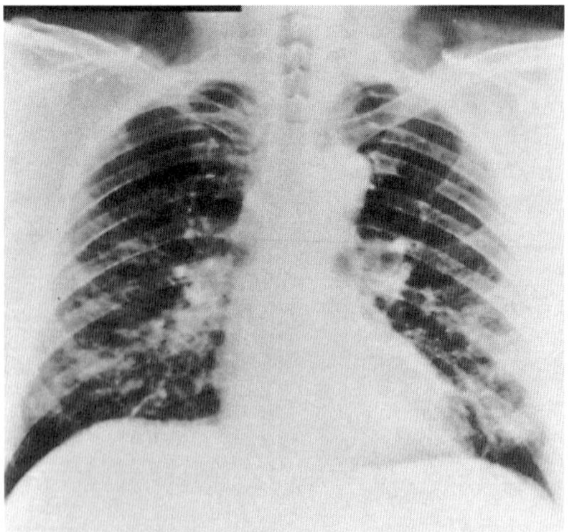

**FIG. 3.** ILO standard radiograph—profusion 2/2 *t/t*.

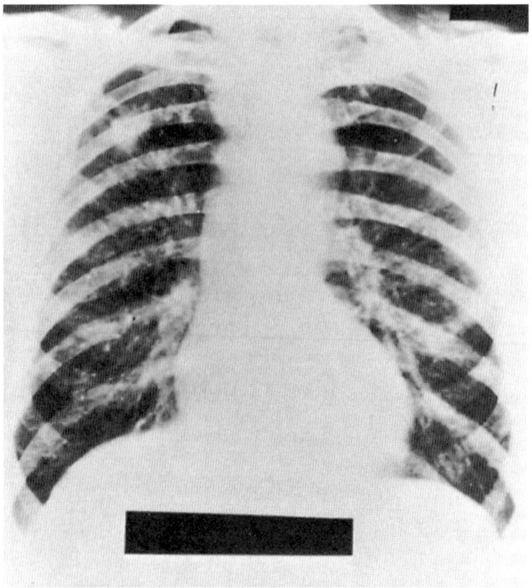

**FIG. 5.** ILO standard radiograph—category A.

Large opacities thought not to be consistent with pneumoconiosis should be described in the Symbol and Comment sections of the reading form.

### Classification of Pleural Abnormalities

Recognition of the physiologic importance of pleural disease arising from asbestos exposure has led to a more detailed scheme for categorizing pleural abnormalities in the ILO 1980 classification (Fig. 6). Recent clinical and epidemiologic studies have demonstrated that pleural fibrosis (pleural plaques and diffuse pleural thickening) is associated with significant functional impairment (7,8). As a result there is considerable interest in further assessment of the classification of pleural abnormalities. A detailed grading scheme is provided by the ILO to assess these changes.

#### *Site*

Should the radiograph show any pleural changes, three major sites must be assessed: the chest wall, the diaphragm, and the costophrenic angles. In assessing the chest wall it is necessary to determine the width and extent of pleural thickening and whether the thickening is diffuse, circumscribed, or both. The diaphragm is assessed as to whether plaque formation is present or absent on the right or left surface, or both diaphragmatic surfaces. A diaphragmatic plaque is illustrated in the standard films. Costophrenic angle obliteration (on the right, left, or both sides) is noted separately from the chest wall assessment. The lower limit of such obliteration to be recorded is found on the standard film illustrating profusion category 1/1 *t/t* (see Fig. 2). If obliteration of the angle extends up the chest wall, both costophrenic angle obliteration and pleural thickening (grade 1 or more) should be recorded.

#### *Pleural Thickening*

It is often difficult to determine whether chest wall pleural thickening is circumscribed or diffuse, but this category was added to the ILO 1980 classification because it is thought that these abnormalities may have a different etiology and natural history. A convention adopted by the American College of Radiology Task Force in Pneumoconiosis, which we recommend, is to define diffuse pleural thickening as pleural thickening that involves the costophrenic angle. By this convention, other pleural thickening of the chest wall is considered circumscribed. This is a departure from the 1980 ILO classification. The site (right, left, or both sides) is

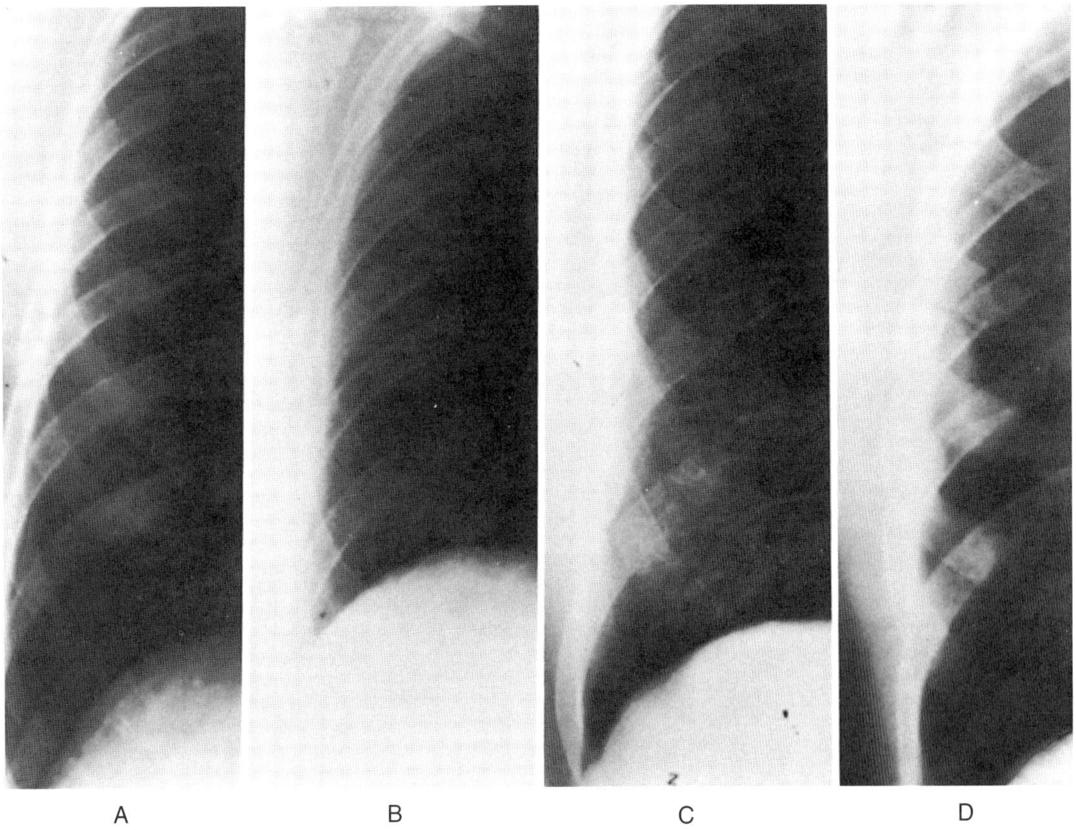


**FIG. 6.** Four different patients demonstrating normal pleura **(A)** and pleural plaques **(B, C, D)** with increasing grades of severity, from left to right, along middle of the chest wall laterally.

recorded. Width is judged by the maximum width of the pleural thickening from the inner margin of the chest wall to the inner margin of the pleural shadow:

Width A. Maximum width 5 mm or less
Width B. Maximum width greater than 5 mm but no greater than 10 mm
Width C. Maximum width greater than 10 mm

For face-on (en face) shadows, width cannot be measured. Extent is defined by the length of chest wall involvement as judged by the sum of the maximal lengths seen in profile or face on:

Extent 1. Length up to one-fourth the lateral chest wall
Extent 2. Length between one-fourth and half the lateral chest wall
Extent 3. Length exceeding half the lateral chest wall

#### *Pleural Calcification*

The classification calls for categorization of pleural calcification, which is frequently observed, in terms of site (chest wall, diaphragm, or other, including mediastinal and pericardial pleura) and extent. Extent is graded as follows:

Extent 1. An area, or number of areas, whose total diameter(s) of calcified pleura does not exceed 20 mm
Extent 2. An area, or number of areas, whose total diameter(s) of calcified pleura is between 20 mm and 100 mm
Extent 3. An area, or number of areas, whose total diameter(s) of calcified pleura exceeds 100 mm.

### Obligatory Symbols

Symbols, which are obligatory, are next recorded. Several examples are provided by the standard radiographs. These findings are taken as being suspect or suggestive of:

ax: coalescence of small pneumoconiotic opacities
bu: bulla
ca: cancer of lung or pleura
cn: calcification in small pneumoconiotic opacities
co: abnormality of cardiac size or shape
cp: cor pulmonale
cv: cavity
di: marked distortion of the intrathoracic organs
ef: effusion
em: definite emphysema
es: eggshell calcification of hilar or mediastinal lymph nodes
fr: fractured rib(s)
hi: enlargement of hilar or mediastinal nodes
ho: honeycomb lung
id: ill-defined diaphragm
ih: ill-defined heart
kl: septal (Kerley) lines
od: other significant abnormality
pi: pleural thickening in the interlobar fissure or mediastinum
px: pneumothorax
rp: rheumatoid pneumoconiosis
tb: tuberculosis

### Other Comments

Finally, and very important, comments are to be recorded at the bottom of the reading form to bring attention to abnormalities, particularly those thought to be clinically relevant but not caused by pneumoconiosis. This section is also the proper place for specific comments on film quality. Many standard forms also include a box for the interpreter to check if the radiograph suggests an abnormality for which the subject should seek immediate medical advice.

## EPIDEMIOLOGIC CONSIDERATIONS IN THE USE OF RADIOGRAPHIC CLASSIFICATIONS

### Interreader Variability

Categorization of the pneumoconioses is necessarily based on subjective interpretation of the radiograph. The resulting disagreement between observers, and between the first and subsequent readings by the same observer, is well documented (9–13). Fletcher and Oldham (10) observed that readers differed to a remarkable degree, both among themselves and, to a lesser extent, from one occasion to another. Divergence of opinion among consultant radiologists was as great as among other observers. Reger and colleagues (11,12) showed that, despite the use of experienced readers, there was a marked divergence of opinion in the assessment of both simple and complicated coal worker's pneumoconiosis. Felson and colleagues (9) studied the influence of multiple readings on the problem of detecting and evaluating coal worker's pneumoconiosis. There was an unexpected disagreement among three groups of readers based on (a) poor film quality, (b) inexperience with the classification systems employed, and (c) unfamiliarity with the radiographic manifestations of coal worker's pneumoconiosis. A review in 1976 by Weill and Jones (13) pointed out that at least three experienced readers should be used to minimize observer variability, and the comparability of their observations should be established initially and checked periodically. In addition, all readers should use standard films constantly for reference. Chest films of unexposed workers should be included for purposes of control, and a proportion of films should be reissued to the reader periodically to check repeatability.

### Assessment of Progression

The methodology to assess radiographic progression of the pneumoconioses has been debated for many years. Although there were a few early attempts at comparing different methods, the studies have little value by today's standards (14,15). Liddell and Morgan (16) pointed out that the early work utilized the four-point ILO scale, which has been shown to be inadequate (17,18). Moreover, the studies relied mainly on some form of joint assessment, a process that has been abandoned for scientific reasons. The most comprehensive review of this subject evaluated data from seven contemporary trials (16). All compared side-by-side reading, with the order known, to an independent randomized approach. Consistency, differentiability, signal-to-noise ratio, specificity, and validity were investigated. It was concluded from Canadian and British sources that side-by-side interpretation was the method of choice, but how change was recorded depended on the objective of the study. The American evidence indicated little difference between methods, but the side-by-side method was often preferred, principally because of training and simplicity (19). On the other hand, some studies and notes point to an uncontrollable bias being introduced by reading serial films for research purposes (20,21; M. Jacobsen, Edinburgh, Scotland, personal communication). Reger and colleagues (21) demonstrated that the assumed chronologic sequence of films significantly influenced the assessment of change in tuberculosis and sarcoidosis. Further, it was demonstrated for coal workers that the assumed chronologic sequence (i.e., the position), as well as the disease stage existing for a given pair member, affected the categorization process (20). Even when the reader was faced with the obvious, there was a marked reluctance to diagnose regression of pneumoconiosis. Jacobsen argues, supporting Liddell and May (18), that side-by-side readings that differ markedly from those determined by independent interpretation should be viewed with caution. Finally, Jacobsen (22) published a rather exhaustive account relating to the quantification of radiographic changes in simple pneumoconiosis. He concluded that there are many useful ways of handling data arranged in ordered categories when the ordering is based on subjective assessments. He surmised that the procedure adopted should depend largely on the information being sought from the data.

### Certification of Readers

Since passage of the Coal Mine Health and Safety Act of 1969, application of good radiographic technique, adoption of the ILO classification, and attention to the lessons learned from epidemiologic studies have been incorporated into the NIOSH National Coal Workers' Health Surveillance Program. Many of these applications have arisen from the American College of Radiology Task Force on Pneumoconiosis and have been codified into regulations used to administer this program. As a result, radiographic equipment and technique have improved in the several hundred clinics and hospitals that participate in this program, and an active training program for physicians has emerged in the form of annual seminars provided by the American College of Radiology and NIOSH (NIOSH confers the status of "A reader" on those who attend). The NIOSH Surveillance Program relies on A readers to screen the radiograph for serious abnormalities among underground coal miners at the initiating clinic or hospital and to classify the radiograph for pneumoconiosis using the ILO 1980 classification. These radiographs are all then reread by at least one B reader, who is a physician who has passed a comprehensive examination given by NIOSH and based on 120 radiographs and the ILO 1980 classification. In many respects, the National Coal Workers' Health Surveillance Program has served as a useful model. Many of the aspects of this program have now been incorporated into Department of Labor standards and regulations and are utilized by the U.S. Navy, unions, and industry in their surveillance programs.

## COMPUTED TOMOGRAPHY

Although chest radiography is currently the cornerstone of our diagnostic armamentarium for the pneumoconioses, the chest x-ray is neither a highly sensitive nor specific method for identifying the pleural and parenchymal manifestations of these diseases. For example, 15% to 20% of persons with pathologic evidence of either pleural plaques (23) or asbestosis (24) have normal appearing chest radiographs. Additionally, chest CT appears to distinguish effectively between subpleural fat and asbestos-induced pleural fibrosis (25), thus enhancing the specificity of this diagnosis. In this context, CT of the chest represents a particularly important advance that may substantially improve our ability to noninvasively identify and quantify pleural and parenchymal lesions caused by inhalation of inorganic dusts (26). Furthermore, the chest CT may prove useful in identifying these diseases at an earlier, potentially reversible, stage.

### Parenchymal Abnormalities

Asbestos-induced interstitial lung disease is perhaps the best-studied pneumoconiosis in terms of CT. This diagnosis is usually based on an appropriate exposure history and evidence of parenchymal changes on the routine chest radiograph, but for asbestos-exposed workers who have a normal chest radiograph and either respiratory symptoms or restrictive lung function, high-resolution chest CT (HRCT) may provide useful diagnostic information (26).

While conventional CT images use 8- to 10-mm slices through the chest, HRCT images use 1- to 3-mm slices and a different reconstruction algorithm to improve spatial resolution. Specific parenchymal abnormalities identified on the HRCT scan that appear to be relevant to asbestosis include thickened interlobular septal lines, curvilinear subpleural lines, parenchymal bands, and honeycombing (26,27) (Fig. 7). However, it is very clear that other, possibly more subtle changes, such as ground-glass infiltrates (Fig. 8), may be relevant to this and other interstitial inflammatory processes. Moreover, the different appearance of the HRCT may provide useful prognostic, as well as diagnostic, information. An important point: these parenchymal abnormalities are specific for interstitial lung disease only if they are demonstrated in the nondependent portions of the lung (27); therefore, prone, and possibly supine, positioning is necessary to precisely identify the cause of the parenchymal abnormalities.

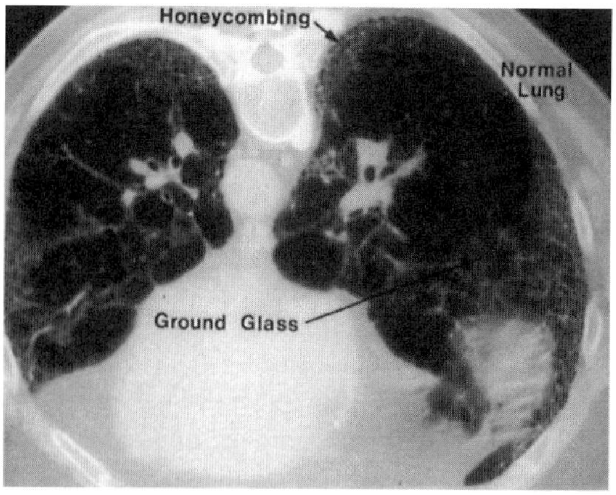


**FIG. 8.** HRCT scan from a patient with severe asbestosis demonstrating peripheral, posterior-based honeycombing and an area of ground-glass infiltrate.

Although a systematic investigation of the pathologic or anatomic features identified on HRCT has not yet been undertaken, several studies (28–30) indicate that the findings on HRCT are indicative of histologic evidence of parenchymal inflammation and fibrosis. In idiopathic pulmonary fibrosis the reticular patchy densities in the lung periphery have been found to correspond to histologic evidence of inflammation and irregular fibrosis (30). In addition, the cystic (2- to 20-mm) subpleural findings on HRCT appear to represent regions of diffuse fibrosis with honeycombing (30,31). In asbestosis, case reports indicate that peribronchial fibrosis, focal thickening of the interalveolar septa, thickened septal tissue (i.e., parenchymal bands), and honeycombing can be identified on HRCT. Moreover, these findings appear to correlate with specific histologic findings from pathologic specimens (28,29). Recently, Akira and co-workers (28) have identified a variety of histologic features that correlate with specific HRCT findings in patients with asbestosis. In aggregate, these studies suggest that HRCT can effectively identify regions of abnormal lung tissue that appear to be associated with diffuse forms of interstitial fibrosis.

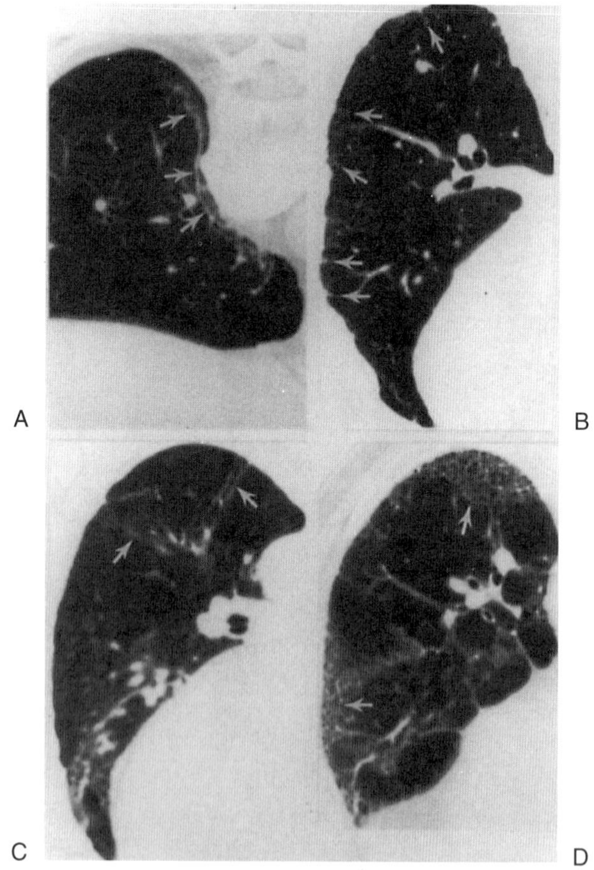


**FIG. 7.** Single HRCT sections from four patients with asbestosis with *arrows* demonstrating curvilinear subpleural lines **(A)**, thickened interlobular septal lines **(B)**, parenchymal bands **(C)**, and honeycombing **(D)**.

Silicosis and coal worker's pneumoconiosis are characterized by small rounded nodules in the middle and upper lung zones that appear similar on chest radiographs and HRCT (Fig. 9). However, the HRCT may help to define the interstitial process, since it appears to detect the early coalescence of nodules that are not fully appreciated on the radiograph (32). The absence of a correlation between the nodules on the HRCT and lung function of patients with silicosis (32,33) probably relates more to the histologically distinct nodules in silicosis than to the specificity of the HRCT findings in this disease. Further studies are needed to identify the physiologic importance of specific findings on the HRCT in patients with either silicosis or coal worker's pneumoconiosis.

Although the HRCT can identify parenchymal abnormalities that are not evident on the standard chest radiograph, the clinical and pathologic relevance of these

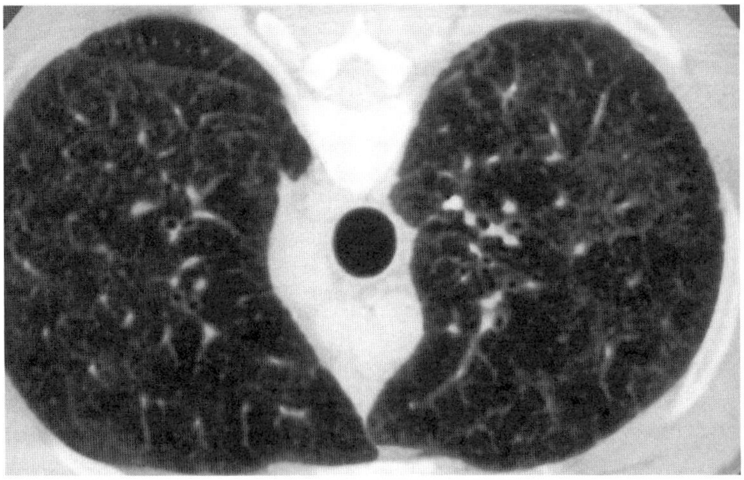

**FIG. 9.** HRCT scan from a patient with silicosis demonstrating numerous, small bilateral nodules.

radiographic abnormalities is still not entirely clear (34). We recently found that among asbestos-exposed patients with normal parenchyma on plain chest radiographs, patients with pleural disease are more likely than those with normal pleura to have interstitial abnormalities on the HRCT (8). Although these interstitial abnormalities were associated with reduced lung volumes and abnormal gas exchange, the differences were not statistically significant (8). Similarly, Staples and associates (35) reported that among asbestos-exposed workers with normal parenchyma on the plain chest film, approximately a third have HRCT findings suggestive of interstitial fibrosis. Workers who had interstitial changes on HRCT were more dyspneic, had a lower vital capacity, and less gas exchange than those whose HRCT findings were normal (35). Moreover, the computer-derived density of the lung parenchyma on the HRCT scan appears to be a valid, clinically meaningful, and objective measure of interstitial lung disease (36). Clearly, prospective, controlled studies are needed to determine the prognostic significance of these abnormalities on HRCT among exposed persons with normal-looking parenchyma on chest radiographs.

### Pleural Abnormalities

Findings of autopsy (23,37) and CT studies (25,27,38, 39) indicate that the chest radiograph is neither a sensitive nor a specific method of identifying asbestos-induced pleural fibrosis. These studies indicate that the standard chest radiograph is able to demonstrate some 50% to 80% of the pleural plaques that are actually present. In comparison to conventional CT, the standard chest radiograph has a specificity of 71% for pleural fibrosis (25). CT can distinguish between subpleural fat (Fig. 10) and pleural fibrosis (Fig. 11), whereas in obese patients this distinction is not always clear on the chest radiograph. In addition, the CT scan can quantify the amount of pleural fibrosis, which has recently been reported to be independently associated with restrictive lung function (40). Therefore, CT can be helpful in identifying and quantifying pleural disease when chest radiographic findings are suggestive but not diagnostic, and it can distinguish pleural fat from pleural fibrosis in obese patients.

### Clinical Indications for CT Examination

The clinician is faced with a dilemma: the chest radiograph is the accepted standard for the assessment of the pneumoconioses, but conventional CT and HRCT appear to provide more accurate information for the diagnosis of parenchymal and pleural abnormalities. Although this statement is solidly supported by multiple clinical studies, only a small percentage of persons exposed to inorganic dusts actually benefit from the more costly studies.

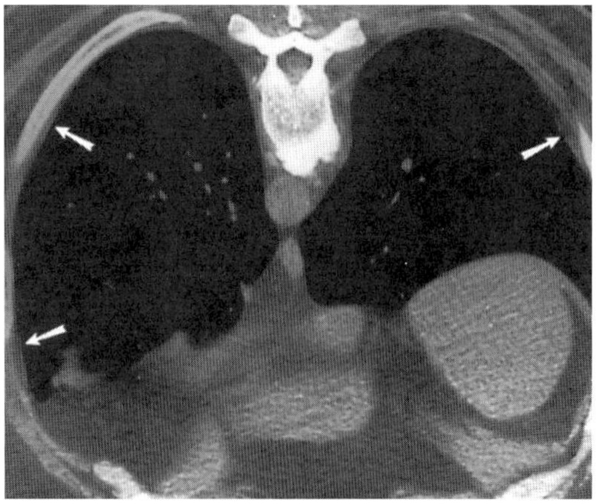

**FIG. 10.** Conventional CT scan from an asbestos-exposed patient demonstrating bilateral pleural fat *(arrows)*. Note the smooth, low-density quality of the chest wall lesions.

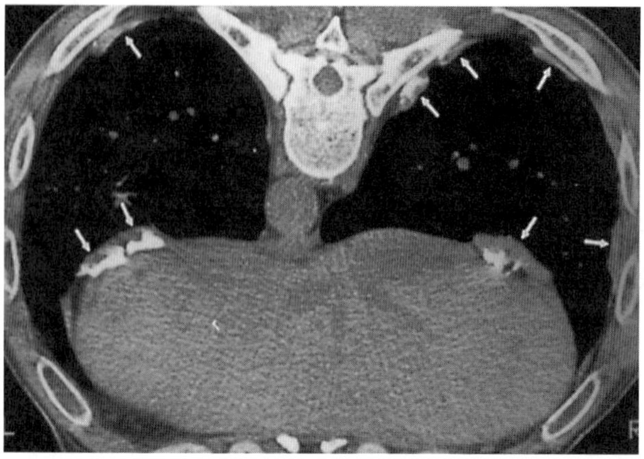

**FIG. 11.** Conventional CT scan from a patient with asbestos-induced pleural fibrosis *(arrows)*. Note the symmetric quality of these lesions and their presence on both diaphragms.

If the radiographic changes of asbestosis, silicosis, or coal worker's pneumoconiosis are clear on the chest radiograph, currently there is no indication to confirm the diagnosis with CT. Alternatively, if the parenchymal features on the chest radiograph are equivocal or if a patient has unexplained respiratory symptoms or lung function abnormalities suggestive of interstitial fibrosis, HRCT scans may be very helpful in identifying interstitial changes, which may account for the pulmonary symptoms and functional changes. Thus, HRCT can be used to confirm the diagnosis of asbestosis, silicosis, or coal worker's pneumoconiosis when the standard chest radiograph is not diagnostic, but it does not appear to be necessary when clinical and radiographic findings are conclusive. In comparison to the chest radiograph, HRCT appears to improve the sensitivity, but not the specificity, of the diagnosis of occupationally induced interstitial fibrosis.

In some cases diagnosis of asbestos-induced pleural disease may be problematic when the standard chest radiograph alone is used. Only a small proportion of patients, however, need conventional CT to confirm the diagnosis. In cases when the pleural findings are not clearly characteristic of asbestos-induced disease or in obese patients with unusual pleural shadows, conventional CT may markedly improve the certainty of the diagnosis. Otherwise, the standard chest radiograph should be used to definitively identify the different types of asbestos-induced pleural disease.

## REFERENCES


1. Collis EL, Gilchrist JC. Effects of dust upon coal trimmers. *J Ind Hyg* 1928;10:101.
2. Guidelines for the Use of ILO International Classification of Radiographs of Pneumoconioses. Occupational Safety and Health Series 22, Rev. 80. Geneva, Switzerland: International Labour Office, 1980.
3. Van Ordstrand HS. Pneumoconioses and their masqueraders. *J Occup Med* 1977;19:747–753.
4. Lyons JP, Ryder RC, Campbell H, et al. Significance of irregular opacities in the radiograph of coal workers' pneumoconiosis. *Br J Ind Med* 1974;31:36–44.
5. Code of Federal Regulation. Title 42, Part 37, Vol. 43, No. 148, August 1, 1978, and Vol. 44, No. 76, April 18, 1979.
6. Morgan R. *Radiology:* NIOSH Occupational Respiratory Disease Report. DHHS publication. Washington, DC: U.S. Government Printing Office, 1991.
7. Schwartz DA, Fuortes LJ, Galvin JR, et al. Asbestos-induced pleural fibrosis and impaired lung function. *Am Rev Respir Dis* 1990;141: 321–326.
8. Schwartz DA, Galvin JR, Dayton CS, et al. Determinants of restrictive lung function in asbestos-induced pleural fibrosis. *J Appl Physiol* 1990; 68:1932–1937.
9. Felson B, Morgan WKC, Bristol LJ, et al. Observations on the results of multiple readings of chest films in coal miners' pneumoconiosis. *Radiology* 1973;109:19–23.
10. Fletcher CM, Oldham PD. The problems of consistent radiological diagnosis in coal miners' pneumoconiosis. *Br J Ind Med* 1949;6: 168–183.
11. Reger RB, Amandus HE, Morgan WKC. On the diagnosis of coal workers' pneumoconiosis: Anglo-American disharmony. *Am Rev Respir Dis* 1973;108:1186.
12. Reger RB, Morgan WKC. On the factors influencing consistency in the radiological diagnosis of pneumoconiosis. *Am Rev Respir Dis* 1970; 102:905.
13. Weill H, Jones R. The chest roentgenogram as an epidemiologic tool: reply. *Arch Environ Health* 1976;31:270.
14. Cochrane AL. The attack rate of progressive massive fibrosis. *Br J Ind Med* 1962;19:52–64.
15. Wise ME, Oldham PD. Estimating progression of coal-workers' simple pneumoconiosis from readings of radiological categories. *Br J Ind Med* 1963;20:124–144.
16. Liddell FDK, Morgan WKC. Methods of assessing serial films of the pneumoconioses: a review. *J Soc Occup Med* 1978;28:6–15.
17. Liddell FDK. Assessment of radiological progression of simple pneumoconiosis in individual miners. *Br J Ind Med* 1974;31:185–195.
18. Liddell FDK, May JD. *Assessing the radiological progression of simple pneumoconiosis.* Medical Research Memorandum 4. London: National Coal Board Medical Service, 1966.
19. Amandus HE, Reger RB, Pendergrass EP, et al. The pneumoconioses: methods of measuring progression. *Chest* 1973;63:736.
20. Reger RB, Butcher DF, Morgan WKC. Assessing change in the pneumoconioses using serial radiographs. *Am J Epidemiol* 1973;98: 243–254.
21. Reger RB, Petersen MR, Morgan WKC. Variation in the interpretation of radiographic change in pulmonary disease. *Lancet* 1974;1:111–113.
22. Jacobsen M. Quantifying radiological changes in simple pneumoconiosis. *Appl Stat* 1975;24:229–249.
23. Hillerdal G, Lingran A. Pleural plaques: correlation of autopsy findings to radiographic findings and occupational history. *Eur J Respir Dis* 1980;61:315–319.
24. Kipen HM, Lilis R, Suzuki Y, et al. Pulmonary fibrosis in asbestos insulation workers with lung cancer: a radiological and histopathological evaluation. *Br J Ind Med* 1987;44:96–100.
25. Friedman AC, Fiel SB, Fisher MS, et al. Asbestos-related pleural disease and asbestosis: A comparison of CT and chest radiography. *Am J Radiol* 1988;150:269–275.
26. Muller NL, Miller RR. Computed tomography of chronic diffuse infiltrative lung disease. *Am Rev Respir Dis* 1990;142:1206–1215, 1440–1448.
27. Aberle DR, Gamsu G, Ray CS, et al. Asbestos-related pleural and parenchymal fibrosis: Detection with high-resolution CT. *Radiology* 1988;166:729–734.
28. Akira M, Yamamoto S, Yokoyama K, et al. Asbestosis: high-resolution CT—pathologic correlation. *Radiology* 1990;176:389–394.
29. Lynch DA, Gamsu G, Aberle DR. Conventional and high-resolution computed tomography in the diagnosis of asbestos-related diseases. *Radiographics* 1989;9:523–551.
30. Muller NL, Miller RR, Webb WR, et al. Fibrosing alveolitis: CT-pathologic correlation. *Radiology* 1986;160:585–588.
31. Staples CA, Muller NL, Vedal S, et al. Usual interstitial pneumonia: Correlation of CT with clinical, functional, and radiologic findings. *Radiology* 1987;162:377–381.
32. Bergin CJ, Muller NL, Vedal S, et al. CT in silicosis: correlation

with plain films and pulmonary function tests. *AJR* 1986;146: 477–483.
33. Kinsella M, Muller NL, Vedal S, et al. Emphysema in silicosis: a comparison of smokers with nonsmokers using pulmonary function testing and computed tomography. *Am Rev Respir Dis* 1990;141: 1497–1500.
34. McCloud TC. Critical review. *Invest Radiol* 1989;24:636–637.
35. Staples CA, Gamsu G, Ray CS, et al. High-resolution computed tomography and lung function in asbestos-exposed workers with normal chest radiographs. *Am Rev Respir Dis* 1989;139:1502–1508.
36. Hartley PG, Galvin JR, Hunninghake GW, et al. High-resolution CT-derived measures of lung density are valid indexes of interstitial lung disease. *J Appl Physiol* 1994;76:271–277.
37. Hourihane D O'B, Lessof L, Richardson PC. Hyaline and calcified pleural plaques as a index of exposure to asbestos: a study of radiological and pathological features of 100 cases with a consideration of epidemiology. *Br Med J* 1966;1:1069–1074.
38. Aberle DR, Gamsu G, Ray CS. High-resolution CT of benign asbestos-related diseases: clinical and radiographic correlation. *AJR* 1988;151: 883–891.
39. Sargent EN, Boswell WD, Ralls PW, et al. Subpleural fat pads in patients exposed to asbestos: distinction from noncalcified pleural plaques. *Radiology* 1984;152:273–277.
40. Schwartz DA, Galvin JR, Yagla SJ, Speakman SB, Merchant JA, Hunninghake GW. Restrictive lung function and asbestos-induced pleural fibrosis: a quantitative approach. *J Clin Invest* 1993;91:2685–2692.

*Environmental and Occupational Medicine, Third Edition,* edited by William N. Rom.
Lippincott–Raven Publishers, Philadelphia © 1998.

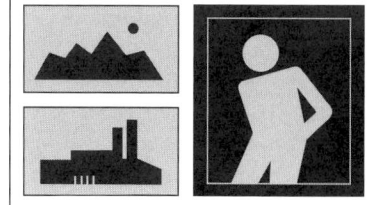

CHAPTER 22

# Molecular Mechanisms of Particle-Induced Lung Disease

Gilbert F. Morris and Arnold R. Brody

Environmental lung disease is manifested in multiple forms, depending on the offending agent inhaled and the anatomic region involved. This text includes complete descriptions of a number of lung diseases known to be caused by inhaled particles. For example, asthma clearly can be induced by inhaling gases such as toluene diisocyante (1,2) and is exacerbated by oxidant gases like ozone (3) and sulfur dioxide (4,5). Whether asthma is caused by immune mechanisms consequent to inhaling antigens or by irritant gases, the fundamental processes that result in airway hyperresponsiveness and eventual remodeling are likely to be the same. Similarly, pneumoconiosis is the fibrogenic lung disease caused by inhaling a variety of minerals, including silica and asbestos. Finally, lung cancer and mesothelioma are neoplastic diseases clearly associated with the inhalation of environmental agents, e.g., cigarette smoke with bronchogenic carcinoma and asbestos with mesothelioma.

We are focusing here on the molecular mechanisms through which inorganic particles are thought to initiate fibroproliferative lung disease and induce early carcinogenic events. While a number of inhaled particles induce lung fibrosis, the interstitial fibroproliferative process that culminates in fibrosis is likely to be mediated, at least in part, by numerous cytokines and growth factors. These interact with specific receptors, signaling elements, and transcription factors that control cell proliferation and extracellular matrix production, the hallmarks of lung fibrosis.

G. F. Morris: Department of Pathology and Laboratory Medicine, Tulane University Medical Center, New Orleans, Louisiana 70118.

A. R. Brody: Department of Pathology, Tulane University Medical Center, New Orleans, Louisiana 70112.

## CELLULAR AND MOLECULAR BIOLOGY OF PARTICLE-INDUCED LUNG DISEASE IN HUMANS

Although an understanding of the molecular mechanisms of environmental lung disease relies principally on animal models, in general, clinical findings relate well to experimental systems. However, comparisons between experimental and clinical studies in environmental lung disease can be complicated by differences in the levels of exposure and in the periods of analysis. Animal models generally must be exposed to high doses of a given agent for short periods, and observations from these exposures are extrapolated to the chronic, low-level exposures frequently experienced by humans. Moreover, clinical findings are generally restricted to a period well after the onset of disease. Despite these differences, the utility of animal models is illustrated by the observation that particle and fiber-induced lung diseases in animals closely approximate those observed in humans (6–11).

In general, the pulmonary response to inhaled particles is an inflammatory process that leads to alterations of the small airways and parenchyma (12–15). Peribronchiolar fibrosis and epithelial metaplasia of alveolar spaces and small airways are frequently observed (16). Experimental models and bronchoalveolar lavage (BAL) analyses of asbestos-exposed individuals indicate that alveolitis develops subsequent to inhalation, dominated by macrophage accumulation (14,17,18), although lymphocytes (19,20), neutrophils (21,22), and eosinophils (22) may participate in the inflammatory response. The alveolitis stimulates the accumulation of fibroblasts and deposition of extracellular matrix that becomes clinically significant when the disease becomes diffuse and fibrosis extends between the airways [e.g., grade 2 or more of pathologic asbestosis (23)].

Macrophage-derived cytokines and growth factors appear to be central in the pulmonary response to inhaled particles, with asbestos providing most of the examples documented (14,15,24–27). Alveolar macrophages (AMs) recovered by BAL from diseased and normal individuals can be assessed for expression of specific cytokines; however, variability is encountered in this approach due to different adherent properties and differential extraction of AM from normal and diseased individuals (28). Analyses of the BAL fluid from asbestos-exposed individuals are consistent with chronic inflammation (14). The AM recovered from humans chronically exposed to asbestos release elevated amounts of inflammatory cytokines and mediators of the immune response including interleukin-1β (IL-1β), tumor necrosis factor-α (TNF-α), interleukin-6 (IL-6), and prostaglandin $E_2$ ($PGE_2$) (25,29). In contrast, acute *in vitro* exposure of human AM isolated from normal individuals to asbestos results in activation of only TNF-α from this panel of four cytokines (25). Thus, secretions *in vitro* must be interpreted with caution. Moreover, TNF-α and IL-6 levels increase in AM recovered from individuals with pneumoconioses of other etiologies (30–34), and this increase in TNF-α can be observed in circulating monocytes from patients with particle-induced lung disease (35). However, one study of workers exposed to asbestos reveals no association between AM release of TNF-α and asbestos-induced disease state (28), and another indicates that higher serum TNF-α levels correlates with tumorigenesis rather than severity or progression of asbestosis (36). Other studies confirm an increase in IL-1β in AM from workers occupationally exposed to asbestos and demonstrate that the ratio of IL-1β to IL-1 receptor antagonist (IL-1ra) is greater in individuals with disease compared to normal volunteers (37). IL-1ra binds to, but does not activate, the IL-1 receptor (38). Therefore, a higher ratio of IL-1β to IL-1ra in affected individuals is consistent with ongoing inflammation. At least two inflammatory mediators may account for the twofold increase in the percent neutrophils in the BAL fluid of asbestos-exposed individuals (21). The proinflammatory cytokine and neutrophil chemotaxin interleukin-8 (IL-8) appears in AM from asbestos-exposed workers. Additionally, asbestos stimulates IL-8 release from monocytes *in vitro* (21). AM of patients with asbestosis release another potent chemotactic factor for neutrophils, leukotriene $B_4$, which is an arachidonic acid metabolite (39). In contrast, the Clara cell protein (CC16) is a purported pulmonary antiinflammatory agent, and decreases in serum levels of CC16 are suggested as an early marker for pneumoconiosis (40).

In addition to these mediators of inflammatory responses, BAL fluid and AM from individuals with pneumoconiosis possess increased amounts of the profibrogenic cytokines, platelet-derived growth factor (PDGF), transforming growth factor-β (TGF-β), and type 1 insulin-like growth factor (IGF-1) (41). Indeed, serum levels of PDGF appear to be a marker for the severity of the two major types of pneumoconiosis—asbestosis and silicosis (42). As a potent mesenchymal cell mitogen, PDGF may be integral to proliferation of interstitial cells subsequent to particle deposition (see below). The PDGF-AA and -AB isoforms can be recovered by BAL of normal individuals, whereas the PDGF-BB isoform is undetectable in these same preparations (43). BAL from patients with interstitial lung disease contains increased amounts of both the PDGF-A (44) and the PDGF-B isoforms (44,45). In addition to the AM, in situ hybridization indicates that PDGF-B and PDGF-β receptor messenger RNSa (mRNAs) are transcribed in alveolar type II cells, and PDGF-mRNA–positive interstitial macrophages increase in patients with idiopathic pulmonary fibrosis (IPF) (44,46). In pneumoconiosis, expression of PDGF and IGF-1 is higher in more severe cases of the disease, while increases in TGF-β levels correlate with less severe disease (41). However, in related clinical studies of idiopathic pulmonary fibrosis, higher levels of TGF-β from BAL correlates with a more aggressive disease and a poorer prognosis (47). TGF-β is a potent inducer of extracellular matrix deposition by mesenchymal cells, and it can regulate proliferation of these cells (48). Thus, it is significant that TGF-β colocalizes with sites of procollagen 1 and fibronectin synthesis in patients with pulmonary fibrosis (49) and appears to be associated with silicotic nodules and the development of progressive massive fibrosis in silicosis (50). Serum levels of transforming growth factor-α (TGF-α), a potential mediator of the observed epithelial hyperplasia, also appear to increase in patients with asbestosis (51). Heightened levels of fibronectin and procollagen in BAL fluid and serum from individuals with pneumoconiosis are consistent with the enhanced deposition of extracellular matrix (34,52–54) and expression of TGF-β.

The incidence of lung cancer is elevated in cohorts occupationally exposed to asbestos (55–57). Nevertheless, the spectrum of lung cancer types associated with asbestos exposure is not significantly different from that observed in unexposed individuals (58–61). Although this lack of specific pathologic features of asbestos-associated lung cancers reduces the certainty of a causal relationship in every case, epidemiologic evidence suggests that asbestos exposure alone increases the risk of lung cancer approximately fivefold (62). Investigations are ongoing for any pattern of mutations in proto-oncogenes or tumor suppressor genes in asbestos-associated lung cancers and mesothelioma in humans (63). In a prospective study, a significant number of pneumoconiosis patients who subsequently developed cancers of various types possess increased serum levels of the *ras* oncoprotein (42). Serum levels of the extracellular domain of the *erb*B-2 receptor increase in asbestosis (51), and a correlation may exist between serum levels of *erb*B-2 receptor and tumor progression in pneumoconiosis patients (64). Mutations in p53 and p53 accumulation occur in lung cancers associated with asbestos exposures (65,66), and these higher amounts of pulmonary p53 expression may be observed in the serum of patients with asbestosis (51,67). Glutathione S-transferase, which may assist in detoxification of reactive oxygen species, is increased in lung cancer patients exposed to asbestos, but not to other mineral fibers (68). Studies suggest that the pattern of glutathione S-transferase expression correlates with mutations in p53 in lung cancers (69,70).

Epidemiologic studies of malignant mesothelioma indicate that 75% to as high as 90% are associated with prior asbestos exposure (71–74). Cytogenetic analyses of malignant mesothelioma reveal a recurring pattern of chromosomal abnormalities, but identification of a preferred subset of genes mutated in mesothelioma remains elusive (75–82). Mutations in p53 do not appear to contribute significantly to the pathogenesis of mesothelioma (83,84). Overexpression of PDGF occurs in some human mesotheliomas (85–87), an observation that is consistent with oncogenic potential of PDGF (88). In addition, asbestos may activate mesenchymal cell proliferation via an autocrine loop mediated by PDGF (see below). Sequences with homology to an oncogenic DNA virus, SV40, can be found in mesothelioma samples, yet not in areas of unaffected lung that contain asbestos fibers (89).

## ANIMAL MODELS OF PARTICLE-INDUCED LUNG DISEASE

Animal models of pneumoconiosis are essential to investigate the early events associated with development of disease. The degree of fibrogenic disease induced by inhaled particles is dose related (90,91), but the process is initiated by repeated injury to the pulmonary epithelium, followed by accumulation and activation of AM, fibroblast proliferation, and deposition of extracellular matrix (15,26,52). Inhalation exposure of rodents to fibrogenic particles produces a pattern of disease that mimics that observed in humans (9,92–94), primarily because the deposition and translocation of inhaled particles are similar in experimental models to what is found in humans (95). Transgenic technology and the availability of animals of defined genetic backgrounds accentuate the use of mouse models of pneumoconiosis; however, variable strain-specific pulmonary responses to particles (96) complicate the interpretation of experimental results obtained using mice. These and other issues central to the molecular mechanisms of disease development in model systems are discussed below. But first, a brief description of the earliest cellular responses to particle deposition in rodent models of fibroproliferative disease is presented.

### Particle Deposition and Uptake

The majority of inhaled fibers depositing in the upper airways are quickly transported out of the lung by the mucociliary escalator, while fibers depositing in the peripheral lung can be retained for the lifetime of the animal or human exposed (97). The biopersistence of the inhaled fibers in the lung (reviewed in ref. 98) govern many of the pathologic consequences. The aerodynamic properties of inhaled fibers (i.e., particles with a length/diameter ratio greater than 3:1) determine whether or not they reach the gas exchange region of lung (94,97,99). Shorter fibers are cleared from the lung faster than longer fibers (100,101), the latter of which are more likely to induce lung disease (94,102). Indeed, it appears that clearance of fibers longer than 15 μm is too slow to be measured during the first few months after exposure (102). Chrysotile asbestos may split longitudinally and thereby increase the number of pathogenic fibers (102). Fragmentation and dissolution of chrysotile reduces its biopersistence (103), but the severity of asbestos-induced lung disease is similar for all the asbestos varieties (104). Fibers that are small enough to pass through the conducting airways deposit at the ends of the terminal bronchioles at the bifurcations of the bronchiolar-alveolar ducts (105,106) in central and peripheral regions with some lobe preference (106). Deposited fibers interact with sialic acid moieties (107,108) and integrins and become bound to the cell surfaces (109). Type I alveolar epithelial cells actively internalize the fibers (110–112), and a portion are translocated by actin-containing microfilaments (113) across the epithelium and into the interstitial compartment (111,114). Approximately 20% of the fiber mass reaching the alveolar level is retained in the lung for more than 6 months postexposure (114). These initial events of particle deposition are documented best for asbestos, but appear to be identical for fibrogenic silica as well (115). Carbonyl iron, a nuisance dust, deposits in a similar pattern, but few particles are transported to the lung interstitium, and it does not cause cell injury (15). Thus, initial injury is induced consequent to particle deposition and translocation as genes are activated and the cascades of inflammatory mediators, growth factors, and cytokines are released.

### Particle-Induced Injury

Injury to the pulmonary epithelium and subsequent exposure of the interstitial cells to the inflammatory milieu are believed to be integral parts of the fibrotic response initiated by particle deposition (116,117). Levels of lactate dehydrogenase and total protein in BAL fluid of asbestos-exposed rats increase postexposure, indicating cytotoxicity and enhanced epithelial permeability (118). Reactive oxygen species (ROS) generated by redox reactions of molecular oxygen in the catalytic environment provided by the fiber surface (119), or by interactions of the fibers with the surface of a various cell types (15), or by inflammatory cells that become activated after phagocytosis of the fibers (120) are likely to mediate some of the cytotoxic effects (15,112,121,122). Thus, leukocytes recovered from quartz-exposed animals by BAL damage extracellular matrix components and injure epithelial cells *in vitro* (123). The cause of injury associated with activated inflammatory cells appears to be mediated, in part, by the release of ROS. Although AMs dominate the inflammatory response to inhaled particles, other inflammatory cells, such as polymorphonuclear leukocytes (PMNs), produce reactive oxygen (123,124) and PMN-derived proteases (125) that contribute to epithelial injury induced by inhaled particles. Electron spin resonance studies indicate that exposure of inflammatory cells to particles *in vitro* stimulates the release of oxygen free radicals (126). Furthermore, release of ROS can be observed *in vivo* by intratracheal instillation of asbestos into rats, which produces increased amounts of hydroxyl radical production in the lung (127). Similarly, intratracheal instillation of silica into rats creates products of lipid peroxidation, a consequence of the generation of ROS in the lung (128). In contrast to silica, inhalation exposure of rats to asbestos increases the pulmonary levels of enzymes that alleviate oxidant stress (129,130). These data suggest that the degree of injury or the mechanisms of silica-induced lung injury are distinct from that due to exposure to asbestos. In accord with this observation, inhaled glass fibers do not produce the pulmonary disease in rats that is observed in similar exposures to chrysotile (11), but inhalation of mixtures of quartz and chrysotile exacerbates the extent of pulmonary disease in rats (131). The observation that lung injury induced by intratracheal instillation of enzymes that generate ROS produces fibrotic lesions similar to those induced by asbestos is consistent with the postulate that ROS mediate the injury caused by inhaled fibers (14,132).

Cell culture models may be employed to demonstrate the cytotoxic potential of particles (133), but the choice of cell type may significantly affect findings of fiber pathogenesis (134). Asbestos fibers are cytotoxic to cells in culture, with chrysotile being one of the most toxic particles in these assays (135,136). Both long and short asbestos fibers are toxic to cells *in vitro*, and the addition of iron chelators or enzymes that scavenge reactive oxygen reduce the cytotoxic effects of asbestos (137). Consistent with a cellular response to ROS incited by fiber addition, asbestos exposure of cells in culture produces enhanced cellular levels of antioxidant enzymes (138). The fiber-initiated generation of ROS can damage the inner mitochondrial membrane and interfere with energy metabolism that leads ultimately to the loss of cell viability (139). In addition, cytotoxic effects of asbestos may be independent of the generation of ROS, e.g., mechanical disruption of both the membrane and the mitotic apparatus (140,141).

One of the principal targets of ROS is the cellular DNA (139). Consistent with this view, antioxidant enzymes, iron chelators, and oxygen radical scavengers inhibit the mutagenic and cytotoxic effects of asbestos *in vitro* (142–145). Iron intrinsic to some fiber types or adsorbed to the fiber surface can catalyze production of ROS and thereby produce single-strand breaks in DNA *in vitro* (146–148). Cell culture experiments indicate that longer asbestos fibers elicit more DNA damage than do shorter fibers and that reduction of cellular glutathione levels exacerbates the chromosomal damage induced by asbestos (149). Further evidence that asbestos causes DNA damage in cells is suggested by cellular responses to the fibers. Asbestos promotes unscheduled DNA synthesis in cells exposed in culture (150) and activates expression of poly-(ADP-ribose)-polymerase (PARP), a DNA repair protein (151). Addition of inhibitors of PARP do not augment the cytotoxicity of asbestos, thereby suggesting that the toxic effects of asbestos are not mediated via DNA damage (151). These observations are consistent with the postulate that the oxidant stress induces some of the chromosomal abnormalities associated with asbestos exposure (see below). In cells exposed to asbestos, induction of DNA strand breaks may be a consequence of nucleolytic cleavage by calcium-dependent nucleases that become activated by the ROS-initiated release of intracellular calcium (152). Increases in cellular calcium levels and DNA strand breaks are hallmarks of programmed cell death (apoptosis) (153), and recent studies show that exposure of cells in culture to asbestos can cause apoptosis (154).

## CELL PROLIFERATION AND DEPOSITION OF EXTRACELLULAR MATRIX

Inhaled fibers activate cell proliferation at the original sites of particle deposition as described above. Peripheral tissues remain relatively unaffected unless there are repeated exposures (16,90,155–159). We have shown in a number of studies that cell proliferation in exposed rodents increases 10- to 40-fold at the bronchiolar-alveolar duct bifurcations (160), where fibrotic lesions consequently develop (16,156,161). In addition, it has been postulated that cytokines released by activated interstitial macrophages may diffuse across the interstitium to activate mesothelial cell proliferation (90,162–164). Exposure of rodents to fibrous particles induces DNA replication as measured by incorporation of deoxynucleotide analogs into nuclei of AM (165), epithelial (90,156,158, 161,164,166,167), interstitial (90,156,167), and endothelial (155,164) cells. Consistent with these findings, inhalation exposure of rats to asbestos elevates pulmonary levels of the mRNA encoding the proliferating cell nuclear antigen (PCNA), a DNA replication and repair protein (168,169). Furthermore, the temporal and spatial pattern of immunohistochemical detection of PCNA (Fig. 1) appears to coincide with analyses of deoxynucleotide incorporation in asbestos-exposed rats (168,169). Similarly, intratracheal administration of silica induces PCNA expression in a variety of cell types associated with granulomatous lesions that precede interstitial fibrosis (170). Asbestos-associated increases in pulmonary cell proliferation and in the lung content of the mRNAs encoding c-*jun* and ornithine decarboxylase, two markers of cell proliferation, appear to depend on fiber type (90,91,167).

Cell proliferation is likely to play a central role in the development of fibroproliferative lesions. Thus, it is essential that investigators understand the mechanisms controlling the proliferative response. Cell division could be mediated, in large part, by growth factors secreted by particle-activated AM (13,171–173). In addition, fibroblasts could accumulate at the sites of fiber deposition without dividing since chemoattractant factors such as PDGF and fibronectin are released from activated AM at sites of injury (174,175). Asbestos translocated to the interstitial compartment may also stimulate lung fibroblast proliferation directly via an autocrine mechanism that involves induction of both the ligand and the receptor for PDGF (176,177). Interestingly, isolated lung mesenchymal cells maintain the proliferative response to lung injury in cell culture and constitutively express the c-*fos* and c-*jun* genes at higher levels than do mesenchymal cells isolated from normal lungs (178). Accordingly, activation of c-*jun* and c-*fos* in isolated rat pleural mesothelial (RPM) cells *in vitro* by asbestos is consistent with a proliferative response (179,180), but asbestos also causes apoptosis of RPM cells (154). Thus, asbestos-associated induction of c-*jun* and c-*fos* in RPM cells concomitantly with apoptosis may indicate activation of the stress-activated protein kinase pathway (181–184). Similarly, activation of growth-responsive genes in isolated pulmonary epithelial cells in culture by asbestos (179,180,185) may reflect a cytotoxic (136) as well as proliferative (185) response in these cells. *In vivo* it is not clear whether cytokines secreted by AM and neighboring cells can prevent apoptosis of cells exposed to asbestos (186–188).

A collagenous scar develops at the duct bifurcations and along the alveolar duct walls between 48 hours and 1 month postexposure to asbestos (16). Particle-induced deposition of extracellular matrix (16) correlates with elevated synthesis of both types I and III collagen and reduced collagen degradation (189–192). Enhanced type I procollagen synthesis colocalizes with granulomatous lesions and TGF-β synthesis in silicotic rats (189), whereas increased tropoelastin expression in silica-exposed rats is restricted to interstitial cells in nongranulomatous regions (193). The lung content of hydroxyproline, an indicator of collagen synthesis, increases in rodent models of fiber-induced lung disease (91,96,118, 194), and trichrome staining has been used to identify fibrogenic responses to inhaled fibers in chronic exposures (118), as well as after brief, 3-day exposures (160). Asbestos also stimulates production of fibronectin in the lung (14,53,195) which colocalizes with accumulated AM that stain positively for TGF-β synthesis (195). It has

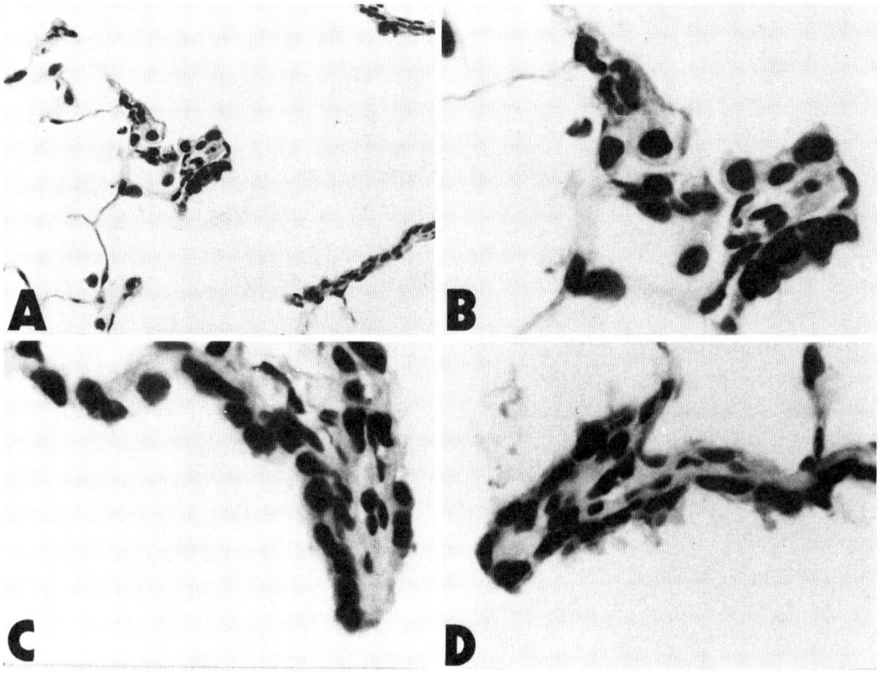


**FIG. 1.** Asbestos induces PCNA expression at the sites of fiber deposition. Rats were exposed 5 hours to an aerosol of asbestos at 10 mg/m$^3$ **(A and B)**, exposed 5 hours to an aerosol of carbonyl iron at a concentration of 50 mg/m$^3$ **(C)**, or unexposed **(D)**. Four days postexposure the animals were sacrificed and the left lung of each animal was perfused with fixative. Histologic sections were prepared and immunostained with a monoclonal antibody specific for PCNA. Panel A identifies a fiber deposition site—the bronchiolar-alveolar duct bifurcation at low magnification (200×). Panels B through D are at higher magnification (1000×) to demonstrate PCNA immunostaining in the three exposure groups—asbestos (B), iron (C), and unexposed (D). Inhalation exposure of rats to asbestos induces PCNA expression rapidly at the fiber deposition sites (see ref. 169 for details). *See color plate between pages 344 and 345.*

been proposed that enhanced production of fibronectin by AM is a predictive marker of increased collagen deposition and pulmonary fibrosis (118).

## FACTORS ELICITED BY PARTICLE-INDUCED LUNG INJURY

Cytokines released primarily from pulmonary macrophages dominate the response of the lung to inhaled particles (15,27,52,104). Additionally, direct cell contacts between the pulmonary epithelium and interstitial cells influence the response of the lung to injury as well (196,197). Cytokines affect multiple functions and the expression of other cytokines, complicating analyses to determine the role of specific cytokines elaborated in particle-induced lung injury (198). Initially, macrophages are recruited to the site of injury (17,199) by asbestos-mediated activation of complement via the alternative pathway (95,117,200,201) and by the particle-induced release of chemokines by pulmonary epithelial cells (202,203). Particle-induced injury to the vasculature can promote platelet trapping, which appears to be a central component of fibrosis instigated by bleomycin (204,205). The α granules of platelets are rich in PDGF (206), which may play a key role in fibrogenesis (see below). The AMs phagocytose the fibers on the bifurcation surface and interstitial macrophages and fibroblasts phagocytose the fibers in the interstitium (157). T lymphocytes appear to reduce the inflammatory and fibrogenic responses of the lung induced by asbestos (207). Among the cytokines released by activated macrophages, PDGF, TGF-α, TGF-β, and TNF-α can directly regulate epithelial and fibroblast proliferation as well as extracellular matrix deposition, the hallmarks of fibroproliferative lung disease (12,15,173,208). Biochemical and molecular aspects of these four potent factors are discussed below in some detail along with consideration of the potential roles they may play in fibroproliferative lung disease.

### Platelet-Derived Growth Factor

Platelet-derived growth factor is the major mesenchymal cell mitogen in serum (206), and it has been proposed in several settings that this potent peptide plays a central role in lung development (209–211), wound healing (212), and atherosclerosis (213). PDGF regulates a number of cellular responses that are relevant to pulmonary fibrogenesis, including chemotaxis, adhesion to fibronectin, cellular survival, induction of DNA synthesis, and actin cytoskeleton rearrangement (214,215). PDGF exists in three different isoforms, PDGF-AA, -AB, and -BB, which are homo- and heterodimers formed via disulfide bonds between two related polypeptides, PDGF-A and PDGF-B (206,216). The different isoforms of PDGF bind and promote formation of homo- and heterodimers of the two PDGF receptor polypeptides, α and β (215). Homodimers of the α receptor will bind all three PDGF isoforms, whereas homo- or heterodimers containing the β polypeptide will not bind the PDGF-AA isoform (215). PDGF binding to the extracellular domain of the PDGF receptor causes dimerization leading to autophosphorylation and activation of a tyrosine kinase in the intracellular domain (217). The phosphorylated receptor binds intracellular signal transduction proteins via Src homology 2 (SH2) domains (217). Among the proteins that bind the activated receptor are a variety of enzymes that can generate second messengers such as phospholipase Cγ, phosphatidylinositol 3′-kinase, protein kinases (Src and Raf), and phosphatases (protein tyrosine phosphatase-1D), and adapter proteins such as Shc that can link the activated receptor to signal transduction via the Ras pathway (215). The particular signal elicited by PDGF binding varies in a cell type–dependent manner (214,215). In the nucleus, PDGF can activate expression of growth regulatory transcription factors such c-*fos* (218), c-*jun* (219), and c-*myc* (220). In addition to its mitogenic effects, PDGF regulates interactions with the extracellular matrix (ECM). As an illustration, human foreskin fibroblasts exposed to PDGF contract collagen gels (221), and PDGF also alters the adherent properties of smooth muscle cells in culture. The altered adherence could occur by rearranging the distribution of integrins, i.e., cell surface receptors for ECM components (222). Moreover, PDGF can influence mesenchymal cell interactions with the ECM by altering integrin expression. For example, exposure of fibroblasts in culture to PDGF activates expression of $\alpha_2$-integrin via the protein kinase C-zeta isoform (223). This modulation of cellular interactions with the ECM by PDGF may be an essential aspect of the proliferative response, since the ECM has been shown to influence PDGF-induced cell division (224).

In a rat model of asbestos-induced fibroproliferative lung disease, we have shown that unexposed animals express little PDGF in the lung and that activation of pulmonary expression of PDGF by inhaled fibers is very rapid (Figs. 2 and 3) (225). PDGF-A and -B mRNA levels increase significantly during a 5-hour exposure to asbestos, and in situ hybridization demonstrates that elevated expression of both PDGF-B (Fig. 2C) and PDGF-A (Fig. 3A) mRNAs is primarily restricted to the bronchiolar-alveolar duct regions where asbestos-induced injury is initiated (225). In agreement with these findings, PDGF-B (Fig. 2D) and -A proteins (Fig. 3B) are detected immunohistochemically in macrophages and epithelial and interstitial cells at the sites of developing fibroproliferative lesions (225). These findings correlating PDGF expression with injury and repair in the rat agree with similar findings in humans (see above). Accordingly, AM and fluid recovered by BAL of humans and sheep in the early stages of silicosis or asbestosis contain elevated amounts of PDGF (171,172). The temporal and spatial

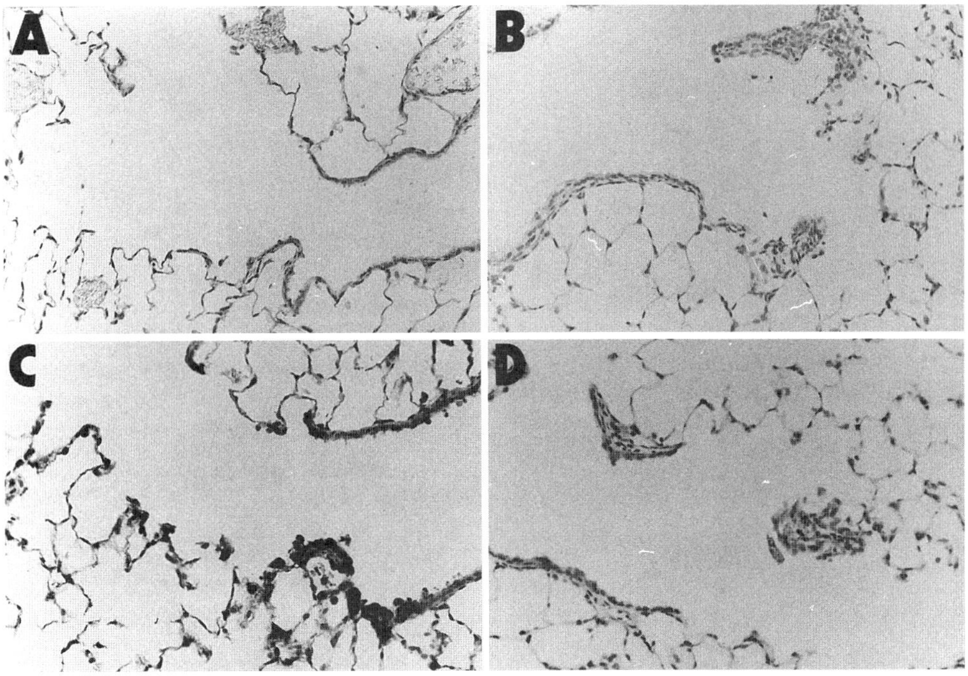


**FIG. 2.** Activation of PDGF-B expression at sites of lung injury and repair after inhalation exposure to asbestos. Rats were unexposed **(A)** or exposed for 5 hours to an aerosol of asbestos **(B–D)**. Two days postexposure the animals were sacrificed and formalin-fixed lung sections were analyzed for PDGF-B expression by *in situ* hybridization and immunohistochemistry. Panel A is a lung section from an unexposed animal probed with an antisense sequence to PDGF-B mRNA. The absence of significant bluish-black staining (compare to panel C) indicates the relative lack of PDGF-B mRNA in the lungs of normal animals. Panel B is a lung section from an exposed rat probed with a sense sequence to PDGF-B mRNA. Again, there is little bluish-black staining, an observation that suggests that the *in situ* hybridization assay is specific for PDGF-B mRNA. Panel C is the same as panel B except that an antisense sequence to PDGF-B mRNA was employed in the assay. The strong bluish-black staining at the ends of the terminal bronchiole indicates that inhaled asbestos has activated PDGF-B expression at these sites. Consistent with these results, the brown stain in panel D indicates immunohistochemical detection of the PDGF-B protein after inhalation of asbestos. Little immunohistochemical detection of PDGF-B is observed in the lungs of unexposed animals (not shown). Each section was counterstained with Mayer's hematoxylin (blue color) with a magnification of 200×. (See ref. 225 for further information.)

correlation of PDGF expression with fibrogenesis and the ability of PDGF to stimulate mesenchymal cell proliferation discussed above suggest a significant role for this factor in fibroproliferative lung disease. Additional experimental findings in cell culture bolster the postulate that PDGF promotes expansion of the interstitium in fiber-induced lung disease. For example, lung fibroblasts respond in a concentration-dependent fashion to PDGF in culture with enhanced proliferation and migration (226,227). Early passage lung fibroblasts express the PDGF-A isoform (228), but do not express detectable amounts of the PDGF-B isoform (228) or PDGF-α receptor (229,230). Nevertheless, all three isoforms of PDGF promote proliferation of fetal and adult lung fibroblasts in cell culture during a 7-day exposure period (231). Diverse agents such as asbestos (230), dexamethasone, and lipopolysaccharides (232) can induce PDGF-α receptor expression in these cells. Indeed, asbestos exposure of lung fibroblasts in cell culture activates expression of PDGF-A (176), PDGF-α receptor (230), and cell proliferation (177). Once PDGF-A expression is activated in lung fibroblasts by asbestos, it can transcriptionally activate its own expression through a *cis*-acting serum response element in its promoter (233). These results show that asbestos can initiate autocrine stimulation of cell proliferation *in vitro* in lung mesenchymal cells and suggest that a similar process contributes to fibroproliferative lung disease (176,177). In support of this view, addition of an antibody to PDGF blocks proliferation of rat lung fibroblasts exposed in serum-free media to asbestos (176). Although direct exposure of fibroblasts to asbestos can initiate this autocrine loop, the AM appears to be a major source of PDGF elicited by fiber exposure. Exposure of isolated AM in culture to particles induces secretion of PDGF (234,235), and activated alveolar macrophages (236) and interstitial macrophages (237) stimulate rat lung fibroblast proliferation *in vitro* via a growth factor with the characteristics of PDGF. *In vivo*, release of

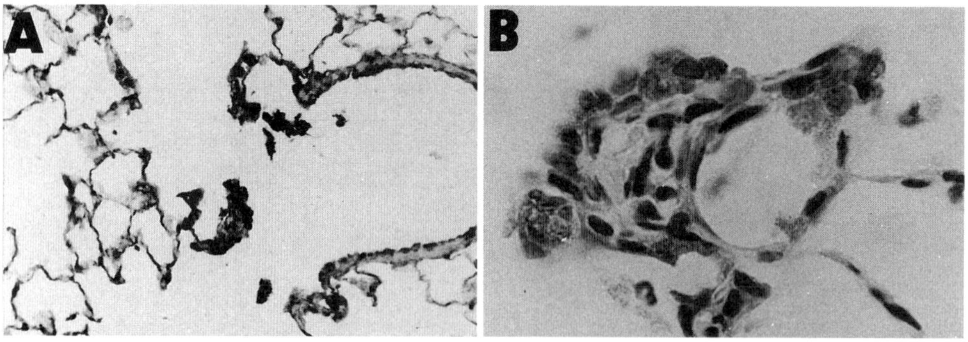

**FIG. 3.** PDGF-A expression in asbestos-exposed rats. **A:** In analyses similar to that depicted in Fig. 2, PDGF-A mRNA expression was detected by *in situ* hybridization in lung sections from rats 2 days postexposure to asbestos (200× magnification). Dark-staining cells are positive for PDGF mRNA. Negative control assays appeared similar to those for PDGF-B shown in Fig. 2. **B:** Immunohistochemical detection (by the DAB method, brown stain) of PDGF-A protein in the lungs of rats 2 days postexposure to asbestos (1000× magnification) (see ref. 225 for details). *See color plate between pages 344 and 345.*

macrophage-derived PDGF is augmented by macrophage accumulation at the sites of injury. The observation that vascular smooth muscle cells stimulated with PDGF secrete monocyte chemoattractant protein-1 (MCP-1) suggests a mechanism whereby PDGF participates in the accumulation of AM at the sites of lung injury and fibroproliferative lesions (238).

Analyses of animal models directly implicate PDGF as a controlling factor in mesenchymal cell proliferation in the lung. Intratracheal instillation of recombinant human PDGF-BB into the lungs of rats produces transient characteristics of fibrogenesis, including proliferation of airway epithelial cells, but intravenous administration of PDGF-BB produces no effect in the lung (239). In a similar experiment, elevated pulmonary expression of PDGF-B by intratracheal instillation of a recombinant adenovirus expression vector produces enhanced deposition of collagen and fibroblast proliferation that approximates the histology of IPF (240). A prominent role for PDGF in pulmonary wound healing agrees with the essential roles of PDGF-B in embryonic lung growth (209) and PDGF-A in lung morphogenesis (210,211). Phenotypic changes of fibroblasts during fibrogenesis parallels that observed during embryogenesis, i.e., fibroblasts derived from adult fibrotic tissue and neonatal fibroblasts respond similarly to PDGF and possess enhanced growth characteristics, while fibroblasts from normal adult lung tissue exhibit more limited growth *in vitro* (241). A description of the lung histology of mice harboring a transgene that expresses PDGF-B from the surfactant protein-C promoter may further implicate PDGF in fibroproliferative lung disease (242).

### Transforming Growth Factor-β

Transforming growth factor-β controls cell proliferation and migration and is a potent stimulator of extracellular matrix deposition (see refs. 48 and 243–246 for recent reviews). TGF-β1 is the most abundant member of this cytokine family, which consists of three isoforms with similar but nonoverlapping activities (244). TGF-β is secreted in a latent form as a high molecular weight complex (247) that can be converted to the mature, active form of TGF-β by proteolytic cleavage (248). Active TGF-β inhibits proliferation of epithelial cells, while producing variable effects on mesenchymal cell proliferation (249). Inhibition of cellular proliferation by TGF-β correlates with induction of two inhibitors of cell cycle progression, cyclin-dependent kinase inhibitors $p27^{KIP-1}$ and $p15^{INK4b}$ (250). Stimulation of fibroblast proliferation by TGF-β appears to be mediated via induction of connective tissue growth factor, a peptide with PDGF-like activities (251). TGF-β isoforms signal via binding dimerized transmembrane receptors of two subtypes (type I and type II) with unique serine/threonine kinase activity (252). Ligand binding is not required for type II receptor kinase activity; rather, it appears that ligand binding initiates signaling by promoting the association of type II with type I receptors (245). TGF-β–induced transcriptional regulation appears to be mediated via phosphorylation and nuclear localization of the Mad family of transcription factors (245).

Studies of lung development and transgenic mouse models indicate essential roles for TGF-β in immune regulation and lung morphogenesis. Genetically altered mice lacking the TGF-β1 gene die with chronic multifocal inflammation (253,254). The relevance of TGF-β to lung biology is indicated by the observation that TGF-β1 inhibits branching morphogenesis of the embryonic mouse lung (255,256), and mice lacking the TGF-β3 isoform die shortly after birth with abnormally developed lungs (257,258). Corticosteroids may enhance lung morphogenesis by upregulating TGF-β3 synthesis in fetal lung fibroblasts (259), although corticosteroids decrease

TGF-β3 mRNA levels in the total lung (260). This association of TGF-β with immune regulation and lung development suggests that it is a factor in chronic inflammatory lung disease induced by inhaled fibrogenic particles.

Several studies demonstrate an association between high levels of TGF-β expression, deposition of extracellular matrix (ECM), and fibrotic lung disease (195, 261–263). TGF-β stimulates synthesis and deposition of the ECM components, collagen of various types and fibronectin, in a number of tissues, including the lung (264–273). Moreover, TGF-β may stimulate matrix production by inhibiting the production of proteases (272, 274). Exposure of alveolar type II cells in culture to TGF-β1 increases fibronectin, laminin, and proteoglycan synthesis and modulates integrin and surfactant protein C expression, thereby suggesting TGF-β–mediated regulation of pulmonary cell ECM deposition and differentiation (275–277). Furthermore, TGF-β blocks proliferation of cultured alveolar type II cells exposed to TGF-α or epidermal growth factor (278). Inhibition of proliferation of an alveolar epithelial cell line by TGF-β correlates with enhanced synthesis of insulin-like growth factor–binding protein 2 (279). Stimulation of matrix components by TGF-β does not require altered cell proliferation (280), but the structure and composition of matrix components may regulate mesenchymal cell proliferation (281,282). Thus, TGF-β–mediated regulation of the ECM can also affect cell proliferation. Exposure of a fetal rat lung epithelial cell line to TGF-β induces synthesis and secretion of types I and III collagen (283). Other factors that stimulate deposition of the ECM by fibroblasts may stimulate endogenous expression of TGF-β. For example, elevation of 1-alpha (I) procollagen mRNA levels in isolated rat lung fibroblasts treated with monocyte chemotactic protein-1 appears to be mediated via activation of endogenous TGF-β1 expression (284).

Regulation of ECM deposition by TGF-β correlates with transcriptional regulation of the genes encoding components of the ECM. Transcriptional stimulation of type IV collagen by TGF-β occurs rapidly in cell culture, becoming detectable 2 to 4 hours after treatment (269). TNF-α counteracts TGF-β–induced stimulation of transcription of the human alpha-1 (I) collagen gene through overlapping *cis*-acting elements including an Sp1-binding site in the promoter (266) or through an activating protein (AP)-1–binding site that is more promoter proximal (267). In arterial smooth muscle cells, TGF-β stimulates PDGF synthesis (285) and cooperates with PDGF to induce synthesis of 1-alpha (I) procollagen expression (268). Stimulation of PDGF in smooth muscle cells occurs at low concentrations of TGF-β, which also promotes DNA synthesis that can be blocked with an antibody to PDGF (285). At higher concentrations of TGF-β, cell proliferation is inhibited and PDGF-α receptor levels decrease (285).

Intratracheal instillation of silica in rats induces TGF-β expression in fibroblasts, macrophages, and hyperplastic alveolar type II cells that is associated with silicotic granulomas (189,286) and colocalizes with type I procollagen synthesis (189). Similarly, inhalation exposure of rats to asbestos produces enhanced TGF-β and fibronectin expression at the sites of fiber deposition (195), which correlates with elevated levels of ECM detected by morphometry at times postexposure (16). During the early stages of lung injury and repair after asbestos exposure, TGF-β is found primarily in alveolar macrophages and in pulmonary epithelial cells (287). This pattern also is seen in the later stages of a fibrogenic response produced by bleomycin (261). The biologic effects of TGF-β are amplified by autocrine stimulation in AM (288) or in fibroblasts (289). Isolated fetal rat lung fibroblasts elaborate all three TGF-β isoforms and lung epithelial cells synthesize isoforms 1 and 3 (290). Whereas the TGF-β2 and -β3 isoforms appear to be constitutively expressed throughout the lung, TGF-β1 localizes in areas of fibrotic lung disease (49,291). Introduction via the trachea of a recombinant adenovirus expressing TGF-β1 causes histopathologic changes consistent with pulmonary fibrosis in rats (240). These observations suggest a pathogenic role for TGF-β in animal models of particle-induced lung disease and agree with the observations of elevated TGF-β in patients with silicosis (50), asbestosis (291), and idiopathic pulmonary fibrosis (261).

### Transforming Growth Factor-α

Transforming growth factor-α (TGF-α) is a powerful epithelial cell mitogen and a member of a large family of ligands that bind the epidermal growth factor receptors (EGF-R) (292). It is synthesized as a biologically active integral membrane glycoprotein that is released from the cell surface by proteolytic cleavage (293). Despite having common receptors, different biologic responses, including proliferation, migration, and differentiation, are mediated by individual members of the EGF family in diverse cell types of different tissues (292). Ligand binding activates an intrinsic tyrosine kinase of the EGF-R and transduces a signal to the nucleus through the *ras*/mitogen-activated protein (MAP) kinase pathway (294–296). Despite the potent biologic activities of TGF-α, disruption of the gene encoding it in mice produces phenotypic alterations only in the skin and eyes (297,298). This observation is consistent with the redundancy in the TGF-α signaling system. Expression of a TGF-α transgene in mice is associated with tumor formation (299,300), and induction of TGF-α frequently occurs in a variety of neoplasias, including lung tumors (292). TGF-α expression can be activated by a positive autoregulatory pathway through protein kinase C signaling (301,302) and by TNF-α (303).

Transforming growth factor-α is expressed in the lung during development in animals (304,305) and humans

(306), where it appears to influence branching morphogenesis and differentiation (307). Consistent with the proposed role for EGF-like proteins in pulmonary epithelial cell proliferation and lung development, infusion of EGF causes epithelial hyperplasia and maturation in the lungs of fetal lambs (308). Expression of the EGF-R (309) and TGF-α (305) by lung epithelial cells suggests that proliferation of these cells may be stimulated via an autocrine mechanism (310). Addition of TGF-α to type II alveolar epithelial cells in culture stimulates cellular proliferation (278,311) that can be blocked by the prior addition of TGF-β (278,312) or inhibitors of tyrosine kinases (312).

Transforming growth factor-α expression is frequently associated with inflammatory responses in cell culture and in animal models of chronic inflammation and fibrosis. AMs stimulated with lipopolysaccharide (LPS) in culture synthesize TGF-α mRNA and secrete TGF-α protein (313), and lung fibroblasts secrete TGF-α after injury (314). Consistent with these observations, AMs exposed to silica in cell culture release soluble factors that stimulate alveolar type II cell proliferation (172). In bleomycin-induced lung injury and fibrosis, increased amounts of TGF-α correlate with sites of cell proliferation (315). Fiber-induced lung injury and repair also correlate with TGF-α expression. Inhalation exposure of rats to cristabolite elevates TGF-α levels in the BAL fluid and in lung macrophages for an extended period, 16 to 20 weeks postexposure (316). Similarly, mice that inhale quartz dust elaborate an EGF-like activity in the BAL fluid that is able to bind EGF receptors on pulmonary fibroblasts and stimulate their proliferation *in vitro* (317). In our model of asbestosis in rats, inhalation of asbestos rapidly upregulates TGF-α mRNA and protein expression at the sites of the developing fibroproliferative lesions (Fig. 4) (168), while inhaled nonfibrogenic iron particles do not produce this response (168). The temporal and spatial pattern of TGF-α expression coincides with the appearance of PCNA (compare Figs. 1 and 4), thereby indicating an association of TGF-α with a proliferating population of cells during fibrogenesis (168). These associations of TGF-α expression with developing fibrotic lesions in animal models are supported by observations with transgenic mice indicating a causative role for TGF-α in fibroproliferative lung disease, i.e., pulmonary overexpression of a transgene encoding TGF-α

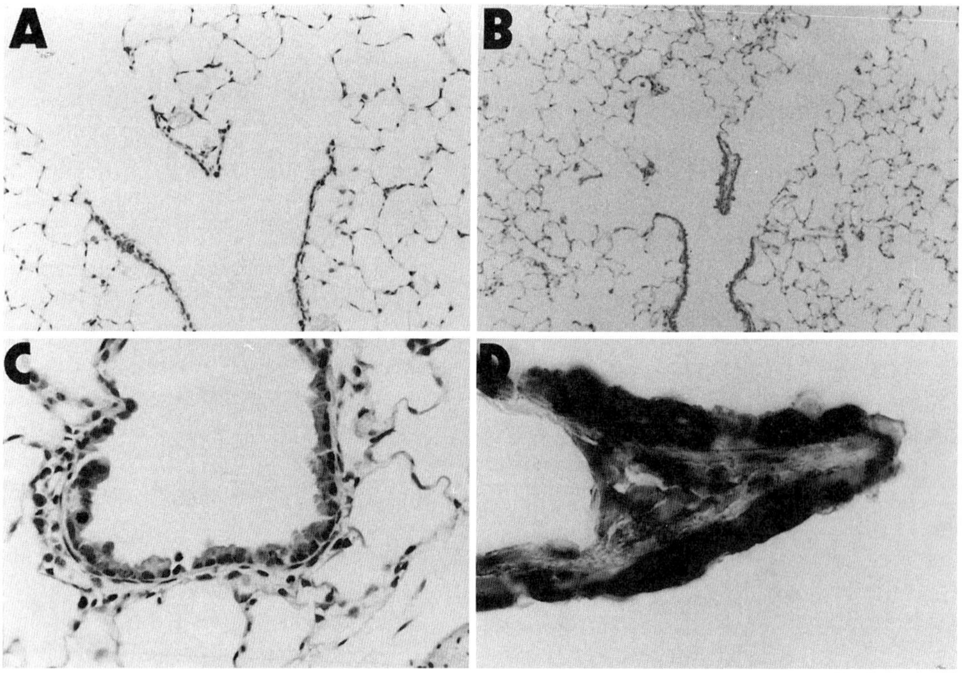

**FIG. 4.** Expression of TGF-α in developing fibroproliferative lesions. As described in Fig. 2, rats were unexposed or exposed to an aerosol of asbestos. At various times postexposure the animals were sacrificed and histologic sections of the lung were assessed for TGF-α protein by immunohistochemistry. The lung parenchyma of an unexposed animal does not express detectable TGF-α **(A)** (100× magnification). In contrast, clear brown staining indicating the presence of TGF-α appears in the lung section from the exposed animal at the 2-day time point **(B)** (100× magnification). TGF-α can also be immunohistochemically detected in the terminal bronchioles of asbestos-exposed animals at 1-day postexposure **(C)** (400× magnification). In agreement with this finding, TGF-α mRNA is detected by *in situ* hybridization primarily in the pulmonary epithelium (dark-staining cells are positive) at the 1-day time point **(D)** (1000× magnification) (see ref. 168 for details).

from the human surfactant protein C promoter in mice produces disrupted alveoli and fibrosis (318). Moreover, this fibrotic response to TGF-α in the lung does not require infiltration of inflammatory cells (318).

### Tumor Necrosis Factor-α

A variety of cell types produce TNF-α, a potent proinflammatory cytokine with a major role in endotoxic shock (see refs. 319 and 320 for recent reviews), but activated macrophages are the primary source (321). TNF is synthesized as a precursor and becomes a biologically active integral membrane protein of 26-kd that can be released by proteolytic cleavage as a soluble active 17-kd form (322). The three-dimensional structure of TNF reveals a trimer of identical subunits (323) that dissociates to inactive monomers in mild detergents (324). TNF binds two distinct receptors, TNF-R55 and TNF-R75, and thereby mediates such diverse responses as apoptosis and cell proliferation (319). Receptor activation by TNF appears to occur by clustering to transduce an intracellular signal that varies according to cell type (325), and concomitant signal transduction apparently is mediated by phosphorylation of the receptor by an associated kinase (326) and by a number of proteins that interact with the cytoplasmic domain of the TNF-R (319,327). Mice genetically altered to lack TNF-R55 or TNF-R75 resist lethal doses of lipopolysaccharide, but succumb to infection easily (327,328). In the nucleus, TNF effects are mediated by a number of transcription factors including nuclear factor κB (NF-κB), AP-1, interferon-regulator factor-1, nuclear factor–IL-6, adenosine 3′,5′-cyclic monophosphate (cAMP) response element binding protein, and serum response factor (329). The recent finding that NF-κB prevents TNF-induced cell death suggests a means of enhancing the cytotoxic potential of TNF in cancer therapy (330–332). Glucocorticoids, prostaglandin $E_2$, interleukin-4, TGF-β, and interleukin-10, all elaborated in developing lung disease, are among a number of endogenous molecules that suppress induction of TNF (333). Transgenic expression of TNF in mice suggests its role in such diverse inflammatory and immune-mediated diseases as rheumatoid arthritis and multiple sclerosis (320).

Pulmonary fibrosis appears to be a consequence of prolonged TNF expression in the lung. Constitutive expression of TNF-α in the lung from the human surfactant protein-C promoter in transgenic mice produces pulmonary pathology that resembles fibrotic lung disease in humans (334). Intratracheal instillation of TNF-α causes infiltration of inflammatory cells into the lung (335), and concomitant stimulation of adhesion molecule expression and of chemokine release by TNF may enhance pulmonary recruitment of inflammatory cells (94). In addition to this proinflammatory role, the observation that TNF-α stimulates production of types I and III collagen and fibronectin in human diploid fibroblasts (29), suggests its direct influence on deposition of extracellular matrix. However, in apparent contrast to the *in vitro* studies, chronic expression of TNF-α in mice decreases both synthesis of collagen and transcription of a human alpha-1 (I) collagen transgene while also inhibiting TGF-β expression (336). Another aspect of fibrogenesis mediated by TNF is mesenchymal cell proliferation and recruitment. Stimulation of fibroblast proliferation by TNF in cell culture includes a transient induction of PDGF-A expression, but additional factors appear to participate in fibroblast mitogenesis after exposure to TNF (337). Recombinant TNF and TNF-related peptides elicit migration of fibroblasts in culture, and activated macrophages secrete a chemotactic factor for fibroblasts that can be blocked with an antibody to TNF (338).

A number of observations implicate TNF as a key component of fiber-induced lung fibrosis. A single intratracheal administration of silica elicits a marked increase in the level of TNF-α mRNA in the lung for a prolonged period (339). The significance of this observation becomes apparent through the finding that antibodies to TNF inhibit deposition of collagen (339) and histopathologic changes (340) associated with silica exposure. Moreover, infusion of recombinant TNF augments the silica-induced fibrogenesis in the murine model (339). Intratracheal instillation of asbestos also causes elevated production of TNF-α in BAL fluid (341) with maximal expression 3 days postexposure (118). Consistent with this finding, silica or asbestos fibers stimulate the release of TNF-α *in vitro* from AM (25,341–343) and a murine macrophage-like cell line (344). Longer fibers or fibers coated with immunoglobulin G (IgG) stimulate greater release of TNF-α from AM in culture than do short, untreated fibers (345). If iron chelators or hydroxyl radical scavengers are added simultaneously with asbestos to AM in culture, the induction of TNF-α is inhibited (343). These data suggest that activation of TNF-α expression in AM is mediated by the asbestos-associated production of ROS discussed previously. This supposition is supported by the finding that pretreatment of rats with a free radical scavenger decreases the production of TNF-α mRNA in AM isolated after intratracheal instillation of silica (340). In addition, the free radical scavenger prevented formation of granulomatous lesions in rats exposed to silica (340). Consistent with the postulate that oxidative stress induces TNF-α and consequent lung histopathologic changes after silica exposure, a strain of ozone-resistant mice elaborates less TNF-α and histopathologic changes postexposure to silica than does a similarly exposed ozone-sensitive strain (96). Although AM extracted from silica-exposed rats secrete elevated amounts of TNF-α, altered metabolism of leukotrienes and prostaglandins suggests ongoing modulation of the immune response (346,347). Thus, AM isolated 1 and 3 weeks postexposure of rats to silica or asbestos express lower amounts of

TNF-α than AM from unexposed animals after a challenge with lipopolysaccharide *in vitro* (348,349). Experiments with a myelomonocytic cell line suggest that silica enhances TNF synthesis and secretion by transcriptionally activating the TNF gene (350).

### Other Cytokines

In addition to the cytokines and growth factors discussed above, a variety of other molecules are expressed in animal models of pneumoconiosis, but an association with fibrogenesis is not as clearly demonstrated. As a proinflammatory cytokine, many of the effects of interleukin-1 (IL-1) overlap with those of TNF (351). IL-1 exists in both a predominant β form and a less prevalent α form, which are encoded by distinct genes (352). Since both forms bind a common receptor, their biologic effects are similar (198). Intratracheal instillation of crocidolite in rats elicits a transient decrease in IL-1 in BAL fluid at early times (1 to 14 days) postexposure and elevated levels at later times (341). Pleural leukocytes also exhibit a transient decrease in IL-1 production after intratracheal instillation of crocidolite (353). Asbestos-induced alterations in IL-1 expression may be dose-dependent since it was shown that a high dose of instilled crocidolite induces rapid increases of IL-1 in BAL fluid and increased production of IL-1 in AM from exposed animals (118). Similarly, AM recovered from rats instilled with chrysotile produce enhanced amounts of IL-1 (349). An association with macrophage activation by fibers and release of IL-1 can also be demonstrated in cell culture. Increasing amounts of IL-1 mRNA are observed in a macrophage cell line exposed to silica (354). Enhanced release of IL-8, a potent chemoattractant for neutrophils, by pleural mesothelial cells exposed to asbestos appears to be mediated by IL-1 (355). An influx of neutrophils and release of IL-8 characterizes a rabbit model of pleurisy induced by asbestos (356). In addition, asbestos triggers release of IL-8 in A549 cells, a type II cell line, without prior release of IL-1 (357). The potent mitogenic activity of PDGF discussed above is augmented by the production of IGF-1 in particle-induced lung disease (351). AMs exposed to silica release IGF-1 (172,358), and AMs recovered from silicotic rats elaborate increased amounts of IGF-1 (359). The discussion above presents a limited number of cytokines as potential mediators of particle-induced lung disease. Although not discussed here, the effect of these cytokines in the lung will be subject to the activities of cytokine-binding proteins that interact with cytokines and thereby regulate their effective extracellular levels (360). Recent review articles present additional views (12,52,361).

## PARTICLE-INDUCED NUCLEAR SIGNALING

Although inhaled fibers may vary the pattern of gene expression in the lung via multiple mechanisms, the clear association with oxidative stress and growth stimulation indicate an altered pattern of transcription. The intracellular redox state affects the activity of at least three growth regulating transcription factors implicated in fiber-induced effects: NF-κB, AP-1, and p53 (362). In the inactive state, NF-κB, which includes the *rel* oncogene family, exists in a cytoplasmic complex with a member from the IκB family of inhibitor proteins (363). A number of stimuli, including oxidative stress, activate NF-κB by triggering reactions that lead to proteolysis of IκB followed by translocation of NF-κB to the nucleus (362). Furthermore, NF-κB activation in a human T cell line by such diverse agents as TNF, phorbol ester, calcium ionophore, and lectins is blocked by antioxidants, thus suggesting that reactive oxygen intermediates mediate NF-κB activation by a variety of effectors (364). Nuclear NF-κB binds to specific DNA sequences as a homo- or heterodimer and activates transcription of a wide variety of genes, including those encoding inflammatory mediators (365). Of the proposed cytokine mediators of fibrogenesis described above, NF-κB can transcriptionally activate expression of PDGF (366) and TNF (367) and indirectly activate synthesis of TGF-β (368). Since both TNF (365,369) and PDGF (370,371) induce NF-κB activity, autocrine stimulation may amplify the cellular responses to these cytokines. In contrast, TGF-β appears to inhibit the activity of NF-κB by transcriptionally activating expression of IκB (372). Whether or not inhaled particles can activate NF-κB in the lung remains to be determined; however, addition of asbestos to A549 cells, a type II–like epithelial cell line, or to primary pulmonary epithelial cells in culture induces NF-κB activity (373, 374) and addition of antioxidants or protein kinase inhibitors suppress that activation (374). Moreover, inhibition of NF-κB activation by stabilizing IκB reduces silica-induced expression of TNF in a macrophage cell line (354).

Similar to NF-κB, AP-1 regulates cell growth and mediates a nuclear response to oxidative stress (362,375, 376). Products of the *jun* and *fos* family of proto-oncogenes dimerize via "leucine zipper" motifs to form AP-1, which binds specific DNA sequences and regulates transcription (375). The various factors that form AP-1 possess different degrees of transcription activation strength and DNA binding may occur only with certain dimerization partners (375). Moreover, phosphorylation of AP-1 at specific sites enhances transcriptional activation; thus, DNA binding does not indicate the potential to activate transcription by AP-1 (377). In addition to oxidative stress, growth factors and UV irradiation are among the various stimuli that induce AP-1 activity (375). A number of studies indicate that oxidative stress of cultured cells induces c-*fos* and c-*jun*, the major components of AP-1 (362). Induction of AP-1 by mitogens can be inhibited by antioxidants (378), thereby suggesting that reactive oxygen intermediates mediate mitogenic stimulation of AP-1. Exposure of hamster tracheal epithelial cells in culture to asbestos fibers produces a prolonged increase in cellular levels of c-*jun* mRNA and AP-1 activity (180) and introduction of a c-*jun* expression construct into these cells increases their proliferation (185). Asbestos also causes prolonged induction of AP-1 in cultured rat pleural mesothelial cells accompanied by elevated cellular levels of the mRNAs encoding c-*fos* and c-*jun* (180). A connection to oxidative stress is suggested by the observation that the induction of c-*fos* and c-*jun* is diminished by the addition of a reducing agent, *N*-acetyl-L-cysteine (379). Autocrine stimulation of cell proliferation may occur via AP-1 mediated activation of PDGF (380), which can, in turn, enhance expression of the AP-1 components, c-*fos* (218) and c-*jun* (219). In addition, AP-1 can mediate TGF-β–induced stimulation of the alpha-2 (I) collagen (COL1A2) promoter in human dermal fibroblasts, which can be blocked by overexpression of c-*jun* (267). TNF-α antagonizes TGF-β–associated stimulation of the COL1A2 promoter through promoter sequences that include the AP-1 motif (267). Thus, an AP-1 site transduces opposing cellular responses to the profibrogenic cytokines cited above. An illustration of the complexity of this system is provided by the observation that, in other cell types, TGF-β induces phosphorylation of the *fos* family member *Fra-2,* which appears to mediate transcriptional repression of the osteocalcin gene (381). In an experimental model of regenerating liver, addition of antibodies to TNF-α prevents activation of jun nuclear kinase and accumulation of c-*jun* in the nucleus leading to alterations in DNA binding by AP-1 (382). Similarly, TNF-α stimulates the jun kinase in human fibroblasts and enhances expression of c-*jun* (383). In a human astrocytoma cell line, IL-1β elevates cellular levels of TNF-α mRNA via a protein kinase C–dependent pathway that includes AP-1 (384). This indication that AP-1 regulates expression of the TNF-α gene coupled with the observation that TNF-α stimulates AP-1 activity suggests autocrine activation of TNF-α expression via AP-1 in some cells.

The p53 tumor suppressor is a nuclear phosphoprotein that regulates cell cycle progression and viability (see refs. 385–388 for review). The significance of p53 to tumor suppression is illustrated by the observations that the gene encoding p53 is frequently mutated in a wide array of human cancers (389) and mice lacking a functional p53 gene develop cancer at an early age (390). Although a role for p53 in regulation of translation must be considered (391), the biologic activities of p53 appear to correlate primarily with its ability to activate or repress transcription (385,387). Among the genes transcriptionally activated by p53 are p21/WAF (392), a cyclin-dependent kinase inhibitor, and bax (393), a homolog of bcl-2. The former arrests cell cycle progression (394,395), while the latter appears to mediate the pro-apoptotic effects of p53 (396). Transcriptional repression may involve direct binding to the TATA-binding protein of the transcription initiation complex (387). Among the genes transcriptionally repressed by p53 are c-*fos* and c-*jun* of the AP-1 family of transcription factors discussed above (386). The complex regulation of p53 activity stems from interactions with viral and cellular proteins, posttranslational modifications, and allosteric mechanisms (385). Agents that damage DNA, including hydrogen peroxide, increase cellular levels of p53 protein via a posttranslational mechanism (397,398), and DNA strand breaks are sufficient to induce p53-mediated cell cycle arrest (399). Indeed, p53 may be involved in the direct recognition of DNA damage (400,401) and in the induction of DNA repair (402). The association of asbestos with oxidative stress (discussed above) and DNA damage (see below), is consistent with the recent observation that inhaled asbestos induces p53 expression at the sites of fiber deposition (Fig. 5A) (169). In addition, detection of p53 coincides temporally and spatially with immunodetection of PCNA (Fig. 5A), a DNA replication and repair protein that is transcriptionally regulated by p53 (403,404). Coexpression of these two proteins suggests a cellular response to asbestos-induced DNA damage whereby p53 activates PCNA expression for purposes of DNA repair (122).

Whether or not p53 mediates the apoptotic response of cells exposed in culture to asbestos (154) is not known. In a swine model of wound healing, PDGF is expressed at early times after injury, while p53 is expressed later (405). This reciprocal pattern of expression indicates potential roles for the proteins in activation and suppression, respectively, of cell proliferation during the healing process, but higher levels of p53 in proliferating tissues may not be active (406). A similar delayed pattern of p53 expression also occurs in asbestos-exposed rats (Fig. 5B) (169). In contrast, p53 may be involved in the proliferative response to replace damaged cells by transcriptionally activating the TGF-α gene (407). Although inhibition of epithelial cell proliferation by TGF-β is p53-independent (408), cell cycle localization of p53 (409) and p53-mediated inhibition of cyclin-dependent kinase 4 mRNA translation (410) correlate with TGF-β treatment. Thus, growth inhibition by p53 or TGF-β appears to be signaled via separate but interacting pathways (411,412). Similarly, p53 may mediate some of the growth inhibitory effects of TNF in a leukemia cell line (413) and in a breast cancer cell line (414). Consistent with this view, TNF produces increases in cellular levels of p53 mRNA (415) and activation of the p53 promoter by NF-κB is inducible by TNF (416). Nevertheless, TNF-associated increases in cellular levels of the p21/WAF1 cyclin-dependent kinase inhibitor are independent of p53 (417,418). In contrast to these findings, TNF stimulation of a T cell line induces a conformational change in p53, and the altered form of protein mediates transcriptional activation of the human immunodeficiency virus long terminal repeat (419). Thus, p53 appears to be involved in both proliferative and antiproliferative responses to TNF.

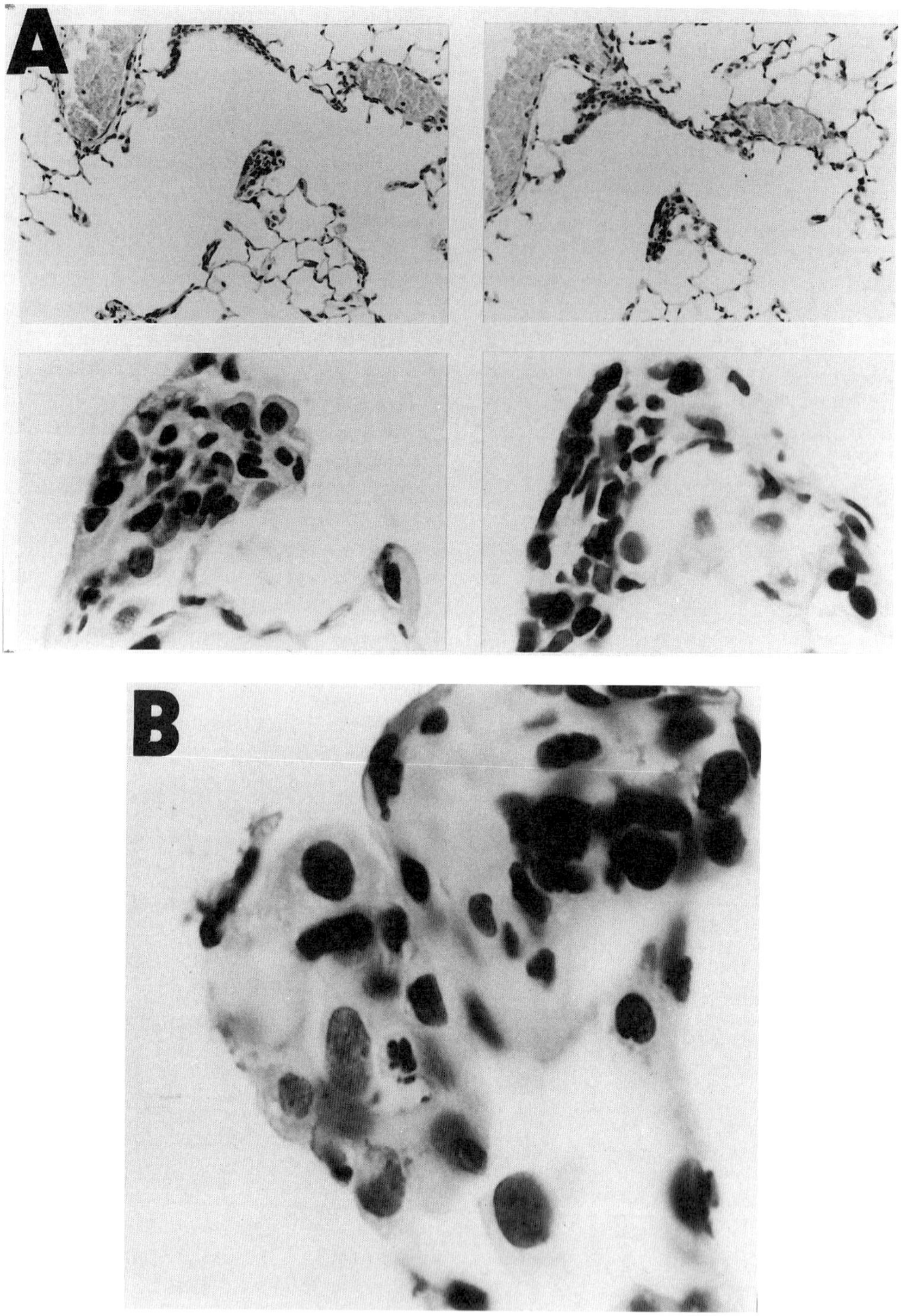


**FIG. 5. A:** Coexpression of PCNA and p53 postexposure to asbestos. As in Fig. 1, rats were exposed 5 hours to an aerosol of asbestos at 10 mg/m$^3$. Two days postexposure the animals were sacrificed, and histologic sections were prepared and immunostained with a monoclonal antibody specific for p53 *(left panels)* and PCNA *(right panels)*. Common features in the two *top panels* indicate that the sections are derived from the same anatomic site in the lung. The *lower panels* indicate that this location is positive for both p53 *(lower left)* and PCNA *(lower right)*. **B:** Prolonged p53 expression in asbestos-exposed rats. p53 immunostaining in rat lung sections from animals 8 days postinhalation exposure to asbestos. The micrograph (1000×) reveals high levels of p53 immunostaining. A variety of cell types are p53-positive including probable macrophages, epithelial, and interstitial cells. *See color plate between pages 344 and 345.*

## MOLECULAR BIOLOGY OF CANCER CAUSED BY INORGANIC PARTICLES

Intratracheal instillation or inhalation of fibrous particles produces tumors in experimental models (9,286, 420). Although the molecular mechanisms associated with tumor formation induced by asbestos remain unclear, it seems likely that the effects of fibers discussed above, i.e., fiber-induced formation of ROS and cell proliferation mediated by release of inflammatory cytokines, contribute to tumorigenesis (63). Asbestos is not classified as a mutagen in the Ames test (421), but it appears to be genotoxic in cell culture studies that are complicated by cell type and species-specific differences (136,422). Asbestos can induce both DNA strand breaks (144–147, 423) and DNA repair proteins (151,169). An association with reactive oxygen is suggested by the observation that the genotoxic potential of asbestos in cell culture is ameliorated by antioxidants (143). As discussed above, DNA cleavage induced by asbestos and initiated by ROS may be associated with the release of intracellular calcium and the induction of apoptosis. Similar to the observations with asbestos, incubation of DNA with silica in aqueous solution promotes strand breaks that can be inhibited by catalase or free radical scavengers (424). In cell culture, crystalline silica produces neoplastic transformation of a mouse cell line or fetal rat epithelial cells, and the transformed cells are tumorigenic in nude mice (425,426). Oncogenic conversion of epithelial cells by silica correlates with a loss of TGF-β1 expression (425). In addition to DNA damage that may be caused by fiber-induced generation of ROS (63,122), internalized fibers cause chromosomal aberrations by disruption of the mitotic apparatus (134,427–429) or by fiber adherence to chromosomes (430). In concert with chromosomal alterations, clonal expansion through sustained elaboration of cytokines (431) and chronic induction of growth-related transcription factors (91,180) will increase the number of target cells that can accumulate the additional mutations needed for tumor progression (432–434). In this proposed scenario, asbestos acts as a complete carcinogen that can initiate and promote tumor progression (435). Asbestos also exacerbates the carcinogenic potential of other agents. The surface of asbestos fibers adsorb carcinogens (436) and DNA (437) and thereby promotes uptake of these agents upon internalization by various cell types.

There is not a consistent pattern of genomic mutations in asbestos-associated tumors (63). In a rat model of asbestos-induced mesothelioma, higher levels of TGF-α are observed (94). Furthermore, antibodies to TGF-α inhibit proliferation of asbestos-transformed rat mesothelial cells in culture (438), but it is not known whether TGF-α is overexpressed in human mesotheliomas. There may be species specificity in the pathogenesis of mesothelioma. PDGF is overexpressed in some human mesotheliomas (see above) and overexpression of the PDGF-A gene enhances the tumorigenicity of a human mesothelial cell line (439), but no alterations of PDGF expression occur in a rat mesothelioma model (440). A potent repressor of PDGF-A expression (441), the Wilms' tumor gene, WT1, is expressed in rat and human mesotheliomas, but it is not frequently mutated (442,443). Deletion of the neurofibromatosis type 2 gene, which encodes a protein presumed to be involved in signal transduction, occurs with significant frequency in mesothelioma (444) and may by a consequence of the disruption of DNA segregation by asbestos (445).

## THERAPEUTIC APPROACHES

The prognosis of patients with fibrotic lung disease is poor, and current therapies have little positive effect (446). Strategies to prevent disease progression focus on the basic molecular mechanisms of the disease process discussed above, i.e., prevention of tissue injury by ROS and suppression of the inflammatory response (see refs. 447 and 448 for reviews). To reduce inflammation, glucocorticoids might be administered, but AMs from IPF patients treated with glucocorticoids continue to secrete elevated amounts of cytokines (449). In particular, dexamethasone does not reduce TGF-β1 secretion by activated AMs in cell culture (450), and levels of TGF-β3 in fetal lung fibroblasts increase with exposure to glucocorticoids (259). Cyclophosphamide, a DNA alkylating immunosuppressive drug, may enhance glucocorticoid therapy of IPF (451), and colchicine can inhibit the release of growth factors by alveolar macrophages *in vitro* (452), but *in vivo* the levels necessary to produce reduction of growth factor expression could produce adverse effects (453).

As discussed above, inhaled fibers generate ROS in the lung, which contributes to lung injury. To correct undesirable redox changes observed in patients with fibrotic lung disease, aerosolized antioxidants, such as glutathione, have been employed (454). In addition, the observed deficits in lung glutathione levels in patients with pulmonary fibrosis might be corrected by intravenous administration of *N*-acetylcysteine with no harmful side effects (455). However, the short half-life of antioxidants (456) becomes problematic in the treatment of chronic disease. Antioxidant therapy may produce the added benefit of blocking cytokine gene expression by inhibiting activation of the transcription factors (described above) that mediate induction of fibrogenic gene products (457). In this regard, the antioxidant dehydroepiandrosterone can block production of ROS by alveolar macrophages lavaged from asbestos workers (458) and by human peripheral blood monocytes activated by LPS or silica (459). In the latter case, antioxidants reduced the LPS-associated increase in cellular TNF-α mRNA levels and reduced transcription of cytokine genes (459). Prevention of NF-κB and AP-1 activation appears to be the molecular mechanism of antioxidant alterations of cytokine expression (362,457,459). Whether or not antioxidants prevent cytokine expression in cell types other than macrophages remains to be determined (457). Exposure of human fibroblasts in cell culture to antioxidants reduces the steady-state levels of procollagen alpha-1 (I) mRNA and the transcription of the procollagen alpha-1 (I) gene (460). The therapeutic utility of antioxidants is suggested by the palliative effect of intratracheal instillation of polyethylene glycol-conjugated catalase in a rat asbestosis model (461). In addition, oral administration of *N*-acetylcysteine reduces collagen deposition in a mouse model of bleomycin-induced fibrosis (462). Despite these apparent benefits of antioxidant therapy, a clinical trial employing antioxidants in the form of β carotene and retinyl palmitate to reduce cancer risk was aborted due to increased cancer incidence in the experimental group (463).

The link between TNF-α and fibrogenic lung disease discussed above suggests a therapeutic approach designed to inhibit production or effects of TNF-α. Anti-TNF antibodies prevent silicosis in mice (339) and produce efficacious results in patients with other chronic inflammatory diseases, rheumatoid arthritis (464), and Crohn's disease (465). However, the antigenicity of monoclonal antibodies, complications due to excessive formation of immune complexes, and high titers of antibody required to achieve neutralization preclude their use in long-term therapies for chronic diseases (319). Another approach to prevent the adverse effects of TNF is to inhibit its synthesis by blocking the activity of the protease involved in maturation and release of mature TNF (446). However, it is unclear whether or not the protease that cleaves TNF can be specifically inhibited. Bicyclic imidazoles, a class of pharmacologic inhibitors of CSBP/p38 MAP kinase, block LPS-induced synthesis of TNF-α by interfering with translation of the TNF-α mRNA (466). Furthermore, the drug selectively inhibits NF-κB–mediated stimulation of transcription associated with TNF-α treatment without interfering with the cytotoxic effect of TNF-α (467). Although the efficacy of the CSBP/p38 MAP kinase inhibitor in fibrotic lung disease remains unknown, an analog reduces edema in a rat model of arthritis (468). Ongoing research efforts are designed to identify derivatives of the bicyclic imidazoles with less toxicity (457). Another antiinflammatory drug, acanthoic acid, inhibits TNF and IL-1 production by human macrophages exposed to silica *in vitro* (469). Furthermore, in a rat silicosis model, acanthoic acid suppressed formation of granulomatous lesions and fibrosis (469). These observations suggest that reduction of TNF and IL-1 production is therapeutically beneficial in silicosis and perhaps in other diseases characterized by chronic inflammation (469). In a mouse silicosis model, a soluble form of the human TNF receptor prevents the increase in lung hydroxyproline and the formation of collagen rich nodules associated with silica exposure (194). Furthermore, administration of the soluble TNF receptor at later times reverses fibrogenic alterations and reduces the amount of collagen in the lung (194). Formation of chimeras between the soluble TNF receptor and an immunoglobulin heavy chain fragment may improve the stability of the TNF receptor and thereby enhance its therapeutic use (470). Whether or not inhibition of TNF benefits patients with pneumoconiosis will likely be determined soon.

Antiinflammatory cytokines may also be employed to subdue the chronic inflammation that leads to excessive connective tissue production (208). TGF-β can inhibit macrophage activation (471), but its profibrogenic effects described above preclude its use. In cultures of human monocytes, antioxidants appear to antagonize the effects of the proinflammatory cytokines by increasing production of IL-1 receptor antagonist (IL-ra), a potent antiinflammatory factor (472). In mouse models of pulmonary fibrosis induced by intratracheal instillation of silica or bleomycin, preadministration of IL-1ra prevents lung injury and accumulation of hydroxyproline, and postadministration reverses the course of established pulmonary disease (473). The antifibrotic effects of granulocyte-macrophage colony-stimulating factor (GM-CSF) in a mouse model of bleomycin-induced fibrosis (474) may be mediated via increased production of IL-1ra (448). Thus, IL-1ra may abrogate chronic inflammation and the fibroproliferative response to inhaled fibers. IL-4 is an antiinflammatory cytokine that represses cellular levels of proinflammatory cytokine mRNAs in human monocytes (475,476). However, the use of IL-4 to reduce chronic inflammation in fibrogenesis is compromised by the undesirable profibrogenic effects of stimulating synthesis of both collagen (477) and MCP-1/JE (478). In addition, induction of immunoglobulin E synthesis by IL-4 could lead to allergic reactions (457). IL-10 is a potent antiinflammatory cytokine that appears with a delayed onset after monocyte activation, and its activity appears to downregulate the inflammatory response of stimulated macrophages (479). IL-10 inhibits production of inflammatory cytokines (TNF, IL-1, IL-8, and IL-6) by human AM exposed in culture to LPS (480). Whether or not IL-10 can reduce chronic inflammation in the lung and the severity of lung disease produced by inhaled fibers is not known (208,457). Interferon-γ diminishes fibroblast proliferation and collagen synthesis in cell culture (481,482). Human AM exposed to interferon-γ release more of the soluble form of the TNF-receptor (483). As indicated above, the soluble form of the TNF-receptor would produce antiinflammatory effects by binding TNF. In animal models, interferon-γ, or an interferon inducer, decreases fibrogenesis induced by bleomycin in mice (484,485) and in rats (486). Although interferon-γ prevents PDGF production by stimulated monocytes (487), production of PDGF and cytokine synthesis is generally enhanced by exposure of pulmonary macrophages to interferon-γ (488,489). Thus, interferon-γ appears to possess both pro- and antifibrogenic activities. The approach to target proinflammatory cytokines as a means to prevent progressive fibroproliferative lung disease contrasts with immunostimulatory treatment of established neoplastic lung disease (86).

The association of growth factor expression with fiber-induced lung disease described above suggests that inhibition of their function would be of therapeutic value. Due to its potent mitogenic effect on mesenchymal cell proliferation, a variety of therapies target the synthesis and activities of PDGF. An observation suggesting the therapeutic utility of blocking PDGF in fibrotic lung disease is that antibodies to PDGF block proliferation of lung fibroblasts exposed to asbestos in culture (176). Since biologically active PDGF is a dimer, inhibition may be achieved by forcing dimerization of the wild-type protein with an inactive mutant, having a so-called dominant negative phenotype. Dominant negative mutants of PDGF can inhibit its function in cell culture (490) and cause phenotypic reversion of transformed cell lines that overexpress PDGF (491). Similarly, a chimera between PDGF and VEGF that can dimerize, but fails to bind the PDGF receptor, exhibits a dominant negative phenotype (492). This chimera causes reversion of transformed cells that overexpress PDGF-B (492). Methods to block synthesis of PDGF include means to prevent accumulation and translation of PDGF mRNA. A ribozyme designed to specifically cleave the PDGF mRNA can repress proliferation of a mesothelioma cell line that overexpresses PDGF (493). Antisense oligonucleotides to PDGF are also an effective means of preventing mesenchymal cell proliferation (209). A polyanionic drug, suramin, can bind to PDGF in the extracellular space and thereby prevent its activity (198). These observations suggest potential means of inhibiting the activity of PDGF and thereby disrupting the autocrine loop (see above) that appears to drive some of the excessive mesenchymal cell proliferation that characterizes the fiber-induced fibrotic and neoplastic diseases of the lung.

Reduction of collagen biosynthesis and maturation may be a useful means of reducing fibrogenesis (447,448). As a potent inducer of collagen deposition, inhibition of the synthesis or activity of TGF-β might be a therapeutic approach in fiber-induced lung disease. The strategies discussed above for inhibition of PDGF would be useful for inhibiting TGF, but more complicated due to the different isoforms of TGF-β (447). Antibodies to TGF-β reduce collagen deposition in a mouse model of bleomycin-induced fibrosis (494). However, the antiinflammatory activity of TGF-β may be vital in suppression of the inflammatory response (253,254). The observation that pretreatment with retinoids reduces synthesis of types I and III collagen by TGF-β–exposed human lung fibroblasts suggests an alternative means of inhibiting ECM deposition while retaining the antiinflammatory properties of TGF-β (495). Another means of inhibiting collagen deposition could be with $PGE_2$, which reduces collagen production by fibroblasts in cell culture (448). Systemic administration of $PGE_2$ can produce undesirable side effects, but aerosolized $PGE_2$ can lead to effectively increased levels in the epithelial lining fluid of the lung (496). $PGE_2$ may produce a variety of responses (447) that differ between rodents and humans (448). A plant alkaloid, halfuginone, also inhibits collagen type I synthesis by mouse fibroblasts in cell culture (497) and reduces collagen deposition in the lungs of rats exposed to bleomycin (498).

The airways offer a unique access that cannot be achieved in other organs, yet effective therapies for a number of lung diseases are lacking. Thus, more gene therapy protocols are approved for the lung than any other organ (499). Both viral and nonviral modes of gene delivery can successfully transduce pulmonary cells *in vivo*, but a number of obstacles must be overcome before lung gene therapy is commonly employed (499). Of the viral vectors, adenovirus is the most efficient at gene delivery, but an inflammatory response to the virus limits the effectiveness of recombinant adenovirus (499). Adenoviruses lacking additional portions of the viral genome may circumvent problems with the immunogenicity of the virus (500). A recombinant adenovirus containing the human catalase cDNA protects human endothelial cells from oxidant stress *in vitro* (501). This virus might be employed to protect endothelial cells of the lung from oxidant injury associated with inhaled fibers (see above). To suppress the inflammatory response in the lung, intravenous injection of cationic liposomes containing the prostaglandin G/H synthase gene can elevate levels of $PGE_2$ and prostacyclin in the lung (502). The lungs of rabbits transduced with the prostaglandin G/H synthase gene resist injury induced by infusion of endotoxin (502). Another means to suppress inflammation in the lung involves a recombinant adenovirus that expresses a soluble form of the TNF receptor (503). Mice treated with TNF-receptor adenovirus resist intratracheal instillation of silica, but become susceptible to infection by *Listeria monocytogenes* (503). These studies contrast with gene therapy approaches designed for proinflammatory responses to treat lung cancer and mesothelioma (499). Gene therapy holds some promise in the treatment of human pulmonary disease, but problems that limit this technology remain to be solved.

## SUMMARY AND CONCLUSIONS

The diseases caused by inhaled inorganic particles have been with us for centuries, but we are just now beginning to understand the basic molecular mecha-

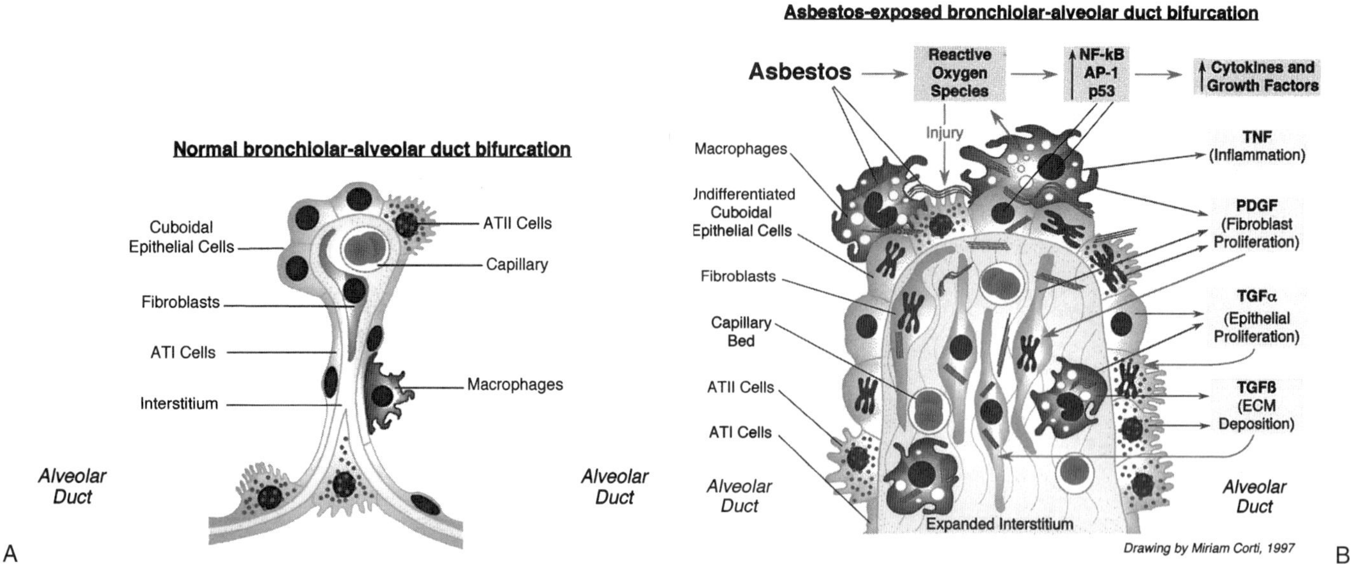


**FIG. 6.** A model of particle-induced fibrosis. This diagram illustrates many of the responses of the lung to inhaled particles that are described in the text. **A:** A schematic of a normal bronchiolar-alveolar duct bifurcation. **B:** Asbestos induces signaling leading to cytokine release that promotes fibroproliferative lung disease. *See color plate between pages 344 and 345.*

nisms that mediate the processes involved. Fig. 6 provides a simple overview of some of the molecular mechanisms discussed in the text. It is becoming apparent that initial injury to lung cells is caused by reactive oxygen species that, in turn, open several doors to the elaboration of multiple growth factors, cytokines, and inflammatory mediators. Here we have attempted to describe a small segment of this rapidly growing field of study by dealing with several of the molecular pathways through which PDGF, TGF-α, TGF-β, and TNF might exert their potent effects during development of fibroproliferative lung disease. Neoplastic disease depends on cell proliferation and clearly is caused by inhaled particles. Thus, any discussion of growth factor biology would be incomplete without some consideration of how the factors can influence lung cell growth during carcinogenesis.

It is our hope that with an understanding of the fundamental mechanisms of fibrosis and a few thoughts on emerging attempts at therapeutic intervention of fibrogenic lung disease, new molecular technologies can be applied in the struggles to successfully treat interstitial fibroproliferative lung disease.

## ACKNOWLEDGMENTS

The authors are grateful to the National Institutes of Health for research grants R29 ES07856 and R03 ES08628 to GFM and R01 ES06766 and R01 HL/ES60532 to ARB, and to the Tulane/Xavier Center for Bioenvironmental Research.

## REFERENCES

1. Maestrelli P, di Stefano A, Occari P, et al. Cytokines in the airway mucosa of subjects with asthma induced by toluene diisocyanate. *Am J Respir Crit Care Med* 1995;151(3 Pt 1):607–612.
2. Mapp CE, Lapa e Silva JR, Lucchini RE, Chitano P, Rado V, Saetta M, Pretolani M, Karol MH, Maestrelli P, Fabbri LM. Inflammatory events in the blood and airways of guinea pigs immunized to toluene diisocyanate. *Am J Respir Crit Care Med* 1996;154(1):201–208.
3. Koenig JQ. Effect of ozone on respiratory responses in subjects with asthma. *Environ Health Perspect* 1995;103(suppl 2):103–105.
4. Barnes PJ. Air pollution and asthma. *Postgrad Med J* 1994;70(823): 319–325.
5. Bates DV. Observations on asthma. *Environ Health Perspect* 1995; 103(Suppl 6):243–247.
6. Bozelka BE, Sestini P, Gaumer HR, Hammad Y, Heather CJ, Salvaggio JE. A murine model of asbestosis. *Am J Pathol* 1983;112: 326–337.
7. Brody AR. Inhaled particles in human disease and animal models: use of electron beam instrumentation. *Environ Health Perspect* 1984;56: 149–162.
8. Filipenko D, Wright JL, Churg A. Pathologic changes in the small airways of the guinea pig after amosite asbestos exposure. *Am J Pathol* 1985;119(2):273–278.
9. Davis JMG, Cowie HA. The relationship between fibrosis and cancer in experimental animals exposed to asbestos. *Environ Health Perspect* 1990;88:305–309.
10. Mossman BT, Janssen YM, Marsh JP, et al. Development and characterization of a rapid-onset rodent inhalation model of asbestosis for disease prevention. *Toxicol Pathol* 1991;19(4 Pt 1):412–418.
11. Hesterberg TW, Miller WC, McConnell EE, Chevalier J, Hadley JG, Bernstein DM. Chronic inhalation toxicity of size-separated glass fibers in Fischer 344 rats. *Fundam Appl Toxicol* 1993;20(4):464–476.
12. Allison AC. Fibrogenic and other biological effects of silica. *Curr Top Microbiol Immunol* 1996;210:147–158.
13. Lapp NL, Castranova V. How silicosis and coal workers' pneumoconiosis develop—a cellular assessment. *Occup Med* 1993;8(1):35–56.
14. Rom WN, Bitterman PB, Rennard SI, Cantin AC, Crystal RG. Characterization of the lower respiratory tract inflammation of nonsmoking individuals with interstitial lung disease associated with chronic inhalation of inorganic dusts. *Am Rev Respir Dis* 1987;136: 1429–1434.

15. Brody AR. Asbestos-induced lung disease. *Environ Health Perspect* 1993;100:21–30.
16. Chang LY, Overby LH, Brody AR, Crapo JD. Progressive lung cell reactions and extracellular matrix production after a brief exposure to asbestos. *Am J Pathol* 1988;131:156–170.
17. Warheit DB, Chang LY, Hill LH, Hook GER, Crapo JD, Brody AR. Pulmonary macrophage accumulation and asbestos-induced lesions at sites of fiber deposition. *Am Rev Respir Dis* 1984;129:301–310.
18. Begin R, Rola-Pleszczynski M, Masse S, et al. Asbestos-induced lung injury in the sheep model: the initial alveolitis. *Environ Res* 1983; 30(1):195–210.
19. Sprince NL, Oliver LC, McLoud TC, Ginns LC. T-cell alveolitis in lung lavage of asbestos-exposed subjects. *Am J Ind Med* 1992;21: 311–319.
20. Rom WN, Travis WD. Lymphocyte-macrophage alveolitis in non-smoking individuals occupationally exposed to asbestos. *Chest* 1992; 101:779–786.
21. Broser M, Zhang Y, Aston C, Harkin T, Rom WN. Elevated interleukin-8 in the alveolitis of individuals with asbestos exposure. *Int Arch Occup Environ Health* 1996;68:109–114.
22. Robinson BWS, Rose AH, James A, Whitaker D, Musk AW. Alveolitis of pulmonary asbestosis. *Chest* 1986;90:396–402.
23. Begin R, Ostiguy G, Filion R, Groleau S. Recent advances in the early diagnosis of asbestosis. *Semin Roentgenol* 1992;27:121–139.
24. Lasky JA, Bonner JC, Brody AR. The pathobiology of asbestos-induced lung disease: a proposed role for macrophage-derived growth factors. *Ann NY Acad Sci* 1991;643:239–244.
25. Perkins RC, Scheule RK, Hamilton R, Gomes G, Freidman G, Holian A. Human alveolar macrophage cytokine release in response to *in vitro* and *in vivo* asbestos exposure. *Exp Lung Res* 1993;19(1):55–65.
26. Rom WN, Travis WD, Brody AR. Cellular and molecular basis of the asbestos-related diseases. *Am Rev Respir Dis* 1991;143(2):408–422.
27. Driscoll KE, Maurer JK, Hassenbein D, et al. Contribution of macrophage-derived cytokines and cytokine networks to mineral dust-induced lung inflammation. In: Dungworth D, Mohr U, Mauderly J, Oberdoerster G, eds. *Toxic and carcinogenic effects of solid particles in the respiratory tract.* Washington, DC: ILSI Press, 1994;177–190.
28. Schwartz DA, Galvin JR, Frees KL, et al. Clinical relevance of cellular mediators of inflammation in workers exposed to asbestos. *Am Rev Respir Dis* 1993;148(1):68–74.
29. Zhang Y, Lee TC, Guillemin B, Yu MC, Rom WN. Enhanced IL-1 beta and tumor necrosis factor alpha release and messenger RNA expression in macrophages from idiopathic pulmonary fibrosis or after asbestos exposure. *J Immunol* 1993;150:4188–4196.
30. Vanhee D, Gosset P, Marquette CH, et al. Secretion and mRNA expression of TNF alpha and IL-6 in the lungs of pneumoconiosis patients. *Am J Respir Crit Care Med* 1995;152(1):298–306.
31. Bost T, Newman L, Riches D. Increased TNF-alpha and IL6 mRNA expression by alveolar macrophages in chronic beryllium disease. *Chest* 1993;103(2 suppl):138S.
32. Lesur OJ, Mancini NM, Humbert JC, Chabot F, Polu JM. Interleukin-6, interferon-gamma, and phospholipid levels in the alveolar lining fluid of human lungs. Profiles in coal worker's pneumoconiosis and idiopathic pulmonary fibrosis. *Chest* 1994;106(2):407–413.
33. Schins RP, Borm PJ. Epidemiological evaluation of release of monocyte TNF-alpha as an exposure and effect marker in pneumoconiosis: a five year follow up study of coal workers. *Occup Environ Med* 1995;52(7):441–450.
34. Borm PJ, Schins R, Janssen YM, Lenaerts L. Molecular basis for differences in susceptibility to coal workers' pneumoconiosis. *Toxicol Lett* 1992;64-65:767–772.
35. Borm PJ, Palmen N, Engelen JJ, Buurman WA. Spontaneous and stimulated release of tumor necrosis factor-alpha (TNF) from blood monocytes of miners with coal workers' pneumoconiosis. *Am Rev Respir Dis* 1988;138(6):1589–1594.
36. Partanen R, Koskinen H, Hemminki K. Tumor necrosis factor-alpha (TNF-alpha) in patients who have asbestosis and develop cancer. *Occup Environ Med* 1995;52:316–319.
37. Kline JN, Schwartz DA, Monick MM, Floerchinger CS, Hunninghake GW. Relative release of interleukin-1 beta and interleukin-1 receptor antagonist by alveolar macrophages. A study in asbestos-induced lung disease, sarcoidosis, and idiopathic pulmonary fibrosis. *Chest* 1993; 104(1):47–53.
38. Hannum CH, Wilcox CJ, Arend WP, et al. Interleukin-1 receptor antagonist activity of a human interleukin-1 inhibitor. *Nature* 1990; 343(6256):336–340.
39. Garcia JGN, Griffith DE, Cohen AB, Callahan KS. Alveolar macrophages from patients with asbestos exposure release increased levels of leukotriene B4. *Am Rev Respir Dis* 1989;139:1494–1501.
40. Bernard AM, Gonzalez-Lorenzo JM, Siles E, Trujillano G, Lauwerys R. Early decrease of serum clara cell protein in silica-exposed workers. *Eur Respir J* 1994;7:1932–1937.
41. Vanhee D, Gosset P, Wallaert B, et al. Mechanisms of fibrosis in coal workers' pneumoconiosis. Increased production of platelet-derived growth factor, insulin-like growth factor type I, and transforming growth factor beta and relationship to disease severity. Clinical relevance of cellular mediators of inflammation in workers exposed to asbestos. *Am J Respir Crit Care Med* 1994;150(4):1049–1055.
42. Brandt-Rauf PW, Smith S, Hemminki K, Koskinen H, Vainio H, Niman H, Ford J. Serum oncoproteins and growth factors in asbestosis and silicosis patients. *Int J Cancer* 1992;50(6):881–885.
43. Allam M, Martinet N, Gallati H, Vaillant P, Hosang M, Martinet Y. Platelet-derived growth factor AA and AB dimers are present in normal human epithelial lining fluid. *Eur Respir J* 1993;6(8):1162–1168.
44. Homma S, Nagaoka I, Abe H, Takahashi K, Seyama K, Nukiwa T, Kira S. Localization of platelet-derived growth factor and insulin-like growth factor I in the fibrotic lung. *Am J Respir Crit Care Med* 1995; 152(6 Pt 1):2084–2089.
45. Shaw RJ, Benedict SH, Clark RAF, King TE. Pathogenesis of pulmonary fibrosis in interstitial lung disease. *Am Rev Respir Dis* 1991; 143:167–173.
46. Vignaud JM, Allam M, Martinet N, Pech M, Plenat F, Martinet Y. Presence of platelet-derived growth factor in normal and fibrotic lung is specifically associated with interstitial macrophages, while both interstitial macrophages and alveolar epithelial cells express the c-sis oncogene. *Am J Respir Cell Mol Biol* 1991;5:531–538.
47. DiGiovine B, Lynch JP, Martinez FJ, et al. The presence of profibrotic cytokines correlate with outcome in patients with idiopathic pulmonary fibrosis. *Chest* 1996;109:24S.
48. Polyak K. Negative regulation of cell growth by TGF beta. *Biochim Biophys Acta* 1996;1242(3):185–199.
49. Broekelmann TJ, Limper AH, Colby TV, MacDonald JA. Transforming growth factor-β1 is present at sites of extracellular matrix gene expression in human pulmonary fibrosis. *Proc Natl Acad Sci USA* 1991;88:6642–6646.
50. Jagirdar J, Begin R, Dufresne A, Goswami S, Lee TC, Rom WN. Transforming growth factor-β in silicosis. *Am J Respir Crit Care Med* 1996;154:1076–1081.
51. Partanen R, Koskinen H, Oksa P, et al. Serum oncoproteins in asbestosis patients. *Clin Chem* 1995;41:1844–1847.
52. Vanhee D, Gosset P, Boitelle A, Wallaert B, Tonnel AB. Cytokines and cytokine network in silicosis and coal workers' pneumoconiosis. *Eur Respir J* 1995;8(5):834–842.
53. Begin R, Martel M, Desmarais Y, et al. Fibronectin and procollagen 3 levels in bronchoalveolar lavage of asbestos-exposed human subjects and sheep. *Chest* 1986;89:237–243.
54. Rom WN. Relationship of inflammatory cytokines to disease severity in individuals with occupational inorganic dust exposure. *Am J Ind Med* 1991;19:15–27.
55. McDonald JC. Asbestos and lung cancer: Has the case been proven? *Chest* 1980;67:374–376.
56. Doll R. Mortality from lung cancer in asbestos workers. *Br J Ind Med* 1955;12:81–86.
57. Stayner LT, Dankovic DA, Lemen RA. Occupational exposure to chrysotile asbestos and cancer risk: a review of the amphibole hypothesis. *Am J Public Health* 1996;86:179–186.
58. de Klerk NH, Musk AW, Eccles JL, Hansen J, Hobbs MST. Exposure to crocidolite and the incidence of different histological types of lung cancer. *Occup Environ Med* 1996;53:157–159.
59. Churg A. Lung cancer cell type and asbestos exposure. *JAMA* 1985; 253:2984–2985.
60. Jarrholm B. Incidence of lung cancer by histological type among asbestos cement workers in Denmark [letter; comment]. *Br J Ind Med* 1993;50(8):767.
61. Mollo F, Pira E, Piolatto G, et al. Lung adenocarcinoma and indicators of asbestos exposure. *Int J Cancer* 1995;60(3):289–293.
62. Selikoff IJ, Hammond EC, Seidman H. Morality experience of insulation workers in the United States and Canada, 1943–1976. *Ann NY Acad Sci* 1979;330:473–490.

63. Mossman BT, Kamp DW, Weitzman SA. Mechanisms of carcinogenesis and clinical features of asbestos-associated cancers. *Cancer Invest* 1996;14:466–480.
64. Brandt-Rauf PW, Luo J-C, Carney WP, et al. Detection of increased amounts of the extracellular domain of the c-erbB-2 oncoprotein in serum during pulmonary carcinogenesis in humans. *Int J Cancer* 1994;56:383–386.
65. Wang X, Christiani DC, Wiencke JK, et al. Mutations in the p53 gene in lung cancer are associated with cigarette smoking and asbestos exposure. *Cancer Epidemiol Biomarkers Prevent* 1995;4(5):543–548.
66. Nuorva K, Makitaro R, Huhti E, et al. p53 protein accumulation in lung carcinomas of patients exposed to asbestos and tobacco smoke. *Am J Respir Crit Care Med* 1994;150:528–533.
67. Hemminki K, Partanen R, Koskinen H, Smith S, Carney W, Brandt-Rauf PW. The molecular epidemiology of oncoproteins. Serum p53 protein in patients with asbestosis. *Chest* 1996;109(3 suppl):22S–26S.
68. Anttila S, Luostarinen L, Hirvonen A, et al. Pulmonary expression of glutathione S-transferase in lung cancer patients: association with GSTM1 polymorphism, smoking and asbestos exposure. *Cancer Res* 1995;55:3305–3309.
69. Ryberg D, Kure E, Lystad S, et al. p53 mutations in lung tumors. Relationship to putative susceptibility markers for cancer. *Cancer Res* 1994;54:1551–1555.
70. Ryberg D, Hewer A, Phillips DH, Haugen A. Different susceptibility to smoking-induced DNA damage among male and female lung cancer patients. *Cancer Res* 1994;54(22):5801–5803.
71. Greenberg M, Lloyd Davies TA. Mesothelioma register 1967–1968. *Br J Ind Med* 1974;31:91.
72. Milne JEH. Thirty-two cases of mesothelioma in Victoria, Australia: a retrospective survey related to asbestos exposure. *Br J Ind Med* 1976; 33:195.
73. Hammar SP. Pleural diseases. In: Dail DH, Hammar SP, eds. *Pulmonary pathology.* New York: Springer-Verlag, 1994;1463–1579.
74. Whitwell F, Scott J, Grimshaw M. Relationship between occupations and asbestos fibre content of the lungs in patients with pleural mesothelioma, lung cancer, and other diseases. *Thorax* 1977;32:377.
75. Precerutti JA, Mayorga M, Dalurzo L, Pallotta G, de la Canal A. Is there a "genetic model" in the genesis of malignant pleural mesothelioma? [letter; comment]. *Hum Pathol* 1990;21(9):983.
76. Popescu NC, Chahinian AP, DiPaolo JA. Nonrandom chromosome alterations in human malignant mesothelioma. *Cancer Res* 1988; 48(1):142–147.
77. Tiainen M, Tammilehto L, Mattson K, Knuutila S. Nonrandom chromosomal abnormalities in malignant pleural mesothelioma. *Cancer Genet Cytogenet* 1988;33(2):251–274.
78. Tiainen M, Tammilehto L, Rautonen J, Tuomi T, Mattson K, Knuutila S. Chromosomal abnormalities and their correlations with asbestos exposure and survival in patients with mesothelioma. *Br J Cancer* 1989;60(4):618–626.
79. Hagemeijer A, Versnel MA, Van Drunen E, et al. Cytogenetic analysis of malignant mesothelioma. *Cancer Genet Cytogenet* 1990;47(1): 1–28.
80. Gibas Z, Li FP, Antman KH, Bernal S, Stahel R, Sandberg AA. Chromosome changes in malignant mesothelioma. *Cancer Genet Cytogenet* 1986;20(3-4):191–201.
81. Flejter WL, Li FP, Antman KH, Testa JR. Recurring loss involving chromosomes 1, 3, and 22 in malignant mesothelioma: possible sites of tumor suppressor genes. *Genes Chromosomes Cancer* 1989;1(2): 148–154.
82. Taguchi T, Jhanwar SC, Siegfried JM, Keller SM, Testa JR. Recurrent deletions of specific chromosomal sites in 1p, 3p, 6q, and 9p in human malignant mesothelioma. *Cancer Res* 1993;53(18):4349–4355.
83. Huncharek M, Wang X, Wain J, Mark E, Kelsey K. Absence of p53 mutations in malignant pleural mesothelioma. *Chest* 1996;110:11S.
84. Metcalf RA, Welsh JA, Bennett WP, et al. p53 and Kirsten-ras mutations in human mesothelioma cell lines. *Cancer Res* 1992;52: 2610–2615.
85. Versnel MA, Hagemeijer A, Bouts MJ, van der Kwast TH, Hoogsteden HC. Expression of c-sis (PDGF B-chain) and PDGF A-chain genes in ten human malignant mesothelioma cell lines derived from primary and metastatic tumors. *Oncogene* 1988;2(6):601–605.
86. Garlepp MJ, Leong CC. Biological and immunological aspects of malignant mesothelioma. *Eur Respir J* 1995;8:643–650.
87. Fitzpatrick DR, Peroni DJ, Bielefeldt-Ohmann H. The role of growth factors and cytokines in the tumorigenesis and immunobiology of malignant mesothelioma. *Am J Respir Cell Mol Biol* 1995;12: 455–460.
88. Westermark B, Heldin CH. Platelet-derived growth factor. Structure, function and implications in normal and malignant cell growth. *Acta Oncol* 1993;32:101–105.
89. Carbone M, Pass HI, Rizzo P, et al. Simian virus 40-like DNA sequences in human pleural mesothelioma. *Oncogene* 1994;9(6): 1781–1790.
90. Quinlan TR, BeruBe KA, Marsh JP, et al. Patterns of inflammation, cell proliferation, and related gene expression in lung after inhalation of chrysotile asbestos. *Am J Pathol* 1995;147(3):728–739.
91. Quinlan TR, Marsh JP, Janssen YMW, et al. Dose-responsive increases in pulmonary fibrosis after inhalation of asbestos. *Am J Respir Crit Care Med* 1994;150:200–206.
92. Hesterberg TW, Miiller WC, Thevenaz P, Anderson R. Chronic inhalation studies of man-made vitreous fibres: characterization of fibres in the exposure aerosol and lungs. *Ann Occup Hyg* 1995;39(5):637–653.
93. Mast RW, Hesterberg TW, Glass LR, McConnell EE, Anderson R, Bernstein DM. Chronic inhalation and biopersistence of refractory ceramic fiber in rats and hamsters. *Environ Health Perspect* 1994; 102(Suppl 5):207–209.
94. Warheit DB, Driscoll KE, Oberdoerster G, Walker C, Kuschner M, Hesterberg TW. Contemporary issues in fiber toxicology. *Fundam Appl Toxicol* 1995;25:171–183.
95. Warheit DB, Hartsky MA. Role of alveolar macrophage chemotaxis and phagocytosis in pulmonary clearance responses to inhaled particles: comparisons among rodent species. *Microsc Res Tech* 1993; 26(5):412–422.
96. Ohtsuka Y, Munakata M, Ukita H, et al. Increased susceptibility to silicosis and TNF-alpha production in C57BL/6J mice. *Am J Respir Crit Care Med* 1995;152(6 Pt 1):2144–2149.
97. Morgan A. Deposition of inhaled asbestos and man-made mineral fibres in the respiratory tract. *Ann Occup Hyg* 1995;39(5):747–758.
98. Bignon J, Saracci R, Touray J-C. INSERM-IARC-CNRS Workshop on biopersistence of respirable synthetic fibers and minerals. *Environ Health Perspect* 1994;102(suppl 5):3–284.
99. Lippmann M. Nature of exposure to chrysotile. *Ann Occup Hyg* 1994;38:459–467.
100. Morgan A, Holmes A. The deposition of MMMF in the respiratory tract of the rat, their subsequent clearance, solubility *in vivo* and protein coating. In: *Biological effects of man-made fibers.* Copenhagen, Denmark: World Health Organization, 1984.
101. Roggli VL, George MH, Brody AR. Clearance and dimensional changes of crocidolite asbestos fibers isolated from the lungs of rats following short-term exposure. *Environ Res* 1987;42:94–105.
102. Coin PG, Roggli VL, Brody AR. Persistence of long, thin chrysotile asbestos fibers in the lungs of rats. *Environ Health Perspect* 1994; 102(suppl 5):197–199.
103. Churg A. Deposition and clearance of chrysotile asbestos. *Ann Occup Hyg* 1994;38(4):424–425,625–633.
104. Oberdorster G. Macrophage-associated responses to chrysotile. *Ann Occup Hyg* 1994;38(4):421–422,601–615.
105. Brody AR, Roe MW. Deposition pattern of inorganic particles at the alveolar level in the lungs of rats and mice. *Am Rev Respir Dis* 1983; 128:724–732.
106. Pinkerton KE, Plopper CG, Mercer RR, et al. Airway branching patterns influence asbestos fiber location and the extent of tissue injury in the pulmonary parenchyma. *Lab Invest* 1986;55(6):688–695.
107. Kouzan S, Gallagher J, Eling T, Brody AR. Particle binding to sialic acid residues on macrophage plasma membranes stimulates arachidonic acid metabolism. *Lab Invest* 1985;53:320–327.
108. Gallagher JE, George F, Brody AR. Sialic acid mediates the initial binding of positively-charged inorganic particles to alveolar macrophage membranes. *Am Rev Respir Dis* 1987;135:1345–1352.
109. Boylan AM, Sanan DA, Sheppard D, Broaddus VC. Vitronectin enhances internalization of crocidolite asbestos by rabbit pleural mesothelial cells via the integrin alpha v beta 5. *J Clin Invest* 1995;96(4):1987–2001.
110. Brody AR, Hill LH, Adkins B, O'Connor B. Chrysotile asbestos inhalation in rats: deposition pattern and reaction of alveolar epithelium and pulmonary macrophages. *Am Rev Respir Dis* 1981;123: 670–679.
111. Pinkerton KE, Pratt PC, Brody AR, Crapo JD. Fiber localization and

its relationship to lung reaction after chronic inhalation of chrysotile asbestos. *Am J Pathol* 1984;117:484–498.
112. Churg A. The uptake of mineral particles by pulmonary epithelial cells. *Am J Respir Crit Care Med* 1996;154:1124–1140.
113. Brody AR, Hill LH, Adler KB. Actin-containing microfilaments of pulmonary epithelial cells provide a mechanism for translocating asbestos to the interstitium. *Chest* 1983;83:11–12.
114. Roggli V, Brody AR. Changes in numbers and dimensions of chrysotile asbestos fibers in lungs of rats following short-term exposure. *Exp Lung Res* 1984;7:133–147.
115. Brody AR, Roe MW, Evans JN, Davis GS. Deposition and translocation of inhaled silica in rats. Quantification of particle distribution, macrophage participation, and function. *Lab Invest* 1982;47(6): 533–542.
116. Gross TJ, Cobb SM, Peterson MW. Asbestos exposure increases paracellular transport of fibrin degradation products across human airway epithelium. *Am J Physiol* 1994;266:L287–L295.
117. Warheit DB, Hill LH, George G, Brody AR. Time course of chemotactic factor generation and the corresponding macrophage response to asbestos inhalation. *Am Rev Respir Dis* 1986;134:128–133.
118. Driscoll KE, Maurer JK, Higgins J, Poynter J. Alveolar macrophage cytokine and growth factor production in a rat model of crocidolite-induced pulmonary inflammation and fibrosis. *J Toxicol Environ Health* 1995;46:155–169.
119. Pezerat H, Zalma R, Guignard J, Jaurand MC. Production of oxygen radicals by the reduction of oxygen arising from the surface activity of mineral fibres. *IARC Sci Publ* 1989(90):100–111.
120. Hansen K, Mossman BT. Generation of superoxide from alveolar macrophages exposed to asbestiform and nonfibrous particles. *Cancer Res* 1987;47:1681–1688.
121. Quinlan TR, Marsh JP, Janssen YMW, Borm PA, Mossman BT. Oxygen radicals and asbestos-mediated disease. *Environ Health Perspect* 1994;102(suppl 10):107–110.
122. Moyer VD, Cistulli CA, Vaslet CA, Kane AB. Oxygen radicals and asbestos carcinogenesis. *Environ Health Perspect* 1994;102(suppl 10): 131–136.
123. Donaldson K, Brown GM, Brown DM, Slight J, Li X-Y. Epithelial and extracellular matrix injury in quartz-inflamed lung: role of the alveolar macrophage. *Environ Health Perspect* 1992;97:221–224.
124. Kamp DW, Dunn MM, Sbalchiero JS, Knap AM, Weitzman SA. Contrasting effects of alveolar macrophages and neutrophils on asbestos-induced pulmonary epithelial cell injury. *Am J Physiol* 1994;266(1 Pt 1):L84–91.
125. Kamp DW, Dunne M, Dykewicz MS, Sbalchiero JS, Weitzman SA, Dunn MM. Asbestos-induced injury to cultured human pulmonary epithelial-like cells: role of neutrophil elastase. *J Leukoc Biol* 1993; 54(1):73–80.
126. Vallyathan V, Mega JF, Shi X, Dalal NS. Enhanced generation of free radicals from phagocytes induced by mineral dusts. *Am J Respir Cell Mol Biol* 1992;6(4):404–413.
127. Schapira RM, Ghio AJ, Effros RM, Morrisey J, Dawson CA, Hacker AD. Hydroxyl radicals are formed in the rat lung after asbestos instillation *in vivo*. *Am J Respir Cell Mol Biol* 1994;10(5):573–579.
128. Guo WX, Li GH, Zheng SQ, Lin ZN. Effects of silica on serum phospholipid, lipid peroxide and morphological characteristics of rat lung. *Biomed Environ Sci* 1995;8:169–175.
129. Janssen YM, Marsh JP, Assher MP, et al. Expression of antioxidant enzymes in rat lungs after inhalation of asbestos or silica. *J Biol Chem* 1992;267(15):10625–10630.
130. Janssen YM, Marsh JP, Absher M, Borm PJ, Mossman BT. Increases in endogenous antioxidant enzymes during asbestos inhalation in rats. *Free Rad Res Commun* 1990;11:53–58.
131. Davis JM, Jones AD, Miller BG. Experimental studies in rats on the effects of asbestos inhalation coupled with inhalation of titanium dioxide or quartz. *Int J Exp Pathol* 1991;72:501–525.
132. Hyde DM, Nakasima JM, Harris JA, Giri SN. Epithelial injury is a critical factor in the development of pulmonary fibrosis following multiple episodes of inflammation. *Chest* 1991;99:28S.
133. Mossman BT, Sesko AM. *In vitro* assays to predict the pathogenicity of mineral fibers. *Toxicology* 1990;60:53–61.
134. Hart GA, Kathman LM, Hesterberg TW. *In vitro* cytotoxicity of asbestos and man-made vitreous fibers: roles of fiber length, diameter and composition. *Carcinogenesis* 1994;15(5):971–977.
135. Koshi K, Kohyama N, Myojo T, Fukuda K. Cell toxicity, hemolytic action and clastogenic activity of asbestos and its substitutes. *Ind Health* 1991;29:37–56.
136. Kodama Y, Boreiko CJ, Maness SC, Hesterberg TW. Cytotoxic and cytogenetic effects of asbestos on human bronchial epithelial cells in culture. *Carcinogenesis* 1993;14(4):691–697.
137. Goodglick LA, Kane AB. Cytotoxicity of long and short crocidolite asbestos fibers *in vitro* and *in vivo*. *Cancer Res* 1990;50:5253–5163.
138. Janssen YM, Marsh JP, Absher MP, et al. Oxidant stress responses in human pleural mesothelial cells exposed to asbestos. *Am J Respir Crit Care Med* 1994;149:795–802.
139. Farber JL. Mechanisms of cell injury by activated oxygen species. *Environ Health Perspect* 1994;102(suppl 10):17–24.
140. Kinnula VL, Aalto K, Raivio KO, Walles S, Linnainmaa K. Cytoxicity of oxidants and asbestos fibers in cultured human mesothelial cells. *Free Radic Biol Med* 1994;16(2):169–176.
141. Pelin K, Husgafvel-Pursianen K, Vallas M, Vanhala E, Linnainmaa K. Cytoxicity and anaphase aberrations induced by mineral fibers in cultured human mesothelial cells. *Toxicol In Vitro* 1992;6:445–450.
142. Korkina LG, Durnev AD, Suslova TB, Cheremisina ZP, Daugel-Dauge NO, Afanas'ev IB. Oxygen radical-mediated mutagenic effect of asbestos on human lymphocytes: suppression by oxygen radical scavengers. *Mutat Res* 1992;265(2):245–253.
143. Hei TK, He ZY, Suzuki K. Effects of antioxidants on fiber mutagenesis. *Carcinogenesis* 1995;16(7):1573–1578.
144. Dong H, Buard A, Renier A, Levy F, Saint-Etienne L, Jaurand MC. Role of oxygen derivatives in the cytotoxicity and DNA damage produced by asbestos on rat plerual mesothelial cells *in vitro*. *Carcinogenesis* 1994;15(6):1251–1255.
145. Kamp DW, Israbian VA, Preusen SE, Zhang CX, Weitzman SA. Asbestos causes DNA strand breaks in cultured pulmonary epithelial cells: role of iron-catalyzed free radicals. *Am J Physiol* 1995;268(3 Pt 1):L471–480.
146. Hardy JA, Aust AE. The effect of iron binding on the ability of crocidolite asbestos to catalyze DNA single-strand breaks. *Carcinogenesis* 1995;16(2):319–325.
147. Lund LG, Aust AE. Iron mobilization from crocidolite asbestos greatly enhances crocidolite-dependent formation of DNA single-strand breaks in phi X174 RFI DNA. *Carcinogenesis* 1992;13(4): 637–642.
148. Lund LG, Aust AE. Iron-catalyzed reactions may be responsible for the biochemical and biological effects of asbestos. *Biofactors* 1991;3: 83–89.
149. Donaldson K, Golyasnya N. Cytogenetic and pathogenic effects of long and short amosite asbestos. *J Pathol* 1995;177(3):303–307.
150. Renier A, Levy F, Pilliere F, Jaurand MC. Unscheduled DNA synthesis in rat pleural mesothelial cells treated with mineral fibres. *Mutat Res* 1990;241(4):361–367.
151. Dong HY, Buard A, Levy F, Renier A, Laval F, Jaurand MC. Synthesis of poly(ADP-ribose) in asbestos treated rat pleural mesothelial cells in culture. *Mutat Res* 1995;331(2):197–204.
152. Faux SP, Michelangeli F, Levy LS. Calcium chelator Quin-2 prevents crocidolite-induced DNA strand breakage in human white blood cells. *Mutat Res* 1994;311(2):209–215.
153. Ueda N, Shah SV. Apoptosis. *J Lab Clin Med* 1994;124:169–177.
154. BeruBe KA, Quinlan TR, Fung H, et al. Apoptosis is observed in mesothelial cells after exposure to crocidolite asbestos. *Am J Respir Cell Mol Biol* 1996;15:141–147.
155. McGavran PD, Moore LM, Brody AR. Inhalation of chrysotile asbestos induces rapid cellular proliferation in small pulmonary vessels of mice and rats. *Am J Pathol* 1990;136:695–705.
156. Brody AR, Overby LH. Incorporation of tritiated thymidine by epithelial and interstitial cells in bronchiolar-alveolar regions of asbestos-exposed rats. *Am J Pathol* 1989;134:133–140.
157. Brody AR, Hill LH. Interstitial accumulation of inhaled chrysotile asbestos fibers and consequent formation of microcalcifications. *Am J Pathol* 1982;109:107–114.
158. Miller BE, Hook GER. Hypertrophy and hyperplasia of alveolar type II cells in response to silica and other pulmonary toxicants. *Environ Health Perspect* 1990;85:15–23.
159. Gardner S, Brody AR. Incorporaton of bromodeoxyuridine as a method to quantify cell proliferation in bronchiolar-alveolar duct regions of asbestos-exposed mice. *J Inhal Toxicol* 1995;7:215–224.
160. Coin PC, Osornio-Vargas A, Moore L, Brody AR. Three consecutive exposures to chrysotile asbestos induces prolonged cell proliferation

and a fibrogenic lesion of the alveolar duct walls. *Am J Respir Crit Care Med* 1996;154:1511–1519.
161. McGavran PD, Brody AR. Chrysotile asbestos inhalation induces tritiated thymidine incorporation by epithelial cells of distal bronchioles. *Am J Respir Cell Mol Biol* 1990;1:231–235.
162. Adamson IY, Bakowska J, Bowden DH. Mesothelial cell proliferation after instillation of long or short asbestos fibers into the mouse lung. *Am J Pathol* 1993;142:1209–1216.
163. Adamson IY, Bakowska J, Bowden DH. Mesothelial cell proliferation: a nonspecific response to lung injury associated with fibrosis. *Am J Respir Cell Mol Biol* 1994;10:253–258.
164. Sekhon H, Wright J, Churg A. Effects of cigarette smoke and asbestos on airway, vascular and mesothelial cell proliferation. *Int J Exp Pathol* 1995;76(6):411–418.
165. Prieditis H, Adamson IY. Alveolar macrophage kinetics and multinucleated giant cell formation after lung injury. *J Leukoc Biol* 1996; 59(4):534–538.
166. Panos RJ, Mason RJ. Hypertrophic alveolar cells isolated after silica-induced lung injury are proliferating. *Am Rev Respir Dis* 1990;141: A630.
167. BeruBe KA, Quinlan TR, Moulton G, et al. Comparative proliferative and histopathologic changes in rat lungs after inhalation of chrysotile or crocidolite asbestos. *Toxicol Appl Pharmacol* 1996;137:67–74.
168. Liu J-Y, Morris GF, Lei W-H, Corti M, Brody AR. Upregulated expression of transforming growth factor alpha in the bronchiolar-alveolar duct regions of asbestos-exposed rats. *Am J Pathol* 1996;149:205–217.
169. Mishra A, Liu JY, Brody AR, Morris GF. Inhaled asbestos fibers induce p53 expression in the rat lung. *Am J Respir Cell Mol Biol* 1997;16:479–485.
170. Kawanami O, Jiang H-X, Mochimaru H, et al. Alveolar fibrosis and capillary alteration in experimental silicosis in rats. *Am J Respir Crit Care Med* 1995;151:1946–1955.
171. Lesur O, Melloni B, Cantin AM, Begin R. Silica-exposed lung fluids have a proliferative activity for type II epithelial cells: a study on human and sheep alveolar fluids. *Exp Lung Res* 1992;18(5):633–654.
172. Rom WN. Activated alveolar macrophages from individuals with asbestosis release peptide growth factors. In: Harris CC, Lechner JF, Brinkley BR, eds. *Cellular and molecular aspects of fiber carcinogenesis.* Cold Spring Harbor, NY: Cold Spring Harbor Press, 1991; 103–114.
173. Brody AR. Control of lung fibroblast proliferation by macrophage-derived platelet-derived growth factor. *Ann NY Acad Sci* 1994;275: 193–206.
174. Kullmann A, Vaillant P, Muller V, Martinet Y, Martinet N. *In vitro* effects of pentoxifylline on smooth muscle cell migration and blood monocyte production of chemotactic activity for smooth muscle cells: potential therapeutic benefit in the adult respiratory distress syndrome. *Am J Respir Cell Mol Biol* 1993;8(1):83–88.
175. Inamoto T, Georgian MM, Kagan E, Ogimoto K. Enhanced release of an alveolar macrophage-derived chemoattractant for fibroblasts in rats after asbestos inhalation. *J Vet Med Sci* 1993;55(2):195–201.
176. Lasky JA, Coin PG, Lindroos PM, Ostrowski LE, Brody AR, Bonner JC. Chrysotile asbestos stimulates platelet-derived growth factor-AA production by rat lung fibroblasts *in vitro*: evidence for an autocrine loop. *Am J Respir Cell Mol Biol* 1995;12(2):162–170.
177. Lasky JA, Bonner JC, Tonthat B, Brody AR. Chrysotile asbestos induces PDGF-A chain-dependent proliferation in human and rat lung fibroblasts *in vitro*. *Chest* 1996;109:26S–28S.
178. Chen B, Polunovsky V, White J, et al. Mesenchymal cells isolated after acute lung injury manifest an enhanced proliferative phenotype. *J Clin Invest* 1992;90(5):1778–1785.
179. Janssen YMW, Heintz NH, Marsh JP, Borm PJA, Mossman BT. Induction of c-*fos* and c-*jun* in target cells of the lung and pleura by carcinogenic fibers. *Am J Respir Cell Mol Biol* 1994;11:522–530.
180. Heintz NH, Janssen YM, Mossman BT. Pesistent induction of c-*fos* and c-*jun* expression by asbestos. *Proc Natl Acad Sci USA* 1993;90: 3299–3303.
181. Verheij M, Bose R, Lin XH, et al. Requirement for ceramide-initiated SAPK/JNK signalling in stress-induced apoptosis. *Nature* 1996; 380(6569):75–79.
182. Yan M, Dai T, Deak JC, et al. Activation of stress-activated protein kinase by MEKK1 phosphorylation of its activator SEK1. *Nature* 1994;372(6508):798–800.
183. Kyriakis JM, Banerjee P, Nikolakaki E, et al. The stress-activated protein kinase subfamily of c-*jun* kinases. *Nature* 1994;369(6476): 156–160.
184. Moriguchi T, Kawasaki H, Matsuda S, Gotoh Y, Nishida E. Evidence for multiple activators for stress-activated protein kinase/c-*jun* amino-terminal kinases. Existence of novel activators. *J Biol Chem* 1995; 270(22):12969–12972.
185. Timblin CR, Janssen YW, Mossman BT. Transcriptional activation of the proto-oncogene c-*jun* by asbestos and H2O2 is directly related to increased proliferation and transformation of tracheal epithelial cells. *Cancer Res* 1995;55:2723–2726.
186. Otani H, Erdos M, Leonard WJ. Tyrosine kinase(s) regulate apoptosis and bcl-2 expression in a growth factor-dependent cell line. *J Biol Chem* 1993;268(30):22733–22736.
187. Vaux DL, Aguila HL, Weissman IL. Bcl-2 prevents death of factor-deprived cells but fails to prevent apoptosis in targets of cell mediated killing. *Int Immunol* 1992;4(7):821–824.
188. Yao R, Cooper GM. Growth factor-dependent survival of rodent fibroblasts requires phosphatidylinositol 3-kinase but is independent of pp70S6K activity. *Oncogene* 1996;13(2):343–351.
189. Mariani TJ, Roby JD, Mecham RP, Parks WC, Crouch E, Pierce RA. Localization of type I procollagen gene expression in silica-induced granulomatous lung disease and implication of transforming growth factor-beta as a mediator of fibrosis. *Am J Pathol* 1996;148:151–164.
190. Arden MG, Adamson IYR. Collagen synthesis and degradation during the development of asbestos-induced pulmonary fibrosis. *Exp Lung Res* 1992;18:9–20.
191. Liu BC, He YX, Miao Q, Wang HH, You BR. The effects of tetrandrine (TT) and polyvinylpyridine-N-oxide (PVNO) on gene expression of type I and type III collagens during experimental silicosis. *Biomed Environ Sci* 1994;7(3):199–204.
192. Montano M, Ramos C, Pardo A, Selman M. Comparison between lung parenchyma and bronchoalveolar lavage collagenolytic activity. *Lung* 1993;171(2):87–93.
193. Mariani TJ, Crouch E, Roby JD, Starcher B, Pierce RA. Increased elastin production in experimental granulomatous lung disease. *Am J Pathol* 1995;147:988–1000.
194. Piguet PF, Vesin C. Treatment by human recombinant soluble TNF receptor of pulmonary fibrosis induced by bleomycin or silica in mice. *Eur Respir J* 1994;7(3):515–518.
195. Perdue TD, Brody AR. Distribution of transforming growth factor-beta 1, fibronectin, and smooth muscle actin in asbestos-induced pulmonary fibrosis in rats. *J Histochem Cytochem* 1994;42(8):1061–1070.
196. Adamson IYR, Hedgecock C, Bowden DH. Epithelial cell-fibroblast interactions in lung injury and repair. *Am J Pathol* 1990;137:385–392.
197. Adamson IYR, Young L, King GM. Reciprocal epithelial: fibroblast interactions in the control of fetal and adult rat lung cells in culture. *Exp Lung Res* 1991;17:821–835.
198. Kelley J. Cytokines of the lung. *Am Rev Respir Dis* 1990;141: 765–788.
199. Spurzem JR, Saltini C, Rom W, Winchester RJ, Crystal RG. Mechanisms of macrophage accumulation in the lungs of asbestos-exposed subjects. *Am Rev Respir Dis* 1987;136:276–280.
200. McGavran PD, Butterick CJ, Brody AR. Tritiated thymidine incorporation and the development of an interstitial lesion in the bronchiolar-alveolar regions of normal and complement-deficient mice after inhalation of chrysotile asbestos. *J Environ Pathol Toxicol Oncol* 1990;6:377–388.
201. Warheit DB, George G, Hill LH, Snyderman R, Brody AR. Inhaled asbestos activates a complement-dependent chemotactic factor for macrophages. *Lab Invest* 1985;52:505–514.
202. Driscoll KE, Hassenbein DG, Carter J, et al. Macrophage inflammatory proteins 1 and 2: expression by rat alveolar macrophages, fibroblasts, and epithelial cells and in rat lung after mineral dust exposure. *Am J Respir Cell Mol Biol* 1993;8:311–318.
203. Driscoll KE, Howard BW, Carter JM, et al. Alpha-quartz-induced chemokine expression by rat lung epithelial cells. *Am J Pathol* 1996; 149:1627–1637.
204. Piguet PF, Vesin C. Pulmonary platelet trapping induced by bleomycin: correlation with fibrosis and involvement of the beta 2 integrins. *Int J Exp Pathol* 1994;75(5):321–328.
205. Piguet PF, Vesin C, Thomas F. Bombesin down modulates pulmonary fibrosis elicited in mice by bleomycin. *Exp Lung Res* 1995;21(2): 227–237.

206. Ross R, Raines EW, Bowen-Pope DF. The biology of platelet-derived growth factor. *Cell* 1986;46:155–166.
207. Corsini E, Luster MI, Mahler J, Craig WA, Blazka ME, Rosenthal GJ. A protective role for T lymphocytes in asbestos-induced pulmonary inflammation and collagen deposition. *Am J Respir Cell Mol Biol* 1994;11:531–539.
208. Kovacs EJ, DiPietro LA. Fibrogenic cytokines and connective tissue production. *FASEB J* 1994;8:854–861.
209. Souza P, Sedlackova L, Kuliszewski M, et al. Antisense oligodeoxynucleotides targeting PDGF-B mRNA inhibit cell proliferation during embryonic rat lung development. *Development* 1994;120:2163–2173.
210. Bostrom H, Willetts K, Pekny M, et al. PDGF-A signaling is a critical event in lung myofibroblast development and alveogenesis. *Cell* 1996;85:863–873.
211. Souza P, Kuliszewski M, Wang J, Tseu I, Tanswell AK, Post M. PDGF-AA and its receptor influence early lung branching via an epithelial-mesenchymal interaction. *Development* 1995;121:2559–2567.
212. Meyer-Ingold W. Wound therapy: growth factors as agents to promote healing. *Trends Biotech* 1993;11(9):387–392.
213. Schwartz SM, Reidy MA, O'Brien ER. Assessment of factors important in atherosclerotic occlusion and restenosis. *Thromb Haemost* 1995;74(1):541–551.
214. Bornfeldt KE, Raines EW, Graves LM, Skinner MP, Krebs EG, Ross R. Platelet-derived growth factor. Distinct signal transduction pathways associated with migration versus proliferation. *Ann NY Acad Sci* 1995;766:416–430.
215. Claesson-Welsh L. Platelet-derived growth factor receptor signals. *J Biol Chem* 1994;269:32023–32026.
216. Heldin CH, Westermark B. Platelet-derived growth factor and autocrine mechanisms of oncogenic processes. *Crit Rev Oncogen* 1991;2(2):109–124.
217. Kazlauskas A. Receptor tyrosine kinases and their targets. *Curr Opin Genet Dev* 1994;4(1):5–14.
218. Greenberg ME, Ziff EB. Stimulation of 3T3 cells induces transcription of the c-*fos* proto-oncogene. *Nature* 1984;311:433–438.
219. Rauscher FJ, Cohen DR, Curran T, et al. Fos-associated protein p39 is the product of the *jun* proto-oncogene. *Science* 1988;240:1010–1016.
220. Kelly K, Cochran BH, Stiles CD, Leder P. Cell-specific regulation of the c-myc gene by lymphocyte mitogens and platelet-derived growth factor. *Cell* 1983;35:603–610.
221. Clark RA, Folkvord JM, Hart CE, Murray MJ, McPherson JM. Platelet isoforms of platelet-derived growth factor stimulate fibroblasts to contract collagen matrices. *J Clin Invest* 1989;84(3):1036–1040.
222. Fujio Y, Yamada F, Takahashi K, Shibata N. Altered fibronectin-dependent cell adhesion by PDGF accompanies phenotypic modulation of vascular smooth muscle cells. *Biochem Biophys Res Commun* 1993;196(2):997–1002.
223. Xu J, Zutter MM, Santoro SA, Clark RA. PDGF induction of alpha 2 integrin gene expression is mediated by protein kinase C-zeta. *J Cell Biol* 1996;134:1301–1311.
224. Rhudy RW, McPherson JM. Influence of the extracellular matrix on the proliferative response of human skin fibroblasts to serum and purified platelet-derived growth factor. *J Cell Physiol* 1988;137(1):185–191.
225. Liu JY, Morris G, Lei WH, Hart C, Lasky J, Brody A. Rapid activation of PDGF-A and -B expression at sites of lung injury in asbestos-exposed rats. *Am J Respir Cell Mol Biol* 1997;17:129–140.
226. Osornio-Vargas AR, Kalter VG, Badgett A, Hernandez-Rodriguez N, Aguilar-Delfin I, Brody AR. Early-passage rat lung fibroblasts do not migrate *in vitro* to transforming growth factor-beta. *Am J Respir Cell Mol Biol* 1993;8(5):468–471.
227. Suganuma H, Sato A, Tamura R, Chida K. Enhanced migration of fibroblasts derived from lungs with fibrotic lesions. *Thorax* 1995;50(9):984–989.
228. Fabisiak JP, Absher M, Evans JN, Kelley J. Spontaneous production of PDGF-A chain homodimer by rat lung fibroblasts *in vitro*. *Am J Physiol* 1992;263:L185–L193.
229. Caniggia I, Liu J, Han R, et al. Fetal lung epithelial cells express receptors for platelet-derived growth factor. *Am J Respir Cell Mol Biol* 1993;9:54–63.
230. Bonner JC, Goodell AL, Coin PG, Brody AR. Chrysotile asbestos upregulates gene expression and production of alpha-receptors for platelet-derived growth factor (PDGF-AA) on rat lung fibroblasts. *J Clin Invest* 1993;92(1):425–430.
231. Clark JG, Madtes DK, Raghu G. Effects of platelet-derived growth factor isoforms on human lung fibroblast proliferation and procollagen gene expression. *Exp Lung Res* 1993;19(3):327–344.
232. Coin PG, Lindroos PM, Bird GS, Osornio-Vargas AR, Roggli VL, Bonner JC. Lipopolysaccharide up-regulates platelet-derived growth factor (PDGF) alpha-receptor expression in rat lung myofibroblasts and enhances response to all PDGF isoforms. *J Immunol* 1996;156(12):4797–4806.
233. Lin X, Wang Z, L. G, Deuel TF. Functional analysis of the human platelet-derived growth factor A-chain promoter region. *J Biol Chem* 1992;267:25614–25619.
234. Bauman MB, Jetten AM, Bonner JC, Kuman RK, Bennett RA, Brody AR. Secretion of platelet-derived growth factor homologue by rat alveolar macrophages exposed to particulates *in vitro*. *Eur J Cell Biol* 1990;51:327–334.
235. Schapira RM, Osornio-Vargas AR, Brody AR. Inorganic particles induce secretion of a macrophage homologue of platelet-derived growth factor in a density and time-dependent manner. *Exp Lung Res* 1991;17:1011–1024.
236. Bonner JC, Osornio-Vargas AR, Badgett A, Brody AR. Differential proliferation of rat lung fibroblasts induced by platelet-derived growth factor -AA, -AB, and -BB isoforms secreted by alveolar macrophages. *Am J Respir Cell Mol Biol* 1991;5:539–547.
237. Brody AR, Bonner JC, Overby LH, et al. Interstitial pulmonary macrophages produce platelet-derived growth factor that stimulates rat lung fibroblast proliferation *in vitro*. *J Leukoc Biol* 1992;51(6):640–648.
238. Poon M, Hsu WC, Bogdanov VY, Taubman MB. Secretion of monocyte chemotactic activity by cultured rat aortic smooth muscle cells in response to PDGF is due predominantly to the induction of JE/MCP-1. *Am J Pathol* 1996;149:307–317.
239. Yi ES, Lee H, Yin S, et al. Platelet-derived growth factor causes pulmonary cell proliferation and collagen deposition. *Am J Pathol* 1996;149:539–548.
240. Yoshida M, Sakuma J, Hayashi S, et al. A histologically distinctive interstitial pneumonia induced by overexpression of the interleukin 6, transforming growth factor beta 1, or platelet-derived growth factor B gene. *Proc Natl Acad Sci USA* 1995;92(21):9570–9574.
241. Torry DJ, Richards CD, Podor TJ, Gauldie J. Anchorage-independent colony growth of pulmonary fibroblasts derived from fibrotic human lung tissue. *J Clin Invest* 1994;93(4):1525–1532.
242. Fox JM, Conklin K, Chiang L, et al. Acute lung injury. A transgenic murine model of intra-alveolar fibrosis. *Chest* 1994;195:121S-122S.
243. Brand T, Schneider MD. Transforming growth factor-beta signal transduction. *Circ Res* 1996;78(2):173–179.
244. Letterio JJ, Roberts AB. Transforming growth factor-beta1-deficient mice: identification of isoform-specific activities *in vivo*. *J Leukoc Biol* 1996;59(6):769–774.
245. Massague J. TGFbeta signaling: receptors, transducers, and Mad proteins. *Cell* 1996;85(7):947–950.
246. Serra R, Moses HL. Tumor suppressor genes in the TGF-beta signaling pathway? *Nature Med* 1996;2(4):390–391.
247. Harpel JG, Metz CN, Kojima S, Rifkin DB. Control of TGF-β activity: latency vs activation. *Prog Growth Factor Res* 1992;4:321–335.
248. Odekon LE, Blasi F, Rifkin DB. Requirement for receptor bound urokinase in plasmin-dependent cellular conversion of latent TGF-β to TGF-β. *J Cell Physiol* 1994;158:398–407.
249. Massague J, Chiefetz S, Laiho M, Ralph DA, Weis FMB, Zentella A. Transforming growth factor-β. *Cancer Surv* 1992;12:81–103.
250. Reynisdottir I, Polyak K, Iavarone A, Massague J. Kip/Cip and Ink 4 Cdk inhibitors cooperate to induce cell cycle arrest in response to TGF-β. *Genes Dev* 1995;9:1831–1845.
251. Igarashi A, Okochi H, Bradham DM, Grotendorst GR. Regulation of connective tissue growth factor gene expression in human skin fibroblasts and during wound repair. *Mol Biol Cell* 1993;4(6):637–645.
252. Wrana JL, Attisano L, Wieser R, Ventura F, Massague J. Mechanism of activation of the TGF-beta receptor. *Nature* 1994;370(6488):341–347.
253. Shull MM, Ormsby I, Kier AB, et al. Targeted disruption of the mouse transforming growth factor-β1 gene results in chronic multifocal inflammatory disease. *Nature* 1992;359:693–699.
254. Diebold RJ, Eis MJ, Yin M, et al. Early-onset multifocal inflammation

in the transforming growth factor beta 1-null mouse is lymphocyte mediated. *Proc Natl Acad Sci USA* 1995;92(26):12215–12219.
255. Serra R, Moses HL. pRb is necessary for inhibition of N-myc expression by TGF-β1 in embryonic lung organ cultures. *Development* 1995;121:3057–3066.
256. Zhou L, Dey CR, Wert SE, Whitsett JA. Arrested lung morphogenesis in transgenic mice bearing an SP-C-TGF-beta 1 chimeric gene. *Dev Biol* 1996;175(2):227–238.
257. Kaartinen V, Voncken JW, Shuler C, et al. Abnormal lung development and cleft palate in mice lacking TGF-beta 3 indicates defects in epithelial-mesenchymal interaction. *Nature Genet* 1995;11: 415–421.
258. Proetzel G, Pawlowski SA, Wiles MV, et al. Transforming growth factor-beta 3 is required for secondary palate fusion. *Nature Genet* 1995; 11(4):409–414.
259. Wang J, Kuliszewski M, Yee W, et al. Cloning and expression of glucocorticoid-induced genes in fetal rat lung fibroblasts. Transforming growth factor-beta 3. *J Biol Chem* 1995;270(6):2722–2728.
260. Jaskoll T, Choy HA, Melnick M. The glucocorticoid-glucocorticoid receptor signal transduction pathway, transforming growth factor-beta, and embryonic mouse lung development *in vivo*. *Pediatr Res* 1996;39(5):749–759.
261. Khalil N, O'Connor RN, Unruh HW, et al. Increased production and immunohistochemical localization of transforming growth factor-β in idiopathic pulmonary fibrosis. *Am J Respir Cell Mol Biol* 1991;5: 155–162.
262. Denis M, Ghadirian E. Transforming growth factor-beta is generated in the course of hypersensitivity pneumonitis: contribution to collagen synthesis. *Am J Respir Cell Mol Biol* 1992;7:156–160.
263. Limper AH, Colby TV, Sanders MS, Asakura S, Roche PC, DeRemee RA. Immunohistochemical localization of transforming growth factor-β1 in the nonnecrotizing granulomas of pulmonary sarcoidosis. *Am J Respir Crit Care Med* 1994;149:197–204.
264. Raghow R, Postlethwaite AE, Keski-Oja J, Moses HL, Kang AH. Transforming growth factor-β increases steady state levels of type-1 procollagen and fibronectin mRNAs post-transcriptionally in cultured human dermal fibroblasts. *J Clin Invest* 1987;79:1258–1288.
265. D'Souza RN, Niederreither K, de Crombrugghe B. Osteoblast-specific expression of the alpha 2(I) collagen promoter in transgenic mice: correlation with the distribution of TGF-beta 1. *J Bone Miner Res* 1993;8(9):1127–1136.
266. Inagaki Y, Truter S, Tanaka S, Di Liberto M, Ramirez F. Overlapping pathways mediate the opposing actions of tumor necrosis factor-alpha and transforming growth factor-beta on alpha 2(I) collagen gene transcription. *J Biol Chem* 1995;270(7):3353–3358.
267. Chung KY, Agarwal A, Uitto J, Mauviel A. An AP-1 binding sequence is essential for regulation of the human alpha2(I) collagen (COL1A2) promoter activity by transforming growth factor-beta. *J Biol Chem* 1996;271(6):3272–3278.
268. Halloran BG, So BJ, Baxter BT. Platelet-derived growth factor is a cofactor in the induction of 1 alpha(I) procollagen expression by transforming growth factor-beta 1 in smooth muscle cells. *J Vasc Surg* 1996;23(5):767–773; discussion 774.
269. Grande J, Melder D, Zinsmeister A, Killen P. Transforming growth factor-beta 1 induces collagen IV gene expression in NIH-3T3 cells. *Lab Invest* 1993;69(4):387–395.
270. Heckmann M, Aumailley M, Chu ML, Timpl R, Krieg T. Effect of transforming growth factor-beta on collagen type VI expression in human dermal fibroblasts. *FEBS Lett* 1992;310(1):79–82.
271. Ohji M, SundarRaj N, Thoft RA. Transforming growth factor-beta stimulates collagen and fibronectin synthesis by human corneal stromal fibroblasts *in vitro*. *Curr Eye Resh* 1993;12(8):703–709.
272. Keski-Oja J, Raghow R, Sawdey M, et al. Regulation of mRNAs for type-1 plasminogen activator inhibitor, fibronectin, and type I procollagen by transforming growth factor-β. Divergent responses in lung fibroblasts and carcinoma cells. *J Biol Chem* 1988;263:3111–3115.
273. Ignotz RA, Massague J. Transforming growth factor-β stimulates the expression fof fibronectin and collagen and their incorporation into the extracellular matrix. *J Biol Chem* 1986;261:4337–4345.
274. Edwards DR, Murphy G, Reynolds JJ, et al. Transforming growth factor beta modulates the expression of collagenase and metalloproteinase inhibitor. *EMBO J* 1987;7:1899–1904.
275. Maniscalco WM, Sinkin RA, Watkins RH, Campbell MH. Transforming growth factor-beta 1 modulates type II cell fibronectin and surfactant protein C expression. *Am J Physiol* 1994;267(5 Pt 1): L569–577.
276. Maniscalco WM, Campbell MH. Transforming growth factor-beta induces a chondroitin sulfate/dermatan sulfate proteoglycan in alveolar type II cells. *Am J Physiol* 1994;266(6 Pt 1):L672–680.
277. Kumar NM, Sigurdson SL, Sheppard D, Lwebuga-Mukasa JS. Differential modulation of integrin receptors and extracellular matrix laminin by transforming growth factor-beta 1 in rat alveolar epithelial cells. *Exp Cell Res* 1995;221(2):385–394.
278. Ryan RM, Mineo-Kuhn MM, Kramer CM, Finkelstein JN. Growth factors alter neonatal type II alveolar epithelial cell proliferation. *Am J Physiol* 1994;266(1 Pt 1):L17–22.
279. Cazals V, Mouhieddine B, Maitre B, et al. Insulin-like growth factors, their binding proteins, and transforming growth factor-beta 1 in oxidant-arrested lung alveolar epithelial cells. *J Biol Chem* 1994; 269(19):14111–14117.
280. Shi DL, Savona C, Chambaz EM, Feige JJ. Stimulation of fibronectin production by TGF-beta 1 is independent of effects on cell proliferation: the example of bovine adrenocortical cells. *J Cell Physiol* 1990; 145:60–68.
281. Koyama H, Raines EW, Bornfeldt KE, Roberts JM, Ross R. Fibrillar collagen inhibits arterial smooth muscle proliferation through regulation of CDK 2 inhibitors. *Cell* 1996;87:1069–1078.
282. Bitterman PB, Rennard SI, Adelberg S, Crystal RG. Role of fibronectin as a growth factor for fibroblasts. *J Cell Biol* 1983;97: 1925–1932.
283. DiMari SJ, Howe AM, Haralson MA. Effects of transforming growth factor-β on collagen synthesis by fetal rat lung epithelial cells. *Am J Respir Cell Mol Biol* 1991;4:455–462.
284. Gharaee-Kermani M, Denholm EM, Phan SH. Costimulation of fibroblast collagen and transforming growth factor beta 1 gene expression by monocyte chemoattractant protein-1 via specific receptors. *J Biol Chem* 1996;271:17779–17784.
285. Battegay EF, Raines EW, Seifert RA, Bowen-Pope DF, Ross R. TGF-β induces bimodal proliferation of connective tissue cells via complex control of autocrine PDGF loop. *Cell* 1990;63:515–524.
286. Williams AO, Flanders KC, Saffiotti U. Immunohistochemical localization of transforming growth factor-beta 1 in rats with experimental silicosis, alveolar hyperplasia, and lung cancer. *Am J Pathol* 1993; 142:1831–1840.
287. Lee TC, Gold LI, Reibman J, et al. Immunohistochemical localization of transforming growth factor-β and insulin-like growth factor-I in asbestosis in the sheep model. *Int Arch Occup Environ Health* 1997; 69:157–164.
288. Van Obberghen-Schilling E, Roche NS, Flanders KC, Sporn MB, Roberts AB. Transforming growth factor β1 positively regulates its own expression in normal and transformed cells. *J Biol Chem* 1988; 263:7741–7746.
289. Kelley J, Shull S, Walsh JJ, Cutroneo KR, Absher M. Auto-induction of transforming growth factor-beta in human lung fibroblasts. *Am J Respir Cell Mol Biol* 1993;8(4):417–424.
290. de Bortoli C, Chailley-Heu B, Bourbon JR. Production of transforming growth factor (TGF) beta by fetal lung cells. *Biol Cell* 1995;84(3): 215–218.
291. Khalil N, O'Connor RN, Flanders KC, Unruh H. TGF-β1, but not TGF-β2 or TGF-β3, is differentially present in epithelial cells of advanced pulmonary fibrosis: an immunohistochemical study. *Am J Respir Crit Care Med* 1996;14:131–138.
292. Lee DC, Fenton SE, Berkowitz EA, Hissong MA. Transforming growth factor alpha: expression, regulation, and biological activities. *Pharmacol Rev* 1995;47(1):51–85.
293. Derynck R, Roberts AB, Winkler ME, Chen EY, Goeddel DV. Human transforming growth factor alpha: precursor structure and expression in *E. coli*. *Cell* 1984;38:287–297.
294. Moodie SA, Willumsen BM, Weber MJ, Wolfman A. Complexes of ras GTP with Raf-1 and mitogen activated protein kinase. *Science* 1993;260:1658–1661.
295. Ullrich A, Schlessinger J. Signal transduction by receptors with tyrosine kinase activity. *Cell* 1990;61:203–212.
296. Buday L, Downward J. Epidermal growth factor regulates p21ras through the formation of a complex or receptor, Grb2 adapter protein, and Sos nucleotide exchange factor. *Cell* 1993;73:611–620.
297. Mann GB, Fowler KJ, Gabriel A, Nice EC, Williams RL, Dunn AR. Mice with a null mutation of the TGF-alpha gene have abnormal skin

architecture, wavy hair, and curly whiskers and often develop corneal inflammation. *Cell* 1993;73:249–261.
298. Lukette NC, Qiu TH, Oliver P, Smithies O, Lee DC. TGF-alpha deficiency results in hair follicle and eye abnormalities in targeted and waved-1 mice. *Cell* 1993;73:263–278.
299. Matsui Y, Halter SA, Holt JT, Hogan BLM, Coffey RJ. Development of mammary hyperplasia and neoplasia in MMTV-TGF alpha transgenic mice. *Cell* 1990;61:1147–1155.
300. Sandgren EP, Luetteke NC, Palmiter RD, Brinster RL, Lee DC. Overexpression of TGF alpha in transgenic mice: induction of epithelial hyperplasia, pancreatic metaplasia, and carcinoma of the breast. *Cell* 1990;61:1121–1135.
301. Coffey RJ, Derynck R, Wilcox JN, Bringman TS, Goustin AS, Moses HL, Pittelkow MR. Production and autoinduction of transforming growth factor alpha in human keratinocytes. *Nature* 1987;328: 817–820.
302. Coffey RJ, Graves-Deal R, Dempsey PJ, Whitehead RH, Pittelkow MR. Differential regulation of transforming growth factor alpha autoinduction in a nontransformed and transformed epithelial cell. *Growth Diff* 1992;3:347–354.
303. Kalthoff H, Roeder C, Brockhaus M, Thiele HG, Schmiegel W. Tumor necrosis factor (TNF) up-regulates the expression of p75 but not p55 TNF receptors, and both receptors mediate, independently of each other, up-regulation of transforming growth factor alpha and epidermal growth factor receptor mRNA. *J Biol Chem* 1993;268(4): 2762–2766.
304. Lee DC, Rochford R, Todaro GJ, Villarreal LP. Developmental expression of rat transforming growth factor alpha mRNA. *Mol Cell Biol* 1985;5:3644–3646.
305. Strandjord TP, Clark JG, Madtes DK. Expression of TGF-alpha, EGF, and EGF receptor in fetal rat lung. *Am J Physiol* 1994;267(4 Pt 1): L384–389.
306. Strandjord TP, Clark JG, Hodson WA, Schmidt RA, Madtes DK. Expression of transforming growth factor-alpha in mid-gestation human fetal lung. *Am J Respir Cell Mol Biol* 1993;8(3):266–272.
307. Ganser GL, Stricklin GP, Matrisian LM. EGF and TGF alpha influence *in vitro* lung development by the induction of matrix-degrading metalloproteinases. *Int J Dev Biol* 1991;35:453–461.
308. Sundell HW, Gray ME, Serenius FS, Escobedo MB, Stahlman MT. Effects of epidermal growth factor on lung maturation in fetal lambs. *Am J Pathol* 1980;100:707–719.
309. Johnson MD, Gray ME, Carpenter G, Pepinsky RB, Sundell H, Stahlman MT. Ontogeny of epidermal growth factor receptor/kinase and of lipocortin-1 in the ovine lung. *Pediatr Res* 1989;25:535–541.
310. Strandjord TP, Clark JG, Guralnick DE, Madtes DK. Immunolocalization of transforming growth factor-alpha, epidermal growth factor (EGF), and EGF-receptor in normal and injured developing human lung. *Pediatr Res* 1995;38(6):851–856.
311. Kheradmand F, Folkesson HG, Shum L, Derynk R, Pytela R, Matthay MA. Transforming growth factor-alpha enhances alveolar epithelial cell repair in a new *in vitro* model. *Am J Physiol* 1994;267(6 Pt 1): L728–738.
312. Chess PR, Ryan RM, Finkelstein JN. Tyrosine kinase activity is necessary for growth factor-stimulated rabbit type II pneumocyte proliferation. *Pediatr Res* 1994;36(4):481–486.
313. Madtes DK, Raines EW, Sakariassen KS, et al. Induction of transforming growth factor-alpha in activated human alveolar macrophages. *Cell* 1988;53:285–293.
314. Vivekananda J, Lin A, Coalson JJ, King RJ. Acute inflammatory injury in the lung precipitated by oxidant stress induces fibroblasts to synthesize and release transforming growth factor-alpha. *J Biol Chem* 1994;269(40):25057–25061.
315. Madtes DK, Busby HK, Strandjord TP, Clark JG. Expression of transforming growth factor-alpha and epidermal growth factor receptor is increased following bleomycin-induced lung injury in rats. *Am J Respir Cell Mol Biol* 1994;11(5):540–551.
316. Absher M, Sjostrand M, Baldor LC, Hemenway DR, Kelley J. Patterns of secretion of transforming growth factor alpha (TGF-alpha) in experimental silicosis. Acute and subacute effects of cristobalite exposure in rats. *Reg Immunol* 1993;5:225–231.
317. Kumar RK, Velan GM, O'Grady R. Epidermal growth factor-like activity in bronchoalveolar lavage fluid in experimental silicosis. *Growth Factors* 1994;10:163–170.
318. Korfhagen TR, Swantz RJ, Wert SE, et al. Respiratory epithelial cell expression of human transforming growth factor-alpha induces lung fibrosis in transgenic mice. *J Clin Invest* 1994;93(4):1691–1699.
319. Bazzoni F, Beutler B. The tumor necrosis factor ligand and receptor families. *N Engl J Med* 1996;334:1717–1725.
320. Probert L, Akassoglou K, Alexopoulou L, et al. Dissection of the pathologies induced by transmembrane and wild-type tumor necrosis factor in transgenic mice. *J Leukoc Biol* 1996;59(4):518–525.
321. Beutler B, Cerami A. The biology of cachectin/TNF - a primary mediator of the host response. *Annu Rev Immunol* 1989;7:625–655.
322. Perez C, Albert I, DeFay K, Zachariades N, Gooding L, Kriegler M. A nonsecretable cell surface mutant of tumour necrosis factor (TNF) kills by cell-to-cell contact. *Cell* 1990;63:251–258.
323. Jones EY, Stuart DI, Walker NPC. Structure of tumour necrosis factor. *Nature* 1989;338:225–228.
324. Smith RA, Baglioni C. The active form of tumor necrosis factor is a trimer. *J Biol Chem* 1987;262:6951–6954.
325. Vandenabeele P, Declercq W, Beyaert R, Fiers W. Two tumour necrosis factor receptors: structure and function. *Trends Cell Biol* 1995;5: 392–399.
326. Darnay BG, Reddy SAG, Aggarwal BB. Identification of a protein kinase associated with the cytoplasmic domain of the p60 tumor necrosis factor receptor. *J Biol Chem* 1994;269:19687–19690.
327. Rothe M, Wong SC, Hensel WF, Goeddel DV. A novel family of putative signal transducers associated with the cytoplasmic domain of the 75 kDa tumor necrosis factor receptor. *Cell* 1994;78:681–692.
328. Erickson SL, de Sauvage FJ, Kikly K. Decreased sensitivity to tumour-necrosis factor but normal T-cell development in TNF receptor-2 deficient mice. *Nature* 1994;372:560–563.
329. Fiers W. Biologic therapy with TNF: preclinical studies. In: DeVita VT, Hellman S, Rosenberg SA, eds. *Biologic therapy of cancer,* 2nd ed. Philadelphia: Lippincott, 1995;295–327.
330. Beg AA, Baltimore D. An essential role for NF-κB in preventing TNF-alpha-induced cell death. *Science* 1996;274:782–784.
331. Van Antwerp DJ, Martin SJ, Kafri T, Green DR, Verma IM. Suppression of TNF-alpha-induced apoptosis by NF-κB. *Science* 1996;274: 787–789.
332. Wang C-Y, Mayo MW, Baldwin AS. TNF- and cancer therapy-induced apoptosis: potentiation by inhibition of NF-κB. *Science* 1996;274: 784–786.
333. Brouckaert P, Fiers W. Tumor necrosis factor and the systemic inflammatory response syndrome. *Curr Top Microbiol Immunol* 1996;216: 167–187.
334. Miyazaki Y, Araki K, Vesin C, et al. Expression of a tumor necrosis factor-alpha transgene in murine lung causes lymphocytic and fibrosing alveolitis. A mouse model of progressive pulmonary fibrosis. *J Clin Invest* 1995;96(1):250–259.
335. Ulich TR, Watson LR, Yin S, Guo K, Wang P, Thang H, del Castillo J. The intratracheal administration of endotoxin and cytokines: 1. Characterization of LPS-induced IL-1 and TNF mRNA expression and the LPS-, IL-1, and TNF-induced inflammatory infiltrate. *Am J Pathol* 1991;138:1485–1491.
336. Buck M, Houglum K, Chojkier M. Tumor necrosis factor-alpha inhibits collagen alpha1(I) gene expression and wound healing in a murine model of cachexia. *Am J Pathol* 1996;149(1):195–204.
337. Paulsson Y, Austgulen R, Hofsli E, Heldin CH, Westermark B, Nissen-Meyer J. Tumor necrosis factor-induced expression of platelet-derived growth factor A-chain messenger RNA in fibroblasts. *Exp Cell Res* 1989;180:490–496.
338. Postlethwaite AE, Seyer JM. Stimulation of fibroblast chemotaxis by human recombinant tumor necrosis factor alpha and a synthetic tumor necrosis factor alpha peptide. *J Exp Med* 1990;172:1749–1756.
339. Piguet PF, Collart MA, Gram GE, Sappino AP, Vassali P. Requirement of tumor necrosis factor for development of silica-induced pulmonary fibrosis. *Nature* 1990;344:245–247.
340. Gossart S, Cambon C, Orfila C, et al. Reactive oxygen intermediates as regulators of TNF-alpha production in rat lung inflammation induced by silica. *J Immunol* 1996;156(4):1540–1548.
341. Li XY, Lamb D, Donaldson K. The production of TNF-alpha and IL-1-like activity by bronchoalveolar leukocytes after intratracheal instillation of crocidolite asbestos. *Int J Exp Pathol* 1993;74:403–410.
342. Dubois CM, Bissonnette E, Rola-Pleszczynski M. Asbestos fibers and silica particles stimulate rat alveolar macrophages to release tumor necrosis factor. *Am Rev Respir Dis* 1989;139:1257–1264.
343. Simeonova PP, Luster MI. Iron and reactive oxygen species in the

asbestos-induced tumor necrosis factor-alpha response from alveolar macrophages. *Am J Respir Cell Mol Biol* 1995;12(6):676–683.

344. Claudio E, Segade F, Wrobel K, Ramos S, Lazo PS. Activation of murine macrophages by silica particles *in vitro* is a process independent of silica-induced cell death. *Am J Respir Cell Mol Biol* 1995; 13(5):547–554.
345. Donaldson K, Li XY, Dogra S, Miller BG, Brown GM. Asbestos-stimulated tumour necrosis factor release from alveolar macrophages depends on fibre length and opsonization. *J Pathol* 1992;168:243–248.
346. Mohr C, Davis GS, Graebner C, Amann S, Hemenway DR, Gemsa D. Reduced release of leukotrienes B4 and C4 from alveolar macrophages of rats with silicosis. *Am J Respir Cell Mol Biol* 1992;7(5): 542–547.
347. Mohr C, Davis GS, Graebner C, Hemenway DR, Gemsa D. Enhanced release of prostaglandin E2 from macrophages of rats with silicosis. *Am J Respir Cell Mol Biol* 1992;6(4):390–396.
348. Ouellet S, Yang H, Aubin RA, Hawley RG, Wenckebach GF, Lemaire I. Bidirectional modulation of TNF-alpha production by alveolar macrophages in asbestos-induced pulmonary fibrosis. *J Leukoc Biol* 1993;53:279–286.
349. Lemaire I, Ouellet S. Distinctive profile of alveolar macrophage-derived cytokine release induced by fibrogenic and nonfibrogenic mineral dusts. *J Toxicol Environ Health* 1996;47(5):465–478.
350. Savici D, He B, Geist LJ, Monick MM, Hunninghake GW. Silica increases tumor necrosis factor (TNF) production, in part, by upregulating the TNF promoter. *Exp Lung Res* 1994;20(6):613–625.
351. Martinet Y, Menard O, Vaillant P, Vignaud J-M, Martinet N. Cytokines in human lung fibrosis. *Arch Toxicol Suppl* 1996;18:127–139.
352. March CJ, Mosley B, Larsen A, et al. Cloning, sequence and expression of two distinct human interleukin-1 complementary DNAs. *Nature* 1985;315(6021):641–647.
353. Li XY, Lamb D, Donaldson K. Production of interleukin 1 by rat pleural leucocytes in culture after intratracheal instillation of crocidolite asbestos. *Br J Ind Med* 1993;50:90–94.
354. Chen F, Sun SC, Kuh DC, Gaydos LJ, Demers LM. Essential role of NF-kappa B activation in silica-induced inflammatory mediator production in macrophages. *Biochem Biophys Res Commun* 1995;214(3): 985–992.
355. Griffith DE, Miller EJ, Gray LD, Idell S, Johnson AR. Interleukin-1-mediated release of interleukin-8 by asbestos-stimulated human pleural mesothelial cells. *Am J Respir Cell Mol Biol* 1994;10: 245–252.
356. Boylan AM, Ruegg C, Kim KJ, et al. Evidence of a role for mesothelial cell-derived interleukin 8 in the pathogenesis of asbestos-induced pleurisy in rabbits. *J Clin Invest* 1992;89:1257–1267.
357. Rosenthal GJ, Germolec DR, Blazka ME, et al. Asbestos stimulates IL-8 production from human lung epithelial cells. *J Immunol* 1994; 153:3237–3244.
358. Melloni B, Lesur O, Bouhadiba T, Cantin A, Martel M, Begin R. Effect of exposure to silica on human alveolar macrophages in supporting growth activity in type II epithelial cells. *Thorax* 1996;51(8): 781–786.
359. Chen F, Deng HY, Ding GF, Houng DW, Deng YL, Long ZZ. Excessive production of insulin-like growth factor-I by silicotic rat alveolar macrophages. *APMIS* 1994;102(8):581–588.
360. Bonner JC, Brody AR. Cytokine-binding proteins in the lung. *Am J Physiol* 1995;268(6 Pt 1):L869–878.
361. Rudd RM. New developments in asbestos-related pleural disease. *Thorax* 1996;51(2):210–216.
362. Sen CK, Packer L. Antioxidant and redox regulation of gene transcription. *FASEB J* 1996;10:709–720.
363. Thanos D, Maniatis T. NF-κB a lesson in family values. *Cell* 1995;80: 529–532.
364. Schreck R, Rieber P, Baeuerle PA. Reactive oxygen intermediates as apparently widely used messengers in the activation of the NF-kappa B transcription factor and HIV-1. *EMBO J* 1991;10(8):2247–2258.
365. Baeuerle PA, Henkel T. Function and activation of NF-κB in the immune system. *Annu Rev Immunol* 1994;12:141–179.
366. Khachigian LM, Resnick N, Gimbrone MA Jr, Collins T. Nuclear factor-kappa B interacts functionally with the platelet-derived growth factor B-chain shear-stress response element in vascular endothelial cells exposed to fluid shear stress. *J Clin Invest* 1995;96(2): 1169–1175.
367. O'Connell MA, Cleere R, Long A, O'Neill LA, Kelleher D. Cellular proliferation and activation of NF kappa B are induced by autocrine production of tumor necrosis factor alpha in the human T lymphoma line HuT 78. *J Biol Chem* 1995;270(13):7399–7404.
368. Perez JR, Higgins-Sochaski KA, Maltese JY, Narayanan R. Regulation of adhesion and growth of fibrosarcoma cells by NF-kappa B RelA involves transforming growth factor beta. *Mol Cell Biol* 1994;14(8):5326–5332.
369. Adam D, Kessler U, Kronke M. Cross-linking of the p55 tumor necrosis factor receptor cytoplasmic domain by a dimeric ligand induces nuclear factor-kappa B and mediates cell death. *J Biol Chem* 1995;270(29):17482–17487.
370. Freter RR, Alberta JA, Hwang GY, Wrentmore AL, Stiles CD. Platelet-derived growth factor induction of the immediate-early gene MCP-1 is mediated by NF-kappaB and a 90-kDa phosphoprotein coactivator. *J Biol Chem* 1996;271(29):17417–17424.
371. Olashaw NE, Kowalik TF, Huang ES, Pledger WJ. Induction of NF-kappa B-like activity by platelet-derived growth factor in mouse fibroblasts. *Mol Biol Cell* 1992;3(10):1131–1139.
372. Arsura M, Wu M, Sonenshein GE. TGF beta 1 inhibits NF-kappa B/Rel activity inducing apoptosis of B cells: transcriptional activation of I kappa B alpha. *Immunity* 1996;5(1):31–40.
373. Janssen YM, Barchowsky A, Treadwell M, Driscoll KE, Mossman BT. Asbestos induces nuclear factor kappa B (NF-kappa B) DNA-binding activity and NF-kappa B-dependent gene expression in tracheal epithelial cells. *Proc Natl Acad Sci USA* 1995;92:8458–8462.
374. Simeonova PP, Luster MI. Asbestos induction of nuclear transcription factors and interleukin 8 gene regulation. *Am J Respir Cell Mol Biol* 1996;15:787–795.
375. Angel P, Karin M. The role of Jun, Fos and the AP-1 complex in cell proliferation and transformation. *Biochim Biophys Acta* 1991;1072: 129–157.
376. Pahl HL, Baeuerle PA. Oxygen and the control of gene expression. *Bioessays* 1994;16:497–502.
377. Karin M. The regulation of AP-1 activity by mitogen-activated protein kinases. *J Biol Chem* 1995;270:16483–16486.
378. Goldstone SD, Fragonas J-C, Jeitner TM, Hunt NH. Transcription factors as targets for oxidative signaling during lymphocyte activation. *Biochim Biophys Acta* 1995;1263:114–122.
379. Janssen YM, Heintz NH, Mossman BT. Induction of c-*fos* and c-*jun* proto-oncogene expression by asbestos is ameliorated by N-acetyl-L-cysteine in mesothelial cells. *Cancer Res* 1995;15:2085–2089.
380. Bandyopadhyay RS, Phelan M, Faller DV. Hypoxia induces AP-1-regulated gens and AP-1 transcription factor binding in human endothelial and other cell types. *Biochim Biophys Acta* 1995;1264:72–78.
381. Banerjee C, Stein JL, Van Wijnen AJ, Frenkel B, Lian JB, Stein GS. Transforming growth factor-beta 1 responsiveness of the rat osteocalcin gene is mediated by an activator protein-1 binding site. *Endocrinology* 1996;137(5):1991–2000.
382. Diehl AM, Yin M, Fleckenstein J, et al. Tumor necrosis factor-alpha induces c-*jun* during the regenerative response to liver injury. *Am J Physiol* 1994;267(4 Pt 1):G552–561.
383. Westwick JK, Weitzel C, Minden A, Karin M, Brenner DA. Tumor necrosis factor alpha stimulates AP-1 activity through prolonged activation of the c-*jun* kinase. *J Biol Chem* 1994;269(42):26396–26401.
384. Lieb K, Kaltschmidt C, Kaltschmidt B, et al. Interleukin-1 beta uses common and distinct signaling pathways for induction of the interleukin-6 and tumor necrosis factor alpha genes in the human astrocytoma cell line U373. *J Neurochem* 1996;66(4):1496–1503.
385. Gottlieb TM, Oren M. p53 in growth control and neoplasia. *Biochim Biophys Acta* 1996;1287:77–102.
386. Donehower LA, Bradley A. The tumor suppressor p53. *Biochim Biophys Acta* 1993;1155:181–205.
387. Ko LJ, Prives C. p53: puzzle and paradigm. *Genes Dev* 1996;10(9): 1054–1072.
388. Kastan MB. Signalling to p53: where does it all start? *Bioessays* 1996; 18(8):617–619.
389. Hollstein M, Sidransky D, Vogelstein B, Harris CC. p53 mutations in human cancers. *Science* 1991;252:49–53.
390. Donehower LA, Harvey M, Slagle BL, McArthur MJ, Montgomery CA, Butel JS, Bradley A. Mice deficient for p53 are developmentally normal but are susceptible to spontaneous tumors. *Nature* 1992;356: 215–221.
391. Ewen ME, Miller SJ. p53 and translational control. *Biochim Biophys Acta* 1996;1242(3):181–184.

392. El-Deiry W, Tokino T, Velculescu VE, et al. WAF1, a potential mediator of p53 tumor suppression. *Cell* 1993;75:817–825.
393. Miyashita T, Reed JC. Tumor suppressor p53 is a direct transcriptional activator of the human bax gene. *Cell* 1995;80(2):293–299.
394. Harper JW, Adami GR, Wei N, Keyomars K, Elledge SJ. The p21 Cdk-interacting protein Cip1 is a potent inhibitor of G1 cyclin-dependent kinases. *Cell* 1993;75:805–816.
395. Xiong Y, Hannon GJ, Zhang H, Casso D, Kobayashi R, Beach D. p21 is a universal inhibitor of cyclin kinases. *Nature* 1993;366(6456): 701–704.
396. Oltvai ZN, Milliman CL, Korsmeyer SJ. Bcl-2 heterodimerizes *in vivo* with a conserved homolog, Bax, that accelerates programmed cell death. *Cell* 1993;74(4):609–619.
397. Kastan MB, Onyekwere O, Sidransky D, Vogelstein B, Craig RW. Participation of p53 protein in the cellular response to DNA damage. *Cancer Res* 1991;51:6304–6311.
398. Tishler RB, Calderwood SK, Coleman CN, Price BD. Increases in sequence specific DNA binding by p53 following treatment with chemotherapeutic and DNA damaging agents. *Cancer Res* 1993;53: 2212–2216.
399. Huang L-C, Clarkin KC, Wahl GM. Sensitivity and selectivity of the DNA damage sensor responsible for activating p53-dependent G1 arrest. *Proc Natl Acad Sci USA* 1996;93:4827–4832.
400. Reed M, Woelker B, Wang P, Wang Y, Anderson ME, Tegtmeyer P. The C-terminal domain of p53 recognizes DNA damaged by ionizing radiation. *Proc Natl Acad Sci USA* 1995;92:9455–9459.
401. Lee S, Elenbaas B, Levine AJ, Griffith J. p53 and its 14 kDa C-terminal domain recognize primary DNA damage in the form of insertion/deletion mismatches. *Cell* 1995;81:1013–1020.
402. Smith ML, Fornace AJ Jr. The two faces of tumor suppressor p53. *Am J Pathol* 1996;148(4):1019–1022.
403. Shivakumar CV, Brown DR, Deb S, Deb SP. Wild-type human p53 transactivates the human proliferating cell nuclear antigen promoter. *Mol Cell Biol* 1995;15:6785–6793.
404. Morris GF, Bischoff JR, Mathews MB. Transcriptional activation of the human proliferating cell nuclear antigen promoter by p53. *Proc Natl Acad Sci USA* 1996;93:895–899.
405. Antoniade HN, Galanopoulos T, Neville-Golden J, Kiritsy CP, Lynch SE. p53 expression during normal tissue regeneration in response to acute cutaneous injury in swine. *J Clin Invest* 1994;93:2206–2214.
406. Weinberg WC, Azzoli CG, Chapman K, Levine AJ, Yuspa SH. p53-mediated transcriptional activity increases in differentiating epidermal keratinocytes in association with decreased p53 protein. *Oncogene* 1995;10(12):2271–2279.
407. Shin TH, Paterson AJ, Kudlow JE. p53 stimulates transcription from the transforming growth factor alpha promoter: a potential growth-stimulatory role for p53. *Mol Cell Biol* 1995;15:4694–4701.
408. Datto MB, Li Y, Panus JF, Howe DJ, Xiong Y, Wang XF. Transforming growth factor beta induces the cyclin-dependent kinase inhibitor p21 through a p53-independent mechanism. *Proc Natl Acad Sci USA* 1995;92(12):5545–5549.
409. Suzuki K, Ono T, Takahashi K, et al. Inhibition of DNA synthesis by TGF-beta 1 coincides with inhibition of phosphorylation and cytoplasmic translocation of p53 protein. p53-dependent repression of CDK4 translation in TGF-beta-induced G1 cell-cycle arrest. *Biochem Biophys Res Commun* 1992;183(3):1175–1183.
410. Ewen ME, Oliver CJ, Sluss HK, Miller SJ, Peeper DS. p53-dependent repression of CDK4 translation in TGF-beta-induced G1 cell-cycle arrest. *Genes Dev* 1995;9:204–217.
411. Gerwin BI, Spillare E, Forrester K, et al. Mutant p53 can induce tumorigenic conversion of human bronchial epithelial cells and reduce their responsiveness to a negative growth factor, transforming growth factor beta 1. *Proc Natl Acad Sci USA* 1992;89(7):2759–2763.
412. Blaydes JP, Schlumberger M, Wynford-Thomas D, Wyllie FS. Interaction between p53 and TGF beta 1 in control of epithelial cell proliferation. *Oncogene* 1995;10(2):307–317.
413. Ehinger M, Nilsson E, Persson AM, Olsson I, Gullberg U. Involvement of the tumor suppressor gene p53 in tumor necrosis factor-induced differentiation of the leukemic cell line K562. *Cell Growth Diff* 1995;6(1):9–17.
414. Jeoung DI, Tang B, Sonenberg M. Effects of tumor necrosis factor-alpha on antimitogenicity and cell cycle-related proteins in MCF-7 cells. *J Biol Chem* 1995;270(31):18367–18373.
415. Jacobsen FW, Dubois CM, Rusten LS, Veiby OP, Jacobsen SE. Inhibition of stem cell factor-induced proliferation of primitive murine hematopoietic progenitor cells signaled through the 75-kilodalton tumor necrosis factor receptor. Regulation of c-kit and p53 expression. *J Immunol* 1995;154(8):3732–3741.
416. Wu H, Lozano G. NF-kappa B activation of p53. A potential mechanism for suppressing cell growth in response to stress. *J Biol Chem* 1994;269(31):20067–20074.
417. Akashi M, Hachiya M, Osawa Y, Spirin K, Suzuki G, Koeffler HP. Irradiation induces WAF1 expression through a p53-independent pathway in KG-1 cells. *J Biol Chem* 1995;270(32):19181–19187.
418. Shiohara M, Akashi M, Gombart AF, Yang R, Koeffler HP. Tumor necrosis factor alpha: posttranscriptional stabilization of WAF1 mRNA in p53-deficient human leukemic cells. *J Cell Physiol* 1996; 166(3):568–576.
419. Gualberto A, Hixon ML, Finco TS, Perkins ND, Nabel GJ, Baldwin AS Jr. A proliferative p53-responsive element mediates tumor necrosis factor alpha induction of the human immunodeficiency virus type 1 long terminal repeat. *Mol Cell Biol* 1995;15(6):3450–3459.
420. Lippmann M. Deposition and retention of inhaled fibres: effects on incidence of lung cancer and mesothelioma. *Occup Environ Med* 1994;51:793–798.
421. Shelby MD. The genetic toxicity of human carcinogens and its implications. *Mutat Res* 1988;204:3–15.
422. Pelin K, Kivipensas P, Linnainmaa K. Effects of asbestos and man-made vitreous fibers on cell division in cultured human mesothelial cells in comparison to rodent cells. *Environ Mol Mutagen* 1995;25(2): 118–125.
423. Mahmood N, Khan SG, Athar M, Rahman Q. Differential role of hydrogen peroxide and organic peroxides in augmenting asbestos-mediated DNA damage: implications for asbestos induced carcinogenesis. *Biochem Biophys Res Commun* 1994;200(2):687–694.
424. Daniel LN, Mao Y, Saffiotti U. Oxidative DNA damage by crystalline silica. *Free Radic Biol Med* 1993;14:463–472.
425. Williams AO, Knapton AD, Ifon ET, Saffiotti U. Transforming growth factor beta expression and transformation of rat lung epithelial cells by crystalline silica (quartz). *Int J Cancer* 1996;65:639–649.
426. Saffiotti U, Ahmed N. Neoplastic transformation by quartz in the BALB/3T3/A31-1-1 cell line and the effects of associated minerals. *Teratogenesis Carcinogen Mutagen* 1995;15(6):339–356.
427. Ault JG, Cole RW, Jensen CG, Jensen LC, Bachert LA, Rieder CL. Behavior of crocidolite asbestos during mitosis in living vertebrate lung epithelial cells. *Cancer Res* 1995;55(4):792–78.
428. Both K, Turner DR, Henderson DW. Loss of heterozygosity in asbestos-induced mutations in a human mesothelioma cell line. *Environ Mol Mutagen* 1995;26(1):67–71.
429. Yegles M, Saint-Etienne L, Renier A, Janson X, Jaurand MC. Induction of metaphase and anaphase/telophase abnormalities by asbestos fibers in rat pleural mesothelial cells *in vitro*. *Am J Respir Cell Mol Biol* 1993;9(2):186–191.
430. Hei TK, Piao CQ, He ZY, Vannais D, Waldren CA. Chrysotile fiber is a strong mutagen in mammalian cells. *Cancer Res* 1992;52(22): 6305–6309.
431. Brody AR. Production of cytokines by particle-exposed lung macrophages. In: Brinkley W, Lechner J, Harris C, eds. *Cellular and molecular aspects of fiber carcinogenesis.* Cold Spring Harbor, NY: Cold Spring Harbor Laboratory Press, 1991, 83–102.
432. Yuspa SH. The pathogenesis of squamous cell cancer: lessons learned from studies of skin carcinogenesis. *Cancer Res* 1994;54:1178–1189.
433. Fearon ER, Vogelstein B. A genetic model of colorectal tumorigenesis. *Cell* 1990;61:751–767.
434. Ames BN, Gold LS. Mitogenesis increases mutagenesis. *Science* 1990;249:970–971.
435. Barrett JC, Lamb PW, Wiseman RW. Hypotheses on the mechanisms of carcinogenesis and cell transformation by asbestos and other mineral dusts. In: Bignon J, ed. *Health related effects of phyllosilicates,* vol G21. NATO ASI. Berlin: Springer Verlag 1990:292–307.
436. Eastman A, Mossman BT. Influence of asbestos on the uptake of benzo [a] pyrene and DNA alkylation in hamster tracheal epithelial cells. *Cancer Res* 1983;43:1251–1255.
437. Appel JD, Fasy TM, Kohtz DS, Kohtz JD, Johnson EM. Asbestos fibers mediated transformation of monkey cells by exogenous plasmid DNA. *Proc Natl Acad Sci USA* 1988;85:7670–7674.
438. Walker C, Everitt J, Ferriola PC, Stewart W, Mangum J, Bermudez E. Autocrine growth stimulation by transforming growth factor alpha in

asbestos-transformed rat mesothelial cells. *Cancer Res* 1995;55(3): 530–536.
439. Van der Meeren A, Seddon MB, Betsholtz CA, Lechner JF, Gerwin BI. Tumorigenic conversion of human mesothelial cells as a consequence of platelet-derived growth factor-A chain overexpression. *Am J Respir Cell Mol Biol* 1993;8:214–221.
440. Walker C, Bermudez E, Stewart W, Bonner J, Molloy CJ, Everitt J. Characterization of platelet-derived growth factor and platelet-derived growth factor receptor expression in asbestos-induced rat mesothelioma. *Cancer Res* 1992;52:301–306.
441. Wang ZY, Madden SL, Deuel TF. The Wilms' tumor gene product, WT1, represses transcription of the platelet-derived growth factor A-chain gene. *J Biol Chem* 1992;267:21999–22002.
442. Walker C, Rutten F, Yuan X, Pass H, Mew DM, Everitt J. Wilms' tumor suppressor gene expression in rat and human mesothelioma. *Cancer Res* 1994;54(12):3101–3106.
443. Park S, Schalling M, Bernard A, et al. The Wilms tumour gene WT1 is expressed in murine mesoderm-derived tissues and mutated in a human mesothelioma. *Nature Genet* 1993;4(4):415–420.
444. Knudson A. Asbestos and mesothelioma: genetic lessons from a tragedy. *Proc Natl Acad Sci USA* 1995;92:10819–10820.
445. Hesterberg TW, Barrett JC. Induction by asbestos fibers of anaphase abnormalities: mechanism for aneuploidy induction and possible carcinogenesis. *Carcinogenesis* 1985;6:2170–2178.
446. Hunninghake GW, Kalica AR. Approaches to the treatment of pulmonary fibrosis. *Am J Respir Crit Care Med* 1995;151:915–918.
447. Phan SH. New strategies for treatment of pulmonary fibrosis. *Thorax* 1995;50:415–421.
448. Goldstein RH, Fine A. Potential therapeutic initiatives for fibrogenic lung diseases. *Chest* 1995;108:848–855.
449. Lacronique JG, Rennard SI, Bitterman PB, Ozaki T, Crystal RG. Alveolar macrophages in idiopathic pulmonary fibrosis have glucocorticoid receptors, but glucocorticoid therapy does not suppress alveolar macrophage release of fibronectin and alveolar macrophage derived growth factor. *Am Rev Respir Dis* 1984;130:450–456.
450. Khalil N, Whitman C, Zuo L, Danielpour D, Greenberg A. Regulation of alveolar macrophage transforming growth factor-beta secretion by corticosteroids in bleomycin-induced pulmonary inflammation in the rat. *J Clin Invest* 1993;92(4):1812–1818.
451. Johnson MA, Kwan S, Snell NJC, Nunn AJ, Darbyshire JH, Turner-Warwick M. Randomised controlled trial comparing prednisolone alone with cyclophosphamide and low dose prednisolone in combination in crypotogenic fibrosing alveolitis. *Thorax* 1989;44:280–288.
452. Rennard SI, Bitterman PB, Ozaki T, Crystal RG. Colchicine suppresses the release of fibroblast growth factors from alveolar macrophages *in vitro*: the basis of a possible therapeutic approach to the fibrotic disorders. *Am Rev Respir Dis* 1988;137:181–185.
453. Crystal RG, Ferrans VJ, Basset F. Biologic basis of pulmonary fibrosis. In: Crystal RG, West JB, eds. *The lung:* scientific foundations. New York: Raven Press, 1991:2031–2046.
454. Borok Z, Buhl R, Grimes GJ, et al. Effect of glutathione aerosol on oxidant-antioxidant imbalance in idiopathic pulmonary fibrosis. *Lancet* 1991;338(8761):215–216.
455. Meyer A, Buhl R, Kampf S, Magnusssen H. Intravenous N-acetylcysteine and lung glutathione of patients with pulmonary fibrosis and normals. *Am J Respir Crit Care Med* 1995;152:1055–1060.
456. Bridgeman MME, Marsden M, MacNee W, Flenley DC, Ryle AP. Cysteine and glutathione concentrations in plasma and bronchoalveolar lavage fluid after treatment with N-acetylcysteine. *Thorax* 1991; 46:39–42.
457. Allison AC, Lee JC, Eugui EM. Pharmacological regulation of the production of the proinflammatory cytokines TNF-alpha and IL-1beta. In: Aggarwal BB, Puri RK, eds. *Human cytokines:* their role in disease and therapy. Cambridge, MA: Blackwell Science, 1995, 689–713.
458. Rom WN, Harkin T. Dehydroepiandrosterone inhibits the spontaneous release of superoxide radical *in vitro* by alveolar macrophages in asbestosis. *Environ Res* 1991;55:145–156.
459. Eugui EM, DeLustro B, Rouhafza S, et al. Some antioxidants inhibit, in a co-ordinate fashion, the production of tumor necrosis factor-alpha, IL-beta, and IL-6 by human peripheral blood mononuclear cells. *Int Immunol* 1994;6(3):409–422.
460. Houglum K, Brenner DA, Chojkier M. d-alpha-tocopherol inhibits collagen alpha 1(I) gene expression in cultured human fibroblasts. Modulation of constitutive collagen gene expression by lipid peroxidation. *J Clin Invest* 1991;87(6):2230–2235.
461. Mossman BT, Marsh JP, Sesko A, et al. Inhibition of lung injury, inflammation, and interstitial pulmonary fibrosis by polyethylene glycol-conjugated catalase in a rapid inhalation model of asbestosis. *Am Rev Respir Dis* 1990;141(5 Pt 1):1266–1271.
462. Shahzeidi S, Sarnstrand B, Jeffery PK, McAnulty RJ, Laurent GJ. Oral N-acetylcysteine reduces bleomycin-induced collagen deposition in the lungs of mice. *Eur Respir J* 1991;4(7):845–852.
463. Omenn GS, Goodman G, Thornquist M, et al. The beta-carotene and retinol efficacy trial (CARET) for chemoprevention of lung cancer in high risk populations: smokers and asbestos-exposed workers. *Cancer Res* 1994;54(7 suppl):2038s–2043s.
464. Elliott MJ, Maini RN, Feldmann M, Long-Fox A, Charles P, Bijl H, Woody JN. Repeated therapy with monoclonal antibody to tumour necrosis factor alpha (cA2) in patients with rheumatoid arthritis. *Lancet* 1994;344(8930):1125–1127.
465. van Dullemen HM, van Deventer SJ, Hommes DW, et al. Treatment of Crohn's disease with anti-tumor necrosis factor chimeric monoclonal antibody (cA2). *Gastroenterology* 1995;109(1):129–135.
466. Lee JC, Laydon JT, McDonnell PC, et al. A protein kinase involved in the regulation of inflammatory cytokine biosynthesis. *Nature* 1994; 372(6508):739–746.
467. Beyaert R, Cuenda A, Vanden Berghe W, et al. The p38/RK mitogen-activated protein kinase pathway regulates interleukin-6 synthesis response to tumor necrosis factor. *EMBO J* 1996;15(8):1914–1923.
468. Boehm JC, Smietana JM, Sorenson ME, et al. 1-substituted 4-aryl-5-pyridinylimidazoles: a new class of cytokine suppressive drugs with low 5-lipoxygenase and cyclooxygenase inhibitory potency. *J Med Chem* 1996;39(20):3929–3937.
469. Kang H-S, Kim Y-H, Lee C-S, Lee J-J, Choi I, Pyun K-H. Suppression of interleukin-1 and tumor necrosis factor alpha production by acanthoic acid, (-)-pimara-9(11),15-dien-19-oic acid, and its antifibrotic effects *in vivo*. *Cell Immunol* 1996;170:212–221.
470. Peppel K, Crawford D, Beutler B. A tumor necrosis factor (TNF) receptor-IgG heavy chain chimeric protein as a bivalent antagonist of TNF activity. *J Exp Med* 1991;174:1483–1489.
471. Tsunawaki S, Sporn M, Ding A, Nathan CF. Deactivation of macrophages by transforming growth factor beta. *Nature* 1988;334:260–262.
472. Waters RV, Allison AC. Mycophenolic acid and some anti-oxidants induce differentiation of monocytic lineage cells and augment production of the IL-1 receptor antagonist (IL-1ra). *Ann NY Acad Sci* 1993;696:185–196.
473. Piguet PF, Vesin C, Grau GE, Thompson RC. Interleukin 1 receptor antagonist (IL-1ra) prevents or cures pulmonary fibrosis elicited in mice by bleomycin or silica. *Cytokine* 1993;5:57–61.
474. Piguet PF, Grau GE, de Kossodo S. Role of granulocyte-macrophage colony stimulating factor in pulmonary fibrosis induced in mice by bleomycin. *Exp Lung Res* 1993;19:515–518.
475. Hart PH, Vitti GF, Burgess DR, Whitty GA, Piccoli DS, Hamilton JA. Potential anti-inflammatory effects of interleukin 4: suppression of human monocyte tumor necrosis factor alpha, interleukin-1 and prostaglandin E2. *Proc Natl Acad Sci USA* 1989;86:3803–3807.
476. te Velde AA, Huijben RJF, Heije K, de Vries JE, Figdor CG. Interleukin 4 (IL-4) inhibits secretion of IL-1 beta, tumor necrosis factor alpha, and IL-6 by human monocytes. *Blood* 1990;76:1392–1397.
477. Postlethwaite AE, Holness MA, Katai H, Raghow R. Human fibroblasts synthesize elevated levels of extracellular matrix proteins in response to interleukin-4. *J Clin Invest* 1992;90:1479–1485.
478. Rollins BJ, Pober JS. Interleukin-4 induces the synthesis and secretion of MCP-1/JE by human endothelial cells. *Am J Pathol* 1991;138: 1315–1319.
479. de Waal Malefyt R, Abrams J, Bennett B, Figdor CG, de Vries JE. Interleukin 10 (IL-10) inhibits cytokine synthesis by human monocytes: an autoregulatory role of IL-10 produced by monocytes. *J Exp Med* 1991;174:1209–1220.
480. Thomassen MJ, Divis LT, Fisher CJ. Regulation of human alveolar macrophage inflammatory cytokine production by interleukin-10. *Clin Immunol Immunopathol* 1996;80(3 Pt 1):321–324.
481. Elias JA, Jimenez SA, Freundlich B. Recombinant gamma, alpha and beta interferon regulation of human lung fibroblast proliferation. *Am Rev Respir Dis* 1987;135:62–65.
482. Varga J, Olsen A, Herhal J, Constantine G, Rosenbloom J, Jimenez SA. IFN-gamma reverses the stimulation of collagen but not

fibronectin gene expression by TGF beta. *Eur J Clin Invest* 1990;20: 487–492.

483. Galve-de Rochemonteix B, Nicod LP, Dayer JM. Tumor necrosis factor soluble receptor 75: the principal receptor form released by human alveolar macrophages and monocytes in the presence of interferon (gamma). *Am J Respir Cell Mol Biol* 1996;14(3):279–287.
484. Giri SN, Hyde DM, Marifino BJ. Ameliorating effect of murine interferon -gamma on bleomycin induced lung collagen fibrosis in mice. *Biochem Med Metabol Biol* 1986;36:194–197.
485. Hyde DM, Giri SN. Polyinosinic-polycytidylic acid, as interferon inducer, ameliorates bleomycin-induced lung fibrosis in mice. *Exp Lung Res* 1990;16:533–546.
486. Okada T, Sugie I, Aisaka K. Effects of gamma-interferon on collagen and histamine content in bleomycin-induced lung fibrosis in rats. *Lymphokine Cytokine Res* 1993;12:87–91.
487. Kosaka C, Masuda J, Shimakado K, et al. Interferon-gamma suppresses PDGF production from THP-1 cells and blood monocyte-derived macrophages. *Atherosclerosis* 1992;97:75–87.
488. Kovacs EJ, Kelley J. Lymphokine regulation of macrophage-derived growth factor secretion following pulmonary injury. *Am J Pathol* 1985;121:261–268.
489. Badgett A, Bonner JC, Brody AR. Interferon-gamma modulates lung macrophage production of PDGF-BB and fibroblast growth. *J Lipid Mediat Cell Signal* 1996;13(1):89–97.
490. Mercola M, Deininger PL, Shamah SM, Porter J, Wang CY, Stiles CD. Dominant-negative mutants of a platelet-derived growth factor gene. *Genes Dev* 1990;4(12B):2333–2341.
491. Shamah SM, Stiles CD, Guha A. Dominant-negative mutants of platelet-derived growth factor revert the transformed phenotype of human astrocytoma cells. *Mol Cell Biol* 1993;13(12):7203–7212.
492. Vassbotn FS, Andersson M, Westermark B, Heldin CH, Ostman A. Reversion of autocrine transformation by a dominant negative platelet-derived growth factor mutant. *Mol Cell Biol* 1993;13(7): 4066–4076.
493. Dorai T, Kobayashi H, Holland JF, Ohnuma T. Modulation of platelet-derived growth factor-beta mRNA expression and cell growth in a human mesothelioma cell line by a hammerhead ribozyme. *Mol Pharmacol* 1994;46:437–444.
494. Giri SN, Hyde DM, Hollinger MA. Effect of antibody to transforming growth factor beta on bleomycin induced accumulation of lung collagen in mice. *Thorax* 1993;48(10):959–966.
495. Redlich CA, Delisser HM, Elias JA. Retinoic acid inhibition of transforming growth factor-beta-induced collagen production by human lung fibroblasts. *Am J Respir Cell Mol Biol* 1995;12(3):287–295.
496. Borok Z, Gillissen A, Buhl R, et al. Augmentation of functional prostaglandin E levels on the respiratory epithelial surface by aerosol administration of prostaglandin E. *Am Rev Respir Dis* 1991;144(5): 1080–1084.
497. Granot I, Hurwitz S, Halevy O, Pines M. Halofuginone: and inhibitor of collagen type I synthesis. *Biochim Biophys Acta* 1993;1156: 107–112.
498. Nagler A, Firman N, Feferman R, Cotev S, Pines M, Shoshan S. Reduction in pulmonary fibrosis *in vivo* by halofuginone. *Am J Respir Crit Care Med* 1996;154:1082–1086.
499. Curiel DT, Pilewski JM, Albelda SM. Gene therapy approaches for inherited and acquired lung diseases. *Am J Respir Cell Mol Biol* 1996; 14:1–18.
500. Yang Y, Nunes FA, Berencsi K, Gonczol E, Engelhardt JF, Wilson JM. Inactivation of E2a in recombinant adenoviruses improves the prospect for gene therapy in cystic fibrosis. *Nature Genet* 1994;7(3):362–369.
501. Erzurum SC, Lemarchand P, Rosenfeld MA, Yoo JH, Crystal RG. Protection of human endothelial cells from oxidant injury by adenovirus-mediated transfer of the human catalase cDNA. *Nucleic Acids Res* 1993;21(7):1607–1612.
502. Conary JT, Parker RE, Christman BW, et al. Protection of rabbit lungs from endotoxin injury by *in vivo* hyperexpression of the prostaglandin G/H synthase gene. *J Clin Invest* 1994;93(4):1834–1840.
503. Kolls J, Peppel K, Silva M, Beutler B. Prolonged and effective blockade of tumor necrosis factor activity through adenovirus-mediated gene transfer. *Proc Natl Acad Sci USA* 1994;91(1):215–219.

*Environmental and Occupational Medicine, Third Edition,* edited by William N. Rom.
Lippincott–Raven Publishers, Philadelphia © 1998.

# CHAPTER 23

# Fiber Analysis

Victor L. Roggli

The inhalation of asbestos fibers has been associated with the subsequent development of a variety of diseases. An important determinant of the development of an asbestos-related disease is the accumulation and distribution of asbestos in the respiratory tract. Therefore, there has been increasing interest in the analysis of tissue mineral fiber content and its relation to the various asbestos-associated diseases. Because a variety of studies have shown that some asbestos fibers can be found in the lungs of virtually all adults in the general population (1–7), the mere identification of asbestos in human lung tissue samples has little significance, and quantitative techniques are necessary.

Aerosolized asbestos fibers may be deposited at any site in the respiratory tract. In the upper airway, fibers landing on the respiratory epithelium of the larynx or trachea may be transported across the epithelium into the underlying connective tissues (8). Similarly, fibers deposited on the surfaces of bronchi and bronchioles may be translocated into the peribronchial or peribronchiolar connective tissues (9). Fibers that reach the gas-exchange portions of the lung tend to be deposited primarily at the first alveolar duct bifurcations (10). Transepithelial migration of fibers results in their accumulation in the interstitium of alveolar duct and alveolar septal walls. From this location, fibers may find their way into the pulmonary lymphatic system and subsequently be transported to the pleura or to mediastinal and hilar lymph nodes (11,12). In addition, fiber deposition on the surfaces of alveolar ducts results in the local accumulation of alveolar macrophages, which then proceed to phagocytose the fibers (10,13). Accumulation of sufficient numbers of fibers at any of these sites in the respiratory tract can result in asbestos-related tissue injury. A variety of factors influence the accumulation of the fibers within the respiratory tract, including intensity and duration of exposure, fiber size and chemical composition, host factors such as efficiency of clearance mechanisms and intensity of the inflammatory response, and other factors such as cigarette smoking (14).

In some instances the interaction of alveolar macrophages with asbestos fibers results in the formation of unique structures referred to as asbestos bodies. These structures consist of a central core fiber and a coating of iron-protein-mucopolysaccharide material deposited by the macrophages (15,16). The coating material gives the asbestos body its characteristic golden brown segmented appearance and dumbbell or javelin shape (Fig. 1). The primary determinant of whether an asbestos body forms from a phagocytosed fiber is fiber length; most asbestos bodies are 20 μm or longer. Additional factors, including fiber diameter, surface features, and fiber type, also affect asbestos body formation (15–17). Asbestos bodies are an irrefutable marker of past asbestos exposure, although only a small proportion of fibers retained in the lung become coated to form asbestos bodies (15,18).

This chapter reviews the techniques that have been developed for the analysis of tissue mineral fiber content. In addition, the relationship between quantitative determinations of mineral fiber content and the various asbestos-related diseases in series of patients is explored, along with the correlation between fiber content and various occupational and paraoccupational exposures. Finally, the chapter concludes with a review of the relationship between fiber type and accumulation within the lung.

V. L. Roggli: Department of Pathology, Duke University Medical Center, Durham, North Carolina 27705.

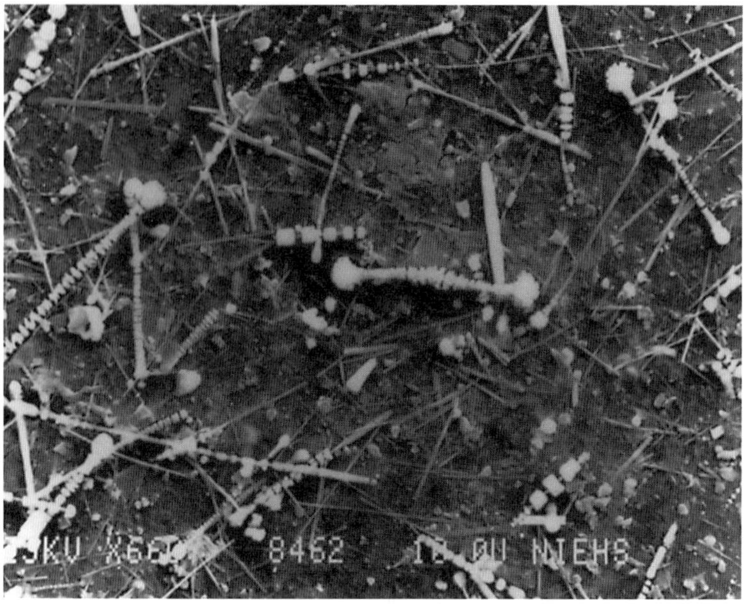


**FIG. 1.** Scanning electron micrograph of Nuclepore filter preparation of lung tissue from an asbestos insulator with malignant pleural mesothelioma and asbestosis. Numerous asbestos bodies and uncoated asbestos fibers are visible. Magnified ×660.

## METHODS FOR ANALYSIS OF FIBER CONTENT

Asbestos is not a single mineral substance but a group of minerals with the common properties of thermal and chemical resistance and high tensile strength. Asbestos minerals are divided into two large groups: serpentine and amphibole. The sole member of the serpentine group of asbestiform minerals is chrysotile, also known as white asbestos. The amphiboles include five separate mineral species: amosite, crocidolite, tremolite, anthophyllite, and actinolite (Table 1). Two of these are commercially valuable forms: amosite, or brown asbestos, and crocidolite, or blue asbestos. The other three amphibole minerals are mainly important as contaminants of other materials such as talc, vermiculite, and chrysotile asbestos. Each of these types of asbestos has morphologic, chemical, and crystalline properties that aid in its specific identification. For example, chrysotile is a hydrated magnesium silicate with a unique structure characterized as a sheet rolled up to form a tube or scroll. Long chrysotile fibers tend to have a curved appearance and splayed ends. These fibers fragment readily *in vivo* (19). The amphiboles are chain silicates with a straight line rather than curved morphology. They have various cations in their crystal structure (magnesium, iron, calcium, sodium), and the various amphiboles can be distinguished on the basis of their chemical composition (5). Asbestiform minerals also occur in a nonasbestiform habit; the chemical structure is identical but they lack the fibrous structure of their asbestiform counterparts (20). In addition, a wide variety of nonasbestos mineral fibers have been recovered from human tissues (21,22).

**TABLE 1.** *Types of asbestos*

| |
|---|
| Serpentine |
| Chrysotile (white asbestos) |
| Amphibole |
| Amosite (brown asbestos) |
| Crocidolite (blue asbestos) |
| Tremolite |
| Anthophyllite |
| Actinolite |

The identification and quantification of mineral fibers in human tissues generally requires a method of extracting the fibers from the organic matrix in which they are embedded. Various digestion procedures have been employed for this purpose, including chemical dissolution of tissue and ashing in a furnace (23). Theoretically, any type of tissue could be analyzed in this manner; however, the vast majority of available data relates to the fiber content of lung parenchyma. Sample selection is important in this regard. Adequacy of sample size requires, at minimum, open or thoracoscopic lung biopsy, and more selective sampling may be obtained from lobectomy or pneumonectomy specimens. Autopsy specimens are ideal for obtaining representative samples. Transbronchial biopsy is inadequate because of the variability of sampling and the relatively small numbers of fibers recovered. Results of tissue digestion are usually expressed as a concentration of fibers per gram of wet or dry lung tissue. Therefore, consideration must be given to factors that would effect the denominator (i.e., tissue weight) in these calculations, so areas of tumor, consolidation, or congestion should be avoided as much as possible (23). Bronchoalveolar lavage samples may provide useful information as well (24–27), and studies have shown a good correlation between asbestos content of lung tissue and bronchoalveolar lavage fluid. Results are usually expressed as bodies or fibers per milliliter of lavage fluid recovered.

Once a sample has been selected, the digestion procedure requires a dissolution step and a recovery step. Wet chemical digestion is the procedure most often used for tissue dissolution, although low-temperature plasma ashing works just as well (23). In the past, formamide, hydrogen peroxide, or proteolytic enzymes were used for chemical digestion; however, today the most widely used reagents are sodium or potassium hydroxide and sodium hypochlorite solution (commercial bleach). Once digestion is complete, the inorganic residues are collected on the surface of an acetate or polycarbonate filter. Filter pore size is important in this regard: filters with the smallest pore size retain the smallest fibers (28).

Analysis of fiber content requires examination of the filter preparation by some form of microscopy—conventional bright-field light microscopy, phase-contrast light microscopy (PCLM), scanning electron microscopy (SEM), or transmission electron microscopy (TEM). Each technique has its own advantages and limitations (23). Conventional light microscopy is perfectly adequate for quantification of asbestos bodies. PCLM permits detection of uncoated fibers as well but is limited to fibers with a diameter of at least 0.2 μm. SEM allows detection of smaller fibers as well as identification of fiber type as determined by energy dispersive x-ray analysis (EDXA) of the elemental composition. TEM detects the smallest fibrils and also permits identification of crystalline structure by means of selected area electron diffraction (SAED). Whichever form of microscopy is used, the fiber density (fibers per square millimeter) on the surface is determined, from which the total fiber count on the filter may be calculated. The final result can then be expressed as fibers per gram of wet or dry lung tissue or per cubic centimeter of lung. As a general rule of thumb, 1 fiber/g wet lung ≅ 1 fiber/cm$^3$ ≅ 10 fibers/g dry lung (23).

**TABLE 2.** *Factors affecting fiber burden data*

| |
|---|
| Digestion procedure |
| Wet chemical digestion (alkali, enzymes) |
| Low temperature plasma ashing |
| Number of sites sampled |
| Recovery procedure |
| Use of centrifugation step |
| Use of a sonication step |
| Filtration step (type of filter, pore size) |
| Analytical procedure |
| Microscopic technique (LM, PCLM, SEM, TEM) |
| Magnification used |
| Sizes of fibers counted and other counting rules |
| Numbers of fibers or fields actually counted |
| Reporting of results |
| Asbestos bodies or fibers (or both) |
| Sizes of fibers counted |
| Concentration of fibers (per g wet or dry lung or per cm$^3$) |

LM, light microscopy; PCLM, phase contrast light microscopy; SEM, scanning electron microscopy; TEM, transmission electron microscopy.

Reprinted from ref. 23.

The actual analytic result obtained on any one sample can be profoundly influenced by the steps employed in the analytic procedure (Table 2). Therefore, extrapolations of results from one laboratory to another should be made with great caution (23,29). In addition, site-to-site variation among samples obtained from the same lung may yield analytic results that vary by a factor of 5, or even 10 (30,31). Also, the analysis occurs at a single point in time, usually when advanced disease is present, and the fiber burden at that time may or may not relate to the tissue fiber content when disease was actively evolving (23).

## ASBESTOS CONTENT OF LUNG TISSUE IN ASBESTOS-ASSOCIATED DISEASES

### Asbestosis

Asbestosis is defined as pulmonary interstitial fibrosis secondary to the inhalation of asbestos fibers. The pathologic features of asbestosis have been well defined (32,33). Studies have shown that asbestosis generally follows prolonged, direct, often intense exposure to aerosolized asbestos fibers (34,35). These observations are in good agreement with the results of lung fiber burden analysis in series of patients with asbestosis (2,33,36–39) (Table 3). Although they employed a variety of preparatory and analytic techniques, they report remarkably similar findings: the vast majority of patients with asbestosis have a markedly elevated pulmonary fiber burden. As summarized in Table 3, the median uncoated fiber count exceeds 1 million fibers per gram of dried lung tissue in all six studies. For comparative purposes, the fiber burden data from the author's laboratory for patients with asbestosis, other asbestos-related diseases, and normal lungs are summarized in Table 4.

Asbestos bodies are the histologic hallmark of asbestos exposure (18) and an important criterion for the pathologic diagnosis of asbestosis (32,33). The asbestos body content, which correlates well with the concentration of amphibole fibers longer than 5 μm in the lung, is markedly elevated in most patients with asbestosis (5,33). Asbestos body counts exceeded 1,700 per gram of wet lung in 90% in the author's series of 148 asbestosis cases; the median number of asbestos bodies per gram exceeds 15,000 (Table 4). Consequently, asbestos bodies are present in most histologic sections from patients with asbestosis (40), although it may require careful searching and special histologic stains (e.g., Prussian blue) to identify them. Studies have shown that, in addition to histologic criteria, analysis of asbestos body and uncoated fiber content provides useful information for distinguish-

**TABLE 3.** *Asbestos content of lung tissue in reported series of patients with asbestosis*

| No. cases | Method | Fibers/gram dried lung (×10⁶)[a] | Reference |
|---|---|---|---|
| 23 | PCLM | 8 (1.0–70) | 2 |
| 22 | PCLM | 32 (1.3–493) | 36 |
| 22 | TEM | 5.68 (1.6–121) | 37 |
| 100 | PCLM | 1.5 (0.001–31.6) | 38 |
| 170 | TEM | 372 (<1.0–10,000) | 38 |
| 23 | TEM | 10[b] | 39 |

[a]Values reported as median counts for millions ($10^6$) of fibers per gram of dried lung tissue, with ranges indicated in parentheses (refs. 2, 36, 37) or mean fiber count (ref. 38) or geometric mean count (ref. 39).
[b]Range not reported.
PCLM, phase contrast light microscopy; TEM, transmission electron microscopy.
Modified from ref. 33.

ing between asbestosis and idiopathic pulmonary fibrosis (5,33,41).

One of the goals of fiber burden analysis is to determine the mineralogic correlates of severity of pulmonary fibrosis. In this regard, several studies have shown a correlation between the severity of pulmonary fibrosis and the concentration of mineral fibers per gram of lung tissue (2,5,33,36,38), but the correlation is imperfect and the data widely scattered. More recently, investigators have reported a correlation between severity of fibrosis and the total surface area of retained mineral fibers (42,43). Detailed studies by Churg and co-workers of workers exposed to predominately chrysotile asbestos (44) or to a mixture of amosite and chrysotile (45) showed a very significant correlation between severity of fibrosis and concentration of fibers in the fibrotic lung. These authors also noted an inverse correlation between severity of fibrosis and mean fiber length. This observation is surprising in light of animal studies that show that it is principally fibers longer than 5 μm that are responsible for tissue injury and subsequent fibrosis (19). One possible explanation for the inverse correlation between fibrosis and mean fiber length is that short fibers that are cleared readily from normal lungs are removed ineffi-

**TABLE 4.** *Asbestos content of lung tissue in asbestos-associated disease*[a]

| | N | AB | AF | AC | TAA | Chrys |
|---|---|---|---|---|---|---|
| Asbestosis[b] | 40 | 18,800 (250–1,400,000) | 252,0000 (6,240–7,530,000) | 194,000 (2,040–7,530,000) | <47,000 (<860–471,000) | (<20,300) (<860–68,000) |
| Pleural mesothelioma | | | | | | |
| +Asbestosis[c] | 30 | 15,900 (1,570–1,600,000) | 121,000 (9,220–11,900,000) | 94,500 (6,620–11,900,000) | <10,500 (<1,770–45,000) | <5,560 (<610–42,900) |
| +PPP | 63 | 900 (2.6–74,500) | 23,200 (370–933,000) | 17,500 (120–933,000) | 2,820 (250–28,300) | <1,510 (<120–124,000) |
| Other[d] | 62 | 49 (<0.2–15,100) | 4,640 (<490–460,000) | 2,460 (<310–460,000) | 1,740 (280–32,300) | <1,060 (<280–11,000) |
| Peritoneal mesothelioma | | | | | | |
| +Asbestosis[c] | 8 | 127,000 (370–684,000) | 604,000 (38,600–1,960,000) | 604,000 (36,700–1,960,000) | <26,000 (<1,900–<98,000) | <26,000 (<1,410–<98,000) |
| +PPP | 2 | 11,600 (29–23,100) | 122,000 (260–244,000) | 106,000 (230–213,000) | <4580 (26–9,160) | 15,400 (<26–30,800) |
| Other[d] | 5 | 3.3 (1.0–590) | 680 (490–10,100) | <660 (<300–2,920) | 610 (<340–7,170) | <490 (<300–1,030) |
| Lung cancer | | | | | | |
| +Asbestosis[c] | 70 | 27,300 (150–343,000) | 253,000 (14,600–8,540,000) | 253,000 (11,200–8,540,000) | <22,000 (1,460–149,000) | <22,000 (910–63,900) |
| +PPP | 44 | 710 (<3–18,900) | 14,000 (<510–142,000) | 8,140 (<490–118,000) | 2,180 (180–48,900) | <2,000 (180–8,600) |
| Other[d] | 120 | 80 (2.6–45,800) | 4,990 (370–157,000) | 3,490 (<370–113,000) | 2,110 (170–144,000) | 1,800 (<310–<14,000) |
| Reference population | 19 | 2.9 (0.2–22) | <600 (<170–2,540) | <600 (<100–<2,540) | <600 (<170–2,540) | <600 (<100–<2,540) |

[a]Values presented are the median with ranges indicated underneath.
[b]Excluding cases with lung cancer or mesothelioma.
[c]Includes 28 cases with PPP, 6 without, and 4 unknown.
[d]Neither plaques nor asbestosis.
N, number of cases in each catagory; PPP, parietal pleural plaques; <, below limits of deduction for that case; AB, asbestos bodies per gram of wet lung tissue as determined by light microscopy; AF, total (coated+uncoated) asbestos fibers ≥5 μm in length per gram of wet lung, as determined by scanning electron microscopy; AC, amosite+crocidolite fibers (subgroup of AF); TAA, tremolite+anthophyllite+actinolite fibers; Chrys, chrysotile fibers.

ciently from fibrotic lungs owing to impairment of clearance mechanisms. Alternatively, short fibers may be less injurious because they are more readily cleared, but when clearance mechanisms break down and short fibers accumulate they too may contribute to overall tissue injury (46).

In patients with asbestosis who are exposed to a mixture of chrysotile and amphibole asbestos fibers, it is principally the amphiboles that are found in the lung at the time of fiber analysis (33,38,39,45). This is because the amphiboles accumulate progressively in lung tissue with continuous exposure, whereas chrysotile reaches a plateau after a few months and the concentration remains steady thereafter in spite of continued exposure (47). Therefore, with heavy tissue burdens chrysotile is diluted by the amphibole accumulation and so may be difficult to detect.

### Mesothelioma

Malignant pleural mesothelioma is considered a signal neoplasm that is strongly associated in epidemiologic studies with a history of asbestos exposure (34,48,49). Although most cases occur in persons who are exposed occupationally to asbestos, some result from indirect exposure, such as in household contacts of asbestos workers (50,51) or persons who live near an asbestos mine or manufacturing plant (34,48). Relatively low-level exposures may also be identified in some persons who, decades later, present with the clinical findings of pleural mesothelioma. Peritoneal and pericardial mesotheliomas also occur following exposure to asbestos (52). These observations fit well with the results of lung fiber burden analyses in series of patients with malignant mesothelioma (2,4,7,39,53–57) (Table 5). These studies show that patients with malignant mesothelioma often have a lung fiber burden greater than that of the general population, and sometimes as great as those of patients with asbestosis. Indeed, about 20% of patients with malignant pleural mesothelioma also have clinically or histologically documented asbestosis (52,58). For peritoneal mesotheliomas, as many as 50% also have asbestosis (58).

**TABLE 5.** *Asbestos content of lung tissue in reported series of patients with mesothelioma*

| No. cases | Method | Fibers/ gram dried lung ($\times 10^6$)[a] | Reference |
|---|---|---|---|
| 100 | PCLM | 0.75 (0–70) | 2 |
| 27 | TEM | 4.9 (0.57–137) | 53 |
| 10 | TEM | 3.5 (0.1–85.2) | 54 |
| 6 | TEM | 238 (52–2,190) | 55 |
| 20 | TEM | 18[b] | 7 |
| 83 | TEM | 0.92[b] | 39 |
| 14 | SEM | 2.4 (0.4–37) | 4 |
| 15 | SEM | 11 (2–490) | 57 |

[a]Values reported as median counts for millions ($10^6$) of fibers per gram of dried lung tissue, with ranges indicated in parentheses (2,4,53–55,57) or mean fiber count (7) or geometric mean count (39).

[b]Ranges not reported

PCLM, phase contrast light microscopy; TEM, transmission electron microscopy; SEM, scanning electron microscopy.

Modified from ref. 23.

Evaluation of the asbestos body content of lung tissue in patients with mesothelioma provides some interesting information. The distributions of asbestos body counts observed in 170 cases of malignant pleural mesothelioma from the author's consultation files is shown in Fig. 2A. In 79% of pleural cases, the asbestos body content exceeds that of our previously established normal range (0 to 20 per gram of wet lung), whereas in the remainder of cases the values overlap with the normal range. In addition, the distribution for pleural mesothelioma cases appears to be bimodal, suggesting that there are two distinct populations (56). These data agree with clinical observations that 70 to 80% of patients with mesothelioma have an identifiable exposure to asbestos by history, whereas 20 to 30% do not (59). Some patients with asbestos body counts within the normal range can be shown by electron microscopy to have an elevated asbestos fiber count and thus are probably asbestos related. Cases with background range fiber counts are most likely spontaneous or background mesotheliomas, and the etiology of most of these cases is unknown (2,56). These cases represent approximately 11% of cases in the author's consultation files (Fig. 3).

The median asbestos body count in patients with mesothelioma is considerably less than that in patients with asbestosis (see Table 4); however, the median concentration of asbestos bodies in the lungs of 30 pleural mesothelioma patients who had histologically documented asbestosis (15,900 bodies per gram wet lung) is not significantly different from that of 40 patients with asbestosis who had neither lung cancer nor mesothelioma (18,800 per gram wet lung) studied in the author's laboratory. When patients with asbestosis are excluded, the median count in 63 pleural mesothelioma patients who also had parietal pleural plaques (see below) was 900 bodies per gram wet lung, whereas the count in 62 mesothelioma patients without plaques was only 49 bodies per gram. Asbestos bodies can be identified in histologic sections of lung parenchyma (hematoxylin and eosin or iron-stained sections) in about 57% of cases (Fig. 3). They are not observed in sections of pleural tumor.

The distribution of asbestos body counts in 21 patients with peritoneal mesothelioma is shown in Fig. 2B. The asbestos body counts exceed those of our reference population in only 62% of cases, as compared to 79% of pleural cases. However, the peritoneal mesothelioma cases had the highest asbestos content of any group when

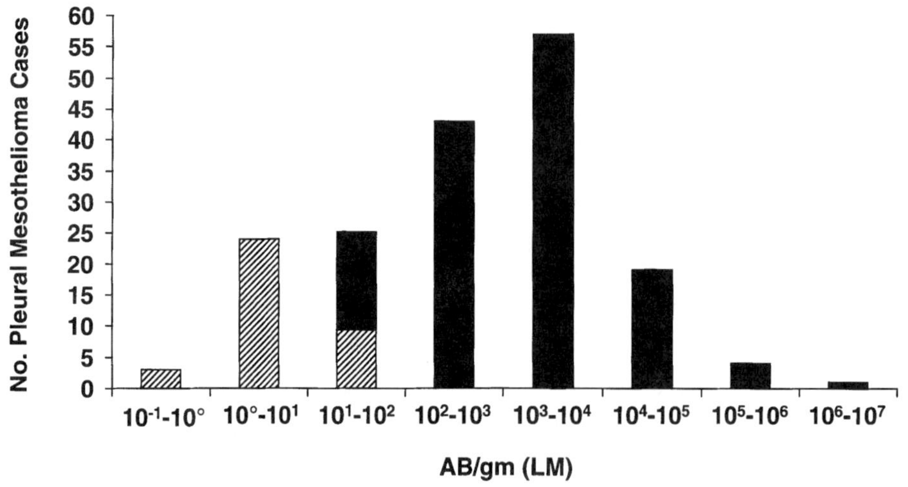


A

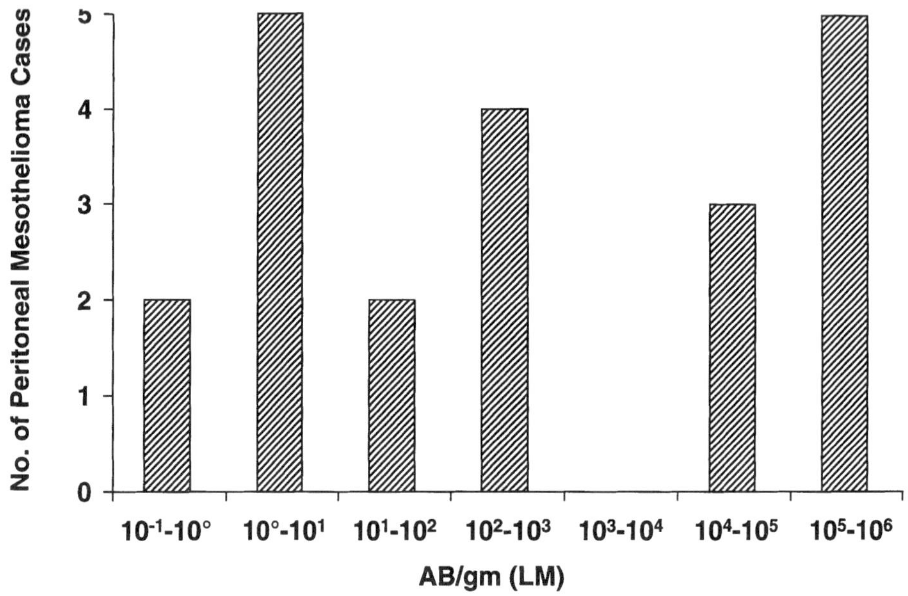


B

**FIG. 2. A:** Distribution of asbestos body counts in 170 patients with malignant pleural mesothelioma. The *lightly shaded areas* show cases with counts within our background range of 0 to 20 asbestos bodies per gram of wet lung (AB/g). Note the logarithmic scale, with values ranging from 0.1 ($10^{-1}$) to 10 million ($10^7$) AB/g. The data are consistent with a biphasic log normal distribution with 18% of cases having a mean of 3.1 AB/g (SD 2.6), while 82% of cases have a mean of 1,170 AB/g (SD 11.4). The *p* value for goodness of fit for a bimodal distribution is .50, whereas the unimodal distribution is rejected with a *p* value of .0016. **B:** Distribution of asbestos body counts in 21 patients with malignant peritoneal mesothelioma; 38% of these cases have asbestos body counts within our normal range of 0 to 20 AB/g.

stratified according to the presence or absence of asbestosis or pleural plaques (Table 4). When taken together, these findings imply that more asbestos is needed to produce peritoneal as compared to pleural mesotheliomas, and a smaller percentage of peritoneal mesotheliomas are asbestos related. Since previous studies from our laboratory have shown no significant difference in the duration of exposure to asbestos between pleural and peritoneal cases (60), it follows that the intensity of exposure is, on average, greater for peritoneal mesotheliomas.

About 8.0% of mesotheliomas in the author's consultation files arose in women, with 86% having a pleural origin. Asbestosis was found in 16% of cases. More than half of the patients were household contacts of asbestos workers. Occupational exposure to asbestos was identified in only 19% of cases. An elevated tissue asbestos burden was noted in 70% of women for whom lung tissue was available for analysis; 58% had an asbestos body count exceeding our normal range, with a median asbestos body count of 31 per gram (range: 2.0–8,200) (61).

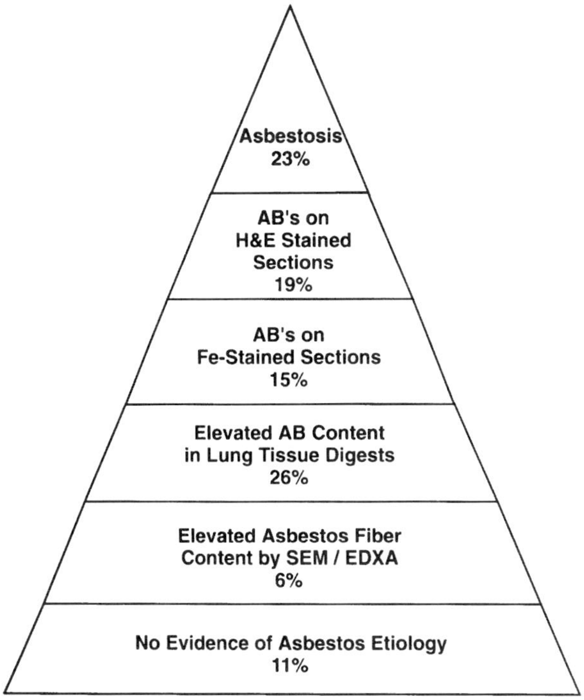


**FIG. 3.** Pyramid showing the relationship between asbestos exposure and mesothelioma. At the upper range of exposures, 23% of patients have histologically confirmed asbestosis. An additional 34% have asbestos bodies on hematoxylin and eosin (H&E) or iron-stained sections. At the next level, 26% of patients will have an elevated pulmonary asbestos body content even though asbestos bodies are not observed in histologic sections. A further 6% will have an elevated lung fiber burden as determined by scanning electron microscopy even though asbestos body counts are within the background range of 0 to 20 AB/g. Finally, in 11% of cases, there is no pathologic evidence for an asbestos etiology.

Evidence has accumulated that indicates that the various asbestos fiber types (Table 1) are not equally potent inducers of malignant mesothelioma (62). Some of this evidence derives from studies of the fiber content of the lung in patients with mesothelioma. Cases of mesothelioma patients whose predominant exposure was to the amphibole amosite had considerably smaller fiber burdens than those exposed to chrysotile mine dust (54,55) (see Table 5). Furthermore, analysis of the fiber content of the lung parenchyma in mesothelioma patients with mixed serpentine and amphibole exposure shows principally amphibole fibers; chrysotile was present in concentrations indistinguishable from "background" (7,63, 64). Even among patients exposed to chrysotile mine dust, the amphibole tremolite accounts for more than half of the fiber burden in these patients' lungs, despite the fact that tremolite accounts for only a small percentage of the fibers in the mine dust (65). Consequently, some investigators believe that the amphibole fibers are principally responsible for the production of malignant mesothelioma (38,55,64). Fiber size is undoubtedly important in this regard: long, thin fibers pose the greatest hazard (43,66). Studies have shown that the average fiber length of amosite or crocidolite recovered from the lungs of patients with mesothelioma is greater than the average length of chrysotile or tremolite fibers (54,55). Nonetheless, it should be remembered that inhaled chrysotile asbestos can produce mesotheliomas in experimental animals (47) and that chrysotile is a potent producer of asbestosis even though chrysotile fibers do not accumulate as readily as amphiboles in lung parenchyma (67).

## Benign Asbestos-Related Pleural Diseases

A variety of benign pleural abnormalities are associated with exposure to aerosolized asbestos fibers: parietal pleural plaques, diffuse pleural fibrosis, benign asbestos effusion, and rounded atelectasis (68). Parietal pleural plaques, the most common abnormality associated with asbestos exposure, may result from brief or low-level exposure. These observations are in close agreement with the results of lung fiber burden analyses in series of patients with benign asbestos-related pleural diseases (57,69,70) (Table 6). These studies and others have shown that the lung fiber burden of patients with parietal pleural plaques is intermediate between that of the general population (background levels) and that of patients with asbestosis (Table 4). The few patients with diffuse pleural fibrosis who have been studied had lung fiber burdens between those of patients with plaques and those of patients with asbestosis (71) (Table 6).

Evaluation of the asbestos body content of lung tissue in 65 cases of parietal pleural plaques and malignant mesothelioma and 44 cases of plaques and lung cancer from the author's consultation files yielded median

**TABLE 6.** *Asbestos content of lung tissue in reported series of patients with benign asbestos-related pleural diseases*[a]

| No. cases | Method | Fibers/ gram dried lung ($\times 10^6$)[a] | Reference |
|---|---|---|---|
| 29 | TEM | 1.14[c] | 69 |
| 20 | TEM | 0.54 (0.018–71) | 70 |
| 14 | SEM | 2.2 (0.1–13) | 57 |
| 7 | PCLM | 0.131 (0.029–0.378) | 71 |
| | TEM | 28.9 (9.2–83.5) | 71 |
| 5 | SEM | 1.14 (0.087–1.89) | 77 |

[a]Diseases reported include parietal pleural plaques (57,69,70), diffuse visceral pleural fibrosis (71), and rounded atelectasis (77).

[b]Values reported as median counts for million ($10^6$) of fibers per gram of dried lung tissue, with ranges indicated in parentheses (57,70,71,77) or mean fiber count (69).

[c]Range not reported.

Modified from ref. 23.

asbestos body counts of 900 and 710 per gram of wet lung tissue, respectively (Table 4), with a range of 2.6 to 74,500 (normal range: 0–20 asbestos bodies per gram). The median count for the plaque cases is considerably less than that of patients with asbestosis. The median asbestos body count tends to be higher in patients with bilateral plaques than in those with unilateral plaques (5). The author has also examined the asbestos body content of five patients with rounded atelectasis. The median count was 1,150 per gram, which is similar to that of patients with pleural plaques. The asbestos content of lung tissue in patients with benign asbestos effusion has not been reported.

It should be noted that almost all the studies of fiber burdens in patients with benign or malignant asbestos-related pleural disease have examined lung parenchyma. It is reasonable to assume that fibers that actually reach the pleura are the ones responsible for pleural disease, and that the dimensions and types of fibers that accumulate in the pleura are not necessarily similar to those that accumulate in the lung (23). Some investigators have observed that the fibers that accumulate in the pleura are principally short, chrysotile fibers, whereas those that accumulate in lung parenchyma are longer amphibole fibers (73). Three more recent studies have investigated the asbestos fiber content of parietal pleural plaques (74), diffuse visceral pleural fibrosis (75), and pigmented spots observed at time of thoracoscopy on the parietal pleura (76). In addition to chrysotile fibers, each of these studies has demonstrated the presence of long (>5 μm) amphibole fibers within the pleural tissues. In some instances, the concentration of fibers in the parietal pleura exceeded that in the adjacent lung tissues (74,76). These studies have unequivocally shown that chrysotile and amphibole fibers with dimensions that have shown the greatest degree of carcinogenic potential do in fact reach the pleural space.

**TABLE 7.** *Asbestos content of lung tissue in reported series of patients with carcinoma of the lung*

| No. cases | Method | Fibers/ gram dried lung (×10$^6$)[a] | Reference |
|---|---|---|---|
| 100 | PCLM | 0.009 (0–0.115) | 2 |
| 40 | TEM | 16[b] | 7 |
| 9 | TEM | 5.83 (3.10–73.3) | 37 |
| 75 | TEM | 2.18 (0.077–97) | 79 |
| 32 | TEM | 1.34[b] | 39 |

[a]Values reported as median counts for millions (X 10$^6$) of fibers per gram of dried lung tissue, with ranges indicated in parentheses (2,37,79) or mean fiber count (7) or geometric mean count (39).
[b]Ranges not reported.

## Carcinoma of the Lung

Asbestos exposure has been shown to increase the risk of lung cancer, especially among persons who also smoke cigarettes (49). Although the risk appears to be substantially increased among some groups of asbestos workers, it has been conservatively estimated that perhaps 2% of the lung cancers that occur every year in the United States may be attributable to asbestos (78). It is therefore interesting to examine the results of fiber analysis in various populations with carcinoma of the lung (Table 7).

As might be expected, the results of fiber analysis in series of patients with lung cancer depend on what criteria are used to select the cases. In the first two studies listed in Table 7 the patients selected were consecutive lung cancer cases from the general population (23). In such unselected populations there is no evidence of an abnormal pulmonary mineral fiber burden, and thus no evidence for a contributing role for asbestos in any lung cancers that occur. The next two studies listed in the table examined the asbestos content of the lung in groups of patients who had a history of substantial asbestos exposure (37,79). In fact, asbestosis was confirmed in 78% and 19% of the patients examined, respectively. These authors argued that the fiber burden in the lung, rather than the presence or absence of asbestosis, should be used as an indicator that a lung cancer may be asbestos related (79). Karjalainen et al. (80) studied the pulmonary concentration of asbestos fibers in 113 surgically treated male lung cancer patients and 297 autopsy cases among men serving as referents. The odds ratio for lung cancer risk was 1.7 [confidence interval (CI) 0.9–3.2] for patients with more than 1 million amphibole fibers per gram of dry lung as determined by scanning electron microscopy, and 5.3 (CI 1.9–14.8) for patients with more than 5 million amphibole fibers per gram. This is an important study, since it is the first to demonstrate an increased lung cancer risk based on the pulmonary asbestos fiber burden, independent of pathologic asbestosis and smoking.

The author has examined the fiber content of lung parenchyma in 234 patients with carcinoma of the lung (Table 4). Seventy of these patients had histologically documented asbestosis, 44 had parietal pleural plaques without asbestosis, and 120 had neither plaques nor asbestosis. All alleged some degree of asbestos exposure. Smoking histories were available for two-thirds of the cases, and all but 11 were smokers or former smokers. The median asbestos body count of patients with asbestosis was more than 35 times that of those who had pleural plaques and more than 300 times that of those who had neither plaques nor asbestosis (see Table 4). Similarly, asbestosis patients had a median asbestos fiber content nearly 20 times that of the "plaque patients" and more than 50 times that of subjects with neither plaques nor asbestosis. About 10% of the lung cancer patients with pleural plaques alone and about 5% of those with neither plaques nor asbestosis had an amphibole fiber count

**TABLE 8.** *Asbestos content of lung tissue in reference or control populations*

| No. cases | Method | Fibers/ gram dried lung ($\times 10^6$)[a] | Reference |
|---|---|---|---|
| 100 | PCLM | 0.007 (0–0.521) | 2 |
| 20 | TEM | 1.29 (0.260–7.55) | 3 |
| 23 | TEM | 0.62[b] | 6 |
| 20 | TEM | 11.2[b] | 7 |
| 28 | SEM | 0.25 (0–4.8) | 4 |

[a]Values reported as median counts for millions (X $10^6$) of fibers per gram of dried lung tissue, with ranges indicated in parentheses.
[b]Ranges not reported.
PCLM, phase content light microscopy; TEM, transmission electron microscopy; SEM, scanning electron microscopy.

within the range of values associated with an increased risk of lung cancer as determined by Karjalainen et al. (80).

### Normal Lungs (Unexposed Persons)

Several studies have reported the ranges of fiber burdens identified in control or reference populations (2–4,6,7). The results of these studies are compared in Table 8 and may be compared to the results from the author's laboratory in Table 4. The values differ somewhat from study to study, depending on the selection criteria for cases, the analytic technique, and the sizes of fibers counted. In any analysis of fiber burden for a population with a given disease it is critically important to compare the findings with those of an appropriate reference or control population for which an identical analytic technique was employed (23).

## ASBESTOS CONTENT OF LUNG TISSUE BY EXPOSURE CATEGORY

Relatively few studies have attempted to correlate tissue fiber burdens with occupational exposure history. Whitwell and coworkers (2) reported that the number of fibers found in the lungs correlated closely with a patient's occupation but not with the home environment. Sebastien and associates (73) described the tissue asbestos content in six workers with heavy asbestos exposure, six subjects who handled small amounts of asbestos during their professional lives, and six randomly selected workers who had no known exposure to asbestos. The tissue fiber burdens, as determined by PCLM and TEM, correlated well with the three occupational categories; however, the fiber counts by PCLM separated the three groups to a greater degree than did the counts by TEM. Churg and Warnock (81) reported pulmonary asbestos body counts in 252 urban patients older than 40 years and found that 32% of blue-collar men but fewer than 12% of white-collar men and blue- or white-collar women had more than 100 asbestos bodies per gram of wet lung tissue. The author has examined the pulmonary mineral fiber content in more than 200 patients whose occupational category was known. The results of these analyses are summarized by occupational category in the following sections and in Table 9.

### Insulators

A high prevalence of asbestos-associated disease has been reported among asbestos insulators (49). These patients, whose jobs include insulator, pipe fitter, pipe coverer, boilermaker, asbestos sawer, and asbestos plasterer, have the highest tissue asbestos contents of any of the occupational categories examined. The median asbestos body content among 59 insulators was 20,400 bodies per gram of wet lung, and the uncoated fiber content was 224,000 fibers 5 μm or longer per gram of wet lung. Thirty of these 59 insulators had histologically confirmed asbestosis.

### Shipyard Workers Other than Insulators

Large numbers of workers were exposed to asbestos while constructing ships during World War II, and United States shipyards have continued to be a source of asbestos

**TABLE 9.** *Asbestos content of lung tissue by exposure category*[a]

| | No. cases | AB/g (LM) | UF/g (SEM) |
|---|---|---|---|
| Insulators | 59 | 20,400 (16–1,600,000) | 224,000 (1,660–12,500,000) |
| Shipyard workers (other than insulators) | 60 | 3,600 (1.0–436,000) | 37,000 (680–1,890,000) |
| Railroad workers | 10 | 55 (<5–5,700) | 28,800 (3,470–90,000) |
| Brake-line work or repair | 8 | 50 (2.6–7740) | 15,400 (1,220–54,100) |
| Other asbestos | 24 | 2,360 (<3–322,000) | 68,800 (1,750–901,000) |
| Household contacts | 16 | 410 (2.0–8,200) | 23,900 (2,920–120,000) |
| Building occupants | 4 | 1.9 (<0.2–14) | 9,680 (6,120–25,000) |

[a]Values reported are the median values for asbestos bodies (AB) (as determined by light microscopy) or uncoated fibers (as determined by scanning electron microscopy) per gram of wet lung tissue, with ranges indicated in parentheses. Uncoated fibers (UF) were counted at a magnification of 1000× enumerating only fibers that were ≥5 μm in length; asbestos bodies were counted at a magnification of 400×.

exposure in the ensuing decades. The author has had the opportunity to examine the tissue asbestos content of 60 shipyard workers other than insulators—joiners, welders, riggers, sandblasters, fitters, shipwrights, electricians, draftsmen, handymen, engineers, and estimators. For the group, the median asbestos content was almost an order of magnitude lower than that of the insulators: median asbestos body and uncoated fiber counts were 3,600 and 37,000 per gram of wet lung, respectively (see Table 9). Many of these would be considered "bystander" exposures, since workers in this category often did not work directly with materials containing asbestos. Nineteen of these 60 shipyard workers had histologically confirmed asbestosis.

### Railroad Workers

During the steam engine era, railroad workers often were exposed to asbestos in their jobs, especially workers in the machine shops and those involved with ripping out old insulation from the steam boilers and replacing it with new insulation (82,83). Such exposure virtually disappeared when diesel engines replaced steam locomotives. The author has examined the tissue asbestos content in ten workers whose only known exposure to asbestos was in the railroad yards during the steam engine era. The median uncoated fiber content for these workers (28,800 fibers per gram) was similar to that of the shipyard workers who were not insulators, but the median asbestos body count (55 per gram) was considerably less (see Table 9). The latter finding is probably related to the predominant use of chrysotile asbestos in the railroad yards (82,83). Only one of the ten workers had histologically confirmed asbestosis.

### Brake Repair Workers

Large numbers of workers are involved with the repair and replacement of brake linings and clutch facings in the course of their daily work. Since these friction products contain asbestos, there has been some concern that the workers are at risk of developing asbestos-related disease. The author has examined the tissue asbestos content in eight brake-line repair workers, none of which satisfied histologic criteria for the diagnosis of asbestosis (33). The median uncoated fiber content for the group was 15,400 fibers 5 μm or longer per gram of wet lung, and the median asbestos body count was 50 per gram (see Table 9). The low risk of asbestos-related diseases among brake repair workers, and their relatively low pulmonary asbestos content, are apparently related to the nature of brake dust. The asbestos content of the dust is low (about 1%), most of which is chrysotile fibers (less than 1.0 μm in length), and the crystalline structure of much of the chrysotile in the dust has been altered by the heat generated during braking (84).

### Other Asbestos Workers

Persons in this category include asbestos cement workers, asbestos textile workers, chemical maintenance workers, welders (other than shipyard), machinists, asbestos filter manufacturers, roofing plant workers, refinery workers, sheet metal workers, and others exposed in industry to asbestos but not further specified. The 24 workers in this category had median asbestos body and uncoated fiber counts of 2,360 and 68,000 per gram, respectively (Table 9). These values are similar to those among the 60 shipyard workers but considerably less than those observed among the 59 insulators. Six of the 24 asbestos workers in this category had histologically confirmed asbestosis.

### Household Contacts

An increased risk of developing asbestos-related disease has been reported among household contacts of asbestos workers (50,51), apparently owing to asbestos fibers brought home on the worker's clothing. Few studies have analyzed the fiber content of lung tissue from household contacts (7,85,86), and in general their lung fiber burdens were similar to those of asbestos workers who suffered mild to moderate exposures. The author has examined the pulmonary asbestos content in 16 household contacts of asbestos workers. Seven housewives, five daughters, and one mother had malignant mesothelioma (11 pleural and two peritoneal), and the remaining three housewives of asbestos workers had lung cancer. Two of the 16 subjects had histologically confirmed asbestosis. The median asbestos body content for these 16 household exposures was 410 bodies per gram, and the median uncoated fiber count was 23,900 fibers per gram of wet lung (Table 9). The asbestos body counts in these cases are intermediate between those of railroad workers with an asbestos exposure history and shipyard workers other than insulators.

### Building Occupants

There has been considerable scientific and public debate about the possible risks of asbestos-related disease resulting from living or working (or attending school) in buildings containing asbestos (87,88). The measured fiber levels in buildings are extremely low (89). There is a single case report in the literature of a pleural mesothelioma occurring in a woman who was an office worker in a building whose ceiling material contained amosite asbestos, and considerable numbers of amosite fibers were identified in this patient's lung tissues (90). The author has examined the pulmonary asbestos content of four patients whose only known exposure to asbestos was in buildings with asbestos insulation. Two patients had pleural mesothelioma, one peritoneal mesothelioma, and

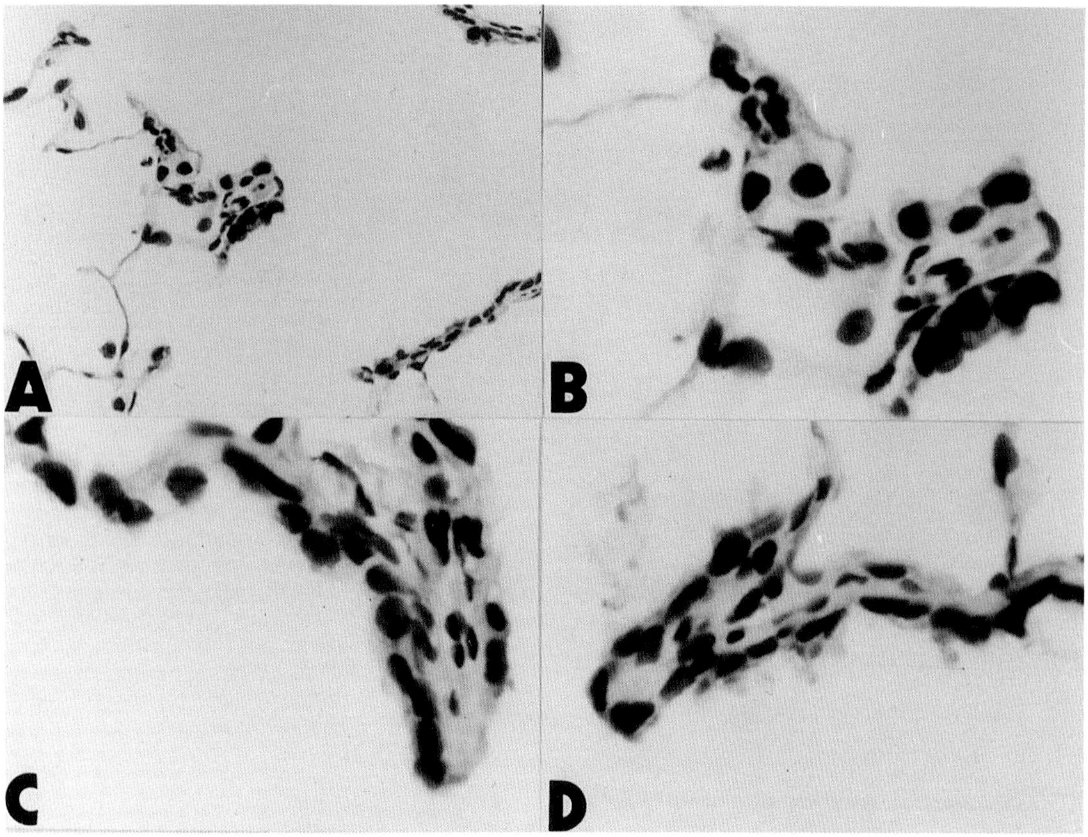


**COLOR PLATE 22–1.** Asbestos induces PCNA expression at the sites of fiber deposition. Rats were exposed 5 hours to an aerosol of asbestos at 10 mg/m$^3$ **(A** and **B)**, exposed 5 hours to an aerosol of carbonyl iron at a concentration of 50 mg/m$^3$ **(C)**, or unexposed **(D)**. Four days postexposure the animals were sacrificed and the left lung of each animal was perfused with fixative. Histologic sections were prepared and immunostained with a monoclonal antibody specific for PCNA. Panel A identifies a fiber deposition site—the bronchiolar-alveolar duct bifurcation at low magnification (200×). Panels B through D are at higher magnification (1000×) to demonstrate PCNA immunostaining in the three exposure groups—asbestos (B), iron (C), and unexposed (D). Inhalation exposure of rats to asbestos induces PCNA expression rapidly at the fiber deposition sites (see ref. 169 for details).

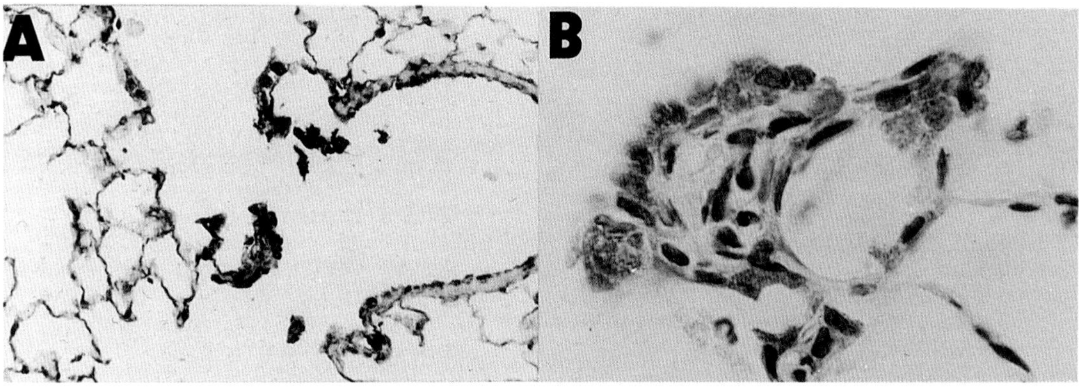


**COLOR PLATE 22–3.** PDGF-A expression in asbestos-exposed rats. **A:** In analyses similar to that depicted in Fig. 2 (of Chapter 22), PDGF-A mRNA expression was detected by *in situ* hybridization in lung sections from rats 2 days postexposure to asbestos (200× magnification). Dark-staining cells are positive for PDGF mRNA. Negative control assays appeared similar to those for PDGF-B shown in Fig. 2. **B:** Immunohistochemical detection (by the DAB method, brown stain) of PDGF-A protein in the lungs of rats 2 days postexposure to asbestos (1000× magnification) (see ref. 225 for details.)

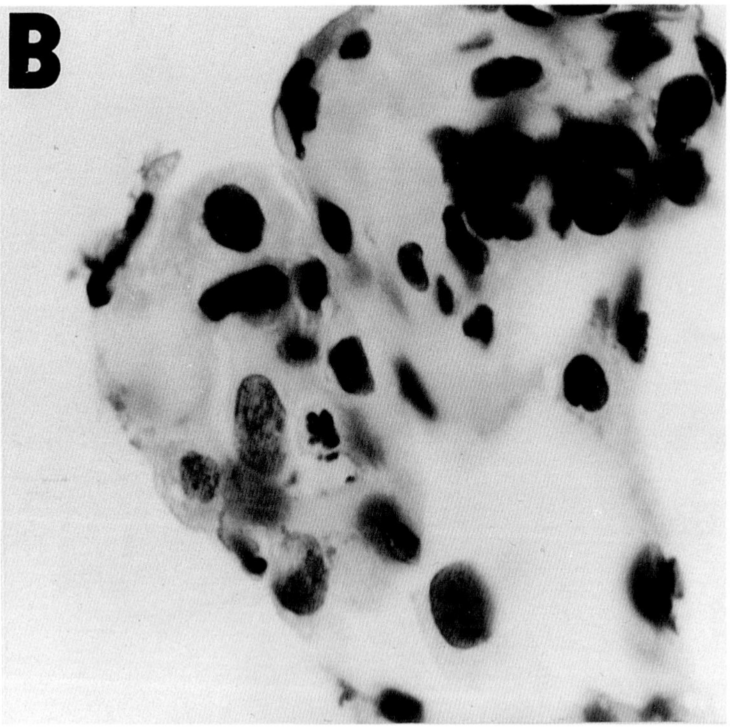


**COLOR PLATE 22–5B.** Prolonged p53 expression in asbestos-exposed rats. p53 immunostaining in rat lung sections from animals 8 days postinhalation exposure to asbestos. The micrograph (1000×) reveals high levels of p53 immunostaining. A variety of cell types are p53-positive including probable macrophages, epithelial, and interstitial cells.

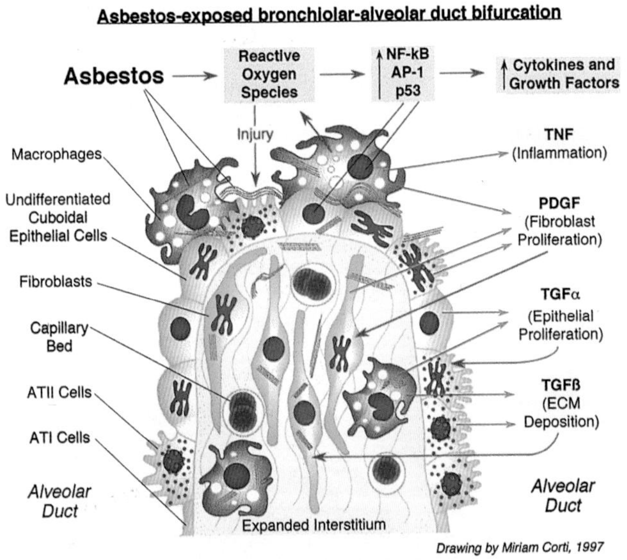


**COLOR PLATE 22–6B.** A model of particle-induced fibrosis. This diagram illustrates many of the responses of the lung to inhaled particles that are described in the text. Asbestos induces signaling leading to cytokine release that promotes fibroproliferative lung disease.

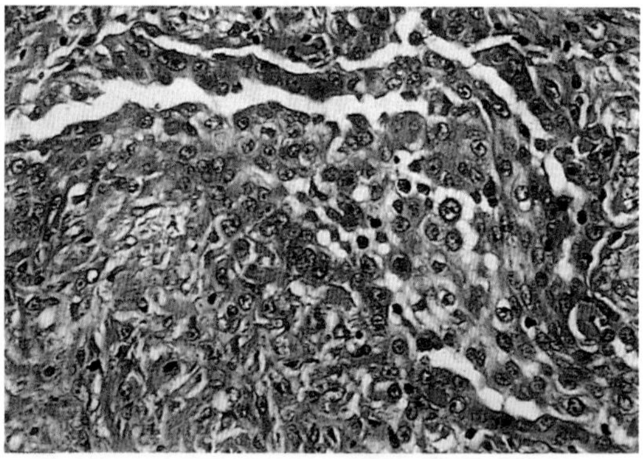

**COLOR PLATE 24–22.** Light microscopy of the tumor with hematoxylin-phloxin-saffron (HPS) staining demonstrates malignant mesothelioma with mixed epithelial and sarcomatous features (780×). (Courtesy of Gurdip Sidhu, M.D., and Rosemary Wieczorek, M.D.)

one (not a smoker) pulmonary adenocarcinoma. The median asbestos body and uncoated fiber content for these four cases was 1.9 bodies per gram and 9,680 fibers per gram wet lung, respectively (Table 9). One patient with a normal asbestos body count was a teacher's aide for 18 years who developed pleural mesothelioma and parietal pleural plaques. Her lung tissues contained chrysotile and tremolite asbestos, talc, and other nonfibrous minerals, which were also identified in acoustic ceiling tile in the building where she worked (91). Although limited data are available on this controversial topic, the asbestos content of the lungs of patients exposed in buildings is generally in the range of background levels (see Table 4).

## IDENTIFICATION OF FIBER TYPES

A number of studies have found that when humans are exposed to a mixture of chrysotile and amphibole asbestos fibers it is principally the amphibole fibers that accumulate in the lung parenchyma (5,38,39,55,63, 64,69,70). In some studies, the chrysotile content in the exposed population was not different from that of a reference population (63,64). These observations are in agreement with findings of experimental animal studies, which show preferential accumulation of amphiboles in the lungs of rats (47) and a tendency for chrysotile to be broken down into smaller components that can ostensibly be removed by clearance mechanisms (19). The author has examined the chemical composition of more than 3,400 fibers from more than 250 patients by means of energy dispersive spectrometry, and these studies show that as the pulmonary asbestos burden increases, the proportion of commercial amphiboles (amosite or crocidolite) also increases (5,33,56,67,72,92). Uncoated commercial amphibole fibers are generally undetectable in patients from the general population but account for as much as 100% of the fiber burden among individuals with asbestosis (see Table 4) (56). Noncommercial amphiboles (tremolite, anthophyllite, actinolite) and chrysotile together accounted for only 2.5% of fibers 5 μm or longer that were isolated from the lungs of patients with asbestosis but for 16% of fibers from control lungs and 10% from patients with malignant mesothelioma (67). The vast majority of asbestos bodies have an amosite or crocidolite core (93–95). Chrysotile asbestos bodies do occur (92,95), but they are distinctly uncommon.

A substantial percentage of commercial amphibole fibers isolated from human lung samples are long (>8 μm) and thin (<0.25 μm). These are the dimensions that are associated with the greatest carcinogenic and fibrogenic potential (66,93,96). Commercial amphiboles accounted for as much as 5% to 10% of asbestos imported into the United States in the past (20). Although small amounts of crocidolite were imported, most of this was incorporated into cement for the manufacture of water and sewage pipes.

A variety of nonasbestos mineral fibers have also been identified in human lung tissue samples (21,22). Among members of the general population, nonasbestos mineral fibers actually outnumber asbestos fibers by a ratio of about 4:1. The most commonly encountered fibers are talc, silica, rutile, kaolinite, mica or feldspar, other silicates, and various metal oxides. Calcium phosphate (apatite) fibers were common in the TEM study of Churg (21) but not in the SEM study of Roggli (22). Various manmade mineral fibers may also be occasionally detected in human lung samples. Although nonasbestos mineral fibers enumerated in the previous studies meet the regulatory definition of a fiber—i.e., a mineral particle with a length-to-diameter ratio of at least 3:1 and roughly parallel sides—from a mineralogic perspective, many of these are actually cleavage fragments derived from nonfibrous minerals. Some ferruginous bodies also have nonasbestos mineral fiber cores, and these have been referred to as pseudoasbestos bodies or nonasbestos ferruginous bodies (15,92,95).

## REFERENCES


1. Smith MJ, Naylor B. A method of extracting ferruginous bodies from sputum and pulmonary tissues. *Am J Clin Pathol* 1972;58:250–254.
2. Whitwell F, Scott J, Grimshaw M. Relationship between occupations and asbestos fibre content of the lungs in patients with pleural mesothelioma, lung cancer, and other diseases. *Thorax* 1977;32:377–386.
3. Churg A, Warnock ML. Asbestos fibers in the general population. *Am Rev Respir Dis* 1980;122:669–678.
4. Mowé G, Gylseth B, Hartveit F, Skaug V. Fiber concentration in lung tissue of patients with malignant mesothelioma: a case-control study. *Cancer* 1985;56:1089–1093.
5. Roggli VL, Pratt PC, Brody AR. Asbestos content of lung tissue in asbestos-associated diseases: a study of 110 cases. *Br J Ind Med* 1986; 43:18–28.
6. Case BW, Sebastien P. Environmental and occupational exposures to chrysotile asbestos: a comparative microanalytic study. *Arch Environ Health* 1987;42:185–191.
7. Gaudichet A, Janson X, Monchaux G, et al. Assessment by analytical microscopy of the total lung fibre burden in mesothelioma patients matched with four other pathological series. *Ann Occup Hyg* 1988; 32:213–223.
8. Mossman BT, Kessler JB, Levy BW, Craighead JE. Interaction of crocidolite asbestos with hamster respiratory mucosa in organ culture. *Lab Invest* 1977;36:131–139.
9. Churg A. The uptake of mineral particles by pulmonary epithelial cells. *Am J Respir Crit Care Med* 1996;154:1124–1140.
10. Brody AR, Hill LH, Adkins B, O'Connor RW. Chrysotile asbestos inhalation in rats: deposition patterns and reaction of alveolar epithelium and pulmonary macrophages. *Am Rev Respir Dis* 1981;123: 670–679.
11. Holt PF. Transport of inhaled dust to extrapulmonary sites. *J Pathol* 1981;133:123–129.
12. Roggli VL, Benning TL. Asbestos bodies in pulmonary hilar lymph nodes. *Mod Pathol* 1990;3:513–517.
13. Warheit DB, Chang LY, Hill LH, Hook GE, Crapo JD, Brody AR. Pulmonary macrophage accumulation and asbestos-induced lesions at sites of fiber deposition. *Am Rev Respir Dis* 1984;129:301–310.
14. Green GM, Jakab GJ, Low RB, Davis GS. Defense mechanisms of the respiratory membrane. *Am Rev Respir Dis* 1977;115:479–514.
15. Churg A, Warnock ML. Asbestos and other ferruginous bodies: their formation and clinical significance. *Am J Pathol* 1981;102:447–456.

16. Morgan A, Holmes A. The enigmatic asbestos body: its formation and significance in asbestos-related disease. *Environ Res* 1985;38:283–292.
17. Dodson RF, O'Sullivan MF, Williams MG, Jr., Hurst GA. Analysis of cores of ferruginous bodies from former asbestos workers. *Environ Res* 1982;28:171–178.
18. Greenberg SD. Asbestos. In: Dail DH, Hammar SP, eds. *Pulmonary pathology.* New York: Springer-Verlag, 1988;619–635.
19. Coin PG, Osornio-Vargas AR, Roggli VL, Brody AR. Pulmonary fibrogenesis after three consecutive inhalation exposures to chrysotile asbestos. *Am J Respir Crit Care Med* 1996;154:1511–1519.
20. Roggli VL, Coin P. Mineralogy of asbestos. In: Roggli VL, Greenberg SD, Pratt PC, eds.*Pathology of asbestos-associated diseases.* Boston: Little, Brown, 1992;1–17.
21. Churg A. Nonasbestos pulmonary mineral fibers in the general population. *Environ Res* 1983;31:189–200.
22. Roggli VL. Nonasbestos mineral fibers in human lungs. In: Russell PE, ed. *Microbeam analysis—1989.* San Francisco: San Francisco Press, 1989;57–59.
23. Roggli VL. Human disease consequences of fiber exposures—a review of human lung pathology and fiber burden data. *Environ Health Perspect* 1990;88:295–303.
24. Roggli VL, Coin PG, MacIntyre NR, Bell DY. Asbestos content of bronchoalveolar lavage fluid: a comparison of light and scanning electron microscopic analysis. *Acta Cytol* 1994;38:502–510.
25. Rom WN, Churg A, Leapman R, Fiori C, Swyt C. Evaluation of alveolar macrophage particle burden in individuals occupationally exposed to inorganic dusts. *J Aerosol Med* 1990;3:543–556.
26. Karjalainen A, Piipari R, Mantyla T, et al. Asbestos bodies in bronchoalveolar lavage in relation to asbestos bodies and asbestos fibres in lung parenchyma. *Eur Respir J* 1996;9:1000–1005.
27. DeVuyst P, Dumortier P, Moulin E, et al. Asbestos bodies in bronchoalveolar lavage reflect lung asbestos body concentration. *Eur Respir J* 1988;1:362–367.
28. O'Sullivan MF, Corn CJ, Dodson RF. Comparative efficiency of Nuclepore filters of various pore sizes as used in digestion studies of tissue. *Environ Res* 1987;43:97–103.
29. Gylseth B, Churg A, Davis JMG, et al. Analysis of asbestos fibers and asbestos bodies in tissue samples from human lung: an international interlaboratory trial. *Scand J Work Environ Health* 1985;11:107–110.
30. Morgan A, Holmes A. The distribution and characteristics of asbestos fibers in the lungs of Finnish anthophyllite mine workers. *Environ Res* 1984;33:62–75.
31. Morgan A, Holmes A. Distribution and characteristics of amphibole asbestos fibres in the left lung of an insulation worker measured with the light microscope. *Br J Ind Med* 1983;40:45–50.
32. Craighead JE, Abraham JL, Churg A, et al. Pathology of asbestos-associated diseases of the lungs and pleural cavities: diagnostic criteria and proposed grading schema. *Arch Pathol Lab Med* 1982;106:544–596.
33. Roggli VL. Pathology of human asbestosis: a critical review. In: Fenoglio-Preiser CM, ed. *Advances in pathology.* Chicago: Year Book, 1989;2:31–60.
34. Becklake MR. Asbestos-related diseases of the lung and other organs: their epidemiology and implications for clinical practice. *Am Rev Respir Dis* 1976;114:187–227.
35. Craighead JE, Mossman BT. Pathogenesis of asbestos-associated diseases. *N Engl J Med* 1982;306:1446–1455.
36. Ashcroft T, Heppleston AG. The optical and electron microscopic determination of pulmonary asbestos fibre concentration and its relation to the human pathological reaction. *J Clin Pathol* 1973;26:224–234.
37. Warnock ML, Kuwahara TJ, Wolery G. The relation of asbestos burden to asbestosis and lung cancer. *Pathol Annu* 1983;18:109–145.
38. Wagner JC, Moncrief CB, Coles R, Griffiths DM, Munday DE. Correlation between fibre content of the lungs and disease in naval dockyard workers. *Br J Ind Med* 1986;43:391–395.
39. Churg A, Vedal S. Fiber burden and patterns of asbestos-related disease in workers with heavy mixed amosite and chrysotile exposure. *Am J Respir Crit Care Med* 1994;150:663–669.
40. Roggli VL, Pratt PC. Numbers of asbestos bodies on iron-stained tissue sections in relation to asbestos body counts in lung tissue digests. *Hum Pathol* 1983;14:355–361.
41. Roggli VL. Scanning electron microscopic analysis of mineral fiber content of lung tissue in the evaluation of diffuse pulmonary fibrosis. *Scanning Microsc* 1991;5:71–83.
42. Timbrell V, Ashcroft T, Goldstein B, et al. Relationships between retained amphibole fibers and fibrosis in human lung tissue specimens. *Ann Occup Hyg* 1988;32:323–340.
43. Lippmann M. Asbestos exposure indices. *Environ Res* 1988;46:86–106.
44. Churg A, Wright JL, De Paoli L, Wiggs B. Mineralogic correlates of fibrosis in chrysotile miners and millers. *Am Rev Respir Dis* 1989;139: 891–896.
45. Churg A, Wright J, Wiggs B, De Paoli L. Mineralogic parameters related to amosite asbestos—induced fibrosis in humans. *Am Rev Respir Dis* 1990;142:1331–1336.
46. Goodglick LA, Kane AB. Cytotoxicity of long and short crocidolite asbestos fibers *in vitro* and *in vivo*. *Cancer Res* 1990;50:5153–5163.
47. Wagner JC, Berry G, Skidmore JW, Timbrell V. The effects of inhalation of asbestos in rats. *Br J Cancer* 1974;29:252–269.
48. Wagner JC, Sleggs CA, Marchand P. Diffuse pleural mesothelioma and asbestos exposure in the North Western Cape Province. *Br J Ind Med* 1960;17:260–271.
49. Selikoff IJ, Lee DH. *Asbestos and disease.* New York: Academic Press, 1978.
50. Newhouse ML, Thompson H. Mesothelioma of pleura and peritoneum following exposure to asbestos in the London area. *Br J Ind Med* 1965; 22:261–269.
51. Anderson HA, Lillis R, Daum SM, Selikoff IJ. Asbestosis among household contacts of asbestos factory workers. *Ann NY Acad Sci* 1979; 330:387–399.
52. Roggli VL, Sanfilippo F, Shelburne JD. Mesothelioma. In: Roggli VL, Greenberg SD, Pratt PC, eds. *Pathology of asbestos-associated diseases.* Boston: Little, Brown, 1992;109–164.
53. Warnock ML. Lung asbestos burden in shipyard and construction workers with mesothelioma: comparison with burdens in subjects with asbestosis or lung cancer. *Environ Res* 1989;50:68–85.
54. Churg A, Wiggs B. Fiber size and number in amphibole asbestos—induced mesothelioma. *Am J Pathol* 1984;115:437–442.
55. Churg A, Wiggs B, De Paoli L, Kampe B, Stevens B. Lung asbestos content in chrysotile workers with mesothelioma. *Am Rev Respir Dis* 1984;130:1042–1045.
56. Srebro SH, Roggli VL, Samsa GP. Malignant mesothelioma associated with low pulmonary tissue asbestos burdens: a light and scanning electron microscopic analysis of 18 cases. *Mod Pathol* 1995;8:614–621.
57. Gylseth B, Mowé G, Skaug V, Wannag A. Inorganic fibers in lung tissue from patients with pleural plaques or malignant mesothelioma. *Scand J Work Environ Health* 1981;7:109–113.
58. Antman KH. Malignant mesothelioma. *N Engl J Med* 1980;303: 200–202.
59. Chahinian AP, Pajak TF, Holland JF, Norton L, Ambinder RM, Mandel EM. Diffuse malignant mesothelioma: prospective evaluation of 69 patients. *Ann Intern Med* 1982;96:746–755.
60. Roggli VL. Malignant mesothelioma and duration of asbestos exposure: correlation with tissue mineral fiber content. *Ann Occup Hyg* 1995;39:363–374.
61. Roggli VL, Oury TD, Moffatt EJ. Malignant mesothelioma in women, In: Rosen PP, Fechner RE, eds. *ASCP reviews of pathology.* Chicago: ASCP Press (in press, 1998).
62. Rom WN, Travis WD, Brody AR. Cellular and molecular basis of the asbestos-related diseases. *Am Rev Respir Dis* 1991;143:408–422.
63. McDonald AD, McDonald JC, Pooley FD. Mineral fibre content of lung in mesothelial tumours in North America. *Ann Occup Hyg* 1982;26:417–422.
64. McDonald JC, Armstrong B, Case B, et al. Mesothelioma and asbestos fiber type: evidence from lung tissue analyses. *Cancer* 1989;63: 1544–1547.
65. Dufresne A, Begin R, Churg A, Masse S. Mineral fiber content of lungs in patients with mesothelioma seeking compensation in Quebec. *Am J Respir Crit Care Med* 1996;153:711–718.
66. Stanton MF, Layard M, Tegeris A, et al. Relation of particle dimension to carcinogenicity in amphibole asbestoses and other fibrous minerals. *J Natl Cancer Inst* 1981;67:965–975.
67. Roggli VL, Pratt PC, Brody AR. Asbestos fiber type in malignant mesothelioma: an analytical electron microscopic study of 94 cases. *Am J Ind Med* 1993;23:605–614.
68. Schwartz DA. New developments in asbestos-induced pleural disease. *Chest* 1991;99:191–198.
69. Churg A. Asbestos fibers and pleural plaques in a general autopsy population. *Am J Pathol* 1982;109:88–96.
70. Warnock ML, Prescott BT, Kuwahara TJ. Numbers and types of

asbestos fibers in subjects with pleural plaques. *Am J Pathol* 1982; 109:37–46.
71. Stephens M, Gibbs AR, Pooley FD, Wagner JC. Asbestos-induced diffuse pleural fibrosis: pathology and mineralogy. *Thorax* 1987;42: 583–588.
72. Roggli VL. Analytical electron microscopy of mineral fibers from human lungs. In: Bailey GW, ed. *Proceedings of the 45th Annual Meeting of the Electron Microscopy Society of America.* San Francisco: San Francisco Press, 1987;666–669.
73. Sebastien P, Fondimare A, Bignon J, Monchaux G, Desbordes J, Bonnaud G. Topographic distribution of asbestos fibers in human lung in relation to occupational and nonoccupational exposure. In: Walton WH, McGovern B, eds. *Inhaled particles IV.* Oxford: Pergamon Press, 1977; 435–444.
74. Dodson RF, Williams MG, Corn CJ, Brollo A, Bianchi C. Asbestos content of lung tissue, lymph nodes, and pleural plaques from former shipyard workers. *Am Rev Respir Dis* 1990;142:843–847.
75. Gibbs AR, Stephens M, Griffiths DM, Blight BJN, Pooley FD. Fibre distribution in the lungs and pleura of subjects with asbestos related diffuse pleural fibrosis. *Br J Ind Med* 1991;48:762–770.
76. Boutin C, Dumortier P, Rey F, Viallat JR, De Vuyst P. Black spots concentrate oncogenic asbestos fibers in the parietal pleura. *Am J Respir Crit Care Med* 1996;153:444–449.
77. Roggli VL. Fiber analysis. In: Rom WN, ed. *Environmental and occupational medicine,* 2nd ed. Boston: Little, Brown, 1992;255–267.
78. Gaensler EA, McLoud TC, Carrington CB. Thoracic surgical problems in asbestos-related disorders. *Ann Thorac Surg* 1985;40:82–96.
79. Warnock ML, Isenberg W. Asbestos burden and the pathology of lung cancer. *Chest* 1986;89:20–26.
80. Karjalainen A, Anttila S, Vanhala E, Vainio H. Asbestos exposure and the risk of lung cancer in a general urban population. *Scand J Work Environ Health* 1994;20:243–250.
81. Churg A, Warnock ML. Correlation of quantitative asbestos body counts and occupation in urban patients. *Arch Pathol Lab Med* 1977; 101:629–634.
82. Mancuso TF. Mesothelioma among machinists in railroad and other industries. *Am J Ind Med* 1983;4:501–513.
83. Mancuso TF. Relative risk of mesothelioma among railroad machinists exposed to chrysotile. *Am J Ind Med* 1988;13:639–657.
84. Williams RL, Muhlbaier JL. Asbestos brake emissions. *Environ Res* 1982;29:70–82.
85. Huncharek M, Capotorto JV, Muscat J. Domestic asbestos exposure, lung fibre burden, and pleural mesothelioma in a housewife. *Br J Ind Med* 1989;46:354–355.
86. Gibbs AR, Griffiths DM, Pooley FD, Jones JSP. Comparison of fibre types and size distributions in lung tissues of paraoccupational and occupational cases of malignant mesothelioma. *Br J Ind Med* 1990; 47:621–626.
87. Mossman BT, Bignon J, Corn M, Seaton A, Gee JBL. Asbestos: scientific developments and implications for public policy. *Science* 1990; 247:294–301.
88. Gaensler EA. Asbestos exposure in buildings. *Clin Chest Med* 1992; 13:231–242.
89. Crump KS, Farrar DB. Statistical analysis of data on airborne asbestos levels collected in an EPA survey of public buildings. *Regul Toxicol Pharmacol* 1989;10:51–62.
90. Stein RC, Kitajewska JY, Kirkham JB, Tait N, Sinha G, Rudd RM. Pleural mesothelioma resulting from exposure to amosite asbestos in a building. *Respir Med* 1989;83:237–239.
91. Roggli VL, Longo WE. Mineral fiber content of lung tissue in patients with environmental exposures: household contacts vs. building occupants. *Ann NY Acad Sci* 1991;643:511–518.
92. Roggli VL. Scanning electron microscopic analysis of mineral fibers from human lungs. In: Ingram P, Shelburne JD, Roggli VL, eds. *Microprobe analysis in medicine.* Washington, DC: Hemisphere, 1989; 97–110.
93. Roggli VL, Brody AR. Imaging techniques for application to lung toxicology. In: Gardner DE, Crapo JD, Massaro EJ, eds. *Toxicology of the lung.* New York: Raven Press, 1988;117–145.
94. Roggli VL, Pratt PC, Brody AR. Analysis of tissue mineral fiber content. In: Roggli VL, Greenberg SD, Pratt PC, eds. *Pathology of asbestos-associated diseases.* Boston: Little, Brown, 1992;299–345.
95. Roggli VL. Asbestos bodies and non-asbestos ferruginous bodies. In: Roggli VL, Greenberg SD, Pratt PC, eds. *Pathology of asbestos-associated diseases.* Boston: Little, Brown, 1992;39–75.
96. Roggli VL, Brody AR. Experimental models of asbestos-related diseases. In: Roggli VL, Greenberg SD, Pratt PC, eds. *Pathology of asbestos-associated diseases.* Boston: Little, Brown, 1992;257–297.

*Environmental and Occupational Medicine, Third Edition,* edited by William N. Rom.
Lippincott–Raven Publishers, Philadelphia © 1998.

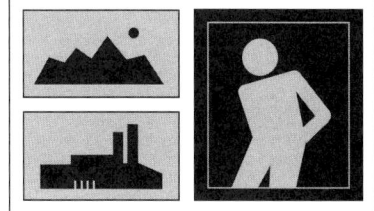

# CHAPTER 24

# Asbestos-Related Diseases

William N. Rom

## HISTORY

Asbestos is a fibrous hydrated magnesium silicate with over 3,000 commercial uses due to its indestructible nature, fire resistance, and spinnability. It has been used since ancient times with Plutarch (46–120 A.D.) commenting on its use as a wick for oil lamps and use as napkins that can be cleansed in a fire (1). This property led the Greeks to call asbestos *amiantos* (1). Mining and milling began in the late 19th century with asbestos being used in textiles and insulation materials. W. E. Cooke described the first case of asbestosis in 1924 in a 33-year-old textile worker exposed since 1899 who had extensive pulmonary fibrosis (1).

## PHYSICAL PROPERTIES

Approximately 95% of United States consumption has been chrysotile, a serpentine form of asbestos. Other asbestos types are the amphiboles, notably amosite mined in South Africa and crocidolite mined in the Cape Province of South Africa and western Australia. Anthophyllite had minimal commercial use in Finland. These asbestos fiber types have strikingly different physical characteristics with chrysotile tending to be wavy and long, and it occurs in bundles (Fig. 1); crocidolite is needle-shaped with many long fibers; and amosite is similar to crocidolite but generally thicker (Fig. 2). A fiber is defined as being at least three times as long as it is wide.

W. N. Rom: Division of Pulmonary and Critical Care Medicine, Departments of Medicine and Environmental Medicine; and Chest Service, Bellevue Hospital Center, New York University Medical Center, New York, New York 10016.

## USE IN INDUSTRY

The physical properties of asbestos that resulted in its widespread use are (a) insulation against heat, cold, and noise; (b) incombustibility; (c) good dielectric properties; (d) great tensile strength; (e) flexibility; and (f) resistance to corrosion by alkalis and most acids. Asbestos was initially woven extensively into fireproof textiles followed by insulation uses for boilers and pipes. Asbestos was used for yarn, felt, paper, millboard, shingles, paints, cloth, tape, filters, and wire insulation. More recently asbestos has been used in cement pipes for potable water, gaskets and friction materials including brake linings, and roofing and floor products. Asbestos was extensively used for ship construction during World War II. Approximately 2.7 million tons were produced in 1994 and world mine production, in order of output, was based in Russia, Canada, Kazakhstan, China, and Brazil. World production has declined in the 1990s to approximately 50% of that of the peak in 1973. United States consumption was less than 27,000 metric tons in 1994. Asbestos in the United States increased after 1941, and during the 1950s and 1960s averaged 625,000 tons of chrysotile, 16,000 tons of amosite, and 18,000 tons of crocidolite per year.

## TYPES OF EXPOSURE

Primary exposures occurred to miners and millers followed by secondary exposures in manufacturing plants producing textiles, friction materials, tiles, and insulation materials. Epidemiologic studies could focus on cohorts in these plants since asbestos fiber type was often specified and dust measurements obtained. However, the construction trades endured the most significant exposures. These trades included asbestos insulators (called laggers in the United Kingdom) who mixed asbestos cement on site to

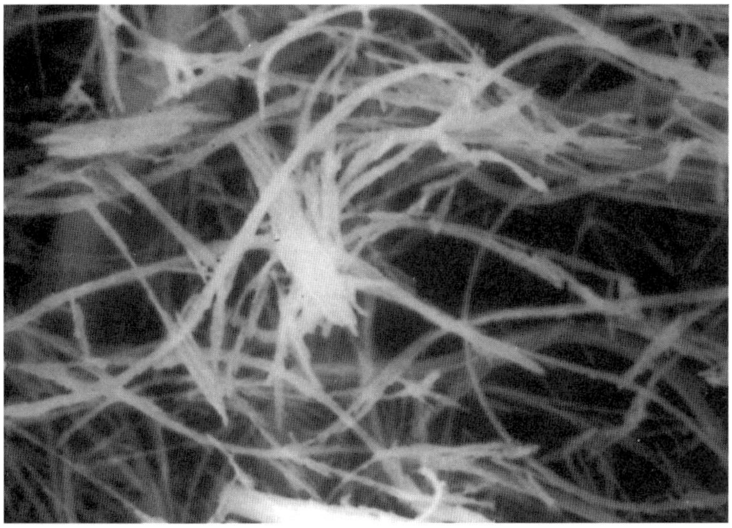

**FIG. 1.** Electron micrograph of National Institute of Environmental Health Sciences intermediate-length chrysotile (×3,000). (Courtesy of T. Takemura, M.D.)

insulate joints and elbows on pipes, boilermakers and sheet-metal workers who worked adjacent to the asbestos workers, and electricians, carpenters, plumbers, and others who worked in the vicinity of asbestos work. Seldom were any measurements of airborne exposure made. Asbestos workers and other construction workers wore their asbestos-covered clothes home and their wives and children were exposed upon greeting them or washing their work clothes. These household contact exposures are often referred to as indirect exposures, and those exposed while working near asbestos insulators received bystander exposure. Lilis and colleagues (2) compared directly asbestos insulation workers ($n$ = 1,584) to sheet-metal workers ($n$ = 1,330), finding a remarkable difference in asbestosis with 83.5% abnormal radiographs (55% parenchymal opacities) among the insulators but only 42% abnormal radiographs (17% parenchymal opacities) in the sheet-metal workers. These variations in prevalence likely result from their differences in intensity and duration of exposure. Approximately 14 million persons were exposed to asbestos at 2 to 3 fiber/ml concentrations in their U.S. workplace from 1940 to 1979 and were alive in 1980 (3). From this cohort, estimates have been made that there would be a peak incidence of approximately 3,000 mesothelioma deaths and 5,000 asbestos-related lung cancer deaths by the late 1990s. Pleural fibrosis remains a relatively common finding among asbestos-exposed blue collar workers, whereas asbestosis is becoming increasingly uncommon.

## PLEURAL FIBROSIS, ROUNDED ATELECTASIS, AND PLEURAL EFFUSION

### Pathology

Pleural disease is the most common manifestation of asbestos exposure and is subdivided into circumscribed

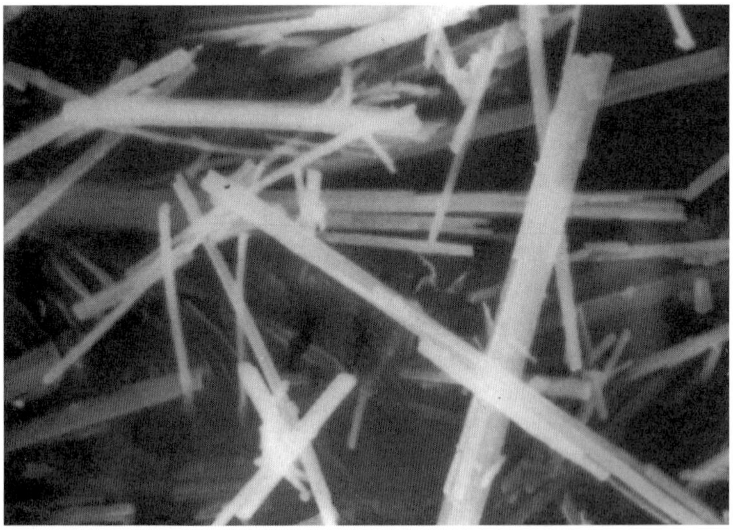

**FIG. 2.** Electron micrograph of International Union Against Cancer standard sample of amosite (×3,000). (Courtesy of T. Takemura, M.D.)

pleural plaques and diffuse pleural thickening. Circumscribed pleural plaques are discontinuous, whereas diffuse pleural thickening is a continuous sheet, usually 5 to 10 cm in craniocaudal extent and in 90% of the cases involves the costophrenic angle. In about one-third of the cases, diffuse pleural thickening can be related to a prior benign, asbestos-related pleural effusion diagnosed by thoracentesis or on serial chest radiographs (4). In another third, confluent plaques give rise to diffuse thickening. Pleural calcifications develop in fibrohyaline lesions as onset from exposure increases.

The histology is characterized by a paucity of cells with extensive collagen fibrils arranged in a basket weave pattern. The parietal pleura is uniformly involved with minimal thickening of the visceral pleura. There is an absence of adhesions between the two pleural surfaces.

*In vitro* culture of pleural mesothelial cells has demonstrated their capability of synthesizing collagens types I, III, and IV, elastin, laminin, and fibronectin (5). Interestingly, these cells in culture were able to organize these macromolecular connective tissue components into an assemblage of extracellular matrix limited to the base of the cell. Pleural mesothelial cells internalize asbestos via the $\alpha v\beta 5$ integrin receptor, which recognizes vitronectin (6).

### Natural History

Diffuse pleural fibrosis may be preceded by a pleural effusion years earlier and is accompanied by blunting of the costophrenic angle. Circumscribed pleural plaques are not associated with a pleural effusion and occur most frequently along the posterior ribs and on top of the diaphragm. They increase in size very slowly, usually decades, and do not give rise to diffuse malignant mesothelioma.

### Epidemiology

Hyaline and calcified pleural plaques were noted in the 1960s to be an index of exposure to asbestos (Fig. 3). Shipyard workers were found to have pleural abnormalities ten times more frequently than parenchymal disease (7). The higher the exposure, the more likely there will be extensive calcified pleura plaques as well as parenchymal fibrosis. Among British shipyard workers, 36% of those with continuous exposure as laggers developed pleural plaques, extensive pleural thickening (5%), or pulmonary fibrosis (7%). Those with intermittent exposure had a 6% prevalence of plaques and no pulmonary fibrosis. Interestingly, the prevalence of pleural plaques increased from 17% at 10 years since first exposure to 70% at 30 years from onset among those with continuous exposure, and from 1% at 10 years to 16% at 30 years for those with intermittent exposure.

### Clinical and Physiologic Features

Pleural plaques by themselves are generally considered to be asymptomatic without pleural rubs or rales on auscultation of the chest.

Pleural disease has been known to reduce pulmonary function since the 1970s. Among 998 shipyard workers in Groton, Connecticut, with 15 or more years of asbestos exposure, 122 had pleural changes without parenchymal abnormalities and 484 had normal films (8); 17% of those with pleural changes had forced vital capacity (FVC)<80% predicted compared to 9% of normal chest x-rays ($p<0.05$). However, all spirometric values were significantly reduced only among smokers and ex-smokers in both groups. Diffuse pleural thickening may reduce FVC and carbon monoxide diffusing capacity of the lungs ($D_LCO$) percent predicted even in the radiologic

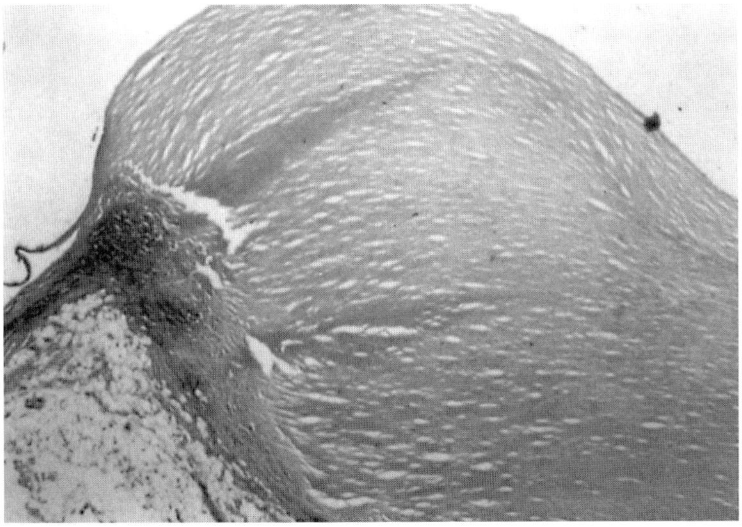

**FIG. 3.** Pleural plaque illustrates basket-weave pattern from a person with asbestosis who died of malignant mesothelioma.

categories 0/0 to 0/1 among occupationally exposed asbestos workers (4).

Circumscribed pleural plaques have been considered to have little or no effect on pulmonary function, yet can be of varying thickness and extent occurring on top of the diaphragm, along the chest wall in profile, face on, or mediastinal. For these reasons, Lilis and colleagues (9) developed an integrated pleural index to study 1,584 asbestos insulation workers of whom 75% had pleural fibrosis. Stepwise regression analysis indicated that there was a significant inverse relationship between FVC and the integrative pleural index for the circumscribed plaque subgroup. Even among these with pleuroparenchymal abnormalities, the pleural index was found to make a significant contribution, independent of that of parenchymal abnormalities, to decrements in FVC. Flow rates [forced expiratory volume in 1 second ($FEV_1$), and forced expiratory flow 25% to 75% and 75% to 85% of vital capacities have been expelled ($FEF_{25-75}$ and $FEF_{75-85}$)] have been reported to be reduced in nonsmoking asbestos workers with circumscribed or diaphragmatic pleural plaques (10,11). In an epidemiologic study of 1,211 sheet metal workers, pleural fibrosis was detected in 334 associated with age, duration of exposure, more pack-years of smoking, and presence and degree of interstitial fibrosis (12). After controlling for these confounders, multivariate regression found that both plaques and diffuse thickening were independently associated with decrements in FVC, but not with decrements in $FEV_1$/FVC ratio. Furthermore, the effect of diffuse pleural thickening on decrements in FVC was twice as great as that seen in circumscribed pleural plaques. After such confounding variables as age, height, smoking status, and the presence of parenchymal abnormality as assessed by chest radiography and gallium scintigraphy were taken into account, there was a significant decrease in $FEV_1$ and FVC (222 and 402 ml, respectively) among construction insulators who had pleural plaques or diffuse pleural fibrosis (13). The determinants of this restriction have been postulated to be reduced compliance due to visceral pleural fibrosis contributing to an increased $V_D$ (dead space) to $V_T$ (tidal volume) ratio, or to interstitial and peribronchial inflammation (alveolitis) (12). Using high-resolution computed tomography (HRCT) to construct three-dimensional models of pleural fibrosis in 29 sheet-metal workers, the volume of the pleural lesion varied from 0.01% to 7.11% (0.5 to 260 ml) of the total chest cavity (14). Total lung capacity (TLC) correlated inversely with pleural fibrosis after controlling for age, smoking, and parenchymal fibrosis.

Benign asbestos-induced pleural effusion occurred in 34 of 1,135 (3%) asbestos workers followed serially (15). Latency may be short (<20 years), with a mean of 12 years in one series compared to over 25 years for malignant mesothelioma (16). Other series have reported benign asbestos pleural effusions to occur after 30 years' mean latency (17). Almost half are asymptomatic, and in those with symptoms, pain, fever, cough, and dyspnea are most common. Half are hemorrhagic and one-fourth are eosinophilic. Two-thirds have mesothelial cells identified, and biochemically the fluid is an exudate with a normal glucose level. The duration of pleural effusion may extend to 6 months or longer. The latent period for benign asbestos pleural effusion is inversely related to total cumulative exposure, and its appearance is a risk factor for subsequent pleural thickening, especially diffuse pleural fibrosis and blunting of the costophrenic angle. Follow-up is recommended to rule out malignant mesothelioma.

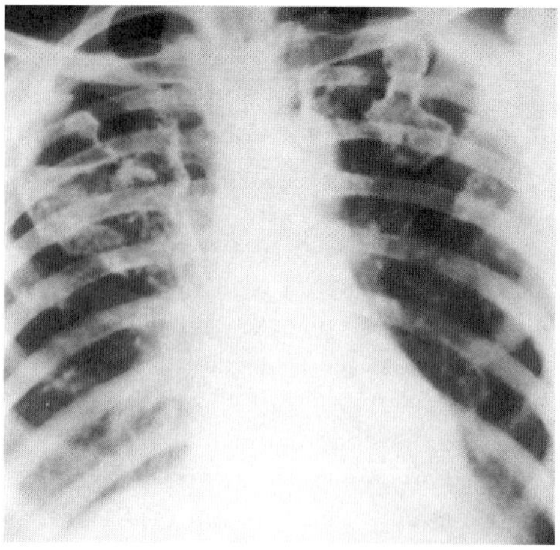

**FIG. 4.** Calcification of bilateral en face pleural plaques with the holly-leaf appearance in a South African asbestos miner. (Courtesy of P. E. S. Palmer, M.D.)

### Radiographic Features

Pleural plaques can be viewed in profile along the lateral chest wall or en face with a rolled or holly leaf pattern, especially if calcified (Figs. 4–7). The thickness and

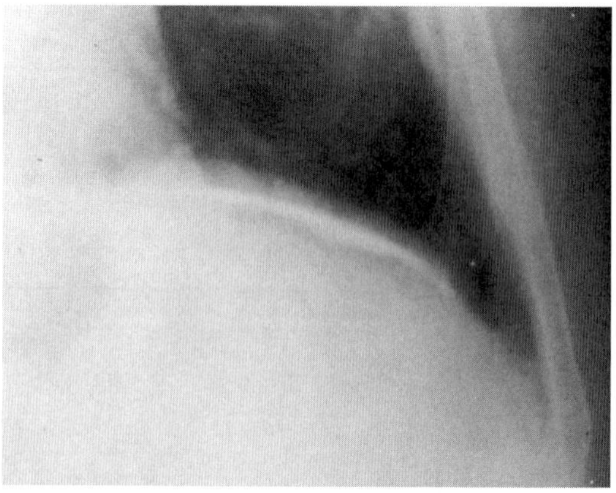

**FIG. 5.** Calcification of a pleural plaque on top of the diaphragm. Other causes of this finding are rare: trauma, tuberculosis, scleroderma, and free barium in the abdomen. (From ref. 185.)

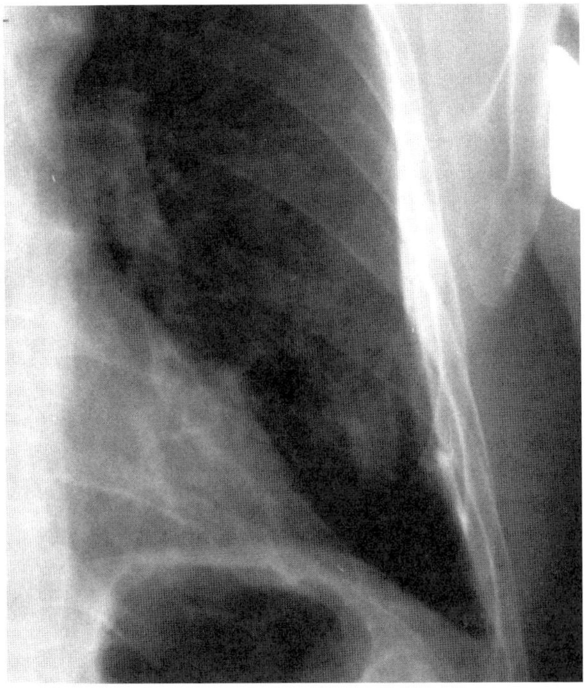

**FIG. 6.** Close-up view of circumscribed pleural plaques seen en face and in profile in an asbestos insulator.

extent of pleural lesion can be quantified. The HRCT scan of the chest has increased sensitivity in determining the extent of the plaque and high specificity in differentiating pleural fat from hyaline plaque.

Rounded atelectasis or folded lung due to pleural fibrosis with cicatrization resulting in a trapped lung segment or subsegment may mimic a lung cancer. HRCT scans can noninvasively demonstrate contiguity to areas of diffuse pleural thickening, evidence of volume loss in the adjacent lung, or a characteristic comet tail of vessels and bronchi sweeping into a wedge-shaped mass (18). Most importantly, stability over time from 9 months to 2 years supports a benign lesion. Other focal lung masses identified by CT scan are visceral pleural plaques that are usually multiple and associated with extensive parietal pleural disease (Fig. 8). In one clinical series of 74 patients with rounded atelectasis, 64 had significant asbestos exposure and the lingula or right middle lobe was affected in 49 (66%) of the cases (19). HRCT scans localized most rounded atelectases to the lower, posterior portion of the lungs, and in one-third of cases they may be multiple (20). In 39 patients the rounded atelectasis occurred suddenly on a background of only plaques or a normal chest x-ray; in 13 there was a slowly increasing pleural effusion. If the benign nature of the lesion cannot be assured with chest radiography, the patient may require a fiberoptic bronchoscopy with a transbronchial biopsy or a transthoracic needle aspiration to rule out a malignant process. Bronchoalveolar lavage (BAL) found >1 asbestos body per ml in 12 of 18 patients in one series (20).

### Diagnosis

Pleural plaques due to asbestos exposure are usually bilateral (80% of the time), whereas unilateral pleural plaques may be due to trauma, previous tuberculosis, or rarely, to other causes such as collagen vascular disease. The lesions are stable and will remain the same size for months, which should differentiate plaques from pleural tumors. Obtaining tissue is not necessary for diagnosis.

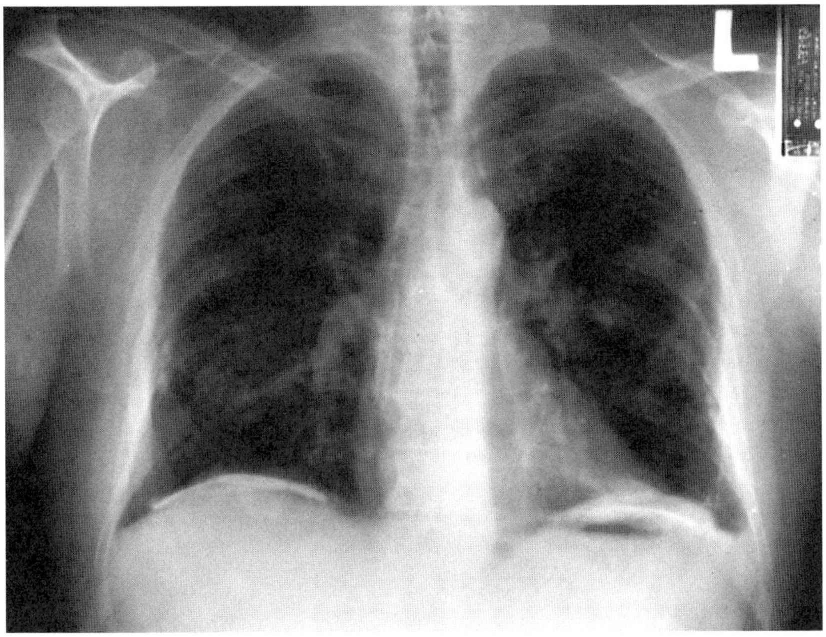

**FIG. 7.** Discrete circumscribed pleural plaques with calcification along both chest walls and on top of the diaphragm in a worker exposed for 2 years in a World War II shipyard.

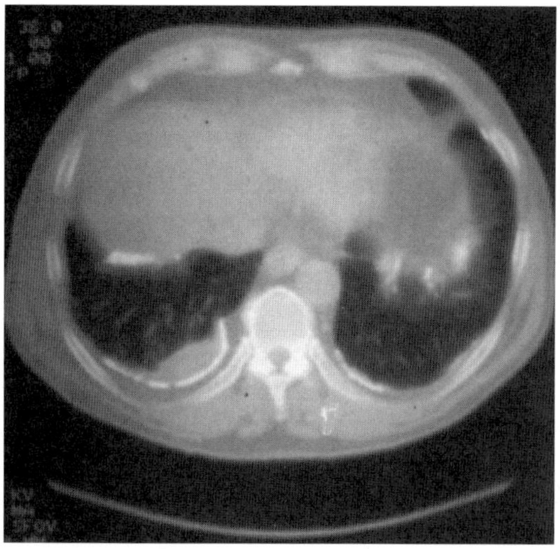

**FIG. 8.** Chest CT illustrates calcified pleural plaques on top of the diaphragm and clacified diffuse pleural thickening in the posterior parietal pleura bilaterally.

### Treatment and Prognosis

No treatment is necessary, although there are markers for asbestos-related diseases that may develop in the future. For these reasons, medical surveillance is recommended including periodic chest radiographs. Diffuse pleural thickening has been reported to reduce FVC and $D_LCO$ percent predicted even in the absence of parenchymal fibrosis among occupationally exposed asbestos workers (12). Severe restrictive impairment may accompany advanced pleural fibrosis and may require pleurectomy to prevent or treat ventilatory failure (21). Interestingly, progression of diffuse pleural thickening has been noted to level off 15 years after onset in heavily exposed crocidolite asbestos miners (22).

## ASBESTOSIS

### Pathology

Asbestos fibers deposit at airway bifurcations and respiratory bronchioles by impaction, sedimentation, and interception. Alveolar macrophages (AMs) accumulate in the alveolar ducts, peribronchiolar interstitium, and alveolar spaces constituting an alveolar macrophage alveolitis (23). Initial events occurring after asbestos inhalation are concentrated on the AMs found free in the alveolar spaces (24). Multinucleation is more than twice as frequent as in normal subjects, and multinucleated macrophages have enhanced phagocytic capability. Mitoses are seen in a mean of 3.7% ± 0.2% of AMs in asbestosis versus 1.4% ± 0.2% in control subjects consistent with *in vivo* macrophage replication in the inflammation of the lower respiratory tract. Moreover, AM surfaces showed a striking increase in rufflings including long, threadlike filopodia reaching to engulf long fibers. Surface blebs and pinocytotic vesicles are increased on the surface, and lysosomes and phagolysosomes are increased per unit area of cytoplasm. In asbestosis, AMs exhibit a morphologic phenotype of activation, and increased numbers accumulate at sites of fiber deposition from chemotaxis, in situ replication, and monocyte recruitment from the blood (25).

In human lung specimens, asbestosis may be patchy in that the interstitial fibrosis tends to primarily affect the lower lobes and subpleural regions of the lung (Figs. 9 and 10). Early lesions are characterized by discrete areas of fibrosis in the walls of respiratory bronchioles, which are sometimes accompanied by asbestos bodies. The septa adjacent to the respiratory bronchioles are often thickened, and the fibrosis sometimes appears to spread outward from the bronchioles. In addition to peribronchiolar fibrosis, there is an intense peribronchiolar cellular

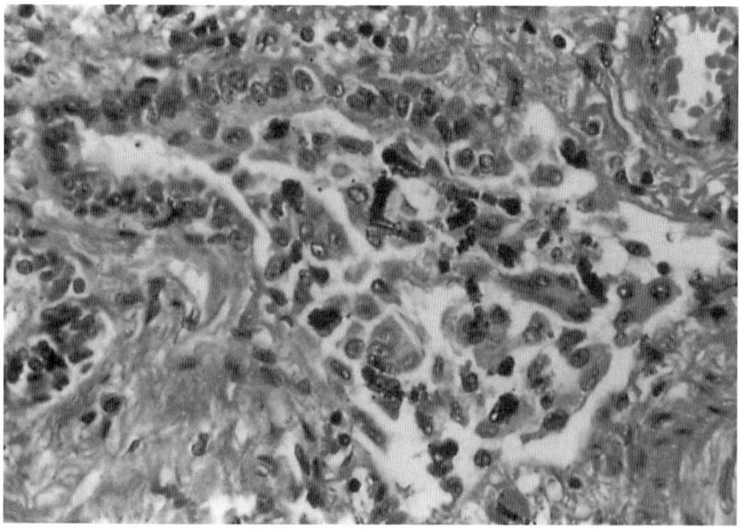

**FIG. 9.** Histologic section of lung from an insulator with asbestosis illustrating accumulation of alveolar macrophages in respiratory bronchiole and alveolar spaces with asbestos bodies, proliferation of alveolar epithelial cells and denudation of epithelial lining, and thickening of peribronchiolar and alveolar interstitium with mesenchymal cells and collagen.

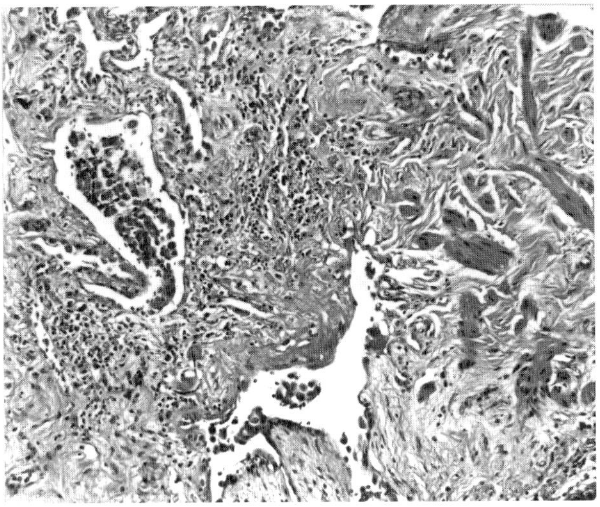

**FIG. 10.** The severe interstitial fibrosis in this section is associated with smooth muscle proliferation as well as chronic inflammation and distorted air spaces containing numerous macrophages. (Reprinted with permission from ref 27.)

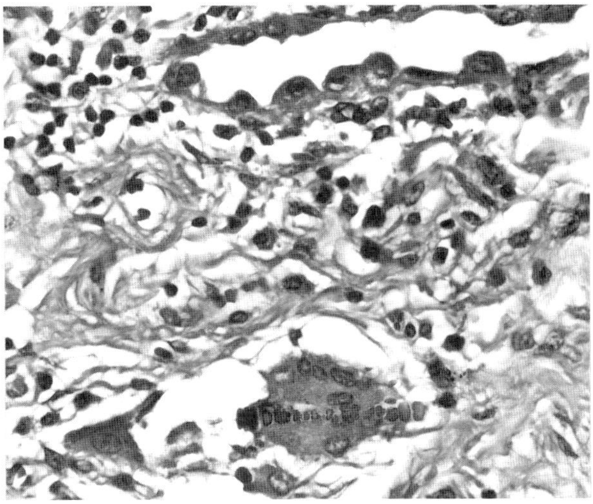

**FIG. 11.** A ferruginous body with the characteristic beaded appearance and club-shaped ends is present within the cytoplasm of this giant cell. The adjacent lung is fibrotic and contains an alveolar space lined by hyperplastic pneumocytes. (Reprinted with permission from ref. 27.)

reaction that may narrow and obstruct the airway lumen. As the fibrosis progresses, the architecture of the lung undergoes extensive remodeling and eventually results in honeycomb changes. Collections of lymphocytes are occasionally observed in the interstitium (26). Histologic asbestosis is characterized by peribronchiolar fibrosis, interstitial chronic inflammation, macrophage accumulation in air spaces, and type II pneumocyte proliferation. Smooth muscle proliferation may be prominent in the thickened interstitium (27). Intraalveolar buds of loose connective tissue may be observed.

Pathologic classification of human asbestosis is based on extent and severity of parenchymal lung involvement. The extent is graded as A (occasional respiratory bronchioles involved), B (greater than occasional but less than 50%), or C (greater than 50%). The severity is graded 1 (peribronchiolar fibrosis extending into alveolar walls), 2 (also involving alveolar ducts and two or more alveolar septa), and 3 (dense fibrosis of all alveoli between two adjacent bronchioles) (28).

Asbestos bodies (ABs) are characteristically observed in tissue sections (Fig. 11). The number of bodies per gram dry lung tissue in the general population is generally fewer than 500, but twice as many are found in the lungs of blue-collar males. Persons with pleural plaques have 10,000 to 20,000 bodies per gram and persons with parenchymal asbestosis more than 100,000—and usually more than a million per gram of lung, which correlates with the dictum of observing at least one asbestos body per high-power field (29,30). Sebastién and coworkers (31) estimated that recovery by BAL of 1 AB per milliliter correlated with 1,000 to 3,000 AB per gram dry lung parenchyma. ABs form around amphibole fibers in preference to chrysotile and contain iron with the morphologic appearance of hemosiderin (32). Analysis of the coating identifies a ferritin core containing ferric oxyhydroxide, hydrous ferric oxides, acid mucopolysaccharides in the matrix protein, and calcium and phosphorus. Only a small proportion of the total fiber burden in the lung ever becomes coated, probably not more than 1%, and the proportion increases with fiber length. Coated fibers are less toxic to alveolar macrophages than uncoated ones (33).

## Natural History

Asbestosis differs from idiopathic pulmonary fibrosis (IPF) in that the clinical-physiologic parameters demonstrate milder impairment, and more important, the progression of the fibrosis is slower. In some individuals, there may even be improvement in symptoms following removal from exposure. Since exposures are very low in current workplaces, one approach to evaluate risk from low levels of exposure is outcome from short-term exposure; for example, in an amosite asbestos factory, employment for even 1 month resulted in a subsequent prevalence of 20% parenchymal opacities ≥1/0 (34,35). One-third reported to have pleural abnormalities after 20 years' follow-up (35). Importantly, both "first attacks" and progression of established radiologic abnormalities occurred 20 and more years after exposure had ceased in this cohort. Radiographic studies of western Australian crocidolite workers found a median of 14 years before asbestosis was detectable (range 2–34 years) (36). The "attack rate" among retired Quebec chrysotile miners and millers for pleuroparenchymal lesions was 31%, progression of parenchymal opacities occurred in 9.3%, and the increase was confined to the more heavily exposed group (37).

### Epidemiology

The prevalence of parenchymal asbestosis increases as the length of employment increases among cohorts of asbestos workers. In one of the earliest reports, Selikoff and coworkers (1,38) analyzed chest radiographs of 1,117 New York and New Jersey asbestos insulation workers. They found asbestosis in 10% of those who worked 0 to 9 years, 44% of those who worked 10 to 19 years, 73% in those who worked 20 to 29 years, 87% of those who worked 30 to 39 years, and 92% in those who worked 40 or more years. Approximately 15% of asbestos miners and millers have radiographic evidence of asbestosis by age 65 years (39). There was also a dose-response for asbestosis with dust exposure in the asbestos cement industry, and the correlation had a better fit than years of exposure (40). These three groups (asbestos insulators, miners and millers, and asbestos cement workers) were directly exposed to asbestos, and a national survey evaluated radiographic changes among "bystanders" who were sheet-metal workers who worked in close proximity to insulation workers (41). In the United States 9,605 workers who were employed in the trade at least 20 years participated. The overall prevalence of asbestos-related changes was 31% including 19% pleural abnormalities alone and 12% parenchymal abnormalities ≥1/0 (half of these had combined pleural and parenchymal abnormalities). Among those with 40 years or more in the trade, 41.5% had radiographic signs of asbestos-related disease.

Cigarette smoking has been noted to increase the prevalence of irregular opacities on the chest radiograph (42). Although smokers without dust exposure may have few irregular opacities likely representing acute or chronic bronchitis or bronchiectatic changes in the lung parenchyma, more likely cigarette smoking interferes with clearance of the inhaled dust potentiating the dust's effects on the lung. Both smokers and ex-smokers had a higher prevalence of asbestos-related radiologic lesions than nonsmokers in British shipyard workers (43). Lilis and coworkers (44) studied 1,117 asbestos insulation workers, finding a higher prevalence of small opacities among smokers, which was more pronounced at the lower International Labor Organization (ILO) grades of roentgenographic small opacities (44). No effect of smoking was noted on pleural fibrosis. Selikoff and Hammond (42) have noted that the mortality rate from asbestosis was 2.8 times higher in asbestos insulators who smoked compared to nonsmoking insulators, and that this risk declined if the worker quit smoking.

### Clinical and Physiologic Features

The two most important clinical findings are the symptom of dyspnea on exertion and end-inspiratory crackles or rales on auscultation of the chest. In a cross-sectional survey of 816 asbestos-exposed workers using the American Thoracic Society respiratory symptoms questionnaire, cough, phlegm, wheeze, and dyspnea were inversely related to pulmonary function (45); 81% of this cohort had profusion of irregular opacities ≥1/0 with 48% of the cohort having pleural thickening. Cough, phlegm, and chronic bronchitis were associated with a 2% to 8% reduction in FVC and $FEV_1$ percent predicted; wheeze and dyspnea were clinically more significant with an 11% to 17% reduction ($p < 0.001$). Dyspnea had an odds ratio of 2.58 for restrictive impairment and statistically was associated with an estimated FVC loss of –0.4 L ($p < 0.001$). Using the British Medical Research Council (MRC) questionnaire for dyspnea (grade 3), Lilis and colleagues (46) evaluated data on 2,907 asbestos insulators. Grade 3 dyspnea prevalence among asbestos insulators with parenchymal/pleural abnormalities increased in a stepwise fashion from 19.4% in category 1 profusion (1/0 to 1/2) of small opacities to 34.5% for category 2 to 49.4% for category 3.

Rales in asbestosis are usually bilateral, and late to pan-inspiratory crackles at the posterior lung bases that are not cleared by coughing. They differ in quality and timing from the crackles of bronchitis which tend to be fewer in number and earlier in timing. The crackles of asbestosis appear first at the bases in the mid-axillary lines and tend to spread toward the posterior bases. In prevalence surveys, higher radiographic categories of asbestosis (≥1/1) usually have the same percentage (83%) of bilateral rales heard by a technician as by a physician (47). In 42 patients with the clinical diagnosis of asbestosis, 40 had a chest x-ray ≥1/0 profusion of irregular opacities, 36 had rales, 36 had dyspnea, and 22 had clubbing (48). Rales and clubbing were almost as common among those with less as those with more advanced categories of asbestosis.

The characteristic pulmonary function changes of asbestosis are a restrictive impairment with a reduction in lung volumes, especially FVC, TLC, $D_LCO$, and hypoxemia. Large airway function as reflected in the $FEV_1$/FVC ratio is generally well preserved. Eight asbestos workers had a reduced FVC in one of the earliest studies and vital capacity decreased by a mean of 18% predicted over the next 10 years (49). Among the 1,117 asbestos insulators in New York and New Jersey examined in 1963, the prevalence of abnormal FVC increased to over half the workers by 25 years since onset (50). In a larger cohort of 2,611 asbestos insulators, FVC percent predicted declined with greater profusion of irregular opacities, and pleural thickening exaggerated the decline for each category of profusion (51). Diffuse pleural thickening caused a further ≥10% decrease in percent predicted FVC compared to circumscribed plaques for each radiographic category of profusion. For cigarette smoking, the FVC percent predicted was higher for nonsmokers than current smokers and ex-smokers, and for each radiographic category. Interestingly, there was no difference between categories 0/1 and 1/0 for FVC percent predicted. In 684 male plumbers and pipe fitters, 7.8% had restrictive impairment and 21.7% obstructive defects (52).

The peribronchiolar fibrosis that develops as the early lesion of asbestosis may have an obstructive component. In a group of 17 lifelong nonsmoking asbestos miners with an average 28 years' exposure, 7 had abnormal radiographs and had a restrictive pattern of lung function, increased isoflow volume, and increased upstream resistance at low lung volumes (53). Open lung biopsies from three patients showed peribronchiolar infiltrates with macrophages and fibrosis that extended into the adjacent interstitium.

### Radiographic Features

The standard posterior-anterior chest radiograph reveals bilateral diffuse reticulonodular opacities predominantly in the lower lung zones. The 1980 International Classification of the Radiographs of the Pneumoconioses has devised a 12-point scale of profusion of irregular opacities, with category 0, normal; 1, mild asbestos; 2, moderate asbestosis; and 3, advanced asbestos. As duration from onset and intensity of exposure increase, there is an increase in prevalence and severity of asbestosis on the chest radiograph.

The radiographic appearance of asbestosis is characterized by irregular opacities in the lower two-thirds of both lung fields. When densely profuse these opacities may obscure the cardiac outline (hence the term *shaggy heart* of asbestosis) or even the dome of the diaphragm (Fig. 12). A ground-glass appearance may be noted, particularly when the pulmonary fibrosis is overlaid en face by a pleural plaque. The large opacities seen in the progressive massive fibrosis (PMF) of silicosis or coal worker's pneumoconiosis are rare. Progression has been observed after exposure was discontinued. One-third of asbestos laggers and factory workers followed at least 6 years demonstrated radiographic progression (54). Radiographic evidence of asbestosis should prompt avoidance of further exposure to asbestos dust.

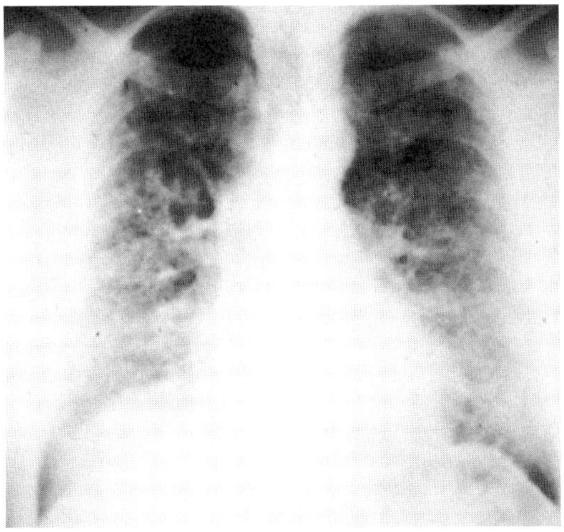

**FIG. 12.** Asbestosis with extensive pulmonary fibrosis, profusion, and category 3/3 irregular opacities. The heart and diaphragmatic borders are ill-defined. The heart is enlarged. The worker had been employed in a small asbestos products factory, where he seldom could see across the room because of the heavy concentration of dust.

The use of CT scanning has remarkably improved the sensitivity for detecting asbestos-related lesions by eliminating superimposition of pleural disease over parenchymal lesions and enhancing attenuation discrimination for parenchymal opacities. In evaluating more than 300 individuals with asbestos exposure, Gamsu's group (55) identified five major features for HRCT: curvilinear subpleural lines, increased interlobular septa, dependent opacity, parenchymal bands and intralobular core structures, and honeycombing (55). These changes have recently been corroborated with histologic examination in 30 individuals (56). This spectrum of radiographic characteristics are in contrast to the fine irregular opacities deemed to be so prominent on the posteroanterior (PA) chest radiograph. Importantly, when abnormal and suggestive of asbestosis, HRCT correlated with reduced vital capacity and diffusing capacity compared to a group with normal HRCT in a population of 133 asbestos-exposed workers with chest radiographs in the ILO <1/0 category (57). Using quantitative grid scoring for HRCT and the 12-point ILO scores for the PA chest radiograph, concordant abnormality on both in a group of 37 asbestos workers was consistent with asbestosis with significant duration from onset, elevated dyspnea score, highly significant reduced diffusion capacity, and alveolitis on BAL (58).

### Diagnosis

Asbestosis is defined as parenchymal fibrosis with or without pleural thickening and is usually associated with dyspnea, bibasilar crackles (rales), and pulmonary function changes (59). The PA chest radiograph and its interpretation are the most important factors in the diagnosis of asbestosis and asbestos-induced pleural changes. In 1980, the ILO revised the International Classification of Radiographs of the Pneumoconioses. This schema categorizes irregular or rounded opacities found on PA chest radiographs according to size and expresses profusion on a 12-point scale. Typically, asbestosis is defined using a profusion of irregular opacities at the level of 1/0 as the breakpoint between normal and abnormal. The diagnosis of asbestosis must take clinical factors into consideration in addition to the chest x-ray, including duration, onset and type of exposure, symptoms (especially dyspnea), physical findings, and pulmonary function tests. Convincing occupational exposures include manufacturing asbestos products, asbestos mining and milling, construction trades (insulator, sheet-metal worker, electrician, plumber, pipe fitter, boilermaker, carpenter), power plant worker, and shipyard worker. Duration depends in part on intensity, e.g., short-term shipyard exposure may be especially hazardous when workers remove asbestos insulation and create high exposures in contained areas for brief periods. Also, apprentice asbestos insulators would unload asbestos sacks into troughs and mix the asbestos cement, generating dense clouds of dust. Short exposures for several months or 1 to 2 years would be sufficient in these instances to cause asbestos-related disease, but exposure over 10 to 20 years is usually necessary. Exposure onset is relevant because industrial hygiene controls in the 1950s and 1960s, especially in the construction trades, were not widely applied or enforced. Cohort studies have identified latency to be an important factor, with the prevalence of asbestosis increasing as time since onset of exposure increases. The specificity of the diagnosis of asbestosis increases as the number of clinical criteria (symptoms, signs, chest radiograph, pulmonary function) increases. Misclassification and diagnostic difficulty occur in those with a heavy cigarette smoking history and concurrent emphysema, which also reduces the diffusing capacity. Patients with IPF may have an asbestos exposure history, but these patients tend to be younger and asbestos exposure is usually casual, brief, recent, and often can be discounted. Since patients with IPF require an open lung biopsy for confirmatory diagnosis, an asbestos fiber count per milligram dry lung can be helpful (60). Since 18% of asbestos workers had histologic asbestosis with a normal PA chest radiograph in one series (61), the history of occupational exposure has been usually considered the necessary criterion for diagnosis.

Asbestos bodies (ABs) in BAL fluid correlate with heavy exposure and asbestosis (Fig. 13). In a large series of 563 patients, those with asbestosis had a mean of 120 AB/ml, pleural disease 5 AB/ml, and malignant mesothelioma or lung cancer 8 AB/ml (62). Of 49 patients with more than 100 AB/ml, 30 had asbestosis, 8 had pleural disease, 13 had mesothelioma or lung cancer, and 3 were exposed only (2 had worked in a brake-lining factory). In assessing fiber type, mean amphibole correlation in BAL correlated positively with tissue burden, whereas chrysotile did not (63). This reflects the fact that chrysotile is preferentially carried to the pleura by lymphatic drainage and that chrysotile tends to break down in tissue. Importantly, in U.S. asbestos insulators, electron microscopy has identified one chrysotile fiber per 35 macrophages and one amosite fiber per 215 macrophages (64). No crocidolite was observed in any cells lavaged from 29 consecutive U.S. asbestos insulators, and small amounts of tremolite were detected in two controls and two workers. Thus these workers, who had the highest incidences of asbestos-related diseases, were not exposed to crocidolite. Asbestos workers had a significantly increased fiber burden per $10^6$ alveolar macrophages (chrysotile $28.2 \times 10^3$ versus $1.1 \times 10^3$ in normals, and amosite $4.7 \times 10^3$ versus $0.3 \times 10^3$ in normals, $p < .01$ both comparisons) (Fig. 14).

### Treatment and Prognosis

Asbestosis has no established treatment and because of the risk for lung cancer or mesothelioma, periodic chest radiographs are recommended. Although corticosteroids or colchicine have been used for the treatment of IPF, they have not been demonstrated to benefit asbestosis.

Longitudinal observation of asbestos-exposed trades workers have demonstrated accelerated declines in pul-

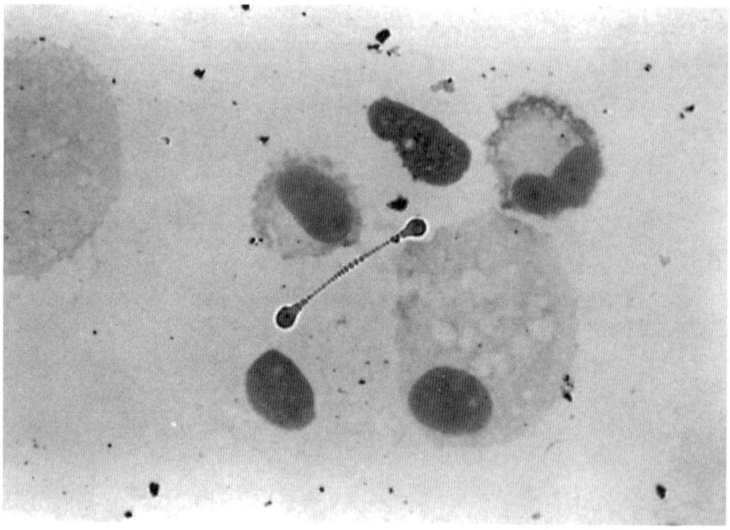

**FIG. 13.** BAL cytospin specimen from a nonsmoking shipyard worker illustrating macrophages and a beaded asbestos body (×400). (Courtesy of T. Takemura, M.D.)

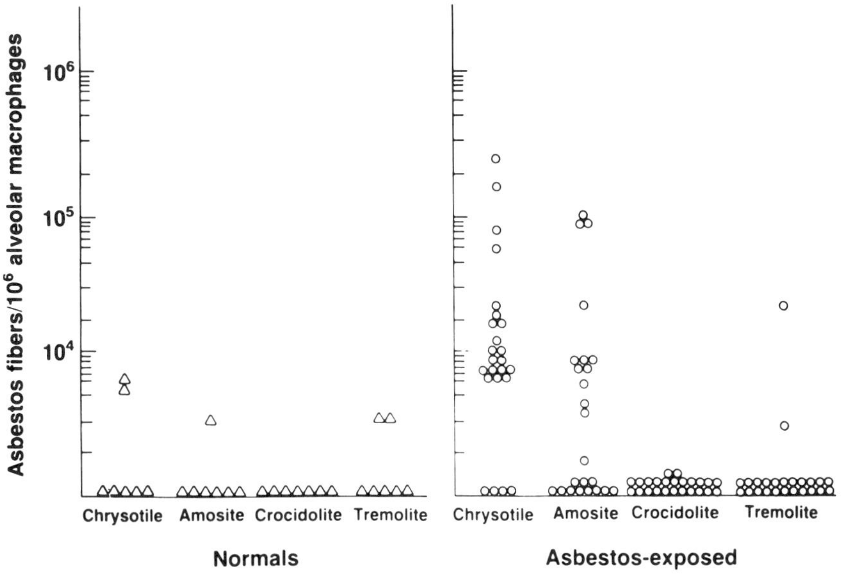


**FIG. 14.** Number of asbestos fibers identified as chrysotile, amosite, crocidolite, or tremolite using analytical optical electron microscopy per $10^6$ alveolar macrophages in normal ($n$ = 7) or asbestos-exposed ($n$ = 24) individuals. More chrysotile and amosite fibers were identified in the asbestos-exposed ($n$ = 24) individuals. More chrysotile and amosite fibers were identified in the asbestos-exposed (both $p$ <0.01). Δ, normal; O, asbestos-exposed individuals. (Reprinted with permission from ref. 64.)

monary function. In one study of 77 workers with a mean of three visits and 31 ± 1 years of occupational exposure, vital capacity and total lung capacity percent predicted correlated strongly with irregular opacities on the chest x-ray and rales, whereas $D_LCO$ did not (65). Linear regression determined mean annual declines to be FVC −92 ± 28 ml/yr, $FEV_1$ −66 ± 22 ml/yr, and TLC −14 ± 53 ml/yr. In a similar study of asbestos trades workers, there was an average annual decline of 1.5% in TLC and 2.5% for $D_LCO$ with strong correlations using multiple regression for dyspnea, smoking, honeycombing on CT scan, and BAL cellularity (66).

## MALIGNANT MESOTHELIOMA

### Pathology

Mesotheliomas are conventionally classified into three histologic patterns: (a) epithelial, (b) sarcomatous, or (c) mixed or biphasic. These patterns occur in approximately 50%, 20%, and 30% of cases, respectively. The epithelial variant is most easily confused with metastatic adenocarcinoma with neoplastic cells arranged in papillary, tubular, or solid nest configurations. The sarcomatous variant has spindle-shaped cells that may be pleomorphic with considerable mitotic activity.

Histochemistry differentiates adenocarcinoma from mesothelioma since adenocarcinoma has neutral mucin that is periodic acid-Schiff (PAS) stain positive and diastase resistant. Diastase may remove glycogen found in some epithelial mesotheliomas. Hyaluronic acid is the major acid mucopolysaccharide in mesothelioma and can be identified with the alcian blue or colloidal iron stains. Removal by prior digestion with hyaluronidase increases the specificity of the reaction.

Mesothelial cells contain cytoskeletal filaments including cytokeratin and vimentin, and staining for these is useful but not specific since other tumor types are also positive. Carcinoembryonic antigen (CEA) is absent in malignant mesothelioma yet present in adenocarcinomas (67). The monoclonal antibody B72.3 generated against a membrane fraction of human metastatic breast cancer was positive in 19 of 22 pulmonary adenocarcinomas but in none of 20 mesotheliomas (68). Another monoclonal antibody reported to be nonreactive with mesothelioma is Leu MI, and it is frequently positive in lung carcinoma (69).

Ultrastructural features of malignant mesothelioma are abundant intermediate filaments often organized into perinuclear tonofibrillar bundles, and long, sinuous, slender surface microvilli (70). The microvilli sometimes show secondary and tertiary branching. Microvilli may be interdigitated with stromal collagen. Collagen production occurs from malignant mesothelial cells and is prominent in the sarcomatous variant.

### Natural History

Malignant mesothelioma is locally invasive, spreading along the pleural wall and invading lung and mediastinal lymph nodes. At autopsy, tumor may be found in the diaphragm, heart, liver, spleen, adrenals, gastrointestinal tract serosa, bone, pancreas, and kidneys with 50% to 80% of cases having metastases. Isolated pleural nodules of tumor have been reported. Survival is approximately 10% at 24 months despite therapy. Survival is significantly better for patients with an epithelial subtype, with pleural versus peritoneal mesothelioma, and for those under 65 years of age (71). The incidence of mesothelioma is increasing since the cohort exposed from 1940 to 1970 is peaking in the 1990s. Incidence rates in the United States is approximately 11 to $13/10^6$/year. Although the peak incidence in the United States may have passed since imports declined after 1945, peak asbestos imports in the United Kingdom occurred in the 1960s to 1970s with an expected peak of mesothelioma deaths in 2020, when up to 1% of men may die of the disease (72). Chrysotile was their major import by far, and half went into the construction industry; amosite was the leading amphibole and most was mixed with chrysotile, giving workers in the construction industry the greatest risk similar to that in the United States.

The question of whether pleural plaques constitute a risk factor for mesothelioma on lung cancer was ably addressed in a prospective study by Hillerdal (73). He followed 1,596 men in Uppsala County, Sweden, from 1963 to 1985 to assess the risk for asbestos-related disease among those with bilateral circumscribed pleural plaques that did not involve the costophrenic angle; 89% of these men had an occupational exposure to asbestos. There were 50 bronchogenic cancers with 32.1 expected after correcting for smoking. The increase was 1.4 for those without asbestosis and 2.3 for those with asbestosis (both statistically significant), consistent with a greater exposure (dose) for those with asbestosis and greater risk for lung cancer. There were 9 mesotheliomas observed and 0.8 expected.

**Epidemiology**

The majority of patients with malignant mesothelioma have a history of occupational or environmental exposure to asbestos. The exposure history may be brief and forgotten, e.g., just a few months as a lagger's helper in a shipyard over 40 years ago. Mesothelioma is more common in the pleura than peritoneum. Cigarette smoking is not related to malignant mesothelioma.

Wagner and colleagues (74) reported the first case series of histologically confirmed malignant mesothelioma. They reported 33 cases, with 28 exposed in the crocidolite mining region and 4 exposed in asbestos factories from South Africa. They observed that mesothelioma occurred 20 to 40 years after exposure to asbestos dust, and found asbestosis or asbestos bodies in 8 of 10 specimens that also had lung tissue. Subsequently Wagner expounded the view that crocidolite asbestos was the major asbestos type that could cause mesothelioma. Immediately the question of chrysotile and/or amosite asbestos exposure was queried by Selikoff and colleagues (75) in the United States, where crocidolite constituted <3% of asbestos imports and the use was relatively recent. Crocidolite was not used in insulation materials, although it was used in asbestos-cement pipes with a smaller amount used for gaskets and filters. They searched 2,500 consecutive autopsies from 1953 to 1964 finding 26 cases of asbestosis with 7 having malignant mesothelioma. They reported 10 mesotheliomas as the cause of death among 307 consecutive asbestos insulator deaths between 1943 and 1964 from Asbestos Insulator Locals 12 and 32 in New York City and Newark, New Jersey. They concluded that malignant mesothelioma was a risk from asbestos exposure in general, confirmed that indirect exposure could also be important, and demonstrated that chrysotile/amosite asbestos could also be a major risk factor for mesothelioma.

At about the same time, Newhouse and Thompson (76) collected 83 mesothelioma cases from the London Hospital and compared them to two inpatient control groups based on age, another disease, and date of admission. There were 53% of cases versus 12% of controls ($p$ <0.001) with an occupational or household contact exposure to asbestos and 31% of cases versus 8% of controls ($p$ <0.01) lived within half a mile of an asbestos factory. Two-thirds had asbestos bodies or asbestosis on lung tissue examination.

Further epidemiologic studies focused on fiber type, especially the amphibole hypothesis, which pitted authors such as Mossman, Gee, McDonald, and Wagner (77–81) favoring crocidolite against Selikoff, Smith, Cullen and others who stated that all commercial asbestos types could cause mesothelioma (82–85). The evidence against the amphibole hypothesis was the impressive association of asbestos-related disease with the exposures of North American insulators, and the lack of finding crocidolite in their BAL cells or lung tissues (64,86). Importantly, Johns-Manville captured half of the insulation material market and only mixed amosite with chrysotile, not crocidolite, in their insulation manufacture. In a tour of their facility at Manville, New Jersey, in 1973, company officials stressed that crocidolite was being used in asbestos cement for potable water pipes exclusively. The amphibole hypothesis began in South Africa where most mesotheliomas were described in workers of the crocidolite mining district where the mines were old, the ore was hand-cobbed, and conditions were described as extraordinarily dusty in the workplace and environs (74). McDonald and McDonald (80) reported surprisingly low prevalences of asbestosis, lung cancer, and mesothelioma in Quebec asbestos miners and millers, but mortality of Quebec miners and millers with >20 years of exposure from lung cancer was as high as that of insulators (85). The mines and mills of Quebec are highly mechanized with extensive dust controls. However, when chrysotile fiber bundles are broken up in manufacturing processes, there are high mortality rates due to lung cancer [see Dement et al. (126) cited in Lung Cancer, below]. Bégin and colleagues (87) reviewed the 120 cases of malignant mesothelioma that came before the Worker's Compensation Board of Quebec from 1967 to 1990. The 49 cases from the chrysotile mining area were compared to 50 cases in manufacturing and construction (mixed exposure). The former had a mean age that was significantly older (62 vs. 57 years), with longer exposure time (31 vs. 22 years) and different distribution of exposure (15% <10 years vs. 29% <10 years). In the mining towns of Thetford and Asbestos, the incidence of mesothelioma was proportional to the work force, suggesting that the greater tremolite contamination in Thetford (7.5-fold) was not a significant factor in causing mesothelioma. Bégin and colleagues reported an incidence of 62.5 cases/$10^6$/year, which was similar to the incidence in western Australian crocidolite miners, providing additional evidence against the amphibole hypothesis. They also found the incidence increasing in the 1960s to 1990s, a time during which most of the McDonald cohort was deceased, suggesting that McDonald's cohort definition had missed the peak incidence of mesothelioma in Quebec (80). The Bégin et al. study is remarkable because one tenet of the amphibole hypothesis was that mesothelioma was rare among Quebec chrysotile miners and millers. Smith and Wright (82) reviewed the epidemiologic and animal data comparing crocidolite and chrysotile, concluding emphatically that chrysotile was the main cause of pleural mesothelioma.

Epidemiologists have attempted to locate cohorts with documented single exposure to either crocidolite or chrysotile to differentiate mesothelioma risk by fiber type. During World War II, women had worked in gas mask factories for brief periods of time, and type of asbestos was usually specified. In Canada, a crocidolite gas mask factory operated from 1939 to 1942 employing 199 persons (88). By 1975, 56 had died including 9 from malignant mesothelioma, and the mortality rate for lung cancer was double that for Quebec chrysotile miners. Mortality studies of two gas mask factories in the United Kingdom have placed practically all of the mesothelioma cases at the plant where crocidolite had been used (89). Smith and Wright (82) point out that crocidolite manufacturing plants were very dusty, whereas the chrysotile plants were mechanized with better dust control. From 1951 to 1957 a cigarette filter manufacturing company near Boston imported crocidolite asbestos for exclusive use (90). Among 33 men traced, there were 11 lung cancers (0.7 expected, ratio 15.1), 5 mesotheliomas, and 5 who died of asbestosis. All of the lung cancer cases were smokers, and asbestosis had been diagnosed in 19 workers. This was a particularly dusty factory with crocidolite asbestos on window sills and in the corners, and 16 years after the plant closed, this author found an open burlap bag half full of crocidolite asbestos in the middle of the plant floor. Environmental risk continues to be of concern since 24 mesotheliomas have now been recorded in a cohort of about 5,000 residents of Wittenoom, Western Australia, near the crocidolite mines (91). None had ever worked in the mines or mills.

In summary, the amphibole hypothesis arose from confusion about exposure where high exposures in crocidolite mines and shipyards caused much asbestos-related disease, but ignored the fact that asbestos insulators exposed to chrysotile and amosite had as much or more asbestos-related disease. Also, epidemiologic studies confounded the situation with narrowly defined entry periods, large cohorts with little exposure that found little asbestos-related diseases, or well-controlled exposures in factories or mines that would indict a specific fiber type or exonerate another. Cullen (84) had it exactly right when he paraphrased Shakespeare's *Julius Caesar,* "The evil that theories do lives after them; the good is oft interred with their bones."

### Clinical and Physiologic Features

Pleural mesotheliomas are mainly found in males (3–4:1) and are commonly diagnosed at ages 50 to 70. The most common symptom is chest pain followed by dyspnea. Less common symptoms are cough, weight loss, and fever. Pleural effusion is usually present and can be massive. Malignant mesothelioma is locally invasive, spreading along the pleural wall and invading lung and mediastinal lymph nodes. At autopsy tumor may be found in diaphragm, heart, liver, spleen, adrenals, gastrointestinal tract serosa, bone, pancreas, and kidneys with 50% to 80% of cases having metastases. Isolated pleural nodules of tumor have been reported. The effusion is an exudate and can be hemorrhagic (92). Rare features are syndrome of inappropriate antidiuretic hormone (ADH) secretion, clubbing, or hypoglycemia. Thrombocytosis has been reported to occur in 90% in one series and thromboembolic complications can occur (93). Ascites and weight loss characterize peritoneal mesothelioma.

Analysis of lung or tumor tissue for asbestos fibers has shown a clear increase in asbestos-exposed workers compared to control groups, and generally has supported the notion that amphibole fibers are more persistent in tissue. One of the first reports (94) used phase contrast microscopy to estimate asbestos fibers per gram dry lung, finding 83 out of 100 mesothelioma patients to have $>10^5$ fibers/g dry lung compared to $<2 \times 10^5$ fibers/g lung in 71 out of 100 controls. Churg et al. (95–97) have extensively reported asbestos fiber number, type, and size from Canadian asbestos-exposed cohorts. In lung tissue of mesothelioma cases from Quebec chrysotile mining regions, they observed high median fiber concentrations ($280 \times 10^6$ fibers/g dry lung) that were 400 times higher than shipyard amphibole-associated cases and higher than asbestosis cases. Also, they found tremolite in the specimens, but the fibers were short (geometric mean 2 mm) and had a low aspect ratio (length:width). They concluded that it took very high concentrations of chrysotile to cause mesothelioma, which is consistent with longer exposure duration of mesothelioma cases reported by Bégin et al. (87). Analysis of fibers from lung samples from 78 Canadian mesothelioma patients demonstrated a high odds ratio for amphibole fibers >8 μm in length. Becklake (98) has integrated data on fiber quantitation, stating that tremolite was sixfold greater in Quebec mining mesothelioma cases than chrysotile, suggesting weaker biopersistence of chrysotile given the fact that tremolite is merely a contaminant in the ore. For example, only $10^6$ amosite fibers were found in the lung of mesothelioma patients in shipyards compared to $4 \times 10^3$ chrysotile fibers (geometric means). In the United States, amosite is the predominant amphibole found in lung tissue; Roggli and colleagues (99) reported amosite asbestos was identified in lung tissue in 81% of 90 cases of mesothelioma and accounted for 58% of all fibers 5 mm or greater in length. Chrysotile was identified in 21% of cases and accounted for 3% of fibers exceeding 5 mm in length. The numbers of fibers per gram dry lung tissue ranged from 0.5 to $370 \times 10^6$ fibers and usually (80% of the time) the fiber concentration exceeded $10^6$ fibers/g dry lung. Roggli (99) has reported asbestos body counts from lungs of mesothelioma cases, observing a median of 3,350 asbestos bodies/g with about 20% overlapping the normal range of up to 200 asbestos bodies/g dry lung. There was a log increase in those individuals who also had asbestosis.

In U.S. asbestos insulators whose exposure was mainly to chrysotile with small amounts of amosite and virtually no crocidolite, analysis of asbestos fibers in lung, mesothelioma tissue, and pleural plaques revealed similar amounts of amosite and chrysotile in the lung, but a preponderance of chrysotile in plaque and mesothelioma tissue (86). The chrysotile fibers tended to be thinner <0.1 μm) than the amosite when translocated to the pleura. No tremolite was detected in the pleural tissues. Crocidolite was at the limit of detection and was found only in lung tissue in fewer than half of the specimens.

The Australian Mesothelioma Surveillance Program collected 221 definite or probable cases from 1980 to 1985, and compared fibers per gram dry lung tissue to 359 controls (100). There was a linear relationship between the log of the odds ratio and log of the fiber concentration. Odds ratios for tenfold increases in fiber concentration were crocidolite ≥10 μm, 29.4; chrysotile <10 μm, 15.7; and amosite <10 μm, 2.3. These data are consistent with greater risk for amphiboles and fiber length, although a small group with only chrysotile found in their lungs had a statistically significant association of increasing risk for mesothelioma with increasing lung fiber content. Surprisingly, the crocidolite asbestos mines only contributed 5% of the mesothelioma cases.

Analysis of asbestos fibers in pleural plaques from the parietal pleura compared to lung parenchyma has shown chrysotile to be preferentially translocated to the pleura (101). Lymphatic transport of chrysotile to the pleura is one possible explanation of why smaller amounts of chrysotile are found in the lung tissue compared to the amounts inhaled. Asbestos fibers in parietal pleura and plaques of former shipyard workers are predominantly short <5 μm) chrysotile (102).

**Radiographic Features**

The chest radiograph typically reveals a thick pleural peel along the lateral chest wall that extends to the apex. There typically is a pleural effusion, and this is the usual presenting sign. The HRCT scan differentiates pleural effusion from tumor, and can evaluate the extent of tumor. Asbestosis or pleural plaques on the opposite side of the tumor may be present.

**Diagnosis**

Cytologic diagnosis of the pleural exudate is difficult because reactive mesothelial cells and tumor cells are not easy to distinguish. Biopsy is required, and because mesothelioma may invade a needle track in 10% to 20% of cases, an open procedure is recommended. Thoracoscopy is probably the best procedure with diagnostic rates greater than 80%, similar to open pleural biopsy. Local radiation significantly reduces spread in needle tracks or incisions.

Gallium-67 lung scans demonstrate increased uptake in areas affected by malignant mesothelioma (103) (Figs. 15 and 16). Pleural plaques are usually negative, although there are occasional instances where increased gallium-67 uptake is noted near the lung periphery that could be due to plaque or subpleural alveolitis. In one large series, 43 of 49 (88%) of mesothelioma patients had a positive gallium-67 scan, and 3 of 16 (19%) with benign asbestos-related pleural disease had a positive scan.

Environmental exposure to tremolite asbestos in Turkey and Cyprus has been associated with mesothelioma; the asbestos is used as a whitewash or stucco and usually is a mixture of tremolite and chrysotile (104). Tremolite contamination of vermiculite has resulted in several mesothelioma cases among vermiculite miners and millers (105). In six mesothelioma cases from Finland, anthophyllite was the main fiber type (106). In the central Anatolian Cap-

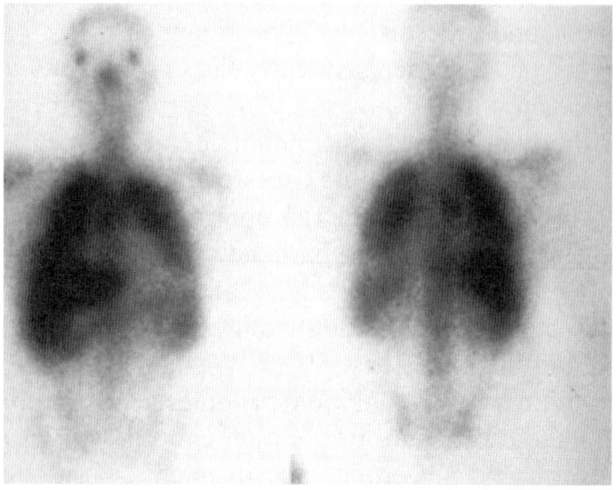

**FIG. 15.** Gallium-67 scintigram of a lung involved with pneumoconiosis shows diffusely increased uptake in the lung parenchyma [anterior *(left)* and posterior *(right)* views].

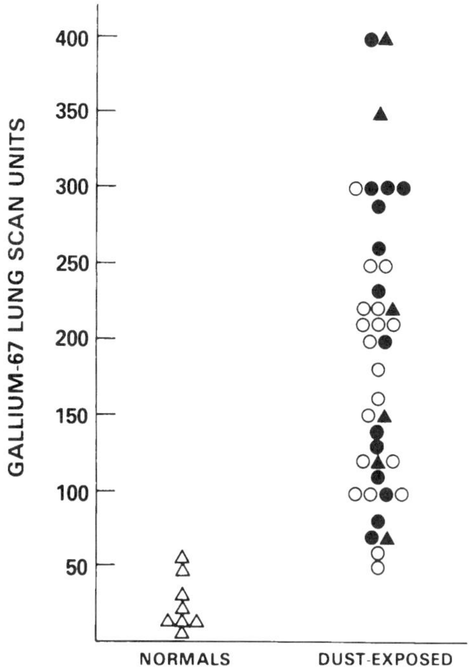


**FIG. 16.** Gallium lung scan units in individuals with inorganic dust exposure (asbestos ○, coal ●, silica ▲) are significantly increased compared to normals Δ ([see Rom and co-workers (23) for description of gallium lung scan units]).

padocia region of Turkey, three villages have high rates of mesothelioma (107). Karain had 249 deaths from 1970 to 1990 and 126 (51%) were due to mesothelioma. Villagers lived in houses carved from a volcanic tuff known as erionite. Erionite is an aluminum silicate but occurs as long, narrow fibers in a similar size distribution as crocidolite.

### Treatment and Prognosis

Median survival time is approximately 8 to 12 months for all patients with malignant mesothelioma, with less than 20% of patients alive at 2 years. Pleurectomy or pneumonectomy combined with radiation therapy has failed to significantly influence survival, and chemotherapy with doxorubicin (Adriamycin) has shown variable response without improvement in survival (108).

Experimental therapies with cytokines or gene therapy may have potential. Intrapleural instillation of interferon-γ twice weekly for 8 weeks resulted in eight histologically confirmed complete responses and nine partial responses with at least a 50% reduction in tumor size in 89 patients (109). The overall response rate was 20%, increasing to 45% in stage I disease. Asbestos added *in vitro* suppresses human natural killer (NK) cell activity, and NK activity can be restored by recombinant interleukin-2 (rIL-2); several malignant mesothelioma cell lines are lysed by NK cells (110,111). A phase I clinical trial of continuous pleural infusion of rIL-2 for 5 days to 15 patients when evaluated at 36 days postinfusion revealed one complete remission and six partial remissions (112). The main side effect was fluid retention in one-third of the patients, which never exceeded 10% of body weight. Gene therapy using replication defective adenovirus carrying the Herpes simplex–thymidine kinase gene followed by the antiviral drug ganciclovir has been successful in treating human malignant mesothelioma in severe combined immune deficient (SCID) mice (113). Significant antitumor effect has been noted with dose-response of virus and ganciclovir, with effects seen even in bulky tumors at clinically achievable dose ranges. There was no dissemination of virus from the serosal cavity following instillation. In a subcutaneous model of mesothelioma, tumor regression was seen when only 10% of cells were infected consistent with a bystander effect *in vivo*. A phase I clinical trial has shown this therapy to be safe, but humoral and cell-mediated immune responses developed against viral surface proteins. Also, there was no evidence of mesothelial cell transduction with the thymidine kinase gene *in vivo* using the adenoviral vector only at the highest viral titer.

## LUNG CANCER

### Pathology

All histologic types of lung cancer occur in asbestos-exposed workers, but adenocarcinoma has the highest percentage. In the United States–Canada insulators' cohort mortality study, there have been 544 deaths due to bronchogenic carcinoma in whom specimens were available for histologic evaluation (114). Most (467 out of 471) of the asbestos workers had a history of cigarette smoking. Lung tissue not involved with carcinoma was available from 356, and all but one had histologic evidence of fibrosis; in 90.7% of cases it was moderate to severe. Asbestos bodies were found in 344 of 356.

### Natural History

There is approximately a fivefold increase in risk for lung cancer among asbestos workers exposed directly to asbestos, and this risk is almost entirely borne by those who have a history of cigarette smoking (1). Cancer of the larynx has also been reported to be associated with asbestos exposure in case-control cohort studies, and substantiated by meta-analysis of the evidence (115,116). Asbestos has been found in laryngeal tissue, and as in cancer of the lung, cigarette smoking has a strong association with this disease.

### Epidemiology

Case reports of lung cancer in asbestos workers occurred as early as 1935 with collected series being mentioned by 1947, usually among asbestosis cases coming to autopsy. Sir Richard Doll (117) published an epidemiologic cohort study in 1955 of 113 men exposed to asbestos for 20 years in "scheduled areas" subject to the 1931 asbestos industrial hygiene measures. He found 11 deaths due to lung cancer with 0.8 expected, and all lung cancer patients had evidence of asbestosis. Selikoff and colleagues (118) obtained union records of two asbestos insulator unions in New York (Local 12) and Newark, New Jersey (Local 32), and published a retrospective cohort study in 1964. The 42 deaths from lung cancer were 6.8 times the expected rate and three malignant mesotheliomas were found; Selikoff et al. observed also that lung cancer increased with latency, and they speculated that work mates in other trades may also be at risk. In 1968 the same authors reported on the follow-up of 370 men of the original cohort with data on smoking habit (119). Of 87 nonsmokers, none died of lung cancer, whereas of 283 with a history of regular cigarette smoking, 24 died of lung cancer, consistent with a synergism between the two exposures.

In evaluating epidemiologic mortality studies, the North American asbestos insulator cohort assembled in 1967 by Selikoff and Seidman (120) contains the largest number of asbestos-related deaths among any group of asbestos workers evaluated. The mortality experience of 17,800 insulation workers was studied prospectively from January 1, 1967 to December 31, 1986. The standardized mortality ratio (SMR) for all causes of death was 143 ($p < 0.001$) with a threefold excess of all cancer deaths that was due principally to lung cancer: 1,168 cases observed with 269 expected, ratio 4.35. The number of mesotheliomas observed was 458. Mesothelioma represented 9% of all deaths; an exposure gradient of the chrysotile/amosite mixture was more than twice as potent in causing mesothelioma as South African crocidolite. Comparatively few excess deaths were observed among those with fewer than 20 or more years from onset of exposure. Lung cancer and mesothelioma peaked at 30 to 40 years' latency, whereas asbestosis death rates progressively increased with latency. Using data collected early on in the prospective follow-up of this cohort, the multiplicative effect of smoking plus asbestos exposure on lung cancer risk was confirmed. They reported the mortality for lung cancer per $10^5$ person-years to be 11.3 for nonsmoking controls, 58.4 for nonsmoking asbestos workers, and 122.6 for smoking controls; the sum of these three groups (192.3) was less than a third of the death rate for smoking asbestos workers (601.6), demonstrating the synergistic effect of smoking and asbestos exposure. Lung cancer mortality dropped by almost two-thirds for the asbestos insulators who subsequently stopped smoking.

Amosite asbestos was imported and processed exclusively at a Paterson, New Jersey, manufacturing facility from 1941 to 1954. An epidemiologic follow-up to 1982 of 820 men who had no subsequent or previous exposure revealed excess mortality (629 deaths observed, 375 expected), a fivefold increase in lung cancer, 17 mesotheliomas, and 33 asbestosis deaths (34). The exposure level was approximately 50 fibers per milliliter, and the long follow-up led to several observations: (a) there was a latency period of about 20 years before the increase in cancer was noted; (b) the greater the dose or the longer the exposure period, the greater the risk for developing lung cancer (dose-response); and (c) the greater the dose or exposure time, the shorter the induction time until the development of a tumor (dose-induction period). Wives and children of these asbestos factory workers were exposed to asbestos in the household primarily from asbestos brought home on work clothes; several developed malignant mesothelioma and a third exhibited pleural or parenchymal abnormalities on radiographs (121). Surprisingly, men employed less than 1 month during the period 1941 to 1945 had a lung cancer SMR of 267.

In New Jersey there was a large asbestos factory at Manville producing asbestos textiles, insulation, rigid shingles and sheets, and asbestos cement pipes. A mortality report of 1,075 men who were retired or had reached age 65 and were employed during 1941 to 1967 and followed through 1973 found increased rates of digestive and respiratory tract cancer (122). The respiratory tract cancers had a simple, linear dose-response relationship. A higher SMR for lung cancer was found in the pipe department, where both chrysotile and crocidolite were used. Interestingly, this study missed practically all of the 72 mesotheliomas reported by a thoracic surgeon in the nearby community hospital because of exclusion criteria in the initial design of the cohort; most of these patients had developed mesothelioma before age 65 (123).

Chrysotile asbestos is mined primarily in Quebec, Canada, with smaller mines in Italy, Rhodesia (now Zimbabwe), Russia, and other countries. An asbestos textile plant in Rochdale, England used chrysotile (crocidolite was used in 2% to 5% of operations) and instituted extensive industrial hygiene controls in 1933, 1951, and thereafter. The Rochdale factory formed the basis of Doll's original epidemiologic study and asbestos fiber measurements from the early 1950s onward enabled epidemiologists to construct dose-response relationships. A linear dose-response for lung cancer was found with a twofold increase noted at a cumulative exposure of 100 fibers/ml. Although SMRs decreased after industrial hygiene regulations in 1933 and again in 1951, there was still a dose-response with a clear latency in workers followed until the early 1980s (124). At lower exposure levels of 5 fibers/ml and with up to 10 years of exposure (50 fibers/ml-years), there was no increase in lung cancer risk. Mortality in over 11,000 miners and millers in the Quebec chrysotile townships showed excess mortality due to lung cancer and asbestosis, also with a linear dose response (125). Eleven pleural malignant mesotheliomas occurred in this cohort [Bégin et al. (87) reported 49 mesotheliomas in Quebec asbestos miners and millers].

Chrysotile asbestos from Quebec or Rhodesia was imported by a South Carolina textile plant that had begun operations in 1895 producing gaskets and packings with textile processes introduced in 1909. Mortality studies of this South Carolina plant demonstrated a 50-fold steeper linear dose-response relationship for lung cancer than for miners and millers (126,127). For example, lung cancer SMRs for textile workers increased from 207 to 728 as duration of employment increased from less than 5 years to more than 20 years, whereas for miners and millers it increased only from 91 to 161. There were 21 deaths due to asbestosis in the textile workers cohort (out of 863 deaths) and 46 deaths due to asbestosis in the miners (out of 4,463 deaths). Only one mesothelioma death occurred in the textile workers. The striking increase in lung cancer dose response is likely due to a process whereby manufacturing may result in high, brief exposure in opening the asbestos bags, followed by traumatic separation of the fibers leading to dispersal of chrysotile fibrils from larger fiber bundles. These fine fibers may pose a greater risk for pulmonary fibrosis and lung cancer but a far smaller risk for malignant mesothelioma.

Newhouse et al. (128) studied an English asbestos factory to provide corroborating data on mortality, fiber type, and dose. The East London factory used amosite, crocidolite, and chrysotile asbestos, exposing 4,200 male workers with most (83%) followed up for at least 20 years. Lung cancer mortality increased significantly with duration of follow-up, length of exposure, and severity of exposure; 7.5% of the deaths were due to malignant mesothelioma and 24 deaths (2%) were due to asbestosis. The mesothelioma death rate showed a consistent rise with duration and severity of exposure. Among those with heavier exposure and/or asbestos-induced disease, amosite and crocidolite constituted 60% to 87% of recovered fibers in the lung (129).

Since 85% of asbestos demand is for asbestos cement pipe products, especially in developing countries, numerous mortality studies have evaluated such workers. Weill's (130) group studied two plants in Louisiana that used predominantly chrysotile with 5,492 employees and 1,351 deaths. Only plant 2 had significantly increased risk of lung cancer mortality, and this plant had one of four buildings that consistently added crocidolite to the asbestos cement pipe mixture. Employees who worked in the asbestos cement pipe building (crocidolite exposed) were compared to those who were never assigned there (chrysotile exposed). Interestingly, both groups showed an increase in lung cancer risk with cumulative exposure, and the slopes of the dose-response relationships were similar. Ten mesotheliomas occurred and eight were in the plant that also used crocidolite. A nested case-control study of these subjects revealed a significant proportion of time in the pipe area for these cases. Only seven deaths were attributed to asbestosis, suggesting asbestos exposure may not have been particularly intense in comparison to asbestos insulator cohorts, for example. Finkelstein (131) reported on 201 men who had 1 year of exposure in an asbestos cement factory and 15 years' latency with 70 certified as having asbestosis. Mortality of the whole cohort with at least 1 years' exposure revealed a fivefold increase for both mesothelioma and lung cancer at 20 years' latency at an average cumulative exposure of about 60 fibers/ml-year. This estimate exceeds by almost one log the lung cancer risk estimated by Hughes et al. (130) in the New Orleans asbestos cement factory. These differences are most likely related to the difficulty in modeling exposures based on crude measures of exposure although it appears that the Canadian plant had more crocidolite exposure. In contrast to this study, Doll and Peto (132) made cross-study comparisons of 22 cohort studies, and argued that there was a difference in lung cancer risk for fiber type, with risk of lung cancer increasing with the relative amount of amphibole fiber used (132). A similar fivefold increase in lung cancer was reported for crocidolite asbestos miners and millers at 60 fibers/ml-year in Australia (133,134).

## Clinical and Physiologic Features

Lung cancer presents similarly among asbestos workers as in other high-risk groups with changes in cough or sputum production, chest pain, and weight loss being common features. However, a more vexing question is whether asbestosis is necessary for classification as a high-risk group. Most, but not necessarily all, cases of lung cancer in the Quebec asbestos mining district have small parenchymal opacities before death (135). In the North American insulator cohort, there were 544 lung cancer deaths with tissue provided for analysis. On review of chest radiographs from 138 with lung tissue and evidence of fibrosis, 25 (18%) had no radiographic evidence of parenchymal fibrosis (61). In a study of 75 lung cancers from a shipyard worker cohort, 60 had moderate to large numbers asbestos fibers in lung tissue and 50 of the 60 had microscopic fibrosis, particularly in subpleural areas of the lower lobes (136). Amphibole miners from South Africa with bronchial cancer were evaluated for exposure variables by stepwise regression; asbestosis was by far the most significant variable and there was a dose relationship with increase severity of asbestosis (137). Smoking was also significantly associated but cumulative exposure expressed as fiber years had no significant effect. In a mortality study of 839 asbestos cement workers, those with small opacities ≥1/0 by ILO classification) experienced a significantly raised risk of lung cancer (9 observed versus 2.1 expected) (138). By contrast, no excess of lung cancer was found among workers without radiographically lung fibrosis, even among long-term workers (≥21.5 years). Also, there was no relationship of lung cancer with level of cumulative exposure among these latter workers. In a case-control

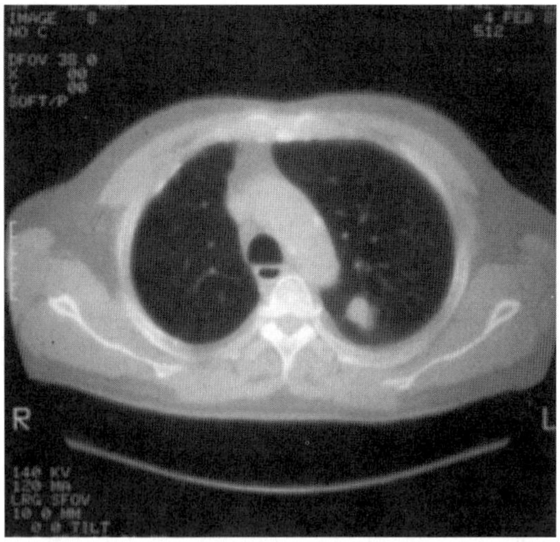

**FIG. 17.** Chest CT illustrating solitary pulmonary nodule in the left upper lobe.

study of 271 lung cancer patients and 678 controls (279 with other respiratory disease and 399 with cardiac disease), 34.3% of cases had worked in an occupation with definite or probable asbestos exposure compared to 25.8% of the controls [odds ratio 1.49, confidence interval (CI) 1.09–2.04] (139). The odds ratio for ≥1/0 small parenchymal opacities was 2.03 (CI 1.00–4.13) and ≤0/1 was 1.56 (CI 1.02–2.39). This study indicated that asbestos exposures that do not cause small opacities on the chest radiograph may nonetheless increase the risk of lung cancer. Further corroboratory evidence came from a study of Wittenoom crocidolite miners in Australia in which chest x-rays were compared between 39 cases and 718 controls (140). After controlling for smoking, there was a significant exposure-response relationship for cancer, even in subjects with no radiographic evidence of asbestosis. Radiographic fibrosis did not confer additional risk.

### Radiographic Features

Lung cancer in asbestos-exposed workers presents as a mass lesion on the chest radiograph (Figs. 17 and 18). Confusion may rise from en face pleural plaques or rounded atelectasis, but these abnormalities are stable over time. Newer technologies such as the helical CT scan, which can scan the chest on a single breath, may increase the early detection rate of lung cancer in high-risk groups.

### Diagnosis

Diagnosis of lung cancer in asbestos workers requires tissue or cytologic specimens obtained via fiberoptic bronchoscopy with lavage, brushing, or biopsy. Peripheral lesions, especially adenocarcinomas, may be best reached with fine needle transthoracic aspiration.

### Treatment and Prognosis

Surgical extirpation of non–small cell carcinomas can achieve greater than 50% 5-year survival rates, but overall, lung cancer remains a dismal prognosis with an 8% to 10% 5-year survival. Significant advances are being made in the molecular pathogenesis of lung cancer, and gene therapy approaches with specific targeting by altering surface and attachment properties of vectors that deliver therapeutic toxic genes to cancer cells show promise.

## PATHOGENESIS

### Asbestosis

#### *Clinical Studies*

Bronchoalveolar lavage (BAL) studies of asbestos insulators, and other trades workers who were nonsmok-

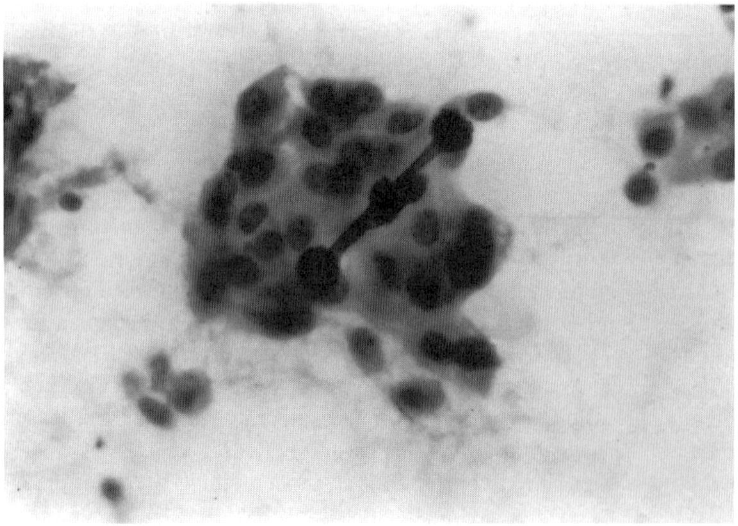

**FIG. 18.** Transthoracic needle biopsy of the nodule recovered adenocarcinoma cells and asbestos body.

ers or ex-smokers >5 years, demonstrated an alveolar macrophage (AM) alveolitis with a slight, albeit significant, increase in neutrophils (23). Those with more advanced fibrosis and respiratory impairment had a higher percent neutrophils in the BAL differential. In 52 Spanish asbestos cement workers, including 42 who had a history of smoking and 27 with radiographic asbestosis, there was a significant increase in neutrophils (7.8% ± 5%) that correlated with the presence of crackles, $PaO_2$ and $AaPO_2$ at rest values (141). In a large cross-sectional clinical study of 217 Quebec chrysotile asbestos miners and millers, most had positive gallium-67 lung scans and AM alveolitis diagnosed by BAL, with those with more advanced asbestosis having a slight increase (5%) in BAL neutrophils (142). Alveolar macrophages lavaged from asbestos workers spontaneously release increased amounts of the α-chemokine interleukin-8 (IL-8), an 8-kd potent neutrophil chemotaxin, into culture supernatants compared to normal controls (143). In addition, they had a significant increase in IL-8 gene expression by reverse transcriptase–polymerase chain reaction compared to β-actin, a housekeeping gene.

The alveolar macrophage is a key cell in stimulating intraalveolar and interstitial inflammation and developing fibrosis. Alveolar macrophages spontaneously release mesenchymal cell growth activity that stimulates human diploid lung fibroblasts to synthesize DNA and proliferate (Fig. 19) (23). The growth factor activity consists of both "competence" activity that signals quiescent fibroblasts in $G_0$ to enter $G_1$ and "progression" activity that acts later in $G_1$ to signal competence-primed fibroblasts to complete $G_1$ and enter the S phase or DNA synthesis phase of the cell cycle.

Alveolar macrophages stimulated with asbestos *in vitro* and lavaged from asbestosis patients release increased amounts of platelet-derived growth factor (PDGF), especially the B chain (144,145). PDGF is not only a potent growth factor for fibroblasts, it is chemotactic for them as well (146). Using a specific polyclonal antibody to fibronectin, significantly increased amounts were spontaneously released by AM from those with asbestosis compared with unexposed control subjects (23). Fibronectin, a 440-kd glycoprotein, is another chemoattractant for lung fibroblasts, and it provides a mechanism to attach the fibroblasts to the connective tissue matrix. In addition to competence activity, macrophage supernatants from patients with asbestosis contain significantly increased amounts of progression growth activity termed *alveolar macrophage-derived growth factor* (AMDGF) (23). AMDGF is a tissue-type insulin-like growth factor-I (IGF-I) with a molecular weight of 25 kd that was identified to be IGF-I by purification of asbestos-activated macrophage supernatants by ion exchange and molecular sieve chromatography, interaction with polyclonal and monoclonal IGF-I antibodies, competition with labeled recombinant IGF-I for the receptor, and mRNA expression in macrophages (147). Both fibronectin and AMDGF release are higher in those with asbestosis and respiratory impairment, although release of these mediators is less than that observed from BAL cells recovered from patients with idiopathic pulmonary fibrosis (148). Alveolar macrophages from asbestos-exposed individuals release significantly increased amounts of tumor necrosis factor-α (TNF-α) and interleukin-1β (IL-1β) than unexposed controls, and upregulate their respective mRNAs (149). Amosite, crocidolite, and chrysotile asbestos stimulate the release of both cytokines from peripheral blood monocytes. Both cytokines stimulated the mRNAs for collagens I and III and fibronectin in human lung fibroblasts in short-term culture, and are thus involved in the accumulation of extracellular matrix.

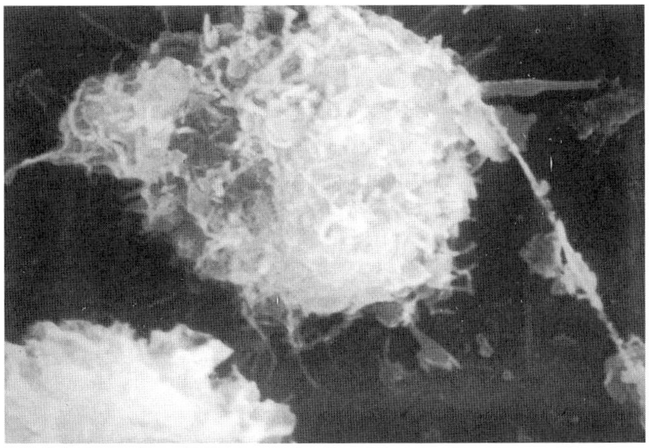

**FIG. 19.** Scanning electron micrograph of alveolar macrophages from a nonsmoking asbestos-exposed individual. The macrophages are attempting to phagocytose an asbestos fiber, and the macrophage surfaces show ruffling and increased filopodia (×3,000). (Courtesy of T. Takemura, M.D.)

Inflammatory cells recovered by BAL spontaneously release significantly increased amounts of superoxide anion and hydrogen peroxide from nonsmoking patients with asbestosis (23). Because these patients have few neutrophils in their BAL, this oxidant burden was most likely from AM; furthermore, after adherence, there was a persistent exaggerated oxidant release. The mechanisms of toxicity of oxidant species to alveolar walls may be direct cytotoxicity or through lipid peroxidation of membrane components. Prolonged administration of oxidant scavengers, e.g., polyethylene glycol-linked catalase, can inhibit several biochemical parameters of asbestosis in rats, suggesting this or other antioxidants as potential therapies (150).

### *Animal Studies*

Inhalation studies have been performed in baboons with amosite, chrysotile, or crocidolite (151). Four animals developed pleural mesothelioma (2 amosite and 1 crocidolite) with 1 of the peritoneum (crocidolite). All asbestos types induced pulmonary fibrosis with severity directly related to cumulative dose. Amphibole asbestos types demonstrated clearing of short fibers during recovery after exposure since the geometric fiber length increased; in contrast, fiber width decreased for chrysotile over time, suggesting that fiber bundles had separated into thin fibrils. There were long, thin fibers detected in mesothelioma tissue, but the chrysotile-exposed baboons died too early to develop mesothelioma and the report only evaluated amosite and crocidolite. Asbestos bodies were formed around all three fiber types, although chrysotile was less.

Two additional animal models have provided increased understanding of the mechanisms of fibrosis using inhalation or intratracheal injection of chrysotile in the rat and sheep, respectively. Brody's group (152) showed that brief inhalation of chrysotile asbestos resulted in deposition at the bifurcations of alveolar ducts, where complement activation via the alternate pathway attracted alveolar macrophages to these sites, and in the adjacent interstitium where the fibers were phagocytosed. Asbestos fibers were taken up by the type I alveolar epithelium, and transepithelial migration from the airspace to the interstitium occurs. Actin microfilaments were active in intracellular transport in the translocation of chrysotile through alveolar epithelial cells. A 10- to 20-fold increase in thymidine incorporation in adjacent bronchial and alveolar epithelial cells and interstitial cells consistent with cellular proliferation occurred (153). Morphometry demonstrated that the bifurcations were increased in volume because of excess connective tissue matrix. Interstitial matrix and cells accumulated after 3 months' exposure with a striking increase in the number and volume of type II alveolar epithelial cells with a 58% increase in the interstium including cells and matrix (154). Even a 1-hour exposure followed up at 1 month revealed a 67% expansion of the interstitium at sites of deposition with accumulation of interstitial macrophages, myofibroblasts/smooth muscle cells, and connective tissue matrix (155). Important to the development of these lesions were PDGF produced by alveolar macrophages and fibroblasts responsible for cell proliferation, and transforming growth factor-β (TGF-β) produced by macrophages, fibroblasts, and epithelial cells stimulating fibroblasts to produce increased amounts of collagens, fibronectins, and other matrix molecules (146,156).

Bégin and colleagues (157) developed a sheep model where they could sequentially monitor the development of asbestosis after instilling chrysotile through a bronchoscope with BAL, physiology, and histology. The initial lung events after three monthly doses were increases in BAL macrophages and lymphocytes with no changes in histology or pulmonary function. Increased dosage to 128 mg monthly for 6 months followed by weekly doses for 6 months resulted in a macrophage alveolitis, peribronchiolar fibrosis, and restrictive lung function (158). Extending asbestos exposure to 3 years separated sheep into a more severe fibrosis group compared to an airway-disease-only group with significantly fewer (fourfold) asbestos fibers recovered per milliliter BAL fluid (159). No differences were noted in fiber length. Evaluation of BAL from asbestosis sheep revealed increased protein, lactic dehydrogenase, fibronectin, procollagen 3, and BAL cells had an enhanced capacity to release superoxide anion and a fibroblast growth factor (160–162). Asbestotic lung lesions were strikingly positive by immunostaining for TGF-β1, 2, and 3, and they localized to zones of extracellular matrix with little staining of interstitial cells. IGF-I immunostaining was detected in macrophages in peribronchial fibrosis and in fibroblasts along the periphery of and within lesions, but not in the extracellular matrix (163). This pattern suggested a complementary role for the growth factors in stimulating interstitial fibroblast proliferation and new collagen deposition in areas of active fibrosis.

Further animal studies explored the issue of fiber length in causing fibrosis, and the data tend to indict longer fibers as being more fibrogenic. Inhalation of short amosite with >99% fibers <5 μm in length produced virtually no fibrosis in rats compared with long amosite with 11% >10 μm that produced extensive interstitial fibrosis at 12 months (164). Inhalation of long chrysotile fibers >20 μm was associated with greater lung fibrosis in the rat while attempting to control for fiber mass and type (165).

Both long and short crocidolite asbestos stimulated reactive oxygen intermediates when incubated with macrophages *in vitro*, but the long crocidolite was more active in the rat peritoneal cavity (166). Intratracheal injection of crocidolite asbestos >20 μm in length produced a vigorous fibroblastic proliferation and inflammation at peribronchiolar regions of the mouse lung compared to a minimal alveolar reaction elicited by short (<1 μm) crocidolite (167). The crocidolite also increased DNA synthesis in mesothelial cells and submesothelial cells one week after injection. Angiogenesis surrounding mesothelial nodules occurred in 58% of the lesions following long crocidolite versus 10% with short crocidolite following intraperitoneal injection (168).

### Molecular Mechanisms of Malignant Mesothelioma

One theory of carcinogenesis by asbestos is that fibers become entangled in the mitotic spindle during interphase, resulting in chromosomal abnormalities. Fibers observed by electron microscopy (EM) are seen to penetrate between multiple lobes of the nucleus and are associated along their length with the outer surface of the nuclear envelope. Structural chromosomal abnormalities in mesothelioma are clonal, complex, and include both chromosomal gains (chromosome 22) and losses (chromosome 7). Deletions of the short arm of chromosome 3, breakpoint 1p11-p22, and structural and numerical changes involving chromosome 7 are common findings (169,170). Asbestos insulators have been shown to have increased sister-chromatid exchanges in circulating lymphocytes (171). Larger chromosomes were more susceptible, and in the largest chromosome group there was a significant interactive effect of asbestos exposure and smoking.

Cell lines established from malignant mesotheliomas have been shown to constitutively upregulate the PDGF B-chain gene (c-*sis)* and to a lesser extent the PDGF A-chain gene (172). High levels of TGF-β1–3 mRNA and bioactivity have been reported for cell lines derived from malignant mesothelioma (173). TGF-β may be involved in the considerable matrix formation that accompanies mesothelial tumors. In conjunction with PDGF and TGF-β, mesothelioma cell lines release IGF-I and express mRNA for IGF-I and its receptor, consistent with an additional autocrine loop for cell proliferation (174). Deletions in chromosome 17 have also been observed in malignant mesothelioma, and the tumor suppressor gene p53, located in the region of 17p13, has been reported to be mutated in mesothelioma (175).

### Cellular and Molecular Mechanisms of Asbestos-Induced Lung Cancer

In the inflammatory local milieu surrounding asbestos fibers, there may be damaged DNA that can upregulate proto-oncogenes or inactivate tumor suppressor genes that control growth processes, lead to enhanced cell growth, and initiate carcinogenesis. Transfection of highly fragmented DNA into cells may occur in the lung, e.g., bronchial epithelial cells and mesothelial cells. DNA, RNA, and chromatin bind to asbestos, with chrysotile having greater avidity than the amphiboles because of its positive surface charge (176). Using a plasmid with p53 linked to the SV40 early region promoter enhancer, gene expression was observed after chrysotile asbestos transfection by fluorescence microscopy using a double-antibody technique with a specific anti-p53 monoclonal antibody. Crocidolite asbestos plus cigarette smoke synergistically increased DNA strand breaks measured by fluorescent spectroscopy from 4.3% (crocidolite) and 9.8% (smoking), respectively, to 78% ± 12% together (177). Hydroxyl radical release was measured by electron paramagnetic resonance, and oxidant scavengers such as mannitol, catalase, iron chelators, and dimethylsulfoxide prevented the DNA damage. Asbestos induces nuclear factor κB DNA-binding activity in tracheal epithelial cells *in vitro* and NF-κB is an important transcription factor for cytokines, growth factors, and proto-oncogenes (178).

There is a striking increase in neoplasms when chrysotile asbestos plus benzo[*a*]pyrene are instilled into experimental animals. Tracheal organ cultures incubated with crocidolite asbestos with adsorbed 3-methylcholanthrene for 1 month, and implanted subcutaneously into syngeneic hamsters, produced carcinomas in 12 to 52 weeks, whereas neoplasms did not occur after implantation with organ cultures exposed to crocidolite alone (179). Both crocidolite and amosite promote epithelial hyperplasia and an increase in the incorporation of [$^3$H]thymidine by tracheal epithelium *in vitro* (180). Furthermore, crocidolite asbestos with adsorbed polycyclic aromatic hydrocarbon is transported into the cell, induces the aryl hydrocarbon hydroxylase system, producing active metabolites of the hydrocarbon that can interact with DNA facilitating the process of carcinogenesis. Adsorption of polycyclic aromatic hydrocarbons onto asbestos fibers is probably an indirect process whereby adsorption of surfactant phospholipids onto the fibers creates a continuous lipid phase along the fiber surface within which lipophilic substances such as polycyclic aromatic hydrocarbons can be solubilized. Aryl hydrocarbon hydroxylase (AHH) is a ubiquitous enzyme involved in the early metabolism of aromatic hydrocarbons and is inducible by asbestos *in vitro*. Studies of blood lymphocytes from long-term asbestos workers reveal increased inducibility by 3-methylcholanthrene and dibenz[*a,h*]anthracene (181).

Animal experimentation using several asbestos types and routes of administration have been successful at reproducing asbestosis, lung cancers, and mesotheliomas in a variety of animal species. Wagner and colleagues (182) exposed rats by inhalation to asbestos (amosite, anthophyllite, crocidolite, and Canadian or Rhodesian chrysotile) for periods ranging from 1 day to 24 months. There was an increase of asbestosis with exposure to all of the dusts. All of the asbestos types produced adenocarcinoma or squamous carcinomas of the lung in approximately one-third of the animals in each group with a clear dose-response related to duration of exposure. Importantly, all asbestos types caused mesothelioma (one amosite, two anthophyllite, four crocidolite, and four Canadian chrysotile). Fiber type and fiber size were evaluated in greater depth with intrapleural inoculation (183). Asbestos fibers were also carcinogenic with intrapleural inoculation, and a narrow fiber size range could induce pleural tumors including fibrous glass, erionite, and aluminum silicate fibers. Stanton and colleagues (184) implanted a variety of fibers and fiber sizes but predominantly asbestos onto pledgets that were surgically inserted into the pleural cavity, and enumerated the number of mesotheliomas according to the length and width of the fiber. The most carcinogenic fiber size was less than or equal to 0.25 μm in diameter and greater than 8 μm in length (later known as the Stanton hypothesis).

### Efforts at Asbestos Control

To control asbestos exposure risk, the U.S. Occupational Safety and Health Administration (OSHA) regulates all asbestos types requiring employers to meet an 0.1 fiber/ml 8 hour time-weighted average for fibers >5 μm length with a 3:1 aspect ratio using phase contrast microscopy. A 30-minute excursion level proscribes exposures over 1 fiber/ml.

Industrial hygiene efforts at controlling exposure have focused on engineering controls including enclosing process lines especially where asbestos is introduced into a system, increased ventilation, and wet manufacturing methods. Personal respirators are a last resort in achieving workplace exposure control. Most of the insulation manufacturing industry has switched to alternate materials, especially fibrous grass, rock and slag wool, and refractory ceramic fibers. Animal experiments have generally shown these asbestos substitutes to be safe, except that refractory ceramic fibers were able to produce mesotheliomas in hamsters. Asbestosis and asbestos-related cancers may occur at increased rates in the future due to the increased use of asbestos in developing countries.

## CASE STUDY 1. ADENOCARCINOMA IN AN INSULATOR WITH ASBESTOSIS

A 64-year-old white male insulator had been employed from 1942 to 1988 (46 years) insulating powerhouses and government buildings without wearing respiratory tract protection. He mixed asbestos "mud" as a helper in the 1940s. He had smoked one pack of cigarettes per day from age 19 to 53. He had no symptoms of dyspnea, cough, phlegm, or hemoptysis. Bibasilar end-inspiratory rales were ausculated, and he had no clubbing. His posteroanterior chest radiograph was read according to the 1980 International Classification of the Radiographs of the Pneumoconioses as a 2/3 profusion of irregular opacities in the four lower lung zones with bilateral circumscribed and diffuse pleural thickening with calcifications. The pulmonary parenchyma was diffusely positive on a gallium-67 lung scintigraphy. Pulmonary function tests revealed a vital capacity of 73% of predicted, total lung capacity 68%, forced expired volume in 1 second 77%, and diffusion capacity 57%; this picture was consistent with restrictive impairment. Bronchoalveolar lavage revealed 355,000 cells per milliliter—81% macrophages, 10% lymphocytes, 7% neutrophils, and 2% eosinophils with many asbestos bodies. After one year's follow-up, a solitary nodule was observed in the left upper lung field that contained adenocarcinoma cells on needle biopsy (Figs. 17 and 18). Lobectomy was performed to remove the tumor.

## CASE STUDY 2. MALIGNANT MESOTHELIOMA OF THE PLEURA

A 72-year-old white male was referred for evaluation of a freely flowing right-sided pleural effusion. He had been in good health his entire life and effusion was discovered on screening chest radiography. He was asymptomatic. Findings on physical examination were within normal limits, except for decreased breath sounds with dullness to percussion at the right lung base posteriorly. There was no adenopathy, clubbing, hoarseness, or organomegaly. The patient had been employed at the Brooklyn Navy Yard for 38 years before retiring at age 65. He had maintained boilers and had operated generators at the shipyard. He was an ex-smoker.

A diagnostic thoracentesis yield straw-colored exudative fluid with a pH of 7.18, a glucose value of 11 mg/dl, protein of 5 mg/dl, and lactic dehydrogenase of 680 mg/dl. The leukocyte count was 1,241 per milliliter with 7% segmented forms, 38% lymphocytes, and 55% macrophages. The red blood cell count was 1,370 per microliter. No malignant cells were observed on cytologic examination. A pleural biopsy specimen demonstrated fibrinous inflammation. CT of the chest revealed

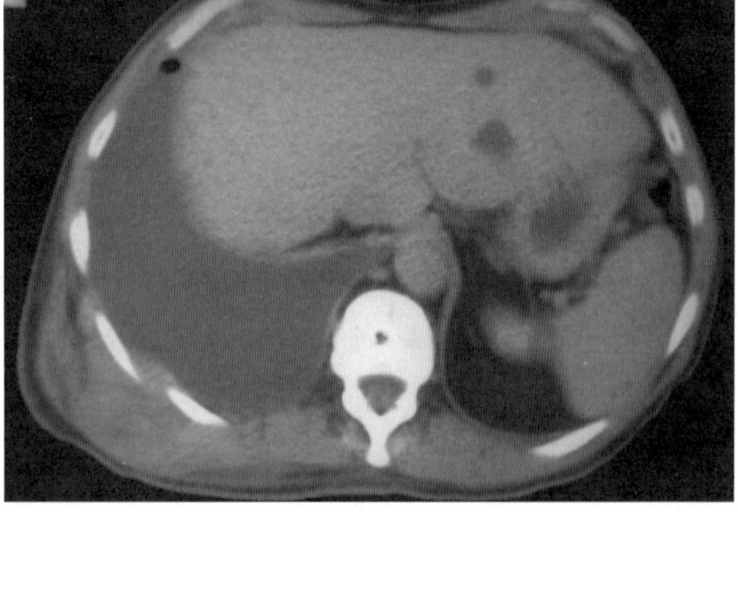

**FIG. 20.** CT of the chest demonstrates local extension of the malignant mesothelioma through the posterior chest wall. Compare the area of soft tissue density on the right to that on the left. Air within the tumor is secondary to the diagnostic biopsy.

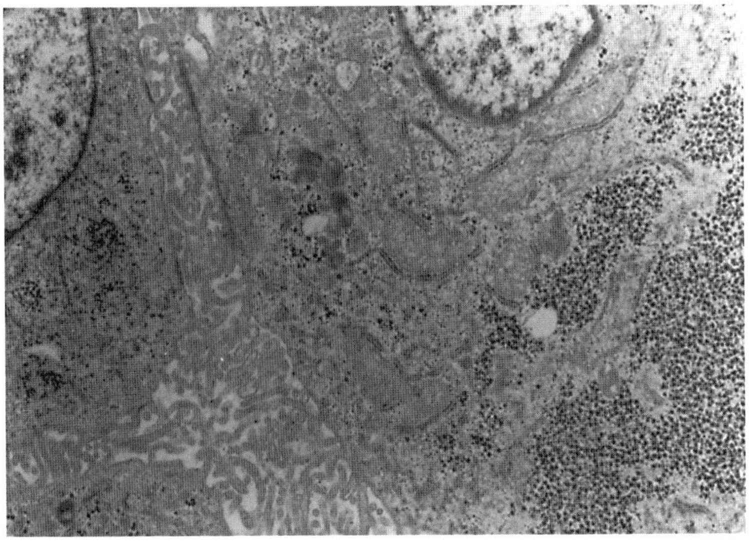

**FIG. 21.** Malignant mesothelioma: electron microscopy revealed long microvilli with length-to-diameter ratio of approximately 1:10. Tonofibrils are also prominent (13,200×). (Courtesy of Gurdip Sidhu, M.D.)

normal lung parenchyma, a small right-sided pleural effusion, pleural thickening, and pleural calcification. Beginning approximately 8 weeks after the initial evaluation, the patient noted a painless lump along the posterior chest wall. The lump enlarged steadily and the patient developed anorexia and fatigue. Physical examination again demonstrated a pleural effusion. In addition, there was a new palpable, irregularly shaped right-sided mass. The mass was hard, nontender, and approximately 5 by 9 cm in size. Chest radiography demonstrated an increase in the size of the right pleural effusion, areas of thickening and lobulation, and normal lung parenchyma. An area of soft tissue density extended from the lower right posterior chest wall into the right flank and had not been present on the scan performed 4 months earlier (Figs. 19 and 20). The patient was not a surgical candidate because of the local spread of the tumor, and he elected chemotherapy with Adriamycin and cisplatin (Figs. 21 and 22).

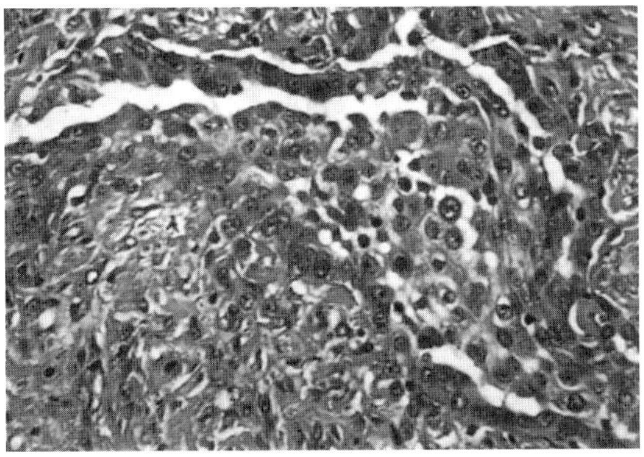

**FIG. 22.** Light microscopy of the tumor with hematoxylin-phloxin-saffron (HPS) staining demonstrates malignant mesothelioma with mixed epithelial and sarcomatous features (780×). (Courtesy of Gurdip Sidhu, M.D., and Rosemary Wieczorek, M.D.) *See color plate between pages 344 and 345.*

## REFERENCES


1. Selikoff IJ, Lee DHK. *Asbestos and disease.* New York: Academic Press, 1978;3–32.
2. Lilis R, Miller A, Godbold J, Benkert S, Wu X, Selikoff IJ. Comparative quantitative evaluation of pleural fibrosis and its effects on pulmonary function in two large asbestos-exposed occupational groups-insulators and sheet metal workers. *Environ Res* 1992;59:49–66.
3. Nicholson WJ, Perkel G, Selikoff IJ. Occupational exposure to asbestos: population at risk and projected mortality—1980–2030. *Am J Ind Med* 1982;3:259–311.
4. McLoud TC, Woods BO, Carrington CB, Epler GR, Gaensler EA. Diffuse pleural thickening in an asbestos-exposed population: prevalence and causes. *AJR* 1985;144:9–18.
5. Rennard SI, Jaurand MC, Bignon J, et al. Role of pleural mesothelial cells in the production of submesothelial connective tissue matrix lung. *Am Rev Respir Dis* 1984;130:267–274.
6. Boydan M, Sanan DA, Sheppard D, Broaddus VC. Vitronectin enhances internalization of crocidolite asbestos by rabbit pleural mesothelial cells via the integrin $\alpha v\beta 5$. *J Clin Invest* 1995;96:1987–2001.
7. Sheers G, Templeton AR. Effect of asbestos on dockyard workers. *Br Med J* 1968;3:574–579.
8. Rom WN, Thorton J, Miller A, Lilis R, Selikoff IJ. Abnormal spirometry in shipyard workers with pleural disease. *Am Rev Respir Dis* 1977;115:239A.
9. Lilis R, Miller A, Godbold J, Chan E, Selikoff IJ. Pulmonary function and pleural fibrosis: quantitative relationships with an integrative index of pleural abnormalities. *Am J Ind Med* 1991;20:145–161.
10. Kilburn KH, Warshaw RH. Abnormal pulmonary function associated with diaphragmatic pleural plaques due to exposure to asbestos. *Br J Ind Med* 1990;47:611–614.
11. Kilburn KH, Warshaw RH. Pulmonary functional impairment associated with pleural asbestos disease. *Chest* 1990;98:965–972.
12. Schwartz DA, Fuortes LJ, Galvin JR, et al. Asbestos-induced pleural fibrosis and impaired lung function. *Am Rev Respir Dis* 1990;141:321–326.
13. Bourbeau J, Ernst P, Chrome J, Armstrong B, Becklake MR. The relationship between respiratory impairment and asbestos-related pleural abnormality in an active work force. *Am Rev Respir Dis* 1990;142:837–842.
14. Schwartz DA, Galvin JR, Yagla SJ, Speakman SB, Merchant JA, Hunninghake GW. Restrictive lung function and asbestos-induced pleural fibrosis. *J Clin Invest* 1993;91:2685–2692.
15. Epler GR, McLoud TC, Gaensler EA. Prevalence and incidence of benign asbestos related pleural effusion in a working population. *JAMA* 1982;247:617–622.
16. Cookson WOCM, de Klerk NH, Musk AW, Glancy JJ, Armstrong BK, Hobbs MST. Benign and malignant pleural effusions in former Wit-

tenoom crocidolite millers and miners. *Aust NZ J Med* 1985;15: 731–737.
17. Hillerdal G, Ozesmi M. Benign asbestos pleural effusion: 73 exudates in 60 patients. *Eur J Respir Dis* 1987;71:113–121.
18. Lynch DA, Gamsu G, Ray CS, Aberle DR. Asbestos-related focal lung masses: manifestations on conventional and high-resolution CT scans. *Radiology* 1988;169:603–607.
19. Hillerdal G. Rounded atelectasis. *Chest* 1989;95:836–841.
20. Voisin C, Fisekci F, Saltiel SV, Ameille J, Brochard P, Pairon JC. Asbestos-related rounded atelectasis. *Chest* 1995;107:477–481.
21. Miller A, Teirstein AS, Selikoff IJ. Ventilatory failure due to asbestos pleurisy. *Am J Med* 1983;75:911–919.
22. de Klerk NH, Cookson WOCM, Musk AW, Armstrong BK, Glancy JJ. Natural history of pleural thickening after exposure to crocidolite. *Br J Ind Med* 1989;46:461–467.
23. Rom WN, Bitterman PB, Rennard SI, Cantin AC, Crystal RG. Characterization of the lower respiratory tract inflammation of non-smoking individuals with interstitial lung disease associated with chronic inhalation of inorganic dusts. *Am Rev Respir Dis* 1987;136:1429–1434.
24. Takemura T, Rom WN, Ferrans VJ, Crystal RG. Morphological characterization of alveolar macrophages from individuals with occupational exposure to inorganic particles. *Am Rev Respir Dis* 1989;140: 1674–1685.
25. Spurzem JR, Saltini C, Rom WN, Winchester RJ, Crystal RG. Mechanisms of macrophage accumulation in the lungs of asbestos-exposed individuals. *Am Rev Respir Dis* 1987;136:276–280.
26. Rom WN, Travis WD. Lymphocyte-macrophage alveolitis in non-smoking individuals occupationally exposed to asbestos. *Chest* 1992; 101:779–786.
27. Rom WN, Travis WD, Brody AR. Cellular and molecular basis of the asbestos-related diseases. State of the Art. *Am Rev Respir Dis* 1991; 143:408–422.
28. Craighead JE, Abraham JL, Churg A, et al. The pathology of asbestos-associated diseases of the lungs and pleural cavities: diagnostic criteria and proposed grading schema. *Arch Pathol Lab Med* 1982;106:544–596.
29. Churg A. Fiber counting and analysis in the diagnosis of asbestos-related disease. *Hum Pathol* 1982;13:381–392.
30. Dodson RF, Greenberg SD, Williams MG Jr, Corn CJ, O'Sullivan MF, Hurst GA. Asbestos content in lungs of occupationally and nonoccupationally exposed individuals. *JAMA* 198;252:68–71.
31. Sebastién P, Armstrong B, Monchaux G, Bignon J. Asbestos bodies in bronchoalveolar lavage fluid and in lung parenchyma. *Am Rev Respir Dis* 1988;137:75–8.
32. Suzuki Y, Churg J. Structure and development of the asbestos body. *Am J Pathol* 1969;55:79–107.
33. McLemore TL, Roggli V, Marshall MV, Lawrence EC, Greenberg SD, Stevens PM. Comparison of phagocytosis of uncoated versus coated asbestos fibers by cultured human pulmonary alveolar macrophages. *Chest* 1981;80:39S–41S.
34. Seidman H, Selikoff IJ, Gelb SK. Mortality experience of amosite asbestos factory workers: dose-response relationships 5 to 40 years after onset of short term work exposure. *Am J Ind Med* 1986;10:479–514.
35. Ehrlich R, Lilis R, Chan E, Nicholson WJ, Selikoff IJ. Long term radiological effects of short term exposure to amosite asbestos among factory workers. *Br J Ind Med* 1992;49:268–275.
36. Cookson WOCM, de Klerk N, Musk AW, Glancy JJ, Armstrong B, Hobbs M. The natural history of asbestosis in former crocidolite workers of Wittenoom Gorge. *Am Rev Respir Dis* 1986;133:944–998.
37. Becklake MR, Liddell FDK, Manfreda J, McDonald JC. Radiological changes after withdrawal from asbestos exposure. *Br J Ind Med* 1979;36:23–28.
38. Selikoff IJ, Bader RA, Bader ME, et al. Asbestosis and neoplasia. *Am J Med* 1967;42:487–496.
39. Liddell FDK, McDonald JC. Radiological findings as predictors of mortality in Quebec asbestos workers. *Br J Ind Med* 1980;37:257–267.
40. Weill H, Waggenspack C, Bailey W, Ziskind M, Rossiter C. Radiographic and physiologic patterns among workers engaged in manufacture of asbestos cement products. *J Occup Med* 1973;15:248–252.
41. Welch LS, Michaels D, Zoloth SR. The national sheet metal worker asbestos disease screening program: radiologic findings. *Am J Ind Med* 1994;25:635–648.
42. Selikoff IJ, Hammond ED. Asbestos and smoking. *JAMA* 1979;242: 458–459.
43. McMillan GHG, Pethybridge RJ, Sheers G. Effect of smoking on attack rates of pulmonary and pleural lesions related to exposure to asbestos dust. *Br J Ind Med* 1980;37:268–272.
44. Lilis R, Selikoff IJ, Lerman Y, et al. Asbestosis: interstitial pulmonary fibrosis and pleural fibrosis in a cohort of asbestos insulation workers: influence of cigarette smoking. *Am J Ind Med* 1986;10:459–470.
45. Brodkin CA, Barnhart S, Anderson G, Checkoway H, Omenn GS, Rosenstock L. Correlation between respiratory symptoms and pulmonary function in asbestos-exposed workers. *Am Rev Respir Dis* 1993;148:32–37.
46. Lilis R, Miller A, Godbold J, Chan E, Selikoff IJ. Radiographic abnormalities in asbestos insulators: effects of duration from onset of exposure and smoking. Relationships of dyspnea with parenchymal and pleural fibrosis. *Am J Ind* Med 1991;20:1–15.
47. Murphy RLH, Gaensler EA, Holford SK, Del Bono EA, Epler G. Crackles in the early detection of asbestosis. *Am Rev Respir Dis* 1984;129:375–379.
48. Picado C, Rodriguez Roisin R, Sala H, Agusti Vidal A. Diagnosis of asbestosis. *Lung* 1984;162:325–335.
49. Bader ME, Bader RA, Teirstein AS, Selikoff IJ. Pulmonary function in asbestosis: serial tests in a long-term prospective study. *Ann NY Acad Sci* 1965;132:391–405.
50. Lerman Y, Seidman H, Gelb S, Miller A, Selikoff IJ. Spirometric abnormalities among asbestos insulation workers. *J Occup Med* 1988;30:228–233.
51. Miller A, Lilis R, Godbold J, Chan E, Selikoff IJ. Relationship of pulmonary function to radiographic interstitial fibrosis in 2611 long term asbestos insulators. *Am Rev Respir Dis* 1992;145:263–270.
52. Rosenstock L, Barnhart S, Heyer NJ, Pierson DJ, Hudson LD. The relation among pulmonary function, chest roentgenographic abnormalities, and smoking status in an asbestos-exposed cohort. *Am Rev Respir Dis* 1988;138:272–277.
53. Bégin R, Cantin A, Berthiaume Y, Boileau R, Piloquin S, Massé S. Airway function in lifetime-nonsmoking older asbestos workers. *Am J Med* 1983;75:631–638.
54. Gregor A, Parkers RW, du Bois R, Turner-Warwick M. Radiographic progression of asbestosis: Preliminary report. *Ann NY Acad Sci* 1979; 330:147–156.
55. Lynch DA, Gamsu G, Aberle DR. Conventional and high resolution computed tomography in the diagnosis of asbestos-related diseases. *Radiographics* 1989;9:523–551.
56. Gamsu G, Salmon CJ, Warnock ML, Blanc PD. CT quantification of interstitial fibrosis in patients with asbestosis: a comparison of two methods. *AJR* 1995;164:63–68.
57. Staples CA, Gamsu G, Ray CS, Webb NR. High resolution computed tomography and lung function in asbestos-exposed workers with normal chest radiographs. *Am Rev Respir Dis* 1989;139:1502–1508.
58. Harkin TJ, McGuinness G, Goldring R, et al. Differentiation of the ILO boundary chest x-ray (0/1–1/0) in asbestosis by high resolution CT scan, alveolitis, and respiratory impairment. *J Occup Environ Med* 1996;38:46–52.
59. American Thoracic Society Statement. The diagnosis of non-malignant diseases related to asbestos. *Am Rev Respir Dis* 1986;134:363–368.
60. Gaensler EA, Jederlinc PJ, Churg A. Idiopathic pulmonary fibrosis in asbestos-exposed workers. *Am Rev Respir Dis* 1991;144:689–696.
61. Kipen HM, Lilis R, Suzuki Y, Valciukas JA, Selikoff IJ. Pulmonary fibrosis in asbestos insulation workers with lung cancer: a radiological and histopathological evaluation. *Br J Ind Med* 1987;44:96–100.
62. de Vuyst P, Dumortier P, Moulin E, Yourassowsky N, Yernault JC. Diagnostic value of asbestos bodies in bronchoalveolar lavage fluid. *Am Rev Respir Dis* 1987;136:1219–1224.
63. Teschler H, Friedrichs KH, Hoheisel GB, et al. Asbestos fibers in bronchoalveolar lavage and lung tissue of former asbestos workers. *Am J Respir Crit Care Med* 1994;149:614–645.
64. Rom WN, Churg A, Leapman R, Fiori C, Swyt C. Evaluation of alveolar macrophage particle burden in individuals occupationally exposed to inorganic dusts. *J Aerosol Med* 1990;3:s43–s56.
65. Rom WN. Accelerated loss of lung function and alveolitis in a longitudinal study of non-smoking individuals with occupational exposure to asbestos. *Am J Ind Med* 1992;21:835–844.
66. Schwartz DA, Davis CS, Merchant JA, et al. Longitudinal changes in lung function among asbestos-exposed workers. *Am J Respir Crit Care Med* 1994;150:1243–1249.
67. Wang NS, Huang SN, Gold P. Absence of carcinoembryonic antigen-like material in mesothelioma. *Cancer* 1979;44:937–943.

68. Szpak CA, Johnston WN, Roggli V, et al. The diagnostic distinction between malignant mesothelioma of the pleura and adenocarcinoma of the lung as defined by a monoclonal antibody (B72.3). *Am J Pathol* 1987;122:252–260.
69. Warnock ML, Stoloff A, Thor A. Differentiation of adenocarcinoma of the lung from mesothelioma: periodic acid Schiff, monoclonal antibodies B72.3, and Leu MI. *Am J Pathol* 1988;133:30–38.
70. Coleman M, Henderson DW, Mukherjee TM. The ultrastructural pathology of malignant pleural mesothelioma. *Pathol Annu* 1989;24: 303–353.
71. Sridhar KS, Doria R, Raub WA, Thurer RJ, Saldana M. New strategies are needed in diffuse malignant mesothelioma. *Cancer* 1992;70: 2969–2979.
72. Peto J, Matthews FE, Hodgson JT, Jones JR. Continuing increase in mesothelioma mortality in Britain. *Lancet* 1995;345:535–539.
73. Hillerdal G. Pleural plaques and risk for bronchial carcinoma and mesothelioma. *Chest* 1994;105:144–150.
74. Wagner JC, Sleggs CA, Marchand P. Diffuse pleural mesothelioma and asbestos exposure in the northwestern Cape province. *Br J Ind Med* 1960;17:260–271.
75. Selikoff IJ, Churg J, Hammond EC. Relation between exposure to asbestos and mesothelioma. *N Engl J Med* 1965;272:560–565.
76. Newhouse ML, Thompson H. Mesothelioma of pleura and peritoneum following exposure to asbestos in the London area. *Br J Ind Med* 1965;22:261–266.
77. Mossman BT, Gee JBL. Asbestos-related diseases. *N Engl J Med* 1989;320:1721–1730.
78. Mossman BT, Bignon J, Corn M, Seaton A, Gee JBL. Asbestos: scientific developments and implications for public policy. *Science* 1990;247:294–301.
79. Morgan WKC, Gee JBL. Asbestos-related diseases. In: Morgan WKC, Seaton A, eds. *Occupational lung disease,* 3rd ed. Philadelphia: WB Saunders, 1995;308–373.
80. McDonald JC, McDonald AD. The epidemiology of mesothelioma in historical context. *Eur Respir J* 1996;9:1932–1942.
81. Wagner JC. The discovery of the association between blue asbestos and mesotheliomas and the aftermath. *Br J Ind Med* 1991;48:399–403.
82. Smith AH, Wright CC. Chrysotile asbestos is the main cause of pleural mesothelioma. *Am J Ind Med* 1996;30:252–266.
83. Stayner LT, Dankovic DA, Lemen RA. Occupational exposure to chrysotile asbestos and cancer risk: a review of the amphibole hypothesis. *Am J Public Health* 1996;86:179–186.
84. Cullen MR. Annotation: The amphibole hypothesis of asbestos-related cancer-gone but not forgotten. *Am J Public Health* 1996;86:158–159.
85. Nicholson WJ, Landrigan PJ. The carcinogenicity of chrysotile asbestos. *Adv Med Environ Toxicol* 1994;22:407–423.
86. Kohyama N, Suzuki Y. Analysis of asbestos fibers in lung parenchyma, pleural plaques and mesothelioma tissues of North American insulation workers. *Ann NY Acad Sci* 1991;643:27–52.
87. Bégin R, Guntier JJ, Desmeules M, Ostiguy G. Work-related mesothelioma in Quebec, 1967–1990. *Am J Ind Med* 1992;22:531–542.
88. McDonald AD, McDonald JC. Mesothelioma after crocidolite exposure during gas mask exposure. *Environ Res* 1978;17:340–346.
89. Acheson ED, Gardner MJ, Pippard EC, Grime LP. Mortality of two groups women who manufactured gas masks from chrysotile and crocidolite asbestos: a 40-year follow-up. *Br J Ind Med* 1982;39: 344–348.
90. Talcott JA, Thurber WA, Kantor AF, et al. Asbestos-associated diseases in a cohort of cigarette-filter workers. *N Engl J Med* 1989;321:1220–1223.
91. Hansen J, de Klerk NH, Eccles JL, Musk AW, Hobbs MST. Malignant mesothelioma after environmental exposure to blue asbestos. *Int J Cancer* 1993;54:578–581.
92. Hillerdal G. Malignant mesothelioma 1982: review of 4710 published cases. *Br J Dis Chest* 1983;77:321–339.
93. Chahinian AP, Pajak TF, Holland JF, Norton L, Ambinder RM, Mandel EM. Diffuse malignant mesothelioma. *Ann Intern Med* 1982;96: 746–755.
94. Whitwell F, Scott J, Grimshaw M. Relationship between occupations and asbestos fibre content of the lungs in patients with pleural mesothelioma, lung cancer, and other disease. *Thorax* 1977;32: 377–386.
95. Churg A. Chrysotile, tremolite, and malignant mesothelioma in man. *Chest* 1988;93:621–628.
96. Churg A, Wright JL, Vedal S. Fiber burden and patterns of asbestos-related disease in chrysotile miners and millers. *Am Rev Respir Dis* 1993;143:25–31.
97. Churg A, Vedal S. Fiber burden and patterns of asbestos-related disease in workers with heavy mixed amosite and chrysotile exposure. *Am J Respir Crit Care Med* 1994;150:663–669.
98. Becklake M. Fiber burden and asbestos-related lung disease: determinants of dose-response relationships. *Am J Respir Crit Care Med* 1994;150:1488–1492.
99. Roggli V, Pratt PC, Brody AR. Asbestos fiber type in malignant mesothelioma: an analytical scanning electron microscopic study of 94 cases. *Am J Ind Med* 1993;23:605–614.
100. Rogers AJ, Leigh J, Berry G, Ferguson DA, Mulder HB, Ackad M. Relationship between lung asbestos fiber type and concentration and relative risk of mesothelioma. *Cancer* 1991;67:1912–1920.
101. Sebastién P, Jonson X, Gaudichet A, Hirsch A, Bignon J. Asbestos retention in human respiratory tissues: comparative measurements in lung parenchyma and in parietal pleura. In: Wagner JC, ed. *Biological effects of mineral fibers.* Lyon: IARC Science (publication #30), 1980;237–246.
102. Dodson RF, Williams MG, Corn CJ, Brollo A, Bianchi C. Asbestos content of lung tissue, lymph nodes, and pleural plaques from former shipyard workers. *Am Rev Respir Dis* 1990;142:843–847.
103. Teirstein AS, Chahinian P, Goldsmith SJ, Sorek M. Gallium scanning in differentiating malignant from benign asbestos-related pleural disease. *Am J Ind Med* 1986;9:487–494.
104. Selcuk ZT, Coplu L, Ernri S, Kalyoncu AF, Sakin AA, Baris YI. Malignant pleural mesothelioma due to environmental mineral fiber exposure in Turkey. *Chest* 1992;102:790–796.
105. McDonald JC, McDonald AD, Sebastien P, Moy K. Health of vermiculite miners exposed to trace amounts of fibrous tremolite. *Br J Ind Med* 1988;45:630–634.
106. Tuomi T, Konttinen MS, Tammilehto L, Tossavainen A, Vanhala E. Mineral fiber concentration in lung tissue of mesothelioma patients in Finland. *Am J Ind Med* 1989;16:247–254.
107. Baris YI, Saracci R, Simonato L, Skidmore JW, Artvivli M. Malignant mesothelioma and radiological chest abnormalities in two villages in central Turkey. *Lancet* 1981;1:984–987.
108. Brancatisano RP, Joseph MG, McCaughan BC. Pleurectomy for mesothelioma. *Med J Aust* 1991;154:455–460.
109. Boutin C, Nussbaum E, Monnet I, et al. Intrapleural treatment with recombinant gamma interferon in early stage malignant pleural mesothelioma. *Cancer* 1994;74:2460–2467.
110. Robinson BWS. Asbestos and cancer: human natural killer cell activity is suppressed by asbestos fibers but can be restored by rIL-2. *Am Rev Respir Dis* 1989;139:897–901.
111. Manning CS, Bowman RV, Darby SB, Robinson BWS. Lysis of human malignant mesothelioma cells by natural killer and lymphokine activated killer cells. *Am Rev Respir Dis* 1989;139:1369–1374.
112. Astoul P, Viallat JR, Laurent JC, Brandely M, Boutin C. Intrapleural recombinant IL-2 in passive immunotherapy for malignant pleural effusion. *Chest* 1993;103:209–213.
113. Huang HC, Smythe WR, Elshami AA, et al. Gene therapy using adenovirus carrying the Herpes simplex-thymidine kinase gene to treat *in vivo* models of human malignant mesothelioma and lung cancer. *Am J Respir Cell Mol Biol* 1995;13:7–16.
114. Suzuki Y, Selikoff IJ. Pathology of lung cancer among asbestos insulation workers. *Fed Proc* 1986;45:744A.
115. Stell PM, McGill T. Asbestos and laryngeal carcinoma. *Lancet* 1973; 1:416–417.
116. Smith AH, Handley MA, Wood R. Epidemiological evidence indicates asbestos causes laryngeal cancer. *J Occup Med* 1990;32:499–507.
117. Doll R. Mortality from lung cancer in asbestos workers. *Br J Ind Med* 1955;12:81–86.
118. Selikoff IJ, Churg J, Hammond EC. Asbestos exposure and neoplasia. *JAMA* 1964;188:22–26.
119. Selikoff IJ, Hammond EC, Churg J. Asbestos exposure, smoking and neoplasia. *JAMA* 1968;204:106–112.
120. Selikoff IJ, Seidman H. Asbestos-associated deaths among workers in the United States and Canada, 1967–1987. *Ann NY Acad Sci* 1991; 643:1–14.
121. Anderson HA, Lilis R, Daum SM, et al. Asbestosis among household contacts of asbestos factory workers. *Ann NY Acad Sci* 1979;330: 387–399.

122. Henderson VL, Enterline PE. Asbestos exposure: factors associated with excess cancer and respiratory disease mortality. *Ann NY Acad Sci* 1979;330:117–126.
123. Borow M, Conston A, Livornese L, et al. Mesothelioma following exposure to asbestos: A review of 72 cases. *Chest* 1973;64:641–646.
124. Peto J, Doll R, Hermon C, Binns N, Clayton R, Goffe T. Relationship of mortality to measures of environmental asbestos pollution in an asbestos textile factory. *Ann Occup Hyg* 1985;29:305–355.
125. McDonald JC, Liddell FD, Gibbs GW, Eyssen GE, McDonald AD. Dust exposure and mortality in chrysotile mining 1919–1975. *Br J Ind Med* 1980;37:11–24.
126. Dement JM, Harris RL, Symons MJ, Shy CM. Exposures and mortality among chrysotile asbestos workers. Part II. Mortality. *Am J Ind Med* 1983;4:421–433.
127. McDonald AD, Fry JS, Wooley AJ, McDonald J. Dust exposure and mortality in an American chrysotile textile plant. *Br J Ind Med* 1983; 40:361–367.
128. Newhouse ML, Berry G, Wagner JC. Mortality of factory workers in east London 1933–80. *Br J Ind Med* 1980;42:4–11.
129. Wagner JC, Newhouse ML, Corrin B, Rossiter CER, Griffiths DM. Correlation between fibre content of the lung and disease in east London asbestos factory workers. *Br J Ind Med* 1988;45:305–308.
130. Hughes JM, Weill H, Hammad YY. Mortality of workers employed in the asbestos cement manufacturing plants. *Br J Ind Med* 1987;44: 161–174.
131. Finkelstein MM. Mortality among employees of an Ontario asbestos cement factory. *Am Rev Respir Dis* 1984;129:754–761.
132. Doll R, Peto J. *Effects on health and exposure to asbestos.* London: Health and Safety Commission, HMSO, 1985.
133. Armstrong BK, de Klerk NH, Musk AN, Hobbs MST. Mortality in miners and millers of crocidolite in Western Australia. *Br J Ind Med* 1988;45:5–13.
134. de Klerk NH, Armstrong BK, Musk AN, Hobbs MST. Cancer mortality in relation to measures of occupational exposure to crocidolite at Wittenoom Gorge in western Australia. *Br J Ind Med* 1989;46: 529–536.
135. Liddell FDK, McDonald JC. Radiological findings as predictors of mortality in Quebec asbestos workers. *Br J Ind Med* 1980;37: 257–267.
136. Warnock ML, Isenberg W. Asbestos burden and the pathology of lung cancer. *Chest* 1986;89:20–26.
137. Sluis-Cremer GK, Bezuidenhout BN. Relation between asbestosis and bronchial cancer in amphibole asbestos miners. *Br J Ind Med* 1989; 46:537–540.
138. Hughes JM, Weill H. Asbestosis as a precursor of asbestos related lung cancer: results of a prospective mortality study. *Br J Ind Med* 1991;48:229–233.
139. Wilkinson P, Hansell DM, Janssens J, et al. Is lung cancer associated with asbestos exposure when there are no small opacities on the chest radiograph? *Lancet* 1995;345:1074–1078.
140. de Klerk NH, Musk AW, Glancy JJ, Pang SC, Hobbs MST. Incidence of lung cancer in subjects with and without radiographic asbestosis in subjects exposed to crocidolite. 9th International Colloquium on Pulmonary Fibrosis, Oaxaca, Mexico, 1996.
141. Xaubet A, Rodriguez-Roisin R, Bombi JA, Marin A, Roca J, Agusti-Vidal A. Correlation of bronchoalveolar lavage and clinical and functional findings in asbestosis. *Am Rev Respir Dis* 1986;133:848–54.
142. Bégin R, Cantin A, Berthiaume Y, et al. Clinical features to stage alveolitis in asbestos workers. *Am J Ind Med* 1985;8:521–36.
143. Broser M, Zhang Y, Aston C, Harkin T, Rom WN. Elevated interleukin-8 in the alveolitis of individuals with asbestos exposure. *Int Arch Occup Environ Health* 1996;68:109–114.
144. Schapira RM, Osornio-Vargas AR, Brody AR. Inorganic particles induce secretion of PDGF by macrophages in a density and time-dependent manner *in vitro*. *Exp Lung Res* 1991;17:1011–1024.
145. Rom WN. Activated alveolar macrophages from individuals with asbestosis release peptide growth factors. In: Harris CC, Lechner JF, Brinkley BR, eds. *Cellular and molecular aspects of fiber carcinogenesis.* Cold Spring Harbor, NY: Cold Spring Harbor Laboratory Press, 1991;103–114.
146. Osornio-Vargas AR, Bonner JC, Budgette A, Brody AR. Rat alveolar macrophage-derived PDGF is chemotactic for rat lung fibroblasts. *Am J Respir Cell Mol Biol* 1990;3:595–602.
147. Rom WN, Basset P, Fells G, Nukiwa T, Trapnell BC, Crystal RG. Alveolar macrophages release an insulin-like growth factor I-type molecule. *J Clin Invest* 1988;87:1685–1693.
148. Rom WN. Relationship of inflammatory cell cytokines to disease severity in individuals with occupational inorganic dust exposure. *Am J Ind Med* 1991;19:15–27.
149. Zhang Y, Lee TC, Guillemin B, Yu MC, Rom WN. Enhanced interleukin-1b and tumor necrosis factor-a release and mRNA expression in macrophages from idiopathic pulmonary fibrosis or following asbestos exposure. *J Immunol* 1993;150:4188–96.
150. Mossman BT, Marsh JP, Sesko A, et al. Inhibition of lung injury, inflammation, and interstitial pulmonary fibrosis by polyethylene-glycol-conjugated catalase in a rapid inhalation model of asbestosis. *Am Rev Respir Dis* 1990;141:1266–71.
151. Hiroshima K, Murai Y, Suzuki Y, Goldstein B, Webster I. Characterization of asbestos fibers in lungs and mesotheliomatous tissues of baboons following long term inhalation. *Am J Ind Med* 1993;23: 883–901.
152. Warheit DB, George G, Hill LH, Synderman R, Brody AR. Inhaled asbestos activates a complement dependent chemotactic factor for macrophages. *Lab Invest* 1985;52:505–514.
153. Brody AR, Overby LH. Incorporation of $^{3}$H-thymidine by epithelial and interstitial cells of asbestos exposed rats. *Am J Pathol* 1989;134: 133–140.
154. Barry BE, Wong KC, Brody AR, Crapo JD. Reaction of rat lungs to inhaled chrysotile asbestos following acute and subchronic exposures. *Exp Lung Res* 1983;5:1–22.
155. Chang LY, Overby LH, Brody AR, Crapo JD. Progressive lung cell reactions and extracellular matrix production after brief exposure to asbestos. *Am J Pathol* 1988;131:156–170.
156. Perdue TD, Brody AR. Distribution of transforming growth factor-b1, fibronectin, and smooth muscle actin in asbestos-induced pulmonary fibrosis in rats. *J Histochem Cytochem* 1994;42:1061–1070.
157. Bégin R, Rola-Pleszczynski M,. Sirois P, et al. Early lung events following low-dose asbestos exposure. *Environ Res* 1981;26:392–401.
158. Bégin R, Massé S, Bureau MA. Morphologic features and function of the airways in early asbestosis in the sheep model. *Am Rev Respir Dis* 1982;126:870–875.
159. Bégin R, Massé S, Sebastién P, et al. Asbestos exposure and retention as determinants of airway disease and asbestos alveolitis. *Am Rev Respir Dis* 1986;134:1176–1181.
160. Bégin R, Martel M, Desmarais Y, et al. Fibronectin and procollagen 3 levels in bronchoalveolar lavage of asbestos-exposed human subjects and sheep. *Chest* 1986;89:237–242.
161. Cantin A, Dubois F, Bégin R. Lung exposure to mineral dusts enhances the capacity of lung inflammatory cells to release superoxide. *J Leukoc Biol* 1988;43:299–303.
162. Lemaire I, Rola-Pleszczynski M, Bégin R. Asbestos exposure enhances the release of fibroblast growth factor by sheep alveolar macrophages. *J Reticuloendothel Soc* 1983;33:275–285.
163. Lee TC, Gold LI, Reibman J, et al. Immunohistochemical localization of transforming growth factor-β and insulin-like growth factor-I in asbestosis in the sheep model. *Int Arch Occup Environ Health,* 1997; 69:157–164.
164. Davis JMG, Addison J, Bolton RE, Donaldson K, Jones AD, Smith T. The pathogenicity of long versus short fibre samples of amosite asbestos administered to rats by inhalation and intraperitoneal injection. *J Exp Pathol* 1986;67:415–430.
165. Davis JMG. Current concepts in asbestos fiber pathogenicity. In: Lemen R, Dement JM, eds. *Dusts and disease.* Park Forest South, IL: Pathotox, 1979;45–49.
166. Goodglick LA, Kane AB. Cytotoxicity of long and short crocidolite asbestos fibers *in vitro* and *in vivo*. *Cancer Res* 1990;50:5153–5163.
167. Adamson IYR, Bakowska J, Bowden DH. Mesothelial cell proliferation after instillation of long or short asbestos fibers into mouse lung. *Am J Pathol* 1993;142:1209–1216.
168. Branchaud RM, MacDonald JL, Kane AB. Induction of angiogenesis by intraperitoneal injection of asbestos fibers. *FASEB J* 1989;3: 1747–1752.
169. Tiainen M, Tammilehto L, Rantonen J, Tuomi T, Mattson K, Knuutila S. Chromosomal abnormalities and their correlations with asbestos exposure and survival in patients with mesothelioma. *Br J Cancer* 1989;60:618–626.
170. Yegles M, Saint-Etienne L, Renier A, Janson Y, Jaurand MC. Induction of metaphase and anaphase/telophase abnormalities by asbestos

fibers in rat pleural mesothelial cell *in vitro*. *Am J Respir Cell Mol Biol* 1993;9:186–191.
171. Rom WN, Livingston GK, Casey KR, et al. Sister chromatid exchange frequency in asbestos workers. *J Natl Cancer Inst* 1983; 70:45–48.
172. Van der Meeren A, Seddon MB, Betsholtz CA, Lechner JF, Gerwin BI. Tumorigenic conversion of human mesothelial cells as a consequence of platelet-derived growth factor-A chain overexpression. *Am J Respir Cell Mol Biol* 1993;8:214–221.
173. Gerwin BI, Lechner JF, Reddel RR, et al. Comparison of production of transforming growth factor-b and platelet-derived growth factor by normal human mesothelial cells and mesothelioma cell lines. *Cancer Res* 1987;47:6180–6184.
174. Lee TC, Zhang Y, Aston C, et al. Normal human mesothelial cells and mesothelioma cell lines express insulin-like growth factor I (IGF-I) and associated molecules. *Cancer Res* 1993;53:2858–2864.
175. Cote RJ, Jhanwar SC, Novick S, Pellicer A. Genetic alterations of the p53 gene are a feature of malignant mesotheliomas. *Cancer Res* 1991; 51:5410–5416.
176. Appel JD, Fasy TM, Kohtz DS, Kohtz JD, Johnson EM. Asbestos fibers mediate transformation of monkey cells by exogenous plasmid DNA. *Proc Natl Acad Sci USA* 1988;85:7670–4.
177. Jackson JH, Schraufstatter IU, Hyslop PA, et al. Role of oxidants in DNA damage. Hydroxyl radical mediates the synergistic DNA damaging effects of asbestos and cigarette smoke. *J Clin Invest* 1987;80:1090–1095.
178. Janssen YMW, Barchowsky A, Treadwell M, Driscoll KE, Mossman BT. Asbestos induces nuclear factor κB (NF-κB) DNA binding activity and NF-κB-dependent gene expression in tracheal epithelial cells. *Proc Natl Acad Sci USA* 1995;92:8458–8462.
179. Mossman BT, Craighead JE. Mechanisms of asbestos carcinogenesis. *Environ Res* 1981;25:269–280.
180. Mossman BT, Craighead JE, MacPherson BV. Asbestos-induced epithelial changes in organ cultures of hamster trachea: inhibition by retinyl methyl ether. *Science* 1980;207:311–313.
181. Naseem SM, Tischler PV, Anderson HA, Selikoff IJ. Aryl hydrocarbon hydroxylase in asbestos workers. *Am Rev Respir Dis* 1978;118: 693–700.
182. Wagner JC, Berry G, Skidmore JW, Timbrell V. The effects of the inhalation of asbestos in rats. *Br J Cancer* 1974;29:252–269.
183. Wagner JC, Berry G, Timbrell V. Mesotheliomata in rats after inoculation with asbestos and other materials. *Br J Cancer* 1973;28:173–185.
184. Stanton MF, Layard M, Tegeris A, et al. Relation of particle dimension to carcinogenicity in amphibole asbestos and other fibrous minerals. Mechanisms of mesothelioma induction with asbestos and fibrous glass. *J Natl Cancer Inst* 1981;67:965–975.
185. Rom WN, Palmer PES. The spectrum of asbestos-related diseases. *West J Med* 1974;121:10–21.

*Environmental and Occupational Medicine,*
*Third Edition,* edited by William N. Rom.
Lippincott–Raven Publishers, Philadelphia © 1998.

CHAPTER 25

# Animal Models of Malignant Mesothelioma

Agnes B. Kane

## HISTORICAL BACKGROUND

Diffuse malignant mesothelioma is a rare neoplasm that arises from the mesothelial lining of the pleural, peritoneal, or pericardial cavities (1). The first case series of human mesotheliomas associated with occupational and environmental exposure to crocidolite, an amphibole asbestos fiber, was published by Wagner et al. in 1960 (2). Prior to this case series, isolated examples of human malignant mesotheliomas had been described; however, the origin and diagnosis of these tumors was disputed among pathologists (1,3). Wagner and other investigators (3–5) developed animal models to investigate the carcinogenicity of mineral fibers using direct intrapleural or intraperitoneal injection. As described in detail below, these animal models closely resembled the human disease (reviewed in refs. 6,7). These models also established an etiologic relationship between the dimensions of mineral fibers and their potency in inducing malignant mesotheliomas (4,8). This relationship is called the Stanton hypothesis and raises the possibility that exposure to any long, thin fiber, whether natural or man-made, may lead to the development of mesothelioma (4,5,8,9). Direct intracavitary injection of fibers is an unnatural route of exposure and bypasses the natural clearance mechanisms of the lungs (10). Early rodent inhalation assays using whole-body exposure to a variety of fibers produced a low incidence of mesotheliomas, with the exception of erionite, a nonasbestiform fiber (11). Recent rodent inhalation assays using new aerosol generating techniques and nose-only inhalation are more reproducible in generating malignant mesotheliomas. These recent inhalation assays have provided evidence that fiber persistence in the lungs, in addition to fiber dimensions, is a critical determinant of fiber carcinogenicity (12).

Despite nearly 30 years of intense investigation, the mechanisms responsible for the development of diffuse malignant mesothelioma are unknown (reviewed in 13). Because these neoplasms are usually diagnosed at an advanced stage after a long latency period, and because no precursor lesions have been clearly defined (14), animal models are the only alternative for studying the pathogenesis of malignant mesothelioma. Recent mechanistic studies in animal models and comparative molecular analysis of human and rodent mesotheliomas are beginning to provide some clues about the pathogenesis of this neoplasm (13). It is anticipated that short-term screening assays for asbestos fiber substitutes will be developed based on this new mechanistic information (15).

The availability of immunodeficient mice as hosts for xenografts of human malignant mesotheliomas has provided the opportunity to test new therapeutic approaches, including novel drug combinations and photodynamic therapy (16). Murine models of malignant mesothelioma have been especially useful in exploring the feasibility of immunotherapy (17). Finally, the potential of gene therapy for malignant mesothelioma is under investigation (18).

## HISTOPATHOLOGY AND NATURAL HISTORY OF RODENT MESOTHELIOMAS

Rodent models of diffuse malignant mesothelioma have been produced by direct intrapleural or intraperitoneal injection or, at a lower frequency, following inhala-

A. B. Kane: Department of Pathology and Laboratory Medicine, Brown University School of Medicine, Providence, Rhode Island 02912.

tion of asbestos fibers or erionite (10). Although direct delivery of fibers into the pleural or peritoneal spaces is an unnatural route of exposure, the histopathology, pattern of growth, and natural history are identical to human diffuse malignant mesothelioma (1). Using this model system, Stanton and other investigators discovered that long, thin mineral fibers are more likely to produce pleural or peritoneal mesotheliomas than short fibers (4,8,19). These studies used samples of short fibers prepared by milling, which may alter the surface properties and biologic reactivity of fibers (20). Short mineral fibers or particulate materials are more readily cleared from the lungs and pleural or peritoneal spaces (19). After a single intraperitoneal injection of crocidolite asbestos fibers in mice, long fibers are trapped at lymphatic stomata located on the inferior surface of the diaphragm and within milky spots or Kampmeir's foci in the intestinal mesenteries. Short asbestos fibers or particulate minerals are successfully cleared through these lymphatic stomata and accumulate in mesenteric lymph nodes. The diameter of lymphatic stomata (8–12 μm in mice) appears to be a critical factor that limits clearance of long fibers (21).

Malignant mesotheliomas are identified histologically after a latency period of 9 to 24 months. These tumors most commonly spread diffusely over the peritoneal lining in multiple layers. These tumors have a variable histologic appearance: epithelioid (Fig. 1), fibroblastic or sarcomatous (Fig. 2), or mixed morphology. The malignant cells express cytokeratins as demonstrated by immunohistochemistry. Rarely, malignant mesotheliomas have areas of osteoid and bone formation. Cystic areas containing hyaluronic acid are present, especially in the mixed tumors. Few asbestos fibers are seen within these tumors when examined under dark-field illumination. Angiogenesis is not a common feature of these superficial tumors. Small detached tumorlets or spheroids of malignant mesothelioma cells are found in some animals. The central areas of these spheroids often contain abundant hyaluronic acid. Rarely, sheets and masses of malignant mesothelioma cells invade locally into skeletal muscle or mesenteric fat. In contrast to the tumors spreading over the serosal surfaces, these locally invasive mesotheliomas elicit a prominent angiogenic response (reviewed in 7).

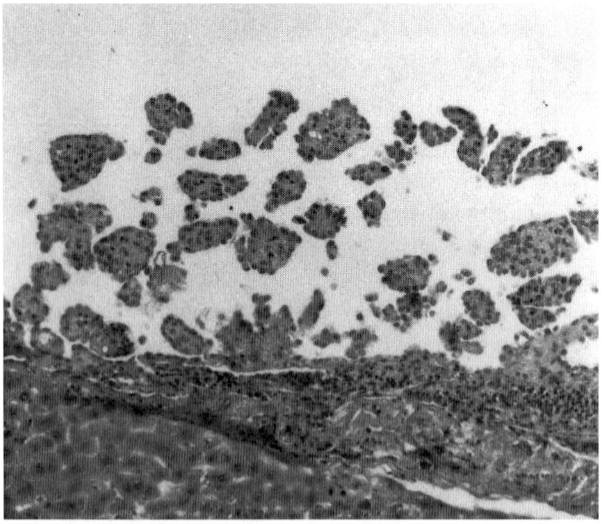

**FIG. 1.** Diffuse malignant mesothelioma, epithelioid type, growing as spheroids within the abdominal cavity. H&E original magnification, 200×.

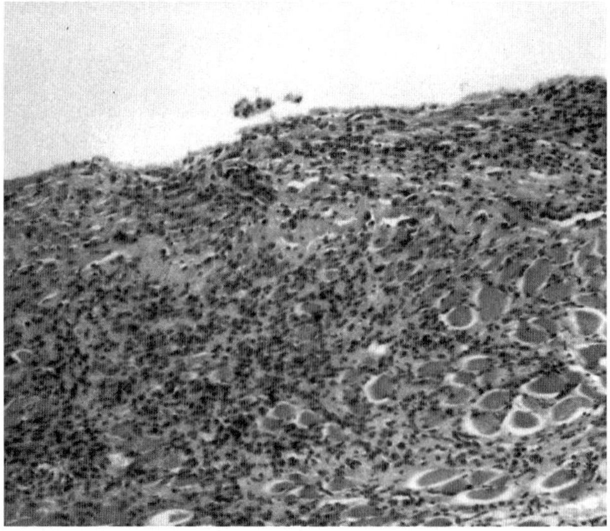

**FIG. 2.** Diffuse malignant mesothelioma, sarcomatous type, infiltrating into skeletal muscle of the abdominal wall. H&E original magnification, 200×.

The earliest response described after intraperitoneal injection of asbestos fibers is mesothelial cell proliferation (21,22). This is evident within 1 week and is accompanied by accumulation of activated macropahges at sites of fiber deposition. In experiments using a high dose (50 mg) of chrysotile or crocidolite asbestos in rats, cuboidal regenerating mesothelial cells were observed covering large areas of previously denuded mesothelium (23). Superficial growth of reactive proliferating mesothelial cells on the surface of the omentum has been described as "malignant mesothelioma *in situ*" by one investigator (22). Fibrous scarring of the peritoneal lining develops 12 to 22 weeks after injection of asbestos fibers; this fibrosis is usually accompanied by granulomas containing asbestos fibers, macrophages, and multinucleated giant cells (7). Although peritoneal fibrosis is not considered a precursor lesion leading to development of diffuse malignant mesothelioma, some investigators have observed that sarcomatous mesotheliomas appear to develop adjacent to these fibrotic lesions (23–25).

Recognition of distinct morphologic stages in the development of malignant mesotheliomas induced by crocidolite asbestos fibers has both mechanistic and diagnostic implications. Carcinogenesis is recognized as a multistage process characterized by progressive accumulation of molecular alterations in a target cell population. In contrast to the recent progress that has been achieved in other carcinomas of the lung (26), little is known about the molecular events leading to the development of human malignant mesotheliomas. This neoplasm is usually diagnosed at a late stage when the tumor has already spread diffusely over the serosal surfaces; no specific histopathologic precursor lesion has been identified (14). However, with the recent introduction of new diagnostic procedures such as thoracoscopy, malignant mesotheliomas are being diagnosed at earlier stages (27). The rodent model systems described here provide an opportunity to identify specific molecular alterations that occur during the development of malignant mesotheliomas induced by mineral fibers. These molecular alterations can then be correlated with specific precursor lesions such as described in these rodent models and may serve as markers to permit earlier diagnosis of this tumor. Recognition of a stage in the development of malignant mesothelioma where tumor growth is confined to the serosal surfaces and has not yet elicited angiogenesis or acquired the ability to invade locally (7) is important because tumors at this stage may be more susceptible to chemotherapy or immunotherapy (16,17).

## LIMITATIONS OF ANIMAL MODELS

There are several shortcomings of the intrapleural or intraperitoneal injection models. First, most protocols require a large dose of mineral fibers (10–40 mg) in order to produce tumors in a high percentage of animals. A single, large injection or implant is usually associated with extensive fibrosis and may become walled off in the omentum (13). Repeated exposures to smaller doses would theoretically allow more fibers to come into contact with the target tissue. Second, most investigators have studied these tumors after they have formed grossly visible masses near the end of the rodent life span (28). Few investigators have systematically described the early reactions of the pleural or peritoneal linings to asbestos fibers in an attempt to identify preneoplastic lesions of the mesothelial lining. Third, high doses of mineral fibers used to induce mesotheliomas in these rodent models raise the possibility that mesotheliomas produced by direct exposure of the peritoneum to high doses of fibers occur by a different mechanism than mesotheliomas that occur after inhalation (29,30). Recent inhalation studies have shown differences in the biopersistence of natural and man-made fibers in the lungs (12). Direct intraperitoneal injection of fibers bypasses the normal defenses of the respiratory tract. Intraperitoneal injection of high doses of fibers that persist for only a short time in the lung become surrounded by a fibrotic, granulomatous inflammatory response that limits fiber dissolution and clearance (31). Lower doses of fibers delivered by intraperitoneal or intrapleural injection may provide a better estimate of biopersistence in the mesothelial lining (32).

Recent rodent inhalation models are more reproducible in induction of pleural mesotheliomas in comparison with earlier studies (33,34). Direct comparison of rats and hamsters exposed to refractory ceramic fibers showed an increased tumor incidence in hamsters (35). Increased sensitivity of hamsters to development of mesothelioma may provide a more sensitive assay to identify potentially carcinogenic asbestos-fiber substitutes (15).

## MECHANISTIC STUDIES

Several mechanisms have been proposed for induction of malignant mesothelioma by exposure to mineral fibers (36). Fiber dimensions, surface reactivity, chemical composition, and biopersistence at the target tissue are important physicochemical properties that are related to the biologic activity of mineral fibers (13). Animal models provided the initial evidence for the importance of fiber dimensions in induction of mesotheliomas by direct intrapleural or intraperitoneal instillation of mineral fibers (3). Inhalation studies suggest that biopersistence and surface reactivity are also important parameters (12). Subchronic inhalation studies have also demonstrated that fibers can migrate to the pleura and induce chronic inflammatory and proliferative responses after inhalation (37). These responses were associated with accumulation of short fibers in the pleural space, raising questions about the potential biologic activity of short fibers (38–40).

*In vitro* studies using direct exposure of target cell populations to mineral fibers also suggest that the biologic activity of fibers depends on both physical and chemical factors (13). Two mechanisms have been proposed for fiber-induced carcinogenesis: physical interference of fibers with the mitotic apparatus (41) and generation of reactive oxygen and nitrogen intermediates (42–44). Video microscopy of living cells has demonstrated physical interference of long asbestos fibers with the mitotic splindle and cleavage furrow of mitotic cells. This mechanism has been proposed to explain induction of aneuploidy, polyploidy, and binucleate cells in a variety of target cells exposed to mineral fibers *in vitro* (45). Cytogenetic analyses of human and rodent mesotheliomas have also shown multiple chromosomal alterations (46,47). No studies have investigated whether these cytogenetic alterations are directly related to the physical presence of fibers within proliferating, preneoplastic mesothelial cell populations.

Alternatively, mineral fibers may catalyze the generation of reactive oxygen and nitrogen intermediates, either directly from molecular oxygen or indirectly from oxidants produced by inflammatory cells or other target cells (13). The availability of iron at the surface of mineral fibers is an important factor leading to generation of reactive oxygen and nitrogen intermediates (44,48–50). Ferric and ferrous cations are major components of amphibole asbestos fibers. Iron may also be present as surface impurities on serpentine asbestos or man-made fibers. Other mineral fibers such as erionite may acquire iron from the biologic medium, depending on the availability of reducing agents or chelators (43). Acute exposure of rats to asbestos fibers by inhalation induces antioxidant defenses (51). Exogenous catalase protected against the acute inflammatory response and tissue injury induced by asbestos in this inhalation model (52). A similar protective effect was observed for acute mesothelial cell injury induced by direct intraperitoneal injection of crocidolite asbestos in mice. These studies provide *in vivo* evidence that acute toxicity induced by asbestos fibers is mediated in part by oxidants such as hydrogen peroxide and hydroxyl radicals (42).

Reactive oxygen and nitrogen intermediates have the potential to damage DNA, activate intracellular signaling cascades, alter gene expression, and stimulate cell proliferation or death by apoptosis (13). All of these biologic end points have been observed in human or rodent mesothelial cells exposed to asbestos and other mineral fibers *in vitro* (53). Activation of transcription factors (NF-κB and AP-1) and induction of proto-oncogene expression (c-*fos* and c-*jun*) are important regulators of inflammation and cell proliferation (54,55). Increased expression of c-*fos* and c-*jun* has been shown in rat lungs after acute inhalation of crocidolite asbestos fibers (56). Upregulation of these proto-oncogenes may be responsible for chronic mesothelial cell proliferation induced by mineral fibers that persist in the target tissue. Enhanced mesothelial cell proliferation was induced by intrapleural injection of man-made fibers in hamsters in comparison with rats; this enhanced proliferative response may be one factor contributing to the increased sensitivity of hamsters to development of mesotheliomas following inhalation (57). Persistent proliferation of mesothelial cells would increase the risk of accumulating spontaneous genetic mutations or DNA breaks, deletions, rearrangements, and altered patterns of methylation induced by reactive oxygen and nitrogen intermediates (13).

Comparative molecular and cytogenetic analyses have been carried out using cell lines derived from human or rodent malignant mesotheliomas. Most of the rodent mesotheliomas were induced by intraperitoneal injection of asbestos fibers; a few cell lines were spontaneously immortalized *in vitro* or obtained from aged male Fischer 344 rats that spontaneously develop mesotheliomas. Most of the human malignant mesothelioma cell lines were derived from patients who had a history of asbestos exposure. In some experiments, the results of *in vitro* studies have been confirmed by immunohistochemistry or in situ hybridization performed directly on human tissues (13).

Tumors show autonomous proliferation with reduced differentiation. In advanced stages, tumors acquire the ability to invade locally and to metastasize to distant sites. These altered growth characteristics are associated with alterations in growth regulatory genes, including growth factors and their receptors, and cell cycle regulatory genes. Increased expression of growth factors and their receptors may result from constitutive overexpression or increased expression resulting from gene amplification. Proto-oncogenes regulate the cell cycle; amplification or point mutations of proto-oncogenes converts them to oncogenes that stimulate cell cycle progression and tumor cell growth. Tumor suppressor genes frequently block cell cycle progression; inactivation by point mutation, deletion, rearrangement, or association with viral oncoproteins eliminates normal cell cycle controls and also contributes to tumor cell growth. Specific alterations in some of these growth regulatory pathways have been described in human and rodent malignant mesothelioma cell lines (reviewed in 58). The mechanisms leading to these alterations are speculative (see below).

### Growth Factors

Growth factors may influence tumor cell growth by paracrine or autocrine mechanisms. Paracrine growth stimulation results from local release of growth factors by neighboring normal cells that modulate growth of tumor cells (59). Asbestos and man-made fibers stimulate synthesis and release of cytokines and growth factors by a variety of target cells. In the pleural and peritoneal spaces, macrophages are an important target for fibers that translocate to that location. Fibers stimulate release of chemotactic factors and cytokines that amplify a localized inflammatory reaction and upregulate production of inflammatory mediators by mesothelial cells. Some of these inflammatory mediators may stimulate mesothelial cell proliferation. Transient mesothelial cell proliferation has been observed in a variety of rodent models after intratracheal instillation, inhalation, or direct intrapleural (57) or intraperitoneal (21) instillation of asbestos or man-made fibers. In some cases, focal regions of persistent mesothelial cell proliferation were observed in response to highly biopersistent fibers such as crocidolite asbestos (32). It is hypothesized that local, paracrine release of cytokines and growth factors from activated macrophages in the adjacent alveolar spaces or in the pleural or peritoneal spaces could sustain mesothelial cell proliferation and contribute to the initial steps in the development of malignant mesothelioma (30). This hypothesis has not yet been tested critically; although transgenic mice that overexpress or are deficient in various cytokines or growth factors have been genetically engineered. A major obstacle in designing experiments with transgenic mice is that mesothelial cells respond to a wide variety of cytokines and growth factors; there is considerable redundancy in the mediators involved in pleural inflammation and healing.

**TABLE 1.** *Expression of growth factors by human, rat, and murine malignant mesothelioma cell lines*

| | Mesothelioma cell line | | |
|---|---|---|---|
| Growth factor | Human | Rat | Murine |
| PDGF | + | – | + |
| TGF-α | + | + | + |
| TGF-β1, β2 | + | ? | + |
| IGF-I | + | Rare | ? |
| IGF-II | ? | +/– | ? |
| bFGF | + | ? | ? |

bFGF, basic fibroblast growth factor; IGF, insulin-like growth factor; PDGF, platelet-derived growth factor; TGF, transforming growth factor.

Once malignant mesotheliomas have fully developed, the tumor cells themselves constitutively overexpress several growth factors and their receptors as summarized in Table 1. Platelet-derived growth factor (PDGF) has been suggested to be an important autocrine growth factor for human (60) or murine (59) mesothelioma cells, but not for rat mesothelioma cells (61). Transforming growth factor-α (TGF-α) is an important autocrine growth factor for all malignant mesothelioma cells (59). Other growth factors, including TGF-β1 and -β2, insulin-like growth factor-II (IGF-II), and basic fibroblast growth factor (bFGF), are also produced by malignant mesothelioma cells (59,62,63). Normal mesothelial cells and malignant mesotheliomal cells express IGF-I, IGF-I receptor, and IGF-binding protein-3 (63).

Autocrine production of growth factors can stimulate autonomous proliferation of tumor cells; at the same time, local or systemic release of growth factors and cytokines can have important clinical consequences (59). While TGF-β1 and -β2 stimulate mesothelial cell growth, local release of the active form of this growth factor downregulates immune responses to this tumor. Deactivation of lymphocytes and macrophages infiltrating malignant mesotheliomas has been demonstrated in a murine model system (17). Strategies to circumvent this downregulation of the immune response to developing malignant mesotheliomas will be discussed subsequently. Some human and murine malignant mesothelioma cell lines constitutively release multiple cytokines including interleukins IL-1α and β, colony-stimulating factors (CSFs), IL-8, and IL-6. Some of these cytokines, especially IL-6, may be responsible for the systemic manifestations of advanced malignant mesotheliomas such as weight loss, anorexia, and thrombocytosis. The insulin-like growth factors (IGF-I and -II) may be responsible for hypoglycemia (7,17,59).

### Oncogenes and Tumor Suppressor Genes

Few alterations in oncogenes have been identified in human or rodent mesotheliomas. No point mutations have been identified in K-*ras* in human or rat mesothelioma cell lines (58). Acute exposure of rat pleural mesothelial cells to asbestos fibers *in vitro* induces prolonged expression of the proto-oncogenes c-*fos* and c-*jun*. It is hypothesized that coordinated overexpression of these proto-oncogenes activates transcription factors leading to mesothelial cell proliferation (54). Constitutive overexpression of c-*fos* and c-*jun* has been observed in two murine malignant mesothelioma cell lines induced by intraperitoneal injections of crocidolite asbestos fibers; these tumors had a highly invasive phenotype (Kane, unpublished observations).

In contrast to the absence of oncogene alterations in human or rodent mesotheliomas, alterations in four tumor suppressor genes have been reported in human or rodent mesotheliomas. As summarized in Table 2, there are some differences between the results obtained with human, rat, and murine mesothelioma cell lines. An important caveat to be considered in all of these studies is that human mesotheliomas usually develop after a long latency period during which inhaled fibers are presumably translocated to the pleural or peritoneal linings. In contrast, all of the comparative molecular analyses of rodent mesotheliomas use tumors produced within 1 or 2 years after direct intrapleural or intraperitoneal instillation of fibers (30).

The *p53* tumor suppressor gene has multiple functions, including regulation of cell proliferation, apoptosis, and induction of cell cycle arrest and repair in response to DNA damage. The *p53* gene is frequently inactivated in a wide range of human neoplasms, usually by point mutations in exons 5 to 8 (64). Analysis of two series of human

**TABLE 2.** *Tumor suppressor gene alterations in human, rat, and murine malignant mesothelioma cell lines*

| | Mesothelioma cell line | | |
|---|---|---|---|
| Gene | Human | Rat | Murine |
| *p53* | Overexpressed, no point mutations | No point mutations | Not expressed (30%), no point mutations |
| *WT1* | Expressed, no point mutations | Expressed, no point mutations | Expressed |
| *NF2* | Multiple mutations | No mutations | ? |
| *Rb* | No alterations | ? | ? |
| $p16^{INK4a}$ | Deleted | ? | Deleted |
| $p15^{INK4b}$ | Deleted | ? | Deleted |

mesothelioma cell lines revealed point mutations or deletions in only 25% (65). In contrast, no point mutations were found in rat (Pylev, unpublished observations) or murine mesothelioma cell lines, although no *p53* expression was detected in 30% of murine mesothelioma cell lines (66). However, in most human mesotheliomas, p53 protein is overexpressed as assessed by immunohistochemistry (67,68). The mechanism responsible for p53 overexpression is unknown; in some cases, SV40 viral sequences have been detected (69). The presence of SV40 T-antigen inactivates normal p53 function in the absence of point mutation and prolongs the half-life of the protein (64).

Inherited mutations in the Wilms' tumor suppressor gene *(WT1)* are associated with development of kidney tumors in early childhood; survivors of this tumor have been reported to have an increased risk of developing malignant mesotheliomas as adults (70,71). In contrast to most adult tissues, both normal and neoplastic mesothelial cells express *WT1*; no point mutations have been detected in human or rat cell lines derived from diffuse malignant mesotheliomas (72).

Neurofibromatosis type 2 is an inherited autosomal dominant disease characterized by tumors of the central nervous system. The *NF2* gene product is called merlin, a protein that is hypothesized to link the cytoskeleton to the plasma membrane. Multiple genetic alterations in *NF2* have been identified in approximately 40% of human malignant mesotheliomas; no alterations were detected in rat malignant mesotheliomas (73–75).

The most frequently altered tumor suppressor gene in human malignant mesotheliomas is *p16*; it has been reported to be inactivated in 70% to 100% of cases, usually by co-deletion involving *p15*, a closely linked gene on human chromosome 9p (76–79). Inherited mutations in the *p16* tumor suppressor gene are associated with the development of malignant melanoma or pancreatic cancer. The *p16* tumor suppressor gene is one of a family of cyclin-dependent kinase (CDK) inhibitors named INK4 proteins that bind to cyclins to regulate phosphorylation of the retinoblastoma gene (Rb) product. The cyclin D1, CDK4, p16, Rb complex is a frequent functional target for inactivation in human tumors (80). Inactivation of one component of the complex apparently confers a significant proliferative advantage to tumor cells; for example, *p16* is inactivated in almost all mesotheliomas (79), *cyclin D1* is rarely overexpressed, and no *Rb* mutations have been found (65,77). Inactivation of *p16* has also been found in 80% of murine mesothelioma cell lines (Kane, unpublished observations).

## Genetically Engineered Mice

The technique of gene transfer by implanting embryonic stem cells into developing mouse blastocysts has been developed to overexpress or inactivate specific genes in the offspring (81). Mice that overexpress a specific oncogene or are deficient in a tumor suppressor gene show increased development of spontaneous tumors and increased susceptibility to chemical and physical carcinogens (82). Genetically engineered mice have also been developed that have altered levels of antioxidant defense enzymes or abnormalities in DNA repair pathways. Increasing availability of these mouse strains will allow investigators to dissect the steps leading to asbestos-induced mesotheliomas at the molecular level (81).

Initial studies using mice with homozygous or heterozygous disruption of the *p53* tumor suppressor gene have been described (81). These mice are susceptible to spontaneous development of sarcomas and lymphomas and show increased sensitivity to induction of lymphomas by ionizing radiation (83). DNA damage induced by ionizing radiation and asbestos fibers activates a cell cycle checkpoint that arrests cells in G1. Increased expression of the p53 protein initiates this checkpoint and induces expression of additional genes that prevent cell cycle progression and initiate DNA repair. Cells lacking functional p53 protein as a result of gene deletion or disruption, point mutation, or inactivation by viral proteins are defective in cell cycle arrest triggered by DNA-damaging agents (64). A murine mesothelial cell line that spontaneously acquired a point mutation in the *p53* gene did not arrest at the G1 checkpoint after exposure to ionizing radiation. This cell line also showed increased sensitivity to induction of micronuclei by exposure to ionizing radiation or crocidolite asbestos fibers *in vitro*. Failure of the G1 cell cycle checkpoint allows cells to enter S phase without repair of damaged DNA, resulting in DNA fragments that form micronuclei during the subsequent mitosis (84). Micronuclei are also a marker of genetic damage *in vivo*: *p53*-deficient mice show increased formation of micronuclei after exposure to ionizing radiation (83). A single intraperitoneal injection of crocidolite asbestos fibers induces micronuclei in proliferating mesothelial cells. The number of micronuclei was increased threefold in homozygous *p53*-deficient mice. Therefore, it is hypothesized that *p53*-deficient mice would show increased susceptibility to induction of malignant mesothelioma by asbestos fibers (85).

Homozygous or heterozygous *p53*-deficient and wild-type mice were injected weekly with 200 μg of crocidolite asbestos fibers for 35 weeks. The time course for induction of malignant mesotheliomas was significantly reduced in *p53*-deficient mice; homozygous *p53*-deficient mice developed mesotheliomas after only 10 weeks. The mean latency period for induction of tumors in heterozygous *p53*-deficient mice was 44 weeks in comparison to 67 weeks in wild-type mice. Focal tumors limited to the serosal surfaces were the earliest mesotheliomas observed in the heterozygous or wild-type mice. In the homozygous *p53*-deficient mice and in 50% of the heterozygous mice, invasive mesotheliomas were found.

These tumors were large, with regions of central necrosis. They showed lymphatic invasion and penetration through the diaphragm to involve the pleura. Microdissection of these invasive tumors in heterozygous *p53*-deficient mice and genotyping of isolated DNA showed loss of the wild-type allele. These highly invasive tumors also showed increased anaplasia with binucleate and multinucleated tumor cells and abnormal mitotic figures (85).

The *p53* tumor suppressor gene has multiple functions. In addition to induction of cell cycle arrest and repair in response to DNA damage, p53 protein also induces apoptosis (64). Tumor cells that are deficient in *p53* function are resistant to apoptosis; this resistance may contribute to aggressive growth of tumors in late stages of tumor progression (86). It is hypothesized that *p53*-deficient mesothelial cells would be resistant to induction of apoptosis. The chemotherapeutic drug camptothecin binds to topoisomerase I and induces DNA strand breaks during S phase. Camptothecin induces apoptosis in wild-type murine mesothelioma cell lines *in vitro*, but not in *p53*-deficient mesothelioma cell lines (85). Crocidolite asbestos fibers also induce apoptosis in rat, rabbit, and human mesothelial cells *in vitro* (87,88); this response is induced in wild-type murine mesothelioma cells, but not in *p53*-deficient mesothelioma cells (85).

A working hypothesis for the development of malignant mesothelioma by asbestos fibers is outlined in Fig. 3. The initial response of the mesothelial lining to asbestos fibers is proliferation in response to injury (21) or activation of mitogenic signaling pathways (53). Production of oxidants by macrophages at sites of deposition of long fibers on the mesothelial surface has been demonstrated in situ (89). It is hypothesized that macrophages release reactive oxygen and nitrogen intermediates that induce DNA damage (44) and apoptosis (87,88) in proliferating mesothelial cells. Oxidants may also contribute to altered methylation and deletion of the *p16* tumor suppressor gene (90,91). Functional inactivation of *p53* by viral proteins such as SV40 T-antigen in humans (69) or by targeted deletion in *p53*-deficient mice (85) results in loss of cell cycle checkpoints, genetic instability, and resistance to apoptosis (64). Inactivation of *p53* or other components of the G1 cell cycle checkpoint such as *mdm2* (92) accelerates late stages in progression and invasion of malignant mesotheliomas.

## PRACTICAL APPLICATIONS OF ANIMAL MODELS

### Drug Sensitivity of Human Mesothelioma Xenografts

Diffuse malignant mesothelioma is a rare neoplasm in humans and clinical trials to evaluate new therapeutic strategies are difficult to conduct. An alternate approach to test new combination therapies is transplantation of human mesothelioma cells into immunodeficient mice. Athymic nude mice deficient in T cells have been used most commonly as recipients of mesothelioma xenografts. Human mesothelioma cell lines maintained as xenografts retain their original histologic characteristics and karyotype. Treatment with single chemotherapeutic agents such as 5-azacytidine, 5-fluorouracil, methotrexate, and vincristine was ineffective, confirming previous clinical observations. In some human mesothelioma cell lines, a partial response to combination chemotherapy (cisplatin plus mitomycin or doxorubicin) was demonstrated in the xenografts. This animal model is useful to test additional novel therapeutic approaches including the combination of interferon-α (IFN-α) with mitomycin and cisplatin. Novel treatments such as photodynamic therapy were tested in nude mice followed by phase I clinical trials (16).

### Immunotherapy

A novel approach to cancer therapy is to activate the host immune response to kill tumor cells. Mice are an ideal animal model to investigate this strategy because the immune system of inbred strains has been well characterized. Both human and murine mesothelioma cell

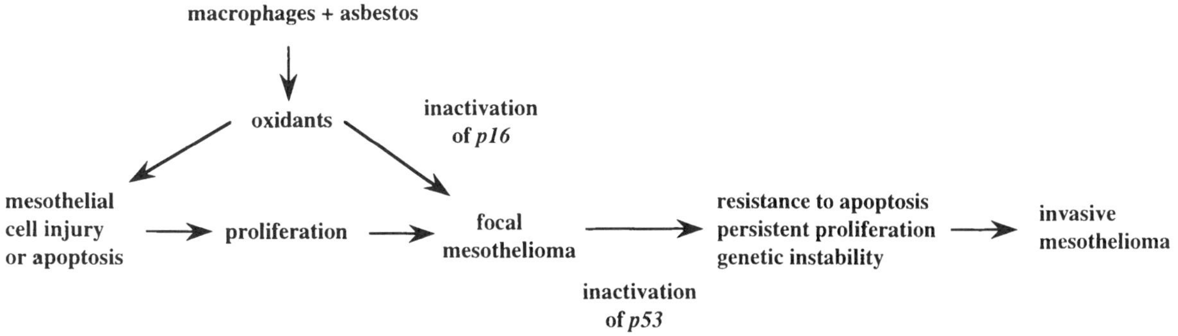


**FIG. 3.** Proposed mechanisms leading to the development of malignant mesothelioma induced by asbestos fibers.

lines can be lysed by lymphokine-activated killer cells or gamma-delta T lymphocytes, but not by natural killer cells, *in vitro*. Mesothelioma cell lines express class I major histocompatibility complex (MHC) molecules. Transfection of a co-stimulatory gene B7-1 into a murine mesothelioma cell line slows growth of cells transplanted *in vivo*. Both lymphocytes and macrophages infiltrate transplanted mesothelioma cells initially; eventually, they show downregulation of surface markers. It is hypothesized that TGF-β produced by the tumor cells deactivates the local immune response to malignant mesothelioma. New strategies to enhance the local immune response have been developed using gene transfer techniques (described below) or cytokines such as IFN-γ and IL-2 (17).

## Gene Therapy

As described earlier, human and rodent mesotheliomas grow diffusely over the pleural and peritoneal linings (7). Local delivery of chemotherapeutic agents and cytokines to these spaces may arrest tumor growth before invasion and metastases develop. Some combination therapies have shown promise in murine models; however, they have not yet been shown to eradicate human malignant mesotheliomas (16). New protocols using delivery of genes to pleural or peritoneal mesotheliomas are in progress. So far, viral gene transfer vectors have been tested in murine mesotheliomas and human mesothelioma xenografts (92,93). The first approach was to enhance the local immune response to murine mesotheliomas by transfecting class I or class II MHC genes plus the co-stimulatory molecule B7-1 (17). The transfection efficiency of viral gene vectors is low; however, successful transfection of a small number of tumor cells may be sufficient to augment the host immune response and eradicate the entire tumor. Additional studies using antisense TGF-β vectors may be required (18).

Replacement of inactivated tumor suppressor genes by viral vectors is an alternate approach to gene therapy (18). Deletion of the *p16* tumor suppressor gene is common in human and murine malignant mesotheliomas. Replacement of the *p16* gene in human mesothelioma cell lines slowed their growth and colony formation *in vitro* (77,79). This approach could be applied to murine mesotheliomas or human mesothelioma xenografts.

Molecular chemotherapy is another promising approach to deliver enzymes to cancer cells that convert nontoxic agents to a toxic metabolite. This approach uses retroviral, adenoviral, or modified herpes simplex viruses to deliver the herpes simplex thymidine kinase gene (HSVtk) into tumor cells. HSVtk converts the nontoxic nucleoside analog, ganciclovir, into a toxic metabolite. The toxic metabolite is transferred to adjacent nontransfected cells resulting in a "bystander effect" and killing of the majority of tumor cells (18). This therapeutic approach has been successfully tested in human malignant mesotheliomas transplanted intraperitoneally into severe combined immunodeficiency disease (SCID) mice (93,94). The next step is to test this new therapeutic strategy in clinical trials of human malignant mesothelioma.

## ACKNOWLEDGMENT

The research conducted in the author's laboratory was supported by grants from the National Institute of Environmental Health Sciences (R01 ES03721 and R01 ES05712).

## REFERENCES

1. Craighead JE. Current pathogenetic concepts of diffuse malignant mesothelioma. *Hum Pathol* 1987;18:544–557.
2. Wagner JC, Sleggs CA, Marchand P. Diffuse pleural mesothelioma and asbestos exposure in the Northwestern Cape Province. *Br J Ind Med* 1960;17:260–271.
3. Wagner JC. Historical background and perspectives of mesothelioma. In: Jaurand M-C, Bignon J, eds. *The mesothelial cell and mesothelioma.* New York: Marcel Dekker, 1994;1–18.
4. Stanton MF, Wrench C. Mechanisms of mesothelioma induction with asbestos and fibrous glass. *J Natl Can Inst* 1972;48:797–821.
5. Pott F, Friedrichs KH. Tumours in rats after intraperitoneal injection of asbestos dusts. *Naturwissenschaften* 1972;59:318–320.
6. Davis JMG. Experimental and spontaneous mesotheliomas. In: Jaurand M-C, Bignon J, eds. *The mesothelial cell and mesothelioma.* New York: Marcel Dekker, 1994;187–206.
7. Craighead JE, Kane AB. The pathogenesis of malignant and nonmalignant serosal lesions in body cavities consequent to asbestos exposure. In: Jaurand M-C, Bignon J, eds. *The mesothelial cell and mesothelioma.* New York: Marcel Dekker, 1994;79–102.
8. Stanton MF, Layard M, Tegeris A, et al. Relation of particle dimension to carcinogenicity in amphibole asbestos and other fibrous minerals. *J Natl Can Inst* 1981;67:965–975.
9. Wagner JC, Griffiths DM, Hill RJ. The effect of fibre size on the *in vivo* activity of UICC crocidolite. *Br J Cancer* 1984;49:453–458.
10. Johnson NF. The limitations of inhalation, intratracheal, and intracoelomic routes of administration for identifying hazardous fibrous materials. In: Jaurand M-C, Bignon J, eds. *The mesothelial cell and mesothelioma.* New York: Marcel Dekker, 1994;43–72.
11. Meek ME, Long G. Man-made vitreous fibres. *Environ Carcinogen Ecotox Rev* 1994;C12:361–387.
12. Hesterberg TW, Miller WC, Musselman RP, Kamstrup O, Hamilton RD, Thevenaz P. Biopersistence of man-made vitreous fibers and crocidolite asbestos in rat lung following inhalation. *Fundam Appl Toxicol* 1996;29:267–279.
13. Kane AB. Mechanisms of mineral fibre carcinogenesis. In: Kane AB, Boffetta P, Saracci R, Wilbourn JD, eds. *Mechanisms of fibre carcinogenesis.* Lyon: IARC Scientific Publications (No. 140), 1996;11–34.
14. McCaughey WTE, Al-Jabi M. Differentiation of serosal hyperplasia and neoplasia in biopsies. *Pathol Ann* 1986;21:271–294.
15. Vu V, Barrett JC, Roycroft J, et al. Chronic inhalation toxicity and carcinogenicity testing of respirable fibrous particles. *Reg Toxicol Pharmacol* 1996;24:202–212.
16. Chahinian AP. Therapeutic studies of malignant mesothelioma in nude mice. In: Jaurand M-C, Bignon J, eds. *The mesothelial cell and mesothelioma.* New York: Marcel Dekker, 1994;285–296.
17. Bielefeldt-Ohmann H, Jarnicki AG, Fitzpatrick DR. Molecular pathobiology and immunology of malignant mesothelioma. *J Pathol* 1996;178:369–378.
18. Curiel DT, Pilewski JM, Albelda SM. Gene therapy approaches for inherited and acquired lung diseases. *Am J Respir Cell Mol Biol* 1996; 14:1–18.
19. Davis JMG, Addison J, Bolton RE, Donaldson K, Jones AD, Smith S.

The pathogenicity of long versus short fibre samples of amosite asbestos administered to rats by inhalation and intraperitoneal injection. *Br J Exp Pathol* 1986;67:415–430.
20. Harington JS. Fiber carcinogenesis: epidemiologic observations and the Stanton hypothesis. *J Natl Cancer Inst* 1981;67:977–989.
21. Moalli PA, Macdonald JL, Goodglick LA, Kane A. Acute injury and regeneration of the mesothelium in response to asbestos fibers. *Am J Pathol* 1987;128:426–445.
22. Friemann J, Müller KM, Pott F. Mesothelial proliferation due to asbestos and man-made fibres. Experimental studies on rat omentum. *Pathol Res Pract* 1990;186:117–123.
23. Shin ML, Firminger HI. Acute and chronic effects of intraperitoneal injection of two types of asbestos in rats with a study of the histopathogenesis and ultrastructure of resulting mesotheliomas. *Am J Pathol* 1973;70:219–314.
24. David JMG. Histogenesis and fine structure of peritoneal tumors produced in animals by injections of asbestos. *J Natl Cancer Inst* 1979; 52:1823–1837.
25. Craighead JE, Akley NJ, Gould LB, Libbus BL. Characteristics of tumors and tumor cells cultured from experimental asbestos-induced mesotheliomas in rats. *Am J Pathol* 1987;129:448–462.
26. Viallet J, Minna JD. Dominant oncogenes and tumor suppressor genes in the pathogenesis of lung cancer. *Am J Respir Cell Mol Biol* 1990;2:225–232.
27. Boutin C, Rey R. Thoracoscopy in pleural malignant mesothelioma: a prospective study of 188 consecutive patients. Part 1: Diagnosis. *Cancer* 1993;72:389–393.
28. Pott F, Ziem U, Reiffer F-J, Huth F, Ernest H, Mohr U. Carcinogenicity studies on fibres, metal compounds, and some other dusts in rats. *Exp Pathol* 1987;32:129–152.
29. Warheit DB, Driscoll KE, Oberdoerster G, Walker C, Kuschner M, Hesterberg TW. Contemporary issues in fiber toxicology. *Fundam Appl Toxicol* 1995;25:171–183.
30. Consensus report. In: Kane AB, Boffetta P, Saracci R, Wilbourn JD, eds. *Mechanisms of fibre carcinogenesis.* Lyon: IARC Scientific Publications (No. 140), 1996;1–9.
31. Collier CG, Morris KJ, Launder KA, et al. The behavior of glass fibers in the rat following intraperitoneal injection. *Reg Toxicol Pharmacol* 1994;20: S89–S103.
32. Macdonald JL, Kane AB. Mesothelial cell proliferation and biopersistence of wollastonite and crocidolite asbestos fibers. *Fundam Appl Toxicol* 1997;38:173–183.
33. McConnell EE, Kamstrup O, Musselman R, et al. Chronic inhalation study of size-separated rock and slag wool insulation fibers in Fischer 344/N rats. *Inhalation Toxicol* 1994;6:571–614.
34. Mast RW, McConnell EE, Anderson R, et al. Studies on the chronic toxicity (inhalation) of four types of refractory ceramic fiber in male Fischer 344 rats. *Inhalation Toxicol* 1995;7:425–467.
35. McConnell EE, Mast RW, Hesterberg TW, et al. Chronic inhalation toxicity of a kaolin-based refractory ceramic fiber in Syrian golden hamsters. *Inhalation Toxicol* 1995;7:503–532.
36. Walker C, Everitt J, Barrett JC. Possible cellular and molecular mechanisms for asbestos carcinogenicity. *Am J Ind Med* 1992;21:253–273.
37. Gelzleichter TR, Bermudez E, Mangum JB, Wong BA, Everitt JI, Moss OR. Pulmonary and pleural responses in Fischer 344 rats following short-term inhalation of a synthetic vitreous fiber. I. Quantitation of lung and pleural fiber burdens. *Fundam Appl Toxicol* 1996;30:31–38.
38. Oehlert GN. A re-analysis of the Stanton et al pleural sarcoma data. *Environ Res* 1991;54:L194–205.
39. Dunnigan J. Biological effects of fibers: Stanton's hypothesis revisited. *Environ Health Perspect* 1984;57:333–337.
40. Churg A, Wiggs B. Fiber size and number in amphibole asbestos-induced mesothelioma. *Am J Pathol* 1984;115:437–442.
41. Hesterberg T, Barrett J. Induction by asbestos fibers of anaphase abnormalities: mechanisms for aneuploidy induction and possibly carcinogenesis. *Carcinogenesis* 1985;6:473–475.
42. Moyer VD, Cistulli CA, Vaslet CA, Kane AB. Oxygen radicals and asbestos carcinogenesis. *Environ Health Perspect* 1994;102:131–136.
43. Hardy JA, Aust AE. Iron in asbestos chemistry and carcinogenicity. *Chem Rev* 1995;95:97–118.
44. Chao C-C, Park S-H, Aust AE. Participation of nitric oxide and iron in the oxidation of DNA in asbestos-treated human lung epithelial cells. *Arch Biochem Biophys* 1996;326:152–157.
45. Ault JG, Cole RW, Jensen CG, Jensen LCW, Bachert LA, Reider CL. Behavior of crocidolite asbestos during mitosis in living vertebrate lung epithelial cells. *Cancer Res* 1995;55:792–798.
46. Libbus BL, Craighead JE. Chromosomal translocations with specific breakpoints in asbestos-induced rat mesotheliomas. *Cancer Res* 1988; 48:6455–6461.
47. Knuutila S, Tammilehto L, Mattson K. Chromosomal abnormalities in human malignant mesothelioma. In: Jaurand M-C, Bignon J, eds. *The mesothelial cell and mesothelioma.* New York: Marcel Dekker, 1994; 145–252.
48. Weitzman SA, Graceffa P. Asbestos catalyzes hydroxyl and superoxide radical release from hydrogen peroxide. *Arch Biochem Biophys* 1984;22:373–376.
49. Bonneau L, Marlard C, Pezerat H. Studies on surface properties of asbestos. *Environ Res* 1986;41:268–275.
50. Gulumian M, Van Wyk JA. Hydroxyl radical production in the presence of fibres by a Fenton-type reaction. *Chem Biol Interact* 1987;62:89–97.
51. Janssen YMW, Marsh JP, Absher MP, et al. Expression of antioxidant enzymes in rat lungs after inhalation of asbestos or silica. *J Biol Chem* 1992;267:10625–10630.
52. Mossman BT, Marsh JP, Gilbert R, et al. Inhibition of lung injury, inflammation, and interstitial pulmonary fibrosis by polyethylene glycol-conjugated catalase in a rapid inhalation model of asbestosis. *Am Rev Resir Dis* 1990;141:1266–1271.
53. Mossman BT, Faux S, Janssen Y, et al. Cell signaling pathways elicited by asbestos. *Environ Health Perspect* 1997;105(suppl 5):1121–1126.
54. Heintz NH, Janssen YM, Mossman BT. Persistent induction of c-*fos* and c-*jun* expression by asbestos. *Proc Natl Acad Sci USA* 1993; 90:3299–3303.
55. Janssen YMW, Heintz NH, Mossman BT. Inductions of c-*fos* and c-*jun* proto-oncogene expression by asbestos is ameliorated by *N*-acetyl-L-cysteine in mesothelial cells. *Cancer Res* 1995;55:2085–2089.
56. Quinlan TR, Bérubé KA, Marsh JP, et al. Patterns of inflammation, cell proliferation, and related gene expression in lung after inhalation of chrysotile asbestos. *Am J Pathol* 1995;147:728–739.
57. Rutten AAJJL, Bermudez E, Mangum JB, Wong BA, Moss OZR, Everitt JI. Mesothelial cell proliferation induced by intrapleural instillation of man-made fibers in rats and hamsters. *Fundam Appl Toxicol* 1994;23:107–116.
58. Lechner JF, Tesfaigzi J, Gerwin BI. Oncogenes and tumor suppressor genes in mesothelioma—a synopsis. *Environ Health Perspect* 1997;105 (suppl 5):1061–1068.
59. Fitzpatrick DR, Peroni DJ, Bielefeldt-Ohmann H. The role of growth factors and cytokines in the tumorigenesis and immunobiology of malignant mesothelioma. *Am J Respir Cell Mol Biol* 1995;12:455–460.
60. Versnel MA, Hagemeijer A, Bouts JJ, van der Kwast TH, Housteden HC. Expression of c-sis (PDGF B-chain) and PDGF A-chain genes in ten human malignant mesothelioma cell lines derived from primary and metastatic tumors. *Oncogene* 1998;2:601–606.
61. Walker C, Bermudez E, Steward W. Characterization of platelet-derived growth factor and platelet-derived growth factor receptor expression in asbestos-induced rat mesothelioma. *Cancer Res* 1992;52:301–306.
62. Gerwin BI, Lechner JF, Reddel RR, et al. Comparison of production of transforming growth factor-b and platelet-derived growth factor by normal human mesothelial cells and mesothelial cell lines. *Cancer Res* 1987;47:6180–6184.
63. Lee TC, Zhang Y, Aston C, et al. Normal human mesothelial cells and mesothelioma cell lines express insulin-like growth factor-I (IGF-I) and associated molecules. *Cancer Res* 1993;53:2858–2864.
64. Ko LJ, Prives C. p53: Puzzle and paradigm. *Genes Dev* 1996;10: 1054–1072.
65. Metcalf RA, Welsh JA, Bennett WP, et al. *p53* and Kirsten-*ras* mutations in human mesothelioma cell lines. *Cancer Res* 1992;52:2610–2615.
66. Cora EM, Kane AB. Alterations in a tumor suppressor gene, *p53*, in mouse mesotheliomas induced by crocidolite asbestos. *Eur Respir Rev* 1993;3:148–150.
67. Kafiri G, Thomas DM, Shepherd NA, Krausz T, Lane DP, Hall PA. *p53* expression is common in malignant mesothelioma. *Histopathology* 1992;21:331–334.
68. Mayall FG, Goodard H, Gibbs AR. The frequency of p53 immunostaining in asbestos-associated mesotheliomas and non-asbestos-associated mesotheliomas. *Histopathology* 1993;22:383–386.
69. Carbone M, Pass HI, Rizzo P, et al. Simian virus 40-like DNA sequences in human pleural mesothelioma. *Oncogene* 1994;9: 1781–1790.

70. Antman KH, Ruxer RL, Aisner J, Vawter G. Mesothelioma following Wilms' tumor in childhood. *Cancer* 1984;54:367–369.
71. Austin MB, Fechner RE, Roggli VL. Pleural malignant mesothelioma following Wilms' tumor. *Am J Clin Pathol* 1986;86:227–230.
72. Walker C, Rutten F, Yuan X, Pass H, Mew DH, Everitt J. Wilms' tumor suppressor gene expression in rat and human mesothelioma. *Cancer Res* 1994;54:3101–3106.
73. Bianchi AB, Mitzunaga S-I, Cheng JQ, et al. High frequency of inactivating mutations in the neurofibromatosis type 2 gene (*NF2*) in primary malignant mesotheliomas. *Proc Natl Acad Sci USA* 1995;92: 10854–10858.
74. Sekido Y, Pass HI, Bader S, et al. Neurofibromatosis type 2 (*NF2*) gene is somatically mutated in mesothelioma but not in lung cancer. *Cancer Res* 1995;55:1227–1231.
75. Kleymenova EV, Bianchi AA, Kley N, Pylev LN, Walker CL. Characterization of the rat neurofibromatosis 2 gene and its involvement in asbestos-induced mesothelioma. *Mol Carcinogen* 1997;18:54–60.
76. Cheng JQ, Jhanwar SC, Klein WM, et al. *p16* Alterations and deletion mapping of 9p21-p22 in malignant mesothelioma. *Cancer Res* 1994; 54:5547–5551.
77. Okamoto A, Demetrick DJ, Sillare EA, et al. Mutations and altered expression of $p16^{INK4}$ in human cancer. *Proc Natl Acad Sci USA* 1994; 91:11045–11049.
78. Xiao S, Li D, Vijg J, Sugarbaker DJ, Corson JM, Fletcher JA. Codeletion of p15 and p16 in primary malignant mesothelioma. *Oncogene* 1995;11:511–515.
79. Kratzke RA, Otterson GA, Lincoln CE, et al. Immunohistochemical analysis of the $p16^{INK4}$ cyclin-dependent kinase inhibitor in malignant mesothelioma. *J Natl Cancer Inst* 1995;87:1870–1875.
80. Sherr CJ. Cancer cell cycles. *Science* 1996;274:1672–1677.
81. Sands A, Donehower LA, Bradley A. Gene-targeting and the p53 tumor-suppressor gene. *Mutat Res* 1994;307:557–572.
82. Tennant RW, French JE, Spalding JW. Identifying chemical carcinogens and assessing potential risk in short-term bioassays using transgenic mouse models. *Environ Health Perspect* 1995;103:942–950.
83. Lee JM, Abrahamson JLA, Kandel R, Donehower LA, Bernstein A. Susceptibility to radiation-carcinogenesis and accumulation of chromosomal breakage in p53 deficient mice. *Oncogene* 1994;9: 3731–3736.
84. Cistulli CA, Sorger T, Marsella JM, Vaslet CA, Kane AB. Spontaneous *p53* mutation in murine mesothelial cells: increased sensitivity to DNA damage induced by asbestos and ionizing radiation. *Toxicol Appl Pharmacol* 1996;141:264–271.
85. Marsella JM, Liu BL, Vaslet CA, Kane AB. Susceptibility of *p53*-deficient mice to induction of mesothelioma by crocidolite asbestos fibers. *Environ Health Perspect* 1997;105(suppl 5):1069–1072.
86. Symonds H, Krall L, Remington L, et al. p53-Dependent apoptosis suppresses tumor growth and progression *in vivo*. *Cell* 1994;78:703–711.
87. Broaddus VC, Yang L, Scavo LM, Ernst JD, Boylan AM. Asbestos induces apoptosis of human and rabbit pleural mesothelial cells via reactive oxygen species. *J Clin Invest* 1996;89:20050–20059.
88. Bérubé KA, Quinlan TR, Fung H, et al. Apoptosis is observed in mesothelial cells after exposure to crocidolite asbestos. *Am J Respir Cell Mol Biol* 1996;15:141–147.
89. Goodglick LA, Kane A. Cytotoxicity of long and short crocidolite fibers *in vitro* and *in vivo*. *Cancer Res* 1990;50:5153–5163.
90. Weitzman SA, Turk PW, Milkowski DH, Kozlowski K. Free radical adducts induce alterations in DNA cytosine methylation. *Proc Natl Acad Sci USA* 1994;91:1261–1264.
91. Costello JF, Berger MS, Huang H-JS, Cavenee W. Silencing of p16/CDKN2 expression in human gliomas by methylation and chromatin condensation. *Cancer Res* 1996;56:2405–2410.
92. Sergers K, Backhovens H, Singh SK, et al. Immunoreactivity for p53 and mdm2 and the detection of p53 mutations in human malignant mesothelioma. *Virchows Arch* 1995;427:431–436.
93. Hwang HC, Smythe WR, Elshami AA, et al. Gene therapy using adenovirus carrying the herpes simplex-thymidine kinase gene to treat *in vivo* models of human malignant mesothelioma and lung cancer. *Am J Respir Cell Mol Biol* 1995;13:7–16.
94. Kucharczuk JC, Randazzo B, Chang MY, et al. Use of a "replication-restricted" herpes virus to treat experimental human malignant mesothelioma. *Cancer Res* 1997;57:466–471.

*Environmental and Occupational Medicine, Third Edition,* edited by William N. Rom.
Lippincott–Raven Publishers, Philadelphia © 1998.

# CHAPTER 26

# Asbestos in Public Buildings

L. Christine Oliver

Adverse health effects of occupational exposure to asbestos include asbestosis, lung cancer, malignant mesothelioma, and, in some populations, gastrointestinal and laryngeal cancer (1,2). These effects have been described in workers in asbestos mining and milling; in the manufacture of asbestos-containing products such as insulation and textile materials, cement, and ceiling and floor tile; and in the construction and renovation of buildings and ships (1–5). Asbestos-related disease has also been reported in association with bystander, household, and residential exposures (6,7). In addition, occupational and environmental exposures resulting from asbestos-containing materials (ACM) in buildings have been associated with an increase in risk for asbestos-related disease.

The potential for asbestos exposure from ACM in buildings exists for skilled craftspeople involved in structural renovation and repair work, custodial and maintenance personnel, asbestos abatement workers, and building occupants, including children in schools. The extent to which each of these groups is exposed to asbestos varies, as does the likely consequent risk. Issues at the crux of the problem of what to do with in-place asbestos in buildings include (a) determinants of exposure, (b) risk from "low level" exposure to asbestos, (c) toxicity of chrysotile asbestos, and (d) the relative risks of removal versus containment. There has been an ongoing struggle to come to grips with these issues by policymakers, government regulators, building owners, managers, developers, labor organizations, scientists, and the general public.

L. C. Oliver: Department of Medical Services, Pulmonary and Critical Care Unit, Massachusetts General Hospital; and Harvard Medical School, Boston, Massachusetts 02114.

## SCOPE OF THE PROBLEM

Asbestos has been used in public, residential, and commercial buildings in pipe and boiler insulation, in surface materials such as acoustic and decorative plaster, and on structural beams to prevent building collapse in the event of fire. The average percentage of asbestos has varied by product: floor tile, 20%; corrugated pipe wrap, 80%; preformed pipe wrap, 50%; sprayed- and troweled-on insulation, 50% and 70%, respectively; and boiler insulation, 10% (8). Its first use in building construction in the United States was in 1890 in boiler insulation. In 1910 its use in buildings was expanded to include pipe wrap; and in 1935, sprayed- and troweled-on insulation (8). The Environmental Protection Agency (EPA) banned its use in preformed pipe wrap in 1975 and in sprayed- and troweled-on insulation in 1978. In the summer of 1996, the minister of labor, health, and social affairs of France banned the manufacture, import, and use of asbestos fiber and asbestos-containing products in France, effective January 1, 1997 (9). The imposition of the ban followed by one day the June 1996 publication of a report entitled "Effects on Health of the Main Types of Exposure to Asbestos" written by 11 experts working on behalf of the French Medical Research Council (INSERM).

A nationwide survey was conducted in 1984 in the United States by the EPA to determine the prevalence and types of ACM in buildings. The survey produced the following estimates: approximately 733,000 buildings (20% of all buildings exclusive of schools and residential apartment buildings of fewer than ten units) contain friable ACM; 5% have sprayed- or troweled-on friable asbestos, and 16%, asbestos-containing pipe and boiler insulation (10). Of the asbestos identified in this survey, 70% was in pipe and boiler insulation, 14% in sprayed- or troweled-on friable material, and 3% in ceiling tile. Older buildings

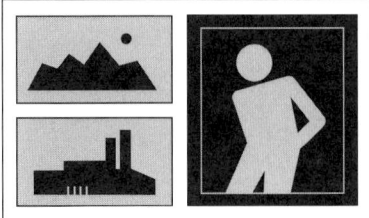

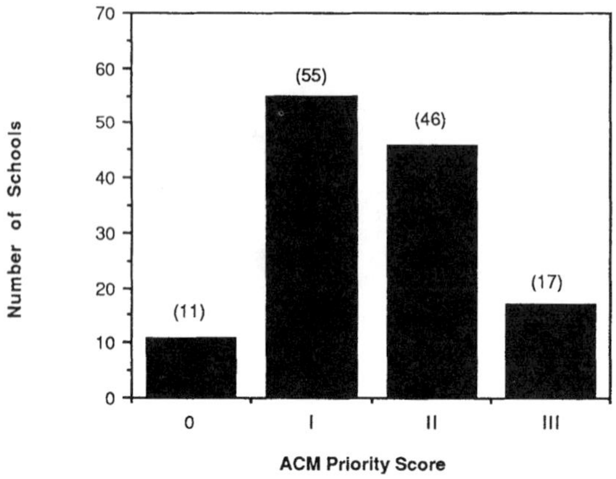


**FIG. 1.** Distribution of Boston public schools by priority category of ACM (Hygeia, 1983).

were more likely to have ACM in pipe and boiler insulation, whereas buildings constructed in the 1960s were more likely to have sprayed- or troweled-on ACM.

On a smaller scale, municipalities have conducted similar surveys targeted to more specific types of public buildings. In Boston, Massachusetts, for example, a 1983 survey of the public schools was done to determine the extent and quality of ACM (11). Each room of each school was visited and the presence and condition of any sprayed-on fireproofing, pipe covering, or acoustical plaster possibly containing asbestos was recorded. Bulk samples were analyzed by polarized light microscopy to confirm the presence of asbestos. Schools were then prioritized on the basis of presence, type, location, and condition of ACM (Fig. 1). Of the 129 schools inspected, 55 (42.6%) had ACM in serious disrepair, requiring prompt corrective action. In 46 (35.7%) asbestos was damaged but isolated, and in 17 (13.2%) ACM was intact and stable. Only 11 schools (8.5%) were free of identified ACM.

## THE ISSUES

### Determinants of Exposure

Asbestos that remains in place is not a threat to health. Asbestos that becomes airborne carries with it the risk for asbestos-related disease. Determinants of exposure (i.e., of the likelihood the asbestos will become airborne and inhalable) include friability, accessibility, condition, airflow patterns (pathways), and potential for disturbance (12) (Table 1). Friable ACM is ACM capable of being crushed by hand pressure. The more friable the material, the greater the potential for asbestos release. For example, corrugated paper pipe wrap is more friable and therefore poses a greater risk than preformed pipe wrap. Although nonfriable ACM is capable of releasing asbestos fibers under certain conditions (e.g., sanding vinyl asbestos floor tile), it is not likely to do so under normal circumstances.

**TABLE 1.** *Asbestos-containing material in buildings: determinants of exposure*

| |
|---|
| Friability |
| Accessibility |
| Condition |
| Patterns of air flow (pathways) |
| Potential for disturbance |

Accessibility of ACM to building occupants determines the likelihood of accidental disturbance and fiber release. Accessibility and the presence or absence of appropriate identifying and warning labels determines the likelihood of worker exposure. ACM that is accessible to custodians and skilled craftspeople is not necessarily accessible to other building occupants. An example is ACM in boiler rooms. Asbestos-covered pipes above dropped ceilings pose a risk for workers and occupants as well if it is not properly identified and appropriate precautions taken when ceiling tiles are removed for any reason. ACM that has been damaged by water or trauma is capable of fiber release, regardless of whether it is disturbed further. Airflow patterns in a building and pathways between ACM and occupied areas may determine both the extent to which damaged material releases fibers and the extent to which these fibers reach occupants.

Finally, the potential for accidental, unpredictable, and unintentional disturbance is an important risk factor for exposure. Disturbance of ACM may take several forms: predictable or episodic but intentional (e.g., routine maintenance), accidental (e.g., pipe leak requiring repair), episodic and intentional but unpredictable (e.g., vandalism), and continuous (e.g., building vibration). Predictable episodic and continuous disturbance can be taken into account in planning operations and maintenance (O&M) programs; but accidental and unpredictable or unintentional disturbances are more difficult to control, particularly in situations in which the ACM is accessible to building occupants.

### Risks from "Low Level" Exposure

Asbestos exposure from ACM in buildings is generally considered to be low level relative to occupational exposures that occurred historically in other occupational settings, such as building construction or shipyard work. In 1987 the EPA conducted air sampling in 49 public buildings to determine airborne asbestos levels (13). These buildings included six buildings without ACM (category 1), six buildings with all or most of the ACM in good condition (category 2), and 37 buildings with at least one area of significantly damaged ACM or several areas of moderately damaged ACM (category 3). Samples were analyzed for total structures count using transmission electron microscopy and the direct transfer method. Structures included but were not limited to fibers with an aspect ratio of 3:1. Mean levels, measured in structures per cubic centimeter (s/cm$^3$) were as follows: category 1, 0.00099 (±0.00198 SD); category 2, 0.00059 (±0.00052); category 3, 0.00073 (±0.00072). Using summary statistics for building averages, the levels measured by the EPA are 10 times lower than those reported by other investigators in nonschool buildings: EPA, 0.0007 s/cm$^3$; Pinchin (14), 0.0245 s/cm$^2$; Chatfield (15), 0.0087 s/cm$^3$; Burdett and Jaffrey (16), 0.0043 s/cm$^3$. By comparison, average background concentration of asbestos fibers in the air of U.S. cities has been estimated at 0.00007 fibers (f)/cm$^3$ by the EPA (10). Several factors must be considered in evaluating the significance of these findings with regard to risk for asbestos-related disease.

First, results of short-term air sampling may not reflect long-term fiber levels in ambient air in buildings. They do not reflect episodic disturbance of ACM in place, reentrainment of fibers that have been released and settled onto surfaces, or levels encountered by custodians or maintenance personnel during the performance of routine tasks, or by skilled craftspeople called in to perform specific and specialized tasks. Further, the act of sampling itself alters the reality of day-to-day building activities.

Second, asbestos exposure for custodians doing janitorial work, skilled craftspeople doing repair or maintenance work, and bystanders is not necessarily low level. For example, dusting in a university library with a damaged sprayed asbestos ceiling produced an average level of 4.0 f/cm$^3$ for custodians and 0.3 f/cm$^3$ for proximate library users (17). Under quiet conditions in a university building, fallout from friable ceilings containing 20% asbestos resulted in levels of 0.02 f/cm$^3$ (17). Cleaning and moving books produced levels of 15.5 f/cm$^3$; removing a ceiling section, levels of 2.7 f/cm$^3$; and sweeping and dry dusting, levels of 1.6 f/cm$^3$ (17). Although Sawyer, who participated in the collection of these data, reported at the rule-making hearing for the present Occupational Safety and Health Administration's (OSHA) asbestos standard that the building in which the samples were taken was not representative of other buildings in the United States, the results nevertheless are far in excess of OSHA's current permissible exposure level (PEL) of 0.1 f/cm$^3$ (18).

The results of more recently collected data are cited by OSHA in the preamble to its present asbestos standard. These include the results of personal air sampling carried out during a variety of maintenance activities in buildings (18). Results of air samples taken by Hygienetics, Inc. during the course of its management of an operations and maintenance program for a large hospital in the United States between 1988 and 1990 were included in the 1992 report of the Health Effects Institute–Asbestos Research and provided to OSHA during the comment period for the present standard (18,19). The National Institute for Occupational Safety and Health (NIOSH) 7400 phase contrast microscopy method was used to determine airborne asbestos fiber levels for the following tasks: air handling unit preventive maintenance 0.0942 (0.0087–0.6805); miscellaneous repair 0.1272 (0.0039–0.5496); miscellaneous installation 0.1742 (0.0049–0.8395); cleanup of ACM debris 0.2030 (0.0414–0.6246); cable pulling 0.0544 (0.0240–0.0985); relamping 0.0469 (0.0205–0.0929); generator testing 0.0843 (0.0075–0.2261); and fire alarm testing 0.1654 (0.0836–0.2693) (18) (Table 2). A total of 203 samples were collected. With the exception of relamping, means for all tasks were close to or in excess of the existing standard.

Kaselaan and d'Angelo measured fiber levels in five commercial buildings during "small-scale, short duration" operations (18). Average exposures in the 176 samples taken ranged from 0.02 to 0.073 f/cm$^3$, while 8-hour time-weighted averages ranged from 0.003 to 0.025 f/cm$^3$. The activities were carried out by "trained and experienced asbestos abatement workers," however, not the usual building maintenance workers.

Third, these "low" levels of airborne asbestos can cause disease. The risk of developing asbestos-related disease is a function of asbestos dose, and dose is a function of both level and duration of exposure. Thus, long-term work or occupancy in an area with low levels of airborne asbestos can result in a cumulative dose sufficient to cause disease. Aroesty and Wolf (20) estimated risk

**TABLE 2.** *Asbestos fiber levels during various maintenance activities*

| | Personal samples (PCM:f/cm$^3$) | | |
|---|---|---|---|
| Type of work | No. of samples | Mean | Range |
| Air handling unit preventive maintenace | 87 | 0.0942 | 0.0087–0.6805 |
| Miscellaneous repair | 48 | 0.1272 | 0.0039–0.5496 |
| Miscellaneous installation | 20 | 0.1742 | 0.0049–0.8395 |
| Cleanup of ACM debris | 8 | 0.2030 | 0.0414–0.6246 |
| Cable pulling | 9 | 0.0544 | 0.0240–0.0985 |
| Relamping | 9 | 0.0469 | 0.0205–0.0929 |
| Generator testing | 18 | 0.0843 | 0.0075–0.2261 |
| Fire alarm testing | 4 | 0.1654 | 0.0836–0.2693 |

for lung cancer and for malignant mesothelioma at 0.0004 f/cm$^3$ (a median dose) and at 0.002 f/cm$^3$ (a high dose). For malignant mesothelioma, estimated individual lifetime risks ($\times 10^6$) were 156 and 780, respectively. For lung cancer in male smokers, risks were 292 and 1,459, respectively; and for male nonsmokers, 27 and 132.

Asbestosis and malignant mesothelioma have been reported in household contacts of asbestos workers (6). Malignant mesothelioma has been reported in teachers, office workers, residents living within a half mile of an asbestos source, and in building maintenance workers whose only known exposure to asbestos was to ACM in place in buildings (7,21–23).

Indicative of its concern about the health effects of low-level exposure to asbestos, OSHA lowered the asbestos PEL in 1994 from 0.2 f/cm$^3$ to its present 0.1 f/cm$^3$, acknowledging that even at this level a significant risk remains (18). OSHA, the EPA, and the National Research Council (NRC) of the National Academy of Sciences have estimated risk for lung cancer and malignant mesothelioma from occupational and nonoccupational exposure to asbestos at levels less than or equal to 0.1 f/cm$^3$. OSHA used a minimum fiber concentration of 0.1 f/cm$^3$, the current standard (18,24). The EPA estimated lifetime risk on the basis of assumed exposures of 0.01 f/cm$^3$, the clearance concentration following asbestos removal (22). And the NRC estimated risk over a lifetime from nonoccupational exposure, assuming exposure levels of 0.0004 f/cm$^3$ (26). All show significant occurrence of disease at low levels of exposure.

Fourth, risk is affected by variables other than the asbestos itself. These include cigarette smoking, age at first exposure, and host factors. Although risk of asbestos-related lung cancer is increased for exposed nonsmokers, the risk is higher by tenfold for smokers (27). The younger the age at first exposure, the longer the subsequent life span and therefore the longer the period available for development of asbestos-related disease. This variable is particularly important for malignant mesothelioma because of its long latency period, 35 to 45 years on average (1). Physiologic parameters influence dose. Number of fibers inhaled and deposition patterns in the lung vary with respiratory rate and depth of inhalation. Fiber quantity increases with increase in respiratory rate, and deeper inhalation is likely to result in deeper penetration of fibers into the lung. Risk to schoolchildren is affected both by age and by the fact that their respiratory rate is likely to be higher than that of adult occupants of buildings. In addition, children are at greater risk for exposure resulting from reentrainment of settled fibers because of long hours spent at desks underneath and adjacent to ACM in schools, and short stature, which results in inhalation of air closer to the floor.

**Toxicity of Chrysotile Asbestos**

Asbestos fiber type is a putative determinant of risk for disease from ACM in buildings. Epidemiologic data suggest there may be a difference in terms of carcinogenic potential for the two fiber types most commonly used in building construction in the United States, with amosite being a more potent inducer of malignant mesothelioma than chrysotile (1). However, OSHA has concluded that the data are insufficient to show that chrysotile "does not present a significant mesothelioma risk to exposed employees," and further that it has the same potential as other fiber types to cause lung cancer and asbestosis (18). Accordingly, OSHA has regulated all fiber types as one. The ban on the manufacture, import, and use of asbestos fiber and asbestos-containing products imposed in France included chrysotile, over protests from Canadian scientists and trade and mining representatives (9).

Chrysotile has accounted for more than 90% of the asbestos sold and is the predominant fiber type used in buildings in the United States (8). Its carcinogenic potential has been demonstrated in both animals and humans. In inhalation experiments with SPF Wistar rats, Wagner et al. (28) observed excess rates of lung cancer, malignant mesothelioma, and asbestosis associated with exposure to chrysotile. Tumor prevalence was similar for rats exposed to chrysotile and for those exposed to amphibole fibers. Other inhalation studies have confirmed the carcinogenicity of chrysotile in animals (26,29).

That chrysotile asbestos causes lung cancer and malignant mesothelioma in occupationally exposed human populations has been confirmed in a number of published studies looking at various types of exposed populations. In a longitudinal cohort study of 11,379 workers exposed to chrysotile asbestos during the course of mining and milling, McDonald et al. (4) observed a linear dose-response relationship between cumulative dust exposure to age 45 years and standardized mortality ratios (SMR) for lung cancer. Excess lung cancer deaths were demonstrated in nonsmokers as well as smokers. Eleven deaths from malignant mesothelioma occurred in this cohort. Dement et al. (3) reported a significantly elevated SMR of 315 for lung cancer in 1,261 workers exposed to chrysotile asbestos in the manufacture of asbestos textile products. A linear dose-response relationship was observed for those with at least 15 years' latency. In a more recently published study examining the same population, with the addition of white females and black males and controlling for mineral oil exposure as a possible confounder, Dement et al. (30) confirmed his earlier findings for white males and females. Data demonstrated an increase in relative risk for lung cancer of 2% to 3% for each f/cc-yr of cumulative chrysotile asbestos exposure.

Finkelstein (31) reported an increase in lung cancer risk (SMR 221) in men exposed to chrysotile asbestos in the manufacture of electrical conduit pipe. Case-control analysis revealed that men who had worked as beater operators mixing raw materials had relative risk of 7.2 [95% confidence interval (CI) 2.25–23.3], compared to men who had never worked at that job. In a study of 7,887 men and 576 women chrysotile asbestos cement workers in Denmark, Raffn et al. (32) observed a standardized incidence ratio of 1.23 (95% CI 1.01–1.48) for colorectal cancer in the entire cohort, with a total of 857 incident cases occurring during the 22-year follow-up period. In a group of retired asbestos workers who had been exposed to chrysotile asbestos only, Enterline and Henderson (33) observed an SMR of 237.7 for lung cancer, adjusting for cumulative dust exposure. Products manufactured and jobs performed by these workers varied.

Selikoff et al. (2) reported a fourfold increase in lung cancer deaths (based on death certificate diagnosis) in a group of 17,800 asbestos insulation workers in the United States: 429 compared to 105.6 expected. The number of malignant mesotheliomas, using best available evidence, was 175. Prior to 1943 this group was exposed predominantly to chrysotile asbestos. The mortality experience of these insulators is important because they installed much of the ACM present in public buildings today.

Smith and Wright (34) carried out an extensive review of the scientific literature on malignant pleural mesothelioma. Published studies of asbestos-exposed cohorts were examined to determine number of pleural mesothelioma deaths per 1,000 deaths and the ratio of pleura mesotheliomas to excess lung cancer deaths, as well as primary and secondary (if any) types of asbestos exposure. Cohorts were rank ordered from highest to lowest based on the number of pleural mesotheliomas per 1,000 deaths. Chrysotile was the principal fiber type in at least two of the ten top-ranking cohorts and a contributing exposure in an additional six. Based on these data and the fact that chrysotile has been the predominant type of asbestos produced and used worldwide, the authors concluded that chrysotile asbestos is the most common cause of malignant pleural mesothelioma in humans.

### Risk of Removal Versus Containment

What should be done with ACM presently in buildings? Arguments set forth in favor of containment and in opposition to removal have changed little since debate began in the late 1980s. These are based on the following assumptions: (a) Removal itself creates a hazard for abatement workers and for building occupants. (b) ACM in buildings in the United States is not a serious threat to health. (c) Removal is too costly and the monies spent for removal could be better spent in other ways, such as promoting smoking cessation (35). Implicit is the assumption that containment is achievable.

There are several counterarguments. Removal itself creates a hazard only if it is done improperly. Regulations to control the hazard exist on both federal and state levels. For the construction and shipbuilding industries, the OSHA standard classifies work activities into four categories based on the nature of the work and the risk: class I—activities involving removal of ACM or presumed ACM (PACM) that is "high risk"; class II—activities involving removal of ACM or PACM that is not "high risk"; class III—repair and maintenance work where ACM and PACM is disturbed; and class IV—maintenance and custodial activities involving contact with ACM or PACM, including cleanup of waste and debris containing or presumed to contain asbestos (18). On the belief that the type and condition of the materials themselves and the work practices used are important determinants of risk, along with scale and duration of the job, OSHA has deleted from its current asbestos standard special attention or reference to "small scale, short duration" activities. Conditions under which negative-pressure enclosure (NPE) of work is required are defined, as are procedures for decontamination of workers before they leave the regulated area, and training and certification of abatement workers and supervisory personnel with regard to physical characteristics of ACM, associated health hazards, and proper work practices.

The EPA has extended the OSHA standard to state and local government employees (36). NPE is required before beginning removal, demolition, or renovation work. General and exhaust ventilation, wet methods, and high-efficiency particulate air (HEPA) filter dust-collecting systems and vacuuming are mandated to reduce employee exposure. The EPA has also mandated the training of school employees in the recognition and inspection of ACM (37). The Asbestos School Hazard Abatement Reauthorization Act of 1990 amends the Toxic Substances Control Act to apply accreditation requirements to contractors working with asbestos in public or commercial buildings (38). This act also includes provisions to increase the minimum number of hours of training required for asbestos abatement workers and prescribes civil penalties for contractors who perform specified abatement activities without accreditation.

ACM in buildings does not pose a threat to the health of occupants as long as it remains in place. Theoretically, containment of ACM in public buildings is achievable. That it will be achieved in even the majority of buildings with friable ACM is not clear. Ongoing building maintenance and repair requirements result in disruption of ACM. As a result of these episodic disturbances, asbestos fibers become airborne and may be inhaled by occupants as well as by workers. Accessibility of ACM directly affects the likelihood of disturbance and damage. Effective containment requires commitment to a rigorous and ongoing inspection and O&M programs. Critically important are the identification and proper labeling of ACM, the notification and education of potentially exposed individuals and groups, and periodic reinspection. If done properly, containment is not a cheap alternative to removal.

## HEALTH EFFECTS OF EXPOSURE

At risk for exposure to asbestos in public buildings are skilled craftspeople responsible for major installation, repair, and renovation work; custodial and maintenance personnel, responsible for day-to-day care and maintenance of buildings; and occupants, including other employees and tenants. Levels of asbestos exposure for skilled craftspeople resemble those associated with similar work in other occupational settings. Asbestos exposures and related health effects among building custodians and employees have been less well examined and described. Reported results of studies of health effects associated with maintenance or custodial work on or around ACM in buildings are summarized in Fig. 2 and below.

### Effects on Custodians and Maintenance Personnel

Investigations of ACM-related health effects among custodians and maintenance personnel in public buildings include four studies of school custodians, which were carried out in Massachusetts, New York, Wisconsin, and California by four different teams of investigators (21,39–41). A cross-sectional prevalence study of 120 Boston public school custodians carried out in 1987 and 1988 included medical and occupational histories, chest radiographs (four views), and pulmonary function tests consisting of flow-volume loops and single-breath diffusing capacity for carbon monoxide ($D_LCO$) (39). Information was obtained about intervals and duration of employment at schools previously surveyed and characterized with regard to the presence and condition of ACM (11). Frequency of specific custodial tasks, such as sweeping and dusting, patching or removing torn pipe or boiler insulation, and boiler maintenance was queried. Fifty-seven (47.5%) reported no significant exposure to asbestos outside their usual work as a school custodian. Mean age for this group was 55.2 years; mean duration of employment, 25.7 years; and mean latency, 26.8 years. Chest radiography demonstrated pleural plaques in 12 (21%) of this group and in 40 (33%) of the group overall. [By comparison, pleural plaques were observed on chest radiographs in 0.7% of 711 laboratory, maintenance, and grounds personnel in a large university in Boston who had no known exposure to asbestos at those or prior jobs (42).] Three school custodians (2.5%) had small irregular opacities, International Labor Organization (ILO) profusion category at least 1/0.

Restriction [forced vital capacity (FVC) less than 80% of predicted value and $FEV_1/FVC$ ratio at least 70%] on lung function testing occurred in 10 (17%) of those who had no outside exposure. Both pleural plaques and restriction were significantly associated with duration of work as a school custodian ($p < .05$). The $D_LCO$ was lower in the group with restriction than in those without this defect, and decrement in $D_LCO$ was associated with restriction in multivariate analysis, controlling for smoking. These results reveal pleural plaques attributable to asbestos exposure during the course of work as a custodian in public schools and suggest the occurrence of occult interstitial fibrosis of the lung associated with this work.

Selikoff and Levin (40) surveyed a group of 666 custodians employed by the New York City Board of Education over the period 1985 to 1987. More than 60% of the New York City custodians had worked at least 20 years. The number of subjects who had no significant exposure to asbestos outside of work as a custodian in public schools was 247 (37%). Of this group, 27% had abnormal chest radiographs: 17% small opacities ILO profusion category ≥ 1/0; 7% pleural plaques; and 3% both. The occurrence of asbestos-related radiographic abnormalities was directly related to duration of work as a custodian. Of those with at least 35 years' employment, 53% had abnormal chest x-ray findings. Work histories indicated that the general activities of these custodians placed them at increased risk of having x-ray evidence of pleural and interstitial fibrosis.

Only 17 (2.5%) were retired at the time of their examination. Eighteen (15%) of those examined in Boston were retired at examination. Both groups thus appear to be "survivor" populations. The extent to which observed results may have underestimated the true occurrence of disease is uncertain.

As part of a consultation program of the Wisconsin Division of Health, Anderson et al. (21) interpreted chest radiographs of 457 school maintenance employees. The radiographs were taken as part of clinical examinations performed in compliance with the Asbestos Hazard Emergency Response Act (AHERA) regulations. Duration of work as a school maintenance person ranged from 1 to 42 years. Eighty-five (19%) had worked in this

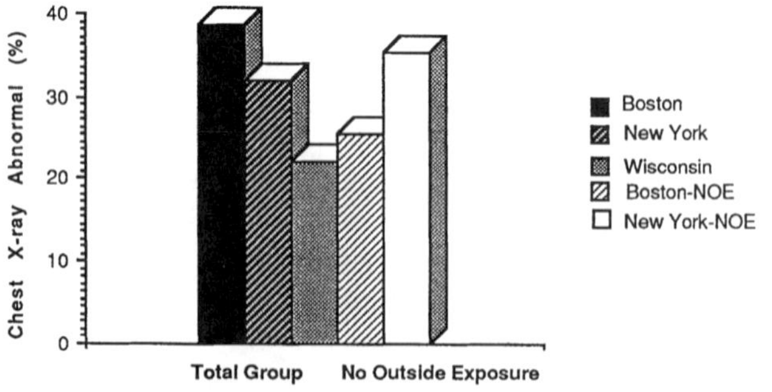


**FIG. 2.** Prevalence of radiographic chest abnormalities in public school custodians with at least 20 years' employment: total group and those who had no outside exposure (NOE).

capacity for at least 20 years. Of this group, 19 (22%) had evidence of asbestos-related disease on x-ray: 3.5% interstitial fibrosis; 17.6% pleural plaques; and 1% both abnormalities. The occurrence of pneumoconiosis was significantly associated with duration of work in school maintenance.

Balmes et al. (41) examined 673 school district employees in California as part of a state-mandated medical surveillance program. Sixty-three percent (422) reported no previous exposure to asbestos. For 102 (24.2%) their job was classified as custodial or building maintenance. Pleural and/or parenchymal fibrosis on chest radiograph occurred in nine (8.8%) of these workers. For the group overall, the relative risk of having asbestos-related disease was approximately 1.3 times greater for those with more than 10 years' school employment.

The data of Oliver and Anderson reveal pleural plaque as the predominant asbestos-related radiographic abnormality. Pleural plaques are a marker of asbestos exposure. But in addition, pleural plaques have been associated with increased mortality from lung cancer in asbestos-exposed populations and with loss of lung function. Fletcher (43) observed a twofold increase in lung cancer mortality in British dockyard workers who had pleural plaques on chest radiographs compared to those without pleural abnormalities. Finkelstein and Vingilis (5) reported mortality rates (deaths per 1,000 person-years exposure) of 103.4 for all causes and 34.5 for lung cancer in asbestos cement workers with 25 to 27 years' latency and bilateral pleural thickening, compared to 49.6 and 10.6, respectively, for those with similar latency and no pleural thickening.

Selikoff et al. (44) examined relationships between mortality experience and initial chest radiography results in 1,117 New York and New Jersey insulators followed from 1963 through 1989. Among the 195 who had pleural fibrosis as the only x-ray abnormality, observed deaths from lung cancer were increased compared to the expected number based on age- and year-specific death rates for white males of the U.S. National Center for Health Statistics. In the group with pleural plaques, percentages of deaths due to lung cancer and malignant mesothelioma were increased compared to the group of 500 insulators without pleural (or parenchymal) fibrosis on chest x-ray: for lung cancer, 22.2% versus 13.0%; for malignant mesothelioma, 17.8% versus 8.3%.

Hillerdal (45) carried out a population-based study of 1,596 males with pleural plaques followed prospectively for 16,369 person-years. Taking smoking into account, a statistically significant 40% increase in risk for lung cancer was observed in the group with pleural plaques as the only asbestos-related abnormality on chest x-ray, compared to the group with no asbestos-related abnormality (45). Additionally, nine mesotheliomas were observed in this group, compared to 0.8 expected. In the population studied, 88.7% had a history of occupational exposure to asbestos. Building and construction workers constituted 51.6% of those occupationally exposed; custodians, 8%; and municipal employees, 3%.

Associations between pleural plaques on chest radiograph and decrement in lung function have been reported by Oliver, Baker, Jarvholm, Bourbeau, and Schwartz (46–50). In Oliver et al.'s (46) study of 383 railroad workers exposed to asbestos, pleural plaques, defined as present-absent or by quantitative pleural score, were associated with decrement in FVC and with restriction. Baker et al. (47) reported a significant association between pleural plaques and decrement in FVC in 314 sheet-metal workers. In a cross-sectional study of 202 nonsmoking shipyard workers, Jarvholm and Sanden (48) observed decrements in FVC associated with pleural plaques. In a study of 110 active Canadian construction insulators, Bourbeau et al. (49) reported average decreases of 222 ml for $FEV_1$ and 350 ml for FVC ($p < 0.05$) in those with pleural plaques on chest radiographs compared to those without this abnormality. The difference was significant, taking into account age, height, smoking, and the presence of interstitial lung fibrosis on chest radiograph or gallium-67 lung scan. Using computed tomography (CT) scan of the chest to control for asbestos-related interstitial fibrosis of the lung not visible on chest X-ray, Schwartz et al. (50) observed associations between pleural plaques on chest radiograph and decrement in FVC and total lung capacity in sheet-metal workers in the midwestern United States.

In Balmes et al.'s (41) study of California school district employees, mean values for $FEV_1$ and FVC were significantly lower in those with pleural plaques than in those without plaques. Preliminary results of analysis of 227 Boston public school custodians examined from 1987 to 1990 reveal restriction in 28.8% of those with pleural plaques, compared to 14.9% of those without plaque ($p < 0.02$) (51). Decrement in FVC was associated with pleural plaques and duration of work as a custodian ($p < 0.02$).

### Effects on Other Public Building Employees

In addition to a cross-sectional prevalence study of radiographic abnormalities in school maintenance personnel, Anderson et al. (21) conducted a case-control study of malignant mesothelioma in Wisconsin males. The study used data from a statewide population-based cancer registry. Elevated sex-specific, age-adjusted odds ratios (OR) were observed for schools (OR, 3.5; 95% CI, 1.5–8.3) and for janitors (OR, 2.83; 95% CI, 1.4–6). Case identification and exposure histories revealed 29 malignant mesotheliomas in building maintenance workers and 12 in school teachers. Of the maintenance workers, 10 worked in public schools; seven, in other public buildings; five, in private building maintenance; and seven, in industrial maintenance. Of the total, 10 (34%) maintenance workers had no known exposure to asbestos outside of their work in buildings. Nine (75%) of the 12 school teachers had no known asbestos exposure outside of school employment. Lilienfeld (22) reported four cases of malignant mesothelioma in schoolteachers in different parts of the country. All taught in schools with ACM. None had known exposure to asbestos outside of their work as a schoolteacher, although one had served in the United States Navy as a radar man for 1½ to 2 years.

Malignant mesothelioma has been reported in other workers exposed to friable ACM in buildings. A Boston public school custodian examined in 1987 subsequently developed mesothelioma (39). In addition to his work for 32 years as a school custodian, he had worked as a sheet-metal worker in a naval shipyard for 6 months in 1942. His chest radiograph revealed bilateral pleural plaques. Stein et al. (23) reported malignant mesothelioma in a female office worker exposed to asbestos from friable ceiling ACM.

## CONCLUSIONS AND RECOMMENDATIONS

Friable ACM remains widespread in public, residential, and commercial buildings in the United States, despite ongoing abatement efforts. In intact, stable condition it is unlikely to pose a threat to health. In damaged, deteriorated condition friable ACM releases fibers into the air. Disturbance of ACM results in fiber release, even in stable, intact material. Once asbestos fibers become airborne, they are capable of causing disease. At greatest risk are building custodians and maintenance personnel, but related disease has been reported in building occupants as well.

Available data indicate a need for careful and ongoing medical surveillance and training of custodial and maintenance personnel in buildings that have friable ACM, and for notification and education of all building occupants at risk for exposure to asbestos from these materials. Regulations governing abatement workers and the abatement process, as well as custodial and maintenance work, must be enforced to prevent related asbestos exposure, not only in these workers but also in other building employees and occupants.

A prudent approach to the management of friable ACM currently in place in buildings is on a case-by-case basis. Damaged, deteriorating, or highly accessible ACM should be removed. Intact, stable ACM that is unlikely to be disturbed can be left in place and managed under an O&M program. To be effective such a program must be rigorous and ongoing. It will not be cheap. Methods of managing ACM in buildings have been described (12). The EPA has mandated a program for the nation's public and private schools through AHERA (52).

Tenets of effective management likely to be protective of individual and public health are shown in Table 3. The described approach is a sensible, straightforward one that embraces neither the extreme of wholesale removal nor that of "containing" and managing all ACM. Some ACM in buildings must be removed to prevent asbestos-related disease. Some can safely be left in place and maintained. In either case, there must be controls to protect the health of those potentially at risk for asbestos exposure.

**TABLE 3.** *Management of asbestos-containing materials in buildings*

| | |
|---|---|
| I. | Building inspection to determine the following:<br>Presence and location of ACM<br>Condition of ACM<br>Accessibility of ACM<br>Pathways or routes of exposure for building workers and occupants<br>Potential for and nature of ACM disturbances |
| II. | Written notification of building workers and occupants with regard to inspection results |
| III. | Development of an operations and maintenance program:<br>Identification of ACM that must be removed<br>Development and implementation of a prioritized plan for safe removal<br>Development and implementation of an O&M<br>Program for ACM left in place; to be included are plans for (1) periodic inspection, (2) containment in the event of predictable and unpredictable disturbance, and (3) medical surveillance and training of custodial and maintenance personnel, and of other building occupants and employees as indicated |
| IV. | Written notification of building workers and occupants of the abatement plan, including both removal and O&M for ACM left in place |

O&M, operations and maintenance.

## REFERENCES


1. Becklake MR. Asbestos-related diseases of the lung and other organs: Their epidemiology and implications for clinical practice. *Am Rev Respir Dis* 1976;114:55–95.
2. Selikoff IJ, Hammond EC, Seidman H. Mortality experience of insulation workers in the United States and Canada, 1943–1976. *Ann NY Acad Sci* 1979;330:91–116.
3. Dement JM, Harris RL, Symons MJ, Shy CM. Exposures and mortality among chrysotile asbestos workers. Part II: Mortality. *Am J Ind Med* 1983;4:421–433.
4. McDonald JC, Liddell FDK, Gibbs GW, Eyssen GE, McDonald AD. Dust exposure and mortality in chrysotile mining, 1910–75. *Br J Ind Med* 1980;37:11–24.
5. Finkelstein MM, Vingilis JJ. Radiographic abnormalities among asbestos-cement workers. An exposure-response study. *Am Rev Respir Dis* 1984;129:17–22.
6. Epler GR, Fitzgerald MX, Gaensler EA, Carrington CB. Asbestos-related disease from household exposure. *Respiration* 1980;39: 229–240.
7. Newhouse ML, Thompson H. Mesothelioma of pleura and peritoneum following exposure to asbestos in the London area. *Br J Ind Med* 1965;22:261–269.
8. Oppenheim-McMullen J, Turner B. Facing the asbestos menace. Progressive Builder, 1986. In: Spengler JD, Ozkaynak H, McCarthy JF, Lee H, eds. *Summary of Symposium on Health Aspects of Exposure to Asbestos in Buildings Proceedings.* Boston: Harvard University Energy and Environmental Policy Center, 1989, 21–22.
9. Asbestos banned by France. *British Asbestos Newsletter* 1996;25:1–2.

10. *EPA study of asbestos-containing materials in public buildings.* A report to Congress. Washington, DC: US Environmental Protection Agency, 1988.
11. *Survey for friable asbestos-containing materials in the city of Boston public schools.* Boston: Hygeia, 1983.
12. Oliver LC, Page T, Ellenbecker MJ, Wegman DH, Bacow L. *Asbestos management in commercial buildings.* Task force report. Boston: Beacon Management Company, 1989.
13. Chesson J, Hatfield J, Schultz B, Dutrow E, Blake J. Airborne asbestos in public buildings. *Environ Res* 1990;51:100–107.
14. Pinchin DJ. *Asbestos in buildings.* Study no. 8. Toronto: Royal Commission on Matters of Health and Safety Arising from the Use of Asbestos in Ontario, 1982.
15. Chatfield EJ. Airborne asbestos levels in Canadian public buildings. In: Chatfield EJ, ed. *Asbestos fibre measurements in building atmospheres, Proceedings.* Mississauga, Ontario: Ontario Research Foundation, 1986.
16. Burdett GJ, Jaffrey SAMT. Airborne asbestos concentrations in buildings. *Ann Occup Hyg* 1986;30:185–199.
17. Sawyer RN, Spooner CM. *Sprayed asbestos-containing materials in buildings.* A guidance document. EPA publication 450/2-78-014., Washington, DC: U.S. Environmental Protection Agency, 1978.
18. Occupational exposure to asbestos; final rule. Part II. 29 CFR Parts 1910, et al. Federal Register 1994;59:40964–41158.
19. Hygienetics, Inc. *In asbestos in public and commercial buildings:* supplementary analyses of selected data previously considered by the literature review panel. Cambridge, MA: Health Effects Institute-Asbestos Research, 1992.
20. Aroesty J, Wolf K. Risk from exposure to asbestos. Letters. *Science* 1986;234:923.
21. Anderson HA, Hanrahan LP, Schirmer J, Higgins D, Sarow P. Mesothelioma among employees with likely contact with in-place asbestos-containing building materials. *Ann NY Acad Sci* 1991;643:550–572.
22. Lilienfeld DE. Asbestos-associated pleural mesothelioma in school teachers: a discussion of four cases. *Ann NY Acad Sci* 1991;643: 454–458.
23. Stein RC, Kitajewski JY, Kirkham JB, Tait N, Shinha G, Rudd RM. Pleural mesothelioma resulting from exposure to amosite asbestos in a building. *Respir Med* 1989;83:237–239.
24. Occupational exposure to asbestos, tremolite, anthophyllite, and actinolite. Federal Register. 29 CFR § 1910, 1986.
25. Sebastien P, Billion-Guilland MA, Dufour G, Bignon J. *Measurement of asbestos air pollution inside buildings sprayed with asbestos.* USEPA report EPA-560/13-80-026. Washington, DC: U.S. Environmental Protection Agency, 1980.
26. National Research Council/National Academy of Sciences. *Asbestiform fibers-nonoccupational health risks.* Washington, DC: National Academy Press, 1984.
27. Hammond EC, Selikoff IJ, Seidman H. Asbestos exposure, cigarette smoking and death rates. *Ann NY Acad Sci* 1979;330:473–490.
28. Wagner JC, Berry G, Skidmore JW, Timbrell V. The effects of the inhalation of asbestos in rats. *Br J Cancer* 1974;29:252–269.
29. Davis JMG, Addison J, Bolton RE, Donaldson K, Jones AD. Inhalation and injection studies in rats using dust samples from chrysotile asbestos prepared by a wet dispersion process. *Br J Exp Pathol* 1986;67: 113–129.
30. Dement JM, Brown DP, Okun A. Follow-up study of chrysotile asbestos textile workers: cohort mortality and case-control analyses. *Am J Ind Med* 1994;26:431–447.
31. Finkelstein MM. Mortality among employees of an Ontario factory that manufactured construction materials using chrysotile asbestos and coal tar pitch. *Am J Ind Med* 1989;16:281–287.
32. Raffn E, Villadsen E, Lynge E. Colorectal cancer in asbestos cement workers in Denmark. *Am J Ind Med* 1996;30:267–272.
33. Enterline PE, Henderson V. Type of asbestos and respiratory cancer in the asbestos industry. *Arch Environ Health* 1973;27:312–317.
34. Smith AH, Wright CC. Chrysotile asbestos is the main cause of pleural mesothelioma. *Am J Ind Med* 1996;30:252–266.
35. Mossman BT, Bignon J, Corn M, Seaton A, Gee JBL. Asbestos: scientific developments and implications for public policy. *Science* 1990; 247:294–301.
36. Asbestos abatement projects; worker protection; final rule. Federal Register. 40 CFR §763,1987.
37. Asbestos-containing materials in schools; final rule and notice. Federal Register. 40 CFR §763,1987.
38. Asbestos School Hazard Abatement Reauthorization Act of 1990 Pub. L. 101-637, S.1893, 1990.
39. Oliver LC, Sprince NL, Greene R. Asbestos-related disease in public school custodians. *Am J Ind Med* 1991;19:303–316.
40. Selikoff IJ, Levin SM. Radiological abnormalities and asbestos exposure among custodians of the New York City Board of Education. *Ann NY Acad Sci* 1991;643:530–539.
41. Balmes JR, Daponte A, Cone JE. Asbestos-related disease in custodial and building maintenance workers from a large municipal school district. *Ann NY Acad Sci* 1991;643:540–549.
42. Epler GR, McLoud TC, Gaensler EA. Prevalence and incidence of benign asbestos pleural effusion in a working population. *JAMA* 1982; 247:617–622.
43. Fletcher DE. A mortality study of shipyard workers with pleural plaques. *Br J Ind Med* 1972;29:142–145.
44. Selikoff IJ, Lilis R, Seidman H. Predictive significance of parenchymal and/or pleural fibrosis for subsequent death of asbestos-associated diseases. Entered into OSHA docket at hearings: OSHA's Proposed Standard for Occupational Exposure to Asbestos, Tremolite, Anthophyllite, and Actinolite, January, 1991.
45. Hillerdal G. Pleural plaques and risk for bronchial carcinoma and mesothelioma. *Chest* 1994;105:144–150.
46. Oliver LC, Eisen EA, Greene F, Sprince NL. Asbestos-related pleural plaques and lung function. *Am J Ind Med* 1988;14:649–656.
47. Baker EL, Dagg T, Greene RE. Respiratory illness in the construction trades. I. The significance of asbestos-associated pleural disease among sheet metal workers. *J Occup Med* 1985;27:483–489.
48. Jarvholm B, Sanden A. Pleural plaques and respiratory function. *Am J Ind Med* 1986;10:419–426.
49. Bourbeau J, Ernst P, Chrome J, Armstrong B, Becklake MR. The relationship between respiratory impairment and asbestos-related pleural abnormality in an active work force. *Am Rev Respir Dis* 1990;142: 837–842.
50. Schwartz DA, Galvin JR, Dayton CS, et al. Determinants of restrictive lung function in asbestos-induced pleural fibrosis. *Am Physiol Soc* 1990;161:1932–1937.
51. Oliver LC, Eisen EA, Sprince NL, Greene R. Asbestos-related abnormalities in school custodians: an on going study. *Am Rev Respir Dis* 1992;145:A330.
52. Asbestos Hazard Emergency Response Act. Pub. L. 99-519, 100 S. 2970, 1986, 15 USC, Section 2641 *et seq.*

## FURTHER READING

Asbestos in public and commercial buildings: a literature review and synthesis of current knowledge. Cambridge, MA: Health Effects Institute-Asbestos Research, 1991.

*Environmental and Occupational Medicine,*
*Third Edition,* edited by William N. Rom.
Lippincott–Raven Publishers, Philadelphia © 1998.

CHAPTER 27

# Man-Made Vitreous Fibers, Vermiculite, and Zeolite

James E. Lockey and Nancy K. Wiese

## MAN-MADE VITREOUS FIBERS

Although man-made vitreous fibers (MMVFs) have been used for insulation purposes for over 60 years, they have played an increasingly important role as an asbestos substitute since the banning of most asbestos products in the United States. MMVFs are amorphous silicates with a length-to-diameter ratio greater than 3:1. They are made primarily from rock, slag, glass, or kaolin clay. These fibers, also known as man-made mineral fibers or synthetic vitreous fibers, can be divided into three general groups (Fig. 1): mineral wool (including rock wool and slag wool), glass fibers (including glass wool, continuous glass filament, and special-purpose glass fibers), and ceramic fibers (including ceramic textile fibers and refractory ceramic fibers). They possess physical properties such as high tensile strength, perfect elasticity, thermal and electrical properties, and moisture and corrosion resistance. These properties make them useful for more than 35,000 applications, including all types of thermal and acoustic insulation, filtration medium, woven fabric, and reinforcement of plastics (1,2).

### Terminology

*Man-made mineral fibers* (MMMF) was a term widely used in governmental, trade, and medical literature. However, *man-made vitreous fibers* and *synthetic vitreous fibers* are a more appropriate terms for two reasons. First, a mineral is defined as a naturally occurring inorganic compound with a crystalline structure and, so, cannot be man-made. Second, when glass, mineral, and ceramic materials are melted and subsequently rapidly solidified into fibers, the atomic arrangement remains disordered, not crystalline, which by definition makes it a vitreous rather than a mineral substance (3).

Man-made vitreous fibers are named for the raw materials from which they are made. Rock wool and slag wool, collectively known as mineral wool, are made by melting and fiberizing naturally occurring rock or slag, a by-product of the smelting of metal ores such as iron or furnace slag (4). In the United States the term *mineral wool* includes rock wool and slag wool, but in Europe it includes glass wool, rock wool, and slag wool. Glass fibers are manufactured from typical glass-making raw materials such as silicon dioxide and oxides of aluminum, calcium, magnesium, sodium, potassium, and boron (2). There are three distinct types of commercial glass fiber products: glass wool, an entangled mass of interlocking fibers; continuous glass filament, a product with a more ordered arrangement of fibers; and special-purpose glass fibers, small-diameter fibers (less than 3 μm) (3). Glass fibers are sometimes referred to as fibrous glass or fiberglass. Ceramic fibers are typically produced from molten masses of raw materials such as kaolin clays, alumina-silica, or alumina-silica-zirconia and are characterized by their excellent refractory properties (stability up to 2,600°F). There are two types of alumina-silica ceramic fibers: ceramic textile fibers and ceramic refractory fibers. The two differ mainly in size, ceramic textile fibers being longer, typically 155 to 250 mm with diam-

J. E. Lockey: Department of Environmental Health, University of Cincinnati College of Medicine, Cincinnati, Ohio 45267-0182.
N. K. Wiese: Department of Occupational Health Services, Cigna Health Care of Arizona, Phoenix, Arizona 85006.

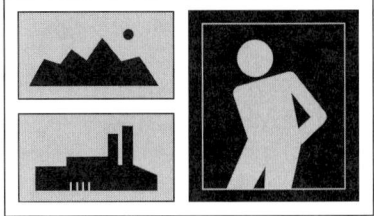

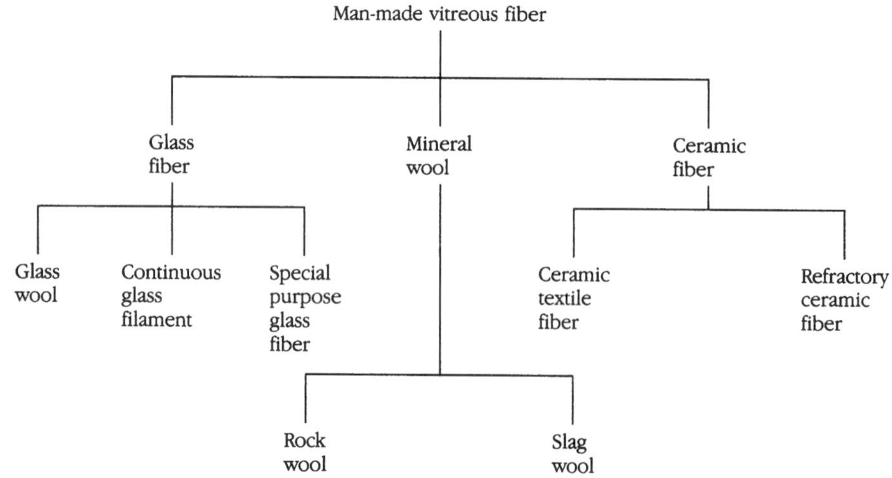


**FIG. 1.** Categorization of man-made vitreous fibers.

eters of 11 to 20 μm. Ceramic refractory fibers are thinner (average diameter 2.2 to 5.0 μm) and shorter (40 to 250 mm). More than 90% of the ceramic fibers produced in the United States are the refractory type (2,3).

## History

### *Mineral Wool*

The natural formation of mineral wool fibers (Pele's hair) can occur when strong gas jets fiberize lava during volcanic eruptions. This process was imitated by the first commercial manufacturers of slag wool in the 1880s, when steam jets were directed against molten blast furnace slag, resulting in the formation of coarse fibers (5). The first successful commercial manufacture of slag wool was in Manchester, England, in about 1885. Rock wool was first manufactured in 1897 in Alexandria, Indiana, by C. C. Hall using limestone as the raw material (4). At first the use of rock- or slag wood was limited to industrial insulation of boilers and pipes. Buildings at that time were generally insulated with ashes, cork, or sawdust; however, the mineral wool industry began to grow after World War I, providing insulation for a more diverse market (5). The number of mineral wool plants in the United States probably peaked in the 1950s at approximately 80 or 90 plants (4). After that, the industry declined because the glass fiber industry, which started in 1938, steadily garnered a greater share of the insulation market.

The manufacture of mineral wool in the early stages involved melting rock or slag in a cupola; a coke-fed, water-cooled, air-fed shaft furnace that can generate tem-

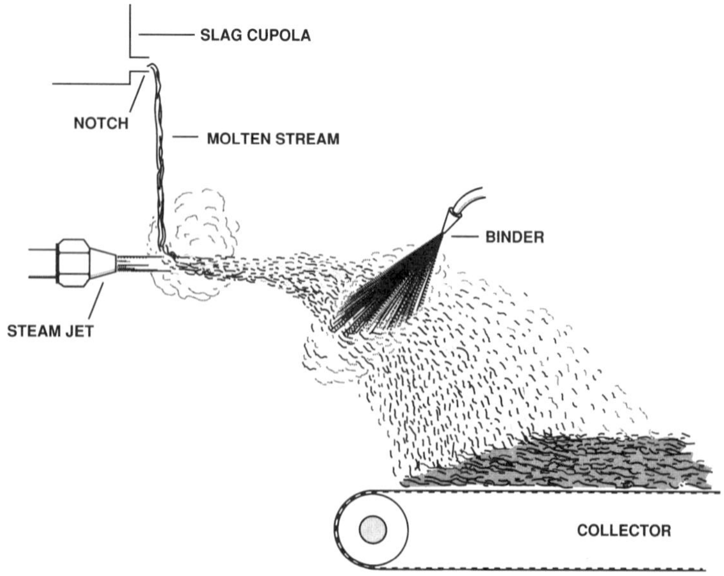


**FIG. 2.** Steam jet fiberization.

peratures of about 4,000°F. Although iron slag was used commonly at first, other metal slags such as chrome, lead, and copper (sometimes contaminated with arsenic) were used later. Common raw materials for early rock wool included granite, limestone, and slate. Today, basalt, limestone, clay, and feldspar are used.

In the early process, a molten stream of rock or slag flowed out a hole in the bottom of the cupola and passed in front of a high-pressure steam jet that fiberized the material (4) (Fig. 2). The fibers were then blown into a chamber, where they settled to the floor. When the chamber was filled to a sufficient level, workers cut the wool into blocks and removed it from the chamber. Later, a conveyor belt and fans were used to empty the chamber, helping to speed production and improve ventilation. Another advancement in the process was the spraying of binders and oils on the fibers immediately after fiberization. This improved the mechanical handling properties of the wool, reduced fiber breakage, and decreased dust formation (2,3). Various early binders included natural resins, sulfite, lye, and tars. With the introduction of phenol formaldehyde resins in the late 1940s, a curing process was instituted that involved heating the resin-coated wool until the resin polymerized.

Today, raw fibers are sprayed with binder and a lubricating oil. Binder solutions include urea-formaldehyde, phenol-formaldehyde, melamine resins, silicone compounds, soluble and emulsified oils, surfactants, extenders, and stabilizers (2).

Steam-jet fiberization left a high percentage of unfiberized material called shot and produced fibers in a wide range of diameters. Shot is undesirable because it interferes with insulation efficiency (5). In the 1940s, the Powell process was developed to reduce the amount of shot in the final product. The Powell process (Fig. 3) uses a group of high-speed rotors to fiberize slag by forcing the molten slag over its surface and casting it off with centrifugal force. The Downey process, developed approximately at the same time, uses steam attenuation and a concave rotor. The molten stream is flung out from the edge of the rotor and then is acted upon by high-velocity steam or air jets surrounding the rotor (Fig. 4). These two processes were an improvement over the steam-jet method but still produced fibers with a wide range of diameters and a relatively high percentage of shot. Most of the mineral wool produced in the United States today has an average diameter between 3.5 and 7.0 μm and is made by a variation of the Downey process (4).

Mineral wool without binder is used for blown insulation or in the manufacture of ceiling tile. Mineral wool with binder is used principally for industrial and some residential purposes in the form of insulation batts, board, blankets, and pipe coverings (3).

### *Glass Fibers*

The fiber-forming capacity of molten glass has been known for centuries. Thin threads of glass were used by Venetian craftsmen in the 17th century to decorate vases and a glass fiber dress was made for the Empress Eugénie, wife of Napoleon III, in the 1800s (3).

### *Glass Wool*

The glass wool industry started in Europe circa 1900 and was based on existing glass-melting technology. Glass raw materials were melted in a furnace and then allowed to flow out through the forehearth to a fiberization device. Production was limited until 1929, when the Hager process was developed, which used scrap glass, an early example

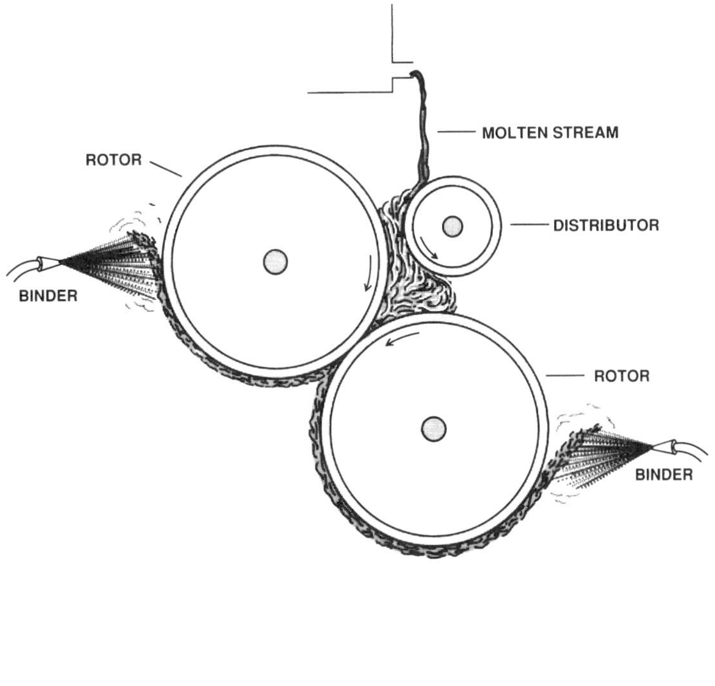


**FIG. 3.** Powell process.

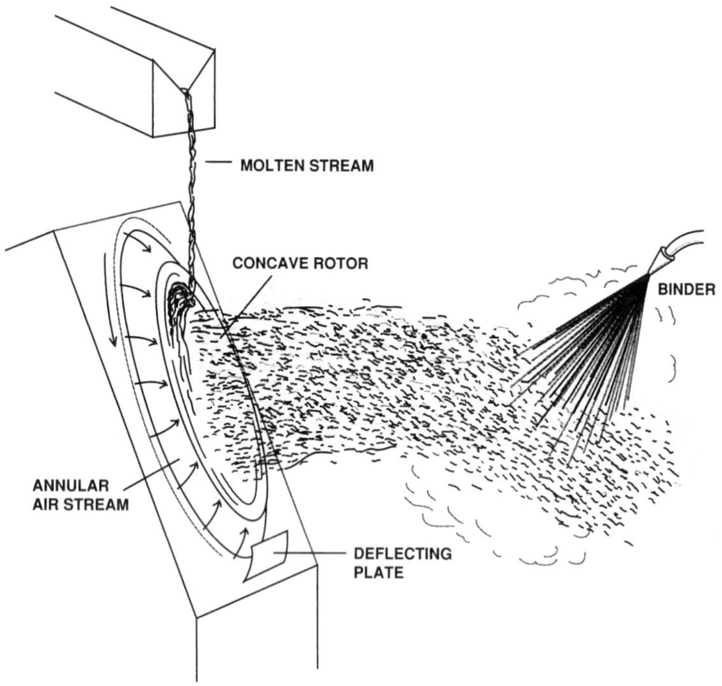


**FIG. 4.** Downey process.

of recycling. The glass was melted in a gas- or oil-heated furnace and streamed onto a rotating horizontal ceramic disk where it flowed outward and became fiberized as it left the disk. A coarse wool was produced with an average fiber diameter of 15 to 25 μm and a wide range of fiber diameters (from less than 1 μm to more than 40 μm) (4).

The Owens process, a steam-blowing process developed in the United States in the 1930s, produced a finer glass wool. Glass melted in a tank furnace was forced through a row of electrically heated platinum tanks, called bushings, and was fiberized by a steam blower.

Flame attenuation of glass fibers was accidentally discovered in 1932 when an attempt was made to weld together two glass blocks using glass rods as the filler. Extremely fine diameter glass fibers were produced, and by 1938 a machine was developed to produce flame-attenuated fine glass fibers commercially (3) (Fig. 5). This process has made it possible to produce fibers with various diameters (approximately 0.05 to 7 μm) (6).

By 1958, Owens-Corning Fiberglas Company had combined the Owens method with a rotary process that used a rotating perforated cup to feed molten streams of glass

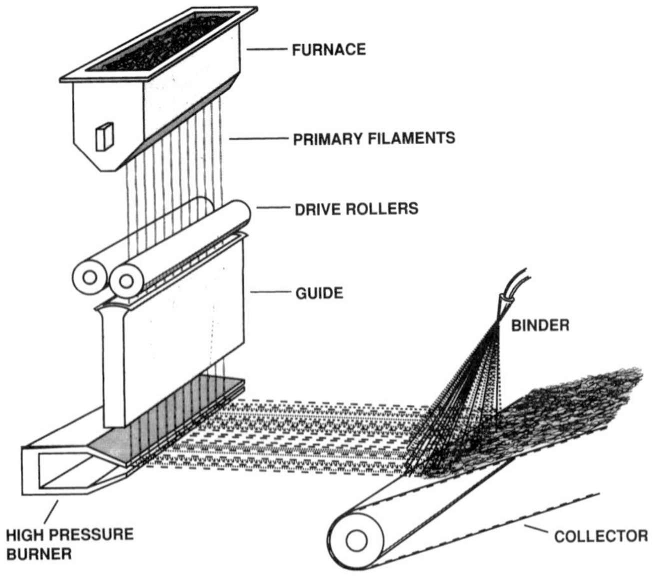


**FIG. 5.** Flame-attenuation process.

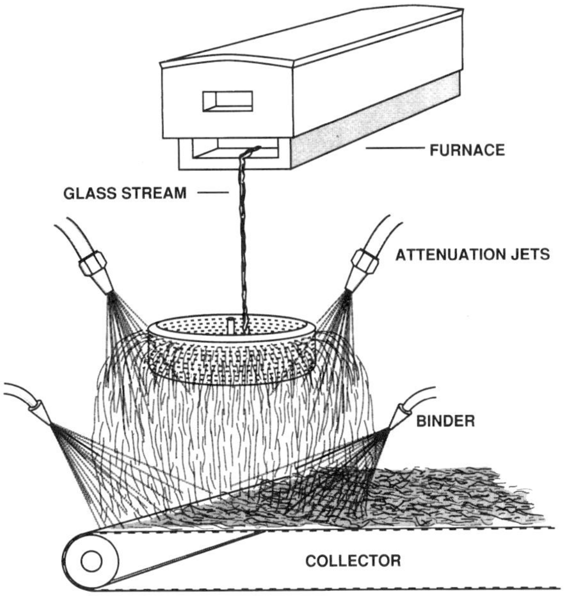


**FIG. 6.** Rotary process.

through a flame attenuator. This combined technique (Fig. 6) afforded better control over fiber diameter and range, raised productivity, and lowered costs. The majority of glass wool produced today is made by a modification of this process and has an average diameter of 4 to 15 μm, depending on the end use. Most glass fiber products, with the exception of some special-purpose ones, are coated with binders, sizing, and lubricants similar to those used on mineral wool fibers. The end product is used primarily for residential and commercial thermal insulation in the form of batts, blankets, boards, or as a loose-fill product (3).

### *Special-Purpose Glass Fibers*

Special-purpose glass fibers are produced by flame attenuation and have a mean diameter smaller than 3 μm. These fibers are costly to produce but are more efficient insulators than larger-diameter fibers. They are used for specialized high-temperature insulation in aircraft and space vehicles and as high-efficiency filtration media (3).

### *Continuous Glass Filament*

The continuous glass filament process differs from the glass-rock-slag wool process in that it allows very accurate sizing of the fibers with little variation in the diameter of the product. Molten glass flows from a furnace into a series of small platinum bushings. These bushings have hundreds of very small holes in the bottom through which the glass is drawn. The individual filaments are collected together in a strand, sprayed with binder, and wound upon a rotating drum (4) (Fig. 7). Continuous glass filaments have a greater strength-to-weight ratio than steel and average diameters of 3.0 to 25 μm, depending on the end use of the product (3). Some of the filament is chopped and chemically bound into chopped-strand mat, and some is twisted into a yarn product that can be made into cord or woven into cloth. Glass fiber cord is used for tire reinforcement and glass fiber cloth for high-quality circuit boards, airplane structures, and fire-proof textiles. Plastic reinforced with chopped-strand mat is used for a wide variety of products, including boat hulls and automobile parts. Chopped fibers are used for roofing mat and as filler for polyurethane in reaction injection molding (2).

### *Ceramic Fibers*

Ceramic fiber production started about 30 years ago and constitutes 1% to 2% of MMVF production worldwide (3,7). The fibers are produced principally by steam-blowing or spinning a melt of kaolin clay or alumina and silica. Ceramic fibers for special applications are produced in smaller quantities by colloidal evaporation,

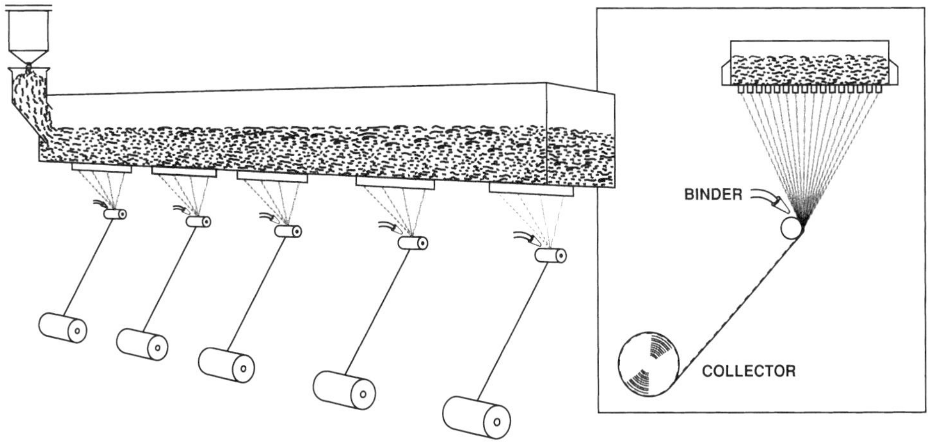


**FIG. 7.** Continuous-filament process.

vapor-phase deposition, and continuous filamentation. The final product is in the form of blankets, boards, felts, bulk fibers, vacuum-formed or cast-shapes, and paper or textile products. Most of the ceramic fibers are used for lining furnaces and kilns. Twenty percent of the ceramic fibers produced are mixed in an aqueous suspension with clays, colloidal metal oxide particles, and organic binders, and then cast into various shapes. Cast-shaped ceramic tiles are used to cover the body of the space shuttle because they can withstand temperatures up to 2,300°F (2). Ceramic fibers that have been used at temperatures above 1,832°F undergo partial conversion to cristobalite. The amount formed is a function of the temperature and length of time the fibers have been heated. These cristobalite fibers should be handled as a potential source of exposure to crystalline silica (2,3).

The average diameter of MMVF can be varied, depending on the end use of the product. Fibers produced by the steam-blowing, flame attenuation or a spinning process contain a wide range of diameters, some of which are in the respirable range (less than 3.5 µm diameter and less than 200 µm length) (8). The continuous filament process allows for accurate sizing of fibers with a narrower range of diameters and is not associated with measurable levels of respirable fibers.

### Experimental Data *in Vitro*

It has been well documented that exposure to asbestos fibers can result in pulmonary interstitial fibrosis and pleural thickening as well as pulmonary carcinoma and mesothelioma in humans. Because materials used as asbestos substitutes can have a fibrous configuration, there has been much interest in determining whether they represent a potential health hazard to humans (9).

Glass fibers have been demonstrated to be toxic to peritoneal and pulmonary macrophages (10,11). Tilkes and Beck (11) demonstrated that toxicity of glass fibers in rat and guinea pig lung macrophages is dose-dependent and is related to increasing fiber length. The chemical composition of MMVF also has been related to the toxicity of fibers (12). Testing in vitro with macrophages or other phagocytic cells is generally considered to be predictive of initial toxic effects, and perhaps fibrogenicity, but is not necessarily indicative of carcinogenicity (9).

Structural chromosome alterations were demonstrated in mammalian cells (13–15) with glass fibers. Hesterberg and Barrett (15) reported that thin glass fibers (average diameter 0.13 µm) were 20 times more potent in producing preneoplastic morphologic changes in cultured Syrian hamster embryo cells than thicker diameter fibers. Howden and Faux (16) demonstrated that DNA adduct formation in *Salmonella typhimurium* and rat lung fibroblasts has been directly related to the amount of iron mobilized from the surface of MMVF. The role of iron at the surface of fibers and the generation of hydroxyl free radical activity with resultant DNA damage needs further investigation (17). MMVFs have also been associated with a significant increase in the number of binucleate cells in a human mesothelial cell line (18). Development of bioassays that focus on fiber-induced malignant mesothelioma may be a short-term approach for assessing the potential toxicity of new synthetic fibers (19).

The durability of various MMVFs has been tested in vitro by observing fiber dissolution rates in Gamble's solution, an artificial extracellular physiologic solution resembling blood plasma (20–22). Glass fiber durability after 180 days in Gamble's solution is determined by monitoring changes in total specimen weight, surface area, and surface morphology. Three borosilicate fibers with different chemical constituents demonstrated silica solubility rates from 650 to 17,000 times greater than chrysotile asbestos. The surface area of the borosilicate fibers increased 1,800% and 22,000% due to pitting, cracking, breaking, or segmenting, while the chrysotile increased 8%. Significant surface area separation and round grape-like clusters were noted on the surface of the borosilicate fibers by scanning electron microscopy (23). In general, glass fibers were found to be the most soluble by Leineweber (22), followed by mineral wool, then refractory ceramic fibers. Klingholz and Steinkopf (21) found slag wool to be the most soluble, followed by glass wool, rock wool, and basalt wool. Figure 8 is a scanning electron micrograph of MMVF before and after subjection to leaching for 180 days in modified Gamble's solution.

The dissolution of MMVF can be influenced by the pH of the surrounding solution. According to de Meringo et al. (24), the best *in vitro* test method uses Gamble's solution with a pH of 7.5 and MMVF with a diameter of 1 µm and mean length of 20 µm. A pH of 7.5 matches that of the extracellular milieu where increased fiber solubility has been demonstrated with glass wool. At pH 4.5, simulating intracellular phagolysosomes milieu, these same fibers can demonstrate decreased solubility, whereas fibers with high aluminum content can demonstrate increased solubility (25). The solubility of MMVF is complex and dependent not only on chemical composition but also most likely on the production process and fiber surface characteristics (24).

### Experimental Data *in Vivo*

Solubility *in vivo* and clearance rates of MMVF in lung tissue have been demonstrated by intratracheal injection (26–28) and inhalation experiments (29–31) in rats. Studies *in vivo* have found MMVF to be quite soluble: in general, glass fibers most soluble, followed by rock wool, then refractory ceramic fibers. Glass fibers by intratracheal injection have caused pulmonary tumors in rats and hamsters and fibers greater than 10 µm in length produced

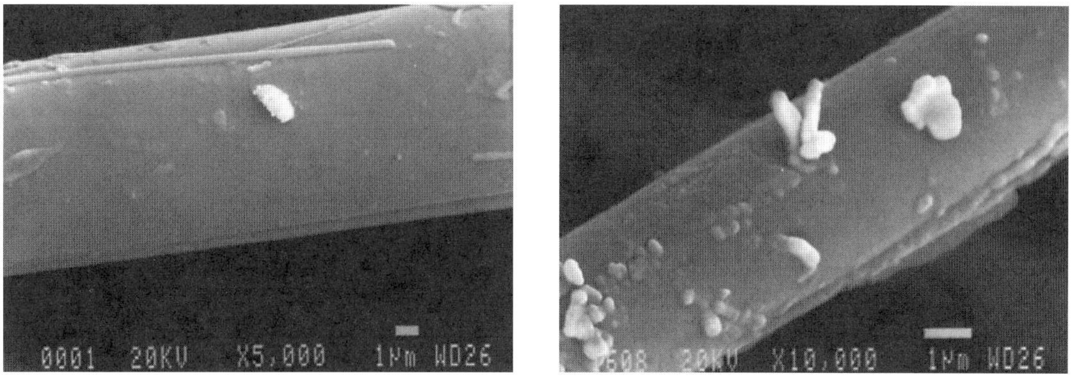


**FIG. 8. A:** SEM photomicrograph of mineral wool fiber before leaching. **B:** SEM photomicrograph of mineral wool fiber after 180 days in modified Gamble's solution. (Courtesy of Bruce Law, R. Hamilton, Ph.D., and T. Hesterberg, Ph.D., Manville Corporation.)

fibrosis in guinea pigs (32,33). Intratracheal injection studies of ceramic fibers have been negative (34).

Stanton and Wrench (35) in 1972 performed experiments in which three types of asbestos, six types of glass fibers, two types of silica, and two types of metal particles were implanted in the pleura of rats. Fine-diameter glass fibers milled to the length of asbestos fibers produced an incidence of mesothelioma in the range of 12% to 18%. The authors concluded, "Carcinogenicity of asbestos and fibrous glass seems primarily related to the structural shape of these materials rather than to physicochemical properties."

In a later report, Stanton and co-workers (36) described 72 pleural implantation experiments utilizing minerals of wide chemical and structural variety. They concluded that a long, thin, fibrous structure is critical to the carcinogenicity of these materials: "The probability of pleural sarcoma correlated best with the number of fibers that measured 0.25 μm or less in diameter and more than 8 μm in length, but relatively high correlations were also noted with fibers in other size categories having diameters up to 1.5 μm and lengths greater than 4 μm." These findings stimulated a large amount of new experimental work on the effects of MMVF (9). Pott and co-workers (33,37,38), Wagner and co-workers (39), and Davis (40) confirmed that glass fibers are carcinogenic when injected into the pleural or peritoneal cavity of experimental animals. Stanton's hypothesis that long, thin fibers are the most carcinogenic was corroborated by intraperitoneal experiments done by Pott and co-workers (38). They suggested that fiber durability *in vivo* is also important in determining carcinogenicity. Slag wool with a high proportion of long, thin fibers failed to produce the expected high tumor rate when implanted in the peritoneum of rats. There was considerable corrosion of the slag wool fibers after 20 months' implantation in the rat species when examined by electron microscopy. This led to the conclusion that slag wool's failure to produce tumors was due to lack of durability within the tissue.

Animal inhalation studies offer the most realistic means of determining the pathogenicity of MMVF because they do not artificially bypass the normal respiratory defense mechanisms (41). Animal inhalation studies with glass wool, rock wool, and slag wool have not shown any statistically significant increase in the incidence of respiratory tumors (30,34,39,42,43). One study did demonstrate focal peribronchiolar fibrosis in baboons after 18 to 30 months of glass fiber exposure (42). A more recent inhalation study in rats of two types of glass wool commercial insulation at 30, 150, and 240 fibers/cm$^3$ demonstrated a partially reversible cellular response. Similar findings were seen with slag wool. Rock wool induced minimal fibrosis at 145 and 247 fibers/cm$^3$ (43,44). One study with ceramic fibers, Davis et al. (45), produced three pulmonary carcinomas, one benign pulmonary adenoma, and four histiocytomas involving primarily lung tissue in 48 rats exposed by inhalation. One peritoneal mesothelioma was also found. Six animals sacrificed at the end of the study showed interstitial fibrosis, in 5% of the lung area on average. Two other studies with ceramic fibers failed to demonstrate any increased incidence of pulmonary tumors except for one mesothelioma in a hamster (34). More recent inhalational studies of refractory ceramic fibers at a maximum tolerated dose of 220 fibers/cm$^3$ demonstrated mesothelioma and pulmonary and pleural fibrosis in hamsters and mesothelioma, lung cancer, and pulmonary and pleural fibrosis in rats (43,46,47). A follow-up multidose study demonstrated a pulmonary cellular response at 36 fibers/cm$^3$, a mesothelioma at 91 fibers/cm$^3$, and minimal fibrosis at 91 and 162 fibers/cm$^3$ (48). There have been no inhalation studies using continuous glass filament because the fibers are not considered to be respirable owing to their large diameter.

Fibers that are short enough to be engulfed by alveolar macrophages are translocated from the epithelial surface (a) to dust foci at the respiratory bronchioles, (b) onto the ciliated epithelium at the terminal bronchioles, or (c) through the epithelium into interstitial storage sites or lymphatic drainage pathways (49).

Disintegration refers to subdivision of fibers into shorter segments, dissolution of the components of the matrix, and surface etching. MMVF differs from asbestos fibers in several ways that result in less deposition in the lungs and more rapid elimination of fibers that are deposited. First, in general, MMVFs tend to have a smaller proportion of respirable-sized fibers than asbestos, except for special-purpose glass fibers and refractory ceramic fibers, which have a significant proportion with diameters smaller than 3.5 µm. Second, MMVFs rarely split lengthwise but are more likely to break into shorter segments. Third, MMVFs are less durable and more soluble in the lung than asbestos fibers.

The potential toxicity of MMVF is related to the dose delivered to the target organ, fiber dimensions, and fiber durability within the chest cavity and pulmonary parenchyma. Other factors such as chemical composition and surface characteristics also play a role. An important factor is the recognition that MMVF can differ significantly both qualitatively and quantitatively in their chemical composition. All these factors have to be taken into consideration on a fiber-type by fiber-type basis in regard to potential toxicity.

### Clinical

Man-made vitreous fibers can induce skin and upper respiratory tract irritation. Possick and co-workers (50) investigating approximately 4,000 glass fiber workers in manufacturing plants in four states found that 5% of all new workers leave within the first 2 weeks because of skin irritation or discomfort. Most workers experience skin irritation in the first week of employment but notice improvement with further exposure. This phenomenon, called "hardening," is not well understood (50).

Pruritus without objective evidence of dermatitis is the most common clinical presentation of glass fiber irritation, the arms, face, and neck being most commonly affected. If dermatitis is present, the primary lesion is a tiny erythematous papule. Other morphologic types of dermatitis have been described but are probably secondary to scratching stimulated by intense pruritus. The most likely mediator of the pruritus is release of histamine or kinins when glass fibers pierce the epidermis. Hot, humid weather generally exacerbates the dermatitis (50). Glass fibers with diameters greater than 5.3 µm are more likely to cause skin irritation than smaller-diameter fibers. Two people who exhibited dermographism developed severe urticarial reactions when exposed to glass fibers in a study by Heisel and Mitchell (51). This finding prompted the authors to suggest that the simple test for dermographism may be a worthwhile preplacement test for glass fiber workers.

Skin irritation from glass fibers is due to mechanical irritation. There is no evidence of allergic sensitization in animal or human subjects. There have been reports of allergic sensitization to the binder that coats the fibers (52,53). Despite the common use of binders on glass and mineral fibers, allergic sensitization is rare, probably because the resins are fully cured prior to human exposure (24).

Glass fiber dermatitis usually is easily differentiated from other causes of dermatitis by its appearance in new workers, the fact that it is transient, and the marked disproportion between objective findings and complaints of itching. The presence of glass fibers can possibly be determined by pressing cellophane tape against skin rinsed of gross contamination and then examining the tape under the microscope for very uniform rod-like fibers.

Although most of the studies on cutaneous reaction to MMVF have been done with glass fibers, some have been done with rock wool and have demonstrated a similar mechanical dermatitis without evidence of allergic sensitization.

Pruritis and dermatitis may result from the wearing of clothes that have been laundered in the same washing machine with glass fiber fabrics. When laundered, glass fiber cloth sheds a large number of glass spicules, which may cross-contaminate clothing.

Preventing skin irritation from glass fibers is an important consideration in the industrial setting. New workers should be advised that skin irritation is common. Work clothing should be long sleeved and loose fitting; the clothes should be changed daily and laundered separately from the family clothes; showering at the end of each work shift is also recommended. The effectiveness of barrier creams in preventing skin irritation from glass fibers has not been established (50).

Eye irritation from MMVF has been suspected, but there have been few reports of eye irritation in the literature. Stokholm and co-workers (54) found a statistically significant increase in eye symptoms in 15 workers exposed to rock wool. Upper respiratory tract irritation from MMVF is uncommon, but some nasal and pharyngeal irritation has been reported under unusually dusty conditions (55).

### Epidemiology

There have been few case reports of pulmonary disease due to exposure to MMVF despite the fact that large populations have been exposed to them since the start of production of rock/slag wool in the late 1800s and glass fibers in the 1930s. In the small number of reported cases, infection played a prominent role, and no consistent trends have been identified (56,57).

There have been extensive epidemiologic investigations, most involving workers in MMVF manufacturing, and to a much lesser extent product manufacturers using MMVF and end users. These studies have been aimed at identifying adverse human effects analogous to those associated with asbestos exposure (56).

Morbidity studies of chest x-ray findings, respiratory symptoms, and lung function in workers exposed to MMVF (58,59) have been generally negative. Weill, Hughes, and co-workers' (60) study of seven glass and mineral wool plants reported no increase in interstitial changes on chest radiographs in comparison to a regional comparison group. In addition, there were no changes noted in spirometric measurements or in upper and lower respiratory tract symptoms. Of chest radiograph changes noted in 23 of 1,435 workers, the majority were irregular opacities and all were at profusion level 1/0 and 1/1. These occurred (21/23) in two glass wool manufacturing plants that produced ordinary (average fiber diameter over 3 μm), fine diameter (1 to 3 μm), and very fine diameter (less than 1 μm) glass wool. There was no consistent association with exposure indices. No relationship was seen between exposure indices and radiographic findings or spirometric measurements (60,61).

Refractory ceramic (RCF) manufacturing employees in the United States are participating in an ongoing respiratory morbidity study and mortality registry. An initial review of posteroanterior (PA) chest radiographs of current workers at three RCF manufacturing plants and current and former workers at two RCF manufacturing plants demonstrated a significant relationship between pleural changes and time since first RCF production job (62). Further analysis using PA and oblique chest radiographs of current and former workers at two plant locations demonstrated a relationship between pleural plaques and years since first fiber production job, years in fiber production, and cumulative fiber exposure. No significant increase in parenchymal changes was noted (63).

Engholm and von Schmalensee (64) found an association between bronchitis and exposure to MMVF in the construction industry in a questionnaire survey of 135,000 Swedish construction workers. An ongoing prospective cohort study of the same population (65) has revealed that a large percentage of the user population is exposed to asbestos and MMVF. Kilburn et al. (66) in a study of workers using rotary spun fiberglass for 15 years or more as an insulation for appliances demonstrated a prevalence of irregular opacities, profusion 1/0 to 2/1, of 3.5%. Historical exposure information was insufficient to calculate cumulative dose and airborne asbestos fibers were reportedly previously measured in the production facility (67). Because it is difficult to separate the effects of asbestos and MMVF exposures, there are insufficient data to evaluate the risks associated with the inhalation of MMVF in the end user trade.

A postmortem study of the lungs of 20 fiberglass workers exposed to fiberglass dust for 16 to 32 years failed to show any statistical difference in average total amount of dust, total number of fibers per gram, and average dimensions of the fibers when compared to a similar study of the lungs of 26 urban dwellers (68).

Several mortality studies have included very large populations. Marsh, Enterline, and co-workers (69,70) have reported on an ongoing retrospective cohort study involving 16,661 workers in 17 glass fiber and mineral wool plants in the United States who were employed for at least 1 year between 1945 and 1963. In the most recent update (70) there is a small but statistically significant increase in all malignant neoplasms [standard mortality ratio (SMR) 108.3] and in respiratory system cancer (SMR 112.1) based on local death rates. The SMRs for respiratory cancer for 20 years or more since first employment in the glass production process are 113.5 and 134.2, respectively (71). The excess risk, however, is not associated with surrogate measures of exposure such as process, plant, duration of exposure, or estimates of worker fiber exposure. A subsequent case-control study of one of the glass fiber manufacturing plants with excessive lung cancer reported the excess may have been due to smoking prevalence differences in the local community versus the United States (72). An interplant difference in SMR for mineral wool workers identified in the Marsh and Enterline study (70) may be related to the use of slag possibly contaminated with arsenic and other metals. A more recent case-control study of nine U.S. slag wool plants found an excess of lung cancer secondary to smoking but not slag wool exposure (73).

In a large multinational historical cohort study involving 25,000 MMVF workers at 13 European production plants in seven countries, Saracci, Simonato, and co-workers (74) reported a statistically significant increased risk of lung cancer in workers with 30 years or more employment (SMR 192). In a follow-up study of the same cohort, Simonato et al. (75) reported that lung cancer mortality increased with time since first exposure only in rock or slag wool production workers. Lung cancer mortality excess in rock or slag wool production was associated with employment in the early technologic phase. The early phase was associated with poor ventilation, use of slag probably contaminated with arsenic and other metals, and exposure to the highest levels of fibrous dust. After the introduction in the production process of dust-suppressing agents such as binders and oils, no lung cancer excess was found. There was no consistent mortality excess for other cancers or nonmalignant respiratory disease.

Environmental surveys done in conjunction with these two large cohort studies demonstrated a wide variation in the concentration of airborne fibers within and between the plants surveyed but the airborne concentration was generally low—less than 2.5 mg/m$^3$ total concentration and less than 0.5 respirable fibers/cm$^3$ (76,77). The smaller the average diameter of the fibers being produced, the greater the airborne concentration of respirable size fibers. For example, during production of fibers with average diameters less than 3 µm, approximately 50% to 90% of airborne fibers are respirable.

Shannon and co-workers (78) in a historical prospective mortality study of 2,557 men at a glass wool plant in Ontario, Canada, reported a statistically significant increase in mortality from lung cancer with an SMR 199 ($p < 0.05$). There was, however, no correlation between lung cancer and time since first employment or duration of exposure. A study of three Swedish MMVF plants by Plato et al. (79) demonstrated an overall low number of lung and stomach cancer cases. There was a significant increase in lung cancer risk with a latency of 30 years but not with increasing duration of exposure to MMVF.

The International Agency for Research on Cancer (IARC), in its summary of the carcinogenic risk to humans from MMVF (2), reviewed studies that reported associations between cancer at sites other than the lungs and exposure to MMVF (75,80–82). The IARC Working Group "could not regard any of these associations as established due to their relatively weak strength, lack of consistency and to the unaccounted role of other exposures such as alcohol and tobacco smoking." In their overall evaluation, IARC classified glass wool, rock wool, slag wool, and ceramic fibers as group 2B (possibly carcinogenic to humans). Continuous glass filament is classified group 3 (not classifiable as to carcinogenicity to humans) (2).

Experimental data in vitro and in vivo have correlated MMVF toxicity with dose to the target organ, dimension of the fiber, and fiber durability. There is greater toxic potential for fibers that are durable in physiologic fluids and are of respirable size with a high aspect ratio. Animal inhalation studies have generally not been able to demonstrate respiratory tumors or interstitial fibrosis with MMVF except in rats and hamsters exposed to refractory ceramic fibers. Human morbidity and mortality studies have not been able to demonstrate an increased risk of respiratory cancer or interstitial fibrosis that correlates with surrogate measures of exposure, except for increased lung cancer mortality of workers in the European cohort exposed to rock or slag wool in the early technological phase. MMVF, therefore, appears to constitute a substantially lower order of health risk to humans than asbestos exposure.

Under current Occupational Safety and Health Administration (OSHA) standards, MMVF is treated as a nuisance dust with a permissible exposure limit (PEL) of 5.0 mg/m$^3$ for respirable dust and 15.0 mg/m$^3$ for total dust. The National Institute for Occupational Safety and Health (NIOSH) (83) has recommended that no worker be exposed to an MMVF airborne [time-weighted average (TWA)] concentration greater than 3 fibers/cm$^3$ with a diameter not more than 3.5 µm and a length not less than 10 µm as determined by phase-contrast optical microscopy. In addition, total MMVF dust should not exceed a TWA of 5 mg/m$^3$ by gravimetric analysis. Some manufacturers of MMVF have established their own recommended exposure guidelines for work force exposure in the range of 1 fiber/cm$^3$ as a TWA. The permissible exposure limit (PEL) for MMVF is under review by OSHA. The current recommended standard for MMVF within the United Kingdom is 2 fibers/cm$^3$, Sweden 1 fiber/cm$^3$, and Australia 0.5 fiber/cm$^3$ for a full working day (84). The World Health Organization reference method for measuring airborne MMVF calls for the use of scanning electron microscopy, which is a more exacting technique for accurate identification and sizing of airborne MMVF (85).

The animal and human studies currently in progress will continue to redefine the database on the potential health risks of MMVF exposure. In the interim, levels of MMVF should be kept at or below 1 fiber/cm$^3$, both in the manufacturing process and in the secondary and end uses of the products. This is especially applicable to durable fibers that are respirable in size and have high aspect ratios such as special purpose glass fibers and refractory ceramic fibers. Ongoing industrial hygiene monitoring for fiber identification, sizing, and counting will characterize the potential for occupational exposure and allow for proper environmental control measures and personal protective equipment. These measures are especially important for workers who fabricate products from MMVF and for end users, because the quality of worker protection and training methods can vary widely.

## VERMICULITE

Vermiculite is the geologic name given to a group of hydrated, laminar, aluminum-iron-magnesium silicate minerals. They were first named and described in 1824 by Thomas H. Webb, from a deposit near Worchester, Massachusetts. The first significant domestic vermiculite deposit was found near Libby, Montana, in 1916. Commercial production of vermiculite began in 1921 and is currently done in the Enoree region of South Carolina and in Louisa County, Virginia. The mine and mill at Libby, Montana, were closed in 1990. Outside the United States, the major source of vermiculite is from mining operations at Phalaborwa, northeastern Transvaal, Republic of South Africa (86).

Vermiculite has the unique property of expanding to as much as 12 times its original size with the application of heat between 400° and 1,100°C. This property is dependent on the presence of water molecules in the space between the layers. Heat converts the water to steam, forcing apart the thin, flexible, laminar plates to form a worm-like configuration. The name *vermiculite* comes from *vermicular,* meaning "to produce worms." The ore is transported in unexpanded form and is heated at regional expanding plants (1,86).

Most of the uses of vermiculite are for the expanded form, which is lightweight, noncombustible, chemically inert, and has a large surface area with ion-exchange capacity. These properties make it useful for construction purposes: loose-fill insulation; lightweight aggregates with setting materials such as gypsum, Portland cement, or acoustic plaster formulations; and as components in rigid board or tile products. Nonconstruction uses include inert carrier for pesticides, herbicides, and fertilizer; insulation of appliances; absorptive material used in water purification and chemical industries; animal bulking agent; and soil conditioner (86).

Investigation of vermiculite has demonstrated a potential for contamination with asbestiform minerals. Moatamed and co-workers (86) reported that unexpanded vermiculite shipped to a local expander plant from Libby, Montana, contained a maximum concentration of 2.0% fibrous actinolite (an amphibole) with a high aspect ratio (more than 10:1 length-to-width). The actinolite persisted in the expanded ore at a maximum concentration of 0.6%. Virginia vermiculite ore was found to contain actinolite contamination but in a lower concentration and mostly as cleavage fragments with low length-to-width ratios. South African vermiculite contains only rare fibers, mostly anthophyllite with low aspect ratios.

Environmental sampling at a plant that utilized Montana vermiculite ore revealed airborne fibers believed to be tremolite, an amphibole that differs from actinolite only in iron content. A cluster of benign, bloody, pleural effusions was reported at the same plant. Lockey and coworkers (87) in a cross-sectional epidemiologic study of 512 employees at the plant reported an association between dyspnea on exertion, pleuritic chest pain, pleural changes on chest radiograph, and cumulative tremolite fiber exposure. There were no significant abnormalities in spirometry or single-breath diffusion capacity.

Workers at the vermiculite mine in Libby, Montana, have been shown to have excess mortality from respiratory cancer (including four mesotheliomas) and nonmalignant respiratory disease in two separate but parallel studies. An increased prevalence of parenchymal and pleural radiographic abnormalities analogous to those produced by commercial asbestos exposure was also found (88–91). The increase in respiratory cancer in both studies was related to cumulative fiber exposure. The Libby, Montana vermiculite ore is contaminated with fibrous tremolite-actinolite estimated at 5% to 10% by bulk weight (92). These mining areas have subsequently been closed. A cohort of 194 men exposed to currently low levels of tremolite-actinolite in the mining and milling of vermiculite in the Enoree region, South Carolina, had a lung cancer SMR of 121, but three of the four lung cancer deaths were in the lowest fiber exposure category. No deaths were reported from mesothelioma or pneumoconiosis. The incidence of parenchymal (profusion at least 1/0) and pleural changes in 86 current and recent employees was 4.0% and 8.1%, respectively. The authors reported similar radiographic findings in an unexposed comparison group (93).

Workers mining and processing South African vermiculite containing low levels of nonfibrous anthophyllite and possibly small amounts of tremolite were not shown to be at an increased risk for pneumoconiosis, lung function impairment, or increased respiratory symptoms in a study of 172 workers in 1989 (94), when compared to a nonvermiculite exposed comparison group. Within the vermiculite-exposed group parenchymal changes (profusion 1/0 or greater) were demonstrated in 1.2%, pleural changes in 3.5%, and pleural calcifications in 1.7%.

The health effects of vermiculite exposure are related to the degree of contamination of the ore, mostly by fibrous tremolite-actinolite. The level of contamination appears to depend on the source of the ore. A continuous monitoring program of bulk vermiculite as well as airborne dust levels during the mining, milling, and end use of the product will help identify any potential for asbestiform mineral contamination and provide the opportunity for proper environmental controls.

## ZEOLITES

Zeolites are hydrated aluminum silicate minerals with a structure that contains large pores, channels filled with water, and exchangeable cations. Zeolites, derived from the ancient Greek word meaning "boiling stone," liberate water at 200°C that can be reabsorbed at room temperature without disrupting the basic structural framework (95).

Approximately 40 distinct fibrous and nonfibrous zeolite species have been identified. The fibrous zeolites, erionite and mordenite, are crystalline in structure and with milling can splinter to form long, thin fibers with extreme aspect ratios of respirable size (96). The main deposits of natural zeolites in the United States are along the margins of the Great Basins in the West (97). Currently, there is little commercial mining of the mineral (95).

The uses of zeolite are related to its selective absorption capabilities, hydrophilic nature, and ion-exchange capabilities. The mineral is used in the petrochemical, wastewater treatment, and water filtration industries. It is also used in pozzolanic cement, in animal litter, and as an animal dietary supplement. The majority of the United States' commercial needs are met by domestic production of nonfibrous synthetic zeolites (95) for which there are no currently identifiable health risks.

The fibrous zeolite, erionite, has been identified as the causal agent in the increased incidence of malignant pleural mesothelioma in the villages of Karain, Tuzköy, and Sarihidir, in the Cappadocia region of Central Anatolia, Turkey. These villages are well known to tourists because of the picturesque rock dwellings called "fairy chimneys." These dwellings are carved out of volcanic tuff composed of the fibrous zeolite, erionite. It has been

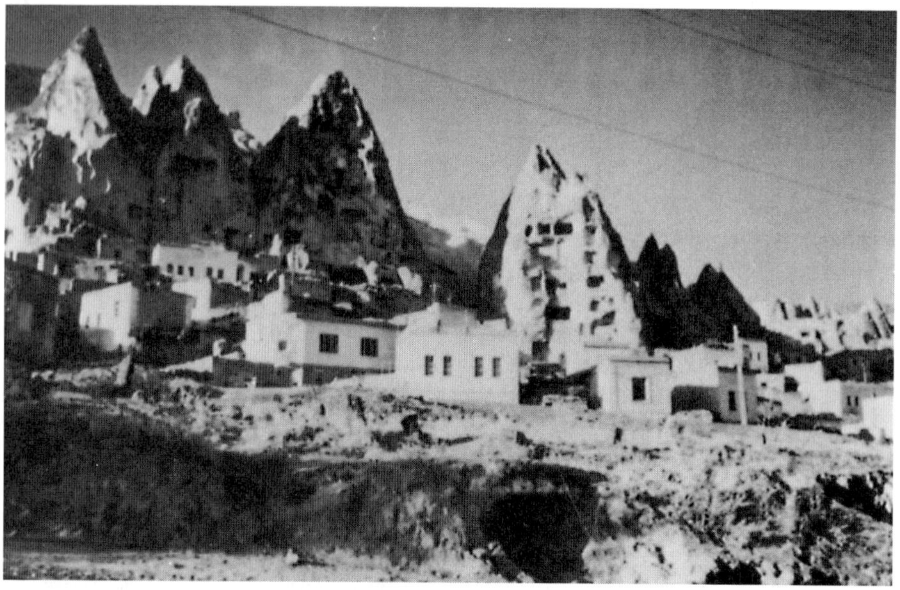

**FIG. 9.** Karain, a town in the Cappadocia region of Turkey, where an outbreak of diffuse malignant mesothelioma and pleural chest disease has been associated with environmental dust exposure containing a fibrous zeolite, erionite, as well as small amounts of tremolite and chrysotile. (Courtesy of Art Rohl, Ph.D.)

known for a long time that people of Karain die of cancer. The local saying goes, "The peasant of Karain falls ill with pain in the chest and belly, the shoulder drops, and he dies" (98) (Figs. 9 and 10).

An epidemiologic study of Tuzköy demonstrated an estimated annual incidence of malignant pleural mesothelioma of 6.5 cases, or 22 cases per 10,000 persons. The prevalence of pleural calcification was 17%, pleural thickening 10.5%, obscured costophrenic angle 15%, and interstitial fibrosis 12.1% (99). A comparative study in the village of Karain demonstrated a 70% to 80% excess in adult mortality, shortened life expectancy, and

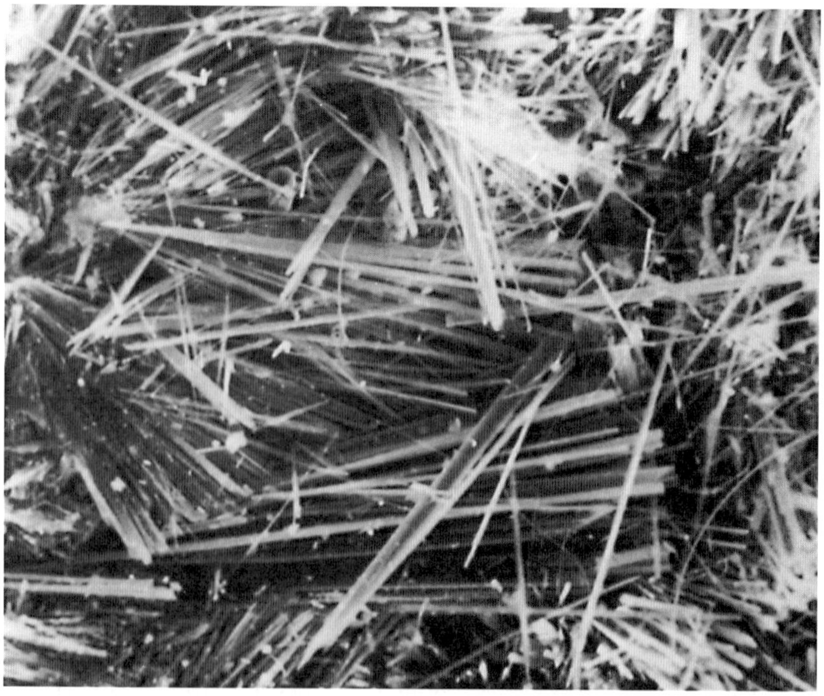

**FIG. 10.** SEM micrograph of zeolite sample from Tuzköy, Turkey (×700). (Courtesy of Farhad Moatamed, M.D.)

an excess of pleural radiographic abnormalities (100). Between 1970 and 1990, there were 249 deaths in Karain, of which 50.6% were due to malignant mesothelioma. In Tuzköy between 1980 and 1990, there were 347 deaths, of which 23.1% were due to malignant mesothelioma. The incidence of malignant mesothelioma in these three villages are 1,000 times greater than the general populations (101,102). Erionite fibers were found in the soil and building stones, in air samples, and within the lung tissue of the villagers. Eighty percent of the respirable fibers in Karain were found to be erionite, but the average concentration was low, generally less than 0.01 fiber/$cm^3$. Indoor samples obtained within the family cave dwellings during cleaning operations ranged from less than 0.01 to 1.38 fibers/$cm^3$ (100). Subsequently, small amounts of tremolite and chrysotile have been identified in the local environment and in lung tissue from local residents (103). In other areas of Central and Eastern Anatolia, soil contaminated with either tremolite or chrysotile asbestos has been used as whitewash or plaster material and has been linked to an environmental cause of malignant mesothelioma (101).

Lung tissue of a heavy equipment operator from Nevada was found to have histologic findings similar to those commonly associated with asbestos exposure. Scanning electron microscopy with energy-dispersive x-ray analysis of the mineral content of the tissue identified an analytic pattern similar to fibrous erionite and the absence of asbestos fibers (104).

Animal studies have demonstrated a definite carcinogenic effect for fibrous erionite reported to be asbestos free obtained from the village of Karain and for fibrous erionite obtained from Nevada and Colorado. The carcinogenic and fibrogenic effects when injected intraperitoneally into mice were similar to those of chrysotile or amosite asbestos (105,106).

There is significant evidence that the fibrous zeolite, erionite, has definite tumorigenic and fibrogenic potential. Proper environmental measurements, including bulk ore analysis and air sampling, should be taken whenever mining or construction work is done in an area where there may be deposits of fibrous zeolites. Erionite should be handled using the same environmental control standards currently in place for asbestos.

## ACKNOWLEDGMENT

The authors wish to express their appreciation to Don Miller for typing the manuscript, and to Patricia Lee and Sherrie Klein for their expertise and dedication in obtaining the references needed to write this chapter.

## REFERENCES

1. Lockey JE. Nonasbestos fibrous minerals. *Clin Chest Med* 1981;2: 203–218.
2. IARC. *Man-made mineral fibres and radon*. Lyon: International Agency for Research on Cancer, 1988.
3. *Health and safety aspects of man-made vitreous fibers*. Stamford, CT: TIMA, 1990.
4. Pundsack FI. Fibrous glass manufacture, use and physical properties. In: LeVee WN, ed. *Occupational exposure to fibrous glass*. NIOSH publication 76-151. Washington, DC: DHEW, 1976;11–18.
5. Hartung WJA. Technical history of MMMF with particular reference to fibre diameter and dustiness. In: Guthe T, ed. *Biological effects of man-made mineral fibres*. Copenhagen: World Health Organization, Regional Office for Europe 1984;1:12–19.
6. Dement JM. Environmental aspects of fibrous glass production and utilization. *Environ Res* 1975;9:295–312.
7. Esmen NA, Hammad YY. Recent studies of the environment in ceramic fibre production. In: Guthe T, ed. *Biological effects of man-made mineral fibres*. Copenhagen: World Health Organization, Regional Office for Europe, 1984;1:222–231.
8. Timbrell V. Aerodynamic considerations and other aspects of glass fiber. In: LeVee WN, ed. *Occupational exposure of fibrous glass*. NIOSH publication 76-151. Washington, DC: DHEW, 1976;33–50.
9. Davis JMG. A review of experimental evidence for the carcinogenicity of man-made vitreous fibers. *Scand J Work Environ Health* 1986; 12:12–17.
10. Davies R. The effect of mineral fibres on macrophages. In: Wagner JC, ed. *Biological effects of mineral fibres*. Lyon: IARC, 1980;1: 419–425.
11. Tilkes F, Beck EG. Macrophage functions after exposure to miner fibers. *Environ Health Perspect* 1983;51:67–72.
12. Ririe DG, Hesterberg TW, Barrett JC, et al. Toxicity of asbestos and glass fibers for rat tracheal epithelial cells in culture. In: Beck EG, Bignon J, eds. *In vitro effects of mineral dusts*. NATO ASI Series, Vol G3. Berlin: Springer, 1985;177–184.
13. Sincock AM, Delhanty JDA, Casey G. A comparison of the cytogenic response to asbestos and glass fibre in Chinese hamster and human cell lines. *Mutat Res* 1982;101:257–268.
14. Oshimura M, Hesterberg TW, Tsutsui T, Barrett JC. Correlation of asbestos-induced cytogenetic effects with cell transformation of Syrian hamster embryo cells in culture. *Cancer Res* 1984;44:5017–5022.
15. Hesterberg TW, Barrett JC. Dependence of asbestos- and mineral dust-induced transformation of mammalian cells in culture on fiber dimension. *Cancer Res* 1984;44:2170–2180.
16. Howden PJ, Faux SP. Fibre-induced lipid peroxidation leads to DNA adduct formation in Salmonella typhimurium TA104 and rat lung fibroblasts. *Carcinogenesis* 1996;17:413–419.
17. Gilmour PS, Beswick PH, Brown DM, et al. Detection of surface free radical activity of respirable industrial fibres using supercoiled phiX174RFI plasmid DNA. *Carcinogenesis* 1995;16:2973–2979.
18. Pelin K, Kivipensas P, Linnainmaa K. Effects of asbestos and man-made vitreous fibers on cell division in cultured human mesothelial cells in comparison to rodent cells. *Environ Mol Mutagen* 1995;25: 118–125.
19. Everitt JI, Bermudez E, Mangum JB, Ferriola PC. Malignant mesothelioma: a legacy of asbestos that effects the safety evaluation of synthetic vitreous fibers. *Chem Ind Inst Toxicol* 1996;16:1–8.
20. Förster H. The behaviour of mineral fibres in physiological solutions. In: Guthe T, ed. *Biological effects of man-made mineral fibres*. Copenhagen: World Health Organization, Regional Office for Europe, 1984;2:27–59.
21. Klingholz R, Steinkopf B. The reactions of MMMF in a physiological model fluid and in water. In: Guthe T, ed. *Biological effects of man-made mineral fibres*. Copenhagen: World Health Organization, Regional Office for Europe, 1984;2:60–86.
22. Leineweber JP. Solubility of fibres in vitro and in vivo. In: Guthe T, ed. *Biological effects of man-made mineral fibres*. Copenhagen: World Health Organization, Regional Office for Europe, 1984;2:87–101.
23. Law BD, Bunn WB, Hesterberg TW. Solubility of polymeric organic fibers and man-made vitreous fibers in Gamble's solution. *Inhal Toxicol* 1990;2:321–339.
24. de Meringo A, Morscheidt C, Thelohan S, Tiesler H. In vitro assessment of biodurability: acellular systems. *Environ Health Perspect* 1994;102:47–53.
25. Luoto K, Holopainen M, Savolainen K. Durability of man-made vitreous fibers as assessed by dissolution of silicon, iron, and aluminum in rat alveolar macrophages. *Ann Occup Hyg* 1995;32:855–867.

26. Luoto K, Holopainen M, Kangas J, et al. The effects of fiber length on the dissolution by macrophages of rockwool and glasswool fibers. *Environ Res* 1995;70:51–61.
27. Bernstein DM, Drew RT, Schidlovsky G, Kuschner M. Pathogenicity of MMMF and the contrasts with natural fibres. In: Guthe T, ed. *Biological effects of man-made mineral fibres.* Copenhagen: World Health Organization, Regional Office for Europe, 1984;2:169–195.
28. Bellmann B, Muhle H, Pott F, et al. Persistence of man-made mineral fibres (MMMF) and asbestos in rat lungs. *Ann Occup Hyg* 1987;31: 693–709.
29. Johnson NF, Griffiths DM, Hill RJ. Size distribution following long-term inhalation of MMMF. In: Guthe T, ed. *Biological effects of man-made mineral fibres.* Copenhagen: World Health Organization, Regional Office for Europe, 1984;2:102–125.
30. Le Bouffant L, Henin JP, Martin JC, et al. Distribution of inhaled MMMF in the rat lung—long-term effects. In: Guthe T, ed. *Biological effects of man-made mineral fibres.* Copenhagen: World Health Organization, Regional Office for Europe, 1984;2:143–168.
31. Hammad YY. Deposition and elimination of MMMF. In: Guthe T, ed. *Biological effects of man-made mineral fibres.* Copenhagen: World Health Organization, Regional Office for Europe, 1984;2:126–142.
32. Wright GW, Kuschner M. The influence of varying lengths of glass and asbestos fibers on tissue response in guinea pigs. In Walton WH, ed. *Inhaled particles* IV, part 2. New York: Pergamon, 1977;455–472.
33. Pott F, Ziem U, Reiffer F-J, et al. Carcinogenicity studies on fibres, metal compounds, and some other dusts in rats. *Exp Pathol* 1987;32: 129–152.
34. Smith DM, Ortiz LW, Archuleta RF, Johnson NF. Long-term health effects in hamsters and rats exposed chronically to man-made vitreous fibres. *Ann Occup Hyg* 1987;31:731–754.
35. Stanton MF, Wrench C. Mechanisms of mesothelioma induction with asbestos and fibrous glass. *J Natl Cancer Inst* 1972;48:797–821.
36. Stanton MF, Layard M, Tegeris A, et al. Relation of particle dimension to carcinogenicity in amphibole asbestoses and other fibrous minerals. *J Natl Cancer Inst* 1981;67:965–975.
37. Pott F, Huth F, Friedrichs KH. Results of animal carcinogenesis studies after application of fibrous glass and their implications regarding human exposure. In: LeVee WN, ed. *Occupational exposure of fibrous glass.* NIOSH publication 76-151. Washington, DC: DHEW, 1976; 183–191.
38. Pott F, Schlipköter HW, Ziem U, et al. New results from implantation experiments with mineral fibres. In: Guthe T, ed. *Biological effects of man-made mineral fibres.* Copenhagen: World Health Organization, Regional Office for Europe, 1984;2:286–302.
39. Wagner JC, Bery GB, Hill RJ, et al. Animal experiments with MMM(V)F—effects of inhalation of intrapleural inoculation in rats. In: Guthe T, ed. *Biological effects of man-made mineral fibres.* Copenhagen: World Health Organization, Regional Office for Europe, 1984; 2:209–233.
40. Davis JMG. Pathological aspects of the injection of glass fiber into the pleural and peritoneal cavities of rats and mice. In: LeVee WN, ed. *Occupational exposure of fibrous glass.* NIOSH publication 76-151. Washington, DC: DHEW, 1976;141–149.
41. Bernstein DM, Thevenaz P, Fleissner H, et al. Evaluation of the oncogenic potential of man-made vitreous fibers: the inhalation model. *Ann Occup Hyg* 1995;39:661–672.
42. Goldstein B, Rendall REG, Webster I. A comparison of the effects of exposure of baboons to crocidolite and fibrous-glass dusts. *Environ Res* 1983;32:344–359.
43. Bunn WB, Bender JR, Hesterberg TW, et al. Recent studies of man made vitreous fibers: chronic animal inhalation studies. *J Occup Med* 1993;35:101–113.
44. Hesterberg TW, Miller WC, Thevenaz P, Anderson R. Chronic inhalation studies of man-made vitreous fibers: characterization of fibres in the exposure aerosol and lungs. *Ann Occup Hyg* 1995;39:637–653.
45. Davis JMG, Addison J, Bolton RE, et al. The pathogenic effects of fibrous ceramic aluminum silicate glass administered to rats by inhalation or peritoneal injection. In: Guthe T, ed. *Biological effects of man-made mineral fibres.* Copenhagen: World Health Organization, Regional Office for Europe, 1984;2:303–322.
46. Mast RW, McConnell EE, Anderson R, et al. Studies on the chronic toxicity (inhalation) of four types of refractory ceramic fiber in male Fischer 344 rats. *Inhal Toxicol* 1995;7:425–467.
47. McConnell EE, Mast RW, Hesterberg TW, et al. Chronic inhalation toxicity of a kaolin-based refractory ceramic fiber in Syrian golden hamsters. *Inhal Toxicol* 1995;7:503–532.
48. Mast RW, McConnell EE, Hesterberg TW. Multiple-dose chronic inhalation toxicity study of size-separated kaolin refractory ceramic fiber in male Fischer rats. *Inhal Toxicol* 1995;7:469–502.
49. Lippmann M. Man-made mineral fibers (MMMF): human exposures and health risk assessment. *Toxicol Ind Health* 1990;6:225–246.
50. Possick PA, Gellin GA, Key MM. Fibrous glass dermatitis. *Am Ind Hyg Assoc J* 1970;31:12–15.
51. Heisel EB, Mitchell JH. Cutaneous reaction to fiberglass. *Ind Med Surg* 1957;26:547–550.
52. Kalimo K, Saarni H, Kytta J. Immediate and delayed type reactions to formaldehyde resin in glass wool. *Contact Dermatitis* 1989;6:496.
53. Holness DL, Nethercott JR. Occupational contact dermatitis due to epoxy resin in a fiberglass binder. *J Occup Med* 1989;31:87–89.
54. Stokholm J, Norn M, Schneider T. Ophthalmologic effects of man-made mineral fibers. *Scand J Work Environ Health* 1982;8:185–190.
55. Milby TH, Wolf CR. Respiratory tract irritation from fibrous glass inhalation. *J Occup Med* 1969;11:409–410.
56. Hill JW. Review of the epidemiology of man-made mineral fibres. In: Wagner JC, ed. *Biological effects of mineral fibres.* Lyon, France: IARC, 1980;979–983.
57. Takahashi T, Munakata M, Takekawa H, et al. Pulmonary fibrosis in a carpenter with long lasting exposure to fiberglass. *Am J Ind Med* 1996;30:596–600.
58. Wright GW. Airborne fibrous glass particles: chest roentgenograms of persons with prolonged exposure. *Arch Environ Health* 1968;16: 175–181.
59. Nasr ANM, Ditchek T, Scholtens PA. The prevalence of radiographic abnormalities in the chests of fiber glass workers. *J Occup Med* 1971; 13:371–376.
60. Weill H, Hughes JM, Hammad YY, et al. Respiratory health in workers exposed to man-made vitreous fibers. *Am Rev Respir Dis* 1983; 128:104–112.
61. Hughes JM, Jones RN, Glindmeyer HW, et al. Follow up study of workers exposed to man made mineral fibres. *Br J Ind Med* 1993;50: 658–667.
62. Lemasters G, Lockey J, Rice C, et al. Radiographic changes among workers manufacturing refractory ceramic fiber and products. *Ann Occup Hyg* 1994;38:745–751.
63. Lockey J, Lemasters G, Rice C, et al. Refractory ceramic fiber exposure and pleural plaques. *Am J Respir Crit Care Med* 1996;154: 1405–1410.
64. Engholm G, von Schmalensee G. Bronchitis and exposure to man-made mineral fibres in non-smoking construction workers. *Eur J Respir Dis* 1982;63:73–78.
65. Engholm G, Englund A, Fletcher AC, Hallin N. Respiratory cancer incidence in Swedish construction workers exposed to man-made mineral fibres and asbestos. *Ann Occup Hyg* 1987;31:663–675.
66. Kilburn KH, Powers D, Warshaw RH. Pulmonary effects of exposure to fine fiberglass: irregular opacities and small airway obstruction. *Br J Ind Med* 1992;49:714–720.
67. Bender JR. Pulmonary effects of exposure to fine fiberglass: irregular opacities and small airway obstruction. *Br J Ind Med* 1993;50:381–382.
68. Gross P, Tuma J, DeTreville RTP. Lungs of workers exposed to fiber glass. *Arch Environ Health* 1971;23:67–76.
69. Enterline PE, Marsh GM, Henderson V, Callahan C. Mortality update of a cohort of U.S. man-made mineral fibre workers. *Ann Occup Hyg* 1987;31:625–656.
70. Marsh GM, Enterline PE, Stone RA, Henderson VL. Mortality among a cohort of U.S. man-made mineral fiber workers: 1985 follow-up. *J Occup Med* 1990;32:594–604.
71. Enterline PE. Carcinogenic effects of man-made vitreous fibers. *Annu Rev Public Health* 1991;12:459–480.
72. Chiazze L, Watkins DK, Fryar C. A case-control study of malignant and non-malignant respiratory disease among employees of a fiberglass manufacturing facility. *Br J Ind Med* 1992;49:326–331.
73. Wong O, Foliart D, Trent LS. A case-control study of lung cancer in a cohort of workers potentially exposed to slag wool fibres. *Br J Ind Med* 1991;48:818–824.
74. Saracci R, Simonato L, Acheson ED, et al. Mortality and incidence of cancer of workers in the man-made vitreous fibres producing industry: an international investigation at 13 European plants. *Br J Ind Med* 1984;41:425–436.

75. Simonato L, Fletcher AC, Cherrie JW, et al. The International Agency for Research on Cancer historical cohort study of MMMF production workers in seven European countries: extension of the follow-up. *Ann Occup Hyg* 1987;31:603–623.
76. Esmen N, Corn M, Hammad Y, et al. Summary of measurements of employee exposure to airborne dust and fiber in sixteen facilities producing man-made mineral fibers. *Am Ind Hyg Assoc J* 1979;40: 108–117.
77. Oltery J, Cherrie JW, Dodgson J, Harrison GE. A summary report on environmental conditions at 13 European MMMF plants. In: Guthe T, ed. *Biological effects of man-made mineral fibres.* Copenhagen: World Health Organization, 1984;1:83–117.
78. Shannon HS, Jamieson E, Julian JA, et al. Mortality experience of Ontario glass fibre workers—extended follow-up. *Ann Occup Hyg* 1987;31:657–662.
79. Plato N, Westerhom P, Gustavsson P, et al. Cancer incidence, mortality and exposure-response among Swedish man-made vitreous fiber production workers. *Scand J Work Environ Health* 1995;21:353–361.
80. Robinson CF, Dement JM, Ness GO, Waxweiler RJ. Mortality patterns of rock and slag mineral wool production workers: an epidemiological and environmental study. *Br J Ind Med* 1982;32:45–53.
81. Moulin JJ, Mur JM, Wild P, et al. Oral cavity and laryngeal cancers among man-made mineral fiber production workers. *Scand J Work Environ Health* 1986;12:27–31.
82. Bertazzi PA, Zocchetti C, Riboldi L, et al. Cancer mortality of an Italian cohort of workers in man-made glass-fiber production. *Scand J Work Environ Health* 1986;12:65–71.
83. NIOSH. *Criteria for a recommended standard . . . occupational exposure to fibrous glass.* NIOSH publication 77–152. Washington, DC: DHEW, 1977.
84. *Synthetic mineral fibres, National standard and national code of practice.* B590/21544 Cat. No. 90 1601X. Canberra: Australian Government Publishing Service, May 1990.
85. The WHO/EURO man-made mineral fiber reference scheme. *Scand J Work Environ Health* 1985;11:123–129.
86. Moatamed F, Lockey JE, Parry WT. Fiber contamination of vermiculites: a potential occupational and environmental health hazard. *Environ Res* 1986;41:207–218.
87. Lockey JE, Brooks SM, Jarabek AM, et al. Pulmonary changes after exposure to vermiculite contaminated with fibrous tremolite. *Am Rev Respir Dis* 1984;129-952–958.
88. McDonald JC, Sebastien P, Armstrong B. Radiological survey of past and present vermiculite miners exposed to tremolite. *Br J Ind Med* 1986;43:445–449.
89. McDonald JC, McDonald AD, Armstrong B, Sebastien P. Cohort study of mortality of vermiculite miners exposed to tremolite. *Br J Ind Med* 1986;43:436–444.
90. Amandus HE, Althouse R, Morgan WKC, et al. The morbidity and mortality of vermiculite miners and millers exposed to tremolite-actinolite: part III. Radiographic findings.*Am J Ind Med* 1987;11:27–37.
91. Amandus HE, Wheeler R. The morbidity and mortality of vermiculite miners and millers exposed to tremolite-actinolite: part II. Mortality. *Am J Ind Med* 1987;11:15–26.
92. Amandus HE, Wheeler R, Jankovic J, Tucker J. The morbidity and mortality of vermiculite miners and millers exposed to tremolite-actinolite: part I. Exposure estimates. *Am J Ind Med* 1987;11:1–14.
93. McDonald JC, McDonald AD, Sebastien P, Moy K. Health of vermiculite miners exposed to trace amounts of fibrous tremolite. *Br J Ind Med* 1988;45:630–634.
94. Hessel PA, Sluis-Cremer GK. X-ray findings, lung function, and respiratory symptoms in black South African vermiculite workers. *Am J Ind Med* 1989;15:21–29.
95. Sand IB, Mumpton FA, eds. *Natural zeolites, occurrence, properties, use.* Oxford: Pergamon, 1978.
96. Wright WE, Moatamed F, Rom WN. Characterization of zeolite fiber sizes using scanning electron microscopy. *Arch Environ Health* 1983; 38:99–103.
97. Rom WN, Casey KR, Parry WT, et al. Health implications of natural fibrous zeolites for the Intermountain West. *Environ Res* 1983;30:1–8.
98. Baris YI, Sahin AA, Özesmi M, et al. An outbreak of pleural mesothelioma and chronic fibrosing pleurisy in the village of Karain/Ürgüp in Anatolia. *Thorax* 1978;33:181–192.
99. Artvinli M, Baris YI. Malignant mesotheliomas in a small village in the Anatolian region of Turkey: an epidemiologic study. *J Natl Cancer Inst* 1979;63:17–20.
100. Baris YI, Saracci R, Simonato L, et al. Malignant mesothelioma and radiological chest abnormalities in two villages in central Turkey. *Lancet* 1981;1:984–987.
101. Selçuk ZT, Lütfi Ç, Emri S, et al. Malignant pleural mesothelioma due to environmental mineral fiber exposure in Turkey. *Chest* 1992;102: 790–796.
102. Sahin AA, Çöplü L, Selcuk ZT, et al. Malignant pleural mesothelioma caused by environmental exposure to asbestos or erionite in rural Turkey: CT findings in 84 patients. *Am J Roentgenol* 1993;161:533–537.
103. Rohl AN, Langer AM, Moncure G, et al. Endemic pleural disease associated with exposure to mixed fibrous dust in Turkey. *Science* 1982;216:518.
104. Casey KR, Shigeoka JW, Rom WN. Moatamed F. Zeolite exposure and associated pneumoconiosis. *Chest* 1985;87:837–840.
105. Suzuki Y, Kohyama N. Malignant mesothelioma induced by asbestos and zeolite in the mouse peritoneal cavity. *Environ Res* 1984;35:277–292.
106. Özesmi M, Patiroglu TE, Hillerdal G, and Özesmi C. Peritoneal mesothelioma and malignant lymphoma in mice caused by fibrous zeolite. *Br J Ind Med* 1985;42:746–749.

*Environmental and Occupational Medicine, Third Edition,* edited by William N. Rom.
Published by Lippincott–Raven Publishers, Philadelphia, 1998.

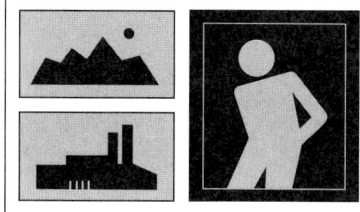

# CHAPTER 28

# Respiratory Disease in Coal Miners

Michael D. Attfield and Gregory R. Wagner

Coal miners develop a variety of lung diseases as a result of their workplace exposures. Of these, coal worker's pneumoconiosis (CWP) has received the most attention, perhaps because of its clear occupational association. Bronchitis and emphysema resulting from coal mine dust exposure, clinically indistinguishable from their nonoccupational analogues, are more prevalent and are associated with significant morbidity among coal miners. The group of lung diseases for which miners are at increased risk have been called "black lung" in coal mining communities and in United States federal compensation legislation. To date, most scientific investigations and preventive efforts have been directed toward the control of CWP.

Although a disease attributed to coal dust inhalation was reported following the autopsy of a Scottish miner in 1831 (1) the nature of coal miners' lung diseases was debated for the next 150 years. CWP was not recognized as an entity distinct from silicosis in Great Britain until around 1940 (2,3). Coal mining has been an important industry in the United States since the early 19th century, but official recognition that coal mine dust causes chronic lung disease, premature disability, and death did not occur until the final third of the 20th century. The disastrous Farmington, West Virginia, mine explosion and fire, in which 78 miners died, combined with findings of U.S. Public Health Service studies and a significant level of political activism among coal miners (4) led to passage of the Federal Coal Mine Health and Safety Act of 1969. This act (5), amended in 1977 (6), directs the secretary of labor to set standards for exposure to toxic materials so that "no miner will suffer material impairment of health or functional capacity even if such miner has regular exposure to the hazards dealt with by such standard for the period of his working life." Specifically, health standards for exposure to coal mine dust were established with the intent "to permit each miner the opportunity to work underground during the period of his entire adult working life without incurring any disability from pneumoconiosis or any other occupation-related disease." A respirable coal mine dust standard (3 $mg/m^3$ air, later reduced to 2 $mg/m^3$) was established. The act also provided for rigorous inspection procedures; medical examinations for working miners and autopsies for deceased miners; a federally administered compensation program for miners with disabling lung diseases; and right of entry for research to advance understanding of the health effects of mining.

Coal worker's pneumoconiosis is a well-defined medical entity resulting from the deposition of coal mine dust in the lung and from the reaction to the deposited dust resulting in coal macules, coal nodules, and progressive massive fibrosis (PMF). Because of the nonspecific nature of chronic obstructive pulmonary disease (COPD) and the frequent concurrent presence of multiple risk factors such as dust exposure and cigarette smoking, the diagnosis of lung diseases related to coal mine dust has led to disagreement and controversy over the definition and diagnosis of black lung (7). Ongoing epidemiologic, pathologic, and clinical studies have provided important information, helping to resolve some of these questions.

The United States has extensive coal deposits (Fig. 1). Owing to the increasing scarcity and cost of petroleum as a fuel, coal will continue to be an essential energy source. It is impossible to extract coal without some dust exposure, so it is critical to understand the relationships between coal

M. D. Attfield: Epidemiology Investigations Branch, National Institute for Occupational Safety and Health, Morgantown, West Virginia 26505-2888.
G. R. Wagner: Division of Respiratory Disease Studies, National Institute for Occupational Safety and Health, Morgantown, West Virginia 26505-2888.

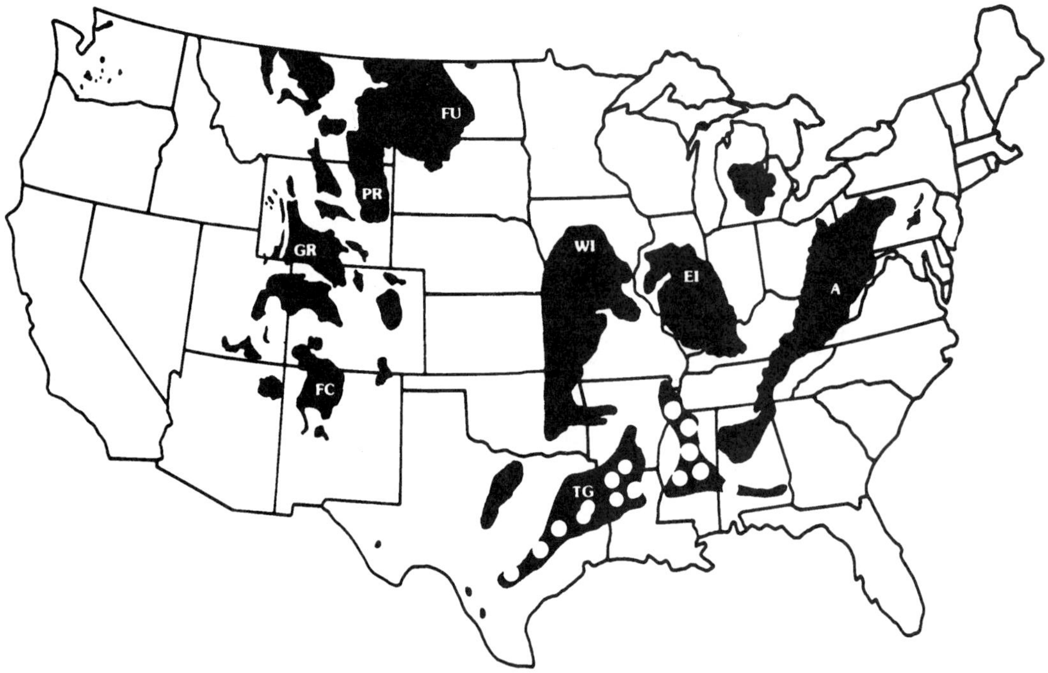


**FIG. 1.** Coal deposits in the United States mainland. *Completely filled areas* have coal deposits; *partially filled areas* have scattered coal deposits. A, Appalachia; EI, eastern interior; WI, western interior; TG, Texas Gulf; PR, Powder River; FU, Fort Union; GR, Green River; FC, Four Corners. (Adapted from ref. 211.)

mine dust exposure and the development of respiratory diseases in order to diagnose, treat, and prevent them.

## EPIDEMIOLOGY

Perhaps more investigation has been directed toward lung diseases of coal miners than toward any other occupational disease. Meiklejohn (8–10), for example, cites more than 100 reports and articles published before 1950 on the health of coal miners. These early works helped to reveal the extent and nature of respiratory disease in miners but were unable to quantify the effects of coal dust because they lacked reliable exposure estimates. More recently, analyses of large epidemiologic studies with comprehensive exposure measurement components, such as the British Pneumoconiosis Field Research (11) have permitted the establishment of exposure-response relationships for a number of medical conditions. The results of these have been applied to the setting of dust control standards around the world. In addition, these intensive multifaceted studies have clarified many aspects of the causation and significance of lung disease in coal miners.

### General Morbidity

Recognition that coal miners were at risk of lung disease due to their work came late to the United States. As a consequence, active epidemiologic investigation of coal miners did not start until after 1960. Between 1960 and 1970, however, seven studies were undertaken in various regions of the country (12–18). The findings from these showed that a risk of CWP existed in all regions studied, but that it varied considerably, depending on rank of coal (Fig. 2). (Coal rank is associated with the degree of metamorphosis of the coal due to heat and pressure and is often measured by the percentage of carbon. Anthracite has the highest percentage of carbon and gives rise to the most severe disease.)

A significant restriction on respirable dust levels in U.S. coal mines was mandated by the 1969 Federal Coal Mine Health and Safety Act (5). CWP prevalence rates from 1970 to the present are shown in Table 1. These figures were derived from a large, long-term, nationwide study of lung diseases of coal miners in the United States (19) and standardized to a common tenure distribution obtained from a survey of coal mine employment in 1986 (20). Standardized rates derived from data collected by the federally operated Coal Worker's X-Ray Surveillance Program (CWXSP) (21) are also shown in the table. Both sets of information indicate a declining trend in prevalence. The observed trends may not be due solely to the lower dust levels, as miner participation in these programs has been suboptimal.

Coal miners tend to report more respiratory symptoms and have poorer lung function than control groups (17,22–25). In some cases a parallel effect has also been seen when miners' wives were compared to wives of the nonminer control group, suggesting that environmental

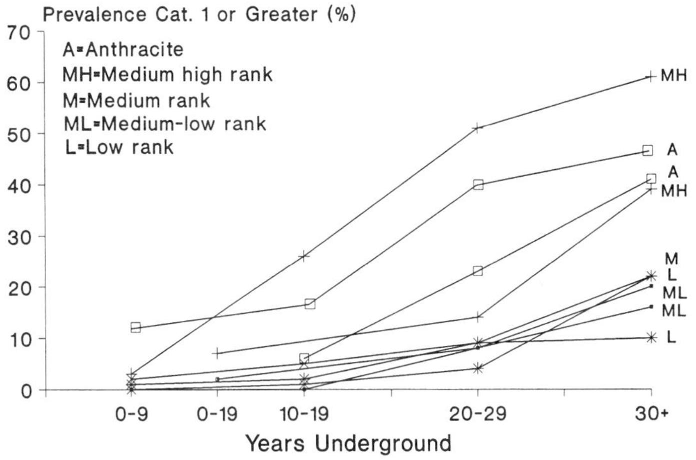


**FIG. 2.** Prevalence of category 1 or greater small rounded opacities against tenure in mining by coal rank group for seven studies (one including three regions) undertaken before 1970 in the United States.

and social factors may also be involved (22,24). Higgins (23) reviewed findings from both the United States and Britain and concluded that there was consistent evidence of greater prevalence of respiratory symptoms and lower average lung function in miners and ex-miners than in nonminers.

## General Mortality

Mortality patterns among coal miners have been studied systematically for about 100 years, beginning with British occupational mortality statistics for 1890 to 1892. These studies have generally shown increased standard mortality rates (SMRs) for accidents, respiratory disease, respiratory tuberculosis, and stomach cancer. Overall, SMRs from all causes have varied somewhat, from a high of 195 in an early study (26) to levels slightly above 100 in a number of more recent large analyses (27–30). The later studies reveal evidence of healthy worker selection effects, some reports showing statistically significant elevations in SMR for ex-miners and for current miners who likely moved to surface jobs because of ill health.

Standardized rates for death from pneumoconiosis have consistently shown increased risks associated with progressive massive fibrosis (PMF) (29–36). Most of the studies, however, failed to detect any elevation in mortality risk associated with the presence of simple CWP. Miller and Jacobsen (30) found that simple CWP was associated with a 2% to 3% reduction in 22-year survival rates, but there was no apparent association with the category of simple CWP. They also reported that the relative risk of death over a 22-year period for miners who developed PMF while young (age 25 to 34 years) was 3.5 compared to those without CWP.

Elevated death rates due to lung disease other than CWP have also been reported. Rockette (27) found increased rates of emphysema, influenza, asthma, and tuberculosis, whereas Miller and Jacobsen (30) concluded that miners exposed to excessive amounts of respirable dust are at elevated risk of death from chronic bronchitis or emphysema. An SMR of 426 was recently reported for nonmalignant respiratory disease among Dutch coal miners (37).

Two consistent features of coal miner death rates relate to cancers of the lung and stomach. In the former case the standardized rates typically have been low (38), and no obvious relationship of lung cancer mortality with dust exposure has been detected (39). An excess of deaths due

**TABLE 1.** *Rate of category 1/0 or greater, and 2/1 or greater small rounded opacities standardized to a common tenure distribution representing the work force distribution in 1986 for the NSCWP and CWXSP*

| | | Adjusted summary prevalence | | | |
|---|---|---|---|---|---|
| | Category | 1970–72 | 1973–75 | 1977–81 | 1985–88 |
| Epidemiologic data (NSCWP) | | | | | |
| Common tenure | 1/0+ | 6.6 | 5.1 | 3.6 | 2.3 |
| Distribution (%) | 2/1+ | 1.5 | 1.2 | 0.5 | 0.3 |
| Surveillance data (CWXSP) | | | | | |
| Common tenure | 1/0+ | 10.7 | 9.9 | 7.3 | 3.6 |
| Distribution (%) | 2/1+ | 2.4 | 1.2 | 0.7 | 0.4 |

NSCWP, National Study of Coal Workers' Pneumoconioses; CWXSP, Coal Worker's X-Ray Surveillance Program.
Note: Rates from the CWXSP are for the second readers (all B readers).

to stomach cancer has been seen among miners in Britain (28,40), the United States (27,41), Holland (37,42), and Japan (43). There is a suggestion that stomach cancer risk is related to exposure to coal mine dust (30). Ames (44) describes a number of hypotheses that could explain the higher gastric cancer mortality in coal miners. Among these is Meyer et al.'s (45) hypothesis that stomach cancer incidence would be greater in miners with good lung clearance, since the dust would be transported from the lungs and then swallowed. Some findings of Dutch coal miners support this view (42), although it was not found for U.S. coal miners (39).

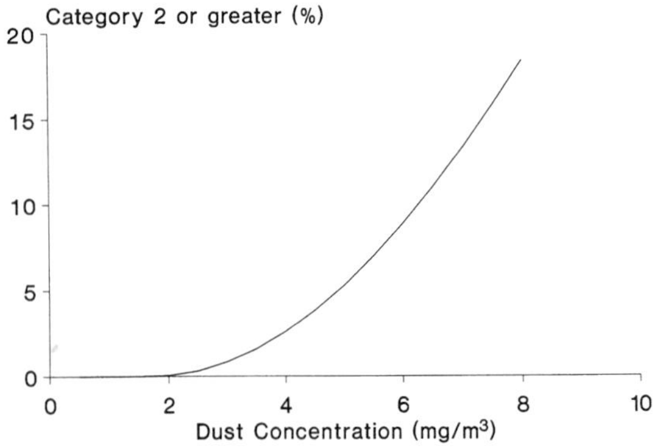


**FIG. 3.** British miners' predicted risk of contracting category 2 or greater small rounded opacities over 35 years plotted against dust concentration.

## Morbidity, Coal Mine Dust Exposure, and Other Risk Factors

### *Coal Worker's Pneumoconiosis*

British epidemiologic studies of the relationship between prevalence and incidence of CWP and environmental measurements have consistently revealed that the predominant adverse exposure factor is respirable mixed coal mine dust (46–50). Coal rank has also been found to play a role in that risk increases with the carbon content of the coal. Quartz (silica), on the other hand, was found to be a minor contributor to CWP development in general, although the environmental levels were low on average (46,47). However, quartz was implicated in a study of a group of cases of unusually rapid progression of simple pneumoconiosis (51). In addition, miners with a particular form of PMF that appeared to consist of conglomerations of the larger nodules of simple CWP (type *r* (123) opacities) had received higher exposures to quartz than had their controls (52).

Among nonoccupational factors, smoking was not found to affect simple CWP development (53), nor did bronchitis appear to play a role (54). However, an important risk factor for the development of PMF is presence of simple CWP (49,55,56), and risk increases with category of disease. There are also indications that body mass and breathlessness may be positively related to future development of PMF (57). [The latter result agrees with pathologic findings that show widespread emphysema in miners with PMF (58).] No other important factors have emerged, and considerable unexplained variation remains in the data. A detailed study of eight "anomalous" mines (i.e., ones with much higher or much lower rates of simple CWP than expected for measured dust levels) was able to account for only part of the variation in five, and for none at all in the remaining three (59).

The current coal mine dust exposure limit for underground coal mines in the United States relies substantially on estimates of exposure-response relationships for CWP obtained from study of British miners (46). Figure 3 shows the relevant curve, which relates the estimated 35-year risk of category 2 or higher small rounded opacities to the concentration of respirable mixed coal mine dust. Category 2 was chosen as the response following the advice of Cochrane (55), who, noting that the incidence rate of PMF increased markedly among miners with simple CWP of category 2 or higher, argued that the logical way to control the appearance of progressive massive fibrosis is to concentrate on preventing miners from reaching category 2 of simple pneumoconiosis. Since the curve predicts zero incidence of category 2 or greater at 2 mg/m$^3$, that dust concentration was adopted as the federal standard.

Recent British analyses of exposure and response have concentrated on PMF as the response variable(49) (Fig. 4). These findings were derived from study of 52,264 5-year intervals of risk for more than 30,000 British miners. Probabilities of contracting simple CWP or PMF, or of progressing from one category of simple CWP to another, were modeled against initial category, dust exposure, coal rank, and worker's age. The results were used to obtain predicted probabilities for 5-year periods, and these predictions were then compounded into 40-year risks. Clear

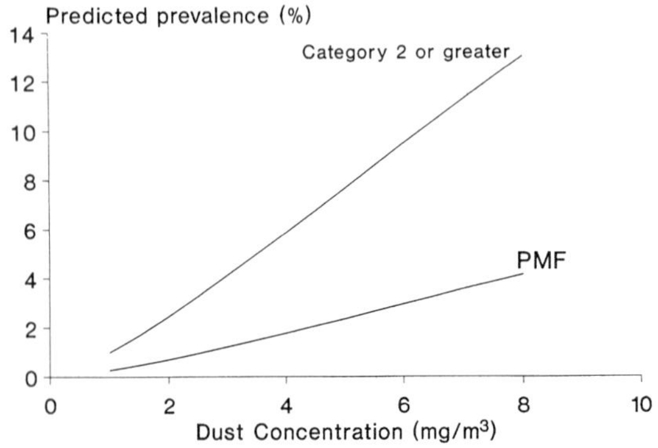


**FIG. 4.** British miners' predicted risks of contracting category 2 or greater small rounded opacities and PMF after 40 years work plotted against dust concentration.

exposure-response relationships were found for dust and coal rank, the predictions of risk being somewhat greater than those from earlier analyses. Although these investigations confirmed that the risk of contracting PMF increases with category of simple CWP, they also showed that PMF could develop over 5 years in miners whose initial chest radiograph was normal. This risk appeared to be dependent on the degree of previous dust exposure. This implies that PMF could not be eliminated exclusively through control of simple CWP.

Exposure-response relationships have been reported among miners from countries other than Britain. Reisner (60,61) has demonstrated clear exposure-related effects of dust and coal rank in German miners. German studies of exposure-response indicate a risk between 1% and 14% for category 2 or greater over 35 years at 4 mg/m$^3$, and less than 4% for 2 mg/m$^3$ (62).

In the United States, data collected in the last few years, before federal regulation caused a reduction in dust levels, were used to compute retrospective dust exposures for miners working at round 1 of the National Study of Coal Workers' Pneumoconiosis (NSCWP) (63) and then applied to estimation of exposure-response for CWP (64). Clear effects of dust exposure, coal rank, and age on prevalence of CWP (small rounded opacities and PMF) were seen. The results are shown in Fig. 5, which provides predicted prevalences of category 1 or greater, 2 or greater, and PMF for a range of dust exposures. These predictions tend to be somewhat higher than those derived from studies of British and German miners (49,62). These findings were confirmed in another study involving U.S. underground coal miners and ex-miners medically examined between 1985 and 1988 (65).

Most of the studies noted above were undertaken on working miners and were therefore vulnerable to bias induced by ignoring miners in poor health who left mining. Such a bias was apparent in older, higher dust exposed miners (66), while Attfield and Seixas (65) showed that miners who reported leaving work because of their health had higher levels of abnormality than their colleagues who remained at work. However, a study of exposure-response in groups of ex-miners and current miners led the authors to conclude, "Estimates of risk of simple pneumoconiosis in relation to exposure to mixed respirable dust in working miners adequately describe the relation found in men who have been miners but have left the industry" (67). A similar observation was made regarding development of PMF in current and ex-miners (68). (These observations should be contrasted with those for ventilatory function discussed below, where there appears to be evidence of more extreme effects of dust on those who leave coal mining.)

Although most exposure-response assessments for CWP have employed a logistic-type of model using cumulative exposure as a predictor, some information exists on alternative approaches. The findings of Reisner (60) support the concept of a "residence time" effect, an observation confirmed to some extent by Hurley and colleagues (48). In an exploration of modeling approaches, Attfield et al. (66) found little evidence for a threshold in exposure-response for CWP. Rather, a nonzero prevalence at zero exposure was indicated, consistent with a background level of detected abnormality probably due to diseases other than CWP as well as artifactual causes of chest radiographic abnormalities.

In summary, the main environmental factors involved in the development of simple CWP are coal mine (mixed) dust exposure and coal rank. Age, quartz exposure, and dust residence time probably also play a role, although these effects appear to have secondary importance. Category of simple CWP remains a strong predictor of PMF development, but occurrence of PMF has been found to be related to dust in the absence of simple CWP. Recently developed exposure-response relationships indicate that CWP incidence for dust levels of 2 mg/m$^3$ air or less may be greater than was predicted in the past.

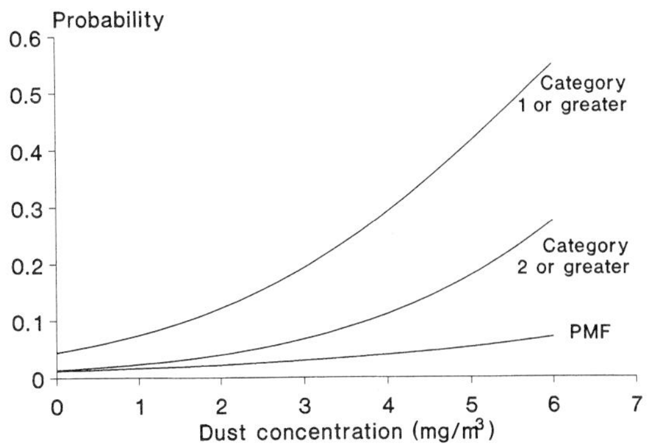


**FIG. 5.** U.S. miners' predicted risk of contracting category 1 or greater small rounded opacities, 2 or greater small rounded opacities, or PMF after 40 years work in coal mining.

### *Small Irregular Opacities*

Epidemiologic researchers in the United States have tended to define simple CWP in terms of the so-called combined opacity-profusion determinations. That is, they took into account both rounded and irregular types of opacity. British studies, in contrast, have generally treated simple pneumoconiosis as being synonymous with small rounded opacities (69). Recently, however, there has been increasing interest in the relationship of irregular opacities per se to both dust exposure and to symptoms and lung function.

As with small rounded opacities, the prevalence of small irregular opacities increases with occupational dust exposure and is linked to reduced lung function (58,70,71). Elevated respiratory symptom levels have also been observed in miners who have irregular opacities (71), but epidemiologic study of the medical implications of the type of opacity (irregular versus rounded) is confounded by reader disagreement on opacity type. The latest information on British miners indicates little difference between the prognostic implications of the two types of opacity for future ill health (69), so opacity profusion rather than opacity type should remain the primary radiographic variable of interest.

### *Other Lung Diseases*

Correlation of measured dust exposures with indicators of lung disease other than pneumoconiosis have consistently revealed clear relationships with both respiratory symptoms and lung function. In the first of such studies, associations were found between the prevalence and incidence of respiratory symptoms and dust levels for workers who had never smoked and for those who currently were smokers, but this was apparent only for the younger miners (72). Findings for United States, Australian, German, and Sardinian coal miners support these observations (73–76).

Cross-sectional studies of 1-minute forced expiratory volume ($FEV_1$) undertaken in a number of countries have consistently shown it to be inversely related to cumulative dust exposure (or work in coal mining) after allowance is made for age, height, and smoking history (67,73,77–83). In general, results from these studies have revealed dust exposure effects comparable to those due to smoking. Dust exposure effects have been seen among current, former, and nonsmokers, but smoking was not found to potentiate the effect of dust. After adjustment for dust exposure, no additional effect of presence of CWP on $FEV_1$ was noted. Some suggestion of a greater dust exposure effect among ex-miners has been reported, but this observation could have been due to chance (67). Ex-miners in this study did have lower overall ventilatory function than current miners.

Several studies have shown that forced vital capacity (FVC), like $FEV_1$, is inversely related to dust exposure and that both lung function variables tended to decline somewhat in parallel. This finding, some have suggested, implies that dust-induced lung damage has a different physiologic basis than that due to smoking. Despite the tendency to parallelism, an inverse relationship between the $FEV_1$/FVC ratio and dust exposure has also been reported (78), although the association was weaker than those for $FEV_1$ and FVC.

Findings from a joint analysis of ventilatory function and respiratory symptoms among British miners led the authors to conclude that both smoking and dust exposure can lead to clinically important respiratory dysfunction (84). Logistic models fitted to responses based on reports of persistent cough and phlegm, $FEV_1$ less than 80% of predicted value, reduced $FEV_1$ and cough and phlegm, and $FEV_1$ less than 65% of predicted all showed significant relationships to dust exposure. The prevalence of the four responses at high dust exposures was found to be close to that among smokers who had hypothetically zero dust exposure (Fig. 6).

Longitudinal changes in ventilatory function in coal miners have also been linked with dust exposure (69,76,85–89). However, the relationship is complex, and varies depending on the age (or, more likely, prior mining tenure) of the miners (89). New miners appear to suffer a fairly severe initial decline after beginning work in mining (89–91). This loss is then ameliorated, but it is still detectable in experienced miners (85,86). In a study of young miners by Carta and colleagues (76), annual decline in $FEV_1$ was significantly related to concurrent dust exposure, but was inversely associated with prior dust exposure. This effect might be attributed to worker selection, whereby those able to withstand the higher dust exposures remain in the dusty jobs. Support for this is found in the study by Petsonk and colleagues (92), which showed that miners with greater airway responsiveness were less likely to work in dusty jobs.

The general effect of dust exposure on $FEV_1$ seems to lie around 0.7 ml of $FEV_1$ per gram-hours/$m^3$ (about 5 ml per year for a dust exposure of 4 mg/$m^3$—twice the current U.S. compliance level). Although it is tempting to dismiss this apparently small effect of dust exposure, it must be remembered that it is being observed in a relatively healthy population fit enough to work in an arduous job. If a close look is taken at the average effect of smoking reported in the various studies on coal miners, it will be seen that the coefficients are also small, e.g., about 5 ml per year per pack smoked (19). Although this decrement is also apparently of little clinical importance, it is known that smoking is a major cause of lung disease. Hence, rejection of an effect just because its average magnitude is not clinically significant can be misleading.

Comparison of average effects of smoking and dust exposure has been said to paint a misleading picture of

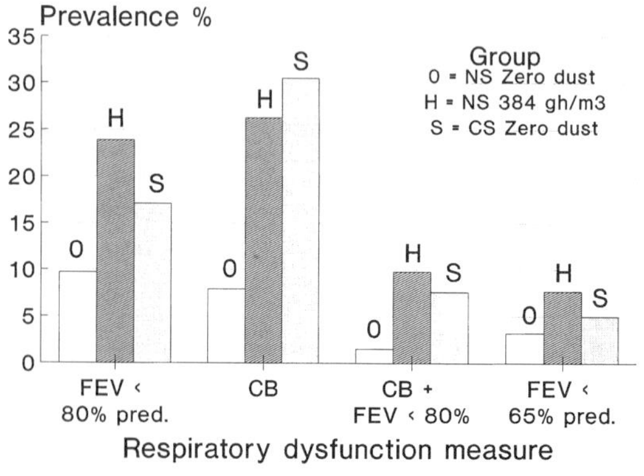


**FIG. 6.** Predicted prevalence of four indices of respiratory dysfunction for never smokers at 0 and 384 gh/$m^3$ (gram-homs/cubed meter) air and current smokers at 0 gh/$m^3$.

their true effects (93). It has been argued that the similar average effects seen in the various studies involving regression modeling of $FEV_1$ (78) arose through different mechanisms, the average decrement associated with smoking being due to a subset of severely affected smokers, and the dust exposure effect arising from a small general shift in all exposed miners. If this argument were true, it would imply that dust exposure is of trivial significance, and that its effect should not be equated with that arising from exposure to tobacco smoke.

There is little evidence to support this conjecture. First, no sign of excess numbers of severely affected smokers (compared to those who never smoked) was seen in an analysis that looked at the distribution of $FEV_1$ values for a group of working U.S. coal miners for whom a definite dust exposure effect had been previously established (65). Rather, the results indicated that the miners were reacting similarly (in terms of $FEV_1$) to exposure to tobacco smoke and to dust. Second, a study of British miners identified a group of ex-miners who apparently had suffered a severe response to their dust exposure (67,94). The authors concluded that this indicates that dust exposure can give rise to severe respiratory impairment in the absence of PMF. Lastly, in an analysis of autopsy material on coal miners, Leigh and coworkers (95) found a clear inverse relationship between extent of emphysema and $FEV_1$ in both smokers and nonsmokers, while emphysema and lung dust content were positively related. These results suggest a dust-related loss in $FEV_1$ not of trivial significance.

In contrast to the study of exposure-response for CWP, where extensive exploration of various dust composition parameters (e.g., coal rank, silica content) has taken place, investigation of exposure-response for other lung diseases has concentrated almost exclusively on mixed mine dust exposure. This has resulted from lack of any convincing evidence to the contrary, an understanding confirmed by the results of Coggon and colleagues (96). These show wide variations in the PMR for CWP across Britain (mainly trending with coal rank), but a relatively uniform excess PMR for chronic bronchitis and emphysema over the different coalfields.

In contrast to the wealth of information available on CWP, bronchitis, obstructive lung disease, and emphysema in coal miners, little attention has been paid to other lung diseases in coal miners. In this respect, one case report exists concerning a miner reported to have occupational asthma due to *Rhizopus nigricans* (97). Mold colonies were found extensively in the mine in which the case worked, including *Rhizopus nigricans* and other genera.

In summary, clear relationships between various measures of ventilatory function and dust exposure have been found in various unrelated groups of underground coal miners. For miners working where dust levels are not well controlled, there is evidence that some may experience nontrivial affects to their health.

#### Mortality, Coal Mine Dust Exposure, and Other Risk Factors

In two studies looking at mortality in association with quantitative measures of cumulative dust exposure (30,98), mortality from pneumoconiosis increased with extent of dust exposure. Additionally, and importantly, mortality from bronchitis and emphysema was also related to dust exposure in both studies ($p < 0.001$ and $< 0.01$, respectively). The relationship with bronchitis and emphysema implies that dust exposure per se, even in the absence of radiographic abnormality, gives rise to excess mortality.

### Surface Coal Miners

Compared to the sizable number of studies and reports on underground coal miners, surface miners have been neglected. This may be due to the generally lower dust exposure they experience and, until recently, their fewer numbers. Despite their lower level of occupational dust exposure in general, severe disease can and has occurred in surface miners. Also, many coal miners often spend time working in both surface and underground mines, and so experience dust exposure from both sources.

Studies of U.S. surface coal miners have revealed an overall level of respiratory disease that is considerably lower than that seen generally in underground coal miners (99,100). In an initial study (99), 4% of the workers showed signs of CWP but only 7 of 1,438 had category 2 disease or worse. Obvious signs of excessive lung disease other than CWP were not seen. However, the impression that work in strip mining was relatively benign was upset by subsequent reports of acute silicosis among surface miners working in drilling operations (101). The hazards of drilling were fully revealed in a later study in which almost half of the cases occurred in the minority of miners who had worked in drilling. In addition, the drillers' disease was more severe and included one case of PMF. These findings confirmed that overexposure to quartz remains a hazard for surface coal miners.

## RADIOGRAPHY

A diagnosis of CWP is generally based on chest x-ray findings combined with an occupational history of significant coal mine dust exposure. The chest radiograph, however, appears to be an insensitive tool for detecting CWP compared to pathologically diagnosable early signs (25% sensitivity when macules only are recorded; 40% for macules or mild degrees of micronodules), although its specificity appears to be good [90% specific for ten films with no observed pathologic abnormalities related to CWP (102,103)]. Other dust diseases of miners are usually undetectable by plain chest radiography (104). This discussion of radiography, therefore, applies only to the use of plain films in the recognition of CWP. Other diagnostic methods must be employed to identify the other diseases related to coal mine dust exposure.

Coal mine dust can produce a pattern of chronic interstitial fibrosis, most often nodular, but frequently mixed nodular and irregular, and occasionally exclusively irregular. Fibrosis is usually noted first in the upper or middle lung zones and predominates there, but potentially it is visible anywhere. In simple CWP, opacities vary in size from 1 mm to 1 cm. By radiographic convention nodular opacities 1 cm and larger are defined as PMF.

Smoking and aging are thought by some to influence the profusion of irregular opacities (105), although in the absence of dust exposure interstitial opacities are rarely found in healthy workers (106,107). A radiograph with predominantly irregular opacities in a coal miner raises the possibility of previous exposure to occupational hazards such as asbestos or talc or of a nonoccupational interstitial lung disease. The large opacities of PMF almost invariably occur on a background of simple CWP. They are usually rounded, may be multiple in number, and are most often found posteriorly in the upper lung zones. PMF may affect an entire lobe (Fig. 7).

The differential diagnosis of the small opacities of simple pneumoconiosis includes (1) diseases that produce acute nodular lesions, such as miliary tuberculosis and viral pneumonia; and (2) diseases that produce chronic nodular patterns such as other pneumoconioses, metastatic disease, tuberculosis, and other granulomas. Silicosis presents with the same radiographic pattern as CWP and so can be differentiated only by occupational history or pathologic examination. The large opacities of PMF must be differentiated from malignancies, granulomatous diseases, and other less common causes.

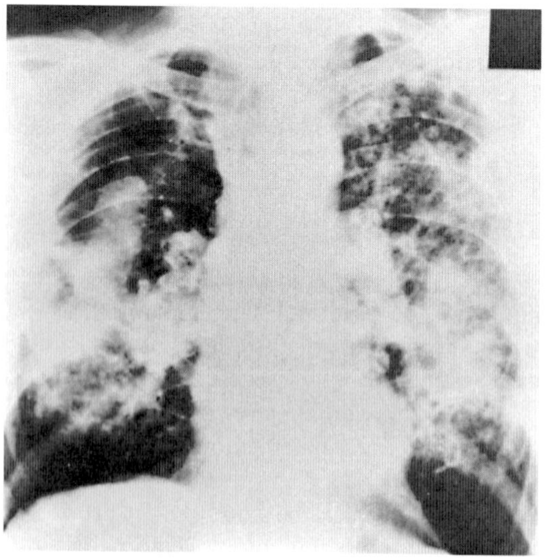

**FIG. 7.** Progressive massive fibrosis, category C, of coal worker's pneumoconiosis.

To improve recognition and reporting of CWP and other pneumoconioses, international standards have been adopted. These classification methods have contributed materially to epidemiologic studies of coal miners, to medical surveillance programs, and to clinical assessment of CWP.

The need for consistency and accuracy in the interpretation of chest radiographs for surveillance purposes led to the development of a program of training and certification of readers by the National Institute for Occupational Safety and Health (NIOSH). Trained readers who pass a competency examination are designated as B readers. Their interpretations are generally more consistent with one another and are given more weight in both epidemiologic investigations and legal proceedings. Nevertheless, there remains significant inter- and intrareader variability, particularly with mild disease (108–110).

More technologically advanced imaging methods such as high-resolution computed tomography (HRCT) have been promoted by some for the diagnosis of coal worker's lung diseases (111,112). To date there is no standardization of interpretation of the changes identified on CT, nor has epidemiologic investigation been sufficient to establish relationships between levels of exposure to coal mine dust and CT abnormalities (113,114). For now, CT should be utilized when there are specific clinical indications or when it is part of a research protocol; routine use for surveillance of miners is not indicated. Use of gallium-67 citrate imaging should be similarly limited (115).

## PATHOLOGIC FEATURES

The descriptive work of Heppleston (116) and Gough and coworkers (117) helped define the characteristic pathologic features of CWP as an entity distinct from silicosis. With the widespread practice of fixing lungs in inflation for investigation has come better definition of the pathologic changes in CWP. It is now generally recognized that the primary lesion of CWP, the macule, occurs specifically among workers exposed to coal mine dust, regardless of geographic location, rank of coal, or type of dust. The characteristic lesion of CWP has been defined by the pneumoconiosis committee of the College of American Pathologists as follows: "A focal collection of coal dust-laden macrophages at the division of the respiratory bronchioles that may exist within alveoli and extend into the peribronchiolar interstitium with associated reticulin deposits and focal emphysema" (118). Other lesions specific to coal mine dust exposure are the well-recognized nodular lesions of simple CWP, PMF, and Caplan's lesions. Emphysema and bronchitis resulting from coal mine dust exposure do not have pathognomonic lesions that identify the occupational cause.

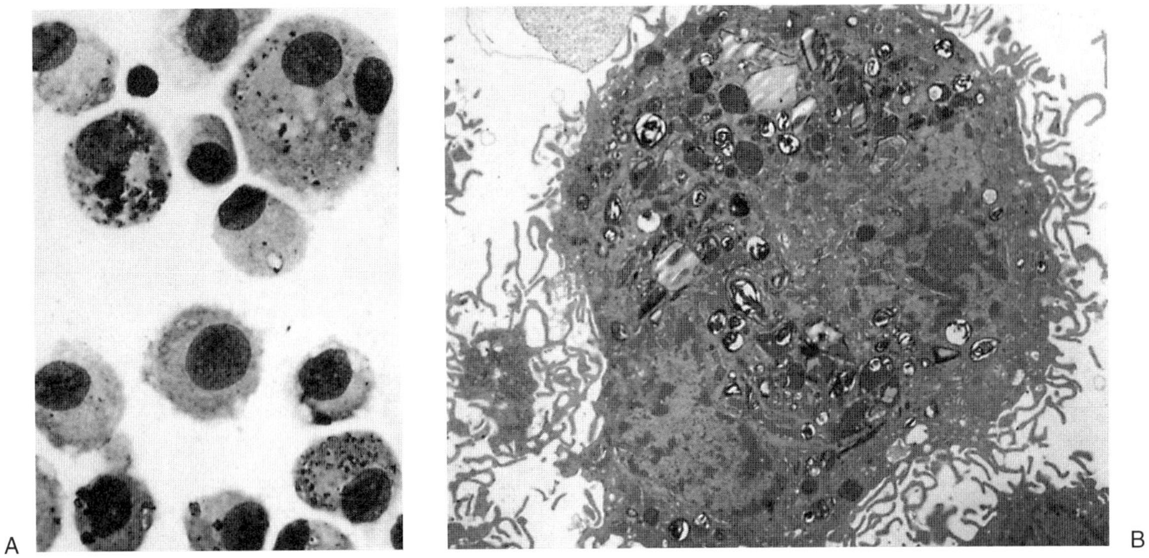


**FIG. 8.** Coal-laden macrophages recovered by bronchoalveolar lavage (BAL) from an active coal miner. **A:** Variably shaped dark particles in light microscopic study of alveolar macrophages (×400). **B:** TEM study of alveolar macrophage from a coal miner shows particles in phagolysosomes (×4,200). (Courtesy of T. Takemura, M.D., and V. Ferrans, M.D.)

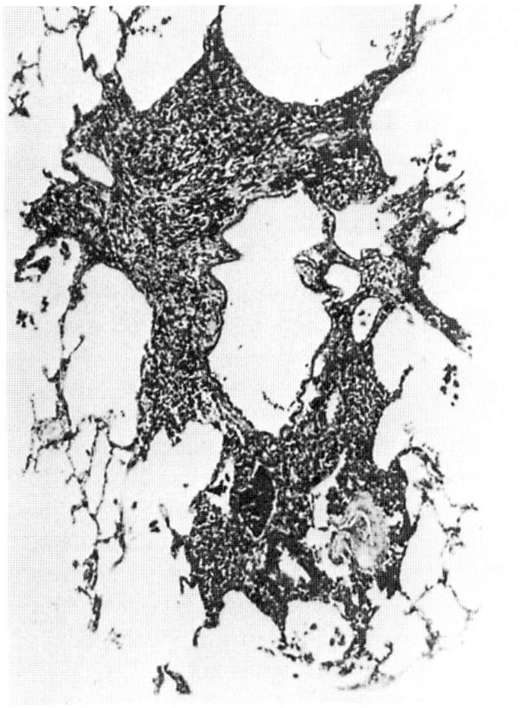

**FIG. 9.** The coal macule surrounding a dilated respiratory bronchiole.

Macrophages laden with coal mine dust are found free in the alveoli of anyone who inhales coal mine dust; they have no specific pathologic meaning (Fig. 8). The coal macule is similar in appearance to dust macules found in urban dwellers and smokers, but coal macules are more profuse. Macules range in size from 1 to 5 mm and may be rounded, irregular, or stellate. The coal macule is typically found together with a 1- to 2-mm zone of enlarged air space referred to as focal emphysema (Fig. 9). Histologically the coal macule consists of dust-laden macrophages that surround the first-, second-, and third-order respiratory bronchioles, extending into alveoli and interspersed with fine reticulin and a variable amount of collagen. Since the lesion may occur with other occupational and environmental exposures (e.g., graphite and carbon black), it is important to identify the nature of the dust particles (119–121). Bituminous and anthracite coal can usually be distinguished by light microscopy (122).

The nodular lesions of CWP have been classified as micronodules (up to 7 mm diameter) and macronodules (7 to 20 mm diameter) (118). These lesions are almost invariably seen on a background of coal macules, are usually rounded black lesions, and may be surrounded by enlarged air spaces. Nodules, unlike macules, are firm to palpation. They are usually found in the region of the respiratory bronchiole and may coalesce to form PMF. Histologically, nodules consist of dust-laden macrophages in a stroma consisting of collagen and reticulin (Fig. 10). Degenerative changes, including calcification, cholesterol crystallization, blood vessel obliteration, and infarction, are commonly observed.

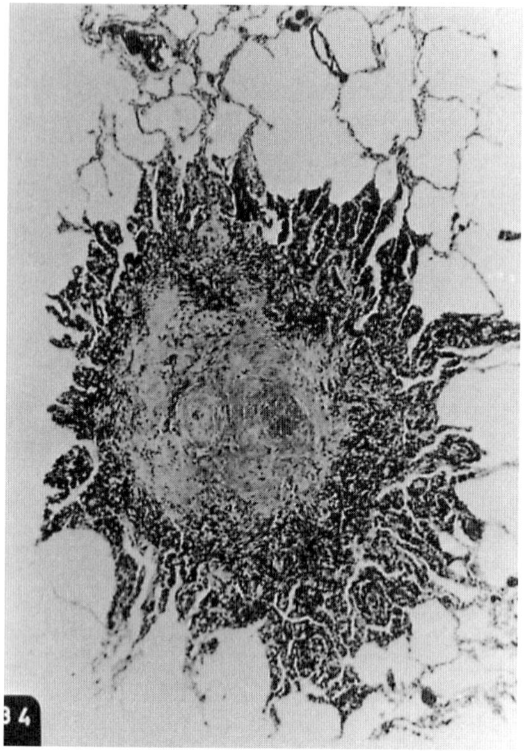

**FIG. 10.** A macronodular lesion of coal worker's pneumoconiosis has a center that is becoming hyalinized.

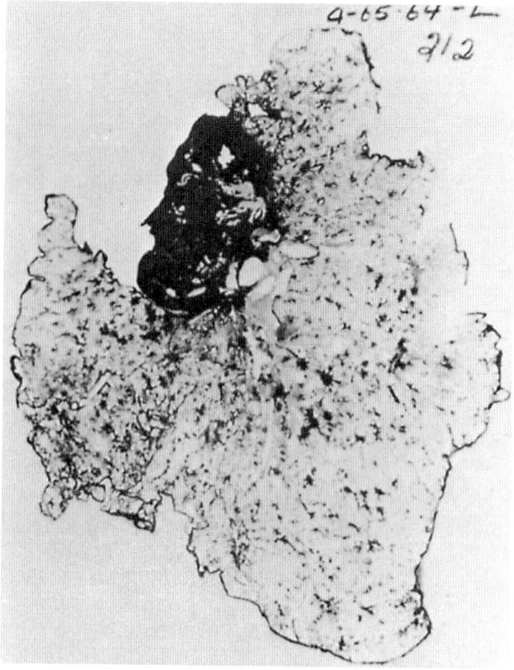

**FIG. 11.** This whole lung section shows progressive massive fibrosis of coal worker's pneumoconiosis against a background of nodules, macules, and focal emphysema.

The pathologic definition of PMF is arbitrarily based on the diameter of lesions. Fibrotic pneumoconiotic lesions greater than 1 cm have been accepted as radiographic evidence of PMF. This definition was adopted in the regulations of the National Coal Workers' Autopsy Study mandated by the 1969 Federal Coal Mine Health and Safety Act. However, the pneumoconiosis committee of the College of American Pathologists recommended a minimum diameter of 2 cm for morphologic investigations (118) despite the radiographic definition of PMF as nodules 1 cm or greater in diameter (123).

The PMF lesions may be unilateral or bilateral often in the upper and posterior regions of the lung. They may be rounded or irregular and frequently cross lobar fissures. The lesions tend to retract toward the hilum, and in so doing destroy blood vessels and airways and greatly distort lung architecture (Fig. 11). The larger PMF lesions tend to cavitate, sometimes discharging a black liquid into a communicating airway. Histologically, the tissues are composed of bundles of irregularly arranged collagen or reticulin, coal dust, and coal dust-engorged macrophages. Less collagen is found toward the center of the lesions, and an obliterative vasculitis is observed in peripheral areas (124).

Rheumatoid pneumoconiosis (Caplan's syndrome) is characterized by large (1 to 5 cm) nodules that typically have smooth rounded borders, concentric internal lamination, and (relative to PMF lesions) little coal dust. The characteristic histiocytic palisading and necrobiosis found in most rheumatoid nodules is usually peripheral and focal.

Silicotic nodules are frequently found in coal miners' lungs and arise from free silica exposure, usually a reflection of the silicaceous rock surrounding the coal seams. These nodules are usually found incidentally in conjunction with coal macules and nodules. They are typically rounded and firm, and they have smooth borders and pale centers that are relatively free of coal dust. They also tend to coalesce, forming PMF or conglomerate silicosis. Histologically, silicosis nodules have characteristically concentric lamination of collagen fibers about a hyalinized center (Fig. 12). A study of 3,365 U.S. underground coal miners' autopsies revealed that about 12% had classic silicosis nodules. A relationship was seen between tenure in mining and prevalence and severity of silicosis. In addition, job category and geographic locality were important determinants of silicosis prevalence (125).

The relationship between pathologic findings, the weight and composition of dust retained in the lungs, and radiographic information has long interested researchers. Early studies showed that there was a clear and direct link between the weight of dust in the lung and the radiographic category of pneumoconiosis (126–128). Weight for weight, the mineral (noncoal) portion of the dust appeared to be more responsible for the radiographic opacities than the coal fraction. This implies that miners in high-rank coal mines would have to retain appreciably

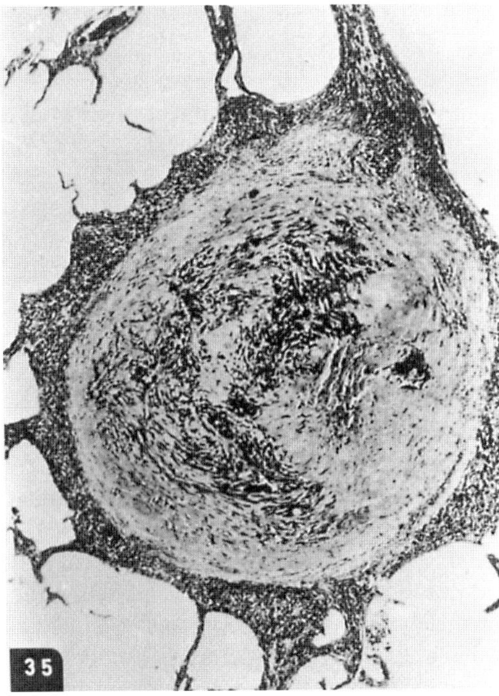

FIG. 12. Silicosis nodule with paracicatricial emphysema in a coal worker's lung.

more dust in their lungs to attain the same radiographic classification (the ratio of coal to ash in the mixed mine dust in high-rank mines is usually much greater than that in low-rank mines). Since lung collagen content did not relate to opacity profusion after adjustment for lung dust (127), it was suggested (128) that radiographic changes are related simply to dust accumulation.

Additional work has supported the link between amount and composition of retained dust and opacity profusion on radiographs (129). It also revealed that the relationships between radiographic data, lung content, and lung disease are rather more complex than was originally supposed. In this respect, it is clear that the size (radiographic type) of the opacity must be taken into consideration. In both high- and low-coal rank areas, miners with the smallest type of rounded opacities (type *p*) had greater lung dust weights than miners with type *r* opacities, after the data was controlled for degree of profusion (129). An explanation for this may be that type *p* opacities may be the manifestation of the summation effect of very many small dust deposits, whereas larger opacities are often individually radiopaque. The relationship between lung dust weight and profusion of opacities was much more evident among those miners with predominantly type *p* opacities than for type *q* or *r* (130). For the largest type (*r*) and a high proportion of ash in the retained dust, no association between profusion and dust weight was found (130), although the number of cases was small.

A detailed study of the pathologic lesions of pneumoconiosis and opacity type showed that lungs of miners with predominantly type *p* opacities contained mostly dust macules and pinhead nodules [smaller than 1 mm diameter but offering resistance to a needle (130)]. For these miners, the only pathologic lesion that correlated with radiologic profusion was the number of pinhead nodules; in fact, total lung dust correlated even better. Opacity profusion in miners with predominantly type *q* opacities related best to numbers of small nodules (1 to 3 mm), though nodules of >3 to 9 mm also played a role. In these cases, lung dust weight correlated weakly with profusion. In the few type *r* cases, association between profusion and the largest size nodules was poor, as was that with dust content.

All in all, these findings support the view that profusion of type *p* opacities is a reflection of numbers of macules and very small nodules, and that it relates mostly to coal dust deposition per se, particularly for high-rank coals. Type *q* and *r* opacities are seen in miners with the larger lung nodules. The presence of these types of small opacities on the radiographs seems linked more to the ash content of the dust than to the coal fraction; the correlation between radiographic profusion and weight of dust is less clear. The possibility that the dust associated with coals of different rank gives rise to different disease processes is suggested by radiographic findings (52) and pathologic data (131). A study undertaken to compare radiographic and pathologic appearances of PMF provided some support for this hypothesis (132).

There is a clear correlation between dust exposures and retained dust in the lung (133,134), between retained dust and presence and severity of pathologic lesion (133,134), and between dust exposure and presence and severity of pathologic lesion (134). Pathologic abnormality was better predicted by retained dust than using dust exposure (134). Miners with PMF appeared to have retained more dust per unit of exposure than those without PMF (133). With regard to dust composition, coal miners from high-rank mines had been exposed to low levels of ash and had low levels of ash in their retained dust. In contrast, low-rank coal miners had higher levels of ash in the retained dust, the ash content being greater proportionately than it was in the mines (133). It is not clear how this excess occurred, although differential deposition or retention is an obvious hypothesis.

Pathologic studies of emphysema in different groups of coal workers have repeatedly shown an excess over levels in controls (135–137). Much discussion has centered on the implications of this finding. Questions center around the nature, cause, and significance of the emphysema, and on the potential for bias in the selection of coal miner cases in some of the studies. Recent work has clarified some of the outstanding issues (58,138,139). Not only was the excess of emphysema among coal workers confirmed in a study that controlled well for bias (58), but emphysema was also found to be related to both dust retained in the lungs (58,129) and to pathologic measurements of pneumoconiosis (129). The finding that miners with PMF also have elevated amounts of emphysema unrelated to the PMF lesions(58) is consistent with the epidemiologic finding that dyspneic miners were at greater risk of PMF development (57). Importantly, the presence of emphysema was related to dust exposure during life (129), particularly the coal rather than the silica component (139), and to $FEV_1$ percent predicted (95,139). These findings therefore indicate a causal relationship between dust exposure and emphysema, and the potential for ensuing disability. There is some indication that irregular opacities on chest radiographs are associated with pathologic signs of emphysema and interstitial fibrosis (58).

Despite the clear association between occupational exposure and chest symptoms reported by Rae and coworkers (72), results from the few pathologic studies of bronchitis have been mixed. Leigh and colleagues found no evidence of an association between bronchial mucous gland-wall ratio and years worked underground (139), even though other studies of Australian miners had shown correlations between gland-wall ratio and various symptoms and signs of bronchitis (140,141). However, a study using measured dust exposures rather than the surrogate years underground (142) found that maximum mucous gland-wall ratio did correlate with lifetime occupational exposure. Douglas and colleagues (142) said their results "lend support to the view that irritants encountered in an occupational environment may play an important part in the development of hypersecretion of mucus."

## DISEASE MECHANISMS

Elucidation of the mechanisms involved in the development and progression of coal mine dust–induced pulmonary disease has been a topic of extensive investigation. Most theories on the cause of mineral dust–induced lung injury involve the role of free radicals and oxidative damage (143). It has been shown *in vivo* that exposure of rats to mineral dust enhanced the release of reactive oxygen species from pulmonary phagocytes and was associated with oxidant damage to the lung parenchyma (144,145). Indeed, treatment *in vivo* of animals with scavengers of superoxide, hydrogen peroxide, and hydroxyl radical was effective in decreasing lipid peroxidation and edema associated with pulmonary inflammation (146). In addition, superoxide secretion from alveolar macrophages has been shown to decrease $\alpha_1$-antiprotease activity, which may represent an alternative mechanism that renders the lung subject to elastase damage and emphysema (147). Inhalation of coal dust has also been shown to increase the production of the reactive nitrogen species (nitric oxide) and to enhance messenger RNA (mRNA) levels for the inducible form of the nitric oxide synthase enzyme (148).

Studies *in vitro* indicate that coal dust was lytic and resulted in the release of lysosomal enzymes from alveolar macrophages (149). In addition, *in vivo* exposure of alveolar macrophages to coal dust resulted in release of inflammatory mediators that have been characterized by abnormal gallium lung scans and clearance of inhaled technetium diethylenetriamine pentaacetic acid (DFTPA) aerosol (150). In general, studies *in vitro* suggest that coal dust is a less potent stimulant than silica. Such a relationship correlates with the pathogenicity of these dusts *in vivo*.

Lebeder and co-workers (151) have reported that crushing coal resulted in the generation of free radicals on the cleavage planes. The presence of these coal radicals has been associated with the lytic potential of the dust (152). Freshly fractured, but not aged, coal dust has been shown in vitro to increase the release of proinflammatory metabolites of arachidonic acid, such as prostaglandin $E_2$ ($PGE_2$) and thromboxane $A_2$ ($TXA_2$) (153). A relationship has also been found between the pathogenicity of anthracite versus bituminous coal and the reactivity of radicals generated after grinding coal of different ranks (152). Pathologic studies of coal miners' lungs indicate that lungs with PMF contained higher levels of coal free radicals than less severely diseased lungs (152). This may be due in part to higher levels of retained dust in lungs with more extensive disease.

Animal studies also support the theory that exposure to coal dust results in excess oxidant load in the lungs. Inhalation exposure of rats to coal dust (2 mg/m$^3$, 7 hours per day, 5 days a week, for 2 years) resulted in the activation of alveolar macrophages. Activation was expressed as an increase in surface ruffling and cell spreading and enhancement of the spontaneous and particle-stimulated levels of chemiluminescence (an indicator of production of reactive species) (154). Animal studies also indicate that inhalation of coal dust increases the number of alveolar macrophages (154–156) and neutrophils (157) obtained by bronchoalveolar lavage. Elevated levels of blood and interstitial monocytes have also been noted following animal exposure to coal dust (158). This recruitment of phagocytes may be due to the coal dust-induced release of leutotriene $B_4$ from alveolar macrophages (159).

Such activation of alveolar macrophages has also been reported in coal miners with pneumoconiosis. Wallaert and colleagues (160) reported that bronchoalveolar lavage yielded more alveolar macrophages from coal miners with pneumoconiosis than from controls. In addition, chemiluminescence was elevated in miners with measurable pulmonary disease. The relationship between CWP and activity of alveolar macrophages was also reported by Rom and co-workers (161,162). Their results indicate that CWP was associated with enhanced secretion of superoxide anion and hydrogen peroxide from alveolar macrophages. Elevated levels of elastase complexed with $\alpha_1$-antitrypsin and increased secretion of fibroblast proliferative factors (fibronectin and alveolar macrophage-derived growth factor) were also noted (161,162). Morphologic studies also support the hypothesis that alveolar macrophages are activated in CWP (163). Cells contained more particles; exhibited more ruffling, filopodia, and phagolysosomes; and demonstrated more cell fusion and mitosis. It is interesting that the number of coal dust particles within each phagocytic cell was not different for currently exposed miners and those who had not been exposed for at least a year (163). This suggests that lung burden in lifelong coal miners can remain high long after occupational exposure has ceased.

There is evidence that the magnitude of activation of alveolar macrophages in coal miners is directly related to the extent of pulmonary injury. Wallaert and coworkers (160) reported that macrophages from coal miners with progressive massive fibrosis generated more chemiluminescence than macrophages from miners with simple pneumoconiosis. Rom (164) reported that macrophages harvested from individuals with mineral dust exposure but no impairment secreted significantly lower levels of fibronectin, alveolar macrophage-derived growth factor, superoxide, and hydrogen peroxide than those with radiographic and spirometric evidence of disease. Lapp and colleagues (165) reported that although asymptomatic coal miners did not exhibit enhanced chemiluminescence, their alveolar macrophages were significantly more ruffled, suggesting some level of activation.

Recent studies with coal miners have concerned the identification of cytokines and growth factors, which correlate with disease severity. Lapp et al. (166) reported that bronchoalveolar lavage fluid levels of tumor necrosis factor (TNF-$\alpha$) are decreased in coal miners without CWP. In contrast, miners with CWP exhibited elevated release of TNF-$\alpha$ from alveolar macrophages and blood monocytes (167,168). In addition, mRNA levels for TNF-$\alpha$ are elevated in alveolar macrophages of miners with CWP (169). TNF-$\alpha$ is an initiating cytokine that has been correlated with the release of chemoattractants and fibroblast growth factors (170,171). Therefore, it is not surprising that antibodies to TNF-$\alpha$ have been shown to suppress fibrosis in animal models (172) and that TNF-$\alpha$ secretion from alveolar macrophages correlates with disease severity in coal miners.

The production of fibrogenic factors by alveolar macrophages has also been reported for coal miners with pneumoconiosis. Both type I insulin-like growth factor (a progression factor) and platelet-derived growth factor (a competence factor) are elevated in miners with CWP and to a greater extent in coal workers with PMF (173). In contrast, interleukin-6, a cytokine that may be antifibrogenic (174), is elevated in asymptomatic miners (166) and tends to decrease with increasing disease severity (169). These data suggest that the balance between protective and damaging cytokines controls the initiation and progression of disease.

## PULMONARY PHYSIOLOGY

Cross-sectional and longitudinal epidemiologic investigations, reviewed above, have provided most of the information currently available concerning pulmonary changes resulting from exposure to coal mine dust. A limited number of clinical investigations have extended our knowledge in this area. Studies of coal miners have consistently shown a relatively high prevalence of dyspnea, chronic bronchitis, and chronic obstructive pulmonary disease in addition to CWP. Pathology investigations demonstrate elevated levels of emphysema in miners (175). Coal mine dust exposure and cigarette smoking have both been found to be unambiguous risk factors in airways obstruction among coal miners, although they do not appear to be synergistic.

No single pattern of pulmonary response has been identified that uniquely differentiates the physiologic derangement of miners from that of others without coal mine dust exposure. Some confusion has resulted from studies comparing lung function among coal miners with radiographic evidence of simple CWP to those without CWP (78,176). These studies attempt to correlate two different effects of coal mine dust exposure: development of CWP and changes in pulmonary function. Since both groups studied have had significant coal mine dust exposure, it is not surprising that such studies often show little or no difference in pulmonary function tests (15,177). Nevertheless, a matched sample analysis of a large number of American bituminous coal miners, regardless of category of simple CWP, has shown that both bronchitis and cigarette smoking are significant factors that influence both lung volumes and flow rates (178). $FEV_1$ and $FEV_1$/FVC ratio were found to be the measures that best discriminated between smoking and nonsmoking groups and between groups with and without bronchitis. PMF is associated with significant decrease in lung function, particularly in category B and C of that disorder (15,177, 179,180). Coal mine dust exposure per se has been associated with accelerated loss of $FEV_1$ in longitudinal studies and reduced $FEV_1$ in both cross-sectional field studies and in laboratory investigations (see other lung diseases in Epidemiology, above).

Studies of lung volume in coal miners have revealed a slight increase in total lung capacity (TLC) among obstructed and nonobstructed miners (181). Those without airways obstruction have been found to have consistent increases in residual volume (RV), which tended to increase with the radiographic category of CWP. Similarly, studies of dynamic compliance, thought to reflect narrowing or closure of small airways, found that most nonobstructed miners who had category 2 or 3 CWP had significant decreases, as did some category 0 or 1 subjects (176). The clinical significance of these early physiologic changes is not yet clear.

Diffusing capacity has been found to be reduced among those with predominately type *p* opacities of simple CWP, among these with category B and C of PMF, and among smoking miners. Nonsmoking miners have generally been found to have diffusing capacity measurements within the normal range (182–184)

Among working miners resting arterial blood gas tension ($PaO_2$) has generally been found to be within the normal range or minimally reduced. Miners with airway obstruction tend to show lower $PaO_2$ during exercise than those without obstruction (185). Significant decreases in $PaO_2$ with exercise have been found among miners with PMF (186). Nonsmoking miners have been found to have a lower $PaO_2$ and higher alveoloarterial oxygen difference than nonsmoking nonminers, both at rest and with exercise (83).

## CLINICAL EVALUATION AND MANAGEMENT

### Evaluative Examinations

Because there is a federal compensation and benefits program directed exclusively toward miners with lung disease, patients may seek care initially to determine their eligibility for these benefits. It is therefore important that physicians understand not only the disease process and its diagnosis and management but also the provisions of state and federal law that apply in these cases (7). Physicians who provide information to disability or benefits systems should determine the specific type of information required, provide it if possible, or indicate how the information might be generated. Ultimately, nonphysicians make administrative decisions concerning benefits eligibility utilizing the physician report in addition to other information. It is therefore critical that all reports be complete and accurate. A carefully elicited and recorded occupational and medical history can be invaluable in planning care, ascertaining progress, and ensuring fairness and consistency in benefits eligibility determinations. Examiners should inquire not only into current work but also into past jobs and the reasons for job change. People may switch jobs when poor health precludes continuing their normal occupation. This may be a significant fact, as a judgment is made during federal black lung benefits determinations as to whether the applicant was capable of performing his or her normal coal mine job.

A history of chest infections or chest trauma may be important. Medical records, especially previous chest radiographs and lung function tests, are often helpful to the medical assessment. Harmful respiratory tract exposures (e.g., asbestos, silica) in the home or in prior workplaces may be important. Smoking is a major risk factor that must be fully defined in terms of time of onset, duration, amount, type and manner of smoking, and (if discontinued) reason for stopping. A subjective measure of dyspnea, cough, and phlegm is useful. Questioning what kinds of avocational activities may have been modified as a result of progressive dyspnea, and the timing of these life changes, is often illuminating.

Dyspnea is the symptom that most often correlates with respiratory impairment. It may be graded via standard questions published in the American Thoracic Society's Epidemiologic Standardization Project Questionnaire (187), which also contains questions aimed at assessing cough, phlegm, and wheezing. It is designed to be administered by a trained interviewer, such as an office nurse, and provides a very useful basis for further questioning of the patient. The questionnaire does not provide information on the relationship between symptoms and mining or other exposures, nor does it permit characterization of nonrespiratory symptoms. It affords no insight into the consequences of dyspnea (for example, the need to abandon activities such as hunting). Also, unless the subject is questioned specifically, frequent consequences of dyspnea such as sexual dysfunction will be overlooked. It is important to thoroughly explore cardiovascular symptoms and signs such as chest pain, orthopnea, ankle swelling, rapid weight gain, and nocturnal dyspnea.

The evaluative examination provides an opportunity to look broadly at the health of the miner and to plan future interventions. For example, since occupationally induced hearing impairment, musculoskeletal trauma, and dermatitis are common in coal miners, it is reasonable to assess these histories carefully.

The physical examination should be thorough, but with a focus on pulmonary, cardiac, and musculoskeletal function. The examiner should seek evidence of coughing and note whether the patient produces phlegm (if so, the nature of the specimen should be noted). The patient's breathing pattern, breath sounds, and respiratory rate should be observed and recorded. The cardiovascular examination should include inspection for neck vein distention and pulsation; palpation for the presence of a right ventricular lift or heave; and auscultation for determination of the pulmonic closure sound, variation of heart sounds with respiration, and gallop rhythm. If present, liver distention or pulsation and pedal edema should be noted.

A clinical assessment of hearing ability is important; audiometric testing is suggested if diminished capacity is suspected. Special attention should be given to assessment of joint and muscle function and to any evidence of trauma.

Laboratory investigations should include, at a minimum, posteroanterior and lateral chest radiographs, spirometry, and a hematocrit determination. An electrocardiogram may also be useful. The chest radiographs should be interpreted in light of the history and physical examination. If possible, previous radiographs should be obtained and evaluated together with the current radiograph using the current International Labour Organization (ILO) classification to assess pneumoconiosis, while paying particular attention to other thoracic abnormalities. The electrocardiogram (ECG) should be evaluated if exercise testing is contemplated, if there is an irregularity of heart rhythm, or if right heart strain is suspected.

Spirometry is the single most important test in evaluating a miner's lung function. Test procedures and published standards are available and have been incorporated into black lung disability determination standards promulgated by the U.S. Department of Labor (188). The $FEV_1$ is the single most useful measurement of the spirogram. It is reasonably reproducible, less effort dependent than the FVC or maximal voluntary ventilation (MVV), and has proved to be the test that correlates best with severe impairment and mortality. The FVC and ratio of $FEV_1$ to FVC are also important, but dependent on a full and reproducible FVC. The MVV is a difficult test to perform, particularly for patients with significant impairment; however, it remains part of some standard disability determination protocols.

It should be borne in mind that these tests may be influenced by intercurrent infection and by the use of bronchodilators. Some miners have a reversible component to their airways disease. In these cases, repeat spirometry following bronchodilation may be of some benefit in planning clinical interventions. An improvement of 10% to 15% supports a trial of bronchodilators; however, many clinicians opt for a clinical trial in the absence of such data. Spirometry results should be compared with available population standards, one of which is incorporated into the current federal black lung standards. Since predicted values vary with age, gender, height, and race, these factors should be taken into consideration when interpreting results (189–191). Also worth considering is that working people as a rule are healthier than the average person when they begin employment (192). It is therefore not unexpected for miners to be cognizant of a loss of exercise capacity, even when their spirometry values do not fall below an arbitrary level of abnormality. Comparison of results of a current spirometry examination with one performed in the past can give some indication of relative loss over time (193). Recent analyses have highlighted the fact that impaired workers may have more variable spirometric findings than healthier ones (194). All available measurements for a miner should be assessed, and care must be taken not to ignore information merely because it does not meet reproducibility guidelines.

Measurement of diffusing capacity can be helpful in assessing interstitial lung disease or emphysema. Some of these patients may have relatively normal spirometric findings. Recommended methods for performing diffusing capacity test have been published and should be followed (187). Reliable prediction equations are available (195).

Arterial blood gas measurement may be useful, particularly if there is some question about the degree of impairment indicated by spirometry. For patients with mild dysfunction or those with marked impairment by spirometry, arterial blood gas studies are not needed to assess impairment. The decision to obtain blood gas analysis should be made only after assessment of other examination data. One should remain mindful of the potential for associated morbidity and of technical factors that are important for obtaining a valid result. Equipment calibration, refrigeration, expedient analysis, breath holding or hyperventilation prior to the test, and the patient's position can all result in invalid measurements. Patients with significant interstitial disease may have a normal resting $PaO_2$, which becomes abnormal with exercise. Patients with marked airway obstruction may also have a normal resting $PaO_2$ that, in the absence of myocardial disease, may increase with exercise. Federal standards for $PaO_2$, adjusted for altitude, have been published (188). The significance of hypoxemia is often most obvious when it results in polycythemia, pulmonary hypertension, and cor pulmonale.

Maximum exercise testing is time-consuming and expensive but may be helpful in assessing the patient's ability to tolerate relatively brief high-energy demands. This test is often difficult for the patient and may be dangerous, especially for older patients. Furthermore, it is difficult to model the job energy demand. To avoid these problems, submaximal exercise may be used to estimate the maximum oxygen consumption per minute ($VO_2$) from observation of heart rate and $VO_2$ (196). In the patient with both cardiovascular disease and lung impairment, these tests may be indicative of potential work capacity but they do not define cause.

### *Clinical Care*

Clinical management of coal miners with lung impairment is the same as for other patients with airways obstruction or interstitial disease. The care plan must be designed and adjusted individually with a goal of maintaining maximal function with minimal disability. The miner and his family must be educated about his disease and about how to treat it. Exertional dyspnea—the hallmark of pulmonary disability—can significantly reduce quality of life. The psychological effects of pulmonary disability on the patient and family should be explored and treated supportively. Sexual dysfunction may develop early and have devastating consequences. Any additional factors that lead to social isolation and diminished quality of life should be identified and treated where possible. For example, hearing loss may be partially overcome through use of properly prescribed and fitted aids.

Reduced strength resulting from chronic inactivity can be countered through graded exercise programs. Smoking miners must be directed to stop smoking and aided in the endeavor with appropriate support, referral, or pharmacologic measures. Techniques of energy conservation and breathing retraining help dyspneic patients avoid a sense of helplessness and loss of control. Pulmonary rehabilitation programs have been of significant benefit to patients with COPD and their families (197,198). Such programs utilizing multidisciplinary teams for education and treatment of miners and their families have been developed and supported in coal mining areas by the U.S. Department of Labor.

For miners with bronchitis and airway obstruction, good hydration and postural drainage together with bronchodilators and, if indicated, a trial with steroids often prove helpful. Early empiric antibiotic therapy may be helpful when there is evidence of pulmonary infection. Influenza and antipneumococcal vaccines should be given at prescribed intervals. Continuous low-flow oxygen (1 to 3 L per minute) is indicated for patients with chronic hypoxemia (199). Sedatives and tranquilizers should be avoided, especially in patients with COPD. Congestive right-sided heart failure (cor pulmonale), a potential complication of advanced CWP, should be watched for and treated promptly. Finally, evidence of respiratory failure should be monitored closely.

Reduction of lung dust burden by whole-lung lavage is a therapeutic technique routinely practiced in China but only as yet attempted as an exploratory technique in the United States. Though it appears to remove considerable amounts of deposited dust, cells, and other materials from the lungs, its long-term benefit to the miner has yet to be demonstrated (200).

Miners partially or totally disabled from their normal coal mine employment may be eligible for participation in state or federal benefits and compensation programs. Benefits may include limited or permanent income replacement as well as payment for medical expenses resulting from the pulmonary disability. The health care provider should facilitate referral to a knowledgeable counselor or agency able to inform the miner and his family about these programs.

## PREVENTION

The means to prevent CWP and coal dust–related respiratory disease were provided in the Coal Mine Health and Safety Act of 1969 (5). These include primary prevention through dust control and secondary prevention through the use of medical screening.

The Mine Safety and Health Administration of the Department of Labor is mandated to conduct regular mine inspections and monitor results from the operator dust sampling program. Since passage of the act, marked reductions in average dust levels appear to have been achieved, well below the current standard (Fig. 13) (201–203). The exception to this is in the highly productive growing number of long-wall mines, where dust control presents significant engineering challenges (204), and it has been difficult to attain mandated levels.

The dust standard of 2 mg/m$^3$ air was established to prevent the progression of simple CWP to PMF (205). A recent comprehensive review of the successes and limitations of this prevention strategy resulted in a new set of recommendations for NIOSH issued as a criteria document (206). This document noted progress in prevention but the persistent risk to miners of CWP and other pulmonary diseases. Updated recommendations were made to reduce dust exposure, improve hazard surveillance and exposure limit enforcement, expand medical surveillance to include baseline and periodic tests of lung function, as well as provide chest radiographs for all miners. The NIOSH recommendation as well as others were considered by an advisory panel on the elimination of pneumoconiosis empaneled by the secretary of labor (207). This committee issued findings and recommendations:

- Improved methods for inspection and enforcement of dust limits
- Enforcement of separate exposure limits for coal mine dust and silica that are lower than current levels
- Improved hazard surveillance
- Expanded health screening and surveillance to include lung function for all miners
- Improved and expanded training in dust control.

Until the next century, however, many retiring miners will have experienced dust exposure prior to 1972 and will therefore be at increased risk for disease. Also, concerns are periodically raised about whether the dust samples analyzed by the Mine Safety and Health Administration (MSHA) accurately reflect dust conditions in the mines (208,209). Thus the risk of disease remains uncertain and preventive interventions are critical.

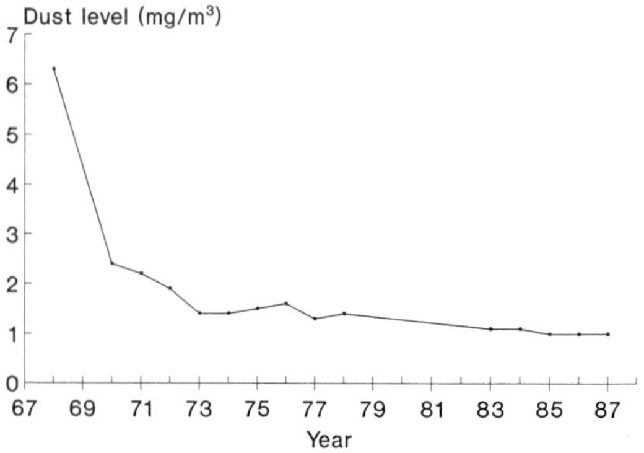


**FIG. 13.** Reported trends in dust levels for continuous miner operators 1968 to 1987. (Data taken from three reports.)

Working miners with evidence of CWP as identified under the NSCWP administered by NIOSH are entitled to work in a low-dust area within the mine (currently less than 1 mg/m$^3$ air) (210). In this program, miners receive a mandatory chest radiograph on entry into the work force and after 3 years. Thereafter, voluntary radiography is offered every 5 years. Films are interpreted by trained readers, and results are sent to the miner and a personal physician if one is designated, but not to the employer. If a job transfer to a low-dust area of the mine is necessary, there is no immediate loss of pay for the miner. Miners should be encouraged to participate in the surveillance program and exercise the transfer option when eligible, as this is the only currently available preventive intervention.

## REFERENCES


1. Gregory JC. Case of peculiar black infiltration of the whole lungs, resembling melanosis. *Edinburgh Med Surg J* 1831;36:391.
2. Medical Research Council of Great Britain. *Chronic pulmonary diseases in South Wales coal miners.* Special report series 243. London: Medical Research Council of Great Britain, 1942.
3. Medical Research Council of Great Britain. *Chronic pulmonary diseases in South Wales coal miners.* Special report series 244. London: Medical Research Council of Great Britain, 1943.
4. Smith BE. *Digging our own graves:* coal miners and the struggle over black lung diseases. Philadelphia: Temple University Press, 1987.
5. Federal coal mine health and safety act. Publ. L No. 91-173, 2917. 1969.
6. Federal mine safety and health act of 1977. Publ. L No. 91-173. Amended by Publ. L No 95-164, 101. 1977.
7. Weeks JL, Wagner GR. Compensation for occupational disease with multiple causes: the case of coal miners' respiratory diseases. *Am J Public Health* 1985;76:58–61.
8. Meiklejohn A. History of lung diseases of coal miners in Great Britain: part I, 1800–1875. *Br J Ind Med* 1951;8:127–137.
9. Meiklejohn A. History of lung diseases of coal miners in Great Britain: part II, 1875–1920. *Br J Ind Med* 1952;9:93–98.
10. Meiklejohn A. History of lung diseases of coal miners in Great Britain: part III, 1920–1952. *Br J Ind Med* 1952;9:208–229.
11. Fay JWJ, Rae S. The pneumoconiosis field research of the National Coal Board. *Ann Occup Hyg* 1959;1:149–161.
12. McBride WW, Pendergrass EG, Lieben J. Pneumoconiosis study of Pennsylvania anthracite miners. *J Occup Med* 1966;8:365–376.
13. Tokuhata CK, Dessauer P, Pendergrass EP, Hartman T, Digon E, Miller W. Pneumoconiosis among anthracite coal miners in Pennsylvania. *Am J Public Health* 1970;60:441–451.
14. Lieben J, Pendergrass E, McBride WW. Pneumoconiosis study in central Pennsylvanian coal miners. *J Occup Med* 1961;5:376–388.
15. Hyatt RE, Kistin AD, Mahan TK. Respiratory disease in southern West Virginia coal miners. *Am Rev Respir Dis* 1964;89:387–401.
16. McBride WW, Pendergrass E, Lieben J. Pneumoconiosis study of western Pennsylvania bituminous-coal miners. *J Occup Med* 1963;5:376–388.
17. Higgins ITT, Higgins MW, Lockshin MD, Canale N. Chronic respiratory disease in mining communities in Marion county, West Virginia. *Br J Ind Med* 1968;25:165–175.
18. Lainhart WS. Roentgenographic evidence of coal workers' pneumoconiosis in three areas in the United States. *J Occup Med* 1969;11: 399–408.
19. Attfield MD, Castellan RM. Epidemiological data on US coal miners' pneumoconiosis, 1960 to 1988. *Am J Public Health* 1992;82:964–970.
20. Butani SJ, Bartholomew AM. *Characterization of the 1986 coal mining workforce.* Bureau of Mines information circular IC 9192. Washington, DC: US Bureau of Mines, 1988.
21. Attfield MD, Althouse RB. Surveillance data on US coal miners' pneumoconiosis, 1970 to 1986. *Am J Public Health* 1992;82:971–977.
22. Enterline PE, Lainhart WS. The relationship between coal mining and chronic nonspecific respiratory disease. *Am J Public Health* 1967;57: 484–495.
23. Higgins ITT. Chronic respiratory disease in mining communities. *Ann N Y Acad Sci* 1972;200:197–210.
24. Higgins ITT, Cochrane AL. Chronic respiratory disease in a random sample of men and women in Rhondda Fach in 1958. *Br J Ind Med* 1961;18:93–102.
25. Higgins ITT, Oh MS, Whittaker DE. *Chronic respiratory disease in coal miners.* DHHS (NIOSH) publication 81-109. Washington, DC: US Department of Health and Human Services, 1981.
26. Enterline PE. Mortality rates among coal miners. *Am J Public Health* 1964;54:758–768.
27. Rockette H. *Mortality among coal miners by the UMWA health and retirement funds.* DHEW (NIOSH) publication 77-155. Washington, DC: US Department of Health, Education, and Welfare, 1977.
28. Liddell FDK. Mortality of British coal miners in 1961. *Br J Ind Med* 1973;30:1–14.
29. Ortmeyer CE, Costello J, Morgan WKC, Swecker S, Petersen MR. The mortality of Appalachian coal miners. *Arch Environ Health* 1974;29:67–72.
30. Miller BG, Jacobsen M. Dust exposure, pneumoconiosis, and mortality of coal miners. *Br J Ind Med* 1985;42:723–733.
31. Cochrane AL, Carpenter RG, Moore F, Thomas J. The mortality of miners and ex-miners in the Rhondda Fach. *Br J Ind Med* 1964;21: 38–45.
32. Cochrane AL. Relation between radiographic categories of coalworkers' pneumoconiosis and expectation of life. *Br J Ind Med* 1973;2: 532–534.
33. Cochrane AL, Haley TJL, Moore F, Hold D. The mortality of men in the Rhondda Fach, 1950–79. *Br J Ind Med* 1979;36:15–22.
34. Cochrane AL, Moore F. Preliminary results of a twenty-year follow-up of a random sample of an industrial town. *Br Med J* 1978;35: 411–412.
35. Cochrane AL, Moore F. A 20-year follow-up of men aged 55–64 including coal-miners and foundry workers in Staveley, Derbyshire. *Br J Ind Med* 1980;37:226–229.
36. Ortmeyer CE, Baier EJ. Life expectancy of Pennsylvania coal miners compensated for disability. *Arch Environ Health* 1973;27:227–230.
37. Meijers JMM, Swan GMH, Slangen JJM, van Vliet K, Sturmans F. Long-term mortality in miners with coal workers' pneumoconiosis in the Netherlands. *Am J Ind Med* 1991;19:43–50.
38. Goldman KP. Mortality of coal-miners from carcinoma of the lung. *Br J Ind Med* 1965;22:72–77.
39. Ames RG, Amandus H, Attfield M, Green FY, Vallyathan V. Does coal mine dust present a risk for lung cancer? A case-control study of U.S. coal miners. *Arch Environ Health* 1983;38:331–333.
40. Stocks P. On the death rates from cancer of the stomach and respiratory diseases in 1949–53 among coal miners and other residents in counties of England and Wales. *Br J Cancer* 1962;16:592–598.
41. Matolo NM, Klauber MR, Gorishek WM. High incidence of gastric carcinoma in a coal mining region. *Cancer* 1972;29:733
42. Swaen GMH, Meijers JMM, Slangen JJM. Risk of gastric cancer in pneumoconiotic coal miners and the effect of respiratory impairment. *Occup Environ Med* 1995;52:606–610.
43. Une H, Esaki H, Osajima K, Ikui H, Kodama K, Hatada K. A prospective study on mortality among Japanese coal miners. *Ind Health* 1995;33:67–76.
44. Ames RG. Gastric cancer in coal miners: some hypotheses for investigation. *J Soc Occup Med* 1982;32:73–81.
45. Meyer MB, Luk GD, Sotelo JM, Cohen BH, Menkes HA. Hypothesis: the role of the lung in stomach carcinogenesis. *Am Rev Respir Dis* 1980;121:887–892.
46. Jacobsen M, Rae S, Walton WH, Rogan JM. The relation between pneumoconiosis and dust exposure in British coal mines. In: Walton WH, ed. *Inhaled particles* III. Old Woking, England: Unwin Brothers, 1971:903–919.
47. Walton WH, Dodgson J, Hadden GG, Jacobsen M. The effect of quartz and other non-coal dusts in coalworkers' pneumoconiosis. In: Walton WH, ed. *Inhaled particles* IV, vol 2. Old Woking, England: Unwin Brothers, 1977:669–689.
48. Hurley JF, Burns J, Copland L, Dodgson J, Jacobsen M. Coalworkers' simple pneumoconiosis and exposure to dust at 10 British coalmines. *Br J Ind Med* 1982;39:120–127.

49. Hurley JF, Maclaren WM. *Dust-related risks of radiological changes in coalminers over a 40-year working life.* Report on work commissioned by NIOSH. Edinburgh, Scotland: Institute of Occupational Medicine, 1987.
50. Hurley JF, Alexander WP, Hazledine DJ, Jacobsen M, Maclaren WM. Exposure to respirable coalmine dust and incidence of progressive massive fibrosis. *Br J Ind Med* 1987;44:661–672.
51. Jacobsen M, Maclaren WM. Unusual pulmonary observations and exposure to coalmine dust: a case-control study. *Ann Occup Hyg* 1982;26:753–765.
52. Soutar CA, Collins HPR. Classification of progressive massive fibrosis of coalminers by type of radiographic appearance. *Br J Ind Med* 1984;41:334–339.
53. Jacobsen M, Burns J, Attfield MD. Smoking and coalworkers' simple pneumoconiosis. In: Walton WH, ed. *Inhaled particles* IV. Oxford: Pergamon Press, 1977;759–772.
54. Muir DCF, Burns J, Jacobsen M, Walton WH. Pneumoconiosis and chronic bronchitis. *Br J Ind Med* 1977;2:424–427.
55. Cochrane AL. The attack rate of progressive massive fibrosis. *Br J Ind Med* 1962;19:52–64.
56. McLintock JS, Rae S, Jacobsen M. The attack rate of progressive massive fibrosis in British miners. In: Walton WH, ed. *Inhaled particles* III. Old Woking: Unwin Brothers, 1971;933–952.
57. Maclaren WM, Hurley JF, Collins HPR, Cowie AJ. Factors associated with the development of progressive massive fibrosis in British coalminers: a case-control study. *Br J Ind Med* 1989;46:597–607.
58. Cockcroft AE, Wagner JC, Seal EME, Lyons JP, Campbell MJ. Irregular opacities in coalworkers' pneumoconiosis—correlation with pulmonary function and pathology. *Ann Occup Hyg* 1982;26:767–787.
59. Crawford NP, Bodsworth FL, Dodgson J. A study of the apparent anomalies between dust levels and pneumoconiosis at several British collieries. *Ann Occup Hyg* 1982;26:725–744.
60. Reisner MTR. Results of epidemiological studies of pneumoconiosis in West German coal mines. In: Walton WH, ed. *Inhaled particles* III. Old Woking, England: Unwin Brothers, 1971;921–931.
61. Reisner MTR, Robock K. Results of epidemiological, mineralogical, and cytotoxicogical studies on the pathogenicity of coal-mine dusts. In: Walton WH, ed. *Inhaled particles* IV. Oxford: Pergamon Press, 1977;703–716.
62. Breuer H, Reisner MTR. Criteria for long-term dust standards on the basis of personal dust exposure records. *Ann Occup Hyg* 1988;32:523–527.
63. Attfield MD, Morring K. The derivation of estimated dust exposures for U.S. coal miners working before 1970. *Am Ind Hyg Assoc J* 1992;53:248–255.
64. Attfield MD, Morring K. An investigation into the relationship between coal workers' pneumoconiosis and dust exposure in U.S. coal miners. *Am Ind Hyg Assoc J* 1992;53:486–492.
65. Attfield MD, Seixas NS. Prevalence of pneumoconiosis and its relationship to dust exposure in a cohort of U.S. bituminous coal miners and ex-miners. *Am J Ind Med* 1995;27:137–151.
66. Attfield M, Kuempel E, Wagner G. Exposure-response for coal workers' pneumoconiosis in underground coal miners: a discussion of issues and findings. *Ann Occup Hyg* 1997;41(suppl 1):341–345.
67. Soutar CA, Hurley JF. Relation between dust exposure and lung function in miners and ex-miners. *Br J Ind Med* 1986;43:307–320.
68. Hurley JF, Maclaren WM. Factors influencing the occurrence of progressive massive fibrosis (PMF) in miners and ex-miners. *Ann Occup Hyg* 1988;32:575–583.
69. Miller BG, Campbell SJ, Cowie HA, et al. *The natural history and implications of irregularly-shaped small shadows on coalminers' chest radiographs.* Edinburgh: Institute of Occupational Medicine, 1990.
70. Amandus HE, Lapp NL, Jacobson G, Reger RB. Significance of irregular small opacities in radiographs of coalminers in the USA. *Br J Ind Med* 1976;33:13–17.
71. Collins HPR, Dick JA, Bennett JG, et al. Irregularly shaped small shadows on chest radiographs, dust exposure, and lung function in coalworkers' pneumoconiosis. *Br J Ind Med* 1988;45:43–55.
72. Rae S, Walker DD, Attfield MD. Chronic bronchitis and dust exposure in British coalminers. In: Walton WH, ed. *Inhaled particles* III. Old Woking, England: Unwin Brothers, 1971;883–896.
73. Kibelstis JS, Morgan EJ, Reger R, Lapp NL, Seaton A, Morgan WKC. Prevalence of bronchitis and airway obstruction in American bituminous coal miners. *Am Rev Respir Dis* 1973;108:886–893.
74. Leigh J, Wiles AN, Glick M. Total population study of factors affecting chronic bronchitis prevalence in the coal mining industry of New South Wales, Australia. *Br J Ind Med* 1986;43:263–271.
75. Schmidt U. Dust and non-specific respiratory disorders in foundry workers and coal miners in the Rhine-Ruhr area. *Rev Inst Hyg Mines* 1979;34:70–76.
76. Carta P, Aru G, Barbieri MT, Avataneo G, Casula D. Dust exposure, respiratory symptoms, and longitudinal decline in lung function in young coal miners. *Occup Environ Med* 1996;53:312–319.
77. Rogan JM, Attfield MD, Jacobsen M, Rae S, Walker DD, Walton WH. Role of dust in the working environment in development of chronic bronchitis in British coal miners. *Br J Ind Med* 1973;30:217–226.
78. Hankinson JL, Reger RB, Fairman RP, Lapp NL, Morgan WKC. Factors influencing expiratory flow rates in coal miners. In: Walton WH, ed. *Inhaled particles* IV. Oxford: Pergamon Press, 1977;737–755.
79. Attfield MD, Hodous TK. Pulmonary function of U.S. coal miners related to dust exposure estimates. *Am Rev Respir Dis* 1992;14:605–609.
80. Leigh J, Wiles AN. Factors affecting prevalences of mucus hypersecretion and airflow obstruction in the coal industry of New South Wales, Australia. *Ann Occup Hyg* 1988;32(suppl 1):1186–1188.
81. Jain BL, Patrick JM. Ventilatory function in Nigerian coal miners. *Br J Ind Med* 1981;38:275–280.
82. Seixas NS, Robins TG, Attfield MD, Moulton LH. Exposure-response relationships for coal mine dust and obstructive lung disease following enactment of the Federal Coal Mine Health and Safety Act of 1969. *Am J Ind Med* 1992;21:715–734.
83. Nemery B, Veriter C, Brasseur L, Frans A. Impairment of ventilatory function and pulmonary gas exchange in non-smoking coalminers. *Lancet* 1987;2(8573):1427–1430.
84. Marine WM, Gurr D, Jacobsen M. Clinically important respiratory effects of dust exposure and smoking in British coal miners. *Am Rev Respir Dis* 1988;137:106–112.
85. Love RG, Miller BG. Longitudinal study of lung function in coal miners. *Thorax* 1982;37:193–197.
86. Attfield MD. Longitudinal decline in $FEV_1$ in United States coalminers. *Thorax* 1985;40:132–137.
87. Bates DV, Pham QT, Chau N, Pivoteau C, Dechoux J, Sadoul P. A longitudinal study of pulmonary function in coal miners in Lorraine, France. *Am J Ind Med* 1985;8:21–32.
88. Dimich-Ward H, Bates DV. Reanalysis of a longitudinal study of pulmonary function in coal miners in Lorraine, France. *Am J Ind Med* 1994;25:613–623.
89. Henneberger PK, Attfield MD. Coal mine dust exposure and spirometry in experienced miners. *Am J Respir Crit Care Med* 1996;153:1560–1566.
90. Hodous TK, Hankinson JL. Prospective spirometric study of new coal miners. In: *Proceedings of the International Symposium on Pneumoconiosis, 1988.* Shenyang, PRC: Chinese Society of Preventive Medicine, 1990, 206–211.
91. Seixas NS, Robins TG, Attfield MD, Moulton LH. Longitudinal and cross sectional analyses of exposure to coal mine dust and pulmonary function in new miners. *Br J Ind Med* 1993;50:929–937.
92. Petsonk EL, Daniloff EM, Mannino DM, Wang ML, Short SL, Wagner GR. Airway responsiveness and job selection: a study in coal miners and non-mining controls. *Occup Environ Med* 1995;52:745–749.
93. Morgan WKC, Seaton A. *Occupational lung diseases,* 3rd ed. Philadelphia: WB Saunders, 1995.
94. Hurley JF, Soutar CA. Can exposure to coalmine dust cause a severe impairment of lung function? *Br J Ind Med* 1986;43:150–157.
95. Leigh J, Driscoll TR, Cole BD, Beck RW, Hull BP, Yang J. Quantitative relation between emphysema and lung mineral content in coalworkers. *Br J Ind Med* 1994;51:400–407.
96. Coggon D, Inskip H, Winter P, Pannett B. Contrasting geographical distribution of mortality from pneumoconiosis and chronic bronchitis and emphysema in British coal miners. *Occup Environ Med* 1995;52:554–555.
97. Gamboa PM, Jáuregui I, Urrutia I, Antépara I, González G, Múgica V. Occupational asthma in a coal miner. *Thorax* 1996;51:867–868.
98. Kuempel ED, Stayner LT, Attfield MD, Buncher CR. Exposure-response analysis of mortality among coal miners in the United States. *Am J Ind Med* 1995;28:167–184.
99. Fairman RP, O'Brien RJ, Swecker S, Amandus HE, Shoub EP. Respiratory status of surface coal miners in the United States. *Arch Environ Health* 1977;32:211–215.

100. Amandus HE, Hanke W, Kullman G, Reger RB. A re-evaluation of radiological evidence from a study of U.S. strip coal miners. *Arch Environ Health* 1984;39:346–351.
101. Banks DE, Bauer MA, Castellan RM, Lapp NL. Silicosis in surface coalmine drillers. *Thorax* 1983;38:275–278.
102. Attfield MD, Vallyathan V, Green FHY. Radiographic appearances of small opacities and their correlation with pathology grading of macules, nodules, and dust burden in the lungs. *Ann Occu HYG* 1994; 38(suppl 1):783–789.
103. Vallyathan V, Brower PS, Green FHY, Attfield MD. Radiographic and pathologic correlation of coal workers' pneumoconiosis. *Am J Respir Crit Care Med* 1996;154:741–748.
104. Wagner GR, Attfield MD, Parker JE. Chest radiography in dust-exposed miners: promise and problems, potential and imperfections. In: Banks DE, ed. *Occupational medicine:* state of the art reviews, vol 8, no. 1. Philadelphia: Hanley and Belfus, 1993;127–141.
105. Weiss W. Smoking and pulmonary fibrosis. *J Occup Med* 1988;30: 33–39.
106. Castellan RM, Sanderson WT, Petersen MP. Prevalence of radiographic appearances of pneumoconiosis in an unexposed blue collar population. *Am Rev Respir Dis* 1985;131:684–686.
107. Blank PD, Gamsu G. Cigarette smoking and pneumoconiosis: structuring the debate (editorial). *Am J Ind Med* 1989;16:1–4.
108. Ducatman AM, Yang WN, Forman SA. "B-Readers" and asbestos medical surveillance. *J Occup Med* 1988;30:644–647.
109. Attfield MD, Althouse RB, Reger RB. An investigation of inter-reader variability among X-ray readers employed in the underground coal miner surveillance program. *Ann Am Conf Gov Ind Hyg* 1986;14: 401–409.
110. Bourbeau J, Ernest P. Between and within reader variability in the assessment of pleural abnormality using the ILO 1980 international classification of pneumoconiosis. *Am J Ind Med* 1988;14:537–543.
111. Remy-Jardin M, Degreef JM, Beuscart R, Voisin C, Remy J. Coal worker's pneumoconiosis: CT assessment in exposed workers and correlation with radiographic findings. *Radiology* 1990;177:363–371.
112. Akira M, Higashihara T, Yokoyama K, et al. Radiographic type p pneumoconiosis: high resolution CT. *Radiology* 1989;171:117–123.
113. Harkin TJ, McGuiness G, Goldring R, et al. Differentiation of the ILO boundary chest roentgenograph (0/1 to 1/0) in asbestosis by high-resolution computed tomography scan, alveolitis, and respiratory impairment. *J Occup Environ Med* 1996;38:46–52.
114. Remy-Jardin M, Remy J, Farre I, Marquette CH. Computed tomographic evaluation of silicosis and coal workers' pneumoconiosis. *Radiol Clin North Am* 1992;30:1155–1176.
115. Kanner RE, Barkman HW Jr, Rom WN, Taylor AT Jr. Gallium-67 citrate imaging in underground coal miners. *Am J Ind Med* 1985;8: 49–55.
116. Heppleston AG. Essential lesion of pneumoconiosis in Welsh coal workers. *J Pathol Bacterial* 1947;59:453–460.
117. Gough J, James WRL, Wentworth JE. A comparison of the radiological and pathological changes in coal workers' pneumoconiosis. *J Fac Radiol* 1949;1:28–60.
118. Kleinerman J, Green FHY, Laqueur W, et al. Pathology standards for coal workers' pneumoconiosis. *Arch Pathol Lab Med* 1979;103: 375–432.
119. Miller AA, Ramsden F. Carbon pneumoconiosis. *Br J Ind Med* 1961;18:103–113.
120. Watson AJ, Black J, Doig AT, Nagelschmidt G. Pneumoconiosis in carbon electrode makers. *Br J Ind Med* 1959;16:274–385.
121. Zahorski W. Pneumoconiosis dans l'industrie du graphite artificiel. In: *Proceedings of the XIII International Congress on Occupational Health.* New York: Book Craftsmen Associates, Inc., 1961;828–832.
122. Green FHY, Laqueur WA. Coal workers' pneumoconiosis. *Pathology* 1980;15:333–410.
123. International Labour Office. *International classification of radiographs of pneumoconiosis,* rev. ed. Occupational Safety and Health Series no. 22, rev. 80. Geneva: International Labour Office, 1980.
124. Wagner JC, Wusteman FS, Edwards JH, Hill RJ. The composition of massive lesions in coal miners. *Thorax* 1975;30:382–388.
125. Green FHY, Althouse R, Weber KC. Prevalence of silicosis at death in underground coal miners. *Am J Ind Med* 1989;16:605–615.
126. Rivers D, Wise ME, King EJ, Nagelschmidt G. Dust content, radiology, and pathology in simple pneumoconiosis of coalworkers. *Br J Ind Med* 1960;17:87–108.
127. Rossiter CM, Rivers D, Bergman C, Casswell C, Nagelschmidt G. Dust content, radiology, and pathology in simple pneumoconiosis of coal workers. In: Davies CN, ed. *Inhaled particles and vapours* II. Oxford: Pergamon, 1967;419–437.
128. Rossiter CM. Relation of lung dust content to radiological changes in coalworkers. *Ann NY Acad Sci* 1972;200:465–477.
129. Ruckley VA, Fernie JM, Chapman JS, et al. Comparison of radiographic appearances with associated pathology and lung dust content in a group of coalworkers. *Br J Ind Med* 1984;41:459–467.
130. Fernie JM, Ruckley VA. Coalworkers' pneumoconiosis: correlation between opacity profusion and number and type of dust lesions with special reference to opacity type. *Br J Ind Med* 1987;44:273–277.
131. Davis JMG, Chapman J, Collings P, et al. Variations in the histological patterns of the lesions of coal workers' pneumoconiosis in Britain and their relationship to lung dust content. *Am Rev Respir Dis* 1983; 128:118–124.
132. Douglas AN, Colline HPR, Fernie JM, Soutar CA. The relationship between radiographic and pathological appearances of progressive massive fibrosis. *Ann Occup Hyg* 1988;1:561–566.
133. Douglas AN, Robertson A, Chapman JS, Ruckley VA. Dust exposure, dust recovered from the lung, and associated pathology in a group of British coalminers. *Br J Ind Med* 1986;43:795–801.
134. Kuempel ED, O'Flaherty EJ, Stayner LT, Attfield MD, Green FHY, Vallyathan V. Relationships between lung dust burden, pathology, and lifetime exposure in an autopsy study of U.S. coal miners. *Ann Occup Hyg* 1997;41(suppl 1):384–389.
135. Ryder RC, Lyons JP, Campbell H, Gough J. Emphysema and coal workers' pneumoconiosis. *Br Med J* 1970;3:481–487.
136. Naeye RI, Mahon JK, Dellinger WS. Effects of smoking on lung structure of Appalachian coalminers. *Arch Environ Health* 1971;22:190–193.
137. Lamb D. A survey of emphysema in coal workers and the general population. *Proc R Soc Med* 1976;69:14.
138. Ruckley VA, Gauld SJ, Chapman JS, et al. Emphysema and dust exposure in a group of coal workers. *Am Rev Respir Dis* 1984;129: 528–532.
139. Leigh J, Outhred KG, McKenzie HI, Glick M, Wiles AN. Quantified pathology of emphysema, pneumoconiosis, and chronic bronchitis in coal workers. *Br J Ind Med* 1983;40:258–263.
140. Glick M, Outhred KG, McKenzie HI. Pneumoconiosis and respiratory disorders of coal mine workers in New South Wales, Australia. *Ann NY Acad Sci* 1972;200:316–334.
141. Leigh J, Outhred KG, McKenzie HI, Wiles AN. Multiple regression analysis of quantified aetiological, clinical and post-mortem pathological variables related to respiratory disease in coal workers. *Ann Occup Hyg* 1982;26:383–400.
142. Douglas AN, Lamb D, Ruckley VA. Bronchial gland dimensions in coalminers: influence of smoking and dust exposure. *Br J Ind Med* 1982;37:760–764.
143. Brighan KL. Role of the free radical in lung injury. *Chest* 1986;89: 859–863.
144. Johnson KJ, Fantone JC, Kaplan J, Ward PA. In vivo damage of rat lungs by oxygen metabolites. *J Clin Invest* 1981;68:1277–1288.
145. Martin WJ, Gadek JE, Hunninghake GW, Crystal RG. Oxidant injury of lung parenchymal cells. *J Clin Invest* 1981;67(4):983–993.
146. Kuroda M, Murakami K, Ishikawa Y. Role of hydroxyl radicals derived from granulocytes in lung injury induced by phorbol myristate acetate. *Am Rev Respir Dis* 1987;136:1435–1444.
147. Hubbard RC, Ogushi F, Fells GA, et al. Oxidants spontaneously released by alveolar macrophages of cigarette smokers can inactivate the active site of $\alpha$-antitrypsin rendering it ineffective as an inhibitor of neutrophil elastase. *J Clin Invest* 1987;80:1289–1295.
148. Blackford J, Castranova V, Jones W, Dey R. Induction of the inducible nitric oxide synthase gene by intratracheal instillation of silica, coal, titanium dioxide, and carbonyl iron. *FASEB J* 1995;9:767.
149. Vallyathan V, Schwegler D, Reasor M, Stettler L, Green FHY. Comparative in vivo cytotoxicity and relative pathogenicity of mineral dusts. In: Dodgson J, McCallum RI, Bailey MR, Fisher DR, eds. *Inhaled particles* VI. Oxford: Pergamon, 1988;279–289.
150. Susskind H, Rom WN. Lung inflammation in coal miners assessed by uptake of $^{67}$Ga citrate and clearance of inhaled $^{99m}$Tc DTPA aerosol. *Am Rev Respir Dis* 1992;148:47–52.
151. Lebeder VV, Khrenkova TM, Goldenko NL. The formation of paramagnetic centers during crushing of coal. *Solid Fuels Chem* 1978;12: 117–119.

152. Dalal NS, Suryan MM, Vallyathan V, Green FHY, Jafari B, Wheeler R. Detection of reactive free radicals in fresh coal mine dust and their implication for pulmonary injury. *Ann Occup Hyg* 1989;33:79–84.
153. Kuhn DC, Demers LM. Influence of mineral dust surface chemistry on eicosanoid production by the alveolar macrophage. *J Toxicol Environ Health* 1992;35:39–50.
154. Castranova V, Bowman L, Reason MJ, Lewis T, Tucker J, Miles PR. The response of rat alveolar macrophages to chronic inhalation of coal dust and/or diesel exhaust. *Environ Res* 1985;36:405–419.
155. Brain JD. The effect of increased particles on the number of alveolar macrophages. In: Walton WH, ed. *Inhaled particles* III. Old Woking, England: Unwin Brothers, 1971;209–233.
156. Bingham E, Barkley W, Murthy R, Vassalo C. Investigation of alveolar macrophages from rats exposed to coal dust. In: Walton WH, ed. *Inhaled particles* IV. Oxford: Pergamon, 1977;543–550.
157. Bowden DH, Adamson IYR. Adaptive responses of the pulmonary macrophagic system to carbon. I. Kinetic studies. *Lab Invest* 1978;38:422–429.
158. Adamson IYR, Bowden DH. Adaptive responses of the macrophagic system to carbon. II. Morphologic studies. *Lab Invest* 1978;38: 430–438.
159. Kuhn DC, Standley CFS, Ayouby NEI, Demers LM. Effect of *in vivo* coal dust exposure on arachidonic acid metabolism in the rat alveolar macrophage. *J Toxicol Environ Health* 1990;29:157–168.
160. Wallaert B, Lassalle P, Fortin F. Superoxide anion production by alveolar inflammatory cells in simple pneumoconiosis and in progressive massive fibrosis of nonsmoking coal workers. *Am Rev Respir Dis* 1990;141:129–133.
161. Rom WN, Bitterman PB, Rennard SI, Cantin A, Crystal RG. Characterization of the lower respiratory tract inflammation of non-smoking individuals with interstitial lung disease associated with chronic inhalation of inorganic dusts. *Am Rev Respir Dis* 1987;136: 1429–1434.
162. Rom WN. Basic mechanisms leading to focal emphysema in coal workers' pneumoconiosis. *Environ Res* 1990;53:16–28.
163. Takemura T, Rom WN, Ferrans VJ, Crystal RG. Morphologic characterization of alveolar macrophages from subjects with occupational exposure to inorganic particles. *Am Rev Respir Dis* 1989;140: 1674–1685.
164. Rom WN. Relationship of inflammatory cell cytokines to disease severity in individuals with occupational inorganic dust exposure. *Am J Ind Med* 1991;19:15–27.
165. Lapp NL, Lewis D, Schwegler-Berry D, Castranova V, Abrons H, Kung M. Bronchoalveolar lavage in asymptomatic underground coal miners. 56th Meeting of American College of Chest Physicians, Toronto, Canada 1990(abstr).
166. Lapp NL, Weber SL, Vallyathan V, Castranova V, Shumaker J. Cytokine profiles in bronchoalveolar fluid of asymptomatic coal miners: natural defense mechanisms. *Am J Respir Crit Care Med* 1995; 151:A571
167. Lassalle P, Gosset P, Aerts C, et al. Alveolar macrophages secretory dysfunction in coal workers' pneumoconiosis. Comparison between simple pneumoconiosis and progressive massive fibrosis. In: Mossman BT, Begin RO, eds. *Effects of mineral dusts on cells.* Berlin: Springer-Verlag, 1984;65–71.
168. Borm PJA, Meijers JMM, Swaen GMH. Molecular epidemiology of coal workers' pneumoconiosis: application to risk assessment of oxidant and monokine generation by mineral dusts. *Exp Lung Res* 1990; 16:57–71.
169. Vanhee D, Gosset P, Marquette CH, et al. Secretion and mRNA expression of TNF-$\alpha$ and IL-6 in alveolar macrophages and in lung of pneumoconiotic patients. *Am Rev Respir Dis* 1993;147:906A.
170. Driscoll KE, Hassenbein DG, Carter JM, Kunkel SL, Quinlan TR, Mossman BT. TNF-$\alpha$ and increased chemokine expression in rat lung after particle exposure. *Toxicol Lett* 1995;82/82:483–489.
171. Hajjar KA, Hajjar DP, Silverstein RL, Nachman RL. Tumor necrosis factor-mediated release of platelet derived growth factor from endothelial cells. *J Exp Med* 1987;166:235–241.
172. Piguet PF, Collart MA, Grau GE, Sappino A, Vassili P. Requirement for tumor necrosis factor for development of silica-induced pulmonary fibrosis. *Nature* 1990;344:245–251.
173. Vanhee D, Gosset P, Wallaert B, Voisin C, Tonnel AB. Mechanisms of fibrosis in coal workers' pneumoconiosis; Increased production of platelet-derived growth factor, insulin-like growth factor Type I, and transforming growth factor beta and relationship to disease severity. *Am J Respir Crit Care Med* 1994;150:1049–1055.
174. Kelley J. Cytokines of the lung. *Am Rev Respir Dis* 1990;141:765–781.
175. Worth G. Emphysema in coal workers. *Am J Ind Med* 1984;6: 401–403.
176. Morgan WKC, Handelsman L, Kibelstis JS, Lapp NL, Reger R. Ventilatory capacity and lung volumes of US coal miners. *Arch Environ Health* 1974;28:182–189.
177. Rogan JM, Ashford JR, Chapman PJ, Duffield KP, Fay JWJ, Rae S. Pneumoconiosis and respiratory symptoms in miners at eight collieries. *Br Med J* 1961;1:1337–1342.
178. Hankinson JL, Reger RB, Morgan WKC. Maximal expiratory flows in coal miners. *Am Rev Respir Dis* 1977;116:175–180.
179. Cochrane AL, Higgins ITT, Thomas J. Pulmonary ventilatory functions of coalminers in various areas in relation to the x-ray category of pneumoconiosis. *Br J Prev Soc Med* 1961;15:1–11.
180. Morgan WKC, Lapp NL, Morgan EJ. The early detection of occupational lung disease. *Br J Dis Chest* 1974;68:75–85.
181. Morgan WKC. Hyperinflation of the lungs in coal miners. *Thorax* 1971;26:585–590.
182. Cotes JE, Field GB. Lung gas exchange in simple pneumoconiosis of coal workers. *Br J Ind Med* 1972;29:268–273.
183. Seaton A, Lapp NL, Morgan WKC. Relationship of pulmonary impairment in simple coalworkers' pneumoconiosis to type of radiologic opacity. *Br J Ind Med* 1972;29:50–55.
184. Ulmer WT, Reichel G. Functional impairment in coal workers' pneumoconiosis. *Ann NY Acad Sci* 1972;200:405–412.
185. Lapp NL, Seaton A. Pulmonary function in coal workers' pneumoconiosis. In: Key MM, Kew LE, Bundy M, eds. *Pulmonary reactions to coal dust.* New York: Academic Press, 1971;153–185.
186. Rasmussen DL, Laqueur WA, Futterman HD. Pulmonary impairment in Southern West Virginia coal miners. *Am Rev Respir Dis* 1968;98:658–667.
187. Ferris BG. Epidemiology standardization project: part II. *Am Rev Respir Dis* 1978;suppl 118:1–120.
188. U.S.Department of Labor. *Federal regulations:* parts 718,722,725, *726 and 727:* black lung benefits. Washington, DC: U.S. Department of Labor, 1991.
189. Lanese RR, Keller MD, Foley MF, Underwood EH. Differences in pulmonary function tests among whites, blacks, and american indians in a textile company. *J Occup Med* 1978;20:39–44.
190. Lapp NL, Amandus HE, Hall R, Morgan WKC. Lung volumes and flow rates in black and white subjects. *Thorax* 1974;29:185–188.
191. Rossiter CE, Weill H. Ethnic differences in lung function: evidence for proportional differences. *Int J Epidemiol* 1974;3:55–61.
192. Sorlie PD, Rogot E. Mortality status in the national longitudinal mortality study. *Am J Epidemiol* 1990;132:983–992.
193. Hankinson JL, Wagner GR. Medical screening using periodic spirometry for detection of chronic lung diseases. *Occup Med State Art Rev* 1993;8:353–362.
194. Eisen EA, Oliver LC, Christiani DC, Robins JM, Wegman DH. Effects of spirometry standards in two occupational cohorts. *Am Rev Respir Dis* 1985;132:120–124.
195. Crapo RO, Morris AH, Gardner RM. Reference spirometric values using techniques and equipment that meet the ATS recommendations. *Am Rev Respir Dis* 1981;123:659–664.
196. Astrand PO, Rhyming I. A nomogram for calculation of aerobic capacity (physical fitness) from pulse rate during submaximal work. *J Appl Physiol* 1954;7:218–221.
197. Hodgkin J. Pulmonary rehabilitation. *Clin Chest Med* 1990;11: 447–454.
198. American Thoracic Society. Pulmonary rehabilitation. American Thoracic Society position statement. *Am Rev Respir Dis* 1981;124:663–666.
199. Tiep BL. Long-term home oxygen therapy. *Clin Chest Med* 1990;11: 505–522.
200. Wilt JL, Banks DE, Weissman DN, et al. Reduction of lung dust burden in pneumoconiosis by whole-lung lavage. *J Occup Environ Med* 1996;38:619–624.
201. Jacobson M. Respirable dust in bituminous coal mines in the U.S. In: Walton WH, ed. *Inhaled particles* III. Old Woking, England: Unwin Brothers, 1971;903–917.
202. Parobeck PS, Jankowski RA. Assessment of the respirable dust levels

in the nation's underground and surface coal mining operations. *Am Ind Hyg Assoc J* 1979;40:910–915.

203. Watts WF. Respirable dust trends in coal mines with longwall or continuous miner sections. In: *Proceedings of the VIIth International Pneumoconiosis Conference,* Pittsburgh, August 1988. DHHS (NIOSH) publication 90-108. Washington, DC: DHHS, 1990;94–99.
204. Weeks JL. Characteristics of chronically dusty longwall mines in the U.S. In: *Proceedings of the VIIth International Pneumoconiosis Conference,* Pittsburgh, August 1988. DHHS (NIOSH) publication 90-108. Washington, DC: DHHS, 1990;76–80.
205. Key MM. Health standards and standard setting in the United States. *Ann NY Acad Sci* 1972;200:707–711.
206. National Institute for Occupational Safety and Health. *Criteria for a recommended standard:* occupational exposure to coal mine dust. Cincinnati, OH: National Institute for Occupational Safety and Health, 1995.
207. U.S.Department of Labor. *Report of the secretary of labor's advisory committee on the elimination of pneumoconiosis among coal mine workers.* Washington, DC: U.S. Department of Labor, 1996.
208. Boden LI, Gold M. The accuracy of self-reported regulatory data: the case of coal mine dust. *Am J Ind Med* 1984;6:427–440.
209. Mine Safety and Health Administration. *Report of the statistical task team of the coal mine respirable dust task group.* Washington DC: US Department of Labor, 1993.
210. Specifications for medical examinations of underground coal miners. *Federal Register* 1973;38:20076–20081.
211. *U.S. geological survey.* Washington, DC: U.S. Government Printing Office, 1975.

*Environmental and Occupational Medicine, Third Edition,* edited by William N. Rom.
Lippincott–Raven Publishers, Philadelphia © 1998.

# CHAPTER 29

# Silicosis

Marvin R. Balaan and Daniel E. Banks

Silicosis refers to a spectrum of pulmonary diseases attributed to the inhalation of various forms of free crystalline silicon dioxide or silica. A man-made disease, it is probably as old as human history and was known to the ancient Egyptians and Greeks (1,2). Although the prevalence of silicosis apparently peaked in the late 19th and early 20th century when mechanized industry was just beginning, even in developed countries today sporadic yet preventable cases of silicosis occur.

Silicon dioxide or silica is the most abundant mineral on earth. It is formed from the elements silicon and oxygen under conditions of increased heat and pressure. Silica exists in the crystalline and amorphous forms. Crystalline forms are based on a tetrahedral structure in which the central atom is silicon, and the corners are occupied by oxygen. The structure of the crystal is such that two adjacent tetrahedrons share two oxygen atoms. Examples of crystalline silica are quartz, cristobalite, and tridymite. The most common form is quartz, a typical component of rocks. Some of the common quartz-containing materials in industry are granite, slate, and sandstone. Granite contains about 30% free silica, slate about 40%, and sandstone is almost pure silica (3). Crystobalite and tridymite occur naturally in lava and are formed when quartz or amorphous silica is subjected to very high temperatures. They may also be formed in silica bricks (refractory bricks) used in industrial furnaces. Amorphous silica is noncrystalline and has relatively nontoxic pulmonary properties. It occurs as diatomite (skeletons of prehistoric marine organisms) or as vitreous silica (the result of carefully melting and then quickly cooling crystalline silica). Heating diatomite with or without alkali (a process known as calcining) forms cristobalite, a material that has the potential to be more toxic than quartz.

Crystalline silica that is not bound to other minerals is referred to as “free”; when it is bound to other minerals it is referred to as “combined.” The latter are also known as silicates. Examples of silicates that have been widely used in industry include asbestos, talc [$(Mg_3Si_4)O_{10}(OH)_2$], and kaolinite ($Al_2O_3SiO_2H_2O$), a major component of china clay, or kaolin.

## WORKERS AT RISK FOR SILICOSIS

The knowledge that silicosis is associated with certain occupations is rooted in antiquity. Hippocrates reported that miners developed dyspnea with exertion. Ramazzini and Agricola were instrumental in recognizing the relationship between rock dust exposure and the development of dyspnea in those who worked in this trade (2).

The worst outbreak of silicosis in the United States occurred during the construction of the Gauley Bridge tunnel in West Virginia in 1930 and 1931. In this unfortunate but preventable disaster, more than 400 men of the estimated 2,000 engaged in rock drilling died, and about 1,500 contracted silicosis and were eventually disabled (2).

Occupations known to carry increased risk for silicosis and the pertinent sources of exposure in these trades are enumerated in Table 1. It is difficult to obtain precise estimates of the prevalence of silicosis because of the many different occupations involved, the participation of tran-

M. R. Balaan: Section of Pulmonary and Critical Care Medicine, Department of Medicine; and Respiratory Care and Pulmonary Function Laboratory, Robert C. Byrd Health Sciences Center, West Virginia University School of Medicine, Morgantown, West Virginia 26506-9166.

D. E. Banks: Section of Pulmonary and Critical Care Medicine, Department of Medicine, Robert C. Byrd Health Sciences Center, West Virginia University School of Medicine, Morgantown, West Virginia 26506-9166.

**TABLE 1.** *Workers at risk for silicosis*

| Occupation | Exposure hazard |
|---|---|
| Sandblaster | Shipbuilding and iron-working are important industries |
| Miner or tunneler | Underground miners are at risk during roof bolting, shot firing, and drilling; surface coal mine drillers are at high risk |
| Miller | Finely milled silica for fillers and abrasives; "silica flour workers" |
| Pottery workers | Crushing flint and fettling are the major exposures |
| Glassmaker | Sand used for polishing and enameling |
| Foundry worker | Silica is essential during mold making; exposure is during fettling |
| Quarry worker | Slate, sandstone, granite |
| Abrasives worker | Finely ground particles |

sient workers, and the variability of disease detection methods (e.g., autopsy versus compensation or screening data) and reporting practices from place to place. In 1956 Trasko (4) obtained estimates of silicosis prevalence by examining records of workers in 20 states who were compensated for silicosis. About 6,000 cases were identified. The largest numbers of silicosis cases were found among metal miners (1,637) and foundry workers (1,645). Because of the nature of case identifications, these numbers most likely underestimate the actual frequencies. Autopsy records of 3,365 underground miners submitted to the U.S. National Coal Workers' Autopsy Study between 1971 and 1980 revealed the presence of classical silicotic nodules in the lungs of 12.5% of the cases (5). In an investigation of worker health at two silica flour mills, 16 (26%) of the 61 workers who were exposed to microcrystalline silica had radiographic evidence of simple silicosis, and 7 (11%) had progressive massive fibrosis (6).

In the United States, it is estimated that 200,000 miners and 1.7 million workers outside of the mining industry are potentially exposed to crystalline silica (7). Compared to working conditions of 20 years ago, better methods of dust suppression and ventilation as well as respiratory protection have diminished the attack rate among workers. However, new cases of silicosis are still reported sporadically in both developed and developing countries, and silicosis is still very much a disease of the 1990s (8). Rosenman et al. (9) recently reported 577 workers who were identified between 1987 and 1995 through a state surveillance system. Ten new cases of silicosis were reported in a sandblasting facility in Texas (10). One of these cases was fatal acute silicoproteinosis. Abrasive sandblasting and hard rock drilling continue to be significant sources of morbidity from silicosis in the United States. Sandblasting has been prohibited in Great Britain. Figure 1 shows how sandblasting can expose the worker to tremendous amounts of respirable silica.

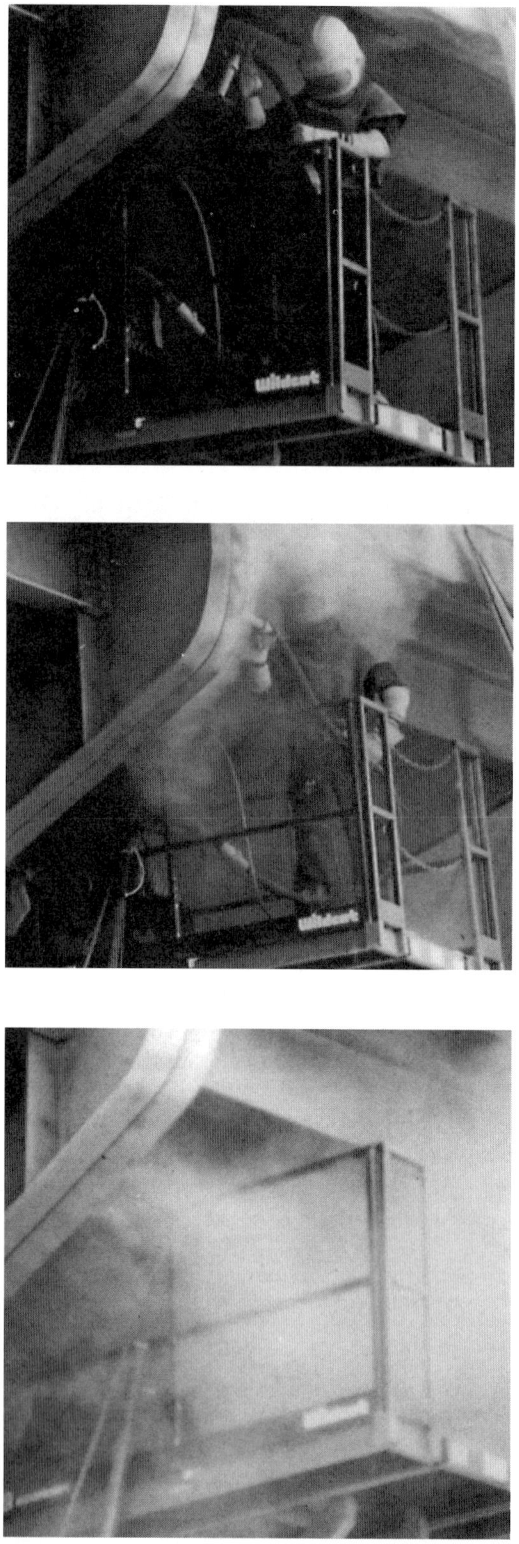

**FIG. 1.** A worker prepares the steel surface of an overpass for painting by sandblasting. This series of photographs illustrates how this practice may expose workers to high concentrations of respirable silica. (Courtesy of R. N. Jones, M.D.)

## PATHOLOGY

The gross and microscopic pathology of silicosis are described in detail in a publication of the silicosis and silicate disease committee of the National Institute for Occupational Safety and Health (NIOSH) (11).

On inspection, the silicotic lung is firm and blacker than normal. The surface is coarse and nodular. The visceral pleura has areas of fibrosis and may be covered by plaquelike lesions. Peribronchial and hilar lymph nodes are typically enlarged. On sectioning, these enlarged nodes show concentrically arranged fibrous tissue. Cutting the lung reveals palpable intrapulmonary nodules, especially in the upper lobes (Fig. 2). In simple silicosis these nodules are usually 2 to 6 mm in diameter. In conglomerate silicosis or progressive massive fibrosis, the lesions are typically 10 to 20 mm diameter, a result of the coalescence of smaller nodules. Nodules vary in color depending on the presence of other dusts. The extent of nodule calcification is also variable.

The earliest parenchymal lesion in workers with relatively low-dose, chronic exposure to free crystalline silica is a collection of dust-laden macrophages and loose reticulin fibers in the peribronchial, perivascular, and paraseptal or subpleural areas. Later, these lesions become more organized and may appear whorled. The silicotic nodule, the pathologic hallmark of silicosis, has a histologic appearance analogous to tornado (Fig. 3). The central zone, like the eye of the storm, shows little activity. It is hyalinized and composed of concentrically arranged collagen fibers. The peripheral zone is whorled and becomes less organized toward the edges. It contains macrophages, lymphocytes, and lesser amounts of loosely formed collagen. Under polarized light microscopy, a few weakly birefringent particles may be seen in the center of the nodule, likely the result of trapped crystalline silica mixed with other dusts. In the periphery of the nodule, the amount of dust and the degree of birefringence differ dramatically. Needle-shaped, strongly birefringent material is easily seen intermingled with cells and dust. The strongly birefringent crystals are silicates. This is the site of active enlargement of the nodule and of ongoing inflammation. As the disease progresses, the periphery of the silicotic nodule moves farther from the hyalinized center, enmeshing small airways, pleura, and blood and lymphatic vessels in the fibrotic process.

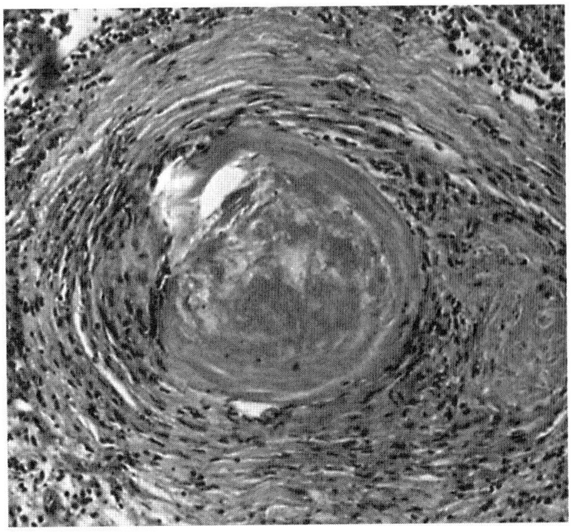

**FIG. 3.** Photomicrograph of a well-developed silicotic nodule (×180). An acellular, hyalinized center is surrounded by concentrically arranged collagen fibers and a peripheral rim of dust-containing macrophages. (Courtesy of V. Vallyathan, Ph.D.)

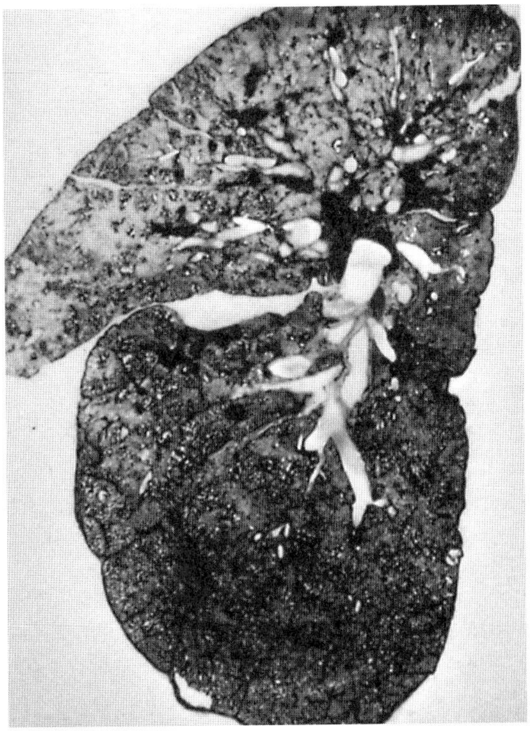

**FIG. 2.** Gough-Wentworth whole lung section of an underground coal miner who worked as a motorman for 30 years shows simple silicosis with nodules predominantly located in the upper lobe and a few in the lower lobe. (Courtesy of V. Vallyathan, Ph.D.)

Coalescence of silicotic nodules form the progressive massive fibrotic (PMF) lesion, a mass of dense, hyalinized connective tissue with minimal silica content, a small amount of anthracotic pigment, minimal cellular infiltrate, and negligible vascularization. Typically, the centers of these conglomerate lesions cavitate, the result of mycobacterial infection or ischemic necrosis when they exceed a certain size.

The histologic pattern of acute silicosis differs from that of chronic silicosis. Silicotic nodules are rarely seen, and, if identified, are usually poorly developed. The interstitium is thickened with inflammatory cells. There is alveolar filling with proteinaceous material consisting largely of phospholipids or surfactant (or surfactant-like material) which stain with periodic acid-Schiff (PAS) reagent. Since the histologic appearance resembles that of idiopathic alveolar preteinosis, this process occurring in a clinical background of overwhelming silica exposure has also been called *silicoproteinosis,* a term coined by Buechner and Ansari (12). On electron microscopic examination the alveoli are lined by prominent epithelial cells, the majority of which are hypertrophic type II pneumocytes(13). The alveolar exudate is most likely the result of overproduction of phospholipids and surfactant-associated proteins by these hypertrophic type II cells. In addition, desquamated pneumocytes, macrophages, and silica particles are found in the alveolar spaces. Typically a minimal amount of pulmonary fibrosis is present. Therefore, although the term *silicoproteinosis* may reflect one of the pathologic changes present, other features of acute alveolar damage syndromes and even of desquamative interstitial pneumonitis are a part of the recognized lung injury.

## PATHOGENESIS

The majority of the existing information regarding the pulmonary cellular and molecular responses to silica comes from experimental animal models. Silicosis is induced in these models by tracheal instillation of silica or by inhalational exposure of animals over a few weeks to months. One therefore has to be concerned about correlates drawn between the development of the silicotic nodules in experimental animals after only 6 or 8 months' exposure to silica and the development of classic silicosis over 20 or more years in humans. The applicability of this information to humans is subject to speculation. Nevertheless, animal work has provided much insight into the pathogenesis of the illness.

The pathogenesis of silicosis begins with the inhalation of crystalline silica particles that have favorable characteristics for deposition in the alveolar spaces. The most important of these is size. Particles of a diameter smaller than 3 μm and greater than 0.5 μm have the best chances of entering and being retained in the pulmonary acini. The key event in the genesis of silicosis is the interaction between the silica particle and the alveolar macrophage, the main phagocytic cell in the alveolar space. Early work on the pathogenesis of silica-induced lung injury focused on the injury and cell death that occurred after ingestion of silica by alveolar macrophages in vitro (14) and *in vivo* (15). Lung injury was believed to be related to the release of intracellular proteolytic enzymes following the disruption of the alveolar macrophage. Intracellular silica released in this process was taken up by other macrophages. The recurrent cycle of macrophage phagocytosis, cell death, release of intracellular enzymes, and reuptake of silica perpetuated the inflammatory process. More recent studies suggest that cell injury may be a more crucial factor than cell death in the pathogenesis of silicosis.

The fibrogenic effect of silica may be due to elaboration of several inflammatory mediators by alveolar macrophages that have been activated by silica exposure or ingestion. The data supporting this come mainly from experiments wherein alveolar macrophages are harvested by bronchoalveolar lavage (BAL) from subjects or animals exposed to silica particles *in vivo,* or are collected directly after being exposed to silica particles *in vitro.* Lugano and coworkers (16) demonstrated increased chemotaxis of neutrophils and macrophages when these cells were exposed to BAL fluid supernatant of silica-exposed guinea pigs. The recruitment of cells to the sites of particle deposition and cell injury promotes the amplification of the inflammatory response. Enhanced production of fibrogenic factors (17), specifically interleukin-1 (IL-1) (18,19), tumor necrosis factor (TNF) (20), and transforming growth factor-β (21), by silica-activated alveolar macrophages has been shown.

Recent work suggests that TNF may play an important role in the pathogenesis of silicosis. Piquet and coworkers (20) found increased levels of lung TNF messenger RNA (mRNA) in mice instilled with silica. The deposition of collagen, measured by an increase in hydroxyproline, was prevented by pretreating the mice with anti-TNF antibodies. Administration of human recombinant soluble TNF receptors, which bound TNF in lungs of silica-treated mice, not only prevented collagen deposition but also reduced lung collagen content in established fibrosis (22). Silicotic nodules were less dense and contained fewer microfibrils. Inbred strains of TNF-deficient mice show less inflammation and collagen accumulation in the lungs after instillation of silica, as compared to TNF-producing strains of mice (23). It is postulated that silica increases TNF production by upregulation of the TNF promoter in the TNF gene (24). The secretion of TNF can be induced with a small load of silica particles that does not induce cell death (25).

Other investigators have found a role for transforming growth factor-β (TGF-β) in experimental silicosis using immunohistochemical techniques (26). TGF-β has been localized in peribronchiolar fibrotic lesions, hyaline centers of nodules, PMF lesions, fibroblasts, and alveolar macrophages of human silicotic lungs (27). TGF-β apparently participates in the genesis of silicosis by stimulating the production of profibrotic factors, collagen and fibronectin, and factors that inhibit breakdown of these substances. Other cytokines and cytokine networks may participate in processes that initiate or perpetuate inflammation and fibrogenesis (28).

Several studies have examined the human pulmonary cellular responses in silicosis. BAL performed in sandblasters with complicated silicosis showed no difference in cell numbers, viability, or adherence of macrophages when compared to controls (29). Similar findings were shown in a study of BAL fluid obtained from healthy granite workers (30). In this study the majority of alveolar macrophages contained granite dust, as demonstrated by polarized light microscopy. The identity of the particles was subsequently confirmed by scanning electron microscopy and x-ray energy spectrometry to be silicon. In another study of workers exposed to silica, intracellular dust particles, increased ruffling, and filopodia were demonstrated in alveolar macrophages obtained by BAL (31). It is thought that these morphologic changes in the macrophages represent cell activation following ingestion of these inorganic particles.

Since pulmonary fibrosis is not a prominent feature of acute silicosis, the pathogenesis of the diseases may be different from that of classic or chronic silicosis. In acute silicosis, the alveoli fill with an amorphous lipoproteinaceous exudate. Animal models of this condition show a dramatic increase in the amounts of intracellular and extracellular phospholipids (32–34). The composition of lung surfactant is also altered (35). A distinct population of hypertrophic type II pneumocytes has been observed in experimental acute silicosis. These cells appear to be responsible for the marked increase in the amount of pulmonary surfactant in the silica-treated animals (36,37). In addition to the increased activity of metabolic pathways involved in surfactant production, increased biosynthesis of surfactant protein A (SP-A) and augmented levels of SP-A messenger ribonucleic acid (mRNA) have also been shown (38)

It is interesting to speculate on why exposure to silica can produce different responses in animals and humans (i.e., why some develop nodules and fibrosis alone while others develop a more extensive and clinically serious form of silicosis such as silicoproteinosis). There may be host factors that are not yet identified. For example, in one study experimental exposure to a high concentration of quartz dust produced an alveolar proteinosis response in specific pathogen-free (SPF) rats, but resulted in the typical granulomatous and fibrotic changes in ordinary stock rats (39). The only difference seemed to be an inadequately developed lymphatic system in the SPF rats. Whether this has any human correlates or whether it has significance in the pathophysiology of acute silicosis is not known. On the other hand, the difference in the histopathologic and clinical responses may be due to certain characteristics of the inhaled material itself. For example, using techniques that measure electron spin resonance (ESR), it has been shown that much higher concentrations of silicon-based radicals (SiO and Si) are generated by freshly crushed silica than by aged silica (40). These silicon-based radicals react with water to form hydroxyl radicals, which are well known to be reactive oxygen species (along with superoxide, hydrogen peroxide, and singlet oxygen) that play an important role in the pathogenesis of many forms of oxidant-induced lung injury (41). Indeed, freshly crushed silica was more cytotoxic, produced more lipid per-oxidation, and induced alveolar macrophages to produce more superoxide and hydrogen peroxide than did stored silica (40). These findings may be relevant to the observation that acute silicosis is seen more frequent in industrial activities where silica is fractured or crushed, such as sandblasting and hard rock drilling.

## CLINICAL PRESENTATION, DIAGNOSIS, AND NATURAL HISTORY

The clinical diagnosis of silicosis has three requisites: first, the recognition by the physician that silica exposure adequate to cause this disease has occurred; second, the presence of chest radiographic abnormalities consistent with silicosis; and third, the absence of other illnesses that may mimic silicosis. For example, miliary tuberculosis or pulmonary fungal infection may appear radiographically identical to silicosis. In such cases, an extensive history and microbiologic workup to identify infectious pathogens could help better understand the cause of the radiographic abnormalities. Open lung biopsy is not needed to make the diagnosis of silicosis in the great majority of cases. However, in cases where the exposures and clinical presentations are atypical, biopsy, BAL, and scanning electron microscopy combined with analytic techniques such as energy-dispersive x-ray analysis may be needed for accurate diagnosis of the disease (42). Figure 4 shows a scanning electron micrograph of silica particles.

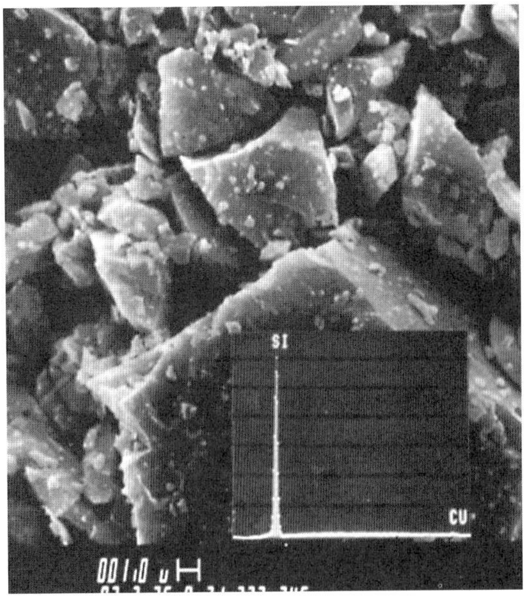


**FIG. 4.** Scanning electron micrograph of silica particles, which are irregular and sharp. *Inset* shows the silicon peak on energy dispersive x-ray analysis.

The presentation and severity of silicosis are influenced by multiple factors, principally the concentration of free crystalline silica in the workplace, the duration of exposure, and the physical characteristics and innate fibrogenic properties of the respirable dust (i.e., the fraction of crystalline silica in the dust). Genetic factors, cigarette smoking (43), and additional complicating pulmonary diseases are among the host factors that interact with the environment in an apparently complex and poorly understood fashion resulting in a spectrum of disease presentations. For these reasons it is critical to recognize the features of classic silicosis, acute silicosis, and accelerated silicosis.

### Classic Silicosis

Classic silicosis is the most frequently recognized clinical presentation of silicosis. This results from low to moderate exposure to silica dust for 20 years or more, although cases where the exposure occurred for 10 years or less have been reported (9). The extent of classic silicosis is described by the degree of radiographic chest involvement (see below). In the lesser radiographic categories, silicosis does not typically cause impairment, although patients may complain of cough, sputum production, and dyspnea as a result of industrial bronchitis or concurrent cigarette smoking. Only in the most advanced radiographic categories of classic silicosis without progressive massive fibrosis is respiratory impairment attributable to silica exposure. The primary health concerns associated with mild classic silicosis are a predisposition to mycobacterial infections and disabling progressive massive fibrosis.

Progressive massive fibrosis typically causes respiratory impairment. Large opacities develop in the upper lung zones, usually on an extensive background of small, rounded nodules. The result is restriction of lung volumes, decreased pulmonary compliance, and diminution of gas transfer. Initially dyspnea occurs with exercise, but the condition progresses to dyspnea at rest as more lung is involved. Cor pulmonale develops as the illness progresses. Mycobacterial infection is always a concern. Development of such an infectious process in this clinical setting can radically worsen chest symptoms, accelerate lung function decline, and alter the chest radiograph.

The stiff lungs and basilar emphysema associated with progressive massive fibrosis increase the risk of developing spontaneous pneumothorax. This can result in a precipitous worsening of preexisting hypoxemia and could be life threatening. The problem is exacerbated by the impaired ability of the poorly compliant lung to reexpand. In complicated silicosis, death is commonly attributable to progressive respiratory insufficiency.

### Accelerated Silicosis

Accelerated silicosis results from exposure to higher concentrations of silica over a period of 5 to 10 years (Fig. 5). Progression is virtually certain, even if the worker is removed from the workplace. Furthermore, antinuclear antibodies and clinical autoimmune connective tissue diseases such as scleroderma, rheumatoid arthritis, and systemic lupus erythematosus are frequently associated with accelerated silicosis.

### Acute Silicosis

Acute silicosis, the least frequent yet the most devastating form of this disease, results from exposure to over-

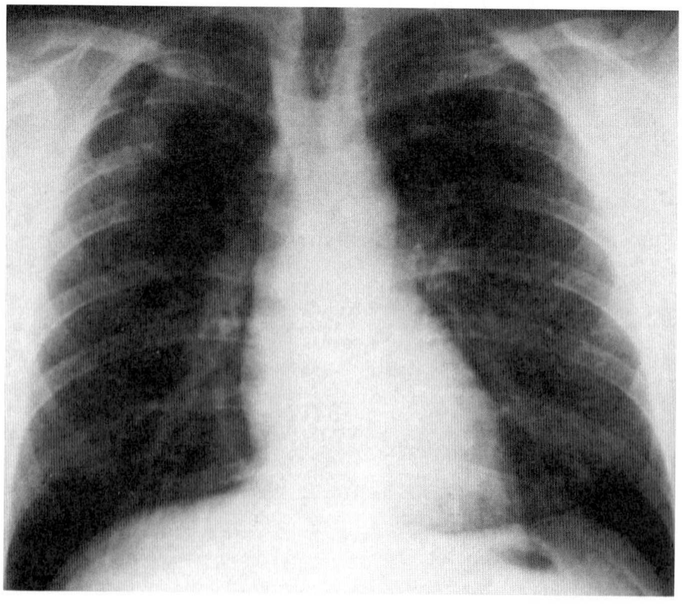

**FIG. 5.** Chest radiograph of a 31-year-old man who worked as a surface driller for 5 years. The clinical presentation was that of accelerated silicosis. Aside from a background of small rounded opacities, note the appearance of conglomerate opacities in the outer portions of both lung fields.

whelmingly excessive concentrations of free crystalline silica for as little as a few years or even 1 year. It was described in Britain by Middleton (44) in 1929 as a syndrome of rapidly progressing respiratory illness occurring after 2½ to 4 years' exposure to silica dust. In 1930, MacDonald et al. (45) reported on two young women in a London factory who packed a kind of cleaning powder containing ground silica. Both had also worked for brief periods (2¾ years and 4¼ years) in this industry and they died from silica-induced respiratory failure. At autopsy the patients' lungs were noted to be heavy. Microscopic examination revealed that the alveoli were filled with desquamated cells and an "albuminous" exudate. The authors proposed that the histologic changes resulted from the formation of colloidal silica and insoluble silicates. Soon after these reports, similar cases of pneumoconiosis occurring after brief exposures in the abrasive soap manufacturing industry were published in the United States (46,47), culminating in a review by Ritterhoff (48) in 1941. In 1969, Buechner and Ansari (12) described four sandblasters who worked for 3 to 6 years and developed progressive air space disease characterized by intraalveolar deposits of a proteinaceous, PAS-staining exudate, and they used the term *silicoproteinosis* to describe the lesions. Since then, there have been reports of acute silicosis in other silica-exposed workers such as tombstone sandblasters (49), surface drillers (50), silica flour workers (51), and oil pipe sandblasters (10). All affected workers had a very excessive exposure to crystalline silica over a relatively short period.

The invariable downhill clinical course of acute silicosis includes relentless dyspnea, cor pulmonale, and pulmonary cachexia. Serial lung function tests show progressive restriction of lung volumes and impairment of diffusing capacity. This form of silicosis is fatal, and death is typically attributable to respiratory failure within several years of beginning exposure.

## RADIOLOGY

The clinical presentation of silicosis (classic, accelerated, or acute) is based on the time course necessary for the development of disease. The type of chest radiographic lesions, however, does not seem to correlate well with the duration of exposure. For example, conglomerate lesions may be found in a worker exposed for only 5 years, whereas small rounded opacities may be the only radiographic lesions in a worker who has been exposed for more than 20 years.

The characteristic radiographic pattern of simple silicosis is the presence of rounded opacities that range in size from 1 to 10 mm (Fig. 6). Using the 1980 convention described by the International Labour Organization's (ILO) International Classification of Radiographs of the Pneumoconioses, these small rounded opacities are grouped into three diameter ranges designated as $p$ (up to 1.5 mm), $q$ (exceeding 1.5 and up to 3 mm), and $r$ (exceeding 3 and up to 10 mm) (52). In the lower-profusion categories these opacities are most often in the upper lung zones. In the more advanced stages of the disease, the middle and lower lung zones typically are also involved.

In complicated or conglomerate silicosis, also described as progressive massive fibrosis, smaller lesions coalesce into large ones and opacities exceeding 10 mm in diameter are recognized on the chest radiograph (Fig. 7). The 1980 ILO classification categorizes these as A (10 to 50 mm diameter or several opacities

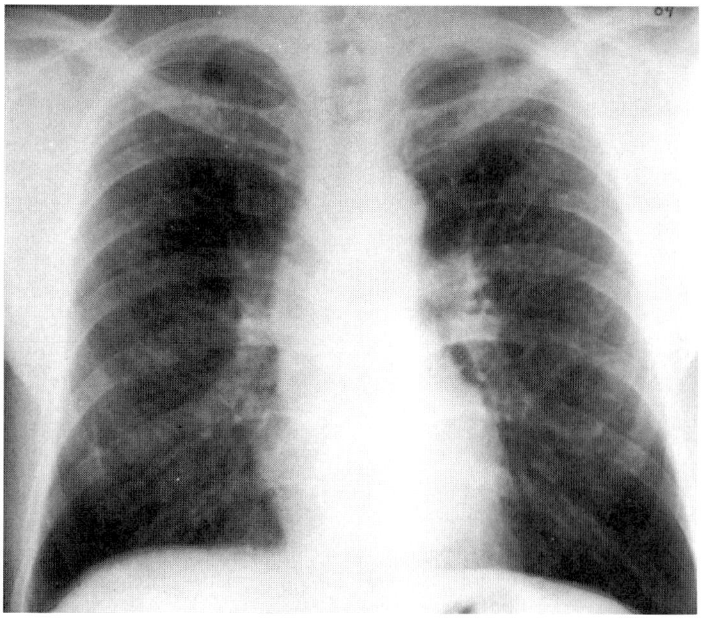

**FIG. 6.** Chest radiograph in a 56-year-old surface miner shows simple silicosis. The radiographic lesions consist principally of small rounded opacities distributed throughout the upper, middle, and most of the lower lung zones. Bilateral hilar prominence.

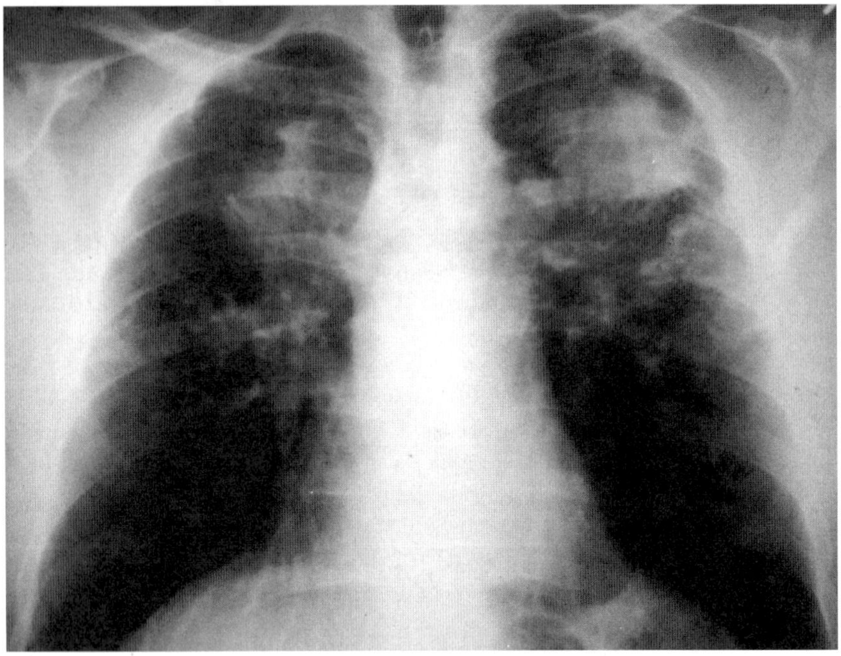

**FIG. 7.** Chest radiograph shows progressive massive fibrosis in silicosis. Large mass-like opacities are present in both upper lobes. There is bilateral hilar retraction and basilar hyperlucency.

greater than 10 mm but less than 50 mm aggregate diameter), B (one or more opacities larger or more numerous than category A but not exceeding the equivalent of the right upper zone), and C (one or more large opacities whose combined area exceeds the equivalent of the right upper zone). These large opacities tend to retract toward the hilus, resulting in subpleural areas of air space enlargement. The clear area between the lateral border of the opacity and the chest wall appears as a bulla. Since coalescence of these nodules occurs in the upper zones, the result is loss of upper zone volume, elevation of both hila, and the development of basilar emphysematous changes. While cavitation of these coalesced lesions may be explained by ischemia, tuberculosis or carcinoma with necrosis should also be considered in the differential diagnosis. These distinctions are not always easy to make on a clinical basis.

Enlargement of hilar lymph nodes is common. In 5% to 10% of cases, the hilar nodes calcify circumferentially, producing the so-called eggshell pattern of calcification. This is not pathognomonic of silicosis, as it has also been described in sarcoidosis, postirradiation Hodgkin's disease, blastomycosis, scleroderma, amyloidosis, and histoplasmosis (53). However, the presence of eggshell hilar

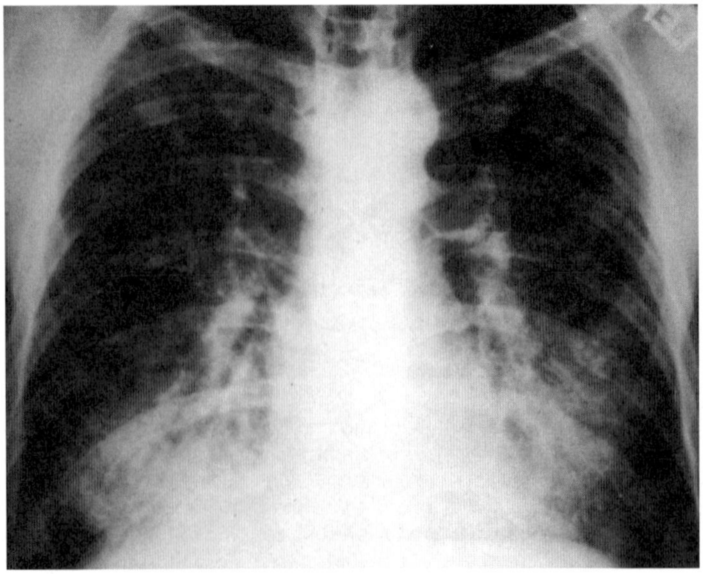

**FIG. 8.** Radiographic appearance of acute silicosis. Air space densities with bronchograms are seen in both lower lung zones.

calcifications in the presence of typically distributed nodular parenchymal opacities reinforces the clinical impression of silicosis when there is an appropriate exposure history.

Acute silicosis or silicoproteinosis presents radiographically with varying degrees of air space filling (Fig. 8). The radiographic differential diagnosis includes pneumonias and other pulmonary infections, pulmonary edema, alveolar hemorrhage, alveolar cell cancer, and idiopathic alveolar proteinosis. Several studies have examined the role of computed tomography (CT) of the thorax in the diagnosis of silicosis. Begin et al. (54) studied a group of 58 granite or foundry workers in Quebec and compared conventional chest radiography and CT. There was a good correlation between the two techniques for parenchymal profusion scores, although some workers without CT changes showed minimal parenchymal opacities on the chest radiograph. The advantage of CT scan was its ability to demonstrate conglomerate densities that were not detectable on the routine chest radiograph. Bergin et al. (55) and Kinsella et al. (56) showed the same findings and demonstrated that decrements in pulmonary function correlated with the degree of emphysema and not with the profusion of parenchymal opacities attributable to silica exposure.

## PULMONARY FUNCTION

It is difficult to make definitive conclusions about the alterations in pulmonary function in workers with silicosis, since considerable variability in individual cases may be present, probably because of the multifactorial effects of concurrent cigarette smoking, the type of dusts involved in the exposure (mixed versus pure), the dose of dust and duration of exposure, and the presence of other pulmonary diseases such as tuberculosis.

In general, when the radiographs show only small rounded opacities of low profusion, no significant impairment in ventilatory capacity is associated. Abnormalities in spirometry can usually be explained by concurrent cigarette smoking or dust-induced bronchitis. Studies of different groups of workers tend to support this generalization, especially when care is taken to choose appropriate controls or to account for the effects of coexisting factors such as those mentioned above. When these precautions were taken, for example, no significant differences in forced vital capacity (FVC) or forced expiratory volume in 1 second ($FEV_1$) were demonstrated in South African gold miners who had radiographic evidence of silicosis and those who did not (57). In a study of silicotic pottery workers in Hong Kong, there was no statistically significant gradient in percentage of predicted $FEV_1$ among the radiographic categories of simple silicosis in workers with and without symptoms of chronic bronchitis, although $FEV_1$ was lower in those with symptoms (58). $FEV_1$ was significantly lower as a percent predicted in those with conglomerate silicosis of B and C types compared to those who had simple silicosis. These trends were similar for those who had bronchitis and those who did not, though values were significantly lower for the former group. In this study, as in many others, significant impairment in total lung capacity, residual volume, and diffusion capacity tended to be associated with conglomerate disease. A similar patterns of pulmonary function abnormality was also shown in a study of silicotic sandblasters in Louisiana by Jones et al. (59). Studies of lung mechanics in silicosis patients show abnormalities in lung compliance, which tends to decrease as the severity of radiographic involvement increases (60).

As a rule, rapid and progressive decline in pulmonary function accompanies acute silicosis. This is well illustrated in the case of a 34-year-old surface coal mine driller who presented with progressive dyspnea, cough, weight loss, and bibasilar alveolar filling on the chest radiograph (50). His initial FVC was 3.47 L (63% of predicted), and the single-breath transfer factor was 6.32 ml/min/mm Hg (18% of predicted). After 10 months, the FVC had further decreased to 1.77 L, and the patient was unable to perform the diffusing capacity test due to dyspnea. A radiographic picture of progressive massive fibrosis had developed from the initial alveolar pattern. This man died 26 months after his initial presentation.

## COMPLICATIONS

### Mycobacterial Infections

The association between silicosis and pulmonary tuberculosis is well accepted. Epidemiologic studies suggest that the risk of pulmonary and extrapulmonary tuberculosis is increased about threefold in workers who have silicosis compared to those who do not (61,62). The incidence of tuberculosis increases with the profusion of radiographic opacities. One study an increased incidence of pulmonary tuberculosis in foundry workers who did not have radiographic evidence of silicosis but were employed in the industry longer than 25 years (61).

Mycobacterial infection should always be suspected when a silicosis patient experiences worsening of respiratory symptoms or chest radiographs (Fig. 9). Yearly tuberculin tests are important in the follow-up of patients with silicosis. A positive result on an intermediate purified protein derivative (PPD) test or radiographic evidence of progression of the silicotic abnormalities mandates a search for mycobacteria. If acid-fast smears are negative in the presence of a positive tuberculin test, the American Thoracic Society and the Centers for Disease Control recommend treatment with 300 mg of isoniazid daily for a year or a 4-month course of a mutlidrug regimen (63). Poor compliance and the concern of isoniazid resistance has generated interest in shorter, multidrug chemopro-

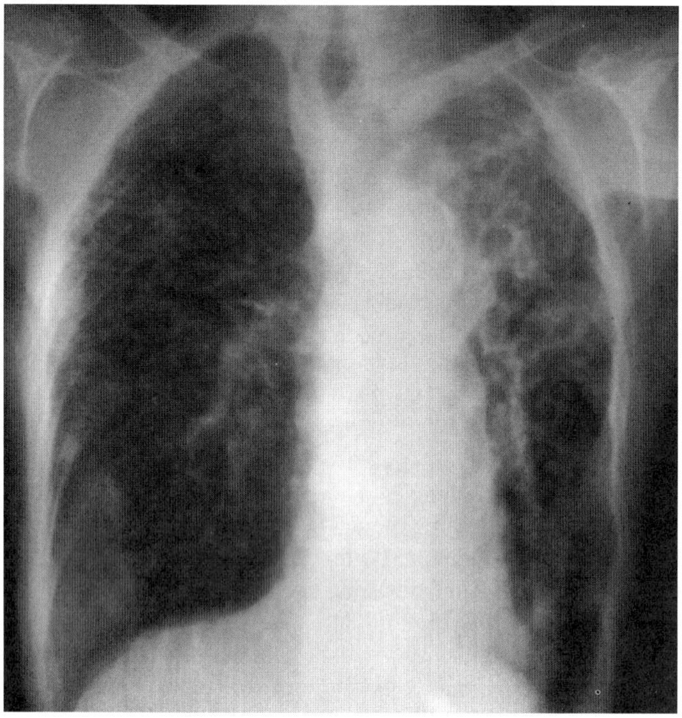

**FIG. 9.** Chest radiograph on an 80-year-old woman who worked in a pottery factory for 40 years. She was known to have simple silicosis for many years but developed increasing dyspnea and a deteriorating appearance on chest radiographs. Acid-fast bacilli were seen in the sputum smears and were identified later as *Mycobacterium tuberculosis.*

phylaxis regimens, and recent studies have highlighted the importance of directly observed therapy (64).

Smear or culture-positive silicotics should be treated with multiple antituberculous drugs. Effective regimens generally contain isoniazid, rifampin, and pyrazinamide. Older studies suggest that antituberculous chemotherapy should be given for an extended period, ranging from more than a year to a lifetime (65). Recent articles show successful outcomes and acceptable relapse rates with shorter treatment regimens (66,67). One study suggested that silicotics with tuberculosis do better when the usual multidrug regimen is given for 8 months (68). It is prudent, however, to guide therapy by frequent clinical and radiographic examinations as well as smear and culture responses.

Infections with atypical mycobacteria such as *Mycobacterium kansasii* and *Mycobacterium avium-intracellulare* have also been reported (69). The frequency at which these atypical mycobacterial infections are found is probably related to the geographic distribution of the organisms.

### Immune-Mediated Complications

Associations between silicosis and progressive systemic sclerosis scleroderma or rheumatoid arthritis are well described in the literature (70–72). Serologic studies show a high prevalence of antinuclear antibodies, rheumatoid factor, and other markers of an activated humoral immune system such as immune complexes and immunoglobulins (73,74). Whether and how these factors, or the immune system in general, plays a direct role in the genesis of silicotic lesions, and whether tissue injury related to silicosis predisposes a person to autoimmune disease are matters of speculation.

### Renal Complications

A variety of renal complications have been described in association with silicosis. The clinical spectrum of silicon nephropathy includes glomerulonephritis, nephrotic syndrome, end-stage renal disease requiring dialysis, and in one report a presentation mimicking Fabry's disease (75,76). On light microscopy, glomerular sclerosis, hypercellularity, crescents, cellular inflammatory infiltrates, and tubule damage have been seen. Electron microscopic lesions include obliteration of foot processes, cytoplasmic dense lysosomes, electron-dense deposits, and myelinlike bodies. Evidence of immune system activation is frequently present in serum and in the glomeruli.

### Cancer

Many animal and human epidemiologic studies have addressed the issue of whether exposure to crystalline silica plays a role in the development of pulmonary neoplasms. Animal studies have shown that rats given intrapleural silica develop malignant histiocytic lymphoma (77,78), and intratracheal administration can result in respiratory neoplasms that resemble human bronchogenic carcinoma (79). Older epidemiologic data reached conflicting conclusions regarding the association of silica exposure and lung cancer (80). The discrepancies in conclusions from these studies were thought to be related to sampling methods or to the fact that many of these studies did not account for the effects of cigarette smoke or radon exposure in underground mines. Based on such information, the International Agency for Research on Cancer (IARC) working group met in 1986 and concluded that there was sufficient evidence for the carcinogenicity of crystalline silica in experimental animals but only limited evidence in human beings (81). Crystalline silica was classified as 2A—probably carcinogenic to humans (82).

Since 1986, additional studies have addressed the issue of whether silicosis predisposes to lung cancer (83–88). These and other studies have been analyzed in a review written by Weill and McDonald (89) and by the American Thoracic Society (90). Like the older studies, the strength of the association is weakened by potential confounding exposures to other environmental carcinogens. The studies on refractory brick manufacturers in Genoa, Italy, and diatomaceous earth miners in California provide strong clues that exposure to crystalline silica itself may be linked to excess deaths from respiratory neoplasms (91,92). These epidemiologic studies led to the reclassification of silica in 1996 as a group I substance by the IARC, i.e., inhaled crystalline silica in the form of quartz or cristobalite from occupational sources is carcinogenic to humans (90,93).

## TREATMENT

The diagnosis of silicosis, especially if it is progressive, is always a source of tremendous frustration for both clinician and patient, since there is no proven effective therapy for this disease. Symptomatic airflow obstruction is treated with inhaled bronchodilators. Antibiotics are empirically given to patients with acute bronchitis. Oxygen is used to manage hypoxemia and the associated pulmonary hypertension.

Numerous investigators have attempted to deal therapeutically with the primary problem in silicosis, the presence of free crystalline silica in the lung and the resulting inflammatory cascade, which is aggravated or perpetuated by cells or the fibrogenic mediators they produce. In an attempt to reduce the dust burden and the number of activated macrophages and other effector cells, Mason and colleagues (94) performed a whole lung lavage (WLL) in a foundry worker. This patient improved symptomatically, although no significant changes in pulmonary function were measured. Chinese investigators have the largest series of cases of workers with coal workers' pneumoconiosis treated with WLL (95). Their technique involves the use of general anesthesia and the use of a double-lumen endotracheal tube to lavage one lung with 1,000- to 2,000-ml aliquots of saline 10 to 15 times while ventilating the other lung. In patients with minimal disease, both lungs are lavaged sequentially in the same session. Those with more severe disease have each lung lavaged in separate sessions. Close auscultatory monitoring of the ventilated lung to prevent and detect overflow from the lung being lavaged, as well as positive pressure bag ventilation with 100% oxygen after infusion, are important safety measures.

More recent use of WLL in silicosis in the United States is reported by Wilt and colleagues (96,97). These investigators estimated that nearly 2 g of dust was removed from a lung of a coal miner with category 2 pneumoconiosis. This amount of dust is thought to approximate the mineral dust burden in the ashed lungs of coal miners with a similar extent of pneumoconiosis profusion score (98). While published work of WLL as a modality in the treatment of pneumoconiosis shows that the procedure itself is safe, it is too early to speculate on whether it has significant and long-lasting therapeutic benefit, or whether it alters the natural history of the disease.

Corticosteroids and immunosuppressive agents have been used to treat accelerated and acute silicosis. Although there is a suggestion that the inflammatory process is at least lessened, whether this pharmacologic approach affects long-term outcome is not clear. If steroid therapy is instituted, tuberculosis prophylaxis with isoniazid is probably prudent until cultures definitely show the absence of mycobacterial infection (99). In a 6-month trial of prednisolone for the treatment of chronic simple and complicated silicosis in 34 patients in northern India, there were statistically significant (although not clinically significant) improvements in lung volumes, diffusing capacity ($D_LCO$), and partial pressure of arterial oxygen ($PaO_2$), and a decrease in total cell count in BAL fluid (100).

Other therapies investigated in animal models and humans include inhalation of aluminum, and inhalational or parenteral administration of a polymer, polyvinyl pyridine N-oxide (PVNO) (101–103). Inhaled aluminum has not been shown to be effective in human disease and in a sheep model of chronic silicosis (104). While PVNO was shown to have some beneficial effects in some experimental models, there is some concern that it could be carcinogenic. More aggressive therapies have also been tried. A case of unilateral lung transplantation in a 23-year-old man with acute silicosis was reported in 1972 (105). Lung function and gas exchange improved and the patient survived 10 months. With the current advances in transplantation medicine, this option should therefore be considered seriously for individuals with far advanced silicosis.

In Chinese traditional medicine *hanfangji,* an extract of the root of the plant *Stephania tetrandria,* has been used to treat rheumatic diseases. The principal active component of the extract is tetrandrine, a bisbenzylisoquinoline with the empirical formula $C_{38}H_{42}O_6N_2$. Tetrandrine has been shown to inhibit and even reverse pulmonary lesions in experimental silicosis (106). An open clinical trial showed clinical and radiographic improvement in patients with pulmonary fibrosis from silica inhalation (107). While the exact mechanism of the antifibrotic properties of tetrandrine is not established, it has in vitro antiphagocytic and antioxidant properties (108) and inhibits human neutrophil and monocyte adherence (109). More recent work has demonstrated that tetrandrine is a potent inhibitor of particle-stimulated oxygen consumption, superoxide release, and hydrogen peroxide production by rat alveolar macrophages. The inhibition of these inflammatory mechanisms is strongly correlated with tetrandrine's binding affinity to alveolar macrophages (110).

Finally, the only reasonable way to deal with this man-made illness is to prevent it. As a consequence of reduced dust standards and better industrial hygiene practices, silicosis afflicts far fewer people that it did before. The Occupational Safety and Health Administration (OSHA) has set the permissible exposure limit (PEL) for respirable silica at 10 mg/m$^3$ divided by (%$SiO_2$ + 2) or 250 million particles per cubic foot divided by (%$SiO_2$ + 5), superseding the previous standard of 0.1 mg/m$^3$ respirable silica (111). Adherence to this standard will undoubtedly reduce the number of new cases, although some studies suggest that this exposure level may still be unacceptably high (112,113). A lower PEL standard of 0.05 mg/m$^3$ is recommended by the National Institute for Occupational Safety and Health (NIOSH) (114). In places where microcrystalline silica is handled, special attention to the proper use of respiratory protection devices will have a tremendous impact on preventing this disease. The fact that this can be overlooked is seen in Fig. 10. Prohibition of abrasive blasting with silica-containing material might be the more pragmatic and only effective way of decreasing the incidence of this disease in this population of workers. The NIOSH has circulated a number of publications addressing the prevention of silicosis by focusing on an awareness of silica as a workplace hazard, environmental controls, personal protection, and medical monitoring (115–117).

Silicosis is preventable. The extent to which this can be realized depends on education of employers and employees, strict enforcement of industrial hygiene practices, and vigilance for circumstances where unacceptable exposures to respirable silica may happen. Further research on the mechanism of lung injury in silicosis and its modulation by pharmacologic agents will contribute to our therapeutic armamentarium for this disease.

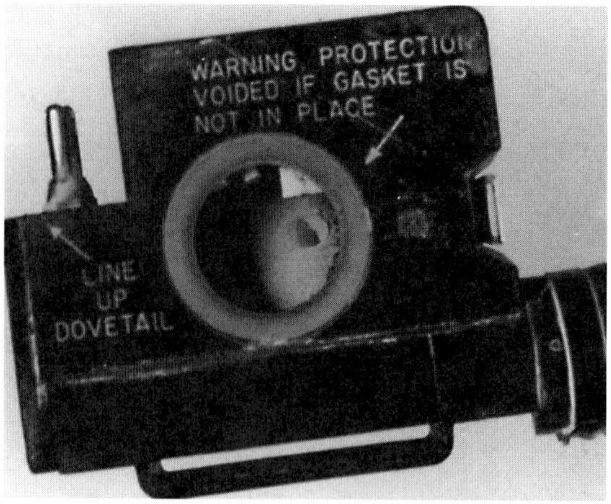


**FIG. 10.** This improperly used and maintained respiratory protection device shows fine silica particles inside the apparatus. It illustrates how even sophisticated technologic protective devices are sometimes inadequate in preventing workers from being exposed to respirable fine silica particles.

## ACKNOWLEDGMENTS

This work is supported in part by the National Institute for Occupational Safety and Health (NIOSH) grants U60/CCU306149-01, U60/CCU313020-01, and U.S. Bureau of Mines grant G1105142.

## REFERENCES

1. Holt P. Silicosis. In: Holt P, ed. *Inhaled dust and disease.* New York: Wiley, 1987;46–85.
2. Corn J. Historical aspects of industrial hygiene-silicosis. *Am Ind Hyg Assoc J* 1980;41:125–132.
3. Lapp N. Lung disease secondary to inhalation of nonfibrous minerals. *Clin Chest Med* 1981;2:219–233.
4. Trasko V. Some facts on the prevalence of silicosis in the United States. *Arch Ind Health* 1956;14:379–387.
5. Green F, Althouse R, Weber K. Prevalence of silicosis at death in underground coal miners. *Am J Ind Med* 1989;16:605–615.
6. Banks D, Morring K. Silicosis in the 1980's. *Am Ind Hyg Assoc J* 1981;42:77–89.
7. NIOSH. *Work-related lung diseases surveillance report* 1991. DHHS (NIOSH) publication 91-113.
8. Banks D, Balaan M, Wang M. Silicosis in the 1990s, Revisited. *Chest* 1997;111:837–838.
9. Rosenman K, Reilly M, Kalinowsky D. Silicosis in the 1990s. *Chest* 1997;111:779–86.
10. Silicosis: cluster in sandblasters—Texas and occupational surveillance of silicosis. *MMWR* 1990;39(5).
11. Silicosis and Silicate Disease Committee. Diseases associated with exposure to silica and nonfibrous silicate minerals. *Arch Pathol Lab Med* 1988;112:673–720.
12. Buechner H, Ansari A. Acute silicosis. *Dis Chest* 1969;55:274–284.
13. Hoffman E, Lamberry, Pizzolato P, Coover J. The ultrastructure of acute silicosis. *Arch Pathol* 1973;96:104–107.
14. Allison A, Harrington J, Birbeck M. An examination of the cytotoxic effects of silica on macrophages. *J Exp Med* 1966;124:141–154.
15. Bowden D, Adamson L. The role of cell injury and the continuing inflammatory response in the generation of silicotic pulmonary fibrosis. *J Pathol* 1981;144:149–161.
16. Lugano E, Dauber J, Danielle R. Acute experimental silicosis. *Am J Pathol* 1982;109:27–36.
17. Heppleston A, Styles J. Activity of a macrophage factor in collagen formation by silica. *Nature* 1967;214:521.

18. Schmidt J, Oliver C, Lepe-Zuniga J, Gery I. Silica-stimulated monocytes release fibroblast proliferation factors identical to interleukin 1. A potential role for interleukin 1 in the pathogenesis of silicosis. *J Clin Invest* 1984;73:1462–1472.
19. Oghiso Y, Kubota Y. Enhanced interleukin 1 production by alveolar macrophages in Ia-positive lung cells in silica-exposed rats. *Microbiol Immunol* 1986;30:1189–1198.
20. Piquet P, MACollart, Grau J, Sappino A, Vassalli P. Requirement of tumour necrosis factor for development of silica-induced pulmonary fibrosis. *Nature* 1990;344:245–247.
21. Dubois C, Bissonette E, Rola-Pleszynski M. Asbestos fibers and silica particles stimulate rat alveolar macrophages to release tumor necrosis factor. *Am Rev Respir Dis* 1989;139:1257–1264.
22. Piquet P, Vesin C. Treatment by human recombinant soluble TNF receptor of pulmonary fibrosis induced by bleomycin or silica in mice. *Eur Respir J* 1994;7:515–518.
23. Davis G, Hill-Eubanks L, Pfeiffer L, Leslie K, Hemenway D. Reduced silicosis in C3H/HeJ-LPSd mice: an implied role for cytokine production deficiency. *Am Rev Respir Dis* 1992;145:A325.
24. Savici D, He B, Geist L, Monick M, Hunninghake G. Silica Increases tumor necrosis factor (TNF) production, in part, by upregulating the TNF promoter. *Exp Lung Res* 1994;20:613–625.
25. Claudio E, Segade F, Wrobel K, Ramos S, Lazo P. Activation of Murine Macrophages by Silica Particles In vitro Is a Process Independent of Silica-induced Cell Death. *Am J Respir Cell Mol Biol* 1995;13:547–554.
26. Williams AO, Flanders KC, Saffiotti U. Immunohistochemical localization of transforming growth factor-beta 1 in rats with experimental silicosis, alveolar type II hyperplasia, and lung cancer. *Am J Pathol* 1993;142(6):1831–40.
27. Jagirdar J, Begin R, Dufresne A, Goswami S, Lee T, Rom W. Transforming growth factor-β in silicosis. *Am J Respir Crit Care Med* 1996; 154:1076–81.
28. Vanhee D, Gosset P, Boitelle A, Wallaert B, Tonnel A. Cytokines and cytokine network in silicosis and coal workers' pneumoconiosis. *Eur Respir J* 1995;8:834–842.
29. Schuyler M, Gaumer H, Stankus R, Kaimal J, Hoffman E, Salvaggio J. Bronchoalveolar lavage in silicosis. *Lung* 1980;157:95–102.
30. Christman J, Emerson R, Graham W, Davis G. Mineral dust and cell recovery from the bronchoalveolar lavage of healthy Vermont granite workers. *Am Rev Respir Dis* 1985;132:393–399.
31. Takemura T, Rom W, Ferrans V, Crystal R. Morphologic characterization of alveolar macrophages from subjects with occupational exposure to inorganic particles. *Am Rev Respir Dis* 1989;140:1674–1685.
32. Heppleston A, Fletcher K, Wyatt I. Changes in the composition of lung lipids and the turnover of dipalmitoyl lecithin in experimental alveolar lipoproteinosis induced by inhaled quartz. *Br J Exp Pathol* 1974;55:384–395.
33. Gabor S, Zugravu E, Kovats A, Bohm B, Andrasoni D. Effects of quartz on lung surfactant. *Environ Res* 1978;16:443–448.
34. Dethloff L, Gilmore L, Brody A, Hook G. Induction of intra- and extracellular phospholipids in the lungs of rats exposed to silica. *Biochem J* 1986;233:111–118.
35. Kawada H, Horiuchi T, Shannon J, Kuroki Y, Voelker D, Mason R. Alveolar type II cells, surfactant protein A (SP-A), and the phospholipid components of surfactant in acute silicosis in the rat. *Am Rev Respir Dis* 1989;140:460–470.
36. Miller B, Dethloff L, Hook G. Silica-induced hypertrophy of type II cells in the lungs of rats. *Lab Invest* 1986;55:153–163.
37. Miller B, Dethloff L, Gladen B, Hook G. Progression of type II cell hypertrophy and hyperplasia during silica-induced pulmonary inflammation. *Lab Invest* 1987;57:546–554.
38. Miller B, Bakewell W, Katyal S, Singh G, Hook G. Induction of surfactant protein A (SP-A) biosynthesis and SP-A mRNA in activated type II cells during acute silicosis in rats. *Am J Respir Cell Mol Biol* 1990;3:217–226.
39. Eden K, Seebach Hv. Atypical dust-induced pneumoconiosis in SPF rats. *Virchows Arch (Pathol Anat)* 1976;372:1–9.
40. Vallyathan V, Xianglin S, Dalal N, Irr W, Castranova V. Generation of free radicals from freshly fractured silica dust. *Am Rev Respir Dis* 1988;138:1213–1219.
41. Heffner J, Repine J. Pulmonary strategies of oxidant defense-state of the art. *Am Rev Respir Dis* 1989;140:531–554.
42. Nugent K, Dodson R, Idell S, Devillier J. The utility of bronchoalveolar lavage and transbronchial lung biopsy combined with energy-dispersive x-ray analysis in the diagnosis of silicosis. *Am Rev Respir Dis* 1989;140:1438–1441.
43. Kreiss K, Greenberg L, Kogut S, Lezotte D, Irvin C, Cherniack R. Hard-rock mining exposures affect smokers and nonsmokers differently. *Am Rev Respir Dis* 1989;139:1487–1493.
44. Middleton E. The present position of silicosis in industry in Britain. *Br Med J* 1929;2:485–489.
45. McDonald G, Piggot A, Gilder F. Two cases of acute silicosis. *Lancet* 1930;2:846–847.
46. Chapman E. Acute silicosis. *JAMA* 1932;98:1439–1441.
47. Kilgore E. Pneumoconiosis-an unusually acute form. *JAMA* 1932;99: 1414–1416.
48. Ritterhoff R. Acute silicosis. *Am Rev Tuber* 1941;43:117–131.
49. Suratt P, Winn W, Brody A, Bolton W, Giles R. Acute silicosis in tombstone sandblasters. *Am Rev Respir Dis* 1977;115:521–529.
50. Banks D, Bauer M, Castellan R, Lapp N. Silicosis in surface coalmine drillers. *Thorax* 1983;38:275–278.
51. Banks D, Morring K, Boehlecke B, Althouse R, Merchant J. Silicosis in silica flour workers. *Am Rev Respir Dis* 1981;124:445–450.
52. International Labour Organization. *Guidelines for the use of ILO international classification of radiographs of pneumoconioses,* rev. ed. Occupational Safety and Health Series No. 2. Geneva: International Labour Office, 1980.
53. Gross B, Schneider H, Proto A. Eggshell calcification of lymph nodes: an update. *AJR* 1980;135:1265–1268.
54. Begin R, Bergeron D, Samson L, Boctor M, Cantin A. CT assessment of silicosis in exposed workers. *AJR* 1987;148:509–514.
55. Bergin C, Muller N, Vedal S, M C-Y. CT in silicosis: correlation of plain films and pulmonary function tests. *AJR* 1986;146:477–483.
56. Kinsella M, Muller N, Vedal S, Staples C. Emphysema in silicosis. A comparison of smokers with nonsmokers using pulmonary function and computed tomography. *Am Rev Respir Dis* 1990;141:1497–1500.
57. Irwig L, Rocks P. Lung function and respiratory symptoms in silicotic and nonsilicotic gold miners. *Am Rev Respir Dis* 1978;117: 429–435.
58. Prowse K, Allen M, Bradbury S. Respiratory symptoms and pulmonary impairment in male and female subjects with pottery workers'silicosis. *Ann Occup Hyg* 1989;3:375–385.
59. Jones R, Weill H, Ziskind M. Pulmonary function in sandblasters' silicosis. *Bull Physiopathol Respir* 1975;11:589–595.
60. Teculescu D, Stanescu D, Pilat L. Pulmonary mechanics in silicosis. *Arch Environ Health* 1967;14:461–468.
61. Sherson D, Lander F. Morbidity of pulmonary tuberculosis among silicotic and nonsilicotic foundry workers in Denmark. *J Occup Med* 1990;32:110–113.
62. Cowie R. The Epidemiology of Tuberculosis in Gold Miners with Silicosis. *Am J Respir Crit Care Med* 1994;150:1460–2.
63. American Thoracic Society. Treatment of tuberculosis and tuberculous infection in adults and children. *Am J Respir Crit Care Med* 1994;149:1359–1374.
64. Cowie R. Short course chemoprophylaxis with rifampicin, isoniazid and pyrazinamide for tuberculosis evaluated in gold miners with chronic silicosis: a double-blind placebo controlled trial. *Tuberc Lung Dis* 1996;77:239–243.
65. Morgan E. Silicosis and tuberculosis. *Chest* 1979;75:202–203.
66. Lin T-P, Suo J, Lee C-N, Yang S. Short course chemotherapy for pulmonary tuberculosis in pneumoconiotic patients. *Am Rev Respir Dis* 1987;136:808–810.
67. Cowie R. Silicotuberculosis: long term outcome after short-course chemotherapy. *Tuberc Lung Dis* 1995;76:39–42.
68. Hong Kong Chest Service/Tuberculosis Research Centre MBMRC. A controlled clinical comparison of 6 and 8 months of antituberculosis chemotherapy in the treatment of patients with silicotuberculosis in Hong Kong. *Am Rev Respir Dis* 1991;143:262–267.
69. Bailey W, Brown M, Buechner H, Weill H, Ichinose H, Ziskind M. Silicomycobacterial disease in sandblasters. *Am Rev Respir Dis* 1974; 110:115–125.
70. Rodnan G, Benedek R, Medsger T, Cammarata R. The association between progressive systemic sclerosis (scleroderma) with coal miners' pneumoconiosis and other forms of silicosis. *Ann Intern Med* 1967;66:323–334.
71. Sluis-Cremer G, Hessel P, Hnizdo E, Churchill A. The relationship between silicosis and rheumatoid arthritis. *Thorax* 1986;41:596–600.

72. Steenland K, Goldsmith D. Silica Exposure and Autoimmune Diseases. *Am J Ind Med* 1995;28:603–608.
73. Jones R, Turner-Warwick M, Ziskind M, Weill H. High prevalence of antinuclear antibodies in sandblasters' silicosis. *Am Rev Respir Dis* 1976;113:393–395.
74. Doll N, Stankus R, Hughes J. Immune complexes and autoantibodies in silicosis. *J Allergy Clin Immunol* 1981;68:281–285.
75. Bolton W, Suratt P, Surgill B. Rapidly progressive silicon nephropathy. *Am J Med* 1981;71:823–828.
76. Banks D, Multinovic J, Desnick R, Grabowski G, Lapp N, Boehlecke B. Silicon nephropathy mimicking Fabry's disease. *Am J Nephrol* 1983;3:279–284.
77. Wagner M, Wagner J. Lymphomas in the Wistar rat after intrapleural inoculation of silica. *J Natl Cancer Inst* 1972;49:89–91.
78. Wagner M, Wagner J, Davies R, et al. Silica-induced malignant histiocytic lymphoma: incidence linked with strain of rat and type of silica. *Br J Cancer* 1980;41:908–917.
79. Muhle H, Takenaka S, Mohr U, Dasenbrock C, Marmelstein R. Lung tumor induction upon long-term low-level inhalation of crystalline silica. *Am J Ind Med* 1989;15:343–346.
80. McDonald JC. Silica, silicosis, and lung cancer. *Br J Ind Med* 1989; 46(5):289–91.
81. International Agency for Cancer Research (IARC). Silica and some silicates 1987;42:39–143.
82. International Agency for Cancer Research (IARC). *Overall evaluations of carcinogenicity:* an updating of IARC monographs, vol 1-42. Lyon: World Health Organization (WHO), 1987(suppl 7).
83. Forastiere F, Lagorio S, Michelozzi P, et al. Silica, silicosis and lung cancer among ceramic workers: a case-referent study. *Am J Ind Med* 1986;10(4):363–370.
84. Mehnert WH, Staneczek W, Mohner M, et al. A mortality study of a cohort of slate quarry workers in the German Democratic Republic. *IARC Sci Publ* 1990(97):55–64.
85. McLaughlin J, Jing-Qiong C, Dosameci M, et al. A nested case-control study of lung cancer among silica exposed workers in China. *Am J Ind Med* 1992;49:167–171.
86. Mastrangelo G, Zambon P, Simonato L, Rizzi P. A case-referent study investigating the relationship between exposure to silica dust and lung cancer. *Int Arch Occup Environ Health* 1988;60(4):299–302.
87. Amandus H, Costello J. Silicosis and lung cancer in U.S. metal miners. *Arch Environ Health* 1991;46(2):82–89.
88. Amandus HE, Castellan RM, Shy C, Heineman EF, Blair A. Reevaluation of silicosis and lung cancer in North Carolina dusty trades workers. *Am J Ind Med* 1992;22(2):147–153.
89. Weill H, McDonald J. Exposure to crystalline silica and risk of lung cancer: the epidemiological evidence. *Thorax* 1996;51(1):97–102.
90. American Thoracic Society. Adverse effects of crystalline silica exposure. *Am J Respir Crit Care Med* 1997;155:761–765.
91. Merlo F, Doria M, Fontana L, Ceppi M, Chesi E, Santi L. Mortality from specific causes among silicotic subjects: a historical prospective study. *IARC Sci Publ* 1990;97:105–111.
92. Checkoway H, Demers P, Breslow N. Mortality among workers in the diatomaceous earth industry. *Br J Ind Med* 1993;50:586–597.
93. International Agency for Research on Cancer (IARC). *Silica, some silicates, dusts, and organic fibres.* Lyon: IARC, October 1996.
94. Mason G, Abraham J, Hoffman L, Cole S, Lippmann M, Wasserman K. Treatment of mixed-dust pneumoconiosis with whole lung lavage. *Am Rev Respir Dis* 1982;126:1102–1107.
95. Liang Y, sun U, Chen C, et al. Clinical evaluation of massive whole lung lavage for treatment of coal workers' pneumoconiosis. *He Bei Liao Yang (J Hebei Convalescence)* 1992;1:1–9.
96. Wilt J, Banks D, Lapp N, et al. Whole lung lavage for the treatment of silicosis. *Am Rev Respir Dis* 1994;149:A404.
97. Wilt J, Banks D, Weissman D, et al. Reduction of lung dust burden in pneumoconiosis by whole lung lavage. *J Occup Environ Med* 1996; 38:619–624.
98. Rivers D, Wise M, King E, Nagelschmidt G. Dust content, radiology, and patholoptions in simple pneumoconiosis of coalworkers. *Br J Ind Med* 1960;17:87–108.
99. Lapp N, Goodman G, Castranova V, Pailes W, Kaplan P, Stachura I. Acute silicosis responding to corticosteroid therapy. *Chest* 1990;98: 67S.
100. Sharma S, Pande J, Verma K. Effect of prednisolone treatment in chronic silicosis. *Am Rev Respir Dis* 1991;143:814–821.
101. Kennedy M. Aluminum powder inhalation in the treatment of silicosis. *Br J Ind Med* 1956;13:85–101.
102. Jinduo Z, Jingde L, Guizhi L. Long-term follow-up observations of the therapeutic effects of PVNO. *Zentralbl Bakteriol Hyg Abt Orig* 1983;B178:259–262.
103. Dubois F, Begin R, Cantin A, et al. Aluminum inhalation reduces silicosis in a sheep model. *Am Rev Respir Dis* 1988;137:1172–1179.
104. Begin R, Masse S, Dufresne A. Further information on aluminum inhalation in silicosis. *Occup Environ Med* 1995;52:788–780.
105. Vermeire P, Tasson J, F Lamont et al. Respiratory function after lung homotransplantation with a 10 month survival in man. *Am Rev Respir Dis* 1972;106:515–527.
106. Yu X, Zou C, Lin M. Observation of the effect of tetrandrine on experimental silicosis in rats. *Exotoxicol Environ Safety* 1983;7: 306–312.
107. Li Q, Xu Y, Zhon Z, et al. The therapeutic effect of tetrandrine on silicosis. *Chin J Tuberc Respir Dis* 1981;4:321–324.
108. Seow W, Ferrante A, Li S-Y, Thong Y. Antiphagocytic and antioxidant properties of plant alkaloid tetrandrine. *Int Arch Allergy Appl Immunol* 1988;85:404–409.
109. Seow W, Li S-Y, Thong Y. Inhibitory effects of tetrandrine on human neutrophil and monocyte adherence. *Immunol Lett* 1986;13:83–88.
110. Castranova V, Kang J, Ma J, et al. Effects of bisbenzylisoquinoline alkaloids on alveolar macrophages: correlation between binding affinity, inhibitory potency, and antifibrotic potential. *Toxicol Appl Pharmacol* 1991;108:242–252.
111. Office of the Federal Register, National Archives and Records Administration. U.S. Govt Printing Office. 29 CFR (United States Code of Federal Regulations) 1910.1000 1994.
112. Steenland K, Brown D. Silicosis among gold miners: exposure-response analyses and risk assessment. *Am J Public Health* 1995;85: 1372–1377.
113. Kreiss K, Zhen B. Risk of silicosis in a Colorado mining community. *Am J Ind Med* 1996;30:529–539.
114. NIOSH. (US Department of Health, Education and Welfare, Public Health Service, Center for Disease Control, National Institute for Occupational Safety and Health). *Criteria for a recommended standard:* occupational exposure to crystalline silica 1974. HEW Publication Np (NIOSH) 75-120.
115. DHHS (NIOSH). *Request for assistance in preventing silicosis and deaths in rock drillers.* NIOSH Alert. August 1992. Publication No. 92-107.
116. DHHS (NIOSH). *Request for assistance in preventing silicosis and deaths from sandblasting.* NIOSH Alert. August 1992. Publication No. 92-102.
117. DHHS (NIOSH). *Request for assistance in preventing silicosis and deaths in construction workers.* NIOSH Alert. May 1996. Publication No. 96-112.

*Environmental and Occupational Medicine, Third Edition,* edited by William N. Rom.
Lippincott–Raven Publishers, Philadelphia © 1998.

CHAPTER 30

# Byssinosis and Other Diseases of Textile Workers

Kaye H. Kilburn

Awareness of byssinosis in processors of cotton, flax, and soft hemp goes back at least to Ramazzini (1), the father of occupational medicine, who in 1700 described the "foul and mischievous dust" from flax retting as a major occupational health problem. Subsequently, many investigators, including Thackrah, Kay, Prausnitz, and Hill, and the team of Schilling, McKerrow, and Roach, contributed understanding about progressive respiratory impairment coupled to Monday morning chest tightness and shortness of breath, so-called Monday morning asthma, which is the clinical hallmark of this entity (2–4). Workers compensation for byssinosis began in Great Britain in 1941 for workers who had been in the trade 20 years and were totally disabled. Schilling, McKerrow, and Roach contributed the epidemiologic method, the physiologic understanding, and the capacity to measure total dust, and they developed dose-response relationships for the Lancashire cotton mills by the mid-1950s (5,6). It is essential to realize that the term *byssinosis* has been applied both to the acute response to inhalation of cotton dust and to the permanent dyspnea with impaired function that develops after years of exposure. Although a link of pathogenesis between the two is logically assumed and is supported by findings of impairment in textile workers not exposed to other hazards such as cigarette smoke, longitudinal studies have been done only recently.

Inhalation of cotton textile dust (or flax dust or soft hemp dust) produces gradual awareness of chest tightness or difficulty getting air into the chest. This generally occurs 3 or 4 hours after entering the cotton textile working area. It is accompanied by shortness of breath during periods of exertion and frequently by cough, usually without phlegm production. Because more dust is generated in the preparation areas of picking, blending, and carding, the prevalence of byssinosis is highest among workers in these areas. As the making of thread proceeds, less dust is normally generated, so that the spinning operations, winding and twisting, and weaving generally have progressively less dust. Processing of cloth is practically free of cotton dust, as is manufacturing of denim, which is washed during dyeing before thread is spun. Body temperature rises, usually about 1.0°F, although this is infrequently appreciated by the worker, and the leukocyte count in peripheral blood rises by 20% to 30% (practically all polymorphonuclear leukocytes) (7,8). Also, an ill-defined malaise is frequently experienced. Thus, there are systemic as well as pulmonary effects from inhalation of cotton dust.

Pulmonary function tests show that expiratory airflow decreases during work shift exposure as compared with the baseline values before exposure (9). This is best shown by a decrease in forced vital capacity (FVC) and forced expiratory volume in 1 second ($FEV_1$) (Fig. 1). In general, the decrease is less in workers without symptoms than in symptomatic ones. The larger response on Monday is due to a higher baseline. Thus, the 16-hour period of no exposure appears to be insufficient to restore the baseline on the other days of the week. Airway resistance rises, as does closing volume in some workers.

This response is difficult to distinguish from "mill fever," card room fever," or "heckling fever"–classically

K. H. Kilburn: Department of Internal Medicine, University of Southern California School of Medicine, Los Angeles, California 90033.

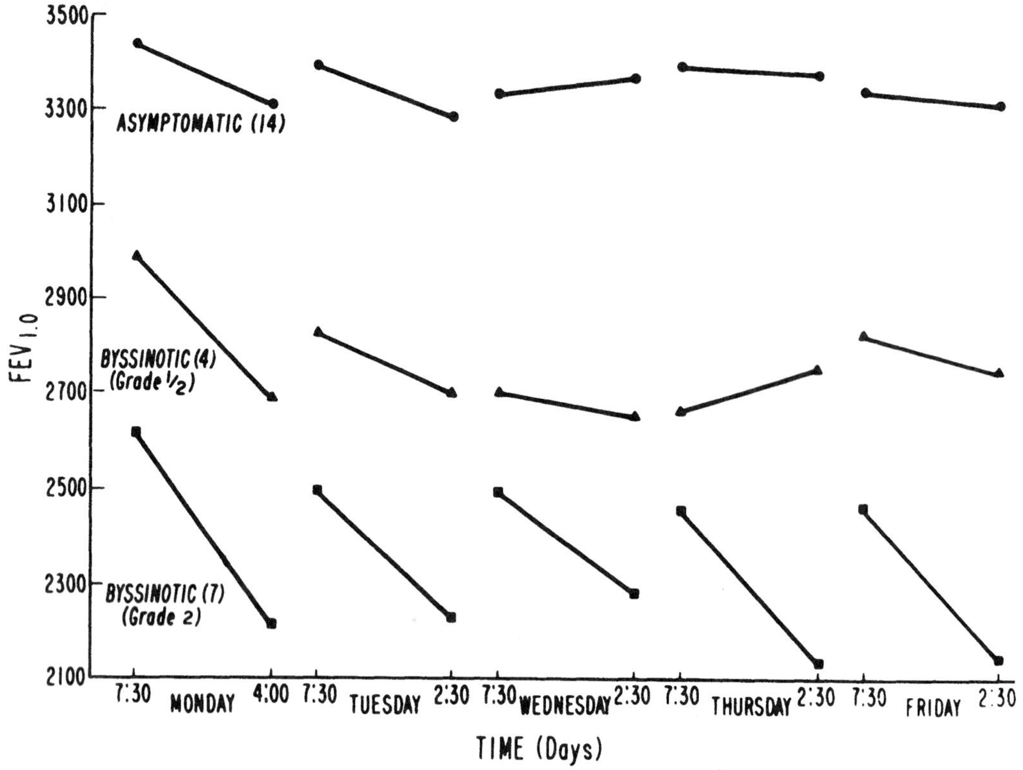


**FIG. 1.** Changes in $FEV_1$ during 5 consecutive days of workplace exposure of 25 card room workers are greater on the first day because the initial baseline is not recovered in 16 hours between shifts. (From ref. 61.)

defined as malaise, fever, chills, upper respiratory tract symptoms, and cough occurring in naive, unaccustomed individuals on the first day of exposure—and the difference may be one of degree, not kind (2). Because tolerance is said to develop to dust exposure, symptoms become less severe as days pass. However, after a break in exposure of several days, symptoms are more severe on the next day of exposure. Pernis and coworkers (10) pointed out the similarity of this syndrome to that produced by inhalation of endotoxin from gram-negative bacilli. The syndrome has been observed in sewer workers and others who work with decaying plant material. From recent studies it seems likely that the mechanism of byssinosis involves stimulation of the same inflammatory receptors by endotoxin and by cotton dust (11–19). Endotoxin activity had a higher coefficient of correlation ($r^2$) with acute reduction in $FEV_1$ in the model card room than did respirable cotton dust, airborne concentrations of fungi, total bacteria, and gram-negative bacteria (14,15). Pooled data from 108 model card room exposure sessions showed an $r^2 = -0.74$ ($p < 0.0001$) for endotoxin; log transformation of endotoxin was better ($r^2 = -0.85, p < 0.0001$) than dust concentration ($r^2 = -0.08, p = .43$) (16). Cross-sectional dose-response relations confirmed a correlation between decrease in $FEV_1$ and current endotoxin level but not respirable dust (17). Confirmation was provided in wool carpet weavers exposed to endotoxin-contaminated wool but not to cotton; 22% showed symptoms of byssinosis and reductions in forced expiratory volume after 1 sec and forced expiratory flow between 25 and 75% of expiration ($FEV_1$ and $FEF_{25-75}$) had been expelled (18). One-fourth of French flax scutching workers suffer from chronic phlegm production, but only an eighth of these have byssinosis despite exposure to enormous levels of airborne dust and gram-negative bacteria (19). This suggests less endotoxin in flax-associated bacteria as well as a difficulty of translating chest tightness.

Similar symptoms follow inhalation of fungal spores, especially of *Aspergillus* or *Micropolyspora faeni,* but the interval between exposure and onset of symptoms is usually longer. In this disorder, which is called acute farmer's lung, the offending particle may be so large (7 μm) as to have only airway effects, as with *Aspergillus,* or small enough (1 μm) to cause alveolar changes as well, as with *Micropolyspora* (20). The alveolar changes primarily involve edema, resulting in decreased diffusing capacity and reduced arterial blood oxygen tension ($PaO_2$). In addition, measurable airway obstruction occurs in all these disorders. Systemic manifestations include fever, malaise, chills, retrosternal discomfort, and headache. Episodes following exposure to "stained" cotton have been recorded as *mattress maker's fever* (21). A similar illness pattern was observed during a survey of several North Carolina textile mills. One weaving room had a high prevalence of symptoms of chest tightness, shortness of breath, malaise, and cough, despite rather low dust levels. The humidity was maintained by nebulizers that recycled water that had condensed on the walls of the workroom. The water contained a myriad of fungi and bacteria. The problem was solved by putting fresh water rather than recycled water through the nebulizers.

Demonstrations that byssinosis with impaired function posed a serious health problem in United States textile mills emerged during the 1970s. Much of the data were assembled by a cooperative problem-solving team of participants from Duke University Medical School, the North Carolina State Board of Health, the National Institute for Occupational Safety and Health, and Burlington Industries, a major cotton manufacturer. This study of more than 3,000 textile workers produced a carefully graded comparison of exposure to respirable dust (measured by a specially designed vertical elutriator developed by Lumsden and Lynch) with the prevalence of symptoms of byssinosis during work coupled with exposure versus the across the shift decrement in $FEV_1$ (22). These data points formed a linear dose-response relationship that was used to recommend the United States cotton dust standard (Fig. 2).

No differences were attributable to age, and men and women had a similar prevalence of byssinosis. Also, work areas that had similar cotton dust levels produced similar effects. Linear regression and fitted probate dose-response curves (Fig. 2) showed that, for respirable dust

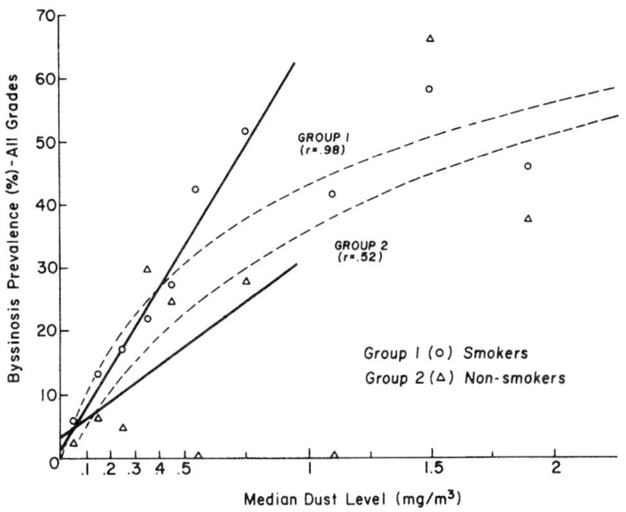


**FIG. 2.** Byssinosis prevalence (ordinate) by median respirable dust level measured by vertical elutriator among cotton preparation and yarn production workers, current smokers, and those who never smoked [North Carolina textile workers, 1970 to 1971 (22)]. The *dark lines* are linear regressions and the *broken lines* are fitted probit dose-response curves. (From ref. 61.)

levels from 0.1 to 0.75 mg/m$^3$, the human response or byssinosis prevalence was a straight line, rising from 5% to 24% in nonsmokers and from 8% to 53% in cigarette smokers (23). The work shift decrement in $FEV_1$ showed a similar straight line up to a dust level of 0.9 mm$^3$. The curving off of the relationship is attributable to the small size of groups of survivors, which then resulted in a smaller number of susceptible individuals at these levels. The study also identified workers with serious pulmonary impairment and thus reinforced the growing awareness that byssinosis is an important occupational chronic bronchitis that leads to progressive pulmonary impairment, not merely a disorder that leads to hypersecretion (that is, cough and sputum production). Thus, disability is associated with shortened working career and premature retirement. A cotton textile mill community study matched 645 current and retired male and female workers with an average of 35 years exposure to a control group of 1,160 unexposed persons from nearby communities (24). The cotton textile workers had an excess of chronic cough, dyspnea, and wheezing, and greater losses of pulmonary function when matched for cigarette smoking, sex, and age. Premature retirement also occurred more frequently in the exposed group.

Pulmonary emphysema does not occur in textile workers more frequently than would be attributable to cigarette smoking. Studies by Edwards and colleagues (25) in England, and by Pratt and coworkers (26) in North Carolina confirm that the pathologic findings in the airways of workers who are chronically exposed to cotton dust are identical to those of patients with chronic bronchitis. Findings included goblet cell hyperplasia, mucous gland hyperplasia, and epithelial leukocytic infiltration in larger airways. Experimental exposure of hamsters to cotton dust and extracts of it produces leukocyte recruitment to small airways (27). Thus, this bronchitis, with its concomitant airway obstruction, is indistinguishable from that resulting from cigarette smoking or from occupational dust exposure in smelters, foundries, grain elevators, plastics manufacture, and pottery making. Therefore, the recognition of a specific response to cotton dust, which defines byssinosis, still depends on tightness in the chest and shortness of breath occurring within a few hours after an exposure following isolation from cotton dust for at least 48 hours or occurring on initial exposure. The second dependable criterion is the demonstration of a reduction in ventilatory capacity or $FEV_1$ after a similar absence from exposure. The acute airway narrowing can be temporarily ameliorated by bronchodilator drugs, but there is probably no effect on permanent changes.

These observations stimulated the building of a model card room containing a single carding engine as a dust generator. In this laboratory, in the textile mill, 12 male card room workers who reacted to cotton dust were test subjects. Dust in the room from carding cotton was sampled carefully with a cyclone separator and the vertical elutriator. Studies, which were done on Monday (after the subjects had been away from work 2 days), consisted of baseline measurements of $FEV_1$ and interview for symptoms of tightness of the chest and shortness of breath (dyspnea) done before exposure and every 2 hours during exposure to cotton that was untreated or specially handled. To validate the decrease in $FEV_1$ as a measure of byssinosis in comparison to the symptoms, spirometry was repeated during exposure to various grades of cotton: heated cotton, washed cotton, steamed cotton, and a synthetic fiber control (Fig. 3). The mean decrease in $FEV_1$ as a percentage of the control showed a clear correlation with the number of workers with symptoms ($r^2 = .95$, $p < 0.005$). This validated the 6-hour or work shift decrease in $FEV_1$ as an objective measure of response to dust. It had the advantage not only of being objective but of being quantitative.

Decreases in $FEV_1$ and the concentration of respirable dust in the model card room were correlated. Heating cotton caused larger decreases and increased amounts of dust. In this panel of workers, respirable dust below 0.10 mg/m$^3$ prevented decreases. Washing cotton in water and steaming cotton reduced the decrease in $FEV_1$. Washing did so by removing dust. Although steaming appeared to have inactivated an agent in the dust that dry heating had appeared to activate, it simply bound dust to fiber. Steamed cotton could be manufactured into thread, but washed cotton was difficult to spin. As steaming appeared to be a practical solution to the problem, it advanced to a pilot textile mill study, where it was found steaming moved the dust from the carding room into the winding and spinning rooms, where more workers are exposed (28,29). Apparently, steam heat made fine dust particles adhere to cotton fibers so their displacement into the air occurred further along in the manufacturing process, which is not a solution. Dust reduction was needed.

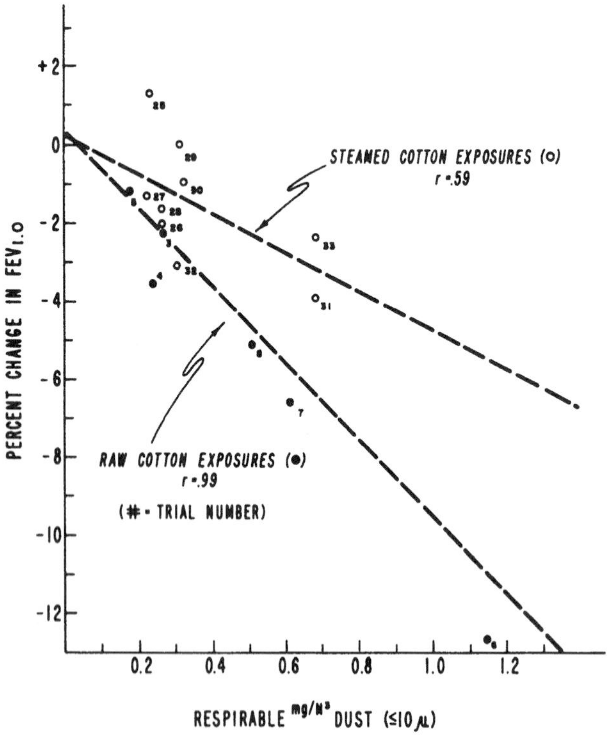


**FIG. 3.** Percentage change in $FEV_1$ by respirable dust level in a 16-man panel of cotton card room workers exposed to raw cotton and steamed cotton, 1971 to 1972 (30). Washed cotton was identical to points 28 to 30.

In 1971, North Carolina revised its occupational health act and simplified the wording by adopting the principle of impairment of function due to work-related exposure. Also, the state revised its workers' compensation benefits and tied these to the median blue-collar wage. Other states lagged in revising their acts to compensate the victims of byssinosis and in adopting benefit levels that permit retirement for disability without such severe economic impoverishment as to be practically impossible. Only 350 of an estimated 30,000 workers with disability caused by byssinosis in the United States had received workers' compensation by 1987, most of these in North Carolina.

The 1968 to 1971 North Carolina cotton dust study that was turned over to the National Institute for Occupational Safety and Health (NIOSH) in November 1971 formed the basis of criteria for exposure to cotton dust. Developing the standard took until 1977, owing to a series of delays. The recommendation was for a standard of 0.1 mg/m$^3$ of vertically elutriated dust, but the presence of an ambient dust level nearly this high at one urban site ultimately resulted in a standard of 0.2 mg/m$^3$ of vertically elutriated dust, which was reached by gradual steps over several years. Industry labeled the cost of meeting the standard as practically confiscatory. However, this was untrue and exhaust ventilation and similar air filtering measures cleaned up many textile mills and factories.

The cotton dust standard of 0.2 mg/m$^3$ of respirable dust was considered tentative, which may need lowered depending on monitoring workers' annual decrements in pulmonary function. Also it was thought that decrements in flows across the work shift would predict the annual decrement in function. Several studies in the 1980s and 1990s confirmed that excessive annual decrements occur in cotton textile works with dust exposures at or below the standard (30–35). These studies also confirmed that the dose-response curve goes through zero, that cigarette smoker decrements exceed those of nonsmokers and ex-smokers, and that across-shift decrements predict annual ones. Other factors that relate to specific environments influence annual decrements. Aside from these details, the standard needs to be reduced to 0.1 mg (100 µg) per m$^3$ or less to protect cotton textile workers. Variations in these limited data (32–34) and caveats needed due to noncomparability of data from China and Croatia show that opportunities were lost by neglecting industrywide monitoring of the annual decrements mandated in the cotton dust standard.

Industry took legal and legislative countermeasures to oppose to cotton dust standard. The United States Court of Appeals for Washington, D.C., found no substantial reason for delaying the adoption of the standard and, thus, it was in place as of March 27,1980, 8½ years after producing the dose-response curve. Full compliance with the 0.2 mg/m$^3$ level occurred by March 27, 1984. Byssinosis has been practically abolished in the United States, so atopic subjects may work in cotton textile factories (36). In Great Britain byssinosis fell from a prevalence of 51% in the 1950s, to 38% in the 1960s, 18% in the 1970s, and 13.8% in the 1980s, which was attributed to reduced dust and bacteria in workroom air (37).

Other sites of cotton use have also been investigated for byssinosis. The data of Palmer and colleagues on 29 cotton gins in Texas and New Mexico supported inclusion of gin workers in the same dose-response curve as cotton textile workers, as did data from Egypt and the Sudan (38,39). Mean dust levels by vertical elutriator ranged from 0.63 to 1.52 mg/m$^3$, and peaks reached almost 5 mg/m$^3$. Decrements in $FEV_1$ were measured in 44% of 203 gin workers. In light of these data, the finding of a 5% or greater decrement in $FEV_1$ in only 16% of 178 California gin workers, compared to 14% of 117 controls, is probably explained by less dust in long fiber length ALCALA (a variety of long style cotton grown exclusively in California) cotton and the absence of dust levels (40). The waste cotton-reclaiming or "willowing" industry has elevated byssinosis and chronic bronchitis rates, combined with cross shift-decrements in $FEV_1$ (41–43).

The cottonseed and oil industries have a byssinosis problem, although the contribution of seed hull and even oil to the total measured dust dilutes the byssinosis factor to reduce worker response and makes a different dose-response curve to dust than in the textile mills and gins (44).

In contrast, cotton fiber reuse industries (exemplified by garnetting workers) do not have byssinosis, and it is absent from the production of medical cotton although chronic bronchitis may be increased, especially if cotton is alkali washed (45,46).

Synthetic fibers have produced mild ventilatory impairment and granulomas and fibrosis with varied symptoms (47). In one study, polyacrylonitrile fiber workers with concentrations of respirable dust of 0.53 mg/m$^3$ had about 25% of the reduction in $FEV_1$, of hemp workers at a respirable dust level of 1.54 mg/m$^3$, so the effects are minor (48). Rayon, in contrast, did not cause pulmonary symptoms and or reduce ventilatory function. Respirable dust levels were below the background levels of 0.05 mg/m$^3$ in the model card room.

What is the future for cotton as a fiber and food crop? Polyester fabrics are made of petrochemicals while cotton is economical and ecologically sound (49). It is also a comfortable and nontoxic fiber that clothes a substantial majority of the world's people, and comes from an annually renewed supply with a moderate energy cost for production and manufacture. The data of Henderson and Enterline (50) showed cotton textile workers had a lower than expected rate of lung cancer.

Questions remain. Quercetin, a product identified in cotton in 1973, is mutagenic for bacteria (51), while in contrast a sesquiterpene found in cotton has antitumor properties (52). Gossypol, which is a polyphenolic product of the cotton gossypol glands, inhibits some insect pests, and gives cotton its generic name, has been shown by the Chinese to inhibit spermatogenesis and to have possible contraceptive use (53). These agents in cotton dust narrow airways as does inhaled endotoxin. Their identity has not changed the strategy for control of cotton dust disease. Thus the anticipation that possibilities such as removal of the causal agent(s) through plant breeding, or their removal after cotton is ginned, by washing or by absorption on cholestyramine or other anion exchange resins, have not become practical (54). It is even conceivable that an antidote to cotton dust could be developed, although this would be less desirable than removal from the plant source or in early manufacturing before worker exposure. Consideration of the pathophysiology of the response to cotton chemicals affirmed additional mechanisms of toxicity for tannins and glycans that were isolated in the 1970s (55–59).

The remaining problems require decisions to break into the equation that human exposure to cotton dust causes pulmonary impairment; they require action. First, screening may eliminate highly susceptible potential workers from exposure. It appears that the most susceptible are atopic or have hypersensitive airways who were eliminated in the past by their intolerance to the first day's exposure to the cotton dust. Subjects with marked reactivity to dust should be removed by preemployment screening, as it now appears they have larger than average annual decrements in function during exposure. Second, the dust levels for current workers must be reduced to 100 μg/m$^3$ so that the vast majority, at least 95% of workers who are employed beyond their first shift, will not have functional deterioration from their work exposure, in excess of that attributable to age. Workers must be informed of the additive effects of cigarette smoking, but in no way must this become a means of evading the employers responsibility to clean the workplace or to attribute a reasonable share of impairment to cotton dust. Third, the small number of workers who show or develop hypersusceptibility or reactivity during work exposure must be relocated into essentially dust-free areas so as to avoid deterioration. Fourth, all workers with byssinosis-related pulmonary impairment, must have an adequate, fair, and rapid workers' compensation system adjusted for cost of living.

North Carolina's occupational health act has been a good model, because it avoids the difficulties of making a specific diagnosis, the criteria for which may change (60). Thus, it does not run the risk of discriminating against the worker who does not develop tightness in the chest or shortness of breath despite showing deterioration of pulmonary function during months or years of exposure. The strategy for evaluation is simple. First, there must have been exposure to the agent in question. This exposure is to cotton dust or to endotoxin as determined gravimetrically by weighing it on filters. Second, there must be pulmonary impairment. The impairment may be obvious and easily documented, but it is shown best by accelerated functional deterioration with time. This process takes at least two, and preferably three, measured points obtained 6 months or a year apart. Of course, when impairment for doing one's job is already present, this observation of accelerated deterioration is not essential. The question is whether cotton dust exposure has contributed to the specific worker's respiratory impairment. As more workplaces are monitored for dust level, it will be easier to ascertain what the last levels of exposure were, but the problem that characterizes other occupational exposures will persist in that exposures that are remote in time can only be estimated. Then solid evidence of longitudinal observations in the same groups of workers will confirm the link between acute response and subsequent impairment.

Evidence since 1700 that cotton dust impairs lung function, probably by the obstruction and obliteration of small airways as shown in the 1970s, sustains this impression not only in the United Kingdom and the United States but in India, China, Ethiopia, Russia, and Croatia. Even if workers' compensation becomes faster and more equitable, experience will confirm that this disease is preventable by dust control, particularly in preparation, carding, and spinning, at modest cost.

## ACKNOWLEDGMENTS

This work was funded by the National Institute for Occupational Safety and Health, National Institute for Environmental Health Sciences, U.S. Department of Agriculture, and Cotton Incorporated.

## REFERENCES


1. Ramazzini B. *A treatise on the diseases of tradesmen.* London: Bell, 1705.
2. Harris TR, Merchant JA, Kilburn KH, Hamilton JD. Byssinosis and respiratory diseases of cotton mill workers. *J Occup Med* 1972;14:199–206.
3. Prausnitz C. *Investigations on respiratory dust disease in operatives in the cotton industry.* London: His Majesty's Stationery Office, 1936.
4. Roach SA, Schilling RSE. A clinical and environmental study of byssinosis in the Lancashire cotton industry. *Br J Ind Med* 1960;17:1–9.
5. McKerrow CB, McDermott M, Gilson IC, Schilling RSF. Respiratory function during the day in cotton workers: a study in byssinosis. *Br J Ind Med* 1958;15:75–83.
6. McKerrow CB, Roach SA, Gilson IC, Schilling RSF. The size of the cotton dust particles causing byssinosis: an environmental and physiological study. *Br J Ind Med* 1962;19:1–8.
7. Bouhuys A, Van Duyn I Van Lennep HJ. Byssinosis in flax workers. *Arch Environ Health* 1961;3:499–509.
8. Merchant JA, Halprin GM, Hudson AR, et al. Evaluation before and after exposure: the pattern of physiological response to cotton dust. *Ann NY Acad Sci* 1974;22(1):38–43.
9. Merchant JA, Halprin GM, Hudson AR, et al. Responses to cotton dust. *Arch Environ Health* 1975;30:222–229.
10. Pernis B, Vigliani EC, Cavagna C, Finulli M. The role of bacterial endotoxins in occupational diseases caused by inhaling vegetable dusts. *Br J Ind Med* 1961;18:120–129.
11. Antweiler H. Histamine liberation by cotton dust extracts: evidence against its causation by bacterial endotoxins. *Br J Ind Med* 1961;18:130–132.
12. Cavagna C, Foa V, Vigliani, EC. Effects in man and rabbits of inhalation of cotton dust or extracts and purified endotoxins. *Br J Ind Med* 1969;26:314–321.
13. Cinkotai FF, Lockwood MG, Rylander R. Airborne microorganisms and prevalence of byssinotic symptoms in cotton mills. *Am Ind Hyg Assoc J* 1977;38:554–559.
14. Castellan RM, Olenchock SA, Hankinson JL, et al. Acute bronchoconstriction induced by cotton dust: dose-related responses to endotoxin and other dust factors. *Ann Intern Med* 1984;101:157–163.
15. Rylander R, Haglind P, Lundholm M. Endotoxin in cotton dust and respiratory function decrement among cotton workers in an experimental cardroom. *Am Rev Respir Dis* 1985;131:209–213.
16. Castellan RM, Olenchock SA, Kinsley KB, Hankinson JL. Inhaled endotoxin and decreased spirometric values: a response relation from cotton dust. *N Engl J Med* 1987;317:605–610.
17. Kennedy SM, Christiani DC, Elsen EA, et al. Cotton dust and endotoxin exposure-response relationships in cotton textile workers. *Am Rev Respir Dis* 1987;135:194–200.
18. Ozesmi M, Asian H, Hillerdahl G, Rylander R, Ozesmi C. Byssinosis in carpet weavers exposed to wool contaminated, with endotoxin. *Br J Ind Med* 1987;44:479–483.
19. Cinkotai FF, Emo P, Gibbs AC, Caillard J-F, Jollany J-M. Low prevalence of byssinotic symptoms in 12 flax scutching mills in Normandy, France. *Br J Ind Med* 1988;45:325–328.
20. Pepys J. Hypersensitivity disease of the lungs due to fungi and organic dusts. *Monogr Allergy* 1969;4:147–153.
21. Neal PA, Schneiter R, Carminita BH. Report on acute illnesses among rural mattress makers using low-grade stained cotton. *JAMA* 1942;119:1074–1082.
22. Merchant JA, Lumsden JC, Kilburn KH, et al. Dose-response studies in cotton textile workers. *J Occup Med* 1973;15:222–230.
23. Merchant JA, Lumsden JC, Kilburn KH, et al. An industrial study of the biological effects of cotton dust and cigarette smoke exposure. *J Occup Med* 1973;15:212–221.
24. Bouhuys A, Schoenberg JB, Beck GJ, Schilling RSF. Epidemiology of chronic lung disease in a cotton mill community. *Lung* 1977;154:167–186.
25. Edwards C, Macartney J, Rooke G, Ward F. The pathology of the lung in byssinotics. *Thorax* 1975;30:612–623.
26. Pratt PC, Vollmer RT, Miller JA. Epidemiology of pulmonary lesions in nontextile and cotton textile workers: a retrospective autopsy analysis. *Arch Environ Health* 1980;35:133–138.
27. Kilburn KH, Lynn WS, Tres L, McKenzie WN. Leukocyte recruitment through airway walls by condensed tannins and quercetin. *Lab Invest* 1973;28:55–59.
28. Merchant JA, Lumsden JC, Kilburn KH, et al. Preprocessing cotton to prevent byssinosis. *Br J Ind Med* 1973;30:237–247.
29. Merchant JA, Lumsden JC, Kilburn KH, et al. Intervention studies of cotton steaming to reduce biological effects of cotton dust. *Br J Ind Med* 1974;31:261–274.
30. Sepulveda MJ, Castellan RM, Hankinson JL, Cocke JB. Acute lung function response to cotton dust in atopic and nonatopic individuals. *Br J Ind Med* 1984;41:487–491.
31. Cinkotai FF, Rigby A, Pickering CAC, Seaborn D, Faragher E. Recent trends in the prevalence of byssinosis symptoms in the Lancashire textile industry. *Br J Ind Med* 1988;45:782–789.
32. Zuskin E, Ivankovic D, Schachter EN, Witek TJ Jr. A ten-year follow-up study of cotton textile workers. *Am Rev Respir Dis* 1991;143:301–305.

33. Glindmeyer HW, Lefante JJ, Jones RN, Rando RJ, Abdel Kader HM, Weill H. Exposure-related deciles in the lung function of cotton textile workers. *Am Rev Respir Dis* 1991;144:675–683.
34. Glindmeyer HW, Lefante JJ, Jones RN, Rando RJ, Weill H. Cotton dust and across-shift change in $FEV_1$ as predictors of annual change in $FEV_1$. *Am J Respir Crit Care Med* 1994;149:584–590.
35. Christiani DC, Wegman DH, Eisen EA, Dai H, Lu P. Pulmonary function among cotton textile workers. *Chest* 1994;105:1713–1721.
36. Sepulveda MJ, Castellan RM, Hankinson JL, Cocke JB. Acute lung function response to cotton dust in atopic and nonatopic individuals. *Br J Ind Med* 1984;41:487–491.
37. Cinkotai FF, Rigby A, Pickering CAC, Seaborn D, Faragher E. Recent trends in the prevalence of byssinosis symptoms in the Lancashire textile industry. *Br J Ind Med* 1988;45:782–789.
38. Khogali M. Byssinosis. A follow-up study of cotton ginnery workers in the Sudan. *Br J Ind Med* 1976;33:166–174.
39. Palmer A, Finnegan W, Herwitt P, Waxweiler R, Jones I. Byssinosis and chronic respiratory disease in U.S. cotton gins. *J Occup Med* 1978;20: 96–102.
40. Larson RK, Barman ML, Smith DN. Study of the respiratory effects of short- and long-term cotton gin exposure. *Chest* 1981;79:225–235.
41. Chinn DI, Cinkotai FF, Lockwood MG, Logan SHM. Airborne dust, its protease content and byssinosis in "willowing" mills. *Ann Occup Hyg* 1976;19:101–108.
42. Dingwall-Fordyce I, O'Sullivan IG. Byssinosis in the waste cotton industry. *Br J Ind Med* 1966;23:53–57.
43. Engelberg AL, Piacitelli GM, Peterson M, et al. Medical and industrial hygiene characterization of the cotton waste utilization industry. *Am J Ind Med* 1985;7:93–108.
44. Jones RN, Carp I, Glindmeyer H, Weill H. Respiratory health and dust levels in cottonseed mills. *Thorax* 1977;32:281–286.
45. El Batawi MA, El-Din Sash S. An epidemiological study on aetiological factors in byssinosis. *Arch Gewerbathol Gewerbehyg* 1962;19: 393–399.
46. Rom W, Thornton I, Einstein K. Pulmonary function abnormalities in garnetting workers exposed to synthetic fibers. Presented to the 43rd Scientific Assembly of the American College of Chest Physicians, Las Vegas, Nevada, November 1, 1977.
47. Pimentel JC, Avila R, Lourenco AG. Respiratory diseases caused by synthetic fibres: a new occupational disease. *Thorax* 1975;30:204–219.
48. Valic F, Zuskin, E. Respiratory function changes in textile workers exposed to synthetic fibers. *Arch Environ Health* 1977;32:283–287.
49. Van Winkle TL, Edeleanu J, Prosser RA. Cotton versus polyester. *Am Sci* 1978;66:280–289.
50. Henderson V, Enterline PE. An unusual mortality experience in cotton textile workers. *J Occup Med* 1973;15:717–719.
51. Beldanes LF, Change GW. Mutagenic activity of quercetin and related compounds. *Science* 1977;197:577–578.
52. Lee ICH, Hall lH, Mar EC, et al. Sesquiterpene antitumor agents: inhibitors of cellular metabolism. *Science* 1977;196:533–535.
53. National Coordinating Group for Male Contraceptives. A new male contraceptive-gossypol. *Chin Med J (Peking)* 1978;8:455–458.
54. Nolan JP, McDevitt JJ, Goldmann GS. Endotoxin binding by charged and uncharged resins. *Proc Soc Biol Med* 1975;149:766–770.
55. Cloutier MM, Guernsey L. Tannin inhibition of protein kinase C in airway epithelium. *Lung* 1995;173:307–319.
56. Bates PJ, Ralston NV, Vuk-Pavlovic Z, Rohrbach MS. Calcium influx is required for tannin-medicated arachidonic acid release from alveolar macrophages. *Am J Physiol* 1995;268:33–40.
57. DeLucca AJ 2nd, Brogden KA, French AD. Agglutination of lung surfactant with glucan. *Br J Ind Med* 1992;49:755–760.
58. Kreofsky TJ, Russell JA, Rohrbach MS. Inhibition of alveolar macrophage spreading and phagocytosis by cotton bract tannin. A potential mechanism in the pathogenesis of byssinosis. *Am J Pathol* 1990;137:263–274.
59. Gordon T, Harkema JR. Effect of inhaled endotoxin on intraepithelial mucosubstances in F344 rat nasal and tracheobronchial airways. *Am J Respir Cell Mol Biol* 1994;10:177–183.
60. Laws of North Carolina (annotated). An act to amend GS97-53 relating to occupational diseases. March 24, 1971.
61. Last J. *Preventive medicine and public Health.* New York: Appleton-Century-Crofts, 1980.

*Environmental and Occupational Medicine, Third Edition,* edited by William N. Rom.
Lippincott–Raven Publishers, Philadelphia © 1998.

# CHAPTER 31

# Hypersensitivity Pneumonitis

Yvon Cormier

Hypersensitivity pneumonitis (HP) is a relatively common disease that is probably present in different forms in all parts of the world. Although its etiologies and clinical presentations have been well described, the diagnosis of HP is most often confirmed only after repeated bouts of acute manifestations or when irreversible damage to the lungs has already occurred. In our experience almost all cases that we see have been treated for a presumed infectious process or chronic bronchitis before the diagnosis is clearly established. Milder or indolent cases probably go undiagnosed. It is also very likely that some patients with unexplained residual lung disease, restrictive, obstructive, or a combination of both, are in fact old cases of never-diagnosed HP.

There are numerous reasons for the difficulties in diagnosing HP. Among these is that HP can mimic more frequent respiratory ailments such as lung infections. Another important factor is the wide range of settings and antigens responsible for the disease. Also, the fact that the symptoms occur only 3 to 8 hours after the exposure makes the etiologic link less obvious. The keys to the diagnosis of HP is awareness of its varied clinical manifestations and etiologic agents. The responsible allergen can be in the workplace, in the home, at recreational facilities, at friends' houses, in cars, in the outside environment, etc. It is important to always keep HP in the differential diagnosis of febrile reactions and parenchymal lung diseases. The importance of a detailed history of the patient's environment, an integral part of the evaluation of all patients with respiratory diseases, cannot be overemphasized in the case of HP.

Y. Cormier: Department of Medicine, Hospital and Université Laval, Ste. Foy, Québec G1V 4G5, Canada.

This chapter emphasizes clinical characteristics of HP, its diagnostic criteria, evaluation, treatment, and outcome. A summary of current pathophysiological understanding and epidemiology of HP is also presented.

## DEFINITION

There is no formally recognized definition of HP. It is an interstitial lung-limited disease caused by an immune (hypersensitive) response to inhaled antigenic particles. The type of immune response is different than the more common immediate response of type 1 immunoglobulin E (IgE)-mediated allergy implicated in atopy, allergic rhinitis, and asthma. The specific serum antibodies in HP are of the IgG class and the response is not immediate but delayed by 3 to 8 hours. Although systemic manifestations like fever, fatigue, and general malaise are present in acute HP, the lung is the only end organ of the disease. Its hypersensitive nature is supported by the observation that all subjects exposed to a given antigen do not get the disease, the type of lung pathology found, and its transferability by primed lymphocytes in an animal model (1). The antigen-specific IgG antibodies are present in the serum and in the lungs where specific IgA is also present (2). Responsible antigens are usually of bacterial, fungal, or animal protein origin. However, inorganic substances, such as toluene diisocyanate (TDI), can act as haptens and bind to serum protein to create an antigenic complex that can then induce HP (3).

## HISTORY

The original description of HP is attributed to Ramazzini (4), who, in 1713, reported a lung disease in grain

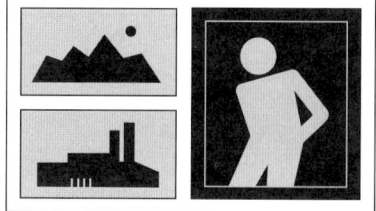

**TABLE 1.** *Most frequent causes of hypersensitivity pneumonitis by inhaled antigens*

| Disease | Source of antigens | Probable antigen |
|---|---|---|
| Plant products | | |
| Farmer's lung | Moldy hay | Thermophilic actinomycetes: *Faenia rectivirgula, Thermoactinomyces vulgaris, Aspergillus* species |
| Bagassosis | Moldy pressed sugarcane (bagasse) | Thermophilic actinomycetes: *F. rectivirgula, T. vulgaris* |
| Mushroom-worker's disease | Moldy compost | Thermophilic actinomycetes: *F. rectivirgula, T. vulgaris, mushroom* |
| Malt-worker's lung | Contaminated barley | *Aspergillus clavatus* |
| Maple bark disease | Contaminated maple logs | Cryptostroma corticale |
| Sequoiosis | Contaminated wood dust | *Graphium* species, *Pullularia* species |
| Wood pulp-worker's disease | Contaminated wood pulp | *Alternaria* species |
| Humidifier lung | Contaminated humidifiers, dehumidifiers, air conditioners | Thermophilic actinomycetes: *Thermoactinomyces candidus, Thermoactinomyces vulgaris, Penicillium* species, *Cephalosporium* species, Amoeba |
| Familial HP | Contaminated wood dust in walls | Bacillus *subtilis* |
| Compost lung | Compost | *Aspergillus* |
| Cheese-washer's disease | Cheese casings | *Penicillium* species |
| Wood-trimmer's disease | Contaminated wood trimmings | *Rhizopus* species, *Mucor* species |
| Thatched roof disease | Dried grasses and leaves | Sacchoromonospora viridis |
| Tea-grower's disease | Tea plants | Unknown |
| Coffee-worker's lung | Green coffee beans | *Unknown* |
| Streptomyces albus HP | Contaminated fertilizer | *S. albus* |
| *Cephalosporium* HP | Contaminated basement (sewage) | *Cephalosporium* |
| Sauna-taker's disease | Sauna water | *Pullularia* species |
| Detergent-worker's disease | Detergent | *Bacillus subtilis* enzymes |
| Paprika-splitter's lung | Paprika dust | *Mucor stolonifer* |
| Japanese summer house HP | House dust; ? bird droppings | *Trichosporon cutaneum* |
| Dry rot lung | Infected wood | *Merulius lacrymans* |
| Office-worker's or home HP | Dust from ventilation or heating systems | Unknown (probably multiple) |
| Car air conditioner HP | Dust from air conditioner | *T. candidus* ? |
| Potato-riddler's lung | Moldy straw around potatoes | Thermophilic actinomycetes: *F. rectivirgula, T. vulgaris, Aspergillus* species |
| Tobacco-worker's disease | Mold on tobacco | *Aspergillus* species |
| Hot tub lung | Mold on ceiling | *Cladosporium* species |
| Tap water lung | Contaminated water | Bacteria or fungi |
| Wine-grower's lung | Mold on grapes | *Botrytis cinerea* |
| Suberosis | Cork dust | *Penicillium* |
| Woodman's disease | Mold on bark | *Penicillium* |
| Saxophone lung | Saxophone mouthpiece | *Candida albicans* |
| Grain-worker's lung | Grain dust | *Erwinia herbicola* |
| Fish meal-worker's lung | Fish meal dust | Unknown |
| Animal products | | |
| Pigeon-breeder's disease | Pigeon droppings | Altered pigeon serum (probably IgA) |
| Duck fever | Duck feathers | Duck proteins |
| Turkey-handler's lung | Turkey products | Turkey proteins |
| Bird-fancier's lung | Bird products | Bird proteins |
| Dove-pillow's lung | Bird feathers | Bird proteins |
| Laboratory-worker's HP | Rat fur | Male rat urine |
| Pituitary snuff-taker's disease | Pituitary powder | Bovine and porcine proteins |
| Mollusk shell HP | Mollusk shells | Animal proteins |
| Insect products | | |
| Miller's lung | Wheat weevils | *Sitophilus granarius* |
| Reactive simple chemicals | | |
| TDI HP | Toluene diisocyanate | Altered proteins (albumin and others |
| TMA HP | Trimetallic anhydride | Altered proteins |
| MDI HP | Diphenylmethane diisocyanate | Altered proteins |
| Epoxy resin lung | Heated epoxy resin | Phthalic anhydride |
| Pauli's HP | Pauli's reagent | Sodium diazobenzene-sulfonate |

workers that was probably HP. In 1932 Campbell (5) gave a clear description of farmer's lung, still one of the most common forms of HP. The immune etiology of this disease and the agents responsible for farmer's lung were described 30 years later by Pepys et al. (6). Since then it has been recognized that HP can afflict not only subjects exposed to the farm, but also individuals exposed to an ever-increasing number of environments.

## CLINICAL PRESENTATIONS

The most frequent presentation of HP is a recurrent febrile episode late in the afternoon or early evening. The fever can be high (40°C) and accompanied by shortness of breath, chest tightness, chills, and general malaise. The timing of the symptoms depends on the time of exposure—evening chills correspond to morning exposure. These symptoms will be present for a few hours and by the next morning dyspnea is the only symptom that sometimes persist. The symptoms recur as often as exposure is repeated. This classical presentation, however, does not always occur. In many cases the disease manifests itself as a low-grade progressive dyspnea and cough, with no systemic reactions and no obvious oscillations of the symptoms. The reasons for the different modes of presentations are not clear, but could reflect the degree and continuity of exposure or individual susceptibility to the offending agent.

Classically, the clinical presentations of HP have been described as acute, subacute, and chronic. These subdivisions are somewhat arbitrary and do not represent clear clinical entities but an overlapping continuum. The exact meaning of each of these terms varies between authors; for some, subacute is an indolent progression that is classified as chronic by others (7–9). Chronic is sometimes used to describe sequelae of the disease that may no longer be active (10). These subclassifications are therefore of little usefulness; what is important is to understand that the clinical presentation of HP is extremely varied.

Even more difficult to define is the presence of irreversible lung scarring with fibrosis and emphysema resulting from chronic HP that may no longer be present and may never have been diagnosed during the disease activity. Therefore, for any subject presenting with dyspnea and cough, with or without recurrent fever, chest tightness, and weight loss, for whom there is no obvious diagnosis, the possibility of HP should be considered. Once the diagnosis is suspected, a careful history will usually identify the potential offending contact. In some cases, for example bird fancier's or farmer's lung, the responsible environment will be obvious. In other cases it may not.

## CLINICAL SETTINGS AND RESPONSIBLE ANTIGENS

An exhaustive, but still incomplete, list of settings and antigens known to be associated with HP has recently been published (Table 1) (11). Any such list can never be complete since new environments continue to be identified. The longer the list the less useful it becomes. More important is the realization that exposure to an environment where the air is contaminated with bacteria, molds, animal proteins, or some inorganic substances like isocyanates can induce HP. All bacteria, molds, and proteins, however, do not have the same antigenicity. For example, pigeon protein is associated with HP, while cat and dog allergens are associated with asthma. The most frequent forms of HP are farmer's lung, bird fancier's disease (including pigeon breeders), humidifier lung, and summer-type HP.

Farmer's lung is caused by bacteria or fungi found in moldy hay, straw, or grain. The bacteria most frequently involved is now classified as a thermophilic actinomyces and named *Saccharopolyspora rectivirgula* (12). Until recently this bacteria was known as *Micropolyspora faeni*. Any bird or bird product in the home or the workplace can induce HP. Feathers, frequently used in pillows, blankets, and clothing, constitute a potential source of antigen. *Penicillium* sp. can be responsible for HP in a number of settings including humidifier lung, and in workers such as compost workers, saw mill workers, mushroom workers, etc. Summer-type HP is caused by *Trichosporon cutanuum,* a mold found in rotting wood in the homes. This type of HP is prevalent in Japan, where it accounts for two-thirds of all cases of HP (13) and has been described in South Africa (14).

## DIAGNOSTIC CRITERIA

Diagnostic criteria for HP have previously been proposed (9,15,16). Based on these, and adding more recent information on the subject, the following diagnostic criteria that do away with the designation of acute, subacute, and chronic, could be used (Table 2). Another advantage of the proposed criteria is that they are applicable to all cases of HP, not only its acute phase. With two or more

**TABLE 2.** *Suggested diagnostic criteria for new, recurrent, or progressive disease*

| |
|---|
| Required (because these findings are always present, the diagnosis cannot be maintained in their absence) |
| Appropriate exposure |
| Dyspnea on exertion |
| Inspiratory crackles |
| Lymphocytic alveolitis (if BAL is done) |
| Supportive |
| Recurrent febrile episodes |
| Infiltrates on chest x-rays |
| Decreased carbon monoxide diffusing capacity of the lungs ($D_LCO$) |
| Precipitating antibodies to causative antigens |
| Granulomas on lung biopsy (usually not required) |
| Improvement with contact avoidance |

supportive criteria, the confirmation of a bronchoalveolar lymphocytosis may not be required. The diagnosis of residual disease can sometimes only be made or suspected by an appropriate history and compatible lung sequelae (see Prognosis, below). All published and proposed diagnostic criteria, however, remain to be validated.

## DIAGNOSTIC PROCEDURES

Once the diagnosis of HP is suspected, the following investigation should be considered to establish the diagnosis and quantify the degree of involvement (Table 3).

The clinical history must clearly describe the presenting symptoms, their timing, and most importantly include a thorough query on the patient's environment. The physical examination is unremarkable. If the patient is seen outside of the peak febrile reaction, which is often the case, body temperature will be normal. Inspiratory crackles are invariably present, but nonspecific (17) and digital clubbing has been reported in chronic cases (18).

Chest x-rays are abnormal in 80% of cases (19) and in acute and subacute disease show fine diffuse interstitial infiltrates (Fig. 1). In chronic disease typical sequelae can take the form of lung fibrosis (20), emphysema (21), or a combination of the two. High-resolution computed tomography (HRCT) is not required in most cases of HP. Its use is justified in cases where the chest x-ray is normal or when the diagnosis of HP is uncertain. The findings on HRCT in active disease are quite characteristic with patchy alveolar infiltrates (22) (Fig. 2). HRCT may also be useful in confirming the presence of emphysema or lung fibrosis as a result of prior HP (21) (Fig. 3).

Lung volumes and forced expiratory flows may be normal in HP. Typical findings in active disease, however, are those of a restrictive pattern (decreased total lung capacity and vital capacity) with a normal or increased residual volume (23–25). In chronic or residual disease a restrictive or an obstructive pattern can be seen. Farmer's lung seems to evolve more toward emphysema (21), while pigeon breeders develop lung restriction (20). Lung diffusion capacity is the most severely affected physiologic parameter and is probably always decreased. Hypoxemia with a normal or decreased $PCO_2$ is the usual finding on blood gas analysis.

**TABLE 3.** *Factors to consider in the investigation of a case suspected of HP*

| |
|---|
| Clinical history |
| Physical examination |
| PA and lateral chest radiographs |
| High-resolution computed tomography (HRCT) |
| Lung functions (volumes, flows, $D_LCO$, blood gas analysis) |
| Serum precipitins analysis |
| Bronchoalveolar lavage (BAL) |
| Transbronchial lung biopsy (TBB) |

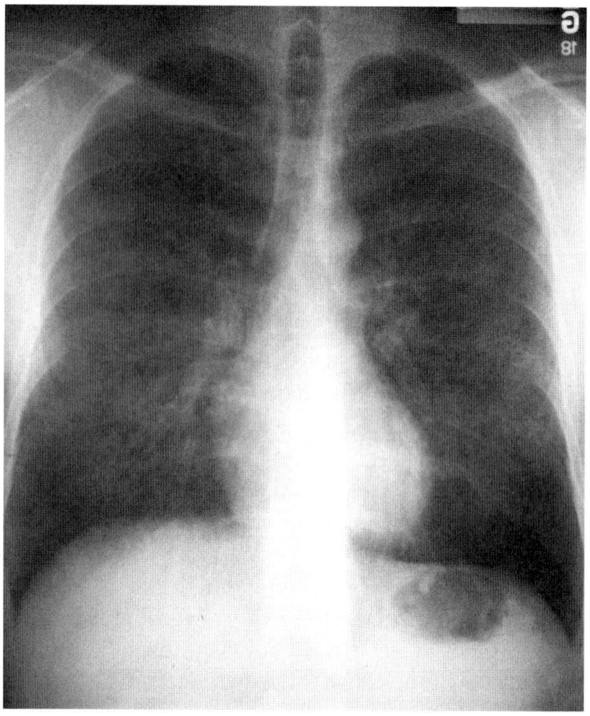

**FIG. 1.** Posteroanterior chest radiograph showing the typical diffuse, fine, and poorly defined interstitial infiltrates in a case of recent-onset hypersensitivity pneumonitis.

Serum analysis for specific IgG "precipitins" antibodies against suspected antigens should be obtained. The presence of precipitins is only a supportive criterion. Many exposed individuals have serum precipitins without having the disease (26–28). Most cases of pigeon fancier's disease have positive precipitins to bird antigens; however, 30% to 40% of patients with farmer's lung have no precipitins to commonly tested farmer's lung antigens *(Saccharopolyspora rectivirgula, Aspergillus,* and *Thermoactinomyces vulgaris)* (25). One possible explanation is that other antigens present in moldy hay could be responsible for farmer's lung.

Bronchoalveolar lavage (BAL) is a very important technique for research in the understanding of the pathophysiology of HP, but its role in the diagnosis of HP is less clear. The cellular findings in the BAL fluid of HP have been clearly described (25,29–35). A lymphocytic alveolitis (lymphocytes accounting for more than 20% of total BAL cells) is always present in active disease; therefore, the absence of increased lymphocytes in BAL would rule out the diagnosis of current HP (25). Although lymphocytosis can persist for a prolonged period of time, at least up to 2 years (17) after the cessation of exposure to the offending agent, BAL lymphocytes will eventually return to normal; therefore, their

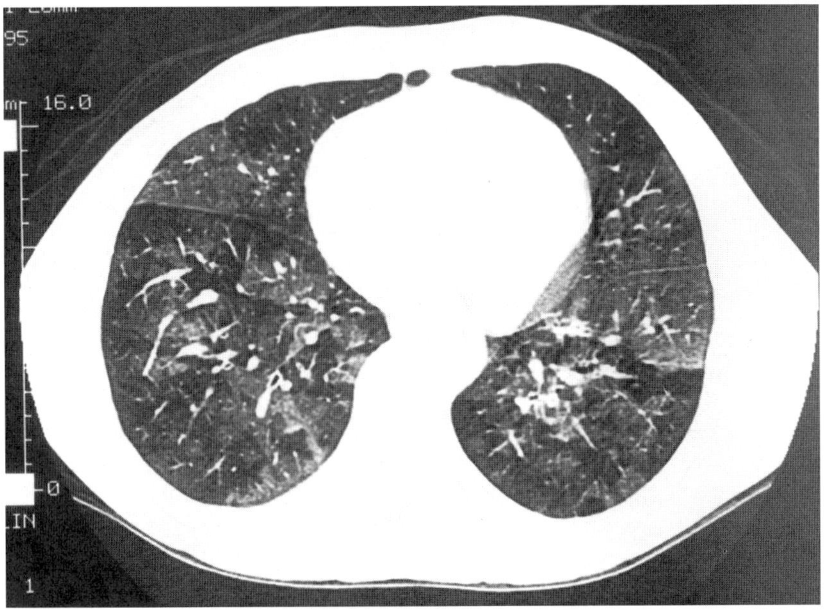


**FIG. 2.** Sample section of high-resolution computed radiograph of a dairy farmer who had presented typical symptoms of recurrent fever, dyspnea, and fatigue, daily over the 2 weeks preceding the radiograph.

absence does not rule out residual disease. However, asymptomatic subjects exposed to an environment that can induce HP (e.g., dairy barns) sometimes have a lymphocytic alveolitis. Therefore, the presence of a lymphocytosis in BAL fluid does not confirm the presence of disease even in exposed subjects (36).

The pathology of HP has been well described (37). Typical findings are those of a mononuclear cellular infiltrate with loosely formed granulomas (Fig. 4). Lung fibrosis is not present in the early phase but can progressively develop. Lung biopsy, however, is rarely needed to establish the diagnosis of HP. Transbronchial biopsies can give supportive pathologic findings, but do not always provide positive or specific results (38). Open lung biopsy is not recommended for routine use, but can sometimes be justified in atypical cases, especially when a careful history fails to uncover a causative agent and other diagnosis cannot be excluded.

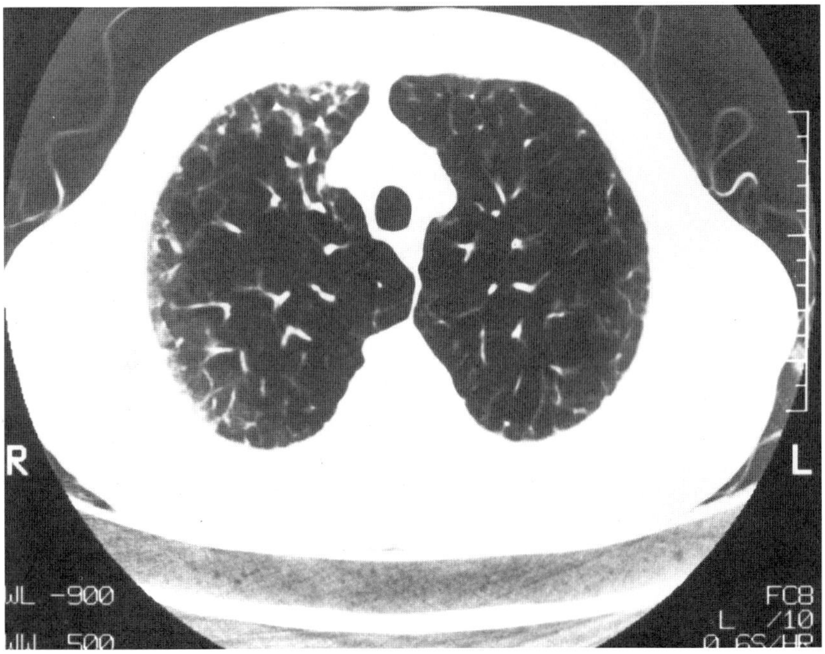


**FIG. 3.** High-resolution computed radiography section obtained in a lifetime nonsmoker with a long-term history of farmer's lung showing diffuse emphysema.

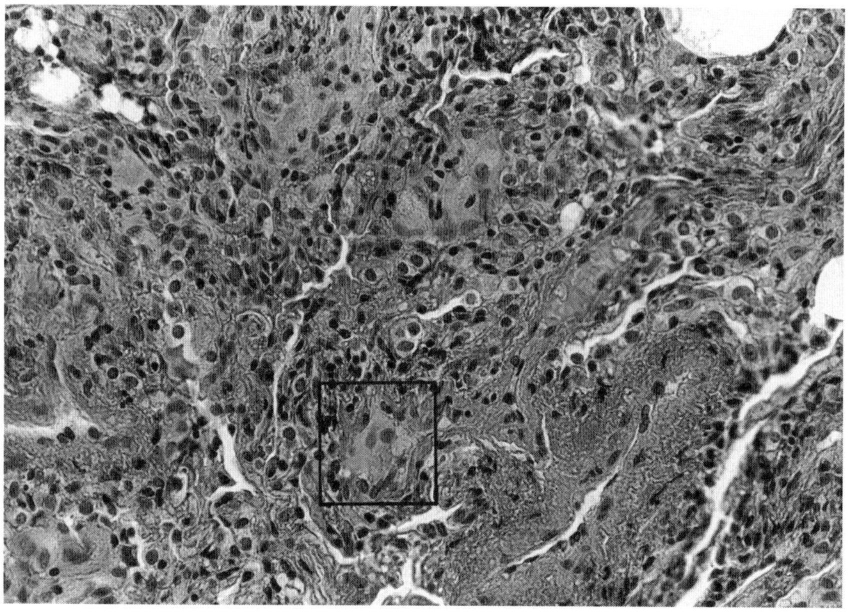

**FIG. 4.** Specimen of a transbronchial biopsy obtained from a case of active HP showing the typical early or loosely formed granulomas and interstitial mononuclear infiltrate (hematoxylin-eosin staining, ×300). Note that transbronchial biopsy only reveals this type of typical pathology in only a third of cases of HP.

## PATHOPHYSIOLOGY

Hypersensitivity pneumonitis is believed to represent a cellular immune response to the offending antigens. In the Gell and Coombs (39) classification the disease cannot be classified in either a type 3 or a type 4 immune response. The appearance of symptoms 3 to 8 hours after exposure suggests a type 3 response; the granulomatous lesions and the cellular participation are more suggestive of a type 4 allergy.

Our understanding of the pathophysiology of HP has recently been improved by studies looking at the lung response by the use of BAL. All studied cellular subsets in the bronchoalveolar fluid are increased in number. Neutrophils are increased early after contact with the antigen (40). Their role is unclear. These cells may contribute to cytokine release and to elastase production that could account for the observed emphysema in some chronic cases of HP (21). The neutrophilic influx is followed by a massive recruitment of lymphocytes, which are the most increased cells in the BAL fluid of HP patients. Normally they constitute less than 20% of BAL, while in HP they often account for 60% to 80% of the recovered cells (25,41). Their number is higher than in other lymphocytic diseases like sarcoidosis (30). BAL lymphocytes are polyclonal (32), predominantly suppressor/cytotoxic $CD8_+$ type (in opposition to sarcoidosis where they are mostly of the helper $CD4_+$ subset) (35). Removal from the offending antigen results in a decrease of $CD8_+$ T cells and an increase of the helper $CD4_+$ cells (33). The ratio CD4/CD8 is therefore a good marker of cellular activation. A high natural killer (NK) cell activity was also found in the BAL of patients with acute HP, correlating with an increasing number of cells bearing the NK-specific $CD56_+$ cell marker (42). The NK activity decreases following corticosteroid treatment or antigen contact avoidance (42,43). Pulmonary memory T cells (CD45 RO) are also increased in HP (44). In an animal model, lymphocytes can transfer sensitization to naive animals, confirming the memory function of these cells (1).

Hypersensitivity pneumonitis alveolar macrophages (AMs) are also activated [increased expression of adhesion molecules intercellular adhesion molecule (ICAM)-1] and are able to release proinflammatory cytokines such as tumor necrosis factor-α (TNF-α) and interleukin-1 (IL-1) *in vitro* (45) as well as IL-8 and macrophage inflammatory protein-1α (MIP-1α). These mediators are decreased after treatment (43). AMs have also lost their normal immunosuppressive function (46) and actually have an enhancing effect on lymphocyte proliferation. When patients with HP are exposed to the responsible antigen, these cells express CD14 antigen, confirming the direct involvement of AM in the immune response (47). Soluble CD14 (sCD14) is also released in the serum. Another useful indicator of AM activation is the expression of interleukin-2 receptor (IL-2R) on the cell surface and the concomitant increase of soluble serum IL-2R (48); both parameters decrease upon immunosuppressive treatment. Mast cell are also increased in BAL of HP patients (49). Their role is controversial (50,51).

Increased levels of immunoglobulins, inflammatory mediators, antiproteases, growth factors, and profibrotic factors are present in BAL fluid. Acute-phase cytokines like TNF-α, IL-1, -2, -5, -6, and -8, and interferon-γ (IFN-γ) are increased in the BAL fluid (52). Monocyte chemotactic protein-1 (MCP-1) and granulocyte-monocyte colony-stimulating factor (GM-CSF) are also increased (46,53). Platelet aggregating factor (PAF) and leukotrienes also participate (54,55). As in many other diseases, the exact role of cytokines and arachidonic acid derivatives in HP is unclear. Many of these substances have a chemotactic and activation role for inflammatory cells.

Specific IgA and IgG are present in BAL fluid (2). It is still unknown if these antibodies, like those found in the serum, are involved in the pathogenesis of HP or if their presence in BAL fluid is only a marker of environmental exposure (56).

Surfactant is altered in HP (57–59). These alterations could play a dual role in HP, both in the modified lung functions and in the immunopathology of the disease process. A decrease in normal surface tension–lowering property of surfactant could contribute to the restrictive lung function of the acute disease. At this time there is usually no lung fibrosis, and the restrictive pattern is reversible and not associated with lung cellular infiltration, which persists after the lung volumes have returned to normal (60). Surfactant and its component have immune-modulator functions (61–63). Surfactant protein A, which enhances the immune response, is increased in the BAL fluid of HP (64,65). Normal surfactant can restore the loss of immunosuppressive function of AMs in HP, while surfactant from patients with the disease has lost this capacity (66).

Hyaluronic acid, fibronectin, vitronectin, fibroblast growth factors, and type III procollagen are all increased in the lungs of HP patients (67–69). Some of these may be markers of disease activity (67) but do not predict long-term outcome (21). High levels of antiproteases have also been reported in the BAL fluid. Although their quantity is increased, their activity may be insufficient to control the increased load of proteases released by local inflammatory cells (neutrophils) explaining the possible emphysematous outcome, or tip the protease/antiprotease balance to favor lung fibrosis.

## EPIDEMIOLOGY

The worldwide prevalence of HP is unknown. Epidemiologic surveys on farmer's lung and pigeon breeders have been reported; even in these two most prevalent forms of HP the data are difficult to interpret. Wide differences in the prevalence of farmer's lung between studies can be explained by differences in climatic conditions in countries where the studies were performed and by differences in the definitions of farmer's lung used (70–73). The best estimates are that farmer's lung afflicts about 3/1,000 farmers in countries where this disease is endemic. Up to 10% to 15% of individuals chronically exposed to pigeons will develop HP (74). HP can occur at all ages and has been described in young children (75). A number of studies have looked for genetic markers of the susceptibility to develop HP (76,77); the issue remains controversial, and it is most likely that familial incidence represents contact with the same environment as in a familial predisposition to the disease. Both the prevalence of serum precipitins and HP are lower in smokers than in nonsmokers (78). Since the number of AMs is increased in the lung of smokers, it is possible that this cell is involved in this protective effect.

## TREATMENT

The best treatment of HP is total avoidance of the offending antigen. This is not always possible or acceptable to the patient; for example, farmers are often reluctant to give up their farm and bird fanciers their hobby. When avoidance is not possible, respiratory protective devices can be useful (79,80). These have to offer an efficient filtration of all contaminating dusts. Many carbon filters and facial masks offer such protection, but they have to be worn continuously when exposed. Small surgical mask–type paper filters are insufficient (81).

Oral corticosteroids are effective in controlling the manifestations of HP. This is the only medical treatment of HP. Recommended doses range from daily administration of 20 mg to 1 mg/kg daily of oral prednisolone (60). In a small short-term study, 20 mg of predinsone daily was as effective as contact withdrawal in improving symptoms, lung infiltrations, and lung functions (60). This medication, however, does not modify the long-term outcome of the disease (82). A reasonable approach is to give oral prednisone (20–25 mg/day) until an adequate control of the environment can be achieved and a higher dose (50 mg/day) for a short course (1 week) in severely affected hypoxic patients. Even if contact can be avoided, corticosteroids will accelerate the initial clinical improvement in most cases.

## PROGNOSIS

The long-term outcome after an attack of HP is extremely variable. It depends on the duration of the disease, the number of recurrences, the persistence of exposure, and probably on undefined intrinsic host factors. It is quite unlikely that one short bout of HP would leave significant sequelae. Fifty percent of farmers with a history of farmer's lung have no residual disease; those who do, often have an obstructive defect due to emphysema (21). Pigeon breeders have a higher risk of developing a fibrotic restrictive lung disease (20). Their 5-year survival may be as low as that of subjects with idiopathic lung fibrosis (20).

## REFERENCES


1. Schuyler M, Subramanyan S, Hassan M. Experimental hypersensitivity pneumonitis: transfer with cultured cells. *J Lab Clin Med* 1987;109: 623–630.
2. Solal-Céligny Ph, Laviolette M.Hébert J, Cormier Y. Immune reactions

in the lungs of asymptomatic dairy farmers. *Am Rev Respir Dis* 1982; 126:964–967.
3. Charles J, Bernstein A, Jones B. Hypersensibility pneumonitis after exposure to isocyanates. *Thorax* 1976;31:127–136.
4. Ramazzini B. *Disease of workers*. Translated by Wright WC, from *De Morbis Artificum Diatriba,* 1713. New York: Hafner, 1964.
5. Campbell JM. Acute symptoms following work with hay. *Br Med J* 1932;2:1143–1144.
6. Pepys J, Jenkins PA, Festenstein GN, et al. Farmer's lung: Thermophilic actinomycetes as a source of farmer's lung hay antigen. *Lancet* 1963;2: 607–611.
7. Fuller CJ. Farmer's lung: a review of present knowledge. *Thorax* 1953; 8:59–64.
8. Emanuel DA, Wenzel FJ, Bowerman CI, Lawton BR. Farmer`s lung, clinical, pathologic, and immunologic study of twenty-four patients. *Am J Med* 1964;37:392–401.
9. Richerson HB, Bernstein IL, Fink JN, et al. Guidelines for the clinical evaluation of hypersensitivity pneumonitis. *J Allergy Clin Immunol* 1989;84:839–844.
10. Boyd G. Clinical and immunological studies in pulmonary extrinsic allergic alveolitis. *Scott Med J* 1978;23:267–276.
11. Cormier Y, Schuyler M. Interstitial lung disease. In: Bone RC, ed. *Hypersensitivity pneumonitis textbook of pulmonary medicine,* vol 2. St. Louis, MO: Mosby-Year Book, 1992;1–9.
12. Korn-Wendisch, F, Kempf A, Grund E, Kroppenstedt, Kutzner HJ. Transfer of faenia rectivirgula kurup and agre to the genus *Saccharopolyspora lacey* and Goodfellow 1975, elevation of *Saccharopolyspora hirsuta* subsp. taberi Labeda 1987 to species level, and emended description of the genus *Saccharopolyspora. Int J Syst Bacteriol* 1989;39:430–441.
13. Yoshida K, Suga M, Nishiura Y, et al. Occupational hypersensitivity pneumonitis in Japan: data on a nationwide epidemiological study. *Occup Environ Med* 1995;52:570–574.
14. Swingler G. Summer-type hypersensitivity pneumonitis in South Africa. *S Afr Med J* 1990;77:104–107.
15. Chemlik F, Dolico G, Reed CE, Dickie H. Farmer's lung. *J Allergy Clin Immunol* 1975;54:180–188.
16. Terho EO. Diagnostic criteria for farmer's lung disease. *Am J Ind Med* 1986;10:329.
17. Leblanc P, Bélanger J, Laviolette M, Cormier Y. Farmer's lung disease: Relationship between continued exposure, alveolitis, and clinical status. *Arch Intern Med* 1986;146:153–157.
18. Sansores R, Salas J, Chapela R et al . Clubbing in hypersensitivity pneumonitis: its prevalence and possible prognostic role. *Arch Intern Med* 1990;150:1849–1851.
19. Hodgson MJ, Parkinson DK, Karpf M. Chest x-rays in hypersensitivity pneumonitis: a meta-analysis of secular trend. *Am J Ind Med* 1989;16: 45–53.
20. Pérez-Padilla R, Salas J, Chapela R, et al. Mortality in Mexican patients with chronic pigeon breeder's lung compared to those with usual interstitial pneumonitis. *Am Rev Respir Dis* 1993;148:49–53.
21. Lalancette M, Carrier G, Ferland S, et al. Long term outcome and predictive value of bronchoalveolar lavage fibrosing factors in farmer's lung. *Am Rev Respir Dis* 1993;148:216–221.
22. Silver SF, Müller Nl, Miller RR, et al. Computed tomography in hypersensitivity pneumonitis. *Radiology* 1989;173:441–445.
23. Hapke EJ, Seal REM, Thomas GO, et al. Farmer's Lung: a clinical, radiological, functional, and serological correlation of acute and chronic stages. *Thorax* 1968;23:451–468.
24. Braun SR, doPico GA, Tsiatis A, Horvath E, Dickie HA, Rankin J. Farmers's lung disease: a long-term clinical and physiological outcome. *Am Rev Respir Dis* 1979;119:185–191.
25. Cormier Y, Bélanger J, Leblanc P, et al. Bronchoalveolar lavage in farmer's lung disease: diagnosis and physiological significance. *Br J Ind Med* 1986;43:401–405.
26. Salvaggio J. Diagnostic significance of serum precipitins in hypersensitivity pneumonitis. *Chest* 1972;62:242.
27. Cormier Y, Bélanger J, Durand P. Factors influencing the development of serum precipitins to farmer's lung antigen in Quebec dairy farmers. *Thorax* 1985;40:138–142.
28. Roberts RC, Wenzelo FJ, Emanuel DA. Precipitating antibodies in midwest dairy farming population toward the antigens associated with farmer's lung disease. *J Allergy Clin Immunol* 1976;57:518–524.
29. Agostini C, Trentin L, Zambello R, et al. Pulmonary alveolar macrophages in patients with sarcoidosis and hypersensitivity pneumonitis: characterization by monoclonal antibodies. *J Immunol* 1987;7: 64–69.
30. Godard P, Clot J, Jonquet O, et al. Lymphocyte subpopulations in bronchoalveolar lavage of patients with sarcoidosis and hypersensitivity pneumonitis. *Chest* 1981;80:447–452.
31. Robinson BWS, Thompson PJ, Rose AH, Hey A. Comparison of bronchoalveolar lavage helper/suppressor t-cell ratios in sarcoidosis versus other interstitial lung diseases. *Aust NZ J Med* 1987;17:9–15.
32. Mornex JF, Cordier G, Pages J, et al. Activated lung lymphocytes in hypersensitivity pneumonitis. *J Allergy Clin Immunol* 1984;74: 719–727.
33. Trentin L, Migone N, Zambello R, et al. Mechanisms accounting for lymphocytic alveolitis in hypersensitivity pneumonitis. *J Immunol* 1990;154:2147–2154.
34. Semanzato G, Agostini C, Zambello R, et al. Lung T cells in hypersensitivity pneumonitis: phenotypic and functional analysis. *J Immunol* 1986;137:1164–1172.
35. Costabel U, Bross KJ, Marxen J, et al. T-lymphocytes in bronchoalveolar lavage fluid of hypersensitivity pneumonitis. *Chest* 1984;4: 514–518.
36. Cormier Y, Bélanger J, Beaudoin J, Laviolette M, Beaudoin R, Hébert J. Abnormal bronchoalveolar lavage in asymptomatic dairy farmers: a study of lymphocytes. *Am Rev Respir Dis* 1984;130:1046–1049.
37. Seal RME, Hapke EJ, Thomas GO, Meek JC, Hayes M. The pathology of the acute and chronic stages of farmer`s lung. *Thorax* 1968;23: 469–489.
38. Lacasse Y, Fournier M, Carrier G, Cormier Y. Transbronchial biopsy in diagnosis of acute farmer's lung disease. *Am Rev Respir Crit Care Med* 1994;149:A79.
39. Gell PGH, Coombs RRA. Classification of allergic reactions responsible for clinical hypersensitivity and disease. In: Gell PGH, Coombs RRA, eds. *Clinical aspects of immunology*. Oxford and Edinburgh: Blackwell, 1968;575–596.
40. Fournier E, Tonnel AB, Gosset PH, et al. Early neutrophil alveolitis after antigen inhalation in hypersensitivity pneumonitis. *Chest* 1985; 88:563–566.
41. Laviolette M. Lymphocyte fluctuation in bronchoalveolar lavage of normal volunteers. *Thorax* 1985;40:651–656.
42. Keller RH, Swartz S, Schlueter DP, Bar-Sela S, Fink JN. Immunoregulation in hypersensitivity pneumonitis: phenotypic and functional studies of bronchoalveolar lavage lymphocytes. *Am Rev Respir Dis* 1984; 130:766–771.
43. Denis M, Bédard M, Laviolette M, Cormier Y. A study of monokine release and natural killer activity in the bronchoalveolar lavage of subjects with Farmer's lung. *Am Rev Respir Dis* 1993;147:934–939.
44. Furaro S, Berman JS. The relation between cell migration and activation in inflammation: Beyond adherence. *Am J Respir Cell Mol Biol* 1992;7:248–250.
45. Denis M, Cormier Y, Tardif J, Ghadirian J, Laviolette M. Hypersensitivity pneumonitis: *Micropolyspora faeni* or antigens thereof stimulate the release of proinflammatory cytokines from macrophages. *Am J Respir Cells Mol Biol* 1991;5:198–203.
46. Dakhama A, Israël-Assayag E, Cormier Y. Altered immunosuppressive activity of alveolar macrophages in farmer's lung. *Eur Respir J* 1996;9: 1456–1462.
47. Pforte A, Schiessler A, Gais P, et al. Increased expression of the monocyte differentiation antigen CD14 in extrinsic allergic alveolitis. *Monaldi Arch Chest Dis* 1993;48:607–612.
48. Pforte A, Brunner A, Gais P, et al. Increased levels of soluble serum interleukin-2 receptor in extrinsic allergic alveolitis correlate with interleukin-2 receptor expression on alveolar macrophages. *J Allergy Clin Immunol* 1994;94:1059–1064.
49. Solar P, Nioche S, Valeyre D, et al. Role of mast cells in the pathogenesis of hypersensitivity pneumonitis. *Thorax* 1987;42:565–572.
50. Bjermer L, Engstrom-Laurent A, Lundgren R, Rosenhall L, Hallgren R. Bronchoalveolar mastocytosis in farmer's lung is related to disease activity. *Arch Invest Med* 1988;148:1362–1365.
51. Laviolette M, Cormier Y, Loiseau A, Soler P, Leblanc P, Hance AJ. Role of mast cell in extrinsic allergic alveolitis. *Am Rev Respir Dis* 1991; 144:855–860.
52. Walker C, Bauer W, Braun RK, et al. Activated T cells and cytokines in bronchoalveolar lavages from patients with various lung diseases associated with eosinophilia. *Am J Respir Crit Care Med* 1994;150:1038–1048.

53. Sugiyama Y, Kasahara T, Mukaida N, Matsushima K, Kitamura S. Chemokines in bronchoalveolar lavage fluid in summer-type hypersensitivity pneumonitis. *Eur Respir J* 1995;8:1084–1090.
54. Tremblay GM, Assayag E, Sirois P, Cormier Y. Evidence for a role of ecosanoids and platelet activating factor (PAF) in murine hypersensitivity pneumonitis (HP). *Immuno Invest* 1993;22:341–352.
55. Selman M, Barquin N, Sansores R, et al. Increased levels of leukotriene C4 in bronchoalveolar lavage from patients with pigeon breeder's disease. *Arch Invest Med (Mex)* 1988;19:127–131.
56. Burrell P, Rylander R. A critical review of the role of precipitins in hypersensitivity pneumonitis. *Eur J Respir Dis* 1981;62:332–343.
57. Lesur O, Mancini NM, Janot C, Chabot F, Polu JM, Gérard H. Loss of lymphocyte modulatory control by surfactant lipid extract from acute hypersensitivity pneumonitis: comparison with sarcoidosis and idiopathic pulmonary fibrosis. *Eur Respir J* 1994;7:1944–1949.
58. Jouanel P, Motta C, Brun J, et al. Phospholipids and microviscosity in broncho-alveolar lavage fluid from control subjects and from patients with extrinsic allergic alveolitis. *Clin Chim Acta* 1981;115:211–221.
59. Schmitz-Schumann M, Costabel U, Ferber E, et al. Composition of surfactant phospholipids in bronchoalveolar lavage fluid from patients with extrinsic allergic alveolitis and sarcoidosis. *Prax Klin Pneumol* 1986;40:216–218.
60. Cormier Y, Desmeules M. Treatment of hypersensitivity pneumonitis (HP): comparison between contact avoidance and corticosteroids. *Can Respir J* 1994;1:223–228.
61. Ansfield MJ, Kaltreider HB, Benson BJ, Caldwell JL. Immunosuppressive activity of canine pulmonary surface active material. *J Immunol* 1979;122:1062–1066.
62. Pison U, Max M , Neuendank A, Weiβbach S, Pietschmann S. Host defence capacities of pulmonary surfactant: evidence for non-surfactant functions of the surfactant system. *Eur J Clin Invest* 1994;24:586–599.
63. Catanzaro A, Richman P, Batcher S, Hallman M. Immunomodulation by pulmonary surfactant. *J Lab Clin Med* 1988;112:727–734.
64. Guzman J, Wang YM, Kalycioglu O, et al. Increased surfactant protein A content in human alveolar macrophages in hypersensitivity pneumonitis. *Acta Cytol* 1992;36:668–673.
65. Cormier Y, Israël-Assayag E, Desmeules M, Lesur O. Bronchoalveolar lavage surfactant protein A (SP-A) in subjects with farmer's lung and asymptomatic farmers: effect of treatment. *Thorax* 1996;51:1210–1215.
66. Israël-Assayag E, Bellemare F, Cormier Y. Surfactant from patients with hypersensitivity pneumonitis (HP) is unable to restore the altered suppressive activity of alveolar macrophages in HP. *Am J Respir Crit Care Med* 1996;153:A663.
67. Bjermer L, Engström-Laurent, Lundgren R, Rosenhall L, Hällgren R. Hyaluronate and type III procollagen peptide concentrations in bronchoalveolar lavage fluid as markers of disease activity in farmer's lung. *Br Med J* 1987;295:803–806.
68. Teschler H, Pohl WR, Thompson AB, et al. Elevated levels of bronchoalveolar lavage vitronectin in hypersensitivity pneumonitis. *Am Rev Respir Dis* 1993;147:332–337.
69. Cormier Y, Tremblay G, Cantin A, Laviolette M, Bégin R. Markers of fibrosis in bronchoalveolar lavage fluid in different states of farmer's lung. *Chest* 1993;104:1038–1042.
70. Terho EO, Heinonen OP, Lammi S. Incidence of clinically confirmed farmer's lung disease in Finland. *Am J Ind Med* 1986;10:330.
71. Madsen D, Klock LE, Wenzel FJ, Robbins JL, Schmidt CD. The prevalence of farmer's lung in an agricultural population. *Am Rev Respir Dis* 1976;113:171–174.
72. Gump DW, Babbott FL, Holly C, Sylwester DL. Farmer's lung disease in Vermont. *Respiration* 1979;37:52–60.
73. Stanford CF, Hall G, Chivers A, Martin B, Nicholls DP, Evans J. Farmer's lung in Northern Ireland. *Br J Ind Med* 1990;47:314–316.
74. Fink JN. Epidemiologic aspects of hypersensitivity pneumonitis. *Monogr Allergy* 1987;21:59–69.
75. Bureau MA, Fecteau C, Patriquin H, Rola-Pleszczynski M, Masse S, Bégin R. Farmer's lung in early childhood. *Am Rev Respir Dis* 1979; 119:671–675.
76. Terho EO, Koshimies S, Heinonen OP, Mäntyjärvi R. HLA and farmer's lung. *Eur J Respir Dis* 1981;63:361–362.
77. Flaherty DK, Braun SR, Marx JL, Blank JL, Emanuel DA, Rankin J. Serologically detectable HLA-A, B and C loci antigens in farmer's lung disease. *Am Rev Respir Dis* 1980;122:437–443.
78. Warren CPW. Extrinsic allergic alveolitis: a disease commoner in nonsmokers. *Thorax* 1977:32:567–569.
79. Hendrick DJ, Marshall R, Faux JA, et al. Protective value of dust respirators in extrinsic allergic alveolitis: clinical assessment using inhalation provocation tests. *Thorax* 1981;36:917–921.
80. Kusaka H, Ogasawara H, Munakata M, et al. Two-year follow-up on the protective value of dust masks against farmer's lung disease. *Intern Med* 1993;32:106–111.
81. Dalphin JC, Pernet D, Roux C, et al. Investigation of the protective value of breathing masks on thermophilic actinomycetes. *Am Rev Respir Dis* 1993;147:A903.
82. Kokkarinen JI, Tukiainen HO, Terho EO. Effect of corticosteroid treatment on the recovery of pulmonary function in farmer's lung. *Am Rev Respir Dis* 1992;145;3–5.

*Environmental and Occupational Medicine,*
*Third Edition,* edited by William N. Rom.
Lippincott–Raven Publishers, Philadelphia © 1998.

# CHAPTER 32

# Inhalation Fever

Cecile S. Rose and Paul David Blanc

## BACKGROUND

A variety of inhalational exposures occurring in disparate occupational and environmental settings can induce flu-like symptoms that are self-limited, although temporarily debilitating. Inhalational exposures to microbially contaminated humidifiers, zinc oxide fumes from welding, pyrolysis products of polytetrafluoroethylene, moldy grain dust from silo unloading, and bubbling whirlpool aerosols contaminated with *Legionella* organisms have all been associated with similar febrile, flu-like responses. Because these syndromes are so similar clinically despite their heterogeneous causes, they have come to be known collectively as "inhalation fevers." The unifying concept of inhalation fever was first proposed in 1978, but did not come into wider use until the last 10 years, when a number of investigators began to focus renewed research interest in the shared mechanisms potentially linking similar syndromes so different in etiology (1–7).

Table 1 summarizes the major documented causes of inhalation fever grouped by broader categories of exposure. The diversity of these exposures is matched by their often colorful names. The varied causes of inhalation fever and its many appellations have led to nosologic imprecision and clinical confusion.

This is complicated further because many of the causes of inhalation fever are capable of eliciting other, less benign clinical syndromes. A key algorithmic branch point requires differentiating between inhalation fever and acute lung injury. In certain aspects these two distinctly different patterns of pulmonary response may appear quite similar (Table 2). Both are manifest within hours of exposure. Fever, the sine qua non of inhalation fever, nonetheless can be present in acute lung injury due to toxic inhalation (8–12). Moreover, the exposure scenarios for both inhalation fever and acute lung injury may be disturbingly similar. Welding may involve zinc oxide inhalation, causing metal fume fever, or may be associated with cadmium fume or nitrogen dioxide gas exposure (13,14). Either of these latter two toxins cause acute lung injury following high-intensity exposure. Thermal breakdown of fluoropolymers may release by-products that cause polymer fume fever or, with higher temperatures, release hydrofluoric acid and other irritant aerosols that can cause acute injury (15). Damp and moldy organic materials that typically cause inhalation fever (organic dust toxic syndrome) can occasionally be contaminated with poorly characterized fungal by-products that appear to act as potent toxins leading to lung injury (16). Fresh silage may release nitrogen dioxide (silo filler's disease); stored silage contaminated with thermophylic bacteria and molds can cause inhalation fever (silo unloader's disease) (9,17). Despite all of these similarities and overlapping exposure scenarios, inhalation fever is quite distinct from acute lung injury, as Table 2 delineates. Inhalation fever is self-limited and should not be complicated by significant respiratory compromise. In contradistinction, the hallmarks of toxin-related acute lung injury are chest radiographic infiltrates, hypoxemia, and, at the severe end of the spectrum, adult respiratory

C. S. Rose: Division of Environmental and Occupational Health Sciences, Department of Medicine, National Jewish Medical and Research Center; and Division of Pulmonary Sciences and Critical Care Medicine, Department of Medicine, University of Colorado Health Sciences Center, Denver, Colorado 80206.

P. D. Blanc: Division of Occupational and Environmental Medicine, Department of Medicine, University of California, San Francisco, San Francisco, California 94117.

**TABLE 1.** *The heterogeneous causes of inhalation fever*

| Exposure | Syndrome name |
|---|---|
| Metal fumes | Metal fume fever |
| Zinc oxide | Spelter shakes, Monday morning fever |
| Magnesium oxide | |
| Contaminated water sources | No generic name |
| Humidifiers and air conditioners | Humidifier fever |
| Fountains, whirlpools, cooling systems | Pontiac fever (*Legionella*) |
| Bath water | Bath water fever |
| Water sumps | Sump fever |
| Sewage | |
| Contaminated vegetable matter/agricultural dusts | Organic dust toxic syndrome |
| Hemp, jute, or flax dust | Heckling fever (flax) |
| Cotton dust | Mill fever, Monday morning fever |
| Grain dust (wheat, sorghum, others) | Grain fever |
| Animal confinement work | Swine fever |
| Silage or straw | Silo-unloader's disease |
| Composted leaves or wood chips | |
| Wood (lumber) trimmings | Wood-trimmer's disease |
| Other causes | No generic name |
| Fluoropolymer breakdown | Polymer fume fever |
| Poultry processing | Duck fever |
| Xanthan gum manufacture | |

distress syndrome (ARDS). In the presence of the symptoms or signs of acute lung injury, the diagnosis of inhalation fever should not be invoked; rather, exposure to a toxic inhalant should be suspected. Terminology such as "severe organic dust toxic syndrome," "serious fume fever," or "toxic dust pneumonitis" obfuscate rather than illuminate the important differences between the inhalation fever syndromes and the acute lung injury response. Such terminology should be avoided where possible.

Differentiation from acute lung injury is not the only diagnostic challenge in assessing inhalation fever. Almost every generic cause of inhalation fever can also be associated with other respiratory responses that are important to recognize and to treat. These include most prominently hypersensitivity pneumonitis (allergic alveolitis) from organic dusts and bioaerosols; invasive respiratory infection, particularly due to some of the same *Legionella* species that are also associated with inhalation fever without invasive disease; and bronchospasm, caused by organic dusts or fibers contaminated with bacteria (as a source of endotoxin) or fungus (point source exposure to *Aspergillus)* or, rarely, bronchospasm due to zinc oxide. Because these alternative diagnoses are more exposure-specific, we will deal with each, in turn, in the discussion of the appropriate exposure group.

**TABLE 2.** *Inhalation fever in contrast to acute lung injury*

| Characteristics | Inhalation fever | Acute lung injury |
|---|---|---|
| Acute, high intensity exposure | ++++ | ++++ |
| Fever | ++++ | +++ |
| Onset within hours of exposure | ++++ | ++++ |
| Dyspnea | + | ++++ |
| Chest radiographic infiltrates | – | ++++ |
| Hypoxemia | – | ++++ |
| Peripheral leukocytosis | ++++ | +++ |
| Lung inflammatory cellular influx | +++ | ++++ |
| Acute mortality risk | – | ++++ |
| Chronic physiologic sequelae | – | ++ |

+, reflects presence and intensity of association; –, no association.

These diagnostic difficulties create additional uncertainty in the already error-prone estimates of the incidence and prevalence of inhalation fever. Although precise data are not available, inhalation fever is certainly not a rare event among those exposed to the materials listed in Table 1. National Poison Control Center surveillance data capture approximately 1,000 cases of metal fume fever a year, just one syndrome among the multiple causes of inhalation fever (18). Among the 35 million agricultural workers in the United States, inhalation fever is more common than hypersensitivity pneumonitis, although far less well recognized, even by respiratory disease specialists. The National Institute for Occupational Safety and Health (NIOSH), recognizing the importance of the problem, issued a special workplace hazard alert in 1994, "Request for Assistance in Preventing Organic Dust Toxic Syndrome" (19).

The precise pathogenic mechanisms of the various inhalation fever syndromes remain poorly understood. Our limited understanding of the mechanisms underlying inhalation fever in large part stems from the very heterogeneity of its causes. However, a number of mechanistic insights have seen suggested by the long-recognized, shared epidemiologic aspects of the different inhalation fever syndromes. These insights have been further enriched by observations from experimental laboratory animal and human exposure studies. Together, these data point to the lung as the key target organ in inhalation fever, serving not only as a portal of entry, but also as the source of biochemical messengers mediating the syndrome's systemic features (5).

The critical epidemiologic and experimental features of inhalation fever are summarized in Table 3. Universally, the inhalation fever syndromes are notable for very high attack rates among those heavily exposed, even if previously naive to the inhalant. This weighs convincingly against an amnestic response associated with humoral or cellular immunity resulting from sensitization. The high attack rate in inhalation fever, which can exceed 90% in Pontiac fever or fall in a similar range with heavy dust exposure (for example, an "indoor" hay ride with damp and moldy straw), also argues against a pathogenic mechanism requiring a genetically determined or idiosyncratic response (20,21).

In contrast to the lack of required sensitization, the inhalation fever syndromes commonly manifest tachyphylaxis following frequent repeated exposure. Such daily exposures are unlikely in environmental outbreaks, but are prominent in certain occupational scenarios such as brass foundries and textile mills. Not surprisingly, in both of these settings the name *Monday morning fever* was applied to inhalation fever, recognizing that employees were most likely to be symptomatic on return to the workplace after a weekend or other period of absence (22,23).

In both animal models and in volunteer human subjects, experimental data have shown that agents known or suspected of causing inhalation fever induce a marked neutrophil influx in the lung. For example, bronchoalveolar lavage (BAL) 1 day after zinc oxide inhalation has shown 35% polymorphonuclear leukocytes; studies of grain and swine-room dust inhalation have identified comparable BAL findings (24–26). Similar experimental approaches to inhalation fever have found exposure dose- and time-dependent increases in proinflammatory cytokines, particularly tumor necrosis factor (TNF), interleukin-6, and the neutrophil chemotactic factor interleukin-8 in the lung (27–29). Indeed, inhalation fever is arguably one of the best experimental models for cytokine networking in the lung. Such networking is thought to be pivotal to the inflammatory response generally (30).

Many important pathogenic questions related to inhalation fever remained to be addressed. In particular, the underlying mechanism of tachyphylaxis in inhalation fever and the reasons for the ultimately benign nature of the syndrome despite its impressive inflammatory cellular component have not yet been elucidated (antiinflammatory negative feedback from inhibitory cytokines remains a distinct possibility). Future epidemiologic and experimental research may answer these intriguing questions.

**TABLE 3.** *Unifying pathogenic characteristics of the inhalation fever syndromes*

1. Sensitization not required
2. High attack rates with heavy exposure
3. Blunted response with repeated exposure (tachyphylaxis)
4. Lung is portal of entry and target organ mediating response
5. Inflammatory cellular pulmonary infiltrate (polymorphonuclear leukocytes)
6. Proinflammatory cytokines appear to play a pivotal role

## METAL FUMES

### Zinc Oxide

Zinc oxide–caused metal fume fever is the inhalation fever syndrome longest recognized historically. Over the years, it has been well characterized in multiple case reports and extensively studied epidemiologically and experimentally. The syndrome was first reported by Thackrah (31) over 150 years ago in association with zinc oxide fume from brass foundry work. By the mid-Victorian era, the role of zinc oxide in metal fume fever (one of its terms was *brass founder's ague)* and the principal clinical aspects of the syndrome were well established.

The best early description of the syndrome, which is instructive to cite at some length, was documented by Greenhow (32) in 1862 who wrote,

> Brass-casters who have personal experience of the disease entirely agree in their account of its symptoms, more than seventy of them having described the disorder in almost identical terms. These symptoms are a sense of malaise and weariness...a feeling of constriction or tightness in the chest, and, in some rare cases, nausea commencing during the afternoon of a day employed in casting, followed towards evening, or at the latest when getting into bed, by shivering, sometimes succeeded by an indistinct hot stage....Regular casters who have been absent from work for a few days are reported to be more liable to suffer from this disease....And now as regards the cause of this curious malady. The men themselves attribute it to inhaling the fumes of deflagrating zinc or spelter....The quantity of fumes given off depends mainly upon the proportion of zinc employed in making the brass, which varies with the purpose for which the brass is intended. Moreover, a much greater quantity is given off when the metals are mixed to make brass than when brass ingots are merely remelted....I may add, in conclusion, that this disease is unknown among operatives, such as makers of galvanized iron, who work over molten zinc when the temperature is not high enough to cause deflagration and oxidation of the metal.

A modern text has little to do but reiterate the key features noted above: the syndrome is associated with high levels of exposure to zinc oxide fume [lower exposure concentrations such as encountered in routine galvanizing (dipping steel in molten zinc) or dust from grinding operations do not typically lead to metal fume fever]; chills, fever, and malaise are the predominant symptoms but minor respiratory and gastrointestinal complaints can accompany the syndrome; and tachyphylaxis occurs with repeated exposure. Wisely, there has also been little change in the clinical management of this self-limited condition, which is predicated on supportive care (rest and fluids) and avoidance of further overexposure. The use of milk as a preventive measure is a widely invoked folk treatment among those exposed. Although this remedy dates back at least to the 19th century, its efficacy has never been formally evaluated.

Early reports of metal fume fever in the brass industry questioned whether the syndrome truly was due to zinc oxide or might rather represent a response to copper or even trace contaminants such as lead or arsenic. This question was effectively put to rest early in the 20th century when a series of experimental human studies conclusively established zinc oxide as the cause of metal fume fever in brass foundry workers (33–36). The first modern review of the scientific literature on metal fume fever appeared in German in 1906 (37); the first English language review was by Drinker (38) in 1922.

The epidemiology of metal fume fever has reflected the shifting industrial exposure patterns to zinc oxide fume. For example, the largest cohort study of metal fume fever was carried out in the 1920s under the aegis of the United States Public Health Service and included 22 brass foundries (22). Of the cohort studied, 30% had experienced at least one attack of metal fume fever and more than one-third of these experienced attacks as often as once a week. The latency from first exposure until symptom onset was documented to be 4 to 6 hours.

By mid-century, the epidemiologic focus shifted to a new occupationally exposed group: welders of galvanized steel. In particular, the shipyard industry has been the source of many reports of metal fume fever in welders (39–43). Other work practices of note have included flame-cutting of galvanized metal and high-temperature zinc coating processes (44–48). These various reports and small case series have documented that leukocytosis is common in the condition (often exceeding 15,000 leukocytes per cubic millimeter of blood) and that radiographic abnormalities in classic zinc-caused metal fume fever are atypical and, if present at all, are minimal and transitory.

Other insights have been gained from case reports of zinc oxide as well. It is often stated that only zinc oxide fume freshly formed from vaporized metal can induce an inhalation fever response. However, case reports have documented fume fever following heavy exposure to finely ground dust without the presence of fume itself (41,44). It has also been shown that although classic inhalation fever is its principal exposure response, other syndromes may also occur rarely after zinc oxide inhalation. There have been well-documented cases of bronchospasm, contact urticaria, and hypersensitivity-like responses associated with exposure to zinc oxide fume (49–56). Case reports have also shown that acute overexposure to zinc oxide via ingestion (e.g., when acidic food materials are inappropriately prepared in galvanized containers) causes a severe gastroenteritis, but not metal fume fever (57,58). There is at least one case report of toxic parenteral overexposure to zinc without a febrile response, reinforcing the concept of the lung as a key mediator of inhalation fever (59).

Although case reports and epidemiologic studies have firmly established the signs and symptoms of inhalation fever associated with zinc oxide fume exposure, more recently the pathophysiology of the syndrome has been clarified by a series of experimental studies in laboratory animals and in human subjects. Inhalation and intratracheal installation of zinc oxide have both been shown to produce a marked inflammatory cellular response in laboratory animals, as well as inducing a temporary decrement in lung function (60–63). Unfortunately, it has been difficult to develop a animal model of zinc oxide inhalation in which a febrile response mimicking the human syndrome can be induced.

Human experimental exposure studies have also documented an impressive time-dependent inflammatory cellular response in the lung paralleling the animal findings, but also accompanied by the full clinical syndrome with sufficiently heavy exposure (24,64). Moreover, further studies have strongly implicated TNF and interleukin-8 as likely key cytokine mediators of metal fume fever (27,65). Interestingly, these data have not shown a consistent pulmonary function decrement even following heavy zinc oxide fume inhalation, suggesting that neither airflow obstruction nor a restrictive ventilatory deficit is a necessary physiologic correlate of metal fume fever. These studies have also failed to show a role of acute serum zinc levels in assessing exposure, although this was suggested as a clinically useful test in one widely cited case report (66).

### Other Metals

It is often stated that, in addition to zinc oxide, any number of metals cause metal fume fever. Frequently cited metals include magnesium, copper, cadmium, chromium, antimony, and iron. In humans, the only strong experimental association is with magnesium oxide, although this is based on data from the 1920s (67). There is also some limited epidemiologic data to support this association, although significant industrial exposure to magnesium oxide fume is extremely uncommon, limiting the opportunities for field investigation (68). Unfortunately, a recent human exposure model has failed to produce a metal fume fever response with magnesium oxide inhalation (69).

Copper is a potential cause of metal fume fever. However, there are only a handful of citations in the scientific literature describing a copper-associated febrile reaction. In none is sufficient industrial hygiene data available together with clinical information convincingly supporting a causal relationship (70–73). Cadmium inhalation is an established cause of acute lung injury, which can be accompanied by fever (10,74–78). Even though the term *cadmium fume fever* is sometimes used for this condition, this designation is inappropriate. In contrast to metal fume fever, lung injury following cadmium inhalation is not self-limited but progressive and often fatal (see Table 2). As noted previously, respiratory compromise is not consistent with inhalation fever and suggests an alternative diagnostic entity. Because welding or flame cutting of sheet metal or of previously soldered metals can lead to significant cadmium fume exposure (silver solder can be cadmium-based), cadmium pneumonitis should be considered in the differential diagnosis of lung injury associated with welding. Zinc chloride, as opposed to zinc oxide fume, is also a cause of severe lung injury but not of metal fume fever. Exposure can occur through the use of zinc chloride–containing smoke bombs in military or police training exercises (79,80).

Aside from one report of fever among ferrochromium smelter workers (81), there are no published studies indicating that metal fume fever occurs with either iron or chromium. There are no data at all to support other metal oxides as causes of inhalation fever, suggesting that zinc oxide acts in a fairly specific rather than generic fashion. This may have important mechanistic implications that await further experimental elucidation.

## CONTAMINATED WATER SOURCES

### Humidifier Fever

Many individual cases and outbreaks of humidifier-related inhalation fever have been reported since such episodes were first linked together in a 1976 Medical Research Council symposium (82). Humidifier fever (HF) is an influenza-like illness with constitutional symptoms of fever, chills, headache, malaise, and, less prominently, respiratory tract symptoms. The syndrome occurs 4 to 12 hours after exposure to aerosols generated from forced-air conditioning and humidification systems. Attack rates of HF among heavily exposed populations are high and consistent with the pattern of inhalation fever from other causes. Humidifier fever is also associated with return to work after some time away from the contaminated environment (so-called Monday miseries), and with improvement in symptoms over the workweek. Nonetheless, HF presents a diagnostic challenge because nearly identical exposure conditions can lead to a similarly named but quite different syndrome, humidifier lung.

Humidifier lung (HL) is a form of hypersensitivity pneumonitis with prominent, often chronic, respiratory symptoms associated with typical findings of radiographic infiltrates, hypoxemia, and granulomatous pneumonitis on lung biopsy. However, there is important overlap between HL and HF. In HF, a majority of symptomatic workers have demonstrated multiple serum precipitins to extracts of humidifier sludge or water, similar to HL. A significant percentage of asymptomatic exposed workers have also been shown to have precipitating antibodies to the humidifier contaminants, reflecting the role of these precipitins as markers of exposure. Specific precipitating antibodies against individual species of bacteria and fungi isolated from contaminated humidifiers have been consistently negative, except for precipitins to amebae that were identified in some of the early reported outbreaks of HF (83). Bronchial challenge with extracts of contaminated water has been shown to reproduce the symptoms of HF in affected workers but not in unexposed controls (84). Moreover, as with hypersensitivity pneumonitis, HF more often affects nonsmokers than cigarette smokers (85,86). The similarities and differences between HF and HL are summarized in Table 4. It may be that in some individuals both illnesses occur simultaneously. In addition to HL and HF, humidifier exposures may also lead to asthma-like symptoms and airflow obstruction.

The specific pathogenic factors leading to HF remain to be identified, but the excessive growth of microorganisms within humidification systems seems to be common to all outbreaks. Implicated organisms include *Naegleria gruberi, Pseudomonas* species, and other gram-negative bacteria. In some outbreaks, endotoxins from gram-negative bacteria may play a pivotal role in the pathogenesis of HF (87), but this has not been established as a universal factor in all HF episodes.

If the pathophysiology of HF is poorly understood, the industrial hygiene parameters of exposure are better elucidated. Humidity control requires the introduction of water into a moving current of air. Baffle plates are often installed in humidification systems in order to eliminate large water droplets. Organic dust may be drawn into the system where it settles on the baffle plates and serves as a biomass for microorganisms entering from the air and water supply. The greatest threat is from humidifiers that draw contaminated water from large and relatively stagnant sources, which is then nebulized through forced-air ventilation systems. The microorganisms probably originate from ambient air and proliferate on nutrients of the water reservoirs. In some cases, a heavily contaminated slime or sludge accumulates within the humidifier. HF occurs principally in winter months, probably owing to the greater use of humidification when air intake to the ventilation

**TABLE 4.** *Inhalation fever in contrast to hypersensitivity pneumonitis*

| | Inhalation fever | Hypersensitivity pneumonitis |
|---|---|---|
| Examples | Humdifier fever<br>ODTS | Humidifier lung<br>Farmer's lung |
| Exposure | Single, high concentration | Repeated |
| Attack rates | High | Often low |
| Symptom latency | 4 to 8 hours, even without previous exposure | Weeks to years following first exposure |
| Symptoms | Systemic symptoms predominate | Respiratory and systemic symptoms |
| Tolerance | Often occurs | Not described |
| Physical examination | Fever; lung exam normal | May have crepitant rales |
| Laboratory findings | | |
| WBC count | Increased | Usually normal, except in "acute" illness |
| Precipitins | Negative | Often positive |
| Chest radiograph of HRCT | Normal | Diffuse reticulonodular infiltrates (may be normal) |
| Pulmonary function | Normal | Restriction, obstruction, or mixed abnormalities, often with decreased $DL_{CO}$ (may be normal) |
| BAL | Neutrophilia | Lymphocytosis |
| Histopathology | Bronchiolar neutrophilic and histiocytic underlying inflammation (few cases) | Monuclear interstitial inflammation, peribronchiolar granulomas |
| Natural history | Complete recovery within 3 days | Recurrent acute or progressive subacute symptoms with ongoing exposure |

system is coolest. However, intermittent humidification during the summer may lead to symptoms that erroneously do not appear to be work related because exposure to humidified air is intermittent (88).

The printing industry has been particularly associated with HF outbreaks, as the process generates paper dust, which appears to provide an ideal organic substrate for microbial proliferation, and optimal printing requires a constant level of ambient humidity (89). Outbreaks have been described in a variety of other occupational and nonoccupational environments, including microprocessor and synthetic textile manufacturing, offices, hospital operating rooms, and from exposure to contaminated home heating units and even tap water (82,85,86,88,90–95). Remedial actions to prevent HF include regular and frequent cleaning of the humidification or cooling systems, modification of the baffle plates to reduce biomass accumulation, installation of prefilters to remove organic nutrients and reduce microbial inoculum, and elimination or decontamination of recirculating water (96).

## PONTIAC FEVER

Pontiac fever is a severe, self-limited, influenza-like illness associated with exposure to aerosols of contaminated water. It bears exposure similarities to HF but is associated with a single pathogen. The causative agent, the bacterium *Legionella pneumophila,* was first isolated in 1977 as the cause of Legionnaires' disease, a clinically and epidemiologically distinct illness from Pontiac fever. Legionnaires' disease, as it occurred in Philadelphia in 1976 and elsewhere, is a multisystem invasive illness involving the lungs (most prominently), kidneys, gastrointestinal tract, and central nervous system (97,98). The incubation period averages 5 to 6 days from exposure. From 1% to 5% of exposed persons develop illness, and the case-fatality rate can be 15% or higher. In contrast, the attack rate for Pontiac fever is high, usually 95% to 100%, and the incubation period short, 5 hours to less than 3 days. The cardinal symptoms include fever, chills, myalgias, headache, and malaise. Nonproductive cough, diarrhea, nausea, vomiting, chest pain, dizziness, and sore throat are also commonly reported in outbreaks of Pontiac fever. Physical examination is generally unremarkable except for fever and tachypnea. The chest radiograph is normal. Leukocytosis is frequently found, with leftward shift on differential examination as with other inhalation fever syndromes. The illness is benign and self-limited, with spontaneous resolution after 1 to 5 days.

Several outbreaks of Pontiac fever have been identified as such only retrospectively. The first recognized and eponymous outbreak occurred in a county health department building in Pontiac, Michigan in July 1968 and was later traced to the airborne spread of *L. pneumophila,* serogroup 1, from a contaminated air-conditioning system (99). Seroconversion to this *Legionella* strain was shown in symptomatic persons but not in controls. The organism was isolated retrospectively from stored frozen samples of condenser water and from lung tissue of guinea pigs exposed to an aerosol of evaporative condenser water. Since this initial outbreak was recognized, several other common-source outbreaks of Pontiac fever have been documented. An outbreak in office workers was traced to contaminated cooling tower water that was used to air-cool the office building. *L. pneumophila* serogroup 1 antigen was detected in the urine of two patients, suggesting that *Legionella* antigen testing of urine may be helpful in the diagnosis of acute-stage legionellosis (100). Pontiac fever due to *L. pneumophila* serogroup 7 was traced to aerosols from a nearby cooling tower and affected all occupants of a Japanese building (101). In 1973, ten men who used compressed air to clean a steam turbine condenser developed an explosive, influenza-like syndrome that resolved rapidly. The pathogenic agent was not isolated, but five of the ten showed seroconversion to *L. pneumophila* serogroup 1, and three others had convalescent-phase titers greater than 64 (20). A different *Legionella* species, *Legionella feeleii* species nova, was found to be the causative agent for a 1981 outbreak of Pontiac fever affecting 317 automobile assembly plant workers (102). The organism, which did not react with antisera against other *Legionella* species, was isolated from a water-based coolant and was probably spread via aerosols generated by machining and grinding operations. Attack rates by department decreased linearly with the department's distance from the implicated coolant system.

Whirlpools and leisure pools have also been implicated as reservoirs of *Legionella* species, causing nonpneumonic legionellosis, probably due to the generation of respirable droplets from air injection and bubbling of the water (103,104). In 1982, 14 of 23 female church groups members who used a whirlpool developed an acute, self-limited illness characterized by fever, chills, cough, chest pain, and nausea (105). Nine of the 14 showed seroconversion to *L. pneumophila* serogroup 6, and the organism was isolated from the whirlpool and its filter. *Legionella micdadei* was isolated from whirlpool bath water and identified as the causative agent for a large outbreak of Pontiac fever affecting 170 people in Lochgoilhead, Scotland (106). The attack rate in this outbreak was 91%. Aerosols of *Legionella anisa* from a decorative fountain in a hotel lobby were the source of an outbreak of Pontiac fever in 34 conference attendees, suggesting that decorative fountains in enclosed areas such as shopping malls, hotels, and indoor swimming pools may be a source for outbreaks of legionellosis (107).

Pontiac fever should be suspected in circumstances where patients present with a flu-like illness following exposure to aerosolized water. The temperature of water in cooling towers, evaporative condensers, and whirlpools where outbreaks have been reported is usually 33°C to 37°C, the temperature at which *Legionella* organisms grow well. Diagnostic confirmation of Pontiac fever rests on the finding of typical symptoms, symptom onset after a short incubation period, short illness duration, the absence of pneumonia, and, in an outbreak setting, the demonstration of seroconversion. Seroconversion may be delayed as long as 6 weeks after onset of symptoms, which may explain the failure to demonstrate increased antibody titers for all those ill in some reported outbreaks. Antibody titers to *Legionella* have been noted to decrease more than fourfold within 18 months after an outbreak (103). Symptom-free but exposed persons have also been reported to have positive *Legionella* serologic tests.

The factors that determine whether a *Legionella* species will cause Legionnaires' disease or Pontiac fever are not known. Dose alone is unlikely to explain the difference, as one would expect larger doses to produce more severe disease after a shorter incubation period. Bacterial strain differences have been postulated to explain the different outcomes, but no important differences, including the presence of toxins, have been found in laboratory testing of strains of *L. pneumophila* that have caused both patterns of illness. Host factors may play an important role. Alcohol abuse, chronic lung disease, and other immunosuppressive states appear to increase the risk for both infection and mortality from Legionnaires' disease. An outbreak of both Pontiac fever and Legionnaires' disease after a point source exposure to *L. pneumophila* from a hot tub aerosol supports the view that the spectrum of illness is influenced by the immune status of the host, as the one case of legionella pneumonia occurred in an individual with insulin- dependent diabetes mellitus (108). As with other inhalation fevers, an anamnestic mechanism for Pontiac fever seems unlikely given the high attack rate even for persons without prior exposure. A toxic effect from inhaling live organisms is the most probable pathogenic mechanism for Pontiac fever (109), and provides a pathogenic link to inhalation fever syndromes associated with other, nonlegionella contaminated water sources such as HF.

### Other Water Sources

In addition to HF and Pontiac fever, other inhalation fever outbreaks have been linked to water-borne aerosols not easily classifiable to either category. An outbreak of recurrent fever, chills, myalgias, and profound cough beginning 4 hours after a hot bath occurred in 56 individuals sharing a public water source (110). Attacks were brief, self-limited, and had short incubation periods. Twenty symptomatic workers exposed to an aerosol containing predominantly *Pseudomonads* and bacterial endotoxin from recirculated water pumps developed an inhalation fever termed *sump bay fever* (111). Replacing and disinfecting the water led to complete resolution of attacks. An investigation at six sewage treatment plants and three drinking water plants found high concentrations of airborne gram-negative organisms in areas of sewage water agitation and higher rates of gastrointestinal symptoms and fever among exposed workers (112).

## CONTAMINATED VEGETABLE MATTER AND AGRICULTURAL DUSTS

### Mill Fever

Mill fever, card room fever, heckling fever, and mattress maker's fever are syndromes characterized by fever, chills, malaise, nausea, cough, and rhinitis that occur in workers newly exposed to vegetable fiber dusts of cotton, flax, soft hemp, or kapok (113). Of these, cotton dust-related symptoms are the best studied. The acute symptoms of mill fever due to cotton dust occur within 1 to 6 hours of the initial exposure and resolve within hours to a few days. The prevalence among new cotton mill workers is not known, but estimates range from 10% to 80% (114). As with other inhalation fever syndromes, tolerance develops, and symptoms cease with continued exposure (tachyphylaxis). Mill fever differs from byssinosis in that the latter occurs several years (usually more than 10) after working in the industry and is manifested by respiratory symptoms of chest tightness or dyspnea that initially occur at the beginning of the workweek (Monday chest tightness). In byssinosis, evidence of airways obstruction over progressively longer periods of the workweek occurs with continued exposure and may lead to permanent respiratory impairment from reduced ventilatory capacity. There is some evidence to suggest that cotton workers who have had mill fever are more prone to develop byssinosis than those who have not, which may point to common etiologic factors (115,116). The precise cause or causes of mill fever and byssinosis in cotton card rooms are unclear, but evidence suggests a role for gram-negative bacterial endotoxins contaminating the vegetable dusts (117–119).

The best model of mill fever historically is the outbreak of mattress makers' fever linked to the use of "stained" cotton as a cottage industry of mattress making during World War II. The cotton was stained from microorganism overgrowth, and the dusty manufacturing process led to a very high attack rate of inhalation fever. This, in turn, was linked epidemiologically and experimentally to the inhalation of gram-negative bacteria, further supporting the hypothesized role of endotoxin (113). More recently, experimental animal data have shown an inflammatory response in the lung following cotton dust extract inhalation linked to increased TNF, a finding also consistent with an endotoxin-mediated syndrome.

### Organic Dust Toxic Syndrome

*Organic dust toxic syndrome* (ODTS) is a term that subsumes inhalation fever syndromes following the inhalation of organic dusts from moldy or damp silage, hay, or other agricultural dusts or similarly contaminated wood chips from mulching processes. Agricultural organic dusts are complex mixtures that contain bacteria, bacterial products, fungal spores and hyphae, feed grains, hay, silage, animal danders, pollens, insect parts, and chemical residues, among many other things, and that vary in composition depending on growing conditions and methods of harvest, storage, and processing (120). ODTS was at one time called "pulmonary mycotoxicosis" owing to the large component of microbial spores and hyphae found in the dust, and has also been known as "silo unloader's syndrome" owing to the association of illness with this specific agricultural activity (121,122).

Attacks of ODTS in the agricultural environment occur most commonly in the summer and fall seasons, when farmers report exposure to large amounts of extremely moldy material. Grain shoveling, threshing and crushing, cleaning bins where moldy grain has been stored, unloading or uncapping silos, and shoveling moldy wood chips have all been reported to induce the illness. ODTS has also been reported in nonoccupational settings. An explosive outbreak of a febrile respiratory illness occurred in 55 of 67 college fraternity members who attended a party where there was dense airborne dust from straw laid on the floor (21); a similar cluster of 21 ODTS-like illnesses was described in persons exposed to dusty grass during a hayride (123).

Organic dust toxic syndrome is reported to be a relatively frequent condition that is probably underrecognized owing to its similarity to other flu-like illnesses and its generally self-limited course. A Swedish survey estimated the annual incidence to be 1 per 100 farmers, which was 30 to 50 times higher than the incidence of hypersensitivity pneumonitis in the same group (estimated at 2 to 3 per 10,000 farmers) (124). The differential diagnosis between ODTS and farmer's lung hypersensitivity pneumonitis (HP) presents the same challenge as the distinction between humidifier fever and humidifier lung HP.

Clinically, the patient with ODTS usually presents 4 to 12 hours after exposure with symptoms of fever, chills, cough, minimal dyspnea, chest tightness, myalgias, malaise, nausea, and headache. The afflicted individual often reports onset of symptoms of eye and mucous membrane irritation and dry cough during the exposure and preceding the severe constitutional symptoms. Similar to other inhalation fever syndromes, lung examination is usually normal, though scattered rhonchi and inspiratory crepitant rales have been reported. A peripheral leukocytosis with granulocyte predominance is commonly present. Serum precipitins to thermophiles and mold species are typically negative. The chest radiograph and tests of pulmonary function are usually normal, although airways obstruction may be present. Since attacks are self-limited, treatment is supportive and no role for steroids has been identified.

There is little information on the natural history or long-term sequelae of this syndrome. Among 80 patients with ODTS identified by questionnaire in the Swedish survey, only 40% were free of respiratory symptoms even though years had elapsed since the last acute attack in some cases

(125). However, overlap with HP and other agricultural dust-related syndromes such as asthma and chronic bronchitis is difficult to exclude. In a small survey of ten farmers with ODTS occurring 5 years prior to evaluation, no differences were found in respiratory symptom scores, resting pulmonary function, or methacholine reactivity compared to control farmers without previous episodes of ODTS (126). A cross-sectional respiratory symptom survey of 352 Midwestern farmers found an increased risk of persistent respiratory symptoms, especially cough and sputum, in those reporting previous episodes of ODTS (127).

The precise cause or causes of ODTS have yet to be identified. Certain fungal toxins can cause acute lung injury, which may explain occasional reports of a severe illness after exposure to agricultural materials. One case report describes a patient who developed acute pulmonary edema after exposure to high levels of *Penicillium* contaminating moldy oranges in a storehouse. Since HP was not found, the authors attribute her illness to an unusually severe form of ODTS, though acute lung injury from a mycotoxin contaminant cannot be excluded (16). It has been suggested that microbial proteinases released from thermophilic organisms may play a role in the inflammatory response (128). Studies with rabbits have shown that high concentrations of aerosolized colonies of *Aspergillus fumigatus* and *Aspergillus terreus* cause acute hypoxemia and hypocomplementemia (129). Rabbits exposed to soluble extracts of silage dust developed an increase in BAL fluid neutrophils; prior immunization had little effect on this inflammatory response (130). Agricultural organic dusts also contain lipopolysaccharides, which may activate alveolar macrophages to release interleukin-1, and possibly contribute to the febrile reaction following massive exposures (131). B-(1–3)-d-glucans are structural components of some fungal cells walls, are potent T-cell adjuvants, and may also be contained in agricultural aerosols; soluble glucans appear to have effects similar to endotoxin, and can activate neutrophils, macrophages, and complement (132,133). Agricultural dusts contain many potential allergens, and it is possible that immune mechanisms contribute to the febrile reactions seen in ODTS. As with mill fever and as will be discussed for grain fever, an endotoxin-dependent mechanism is still viewed as the most likely candidate to explain the signs and symptoms of ODTS.

### Grain Fever

Grain fever is an acute febrile illness occurring during or shortly after exposure to massive concentrations of grain dust. Similar to other inhalation fevers, the clinical findings include chills, fever, malaise, cough, and headache. Symptoms have been reproduced in subjects exposed to grain dusts experimentally. Symptoms typically subside after several hours but occasionally last for several days. Risk for grain fever is associated with exposure to high concentrations of grain dust as occurs with shoveling, threshing, crushing, and cleaning bins, especially where contaminated grain has been stored(134). Grain harvested while still damp, then dried and stored, is most commonly associated with symptoms, circumstances that probably support microbial amplification (135). Grain fever has been reported by 6% to 30% of grain handlers (136).

Forty percent of the particulate matter in grain dust consists of respirable particles of mass median diameter less than 5 μm. The four principal constituents of grain dust are grain extracts, bacterial endotoxins, storage mites, and fungi. Given these constituents, it is not surprising that both nonimmunologic injury with neutrophilic inflammation and immunologic lung injury might occur from grain dust exposures (26). In grain workers, nonspecific bronchial hyperresponsiveness (NSBHR) does not correlate with atopy but is associated with dust exposure levels and with cumulative exposure. Interestingly, NSBHR also increases during the first week of employment for grain workers, suggesting a nonallergic response (28,137). Chronic bronchitis and airways obstruction are associated with chronic grain dust exposure, but the relationship between this and acute febrile episodes is as unclear as the relationship between Monday morning fever and subsequent byssinosis from cotton dust exposure.

### Animal Confinement Work

Farmers differ from grain workers in having more diverse organic dust exposures, often including work in animal confinement units. Since the 1960s, these confinement units have been commonly used to raise swine, cattle, sheep, and poultry, and are typically characterized by high animal density and often poor ventilation. Dust and vapor exposures are variable and complex, reflecting the type of animal housed, feed and waste handling practices, and building ventilation (138). Respiratory health effects from confinement work include acute and chronic bronchitis, airways hyperreactivity, hypersensitivity pneumonitis, asphyxiation from exposure to toxic gases, and ODTS. ODTS rates in swine confinement workers from the United States, Canada, and Sweden are similar, ranging from 10% to 30%. Symptoms of swine confinement ODTS, including fever, chills, malaise, myalgias, headache, cough, and chest tightness, occur 4 to 6 hours after exposure in the confinement house, particularly following dusty operations such as handling, moving, or sorting animals. BAL studies of healthy, previously unexposed subjects exposed to swine dust showed an intense neutrophilia accompanied by increased fibronectin and albumin concentrations (25). Endotoxin levels have shown the strongest and most consistent relationship to symptoms of ODTS (139).

### Wood Dusts

Sawmill workers, pulp and papermill workers, and workers handling contaminated wood chips are at risk for both inhalation fever and hypersensitivity pneumonitis. Wood trimmer's disease describes an inhalation fever occurring in sawmill workers exposed to dust from dried, microbially contaminated wood (140). In a questionnaire survey of over 1,500 sawmill workers from 233 Swedish sawmills, 22% reported work-related febrile attacks, similar to rates reported by Swedish farmers, with rare cases of confirmed allergic alveolitis (141). An outbreak of inhalation fever occurred among workers at a municipal golf course after they manually unloaded moldy wood chips from a trailer (142). As with other inhalation fevers studied, controlled exposure to wood mulch by routine shoveling leads to an inflammatory cellular response characterized by BAL neutrophilia and increased levels of IL-8 and IL-6 (143).

## OTHER EXPOSURES ASSOCIATED WITH INHALATION FEVER

### Polymer Fume Fever

First described in 1951 (144), polymer fume fever is an influenza-like illness caused by inhalation of the pyrolysis products of tetrafluoroethylene resins, most notably polytetrafluoroethylene (PTFE; trade names Fluon, Teflon, Halon) and polyvinyl fluoride. The properties of PTFE such as its chemical inertness, strength, plasticity, lubricity, and thermal stability account for its widespread use in insulation materials, gaskets, wire coatings, self-lubricating bearings, food manufacturing machinery, nonstick cooking utensils, radio and other electrical apparatus, and as a parting compound, dirt-repellent spray starch, and mold-release agent.

When the polymer is heated between 300° and 750°, numerous degradation products have been identified including octafluoroisobutylene, tetrafluoroethylene, hexafluoropropylene, oxygen difluoride, carbonyl fluoride, carbon tetrachloride, and a complex mixture of fluorinated acids and olefins (145,146). Circumstances in which these degradation products occur include welding or flame cutting of metal coated with PTFE, operating molding or extruding machines, high-speed machining of components, and smoking cigarettes contaminated with the polymer. The average temperature of the burning zone of a cigarette is 884°, more than enough to degrade the most stable polymer, and multiple case reports of polymer fume fever have implicated contaminated cigarettes as the source of exposure (147–149). Studies in which volunteers smoked cigarettes spiked with varying amounts of PTFE showed that as little as 0.4 mg of the polymer caused polymer fume fever in nine of ten volunteers (150). Exposure of cigarette-smoking family members to PTFE-contaminated clothes may also precipitate episodes of polymer fume fever (74), probably from polymer contamination of the cigarette via skin contact.

The clinical presentation of polymer fume fever parallels that of other inhalation fevers. Attacks of polymer fume fever occur several hours after exposure, often toward the end of the work shift or in the evening after work. Chest pain or tightness associated with dyspnea and sometimes cough are followed by malaise, myalgias, fever, chills, sweats, nausea, headache, and sore throat. Physical examination reveals fever, tachycardia, tachypnea, and occasionally pulmonary rales. Leukocytosis with leftward shift is often described. The chest radiograph is usually normal, and no consistent pattern of pulmonary function abnormalities has been described. Resolution of symptoms is usually complete within 12 to 48 hours, although more prolonged constitutional symptoms of fever, chills, headache, and photophobia were reported in one case after inhalation of multiple pyrolysis products (151).

Long-term adverse sequelae of classic polymer fume fever are poorly characterized and have been limited to rare case reports (152). Recurrent episodes of polymer fume fever resulted in marked symptomatic deterioration from obstructive pulmonary disease in a carding machine operator in a synthetic fabric plant (153). More importantly, a number of reports of severe, acute pulmonary edema have been described following inhalation of high concentrations of PTFE pyrolysis products from higher temperature combustion (74,154,155). It appears that at these temperatures, acid aerosol irritants leading to an acute lung injury pattern are released (see Table 2). Given the frequency of mixed exposures, cases of suspected polymer fume fever should be followed closely for 24 to 48 hours for signs of noncardiogenic pulmonary edema (15).

The pathogenesis of polymer fume fever is unknown. Unlike metal fume fever and mill fever, no tolerance phenomenon has been established (156). Rats exposed to PTFE pyrolysis products at 450° developed severe epithelial damage to alveolar lining cells, with marked septal edema and necrosis of the tracheobronchial epithelium. An experimental model of polymer fume fever in rabbits exposed to particulate (but not vapor) phase PTFE pyrolysis products manifest delayed-onset fever; transfusion of serum from febrile to control animals produced fever in the latter, which the authors speculate may be due to the release of endogenous pyrogens stimulated by the polymer fumes (157). Deaths from hemorrhagic pneumonitis of caged pet birds associated with accidental overheating of PTFE-lined pans have been described, consistent with an acute lung injury pattern of high-temperature breakdown products rather than inhalation fever (158).

Where PTFE is heated above 300°, adequate ventilation is essential to prevent fume fever; when PTFE is heated above 450°, the risk of acute lung injury among those exposed mandates engineering controls appropriate to that degree of hazard. Because of the association between cigarette smoking and exposure to PTFE pyrolysis products, mandatory hand washing before breaks and elimination of smoking in the work area have been successful in eliminating occupational episodes of polymer fume fever. Not only fume fever but acute lung injury as well has been associated with cigarette-PTFE pyrolysis (159). A recent outbreak of respiratory illness associated with an unheated aerosol containing fluorocarbons included fever but was more consistent with an acute lung injury pattern than inhalation fever (12,159).

### Other Causes of Inhalation Fever

The preceding sections covered the major causes of inhalation fever outlined in Table 1. Nonetheless, there have been other, unusual outbreaks and case reports that fit the overall pattern of inhalation fever but with poorly characterized or heterogeneous exposures. In 1960, Plessner (160) described *"la fievre de canard,"* inhalation fever in geese pluckers cleaning feathers for use in bed covers and sleeping bags. There are sporadic reports of flu-like illness occurring in new workers handling xanthan gum powder, a high molecular weight polysaccharide widely used in the food, cosmetic, and pharmaceutical industries and in oil drilling as a lubricant (161). Construction workers exposed to dusts from alkaline fireproofing materials contaminated with *Penicillium* developed a recurrent flu-like respiratory illness with characteristics of an inhalation fever (162).

## SUMMARY

An increasing array of diverse exposures (including metals, microbial bioaerosols, organic dusts, and polymers) are associated with the nonallergic, noninfectious inhalation fever syndromes. Attack rates for these syndromes are high, suggesting that host factors are relatively unimportant, and evidence exists to suggest a dose-related risk. Pathogenic features of the inhalation fever syndromes include an intense pulmonary neutrophilic inflammatory cellular response and activation of proinflammatory cytokine networks. Unlike acute lung injury and hypersensitivity lung diseases, long-term sequelae are rare. It is thus important to distinguish the inhalation fevers from other illnesses associated with the same or similar exposure circumstances but with very different prognostic and therapeutic implications. Perhaps because of their apparently benign and self-limited nature, preventive interventions (including studies of the efficacy of engineering controls, work practices, and respiratory protection) have received little attention. Yet the inhalation fever syndromes cause significant short-term morbidity and may also serve as markers for more serious disease risk (including hypersensitivity pneumonitis, asthma, chronic bronchitis, airflow limitation, and acute lung injury) requiring aggressive abatement efforts. Future research will be enhanced by more accurate disease recognition, and should lead to better understanding of the epidemiology, pathogenesis, and prevention of these intriguing syndromes.

## REFERENCES

1. Inhalation fevers (editorial). *Lancet* 1978;1:249–250.
2. Taylor G. Acute systemic effects of inhaled occupational agents. In: Merchant JA, ed. *Occupational respiratory diseases.* Pub. No. DHHS (NIOSH) 86-102. Cincinnati: U.S. Department of Health and Human Service: National Institute for Occupational Safety and Health, 1986; 607–625.
3. Rask-Anderson A, Pratt DS. Inhalation fever: A proposed unifying term for febrile reactions to inhalation of noxious substances (letter). *Br J Ind Med* 1992;49:40.
4. Rose C. Inhalation fevers. In: Rom W, ed. *Environmental and occupational medicine,* 2nd ed. Boston: Little, Brown, 1992;373–391.
5. Blanc P, Boushey HA. The lung in metal fume fever. *Semin Respir Med* 1993;14:212–225.
6. Pratt DS, Rask-Anderson A. Inhalation fever: A proposed unifying term for febrile reactions to inhalation of noxious substances (letter). *Br J Ind Med* 1993;50:287.
7. Rask-Anderson A. Inhalation fever. In: Harber P, Schenker M, Balmes J, eds. *Occupational and environmental respiratory diseases.* St. Louis: Mosby, 1995;243–258.
8. Zhicheng S. Acute nickel carbonyl poisoning: A report of 179 cases. *Br J Ind Med* 1986;43:422–424.
9. Douglas WW, Hepper NGG, Colby TV. Silo filler's disease. *Mayo Clin Proc* 1989;64:291–304.
10. Fuortes L, Leo A, Ellergeck PG, Friell LA. Acute respiratory fatality associated with exposure to sheet metal and cadmium fumes. *Clin Toxicol* 1991;29:279–281.
11. Rowens B, Guerrero-Betencourt D, Gottlieb CA, Boyes RJ, Eichenhorn MS. Respiratory failure and death following acute inhalation of mercury vapor. *Chest* 1991;99:185–190.
12. Centers for Disease Control. Severe acute respiratory illness linked to use of shoe sprays (Colorado, November 1993). *MMWR* 1993;42: 885–887.
13. Burgess WA. *Recognition of health hazards in industry:* a review of materials and processes. New York: Wiley, 1981;117–136.
14. National Institute for Occupational Safety and Health. *Criteria for a recommended standard:* welding, brazing, and thermal cutting. Cincinnati: U.S. Department of Health and Human Services, 1988.
15. Shusterman D. Polymer fume fever and other fluorocarbon pyrolysis-related syndromes. *J Occup Med* 1993;8:519–531.
16. Yoshida K, Masayki A, Araki S. Acute pulmonary edema in a storehouse of moldy oranges: A severe care of the organic dust toxic syndrome. *Arch Environ Health* 1989;44:382–384.
17. May JJ, Stallones L, Darrow D, Pratt DS. Organic dust toxicity (pulmonary mycotoxicosis) associated with silo unloading. *Thorax* 1986; 41:919–923.
18. Litovitz TL, Felberg L, White S, Klein-Schwartz W. 1995 annual report of the American Association of Poison Control Centers toxic exposure surveillance system. *Am J Emerg Med* 1996;14:487–548.
19. Centers for Disease Control, National Institute for Occcupational Safety and Health. *NIOSH allergy:* preventing organic dust toxic syndrome. DHHS Publication No. 94-102. Cincinnati: U.S. Department of Health and Human Services, Public Health Service, 1994.
20. Fraser DW, Deubner DC, Hill DL, Gilliam DK. Non-pneumonic, short-incubation period legionellosis (Pontiac fever) in men who cleaned a steam turbine condenser. *Science* 1979;205:690–691.
21. Brinton WT, Vastbinder EE, Greene JW, Marx JJ, Hutcheson RH, Schaffner W. An outbreak of organic dust toxic syndrome in a college fraternity. *JAMA* 1987;258:1210–1212.
22. Turner JA, Thompson LR. Health hazards of brass foundries. *Public Health Bull* 1925;157:1–71.
23. Schilling RSR. Bysinossis in cotton and other textile workers. *Lancet* 1956;271:319–324.
24. Blanc P, Wong H, Bernstein MS, Boushey HA. An experimental model of metal fume fever. *Ann Intern Med* 1991;114:930–936.
25. Larsson KA, Eklund AG, Lars-Olof H, Isaksson B-M, Malmberg PO.

Swine dust causes intense airways inflammation in healthy subjects. *Am J Respir Crit Care Med* 1994;150:973–977.
26. Von Essen SG, O'Neill DP, McGranagham S, Olenchock SA, Rennard SI. Neutrophilic respiratory tract inflammation and peripheral blood neutrophils after grain sorghum dust extract exposure. *Chest* 1995; 108:425–433.
27. Blanc PD, Boushey HA, Wong H, Wintermeyer SF, Bernstein MS. Cytokines in metal fume fever. *Am Rev Respir Dis* 1993;147:134–139.
28. Clapp WD, Becker S, Quay J, et al. Grain dust-induced airflow obstruction and inflammation of the lower respiratory tract. *Am J Respir Crit Care Med* 1994;150:611–617.
29. Wang Z, Malmberg P, Larsson P, Larsson B-M, Larsson KA. Time course of interleukin-6 and tumor necrosis factor-alpha increase in serum following inhalation of swine dust. *Am J Respir Crit Care Med* 1996;143:147–152.
30. Elias JA, Zitnik RJ. Cytokine-cytokine interactions in the context of cytokine networking. *Am J Respir Cell Mol Biol* 1992;7:365–367.
31. Thackrah CT. *The effects of arts, trades, and professions and of civic states and habits of living on health and longevity,* 2nd ed. London: Longman, Rees, Orme, Brown, Green, and Longman, 1832;101–102.
32. Greenhow EH. On brass-founders ague. *Med Chir Tr* 1862;54: 177–187.
33. Arnstein A. Beitrag zur kenntnis des giesfiebers. *Wiener Arbeiten aus dem Gebiete der Sozialen Medizin* 1910;1:49–58.
34. Lehmann KB. Studien uber technisch und hygienisch wichtige Gase und Dampfe: XIV Das giess-oder zinkfieber. *Arch Hyg* 1910;72: 358–381.
35. Bernstein AY. Lychoradka medno-lyteyeshkov (Brassfounders' Ague). *Gigiena Truda* 1925;7:17–41.
36. Sturgis CC, Drinker P, Thomson RM. Metal fume fever: I. Clinical observations on the effect of the experimental inhalation of zinc oxides. *J Ind Hyg* 1927;9:88–97.
37. Sigel J. Das giesfieber und seine bekamfung der verhaltnisse in Wuttemberg (Part 1). *Vierteljahrsschrift fur gerichtliche medizin und offentliches sanitatswesen (Berlin)* 1906;32:174–187.
38. Drinker P. Certain aspects of the problem of zinc toxicity. *J Ind Hyg* 1922;4:177–197.
39. Kuh JR, Collen MF, Kuhn C. Metal fume fever. *Perm Found Med Bull* 1946;4:145–151.
40. Raine JWE. Metal fume fever. *NZ Med J* 1948;47:24–28.
41. Rohrs LC. Metal fume fever from inhaling zinc oxide. *Arch Intern Med* 1957;100:44–48.
42. Papp JP. Metal fume fever. *Postgrad Med* 1968;43:160–163.
43. Jaremin B. Clinical picture of the "zinc fever." *Biul Inst Med [Gdansku]* 1973;24:233–242.
44. Batchelor RP, Fehnel JW, Thomson RM, Drinker KR. A clinical and laboratory investigation of the effect of metallic zinc, of zinc oxide, and of zinc sulphide upon the health of workmen. *J Ind Hyg* 1926;8: 322–363.
45. Swiller AI, Swiller HE. Metal fume fever. *Am J Med* 1957;22:173–174.
46. Anseline P. Zinc-fume fever. *Med J Aust* 1972;2:316–318.
47. Brown JJL. Zinc fume fever. *Br J Radiol* 1988;61:327–329.
48. Heydon JL. Metal fume fever (letter). *NZ Med J* 1990;103:52.
49. Farrell FJ. Angioedema and urticaria as acute and late phase reactions to zinc fume exposure, with associated metal fume fever-like symptoms. *Am J Ind Med* 1987;12:331–337.
50. Malo JL, Cartier A. Occupational asthma due to fumes of galvanized metal. *Chest* 1987;92:375–377.
51. Kawane H, Soejima R, Umeki S. Metal fume fever and asthma (letter). *Chest* 1988;93:116.
52. Malo J-L, Malo J, Cartier A, Dolovich J. Acute lung reaction to zinc inhalation. *Eur Respir J* 1990;3:111–114.
53. Langley RL. Fume fever and reactive airways dysfunction syndrome in a welder. *South Med J* 1991;84:1034–1036.
54. Nemery B, Demedts M. Respiratory involvement in metal fume fever. *Eur Respir J* 1991;4:764–765.
55. Ameille J, Brochard P, Dore MF. Occupational hypersensitivity pneumonitis in a smelter exposed to zinc fumes. *Chest* 1992;101:862–863.
56. Castet D, Bouillard J. Pneumopathie aigue au cours d'une exposition a l'oxyde de zinc. *Rev Mal Respir* 1992;9:632–633.
57. Callender GR. Acute poisoning by the zinc and antimony content of limeade prepared in a galvanized iron can. *Milit Sur* 1937;80:67–71.
58. Murphy JV. Intoxication following ingestion of elemental zinc. *JAMA* 1970;212:2119–2220.
59. Brocks A, Reid H, Glazer RG. Acute intravenous zinc poisoning. *Br Med J* 1977;212:1390–1391.
60. Conner MW, Flood WH, Rogers AE, Amdur MO. Lung injury in guinea pigs caused by multiple exposures to ultrafine zinc oxide. *J Toxicol Environ Health* 1988;25:57–69.
61. Lam HF, Chen LC, Ainsworth D, Peoples S, Amdur MO. Pulmonary function of guinea pigs exposed to freshly generated ultrafine zinc oxide with and without spike concentrations. *Am Ind Hyg Assoc J* 1988;49:333–341.
62. Hirano S, Higo S, Tsukamoto N, Kobayashi E, Suzuki KT. Pulmonary clearance of zinc oxide instilled into the rat lung. *Arch Toxicol* 1989; 63:336–342.
63. Gordon T, Chen LC, Fine JM, et al. Pulmonary effects of inhaled zinc oxide in human subjects, guinea pigs, rats, and rabbits. *Am Ind Hyg Assoc J* 1992;53:503–509.
64. Volgelmeier C, Konig G, Bencze K, Fruhman G. Pulmonary involvement in zinc fume fever. *Chest* 1987;92:946–948.
65. Kuschner WG, D'Alessandro A, Wintermeyer SF, Wong H, Boushey HA, Blanc PD. Pulmonary responses to purified zinc oxide fume. *J Invest Med* 1995;43:371–378.
66. Noel NE, Ruthman JC. Elevated serum zinc levels in metal fume fever. *J Emerg Med* 1988;6:609–610.
67. Drinker P, Thomson RM, Finn JL. Metal fume fever: III. The effects of inhaling magnesium oxide fume. *J Ind Hyg* 1927;9:187–192.
68. Hartmann AL, Hartmann W, Buhlmann AA. Magnesiumoxide als ursache des Metallrauchfebers (Magnesium oxide as cause of metal fume fever). *Sweiz Med Wschr* 1983;113:776–770.
69. Kuschner WG, D'Alessandro A, Wong H, Blanc PD. Pulmonary responses to inhalation of magnesium oxide fume. *Am J Respir Crit Care Med* 1996;153:A470.
70. Koelsch F. Metal-fume fever. *J Ind Hyg* 1923;5:87–91.
71. Gleason RB. Exposure to copper dust. *Am Ind Hyg Assoc J* 1968;29: 461–462.
72. Hooper W. Case report metal fumes fever. *Postgrad Med* 1978;63: 123–127.
73. Armstrong CW, Moore LW Jr, Hackler RL, Miller GB Jr, Stroube RB. An outbreak of metal fume fever: Diagnostic use of urinary copper and zinc determinations. *J Occup Med* 1983;25:886–888.
74. Brubaker RE. Pulmonary problems associated with the use of polytetrafluoroethylene. *J Occup Med* 1977;19:693–695.
75. Anthony JS, Zamel N, Aberman A. Abnormalities in pulmonary function after brief exposure to toxic metal fumes. *J Can Med Assoc* 1978; 119:586–588.
76. Johnson JS, Kilburn KH. Cadmium-induced metal fume fever: Results of inhalation challenge. *Am J Ind Med* 1983;4:533–540.
77. Barnhart S, Rosenstock L. Cadmium chemical pneumonitis. *Chest* 1984;86:789–791.
78. Blount BW. Two types of metal fume fever: Mild vs. serious. *Milit Med* 1990;155:372–377.
79. Evans EH. Casualties following exposure to zinc chloride smoke. *Lancet* 1945;2:368–370.
80. Schenker MR, Speizer FE, Taylor JO. Acute upper respiratory symptoms resulting from exposure to zinc chloride aerosol. *Environ Res* 1981;25:317–324.
81. Stoke J. Metal fume fever in ferro-chrome workers. *Cent Afr J Med* 1977;23:25–28.
82. Humidifier fever: MRC symposium. *Thorax* 1977;32:653–663.
83. Edwards JH. Microbial and immunological investigations and remedial action after an outbreak of humidifier fever. *Br J Ind Med* 1980; 37:55–62.
84. Friend JAR, Gaddie J, Palmer KNV, Pickerin GCA, Pepys J. Extrinsic allergic alveolitis and contaminated cooling water in a factory machine. *Lancet* 1977;1:297–300.
85. Belin L. Prevalence of symptoms and immunoresponse in relation to exposure to infected humidifiers. *Eur J Respir Dis* 1980;107(suppl): 155–162.
86. Cockcroft A, Edwards J, Bevan C, et al. An investigation of operating theatre staff exposed to humidifier fever antigens. *Br J Ind Med* 1981; 38:144–151.
87. Rylander R, Haglind P, Lundholm M, Mattsby I, Stenqvist K. Humidifier fever and endotoxin exposure. *Clin Allergy* 1978;8:511–516.
88. Anderson K, Watt AD, Sinclair D, Lewis C, McSharry CP, Boyd G. Climate, intermittent humidification, and humidifier fever. *Br J Ind Med* 1989;46:671–674.

89. Mamolen M, Lewis DM, Blanchet MA, Satink FJ, Vogt RL. Investigation of an outbreak of "humidifier fever" in a print shop. *Am J Ind Med* 1993;23:483–490.
90. Pickering CAC, Moore WKS, Lacey J, Holford-Strevens V, Pepys J. Investigation of a respiratory disease associated with an air-condition system. *Clin Allergy* 1976;6:109–118.
91. Campbell IA, Cockcroft AE, Edwards JH, Jones M. Humidifier fever in an operating theatre. *Br Med J* 1979;2:1036–1037.
92. Ganier M, Lieberman P, Fink J, Lockwood DG. Humidifier lung: An outbreak in office workers. *Chest* 1980;77:183–187.
93. Ashton I, Axford AT, Bevan C, Cotes JE. Lung function of office workers exposed to humidifier fever antigen. *Br J Ind Med* 1981;38:34–37.
94. Muittari A, Kuusisto P, Sovijarvi A. An epidemic of bath water fever: Endotoxin alveolitis. *Eur J Respir Dis* 1982;123(suppl):108–116.
95. McSharry C, Anderson K, Boyd G. Serological and clinical investigation of humidifier fever. *Clin Allergy* 1987;17:15–22.
96. Marinkovich VA, Novey HS. Humidifier lung. *Clin Rev Allergy* 1983; 1:533–536.
97. Fraser DW, Tsai T, Orenstein W. Legionnaires' disease: Description of an epidemic of pneumonia. *N Engl J Med* 1977;297:1189–1197.
98. Klaucke DN, Vogt RL, LaRue D. Legionnaires' disease: The epidemiology of two outbreaks in Burlington, Vermont, 1980. *Am J Epidemiol* 1984;119:382–391.
99. Glick TH, Gregg MB, Berman B, Mallison G, Rhodes WW, Kassanoff I. Pontiac fever: An epidemic of unknown etiology in a health department: I. Clinical and epidemiologic aspects. *Am J Epidemiol* 1978; 107:149–160.
100. Friedman S, Spitalny K, Barbaree J, Faur Y, McKinney R. Pontiac fever outbreak associated with a cooling tower. *Am J Public Health* 1987;77:568–572.
101. Mori M, Hoshino K, Sonoda H, et al. An outbreak of Pontiac fever due to *Legionella pneumophila* serogroup 7: I. Clinical aspects [Japanese]. *Kansenshogaku Zasshi* 1995;69:646–653.
102. Herwaldt LA, Gorman GW, McGrath T, et al. A new *Legionella* species, *Legionella feeleii* species nova, causes Pontiac fever in an automobile plant. *Ann Intern Med* 1984;100:333–338.
103. Spitalny KC, Vogt RL, Orciari LA, Witherell LE, Etkind P, Novick LF. Pontiac fever associated with a whirlpool spa. *Am J Epidemiol* 1984; 120:809–817.
104. Baron PA, Willeke K. Respirable droplets from whirlpools: Measurements of size distribution and estimation of disease potential. *Environ Res* 1986;39:8–18.
105. Mangione EJ, Remis RS, Tait KA, et al. An outbreak of Pontiac fever related to whirlpool use (Michigan 1982). *JAMA* 1982;253:535–539.
106. Goldberg DJ, Wrench JG, Collier PW, et al. Lochgoilhead fever: Outbreak of non-pneumonic legionellosis due to *Legionella micdadei*. *Lancet* 1989;1:316–318.
107. Fenstersheib MD, Miller M, Diggins C, et al. Outbreak of Pontiac fever due to *Legionella anisa*. *Lancet* 1990;336:35–37.
108. Thomas DL, Mundy LM, Tucker PC. Hot tub legionellosis: Legionnaires' disease and Pontiac fever after a point-source exposure to Legionella pneumophila. *Arch Intern Med* 1993;153:2597–2599.
109. Kaufman AF, McDade JE, Patton CM, et al. Pontiac fever: Isolation of the etiologic agent (*Legionella pneumophila)* and demonstration of its mode of transmission. *Am J Epidemiol* 1981;114:337–347.
110. Atterholm I, Halberg T, Ganrot-Norlin K, Ringertz O. Unexplained acute fever after a hot bath. *Lancet* 1997:684–686.
111. Anderson K, McSharry CP, Clark C, Clark CJ, Barclay GR, Morris GP. Sump bay fever: Inhalational fever associated with a biologically contaminated water aerosol. *Occup Environ Med* 1996;53:106–111.
112. Lundholm M, Rylander R. Work related symptoms among sewage workers. *Br J Ind Med* 1983;40:325–329.
113. Neal PA, Schneiter R, Carminita BH. Report on acute illnesses among rural mattress makers using low-grade stained cotton. *JAMA* 1942; 119:1074.
114. Uragoda CG. An investigation into the health of kapok workers. *Br J Ind Med* 1977;34:181–185.
115. Gill CIC. Byssinosis in the cotton trade. *Br J Ind Med* 1947;4:48–55.
116. Harris TR, Merchant JA, Kilburn KH, Hamilton JD. Byssinosis and respiratory diseases of cotton mill workers. *J Occup Med* 1972;14: 199–206.
117. Rylander R, Haglind P, Lundholm M. Endotoxin in cotton dust and respiratory function decrement among cotton workers in an experimental cardroom. *Am Rev Respir Dis* 1985;131:209–213.
118. Castellan RM, Olenchock SA, Kinsley KB, Hankinson JL. Inhaled endotoxin and decreased spirometric values: An exposure-response relation for cotton dust. *N Engl J Med* 1987;317:605–610.
119. Kennedy SM, Christiani DC, Eisen EA, et al. Cotton dust and endotoxin exposure-response relationship in cotton textile workers. *Am Rev Respir Dis* 1987;135:194–200.
120. Donham KJ. Hazardous agents in agricultural dusts and methods of evaluation. *Am J Ind Med* 1986;10:205–220.
121. Emanuel DA, Wenzel FJ, Lawton BR. Pulmonary mycotoxicosis. *Chest* 1975;67:293–297.
122. Pratt DS, May JJ. Feed-associated respiratory illness in farmers. *Arch Environ Health* 1984;39:43–48.
123. Feldman G, Gordon VH. Hypersensitivity pneumonitis. *South Med J* 1975;68:952–957.
124. Malmberg P, Rask AA, Hoglund S, Kolmodin HB, Read GJ. Incidence of organic dust toxic syndrome and allergic alveolitis in Swedish farmers. *Int Arch Allergy Appl Immunol* 1988;87:47–54.
125. Rask-Anderson A. Organic dust toxic syndrome among farmers. *Br J Ind Med* 1989;46:233–238.
126. May JJ, Marvel LH, Pratt DS, Coppolo DP. Organic dust toxic syndrome: A follow-up study. *Am J Ind Med* 1990;17:111–113.
127. Nowakowski BL, Fryzek J, Eberspacher H, Smith M, Bolin N, Von Essen S. Organic dust toxic syndrome and respiratory symptoms in a farming environment (abstr). *Am J Respir Crit Care Med* 1997;155: A813.
128. Roberts RC, Nelles LP, Treuhaft MW, Marx JJ. Isolation and possible relevance of Thermoactinomyces candidus proteinases in farmer's lung disease. *Infect Immunol* 1983;40:553–562.
129. Olenchock SA, Burrell R. The role of precipitins and complement activation in the etiology of allergic lung disease. *J Allergy Clin Immunol* 1976;58:76–88.
130. Marx JJ, Arden-Jones MP, Treuhaft MW, Gray RL, Motszko CS, Hahn FF. The pathogenetic role of inhaled microbial material in pulmonary mycotoxicosis as demonstrated in an animal model. *Chest* 1981;80: 765–785.
131. Rylander R. Lung diseases caused by organic dusts in the farm environment. *Am J Ind Med* 1986;10:221–227.
132. Adachi Y, Ohno N, Yadomae T. Preparation and antigen specificity of an anti-1-3-b D glucan antibody. *Biol Pharm Bull* 1994;17: 1508–1512.
133. Fogelmark B, Sjÿ94strand M, Rylander R. Pulmonary inflammation induced by repeated inhalations of beta(1,3)-D-glucan and endotoxin. *Int J Exp Pathol* 1994;75:85–90.
134. Yach D, Myers J, Bradshaw D, Benatar SR. A respiratory epidemiologic survey of grain mill workers in Cape Town, South Africa. *Am Rev Respir Dis* 1985;131:505–510.
135. Williams N, Skoulas A, Merriman JE. Exposure to grain dust: I. A survey of the effects. *J Occup Med* 1964;6:319–327.
136. doPico GA, Flaherty D, Bhansali P, Chavaje N. Grain fever syndrome induced by inhalation of airborne grain dust. *J Allergy Clin Immunol* 1982;69:435–443.
137. James AL, Zimmerman MJ, Ee H, Ryan G, Musk AW. Exposure to grain dust and changes in lung function. *Br J Ind* Med 990;47:466–472.
138. Donham KJ. Respiratory disease hazards to workers in livestock and poultry confinement structures. *Semin Respir Med* 1993;14:49–59.
139. Donham KJ. Health effects from work in swine confinement buildings (review). *Am J Ind Med* 1990;17:17–25.
140. Belin L. Clinical and immunological data on "wood trimmer's disease" in Sweden. *Eur J Respir Dis* 1980;107(suppl):169–176.
141. Rask-Anderson A, Land CJ, K. E, Lundin A. Inhalation fever and respiratory symptoms in the trimming department of Swedish sawmills. *Am J Ind Med* 1994;25:65–67.
142. Acute respiratory illness following occupational exposure to wood chips. *MMWR* 1986;35:483–484,489–490.
143. Wintermeyer SF, Kuschner WG, Wong H, D'Allessandro A, Blanc PD. Pulmonary responses following wood chip mulch exposure. *J Occup Environ Med* 1997;4:308–314.
144. Harris DK. Polymer fume fever. *Lancet* 1951;2:1008–1011.
145. Coleman WE, Scheel LD, Kupel RE, Larkin RL. The identification of toxic compounds in the pyrolysis products of polytetrafluoroethylene (PTFE). *Am Ind Hyg Assoc J* 1968;29:33–40.
146. Waritz RS, Kwon BK. The inhalation toxicity of pyrolysis products of polytetrafluoroethylene heated below 500°. *Am Ind Hyg Assoc J* 1968; 29:19–26.

147. Williams N, Smith FK. Polymer fume fever: An elusive diagnosis. *JAMA* 1972;219:1587–1589.
148. Wegman DH, Peters JM. Polymer fume fever and cigarette smoking. *Ann Intern Med* 1974;81:55–57.
149. Albrecht WN, Bryant CJ. Polymer fume fever associated with smoking and use of a mold-release spray containing polytetrafluoroethylene. *J Occup Med* 1987;29:817–819.
150. Clayton JW. The toxicity of fluorocarbons with special reference to chemical constitution. *J Occup Med* 1962;4:262–273.
151. Shusterman D, Neal E. Prolonged fever associated with inhalation of multiple pyrolysis products. *Ann Emerg Med* 1986;15:831–833.
152. Williams N, Atkinson W, Patchefsky AS. Polymer fume fever: Not so benign. *J Occup Med* 1974;16:519–522.
153. Kales SN, Christiani DC. Progression of chronic obstructive pulmonary disease after multiple episodes of an occupational inhalation fever. *J Occup Med* 1994;36:75–78.
154. Robbins JJ, Ware RL. Pulmonary edema from teflon fumes: Report of a case. *N Engl J Med* 1964;271:360–361.
155. Evans EA. Pulmonary edema after inhalation of fumes from polytetrafluoroethylene (PTFE). *J Occup Med* 1973;15:599–601.
156. Kuntz WD, McCord CP. Polymer fume fever. *J Occup Med* 1974;16:480–482.
157. Cavagna G, Funulli G, Vigliani EC. Studio sperimentale sulla patogenesi della febbre da inalazione di fumi di Teflon (politetrafluoroetilene). *Med Lav* 1961;52:251–261.
158. Wells RE, Slocombe RF, Trapp AL. Acute toxicosis of budgerigars (Melopsittacus undulatus) caused by pyrolysis products from heated polytetrafluoroethylene: Clinical study. *Am J Vet Res* 1982;43:1238–1248.
159. Centers for Disease Control. Acute respiratory illness linked to use of aerosol leather condition (Oregon, December 1992). *MMWR* 1993;41:995–997.
160. Plessner MM. Une maladie des trieurs de plumes: La fievre de canard. *Arch Mal Profession* 1960;21:67–69.
161. Sargent EV, Adolph J, Clemmons MK, Kirk GD, Pena B, Fedoruk MJ. Evaluation of flu-like symptoms in workers handling xanthan gum powder. *J Occup Med* 1990;32:625–630.
162. Epling CA, Rose CS, Martyny JW, et al. Endemic work-related febrile respiratory illness among construction workers. *Am J Ind Med* 1995;28:193–205.

*Environmental and Occupational Medicine, Third Edition,* edited by William N. Rom.
Lippincott–Raven Publishers, Philadelphia © 1998.

CHAPTER 33

# Occupational and Environmental Asthma

Stuart M. Brooks

Dramatic advancements in the understanding of bronchial asthma have taken place over the past decade, especially regarding the role of airway inflammation in asthma. However, for a longer period of time, a better cognition of asthma was evolving. There was stipulation of bronchial asthma as a distinct pulmonary entity, and different from other common lung conditions in 1688 (1). In 1713, more than a quarter of a millennium ago, Ramazzini chronicled occupational asthma when observing urticaria and shortness of breath among grain sifters exposed to organic dusts (2). Over the next 200 years, and until the beginning of the 20th century, there was a paucity of publications concerning occupational asthma. In 1911, there was the recognition of asthma due to platinum salts among photographic workers (3). There were recordings of asthma among workers producing oil from castor beans in 1928 (4). More interest in the association between the workplace and asthma evolved in the late 1960s and 1970s (5). Clinical and research interests in occupational asthma substantially heightened in the 1980s. In the 1990s, occupational asthma is the most common type of occupational lung disease in the United States and in many other countries. The supporting data comes from information on morbidity, disability, and the occurrence of the total number of cases (6–8). The interest in occupational asthma will continue into the 21st century, especially as new chemicals are introduced into industries and new technologies evolve.

Bronchial asthma affects approximately 5% of persons of all ages in the general population, perhaps 11 to 12 million individuals in the United States. Asthma in the workplace afflicts as many as 400,000 to 3 million workers in the United States (6) (Table 1). These numbers may be an underestimation if we also consider workplace exacerbation of preexisting asthmatic states. Moving into the 21st century we are gleaning new scientific information to better explain asthma mechanisms and pathogenesis, especially the roles of bronchial mucosal injury and airway inflammation.

When we consider occupational asthma on a clinical basis, a conclusive diagnosis must be based on objective information that combines clinical, physiologic, and laboratory findings. Prevention of occupational asthma is paramount and involves a variety of strategies, most importantly eliminating further workplace exposures of sensitized workers. A key socioeconomic concern is the attempt to preserve the worker's long-term ability to be productive and financially provide for his/her family. An important goal is to try to return affected workers to their workplace in a timely and prudent manner.

## DEFINITION OF OCCUPATIONAL ASTHMA

Occupational asthma is an inflammatory disorder of the airways. There is episodic airflow limitation, usually accompanied by nonspecific bronchial hyperresponsiveness. The initiation of occupational asthma occurs after the inhalation of a substance or material that a worker may manufacture, use directly, or be exposed to incidentally at the work site. More than 200 different agents cause allergic sensitization and specific airway hyperresponsiveness. Nonallergic mechanisms also operate in the initiation of asthma. Thus, irritant exposures may initiate asthma and the induction of nonspecific airway hyperresponsiveness.

There has been difficulty formulating a precise definition of occupational asthma that is acceptable to the different groups and institutions having different agendas and requirements. A definition of use as a surveillance

S. M. Brooks: Department of Environmental and Occupational Health, College of Public Health, University of South Florida, Tampa, Florida 33612-3805.

**TABLE 1.** *Occupations that can carry risk of occupational asthma*

| Industry/occupation | Agent(s) | Workers potentially exposed (no.) |
|---|---|---|
| Animal breeding/handling | Animal antigens | 2,000,000 |
| Baking | Flour, insects, mite debris | 230,000 |
| Hairdresser | Sodium/potassium persulfate | 13,500 |
| Coffee processor | Green coffee beans | 12,900 |
| Detergent enzyme worker | Proteases | 5,700 |
| Farm workers | Animal antigens, vegetable dusts | 4,500,000 |
| Food additive worker | Tartrazine | 14,000 |
| Grain handler | Grain, insect debris dust | 97,000 |
| Laboratory worker | Animal antigens | 10,000 |
| Leather worker | Formalin | 11,000 |
| | Chromium salts | 2,000 |
| Lumber and woodworking | Wood dusts | 1,646,000 |
| Milling | Flour, insects, mite debris | 16,000 |
| Paper product manufacture | Natural glues | 130,000 |
| Pharmaceutical worker | Penicillin, ampicillin | 8,000 |
| Plastics industry | Diisocyanates (TDI, HDI, MDI) | 11,500 |
| | Anhydrides (PA, TCPA) | 4,020 |
| | Diethylene tri- and tetramine | 5,100 |
| Platinum refiner | Platinum salts | 300 |
| Printer | Vegetable gums | 6,000 |
| Veterinarian | Animal antigens | 23,000 |
| Vegetable oil production | Flaxseed, cottonseed castor bean | 6,700 |

strategy and triggering public health investigation or intervention is less restrictive than a definition appropriate for workers' compensation or legal purposes (2). Due to a diversity of opinions, various definitions of occupational asthma are propounded (8–15).

A simple definition of occupational asthma is "variable airflow limitation caused by a specific agent in the workplace" (16). A definition stressing allergic pathogenesis is "variable airflow limitation caused by sensitization to a specific agent encountered at work and excluding other occupational causes of variable airflow limitation not due to sensitization" (6). The Industrial Injuries Advisory Council in Great Britain defines occupational asthma as "asthma which develops after a variable period of symptomless exposure to a sensitizing agent at work" (7). There are limits to the consideration of what is an acceptable sensitizing agent when the definition is applied for compensation purposes. Smith (17) formulated a medico-legal definition of occupational asthma.

A definition of occupational asthma emphasizing a mechanism propounds that allergic occupational asthma is allergic/immunologic sensitization to a substance or material present in the work site. There is variable and work-related airflow limitation and the presence of both specific and nonspecific airway hyperresponsiveness. For this type of occupational asthma, a key clinical feature is that asthma develops after the passage of a latent period, or a time span. During the latent period, exposure continues and allergy evolves. Eventually, there is the clinical manifestation of work-related airflow limitation and specific and nonspecific airway hyperresponsiveness. The specific airway hyperresponsiveness relates to allergic/immunologic influences; the nonspecific airway hyperresponsiveness appears to be the sequela of bronchial mucosal injury and airway inflammation.

Nonspecific airway hyperresponsiveness is such a characteristic feature of allergic and nonallergic occupational asthma that its absence brings into question the very diagnosis of asthma. Nonetheless, there are cases of allergic-type occupational asthma without nonspecific airway hyperresponsiveness (18–20). There are also examples of allergic occupational asthma where latency is not a feature. In such single-exposure cases, both allergic and nonallergic mechanisms seem operative (21). Recurrent nocturnal attacks of asthma are reported after a single exposure to Western red cedar in a sensitized worker (22).

Nonallergic occupational asthma occurs after a high-level, workplace irritant exposure and develops abruptly and without a significant latent period. The exposure is characteristically singular and intense (23). Asthma also occurs after lesser exposures and over a longer (months to years) period of time (24). The absence of a latent period is a critical clinical feature, because it supports the contention that an allergic mechanism is not operative.

## TYPES OF OCCUPATIONAL ASTHMA

There are two types of occupational asthma, depending on the presence or absence of a preceding latency period before asthma develops (15). The first, occupational asthma with a latency period, encompasses instances of occupational asthma for which an allergic/immunologic mechanism are identified. The second, occupational asthma without a latency period, includes asthma developing rather suddenly and is best illustrated by the reactive airways dysfunction syndrome (RADS). Work-aggravated asthma, on the other hand, is not considered occupational asthma but refers to the presence of concurrent asthma worsened by irritants or physical stimuli in the workplace.

## PREVALENCE

Bronchial asthma is the most important pulmonary disorder of Western countries. In the United States, estimates of the prevalence of occupational asthma vary, but one conservative estimate is 2% of all cases of bronchial asthma (25). An analysis of data from the 1978 U.S. Social Security Disability Survey attests that 15% of all asthma cases are work related (26). A conservative estimate of occupational asthma occurrence is 220,000 to 1.7 million cases in the United States (6). An estimation of morbidity associated with occupational asthma is 130,000 to 975,000 physician visits, 10,000 to 75,000 hospital admissions, and a conservative 20,000 to 150,000 days' work lost per year (6).

In Canada, occupational asthma is the most frequently compensated occupational lung disease (27). Occupational asthma is the most frequently diagnosed occupational lung disease reported to the SWORD (Surveillance of Work-Related and Occupational Respiratory Disease) (28). The prevalence of occupational asthma varies among countries and accounts for 2% to 6% of adult asthma cases in the United Kingdom (29) and 5.0% to 6.7% in Spain (30).

The true prevalence of irritant-induced asthma (e.g., asthma without latency) is unknown but is more common than previously perceived (31–34). In one investigation, 6% of workers assessed for occupational asthma had irritant-induced asthma (i.e., RADS) compared to 32% with allergic occupational asthma (24). Data from a community-based random sample of 3,606 adults, 40 to 69 years of age, residing in Beijing, China, examined the relationship between occupational exposures to dusts and irritant gases/fumes and physician's diagnosis of asthma (35). After adjusting for sex, age, education, residential areas, indoor coal combustion, and smoking status, the attributable risks of dust-related asthma was 1.7%, while the risk for asthma from irritant gases/fumes was 1.2%. Another study addressed several hundred adult patients with bronchial asthma belonging to three major races (Chinese, Malay, and Indian) and observed in five outpatient primary care polyclinics (36). The risks of asthma were generally elevated for service and manufacturing production workers, especially municipal cleaners and sweepers, textile workers, garment markers, electrical and electronic production workers, printers, and construction/renovation workers. Nonspecific irritation effects are more common than sensitization as the cause of work-related asthmatic symptoms in flour milling, baking, and other flour-based industries (37). Nonspecific respiratory irritation was the cause of asthma symptoms in 2.6% of workers, while sensitization was responsible for symptoms in 0.3%.

The Sentinel Event Notification System for Occupational Risks (SENSOR) Program, launched by the National Institute for Occupational Safety and Health (NIOSH) in 1987, provides state-based surveillance and intervention programs for occupational asthma (38). From 1988 through 1992, 328 cases met the SENSOR surveillance case definition for occupational asthma. There were 128 cases classified as possible occupational asthma; 42 were RADS; and 37 cases were work-aggravated asthma. In Michigan, more than 40% of the asthma case-patients worked in transportation equipment manufacturing. In another investigation, the prevalence of occupational asthma in Michigan was estimated to be between 3% and 20.2% (39). In New Jersey, 15% of asthma case-patients worked in manufacturing of chemicals and allied products (38). The SENSOR data confirmed that isocyanates are the most frequently reported asthma-causing agents (19.4% of cases).

The prevalence of occupational asthma varies with the extent of exposure and with occupation. For example, investigations note that approximately 4% of workers exposed to Western red cedar develop asthma (40); the prevalence for Eastern red cedar is 3.8% to 7% (41). About 4% to 5% of workers exposed to isocyanates develop occupational asthma (14). Asthma from the proteolytic enzymes occurs in 10% to 45% of workers. Occupational asthma caused by latex evolves in 2.5% of hospital employees (42). Wheat flour allergy appears in 25% of bakers and pastry cooks (43). About 9% of the bakery workers show positive skin prick tests to fungal amylase and 8% demonstrate elevated amylase-specific immunoglobulin E (IgE) antibodies (44). About 41% of technicians report work-related symptoms provoked by laboratory animals (45). The prevalence of work-related asthma among factory employees manufacturing flux-cored solder containing colophony is 21% in the highest exposure group and is 4% in the lower exposure group (46). Malo and associates (47) report that 23% of employees at a carpet-manufacturing plant that used guar gum to adhere the dye to the fiber have a history suggestive of occupational asthma. An investigation of asthma conducted on 619 cedar sawmill, 724 grain elevator, 399 pulp mill, 798 aluminum smelter, and 1,127 unexposed workers shows an overall prevalence of physician-diagnosed asthma of 4.6%. The prevalence of asthma is 3.9 times higher in cedar sawmill workers, 2.2 times higher in pulp mill and aluminum smelter workers, and 1.7 times higher in grain elevator workers compared with unexposed workers (48).

## RISK FACTORS FOR THE DEVELOPMENT OF OCCUPATIONAL ASTHMA

### Exposure Characteristics

A variety of exposure characteristics influence asthma development or aggravate the disease once it is present. The chemical characteristic of an allergen influences its antigenicity and its ability to cause asthma. Such relevant characteristics as chemical type and reactivity, chemical sources, and concentration of an exposure are pertinent. The intensity of an exposure is critical. High levels are implicated in the pathogenesis of both types of occupational asthma, with and without latency. Massive exposures occur with RADS. Intermittent, high-level exposures are important in the pathogenesis of toluene 2,4-diisocyanate (TDI)-induced asthma (21), but also asthma without latency (49,50). Workers who are more frequently exposed to spills are more likely to report asthma symptoms and show alterations in lung function testing.

An unmistakable dose-response relationship exists for an exposure and the prevalence of allergic sensitization. This association is reported for Western red cedar (51,52), Eastern red cedar, isocyanates (53), colophony (46), baking products (54), and acid anhydrides. Symptoms of work-related asthma in red cedar workers are more common after 10 years of exposure, and levels of pulmonary function are lower with higher wood dust exposures (51).

Cumulative exposure may be important, as exemplified by the investigation of Jones and associates (55) for TDI. The duration of an exposure may be influential as ascertained by the investigation of Di Stefano et al. (56). In the latter study, comparisons of lobar bronchial biopsies findings between two TDI groups show that workers who develop asthma after a short-term exposure (e.g., $2.4 \pm 0.4$ years) show significantly higher numbers of mast cells in the airway mucosa compared to the subjects who develop asthma after long-term exposure to TDI (e.g., $21.6 \pm 3.1$ years). Exposure indices may also be tied to the type of asthmatic response noted. The presence of a late asthmatic-response is shown to have a linear relationship to the logarithm of tetrachlorophthalic anhydride air exposure. The immediate asthmatic response does not closely relate to tetrachlorophthalic anhydride air exposure (57).

Poor working conditions are a good predictor for the development of adverse pulmonary outcomes. For example, work activity in a small, poorly regulated hemp mill, where there are routinely very high dust levels, is associated with reduced pulmonary function testing (58). An accelerated decline in forced expiratory volume in 1 second ($FEV_1$) is noted in women workers, who are predominantly nonsmokers; this observation suggests an independent effect of hemp on the airways.

Exposures may be monitored using biomarkers. Thus, bronchial responsiveness in aluminum pot-room workers with asthma appear related to plasma levels of fluoride (59). Trimellitic anhydride (TMA) workers showing late-occurring asthma or late respiratory systemic syndrome improve after moving to lower exposure jobs. However, elevated IgE against TM-HSA is considered to be a marker for a subpopulation of workers with asthma and rhinitis that do not improve (60).

An industry factor is observed with TDI. Asthma is reported more often by workers employed in polyurethane processing than by employees of TDI manufacturing (61). A mill effect or plant effect is described to explain differences in the frequency of byssinosis, and possibly of TDI asthma among workers with similar exposure (62). Hexamethylene diisocyanate (HDI) and TDI display the same vapor pressures and are relatively volatile at room temperature; MDI has a lower vapor pressure and is not volatile at room temperature. MDI becomes volatile and is more likely to lead to asthma after heating when its vapor pressure increases. This circumstance is observed in such industrial processes as foundry work (63). The specific type of industrial process may influence the development of asthma. For example, asthma appears in about 5% of workers exposed to isocyanates; 10% to 45% of workers exposed to proteolytic enzymes; and 2% to 40% of workers exposed to grain dust, including millers and bakers.

### Geographic and Climatic Factors

Weather conditions such as wind direction and humidity may be influential. In Barcelona, Spain grain dusts released by unloading soybeans caused asthma outbreaks (64). Apparently, the unloading of the soybeans gives rise to sudden, massive release of soybean dust that reaches the urban area owing to appropriate meteorological conditions and causes the epidemic. Asthma from red cedar is seen in the western United States. In the Great Lakes area, grain dusts and flour frequently cause asthma. Chemicals are indigenous to many areas, especially the industrial East and Midwest. Working in a cold environment may have an adverse effect on asthmatics who exert themselves.

### Atopy

The presence of the atopic status may influence how an individual worker respond to a workplace allergen (8,15,65). The relationship between atopy and allergic sensitization is best established for agents of higher molecular weight (≥1,000 daltons) (8,15,66). This includes the detergent enzymes (67), laboratory animal allergens (45,68,69), certain insect proteins, and products such as gum acacia and flour (70,71). In a cross-sectional study, involving 178 bakery workers, α-amylase exposure and atopy were the most important determinants of α-amylase skin sensitization (44).

Atopy may also be important for certain low-molecular weight (≤1,000 daltons) compounds such as platinum salts (8,9,72), ethylene diamine (73), and dimethyl ethanolamine (74). Other low molecular weight agents, such as TDI, Western red cedar (75), trimellitic anhydride, phthalic anhydride, and formaldehyde, do not seem to be influenced by the atopic state. The conflicting data on atopic sensitization and an agent's molecular size suggest that other factors are important in determining allergic sensitization.

### Cigarette Smoking

Cigarette smoking predisposes workers to allergic sensitization. There is a connection between cigarette smoking and increased IgE levels (71,76–83). A higher total IgE concentration is noted in smokers' serum (84). Tobacco smoke provokes an increase in serum IgE and enhances respiratory sensitization to ovalbumin in animals studies (85). An association between atopy, cigarette smoking, and allergic sensitization to a workplace exposure is reported for workers exposed to green coffee beans, tetrachlorophthalic anhydride (TCPA), and platinum salts (76,77). In a study of TCPA-exposed workers, 20 of 24 subjects with specific IgE antibodies to a TCPA-HSA were currently smokers (78). Both smoking and the intensity of platinum salts exposure are associated with development of platinum salt sensitivity among South African platinum refinery workers (76).

One proposed mechanism to explain the connection between cigarette smoking and allergic sensitization suggests that inhalation of cigarette smoke injures the bronchial epithelium. As a result of the injury, there may be widening of the tight junctions between epithelial cells that heightens bronchial epithelial permeability; this results in greater penetration of antigen through the epithelial layer (86). The alteration affords more direct access for allergen to the immune machinery in the subepithelium and vasculature (76,87). It is also possible that there may be the release of different mediators in smokers compared to nonsmokers.

### Exposures to Low-Level Airborne Workplace Irritants

Industrial operations that include agents possessing irritant properties are potentially dangerous because of the risk of heavy exposures from spills and accidents (88). However, cumulative lower-level exposures to airborne irritants may produce bronchial epithelium injury and consequences that are similar to cigarette smoking (89,90). Irritant gases such as chlorine and ammonia, which are indigenous to the platinum-refining industry, may inaugurate bronchial epithelial injury (72). Biagini and associates (91) suggested that before platinum salts could cause allergic sensitization in monkeys, it required concurrent exposure to 1 part per million (ppm) ozone. Platinum salts are also irritating and have been reported to induce nonallergic basophil histamine release (91).

Animal studies further document that antecedent exposure to an airborne irritant enhances allergic sensitization to an allergen. Exposure to low levels of sulfur dioxide ($SO_2$) promotes allergic sensitization in guinea pigs (92); a similar mechanism is reported for ozone (93) and nitrogen dioxide ($NO_2$). There are similarities between $NO_2$ and $SO_2$ time-kinetic bronchoalveolar lavage (BAL) inflammatory responses especially for mast cells and lymphocytes; their levels peak 8 to 24 hours after exposure.

The scope of the irritant exposures include not only gases, vapors, and fumes, but also dusts that possess the potential for allergic sensitization. In occupational settings that expose workers to irritant dusts (e.g., red cedar and trimellitic anhydride) or dust having enzymatic properties (e.g., subtilisin, esperase, proteases, papain, amylase) allergic sensitization may ensue. This phenomenon transpires because the dusts inherent irritant qualities somehow damages the bronchial epithelium and perhaps increases permeability or causes bronchial mucosal inflammation. In humans, exposure to irritant gases may lead to lower airway inflammation, which may then lead to bronchial hyperresponsiveness. An investigation of competitive swimmers showed 11 of 14 exhibited bronchial hyperresponsiveness to methacholine and positive radioallergosorbent test (RAST) or skin tests compared to 5 of 14 control subjects (94). It was hypothesized that the higher prevalence of skin and bronchial reactivity among swimmers was due to frequent exposure to chlorine gas and its components in swimming pools.

Various investigations report reductions in serial lung function testing of various occupational groups exposed to irritants. A review by Rylander and co-workers (95) of 11 epidemiologic investigations of a population of more than 1,000 workers exposed to irritant and biologically active agents in swine confinement buildings (e.g., endotoxin, hydrogen sulfide, ammonia) revealed widespread respiratory symptoms in 15% to 55%; there was across-shift decrements in lung function tests in 15% to 20%; and there was a suggestion of a dose-response relationship between lung function changes and exposure (95).

### Nonspecific Bronchial Hyperresponsiveness

Airway hyperresponsiveness, a characteristic of asthma, has been studied under various environmental and occupational settings (96–98). It may be present in seemingly normal persons (96,97). The rate is 6% to 20% in the Norwegian general population, depending on the concentration of methacholine that is deemed to yield a positive result (i.e., ≤8 or ≤32 mg/ml air) (99); about 11% of rural Australians show bronchial hyperreactivity (100). In the Normative Aging Study, 30% of subjects show a positive reaction to methacholine challenge (101). Additionally, airway hyperresponsiveness is reported in 47% of persons with cough and no other chest symptom; in 40% of patients with rhinitis and vague chest symptoms that are not by themselves diagnostic of asthma; and in 22% of persons having rhinitis and no chest symptoms (102). Increased nonspecific bronchial reactivity is also seen in cigarette smokers with normal lung function. The presence of nonspecific bronchial hyperresponsiveness is not uncommon among younger persons (99). A high prevalence of bronchial hyperresponsiveness is noted among highly trained athletes at the University of Iowa (103): 76 of 151 (50%) college football players, 4 of 16 (25%) basketball players, and 69 of 167 (41%) students reveal positive methacholine challenge tests; 47%, 25%, and 37% of these groups, respectively, report minimal or no symptoms.

Individuals with asthma may show pathologic and BAL alterations in the absence of significant asthmatic symptoms. The airways of asthmatics are more "leaky" and demonstrate more inflammatory cells to be present in BAL (104–106).

Nonspecific bronchial hyperresponsiveness is not a predisposing host factor for the initiation of occupational asthma; it evolves in parallel with the development of occupational asthma and is not present in the worker beforehand (107). Asthma symptoms and the degree of bronchial reactivity often decrease after a workers is removed from exposure and increases following reexposure (108,109). Following cessation of exposure, a peak of improvement of spirometric values is reached at 1 year and for bronchial hyperresponsiveness at 2 years (109,110).

Airway inflammation plays a crucial role in the evolution of nonspecific airway hyperresponsiveness and leads to many of the clinical manifestations of asthma (111–116).

Bronchial hyperresponsiveness is documented by the inhalation of a drug such as methacholine, histamine, or carbachol; inhalation of cold-air; and exposures to various hypo-osmolar and acid aerosols (72,117). Methacholine challenge testing is influenced by suggestion, deep inspiration, adequacy of aerosol deposition, pretest pulmonary function status, selection of the proper physiologic parameter to monitor the airways response, a number of infectious, environmental, and clinical factors, the patient's ability to cope with the disease, and emotional lability (118). Investigators report correlations between a greater sensitivity to methacholine or histamine and worsening clinical features of asthma; this includes wider diurnal variation in flow rates, more exercise-induced bronchospasm, more medication required for asthma control, and greater bronchial response to allergens (119,120).

A questionnaire focusing on symptoms of bronchial irritability (respiratory symptoms that develop in response to a number of common irritants) reveals a correlation between a clinical response and physiologic documentation (121). The designation "bronchial irritability syndrome" applies to persons reporting bronchial irritability symptoms and who demonstrate an increase in histamine reactivity, with $PC_{20}$, a provocative concentration of histamine that causes a 20% fall in $FEV_1$. of less than 0.5 g/L. No asymptomatic subjects show a $PC_{20}$ value below 0.5 g/L. About 27% of these subjects have a physician's diagnosis of asthma. Another investigation assessed airway responsiveness both clinically and physiologically (122). In 24 subjects with stable chronic bronchial asthma, disease severity was determined by a disease severity score (DSS) that described six clinical or therapeutic parameters. Airways hyperresponsiveness was assessed in two ways: (1) airway reactivity score (ARS), which is based on the number of positive responses to a question about exposure to 22 nonspecific inhaled irritants; (2) a challenge test, which determines the cumulative dose of methacholine that causes a 20% reduction in $FEV_1$ ($CMD_{20}$). A significant correlation was seen between DSS and $CMD_{20}$ and between DSS and ARS. Significant correlations for ARS with $CMD_{20}$ suggest the consistency with which the ARS estimated methacholine hyperresponsiveness. The findings attest to the important influence of airway hyperresponsiveness on disease severity.

## Sensitive Subpopulation?

An appropriate question is whether there is a sensitive subpopulation at greater risk for developing allergic or irritant-induced occupational asthma. The hypothetical scenario proposes there is a sensitive subpopulation consisting of persons who have inherent injured bronchial epithelium. Such persons may manifest airway hyperresponsiveness but do not report symptoms, seek medical assistance, or receive antiasthma medications. If the opportunity is made available, pathologic changes may show airway injury and epithelial damage are found on bronchial biopsy specimens.

The sensitive population may represent a proportion of both symptomatic and asymptomatic atopic individuals. The sensitive population consists of asthmatics and some atopic persons who are more sensitive to low levels of irritant gases, such as sulfur dioxide. These atopic persons show altered airways that may respond more intensely to airborne irritants. Because irritant gases induce airway inflammation in normal volunteers, a similar exposure may cause more dramatic changes in the airways of asthmatics and atopic persons. Spontaneous mast cell degranulation is characteristic of asthma and is sometimes associated with atopy (123). Perhaps mast cell degranulation is heightened after irritant exposures in sensitive persons. Bronchial epithelial cell alterations appear in asthmatic subjects, even subjects reporting minimal symptoms and who require little or no medication. Shedding of the ciliated respiratory epithelium, collagen deposition beneath the epithelial basement membrane, partial mast cell degranulation, and eosinophil infiltration of the lamina propria are characteristic features of bronchial biopsy specimens of asthmatic subjects (124,125). Similar findings may be present in sensitive persons.

An important consideration is that the airways of asthmatics, and perhaps of some atopics, are leaky. In a study by Van De Graaf and co-workers (106), patients with stable bronchial asthma demonstrate an increase in plasma exudation into the airways. The exudation correlates with bronchial hyperresponsiveness to histamine, and it decreases after corticosteroid therapy. Using rigid tube bronchoscopy, Laitinen and colleagues (126) observed various degrees of epithelial damage in fresh biopsy specimens from eight patients with asthma of varying degrees of severity. The tissue shows changes at all airway levels, including epithelial cell destruction. Occasional mast cells appear within the damaged areas of the epithelium and superficial nerves.

Workers with hyperresponsive airways find it difficult to work in dusty environments, and so they avoid them or quit work early. Worker turnover is more frequent in dusty jobs (foundry work, grain elevators). Airway hyperresponsiveness may lead to a self-protective decrease in exposure to a dusty work environment and promote exclusion of these persons from this type of work (127).

Thus, a body of information suggests: (a) low-level exposures to irritants can cause airway inflammation; (b) a segment of the population may be more responsive to low levels of irritants; (c) a segment of the population appears to be more susceptible to developing workplace allergic sensitization because of certain host factors (i.e., atopy, cigarette smoking), possibly because of exposure to airborne irritants indigenous to the workplace environment; (d) nonspecific airway hyperresponsiveness is more common than was previously appreciated, is common in young persons, and may be present with few symptoms or none; (e) persons with hyperreactive airways, including asthmatics, are more responsive to irritants; and (f) pathologic evidence of bronchial epithelial damage is observed in asthmatics who have few or no respiratory tract complaints. Thus, a population more susceptible to workplace sensitization may include workers with host factors of atopy, asymptomatic hyperresponsive airways, or underlying nonoccupational asthma.

## ALLERGIC AND IMMUNE MECHANISMS

The current thinking is that agents that cause occupational asthma with a latency period (e.g., allergic type) do so either through the production of specific IgE antibodies or through some not yet clearly identified immunologic mechanism (5,8,128).

### IgE Antibody Production in Occupational Asthma

A number of investigations point out the essential role of IgE in many types of occupational asthma. Bronchial epithelial cells of asthmatic patients may be directly activated by an IgE-mediated mechanism (129). In fact, the role of IgE in the pathogenesis of allergic asthma is paramount, and many surveys disclose elevated serum concentrations of IgE in association with a variety of occupational exposures. Table 2 lists some examples of specific agents reported to be associated with IgE mechanisms.

IgG antibodies have also been incriminated in certain instances of occupational asthma (130,131).

### Cellular Immunity

Cellular immune responses in occupational asthma may be more important than was previously suspected (132). The finding of T lymphocytes in the airways of sensitized workers, as observed by bronchial biopsies and BAL, suggests that T-cell–mediated immune responses play an important role in TDI asthma. Distinct T-cell activation leads to different spectra of cytokines production. Allergic asthmatics show increased numbers of $CD4^+$ interleukin (IL)-$2R^+$ T cells in peripheral blood and BAL; T-cell activation closely correlates with numbers of low-affinity IgE receptor (CD23) bearing B cells. In contrast, in nonallergic asthmatics, both $CD4^+$ and $CD8^+$ T cells from blood and BAL possess increased expression of IL-2R, human leukocyte antigen (HLA)-DR, and very late activation antigen (VLA)-1; $CD8^+$ T cells are decreased in blood but increased in BAL.

### Genetic Influences

Genetic factors seem important in the immunopathology of diisocyanate-induced asthma. HLA typing of subjects with TDI asthma (confirmed by inhalation challenge) was carried out by the polymerase chain reaction–restriction fragment length polymorphism (PCR-RFLP) method, which allowed discrimination of most HLA DQA1, DQB1, DPB1, and DRB alleles (133). Allele DQB1*0503 and allelic combination DQB1*0201/0301 were associated with susceptibility to developing TDI asthma. Conversely, allele DQB1*0501 and the DQA1*0101-DQB1*0501-DR1 haplotype conferred significant protection to exposed healthy control subjects. In another study involving HLA class genetic markers, Balboni et al. (134) provided evidence that HLA-DQB1*0503 has a role in conferring susceptibility to

**TABLE 2.** *Examples of occupational asthma with specific IgE antibodies*

| Occupation | Causal agent |
|---|---|
| Animal handler | Urine protein, dander |
| Antibiotics worker | Penicillin, spiramycin |
| Baker | Wheat, rye, buckwheat; mites, α-amylase, hemicellulase, gluco-amylase, papain, soybean |
| Chemical worker | Sulfonechloramides, azo dyes, ethylenediamine, anthraquinone |
| Coffee or tea worker | Green coffee, tea dust |
| Detergent worker | *Bacillus subtilis,* esperase |
| Entomologists | Locusts, blowfly |
| Fishery worker | Sea squirts, prawns |
| Oil extractor, crusher | Castor beans |
| Pharmaceutical worker | Pepsin, flaviastase, penicillin, cephalosporins, phenyl-glycine acid chloride, spiramycin |
| Plastic worker | Phthalic anhydride, trimellitic anhydrides, diisocyanates |
| Printer | Arabic gum, gum acacia |
| Processor | Prawns, hoya, egg powder, tobacco leaf |
| Spice or enzyme worker | Garlic powder, papain, pectinase, trypsin, karaya gum, maiko |
| Woodworker | Quillaja bark, red cedar, Douglas fir, African zebra-wood, iroko |
| Insect handler | Bee moth, cockroach, river flies, locust, mealworm, screwworm |
| Metal processor | Platinum salts, cobalt, nickel |

TDI-induced asthma and that residue 57 of HLA-DQB1 is a potentially critical location.

Atopy provides the predisposition to develop IgE and immediate-type hypersensitivity to common antigens. Occupational asthma due to large molecular weight compounds is often influenced by the atopic status. The atopic status is believed to be under genetic control (135–137). Some pedigree studies of atopy suggest linkage with the high-affinity IgE receptor gene on chromosome 11q13, but others find no linkage (137). The work of van Herwerden et al. (137) provides evidence of significant linkage of a highly polymorphic microsatellite marker in the fifth intron of the Fc-ε RI-β gene to the presence of asthma and to airway hyperresponsiveness. Atopy in the absence of airway hyperresponsiveness did not show significant linkage to the Fc-ε RI-β gene. The findings of Doull et al. (138) support the view that both chromosomes 5 and 11 may contain genes relevant to asthma and atopy, a possible candidate being the IL-4 gene cluster. The work of Postma and colleagues (139) demonstrates that a trait for an elevated serum total IgE is co-inherited with a trait for airway hyperresponsiveness and that a gene governing airway hyperresponsiveness is located near a major locus that regulates serum IgE levels on chromosome 5q. These findings suggest the existence of one or more genes on chromosome 5q31-q33 causing susceptibility to asthma. On the other hand, Lympany et al. (140), who studied nine families of two and, in many instances, three generations, with the index case having asthma and/or atopy, were unable to confirm a significant link between region D11S97 of chromosome 11q and either atopy or airway hyperresponsiveness to methacholine.

Further investigations are necessary to fully appreciate the interrelationships between genetic influences, atopy, IgE production, and airway hyperresponsiveness (135). However, a better understanding can provide important benefits and may open a number of potential preventive, diagnostic, and therapeutic avenues (136). For example, the identification of the specific mutations that alter the immune response may provide targets for gene therapy. However, in the short run this may not be feasible because the risks and costs associated with gene therapy do not presently justify application to alleviate the relatively nonlethal manifestations of an occupational disease. Another potential avenue may be in the development of specific drug treatment regimens based on genetic profiles. However, it is possible that redundancy in the immune and inflammatory responses, coupled with the likelihood of multiple gene involvement, will make such targeting difficult. A third outcome is that of identifying genetic variants that predispose to occupational asthma and allergic sensitization in the workplace and thus incorporate screening programs for these variations (136). Possibly, genetic screening of workers who are atopic may allow more precise identification of those carrying atopy genes, and this could allow a better attempt at workplace modification that may prove to be an effective strategy for occupational asthma prevention.

## AIRWAY INFLAMMATION

Airway changes in asthma is characterized by peribronchial eosinophil accumulation of the submucosa, there is epithelial edema and desquamation and subepithelial deposition of collagen and fibronectin (141). There are increased numbers of activated eosinophils, CD25-positive T-lymphocytes, and immature macrophages. An increased expression of HLA class II is present on epithelium, macrophages, and other infiltrating cells. The inflammatory sequence of events following an allergen challenge can be studied by the technique of local endobronchial allergen challenge and direct airway sampling of the airway milieu (141a). These studies identify allergen-mast cell interaction as the initial airway event, with mediator release inducing bronchoconstriction and enhancing vascular permeability. Preformed mast cell cytokines are released and initiate endothelial cell activation. There is up-regulation of cell adhesion molecules, and tissue cell recruitment. Subsequent cytokine elaboration from airway macrophages and T-lymphocytes perpetuate this response. In chronic asthma, T-lymphocytes, mast cells, matrix tissue, epithelial cells, and eosinophils contribute to the cytokine pool within the airways and to the regulation of inflammatory cell migration and activation.

The late-phase asthmatic reaction is a continuation of the IgE-mediated allergic response and appears to be critical for the development of hyperresponsive airways (225). In occupational asthma there are subpopulations of $CD4^-$ lymphocytes and Th2 subtypes. These lymphocytes produce a family of cytokines that favor IgE production and the growth and activation of mast cells and eosinophils; this alteration arms the airways with the mechanisms of response to subsequent reexposure to the allergen. Allergen-specific T-lymphocytes present in the peripheral blood of allergic patients are of Th1 and Th2 subtypes. Their stimulation appears to lead to the activation of endothelial cells and thereby participate in leukocyte recruitment towards the inflammatory site. Because the inflammatory response develops over hours, various inflammatory cells influence the later and more persistent bronchial obstruction. The consequence of this multiple cell and multiple proinflammatory product interaction is the establishment of a self-perpetuating, redundant inflammatory process by which asthma severity increases (115). Irritant-induced asthma (RADS) may have a similar pathogenesis as viral infections which seemingly involves activation of different pathways. Viral infection activates production of cytokines by airway epithelial cells (141b). Damage to airway epithelial cells may also occur after the inhalation of high levels of irritant agents.

## CLINICAL FEATURES OF OCCUPATIONAL ASTHMA

Symptomatically, persons with occupational asthma with latency manifest asthmatic symptoms within the first few years, and sometimes within a few months of beginning work and having an allergen exposure. The worker's symptoms occur because he/she has become sensitized to an antigen present in the workplace. The clinical manifestations typically appear related to work. Antigen exposure induces an acute asthmatic response. The asthmatic symptoms improve when the individual is away from work, especially during the weekends or vacations, but resume when the individual returns to the workplace. Cough may be the predominant complaint, and an incorrect diagnosis of bronchitis is often entertained. Coughing occurs during the day but also at night, which may interfere with sleep.

In a laboratory setting, when bronchial inhalation testing is conducted employing a specific antigen and under carefully controlled conditions, several distinct patterns of bronchospastic reactions are observed. The types of reactions fall into three major groups: immediate or early; nonimmediate or late; and dual or combined reactions, during which both immediate and late reactions occur (Fig. 1). The immediate reaction develops rapidly (15 to 30 minutes) and is relatively short lived. IgE antibody response is thought to be important for the immediate or type I–mediated allergy. The degree of underlying nonspecific bronchial hyperreactivity influences the allergic response to the antigen. The nonacute or late asthmatic reaction begins about 1 hour after antigen challenge, generally peaks by 3 to 5 hours, and lasts 12 to 24 hours. If the reaction occurs about an hour after antigen challenge, recovery may be swift, within 2 to 3 hours. Some reactions begin after 3 to 4 hours, peak at 5 to 8 hours, and last 24 to 36 hours. There are also reports of reactions beginning early in the morning that can recur for several days after challenge even though measurements of $FEV_1$ return to pretest levels during the day. Although the various patterns of late reactions seem to occur in the absence of IgE antibody, late responses follow early reactions in about 50% of cases.

The lung function changes recorded in the laboratory translate into different clinical presentation of asthma following an allergen exposure in the workplace. Progressive lung function deterioration throughout the work week is characterized by more severe symptoms and poorer ventilatory test values at the end of the week than at the beginning. Usually it takes a few days for recovery to occur. In other cases, symptoms and spirometric changes occur during each work shift but improve rapidly after the patient leaves work and recovery is complete by the next work day. Progressive week-by-week deterioration has been documented in some cases, particularly when the recovery takes longer than 3 days and the worker returns to work at the beginning of each week, while lung function is still reduced. Occasionally the pattern is maximal deterioration on the first day of the week and recovery during the remainder of the week.

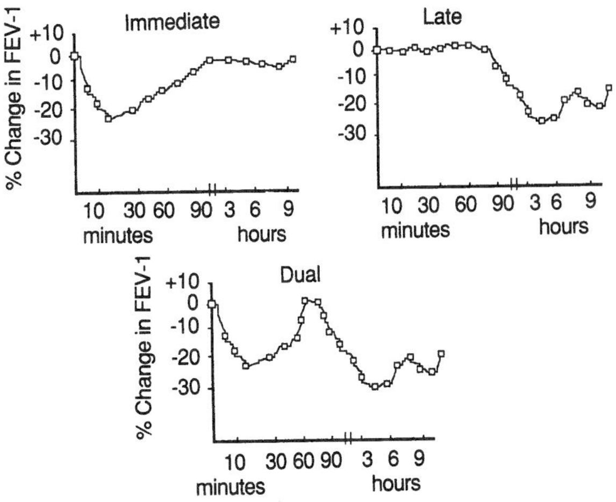


**FIG. 1.** The immediate reaction develops within 15 to 30 minutes and is relatively short lived. The nonimmediate or late asthmatic reaction begins about 1 hour after antigen challenge, generally reaches a maximum by 3 to 5 hours, and lasts 12 to 24 hours.

In the case of occupational asthma without latency, the onset of asthma is relatively sudden and the clinical manifestations are due mainly to the persistent nonspecific airway hyperresponsiveness (see below).

## OCCUPATIONAL ASTHMA WITHOUT LATENCY (IRRITANT-INDUCED ASTHMA)

### Background

Harkonen and colleagues (142) followed seven mine workers involved in a pyrite dust explosion who sustained $SO_2$-induced lung injury. The exact concentration of the gas was estimated to have been between 300 and 1,600 ppm. The authors concluded that nonspecific airways hyperresponsiveness was a frequent sequela of high-level $SO_2$ exposure and that this condition could persist for years. Charan and co-workers (143) described five cases of accidental high-level $SO_2$ exposure with three survivors developing severe airway obstruction. Serial pulmonary function tests performed on a 50-year-old man, who inhaled substantial quantities of concentrated ammonia vapors, over a 5-year period revealed development of an obstructive lung disorder (144). While methacholine challenge was not performed, the authors indicated that hyperreactive airways were present and were likely the direct result of the inhalation injury. Donham and co-workers (145) described an acute toxic exposure to high levels of hydrogen sulfide after agitation of liquid manure. One survivor's respiratory symptoms persisted more than 2 months after the incident. Other reports of persistent obstructive airways disease after high-level exposures included the studies of Murphy and associates (146) on a patient who inhaled vapors liberated when several drain cleaning agents were mixed, and the reports of chlorine gas exposures (147–150). A majority of persons involved in a single severe exposure to TDI developed respiratory symptoms within 24 hours, which persisted for as long as 4 years (151–153).

### Reactive Airways Dysfunction Syndrome–High-Level Exposure

In 1985, Brooks and colleagues (23) reported the clinical and pathologic descriptions of sudden-onset asthma, which develops after a high-level irritant gas, vapor, or fume exposure and is designated as the reactive airways dysfunction syndrome (RADS) (23). In this report, seven men and three women of an average age of 36 years developed an asthma-like illness after a single exposure to high levels of an irritating vapor, fume, gas, or smoke. The duration of exposure ranged from a few minutes to as long as 12 hours. For seven subjects there was an interval between exposure and the appearance of symptoms (mean was 8.9 hours); for three the reaction was immediate. In almost all instances, the exposure was the result of an accident or of poor ventilation and limited air exchange in the area. All subjects had a positive reaction to methacholine challenge. There was no evidence of a preexisting respiratory complaint in any patient; two subjects were found to be atopic but no evidence of allergy was identified for the others. There were six cigarette smokers, who together averaged about 16 pack-years' smoking. Pulmonary function was normal in three of ten, and seven showed airflow limitation. All subjects had negative chest radiographs. Respiratory symptoms and nonspecific airways hyperresponsiveness persisted in all subjects an average of nearly 3 years since the initial exposure. One person's disease was documented to have persisted at least 12 years. Eight of ten were taking anti-asthma medications. As part of the 1985 report, Brooks et al. provided the diagnostic criteria for RADS as shown in Table 3.

**TABLE 3.** *Criteria for reactive airways dysfunction syndrome*

| |
|---|
| No history of asthma-like respiratory disease |
| Onset follows a high-level exposure, usually an accident |
| Toxicant is an irritant gas, vapor, fume, aerosol, or dust in high concentration |
| Onset of symptoms is abrupt, developing within minutes or hours, but always within 24 hours |
| The clinical picture simulates asthma, with unremitting cough, "bronchial irritability" complaints, and wheezing |
| Results of pulmonary function tests may be normal or show reversible air flow limitation |
| Results of challenge with methacholine (or other agents) is positive in the range typical of asthma (i.e., <8 mg/ml) |
| Other respiratory disorders that simulate asthma are ruled out |

The causative agents varied in each case, but all were irritants: uranium hexafluoride gas, floor sealant, spray paint containing significant concentrations of ammonia, heated acid, 35% hydrazine, fumigating fog, metal coating remover, and smoke. In two cases bronchial biopsy documented bronchial epithelial cell injury and bronchial wall inflammation; lymphocytes and plasma cells were present but no eosinophilia was observed. Desquamation of respiratory epithelium was seen in one specimen and goblet cell hyperplasia in another. There was no evidence of mucous gland hyperplasia, basement membrane thickening, or smooth muscle hypertrophy.

In patients with RADS who exhibit nonspecific bronchial hyperresponsiveness, the airways narrow too easily and too much, compared to how a normal person responds. Thus, seemingly innocuous environmental/occupational stimuli to most persons will cause acute attacks of bronchospasm in persons with RADS. The exact reasons for the reflex acute bronchoconstrictor response in RADS is not known but it seems to be related to the presence of chronic airway inflammation, similar to asthma with latency. After an irritant or physical trigger, the resultant acute change in airflow limitation occurs either because there is direct stimulation of airway smooth muscle by the inciting trigger (e.g., pharmacologic stimuli such as methacholine and histamine); indirectly due to the release of biologically active mediators that have been secreted from cells, such as mast cells (provoked by exercise or hyper- and hypo-osmolar aerosols); from nonmyelinated sensory neurons (e.g., in response to agents such as sulfur dioxide or bradykinin); or perhaps a combination of mechanisms.

### Other Published Cases of RADS (Irritant-Induced Asthma)

Following the 1985 description of RADS, other examples of RADS were published (Table 4): sulfuric acid/$SO_2$ (154); smoke inhalation (155); locomotive/diesel exhaust (156); hydrochloric acid; floor sealant; anhydrous ammonia fumes (157); silo gas (158); acetic acid; burned paint fumes; zinc chloride; chlorine gas (159–162); welding fumes; phosphoric acid/disinfectant; phosgene; anticorrosive agent, 2-diethylaminoethanolamine (163); bleaching agents; constituent of free-base cocaine; sodium hydroxide/silicon tetrachloride/tichlorosilane exposure (164); burning paint fumes; TDI (165); metam sodium pesticide environmental spill (166); irritant gas containing chromate nonspecified irritants; and tear gas (167). Kern (168) noted a dose-response relationship for RADS development occurring among hospital workers exposed to a spill of 100% glacial acetic acid. The Patient Data Base System of Health History questionnaire addressed the health status of the exposed persons prior to the spill. Eight workers developed an asthma-like illness within 24 hours, and four continued to show evidence of RADS for nearly a year after the accident. Those subjects with

**TABLE 4.** *Some reported causes of RADS*

| |
|---|
| Sulfuric acid/$SO_2$ |
| Smoke inhalation |
| Locomotive/diesel exhaust |
| Hydrochloric acid |
| Floor sealant |
| Anhydrous ammonia fumes |
| Silo gas |
| Acetic acid |
| Burned paint fumes |
| Zinc chloride |
| Chlorine gas |
| Welding fumes |
| 2-Diethylaminoethanolamine |
| Bleaching agents |
| Constituent of free-base cocaine |
| NaOH/silicon CL4/tichlorosilane |
| Burning paint fumes |
| TDI |
| Metam sodium pesticide spill |
| Gas-containing chromate |
| Nonspecified irritants |
| Tear gas |
| Phosgene |
| Phosphoric acid/disinfectant |

RADS appeared to have suffered the higher dose exposures and were closer to the spill.

Chan-Yeung et al. (50) reported on pulp mill workers with a history of multiple "gassing" episodes occurring over a period of years. The results of immunohistology of bronchial mucosal biopsy of these subjects were compared with those of patients with allergic asthma and patients with Western red cedar–induced asthma. Subjects with RADS had a greater density of activated eosinophils and fewer T lymphocytes, suggesting that cell-mediated immune mechanisms were not involved in the pathogenesis of RADS. Another study of workers with repeated exposures to chlorine in pulp mills was provided by Malo and associates (49). The study population consisted of 20 subjects who demonstrated airway hyperresponsiveness to methacholine when they were first assessed, 18 to 24 months after repeatedly inhaling "puffs" of high concentrations of chlorine in a paper mill over a 3-month period. Although changes in spirometry induced by repeated exposure to chlorine persisted, bronchial hyperresponsiveness improved significantly in those with normal airway caliber, which suggested that less pronounced bronchial alterations induced by repeated exposures to chlorine may be reversible.

There appear to be cases of irritant-induced asthma that do not conform to the original RADS diagnostic criteria (169). A retrospective analysis of 86 asthmatic subjects, performed by Brooks et al. (170) identified 54 subjects discerned to have irritant-induced asthma (170). Two distinct clinical scenarios were recognized in 54 patients the first was sudden-onset in origin, with onset within 24 hours (29 subjects), while the second group was considered not-so-sudden in onset (25 subjects), whereby asthma took longer to develop (≥24 hours). Sudden-onset, irritant-induced asthma was found to be analogous to RADS. Clinical manifestations began immediately or within a few hours (always within 24 hours) following a brief, massive exposure, usually accidental in origin. In contrast, for not-so-sudden-onset asthma, the causative irritant exposure was not brief, it was often not massive, it continued for more than 24 hours, and initiation of asthma took longer to evolve.

There were 88% of individuals with not-so-sudden asthma who displayed an atopy/allergy status, a prevelance found to be statistically significant ($p$ <0.01). Besides atopy/allergy, some subjects with presumed new-onset asthma, in actuality, were found to suffer pre-existing asthma that was clinically quiescent for at least one year before the exposure occurred (16 persons). The investigation clarifies the role of host factors in the initiation of asthma following irritant exposures not considered to be massive. The study underscores the critical interaction between environmental and host factors in the pathogenesis of asthma

RADS likely exemplifies the extreme end of the spectrum of an irritant effect on the airways. For the not-so-sudden asthma cases, it is perplexing to explain why an irritant exposure, not adjudged to be massive or high-level, could result in sufficient injury to cause persistent airway inflammation and continued airway hyperresponsiveness. A longer duration of exposure is likely for the not-so-sudden group because the level of the irritant exposure is lesser than that noted for RADS; the patient tolerated the exposure longer. To explain the disparity between the lower level of the irritant exposure and asthma initiation necessitates considering mechanisms other than solely airway damage induced by the irritant exposure. Pre-exiting host susceptibility, such as pre-existing asthma or atopy, with its associated inherent biochemical and pathological consequences, is most likely. Atopic individuals are at an increased risk for developing asthma. They more often show serial accelerated declines in lung function tests, and atopics appear to display exaggerated responses to irritants IgE, paramount to the atopic state, seems linked to bronchial hyperresponsiveness. Atopic persons and possibly individuals with a genetic tendency for allergies (but without overt atopic manifestations) may be unique in their responses to irritants. Bronchial epithelial cells of atopics may react differently to irritant exposures because of IgE bound to its surface (129). Perhaps an irritant exposure, occurring in an atopic individual, consummates in enhanced bronchial mucosal permeability. This alteration allows greater entrance, into the airway mucosa, of common environmental aeroallergens. In an atopic person, previously sensitized to these aeroallergens, an increase in allergen penetration causes a more pronounced allergenic response and mediator release, eventuating into clinically new-onset asthma. An irritant exposure may lead to mediator release from airway sources causing inflammation and airway hyperresponsiveness. An alternative interpretation is that airway sensitivity to an allergen becomes augmented by an irritant exposure, a proposed scenario supported by works of Molfino et al. and Jorres and colleagues, which demonstrate enhanced specific bronchial airway responsiveness to aeroallergens after pre-exposure to low-levels of ozone (170a,170b). There is likely a complex interplay between irritant-induced airway injury, airway inflammation, IgE-mediated mechanisms, and asthma onset, of which much is not known.

## AGENTS FOR WHICH ASTHMA IS QUESTIONABLE OR RARE

### Meat Wrapper's Asthma

In 1973 three cases were reported of workers employed as meat wrappers who developed respiratory symptoms when they were exposed to fumes of polyvinyl chloride (PVC) film cut with a hot wire (171). This entity was called meat wrapper's asthma. Subsequently, a number of other reports were published with diverse symptoms reported, including rhinorrhea, cough, tightness of the chest, sore throat, exhaustion, and wheezing. Some investigators concluded that the emission from thermally activated price labels was the principal cause of meat wrapper's asthma. Subsequent investigations failed to confirm that any major airways condition affected meat wrappers who were surveyed (172,173). For instance, in one study, lower respiratory tract complaints were observed in a third of the meat wrappers, but no across-shift change in $FEV_1$ was discerned, even in the most symptomatic workers (173). Other studies supported the observation that there is no major chronic respiratory hazard to meat wrappers (174).

The major emissions from the PVC meat wrapping film are di-2-ethylhexyl adipate and hydrogen chloride, both shown to be irritants (173). As far as the emissions from the thermal activation of price labels is concerned, the major ingredient of price label adhesives is dicyclohexyl phthalate. Cyclohexyl ether (dicyclohexyl ether) and cyclohexyl benzoate (cyclohexyl ether of benzoic acid) are the major emission products of dicyclohexyl phthalate. The effects of cyclohexanol, another constituent, at moderate and low exposure levels are basically irritating. A potential sensitizer identified is phthalic anhydride, a stipulated emission from the heated label, but whether this is truly so and whether it remains stable during heating is not known. When tested in the meat-wrapping workplace, phthalic anhydride has not been detected in the vicinity of the heated price label emissions (172). Occupational asthma was said to occur in workers exposed to the plastics blowing agent, azodicarbonamide. Azodicarbonamide most likely acted by causing sensitization and not by irritation.

### Pesticides

The case for pesticides causing asthma is weak. Importantly, there are numerous types of pesticides with varying chemical structures and different modes of action. There are few well-documented cases of pesticides causing allergic sensitization, especially the organophosphate pesticides; most of the cases appear in the older literature. If pesticides do cause occupational asthma, it is rare.

### Formaldehyde

There are reports of respiratory disease among workers exposed to the formaldehyde (175,176). Most respiratory complaints are due to the irritative effects of formaldehyde. Exposure to low levels of indoor formaldehyde rarely if ever leads to specific IgE antibody production. Asthma is reported in workers exposed to higher levels of formaldehyde, such as pathologists and nurses working in a dialysis unit. Current evidence suggests, however, that occupational asthma from formaldehyde is rare (177).

### Machining Fluids

Several investigations have addressed machining fluids and the possibility of occupational asthma (178,179). Kennedy and associates (179) reported an across-shift $FEV_1$ response ( $\geq 5\%$ decrease in $FEV_1$) in 23.6% of machinists exposed to machining fluids. The exact ingredient of machining fluids that is responsible for the acute $FEV_1$ changes is not clear, but it appears to be an irritant response. Microbial contamination with endotoxin from gram-negative bacteria or chemical irritants are speculated as potential causes. There have been reports of occupational asthma from some of the individual additives of machining fluids, such as ethanolamine (180).

## CAUSES OF OCCUPATIONAL ASTHMA WITH LATENCY (ALLERGIC-TYPE ASTHMA)

In this review, causes of occupational asthma with latency are classified as animal, vegetable, or chemical.

### Substances of Animal Origin

#### *Laboratory and Other Animal Allergies*

Animal allergy is common and is associated with encountering specific IgE antibodies to the animal allergen (Table 5). Allergy develops in workers such as shepherds, farmers, jockeys, laboratory and research technicians, animal handlers, veterinarians, and grooms, who come in contact with animals, particularly in poorly ventilated areas. Some workers develop allergies to more than one species. Potential allergens include animal hair, urine or saliva proteins, epidermal squamae, mites, small insects, molds, dander, bacteria, and protein dust. Animal hair and dander and epidermal squamae can themselves be the causal agents, but mites and other small insects and molds in the work environment have also been implicated. Low molecular weight urine proteins, an $\alpha_2$-globulin of rats, and a prealbumin of mice are identified as the specific offending agents in these animals.

The prevalence of laboratory animals allergy (LAA) ranges between 11% and 30%. In another survey conducted in a large medical center, 15% of those with regular exposure to laboratory animals had allergic symptoms, mainly persons with previously known allergies, especially to domestic pets (181). Atopy is a risk factor for developing LAA.

Symptoms of LAA generally manifest within a few months of the first exposure; nasal symptoms usually antedate pulmonary ones. However, in a prospective investigation by Newill et al. (182), who studied a group of 178 young adults working with laboratory animals, there were 74% who showed a negative while 30% had a positive methacholine challenge at the time of their entry into the study. Methacholine response was relatively stable during the course of a year in laboratory animal workers who remain at their jobs; the presence of a positive skin test response to laboratory animals or of chest symptoms did not change the pattern of stable responsiveness. Another prospective study conducted by Renstrom and associates (183) investigated the prognostic value of methacholine provocation in LAA. An elevated preemployment total IgE was predictive of developing animal allergy but the level of preemployment bronchial responsiveness or lung function did not predict future sensitization. Workers exposed to laboratory animal allergens are more likely to have

**TABLE 5.** *Substances of animal origin that may cause asthma*

| Agent | Occupation |
|---|---|
| Animals | |
| Laboratory animals (hair, epidermal squamae, mite dander, urine, and serum protein) | Handler of laboratory animal (rats, mice, guinea pigs, rabbits) |
| Domestic animals | Farmers, veterinarians, meat processors and inspectors |
| Animal organ extracts [adrenocorticotropin hormone (ACTH), pituitary peptone powders] | Pharmaceutical worker |
| Wool | Wool worker |
| Birds | |
| Birds (feathers, serum, droppings, egg products) | Bird fancier, poultry breeder or processor, plucker, egg processor |
| Aquatic | |
| Sea squirt fluid | Oyster or pearl gatherer, oyster shucker |
| Prawns | Prawn processor |
| Culture oysters (marine organisms) | Oyster shucker |
| Crabs | Crab processor |
| Hoya | Oyster farmer |
| Pearl shell dust | Pearl shell opener |
| Amebas and other organisms | Printer (from contaminated water) |
| Animal enzymes | |
| Hot trypsin, pancreatic extract, flaviastase, amylase | Medical or pharmaceutical laboratory worker, plastic polymer processor, pharmaceutical worker, enzyme processor worker or messenger, pharmacist |
| *Bacillus subtilis* | Detergent enzyme worker |
| Esperase | Detergent enzyme worker |
| Glue (fish) | Bookbinder, postal worker |
| Human hair | Hairdresser |
| Insects | |
| Beetles *(Coleoptera)* | Zoo curator |
| Grain weevils | Grainery worker, dock worker, millworker |
| Grain storage mites | Farmer, dock worker |
| Locusts | Laboratory worker, schoolchild or teachers |
| Mexican bean weevil | Pea or bean sorter |
| Moths, butterflies | Entomologists |
| Silkworms (larva, hair, silk glue, sericin) | Silkworm cutter |
| Stick insects | Field worker, laboratory worker, student |
| Cockroaches | Laboratory worker, student, field worker |
| Crickets | Outside worker |
| Housefly maggots | Angler |
| River flies | Outdoor worker |
| Sewerworm flies | Outdoor worker |
| Sewage flies | Outdoor worker |

worked with animals in the past; to show positive skin responsiveness to animal allergens; and to demonstrate nonspecific airway hyperresponsiveness, especially those with positive skin-test responses to animal allergen testing.

An active controversy deals with the preemployment placement examination and whether atopy should be used as an exclusionary basis for determining employment or placement. In the preemployment screening of susceptible individuals, two important atopy selection criteria emerge as being important. They are a family history of allergy and positive skin prick reactions against environmental allergens. While a personal history of allergy showed no statistically significant association with developing laboratory animal allergy in this latter investigation, Slovak and Hill (184) report a statistically significant association. Results of skin prick testing depend on what was defined as a positive reaction. Small reactions (≤1 mm) are sensitive (predictive value 60%) but their clinical significance and reliability are open to question. Definitely positive skin reactions (≥3 mm) are not very sensitive and are observed in a third of subjects with developing LAA. In fact, workers developing laboratory animal asthma seem different from those with developing laboratory animal rhinitis; the former more frequently report a history of allergy and more often display positive skin prick reactions to environmental allergens, and a majority show elevated total serum IgE levels. The data seem consistent with a hypothesis that developing laboratory animal asthma is immunologically different from developing laboratory animal rhinitis (185).

#### *Proteolytic Enzymes*

The discovery that the enzymes used in biologic washing powders are asthma-causing sensitizers derives initially from the concern of an occupational medicine physician (67). Proteases (subtilisin or subtilopetidases) obtained from strains of *Bacillus subtilis* exhibit enzyme activity over a wide range of pH and temperature and are ideally suited for incorporation into household cleaning agents. Occupational exposure occurs among workers who handle drums or paper sacks of enzyme, prepare the enzyme, and package the powders. The risk of sensitization is said to occur even with domestic use.

Asthma is associated with positive scratch and intradermal test reactions to the enzyme extract and the presence of IgE antibodies (186). In some series between 40% and 50% of the workers with moderate to heavy exposure to enzyme dust became sensitized. Atopic persons appear more likely to develop asthma or positive skin test reactions to enzyme extract, but symptoms also occur in nonatopic persons and in those who do not have skin test reactivity.

Papain inhalation causes allergic reactions (187). Milne and Brand (188) studied four food technologists occupationally exposed to heavy concentrations of papain dust who developed asthma.

#### *Insects*

Insects such as mushroom fly, aphid, bedbug, locust, bee, cockroach, housefly, daphnia, Mexican bean weevil, moths, butterflies, sewage filter fly, blowfly, honey bee, and larval of silkworm cause occupational asthma (189). Sensitizing materials include scales and hairs that may be rubbed off in flight from the wings or body and become airborne. Occupational exposure to insect emanations occurs in entomologists, beekeepers, laboratory workers, and mushroom workers. In some instances the majority of workers exposed to insect products become sensitized. Workers in power plants along the Mississippi River became sensitized to river flies and developed rhinitis and asthma.

#### *Birds*

Asthma from pigeons, chickens, and budgerigars is observed. Occupational asthma from airborne egg proteins is described. Exposures include raw egg aerosol and dried egg products in the egg-processing industry. An IgE-mediated sensitivity is demonstrated in this group of workers. Bakery workers using an aqueous egg solution as a glaze for meat rolls also experience asthma-like symptoms.

#### *Aquatic and Microscopic Organisms*

Asthma occurs in seasonal workers who crush oyster shells to obtain the meat. Investigations of workers handling clam and shrimp show a prevalence of occupational asthma due to clam of 4% and 2% for shrimp (189a). There is a significant association between immunologic reactivity to both clam and shrimp, as well as to crab and lobster. Asthma due to snow crabs, prawns, and sea squirts is also observed. A 15.6% prevalence of occupational asthma is noted in two snow crab–processing industries (189b). Positive skin tests to crab and, to a lesser degree, smoking history but not atopy are related to the presence of occupational asthma. In another study of crab workers, Hudson et al. (190) examined 31 subjects having occupational asthma due to crab allergen after there was cessation of their exposure at work for mean periods of 24.5 ± 18.7 months. While significant improvement in bronchial responsiveness to histamine is noted, subjects with occupational asthma caused by crab may continue to complain of symptoms and demonstrate persistent airway obstruction and hyperresponsiveness for years after cessation of exposure.

### Substances of Vegetable Origin

Substances of vegetable origin are commonly reported to cause occupational asthma, including sensitization to wood or wood products, cotton, flax, hemp, grain, flour, maiko, mold, castor beans, green coffee beans, garlic, and kapok (Table 6).

### *Wood*

A multitude of wood dusts have been reported to cause asthma, including California redwood, cedar of Lebanon, African zebra wood, iroko, cocabolla, oak, abiruana, *Tanganyika,* central American walnut, Kejaat and Quilla bark, *Balfourodendron riedelianum* (Pau Marfim), palisander wood dust *(Dalbergia nigra)*, ebony, African maple *(Triplochiton scleroxylon)*, Ramin, cabreuva wood dust *(Myrocarpus fastigiatus*), imbuia wood dust, ash wood dust *(Fraxinus americana)*, rimu *(Dacrydium cupressinum)*, *Tanganyika aningre,* obeche *(Triplochiton scleroxylon)*, *Chrysonilia sitophila,* possibly cinnamon, derived from the bark of the *Cinnamomum zeylanicum* tree and contains cinnamic aldehyde, and Western red cedar (191–197).

Localized epidemics of rhinitis and asthma were first reported in 1926 among Japanese carpenters using Western red cedar (198). Occupational asthma due to Western red cedar is likely the most common form of occupational asthma in the Pacific Northwest and affects 4% to 13.5% of the exposed population (75). Siracusa et al. (48) examined predictors for asthma by investigating 619 cedar sawmill, 724 grain elevator, 399 pulp mill, 798 aluminum smelter, and 1,127 unexposed workers who took part in health studies for assessment of chronic respiratory effects of various workplace exposures between 1979 and 1982. The prevalence of asthma after employment in the current industry, as a surrogate for work-related asthma, was 3.9 times higher in cedar sawmill workers, 2.2 times higher in pulp mill and aluminum smelter workers, and 1.7 times higher in grain elevator workers compared with unexposed workers. Within specific work groups, the prevalence of atopy was significantly higher among pulp mill workers with asthma than those without asthma. Conversely, cedar sawmill workers who had asthma tended to be nonatopic and nonsmokers.

Western red cedar differs from other wood in its unusually large component of water-soluble compounds—tannin, dyes, pitch, resins, and lignins (199). Plicatic acid, a major fraction, is a unique component of Western red cedar and has not been identified in any other wood. In provocation tests, plicatic acid produces bronchial reactions similar to that produced by a whole extract and is believed to be the causative agent (200,201). Specific IgE antibodies to plicatic acid-serum human albumin conjugate have been identified in as many as 40% of subjects evaluated (202). Recurrent nocturnal asthma following a single exposure to Western red cedar sawdust has been documented by measurements of peak flow rates in sensitized subjects (22). Bronchial hyperresponsiveness to histamine precede the changes in airway caliber after an antigen challenge and may persist for up to 2 weeks after the challenge. An apparent dose-response effect between total Western red cedar dust level and prevalence of asthma is reported; the prevalence of asthma is higher among workers in jobs with the greatest dust exposure, such as sawyers, packers, chippers, and splitters. Cigarette smokers show a greater change in pulmonary function test values than do nonsmokers.

The mechanism of asthma induced by plicatic acid is not known, as specific IgG antibodies are found only in about 20% of patients (200,203,204). Sera from patients with red cedar asthma fail to passively sensitize human lung fragments of human basophils. Basophils from patients with cedar asthma release histamine when challenged directly with plicatic acid. Bronchial inhalation challenges in red cedar–sensitive persons document that a late asthmatic reaction is associated with a transient increase in bronchial hyperresponsiveness; at the same time, BAL shows an increase of neutrophils followed by appearance of eosinophils, leukotriene $B_4$, and albumin concentration in BAL fluid (98). There are similar proportions of neutrophils, mast cells, lymphocytes, and macrophages in BAL samples taken from red cedar asthma, atopic asthmatics, and nonatopic, nonasthmatic control subjects, but the numbers of eosinophil are elevated in patients with cedar asthma, as well as in atopic asthmatic subjects (98,104). There are no major histologic differences between atopic asthma and red cedar asthma. Bronchial mucosal biopsies reveal that both cedar asthma and atopic asthmatics show increased numbers of T cells and activated eosinophils in the bronchial mucosa. Besides eosinophilia, BAL fluid during a late asthmatic reaction is characterized by the presence of sloughing of bronchial epithelial cells and an increase in degenerated epithelial cells and alveolar macrophages (98). There is an increase in vascular permeability as reflected by an increase in albumin in the lavage fluid.

The outcome and prognosis of Western red cedar asthma has been explored (205). Survival analysis of subjects with occupational asthma due to various agents was performed. Almost 40% of subjects with asthma due to Western red cedar or isocyanates subjects become symptomatic within 1 year of exposure. After 5 years of exposure, the rate of sensitization becomes slower for subjects with Western red cedar and isocyanate asthma as compared with asthma from high molecular weight agents. Having a nonimmediate reaction at the time of specific inhalation challenges, being continuously exposed, and being younger slightly increase the risk at each time point on the curve of developing asthma. These data suggest that the natural history for onset of occupational asthma is different depending on the sensitizing agent. Factors such as age, type of exposure, and pattern of reaction on exposure to the agent also modulate the rate of development of this condition. The severity of asthma is not the main determinant of working status. Socioeconomic factors appear important in determining the working status of subjects with red cedar asthma. Subjects who continue to work, although sensitized to red cedar, tend to be younger and have a larger number of dependents than do

**TABLE 6.** *Substances of vegetable origin that may cause asthma*

| Agent | Occupation |
|---|---|
| Plants | |
| Flour, grain dust | Grain elevator worker, baker, miller, grain worker |
| Wheat flour | Baker |
| Rye flour | Baker |
| Buckwheat | Baker |
| Wheat gluten derivative | Baker |
| Hops | Brewery worker, farmer |
| Soybean flour and dust | Soybean processor |
| Garlic powder | Spice factory worker |
| Tamarind seeds | Miller |
| Tea fluff | Tea maker, sifter, packer |
| Green leaf tobacco | Tobacco worker or processor |
| Green leaf tea | Tea worker |
| Green and masted coffee beans | Coffee worker |
| Castor beans | Farmer, miller, chemist, bagger |
| Maiko | Japanese food worker, miller |
| Cottonseed | Baker, fertilizer worker |
| Linseed | Oil extractor |
| Flaxseed | Flax worker |
| Psyllium seed | Pharmaceutical worker |
| *Lycopodium clavatus* | Dentist |
| Gum acacia | Printer |
| Gum tragacanth | Printer, candy and gum worker |
| Strawberry pollen | Strawberry grower |
| Potatoes | Housewife |
| Wood | |
| Western red cedar | Woodworker, carpenter |
| African zebrawood | Joiner |
| Cedar of Lebanon | Shuttle marker |
| South African boxwood | Pattern maker |
| Oak | Wood finisher |
| Mahogany | Wood machinist |
| Mansonia | Sawmill worker, carpenter, wood finisher |
| Abiruana | Sawmill worker, carpenter, wood finisher |
| Cocaballa | Sawmill worker, carpenter, wood finisher |
| Kejaat | Sawmill worker, carpenter, wood finisher |
| California redwood | Sawmill worker, carpenter, wood finisher |
| Ramin | Sawmill worker, carpenter, wood finisher |
| Quillaja bark | Manufacturer of saponin |
| Iroko | Sawmill worker |
| Mulberry | Sawmill worker |
| Latex | Operating room nurse |
| Plant enzymes | |
| Papain | Food technologist |
| Diastase | Food handler |
| Pectinase | Pharmaceutical worker |
| Bromelain | Pharmaceutical worker |
| Vegetable gums | |
| Karaya | Food processor |
| Arabic | Printer |
| Acacia | Printer |
| Tragacanth | Printer |
| Fungi, molds | |
| *Alternaria* and *Aspergillus* | Baker |
| Spores of *Cladosporium, Verticillium,* and *Paecilomyces* | Farm worker |
| *Merulius lacrymans* | Domestic worker, paprika splitter |
| Pink rot fungus | Celery picker |
| Mushroom molds | Mushroom worker |
| Molds | Mortician |
| Fungal amylase | Enzyme processor |

the subjects who are not working at the time of the follow-up examination.

### *Flour and Grains*

Besides asthma, studies of workers exposed to cereal grain dusts show an increased prevalence of other types of respiratory disease (206). Exposure to grain dust in lifelong-nonsmoking grain workers is associated with an increased prevalence of chronic bronchitis and evidence of airflow obstruction (207). Airway hyperresponsiveness is described in grain workers (206). In a study of 610 workers in five grain elevators in British Columbia, an additive, but not potentiating, effect is demonstrated for smoking and exposure to grain dust (208). Nonspecific irritation is considerably more common than sensitization as the cause of work-related asthmatic symptoms in flour milling, baking, and other flour-based industries (37).

The magnitude of the dust exposure levels in a modern British bakery was described by Musk and associates (54). Total dust measurements are elevated in the production area, especially in the ingredients, preparation, and manufacturing areas. Levels are as high as 37.6 mg/m$^3$ among staff attending ovens, 16.8 mg/m$^3$ for bakery cleaning staff, 14.1 mg/m$^3$ for doughnut makers, and 12.0 mg/m$^3$ among staff preparing ingredients in confectionery bakery. A positive relationship between greater methacholine sensitivity (reduced $PC_{20}$) and higher dust levels was identified. Sodium dodecyl sulfate–polyacrylamide gel electrophoresis (SDS-PAGE) shows different flours contain proteins of molecular weight similar to those present in air sample eluates. Assays identify airborne proteins from several flours with a detection limit of 1 μg/ml$^{-1}$.

Flour and grains cause allergy and asthma, especially among millers, bakers, farm workers (37,48,209). Among millers and bakers, the prevalence of asthma ranges from 2.1% in a study from the Netherlands to 30% in Yugoslavia; other studies indicate rates of sensitization as high as 50% (37,48,206,209,210). Outbreaks of asthma occur in people exposed to a prevailing wind carrying grain dust from neighboring mills. A similar type of asthma epidemic is described for soybean dust (211).

The specific antigen responsible for wheat allergy is elusive but may be a component of the wheat parasitic fungi such as smut or rust, saprophytes such as *Aspergillus,* organisms such as wheat weevil and mite, gram-negative bacteria, or additives such as α- and β-amylase and soybean-lecithin (209,212–214). An atopic predisposition increases the risk for sensitization. *Aspergillus*-derived enzymes used as flour additives can elicit IgE-mediated respiratory allergy. The most important source of exposure to fungal amylase is the debagging, sieving, weighing, and mixing of bread improvers (37). The fungal amylase functions as sole causative allergen or as an addition with other allergens used in the baking industry (212).

There are observations of bakers with asthma who do not exhibit sensitization to common flour antigens even though they develop complaints when in contact to flour. The report by Baur and colleagues (215) points out the importance of testing for other baking additives. The study on 216 symptomatic persons employed in the bakery industry identifies sensitization to various additives and enzymes, including α-amylase, hemicellulase, and glucoamylase; papain; *B. subtilis* protease; and soybean flour. Alkaline hydrolysis of wheat gluten derivative that is incorporated into marshmallows causes occupational asthma (216). The study emphasizes the principle of reactivity generated by alteration of a food component because the subject's asthma was due not to gluten but to the modified gluten produced by the hydrolysis treatment; the treatment causes loss of antigenic reactivity and development of novel epitopes. Asthma was induced by occupational exposure to egg used to spray cakes before baking (216a). A chocolate-candy worker was diagnosed as having occupational asthma and rhinoconjunctivitis (216b). Positive conjunctival and bronchial challenge tests with lactalbumin show that this protein is the pathogenetic agent. A case of occupational asthma due to barley grain dust, species *Hordeum vulgare L,* was reported in a 32-year-old storeman of a trading company's department that deals with packaging of flour, barley, and peanuts (216c).

Storage mite is the ordinary name for a variety of non-pyroglyphid mites of the genera *Acarus, Lepidoglyphus, Tyrophagus,* and *Glycyphagus.* These four genera are often encountered in ecological studies of hay, straw, grain, and other vegetable products. Occasionally, storage mites live in ordinary house dust, especially damp houses. Storage mites growth is dependent on humidity, and they are found in grain grown in the United Kingdom but not in imported grain. Allergy to storage mites is reported to cause asthma and rhinitis among farmers, grain elevator operators, and bakers (217). Another investigation conducted by Revsbech and Dueholm (218) on 23 bakers documents that almost all the bakers with IgE sensitivity to flour show similar IgE-related sensitivity to storage mites. The investigators hypothesized that a baker who develops allergy to flour (gluten, whole wheat, and rye) will be more prone to develop IgE sensitivity to storage mites. The data are interpreted as indicating that storage mite allergy may be more prevalent among bakers with flour allergy than previously believed, and that storage mite allergy without flour allergy is probably rare.

The prognosis for sensitized bakers varies. Often asthma is sufficiently mild to allow workers to continue working. In almost 50%, symptoms improve, or even disappear, with continued work exposure, which suggests that spontaneous desensitization may occur. Treatment with medication such as disodium cromoglycate controls symptoms in the workplace. Preemployment screening of persons considering working as bakers or with grain products is useful and allows for counseling. The presence of asthma, or of another allergic disease in a severe form, is suggested as a criterion for excluding persons from training as bakers. There is a case of baker's asthma with a fatal outcome (219).

### *Latex and Rubber*

Immunoglobulin E-mediated sensitization to protein allergens of natural rubber latex induces immediate hypersensitivity reactions ranging from mild urticaria to life-threatening anaphylaxis after cutaneous, mucosal, or visceral exposure (220). Asthma is a frequent manifestation of natural rubber latex allergy among workers manufacturing natural rubber latex materials and among health care providers using natural rubber latex products. Elutable allergens from natural rubber latex gloves absorb to the cornstarch powder particles, become airborne, and have the potential to cause respiratory reactions. The prevalence of occupational asthma due to latex gloves among health care workers is found to be 2.5% of hospital employees (42). A survey of 81 workers in a surgical glove-manufacturing plant revealed that 6% of the workers show findings consistent with occupational asthma (221). A case has been described of occupational asthma caused by indirect exposure to airborne latex allergens in an administrative hospital employee who never used latex gloves (222).

Latex hypersensitivity with anaphylactoid-type reaction has been examined by a number of investigators (42, 221–226). A study on the use of hypoallergenic gloves concludes they may be an effective alternative method of reducing the risk of asthmatic reactions in health care workers with latex-induced asthma when complete avoidance cannot be achieved. Skin prick tests and RAST confirm the presence of specific IgE to latex in most patients.

Gum acacia and tragacanth, used in the past in the printing industry and gum manufacturing, causes occupational asthma. Malo et al. (47) surveyed the employees of a carpet-manufacturing plant in which guar gum was used to adhere the dye to the fiber.

## Leafy Plants, Vegetables, and Fruits

Allergies to vegetables and fruits occur (227–230). Two atopic housewives developed asthma attacks while peeling white potatoes (231). Tea dust causes asthma in some workers (229,230). Exposure to *Limonium tataricum* as dried flowers, and used for semipermanent floral arrangements, causes asthma in a floral industry worker. Blanco et al. (232) report a case of occupational asthma and rhinoconjunctivitis caused by *Phoenix canariensis* pollen; the pollen originated from the canary palm, a type of palm tree, belonging to the Arecaceae family and that is widely distributed in frost-free regions as an ornamental tree. An atopic gift-shop owner developed daily asthmatic attacks when he began working with the dried plant, baby's breath *(Gypsophilia panniculata)*. In another case report, an atopic woman developed asthma after inhaling the vapor from boiling Swiss chard (227). Subiza et al. (233) report a patient who developed asthma after exposure to *Pfaffia paniculata* root powder used in the manufacturing of Brazil ginseng capsules. A worker in a beet sugar processing plant developed asthma after exposure to moldy sugar beet pulp (234).

### *Spices*

Various spices have been shown to cause asthma (235,236) and anaphylaxis. A 27-year-old man developed rhinitis and asthma symptoms 1 year after starting to prepare a certain kind of sausage (235). He showed positive immediate skin prick tests for paprika (dry powder of *Capsicum annuum*), coriander *(Coriandrum sativum)*, and mace (shell of nutmeg, *Myristica fragrans*) as well as serum-specific IgE antibodies to paprika, coriander, and mace as demonstrated by enzyme-linked immunosorbent assay (ELISA). Specific bronchial inhalation challenges showed an immediate asthmatic reaction to extracts from paprika, coriander, and mace, with no late asthmatic reactions noted. Positive skin prick test results to various spices, such as curry, coriander, and mace, and RAST as well as specific IgE antibodies for coriander, curry, mace, ginger, and paprika powder were reported. Repeated exposure to garlic dust induced severe asthma in an atopic patient (236). Subsequently, the patient also developed marked adverse responses after ingestion of garlic. Results of an inhalation and a controlled oral challenge test to garlic dust were both positive.

## Substances of Chemical Origin

A variety of chemicals both simple and complex, such as chloramine, ethylenediamine, paraphenylenediamine, formaldehyde, sulfathiazole, tannic acid, aliphatic polyamines, sulfonechloramides, amprolium hydrochloride, polyglycine acid chloride, diazonium salts; metals, such as chromium, vanadium, platinum; heated freon; furan-based binder; and other substances including spiramycin, phenylglycerine, phthalic anhydride (also trimellitic, himic, tetrachlorophthalic, and hexahydrophthalic anhydride), epoxy resins, soldering fluxes, and isocyanates are associated with occupational asthma (Table 7).

### *Isocyanates*

Isocyanates are used in the manufacture of plastics, foam surface coating, elastomers, adhesives, fibers, and in the production of polyurethane foam (237). NIOSH estimated that between 50,000 and 100,000 workers in the United States are exposed to diisocyanates. Perhaps 5% develop adverse respiratory responses. The four most common isocyanates are toluene diisocyanate (TDI), diphenylmethane diisocyanate (MDI), hexameth-

**TABLE 7.** *Substances of chemical origin that may cause asthma*

| Agent | Occupation |
|---|---|
| Metallic salts | |
| Platinum | Platinum refiner, chemist |
| Nickel | Plater, chemical engineer |
| Aluminum (or fumes) | Chemical worker, pot-room worker |
| Vanadium | Boiler and gas turbine cleaner, mineral ore processor |
| Cobalt | Refinery and alloy worker, diamond cutter |
| Stainless steel | Welder |
| Chromium | Chrome polisher, chemical worker, cement tanning worker |
| Tungsten carbide | Hard metals grinder |
| Vanadium | Metal grinder |
| Chemicals | |
| Alkyl cyanoacrylate | Hobbies, home repair |
| Paraphenylenediamine | Fur dyer, chemical worker |
| Piperazine | Chemical process worker |
| Formaldehyde | Nurse, pathologist, laboratory worker |
| Phenol | Chemical worker, laboratory worker |
| Chloramine | Brewery worker |
| Hexachlorophene | Hospital worker |
| Sulfathiazole | Manufacturer |
| Sulfonechloramide | Manufacturer |
| Tannic acid | Sunburn spray user |
| Orris root derivatives | Cosmetic worker, hairdresser |
| Triethyltetramine | Manufacturer of aircraft filters |
| Dimethyl ethanolamine | Spray painter |
| Aminoethanolamine | Aluminum solderer |
| Ethylenediamine | Rubber, shellac manufacturer, photographer |
| Pyrethrins | Fumigator |
| Diisocyanates | Chemical worker, polyurethane foam manufacturer |
| Phthalic anhydrides, trimellitic anhydride | Chemical worker, epoxy resin worker, tool setter, paint manufacturer |
| Ammonium thioglycate | Beauty operator, cosmetic manufacturer |
| Azodicarbonamide | Rubber worker |
| Dioazonium salt | Photocopier |
| Colophony | Electronic manufacturer |
| Resin binder systems | Foundry moldmaker (MDI, furan-based resins) |
| Reactive dyes | Dye weigher |
| Persulfate salts, extract of henna | Hairdresser, chemical worker |
| Reactive dyes | Textile dyer |
| Paraphenylene diamine | Fur dyer |
| Pharmaceuticals | |
| Psyllium | Laxative maker, nurse |
| Amprodium hydrochloride | Poultry feed mixer |
| Penicillin | Pharmaceutical worker |
| Pesticides, insecticides | Manufacturer, farmer, fumigator |
| Tylosin | Pharmaceutical worker |
| Hydrazine | Pharmaceutical worker |
| Spiramycin | Pharmaceutical worker |
| Phenylglycine acid chloride | Pharmaceutical worker |
| Cephalosporins | Pharmaceutical worker |
| Methyl dopa | Pharmaceutical worker |
| Salbutamol intermediate | Pharmaceutical worker |
| Tetracycline | Pharmaceutical worker |
| Sulfone chloramides | Brewery worker |

ylene diisocyanate (HDI), and naphthalene diisocyanate (NDI). HDI and TDI, which have about the same vapor pressure, are relatively volatile at room temperature; MDI, with a relatively lower vapor pressure is not. MDI becomes more volatile and dangerous when it is heated, as in foundry work. Spray painting is a particularly dangerous form of exposure, since vapors (HDI, TDI) and particulates (MDI) are airborne and may be present in high concentrations. Auto body spray painting carries a high risk of occupational asthma and hypersensitivity pneumonias, because of the great potential for exposure to high levels of isocyanates, especially HDI.

### *Acid Anhydrides*

The major commercial acid anhydrides include phthalic anhydride (PA), hexahydrophthalic anhydride (HHPA), himic anhydride (HA), tetrachlorophthalic anhydride (TCPA), trimellitic anhydride (TMA), maleic anhydride (MA), and methyltetrahydrophthalic anhydride (MTHPA). There is cross-immunoreactivity among the various anhydrides (238). Development of immunologically mediated disease depends on the exposure level of the anhydride. A variety of immunologic and nonimmunologic responses are described for the anhydrides (14,60,238–244).

Phthalic anhydride and other anhydrides produce IgE-mediated asthma (245). MA causes a hemolytic anemia syndrome (246). PA has been incriminated as a cause for meat-wrapper's asthma. A case of RADS has been reported for an exposure to high levels of gaseous PA. Nasal rhinitis, nasal mucosal erosion, and epistaxis have been reported for workers exposed to high levels of HHPA. A new acid anhydride, pyromellitic dianhydride (PMDA), behaves as a respiratory irritant and causes immediate-type sensitization (239).

Trimellitic anhydride induces a number of clinical syndromes including an irritant reaction, a late respiratory systemic syndrome, immediate rhinitis and asthma, and pulmonary disease—anemia syndrome. Total TMA antibody levels do not discriminate symptomatic workers from asymptomatic workers. *In vitro* TMA reacts rapidly with protein to form a TMA-protein complex that is used to evaluate various classes of antibodies using radioimmunoassay techniques. Exposure to TMA powder, which occurs in TMA production, causes IgE-mediated asthma in some workers and allergic alveolitis in others (60,247). In a retrospective comparison of two worker cohorts having elevated total antibody against TMA conjugated to human serum albumin, no statistically significant differences in levels of IgG subclass between 19 workers with and 12 workers without TMA-induced immunologic lung disease was observed (247). An extensive and more serious infiltrative pulmonary process with anemia occurs after exposure to TMA fumes without exposure to the dust. This pulmonary disease–anemia syndrome that follows inhalation of TMA fumes consists of cough, hemoptysis, dyspnea, pulmonary infiltrates, a restrictive lung defect, hypoxemia, and anemia. Workers with TMA pulmonary disease–anemia syndrome show no differences in antibody concentrations than workers with other types of TMA-immune lung disease. The pathogenesis of the pulmonary disease–anemia syndrome appears to be a complex interaction between the chemical toxicity of TMA fumes, immune reaction against TMA-haptenized proteins by cells of the respiratory tract, and the degree of exposure to TMA fumes.

Workers with late asthma, late respiratory systemic syndrome, or both, or with late respiratory systemic syndrome and asthma rhinitis report improvement in their symptoms, show better pulmonary functions, and display lower total antibody against TM-HSA. Although TMA workers with late asthma or late respiratory systemic syndrome improve when moved to lower-exposure jobs, only about half of the workers with asthma rhinitis improve; elevated IgE against TM-HSA appears to be a marker for a subpopulation of workers with asthma rhinitis that do not improve after removal from exposure.

### *Colophony*

Pulmonary disease from colophony has been reported (14,46,248,249). Colophony (rosin) is a widespread natural product obtained from species of the pine family Pinaceae (249). One of the most important uses of unmodified rosin is in electronic solder fluxes. The main areas of use of chemically modified rosin are paper sizing, adhesives, paints, varnishes, printing inks, and plasticizers. The flux containing colophony, when heated, exposes workers to colophony fumes. Colophony is well recognized as a skin sensitizer and is also the third highest cause of occupational asthma. It also has irritant properties. The specific allergens involved in occupational asthma have not been identified.

In an early paper by Burge et al. (46), the prevalence of colophony-induced asthma among factory employees manufacturing flux-cored solder was 21% for the high-exposure groups (1.92 mg/m$^3$) and 4% for a lower-exposure group (less than 0.01 mg/m$^3$). Burge et al. stated that the threshold limit value for colophony should be based on the resin acid content of the fume, and not the aldehyde content. They popularized the use of serial peak expiratory flow rate (PEFR) for detecting occupational asthma. They showed the value of this type of testing while conducting their studies on colophony-related asthma. They showed that PEFR records correlated with bronchial provocation testing and provided a suitable alternative to bronchoprovocation testing for the diagnosis of occupational asthma (250).

### *Acrylates*

There are several reports dealing with sensitization to acrylates including methyl methacrylate (250), polyfunctional aziridine hardener (251), and instant glues containing cyanoacrylate esters (252). The cyanoacrylate ester-based glues are used extensively in home repairs and hobbies. Local application of instant glue by catheter injection has been used medically to treat intracerebral berry aneurysms, providing an alternative to surgery. The cyanoacrylate ester possesses irritant properties and has been shown to cause allergic reactions and asthma (252,253). Kopp and co-workers (252), the first to report on their sensitizing properties, reported on a 32-year-old atopic patient with asthma who used Super Glue for building radio-controlled model planes. Bronchial provocation with glue vapors in a manner that simulated his home exposure resulted in a late-phase asthmatic response, with rhinorrhea and lacrimation. An increase in airway hyperresponsiveness to methacholine occurred after the bronchial challenge and persisted for several weeks. Complete resolution of asthma symptoms and reversion to a negative response to methacholine challenge occurred after 6 months of continued avoidance of the glue.

### *Persulfate Salts/Senna*

Persulfate salts are common constituents of hair bleaches and have occasionally caused occupational asthma in hairdressers and other exposed persons (254–256). Blainey et al. (254) identified four of 23 workers employed in a hairdressing salon who developed occupational asthma from the persulfate salts contained in hair bleaches. Early- and late-type asthmatic reactions may occur with persulfate salts (256). Merget et al. (255) conducted a cross-sectional study of 33 employees at a persulfate-producing chemical plant and measured workplace concentrations of ammonium and sodium persulfate. Levels within the bagging plant were below 1 $mg/m^3$; the maximal concentrations found were 1.4 and 3.6 $mg/m^3$. It appears that workplace concentration of ammonium and sodium persulfate of about 1 $mg/m^3$ is not associated with a risk of occupational asthma (255).

Senna also causes occupational asthma (257,258). A 21-year-old male atopic factory worker developed IgE-mediated asthma and rhinoconjunctivitis 5 months after exposure to senna while working for a company manufacturing hair dyes (257). The bronchial challenge test, skin prick test to senna and RAST with senna were positive. The patient became symptom-free after he had changed his job within the company.

### *Reactive Dyes*

Reactive dyes were introduced in 1956 and rapidly became popular for the dyeing of cotton textiles. The advantage of the dyes are lower dyeing temperature and better color fastness in the final product. Because they are highly reactive chemicals, they have the potential to cause sensitization and production of specific IgG and IgE antibodies (259,260). IgE-mediated occupational asthma occurs from exposures to the reactive dyes. More reactions are noted for the yellow, orange, and red dye conjugates than for the blue and brown dyes. Hong and Park (261) studied RAST and RAST inhibition tests to Black GR, the most frequent sensitizer among several reactive dyes. The results suggested that the IgE response to black GR-HSA conjugates were heterogeneous, and cross-reactivity between two reactive dyes differs from one patient to another. The prevalence of specific IgE antibodies in the neighboring factories was higher than in the reactive dye factory. The prevalence of specific IgG was highest in the reactive dye factory, and those of the neighboring factories were markedly lower. The results suggested that IgE-mediated sensitization to reactive dye could occur in employees who were working in neighboring factories. The prevalence of reactive dye-specific IgG antibody can be used as an indirect method of assessing the exposure of workers to reactive dye. A survey conducted at 15 textile plants with dye houses in western Sweden showed IgE-mediated allergy to reactive dyes as being an important cause of respiratory and nasal symptoms among employees (260).

### *Ethanolamine*

Amino alcohols are used in various industries, often as minor constituents of compounds to modify the properties of the compound. Generally, they are considered to be safe, but they have been known to cause local skin irritation at higher concentrations in solutions. Savonius et al. (180) reported on three cases of occupational asthma caused by ethanolamines: two metal workers exposed to a cutting fluid containing triethanolamine, and one cleaner exposed to a detergent containing monoethanolamine. Persistence of the symptoms after exposure ended was a common feature of the three cases. Kennedy et al. (179) reported an acute fall in $FEV_1$ in workers exposed to machining fluids containing ethanolamine.

## Metals

### *Chromium/Welding*

Chromium is a potent sensitizer used in the manufacture of pigments and in tanning and is reported to cause bronchial asthma (262). The hexavalent compound is the most active one chemically and the most widely encountered in occupational health problems. Asthma is reported not only for stainless steel but also mild steel welding (263). The incidence of welding-associated asthma is 5% for stainless steel and 7% for mild steel welders per 1,000 welding–years (263).

### *Aluminum*

The problem with the pot-room environment is well illustrated by a case reported by Desjardins et al. (264). In this example, a 35-year-old male lifelong nonsmoker, with no history of asthma or atopy, was hired by an aluminum plant that began its operation in 1986. Preemployment screening, consisting of spirometry and a chest radiograph, was normal. During his 12-hour shifts, he replaced 10 to 20 anodes (prebake type) and spent about 5 minutes each time adjacent to open pots releasing hot fumes. The patient eventually experienced episodes of cough and dyspnea, which resolved during withdrawal from work in January and December 1991. He resumed work in the pot rooms in March 1992 and his dyspnea recurred at work and at night. There was a 25% drop in PEFR associated with mild-to-moderate nonspecific bronchial hyperresponsiveness. An assessment of the bronchial response to the occupational exposure in pot rooms was carried out in November 1992 and revealed a dual asthmatic response; there was a parallel drop in methacholine $PC_{20}$. A similar pattern was seen again during repeat workplace challenges performed 3 weeks later. Spirometry obtained on control days was stable.

Pot-room workers and aluminum smelter workers can develop occupational asthma (48,59,89,264–269). An irritant response from high-level exposure of pot-room fumes is believed to be the likely cause of the observed immediate bronchospastic response, while a late reaction probably is probably immune mediated. The late response characteristically develops 4 to 12 hours after exposure and may affect workers during the night while they are at home. Dual responses are also reported. Sometimes removal from exposure improves respiratory symptoms and reduces the degree of methacholine reactivity (269).

There is evidence of persistent nonspecific airway hyperresponsiveness in affected workers (268). A nested, case-control study, carried out in two Dutch aluminum producing plants, revealed that workers without respiratory symptoms and with normal lung function and normal bronchial responsiveness before employment can develop pot-room asthma (266).

The etiology of pot-room asthma is unclear (48,59,89). One recurrent theory about pathogenesis is that asthma in aluminum pot-room workers is related to plasma levels of fluoride. There is a positive association between bronchial responsiveness and plasma fluoride levels (59); an increase in the plasma fluoride level of 10 ng/ml is associated with an increase in the dose-response slope by a factor of 1.11. Plasma fluoride levels are found to be associated with the total atmospheric fluoride concentration in $mg/m^3$ but not with total particulates in the environment. A significant dose-response relationship between current fluoride exposure and work-related asthmatic symptoms has been observed

### *Platinum*

Allergic sensitization to platinum salts results in both upper and lower respiratory tract symptoms, a syndrome formerly referred to as platinosis (5,14,16,66). The allergic potential of platinum salts is so great that in some studies as many as 60% to 100% of exposed persons developed allergy. For most cases of platinum salt asthma, sensitization develops within 6 to 7 months. However, allergy may occur as quickly as 10 days or may not appear until after 25 years' employment. Persistence of asthma, elevated levels of IgE, and hyperresponsive airways are reported in workers who are not exposed for several years (72). Cigarette smoking places the worker at an increase risk for developing sensitization to platinum salts (72,270). While asthma is reported in workers exposed to the halide salts of platinum in the platinum refinery industry, the prevalence of asthma in this industry is reported to be decreasing in the United Kingdom because of a policy of removing employees from exposure once a positive platinum skin reaction is identified by surveillance testing.

Asthmatic reactions from platinum salts may be immediate, late, or dual in type; late asthmatic reactions are inhibited by cromolyn sodium. Skin prick tests with low concentrations of chloroplatinates give immediate positive reactions; RAST testing shows increased IgE antibodies to platinum chloride complexes among sensitized workers (271). Other studies confirm the presence of heat-stable, short-term sensitizing antibodies, presumably short-term sensitizing–IgE antibodies to platinum salts. Merget et al. (272) reported that there was no significant correlation between methacholine responsiveness and bronchial responsiveness to platinum salt. However, the platinum salt skin prick test correlated with bronchial response to platinum salt.

In an investigation of 107 current and 29 terminated platinum refinery workers, cold-air challenges were employed to identify the nonspecific bronchial hyperresponsiveness, and platinum skin testing was provided to document allergy to the salts (72). The cold-air challenge testing was positive in 11% of the current workers and 31% of the terminated ones. More than a third of the current workers with positive cold-air responses and half of the terminated employees with positive cold-air responses had positive skin reactions to platinum salt. In a follow-up investigation, three persons who initially show a positive cold-air challenge and negative platinum skin tests are found to convert their platinum skin test reaction 1 year later in the absence of further exposure. This finding suggested that in some cases, nonspecific bronchial reactivity may antedate immune manifestations. This observation suggests the importance of a surveillance program for certain allergens that includes preemployment and serial testing for nonspecific bronchial responsiveness.

While it is generally believed that asthma resolves in platinum refinery workers who cease exposure, the investigation of Brooks et al. (72) document persistence of asthma an average of 5 years after workers leave the industry. Persistence of asthma following cessation of exposure is also documented by Merget et al. (273,274). While bronchial responsiveness to methacholine, $FEV_1$ values, skin test reactivity to platinum salts, and bronchial responsiveness to platinum salt may not change after cessation of exposure, a reduction in total serum IgE is observed. Merget et al. also reported that neither histamine release from basophils with chloroplatinate salt nor RAST measuring specific IgE to the chloroplatinate salt are helpful in the diagnosis of platinum salt asthma. Work-related symptoms develop within 4 months (median) after the onset of exposure and is associated with a positive skin test to chloroplatinate salt. Histamine release with chloroplatinate salt is found in all groups, including asymptomatic workers and controls; it is highest in atopic controls. Histamine release with chloroplatinate salt and histamine release with anti-IgE show an excellent correlation, suggesting a similar release mechanism of chloroplatinate salt and anti-IgE. In skin-test positive subjects, high cutaneous chloroplatinate salt sensitivity is linked to high histamine release with chloroplatinate salt or anti-IgE, supporting the concept of a role of cell surface IgE or IgE-Fc-receptor in the release process with platinum salts. However, high specificity of cutaneous reactions contrasts with the low specificity of in vitro tests with chloroplatinate salt.

#### *Nickel Sulfate*

Nickel sulfate is reported to cause asthma in nonatopic workers involved in nickel plating (275,276). Occupational asthma from nickel sensitivity was confirmed in a male worker by allergy skin tests and inhalational challenge (275). A 28-year-old man developed asthma shortly after being exposed to nickel sulfate in a metal-plating factory. In another study, a worker with occupational exposure to nickel developed asthma a few months after starting work. Inhalation challenge with nickel sulfate induced a late asthmatic reaction, starting 3 hours after the exposure and leading to a severe nocturnal attack. A worker developed asthma after plating with nickel and chromium but not other metals. He developed acute asthma to chromium sulfate and a biphasic asthma-like response to nickel sulfate. Radioimmunoassays incorporating the challenge materials revealed specific IgE antibodies to the nickel sulfate and chromium sulfate but not to another metal, gold, which he can tolerate.

#### *Cobalt*

Hard metal is an alloy of tungsten carbide (80% to 95%) with cobalt (5% to 20%) as a matrix. Sometimes other metals, such as titanium, tantalum, vanadium, nickel, and chromium, are added in the carbide form. Workers exposed to hard metal dusts may develop a spectrum of pulmonary diseases: (a) There are irritation effects that may be mild and transient or severe enough to cause noncardiac pulmonary edema and adult respiratory distress syndrome. The irritant effect is dose-dependent and occurs in all subjects exposed to sufficiently high atmospheric concentrations. (b) Occupational asthma may develop and is related to an IgE mechanism; there is a positive RAST for specific IgE to cobalt (277,278). Cell-mediated immunity may also be involved. Asthma may be reversible but can persist after stopping the exposure. Asthma occurs in a relatively low percentage of exposed subjects. (c) There is a form of alveolitis, either lymphocytic alveolitis with inverted helper/suppressor ratio, or giant cell alveolitis [the pathognomonic, giant cell interstitial pneumonia (GIP)], with or without interstitial fibrotic changes. Sometimes alveolitis and asthma appear together (279). (d) There may be an interstitial fibrosis, associated with or without an alveolitis component. Exposure levels to cobalt may be relatively low and still cause disease. Sprince and associates (280) surveyed 1,039 tungsten carbide production workers. About 11% reported wheezing, and workers exposed to more than 50 μg/m$^3$ were 2.1 times more likely to have work-related wheezing.

### Pharmaceuticals

#### *Ispaghula or Psyllium*

The husks and seed of *Pantago ovato,* also known as ispaghula or psyllium, are hydrophilic and capable of absorbing as much as 40 times their own weight in water. Because of this property, they form a mucilaginous material that is an effective bulk laxative. Inhalation of dusts from pharmaceutical preparations manufactured from husks caused IgE-mediated allergic respiratory tract symptoms in exposed workers such as nurses, process workers, and home users (281,282). In the Nelson's (281) study, 18% of the subjects reported allergic reactions and 5% described dyspnea, wheezing, or hives within 30 minutes of preparing the laxative. A cross-sectional study of 125 pharmaceutical workers engaged in the manufacture of bulk laxatives based on ispaghula husks (e.g., psyllium) and senna pods was conducted (258). Skin prick tests with extracts of these components revealed that 7.6% were allergic to ispaghula and 15.3% were allergic to senna. There were four (3.2%) cases of occupational asthma.

#### *Antibiotics*

Tylosin, a macrolide antibiotic, is widely used as an animal health and growth agent, and may cause occupational asthma in pharmaceutical workers (283). Cases of bronchial asthma due to spiramycin and adipic acid occurred in workers of a pharmaceutical factory. Piperacillin sodium is reported to cause occupational asthma (284). A mechanic working in the antibiotic capsuling section of a pharmaceutical company developed occupational asthmatic from tetracycline. Other causes of occupational asthma described in the pharmaceutical industry include guar gum, salbutamol processing, bromelain, hen egg white-derived lysozyme, *Papaver somniferum* extract used to manufacture morphine and other alkaloids, hydrazine, and ginseng (285).

## PROGNOSIS AND NATURAL HISTORY

The most important aggravating factor for occupational asthma is continued exposure to an allergen to which the person is sensitized; the induced asthmatic attack, especially if associated with a late-asthmatic response, increases airway inflammation and the degree of nonspecific bronchial hyperresponsiveness (286,287). In contrast, irritant and physical triggers, such as exercise, cold air, irritant gases, weather changes, and extreme emotional expression, activate an exaggerated bronchoconstrictor response; they do not induce significant airway inflammation nor promote nonspecific bronchial responsiveness. The irritant and physical triggers do not cause asthma attacks, but lead to exacerbation of asthma that is present. Causal factors and triggers vary from person to person and from time to time.

Persistence of asthma symptoms after termination of exposure is common and may occur in 50% to 90% of cases. It is best documented for isocyanates and Western red cedar asthma, but also for other agents. The persistence of asthmatic manifestations is due mainly to continued nonspecific airway hyperresponsiveness. Repeated allergen exposure in a sensitized individual may explain the apparent irreversible airways obstructive disease and persistent airway hyperresponsiveness noted in some workers who are no longer working. Cessation of exposure to the inciting antigen, such as diisocyanates, is associated with improvement in airway inflammation and reduction in subepithelial fibrosis (288,289). Despite the removal from TDI exposure, occupational asthma can lead to permanent disability with significant socioeconomic consequences.

Following termination of an exposure, clinical improvement in asthma occurs concurrent with reduction in nonspecific airways hyperreactivity (290). Pronounced airway hyperresponsiveness (as determined by methacholine/histamine challenge testing) is not the sole indicator for confirming the severity of the asthma. In some cases, the degree of bronchial reactivity decreases after removal from exposure and then increases again after reexposure to Western red cedar, California redwood, grain dust, or isocyanates (290).

The determinants of a more unfavorable prognosis of occupational asthma are a longer duration of exposure before the onset of asthma, a longer duration of symptoms before diagnosis, the finding of airway obstruction at the time of baseline study, the development of a dual response after specific inhalation challenge testing, the persistence of markers of airway inflammation as reflected in BAL fluid and bronchial biopsy, and more rapid than normal annual decline in lung function tests.

Continued occupational exposure in sensitized subjects may lead to worsening of asthma, even when the exposure is to a low concentration of the sensitizing agent. Bronchial sensitivity to TDI can disappear with time, but nonspecific airway hyperresponsiveness often persists unchanged. These observations suggest a permanent change in the airways. Lemiere et al. (108) report a decrease in specific airway responsiveness in sensitized subjects after removal from exposure, evidently because of a loss of immunologic and/or nonspecific bronchial reactivity. Following cessation of exposure, a plateau of improvement for spirometry is reached by 1 year and for airway hyperresponsiveness by 2 years (109). Inhaled corticosteroids, in addition to withdrawal from the workplace exposure, improve the clinical and functional recovery from occupational asthma. The beneficial effect of the inhaled steroids is more pronounced if inhaled steroids are given early after diagnosis (291).

## AGGRAVATING FACTORS AFFECTING PROGNOSIS

A number of environmental factors retain the potential to temporarily or permanently aggravate existing occupational asthma. Considering such factors is important for disability and causation considerations.

### Indoor Home Allergens

The domestic mites, deposited in floors and buried deep within carpets, mattresses, and soft furnishings are a major cause of asthma worldwide. Sensitization to cockroach allergens is a risk factor for asthma, especially among lower socioeconomic groups and minority populations. Household warm-blooded animals are another important source of indoor allergens. Pets create allergens from secretions (saliva), excretions (urine, feces), and danders. Cat allergens are liberated as small respirable particles, chiefly from the saliva, pelt, and sebaceous secretions. Up to 30% of allergic individuals show positive skin tests to dog extracts (292). Pet rodents can be a source of airborne allergens. Additionally, in inner-city areas wild mice or rats represent an important animal allergen pool. In some locations and among some ethnic groups, sensitization to cockroach allergen is more common than to the domestic mite. Molds and yeasts are indoor airborne allergens, especially *Alternaria,* which is a known risk factor for asthma and is associated with the risk of asthma death in the United States (293).

### Outdoor Allergens

Pollens and fungi are the most common outdoor allergens that cause asthma. The air concentration of pollens originates from trees, grasses, and weeds; it varies with location and atmospheric condition. In general, tree pollens predominate in the early spring; grass pollens increase in the late spring and summer; and, higher levels of weed pollens appear during summer and fall. Molds and yeasts are also outdoor airborne allergens.

### Drugs and Food Additives

Asthmatic adults with nasal polyps and sinusitis may be sensitive to aspirin and nonsteroidal antiinflammatory drugs (294). Some foods and food preservatives, monosodium glutamate, and some food coloring agents may cause asthma exacerbations.

### Active and Passive Smoking

More than 4,500 compounds and contaminants are present in tobacco smoke, including respirable particles, polycyclic hydrocarbons, carbon monoxide, carbon dioxide, nitric oxide, nitrogen oxides, nicotine, and acrolein. Children exposed to the involuntary passive smoke of their parents who smoke, especially mothers, have an increased risk of asthma and exacerbations of asthma, especially during the first 2 years of life. Smoking increases the risk of developing occupational asthma in workers exposed to some occupational sensitizers such as platinum salts and tetrahydrophthalic anhydride.

### Community Air Pollution

The prevalence of asthma correlates with urbanization and migration from country to city centers. Epidemiologic investigations, however, which strive to couple the rising trend of asthma with ambient air pollution, such as ozone, nitrogen oxides, acidic aerosols, and particulate matter, have not been persuasive (295,296). Pollutants such as $SO_2$, ozone, and nitrogen oxides, at concentrations found in heavily polluted cities, can trigger bronchoconstriction, transiently increase airway responsiveness, and enhance allergic responses. $SO_2$ triggers a dose-dependent airflow limitation in exercising patients with asthma, although it has no effect on the airways of normal subjects up to very high concentrations (295,296).

Ozone plays a significant role in the exacerbation of asthma, either by priming the airway mucosa such that cellular responses to allergen are enhanced or by exerting an intrinsic effect on airway inflammation. Ozone exposure also has a priming effect on allergen-induced responses and intrinsic inflammatory action on the nasal airways of perennially allergic asthmatics. Asthmatic individuals appear to be more sensitive to the acute inflammatory effects of ozone than nonasthmatic individuals (297).

Because residents of developed countries spend 90% to 95% of their time indoors, indoor pollutants are important to consider. Some data suggest that indoor pollutants may contribute to the development of asthma, but further studies are needed (296).

### Viral Respiratory Infections

There is evidence to show a temporal relationship between viral respiratory infections and the development of asthma in childhood, but there is no evidence that viral respiratory infections directly cause the development of asthma in adults. Viral infections cause bronchial epithelial cellular damage and airway inflammation; both events influence asthma symptoms. Virus-specific IgE antibody have been identified for the respiratory syncytial virus and for the parainfluenza virus. Viruses may potentiate an allergic response to allergens by increasing the release of inflammatory mediators and may stimulate the cascade of inflammatory events characteristic of asthma.

### Exercise and Hyperventilation

The mechanisms of exercise-induced bronchospasm relates to the associated hyperventilation that occurs with exercise. Like exercise, hyperventilation seems to be a specific trigger for asthma (298). It is believed that the bronchoconstriction response relates to either cooling or rewarming (298–300), or changes in osmolarity of the fluid lining the airway mucosa.

### Emotional Stress

While asthma is not a psychosomatic disorder, emotional distress, and extreme expressions of laughing, crying, anger, or fear can lead to hyperventilation and hypocapnia, which cause airway narrowing and thus may trigger asthma. Panic attacks that may occur in some patients with asthma have a similar effect.

## DIAGNOSIS OF OCCUPATIONAL ASTHMA

To confirm the diagnosis of occupational asthma, the clinician must address the cardinal features of bronchial asthma as well as the feature of work-relatedness. The important diagnostic parameters are (a) documentation of work-relatedness of airflow limitation; (b) presence of reversible airflow limitation; (c) documentation of sensitization if an allergic process is operative (i.e., specific airway hyperresponsiveness); and (d) preferably, confirming the presence of nonspecific airway hyperresponsiveness. The latter is characteristic of both allergic and nonallergic asthma. The clinician, considering the diagnosis of occupational asthma, must obtain information documenting a workplace exposure to an agent known to give rise to occupational asthma. Additional information includes either work-related changes in $FEV_1$ or peak expiratory flow (PEF) and/or a work-related changes in bronchial responsiveness. When possible, a positive response to specific inhalation challenge tests is confirmatory.

The consideration of irritant-induced asthma is appropriate when asthma onset demonstrates a clear association with a high-level irritant exposure in the workplace.

For epidemiologic purposes, the surveillance case diagnosis of occupational asthma requires the documentation of asthma and a clear relationship between the claimed symptoms of asthma and the workplace exposure (301).

The use of lung function testing ($FEV_1$, PEF) documents a number of key features of occupational asthma, including work-relatedness of the airflow limitation and reversible airflow limitation. The use of immunologic testing, biomarkers, and other testing affords evidence of an allergic process. Special testing with lung function and pharmacologic/physical agents (methacholine, histamine, cold air, distilled water) indicates nonspecific airway hyperresponsiveness. Finally, combinations of lung function testing, BAL, biomarkers, and other tests contribute information that indirectly reflects airway inflammatory changes and the presence of specific airway hyperresponsiveness. Chan-Yeung (302) described an approach to the diagnosis of asthma and occupational asthma.

### Obtaining the Necessary History

An important clue for occupational asthma is the observation of the onset of asthma in an adult with no history of allergic disease. Characteristically, asthma with latency is characterized by asthma that evolves after repeated exposures to an agent at work; usually the onset occurs within several months or years of exposure. Many times the patient is unable to pinpoint the exact date of onset of the disease, but generally can recall the year, the season, and possibly the month. It is not likely that the onset of the asthma can be isolated to a specific day or hour. However, a sudden onset of asthma, after a high-level irritant gas, vapor, or fume exposure is characteristic of RADS. In this situation, the worker will often be able to identify the exact date and frequently provide the specific time of asthma onset.

A difficult call is differentiating nonoccupational asthma with existing nonspecific airway hyperresponsiveness that is exacerbated by irritating substances at work (e.g., work-aggravated asthma). Sometimes the investigation elicits a history of asthma during childhood or before employment. Usually, only a small proportion of exposed workers develop asthma from specific sensitizers. For occupational asthma without latency (i.e., RADS) the onset of symptoms is dramatic and is related to a specific intense exposure event. Occasionally, in atopic persons, the irritant exposure may be more prolonged, intermittent in nature, or of moderate intensity before there is initiation of asthma. Once asthma symptoms develop, the patient suffers bronchial irritability symptoms and responds to many and varied nonspecific environmental and occupational irritant stimuli.

While the occupational/environmental history is essential, an accurate medical and respiratory history is indispensable to exclude non-occupationally related pulmonary conditions. It is important to inquire about the time the symptoms commenced, previous medical and respiratory illnesses (including respiratory infections), hospitalizations, use of drugs and medications, cigarette consumption, pets at home, hobbies, and allergic background.

### Exposure History

Important goals of the occupational history is to determine four essential aspects of the exposure information. First, it is essential that an exact identification of the incriminated material or agent in the workplace be made. Designation of exposures as "dusty" or "lots of fumes and smoke" is not adequate. The worker must be queried as to specifics. Sometimes only a trade name of a material is known. Generic identification of the material or agent is imperative and this specific information must be pursued.

The second important piece of information concerns the duration of the exposure. Is the exposure to a specific agent short-termed and lasting a few days, weeks, or months, or does the exposure last for several years? A transient or brief exposure, unless it's to a very toxic gas or fume and in high concentrations, such as with RADS, rarely causes persistent disease.

The third important information component is the intensity or extent of an exposure. A basic toxicologic supposition is one of "dose and response." The intensity of an exposure represents the "dose" part of the dose-response relationship. It is important to determine whether an exposure is meaningful. Accurately approximating the extent of an exposure can be formidable and is limited without actual industrial hygiene measurements. There are some clues to this type information, for example, the type of job.

The fourth piece of information concerns whether there is a relationship between the workplace and symptoms. This is especially pertinent for occupational asthma, where improvement in symptoms may be discerned during times away from work, such as on weekends and vacations.

### Physical Examination

Examination of the worker in the office may not be fruitful, but examination at work during exposure may be. At work, the employee may report cough or chest tightness; inspiratory wheezes may become audible shortly after the exposure begins or several hours later. It is important to remember that the physical finding of wheeze, by itself, is nonspecific and not diagnostic.

### Material Safety Data Sheets (MSDS)

The material safety data sheets (MSDS) are a first step in gaining information on the hazardous exposure. At least the MSDS identifies specific chemicals used in the workplace. The Occupational Safety and Health Administration (OSHA) requires suppliers to include MSDS with each shipment of an industrial material or chemical. These data sheets generically identify the agent supplied and provide cursory but important toxicological information and recommended safety and emergency procedures. OSHA requires the employer to maintain MSDS and make them available to physicians and workers. It is also possible to acquire MSDS information by telephone, by written request to either the employer, the supplier, or through internet search engines. Once an agent is identified, standard text books and publications provide more in depth information.

### Employee Documents

Gaining access to the employer's health surveillance or industrial hygiene records provides another source of information. In order to obtain this type of information, it is necessary to question the patient about companies and employers that they worked for in the past. It is altogether appropriate for a physician to request, from the employer, records pertaining to a patient's past health status. If there are records available of sick leave, accidents, and job performance, this information may be important. The person in charge of the company's health and safety program is usually the individual to contact and the most suitable person to approach for this information. When available, information could also be gained from the worker's compensation insurance underwriter files, which recount medical care rendered to the patient for previous occupational illnesses. This usually necessitates cooperation from the employer, but if there is a reluctance of the company to provide the physician with the requested records, the clinician can point out that persons with a demonstrated "need to know" are permitted access to otherwise confidential health records. Results of employer-sponsored surveillance testing may also supply information, such as annual chest roentgenograms or pulmonary function tests; these can be compared with the more recent tests. Information encompassed in pre-employment health questionnaires may document previous respiratory complaints.

### Industrial Hygiene Assessment

When available, industrial hygiene information is crucial. Industrial hygienists are professionals trained to measure and control the levels of exposures of workers to toxic materials, physical hazards, and infectious agents. Monitoring of workplace pollutants furnishes a quantitative appraisal of dusts, gases, vapors, or aerosols in the environment and is a relatively precise way to identify and analyze exposures in an occupational setting. Moreover, for dusts or aerosols, special testing is a criterion for establishing whether the dust or aerosol is respirable.

Environmental assessment provides important information: several measurements of the workplace environment may reveal that the concentration of an allergen varies; environmental monitoring may measure the effectiveness of interventions aimed at reducing exposure; and, environmental measurements provide information on exposure-response relationships. Methods are available for quantifying airborne allergens using standard analytic industrial hygiene sampling principles and immunoassays (302a). Simply, a known volume of air is sampled using high-volume samplers. The airborne particles are captured on a filter. It is particularly important to use a filter medium that permits high flow rates and efficient elution of the allergens in small volumes of buffer. The soluble allergens are extracted from the filter, and the amount of retained allergen is assayed by sensitive radioimmunoassays (RAST, ELISA).

The safety officer in the plant is the person to contact for information on industrial hygiene data. By law, all companies are required to have a designated safety officer at every office or plant. In smaller companies, this individual usually has very little formal training in safety matters and almost invariably other responsibilities. In larger companies, the safety professional is customarily better trained and deals entirely with health and safety matters. Some companies are large enough to employ not only an industrial hygienist, but also a physician and a nurse. Industrial hygiene information can be made available to smaller companies by consultants or by industrial hygienists from a workers' compensation insurance carrier.

### Factors Outside the Workplace

It is important to examine factors concerning the home environment. It is now clear that, the home environment can be a source of contaminants, especially biological agents, and may be even dirtier than the workplace (see Aggravating Factors, above).

### Walk-Through

Plant walk-through evaluations (i.e., a guided tour of the worksite) are helpful in understanding the context of the exposure and the neighboring activities that are unique to each worksite. In some situations the worksite visit may provide exposure information that is not fully described by routine air sampling. Workers may become sensitized to particular substances, such as isocyanates, following a spill and subsequent exposure levels may be well below the detectable limits of the sampling device.

## LABORATORY TESTS

### Chest Radiography

Chest x-ray findings are normal and of no value in the vast majority of subjects with occupational asthma. The most frequent positive findings are hyperexpansion, changes in thoracic configuration, decrease in size of the heart associated with attenuation of peripheral pulmonary vessels, and prominence of the main hilar arteries. Pulmonary infiltrates suggest mechanisms other than asthma, which may have an immune basis.

### Lung Function Testing

Pre- and postshift changes in $FEV_1$ measurements performed on a Monday or after absence from work may be revealing. This type of approach may lack specificity, since as many as 10% of unexposed and nonsensitized workers demonstrate significant postshift $FEV_1$ changes. In one study of colophony sensitivity, only 20% of patients who were found to have occupational asthma showed a postshift $FEV_1$ greater than 10% (13,46). The diurnal variation of $FEV_1$ is small, perhaps not more than 2% to 3%. Decrements more than 200 ml (from 8:00 A.M. to 4:00 P.M.) are reported in some cases of occupational asthma. Malingering can usually be excluded if multiple measurements vary less than 50 ml, provided the test is performed by an experienced technician with a well-calibrated spirometer. The bronchodilator response helps identify cases of asthma, but failure to respond to bronchodilators does not exclude asthma. In some instances, the before-work and after-work $FEV_1$ values are only slightly different (less than 200 ml). In these cases, a greater than 25% change in forced expiratory flow after 25% to 75% of vital capacity has been expelled ($FEF_{25–75}$) may be helpful.

### *Immunologic Studies*

Immunologic tests are of value in the evaluation of cases of occupational asthma. A positive immune response, taken alone, does not confirm the presence of occupational asthma in a symptomatic worker, but is strong evidence of the allergic nature of the asthma. Immune reactions such as a positive Prausnitz–Kustner reaction in the case of castor bean exposure, or demonstration of an elevated level of specific IgE as with platinum or phthalic anhydride, provides a strong confirmation of the allergic nature of the work-related asthma. Complement fixation tests, precipitating antibody assays, and lymphocyte studies are other tests that may be helpful in confirming sensitization. The use of a combination of tests may add sensitivity to the evaluative process but not necessarily specificity. In the study by Rasanen et al., three imunologic tests, skin prick test, RAST, and basophil histamine-release test are compared to specific bronchoprovocation challenge (303). The sensitivity and specificity, respectively, of the tests are: skin prick test, 74% and 89%; RAST, 57% and 86%; and, basophil histamine-release test, 78% and 93%. The average sensitivity and specificity of the panel of the three tests are 70% and 91%.

### *Prick Skin Testing*

Skin testing with common aeroallergens will identify atopic persons. Skin tests for specific occupational allergens are not always available or reliable. On occasion they may produce false positive or false negative results. Examples of occupational allergens to which prick skin testing is applied are shown in Table 8.

### *Radioallergosorbent (RAST) Testing*

Radioallergosorbent (RAST) testing has been used to detect circulating specific IgE antibodies against occupational allergens. Some examples of occupational allergens to which RAST is applied are shown in Table 9.

### *Specific IgG Antibodies*

Investigations of allergens utilizing enzyme-linked immunosorbent assay (ELISA) or immunoblotting procedures have been adopted for detecting specific IgG (and sometimes IgE) antibodies.

### *Use of Peak Expiratory Flow Monitoring*

Peak expiratory flow measurements can monitor, diagnose, and/or evaluate subjects with suspected or confirmed occupational and nonoccupational asthma. PEF measurements may reflect hazards or events in the workplace that represents essential information for proper employee job placement. Epidemiologic studies utilizing serial PEFR act as a tool to identify cases, describe prevalence, and compare the mean diurnal variation in PEFR with an unexposed control group. Multiple sequential readings of PEF provide a simple way to express the airway variability of all subjects studied. Serial PEFR is a useful additional tool to the respiratory questionnaire and spirometry as it measures airway variability. It may be a practical alternative to histamine or methacholine inhalation testing. PEF recordings in the workplace correlate with laboratory bronchial provocation testing. As such, PEF testing represents a suitable alternative to the more

**TABLE 8.** *IgE sensitization determined by skin prick testing*

| |
|---|
| Crab/snow crab-meat extracts |
| Nickel sulfate |
| Wheat flour |
| Egg protein |
| Barley flour |
| α-Amylase |
| Laboratory animal extracts |
| Sewer flies |
| Pau Marfim |
| Various spices |
| Lactalbumin from cow's milk |
| Chloramine T |
| Canary palm pollen, *Phoenix canariensis* |
| Poultry antigens |
| Bromelain-pineapple *(Ananas comosus)* |
| Sunflower pollen |
| Mealworms larvae |
| Papain |
| Baby's breath *(Gypsophila paniculata)* |
| Latex |
| Pepsin |
| Beneficial arthropods |
| Swiss chard |
| Detergent enzymes |
| Various insects |
| Silkworm cocoon and pupal allergens |
| Alkaline hydrolysis wheat gluten |
| Northern fowl mite in poultry workers |
| Platinum salts |
| *Papaver somniferum* |
| Honey bee body extract |
| Wood dust, *Tanganyika anigre* |
| Reactive dyes |
| Cockroach antigen |
| Raw potato extract |
| Contaminated water—trout processing factory |
| Cobalt |
| Cellulase and xylanase enzymes |
| Green coffee bean |
| *Aspergillus niger* |
| Red spider mite, *Tetranychus urticae* |
| Clam and shrimp products |
| Methyltetrahydrophthalic anhydride |
| Hexahydrophthalic anhydride |
| MDI-human serum albumin (intradermal) |

**TABLE 9.** *Causes of IgE sensitization determined by RAST*

| | |
|---|---|
| *Anopheles stephensi*—mosquito | Psyllium-containing bulk laxative |
| Various laboratory animals | Rat urinary aeroallergen |
| Latex | *Candida albicans* |
| Wheat flour | Extracts of various insects |
| Barley flour | Silkworm cocoon/pupal extracts |
| Rye flour | Senna |
| α- and β-Amylase | Reactive dyes, black GR/orange 3R |
| Extracts weeping fig | Mouse dander |
| Whole flours | Storage mite |
| Poultry antigens | Sea squirt |
| Papain | Konnyaku asthma |
| Lactalbumin from cow's milk | Alkaline hydrolysis wheat gluten |
| mealworms larvae—*Tenibrio molitor* | Soybean lecithin |
| Egg protein | Diazonium tetrafluoroborate |
| Canary palm pollen | Northern fowl mite |
| Chloramine T | Garlic |
| Sunflower pollen | *Cladosporium* |
| Latex | Ispaghula dust |
| Soybean flour | Platinum salts |
| P-tolyl monoisocyanate—HSA | *Papaver* somniferum |
| Various diisocyanates | Remazol dyes |
| MDI-HSA | *Alternaria* tenius |
| Toluene diisocyanate | Honey bee body extract |
| Pepsin | Korean Artemisia pollen extracts |
| Latex and bananas | Reactive dyes |
| Beneficial arthropods | Bahia grass pollen |
| Castor-bean extract | Cockroach antigen |
| Swiss chard | Raw potato extract |
| Red spider mite | Dried flowers of *Limonium tataricum* |
| Clam and shrimp | Carmine-Dactylopius coccus |
| Methyltetrahydrophthalic anhydride | Quillaja bark (soapbark) |
| Tetrachlorophthalic anhydride | Laboratory animals |
| *Aspergillus niger* | Baby's breath |
| Western red cedar | Cellulase and xylanase enzymes |
| Various spices | Green coffee bean |
| Insoluble wheat grain proteins | Cobalt |
| Piperazine and *N*-methyl-piperazine detergent enzymes | |

formal, laboratory-based bronchoprovocation testing procedure (250). PEF measurements are of particular use for screening out workers whose symptoms are not due to the workplace exposures. Some examples of various causes of asthma where PEFR measurements are employed are shown in Table 10.

The recommended approach is for the worker to perform and record PEFR measurements every 2 hours. The recordings should encompass 2 to 3 weeks at work and at least 10 days off work. The monitoring protocol should be standardized, and some criteria for validity should be preselected. Factors that may affect diurnal variation in PEFR such as age, sex, smoking, race, and the mean or maximum PEFR, should be taken into account when comparing with control subjects during epidemiologic investigations. While the exact criteria for a positive test need to be better defined, a consistent pattern of a change in PEFR which is greater than 25% at work suggests a work-related process. Greater diurnal variation in PEFR values occurring at work than at home may constitute important information (Fig. 2). Inclusion of a personal symptom diary at the time of PEFR measurements helps with the interpretation of the PEFR measurements. PEFR evaluated using the kind of statistical analyses employed in the field of biologic rhythm research may furnish a more objective approach to data analysis.

Even with careful instructions and detailed protocol, there continues to be a concern about unsupervised PEFR measurements (304,305). Investigations have assessed the reliability of PEF monitoring using a portable computerized peak flow meter, the VMX Minilog. Subjects were requested to monitor their PEF six times daily using the VMX Mini-Log for 2 weeks at work and at least 10 days away from work. They were unaware that their readings were stored by the flow meter in addition to the digital readout. The digital readout results were supposed to be recorded by the subjects, and then the investigators compared the workers recorded results with the results recorded by the VMX. Of those workers who completed the monitoring, only 55.3% of the records were considered completely accurate in terms of the value and the timing of the measurements; 23.3% were inaccurate either in terms of the recorded value or of the timing of the measurement; and the remainder were fabricated results (not recorded by the Mini-Log). These studies concluded that PEF monitoring, using ordinary peak flow meters for assessment of work-relatedness of asthma, has limitations and is not reliable.

### *Testing for Nonspecific Airway Responsiveness*

Methacholine, histamine, or carbachol inhalation challenges may be helpful in evaluating an individual worker with suspected occupational asthma with normal spirometry or during a symptom-free interval. Guidelines for performing bronchial inhalation challenges with pharmacologic and antigenic agents have been reported (117, 306). The increase in nonspecific bronchial hyperresponsiveness acts as a marker for an allergic bronchial response to an occupational agent. The increase in nonspecific bronchial hyperresponsiveness after a specific inhalation challenge is found to be an early and sensitive marker of a bronchial response to occupational allergen, especially in subjects removed from workplace exposure for a long period of time.

Perhaps the occupational exposure terminated months or years before the evaluation. The worker is completely without symptoms and has normal results on pulmonary functions tests. The demonstration of hyperreactive airways supports the history of a previous asthmatic condition, now either in remission or recovering. Methacholine or histamine challenge can also be helpful in following a patient with occupational asthma after exposure has been terminated and may offer a clue to prognosis. Serial studies demonstrate loss of airway hyperresponsiveness and recovery from disease. Malo and colleagues (109) report that a plateau of improvement for bronchial hyperresponsiveness occurs by 2 years after termination of exposure. It is not yet conclusively known whether serial testing of workers, as part of a surveillance program, affords a preventive health benefit. Such testing may identify employees with hyperreactive airways, who are at greater risk for disease, or workers who are in the process of developing asthma but who have not yet become symptomatic. The studies of platinum refinery workers suggest that in some cases signs of nonspecific bronchial reactivity precede immune manifestations (72,274). Airway hyperreactivity by itself is not likely to be disqualifying, since some subjects with asthma can work without difficulty with allergenic agents. Furthermore, sensitization can be present in the absence of airway hyperreactivity.

**TABLE 10.** *Examples using PEFR for the diagnosis of occupational asthma*

| |
|---|
| Dried flowers of Limonium tataricum |
| Aluminum pot-room asthma |
| Aluminum workers |
| Pharmaceutical company processing psyllium |
| Glutaraldehyde and formaldehyde in endoscopy and x-ray departments |
| Technologist exposed to glutaraldehyde |
| Endotoxin exposure–response in a fiberglass manufacturing facility |
| Latex gloves with a lower protein content |
| Heated polypropylene |
| New Zealand wood workers |
| Occupational exposure to persulfates |
| Chemical workers exposed to aliphatic polyamines |
| Sauna builder's asthma–obeche *(Triplochiton scleroxylon)* dust |
| Overexposure to locomotive exhaust |
| Inhaled egg protein |
| Exposure to 2.0 ppm formaldehyde in occupationally exposed workers |
| Tea-dust induced asthma |
| Oil mists |
| Soft corrosive soldering fluxes containing zinc chloride/ammonium chloride |
| Ash wood dust *(Fraxinus americana)* |
| Common house dust mite, *Dermatophagoides pteronyssinus* |
| Pharmaceutical company processing spiramycin |
| Laboratory animals |
| Breakout of asthma in a steel coating plant |
| Nickel sulfate |
| Dietary supplement with fish oil lipids |
| Egg lysozyme |
| MDI and TDI |
| Autobody shop workers exposed to isocyanate-containing spray paint |
| Contaminated humidifier |
| Lauryl dimethyl benzyl ammonium chloride used in a floor cleaner |
| Pepsin |
| Snow crab-processing workers |
| Eastern white cedar *(Thuja occidentalis)* |
| Grain elevator and mill workers |
| First confirmed case of baker's asthma in Singapore |
| Western red cedar |
| Formaldehyde |
| Styrene |
| Air infiltration incorporating high efficiency particulate air filter |
| Inhaled steroids on recovery after cessation of exposure |
| Children living in a coastal town near two power stations |
| Colophony |

### *Combining Repeat Methacholine and Peak Expiratory Flow Rate*

The use of testing that combines nonspecific bronchial responsiveness and PEFR is reported to be a reliable way of confirming a diagnosis of occupational asthma (306, 307). A number of modifications of the stop–resume work test have been published that can be utilized in suspected cases of occupational asthma (308). A worker's personal symptom diary may help elucidate the interpretation of test results. It seems best to perform at least two or three methacholine challenge studies while the worker is away from work and at least two or three tests during the period at work.

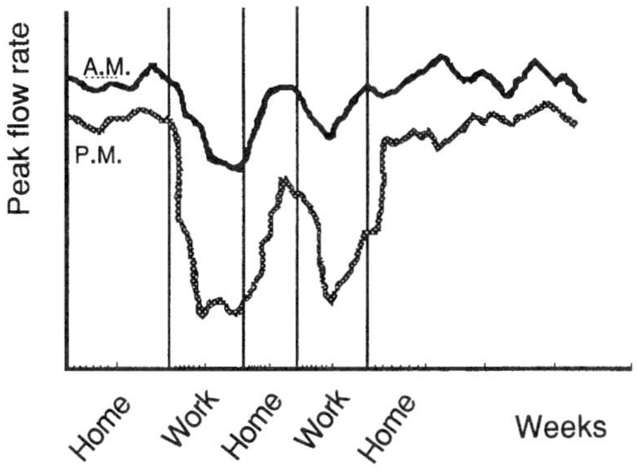


**FIG. 2.** A greater diurnal variation in PEFR values at work than at home may provide confirmatory evidence of occupational asthma.

Combining PEFR and methacholine/histamine challenge confirms that an immunologic-based, asthmatic-inducing process is taking place the workplace; it does not identify the specific agent as does specific inhalation challenge testing performed in a laboratory. A reduction of PEF measurements at work and not at home confirms reversible work-related bronchoconstriction (Fig. 3). Enough time for recovery and response must be considered. Therefore, multiple PEFR recordings are recommended for 2 to 3 weeks at work and at least 10 days off work. The information that a fall in methacholine $PC_{20}$ interjects is that the bronchoconstriction is likely due to an allergic mechanism rather than caused by a reflex irritant response (Fig. 3). The decrease in $PC_{20}$ after a specific inhalation challenge is an early and sensitive marker of a bronchial response to occupational allergen, especially in subjects who are removed from the workplace exposure for a longer period of time.

### *Specific Inhalation Challenges*

Bronchial provocation testing is an extremely important diagnostic application. The indications for bronchial provocation testing include identifying causative agents for which skin testing is not reliable; identifying new allergens for which serum or skin testing have not yet been validated; obtaining evidence to persuade a patient that an allergen is or is not causing asthma; confirming the importance of unavoidable inhalant allergens before committing a patient to immunotherapy; and, on occasion, collecting evidence for medicolegal matters. When the tests are carefully controlled, a positive response establishes a diagnosis of occupational asthma. A negative result while a worker is employed or shortly after employment ceases provides strong evidence against a diagnosis of occupational asthma.

Recent evidence suggests this type of testing may not always be the definitive "gold standard." A significant number of nonreactors give good clinical and work histories for occupational asthma. A negative specific inhalation challenge test does not rule out a diagnosis of occupational asthma; other chemicals that may induce asthma and that are not tested may be present in the workplace, and such agents may be the cause of the asthma. It is also possible that the inhaled dose of the allergen used for the challenge testing is too small. When performing inhalation challenge tests, careful control of the inhaled dose is necessary to avoid dangerous side effects. Controlling the exposure also assesses the contribution of any nonspecific irritant or bronchoconstrictor property of the agent. This is particularly important if the tested subject has a high degree of nonspecific airway hyperresponsiveness (309). Retrospective evaluation of workers who show a negative response but who experience no further exposure may simply reflect the loss of sensitivity to the agent. Importantly, the skills and resources necessary for successful inhalation challenge testing are limited to only a few facilities and are not available to the vast majority of practitioners. Furthermore, with the advent of managed care, it is unlikely that HMOs or workers' compensation groups will pay for inhalation challenge testing.

Testing should be performed under hospital conditions and when the patient is relatively symptom free. While pharmacologic agents can be aerosolized by a proper nebulizer and generating system, challenge with occupational materials is more difficult. When solutions are available for use (e.g., animal, wheat, or grain antigens), they can be aerosolized using methods similar to those for pharmacologic challenges. Correlations with results of prior skin test may suggest what is a safe initial concentration of aerosol to use (309). Vapors such as TDI can be monitored using a continuous rapid-reading monitor as well as standard analytic procedures. Various testing procedures have been reported for vapors (310) and dusts (311). It is important to recognize that MDI exists as both an aerosol and a vapor and creates difficulties for challenge atmospheres. There may be differences in reactivity among isomers—more intense reactions to the 2,6 isomer than the 2,4 isomer for TDI challenges. Dust generation is difficult to standardize and quantify but new methods are available (310,311). Generally, mixing dust with lactose provides a means for diluting it to different concentrations.

### *Use of Biological Markers*

Biological markers can be used to monitor physiological, biochemical and anatomical parameters and may represent indirect indicators of an asthmatic process. A variety of biological markers may be considered for occupational asthma.

### *Sputum Examination*

Sputum analysis provides a noninvasive method of examining the airway secretions of subjects with asthma

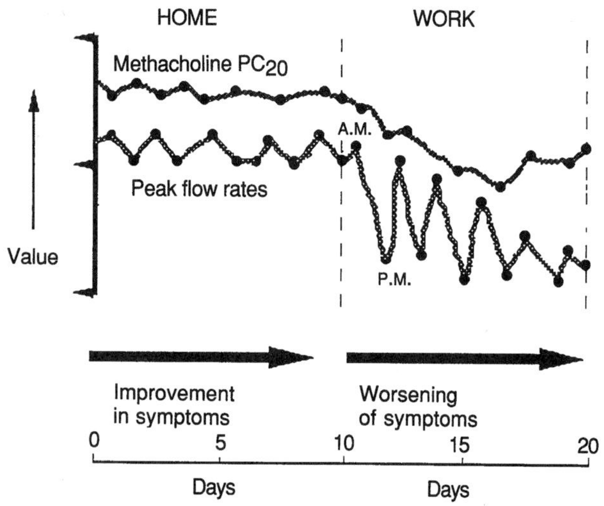


**FIG. 3.** Objective information provided by noting an increased responsiveness to methacholine with documented falls in $PC_{20}$ suggests the response is likely allergic in origin and thus indirectly documents sensitization. It is an indirect indicator of a late asthma attack. PEFR measurements objectively document the occurrence of reversible airflow limitation and the specific work-relatedness of that limitation.

in order to better understand the inflammatory process. Eosinophils are markers of an allergic process. Eosinophilia, in sputum or peripheral blood, is a clinical tool that may be helpful in confirming an allergic process (312). Monitoring blood and sputum eosinophilia during a stop–resume work test is used to help differentiate occupational and nonoccupational allergic causes. Sputum eosinophils are recognized rapidly and reliably on unstained specimens. Often 15% or more of all cells in the sputum of asthmatics are eosinophils; the numbers even bear a rough relation to the severity of the attack. Several days away from the offending workplace allergen may result in a decrease in total blood eosinophil count or sputum eosinophilia. This can be coupled with spirometry or PEF for more definitive results. When airway obstruction becomes chronic, the presence of eosinophilia is helpful in confirming allergic airway obstructive disease. Peripheral blood eosinophilia may also be present in bronchial asthma from nonoccupational causes.

### *Histamine Releasing Factor*

The procedure of activating peripheral blood monocytes in order to increase their spontaneous release of cytokines (e.g., tumor necrosis factor and histamine releasing factor) has been examined in asthma (313). The technique of determining histamine release involves isolating peripheral blood mononuclear cells from venous blood samples and then culturing purified cell populations using different histamine releasing factors stimulating agents, including an antigen to be studied. The evocation of histamine releasing factors correlates with circulating IgE to inhalant allergens, positive RAST, and bronchial sensitivity to histamine (314). Investigations have reported positive tests for such agents as dust mites, flour allergens, trimellitic anhydride, alpha amylase, platinum salts, persulphates, Swiss chard, plicatic acid, chloramine-T, and raw potatoes.

Herd et al. investigated eight individuals with diisocyanate-induced asthma utilizing histamine releasing factor and seven of eight showed a positive response (315). Peripheral blood mononuclear cells of workers with diisocyanate-asthma reveal significantly greater production of antigen-specific histamine releasing factor activity and monocyte chemo-attractant protein-1 compared to the diisocyanate-exposed asymptomatic workers (316). Subjects with asthma after short-term exposure to TDI show increased numbers of mast cells in the airway mucosa (317). Zeiss et al. reports leukocyte histamine release to TMA-human serum albumin (TMA-HSA) in one asthmatic worker with high levels of specific IgE antibody for TMA-HSA (318). Plicatic acid triggers histamine release from bronchial biopsy specimens and BAL samples of patients with western red cedar asthma (319). A plicatic acid response of some normal subjects suggests that plicatic acid has both specific and nonspecific actions on mast cells and basophils.

### *Bronchoalveolar Lavage*

Bronchoalveolar lavage (BAL) provides an *in vivo* way of investigating airway inflammation in occupational asthma as well as the sequence of events after allergen challenge. BAL, in actuality, represents only an indirect estimation of the bronchial inflammation. BAL has been considered an important research tool for assessing the effectiveness of intervention and preventive strategies. When BAL is employed with endobronchial biopsy, pathological observations may enhance the BAL fluid interpretation. BAL samples the contents of large and small airways and alveoli and is generally considered a safe procedure when properly performed, even in severe asthmatic patients. Before performing BAL, the clinical status of the patients is ascertained. It is important that BAL investigations make use of appropriate cellular and biochemical parameters (320): (1) markers should be released by cells that are pertinent to airways inflammation (and reparation) in asthma, and, if possible, they should be specific of a single cell type, (2) the enumeration of cells or titration of the marker or of its metabolites should be specific and sensitive, (3) if possible, the titration should not be modified by the sampling procedure, (4) pilot studies should demonstrate that the cell is increased or the secretory product is released during challenge in asthmatic subjects, (5) studies in a large number of patients demonstrated that the levels of the marker are increased in chronic asthmatics, that these levels correlate with the severity of the disease and are decreased during effective anti-inflammatory treatment, and (6) if possible, the cell or marker should be specific to asthma. At present, there is no such cell or marker, but eosinophils and granule secretory products follow most of these requirements.

### *Bronchial Biopsy*

Bronchial biopsies allows better understanding of the pathobiology of occupational and non-occupational asthma. Information gained includes: evaluation of subepithelial fibrosis, basement membrane, and underlying collagen changes in asthma (321); bronchial mucosa changes before and after ten years of daily treatment with inhaled steroids (189b); estimation of the degree of airway inflammatory changes (322); morphologic outcomes of TDI asthma after cessation of occupational exposure of different durations (74,323,324); relationship between eosinophilic infiltration and persistent nonspecific airway hyperresponsiveness in TDI asthma after cessation of exposure (323); role of basophils and mast cells (325); pathologic changes in RADS (326); quantitative analysis of bronchial biopsies (327); bronchial eosinophils and lymphocytes-induced changes (328); histopathology of asthmatic airways removed at postmortem and by bronchial biopsy (329); pathological changes of western red cedar asthma (330); pathological changes of western red cedar asthma after *in vitro* challenge with plicatic acid-human serum albumin conjugate (319); mast cells changes after short-term exposure to TDI (317); bronchial biopsies changes due to either high molecular weight or low molecular weight agents (69).

### *Biologic Metabolites*

Liquid chromatography can be used to measure isocyanate levels in the air of a factory using a glue containing MDI (331). Although air concentrations of isocyanates are low, MDI metabolites are detected in the plasma and urine from all employees. There appears to be some correlation between the estimate of the air exposure level and the metabolite concentration, especially for workers with heavy exposures.

### *Phospholipid Products*

High levels of lyso-phospholipids and 1-hexadecyl-2-lyso-phospholipids are identified in airways of subjects challenged with antigen (332). A much closer examination of 1-radyl-2-lyso-sn-glycero-3-phosphocholine (GPC) reveals that 1-palmitoyl-2-lyso-GPC, 1-myristoyl-2-lyso-GPC, and 1-hexadecyl-2-lyso-GPC are three major molecular species generated after antigen challenge. The exact ramifications of these high levels of lyso-phospholipids on airway function and in occupational asthma are unknown.

### *Reactive Radicals*

Blood phagocytes from patients with asthma not treated with anti-inflammatory drugs show an increased capacity to produce reactive oxygen metabolites which can be identified using the technique of whole blood chemiluminescence (333). There is no difference in chemiluminescence values between patients with stable asthma without airway obstruction and healthy control subjects. The patients with asthma and current airway obstruction have significantly higher chemiluminescence responses than both the patients with non-obstructive asthma and the healthy control subjects. When the chemiluminescence values are corrected for the number of phagocytes present in the reactions, the patients with non-obstructive asthma show significantly lower values than the healthy control subjects. The data suggest that the chemiluminescence values of the patients with non-obstructive asthma reflect the result of effective anti-inflammatory treatment and that whole blood chemiluminescence may be useful as a systemic parameter in the follow-up of the inflammatory process in asthma.

### *Antibody Titers*

Workers exposed to hexahydrophthalic anhydride (HHPA) have specific IgE and IgG antibody titers to an HHPA-human serum albumin conjugate by an ELISA technique (334). Optimal discriminate analysis shows that the optimal titers for predicting workers with HHPA-induced disease is an IgE titer of more than 1:5 and an IgG titer of more than 1:10. The IgG cutoff correctly classifies 62 of 81 workers; there is a sensitivity of 100%, a predictive value of 67%, a specificity of 91% and a negative predictive value of 97%. Very high levels of specific IgE (≥ 1:50) or IgG (≥ 1:100) indicate a likelihood of immunologically-mediated respiratory disease to HHPA.

## ALLOCATING CAUSE AND EFFECT

In the best setting, the determination of an occupational or environmental pulmonary disorder necessitates a multidisciplinary approach. The medical examination may encompass an individual patient or a large working population. While each requires a somewhat different approach, both essentially utilize the same techniques and procedures: history, pulmonary function testing, and special tests. Industrial hygiene information is crucial. When specific quantitative information is not available, the detailed occupational history is a substitute. Explicit identification of materials by occupational history is particularly critical to determine past exposures and to gain information not available from industrial hygiene results. Since the physician may not be familiar with a process or an industrial material, the use of various informational resources to learn more about the agent or the industrial process is necessary. Standard textbooks, library and governmental sources, as well as industry consultations are important resources. Laboratory tests aid in substantiating a diagnosis. The results of workplace PEF measurements with or without methacholine/histamine challenges add to the information obtained. The results of a specific inhalation challenge may be helpful, especially when the test is positive. Immunologic testing and biomarkers provide important information.

The criteria for establishing a cause-and-effect relationship for the diagnosis of occupational asthma include (Table 11): (a) typical medical and occupational history (i.e., asthma symptoms related to work); (b) specific identification of the offending agent; (c) documentation that the agent can actually cause asthma (i.e., finding similar cases in the literature); (d) presence or induction of nonspecific bronchial hyperresponsiveness; (e) documentation of immune sensitization for allergic reactions; (f) documentation of work-related changes in pulmonary function; and (g) positive response to bronchial inhalation challenge (in hospital or at work). When the subject is no longer working or has no possibility of returning to work, certain pieces of information take on more significance (i.e., the first five factors listed above). A diagnosis cannot be made objectively if the only criterion utilized is a history of work-related symptoms.

## MANAGEMENT OF OCCUPATIONAL ASTHMA

The important goals in the management of the worker with occupational asthma are to: (1) confirm the diagnosis of occupational asthma, (2) gauge the severity of disease, (3) identify aggravants and trigger factors, (4) provide appropriate treatment; the goal of treatment is to curb and reverse the airway inflammation (5) put a high priority on returning the worker back to work, in some capacity, as soon as possible, (6) decide on the best disposition for the worker which may include complete removal from exposure and change to a new job or site, (7) monitor the disease course and insure patient guidance; and, (8) educate patients to develop a partnership in asthma management.

Medical management for asthma should provide such optimal control that: (1) the patient suffers no or few chronic symptoms, especially nocturnal symptoms and symptoms at work; (2) has minimal or infrequent acute exacerbations of bronchospasm at work and at home; (3) requires no emergency visits for treatment of acute attacks; (4) does not require or has minimal need for as needed beta2-agonist; (5) there is no limitations on daily life activities, including exercise; (6) there is normal or near normal PEF at work and at home; (7) peak expiratory flow circadian variation are less than 20 percent (morning PEF versus evening PEF); and, (8) there are minimal or no adverse effects from medicine. It is important to work closely with the employer, insurance carrier, risk manager, patient and other interested parties to insure continued worker employment with no loss of financial status.

Attempts to return subjects rapidly and efficiently to the workplace is the preferable option to discontinuation of work. Occupational asthma generally affects the younger workers, and a diagnosis of this condition has significant economic consequences for workers. However, with this philosophy emphasized, it is very important that persons found to have occupational asthma be separated from the offending agent as soon as possible. Prognosis is more favorable with a shorter period of symptoms before occupational asthma is diagnosed, maintenance of normal pulmonary function, and milder nonspecific airway hyperresponsiveness at diagnosis. There are also at least three other reasons for prompt removal of sensitized persons. (1) Low concentrations, even below governmental permissible levels, can provoke a serious asthmatic reaction. (2) Repeated low-level exposures can lead to irreversible airways obstructive disease in a sensitized person. (3) High concentrations of the material, such as those occuring after accidental spills, can provoke cases of nonallergic occupational asthma, acute severe asthmatic reactions, and possibly death in sensitized persons. Once sensitization occurs, a worker should be protected from any further exposure. The situation is different for irritant-induced occupational asthma where removal from exposure may not be required if the risk for recurrent exposure to high levels is not present. However, if the risk for recurrent high levels of exposure is high, removal is the treatment of choice.

The enlistment of the worker as an active participant in his or her asthma management is paramount for the proper control of asthma. This task requires that the physician insures substantial worker education on the role of trigger factors in the workplace and home environment; avoidance of allergens; explanation of the significance of environmental controls; and, the importance of compliance with prescribed medications usage, especially maintaining the regular use of inhaled corticosteroids. The use of pulmonary function studies is key for assessing the severity of asthma. PEF measurements provide a way to assess severity; appraise degree of diurnal variation in lung function; monitor response to therapy during an acute exacerbation; detect asymptomatic dete-

**TABLE 11.** *Criteria for establishing cause and effect*

| |
|---|
| Typical medical and occupational history (i.e., asthma related to work) |
| Specific identification of the offending agent |
| Documentation that the agent can actually cause asthma (i.e., similar cases in the literature) |
| Presence and/or induction of nonspecific bronchial hyperresponsiveness |
| Documentation of immune sensitization, if allergic in nature |
| Documenting work-related changes in pulmonary function testing |
| Positive bronchial inhalation challenge (in hospital or naturally at work) to confirm allergic cause |

rioration of lung function in the workplace and intervene before it becomes more serious; monitor response to chronic therapy and provide objective justification for change in job location; justify type of therapy to the patient; and identify triggers and occupational sensitizers.

Effective control of asthma can be better insured by educating patients to develop a partnership in asthma management; make sure there is the regular assessing and monitoring of asthma severity (symptom reports and measurements of lung function); encourage avoidance or control of asthma trigger factors; promote establishing an individual medication plan for long-term management. Education of the worker, his or her supervisors, and the coworkers about methods of control and how to deal with emergency situations, such as a spill, can be accomplished.

It is important to recognize triggers such as workplace aggravants, indoor and outdoor air pollutants, changes in environmental temperature or humidity, and physical changes such as exercise, cold air, and influential emotional expression. Thus, a strategy of attacking several exposure environments (including the workplace) at once is preferable. Thus, the practitioner may press the patient for efforts to reduce workplace irritant exposures; decrease indoor allergen exposures; avoid passive smoking; and, limit vehicle emission and outdoor air pollution. In some instances, the use of a respirator (personal protective device) may reduce exposure levels to acceptable values. Strategies such as the continued use of respiratory protective devices are not medically ethical for an already sensitized individual. The use of respiratory protective devices may be part of a comprehensive program involving selection, maintenance, training for use, and periodic testing. The value of immunotherapy and aggressive medication programs to allow a worker to continue employment in the same job or worksite needs to be evaluated on an individual basis. The practitioner must weigh the cost-benefit issues; the desire of the patient; be assured of the cooperation of the employer; and, make sure the patient is very closely and objectively (e.g., PEFR, methacholine, etc.) followed.

Underestimating the severity of a patient's asthma and inadequate treatment contributes to greater morbidity from workplace asthma exacerbations. Important historical information is the frequency of attacks occurring during the day at work and awakening the patient at night; the need for additional bronchodilator therapy by metered dose inhalers; the frequency of emergency room or physician's office visits because of acute attacks; and, whether oral corticosteroids are required to control asthma. Objective data include PEF records, personal diaries, serial methacholine/histamine challenges and perhaps various biomarkers. Preventing or minimizing asthmatic attacks through therapy need not take preference over preventive measures that reduces airway inflammation, such as the removal of the individual from allergen exposures or trigger situations.

The pharmacological treatment of patients with occupational asthma is not different from treatment of patients with non-occupational asthma. The recommendations of the National Asthma Expert Panel (NAEP) of the United States or similar treatment guidelines in other countries can be followed (335). Medications for occupational asthma can be divided into controller-type medications which are taken daily and on a long-term basis. They include anti-inflammatory agents and long-acting bronchodilators. These medications are useful in keeping persistent asthma under control. Inhaled corticosteroids are at present the most effective controllers. The other category of medications can be considered relievers, quick relief medicine, or rescue medicine (335). They include short-acting bronchodilator medications that act quickly to relieve bronchoconstriction and its accompanying acute symptoms. Although bronchodilators reverse and/or inhibit bronchoconstriction and related symptoms of acute asthma, they do not reverse airway inflammation and airway hyperresponsiveness.

## MANAGED CARE

Many states have incorporated managed care into workers' compensation. Few diagnoses offer managed care more return for the investment than do occupational asthma. In the future, physicians may be beset by the state or managed care organizations' requirement of best care practices. There may be a demand to use more anti-inflammatory therapy, peak flow meters, spacer devices, and written step care plans, including return to work instructions. The managed care system provides an organization and resource approach for primary care physicians on the front line and perhaps worker care without the necessary skills of the specialists. Whether the primary care physician, who is the case coordinator, will possess the knowledge and interest, or be allowed the necessary time and opportunity to undertake complicated diagnostic protocols for occupational asthma (serial PEFs at work and home; repeated methacholine challenges; supervising a workplace natural challenge) can not be discerned at this time in the evolution of state managed care initiatives. Important for the institution of a managed care approach to occupational asthma will include details of: (1) physician education, (2) the co-management concept, (3) patient education, (4) cost-effectiveness, (5) diagnostic and intervention protocols, and (6) implementation of managed care arrangements for workers' compensation.

## OCCUPATIONAL ASTHMA OUTCOMES

With the shrinkage of the health care dollar, more attention will be given to cost-effective treatment and management of occupational asthma and for quality outcomes (336). A variety of outcomes can be used for assessing occupational asthma. However, this disease has been poorly studied in the past and little definitive information is available. For example, the effectiveness of occupational asthma interventions may be objectively measured by the physiologic tests that identify the characteristic variable airway obstruction. Severity of occupational asthma is assessed in two dimensions. First, there is the baseline function, which provides a snapshot of current disease status. Second, there is disease lability or airway twitching, reactivity, and responsiveness, which relate to the potential for or the frequency of exacerbation. Baseline spirometry provides a high accuracy of asthma severity and degree of airway obstruction; the $FEV_1$ is the most reproducible pulmonary function test parameter. The post-bronchodilator $FEV_1$ measures the best lung function that is achievable by a bronchodilator therapy on the day of the evaluation. It is a more stable measure for comparing visit-to-visit baseline $FEV_1$. Ambulatory monitoring of PEFR at home and at work assesses the worker's degree of airway obstruction at work and at home both on a daily or weekly basis. Airway responsiveness (e.g., methacholine) assesses the degree to which an individual reacts to nonspecific stimuli that can trigger asthmatic attacks. Serial changes in airway responsiveness has been used to provide an indirect assessment of changes in airway inflammation induced by occupational or environmental exposures. The methacholine/histamine $PC_{20}$ may be improved by long-term inhaled steroids and in some cases by cessation of exposure.

More recently, quality of life, role performance, and functional status measures have been introduced as outcome parameters. Interventions and treatment measures can modify occupational asthma significantly. Therefore, assessment with outcomes measures may be incomplete without information about intervention or treatment. For occupational asthma, with its potential socioeconomic impact, the management of occupational asthma by the worker and his/her family becomes important to consider because it relates to drug treatment compliance, avoidance of allergens and irritants, and other avoidance behaviors (e.g., stop smoking). There is little reliable research information available on this subject for occupational asthma.

Occupational asthma usually is reasonably well controlled if the worker is moderately compliant with their recommended regimens and are removed from exposures to sensitizing agents and consequential irritant gases, fumes, and vapors. Outcome assessment for occupational asthma may combine asthma-specific measures with more generic measures. Asthma-specific measures for occupational asthma may emphasize the incidence and impact of asthma symptoms such as coughing, wheezing, sputum production, and shortness of breath, but can also include questions dealing with loss of income, reduced job satisfaction because of change or removal from work, abilities of performing activities of daily life, and capacity to work .

Burge (248) evaluated 39 electronics workers with colophony-induced asthma who were followed for 1 to 4 years. Most of the workers had a considerable reduction in their quality of life because of continuing asthma. Malo et al. (337) found the quality of life of subjects with occupational asthma who were removed from exposure to be worsened. The Quebec system of compensation for occupational asthma includes assessment of the functional and social outcomes of claimants and estimates the efficiency and cost. At the time of assessment, 2 years and more after the diagnosis, 93% of participants still demonstrated significant bronchial hyperresponsiveness and 84% required antiasthma medication. None of the participants remained exposed to the offending agent. Quality of life was mildly affected. The mean interval between the time claims were addressed and the first medicolegal decision was 8 months. The mean total cost (including temporary and permanent disability indemnities, and medical and technical costs) was $49,200 Canadian (minimum and maximum values of $2,100 and $330,900).

## PREVENTION

Removal from exposure can come about by a change of employment, a transfer within the same company to another facility without exposure, or to another job within the same plant without exposure. Because very low level exposures (e.g., in the parts per billion range) can trigger attacks in sensitized individuals, workers who remain in the same plant must be assured that they do not even transiently enter areas where the sensitizer is in use. In some instances, the patient may wish to remain in the same workplace. It is important that the workplace be altered in such a way that exposure can be drastically reduced.

When control of high level of exposures, rather than complete removal, is the goal, several methods may be used. Process changes can control exposures, for example, use of enclosed rather than open tanks of chemicals. Sensitizing chemicals at times can be replaced by less sensitizing or less volatile ones. Local exhaust ventilation, in which air is exhausted directly from the point of generation, may be effective if properly used. General dilution ventilation (increasing the overall ventilation to a room) is usually ineffective. Whenever there is unavoidable aerosolization, the aerosol should be contained at the source of generation by exhaust. Close attention to preventive maintenance of equipment may help to avoid spills. The level of exposure can be monitored continuously or intermittently.

Control options can include substituting another agent for one that causes sensitization. In the cotton industry, for example, experimental alterations of manufacturing processes such as washing and steaming of cotton before its early processing reduce disease. Changing the product formulation can reduce exposure to inhalants, as in the detergent industry, which encapsulated the proteolytic enzyme portion of the product to make it less dusty. Engineering dust and vapor suppression is the most effective way of lowering the average concentration of an inhalant. Of course, the most difficult kind of exposure to control is short, intermittent, peaks, which generally occur after some equipment or operational malfunction. While respiratory protection is useful under these circumstances, it is usually not possible to apply it before such an exposure occurs.

Medical surveillance programs, the keystone of prevention, should identify workers at increased risk for developing occupational asthma and detect disease at an early stage, when interventions are likely to be successful. An occupational health surveillance program may include preemployment and periodic medical examinations, immune status monitoring, and periodic spirometric or peak flow surveys. At this point in time, tests that measure nonspecific bronchial hyperresponsiveness should not be used as preemployment screening to exclude persons who might be at risk. There is no decisive evidence that preexisting bronchial hyperresponsiveness is a risk factor for development of occupational asthma. Nor is it appropriate to exclude atopic persons from employment. Finally, a smoking cessation program is an important option to consider.

## IMPAIRMENT AND DISABILITY

Because of the significant medical, medicolegal, social, and financial consequences, it is important that the diagnosis of occupational asthma be proven by objective means. The patient should be advised that he or she may be eligible for workers' compensation or similar benefits. Report to workers' compensation boards or similar agencies is often necessary for the patient to be able to leave exposure and should only take place after discussion with the patient. In the United States, the Americans with Disabilities Act mandates that employers make efforts toward "reasonable accommodation" of workers with disabilities.

Once a specific work-related cause of asthma is established, no further exposure is appropriate. A person so affected is usually considered 100% impaired on a permanent basis for the job that caused the asthma and for any job that involves exposure to the causative agent. This point emphasizes the importance of identifying the specific agent that is causing the asthma. The patient, however, is actually temporarily impaired once the diagnosis is established and removal from exposure ensues. Appropriate options for such workers may be vocational rehabilitation, job transfer (with wage retention), and possibly job modification. Retraining should be offered if necessary. Proper therapy should be instituted. Inadequate compensation may contribute to the workers' decision to remain exposed after diagnosis (336). Determining disability for occupational asthma may be difficult.

The level of permanent impairment usually can be assessed by 2 years after discontinuation of exposure, since the disease seems to plateau by that time. This may not be true for all subjects. For asthma without latency, where asthma onset is related to an accident or high-level irritant exposure, no specific workplace exposure is identifiable. Rather, avoidance or reduction of the levels of workplace irritants seems to be an appropriate option. Unfortunately, very little valid guidance is available on assessment of impairment and disability in subjects with occupational asthma (338).

The determination of impairment can be based on two parameters: (a) pertinent clinical parameters (e.g., frequency of symptoms; degree of limitation; frequency of acute exacerbations as defined by objective indicators such as medication, physician visits, emergency room visits, and hospitalizations; amount of medication needed to control asthma; duration of asthma; severity as perceived by patient); and (b) physiologic parameters such as spirometry before and after bronchodilators and measurement of nonspecific bronchial responsiveness (with calculation of $PC_{20}$). Exercise testing and carbon monoxide diffusions and lung volumes probably are not required in well-established cases of occupational asthma (338).

Accurate categorization and early removal of those with occupational asthma from a sensitizer offers the best prognosis. This conclusion was based on the findings of Tarlo et al. (34), who reported that the Ontario Workers' Compensation Board reached a decision on 609 claims submitted to the Board between 1984 and 1988; occupational asthma was determined in 39% of claims, mostly to isocyanates; another 39% were accepted for aggravation of asthma from irritant exposures. Forty percent of persons with aggravation of asthma from irritant exposures were attributed to a spill or accidental exposure and 68% had preceding asthma. Those with aggravation of asthma from irritant exposures were more likely to have clearing of symptoms and were more likely to have remained in the same work. Of 200 occupational asthma (from a sensitizer), outcome was best for cases where there was early diagnosis and removal from exposure and milder impairment of pulmonary function at initial assessment.

## REFERENCES


1. Sakula A. Sir John Floyer's treatise of the asthma (1698). *Thorax* 1984;39:248–254.
2. Alberts WM, Brooks SM. Advances in occupational asthma. *Clin Chest Med* 1992;13(2):281–302.
3. Karasek S, Karasek M. Preliminary reports on the injurious effects of metal platinum, chromates, cyanides, hydrofluoric acid and amterial used by silver miners. 1911.
4. Figley K, Elrod R. Endemic asthma due to castor bean dust. *JAMA* 1928;90:79.
5. Chan-Yeung M, Malo JL. Occupational asthma. *Chest* 1987;91(6 suppl):130S–136S.
6. Task Force ACCP. Workshop on environmental and occupational asthma. *Chest* 1990;98(suppl):145S–252S.

7. Hendrick D, Fabbri L. Compensating occupational asthma. *Thorax* 1981;36:881–884.
8. Chan-Yeung M. Occupational asthma. *Environ Health Perspect* 1995; 103(suppl 6):249–252.
9. Canadian Thoracic Society. Occupational asthma: recommendation for diagnosis, management, and assessment of impairment. *Can Med Assoc J* 1989;140:1989.
10. Subcommittee on Occupational Allergy of the European Academy of Allergology and Clinical Immunology. Guidelines for the diagnosis of occupational asthma. *Clin Exp Allergy* 1992;22(1):103–108.
11. Bernstein D, Cohn J. Guideline for the diagnosis and evaluation of occupational lung disease: preface. *J Allergy Clin Immunol* 1988;84: 1989–1993.
12. Bright P, Burge PS. Occupational lung disease. 8. The diagnosis of occupational asthma from serial measurements of lung function at and away from work. *Thorax* 1996;51(8):857–863.
13. Burge PS. Diagnosis of occupational asthma. *Clin Exp Allergy* 1989; 19(6):649–652.
14. Newman Taylor AJ. Occupational asthma. *Postgrad Med J* 1988;64 (753):505–510.
15. Chan-Yeung M, Brooks SM, Alberts WM, et al. Consensus Statement of the American College of Chest Physicians. Assessment of asthma in the workplace. *Chest* 1995;108(4).
16. Chan-Yeung M. Occupational asthma. *Chest* 1990;98:148S–161S.
17. Smith D. Medical-legal definition of occupational asthma. *Chest* 1990;98:1007–1011.
18. Smith A, Brooks S. Absence of airway hyperreactivity to methacholine in worker sensitized to toluene diisocyanate (TDI). *J Occup Med* 1980;22:327–331.
19. Banks DE, Rando RJ, Barkman HW Jr. Persistence of toluene diisocyanate-induced asthma despite negligible workplace exposures. *Chest* 1990;97(1):121–125.
20. Hargreave FE, Ramsdale EH, Pugsley SO. Occupational asthma without bronchial hyperresponsiveness. *Am Rev Respir Dis* 1984;130(3): 513–515.
21. Moller D, McKay R, Bernstein I, Brooks S. Persistent airways disease caused by toluene diisocyanante. *Am Rev Respir Dis* 1986;134:175–176.
22. Cockcroft DW, Hoeppner VH, Werner GD. Recurrent nocturnal asthma after bronchoprovocation with Western Red Cedar sawdust: association with acute increase in non-allergic bronchial responsiveness. *Clin Allergy* 1984;14(1):61–68.
23. Brooks SM, Weiss MA, Bernstein IL. Reactive airways dysfunction syndrome (RADS): persistent asthma syndrome after high level irritant exposure. *Chest* 1985;88:376–384.
24. Tarlo SM, Broder I. Irritant-induced occupational asthma. *Chest* 1989;96(2):297–300.
25. Brooks SM. Bronchial asthma of occupational origin: a review. *Scand J Work Environ Health* 1977;3(2):53–72.
26. Blanc P. Occupational asthma in a national disability survey. *Chest* 1987;92:613–617.
27. Malo J-L. Compensation for occupational asthma in Quebec. *Chest* 1990;98:236S–239S.
28. Axon EJ, Beach JR, Burge PS. A comparison of some of the characteristics of patients with occupational and non-occupational asthma. *J Occup Med* 1995;45(2):109–111.
29. Meredith S, Nordman H. Occupational asthma: measures of frequency from four countries. *Thorax* 1996;51(4):435–440.
30. Kogevinas M, Anto JM, Soriano JB, Tobias A, Burney P. The risk of asthma attributable to occupational exposures. A population-based study in Spain. Spanish Group of the European Asthma Study. *Am J Respir Crit Care Med* 1996;154(1):137–143.
31. Antti-Poika M, Nordman H, Koskenvuo M, Kaprio J, Jalava M. Role of occupational exposure to airway irritants in the development of asthma. *Int Arch Occup Environ Health* 1992;64(3):195–200.
32. Kremer AM, Pal TM, Boleij JS, Schouten JP, Rijcken B. Airway hyper-responsiveness and the prevalence of work-related symptoms in workers exposed to irritants. *Am J Ind Med* 1994;26(5):655–669.
33. Taylor AJ. Respiratory irritants encountered at work. *Thorax* 1996; 51(5):541–545.
34. Tarlo SM, Liss G, Corey P, Broder I. A workers' compensation claim population for occupational asthma. Comparison of subgroups. *Chest* 1995;107(3):634–641.
35. Xu X, Christiani DC. Occupational exposures and physician-diagnosed asthma. *Chest* 1993;104(5):1364–1370.
36. Ng TP, Hong CY, Goh LG, Wong ML, Koh KT, Ling SL. Risks of asthma associated with occupations in a community-based case-control study. *Am J Ind Med* 1994;25(5):709–718.
37. Smith TA, Lumley KP. Work-related asthma in a population exposed to grain, flour and other ingredient dusts. *Occup Med (Oxf)* 1996; 46(1):37–40.
38. Reilly MJ, Rosenman KD, Watt FC, et al. Surveillance for occupational asthma—Michigan and New Jersey, 1988–1992. *MMWR CDC Surveill Summ* 1994;43(1):9–17.
39. Timmer S, Rosenman K. Occurrence of occupational asthma. *Chest* 1993;104(3):816–820.
40. Chan-Yeung M, Vedal S, Kus J, et al. Symptoms, pulmonary function and airway hyperreactivity in Western red cedar compared to those in the office workers. *Am Rev Respir Dis* 1984;130:1038–1042.
41. Malo JL, Cartier A, L Archeveque J, Trudeau C, Courteau JP, Bherer L. Prevalence of occupational asthma among workers exposed to eastern white cedar. *Am J Respir Crit Care Med* 1994;150(6 Pt 1): 1697–1701.
42. Vandenplas O, Delwiche JP, Evrard G, et al. Prevalence of occupational asthma due to latex among hospital personnel. *Am J Respir Crit Care Med* 1995;151(1):54–60.
43. Armentia A, Martin-Santos JM, Quintero A, et al. Bakers' asthma: prevalence and evaluation of immunotherapy with a wheat flour extract. *Ann Allergy* 1990;65(4):265–272.
44. Houba R, Heederik DJ, Doekes G, van Run PE. Exposure-sensitization relationship for alpha-amylase allergens in the baking industry. *Am J Respir Crit Care Med* 1996;154(1):130–136.
45. Agrup G, Belin L, Sjostedt L, Skerfving S. Allergy to laboratory animals in laboratory technicians and animal keepers. *Br J Ind Med* 1986;43(3):192–198.
46. Burge PS, Edge G, Hawkins R, White V, Taylor AJ. Occupational asthma in a factory making flux-cored solder containing colophony. *Thorax* 1981;36(11):828–834.
47. Malo JL, Cartier A, L Archeveque J, et al. Prevalence of occupational asthma and immunologic sensitization to guar gum among employees at a carpet-manufacturing plant. *J Allergy Clin Immunol* 1990;86(4 Pt 1):562–569.
48. Siracusa A, Kennedy SM, DyBuncio A, Lin FJ, Marabini A, Chan-Yeung M. Prevalence and predictors of asthma in working groups in British Columbia. *Am J Ind Med* 1995;28(3):411–423.
49. Malo JL, Cartier A, Boulet LP, et al. Bronchial hyperresponsiveness can improve while spirometry plateaus two to three years after repeated exposure to chlorine causing respiratory symptoms. *Am J Respir Crit Care Med* 1994;150(4):1142–1145.
50. Chan-Yeung M, Lam S, Kennedy SM, et al. Persistent asthma after repeated exposure to high concentrations of gases in pulpmills. *Am J Respir Crit Care Med* 1994;149:1676–1680.
51. Vedal S, Chan-Yeung M, Enarson D, et al. Symptoms and pulmonary function in Western red cedar workers related to duration of employment and dust exposure. *Arch Environ Health* 1986;41(3):179–183.
52. Brooks SM, Edwards JJ, Edwards FH. An epidemiologic study of workers exposed to Western red cedar and other dusts. *Chest* 1981;80: 30S–32S.
53. Wegman DH, Pagnotto LD, Fine LM, Peters JM. A dose-response relationship in TDI workers. *J Occup Med* 1974;16:258–260.
54. Musk A, Venables K, Crooks B, et al. Respiratory symptoms, lung function and sensitization to flour in a British bakery. *Br J Ind Med* 1989;46:636–642.
55. Jones RN, Rando RJ, Glindmeyer HW, et al. Abnormal lung function in polyurethane foam producers. Weak relationship to toluene diisocyanate exposures. *Am Rev Respir Dis* 1992;146(4):871–877.
56. Di Stefano A, Saetta M, Maestrelli P, et al. Mast cells in the airway mucosa and rapid development of occupational asthma induced by toluene diisocyanate. *Am Rev Respir Dis* 1993;147(4):1005–1009.
57. Venables KM, Newman Taylor AJ. Exposure-response relationships in asthma caused by tetrachlorophthalic anhydride. *J Allergy Clin Immunol* 1990;85(1 Pt 1):55–58.
58. Zuskin E, Mustajbegovic J, Schachter EN. Follow-up study of respiratory function in hemp workers. *Am J Ind Med* 1994;26(1):103–115.
59. Soyseth V, Kongerud J, Ekstrand J, Boe J. Relation between exposure to fluoride and bronchial responsiveness in aluminum potroom workers with work-related asthma-like symptoms. *Thorax* 1994;49(10): 984–989.
60. Grammer LC, Shaughnessy MA, Henderson J, et al. A clinical and

immunologic study of workers with trimellitic-anhydride-induced immunologic lung disease after transfer to low exposure jobs. *Am Rev Respir Dis* 1993;148(1):54–57.
61. Diem JE, Jones RN, Hendricks DJ, et al. Five-year longitudinal study in a new toluene diisocyanate manufacturing plant. *Am Rev Respir Dis* 1982;126:420–428.
62. Jones RN, Diem JE, Glindmeyer H, et al. Mill effect and dose-response relationship in byssinosis. *Br J Ind Med* 1979;36:305–313.
63. Johnson A, Chan-Yeung M, MacLean L, et al. Respiratory abnormalities among workers in an iron and steel foundry in Vancouver. *Br J Ind Med* 1985;42:94–100.
64. Anto J, Sunyer J, Rodriguez-Roisin R, Suarez-Cervera ML. Community outbreak of asthma associated with inhalation of soybean dust. *N Engl J Med* 1989;320:1097–1102.
65. Nordman H. Atopy and work. *Scand J Work Environ Health* 1984;10: 481–485.
66. Bernstein DI. Occupational asthma. *Med Clin North Am* 1992;76(4): 917–934.
67. Flindt ML. Biological miracles and misadventures: identification of sensitization and asthma in enzyme detergent workers. *Am J Ind Med* 1996;29(1):99–110.
68. Sjostedt L, Willers S, Orbaek P. A follow-up study of laboratory animal exposed workers: the influence of atopy for the development of occupational asthma. *Am J Ind Med* 1993;24(4):459–469.
69. Newill CA, Prenger VL, Fish JE, et al. Risk factors for increased airway responsiveness to methacholine challenge among laboratory animal workers. *Am Rev Respir Dis* 1992;146(6):1494–1500.
70. De Zotti R, Molinari S, Larese F, Bovenzi M. Pre-employment screening among trainee bakers. *Occup Environ Med* 1995;52(4):279–283.
71. De Zotti R, Larese F, Bovenzi M, Negro C, Molinari S. Allergic airway disease in Italian bakers and pastry makers. *Occup Environ Med* 1994;51(8):548–552.
72. Brooks SM, Baker DB, Gann PH, et al. Cold air challenge and platinum skin reactivity in platinum refinery workers. Bronchial reactivity precedes skin prick response. *Chest* 1990;97(6):1401–1407.
73. Lam S, Chan-Yeung M. Ethylenediamine-induced asthma. *Am Rev Respir Dis* 1980;121:151–155.
74. Vallieres M, Cockcroft DW, Taylor DM, et al. Dimethyl ethanolamine-induced asthma. *Am Rev Respir Dis* 1977;115:867–871.
75. Chan-Yeung M. Mechanism of occupational asthma due to Western red cedar *(Thuja plicata)*. *Am J Ind Med* 1994;25(1):13–18.
76. Calverley AE, Rees D, Dowdeswell RJ, Linnett PJ, Kielkowski D. Platinum salt sensitivity in refinery workers: incidence and effects of smoking and exposure. *Occup Environ Med* 1995;52(10):661–666.
77. Beckett WS. The epidemiology of occupational asthma. *Eur Respir J* 1994;7(1):161–164.
78. Venables K, Topping M, Howe W, et al. Interaction of smoking and atopy in producing specific IgE antibody against a hapten-protein conjugate. *Br Med J* 1985;290:210–204.
79. Frew AJ, Kennedy SM, Chan-Yeung M. Methacholine responsiveness, smoking, and atopy as risk factors for accelerated FEV1 decline in male working populations. *Am Rev Respir Dis* 1992;146(4):878–883.
80. Brooks SM. Occupational asthma. *Toxicol Lett* 1995;82-83:39–45.
81. Douglas JD, McSharry C, Blaikie L, Morrow T, Miles S, Franklin D. Occupational asthma caused by automated salmon processing. *Lancet* 1995;346(8977):737–740.
82. Mapp CE, Corona PC, De Marzo N, Fabbri L. Persistent asthma due to isocyanates. A follow-up study of subjects with occupational asthma due to toluene diisocyanate (TDI). *Am Rev Respir Dis* 1988; 137(6):1326–1329.
83. Vedal S, Enarson DA, Chan H, Ochnio J, Tse KS, Chan-Yeung M. A longitudinal study of the occurrence of bronchial hyperresponsiveness in Western red cedar workers. *Am Rev Respir Dis* 1988;137(3): 651–655.
84. Burrows B, Halonen M, Barbee RA, Lebowitz MO. The relationship of serum immunoglobulin E to cigarette smoke. *Am Rev Respir Dis* 1981;124:523–525.
85. Zetterstrom O, Nordvall S, Bjorksten B, et al. Increased IgE responses in rats exposed to tobacco smoke. *J Allergy Clin Immunol* 1985;75: 594–598.
86. Goldie RG, Pedersen KE. Mechanisms of increased airway microvascular permeability: role in airway inflammation and obstruction. *Clin Exp Pharmacol Physiol* 1995;22(6-7):387–396.
87. Fabbri LM, Saetta M, Picotti G, Mapp CE. Late asthmatic reactions, airway inflammation and chronic asthma in toluene-diisocyanate-sensitized subjects. *Respiration* 1991;58(suppl 1):18–21.
88. Moller DR, Brooks SM, McKay RT, Cassedy K, Kopp S, Bernstein IL. Chronic asthma due to toluene diisocyanate. *Chest* 1986;90(4): 494–499.
89. Kongerud J, Soyseth V, Burge S. Serial measurements of peak expiratory flow and responsiveness to methacholine in the diagnosis of aluminum potroom asthma. *Thorax* 1992;47(4):292–297.
90. Newman LS. Occupational asthma. Diagnosis, management, and prevention. *Clin Chest Med* 1995;16(4):621–636.
91. Biagini RE, Moorman WJ, Lewis TR, Bernstein IL. Ozone enhancement of platinum asthma in primate model. *Am Rev Respir Dis* 1986; 134:719–725.
92. Reidel F, Krammer M, Scheibenbogen C, Geiger C. Effects of SO2 exposure on allergic sensitization in the guinea pig. *J Allergy Clin Immunol* 1988;82:527–534.
93. Osebold J, Gershwin L, Zee Y. Studies on the enhancement of allergic sensitization by the inhalation of ozone and sulfuric acid aerosol. *J Environ Pathol Toxicol Oncol* 1990;3:221–234.
94. Zwick H, Popp W, Budick G, et al. Increased sensitization to aero-allergens in competitive swimmers. *Lung* 1990;168:111–115.
95. Rylander R, Donham KJ, Hjort C, Brouwer R, Heederik D. Effect of exposure to dust in swine confinement building- a working group report. *Scand J Work Environ Health* 1989;15:309–312.
96. Zhong NS, Chen RC, Yang MO, Wu ZY, Zheng JP, Li YF. Is asymptomatic bronchial hyperresponsiveness an indication of potential asthma? A two-year follow-up of young students with bronchial hyperresponsiveness. *Chest* 1992;102(4):1104–1109.
97. Jones A. Asymptomatic bronchial hyperreactivity and the development of asthma and other respiratory tract illnesses in children. *Thorax* 1994;49(8):757–761.
98. Lam S, LeRiche J, Phillips D, Chan-Yeung M. Cellular and protein changes in bronchial lavage fluid after late asthmatic reaction in patients with red cedar asthma. *J Allergy Clin Immunol* 1987;80(1):44–50.
99. Bakke P, Baste V, Gulsvik A. Bronchial responsiveness in a Norwegian Community. *Am Rev Respir Dis* 1991;143:317–322.
100. Woolcock A, Peat J, Salome C, et al. Prevalence of bronchial responsiveness and asthma in a rural adult population. *Thorax* 1987;42: 361–368.
101. Sparrow D, O'Connor G, Colton T, Barry CL, Weiss ST. The relationship of nonspecific bronchial responsiveness to the occurrence of respiratory symptoms and decreased levels of pulmonary function. *Am Rev Respir Dis* 1987;135:1255–1260.
102. Cockcroft D, Killian D, Mellon J, Hargreave F. Bronchial reactivity to inhaled histamine. A method and clinical survey. *Clin Allergy* 1977;7: 235–243.
103. Weiler JM, Metzger WJ, Donnelly AL, Crowley ET, Sharath MD. Prevalence of bronchial hyperresponsiveness in highly trained athletes. *Chest* 1986;90(1):23–28.
104. Frew AJ, Chan H, Lam S, Chan-Yeung M. Bronchial inflammation in occupational asthma due to Western red cedar. *Am J Respir Crit Care Med* 1995;151(2 Pt 1):340–344.
105. Boulet LP, Boutet M, Laviolette M, et al. Airway inflammation after removal from the causal agent in occupational asthma due to high and low molecular weight agents. *Eur Respir J* 1994;7(9):1567–1575.
106. Van De Graaf E, Out T, Roos C, Jansen H. Respiratory membrane permeability and bronchial hyperreactivity in patients with stable asthma. Effects of therapy with inhaled steroids. *Am Rev Respir Dis* 1991;143: 362–368.
107. Chan-Yeung M, Desjardins A. Bronchial hyperresponsiveness and level of exposure in occupational asthma due to Western red cedar *(Thuja plicata)*. Serial observations before and after development of symptoms. *Am Rev Respir Dis* 1992;146(6):1606–1609.
108. Lemiere C, Cartier A, Dolovich J, et al. Outcome of specific bronchial responsiveness to occupational agents after removal from exposure. *Am J Respir Crit Care Med* 1996;154(2 Pt 1):329–333.
109. Malo J-L, Cartier A, Ghezzo H, Lafrance M, McCants M, Lehrer SB. Patterns of improvement in spirometry, bronchial hyperresponsiveness and specific IgE antibody levels after cessation of exposure in occupational asthma caused by crab processing. *Am Rev Respir Dis* 1988;138:807–812.
110. Paggiaro PL, Vagaggini B, Dente FL, et al. Bronchial hyperresponsiveness and toluene diisocyanate. Long-term change in sensitized asthmatic subjects. *Chest* 1993;103(4):1123–1128.

111. Laitinen L, Laitinen A, Haahtela T. Airway mucosal inflammation even in patients with newly diagnosed asthma. *Am Rev Respir Dis* 1993;147:697–704.
112. Saetta M, Di Stefano A, Maestrelli P, et al. Airway mucosal inflammation in occupational asthma induced by toluene diisocyanate. *Am Rev Respir Dis* 1992;145(1):160–168.
113. Maestrelli P, Del Prete GF, De Carli M, et al. CD8 T-cell clones producing interleukin-5 and interferon-gamma in bronchial mucosa of patients with asthma induced by toluene diisocyanate. *Scand J Work Environ Health* 1994;20(5):376–381.
114. Mapp CE, Lapa E, Silva JR, et al. Inflammatory events in the blood and airways of guinea pigs immunized to toluene diisocyanate. *Am J Respir Crit Care Med* 1996;154(1):201–208.
115. Busse WW, Calhoun WF, Sedgwick JD. Mechanism of airway inflammation in asthma. *Am Rev Respir Dis* 1993;147(6 Pt 2):S20–24.
116. Fabbri LM, Boschetto P, Zocca E, et al. Bronchoalveolar neutrophilia during late asthmatic reactions induced by toluene diisocyanate. *Am Rev Respir Dis* 1987;136(1):36–42.
117. Braman SS, Corrao WM. Bronchoprovocation testing. *Clin Chest Med* 1989;10(2):165–176.
118. Leff A. State of the art. Endogenous regulation of bronchomotor tone. *Am Rev Respir Dis* 1988;137:1198–1216.
119. Burrows B, Sears MR, Flannery EM, Herbison GP, Holdaway MD, Silva PA. Relation of the course of bronchial responsiveness from age 9 to age 15 to allergy. *Am J Respir Crit Care Med* 1995;152(4 Pt 1): 1302–1308.
120. Lebowitz MD, Bronnimann S, Camilli AE. Asthmatic risk factors and bronchial reactivity in non-diagnosed asthmatic adults. *Eur J Epidemiol* 1995;11(5):541–548.
121. Mortagy A, Howell J, Waters W. Respiratory symptoms and bronchial reactivity: identification of a syndrome and its relation to asthma. *Br Med J* 1986;293:525–529.
122. Brooks SM, Bernstein IL, Raghuprasad PK, Maccia CA, Mieczkowski L. Assessment of airway hyperresponsiveness in chronic stable asthma. *J Allergy Clin Immunol* 1990;85(1 Pt 1):17–26.
123. Friedman M, Kaliner M. Symposium on mast cells and asthma: human mast cells and asthma. *Am Rev Respir Dis* 1987;135:1157–1164.
124. Lozewicz S, Wells C, Gomez E, et al. Morphological integrity of the bronchial epithelium in mild asthma. *Thorax* 1990;45(1):12–15.
125. Lundgren R, Soderberg M, Horstedt P, Stenling R. Morphological studies of bronchial mucosal biopsies from asthmatics before and after ten years of treatment with inhaled steroids. *Eur Respir J* 1988; 1(10):883–889.
126. Laitinen L, Heino M, Laitinen A, Kava T, Haahtela T. Damage of the airway epithelium and bronchial reactivity in patients with asthma. *Am Rev Respir Dis* 1985;131:599–606.
127. Ernst P, Dales R, Nunes F, Becklake M. Relationship of airway responsiveness to duration of work in a dusty environment. *Thorax* 1989;44:116–120.
128. Fabbri LM, Maestrelli P, Saetta M, Mapp CM. Mechanisms of occupational asthma. *Clin Exp Allergy* 1994;24(7):628–635.
129. Campbell AM, Vignola AM, Chanez P, Godard P, Bousquet J. Low-affinity receptor for IgE on human bronchial epithelial cells in asthma. *Immunology* 1994;82(4):506–508.
130. Cartier A, Grammer L, Malo JL, et al. Specific serum antibodies against isocyanates: association with occupational asthma. *J Allergy Clin Immunol* 1989;84(4 Pt 1):507–514.
131. Machiels JJ, Somville MA, Lebrun PM, Lebecque SJ, Jacquemin MG, Saint-Remy JM. Allergic bronchial asthma due to Dermatophagoides pteronyssinus hypersensitivity can be efficiently treated by inoculation of allergen-antibody complexes. *J Clin Invest* 1990;85(4):1024–1035.
132. Maestrelli P, di Stefano A, Occari P, et al. Cytokines in the airway mucosa of subjects with asthma induced by toluene diisocyanate. *Am J Respir Crit Care* Med 1995;151(3 Pt 1):607–612.
133. Bignon JS, Aron Y, Ju LY, et al. HLA class II alleles in isocyanate-induced asthma. *Am J Respir Crit Care Med* 1994;149(1):71–75.
134. Balboni A, Baricordi OR, Fabbri LM, Gandini E, Ciaccia A, Mapp CE. Association between toluene diisocyanate-induced asthma and DQB1 markers: a possible role for aspartic acid at position 57. *Eur Respir J* 1996;9(2):207–210.
135. Boguniewicz M, Hayward A. Atopy, airway responsiveness, and genes. *Thorax* 1996;51(suppl 2):S55–59.
136. Sandford A, Weir T, Pare P. The genetics of asthma. *Am J Respir Crit Care Med* 1996;153(6 Pt 1):1749–1765.
137. van Herwerden L, Harrap SB, Wong ZY, et al. Linkage of high-affinity IgE receptor gene with bronchial hyperreactivity, even in absence of atopy. *Lancet* 1995;346:1262–1265.
138. Doull IJ, Lawrence S, Watson M, et al. Allelic association of gene markers on chromosomes 5q and 11q with atopy and bronchial hyperresponsiveness. *Am J Respir Crit Care Med* 1996;153(4 Pt 1): 1280–1284.
139. Postma DS, Bleecker ER, Amelung PJ, et al. Genetic susceptibility to asthma—bronchial hyperresponsiveness coinherited with a major gene for atopy. *N Engl J Med* 1995;333(14):894–900.
140. Lympany P, Welsh K, MacCochrane G, Kemeny DM, Lee TH. Genetic analysis using DNA polymorphism of the linkage between chromosome 11q13 and atopy and bronchial hyperresponsiveness to methacholine. *J Allergy Clin Immunol* 1992;89(2):619–628.
141. Arm JP, Lee TH. The pathobiology of bronchial asthma. *Adv Immunol* 1992;51:323–382.
141a. Howarth PH. The airway inflammatory response in allergic asthma and its relationship to clinical disease. *Allergy* 1995;50:13–21.
141b. Fraenkel DJ, Bardin PG, Sanderson G, Lampe F, Johnston SL, Holgate ST. Lower airways inflammation during rhinovirus colds in normal and in asthmatic subjects. *Am J Respir Crit Care Med* 1995;151: 879–886.
142. Harkonen H, Meyers C, Korhonen O, Winblad I. Long-term effect from exposure to sulfur dioxide: lung function four years after a pyrite dust explosion. *Am Rev Repir Dis* 1983;128:840–847.
143. Charan N, Meyer C, Lakshminarayan S, Spencer T. Pulmonary injuries associated with acute sulfur dioxide inhalation. *Am Rev Respir Dis* 1979;119:555–560.
144. Flury K, Ames D, Rodarte J, Rodgers R. Airway obstruction due to ammonia. *Mayo Clin Proc* 1989;58:389–393.
145. Donham K, Knapp L, Monson R, Gustafson K. Acute toxic exposure to gases from liquid manure. *J Occup Med* 1982;24:142–145.
146. Murphy D, Fairman R, Lapp NL. Severe airways disease due to the inhalation of fumes from cleaning agents. *Chest* 1976;69:372–376.
147. Hasan F, Gehshan A, Fulechan F. Resolution of pulmonary dysfunction following acute chlorine exposures. *Arch Environ Health* 1983; 38:76–80.
148. Kennedy S, Enarson D, Janssen R, Chan-Yeung M. Lung health consequences of repeated accidental chlorine gas exposure among pulp mill workers. *Am Rev Respir Dis* 1991;143:545–558.
149. Kowitz T, Reba R, Parker R, Spicer W. Effects of chlorine gas on respiratory function. *Arch Environ Health* 1967;14:545–558.
150. Kaufman J, Burkons D. Clinical, roentgenologic and physiologic effects of acute chlorine exposure. *Arch Environ Health* 1971;23: 29–34.
151. Axford A, McKerrow C, Jones A, Lequesne P. Accidental exposure to isocyanate fumes on a group of firemen. *Br J Ind Med* 1967;33:65–71.
152. Boulet L-P. Increases in airway responsiveness following acute exposure to respiratory irritants. Reactive airway dysfunction syndrome or occupational asthma? *Chest* 1988;94(3):476–481.
153. Luo J-CJ, Nelsen K, Fischbein A. Persistent reactive airway dysfunction after exposure to toluene diisocyanate. *Br J Ind Med* 1988;47:239–241.
154. Alford PT, McLees BD, Case LD, et al. Reactive airways dysfunction syndrome (RADS) in workers post exposure to sulfur dioxide (SO2). *Chest* 1988;94:87S.
155. Moisan TC. Prolonged asthma after smoke inhalation: a report of three cases and a review of previous reports. *J Occup Med* 1991;33: 458–461.
156. Wade JFD, Newman LS. Diesel asthma. Reactive airways disease following overexposure to locomotive exhaust. *J Occup Med* 1993;35(2): 149–154.
157. Bernstein IL, Bernstein DI. Reactive airways dysfunction syndrome (RADS) after exposure to toxic ammonia fumes. *J Allergy Clin Immunol* 1989;83:173–179.
158. Gilbert R, Auchincloss J Jr. Reactive airways dysfunction syndrome presenting as a reversible restrictive defect. *Lung* 1989;167:55–61.
159. Bherer L, Cushman R, Courteau JP, et al. Survey of construction workers repeatedly exposed to chlorine over a 3 to 6 month period in a pulpmill: II. Follow-up of affected workers by questionnaire, spirometry, and assessment of bronchial responsiveness 18 to 24 months after exposure ended. *Occup Environ Med* 1994;51:225–228.
160. Gautrin D, Boulet LP, Boutet M, et al. Is reactive airways dysfunction syndrome a variant of occupational asthma? *J Allergy Clin Immunol* 1994;93(1 Pt 1):12–22.

161. Moore B, Sherman M. Chronic reactive airways disease following acute chlorine gas exposure in an asymptomatic atopic patient. *Chest* 1991;100:855–856.
162. Schwartz DA, Smith DD, Lakshminarayan S. The pulmonary sequelae associated with accidental inhalation of chlorine gas. *Chest* 1990; 97:820–825.
163. Gadon ME, Melius JM, McDonald CJ, et al. New onset asthma after exposure to the steam system additive 2-diethylaminoethanolamine. *J Occup Med* 1994;36:623–626.
164. Promisloff R, Phan A, Lenchner G, Chichelli A. Reactive airways dysfunction syndrome in three police officers following a roadside chemical spill. *Chest* 1990;98:928–929.
165. Palczynski C, Gorski P, Jakubowski J. The case of TDI-induced reactive airways dysfunction syndrome with the persistence of specific IgE antibodies. *Allerg Immunopathol* 1994;22:80–82.
166. Cone JE, Wugofski L, Balmes JR, et al. Persistent respiratory health effects after metam sodium pesticide spill. *Chest* 1994;106:500–508.
167. Hu H, Christiani D. Reactive airways dysfunction syndrome after exposure to teargas. *Lancet* 1992;339:1535.
168. Kern DG. Outbreak of the reactive airways dysfunction syndrome after a spill of glacial acetic. *Am Rev Respir Dis* 1991;144:1058–1064.
169. Alberts WM, do Pico GA. Reactive airways dysfunction syndrome. *Chest* 1996;109:1618–1626.
170. Brooks SM, Hammad Y, Richards I, Giovinco J, Jenkins K. The spectrum of irritant-induced asthma: sudden and not-so-sudden and the role of allergy. *Chest* 1998 (in press).
170a. Molfino N. Wright S, Katz I, et al. Effect of low concentrations of ozone on inhaled allergen responses in asthmatic subjects. *Lancet* 1991;338:199–203.
170b. Jorres R, Nowak D, Magnussen H, et al. The effect of ozone exposure on allergen responsiveness in subjects with asthma or rhinitis. Short-term $O_3$ increases bronchial allergen response with mild allergic asthma or rhinitis without asthma. *Am J Respir Crit Care Med* 1996;153:56–64.
171. Sokol WN, Aelony Y, Beall GN. Meat wrapper's asthma: an appraisal of a new occupational syndrome. *J Allergy Clin Immunol* 1973;226: 448–454.
172. Vandervort R, Brooks SM. Polyvinyl chloride film thermal decomposition products as an occupational illness of meat wrappers: I. Environmental exposures and toxicology. *J Occup Med* 1977;19:189–191.
173. Brooks SM, Vandervort R. Polyvinyl chloride film thermal decomposition products as an occupational illness of meat wrappers: II. Clinical studies. *J Occup Med* 1977;19:192–196.
174. Jones RN, Weill H. Respiratory health and polyvinyl chloride fumes. *JAMA* 1977;237:1826–1829.
175. Schachter EN, Witek TJ Jr, Brody DJ, Tosun T, Beck GJ, Leaderer BP. A study of respiratory effects from exposure to 2.0 ppm formaldehyde in occupationally exposed workers. *Environ Res* 1987;44(2):188–205.
176. Uba G, Pachorek D, Bernstein J, et al. Prospective study of respiratory effects of formaldehyde among healthy and asthmatic medical students. *Am J Ind Med* 1989;15:91–101.
177. Grammer LC, Harris KE, Cugell DW, Patterson R. Evaluation of a worker with possible formaldehyde-induced asthma. *J Allergy Clin Immunol* 1993;92(1 Pt 1):29–33.
178. Jarvholm B, Ljungkvist G, Lavenius B, Rodin N, Peterson C. Acetic aldehyde and formaldehyde in cutting fluids and their relation to irritant symptoms. *Ann Occup Hyg* 1995;39(5):591–601.
179. Kennedy SM, Greaves IA, Kriebel D, Eisen EA, Smith TJ, Woskie SR. Acute pulmonary responses among automobile workers exposed to aerosols of machining fluids. *Am J Ind Med* 1989;15(6):627–641.
180. Savonius B, Keskinen H, Tuppurainen M, Kanerva L. Occupational asthma caused by ethanolamines. *Allergy* 1994;49(10):877–881.
181. Gross NJ. Allergy to laboratory animals: epidemiologic, clinical and physiologic aspects, and a trial of cromolyn in its management. *J Allergy Clin Immunol* 1980;66:158–162.
182. Newill CA, Eggleston PA, Prenger VL, et al. Prospective study of occupational asthma to laboratory animal allergens: stability of airway responsiveness to methacholine challenge for one year. *J Allergy Clin Immunol* 1995;95(3):707–715.
183. Renstrom A, Malmberg P, Larsson K, Larsson PH, Sundblad BM. Allergic sensitization is associated with increased bronchial responsiveness: a prospective study of allergy to laboratory animals. *Eur Respir J* 1995;8(9):1514–1519.
184. Slovak A, Hill R. Does atopy have a predictive value for laboratory animal allergy? A comparison of different concepts of atopy. *Br J Ind Med* 1987;44:129–132.
185. Newman-Taylor A, Meyers JR, Longbottom JL, Spackman D, Slovak AJM. Immunological differences between asthma and other allergic reactions in laboratory animal workers. *Thorax* 1981;36:329–334.
186. Franz T, McMurrain KD, Brooks SM, Bernstein IL. Clinical, immunologic and physiologic observations in factory workers exposed to B. subtilis dust. *J Allergy* 1971;47:170–180.
187. Novey HS, Marchioli LE, Sokol WN, Wells ID. Papain-induced asthma—physiological and immunological features. *J Allergy Clin Immunol* 1979;63(2):98–103.
188. Milne J, Brand S. Occupational asthma after inhalation of dust of the proteolytic enzyme, papain. *Br J Ind Med* 1975;32:302–307.
189. Wu CH, Lee MF, Liao SC, Luo SF. Sequencing analysis of cDNA clones encoding the American cockroach Cr-PI allergens. Homology with insect hemolymph proteins. *J Biol Chem* 1996;271(30):17937–17943.
189a. Desjardins A, Malo JL, J LA, Cartier A, McCants M, Lehrer SB. Occupational IgE-mediated sensitization and asthma caused by clam and shrimp. *J Allergy Clin Immunol* 1995;96:608–617.
189b. Cartier A, Malo JL, Forest F, et al. Occupational asthma in snow crab-processing workers. *J Allergy Clin Immunol* 1984;74:261–269.
190. Hudson P, Cartier A, Pineau L, et al. Follow-up of occupational asthma caused by crab and various agents. *J Allergy Clin Immunol* 1985;76(5):682–688.
191. Malo JL, Cartier A. Occupational asthma caused by exposure to ash wood dust *(Fraxinus americana)*. *Eur Respir J* 1989;2(4):385–387.
192. Enarson DA, Chan-Yeung M. Characterization of health effects of wood dust exposures. *Am J Ind Med* 1990;17(1):33–38.
193. Malo JL, Cartier A, Desjardins A, Van de Weyer R, Vandenplas O. Occupational asthma caused by oak wood dust. *Chest* 1995;108(3): 856–858.
194. Malmberg PO, Rask-Andersen A, Larsson KA, Stjernberg N, Sundblad BM, Eriksson K. Increased bronchial responsiveness in workers sawing Scots pine. *Am J Respir Crit Care Med* 1996;153(3):948–952.
195. Reijula K, Kujala V, Latvala J. Sauna builder's asthma caused by obeche (Triplochiton scleroxylon) dust. *Thorax* 1994;49(6):622–623.
196. Tarlo SM, Wai Y, Dolovich J, Summerbell R. Occupational asthma induced by Chrysonilia sitophila in the logging industry. *J Allergy Clin Immunol* 1996;97(6):1409–1413.
197. Chan-Yeung M, Malo JL. Aetiological agents in occupational asthma [see comments]. *Eur Respir J* 1994;7(2):346–371.
198. Selki K. Asthma attack among carpenters using Western red cedar lumber. *Jpn Soc Intern Med* 1926;13:884–887.
199. Chan-Yeung M, Barton GM, MacLean L, Gryzbowski S. Occupational asthma and rhinitis due to Western red cedar *(Thuja plicata)*. *Am Rev Respir Dis* 1973;108:1094–1102.
200. Chan-Yeung M. Immunologic and nonimmunologic mechanisms in asthma due to Western red cedar *(Thuja plicata)*. *J Allegy Clin Immunol* 1982;70:32–37.
201. Cartier A, Chan H, Malo JL, Pineau L, Tse KS, Chan-Yeung M. Occupational asthma caused by eastern white cedar (Thuja occidentalis) with demonstration that plicatic acid is present in this wood dust and is the causal agent. *J Allergy Clin Immunol* 1986;77(4):639–645.
202. Tse KS, Chan H, Chan-Yeung M. Specific IgE antibodies in workers with occupational asthma due to Western red cedar. *Clin Allergy* 1982; 12(3):249–258.
203. Vedal S, Chan-Yeung M, Enarson DA, Chan H, Dorken E, Tse KS. Plicatic acid-specific IgE and nonspecific bronchial hyperresponsiveness in Western red-cedar workers. *J Allergy Clin Immunol* 1986; 78(6):1103–1109.
204. Frew A, Chan H, Dryden P, Salari H, Lam S, Chan-Yeung M. Immunologic studies of the mechanisms of occupational asthma caused by Western red cedar. *J Allergy Clin Immunol* 1993;92(3):466–478.
205. Malo JL, Ghezzo H, D Aquino C, L Archeveque J, Cartier A, Chan-Yeung M. Natural history of occupational asthma: relevance of type of agent and other factors in the rate of development of symptoms in affected subjects. *J Allergy Clin Immunol* 1992;90(6 Pt 1):937–944.
206. Enarson DA, Chan-Yeung M, Tabona M, Kus J, Vedal S, Lam S. Predictors of bronchial hyperexcitability in grainhandlers. *Chest* 1985; 87(4):452–455.
207. Dosman JA, Cotton DJ, Graham BL, et al. Chronic bronchitis and decreased forced expiratory flow rates in lifetime nonsmoking grain workers. *Am Rev Respir Dis* 1980;121:11–16.
208. Chan-Yeung M, Schulzer M, MacLean L, et al. Epidemiologic health

survey of grain elevator workers in British Colombia. *Am Rev Respir Dis* 1980;115:915–927.
209. Gimenez C, Fouad K, Choudat D, Laureillard J, Bouscaillou P, Leib E. Chronic and acute respiratory effects among grain mill workers. *Int Arch Occup Environ Health* 1995;67(5):311–315.
210. Prichard MG, Ryan G, Walsh BJ, Musk AW. Skin test and RAST responses to wheat and common allergens and respiratory disease in bakers. *Clin Allergy* 1985;15(2):203–210.
211. Sunyer J, Anto JM, Sabria J, et al. Risk factors for soybean epidemic asthma. *Am Rev Respir Dis* 1992;145:1098–1102.
212. Valdivieso R, Subiza J, Subiza JL, Hinojosa M, de Carlos E, Subiza E. Bakers' asthma caused by alpha amylase. *Ann Allergy* 1994;73(4): 337–342.
213. Lavaud F, Perdu D, Prevost A, Vallerand H, Cossart C, Passemard F. Baker's asthma related to soybean lecithin exposure [see comments]. *Allergy* 1994;49(3):159–162.
214. Sandiford CP, Tee RD, Taylor AJ. The role of cereal and fungal amylases in cereal flour hypersensitivity. *Clin Exp Allergy* 1994;24(6):549–557.
215. Baur XS, Weiss W, Fruhmann W. Inhalant allergens in modern baking industry. *Immunol Allergy Pract* 1989;11:13–15.
216. Lachance P, Cartier A, Dolovich J, Malo JL. Occupational asthma from reactivity to an alkaline hydrolysis derivative of gluten. *J Allergy Clin Immunol* 1988;81(2):385–390.
216a. Blanco Carmona JG, Juse Picon S, Garces Sotillos M, Rodriguez Gaston P. Occupational asthma in the confectionary industry caused by sensitivity to egg. *Allergy* 1992;47:190–191.
216b. Bernaola G, Echechipia S, Urrutia K, Fernandez E, Audicana M, Fernandez de Corres L. Occupational asthma and rhinoconjunctivitis from inhalation of dried cow's milk caused by sensitization to alpha-lactalbumin. *Allergy* 1994;49:189–191.
216c. Yap JC, Chan CC, Wang YT, Poh SC, Lee HS, Tan TK. A case of occupational asthma due to barley grain dust. *Ann Acad Med Singapore* 1994;23:734–736.
217. Blainey A, Topping M, Olliers S, Davies R. Allergic respiratory disease in grain workers: the role of storage mites. *J Allergy Clin Immunol* 1989;84:296–303.
218. Revsbech P, Dueholm M. Stoage mite allergy among bakers. *Allergy* 1990;45:555–564.
219. Ehrlich RI. Fatal asthma in a baker: a case report. *Am J Ind Med* 1994; 26(6):799–802.
220. Vandenplas O. Occupational asthma caused by natural rubber latex. *Eur Respir J* 1995;8(11):1957–1965.
221. Tarlo SM, Wong L, Roos J, Booth N. Occupational asthma caused by latex in a surgical glove manufacturing plant. *J Allergy Clin Immunol* 1990;85(3):626–631.
222. Vandenplas O, Delwiche JP, Sibille Y. Occupational asthma due to latex in a hospital administrative employee. *Thorax* 1996;51(4):452–453.
223. Brugnami G, Marabini A, Siracusa A, Abbritti G. Work-related late asthmatic response induced by latex allergy. *J Allergy Clin Immunol* 1995;96(4):457–464.
224. Hunt LW, Fransway AF, Reed CE, et al. An epidemic of occupational allergy to latex involving health care workers. *J Occup Environ Med* 1995;37(10):1204–1209.
225. Orfan NA, Reed R, Dykewicz MS, Ganz M, Kolski GB. Occupational asthma in a latex doll manufacturing plant. *J Allergy Clin Immunol* 1994;94(5):826–830.
226. Pisati G, Baruffini A, Bernabeo F, Stanizzi R. Bronchial provocation testing in the diagnosis of occupational asthma due to latex surgical gloves. *Eur Respir J* 1994;7(2):332–336.
227. de la Hoz B, Fernandez-Rivas M, Quirce S, et al. Swiss chard hypersensitivity: clinical and immunologic study. *Ann Allergy* 1991;67(5): 487–492.
228. Kraut A, Peng Z, Becker AB, Warren CP. Christmas candy maker's asthma. IgG4-mediated pectin allergy [see comments]. *Chest* 1992; 102(5):1605–1607.
229. Cartier A, Malo JL. Occupational asthma due to tea dust. *Thorax* 1990;45(3):203–206.
230. Roberts JA, Thomson NC. Tea-dust induced asthma. *Eur Respir J* 1988;1(8):769–770.
231. Quirce S, Diez Gomez ML, Hinojosa M, et al. Housewives with raw potato-induced bronchial asthma. *Allergy* 1989;44(8):532–536.
232. Blanco C, Carrillo T, Quiralte J, Pascual C, Martin Esteban M, Castillo R. Occupational rhinoconjunctivitis and bronchial asthma due to Phoenix canariensis pollen allergy. *Allergy* 1995;50(3):277–280.
233. Subiza J, Subiza JL, Escribano PM, et al. Occupational asthma caused by Brazil ginseng dust. *J Allergy Clin Immunol* 1991;88(5):731–736.
234. Rosenman KD, Hart M, Ownby DR. Occupational asthma in a beet sugar processing plant. *Chest* 1992;101(6):1720–1722.
235. Sastre J, Olmo M, Novalvos A, Ibanez D, Lahoz C. Occupational asthma due to different spices. *Allergy* 1996;51(2):117–120.
236. Lybarger JA, Gallagher JS, Pulver DW, Litwin A, Brooks S, Bernstein IL. Occupational asthma induced by inhalation and ingestion of garlic. *J Allergy Clin Immunol* 1982;69(5):448–454.
237. Baur X. Occupational asthma due to isocyanates. *Lung* 1996;174(1): 23–30.
238. Lowenthal M, Shaughnessy MA, Harris KE, Grammer LC. Immunologic cross-reactivity of acid anhydrides with immunoglobulin E against trimellityl-human serum albumin. *J Lab Clin Med* 1994; 123(6):869–873.
239. Baur X, Czuppon AB, Rauluk I, et al. A clinical and immunological study on 92 workers occupationally exposed to anhydrides. *Int Arch Occup Environ Health* 1995;67(6):395–403.
240. Drexler H, Weber A, Letzel S, Kraus G, Schaller KH, Lenhert G. Detection and clinical relevance of a type I allergy with occupational exposure to hexahydrophthalic anhydride and methyltetrahydrophthalic anhydride. *Int Arch Occup Environ Health* 1994;65(5): 279–283.
241. Grammer LC, Shaughnessy MA, Lowenthal M. Hemorrhagic rhinitis. An immunologic disease due to hexahydrophthalic anhydride. *Chest* 1993;104(6):1792–1794.
242. Bernstein DI, Patterson R, Zeiss CR. Clinical and immunologic evaluation of trimellitic anhydride-and phthalic anhydride-exposed workers using a questionnaire with comparative analysis of enzyme-linked immunosorbent and radioimmunoassay studies. *J Allergy Clin Immunol* 1982;69(3):311–318.
243. Grammer LC, Shaughnessy MA, Hogan MB, et al. Study of employees with anhydride-induced respiratory disease after removal from exposure. *J Occup Environ Med* 1995;37(7):820–825.
244. Hayes JP, Daniel R, Tee RD, Barnes PJ, Chung KF, Newman Taylor AJ. Specific immunological and bronchopulmonary responses following intradermal sensitization to free trimellitic anhydride in guinea pigs [see comments]. *Clin Exp Allergy* 1992;22(7):694–700.
245. Wernfors M, Nielsen J, Schutz A, Skerfving S. Phthalic anhydride-induced occupational asthma. *Int Arch Allergy Appl Immunol* 1986; 79(1):77–82.
246. Gannon PF, Sherwood Burge P, Hewlett C, Tee RD. Haemolytic anaemia in a case of occupational asthma due to maleic anhydride. *Br J Ind Med* 1992;49(2):142–143.
247. Gerhardsson L, Grammer LC, Shaughnessy MA, Patterson R. IgG subclass antibody against trimellitic anhydride in workers with and without immunologic lung diseases. *J Occup Med* 1992;34(10): 989–992.
248. Burge PS. Occupational asthma in electronics workers caused by colophony fumes: follow-up of affected workers. *Thorax* 1982;37(5): 348–353.
249. Sadhra S, Foulds IS, Gray CN, Koh D, Gardiner K. Colophony—uses, health effects, airborne measurement and analysis. *Ann Occup Hyg* 1994;38(4):385–396.
250. Burge PS, IM OB, Harries MG. Peak flow rate records in the diagnosis of occupational asthma due to colophony. *Thorax* 1979;34(3): 308–316.
251. Kanerva L, Keskinen H, Autio P, Estlander T, Tuppurainen M, Jolanki R. Occupational respiratory and skin sensitization caused by polyfunctional aziridine hardener. *Clin Exp Allergy* 1995;25(5): 432–439.
252. Kopp S, McKay R, Moller D, Cassedy K, Brooks S. Asthma and rhinitis due to ethylcyanoacrylate instant glue. *Ann Intern Med* 1985;102: 613–615.
253. Nakazawa T. Occupational asthma due to alkyl cyanoacrylate. *J Occup Med* 1990;32(8):709–710.
254. Blainey AD, Ollier S, Cundell D, Smith RE, Davies RJ. Occupational asthma in a hairdressing salon. *Thorax* 1986;41(1):42–50.
255. Merget R, Buenemann A, Kulzer R, et al. A cross sectional study of chemical industry workers with occupational exposure to persulphates. *Occup Environ Med* 1996;53(6):422–426.
256. Wrbitzky R, Drexler H, Letzel S. Early reaction type allergies and diseases of the respiratory passages in employees from persulphate production. *Int Arch Occup Environ Health* 1995;67(6):413–417.

257. Helin T, Makinen-Kiljunen S. Occupational asthma and rhinoconjunctivitis caused by senna. *Allergy* 1996;51(3):181–184.
258. Marks GB, Salome CM, Woolcock AJ. Asthma and allergy associated with occupational exposure to ispaghula and senna products in a pharmaceutical work force. *Am Rev Respir Dis* 1991;144(5):1065–1069.
259. Romano C, Sulotto F, Pavan I, Chiesa A, Scansetti G. A new case of occupational asthma from reactive dyes with severe anaphylactic response to the specific challenge. *Am J Ind Med* 1992;21(2): 209–216.
260. Nilsson R, Nordlinder R, Wass U, Meding B, Belin L. Asthma, rhinitis, and dermatitis in workers exposed to reactive dyes. *Br J Ind Med* 1993;50(1):65–70.
261. Hong CS, Park HS. Heterogeneity of IgE antibody response to reactive dye in sera from four different sensitized workers. *Clin Exp Allergy* 1992;22(6):606–610.
262. Park HS, Yu HJ, Jung KS. Occupational asthma caused by chromium. *Clin Exp Allergy* 1994;24(7):676–681.
263. Wang ZP, Larsson K, Malmberg P, Sjogren B, Hallberg BO, Wrangskog K. Asthma, lung function, and bronchial responsiveness in welders. *Am J Ind Med* 1994;26(6):741–754.
264. Desjardins A, Bergeron JP, Ghezzo H, Cartier A, Malo JL. Aluminum potroom asthma confirmed by monitoring of forced expiratory volume in one second. *Am J Respir Crit Care Med* 1994;150(6 Pt 1): 1714–1717.
265. Sorgdrager B, Pal TM, de Looff AJ, Dubois AE, de Monchy JG. Occupational asthma in aluminum potroom workers related to pre-employment eosinophil count. *Eur Respir J* 1995;8(9):1520–1524.
266. Abramson MJ, Wlodarczyk JH, Saunders NA, Hensley MJ. Does aluminum smelting cause lung disease? *Am Rev Respir Dis* 1989;139(4): 1042–1057.
267. Kongerud J, Boe J, Soyseth V, Naalsund A, Magnus P. Aluminum potroom asthma: the Norwegian experience. *Eur Respir J* 1994;7(1): 165–172.
268. Kongerud J, Soyseth V. Methacholine responsiveness, respiratory symptoms and pulmonary function in aluminum potroom workers. *Eur Respir J* 1991;4(2):159–166.
269. Soyseth V, Kongerud J, Aalen OO, Botten G, Boe J. Bronchial responsiveness decreases in relocated aluminum potroom workers compared with workers who continue their potroom exposure. *Int Arch Occup Environ Health* 1995;67(1):53–57.
270. Venables K, Dally MB, Nunn AJ, et al. Smoking and occupational allergy in workers in a platinum refinery. *Br Med J* 1989;299: 939–942.
271. Cromwell O, Pepys J, Parish WE, Hughes EG. Specific IgE antibodies to platinum salts in sensitized workers. *Clin Allergy* 1979;9: 109–117.
272. Merget R, Schultze-Werninghaus G, Bode F, Bergmann EM, Zachgo W, Meier-Sydow J. Quantitative skin prick and bronchial provocation tests with platinum salt. *Br J Ind Med* 1991;48(12):830–837.
273. Merget R, Reineke M, Rueckmann A, Bergmann EM, Schultze-Werninghaus G. Nonspecific and specific bronchial responsiveness in occupational asthma caused by platinum salts after allergen avoidance. *Am J Respir Crit Care Med* 1994;150(4):1146–1149.
274. Merget R, Caspari C, Kulzer R, Breitstadt R, Rueckmann A, Schultze-Werninghaus G. The sequence of symptoms, sensitization and bronchial hyperresponsiveness in early occupational asthma due to platinum salts. *Int Arch Allergy Immunol* 1995;107(1-3):406–407.
275. Dolovich J, Evans SL, Nieboer E. Occupational asthma from nickel sensitivity: I. Human serum albumin in the antigenic determinant. *Br J Ind Med* 1984;41(1):51–55.
276. Nieboer E, Evans SL, Dolovich J. Occupational asthma from nickel sensitivity: II. Factors influencing the interaction of Ni2-, HSA, and serum antibodies with nickel related specificity. *Br J Ind Med* 1984; 41(1):56–63.
277. Shirakawa T, Kusaka Y, Fujimura N, et al. Occupational asthma from cobalt sensitivity in workers exposed to hard metal dust. *Chest* 1989; 95(1):29–37.
278. Gheysens B, Auwerx J, Van den Eeckhout A, Demedts M. Cobalt-induced bronchial asthma in diamond polishers. *Chest* 1985;88(5): 740–744.
279. Van Cutsem EJ, Ceuppens JL, Lacquet LM, Demedts M. Combined asthma and alveolitis induced by cobalt in a diamond polisher. *Eur J Respir Dis* 1987;70(1):54–61.
280. Sprince NL, Oliver LC, Eisen EA, et al. Cobalt exposure and lung disease in tungsten carbide production. *Am Rev Respir Dis* 1988;138: 1220–1226.
281. Nelson WL. Allergic events among health care workers exposed to psyllium laxatives in the workplace. *J Occup Med* 1987;29:497–499.
282. Malo JL, Cartier A, Archeveque J, et al. Prevalence of occupational asthma and immunologic sensitization to psyllium among health personnel in chronic care hospitals. *Am Rev Respir Dis* 1990;142(6 Pt 1): 1359–1366.
283. Lee HS, Wang YT, Yeo CT, et al. Occupational asthma due to tylosin tartrate. *Br J Ind Med* 1989;46:498–499.
284. Moscato G, Galdi E, Scibilia J, et al. Occupational asthma, rhinitis and urticaria due to piperacillin sodium in a pharmaceutical worker. *Eur Respir J* 1995;8(3):467–469.
285. Agius RM, Davison AG, Hawkins ER, Newman Taylor AJ. Occupational asthma in salbutamol process workers. *Occup Environ Med* 1994;51(6):397–399.
286. Muller BA, Leick CA, Suelzer M, Piyamahunt A, Richerson HB. Prognostic value of methacholine challenge in patients with respiratory symptoms. *J Allergy Clin Immunol* 1994;94(1):77–87.
287. Paggiaro PL, Chan Yeung M. Pattern of specific airway response in asthma due to Western red cedar *(Thuja plicata)*: relationship with length of exposure and lung function measurements. *Clin Allergy* 1987;17(4):333–339.
288. Saetta M, Maestrelli P, Di Stefano A, et al. Effect of cessation of exposure to toluene diisocyanate (TDI) on bronchial mucosa of subjects with TDI-induced asthma. *Am Rev Respir Dis* 1992;145(1): 169–174.
289. Saetta M, Maestrelli P, Turato G, et al. Airway wall remodeling after cessation of exposure to isocyanates in sensitized asthmatic subjects. *Am J Respir Crit Care Med* 1995;151(2 Pt 1):489–494.
290. Chan-Yeung M, Lam S, Koener S. Clinical features and natural history of occupational asthma due to Western red cedar *(Thuja plicata)*. *Am J Med* 1982;72(3):411–415.
291. Malo JL, Cartier A, Cote J, et al. Influence of inhaled steroids on recovery from occupational asthma after cessation of exposure: an 18-month double-blind crossover study. *Am J Respir Crit Care Med* 1996; 153(3):953–960.
292. Spitzhauer S, Pandjiatan B, Muhl S, et al. Major cat and dog allergens share IgE epitopes. *J Allergy Clin Immunol* 1997;99:100–106.
293. Nusslein HG, Zimmermann T, Baum M, Fuchs C, Kolble K, Kalden JR. Improved in vitro diagnosis of allergy to Alternaria tenius and *Cladosporium herbarum*. *Allergy* 1987;42(6):414–422.
294. Nasser SM, Pfister R, Christie PE, et al. Inflammatory cell populations in bronchial biopsies from aspirin-sensitive asthmatic subjects. *Am J Respir Crit Care Med* 1996;153(1):90–96.
295. Committee of the Environmental and Occupational Health Assembly of the American Thoracic Society. Health effects of outdoor air pollution. *Am J Respir Crit Care Med* 1996;153(1):3–50.
296. Brooks SM. Host susceptibility to indoor air pollution. *J Allergy Clin Immunol* 1994;94(2 Pt 2):344–351.
297. McBride DE, Koenig JQ, Luchtel DL, Williams PV, Henderson WR, Jr. Inflammatory effects of ozone in the upper airways of subjects with asthma. *Am J Respir Crit Care Med* 1994;149(5):1192–1197.
298. Kaminsky DA, Irvin CG, Gurka DA, et al. Peripheral airways responsiveness to cool, dry air in normal and asthmatic individuals. *Am J Respir Crit Care Med* 1995;152(6 Pt 1):1784–1790.
299. McFadden ER Jr. Exercise-induced airway obstruction. *Clin Chest Med* 1995;16(4):671–682.
300. McFadden ER Jr. The effects of heat and water exchange in the recovery period after exercise in children with asthma [letter;comment]. *Am Rev Respir Dis* 1990;141(3):801–803.
301. Matte TD, Hoffman RE, Rosenman KD, Stanbury M. Surveillance of occupational asthma under the SENSOR model. *Chest* 1990;98 (suppl):173S–178S.
302. Chan-Yeung M. A clinician's approach to determine the diagnosis, prognosis, and therapy of occupational asthma. *Med Clin North Am* 1990;74(3):811–822.
302a. Immunology AAoAa. Guidelines for the diagnosis and evaluation of occupational immunologic lung disease. *J Allergy Clin Immunol* 1989;84:791–838.
303. Rasanen L, Kuusisto P, Penttila M, Nieminen M, Savolainen J, Lehto M. Comparison of immunologic tests in the diagnosis of occupational asthma and rhinitis. *Allergy* 1994;49(5):342–347.
304. Malo JL, Trudeau C, Ghezzo H, L Archeveque J, Cartier A. Do sub-

jects investigated for occupational asthma through serial peak expiratory flow measurements falsify their results? *J Allergy Clin Immunol* 1995;96(5 Pt 1):601–607.
305. Quirce S, Contreras G, Dybuncio A, Chan-Yeung M. Peak expiratory flow monitoring is not a reliable method for establishing the diagnosis of occupational asthma. *Am J Respir Crit Care Med* 1995;152(3): 1100–1102.
306. Balmes JR. Surveillance for occupational asthma. *J Occup Med* 1991; 6(1):101–110.
307. Perrin B, Lagier F, L Archeveque J, et al. Occupational asthma: validity of monitoring of peak expiratory flow rates and non-allergic bronchial responsiveness as compared to specific inhalation challenge. *Eur Respir J* 1992;5(1):40–48.
308. Cartier A, Pineau L, Malo JL. Monitoring of maximum expiratory peak flow rates and histamine inhalation tests in the investigation of occupational asthma. *Clin Allergy* 1984;14(2):193–196.
309. Cockcroft DW, Murdock KY, Kirby J, Hargreave F. Prediction of airway responsiveness to allergens from skin sensitivity to allergen and airway responsiveness to histamine. *Am Rev Respir Dis* 1987;135: 264–267.
310. Vandenplas O, Malo JL, Cartier A, Perreault G, Cloutier Y. Closed-circuit methodology for inhalation challenge tests with isocyanates. *Am Rev Respir Dis* 1992;145(3):582–587.
311. Cloutier Y, Lagier F, Lemieux R, et al. New methodology for specific inhalation challenges with occupational agents in powder form. *Eur Respir J* 1989;2(8):769–777.
312. Pin I, Freitag AP, O'Byrne PM, et al. Changes in the cellular profile of induced sputum after allergen-induced asthmatic responses. *Am Rev Respir Dis* 1992;145(6):1265–1269.
313. Siracusa A, Vecchiarelli A, Brugnami G, Marabini A, Felicioni D, Severini C. Changes in interleukin-1 and tumor necrosis factor production by peripheral blood monocytes after specific bronchoprovocation test in occupational asthma. *Am Rev Respir Dis* 1992;146:408–412.
314. Pasmans SG, Aalbers M, van der Veen MJ, et al. Reactivity to IgE-dependent histamine-releasing activity in asthma or rhinitis. *Am J Respir Crit Care Med* 1996;154:318–323.
315. Herd ZL, Bernstein DI. Antigen-specific stimulation of histamine releasing factors in diisocyanate-induced occupational asthma. *Am J Respir Crit Care Med* 1994;150:988–994.
316. Lummus ZL, Alam R, Bernstein JA, Bernstein DI. Characterization of histamine releasing factors in diisocyanate-induced occupational asthma. *Toxicology* 1996;111:191–206.
317. Wada S, et al. Clinical observation of bronchial asthma in culture oyster workers. *Hiroshima J Med* 1967;16:255–257.
318. Zeiss CR, Patterson R, Pruzansky JJ, Miller MM, Rosenberg M, Levitz D. Trimellitic anhydride-induced airway syndromes: clinical and immunologic studies. *J Allergy Clin Immunol* 1977;60:96–103.
319. Burge PS. New developments in occupational asthma. *Br Med Bull* 1992;48:221–230.
320. Bousquet J, Van Vyve T, Chanez P, Enander I, Michel FB, Godard P. Cells and mediators in bronchoalveolar lavage of asthmatic patients: the example of eosinophilic inflammation. *Allergy* 1993;48:70–75.
321. Roche WR, Beasley R, Williams JH, Holgate ST. Subepithelial fibrosis in the bronchi of asthmatics. *Lancet* 1989;1:520–524.
322. Djukanovic R, Lai CK, Wilson JW, et al. Bronchial mucosal manifestations of atopy: a comparison of markers of inflammation between atopic asthmatics, atopic nonasthmatics and healthy controls. *Eur Respir J* 1992;5:538–544.
323. Paggiaro P, Bacci E, Paoletti P, et al. Bronchoalveolar lavage and morphology of the airways after cessation of exposure in asthmatic subjects sensitized to toluene diisocyanate. *Chest* 1990;98:536–542.
324. Undem BJ. Neuralimmunologic interactions in asthma. *Hospital Practice* (Office Edition) 1994;29:59–65.
325. Koshino T, Arai Y, Miyamoto Y, et al. Airway basophil and mast cell density in patients with bronchial asthma: relationship to bronchial hyperresponsiveness. *J Asthma* 1996;33:89–95.
326. Lemiere C, Malo JL, Boulet LP, Boutet M. Reactive airways dysfunction syndrome induced by exposure to a mixture containing isocyanate: functional and histopathologic behaviour. *Allergy* 1996;51:262–265.
327. Hendrick DJ. Epidemiological measurement of bronchial responsiveness in polyurethane workers. *Bull Eur Physiopathol Respir* 1987;23: 555–559.
328. Ohashi Y, Motohima S, Fukuda T, Makino S. Airway hyperresponsiveness, increased intracellular spaces of bronchial epithelium, and increased infiltration of eosinophils and lymphocytes in bronchial mucosa in asthma [see comments]. *Am Rev Respir Dis* 1992;145: 1469–1476.
329. Raeburn D, Webber SE. Proinflammatory potential of the airway epithelium in bronchial asthma. *Eur Respir J* 1994;7:2226–2233.
330. Nielsen J, Welinder H, Horstmann V, Skerfving S. Allergy to methyltetrahydrophthalic anhydride in epoxy resin workers. *Br J Ind Med* 1992;49:769–775.
331. Skaring G, Dalene M, Svensson B-G, et al. Biomarkers of exposure, antibodies, and respiratory symptoms in workers heating polyurethane glue. *Occup Environ Med* 1996;53:180–187.
332. Chilton FH, Averill FJ, Hubbard WC, Fonteh AN, Triggiani M, Liu MC. Antigen-induced generation of lyso-phospholipids in human airways. *J Exp Med* 1996;183:2235–2245.
333. Nordman SA, Nyberg PW. Whole blood chemiluminescence as a systemic inflammatory parameter in asthma. *J Allergy Clin Immunol* 1994;94:853–860.
334. Grammer LC, Shaughnessy MA, Hogan MB, et al. Value of antibody levels in diagnosing anhydride-induced immunologic respiratory disease. *J Lab Clin Med* 1995;125:650–653.
335. Institute NHLB. *Global strategies for asthma prevention and management.* Washington, DC, 1992.
336. Gannon PF, Weir DC, Robertson AS, Burge PS. Health, employment, and financial outcomes in workers with occupational asthma. *Br J Ind Med* 1993;50(6):491–496.
337. Malo JL, Boulet LP, Dewitte JD, et al. Quality of life of subjects with occupational asthma. *J Allergy Clin Immunol* 1993;91(6):1121–1127.
338. American Thoracic Society. Guidelines for the evaluation of impairment/disability in patients with asthma. *Am Rev Respir Dis* 1993; 147(4):1056–1061.

*Environmental and Occupational Medicine, Third Edition,* edited by William N. Rom.
Lippincott–Raven Publishers, Philadelphia © 1998.

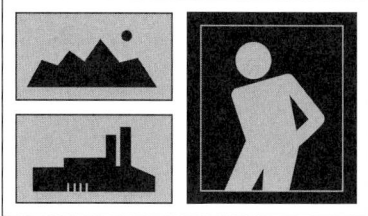

CHAPTER 34

# Inflammatory Mechanisms of Asthma

Joan Reibman and Stuart M. Brooks

Asthma is now recognized as a disease characterized by reversible (completely or incompletely) airway obstruction, hyperreactive airways, airway inflammation, and airway remodeling (1). Experimentally, in sensitized subjects, provocation of the airways produces an early and late phase of airway obstruction associated with the generation of bronchial hyperresponsiveness to nonspecific stimuli. The recognition of the late phase of airway obstruction has aroused an intense interest in understanding the cellular and molecular processes in the airway and has led to our recent understanding of asthma as a disease involving not only airway smooth muscle, but a wide variety of inflammatory cells. The accumulation of these cells results in mechanisms that predispose to immunoglobulin E (IgE)-dependent or -independent airway hyperreactivity. An understanding of the role of specific inflammatory cells, the mechanisms for their recruitment and activation, and the identity of their products will enhance our ability to understand the development of allergic, nonallergic and occupational asthma (Fig. 1).

## SENSITIZATION OF THE AIRWAY

One of the critical questions in asthma is to understand how the airway becomes sensitized. In atopic, IgE-mediated disease there is increasing and exciting information about mechanisms of airway sensitization. Occupational asthma may involve sensitization to high molecular weight particles, a process that may be IgE-mediated, but the mechanisms of sensitization to low molecular weight organic compounds such as plicatic acid are less clear (2). Even less is known about sensitization in nonoccupationally exposed, nonatopic individuals, although the role of environmental factors, including air pollutants and airborne viral infections, is increasingly being considered. Despite the initiating event, evidence is accumulating that local, rather than systemic, responses may direct immune reactions. This concept is critically important for the lung, which may contain within itself all the components for directing a T-cell–mediated and inflammatory response.

The concept of asthma as a T-cell–mediated disease is also now commonly accepted and leads to the obvious question of how the T-cell response to inhaled allergen or protein is initiated. The first question that arises is to understand the identity of the critical antigen-presenting cells (APCs). A variety of cells have been hypothesized as APCs in the airway; however, increasing evidence suggests a critical role for dendritic cells (DCs), which are the most potent APCs (3). These cells are morphologically characterized by the presence of multiple cytoplasmic processes and an irregular and convoluted nucleus (3,4). DCs stain abundantly for major histocompatibility complex (MHC) class-II, CD1c, and/or CD1a, and have low levels of Fc receptors (3).

There is accumulating evidence that DCs participate in airway sensitization. Both human and animal studies have demonstrated that DCs are abundantly distributed in the airway and accumulate in highest number in the upper airway and in locations maximally exposed to inhaled particulates (5–8). In rats, airway DCs display cell processes that extend between epithelial cells and up to epithelial cell tight junctions (9). Indeed, a network of

J. Reibman: Division of Pulmonary and Critical Care Medicine, Department of Medicine, Bellevue Hospital, New York University Medical Center, New York, New York 10016.
S. M. Brooks: Department of Environmental and Occupational Health, College of Public Health, University of South Florida, Tampa, Florida 33612-3805.

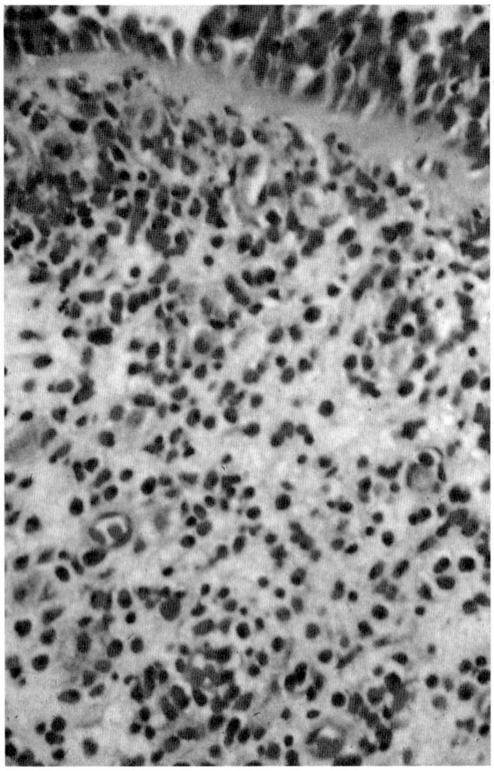

**FIG. 1.** Endobronchial biopsy of a patient with long-standing moderate-severe persistent asthma. Note desquamating epithelium, thickened basement membrane zone, and abundance of inflammatory cells in the submucosa. Inflammatory cells include abundant eosinophils and lymphocytes. (200× magnification).

DCs that comprises up to 700 DC/mm$^2$ has been demonstrated in the airway (8). In addition to their location at the interface with the environment, airway DCs are also primed to serve as critical APCs in the airway because of their rapid mobility; after a primary exposure to antigen, DCs move rapidly from the airway to draining lymph nodes (t1/2 in the airway of less than 2 days) (8,10,11). In humans, airway DCs in the epithelium and subepithelial tissue of the bronchus also form small clusters with T cells (8,12). DCs are also present in the bronchus-associated lymphoid tissue (8,12). Thus they are ideally located to interact with T cells. In addition to MHC class II molecules, airway DCs express accessory molecules for T-cell activation and are effective in presenting both soluble and insoluble antigen to antigen-sensitized T cells (9,13).

Additional cells have been proposed as APCs but their role in this process is less clear. Alveolar macrophages derived from animals or normal human donors have been demonstrated to provide relatively poor antigenic stimulation for T cells. One reason for this relatively poor ability to present antigen has been proposed to be their failure to express co-stimulatory cell surface molecules required for antigen presentation. Human alveolar macrophages derived from normal donors have been demonstrated to express minimal if any B7 and to fail to upregulate accessory molecules B7-1 or B7-2 after interferon-γ (IFN-γ) (14). The expression of B7-1 and B7-2 on alveolar macrophages derived from patients with disease states is less well characterized and may differ from that in the normal. Airway epithelial cells (AECs) have also been proposed as APCs. These cells express MHC class II and in certain circumstances they have been demonstrated to induce an allogeneic T-cell response (15). Although AECs can express MHC class II, their expression of accessory molecules (B7-1, B7-2) has not been well described (16). Indeed, intestinal epithelial cells have been demonstrated to fail to express these molecules (16).

Activation of T cells requires two distinct signals. One signal is delivered via ligation of the T-cell receptor (TcR). An additional signal is delivered by ligation of CD28 and the T cell activation antigen (CTLA)-4 by surface molecules that provide co-stimulatory signals. These molecules include B7-1 (CD80) and B7-2 (CD86) (17). The combined signals delivered by the TcR and CD28 may maximize T-cell signaling, promote T-cell differentiation and expansion, and alter the balance of Th1/Th2 responses during an immune reaction. However, antigen presentation in the absence of these additional co-stimulatory signals may lead to tolerance (17). Recent data suggest that engagement of CD28 and CTLA4 may result in opposing effects; CD28 leads to T-cell activation, whereas CTLA4 may downregulate T cells (18). The importance of these cell surface molecules in the development of airway hyperresponsiveness has been further demonstrated in a murine model using the soluble fusion protein CTLA4-Ig, which blocks the CD28:B7 pathway and primary T-cell–dependent antibody (19). In this model, BALB/c mice sensitized intraperitoneally and subsequently challenged with aerosolized ovalbumin decreased airway hyperresponsiveness to methacholine (18). Histologic evaluation demonstrated that CTLA4-Ig treatment also resulted in a decrease in the accumulation of neutrophils, lymphocytes, and eosinophils in the bronchial mucosa, reduced expansion of the CD4$^+$ and CD8$^+$ T-cell subsets, and reduced serum IgE. Additional molecules such as intercellular adhesion molecule-1 (ICAM-1) may act as co-stimulatory molecules. Indeed, Iwamoto and Nakao's group (20) recently demonstrated in a murine model that sensitization to a soluble antigen in the absence of ICAM-1 [anti-ICAM-1 monoclonal antibody (mAB)] elicited T-cell tolerance.

## ROLE OF T CELLS IN ASTHMA

There is now consensus that asthma is a disease involving activation of specific T-cell subsets. Based predominantly on animal studies, it is now accepted that antigen-specific immune responses evolve from the development of naive CD4$^+$ T cells into functionally distinct T cell subsets termed type 1 (Th1) and type 2 (Th2) (21). Initially described in murine models, these T-cell subsets can be identified by their ability to secrete specific cytokines: Th1 cells release interleukin-2 (IL-2) and IFN-γ, whereas Th2 cells release IL-4, IL-5, and IL-6 but not IFN-γ. Both cell types release IL-3 and granulocyte-macrophage colony-stimulating factor (GM-CSF). Th1 cells are associated with a delayed-type hypersensitivity reaction, whereas Th2 cells are associated with enhanced secretion of Ig, specifically IgE, IgA, IgG1, and IgM (22). The basic concept of T-cell subsets expressing polarized cytokine profiles has been most extensively studied in murine models. In humans, differences between the subsets are somewhat less distinct. Allergen-specific IL-4-producing clones have been isolated; however, these clones may also release IL-2 and IFN-γ (23–25). The cytokine milieu present in the early stages of antigen-driven $CD4^+$ T-cell activation determines the development of the T-cell clone (26). Th1 cells develop when naive T cells are stimulated in the presence of IL-12 and IFN-γ, whereas Th2 cells require IL-4 (26–28). Established Th2 subtypes resist reversal to a Th1/T0 subtype after subsequent exposure to IL-12 because of lack of signaling induced by IL-12, in part due to a failure of these cells to express the IL-12R $\beta_2$ subunit (29,30).

An abundance of lymphocytes have been identified in the intraepithelium and in the lamina propria and submucosa of mucosal biopsies obtained from atopic asthmatics (31–33). These lymphocytes express the IL-2 receptor (CD24+) consistent with T-cell activation and are located in the airway within 15 minutes after an allergen challenge (32,34). The presence of a Th2 T-cell population in atopic asthma in human subjects has been further demonstrated by the evaluation of messenger RNA (mRNA) for specific cytokines in T cells obtained by bronchoalveolar lavage (BAL) from atopic asthmatics (35). In situ hybridization has demonstrated enhanced expression of mRNA for IL-4 and IL-5 in T cells obtained from BAL, suggesting that atopic asthma is associated with a Th2 population (35–38). An accumulation of activated ($CD25^+$) T cells has also been noted in the bronchial mucosa in atopic asthmatics concurrent with an increase in cells expressing IL-5 and GM-CSF (39). Studies employing segmental allergen challenge have also demonstrated a delayed (18-hour) accumulation of activated T cells in BAL as well as a cytokine profile consistent with a Th2 pattern (IL-5). Interestingly, IL-2 was found in these studies as well as IL-2 (40). Recently, using an animal model of eosinophil accumulation in the lung, Kaminuma et al. (41) transferred the late accumulation of eosinophils into the lung by transferring ovalbumin specific Th2 clones and challenging these mice with inhalation of relevant antigen. Their findings further reinforce the critical role of T cells in the eosinophilic accumulation characteristic of asthma.

In humans, the Th2 model of T-cell responses in asthma may be an oversimplification. Th1-type cytokines have also been identified in T cells from subjects with allergic asthma. Using a single-cell technique, Krug et al. (42) identified IL-4 production in only a small proportion of BAL T cells and a selective enhancement of T cells producing IFN-γ (42). In patients with nonatopic asthma, elevated levels of T-suppressor cells expressing class II histocompatibility antigen and very late activation antigen-1 have also been demonstrated as well as elevations in IL-2 (36). Patients with toluene 2,4-diisocyanate (TDI) asthma have also been described to have an increase in $CD8^+$ T cells, which produce both IL-5 and IFN-γ (43).

In additional studies of occupational asthma, a role for T-cell activation has also been demonstrated. Western red cedar has been shown to induce asthma due to sensitization to plicatic acid, a low molecular weight organic compound (44). Studies of subjects with Western red cedar–induced asthma demonstrated an increase in $CD4^+$ T cells in bronchial biopsies in a manner analogous to those of patients with atopic asthma (44). Clinical and functional alterations in asthma induced by TDI are similar to those found in allergen-induced asthma (45). Similarly, activated ($CD25^+$) T cells were abundant in bronchial biopsies of subjects with asthma induced by TDI (46). These data suggest that similar mechanisms may exist for asthma induced by allergen as well as these two occupational exposures.

## MAST CELLS AND EOSINOPHILS AS EFFECTOR CELLS

Whereas T cells are well described as a source of critical cytokines, mast cells and eosinophils are characteristic of the airway inflammatory response in asthma. Mast cells express high affinity immunoglobulin E receptors (FcεRI). Engagement of the FcεRI by IgE elicits the rapid release of preformed mediators including histamine and proteases such as chymase and tryptase. These proteases elicit eosinophil recruitment and increase mucus secretion and microvascular permeability (47). Activation of mast cells also leads to the rapid synthesis of lipid mediators, which include prostaglandin $D_2$ ($PGD_2$) and leukotriene $C_4$ and platelet-activating factor (48). These agents are potent bronchoconstrictors and increase mucus production and microvascular leakage. Mast cells differ not only between tissues, but within the lung. Human lung mast cells express different phenotypes as determined by their content of neutral proteases. Mast cells at mucosal surfaces contain predominantly tryptase, whereas those in the connective tissue also contain chymase, carboxypeptidase A, and cathepsin G (47,49). Elevated levels of degranulating mast cells have been noted in the epithelium and lamina propria of biopsy specimens obtained from patients with stable asthma (50,51).

Mast cells may also participate in the persistence of the asthmatic response through the elaboration of specific cytokines. They are increasingly being recognized as an important source of IL-4, -5, and -6 (52–54). In addition, mast cells synthesize tumor necrosis factor-α (TNF-α), a cytokine that upregulates the expression of multiple adhesion molecules including ICAM-1 and vascular cell adhesion molecule-1 (53). Cells staining for IL-4 have been identified in the submucosa of patients with asthma and are predominantly those mast cells that also stain for tryptase (47,55). Isolated human mast cells synthesize IL-4 in response to cross-linking of the $Fc_{\varepsilon}$ receptor in the presence of stem cell factor (56). In addition, IL-5 immunoreactivity has also been localized to mast cells in the submucosa of both normal as well as asthmatic patients (53,55). Purified human lung mast cells express mRNA for IL-5 and are capable of releasing IL-5 protein in abundance (2,500 pg/$10^6$cells) (54,56). Thus mast cells contain preformed mediators as well as cytokines, all of which may participate in the initiation and perpetuation of airway hyperreactivity. Elevated levels of mast cells have also been described in occupational asthma, specifically in the epithelium of patients with TDI-induced asthma (57).

Both atopic and nonatopic asthma have long been known to be associated with infiltration of the bronchial mucosa with activated eosinophils (58–62). Eosinophilopoiesis can be induced by at least three cytokines: GM-CSF, IL-3, and IL-5 (62). Eosinophils express IgE receptors similar but not identical to the FcεRII (low-affinity IgE receptor). When activated, eosinophils release preformed granular contents including the cationic proteins major basic protein, eosinophil cationic protein, eosinophil peroxidase, and eosinophil-derived neurotoxin. In addition, when activated, eosinophils synthesize lipid mediators including $PGE_2$, $PGD_2$, leukotriene $C_4$, and platelet-activating factor (62,63). Both IL-4 and IL-5 have also been localized to eosinophils in the airway using techniques of in situ hybridization and double immunohistochemistry (55). Ultrastructural studies show that IL-5 localizes to secondary or specific eosinophil granules (64). In addition, eosinophils release GM-CSF, which acts with an autocrine effect to enhance their survival (65). Eosinophils undergo phenotypic alterations once in the airway. After exposure to cytokines in the microenvironment, they become hypodense consistent with a primed phenotype (66).

Allergen challenge of patients with asthma has resulted in an accumulation of eosinophils in BAL (40,67). In addition, BAL fluid displays elevated levels of eosinophils in patients with chronic asthma, with the number of eosinophils correlating with severity (39,50,60,68). Bronchial biopsy specimens have confirmed the finding of elevated numbers of eosinophils in the airway of patients, with asthma with eosinophils abundantly distributed in the epithelium and submucosa of patients with asthma (33,50,50,69). Eosinophil accumulation has been noted in both atopic and nonatopic asthmatics (55). In addition, elevated levels of eosinophils have been found in patients with Western red cedar asthma and in the epithelium and submucosa of patients with occupational asthma induced by TDI (57,70,71). The finding of eosinophils in each of these presentations suggests that although the initial stimulus may differ, the end result of eosinophil recruitment and activation is similar.

## IMMUNOMODULATORY CYTOKINES IN ASTHMA

Interleukin-4 and IL-5 are Th2 T-cell–derived cytokines the elevated presence of which has been extensively reported in asthma (72). IL-4 was initially described by its actions on B lymphocytes (73,74). IL-4 has been demonstrated to elicit type switching of B cells to induce the development of IgG1 and IgE (74). These in vitro studies have been supported by murine models of targeted gene disruption of IL-4 in which mice are incapable of producing IgE (75). IL-4 has subsequently been demonstrated to induce class switching to IgG and IgE by inducing germ-line transcription of Cγ1 and Cε transcripts (76). In addition, IL-4 suppresses IL-2 and IFN-γ production in naive T cells and enhances maturation of naive T cells into Th2 cells (77,78). Thus by a multitude of mechanisms, IL-4 enhances the Th2 type response. IL-4 has additional effects that alter the immune response. These effects include enhancing the expression of CD23 (FcεRII) as well as MHC class II molecules. IL-4 can also enhance heterotypic cell adhesion by selectively increasing the expression of vascular cell adhesion molecule-1 on human umbilical vein endothelial cells (79).

Numerous studies have demonstrated elevated levels of IL-4 in BAL of patients with atopic asthma. Studies of patients with nonatopic asthma compared to atopic asthma have demonstrated conflicting results about the expression of IL-4 and IL-5. Walker et al. (36) demonstrated that whereas IL-2 and IL-5 were elevated in BAL derived from patients with both clinically defined types of asthma, elevated levels of IL-4 were only found in BAL of patients with allergic asthma. However, using semiquantitative reverse transcriptase–polymerase chain reaction amplification, in situ hybridization, and immunohistochemistry in bronchial biopsies, Humbert et al. (55,80) demonstrated equivalent expression of both IL-4 and IL-5.

In conjunction with IL-4, IL-5 has been recognized as a critical cytokine in asthma. IL-5 was initially described as a substance in supernatants of alloreactive T-cell clones, which supported the growth of eosinophils. Subsequent studies demonstrated that purified IL-5 could act on untreated bone marrow cells to exclusively induce eosinophil colony formation (81). In addition, rhIL-5 was demonstrated to selectively activate eosinophils (82). Both blood and tissue eosinophilia induced by *Nippostrongylus brasiliensis* was also dependent on IL-5. Thus the role of IL-5 in eosinophil function and the recognition of asthma as a disease with blood and tissue eosinophilia led to the investigation of IL-5 as an agent in the development of airway hyperreactivity. Extensive studies on BAL fluid and airway biopsies have demonstrated elevated levels of IL-5 protein and mRNA in humans with atopic as well as nonatopic asthma (35,36, 39,40,55,83–86).

Although numerous studies demonstrate an association between the Th2 cytokines IL-4 and IL-5 in the lung in asthma, they do not demonstrate a requirement for the expression of these cytokines for the development of asthma. Murine models in which the inflammatory and eosinophilic response was monitored demonstrated a requirement for IL-4 (87,88). However, studies evaluating the development of hyperreactivity in murine models have demonstrated conflicting results. Using neutralizing antibodies to IL-4, Corry et al. (89) showed that BALB/c mice immunized to ovalbumin required IL-4 during the period of systemic immunization to develop hyperreactivity. In contrast, Hogan et al. (90) used ovalbumin sensitized C57BL/6 $IL4^{-/-}$ mice and demonstrated that these mice developed a pathologic state and a physiologic response that was indistiguishable from $IL\text{-}4^{+/+}$ mice (90). In contrast to Foster (91), Corry et al. also demonstrated that neither IL-5 nor eosinophils were required for their model of airway hyperreactivity. The reason for the discrepancies in these results are unclear; however, the suggestion can be raised that there are multiple ways to develop airway hyperreactivity and that species differences may illustrate some of these differing mechanisms. In addition, the role of IL-13, which has many similar properties to IL-4, may be important.

Despite the heightened interest in IL-4 and IL-5, asthma is a disease involving multiple cytokines. The importance of many of these cytokines in the development of airway eosinophilia and hyperreactivity is only now being delineated.

IL-13, a 132-amino acid unglycosylated protein ($M_r$ 10 kd) is a recently described protein secreted by activated T cells (92,93). Like IL-4, it is encoded on chromosome 5q31 and can be produced by $CD4^+$ as well as $CD8^+$ T cells with Th0, Th1, and Th2 phenotypes (93). IL-13 shares some biologic properties and structural similarities with IL-4, including the ability to induce class switching to IgE (94). In addition, IL-13 inhibits the production of IFN-γ and IL-12 (p35 and p40) (95). In view of the multitude of functions of IL-13, and the similarities to IL-4, it would be likely that IL-13 is also involved in the underlying mechanism of asthma. Indeed, local allergen challenge in atopic patients with asthma results in delayed increase in IL-13, which is associated with elevated eosinophil numbers suggesting that IL-13 is involved in the late asthmatic response in mild asthmatic subjects (96). Granulocyte-macrophage colony-stimulating factor (GM-CSF) has many functions. The human GM-CSF gene has been mapped to chromosome 5q21-q32, a region downstream from IL-3, IL-4, IL-5 and macrophage colony stimulating factor (97–99). The human gene encodes for a 23-kd glycoprotein characterized by a four α-helical bundle topology (100). The functions of GM-CSF are mediated by the binding of GM-CSF to its receptor, a member of a superfamily of growth factor and cytokine receptors that include those for IL-3, IL-4, IL-6, and G-CSF (101).

Original studies of GM-CSF delineated its actions on stimulating the formation of granulocyte, macrophage, and eosinophil cells from progenitor cells (101). In addition, GM-CSF activates mature peripheral blood neutrophils and eosinophils (102,103). GM-CSF also regulates the recruitment, phenotypic differentiation, and activation of dendritic cells (DCs) and Langerhans' cells. One mechanism by which GM-CSF enhances antigen presentation by GM-CSF is its ability to alter the expression of accessory molecules required for antigen presentation (3,4,9,104,105).

Recent work, using mice homozygous for a disrupted GM-CSF gene, has demonstrated normal hematopoiesis in the absence of GM-CSF. Surprisingly, these mice demonstrated marked pulmonary effects with lung abnormalities resembling alveolar proteinosis (106,107). These abnormalities could be reversed with targeted alveolar epithelial cell delivery of the GM-CSF gene (108). Mice with null mutations for the GM-CSF-$\beta_c$ receptor also showed a similar phenotype, with the lungs demonstrating areas of alveolar proteinosis (109). Since circulating levels of GM-CSF have rarely been detected, GM-CSF is most likely a locally acting cytokine with paracrine rather than endocrine effects(101). Elevated levels of GM-CSF have been demonstrated in bronchoalveolar lavage fluid in atopic patients after segmental allergen challenge with ragweed, dust mite, or timothy grass (40,110). GM-CSF may be derived form hematopoietic cells. In addition, airway epithelial cells (AEL) have also been demonstrated to secrete GM-CSF in response to IL-1, TNF-α, IL-4, IL-13, and viruses. Immunostaining of bronchial biopsy specimens has revealed GM-CSF in AECs derived from human subjects with atopic asthma but not in normals (111–117).

Interleukin-11 was initially described as an agent affecting hematopoiesis, particularly the proliferation of plasmacytoma cells (118). However, IL-11 has been recently described to possess additional properties including altering immunoglobulin production. IL-11 is secreted in nasal secretions of children with viral upper respiratory tract infections. Recently, a mouse transgenic with IL-11 targeted to the respiratory tree with a Clara cell 10-kd promoter has been described (119). This mouse demonstrated lymphocytic peribronchiolar inflammation with subepithelial fibrosis and airways obstruction. The role of this cytokine in human disease is intriguing; its importance has yet to be fully delineated.

Whereas IL-4, -5, -11, and -13 may all enhance the responses seen in asthma, specific cytokines may downregulate the responses. These cytokines include IFN-$\gamma$ and IL-12. Although initially described as an antiviral agent, IFN-$\gamma$ has pleiotropic effects. A product of $CD8^+$, Th1 and Th0 $CD4^+$ T cells, and NK cells, its gene is located on human chromosome 12q24.1 (120). IFN-$\gamma$ is induced when T cells are stimulated in the presence of MHC class I or II and can also be induced after engagement of the T-cell receptor/CD3 complex. Production of IFN-$\gamma$ can also be enhanced by IL-2 and leukotrienes $B_4$, $LTC_4$, and $LTD_4$ (120). Recent studies also demonstrate that IL-12 also induces IFN-$\gamma$ gene expression in T cells, whereas IL-10 inhibits its production (121,122). IFN-$\gamma$ functions as a noncovalent homodimer of two mature proteins of 143 amino acids and induces dimerization of its receptor and activation of the Jak/Stat signaling pathway (120). The role of IFN-$\gamma$ as a protective agent or as an agent whose downregulation leads to enhanced IgE-dependent disease is only recently being elucidated. Elevated levels of IFN-$\gamma$ have been described in serum of patients with severe asthma and in some BAL samples (123). However, a more recent study failed to detect elevated levels (55). The potential protective effects of IFN-$\gamma$ are demonstrated by two exciting studies in mice that demonstrate that exogenous IFN-$\gamma$ delivered by nebulization or mucosal delivery of the IFN-$\gamma$ gene inhibits Ag and Th2 cell-induced pulmonary eosinophilia and airway hyperreactivity (30,124). The potential for IFN-$\gamma$ as a treatment for asthma remains intriguing.

Interleukin-12 was initially isolated from human Epstein-Barr virus-transformed B-cell lines that, in the presence of IL-2, induced lymphokine activated killer cells and cytotoxic T lymphocytes (125). Bioactive IL-12 is a heterodimer of two *N*-glycosylated polypeptides, 40 kd (p40) and 35 kd (p35) (126). Although IL-12 is predominantly synthesized by antigen-presenting cells such as monocytes, macrophages, and dendritic cells, murine mast cells have also been identified as a source (126). The production of IL-12 can be suppressed by IL-10 as well as IL-4, IL-13, and transforming growth factor-$\beta$. When IL-12 receptors are upregulated (IL-2, phorbol esters, anti-CD3 mAb), IL-12 exhibits growth promotion for $CD4^+$ and $CD8^+$ T cells. IL-12 has several modulatory roles that may diminish the effects of the proinflammatory cytokines. Recombinant IL-12 has been demonstrated to inhibit the synthesis of IgE after T cells have been stimulated with IL-4. In addition, in contrast to IL-4 and IL-13, stimulation of T cells by IL-12 in the presence of B7 induces the proliferation of Th1 clones and induces the production of IFN-$\gamma$ from resting or activated T cells (68,127). This effect is even greater when in the presence of IL-2 but can be diminished after cells have been differentiated into Th2 cells (29). Thus IL-12 may act as a potent modulator to diminish the immune response in asthma.

## MECHANISMS OF CELL RECRUITMENT

Recruitment of inflammatory cells to the airway involves the release of chemoattractants and the expression of adhesion molecules on leukocytes, vascular endothelium, and airway epithelium. Chemoattractants involved in the airways in asthma include lipid molecules such as $LTB_4$, and cytokines such as IL-2, IL-5, and IL-8. Most recently, the CC chemokine RANTES and monocyte chemotactic protein-3 (MCP-3) have been implicated as a potent chemoattractants involved in asthma, particularly in the regulation of eosinophil recruitment (128). Elevated expression of mRNA for RANTES and MCP-3 has been demonstrated in bronchial biopsies from both atopic and nonatopic asthmatics, although the cellular source of the chemokines is unclear (129). Interestingly, despite the in vitro ability of epithelial cells to synthesize RANTES, epithelial cell expression of RANTES was not detected in this study. Using blocking mAbs to RANTES, the eosinophil chemotactic activity derived from BAL in subjects with asthma has been demonstrated to be due to RANTES (130).

Inflammatory cells express on their surfaces molecules that bind to adhesion proteins on endothelial cells and epithelial cells. The expression of these molecules regulates the migration of these cells. Leukocyte adhesion molecules include the sialylated, fucosylated carbohydrate sialyl Lewis$^x$ (SLe$^x$) which binds to E-selectin (131). In addition, leukocytes express integrins that bind to ligands of the immunoglobulin superfamily. These integrins include members of the $\beta_2$ family of integrins $\alpha_L\beta_2$ [CD11a/CD18, lymphocyte function-associated antigen (LFA-1)], which binds to the first Ig domain of ICAM-1 and ICAM-2, and $\alpha_M\beta_2$ (CD11b/CD18, Mac-1, M0-1, CR3) which binds to the third immunoglobulin domain of ICAM-1 (131,132). These are expressed on neutrophils, eosinophils, and lymphocytes. In contrast, $\alpha_4\beta_1$ (CD49d/CD29; VLA-4) is expressed on eosinophils, basophils, and lymphocytes, but not on neutrophils. This integrin binds to vascular cell adhesion molecule-1, another member of the Ig superfamily (133,134). Mast cells express a number of integrins that enable their recruitment to sites of inflammation. Engagement of Fc$\varepsilon$RI on mast cells upregulates the surface expression of integrins including the $B_1$ integrins CD29/CD49 and VLA-4 (48). Thus the regulation of functional expression of integrins on leukocytes as well as the regulation of expression of adhesion molecules on endothelial cells and epithelial cells may modify the recruitment and inflammatory response in the airway.

E-selectin is an endothelial glycoprotein with the classic C-type lectin domain, the epithelial growth factor

(EGF)-like domain, and six complement-regulatory protein regions that recognizes the sialylated fucosylated carbohydrate moieties on leukocytes (131). E-selectin is rapidly (4 to 6 hours) but transiently expressed in response to cytokines including IL-1 and TNF-α. ICAM-1 (CD54) serves as a counterreceptor to integrins of the $\beta_2$ family. Interestingly, ICAM-1 is also the receptor for rhinovirus (135). ICAM-1, a heavily glycosylated polypeptide ($M_r$ 76,000–114,000), is expressed on endothelial cells and epithelial cells as well as on monocytes/macrophages and lymphocytes (136–140). Expression of ICAM-1 is increased by a variety of cytokines including IL-1, TNF-α, and IFN-γ (137,141). Enhanced expression of E-selectin and ICAM-1 has been demonstrated on endothelial cells in subjects with asthma. ICAM-1 has also been detected by immunolocalization as well as by *in situ* hybridization in endothelial cells and mononuclear cells in bronchial submucosa of asthmatics (142–147). Immunoelectron microscopy revealed ICAM-1 and E-selectin expression along the luminal surface of the endothelial cell (147).

Some selectivity for the recruitment of adhesion molecules is provided by limited expression of integrins. Very late antigen-4 (VLA-4, $\alpha^4\beta_1$, CD49d/CD29), a member of the $\beta_1$ family of integrins, is expressed on lymphocytes, eosinophils, and monocytes but not on neutrophils (148). VLA-4 interacts with vascular cell adhesion molecule-1 (VCAM-1). VCAM-1 ($M_r$ 110,000) is a transmembrane glycoprotein (133,134,149,150). Although initially described as an inducible protein on endothelial cells, it has also been demonstrated in cells of dendritic morphology in follicular centers, in interfollicular zones of peripheral lymph nodes and tonsils, and in splenic and thymic macrophages (151). Its expression can be enhanced by IL-1, IL-4, TNF-α, and endotoxin (134,149). In addition, a synergistic response between IL-4 and IL-1β or TNF-α has been described for the expression of VCAM-1 (79,152,153). Upregulation of VCAM-1 leads to the selective adhesion of eosinophils and basophils, but not neutrophils, to the endothelium (79,152,153). Elevated expression of VCAM-1 has been demonstrated on endothelial cells of patients with asthma in most studies (145,147,154,155). Unlike ICAM-1, expression of VCAM-1 has not been described on bronchial epithelial cells (147). In contrast to studies in asthmatics, one study in subjects with TDI asthma failed to demonstrate in increase in either E-selectin or ICAM-1 expression compared to normals (46).

## AIRWAY REMODELING

The presence and activation of inflammatory cells in the airway results in morphologic changes. These changes include the loss of airway epithelium, an increase in goblet cells compared to ciliated epithelial cells and smooth muscle hypertrophy (156–159). The loss of epithelial cells can be reduced after treatment with corticosteroids, suggesting that it is a direct result of the airway inflammation (157). In addition to these changes, alterations in the structural matrix of the airway may be profound. The extracellular matrix includes glycosaminoglycan and proteoglycan macromolecules with fibrous proteins including collagen (type IV), elastin fibronectin, and laminin (159). The sources of these proteins include epithelial cells (type IV collagen, fibronectin, and laminin), as well as myofibroblasts and fibroblasts. With the advent of endobronchial biopsies in airways of asthmatics, the presence of thickening of the basement membrane under the airway epithelium has been well described as an outcome of asthma (31,157,160,161). These changes have been described now even in patients with mild or early asthma (50,162). Thickening is due to the presence of altered matrix proteins, with an excess of collagen deposition, specifically collagens I, III, and V, as well as fibronectin (160). Neither collagen type IV, a normal component of the basement membrane, nor laminin, is increased. Airway remodeling has been described in patients with occupational asthma as well. Laitinen et al. (162) studied patients exposed to aluminum fluoride, welding fumes, piperazine, methyltetrahydrophthalic anhydride, sulfuric acid aerosols, or isocyanates. These patients also demonstrated abnormal basement membranes with enhanced expression of tenascin. Exposure to toluene diisocyanate has also been demonstrated to result in a thickened subepithelial reticular layer with increased deposition of collagen III (57). Cessation of exposure to TDI led to a reduction in the subepithelial fibrosis (163). In addition, laminin $\alpha_1$ chain is distributed normally in the bronchial subepithelial basement membrane of control subjects and patients with various types of asthma; however, in patients with occupational asthma, an increase in the thickness of the laminin $\alpha_1$ chain is detected (164). The importance of airway remodeling is increasingly being recognized with concern over long-term effects and the development of irreversible airway obstruction.

In summary, in the past decade, exciting new developments in our understanding of the underlying mechanisms of asthma have evolved. From a disease of smooth muscle contraction, we now understand that, in addition, there are a multitude of mechanisms, IgE-dependent or IgE-independent, that result in altered T-cell activity, recruitment and activation of proinflammatory leukocytes, and chronic structural airway alterations. Despite differences in inciting events, the mechanisms of atopic, nonatopic, and occupational asthma are often similar.

## REFERENCES

1. NHLBI/WHO Workshop report. *Global initiative for asthma.* Bethesda, MD: National Institutes of Health, 1995.
2. Chan-Yeung M, Malo J-L. Occupational Asthma. N Eng J Med 1995; 333:107–112.

3. Steinman RM. The dendritic cell system and its role in immunogenicity. *Annu Rev Immunol* 1991;9:271–296.
4. Hance AJ. Pulmonary immune cells in health and disease: dendritic cells and Langerhans' cells. *Eur Respir J* 1993;6:1213–1220.
5. Sertl K, Takemura T, Tschachler E, Ferran VJ, Kaliner MA, Shevach EM. Dendritic cells with antigen-presenting capability reside in airway epithelium, lung parenchyma, and visceral pleura. *J Exp Med* 1986;163:436–451.
6. Soler PG, Moreau A, Basset F, Hance AJ. Cigarette smoking-induced changes in the number and differentiated state of pulmonary dendritic cells/Langerhans' cells. *Am Rev Respir Dis* 1989;139:1112–1117.
7. Holt PG, Schon-Hegrad MA, Oliver J, Holt BJ, McMenamin PG. A contiguous network of dendritic antigen-presenting cells within the respiratory epithelium. *Int Arch Allergy Appl Immunol* 1990;91: 155–159.
8. McWilliam A, Nelson DJ, Holt PG. The biology of airway dendritic cells. *Immunol Cell Biol* 1995;73:405–413.
9. Gong JL, McCarthy KM, Telford J, Tamatani T, Miyasaka M, Schneeberger EE. Intraepithelial airway dendritic cells: a distinct subset of pulmonary dendritic cells obtained by microdissection. *J Exp Med* 1992;175:797–807.
10. Nelson DJ, McMenamin C, McWilliam AS, Brenan M, Holt PG. Development of the airway intraepithelial dendritic cell network in the rat from class II major histocompatibility (Ia)-negative precursors: differential regulation of Ia expression at different levels of the respiratory tract. *J Exp Med* 1994;179:203–212.
11. Xia W, Pinto CE, Kradin RL. The antigen-presenting activities of Ia+ dendritic cells shift dynamically from lung to lymph node after an airway challenge with soluble antigen. *J Exp Med* 1995;181: 1275–1283.
12. Maarten J, van Haarst W, de Wit HJ, Drexhage HA, Hoogsteden HC. Distribution and immunophenotype of mononuclear phagocytes and dendritic cells in the human lung. *Am J Respir Cell Mol Biol* 1994;10: 487–492.
13. Nicod LP, Habre FE. Adhesion molecules on human lung dendritic cells and their role for T-cell activation. *Am J Respir Cell Mol Biol* 1992;7:207–213.
14. Chelen CJ, Fang Y, Freeman GJ, et al. Human alveolar macrophages present antigen ineffectively due to defective expression of B7 costimulatory cell surface molecules. *J Clin Invest* 1995;95:1415–1421.
15. Kalb TH, Chuang MT, Marom S, Mayer L. Evidence for accessory cell function by class II MHC antigen-expressing airway epithelial cells. *Am J Respir Cell Mol Biol* 1991;4:320–329.
16. Bloom S, Simmon D, Jewell DP. Adhesion molecules intercellular adhesion molecule-1 (ICAM-1), ICAM-3 and B7 are not expressed by epithelium in normal or inflamed colon. *Clin Exp Immunol* 1995;101: 157–163.
17. Bluestone JA. New perspective of CD28-B7 mediated T cell costimulation. *Immunity* 1995;2:555–559.
18. Krinzman SJ, De Sanctis GT, Cernadas M, et al. Inhibition of T cell costimulation abrogates airway hyperresponsiveness in a murine model. *J Clin Invest* 1996;98:2693–2699.
19. Linsley PS, Wallace PM, Johnson J, et al. Immunosuppression in vivo by a fusion form of the CTLA-4 T cell activation molecule. *Science* 1992;257:792–795.
20. Nakao A, Nakajima H, Tomioka H, Nishimura T, Iwamoto I. Induction of T cell tolerance by pretreatment with anti-ICAM-1 and anti-lymphocyte function-associated antigen-1 antibodies prevents antigen-induced eosinophil recruitment into the mouse airways. *J Immunol* 1994;153:5819–5825.
21. Mosmann TR, Cherwinski H, Bond MW, Gieldon MA, Coffman RL. Two types of murine helper T cell clones. 1. Definition according to profiles of lymphokine activities and secreted proteins. *J Immunol* 1986;136:2348–2357.
22. Mosmann TR, Coffman RL. Th1 and Th2 cells: different patterns of lymphokine secretion lead to different functional properties. *Annu Rev Immunol* 1989;7:145–173.
23. Wierenga EA, Snoek M, de Groot C, et al. Evidence for compartmentalization of functional subsets of $CD2^+$ T lympocytes in atopic patients. *J Immunol* 1990;144:4651–4656.
24. Parronchi P, Macchia D, Piccinni MP, et al. Allergen- and bacterial antigen specific T-cell clones established from atopic donors show a different profile of cytokine production. *Proc Natl Acad Sci USA* 1991;88:4538–4542.
25. Brinkmann V, Kristofic C. TCR-stimulated naive human $CD4^+$ 45Ro-T cells develop into effector cells that secrete IL-13, IL-5, and IFN-gamma, but no IL-4, and help efficient IgE production by B cells. *J Immunol* 1995;154:3078–3087.
26. Seder RA, Paul WE. Acquisition of lymphokine producing phenotype by $CD4^+$ T cells. *Annu Rev Immunol* 1994;12:635–673.
27. Wenner CA, Guler ML, Macatonia SE, O'Garra A, Murphy KM. Roles of IFN-gamma and IFN-alpha in IL-12 induced T helper cell-1 development. *J Immunol* 1996;156:1442–1447.
28. Le Gros G, Ben-Sasson SZ, Seder RA, Finkelman FD, Paul WE. Generation of interleukin 4 (IL-4)-producing cells in vivo and in vitro: IL-2 and IL-4 are required for in vitro generation of IL-4 producing cells. *J Exp Med* 1990;172:921–929.
29. Hildens CM, Messer G, Tesselaar K, Rietschoten AG, Kapsenberg ML, Wierenga EA. Lack of IL-12 signaling in human allergen-specific Th2 cells. *J Immunol* 1996;157:4316–4321.
30. Szabo SJ, Dighe AS, Gubler U, Murphy KM. Regulation of the interleukin (IL)-12R β2 subunit expression in developing T helper 1 (Th1) and Th2 cells. *J Exp Med* 1997;185:817–824.
31. Jeffrey PK, Wardlaw AJ, Nelson FC, Collins JV, Kay AB. Bronchial biopsies in asthma. *Am Rev Respir Dis* 1989;140:1745–1753.
32. Azzawi M, Bradley B, Jeffery PK, et al. Identification of activated T lymphocytes and eosinophils in bronchial biopsies in stable atopic asthma. *Am Rev Respir Dis* 1990;142:1407–1413.
33. Poston RN, Lacoste JY, Litchfield T, Lee TH, Bousquet J. Immunohistochemical characterization of the cellular infiltration in asthmatic bronchi. *Am Rev Respir Dis* 1992;145:918–921.
34. Gratziou C, Carroll M, Walls A, Howarth PH, Holgate ST. Early changes in T-lymphocytes recovered by BAL following local allergen challenge of asthmatic airways. *Am Rev Respir Dis* 1992;145: 1259–1264.
35. Robinson DS, Hamid Q, Ying S, et al. Predominant Th2-like bronchoalveolar T-lymphocyte population in atopic asthma. *N Engl J Med* 1992;326:298–304.
36. Walker C, Bode E, Boer L, Hansel T, Blaser K, Virchow J-C. Allergic and nonallergic asthmatics have distinct patterns of T-cell activation and cytokine production in peripheral blood and bronchoalveolar lavage. *Am Rev Respir Dis* 1992;146:109–115.
37. Del Prete GF, De Carli M, D'Elios MM, et al. Allergen exposure induces the activation of allergen-specific Th2 cells in the airway mucosa of patients with allergic respiratory disorders. *Eur J Immunol* 1993;23:1445–1449.
38. Marini M, Avoni E, Hollemborg J, Mattoli S. Cytokine mRNA profile and cell activation in bronchoalveolar lavage fluid from nonatopic patients with symptomatic athma. *Chest* 1992;102:661–669.
39. Bentley AM, Meng Q, Robinson DS, Hamid Q, Kay AB, Durham SR. Increases in activated T lymphocytes, eosinophils, and cytokine mRNA expression for Interleukin-5 and granulocyte/macrophage colony-stimulating factor in bronchial biopsies after allergen inhalation challenge in atopic asthmatics. *Am J Respir Cell Mol Biol* 1993;8:35–42.
40. Virchow JC, Walker C, HAfner D, et al. T cells and cytokines in bronchoalveolar lavage fluid after segmental allergen provocation in atopic asthma. *Am J Resp Crit Care Med* 1995;151:960–968.
41. Kaminuma O, Mori A, Ogawa K, et al. Successful transfer of late phase eosinophil infiltration in the lung by infusion of helper T cell clones. *Am J Respir Cell Mol Biol* 1997;16:448–454.
42. Krug N, Madden J, Redington AE, et al. T-cell cytokine profile evaluated at the single cell level in BAL and blood in allergic asthma. *Am J Respir Cell Mol Biol* 1996;14:319–326.
43. Maestrelli P, Del Prete GF, De Carli M. CD-8 T-cells producing interleukin-5 and interferon-gamma in bronchial mucosa of patients with asthma induced by toluene-diisocyanate. *Scand J Work Environ Health* 1994;20:376–381.
44. Chan-Yeung M. Immunologic and nonimmunologic mechanisms in asthma due to Western red cedar *(Thuja plicata)*. *J Allergy Clin Immunol* 1982;70:32–37.
45. Fabbri LM, Maestrelli P, Saetta M, Mapp CE. Airway inflammation during late asthmatic reactions induced by toluene diisocyanate. *Am Rev Respir Dis* 1991;143:37s–38s.
46. Maestrelli P, di Stefano A, Occari P, et al. Cytokines in the airway mucosa of subjects with athma induced by toluene diisocyanate. *Am J Resp Crit Care Med* 1995;151:607–612.
47. Wasserman SI. Mast cells and airway inflammation in asthma. *Am J Resp Crit Care Med* 1994;150:S39–S41.

48. Warner JA, Kroegel C. Pulmonary immune cells in health and disease: mast cells and basophils. *Eur Respir J* 1994;7:1326–1341.
49. Holgate ST. The immunopharmacology of mild asthma. *J Allergy Clin Immunol* 1996;98:S7–S16.
50. Laitinen LA, Laitinen A, Haahtela T. Airway mucosal inflammation, even in patients with newly diagnosed asthma. *Am Rev Respir Dis* 1993;147:697–704.
51. Pesci A, Foresi A, Bertorelli G, Chetta A, Oliveri D. Histochemical characteristics and degranulation of mast cells in epithelium and lamina propria of bronchial biopsies from asthmatic and normal subjects. *Am Rev Respir Dis* 1993;147:684–689.
52. Bradding P, Feather IH, Howarth PH. Interleukin 4 is localized to and released by human mast cells. *J Exp Med* 1992;176:1381–1386.
53. Bradding P, Roberts JA, Britten KM, et al. Interleukin-4, -5, and -6 and tumor necrosis factor-α in normal and asthmatic airways: evidence for the human mast cell as a source of these cytokines. *Am J Respir Cell Mol Biol* 1994;10:471–480.
54. Jaffe JS, Glaum MC, Raible DG, et al. Human lung mast cell IL-5 gene and protein expression: temporal analysis of upregulation following IgE-mediated activation. *Am J Respir Cell Mol Biol* 1995;13: 665–675.
55. Ying S, Humbert M, Barkans J, et al. Expression of IL-4 and IL-5 mRNA and protein product by $CD4^+$ and $CD8^+$ T cells, eosinophils, and mast cells in bronchial biopsies obtained from atopic and nonatopic (intrinsic asthmatics). *J Immunol* 1997;158:3539–3544.
56. Okayama Y, Petit-Frere C, Kassel O. Expression of mRNA for IL-5 and IL-4 in human mast cells in response to Fcε-receptor cross-linking and the presence of stem cell factor. *J Immunol* 1995;155: 1796–1808.
57. Saetta M, di Stefano A, Maestrelli P, et al. Airway mucosal inflammation in occupational asthma induced by toluene diisocyanate. *Am Rev Respir Dis* 1992;145:160–168.
58. Ellis AG. The pathological anatomy of bronchial asthma. *Am J Med Sci* 1908;136:407–429.
59. Filley WC, Holley KE, Kephart GM, Gleich GJ. Identification by immunofluorescence of eosinophil granule major basic protein in lung tissues of patients with bronchial asthma. *Lancet* 1982;2:11–15.
60. Bousquet J, Chanez P, Lacoste JY, et al. Eosinophilic inflammation in asthma. *N Engl J Med* 1990;232:1033–1039.
61. Broide DH, Gleich GJ, Cuomo AJ, et al. Evidence of ongoing mast cell and eosinophil degranulation in symptomatic asthma airway. *J Allergy Clin Immunol* 1991;88:637–648.
62. Kroegel C, Virchow JC, Luttman W, Walker C, Warner JA. Pulmonary immune cells in health and disease: the eosinophil leucocyte. *Eur Respir J* 1994;7:519–543.
63. Wardlaw AJ. Eosinophils in the 1990's: new perspectives on their role in health and disease. *Postgrad Med J* 1994;70:536–552.
64. Moller GM, de Jong TA, Overbeek SE, van der Kwast TH, Postma DS, Hoogsteden HC. Ultrastructural immunogold localization of interleukin 5 to the crystalloid core compartment of eosinophil secondary granules in patients with atopic asthma. *J Histochem Cytochem* 1996;44:67–69.
65. Kita H, Ohnishi Y, Okubu Y, Weller JS, Abrams JS, Gleich GJ. GM-CSF and interleukin-3 release from human peripheral blood eosinophils and neutrophils. *J Exp Med* 1991;174:743–748.
66. Rothenberg ME, Owen WF, Silberstein DS, et al. Human eosinophils have prolonged survival, enhanced functional properties, and become hypodense when exposed to human interleukin 3. *J Clin Invest* 1988; 81:1986–1992.
67. De Monchy JG, Kauffman HK, Venge P, et al. Bronchoalveolar eosinophila during allergen-induced late asthmatic reactions. *Am Rev Respir Dis* 1985;131:373–376.
68. Murphy EE, Terres G, Macatonia SE, et al. B7 and interleukin-12 cooperate for proliferation and interferon gamma production by mouse T helper clones that are unresponsive to B7 costimulation. *J Exp Med* 1994;180:223–231.
69. Ohashi Y, Motojima S, Fukuda T, Makino S. Airway hyperresponsiveness, increased intracellular spaces of bronchial epithelium, and increased infiltration of eosinophils and lymphocytes in bronchial mucosa in asthma. *Am Rev Respir Dis* 1992;145:1469–1476.
70. Bentley AM, Maestrelli P, Fabbri LM, Menz G, Storz C, Bradley B. Activated T lymphocytes and eosinophils in the bronchial mucosa in isocyanate-induced asthma. *J Allergy Clin Immunol* 1992;89: 821–829.
71. Frew AJ, Chan H, Lam S, Chan-Yeung M. Bronchial inflammation in occupational asthma due to Western red cedar. *Am J Resp Crit Care Med* 1995;151:340–344.
72. Romagnani S. Lymphokine production by human T cells in disease states. *Annu Rev Immunol* 1994;12:227.
73. Howard M, Farrar J, Hilfiker M, et al. Identification of a T cell-derived B cell growth factor distinct from interleukin 2. *J Exp Med* 1982;155:914–923.
74. Paul WE. Interleukin-4: a prototypic immunoregulatory lymphokine. *Blood* 1991;77:1859–1870.
75. Kuhn R, Rajewsky K, Muller W. Generation and analysis of interleukin-4 deficient mice. *Science* 1991;254:707–710.
76. Rothman P. Interleukin 4 targeting of immunoglobulin heavy chain class-switch recombination. *Res Immunol* 1993;144:579–583.
77. Tanaka T, Hu-Li J, Seder RA, de St. Groth BF, Paul WE. Interleukin 4 suppresses interleukin 2 and interferon gamma production by naive T cells stimulated by accessory cell-dependent receptor engagement. *Proc Natl Acad Sci USA* 1993;90:5914–5918.
78. Seder RA, Paul WE, Davis MM, Fazekas D, St. Groth B. The presence of interleukin 4 during in vitro priming determines the lymphocyte-producing potential of $CD4^+$ T cells from T cell receptor transgenic mice. *J Exp Med* 1992;176:1091–1098.
79. Masinovsky B, Urdal D, Gallatin WM. IL-4 acts synergistically with IL-1β to promote lymphocyte adhesion to microvascular endothelium by induction of vascular cell adhesion molecule-1. *J Immunol* 1990; 145:2886–2895.
80. Humbert M, Durham SR, Ying S, et al. IL-4 and IL-5 mRNA and protein in bronchial biopsies from patients with atopic and nonatopic asthma: evidence against "intrinsic" asthma being a distinct immunopathologic entity. *Am J Resp Crit Care Med* 1996;154: 1497–1504.
81. Yamaguchi Y, Suda T, Suda J, et al. Purified interleukin 5 supports the terminal differentiation and proliferation of murine eosinophilic precursors. *J Exp Med* 1988;167:43–56.
82. Lopez AF, Sanderson CJ, Gamble JR, Campbell HD, Young IG, Vadas MA. Recombinant human interleukin 5 is a selective activator of human eosinophil function. *J Exp Med* 1988;167:219–224.
83. Hamid Q, Azzawi M, Sun Ying, et al. Expression of mRNA for Interleukin-5 in mucosal bronchial biopsies from asthma. *J Clin Invest* 1991;87:1541–1546.
84. Ying S, Durham SR, Corrigan CJ, Hamid Q, Kay AB. Phenotype of cells expressing mRNA for TH2-type (interleukin 4 and interleukin 5) and TH1-type (interleukin 2 and interferon-γ) cytokines in bronchoalveolar lavage and bronchial biopsies from atopic asthmatic and normal control subjects. *Am J Respir Cell Mol Biol* 1995;12:477–487.
85. Virchow JC, Kroegel C, Walker C, Matthys H. Inflammatory determinants of asthma severity: mediator and cellular changes in bronchoalveolar lavage fluid of patients with severe asthma. *J Allergy Clin Immunol* 1996;98:S27–S40.
86. Shaver JR, Zangrilli JG, Cho S-K, et al. Kinetics of the development and recovery of the lung from IgE-mediated inflammation. *Am J Resp Crit Care Med* 1997;155:442–448.
87. Brusselle GG, Kips JC, Tavernier JH, et al. Attenuation of allergic airway inflammation in IL-4 deficient mice. *Clin Exp Allergy* 1994; 24:73–80.
88. Lukacs NW, Strieter RM, Chensue SW, Kunkel SL. Interleukin-4-dependent pulmonary eosinophil infiltration in a murine model of asthma. *Am J Respir Cell Mol Biol* 1994;10:526–532.
89. Corry DB, Folkesson HG, Warnock ML, et al. Interleukin 4, but not interleukin 5 or eosinophils, is required in a murine model of acute airway hyperreactivity. *J Exp Med* 1996;183:109–117.
90. Hogan SP, Mould A, Kikutani H, Ramsay AJ, Foster PS. Aeroallergen-induced eosinophilic inflammation, lung damage, and airways hyperreactivity in mice can occur independently of IL-4 and allergen-specific immunoglobulins. *J Clin Invest* 1997;99:1329–1339.
91. Foster PS, Hogan SP, Ramsay AJ, Matthaei KI, Young IG. Interleukin 5 deficiency abolishes eosinophilia, airways hyperreactivity, and lung damage in a mouse asthma model. *J Exp Med* 1996;183:195–201.
92. Minty A, Chalon P, Derocq J-M, et al. Interleukin-13 is a new human lymphokine regulating inflammatory and immune responses. *Nature* 1993;362:248–250.
93. McKenzie AN, Culpepper JA, de Waal Malefyt R, et al. Interleukin 13, a T-cell derived cytokine that regulates human monocyte and B-cell function. *Proc Natl Acad Sci USA* 1993;90:3735–3739.

94. Zurawski G, De Vries JE. Interleukin 13, an interleukin 4-like cytokine that acts on monocytes and B cells, but not on T cells. *Immunol Today* 1994;15:19–26.
95. de Waal Malefyt R, Figdor CG, Huijbens R, et al. Effects of IL-13 on phenotype, cytokine production, and cytotoxic function of human monocytes. *J Immunol* 1993;151:6370–6381.
96. Kroegel C, Julius P, Matthys H, Virchow JC, Luttmann W. Endobronchial secretion of interleukin-13 following local allergen challenge in atopic asthma: relationship to interleukin-4 and eosinophil counts. *Eur Respir J* 1996;9:899–904.
97. Miyatake S, Otsuka T, Yokota T, Lee F, Arai K. Structure of the chromosomal gene for granulocyte macrophage colony stimulating factor: comparison of the mouse and human genes. *EMBO J* 1985;4:2561.
98. Heubner K, Isobe M, Croce CM, Golde DW, Daufman SE, Gasson JC. The human gene encoding GM-CSF is at 5q21-q32, the chromosome region deleted in the 5q-anomaly. *Science* 1985;230:1282.
99. Kaushansky K, O'Hara PJ, Berkner K, Segal GM, Hagen FS, Adamson JW. Genomic cloning characterization and multilineage growth-promoting activity of human granulocyte-macrophage colony-stimulating factor. *Proc Natl Acad Sci USA* 1986;83:3101.
100. Diederichs K, Boone T, Karplus PA. Novel fold and putative receptor binding site of granulocyte-macrophage colony-stimulating. *Science* 1991;254:1779–1781.
101. Gasson JC. Molecular physiology of granulocyte-macrophage colony-stimulating factor. *Blood* 1991;77:1131–1145.
102. Weisbart RH, Golde DW, Clark SC, Wong GG, Gasson JC. Human granulocyte-macrophage colony-stimulating factor is a neutrophil activator. *Nature* 1985;314:361–363.
103. Lopez AF, Williamson J, Gamble JR, et al. Recombinant human granulocyte-macrophage colony-stimulating factor stimulates in vitro mature human neutrophil and eosinophil function, surface receptor expression, and survival. *J Clin Invest* 1986;78:1220–1228.
104. Tazi A, Bouchonnet F, Grandsaingne M, Boumsell L, Hance AJ, Soler P. Evidence that granulocyte macrophage-colony-stimulating factor regulates the distribution and differentiated state of dendritic cells/Langerhans cells in human lung and lung cancers. *J Clin Invest* 1993; 91:566–576.
105. Witmer-Pack MD, Olivier W, Valinsky J, Schuler G, Steinman RM. Granulocyte/macrophage colony-stimulating factor is essential for the viability and function of cultured murine epidermal langerhans cells. *J Exp Med* 1987;166:1484–1498.
106. Dranoff G, Crawford AD, Sadelain M, et al. Involvement of granulocyte-macrophage colony stimulating factor in pulmonary homeostasis. *Science* 1994;264:713–716.
107. Stanley E, Lieschke GJ, Grail D, et al. Granulocyte/macrophage colony-stimulating factor-deficient mice show major perturbation of hematopoiesis but develop a characteristic pulmonary pathology. *Proc Natl Acad Sci USA* 1994;91:5592–5596.
108. Huffman JA, Hull WM, Dranoff G, Mulligan RC, Whitsett JA. Pulmonary epithelial cell expression of GM-CSF corrects the alveolar proteinosis in GM-CSF-deficient mice. *J Clin Invest* 1996;97: 649–655.
109. Nishinakamura R, Wiler R, Dirksen U, et al. The pulmonary alveolar proteinosis in granulocyte macrophage colony-stimulating factor/interleukins 3/5 βc receptor-deficient mice is reversed by bone marrow transplantation. *J Exp Med* 1996;183:2657–2662.
110. Kato M, Liu MC, Stealey BA, et al. Production of granulocyte/macrophage colony-stimulating factor in human airways during allergen-induced late-phase reactions in atopic subjects. *Lymph Cytokine Res* 1992;11:287–292.
111. Churchill L, Friedman B, Schleimer RP, Proud D. Production of granulocyte-macrophage colony-stimlating factor by cultured human tracheal epithelial cells. *Immunology* 1992;75:189–195.
112. Cromwell O, Hamid Q, Corrigan CJ, Barkans J, Meng. Q, Collins PD. Expression and generation of interleukin-8, Il-6, and granulocyte-macrophage colony-stimulating factor by bronchial epithelial cells and enhancement by IL-1β and tumour necrosis factor-α. *Immunology* 1992;77:330–337.
113. Marini M, Soloperto M, Mezzetti M, Fasoli A, Mattoli S. Interleukin-1 binds to specific receptors on human bronchial epithelial cells and upregulates granulocyte/macrophage colony-stimulating factor synthesis and release. *Am J Respir Cell Mol Biol* 1991;4:519–524.
114. Nakamura Y, Azuma M, Okano Y, et al. Upregulatory effects of interleukin-4 and interleukin-13 but not interleukin-10 on granulocyte/macrophage colony-stimulating factor production by human bronchial epithelial cells. *Am J Respir Cell Mol Biol* 1996;15:680–687.
115. Marini M, Vittori E, Hollemborg J, Mattoli S. Expression of the potent inflammatory cytokines, granulocyte-macrophage-colony-stimulating factor and interleukin-6 and interleukin-8, in bronchial epithelial cells of patients with asthma. *J Allergy Clin Immunol* 1992;89:1001–1009.
116. Sousa AR, Poston RN, Lane SJ, Nakhosteen JA, Lee TH. Detection of GM-CSF in asthmatic bronchial epithelium and decrease by inhaled corticosteroids. *Am Rev Respir Dis* 1993;147:1557–1561.
117. Ackerman V, Marini M, Vittori E, Bellini A, Bassali G, Mattoli S. Detection of cytokines and their cell sources in bronchial biopsy specimens from asthmatic patients. *Chest* 1994;105:687–686.
118. Paul SR, Bennett JA, Calvetti JA, et al. Molecular cloning of a cDNA encoding interleukin-11, a stromal cell-derived lymphopoietic and hematopoietic cytokine. *Proc Natl Acad Sci USA* 1990;87:7512–7516.
119. Tang W, Geba GP, Zheng T, et al. Targeted expression of IL-11 in the murine airway causes lymphocytic inflammation, bronchial remodeling, and airways obstruction. *J Clin Invest* 1996;98:2845–3853.
120. Farrar MA, Schreiber RD. The molecular cell biology of interferon-γ and its receptor. *Annu Rev Immunol* 1993;11:571–611.
121. Stern AS, Podlaski FJ, Hulmes JD, et al. Purification to homogeneity and partial characterization of cytotoxic lymphocyte maturation factor from human B-lymphoblastoid cells. *Proc Natl Acad Sci USA* 1990; 87:6808–6812.
122. Howard M, O'Garra A. Biological properties of interleukin 10. *Immunol Today* 1992;13:198–200.
123. Cembrzynska-Nowak ME, Szklarz AD, Inglot AD, Teodorczyk-Injeyan JA. Elevated release of tumor necrosis factor-alpha and interferon-gamma by bronchoalveolar leukocytes from patients with bronchial asthma. *Am Rev Respir Dis* 1993;147:291–295.
124. Xiu-Min L, Chopra RK, Chou T-Y, Schofield BH, Wills-Karp M, Huang S-K. Mucosal IFN-γ gene transfer inhibits pulmonary allergic responses in mice. *J Immunol* 1996;157:3216–3219.
125. Wolf SF, Temple PA, Kobayashi M, et al. Cloning of cDNA for natural killer cell stimulatory factor, a heterodimeric cytokine with multiple biologic effects on T and natural killer cells. *J Immunol* 1991;146: 3074–3081.
126. Germann T, Rude E. Interleukin-12. *Int Arch Allergy Immunol* 1995;108:103–112.
127. Seder RA, Gazzinelli R, Sher A, Paul WE. Interleukin 12 acts directly on $CD4^+$ T cells to enhance priming for interferon gamma production and diminishes interleukin 4 inhibition of such priming. *Proc Natl Acad Sci USA* 1993;90:10188–10192.
128. Knol EF, Roos D. Mechanisms regulating eosinophil extravasation in asthma. *Eur Respir J* 1996;22:136s–140s.
129. Humbert M, Ying S, Corrigan C, et al. Bronchial mucosal expression of the genes encoding chemokines RANTES and MCP-3 in symptomatic atopic and nonatopic asthmatics: relationship to the eosinophil-active cytokines interleukin (IL)-5, granulocyte-macrophage colony-stimulating factor, and IL-3. *Am J Respir Cell Mol Biol* 1997;16:1–8.
130. Venge J, Lamplinen M, Hakansson L, Rak S, Venge P. Identification of IL-5 and RANTES as the major eosinophil chemoattractants in the asthmatic lung. *J Allergy Clin Immunol* 1996;97:1110–1115.
131. Carlos TM, Harlan JM. Leukocyte-endothelial adhesion molecules. *Blood* 1994;84:2068–2101.
132. Larson RS, Springer TA. Structure and function of leukocyte integrins. In: *Immunological reviews,* 114th ed. Copenhagen, Denmark: Munksgaard, 1990;181–206.
133. Bevilacqua MP, Pober JS, Mendrick DL, Cotran RS, Gimbrone A. Identification of an inducible endothelial leukocyte adhesion molecule. *Proc Natl Acad Sci USA* 1987;84:9238–9242.
134. Osborn L, Hession C, Tizard R, et al. Direct expression cloning of vascular cell adhesion molecule 1, a cytokine-induced endothelial protein that binds lymphocytes. *Cell* 1989;59:1203–1211.
135. Greve FM, Davis G, Meyer AM, et al. The major human rhinovirus receptor is ICAM-1. *Cell* 1989;56:839–845.
136. Rothlein R, Dustin ML, Marlin SD, Springer TA. A human intercellular adhesion molecule (ICAM-1) distinct from LFA-1. *J Immunol* 1986;137:1270–1274.
137. Dustin ML, Rothlein R, Bhan AK, Dinarello CA, Springer TA. Induction by IL-1 and interferon-gamma: tissue distribution, biochemistry, and function of a natural adherence molecule (ICAM-1). *J Immunol* 1986;137:245–254.
138. Marlin SD, Springer TA. Purified intercellular adhesion molecule-1

(ICAM-1) is a ligand for lymphocyte function-associated antigen-1 (LFA-1). *Cell* 1987;51:813–819.
139. Staunton DE, Marlin SD, Stratowa C, Dustin ML, Springer TA. Primary structure of ICAM-1 demonstrates interaction between members of the immunoglobulin and integrin supergene families. *Cell* 1988;52:925–933.
140. Simmons D, Makgoba MW, Seed B. ICAM, an adhesion ligand of LFA-1 is homologous to the neural cell adhesion molecule NCAM. *Nature* 1988;331:624–627.
141. Rothlein R, Czajkowski M, O'Neill MM, Marlin SD, Mainolfi E, Merluzzi VJ. Induction of intercellular adhesion molecule 1 on primary and continuous cell lines by pro-inflammatory cytokines. *J Immunol* 1988;144:1665–1669.
142. Wegner CD, Gundel RH, Reilly P, Haynes N, Letts LG, Rothlein R. Intercellular adhesion molecule-1 (ICAM-1) in the pathogenesis of asthma. *Science* 1990;247:456–459.
143. Montefort S, Roche WR, Howarth PH, et al. Intercellular adhesion molecule-1 (ICAM-1) and endothelial leucocyte adhesion molecule-1 (ELAM-1) expression in the bronchial mucosa of normal and asthmatic subjects. *Eur Respir J* 1992;5:815–823.
144. Vignola AA, Campbell AM, Chanez P, et al. HLA-DR and ICAM-1 expression on bronchial epithelial cells in asthma and chronic bronchitis. *Am Rev Respir Dis* 1993;148:689–694.
145. Bentley AM, Durham SR, Robinson DS, et al. Expression of endothelial and leukocyte adhesion molecules ICAM-1, E-selectin, and VCAM-1 in the bronchial mucosa in steady state and allergen-induced asthma. *J Allergy Clin Immunol* 1993;92:857–868.
146. Georas SN, Liu MC, Newman W, Beall LD, Stealey BA, Bochner BS. Altered adhesion molecule expression and endothelial cell activation accompany the recruitment of human granulocytes to the lung after segmental allergen challenge. *Am J Respir Cell Mol Biol* 1992;7:261–269.
147. Ohkawara Y, Yamauchi K, Maruyama N, et al. In situ expression of the cell adhesion molecules in bronchial tissues from asthmatics with air flow limitation: in vivo evidence of VCAM-1/VLA-4 interaction in selective eosinophil infiltration. *Am J Respir Cell Mol Biol* 1995; 12:4–12.
148. Lobb RR, Pepinskly B, Leone DR, Abraham WM. The role of alpha 4 integrins in lung pathophysiology. *Eur Respir J* 1996;22:104s–108s.
149. Rice GE, Bevilacqua MP. An inducible endothelial cell surface glycoprotein mediates melanoma adhesion. *Science* 1989;246:1303–1306.
150. Rice GE, Munro JM, Corless C, Bevilacqua MP. Inducible cell adhesion molecule 110 is an endothelial receptor for lymphocytes. A CD11/CD18-independent adhesion mechanism. *J Exp Med* 1990; 171:1369–1374.
151. Cybulsky MI, Fries JW, Williams AJ, et al. Alternative splicing of human VCAM-1 in activated vascular endothelium. *Am J Pathol* 1991;138:815–820.
152. Thornhill MH, Wellicome SM, Mahiouz DL, Lanchbury JS, Kyan-Aung U, Haskard DO. Tumor necrosis factor combines with IL-4 or IFN-γ to selectively enhance endothelial cell adhesiveness for T cells. *J Immunol* 1991;146:592–598.
153. Schleimer RP, Sterbinsky SA, Kaiser J, et al. IL-4 induces adherence of human eosinophils and basophils but not neutrophils to endothelium. *J Immunol* 1992;148:1086–1092.
154. Gosset P, Tillie-Leblond I, Janin A, et al. Expression of E-Selectin, ICAM-1 and VCAM-1 on bronchial biopsies from allergic and non-allergic asthmatic patients. *Int Arch Allergy Immunol* 1995;106:69–77.
155. Fukuda T, Fukushima Y, Numao T, et al. Role of interleukin-4 and vascular cell adhesion molecule-1 in selective eosinophil migration into the airways in allergic asthma. *Am J Respir Cell Mol Biol* 1996;14: 84–94.
156. Laitinen LA, Heino M, Laitinen A, Kava T, Haahtela T. Damage of the airway epithelium and bronchial reactivity in patients with asthma. *Am Rev Respir Dis* 1985;131:599–606.
157. Lundgren R, Soderberg M, Horstedt M, Stenling R. Morphological studies of bronchial mucosal biopsies from asthmatics before and after ten years of treatment with inhaled steroids. *Eur Respir J* 1988; 1:883–889.
158. Dunnill MS, Massarella GR, Anderson JA. A comparison of the quantitative anatomy of the bronchi in normal subjects, in status asthmaticus, in chronic bronchitis, and in emphysema. *Thorax* 1969;24: 176–179.
159. Laitinen LA, Laitinen A. Remodeling of asthmatic airways by glucocorticosteroids. *J Allergy Clin Immunol* 1996;97:153–158.
160. Roche WR, Williams JH, Beasley R, Holgate S. Subepithelial fibrosis in the bronchi of asthmatics. *Lancet* 1989;520–523.
161. Ollerenshaw SL, Woolcock AJ. Characteristics of the inflammation in biopsies from large airways of subjects with asthma and subjects with chronic airflow limitation. *Am Rev Respir Dis* 1992;145:922–927.
162. Laitinen LA, Laitinen A, Altraja A, et al. Bronchial biopsy findings in intermittent or "early" asthma. *J Allergy Clin Immunol* 1996;98: S3–S6.
163. Saetta M, Maestrelli P, Turato G, et al. Airway wall remodeling after cessation of exposure to isocyanates in sensitized asthmatic subjects. *Am J Respir Crit Care Med* 1995;151:489–494.
164. Altraja A, Laitinen A, Virtanen I, et al. Expression of laminins in the airways in various types of asthmatic patients: a morphometric study. *Am J Respir Cell Mol Biol* 1996;15:482–488.

*Environmental and Occupational Medicine,*
*Third Edition,* edited by William N. Rom.
Lippincott–Raven Publishers, Philadelphia © 1998.

CHAPTER 35

# Respiratory Effects of Isocyanates

Daniel E. Banks

Polyurethane foams were first produced in Germany during the Second World War using toluene diisocyanate (TDI), a volatile compound of low molecular weight that exists in the 2,4 and 2,6 isomeric forms. Production of this isocyanate was limited because of technical problems and the recognition of adverse respiratory effects in German production workers during the war (1). Safe commercial production of urethane polymers as flexible foam began in the United States in 1953 (2). Since then, a myriad of uses has been found for flexible polyurethane foam. Applications of flexible foam include thermal insulating materials, upholstery, mattresses, and packaging materials. Of all the isocyanates, TDI has historically been the isocyanate produced in greatest quantity until relatively recently.

With technical improvements, a system for the safe commercial production of rigid foam was developed in the 1950s using methylene diphenyl diisocyanate (MDI), an isocyanate that is markedly less volatile and therefore considered less toxic than TDI. Specifically, because the vapor pressure of MDI is less than TDI, TDI vaporizes at a lesser temperature and therefore provides a greater chance for exposure. For example, at a temperature of 75°C, TDI would have a vapor pressure of 1.0 mm Hg of TDI while MDI would have a vapor pressure of only 0.01 mm Hg. MDI can be injected into enclosed spaces and serves as a good insulating material. It provides moderate tensile strength with the benefit of minimal weight. Rigid polyurethane foam is not appreciably deformed by modest impact and a major use has been as a substitute for automobile body components that previously were made of steel, such as bumpers and, more recently, fenders. Such changes have made possible lighter, and therefore more fuel-efficient, automobiles. The greatest projected growth in MDI usage is anticipated to be in the construction industry and in a relatively newly recognized application, as an adhesive, with automotive, appliance and durable goods close behind.

A third commercially important isocyanate is hexamethylene diisocyanate (HDI), a color-stable aliphatic isocyanate (unlike the aromatic isocyanates MDI and TDI). Because of its stability, HDI is used in paints as an activating agent and is best suited for coating and external finishes. It has a vapor pressure paralleling TDI.

This chapter addresses the respiratory health effects associated with isocyanate exposure. Isocyanates to be considered include those mentioned above and other less frequently used compounds, including naphthalene diisocyanate (NDI) and isophorone diisocyanate (IPDI) (Fig. 1). NDI is heated and used as a curing agent in the production of synthetic rubber.

Since the early days of this industry, utilization of isocyanates has dramatically increased. In 1975, 400 million pounds of TDI and 300 million pounds of MDI were consumed worldwide, with only a few million pounds of the other isocyanates. A more recent estimate of the production of flexible and rigid foam is provided in Table 1 (3). Recent industry estimates project MDI production to grow at a rate of 5% per year and TDI growth to approximate 2% per year through the year 2000. The National Occupational Hazard Survey, conducted by the U.S. Public Health Service between 1972 and 1974, estimated that between 50,000 and 100,000 people had potential workplace exposures to diisocyanates (4). An estimated 34,000 workers were exposed to TDI in the United States during the period of 1981 to 1983 (5). That number is likely greater today.

D. E. Banks: Section of Pulmonary and Critical Care Medicine, Department of Medicine, Robert C. Byrd Health Sciences Center, West Virginia University School of Medicine, Morgantown, West Virginia 26506-9166.

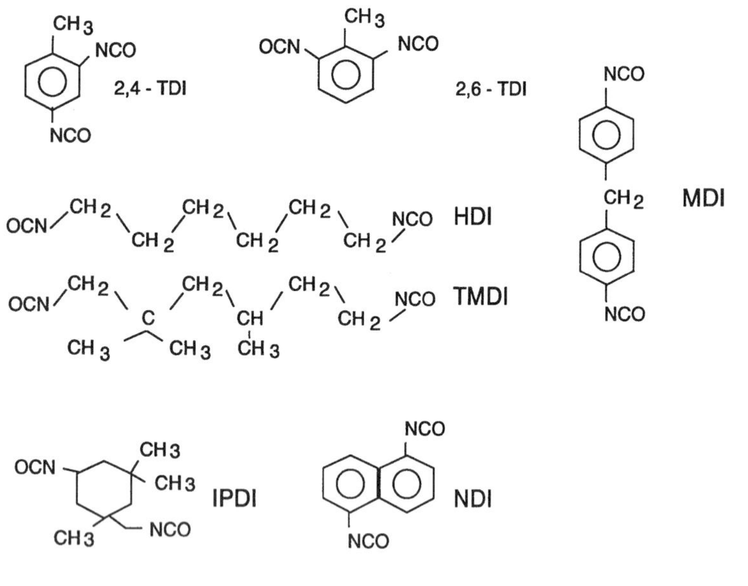


**FIG. 1.** The chemical structures of the 2,4 and 2,6 isomers of TDI, HDI, MDI, and trimeric MDI, IPDI, and NDI. (Courtesy of Roy Rando, D.Sc.)

## PRODUCTION AND CHARACTERISTICS OF ISOCYANATES AND URETHANES

Isocyanates are formed from the mixture of amines with phosgene. A primary aliphatic or aromatic amine is dissolved in a solvent such as xylene or monochlorobenzene and mixed with phosgene dissolved in the same solvent for several hours at high heat. At the end of the reaction fractions of isocyanate, reclaimable phosgene, hydrochloric acid, excess solvent, and waste residues are the result.

Urethanes are formed by a chemical reaction between polyglycols or polyols and diisocyanates. A primary feature of the isocyanates as a class of chemicals is their extreme chemical reactivity. This reactivity is a major asset to their use as chemical agents, but is also responsible for their adverse interactions in the lung. In a controlled chemical reaction, this reactivity allows isocyanate molecules to bind polyol molecules to form a polymeric mass. When water is added to these reacting chemicals, carbon dioxide is released, causing the mixture to carbonate or foam. By adding catalysts such as tin and various amines the chemical reactions are enhanced.

The produced foam is stabilized by adding silicon-based agents. If water is not added to this reaction, there is no foaming. In this instance, this mixture of isocyanates, polyols or polyglycols, and catalyst can then be used as a coating material, sometimes applied by power spraying. Examples of isocyanate-coated materials include waterproof clothes and recreational canvas shoes.

**TABLE 1.** *United States isocyanate demand (millions of pounds)*

| | 1995 | 1996 | 2000[a] |
|---|---|---|---|
| TDI | 870 | 900 | 995 |
| MDI | 1,110 | 1,114 | 1,145 |

[a]Projected values.

The physical characteristics of the individual isocyanates affect the ambient environmental levels and the chance for adverse respiratory effects. While TDI exists as a liquid, NDI and pure MDI are solid at room temperature (although MDI is more often stored as a thick liquid combination of polymerized MDI and acetone). MDI must be pressurized or heated for vapors to be released, although droplets of MDI persist in the atmosphere following aerosolization.

The ability of different isocyanates to be dispersed into the ambient environment is determined by their vapor pressure. As a rule, the lesser-molecular weight isocyanates (TDI, HDI) have similar vapor pressures (4) and are readily volatilized into workplace air. Therefore, unless TDI and HDI are handled with great care, irritating (and potentially sensitizing) concentrations of vapor are the rule. The ultimate use of the isocyanate also plays a role in determining the level of the agent in the environment. For example, the molecular weight of HDI, typically in the biuret or trimeric form (i.e., three molecules of HDI bound together) when used in HDI-based paints, is greater and the result is a diminution of vapor pressure. A lower concentration of isocyanate is likely to be produced by drying of HDI-based than by curing of TDI-based polyurethane foam.

Higher molecular weight compounds such as NDI, IPDI, and MDI exert a fraction of the vapor pressure of TDI or HDI. This realization has driven technology to adapt industrial processes that substitute MDI for TDI. An example of this is in the isocyanate injection molding process used to insulate doors and refrigerators. These changes, as well as the recognition of more uses for rigid foam, are reflected in the slope of increased production of rigid—compared to flexible—foam. Yet, in spraying and in certain foaming operations where isocyanates exist as an aerosol, substitution of higher molecular weight agents for TDI may not effectively reduce exposure. In addition, in poorly ventilated areas these higher molecular weight isocyanates may generate vapor concentrations sufficient to be both irritating and sensitizing.

## ADVERSE RESPIRATORY HEALTH EFFECTS OF ISOCYANATES

Potential adverse respiratory effects associated with isocyanate exposure include acute or long-lasting effects due to a single episode of overexposure, chronic respiratory effects caused by long-term low-level exposure,occupational asthma, and hypersensitivity pneumonitis (5). In addition, a single case of a spray painter with a sporadic history of intravenous drug abuse and recognized exposure to HDI, and likely to TDI, had the acute onset of dyspnea, pulmonary hemorrhage, hematuria, and bilateral pulmonary opacities inducing respiratory failure has been reported. High serum levels of immunoglobulin G (IgG) and IgE against HDI and TDI, both bound to human serum albumin (HSA), were found. An open lung biopsy showed intraalveolar hemorrhage, a minimal number of foreign body giant cells thought attributable to contaminants trapped in the lung from intravenous injections, an increased number of macrophages, and no vasculitis. The clinical and immune system features paralleled those associated with hemorrhagic pneumonia attributable to trimellitic anhydride exposure, and the authors thought this illness was caused by isocyanate exposure. No explanation for the hematuria was put forth. Additional cases have not been reported (6).

The pulmonary response to a single, overwhelming exposure of isocyanate is not predictable. First, like an excessive inhalational exposure to any of a long list of chemicals and gases, such a catastrophic event may precipitate diffuse alveolar damage which, if severe enough, can result in the acute respiratory distress syndrome (ARDS). In such cases, the histologic appearance of the lung is not specific for isocyanate injury and the clinical outcome may be unpredictable (7). Some may develop the histologic features of the proliferative phase of ARDS and persistent respiratory impairment. Second, a brief, overwhelming exposure may lead to reactive airways dysfunction syndrome (RADS) with the previously healthy host developing persistent cough, wheeze, and dyspnea occurring with exposures to nonspecific irritant exposures. Although a single, excessive isocyanate exposure was not among the causes of RADS in Brooks et al.'s (8) initial report, other investigators have described persistent respiratory complaints following a singular excessive exposure (9,10). Finally, others may develop sensitization to isocyanates in association with this single overwhelming exposure (11). This is manifest as isocyanate-induced asthma.

**TABLE 2.** *Clinical features of isocyanate-induced asthma*

| |
|---|
| Typically, the worker has no history of preexisting asthma. |
| The worker has exposure to isocyanates. |
| Recurrent asthma occurs in relation to the workplace. |
| Most often, improvement occurs away from the workplace. |
| Once the worker is sensitized, episodes of asthma recur following exposure to subirritant levels of this agent. |
| In chronic cases, recurrent bouts of asthma can develop with exposure to nonspecific irritants unrelated to isocyanates and away from the workplace. |
| Objective evidence of cause and effect makes the diagnosis certain. |

The predominant respiratory illness attributable to isocyanate exposure is asthma. Inhalational exposure to isocyanate vapors can occur in the production of the chemical, during its transport, or in association with the production of polyurethane foams and coatings. Clinical findings needed for the accurate diagnosis of isocyanate-induced asthma are listed in Table 2.

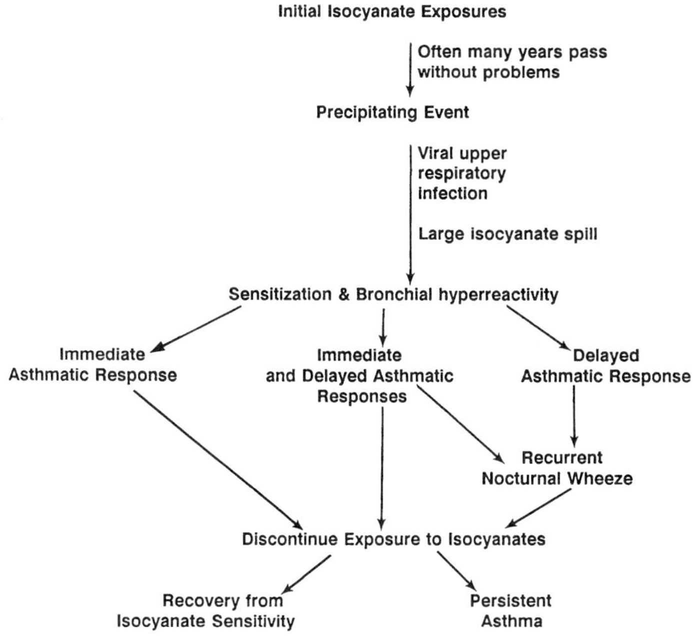


**FIG. 2.** The natural history of isocyanate-induced asthma.

Fuchs and Valade (12) were the first to report a relationship between isocyanate exposure and respiratory disease. In 1951, they reported seven workers with asthma caused by TDI exposure. Although they did not show that TDI provoked chest symptoms by specific challenge testing, they described the now well recognized late asthmatic reaction common in isocyanate-induced asthma. All seven workers had been employed for varying periods in different jobs in the same workplace and had a range of TDI exposure. Typically, asthma began near the end of the workday and continued through the night, improving some in the morning hours, and then recurring in similar temporal fashion following the next workday. Since this initial report, many investigators studying the numerous industries where isocyanates are used have identified workers with isocyanate-induced asthma.

Importantly, not all isocyanate exposures resulting in respiratory illness occur in the traditional setting of the industrialized workplace. Peters and Murphy (13) reported a patient who developed apparent sensitization to TDI following exposure to the fumes released from a do-it-yourself TDI foam kit. Liss et al. (14) reported two sisters who developed asthma while working at home dipping the ends of polyurethane coated wire into molten solder. Two police officers who directed automobile traffic were exposed to a single, excessive exposure to TDI and developed persistent asthma (15). Three clerical workers developed challenge-test–proven TDI sensitivity with asthma following inhalational exposure to TDI from vapors released from an adjacent workplace (16).

Once sensitized, wheezing, shortness of breath, chest tightness, and cough recur in workers following exposure to agents in the workplace, in association with the development of specific and nonspecific bronchial hyperresponsiveness. The clinical pattern and possible outcomes associated with the isocyanate-induced asthma are reported in Fig. 2. Among these clinical features, recurrent nocturnal asthma (i.e., episodes of asthma that occur in those with chronic asthma at or near the same time as the usual late asthmatic episode, independent of whether a worker has isocyanate exposure during that day) remains inadequately explained and frequently causes considerable confusion when attempting to define the etiology of the asthma episodes. In those so sensitized, once the cycle of asthma begins, recurrent episodes of late asthma recur in a circadian pattern (Fig. 3).

In the workplace, episodes of bronchospasm attributable to isocyanates continue to occur with ongoing exposure in sensitized workers. The worker has progressive worsening of respiratory complaints with prolongation of

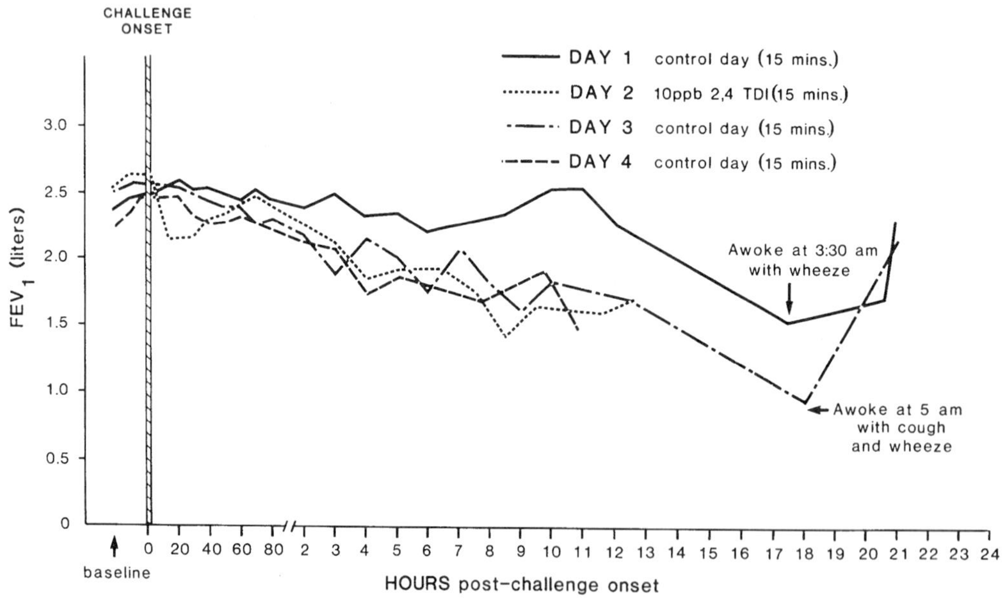


**FIG. 3.** The results of challenge testing performed on a 31-year-old woman who had been employed in a refrigerator-manufacturing facility where TDI was used as an insulant for 9 years. Her chest complaints began about 6 years prior to challenge testing when she developed asthma and dyspnea in association with participating in a recreational basketball program. As time went on she began to relate her respiratory complaints to the workplace. At work, her asthma occurred at the end of the work shift and persisted throughout the night, usually improving in the morning prior to work. Despite these complaints she continued working. At the time of testing she was not wheezing, had normal spirometric parameters, and her level of bronchial hyperresponsiveness to methacholine was moderately increased. She was tested 4 days after her last workplace exposure. On the first day of testing she had evidence of recurrent nocturnal asthma. After a very brief exposure to 0.010 ppm of TDI on day 2 she had progressive late asthma. Day 3 spirometry showed a dramatic recurrent nocturnal decline in FEV1 that awoke the patient and improved in response to albuterol inhalation. (Reprinted with permission from ref. 106.)

the recovery phase with these recurrent isocyanate exposures. This often results in chronic asthma. In this advanced clinical situation, not only isocyanates, but nonspecific irritants such as bleaches, perfumes, tobacco smoke, cold air, and exercise, provoke bronchospasm and occasionally recurrent nocturnal asthma. Workers who develop chronic asthma are the least likely to improve after being removed from the workplace.

Only a small percentage of workers exposed to isocyanates become sensitized. In a 1976 study, five of 112 workers employed in a newly opened TDI production facility developed asthma. A 1977 report of the same population showed 11 of 130 to be sensitized (17). These studies are the origin of the often quoted 5 to 10% prevalence of TDI-induced asthma among exposed workers. Bernstein et al. (18) reported the results of a cross-sectional survey of 243 employees of a polyurethane plant that used MDI exclusively for the 3 years the plant had been in operation. Although, MDI levels were monitored 24 hours per day in multiple sites and no short-term exposure exceeded 0.005 parts per million (ppm), the authors could not rule out excessive short-term exposures occurring outside of the monitored areas. Nine workers (4%) had respiratory complaints consistent with occupational asthma. Three of these nine had peak flow rate variability exceeding 15% over the work shift. If these three are considered to have objective evidence of isocyanate-induced asthma, then the prevalence in this population approximated 1%. This may be one reason why some investigators maintain that there is no safe level of isocyanate exposure.

Bignon et al. (19) have taken the first steps to address whether there is a genetic predisposition leading some workers to develop isocyanate-induced asthma. They sampled blood from workers with isocyanate-induced asthma and from those workers exposed to isocyanates but without symptoms and addressed the role of the human leukocyte antigen (HLA) class II genes in the development of asthma. The products from these genes are involved in the presentation by antigen-presenting cells of peptides derived from endocytosed extracellular antigens to $CD4^+$ T lymphocytes. Different HLA genes or their products appear to protect against or increase the risk for the development of asthma due to sensitization by a specific allergen. Identifiable allelic variations at the

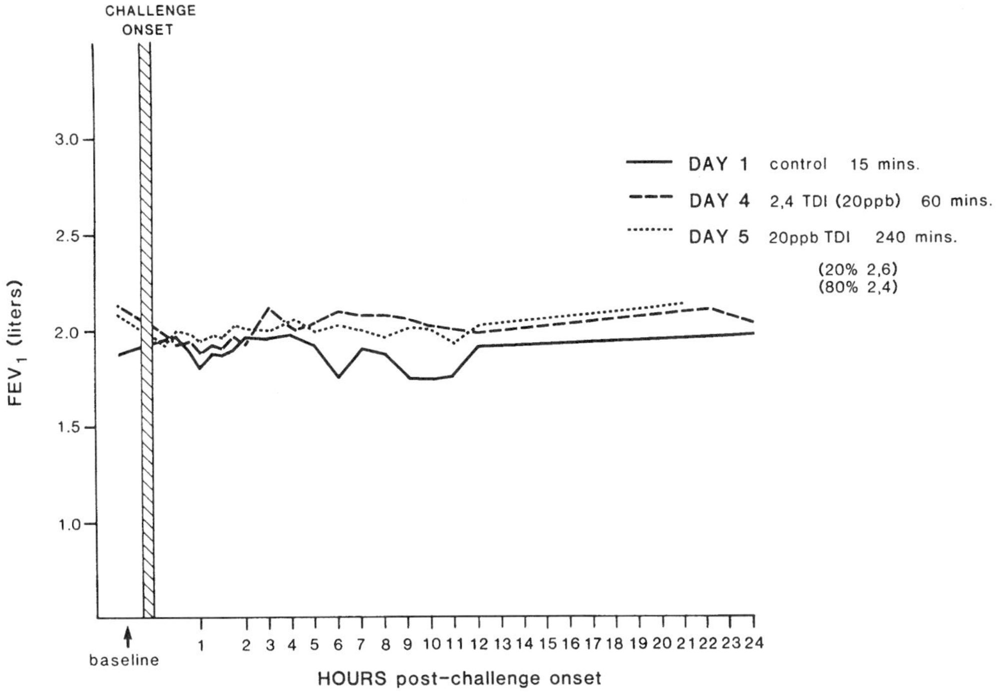


**FIG. 4.** The results of inhalation challenge testing with TDI in a 48-year-old long-time smoker employed for 22 years in a polyurethane foam production plant. He had a history of childhood asthma, which he "outgrew" in his teen years, and currently described seasonal asthma. When he first began work he noted dyspnea and wheeze, most noticeably during spills of TDI. The chest complaints would begin soon after the spill and resolve by the next morning. At this evaluation he reported no clear-cut respiratory complaints associated with TDI exposure but complained of a "subtle" reduction of his exercise tolerance while at work. Findings of the chest examination at the time of testing were not remarkable. Routine spirometry showed moderate obstructive ventilatory impairment and a moderate level of bronchial hyperresponsiveness to methacholine. Two days' exposure to 0.020 ppm of TDI provoked no decline in $FEV_1$. These data show the lack of correlation between the diagnosis of asthma, nonspecific airway hyperresponsiveness, and the diagnosis of isocyanate-induced asthma. (Reprinted with permission from ref. 106.)

same locus were associated with resistance or susceptibility to isocyanate-induced asthma and play a major role in activation of $CD4^+$ T cells.

It should be recognized that asthmatic episodes in workers with isocyanate exposure are not always attributable to isocyanates. Workers with underlying asthma can develop bronchospasm in the workplace following exertion or exposure to environmental or other allergens, irritants, or cold. Alternatively, those with asthma unrelated to isocyanates do not develop respiratory symptoms following subirritant isocyanate exposure (Fig. 4). The diagnosis of isocyanate-induced asthma must be made with care. Every effort should be made to collect objective information linking isocyanate exposure to the development of asthma if the diagnosis is to be made accurately.

Varying periods of isocyanate exposure (months to years) may exist before asthma develops. Although it has been suggested that the development of isocyanate-induced asthma requires about 2 years of exposure, the latency period is often unpredictable (20). In those sensitized, exacerbations of asthma initially occur only in association with isocyanate exposure. Vapor concentrations below the Occupational Safety and Health Administration (OSHA) time-weighted average of 0.005 ppm can provoke bronchospasm. Because of this, even the best attempts to keep isocyanate levels well below this limit will not prevent bronchospasm in sensitized individuals.

Finally, the causes of mortality have been addressed in three populations exposed to TDI. Hagmar et al. (21) demonstrated an increase in rectal cancer and non-Hodgkin's lymphoma in Swedish polyurethane foam manufacturing workers exposed to both MDI and TDI. There was no increase in overall mortality in the cohort. A second mortality study on employees in the United Kingdom flexible foam industry showed an increase in lung and pancreatic cancer in women, neoplasms commonly associated with cigarette smoking. There was no increase in overall mortality (22). In a third report of 4,611 U.S. polyurethane foam industry employees (5), there was no increase in mortality or the rate of cancer. This cohort included workers who had begun their exposure in the late 1950s and worked for at least 3 months until 1987. Mortality was addressed at the end of 1993. It should be noted, however, that the period of follow-up in all three studies was short with relatively few deaths (4.5% of the first cohort, 9.7% of the second cohort, and 7% of the third cohort had died).

## MECHANISMS FOR THE DEVELOPMENT OF ISOCYANATE-INDUCED ASTHMA

Events that lead to the development of isocyanate-induced asthma remain inadequately defined. Two apparently predisposing factors are frequent exposure to large spills of isocyanates and upper respiratory tract infections. In one report, among 332 TDI exposed workers interviewed, 65% were exposed to spills. The prevalence of airway obstruction and questionnaire defined bronchitis and asthma increased in those exposed to 20 or more isocyanate spills (23). Although the report of spills implies an excessive exposure, no one knows what level of exposure induces sensitization. Moreover, in any given worker with a diagnosis of isocyanate-induced asthma, it is often impossible to identify the event(s) that have led to sensitization.

Routine isocyanate workplace exposures may be relevant when attempting to gauge the rate of sensitization of a population. Tarlo et al. (24) reviewed the ambient levels of MDI and TDI in Ontario workplaces and compared isocyanate exposures in workplaces where workers had been compensated for this illness to workplaces where cases were not recognized. Overall, at least one sample of MDI or TDI exposure that exceeded 0.005 ppm occurred more frequently in workplaces with compensated cases of asthma.

Chester et al. (25) showed both isocyanate-specific and non-specific bronchial hyperresponsiveness to be increased following upper respiratory tract viral illnesses. The level of isocyanate exposure needed to induce sensitization is likely to be less in persons with viral infection. Atopy, defined as two or more positive skin prick tests, or underlying asthma unrelated to isocyanates, does not appear to predispose to isocyanate sensitization (17).

An understanding of the cellular and biochemical mechanisms of sensitization remains elusive. Radioisotope methods have made it possible to assess lung injury following a single excessive isocyanate exposure in rats by measuring uptake and clearance of different isocyanates and by identifying molecules bound to labeled isocyanate. Isocyanate exposure resulted in dose-dependent amounts in the blood, minimal epithelial injury, and the recognition that isocyanates bind to laminin, a major component of the basement membrane that is important in epithelial cell adhesion. The interaction between TDI and laminin caused decreased epithelial cell adherence and desquamation of airway lining cells. In addition, an unlabeled unidentified protein appeared in the lung. Increased epithelial permeability attributed to the loss of these protective airway cells may allow airway inflammation and ultimately result in sensitization (26,27). This effect may be most sensitively assessed in the small airways. Hjortsberg et al. (28) studied 20 nonatopic, asymptomatic isocyanate workers and compared their small airway response to a group of unexposed workers and to a small group of workers with isocyanate-induced asthma. The mean volume of trapped gas (VTG) in the workers' lungs was measured before and after methacholine inhalation. Before methacholine inhalation, the VTG was equal in the three groups. After methacholine inhalation, the VTG increased similarly in asthmatics and isocyanate workers. Bronchial hyperresponsiveness was not present in the larger airways of the control group or in the isocyanate workers. The increase in small airway hyperreactivity in isocyanate workers may be a sensitive marker for predicting persons at higher risk for sensitization before clinical findings are overt.

There have been two paths traveled in the investigations of the pathogenesis of isocyanate-induced asthma. Although the early studies focused principally on immune and pharmacologic mechanisms, more recent studies have centered on understanding how the inflammatory process begins and perpetuates asthma due to these agents. Central throughout has been the question of whether isocyanate-induced asthma is mediated by allergic or nonallergic mechanisms. Although many of the clinical features of isocyanate-induced asthma have caused investigators to evaluate IgE-mediated hypersensitivity as the pathogenic mechanism, this illness is not in all respects consistent with an allergic mechanism. Like IgE-mediated asthma, the sensitizing agent causing asthma appears to be clear-cut, there is a symptom-free period of variable time before asthma develops, a small percentage develop the illness, the clinical presentation and the laboratory means of provoking asthma are reproducible, and bronchial hypersensitivity to the offending agent waxes and wanes in relation to exposure. Yet, circulating specific IgE antibodies are seldom found (29). However, unlike IgE-mediated asthma, late asthmatic reactions (occasionally with recurrent nocturnal asthma) appear to be recognized more often and isocyanate-induced asthma may become chronic and persistent despite ceasing exposure to the offending agent (30). Intriguingly, the biologic mechanisms of allergic and nonallergic asthma appear to be different. Walker et al. (31) reported distinct patterns of T-cell activation in the peripheral blood and bronchoalveolar lavage fluid (BAL) of allergic and nonallergic asthmatics. Specifically, the cytokines interleukin-4 and -5 (IL-4 and IL-5) predominate in allergic asthma, and IL-2 and IL-5 predominate in nonallergic asthma. Levels of $CD4^+$ T lymphocytes were similar in asthmatics and normal individuals, but in nonallergic asthmatics there were decreased numbers of $CD8^+$ T cells in the blood and increased numbers of $CD8^+$ T cells in BAL. In addition, results from epidemiologic studies have failed to show a correlation between isocyanate-induced asthma and atopy, a feature typical of IgE-mediated asthma (32).

Since chemicals with molecular weights of less than 1,000 daltons are rarely antigenic by themselves, but may act as haptens, one way to identify mechanisms of isocyanate-induced asthma has been to conjugate isocyanates to protein carrier molecules such as albumin, and then determine the cellular response to this conjugated protein. An assessment of cellular mechanisms has included lymphocyte transformation and mixed lymphocyte reactions. Avery et al. (33,34) were unable to elicit histamine release from washed leukocytes collected from workers sensitized to TDI when the cells were cultured with TDI bound to HSA, but reported TDI-induced lymphocyte transformation in some of those sensitized. As in many of the studies that follow, the presence of an immunologic abnormality did not always correlate with disease and often reflects isocyanate exposure.

Serologic testing has evaluated IgG- and IgE-mediated hypersensitivity reactions. Scheel et al. (35) were the first to show that TDI reacted with protein in vitro and, when bound to HSA, stimulated the rabbit to produce circulating antibodies containing a reactive moiety specific to TDI. Taylor (36) attempted to detect circulating antibodies to TDI in 55 workers with clinical TDI sensitivity. Approximately half had humoral abnormalities, but the different techniques used (complement fixation to TDI bound to bovine serum albumin, passive cutaneous anaphylaxis, and red cell–linked antiglobulin tests) yielded little overlap in those with positive results, implying varying immune function abnormalities or, perhaps more reasonably, inadequate test sensitivity. Furthermore, there was no correlation between positive antibody reactions, respiratory symptoms, and peripheral blood eosinophilia.

Karol et al. (37) conjugated the antigen tolyl monoisocyanate to HSA and demonstrated the presence of these antibodies in the serum of some TDI sensitive workers by radioallergosorbent testing (RAST); however, the prevalence of these antibodies in those with challenge-test–proven isocyanate-induced asthma approximated just 20%. This suggests that it may not be the major antigen responsible for isocyanate-induced asthma or that this antigen–HSA complex was inadequately sensitive. More speculatively, the 20% prevalence of specific IgE antibodies in persons with isocyanate-induced asthma may reflect the fact that antibodies are present in the lung, but are in quantities too small to measure in the peripheral circulation. Moreover, RAST results must be interpreted with great caution, since the same specific IgE antibodies have also been detected in the sera of exposed, asymptomatic persons (38). In these reports, the presence of tolyl-specific serum IgE antibodies was not sensitive or specific enough for use as a diagnostic test for isocyanate-induced asthma.

Preliminary evaluations in humans and guinea pigs suggest that these antibodies may be directed against altered portions of the hapten rather than the isocyanate, suggesting in vivo formation of neoantigens resulting from interaction of isocyanates with body proteins (39). This is consistent with what we know about the extreme reactivity of the isocyanate molecule. Similar findings have been demonstrated with other very reactive industrial chemicals (40).

Cartier et al. (41) demonstrated a correlation (albeit, imperfect) between the presence of specific IgG or IgE antibodies to MDI and HDI and isocyanate-induced asthma. They described an important relationship between specific IgG antibody to isocyanate-HSA (21 of

29 subjects with positive MDI or HDI challenges had increased levels of this antibody, whereas 25 of 33 subjects who were challenge negative did not have the antibody). They concluded that levels of specific IgG bear a satisfactory relationship to be clinically useful in asthma due to these isocyanates. Grammer et al. (42), using sera from the same study population, improved on this correlation. They developed an index that related the worker's antibody levels to specific isocyanates and HSA to the mean antibody levels of the specific isocyanate antibody and to HSA present in the group as a whole. Again, specific IgG levels appeared to correlate better than specific IgE levels.

Karol et al. (43) reported on the relationship between total IgE antibody and airway responsiveness to TDI in a population of workers referred for suspected isocyanate-induced asthma. Thirty-four of 63 were challenge positive. The mean serum IgE values did not differ between the reactors and nonreactors; however, when the group of responders was segregated into early and other temporal reactions, differences were noted. The mean IgE levels from the early responders were greater than the levels from the nonresponders and from those with a late response. IgE to TDI-HSA was present in two workers, one who responded to specific challenge and one who did not. IgG to TDI-HSA was also positive in two workers, again, one challenge positive and the other challenge negative.

In another postulated mechanism, Butcher's group (44) has shown that isocyanates act as pharmacologic inhibitors, reducing the ability of β-adrenergic receptors to produce cyclic adenosine monophosphate (cAMP) levels in quantities necessary to maintain bronchial tone. At one concentration TDI behaved as a partial agonist to lymphocytes to stimulate cAMP production. At lesser concentrations, TDI blocked cAMP stimulation by isoproterenol and prostaglandin $E_1$, but not histamine. Lymphocytes of TDI-sensitive persons have decreased ability to respond to cAMP stimulators such as β-agonists, isoproterenol, prostaglandin $E_1$, and TDI. This in vitro work has been criticized because of the necessity of solubilizing TDI, a hydrophobic agent, by adding the solvent dimethyl sulfoxilide, an agent that may alter the phospholipid characteristics of the cell membrane and make membrane receptors more vulnerable to TDI (45). Yet, this work is consistent with the β-adrenergic blockade theory of asthma and therefore may not be specific to the mechanism by which TDI induces bronchospasm.

Although pathology reports have described inflammation from the lung for nearly 40 years, it has only been in the past 10 to 15 years that asthma has been recognized as an inflammatory process. Although considerable inflammation is apparent in asymptomatic asthmatics with mild disease (46), inflammation is most apparent in the lungs of individuals dying of asthma, regardless of etiology. Postmortem studies of these lungs showed tenacious plugs obstructing the small and large airways, desquamation of epithelial cells, and infiltration of the peribronchial areas with eosinophils and mononuclear cells (47–49). There is increasing evidence that this airway inflammation represents a feature of cell-mediated immunity, where specialized populations of activated lymphocytes interact with other inflammatory cells via a number of cytokines (50). In workers with isocyanate-induced asthma, procedures such as analysis of BAL fluids and bronchial biopsy have provided considerable information regarding the role of inflammation.

Fabbri et al. (51) showed a dramatic early and sustained increase in the number of neutrophils followed by less pronounced eosinophilia in the BAL of those with late asthmatic reactions following a subirritant exposure to TDI. This suggests that both cell types release mediators responsible for a late reaction and the ensuing inflammatory process (30). The suggestion that the late reaction is attributable to airway inflammation is further supported by the fact that late (but not immediate) asthmatic reactions are inhibited by steroid therapy and are associated with increased airway responsiveness to methacholine (52,53).

The inflammatory cellular response in TDI asthma is similar to that identified in allergic asthma. Bentley et al. (54) showed that $CD25^+$ T lymphocytes (activated lymphocytes bearing IL-2 receptors), and total [major basic protein ($MBP^+$) staining] and activated [cells that recognize the cleaved form of eosinophilic cationic protein ($EG2^+$)] eosinophils were increased in the bronchial mucosa of individuals with isocyanate-induced asthma. These same findings have been reported in allergic asthma (46).

Saetta et al. (55) evaluated bronchial biopsies from isocyanate-induced asthmatics and controls not exposed to isocyanates. They found an increased total number of cells, with increased numbers of eosinophils, mast cells, and lymphocytes, most prominent in the epithelial layer in those with isocyanate-induced asthma. Ultrastructural assessment revealed the eosinophils and mast cells to be degranulated only in the asthmatic group. The intercellular spaces between the columnar cells were similar in the asthmatic and nonasthmatic group, but wider in the asthmatics in the basal layers. The asthmatics also had a thicker subepithelial collagen layer. These electron microscopic features are again those reported in allergic asthma (56).

Finally, bronchial biopsies were performed on workers with isocyanate-induced asthma at baseline and several days after inhalation challenge. Immunohistology was performed on the tissue to define the cytokines and cells present in the mucosa. Inflammatory cells (activated T lymphocytes, mast cells, and eosinophils) were increased in the subjects with TDI-induced asthma. Cells staining for IL-1 and tumor necrosis factor (TNF) were significantly increased in the mucosa. The number of activated

T lymphocytes (CD25$^+$ staining cells) was increased and the other cells [very late activation antigen-1 (VLA-1)-staining cells] were also increased and present in relation to the magnitude of the late asthmatic response. The recognition that the activated lymphocytes remained for periods after the last isocyanate exposure is consistent with the notion that continuing inhalation of the sensitizing agent is not needed to maintain inflammation (57).

At this stage in the development of the understanding of the mechanism(s) of isocyanate-induced asthma, it appears that isocyanate-induced asthma is mediated by an immunologic mechanism. Yet, the specific antigenic stimulus for this response remains elusive. In view of the numerous difficulties in identifying IgE or IgG antibodies to isocyanates bound to HSA, it may well be that the most likely antigens could be neoantigens formed by the very reactive isocyanate molecule and proteins on the epithelial cell surfaces. Yet, once a worker becomes sensitized, airway inflammation plays a critical role in maintaining the airway hyperresponsiveness. Most importantly, it appears that the process is often self-perpetuating, and reexposure to the isocyanate molecule (in this case perhaps reasonably described as the preantigen) is not needed for this process to continue. Although specific responsiveness to isocyanates may lessen over time, nonspecific hyperresponsiveness frequently persists relatively unchanged.

## THE NATURAL HISTORY OF ISOCYANATE-INDUCED ASTHMA

Unfortunately, no recognized physiologic markers predict symptom remission or persistence in persons with isocyanate asthma, and the natural history of isocyanate asthma remains to be fully defined. Few reports have been published of long-term follow-up of patients with TDI asthma with repeat challenge testing. Two case reports have shown resolution of airway hyperresponsiveness to TDI by specific inhalation challenge testing. Butcher et al. (58) described a worker who developed and lost symptoms of isocyanate-induced asthma, specific and nonspecific bronchial hyperresponsiveness, and an abnormal cellular adrenergic response 2 years after ceasing isocyanate exposure. Banks and Rando (59) reported a worker who had recovered from the symptoms of TDI-induced asthma after 5 years, and after 11 years had a negative reaction to a specific challenge.

Two studies measuring isocyanate sensitivity at the time of diagnosis and at follow-up have been reported. Lemiere et al. (60) showed that one of seven isocyanate-sensitized workers had less bronchial hyperresponsiveness to methacholine and four of seven isocyanate-sensitized workers had diminished but persistent hyperresponsiveness to isocyanates 2 or more years after leaving the workplace. Mapp et al. (61) reported specific bronchoprovocation testing in a group with isocyanate-induced asthma at a mean follow-up of 10 months. Eight of 30 who had left the workplace lost TDI reactivity at follow-up. Five who remained in the same jobs had persistent asthma. Those who recovered from TDI sensitization had a shorter duration of symptoms prior to diagnosis, were more likely to have an immediate asthmatic reaction to isocyanate exposure, and had less bronchial responsiveness to methacholine and an improved forced expiratory volume in 1 second ($FEV_1$) at follow-up.

Interestingly, among those with Western red cedar asthma, a higher proportion who recovered had a late asthmatic reaction during inhalation provocation testing at the time of diagnosis (62). This leads to the question of whether the natural history of occupational asthma induced by different agents is the same (63). Yet, some suggest that the outcome of occupational asthma is not related to the agent. Allard et al. (64) reported on 28 subjects with asthma due to different workplace agents who were reevaluated at mean intervals of 2.3 and 5.8 years after diagnosis. Ten of the 28 had isocyanate-induced asthma. Only three of 28 required less respiratory medication, had improved lung function, or had less airway hyperresponsiveness at the follow-up examination.

Several investigators have shown that once isocyanate-induced asthma develops, a worker's risk for persistent asthma can be quite high. Paggiaro et al. (65) studied 27 workers with TDI-induced asthma approximately 2 years after diagnosis. Although symptoms of dyspnea and wheeze were less frequent in the 12 who had left the industry, only four were without respiratory symptoms. Just one of 15 who remained in the workplace experienced resolution of respiratory complaints. More than half who remained developed chronic cough with phlegm. No data were provided on whether those who remained in the workplace were moved to jobs associated with less TDI exposure.

Moller et al. (66) reported on seven workers with TDI-induced asthma. In six, asthma persisted as long as 12 years (mean 4.5 years) even though they left the workplace. Lozewicz et al. (67) also suggested that many with isocyanate-induced asthma continue to have respiratory complaints. Forty-one of 50 workers away from isocyanate exposure for at least 4 years continued to have respiratory complaints, and 22 required respiratory medication at least once a week. The frequency of chest complaints was similar among those who had left the workplace and those who had relocated in their original workplace to jobs without recognized direct isocyanate exposures.

Rosenberg et al. (68) reported a somewhat different experience in 31 workers with isocyanate-induced asthma. Four continued in the same job and did poorly. Seven were relocated to jobs with less isocyanate exposure and were reported to have mild to moderate asthma. The remaining 20 were completely removed from exposure. Of these, ten still had symptoms after 19 months. Four reported rare attacks of wheeze while the other six had more severe symptoms. Two of the six had airway obstruction and three required continuing respiratory medication.

In summary, although the outlook for workers with isocyanate-induced asthma varies, it is clear that many workers will continue with respiratory symptoms, nonspecific bronchial hyperresponsiveness, and specific responsiveness to isocyanates, and will require continuing medication for asthma despite leaving the workplace at the time of diagnosis.

## RESPIRATORY EFFECTS OF LOW-LEVEL TDI EXPOSURE

Effects of long-term low-level TDI exposure have been assessed by several groups of investigators. Adams (69) assessed the respiratory health of 180 workers employed from 1 to 11 years in two TDI-manufacturing plants. The mean annual decline in $FEV_1$ and the forced vital capacity (FVC) in these workers was no different from the values measured in a local population not exposed to TDI. In 63 former workers with TDI sensitivity and persistent symptoms followed from 2 to 11 years after leaving the workplace, the mean annual $FEV_1$ decline was only slightly excessive.

McKerrow et al. (70) reported on a group of firemen who suffered an acute overexposure to isocyanates and on a population of workers exposed to TDI who were tested initially and after 6 months. In both groups there was a high attack rate of bronchitis but no evidence of an adverse effect on lung function. A series of longitudinal surveys describing the respiratory health of employees at two polyurethane foam manufacturers using TDI disputed these conclusions. In these reports, accelerated declines of both annual and across-shift $FEV_1$ values were recorded (71–74). Initial work suggested that workplace TDI exposure caused alarmingly large decrements in $FEV_1$ when measured at the start and at the end of a Monday work shift (mean decline 220 ml), which persisted as the workweek progressed, although to a lesser degree. Workers with chest symptoms had greater declines than those without symptoms. After 2 years, the rate of $FEV_1$ decline was approximately twice predicted. Those with excessive across-shift declines had a greater $FEV_1$ decline over time. The annual decline in lung function occurred in the presence of what was considered acceptable peak TDI levels (<0.020 ppm) and independent of the cigarette smoking category.

In another polyurethane production plant where TDI was used, the same group of investigators reported baseline and 6-month follow-up spirometry and questionnaire information (75). Among 111 workers with TDI exposure, significant across-shift decreases in $FEV_1$ occurred and increased with levels of TDI exposure. Accelerated lung function declines occurred even with exposure to 1/10 of the permissible exposure limit of 0.020 ppm. The mean loss of $FEV_1$ across the work shift was apparently independent of age, smoking history, or years of employment. After 2 years, the population was studied again (76). Although only about half the workers remained, those exposed to TDI levels greater than 0.003 ppm had accelerated $FEV_1$ declines. The investigators suggested that long-term occupational exposure to TDI at 0.003 ppm or more was unsafe. In this report, since only mean exposure data were available from a limited number of air samples over 20- to 90-minute periods, it is possible that those with excessive annual declines in lung function were exposed to excessive peak levels of TDI that were not detected. After 5 years, and after MDI had been added to the polyurethane-producing operation at this plant, the very low exposure levels of isocyanates in this workplace were reported to be associated with a mean annual $FEV_1$ decline approximating that expected from aging. Significant $FEV_1$ declines across the work shift were not observed (77).

Concern about the validity of lung function measurements in these polyurethane workers was expressed by Gee and Morgan (78), who studied the workers who remained at this same workplace 10 years after the first study was performed (77). The rate of lung function decline could not be accurately calculated because many of the earlier spirometric efforts were described as inadequate. In those with initial acceptable spirometric curves, the $FEV_1$ decline from the earlier study to the 10-year follow-up was unrealistically small. These authors also criticized the above work for failing to show correlations between the decline in $FEV_1$ over time, the baseline $FEV_1$ values, and smoking categories.

Another report of a longitudinal survey of the ventilatory function of workers engaged in the manufacture of TDI was reported in 1982 (32). This study began at the opening of the isocyanate-producing workplace, and pre-exposure data were collected before TDI manufacturing began. Environmental measurements and physiologic data were obtained longitudinally from nearly 300 workers. Exposure to TDI vapor was determined by personal monitors. More than 2,000 personal samples were collected and broken down among 42 job titles. All employees had some degree of measurable TDI exposure, depending on both job and location. On average, TDI vapor concentrations exceeded 0.020 parts per billion (ppb) approximately 3% of the time. The average annual decline in $FEV_1$ among all in the study was 24 ml, a value comparable to that expected in cross-sectional studies of "normal" populations. The average annual declines in forced expiratory flow after 25% to 75% of vital capacity has been expelled ($FEF_{25-75}$) and $FEF_{50}$ were 93 and 110 ml/L, respectively, larger than what would be expected on the basis of cross-sectional data. After controlling for smoking and atopic status, the annual declines in $FEV_1$, $FEV_1$%, and $FEF_{25-75}$ appeared to depend on TDI exposure and were recognized as excessive even in "never smokers." Among never smokers, there was a 38 ml per year difference in the $FEV_1$ decline between the low- and high-cumulative exposure categories ($p = .001$). In "current smokers," there was no observed difference in the amount of $FEV_1$ decline, regardless of cumulative exposure level. For the low-exposure category, there was a 27 ml per year ($p = .004$) excess decline in $FEV_1$ in current smokers compared to never smokers. TDI exposure correlated well with the annual change in lung function, whether it was determined by cumulative or peak exposure (duration of exposure to more than 0.020 ppm). This study showed a statistically significant effect of TDI exposure on the annual decline in $FEV_1$ in never smokers, similar to that caused by cigarette smoking.

In a recently reported 5-year longitudinal lung function study of 386 polyurethane foam manufacturers, 64 of 254 (25.2%) workers had hyperresponsiveness to methacholine. In 4,845 TDI samples, exposures appeared to be generally low: 9% exceeded 0.005 ppm and 1% exceeded 0.020 ppm (79). Baseline bronchial hyperresponsiveness to methacholine was associated with a baseline $FEV_1$ 8.5% less than predicted and an $FEF_{25-75}$ 20% less than predicted ($p < .001$ for both). In addition, the baseline values showed a significant relationship between higher cumulative TDI exposures to an increased risk of chronic bronchitis and lower levels of lung function. The rate of annual lung function decline was computed for 227 participants. Although the mean annual $FEV_1$ decline was excessive (67 ml for current smokers and 53 ml for never smokers), these differences were not significant by smoking category. TDI exposure, either cumulative or concurrent, had little effect on the slope of the $FEV_1$ decline, despite the effect on baseline $FEV_1$ and an increased number with bronchitis. It may be that exposure to unrecognized workplace agents played an important role in lung function decline; for example, amine catalysts have been suspected of having toxic effects (80,81). Alternatively, or perhaps in addition, important differences in the workers who entered the study and the fraction who completed the study may have affected the results.

In summary, these data have led OSHA to address the reasonableness of the standard for isocyanate exposure, and to implement a more stringent standard for isocyanate exposures. The current standard is a time-weighted average of 0.005 ppm (0.04 $mg/m^3$) for a 10-hour work shift, 40-hour workweek, and a ceiling limit of 0.020 ppm (0.15 $mg/m^3$) for a 15-minute time-weighted average over the working day (4).

## HYPERSENSITIVITY PNEUMONITIS AND ISOCYANATE EXPOSURE

Unlike asthma attributable to TDI exposure, recognition of the induction of hypersensitivity pneumonitis due to isocyanates has been reported relatively less frequently. Charles et al. (82) reported four TDI-exposed workers who had an impairment of respiratory function other than obstruction following TDI exposure. In one of these cases, histologic examination detected pulmonary lesions suggestive of allergic bronchopulmonary aspergillosis. Immune system abnormalities were not found in any of the four exposed to TDI, and the possibility that these changes were related to another inhaled antigen could not be excluded. Fink and Schlueter (83) reported a convincing case of porcelain refinisher's disease attributable to TDI exposure with a clinical presentation of hypersensitivity pneumonitis but no measurable immune response.

Simpson et al. (84) reported an outbreak of hypersensitivity pneumonitis-like reactions and asthma in a 10-week period that followed the introduction into an auto parts manufacturing facility of a paint containing the relatively infrequently used oligomer 1,3-bis (isocyanatomethyl) cyclohexane. Twenty-three of 34 workers developed respiratory complaints over a 2-month period and 9 of 34 (26%) developed an illness consistent with hypersensitivity pneumonitis.

Several groups have reported their experience with hypersensitivity pneumonitis in isocyanate workers exposed to MDI. Zeiss et al. (85) reported two workers with immune system abnormalities associated with MDI exposure: one with MDI-induced asthma and the other with MDI-induced hypersensitivity pneumonitis. Both had specific IgE and IgG antibodies to MDI-HSA, and the worker with hypersensitivity pneumonitis also had precipitating antibodies to MDI-HSA.

Bascom et al. (86) showed a lymphocytic alveolitis and serum and bronchoalveolar fluid IgG antibody to MDI-HSA in a worker with MDI-induced hypersensitivity pneumonitis, suggesting that both humoral and cellular immunity play a role in the pathogenesis of this disease following isocyanate exposure.

Malo et al. (87) described a foundry worker with hypersensitivity pneumonitis following PepSet™ exposure and with serum IgG antibodies to MDI-HSA, and another worker with hypersensitivity pneumonitis and late asthma following HDI workplace exposure, with no history of occupational exposure to MDI (88). Laboratory data in this second case showed IgG antibodies to HDI-HSA and MDI-HSA, implying cross-reactivity to isocyanates (despite the fact that MDI is an aromatic compound and HDI an aliphatic one). This cross-reactivity was thought to be due to the possibility that the isocyanate-protein link is the major antigenic determinant to which antibody is directed. Vandenplas et al. (89) reported eight of 167 (4.8%) workers employed in a plant where MDI resin was used to bind wood chips in the manufacture of particleboard had respiratory and systemic complaints and were shown to have hypersensitivity pneumonitis by challenge testing to MDI. Because the symptoms were so severe, a number of workers had to stop working, and it may be that this lessened the number in the population with this illness. Why such an outbreak occurred in this workplace is not clear; however, the authors suggest that the high levels of MDI within the plant and the mixture of monomeric and a complex mixture of MDI oligomers may have been relevant.

An initial report by Baur et al. (90) described an auto painter with immediate-onset asthma followed by evening complaints consistent with hypersensitivity pneumonitis after MDI-based paint exposure. Although results of RAST to multiple isocyanate antigens were negative, IgG antibodies to HDI, TDI, p-tolyl monoisocyanate, methylene diphenyl monoisocyanate, and HDI bound to HSA were positive. Later, Baur (91) provided perhaps the most comprehensive report of hypersensitivity pneumonitis in isocyanate-exposed workers. He reviewed the records of 1,780 workers from four German car and chemical factories, as well as other workers under medical surveillance for isocyanate related adverse effects. Sixteen (0.9%) had repeated bouts of dyspnea, fever, and malaise several hours following isocyanate exposure. In the 14 who agreed to participate, one was atopic. These workers performed lung function, immunologic testing, BAL, and inhalational challenge testing to MDI. Of the 14, nine had MDI exposure, three were exposed to HDI biuret, and three handled TDI and other isocyanates. Nine of 14 chest radiographs showed abnormalities consistent with hypersensitivity pneumonitis. The FVC was decreased in seven and the diffusing capacity ($D_LCO$) was abnormal in ten subjects. Although ten had significant levels of IgG to isocyanate-HSA, specific IgE was not found. Challenge testing reproduced clinical symptoms in the five in which it was performed. BAL and lung biopsies were also consistent with hypersensitivity pneumonitis. Of interest, compared to the other isocyanates, MDI was the most common isocyanate causing hypersensitivity pneumonitis, although the denominator of cases with different isocyanate exposures was not provided.

In summary, hypersensitivity pneumonitis appears to be a consistently described, although relatively rare, illness that occurs in populations of isocyanate exposed workers. Although the data are not yet clear, it may be that exposures to MDI or HDI may be relatively more likely to induce this illness than TDI.

## ADVERSE RESPIRATORY EFFECTS ASSOCIATED WITH MDI EXPOSURES

A longitudinal assessment of the respiratory effects of long-term low-level MDI exposure has not been reported.

A cross-sectional survey of the respiratory health of 318 workers at two plants employed for at least 1 year with exposures to MDI (with apparent coexisting TDI exposure) in the production of polyurethane foam molding, has been performed (92). After adjusting for both smoking and age, the frequency of bronchitis and bronchial hyperresponsiveness to acetylcholine was found to be increased, and the mean $FEV_1$, FVC, and $D_LCO$ was decreased in men with direct isocyanate exposure. The decline in lung function paralleled years of exposure. The principal problem in interpreting these results is the lack of information on the combination, duration, and cumulative amount of MDI or TDI exposure. Although MDI measurements were reported to occasionally exceed four times the permissible exposure level of 0.020 ppm, no insight into the frequency of such excursions and no information regarding TDI exposure were included.

One of the first discussions of workers with MDI-induced asthma was in a 1970 symposium on isocyanates. Comments by industrial physicians made at this symposium provide evidence that MDI-induced asthma was recognized prior to this meeting (93). The first report of a population survey of workers was published in 1973. Among 57 workers, three had symptoms of MDI-induced asthma, one had complaints consistent with hypersensitivity pneumonitis, and ten had respiratory irritation attributed to MDI inhalation. No airborne MDI measurements were reported (94).

Zammit-Tabonga et al. (95) reported data that challenged the notion that MDI-induced asthma is infrequent. The authors reported six cases of MDI-induced asthma among 78 foundry workers who used PepSet™ (60% MDI, formaldehyde, hydrocarbons, and a pyridine catalyst), a chemical binding system used in mold making. Probably contributing to this high percentage of workers sensitized to MDI was the finding that MDI levels approximated 0.080 ppm (four times the permissible exposure level at the time) in the workplace atmosphere. Immunologically, neither serum IgE nor IgG antibodies to MDI-HSA were specific to those with occupational asthma. Liss et al. (96) reported on a second foundry population where the binding agent was No-Bake, a three-component system that included MDI, hydrocarbon binder, and organometallic catalyst. This material was mixed with silica sand to make the mold. Of the 32 current or previously exposed workers, ten described symptoms consistent with occupational asthma, although only one had an intrashift $FEV_1$ decline exceeding 10%. Elevated levels of specific IgE to MDI-HSA was detected in one worker with clinical symptoms of immediate-onset asthma, rhinitis, and conjunctivitis. Although serum IgG levels to MDI-HSA and total antibodies to MDI-HSA were present in approximately one-fourth of the currently exposed workers, this immune response occurred in both symptomatic and asymptomatic workers.

## ADVERSE RESPIRATORY EFFECTS DUE TO EXPOSURE TO OTHER ISOCYANATES

Although there are occasional reports of respiratory disease resulting from exposure to the less common isocyanates, relatively little is known about the respiratory health risks of these isocyanates. HDI (97) and NDI (98) have been reported to cause asthma, and a case of IPDI-induced respiratory disease was reported by Clarke and Aldons (99).

Alexandersson et al. (100) reported a cross-sectional survey of 23 workers exposed to NDI in tire production. Ambient levels of NDI approximated one-third of the Swedish limit for this agent. Eye irritation occurred in two-thirds of the workers, while cough and dyspnea occurred in one-third of the individuals. Those who cleaned and sprayed the molds used for tire making had the greatest exposures and the most complaints. Although the $FEV_1$ was no different from the controls, the closing volume (a more sensitive measure of small airways obstruction) increased in the exposed workers. A second report suggested that NDI was associated with episodes of bronchitis but no worsening in the rate of lung function decline (101). Fuortes et al. (102) reported an outbreak of seven cases of apparent NDI-induced asthma in a factory where workers hand-applied hot polyurethane (made from NDI) onto metal wheels. The polyurethane was then oven-cured and subjected to a series of grinding and lathe operations for its ultimate use as part of the wheel on fork-lift trucks. Prior to the use of NDI, MDI had been used for a number of years in this workplace, and had not been associated with health problems.

A study of 150 spray painters who used paints containing HDI and trimeric HDI (THDI) has been reported (103). Measurements of ambient isocyanate levels, answers to a respiratory questionnaire, and measurements of the amount of serum antibody to HDI-HSA and THDI-HSA were evaluated. Since these spray painters wore respirators, isocyanate exposure was very low. Although 8% reported respiratory symptoms, only one worker was thought to have symptoms of work-related respiratory disease. Despite the apparently very low exposures, 21% had antibodies to isocyanates. Approximately, 12% had IgG antibodies to one of the two isocyanates (HDI or THDI), while 5% had IgE antibodies to one of the two. There was no significant difference between antibody level by job classification and no significant correlation between isocyanate exposure level and antibody level except in the paint mixer group.

A second publication addressing the respiratory health of automobile painters was reported in the same year (104). Thirty car painters exposed to paints containing HDI polymers were studied for the RAST (IgE) and enzyme-linked immunosorbent assay (ELISA) (IgG) response to HDI-HSA. Although a number of the workers had respiratory complaints, only one was shown to have isocyanate asthma. Although there was variability in individual RAST levels and mean RAST ratios for IgE to HDI (monomer or polymer)-HSA car painters and controls, mean levels of IgG to HDI (monomer)-HSA were not significantly increased in the car painters. Yet, mean IgG to HDI (polymer)-HSA were significantly increased in the car painters, with the greatest value in the worker with occupational asthma. Six of the 30 workers had antibodies of IgG subclass 4 to HDI (monomer)-HSA and 6 to HDI (polymer)-HSA, compared to none of the controls. The role of antibodies in these HDI exposed workers is not clear, as there seemed to be no correlation between antibodies and symptoms (except for the single case of asthma). In addition, the recognition that workers may have antibodies to the HDI monomer or polymer leads one to speculate that the immune system may perceive these as different chemicals.

Dahlquist et al. (105) reported an interesting correlation between the rate of FVC decline over the workweek in car spray painters exposed to HDI-biuret and the long-term rate of lung function decline over a 6-year period.

In summary, although there are occasional reports regarding adverse respiratory effects (primarily asthma) associated with these lesser used isocyanates, the lack of epidemiologic studies and the relative paucity of data regarding the prevalence of respiratory illness in persons exposed to these agents make conclusions regarding the level of risk of respiratory illness associated with exposure to these isocyanates uncertain.

## OBJECTIVE DETERMINATION OF THE DIAGNOSIS OF ISOCYANATE-INDUCED ASTHMA

There is no accurate biochemical method for diagnosing isocyanate-induced asthma. Although clinical evidence can appear to be convincing, the diagnosis can be made with certainty only if asthma occurs following exposure to a subirritant level of isocyanate.

There are different ways to "challenge" a worker suspected of having isocyanate asthma. One is to reproduce the exposure associated with chest symptoms in the workplace. The other is to expose the worker to isocyanates in the controlled environment of a challenge chamber (106). Immediate and late declines in ventilatory function following short-term subirritant isocyanate exposure in sensitized persons can safely be diagnosed by challenge testing (107). Although laboratory-based challenge testing is not necessary for the diagnosis of isocyanate-induced asthma, accurate clinical diagnosis of isocyanate-induced asthma has been shown to be difficult among a referred group of workers who claim isocyanate-induced asthma in the absence of specific challenge testing (108). Regardless of how these objective data are collected, the intent of these challenge tests is to reproduce asthma, and therefore either method carries a healthy risk.

The diagnosis of isocyanate-induced asthma should be entertained when an exposed worker first reports respiratory symptoms, and if possible while the worker is still employed, as then the diagnosis can be made with more confidence because the worker can be carefully and objectively monitored in the workplace. There are few more difficult challenges in the practice of occupational lung disease medicine than attempting to identify isocyanate-induced asthma on the basis of a review of a worker's records. Two important caveats in making the diagnosis of isocyanate-induced asthma are relevant. The first is that isocyanate-induced asthma should be considered in all persons with adult-onset asthma who have an appropriate history of occupational exposure. The second is the recognition that not all isocyanate-exposed workers' asthma is induced by these agents.

Parallels between measuring bronchial hyperresponsiveness to methacholine or histamine and isocyanate challenge testing can reasonably be drawn. In both, collection of objective data (a measured decline in lung function) is the aim. In both, the physician must be close at hand to measure the relevant clinical indices and to intervene in the event of bronchospasm. In both, resolution of the bronchospastic episode following inhaled β-agonist therapy is the norm; yet in isocyanate challenge testing late reactions frequently recur despite appropriate inhaled β-agonist therapy (109) (Fig. 5). Recognizing the possibility of recurrent nocturnal reactions following isocyanate challenge testing is also important.

Before undergoing isocyanate challenge testing, the worker should discontinue respiratory medication for several days and have sufficient baseline lung function to tolerate a clinically important decline in $FEV_1$. A positive response is reasonably accepted to be a decline in $FEV_1$ of 20% or more compared to the baseline value in association with the development of chest symptoms.

The first approach to isocyanate challenge testing, described in the context of this discussion as a "workplace challenge," can provide important diagnostic information about the presence or absence of isocyanate asthma. The worker is tested in the area of the workplace where respiratory symptoms have occurred. Such a challenge can be performed rather easily and inexpensively by measuring peak flow rates or determining the $FEV_1$ value before the workday begins and then serially throughout the workday and evening at and away from work. Since there occasionally can be a priming effect, i.e., no change in lung function for the first several days back to work and then a decline, serial peak flow rates should be monitored for at least 2 weeks at work before any interpretation of the relationship between the work-

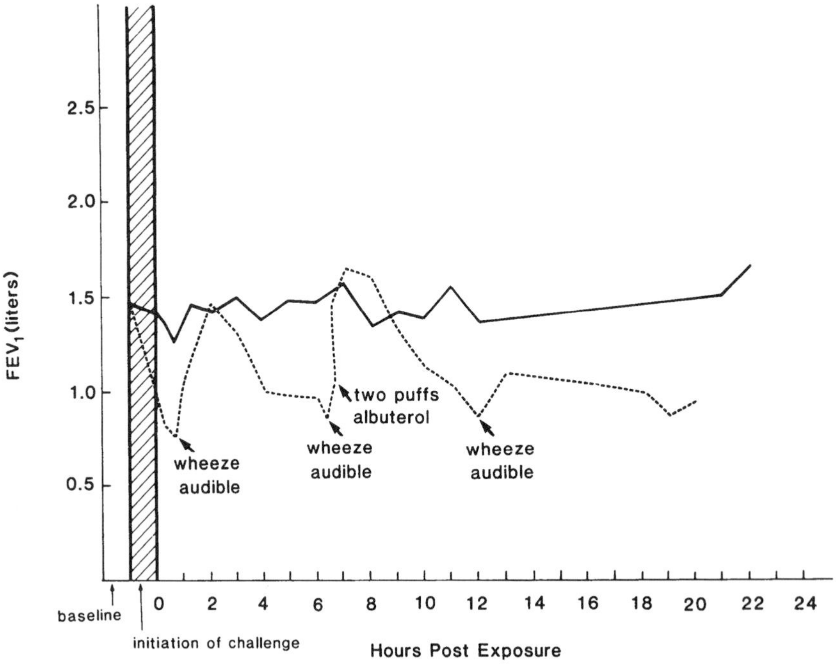


**FIG. 5.** The results of lung function following TDI inhalation challenge testing performed on a 48-year-old woman employed for 16 years in a refrigerator manufacturing plant where polyurethane foam was used as an insulant. She had no problem for the first 12 years, but after changing jobs within the plant to one that resulted in exposure to recently cured foam, she noted dyspnea, wheeze, cough, and chest tightness. Despite these ongoing chest problems and several exacerbations of asthma that resulted in hospitalizations, she continued to work. She had a 26-year smoking history and had not quit smoking despite her respiratory problems. Spirometry prior to TDI challenge testing showed moderate obstructive ventilatory impairment. She had a marked decline in $FEV_1$ following inhalation of a small amount of methacholine. Day 1 *(solid line)* shows a stable baseline $FEV_1$ with no great variation during the day or night. Exposure to 0.010 ppm of TDI for 15 minutes provoked a dramatic immediate and late persistent $FEV_1$ decline *(interrupted line)*, with clinical asthma. Inhalation of bronchodilators only interrupted the late reaction. (Reproduced with permission from ref. 109.)

place and lung function can be inferred. Similarly, since improvement in lung function after stopping work may not be immediately apparent, monitoring should be performed for at least 2 weeks off work.

Peak flow monitoring in isocyanate workers was assessed by Burge et al. (110) in 20 workers who also underwent isocyanate chamber challenges. Twelve of the 20 had positive isocyanate challenges. Peak flow monitoring for at least 2 weeks at work and off work included a period of isocyanate exposure in 15 of 23 records. Three of these were inadequate for interpretation. Thus, the 12 adequate records were interpreted and the results compared with the diagnosis of occupational asthma determined from subsequent outcome at work. With these criteria, when the peak flow measurements were able to be interpreted, they were 100% sensitive and specific for occupational asthma, whereas the chamber challenges were 83% sensitive and 100% specific. Those with peak flow recordings of occupational asthma (eight subjects) generally showed progressive worsening of peak flow values week by week, while improvement away from the workplace usually was frequently delayed 4 to 12 days.

Liss and Tarlo (111) assessed peak flow records in 78 workers with suspected occupational asthma, including 22 isocyanate exposed workers. Results from 28 (36%) were excluded because of unacceptable measurements. In 50 acceptable tests, the information was unhelpful in 13 (26%). Yet, where an accurate objective interpretation could be performed, there was good sensitivity (93%) and specificity (90%) for occupational asthma. Similar high sensitivity and specificity of peak flow recordings were reported in red-cedar workers when peak flow readings and specific challenge results were compared (112). Thus in workers who can perform and accurately record adequate peak flow readings, this approach can be useful.

When asthma is suspected to occur after the work shift is completed, the peak flow meter or portable spirometer can be taken home by the worker to record frequent values. The data are best applied if the physician has been able to assess the worker for respiratory symptoms and correlate them with the adequacy of spirometry efforts. Finally, the assistance of a qualified industrial hygienist to accurately measure isocyanate exposure can be of inestimable value. Overall, with this approach the cost is minimal and hospitalization becomes unnecessary. Yet, important flaws may exist with this approach. As previously noted, episodes of asthma following exposure to common allergens, exertion, or cold may be associated with the workplace environment or the job itself, and result in respiratory symptoms independent of isocyanate exposure. In addition, the workplace atmosphere may not be controllable. It is possible that on one day essentially no isocyanate exposure could occur, in which case the diagnosis of isocyanate-induced asthma would be missed, whereas on another day the isocyanate exposure could be excessive and a decline in lung function and symptoms would be induced by an irritant exposure. To complicate matters further, chemicals other than isocyanates in the workplace may act as respiratory sensitizers or irritants and precipitate asthma. Therefore, although one may be able to make a diagnosis of occupational asthma, this approach does not identify the toxicant, and proving that asthma was induced by isocyanates may be difficult. This is not surprising in the face of information showing that more than 200 agents can induce occupational asthma (113,114).

Finally, routine peak flow measurements are without a "hard copy," and the values recorded may not reflect optimal effort or correct values. A recent report by Quirce et al. (115) emphasized this by addressing the presence or absence of occupational asthma in a group of 17 subjects by use of a portable peak flow monitor that stored the readings in a small, portable computer which also provided a digital readout, as well by asking workers to keep a diary recording the values. The workers were aware of the digital readout, but did not know that the readings were recorded by the monitoring device. Of the 13 who completed the monitoring, only 55% of the records were accurate in recording the value and timing of the measurements, 23% were inaccurate either in terms of the recorded value or timing, and the rest of the tests were fabricated. Similar results were reported by Malo et al. (116), where 21 subjects with suspected occupational asthma to a number of agents were asked to record peak flow rates every two hours during the day for two weeks at work and then two weeks away from the job. Only 52% of the peak flow rate values were accurately recorded. Significantly worse compliance was found in workers referred by the Workers' Compensation Bureau.

These new data complicate the approach to the assessment of the use of the peak flow meter in the assessment of occupational asthma. When available, the use of a computerized instrument (VMX Instrument, Clement Clarke International, Columbus, OH) seems to be very important in this clinical situation.

A second objective method of measuring changes in the lung function is to assay bronchial hyperresponsiveness to methacholine or histamine at the start and the end of the workweek, and then repeat this measurement 10 to 14 days away from isocyanate exposure. A significant improvement in histamine or methacholine reactivity away from work supports the diagnosis of occupational asthma.

The sensitivity and specificity of these paired tests relative to isocyanate challenges has not been reported. In red-cedar workers, however, the sensitivity and specificity was less than that for peak flow monitoring (112). A lack of improvement in methacholine response off work does not exclude occupational asthma since a significant improvement [a greater than threefold improvement in the concentration causing a 20% decline in $FEV_1$ ($PC_{20}$)] may not occur for up to 45 months, if at all (117). In addition, as with peak flow rate changes, a significant worsening of nonspecific bronchial hyperresponsiveness into the asthmatic range with isocyanate exposure may only occur after 10 to 14 days back at work in a sensitized subject whose asthma had resolved off work (118). Similarly, normal methacholine responsiveness has been reported even after definite positive isocyanate challenges (119). Nevertheless, a normal methacholine or histamine response within 24 hours of the worker's usual respiratory symptoms with workplace exposure makes the diagnosis of occupational asthma very unlikely, and correlates well with negative peak flow results (110). Thus paired methacholine tests can be a useful adjunct to serial peak flow monitoring (when it is valid), but interpretation appears to be limited.

In summary, if the measurement of serial peak flow rates or serial methacholine tests do not allow for the clear-cut explanation for the etiology of asthma in an individual with suspected isocyanate sensitivity, a specific chamber challenge test may be the way to define the attributability of the worker's asthma. In addition, at the time of initial assessment, if the patient has left work and cannot or will not return for workplace studies, laboratory challenges to the specific workplace agent may be the only diagnostic option to define the etiology of the worker's asthma.

## LABORATORY-BASED CHALLENGE TEST METHODOLOGY

In view of the potential weaknesses associated with the use of serial peak flow rates in the objective determination of workplace asthma, the importance of the "laboratory method" of provoking isocyanate asthma is of increasing interest (120). This approach utilizes an exposure chamber and sophisticated equipment to generate measured subirritant atmospheres of individual isocyanates. Exposure to nonirritant levels of isocyanates provokes an episode of bronchospasm in a sensitized worker but does not affect those who are not sensitized or those with asthma due to other agents. However, there are several issues relevant to challenging workers with isocyanates that must be noted before testing can be described.

First, an industrial hygienist, or one with comparable skills, must be a part of the working group. These professionals understand how to accurately generate and monitor potentially toxic chemical exposures and have the knowledge required to make the laboratory a safe place.

Second, because some isocyanates are volatile, the chance for an irritant exposure (which may be sensitizing) can occur even with what may be perceived as a minor spill. These agents must be handled in a manner that minimizes exposures to laboratory workers. Exposures must be generated in a way that is capable of provoking an asthmatic response but below the threshold for overt irritation. With that in mind, it is appropriate for an exposure chamber to be built in a relatively remote area of the building (rather than in the pulmonary function laboratory, for example), for all chemicals to be stored safely in appropriate containers and in an enclosed chamber (or under an enclosed hood), and to only open the chemicals under the laboratory hood. Because the greatest chance for spills and excessive exposures occurs when the exposure is being prepared, an isolated, well-ventilated area set aside for the preparation and generation of isocyanate exposure is critical to the safety of the entire system.

Third, the characteristics of the commercially important isocyanates are quite different (Table 3). TDI and HDI are volatile and exist in liquid form at room temperature, and the degree of reactivity increases as the temperature and humidity increase. In contrast, pure MDI exists as a solid at room temperature or as a polymer in liquid state with the addition of acetone. Liquid MDI has a vapor pressure and saturated vapor concentration about three orders of magnitude below that of TDI or HDI. As a result, heating of MDI is necessary to the release of vapors, which tend to condense back to a fine aerosol upon cooling. On the other hand, HDI-biuret and triphenyl-methane triisocyanate are essentially nonvolatile and must be mechanically introduced into the atmosphere as large aerosols.

A fourth factor concerns the isocyanates' reactivity and affinity for surfaces. To minimize absorption onto surfaces, it is necessary to use stainless steel, Teflon, or glass for all parts of the system that come in contact with isocyanates. This includes the chamber and all conduits that carry isocyanates.

**TABLE 3.** *Overview of isocyanate characteristics*

| Isocyanate | Appearance at room temperature | Vapor pressure, mm Hg at 25°C | Saturated vapor concentration, ppm |
|---|---|---|---|
| TDI | Liquid | 0.0167 | 22 |
| HDI | Liquid | 0.05 | 66 |
| MDI | White crystalline solid | $6.3 \times 10^{-6}$ | 0.08 |
| IPDI | Liquid | 0.0003 (at 20°C) | 0.4 (at 20°C) |
| HMDI | Liquid | 0.001 | 1.3 |
| NDI | White to yellow solid | 0.003 (at 24°C) | 4.0 (at 24°C) |
| CHDI | White crystalline solid | 0.004 | 5.3 |

Reprinted with permission from ref. 120.

In addition, there are several principles that guide the generation of atmospheres of a challenge agent. The worker can be exposed by delivering the agent through a mouthpiece or face mask, or by exposure to the agent in a chamber. In the traditional face mask technique, the worker's tight-fitting mask is connected via tubing to the generator. Inspiratory and expiratory one-way valves allow the worker's respiratory movements to act as a demand system. A monitoring system may be placed in-line to provide an assessment of exposure. This method is most useful when the exposure is of short duration or if only a small amount of the material is to be generated. Prolonged sessions where the worker is required to wear a face mask can be quite uncomfortable and are probably best avoided. Other limitations include losses of the agent by absorption, adsorption, and chemical reactions within the valves, tubing, or mask. Furthermore, for those isocyanates that may be primarily in the aerosol phase, such as MDI, significant losses of material occur due to gravitational settling and impaction in the transfer lines. This factor makes application of the face mask technique to the semi- and nonvolatile isocyanates difficult and unreliable.

A whole-body chamber can be operated in the static or dynamic mode. Using the static mode, generating an atmosphere prior to the worker entering the chamber may be limiting. In this context, the worker enters the chamber containing the atmosphere of the agent and the concentration of the agent begins to be used up from that point. This approach is most useful when small amounts of agent are available. Dynamic systems are capable of continuously delivering and blending one or more agents in a constant proportion over a protracted period. This approach is attractive because it delivers volumes of the agent at a precise concentration over a period of time. This is useful for generating unstable gases and vapors, where undesirable products are continuously flushed and replaced by fresh unreacted mixtures. Features such as humidity, temperature, and flow rate controls can be built into the chamber system to reproduce exposures. Yet the use of a whole-body chamber has its own set of drawbacks. Disadvantages include its complexity, the need for large quantities of agent, and the high initial and operational costs.

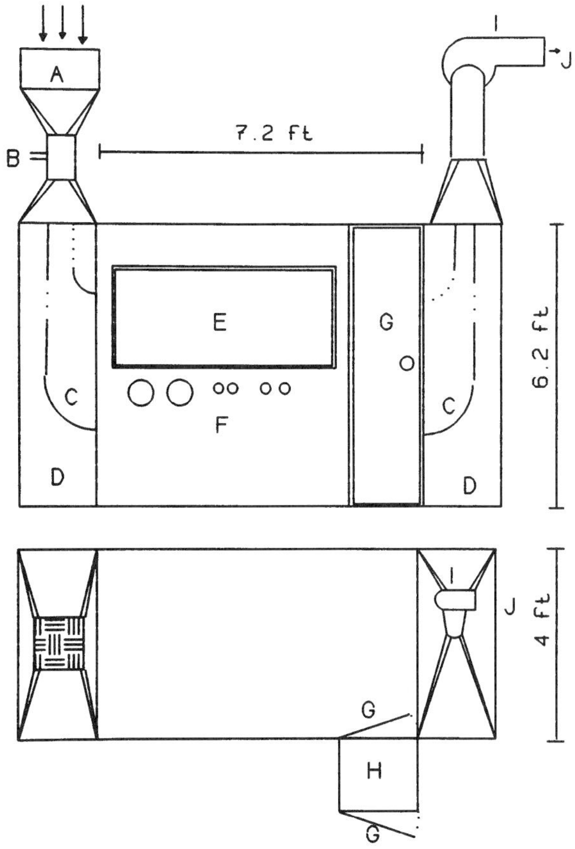


**FIG. 7.** This chamber system at Tulane University has been used to successfully generate numerous isocyanates. The first view is from the side and the second is from the top. *A*, charcoal/HEPA filter box; *B*, pollutant injection port; *C*, splitter vanes; *D*, plenum with diffuser screens; *E*, observation window; *F*, access ports; *G*, door; *H*, air lock; *I*, exhaust blower; *J*, exhaust connection into chemical fume hood system. (Reprinted with permission from ref. 120.)

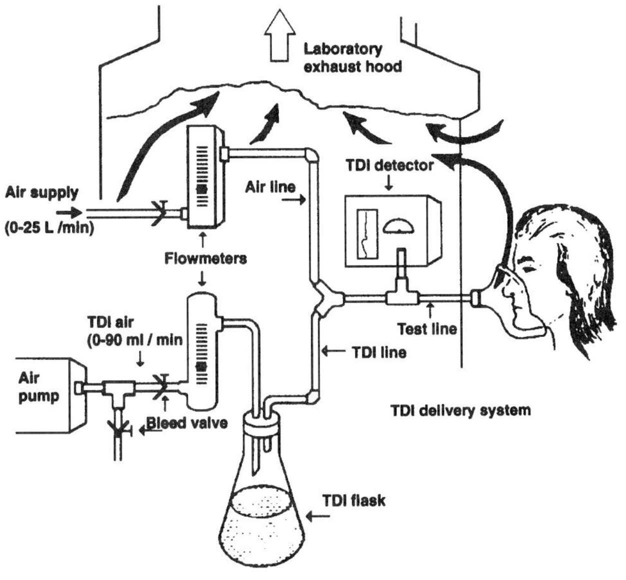


**FIG. 6.** A face mask-type TDI delivery system. The level of TDI exposure delivered to the worker is the result of mixing the TDI-free air, flowing at a high rate, with TDI vapor in the low flow line. Exposure is most easily altered by adjusting the rate of flow in the TDI-free air line. The flow rate of the mixed gases exceeds the resting flow rates of 6 to 9 Lpm. Although somewhat uncomfortable, these higher flow rates ensure that the subject does not inhale room air or rebreathe exhaled air. (Reprinted with permission from ref. 134.)

## APPROACHES TO CHALLENGE TESTING

There are several approaches to laboratory inhalational tests to isocyanates. Pepys et al. (121,107) were among the first to report isocyanate challenge testing methodologies.

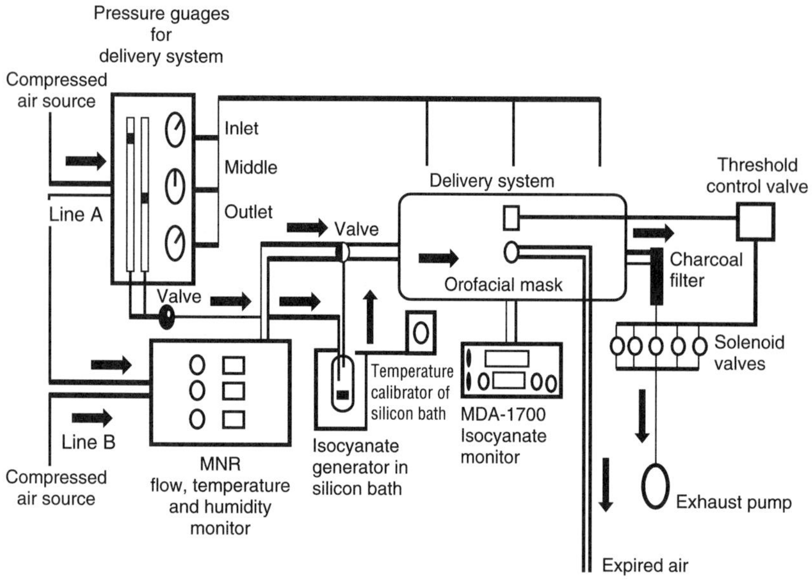


FIG. 8. This self-contained system is attractive because it captures the exhaled volatile isocyanates. (Reprinted with permission from ref. 124.)

In the first method, a two-part polyurethane varnish consisting of an isocyanate activator and a varnish resin is used. On the first day (the control day), the worker paints with the varnish resin in a closed room. On the second day, the worker paints with the varnish resin and TDI (the activator) mixture. Clinical evaluations and lung function tests are performed at regular intervals during the exposures. In the second method, the worker solders and inhales fumes containing TDI arising from burning the polyurethane film wire coating (122). With these approaches, generating an atmosphere of TDI is a simple task, yet determining the amount of varnishing or wire-burning sufficient to provoke an asthmatic response (if such a response is to occur) while keeping the exposure constant and providing a rate of exposure that remains below the permissible exposure limit can be difficult (Fig. 6).

A sophisticated prototype for the inhalation challenge chamber for isocyanates was reported in 1985 (Fig. 7) (123). The stainless steel chamber is 4 feet wide, 6.2 feet high, and 7.2 feet long with a side observation window through which the subject can be observed. Room air enters the chamber through high-efficiency particulate and charcoal filters and is blended with a concentrated amount of the test agent injected at a narrow throat for more complete mixing. The mixture enters the chamber through stainless steel splitter vanes and diffusion screen and sweeps across the chamber to exhaust through another set of screens and splitter vanes. A blower capable of providing flow rates in the range of 100 to 250 cubic feet per minute (cfm) at the site of exhaust drives this flow. These screens and splitter vanes at the inlet and outlet ensure even distribution of the agent in the chamber. The chamber is maintained at a slight negative pressure (0.5–1.5 inches of water) to prevent leakage of the agent into the environment. An air lock for worker entry also lessens the chance for leakage of the material into the environment and disruption of the test environment upon entering the chamber.

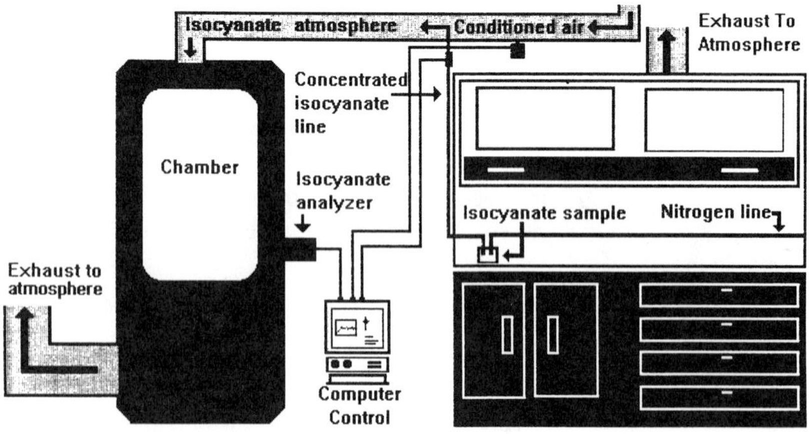


FIG. 9. This chamber system builds on the development of other systems and has incorporated computerized controls to increasingly monitor exposures, air flow rates, pressure, temperature, and humidity. This approach allows for the same values for these variables so that exposures can be easily reproduced and can be used for the generation of other agents besides diisocyanates. (Reprinted with permission from ref. 120.)

An even more sophisticated approach that emphasized safety was put forth by Vandenplas et al. (124) in a recent report; a closed-circuit apparatus was designed to provide TDI atmospheres (Fig. 8). This apparatus provides a combination of face mask delivery characteristics and humidity and temperature controlled TDI treated air. A low flow of air is blown over heated isocyanates in a glass container and mixed with a high flow of air adjusted to a specific humidity and temperature. The concentration of TDI can be altered by changing these flow rates. The combined air flow is then stored in a Teflon-coated plexiglass mixing cylinder. Within the cylinder is a sampling device to monitor TDI concentrations. The pressure within the cylinder is closely monitored and kept at -2 cm $H_2O$ pressure. This negative pressure is maintained by an exhaust pump on line with a solenoid valve system regulated by a threshold control valve. The subject breathes air through a face mask attached to a hole in the cylinder wall. Exhaled air is scrubbed by a charcoal filter and vented from the laboratory.

We have designed and constructed a system that builds on the work of our predecessors and uses a hood, a chamber with antechamber, and a computerized monitoring system to maintain control of the rate of ventilation, humidity, temperature, isocyanate levels, and the chamber pressure (Fig. 9) (120). The isocyanates are handled and the concentrated exposure is generated under a laboratory hood adjacent to the chamber. This serves as the exposure preparation area with a sink and air-gas service. Because the greatest chance for spills and excessive exposures occurs when the exposure is being prepared, this isolated, well-ventilated area for generation of the exposure is critical to the safety of the entire system. To provide an exposure that is relatively free of environmental contaminants, air entering the hood undergoes filtering by a high-efficiency particulate air (HEPA) filter. The hood is vented through the roof by an exhaust fan. Considering the quantities used in the preparation of an exposure, the need for a scrubber at the exhaust was deemed unnecessary. However, for added safety, a charcoal filter was added to absorb isocyanate and organic contaminants leaving the preparation area. This filter is replaced periodically to ensure maximum absorption of contaminants.

## APPROACHES TO GENERATING ISOCYANATE ATMOSPHERES

The design of the generation system is dictated by the physical properties of the particular diisocyanate compound. The more volatile diisocyanates [TDI, HDI, and cyclohexane diisocyanate (CHDI)] are generated at room temperature with a simple saturation technique employing an purge/trap apparatus customized with a coarse glass frit. For the liquid components (TDI, HDI), several milliliters of the diisocyanate are added to the bubbler and dry nitrogen is passed through, resulting in a saturated stream of diisocyanate vapor in the carrier gas, nitrogen. Nitrogen is used, rather than air, because it is clean of contaminants, is chemically inert, and contains no water vapor to react with the isocyanate. Prior to entering the injection line, the vapor stream is passed through a 4- to 7-mm glass fiber filter to remove diisocyanate aerosols generated by the bubbling process.

Cyclohexane diisocyanate, a solid of intermediate volatility, is coated onto 5-mm glass beads by evaporation of a solution of this diisocyanate in acetone. The coated glass beads are then added to the purge/trap. The purge/trap is immersed in a circulating water bath maintained at 40°C. Nitrogen carrier gas is passed through the apparatus and into the heated injection line leading to the chamber inlet port.

For the diisocyanates of low volatility [MDI, dicyclohexylmethane diisocyanate (HMDI), NDI, and IPDI], a high-temperature generator is required to introduce enough vapor into the challenge chamber to attain target concentrations. The diisocyanate solution (neat for HMDI and IPDI; 5% w/v in acetone for MDI and NDI) is metered into a flash evaporator via a syringe pump. The flash evaporator is constructed from a stainless steel "T" fitting connected to a length of copper tubing wrapped with heating tape. The syringe needle is inserted through a high temperature gas chromatograph septum contained in a septum port adapter on one arm of the "T." Temperature in the flash adapter is maintained by regulation of the heating tape with a rheostat.

For both of the systems described above, target concentrations of diisocyanates are attained by manipulation of the nitrogen carrier gas flow rate. This flow rate is generally in the range of 0.5 to 10.0 liters per minute (Lpm), depending on target concentration and chamber dilution flow rate. After the diisocyanate has been blended with nitrogen, a concentrated sample of diisocyanate is generated. This flows into a large ventilation duct to be mixed and diluted with air flowing at a faster rate before reaching the chamber. This mixture then enters the chamber and, by a small fan within the chamber, is adequately mixed.

### Ventilation

The air entering the chamber can be drawn from the central ventilation system of the building (house air) or from a separate roof vent. The second option is an ideal solution but it can be prohibitively costly and, if the air intake is placed near the chamber exhaust vent on the roof, poses a potential risk of contamination of the air entering the chamber. Because the temperature and humidity of ambient air affect the vapor pressure and degradation rate of isocyanates (and therefore the concentration), a heater and humidifier was placed in the ventilation duct to keep these variables constant (around 70°F temperature and 50% humidity).

### Exposure Chamber

The exposure chamber (Respirator Test Chamber, Dynatec Frontier Corp., Albuquerque, New Mexico) is a 125 cubic foot (4 × 4 × 7.8 feet) fiberglass chamber with a small antechamber (73 cubic foot; 2 × 4 × 7.8 feet). The worker enters the chamber through an air lock. This minimizes agent concentration fluctuations. With windows on three sides of the chamber, the subject can be observed during the exposure and claustrophobia can be minimized.

The chamber's environment controller is a microprocessor-based control unit applicable to automated monitoring and control of environmental parameters. In our chamber, the controller has been interfaced with a desktop computer via an RS 232 port. Using company-supplied software, a number of parameters such as diluting air flow, temperature, humidity, and pressure can be manually adjusted. In the case of pressure, the controller monitors input airflow and adjusts exhaust flow to a slightly higher level, thus maintaining negative pressure in the exposure chamber.

The protocol for challenge testing using the "laboratory approach" can require up to a week's hospitalization of the worker. A typical approach would be for the worker with suspected isocyanate asthma to be hospitalized Monday morning and undergo spirometry and methacholine challenge testing on that day. On Tuesday, the worker enters the exposure chamber but receives no isocyanate exposure and a "mock procedure" is undertaken to define the variability in lung function over 24 hours. Wednesday, Thursday, and Friday are isocyanate testing days. The dose and duration of isocyanate exposure is based on the presence of respiratory symptoms, the baseline spirometry values, and the degree of methacholine reactivity. Initial isocyanate exposures are 0.020 ppb for 15 minutes. Additional exposures should approximate 0.005 ppb for 4 hours. Spirometry is performed every hour during the workday in the laboratory. After hours, a spirometer is placed in the hospital room and forced expiratory maneuvers are performed hourly until bedtime. Alternatively, the absence of this decline in FEV1 after 4 hours' isocyanate exposure at the permissible exposure limit on two successive days provides reasonable evidence that a diagnosis of current isocyanate asthma cannot be made.

In conclusion, over the past 25 years, investigators have continued to improve on the approach to providing nonirritant exposures for the accurate diagnosis of isocyanate-induced asthma. Although the technology used in testing has become more sophisticated and may be fairly considered the domain of the bioengineer, the chemist, and the industrial hygienist, the requirements of the physician have remained unchanged. The physician must observe the level of exposure closely and monitor the worker's symptoms and lung function. Direct physician involvement in the testing procedure remains critical to the worker's safety and necessary for the accurate diagnosis of isocyanate-induced asthma.

## THERAPY FOR ISOCYANATE-INDUCED ASTHMA

The cornerstone of therapy of asthma attributable to isocyanates is the removal of the worker from the workplace. Saetta et al. (125) demonstrated structural changes in the airway after the sensitized worker ceased exposure. Bronchial biopsies from ten isocyanate sensitive subjects were taken at the time of diagnosis and 6 to 21 months later. All were away from isocyanates during this time. At follow-up, the asthmatics had a significant decrease in TDI sensitivity, and the airways showed a significant decrease in the thickness of subepithelial fibrosis (likely due to decreased collagen synthesis), and the number of subepithelial fibroblasts, mast cells, and lymphocytes. Yet, nonspecific airway hyperresponsiveness, and the mean numbers of macrophages and eosinophils in the airways walls were unchanged. In addition, therapy with β-agonists and inhaled steroids, as in the therapy of asthma attributable to other agents, plays a role. Maestrelli et al. (126) treated 15 subjects with challenge test proven TDI-induced asthma who were removed from the workplace. Eight received 1 mg of inhaled beclamethasone twice daily and the remaining seven received placebo for 5 months. The mean $FEV_1$ declined to a subirritant exposure of TDI at the start of the study (done to prove isocyanate sensitivity) and after 6 months (done to determine whether the worker had recovered from isocyanate sensitivity) was similar in both groups. At the end of the study, six in the placebo group and four in the treatment group had a less than 20% decline in $FEV_1$ to TDI exposure. Importantly, airway hyperresponsiveness to methacholine, comparable in both groups at the start, became statistically less at 2 months and remained less at 6 months in the treated group, while the untreated group was unchanged. Yet, only one in the placebo group and two in the treated group had a complete recovery. In those with isocyanate sensitivity, beclamethasone inhalation may lessen hyperreactivity in workers who might otherwise become symptomatic with exercise or upon exposure to irritants.

## CLINICAL LESSONS FROM ISOCYANATE CHALLENGE TESTING

Numerous provocative concerns remain about isocyanate-induced asthma. Some are addressed below in an illustrative manner that may help readers better evaluate workers who present with suspected isocyanate-induced asthma.

Is bronchial hyperresponsiveness to methacholine a necessary feature for the diagnosis of isocyanate-induced asthma? The relationship between the presence of airway responsiveness to methacholine and to the isocyanate

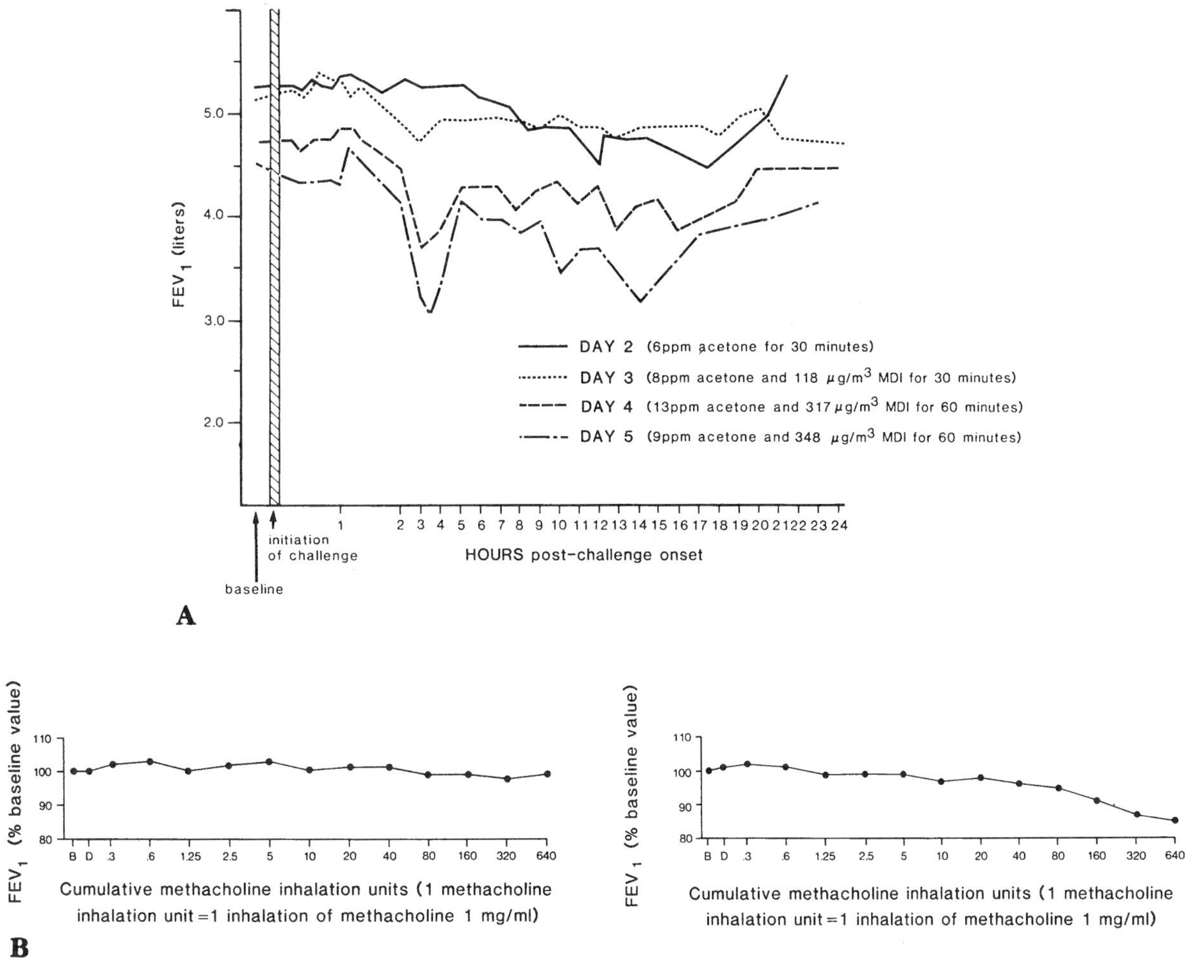


**FIG. 10.** The worker was a 30-year-old technical representative of an isocyanate manufacturer who had an initial massive exposure to MDI over a 2-day period while unloading a railroad car filled with this chemical approximately 5 years earlier. The worker wore no respiratory protection during the unloading and reported that he was unaware of the risks associated with exposure to this agent. After the second day of exposure he developed a severe episode of asthma that required an emergency room visit and a tapering course of oral steroid therapy. Since that first episode, he has occasionally had other exposures to MDI, with resulting late episodes of bronchospasm. He had had no recognized episodes of asthma in association with TDI exposures. After 5 years of these occasional episodes and concern regarding the relationship of MDI exposure and the delayed episodes of bronchospasm, specific challenge testing was undertaken. The physiologic assessment prior to challenge testing showed normal pulmonary function and no increased airway responsiveness to methacholine. **A:** Upon exposure to subirritant doses of MDI, he developed a dose-related decline in $FEV_1$ associated with a clinical picture of IgE-mediated allergy (hives, rhinitis, and generalized pruritis), which progressed over the week of challenge testing. **B:** Bronchial responsiveness to methacholine, although unmeasurable prior to MDI inhalation testing *(left)*, was increased after the week of a controlled MDI exposure *(right)*. Results of RAST to MDI-HSA were negative. (Reprinted with permission from ref. 119.)

suspected of inducing asthma is of interest in the diagnosis of isocyanate-induced asthma.

The presence of bronchial hyperresponsiveness does not always predict isocyanate-induced asthma. In the example given in Fig. 10, the absence of airway responsiveness to methacholine can be explained by the only occasional exposure to MDI. It is likely that this worker would have regained persistent bronchial responsiveness with more frequent and protracted isocyanate exposures.

These data reflect important concepts about the development of isocyanate-induced asthma. To the clinician, the most important is the recognition that the absence of airway hyperresponsiveness to methacholine or histamine does not rule out airway hyperresponsiveness to isocyanates in the proper clinical setting. Collection of additional data is necessary to objectively identify hyperresponsiveness to isocyanates. This concept has been confirmed by several other investigators (127–130). Sec-

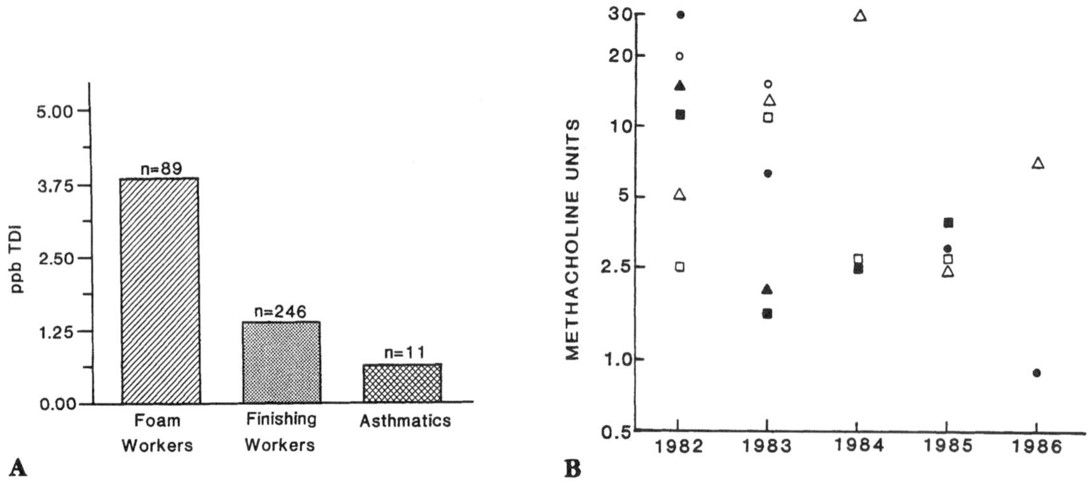


**FIG. 11. A:** Six workers were shown by specific challenge testing to be sensitized to TDI. All continued working in the same workplace but were transferred to areas in the workplace where exposure was negligible. The mean and time-weighted average (TWA) exposure concentration of 12-minute TDI samples for this asthmatic group after transfer was 0.0064 ± 0.0046 ppm, approximately one-twentieth of the allowable ceiling limit, and were significantly less ($p < 0.01$) than the mean TWA exposures for groups of workers typically exposed (foam and finishing workers) in other areas of the plant. Exposures for this asthmatic group were 0.001 ppm or less (undetectable) 88% of the time. **B:** All six had persistent respiratory symptoms and none exhibited improvement in bronchial hyperresponsiveness to methacholine. This figure plots bronchial hyperresponsiveness (as determined by the provocative cumulative dose of methacholine causing a 20% decline in the $FEV_1$ by year for each of the six asthma patients. Worker 1 is denoted by an *open circle;* worker 2 by an *open triangle;* worker 3 by an *open square;* worker 4 by a *closed triangle;* worker 5 by a *closed triangle;* and worker 6 by a *closed triangle.* Not all workers underwent methacholine testing each year. Three had a decline in their $FEV_1$ greater than 15% on one of the days of spirometric testing over the 5-year period (see Table 3). A relevant comment about the collection of these pre- and postshift spirometric data over this period was how infrequent a significant $FEV_1$ decline occurred across the work shift. If this had been the only index used, three of these cases would not have been recognized as isocyanate-induced asthma. TDI asthma persisted despite negligible levels of exposure. Improving the outcome of isocyanate-induced asthma appears to require removing the worker from further workplace exposure. (Reprinted with permission from ref. 131.)

ond, specific airway hyperresponsiveness apparently induces airway responsiveness to methacholine.

Can workers with isocyanate-induced asthma remain in the workplace in areas where isocyanate exposure is negligible or absent? When a worker is found to have TDI-induced asthma, the counseling physician is called upon to assess whether the worker can continue in the workplace. One strategy, without the social and financial implications of discharge and the legal implications to the company, is to move the sensitized worker to a part of the workplace recognized to have a negligible level of TDI or none.

Six polyurethane workers with challenge-test–proven TDI-induced asthma remained in the workplace at jobs where TDI exposure was thought to be negligible or absent (131). These workers were assessed serially over a 5-year period. All continued with respiratory symptoms, none had improvement in bronchial hyperresponsiveness to methacholine, and three had a decline in $FEV_1$ greater than 15% on one of the days of spirometric testing over this period (Fig. 11).

Although we could not have predicted the outcome of asthma had these workers left the workplace and ceased isocyanate exposure entirely, occupational asthma persisted despite negligible ongoing TDI exposures. Exposure to the slightest doses of isocyanates can precipitate an episode of asthma once sensitization occurs. For example, an isocyanate-sensitized worker who is completely isolated from these agents during the workday can develop bronchospasm in the cafeteria around coworkers who have only small amounts on their shoes or clothes. No improvement in respiratory symptoms can be expected unless the sensitized worker completely avoids exposure to isocyanate.

Is isocyanate challenge testing necessary for the accurate diagnosis of isocyanate-induced asthma? Most authors have focused on the clinical history for the diagnosis of occupational asthma. A major tenet of the diagnosis of isocyanate-induced asthma is the recognition that the worker develops symptoms at work and typically improves when away from the workplace. Yet, regardless of cause, workers who feel bad or complain of respiratory problems at work typically feel better away from work.

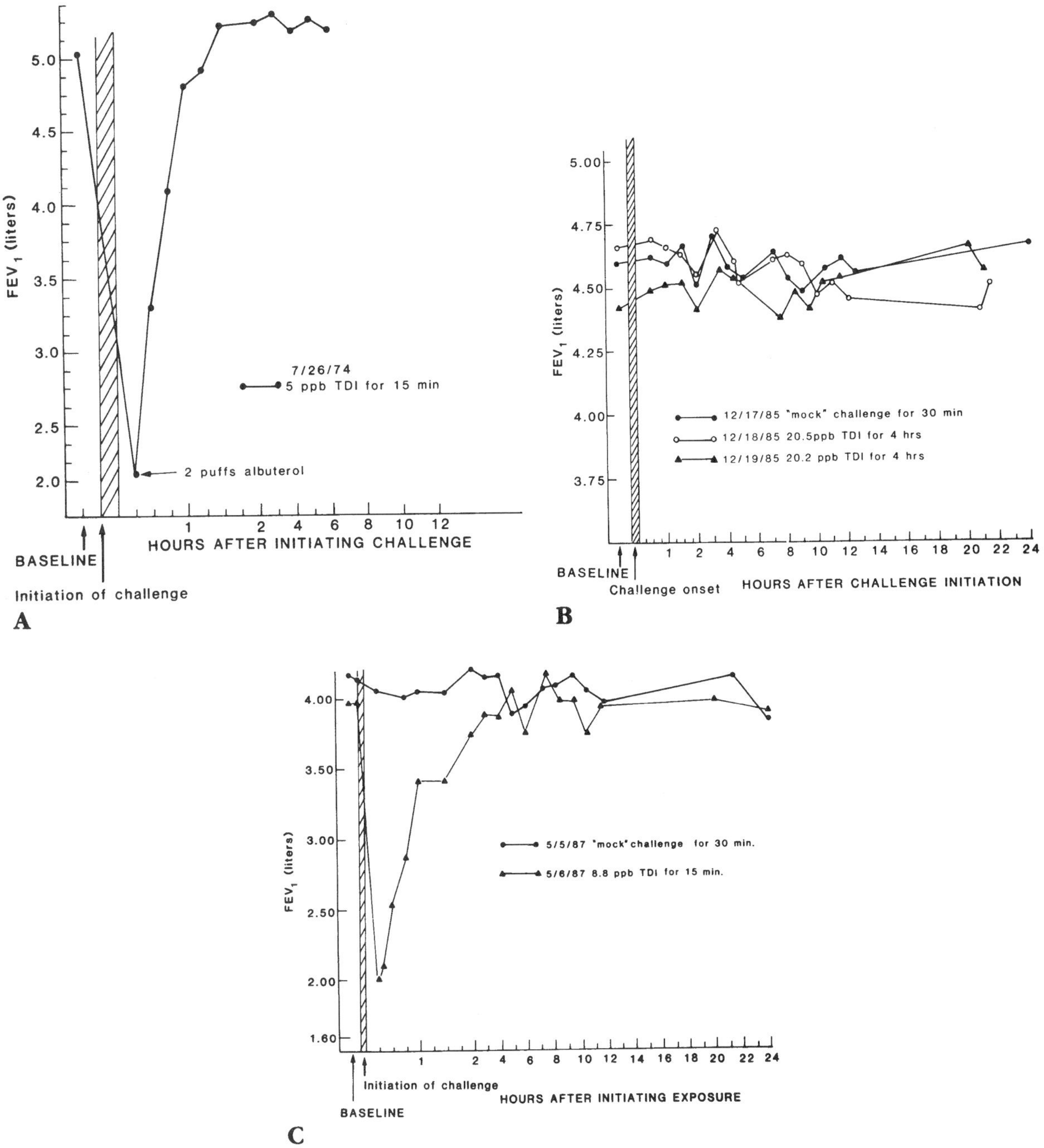


**FIG. 12.** The history of isocyanate-induced asthma in a 27-year-old worker who began employment at a chemical plant where TDI was produced in 1974. He worked for a short time and then developed asthma following exposure to a large spill of TDI. He spent the next 6 months in jobs in this plant where TDI exposure was thought to be negligible. Despite this, he persisted with asthma. **A:** Specific challenge testing to TDI confirmed that the asthma was attributable to this agent. He left this workplace but continued with the same corporation in a chemical-free site. After 5 years he no longer had respiratory symptoms or required respiratory medications. After 11 years, the company closed the chemical-free workplace and he was considered for transfer to the original workplace. **B:** Assessment in 1985 showed normal pulmonary function test results, airway responsiveness to methacholine, and no decline in $FEV_1$ or respiratory symptoms associated with a controlled subirritant exposure to TDI. A decision was made to allow him to return to the original work situation. After 4 months he developed asthma. **C:** A repeat evaluation approximately 18 months after returning to the original workplace in 1987 showed bronchial hyperresponsiveness to methacholine and a vigorous episode of asthma following a short subirritant exposure to TDI.

Concerns about the accurate use of the clinical history to make the diagnosis of isocyanate-induced asthma appear to be well-founded. In one series, 63 workers were referred for isocyanate challenge testing by physicians (108). All had a physician's diagnosis of isocyanate-induced asthma at the time of the referral. Thirty-three were proven to have no airway responsiveness to subirritant levels of isocyanates, yet 88% of this group reported work-related respiratory tract complaints and 97% noted an improvement in chest complaints when away from the workplace. To make the diagnosis even more difficult, 43% of those who did not respond to isocyanate challenge possessed airway hyperresponsiveness to methacholine, confirming the fact that this test may help with the diagnosis of asthma but not help identify the provoking agent.

Why were the results of the clinical evaluation so disparate from those of isocyanate challenge? One possibility was that the referral population was not representative of those with isocyanate-induced asthma. This seems an unlikely explanation for several reasons. First, challenged subjects were referred from different workplaces by different physicians. Second, there was a high prevalence of the same respiratory complaints. This suggests that the clinical data collected by the referring physicians were similar. Importantly, the surprisingly low percentage of positive isocyanate challenge tests in this study (48%) is similar to data reported by others. Mapp et al. (130) reported the largest series of workers undergoing isocyanate challenge testing. Of 165 workers suspected clinically to have TDI asthma, only 56% had a positive response to isocyanate challenge. Moller et al. (66) reported challenge testing results on 12 workers with a clinical and occupational history consistent with isocyanate-induced asthma. Only seven responded to specific challenge. These findings reinforce the concept that the clinical diagnosis of isocyanate-induced asthma is difficult.

Finally, it is not surprising that data from numerous laboratories show that the clinical diagnosis of isocyanate-induced asthma is made more often than it can be proven. Physicians who care for workers exposed to isocyanates recognize the potentially serious health risks to sensitized workers who continue isocyanate exposure. We are aware of two workers with isocyanate-induced asthma who have died due to asthma induced by this agent (133). However, attributing asthma to isocyanate exposure when this is not the case may result in the worker leaving the workplace, when this might not be necessary. Defining the relationship between workplace exposures and the development of asthma in the individual worker has become very important.

Is laboratory based isocyanate challenge testing the "gold standard" for the diagnosis of this illness? When an episode of asthma develops in association with a decline greater than 20% in $FEV_1$ following subirritant isocyanate exposure, the diagnosis of isocyanate-induced asthma is straightforward. The difficulty lies in assessing the degree of confidence that occupational asthma is absent following a negative isocyanate inhalation challenge test (specificity). The answer is not clear. First, because other chemicals that have the potential to induce asthma may be present along with isocyanates in workplaces, a negative response to isocyanate inhalation does not rule out occupational asthma. Second, during a retrospective evaluation, a worker with isocyanate-induced asthma may leave the workplace and lose his or her sensitivity to isocyanates. When that worker is then challenged with subirritant levels to isocyanates, no acute decline in lung function occurs. In the series of 63 workers referred for challenge testing noted above, the mean time from last exposure to challenge testing in the reactor and nonreactor groups was similar (approximately 4 months). Although there is no way to completely rule out the fact that some with isocyanate-induced asthma may have recovered and no longer be demonstrably sensitized to isocyanates, this does not explain the large percentage who do not respond to isocyanate challenge testing.

A negative response to isocyanate inhalation challenge performed while workers are still employed or soon after they leave employment at a workplace where they are exposed to isocyanate conclusively rules out isocyanate-induced asthma. In such a situation other explanations for respiratory symptoms should be investigated.

How long does airway hyperresponsiveness to isocyanates persist? Although investigators have shown that in workers who become sensitized to isocyanates asthma persists even when they leave the workplace, many workers recover and no longer need respiratory medications, are without respiratory symptoms, and no longer exhibit bronchial hyperresponsiveness. Those most likely to recover appear to be those who are diagnosed soon after they develop asthma.

The report of just one case (Fig. 12) showing the recurrence of airway hyperresponsiveness to isocyanates following repeat workplace exposures is an inadequate basis for definite conclusions regarding how long isocyanate-induced asthma may persist. The data, however, are informative, because they strengthen the clinical relationship between isocyanate-induced asthma and an IgE-mediated mechanism of isocyanate-induced asthma. The recovery of airway hyperresponsiveness and its recurrence following repeat isocyanate exposure constitute a pattern similar to allergic asthma, which produces seasonal asthmatic symptoms every year. Although one cannot rule out sensitization anew with repeated exposure, it may well be that isocyanate sensitivity, once developed, is lifelong, and, like allergic asthma, is altered in relation to specific antigen exposure.

## SUMMARY

Over the past 50 years, the presence of isocyanates has improved the quality of life for many around the world. The trade-off has been the development of a number of illnesses that are attributable to these man-made chemicals. The most prominent among them is asthma. A number of questions remain regarding the basic issues associated with sensitization to isocyanates. Of the three key concerns described below, the first is the most worrisome. After approximately 50 years of experience with these chemicals and efforts by health professionals, workplace physicians, industrial hygiene experts, and labor-management groups, we have not yet been able to achieve an illness-free workplace.

1. Even in the most controlled workplace where exposures are continuously below the permissible limit, the use of isocyanates results in chemical sensitization. Is there a level of exposure that is not associated with sensitization? Can these chemicals ever be used safely and the protection of all workers be achieved ?
2. Will changing of industrial processes from TDI to MDI decrease the likelihood of sensitization of isocyanates to workers within the workplace?
3. Although there appears to be an allergic mechanism associated with isocyanate-induced asthma, how can the antigen be identified? If this is identified, can desensitization or other means be developed to alter the natural history of these illnesses?

## REFERENCES


1. Ulrich H. Urethane polymers. In: Kirk-Othmer AC, ed. *Encyclopedia of chemical technology*, 3rd ed. New York: John Wiley; 1983;23: 577–608.
2. Buist JM. Isocyanates in industry. *Proc R Soc Med* 1970;63:365–368.
3. Internet site www.chemexpo.com.
4. Occupational exposure to diisocyanates (NIOSH criteria document for a recommended standard). DHEW publication 78-215. Washington, DC: U.S. Department of Health, Education, and Welfare, 1978.
5. Schnorr TM, Steenland K, Egeland GM, et al. Mortality of workers exposed to toluene diisocyanate in the polyurethane foam industry. *Occup Environ Med* 1996;53:703–706.
6. Patterson R, Nugent KM, Harris KE, et al. Immunologic hemorrhagic pneumonia caused by isocyanates. *Am Rev Respir Dis* 1990;141; 226–230.
7. Tomashefski JF. Pulmonary pathology of the adult respiratory distress syndrome. *Clin Chest Med* 1990;11:593–619.
8. Brooks SM, Weiss MA, Bernstein IL. Reactive airways dysfunction (RADS). Persistent asthma syndrome after high level irritant exposures. *Chest* 1985;88:376–384.
9. Axford AT, McKerrow CB, Jones AP, et al. Accidental exposure to isocyanate fumes on a group of firemen. *Br J Ind Med* 1976;33:65–71.
10. Mastromatteo E. Recent occupational health experience in Ontario. *J Occup Med* 1965;7:502–511.
11. Banks DE, Butcher BT, Salvaggio JE. Isocyanate induced respiratory disease. *Ann Allergy* 1986;57:389–398.
12. Fuchs S, Valade P. Etude clinique et experimentale sur quelques cad d'intoxication par les Desmodur T (diisocyanate de tolylene 1-2-4 et 1-2-6). *Arch mal Profess Med Travail Securite Sociale* 1951;12: 191–196.
13. Peters JM, Murphy RLH. Hazards to health: do it yourself polyurethane foam. *Am Rev Respir Dis* 1971;104:432–433.
14. Liss GM, Halperin WE, Landrigan PJ. Occupational asthma in a home pieceworker. *Arch Environ Health* 1986;41:359–362.
15. Luo J-C L, Nelsen KG, Fischbein A. Persistent airway dysfunction syndrome after exposure to toluene diisocyanate. *Br J Ind Med* 1990; 47:239–241.
16. Carroll KB, Secombe CJP, Pepys J. Asthma due to non-occupational exposure to toluene (tolylene) di-isocyanate. *Clin Allergy* 1976; 6:99–104.
17. Butcher BT, Jones RN, O'Neil CE, et al. Longitudinal study of workers employed in the manufacture of toluene diisocyanate. *Am Rev Respir Dis* 1977;116:411–422.
18. Bernstein DI, Korbee L, Stauder T, et al. The low prevalence of occupational asthma and antibody-dependent sensitization to diphenylmethane diisocyanate in a plant engineered for minimal exposure to isocyanates. *J Allergy Clin Immunol* 1993;92:387–396.
19. Bignon JS, Aron Y, Ju LY, et al. HLA class II alleles in isocyanate-induced asthma. *Am J Respir Crit Care Med* 1994;149:71–75.
20. Burge P. Diagnosis of occupational asthma. *Clin Exp Allergy* 1989; 19:649–652.
21. Hagmar L, Welinder H, Mikoczy Z. Cancer incidence and mortality in the Swedish polyurethane foam manufacturing industry. *Br J Ind Med* 1993;50:537–543.
22. Sorahan T, Pope D. Mortality and cancer morbidity of production workers in the United Kingdom polyurethane foam industry. *Br J Med* 1993;50:528–536.
23. Brooks SM. The evaluation of occupational airways disease in the workplace. *J Allergy Clin Immunol* 1982;70:56–66.
24. Tarlo SM, Liss GM, Dias C, et al. Assessment of the relationship between isocyanate exposure levels and occupational asthma. *Am J Ind Med* (in press).
25. Chester EH, Martinez-Catinchi M, Schwartz HJ, et al. Patterns of airway reactivity to asthma produced by exposure to toluene di-isocyanate. *Chest* 1979;75:S229–231.
26. Kennedy AL, Brown WE. Identification of airway proteins and identification of secondary responses by inhalation exposure to isocyanates. *Am Rev Respir Dis* 1989;139:A37 (abstr).
27. Kennedy AL, Wilson TR, Brown WE. Analysis of functional alterations of laminin modified by isocyanates in vivo and in vitro. *Am Rev Respir Dis* 1990;141:A706 (abstr).
28. Hjortsberg L, Orbaek P, Arborelius M Jr. Small airway hyperreactivity among lifelong nonatopic nonsmokers exposed to isocyanates. *Br J Ind Med* 1987;44:824–828.
29. Grammer LC, Patterson R. Immunologic evaluation of occupational asthma. In: Bernstein DI, Bernstein IL, Chang-Yeung M, Malo J-C, eds. *Asthma in the work place.* New York: Decker, 1993:125–144.
30. Chan-Yeung M, Malo J-L. Occupational asthma. *N Engl J Med* 1995; 333:107–112.
31. Walker C, Bode E, Boer L, et al. Allergic and nonallergic asthmatics have distinct patterns of T-cell activation and cytokine production in peripheral blood and bronchoalveolar lavage. *Am Rev Respir Dis* 1992;146:109–115.
32. Diem JE, Jones RN, Hendrick DJ, et al. Five-year longitudinal study of workers employed in a new toluene diisocyanate manufacturing plant. *Am Rev Respir Dis* 1982;126:420–428.
33. Avery SB, Stetson DM, Pan PM, Mathews IQ. Immunological investigation of individuals with toluene diisocyanate asthma. *Clin Exp Immunol* 1969;4:585–596.
34. Bruckner HC, Avery SB, Stetson DM, Dodson VN, Ronayne JJ. Clinical and immunological appraisal of exposure of workers exposed to isocyanates. *Arch Environ Health* 1968;16:619–625.
35. Scheel LD, Killens R, Josephson A. Immunochemical aspects of toluene diisocyanate (TDI) toxicity. *Am Ind Hyg Assoc J* 1964;25: 179–184.
36. Taylor G. Immune response to toluene diisocyanate (TDI) exposure in man. *Proc R Soc Med* 1970;63:379–380.
37. Karol MH, Ioset HH, Alarie YC. Tolyl-specific IgE antibodies in workers with hypersensitivity to toluene diisocyanate. *Am Ind Hyg Assoc J* 1978;39:454–458.
38. Butcher BT, O'Neil C, Reed MA, Salvaggio JE. Radioallergosorbent testing with p-tolyl monoisocyanate in toluene diisocyanate workers. *Clin Allergy* 1983;13:31–34.

39. Butcher BT, Mapp C, Reed MA, O'Neil C, Salvaggio JE. Evidence for carrier specificity of IgE antibodies detected in sera of isocyanate exposed workers. *J Allergy Clin Immunol* 1982;69:123 (abstr).
40. Zeiss CR, Levitz D, Chacon P, Wolonsky P, Patterson R, Prujansky JJ. Quantitation and new antigenic determinant specificity of antibodies induced by inhalation of trimellitic anhydride in man. *Int Arch Allergy Appl Immunol* 1980;61:380–388.
41. Cartier A, Grammer L, Malo J-L, et al. Specific serum antibodies against isocyanates: association with occupational asthma. *J Allergy Clin Immunol* 1989;84:507–514.
42. Grammer L Cartier C, Harris IE, Malo J-L, Cartier A, Patterson R. The use of an immunoassay index against isocyanate human protein conjugates and application to human isocyanate disease. *J Allergy Clin Immunol* 1990;86:94–98.
43. Karol MH, Tollerud DJ, Campbell TP, et al. Predictive value of airways hyperresponsiveness and circulating IgE for identifying types of responses to toluene diisocyanate inhalation challenge. *Am J Respir Crit Care Med* 1994;149:611–615.
44. Davies RJ, Butcher BT, O'Neil CE, Salvaggio JE. The *in vitro* effect of toluene diisocyanate on lymphocyte cyclic adenosine monophosphate production by isoproterenol, prostaglandin, and histamine. *J Allergy Clin Immunol* 1977;60:223–229.
45. Bernstein IL. Isocyanate-induced pulmonary diseases: a current perspective. *J Allergy Clin Immunol* 1982;70:24–31.
46. Azzawi M, Bradley B, Jeffrey PK, et al. Identification of activated T-lymphocytes and eosinophils in bronchial biopsies in stable atopic asthma. *Am Rev Respir Dis* 1990;142:1407–1413.
47. Houston JC, deNavasquez S, Trounce SR. A clinical and pathological study of fatal cases of status asthmaticus. *Thorax* 1953;8:195–206.
48. Dunhill MS. The pathology of asthma, with special reference to changes in the bronchial mucosa. *J Clin Pathol* 1960;13:27–33.
49. Cardill BS, Pearson RSB. Death in asthmatics. *Thorax* 1959;14: 341–352.
50. Kay AB. Asthma and inflammation. *J Allergy Clin Immunol* 1991;87: 893–910.
51. Fabbri LM, Boschetto P, Zocca E, et al. Bronchoalveolar lavage neutrophilia during late asthma induced by toluene diisocyanate. *Am Rev Respir Dis* 1987;136:36–42.
52. Mapp CE, DiGiacomo GR, Omini C, et al. Late, but nor early, asthmatic reactions induced by toluene diisocyanate are associated with increased airways responsiveness to methacholine. *Eur J Respir Dis* 1986;69:276–284.
53. Fabbri LM, Chiesura-Corona P, Dal Vecchio L, et al. Prednisone inhibits late asthmatic reactions and the associated increase in airways responsiveness induced by toluene diisocyanate in sensitized subjects. *Am Rev Respir Dis* 1985;132:1010–1014.
54. Bentley AM, Maestrelli P, Saetta M, et al. Activated T-lymphocytes and eosinophils in the bronchial mucosa in isocyanate-induced asthma. *J Allergy Clin Immunol* 1992;89:821–829.
55. Saetta M, DiStefano A, Maestrelli P, et al. Airway mucosal inflammation in occupational asthma induced by toluene diisocyanate. *Am Rev Respir Dis* 1992;145:160–166.
56. Jeffrey PK, Wardlaw AJ, Nelson FC, et al. Bronchial biopsies in asthma. An ultrastructural, quantitative study and correlation with hyperreactivity. *Am Rev Respir Dis* 1989;140:1745–1753.
57. Maestrelli P, DiStefano A, Occari P, et al. Cytokines in the airway mucosa of subjects with asthma induced by toluene diisocyanate. *Am J Respir Crit Care Med* 1995;151:607–612.
58. Butcher BT, O'Neil CE, Reed MA, Salvaggio JE, Weill H. Development and loss of toluene diisocyanate reactivity: immunologic, pharmacologic, and provocative challenge studies. *J Allergy Clin Immunol* 1982;70:231–235.
59. Banks DE, Rando RJ. Recurrent asthma induced by toluene diisocyanate. *Thorax* 1988;43:660–662.
60. Lemiere C, Cartier A, Dolovich J, et al. Outcome of specific bronchial responsiveness to occupational agents after removal from exposure. *Am J Respir Crit Care Med* 1996;154:329–333.
61. Mapp CE, Corona PC, Marzo ND, et al. Persistent asthma due to isocyanates: a follow-up study of subjects with occupational asthma due to toluene diisocyanate (TDI). *Am Rev Respir Dis* 1988;137: 1326–1329.
62. Chan-Yeung M, MacLean L, Paggiaro PL. Follow-up study of 232 patients with occupational asthma caused by Western red cedar (*Thuja plicata*). *J Allergy Clin Immunol* 1987;79:792–796.
63. Hudson P, Cartier A, Pineau L, et al. Follow-up of occupational asthma caused by crab and various agents. *J Allergy Clin Immunol* 1985;76:683–685.
64. Allard C, Cartier A, Ghezzo H, et al. Occupational asthma due to various agents: absence of clinical and functional improvement at an interval of four or more years after cessation of exposure. *Chest* 1989; 96:1046–1049.
65. Paggiaro PL, Loi AM, Rossi O, et al. Follow-up study of patients with respiratory disease due to toluene diisocyanate (TDI). *Clin Allergy* 1984;14:462–469.
66. Moller DR, Brooks SM, McKay RT, et al. Chronic asthma due to toluene diisocyanate. *Chest* 1986;90:494–499.
67. Lozewicz S, Assoufi BK, Hawkins R, et al. Outcome of asthma induced by isocyanates. *Br J Dis Chest* 1987;81:14–22.
68. Rosenberg N, Garnier R, Rousselin X, et al. Clinical and socioprofessional fate of isocyanate-induced asthma. *Clin Allergy* 1987;17: 55–61.
69. Adams WGF. Long-term effects on the health of men engaged in the manufacture of tolylene di-isocyanate. *Br J Industr Med* 1975;32: 72–78.
70. McKerrow CB, Davies HJ, Parry Jones A. Symptoms and lung function following acute and chronic exposure to tolylene diisocyanate. *Proc Roy Soc Med* 1970;63:376–378.
71. Peters JM, Murphy RLH, Pagnatto LD, et al. Acute respiratory effects in workers exposed to low levels of toluene diisocyanate (TDI). *Arch Environ Health* 1968;16:642–647.
72. Peters JM, Murphy RLH, Ferris BG Jr. Ventilatory function in workers exposed to low levels of toluene diisocyanate: a 6-month follow-up. *Br J Ind Med* 1969;26:115–120.
73. Peters JM. Studies of isocyanate toxicity. Cumulative pulmonary effects in workers exposed to tolylene diisocyanate. *Proc R Soc Med* 1970;63:372–375.
74. Peters JM, Murphy RLH, Pagnatto LD, et al. Respiratory impairment in workers exposed to safe levels of toluene diisocyanate (TDI). *Arch Environ Health* 1970;20:364–367.
75. Wegman DH, Pagnoto LD, Fine LJ, et al. A dose response relationship in TDI workers. *J Occup Med* 1974;16:258–260.
76. Wegman DH, Peters JM, Pagnotto L, et al. Chronic pulmonary function loss from exposure to toluene diisocyanate. *Br J Ind Med* 1977; 34:196–200.
77. Musk AW, Peters JM, DiBerardinis L, et al. Absence of respiratory effects in subjects exposed to low concentrations of TDI and MDI. *J Occup Med* 1982;24:746–750.
78. Gee JB, Morgan WKC. A 10-year follow-up study of a group of workers exposed to isocyanates. *J Occup Med* 1985;27:15–18.
79. Jones RN, Rando RJ, Glindmeyer HW, et al. Abnormal lung function in polyurethane foam producers: weak relationship to toluene diisocyanate exposures. *Am Rev Respir Dis* 1992;146:871–877.
80. Belin L, Wass U, Audunsson G, et al. Amines: possible causative agents in the development of bronchial hyperreactivity in workers manufacturing polyurethanes from isocyanates. *Br J Ind Med* 1983; 40:251–257.
81. Candura F, Moscato G. Do amines induce occupational asthma in workers manufacturing polyurethane foams? *Br J Ind Med* 1984;41: 552–553.
82. Charles J, Bernstein A, Jones B, et al. Hypersensitivity pneumonitis after exposure to isocyanates. *Thorax* 1976;31:127–136.
83. Fink JN, Schlueter DP. Bathtub refinisher's lung: an unusual response to toluene diisocyanate. *Am Rev Respir Dis* 1978;118: 955–959.
84. Simpson C, Garabant D, Torrey S ,et al. Hypersensitivity pneumonitis-like reaction and occupational asthma associated with 1,3-bis(isocyanatomethyl) cyclohexane pre-polymer. *Am J Ind Med* 1996;30: 48–55.
85. Zeiss CR, Kanellakes TM, BelloneJD, et al. Immunoglobulin E-mediated asthma and hypersensitivity pneumonitis with precipitating antihapten antibodies due to diphenylmethane diisocyanate (MDI) exposure. *J Allergy Clin Immunol* 1980;65:346–352.
86. Bascom R, Kennedy TP, Levitz D, et al. Specific bronchoalveolar lavage IgG antibody in hypersensitivity pneumonitis from diphenylmethane diisocyanate. *Am Rev Respir Dis* 1985;131:463–465.
87. Malo J-L, Ouimet G, Cartier A, et al. Combined alveolitis and asthma due to hexamethylene diisocyanate (HDI), with demonstration of crossed respiratory and immunologic reactivities to dimethyl-

methane diisocyanate (MDI). *J Allergy Clin Immunol* 1983;72: 413–419.

88. Malo J-L, Zeiss CR. Occupational hypersensitivity pneumonitis after exposure to diphenylmethane diisocyanate. *Am Rev Respir Dis* 1982;125:113–116.
89. Vandenplas O, Malo J-L, Dugas M, et al. Hypersensitivity pneumonitis-like reaction among workers exposed to piphenylmethane diisocyanate (MDI). *Am Rev Respir Dis* 1993;147:338–346.
90. Baur X, Dewair M, Rommelt H. Acute airway obstruction followed by hypersensitivity pneumonitis in an isocyanate (MDI) worker. *J Occup Med* 1984;26:285–287.
91. Baur X. Hypersensitivity pneumonitis (extrinsic allergic alveolitis) induced by isocyanates. *J Allergy Clin Immunol* 1995;95:1004–1010.
92. Pham QT, Cavelier C, Mereau P, et al. Isocyanates and respiratory function: a study of workers producing polyurethane foam moulding. *Ann Occup Hyg* 1978;21:121–129.
93. Parkes HG. Isocyanates in industry: environmental control. *Proc R Soc Med* 1970;63:368–372.
94. Tansar AR, Bourke MP, Blandford AG. Isocyanate asthma: respiratory symptoms caused by diphenyl methane diisocyanate. *Thorax* 1973;28: 96–600.
95. Zammit-Tabonga M, Sherkin M, Kijek K, et al. Asthma caused by diphenylmethane diisocyanate in foundry workers. *Am Rev Respir Dis* 1983;128:226–230.
96. Liss GM, Bernstein DI, Moller DR, et al. Pulmonary and immunologic evaluation of foundry workers exposed to methylene diisocyanate (MDI). *J Allergy Clin Immunol* 1988;82:55–61.
97. O'Brien IM, Harries MG, Burge PS, et al. Toluene diisocyanate-induced asthma. I. Reactions to TDI, MDI, HDI, and histamine. *Clin Allergy* 1979;9:1–6.
98. Harries MG, Burge PS, Samson M, et al. Isocyanate asthma: respiratory symptoms due to 1,5- naphthalene diisocyanate. *Thorax* 1979;34: 762–766.
99. Clarke CW, Aldons PM. Isophorone diisocyanate (IPDI)-induced respiratory disease. *Aust NZ J Med* 1981;11:290–292.
100. Alexandersson R, Gustafsson, Hedenstierna G, et al. Exposure to naphthalene-diisocyanate in a rubber plant: symptoms and lung function. *Arch Environ Health* 1986;41:85–90.
101. Hill RN. A controlled study of workers handling organic diisocyanates. *Proc R Soc Med* 1970;63:375.
102. Fuortes LJ, Kiken S, Makowsky M. An outbreak of naphthalene diisocyanate-induced asthma in a plastics factory. *Arch Environ Health* 1995;50:337–340.
103. Grammer LC, Eggum P, Silverstein M, et al. Prospective immunologic and clinical study of a population exposed to hexamethylene diisocyanate. *J Allergy Clin Immunol* 1988;82:627–633.
104. Linder HW, Nielsen J, Bensyrd I, et al. IgG antibodies against polyisocyanates in car painters. *Clin Allergy* 1988;18:85–93.
105. Dahlquist M, Tornling G, Plato N, et al. Effects within the week on forced vital capacity are correlated with long term changes in pulmonary function: reanalysis of studies on car painters exposed to isocyanate. *Occup Environ Med* 1995;52:192–195.
106. Barkman HW Jr, Banks DE. Bronchoprovocation testing in occupational asthma. Folia Allergol Immunol Clin 1985; 32:45-51.
107. Pepys J, Pickering CAC, Breslin ABX, et al. Asthma due to inhaled chemical agents—tolylene diisocyanate. *Clin Allergy* 1972;2: 225–236.
108. Banks DE, Sastre J, Butcher BT, et al. Role of inhalation challenge testing in the diagnosis of isocyanate-induced asthma. *Chest* 1989;95: 414–423.
109. Banks DE, deShazo RD. An overview of occupational asthma: principles of diagnosis and management. *Immunol Allergy Pract* 1985;7: 122–130.
110. Burge PS, O'Brien IM, Harries MG. Peak flow records in the diagnosis of occupational asthma due to isocyanates. *Thorax* 1979;34: 317–323.
111. Liss GM, Tarlo SM. Peak expiratory flow rates in possible occupational asthma. *Chest* 1991;100:63–69.
112. Cote J, Kennedy S, Chan-Yeung M. Sensitivity and specificity of $PC_{20}$ and peak expiratory flow rates in cedar asthma. *J Allergy Clin Immunol* 1990;85:592–598.
113. Newman-Taylor AJ. Occupational asthma. *Thorax* 1980;35:441–444.
114. Venables KM, Chan-Yeung M. Occupational asthma. *Lancet* 1997; 349:1465–1469.
115. Quirce S, Contreras G, Dybuncio A, et al. Peak expiratory flow monitoring is not a reliable method of establishing the diagnosis of occupational asthma. *Am J Respir Crit Care Med* 1995;152:1100–1102.
116. Malo J-L, Trudeau C, Ghezzo H, et al. Do subjects investigated for occupational asthma through serial peak flow measurements falsify their results? *J Allergy Clin Immunol* 1995;96:601–607.
117. Paggiaro PL, Vagaggini B, Dente FL, et al. Bronchial hyperresponsiveness and toluene diisocyanate. Long-term change in sensitized asthmatic subjects. *Chest* 1993;103:1123–1128.
118. Hargreave FE, Ramsdale EH, Pugsley SO. Occupational asthma without bronchial hyperresponsiveness. *Am Rev Respir Dis* 1984;130: 513–515.
119. Banks DE, Barkman HW Jr, Butcher BT, et al. Absence of hyperresponsiveness to methacholine in a worker with methylene diphenyl diisocyanate (MDI) asthma. *Chest* 1986;89:389–393.
120. Banks DE, Tarlo SM, Masri F, et al. Bronchoprovocation tests in the diagnosis of isocyanate-induced asthma. *Chest* 1996;109:1370–1379.
121. Pepys J, Hutchcroft BJ. Bronchial provocation tests in etiologic diagnosis and analysis of asthma. *Am Rev Respir Dis* 1975;112:829–859.
122. Paisley DPG. Isocyanate hazard from wire insulation: an old hazard in a new guise. *Br J Ind Med* 1969;26:79–82.
123. Hammad YY, Rando RJ, Abdel-Kader H. Considerations in the design and use of human inhalation challenge delivery systems. *Folia Allergol Immunol Clin* 1985;32:37–44.
124. Vandenplas O, Malo JL, Cartier A, Perreault G, Cloutier Y. Closed-circuit methodology for inhalation challenge test with isocyanates. *Am Rev Respir Dis* 1992;145:582–587.
125. Saetta M, Maestrelli P, Turato G, et al. Airway wall remodeling after cessation of exposure to isocyanates in sensitized asthmatic subjects. *Am J Respir Crit Care Med* 1995;151:489–494.
126. Maestrelli P, deMarzo N, Saetta M, et al. Effects of inhaled beclomethasone on airway responsiveness in occupational asthma. *Am Rev Respir Dis* 1993;148:407–412.
127. O'Brien IM, Newman-Taylor AJ, Burge PS, et al. Toluene diisocyanate-induced asthma. II. Inhalation challenge tests and bronchial reactivity studies. *Clin Allergy* 1979;9:7–15.
128. Smith AB, Brooks SM, Blanchard J, et al. Absence of airway hyperreactivity to methacholine in a worker sensitized to toluene diisocyanate (TDI). *J Occup Med* 1980;22:327–331.
129. Hargreave FE, Ramsdale EH, Pugsley SO. Occupational asthma without bronchial hyperresponsiveness. *Am Rev Respir Dis* 1984;130: 513–515.
130. Mapp CE, DalVecchio L, Boschetto P, et al. Toluene diisocyanate-induced asthma without airway hyperresponsiveness. *Eur J Respir Dis* 1986;68:89–95.
131. Banks DE, Rando RJ, Barkman HW Jr. Persistence of toluene diisocyanate-induced asthma despite negligible workplace exposures. *Chest* 1990;97:121–125.
132. Mapp CE, DiGiacomo CR, Zedda L, et al. Isocyanate-induced asthma: A review of 165 cases studied in 1983–1985. *J Allergy Clin Immunol* 1986;77:17 (abstr).
133. Fabbri LM, Daniele D, Criscioli S, et al. Fatal asthma in a subject sensitized to toluene diisocyanate. *Am Rev Respir Dis* 1988;137: 1494–1498.
134. Gerblich AA, Horowitz J, Chester EH, Schwartz HJ, Fleming GM. A proposed standardized method for bronchoprovocation tests in toluene diisocyanate-induced asthma. *J Allergy Clin Immunol* 1979;64: 658–661.

*Environmental and Occupational Medicine,*
*Third Edition,* edited by William N. Rom.
Lippincott–Raven Publishers, Philadelphia © 1998.

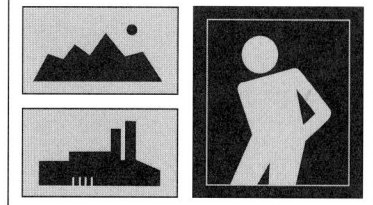

CHAPTER 36

# Agricultural Dust-Induced Lung Disease

Joel N. Kline and David A. Schwartz

Although not widely appreciated, the agricultural worker and possibly those living in rural environments are at increased risk of developing lung disease (1–5). The risk associated with progressive lung disease appears to be more than threefold greater among those who are more heavily exposed to dusts generated in the agricultural environment (3). Interestingly, cigarette smoking does not appear to account for this excess risk, since agricultural workers consistently have lower rates of cigarette smoking than other occupations (6,7). These general epidemiologic observations are supported by an increasing number of exposure-specific studies in agricultural workers, which are reviewed in this chapter. Lung disease caused by agricultural aerosols affects a large population, with more than five million agricultural workers in the United States and over 80% of the work force in developing countries involved in agriculture. Unlike other occupations, the agricultural worker usually lives in the same environment as he/she works in, with exposures occurring throughout the week, and children are commonly involved in agricultural work.

The agricultural worker and those living in a rural environment encounter a variety of inhaled organic dusts suspended in the atmosphere, including molds and pollens in the air, dusts generated in silos and barns, aeroallergens, silica from the soil, and general exposure to animal danders, grain dust, feed additives, and mite dust. While agricultural dusts generally have a large fraction (approximately 30% to 40%) of particles in the respirable range (8,9), these dusts differ tremendously in terms of their individual constituents. Dusts generated in the production of animals are obviously very different than dusts generated in the production and marketing of grain products. In fact, within the animal confinement setting, workers may be exposed to grain dust, gases (ammonia, hydrogen sulfide, and carbon monoxide) generated from the manure pit, microorganisms contaminating the manure, aerosolized fecal material, and animal proteins (10–13). In all cases, these organic dusts are characterized by a complex mixture of vegetable particles and fragments, microorganisms and their toxic products, insects and insect fragments, feed additives including fish meal and antibiotics, avian and rodent proteins, pesticides, and adsorbed gases (8,14). While the vegetable dust and exposures resulting from contamination with microorganisms appear to be the primary respiratory pathogen, specific methods involved in the cultivation and storage of these products influence the type and degree of exposure. For example, irritant gases such as ammonia and oxides of nitrogen are generated in storage silos and may contribute to the respiratory symptoms experienced by these workers (15). Thus, the agricultural aerosol is complex and contains a variable mix of agents that may contribute to the development of lung disease.

This chapter discusses the clinical and occupational features of some of the most common forms of lung disease associated with exposure to agricultural dusts—asthma, chronic airway disease, and interstitial lung disease.

## AGRICULTURAL ASTHMA

Asthma may either be caused or exacerbated by a specific exposure to agents in the agricultural environment. In both cases, agricultural asthma is characterized by

J. N. Kline and D. A. Schwartz: Divisions of Pulmonary and Critical Care and Occupational Medicine, Department of Internal Medicine, University of Iowa College of Medicine, Iowa City, Iowa 52242.

variable and intermittent airflow obstruction initiated by specific exposures in the agricultural environment. The objective signs of airflow obstruction are often associated with symptoms of chest tightness, wheezing, coughing, and dyspnea. Since immediate and delayed (up to 12 hours) airway responses may occur following these exposures, the specific agent causing the onset of airflow obstruction may not always be obvious.

## Exposures

### *Plant-Derived Material*

The largest and perhaps the most clinically relevant category of agents known to cause asthma in the agricultural setting are the plant-derived materials (Table 1). Grain dust (16), cotton dust (17), and dusts generated from teas (18), tobacco (19), mushroom (20), chicory (21), and vegetable gums (22) all represent a complex mixture of vegetable particles and fragments, microorganisms and their products, insects and insect fragments, feed additives including fish meal and antibiotics, avian and rodent proteins, and pesticides. The specific agents most likely to cause or exacerbate asthma from these plant products are the high molecular proteins that can act as allergens. However, other agents in these dusts, such as tannins, mycotoxins, endotoxin, pollens, and insect parts, may also contribute to the development of asthma in these individuals.

### *Animal-Derived Material*

Animal-derived proteins can cause asthma in agricultural workers. This form of asthma is much more common in atopic individuals who are capable of developing an immunoglobulin E (IgE) response to specific aerosolized animal proteins. Animal handlers, especially in sale barns and confinement units, may be intermittently exposed to high concentrations of animal-derived proteins, and are at particularly high risk of developing asthma (23,24). Arthropod-derived material from grain mites (25), honeybees (26), barn mites (27), and other arthropoda have been clearly shown to cause or exacerbate asthma in exposed populations. Since these are IgE-mediated responses, a period of sensitization is needed and onset of wheezing is usually immediate, often accompanied by rhinitis and other allergic symptoms.

### *Irritants*

Low concentrations of irritants may result in airflow obstruction in workers with underlying asthma but do not usually cause asthma. Thus, chemicals common to the agricultural environment, including solvents, ammonia vapors, welding fumes, pesticides, herbicides, and fertilizers, may contribute to the exacerbation of airflow obstruction in individuals with preexisting asthma. An extreme form of irritant-induced asthma may occur following inhalation of high concentrations of fumes or vapors in the agricultural setting. In particular, noxious vapors, such as ammonia, may acutely cause extensive airway injury and result in recurrent episodes of airflow obstruction. Characteristically, irritant-induced asthma occurs only after an overwhelming exposure to irritating gases. The worker should be able to report a specific event where he/she was exposed to a high concentration of fumes that resulted in an acute respiratory illness. These exposures can acutely cause alveolar injury and result in pneumonia or adult respiratory distress syndrome. Subsequent to the acute illness, the worker may develop recurrent episodes of airflow obstruction that are caused by a variety of irritants.

### *Pharmacologic Agents*

Two agents that are thought to cause asthma through pharmacologic mechanisms are organophosphate insecticides (28) and vegetable dusts containing histamine (29). Organophosphates inhibit acetylcholinesterase and result in overstimulation of cholinergic receptors. This is thought to induce bronchospasm by increasing the concentration of guanosine 3′,5′-cyclic monophosphate (cGMP). Although many factors may account for the development of asthma in individuals exposed to cotton dust, cotton dust and other vegetable dusts contain histamine, which may promote an allergic-like inflammatory process in the airway. The inflammatory response to inhaled histamine may, in part, be responsible for the development of asthma following inhalation of vegetable dusts containing histamine.

## Occurrence

The prevalence of asthma caused by exposure to agricultural dusts and fumes is not known. Clearly, the preva-

**TABLE 1.** *Categories of exposure and selected agents known to cause agricultural asthma*

| Category | Occupations | Causative agents |
|---|---|---|
| Organic dusts | Grain and cotton industries, farmers, and lumber industry | Endotoxin, tannins, plant proteins and pollens, mycotoxins, and insect parts |
| Animal-derived material | Farmers and animal handlers | Antigenic proteins |
| Irritants | Farmers and pesticide manufacturers | Pesticides, herbicides, and fertilizers |
| Fumes | Farmers | Ammonia, oxides of nitrogen, and welding fumes |

lence of agricultural asthma depends on the exposure and the setting. However, occupational asthma is estimated to account for between 5% and 15% of the patients who are diagnosed with asthma (30,31). Among farmers, 15% were found to have symptoms consistent with either asthma or allergic rhinitis (27). Interestingly, the prevalence of asthma among grain workers is reported to be similar to a comparative population of unexposed workers (32). This apparent disparity may be explained by the factors that select workers into and out of the grain industry. Despite these inconsistencies, a recent review (33) indicates that most studies in grain workers have shown approximately a twofold excess risk of wheezing among grain workers when compared to unexposed workers. The prevalence of chronic wheezing apart from a cold (37%) (34) and in association with asthma exacerbations (11%) (35) appears to be higher in hog-confinement workers who are exposed to both organic dusts and irritating fumes. Although data are sparse regarding the prevalence of agricultural asthma, absolutely no data are available concerning the incidence of asthma among agricultural workers and their family members who are often exposed to similar bioaerosols. Importantly, the prevalence of asthma among agricultural workers is dose related and appears to be influenced by host factors including preexisting asthma, airway hyperreactivity, and atopy. In addition to these factors, differences in specific products or processing may account for seasonal and geographic differences in the prevalence of asthma among agricultural workers.

### Pathogenesis

The pathogenesis of asthma induced or exacerbated by exposures in the agricultural setting is highly variable and entirely dependent on the specific nature and intensity of the exposure. Airway narrowing caused by inflammation, edema, or hyperreactivity results in acute and reversible decreases in airflow (Fig. 1). Allergic and nonallergic mechanisms of inflammation directly injure the airway epithelia. Recurrent episodes of inflammation may result in chronic remodeling of the conducting airways and could be responsible for the development of progressive airflow obstruction.

Classical allergic mechanisms of airway inflammation involving mast cells, IgE, histamine, eosinophils, and lymphocytes may be responsible for the development of asthma following exposure to animal-derived proteins. In patients with an IgE-mediated response, the symptoms and signs of asthma occur in close temporal proximity to the exposure. Patients can usually identify the specific agent responsible for their symptom, and these individuals have an atopic history. IgE-antigen interactions result in mast cell degranulation with the release of histamine. Importantly, histamine can stimulate bronchial obstruction by enhancing vascular permeability, increasing smooth muscle contraction and mucus secretion, and upregulating the production of prostaglandins (36).

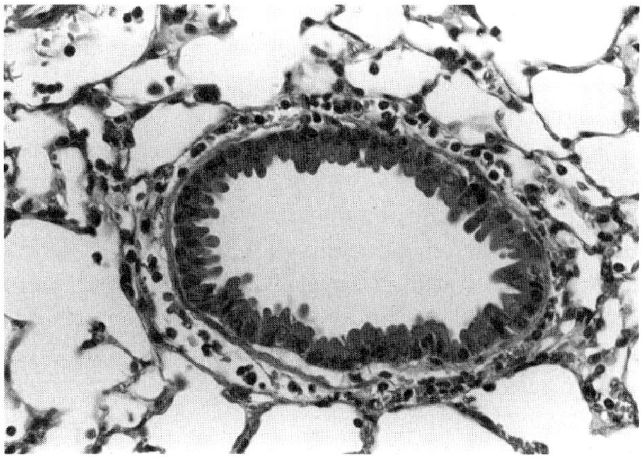

**FIG. 1.** Histologic section of mouse lung following inhalation of corn dust extract. The neutrophilic inflammatory response is localized to the conducting airway (original magnification ×1,000).

Noxious gases and irritants may directly injure the airway epithelia, resulting in edema, inflammation, and cell death. In fact, the airway epithelia may prove to be an important mediator of the inflammatory response by producing and releasing chemotactic factors such as interleukin-8 (37). Sloughing of the airway epithelia and thickening of the subepithelial region is common in asthma and has been reported in asthma associated with agricultural exposures (38). Thus, the airway epithelia may actually contribute to the edema and inflammation following inhalation of particularly irritating stimuli.

Direct pharmacologic effects of agents such as organophosphates and vegetable dusts containing histamine may cause asthma by modulating endogenous pathways associated with bronchial tone or airway inflammation. For instance, cotton dust containing sufficient concentrations of histamine, may have effects similar to endogenously produced histamine and may substantially influence airway inflammation. Similarly, organophosphate insecticides block acetylcholinesterase and can cause airflow obstruction by increasing bronchial tone and decreasing the caliber of the airways.

### Clinical Features

The diagnosis of agricultural asthma is dependent on the demonstration of reversible airflow obstruction that occurs in conjunction with inhalation of specific agents that have been reported to cause or exacerbate asthma. Therefore, the physician should initially focus on the diagnosis of asthma and secondarily determine if there is an occupational etiology. Typical symptoms of asthma include recurrent episodes of a nonproductive cough, chest tightness, wheezing, and dyspnea. These respiratory symptoms may occur immediately after specific exposures or may develop several hours after the toxic exposure. Often these symptoms worsen during the workweek and improve on weekends and vacations.

The diagnosis of asthma is based on the demonstration of reversible airflow obstruction. Standard spirometry, reversible airflow obstruction after bronchodilators, and inducible airflow obstruction with nonspecific airway challenges are considered acceptable physiologic assessments of reversible airflow obstruction. Demonstration of a forced expiratory volume in 1 second ($FEV_1$) to forced vital capacity (FVC) ratio of less than 75% is considered diagnostic of airflow obstruction. A decrease in the $FEV_1$/FVC ratio is usually associated with a low $FEV_1$ (less than 80% predicted or in the bottom tail of the 90% confidence interval) or a low forced expiratory flow after 25% to 75% of vital capacity has been expelled ($FEF_{25-75}$) (less than 60% predicted). Variability in airflow obstruction is usually demonstrated by sequential spirometry but may be documented by improvement in airflow with bronchodilators (at least a 12% improvement in $FEV_1$ is considered significant) or enhanced bronchodilator responsiveness following inhalation of either histamine or methacholine. In many circumstances, spirometric measures of lung function are normal. The demonstration of nonspecific bronchial reactivity is an acceptable, objective measure of reversible airflow obstruction, which is useful in supporting the diagnosis of asthma.

The diagnosis of agricultural asthma requires the demonstration of a clear temporal relationship to specific exposures in the agricultural setting that are known to cause asthma. The history is often helpful in identifying an occupational etiology and should incorporate the following items:

- Presence of asthma-causing agents in the workplace
- New-onset asthma or worsening of previous asthma
- Exposure to an overwhelming concentration of ammonia or oxides of nitrogen
- Worsening of symptoms during times of more intense exposure
- Improvement of symptoms when away from work or seasonally

Agricultural workers usually work and live in the same environment, and some may work seven days a week. Thus, the temporal relationship between exposures and symptoms may be difficult to determine. Physiologic testing, either by spirometry, peak flow measurements, or periodic nonspecific bronchoprovocative challenges, can and should be used to critically evaluate the temporal relationship between occupational exposures and the development of airflow obstruction. For instance, demonstration of consistent decreases in $FEV_1$ of 15% when exposed to a specific agent in the agricultural setting not only helps establish the diagnosis of agricultural asthma, but may assist in identifying the offending agent. Although peak flow measures are dependent on patient cooperation and are less reliable than traditional spirometric measures of airflow, peak flow measurements are the most convenient and often the only feasible approach to investigating work-induced asthma. Specific airway challenges are a definitive method of making the diagnosis of occupational asthma, however, these inhalation challenges are not entirely accurate, and very few centers are equipped to perform these exposure-response studies in a way that minimizes risk. On-site spirometric measures of airflow is the preferable method to establish a temporal relationship between specific exposures in the agricultural setting and the development of asthma.

Several immunologic tests have been proposed to evaluate patients with suspected or proven occupational asthma; however, their clinical utility is limited. Serologic or immunologic testing can assist in determining atopic status with respect to environmental allergens. Reactions to specific allergens are limited to the relatively few that have been completely purified such as extracts of flour and grain dusts, animal products, and certain chemicals. Serum IgG or IgE antibodies may be measured by radioimmunoassay or enzyme-linked immunosorbent assay (ELISA) methods. Unfortunately, these tests lack the sensitivity and specificity required for making a definitive diagnosis, but when used in conjunction with other testing methods and a careful patient history, these tests may help document a specific etiology. In the most limited context, immunologic tests may be helpful in further documenting exposure and identifying the atopic status of the patient.

### Natural History

Among patients with occupational asthma, the majority continue to have asthma despite removal from the exposure (39). Remissions appear to be related to the duration and intensity of the disease, with earlier and less severe forms of asthma more likely to improve. Spontaneous recovery has not been reported among workers who remain exposed to the agent causing asthma (40,41). Thus, among agricultural workers, those with work-related asthma should be encouraged to modify their exposures by either changing jobs or reducing the concentration of inhaled dust and fumes. Although most agricultural workers will not change their occupation, substantial progress can be made by encouraging the use of a two-strap dust mask or, in some cases, using an airstream respirator. In fact, one study (42) indicates that symptoms substantially improve by reducing the ambient concentration of dust through the use of respirators.

The treatment of agricultural asthma is similar to other forms of asthma and depends on the severity and frequency of symptoms. Antiinflammatory medications (preferably inhaled steroids) should be the mainstay of treatment, and bronchodilators should be used as needed.

Importantly, the use of inhaled steroids should be continued for at least 6 months after the patient has been free of any respiratory symptoms. Immunologic testing should not be used to definitively diagnose agricultural asthma.

## CHRONIC AIRWAY DISEASE

Agricultural workers are at excess risk of developing chronic bronchitis and chronic obstructive lung disease. Among agricultural workers, accelerated declines in airflow are significantly related to the concentration of dust and endotoxin in the bioaerosol, and the degree of airflow obstruction across the work shift or after challenge with nonspecific inhalants. Moreover, agricultural workers have a higher mortality from chronic pulmonary diseases than workers from other industrial sectors (4,5,43).

### Occurrence

Chronic exposure to agricultural dusts can cause irreversible and progressive airway disease. Epidemiologic studies performed in North America (44–48), the United Kingdom (49), Egypt (50), and South Africa (51) all demonstrate that workers chronically exposed to agricultural dust are at increased risk of developing chronic cough, phlegm production, wheeze, and dyspnea, irrespective of smoking habits. Moreover, long-term follow-up studies have shown that grain workers (52), as well as other agricultural workers (53,54), have accelerated decline in airflow that is directly related to the concentration of dust or duration of exposure. Although short-term experimental (55) or occupational (56) exposure to grain dust results in reversible airway symptoms and airflow obstruction, long-term occupational exposure to either grain dust (57) or cotton dust (58) causes irreversible and progressive airway disease.

Epidemiologic studies have shown that the acute airway response to grain dust and other organic dusts is predictive of the chronic airway response to these agents. Several epidemiologic studies have shown that the acute work-shift–related declines in airflow are independently associated with accelerated longitudinal declines in lung function among grain handlers (52,59,60), cotton workers (54), and agricultural workers (53). Although the work-shift response to organic dust may simply identify a cohort of individuals with a high intrinsic risk of airway disease, it is equally possible that the acute physiologic and biologic responses to inhaled organic dusts place workers at higher risk of developing progressive airway disease. In a human autopsy report of three grain workers (61), the significant pathologic findings included peribronchiolar fibrosis without bronchiectasis, patchy emphysema, and interstitial fibrosis; however, the smoking histories for these individuals were not mentioned in the report. Among cotton workers (62), chronic pathologic findings attributable to cotton dust include bronchitis and bronchiolitis with mucus gland hyperplasia and goblet cell metaplasia. In aggregate, these findings indicate that agricultural workers chronically exposed to organic dust are at risk for developing chronic airway disease, involving progressive airflow obstruction, persistent airway and alveolar inflammation, and remodeling of the airway architecture.

### Pathogenesis

Animal inhalation studies demonstrate that inhalation of grain dust and other organic dusts cause acute and chronic inflammatory lesions primarily focusing on the airway and involving macrophages, neutrophils, and specific proinflammatory cytokines. Inhalation studies in mice (55,63,64) have shown that following a single exposure to grain dust, neutrophils are rapidly recruited to the lung and proinflammatory cytokines [IL-1β, tumor necrosis factor-α (TNF-α), and IL-6], and chemokines [macrophage inflammatory (MIP)-2] are produced and released for up to 48 hours (55). Swiss mice exposed to grain dust for 16 weeks demonstrated increased neutrophils in the walls and lumin of small bronchi and clusters of neutrophils and macrophages in the ascini (65). Similarly, in rats exposed to grain dust for 8 weeks, histologic changes included subepithelial neutrophils in the bronchi and bronchioli, and dilated respiratory and alveolar ducts (66). In guinea pigs, chronic exposure to cotton dust for 1 year resulted in airflow obstruction (67), anatomic changes of the small airways consisting of hyperplasia of bronchiolar epithelium and type II cells, and thickening of the alveolar ducts and alveolar septa (68,69). A recent study in hamsters showed that 6-week intratracheal dosing with either cotton dust or endotoxin can cause mild centrilobular emphysema (70). However, the pathogenic mechanisms that result in chronic inflammation, irreversible airflow obstruction, and permanent airway remodeling are unknown.

### Clinical Features

The diagnosis of chronic obstructive lung disease (COPD) is based on the physiologic assessment of airflow. Patients with COPD have a reduced $FEV_1$ and a reduced $FEV_1/FVC$ ratio. Although most of the patients with COPD may improve with bronchodilators, improvement in $FEV_1$ is usually less than 15% and the spirometric measures of airflow, by definition, do not normalize. In addition, lung volumes may reveal air trapping and the diffusing capacity may identify those patients with emphysema.

### Natural History

The key, unanswered question is whether effective control of the acute inflammatory response to inhaled agricultural dusts will prevent the development of chronic airway disease. Studies have not been conducted to address this question. However, there is increasing evidence in asthmatics that control of the acute inflammatory response substantially improves airflow and chronic airway inflammation (71–73). Prolonged treatment of newly diagnosed mild asthmatics, chronic stable asthmatics, and severe asthmatics with inhaled corticosteroids resulted in significant improvement in airflow. Our recommendations currently include reducing the concentration of inhaled dust (better hygiene and use of a two-strap respirator) and using inhaled corticosteroids in individuals with recurrent episodes of agricultural dust–induced airflow obstruction.

## INTERSTITIAL LUNG DISEASE

### Exposures

Agricultural workers are exposed to a wide variety of inorganic dusts, depending on their occupation and local geography. Although there is some evidence that asbestosis can be induced by inhalation of dust generated by agriculture in asbestos-mining regions, agricultural dust–associated pulmonary fibrosis is most closely associated with inhalation of inorganic silicate compounds. Most soils contain significant percentages of quartz and other silica dusts. These dusts are aerosolized in processes that disrupt the soil surface, such as tilling, sowing, and harvesting, particularly of root vegetables. Harvesting can also secondarily aerosolize dusts previously deposited on leaves and growing plants in harvesting and processing agricultural products such as grains and cotton. Workers who sort and clean produce following harvest may be at particular risk from secondary silica aerosolization (74). Farming activity causes significant particulate suspension (75), which may be exacerbated by factors such as erosion, flooding, and absent ground cover. The raising of livestock and other animals is also associated with significant dust exposure, caused both by the soil surface disruption and by contamination of livestock feed with inorganic dusts. In addition, silicosis may result from inhalation of biogenic silica. A number of plants are known to produce silica-containing fibers, including sugar cane and grains (76,77); ingestion of these plants is associated with the development of esophageal carcinoma, but no studies have demonstrated silicosis due to these fibers.

### Occurrence

While the relationship between many occupations and pulmonary fibrosis has been closely studied, the association between agricultural exposure and pulmonary fibrosis has been less well examined. Although most studies have focused on the contribution of silicates to pulmonary fibrosis in agricultural settings (76–78), asbestos (79) and biotoxin inhalation (80) can also lead to fibrogenesis in the agricultural setting. Current exposure limits for silica have been set using mining and industrial exposures as benchmarks; the relevance of these limits for agricultural workers has not been established.

## REFERENCES


1. Anto JM, Sunyer J, Rodriguez-Roisin R, Suarez-Cervera M, Vazquez L, and the Toxicoepidemiological Committee. Community outbreaks of asthma associated with inhalation of soybean dust. *N Engl J Med* 1989; 320-1097–1102.
2. Haber L. Disabling effect of chronic diseases and impairment. *J Chronic Dis* 1971;24:482.
3. Carlson M, Peterson G. Mortality of California agricultural workers. *J Occup Med* 1978;20:30–32.
4. Milham S. Occupational mortality in Washington state, 1950–1971, vol 1, NIOSH Research Report. HEW Publication No. (NIOSH) 76-175-A. Cincinnati, OH: HEW, 1976.
5. Peterson G. Occupational mortality in the state of California, 1959–1961. NIOSH Research Report. DHEW (NIOSH) Publication No. 80-104. Cincinnati, OH: HEW, 1980.
6. Pomrehn P, Wallace R, Burmeister L. Ischemic heart disease mortality in Iowa farmers: the influence of life-style. *JAMA* 1982;248:1073–1076.
7. Sterling TK, Weinkam JJ, Smoking patterns by occupation, industry, sex, and race. *Arch Environ Health* 1978;33:313–317.
8. Dosman JA, Cotton DJ. Grain dust and health. IV. Health surveillance programs. *Ann Intern Med* 1978;88:134–135.
9. Parnell CB, Jones AD, Rutherford RD, Goforth KJ. Physical properties of five grain dust types. *Environ Health Perspect* 1986;66:183–188.
10. Haglind P, Rylander R. Occupational exposure and lung function measurements among workers in swine confinement buildings. *J Occup Med* 1987;29:904–907.
11. Donham KJ, Scallon LJ, Popendorf W, Treuhaft MW, Roberts RC. Characterization of dusts collected from swine confinement buildings. *Am Ind Hyg Assoc J* 1986;47:404–410.
12. Donham KJ, Popendorf W, Palmgren U, Larsson L. Characterization of dusts collected from swine confinement buildings. *Am J Ind Med* 1986;10:294–297.
13. Attwood P, Brouwer R, Ruigewaard P, et al. A study of the relationship between airborne contaminants and environmental factors in Dutch swine confinement buildings. *Am Ind Hyg Assoc J* 1987;48: 745–751.
14. Goynes WR, Ingber BF, Palmgren MS. Microscopical comparison of cotton, corn, and soybean dusts. *Environ Health Perspect* 1986;66: 125–133.
15. Schwartz DA. Acute inhalational injury. *State Art Rev Occup Med* 1987;2:297–318.
16. Chan-Yeung M, MacLean L. Respiratory abnormalities among grain elevator workers. *Chest* 1979;75:461–467.
17. Kennedy SM, Christiani DC, Eisen EA, et al. Cotton dust and endotoxin exposure-response relationships in cotton textile workers. *Am Rev Respir Dis* 1987;135:194–200.
18. Blanc PD, Trainor WD, Lim DT. Herbal tea asthma. *Br J Ind Med* 1986;43:137–138.
19. Lander F, Gravesen S. Respiratory disorders among tobacco workers. *Br J Ind Med* 1980;45:500–502.
20. Symington IS, Kerr JW, McLean DA. Type I allergy in mushroom soup processors. *Clin Allergy* 1981;11:43–47.
21. Nemery B, Demedts M. Occupational asthma in a chicory grower. *Lancet* 1980;1:672–673.
22. Bohner CB, Sheldon JM, Trenis JW. Sensitivity to gum acacia, with a report of ten cases of asthma in printers. *J Allergy* 1941;12:290–294.
23. Newman-Taylor AJ, Longbottom JL, Pepys J. Respiratory allergy to urine proteins of rats and mice. *Lancet* 1977;2:847–849.
24. Mantyjarvi J, Ylonen R, Taivainen A, Virtanen T. IgG and IgE antibody responses to cow dander and urine in farmers with cow-induced asthma. *Clin Exp Allergy* 1992;22:83–90.
25. Blainey AD, Topping MD, Ollier S, Davies RJ. Allergic respiratory disease in grain workers: the role of storage mites. *J Allergy Clin Immunol* 1989;84:296–303.
26. Ostrom NK, Swanson MC, Agarwal MK, Yunginger JW. Occupational

allergy to honeybee-body dust in a honey-processing plant. *J Allergy Clin Immunol* 1986;77:736–740.
27. Cuthbert OD, Brostoff J, Wraith DG, Brighton WD. Barn allergy: asthma and rhinitis due to storage mites. *Clin Allergy* 1979;9:229–236.
28. Winer A. Bronchial asthma due to the organic phosphate insecticides. *Ann Allergy* 1961;19:397–401.
29. Butcher BT, O'Neill CE, Jones RN. The respiratory effects of cotton dust. In: Salvaggio JE, Stankus RP, eds. *Clinics in chest medicine,* vol 4.1. Philadelphia: WB Saunders 1983;63–70.
30. Karr RM, David RJ, Butcher BT, et al. Occupational asthma. *J Allergy Clin Immunol* 1978;61:54–64.
31. Blanc P. Occupational asthma in a national disability survey. *Chest* 1987;92:613–617.
32. Chan-Yeung M. Grain dust asthma, does it exist? In: Dosman JA, Cockcroft, eds. *Principles of health and safety in agriculture.* San Diego: Academic Press, 1990;169–174.
33. Chan-Yeung M, Enarson DA, Kennedy SM. The impact of grain dust on respiratory health. *Am Rev Respir Dis* 1992;145:476–487.
34. Donham KJ, Zavala DC, Merchant JA. Respiratory symptoms and lung function among workers in swine confinement buildings: a cross-sectional epidemiological study. *Arch Environ Health* 1984;39:96–100.
35. Iversen M, Dahl R, Korsgaard J, Hallas T, Jensen EJ. Respiratory symptoms in Danish farmers: an epidemiological study of risk factors. *Thorax* 1988;43:872–877.
36. White MV, Kaliner MA. Regulation by histamine. In: Crystal RG, West JB, eds. *The lung—scientific foundations.* Philadelphia: Lippincott-Raven, 1991;927–939.
37. Strieter RM. Interleukin-8. In: Kelley J, ed. *Cytokines of the lung.* New York: Marcel Dekker, 1993.
38. Schwartz DA, Landas SK, Burmeister LF, Hunninghake GW, Merchant JA. Airway injury in swine confinement workers. *Ann Intern Med* 1992;116:630–635.
39. Chan-Yeung M. Occupational asthma. *Chest* 1990;98:148s–161s.
40. Paggiaro Pl, Loi AM, Rossi O, et al. Follow up study of patients with respiratory disease due to toluene diisocyanate (TDI). *Clin Allergy* 1984;14:463–469.
41. Cote J, Kennedy SM, Chan-Yeung M. Outcome of patients with cedar asthma with continuous exposure. *Am Rev Respir Dis* 1989;139:A388.
42. Slovak AJM, Orr RG, Teasdale EL. Efficacy of the helmet respirator in occupational asthma due to laboratory animal allergy (LAA). *Am Ind Hyg Assoc J* 1985;46:411–415.
43. Speizer FE, Fay ME, Dockery DW, Ferris BG. Chronic obstructive pulmonary disease in six U.S. cities. *Am Rev Respir Dis* 1989;140: S49–S55.
44. Becklake MR, Jodoin G, Lefort L, Rose R, Mandl M, Fraser RG. A respiratory health study of grain handlers in St. Lawrence River ports. In: Dosman JA, Cotton DJ, eds. *Occupational pulmonary disease: focus on grain dust and health.* New York: Academic Press, 1980; 239–251.
45. doPico GA, Reddan W, Flaherty D, et al. Respiratory abnormalities among grain handlers. *Am Rev Respir Dis* 1977;115:915–927.
46. Dosman JA, Cotton DJ, Graham BL, Li KYR, Froh F, Barnett GD. Chronic bronchitis and decreased forced expiratory flow rates in lifetime nonsmoking grain workers. *Am Rev Respir Dis* 1980;121:11–16.
47. Cotton DJ, Graham BL, Li KYR, Froh F, Barnett GD, Dosman JA. Effects of grain dust exposure and smoking on respiratory symptoms and lung function. *J Occup Med* 1983;25:131–141.
48. Schwartz DA, Thorne PS, Yagla SJ, et al. The role of endotoxin in grain dust-induced lung disease. *Am J Respir Crit Care Med* 1995;152: 603–608.
49. Blainey AD, Topping MD, Ollier S, Davies RJ. Allergic respiratory disease in grain workers: the role of storage mites. *J Allergy Clin Immunol* 1989:296–303.
50. El Karim MAA, El Rab MOG, Omer AAA, El Haimi YAA. Respiratory and allergic disorders in workers exposed to grain and flour dusts. *Arch Environ Health* 1986;41:297–301.
51. Yach D, Myers J, Bradshaw D, Benatar SR. A respiratory epidemiologic survey of grain mill workers in Cape Town, South Africa. *Am Rev Respir Dis* 1985;131:505–510.
52. Chan-Yeung M, Schulzer M, Maclean L, et al. Follow-up study of the grain elevator workers in the Port of Vancouver. *Arch Environ Health* 1981;36:75–81.
53. Schwartz DA, Donham KJ, Olenchock SA, et al. Determinants of longitudinal changes in spirometric functions among swine confinement operators and farmers. *Am J Respir Crit Care Med* 1995;151:47–53.
54. Christiani D, Ye T-T, Wegman D, Eisen E, Dai H-L, Lu P-L. Cotton dust exposure, across-shift drop in $FEV_1$, and five-year change in lung function. *Am J Respir Crit Care Med* 1994;150:1250–1255.
55. Deetz DC, Jagielo PJ, Quinn TJ, Thorne PS, Bleuer SA, Schwartz DA. The kinetics of grain dust-induced inflammation of the lower respiratory tract. *Am J Respir Crit Care Med* 1997;155:254–259.
56. James AL, Zimmerman MJ, Ee H, Ryan G, Musk AW. Exposure to grain dust and changes in lung function. *Br J Ind Med* 1990;47: 466–472.
57. Kennedy SM, Dimich-Ward H, Desjardins A, Kassam A, Vedal S, Chan-Yeung M. Respiratory health among retired grain elevator workers. *Am J Crit Care Med* 1994;150:59–65.
58. Beck GJ, Schachter EN, Maunder LR, Schilling RSR. A prospective study of chronic lung disease in cotton textile workers. *Ann Intern Med* 1982;97:645–651.
59. James AL, Cookson WOCM, Buters G, et al. Symptoms and longitudinal changes in lung function in young seasonal grain handlers. *Br J Ind Med* 1986;43:587–591.
60. Tabona M, Chan-Yeung M, Enarson D, MacLean L, Dorken E, Schulzer M. Host factors affecting longitudinal decline in lung spirometry among grain elevator workers. *Chest* 1984;85:782–786.
61. Cohen VL, Osgood H. Disability due to inhalation of grain dust. *J Allergy* 1953;24:193–211.
62. Pratt PC, Vollmer RT, Miller JA. Epidemiology of pulmonary lesions in nontextile and cotton textile workers: a retrospective autopsy analysis. *Arch Environ Health* 1980;35:133–138.
63. Schwartz DA, Thorne PS, Jagielo PJ, White GE, Bleuer SA, Frees KL. Endotoxin responsiveness and grain dust-induced inflammation in the lower respiratory tract. *Am J Physiol* 1994;267:L609–L617.
64. Jagielo PJ, Thorne PS, Kern JA, Quinn TJ, Schwartz DA. The role of endotoxin in grain dust-induced inflammation in mice. *Am J Physiol Lung Cell Mol Physiol* 1996;270:L1052–L1059.
65. Armanious M, Cotton D, Wright J, Dosman J, Carr I. Grain dust and alveolar macrophages: an experimental study of the effects of grain dust on the mouse lung. *J Pathol* 1982;136:265–272.
66. Friborsky V, Ulrich L, Tesik L, Malik E. Morphological changes of rat lung after exposure to plant dust. *Acta Morphol Acad Sci Hung* 1972; 20:191–197.
67. Alarie Y, Ellakkani M, Wayel D, Karol M. Respiratory parameters which characterize the response of guinea pigs to inhalation of cotton dust. Tenth Cotton Dust Research Conference, 1986.
68. Ellakkani M, Cockrell B, Thorne P, Karol MH. Histopathology of guinea pigs exposed for 12 months to cotton. Tenth Cotton Dust Research Conference, 1986.
69. Coulombe PA, Filion PR, Cote MG. Histomorphometric study of the pulmonary response of guinea pigs to chronic cotton dust inhalation. *Toxicol Appl Pharmacol* 1986;85:437–449.
70. Milton DK, Godleski JJ, Feldman HA, Greaves IA. Toxicity of intratracheally instilled cotton dust, cellulose, and endotoxin. *Am Rev Respir Dis* 1990;142:184–192.
71. Laitinen LA, Heino M, Laitinen A, Kava T, Haahtela T. Damage of the airway epithelium and bronchial reactivity in patients with asthma. *Am Rev Respir Dis* 1985;131:599–606.
72. Bleecker ER. Airways reactivity and asthma: significance and treatment. *J Allergy Clin* 1985;75:21–24.
73. Cockroft DW. Airway hyperresponsiveness: therapeutic implications. *Ann Allergy* 1987;59:405–414.
74. Jorna TH, Borm PJ, Koiter KD, Slangen JJ, Henderson PT, Wouters EF. Respiratory effects and serum type III procollagen in potato sorters exposed to diatomaceous earth. *Int Arch Occup Environ Health* 1990; 66:217–222.
75. Green F, Yoshida K, Fick G, Paul J, Hugh A, Green W. Characterization of airborne mineral dusts associated with farming activities in rural Alberta, Canada. *Int Arch Occup Environ Health* 1990;62:423–430.
76. Newman RH. Fine biogenic silica fibres in sugar cane: a possible hazard. *Ann Occup Hyg* 1986;30:365–370.
77. Newman R. Association of biogenic silica with disease. *Nutr Cancer* 1986;8:217–221.
78. Sherwin RP, Barman ML, Abraham JL. Silicate pneumoconiosis of farm wokers. *Lab Invest* 1979;40:576–582.
79. Zolov C, Bourilkov T, Babadjov L. Pleural asbestosis in agricultural workers. *Environ Res* 1967;1:287–292.
80. Dvorackova I, Pichova V. Pulmonary interstitial fibrosis with evidence of aflatoxin B1 in lung tissue. *J Toxicol Environ Health* 1986;18: 153–157.

*Environmental and Occupational Medicine, Third Edition,* edited by William N. Rom.
Lippincott–Raven Publishers, Philadelphia © 1998.

CHAPTER 37

# Occupational Exposures as a Cause of Chronic Airways Disease

Margaret R. Becklake

## BURDEN ON POPULATIONS

Chronic airways disease, if associated with airflow limitation, continues to constitute a global health problem and a cause for international (1) and national (2) concern. Men are more frequently affected than women (3), the conditions are not confined to industrialized countries (1), and tobacco smoking has been identified as an important environmental risk factor (1–6). In Canada, for instance, chronic airways disease accounts for proportionately more morbidity, as reflected in consultations with health professionals, than coronary heart disease, which affects five times as many individuals but has a higher fatality rate (5). In the United States in 1986, though chronic obstructive pulmonary disease (COPD) and other chronic respiratory conditions (International Classification of Diseases 490–496) accounted for fewer than 4% of approximately 2 million deaths, they were listed first on the discharge summaries of more than 900,000 hospitalizations, and in 1985 accounted for 16.4% of all office visits to physicians by men aged 55 to 84 and 12.5% of visits by women of the same ages (2). Age-specific mortality attributable to COPD in white men aged 45 to 75 years appears to have stabilized since 1968, but it is increasing in white women and in nonwhites of both sexes (2). The patterns in other industrialized countries are not dissimilar (5,7). Up to 28% of adult asthma cases and up to 14% of COPD cases are estimated to be attributable to occupational exposures (8), and in their 1996 research agenda, the National Institute for Occupational Safety and Health (NIOSH) listed asthma and COPD among eight work-related conditions for which concentrated research efforts have the potential to improve the well-being of large numbers of workers and their families (9).

M. R. Becklake: Department of Medicine and the Joint Departments of Epidemiology and Biostatistics and of Occupational Health, McGill University, Montréal, Québec H3A 1A3, Canada.

## RISK FACTORS

The conditions included under the general rubric of chronic airway disease or COPD are multifactorial in etiology (1–4). Nevertheless, in the 1984 Surgeon General's report (3) in addition to smoking, $\alpha_1$-antitrypsin deficiency was the only other factor accepted as being causally related to COPD, while the list of putative causes included environmental factors such as occupational exposures, low socioeconomic status, and community air pollution, as well as host factors such as atopic status, airway hyperresponsiveness, and past respiratory health. Even in the 1985 Surgeon General's report on cancer and chronic lung disease in the workplace (4), which implicated a number of workplace exposures in the genesis of simple bronchitis, a causal role in disability (and by implication airflow limitation) from chronic airways disease was considered likely for only a few workplace exposures, among which were coal, silica, and cotton dust. Nor, over the ensuing decade, has it been easy to establish the contribution of occupational exposures to the genesis of airway disease. Even now, their role is underestimated (10–14), and underrecognized in the practice of clinical and occupational medicine (15,16). For instance, a recent American Thoracic Society (ATS) statement on standards for the diagnosis and care of patients with COPD recognizes that occupational factors give rise to increased prevalence of chronic airflow obstruction (apparently on the basis of one reference to in vitro studies of $O_3$), but concludes that "smoking effects greatly exceed occupational effects" (16). Reasons include (a) the prevalence of the smoking habit in general populations (2,3,8) and, until recently, of the pneumoconioses in many dusty industries (8–10); and (b) the focus on workplace studies, the study power of which is often limited by the size of the work force. In addition, many workplace studies have been cross-sectional in design; although cross-sectional studies are the most practical for chronic disease, the onset of which is difficult to define, they are seldom able to take account of health selection, either into the workplace (the "healthy" worker effect), which has turned out to be surprisingly strong for airway disease (8,11–14,17), or out of the workplace, the survivor effect (4,11), due to workers who quit for reasons of ill health being lost to view.

Since the previous edition of this book, the publication of the findings from several cohort (longitudinal) studies in exposed work forces, and several community-based studies, which are less compromised by health selection, has greatly strengthened the evidence that occupational exposures are implicated in the genesis of chronic obstructive airway disease, to the point that two recent reviewers judge it to be causal at least for certain exposures (13,14). These include inorganic dusts and certain organic dusts such as grain and cotton as well as certain mixed exposures (13,14). This chapter reviews this evidence and assesses its implications for public health and clinical practice. Causality and attributability of chronic conditions of multifactorial etiology, though susceptible to quantitative assessment in populations, are much less easy to assess in individual subjects (18).

## TERMINOLOGY AND DIAGNOSTIC CRITERIA

### Clinical Conditions Characterized by Airways Dysfunction

Several clinical conditions that are defined by different criteria are usually included under the rubric of COPD (19–25), all characterized by airway dysfunction (Table 1). For instance, asthma is usually defined in clinical terms, and, because of its reversibility, persons who have asthma may at the time of any one examination be without any objective evidence of the condition except the medical history. Nor is bronchial hyperresponsiveness to nonspecific challenge such as methacholine necessarily present between attacks (22), although it is a feature included in some definitions of asthma (20). Chronic bronchitis is defined in terms of reported symptoms consistent with chronic mucus hypersecretion (19,20). By contrast, emphysema, always defined in the past by anatomic pathology (19,20), can now also be defined by computed tomography (CT) (23). In life, airflow limitation of varying degree and reversibility is, or may be, a feature of all these conditions, and since the main symptom of airflow limitation is shortness of breath, a nonspecific symptom for which there are many underlying causes, objective measurements in the form of lung function tests are used to establish its presence in most clinical circumstances. As in many other clinical syndromes there is considerable overlap, but despite concerns over its ambiguity or imprecision, COPD or a similar designation (1,16,20) continues to be widely used by clinicians (1,16,20), probably because it enables them to express their uncertainty about the exact cause and mechanisms, the degree of reversibility of airflow limitation and/or airway hyperreactivity in a given case, and to indicate their recognition of a diagnostic continuum in keeping with what has come to be known as the Dutch hypothesis of the natural history of chronic nonspecific lung disease (24), discussed in more detail below.

Bronchitis (25) and asthma (26) have both been recognized for some time as being potentially work related. However, for various reasons, there is much greater reluctance on the part of clinicians to accept the potential work relatedness of COPD. This chapter focuses on evidence that COPD, and in particular that its cardinal feature, airflow limitation, may also be work related

**TABLE 1.** *Terms and criteria used to describe and/or diagnose airways disease*

| Term | Criteria | Definition |
|---|---|---|
| Asthma | Clinical features | Acute, episodic airflow limitation reversible spontaneously or on treatment[a] |
| Chronic bronchitis | Symptoms | Chronic or recurrent bronchial hypersecretion, e.g., almost daily sputum for 3 months of the year for at least 3 years[b] |
| Emphysema | Pathologic features, chest imaging | Abnormal enlargement of airspaces distal to the terminal bronchiole with destructive changes in the alveolar walls |
| Chronic obstructive pulmonary disease | Airflow obstruction with or without other clinical features | Main feature is chronic airflow limitation, generally progressive, largely irreversible, occurring primarily in peripheral airways |

Based on definitions proposed by the 1959 Ciba Guest Symposium (19), the American Thoracic Society (16), and other sources (14,20–24).

[a]Some definitions included the feature of airway hyperresponsiveness (16).

[b]Assessed by clinical history or respiratory symptoms questionnaire.

(11–14). Other manifestations of airways dysfunction such as bronchitis and asthma are also considered, insofar as they are, or may be, part of the natural history of COPD (8,19,24).

### Diagnostic Criteria

The criteria used to establish the presence of any medical condition necessarily vary in stringency according to the purpose for which a diagnosis is required. Much more stringent criteria are required, for instance, for medicolegal purposes than for epidemiologic studies of working men and women at risk for occupational airway disease in which the focus is on its early manifestations, risk factors, and other determinants. Thus, diagnostic nuances, which often are achieved in a clinical context by taking into account all sources of information (clinical, laboratory, environmental), are seldom possible in the context of population-based studies, which usually use disease markers rather than all the criteria that might be required to attract the same diagnosis in the clinical context. Failure on the part of clinicians to recognize the usefulness, strength, and indeed the validity, of using less than complete clinical criteria to define study outcomes for epidemiologic purposes (27) may be one of the reasons why they have been slow to accept epidemiologic information implicating environmental (including occupational) exposures other than tobacco smoking in the genesis of chronic airflow limitation, and in particular the causal role of some of these exposures.

### Relationship to Occupational Exposure

In relation to the several categories of occupational disease syndromes identified by the World Health Organization (WHO), chronic airways disease is not in the category of diseases that are only occupational in origin, such as silicosis and the other pneumoconioses (28). Chronic airways disease could, however, be considered under one or more of several other categories: diseases in which occupation is (a) one of the causal factors, (b) a contributing factor in a complex situation, or (c) an aggravating, accelerating, or exacerbating factor of a preexisting condition. In the case of conditions like chronic airways disease for which there is a background rate in the general population, the criteria required to establish causality include evidence of association, not attributable to bias, confounding, or chance, evidence of exposure response relationships (i.e., that the more heavily exposed are at greater risk) as well as biologic plausibility and coherence with experimental data. An appropriate and useful framework within which to assess biologic plausibility is the Dutch hypothesis of the natural history of chronic airway disease (24).

## EVIDENCE IMPLICATING OCCUPATIONAL EXPOSURES IN THE GENESIS OF CHRONIC AIRWAYS DISEASE

The evidence that implicates occupational exposure in the genesis of chronic airway disease is mostly epidemiologic, and its strength can be attributed to several features. First is its variety: sources include morbidity data collected in health surveys, mortality statistics, pathologic studies, and case series. Second is its consistency: by far the bulk of the material reviewed shows positive associations between airflow limitation and occupational exposure, despite inevitable imprecision in assessing exposure, which, however detailed, can be only an imperfect characterization of the profile of exposure over a working life. Finally, the evidence is widely based in terms of time, place, and person. Much was gathered in surveys, based either in work forces or in their communities (8–14). Work force–based surveys, the traditional approach to the study of the work-relatedness of disease, have furnished the bulk of the evidence that has recently been subjected to careful review by several authors (8,13,14). However, owing to health selection and survivor effects referred to above, such studies may underestimate work-relatedness. Community-based studies are less likely to be compromised for these reasons, but they inevitably lack precision in the assessment of exposure, which is usually self-reported. Self-reported exposures do, however, usually recognize accurately broad categories of exposure (e.g., dusts, fumes, chemicals), as well as, in some studies, the number of agents to which exposure has occurred. This allows the complex nature of exposures in most modern workplaces to be recognized (13), both conceptually and in analysis. Also, such categories, perhaps because they are broad, may also be more pertinent to the genesis of airways disease than the more usual agent-specific categories; airways are, after all, subject to the effects of the total pollutant load of the air breathed, not to the separate effects of its individual components. For these and other reasons community-based studies are now gaining acceptance as a useful way to assess the long-term effects of occupational exposures on respiratory health status (29).

Evidence from community-based studies of the role of occupational exposure in the genesis of chronic airways disease is reviewed here in some detail because it is less accessible to, and less acceptable among, practitioners in occupational and respiratory medicine than is evidence from work force–based studies; it is also surprisingly strong. Finally, and perhaps most important, the results of community-based studies have challenged the concept of nuisance dusts, a concept that has also recently been rejected by the Chemical Substances Committee of the American Conference of Governmental and Industrial Hygienists (ACGIH) (30), which, in a

**TABLE 2.** *Relationship between occupational exposure and respiratory conditions in selected community-based studies*

| City, country, year, author, (reference) | Number of subjects (age) | Current smokers (%) | Exposure at work (%)[a] | Conditions[b,c] Bronchitis E vs NE | Wheezing E vs NE | Comments 1) Other factors taken into account 2) Exposures implicated |
|---|---|---|---|---|---|---|
| Tucson, AZ,<br>Lebowitz,<br>1977 (31) | 1,195 M<br>(≥18 yr) | ~56 | 57 | 2.21 | 1.31 | 1) Age, smoking<br>2) Test statistics refer to silica exposure; also implicated were solvents and other exposures[d] |
| Six cities, USA,<br>Korn et al.,<br>1987 (32) | 8,515<br>M & W<br>(≥25 yr) | ~36 | ~30 | 1.42 | 1.54 | 1) Age, smoking, gender, city<br>2) Test statistics refer to dusts; also implicated were gases or fumes |
| Seven cities | 8,602 M | ~56 | 34 | 1.53 | 1.63 | 1) Age, smoking, education, socioeconomic class, air pollution |
| France,<br>Krzyzanowski<br>and Kauffmann,<br>1988 (33) | (25–59 yr)<br>7,772 W<br>(25–59 yr) | ~22 | 23 | 2.13 | 1.70 | 2) Exposure to dust, gases or chemicals in most recent occupation vs none |
| Zutphen,<br>Netherlands<br>Heederik,<br>1990 (34) | 804 M<br>(40–59 yr) | ~46 | 54 | 3.13 | 2.41[e] | 1) Age, smoking and socioeconomic status<br>2) Exposure to dust, fumes, or gases (according to exposure matrix) vs none[f] |
| Cracow, Poland,<br>Krzyzanowski and | 1,132 M<br>(19–60 yr) | ~45 | 31 | 2.10 | 2.40 | 1) Age, smoking, education |
| Jedrychowski,<br>1990 (39) | 1,598 W<br>(19–60 yr) | ~17 | 19 | 2.10 | 2.40 | 2) Dusts in men; dust for bronchitis and chemicals for wheezing in women |
| Bergen, Norway,<br>Bakke et al.,<br>1991 (40) | 2,220 M<br>(17–70 yr) | 44 | 46 | 1.60 | 2.00 | 1) Age, smoking, area of residence<br>2) Exposure to dusts or gases |
| | 2,249 W<br>(15–70 yr) | 37 | 12 | 1.70 | 2.20 | |
| Po valley, Italy,<br>Viegi et al.,<br>1991 (44) | 1,027 M<br>(18+ yr) | 60 | 45 | 1.69 | 2.39 | 1) Age, smoking, pack years<br>2) Rockwool, solvents |
| | (18+ yr) | 608 W | 38 | 16 | — | 2.94 1) Age, smoking, pack years<br>2) Acids, insecticides, sawdust, solvents |
| Beijing, China,<br>Xu et al.,<br>1992 (45) | 3,506<br>M & W<br>(40–69 yr) | 64 | 32 | 1.32 | 1.62 | 1) Age, gender, area of residence, smoking, coal heating, education<br>2) Dust in bronchitis, gases/fumes in wheezing |

E, exposed; NE, nonexposed.

Note that all the test statistics cited were significant in the analyses carried out by the authors.

[a]Reported exposures were to dust and/or gases and in some studies chemicals, and in one study blue collar vs white collar jobs (34).

[b]Definitions of bronchitis used: persistent cough and phlegm both morning and other times of the day or night (31); sputum production for 3 or more months of the year (32,40); phlegm almost every day for 3 consecutive months every year (33,44); cough for 3 months or more during a year (40); cough occurring most days for as much as 3 months of the year for 2 years (39,44). Definitions of wheezing used: wheezing most days (31); wheeze on most days or nights (32); attacks of shortness of breath with wheeze, or "Have you ever had asthma? (33); wheeze apart from colds? (39); wheezing ever?" (40).

[c]Test statistics used to compare symptom rates in exposed versus nonexposed were prevalence ratios (31); odds ratios (32,40,44,45); and relative risk of cumulative incidence (39).

[d]Other exposures implicated in wheezing were asbestos, fiberglass, sawdust, smoke, and auto exhaust.

[e]Refers to chronic nonspecific lung disease defined clinically by the examining physician.

[f]Specific exposures implicated in bronchitis were organic and mineral dusts, adhesives and paint; and in chronic nonspecific lung disease organic dusts, solvents, paint, heat, and working outside.

1996 document, expressed the view that exposure to any dusts, if sufficiently heavy, is potentially harmful to human health, a widely held and clinically plausible view. This is further discussed below.

## Community-Based Studies

Evidence from community-based studies supporting a causal role for occupational exposures in the genesis of chronic airways disease is summarized in Tables 2 and 3. The evidence summarized in Table 2 refers to respiratory symptoms and in Table 3 to indices of chronic airflow limitation (31–45). Of the studies reviewed in these tables, two were carried out in the United States (31,32), five in Europe (33–44), and one in China (45); two were confined to men (31,34), and all but one (34) covered the full adult age range. Five studies reported only cross-sectional findings, while longitudinal findings were reported in three, those carried out in the Netherlands (34–36), in Cracow, Poland (37–39), and in Bergen, Norway (40–43).

**TABLE 3.** *Relationship between occupational exposure and ventilatory lung function: results in selected community-based studies*

| City, country, author, year (reference) | Number of subjects[a] | Ventilatory function[b]: Spirometric value | Ventilatory function[b]: Value in NE | Ventilatory function[b]: E vs NE[c] | Comments: 1) Other factors taken into account 2) Exposures implicated |
|---|---|---|---|---|---|
| Tucson, AZ, Lebowitz, 1977 (31) | 1,195 (men at work) | COPD index prevalence (%) | 6.5 | 1.40[d] (any) | 1) Smoking, age, height<br>2) Any vs none; also implicated were some dusts (silica, fiberglass, sawdust) and gases (freon, auto exhaust, smoke), solvents, and construction work |
| Cracow, Poland, Krzyzanowski et al., 1986 (37) | 731 (M)<br>1,038 (W) | Decrease in $FEV_1$ ML/year | -55<br>-38 | -6[d]<br>-1 (W) | 1) Smoking, age, height, $FEV_1$ level<br>2) Effect of exposure to dust shown: also implicated were chemicals in men, variable temperatures in women |
| Six cities, USA, Korn et al., 1987 (32) | 8,515 (M & W) | COPD index prevalence (%) | 14<br>15<br>16 | 1.68[d] (dust)<br>1.19 (fume)<br>1.57[d] (both) | 1) Smoking, age, gender, city<br>2) Exposure to dust only, or both dust and fumes vs none |
| Seven cities, France, Krzyzanowski and Kauffmann, 1988 (33) | 8,692 (M)<br>7,772 (W) | $FEV_1$/FVC (%) | 80.9<br>81.6 | -0.09[d]<br>-0.02 | 1) Smoking, age, height, pollution, socio-economic class, and education<br>2) Any exposure (dusts, gases, chemicals) vs. none in workplaces with only moderate exposure |
| Zutphen, Netherlands, Heederik et al., 1990 (34,35) | 668 (M) | $FEV_1$ L | 2.96 | -0.16[d] | 1) Smoking, age<br>2) Blue- vs white-collar workers; textile, construction, and transport workers also had lower $FEV_1$ than other blue-collar workers |
| Bergen, Norway, Bakke et al., 1991 (42) | 714 (M & W) | COPD index prevalence (%) | 7.2 | 3.60[d] | 1) Smoking, age, gender<br>2) High degree of airborne exposure in longest held job; quartz, metal gases, and aluminum also implicated |
| Po valley, Italy, Viegi et al., 1991 (44) | 763 (M)<br>518 (W) | COPD index prevalence (%) | N/A<br>N/A | 1.45[d] (M)<br>NS (W) | 1) Smoking, age<br>2) Any exposure (dusts, chemicals, fumes) vs none |
| Beijing, China, Xu et al., 1992 (45) | 1,094 (M & W) | $FEV_1$ predicted (%) | 100.7 | -2.9[d] (dust)<br>+2.9[d] (fume)<br>-0.9 (both) | 1) Smoking, age, gender, height, education, area of residence<br>2) Exposure-response relationship for gases and fumes |

[a]Subject characteristics (age, smoking, exposure) for most studies cited are listed in Table 2.

[b]Ventilatory function was assessed by different spirometric values derived from volume-time or volume flow curves, and these in turn were used to calculate the various COPD indices for the different studies: $FEV_1/FVC \leq 0.8$ or $FEV_1$ <75% predicted (31); $FEV_1/FVC \leq 0.6$ (32); $FEV_1/FVC \leq 0.7$ and $FEV_1$ <80% predicted (42); respiratory symptoms and $FEV_1$ % predicted or $FEV_1/FVC \leq 0.7$ (44).

[c]Test statistics used to compare exposed (E) with nonexposed (NE) were: prevalence ratios (31), odds ratios (32,42,44,45), or *t*-tests to compare coefficients of linear regression (37,45).

[d]Significant independent effects of exposure shown in analyses carried out by the authors.

Several points are of note: (a) None of the studies reviewed was designed to examine the effect of occupational exposures. (b) Exposure category in all was based solely on the subject's own impressions reflected in answers to a questionnaire. (c) Exposure misclassification, unless subject to systematic bias, could only have attenuated, not exaggerated, exposure-response relationships (46). (d) Systematic bias, if it occurred, is more likely to have influenced symptom reporting than lung function measurements. Given these facts, the consistency and strength of the relationships to exposure, not only of symptoms but also of lung function deficit, are remarkable. Equally remarkable is the fact that in several studies (31,34,41,43) it was possible to implicate specific exposures, characterization of which, though careful, had also only been on the basis of self-reports and in one study using industrial hygiene expertise to construct a job-exposure matrix based on job title and industry (36).

Thus, all eight community-based studies listed in Table 2 showed that bronchitis and wheezing complaints were work related, individuals exposed to dusts, chemicals, or gases being at greater risk for these complaints than persons not so exposed, after age, smoking, and other potential confounders were taken into account. Furtnermore, in the study carried out in the Netherlands, the 25-year incidence of a clinical diagnosis of COPD (or chronic nonspecific lung disease as it is called in the Netherlands) was greater for persons who had any such exposure than for those who had none (35).

In addition, all the studies listed in Table 3 (all of which were also listed in Table 2) showed that ventilatory function impairment was work related, after taking into account the important potential confounders of smoking and age. Compared to those without, those with occupational exposure exhibited lower lung function levels (33,34,45), or an increased prevalence (31,41), or risk of ventilatory function impairment (37) expressed as a COPD index (31,32,42,44), or a greater annual loss of ventilatory function over time. In a follow-up of the Bergen, Norway, study, the decline in annual forced expiratory volume in 1 second ($FEV_1$) was related directly to the number of agents to which exposure occurred at work (43). The percentage of current smokers varied considerably between the study populations, and ranged from 12% to 23% in women and from 44% to 60% in men, as did the percentage reporting occupational exposures, which ranged from 12% to 23% in women and from 32% to 57% in men (see Table 2). It is therefore not surprising that estimates of the effects of occupational exposure vis-à-vis smoking also showed a wide range, from approximately half (33) to greater than those attributable to current smoking (38), even though the prevalence and level of smoking were particularly high in the inhabitants of Cracow, Poland, the location of the latter study. A later analysis of this study implicated variable temperatures as a more important determinant of $FEV_1$ decline than dust exposure and also noted relatively immediate effects of exposure to chemicals (38).

### Work Force-Based Studies

Until quite recently, most work force-based studies focused on categories of disease that are, for all practical purposes, occupation or agent specific (28), for example the pneumoconioses. Work force-based studies have usually also benefited from industrial hygiene measurements of the pertinent airborne contaminants. As a result, exposure response relationships could be defined and these have provided the scientific basis for recommending industrial hygiene standards. In addition, in recent years spirometric tests of lung function have been widely used in respiratory health surveys and in surveillance of workers at risk for occupationally related lung disease, so a considerable amount of information pertinent to the relationship of occupational exposures to airways disease has been generated, clearly more than can be reviewed in this chapter. Only an overview and summary of these data are presented here. The interested reader is referred to certain earlier reviews (8,10), and to two published recently, both of which are careful, comprehensive, and thoughtful, focusing respectively on the agents causing chronic airflow obstruction, in particular mixed and complex exposures (13), and an update to 1996 of the evidence implicating occupational exposures in the genesis of airway disease (14).

For the most part, findings of work force-based studies have been consistent in implicating occupational exposure in the genesis of chronic airflow limitation. For instance, a 1985 review noted negative effects of occupational exposure on ventilatory function tests, independent of smoking, in 8 of 11 cross-sectional studies carried out in industries that pose risks for pneumoconiosis, mainly mining and quarrying (10). Subsequently, in 1989 a review of ten cohort studies noted significant adverse effects of exposure in seven of eight studies in which the hazard was mainly dusts or dusts and gases, and in one of two studies where exposure was mainly to gases (11). In the 1996 update referred to above, similar conclusions were reached based on 15 studies (4 cohort and 11 cross-sectional) covering over 15,000 workers exposed to inorganic fibrogenic dusts (in hard rock, coal, asbestos, and wollastonite mining) in the United Kingdom, United States, Canada, Australia, and South Africa (14). In several studies, the independent effects of the occupational exposure were comparable in magnitude to, or exceeded the independent effects of currently being a smoker (10,13,14). Also of interest is the evidence implicating mixed exposures to dust in combination with fumes in certain mining environments, in some but not all welding exposures, and in exposure to combustion products (such as in the manufacture of rubber products) and in some studies interacting with smoking (13).

The evidence implicating exposure to gases and vapors or fumes without dust is weaker or less consistent (8,14). In addition to the evidence on affected workers gathered during life, pathologic studies have confirmed the association of emphysema, assessed quantitatively at autopsy, with exposure in coal and in gold mining (11,47–49). Clinical pathologic correlation studies have also furnished evidence that small airways disease occurs in association with exposure to mineral dusts, and to mixed dust and fumes, not dissimilar to that attributable to smoking (21,50). Finally, mortality studies carried out in several of these industries have also shown an increased standardized mortality ratio (SMR) in relation to dust exposure from all causes and from bronchitis and emphysema (11).

## Some Specific Exposures and Occupations Implicated

This section discusses features of the airway conditions, acute and chronic, associated with selected specific exposures. Since several of these exposures also produce agent-specific diseases, dealt with in other chapters of this book, the reader may find it convenient to refer to the relevant chapter(s), depending on his/her focus and interest.

### *Coal Dust*

Exposure to coal dust in mining occupations has been recognized as a cause of chronic bronchitis for some time (4,25). Exposure to coal dust has also been shown to be associated with a deficit in ventilatory function ($FEV_1$) level and with increased annual decrements in ventilatory function independent of smoking, in mining (10,47,48) as well as in other occupations (51). However, the association has only been accepted as causal relatively recently (13,14), in no small part due to the demonstration of dose-response relationships to exposure estimated quantitatively, usually as gram hours per cubic meter, in longitudinal as well as cross-sectional studies of U.S. coal miners (53,54). The effects on ventilatory function are comparable in degree, but independent of the effects of smoking, and, like those of smoking, may lead to clinically important ventilatory impairment (12–14,47). Also like the effects of smoking, not all those exposed are susceptible. The evidence implicating coal dust exposure in ventilatory function loss is also broadly based, with comparable findings being reported for U.S., U.K., and German coal miners (52). The effects also appear to be more marked in the younger and perhaps more susceptible workers (14,54). Coal mining in the United Kingdom has also been shown to be associated with an increased risk of focal emphysema, which is usually associated with the presence of pneumoconiosis (3), and of centrilobular emphysema, which occurs independently of the presence of pneumoconiosis, and is related to exposure to respirable dust, independently of smoking (3,10,47).

More recently, associations between emphysema, measured quantitatively at autopsy, and lung dust burden, also measured quantitatively at autopsy (a measure of lung dose rather than exposure), have been shown in a study of Australian coal miners (48), strengthening the evidence that coal mine dust is a cause of emphysema. Strong associations between $FEV_1$ level and emphysema score in this study indicated that the emphysema was clinically important. In addition, the SMR from all causes has been shown to relate significantly and independently to dust exposure as well as to smoking in the two large cohorts of U.S. and U.K. coal miners, a noteworthy finding considering that smoking, not dust, is a cause of mortality from heart disease and accounts for many more deaths in adult males than lung disease (11).

### *Hard Rock and Other Mining*

Hard rock mining operations invariably exploit orebearing rock with a higher silica content than that exploited in coal mines and, in consequence, must usually conform to more stringent dust control levels. Nevertheless, most studies of persons engaged in this type of mining have shown a ventilatory function deficit related to occupation. These findings, reviewed in more detail elsewhere (3,11,55), are consistent in work force studies from several continents and include cross-sectional studies in South African gold miners, one of which emphasized the work-relatedness of chronic airflow limitation independent of silicosis (56), cross-sectional studies in U.S. and Canadian hard rock miners, and longitudinal studies in iron miners in France and hard rock miners in Canada. Of particular interest was a meta-analysis of three coal mining cohorts (from the United Kingdom, the United States, and Germany) and one gold mining cohort (South Africa) involving over 16,000 men (52). This analysis led to estimates that 80/1,000 nonsmoking and 60/1,000 smoking coal miners would be expected to develop a loss of ventilatory function of 20% or more after 35 years exposed to 2 $mg/m^3$ of coal dust, an exposure not uncommon in coal mining today. In addition, the estimates of ventilatory function loss in gold mining were three times larger for one-fifth of the dust exposure in coal mining, attributed to the higher silica content, an explanation for which there is supporting experimental evidence (50).

Emphysema assessed quantitatively at autopsy has also been shown to be related to years of exposure in high-dust occupations among Witwatersrand gold miners, an effect independent of smoking and of silicosis (49). A subsequent study in the same work force showed panacinar emphysema to be dose related to a qualitative dust exposure index and centriacinar emphysema, by contrast, to be associated with silicosis (57). Mineral dust airways disease occurs in persons exposed to mineral dusts at work (3,13,50), and is characterized by morphologic abnormalities involving respiratory bronchioles in addition to the involvement of membranous bronchioles seen in association with cigarette smoking (50). If sufficiently severe or widespread, these abnormalities may cause airflow limitation, as is the case for smoking-related small airways abnormality (21).

### *Occupational Environments Contaminated by Asbestos Dust*

The powerful fibrogenic potential of asbestos dust, together with heavy airborne contamination of many workplaces during and for some time after World War II, resulted in high prevalences of radiographic abnormalities, parenchymal and pleural, and this complicated the assessment of the independent effects of exposure on airways function. The initial effects of asbestos retention in the lungs are seen at the level of the small airways, and have been well documented by experimental studies in animals, and in observational studies in humans (13,50,58–60). These include abnormalities of small airway function reflected in the single-breath nitrogen test, closing volume, upstream resistance, late expiratory showing on the forced expiratory flow volume curve, and the frequency dependence of compliance (3,13,50,60). The characteristic lesion is peribronchiolar fibrosis similar to that seen in relation to other mineral dust exposure, often with more extensive involvement of the membranous bronchioles (50,61). This may or may not be accompanied by macrophagic alveolitis, which marks the onset of the process that may eventually lead to asbestosis (58).

It has been less easy to determine whether exposure to environments contaminated by asbestos dust also affects large airway function. For instance, in cross-sectional studies obstructive and restrictive pulmonary function profiles were shown to occur, often with comparable frequency, in exposed work forces (61). In one study that took into account smoking, neither function was strongly related to exposure (62). Other cross-sectional studies of miners and of workers in a variety of industries in which asbestos is applied have shown exposure effects and exposure response relationships (13,61), while in longitudinal studies of Italian and Swedish asbestos cement workers annual loss of $FEV_1$ was found to be related to exposure, an effect independent of, but comparable to, that of smoking (63,64). Also of interest is the observation that airflow limitation appears to be associated with pleural as well as parenchymal radiographic changes (14,65). These and other findings strengthen the rather cautious conclusions of an earlier review (11) that exposure to environments contaminated by asbestos dust may affect large as well as small airway function (13,14,65). Thus it appears that asbestosis (and its functional consequences) may coexist with dust-related airway disease (and its functional consequences) in exposed populations as well as in persons to asbestos dust (61). Also of importance is some evidence to suggest that, similar to the findings in coal workers, exposure effects on airways are greater in the earlier years of exposure (and/or in younger workers)than in the later years (and/or in older workers) (13,66) (see also Chapter 24).

### *Cotton Dust*

Exposure to cotton dust may cause the immediate work-related symptoms of byssinosis, including a cross-shift decrease in $FEV_1$, as well as chronic respiratory ill effects, including chronic bronchitis and chronic airflow limitation, both of which are more common in smokers (3,15,67–70). Initially, the evidence linking chronic airflow limitation to exposure came from cross-sectional studies, and later longitudinal studies showed that the annual decline in $FEV_1$ was related to duration and in some studies to level of exposure (67). No clear association has been shown between cotton dust exposure in life and emphysema at autopsy (67). Although there is only inconsistent evidence linking acute responses to exposure (in the form of byssinosis symptoms) with the subsequent development of chronic airflow limitation (67,71), two recent longitudinal studies of cotton operatives in cotton textile mills in the United States and in Shanghai, China, have shown acute cross-shift changes in $FEV_1$ to be related to accelerated decline of $FEV_1$ over time (69,70,72). The study in U.S. mills also showed the annual decline in $FEV_1$ was related to cumulative exposure to cotton dust, even at levels of 200 $\mu g/m^3$, the current Occupational Safety and Health Administration (OSHA) permissible level (70). Byssinosis symptoms appear to be caused by a bioactive component of cotton dust, currently thought to be bacterial endotoxin. However, in the Shanghai study, no variation in symptoms or lung function level or longitudinal lung function decline was found in relation to exposure to endotoxin or to elutriated cotton dust concentrations, and research continues to clarify exposure response relationships to cotton dust and to associated endotoxins (see also Chapter 30).

### *Grain and Wood Dusts*

Acute effects of exposure to grain dust include airway hyperresponsiveness as well as cross-shift and cross-week decreases in $FEV_1$ (71,73), even though work-related respiratory symptoms are less acute and less specific than those of byssinosis. A small proportion of those exposed develop grain dust asthma (74). Exposure to grain dust may also cause chronic bronchitis, chronic wheezing symptoms, a reduction in lung function, and an accelerated annual decline in lung function (74). All these changes have been documented in an integrated series of studies carried out in grain handlers in the Port of Vancouver, British Columbia (74); findings in various other work forces confirm many of those findings (75). In addition, longitudinal studies of Vancouver workers have shown that cross-shift changes in $FEV_1$ predict the subsequent annual decline in $FEV_1$ (74) and are related to exposure level (76). These observations constitute evidence that, in this work force, immediate responses to grain exposure are associated with the development of chronic airflow limitation. In addition, accelerated annual decline of lung function has been shown in young persons who quit the industry within a few years of hire, documenting selection out of the industry on the basis of unfavorable airway responses to exposure (73). Aside from case reports, the relationship between grain exposure and emphysema at autopsy has not been formally studied (74). The prevalence and characteristics of acute and chronic reactions to wood dust exposure are similar to those of grain dust exposure (77), with chronic bronchitis and chronic airflow limitation being most frequent. In addition, airflow limitation initially associated with asthma due to exposure to certain wood dusts, for example Western red cedar, may not remit even when the subject is no longer exposed (26) (see also Chapter 35).

### *Industrial Chemicals*

More than a few of the chemical agents used in modern workplaces have been identified as causes of occupational asthma (26), the isocyanates being among the first to be identified and among the most widely used (26). As with other compounds of small molecular weight that cause asthma, atopy is not always a risk factor, even though allergic as well as pharmacologic mechanisms have been implicated (26,27). There is also evidence that airflow limitation associated with exposure to isocyanates may become chronic, and/or bronchial hyperresponsiveness may become persistent, even when exposure ceased several, if not many, years earlier. Sustained exposure even to low levels may be responsible (12).

### *Particles Not Otherwise Classified*

The American Conference of Government and Industrial Hygienists (ACGIH) is a professional body that has over the past several decades performed an invaluable service by reviewing the pertinent evidence and proposing threshold limits values (TLVs) and permissible exposure limits (PELs) for substances encountered in the workplace for which there is evidence of specific toxic effects for humans. Among the particulates so regulated are silica, asbestos, and coal dust. Particulates for which no such evidence existed had in the past frequently been referred to as nuisance dusts. In their 1996 recommendations, the Chemical Substances TLV Committee of the ACGIH introduced the term *particulates not otherwise classified* (PNOCs) to emphasize that, although these materials may not cause fibrosis or systemic effects, they are not biologically inert (30). The report goes on to say that at high concentrations, otherwise nontoxic particles may cause alveolar proteinosis; at low concentrations they may inhibit alveolar macrophages. This recognition was given substance by their proposal of a TLV of 10 $mg/m^3$ for total and 3 $mg/m^3$ for respirable PNOCs. For instance, OSHA has recently adopted this standard for grain dust, previously rated as a nuisance dust. The strong evidence from community-based studies implicating exposure to dusts in general in the genesis of COPD supports the need for a TLV for PNOCs.

## THE "HEALTHY" WORKER EFFECT

The *"healthy" worker effect* is a term originally coined to describe the lower overall death rates experienced among the employed compared to the general population, which included those who for reasons of ill health are no longer actively employed (78). Recognition of its even greater pertinence in morbidity data has been slow (8,79). Morbidity data relating to pulmonary conditions is particularly susceptible to bias due to the healthy worker effect because the outcome measurements used to assess the ill-health effects of, for example, occupational exposures that are most frequently spirometric, are also not infrequently the characteristics on which health selection into dusty or other blue-collar jobs occurs (8,79).

One of the earliest and most eloquent examples of the "healthy" worker effect is to be found in the data from a longitudinal study conducted in Paris (51) using $FEV_1$ as an indicator of COPD (Fig. 1). Not only did this study show a health selection effect on the basis of $FEV_1$ in subjects exposed occupationally to mineral dusts (the figure is based on 66 men with noticeable exposure to abrasives and silica dust, compared to 196 men with slight or no exposure). The data also illustrate how bias due to health selection resulted in an underestimate of the ill-health consequences of exposure, particularly for younger persons. Thus among persons aged 54 years or older when first studied, $FEV_1$ was, as expected, lower at the initial examination for exposed compared to nonexposed men, and the $FEV_1$ decline over the 12 years was greater. The same was true for men 40 to 45 years of age when they were first examined. By contrast, among workers in their 20s and 30s when first studied, $FEV_1$ level was higher (not lower) at the initial examination for exposed compared to nonexposed workers,

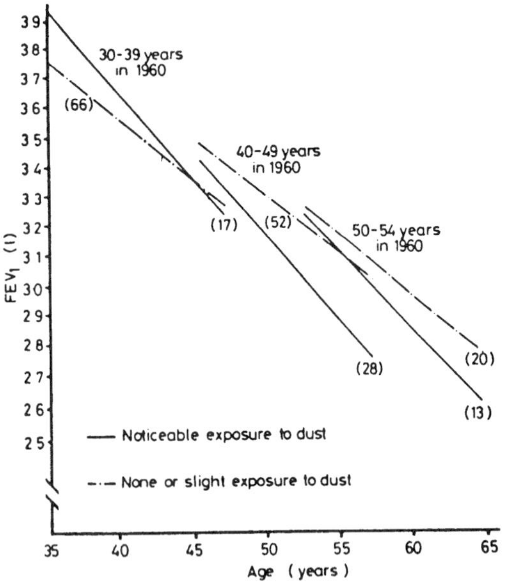


**FIG. 1.** Relationship between $FEV_1$ and age at the time of the first study (1960) and 12 years later (1972) in 66 men with noticeable exposure to silica dust and abrasives and 196 men with slight exposure or none. None of the men had changed jobs between studies. (From ref. 51, with permission.)

apparently owing to health selection into these occupations of persons with above-average ventilatory function. This is referred to as the healthy hire effect (79). In addition, their annual decline in $FEV_1$ was greater than that of nonexposed workers of their own age, and indeed of other workers, consistent with data already cited suggesting that younger individuals are more vulnerable. Clearly, also in this exposed population, cross-sectional studies of workers younger than age 45 years would have failed to identify any ill effects of exposure on $FEV_1$. In older workers, by contrast, underestimation bias was due to the survivor effect, related to age when first studied. Thus the $FEV_1$ level of those 50 to 54 years old when first seen was higher than that of men who were 40 to 45 when first seen when they reached the age of 50 years. Likewise the $FEV_1$ level of those 40 to 45 when first seen was higher than that of those 30 to 39 when first seen when they reached the age of 40 and over.

Evidence of the "healthy" worker effect, due to health selection into (healthy hire) and/or ill health selection out of (survivor) active work forces, has subsequently been shown in a number of other industries and indeed probably operates in many if not most work forces exposed to inhaled pollutants. However, it is likely to be overlooked unless specifically sought in studies of appropriate design (79), as illustrated in the following examples. For instance, in U.S. coal miners the effect of dust exposure on $FEV_1$ level was greater in new miners than in experienced miners (54,80). Also among U.S. coal miners, those in dusty jobs exhibited airway hyperresponsiveness to methacholine less frequently than men not so exposed (81). In grain workers, mention has already been made of the direct evidence of dropout among new hires whose airways are most affected by exposure (73). In other studies of U.S. autoworkers, asthma was found to be least frequent in those most heavily exposed to metal working fluids in grinding operations, suggesting a systematic job change in those whose airways are most affected by this exposure (79). The same phenomenon has been reported in workers at risk for laboratory animal asthma (82). These illustrations of "healthy" worker effect offer a convincing explanation of the consistency of the findings in community-based studies implicating exposure to dust and fumes or gases at work in the genesis of COPD, as reflected in ventilatory function deficit.

## NATURAL HISTORY OF CHRONIC AIRWAY DISEASE

Current concepts of the respective roles of environmental and host factors in the genesis of COPD derive in no small part from two cohort studies conducted during the 1960s and 1970s that led to what came to be known as the British and Dutch hypotheses of the natural history of chronic airways disease (8,19,24). Under the British hypothesis, chronic bronchitis and chronic airflow limitation were regarded as separate and independent processes, unrelated to each other, but both related to an environmental exposure—cigarette smoking. By contrast, the Dutch hypothesis argued for the use of the term *chronic nonspecific lung disease* to replace the asthma COPD complex, in order to imply a diagnostic continuum, and it also emphasized the role of an endogenous or host factor, characterized as an asthmatic tendency (8). Follow-up studies on each cohort provided evidence in favor of the other hypothesis (8), and current views incorporate both (8,83).

In their recent review (24), the Dutch retain the concept that asthma, chronic bronchitis, and emphysema are different expressions of one disease entity in which both host factors (in the form of separately and independently inherited predispositions to develop allergy and airway hyperresponsiveness) modulated by age and gender, and environmental factors (such as exposure to allergens and irritants) play a role. The final common pathway is airway inflammation leading to bronchial obstruction, and the phenotype expression is modulated by coexisting disease, which includes smoking and complications.

Evidence implicating occupational exposure can be readily incorporated into the current view of the natural history of chronic airflow limitation, in the same way that cigarette smoking has been (8): (a) As with cigarette smoking, work-related chronic bronchitis and chronic airflow limitation are independently related to occupational exposure, but not necessarily to each other. (b) Although in general both chronic bronchitis and chronic airflow limitation are related to level and duration of exposure, whether occupational or to cigarettes, not all persons with comparable exposure to either respond by developing either or both clinical conditions. (c) The target site for the initial effects of both exposures and the site of sustained inflammation appear to be the small airways of the lung. (d) An inherited tendency to develop airway hyperresponsiveness may distinguish persons whose airways will respond or have responded to either kind of exposure from persons whose airways will not or have not responded to either—the "healthy" worker effect and the "healthy" smoker effect, respectively.

Bronchial hyperresponsiveness to nonspecific stimuli continues to attract attention as a risk factor for COPD (22). To address this concept in terms of occupational airway disease, the schema illustrated in Fig. 2 was used as the basis of a literature review to see whether it supported the hypothesis that acute airway respiratory responses, immediate and/or delayed, to various occupational exposures or agents (35) are a predictor of chronic airflow limitation (horizontal arrow in Fig. 2). In general, the evidence supports the hypothesis for exposures to organic dusts such as cotton, grain, and wood dust (in particular red cedar), in occupations such as fire fighting and work in swine containment buildings, as well as to chemicals such as the isocyanates. The acute responses implicated range from cross-shift and cross-week decreases in $FEV_1$, and airway hyperresponsiveness to methacholine challenge, to full-blown asthma attacks with persistent airflow limitation after removal from exposure, as in some red cedar and isocyanate workers (26,71). There are less data to review on inorganic dusts. In one study of South African gold miners, acute airway responses in the form of wheezing, recorded at annual surveillance examinations 25 or more years prior to death predicted the presence of significant emphysema at autopsy (49). Acute respiratory responses also occur in relation to coal mining exposure in the form of cross-shift decline in $FEV_1$ and airway hyperresponsiveness to methacholine (81), but whether they predict accelerated decline in $FEV_1$ has not been investigated.

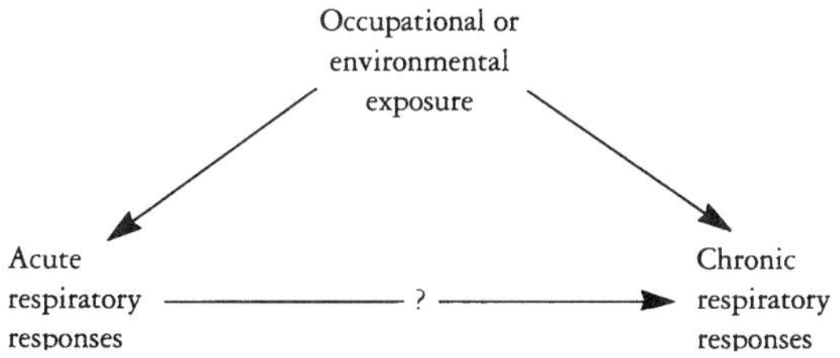


**FIG. 2.** Schematic drawing illustrates the relationships of immediate and delayed airway responses to exposure and possible interrelationships. The *arrows* describe possible associations. For acute responses (e.g., work-related symptoms and cross-shift changes in lung function), there is usually little difficulty in establishing causality. For chronic responses (e.g., symptoms, lung function level, decline over time) certain criteria must be met to establish causality. (From ref. 71.)

## IMPLICATIONS FOR OCCUPATIONAL MEDICINE

### Public Health Implications

The evidence that chronic airflow limitation, a cardinal feature of COPD, may be work related has important implications for public health. Since the publication of the previous edition of this book, the evidence has been greatly strengthened and now implicates not only exposures to organic dusts, and to inorganic dusts in industries at risk for pneumoconiosis, but also to inorganic dusts in industries not at risk for pneumoconiosis. Also implicated are exposures in industries in which exposures are to dusts that are poorly characterized, with or without chemicals, fumes, and vapors as well as extremes of temperature. This evidence comes mainly from community-based studies for which exposures are self-reported. Given the number and variety of exposures and/or agents implicated in work-related chronic airflow limitation, it would not be unreasonable to view with suspicion all exposures sufficiently intense to be reported by those exposed. In addition, the following points merit emphasis:

1. The work-relatedness of chronic airways disease has been underestimated, in no small part because of the "healthy" worker effect, which affects cross-sectional studies due to healthy hire or early dropout effects, and longitudinal studies because of the survivor effect.
2. To protect the airways against the ill-health effects of airborne pollutants requires an integrated view of all exposures that an individual experiences, whether gaseous or particulate, fume or vapor, including potential interactions.
3. The ACGIH has taken an important step in this regard by replacing the concept of nuisance dusts with a view, formulated many years ago, that exposure to any dust if sufficiently intense and for an adequate period, is capable of evoking lung tissue reactions. Chronic inflammation of the airways, whether on an allergic or an irritant basis, has the potential, if unchecked, to set in motion the pathophysiologic processes that may eventually lead to airflow limitation of a progressively irreversible nature.
4. A weakness in the evidence is the absence of quantitative exposure measurements in community-based studies. Nevertheless, these studies provide some of

the strongest evidence for the importance of considering total exposure burden.

5. With smoking rates declining, at least for men, the proportional contribution of occupational exposures to the burden of COPD is likely to increase. In addition, younger workers appear to be at great risk, and should be the target for public health intervention.
6. Important issues for future research include: (a) the development of composite exposure measurements, quantitatively based on industrial hygiene technology, which can predict loss of ventilatory function and could therefore be used to estimate a worker's risk of ill-health effects in the future; (b) an evaluation of the general usefulness of acute airway responses to exposure, in particular cross-shift changes in $FEV_1$, as a marker of susceptibility [this could be done by using surveillance databases as a sampling frame (84)]; and (c) the need to incorporate research on the work-relatedness of chronic airflow into mainstream research into COPD. The occupational model could make an important contribution to our understanding of the epidemiology, population burden, causes, and mechanisms underlying chronic airways disease.

### Clinical Implications

The evidence that chronic airflow limitation (and COPD) may be work related also has important implications for clinical practice, though these are complex, and may explain the reluctance of many health professionals to recognize the strength of the evidence.

The following points merit emphasis:

1. Whatever the difficulties inherent in applying this information in the clinical context, it is important to do so, in fairness both to those who already have work-related chronic airflow limitation (in terms of attributability) and to those who may develop it in the future (in terms of prevention).
2. Despite the strength of the epidemiologic evidence that chronic airflow limitation (or COPD) may be work related, it is not possible to quantify the risk attributable to a given exposure for a given person with COPD, since the condition is multifactorial in etiology and is also common in the general population. Until better composite exposure measurements are developed, numbers of agents involved together with estimates of level and duration should be used to estimate dose, in the same way as pack-years and other indicators are used to estimate cigarette exposure. A major difficulty is taking appropriate account of smoking, a frequent potential confounder, particularly since persons who take up smoking, like those who continue in dusty jobs, may be less susceptible to the effects of both exposures than those who do neither (17).
3. For the moment, attribution will inevitably remain a clinical judgment based on all the facts about a given case tempered by experience. Like so many clinical judgments, it is in the nature of a hypothesis, the best available to explain the facts, but susceptible to revision in the light of new evidence. Proof in the scientific sense, much less in the legal sense, cannot be advanced in individual cases. This should not prevent the physician from doing what is always done in setting prognosis, namely making a reasonable statement of probability.

## REFERENCES


1. Murray JF. Guest ed. Chronic airways disease—distribution and determinants, prevention and control. *Chest* 1989;96:3(suppl):301S.
2. Higgins MW. Chronic airways disease in the United States: trends and determinants. *Chest* 1989;196:3(suppl):328S–334S.
3. US Department of Health and Human Services. *The health consequences of smoking:* a report of the Surgeon General. DHEW Pub. No. (PHS) 84-50205. Washington, DC: U.S. Department of Health, Education, and Welfare, Public Health Service, Office of the Assistant Secretary for Health, Office on Smoking and Health, 1984.
4. US Department of Health and Human Services. *The health consequences of smoking:* cancer and chronic lung disease in the workplace. A report of the Surgeon General. DHEW Pub. No. (PHS) 85-50207. Washington, DC: U.S. Department of Health, Education, and Welfare, Public Health Service, Office of the Assistant Secretary for Health, Office on Smoking and Health, 1985.
5. Manfreda J, Mao Y, Litven W. Morbidity and mortality from chronic obstructive pulmonary disease. *Am Rev Respir Dis* 1989;140:S19–S26.
6. Bégin R, Boileau R, Peloquin S. Asbestos exposure, cigarette smoking and airflow limitation in long term Canadian chrysotile miners and millers. *Am J Ind Med* 1987;11:55–66.
7. Thom TJ. International comparisons in COPD mortality. *Am Rev Respir Dis* 1989;140:S27–S34.
8. Becklake MR. The work relatedness of airways dysfunction. In: *Proceedings of the 9th International Symposium on Epidemiology in Occupational Health.* DHHS (NIOSH) Publication No. 94-112. Cincinnati, OH: U.S. Department of Health and Human Services, Public Health Service, Centers for Disease Control and Prevention, National Institute for Occupational Safety and Health, 1994,1–28.
9. *NIOSH National Occupational Research Agenda.* DHHS (NIOSH) Publication No 96-115. Washington, DC: US Department of Health and Human Services, Public Health Service, Centers for Disease Control, National Institute for Occupational Safety and Health, 1996,10–11.
10. Becklake MR. Chronic airflow limitation: its relationship to work in dusty occupations. *Chest* 1985;88:606–617.
11. Becklake MR. Occupational exposures: evidence for a causal association with chronic obstructive pulmonary disease. *Am Rev Respir Dis* 1989;140:S85–S91.
12. Becklake MR. Occupational pollution. *Chest* 1989;96:372S–378S.
13. Kennedy SM. Agents causing chronic airflow obstruction. In: Schenker M, Balmes JR, Harber P, eds. *Occupational and environmental lung disease.* New York: Mosby-Yearbook, 1995;433–449.
14. Dimich-Ward H, Kennedy SM, Chan-Yeung M. Occupational exposures and chronic airflow limitation. *Can Respir J* 1996;3:133–140.
15. Morgan WKC. Bronchitis, airflow obstruction, and emphysema. In: Parkes WR, ed. *Occupational lung disorders,* 3rd ed. Oxford: Butterworth Heineman, 1994;238–252.
16. American Thoracic Society. Standards for the diagnosis and care of patients with chronic obstructive pulmonary disease. *Am J Respir Crit Care Med* 1995;152(suppl 5):S78–S121.
17. Becklake MR, Lalloo U. The healthy smoker: a phenomenon of health selection. *Respiration* 1990;57:137–144.
18. Chan-Yeung M, Becklake MR, Bleeker ER, et al. Impairment of men and women for work: some scientific issues in evaluation. *Am Rev Respir Dis* 1987;36:1052–1054.
19. Fletcher CM, Pride NB. Definitions of emphysema, chronic bronchitis,

asthma and airflow obstruction: 25 years on from the Ciba Symposium. *Thorax* 1984;39:81–85.
20. Snider GL. What's in a name? Names, definitions, descriptions and diagnostic criteria of diseases with emphasis on chronic obstructive pulmonary disease. *Respiration* 1995;62:297–301.
21. Hogg JC, Macklem PT, Thurlbeck WM. Site and nature of airway obstruction in chronic obstructive lung disease. *N Engl J Med* 1968; 278:1355–1360.
22. Weiss ST, Sparrow D. *Airway responsiveness and atopy in the development of chronic lung disease.* New York: Raven Press, 1989.
23. Thurlbeck WM, Müller NL. Emphysema: definition, imaging and quantification. *AJR* 1994;163:1017–1025.
24. Sluiter HJ, Koeter GH, de Monchy JGR, Postma DS, de Vries K, Orie NGM. The Dutch hypothesis (chronic non specific lung disease) revisited. *Eur Respir J* 1991;4:479–489.
25. Morgan WKC. Industrial bronchitis. *Br J Ind Med* 1978;35:285–291.
26. Bernstein IL, Chan-Yeung M, Malo JL, Bernstein DI, eds. *Asthma in the workplace.* New York: Marcel Dekker, 1993.
27. Becklake MR. Epidemiology and surveillance. In: Environmental and occupational asthma, Merchant JA (guest ed.). *Chest* 1990;98: (suppl):165S–172S.
28. World Health Organization. *Early detection of health impairment in occupational exposure to hazards.* Technical report series 571. Geneva: WHO, 1975.
29. Viegi G, Paoletti P. How to assess long term effects of occupational exposure. *Eur Respir J* 1993;6:1088–1089.
30. American Conference of Governmental and Industrial Hygienists. *Threshold limit values (TLVs) for chemical substances and physical agents. Biological exposure indices (BEIs).* Cincinnati: ACGIH, 1996.
31. Lebowitz M. Occupational exposures in relation to symptomatology and lung function in a community population. *Environ Res* 1977;44: 59–67.
32. Korn RJ, Dockery DW, Speizer FE, Ware JH, Ferris BG. Occupational exposures and chronic respiratory symptoms: a population-based study. *Am Rev Respir Dis* 1987;136:298–304.
33. Krzyzanowski M, Kauffmann F. The relation of respiratory symptoms and ventilatory function to moderate occupational exposure in a general population. *Int J Epidemiol* 1988;17:397–406.
34. Heederik D. *Epidemiologic studies of the relationship between occupational exposures and chronic nonspecific lung disease.* Report no. 1990-404. Wageningen, The Netherlands; Agricultural University, 1990.
35. Heederik D, Kromhout H, Burema J, Biersteker K, Kromhout D. Occupational exposure and 25-year incidence rate of nonspecific lung disease: the Zutphen study. *Int J Epidemiol* 1990;19:945–952.
36. Heederik D, Pouwels H, Kromhout H, Kromhout D. Chronic nonspecific lung disease and occupational exposures estimated by means of a job exposure matrix: the Zutphen study. *Int J Epidemiol* 1989;18: 382–389.
37. Krzyzanowski M, Jedrychowski W, Wysocki M. Factors associated with change in ventilatory function and the development of chronic obstructive pulmonary disease in a 13-yr follow-up of the Cracow study: risk of chronic obstructive pulmonary disease. *Am Rev Respir Dis* 1986;134:1011–1019.
38. Krzyzanowski M, Jedrychowski W, Wysocki M. Occupational exposures and changes in pulmonary function over 13 years among residents of Cracow. *Br J Ind Med* 1988; 45:747–754.
39. Krzyzanowski M, Jedrychowski W. Occupational exposure and incidence of chronic respiratory symptoms among residents of Cracow followed for 13 years. *Int Arch Occup Environ Health* 1990;62:311–317.
40. Bakke P, Eide GE, Hanooa R, Gulsvik A. Occupational dust or gas exposure and prevalence of respiratory symptoms and asthma in a general population. *Eur Respir J* 1991;4:273–278.
41. Bakke P, Gulsvik A, Eide GE, Hanoa R. Smoking habits and lifetime occupational exposure to gases or dusts, including asbestos and quartz in a Norwegian community. *Scand J Work Environ Health* 1990;16: 195–202.
42. Bakke PS, Baste V, Hanoa R, Gulsvik A. Prevalence of obstructive lung disease in a general population: relation to occupational title and exposure to some airborne agents. *Thorax* 1991;46:863–870.
43. Humerfelt S, Gulsvik A, Skjaerven R, et al. Decline in $FEV_1$ and airflow limitation related to occupational exposure in men of an urban community. *Eur Respir J* 1993;6:1096–1103.
44. Viegi G, Prediletto R, Paoletti P, Carozzi L, Di Pede F, Vellutini M, Di Pede C, Giutini C, Lebowitz MD. Respiratory effects of occupational exposure in a general population sample in North Italy. *Am Rev Respir Dis* 1991;143:510–515.
45. Xu X, Christiani D, Dockery DW, Wang L. Exposure-response relationships between occupational exposures and chronic respiratory illness: a community based study. *Am Rev Respir Dis* 1992;146:413–416.
46. Heederik D, Miller B. Weak associations in epidemiology: adjustment for exposure estimation error. *Int J Epidemiol* 1988;17:S970–S974.
47. Soutar CA. Update on lung disease in coal miners. *Br J Ind Med* 1987; 44:145–148.
48. Leigh J, Driscoll TR, Cole BD, Beck RW, Hull BP, Yang J. Quantitative relation between emphysema and lung mineral content in coal workers. *Occup Environ Med* 1994;51:400–407.
49. Becklake MR, Irwig L, Kielkowski D, Webster I, DeBeer M, Landau S. The predictors of emphysema in South African gold miners. *Am Rev Respir Dis* 1987;135:1234–1241.
50. Wright JL, Cagle P, Churg A, Colby TV, Myers J. Diseases of the small airways. *Am Rev Respir Dis* 1992; 146:240–262.
51. Kauffmann F, Drouet D, Lellouch J, Brille D. Occupational exposure and 12 year spirometric changes among Paris area workers. *Br J Ind Med* 1982;39:221–232.
52. Oxman AD, Muir DCF, Shannon HS, Stock SR, Hnzido E, Lange HJ. Occupational exposure and chronic obstructive pulmonary disease. *Am Rev Respir Dis* 1993;148:38.
53. Attfield MD, Houdous TK. Pulmonary function in US coal miners related to dust exposure estimates. *Am Rev Respir Dis* 1992;145: 605–609.
54. Seixas NS, Robbins TG, Attfield MD, Moulton LH. Longitudinal and cross-sectional analyses of coalmine dust and pulmonary function in new miners. *Br J Ind Med* 1993;50:929–937.
55. American Thoracic Society. Adverse effects of crystalline silica exposure. *Am J Respir Crit Care Med* 1997;155:761–765.
56. Cowie RL, Mabena S. Silicosis, chronic airflow limitation and chronic bronchitis in South African gold miners. *Am Rev Respir Dis* 1991;143: 80–84.
57. Hnzido E, Sluis-Cremer GK, Abramowitz JA. Emphysema type in relation to silica dust exposure in South African gold miners. *Am Rev Respir Dis* 1991;143:1241–1247.
58. Bégin R, Massé S, Sébastien P, et al. Asbestos exposure and retention as determinants of airway disease and asbestos alveolitis. *Am Rev Respir Dis* 1986;134:1170–1181.
59. Bégin R, Cantin A, Massé S. Recent advances in the pathogenesis and clinical assessment of mineral dust pneumoconioses: asbestosis, silicosis and coal pneumoconiosis. *Eur Respir J* 1989;2:988–1001.
60. Cotes JE, Steel J. *Work-related lung disorders.* Oxford: Blackwell, 1987.
61. Becklake MR. Asbestos and other fiber-related diseases of the lungs and pleura: distribution and determinants in populations. *Chest* 1991; 100:248–254.
62. Oliver LC, Eisen EA, Greene RE, Sprince NL. Asbestos-related disease in railroad workers: a cross-sectional study. *Am Rev Respir Dis* 1985;131:499–550.
63. Siracusa A, Forcina A, Volpi R, Mollichella E, Cicioni C, Fiordi T. Lung function among asbestos cement factory workers: cross-sectional and longitudinal study. *Am J Ind Med* 1984;5:315–325.
64. Ohlson CG, Bodin L, Rydman T, Hogstedt C. Ventilatory decrements in former asbestos workers: a four-year follow-up. *Br J Ind Med* 1985;42: 612–616.
65. Ernst P, Zejda J. Pleural and airway disease associated with mineral fibers. In: Liddell D, Miller K, eds. *Mineral fibers and human health.* Boca Raton, FL: CRC Press, 1991.
66. Copes R, Thomas D, Becklake MR. Temporal patterns of exposure and non malignant pulmonary abnormality in Quebec chrysotile workers. *Arch Environ Health* 1985;40:80–87.
67. Beck GJ, Schachter EN. The evidence for chronic lung disease in cotton textile workers. *Am Stat* 1983;37:404–412.
68. Zuskin E, Ivankovic D, Schachter EN, Witek TJ. A ten-year follow-up study of cotton textile workers. *Am Rev Respir Dis* 1991;143:301–305.
69. Christiani DC, Ye TT, Wegman DH, Eisen EA, Dai HL, Lu PL. Cotton dust exposure, cross-shift drop in $FEV_1$ and five-year change in lung function. *Am J Respir Crit Care Med* 1994;150:1250–1255.
70. Glindmeyer HW, Lefante JJ, Jones RN, Rando RJ, Weill H. Cotton dust and across-shift change in $FEV_1$ as predictors of annual change in $FEV_1$. *Am J Respir Crit Care Med* 1994;149:584–590.

71. Becklake MR, Bourbeau J, Menzies R, Ernst P. The relationship between acute and chronic airway responses to occupational exposures. In: Simmons DH, ed. *Current pulmonology.* Chicago: Year Book, 1988;9:25–66.
72. Becklake MR. Relationship of acute obstructive airway change to chronic (fixed) obstruction. *Thorax* 1995;50:516–521.
73. Zejda J, Pahwa P, Dosman J. Decline in spirometric variables from the start of employment: differential effect of duration of follow-up. *Br J Ind Med* 1992;46:576–580.
74. Chan-Yeung M, Enarson D, Kennedy S. The impact of grain dust on respiratory health. *Am Rev Respir Dis* 1992;145:476–487.
75. Fonn S, Becklake MR. Documentation of ill health effects of occupational exposure to grain dust through sequential, coherent, epidemiologic investigation. *Scand J Work Environ Health* 1994;20:13–21.
76. Enarson D, Vedal S, Chan-Yeung M. Rapid decline in $FEV_1$ in grain handlers. *Am Rev Respir Dis* 1985;132:814–817.
77. Enarson DA, Chan-Yeung M. Characterization of health effects of wood dust exposure. *Am J Ind Med* 1990;17:33–38.
78. Last JM, ed. *A dictionary of epidemiology,* 3rd ed. New York: Oxford University Press, 1995.
79. Eisen E. Healthy worker effect in morbidity studies. *Med Lav* 1995;2:125–138.
80. Hennenberger PK, Attfield MD. Coal mine dust exposure and spirometry in experienced miners. *Am J Respir Crit Care Med* 1996;153:1560–1566.
81. Petsonk EL, Daniloff EM, Mannino DM, Wang ML, Short SR, Wagner GR. Airway responsiveness and job selection: a study in coal miners and non mining controls. *Occup Environ Med* 1995;52:745–749.
82. Newman Taylor A. Asthma. In: McDonald JC, ed. *Epidemiology of work related diseases.* London: BMJ, 1995;117–142.
83. Burrows B, Bloom JW, Traver GA, Cline MG. The course and prognosis of different forms of chronic airways obstruction in a sample from the general population. *N Engl J Med* 1987;317:1309–1314.
84. Wagner GR. *Screening and surveillance of workers exposed to mineral dusts.* Geneva: World Health Organization, 1996.

*Environmental and Occupational Medicine, Third Edition,* edited by William N. Rom.
Lippincott–Raven Publishers, Philadelphia © 1998.

# CHAPTER 38

# Silicates and Benign Pneumoconioses

William N. Rom

A wide variety of mineral species other than asbestos, coal, and silica may give rise to pneumoconiosis, industrial bronchitis, or obstructive airway disease. Virtually any inorganic dust may elicit some pulmonary reaction; even so-called nuisance dusts may cause bronchitis or respiratory symptoms in some workers. The dusts discussed in this chapter may produce radiographic changes and pulmonary reactions, but the condition seldom progresses to impairment and respiratory disability. Workers employed in mining, milling, ore processing, tunneling, quarrying, or other occupations that expose them to minerals, clays, or rocks may be at risk. The form of the mineral (habit) is important for predicting its biologic effect (e.g., if the habit is fibrous, the mineral may be biologically active).

There are three broad categories of rocks: igneous (90% of the upper 10 miles of the earth's crust), sedimentary (5%), and metamorphic (5%). Igneous rocks are formed by the cooling and subsequent solidification of fluid rock mass called magma. The common minerals in igneous rocks are quartz, cristobalite, tridymite, fibrous mica, tuffs (including those containing zeolites), and olivine. There are two types of igneous rock, intrusive and extrusive; the former type cools beneath the earth's surface, the latter, at or near the surface. Intrusive rocks cool more slowly, and larger crystals are formed. Sedimentary rocks are formed from existing rock masses that are altered through weathering, for example by oxygen, water, and acids. Common minerals in sedimentary rock include quartz and other silica polymorphs, feldspars, micas, clays, carbonate minerals, limestone, shale, and sandstones. Metamorphic rocks form when existing rocks are altered by high pressures and temperatures and by chemical reactions. These rocks are frequently biologically active and include slate, as well as minerals such as silicates, quartz, asbestiform amphiboles and serpentine, graphite, talc, and aluminum silicates.

Mixed-dust pneumoconiosis usually refers to the fact that both irregular and rounded opacities are noted on the chest radiograph, as a result of exposure to more than one type of dust, whether at one time or at different times in the worker's life. Mixed-dust pneumoconiosis is usually noted among miners because of ore-bearing bodies that contain free silica, or are contaminated with a mineral that may have a fibrous habit. An example is "Labrador lung," which occurs in iron ore miners in Labrador who are exposed to silica and asbestos amphiboles in the gangue, or host rock. The best-known mixed pneumoconioses are anthracosilicosis in coal miners who tunnel through siliceous rock, and silicosiderosis in iron foundry workers. Other combinations are silicoaluminosis in alumina abrasive workers, argyriasiderosis in silver finishers, and various combinations of reactions to talc, silica, asbestos, and kaolin. A worker who fashioned molds made up of asbestos and talc with a silicone coating, and who filled them with beryllium-copper alloy, developed silicosis, asbestosis, talcosis, and berylliosis, all confirmed by biopsy (1).

Mixed-dust pneumoconiosis may become more common in the future as new mineral products are introduced in substitution for more toxic varieties such as asbestos. Recently, a shipyard worker with interstitial fibrosis and carcinoma of the lung was noted to have large quantities of mullite in addition to small amounts of asbestos in his lung (2). Mullite is a fibrous aluminum silicate (0.1 μm

W. N. Rom: Division of Pulmonary and Critical Care Medicine, Departments of Medicine and Environmental Medicine; and Chest Service, Bellevue Hospital Center, New York University Medical Center, New York, New York 10016.

wide × 1 to 2 μm long), a component of refractory materials used to line boilers and insulate pipes.

## ANTIMONY

Antimony dust has produced pneumoconiosis in antimony miners (usually a mixed-dust lesion such as silicoantimoniosis) and in men working with stibnite (3). Fine, nodular opacities may be seen, and ventilatory function remains normal. Other findings may include rhinitis, conjunctivitis, bronchitis, dermatitis, and nasal septal perforation. Exposure to metal fumes and oxidized metal powder over many years has been associated with chronic obstructive pulmonary disease (4,5).

## ATTAPULGITE AND SEPIOLITE

Attapulgite and sepiolite are fibrous magnesium-aluminum silicates used in many industries because of their absorbing, water-retentive, and cation-exchanging properties. Attapulgite is used as an antidiarrheal agent and as an absorbent in pet litter, and sepiolite has been used in cigarette filters. Sors and colleagues (6) reported a case of interstitial lung disease in a mining engineer exposed for 2 years to attapulgite during the course of many industrial operations. Electron microscopy of alveolar macrophages showed fibers that were shorter than asbestos fibers and had an energy dispersive x-ray diffraction pattern consistent with attapulgite. Long fibers of attapulgite have been reported to cause mesotheliomas when introduced into the rat pleural cavity, but short attapulgite fibers (100% shorter than 4 μm, mean 0.77 μm) did not (7). Attapulgite did not increase the sister-chromatid exchange rate after incubation with rat pleural mesothelial cells, whereas crocidolite asbestos increased it significantly (8). An epidemiologic mortality study of 2,302 males exposed for 1 month or longer to attapulgite clay mining and milling in the United States over the period 1940 to 1975 found a slight excess of lung cancer that was significant among those with more than 5 years of work in high exposure level jobs (9).

Because sepiolite occurs in a fibrous habit and may be mistaken for fibrous talc or chrysotile (10) it may contaminate consumer talcs and crushed stone products. Baris and associates (11) studied 63 sepiolite trimmers in Turkey; ten showed pulmonary fibrosis. The findings were difficult to attribute to sepiolite, since all ten fibrotic patients smoked and came from dusty rural regions where tremolite and zeolites were also present.

## BARITOSIS

Barium has two main ores, barite ($BaSO_4$) and witherite ($BaCO_3$). Barite is used principally as a constituent of lithopone, a white pigment used in the manufacture of paints. Barite is also used as a filler in textiles, rubber, soaps, cements, and plasters, and in oil drilling. It is highly insoluble and radiopaque, which allows it to be used safely as a radiographic contrast medium.

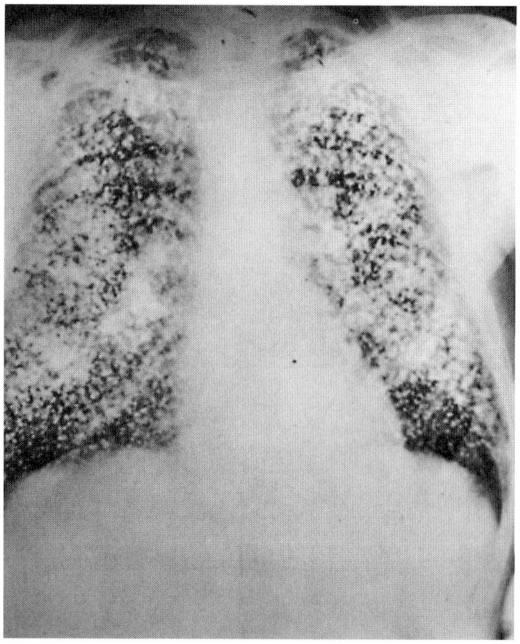

**FIG. 1.** Chest radiograph of an asymptomatic 46-year-old man who packaged lithopone for 10 years. (Courtesy of Ben Felson, M.D., University of Cincinnati.)

Baritosis is a benign pneumoconiosis resulting from the inhalation of barium sulfate or barite ore. In all cases reported there has been no respiratory impairment (12). Pendergrass and Greening (13) reported a case of a worker in a small lithopone plant in Pennsylvania (Fig. 1). The chest radiograph showed a nodular pattern evenly distributed throughout both lung fields. It resembled that of silicosis, but the individual nodules were more radiodense. Barium was identified by chemical and x-ray diffraction analyses from lung tissue. Doig (12) followed five subjects with baritosis over 10 years, observing marked radiographic clearing in all.

## BENTONITE

Bentonite is not a true mineral but is the name given to a group of clays formed by crystallization of vitreous volcanic ashes that were deposited in water. In general, bentonite is defined as rocks that contain at least 75% sodium montmorillonite or beidelite. Its free silica content varies from less than 1% to almost 25% in Wyoming bentonite (14).

Bentonite clays are mined in open pits, and most dust exposure occurs during the milling process. Bagging and loading operations produce the high dust concentrations. The water-retaining properties of bentonite make it useful as a filler in crayons, as a lubricant in oil well drilling, and in the manufacture of concrete.

In the past, control measures were minimal because it was contended that bentonite dust was harmless; however, in the 1960s, radiographic changes consistent with silicosis were noted in workers who had been employed in the bentonite industry for 6 to 10 years and who had no previous silica exposure (14). One of these cases is of historical importance. A 67-year-old man who had been employed in a bentonite milling plant in Wyoming for 10 years underwent open lung biopsy to evaluate severe dyspnea with chest radiographic findings of circumscribed nodules. Chronic granulomatous inflammation consistent with silicosis was documented, and the Industrial Hygiene Committee of the Wyoming State Medical Society began investigating silicosis in Wyoming bentonite workers. This led to legislation and the enactment of health and safety codes to control exposure to bentonite in Wyoming.

## BISMUTH

Bismuth compounds have been used as a skin salve since the 18th century, as a treatment for chronic abscesses especially because it is radio-opaque, and as a treatment for gastritis and other gastrointestinal symptoms. Bismuth subsalicylate (Pepto-Bismol, Proctor and Gamble, Cincinnati, OH) has been reported to be in greater than 60% of homes in the United States and more than 10 billion doses have been consumed. Neurotoxicity has been reported in individuals who have taken an overdose or large doses (1–20 g/day) for long periods (4 weeks to 30 years) for gastrointestinal ailments. A case report of a 39-year-old émigré who presented with radio-opaque punctate metallic opacities on the chest radiograph following intravenous injection of a bismuth compound has been reported (15). Bismuth was identified in his alveolar macrophages with energy dispersive x-ray spectroscopy.

## DENTAL LABORATORY WORKERS' PNEUMOCONIOSIS

Dental laboratory technicians work with a variety of potentially toxic materials including silica in cabinet-style sandblasters and as a constituent (diatomaceous earth) of porcelain, methylmethacrylate used in preparing dentures, and nonprecious metal alloys used in the manufacture of crowns, bridges, and dentures (16). Nonprecious metal alloys used in dental laboratories contain varying quantities of chromium, nickel, cobalt, molybdenum, and beryllium and small amounts of gallium, ruthenium, and aluminum. Kronenberger and colleagues (17) reported a clinical epidemiologic evaluation of 70 German dental laboratory technicians: half complained of respiratory symptoms, and 27 had radiographic evidence of simple pneumoconiosis. Twenty-one underwent fiberoptic bronchoscopy, and interstitial fibrosis was noted on transbronchial biopsy in 12; x-ray elemental microanalysis identified aluminum and silicon related to grinding and polishing materials and chromium, cobalt, nickel, and titanium related to the metal alloys (18). Elemental analyses of bronchoalveolar lavage (BAL) material from two patients identified chromium-cobalt-molybdenum originating from Vitallium prostheses and no silicotic nodules on lung biopsy, implicating metals as the cause of the pulmonary fibrosis (19).

An epidemiologic survey of Utah technicians found eight (4.5%) with simple pneumoconiosis related to duration (mean 28 years) of employment and intensity of exposure (more than 4 hours' grinding per day) (16). Pulmonary function test results were normal. In addition, an index case of acute berylliosis was identified: a worker who had been melting and grinding a nonprecious metal-beryllium alloy 4 to 6 hours a week for 3 months using only a nuisance dust respirator for protection and no local ventilation on the grinder. Another epidemiologic study of Danish dental laboratory technicians found six cases of pneumoconiosis (one advanced) among 31 workers and none among the controls (20). Lung function was slightly reduced in cases of pneumoconiosis, particularly diffusing capacity, and the prevalence of dyspnea was increased in the exposed workers.

Methylmethacrylate resin powder may cause interstitial pneumonitis with vacuolated alveolar macrophages observed in BAL fluid (21). The chest x-ray cleared after exposure ceased. Alginate impression powders were associated with interstitial lung disease in a dentist who used the material frequently to produce impressions of edentulous arches (22). Scanning electron microscopy revealed intraalveolar deposits of mulberry-shaped foreign inclusions. Alginate impression powders contain salts of alginic acid, a polymerized polysaccharide from seaweed whose primary constituents are diatomaceous earth and calcium sulfate.

## DIATOMACEOUS EARTH

Diatomaceous earth is composed of the remains of minute planktonic algae that were deposited millions of years ago and whose skeletons became silicified. Diatomite in nature is an amorphus nonfibrous silicate. In industry, diatomaceous earth is calcined at 800° to 1000°C to a grayish white powder called kieselguhr, which contains fibrogenic cristobalite. Natural diatomite usually contains about 1% cristobalite, but flux-calcined diatomite can contain up to 60% cristobalite (23). Whether or not the raw, unprocessed earth causes silicosis is controversial, but there is some evidence that prolonged exposure may result in mild pneumoconiosis.

Diatomite, often in combination with other substances such as asbestos, is used in insulation materials, polishes, pottery glazes, filters, and other products. Major exposure to cristobalite occurs in the processing mills, where

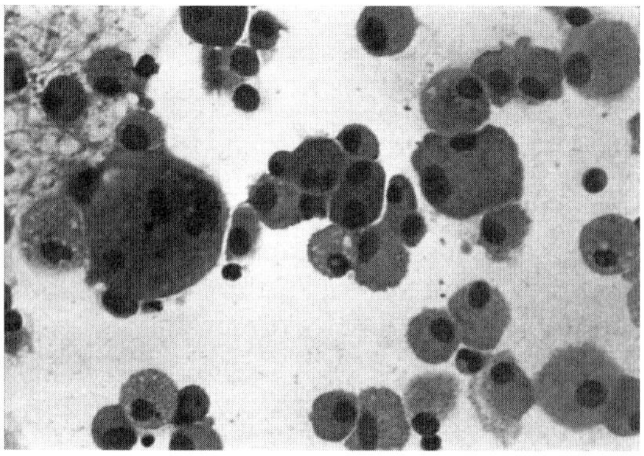

**FIG. 2.** Light microscopic evaluation of bronchoalveolar (BAL) cells from a person with diatomaceous earth pneumoconiosis (400×). There are prominent inflammatory multinucleate giant cells and vacuoles in the alveolar macrophages. *See color plate between pages 632 and 633.*

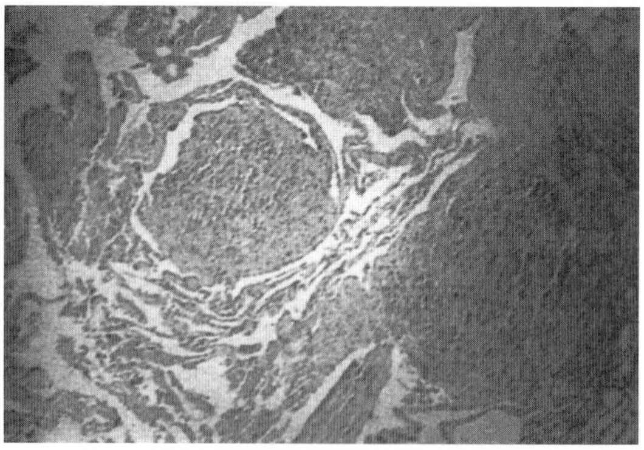

**FIG. 3.** Silicotic nodules in transbrochial lung biopsy specimen from the patient presented in Fig. 2. *See color plate between pages 632 and 633.*

48 of 100 workers who had been employed at least 5 years had pneumoconiosis detectable by chest x-ray in a study done in 1953 (23). In 21 years' follow-up, the incidence of pneumoconiosis in the employees of this plant decreased sharply, to less than 3%, owing to dust control programs and the wearing of respirators. Experimental studies of intratracheal instillation in guinea pigs of calcined diatomaceous earth have shown a neutrophil-macrophage alveolitis with injury to alveolar epithelial cells followed by mild, diffuse fibrosis beginning at 6 months, especially near areas containing the dust material (24). The case reported below illustrates that diatomaceous earth pneumoconiosis is similar to silicosis.

A cohort mortality study was reported from two plants in the diatomaceous earth mining and processing industry in California (25). There were 2,570 men who had 12 months' employment during 1942 to 1987. There were 59 deaths due to lung cancer [standardized mortality ratio (SMR) 143] and 56 deaths due to noninfectious nonmalignant respiratory disease (SMR 259). Increasing gradients of risk were detected for lung cancer and nonmalignant respiratory disease with duration of employment and an index of crystalline silica exposure. Based on a review of available but limited data on cigarette smoking in the cohort and from application of indirect methods for assessing confounding variables, it was considered unlikely that smoking habits could account for all of the

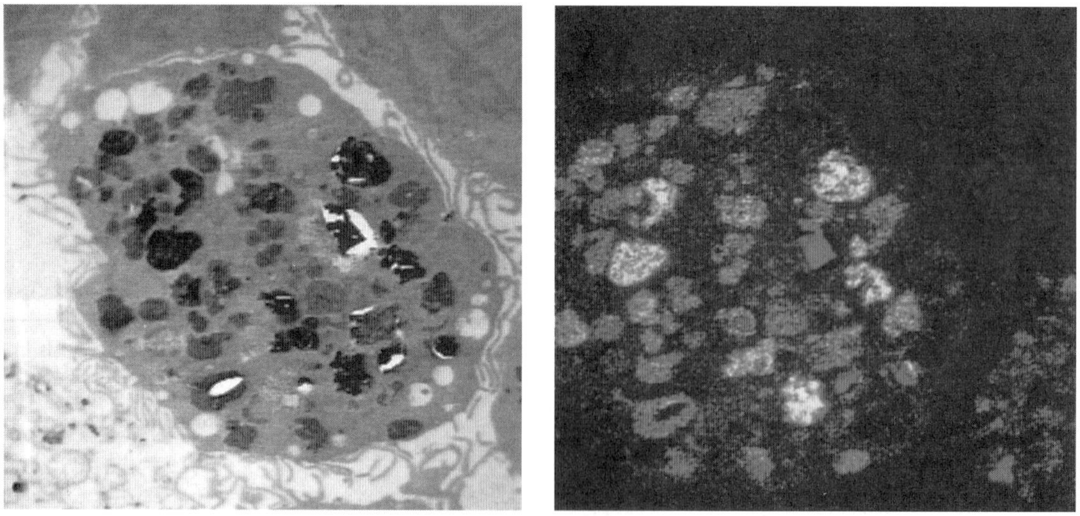

A B

**FIG. 4. A:** Transmission electron micrographs of the same alveolar macrophage from a person with diatomaceous earth pneumoconiosis (4200×). **B:** Energy dispersive x-ray analysis with an electron microprobe computer programmed to raster scan the alveolar macrophage section demonstrates numerous inorganic dust particles. (Courtesy of Richard Leapman, Ph.D., National Institutes of Health.) *See color plate between pages 632 and 633.*

association between exposure to dust and lung cancer. The intense and poorly controlled dust exposures encountered before the 1950s probably were the most etiologically significant contributions to the risks for lung cancer and nonmalignant respiratory disease.

### Case Study: Diatomaceous Earth Pneumoconiosis

A 50-year-old man was evaluated for dyspnea on exertion when walking on level ground with someone his own age. He had never been a smoker. He had worked for 32 years at a dental supply company dumping a white powder (containing diatomaceous earth) into a hopper without wearing dust protection. He worked 50 hours' overtime every 2 weeks. Previously, he had been in good health. Chest radiography revealed nodular opacities in the upper lung fields with complicated pneumoconiosis, category C. Pulmonary function tests showed mild obstructive impairment. BAL fluid revealed multinucleated giant cells (Fig. 2). A transbronchial biopsy contained nodules typical of silicosis from calcined diatomaceous earth (Fig. 3). Elemental analysis of a transmission electron micrograph of an alveolar macrophage (Fig. 4) identified many electron-dense particles in the cytoplasm that consisted of silicon surrounded by iron.

## FULLER'S EARTH

Fuller's earth is a nonfibrous silicate and an adsorbent clay that has been used primarily as a soap and for thickening ("fulling") finished woolen cloth. It consists of calcium montmorillonite (which is different from sodium montmorillonite or bentonite) and contains aluminum, iron, and manganese. Deposits probably originate from volcanic ash or the decomposition of rocks in water and are obtained by open quarrying. Drying and grinding produce "natural" fuller's earth, and chemical treatment produces "activated" fuller's earth. Natural impurities rarely include quartz. Fuller's earth behaves as an amorphous powder, with strong adsorptive, base exchange, and bonding properties. In industry it is useful in refining and lubricating and in edible oils, in oil-well drilling, and in bonding foundry-molding sands (26).

Calcium montmorillonite exposure was regarded as essentially harmless until about 1940, when pulmonary changes were noted among workers who had been employed for 16 to 39 years (26). The pneumoconiosis it produced was soft and patchy, with an appearance quite different from the massive fibrosis of silicosis. The disease is usually benign, related to very long-term exposure and high dust concentrations; it is nonprogressive (27). Sakula (26) described two cases of fuller's earth pneumoconiosis diagnosed by chest radiography; the symptoms were recurrent bronchitis and increasing dyspnea. One of the patients underwent autopsy, which showed reticular fibrosis. These studies indicate that prolonged exposure to the dust of fuller's earth is damaging to the lung but that the resulting pneumoconiosis is more benign than silicosis.

## GRAPHITE

Natural graphite is a crystalline form of carbon and may cause pneumoconiosis. Although graphite mining may involve exposure to free silica, graphite pneumoconiosis secondary to the purified product demonstrated that pure carbon may produce fibrosis. Graphite burns slowly, conducts heat, and remains strong over a wide temperature range. It is used in steel production; in foundry electrotyping and refractory industries; as the core in "lead" pencils; and in lubricants, generator brushes and electrodes, dry cell batteries, dark-pigmented paints, brake linings, and gaskets. Deposits are found in Texas, Alabama, Idaho, Montana, New York, and Pennsylvania, and annual domestic consumption exceeds 70,000 tons.

Graphite pneumoconiosis resembles coal workers' pneumoconiosis, clinically and radiographically. Gaensler et al. (28) studied four electrotypers and found impairment of gas exchange and arterial hypoxemia; radiographically there were fine reticulations and coarse nodulations that progressed in two cases to massive fibrosis. On histologic examination alveolar macrophages were filled with black pigment; postmortem examination revealed interstitial fibrosis, perifocal emphysema, massive fibrosis with graphite cysts, vascular sclerosis, and cor pulmonale. Analysis of the electrotypers' lung tissues revealed no detectable silica in two cases and 5% cristobalite in a third. Okutani and colleagues (29) surveyed 256 graphite electrode workers and found radiographic abnormalities in 43.8%. There were few pulmonary function abnormalities except in patients classified as category 3 and in one worker who had complicated pneumoconiosis. The authors stated that graphite pneumoconiosis occurred early after exposure and progressed rapidly over 4 years' observation. The carbon content was reported to be 99.6%; free silica was less than 0.1%.

## HAIRSPRAY-INDUCED LUNG DISEASE (THESAUROSIS)

Hairspray as a cause of respiratory disease has been debated since the term *thesaurosis* (storage disease) was first coined by Bergmann and co-workers (30) in 1958. At that time they reported two asymptomatic cases of suspected hairspray-induced lung disease. Both women had used hairspray twice a day for 2 to 3 years; they were found to have bilateral hilar lymphadenopathy and interstitial infiltrates on routine chest x-ray examination. The x-ray appearance returned to normal within 5 months after hairspray use stopped. One patient had a scalene node biopsy that showed a foreign body–type granulomatous reaction. Bergmann et al. noted that hairsprays in general contain three types of ingredients: (a) various aromatic oils, perfumes, or lanolin; (b) propellants, including fluorocarbons; and (c) resins, which are the actual hair fixatives. Only the resins could be implicated in the type of lung injury found in their cases.

As a group, resins used in hairspray tend to be chemically inert; consequently, once they enter the body they would be phagocytosed and might incite an inflammatory reaction. Polyvinylpyrrolidone (PVP) is one such commonly used resin. Subcutaneous injection of hairspray into guinea pigs did produce a local granulomatous reaction, and mild interstitial pneumonitis in the lungs. In 1962, Bergmann et al. (31) reported 12 more cases of suspected thesaurosis. This series of patients' hairspray exposure ranged from 1 to 7 years, and the pathologic picture included granulomas or thickening of alveolar walls. Experimental data from animals have uniformly failed to prove any parenchymal lung injury from either acute or chronic exposure to inhaled hairspray (32).

Epidemiologic studies of hairdressers also uniformly failed to show any role for hairspray in the production of parenchymal lung injury (33–38). Of these studies, only Palmer and colleagues (35) performed a randomized, well-controlled study of hairdressers. Although they were unable to identify the presence of thesaurosis, they did find more respiratory symptoms, evidence of small airways obstruction, and increased atypia on sputum cytology in examination of hairdressers compared to controls.

Epidemiologic evidence—an increased rate of lung cancer mortality among beauticians in California—suggested carcinogenic potential for hairspray compounds. A later study detected a higher rate of mortality from multiple myeloma for female beauticians but not for males (39,40). Zuskin and Bouhuys (41) found small airway obstruction after acute exposure to hairspray in normal subjects, but this finding has not been substantiated by others (42,43). Friedman and co-workers (44) documented a decrease in mucociliary transport in normal subjects exposed to hairspray acutely, a finding that may partly explain the increased respiratory tract symptoms of hairdressers. A 37-year-old hairdresser with severely reduced lung function was found to have peribronchial fibrosis on transbronchial lung biopsy (45). The alveolar macrophages contained a lipid material in vacuoles, and increased numbers of lysosomes. A case of hypersensitivity pneumonitis in a Japanese hairdresser with precipitins against *Trichosporum cutaneum* has been reported (46).

Beauticians also have an increased prevalence of skin disorders: nickel allergy from costume jewelry, and dermatitis from various chemicals in hair dyes, bleaches, and permanent waves (47).

## KAOLIN

Kaolin, also known as china clay, is a hydrated aluminum silicate formed by the decomposition of aluminous minerals. The word *clay* does not denote a particular chemical composition, and kaolin ($Al_2O_3 \cdot 2H_2O \cdot 2SiO_2$) is composed chiefly of kaolinite with minute quantities of oxides of iron and titanium and less than 1% respirable free quartz. Kaolin is obtained by open-pit mining, usually being washed from the pits by high-pressure jets of water. Most dust exposure occurs during drying, processing, bagging, and loading of the product, which is an important constituent of china and earthenware pottery, paper, paint, soap, cement, and refractory bricks.

In 1936 Middleton (48) recorded radiographic fine mottling in the lung fields of two china-clay workers but stated that there was "a general belief that no injury to health follows exposure to the dust." In 1978 Lesser and colleagues (49) studied nine kaolin workers from Missouri who had no known exposure to silica or asbestos but had fine nodules and diffuse reticular infiltrates on chest x-ray examination. The appearance of lung tissue from two of them was consistent with silicosis, showing black, brown, and refractile particles within dense fibrosis, and irregular cystic air spaces. The period of kaolin exposure varied from 2 to 48 years among the nine workers. Seven had pulmonary function tests and all had decreased forced expiratory volume in 1 second ($FEV_1$), and four of seven had decreased vital capacity as well.

Several epidemiologic studies have evaluated kaolin workers in Georgia where 70% of commercial U.S. kaolin is strip-mined (50–53). A cross-sectional survey of 459 workers in three kaolin plants representing 85% of the total eligible population had an overall prevalence of simple pneumoconiosis of 9.2%; pneumoconiosis correlated with duration of exposure longer than 15 years in job categories associated with greater dust exposure (50). The pneumoconiosis was not associated with respiratory symptoms and had minimal effect on pulmonary function, even in complicated cases. In a similar study of a single Georgia mill, eight cases of pneumoconiosis (12%) were found and two workers had restrictive lung function (51). Altekuse and colleagues (52) found both $FEV_1$ and forced vital capacity (FVC) percent predicted declined as exposure duration increased and were lower in the workers who had pneumoconiosis. In a larger study of 2,000 Georgia kaolin workers, Morgan and associates (53) found adjusted prevalence rates of 3.2% for simple pneumoconiosis and 0.63% for complicated disease. They concluded that complicated pneumoconiosis had a modest effect on ventilatory function and that reduced $FEV_1$ was seen in calcined clay workers. Evaluation of lungs of Cornish china-clay workers found nodular changes in those exposed to china stone and irregular changes with interstitial fibrosis in those exposed to china clay (kaolinite) (54). The complicated pneumoconiosis progresses more slowly than silicosis; progressive massive fibrosis (PMF), and Caplan's syndrome may also occur (55).

## MICA PNEUMOCONIOSIS

Mica, a nonfibrous silicate, is found in three different forms: muscovite, biotite, and phlogopite. Muscovite is a potassium-aluminum silicate used for stove windows and in powder form for paints and in the rubber industry, to prevent sticking. Biotite is a complex silicate of potassium, aluminum, magnesium, and iron, and is also used in the roofing and rubber industries. Phlogopite is a magnesium-aluminum silicate used principally as an electrical insulator.

Pneumoconiosis has been observed in muscovite grinders. Davies and Cotton (56) reported two cases: one after 6 years of exposure and the other after 8 years. Both had nodular opacities, and in one the nodules were as large as 1.5 cm diameter at postmortem. In addition there was diffuse interstitial fibrosis and focal emphysema, but no pleural disease. Both had progressive respiratory impairment, and mineralogic analysis revealed birefringent particles that constituted as much as 9% of the dry weight of the lung. Thin plates of material were seen with electron microscopy, and potassium, aluminum, and silicon were identified by energy dispersive x-ray analysis.

Epidemiologic surveys of mica workers have largely supported a role for mica in causing pneumoconiosis. Dreessen and colleagues (57) reported a survey of muscovite and biotite workers in North Carolina. Of 57 workers involved in the grinding of quartz-free mica, 10 had chest radiographs consistent with pneumoconiosis. Symptoms of cough and dyspnea were related to the severity of lung involvement as determined by the chest radiograph. In another chest radiographic survey of mica miners and workers, Vestal and associates (58) found 11.4% of those exposed to pure mica had pneumoconiosis. However, Smith (59) surveyed 302 workers exposed to muscovite in the manufacture of electrical insulators and found pleural calcification in five. Pleural calcification was reported also by Kleinfeld (60) in two workers involved in the sawing and sanding of muscovite mica sheets for more than 30 years.

Landas and Schwartz (61) described a 63-year-old mica-exposed worker who had interstitial fibrosis with honeycombing after 5 years of shoveling mica during the 1940s. Bronchoalveolar lavage revealed 20% neutrophils in the lavage fluid with many rectangular flake-like polarizable crystals. Energy dispersive x-ray analysis confirmed the material in an open lung biopsy to have features of mica (61).

## OIL SHALE PNEUMOCONIOSIS

Oil shale exists in large deposits in the western United States, with an estimated 600 billion barrels of recoverable oil in the Piceance and Uinta Basins along the Colorado–Utah border (62). Shale oil has been processed in surface retorts where the crushed oil shale from underground mines had been heated to around 1000°C in experimental facilities in Colorado and production retorts in Scotland. The Scottish industry lasted nearly a century, peaking in the 1920s with approximately 5,000 miners and 2,500 refinery and other workers. Seaton and colleagues (63) reported four cases of PMF in this cohort, and all had developed the disease toward the end of a prolonged lifetime's work in the mines. A mortality study of 6,359 oil shale workers employed between 1950 and 1962 and followed until 1982 found no excess deaths due to respiratory disease, bronchitis/emphysema, or lung cancer (64). A radiographic survey of 47% of this cohort found small opacities in the International Labor Organization (ILO) categories 1 and 2 that correlated with both age and dust exposure (65). Significant reductions in FVC, $FEV_1$, and diffusion capacity occurred in 61 men who had category 1/1 or greater chest x-ray changes when compared to a matched group with category 0/1 or less profusion of small radiologic opacities (66). Although an investigation for shalosis in Colorado oil shale miners found only six chest x-rays in category 1, PMF was not observed and half had other mining experience (67). The risk of pneumoconiosis probably relates to the quartz content of the host rock which ranged from 5% to 20%, and also likely to other silicates including kaolin, mica, and dolomite.

Skin cancers, including both squamous and basal cell carcinomas, have been reported by Scott (68) among early Scottish oil shale workers, and cancer of the scrotum was reported among mule spinners in the early English textile mills when refined oil shale was used to lubricate spindles (69). Shale oil, when painted on the skin of mice, has produced skin cancers in 14/30 mice with a mean latency of 145 days (70). In a morbidity survey of 325 oil shale workers employed in Colorado during the period 1948–1969, Rom and colleagues (71) reported increased keratoses in oil shale workers, but no increase in skin cancers or respiratory symptoms compared to Utah coal miner controls. Sputum and urine cytologies showed more metaplasia in oil shale workers, but allowing for age and pack-years of smoking, no association was then found. Alexander Scott (68) had reported 65 cases of epithelioma from 1900 to 1921 among approximately 5,000 Scottish shale oil workers. Rowland et al. (72) used skin painting to test raw oil shale, spent oil shale, and shale oil resulting in 0/50, 6/50, and 48/50 mice, respectively, with tumors. *In situ* techniques, in which holes are drilled into the oil shale, followed by placing explosives to turn the rock to rubble, igniting the oil shale, and, lastly, extracting the oil from the base of the deposit, may be the safest method in preventing occupational exposures. This industry awaits shortages of crude oil before it would be economic to process oil shale into liquid petroleum products.

## PORTLAND CEMENT

Portland cement (commonly known as cement) is a fine, grayish green powder that is produced by heating ground cement rock or other limestone-bearing materials into a fused clinker that is then ground into a fine powder. Cement is composed of lime ($CaO$), alumina ($M_2O$), and iron oxide ($Fe_2O_3$) in various forms: tricalcium silicate ($3CaO{\cdot}Al_2O_3$), tetracalcium alurninsate ($3CaO{\cdot}Al_2O_3$), dicalcium silicate ($2CaO{\cdot}SiO_2$), and tetracalcium aluminoferrate ($4CaO{\cdot}Al_2O_3{\cdot}Fe_2O_3$), along with trace amounts of magnesium, sodium, potassium, and sulfur compounds. It is mixed with varying proportions of sand, rock, and water to form concrete, which hardens in a curing process. It is the powdery form of cement and the wet form of the concrete that pose a health hazard. Wet concrete is quite irritating to the skin and eyes as a caustic and abrasive material; cement dust is irritating to the eyes and respiratory tract.

Studies of cement workers in Yugoslavia have shown a significant degree of obstructive airway disease (decreased $FEV_1/FVC$ ratio) compared to controls and reduced mean forced expiratory flow during the third quarter of the FVC ($FEF_{50-75}$); these findings suggest the presence of small airway disease (73,74). These cross-sectional surveys also found that the amount of reduction was proportionate to the period of cement factory employment. Saric and colleagues (75) found no spirometric abnormalities during an 8-year longitudinal study. Kalacic (73) has found an increased prevalence of respiratory symptoms (cough, phlegm, dyspnea, wheezing) in the cement workers. Most investigators have not found radiographic abnormalities suggestive of pneumoconiosis among cement workers; however, Maestrelli and associates (76) found radiographic changes of pneumoconiosis among 7.2% of 318 Italian cement workers (all exposed longer than 10 years). An epidemiologic study of Danish cement workers found no lung function changes compared to blue-collar controls (77).

In a nationwide study of 16 randomly selected cement plants in the United States, Abrons and associates (78) studied 2,736 Portland cement workers and 755 unexposed controls in a cross-sectional study. There were no differences in mean pulmonary function values or respiratory symptoms, except that 5.4% of the cement workers had dyspnea compared with 2.7% of the controls. Quartz was detected in 14.4% of 1,011 respirable dust samples. In addition to an increased adjusted odds ratio for dyspnea, cement workers also had increases for rounded and irregular small x-ray opacities and pleural abnormalities (79).

## STANNOSIS

Tin occurs in both organic and inorganic forms. The inorganic forms (except tin oxide) usually produce irritation of the eyes and skin, whereas the organic forms may cause simple eye or skin irritation, or with heavier exposures hepatotoxicity and death. In contrast, tin oxide ($SnO_2$) has been widely used in industry without adverse health effects. Stannosis occurs after inhalation of respirable particles of tin oxide; in its early stages the chest radiographic pattern is indistinguishable from that of silicosis. In later stages the nodules become densely radiopaque owing to the high atomic number of tin (Fig. 5).

Tin oxide is mined as the ore cassiterite, sometimes from underground lodes but more commonly from alluvial deposits formed by the erosion of primary deposits. Tin is mined in Malaysia, Thailand, Bolivia, Nigeria, and Zaire. Miners of tin commonly develop silicosis because of the high silica content of the surrounding rock. Stannosis develops in workers who are exposed to airborne particles of tin oxide whether they originate from dust, as in bagging operations, or from fumes of tin oxide produced in smelting (80). Robertson and Whitaker (81) examined 200 tin smelter workers and found radiographic changes in 121. None of these workers had any clinical signs or symptoms referable to the pneumoconiosis.

Pathologic studies of seven workers with stannosis were reported by Robertson and co-workers (82). All had worked in the same tin smelter in England. None died of pulmonary disease. Aggregates of macrophages contain-

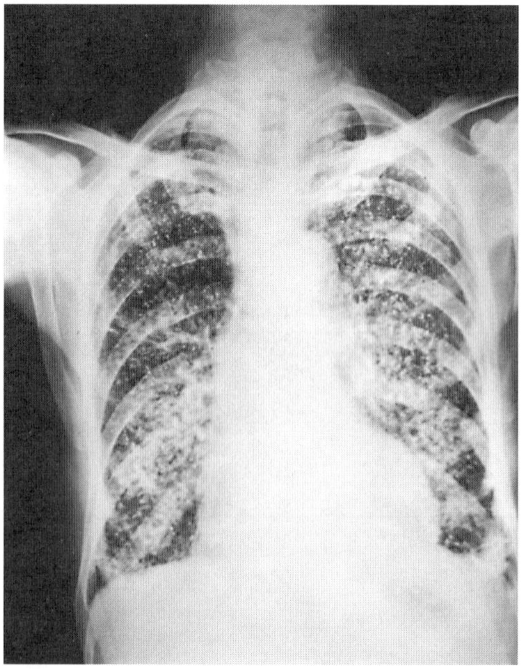

**FIG. 5.** Chest radiograph of a 72-year-old worker with stannosis who had been exposed to stannic oxide dust and fumes for 18 years working near a furnace where tin was recovered from tin scrap by a calcining process. (Courtesy of Ben Felson, M.D., University of Cincinnati.)

ing dust were seen around respiratory bronchioles, and less commonly around segmental bronchi, in the alveoli, in the interlobular septa, and in the prevascular lymphatics. The mild focal emphysema observed was felt to be clinically insignificant and was considerably less severe than that seen in coal workers' pneumoconiosis. No fibrosis was present.

## TALC PNEUMOCONIOSIS

Talc is a crystalline layer-type sheet silicate with the chemical formula $Mg_3Si_4O_{10}(OH)_2$ and is frequently contaminated with asbestos or quartz (83). About a third of all talc produced annually in the world, about 800,000 tons, comes from the United States, mostly from New York, California, Vermont, Texas, North Carolina, and Montana. Canada, France, and Italy account for most of the remaining two-thirds, but deposits are also known to exist in Scandinavia, China, India, Australia, South Africa, and Russia. Talcs from Vermont, Montana, California, France, and Italy are said to be especially pure.

Cosmetic-grade talc is usually more than 90% mineral talc, free of detectable amounts of asbestos or other minerals. In consumer products it is found in pottery, chalk, crayons, cosmetic talcum, deodorants, coating for polished rice, and as a filler in pills and tablets. Industrial-grade talc, which may contain free silica and asbestiform minerals, is used in ceramics, textiles, soaps, paper, plastics, rubber, paints, stucco, spackling and patching compounds, putties, asphalt, roofing material, electrical insulation, enamelware, and shoe polish. Talc insufflation is used to cause pleural adhesions in patients with recurrent pneumothoraces, and as a slurry is introduced into the pleural space to treat malignant or recurrent pleural effusions through pleurodesis.

Talc pneumoconiosis may present as one of four forms: talcosilicosis, talcoasbestosis, talcosis, and following intravenous injection of medications in which talc is a filler (84). This form of exposure causes perivascular inflammation and granulation, proceeding to pulmonary consolidation, nodules, and large masses. Paré and colleagues (85) described six patients that had pinpoint micronodularity on their chest radiographs that progressed to granulomatous inflammation and progressive massive fibrosis despite no further intravenous drug use. The lower lung fields developed bullae and pulmonary function was characterized by obstruction with air trapping. Funduscopic examination of 9 of 15 intravenous drug users revealed a macular concentration of glistening white dots (86).

Epidemiologic studies of Gouverneur talc miners and millers in upstate New York began in the 1940s when 32 of 221 subjects were found to have advanced fibrosis and 14 had pleural plaques (87). The prevalence of pleural thickening was almost 33% in those with at least 15 years' employment. A follow-up of 32 of these men by Kleinfeld and colleagues (88) in 1955 reported that the pneumoconiosis slowly progressed and was disabling in older workers. In an autopsy study, Kleinfeld et al. (89) documented that marked fibrosis may occur and observed asbestos-like bodies, pleural fibrosis, nodular and irregular radiographic opacities, and granulomatous inflammation in the interstitium. Lung function of 43 talc millers revealed a significant reduction in vital capacity in 17 and reduced diffusing capacity in 12 (90). A more recent cross-sectional study of 121 in New York talc miners by the National Institute for Occupational Safety and Health (NIOSH) found decreased vital capacity and flow rates compared to controls (potash miners), but only two individuals with parenchymal opacities and 12% with pleural fibrosis (91). Since the New York talc mines are contaminated with tremolite and anthophyllite, Wegman and colleagues (92) studied 116 Vermont talc miners where the ore was free of asbestos and silica. They found 12 individuals with chest radiographs ≥1/0 profusion of rounded opacities that correlated with exposure but not smoking.

Feigin (84) reviewed 18 cases of talc exposure from the archives of radiologic pathology of the U.S. Armed Forces Institute of Pathology. Pure talc was demonstrated in the tissue in four cases; radiographic abnormalities in all four consisted of small nodules and reticulations, which were diffuse in two cases and predominantly in the lower lung fields in the other two. Minimal pleural thickening was found in one, although no calcifications were present. Pathologic findings were inflammation of the alveolar walls and septa with diffuse talc deposition. Small airways inflammation was also present.

Talcosis closely resembles other pneumoconioses: symptoms consist of chronic productive cough, progressive shortness of breath, diffuse rales, clubbing of the fingers, and eventually weight loss, debility, and cor pulmonale. Chest x-ray examination discloses varying degrees of interstitial infiltration or interstitial reticulation and small nodulation in the mid-lung fields and bases with relative sparing of the apices. Some emphysema with various sized bullae may be seen. A striking feature may be the presence of opaque platelike densities above the diaphragm, and occasionally obscuring the left heart border, representing pleural thickening, often with frank calcification, resembling similar findings in asbestosis and mica pneumoconiosis (93). This diffuse bilateral pattern is characteristic of all pneumoconioses, and radiographic changes produced by talc are not distinctive. Indeed when talc is admixed with silica or asbestos, the radiographic picture may be typical of silicosis or asbestosis. Pulmonary function studies in pure talcosis are not distinctive either; findings include varying degrees of restrictive and obstructive impairment, frequently with reduced diffusion capacity. It is well known that radiographic evidence and abnormal findings on lung function studies may not be associated with symptoms. Furthermore, in the absence of x-ray changes, widespread, but focal, pulmonary lesions may occur (93). More recently it has been shown that applying newer analytic methods, including energy dispersive x-ray analysis of cells obtained by BAL can confirm exposure to talc dust, provide information on heterogeneity of the inhaled dust, and confirm the retention of dust years after exposure has ended (94,95). Three cases of talc pneumoconiosis that had BAL revealed lymphocytic alveolitis with elevated $CD4^+/CD8^+$ ratio and detected asbestos fiber concentrations of 510, 2,039, and 3,392 fibers/ml (96).

Microscopically, three groups of lesions are seen (93). Diffuse interstitial fibrosis with collagen deposition in alveolar walls and with dust-laden macrophages in the alveolar septa and free in the alveoli accompanied by distended small bronchi and bronchioles, and club-shaped asbestos bodies may be seen, particularly where asbestiform fibers have been identified in the tissue (97). A second group of lesions consists of ill-defined nodules containing birefringent particles with some fine reticulin strands but little collagen. These nodules center on medium-sized and small vessels and around small bronchi and bronchioles. They may be whorled as in silicosis, and may coalesce and cavitate. This reaction is more common where more silica is found in the tissue and may be accompanied by collagen formation and the finding of dust-laden macrophages in pulmonary lymph nodes. The third kind of reaction consists of foreign body granulomas composed of epithelioid cells and foreign body giant cells containing birefringent particles. The granulomas may be associated with nodular fibrosis or may occur isolated in the alveolar interstitium with normal alveolar septa intervening. They are also seen in fibrotic and thickened pleura, and in the pulmonary and other vessel walls after intravenous injection. Reactions to pure talc tend to be more cellular and less fibrotic than those to talc contaminated with silica or asbestosis. In fact, if the dust burden is not too great it may be cleared by these cellular reactions with the usual mechanisms of pulmonary defenses and leave little permanent change. If the dust burden is heavy, foreign body granulomas predominate (Fig. 6).

Kleinfeld and colleagues (98) raised the possibility of a cancer potential from talc in a report of 220 New York talc workers with ≥15 years' employment. Causes of death included 9 lung cancers and 1 fibrosarcoma of the pleura, which was a fourfold increase using proportional mortality rates. Later the same workers reported that men employed in the mine after dust levels had been reduced had death rates from malignant disease similar to U.S. white males (99). Stille and Tabershaw (100) found a SMR for respiratory cancer of 163 in the same locale and time frame, but made the point that the 10 lung cancers had extensive employment outside the talc industry with only 2 having >4 years' exposure (100).

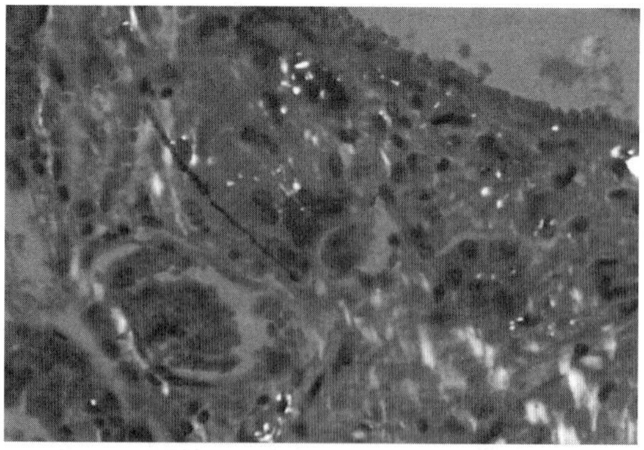

**FIG. 6.** Autopsy lung specimen of New York State talc miner showed talcosis and asbestosis in underlying lung parenchyma. High-power, partially polarized light micrograph shows strongly birefringent talc particles and asbestos body in interstitium. The asbestos body is within a multinucleated giant cell (H&E). (Courtesy of J. Abraham, M.D.) *See color plate between pages 632 and 633.*

Brown and colleagues (101) performed a third retrospective cohort study of 398 New York talc workers employed between 1947 and 1960, finding 9 deaths due to lung cancer (SMR 270). These miners had long latency before developing lung cancer, but five of the mine workers who died of lung cancer had been employed for 1 year or less. Gamble (102) updated this study with 8 more years of follow-up and performed a nested case control analysis of 22 lung cancer cases. No relationship was seen between death from lung cancer and length of talc employment.

In a recent study of 389 workers exposed to nonasbestiform talc, Wergeland and colleagues (103) did not observe an increase in deaths from lung cancer or from all respiratory diseases, even in the one mine and mill with a small percentage of silica in the dust. They cautioned, however, that further follow-up was needed to lessen the healthy worker effect on the data. In a study of 2,055 male pottery workers exposed to both talc and silica over a significant time span, Thomas and Stewart (104) observed an insignificant standardized mortality ratio of 1.37 for men exposed to high concentrations of silica without talc. However, those exposed to nonfibrous talc and also to a high level of silica had a significant standardized ratio of 2.5. The authors suggested that nonfibrous talc was associated with lung cancer, but that silica may be needed as a cofactor or promoter. Thus, the recent literature does not favor a definite association of talc exposure with carcinoma of the lung, but there may be a weak association with mesothelioma, probably related to asbestiform fiber contamination. Another mortality study of 392 Vermont talc miners and millers found 11 who died of nonmalignant respiratory tract disease (105). Of eight whose chest radiographs were located, six had a profusion of small, rounded opacities of 2/1 or greater.

Inhalation of cosmetic talc has resulted in talc pneumoconiosis documented in numerous case reports (106–108). Habitual use of excessive amounts of cosmetic talcum powder can produce significant pulmonary disease in adults (109). Respiratory distress and death from accidental inhalation of talc powder has occurred in infants and children (83).

## TITANIUM DIOXIDE

Titanium dioxide ($TiO_2$) is a white pigment that is considered nontoxic and is used in the manufacture of high-quality white paints and dyes. Its advantages over lead and zinc are its intense whiteness, durability, low cost, and high refracture index. Inhalation studies of rats have not demonstrated any pulmonary toxicity (110). An epidemiologic study of Ceylonese workers in an ilmenite (52% $TiO_2$)-extracting plant detected no pneumoconiosis or increased respiratory symptoms (111). Light and electron microscopic examinations of lung tissue and alveolar macrophages from titanium dioxide workers revealed titanium dioxide particles in phagolysosomes in the cytoplasm. Since the 1960s, silica and aluminum have been added to the manufacturing process to coat titanium dioxide particles (112). Long-term workers have been noted to show slight fibrosis associated with carbon-like collections of particles that are refringent under polarized light (113). These particles are found to contain titanium on energy dispersive x-ray microanalysis.

## TRONA DUST

Trona (sodium sesquicarbonate) is mined from a large underground deposit in Wyoming and processed to soda ash for use in the manufacture of glass, paper, and detergents and in various chemical applications. Trona dust is alkaline (pH 10.5) with potential to irritate the upper airways, mucous membranes, and skin. An epidemiologic study of 142 underground miners and 88 surface workers found no radiographic evidence of pneumoconiosis, but half the workers complained of upper respiratory tract symptoms and eye irritation, and lung function changes included significant declines in $FEV_1$ for ex-smokers related to respiratory dust (114). A shift study among 104 workers revealed a significant 90-ml drop in $FEV_1$ in nonsmokers, but this did not correlate with longitudinal changes in lung function. Half the study participants complained of skin symptoms that were irritant in nature and correlated strongly with increased time in the job (115).

## VOLCANIC ASH

The eruption of the Mount St. Helens volcano in Washington State on May 18, 1980 deposited as much as 40 mm of volcanic ash over much of Washington and parts of Idaho and Montana. Total suspended particulates exceeded national ambient air quality standards for more than a week in many communities, including Yakima. Complaints of irritation to the eyes and upper respiratory tract were common. The ash contained between 4% and 10% free silica. A 4-year longitudinal study of loggers exposed to varying levels of ash found a significant exposure-related decline in $FEV_1$ during the first year and increases in cough, phlegm, and wheeze that largely disappeared over the subsequent 3 years (116). No ash-related changes in chest radiographs were noted at the beginning or the end of the follow-up period. Volcanic ash exhibited modest cytotoxicity compared to that of silica (which was marked in tests in vitro), and the dust was readily phagocytosed by alveolar macrophages (117).

## WOLLASTONITE

Wollastonite is a fibrous monocalcium silicate used as a substitute for many silica-containing minerals in ceramics, as a substitute for asbestos in wallboard, insulation, and brake linings, in water and automobile exhaust purification, and as a dental polishing agent. Wollastonite contains less than 2% free silica, and fibrous particulates at the U.S. deposit have a median diameter of 0.22 μm and a median length of 2.5 μm. Experimental studies have shown that wollastonite fibers activate serum complement in vitro and demonstrate dose-related increases in pulmonary macrophage chemotaxis (118). Hanke and co-workers (119) studied 103 workers at a wollastonite mine and mill in the United States: three individuals had simple pneumoconiosis with rounded opacities and no pleural changes, although their mean duration of exposure was only 9.2 years. There were dust-related changes in $FEV_1$ and $FEV_1/FVC$ ratio, and the annual decline in $FEV_1$ for nonsmokers was 49 ml. In contrast, at the Finnish wollastonite mine, 46 men were surveyed and 14 had mild profusion of irregular opacities and 13 had bilateral pleural thickening (120). Those with radiographic abnormalities had a mean duration of exposure in the quarry of 22 years. The fiber sizes and medical findings were similar to those in the Finnish anthophyllite asbestos mine (120). Studies on chronic inhalation in rats reveal no carcinogenicity with only an alveolar macrophage response (121).

## REFERENCES

1. Mark GJ, Monroe CB, Kazemi H. Mixed pneumoconiosis, silicosis, asbestosis, talcosis, berylliosis. *Chest* 1979;75:726–728.
2. Golden E, Warnock M. Pulmonary fibrosis associated with the aluminum silicate, mullite. *Am Rev Respir Dis* 1983;123:129A.
3. Morgan WKC. Antimony pneumoconiosis. In: Morgan WKC, Seaton A, eds. *Occupational lung disease,* 3rd ed. Philadelphia: WB Saunders, 1995;416–417.
4. Potkonjak V, Pavlovich M. Antimoniosis: a particular form of pneumoconiosis. *Int Arch Occup Environ Health* 1983;51:199–207.
5. Gaillard MCG, Davies JCA, Kilroe-Smith TA. A case of chronic

obstructive pulmonary disease after antimony exposure. *S Afr Med J* 1988;74:426.

6. Sors H, Gaudichet A, Sebastien P, et al. Lung fibrosis after inhalation of fibrous attapulgite. *Thorax* 1979;34:69A.
7. Jaurand MC, Fleury J, Monchaux G, Nebut M, Bignon J. Pleural carcinogenic potency of mineral fibers (asbestos, attapulgite) and their cytotoxicity on cultured cells. *J Natl Cancer Inst* 1987;79:797–804.
8. Archard S, Perderiset M, Jaurand MC. Sister chromatid exchanges in rat pleural mesothelial cells treated with crocidolite, attapulgite, or benzo 3-4 pyrene. *Br J Ind Med* 1987;44:281–283.
9. Waxweiller RJ, Zumwalde RD, Ness GO, Brown DP. A retrospective cohort mortality study of males mining and milling attapulgite clay. *Am J Ind Med* 1988;13:305–315.
10. Germine M. Sepiolite asbestos from Franklin, New Jersey: a case study in medical geology. *Environ Res* 1987;42:386–399.
11. Baris YI, Sahin AA, Erkan ML. Clinical and radiological study in sepiolite workers. *Arch Environ Health* 1980;35:343–346.
12. Doig AT. Baritosis: a benign pneumoconiosis. *Thorax* 1976;31:30–39.
13. Pendergrass EP, Greening RR. Baritosis, report of a case. *Arch Ind Hyg* 1953;7:44–48.
14. Phibbs BP, Sundin RE, Mitchell RS. Silicosis in Wyoming bentonite workers. *Am Rev Respir Dis* 1971;103:1–17.
15. Addrizzo-Harris D, Churg A, Rom WN. Radio-opaque punctate opacities on the chest radiograph following following intravenous injection of a bismith compound. *Thorax* 1997;52:303–304.
16. Rom WN, Lockey JE, Lee JS, et al. Pneumoconiosis and exposure of dental laboratory technicians. *Am J Publ Health* 1984;74:1252–1257.
17. Kronenberger H, Morgenroth K, Tuengerthal S, et al. Pneumoconiosis in dental technicians: clinical, physiological, radiological, and histological findings. *Am Rev Respir Dis* 1981;123:127A.
18. Morgenroth K, Schneider M, Kronenberger H. Histologic features and x-ray microanalysis in pneumoconiosis of dental technicians. *Am Rev Respir Dis* 1981;123:127A.
19. De Vuyst P, Weyer RV, De Coster A, et al. Dental technician's pneumoconiosis. A report of two cases. *Am Rev Respir Dis* 1986;133: 316–320.
20. Sherson D, Maltbaek, Olsen O. Small opacities among dental laboratory technicians in Copenhagen. *Br J Ind Med* 1988;45:320–324.
21. Barrett TE, Pietra GG, Maycock RL, et al. Acrylic resin pneumoconiosis: report of a case in a dental student. *Am Rev Respir Dis* 1989; 139:841–843.
22. Loewen GM, Weiner D, McMahan J. Pneumoconiosis in an elderly dentist. *Chest* 1988;93:1312–1313.
23. Cooper WC, Jacobson GA. A 21-year radiographic follow-up of workers in the diatomite industry. *J Occup Med* 1977;19:563–566.
24. Maeda H, Ford J, Williams MG Jr, Dodson RF. An ultrastructural study of acute and long-term lung response to commercial diatomaceous earth. *J Comp Pathol* 1986;96:307–317.
25. Checkoway H, Heyer NJ, Demers PA, Breslow NE. Mortality among workers in the diatomaceous earth industry. *Br J Ind Med* 1993;50: 586–597.
26. Sakula A. Pneumoconiosis due to fuller's earth. *Thorax* 1961;16: 176–179.
27. Tonning HO. Pneumoconiosis from fuller's earth. *J Ind Hyg Toxicol* 1949;31:41–45.
28. Gaensler EA, Cadigan JB, Sashara AA, et al. Graphite pneumoconiosis of electrotypers. *Am J Med* 1966;41:864–882.
29. Okutani H, Shima S, Sano T. Graphite pneumoconiosis in carbon electrode makers. *Excerpta Medica* 1963;2:626.
30. Bergmann M, Glance IJ, Blumenthal HT. Thesaurosis following inhalation of hairspray. *N Engl J Med* 1958;258:471–476.
31. Bergmann M, Glance IJ, Cruz PT, et al. Thesaurosis due to inhalation of hairspray. *N Engl J Med* 1962;266:750–755.
32. Schepers GWH. Thesaurosis versus sarcoidosis. *JAMA* 1962;181: 635–637.
33. Gowdy JM, Wagstaff MJ. Pulmonary infiltration due to aerosol thesaurosis. A survey of hairdressers. *Arch Environ Health* 1972;25: 101–108.
34. Larson RK. A study of midexpiratory flow rates in users of hair spray. *Am Rev Respir Dis* 1964;91:786–788.
35. Palmer A, Renzetti AD, Gillam D. Respiratory disease prevalence in cosmetologists. *Environ Res* 1979;19:136–153.
36. Renzetti AD, Conrad J, Wantanabe S, et al. Thesaurosis from hairspray exposure: a non-disease. *Environ Res* 1980;22:130.
37. Sharma OP, Williams HW. Thesaurosis: pulmonary function studies in beauticians. *Arch Environ Health* 1966;13:616–618.
38. Tanaka S, Pendergrass EP. A thesaurosis survey. *Arch Environ Health* 1965;10:438–440.
39. Garfinkel J, Selvin S, Brown SM. Possible increased risk of lung cancer among beauticians. *J Natl Cancer Inst* 1977;58:141–143.
40. Spinelli JJ, Gallager RP, Band PR, Threlfall WJ. Multiple myeloma, leukemia, and cancer of ovary in cosmetologists and hairdressers. *Am J Ind Med* 1984;6:97–102.
41. Zuskin E, Bouhuys A. Acute airway responses to hairspray preparations. *N Engl J Med* 1974;290:660–663.
42. Cohen BM. Peripheral airway responses to acute hairspray exposure. *Respiration* 1977;34:270–277.
43. Schlueter DP, Soto RJ, Baretta ED, et al. Airway response to hairspray in normal subjects and subjects with hyperreactive airways. *Chest* 1979;75:544–548.
44. Friedman M, Dougherty R, Nelson SR, et al. Acute effects of an aerosol hairspray on tracheal mucociliary transport. *Am Rev Respir Dis* 1977;116:281–286.
45. Wright JL, Cockcroft DW. Lung disease due to abuse of hairspray. *Arch Pathol Lab Med* 1981;105:363–366.
46. Kawane H, Soejima R. Hypersensitivity pneumonitis in a hairdresser. *Chest* 1987;93:577–578.
47. Heacock HJ, Rivers JK. Occupational disease of hairdressers. *Can J Pub Health* 1986;77:109–113.
48. Middleton EL. Industrial pulmonary disease due to the inhalation of dust. *Lancet* 1936;2:59–64.
49. Lesser M, Zia M, Kilburn KH. Silicosis in kaolin workers and firebrick makers. *South Med J* 1978;71:1242–1246.
50. Kennedy T, Rawlings W Jr, Baser M, Tockman M. Pneumoconiosis in Georgia kaolin workers. *Am Rev Respir Dis* 1983;127:215–220.
51. Sepulveda MJ, Vallythan V, Attfield MD, Piacitelli L, Tucker JH. Pneumoconiosis and lung function in a group of kaolin workers. *Am Rev Respir Dis* 1983;127:231–235.
52. Altekuse EB, Chaudhary BA, Pearson MG, Morgan WKC. Kaolin dust concentrations and pneumoconiosis at a kaolin mine. *Thorax* 1984;39:436–441.
53. Morgan WKC, Donner A, Higgins ITT, Pearson MG, Rawlings W Jr. The effects of kaolin on the lung. *Am Rev Respir Dis* 1988;138:813–820.
54. Wagner JC, Pooley FD, Gibbs A, Lyons J, Sheers G, Moncrieff CB. Inhalation of china stone and china dusts: relationship between the mineralogy of dust retained in the lungs and pathological changes. *Thorax* 1986;41:190–196.
55. Wells IP, Bhatt CV, Flanagan M. Kaolinosis: a radiological review. *Clin Radiol* 1985;36:579–582.
56. Davies D, Cotton R. Mica pneumoconiosis. *Br J Med* 1983;40:22–27.
57. Dreessen WC, Dall Valle JM, Edwards TI, et al. Pneumoconiosis among mica and pegmatite workers. *US Public Health Bull* 1940;240.
58. Vestal TF, Windstead JA, Joliet PV. Pneumoconiosis among mica and pegmatite workers. *Ind Med Surg* 1943;12:11–14.
59. Smith AR. Pleural calcification resulting from exposure to certain dusts. *AJR* 1952;67:375–382.
60. Kleinfeld M. Pleural calcifications as a sign of silicatosis. *Am J Med Sci* 1966;251:215–224.
61. Landas SK, Schwartz DA. Mica-associated pulmonary interstitial fibrosis. *Am Rev Respir Dis* 1991;144:718–721.
62. Rom WN, Lee JS, Craft B. Occupational and environmental health problems of the developing oil shale industry. *Am J Ind Med* 1981; 2:247–260.
63. Seaton A, Lamb D, Brown WR, Sclare F, Middleton WG. Pneumoconiosis of shale miners. *Thorax* 1981;36:412–418.
64. Miller BG, Cowie HA, Middleton WG, Seaton A. Epidemiologic studies of Scottish oil shale workers. III. Causes of death. *Am J Ind Med* 1986;9:433–446.
65. Seaton A, Louw SJ, Cowie HA. Epidemiologic studies of Scottish oil shale workers. I. Prevalence of skin disease and pneumoconiosis. *Am J Ind Med* 1986;9:409–421.
66. Louw SJ, Cowie HA, Seaton A. Epidemiologic studies of Scottish oil shale workers. II. Lung function in shale workers' pneumoconiosis. *Am J Ind Med* 1986;9:423–432.
67. Wright WE, Rom WN. A preliminary report: investigation for shalosis among oil shale workers. In: Rom WN, Archer VE, eds. *Health implications of new energy technologies.* Ann Arbor, MI: Ann Arbor Science, 1980;481–489.

68. Scott A. On the occupational cancer of the paraffin and oil workers of the Scottish shale industry. *Br Med J* 1922;2:1108–1109.
69. Southam AH, Wilson SR. Cancer of the scrotum: the aetiology, clinical features and treatment of the disease. *Br Med J* 1922;1:971–973.
70. Holland JM Rahn RO, Smith LH, Clark BR, Chang S, Stephens TJ. Skin carcinogenicity of synthetic and natural petroleums. *J Occup Med* 1979;21:614–618.
71. Rom WN, Krueger G, Zone J, et al. Morbidity survey of U.S. oil shale workers employed during 1948–1969. *Arch Environ Health* 1985;40: 58–62.
72. Rowland J, Shubik P, Wallcave L, Sellakumar A. Carcinogenic bioassay of oil shale: long-term percutaneous application in mice and intratracheal instillation in hamsters. *Toxicol Appl Pharmacol* 1980;55: 522–534.
73. Kalacic I. Chronic nonspecific lung disease in cement workers. *Arch Environ Health* 1973;26:78–83.
74. Kalacic I. Ventilatory lung function in cement workers. *Arch Environ Health* 1974;29:84–85.
75. Saric M, Kalacic I, Holetic A. Follow-up of ventilatory lung function in a group of cement workers. *Br J Ind Med* 1976;33:18–24.
76. Maestrelli P, Simonato L, Bartolucci GB, et al. Pneumoconiosis and chronic bronchitis in a group of cement workers. *Med Lav* 1979;70: 195–202.
77. Rasmussen FV, Borchsenius P, Holstein B, Sølvsteen P. Lung function and long-term exposure to cement dust. *Scand J Resp Dis* 1977; 58:252–264.
78. Abrons HL, Petersen MR, Sanderson WT, Engelberg AL, Harber P. Symptoms, ventilatory function, and environmental exposures in Portland cement workers. *Br J Ind Med* 1988;45:368–375.
79. Abrons HL, Sanderson WT, Petersen MR. *Respiratory effects of Portland cement dust.* Morgantown, WV: National Institute of Occupational Safety and Health, 1985.
80. Pendergrass EP, Pryde AW. Benign pneumoconiosis due to tin oxide. *J Ind Hyg Toxicol* 1948;30:119–123.
81. Robertson AJ, Whitaker PH. Radiological changes in pneumoconiosis due to tin oxide. *J Fac Rad* 1955;6:224–233.
82. Robertson AJ, Rivers D, Nagelschmidt G, et al. Stannosis: benign pneumoconiosis due to tin oxide. *Lancet* 1961;1:1089–1093.
83. Lockey JE. Nonasbestos fibrous minerals. *Clin Chest Med* 1981;2: 203–218.
84. Feigin DS. Talc: understanding its manifestations in the chest. *AJR* 1986;46:295–301.
85. Paré JAP, Fraser RG, Hogg JC, Howlett JG, Murphy SB. Pulmonary “mainline” granulomatosis: talcosis of intravenous methadone abuse. *Medicine* 1979;58:229–239.
86. Paré JP, Cote G, Fraser RS. Long-term follow-up of drug abusers with intravenous talcosis. *Am Rev Respir Dis* 1989;139:233–241.
87. Segal W, Smith AR, Greenburg L. Study of talc miners and millers in St. Lawrence County. *Ind Bull* 1943;22:468–469.
88. Kleinfeld M, Messite J, Tabershaw IR. Talc pneumoconiosis. *Arch Ind Health* 1955;12:66–72.
89. Kleinfeld M, Giel CP, Majeranowski JF, Messite J. Talc pneumoconiosis. A report of six patients with postmortem findings. *Arch Environ Health* 1963;7:101–115.
90. Kleinfeld M, Messite J, Shapiro J, Kooyman O, Swencicki R. Lung function in talc workers. A comparative physiologic study of workers exposed to fibrous and granular talc dusts. *Arch Environ Health* 1964; 9:559–566.
91. Gamble JF, Fellner W, Dimeo MJ. An epidemiologic study of a group of talc workers. *Am Rev Respir Dis* 1979;119:741–753.
92. Wegman DH, Peters JM, Boundy MG, Smith TJ. Evaluation of respiratory effects in miners and millers exposed to talc free of asbestos and silica. *Br J Ind Med* 1982;39:233–238.
93. Vallyathan NV and Craighead JE. Pulmonary pathology in workers exposed to nonasbestiform talc. *Hum Pathol* 1981;12:28–35.
94. De Vuyst P, Dumortier P, Léophante P, Weyer RV, Yernault JC. Mineralogic analysis of bronchoalveolar lavage in talc pneumoconiosis. *Eur J Respir Dis* 1987;70:150–156.
95. Redondo AA, Ettensohn DB, Kahn M, Kessimian N. Bronchoalveolar lavage in talc-induced lung disease. *Thorax* 1988;43:1019–1021.
96. Scancarello G, Romeo R, Sartorelli. Respiratory disease as a result of talc inhalation. *J Occup Environ Med* 1996;38:610–614.
97. Gibbs AE, Pooley FD, Griffiths DM, Mirtha R, Craighead JE, Ruttner JR. Talc pneumoconiosis: a pathologic mineralogic study. *Hum Pathol* 1992;23:1344–1354.
98. Kleinfeld M, Messite J, Kooyman O, Zaki MH. Mortality among talc miners and millers in New York State. *Arch Environ Health* 1967;14: 663–667.
99. Kleinfeld M, Messite J, Zaki MH. Mortality experience among talc workers: a follow-up study. *J Occup Med* 1974;16:345–359.
100. Stille WT, Tabershaw IR. The mortality experience of upstate New York talc workers. *J Occup Med* 1982;24:480–484.
101. Brown DP, Dement JM, Wagoner JK. Mortality patterns among miners and millers occupationally exposed to asbestiform talc. In Lemen R, Dement JM, eds. *Proceedings of the conference on occupational exposure to fibrosis and particulate dusts and their extension into the environment. Dust and disease.* Park Forest South, IL: Pathotox, 1979; 317–324.
102. Gamble J. A nested case control study of lung cancer among New York talc workers. *Int Arch Occup Environ Health* 1993;64:449.
103. Wergeland E, Andersen A, Baerheim A. Morbidity and mortality in talc-exposed workers. *Am J Ind Med* 1990;17:505–513.
104. Thomas TL, Stewart PA. Mortality from lung cancer and respiratory disease among pottery workers exposed to silica and talc. *Am J Epidemiol* 1987;125:35–43.
105. Selevan SG, Dement JM, Wagoner JK, Frolines JR. Mortality patterns among miners and millers of non-asbestiform talc: preliminary report. *J Environ Pathol Toxicol* 1979;2:273–284.
106. Moskowitz RL. Talc pneumoconiosis: a treated case. *Chest* 1970;58: 37–41.
107. Miller A, Teirstein AS, Bader ME, Bader RA, Selikoff IJ. Talc pneumoconiosis. *Am J Med* 1971;50:395–402.
108. Nam K, Gracey DR. Pulmonary talcosis from cosmetic talcum powder. *JAMA* 1972;221:492–493.
109. Wells IP, Dubbins PA, Whimster WF. Pulmonary disease caused by the inhalation of cosmetic talcum powder. *Br J Radiol* 1979;52:586–588.
110. Christie H, Mackay RJ, Fisher AM. Pulmonary effects of inhalation of titanium dioxide by rats. *Am Ind Hyg Assoc J* 1963;24:42–46.
111. Uragoda CG, Pinto MRM. An investigation into the health of workers in an ilmenite extracting plant. *Med J Aust* 1972;1:167–169.
112. Elo R, Määttä K, Arstila AU. Pulmonary deposits of titanium dioxide in man. *Arch Pathol* 1972;94:417–424.
113. Määttä K, Arstila AU. Pulmonary deposits of titanium dioxide in cytologic and lung biopsy specimens. Light and electron microscopic x-ray analysis. *Lab Invest* 1975;33:342–346.
114. Rom WN, Greaves W, Bang KM, Holthouser M, Campbell D, Bernstein R. An epidemiologic study of the respiratory effects of trona dust. *Arch Environ Health* 1983;38:86–92.
115. Rom WN, Moshell A, Greaves W, et al. A study of dermatitis in trona miners and millers. *J Occup Med* 1983;25:295–299.
116. Buist AS, Vollmer WM, Johnson LR, Bernstein RS, McCamant LE. A four-year prospective study of the respiratory effects of volcanic ash from Mount St. Helens. *Am Rev Respir Dis* 1986;133:526–534.
117. Vallyathan V, Robinson V, Reasor M, Stettler L, Bernstein R. Comparative in vitro cytotoxicity of volcanic ashes from Mount St. Helens, El Chichon, and Galunggung. *J Toxicol Environ Health* 1984;14:641–654.
118. Warheit DB, Hill LH, Brody AR. In vitro effects of crocidolite asbestos and wollastonite on pulmonary macrophages and serum complement. *Scanning Microsc* 1984;II:919–926.
119. Hanke W, Sepulveda MJ, Watson A, Jankovic J. Respiratory morbidity in wollastonite workers. *Br J Ind Med* 1984;41:474–479.
120. Huuskonen MS, Tossavainen A, Koskinen H, et al. Wollastonite exposure and lung fibrosis. *Environ Res* 1983;30:291–304.
121. McConnell EE, Hall L, Adkins B. Studies on the chronic toxicity (inhalation) of Wollastonite in Fischer 344 rats. *Inhalat Toxicol* 1991;3:323–337.

*Environmental and Occupational Medicine, Third Edition*, edited by William N. Rom.
Lippincott–Raven Publishers, Philadelphia © 1998.

# CHAPTER 39

# Ozone

Morton Lippmann

Ozone ($O_3$) exposure affects the structure and functions of the respiratory tract in a variety of ways. A large and reasonably consistent body of knowledge has accumulated on the effects of $O_3$ on respiratory function in humans, especially on transient responses to acute exposure. Other lung function responses to acute and subacute exposure that have been studied, largely in animals, include mucociliary and early alveolar zone particle clearance, functional responses in macrophages and epithelial cells, and changes in lung cell secretions. Structural changes in the smaller conductive airways and the more proximal gas-exchange region have been associated with subchronic and chronic animal exposure protocols; however, the health significance of localized structural changes, and the roles, if any, of the transient functional and cellular responses in the pathogenesis of lung disease, remain speculative. The responses in animals suggest possible links between $O_3$ exposure and respiratory disease in humans, but do not provide clear evidence for such ties. Chronic effects may result from cumulative damage or from the side effects of adaptive responses to repeated daily or intermittent exposure. This chapter summarizes current knowledge on $O_3$ formation and transport, human exposure, and transient and chronic health effects produced by the inhalation of $O_3$. It does not discuss the effects of $O_3$ or its metabolites on nonrespiratory tissues or the health effects of increased ultraviolet radiation resulting from the depletion of stratospheric $O_3$.

M. Lippmann: Department of Environmental Medicine, New York University Medical Center, Tuxedo, New York 10987.

## FORMATION AND TRANSPORT WITHIN THE ATMOSPHERE

Ozone is a product of a series of photochemical reaction sequences that require hydrocarbon vapors (HC), nitrogen dioxide ($NO_2$), and sunlight. The $O_3$ concentration in the ambient atmosphere usually peaks in late morning or afternoon and declines in the evening, owing to $O_3$ loss from reaction with nitric oxide (NO) and terrestrial surfaces. Since hydrocarbon vapors and $NO_2$ remain in the atmosphere, $O_3$ continues to form in the atmosphere far downwind of the sources. The $O_3$ concentrations are often higher in suburbs and rural downwind areas than in cities (1).

## POPULATION EXPOSURES AND EXPOSURE LIMITS

Widespread $O_3$ contamination in ambient air increases both the number of people exposed and the magnitude of their exposure, especially in mild weather, when the largest number of people are outdoors for extended periods. During the period 1983 to 1985 approximately half of the United States population lived in communities where ambient $O_3$ concentrations exceeded 120 parts per billion by volume (ppb) (2,3). More than 10 million people in the United States were estimated to be exposed to such concentrations while exercising at moderate to heavy levels of exertion (3). In 1987 and 1988, $O_3$ concentrations were higher than those in the 1983 to 1985 period, and the population that was heavily exposed was therefore larger. Since 1988, the ambient $O_3$ concentrations have generally declined, as illustrated in Fig. 1.

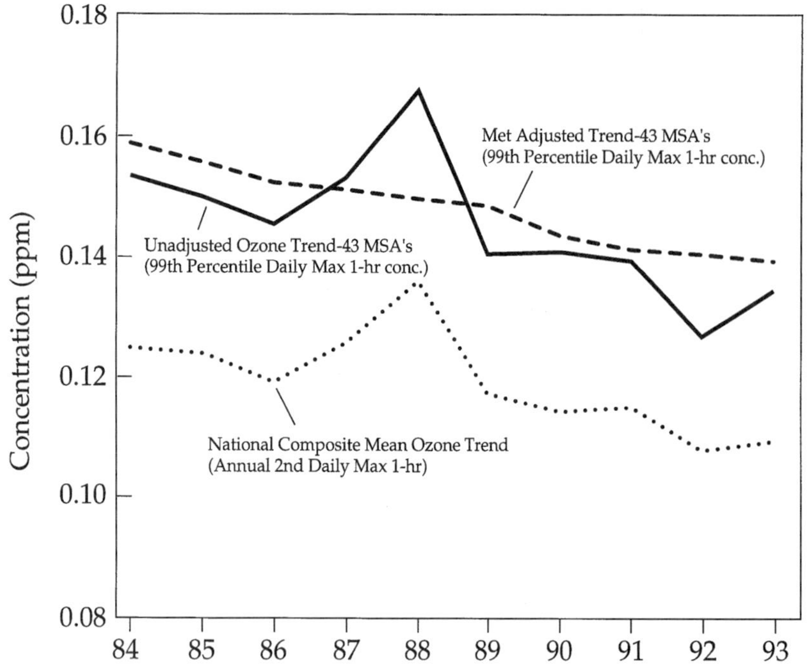


**FIG. 1.** Metropolitan area $O_3$ trends adjusted for meteorological variability, 1984–93.

Indoor sources of $O_3$ include xerographic copy machines and electrostatic air cleaners. A major source of occupational exposure is arc welding. The Occupational Safety and Health Administration's (OSHA) permissible exposure limit (PEL) for $O_3$ is 100 ppb as a time-weighted average for 8 hours per day; the short-term exposure limit is 300 ppb for 15 min (4). The American Conference of Governmental Industrial Hygienists (ACGIH) adopted a threshold limit value of 100 ppb as a ceiling in 1989. In 1996, ACGIH's Notice of Intended Change proposed replacing the ceiling value with an 8-hour time-weighted average values based on work intensity, i.e., 100 ppb for light work, 80 ppb for moderate work, and 50 ppb for heavy work (5).

A U.S. National Ambient Air Quality Standard (NAAQS) of 120 ppb for $O_3$ using a 1-hour averaging time not to be exceeded more than once per year was established in 1979. It was based principally on the expectation that ambient exposure is characterized by relatively sharp afternoon peaks (1). However, it has been shown that ambient $O_3$ concentrations in the Netherlands and New Jersey often have broad daytime peaks—maximum 8-hour averages close to 90% of peak 1-hour levels (6). In the ambient air in the United States as a whole, a 1-hour $O_3$ peak at 120 ppb is, on average, associated with a maximum 8-hour average concentration of ~100 ppb (2). In November 1996, the Environmental Protection Agency (EPA) administrator proposed a revised $O_3$ NAAQS with an 8-hour average concentration limit of 80 ppb, not to be exceeded more than three times a year. The spatial distribution of counties that would have exceeded this proposed limit in the 1991–1993 period is shown in Fig. 2, along with an estimate of the population in these counties (137 million). By contrast, the number of people

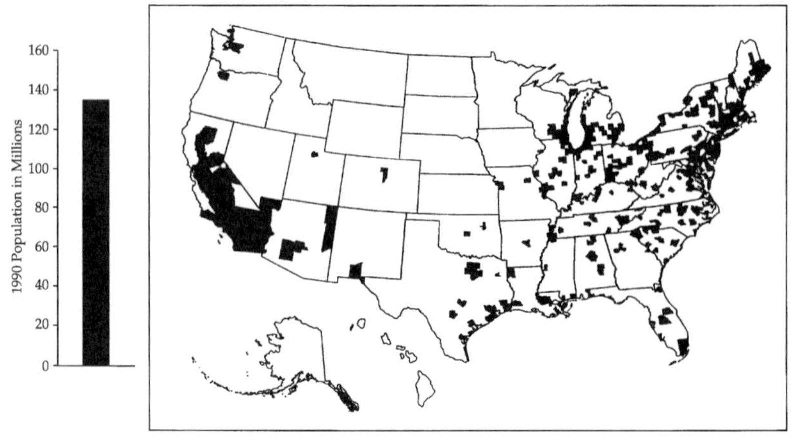


**FIG. 2.** Spatial distribution of counties with 8-hour daily maximum, 1 expected exceedance design value greater than 0.08 ppm based on 1991–93 air quality data.

in counties exceeding the 1-hour, 120 ppb NAAQS for the same period was 60 million.

## TRANSIENT EFFECTS ON RESPIRATORY FUNCTION

It is well established that inhalation of $O_3$ causes concentration-dependent mean decrements in exhaled volume and flow rate during forced expiratory maneuvers, and that the mean decrement increases with increasing depth of breathing (7). There is a wide range of reproducible responsiveness among healthy young adults (8), with no significant differences among groups of men or women or between blacks and whites (9). Functional responsiveness to $O_3$ is no greater, and usually lower, among cigarette smokers (10,11), older adults (12–15), and patients with asthma (16–18), allergic rhinitis (19), or chronic obstructive pulmonary disease (COPD) (20,21). It is also well established that repeated daily 1- or 2-hour exposures, at a level that produces a functional response with a single exposure, results in an enhanced response on the second day, diminishing responses on days 3 and 4, and virtually no response by day 5 (22–24). This functional adaptation to exposure disappears about a week after exposure ceases (25,26). For repeated 6.6 hour/day exposures to 120 ppb $O_3$, the peak functional response occurs on the first day, with progressively lesser responses after the second, third, and fourth days of exposure. However, for these same subjects, their responsiveness to methacholine challenge peaked on the second day, and remained elevated throughout all 5 days of exposure (27).

The persistent elevation of airway responsiveness is one reason to discount the view of some people that the functional adaptation phenomenon indicates that transient functional decrements are not an important health effect. Additional evidence comes from research in animals showing that persistent damage to lung cells accumulates even as functional adaptation takes place. Tepper and colleagues (28) exposed rats to $O_3$—350, 500, or 1,000 ppb—for 2.25 hours on 5 consecutive days. Carbon dioxide (8%) was added to the exposure during alternate 15-minute periods to stimulate breathing and so increase $O_3$ uptake and distribution. The consequences of exposure on pulmonary function, morphology, macrophage phagocytosis, lavageable protein, differential cell counts, and lung tissue antioxidants were assessed. Tidal volume, frequency of breathing, inspiratory time, expiratory time, and maximal tidal flow were affected on day 1 and 2 by all concentrations of ozone. By day 5, the $O_3$ responses were completely adapted at 350 ppb and greatly attenuated at 500 ppb, but showed no signs of adaptation in the group exposed to 1,000 ppb. Unlike the pulmonary function adaptation, light microscopy indicated a pattern of progressive epithelial damage and inflammatory changes associated with the terminal bronchiolar region. Over the 5-day testing period, a sustained 37% increase in lavageable protein and a 60% suppression of macrophage phagocytic activity were observed with exposure to 500 ppb. There were no changes in differential cell counts. Lung glutathione was initially increased, but it was within the control range on days 4 and 5. Lung ascorbate values were elevated significantly above those of controls on days 3 through 5. These data suggest attenuation of the pulmonary functional response at the same time that the tissue response revealed progressive damage.

The first indications that the effects of $O_3$ on respiratory function accumulate over more than 1 hour were the observations of McDonnell et al. (29) and Kulle et al. (30) in chamber exposures of young adults to $O_3$ in purified air for 2 hours, with the volunteer subjects engaged intermittently in vigorous exercise. Significant function decrements observed after 2 hours' exposure were not demonstrated by measurements made after 1 hour.

Spektor and colleagues (31) noted that children at summer camps with active outdoor recreation programs had greater decrements in lung function than children exposed to $O_3$ at comparable concentrations in chambers for 1 or 2 hours (31). Furthermore, their activity levels, although not measured, were known to be considerably lower than those of the children exposed in the chamber studies while performing very vigorous exercise. Since it is well established that functional responses to $O_3$ increase with levels of physical activity and ventilation (7), the greater responses in the camp children had to be caused by other factors, such as greater cumulative exposure, or to the potentiation of the response to $O_3$ by other pollutants in the ambient air. Cumulative daily exposures to $O_3$ were generally greater for the camp children, since they were exposed all day long rather than for 1 or 2 hours.

Similar considerations apply to the studies of Kinney et al. (32) and Hoek et al. (33) of school children. In the Kinney et al. study, in Kingston and Harriman, Tennessee, lung function was measured in school on as many as six occasions during a 2-month period in the late winter and early spring. Child-specific regressions of function versus maximum 1-hour $O_3$ during the previous day indicated significant associations between $O_3$ and function, with coefficients similar to those seen in the summer camp studies of Spektor and colleagues (31). Since children in school may be expected to have relatively low activity levels, the relatively high response coefficients may be due to potentiation by other pollutants or to a low level of seasonal adaptation. Kingston-Harriman is notable for its relatively high levels of aerosol acidity. As shown by Spengler and colleagues (34), Kingston-Harriman has higher annual average and higher peak acid aerosol concentrations than other cities studied (Steubenville, Ohio; St. Louis, Missouri; and Portage, Wisconsin). Alternatively, the relatively high response coefficients could have been due to the fact that the measurements were made in the late winter and early spring. Linn and associates (35) have shown evidence for a seasonal adaptation, and children studied during the summer may not be as responsive as children measured earlier in the year. In a study of children with moderate to severe asthma at a summer camp in the Connecticut River Valley (36), the association between decrements in peak expiratory flow rates associated with ambient $O_3$ concentrations were similar in magnitude to those reported by the same group of investigators for healthy children at other northeastern U.S. summer camps (31). However, the level of physical activity of the asthmatic children, and hence their $O_3$ intake was much lower. Also, the asthmatic children have less reserve functional capacity. Thus, the level of health concern for such comparable functional decrements is much greater.

Field studies of functional responses of adults engaged in recreational activities outdoors in the presence of varying levels of $O_3$ have also been performed. Spektor et al. (37) made pre- and postexercise respiratory function measurements on 30 young adults who were engaged in daily outdoor exercise for about one-half hour per day in an area with regional summer haze but no local point sources. The magnitudes of the functional decrements per unit of ambient $O_3$ concentration was similar to those observed in volunteers exposed while exercising vigorously for 1 or 2 hours in controlled chamber exposure studies. Functional decrements in proportion to ambient $O_3$ concentrations have also been reported for joggers in Houston, Texas (38), competitive cyclists in the Netherlands (39), hikers on Mount Washington, New Hampshire (40), and agricultural workers in British Columbia (41).

In Linn's study (35) in Southern California, a group of adult subjects selected for their relatively high functional responsiveness to $O_3$ exhibited much greater functional decrements in response to 2 hours' exposure (to $O_3$ at 180 ppb with intermittent exercise in a chamber) in the spring than they did the following autumn or winter, and their responses the following spring were equivalent to those of the preceding spring. These findings suggest that some of the variability in response coefficients reported for earlier controlled human exposures to $O_3$ in chambers could have been due to seasonal variations in responsiveness, which, in turn, may be related to a long-term adaptation to chronic $O_3$ exposure.

The observations from the field studies in the children's camps stimulated Folinsbee and colleagues (42) to undertake a 6.6-hr chamber exposure study of adult volunteers to 120 ppb $O_3$. Moderate exercise was performed for 50 minutes every hour, for 3 hours in the morning and again in the afternoon. The investigators found that the function decrements became progressively greater after each hour of exposure, reaching average values of about 400 ml for forced vital capacity (FVC) and about 540 ml for forced expiratory volume in 1 second ($FEV_1$) by the end of the day (Fig. 3). The effects were transient in that there were no residual function decrements on the following day. The decrements in $FEV_1$ after 6.6 hours' exposure to 120 ppb

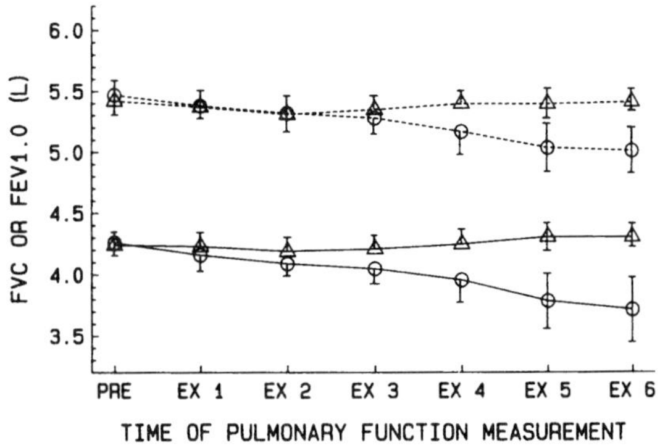


**FIG. 3.** Mean ± SE of FVC *(dashed lines)* and $FEV_1$ *(solid lines)* after each of six 1-hour exercise periods. *Triangles* represent air exposures and *circles* represent ozone exposures. (From ref. 42.)

averaged 13% and were comparable to those seen previously in the same laboratory in similar subjects following 2 hours' intermittent heavier exercise (68 L inhaled per minute for a total exercise time of 60 minutes) at an interpolated concentration of about 215 ppb. Assuming that the rate of ventilation was 10 L per minute between exercise periods, the total amount of $O_3$ inhaled during 2 hours of intermittent heavy exercise at 430 μg/m$^3$ would be (60 min × 0.068 m$^3$/min + 60 min + 0.010 m$^3$/min) + 430 μg/m$^3$ = 2.01 mg $O_3$. The corresponding amount of $O_3$ inhaled during 6.6 hours' intermittent moderate exercise at 235 μg/m$^3$ would be (300 min × 0.040 mg/m$^3$ + 100 min + 0.010 m$^3$/min) + 235 μg/m$^3$ = 3.06 mg $O_3$. Thus, the function deficit accumulates with time but there appears to be a temporal decay of effect going on at the same time. Follow-up studies in the same laboratory involved 6.6-hour exposures at concentrations of 80, 100, and 120 ppb. The results at 120 ppb confirmed the previous findings, whereas those at 80 and 100 ppb showed smaller changes, which however also became progressively greater with duration of exposure (43). These exposures also produced inflammatory responses as determined by analyses of bronchoalveolar lavage (BAL) samples, as discussed in a later section.

Figure 3 demonstrates why the appropriate averaging time for transient functional decrements caused by $O_3$ is at least 6 hours, and why there is no scientific basis for a health-based exposure limit with an averaging time of 1 hour. Since $O_3$ levels in ambient air can have broad peaks and 8-hour averages equal to about 90% of the peak 1-hour averages, the functional decrements associated with ambient concentrations are likely to be much greater than those predicted on the basis of the responses in the chamber studies following 1- or 2-hour exposures.

The results of these studies, and other follow-up studies at the EPA Clinical Research Center in Chapel Hill, North Caroline, as summarized in the recent EPA Criteria Document (1), are illustrated in Fig. 4. They illustrate

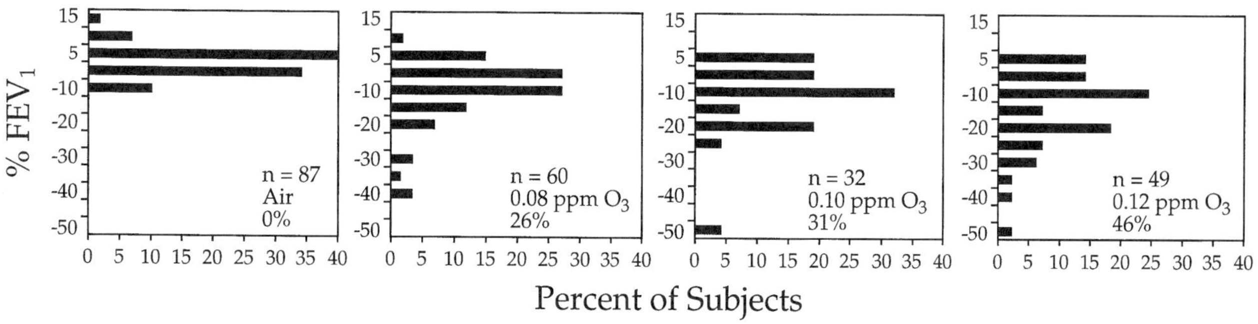


**FIG. 4.** The distribution of response for 87 subjects exposed to clean air and at least one of 0.08, 0.10, or 0.12 ppm ozone ($O_3$) is shown here. The $O_3$ exposures lasted 6.6 hours, during which time the subjects exercised for 50 minutes of each hour with a 35-minute rest period at the end of the third hour. Decreases in forced expiratory volume in 1 second ($FEV_1$) are expressed as percent change from baseline. For example, the bar labeled "-10" indicates the percent of subjects with a decrease in $FEV_1$ of >5% but ≤10%, and the bar labeled "5" indicates improvement in $FEV_1$ of >0% but ≤5%. Each panel of the figure indicates the percentage of subjects at each $O_3$ concentration with a decrease of $FEV_1$ in excess of 10%.

the presence of an overall exposure-response relationship, as well as the extent of interindividual variability of response. At all three exposure levels (80, 100, 120 ppb), there are individuals with little or no response, while others have large functional decrements ($FEV_1$ declines > 40%). McDonnell et al. (15) modeled the data from 68 healthy nonsmoking adults studied using this protocol at the EPA Chapel Hill laboratory and reported that for exposure at 120 ppb for 6.6 hours, 47% [90% confidence interval (CI) = 30–65%) would have an $FEV_1$ decrement ≥10%.

## EFFECTS ON AIRWAY REACTIVITY

Exposure to $O_3$ can also alter the responsiveness of the airways to other bronchoconstrictive challenges as measured by changes in respiratory mechanics. For example, Folinsbee and co-workers (42) reported that for the group of healthy subjects as a whole, airway reactivity to the bronchoconstrictive drug methacholine was approximately doubled following 6.6 hours' exposure to 120 ppb $O_3$. Airway hyperresponsiveness (to histamine) had previously been demonstrated in healthy subjects, but only at $O_3$ concentrations of at least 400 ppb (44,45). On an individual basis, the investigators found no apparent relationship between the $O_3$-associated changes in methacholine reactivity and those in FVC or $FEV_1$. This differs from responses to inhaled sulfuric acid aerosol: in that study changes in function correlated closely to changes in reactivity to carbachol aerosol, a bronchoconstrictive drug (46). Perhaps the $O_3$-associated changes in bronchial reactivity predispose to bronchospasm from other environmental agents such as acid aerosol and naturally occurring aeroallergens.

The follow-up tests by Horstman and co-workers (43) in healthy subjects, involving 6.6-hour exposures to 80, 100, and 120 ppb, indicated 56%, 89%, and 121% increases in methacholine responsiveness, respectively. Increased responsiveness to methacholine was also seen in the Folinsbee and Hazucha (47) study (1 hour at 350 ppb). Increased responsiveness to histamine was seen by Gong and co-workers (48) in one of 17 competitive cyclists exposed to 120 ppb for 1 hour at an expired volume ($\dot{V}_E$) of 89 L per minute followed by 3 to 4 minutes at 150 L per minute. At 200 ppb, responsiveness increased in 9 of the 17 subjects. McDonnell and colleagues (19) found increased histamine responsiveness in 26 young adult males with allergic rhinitis after they breathed ozone at 180 ppb during 2 hours exercise at 64 L per minute. Jorres et al. (49) exposed 24 subjects with mild stable allergic asthma, 12 subjects with allergic rhinitis without asthma, and 10 healthy subjects to 250 ppb $O_3$ or filtered air (FA) for 3 hours with intermittent exercise. They determined the concentration of methacholine ($PC_{20}FEV_1$) and the dose of allergen ($PD_{20}FEV_1$) producing a 20% fall in $FEV_1$. In the subjects with asthma, $FEV_1$ decreased by 12.5% ± 2.2%, $PC_{20}FEV_1$ of methacholine by 0.91% ± 0.19% doubling concentrations, and $PD_{20}FEV_1$ of allergen by 1.74% ± 0.25% doubling doses after $O_3$ compared with FA. The changes in lung function, methacholine, and allergen responsiveness did not correlate with each other. In the subjects with rhinitis, mean $FEV_1$ decreased by 7.8% and 1.3% when $O_3$ or FA, respectively, were followed by allergen inhalation.

The basis for the effect of $O_3$ on airway reactivity was examined by Gordon and associates (50) in guinea pigs exposed for 1 hour to either 100 or 800 ppb $O_3$. Both exposures significantly inhibited lung cholinesterase activity as compared to that of unexposed animals.

The $O_3$-induced responsiveness may be centered in the peripheral lung and be retained long after the $O_3$ exposure ceases. Beckett and co-workers (51) exposed the peripheral lungs of anesthetized dogs to 1,000 ppb $O_3$ for 2 hours using a wedged bronchoscope technique. A contralateral sublobar segment was simultaneously exposed to air as a control. In the ozone-exposed segments, collateral resistance ($R_{cs}$) was increased within 15 minutes and remained elevated about 150% throughout the 2-hour exposure period. Fifteen hours later, the baseline $R_{cs}$ of the $O_3$-exposed sublobar segments was significantly elevated and these segments demonstrated increased responsiveness to aerosolized acetylcholine (100 and 500 μg/ml). There were no differences in neutrophils, mononuclear cells, or mast cells (numbers or degree of mast cell degranulation) between $O_3$- and air-exposed airways at 15 hours. The small airways of the lung periphery thus are capable of remaining hyperresponsive hours after localized exposure to $O_3$ ceases, but this does not appear to depend on the presence of inflammatory cells in the small airway wall.

## SYMPTOMATIC RESPONSES

Respiratory symptoms have been closely associated with group mean pulmonary function changes after brief exposure for adults following controlled exposures to $O_3$ and in ambient air containing $O_3$ as the predominant pollutant. However, Hayes and colleagues (52) found only a weak to moderate correlation between $FEV_1$ changes and symptom severity when the analysis was conducted with individual data.

In controlled 2-hour ozone exposures, McDonnell and associates (29) reported that with vigorous exercise some adult subjects experienced cough, shortness of breath, and pain on deep inspiration at 120 ppb, although the group mean response was statistically significant for cough only. Above 120 ppb, respiratory and nonrespiratory symptoms have included throat dryness, chest tightness, substernal pain, cough, wheeze, pain on deep inspiration, shortness of breath, dyspnea, lassitude, malaise, headache, and nausea.

The recent prolonged exposure studies involving 6.6 hours' exposure to concentrations between 80 and 120 ppb also produced significant increases in respiratory symptoms, including cough and pain on deep inspiration (41,42). Linder and colleagues (53) reported that brief exposures (16 to 28 minutes) at high ventilatory rates (30 to 120 L per minute) produced symptoms of irritation and cough in young adults exposed to 120 to 130 ppb.

While $O_3$ causes symptomatic responses in adults at current peak levels, there are much data to indicate that such responses do not occur in healthy children (54,55). While children aged 8 to 11 years exposed for 2.5 hours to 120 ppb while intermittently exercising ($\dot{V}_E$ = 39 L per minute) showed small but statistically significant decreases in $FEV_1$, they showed no changes in frequency or severity of cough compared to controls (8,56). Similarly, adolescents aged 12 to 15 exercising continuously ($\dot{V}_E$ = 31–33 L per minute) during exposure to 140 ppb mean $O_3$ in ambient air showed no changes in symptoms despite statistically significant decrements in group mean $FEV_1$ (4%), which persisted at least an hour when resting after exposure (54).

These laboratory results are consistent with the results obtained in a series of field studies at children's summer camps, which failed to find any symptomatic responses in healthy children despite the occurrence of relatively large decrements in function, which were proportional to the ambient $O_3$ concentrations (31,57).

Several epidemiologic studies have provided evidence of qualitative associations between ambient oxidant levels greater than 100 ppb and symptoms in children and young adults—throat irritation, chest discomfort, cough, and headache. Thus, symptoms reported in persons exposed to ozone in purified air are similar to those observed for ambient air exposure, except for eye irritation, a common symptom associated with exposure to photochemical oxidants, which has not been reported for controlled exposures to ozone alone. Other oxidants, such as aldehydes and peroxyacetyl nitrate (PAN), are principally responsible for eye irritation and are generally found in atmospheres that contain more ambient $O_3$ (58,59).

Respiratory symptoms in relation to ambient pollution in healthy young women (100 student nurses) in Los Angeles (60) were monitored by Hammer's group. They found associations between photochemical oxidants and respiratory symptoms, but that analysis ignored smoking and serial correlations in the data, used linear regression to model the probability of a respiratory incident, ignored other potentially colinear air pollutants, and assumed that a pollutant would have the same impact on starting an episode of symptoms as on prolonging the episode. Because of limited computational facilities at the time, the data on individual subjects were collapsed to rates per day.

Schwartz and Zeger (61) reexamined the original diaries from this study that contained smoking and allergy histories as well as symptom reports that had never been analyzed. Diaries were completed daily and collected weekly for as long as 3 years. Air pollution was measured at a monitoring location within 4 km of the school. The incidence and duration of a system were modeled separately. Photochemical oxidants were associated with increased risk of chest discomfort [odds ratio (OR) = 1.7, $p < 0.001$] and eye irritation (OR = 1.20, $p < 0.001$).

## RESPIRATORY DISEASE

There have been several reports of associations between ambient photochemical oxidant pollution and exacerbation of asthma (62–64), but the specific role of

$O_3$ and the nature of the exposure-response relationships remain poorly defined.

Associations between ambient air pollutants and respiratory morbidity were examined by Ostro and Rothschild (65) using the Health Interview Survey (HIS), a large cross-sectional database collected by the National Center for Health Statistics. They attempted to determine the separate health consequences of $O_3$ and particulate matter, using six separate years of the HIS. Using a fixed-effects model that controls for intercity differences, results indicate an association between fine particulate and both minor restrictions in activity and respiratory conditions severe enough to result in work loss and "bed disability" for adults. $O_3$, on the other hand, was associated only with the more minor restrictions.

Bates and Sizto (66) examined associations between ambient air pollutants and hospital admissions for respiratory disease in southern Ontario. In summer they found a consistent association between hospital admissions for respiratory disease and daily levels of sulfate ($SO_4^=$), $O_3$, and temperature, but no association for a group of nonrespiratory conditions. Multiple regression analyses showed that all environmental variables together accounted for 5.6% of the variability in respiratory disease admissions and that when temperature was forced into the analysis first, it accounted for only 0.89% of the variability. It was found that daily $SO_4^=$ data collected at one monitoring site in the center of the region were not correlated with admissions for respiratory complaints, whereas the $SO_4^=$ values collected every sixth day, on different days of the week, at 17 stations in the region had the highest correlation for complaints. They concluded that probably neither $O_3$ nor $SO_4^=$ alone was responsible for the observed associations with acute respiratory admissions, but that either some unmeasured species [sulfuric acid ($H_2SO_4$) is the strongest candidate] or some pattern of sequential or cumulative exposure was responsible for the observed morbidity.

Another study of hospital admissions in relation to $O_3$ was performed by Ozkaynak and co-workers (67) in Boston, Springfield, Worcester, New Bedford, and Fall River, Massachusetts. They reported that the associations between daily air pollution levels and admissions due to certain respiratory diagnosis classes were not always positive or significant, perhaps due to sample size limitations or other statistical problems. Nevertheless, the most complete and statistically reliable models indicated positive associations between 1-hour maximum $O_3$ levels in the summer months and the daily admissions for pneumonia and influenza. Thus, in this respect these findings bore some similarity to those obtained by Bates and Sizto (66).

## EFFECTS ON LUNG DEFENSES AND LUNG STRUCTURE

Practical and ethical considerations limit the amounts and kinds of data that can be collected on the effects of $O_3$ on lung defenses and lung structure. Most of the limited body of data on humans that are available relate to the rate of particle clearance from the lungs and to alterations in the constituents of BAL fluid.

### Particle Clearance

Foster and co-workers (68) studied the effect of 2-hour exposures to 200 or 400 ppb $O_3$ with intermittent light exercise on the rates of tracheobronchial mucociliary particle clearance in healthy adult males. The 400-ppb $O_3$ exposure produced a marked acceleration in particle clearance from both central and peripheral airways, as well as a 12% drop in FVC. The 200-ppb $O_3$ exposure produced significant acceleration of particle clearance in peripheral airways but failed to produce a significant reduction in FVC, suggesting that significant changes in the ability of the deep lung to clear deposited particles take place before significant changes in respiratory function.

The effects of $O_3$ on mucociliary particle clearance have also been studied in rats and rabbits. Rats exposed for 4 hours to $O_3$ at concentrations in the range of 400 to 1,200 ppb exhibited slowing of particle clearance at concentrations of 800 ppb and higher but not at 400 ppb (69). Rabbits exposed for 2 hours at 100, 250, and 600 ppb $O_3$ showed a concentration-dependent trend of reduced clearance rate with increasing concentrations, the change at 600 ppb being about 50% and significantly different from that for controls (70). It is not known why the animal tests show only retarded mucociliary clearance in response to $O_3$ exposure, while the human tests show accelerated clearance. In corresponding tests with other irritants ($H_2SO_4$ aerosol and cigarette smoke) both humans and animals have exhibited accelerated clearance at lower exposure levels and retarded clearance at higher levels (71).

The effects of $O_3$ on alveolar macrophage–mediated particle clearance during the first few weeks have also been studied in rats and rabbits. Rats exposed for 4 hours to 800 ppb $O_3$ had accelerated particle clearance (69). Rabbits exposed to 100, 600, or 1,200 ppb $O_3$ once for 2 hours had accelerated clearance at 100 ppb and retarded clearance at 1,200 ppb. Rabbits exposed for 2 hours per day for 13 consecutive days at 100 or 600 ppb $O_3$ had accelerated clearance for the first 10 days and a greater effect at 600 ppb (72).

Kehrl and colleagues (73) have studied the effects of inhaled $O_3$ on respiratory epithelial permeability in healthy, nonsmoking young men. They were exposed for 2 hours to purified air and 400 ppb $O_3$ while performing intermittent high-intensity treadmill exercises. Specific airway resistance ($SR_{aw}$) and FVC were measured before and at the end of exposure. Seventy-five minutes after the exposures, the pulmonary clearance of a radioactive technetium-labeled organic molecule, diethylenetriamine pentaacetic acid ($^{99m}$Tc-DTPA), was measured as an index of epithelial permeability. Ozone exposure caused respiratory symptoms in all eight subjects and was associated with a 14% ± 2.8% (mean ± SE) decrement in FVC ($p < 0.001$), as well as a 71% ± 22% increase in $SR_{aw}$ ($p = 0.04$). Compared with the air exposure day, seven of the eight subjects showed increased $^{99m}$Tc-DTPA clearance after the $O_3$ exposure, and the mean value increased from 0.59% ± 0.08% to 1.75% ± 0.43% per minute ($p = 0.03$). Thus, $O_3$ exposure sufficient to produce decrements in the respiratory function of human subjects also causes an increase in permeability. Increased permeability could facilitate the uptake of other inhaled toxicants or the release of inflammatory cells such as neutrophils onto the airway surfaces.

## Airway Inflammation

Seltzer and co-workers (44) showed that $O_3$-induced airway reactivity to methacholine is associated with polymorphonuclear leukocyte (PMN) influx into the airways and with changes in cyclooxygenase metabolites of arachidonic acid. With 2-hour exposures to $O_3$ at 400 ppb with intermittent exercise, the BAL fluid had increased prostaglandins $E_2$ and $F_{2a}$, and 3 hours after the $O_3$ exposure, thromboxane $B_2$.

Reports of Koren and colleagues (74,75) also described inflammatory and biochemical changes in the airways of healthy subjects following $O_3$ exposure. In their initial studies subjects were exposed to 400 ppb for 2 hours while performing intermittent exercise at a ventilation rate of 70 L per minute in order to examine cellular and biochemical responses in the airways. BAL was performed 18 hours after the $O_3$ exposure. An 8.2-fold increase in PMNs after $O_3$ exposure confirmed the observations of Seltzer and associates (44). Twofold increases in protein, albumin, and immunoglobulin G (IgG) were indicative of increased epithelial permeability, as previously suggested by the $^{99m}$Tc-DTPA clearance studies of Kehrl's group (73). In addition to confirming the previous findings, Koren and colleagues (74) provided evidence of stimulation of fibrogenic processes. They reported that an inflammatory response, as indicated by increased levels of PMNs, was also observed in BAL fluid from subjects exposed to 100 ppb $O_3$ for 6.6 hours (75). The 6.6-hour exposure at 100 ppb produced a 4.8-fold increase in PMNs 18 hours after the exposure. Since the amount of $O_3$ inhaled in the 100-ppb protocol was about 2.5 μg, while in the 400-ppb protocol it was about 3.6 μg, we might have expected an increase in PMNs of $2.5/3.6 \times 8.2 = 5.7$ times. Further studies by Devlin et al. (76) extended the effects range for this exposure protocol down to 80 ppb. The close correspondence of the observed and expected ratio suggests that lung inflammation from inhaled $O_3$ also has no threshold down to ambient background levels.

These studies indicate that the inflammatory process caused by $O_3$ exposure is promptly initiated (44) and persists at least 18 hours (74). The time course of this inflammatory response and the $O_3$ exposures necessary to initiate it, however, have not been precisely determined. Furthermore, these studies demonstrate that, as a result of $O_3$ exposure, cells and enzymes capable of causing damage to pulmonary tissues were increased and levels of proteins that play a role in the fibrotic and fibrinolytic processes were elevated.

Scannell et al. (18) exposed a group of 18 asthmatic subjects to $O_3$ using the same exposure protocol they previously used for 81 healthy subjects. They reported no significant differences in lung function responses and a trend toward higher airway resistance ($p < 0.13$). By contrast, the asthmatic subjects had significantly greater ($p < 0.05$) $O_3$-induced increases in inflammatory end points (percent of neutrophils and total protein) in BAL fluid as compared to 20 of the normal subjects who also underwent bronchoscopy.

Inflammatory reactions occur in the nasal passages as well as in the lungs (77). Graham and Koren (78) compared the cellular changes in nasal lavage (NL) fluid with those detected in BAL fluid from the same individuals. This study demonstrated that PMN counts in the NL could be a useful, inexpensive means of studying the acute inflammatory effect of $O_3$ and monitoring those effects in the lower parts of the lung.

Prolonged inflammatory processes following repetitive exposures to $O_3$ in ambient air were reported by Kinney et al. (79) in terms of reduced release of reactive oxygen species, increased levels of lactate dehydrogenase (LDH), interleukin-8 (IL-8), and prostaglandin $E_2$ ($PGE_2$) in the BAL.

The Overton and Miller (80) model of $O_3$ dosimetry within the lungs predicts similar airway deposition patterns for $O_3$ in rats and humans: deposition is greatest in the vicinity of the respiratory acinus (i.e., the junction between the small conductive airways and the gas-exchange region). A recent extension of this work, based on differences in $O_3$ removal in the upper respiratory tract and in fraction exhaled, suggests that humans have about twice the deposition rate at the respiratory acinus as rats (81). Thus, the effects seen in the long-term inhalation animal studies are likely to be conservative estimates of the effects that occur in humans who live in areas that routinely have high levels of $O_3$, such as Southern California.

Interpretation of the nature and significance of the inflammatory responses following short-term $O_3$ exposures is difficult without knowledge of the cumulative effects that may be triggered by repetitive episodes of lung inflammation. The relation of the inflammatory responses, if any, to the well-studied respiratory function responses also remains unknown. We do know that these responses are poorly correlated. In a recent report, Balmes et al. (82) tested the hypothesis that changes in lung function induced by $O_3$ are correlated with indices of respiratory tract injury/inflammation. They exposed 20 healthy subjects, on separate days, to $O_3$ (0.2 ppm) and filtered air for 4 hours during exercise. Symptom questionnaires were administered before and after exposure, and pulmonary function tests ($FEV_1$, FVC, and $SR_{aw}$) were performed before, during, and immediately after each exposure. Fiberoptic bronchoscopy, with isolated left main bronchus proximal airway lavage (PAL) and BAL (bronchial fraction, the first 10 ml of fluid recovered) of the right middle lobe, was performed 18 hours after each exposure. The PAL, bronchial fraction, and BAL fluids were analyzed for the following end points: total and differential cell counts, and total protein, fibronectin, IL-8, and granulocyte-macrophage colony-stimulating factor (GM-CSF) concentrations. The study population was divided into two groups: least sensitive ($n = 12$; mean $O_3$-induced change in $FEV_1 = -7.0\%$) and most sensitive ($n = 8$; mean $O_3$-induced change in $FEV_1 = -36.0\%$). They found a highly significant $O_3$ effect on $SR_{aw}$ and lower respiratory symptoms for all subjects combined, but no significant differences between the least- and most-sensitive groups. Ozone exposure increased significantly percent neutrophils in PAL; percent neutrophils, total protein, and IL-8 in bronchial fraction ($p < 0.001$, $p < 0.001$, and $p < 0.01$, respectively); and percent neutrophils, total protein, fibronectin, and GM-CSF in BAL for all subjects combined; there were no significant differences, however, between least- and most-sensitive groups. Thus, levels of $O_3$-induced symptoms and respiratory tract injury/inflammation were not correlated with the magnitude of decrements in $FEV_1$ and FVC.

### Lung Infectivity

Studies in vivo and in vitro have demonstrated that $O_3$ can affect the ability of the immune system to defend against infection. Increased susceptibility to bacterial infection has been reported in mice exposed to 80 to 100 ppb $O_3$ for a single 3-hour period (83–85). Related alterations of the pulmonary defenses caused by short-term exposure to $O_3$ include impaired ability to inactivate bacteria in rabbits and mice (86–89), impaired macrophage phagocytic activity, mobility, fragility, and membrane alterations, and reduced lysosomal enzymatic activity. Some of these effects have been shown to occur in a variety of species, including mice, rats, rabbits, guinea pigs, dogs, sheep, and monkeys.

Other studies indicate similar effects for mice after short-term or "subchronic" exposure to $O_3$ combined with pollutants such as $SO_2$, $NO_2$, $H_2SO_4$ and particles (90–92). The activity level of mice exposed to $O_3$ has been shown to play a role in determining the lowest effective concentration that alters immune defenses (93). In addition, the duration of exposure must be considered. In groups of mice exposed to 200 ppb $O_3$ for 1, 3, or 6 hours, superoxide anion radical production decreased 8%, 18%, and 35%, respectively, indicating a progressive decrease in bactericidal capacity with increasing duration of exposure (94). The major limitation of this large body of data on the influence of inhaled $O_3$ on lung infectivity in animals is that it requires interspecies extrapolation in order to estimate the possible effects on infectivity in humans.

## EFFECTS ON LUNG STRUCTURE AND CONTROLLED EXPOSURE STUDIES

Most of the inhaled $O_3$ penetrates beyond the sites in the airways that trigger the functional responses. In this deeper region of the lung, at and just beyond the terminal bronchioles, the effects produced by $O_3$ include changes in biochemical indices, lung inflammation, and airway structure. Furthermore, the effects of $O_3$ exposure in this region appear to be cumulative and persistent, even in animals that have adapted to the exposure in terms of respiratory mechanics (25).

In a series of inhalation studies rats were exposed to $O_3$ at constant concentrations of either 120 or 250 ppb for 12 hours per day for 6 and 12 weeks, or to a daily cycle with a baseline of 60 ppb for 15 hours with a broad peak for 8 hours averaging 180 ppb for a period of 3 to 12 weeks. Huang and colleagues (95) found that hyperplasia of type I alveolar cells in the proximal alveoli was linearly related to the cumulative $O_3$ dose in the four groups. Thus, there is no apparent threshold for cumulative lung damage.

For some chronic effects, intermittent exposure can produce greater effects than continuous exposure and a larger cumulative dose. For example, Tyler and colleagues (96) exposed two groups of 7-month-old male monkeys to 250 ppb $O_3$ for 8 hours per day, either daily or, in the seasonal model, on days of alternate months during a total exposure period of 18 months. A control group breathed only filtered air. Monkeys from the seasonal exposure model, but not those exposed daily, had significantly greater total lung collagen content, chest wall compliance, and inspiratory capacity. All monkeys exposed to $O_3$ had respiratory bronchiolitis with significant increases in related morphometric parameters. The only significant morphometric difference between seasonal- and daily-exposure groups was in the volume fraction of macrophages. Even though the seasonally exposed monkeys were exposed to the same concentration of $O_3$ for only half as many days, they had greater biochemical and physiologic alterations and equivalent morphometric changes to those exposed daily. Lung growth was not completely normal in either exposed group. Thus, long-term effects of oxidant air pollutants that have a seasonal occurrence may depend more on the sequence in which they breathe polluted and clean air than on the total number of days of pollution, and estimates of the risks of human exposure to seasonal air pollutants from effects observed in animals exposed daily may underestimate long-term pulmonary damage.

## STUDIES OF POPULATIONS EXPOSED TO OZONE IN AMBIENT AIR

Epidemiologic studies of populations living in Southern California suggest that chronic oxidant exposure does affect baseline respiratory function. Detels and colleagues (97) compared respiratory function at two points in time 5 years apart in Glendora (a high oxidant community) and in Lancaster (a lower oxidant community, though not low by national standards). Baseline function was lower in Glendora, and there was a greater rate of decline over 5 years. Table 1 shows a comparison of the annual change in lung function in Lancaster and Glendora from the Detels study (97) with that reported for Tucson, Arizona by Knudson and colleagues (98) for a comparable population of Caucasian nonsmokers. The second highest 1-hour $O_3$ concentrations in Tucson in all of 1981, 1982, and 1983 were, respectively, 100, 120, and 110 ppb (1). In Lancaster there were 58 days in 1985 when the 1-hour $O_3$ maximum was greater than 120 ppb, while in Azusa, adjacent to Glendora, there were 117 days in 1985 with a 1-hour $O_3$ maximum greater than 120 ppb. Thus, the three different rates of function decline in Table 1 appear to suggest an exposure-response relationship that may be significant for health. Kilburn and co-workers (99) reported that nonsmoking and ex-smoking wives of Long Beach shipyard workers had significantly lower values for $FEV_1$, midexpiratory flow, terminal expiratory flow, and carbon monoxide-diffusing capacity than those in a matched population from Michigan. The oxidant levels in Long Beach and Michigan are not known, but those in Long Beach are similar to those in Lancaster, whereas those in Michigan are generally much lower. Both of these epidemiologic studies have some serious methodologic deficiencies, but they deserve citation in this discussion because they suggest effects that are consistent with the findings in the chronic animal exposure studies (i.e., they suggest premature aging of the lung, in terms of lung function, which might be expected on the basis of the cumulative changes in lung structure seen in animals in chronic exposure protocols).

Further evidence for chronic effects of $O_3$ were recently reported by Schwartz (100) based on an analysis of pulmonary function data in a national population study in 1976 to 1980, the second National Health and Nutrition Examination Survey (NHANES II). Using ambient $O_3$ data from yearly monitoring sites, he reported a highly significant $O_3$-associated reduction in lung function for people living in areas where the annual average $O_3$ concentrations exceeded 40 ppb.

As discussed previously, asthmatic children may respond to ambient $O_3$ in terms of increased frequency of unscheduled medication usage, increased respiratory symptoms, and decreased peak expiratory flow rates (36). People with preexisting pulmonary disease may also respond to short-term $O_3$ exposures in terms of increased hospital admissions and emergency room visits.

A number of epidemiologic studies have shown a consistent relationship between ambient oxidant exposure and acute respiratory morbidity in the population. Decreased lung function and increased respiratory symptoms, including exacerbation of asthma, occur with increasing ambient $O_3$, especially in children. Modifying factors, such as ambient temperature, aeroallergens, and other co-pollutants (e.g., particles) also can contribute to this relationship. Ozone air pollution can account for a portion of summertime hospital admissions and emergency room visits for respiratory causes. The results of studies conducted in various locations in the eastern United States and Canada, summarized in Table 2, are consistent in terms of showing relationships between ambient $O_3$ concentrations and increased incidence of

**TABLE 1.** *Annual change in lung function in various studies of ozone exposure*

| Population (no.) | $FEV_1$ (ml) | FVC (ml) | $FEF_{25-75}$ (ml/sec) | $\dot{V}_{50}$ (ml/sec) | $\dot{V}_{75}$ (ml/sec) | $O_3$ > NAAQS (d/yr) |
|---|---|---|---|---|---|---|
| Males | | | | | | |
| Tucson (86)[a] | −29 | −30 | −36 | −37 | −23 | ~1[d] |
| Lancaster (153)[b] | −46 | −51 | −47 | −65 | −44 | +58[e] |
| Glendora (168)[b] | −48 | −60 | −89 | −112 | −69 | +117[f] |
| Females | | | | | | |
| Tucson (176)[c] | −19 | −17 | −31 | −24 | −25 | ~1[d] |
| Lancaster (286)[b] | −33 | −38 | −53 | −77 | −41 | +58[e] |
| Glendora (325)[b] | −44 | −44 | −97 | −109 | −76 | +117[f] |

[a]White, non–Mexican-American, younger than 25 years who never smoked (96).
[b]White, non-Spanish surnames only, 19 to 59 years old who never smoked (95). Test results were between baseline and retest 5 years later. None had changed job or residence because of a respiratory problem (97).
[c]White, non–Mexican-American, aged > 20 but < 70 years who never smoked (96).
[d]Second highest 1-hour ozone levels for 1981, 1982, and 1983 were 0.10, 0.12, 0.11 ppm.
[e]Data from ref. 97.
[f]Data for Azusa (3 mi from Glendora) from ref. 97.

**TABLE 2.** *Summary of effect estimates for ozone in recent studies of respiratory hospital admissions*

| Location | Reference | Respiratory admission category | Effect size (± SE) (Admissions/100 ppb $O_3$/ day/$10^6$ persons) | Relative risk (95% CI)[a] (RR of 100 ppb $O_3$, 1-hour max) |
|---|---|---|---|---|
| New York City, NY[b] | Thurston et al. (109) | All | 1.4 (± 0.5) | 1.14 (1.06 to 1.22) |
| Buffalo, NY[b] | Thurston et al. (109) | All | 3.1 (± 1.6) | 1.25 (1.04 to 1.46) |
| Ontario, Canada[b] | Burnett et al. (110) | All | 1.4 (± 0.3) | 1.10 (1.06 to 1.14) |
| Toronto, Canada[b] | Thurston et al. (111) | All | 2.1 (± 0.8) | 1.36 (1.13 to 1.59) |
| Montreal, Canada[c] | Delfino et al. (112) | All | 1.4 (± 0.5) | 1.22 (1.09 to 1.35) |
| Birmingham, AL[d] | Schwartz (113) | Pneumonia in elderly | 0.73 (± 0.54) | 1.11 (0.97 to 1.26) |
| Birmingham, AL[d] | Schwartz (113) | COPD in elderly | 0.83 (± 0.33) | 1.13 (0.92 to 1.39) |
| Detroit, MI[d] | Schwartz (114) | Pneumonia in elderly | 0.82 (± 0.26) | 1.22 (1.12 to 1.35) |
| Detroit, MI[d] | Schwartz (114) | COPD in elderly | 0.90 (± 0.41) | 1.25 (1.07 to 1.45) |
| Minneapolis, MN[d] | Schwartz (115) | Pneumonia in elderly | 0.41 (± 0.19) | 1.117 (1.03 to 1.39) |
| Minneapolis, MN[d] | Schwartz (115) | COPD in elderly | [e] | [e] |

[a]One-way (β ± 1.65 SE).
[b]1-hour daily maximum ozone data employed in analysis.
[c]8-hour daily maximum ozone data employed in analysis.
[d]24-hour daily average ozone data employed in analysis (1 hour/24 hour average ratio = 2.5 assumed to compute effects and RR estimates).
[e]Not reported (nonsignificant).

visits and admissions, even after controlling for modifying factors, as well as when considering only concentrations < 120 ppb $O_3$. It has been estimated from these studies that $O_3$ may account for roughly one to three excess summertime respiratory hospital admissions per 100 ppb $O_3$, per million persons.

Ambient $O_3$ concentrations have also been associated with respiratory disease visits to emergency rooms (ERs) by Cody et al. (101), White et al. (102), and Weisel et al. (103).

There have also been reports of excess daily mortality in association with ambient $O_3$ concentrations in Los Angeles (67) and New York (104), but a subsequent report by Kinney et al. (105), using multiple regression analysis, suggested that the excess mortality was more closely associated with particulate matter than with $O_3$.

## EFFECTS OF OTHER POLLUTANTS ON RESPONSES TO OZONE

An important study that addressed the issue of the potentiation of the characteristic functional response to inhaled $O_3$ by other environmental cofactors was performed in Tuxedo, New York (37). It involved healthy adult nonsmokers engaged in a daily program of outdoor exercise with exposures to an ambient mixture containing low concentrations of acidic aerosols and $NO_2$ as well as $O_3$. Each subject did the same exercise each day, but exercise intensity and duration varied widely between subjects, with minute ventilation ranging from 20 to 153 L (average 79 L) and with duration of daily exercise ranging from 15 to 55 minutes (average 29 minutes). Respiratory function measurements were performed immediately before and after each exercise period. Ozone concentrations during exercise ranged from 21 to 125 ppb. All measured functional indices showed significant ($p < 0.01$) $O_3$-associated mean decrements.

The functional decrements in the adults (37) were similar, in proportion to lung volume, to those seen in children engaged in supervised recreational programs in summer camps (31). As shown in Table 3, the functional decrements in the field studies of the children in the field studies were as large ($FEV_1$) or much larger [FVC, $FEF_{25-75}$, peak expiratory flow rate (PEFR)] than those seen in controlled 2-hour exposures of children in chambers. For the subgroup of seven boys and three girls in the Spektor et al. (31) study who had the most comparable levels of physical activity, the responses in the field study were even greater. Also, since the ambient exposure of the adults who exercised outdoors was about a half hour, as compared to the 1- or 2-hour exposures of the adults in the chamber studies, it was concluded that ambient cofactors potentiate the responses to $O_3$. Thus, it is reasonable to conclude that the results of the exposure in chambers to $O_3$ in purified air are milder than the responses to $O_3$ in ambient air that occur among populations engaged in normal outdoor recreational activity.

The study on exercising adults and earlier studies on children at summer camps (31,57) were not able to demonstrate the specific effect of any of the measured environmental variables, including heat stress and acid aerosol concentration, on the $O_3$-associated responses. The inability to show the individual effects of other environmental cofactors on the response to ambient $O_3$ may be due to inadequate knowledge of the appropriate biologic averaging time for these other factors. However, in the study of functional responses of children to ambient pollution in Mendham, New Jersey, a week-long baseline shift in PEFR was associated with both $O_3$ and $H_2SO_4$

**TABLE 3.** *Mean functional changes per part per billion ozone after moderate or heavy exercise—comparison of results from field and chamber exposure studies*

| Investigator, subjects, age (yr) | Minute ventilation (L) | Exposure (exercise) time (min) | Ozone concentration (ppb) | Mean rate of functional change: FVC (ml/ppb) | FEV$_1$ (ml/ppb) | FEF$_{25-75\%}$ (ml/s/ppb) |
|---|---|---|---|---|---|---|
| Folinsbee (42), 10 M, 18–33 | 40 | 395 (300) | 120[c] | -0.38 | -4.5 | -5.0 |
| McDonnell (29), 22 M, 22.3 ± 3.1[a] | 65 | 120 (60) | 120[c] | -1.4 | -1.3 | -2.9 |
| 20 M, 23.3 ± 2.0[a] | 65 | 120 (60) | 180[c] | -1.8 | -1.6 | -3.0 |
| Kulle (30), 20 M, 25.3 ± 4.1[a] | 68 | 120 (60) | 150[c] | -0.5 | -0.2 | -2.1 |
| Linn (17), 24 M, 18–33 | 68 | 120 (60) | 160[c] | -0.7 | -0.6 | -1.1 |
| Spektor (37), | | | | | | |
| 1 M, 9 F, 28–44 | 38.4 ± 12.3[a] | 34.4 ± 9.9[a] | 21–124[b] | -1.9 | -1.8 | -6.7 |
| 7 M, 3 F, 22–40 | 64.6 ± 10.0[a] | 26.7 ± 8.7[a] | 21–124[b] | -2.9 | -3.0 | -9.7 |
| Spektor (31), 53 M, 38 F, 7–13 | | 150–550 | 19–113[b] | -1.0 | -1.4 | -2.5 |
| Avol (54), 33 M, 33 F, 8–11 | 22 | 60 (60) | 113[b] | -0.3 | -0.3 | |
| Avol (55), 46 M, 13 F, 12–15 | 32 | 60 (60) | 150[c] | -0.7 | -0.8 | -0.7 |
| McDonnell (56), 23 M, 8–11 | 39 | 150 (60) | 120[c] | -0.3 | -0.5 | -0.6 |

[a]Mean ± SD.
[b]Ozone concentration within ambient mixture.
[c]Ozone concentration within purified air.

exposure during a 4-day pollution episode that preceded it (56). A similar response to a brief episode with elevated $O_3$ and a much higher peak 4-hour concentration of $H_2SO_4$ (46 μg/m$^3$) was seen among girls attending a summer camp at Dunnville, Ontario, on the northeast shore of Lake Erie in 1986 (106).

Exposure to $O_3$ can also alter the responsiveness of the airways to other bronchoconstrictive challenges as measured by changes in respiratory mechanics. For example, Folinsbee and colleagues (42) reported that airway reactivity to the bronchoconstrictive drug methacholine for the group of subjects as a whole was approximately doubled following 6.6 hours' exposure to 120 ppb. Airway hyperresponsiveness (to histamine) had previously been demonstrated, but only at ozone concentrations of at least 400 ppb (43,44). On an individual basis, Folinsbee's group found no apparent relationship between the $O_3$-associated changes in methacholine reactivity and those in FVC or $FEV_1$. In contrast, changes in function after inhalation of $H_2SO_4$ aerosol correlated closely with changes in reactivity to carbachol aerosol, a bronchoconstrictive drug (45). Perhaps the $O_3$-associated changes in bronchial reactivity predispose persons to bronchospasm from other environmental agents such as acid aerosol and naturally occurring aeroallergens.

A variety of pollutant interactions that potentiate other characteristic $O_3$ responses have been reported in controlled exposure studies in animals. Last (107) reported synergistic interaction in rats, in terms of a significant increase in lung protein content, following 9 days' exposure at 200 ppb $O_3$ with 20 or 40 μg/m$^3$ $H_2SO_4$, and an insignificant increase for 9 days at 200 ppb $O_3$ with 5 μg/m$^3$ $H_2SO_4$. Pinkerton and co-workers (108) reported that clearance of asbestos fibers from the lungs of rats was reduced when the rats were also exposed to $O_3$. This increased fiber retention could increase the fibrogenic and carcinogenic risks of asbestos.

The ability of $O_3$ and other toxicants to act synergistically indicates that exposure limits for $O_3$ should include an extra margin of safety against the possibility of coexposures to ubiquitous copollutants such as $O_3$, $NO_2$, $H_2SO_4$, and asbestos, which are likely to be found in many work environments.

## EXPOSURE-RESPONSE RELATIONSHIPS

In terms of the transient effects of $O_3$ on respiratory function in individuals, the effects appear to increase in proportion to exposure duration up to 6 hours (41,42) for $O_3$ concentrations down to 60 ppb (31). In terms of populations, there is a broad range of responsiveness among healthy young adults and children, and lesser responses among smokers, older people, and persons with asthma, allergic rhinitis, and chronic obstructive pulmonary disease. On the other hand, among persons with preexisting lung disease milder responses may be more significant because of their reduced respiratory capacity (2).

Dose-response relationships to lasting effects on baseline lung function (95) and structure (93) are less firmly established, but the available data suggest that such effects also increase in proportion to cumulative dose.

## MINIMIZING EFFECTS FROM OZONE

The only two ways to reduce the effects of ambient $O_3$ are to reduce exposure and to reduce activity level during times of peak exposures. Exposure levels are generally much lower inside homes, offices, and commercial buildings than outdoors, since there are few significant indoor sources of $O_3$, and its chemical reactivity causes rapid loss of outdoor $O_3$ that infiltrates indoors. People who exercise outdoors can reduce their $O_3$ uptake by exercising before about 10:00 A.M., when the outdoor $O_3$ concentration begins to rise rapidly.

Occupational environments that warrant examination for excessive exposure include rooms that contain copying machines and the breathing zone of arc welders. Excessive exposures can generally be much reduced by appropriate application of exhaust ventilation.

## ACKNOWLEDGMENTS

This research was supported, in part, by Cooperative Agreement CR811563 from the U.S. Environmental Protection Agency, and Contract HEI 96-1 from the Health Effects Institute. It is part of a Center Program supported by grant ES00260 from the National Institute of Environmental Health Sciences.

## REFERENCES

1. *Air quality criteria for ozone and other photochemical oxidants.* EPA publication 600/P-93/004F. Research Triangle Park, NC: U.S. Environmental Protection Agency, 1996.
2. *Review of the National Ambient Air Quality Standards for Ozone-Preliminary Assessment of Scientific and Technical Information.* OAQPS Staff Paper, June 1996. EPA publication 452/R-96-007.
3. *Urban Ozone and the Clean Air Act:* problems and proposals for change. *Oceans and Environment Program.* OTA publication 20510-8025. Washington, DC: Office of Technology Assessment, U.S. Congress, 1988.
4. Air contaminants; final rule (29 CFR 1910). *Federal Register* 1989;54 (12):2332–2983.
5. *Threshold limit values and biological exposure indices for 1996.* Cincinnati, OH: American Conference of Governmental Industrial Hygienists, 1996.
6. Rombout PJA, van Bree L, Heisterkamp SH, Marra M. The need for an eight-hour standard. In: Schneider T, Lee SD, Wolters GJR, Grant LD, eds. *Atmospheric ozone research and its policy implications.* Nijmegen, The Netherlands: Elsevier, 1989;700–710.
7. Hazucha MJ. Relationship between ozone exposure and pulmonary function changes. *J Appl Physiol* 1987;62:1671–1680.
8. McDonnell WF, Horstman DH, Abdul-Salaam S, House DE. Reproducibility of individual responses to ozone exposure. *Am Rev Respir Dis* 1985;131:36–40.
9. Seal E Jr, McDonnell WF, House DE, et al. The pulmonary response of white and black adults to six concentrations of ozone. *Am Rev Respir Dis* 1993;147:804–810.
10. Kagawa J. Exposure-effect relationship of selected pulmonary function measurements in subjects exposed to ozone. *Int Arch Occup Environ Health* 1984;53:345–358.
11. Shephard RJ, Urch B, Silverman F, Corey PN. Interaction of ozone and cigarette smoke exposure. *Environ Res* 1983;31:125–137.
12. Drechsler-Parks DM, Bedi JF, Horvath SM. Pulmonary function responses of older men and women to ozone exposure. *Exp Gerontol* 1987;22:91–101.
13. Reisenauer CS, Koenig JQ, McManus MS, Smith MS, Kusic G, Pierson WE. Pulmonary response to ozone exposures in healthy individuals aged 55 years or greater. *JAPCA* 1988;38:51–55.
14. McDonnell WF, Muller KE, Bromberg PA, Shy CM. Predictors of individual differences in acute response to ozone exposure. *Am Rev Respir Dis* 1993;147:818–825.
15. McDonnell WF, Stewart PW, Andreoni S, Smith MV. Proportion of moderately exercising individuals responding to low-level, multi-hour ozone exposure. *Am J Respir Crit Care Med* 1995;152:589–596.
16. Koenig JQ, Covert DS, Marshall SG, van Belle G, Pierson WE. The effects of ozone and nitrogen dioxide on pulmonary function in healthy and in asthmatic adolescents. *Am Rev Respir Dis* 1987;136: 1152–1157.
17. Linn WS, Jones MP, Bachmeyer EA, et al. Short-term respiratory effects of polluted air: a laboratory study of volunteers in a high-oxidant community. *Am Rev Respir Dis* 1980;121:243–252.
18. Scannell C, Chen L, Aris RM, et al. Greater ozone-induced inflammatory responses in subjects with asthma. *Am J Respir Crit Care Med* 1996;154:24–29.
19. McDonnell WF, Horstman DH, Abdul-Salaam S, Raggio LJ, Green JA. The respiratory responses of subjects with allergic rhinitis to ozone exposure and their relationship to non-specific airway reactivity. *Toxicol Ind Health* 1987;3:507–517.
20. Linn WS, Shamoo DA, Venet TG, et al. Response to ozone in volunteers with chronic obstructive pulmonary disease. *Arch Environ Health* 1983;38:278–283.
21. Solic JJ, Hazucha MJ, Bromberg PA. The acute effects of 0.2 ppm ozone in patients with chronic obstructive pulmonary disease. *Am Rev Respir Dis* 1982;125:664–669.
22. Farrell BP, Kerr HD, Kulle TJ, Sauder LR, Young JL. Adaptation in human subjects to the effects of inhaled ozone after repeated exposure. *Am Rev Respir Dis* 1979;119:725–730.
23. Folinsbee LJ, Bedi JF, Horvath SM. Respiratory responses in humans repeatedly exposed to low concentrations of ozone. *Am Rev Respir Dis* 1980;121:431–439.
24. Hackney JD, Linn WS, Mohler JG, Collier CR. Adaptation to short-term respiratory effects of ozone in men exposed repeatedly. *J Appl Physiol* 1977;43:82–85.
25. Horvath SM, Gliner JA, Folinsbee LJ. Adaptation to ozone: duration of effect. *Am Rev Respir Dis* 1981;123:496–499.
26. Kulle TJ, Sauder LR, Kerr HD, Farrell BP, Bermel MS, Smith DM. Duration of pulmonary function adaptation to ozone in humans. *Am Ind Hyg Assoc J* 1982;43:832–837.
27. Folinsbee LJ, Horstman DH, Kehrl HR, Harder S, Salaam SA, Ives PJ. Respiratory response to repeated prolonged exposure to 0.12 ppm ozone. *Am J Respir Crit Care Med* 1994;149:98–105.
28. Tepper JS, Costa DL, Lehmann JR, Weber MF, Hatch GE. Unattenuated structural and biochemical alterations in the rat lung during functional adaptation to ozone. *Am Rev Respir Dis* 1989;140:493–501.
29. McDonnell WF, Horstman DH, Hazucha MJ, et al. Pulmonary effects of ozone exposure during exercise: dose-response characteristics. *J Appl Physiol* 1983;54:1345–1352.
30. Kulle TJ, Sauder LR, Hebel JR, Chatham MD. Ozone response relationships in healthy nonsmokers. *Am Rev Respir Dis* 1985;132: 36–41.
31. Spektor DM, Lippmann M, Lioy PJ, et al. Effects of ambient ozone on respiratory function in active normal children. *Am Rev Respir Dis* 1988;137:313–320.
32. Kinney PL, Ware JH, Spengler JD. A critical evaluation of acute ozone epidemiology results. *Arch Environ Health* 1988;43:168–173.
33. Hoek G, Fischer P, Brunekreef B, Lebret E, Hofschreuder P, Mennen MG. Acute effects of ambient ozone on pulmonary function of children in the Netherlands. *Am Rev Respir Dis* 1993;147:111–117.
34. Spengler JD, Keeler GJ, Koutrakis P, Ryan PB, Raizenne M, Franklin CA. Exposures to acidic aerosols. *Environ Health Perspect* 1989;79: 43–51.

35. Linn WS, Avol EL, Shamoo DA, et al. Repeated laboratory ozone exposures of volunteer Los Angeles residents: an apparent seasonal variation in response. *Toxicol Ind Health* 1988;4:505–520.
36. Thurston GD, Lippmann M, Scott MB, Fine JM. Summertime haze air pollution and children with asthma. *Am J Respir Crit Care Med* 1997;155:654–660.
37. Spektor DM, Lippmann M, Thurston GD, et al. Effects of ambient ozone on respiratory function in healthy adults exercising outdoors. *Am Rev Respir Dis* 1988;138:821–828.
38. Selwyn BJ, Stock TH, Hardy RJ, et al. Health effects of ambient ozone exposure in vigorously exercising adults. In: Lee SD, ed. *Evaluation of the scientific basis for ozone/oxidants standards:* Proceedings of an APCA International Specialty Conference, *November 1984, Houston TX.* Pittsburgh, PA: Air Pollution Control Association; 1985;281–296. (APCA International Specialty Conference Transactions: TR-4.)
39. Brunekreef B, Hoek G, Brugelmans O, Leentvaar M. Respiratory effects of low-level photochemical air pollution in amateur cyclists. *Am J Respir Crit Care Med* 1994;150:962–966.
40. Korrick SA, Neas LM, Dockery DW, et al. Respiratory effects of ambient ozone on adults hiking on Mount Washington. *Am J Respir Crit Care Med* 1995;151(4):A497.
41. Brauer M, Blair J, Vedal S. Effect of ambient ozone exposure on lung function in farm workers. *Am J Respir Crit Care Med* 1996;154: 981–987.
42. Folinsbee LJ, McDonnell WF, Horstman DH. Pulmonary function and symptom responses after 6.6 hour exposure to 0.12 ppm ozone with moderate exercise. *JAPCA* 1988;38:28–35.
43. Horstman DH, Folinsbee LJ, Ives PJ, Abdul-Salaam S, McDonnell WF. Ozone concentration and pulmonary response relationships for 6.6-hour exposures with five hours of moderate exercise to 0.08, 0.10, and 0.12 ppm. *Am Rev Respir Dis* 1990;142:1158–1163.
44. Seltzer J, Bigby BG, Stulbarg M, et al. $O_3$-induced change in bronchial reactivity to methacholine and airway inflammation in humans. *J Appl Physiol* 1986;60:1321–1326.
45. Holtzman MJ, Cunningham JH, Sheller JR, Irsigler GB, Nadel JA, Boushey H. Effect of ozone on bronchial reactivity in atopic and nonatopic subjects. *Am Rev Respir Dis* 1979;120:1059–1067.
46. Utell MJ, Morrow PE, Speers DM, Darling J, Hyde RW. Airway responses to sulfate and sulfuric acid aerosols in asthmatics. *Am Rev Res Dis* 1983;128:444–450.
47. Folinsbee LJ, Hazucha MJ. Persistence of ozone-induced changes in lung function and airway responsiveness. In: Schneider T, Lee SD, Wolters GJR, Grant LD, eds. *Atmospheric ozone research and its policy implications.* Nijmegen, The Netherlands: Elsevier, 1989; 483–492.
48. Gong H Jr, Bedi JF, Horvath SM. Inhaled albuterol does not protect against ozone toxicity in nonasthmatic athletes. *Arch Environ Health* 1988;43:46–53.
49. Jorres R, Nowak D, Magnussen H, Speckin P, Koschyk S. The effect of ozone exposure on allergen responsiveness in subjects with asthma or rhinitis. *Am J Respir Crit Care Med* 1996;153:56–64.
50. Gordon T, Taylor BF, Amdur MO. Ozone inhibition of tissue cholinesterase in guinea pigs. *Arch Environ Health* 1981;36:284–288.
51. Beckett WS, Freed AN, Turner C, Menkes HA. Prolonged increased responsiveness of canine peripheral airways after exposure to $O_3$. *J Appl Physiol* 1988;64(2):605–610.
52. Hayes SR, Moezzi M, Wallsten TS, Winkler RL. *An analysis of symptom and lung function data from several human controlled ozone exposure studies (draft final report).* San Rafael, CA: Systems Applications, 1987.
53. Linder J, Herren D, Monn C, Wanner HU. The effect of ozone on physical activity. *Schweiz Z Sportmed* 1988;36:5–10.
54. Avol EL, Linn WS, Shamoo DA, et al. Short-term respiratory effects of photochemical oxidant exposure in exercising children. *JAPCA* 1987;37:158–162.
55. Avol EL, Linn WS, Shamoo DA, Valencia LM, Anzar UT, Hackney JD. Respiratory effects of photochemical oxidant air pollution in exercising adolescents. *Am Rev Respir Dis* 1985;132:619–622.
56. McDonnell WF III, Chapman RS, Leigh MW, Strope GL, Collier AM. Respiratory responses of vigorously exercising children to 0.12 ppm ozone exposure. *Am Rev Respir Dis* 1985;132:875–879.
57. Lioy PJ, Vollmuth TA, Lippmann M. Persistence of peak flow decrement in children following ozone exposures exceeding the national ambient air quality standard. *JAPCA* 1985;35:1068–1071.
58. Altshuller AP. Eye irritation as an effect of photochemical air pollution. *JAPCA* 1977;27:1125–1126.
59. National Research Council. Toxicology. In: *Ozone and other photochemical oxidants.* Washington, DC: National Academy of Sciences, 1977;323–387.
60. Hammer DI, Hasselblad V, Portnoy B, Wehrle PF. Los Angeles student nurse study: daily symptom reporting and photochemical oxidants. *Arch Environ Health* 1974;28:255–260.
61. Schwartz J, Zeger S. Passive smoking, air pollution, and acute respiratory symptoms in a diary study of student nurses. *Am Rev Respir Dis* 1990;141:62–67.
62. Schoettlin CE, Landau E. Air pollution and asthmatic attacks in the Los Angeles area. *Public Health Rep* 1961;76:545–548.
63. Holguin AH, Buffler PA, Contant CF Jr, et al. The effects of ozone on asthmatics in the Houston area. *Trans APCA* TR-4, 1985;262–280.
64. Whittemore A, Korn E. Asthma and air pollution in the Los Angeles area. *Am J Public Health* 1980;70:687–696.
65. Ostro BD, Rothschild S. Air pollution and acute respiratory morbidity: an observational study of multiple pollutants. *Environ Res* 1989; 50:238–247.
66. Bates DV, Sizto R. The Ontario air pollution study: identification of the causative agent. *Environ Health Perspect* 1989;79:69–72.
67. Ozkaynak H, Kinney PL, Burbank B. Recent epidemiological findings on morbidity and mortality effects of ozone. Presented at the annual meeting of Air and Waste Management Association, Pittsburgh, 1990. Preprint 90-150.6.
68. Foster WM, Costa DL, Langenback EG. Ozone exposure alters tracheobronchial mucociliary function in humans. *J Appl Physiol* 1987; 63:996–1002.
69. Kenoyer JL, Phalen RF, Davis JR. Particle clearance from the respiratory tract as a test of toxicity: effect of ozone on short and long term clearance. *Exp Lung Res* 1981;2:111–120.
70. Schlesinger RB, Driscoll KE. Mucociliary clearance from the lungs of rabbits following single and intermittent exposures to ozone. *J Toxicol Environ Health* 1987;20:125–134.
71. Lippmann M, Gearhart JM, Schlesinger RB. Basis for a particle size-selective TLV for sulfuric acid aerosols. *Appl Ind Hyg* 1987;2: 188–199.
72. Driscoll KE, Vollmuth TA, Schlesinger RB. Early alveolar clearance of particles in rabbits undergoing acute and subchronic exposure to ozone. *Fundam Appl Toxicol* 1986;7:264–271.
73. Kehrl HR, Vincent LM, Kowalsky RJ, et al. Ozone exposure increases respiratory epithelial permeability in humans. *Am Rev Respir Dis* 1987;135:1174–1178.
74. Koren HS, Devlin RB, Graham DE, et al. Ozone-induced inflammation in the lower airways of human subjects. *Am Rev Respir Dis* 1989; 139:407–415.
75. Koren H, Devlin RB, Graham D, Mann R, McDonnell WF. The inflammatory response in human lung exposed to ambient levels of ozone. In: Schneider T, Lee SD, Wolters GJR, Grant LD, eds. *Atmospheric ozone research and its policy implications.* Amsterdam, The Netherlands: Elsevier, 1989;745–753.
76. Devlin RB, McDonnell WF, Mann R, et al. Exposure of humans to ambient levels of ozone for 6.6 hours causes cellular and biochemical changes in the lung. *Am J Respir Cell Mol Biol* 1991;4:72–81.
77. Graham D, Henderson F, House D. Neutrophil influx measured in nasal lavages of humans exposed to ozone. *Arch Environ Health* 1988; 43:228–233.
78. Graham DE, Koren HS. Biomarkers of inflammation in ozone-exposed humans: comparison of the nasal and bronchoalveolar lavage. *Am Rev Respir Dis* 1990;142:152–156.
79. Kinney PL, Nilsen DM, Lippmann M, et al. Biomarkers of lung inflammation in recreational joggers exposed to ozone. *Am J Respir Crit Care Med* 1996;154:1430–1435.
80. Overton JH, Miller FJ. Modelling ozone absorption in lower respiratory tract. Presented at the 1987 Annual Meeting of the Air Pollution Control Association, New York, June 1987. Preprint 87-99.4.
81. Gerrity TR, Wiester MJ. Experimental measurements of the uptake of ozone in rats and human subjects. Presented at the 1987 annual meeting of the Air Pollution Control Association, New York, June 1987. Preprint 87-99.3.
82. Balmes JR, Chen LL, Scannell C, et al. Ozone-induced decrements in $FEV_1$ and FVC do not correlate with measures of inflammation. *Am J Respir Crit Care Med* 1996;153:904–909.

83. Coffin DL, Blommer EJ, Gardner DE, Holzman R. Effect of air pollution on alteration of susceptibility to pulmonary infection. In: *Proceedings of the Third Annual Conference on Atmospheric Contamination in Confined Spaces.* Report AMRL-TR-67-200. Springfield, VA: 1967;71–80.
84. Ehrlich R, Findlay JC, Fenters JD, Gardner DE. Health effects of short-term inhalation of nitrogen dioxide and ozone mixtures. *Environ Res* 1977;14:223–231.
85. Miller FJ, Illing JW, Gardner DE. Effects of urban ozone levels on laboratory-induced respiratory infections. *Toxicol Lett* 1978;2:163–169.
86. Coffin DL, Gardner DE, Holzman RS, Wolock FJ. Influence of ozone on pulmonary cells. *Arch Environ Health* 1968;16:633–636.
87. Coffin DL, Gardner DE. Interaction of biological agents and chemical air pollutants. *Ann Occup Hyg* 1972;15:219–235.
88. Goldstein BD, Hamburger SJ, Falk GW, Amoruso MA. Effect of ozone and nitrogen dioxide on the agglutination of rat alveolar macrophages by concanavalin A. *Life Sci* 1977;21:1637–1644.
89. Ehrlich R, Findlay JC, Gardner DE. Effects of repeated exposures to peak concentrations of nitrogen dioxide and ozone on resistance to streptococcal pneumonia. *J Toxicol Environ Health* 1979;5:631–642.
90. Ehrlich R. Interaction between environmental pollutants and respiratory infections. *Environ Health Perspect* 1980;35:89–100.
91. Graham JA, Gardner DE, Blommer EJ, House DE, Menache MG, Miller FJ. Influence of exposure patterns of nitrogen dioxide and modifications by ozone on susceptibility to bacterial infectious disease in mice. *J Toxicol Environ Health* 1987;21:113–125.
92. Grose EC, Richards JH, Illing JW, et al. Pulmonary host defense responses to inhalation of sulfuric acid and ozone. *J Toxicol Environ Health* 1980;10:351–362.
93. Illing JW, Miller FJ, Gardner DE. Decreased resistance to infection in exercised mice exposed to $NO_2$ and $O_3$. *J Toxicol Environ Health* 1980;6:843–851.
94. Amoruso MA, Goldstein BD. Effect of 1, 3, and 6-hour ozone exposure on alveolar macrophages superoxide production. *Toxicologist* 1988;8:197.
95. Huang Y, Chang LY, Miller FJ, Graham JA, Ospital JJ, Crapo JD. Lung injury caused by ambient levels of oxidant air pollutants: extrapolation from animal to man. *Am J Aerosol Med* 1988;1:180–183.
96. Tyler WS, Tyler NK, Last JA, Gillespie MJ, Barstow TJ. Comparison of daily and seasonal exposures of young monkeys to ozone. *Toxicology* 1988;50:131–144.
97. Detels R, Tashkin DP, Sayre JW, et al. The UCLA population studies of chronic obstructive respiratory disease. 9. Lung function changes associated with chronic exposure to photochemical oxidants: a cohort study among never-smokers. *Chest* 1987;92:594–603.
98. Knudson RJ, Lebowitz MD, Holberg CJ, Burrows B. Changes in the normal maximal expiratory flow-volume curve with growth and aging. *Am Rev Respir Dis* 1983;127:725–734.
99. Kilburn KH, Warshaw R, Thornton JC. Pulmonary functional impairment and symptoms in women in the Los Angeles harbor area. *Am J Med* 1985;79:23–28.
100. Schwartz J. Lung function and chronic exposure to air pollution: a cross-sectional analysis of NHANES II. *Environ Res* 1989;50: 309–321.
101. Cody RP, Weisel CP, Birnbaum G, Lioy PJ. The effect of ozone associated with summertime photochemical smog on the frequency of asthma visits to hospital emergency departments. *Environ Res* 1992; 58:184–194.
102. White MC, Etzel RA, Wilcox WD, Lloyd C. Exacerbations of childhood asthma and ozone pollution in Atlanta. *Environ Res* 1994;65:56–68.
103. Weisel CP, Cody RP, Lioy PJ. Relationship between summertime ambient ozone levels and emergency department visits for asthma in central New Jersey. *Environ Health Perspect* 1995;103(suppl 2):97–102.
104. Kinney PL, Ozkaynak H. Associations between ozone and daily mortality in Los Angeles and New York City. *Am Rev Respir Dis* 1992; 145(4), A95.
105. Kinney PL, Ito K, Thurston GD. A sensitivity analysis of mortality/PM-10 associations in Los Angeles. *Inhal Toxicol* 1995;7:59–69.
106. Raizenne ME, Burnett RT, Stern B, Franklin CA, Spengler JD. Acute lung function responses to ambient acid aerosol exposures in children. *Environ Health Perspect* 1989;79:179–185.
107. Last JA. Effects of inhaled acids on lung biochemistry. *Environ Health Perspect* 1989;79:115–119.
108. Pinkerton KE, Brody AR, Miller FJ, Crapo JD. Exposure to low levels of ozone results in enhanced pulmonary retention of inhaled asbestos fibers. *Am Rev Respir Dis* 1989;140:1075–1081.
109. Thurston GD, Ito K, Kinney PL, Lippmann M. A multi-year study of air pollution and respiratory hospital admissions in three New York State metropolitan areas: results for 1988 and 1989 summers. *J Expo Anal Environ Epidemiol* 1992;2:429–450.
110. Burnett RT, Dales RE, Raizenne ME, et al. Effects of low ambient levels of ozone and sulfates on the frequency of respiratory admissions to Ontario hospitals. *Environ Res* 1994;65:172–194.
111. Thurston GD, Ito K, Hayes CG, Bates DV, Lippmann M. Respiratory hospital admissions and summertime haze air pollution in Toronto, Ontario: consideration of the role of acid aerosols. *Environ Res* 1994; 65:271–290.
112. Delfino RJ, Becklake MR, Hanley JA. The relationship of urgent hospital admissions for respiratory illnesses to photochemical air pollution levels in Montreal. *Environ Res* 1994a;67:1–19.
113. Schwartz J. Air pollution and hospital admissions for the elderly in Birmingham, Alabama. *Am J Epidemiol* 1994;139:589–598.
114. Schwartz J. Air pollution and hospital admissions for the elderly in Detroit, Michigan. *Am J Respir Crit Care Med* 1994;150:648–655.
115. Schwartz J. $PM_{10}$, ozone, and hospital admissions for the elderly in Minneapolis, MN. *Arch Environ Health* 1994;49:366–374.

*Environmental and Occupational Medicine, Third Edition,* edited by William N. Rom.
Lippincott–Raven Publishers, Philadelphia © 1998.

CHAPTER 40

# Nitrogen Dioxide/Nitric Oxide

Richard B. Schlesinger

Nitrogen dioxide ($NO_2$) and nitric oxide (NO) belong to a group of gaseous chemicals collectively known as nitrogen oxides ($NO_x$). This categorization also includes nitrous oxide ($N_2O$), nitrogen trioxide ($NO_3$), dinitrogen trioxide ($N_2O_3$), dinitrogen tetroxide ($N_2O_4$), and dinitrogen pentoxide ($N_2O_5$). Except for $N_2O$, the various $NO_x$ are interconvertible and many of them coexist in the atmosphere. However, from an occupational and environmental exposure and health perspective, the materials of most concern are NO and $NO_2$.

Nitric oxide is a water-insoluble, odorless, and colorless gas. Nitrogen dioxide, a stable free radical, is a relatively water-insoluble, reddish-orange-brown gas having a very pungent odor; it is highly corrosive and highly reactive as an oxidizing agent. The health effects database for $NO_2$ is much greater than that for NO, and the former is also more toxic.

## SOURCES AND EXPOSURES

Anthropogenic ambient $NO_x$ emissions, which annually average about 20 million metric tons (1), derive from high temperature combustion processes of both mobile and stationary sources. The major mobile source is the internal combustion engine, while the major stationary source is electric power generation using fossil fuels, with industrial processes a close second.

Under high temperature conditions, nitrogen derived from the combustion air and/or the fuel being used reacts with atmospheric oxygen. Most of the $NO_x$ initially produced is in the form of NO, but this is generally rapidly oxidized to $NO_2$. In some operations, e.g., where nitric acid is used as a reactant in acid dipping processes, much of the $NO_x$ will be released as $NO_2$. Because the conversion rate of NO to $NO_2$ depends on a number of factors, including the initial concentration of NO and the operating temperature of the combustion process, the distribution of NO and $NO_2$ generated from industrial sources is quite variable.

The pattern of outdoor $NO_2$ concentration in urban areas is characterized by a background level superimposed onto which are two daily peaks related to motor vehicle traffic patterns in the morning and afternoon. The atmosphere in areas having significant stationary sources is characterized by baseline $NO_2$ levels that have spikes superimposed on an irregular basis. In areas not impacted by any significant local sources, $NO_2$ levels have little variation on an hourly basis throughout the day, unless there is transport of $NO_2$ into that region.

Annual average outdoor concentrations of $NO_2$ in most regions of the country are in the 0.015 to 0.035 ppm range, with levels in major urban areas tending toward the high end and those in nonmetropolitan or more rural areas toward the low (1). However, some metropolitan areas, most notably Southern California, may show annual averages of about 0.06 ppm. While short-term levels follow a pattern similar to yearly means, with 24-hour average levels generally $\leq$0.17 ppm and 1-hour averages $\leq$0.3 ppm in major metropolitan areas, hourly averages or short-term peaks in many regions can exceed 0.5 ppm at least once during the year. In most areas of the United States, $NO_2$ levels are highest in the summer. However, Southern California is characterized by elevated $NO_2$ throughout the year.

Maximum hourly average NO concentrations range from 0.17 to 1 ppm in metropolitan areas, with annual averages in the range of 0.01 to 0.06 ppm (1). Rural areas

R. B. Schlesinger: Department of Environmental Medicine, New York University School of Medicine, New York, New York 10016.

show maximum hourly averages of 0.01 to 0.4 ppm and annual averages of 0.005 to 0.009 ppm.

Nitrogen dioxide is a widespread indoor pollutant in households. Since nonoccupational indoor concentrations and exposures are generally higher than those outdoors when significant sources, such as gas-fired ranges, kerosene heaters, and improperly or unvented gas space heaters, are present, indoor exposure is commonly the main contributor to total exposure. The indoor/outdoor ratio of $NO_2$, when there are no indoor sources, is 0.5 to 0.6, and is generally lower in winter than in summer (2). On the other hand, when indoor sources are present, the ratio is >1 and is higher in the winter. Nitrogen oxides are also major components of smoke derived from the burning of tobacco products. Cigarette smoke contains high levels of NO, which is oxidized to $NO_2$ as the smoke ages.

Indoor levels of $NO_2$ vary widely depending on strength of the sources and the degree of ventilation. Furthermore, because combustion from indoor sources tends to be episodic, very high short-term concentrations are possible. Daily (24-hour average) levels in homes with gas-fired stoves, ovens, or heaters can average 0.05 to 0.5 ppm and can reach peak levels >1 ppm (1,3–5). Indoor concentrations of NO are not commonly reported and, thus, data are limited. Levels of NO associated with gas cooking may reach daily mean peaks of 0.4 ppm (3), but generally are about 0.1 ppm.

Potential occupational sources of $NO_x$ exposure are diverse. Exposures may occur with welding using oxyacetylene flames; glassblowing; working near internal combustion engines, such as in parking lots; underground blasting operations, such as occur in mining; storage of silage in agricultural operations; manufacture of nitric acid, oxidized cellulose compounds, lacquers and dyes, and rocket propellants and fertilizers; brazing; metal cleaning; textile (rayon) and food bleaching; and fire fighting. At least 1.5 million workers are potentially exposed to $NO_x$ in the course of their occupation.

The amount of $NO_x$ found in occupational settings is very variable, but may reach fairly high values. For example, $NO_2$ concentrations of 50 to 250 ppm may be produced during high-temperature oxyacetylene welding processes, while up to several hundred parts per million may occur in freshly filled agricultural silos due to fermentation of stored silage (6,7). More constant, lower-level exposures may occur in some occupations. For example, railroad workers can be regularly exposed to up to 0.12 ppm $NO_2$ derived from diesel exhaust (8). High concentrations of NO may occur in certain clinical settings when it is used as a therapeutic agent, such as in the treatment of pulmonary hypertension (9,10).

Table 1 lists occupational and environmental exposure limits for NO and $NO_2$.

**TABLE 1.** *Exposure limits for nitrogen oxides*

| Oxide | Limit |
|---|---|
| Nitric oxide | |
| TLV[a] | 25 ppm |
| PEL[b] | 25 ppm |
| REL[c] | 25 ppm |
| IDLH[d] | 100 ppm |
| Nitrogen dioxide | |
| NAAQS[e] | 0.053 ppm |
| PEL[f] | 1 ppm |
| REL[g] | 1 ppm |
| EEGL[h] | 1 ppm |
| TLV[a] | 3 ppm |
| STEL[i] | 5 ppm |
| IDLH[d] | 50 ppm |

[a]Threshold limit value (ACGIH; time weighted average for an 8-hour workday and a 40-hour workweek).
[b]Permissible exposure limit (OSHA; time weighted average for an 8-hour workday).
[c]Recommended exposure limit (NIOSH; time weighted average for an 8-hour workday).
[d]Immediately dangerous to life and health (NIOSH; 30-minute average).
[e]National ambient air quality standard (EPA; annual average).
[f]Permissible exposure limit (OSHA; ceiling for 15-minute exposure).
[g]Recommended exposure limit (NIOSH; ceiling for 15-minute exposure).
[h]Emergency exposure guidance level (NAS; 1-hour exposure).
[i]Short-term exposure limit (ACGIH; ceiling for 15-minute exposure).
ACGIH, American Conference of Governmental Industrial Hygienists; EPA, Environmental Protection Agency; NAS, National Academy of Science; NIOSH, National Institute for Occupational Safety and Health; OSHA, Occupational Safety and Health Administration.

## DOSIMETRY

The exposure route for NO and $NO_2$ is inhalation. A large percentage of inhaled $NO_2$ is removed within the respiratory tract; absorption of up to 90% of the amount inhaled occurs in both humans and laboratory animals. Absorption occurs along the entire tracheobronchial tree and within the respiratory region, but the major dose to tissue is delivered at the transition zone of the lungs, i.e., the junction between the conducting and respiratory (alveolated) airways (11). Beyond this zone, a dramatic falloff in dose delivered to tissue occurs due to the rapid increase in lung surface area.

The primary determinant of $NO_2$ uptake is surface reactivity (12), i.e., direct interaction with airway lining fluid constituents and/or cellular components. While $NO_2$ does not penetrate through the airway epithelium unreacted, the specific substrate(s) with which it initially interacts have not been elucidated with certainty. Dissolution in airway lining fluid followed by hydrolysis could produce nitric ($HNO_3$) and nitrous acids ($HNO_2$), which could then subsequently exert toxic effects due directly to the hydrogen ion or to formation of nitrite ion. On the other hand, the primary reaction of $NO_2$ may be with tissue components such as unsaturated fatty acids, amino acids, and/or proteins, producing nitrite ions or various radicals. Because of these potential tissue substrates, a major target of $NO_2$ is the cell membrane.

The uptake of $NO_2$ within the respiratory tract is influenced by ventilatory factors. Increased ventilation, such as during exercise or certain occupational tasks, reduces uptake in both the upper respiratory tract and tracheobronchial tree, increasing the amount of $NO_2$ delivered to the respiratory region. For example, nasal uptake in humans was noted to be 44% at rest and only 15% with exercise (13).

Little is known about NO absorption, and even less about its subsequent distribution. However, unlike $NO_2$, most absorbed NO crosses epithelial surfaces unreacted. The lower solubility of NO results in greater amounts reaching the respiratory region, where it can diffuse into the blood and react with hemoglobin, producing methemoglobin (14).

Absorbed NO and $NO_2$ are both excreted in the urine, primarily as nitrate ion. Because of the ubiquitous nature of nitrate, there have been various attempts to identify other biologic markers for exposure to $NO_2$ that would allow for determination of dose. Some suggestions are urinary hydroxyproline excretion (15), NO-heme protein complex in bronchial lavage (16), and 3-nitrotyrosine in urine (17). However, because of their lack of sensitivity and/or specificity, there is still no useful marker for environmental $NO_2$ exposure.

## NITROGEN DIOXIDE

### Acute High-Level Exposure

One of the problems in assessing effects of $NO_2$ is that, in many early studies, especially those related to occupational exposure, concentrations have been reported variously as nitrogen oxides, nitrous gases, or even as NO. Thus, it is sometimes difficult to determine actual $NO_2$ exposures for intercomparison between studies. In any case, acute exposure to high concentrations may occur in various occupational situations, and reported illnesses from such exposure clearly indicate toxicity.

Exposure to 1 to 5 ppm $NO_2$ may result in mild intoxication, consisting of transient, nonspecific symptoms, such as cough, headache, fatigue, and nausea, which can dissipate over hours to days postexposure or can last up to 2 weeks. Frank acute respiratory irritation may occur at 15 to 25 ppm, with nausea, cough, irritation of eyes and throat, and dyspnea. Again, such symptoms may persist for days to weeks, or subside a few hours after exposure ends, depending on the concentration. Exposure to 25 to 100 ppm results in pneumonia and bronchiolitis that may be reversible, while exposure at levels >150 ppm is generally fatal, due to laryngospasm or bronchospasm occurring immediately or to bronchiolitis obliterans and pulmonary edema occurring with a delay; 500 ppm produces fatal edema within 48 hours of exposure. Arterial hypoxemia is often observed with $NO_2$ exposure. This results primarily from impaired diffusion capacity due to edema, but can also be due to the production of methemoglobin resulting from the reaction of nitrite ions with hemoglobin (18); however, the extent to which inhaled $NO_2$ results in methemoglobin formation is likely low (19). The clinical presentation following nonlethal exposure to high levels of $NO_2$ can include fever and chills and, because of this, such exposure can simulate other respiratory diseases, such as influenza, pneumonia, or acute bronchitis. Table 2 outlines some clinical features of high-level $NO_2$ exposure.

The clinical presentation following certain exposures to $NO_2$ is commonly characterized by delayed responses. Initial symptoms, including acute pulmonary edema, may be followed by an apparent recovery which is then, in turn, followed in 2 to 3 weeks by dyspnea, fever, cyanosis, and severe, prolonged respiratory distress due to edema and bronchiolitis obliterans. While such delayed responses are very characteristic of acute, high-level exposure, they are also seen with exposure to lower levels, even below 3 ppm (20).

A number of descriptions of the clinical pattern following $NO_2$ inhalation are available. Milne (21) noted that a proportion of patients exposed to "nitrous fumes" (an early term for $NO_x$) exhibited a biphasic clinical pattern. Exposure was followed by a latent period of hours, acute respiratory distress, then apparent recovery over a period of at least 2 to 3 weeks. The final stage was a sudden onset of severe respiratory distress. Some individuals who survive the initial stage may fully recover within 2 to 3 weeks, while others may have impaired pulmonary function that persists for years (18). On the other hand, death from respiratory failure may occur in either the initial or final stages following exposure. Becklake et al.

**TABLE 2.** *Some clinical features of $NO_2$ intoxication*

| Symptom | Time course[a] |
|---|---|
| Nausea, vomiting | Acute |
| Local irritation | Acute |
| Laryngospasm/bronchospasm | Acute |
| Respiratory arrest (reflex) | Acute |
| Shortness of breath | Acute |
| Pulmonary edema | Acute |
| Bronchiolitis obliterans | Chronic |
| Neurologic symptoms | Chronic |
| Dyspnea | Chronic |
| Death | Acute or chronic |

[a]Acute, effects develop in hours to days; chronic, effects develop in weeks to months.

Adapted from ref. 153.

(22) categorized the reaction to $NO_x$ into three types: type 1, acute pulmonary edema, occurring after a latent period of 30 hours with apparent recovery, if not initially fatal; type 2, biphasic, with bronchiolitis obliterans, acute symptoms, then recovery, followed by progressive development of dyspnea; and type 3, chemical pneumonia, with gradual deterioration.

Hospitalization of patients with significant $NO_2$ exposure is indicated. Treatment is supportive therapy, and should include oxygen and ventilatory support; corticosteroids have been used to retard or abort the proliferative cellular phase of inflammatory bronchiolitis. Pulmonary physiologic manifestations of acute high-level exposure involve initial reduction of lung volumes and diffusing capacity, followed by reduced dynamic compliance and normal spirometry characteristic of small airways dysfunction (23). Radiology in the initial stage following exposure may range from normal to evidence of transient lung infiltrates. Miliary mottling is common as effects progress.

Silo-filler's disease is one of the best-known conditions resulting from high-level $NO_2$ inhalation. The conversion of nitrate to nitrite in recently ensiled plant material results in the generation of $NO_2$, as well as other $NO_x$. An individual who enters the silo 18 hours to 10 days after fresh silage has been stored, generally in the late summer or autumn, may complain of being "choked," and later of a "smothered" sensation. Severity of response depends on the $NO_x$ concentration (which can exceed 500 ppm) and duration of exposure. Symptoms, which resemble those of flu, i.e., fever, chills, cough, chest pain, and dyspnea, may be delayed, and death may follow noncardiogenic pulmonary edema or subsequent bronchiolitis obliterans (21,24,25). Chronic pulmonary insufficiency may be present in those who do recover (26).

Oxides of nitrogen may also be hazards from fires. The 1929 Cleveland Clinic fire, which burned thousands of nitrocellulose based x-ray films, released nitric oxide, carbon monoxide (CO), and hydrogen cyanide (HCN). There were 97 workers who died immediately due to CO and HCN; 26 fatalities that occurred more than 2 hours and less than 1 month after the exposure were most likely due to $NO_x$ (27).

Recently, $NO_2$ emissions from indoor ice skating rink resurfacer machines have been suggested as responsible for respiratory symptoms, e.g., cough and dyspnea, in both hockey players and spectators. In one situation, a concentration of 4 ppm $NO_2$ was measured in an ice skating rink when the resurfacer was operating for a half hour (28). Delayed onset pneumonitis ascribed to $NO_2$ exposure during an indoor ice hockey game has also been reported (29).

The odor threshold for $NO_2$ for most people is ~0.5 ppm. Sensitive individuals may detect a level as low as 0.1 ppm.

## Low-Level and Chronic Exposure

### *Toxicology*

The responses that follow acute accidental or occupational exposure clearly show that $NO_2$ has health consequences and have contributed to the understanding of possible effects associated with lower concentrations found in ambient outdoor and indoor air. The largest database concerning the biologic effects of $NO_2$ derives from laboratory animal exposures. While the mechanisms underlying many responses are similar across species and, thus, effects in laboratory animals may have implications for humans, the exposure concentrations needed for comparable responses likely differ between species. The main target for inhaled $NO_2$ is the respiratory tract and various aspects of responses in this organ system have been described.

Effects on lung defense mechanisms have received considerable attention in attempts to ascertain the potential health significance of exposure. The clearance of tracer particles from the tracheobronchial tree (due to mucociliary transport) or respiratory (alveolar) region of the lungs (due to macrophage activity) has been assessed as an index of nonspecific defense function following exposure to $NO_2$. Single acute exposures at ≤10 ppm did not alter mucociliary transport rate from the tracheobronchial tree of laboratory animals (30,31), while repeated exposures for 6 weeks to 6 ppm $NO_2$ resulted in transient depression of mucociliary activity (32). Alveolar clearance rates are altered by short-term repeated exposures to 0.3 ppm (33). The latter may be associated with changes in the function of alveolar macrophages, also seen at similar to higher concentrations (34–37). While both tracheobronchial and alveolar clearance studies support a graded response, whereby low $NO_2$ levels accelerate and high levels retard clearance, most effects of $NO_2$ on clearance seem to begin at higher than ambient levels.

Nitrogen dioxide impairs resistance to infectious agents, i.e., bacteria and viruses, in animals exposed to levels as low as 0.5 ppm for 3 months (35,38). A few infectivity studies involved exposure to a baseline level upon which spikes to a higher level were superimposed, so as to better mimic some ambient exposure conditions. The relative effect of such spikes is not clear, but seems to depend on both spike duration and time between spikes. Miller et al. (39) noted that mortality due to infection was greater in a spike regimen (to 0.8 ppm) than in a baseline-exposed group (0.2 ppm). Others have also found that mortality is influenced by both the number and amplitude of any spikes (40,41). In fact, effects from such exposure excursions may approach those due to more continuous exposure to a lower concentration. This is consistent with the notion that, in general, brief exposures to high $NO_2$ levels are more hazardous than are longer duration exposures to lower concentrations (42).

The effect of $NO_2$ on bacterial infectivity increases with both exposure duration and peak concentration, although the latter seems to have more influence than the former (40). Any differences between intermittent and continuous exposure also seem to disappear as the number of days of exposure increase. Furthermore, as concentration increases, a shorter exposure time is needed for intermittent and continuous exposure regimes to produce similar degrees of effect (43,44). Mortality due to infection is also proportional to exposure duration if the bacterial challenge is given immediately after exposure, but may not be when the challenge is given much later, suggesting that a critical time between $NO_2$ and bacterial exposure is needed for increased susceptibility.

The mechanism(s) underlying $NO_2$-induced increases in microbial infectivity are not known. However, since exposure levels that alter host resistance do not generally affect physical clearance processes, this response to $NO_2$ is likely due to impaired intracellular killing of microbes, probably due to macrophage dysfunction. For example, macrophages are a source of numerous biochemical mediators that are directly involved in antibacterial action; a depression in one of these, namely superoxide anion, has been noted following $NO_2$ exposure (36,45).

While changes in susceptibility to infectious agents are an indirect index of altered immune function, a number of studies have directly examined the effects of $NO_2$ exposure on specific parameters of both humoral and cellular immunity. While immune suppression follows exposure to $NO_2$ above 5 ppm (46,47), there are only a few reports of response to lower levels. These suggest that short-term repeated exposures may result in a reduction in counts of certain lymphocytes in the lungs or spleen, or a depression in antibody responsiveness to particular antigens (48–50). Enhanced immune function or increased immune cell numbers may follow $NO_2$ exposure (51,52), but this is just as detrimental as suppressed function, through overstimulation of response and hypersensitivity. As with other end points, the direction of change in immune system responses appears to depend on exposure concentration. For example, humoral response in monkeys chronically exposed to $NO_2$ was enhanced at a low concentration (1 ppm) but suppressed at a higher level (5 ppm) (53,54).

Exposure to $NO_2$ may affect allergic response. Rats exposed to 5 ppm for 3 hours after sensitization with house dust mite antigen had higher levels of serum IgE and local respiratory tract IgA, IgG, and IgE antibodies than did controls (55). The exposed animals also had increased lymphocyte activity in the spleen and local lymph nodes and showed an increase in respiratory tract inflammatory cells. This suggests that $NO_2$ may enhance immune responsiveness and increase the severity of pulmonary inflammation in sensitized lungs and may, thus, play some role in the exacerbation of immune-mediated respiratory disease (56).

Studies in animal models show that $NO_2$ exposure may produce morphologic alterations in the respiratory tract (57–60). The anatomic region most sensitive to $NO_2$, and within which injury is first noted, is the area encompassing the terminal and respiratory bronchioles and adjacent alveolar ducts and alveoli. Within this region, the ciliated cells of the bronchiolar epithelium and the type 1 cells of the alveolar epithelium are the primary targets. In the alveolar region, acute exposure to $NO_2$ results in hypertrophy and hyperplasia of type 1 cells, followed by death and desquamation of these cells and proliferation of and replacement by type 2 cells. The end result can be a thickened air-blood barrier. Bronchiolar response is characterized by hypertrophy and hyperplasia of epithelial cells, loss of secretory granules and surface protrusions in Clara cells, and loss of ciliated cells or cilia. With chronic exposure, many of these same changes are seen, but there is increased cilia loss over larger areas of epithelium and in more proximal airways and the structure of the remaining cilia may be altered.

The earliest alterations resulting from concentrations ≥2 ppm occur within 24 to 72 hours of continuous exposure. These include increased macrophage aggregation, desquamation of type 1 cells and ciliated bronchiolar cells, and accumulation of fibrin in small airways. Repair of injured tissue and replacement of destroyed cells can, however, begin within 24 to 48 hours of continuous exposure. The new cells in the bronchioli are derived from nonciliated cells, while in the alveoli the damaged type 1 cells are replaced with type 2 cells. These new cells are relatively resistant to any further effects of $NO_2$. Division of type 2 cells is observed within 12 hours after initial $NO_2$ exposure, the rate becoming maximal by about 48 hours and decreasing to preexposure levels by about 6 days, even with continued exposure. In some cases, the resolution of $NO_2$-induced morphologic changes may be complete after exposures end; on the other hand, some lesions may resolve while others remain, even when exposure continues.

Chronic exposure may result in alterations in lung architecture resembling emphysema-like disease, e.g., enlargement of airspaces, an increase in mean linear intercept (a measure of the distance between alveolar walls), and a reduction in the internal surface area of the alveolar region. However, the relationship between exposure and the development of emphysema remains unclear. A problem in evaluating reported emphysematic changes in animal models is the definition of the disease, which has changed over the years and which has been defined differently by various professional groups (61). While long-term exposure to high $NO_2$ concentrations (>10 ppm) are required to produce clearly definable emphysema-like changes (62), there is evidence that lower $NO_2$ levels may result in emphysema, emphysema-like changes, or altered alveolar dimensions if present in complex mixtures of $NO_x$ (63) or administered during lung development (64). However, clear evidence of changes characteristic of human emphysema, i.e., alveolar septal degeneration, enlarged airspaces, and associated functional changes, is absent, especially with exposure at low levels.

While the extent and degree of morphologic alterations induced by $NO_2$ appear to be related to exposure concentration, little is known about effects of other modifying factors, e.g., exposure duration or the temporal pattern of exposure. Concentration appears to play a more important role than exposure time in tissue injury (58,65), consistent with their relative roles in enhancing infectivity. The effect of concentration may be greater with intermittent than with continuous exposure, and the onset of response may also be delayed with intermittent compared to continuous exposure. The relative roles of exposure concentration and duration in eliciting responses may be end-point dependent, and dose rate or cumulative exposure may be more important than peak exposure for some end-points but not for others (66).

In spite of the fact that there is a fairly extensive database concerning morphologic effects of $NO_2$ in animal models, it is still quite difficult to establish a threshold exposure condition for this end-point. This is due to the great complexity of changes occurring with exposure, as well as to large interspecies differences in response. For example, the rat appears to be less sensitive to $NO_2$ compared to other species, such as the guinea pig or monkey. Furthermore, different cell types show differential sensitivity to $NO_2$. In general, morphologic alterations, some of which may be persistent, are found with chronic exposure to concentrations $<1$ ppm. However, long-term exposure to levels $\geq 2$ ppm are generally required to produce more extensive or permanent changes.

Nitrogen dioxide may induce biochemical changes in the lungs, such as oxidation of protein or protein components (67). Of importance in the pathogenesis of chronic lung disease are effects on lung structural proteins, such as elastin and collagen. Thickened collagen fibrils were noted in the lungs of $NO_2$ exposed monkeys (68), while increased rates of lung collagen synthesis, a possible marker for development of fibrosis, has been noted in exposed rats (69). A decrease in elastin may also be associated with the development of emphysema. Chronic exposure at high levels, i.e., about 10 ppm, are needed to increase collagen deposition within the lungs (70). Studies at high-exposure concentrations also suggest that $NO_2$ may reduce elastin content via an increase in the activity of neutrophil elastase, the enzyme responsible for elastin breakdown (71,72).

The effects of $NO_2$ on pulmonary mechanics have been studied in laboratory animals using various standard indices of pulmonary function and with mixed results (39,73,74). Perhaps of greater clinical significance is use of bronchoprovocation challenge testing to assess nonspecific airway responsiveness. However, it appears that exposure to high levels are needed to induce hyperresponsiveness with either acute or continuous exposure regimens (75,76). Thus, at levels that occur in ambient air, $NO_2$ does not seem to alter pulmonary mechanics or bronchial responsiveness in animal models undergoing acute or longer- term exposure; this is consistent with results of controlled clinical studies in humans, as discussed below.

The ability of $NO_2$ to induce cancer has been assessed by some investigators. Although not likely a carcinogen itself, $NO_2$ may modulate tumorogenic processes in the lungs (77). For example, exposure may, in conjunction with a specific carcinogen, be involved in the pathogenesis of small cell lung carcinoma (77); $NO_2$ has been shown to modulate the number of neuroendocrine cells, the precursor cells for this disease (78,79). As another example, an enhancement of tumor colonization in the lungs of mice injected (iv) with tumor (melanoma) cells was noted after exposure to $NO_2$ at 0.4 or 0.8 ppm for 8 hours a day, 5 days a week for 10 to 12 weeks (80). This may be due to injury of lung capillary endothelium by $NO_2$, facilitating metastases of blood-borne cancer cells to the lungs (81), or to suppression of immune system components, as discussed previously. But as with other end points, the database regarding the role of $NO_2$ in carcinogenic processes is conflicting. For example, $NO_2$ was found to actually enhance the cytotoxic response of macrophages (82), which implies greater antitumor defense capabilities. Thus, any role for $NO_2$ in cancer etiology requires further study.

### *Controlled Clinical Tests*

Controlled clinical tests of healthy human volunteers indicate that acute exposure (up to about 2 hours) at rest to $NO_2$ levels $\leq 1$ ppm does not result in any significant changes in pulmonary mechanics (29,83–85). Although there have been some reports showing positive effects at higher levels, there is no consistent pattern of response (86–88). Furthermore, exposures to $\leq 1$ ppm $NO_2$ in conjunction with various degrees of exercise have also resulted in inconsistent effects on the lung function of healthy people; most of the studies showed no effects that could be unequivocally attributed to $NO_2$ (89–91).

Increased nonspecific airway responsiveness in healthy subjects was noted following a 2-hour exposure to 7.5 ppm (86), with 1 hour to 2 ppm (87), and with 3 hours (with intermittent exercise) to 1.5 ppm (91). Again, however, the results are not consistent, with other studies at similar levels and exposure durations finding no such changes. Exposures to $\leq 0.6$ ppm have not produced any change in responsiveness at all (83,91,92). Treatment with an antioxidant may prevent $NO_2$-induced increased airway responsiveness (93), indicating that effects may be due to the oxidative ability of the gas.

Particular subsegments of the population may be especially susceptible to $NO_2$. One such group is asthmatics. A number of investigations have been performed at exposure levels from 0.1 to 4 ppm for durations ranging up to 4 hours, usually with exercise; effects on various aspects of lung mechanical function, such as spirometry or airway resistance, have ranged from none to slight, and all with much inconsistency (83,84,88,94–100). A study that measured pulmonary function in adult asthmatics in their home and monitored indoor $NO_2$ levels suggested that average exposures ≥0.3 ppm produced a decline in certain pulmonary function measures, while inconsistent effects were seen at lower exposure levels (5).

There is evidence that subgroups may exist within the asthmatic population that are especially sensitive to the effects of $NO_2$ (94). That is, the variability in responses may be the result of differences in the severity or type of asthma in the various subjects examined within one study or between studies. Asthmatics also exhibit a wide range of response to external stimuli, so variability may be due, to some extent, to interindividual variation in response to $NO_2$.

Another possibly sensitive subsegment of the population is people with chronic obstructive pulmonary disease (COPD), i.e., chronic bronchitis and emphysema. Increased airway resistance has been found in COPD individuals after exposure to 1.6 ppm in conjunction with exercise (101). On the other hand, no change in airway resistance has been noted in chronic bronchitics exposed to 0.5 ppm for 2 hours with exercise, or in spirometry of COPD patients exposed to 0.5 to 2 ppm for 1 hour, also with exercise (102,103).

The most sensitive pulmonary mechanical response to $NO_2$ in people with airway disease appears to involve changes in airway responsiveness. However, there is much variability in results from different studies and there is also an apparent lack of any dose-response relationship. While some studies have indicated increased responsiveness due to $NO_2$ exposures at 0.14 to 0.5 ppm (83,94,99), others have indicated no effects at similar, or even higher, levels (92,97,98,104,105).

In general, the clinical study database is not robust enough to allow determination of the specific exposure conditions, i.e., concentration, duration, and ventilation, for threshold effects on lung mechanical function in healthy humans with acute exposure. Pulmonary mechanics may, in fact, not be a very sensitive index of response. This is likely due to the tendency of such tests to reflect changes in the larger airways, while the major target for inhaled $NO_2$ is the smaller conducting airways and respiratory region. On the other hand, functional changes may occur in individuals with asthma and/or COPD following exposure to lower levels of $NO_2$ than affect normals. But, again, the results are inconsistent. The lowest $NO_2$ concentrations that have resulted in observed effects, albeit inconsistent, on airway responsiveness in exercising asthmatics are in the range of 0.2 to 0.5 ppm. It should be mentioned, however, that most mild asthmatics are not sensitive to $NO_2$ at ≤0.6 ppm, at least in terms of changes in pulmonary mechanics, while nonspecific airway responsiveness in mild asthmatics may be increased at levels >0.1 ppm. In normals, levels of about 5 ppm may cause bronchoconstriction, but minimum levels of at least 1 to 2 ppm are needed for changes in pulmonary functional parameters.

Controlled clinical studies have also examined effects of $NO_2$ on microbial infectivity. There is some suggestion that $NO_2$ may reduce the ability of the lungs to inactivate inhaled respiratory viruses (106). Increased infectivity in $NO_2$ exposed laboratory animals, together with the above suggestive findings, indicate that $NO_2$ may alter host defenses in humans.

Nitrogen dioxide has been associated with development of emphysema in animal models. A biochemical mechanism underlying the development of emphysema is a deficiency in proteinase inhibitor activity within the lungs, and $NO_2$-related morphologic injury may be mediated via enzyme inactivation. In this regard, humans exposed to 3 to 4 ppm for 3 hours showed a decrease in levels of $\alpha_1$-proteinase inhibitor in lung lavage fluid (107), although the investigators noted that the extent of the decrease was not associated with any increased risk of emphysema. However, as with other end points, these effects of $NO_2$ are not always reproducible, especially at low exposure levels (108). Thus, exposure of normal humans for 3 hours (with intermittent exercise) to 1.5 ppm, or for 3 hours to 0.05 ppm with three 2-ppm peaks, did not result in any change in activity of $\alpha_1$-proteinase inhibitor in lavage fluid (108) while a 3-hour exposure to 0.6 ppm resulted in increased levels of another antiprotease, $\alpha_2$-macroglobulin, in lung lavage (109). Effects of chronic exposures more relevant to ambient situations on these biochemical end points are unknown.

### *Epidemiology*

Epidemiologic studies attempt to directly analyze the role of ambient exposure to $NO_2$ in producing adverse human health effects, generally using indices of respiratory illness and/or changes in pulmonary mechanical function. While most early studies related health end points to outdoor concentrations, the current trend is to also rely on indoor levels. Although many epidemiologic studies are considered to be weak, due largely to a lack of reliable estimates of actual $NO_x$ exposure conditions, small sample sizes, inadequate compensation for the effects of covariates (such as cigarette smoking), and/or misclassification of health end points, they do provide a link between chronic laboratory animal studies and long-term exposure of humans.

In a series of epidemiologic surveys conducted in six cities in the United States (the "Six Cities Study") selected to represent a range of air quality, grade-school children within each community were followed for several years by reporting on questionnaires and by annual measurements of pulmonary function, while outdoor pollution levels were measured at various sites within each community. Indoor levels of $NO_2$ were also measured in selected households. Results of this study from 1974 to 1977 on over 8,000 children aged 6 to 10 years indicated there to be a significant increase in the rate of respiratory illness before age 2 in homes with gas-fired stoves compared to those with electric stoves (110). Estimated levels of exposure were 0.004 to 0.026 ppm $NO_2$. However, examination of the same communities over a longer time period, namely 1974 to 1979, did not show any statistically significant increase in respiratory illness in these young children (111). A later analysis from this study reported results from a sample of over 5,000 children aged 7 to 11 years during the period 1983 to 1986 (112). Marginal significance was noted for physician diagnosed respiratory illness prior to age 2 in homes using gas-fired stoves compared to those using electric stoves; estimated exposures to $NO_2$ were similar to those above.

Ware et al. (111) examined various pulmonary mechanical indices in the above children. The use of gas stoves was associated with significant reductions in parameters of expiratory flow forced [expiratory volume in 1 second ($FEV_1$), forced vital capacity (FVC)] in a first examination, but was found not to be significant in a second. Neas et al. (113), in another analysis of children from the Six Cities Study, noted increasing respiratory symptoms (wheeze, shortness of breath, phlegm) with increasing annual average indoor concentrations of $NO_2$, but no such relationship with pulmonary functional parameters.

A study that examined a sample of over 100 children in Tucson (114) found a borderline significant effect between peak flow reduction in healthy children in homes with gas stoves, while for asthmatics peak flow was highly significantly associated with use of such stoves; no measurements of indoor levels of $NO_2$ were performed. Vedal et al. (115) examined lung mechanics in children at Chestnut Ridge, Pennsylvania. $NO_2$ levels (outdoor) ranged from 0.006 to 0.042 ppm, and no effect on peak expiratory flow was found. Indoor levels were not measured.

Keller et al. (3,116) obtained reports of respiratory illness and symptoms from family members of all ages in various homes in Ohio. No significant difference was found between gas or electric cooking homes, and there was no evidence that the incidence of acute respiratory illness was associated with gas cooking. In another study (117), neither the incidence of lower respiratory tract illness nor the duration of such illness in infants up to 18 months of age residing in Albuquerque, New Mexico could be associated with indoor exposure to $NO_2$.

In a study involving examination of respiratory symptoms in adult women and children (aged 13 years and younger) in Connecticut (118), indoor $NO_2$ levels were measured in most of the homes (0.003 to 0.048 ppm) while personal samplers were also used in some cases to relate actual exposure to measured indoor levels. These two measures were found to be highly correlated. Children under the age of 7 exposed to $\geq$0.016 ppm were found to be at an increased risk of lower respiratory tract symptoms over those who were not so exposed; there was also an increased, but lesser, risk of upper respiratory symptoms. No increased risk was found in older children or adults. This study, however, was characterized by a lack of consistency across age groups, perhaps due to a small sample size.

Comstock et al. (119) noted a relationship between the use of gas stoves and increased prevalence of respiratory symptoms (cough) and reduction in some pulmonary function indices in adults in Maryland. Other studies have found no association between gas stove use and symptoms or lung function changes in children (120,121) or any association between such use and hospitalization for acute respiratory illness in children under 2 years of age (122).

A number of epidemiologic studies have been performed outside the United States. In one, the effects of both indoor and outdoor air pollution on respiratory illness in a cohort of primary-school children from randomly selected areas of Great Britain were examined (123). A gradient of increased respiratory symptoms with increasing indoor levels of $NO_2$ was noted in homes with gas stoves; no actual measurements of $NO_2$ were made. Later assessment (124) also indicated some increase in relative risk in homes with gas stoves, but this was not a consistent finding. In this case, levels of $NO_2$ were measured in bedrooms of gas stove homes, and ranged from 0.003 to 0.017 ppm. In another study (125), children aged 5 to 6 years were sampled from the same communities. No significant relationship was noted between levels of $NO_2$ and the prevalence of respiratory illness; levels of $NO_2$ in the bedrooms of gas stove homes were 0.005 to 0.029 ppm.

Gnehm et al. (126) examined common respiratory symptoms (e.g., cough, sore throat, etc.) in children up to 5 years of age in Switzerland. $NO_2$ was measured both indoors and outdoors. A respiratory symptom score was computed for each child to allow comparison between effects and exposure levels of $NO_2$. There was a statistically significant relationship between outdoor levels and this score, indicating an effect of $NO_2$. Mean levels outdoors were 0.013 to 0.028 ppm, while those indoors ranged from 0.006 to 0.018 ppm. Braun-Fahrlander et al. (128) examined respiratory symptoms in Swiss children, monitoring both indoor and outdoor levels of $NO_2$. The incidence of symptoms was not associated with either indoor or outdoor $NO_2$ concentrations, but the duration of increased symptoms was associated only with outdoor levels.

The effect of $NO_2$ on respiratory health in 6- to 9-year-old Dutch children was examined by Brunekreef et al. (128). Personal exposures to $NO_2$ were measured, as were indoor levels in the home. The prevalence of lung disease was found to be associated with the presence of unvented gas water heaters, with weekly exposures estimated (average) at 0.021 ppm. On the other hand, Dijkstra et al. (129) found no association between symptoms of chronic cough or shortness of breath with indoor $NO_2$ measurements in homes. Koo et al. (130) used personal samples to monitor $NO_2$ exposure in children aged 7 to 13 in Hong Kong. No association was noted between exposure levels (means ranged from 0.013 to 0.023 ppm for a 1-week period) and respiratory symptoms, such as wheeze, running nose, or cough. Moseler et al. (131) concluded that children in Freiburg, Germany with asthmatic symptoms appeared to be more susceptible to having reduced lung function when outdoor average $NO_2$ concentrations exceeded 0.02 ppm. No association was found with children without asthmatic symptoms.

It is not possible to provide any definitive conclusion regarding adverse health effects of $NO_2$ based on the epidemiologic database. This is due, to some extent, to inherent limitations in the methodology of such studies. There have been both positive and negative findings at various levels of $NO_2$ exposure and with various degrees of precision in measuring actual outdoor exposure levels and generally with gas stove use as a surrogate measure of indoor exposure. Some results are suggestive that an increase in acute respiratory illness, especially in young children, may be associated with chronic ambient exposure to $NO_2$ at concentrations generally found in the home or outdoors. But even so, any observed excess risk is quite low. Although this conclusion is by no means definitive, it is consistent with the increased bacterial infectivity found in toxicologic studies. The effects of short-term exposure to ambient peaks on acute respiratory illness are not known.

### Conclusion

While acute high-level exposure to $NO_2$ (or $NO_x$), which may occur accidentally or in occupational settings, has clear health consequences in humans, and exposure to high concentrations for extended periods can produce emphysema-like changes and alterations in anti-microbial defenses in animals, the extent to which adverse health effects may occur with long-term exposure to lower levels more relevant to ambient outdoor or indoor environments has not as yet been resolved. While some epidemiologic studies noted small effects of $NO_2$ on pulmonary function in children, most have not shown such associations, and only a few studies in adults indicate any adverse effect of $NO_2$ on pulmonary function. Furthermore, in many cases, there is inconsistent dose-response data. Although toxicologic studies provide indication of mechanisms of action, controlled clinical and epidemiologic studies have not resulted in a consistent pattern of responses that allows an unequivocal conclusion as to the potential effects on human health of ambient outdoor or indoor exposure to $NO_2$.

## NITRIC OXIDE

Nitric oxide is synthesized endogenously in the cells of many tissues (133). Low concentrations of NO are produced by constitutive enzymes, while higher concentrations are formed by enzymes that increase in amount through their induction upon exposure to certain cytokines or other mediators. Since endogenous NO is involved in numerous processes, such as nervous system signaling, regulation of pulmonary and systemic vascular resistance, and mediation of immune defenses, the impact of inhaled, exogenous NO, especially at low concentrations, is often difficult to evaluate.

The database for health effects of inhaled nitric oxide is not extensive, except for its interaction with blood. One problem is the difficulty in obtaining pure NO without some contamination with $NO_2$. A few studies have examined histologic responses to NO in laboratory animals. While some studies suggest that the lesions are similar to those with $NO_2$, except perhaps that NO levels needed to produce them are higher, i.e., ≥2 ppm with continuous exposure (46,133,134), recent work suggests that NO may actually be more potent than $NO_2$ for some morphologic injury, such as effects in interstitial spaces of alveolar septa (135). While little NO appears to react with lung tissue at exposure concentrations found in ambient outdoor or indoor air, with most diffusing into the blood, chronic exposure of rats to 0.5 ppm (with spikes to 1.5 ppm) produced interstitial lung damage (135).

The specific substrates and reactions that mediate NO toxicity are not clear. Some studies indicate that the toxic effects of NO are different from the membrane damage due to $NO_2$. For example, NO may target fibroblasts that are responsible for the maintenance and repair of the alveolar interstitium (135).

Data concerning physiologic effects of inhaled NO are sparse, and exposure levels used were high. Guinea pigs exposed for 0.5 hour twice weekly for 7 weeks to 5 ppm NO showed an increase in nonspecific airway responsiveness (136). No change in pulmonary mechanical function of guinea pigs exposed for 4 hours to NO at 16 or 50 ppm was found (137). Holt et al. (46) examined immunologic end points in mice exposed to 10 ppm NO for 2 hours a day, 5 days a week for up to 30 weeks. Leukocytosis was evident by 5 weeks of exposure, while a decrease in mean hemoglobin content of red blood cells was found by 30 weeks. The ability of spleen cells to mount a graft versus host reaction was stimulated by 20 weeks of exposure, but suppressed by 26 weeks. When the ability of mice to reject virus-induced tumors was assessed, less of the NO exposed animals survived tumor challenge compared to control; this suggests that NO at high levels may have affected the immunologic competence of the animals. In another study, (138), mice were exposed continuously to 2 ppm NO for 6 hours up to 4 weeks, to assess the effect on resistance to bacterial infection. There was some indication that NO-exposed females showed a significant increase in percentage mortality and a significant decrease in survival time that was not seen in males.

Following a 2-hour exposure of humans to 1 ppm, there appeared to be some variability in pulmonary function response among subjects, but only one of a large battery of tests showed statistical significance (139); it is likely that this effect, if not due to chance, has little biologic significance. On the other hand, vasodilation is a sensitive target for NO, and pulmonary vasodilation has been noted with acute exposure to 5 to 10 ppm in normal animals and humans (140).

Inhaled NO that enters the bloodstream binds to hemoglobin, producing nitrosylhemoglobin (NOHb) (19, 141–143). NOHb is easily and rapidly oxidized to methemoglobin (metHb) in the presence of oxygen (144,145). MetHb is subsequently converted into ferrous Hb by MetHb reductase, an enzyme present in red blood cells (146–148). As long as the activity of MetHb reductase is maintained, the conversion of NOHb to MetHb should, to a large extent, mitigate any toxicity of inhaled NO related to oxygen transport effects.

Nitric oxide appears to stimulate guanylate cyclase, which in turn leads to smooth muscle relaxation and vasodilation and nervous system effects (149). Nitric oxide can also react with thiol-associated iron in enzymes, which is a mechanism for cytotoxicity. Permanent modification of hemoglobin has also been noted due to NO (150). It can also react with superoxide, producing peroxynitrite that can then react with proteins (151). Many of these effects have been noted in vitro and offer potential explanations for effects of NO on host defenses. Whether they can explain any effects of NO inhalation exposure is not clear. There is, however, indication that, at least for some end points, effects of endogenous NO can be mimicked by exposure to exogenous NO (140). Furthermore, individuals with depressed endogenous NO may be more sensitive to inhaled NO.

In summary, a large fraction of inhaled NO reaches the respiratory region of the lungs, where it rapidly diffuses into blood and reacts with hemoglobin; unlike $NO_2$, little NO directly interacts with lung tissue, especially at low concentrations. In spite of any binding with hemoglobin, anoxia of $O_2$-sensitive organs does not seem to occur, at least with NO levels $\leq 10$ ppm. However, methemoglobinemia has been detected in workers exposed to high levels of NO. MetHb levels as high as 44% have been reported among silo fillers, and 2% to 3% among arc welders (the normal level is II <1%) (152). Methemoglobinemia may further complicate hypoxemia due to other responses to inhaled $NO_x$.

## ACKNOWLEDGMENT

The author's work cited in this chapter is part of a Center Program supported by the National Institute of Environmental Health Sciences (ES00260).

## REFERENCES

1. United States Environmental Protection Agency (USEPA). *Air quality criteria for oxides of nitrogen.* EPA/600/8-91/049aF. Washington, DC: USEPA, 1993.
2. Berglund M. Exposure. *Scand J Work Environ Health* 1993;19:14–20.
3. Keller MD, Lanese RR, Mitchell RI, Cote RW. Respiratory illness in households using gas and electricity for cooking. I. Survey of incidence. *Environ Res* 1979;19:495–503.
4. Spengler JD, Cohen MA. Emissions from indoor sources. In: Gammage RB, Kaye SV, eds. *Indoor air and human health.* Chelsea, MI: Lewis, 1985;261–278.
5. Goldstein IF, Lieber K, Andrews LR, et al. Acute respiratory effects of short-term exposures to nitrogen dioxide. *Arch Environ Health* 1988; 43:138–142.
6. Norwood WD, Wisehart DE, Earl CA, Adley FE, Anderson DE. Nitrogen dioxide poisoning due to metal-cutting with oxyacetylene torch. *J Occup Med* 1966;8:301–306.
7. Cummins BT, Ravency FJ, Jesson MW. Toxic gases in tower silos. *Ann Occup Hyg* 1971;14:275–283.
8. Woskie SR, Hammond SK, Smith TJ, Shenker MB. Current nitrogen dioxide exposures among railroad workers. *Am Ind Hyg Assoc J* 1989; 50:346–353.
9. Pepke-Zaba J, Higenbottam TW, Dinh-Xuan AT, Stone D, Wallwork J. Inhaled nitric oxide as a cause of selective pulmonary vasodilation in pulmonary hypertension. *Lancet* 1991;338:1173–1174.
10. Kinsella JP, Neish SR, Shaffer E, Abman SH. Low-dose inhalation nitric oxide in persistent pulmonary hypertension of the newborn. *Lancet* 1992;340:819–820.
11. Miller FJ, Overton JH, Myers ET, Graham JA. Pulmonary dosimetry of nitrogen dioxide in animals and man. In: Schneider T, Grant L, eds. *Air pollution by nitrogen oxides:* Proceedings of the U.S.-Dutch International Symposium. Studies in Environmental Science 21. Amsterdam, The Netherlands: Elsevier Scientific, 1982;377–386.
12. Postlethwait EM, Bidani A. Reactive uptake governs the pulmonary air space removal of inhaled nitrogen dioxide. *J Appl Physiol* 1990;68: 594–603.
13. Mohsenin V. Human exposure to oxides of nitrogen at ambient and supra-ambient concentrations. *Toxicology* 1994;89:301–312.
14. Ewetz L. Absorption and metabolic fate of nitrogen oxides. *Scand J Work Environ Health* 1993;19:21–27.
15. Adgate JL, Reid HF, Morris R, et al. Nitrogen dioxide exposure and urinary excretion of hydroxyproline and desmosine. *Arch Environ Health* 1992;47:376–384.
16. Maples KR, Sandström T, Su Y-F, Henderson RF. The nitric oxide/heme protein complex as a biological marker of exposure to nitrogen dioxide in humans, rats and in vitro models. *Am J Respir Cell Mol Biol* 1991;4:538–543.
17. Oshima H, Friesen M, Brouet I, Bartsch H. Nitrotyrosine as a new marker for endogenous nitrosation and nitration of products. *Food Chem Toxicol* 1990;28:647–652.
18. Horvath EP, doPico GA, Barbee RA, Dickie HA. Nitrogen dioxide-induced pulmonary disease. Five new cases and a review of the literature. *J Occup Med* 1978;20:103–110.
19. Oda H, Nogami H, Nakajima T. Reaction of hemoglobin with nitric oxide and nitrogen dioxide in mice. *J Toxicol Environ Health* 1980;6: 673–678.
20. Rasmussen TR, Kjaergaard SK, Tarp U, Pedersen OF. Delayed effects of $NO_2$ exposure on alveolar permeability and glutathione peroxidase in healthy humans. *Am Rev Respir Dis* 1992;146:654–659.

21. Milne JEH. Nitrogen dioxide inhalation and bronchiolitis obliterans: a review of the literature and report of a case. *J Occup Med* 1969;11:538–547.
22. Becklake MR, Goldman HI, Boxman AR, et al. The long-term effects of exposure to nitrous fumes. *Am Rev Tuber* 1957;76:398–409.
23. Fleming GM, Chester EH, Montenegro HD. Dysfunction of small airways following pulmonary injury due to nitrogen dioxide. *Chest* 1979;75:720–729.
24. Ramirez RJ, Dowell AR. Silo-fillers' disease-nitrogen dioxide-induced lung injury: long-term follow-up and review of the literature. *Ann Intern Med* 1971;74:569–576.
25. Scott EG, Hunt WB. Silo-fillers' disease. *Chest* 1973;63:701–706.
26. Leib GMP, Davis WN, Brown T, et al. Chronic pulmonary insufficiency secondary to Silo-fillers' disease. *Am J Med* 1958;24:471–474.
27. Gregory KL, Malinoski VF, Sharp CR. Cleveland clinic fire survivorship study, 1929–1965. *Arch Environ Health* 1969;18:508–515.
28. Hedberg K, Hedgery CW, Iber C, et al. An outbreak of nitrogen dioxide-induced respiratory illness among ice hockey players. *JAMA* 1989;262:3014–3017.
29. Karlson-Stiber C, Hojer J, Sjoholm A, Bluhm G, Salmonson H. Nitrogen dioxide pneumonitis in ice hockey players. *J Intern Med* 1996;239:451–456.
30. Abraham WM, Welker M, Oliver W Jr, et al. Cardiopulmonary effects of short-term nitrogen dioxide exposure in conscious sheep. *Environ Res* 1980;22:61–72.
31. Schlesinger RB. Comparative toxicity of ambient air pollutants: some aspects related to lung defense. *Environ Health Perspect* 1989;81:123–128.
32. Giordano AM Jr, Morrow PE. Chronic low-level nitrogen dioxide exposure and mucociliary clearance. *Arch Environ Health* 1972;25:443–449.
33. Vollmuth TA, Driscoll KE, Schlesinger RB. Changes in early alveolar particle clearance due to single and repeated nitrogen dioxide exposures in the rabbit. *J Toxicol Environ Health* 1986;19:255–266.
34. Greene ND, Schneider SL. Effects of $NO_2$ on the response of baboon alveolar macrophages to migration inhibitory factor. *J Toxicol Environ Health* 1978;4:869–880.
35. Ehrlich R, Findlay J, Gardner DE. Effects of repeated exposures to peak concentrations of nitrogen dioxide and ozone on resistance to streptococcal pneumonia. *J Toxicol Environ Health* 1979;5:631–642.
36. Suzuki T, Ikeda S, Kanoh T, Mizoguchi I. Decreased phagocytosis and superoxide anion production in alveolar macrophages of rats exposed to nitrogen dioxide. *Arch Environ Contam Toxicol* 1986;15:733–739.
37. Schlesinger RB. Intermittent inhalation of nitrogen dioxide: effects on rabbit alveolar macrophages. *J Toxicol Environ Health* 1987;21:127–139.
38. Rose RM, Fuglestad JM, Skornik WA, et al. The pathophysiology of enhanced susceptibility to murine cytomegalovirus respiratory infection during short-term exposure to 5 ppm nitrogen dioxide. *Am Rev Respir Dis* 1988;137:912–917.
39. Miller FJ, Graham JA, Raub JA, et al. Evaluating the toxicity of urban patterns of oxidant gases. II. Effects in mice from chronic exposure to nitrogen dioxide. *J Toxicol Environ Health* 1987;21:99–112.
40. Gardner DE, Miller FJ, Blommer EJ, Coffin DL. Influence of exposure mode on the toxicity of $NO_2$. *Environ Health Perspect* 1979;30:23–29.
41. Graham JA, Gardner DE, Blommer EJ, House DE, Menache MG, Miller FJ. Influence of exposure patterns of nitrogen dioxide and modifications by ozone on susceptibility to bacterial infectious disease in mice. *J Toxicol Environ Health* 1987;21:113–125.
42. Lehnert BE, Archuleta DC, Ellis T, et al. Lung injury following exposure of rats to relatively high mass concentrations of nitrogen dioxide. *Toxicology* 1994;89:239–277.
43. Ehrlich R, Henry MC. Chronic toxicity of nitrogen dioxide: I. Effect on resistance to bacterial pneumonia. *Arch Environ Health* 1968;17:860–865.
44. Ehrlich R. Interaction between environmental pollutants and respiratory infections. *Environ Health Perspect* 1980;35:89–100.
45. Amoruso MA, Witz G, Goldstein BD. Decreased superoxide anion radical production by rat alveolar macrophages following inhalation of ozone or nitrogen dioxide. *Life Sci* 1981;28:2215–2221.
46. Holt PG, Finlay-Jones LM, Keast D, Papadimitrou JJ. Immunological function in mice chronically exposed to nitrogen oxides ($NO_x$). *Environ Res* 1979;19:154–162.
47. Fujimaki H, Shimizu F. Effects of acute exposure to nitrogen dioxide on primary antibody response. *Arch Environ Health* 1981;36:114–119.
48. Fujimaki H, Shimizu F, Kubota K. Effect of subacute exposure to $NO_2$ on lymphocytes required for antibody response. *Environ Res* 1982;29:280–286.
49. Maigetter RZ, Fenters JD, Findlay JC, Ehrlich R, Gardner DE. Effect of exposure to nitrogen dioxide on T and B cells in mouse spleens. *Toxicol Lett* 1978;2:157–161.
50. Richters A, Damji KS. Changes in T-lymphocyte subpopulations and natural killer cells following exposure to ambient levels of nitrogen dioxide. *J Toxicol Environ Health* 1988;25:247–256.
51. Sandstrom T, Stjernberg N, Eklund A, et al. Inflammatory cell response in bronchoalveolar lavage fluid after nitrogen dioxide exposure of healthy subjects: a dose-response study. *Eur Respir J* 1991;4:332–339.
52. Rubinstein I, Reiss TF, Bigby BG, Stites DP, Boushey HA. Effects of 0.60 ppm nitrogen dioxide on circulating and bronchoalveolar lavage lymphocyte phenotypes in healthy subjects. *Environ Res* 1991;55:18–30.
53. Fenters JD, Ehrlich R, Findlay J, Spangler J, Tolkacz V. Serologic response in squirrel monkeys exposed to nitrogen dioxide and influenza virus. *Am Rev Respir Dis* 1971;104:448–451.
54. Fenters JD, Findlay JD, Port CD, Ehrlich R, Coffin DL. Chronic exposure to nitrogen dioxide: immunologic, physiologic, and pathologic effects in virus-challenged squirrel monkeys. *Arch Environ Health* 1973;27:85–89.
55. Gilmour MI. Interaction of air pollutants and pulmonary allergic responses in experimental animals. *Toxicology* 1995;105:335–342.
56. Kitabatake M, Yamamoto H, Yuan PF, Manjurul H, Murase S, Yamauchi T. Effects of exposure to $NO_2$ or $SO_2$ on bronchopulmonary reaction induced by Candida albicans in guinea pigs. *J Toxicol Environ Health* 1995;45:75–82.
57. Evans MJ, Cabral LJ, Stephens RJ, Freeman G. Transformation of alveolar type 2 cells to type 1 cells following exposure to $NO_2$. *Exp Mol Pathol* 1975;22:142–150.
58. Rombout PJA, Dormans JAMA, Marra M, van Esch FJ. Influence of exposure regimen on nitrogen dioxide-induced morphological changes in the rat lung. *Environ Res* 1986;41:466–480.
59. DeNicola DB, Rebar AH, Henderson RF. Early damage indicators in the lung. V. Biochemical and cytological response to $NO_2$ inhalation. *Toxicol Appl Pharmacol* 1981;60:301–312.
60. Kubota K, Murakami M, Takenaka S, Kawai K, Kyono H. Effects of long-term nitrogen dioxide exposure on rat lung: morphological observations. *Environ Health Perspect* 1987;73:157–169.
61. NIH. National Institutes of Health. The definition of emphysema: report of a National Heart, Lung, and Blood Institute, Division of Lung Diseases Workshop. *Am Rev Respir Dis* 1985;132:182–185.
62. Barth PJ, Muller B, Wagner U, Bittinger A. Quantitative analysis of parenchymal and vascular alterations in $NO_2$-induced lung injury in rats. *Eur Respir J* 1995;8:1115–1121.
63. Hyde D, Orthoefer J, Dungworth D, Tyler W, Carter R, Lum H. Morphometric and morphologic evaluation of pulmonary lesions in beagle dogs chronically exposed to high ambient levels of air pollutants. *Lab Invest* 1978;38:455–469.
64. Rasmussen RE, McClure TR. Effect of chronic exposure to $NO_2$ in the developing ferret lung. *Toxicol Lett* 1992;63:253–260.
65. Stavert DM, Lehnert BE. Concentration versus time is the more important exposure variable in nitrogen dioxide-induced acute lung injury. *Toxicologist* 1988;8:140.
66. Gelzleichter TR, Witschi H, Last JA. Concentration-response relationships of rat lungs to exposure to oxidant air pollutants: a critical test of Haber's law for ozone and nitrogen dioxide. *Toxicol Appl Pharmacol* 1992;112:73–80.
67. Prütz WA, Mönig H, Butler J, Land EJ. Reactions of nitrogen dioxide in aqueous model systems: oxidation of tyrosine units in peptides and proteins. *Arch Biochem Biophys* 1985;243:125–134.
68. Bils RF. The connective tissues and alveolar walls in the lungs of normal and oxidant-exposed squirrel monkeys. *J Cell Biol* 1976;70:318.
69. Last JA, Warren DL. Synergistic interaction between nitrogen dioxide and respirable aerosols of sulfuric acid or sodium chloride on rat lungs. *Toxicol Appl Pharmacol* 1987;90:34–42.
70. Rasmussen RE. Localization of increased collagen in ferret lung tissue after chronic exposure to nitrogen dioxide. *Toxicol Lett* 1994;73:241–248.
71. Kleinerman J, Gordon RE, Ip MPC, Collins A. Structure and function of airways in experimental chronic nitrogen dioxide exposure. In:

Gammage RB, Kaye SV, eds. *Indoor air and human health.* Chelsea, MI: Lewis, 1985;297–301.

72. Kleinerman J, Ip MPC. Effects of nitrogen dioxide on elastin and collagen contents of lung. *Arch Environ Health* 1979;34:228–232.
73. Suzuki AK, Tsubone H, Kubota K. Changes of gaseous exchange in the lung of mice acutely exposed to nitrogen dioxide. *Toxicol Lett* 1982;10:327–335.
74. Tepper JS, Costa DL, Winsett DW, Stevens MA, Doerfler DL, Watkinson WP. Near-lifetime exposure of the rat to a simulated urban profile of nitrogen dioxide: pulmonary function evaluation. *Fundam Appl Toxicol* 1993;20:88–96.
75. Silbaugh SA, Mauderly JL, Macken CA. Effects of sulfuric acid and nitrogen dioxide on airway responsiveness of the guinea pig. *J Toxicol Environ Health* 1981;8:31–45.
76. Kobayashi T, Shinozaki Y. Induction of transient airway hyper-responsiveness by exposure to 4 ppm nitrogen dioxide in guinea pigs. *J Toxicol Environ Health* 1992;37:451–461.
77. Witschi H. Ozone, nitrogen dioxide and lung cancer: a review of some recent issues and problems. *Toxicology* 1988;48:1–20.
78. Palisano JR, Kleinerman J. APUD cells and NEB in hamster lung. Methods, quantitation and response to injury. *Thorax* 1980;35:5–11.
79. Kleinerman J, Marchevsky AM, Thornton J. Quantitative studies of APUD cells in airways of rats. The effects of diethylnitrosamine and $NO_2$. *Am Rev Respir Dis* 1981;124:458–462.
80. Richters A, Kuraitis K. Inhalation of $NO_2$ and blood borne cancer cell spread to the lungs. *Arch Environ Health* 1981;36:36–39.
81. Richters A, Richters V. Nitrogen dioxide ($NO_2$) inhalation, formation of microthrombi in lungs and cancer metastasis. *J Environ Pathol Toxicol Oncol* 1989;9:45–51.
82. Sone S, Brennan LM, Creasia DA. In vivo and in vitro $NO_2$ exposures enhance phagocytic and tumoricidal activities of rat alveolar macrophages. *J Toxicol Environ Health* 1983;11:151–163.
83. Bylin G, Lindvall T, Rehn T, Sundin B. Effects of short-term exposure to ambient nitrogen dioxide concentrations on human bronchial reactivity and lung function. *Eur J Respir Dis* 1985;66:205–217.
84. Koenig JQ, Covert DS, Morgan MS, et al. Acute effects of 0.12 ppm ozone or 0.12 ppm nitrogen dioxide on pulmonary function in healthy and asthmatic adolescents. *Am Rev Respir Dis* 1985;132:648–651.
85. Bascom R, Bromberg PA, Costa DL, et al. Health effects of outdoor air pollution. *Am J Respir Crit Care Med* 1996;153:477–498.
86. Beil M, Ulmer WT. Effect of $NO_2$ in workroom concentrations on respiratory mechanics and bronchial susceptibility to acetylcholine in normal persons. *Int Arch Occup Environ Health* 1976;38:31–44.
87. Mohsenin V. Airway responses to 2.0 ppm nitrogen dioxide in normal subjects. *Arch Environ Health* 1988;43:242–246.
88. Linn WS, Solomon JC, Trim SC, et al. Effects of exposure to 4 ppm nitrogen dioxide in healthy and asthmatic volunteers. *Arch Environ Health* 1985;40:234–239.
89. Folinsbee LJ, Horvath SM, Bedi JF, Delehunt JC. Effect of 0.62 pm $NO_2$ on cardiopulmonary function in young male nonsmokers. *Environ Res* 1978;15:199–205.
90. Hackney JD, Thiede FC, Linn WS, et al. Experimental studies on human health effects of air pollutants. IV. Short-term physiological and clinical effects of nitrogen dioxide exposure. *Arch Environ Health* 1978;33:176–181.
91. Frampton MW, Gibb FR, Speers DM, Morrow PE, Utell MJ. Effects of $NO_2$ exposure on pulmonary function and airway reactivity. *Am Rev Respir Dis* 1989;139:A124.
92. Hazucha MJ, Ginsberg JF, McDonnell WF, et al. Effects of 0.1 ppm nitrogen dioxide on airways of normal and asthmatic subjects. *J Appl Physiol Respir Environ Exercise Physiol* 1983;54:730–739.
93. Mohsenin V. Effects of vitamin C on $NO_2$-induced airway hyperresponsiveness in normal subjects: a randomized double-blind experiment. *Am Rev Respir Dis* 1987;136:1408–1411.
94. Bauer MA, Utell MJ, Morrow PE, Speers DM, Gibb FR. Inhalation of 0.30 ppm nitrogen dioxide potentiates exercise-induced bronchospasm in asthmatics. *Am Rev Respir Dis* 1986;134:1203–1208.
95. Ahmed T, Marchette B, Danta I, et al. Effect of 0.1 ppm $NO_2$ on bronchial reactivity in normals and subjects with bronchial asthma. *Am Rev Respir Dis* 1982;125(suppl.):152S.
96. Rubinstein I, Bigby BG, Reiss TF, Bousley HA. Short-term exposure to 0.3 ppm nitrogen dioxide does not potentiate airway responsiveness to sulfur dioxide in asthmatic subjects. *Am Rev Respir Dis* 1990;381–385.
97. Roger LJ, Horstman DH, McDonnell W, et al. Pulmonary function, airway responsiveness, and respiratory symptoms in asthmatics following exercise in $NO_2$. *Toxicol Ind Health* 1990;6:155–171.
98. Linn WS, Shamoo DA, Avol EL, et al. Dose-response study of asthmatic volunteers exposed to nitrogen dioxide during intermittent exercise. *Arch Environ Health* 1986;41:292–296.
99. Mohsenin V. Airway responses to nitrogen dioxide in asthmatic subjects. *J Toxicol Environ Health* 1987;22:371–380.
100. Morrow PE, Utell MJ, Bauer MA, et al. Pulmonary performance of elderly normal subjects and subjects with chronic obstructive pulmonary disease exposed to 0.3 ppm nitrogen dioxide. *Am Rev Respir Dis* 1992;145:291–300.
101. von Nieding G, Wagner HM. Effects of $NO_2$ on chronic bronchitics. *Environ Health Perspect* 1979;29:137–142.
102. Kerr HD, Kulle TJ, McIlhany ML, Swidersky P. Effects of nitrogen dioxide on pulmonary function in human subjects: an environmental chamber study. *Environ Res* 1979;19:392–404.
103. Linn WS, Shamoo DA, Spier CE, et al. Controlled exposure of volunteers with chronic obstructive pulmonary disease to nitrogen dioxide. *Arch Environ Health* 1985;40:313–317.
104. Avol EL, Linn WS, Peng RC, Valencia G, Little D, Hackney JD. Laboratory study of asthmatic volunteers exposed to nitrogen dioxide and to ambient air pollution. *Am Ind Hyg Assoc J* 1988;49:143–149.
105. Bylin G, Hedenstierna G, Lindvall T, Sundin B. Ambient nitrogen dioxide concentrates increase bronchial responsiveness in subjects with mild asthma. *Eur Resp J* 1988;1:606–612.
106. Frampton MW, Smeglin AM, Roberts NJ Jr, Finkelstein JN, Morrow PE, Utell MJ. Nitrogen dioxide exposure in vivo and human alveolar macrophage inactivation of influenza virus in vitro. *Environ Res* 1989; 48:179–192.
107. Mohsenin V, Gee BL. Acute effect of nitrogen dioxide exposure on the functional activity of alpha-1-protease inhibitor in bronchoalveolar lavage fluid of normal subjects. *Am Rev Respir Dis* 1987;136: 646–650.
108. Johnson DA, Frampton MW, Winters RS, Morrow PE, Utell MJ. Inhalation of nitrogen dioxide fails to reduce the activity of human lung alpha-1 proteinase inhibitor. *Am Rev Respir Dis* 1990;142: 758–762.
109. Frampton MW, Finkelstein JN, Roberts NJ Jr, Smeglin AM, Morrow PE, Utell MJ. Effects of nitrogen dioxide exposure on bronchoalveolar lavage proteins in humans. *Am J Respir Cell Mol Biol* 1989;1: 499–505.
110. Speizer FE, Ferris B Jr, Bishop YMM, Spengler J. Respiratory disease rates and pulmonary function in children associated with $NO_2$ exposure. *Am Rev Respir Dis* 1980;121:3–10.
111. Ware JH, Dockery DW, Spiro A III, Speizer FE, Ferris BG, Jr. Passive smoking, gas cooking, and respiratory health of children living in six cities. *Am Rev Respir Dis* 1984;129:366–374.
112. Dockery DW, Speizer FE, Stram DO, Ware JH, Spengler JD, Ferris BG Jr. Effects of inhalable particles on respiratory health of children. *Am Rev Respir Dis* 1989;139:587–594.
113. Neas LM, Dockery DW, Ware JH, Spengler JD, Speizer FE, Ferris BG Jr. Association of indoor nitrogen dioxide with respiratory symptoms and pulmonary function in children. *Am J Epidemiol* 1991;134: 204–209.
114. Lebowitz MD, Holberg CJ, Boyer B, Hayes C. Respiratory symptoms and peak flow associated with indoor and outdoor air pollutants in the southwest. *J Air Pollut Contr Assoc* 1985;35:1154–1158.
115. Vedal S, Schenker MB, Munoz A, Samet JM, Batterman S, Speizer FE. Daily air pollution effects on children's respiratory symptoms and peak expiratory flow. *Am J Public Health* 1987;77:694–698.
116. Keller MD, Lanese RR, Mitchell RI, Cote RW. Respiratory illness in households using gas and electricity for cooking. II. Symptoms and objective findings. *Environ Res* 1979;19:504–515.
117. Samet JM, Lambert WE, Skipper BJ, et al. Nitrogen dioxide and respiratory illnesses in infants. *Am Rev Respir Dis* 1993;148:1258–1265.
118. Berwick M, Leaderer BP, Stolwijk JA, Zagraniski RT. Lower respiratory symptoms in children exposed to nitrogen dioxide from unvented combustion sources. *Environ Int* 1989;15:369–373.
119. Comstock GW, Meger MB, Helsing KJ, Tockman MJ. Respiratory effects of household exposures to tobacco smoke and gas cooking. *Am Rev Respir Dis* 1981;124:143–148.
120. Schenker MB, Samet JM, Speizer FE. Risk factors for childhood respiratory disease: the effect of host factors and home environmental exposures. *Am Rev Respir Dis* 1983;28:1038–1043.

121. Dodge R. The effects of indoor pollution on Arizona children. *Arch Environ Health* 1982;37:151–155.
122. Ekwo EE, Weinberger MW, Lachenbruch PA, Huntley WH. Relationship of parental smoking and gas cooking to respiratory disease in children. *Chest* 1983;84:662–668.
123. Melia RJW, Florey CV, Altman DG, Swan AV. Association between gas cooking and respiratory disease in children. *Br Med J* 1977;2:149–152.
124. Melia RJW, Florey CDV, Chinn S. The relation between respiratory illness in primary schoolchildren and the use of gas for cooking. I. Results from a national survey. *Int J Epidemiol* 1979;8:333–339.
125. Melia RJW, Florey CDV, Morris RW, et al. Childhood respiratory illness and the home environment: II. Association between respiratory illness and nitrogen dioxide, temperature and relative humidity. *Int J Epidemiol* 1982;11:164–169.
126. Gnehm HE, Ackerman U, Braun C, Rutishauser M, Wanner HU. Significant association of respiratory symptoms in small children with outdoor $NO_2$ air pollution. *Pediatr Res* 1988;23:291A.
127. Braun-Fahrlander C, Ackermann-Liebrich U, Schwartz J, Gnehn HP, Rutishauser M, Wanner HU. Air pollution and respiratory symptoms in preschool children. *Am Rev Respir Dis* 1992;145:42–47.
128. Brunekreef B, Houthuijs D, Boleij J, Dijkstra, L. Indoor nitrogen dioxide exposure and children's pulmonary function. *J Air Waste Manag Assoc* 1990;40:1252–1256.
129. Dijkstra L, Houthuijs D, Brunekreef B, Akkermann I, Boleij JSM. Respiratory health effects of the indoor environment in a population of Dutch children. *Am Rev Respir Dis* 1990;142:1172–1178.
130. Koo LC, Ho JHC, Ho C-Y, et al. Personal exposure to nitrogen dioxide and its association with respiratory illness in Hong Kong. *Am Rev Respir Dis* 1990;141:1119–1126.
131. Moseler M, Hendel-Kramer A, Karmaus W, et al. Effect of moderate $NO_2$ air pollution on the lung function of children with asthmatic symptoms. *Environ Res* 1994;67:109–124.
132. Snyder SH, Bredt DS. Biological roles of nitric oxide. *Sci Am* 1992;266:68–77.
133. Oda H, Nogami H, Kusumoto S, Mukajima T, Kurata A. Lifetime exposure to 2.4 ppm nitric oxide in mice. *Environ Res* 1980;22:254–263.
134. Hugod C. Ultrastructural changes of the rabbit lung after a 5 ppm nitric oxide exposure. *Arch Environ Health* 1979;34:12–17.
135. Mercer RR, Costa DL, Crapo JD. Effects of prolonged exposure to low doses of nitric oxide or nitrogen dioxide on the alveolar septa of the adult rat lung. *Lab Invest* 1995;73:20–28.
136. Murphy SD, Ulrich CE, Frankowitz SH, Xintaras C. Altered function in animals inhaling low concentrations of ozone and nitrogen dioxide. *Am Ind Hyg Assoc J* 1964;25:246–253.
137. Murphy SD. A review of effects on animals of exposure to auto exhaust and some of its components. *J Air Pollut Contr Assoc* 1964;14:303–308.
138. Azoulay E, Bouley G, Blayo MC. Effects of nitric oxide on resistance to bacterial infection in mice. *J Toxicol Environ Health* 1981;7:873–882.
139. Kagawa J. Respiratory effects of 2-hr exposure to 1.0 ppm nitric oxide in normal subjects. *Environ Res* 1982;27:485–490.
140. Gustafsson LE. Experimental studies on nitric oxide. *Scand J Work Environ Health* 1993;19:44–49.
141. Case GD, Dixon JS, Schooley JC. Interactions of blood metalloproteins with nitrogen oxides and oxidant air pollutants. *Environ Res* 1979;20:43–65.
142. Oda H, Kusumoto S, Nakajima T. Nitrosyl-hemoglobin formation in the blood of animals exposed to nitric oxide. *Arch Environ Health* 1975;30:453–456.
143. Nakajima T, Oda H, Kusumoto S, Nogami H. Biological effects of nitrogen dioxide and nitric oxide. In: Lee SD, ed. *Nitrogen oxides and their effects on health.* Ann Arbor, MI: Ann Arbor Science, 1980; 121–141.
144. Chiodi H, Mohler JG. Effects of exposure of blood hemoglobin to nitric oxide. *Environ Res* 1985;37:355–363.
145. Kon K, Maeda N, Shiga T. Effect of NO on the oxygen transport of human erythrocytes. *J Toxicol Environ Health* 1977;2:1109–1113.
146. Kon K, Meada N, Suda T, Shiga T. Reaction between nitrosylhemoglobin and oxygen-methemoglobin formation and hemoglobin degradation. *J Jpn Soc Air Pollut* 1980;15:401–411.
147. Maeda N, Kon K, Imaizumi K, Shiga T. Kinetic study on nitrosylhemoglobin and methemoglobin formation in the blood of rats exposed to nitric oxide. *J Jpn Soc Air Pollut* 1984;19:239–246.
148. Maeda N, Imaizumi K, Kon K, Shiga T. A kinetic study on functional impairment of nitric oxide-exposed rat erythrocytes. *Environ Health Perspect* 1987;73:171–177.
149. Moncada S, Palmer RMJ, Higgs EA. Nitric oxide: physiology, pathophysiology, and pharmacology. *Pharmacol Rev* 1991;43:109–142.
150. Moriguchi M, Manning LR, Manning JM. Nitric oxide can modify amino acid residues in proteins. *Biochem Biophys Res Commun* 1992;183:598–604.
151. Ischiropoulos H, Zhu L, Beckman JS. Peroxy-nitrite formation from macrophage-derived nitric oxide. Arch. *Biochem Biophys* 1992;298:446–451.
152. Fleetham JA, Tunnicliffe BW, Munt PW. Methemoglobinemia and the oxides of nitrogen (letter). *N Engl J Med* 1978;298:1130.
153. Mayorga MA. Overview of nitrogen dioxide effects on the lung with emphasis on military relevance. *Toxicology* 1994;89:175–192.

*Environmental and Occupational Medicine, Third Edition,* edited by William N. Rom.
Lippincott–Raven Publishers, Philadelphia © 1998.

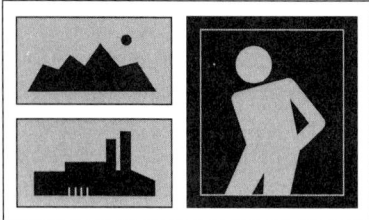

CHAPTER 41

# Sulfur Dioxide and Sulfuric Acid Aerosols

Mark J. Utell and Mark W. Frampton

Exposure to sulfur dioxide ($SO_2$) or acidic particles can occur in the workplace, outdoors, or in the home. Sulfur dioxide and acidic aerosols generally occur together as atmospheric pollutants, formed principally as a result of combustion of sulfur-containing fossil fuels. Although contamination of outdoor air by sulfur dioxide and acidic particles has been the subject of substantial research and of much regulatory concern, pollution of indoor environments by sulfur dioxide and sulfuric acid ($H_2SO_4$) aerosols emitted from kerosene space heaters (1) has only recently been recognized. In the occupational setting, massive exposure to sulfur dioxide has resulted from industrial accidents; exposures to sulfur dioxide and sulfuric acid aerosols may be encountered in industry in petroleum refining, a variety of manufacturing processes, and processes that require the burning of fossil fuel. This chapter reviews the sources of these pollutants, their sites of injury and mechanisms of action, and our current understanding of health effects of inhalation of sulfur dioxide and acidic particles.

## RESPIRATORY SITES OF POLLUTANT EFFECTS

Sulfur dioxide and acidic aerosols exist in the ambient environment in gaseous and particulate forms, respectively. The extent of penetration and retention of pollutant gases within the lungs vary greatly, depending on several factors, including the solubility of the gas, its concentration in inspired air, the duration of exposure, and the pattern of flow during breathing. Sulfur dioxide is a highly soluble, irritating gas that is absorbed quickly and almost entirely in the nose and upper airway of healthy subjects during quiet breathing (2). The mucosal surfaces of the nasal turbinates act as efficient "scrubbers" of sulfur dioxide and thereby reduce levels at the glottis to less than 2% of the concentration measured at the nose. During exercise, when inspiratory flow rate and tidal volume are greater, sulfur dioxide reaches the lower airways.

Pollutants in particulate form are usually found in nature as aerosols (i.e., small liquid droplets or solid particles such as sulfuric acid mists with sufficient stability to remain suspended in the atmosphere). Although deposition of inhaled particles depends on many factors including the aerodynamic properties of the particle (primarily size), airway anatomy, hygroscopic properties, and breathing pattern, several generalizations can be made. Particles larger than 10 μm are effectively filtered out of the nose and nasopharynx. These relatively large particles tend to be deposited rapidly because of impaction against surfaces and gravitational forces. Particles trapped in the nose and nasopharynx are cleared in nasal secretions, coughed out, or swallowed. Particles smaller than 10 μm in aerodynamic diameter may be deposited in the tracheobronchial tree; deposition in the alveoli is maximal for particles of 1 to 2 μm diameter. Particles smaller than 0.5 μm are carried by diffusion to the alveolar level, where brownian movement causes collision with gas molecules and impaction on alveolar surfaces. Removal of particles from the upper airways by mucociliary clearance is efficient and occurs within hours; this rapid clearance contrasts with clearance from the deep lung by alveolar macrophages, which may require days to months.

M. J. Utell and M. W. Frampton: Divisions of Pulmonary/Critical Care and Occupational Medicine, Departments of Medicine and Environmental Medicine, University of Rochester Medical Center, Rochester, New York 14642.

Ambient aerosols are often depicted as bimodal in distribution, with peaks that range in size from 0.05 to 1.0 μm and 2.0 to 8.0 μm (3). Therefore, the wide variability in ambient aerosol particle size presumably results in deposition throughout the respiratory system in upper airways and the tracheobronchial tree as well as in pulmonary parenchyma. Hygroscopic aerosol particles such as sulfuric acid increase in size as they absorb water during transit through the airways. The growth characteristics of these aerosols are such that within a 3-second residence time, submicron particles (i.e., 0.8 μm) may more than triple in size as a function of relative humidity and establish a new mass median aerodynamic diameter (MMAD) greater than 2.0 μm (4,5).

## Sources of Pollutants

### *Environmental*

Atmospheric pollution has been associated with increased rates of respiratory tract illness and mortality, and both sulfur dioxide and particles, including sulfates and sulfuric acid, have been linked with these episodes. The most catastrophic episodes were in the Meuse Valley in Belgium in 1930; Donora, Pennsylvania in 1948 (6); and London, England in 1952 (7). Each was a site of major coal-fired manufacturing or home heating, and the events were preceded by the development of a stagnant, moist air mass over the region. Combustion of fossil fuels oxidized contaminating sulfur to sulfur oxides and sulfuric acid particles. Sulfur oxides released into the atmosphere then reacted with moisture in the presence of metal catalysts to form additional sulfuric acid.

Currently, residents of North America are exposed to sulfur dioxide and acidic aerosol pollutants, although to much lower concentrations than during the historical pollution episodes. Sulfur dioxide emissions generally originate from point sources such as utility power plants, which burn fuels containing sulfur. Metal smelting is another major contributor. Exposure to high concentrations of sulfur dioxide, therefore, is highly localized and in the vicinity (within 20 km) of major point sources. It is dependent on source factors such as stack height, diurnal and seasonal emission patterns, and dispersion patterns. Away from large point sources, urban sulfur dioxide concentrations do not often exceed 0.2 to 0.3 ppm as a 1-hour average (8).

Atmospheric acidity also results from the combustion of sulfur-containing fuels by power-generating plants, predominantly in the Ohio River Valley. The tall stacks designed to reduce local pollution result in release of $SO_2$, $H_2SO_4$, and particles above inversion layers, allowing these pollutants to remain aloft for days, traveling hundreds of miles. In contrast to the pollution disasters in which foggy air masses permitted a rapid reaction with sulfur dioxide to form sulfuric acid, formation of sulfuric acid aerosols in the upper atmosphere is a photochemical process. Nitrogen oxides, reactive hydrocarbons, and ozone from combustion sources combine in the presence of sunlight to form strong oxidizing agents that slowly react with sulfur dioxide to form sulfuric acid aerosols (9). Thus, in North America the highest levels of atmospheric acidity occur in the summer months, and in locations far downwind of the sources in the Ohio River Valley, including the northeastern United States and Canada. Atmospheric acidity, however, may be largely neutralized by ammonia near ground level, which is found both in agricultural and urban regions (9). For example, recent measurements undertaken in Toronto, Canada found the highest levels of particle acidity in the least urbanized areas, due to neutralization by ammonia in the most urbanized areas (10).

Because measurements of atmospheric acidity present technical problems, accurate measurements in the United States and Canada have only recently been undertaken. Twenty-four-hour average concentrations of sulfuric acid aerosols greater than 20 $\mu g/m^3$ have been recorded, and peaks as high as 100 $\mu g/m^3$ (11,12). These figures are probably two to ten times less than those present during the pollution disasters. Concentrations of particle strong acidity are correlated with regions of high sulfur emissions, and are highest in the eastern United States and Canada, but lowest in the western United States (13).

Although outdoor air contamination by sulfur dioxide or acidic aerosols has been the focus of concern, kerosene space heaters are now recognized as an important indoor source of sulfur dioxide, sulfates, and acidic aerosols (1,14). Indoor levels may exceed maximum outdoor levels by 10 times or more. Since most persons spend the majority of time indoors, for many pollutants the indoor environment is a major determinant of total exposure.

### *Occupational*

Sulfur dioxide and sulfuric acid are also common in industry. In 1974 the National Institute for Occupational Safety and Health (NIOSH) estimated that 500,000 workers could be exposed to sulfur dioxide (15). It may be encountered in a variety of industries—the production of paper, refrigeration plants, fruit processing, manufacturing of sodium sulfite, and petroleum refining.

Sulfuric acid is the most commonly used industrial chemical (16), and the potential for exposure to acidic aerosols occurs in more than 200 occupational categories. Approximately 800,000 persons are considered to be at risk who work in the production of fertilizer, petroleum alkylation, iron and steel pickling, uranium processing, and a variety of manufacturing processes (16,17). The highest exposure levels are associated with the manufacture of batteries, principally with forming and charging. In the forming process, lead battery plates are immersed in tanks of dilute sulfuric acid and subjected to an elec-

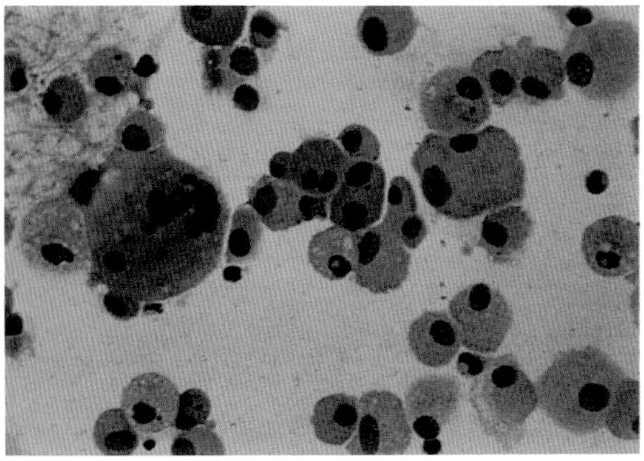

**COLOR PLATE 38–2.** Light microscopic evaluation of bronchoalveolar (BAL) cells from a person with diatomaceous earth pneumoconiosis (400×). There are prominent inflammatory multinucleate giant cells and vacuoles in the alveolar macrophages.

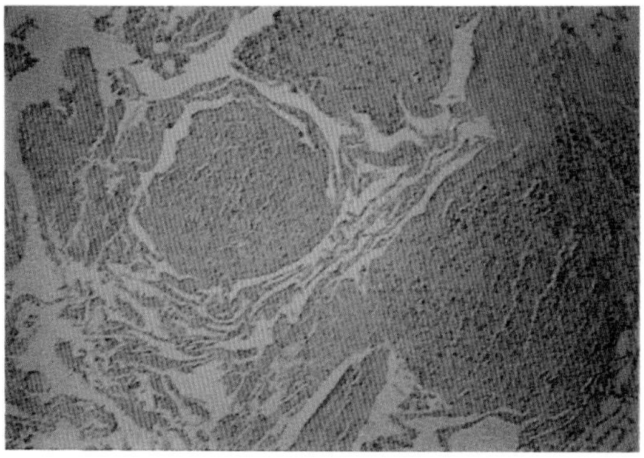

**COLOR PLATE 38–3.** Silicotic nodules in transbrochial lung biopsy specimen from the patient presented in Fig. 2 (of Chapter 38).

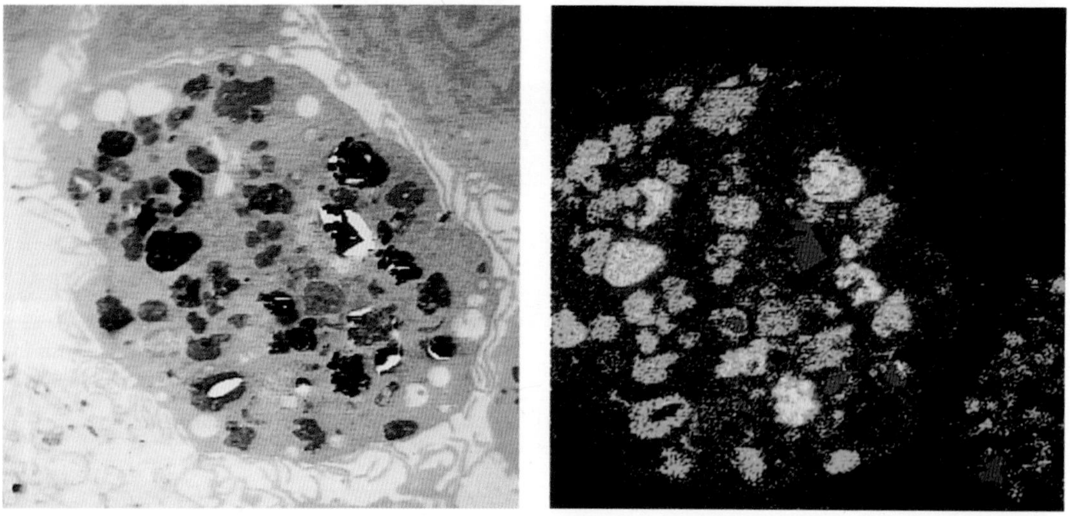

**COLOR PLATE 38–4. A:** Transmission electron micrographs of the same alveolar macrophage from a person with diatomaceous earth pneumoconiosis (4200×). **B:** Energy dispersive x-ray analysis with an electron microprobe computer programmed to raster scan the alveolar macrophage section demonstrates numerous inorganic dust particles (*red*=silicon, *green*=iron). (Courtesy of Richard Leapman, Ph.D., National Institutes of Health.)

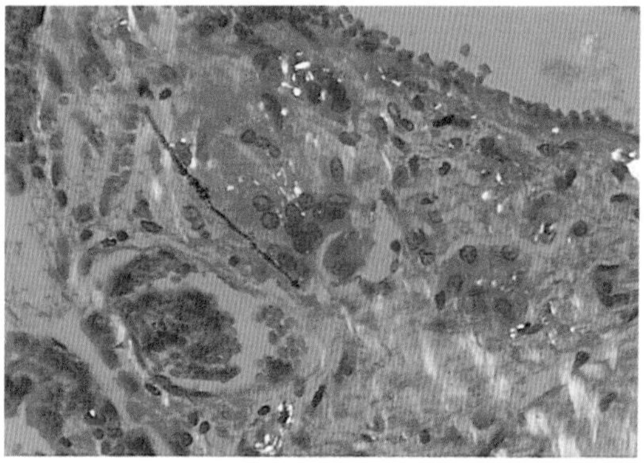

**COLOR PLATE 38–6.** Autopsy lung specimen of New York State talc miner showed talcosis and asbestosis in underlying lung parenchyma. High-power, partially polarized light micrograph shows strongly birefringent talc particles and asbestos body in interstitium. The asbestos body is within a multinucleated giant cell (H&E). (Courtesy of J. Abraham, M.D.)

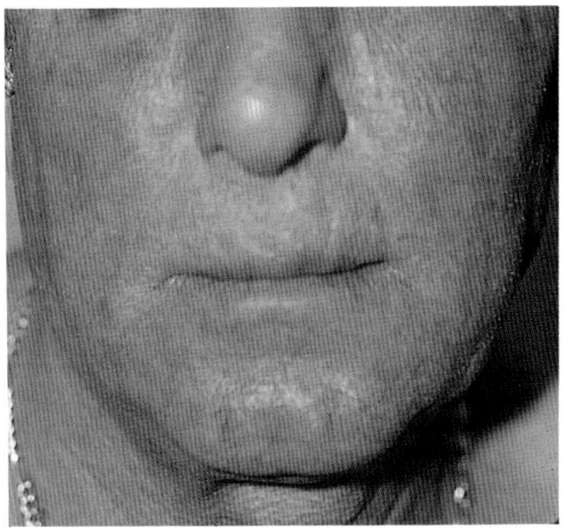

**COLOR PLATE 46–5.** Allergic contact dermatitis to aerosolized epoxy resin in an automotive plant worker.

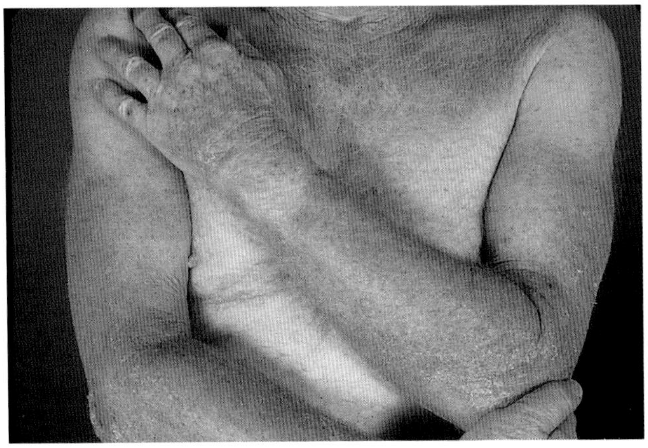

**COLOR PLATE 46–6.** Photoallergic contact dermatitis from a sunscreen. Note the sparing under the watchband and sleeves on the shoulders and chest that were photoprotected by his shirt.

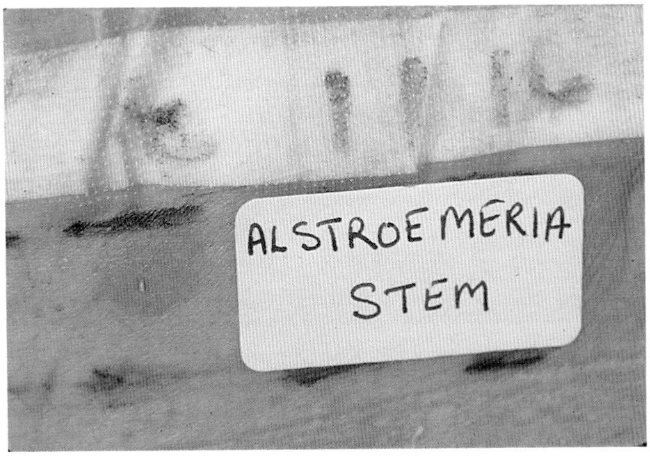


**COLOR PLATE 46–9B.** Positive patch test to Peruvian lily (alstroemeria).

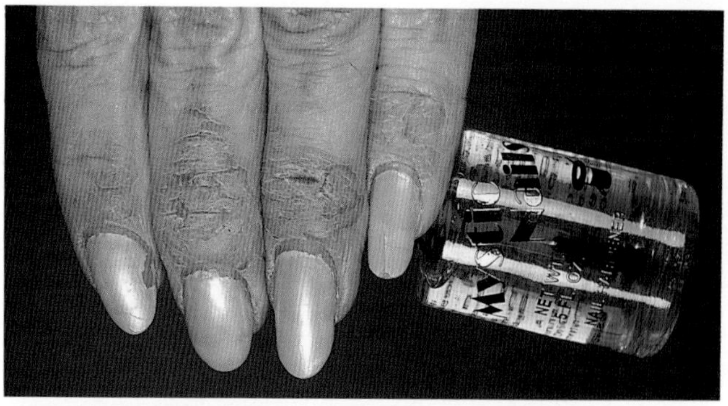

**COLOR PLATE 46–10A.** Allergic contact dermatitis to a nail hardener in a manicurist who also uses the product.

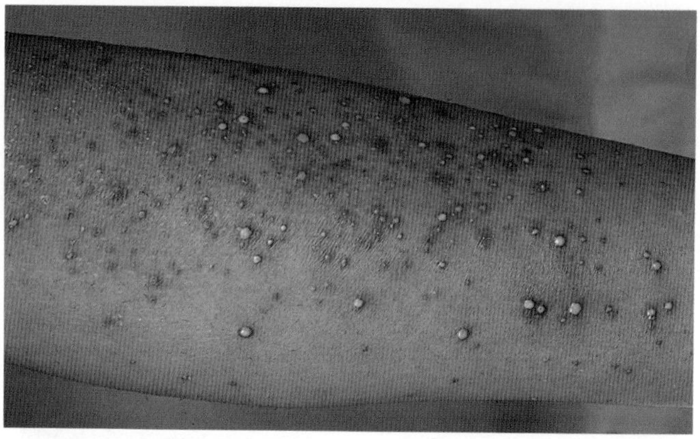

**COLOR PLATE 46–11.** Folliculitis induced by the inadvertent contamination of his clothing with metal cutting oil.

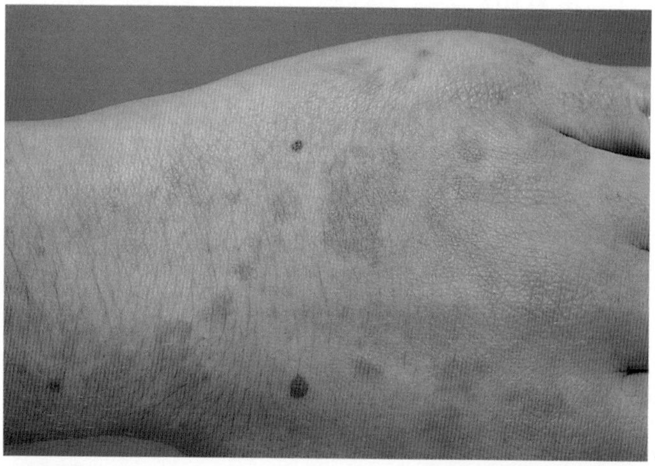

**COLOR PLATE 46–12A.** Contact urticaria to natural latex rubber gloves.

trical current. During this process small gas bubbles carry a spray of acid mist into the atmosphere; a visible fog is often present in this area of the plant. In the charging process, finished batteries are filled with acid and charged with direct current. Because the acid is enclosed during the charging process, less visible acid mist is generated.

Older surveys of battery plants described concentrations well above the current Occupational Safety and Health Administration (OSHA) standard (1 mg/m$^3$). For example, Malcolm and Paul (18) reported levels ranging from 3.0 to 16.6 mg/m$^3$ in the forming area of one plant. El-Sadik and colleagues (19) surveyed two plants in Egypt and measured levels from 13 to 35 mg/m$^3$. A more recent survey of five battery plants in the United States, using personal monitoring techniques, found levels of personal exposure to sulfuric acid aerosols ranging from 0 to 1.7 mg/m$^3$ (20). The highest exposure levels occurred in the charging and forming areas of the plants. Aerosol mass median aerodynamic diameter was within the respirable range—about 5 μm.

## HEALTH EFFECTS

The strongest evidence linking sulfur dioxide and acidic aerosols with adverse health effects is the reported increase in mortality associated with the large-scale, mid-century pollution disasters in Donora, Pennsylvania in 1948 (6) and in London in 1952 (7). During the London fog of 1952, an estimated excess of 4,000 deaths occurred, principally among elders and persons with chronic respiratory tract disease. A recent reexamination of London mortality data for the years 1963 through 1972 showed a correlation between daily mortality rates and sulfuric acid aerosol levels on the previous day (21). Additional evidence that atmospheric sulfuric acid aerosols is associated with adverse health effects comes from Japan. Kitagawa (22) studied residents who lived downwind from a titanium dioxide plant that released large quantities of sulfuric acid particles into the atmosphere. More than 600 cases of respiratory disease, predominantly asthma and bronchitis, were identified between 1960 and 1969 in an area within 5 km of the plant. Mortality rates from asthma increased in the area during the period of greatest pollution; in addition, the rate of mortality from chronic bronchitis increased about 4 or 5 years after the asthma mortality rate did (23). Installation of emission controls resulted in a reduction in respiratory illnesses for both asthma and chronic bronchitis in subsequent years.

Recent epidemiologic studies suggest that exposure to current low levels of particulate matter in the air may have adverse health effects. In a growing number of studies worldwide, significant relationships have been observed between atmospheric particle concentrations and mortality from respiratory and cardiovascular disease (24,25). A recent review of the data by the U.S. Environmental Protection Agency (25) found that a 50 μg/m$^3$ increase in the concentration of particulate matter less than 10 μm ($PM_{10}$) is associated with a 3% to 8% increase in the relative risk of death. Atmospheric particle levels are also linked with respiratory symptoms (26,27), medication use in asthmatics (28), and hospital admissions for respiratory disease (29). The mechanisms mediating these effects have not been elucidated, and causality has not been proven (30). However, current evidence suggests that levels of particulate matter seen in many urban areas may adversely affect the health of some individuals with underlying respiratory or cardiovascular disease.

The degree to which acid aerosols or sulfur dioxide, as part of the burden of atmospheric pollutants, contribute to these adverse effects, is unclear. Relationships between particle exposure and mortality have been observed in communities with very low levels of acidity, indicating that particle acidity is not the sole causative factor. However, evidence links acid aerosol exposure with adverse health outcomes. In southern Ontario, Canada, several studies have demonstrated consistent associations between hospital admissions for respiratory illness and daily levels of sulfate, aerosol strong acidity, and ozone (31,32).

The Six Cities Study, conducted by Harvard University in six eastern and midwestern U.S. cities, demonstrated links between particle exposure and respiratory disease in children (33). Chronic cough and bronchitis symptoms were more closely associated with hydrogen ion concentration, a measure of acidity, than with sulfate or total levels of particles (34). A recent study of 24 cities in the United States and Canada found that long-term exposure to acid aerosols was associated with increased symptoms of bronchitis (35) and adverse effects on lung function (36) in children aged 8 to 12 years. In one of these cities (Uniontown, Pennsylvania), an increment in particle acidity of 125 nmol/m$^3$ was associated with an increase in cough and a decline in peak expiratory flow of 2.5 L/min (27). Increased prevalence of cough and sputum in communities has been associated with annual average sulfur dioxide levels of 0.04 to 0.05 ppm (37).

Determining the relative importance of acid aerosols in the health effects of air pollution is complicated by a paucity of direct measurements of acidic species, the complex nature of the pollutant mix, and the difficulty in separating the relative contribution of the individual pollutants. It remains unclear whether health effects are associated with chronic exposure to low levels of sulfur dioxide/acidic aerosol, or to intermittent exposure to higher concentrations.

Given the findings at very low levels of exposure, it should follow that the considerably higher concentrations that can be found in the workplace would be associated with respiratory tract illness. However, surprisingly few health effects have been associated with occupational exposure to sulfuric acid particles. A number of studies have failed to find acute or chronic effects on pulmonary function or incidence of chronic bronchitis, even in the presence of high levels of exposure (19,38). Williams (39) reported an increase in episodes of respiratory tract illness among exposed workers in a battery plant compared with presumably unexposed workers, but exposure measurements were not reported and smoking habits were not taken into account. Workers with years of exposure to sulfuric acid aerosols show evidence of more erosion and discoloration of dental enamel (18,38), presumably as a result of impaction of larger acidic particles on exposed dental surfaces. Hygroscopic growth of particles generated in the course of industrial processes leads to preferential deposition in the mouth and upper airways, which may minimize pulmonary effects. In contrast, environmental acid aerosols are often smaller than 1 μm aerodynamic diameter (40), and so are more likely to be deposited in distal airways.

The potential for chronic and recurrent irritation of the upper airways in response to occupational exposures to sulfuric acid has raised questions of increased risk for malignancy. A number of studies, recently reviewed by Soskolne and co-workers (41), suggest that workers exposed to acidic aerosols are at increased risk for lung and laryngeal cancers. Because other chemicals and potential carcinogens are generally associated with these aerosols in the workplace, a cause-and-effect relationship between sulfuric acid aerosols and malignancy has been difficult to prove. However, a working group of the International Agency for Research on Cancer has reviewed the evidence and concluded that "occupational exposure to strong-inorganic-acid mists containing sulfuric acid is carcinogenic to humans" (17).

Exposure to sulfur dioxide at concentrations of 10 to 50 ppm for 5 to 15 minutes causes cough; dyspnea; irritation of nose, throat, and eyes; choking; and reflex bronchoconstriction (42). Accidental high-dose exposure to sulfur dioxide may cause severe pulmonary injury or death. An accidental exposure of five workers to high levels of sulfur dioxide in a paper mill resulted in two deaths (43). Two of the three surviving workers demonstrated persistent pulmonary function abnormalities. In 1977, nine workers were exposed to a concentration of sulfur dioxide estimated to be several hundred parts per million as a result of a pyrite dust ($FeS_2$) explosion in an underground mine (44). One worker died and seven of eight workers followed over a 4-year interval with repeated measurements of lung function demonstrated persistent reductions in forced vital capacity (FVC), 1-second forced expiratory volume ($FEV_1$), and maximal midexpiratory flow rate. Four workers also showed airway hyperreactivity based on tests with inhaled histamine 4 years after the accident, suggesting that hyperreactivity is a sequela of high-level exposure.

### Acute Airway Function Responses

Experimental studies of human subjects exposed to sulfur dioxide and acidic aerosols under carefully controlled conditions can demonstrate immediate responses to various levels of these pollutants. The most striking effect of acute exposure to sulfur dioxide at concentrations of 1.00 ppm or less is the induction of bronchoconstriction in asthma patients after only 5 minutes' exposure. In contrast, inhalation of concentrations of sulfur dioxide in excess of 5 ppm was shown to cause only small decrements in airway function in normal subjects (45). Lung function responses to sulfur dioxide in asthma patients are greater when sulfur dioxide exposure is accompanied by increased ventilation, usually stimulated by exercise (46). In a group of seven subjects with mild asthma, inhaling 0.25 and 0.5 ppm sulfur dioxide during mild exercise caused significant bronchoconstriction; most subjects experienced symptoms after inhaling 0.5 ppm sulfur dioxide. The two most sensitive subjects also developed bronchoconstriction after inhaling 0.1 ppm sulfur dioxide (Fig. 1.) Furthermore, sulfur dioxide–induced bronchoconstriction can be exacerbated by breathing cold or dry air and by mouth breathing (47,48). The sulfur dioxide bronchoconstrictor response can be reduced or inhibited in asthma sufferers by anticholinergic agents such as atropine, mast-cell stabilizers such as cromolyn (49), and β-agonist bronchodilators such as metaproterenol (50). Unlike some other pollutants,

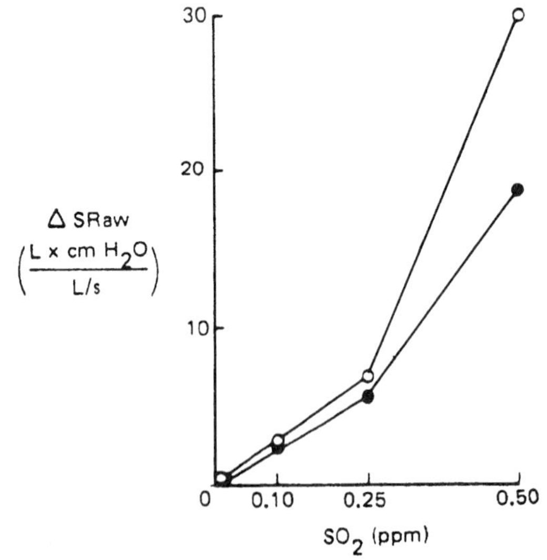


**FIG. 1.** Dose-response to sulfur dioxide inhaled during exercise in two subjects (• and ○). The ΔSRaw is the difference between baseline specific airway resistance and specific airway resistance after inhalation of sulfur dioxide. The subjects exercised on a bicycle for 10 minutes while they breathed air containing 0, 0.1, 0.25, or 0.5 ppm sulfur dioxide through a mouth piece. (From ref. 46.)

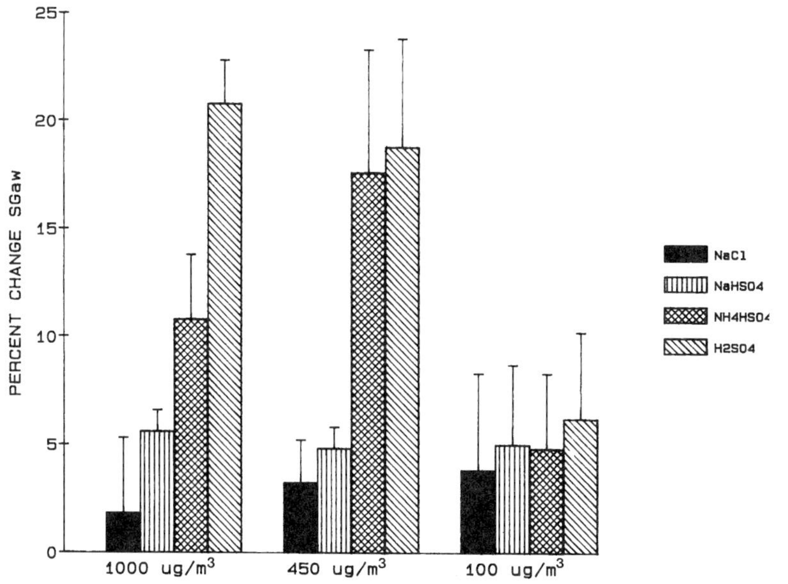


**FIG. 2.** Percentage change in specific airways conductance (SGaw) in 17 asthmatic subjects exposed for 16 minutes to sodium chloride and various sulfate aerosols. (Modified from ref. 4.)

inhalation of sulfur dioxide does not appear to cause pronounced changes in nonspecific airway reactivity (51).

Inhalation of acidic aerosols has generally produced little alteration of pulmonary function in normal subjects even at the threshold limit value of 1 mg/m$^3$ (52). As with sulfur dioxide, asthmatic subjects have been found most susceptible to the effects of acidic aerosol exposure, although different laboratories have found different threshold exposure concentrations (53). In general, however, studies of adult asthma patients have failed to demonstrate alterations in lung function at levels below 200 μg/m$^3$ (4,54). Utell and co-workers (4) exposed asthma patients to sulfuric acid, $NH_4HSO_4$, $NaHSO_4$, and a control sodium chloride aerosol at concentrations of 100, 450, and 1,000 μg/m$^3$ (Fig. 2). Following exposures to the 450- and 1,000-μg/m$^3$ aerosols for 16 minutes, specific airway conductance decreased more or less in relation to the acidity of the aerosol, supporting the hypothesis that airway effects are related to acidity rather than to the sulfate ion.

Recently, respiratory ammonia was identified as a factor influencing responses to sulfuric acid aerosols; by reducing the level of endogenous respiratory ammonia, airway responses of exercising asthmatics to inhalation of 350-μg/m$^3$ sulfuric acid aerosols were enhanced (55), thus providing further evidence that aerosol acidity significantly affected bronchoconstriction caused by inhalation of sulfate aerosols.

In some studies, adolescent asthma patients appear to be more sensitive than asthmatic adults to the effects of acidic aerosols. Functional decrements have been observed in adolescent asthmatics at levels as low as 68 μg/m$^3$ for 40 minutes (56). The apparent difference in sensitivity of adult and adolescent asthmatics may also be due to differences in aerosol size or exposure protocols, but adolescent asthmatics respond to concentrations of sulfuric acid aerosols that are an order of magnitude lower than those that affect normal healthy subjects. In these studies (56), young asthmatics showed functional decrements at exposure levels near peak outdoor levels in the northeastern United States. Field studies of both normal and asthmatic children in summer camps found decrements in pulmonary function during pollution episodes that included increased levels of acidic aerosols (57), reinforcing concern that children and adolescents may be particularly susceptible to effects of acidic atmospheres.

## Mucociliary Clearance

Studies of both humans and animals have demonstrated that exposures to sulfur dioxide and acidic aerosols alter mucociliary clearance. The removal of inhaled particles from the airways depends on the intact function of ciliated epithelium and its overlying mucous layer. Resting exposure to sulfur dioxide levels as low as 1.0 ppm reduced nasal mucous flow rates (58); in contrast, much higher levels (5.0 ppm) during exercise were required to increase tracheobronchial mucociliary clearance rates (59).

Brief (1- to 2-hour) exposures to sulfuric acid aerosols have shown consistent effects on clearance in three species (donkeys, rabbits, humans): low-level (100 to 200 μg/m$^3$) exposure accelerates mucociliary clearance, while higher levels (1,000 μg/m$^3$) delay clearance (60–62). Potency of acidic aerosols is related to acidity, with sulfuric acid aerosols being most potent, and to aerosol size (63). Because prolonged exposures in donkeys (64) and rabbits (65) has resulted in persistent decreases in mucociliary clearance, chronic acid exposure has been considered a potential model of chronic airways disease (66).

One study has examined effects of $H_2SO_4$ aerosols on clearance rates in subjects with asthma (67). Individuals who did not require regular medications for control of their asthma showed a dose-dependent slowing of mucociliary clearance, while medication-dependent asthmatics showed no clear pattern of effects, but the range of responses was large. Insufficient data were available to relate the dose-dependent effects in healthy volunteers with responses in asthmatics.

### Pollutant Mixtures

Epidemiologic studies of the health effects of pollutants frequently involve combined exposures. Pollutants, including ozone, nitrogen dioxide, and reactive hydrocarbons, are present in sulfur dioxide and acidic aerosol atmospheres. Increased rates of respiratory illness and mortality associated with sulfur dioxide and acidic aerosols may be potentiated by other pollutants. This is supported by animal data. For example, exposure of mice to sulfuric acid aerosols at 241 or 483 $\mu g/m^3$ combined with ozone at 196 $\mu g/m^3$ increased susceptibility to respiratory infection with aerosolized bacteria, whereas exposure to sulfuric acid aerosol alone had no effect (68). Prasad and colleagues (69) observed in rats that inhalation of a mixture of pollutants, including acidic droplets, reduced Fc receptor–mediated phagocytosis by alveolar macrophages in bronchoalveolar lavage fluid. Exposure to acidic aerosols potentiated effects of nitrogen dioxide and ozone on lung collagen synthesis in rats (70–72), suggesting a role for pollutant mixtures in lung fibrosis. Finally, Amdur and Chen (73,74) found that small particles present in polluted atmospheres become surface-coated with sulfuric acid, increasing the dose of hydrogen ion to the respiratory epithelium. In these studies, guinea pigs exposed to zinc oxide and sulfuric acid 3 hours per day for 5 days showed alterations in lung volumes, diffusing capacity, bronchial reactivity, and neutrophils in lavage fluid at levels of sulfuric acid as low as 20 $\mu g/m^3$.

Limited studies in healthy humans have not found interactions between sulfuric acid and ozone on pulmonary function (75–78). However, two recent studies suggest that individuals with asthma may be particularly susceptible to effects of acid aerosols in combination with ozone. One study found that a 3-hour exposure to 100 $\mu g/m^3$ $H_2SO_4$ aerosol enhanced the lung function response to 0.18 ppm ozone for 3 hours in asthmatic, but not healthy, subjects (79). In the other study, exposure to 0.12 ppm ozone with 100 $\mu g/m^3$ $H_2SO_4$ for 6.5 hours on two consecutive days caused greater decrements in lung function than either pollutant alone (80). Thus exposure to relatively low concentrations of acid aerosols may enhance responses to ozone in some individuals. Possible effects of pollutant mixtures on mucociliary clearance or alveolar cell function have not yet been studied.

A recent study suggests that sulfur dioxide, in combination with other pollutants, may enhance the airway response of asthmatic subjects to allergen inhalation (81). Ten atopic asthmatics were exposed for 6-hours to air, 0.2 ppm sulfur dioxide, 0.4 ppm nitrogen dioxide, or the combination of gases on separate occasions followed by predetermined concentrations of *Dermatophagoides pteronyssinus* allergen 10 minutes after each exposure. Although the decreases in airway function after exposure to each agent alone were not significant, the exposure to a combination of sulfur dioxide and nitrogen dioxide increased the response to challenge with specific antigen. Thus, for individuals with asthma, ambient pollution could increase the adverse effects of exposure to common indoor allergens, such as those associated with house dust mites, cats, or cockroaches.

## CELLULAR RESPONSES AND MECHANISMS

A convergence of data from epidemiologic, animal, and human exposure studies has led to speculation about the mechanisms by which sulfur dioxide and acidic aerosols may affect respiratory functions. Table 1 summarizes the probable mechanisms associated with health effects of exposure to sulfur dioxide and acidic aerosols.

**TABLE 1.** *Exposure to sulfur dioxide and acidic aerosols: health effects and mechanisms*

| Health effects | Mechanisms | References | |
|---|---|---|---|
| | | $H_2SO_4$ | $SO_2$ |
| Upper airways irritation | Impaction of large droplets on teeth and mucous membranes | 16,19 | 42 |
| Dental erosion | | 18,38 | — |
| Malignancy | Chronic irritation of respiratory epithelium | 41 | — |
| Pulmonary function decrements | Bronchoconstriction | 4,52,54–56 | 46–49 |
| Increased airway reactivity | Airway inflammation | 4,52 | 44,51 |
| | Airway narrowing | | |
| Altered mucociliary clearance | Change in pH of mucus | 59–65 | 58,59 |
| | Change in mucus composition and viscosity | 82–84 | |
| Altered mucus production | Increased number of mucus-secreting cells | 65 | 85 |
| Altered alveolar clearance | Altered function of alveolar macrophages | 69,86,89 | 88 |
| Sensitivity to allergens | | — | 81 |

The chemical mechanisms underlying the bronchoconstrictor effects of sulfur dioxide are not well defined. Sulfur dioxide dissolves in water to form bisulfite ion, sulfite ion, and hydrogen ion. Sheppard (49) has suggested that it is unlikely that the hydrogen ion or sulfite ion mediates sulfur dioxide–induced bronchoconstriction, whereas the bisulfite ion might. In contrast to acidic aerosols, presumably the concentration of hydrogen ion generated by inhalation of levels of sulfur dioxide required to produce bronchoconstriction are too low to cause airway effects (82). It is not clear whether the bronchoconstriction that occurs following oral ingestion of sulfite-containing liquids and foods in some asthmatics is mechanistically linked to sulfur dioxide–induced bronchoconstriction.

Considerable evidence supports the concept that toxic effects of acidic aerosols are related to the total hydrogen ion available to the respiratory epithelium (82). For any of the observed health effects, sulfuric acid is more potent than any of its neutralization products. However, Schlesinger (83) has suggested that the sulfate species of the neutralization products may also play a role in altering lung clearance. The effects of acidic aerosol exposure also may be mediated in part through effects on mucus. Holma (84) has shown that acidity decreases the buffering capacity and increases the viscosity of mucus glycoproteins, which may contribute to the decreased mucociliary clearance observed in animal and human studies. It may also lead to a compensatory increase in mucus production; indeed, animal morphologic studies have shown increases in airway mucus secretory cells in response to sulfuric acid (65). Short-term exposure to sulfur dioxide has also been shown to stimulate secretion from submucosal glands (85).

In addition, exposure to sulfuric acid aerosols may alter the alveolar microenvironment. Following exposure of rabbits to sulfuric acid aerosols, alterations in alveolar clearance of inhaled particles have been detected that parallel the effects on mucociliary clearance (86). Sequential exposures to sulfuric acid particles at 500 μg/m$^3$ impaired release of superoxide anion and killing of bacteria by alveolar macrophages (87). Acidic aerosol exposure in guinea pigs alters intracellular regulation of pH in alveolar macrophages, possibly through effects on membrane $Na^+$-$H^+$ exchange (17).

Bronchoalveolar lavage has been used to evaluate responses to exposure to sulfur dioxide and sulfuric acid aerosols in humans. Exposure to 8 ppm sulfur dioxide for 20 minutes resulted in increases in macrophages, lymphocytes, and mast cells recovered by bronchoalveolar lavage (88). No cellular inflammatory response or effects on alveolar macrophage function were found 18 hours after single 2-hour exposures to 1,000 μg/m$^3$ sulfuric acid aerosol (89). Furthermore, exposure to 1,000 μg/m$^3$ $H_2SO_4$ for 2 hours did not change the glycoprotein profile in mucus collected by bronchoscopy 18 hours after exposure (90). Studies of the effects of repeated exposures in humans have yet to be performed.

## STANDARDS

Recently the OSHA permissible exposure limit for sulfur dioxide was reduced from 5 to 2 ppm (5 mg/m$^3$) as a time-weighted average (TWA) for an 8-hour workday (42). A short-term (15-minute) exposure limit OSHA standard of 5 ppm (10 mg/m$^3$) has also been adopted. NIOSH has recommended a standard of 0.5 ppm to provide a larger margin of safety. The exposure standard for sulfuric acid established by OSHA, a TWA of 1 mg/m$^3$, is based on the known irritative properties of $H_2SO_4$ for the upper respiratory tract. Irritation of the eyes and nose occurs at 1 to 2 mg/m$^3$, and cough results at 5 to 6 mg/m$^3$ (16). However, irritative effects are highly dependent on relative humidity.

For sulfur dioxide, the Environmental Protection Agency (EPA) has set 24-hour (0.14 ppm) and annual (0.3 ppm) primary national ambient air quality standards (NAAQS). Despite the convincing bronchospasm induced in exercising asthmatics by brief exposure to sulfur dioxide, no short-term environmental sulfur dioxide standard has yet been established. Although there is no NAAQS for acidic aerosols, particulate acids are subject to the particulate matter, 10 μm ($PM_{10}$) NAAQS (24-hour, 150 μg/m$^3$; annual, 50 μg/m$^3$). In December 1996, the EPA proposed to change the current particulate matter standards by adding two new primary fine particle standards ($PM_{2.5}$, particles with an aerodynamic diameter of 2.5 μm or less); a $PM_{2.5}$ standard set at 15 μg/m$^3$, annual mean, and a second standard at 50 μg/m$^3$, a 24-hour average. These proposed modifications are based on the concern that the observed association between $PM_{10}$ and health effects may actually be the result of exposures to the fine-particle fraction of $PM_{10}$. At present, the EPA is reexamining monitoring technologies, ambient exposure, and available health effects data for sulfuric acid aerosols; acidic aerosols may be eventually listed for regulation (91).

## ACKNOWLEDGMENT

This work is supported in part by grants ESO2679, RO1HL51701, and RR00044 from the National Institutes of Health.

## REFERENCES

1. Leaderer BP. Air pollutant emissions from kerosene space heaters. *Science* 1982;218:q1113–1115.
2. Frank NR, Yoder RE, Brain JD, Yokoyama E. $SO_2$ ($^{35}$S-labeled) absorption by the nose and mouth under conditions of varying concentration and flow. *Arch Environ Health* 1969;18:315–322.
3. Kadowaki S. Size distribution of atmospheric total aerosols, sulfate, ammonium and nitrate particles in the Nagoya area. *Atmos Environ* 1976;10:39–43.

4. Utell MJ, Morrow PE, Speers DM, Darling J, Hyde RW. Airway responses to sulfate and sulfuric acid aerosols in asthmatics. *Am Rev Respir Dis* 1983;128:444–450.
5. National Research Council: Subcommittee on airborne particles. Effects of sulfur dioxide and aerosols, alone and combined on lung function. In: *Airborne particles.* Baltimore: University Park Press, 1978;154–160.
6. Shrenk HH, Heimann H, Clayton GD, Gafafen W, Wexler H. Air pollution in Donora, Pennsylvania: epidemiology of the unusual smog episodes of October 1948. *Public Health Bull* 1949;306.
7. Logan WPD. Mortality in London fog incident. *Lancet* 1953;1: 336–338.
8. Environmental Protection Agency. *Air quality criteria for particulate matter and sulfur oxides.* U.S. Environmental Protection Agency publication 600/8-82-029. Research Triangle Park, NC: Office of Health and Environmental Assessment, 1987.
9. Dockery DW, Speizer FE. Epidemiological evidence for aggravation and promotion of COPD by acid air pollution. In: Hensley MJ, Saunders NA, eds. *Lung biology in health and disease.* New York: Marcel Dekker, 1989;43:201–225.
10. Thurston GD, Gjorczynski JE Jr, Currie JH, et al. The nature and origins of acid summer haze air pollution in metropolitan Toronto, Ontario. *Environ Res* 1994;65:254–270.
11. Spengler JD, Brauer M, Koutrakis P. Acid air and health. *Environ Sci Technol* 1990;24:946–956.
12. Spengler JD, Keeler GJ, Koutrakis P, Ryan PB, Raizenne M, Franklin CA. Exposures to acidic aerosols. *Environ Health Perspect* 1989;79: 43–51.
13. Spengler JD, Koutrakis P, Dockery DW, Raizenne M, Speizer FE. Health effects of acid aerosols on North American children: air pollution exposures. *Environ Health Perspect* 1996;104:492–499.
14. Leaderer BP, Boone PM, White JB, Hammond KS. Total particle sulfate and acidic aerosol emissions from kerosene space heaters. *Environ Sci Technol* 1990;24:908–912.
15. NIOSH. *Criteria for a recommended standard:* occupational exposure to sulfur dioxide. Washington, DC: U.S. Government Printing Office, 1974.
16. Gamble J, Jones W, Hancock J. Epidemiological-environmental study of lead acid battery workers. II. Acute effects of sulfuric acid on the respiratory system. *Environ Res* 1984;35:11–29.
17. International Agency for Research in Cancer (IARC) . Occupational exposures to mists and vapours from sulfuric acid and other strong inorganic acids. *IARC Monographs on the Evaluation of Carcinogenic Risks to Humans* 1992;54:41–119.
18. Malcolm D, Paul E. Erosion of the teeth due to sulphuric acid in the battery industry. *Br J Ind Med* 1961;18:63–69.
19. El-Sadik YM, Osman AH, El-Gazzar RM. Exposure to sulfuric acid in manufacture of storage batteries. *J Occup Med* 1972;14:224–226.
20. Jones W, Gamble J. Epidemiological-environmental study of lead acid battery workers. I. Environmental study of five lead acid battery plants. *Environ Res* 1984;35:1–10.
21. Thurston GD, Ito K, Lippmann M, Hayes C. Reexamination of London, England, mortality in relation to exposure to acidic aerosols during 1963–1972 winters. *Environ Health Perspect* 1989;79:73–82.
22. Kitagawa T. Cause analysis of the Yokkaichi asthma episode in Japan. *JAPCA* 1984;34:743–746.
23. Imai M, Katsumi Y, Kitagawa M. Mortality from asthma and chronic bronchitis associated with changes in sulfur oxides air pollution. *Arch Environ Health* 1986;41:29–35.
24. Dockery D, Pope A. Epidemiology of acute health effects: summary of time-series studies. In: Wilson R, Spengler J, eds. *Particles in our air:* concentrations and health effects. Cambridge: Harvard School of Public Health, 1996;123–147.
25. Environmental Protection Agency. *Air quality criteria for particulate matter.* U.S. Environmental Protection Agency publication 600//P-95/001bF. Research Triangle Park, NC: Office of Research and Development, 1996.
26. Dockery DW, Speizer FE, Stram DO, Ware JH, Spengler JD, Ferris BG Jr. Effects of inhalable particles on respiratory health of children. *Am Rev Respir Dis* 1989;139:587–594.
27. Neas LM, Dockery DW, Koutrakis P, Tollerud DJ, Speizer FE. The association of ambient air pollution with twice daily peak expiratory flow rate measurements in children. *Am J Epidemiol* 1995;141: 111–122.
28. Pope CA III, Dockery DW, Spengler JD, Raizenne ME. Respiratory health and $PM_{10}$ pollution. *Am Rev Respir Dis* 1991;144:668–674.
29. Pope CA III. Respiratory disease associated with community air pollution and a steel mill, Utah valley. *Am J Public Health* 1989;79: 623–628.
30. Utell MJ, Frampton MW. Particles and mortality: a clinical perspective. *Inhal Toxicol* 1995;7:645–655.
31. Bates DV, Sizto R. Air pollution and hospital admissions in Southern Ontario: the acid summer haze effect. *Environ Res* 1987;43:317–331.
32. Thurston GD, Ito K, Hayes CG, Bates DV, Lippmann M. Respiratory hospital admissions and summertime haze air pollution in Toronto, Ontario: consideration of the role of acid aerosols. *Environ Res* 1994; 65:271–290.
33. Ware JH, Ferris BG Jr, Dockery DW, Spengler JD, Stram DO. Effects of ambient sulfur oxides and suspended particles on respiratory health of preadolescent children. *Am Rev Respir Dis* 1986;133:834–842.
34. Speizer FE. Studies of acid aerosols in six cities and in a new multicity investigation: design issues. *Environ Health Perspect* 1989;79:61–67.
35. Dockery DW, Cunningham J, Damokosh AI, et al. Health effects of acid aerosols on North American children: respiratory symptoms. *Environ Health Perspect* 1996;104:500–505.
36. Raizenne M, Neas LM, Damokosh AI, et al. Health effects of acid aerosols on North American children: pulmonary function. *Environ Health Perspect* 1996;104:506–514.
37. Dodge R, Solomon P, Moyers J, Hayes C. A longitudinal study of children exposed to sulfur oxides. *Am J Epidemiol* 1985;121:730–736.
38. Gamble J, Jones W, Hancock J, Meckstroth RL. Epidemiological-environmental study of lead acid battery workers. III. Chronic effects of sulfuric acid on the respiratory system and teeth. *Environ Res* 1984;35: 30–52.
39. Williams MK. Sickness absence and ventilatory capacity of workers exposed to sulphuric acid mist. *J Ind Med* 1970;27:61–66.
40. Pierson WR, Brachaczek WW, Truex TJ, Butler JW, Korniski TJ. Ambient sulfate measurements on Allegheny Mountain and the question of atmospheric sulfate in the northeastern United States. *Ann NY Acad Sci* 1980;338:145–173.
41. Soskolne CL, Pagano G, Cipollaro M, Beaumont JJ, Giordano GG. Epidemiologic and toxicologic evidence for chronic health effects and the underlying biologic mechanisms involved in sub-lethal exposures to acidic pollutants. *Arch Environ Health* 1989;44:180–191.
42. Occupational exposures to sulfur dioxide. *Federal Register* 1989;54: 2524–2526.
43. Charan NB, Myers CG, Lakshminarayan S, Spencer TM. Pulmonary injuries associated with acute sulfur dioxide inhalation. *Am Rev Respir Dis* 1979;119:555–560.
44. Harkonen H, Nordman H, Korhonen O, Winblad I. Long-term effects of exposure to sulfur dioxide. Lung function after a pyrite dust explosion. *Am Rev Respir Dis* 1983;128:890–893.
45. Nadel JA, Salem H, Tamplin B, Tokiwa G. Mechanism of bronchoconstriction during inhalation of sulfur dioxide. *J Appl Physiol* 1965;20: 164–167.
46. Sheppard D, Saisho A, Nadel JA, Boushey HA. Exercise increases sulfur dioxide-induced bronchoconstriction in asthmatic subjects. *Am Rev Respir Dis* 1981;123:486–491.
47. Sheppard D, Eschenbacher WL, Boushey HA, Bethel RA. Magnitude of the interaction between the bronchomotor effects of sulfur dioxide and those of dry (cold) air. *Am Rev Respir Dis* 1984;130:52–55.
48. Bethel RA, Erle DJ, Epstein J, Sheppard D, Nadel JA, Boushey HA. Effect of exercise rate and route of inhalation on sulfur dioxide-induced bronchoconstriction in asthmatic subjects. *Am Rev Respir Dis* 1983; 128:592–596.
49. Sheppard D. Mechanisms of airway responses to inhaled sulfur dioxide. In: Loke J, ed. *Lung biology in health and disease.* New York: Marcel Dekker, 1988;34:49–65.
50. Linn WS, Avol EL, Shamoo DA, et al. Effect of metaproterenol sulfate on mild asthmatics' response to sulfur dioxide exposure and exercise. *Arch Environ Health* 1988;43:399–406.
51. Hazucha MJ, Kehrl HR, Roger LJ, Horstman DH. Airway responsiveness to methacholine of asthmatics exposed to 0.25, 0.5, and 1.0 ppm $SO_2$. *Am Rev Respir Dis* 1984;129:A145(abstr).
52. Utell MJ, Morrow PE, Hyde RW. Airway reactivity to sulfate and sulfuric acid aerosols in normal and asthmatic subjects. *J Air Pollut Control Assoc* 1984;34:931–935.
53. Aris R, Christian D, Sheppard D, Balmes JR. Lack of bronchoconstric-

tor response to sulfuric acid aerosols and fogs. *Am Rev Respir Dis* 1991;143:744–750.
54. Linn WS, Avol EL, Shamoo DA, Whynot JD, Anderson KR, Hackney JD. Respiratory responses of exercising asthmatic volunteers exposed to sulfuric acid aerosol. *JAPCA* 1986;36:1323–1328.
55. Utell MJ, Mariglio JA, Morrow PE, Gibb FR, Speers DM. Effects of inhaled acid aerosols on respiratory function: the role of endogenous ammonia. *J Aerosol Med* 1989;2:141–147.
56. Koenig JQ, Covert DS, Pierson WE. Effects of inhalation of acidic compounds on pulmonary function in allergic adolescent subjects. *Environ Health Perspect* 1989;79:173–178.
57. Raizenne ME, Burnett RT, Stern B, Franklin CA, Spengler JD. Acute lung function responses to ambient acid aerosol exposures in children. *Environ Health Perspect* 1989;79:179–185.
58. Andersen I, Lundqvist GR, Jensen PL, Proctor DF. Human response to controlled levels of sulfur dioxide. *Arch Environ Health* 1974;28:31–39.
59. Newhouse MT, Dolovich M, Obminski G, Wolff RK. Effect of TLV levels of $SO_2$ and $H_2SO_4$ on bronchial clearance in exercising man. *Arch Environ Health* 1978;33:24–32.
60. Leikauf G, Yeates DB, Wales KA, Spektor D, Albert RE, Lippmann M. Effects of sulfuric acid aerosol on respiratory mechanics and mucociliary particle clearance in healthy nonsmoking adults. *Am Ind Hyg Assoc J* 1981;42:273–282.
61. Spektor DM, Yen BM, Lippmann M. Effect of concentration and cumulative exposure of inhaled sulfuric acid on tracheobronchial particle clearance in healthy humans. *Environ Health Perspect* 1989;79:167–172.
62. Schlesinger RB. The interaction of inhaled toxicants with respiratory tract clearance mechanisms. *Crit Rev Toxicol* 1990;20:257–286.
63. Laube BL, Bowes SM III, Links JM, Thomas KK, Frank R. Acute exposure to acid fog: effects on mucociliary clearance. *Am Rev Respir Dis* 1993;147:1105–1111.
64. Schlesinger RB, Halpern M, Albert RE, Lippmann M. Effect of chronic inhalation of sulfuric acid mist upon mucociliary clearance from the lungs of donkeys. *J Environ Pathol Toxicol* 1979;2:1351–1367.
65. Gearhart JM, Schlesinger RB. Sulfuric acid-induced changes in the physiology and structure of the tracheobronchial airways. *Environ Health Perspect* 1989;79:127–137.
66. Lippmann M. Airborne acidity: estimates of exposure and human health effects. *Environ Health Perspect* 1985;63:63–70.
67. Spektor DM, Leikauf GD, Albert RE, Lippmann M. Effects of submicrometer sulfuric acid aerosols on mucociliary transport and respiratory mechanics in asymptomatic asthmatics. *Environ Res* 1985;37:174–191.
68. Grose EC, Richards JH, Illing JW, et al. Pulmonary host defense responses to inhalation of sulfuric acid and ozone. *J Toxicol Environ Health* 1982;10:351–362.
69. Prasad SB, Rao VS, Mannix RC, Phalen RF. Effects of pollutant atmospheres on surface receptors of pulmonary macrophages. *J Toxicol Environ Health* 1988;24:385–402.
70. Last JA, Warren DL. Synergistic interaction between nitrogen dioxide and respirable aerosols of sulfuric acid or sodium chloride on rat lungs. *Toxicol Appl Pharmacol* 1987;90:34–42.
71. Warren DL, Last JA. Synergistic interaction of ozone and respirable aerosols on rat lungs. III. Ozone and sulfuric acid aerosol. *Toxicol Appl Pharmacol* 1987;88:203–216.
72. Last JA, Gerriets JE, Hyde DM. Synergistic effects on rat lungs of mixtures of oxidant air pollutants (ozone or nitrogen dioxide) and respirable aerosols. *Am Rev Respir Dis* 1983;128:539–544.
73. Amdur MO, Chen LC. Furnace-generated acid aerosols: speciation and pulmonary effects. *Environ Health Perspect* 1989;79:147–150.
74. Amdur MO. Health effects of air pollutants: sulfuric acid, the old and the new. *Environ Health Perspect* 1989;81:109–113.
75. Kulle TJ, Kerr HD, Farrell BP, Sauder LR, Bermel MS. Pulmonary function and bronchial reactivity in human subjects with exposure to ozone and respirable sulfuric acid aerosol. *Am Rev Respir Dis* 1982;126:996–1000.
76. Stacy RW, Seal E Jr, House DE, Green J, Roger LJ, Raggio L. A survey of effects of gaseous and aerosol pollutants on pulmonary function of normal males. *Arch Environ Health* 1983;38:104–115.
77. Horvath SM, Folinsbee LJ, Bedi JF. Combined effect of ozone and sulfuric acid on pulmonary function in man. *Am Ind Hyg Assoc J* 1987;48:94–98.
78. Kleinman MT, Bailey RM, Chang Y-TC, et al. Exposures of human volunteers to a controlled atmospheric mixture of ozone, sulfur dioxide and sulfuric acid. *Am Ind Hyg Assoc J* 1981;42:61–69.
79. Frampton MW, Morrow PE, Cox C, et al. Sulfuric acid aerosol followed by ozone exposure in healthy and asthmatic subjects. *Environ Res* 1995;69:1–14.
80. Linn WS, Anderson KR, Shamoo DA, et al. Controlled exposures of young asthmatics to mixed oxidant gases and acid aerosol. *Am J Respir Crit Care Med* 1995;152:885–891.
81. Devalia JL, Rusznak C, Herdman MJ, et al. Effect of nitrogen dioxide and sulphur dioxide on airway response of mild asthmatic patients to allergen inhalation. *Lancet* 1994;344:1668–1671.
82. Fine JM, Gordon T, Thompson JE, Sheppard D. The role of titrable acidity in acid aerosol-induced bronchoconstriction. *Am Rev Respir Dis* 1987;135:826–830.
83. Schlesinger RB. Factors affecting the response of lung clearance systems to acid aerosols: role of exposure concentration, exposure time and relative acidity. *Environ Health Perspect* 1989;79:121–126.
84. Holma B. Effects of inhaled acids on airway mucus and its consequences for health. *Environ Health Perspect* 1989;79:109–113.
85. Nadel JA. Regulation of bronchial secretions. In: Newball HH, ed. *Lung biology in health and disease.* New York: Marcel Dekker, 1983; 19:109–139.
86. Schlesinger RB. Functional assessment of rabbit alveolar macrophages following intermittent inhalation exposures to sulfuric acid mist. *Fundam Appl Toxicol* 1987;8:328–334.
87. Zelikoff JT, Sisco MP, Yang Z, Cohen MD, Schlesinger RB. Immunotoxicity of sulfuric acid aerosol: effects on pulmonary macrophage effector and functional activities critical for maintaining host resistance against infectious diseases. *Toxicology* 1994;92:269–286.
88. Sandstrom T, Stjernberg N, Andersson M, et al. Cell response in bronchoalveolar lavage fluid after exposure to sulfur dioxide: a time-response study. *Am Rev Respir Dis* 1989;140:1828–1831.
89. Frampton MW, Voter KZ, Morrow PE, et al. Effects of $H_2SO_4$ aerosol exposure in humans assessed by bronchoalveolar lavage. *Am Rev Respir Dis* 1992;146:626–632.
90. Culp DJ, Latchney LR, Frampton MW, Jahnke MR, Morrow PE, Utell MJ. Composition of human airway mucins and effects after inhalation of acid aerosol. *Am J Physiol* 1995;269:L358-L370.
91. Lipfert FW, Morris SL, Wyzga RE. Acid aerosols: the next criteria air pollutant? *Environ Sci Technol* 1989;23:1316–1322.

*Environmental and Occupational Medicine, Third Edition,* edited by William N. Rom.
Lippincott–Raven Publishers, Philadelphia © 1998.

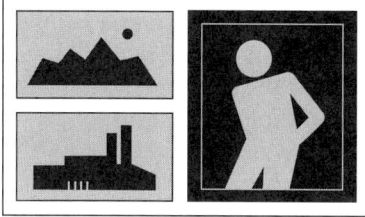

# CHAPTER 42

# Respiratory Tract Irritants

Tee Lamont Guidotti

Respiratory tract irritants are agents that result in an inflammatory response or a physiologic response in the respiratory tract (1), because of either their chemical reactivity or physical properties. Respiratory irritants may be considered strong, weak, or relatively inert for the purposes of this discussion, although this terminology is not standard.

Strong irritants, which are the major emphasis of this chapter, consist of exposures that produce a stereotyped and acute pattern of damage in the respiratory tract; recovery is often associated with major sequelae and sometimes significant respiratory impairment. Strong irritants that are highly reactive are more likely to produce an immediate and sometimes life-threatening response. Examples of strong respiratory irritants, by any standard, would include acrolein, ammonia, chlorine, chlorine dioxide, phosphoric acid, and other chemical exposures described in the final section of this chapter (2,3).

Weak irritants tend to act by inducing chronic symptoms over a prolonged period of time and often by aggravating existing disease such as asthma and chronic bronchitis. It may be difficult to distinguish between sensitization to an agent and airways irritation due to the agent; this is sometimes a clinical problem with the isocyanates, for example (4). Examples of weak irritants include many common solvents (most potently the xylenes), and alcohols.

"Inert" agents are less reactive still and many of their effects are based on physical properties or on a nonspecific host response to foreign agents. Those irritants that are, essentially, chemically inert, such as many of the so-called nuisance dusts or some solvent and petroleum vapors (including cyclohexane and isopropyl alcohol) or air that is extremely dry or cold, may act by triggering inflammatory or physiologic mechanisms that are nonspecific (5), such as particle-induced macrophage overload (6) and protease release (7) or cold-induced bronchoconstriction and bronchial reflexes (8).

T. L. Guidotti: Department of Public Health Sciences, Occupational Health Program, University of Alberta, Edmonton, Alberta T6G 2G3, Canada.

## HOW THE LUNG RESPONDS TO RESPIRATORY IRRITANTS

The lung is highly vulnerable to the effects of respiratory irritants. The respiratory tract is protected by many layers of host defense, but they are primarily effective against infectious agents. Chemical hazards may bypass most of the these in the upper airway and penetrate deeply to airways and alveoli. When this occurs, the effect of the agent on the respiratory tract is governed primarily by the degree of penetration, the characteristics of the agent, and the nature of the host defense mechanisms it encounters at the level affected.

The respiratory tract is saturated with water beyond the carina and is lined with a moist mucosa with a very large surface area. Inhaled gases that are soluble in water to any appreciable extent tend to be dissolved readily and removed from the airway very efficiently. Therefore, gases penetrate the respiratory tract more deeply the less soluble they are in water. Respiratory tract irritants that are chemically reactive but easily neutralized, such as formaldehyde or acetic acid, may induce upper respiratory tract irritation, sinusitis, and sneezing (9) but rarely cause problems deeper in the respiratory tract. Relatively soluble gases, such as ammonia, chlorine, and sulfur dioxide, penetrate poorly and usually cause predominantly airways irritation, which manifests itself as bronchospasm or an acute bronchitis. Occasionally, the concentration at exposure is so high that a soluble gas can penetrate in significant quantities to the alveolar level because of sheer mass, but this is very uncommon. Relatively insoluble gases, such as phosgene, nitrogen dioxide, and ozone penetrate very deeply, to the terminal bronchiolar and alveolar regions. These gases are particularly dangerous because they can induce toxic pulmonary edema, an often-fatal outcome resembling adult respiratory distress syndrome (10,11).

The response to respiratory irritants is highly variable, among the most unpredictable of occupational health outcomes in the individual case. Important factors include the circumstances of exposure, the level of exposure to the agent of interest, the constitutional susceptibility of the host (especially if there is a history of atopy or airways reactivity), recent personal history (such as recent respiratory tract infections), smoking history, and other recent exposures (including environmental tobacco smoke) (2,12). In a few cases, especially involving chronic cough, there may be a behavioral component to the response and the cough itself may perpetuate the response by causing further inflammation. Although documentation appears to be lacking, there is at least an anecdotal impression among some clinicians that persons who smoked cigarettes and then quit are often more susceptible to low-grade airways irritants than persons who never smoked or who continue smoking. Empirical verification of this observation is needed.

Another important aspect of respiratory irritants is that an irritant that primarily affects deep structures often affects proximal structures on the way down. For example, ozone is primarily associated with changes at the level of the terminal bronchiole and alveoli, where it may alter breathing reflexes in addition to a usually low-grade alveolitis. However, ozone may also induce a cough and inflammation in the larger airways and nasal irritation.

## CLINICAL MANIFESTATIONS OF RESPIRATORY TRACT IRRITATION

The clinical effect produced depends on the level of penetration and what happens when the agent encounters the predominant host defense mechanisms at that level.

Gases that are very soluble and dusts that have a large aerodynamic diameter tend to produce upper airways effects, such as sinusitis and nasal irritation. They often aggravate or mimic hay fever and may cause symptoms to be expressed in a previously quiescent atopic individual. Such symptoms are likely to be one important category of the "sick building syndrome" and an important manifestation of indoor air quality. Since approximately 15% of the adult population is atopic, it is clear why this is a common problem. It is perhaps most commonly a result of airborne dust alone. Such symptoms are also aggravated by low humidity, as occurs in northern climates in the winter and particularly indoors in climate-controlled buildings.

Gases that are soluble and dusts that are somewhat larger than 10 μm may have their primary effect on the larger airways of the lower respiratory tract, causing cough or bronchoconstriction. In most cases, this effect is transient or short-lived (13,14). Bronchoconstriction may be manifested as either acute bronchospasm or aggravation of airways reactivity, with more frequent and severe attacks in individuals with asthma (13). Occasionally, airways obstruction or cough may be expressed in an individual without a history of asthma but with a personal or family history of atopy and especially hay fever. In such situations, it is likely that the subclinical airways reactivity is enhanced by an inflammatory response to the irritant (5). This inflammatory response may be very low grade, unlikely to produce a response in an individual who is not susceptible, and rarely resulting in wheezing or productive cough. These responses are very variable, depending on the individual, the exposure situation, and the season, since the person affected may also be responding to allergens.

Dusts of a diameter greater than 10 μm are very important in inducing responses in the upper airway and the larger airways of the lower respiratory tract, especially in inducing bronchospasm in an individual with existing reactive airways. Effects on small airways are usually silent because the cross-sectional area at that level of the respiratory tract is so large that there is a huge functional reserve and no obstruction is clinically apparent. Thus, although there is evidence to suggest that some dusts may induce fibrosis in this region and low-grade small airways disease, this does not seem to be a large effect (15,16). It is certainly a small response compared to that induced by cigarette smoking. However, it may be significant in contributing to chronic obstructive pulmonary disease in the presence of other risk factors (16–18).

Particles that have a diameter less than 10 μm may penetrate to the alveoli, deposit, and induce a pneumoconiosis. "Nuisance dusts," which are also called "particulates not otherwise classified/regulated" (PNOC), are dusts that are rarely associated with obvious clinical disease and for which no separate regulatory standard exists in the United States (16). These dusts do not result in the exuberant fibrosis associated with the clinically important pneumoconioses, such as silicosis and asbestosis, or the dysfunctional immune responses of hypersensitivity pneumonitis or beryllium disease. However, all such dusts may be associated with nonspecific responses at the alveolar level that induce a low-grade response, even small amounts of focal fibrosis.

Gases that penetrate deeply may induce a generalized pattern of diffuse alveolar damage, which resembles the early pathology of adult respiratory distress syndrome (19). This response is very dangerous because it may lead to toxic pulmonary edema, described in greater detail below. This is a response to strong irritants and is clinically the most severe and most often life-threatening effect of respiratory irritants.

## TOXIC INHALATION

Toxic inhalation is a serious pattern of respiratory injury that results from diffuse alveolar damage and associated airway injury in an exposure that involves deep penetration of strong respiratory irritants. The most prominent feature of toxic inhalation is the risk of pulmonary edema. Parenchymal lesions may result in honeycombing (interstitial fibrosis), reflecting abnormally proliferative fibrosis (20,21). Airways effects may be prominent in toxic inhalation, among them acute bronchospasm (12), bronchiolitis obliterans (13), and reactive airways dysfunction syndrome. Toxic inhalation also involves substantial compromise of respiratory host defenses and a risk of infection and complications.

Acute toxic inhalation by irritant, and particularly by oxidant, gases is a complex process involving biochemical, morphologic, and functional changes. The severity and special features of toxic inhalation depend on the concentration inhaled, the duration of exposure, the redox potential and chemical characteristics (especially solubility) of the individual gas, and, as will be seen, other factors (10).

The pulmonary vascular endothelium is the primary target, and compromise of this tissue may lead to pulmonary edema (10). The pulmonary vascular endothelium is a very active tissue that is susceptible to a variety of toxic injuries but is capable of only limited response (22). A specific problem of great complexity in oxidant gas injury is the behavior of fluid following damage to the endothelial barrier. Among the most important functions of the endothelium is the regulation of vascular tone by nitric oxide (NO), which acts as a local hormone on adjacent arterial smooth muscle. Its activity is kept strictly localized. This is an effective means of titrating the vascular response and rapidly adjusting the vascular tone to changing hemodynamics (22,23).

The presence of this endogenous, nitrate-based messenger system for vascular regulation robustly explains the therapeutic vasodilator action of nitrates, the alterations in lung perfusion observed with inhalation of nitrogen dioxide (10), and even the vasoconstriction response of the pulmonary vascular bed during hypoxia, resulting as it does from decreased NO activity. There is some evidence that vascular segments with impaired endothelium may be more sensitive to nitrates and NO-induced vasodilation than intact segments (23).

The apparent sensitivity of the pulmonary capillary endothelium may be a multifactorial phenomenon. The lung is the organ at highest local oxygen tension. The endothelium, despite its low turnover rate, is a very active tissue metabolically (24). Current theory suggests that much of the cytotoxicity induced by agents such as oxidant gases, ionizing radiation, and free radical-forming compounds (e.g., paraquat) is mediated by the superoxide radical. The pulmonary capillary endothelium is thus at maximum risk (10). Furthermore, secondary phenomena of inflammation may result in very localized superoxide injury to the endothelium, an "innocent bystander" effect, after stimulation of adjacent polymorphonuclear leukocytes (PMNs) by activated complement, specifically C5a (10,24). The concept is analogous to but distinct from the release of proteolytic enzymes by phagocytic cells, a process that may set the stage for damage persisting beyond the acute phase (25).

Another possible mechanism of injury is the release of vasoactive humoral factors to which the endothelium is specifically responsive or preferentially exposed by position. In the case of oxygen toxicity such metabolic abnormalities occur before visible evidence of cellular injury. Although humoral factors are undoubtedly involved, it is likely that the release of such factors, including bradykinin and the biogenic amines, contributes to the expression of injury more than the injury itself (10,26).

The presence of specific receptors that increase vascular permeability and induce pulmonary edema may be an important pharmacologic mechanism for the induction of pulmonary edema by toxic gases. This mechanism provides an explanation for ontogenetic and phylogenetic differences in susceptibility, the phenomenon of tolerance, the action of neurogenic pathways, and the sympathetic appearance of edema in the contralateral lung after unilateral embolism. To date, the theory lacks empirical validation (10).

The pulmonary vascular endothelium is not a highly complex structure (22), and its responses to injury are limited by physiologic constraints on its function. Structural endothelial damage by toxic gases such as nitrogen dioxide or ozone or by irradiation include swelling, cytoplasmic changes, proliferation of microvilli, and cell surface redundancy. Vesicles become much more numerous and ultimately large vacuoles form. The cell may retract or slough, even leaving behind denuded areas of basement membrane. The functional results of this injury include loss of control of solute transport across the endothelium, resulting in increased permeability (27). This leads to interstitial and then alveolar edema (10).

Recent exposure to prior toxic inhalation, especially to phosgene, increases relative resistance to a later lethal challenge with another gas (28). This phenomenon of tolerance disappears within days but is remarkably strong while it lasts. Tolerance to repeated exposure to toxic gases, particularly the oxidant gases, is species-specific and inversely correlated with the age of the animal documented. It is usually explained on the basis of the regeneration of type I alveolar epithelial cells by the less susceptible type II cell. However, the role of the endothelium may be more important in the pathophysiology of toxic inhalation than previously realized (10).

The principal structural barrier to the passage of fluid is the alveolar capillary membrane, which may be as thin as 0.5 μm. The lung is highly vulnerable to flooding by plasma-derived fluid. Complex systems to control and contain the passage of fluid through the lungs act to protect it from edema and resultant substantial changes in gas exchange. These mechanisms that protect the lung include (a) the low pressure of the pulmonary circulation, (b) the surfactant system (which reduces intraalveolar surface tension), and (c) the lymphatic drainage system (10). The endothelium is the first barrier component encountered on the capillary side. Plasma water and smaller macromolecules are prevented from passing into the interstitium by intact endothelial junctions (27). These can be disrupted by circulatory overload, which stretches the intercellular junctions (29). Fluid may then enter the interstitium, where there are no barriers, and fluid collects as interstitial edema. At this point the barrier to further penetration is the alveolar epithelium, in which the junctions are tighter, more complex, and less susceptible to alteration by mechanical stress. The final phase of pulmonary edema, that of alveolar flooding, is thought to begin in the corners of greatest curvature of the alveoli at a "critical configuration" of volume and geometry in which inflation pressure no longer balances surface tension and hydrostatic forces (10).

The pathways of resolution of toxic pulmonary edema have not been systematically studied. Most of the work has been done on cardiogenic (hydrostatic) edema and the capillary permeability type caused by sepsis or inflammatory mechanisms (30). The degree to which an irritant gas interferes with the process of resolution and repair may depend on its own intrinsic toxicity to other anatomical elements, particularly to the alveolar epithelium (10,20,21).

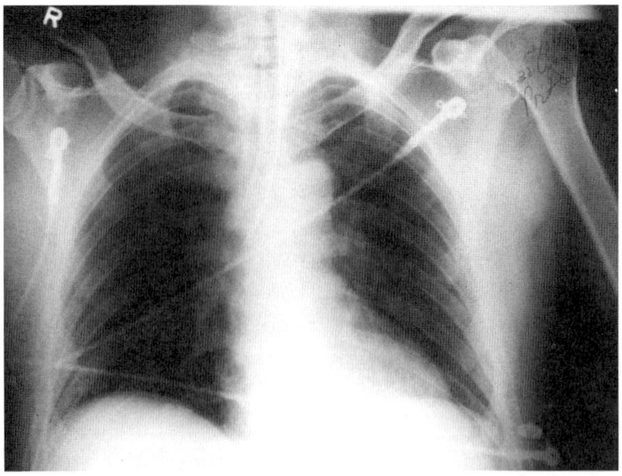


**FIG. 1.** Toxic inhalation in evolution. A 50-year-old never-smoking male insulator who was engaged in repair of a pipe at a fertilizer factory was trapped in a confined space with ammonia and experienced unusually high and prolonged exposure. He experienced dyspnea, cough, eye irritation, and lost consciousness before he was rescued by co-workers wearing self-contained breathing apparatus. This chest film was taken on admission to the nearest intensive care unit approximately 2 hours after the event and is almost normal. Fortunately, he did not experience burns to the face or compromise of his airway, which sometimes happens with exposure to ammonia.

Inhalation of toxic gases produces a more diffuse form of generalized acute lung injury than that generally seen

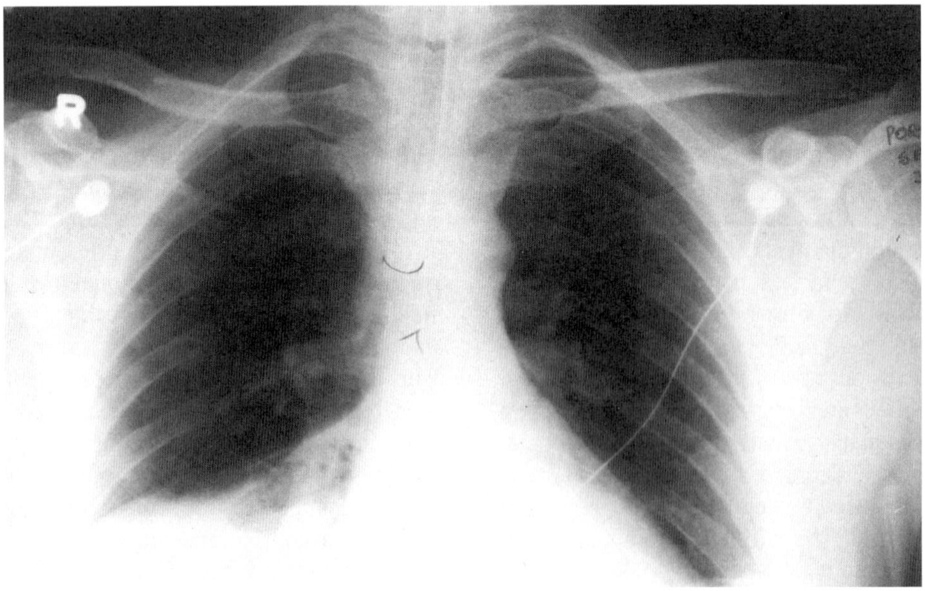


**FIG. 2.** Patient in Fig. 1, 15 hours later, shows bilateral infiltrates, right lower lobe atelectasis, and an effusion on right. He recovered over the next 7 days, after which he also required treatment for chemical burns to the skin. He experienced persistent productive cough, wheezing, and reduced exercise tolerance following discharge, 21 days after the event.

in adult respiratory distress syndrome and involves airway effects as well as injury at the alveolar level. Nitrogen dioxide ($NO_2$) has been well studied as a model for toxic inhalation (10,28).

The clinical presentation of toxic inhalation associated with the risk of pulmonary edema is stereotyped and varies little among the agents that can cause the syndrome. Figures 1 through 3 illustrate some features of this syndrome in a characteristic case (10,11).

There is a stepwise progression of clinical responses that should be anticipated but does not necessarily appear in every case. Patients may survive or skip one phase but encounter trouble in a later phase. Table 1 summarizes these phases (10,11).

Initially, the patient experiences acute bronchospasm and dyspnea, bronchial irritation and cough, and chest pain that may simulate angina pectoris. Alterations in both ventilation and pulmonary perfusion are best documented for nitrogen dioxide. Immediate removal from the source of exposure usually reverses these initial symptoms. Supportive treatment with oxygen and correction of acid/base abnormalities may be necessary. Bronchodilators may be given in persistent bronchospasm. Corticosteroids have been advocated for immediate administration in cases of heavy exposure to prevent the later development of pulmonary edema; although the practice is almost universal, there is little empirical evidence that it is effective. The acute phase of toxic inhalation must be differentiated from an overwhelming anaphylactoid hypersensitivity reaction to organic dusts and from asphyxiation hypoxemia, which may occur in concentrated atmospheres of inert gases (2,11).

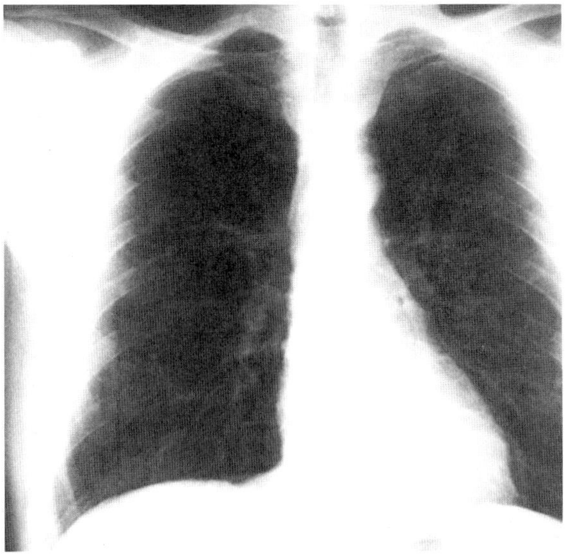

**FIG. 3.** Patient in Fig. 1, 10 months later, shows prominent interstitial markings bilaterally. He experienced a persistent low-grade productive cough, and pulmonary function studies showed moderate airways obstruction reversible with bronchodilators, air trapping, and fixed small airways disease attributed to bronchiolitis obliterans, with a normal diffusing capacity. He was awarded 25% respiratory impairment and returned to work as a stock clerk in a hardware store.

**TABLE 1.** *Clinical phases of response to toxic inhalation*

| |
|---|
| 1. Superacute (rare) |
| 1.1 Severe acute injury |
| 1.2 Acute chemical toxicity in overwhelming exposure (e.g., overwhelming $NO_2$, mixed exposure with CO, CN) |
| 1.3 Asphyxiation |
| 2. Acute (airway irritation) |
| 2.1 Bronchoconstriction |
| 2.2 Cough |
| 2.3 Chest pain |
| 2.4 Systemic symptoms |
| 3. Delayed |
| 3.1 Pulmonary edema |
| 3.2 Respiratory failure |
| 3.3 Superinfection |
| 3.4 Reactive airways dysfunction syndrome |
| 4. Subacute and chronic |
| 4.1 Pneumonitis following exposure |
| 4.2 Bronchitis |
| 4.3 Bronchiolitis obliterans |
| 4.4 Reactive airways dysfunction syndrome (prolonged) |
| 4.5 Interstitial fibrosis (honeycombing) |

Pulmonary edema may follow 12 to 36 hours after acute exposure. The first indication clinically is usually progressive shortness of breath and desaturated arterial blood oxygen, starting several hours after exposure. The chest film often lags behind the progression to respiratory failure but eventually shows patchy infiltrates and, frequently, patchy atelectasis from mucous plugging. The characteristic picture of developing pulmonary edema in a patient several hours after toxic gas exposure is an inhomogeneous chest film with diffuse infiltrates associated with desaturated arterial oxygen tension ($PaO_2$ may be relatively preserved in carbon monoxide toxicity). Oxygen, positive pressure ventilation, and frequent suction are the important supportive measures because of hypersecretion and mucous plugging. The $FIO_2$ should be kept as low as possible to prevent additive oxygen toxicity. Volume and pressure should be maintained with colloid and vasopressors, not fluid loading. The management of toxic pulmonary edema is much like that of other forms of acute lung injury but should not be confused with cardiogenic pulmonary edema or volume overload (10,11,31).

The regeneration of severely damaged bronchial epithelium after 2 to 6 weeks may be dysplastic. Exuberant fibrosis may rarely obstruct small airways as bronchiolitis obliterans proceeds; this is yet a third way by which the patient with acute toxic inhalation can present with shortness of breath and hypoxemia. (Clinically this appears to be a rare sequela of nitrogen dioxide toxicity.) Corticosteroids may once again be used to control this process in the unusual case in which it becomes threatening (32).

Resistance to infection is clearly compromised by toxic inhalation. Host defense mechanisms are greatly compromised following diffuse alveolar damage, and the injured lung is highly susceptible to bacterial infection. Prophylactic antibiotics are often used in acute toxic inhalation but may place the patient at risk for superinfection by resistant organisms (10,11,31).

## AIRWAYS EFFECTS

Toxic injury to airways may also result in the so-called reactive airways dysfunction syndrome (RADS), a partly reversible condition of airways obstruction that seems to be more common—or at least recognized more often—in recent years as a variant of occupational asthma.

Bronchiolitis obliterans, or obliterative bronchiolitis, is a common finding on pathology but uncommon as a clinical outcome to toxic inhalation, and rarely fatal. It probably occurs more often than it is recognized. The condition is easily overlooked in its early stages, when treatment can be effective. As the name implies, it is an inflammatory process of the small airways. The injury leads to fibrosis so severe that airflow is impeded and the airway may be completely closed off and even disappear. Its former location is visible under the microscope only as a few remaining threads of elastin fibers when the tissue is suitably stained (16,33).

Obliterative bronchiolitis develops over a period of weeks following recovery from the acute exposure. It presents clinically as progressive shortness of breath, cough, and an irreversible obstructive defect. As it develops, obliterative bronchiolitis looks like an early pneumoconiosis or interstitial lung disease on x-ray. Later, after the lesions scar to oblivion, the lung may appear hyperinflated or abnormally clear on x-ray (hyperlucent).

A physician may suspect bronchiolitis obliterans on the basis of these findings and a history compatible with exposure to a toxic gas or intense smoke. Confirming the diagnosis is not easy, however, because the characteristic symptoms of cough and dyspnea are very common. The chest film may show hyperlucency and abnormally sharp and early cutoff of pulmonary vessels, but these signs are subtle and require clinical judgment. Pulmonary function tests vary widely and may show restrictive or obstructive changes, or both, of the small airways type because of concomitant interstitial fibrosis, air trapping, and the complete occlusion of injured airways rendering them "silent." Diffusion capacity is likely to be reduced but may be higher than expected because ventilation is cut off to some affected lung units. Lung biopsy presents a histologic picture characterized by the absence of normal vascular and bronchial structures where they should be in the interstitial space, but an open biopsy is required and most physicians are reluctant to take this step in the workup (13,16).

There is no effective treatment for obliterative bronchiolitis once it is established. During its development, the process may be arrested with steroids, which are sometimes required for prolonged periods. Bronchodilators help some patients with mixed airways disease to maintain function of the airways and comfort. Despite the best efforts, some patients with obliterative bronchiolitis become progressively disabled and some die of their complication. Management should be undertaken by a knowledgeable pulmonary specialist, and referral should not be delayed when the condition is suspected (13).

Obliterative bronchiolitis is closely related pathologically to other more familiar conditions such as small airways disease and the early changes associated with cigarette smoking (34). These conditions affect a part of the lung that has enormous functional reserve. The small airways or bronchioles have in the aggregate a much greater cross-sectional area than do the larger airways associated with asthma. There are far more of them. As a result, their obstruction does not interfere significantly with airflow until very many are involved. Conditions that affect them must wipe out a huge number of bronchioles before the consequences are obvious. This means that the disorder is largely silent until the condition is far advanced. Symptoms of cough and shortness of breath may not be associated with the degree of the patient's impairment in pulmonary function. These symptoms relate more closely to the fibrotic changes occurring in the tissue than to the obstruction of the airways (13,33,35).

It appears that the damaged airway epithelium may itself mediate some of the repair process. Airway epithelial cells may migrate chemotactically to remodel the damaged airways' luminal tissue and elaborate transforming growth factor-β (TGF-β) and other cytokines (36). Dysplastic or abnormal repair may lead to permanent airflow obstruction, hyperactivity in bronchial smooth muscle that has "reset" its threshold, and compromised host defenses that may make the damaged airway more susceptible to infection and subsequent injury (1,37–39).

These disorders reflect processes of injury to airways expressed at different levels, with different factors of localization and susceptibility involved. It is possible, for example, that there is a spectrum of airways injury, in which inflammatory changes of the muscular layer result in RADS, whereas those of the epithelium and glandular tissue result in chronic bronchitis, those of the submucosa and fibroblast may lead to obliterative bronchiolitis, and injury followed by heavy seeding by antigen may lead to asthma-like specific airways reactivity. These outcomes may occur in combination and are affected by the chronicity, intensity, and properties of the exposure (37,39).

## STRONG RESPIRATORY IRRITANTS

The strong respiratory irritants of greatest concern are gases (2,3). Table 2 presents the most significant strong irritants and some of their most relevant chemical and physical characteristics (3,40–44). The concentrations in

**TABLE 2.** *Strong respiratory irritants and their characteristics*

| | Formula | Chemistry | Water solubility | Odor threshold | Lethal exposure | Exposure settings | Predominant effects | Unusual Features | OSHA TWA/STEL (1994) |
|---|---|---|---|---|---|---|---|---|---|
| Ammonia | $NH_3$ | Basic | High | 50 ppm | 500 ppm | Refrigeration, agriculture, fertilizer, chemical industry | Local irritation, tissue liquefaction, bronchitis; pulmonary edema unusual | Overwhelming exposure may compromise airway; frostbite | 50 ppm |
| Chlorine | $Cl_2$ | Strong oxidizing agent | High | 3 ppm | 10 ppm | Pulp mills, water disinfection, chemical industry | Bronchitis, persistent airways reactivity | Most common | 1 ppm |
| Chlorine dioxide | $ClO_2$ | Strong oxidizing agent | High | Not available | 5 ppm | Pulp mills (used as bleaching agent to replace $Cl_2$) | Bronchitis, persistent airways reactivity | Introduced as a replacement for $Cl_2$ in pulp mills | 0.1 ppm |
| Hydrogen chloride (hydrochloric acid) | HCl | Acid | High | 5 ppm | 50 ppm | Chemical industry, end uses | Bronchitis, persistent airways reactivity | Skin and mucous membrane irritation | 5 ppm |
| Hydrogen fluoride (hydrofluoric acid) | HF | Acid | High | 3 ppm | 30 ppm | Semiconductor manufacture, glass etching, oilfield stimulation | Severe bronchitis, rapid and deep penetration of skin, risk of hypocalcemia | Deeply necrotic tissue burns on contact require special management; F binds $Ca^{2+}$ | 3 ppm |
| Hydrogen sulfide | $H_2S$ | Reducing agent | Medium | 0.13 ppm | 300 ppm | Oilfields, refining, manure pits, sewer gas | Loss of consciousness, apnea, pulmonary edema, ocular irritation; olefactory paralysis | Neurotoxicity predominates in most cases; sulfide ($S^-$) is the toxic moiety | 20 ppm/ 50 ppm (10 min) |
| Mercury vapor (hot) | Hg | Oxidant | Low | 0.1 mg/m$^3$ | 10 mg/m$^3$ | Rare, usually associated with naive efforts to recover mercury, extract gold, or burn mercury-containing paint | Pulmonary edema, bronchitis, neurotoxicity | Classic mercury intoxication may supervene or occur as a sequela | 0.05 mg/m$^3$ |
| Nitrogen dioxide | $NO_2$ | Acid, oxidant | Low | 5 ppm | 20 ppm | Chemical industry, high-temperature combustion, nitric acid fumes, farms | Classic toxic inhalation, "silo-filler's disease" | Some hemodynamic effects; similar to ozone | 5 ppm |
| Phosgene | $COCl_2$ | Oxidizing agent | Low | 0.5 ppm | 2 ppm | Chemical industry, combustion of plastics, welding in presence of chlorinated hydrocarbon solvents | Classic toxic inhalation | An early chemical warfare agent | 0.1 ppm |
| Ozone | $O_3$ | Strong oxidizing agent | Low | 1 ppm | 5 ppm | Welding on aluminum, water treatment | Classic toxic inhalation | Adsorbs on particulates; short-term adaptation; susceptibility diminishes with age | 0.1 ppm |
| Sulfur dioxide | $SO_2$ | Acid | Medium | 1 ppm | 100 ppm | Chemical industry, sulfur combustion, smelting | Bronchitis | Strongly adsorbs on particulates | 5 ppm |

TWA/STEL, time-weighted average/short-term exposure level.

occupational settings that produce toxic inhalation are generally very high and sustained only in incidents involving confined spaces. However, some of these same compounds are occasionally released in community exposures such as transportation accidents or pipeline leaks.

There are a variety of other strong irritants that are less common or that are encountered only in certain situations. Except where noted, only very high levels of exposure would be expected to produce these effects. Antineoplastic drugs may cause different varieties of pneumonitis in patients receiving them, often in association with radiotherapy. Such agents include bleomycin, carmustine (also known as BCNU), cyclophosphamide, methotrexate, and mitomycin c. The vinca alkyloids may also cause a pneumonitis, but it is a hypersensitivity response. In each case the pulmonary reaction is a local response to exposure from the blood. Some of these responses are idiosyncratic or rare (40).

Cadmium, in addition to its possible role as a cause of metal fume fever, may produce a severe and characteristic toxic pneumonitis associated with renal damage. Exposure settings involve hot metal fumes, such as cutting cadmium-clad metal with an oxyacetylene torch. This acute condition is distinct from chronic systemic cadmium toxicity, which is predominantly renal, and from centrilobular emphysema associated with chronic cadmium inhalation (42).

Chemical warfare agents that are strong pulmonary irritants include chlorine; phosgene and its derivatives diphosgene and phosgene oxime); the alkylating agents (clinically better known for their use as antineoplastic drugs); ricin, a derivative of castor bean that causes a pneumonitis but is primarily an antimetabolic agent interfering with glucose metabolism; chlorpicrin, a strong irritant; and cyanogen chloride, an irritant that metabolizes to cyanide and thereby kills as an asphyxiant. Riot control agents are much less toxic but those in common use before capsaicin, including chloroacetophenone (CN, or Mace) produced airways irritation and even pulmonary edema with overwhelming exposure in a confined space (45). Capsaicin has not been identified as a respiratory hazard to date by the inhalation route, although there are case reports of bronchorrhea following massive ingestion (44).

Osmium tetroxide is a highly reactive metal compound that binds avidly to tissue and irreversibly stains it black. It is most often encountered as a hazard in electron microscopy. It may cause a bronchitis and blindness from corneal staining. The tissue staining may occur at lower exposures (42,46).

Paraquat, a bipyridyl herbicide, induces an intense interstitial inflammatory reaction in the lung when ingested. This may lead to interstitial fibrosis and even end-stage honeycombing and respiratory failure. Although it is possible to produce the effect by the inhalation route in the laboratory, human toxicity seems limited to ingestion (40,44).

Many pesticides have irritant effects, particularly in the upper airway, most notably parathion, lindane, thiram, and dichlorvos. Some pesticides, such as the organophosphates, have specific pulmonary effects and can even induce pulmonary edema as part of a more complex parasympathetic toxicity syndrome. The petroleum vehicles in which these pesticides are diluted are also weak irritants (40,44).

Thiourea compounds produce highly specific endothelial damage and induce toxic inhalation-like pulmonary edema by parenteral routes. These compounds are therefore very popular for research on pulmonary edema. One of these compounds, $\alpha$-naphthylthiourea (ANTU), is used as a rat poison (45).

Trimellitic anhydride may cause protean manifestations when inhaled, among them a hemorrhagic pneumonitis (44).

Vanadium, otherwise a metal with relatively low but unusual systemic toxicity, may cause a bronchitis and may induce occupational asthma. Whether manganese can do the same is controversial (42,46).

Zinc chloride may cause a pneumonitis; other compounds of zinc, most commonly zinc oxide, cause metal fume fever and are much less toxic (42,46).

## MIXTURES

In addition to these specific compounds, there are common exposure situations involving mixtures of respiratory irritants. Environmental tobacco smoke is undoubtedly the most common multiple respiratory irritant. Tobacco smoke consists of a large number of potent respiratory irritants, including acrolein and various aldehydes, in addition to carcinogenic substances, nicotine and carbon monoxide, which tend to receive more attention (37).

Fire and smoke inhalation involves exposure to a mixture of strong respiratory irritants. In such exposures there may be a number of toxic constituents in the smoke, among them acrolein, nitrogen dioxide, sulfur oxides, ammonia, nitriles, and organic compounds such as aldehydes. Wood smoke, while irritating, is relatively much less toxic than smoke from other fuels and mixtures. The presence of polyvinyl chloride and other synthetic materials that serve as chlorine sources in the fuel may result in large amounts of hydrogen chloride, vinyl chloride, and phosgene. Complicating the irritant effect of these compounds is the systemic toxicity of other combustion products such as carbon monoxide and hydrogen cyanide. These may not have pulmonary toxicity but may themselves be lethal. The chronic effects of combustion products has been a matter of great concern in the occupational health of firefighters (47,48).

Certain dusts of low toxicity carry their own standards: starch, boron oxide, barium sulfate, fibrous glass, aluminum oxide (emery), tantalum, molybdenum, zinc oxide, mica, marble, perlite, limestone, kaolin, iron oxide, graphite (synthetic), gypsum and plaster of Paris, soapstone, talc, calcium oxide, calcium carbonate, calcium hydroxide, and wood dust. These compounds and mixtures are regulated as dusts and permissible exposure limits (PELs) for these dusts are generally set at the same level as PNOC (15 mg/m$^3$ total, 5 mg/m$^3$ respirable). Certain dusts treated in the same manner may have a higher potential for toxicity than this approach would warrant—manganese tetroxide, for example.

A wide variety of dusts are regulated only as PNOCs, among them dusts of crustal origin (essentially dirt), fly ash, organic debris, powdered polymeric solids, textile dusts, household or interior dust, paper dust, and diesel exhaust. (Diesel exhaust is implicated in the association of fine particulates ($PM_{10}$) in ambient air pollution with mortality and other health effects and thus represents a special case.)

The rubric of PNOC covers the vast majority of dusts likely to be encountered in the workplace. These dusts are associated with only a small number of claims for workers' compensation or reports of occupational disease. The dusts themselves may be numerous and ubiquitous but as agents of occupational disease they are indeed a residual category. Pneumoconioses caused by these dusts are uncommon and usually confer little or no functional impairment. The traditional view of the contribution of "nuisance dust" to occupational airways disease is that an effect on airways by nonfibrogenic dust can only be related to either bronchitis or emphysema. Recent evidence suggests that the common denominator in the contribution by dust to fixed airflow obstruction is a process of inflammatory change that persists beyond the short-term reversible airways reactivity of asthma (49). This process presumably may be interstitial, in the case of asbestos, or more directly involving airways structures in the case of organic dusts. This process appears to be independent of obvious symptoms of bronchitis such as cough and sputum production, as demonstrated by the rapid reversibility of these symptoms after withdrawal from exposure, compared to the fixed nature of the airflow obstruction.

Chronic inflammation associated with macrophage overloading, either as a direct result or as a dysfunctional perpetuated response following infection or challenge with cigarette smoke, may contribute to local tissue injury by release of proteolytic enzymes and reactive oxygen species (7,8). The result may be a lesion similar to the peribronchial effects of cigarette smoking but much more modest than originally described (34). Thurlbeck and Churg have cautioned that the pathogenesis of smoking-induced emphysema must be much more complicated than the elastase-antielastase model. If this rare complication PNOC lesion occurs, it would probably show up as accelerated loss of the percent of forced expiratory volume in 1 second ($FEV_1$%) and other airflow measures, rather than as clinical chronic obstructive pulmonary disease, as seen in some dust-exposed workers (15,50).

The contribution of PNOC to accelerated decline in airflow that is primarily due to another cause, such as cigarette smoking, is very plausible and probably varies with individual characteristics of susceptibility, exposure, and the chronicity of exposure. That fibrogenic dusts contribute to accelerated airflow obstruction seems clear, but the lesion or lesions responsible appear to be at the level of the parenchyma rather than in the airway itself (20).

## REFERENCES


1. Rylander R. Symptoms and mechanisms—inflammation of the lung. *Am J Ind Med* 1994;25:19–23.
2. Epler GR. Clinical overview of occupational lung disease. *Radiol Clin North Am* 1992;30(C):1121–1133.
3. Barkman HW. Respiratory tract irritants. In: Rom WN, ed. *Environmental and occupational medicine,* 2nd ed. Boston: Little, Brown, 1992;529–533.
4. Fabbri LM, Saetta M, Maestrelli P, Mapp C. Airway inflammation in isocyanate-induced asthma. In: Chrétien J, Dusser D, eds. *Environmental impact of the airways:* from injury to repair. New York: Marcel Dekker, 1996;287–297.
5. Dosman JA, Kania J, Cockroft DW. Occupational obstructive disorders: nonspecific airways obstruction and occupational asthma. *Med Clin North Am* 1990;74:823–835.
6. Mauderly JL, McCunney RJ, eds. *Particle overload in the rat lung and lung cancer:* implications for human risk assessment. Washington DC: Taylor and Francis, 1996.
7. Li K, Keeling B, Churg A. Mineral dusts cause elastin and collagen breakdown in the rat lung: a potential mechanism of dust-induced emphysema. *Am J Respir Crit Care Med* 1996;153:644–649.
8. Burrows B. Airways obstructive diseases: pathogenetic mechanisms and natural histories of the disorder. *Med Clin North Am* 1990;74:547–567.
9. Plavec D, Somogyi-Zalud E, Godnic-Cvar J. Nonspecific nasal responsiveness in workers occupational exposed to respiratory irritants. *Am J Ind Med* 1993;24:525–532.
10. Guidotti TL. Toxic inhalation: diffuse alveolar injury and pulmonary edema. In: Cordasco E Sr, Demeter SL, Zenz C, eds. *Environmental respiratory diseases.* New York: Van Nostrand, 1995;85–114.
11. Cordasco E Sr, Demeter SL. Toxic pulmonary edema: clinical concepts. In: Cordasco E Sr, Demeter SL, Zenz C, eds. *Environmental respiratory diseases.* New York: Van Nostrand, 1995;159–178.
12. Kremer AM, Pal TM, Bolerj JSM, Schouten JP, Rijcken B. Airway hyperresponsiveness, prevalence of respiratory symptoms, and lung function in workers exposed to irritants. *Occup Environ Med* 1994;51:3–13.
13. Blanc PD, Galbo M, Hiatt P, Olson KR, Balmes JR. Symptoms, lung function, and airway responsiveness following irritant inhalation. *Chest* 1993:103:1699–1705.
14. Malo J-L, Cartier A, Boulet L-P, et al. Bronchial hyperresponsiveness can improve while spirometry plateaus two to three years after repeated exposure to chlorine causing respiratory symptoms. *Am J Respir Crit Care Med* 1994;150:1142–1145.
15. Oxman D, Muir DCF, Shannon HS, Stock SR, Hnizdo E, Lange HJ. Occupational dust exposure and chronic obstructive pulmonary disease. *Am Rev Respir Dis* 1993;148:38–48.
16. Guidotti TL. Current clinical practice: attribution of chronic airways disease to occupational dust exposures. *App Occup Environ Hyg* 1998.
17. Xu X, Christiani DC, Dockery DW, Wang LH. Exposure-response relationships between occupational exposures and chronic respiratory illness: a community-based study. *Am Rev Respir Dis* 1992;146:413–418.
18. Burge PS. Occupational and chronic obstructive pulmonary disease (COPD). *Eur Respir J* 1994;7:1032–1034.
19. Windsor ACJ, Mullen PG, fowler AA. Acute lung injury: What have we learned from animal models? *Am J Med Sci* 1993;306:111–116.
20. Snyder LS, Hertz MI, Harmon KR, Bitterman PB. Failure of lung repair following acute lung injury. *Chest* 1990;98:989–993.

21. Bitterman PB. Pathogenesis of fibrosis in acute lung injury. *Am J Med* 1992;92:39S–43S.
22. Davies MG. The vascular endothelium. *Ann Surg* 1993;218:593–609.
23. Busse R, Fleming I. The endothelial organ. *Curr Opin Cardiol* 1993;8: 719–727.
24. Jaffe EA. Cell biology of endothelial cells. *Hum Pathol* 1987;18: 234–239.
25. Rennard SI, Rickard K, Bechmann JD, et al. Protease injury in airways disease. *Ann NY Acad Sci* 1991;624:278–285.
26. Harlan JM. Neutrophil-mediated vascular injury. *Acta Med Scand* 1986;715:123–129.
27. Barrowcliffe MP, Jones JG. Solute permeability of the alveolar capillary barrier. *Thorax* 1987;42:1–10.
28. Mustafa MF, Tierney D. Biochemical and metabolic changes in the lung with oxygen, ozone, and nitrogen dioxide toxicity. *Am Rev Respir Dis* 1978;118:1061–1090.
29. West JB, Mathieu-Costello O. Stress failure of pulmonary capillaries: role in lung and heart disease. Lancet 1992;340:762–767.
30. Matthay MA. Resolution of pulmonary edema—new insights. *West J Med* 1991;154:315–321.
31. Cordasco EM, Piedad O, Kester J, Yarnal J, Sharpe IE, White RE Jr. Acute pulmonary edema with respiratory failure newer concepts in therapy. *Angiology* 1982;33:665–667.
32. Snyder LS, Hertz MI, Harmon KR, Bitterman PB. Failure of lung repair following acute lung injury: regulation of the fibroproliferative response (part 2). *Chest* 1990;98:989–993.
33. Ezri T, Kunichezky S, Eliraz A, Soroker D, Halperin D, Schattner A. Bronchiolitis obliterans—current concepts. *Q J Med* 1994;87:1–10.
34. Thurlbeck WM, Churg AM. *Pathology of the lung.* New York: Thieme, 1995;799.
35. Wright JL, Cagle P, Churg A, Colby TV, Myers J. Diseases of the small airways. *Am Rev Respir Dis* 1992;146:240–262.
36. Rennard SI, Romberger DJ, Sisson JH, et al. Airway epithelial cells: functional role in airway disease. *Am J Respir Crit Care Med* 1994;150: S27–S30.
37. Chrétien J, Dusser D. *Environmental impact on the airways:* from injury to repair. New York: Marcel Dekker, 1996.
38. Holt PG. Inflammation in organic dust-induced lung disease: new approaches for research into underlying mechanisms. *Am J Ind Med* 1990;17:47–54.
39. Landau LI. Bronchiolitis and asthma: Are they related? *Thorax* 1994; 49:293–296.
40. Kehrer JP. Systemic pulmonary toxicity. In: Ballantyne B, Marrs T, Turner P, eds. *General and applied toxicology.* New York: Macmillan, 1993.
41. U.S. National Institute for Occupational Safety and Health. *NIOSH pocket guide to chemical hazards.* DHHS (NIOSH) Publication No. 94-116. Washington DC: U.S. Government Printing Office, 1994.
42. Ross JAS, Seaton A, Morgan WKC. Toxic gases and fumes. In: Morgan WKC, Seaton A, eds. *Occupational lung diseases.* Philadelphia: WB Saunders, 1995;568–596.
43. Declos GL, Carson AI. Acute gaseous exposure. In: Harber P, Schenker MB, Balmes JR, eds. *Occupational and environmental respiratory disease.* St. Louis: Mosby, 1996;514–534.
44. Ellenhorn MJ, Barceloux DG. *Medical toxicology:* diagnosis and treatment of human poisoning. New York: Elsevier Science, 1988; 1239–1240.
45. Urbanetti JS. Battlefield chemical inhalation injury. In: Lake J, ed. *Pathophysiology and treatment of inhalation injuries.* New York: Marcel Dekker, 1988;281–348.
46. Skornik WA. Inhalation toxicity of metal particles and vapors. In: Lake J, ed. *Pathophysiology and treatment of inhalation injuries.* New York: Marcel Dekker, 1988;123–177.
47. Guidotti TL, Clough VM. Occupational health concerns of firefighting. *Annu Rev Public Health* 1992;12:151–171.
48. Loke J, Matthay RA, Smith GJ. The toxic environment and its medical implications with special emphasis on smoke inhalation. In: Lake J, ed. *Pathophysiology and treatment of inhalation injuries.* New York: Marcel Dekker, 1988;453–504.
49. Dimich-Ward H, Kennedy S, Chan-Yeung M. Occupational exposures and chronic airflow limitation. *Can Respir J* 1996;3:133–140.
50. Wang ML, McCabe L, Hankinson JL, et al. Longitudinal and cross-sectional analyses of lung function in steelworkers. *Am J Respir Crit Care Med* 1996;153:1907–1913.

*Environmental and Occupational Medicine, Third Edition,* edited by William N. Rom.
Lippincott–Raven Publishers, Philadelphia © 1998.

# CHAPTER 43

# Simple Asphyxiants

Marc Wilkenfeld

The earth's atmosphere is a mixture of gases, containing by volume about 21% oxygen, 78% nitrogen, 0.94% argon, and 0.04% carbon dioxide, with traces of helium, xenon, krypton, radon, and hydrogen, and varying amounts of ammonia, ozone, and water vapor.

Oxygen ($O_2$) is a colorless, odorless gas with a molecular weight of 32. Mammalian cells are dependent on oxygen so that their mitochondria can perform the energy-producing process of respiration. Asphyxiation, which is synonymous with respiratory failure, can be defined as insufficient oxygenation at the cellular level. Oxygen delivery to the tissues is determined by cardiac output and the oxygen content of the arterial blood, as expressed in these equations:

Oxygen delivery to tissues (in ml $O_2$ per minute):

$$Q_t \times CaO_2 \times 10,$$

$$Q_t \times O_2 \text{ capacity} \times O_2 \text{ saturation} + \text{dissolved } O_2,$$

$$Q_t \times Hgb \times 1.39 \times 10 \times SaO_2 + (0.0031 \times PaO_2),$$

where:

$Q_t$ = cardiac output (in L/min),

$CaO_2$ = oxygen content of arterial blood, (in ml $O_2$/100 ml blood)

10 = conversion factor (from ml $O_2$/100 ml blood to ml $O_2$/liter blood),

Hgb = hemoglobin (in g/100 ml blood),

1.39 = a constant (in ml $O_2$/g Hgb),

$SaO_2$ = saturation of Hgb in arterial blood (in percent), and

$PaO_2$ = partial pressure of $O_2$ in arterial blood (in mm Hg).

Simple asphyxiants are gases that are physiologically inert. They do not suppress cardiac output or alter the function of hemoglobin. Rather, they cause asphyxiation only when present in high enough concentrations to lower the concentration of oxygen in the inspired air to levels at which $SaO_2$ and $PaO_2$ fall, resulting in inadequate oxygen delivery to tissues.

Human beings are asymptomatic while breathing air containing 16.5% to 21% oxygen by volume. Concentrations of oxygen in the inspired air of 12% to 16% cause tachypnea, tachycardia, and slight incoordination. At oxygen levels of 10% to 14%, emotional lability and exhaustion with minimal exertion can be expected. Breathing air containing 6% to 10% oxygen results in nausea, vomiting, lethargic movements, and perhaps unconsciousness. Breathing less than 6% oxygen produces convulsions, then apnea, followed by cardiac standstill. The aforementioned symptoms occur immediately on breathing an oxygen-deficient atmosphere. Since exercise increases the tissue need for oxygen, symptoms occur more quickly during exertion in an oxygen-deficient environment. Should the victim survive the hypoxic insult, some or all organs may show evidence of hypoxic damage, which may or may not be reversible with time, depending on the degree and duration of the hypoxia and the extent of the tissue injury.

M. Wilkenfeld: Department of Environmental Medicine, New York University Medical Center, New York, New York 10016.

## SPECIFIC ASPHYXIANTS

The following substances are simple asphyxiants: smoke, nitrous oxide, argon, hydrogen, helium, nitrogen, methane, ethane, and carbon dioxide. Smoke, in addition to displacing oxygen in inspired air, causes chemical irritation of the airways, and chemical asphyxiation may occur (as in carbon monoxide poisoning). Nitrous oxide ($N_2O$) is an anesthetic, but it can act as an asphyxiant if supplemental oxygen is not added to the inspired air. Health care workers and dentists in particular are at risk for occupational exposure to nitrous oxide (1). Individuals with vitamin $B_{12}$ deficiency appear to be more susceptible to the development of megaloblastosis and/or neuropathy following chronic exposure to nitrous oxide (2). Argon, hydrogen, helium, and nitrogen are inert gases that cause asphyxiation if present in high enough concentrations to dilute oxygen in the inspired air to dangerous levels. Argon and hydrogen gases are not likely to be encountered in excess in nature, medicine, or industry. Inhaled helium-oxygen mixtures are used occasionally when a reduction of turbulent flow in the airways is desired or to prevent decompression sickness.

### Nitrogen

Nitrogen was first recognized as the unrespirable constituent of atmospheric air by Dr. Rutherford of Edinburgh in 1772 (3). Nitrogen is a colorless, odorless gas with a molecular weight of 28.02. Inhalation of nitrogen is toxic only when its presence lowers the available oxygen in the inspired air; inhalation of pure nitrogen has been used in experimental animals to study the effects of anoxia. Although nitrogen bubbles are responsible for decompression sickness, the nitrogen gas itself exerts no toxic effects; rather, the symptoms are due to the mechanical presence of the bubbles in tissues and in blood vessels, which produces local ischemia. Although decompression sickness usually occurs in professional and recreational divers, cases of occupational disease have been reported in compressed air workers involved in construction of tunnels (4). Many of these individuals were exposed to pressures of less than 1 bar. The use of vibrating tools and heavy physical exertion have been suggested as factors that increase the likelihood of developing decompression sickness. Nitrogen gas is used industrially to manufacture synthetic ammonia. Black damp is an asphyxiating combination of 87% nitrogen and 13% carbon dioxide found in coal mines.

### Methane and Ethane

Methane and ethane are members of the saturated aliphatic hydrocarbon series, also called paraffins because of their resistance to chemical reagents (from *parum,* meaning "little," and *affinis,* meaning "akin"). Methane ($CH_4$) is a colorless, odorless, tasteless, inflammable gas with a molecular weight of 16.04 and a vapor density of 0.55 (air = 1.0). Methane is soluble in alcohol ether, benzene, and other solvents. Its solubility in water is 3.5% at 17°C. Because it is biologically inert, toxicity occurs only when its presence reduces or eliminates the oxygen in the environment. Rabbits can inhale a mixture of one volume of oxygen and four volumes of methane for any length of time without showing any ill effects. Methane emanates from decaying organic matter as marsh gas, which is composed almost entirely of methane. "Fire damp" is a combination of methane and air found in mines; as the name implies, this gas tends to explode. Methane is used as an illuminating gas and is widely used for domestic fuel as the principal component of natural gas. Suicide attempts using natural gas most often result in explosion before asphyxiation (5). Since it is lighter than air (specific gravity 0.717), methane accumulates in the upper region of an enclosed space; therefore, collapsing may be therapeutic if the victim begins to inhale less contaminated, better-oxygenated air. Skin contact with methane may produce frostbite due to rapid evaporation.

Ethane ($C_2H_6$) is a colorless, odorless gas with a molecular weight of 30.07 and a vapor density of 1.04. Its chief toxic effect is that of a simple asphyxiant. Ethane has a higher specific gravity than air (1.242 at 25°C) and an odor threshold of 899 ppm. It is soluble in benzene and ethanol. At high concentrations ethane may exert an irritant effect on the upper airways. In addition, when mixed with oxygen, ethane may sensitize cardiac muscle to epinephrine. No symptoms occur in humans breathing an atmosphere containing less than 5% ethane. Ethane is found in illuminating gas and natural gas and is used as a refrigerant. It may also be a component of landfill gas in hazardous waste sites.

### Carbon Dioxide

Carbon dioxide ($CO_2$) is a colorless, odorless, slightly sour-tasting gas with a molecular weight of 44.01 and a vapor density of 1.5. It is toxic as a simple asphyxiant, but also produces the clinical entity of carbon dioxide narcosis; unconsciousness may ensue while breathing concentrations of 7% to 10% carbon dioxide for a few minutes, or while breathing a concentration greater than 10% for less than a minute. Inhalation of carbon dioxide stimulates the respiratory center: at concentrations of 2%, noticeable increases in tidal volume occur; at levels of 5%, the increase in minute ventilation may become distressing to some persons. When dogs, rabbits, guinea pigs, and rats were exposed repeatedly and over long periods to concentrations of carbon dioxide ranging from 1% to 26%, with the oxygen concentration kept normal, they exhibited degenerative changes in the lung, liver, kidney, and brain. Sources of carbon dioxide include animals (as an end product of respiration), fermentation of carbohydrates, volcanic activity, and combustion, including the "afterdamp" (carbon dioxide gas) resulting from the explosion of fire damp in mines. Carbon dioxide is contained in solution in mineral spring water and may be released into the air intermittently.

Industrially, carbon dioxide is released by the burning of lime or by the addition of acid to a carbonate. Carbon dioxide gas is used in textile and leather industries, in water treatment, in the manufacture of drugs and white lead, in fire extinguishers, food preservation, welding, purging pipelines and tanks, and in the manufacture of carbonated drinks. Carbon dioxide gas can be stored at room temperature in liquid form or at low temperatures in solid form (dry ice). Asphyxiation by carbon dioxide produced by fermentation has been reported from entering poorly ventilated brewery vats or silos containing green fodder (5). Deaths have occurred from inhalation of carbon dioxide released when large amounts of dry ice were used as a refrigerant in an inadequately ventilated area. Some victims who survived an explosion of fire damp succumbed to asphyxiation from the afterdamp produced. Because it is heavier than air, carbon dioxide accumulates in the lower region of an enclosed space.

### Mass Extinction of Life Forms as a Result of Carbon Dioxide Exposure

Recently, Knoll et al. (6) have proposed that high concentrations of carbon dioxide played a role in the life changes that occurred on Earth 250 million years ago. These changes are referred to as the Permian mass extinction and involved the disappearance of between one-half and 95% of all life forms on Earth. These changes have been documented by fossil evidence. The Permian period was a time of massive movements of land masses resulting in the aggregation of continents. It appears that the absence of continental ice sheets and the aggregation of continents resulted in low oxygen levels in the deep ocean waters. Photosynthesis and remineralization of organic materials resulted in an increased concentrations of carbon dioxide and hydrogen sulfide in the ocean waters.

Aquatic life differs from land animals in that the level of carbon dioxide in their blood is almost identical to the $PCO_2$ inspired. Even minor changes in the $PCO_2$ could have had a fatal effect on many species of aquatic life. This may also have affected forms of life further up the food chain. The types of organisms made extinct are consistent with the theory of hypercapnia as the causative factor. Then, 250 million years later, water-based production of carbon dioxide created the scenario described below.

### Fatalities from Large-Scale Emission of Carbon Dioxide: The Lake Nyos Disaster

In August 1986, more than 1,700 people died in one of the largest disasters of recent history. A toxic cloud of gas was spontaneously released from Lake Nyos, a volcanic crater lake in Cameroon (7). Clinical, forensic, and environmental testing suggested that carbon dioxide, the simple asphyxiant described above, was contained in this cloud and was responsible for the fatalities. This was not the first such incident. In August 1984, at a nearby crater lake (Lake Monown), more than 35 people were killed by a similar cloud of gas. However, the Lake Nyos disaster received major media coverage throughout the world. In addition to the dead, hundreds were injured, most of whom recovered, and thousands of villagers were displaced and thousands of livestock killed. This unfortunate incident provided a rare opportunity for scientists and physicians to study deaths and injuries from carbon dioxide.

The mechanism of the disaster has been the subject of study and controversy. At first it was thought that an eruption of the volcano beneath the lake had released toxic gases. Further study supported the theory that carbon dioxide from ground water had stratified at the lower levels of the lake. Through an undetermined mechanism, the gas was released all at once from the lake. A similar episode occurred while scientists were studying the lake with gas meters, which revealed increased carbon dioxide, though lower concentrations than those associated with the 1986 disaster (8).

By the force of gravity the cloud was carried down into the settlements in the valley. The unsuspecting population was struck at approximately 9:00 P.M. The absence of any disarray rules out seismic activity, and there was no evidence of any burned clothing or singed foliage, which might be associated with the release of irritant volcanic gases. Close to the source there were few survivors, except inhabitants at higher elevations than the dwellings. Further away the survival rate increased. Humans and animals alike simply fell suddenly to the ground. All insect activity apparently ceased for 24 hours.

Survivors reported falling into a deep coma like sleep for 12 to 36 hours. Some survivors noted a smell of rotten eggs, which suggested the possibility of sulfur dioxide or hydrogen sulfide from a volcanic eruption (8). However, this was most likely olfactory hallucination secondary to carbon dioxide exposure. The depth of unconsciousness is indicated by the fact that the extremities of some survivors who fell landed in cooking fires, where they were seriously burned. This phenomenon was previously reported with carbon monoxide poisoning, but it can occur with any prolonged coma. Injuries among the survivors were limited to orthopedic injuries and thermal burns sustained during falls and to nerve palsies secondary to prolonged immobilization. Almost all of the injured recovered.

Autopsies determined that asphyxiation was the cause of death. Toxicologic studies revealed no significant increase in carboxyhemoglobin, sulfhemoglobin, or methemoglobin. Cyanide and sulfur compounds were ruled out as causes of death.

Chemical studies of the lake revealed high levels of carbon dioxide without increased levels of any other constituents. Although it has been suggested that a small concentration of carbon monoxide may have been present in the cloud, all available evidence supports the notion that the Lake Nyos disaster resulted from carbon dioxide release and subsequent asphyxiation of the inhabitants.

What lesson can be learned from these "killer lake" episodes (9)? Such natural release of carbon dioxide may be more common than is thought and noticeable only when they occur near inhabited areas. The implication of future release has enormous public health implications, and research is needed to protect the lives of inhabitants near crater lakes. The buildup of carbon dioxide is presumably gradual, so some method of prediction, and perhaps intervention, might be developed.

## OXYGEN DEFICIENCY

In addition to displacement or dilution of oxygen by the simple asphyxiants, oxygen deficiency may occur in an environment where oxygen consumption is ongoing but ventilation is inadequate. Such is the case when a child suffocates in a discarded refrigerator or small closet. It was shown that Minneapolis manholes located in low or swampy areas contained soil with an unusually high oxygen demand; this led to varying degrees of oxygen depletion inside the manholes, which caused the asphyxiation death of a plumbing company employee in a manhole that had been entered previously without mishap (10).

## CASE STUDY

On a Utah dairy farm there was a large underground liquid manure storage tank with a ground-level opening (11). The lid had been kicked into the tank by a cow. Having entered the tank previously without consequence, the farmer drained the liquid manure to a depth of 18 inches and descended into the pit to retrieve the lid. Shortly after entering the tank, he fell unconscious. His two sons entered the pit to rescue their father. When one collapsed, the other escaped to find help. The town sheriff and barber responded to the call for help. The barber entered, took one breath (which caused a severe burning sensation in his chest), lifted the still-gasping boy over his shoulder, and was near the opening and safety when he lost consciousness. Both boy and barber plummeted back into the pit. The sheriff entered to save the barber and was quickly overcome. When the town ambulance arrived, the barber was fished out of the tank with a rope looped around his arm and, once above ground, cardiopulmonary resuscitation was instituted. The farmer, his son, and the sheriff were removed from the pit by a fireman wearing a self-contained breathing apparatus and were pronounced dead at the scene.

The barber was transported by air to the Intermountain Respiratory Intensive Care Unit. At the time of admission, his carboxyhemoglobin level was normal at 0.5%. Initially, he displayed hemodynamic instability requiring intravenous fluid and dopamine. He had fulminant adult respiratory distress syndrome, requiring mechanical ventilation with positive end-expiratory pressure. He developed pneumonitis, left maxillary sinusitis, and bacteremia, caused by gram-negative organisms; all were treated successfully with antibiotics. Within 6 weeks he had returned to work and had resumed jogging.

Autopsies on the other victims revealed that the farmer and the sheriff had aspirated massive amounts of liquid manure. The farmer's son had severe pulmonary edema but had not aspirated manure. Measurement of heart blood sulfide ion indicated significant hydrogen sulfide exposure, with levels of 5.0 mg/L (farmer), 3.6 mg/L (sheriff), and 0.8 mg/L (son). A sulfide level was not measured in the survivor. The background levels in control blood are less than 0.05 mg/L, and sulfide values in random autopsy cases, even if the body is badly decomposed, do not exceed 0.4 mg/L (12).

One week after the incident, under different conditions (warmer weather, less concentrated manure), air from the manure storage tank was analyzed. The gases detected were methane (6,360 ppm), carbon monoxide (400 ppm), hydrogen sulfide (76 ppm), ammonia (1.5 ppm), carbon dioxide (2%), and oxygen (18%). It is likely that the gas concentrations were different on the day of the accident. The documented presence of hydrogen sulfide, the rapidity of collapse, and the markedly elevated levels of sulfide ion in the blood of the dead are all consistent with a diagnosis of hydrogen sulfide intoxication. In addition, the presence of simple asphyxiants may have reduced significantly the concentration of oxygen in the pit on the day of the accident. This case illustrates several pertinent points. Potentially unsafe areas, such as liquid manure storage tanks, manholes, or mines, should be checked for safety prior to each entry, since altered conditions may increase the danger. An asphyxiated victim should be removed quickly from the area of exposure; however, a would-be rescuer must avoid becoming a victim himself by wearing a self-contained breathing apparatus and a safety line. Victims should be treated with cardiopulmonary resuscitation, oxygen, mechanical ventilation, and positive end-expiratory pressure, as needed. If the etiologic agent or agents are unknown, they should be identified rapidly, so that definitive therapy can be instituted if necessary.

## ACKNOWLEDGMENT

The author and editor thank Dr. Lida Osbern for contribution to the first edition.

## REFERENCES


1. Donaldson D Maechan J. The hazards of chronic exposure to nitrous oxide: an update. Br Dent J 1995;178(3):95–1005.
2. Louis-Ferdinand RT. Myelotoxic, neurotoxic, and reproductive adverse effects of nitrous oxide. Adv Drug React Toxicol Rev 1994;13 (4):193–206.
3. Witthaus RA. *General medical chemistry for the use of practitioners of medicine.* New York: William Wood, 1981;94–98;157–158; 236–245.
4. How J, Vijayan A, Wong T. Acute decompression sickness in compressed air workers exposed to pressures below 1 bar in the Singapore Mass Rapid Transit Project. *Singapore Med J* 1990;31(2): 104–110.
5. Hamilton A, Hardy HL. *Industrial toxicology,* 3rd ed. Acton, MA: Publishing Sciences Group, 1974;235–237;263–269.
6. Knoll AO, Bambach RK, Canfield DE, Grotzinger JF. Comparative earth history and late Permian mass extinction. *Science* 1996;273:26.
7. Baxter P, Kapila M, Mfonfu D. Lake Nyos disaster Cameroon, 1986. The medical effect of large-scale emission of carbon dioxide. *Br Med J* 1989;298:1437–1441.
8. Wagner GN. Medical evaluation of the victims of the 1986 Lake Nyos disaster. *J Forensic Sci* 1988;33:899–909.
9. Kling GW, Clark MA, Compton HR, et al. The 1986 Lake Nyos gas disaster in Cameroon, West Africa. *Science* 1987;236:169–175.
10. Michaelson GS, Park WE. Asphyxiation in street manholes. *Public Health Rep* 1954;69:29–36.
11. Osbern LN, Crapo RO. Dung lung: a report of toxic exposure to liquid manure. *Ann Intern Med* 1981;95:312–314.
12. McAnalley BH, Lowry WT, Oliver RD, et al. Determination of inorganic sulfide ion electrodes: application to the investigation of hydrogen sulfide and cyanide poisoning. *J Anal Toxicol* 1979;3:111.

*Environmental and Occupational Medicine, Third Edition,* edited by William N. Rom.
Lippincott–Raven Publishers, Philadelphia © 1998.

# CHAPTER 44

# Chemical Asphyxiants

William S. Beckett

Chemical asphyxiants prevent the normal uptake of oxygen by tissues by interfering with specific elements in oxygen delivery and metabolic processes. Simple asphyxiants, discussed in the preceding chapter, are physiologically inert gases that, if present in inhaled gas in sufficient concentration, displace oxygen in the alveoli and lead to tissue hypoxia. Because of the immediate lethality of these gases, only air supplying respiratory protective devices and self-contained breathing apparatus are recommended for use during escape from exposure to these gases.

## CARBON MONOXIDE

### Exposure

Because carbon monoxide is the most frequent cause of poisoning death in the United States, and often goes tragically undiagnosed, early institution of general supportive and oxygen therapy and definitive testing of blood carboxyhemoglobin levels (co-oximetry) should be instituted whenever circumstances indicate a potential significant exposure. Exposure may occur wherever there is fuel-burning, flame, or any kind of combustion. Because poisonings are often associated with poorly vented heating sources and enclosed spaces, they are seasonal, occurring more frequently in winter months.

Carbon monoxide (CO) is a colorless and odorless gas and thus has no warning properties to the exposed. It is the product of incomplete combustion of carbon in oxygen—incomplete burning of wood, furnace oil, kerosene, gasoline, natural gas, propane, or any other carbon-containing material—and is thus frequently produced in everyday circumstances of home heating and industrial processes when ventilation is inadequate or equipment malfunctions so as to burn material less completely. Carbon monoxide is also manufactured for use in industrial chemical processes, and stored and shipped as a nonliquefied or liquefied compressed gas. Highly toxic or fatal exposures frequently occur when motor vehicle exhaust is concentrated in an enclosed space; when gas appliances including gas clothes dryers malfunction and are improperly vented; when fire places or furnaces with faulty flues releases their combustion products into the breathing air of the home or workplace; and when propane-powered equipment such as tow-motors and fork lifts incompletely combust their fuel (1). Unvented kerosene heaters burning improperly are an important source of hazard. Firefighters are frequently exposed to carbon monoxide in their work and should wear air-supplying respirators when in or near an area of combustion, including the smoldering remains of fires.

Cigarette smoke may contain, depending on the make and smoking technique, approximately 400 ppm carbon monoxide. Regular smokers often have 3% to 8% carboxyhemoglobinemia; very heavy smokers may have levels higher than 10%.

### Regulatory Standards

The Occupational Safety and Health Administration (OSHA) permissible exposure limit (PEL) for an 8-hour time-weighted average is 50 ppm, which produces a level of carboxyhemoglobin slightly greater than 6% after 8 hours' exposure at rest, and an equilibrium percent carboxyhemoglobin level of about 8% after 16 hours (Fig. 1); 1,200 ppm is considered immediately dan-

W. S. Beckett: Department of Environmental Medicine, University of Rochester School of Medicine and Dentistry, Rochester, New York 14642.

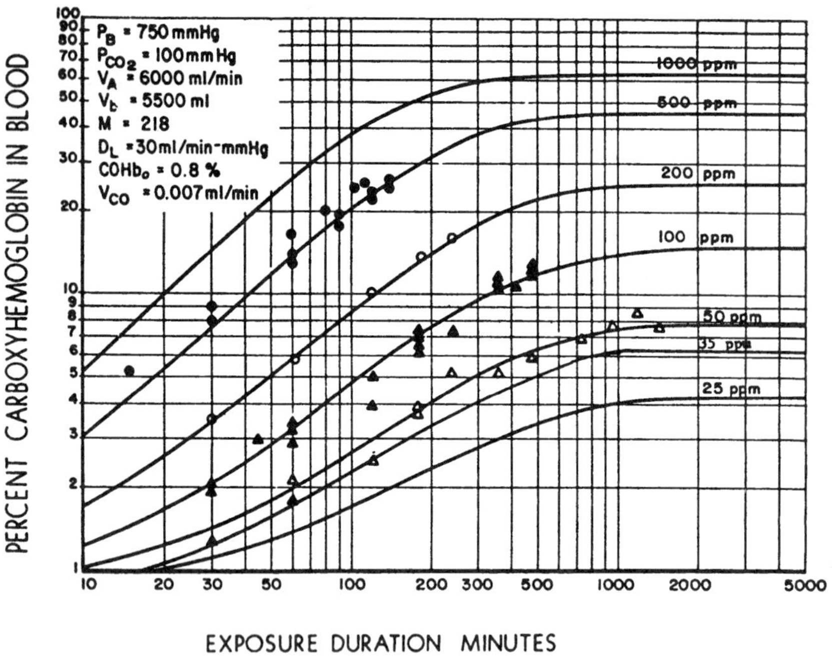


**FIG. 1.** Percent carboxyhemoglobin in blood measured in normal volunteers *(circles and triangles)* and estimated from the Coburn-Forster-Kane equation (25) *(smooth lines)* with inhalation exposure at rest from 25 ppm carbon monoxide to 1,000 ppm (1%) carbon monoxide. These values assume barometric pressure of 750 mm Hg, carbon dioxide tension of 100 mm Hg, resting alveolar ventilation of 6,000 ml per minute, altitude of 218 m above sea level (Milwaukee, WI), a normal diffusing capacity of the lung of 30 ml/min/mm Hg, endogenously produced baseline carboxyhemoglobin level of 0.8%., and $V_{CO}$ (carbon monoxide clearance from the lungs) of 0.007 ml/minute. (Reprinted with permission of R. O. Stewart.)

gerous to life and health (IDLH), a level that is determined to be survivable by healthy adults (without coronary artery disease) without permanent effects for a 30-minute period. This level should be used as indication of urgent need to exit the area immediately. Exposure to 1,000 ppm at rest produces in excess of 25% carboxyhemoglobinemia within an hour.

## Environmental Measurement

Carbon monoxide 1 ppm is equivalent to 1.16 mg/m$^3$; carbon monoxide 1,000 ppm in air is equivalent to a 0.1% carbon monoxide concentration.

Commercially available devices for measuring carbon monoxide in the home include passive chemical colorimetric indicators that sample low levels over a period of days and change color when a limit for an accumulated exposure has been exceeded. Electrically powered audible alarm devices for the home, which sound when air concentrations at the alarm exceed a certain threshold, are now widely available.

For the workplace, indicator tubes for a single sample, electronic short-term testing devices, and continuously monitoring instruments that can be set to alarm at predetermined detection levels can be purchased from industrial hygiene equipment suppliers.

## Pathophysiology

Carbon monoxide diffuses passively across the alveolar membrane, and goes into solution in plasma, where the partial pressure of oxygen dissolved in arterial blood, as measured by $PaO_2$ in arterial blood gases may be normal in spite of a dangerous content of carbon monoxide. Carbon monoxide poisoning may go undetected without measurement of percent carboxyhemoglobin in arterial or venous blood (co-oximetry). (Note that for measurement of carboxyhemoglobin alone without measurement of arterial oxygen, a venous sample usually suffices to establish whether significant carboxyhemoglobinemia is present, since the percent carboxyhemoglobin binding in venous blood is almost the same as in arterial blood.)

From solution in plasma, CO moves rapidly across the red cell membrane. The $Fe^{2+}$ portion of hemoglobin in red cells in the alveolar capillaries binds carbon monoxide with approximately 220 times the affinity of oxygen. Hemoglobin thus acts as a "sink" for carbon monoxide. As carbon monoxide is rapidly removed from solution in plasma, a strong gradient for diffusion of CO from alveoli to plasma is maintained. Thus a low alveolar fraction of carbon monoxide (0.1% in alveolar air) may lead to 25% carbon monoxide saturation of hemoglobin within an hour. The result is a reduction in oxygen-carrying capacity of blood, which is in effect more than proportional to the percent of hemoglobin bound to carbon monoxide (2).

The relationship of inhaled carbon monoxide (in parts per million) to percent blood carboxyhemoglobin in resting adult subjects is shown in Table 1.

Under circumstances of exposure to carbon monoxide greater than 100 ppm, one can estimate the attained percent carboxyhemoglobin as a function of inhaled carbon monoxide (in parts per million), from the duration of exposure, and minute ventilation as follows:

**TABLE 1.** *Carboxyhemoglobin equilibrium at a barometric pressure of one atmosphere*

| CO inhaled (ppm) | Approximate COHb % Saturation |
|---|---|
| 1 | 0.49 |
| 3 | 0.81 |
| 5 | 1.14 |
| 7 | 1.46 |
| 9 | 1.78 |
| 10 | 1.94 |
| 30 | 5.03 |
| 50 | 8 |
| 70 | 11 |
| 90 | 13 |
| 100 | 14 |
| 300 | 33 |
| 500 | 45 |
| 700 | 54 |
| 900 | 60 |
| 1,000 | 62 |
| 3,000 | 83 |

Carbon monoxide 10,000 ppm is equivalent to 1% in air. The values above are based on in vitro equilibration of hemoglobin with gas. In environmental exposures with resting subjects, equilibration occurs after constant exposure for 5 or more hours.

$$\% \, COHb = [CO]_{air} \times \mathrm{KT} \quad [1]$$

where COHb is carboxyhemoglobin, [CO] is the air concentration of carbon monoxide in parts per million, $K$ is a constant that varies with minute ventilation (usually dependent on physical activity) from 0.018 at rest to 0.048 with light work, and $T$ is the duration of exposure in hours. This equation may be used to estimate the air concentration of carbon monoxide when the blood carboxyhemoglobin level and the approximate duration of exposure are known. For instance, in the case of a fatal poisoning of a regular cigarette smoker (whose blood carboxyhemoglobin can be assumed to be no greater than 10%) who was found after 4 hours of exposure with postmortem carboxyhemoglobin level of 75%, the concentration of carbon monoxide inhaled was estimated as follows:

$$[CO]_{\mathrm{exposure}} = 75\%/(0.048)(4 \text{ hours}) = 390 \text{ ppm} \quad [2]$$

Levels of attained carboxyhemoglobin during exposure (and by the same token, rates of excretion when exposure has ceased) are markedly affected by the level of activity of the victim, as seen in Fig. 2.

A second adverse effect is a leftward shift of the oxygen-hemoglobin dissociation curve, making oxygen even less available to tissues in the periphery. Toxic effects may be additionally related to reactions with reduced metallic ions and proteins such as myoglobin, cytochrome oxidase, cytochrome P-450, and others. It is unclear to what degree these other reactions of CO with tissues contribute to the clinical toxicity of the gas, and whether these reactions help to explain the often poor correlation between percent carboxyhemoglobin measured in blood and the clinical outcomes of patients.

Tissue hypoxia leads to an initial compensatory vasodilation and increased cardiac output. Because aortic and carotid chemoreceptors respond to arterial oxygen tension ($PaO_2$) and not to hemoglobin saturation, the chemoreceptor-driven hyperventilation that usually accompanies tissue hypoxia may not occur until relatively late. The rate of dissociation of carbon monoxide from hemoglobin is slow (with a half-life of about 4 hours breathing ambient air at rest). Constant occupational exposure over an 8-hour period may cause buildup of carboxyhemoglobin in blood to levels such that some excess is still present after 16 hours off work and a return to the workplace the following day. Thus an incremental buildup of blood carboxyhemoglobin saturation may take place over the workweek or longer periods of time. Under circumstances with a constant level of exposure, starting from a higher baseline at the beginning of the workday leads to a higher peak level at the end of the day. This may lead to gradually increasing peak levels as the days pass. Levels of carboxyhemoglobin produced by exposures from 25 to 1,000 ppm (0.1%) with varying time periods of constant exposure are shown graphically in Fig. 1 (3).

## Clinical Features

The relationship of symptoms to the percent saturation of blood (COHb%) is shown in Table 2. Fetuses, the elderly, and those with coronary artery disease are more susceptible. Organs with the highest oxygen require-

**TABLE 2.** *Relationship of percent saturation of blood with carbon monoxide (%COHb) to symptoms in carbon monoxide poisoning*

| Percent saturation COHb | Response |
|---|---|
| 0.3–0.7 | None |
| 1–5 | Vasodilation and increased blood flow to certain organs; slightly reduced work time to exhaustion in healthy adults |
| 5–9 | Threshold for visual light detection increased; diminished performance of complex tasks |
| 16–20 | Decreased maximum oxygen uptake during exercise |
| 20–30 | Headache, nausea, impaired manual dexterity, impaired judgment |
| 30–40 | Severe headache, nausea, vomiting, syncope |
| 40–50 | Confusion; collapse on exercise |
| 50–60 | Seizures; coma, loss of consciousness |
| 67–70 | Death if untreated |

Adapted from ref. 3.

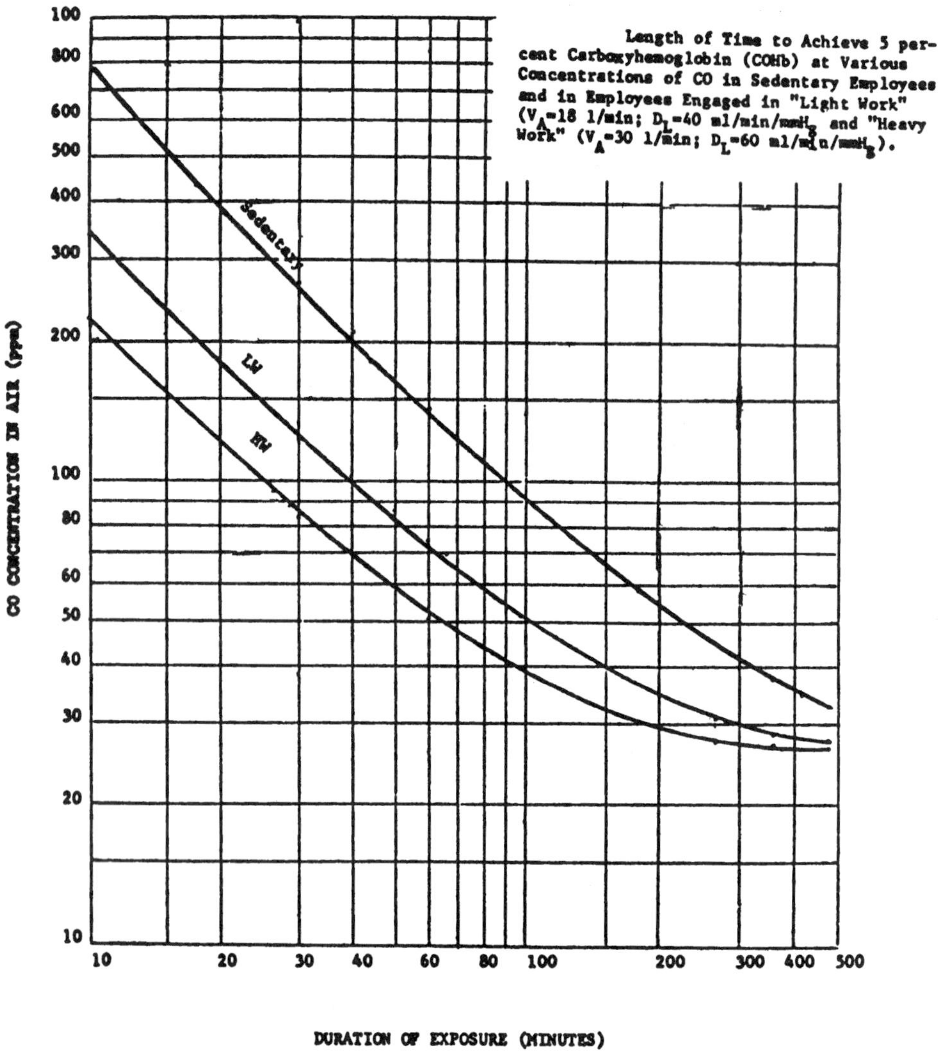


**FIG. 2.** A comparison of the difference in length of time required to acquire blood carboxyhemoglobin levels of 5% with varying inhaled carbon monoxide concentrations in air (10,000 ppm = 1%), durations of exposure (minutes), and levels of exercise (*upper curve* is sedentary, *middle curve* is light work, *lower curve* is heavy work). Increased activity can markedly reduce the concentration needed for a given time, or can reduce the time required at a given concentration. (From NIOSH, *Occupational Exposure to Carbon Monoxide* 1973, with permission.)

ments—brain and heart—are affected first. Early symptoms are nonspecific and related to reduced cerebral oxygen supply—headache, weakness, dizziness, nausea, and impaired vision. Syncope may occur when the peripheral vasodilatory response to tissue hypoxia reduces cerebral oxygen delivery. At higher concentrations of carboxyhemoglobin, hyperventilation, and dyspnea from lactic acidosis, angina (in those with coronary disease), cardiac arrhythmias, seizures, and coma may follow.

Most patients with acute carbon monoxide poisoning have no distinctive physical findings. There may be retinal venous engorgement and retinal flame hemorrhages. Cutaneous bullae or a red coloration of skin and mucous membranes may be present because of the persistent saturation of both arterial and venous hemoglobin with carbon monoxide, making the usual reddish skin tint of saturated hemoglobin even more prominent. The patient's clinical condition is a better indicator of degree of intoxication and prognosis than the blood carboxyhemoglobin level. Focal or global neurologic examination findings or an unstable cardiovascular system may signal impending catastrophic progression of intoxication, and should signal preparations for high levels of medical support such as the institution of mechanical ventilation to protect the airway from aspiration while maintaining minute ventilation and alveolar oxygenation.

For survivors of acute carbon monoxide intoxication, permanent neurologic or other organ dysfunction may result from the anoxic insult. In other cases, after an initial apparent full recovery, delayed neurologic, behavioral, or psychiatric symptoms may appear after 2 to 40 days. Among the many delayed sequelae described in survivors are apathy, disorientation, amnesia, irritability, mood disorders, unusual behavior, irrational speech content, gait and movement disturbances, Parkinsonian-like deficits, urinary or fecal incontinence, hyperreflexia, tremor, flaccid paralysis, or other focal neurologic changes (4). Many but not all of these sequelae may eventually resolve.

### Treatment

Therapy in acute carbon monoxide poisoning is directed to general supportive measures while speeding the dissociation of carbon monoxide from hemoglobin so that oxygen may once again be delivered to organs. Once the patient has been removed from exposure, dissociation is dependent on pulmonary blood flow (carrying carbon monoxide to the alveoli), alveolar ventilation (removing carbon monoxide from alveoli), and the partial pressure of oxygen in the alveoli (competitively binding with carbon monoxide on hemoglobin). Pulmonary blood flow is dependent on cardiac output, initially increased with peripheral vasodilation, but with more extreme poisoning diminished. Alveolar ventilation—the product of the alveolar tidal volume times respiratory rate—may also be initially increased in the patient with lactic acidosis, but diminished with severe poisoning. In the preintensive care setting, the mainstays of therapy are to sustain ventilation if necessary by assisted ventilation (such as with an inflatable bag and oral airway or endotracheal tube) and the administration of 100% oxygen. Administration of 100% oxygen can shorten the half-time for reduction of blood carboxyhemoglobin from approximately 320 minutes to 80 minutes.

Administering 100% oxygen at pressures above atmospheric (e.g., at two atmospheres in a hyperbaric chamber) increases the rate of dissociation of CO from hemoglobin, shortening the half-time even further. Hyperbaric oxygen treatment facilities are available in many regions of the United States for treatment of decompression sickness, osteomyelitis, and carbon monoxide poisoning. Because of the time involved in getting the poisoned individual to a hyperbaric oxygen environment, risks of the hyperbaric treatment itself, the risks related to isolation of a critically ill patient in the chamber, and the lack of controlled trials demonstrating improved outcomes, the indications for hyperbaric oxygen treatment are currently controversial. Circumstances in which hyperbaric oxygen has been most convincingly advocated are those in which the patient is believed to be at risk of permanent neurologic damage or death. Carboxyhemoglobin levels greater than 25% to 40%, transient loss of consciousness, lethargy, stupor, and coma are believed to be indicators of this risk. Opponents cite the lack of controlled trials demonstrating superior outcomes in those who have received hyperbaric oxygen compared with those who have received 100% oxygen at one atmosphere alone, as well as the typical period of tissue hypoxia that usually precedes the institution of hyperbaric therapy (5,6). A recent controlled trial of hyperbaric oxygen in mild to moderately poisoned patients who presented within 6 hours found fewer delayed neurologic sequelae (which are usually transient) in the treatment group (7). Exchange transfusion has recently been suggested as a means to increase oxygen delivery more rapidly than 100% oxygen therapy, but has not been systematically evaluated.

Fetal hemoglobin is more avid for carbon monoxide than adult hemoglobin, resulting in higher percent carboxyhemoglobin levels for the fetus than for the pregnant poisoning patient, and a longer half-life of dissociation. For this reason treatment of the pregnant patient with normobaric 100% oxygen is recommended at lower levels of maternal carboxyhemoglobin, and for more prolonged periods to attain adequate removal of carbon monoxide, than in the nonpregnant patient.

No specific intervention, other than hyperbaric oxygen, to prevent the delayed neurotoxic sequelae is known. Initially it may be difficult to distinguish neuropsychiatric toxicity from the posttraumatic stress disorder, which also may have onset several days after a near-catastrophic poisoning. Pathologically, central nervous system demyelination is seen. Patients who have made a good initial recovery should be alerted about the possibility of delayed neurotoxicity, and when it occurs should receive supportive care and assistance in coping with deficits. Neuropsychological testing may be helpful in identifying and quantifying deficits as an initial stage in developing a supportive treatment plan. For both immediate persistent and delayed neurologic effects, neuropsychological testing coupled with specific adaptive therapy to identified deficits is essential to optimal outcome, and should always be offered the patient. Key elements of such therapy are serial testing to assess the nature of deficits (which may be subtle) and the development of a specific treatment or coping program that will be helpful in relation to the specific deficits identified.

### Studies of Effects of Acute and Chronic Exposure

It is the carbon monoxide in cigarette smoke that is believed to be responsible for much of the mean reduction in birth weight seen in infants born to smoking mothers.

Controlled human chamber studies of exposure to carbon monoxide at levels for which normal subjects are asymptomatic have demonstrated that subjects with coronary disease and stable angina pectoris have a shortened duration of exercise before the onset of angina, arrhythmias, and ischemic ST-segment changes with carbon monoxide exposure that produces 2% carboxyhemoglobinemia (9,10). Case reports of patients with coronary disease suffering myocardial infarction after occupational exposure to carbon monoxide at levels that would not be life threatening for normals have been published and are convincing in relationship to the dose-response effects demonstrated in the chamber studies (9). Epidemiologic mortality studies of occupational groups intermittently or chronically exposed to carbon monoxide (e.g., firefighters and toll collectors in highway tunnels) have investigated whether chronic CO exposure in the absence of acute illness is associated with premature or increased cardiovascular mortality. While some studies have found an association (11,12), other equally high-quality studies have not detected excessive cardiovascular mortality in association with chronic or frequent intermittent occupational exposure to carbon monoxide (13,14). Recent studies have demonstrated a small relative risk in association between ambient carbon monoxide levels in some U.S. and Canadian cities and hospital admissions of elderly people for congestive heart failure (15,16).

## HYDROGEN SULFIDE

Unlike carbon monoxide, which has no warning odor, hydrogen sulfide has a warning smell of rotten eggs and potent respiratory irritant properties. However, usual olfactory adaptive changes and toxic inactivation of the olfactory nerve may render the exposed unable to smell the gas at higher concentrations.

### Exposure

Hydrogen sulfide ($H_2S$) is produced from the decay of organic sulfur-containing material. It is heavier than air and accumulates in low-lying areas. Fatal exposures occur in a variety of industries including petroleum and natural gas extraction and processing, underground coal mines, livestock raising (the agitation of manure in storage and treatment), sewers and human sewage treatment facilities (sewer gas), and where decomposition of fish may occur such as in fish product processing and in the fish-storage holds of fishing vessels. $H_2S$ is shipped for commercial use as a liquefied compressed gas, and used in large quantities to make heavy water for nuclear reactors. It may be encountered environmentally in natural gas deposits and volcanic gases.

Hydrogen sulfide exposures and deaths are a particularly frequent problem in areas where petroleum and natural gas are extracted from the earth, and where the petrochemical industry refines and processes them. In this industry, hydrogen sulfide is known as "sour gas." In the province of Alberta, an area rich in fossil fuel, 221 cases of hydrogen sulfide exposure were traced over a 5-year period. Mortality was 6%, and 65% of cases were admitted to hospital (17).

### Regulatory Standards

The OSHA standard for $H_2S$ is 20 ppm with a 10-minute maximum peak of 50 ppm; 100 ppm is considered immediately dangerous to life and health (1 ppm = 1.42 mg/m$^3$).

### Measurement

Real-time monitoring systems are widely used in the petroleum industry to check for gas during routine maintenance of catalyst beds. They can be attached to alarm systems to warn of rising air levels.

### Pathophysiology

Like cyanide, hydrogen sulfide binds to and inactivates cytochrome oxidase in mitochondria, preventing the cellular metabolism of oxygen. In addition to its asphyxiant effects with initial compensatory tachycardia, hyperpnea, and then respiratory depression, survivors of initial exposures may have delayed noncardiogenic pulmonary edema (the adult respiratory distress syndrome; ARDS) due to the direct irritant effects on the lungs.

Chronic exposure at lower levels may produce chronic conjunctival irritation or corneal ulceration. Chronic exposure may also be toxic to the olfactory system, resulting in complete anosmia, rendering the individual unable to detect the warning odor of the gas with subsequent exposure.

### Clinical Features

With its immediate asphyxiant effects, hydrogen sulfide may cause syncope in one or a group of workers, known in industry as "knockdowns." The exposed may have noticed the sulfurous smell of rotten eggs, and may have conjunctival reddening or other findings of mucous membrane irritation. Victims are often found unconscious in enclosed areas where they have been exposed to gas even transiently, or outdoors where gas has been released into breathing air. At high levels, only a few seconds exposure may be life threatening. When two or more workers are found unconscious, a source of hydrogen sulfide must be considered seriously even if none was previously known to exist. First responders to such poisonings are frequently overcome by the gas while trying to aid victims, and clean air–supplying respiratory protective equipment (usually self-contained breathing apparatus or air packs) must be used for rescue.

Other presenting findings are tachycardia, hyperpnea, and central nervous system depression due to the asphyxiant properties, or the tachypnea, hypoxemia, and chest infiltrates of delayed noncardiogenic pulmonary edema, which appears to be a direct toxic effect of the gas. With higher or more prolonged exposure, the victim may experience central nervous system depression, seizures, cardiovascular instability, respiratory muscle insufficiency, coma, and death. Carbon disulfide exposure has a high mortality rate. In recent years, common circumstances of fatal poisonings include farm workers operating agitating equipment of manure storage tanks, sewer workers, and workers in oilfields and petroleum refineries.

Both delayed (e.g., days to weeks) neurologic and neuropsychiatric deficits and rather severe acute and chronic neurologic and neuropsychiatric deficits have been described in survivors of both apparently minor and obviously severe poisoning (18,19). These deficits have been attributed to anoxic encephalopathy, in some cases exacerbated by circulatory hypoxia from ARDS.

One study has suggested that sewer workers exposed chronically to low levels of carbon disulfide may have a permanent effect on lung function (20).

### Case Report: Hydrogen Sulfide Poisoning

A 27-year-old farm worker entered a 12-foot-deep, 49-inch-diameter hog farm outdoor manure pit to perform repairs on a pump. He descended 9 feet down a ladder, was overcome, and fell into the pit. His uncle descended into the pit to rescue him, was overcome, and fell into the pit. Twenty minutes later rescue personnel equipped with personal protective equipment (self-contained breathing apparatus) removed both men. CPR was initiated and they were transported to a hospital where they were pronounced dead on arrival (21).

### Treatment

In addition to emergency supportive measures for a patient who may undergo very rapid deterioration of cardiovascular, central nervous system, and respiratory function, there are two specific therapies available. The first is 100% oxygen, which could be helpful in cases of pulmonary edema or other circumstances where pulmonary gas exchange is compromised, but would not affect the inhibition of cytochrome oxidase by hydrogen sulfide in metabolizing cells. The second is the use of the first step of the cyanide antidote, sodium nitrite, 300 mg in the average-sized adult, intravenously over 2 to 4 minutes. The purpose is to generate methemoglobin, which competes for hydrogen sulfide by the formation of sulfhemoglobin, freeing and reactivating cytochrome oxidase. Demonstration of the efficacy of this therapy is based on case reports in humans, although animal studies suggest it should be effective if used within a narrow time window after exposure. One potential disadvantage of this therapy is a reduction in the oxygen-carrying capacity of the blood with the formation of sulfhemoglobin.

In patients with persisting neurologic and neuropsychiatric deficits, serial neurologic testing and intensive supportive cognitive behavioral therapy is extremely important in helping the victim to make an optimal adaptation to the often frustrating acquired neurologic deficits that may profoundly affect normal functioning in all spheres of life. Testing by an experienced clinical neuropsychologist can identify the specific areas of cognitive difficulty on which the treatment program can then be focused.

### Prevention

Because of hydrogen sulfide's nearly immediate lethality, aggressive education, warning, and emergency rescue programs should be in place where hydrogen sulfide is used, and in industries where spontaneous exposures may occur. Gas-sensing alarms can be installed. Those working in the area need to be trained in the use of self-contained breathing apparatus, which should be kept available both for escape during gas leaks and for rescue.

## HYDROGEN CYANIDE

### Exposure

Also known as prussic acid, hydrogen cyanide (HCN) is used industrially as an insecticide and rodenticide, in electroplating, and in the manufacture of nylon. Cyanide salts are in the solid state at room temperature. Toxic exposure may occur by inhalation, ingestion, or skin absorption. Firefighters are frequently exposed by inhaling smoke from pyrolysis products of synthetic materials, and patients being treated for smoke inhalation from nonindustrial fires may have had toxic cyanide exposure (22,23). Other common exposures are situations where prussic acid (hydrogen cyanide) has been used as a fumigant to kill rodents and insects in ships or agricultural buildings. Fatal poisonings have occurred with exposure to sodium cyanide and potassium cyanide in metal plating. One of the largest uses of cyanide is as a raw material in the manufacture of nylon.

### Regulatory Standards

The OSHA 8-hour time-weighted average permissible exposure limit is 10 ppm (11 $mg/m^3$). Exposure to 50 ppm is considered immediately dangerous to life and health (Table 3). Air-supplying or self-contained breathing apparatus respirators are the only personal protective equipment recommended for emergency use with exposures above these levels.

**TABLE 3.** *Relation of airborne concentrations of cyanide and time to health effects by the inhalation route*

| Concentration (ppm, in air) and duration | Health effects |
|---|---|
| 7–14, chronic (years) | Vomiting, thyroid enlargement, lacrimation, palpitations, dyspnea |
| 434 (minutes) | Coma |
| 130 (½–1 hour)–524 | Death |

In survivors of an acute poisoning, a delayed neurologic syndrome associated with leukoencephalopathy has been described.

Chronic effects of lower exposure include conjunctival irritation from direct contact, and skin ulceration. Thyroid gland enlargement has been described, particularly in areas where iodine intake is low. Residual symptoms after chronic exposure include a bitter almond taste in the mouth, and headache.

### Measurement

It is difficult to measure hydrogen cyanide in air. To accurately assess exposure, it may be necessary to measure several different cyanide compounds, since HCN can be unstable in the environment. Individual or area exposure measurement are commonly made by drawing air through an impinger containing sodium hydroxide; 1 ppm = 1.12 mg/m$^3$.

Biologic monitoring may also be performed by measuring blood or urine thiocyanate levels, an assay that is widely available from hospital and commercial medical laboratories, because thiocyanate is a toxic metabolite of the therapeutic drug nitroprusside. Biologic monitoring is not recommended as a fundamental routine surveillance tool because of the high toxicity of cyanide, but testing may be helpful in ascertaining the cause of illness in an individual with potential exposure. The time lag in obtaining results usually makes biologic monitoring ineffective in deciding on a treatment course, which in most instances must be chosen rapidly based on the potential for exposure.

### Pathophysiology

Cyanide causes tissue anoxia by rapid binding to the cellular oxygen metabolizing enzyme cytochrome oxidase. This prevents aerobic metabolisms in the affected cells, and causes cell death and organ dysfunction first in those organs most sensitive to anoxia. Exposure appears to affect both aortic and carotid chemoreceptors directly, causing increased firing (and hyperpnea as an early symptom). Death may occur within minutes.

### Clinical Features

Exposed patients may note a bitter almond taste in the mouth. Symptoms of poisoning are nonspecific due to the diffuse nature of the anoxic effects. It may be difficult to distinguish the symptoms of the poisoned patients from the panic of an individual who fears exposure but has not been exposed. Prominent are irritation of mucous membranes, dyspnea, headache, light-headedness, nausea, vomiting, and agitation. Clinical deterioration and apnea often follow rapidly.

### Case Report: Cyanide Poisoning

A man collapsed while cleaning out the residue from the bottom of a 3,500-gallon tank that had contained hydrazodiisobutyronitrile. Thirteen minutes after entering the tank he was removed, and he was given oxygen while en route to hospital. On admission he was comatose with marked conjunctivitis. His skin was decontaminated, and he was given intravenous sodium thiosulfate and was mechanically ventilated; he developed seizures and received diphenylhydantoin, and had other complications including a chest infection and deep venous thrombosis. Two weeks after the event he was discharged from the hospital with residual minor loss in peripheral vision. Hydrogen cyanide was measured in the tank at 500 mg/m$^3$ (24).

### Treatment

Rapid treatment is essential. Antidotes must be administered without delay to have a beneficial effect. If exposure has occurred by ingestion, gastric lavage while protecting the airway and administering antidotes may remove residual cyanide from the stomach. Skin decontamination may be needed. If ventilation is reduced, mechanical ventilation should be administered; 100% oxygen is generally recommended as supportive therapy, but would not be expected to alter the poisoning of cytochrome oxidase in cells.

Two antidotes are used. The commercially available cyanide antidote preparation contains sodium nitrite, sodium thiosulfate, and amyl nitrite. If the patient is breathing spontaneously, amyl nitrite ampules may be administered by inhalation until an intravenous line can be placed and the intravenous regimen begun. The protocol is to rapidly administer sodium nitrite by the intravenous route to generate methemoglobin from hemoglobin. This may produce nitrate-induced vasodilation, which may be treated by placing the patient with the head tilted down (Trendelenburg position) and administering intravenous fluid. The next step of the protocol is to give a slow intravenous infusion of thiosulfate, which converts cyanmethemoglobin to thiocyanate. The thiocyanate, less toxic than cyanide, is excreted in urine.

An alternate treatment regimen that has been used more extensively in Europe is to give an intravenous infusion of hydroxocobalamin (vitamin $B_{12}$), which is meant to form a cyanocobalamin complex that can be excreted in urine.

## Prevention

Skin contact is an important route of exposure to cyanide in plating and other industries, and can be averted by use of gloves, aprons, and face shields. Exposures nonetheless occur, and emergency procedures, including the availability of eyewashes, emergency showers, and antidote kits, are essential to preventing serious illness or death. Ongoing monitoring of air levels in high-risk areas is difficult, and multiroute exposures (skin and inhalation) are common. Thus, strict engineering controls and worker education to recognize early symptoms of toxicity are important preventive measures.

Cyanide poisoning may occur frequently in firefighters with clinically significant smoke inhalation after working near and inside burning residential and commercial buildings. It may be suspected in a clinically unstable firefighter, who may have had a mixed exposure with carbon monoxide, cyanide, and other pyrolysis products. The decision to treat must be made based on the suspicion of exposure, since a rapid bioassay is not available, and therapy must be initiated with the greatest possible speed.

## REFERENCES


1. Fawcett TA, Moon RE, Farcical PJ, Meban GY, Theil DR, Piantadosi CA. Warehouse workers headache. Carbon monoxide poisoning from propane-fueled forklifts. *J Occup Med* 1992;34:12–15.
2. Root WS. Carbon monoxide. In: Fenn WI, Rahn W, eds. *Handbook of physiology:* respiration, vol 2. Bethesda: American Physiological Society, 1977;1087–1098.
3. Stewart RD. The effects of carbon monoxide on humans. *Annu Rev Toxicol* 1975;15:409–423
4. Choi IS. Delayed neurologic sequelae in carbon monoxide intoxication. *Arch Neurol* 1983;40:433–435.
5. Shusterman DJ. Clinical smoke inhalation injury: systemic effects. In: Shusterman DJ, Peters JE, eds. De novo toxicants: combustion toxicology, mixing incompatibilities, and environmental activation of toxic agents. *Occup Med State of the Art Rev* 1993;8:469–503.
6. Gail DR, ed. Hyperbaric oxygen therapy. NHLBI workshop summary. *Am Rev Respir Dis* 1991;1414–1421.
7. Thom SR, Taber RL, Mendiguren IL, Clark JM, Hardy KR, Fisher AB. Delayed neuropsychological sequelae after carbon monoxide poisoning: prevention by treatment with hyperbaric oxygen. *Ann Emer Med* 1995;25:474–480.
8. Allred EN, Bleecker EN, Chaitman BR, et al. Short term effects of carbon monoxide exposure on the exercise performance of subjects with coronary artery disease. *N Engl J Med 1989;*321:1426–1432.
9. Atkins EH, Baker EL. Exacerbation of coronary artery disease by occupational carbon monoxide exposure: a report of two fatalities and a review of the literature. *Am J Ind Med* 1985;7:73–79.
10. Sheps DS, Herbst MC, Hinderliter AL, et al. Production of arrhythmias by elevated carboxyhemoglobin in patients with coronary artery disease. *Ann Intern Med* 1990;113:343–351.
11. Stern FB, Halperin WE, Hornung RW, et al. Heart disease mortality among bridge and tunnel officers exposed to carbon monoxide. *Am J Epidemiol* 1988;128:1276–1288.
12. Stern FB, Lemen RA, Curtis RA. Exposure of motor vehicle examiners to carbon monoxide: a historical prospective mortality study. *Arch Environ Health* 1981;36:59–65.
13. Rosenman KD. Cardiovascular disease and environmental exposure. *Br J Ind Med* 1979;36:85–97.
14. Hansen ES. A cohort study on the mortality of firefighters. *Br J Ind Med* 1990;47:805–809.
15. Burnett RT, Dales RE. Association between ambient carbon monoxide levels and hospitalizations for congestive heart failure in the elderly in 10 Canadian cities. *Epidemiology* 1997;8:162–167.
16. Morris RD, Naumiva EN. Ambient air pollution and hospitalization for congestive heart failure among elderly people in 7 large U.S. cities. *Am J Pub Hlth* 1995;7:1031–1032.
17. Burnett WW, King EG, Grace M, Hall WF. Hydrogen sulfide poisoning: review of 5 years experience. *CMA J* 1977;117:1277–1280.
18. Tvedt B, Skyberg K, Aaserud O, Hobbesland A, Mathiesen T. Brain damage caused by hydrogen sulfide: a follow-up study of six patients. *Am J Ind Med* 1991;20:91–101.
19. Snyder JW, Saffir EF, Summerville GP, Middleberg RA. Occupational fatality and persistent neurological sequelae after mass exposure to hydrogen sulfide. *Am J Emerg Med* 1995;13;199–203.
20. Richardson DB. Respiratory effects of chronic hydrogen sulfide exposure. *Am J Ind Med* 1995;28:99–108.
21. Morbidity & Mortality Weekly Report. *Fatalities attributed to entering manure waste pits*—Minnesota, 1992. *MMWR* 1993;42(17):323–329.
22. Baud FJ, Barriot P, Toffis V, et al. Elevated blood cyanide concentrations in victims of smoke inhalation. *N Engl J Med* 1991;325:1776.
23. Kulig K. Cyanide antidotes and fire toxicology. *N Engl J Med* 1991;325:1801–1802.
24. Bonsall JL. Survival without sequelae following exposure to 500 mg/m$^3$ hydrogen sulfide. *Hum Toxicol* 1984;3:57–60.
25. Coburn RF, Forster RE, Kane PB. Considerations of the physiological variables that determine the blood carboxyhemoglobin concentration in man. *J Clin Invest* 1965;44:1899–1910.

*Environmental and Occupational Medicine, Third Edition,* edited by William N. Rom.
Lippincott–Raven Publishers, Philadelphia © 1998.

# CHAPTER 45

# Rhinitis and Sinusitis

Robert P. Nelson, Jr., and Richard F. Lockey

Rhinitis is a symptom complex consisting of rhinorrhea, sneezing, nasal congestion, and itching, and is usually associated with a general discomfort of the nose and nasal passages (1). Rhinitis occurs secondary to exposure to noninflammatory stimuli such as cold air or from medications, or more commonly results from inflammation caused by infectious organisms, allergens, or chemical irritants. Sinusitis is mucosal inflammation of the sinuses, usually, but not always, caused by an infectious organism and is characterized by symptoms of nasal obstruction, hyposmia, purulent nasal and postnasal secretions, posterior pharyngeal irritation, fetid breath, fatigue, headache. and malaise. Rhinitis and sinusitis often occur together.

Rhinitis, especially allergic rhinitis, predisposes to the development of sinusitis; the symptoms associated with sinusitis may also occur with rhinitis; therefore, sinusitis is often misdiagnosed as rhinitis and rhinitis as sinusitis. The conditions may also coexist, owing to a common etiology such as an infectious organism.

Occupational rhinitis is rhinitis associated with work and can occur concomitantly with occupational asthma (2). Occupational sinusitis is not recognized as a distinct clinical entity in the medical literature. This chapter focuses on rhinitis related to workplace exposure and discusses how rhinitis induced in the workplace may lead to or be involved in the pathogenesis of sinusitis.

R. P. Nelson, Jr.: Division of Allergy and Clinical Immunology, Departments of Medicine and Pediatrics, University of South Florida College of Medicine/All Children's Hospital, St. Petersburg, Florida 33701.

R. F. Lockey: Department of Environmental Health, University of Cincinnati College of Medicine, Cincinnati, Ohio 45267–0182.

## NASAL PHYSIOLOGY AND ALLERGIC RESPONSE

The nose and nasal pharynx filter and alter the temperature and humidity of inspired air. Vibrissae, cilia, and mucus remove larger particulate matter greater than 20 μm in diameter (3,4). The nasal turbinates provide a large mucosal surface area and ensure turbulent airflow, which enhances particle deposition, humidification, and temperature alteration. Inhaled irritants may cause swelling of the nasal mucosa and obstruct the nasal passages, thus decreasing further entry of noxious agents. Sneezing, aided by increased secretions, enhances the expulsion of particulates. The autonomic nervous system, innervating the nasal mucosa, shunts nasal airflow from one air passage to another every 2 to 4 hours throughout the day and night, assisting with the process of nasal cleansing (5).

Plasma proteins, serous cell products, mucus glycoproteins, and inflammatory mediators and cells are present in nasal secretions (Table 1) (6). An increase in nasal secretions is caused by parasympathetic/cholinergic stimulation which is blocked by atropine sulfate. Chemical mediators, such as histamine, increase the protein content and volume of mucus and regulate neuropeptide release; these chemical mediators are also important in regulating the upper and lower airways (7,8).

Macrophages, neutrophils, mast cells, and basophils are present in nasal mucosa. Mast cells and basophils are primarily responsible for the generation of immunoglobulin E (IgE)-mediated anaphylactic inflammatory reactions. These cells contain preformed mediators and can generate newly synthesized mediators, all of which are

**TABLE 1.** *Constituents of human nasal secretions*

| |
|---|
| Mucous cell products |
| Mucous glycoproteins |
| Serous cell products |
| Lactoferrin |
| Lysozyme |
| Secretory IgA and secretory component |
| Neutral endopeptidase |
| Aminopeptidase |
| Uric acid |
| Peroxidase |
| Secretory leukoprotease inhibitor |
| Plasma proteins |
| Albumin |
| Immunoglobulins: IgG, IgA (monomeric) IgM, IgE |
| Carboxypeptidase N |
| Angiotensin-converting enzyme |
| Kallikrein |
| Indeterminate sources |
| Calcitonin gene-related peptide |
| Urea |
| Inflammatory mediators found after allergen challenge |
| Histamine |
| TAME esterase |
| $PGD_2$ |
| Bradykinin |
| $LTC_4$ |
| Tryptase |
| Major basic protein |
| Eosinophil-derived neurotoxin |

Modified from ref. 45.
TAME, tosyl-L-arginine methylesterase; PG, prostaglandin; $LTC_4$, leukotriene $C_4$.

released into the tissue either as a result of bridging by allergen of specific IgE receptors on mast cells and basophils or by nonimmunologic stimuli such as cold air (8). The preformed mediators are released within minutes, causing an immediate-phase reaction, or may require hours for release and generation as occurs during the late-phase reaction (9). Nasal late-phase reactions develop 2 to 12 hours following allergen exposure and are manifested primarily by nasal congestion, and, to a lesser extent, by rhinorrhea and sneezing. Late-phase reactions are characterized physiologically by changes in nasal airway resistance and biologically by influxes of inflammatory cells or generation of mediators from a variety of cells.

Eosinophils begin migrating into the nasal mucosa 3 hours following allergen challenge. Neutrophils, mononuclear cells, and basophils appear next (10). A variety of mediators, including neutrophilic chemotactic factor, platelet-activating factor, eosinophilic cationic protein, eosinophil-derived neurotoxin, major basic protein, prostaglandin $D_2$, kinins, tame esterase, and leukotrienes $LTC_4$, $LTD_4$, and $LTE_4$ attract these cells and initiate and cause the late-phase response (11). The late-phase response results in a priming effect, thus requiring much less allergen to trigger mast cells and basophils. The nasal mucosa is now also more susceptible to nonspecific stimuli, such as noxious irritants and cold air (12).

## ALLERGIC RHINITIS

Allergic rhinitis occurs when airborne allergenic particulates impact on the nasal mucosa and trigger the IgE allergic reaction. Such reactions cause histamine, tame esterase, kininogen, kinins, and other mediators listed above to be released, and the migration of inflammatory cells onto the mucosa of the nasal pharynx (10). With repeated challenges, as occurs with chronic allergen exposure, submucosal sinusoids engorge and blood vessels dilate, leading to nasal congestion, goblet cell hypertrophy, increased glandular secretions, and neutrophilic and eosinophilic infiltration of the mucosa (13). Mast cells, basophils, and eosinophils are present in nasal secretions. Activated lymphocytes can be found in the superficial lamina propria. The major symptoms and responsible mediators are illustrated in Table 2.

## NONALLERGIC RHINITIS

Nonallergic rhinitis includes a heterogeneous group of disorders that should be considered in the differential diagnosis of rhinitis. These include vasomotor rhinitis, nonallergic rhinitis with eosinophils (NARES), rhinitis medicamentosa, atrophic rhinitis, drug-induced rhinitis, rhinitis associated with pregnancy, and hypothyroid-asso-

**TABLE 2.** *Allergic rhinitis: major symptoms and responsible mediators*

| Pathologic event | Symptom elicited | Putative mediator |
|---|---|---|
| Pruritus | Tickling, palatal clicking | Histamine ($H_1$), prostaglandins |
| Mucosal edema, vascular engorgement | Nasal obstruction | Histamine ($H_1$), kinins, eicosanoids |
| Sneezing | Sneezing, urge to sneeze | Histamine ($H_1$), eicosanoids |
| Increased secretions | Runny nose, postnasal drip | Histamine ($H_1$), kinins, eicosanoids |
| Late-phase allergic reactions | Congestion, nasal irritability, hyperresponsiveness | Inflammatory factors and cytokines, chemotactic factors |

Modified from ref. 46.

ciated rhinitis. Some individuals with these forms of rhinitis may be more susceptible to chemical irritants associated with certain working environments, although there is no medical literature on these forms of rhinitis associated with various occupations.

## SINUSITIS

The paranasal sinuses include the maxillary, frontal, ethmoid, and sphenoid sinuses. The sinus mucosa is cleared of infectious organisms by the mucociliary apparatus, which sweeps secretions through ostia into the nasal pharynx. Viral upper respiratory infections cause acute viral-induced sinusitis. Viral-induced sinusitis has been demonstrated by computed axial tomography (CAT) scans obtained during viral-induced upper respiratory infections (URIs) to last several weeks. Retention of secretions, either by reduced ostia patency, ciliary dysfunction, or mucus overproduction, sometimes enable pyogenic bacteria to multiply, often resulting in secondary bacterial sinusitis (14). The maxillary sinuses are the most common site of sinusitis, followed, in order, by the ethmoid, frontal, and sphenoid sinuses (15).

A variety of medical conditions, some of which include anatomical abnormalities of the nasal pharynx, cystic fibrosis, and allergic rhinitis, affect either ostia patency, ciliary function, or quantity or quality of mucus, and predispose individuals to develop sinusitis. The reported prevalence of sinusitis increased between 1982 and 1993. Between 1990 and 1992 approximately 73 million restricted-activity days per year were reported by persons who had sinusitis. This figure represents a 50% increase from the approximately 50 million restricted-activity days reported between 1986 and 1988 (16).

Acute sinusitis is somewhat arbitrarily defined as sinusitis of less than 6 weeks to 3 months. It is characterized by infection by aerobic organisms such as *Streptococcus pneumoniae, Haemophilus influenzae,* and *Moraxella catarrhalis.* Upper respiratory tract symptoms that do not resolve for several weeks following a typical URI may indicate that the patient has acute bacterial sinusitis. Symptoms may include purulent nasal or posterior nasal discharge, facial or tooth pain or discomfort, cough, postnasal drip, and occasionally fever (17). Failure to eliminate the acute infection may lead to chronic sinusitis.

Symptoms of chronic sinusitis may be more subtle and include dull headache, persistent nasal stuffiness, hyposmia, purulent nasal and posterior nasal secretions, foul breath, sore oral pharynx, hoarseness, throat clearing, fatigue, and malaise. Anaerobic organisms, including *Bacteroides* and pepticocci are found with increased frequency in chronic sinusitis (18).

Patients with allergic rhinitis are more susceptible to developing sinusitis, presumably because of inflammation caused by the disease. The sinus ostia or the ostia meatal complex becomes obstructed, leading to retention of secretions and secondary bacterial sinusitis. Allergic individuals, when challenged to an allergen to which they are sensitive, develop radiographic changes such as mucosal thickening and opacification of these sinuses (19).

## DIAGNOSIS OF RHINITIS AND SINUSITIS

The diagnosis of rhinitis or sinusitis is established by the clinical history, physical examination, and appropriate laboratory studies. Symptoms of allergic rhinitis include paroxysms of sneezing, nasal and oral pharyngeal pruritus, rhinorrhea, and nasal congestion with or without postnasal drip. Allergic conjunctivitis, manifested by redness, tearing, and pruritis of the conjunctivae, commonly occurs with allergic rhinitis. Physical findings include periorbital darkening of the skin ("allergic shiners"); pale, edematous nasal turbinates; and clear nasal secretions.

The physical examination of the patient with acute or chronic sinusitis may reveal tenacious, purulent, green or yellow secretions in the nares by anterior nasal rhinoscopy or in the posterior oral pharynx by inspection of the oral pharynx. The nasal mucosa can be hyperemic and edematous and the patient's breath fetid. Purulent discharge from the sinus ostia and anatomical obstruction of the ostia or of the ostia meatal complex often can be visualized by fiber optic rhinoscopy but not by anterior nasal rhinoscopy (20).

An easy to perform and valuable laboratory diagnostic test is the nasal smear. Eosinophils suggest an allergic etiology, while polymorphonuclear cells suggest an infectious etiology (21). Skin testing, via either epicutaneous or intradermal routes, is the most time-efficient, convenient, and inexpensive method to detect specific IgE to environmental allergens. Under special circumstances, such as in a patient with dermatographism, severe atopic eczema, or with scarring of the skin, in vitro assays for specific serum IgE are useful, such as the radioallergosorbent (RAST) test, but these tests are usually more expensive and less sensitive than are skin tests. Endoscopic sinus aspiration through the ostia meatal complex or needle aspiration of a maxillary sinus may help to define the putative infectious organism. Plain radiographs are useful to distinguish sinusitis from rhinitis; the most useful view is the occipitomental or Water's view, which best demonstrates the maxillary sinuses. Radiographic evidence of mucosal thickening of 6 to 8 mm or greater, an air-fluid level, or complete opacification usually indicate bacterial infection of the sinuses (22). Unilateral opacification of a sinus, especially a maxillary sinus, can also mean that the patient has a tumor; thus, appropriate follow-up is necessary to assure resolution. Computed tomography (CT) of the sinuses is

**TABLE 3.** *Work-related allergens that cause rhinitis*

| |
|---|
| Enzyme-containing detergents *(Bacillus subtilis)* |
| Western red cedar *(Thuja plicata)* |
| Ash wood dust *(Fraxinus excelsior)* |
| Laboratory animal exposure |
| Psyllium |
| Guar gum *(Cyamopsis tetragonolobus)* |
| Wheat flour (α-amylase extract) |
| Trimellitic anhydride |
| Isonicotinic acid |

a more sensitive method to identify abnormalities of the sinuses and of the ostia meatal complex; however, its specificity for sinusitis, as with plain radiographs, is unknown (23).

## ETIOLOGY OF OCCUPATIONAL RHINITIS

Symptoms of upper airway disease and its broad differential diagnosis, combined with the high prevalence of URIs, a variety of naturally occurring outdoor and indoor environmental allergens and irritants (pollution), and man-made pollution, make it particularly difficult to establish a cause-and-effect relationship between upper airway symptoms and workplace exposure. Occupational rhinitis is the episodic or continuous occurrence of rhinitis associated with the work environment (2). An individual who has allergic rhinitis and thus a "hair trigger nose" may have heightened nasal mucosal sensitivity when exposed to chemical irritants and other noxious agents. Thus, exposure to coal dust and talc, which are not allergens but irritants, may exacerbate preexisting allergic rhinitis. The allergens or substances for which there is documented evidence for occupational allergic rhinitis are relatively few and are summarized in Table 3.

In 1969 Flindt (24) and Pepys et al. (25) described allergic respiratory symptoms in English workers who manufactured enzyme-containing detergents. Slavin and Lewis (26) investigated a cohort of 238 individuals who worked in a detergent-producing factory. Detailed histories and epicutaneous and intradermal skin tests were performed to an extract containing the *Bacillus subtilis* enzyme. Sixty-six workers (27.7%) had upper and or lower respiratory tract symptoms. Thirty-five (14.7%) had asthma, 26 allergic rhinitis and allergic asthma (10.9%), and five (2.1%) allergic rhinitis alone. The onset of symptoms of allergic rhinitis and allergic asthma varied from a few minutes to 6 to 8 hours following work exposure. Sixty of 66 (90.9%) of the affected workers were classified as atopic and 56 had positive skin tests to the *Bacillus subtilis* enzyme skin test reagent. It is also noteworthy that 58 of 177 unaffected workers who did not have either disease demonstrated significant skin reactivity to the *Bacillus* extract. The skin test reactivity to the enzyme preparation was successfully passively transferred to negative control subjects using sera of three skin test–positive workers, thus indicating that this reaction was most likely IgE mediated. This study demonstrated that work-related allergic rhinitis was associated with specific IgE-mediated hypersensitivity. Comprehensive measures to decrease exposure were successful in reducing symptoms (26).

Occupational asthma occurs due to exposure to Western red cedar *(Thuja plicata)*. Chan-Yeung (27) reported 45 patients with respiratory disease due to exposure to this dust. Twenty-two (49%) of the patients studied had associated allergic rhinitis. Although bronchial challenges were associated with both immediate- and late-phase asthmatic responses, nasal provocation tests were not done. The component of Western red cedar dust that causes asthma is plicatic acid, a small molecular weight compound of 400 daltons (27).

Blainey et al. (28) measured nasal responses to wood dust in two patients with Western red cedar induced asthma, utilizing nasal provocation tests and anterior rhinometry. One patient, who experienced a late-phase reaction with bronchial provocation, had a negative nasal challenge. The second patient, who demonstrated a late-phase asthmatic response following bronchial challenge, experienced a late-phase nasal response when exposed to fine Western red cedar dust in the challenge chamber, similar in timing to the late-phase response of the lower respiratory tract (28).

An 18-year-old man who worked in a furniture factory reported rhinitis and asthma when he was exposed to ash *(Fraxinus excelsior)* wood dust (29). Peak expiratory flow rate (PEFR) variations were found while he was at work. Basal $PC_{20}$ methacholine was 1.41 mg/ml, indicating bronchial hyperreactivity. A bronchial provocation test with ash wood dust extract (1:100 w/v) induced a dual asthmatic response with a 7.5-fold increase of nonspecific bronchial hyperresponsiveness. Intradermal testing with ash wood extract elicited a positive immediate skin test. IgE antibodies against ash wood extract were found in the patient's serum with a RAST value of 0.57 peripheral resistance units per milliliter (PRU/ml). Skin tests, bronchial provocation tests, and RAST with ash wood dust extract performed in control patients were negative, indicating that the patient had IgE-mediated occupational asthma caused by exposure to ash wood dust (29). The authors felt he also had ash wood dust–induced allergic rhinitis, even though he was never challenged nasally with the wood dust or extract.

Platts-Mills et al. (30) documented that patients with occupational asthma and allergic rhinitis related to laboratory rats have specific IgE directed at rat urinary protein. Lutsky and Neuman conducted a survey of twenty medical colleges, seven research institutes and universities, five pharmaceutical manufacturers, three veterinary colleges, two commercial laboratory animal producers, and two hospitals in 1975 to establish the prevalence and clinical profile of patients with laboratory animal–induced allergy; 191 of 1,293 (14.8%) individuals with daily laboratory animal contact reported allergic symptoms, and 30% of the affected subjects were aware of a previous family history of atopy. Clinical symptoms occurred within 1 hour of exposure in all reported cases, and within 10 minutes for 93% of the patients, suggesting that they had an IgE-mediated disease. The frequency of clinical symptoms were as follows: allergic rhinitis with conjunctivitis, 100%; asthma, 71%; cough, 58%; contact urticaria, 58%; and palatal itch, 38%. This study indicates that allergic rhinitis is the most common allergic illness among laboratory animal workers (31).

Schwartz et al. (32) reported the occurrence of rhinitis in a 45-year-old nurse who worked at a skilled health care facility. She developed sneezing, rhinorrhea, watery eyes, postnasal drip, headache, itching and fullness in the ears, cough, chest tightness, and wheezing on the days that she distributed psyllium, a plant fiber powder used as a laxative, to her patients. This nurse had a nonatopic family history, personal evidence of atopy, and a significant elevation of antipsyllium IgE. Only upper and not lower airway challenge studies were positive to psyllium. Symptomatic relief was achieved with cromolyn pretreatment (32).

Guar gum is derived from the vegetable *Cyamopsis tetragonolobus* grown in India. It is incorporated into numerous foods and pharmaceutical products and used as a fixing agent for colors (33). Thirty-seven of 177 subjects (21%) employed at a carpet manufacturing plant had a history suggestive of occupational asthma and 59 (33%) had occupational rhinitis. IgE and IgG antibodies to guar gum were measured in 133 of the 162 (82%) subjects experiencing symptoms. Eight (6%) demonstrated immediate skin test reactivity to guar gum. Eleven (8.3%) had serum IgE antibodies to guar gum. Of four subjects who underwent specific bronchial inhalational challenge, two had typical isolated immediate asthmatic reactions. Thus, some patients with symptoms related to guar gum exposure have specific IgE antibodies, and a relatively high number have symptoms of allergic rhinitis (33).

Valdivieso et al. (34) described four bakers, two with bronchial asthma and two with rhinoconjunctivitis following exposure to wheat flour. Epicutaneous and RAST tests were positive in all four, but nasal and bronchial challenge testing with wheat flour extracts were positive in only one baker with asthma. Epicutaneous, RAST, and nasal or bronchial challenges done with α-amylase, which is a glycolytic enzyme obtained from *Aspergillus oryzae* and used as a flour additive, were positive in all four patients. These data support previous observations that Ramazzini made in 1713, that bakers are susceptible to occupational allergic disease (35), including allergic rhinitis.

Reactive chemical haptens, such as trimellitic anhydride, are associated with complex pulmonary immunologic responses. Trimellitic anhydride (TMA) is an industrial chemical used as a plasticizer and serves as a model for occupational-induced immunologic lung disease. TMA combines with human proteins to form new antigenic determinants, which are probably the most immunogenic forms of the compound. TMA may provoke IgE or IgG antibody production in humans. Sensitization to TMA can present in several forms, including IgE-mediated asthma and rhinitis, hypersensitivity pneumonitis, and an irritated airway syndrome. A late respiratory systemic syndrome (LRSS), which Zeiss et al. (36) described as a complex of cough, malaise, and dyspnea, may also occur 4 to 12 hours following exposure to TMA. This reaction is associated with IgG antibodies against trimellityl–human serum albumin and may represent a variant of hypersensitivity pneumonitis; however, chest x-ray changes have not been documented. Asai et al. (37) described a hospital pharmacist who developed occupational asthma due to isonicotinic acid hydrazine (INH) inhalation after experiencing symptoms of rhinitis.

House dust mites are the most common home environmental allergen in patients with allergic rhinitis and asthma. These organisms produce fecal pellets, which are the source of house dust allergens. Just as house dust mites may trigger symptoms, storage mites are a common cause for allergic rhinitis in farmers and grain elevator operators (38).

## DIAGNOSIS OF OCCUPATIONAL RHINITIS

The diagnosis of occupational allergic rhinitis is based on the history and physical examination. Sneezing, nasal pruritus, rhinorrhea, and nasal stuffiness may occur within a few minutes of exposure to an occupational allergen. The isolated late-phase reaction may not occur until hours following work. Symptoms usually resolve over weekends or holidays, although they may persist for days even if the allergic subject is no longer exposed to the work-related allergen.

Slavin (39) recommends site visits when an occupation is implicated in a disease so that the clinician is familiar with the substances to which the patient is exposed, and to document work-related symptoms. Material safety data sheets, which provide additional information about materials used in the work environment, should also be reviewed.

Where possible, appropriate skin tests should be done in patients with suspected IgE-mediated disease caused by the work environment. A negative skin test to an appropriate allergen usually indicates that the disease is of nonallergic origin; however, positive skin tests do not necessarily indicate that the rhinitis is of allergic origin unless a cause-and-effect relationship can be demonstrated.

Nasal provocation challenges can be done and responses semiquantitated by either symptom score or rhinometry; they are primarily used for research and

**TABLE 4.** *Occupational health measures*

| |
|---|
| Provide adequate ventilation |
| Recognize the offending allergen and understand its source |
| Enclose previously open operations under certain conditions |
| Automate hand operations |
| Supply heavily exposed workers with space suits |
| Provide disposable gloves, uniforms, masks |
| Monitor the concentration of offending substance in the air |
| Monitor selected highly exposed employees with skin testing, serologic testing, and pulmonary function testing when appropriate |

From ref. 26.

require better standardization before they can be recommended for clinical practice (40).

## MANAGEMENT

Management of occupational rhinitis may be best achieved by practicing preventative medicine (39). Environmental control measures that limit exposure to the allergen source and provide adequate ventilation are recommended to prevent occupational rhinitis. Such benefits were realized in the detergent industry by limiting the exposure of workers to *Bacillus subtilis* enzyme. Precautions applicable to work environments are listed in Table 4 (26). Various studies have demonstrated that screening workers before they begin work in a work environment that may induce allergic disease is not beneficial (30). It is also a potential legal problem for the employer and therefore it is not recommended.

In summary, occupational rhinitis is best managed by avoiding the offending allergens, and treating the rhinitis with appropriate pharmaceutical agents and, when necessary, allergen immunotherapy (40–44). Sinusitis, which may complicate rhinitis, is managed by first diagnosing it and then treating it with appropriate medical or surgical therapy (42). Occupational rhinitis rarely, if ever, leads to disability. Chronic sinusitis has not been reported to be associated with the work environment.

## REFERENCES


1. Minotti DA. Allergic rhinitis and sinusitis. In: Virant FS, ed. *Immunology and allergy clinics of North America:* chronic sinus disease. Philadelphia: W. B. Saunders, 1994;14(1):113–128.
2. Salvaggio JE, Taylor G, Weill H. Occupational asthma and rhinitis in occupational respiratory disease. In: Merchant JA, ed. *Occupational and respiratory diseases.* Washington, DC: US Department of Health and Human Services, 1986, 86–102.
3. Geurkink N. Nasal anatomy, physiology, and function. *J Allergy Clin Immunol* 1983;72(2):123–128.
4. Proctor DF. The mucociliary system. In: Proctor DF, Andersen I, eds. *The nose:* upper airway physiology and the atmospheric environment. Amsterdam: Elsevier, 1982.
5. Malm L. Sympathetic influence on the nasal mucosa. Acta Otolaryngol 1977;83(1-2):20–21.
6. Druce HM. Allergic and nonallergic rhinitis. In Middleton E Jr, Reed CE, Ellis EF, Adkinson NF Jr, Yunginger JW, Busse W, eds. *Allergy principles and practice,* vol 2, 4th ed. St. Louis: Mosby Year Book, 1993;1433–1455.
7. Baraniuk JN. Neural control of human nasal secretion. *Pulmon Pharmacol* 1991;4(1):20–31.
8. Schleimer RP, MacGlashan DW Jr, Peters SP, et al. Inflammatory mediators and mechanisms of release from purified human basophils and mast cells. *J Allergy Clin Immunol* 1984;74(4 Pt 1):473–381.
9. Iliopoulos O, Proud D, Norman PS, Lichtenstein LM, Kagey-Sobotka A, Naclerio RM. Nasal challenge with cold, dry air induces a late-phase reaction. *Am Rev Respir Dis* 1988;138(2):400–405.
10. Bascom R, Wachs M, Naclerio RM, et al. Basophil influx occurs after nasal antigen challenge: effects of topical corticosteroid pretreatment. *J Allergy Clin Immunol* 1988;81:580.
11. Lemanske RF Jr, Kaliner MA. Late phase allergic reactions. In: Middleton E Jr, Reed CE, Ellis EF, Adkinson NF Jr, Yunginger JW, Busse W, eds. *Allergy principles and practice,* vol 2, 4th ed. St. Louis: Mosby Year Book, 1993;1433–1455.
12. Connell JT. Quantitative intranasal pollen challenge. II. Effect of daily pollen challenge, environmental pollen exposure, and placebo challenge on the nasal membrane. *J Allergy Clin Immunol* 1968;41:123.
13. Kaliner M, Lemanske R. Rhinitis and asthma. *JAMA* 1992;268(20):2807–2829.
14. Reimer A, von Mecklenburg C, Toremalm NG. The mucociliary activity of the upper respiratory tract. III. A functional and morphological study on human and animal material with special reference to maxillary sinus diseases. Acta Otolaryngol Suppl 1978;356:1–20.
15. Slavin RG. Nasal polyps and sinusitis. In: Middleton E Jr, Reed CE, Ellis EF, Adkinson NF Jr, Yunginger JW, Busse W, eds. *Allergy principles and practice,* vol 2, 4th ed. St. Louis: Mosby Year Book, 1993;1455–1470.
16. Collins JG. Prevalence of selected chronic conditions: United States, 1986–1988. National Center for Health Statistics. *Vital Health Stat* 1993;10:1–87.
17. Ludman H. Paranasal sinus diseases. *Br Med J* 1981;282(6269): 1054–1057.
18. Brook I. Bacteriology of chronic maxillary sinusitis in adults. *Ann Otol Rhinol Laryngol* 1989;98(6):426–428.
19. Pelikan Z, Pelikan-Filipek M. Role of nasal allergy in chronic maxillary sinusitis-diagnostic value of nasal challenge with allergen. *J Allergy Clin Immunol* 1990;86(4 Pt 1):484–491.
20. Rohr A, Hassner A, Saxon A. Rhinopharyngoscopy for the evaluation of allergic-immunologic disorders. *Ann Allergy* 1983;50(6):380–384.
21. Mullarkey MF, Hill JS, Webb DR. Allergic and nonallergic rhinitis: their characterization with attention to the meaning of nasal eosinophilia. *J Allergy Clin Immunol* 1980;65(2):122–126.
22. Evans FO Jr, Sydnor JB, Moore WE, et al. Sinusitis of the maxillary antrum. *N Engl J Med* 1975;293(15):735–739.
23. Cable HR, Jeans WD, Cullen RJ, Bull PD, Maw AR. Computerized tomography of the Caldwell-Luc cavity. *J Laryngol Otol* 1981;95(8): 775–783.
24. Flindt MLH. Pulmonary disease due to inhalation of derivatives of *Bacillus subtilis* containing proteolytic enzyme. *Lancet* 1969;1:1177.
25. Pepys J, Hargreave FE, Longbottom JL, Faux J. Allergic reactions of lungs to enzymes of *Bacillus subtilis. Lancet* 1969;1:1181.
26. Slavin RG, Lewis CR. Sensitivity to enzyme additives in laundry detergent workers. *J Allergy Clin Immunol* 1971;48(5):262–266.
27. Chan-Yeung M. Wood dust hypersensitivity. In: Oehling A, Glaza I, Mathan E, et al., eds. *Advances in allergy and applied immunology.* Oxford, UK: Pergamon Press, 1980;345–353.
28. Blainey AD, Graham VA, Phillips MJ, Davies RJ. Respiratory tract reactions to Western red cedar. *Hum Toxicol* 1981;1(1):41–51.
29. Fernández-Rivas M, Pérez-Carral C, Senent CJ. Occupational asthma and rhinitis caused by ash *(Fraxinus excelsior)* wood dust. *Allergy* 1997;52:196–199.
30. Platts-Mills TA, Longbottom J, Edwards J, Cockroft A, Wilkins S. Occupational asthma and rhinitis related to laboratory rats: serum IgG and IgE antibodies to the rat urinary allergen. J Allergy Clin Immunol 1987;79(3):505–515.
31. Lutsky II, Neuman I. Laboratory animal dander allergy: I. An occupational disease. *Ann Allergy* 1975;35:201–205.
32. Schwartz HJ, Arnold JL, Strobl KP. Occupational allergic rhinitis reaction to psyllium. *J Occup Med* 1989;31:624–626.
33. Malo JL, Cartier A, L'Archeveque J, et al. Prevalence of occupational

asthma and immunologic sensitization to guar gum among employees at a carpet-manufacturing plant. *J Allergy Clin Immunol* 1990;86(4 Pt 1):562–569.
34. Valdivieso R Subiza J, Subiza JL, Hinojosa M, de Carlos E, Subiza E. Bakers' asthma caused by alpha amylase. *Ann Allergy* 1994;73: 337–342.
35. Ramazzini B. *Diseases of workers* (translated by Wright, WC. DeMorbis artificum diatriba). New York: Hafner, 1964.
36. Zeiss CR, Patterson R, Pruzansky JJ, Miller MM, Rosenberg M, Levitz D. Trimellitic anhydride (TMA)-induced airway syndromes: clinical and immunologic studies. *J Allergy Clin Immunol* 1977;60:96–103.
37. Asai S, Shimoda T, Hara K, Fujiwara K. Occupational asthma caused by isonicotinic acid hydrazide (INH) inhalation. *J Allergy Clin Immunol* 1987;80(4):578–582.
38. Terho EO, Husman K, Vohlonen I, Rautalahti M, Tukiainen H. Allergy to storage mites or cow dander as a cause of rhinitis among Finnish dairy farmers. *Allergy* 1985;40(1):23–26.
39. Slavin RG. Occupational rhinitis. *Immunol Allergy Clin North Am* 1992;12:769.
40. Bush RK, Huftel MA, Busse WW. Patient selection. In: Lockey RF, Bukantz SC, eds. *Allergen immunotherapy textbook.* New York: Marcel Dekker, 1991;25–49.
41. Ohman JL. Clinical and immunologic responses to immunotherapy. In: Lockey RF, Bukantz SC, eds. *Allergen immunotherapy textbook.* New York: Marcel Dekker, 1991;209–232.
42. Friedman WH, Slavin RG. Diagnosis and medical and surgical treatment of sinusitis in adults. *Clin Rev Allergy* 1984;2(4):409–428.
43. Druce HM, Schumacher MJ. Nasal provocation challenge. The Committee on Upper Airway Allergy. *J Allergy Clin Immunol* 1990;86(2): 261–264.
44. Druce HM. Allergic and nonallergic rhinitis. In: Middleton E Jr, Reed CE, Ellis EF, Adkinson NF Jr, Yunginger JW, Busse W, eds. *Allergy principles and practice,* vol 2, 4th ed. St. Louis: Mosby Year Book, 1993;1433–1455.
45. Kaliner MA. Human respiratory secretions and host defense. *Am Rev Respir Dis* 1991;144:S52–56.
46. Druce HM, Kaliner MA. Allergic rhinitis. In: Cherniack RM, ed. *Current therapy of respiratory disease,* vol 3. Toronto, Ontario: BC Decker, 1989;16–18.

*Environmental and Occupational Medicine, Third Edition,* edited by William N. Rom.
Lippincott–Raven Publishers, Philadelphia © 1998.

# CHAPTER 46

# Occupational Skin Disease

David E. Cohen

## HISTORICAL PERSPECTIVES

As the largest organ in the body, the skin performs a variety of crucial homeostatic and protective functions. In constant contact with the external environment, the skin is particularly vulnerable to damage by physical and chemical assaults in the workplace. Rather than merely repelling these onslaughts, the skin may compensate by biotransforming potentially hazardous agents to less harmful ones. Yet barrier protection represents only a fraction of the duties performed by the entire integumentary system. In addition to its role as a primary defender against external insult, the skin directly participates in thermal, electrolyte, hormone, and immune regulation. Hence, the skin is far from a passive coat of armor; instead, it is an interactive organ in constant flux with its environment.

The skin's precarious location has rendered it the most commonly injured organ from chemical agents and physical conditions of the workplace. Pathologic responses of the skin can vary from excessive dryness and mild redness to more generalized exfoliative dermatitides that may be life threatening. In addition, neoplasms of the skin may result from primary skin exposures or through systemic absorption of carcinogens. Benign or malignant, such neoplastic events can have catastrophic consequences.

Historically, occupational skin disease has been morphologically documented and often has been accompanied by very descriptive nomenclature that easily identifies the purported causative agent. Examples of such nomenclature commonly used by the work force include asbestos wart, cement burn, chrome holes, fiber glass itch, hog itch, oil acne, rubber rash, and tar smarts. In view of the variety of skin lesions known to result from contactants within the workplace, the term *occupational dermatoses* is preferred because it includes any abnormality of the skin resulting directly from or aggravated by the work environment.

Occupational and environmental illnesses were recognized in historical writings as early as 100 A.D. (1) when Celsus described ulcers of the skin caused by corrosive metals. During later centuries, cutaneous ulcerations remained the major occupational skin disease of record, as such ulcerations were easily recognized, especially among those handling metal salts in mining, smelting, tool and weapon making, glass making, gold and silver coinage, casting, and similar metallics. Little was recorded about occupational skin disease until Ramazzini's (2) historic treatise on diseases of tradesmen in 1700. In this treatise he described skin disorders experienced by bath attendants, bakers, gilders, midwives, millers, and miners, among other tradespeople. Seventy-five years later, Sir Percival Pott (3) published the first account of occupational skin cancer when he described scrotal cancer among chimney sweeps. The industrial revolution and later the chemical age brought enormous numbers of materials, both natural and synthetic, into common industrial and household use, resulting in increased opportunities for domestic and industrial workers to be exposed to an expanding number of potential irritant and allergic chemical contactants.

## EPIDEMIOLOGY

The National Institute for Occupational Safety and Health (NIOSH) (4) has classified skin disease as one of

D. E. Cohen: Department of Dermatology and of Occupational and Environmental Dermatology, New York University Medical Center, New York, New York 10016.

the most pervasive problems facing workers in the United States. Since 1982, skin disease has been listed as one of the top ten work-related diseases based on potential for prevention, incidence and severity. In the 1978 edition of Patty's *Industrial Hygiene and Toxicology*, dermatologic diseases were shown to account for about 40% of all occupational diseases reported to the U.S. Department of Labor. In the 1984 Bureau of Labor Statistics report, dermatologic disease had decreased to 34% of all reported occupational disease. The Bureau of Labor Statistics found a declining trend for occupational skin disease rates from a high in 1972 (16.2 events per 10,000 full-time workers) to a low in 1986 (6.9 events per 10,000 workers). Recently, however, there has been an upward trend in incidence with a rate of 7.9 per 10,000 workers in 1990 or about 61,000 new cases per year. Skin disease resulting from exposures in the agriculture and manufacturing industries were responsible for the greatest number of cases, with incidence rates of 86 and 41 per 10,000 workers, respectively. Although the health care field has a relatively low rate of disease, the large number of workers in this industry results in almost 3,900 cases per year.

Because skin disease is often not life threatening, many believe that the rate at which it is reported to government agencies is underrepresented by 10- to 50-fold. Due to this discrepancy, it is often assumed that the cost of occupational skin disease to society is trivial. It has been estimated that up to 20% to 25% of persons with occupational skin disease lose an average of 11 days of work annually. This translates to an economic loss of $222 million to $1 billion annually.

Occupational skin injuries such as thermal and chemical burns, lacerations, and blunt skin trauma are extremely common. NIOSH estimates that there are approximately 1.07 to 1.65 million skin injuries per year accounting for a rate of 1.4 to 2.2 cases per 100 workers. These potentially disabling injuries are probably the most preventable illnesses and should not be overlooked. The economic costs of injuries to the skin have not been calculated to date.

## STRUCTURE AND FUNCTION OF THE SKIN

Any acute or chronic exposure to chemical or physical agents found in the workplace can result in a skin disease. In the overwhelming majority of cases, the skin is able to adequately compensate for such assaults and thus injury is prevented. These compensatory mechanisms stem from the multifunctional capabilities of the entire integument. As discussed later, the skin is not merely a monomorphous group of cells, but rather it is a dynamic system that closely interacts with almost every other organ system in the body.

Injury to the skin may result from direct toxicity to the cells or through interference of normal homeostatic functions that the skin performs. Only brief interruptions of the skin's thermoregulatory and electrolyte homeostatic mechanisms are compatible with life. Therefore, widespread destruction of the skin may result in immediate breakdown of these mechanisms and death. Such insults include chemical and thermal burns, overexposure to heat and humidity, and prolonged occlusion.

Structurally, the skin has two major anatomical subdivisions: the epidermis and dermis. The more superficial epidermis is composed primarily of keratinocytes that are arranged in a stratified squamous epithelium. Basal cells, the squamous progenitor cells, lie at the base of the epidermis, directly abutting the basement membrane. Together, the basement membrane and basal cells create an interactive, sinuous interface at the dermal/epidermal junction. Keratinocytes constitute the major epidermal cell and begin an upward migration process from the basement membrane with concomitant maturation known as terminal differentiation.

The process begins as a basal cell divides, and a progeny cell separates from the basement membrane, moving into the stratum spinosum and then the stratum granulosum. At the granular layer, keratinocytes are transformed into flattened cells that increase substantially in volume. Lipid granules fuse with the keratinocyte plasma membrane, transforming the intercellular environment from an aqueous to hydrophobic space. In addition, the plasma membranes of these cells become permeable, changing the intracellular environment, which results in extensive disulfide bonding among the keratin proteins. The altered membrane is characterized by the loss of phospholipids and addition of sphingolipids. Cell organelles are degraded and a protein envelope is synthesized immediately beneath the plasma membrane.

This program of terminal differentiation takes approximately 14 days and produces the outermost layer of the skin, the stratum corneum. The mature, nonviable keratinocytes of the stratum corneum contain 80% keratin by weight. These tightly linked fibrous proteins largely replace the cell structure (Fig. 1). An additional 14 days is required for the original corneocyte to traverse the stratum corneum and reach the surface of the skin where it will be sloughed.

The stratum corneum provides a critical barrier that prevents both water and electrolytes from freely entering and exiting the epidermis and provides modest protection against acidic substances. In contrast, it is quite vulnerable to organic and inorganic alkaline materials that denature keratin proteins, and alter keratinocyte cohesion and the capacity to retain water. Physical or chemical stress such as lowered temperature and humidity or repetitive action of soaps, detergents, and organic solvents generally leads to an impairment of the barrier efficiency because of water loss and dryness. Stresses such as friction, pressure, ultraviolet light, and natural light can stimulate a compensatory protective thickening of the stratum corneum in the form of a callous.

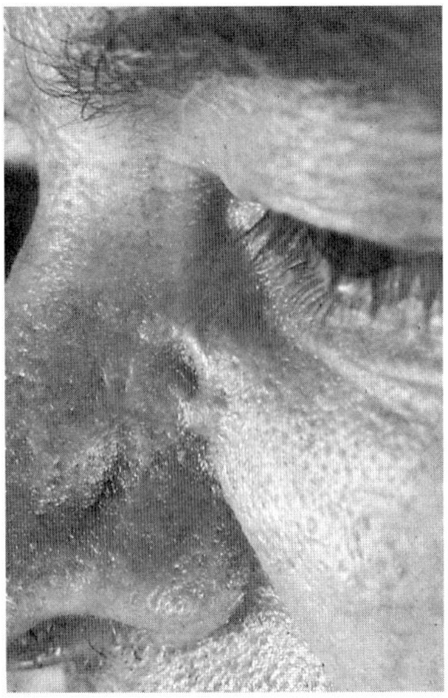

**FIG. 1.** Basal cell carcinoma. Note pearly smooth borders surrounding a crusted erosion.

In addition to keratinocytes, other specialized cells may be found in the epidermis as well. Melanocytes, neuroendocrine-derived cells, are located in the basal layer. They produce melanin and package the pigment into granules (melanosomes) that impart the natural pigmentation to the skin. Variations in the depth of skin pigmentation occur mostly from differences in the melanosome structure rather than from gross quantities of melanin itself. The pigment granules are picked up by the epidermal cells and are eventually shed via keratin exfoliation (5). Melanin serves to protect the skin from ultraviolet light by acting as a broad-spectrum chromophore or light absorber. Certain agents such as coal, tar, pitch, selected aromatic chlorinated hydrocarbons, petroleum products, and trauma can cause excess melanin production, leading to hyperpigmentation. In contrast, members of the quinone family and selected phenolics can inhibit pigment formation following percutaneous absorption by direct action upon the melanin enzymatic system (Fig. 2) (6,7).

Langerhans cells also populate the epidermis; they migrate through the epidermis and function primarily as immune surveillance cells. Thus, they process the chemicals that contact the skin and present them to regional T lymphocytes. These cells allow for primary sensitization and the elicitation of contact dermatitis.

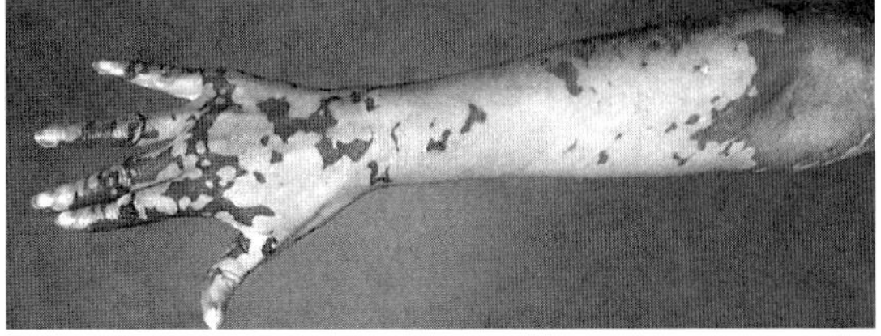

**FIG. 2.** Depigmentation from an alkyl phenol in a worker exposed to antioxidants.

The dermis serves to support the overlying epidermis as well as to house appendageal structures and neurovascular supplies. Fibroblasts, which reside throughout the thickness of the dermis, produce the matrix of this supportive structure consisting primarily of type I collagen and, to a far lesser extent, elastin. Beneath the dermis is the subcutis, or fatty layer, that cushions the skin from physical trauma. In some anatomic sites, appendageal structures may extend into the deeper subcutis. Therefore, from a toxicologic point of view, the subcutaneous fat may serve as a reservoir for percutaneously or systemically absorbed hydrophobic substances.

Traversing the epidermis, ducts of the skin appendages ascend from the deeper dermis. These include eccrine sweat, sebaceous, and apocrine glands. The distribution of these structures are not uniform throughout the entire integument. Rather, there are areas of increased concentration for each type of structure. For example, eccrine glands (sweat glands) predominate on palms, soles, and axillae, while oil-producing sebaceous glands predominate on the face and scalp. Apocrine glands, which perform an incompletely understood function, are present in the axillae and on the areolae.

Thermoregulation is controlled by the central nervous system to maintain a physiologically constant core body temperature despite climatic variations. This is accomplished through modulation in the excretion of eccrine sweat as well as changes in the superficial blood flow. Eccrine sweat, composed primarily of water and electrolytes, participates in temperature control through heat loss via evaporation from the surface. In addition, radiant heat loss is facilitated by the dilatation of the cutaneous blood vessels. The opposite occurs when a decreased core and/or surface temperature causes blood vessels of the skin to constrict and shunt warm blood away from exposed surfaces, thus preserving heat.

Special receptors within the skin are part of a network of nerve fibers that receive and conduct various stimuli. The brain perceives such stimuli as heat, cold, pain, and touch.

## PERCUTANEOUS ABSORPTION

Until the turn of the century, scientists believed the skin to be an impervious barrier to exogenous substances. It was gradually recognized that substances do have the ability to penetrate the skin, albeit slowly. Research in the past 50 years has identified the stratum corneum as the primary barrier (8). Conditions in which this barrier is compromised result in increased uptake of otherwise poorly permeable substances.

Due to its hydrophobic nature, the stratum corneum protects the underlying tissues from water loss by dehydration. Its hydrophobic character is derived from the high lipid content of the intercellular space, composing approximately 15% of the total volume. Sphingolipids, with a high content of long-chain ceramides, compose the majority of these lipids. Removal of these sphingolipids seriously compromises barrier function as measured by transepidermal water loss (9). The hydration of the stratum corneum is due to the water-binding capabilities of the corneocyte proteins. The stratum corneum is typically 20% water, but it can absorb increased amounts upon prolonged immersion, thereby reducing the effectiveness of the barrier to hydrophilic agents.

To understand the consequences of exposure to various environmental agents, it is critical to estimate the rate at which these agents penetrate the skin's barrier. In fact, regulations that permitted bathing in water considered unfit for drinking were revised when it was realized that exposure from dermal/inhalation uptake during bathing could be comparable to that from drinking 2 L of the same water. Uptake through the skin is now incorporated in pharmacokinetic modeling to estimate potential risks from exposures (10). The degree of uptake depends on the details of exposure conditions; it is proportional to solute concentration, time, and amount of skin surface exposed. In addition, two intrinsic factors contribute to the absorption rate of a given compound: its hydrophobicity, which affects its ability to partition into epidermal lipid, and its rate of diffusion through this barrier. A measure of the first property is the commonly used octanol/water partitioning ratio (Kow). An alternative has been to measure the uptake from aqueous solution into powdered human stratum corneum (11). This is particularly relevant for exposure to contaminated water, such as during bathing or swimming. However, partitioning of an agent into the skin is greatly affected by its solubility in or adhesion to the medium in which it is applied. The second property is an inverse function of molecular weight or, more accurately, molecular volume. That is, hydrophobic agents of low molecular weight permeate the skin better than those of high molecular weight or those that are hydrophilic.

Although it is important to estimate the degree of penetration, one must also consider the potency of the agent in question. For example, the hydrophobic organophosphate pesticide parathion (very high potency) can be lethal by skin contact. Considerable empirical information has been collected on compounds of special interest (including pharmaceuticals, pesticides, and pollutants) for use in quantifying these relationships. From such information, relations can be obtained for skin penetration (Pcw) using empirically derived constants (C1, C2, C3) that have the following form (12):

$$\log Pcw = C1 - C2(MW) + C3\log Kow \qquad [1]$$

Such relations describe steady-state conditions, where an agent leaves the stratum corneum at the same rate it enters. Since rates of diffusion are slow, saturation of the stratum corneum provides a depot, which allows for continued penetration into the body for relatively long time periods after the external exposure stops.

Diffusion rates through the epidermis vary considerably depending on the anatomic sites. For example, the following sites are listed in order of decreasing permeability: foot sole > scrotum > palm > forehead > abdomen (8). Surprisingly, the greater thickness of plantar and palmar stratum corneum is more than counterbalanced by alterations in their lipid content. Under ordinary conditions, absorption through the epidermal appendages is generally neglected because their combined surface area is such a small fraction of the total available for uptake. Diffusion rates can be slow on the time scale of exposure variations, however, nonequilibrium conditions often apply, and absorption through the appendages can be appreciable and should be considered (13). In some cases, effects of appendages can even be dominant. For instance, benzo[*a*]pyrene penetrates the skin of haired mice severalfold faster than that of hairless strains (14).

A number of chemicals with or without direct toxic effect on the skin can cause systemic intoxication following percutaneous entry. Once the chemical reaches the upper dermis, it has direct assess to a vascular plexus and the systemic circulation. Examples of chemicals capable

**TABLE 1.** *Percutaneous absorption and target organ systems*

| Chemical | Systemic effects from percutaneous absorption |
|---|---|
| Aniline | Methemoglobinemia, bladder cancer |
| Acrylamide/acrylonitrile | Peripheral neuropathy |
| Benzidine | Bladder cancer |
| Carbon disulfide | Peripheral and central neuropathy, coronary artery disease |
| Carbon tetrachloride | Liver, kidney, CNS disease |
| Chlorinated naphthalenes, biphenyls, and dioxins | Chloracne |
| Ethylene glycol ethers | Aplastic anemia |
| Hydrofluoric acid | Hypocalcemia, hyperkalemia, hypomagnesemia |
| Methyl butyl ketone | Neuropathy |
| Organophosphate pesticides | Inhibition of cholinesterase/acute cardiovascular, respiratory, gastrointestinal, neuromuscular disease |
| Tetrachlorethane | CNS, liver and kidney disease |

of significant percutaneous absorption with demonstrable target organ effects are listed in Table 1.

## METABOLISM

The viable keratinocytes of the lower epidermis have a wide repertoire of biotransformation reactions that render toxic xenobiotics innocuous before reaching the superficial vascular plexus that will carry them inward. The skin possesses most of the phase 1 and phase 2 metabolic enzymes necessary for xenobiotic metabolism and has 2% of the metabolic capacity of the liver. Specific enzyme pathways may also be inducible and result in dramatic increases in enzyme activity. This is particularly important when carcinogenic intermediates are formed in the process of detoxifying certain polycyclic hydrocarbons (15). Animal studies have demonstrated that when skin is exposed to polychlorinated biphenyls or benzo[*a*]pyrene, the activity of the phase 1 enzyme aryl hydrocarbon hydroxylase can be increased to 20% of the total body activity of the enzyme. Integumentary cytochrome P-450 isoenzymes are inducible following exposures to a variety of halogenated hydrocarbons like tetrachlorodibenzo-p-dioxin (TCDD) and polychlorinated biphenyls (PCBs). Hence, under conditions of repeated or significant dermal exposure, the skin detoxifies a marked amount of the chemical. Exposure to procarcinogens on the skin, however, may result in biotransformation to active carcinogens locally, without the aid of hepatic enzymes.

## PATHOLOGIC RESPONSES OF THE SKIN

The skin may produce a variety of different reactions in response to various disease states. An understanding of these responses may lead the clinician to quickly diagnose or suspect a specific illness. Common pathophysiologic responses of the skin are discussed here (see Glossary), but the reader is advised to refer to dermatology texts for more specific or esoteric findings.

## FACTORS INFLUENCING OCCUPATIONAL AND ENVIRONMENTAL SKIN DISEASE

It is critical to analyze the information gathered from the patient via history and physical examination in the context of a potentially relevant occupational and environmental exposure pattern. Work-relatedness may be screened for by using a seven-step approach developed by Mathias (16), who suggests that at least four positive responses are necessary to conclude an occupational relatedness:

1. Is the clinical picture consistent with an occupational dermatosis?
2. Is there exposure at the workplace to an agent capable of causing the dermatosis?
3. Is the location of the dermatosis consistent with the alleged work exposure?
4. Is the onset and time course of the dermatosis consistent with the work exposure?
5. Are nonoccupational exposures reasonably excluded as causes of the dermatosis?
6. Is the activity of the dermatosis consistent with periods of exposure in the working environment?
7. Does testing (patch tests, use tests, potassium hydroxide, biopsy) reveal a likely causative agent?

In determining the cause of an occupationally acquired disease, it is important to recognize other factors that may predispose or aggravate an already-existing dermatosis. Both host and environmental factors should be analyzed (1).

Host factors such as genetic predisposition, preexisting dermatologic disease, and age may be contributing factors in the presentation of an occupationally acquired disease. First, sensitivity to chemical irritants and the development of allergic contact sensitivity are both likely to be genetically determined. Skin type is another genetically determined characteristic that may play a role in the development of occupational skin disease for workers exposed to ultraviolet light. Skin type, which is loosely correlated to the degree of skin pigmentation, refers to the sun reactivity of the skin. The susceptibility of some skin cancers may be linked to those having lower skin types. Sunburn- or ultraviolet-induced skin damage reduces the barrier function of the skin as well as increases sensitivity to irritant chemicals. The use of sunscreen should be encouraged for all workers exposed to ultraviolet light on a regular basis for the prevention of skin cancer. Table 2 illustrates their characteristics (5). Finally, age and work experience may play a role. Young workers, particularly those in the adolescent group, often present with acute contact dermatitis. This may be due to the nature of the work (e.g., fast food, janitorial, car washing) where the exposure is either difficult to prevent or due to lack of experience. Older workers usually are more careful about exposure, but aging skin is often dry and more susceptible to skin injury.

Like host factors, environmental factors, such as temperature, humidity, and season, contribute to the development of an occupationally acquired disease. Seasonal variations can affect the normal physiologic defense mechanisms of the body. Increased temperature coupled with high humidity can overload the normal thermoreg-

**TABLE 2.** *Skin type characteristics*

| Type | Characteristics |
|---|---|
| 1 | Always burns, never tans |
| 2 | Usually burns, tans less than average (with difficulty) |
| 3 | Sometimes burns mildly, tans about average |
| 4 | Rarely burns, tans more than average (easily) |
| 5 | Rarely burns, tans profusely, brown skin |
| 6 | Never burns, tans profusely, black skin |

ulatory mechanisms, resulting in temperature-related diseases such as heat exhaustion and heat stroke. Hot weather may also discourage the use of protective clothing gear, thus exposing more unprotected skin to environmental contactants.

Beneficially, sweat can act to lavage the skin, removing irritant contactants (1,17,18). However, excessive delivery of sweat can cause maceration of the skin at sites where skin surfaces are opposed to each other (e.g., groin, armpits). This can foster the trapping of dusts and suspended particles, allowing percutaneous absorption in this hydrated and occluded environment. Sweat can also partially solubilize nickel, cobalt, and chromium in small amounts, a situation troublesome to those individuals with cutaneous allergy to these metals. Dry chemical agents can be put into aqueous solution, which can be irritating, destructive, or harmful if absorbed. Miliaria, occlusive eccrine sweat gland disease, may produce annoying symptoms such as itching and stinging. Widespread involvement can interfere with temperature regulation secondary to altered sweat pattern (mild forms are known as prickly heat).

Cold weather is associated with dry skin because of decreased temperatures and humidity. Further, the weather may prevent washing directly after work, as exiting the workplace into the cold environment may discourage immediate showering. This creates a situation in which there is prolonged skin contact with potentially dangerous chemicals. Workers with inherently dry skin (xerosis and ichthyosis) usually have a worsening of their condition under the low-humidity conditions of the winter. There is a decreased irritancy threshold when exposed to alkaline agents, acids, detergents, and most solvents.

## OCCUPATIONAL AND ENVIRONMENTAL SKIN DISEASES

Occupational skin disease results primarily from four basic adverse stressors: mechanical (friction and pressure), chemical (organic and inorganic of various pHs), physical (heat, cold, radiation), and biologic (encompassing a legion of infectious agents like bacteria, fungi, viruses, and parasites). Despite the vast array of potentially deleterious exposures to the skin and the corresponding heterogeneity of possible skin lesions that may be produced, occupational skin diseases may be classified in one of three basic disease categories: inflammatory, neoplastic, and infectious. The overwhelming majority of occupational skin disease is due to an inflammatory process.

### Contact Dermatitis

Contact dermatitis is the single most prevalent occupational skin disease, accounting for over 90% of reported causes (19). Irritant and allergic contact dermatitis, two distinct inflammatory processes, result from adverse exposures of the skin. These syndromes have indistinguishable clinical and histologic characteristics. Classically, the clinical picture presents with erythema (redness), induration (thickening and firmness), scaling (flaking), and vesiculation (blistering) on areas directly contacting the chemical agent. Histologically, paraffin-embedded biopsies from affected sites reveal a mixed-cell inflammatory infiltrate of lymphocytes and eosinophils and the hallmark finding of spongiosis (intercellular edema). Unfortunately, these histopathologic features are not sufficient to differentiate between allergic contact dermatitis, irritant contact dermatitis, atopic dermatitis, or certain other common eczematous syndromes. Since their etiology is different, as supported by subtle but clear differences in the inflammatory responses, the two syndromes are presented separately.

### Irritant Contact Dermatitis

As contact dermatitis overwhelmingly represents the majority of occupational skin disease, and approximately 80% of contact dermatitis cases are of the irritant variety, irritant contact dermatitis is singularly the most common occupational disease involving the skin (19). Primary irritant chemicals cause a dermatitis by direct action on normal skin. Irritant dermatitis is not directly mediated by the immune system. Extrinsic variables such as concentration, pH, temperature, duration, repetitiveness of contact, and occlusion impact significantly on the appearance of the eruption. Strongly noxious substances, such as those with extreme pH, can produce an immediate irreversible and potentially scarring dermatitis following a single exposure. This acute irritant phenomenon is akin to a chemical burn and has been described as an "etching" reaction (20).

However, it is more commonly noted that single exposures to potentially irritating chemicals do not produce significant reactions; repeated exposures are necessary to elicit clinically noticeable changes. Such repeated exposures eventually result in either an eczematous dermatitis with clinical and histopathologic changes characteristic of contact dermatitis or a fissured, thickened eruption without a substantial inflammatory component. Chemicals inducing the latter two reactions are termed marginal irritants. Marginal irritation is often associated with contact with soluble metalworking fluids, soap and water, and solvents such as acetone, ketones, and alcohols. Wet work in general is associated with repetitive contact with marginal irritants.

Since the thresholds for irritant reactions vary greatly from person to person, a genetic component to the response has been considered. Monozygotic twins have shown greater concordance than dizygotic twins in their reactions to irritant chemicals like sodium lauryl sulfate and benzalkonium chloride (21). Young individuals with fair complexion appear to be more sensitive to irritant chemicals, and sex does not appear to be a significant factor (20). Attempts to predict the relative irritancy of substances based on their chemical relatedness to other irritants have been unsuccessful.

### *Pathophysiology*

The clinical manifestations of contact irritant dermatitis are readily recognized but not well understood. The behavior of many chemicals used in the laboratory or in industry is fairly well known. For example, organic and inorganic alkalies damage keratin; organic solvents dissolve surface lipids and remove lipid components from the cornified layer; heavy metal salts, notably arsenic and chromium, denature epidermal proteins; salicylic acid, oxalic acid, and urea chemically and physically reduce keratin; and arsenic, tar, methylcholanthrene, and other known carcinogens stimulate abnormal growth patterns. Regardless of the specific agent eliciting an irritant contact dermatitis, multiple chemotactic cytokines are released from both the ailing keratinocytes and neighboring vascular endothelial cells. The cytokines cause an inflammatory cell infiltrate of the epidermis and upper dermis with concomitant edema, resulting in the hallmark dermatitis (1,15,17,18).

Irritant chemicals are commonly used in agriculture, manufacturing, and service pursuits. Hundreds of these agents—classified as acids, alkalies, gases, organic materials, metal salts, solvents, resins, and soaps including synthetic detergents—can cause absolute or marginal irritation (Table 3).

## Chemical Burns

Extremely corrosive and reactive chemicals may produce immediate coagulative necrosis that results in chemical burns characterized by ulceration and sloughing. This substantial tissue damage is distinct from that found in irritant dermatitis, as the lesion is the direct result of the chemical insult and does not rely on secondary inflammation to manifest the cutaneous signs of injury. In addition to the direct tissue damage itself, the necrotic tissue can serve as a chemical reservoir to perpetuate either continued cutaneous damage or percutaneous absorption and systemic injury after exposure. Table 4 lists selected corrosive chemicals that are important clinically.

**TABLE 3.** *Typical primary irritants and chemical classes*

| |
|---|
| Acids |
| Inorganic |
| Organic |
| Alkalies |
| Inorganic |
| Organic |
| Cement |
| Solvents |
| Alcohols |
| Ketones |
| Chlorinated |
| Soaps/detergents/surfactants |
| Petroleum |
| Coal tar |
| Metal salts |
| Antimony trioxide |
| Arsenic trioxide |
| Chromium and alkaline chromates |
| Cobalt sulfate |
| Nickel sulfate |
| Mercuric chloride |
| Zinc chloride |

## Allergic Contact Dermatitis

Allergic contact dermatitis represents a delayed (type IV) hypersensitivity reaction (22). Since this is a true allergy, only minute quantities of material are necessary to elicit overt reactions. This is distinct from irritant contact dermatitis in which the intensity of the reaction is proportional to the dose applied. An estimated 20% of all contact dermatitis reactions is allergic in nature. Currently, over 3,000 chemical agents have been implicated as causal agents in allergic contact dermatitis, and over 65,000 chemicals may produce irritant dermatitis.

### *Pathophysiology*

The elicitation of an allergic contact dermatitis reaction relies on exposure to an allergen to which the individual has already been sensitized. Evidence dating back to the 1940s indicates that the ability to be sensitized to specific agents has a genetic component (23). Recent work has suggested that this genetic component may reside in specific human leukocyte antigen (HLA) alleles that are associated with allergy to nickel, chromium, and cobalt (24). Thus, to mount an immune reaction to an allergen, one must be genetically equipped to become sensitized, have a sufficient contact with a sensitizing chemical, and then have repeated contact later.

In general, low molecular weight chemicals (haptens), most less than 1,000 daltons, are responsible for causing allergic contact dermatitis. Haptens, which may not be

**TABLE 4.** Chemicals capable of severe skin burns

| |
|---|
| Ammonia |
| Calcium oxide |
| Chlorine |
| Ethylene oxide |
| Hydrochloric acid |
| Hydrofluoric acid |
| Hydrogen peroxide |
| Methyl bromide |
| Nitrogen oxide |
| Phosphorus |
| Phenol |
| Sodium hydroxide |
| Potassium hydroxide |
| Toluene diisocyanate |

intrinsically allergenic, must penetrate the stratum corneum and link to epidermal carrier proteins to form a complete allergen (25). The sensitization begins when a Langerhans cell ingests the allergen. These cells display surface HLA class II, which allows the cell to directly present the digested allergen to a helper T lymphocyte. This process activates the lymphocyte and stimulates clonal proliferation in a regional lymph node under the stimulation of cytokines (e.g., interleukin-1 and -2). When these activated cells return to the area of skin that had the original contact with the allergen, they cause a typical dermatitis to form. This initial sensitization may take several days to complete and last a lifetime. Once sensitized, subsequent challenges from the same allergen cause a rapid elaboration of lymphocytes in the dermis and result in a dermatitis within 48 to 96 hours (26).

Clinically, the dermatitis caused by allergic and irritant mechanisms may be indistinguishable. Two critical mechanistic differences exist. First, allergic reactions usually require a longer induction period than occurs with primary irritant effects. Second, cutaneous sensitizers generally do not affect large numbers of workers, except when dealing with select materials that can result in more widespread sensitization. These sensitizers include epoxy resin systems, phenol-formaldehyde plastics, and rhus oleoresins (i.e., poison ivy, oak, and sumac) (18). Table 5 lists common allergens and their likely sources of exposure in the workplace (15).

Many plants and woods cause injury to the skin through direct irritation or allergic sensitization. Although the chemical identity of many plant toxins remains undetermined, it is well known that the irritant or allergic principal can be present in the leaves, stems, roots, flowers, and bark (27). Poison ivy and poison oak are major offenders. They are members of a plant family that includes a number of chemically related allergens (e.g., cashew nut shell oil, Indian marking nut oil, mango)—all with a common chemical allergen pentadecacatechol. Therefore, reactivity to one family member generally confers cross-reactivity to the others. Other plants known to cause dermatitis are carrots, castor beans, celery, chrysanthemum, hyacinth, tulip bulbs, oleander, primrose, ragweed, wild parsnip, and others, including vegetables. High-risk jobs for developing a plant-related occupational skin disease include agricultural workers, construction workers, electric and telephone linemen, florists, gardeners, lumberjacks, pipeline installers, road builders, and others who work outdoors. Photosensitivity may also be a factor in the development of the dermatitis.

As awareness of potential sensitizers grows, hygiene practices and substitution of less allergenic chemicals has resulted in a reduction in the reactivity rates among those with contact dermatitis. Conversely, increased exposure to rubber products in personal protective equipment in the health care field has caused increased reactivity patterns

**TABLE 5.** *Common skin allergens*

- Topical medications
  - Antibiotics
    - Aminoglycosides
    - Bacitracin
    - Neomycin
    - Polymyxin
    - Sulfonamides
  - Therapeutics
    - Benzocaine
    - Corticosteroids
- Preservatives
  - Formaldehyde
  - Methylchloroisothiazolinone
  - Formaldehyde releasers
    - Quarternium 15
    - Imidazolidinyl urea
    - Diazolidinyl urea
    - DMDM hydantoin
- Plants and trees
  - Abietic acid
  - Pentadecylcatechols
  - Balsam of Peru
  - Sesquiterpene lactone
  - Rosin (colophony)
  - Tuliposide A
- Antiseptics
  - Chlorhexidine
  - Chloroxylenol
  - Glutaraldehyde
  - Hexachlorophene
  - Mercurials
  - Thimerosal (merthiolate)
- Rubber products
  - Benzothiazoles
  - Carbamates
  - Diphenylguanidine
  - Hydroquinone
  - Mercaptobenzothiazole
  - p-Phenylenediamine
  - Resorcinol monobenzoate
- Sulfenamides
  - Thioureas
  - Thiurams
- Leather
  - Formaldehyde
  - Potassium dichromate
  - Glutaraldehyde
- Paper products
  - Abietic acid
  - Dyes
  - Formaldehyde
  - Rosin (colophony)
- Glues and bonding agents
  - Acrylic monomers
  - Bisphenol A
  - Cyanocrylates
  - Epichlorohydrin
  - Epoxy
  - Formaldehyde
  - Methacrylates
  - p-(t-butyl)formaldehyde resin
  - Toluene sulfonamide resins
  - Urea formaldehyde resins
- Cement
  - Chromium
- Metals
  - Beryllium
  - Chromium
  - Cobalt
  - Gold
  - Mercury
  - Nickel
  - Palladium
- Others
  - Benzalkonium chloride
  - Cinnamic aldehyde
  - Ethylenediamine
  - Lanolin
  - p-Phenylenediamine
  - Propylene glycol
  - Benzophenones
  - Fragrances
  - Thioglycolates

**TABLE 6.** *Percentage of positive reactors by time period—North American Contact Dermatitis Group (28)*

| Allergen | 1992–1994 | 1985–1989 | 1984–1985 | 1972 |
|---|---|---|---|---|
| Benzocaine | 2.2 | 2.1 | 3.5 | 4.5 |
| Mercaptobenzothiazole | 1.8 | 2.5 | 2.9 | 4.8 |
| Colophony | 1.9 | 2.2 | 1.9 | n/a |
| p-phenylenediamine | 6.3 | 6.4 | 6.9 | 8.1 |
| Imidazolidinyl urea | 1.9 | 1.7 | 1.5 | n/a |
| Cinnamic aldehyde | 2.7 | 3.1 | 5.9 | n/a |
| Wool wax alcohol | 2.9 | 1.5 | 1.2 | 3.1 |
| Carba mix | 4.8 | 3.1 | 3.3 | n/a |
| Neomycin | 9 | 7.2 | 6.6 | 5.9 |
| Thiuram mix | 7.7 | 5.5 | 3.9 | 4.2 |
| Formaldehyde | 7.8 | 6.8 | 6.1 | 3.6 |
| Ethylenediamine dihydrochloride | 2.5 | 3.8 | 5.9 | 7.1 |
| Epoxy resin | 1.8 | 2.1 | 1.9 | n/a |
| Quaternium-15 | 9.6 | 6.2 | 6.7 | n/a |
| p-Tert-butylphenol formaldehyde resin | 1.7 | 1.6 | 0.9 | n/a |
| Mercapto mix | 2.6 | 2.5 | 2.6 | n/a |
| Black rubber mix | 2.1 | 2.1 | 1.4 | n/a |
| Potassium dichromate | 2.0 | 2.4 | 5.2 | 7.6 |
| Balsam of Peru | 7.5 | 5.1 | 3.3 | n/a |
| Nickel sulfate | 14.3 | 10.5 | 9.7 | 11 |

among exposed workers. Table 6 illustrates the trends and reactivity rates of common human sensitizers (28).

## PHYSICAL FINDINGS OF OCCUPATIONAL SKIN DISEASE

The hazardous potential of the work environment is unlimited. Chemical and physical agents may produce a wide variety of clinical presentations that differ in appearance and in histopathologic pattern. The nature of the lesions and the sites of involvement may provide a clue as to the causal materials involved, but only in rare instances does clinical appearance directly identify the culprit (Figs. 3 and 4). With the exception of a few unique findings, the majority of occupational dermatoses can be categorized as acute or chronic eczematous contact dermatitis. Symptoms include itching, burning, and general discomfort; signs include warmth, erythema, swelling, vesiculation, scaling, and oozing. When the forehead, eyelids, ears, face, and neck are involved, one should

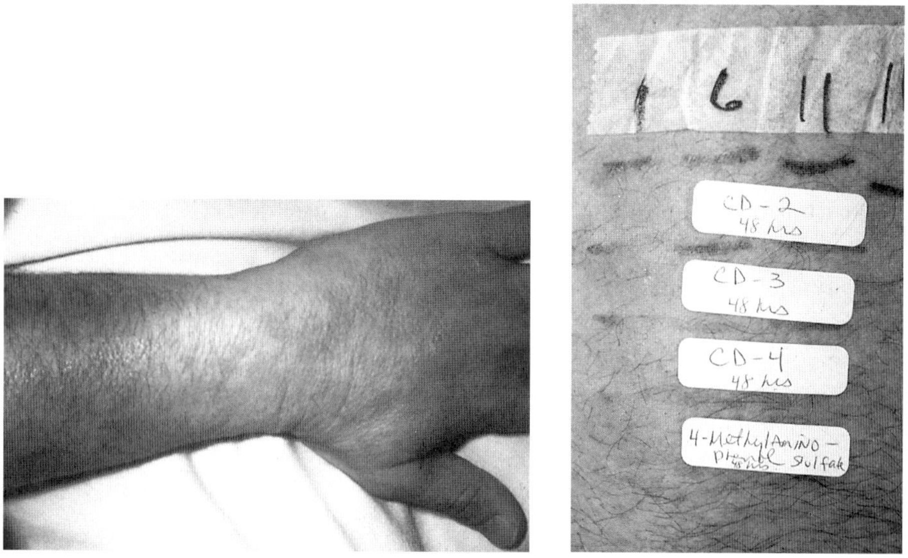


A B

**FIG. 3. A:** Allergic contact dermatitis to color developer. Patient was exposed to film developer chemicals when the machine broke down. He submerged his arm to remove film jammed within a developer tank. **B:** Positive patch tests to color developer and methylamino phenol sulfate, a black and white film developer.

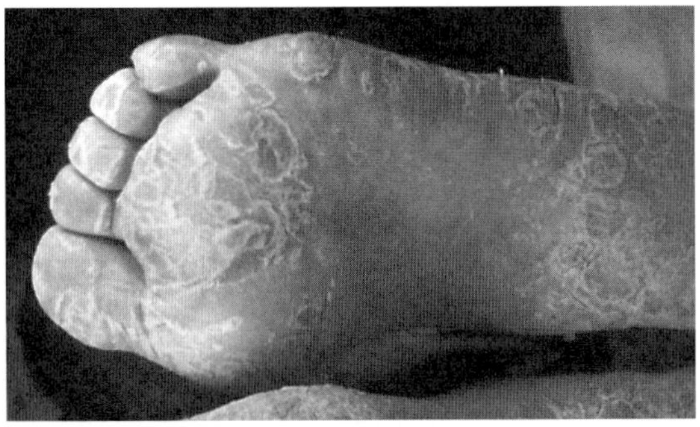

**FIG. 4.** Allergic contact dermatitis to the rubber accelerator d-mercaptobenzothiazole found in this patient's work boots.

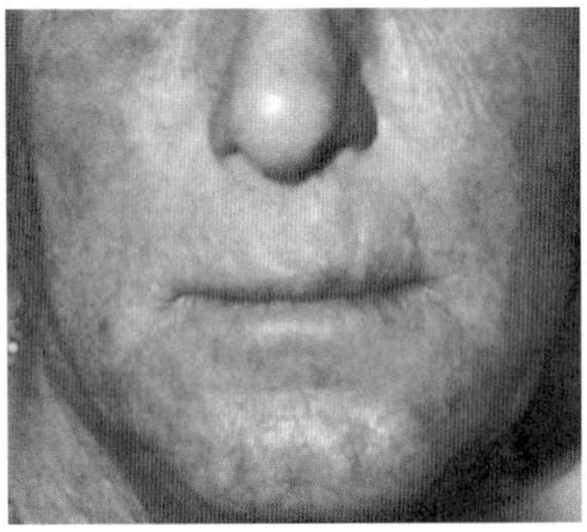

**FIG. 5.** Allergic contact dermatitis to aerosolized epoxy resin in an automotive plant worker. *See color plate between pages 632 and 633.*

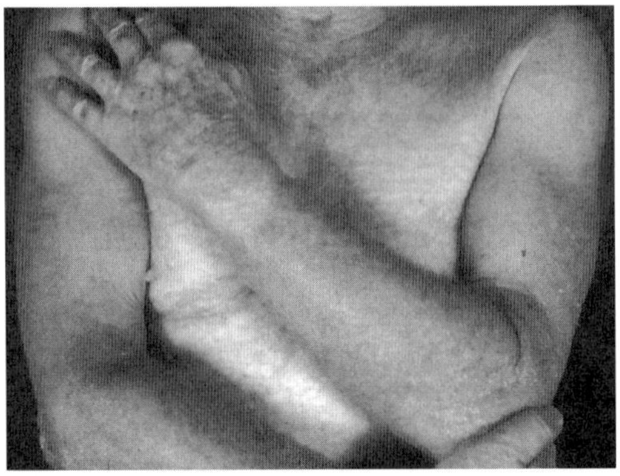

**FIG. 6.** Photoallergic contact dermatitis from a sunscreen. Note the sparing under the watchband and sleeves on the shoulders and chest that were photoprotected by his shirt. *See color plate between pages 632 and 633.*

**TABLE 7.** *Classes of chemicals causing allergic contact dermatitis*

| | |
|---|---|
| Acids, dilute | Metal salts |
| Alkalies, dilute | Plants and woods |
| Anhydrides | Resin systems |
| Detergents | Rubber accelerators |
| Germicides | Rubber antioxidants |
| Herbicides | Soluble emulsions |
| Insecticides | Solvents |
| Liquid fuels | |

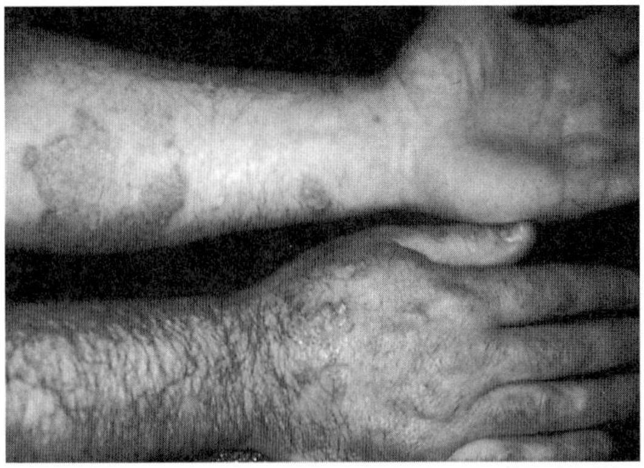

**FIG. 7.** Acute contact dermatitis to chromium in a cement worker.

investigate potential airborne agents (Fig. 5). More subtle clues such as the sparing of the upper lip, posterior ear, and mid-neck suggest a photosensitivity disease, as these areas are usually shielded from exposure to ultraviolet light (Fig. 6). Generalized contact dermatitis may occur from massive exposure, such as the wearing of contaminated clothing, autosensitization from a preexisting dermatitis, or from systemic exposure.

Acute contact dermatitis can be caused by many classes of irritant and sensitizing chemicals, plants, and photoreactive agents. Examples are listed in Table 7.

Chronic eczematous lesions, typically involving the hands, fingers, wrists, and forearms, present with dry, thickened, and scaly skin, with cracking and fissuring of the affected areas (Fig. 7). Concurrent with this skin thickening is lichenification, the process by which normal skin lines and topical features are accentuated. Periodically, acute weeping lesions may appear because of reexposure, imprudent treatment, or secondary infection. Chronic contact dermatitis occurs when exposure is perpetuated to irritant chemicals. Less often, low-level exposure to allergens can produce similar findings. In the latter case, signs and symptoms of acute contact dermatitis persist for long periods before chronic changes occur. A large number of materials (Table 8) have the potential to sustain the symptoms that accompany chronic recurrent skin problems.

**TABLE 8.** *Materials capable of perpetuating chronic contact dermatitis*

| |
|---|
| Abrasive dusts (pumice, sand, fiberglass) |
| Alkalies |
| Cement |
| Chronic fungal infections |
| Cleansers (industrial) |
| Cutting fluids (soluble) |
| Oils |
| Resin systems |
| Solvents |
| Wet work |

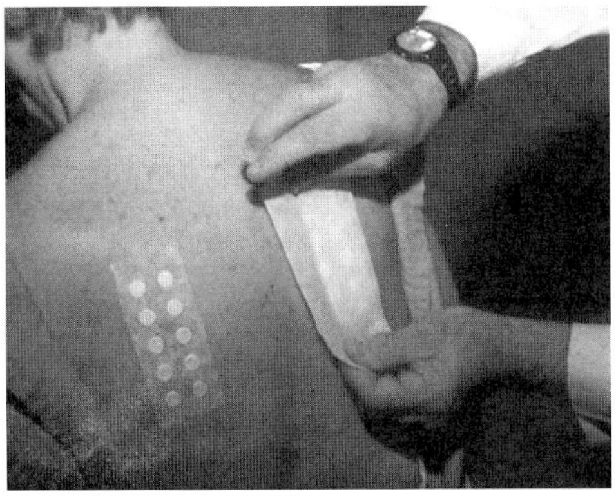

**FIG. 8.** Application of patch tests to the patient's back. The stainless steel disks are filled with potential allergens and left in place for 48 hours. An initial reading will be performed the day the patches are removed. An additional final reading must be performed 24 to 72 hours later.

## DIAGNOSTIC TESTING—THE PATCH TEST

Diagnostic patch testing, properly performed and interpreted, may be used to identify the inciting agent in a worker's acute or chronic eczematous dermatitis. If identified correctly, application of the suspected material to an area of unaffected skin causes an inflammatory (positive) reaction at the site of administration, thereby establishing an allergic sensitivity (Figs. 8 and 9) (18,26).

The patch test is invaluable not only in identifying a causal agent, but also in distinguishing an irritant from an allergic contact dermatitis. To give the test relevance and reliability, one must use concentrations of chemicals known to cause reactions in sensitized individuals and negative results in those not allergic. Hence, ideal test concentrations should be below the threshold necessary to cause an irritant reaction, but above that necessary to cause an allergic reaction. Generally, these concentrations do not overlap for most chemicals. For example, a skin reaction is inevitable if a patch test is conducted with strong or even marginal irritants. Using a diluted formulation of this primary irritant can allow for meaningful patch test results. For reference, published material describes proper patch test concentrations and appropriate vehicles considered safe for skin tests (17,18,29). Furthermore, the clinician performing the tests should have a working knowledge of environmental contactants, particularly those well known as potential cutaneous allergens (Figs. 9 and 10).

The technique of the test is simple. Liquids, powders, or solids are applied in occlusive conditions under stainless steel disks or in a hydrogel suspension to the back. The test panel should include relevant chemicals based on the history and distribution of the rash. A standard allergen panel is not useful since exposure patterns across various occupations are so divergent (30). The North American Contact Dermatitis Group and the International Contact Dermatitis Group advocate standardized test concentrations applied in vertical rows on the back and covered by hypoallergenic tape. Contact with the test material is maintained on the skin for 48 hours, and two readings are made: one at the time of removal, and the second 24 to 72 hours later.

Interpreting the significance of the test reactions is of paramount importance. Reading the reaction and interpreting the results requires experience. True allergic reactions tend to increase in intensity for 24 to 48 hours after patch removal, whereas irritant reactions usually subside within 24 to 48 hours (31,32). When the positive test coincides with a positive history of contact with that chemical, it is considered strong evidence of an allergic etiology. Conversely, the examiner must be aware that clinically irrelevant positive tests can occur if the patient is tested (a) during an active dermatitic phase leading to one or several nonspecific reactions, (b) with a marginal irritant, or (c) with a sensitizer not relevant to the present occupational dermatitis (30). It is important to recognize that a positive result may be due to exposure to both an irritant and a sensitizer. Irritant reactions on a patch test

A

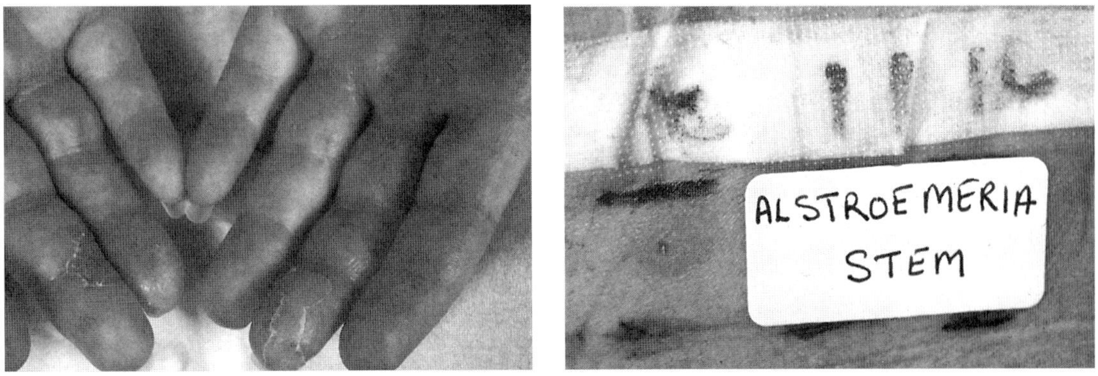


B

**FIG. 9. A:** Allergic contact dermatitis involving the palmar aspects of the hands in a florist. **B:** Positive patch test to Peruvian lily (alstroemeria). *See color plate between pages 632 and 633.*

A 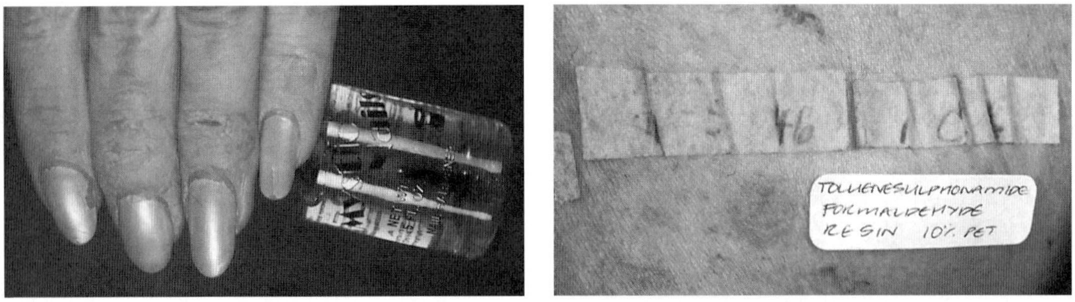 B


**FIG. 10. A:** Allergic contact dermatitis to a nail hardener in a manicurist who also uses the product. *See color plate between pages 632 and 633.* **B:** Positive patch test to toluene sulfonamide formaldehyde resin. Toluene sulfonamide formaldehyde resin is an adhesion promoter for film forming natural and synthetic resins.

should never be correlated with any workplace exposures, as no conclusions regarding the cause of a dermatitis can be drawn. A negative test indicates the absence of an irritant or an allergic reaction. However, a negative reaction can also mean (a) testing omitted an important allergen, (b) insufficient strength and quantity of the test allergen, (c) poor test conditions, or (d) hyporeactivity by the patient at the time of the test.

Performing the patch test with unknown substances the employee has brought to the physician's office can be misleading and potentially hazardous. Useful information concerning unknown materials can be obtained by contacting the plant manager, physician, nurse, industrial hygienist, or safety supervisor (17,31).

## PHOTOTOXICOLOGY

Photoreactive dermatitis is the cutaneous reaction usually resulting from exposure to the ultraviolet (UV) band of the electromagnetic spectrum, spanning from 200 nm to 400 nm. It is further stratified into three sub-bands of light: UV-A, UV-B, and UV-C. Table 9 describes the specific properties of each spectrum (33).

Ultraviolet light may have one of two effects on the skin: phototoxic or photoallergic. Phototoxic reactions result when a chemical, under the influence of ultraviolet light, produces free radicals capable of inducing cell death. The resulting epidermal damage is similar to irritant dermatitis. Outdoor workers in construction, road building, fishing, forestry, gardening, farming, and electric and phone line installing are potentially exposed to both sunlight and photosensitizing chemicals. Additionally, electric furnace and foundry operators, glassblowers, photoengravers, steelworkers, welders, and printers who come in contact with photocure inks are exposed to artificial ultraviolet light (33).

In the coal and tar industry, distillation can potentially expose workers to anthracene, phenanthrene, and acridine—all well-known phototoxic chemical agents. Related products such as creosote, pitch roof paint, road tar, and pipeline coatings have caused hyperpigmentation from the interaction of tar vapors or dusts with sunlight (Table 9) (33).

Occupational photosensitivity is complicated by topical and oral pharmacologic agents that can also produce a phototoxic or photoallergic reaction when exposed to

**TABLE 9.** *Ultraviolet light spectra*

| Waveband | Wavelength | Significance and comments |
|---|---|---|
| UV-C | 200–280 nm | Does not penetrate upper atmosphere |
| | | Artificial sources used for germicidal properties |
| | | Produces sunburn within 8 hours of exposure |
| UV-B | 280–320 nm | Causes significant epidermal damage |
| | | Penetrates epidermis but cannot adequately reach the dermis |
| | | Band most responsible for sunburn |
| UV-A | 320–400 nm | Reaches the earth's surface much more than B light |
| | | Potent stimulator of melanin production |
| | | Can cause DNA damage in keratinocytes |
| | | Results in aging of the skin and likely the most carcinogenic of the UV bands |
| | | Most frequently implicated in photoallergic reactions |
| Visible | 400–760 nm | Rarely produces dermatologic disease |
| | | Blue light (420–490) can photo-isomerize bilirubin |
| Infrared | 760–100,000 | High levels can produce thermal burns |

**TABLE 10.** *Photosensitizing chemical used for testing*

| | | |
|---|---|---|
| 1-(4-isopropylphenyl)-3-phenyl-1,3proandione | Chrysanthemum | Phenanthrene[a] |
| 3-(4-methylbenzylidene) camphor | Cinerariaefolium | Pitch[a] |
| 6-methylcoumarin | Cinoxate | Promethazine |
| Achillea millefolium | Coal tar[a] | Propolis |
| Acridine[a] | Creosote[a] | Pyrethrum |
| Alantolactone | Diallydisulfide | Sandalwood oil |
| A-methylene-Y-butyrolactone | Dichlorophen | Sesquiterpene lactone |
| Anthracene[a] | Diphenhydramine | Sesquiterpene lactone mix |
| Arnica montana | Fentichlor | Sulfanilamide |
| Benomyl | Folpet | Tanacetum vulgare |
| Benzophenone-4 | Hexachlorophene | Taraxacum officinale |
| Bithionol | Lichen acid mix | Thiourea |
| Captafol | Maneb | Tribromosalicylanilide |
| Captan | Methyl anthranilate | Trichlorocarbanilide |
| Certain chlorinated hydrocarbons[a] | Musk ambrette | Triclosan |
| Chamomilla romana | Octyl dimethyl PABA | Zineb |
| Chlorhexidene | Octyl methoxycinnamate | Ziram |
| Chlorpromazine | Permethrin | |

[a]Denotes photosensitizing chemicals not routinely utilized in phototesting protocols.

specific light bands. Examples of such therapeutics include sulfonamide-like drugs, certain antibiotics, phenothiazine tranquilizers, and various phototoxic oils used in fragrances (17,34).

Ultraviolet light exposure may also cause allergic contact dermatitis if there has been prior sensitization to the allergen. In the absence of ultraviolet light, the photoallergens are not allergenic and are incapable of causing a dermatitis in the sensitized individual. It is the exposure of the allergen to the ultraviolet light that renders it allergenic. Phytophotodermatitis is a form of allergic contact dermatitis that results from the combination of a plant photoallergen and ultraviolet light. The photoactive ingredient in these plants are psoralens or furocoumarins, used as therapeutic agents in the treatment of photoresponsive dermatoses such as psoriasis and eczematous dermatitides. Plants known to contain photoallergens include celery infected with pink rot fungus, cow parsnip, dill, fennel, wild carrot, and wild parsnip—all members of the family Umbelliferae (34).

## PHOTOTESTING

To establish photoreactivity to a particular agent, photopatch testing may be performed. Suspected photoallergens are placed on a patient's back in duplicate. One test set is exposed to UV-A light after 24 hours. A positive reaction on the irradiated side with a corresponding negative reaction on the nonirradiated side confirms the diagnosis of photoallergic contact dermatitis. The chemicals listed in Table 10 are capable of causing photoallergic contact dermatitis and may be tested by photopatch testing methods. However, certain agents, such as tar derivative, that typically cause phototoxic reaction are generally not tested in clinical settings since history and physical examination are sufficient for diagnosis. Table 10 outlines potentially photosensitizing chemicals used for photopatch testing (28).

## FOLLICULITIS AND ACNE

Folliculitis, acne, and chloracne are dermatologic conditions caused by exposure to certain chemicals. In fact, folliculitis and acne can often be diagnosed in the same person, as chemicals known to cause one can cause the other. Chloracne, on the other hand, is a distinctive condition linked to exposure to halogenated aromatic hydrocarbons.

Both folliculitis and acne are conditions affecting hair follicles. Folliculitis denotes an inflammation caused by either an irritant chemical or an infection (Fig. 11). The hallmark signs of acne include open and closed comedones (commonly known as blackheads and whiteheads, respectively), papules (raised lesions less than 1 cm), cysts, pustules, and subsequent scars (35). Occupational folliculitis most commonly affects follicles located on the face, neck, forearms, backs of hands, fingers, lower abdomen, buttocks, and thighs in workers with heavy

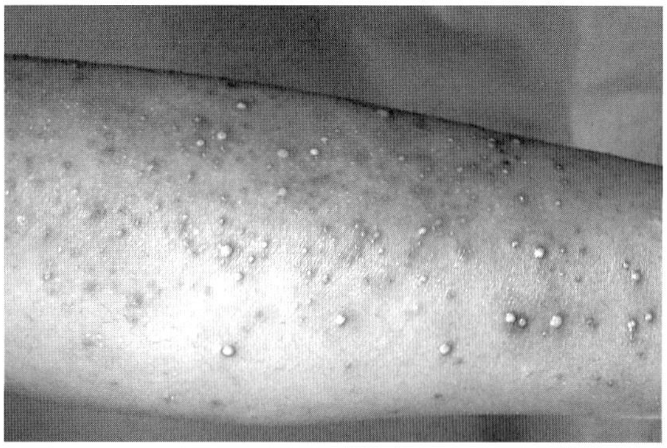

**FIG. 11.** Folliculitis induced by the inadvertent contamination of his clothing with metal cutting oil. *See color plate between pages 632 and 633.*

soilage, such as mechanics, machinists, oil drillers, tar workers, roofers, and tradesmen. The site of exposure also determines the type of follicular disease that clinically appears: acne generally appears on the face, and folliculitis on the arms and legs. Table 11 lists some known causes of folliculitis and acne.

Exposure to halogenated aromatic hydrocarbons (Table 12) can cause chloracne, a unique skin condition also involving the skin follicles. However, the histologic and clinical presentations are quite distinct from folliculitis and acne. Unlike the large and overactive sebaceous glands of acne, the glands of chloracne are conspicuously destroyed (35). There is transition from sebaceous gland cells to keratinizing cells as well as prominent hyperkeratosis in the follicular canal (36). In addition, chemically induced acne and folliculitis resolve without treatment within approximately 1 week, and even sooner with treatment. Chloracne is classically resistant to treatment, including systemic retinoids, and may persist decades after exposure.

Chloracne begins as yellow or straw-colored cysts that appear on the sides of the forehead, around the lateral aspects of the eyelids, and behind the ears. These cysts accompany comedones, pustules, pigmentary disturbances, and subsequent scarring. Areas involved usually include the head, neck, chest, back, groin, and buttocks. Other, less typical areas may be involved if heavily or chronically exposed. Concomitant hypertrichosis (increased hair in atypical locations), hyperpigmentation, brown discoloration of the nails, conjunctivitis, and eye discharge may be present with the chloracne.

Chloracne is a relatively rare disease; however, its recalcitrant nature and preventability make it an important occupational and environmental illness. Chloracne most commonly occurs in the occupational setting from polychlorinated biphenyls (PCBs). While PCBs have not been used since the 1970s, hundreds of millions of pounds escaped into the environment or are still present in electrical transformers (a common use for PCBs prior to the 1970s) in relatively high concentrations. PCB exposure has been reported to be a potential carcinogen as well as the cause for illness in practically every organ system. However, rigorous epidemiologic studies in humans have failed to definitively link PCB exposure with any specific illness other than chloracne. Hence, chloracne remains the only reliable indicator of PCB exposure in humans (37).

**TABLE 11.** *Chemicals capable of inducing acne or folliculitis*

| |
|---|
| Asphalt |
| Creosote |
| Crude oil |
| Greases |
| Insoluble cutting oil |
| Lubricating oil |
| General purpose petroleum oils |
| Heavy plant oils |
| Pitch |
| Tar |

**TABLE 12.** *Chloracnegens*

| |
|---|
| Hexachlorodibenzo-p-dioxin |
| Polybrominated dibenzofurans |
| Polybrominated biphenyls |
| Polychlorinated biphenyls |
| Polychlorinated dibenzofurans |
| Polychloronaphthalenes |
| Tetrachloroazobenzene |
| Tetrachloroazoxybenzene |
| Tetrachlorodibenzo-p-dioxin |

Chloracne was noted soon after industrial accidents and has remained manifest even decades after exposure ceased (38). Some studies have suggested a more frequent association of chloracne with the more highly chlorinated congeners of PCBs than with lower ones (39). Most levels of chlorination, however, have been associated with this skin problem to some degree. Given the high lipid solubility of these chemicals and their recalcitrance to metabolic clearance, their half-life in humans is quite long. Highly chlorinated PCBs can have a serum half-life of 15 years, and less chlorinated PCBs of 5 to 9 years (40). Serum concentrations of PCBs in patients with chloracne are elevated, but the degree of elevation cannot be correlated directly with disease activity.

## MECHANICAL SKIN INJURY

Cutaneous injuries in the workplace account for approximately 35% of occupational injuries for which worker's compensation claims are filed. This translates to almost 1.5 million injuries to workers annually (9). These occupational injuries can be caused by physical trauma, tools, thermal variations, electricity, ultraviolet light (natural and artificial), and various radiation sources that induce cutaneous injury and sometimes systemic effects.

Contact with materials such as spicules of fiber glass, copra, and hemp induce irritation and cause scratching. Skin reacts to repetitive friction by forming a blister or a callus; to pressure, by changing color or becoming thickened or hyperkeratotic; and to shearing by sharp force, by denudation or puncture wound. Any break in the skin may become the site of a secondary infection.

Temperature regulation can play an important role in the initiation of occupational illnesses. In an environment of increased temperatures and humidities, a spectrum of conditions may result. Overexposure may result in miliaria (prickly heat), in which the increase in sweating causes waterlogging of the keratin layer and blockage of the sweat ducts. More seriously, heat exhaustion may result from the worker's failure to thermoregulate. Symptoms include muscle cramping, nausea, vomiting, and syncope. Untreated heat exhaustion can progress to heat stroke, characterized by elevated core temperature, neurologic symptoms, and lack of sweating, which has a high fatality rate if untreated. Aggressive treatment involves fluid and electrolyte replacement as well as core temperature cooling (41). At the other thermal extreme, frostbite results from the intracellular crystallization of water. These ice crystals have sharp points capable of puncturing membranes and fatally disrupting the cells' homeostatic mechanisms. Fingers, toes, ears, and nose, are most commonly injured. Preservation of viable tissue relies on rapid rewarming.

Electrical injury can cause severe cutaneous burns of local or widespread proportions. A ramifying, fern-shaped red lesion emulating the track of the electricity is pathognomonic for high-intensity electrical injury, such as lightning. Less dramatic electric burns can cause local necrosis of skin, similar in nature to a chemical burn.

Modern industry applies ionizing radiation to technologies involved in the production and use of fissionable materials, radioisotopes, x-ray diffraction machines, electron beam operations, industrial x-ray for detecting metal flaws, and various uses in diagnostic and therapeutic radiology. Accidental exposures may result in acute cutaneous and systemic injury depending on the level of radiation received. Lower-level exposures to ionizing radiation may often produce skin changes that manifest years after exposure. Skin thinning, scarring, and ulcerations occurring in sites of previous radiation exposure is termed chronic radiation dermatitis.

## CONTACT URTICARIA

Contact urticaria, or hives, can develop in response to contact with an allergen or nonallergenic chemical urticariant. Allergic contact urticaria represents immediate-type hypersensitivity and requires sensitization to occur.

Occupational contact urticaria has become an extremely important issue, particularly in the health care setting. In response to the recognition of the human immunodeficiency virus and escalating incidence of hepatitis, universal precautions, a standard of personal protection, became obligatory for workers in the health care field. Therefore, the use of protective gloves made of latex became widespread, resulting in a tremendous increase of health care workers using gloves. It is estimated that 5.7 million health care workers use 7 billion pairs of latex gloves yearly (42). Currently, protective gloves come in a variety of forms and are made from pure or hybrid substances. Yet, due to the high-barrier function, form-fitting flexibility, excellent tactile sensation, and affordability of natural latex rubber, it continues to be the major constituent in glove manufacturing. Despite the obvious presence of latex in gloves, medical personnel and potential patients are routinely exposed to nonglove latex because of its ubiquitous presence in modern society.

In the early 1990s, the Food and Drug Administration was notified of deaths in healthy patients who had undergone routine barium enemas with latex-tipped catheters. Investigations revealed that the deaths were related to type I hypersensitivity to natural latex rubber proteins. Since then, latex hypersensitivity has been a well-recognized syndrome with clinical characteristics of contact urticaria, coryza, sneezing, asthma, and, rarely, anaphylaxis and death. This type of hypersensitivity is mediated by immunoglobulin E with the subsequent release of histamine and other mast cell products (Fig. 12A). Proteins derived from latex extracts are not known to cause delayed-type (type IV) hypersensitivity or contact dermatitis.

For health care workers, the main exposure to latex is through rubber gloves. The glove powders, which are known to bind latex protein allergen, become airborne when gloves are removed. Inhaled latex protein can trigger severe allergic reactions as described above. Others at high risk include patients with spina bifida, a history of multiple surgical procedures, or a history of hand dermatitis (43–46). Patients with inexplicable urticaria, angioedema, or type I hypersensitivity reactions following medical procedures should also be suspect for latex hypersensitivity. Such reactions are often mistakenly diagnosed as anesthetic reactions or paradoxical reactions

A 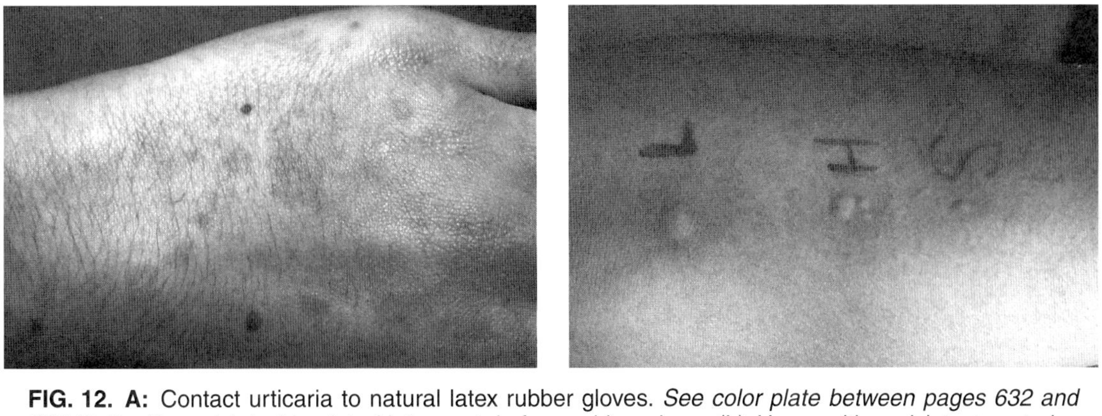 B

**FIG. 12. A:** Contact urticaria to natural latex rubber gloves. *See color plate between pages 632 and 633.* **B:** Positive prick text to eluted latex protein from rubber gloves (L). H, a positive prick test control—histamine; S, a negative control—saline.

to medications. Since dermatitis of the hands is common in many occupational settings, the frequent use of disposable latex gloves should alert health care workers to the sentinel signals of latex allergy.

Health care institutions are now recognizing this problem and are developing strategies to detect latex allergy in employees and cope with them. The suspected latex allergic patient should be carefully questioned regarding symptoms of type I hypersensitivity temporally related to exposure to purported latex agents. Employees are then screened with a latex radioallergosorbent assay (RAST) test to detect latex-specific immunoglobulin E. If negative (as RAST tests may miss over 30% of allergic patients), a "use" test of a latex glove in a supervised setting is performed, first with one finger, then an entire hand. If these tests are negative, eluted latex protein in solution is used for prick or scratch testing (Fig. 12B). The presence of a hive at the test site indicates latex hypersensitivity. If the evaluation proves positive at any point in the evaluation, the workup should be discontinued because generalized hypersensitivity reactions and anaphylaxis might result. If patients exhibit sensitivity, they must be extensively counseled regarding the avoidance of latex products in the home and in the workplace. Depending on the severity of their symptoms, antihistamines, bronchodilators, and an epinephrine autoinjector should be prescribed.

Occupational contact urticaria may also occur from a variety of other allergenic sources such as formaldehyde, guinea pigs, streptomycin, and various foods (including apples, carrots, eggs, fish, beef, chicken, lamb, pork, and turkey). Other sources include products handled by veterinarians or products derived from animal viscera. It is likely that many of these cases are unrecognized and unreported as such (47,48).

## INFECTIOUS OCCUPATIONAL DERMATOSES

Biologic agents may cause a variety of primary and secondary infections of the skin. The skin is too often a portal of entry for infectious agents that can systemically affect the worker. Workers exposed to natural environments and animals are at particular risk for occupationally acquired infections. Infections at work may occur through direct integumentary trauma. However, compromised barrier function secondary to a preexisting skin condition may substantially increase the risk of acquiring a primary cutaneous or systemic infection. Unfortunately, the use of personal protective equipment, particularly gloves, may result in either contact dermatitis from rubber or its constituents or maceration and breakdown, resulting in suboptimal protection against infectious agents. This is a particular problem for health care workers who continuously have infectious fluids in contact with their skin. Following is a discussion of notable infectious agents classically associated with specific occupational exposures.

### Bacteria

Typical human pathogenic bacteria can gain entrance into the skin through routine trauma in almost any occupation. For example, office workers may be susceptible to banal bacterial infections through paper cuts, or they may suffer from folliculitis due to overheated offices resulting in increased perspiration. *Staphylococcus* and *Streptococcus* are the most common agents responsible for routine, trauma-induced cutaneous infections.

Erysipeloid is caused by the gram-positive rod *Erysipelothrix rhusiopathiae* that inhabits the surfaces of fresh and saltwater fish, crustacea, and poultry (especially turkey and quail) (Fig. 13) (49). Fisherman and butchers are at risk following abrasions and puncture wounds in contact with infected animals. In certain parts of the world, it follows eczema as the most common occupational disease of meat packers. A painful, progressively enlarging, well-demarcated purple to erythematous plaque forms at the site of inoculation. Lymphangitis and lymphadenitis with fever and joint pain may occur. Endocarditis has been reported. Spontaneous resolution occurs in 3 to 4 weeks, and penicillin can hasten recovery.

### Fungi

Fungi can produce localized cutaneous disease. Yeast infections *(Candida)* can occur among those employees engaged in wet work (e.g., bartenders, cannery workers, and fruit processors). It is opportunistic on the skin and therefore requires some breakdown of the normal barrier function to establish an entrenched infection. Treatment with topical imidazole antifungals are generally effective, although oral imidazoles may be necessary in recalcitrant cases.

Sporotrichosis, which gains access to the subcutaneous structures through trauma, is seen among garden and landscape workers, florists, farmers, and miners who regularly contact soil and foliage. It begins as painful erythematous nodules that subsequently propagate through lymphatic channels, creating a semilinear row of nodules (Fig. 14). Treatment with systemic imidazole antifungals is effective (50).

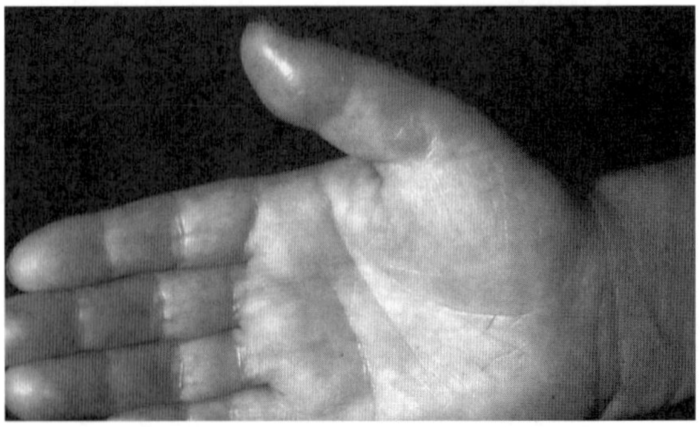

**FIG. 13.** Erysipeloid on the thumb of a fisherman.

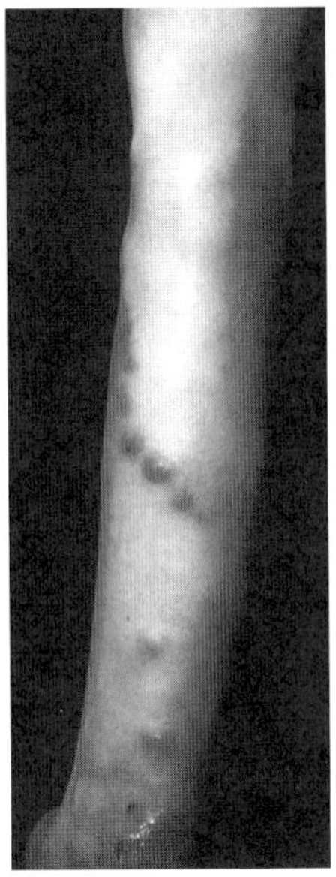

**FIG. 14.** Sporotrichosis in a florist. Note the lymphocutaneous pattern of nodules up the forearm. This distribution is known as a sporotrichoid pattern. It may be seen in other fungal, bacterial, and atypical mycobacterial infections.

## NEOPLASMS

Mutagens are abundant in the workplace and can easily contact the skin under many circumstances. Such cutaneous exposures—as well as systemic exposures—may result in the development of benign or malignant neoplasms in the skin. While often appearing at sites of contact with a suspected carcinogen, the tumors may also occur at distant sites. Asbestos warts and tar papillomas associated with petroleum and tar exposures, respectively, are examples of benign neoplasms associated with repeated contact.

Basal and squamous cell carcinomas (malignant neoplasms) are clearly associated with recurrent ultraviolet light exposure (Figs. 1 and 15) (5). Despite mounting epidemiologic evidence implicating exposure to ultraviolet light (particularly during childhood) as a causal factor in malignant melanoma, controversy still remains. Melanomas may indeed arise in locations classically shielded from ultraviolet light exposure (Fig. 16).

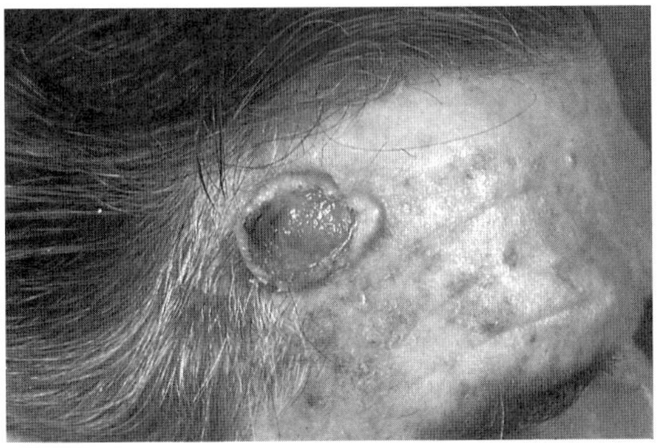

**FIG. 15.** Squamous cell carcinoma. Erosive nodule of an advanced lesion.

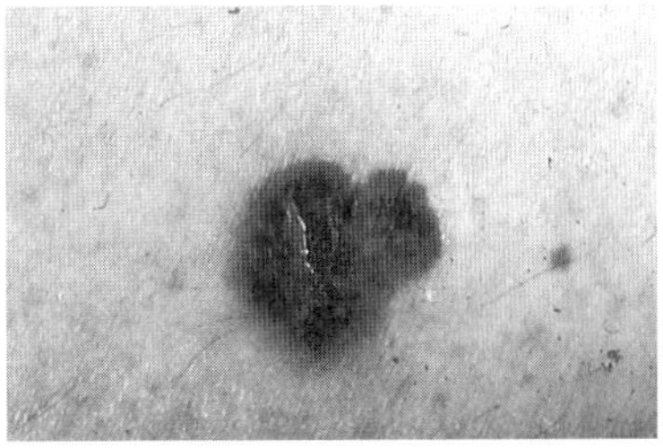

**FIG. 16.** Malignant melanoma. An irregularly pigmented, notched papule.

Several chemical and physical agents are classified as industrial carcinogens, but only a few frequently cause skin cancer (Table 13). Admittedly, more cancers appear on the skin than at any other site; however, the number of these that are of occupational origin is not known. Sunlight is probably the major cause of occupational skin cancer, particularly among those workers engaged in agriculture, construction, fishing, forestry, gardening and landscaping, oil drilling, road building, roofing, and telephone and electric line installing.

In European countries, mule spinners exposed to shale oil and pressmen exposed to paraffin experienced a high frequency of carcinomatous lesions of the scrotum and lower extremities. A similar association with paraffin was observed in the United States, but improved industrial practices and hygienic controls have practically eliminated the problem. In 1984, the International Agency for Research on Cancer determined that mineral oils containing various additives and impurities used in mule spinning, metal machining, and jute processing were carcinogenic to humans. Oils formerly in use that were responsible for cutaneous cancers, including those

**TABLE 13.** *Cutaneous carcinogens*

| |
|---|
| Anthracene |
| Arsenic |
| Benzpyrene |
| Burns |
| Coal tar |
| Coal tar pitch |
| Creosote oil |
| Crude oils |
| Dibenzanthracene |
| Dimethyl benzanthracene |
| Ionizing radiation |
| Methyl cholanthrene |
| Mineral oils containing various additives |
| Shale oil |
| Soot |
| Trauma |
| Ultraviolet light |

affecting the scrotum, were not as well refined as the lubricating oils used today.

Identifying carcinogens involved in systemic exposures is problematic when discussing internal malignancies such as hepatic and pulmonary cancers. For the skin, however, there are relatively few systemic toxins capable of producing malignant neoplasms. The ability of arsenic to cause a variety of benign and premalignant growths as well as basal and squamous cell carcinomas is well known. The clinical and histopathologic appearance of these growths is often so distinct that they have been termed arsenical keratoses and arsenical carcinomas.

## ULCERATIONS

Cutaneous ulcers were the earliest documented skin changes observed among miners and allied craftsmen. In 1827, Cumin (51) reported skin ulcers produced by chromium. Today, the chrome ulcer (hole) caused by chromic acid or concentrated alkaline dichromate is a familiar lesion among chrome platers and chrome reduction plant operators. While these employees may also experience perforation of the nasal septum, the numbers have decreased in the last 30 years due to the fact that many of the operations are now well enclosed (52). Punched out ulcers on the skin can result from contact with arsenic trioxide, calcium arsenate, calcium nitrate, and slaked lime (53).

## NAIL DISCOLORATION AND DYSTROPHY

Chemicals such as alkaline bichromate induce an ochre in nails; tetryl and trinitrotoluene induce yellow coloring; dyes of various colors may change the nail color; and carpenters may have wood stains on their nails. Dystrophy can follow chronic contact with acids, corrosive salts, alkaline agents, moisture exposures, sugars, trauma, and infectious agents. Long-standing contact dermatitis of the fingertips may disrupt the nail matrix and bed, causing dystrophic nail plates to form.

## ACROOSTEOLYSIS

Several years ago, a number of workers involved in cleaning vinyl chloride polymerization reaction tanks incurred a peculiar vascular and bony abnormality involving the digits, hands, and forearms. Bone resorption of the digital tufts was accompanied by Raynaud's syndrome and scleroderma-like changes of the hands and forearms. Removal from the tank cleaning duties led to vascular bone improvement, but the skin changes did not always improve (54). Acroosteolysis has become a rare disease in the United States since the inception of strict exposure standards for vinyl chloride monomer. Polymerized vinyl chloride does not cause this illness.

## DIAGNOSIS, TREATMENT, AND PREVENTION

Although workers may often assume their skin disease is related to their employment, the clinician is responsible for investigating and pinpointing the true nature of the illness. The industrial physician, familiar with both the agents used and the conditions associated within the work environment, has a distinct advantage. Regardless of educational background, however, the physician has a responsibility to satisfy several fundamental tenets in establishing a diagnosis of occupational skin disease. These basic principles include taking a thorough history, performing a complete physical examination, conducting diagnostic tests when necessary, creating a treatment plan, and devising a methodology for prevention of further exposure.

The history is essential, as only thorough questioning can one establish the correct relationship between cause and effect. Areas requiring detailed coverage include family history, allergies, past medical illnesses (particularly past dermatologic illnesses), job titles, nature of work, materials handled, frequency of potential exposures, history and distribution of the skin findings, and any treatments (especially topical drugs) used. Finally, it is important to make inquiries regarding recreational hobbies, because materials used in activities such as gardening, woodworking, painting, and model building may cause skin disease indistinguishable from occupationally acquired conditions.

As a rule, an occupational dermatosis can be expected to disappear or considerably improve within a period of 4 to 8 weeks after initiating treatment. However, follicular or acneiform skin lesions, notably chloracne, are notoriously slow in responding to treatment. Pigmentary change may similarly resist several therapeutic agents and remain active for months. In addition, there are cases that are recalcitrant to appropriate treatment and continue to plague the patient with chronic recurrent episodes. Examples include contact dermatitis caused by chromium, nickel, plastics, and glues. However, all cases of recurrent disease are not necessarily associated with the above materials. The following situations may be operable in prolonged and recurrent disease:

1. Incorrect clinical diagnosis
2. Failure to establish cause
3. Failure to eliminate the cause when direct cause is established
   A. In the workplace (Fig. 17)
   B. At home
4. Improper treatment
   A. Incorrect medicaments/medication vehicles
   B. Inadequate treatment time
   C. Incorrect use of medications
5. Poor hygiene habits at work or home

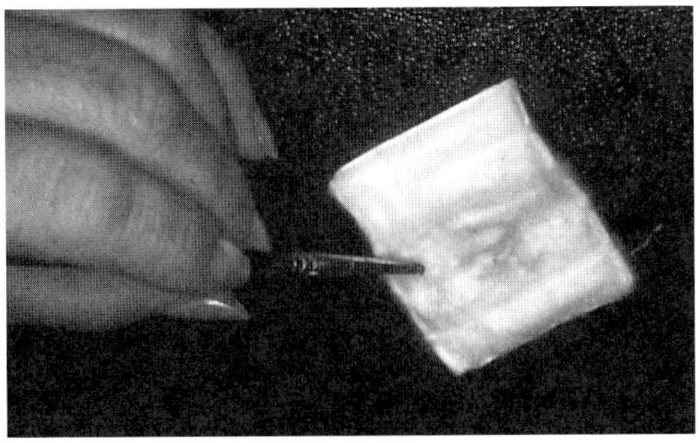

**FIG. 17.** Dimethyl glyoxime test for nickel. A pink color change indicates the presence of available nickel in the metal tip of an artist's brush.

6. Supervening secondary infections
7. Cross-reactions with related chemicals
8. Self-perpetuation for gain
9. Onset of a new unrelated skin disease

Finally, workers in contact with hazardous materials may prevent occupational disease through techniques of personal protection. Personal cleanliness is paramount. Although other protective measures are important in controlling workplace exposures, there is no substitute for washing the hands, forearms, and face. In addition, protective clothing against cold, heat, radiation, and biologic and chemical injury to the skin is advisable. Gloves are a crucial component of protective gear, because the hands are most frequently exposed to chemicals work. Leather gloves offer fairly good protection against mechanical trauma (e.g., friction, abrasion), while cotton gloves may suffice for light work. Neoprene, butadiene-nitrile, and vinyl-dipped cotton gloves are useful in protecting against mechanical trauma, chemicals, solvents, and dusts. Workers exposed to strong solvent chemicals may be unable to find gloves that provide adequate barrier protection under such harsh circumstances. Unlined rubber gloves and plastic gloves can cause further skin disease and are not recommended. In addition to protective clothing, protective creams may also be of value. While there are no protective creams available to prevent contact with irritants and allergens, sunscreens offer incontrovertible protection against sunburn from ultraviolet light exposure. Outdoor workers can use lotions containing diethyltoluamide (DEET) and citronella oil to protect against arthropod assault, although such lotions have the potential to cause allergic contact dermatitis.

Education is the foundation for an effective prevention program against occupational disease, including diseases of the skin. The purpose of these efforts is to acquaint all staff members with the inherent hazards of the workplace and the measures available to control these dangers. A commitment from management, supervisory personnel, and workers is required.

## REFERENCES


1. White RP. *The dermatergoses or occupational affections of the skin,* 4th ed. London: HK Lewis, 1934.
2. Ramazzini B. *Diseases of workers* (translated from the Latin text, De Morbis Artificum, 1713, by WC Wright). New York and London: Hafner, 1864.
3. Pott P. *Cancer scroti.* London: Chirurgical Works, 1775;734; 1790; 257–261.
4. National Institute for Occupational Safety and Health (NIOSH). *National occupational research agenda.* DHHS Publication (NIOSH) 96-115. Cincinnati: US Department of Health and Human Services, 1996.
5. Fitzpatrick TB, Eisen AZ, Wolff K, Freedberg IM, Austen KF, eds. *Dermatology in general medicine,* 4th ed. New York: McGraw-Hill, 1993.
6. Kahn G. Depigmentation caused by phenolic detergent germicides. *Arch Dermatol* 1979;102:177–187.
7. Malten K, Seutter E, Hara I. Occupational vitiligo due to p-tertiary butyl phenol and homologues. *Trans St. John Hosp Dermatol Soc* 1971; 57:115–134.
8. Scheuplein RJ, Blank IH. Permeability of the skin. *Physiol Rev* 1971; 51:702–747.
9. Elias PM. Role of lipids in barrier function of the skin. In: Muktar H, ed. *Pharmacology of the skin.* Boca Raton, FL: CRC Press, 1992; 389–416.
10. McKone TE. Linking a PBPK model for chloroform with measured breath concentrations in showers: implications for dermal exposure models. *J Exp Analysis Environ Epidemiol* 1993;3:339–365.
11. Wester RC, Mobayen M, Maibach HI, et al. In vivo and in vitro absorption and binding to powdered human stratum corneum as methods to evaluate skin absorption of environmental chemical contaminants from ground and surface water. *J Toxicol Environ Health* 1987;21:367–374.
12. Potts RO, et al. Predicting skin permeability. *Pharmacol Res* 1992;9: 663–669.
13. Cleek RL, Bunge AL. A new method for estimating dermal absorption from chemical exposure. 1. General approach. *Pharmacol Res* 1993;10: 497–506.
14. Kao J, et al, In vitro percutaneous absorption in mouse skin: influence of skin appendages. *Toxicol Appl Pharmacol* 1988;94:93–103.
15. Rice RH, Cohen DE. Toxic responses of the skin. In: *Casarett and Doull's toxicology. The basic science of poisons,* 5th ed. New York: Pergamon Press, 1996, 529–546.
16. Mathias CGT. *Contact dermatitis from use and misuse of soaps, detergents, and cleansers in the workplace, occupational medicine- state of art reviews,* vol 1. Philadelphia: Hanley and Belfus, 1986;205–218.
17. Cronin E. *Contact dermatitis.* London: Churchill Livingstone, 1980.
18. Fisher AA. *Contact dermatitis,* 4th ed. Baltimore: Williams & Wilkins, 1995.
19. American Academy of Dermatology. *Proceedings of the National Conference on Environmental Hazards to the Skin.* Schaumburg, IL: American Academy of Dermatology, 1994;61–79.
20. Bjornberg A. Skin reactions to primary irritants in men and women. *Acta Derm Venereol* 1975;55:191–194.
21. Holst R, Moller H. One hundred twin pairs patch tested with primary irritants. *Br J Dermatol* 1975;93:145–149.
22. Landsteiner K, Jacobs J. Studies on the sensitization of animals with simple chemical compounds: II. *J Exp Med* 1935;61:625–639.
23. Chase MW. Inheritance in guinea pigs of the susceptibility to skin sensitization with simple chemical compounds. *J Exp Med* 1941;73: 711–726.
24. Emtestam L, et al. HLA-DR,-DQ, and-DP alleles in nickel, chromium, and/or cobalt-sensitive individuals: genomic analysis based on restriction fragment length polymorphisms. *J Invest Dermatol* 1993;100: 271–274.
25. Baer RL. The mechanism of allergic contact hypersensitivity. In: Fisher AA, ed. *Contact dermatitis,* 3rd ed. Philadelphia: Lea and Febiger, 1986, 1–80.

26. Rietschel RL, Fowler JF, ed. *Contact dermatitis,* 4th ed. Baltimore: Williams and Wilkins, 1995.
27. Lampke KF, Fagerstrom R. *Plant toxicity and dermatitis (a manual for physicians).* Baltimore: William and Wilkins, 1968.
28. Cohen DE, Brancaccio RR. What's new in clinical research in contact dermatitis. *Dermatol Clin* 1997;15:137–148.
29. Maibach HI. *Occupational and industrial dermatology,* 2nd ed. Chicago: Year Book Medical, 1987.
30. Cohen DE, Brancaccio R, Anderson D, Belsito DV. Utility of the Standard Allergen Series alone in the evaluation of allergic contact dermatitis: a retrospective study of 732 patients. *J Am Acad Dermatol* 1997;36:914–918.
31. Marzulli FN, Maibach HI. The use of graded concentrations in studying skin sensitizers: experimental contact sensitization in man. *Food Cosmetics Toxicol* 1974;12(2):219–227.
32. Malten KE, Nater JP, Von Ketel WG. *Patch test guidelines.* Nijmegen, The Netherlands: Dekker Van de Vegt, 1976.
33. Lim H, Soter N, eds. *Clinical photomedicine.* New York: Marcel Dekker, 1993.
34. De Leo V, Harber LC. Contact photodermatitis. In: Fisher AA, ed. *Contact dermatitis.* Baltimore: Williams and Wilkins, 1995.
35. Plewig G, Kligman AM. *Acne and rosacea,* 2nd ed. New York: Springer-Verlag, 1993.
36. Moses M, Prioleau PG. Cutaneous histologic findings in chemical workers with and without chloracne with past exposure to 2,3,7,8-tetrachlorodibenzo-p-dioxin. *J Am Acad Dermatol* 1985;12:497–506.
37. James RC, Busch H, Tamburro CH, et al. Polychlorinated biphenyl exposure and human disease. *J Occup Med* 1993;35:136–148.
38. Urabe H, Asahi M. Past and current dermatological status of Yusho patients. *Environ Health Perspect* 1985;59:11–15.
39. Fischbein A. et al. Dermatological findings in capacitor manufacturing workers exposed to dielectric fluid containing polychlorinated biphenyls. *Arch Environ Health* 1982;37:69–74.
40. Wolff MS, Fishbein A, Selikoff IJ. Changes in PCB serum concentrations among capacitor manufacturing workers. *Environ Res* 1992; 59(1):202–216.
41. De Galan BE, Hoekstra JB. Extremely elevated body temperature: a case report and review of classical heat stroke. *Neth J Med* 1995;47 (6):281–287.
42. Turjanmaa K. Incidence of immediate allergy to latex gloves in hospital personnel. *Contact Dermatitis* 1987;17:270–275.
43. Jaeger D, Kleinhaus D, Czuppon AB, Baur X. Latex-specific proteins causing immediate-type cutaneous, nasal, bronchial, and systemic reactions. *J Allergy Clin Immunol* 1992;89:759–768.
44. Charous BL, Hamilton RG, Yungunger JW. Occupational latex exposure: characteristics of contact and systemic reactions in 47 workers. *J Allergy Clin Immunol* 1994;94:12–18.
45. Tomazic VJ, Shampaine EL, Lamanna A, Withrow TJ, Adkinson NF J, Hamilton RG. Cornstarch powder on latex products is an allergen carrier. *J Allergy Clin Immunol* 1994;93:751–758.
46. Hunt LW, Fransway AF, Reed CE, et al. An epidemic of occupational allergy to latex involving health care workers. *J Occup Environ Med* 1995;37:1204–1209.
47. el Saved F, Seite-Bellezza D, Sans B, Vavie-Lebev P, Marguery MC, Bazex J. Contact urticaria from formaldehyde in a root-canal dental paste. *Contact Dermatitis* 1995;33(5):353.
48. Fisher AA. *Contact urticaria in contact dermatitis,* 4th ed. Baltimore: Williams and Wilkins, 1995.
49. Mutalib A, Keirs R, Austin F. Erysipelas in quail and suspected erysipeloid in processing plant employees. *Avian Dis* 1995;39(1): 191–193.
50. Carrada-Bravo T. Update on sporotrichosis. *Aust Fam Physician* 1995; 24(6):1070–1071,1074.
51. Cumin N. Remarks on the medicinal properties of Madar and on the effects of bichromate of potassium on the human body. *Edinburgh Med Surg J* 1827;28:295–302.
52. Johansen M, Overgaard E, Toft A. Severe chronic inflammation of the mucous membranes in the eyes and respiratory tract due to work-related exposure to hexavalent chromium. *J Laryngol Otol* 1994; 108(7);591–592.
53. Birmingham DJ, Key MM, Holaday DA, Perone VB. An outbreak of arsenical dermatoses in a mining community. *Arch Dermatol* 1964;91: 457–465.
54. Harris DK, Adams WG. Acroosteolysis occurring in men engaged in the polymerization of vinyl chloride. *Br Med J* 1967;3:712–714.

## GLOSSARY

**Apocrine gland**—a gland that secretes a fatty substance with the rest of the discharge secretory product.

**Appendages**—in dermatology, they are applied to internal structures of the skin, like the nail unit, the hair unit, and sweat glands.

**Bulla**—a blister of the skin.

**Bullous**—relating to many blisters.

**Chromophore**—a chemical capable of absorbing various wavelengths of light.

**Comedone**—the classic acne lesion consisting of open and closed varieties commonly referred to in the vernacular as blackheads and whiteheads, respectively.

**Cyst**—a circumscribed nodule filled with fluid or solid matter usually located directly under the skin.

**Cytokines**—chemicals capable of specific cellular action of recruitment and activation.

**Depigmentation**—complete loss of pigment or color.

**Eccrine gland**—a sweat gland.

**Erosion**—loss of epidermis caused by physical, chemical, or metabolic disorders up to the full thickness of the epidermis, but not through the basement membrane.

**Erythema**—relating to redness of the skin.

**Exfoliative dermatitis**—a red, scaling skin rash involving the majority of skin from head to toe. Causes may relate to external exposure or internal disease.

**Granuloma**—an inflammatory response of specific cells intended to wall off infectious or inanimate foreign objects.

**HLA proteins**—human leukocyte antigen proteins on the surface of cells that identify them to the immune system as belonging to self.

**Hyperpigmentation**—excessive coloration of the skin.

**Hypopigmentation**—decreased pigmentation of the skin.

**Ichthyosis**—a genetic disease of marked dryness and scaling of the skin.

**Integument**—a Latin term referring to a covering; in medical use refers to the skin.

**Keratinocyte**—a principal cell making up the epidermis.

**Langerhans cells**—a dendritic cell found in the skin that is capable of processing antigenic material.

**Lichenification**—a compensatory pathologic process marked by accentuation of skin surface markings, usually in the form of a plaque that results from persistent rubbing or scratching.

**Macule**—a flat, nonpalpable discoloration that may be erythematous (red), hyperpigmented (brown or dark), or hypopigmented (lighter in color than the normal skin). Macules are defined as lesions smaller than 1 cm.

**Papule**—a circumscribed, elevated lesion measuring up to 0.5 cm. They may be flesh-colored or dyspigmented. A nodule possesses the same morphologic characteristics as a papule, but is larger than 0.5 cm, but smaller than 1 cm. A tumor, likewise, is a circumscribed lesion larger than 1 cm.

**Patch**—the characteristic findings of the macule with lesions larger than 1 cm in size.

**Plaque**—is an elevated solid lesion that is circumscribed and measures larger than 0.5 cm. It can be formed by a confluence of papules or nodules.

**Stratified squamous**—relating to the stacked nature of epidermal cells.

**Ulcer**—loss of full thickness epidermis and basement membrane with exposure of underlying dermis or subcutis.

**Vesicle**—a circumscribed, fluid-filled elevation smaller than 0.5 cm.

**Xerosis**—relating to dry skin.

*Environmental and Occupational Medicine, Third Edition,* edited by William N. Rom.
Lippincott–Raven Publishers, Philadelphia © 1998.

# CHAPTER 47

# Toxic Peripheral Neuropathy

Margit L. Bleecker

Exposure to neurotoxic compounds frequently affects the peripheral nerves producing nonspecific symptoms of paresthesia in the feet followed by involvement of the hands. If exposure is significant, the health care provider may be alerted to the toxic etiology of the peripheral nerve symptoms by the accompaniment of other features produced by the toxicant, for example, gastrointestinal symptoms with lead or arsenic exposure, or alopecia with thallium exposure. However, since exposure in the occupational and environmental setting is usually not at a level associated with symptoms of acute poisoning, complaints of peripheral nerve pathology tend to occur in isolation and are monotonously similar.

Sometimes a unique clinical presentation surrounding a peripheral neuropathy allows its toxic etiology to be determined. Lead neuropathy classically associated with wristdrop is known to involve nerves that innervate the most metabolically active muscles during exposure. Therefore, lead exposure is found in battery workers and house painters, occupations that require frequent wrist extension, and wristdrop is the clinical expression of lead neuropathy. However, lead exposure while other muscle groups are activated, such as the wrist and finger flexors, does not present with wristdrop. The presence of bladder dysfunction helps to identify the etiology of a sensory neuropathy associated with the plasticizer, β-dimethylaminopropionitrile. The more common presentation of toxic neuropathy, paresthesias in the feet alone, makes the causal connection between symptoms and workplace exposure more difficult to establish.

M.L. Bleecker: Center for Occupational and Environmental Neurology, Children's Hospital, Baltimore, Maryland 21211-1398.

## APPROACH TO THE EVALUATION OF PERIPHERAL NEUROPATHY

In the clinical setting approximately 30% of peripheral neuropathies are found to have no known etiology (1,2). This improves when family members are examined for evidence of mild or subclinical neuropathy. Therefore, finding evidence of peripheral neuropathy in the presence of neurotoxic exposure does not necessarily establish causation. The presence of a preexisting generalized peripheral neuropathy, as in diabetes mellitus, or a focal neuropathy, as in carpal tunnel syndrome, may also alter the clinical expression of a toxic neuropathy.

The adult nervous system constantly undergoes age-related change as reflected in a variety of performance measures (3). It is reasonable to assume based on metabolic changes in the old nervous system that following exposure to a neurointoxicant, structural changes occur more readily and the ability for repair is slowed (4). Therefore, a neurotoxicant is interacting with a different substrate if young and old individuals are exposed (5).

Also, the interaction between entrapment neuropathies and toxic neuropathies from workplace exposure needs to be evaluated. Animal studies support this interaction whereby compression or ischemia of the nerve accentuates the metabolic disturbance of the Schwann cell produced by neurotoxic exposure (6). This "double hit" mechanism has similarities to the double crush syndrome: a proximal nerve compression increases susceptibility of the distal nerve fibers to compression or ischemia, resulting in demyelination and axonal degeneration (7).

Symptoms of peripheral neuropathy are most commonly expressed as sensory change in the feet and hands. These symptoms are expressed as tingling (paresthesia), numbness, burning, pain, or misperception of sensory stimuli (dysesthesia). Motor weakness located in distal muscle groups is frequently accompanied by complaints of cramps. Nonspecific, easy fatigability may accompany proximal weakness suggestive of a myopathy or weakness secondary to neuromuscular junction. Genitourinary, anhidrosis, gustatory hidrosis, and postural hypotension reflect an autonomic neuropathy that may accompany a sensorimotor neuropathy (8).

Standard methods for data collection are vital in order to compare workers with similar exposures and to follow them longitudinally after exposure is reduced or ceases. An occupational history includes all jobs performed and all exposures to chemical and physical agents. Hygienic procedures and the use of personal protective equipment are important factors in estimating the potential for exposure. Duration of exposure and duration of symptoms are needed to establish a temporal association (8).

A Total Neuropathy Score developed by Chaudhry et al. (9) may be used to monitor the development of toxic neuropathy (10). Criteria cumulated for a total score include sensory symptoms, perception of the prickliness of a pin, quantitative sensory testing (QST), motor performance, tendon reflexes, and measurements from nerve conduction tests. Total scores are stratified to indicate severity: 1–7, mild neuropathy; 8–14, moderate neuropathy; and 15–21, severe neuropathy. Sensory symptoms rated are 1 for numbness, tingling, or pain in the feet; 2 for numbness, tingling, or pain in the feet and fingers; and 3 for functionally disabling numbness, tingling, pain, or muscle weakness in arms or legs. Pin sensibility is scored 1 for decreased pin sensibility in the feet from the tip of the great toe up to 10 cm, 2 for decreased pin sensibility in the feet up to 10 to 20 cm or in the finger from the tip of the index finger to less than 10 cm, and 3 for decreased pin sensibility greater then 20 cm in the feet or 10 cm in the finger. Quantitative vibratory threshold is rated 1 for an increased threshold of 25% to 50% in the great toe or less than 25% in the index finger, 2 for an increased threshold of 5% to 100% in the great toe or 25% to 50% in the index finger, and 3 for an increased threshold of greater than 100% in the great toe or greater than 50% in the index finger. Strength is graded 1 for displayed weakness in toe extension, 2 in toe extension and index finger abduction, and 3 for diffuse generalized weakness. Tendon reflexes are graded 1 for reduced or absent ankle jerk, 2 for absent jerk with other reflexes reduced, and 3 for all reflexes absent. From nerve conduction studies, amplitudes of the sural nerve sensory action potential and of the common peroneal compound muscle action potential are rated for decreased amplitude of 10% to 25%, grade 1; of 26% to 50%, grade 2; and greater than 50%, grade 3.

The Total Neuropathy Score developed for large-fiber, dying back axonopathies may be too time-consuming or require skills not present in the workplace where screening for the presence of a neuropathy is needed. Surveillance in the workplace is best accomplished by symptom questionnaire and a QST instrument. QST is a psychophysical test and therefore requires the cooperation of the subject. A psychophysical test involves the central processing of information that is initially perceived by the subject from cutaneous receptors (11). The integrity of large axons, A-beta fibers, those most susceptible to neurointoxicants, is measured either with a quantitative vibration and thermal threshold tool (11) or a current perception threshold (2,000-Hz stimulus) (12) device. QST has the added advantage of providing information about A-delta fibers, medium-sized myelinated fibers, and unmyelinated C fibers using quantitative thermal tests (11) or current perception threshold (250 Hz and 5 Hz stimuli) tests (12). A QST approach that provides good sensitivity and reproducibility is the "method of limits" to approximate the threshold, followed by a more precise threshold determination with a two-alternative forced-choice method (11). In the method of limits, when stimulus intensity increases quickly, much higher thresholds result, as compared to the use of discrete steps of stimulus intensity or a forced-choice algorithm (11,13). Programs now exist for all modalities that are computer administered following a training session.

Electromyography (EMG) is still considered the "gold standard" to document integrity of the peripheral nervous system and consists of nerve conduction studies (NCS) and needle EMG. A standard study examines sensory, motor, and mixed nerve conduction velocities, and amplitudes of responses. Nerve conduction studies examine the largest, most rapidly conducting axons, the A-beta fibers. As long as some large axons are preserved in a toxic axonopathy, conduction velocity studies remain unchanged, but amplitudes are abnormal due to loss of axons. By contrast, demyelinating lesions produce prolonged distal latencies and slowed conduction velocities. Needle EMG provides information about the motor unit function. Numerous proximal and distal muscles are sampled to demonstrate the severity of the underlying pathology. NCS may demonstrate abnormalities especially in sensory fibers at a time when there is no clinically detectable sensory loss (14). Even a clinical presentation of predominantly motor involvement may show more abnormalities in sensory nerves (14).

Performance of NCS requires training along with close attention to skin temperature, electrode placement, distance measurements, and use of supramaximal stimulus. Unfortunately, the same techniques are not used between laboratories. In fact, within a laboratory with different examiners, intraexaminer reliability was high while interexaminer reliability was low (15). Decade-specific norms for each laboratory are needed, but other physical attributes such as extremes of height and weight affect NCS and must be considered for adequate reference values (16). NCS examines a more proximal portion of the nerve when compared to QST, which is able to obtain measurements at the site of initial "dying-back" pathology (see below). NCS does not require subject participation, in contrast to QST, in which it is an integral component of the test. NCS reflects large-fiber function, while QST examines all fiber sizes depending on which modality is used. When the location and underlying pathology is known, NCS can be customized as in the Total Neuropathy Score, where only the amplitude of the sural (sensory) and peroneal (motor) response is used to reflect axonal loss in the lower extremities. Portable EMG machines and use of focused examinations make NCS of large groups feasible; however, these studies require more training to perform than QST.

## NEUROPATHOLOGY

Axonopathies are the most common form of pathology in toxic neuropathies. Axonal degeneration occurs secondary to interference in axonal transport. Protein synthesized in the perikaryon is not transported; therefore, the part of the axon most distant from the cell body degenerates. "Dying-back" refers to this distal pathology in the central and peripheral nervous systems (CNS and PNS) that gradually moves proximally toward the cell body, resulting in a central-peripheral distal axonopathy (17). The longest and largest fibers are most vulnerable. Focal accumulation of neurofilaments on the proximal side of the node of Ranvier produces swellings in the axon (17). Secondary demyelination results from retraction of myelin around this swelling when it becomes large. This pathology is best demonstrated in the hexacarbon neuropathy found in glue sniffers (18). Primary demyelination as found with triethyltin and hexachlorophene is uncommon in toxic neuropathies (19).

Some exposures produce a neuronopathy. Protein synthesis in the cell body is altered particularly in the dorsal root ganglia. It is believed that these sensory ganglia are selectively vulnerable because the blood-nerve barrier is deficient in the dorsal root ganglia. Axonal degeneration follows changes in amino acid incorporation in the perikaryon (19).

## ACRYLAMIDE

Acrylamide monomer is well known for its neurotoxic effects. When polymerized for flocculators and grouting agents, it is not neurotoxic. The monomer may produce significant sensory disturbances in the hands and feet. Another characteristic feature is excessive sweating along with peeling and sloughing of skin in the hands. Muscle weakness in the distal extremities contributes to difficulty walking and frank ataxia; incoordination and tremor is secondary to cerebellar dysfunction. Human nerve biopsy reveals axonal loss of large fibers (20). Acrylamide neuropathy is a good example of the central-peripheral dying-back process in fibers of the CNS and PNS. In the distal end of large myelinated fibers accumulation of 10-nm filaments proximal to the node of Ranvier is found (17). Both motor and sensory fibers are affected; NCS displays no change in motor nerve conduction, but sensory potentials are absent or reduced in amplitude (21). Vibration sensitivity is affected disproportionately to other sensory modalities. QST for vibration is used as a screen for peripheral neuropathy in workers exposed to acrylamide (22). Recovery following removal from exposure is dependent on the severity of the initial clinical presentation. Persistent gait ataxia may result from a less than full recovery of the central lesions.

With acrylamide exposure, hemoglobin adducts are believed to better represent the target dose, the amount of acrylamide that is not detoxified and therefore reaches its target protein (23). A recent study of workers producing acrylamide polymer used hemoglobin adducts as a biomarker for exposure. Hemoglobin adducts predicted acrylamide-induced neuropathy as measured by vibration thresholds (24).

## ARSENIC

Occupational arsenic exposure occurs in the smelting of copper and lead ores, in which arsenic is a by-product. Arsenic is used in pyrotechnics, pigments, and in the manufacture of semiconductors. Herbicides, insecticides, and rodenticides may also contain arsenic. Onset of neuropathy following high arsenic exposure occurs after 7 to 14 days, with numbness and intense paresthesia, spontaneous pain, muscle tenderness, cramps, and increased sweating in the distal lower extremities. Proximal segmental demyelination with subsequent distal sensory axonopathy is found (25). In the occupational setting the common exposure is at a prolonged low level (26). The associated neuropathy is primarily sensory, affecting all modalities but to a greater extent vibration and position sense. Predominant symptoms at the onset are numbness and burning sensations in the feet. If present, distal weakness of intrinsic hand and feet muscles is mild. Other findings with chronic arsenic exposure include hyperkeratoses, Mees' lines, anemia, and cancers of the lung and skin.

The mechanism of arsenic neuropathy is unknown but is similar to the neuropathy of thiamine deficiency (27). As in thiamine deficiency, arsenic inhibits the conversion of pyruvate to acetyl coenzyme A (CoA) and thus blocks the Krebs' cycle. Electrophysiologic studies show absent or reduced amplitude of sensory action potentials. As exposure continues, reduced sensory and motor action potentials are found with only mildly slowed conduction velocities. In these mild cases of neuropathy, recovery is excellent. However, with a severe neuropathy, chelation with bronchoalveolar lavage (BAL) or penicillamine is of little benefit.

Biologic monitoring of workers with the traditional total arsenic in urine can be misleading since urine may contain large quantities of organic arsenic, arsenobetaine, which results from dietary intake and is nonneurotoxic. The only forms of arsenic that are neurotoxic are inorganic arsenic in the trivalent or pentavalent state and the methylated metabolites, monomethylarsonic acid and dimethylarsenic acid (28). To establish a dose effect between arsenic and measures of peripheral nerve function, attention to this aspect of exposure is required.

## CARBON DISULFIDE

Carbon disulfide, a volatile liquid, is used as an industrial solvent in the production of viscose rayon fibers and cellophane films. Significant exposure is commonly associated with mood changes believed to be responsible for an increased suicide rate, memory loss, insomnia, and bad dreams. Parkinsonism and sensorimotor neuropathy are also outcomes. In this case the neuropathy also involves cranial, optic, and auditory nerves. High-frequency hearing loss and optic nerve changes resembling optic neuritis are features of chronic carbon disulfide toxicity (29). Symptoms of polyneuropathy, distal sensory loss, muscle weakness, and pain accompanied by slowed motor and sensory conduction velocities usually are associated with years of exposure at levels greater than 50 ppm (30). If behavioral symptoms are present, evidence of peripheral nerve effects should be found. In fact slowed nerve conduction studies occur prior to clinical symptoms of polyneuropathy with long-term low-level carbon disulfide exposure (31).

A more recently published study found clinical and subclinical neuropathy by examination and NCS at a viscose rayon plant, where the fixed-point air concentrations of carbon disulfide ranged from 12 to 300 ppm in the fiber cutting and spinning areas (32). In another study, complaints of pain, tingling, and fatigue in the lower extremities correlated significantly with diminished motor conduction velocities at exposures of carbon disulfide below the threshold limit value (TLV) (31 $mg/m^3$, 10 ppm) (33).

Animals examined following carbon disulfide inhalation demonstrate slowing in nerve conduction velocities before the development of weakness. The pathology resembles the central-peripheral distal axonopathy with axonal swelling, similar to acrylamide and hexacarbon neuropathy, and alteration in fast axonal transport (34).

Proposed mechanisms for toxicity of carbon disulfide include chelation of essential metals, inhibition of some enzymes, and interference with vitamin $B_6$ metabolism. This latter mechanism is the basis for vitamin $B_6$ supplementation, which only delays the onset and does not prevent the development of carbon disulfide neuropathy (35).

## β-DIMETHYLAMINOPROPIONITRILE

β-Dimethylaminopropionitrile (DMAPN), used as a catalyst in the manufacture of polyurethane, was targeted as the cause of neurogenic bladder dysfunction and a sensory peripheral neuropathy in workers at two sites (36–38). DMAPN was removed following these outbreaks in 1977–1978. Several months after the introduction of DMAPN, symptoms of urinary retention, sensory abnormalities, weakness, sleeping difficulties, and sexual dysfunction had occurred in areas with highest catalyst use. The chemical structure of DMAPN is similar to other known neurotoxins.

In exposed workers, urinary hesitancy and abdominal discomfort were the initial symptoms followed by inability to initiate or maintain an erection. Paresthesia began in the feet and moved proximally. Examination showed diminished perception of the prickliness of a pin, temperature, and light touch in the distal extremities and perianal dermatomes. Autonomic function was normal. Cystometrograms revealed a flaccid neurogenic bladder with residua. Sacral nerve latencies were prolonged. Nerve conduction studies showed diminished amplitudes of sensory potentials and mild slowing of motor nerve conduction velocities that was dose dependent. After DMAPN was removed from the workplace, no new cases developed. In a follow-up study 2 years later, 11 workers had persistence of symptoms. Bladder and sexual dysfunction and sensory neuropathy persisted in a small group (39).

In an index case, gastrocnemius muscle biopsy showed small angular fibers and type grouping suggestive of mild denervation. Sural nerve biopsy revealed axonal loss, and axonal swellings that contained disordered neurofilaments (38). Also, animals exposed chronically to DMAPN developed mild distal axonal changes and diminished urinary function (38,40).

## ETHYLENE OXIDE

Ethylene oxide, a gas used in sterilization of heat-sensitive materials and in production of ethylene glycol, polyesters, and detergents, produces a central-peripheral dying-back axonopathy (41). Impaired neuropsychological performance and an increase in sister-chromatid exchanges (42) is found with chronic ethylene oxide exposure (43,44).

Skin rash accompanies the complaints of hand dysthesias and distal motor weakness with chronic exposure to garments sterilized with ethylene oxide (45). Sensory abnormalities with monofilament testing accounted for impaired touch and pressure perception in almost all the subjects as compared to vibration threshold, the usual screen for toxic neuropathies, in which only 25% of subjects were abnormal.

Sensorimotor polyneuropathy developed within 10 months of daily working with ethylene oxide sterilizers.

Sural nerve biopsy showed mild dropout of large myelinated fibers, mild changes of the myelin sheath, and involvement of unmyelinated fibers (46). Several studies support a sensorimotor polyneuropathy of axonal type, even with only 2 to 8 weeks of exposure (47), which improves when exposure to ethylene oxide ceases or is diminished to acceptable levels (42,43,48).

## *N*-HEXANE AND METHYL *N*-BUTYL KETONE

Hexacarbons used as solvents in many industries are associated with toxic neuropathies following prolonged elevated exposure; however, the most florid neurotoxic sequela occurs with solvent abuse, primarily glue sniffing. In these cases, the peripheral neuropathy, usually attributed to *n*-hexane, consists of distal weakness with muscle atrophy, loss of ankle reflexes, and sensory loss. In extreme cases quadriplegia can develop. As recovery of the peripheral neuropathy ensues, pyramidal tract signs are unmasked. Nerve biopsies reveal multifocal distal axonal swelling filled with 10-nm neurofilaments located proximal to the nodes of Ranvier accompanied by thinning of the overlying myelin sheath (18). It is this effect on the myelin sheath that is responsible for marked slowing in motor conduction velocity; in fact, the severity of the neuropathy correlates with conduction slowing in the motor fibers.

Both *n*-hexane and methyl *n*-butyl ketone are metabolized to 2,5-hexanedione, the active agent believed to be primarily responsible for the neurotoxic effects (19). Proposed toxic mechanisms for the γ-diketone include alterations in axonal transport and formation of a pyrrhol ring that is responsible for cross-linking of neurofilaments (49).

Glue use in the leather shoe industry was responsible for many cases of *n*-hexane neuropathy. Sensory and motor symptoms and signs prevail, with motor features being the most prominent. After removal from exposure, improvement occurred only after several months of further deterioration (50). Three workers in the manufacture of jet engine parts became disabled with progressive extremity weakness 6 months after a change of solvent to 95% *n*-hexane from one containing 2% to 5% *n*-hexane. Electrodiagnostic studies returned to normal 11 to 36 months after exposure ceased (51). *n*-Hexane exposure for 3 years, at approximately 100 ppm measured by personal sampling, produced extremity weakness with motor and sensory changes in NCSs (52). Twenty workers with urinary 2,5-hexanedione concentrations exceeding the biologic exposure index (5 mg/g creatinine) for an average of 8 years demonstrated normal motor and sensory conduction velocity, but the amplitude of the sensory nerve action potential for the sural and median nerves was significantly diminished (53). There is a case report of a worker with low *n*-hexane exposure, 7 to 30 ppm for 30 years, who presented with a sensory neuropathy and sural nerve biopsy and showed accumulation and irregular orientation of neurofilaments in some myelinated axons (54).

Methyl ethyl ketone added to glue potentiated *n*-hexane, resulting in an outbreak of peripheral neuropathy among glue sniffers (55,56). It was believed that methyl ethyl ketone caused a more rapid metabolism of *n*-hexane to the active metabolite 2,5-hexanedione. This same enhanced conversion of the toxic compound probably was responsible for the outbreak of polyneuropathy in a plastic coating–printing plant where methyl *n*-butyl ketone replaced methyl isobutyl ketone in a process that also used methyl ethyl ketone (57,58). After the addition of methyl *n*-butyl ketone, development of symptomatic peripheral neuropathy in a few workers raised concern, and an extensive study of 1,157 workers found 68 with definite peripheral neuropathy and 28 with suspected neuropathy after exclusion of other nonoccupational causes (57,59). After removal from exposure, clinical findings and electrodiagnostic studies deteriorated for several months before improvement began.

Mixtures of solvents is the more common workplace exposure. When working lifetime exposure to a mixture of aliphatic and aromatic hydrocarbons is available, it was possible to demonstrate a dose-effect relationship between exposure and QST measures in the feet before the onset of symptoms (60).

## LEAD

Lead neuropathy, in the older literature, presented with weakness not accompanied by sensory signs. The distribution of weakness reflected the most active motor units during exposure, accounting for greater involvement of the upper extremities (61). Wristdrop in battery workers is due to increased use of wrist extensors in that occupation. In another presentation, lead neuropathy mimics the lower motor neuron form of amyotrophic lateral sclerosis (62). These cases of advanced lead exposure were usually accompanied by other features of lead poisoning, e.g., anemia and abdominal pain.

In humans the underlying pathology as demonstrated by nerve biopsy shows loss of large fibers without demyelination (63,64). By comparison, animal models of lead neuropathy reveal segmental demyelination as the predominant feature (65), except for baboons, which had no neuropathy with chronic lead intoxication (66). Development of lead neuropathy in rats that ingested 6% lead carbonate showed a disruption in the blood-nerve barrier by 7 weeks that was accompanied by an increase in endoneurial fluid pressure secondary to endoneurial edema. Lead moved into the endoneurial compartment, resulting in degenerative changes in the Schwann cells (67,68). Nerve biopsy material from humans affected only by lead without accompanying confounders such as alcoholism or other medical conditions are so limited that it is not possible to rule out the presence of a similar pathology.

Even though lead neuropathy presents with motor abnormalities, nerve conduction studies show the sensory fibers to be altered first (14). Detailed EMG studies of individuals with known lead neuropathy found absent sensory-mixed nerve potentials, sensory conduction slowing, diminished amplitude of sensory potentials and compound motor action potentials, and slowing of motor conduction (63,64,69). An extensive review of lead neuropathy by Ehle (70) in 1986 reports that abnormal EMG activity only correlated with blood lead above 70 g/dl. However, group analysis of lead-exposed workers examined longitudinally with NCS showed no adverse effect for blood lead levels below 40 g/dl (71–73). Thirty-two studies of lead-exposed workers used in a meta-analysis had a mean blood lead ranging from 16 to 70 g/dl, a decrease in nerve conduction velocity (NCV) in 82% of the results, and significant slowing in 60% of median nerve studies as compared to 30% for the ulnar nerve (74). The meta-analysis supported the finding of reduced NCV in lead-exposed workers, with the median motor nerve most frequently involved. There was concern that blood lead was not the appropriate measure of exposure. Conduction velocities were more slowed with longer exposure duration. However, at higher blood lead levels conduction velocities were faster compared to the reference group. This paradoxical relationship may explain the lack of consistent effects between blood lead and peripheral nerve studies. It also emphasizes the need for a more critical examination of dose. Blood lead is not necessarily correlated with past cumulative lead exposure and therefore is not the appropriate index of dose for an outcome that requires months of exposure (75).

Reports of treatment for lead neuropathy include $CaNa_2$ ethylenediaminetetraacetic acid (EDTA) chelation (69,76) and removal from exposure. Muijser et al. (77) followed workers with 5 months of high lead exposure to illustrate that the decreased motor conduction velocity returned to normal 15 months after the cessation of exposure. However, it is unlikely that a lead neuropathy due to blood levels >70 g/dl present for many years would resolve this quickly following removal from exposure, since lead derived from elevated bone lead stores would keep blood lead elevated (75).

## MERCURY

Chloralkali plants, pharmaceuticals, agriculture, mercury switches, and paper and plastics industries use mercury. Elemental mercury and mercury vapor may cause peripheral neuropathy, but it is not clear that the same holds for organic mercury. Cumulative mercury exposure measured as bone burden was related to the presence of polyneuropathy in dentists involved in the preparation of amalgam fillings (78).

Workers with inorganic mercury exposure in chloralkali plants (79,80) have sensory loss by QST for touch-pressure, two-point discrimination, vibration, and pin pain in a distribution involving the distal extremities. Electrodiagnostic evaluation along with the clinical examination showed a sensory neuropathy associated with an elevated urine mercury level. In a second study Albers et al. (81) examined workers 20 to 35 years following occupational elemental mercury exposure. The dose-effect relationship between sensory measures in the extremities and peak urinary mercury levels showed

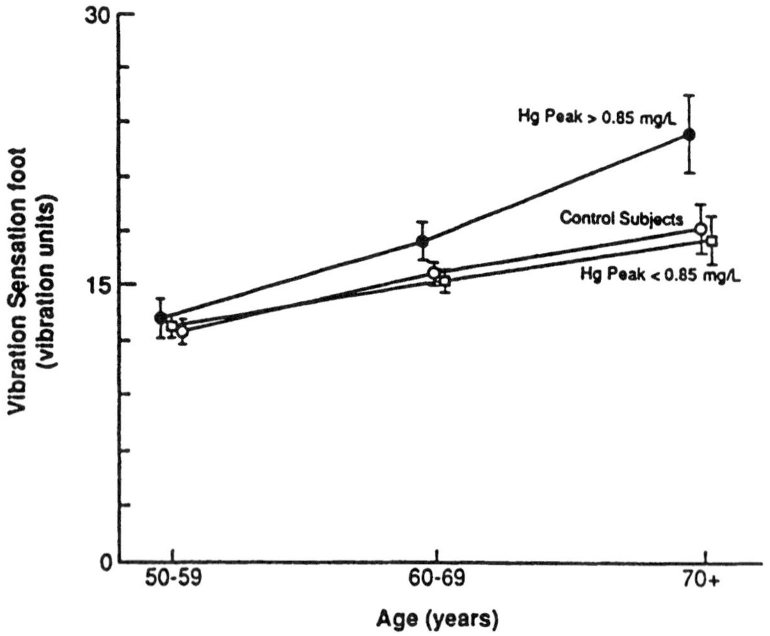


**FIG. 1.** Demonstration of age-mercury interaction. Vibration sensation (foot) as a function of age for control subjects *(open circles)* and subjects with two levels of mercury exposure, peak <0.85 mg/L *(squares)* and peak >0.85 mg/L *(closed circles).* Vibration units are proportional to log-scaled displacement. Standard error is represented by vertical bars. (From ref. 81, with permission.)

27% had equivocal or definite neuropathy in the lowest quartile as compared to 43% in the highest quartile. This is one of the few studies that demonstrates a significant age-exposure interaction (Fig. 1). Significant age-exposure interaction was found for proximal and distal strength, quantitative tremor, touch-pressure sensation (foot), vibration sensation (foot), two-point discrimination, and number of motor nerve abnormalities.

D-penicillamine used for chelation of mercury in the past has raised concerns that in the chelating process more mercury is mobilized into the nervous system.

## METHYL BROMIDE

From the annual use of 66 Gg (1 Gg = $10^9$ g) of methyl bromide as a pesticide, significant environmental contamination from bromine results (82). Its use as a fumigant requires that methyl bromide volatilizes under sealed polyethylene sheeting. Neurologic symptoms related to methyl bromide occur at bromide levels of 2.8 mg/dl, while bromism from inorganic bromides occurs at levels of 50 mg/dl (83). Methyl bromide, as with other heavy metals, is believed to attach to sulfhydryl groups and thereby compromise complex enzyme systems (84).

Acute exposure produces psychiatric disturbances including disorientation, hallucinations, paranoia, anxiety, depression, and euphoria. Visual symptoms are common along with speech abnormalities and myoclonic jerks.

Inhalation of vapor may produce headaches, weakness, muscle tenderness, heaviness of the legs, and paresthesia. Examination shows impaired sensation and strength in the distal extremities, absent reflexes in the legs, very tender calf muscles, and ataxia of gait (85). Follow-up examination after 6 months found a normal neurologic examination.

## NITROUS OXIDE

Nitrous oxide, an inhalational anesthetic, is used by dental practitioners. The greatest exposure occurs from abuse because of its euphoriant properties; compressed nitrous oxide contained in cartridges used to dispense whipped cream is inhaled (86). Chronic exposure may produce a myeloneuropathy; however, even a single exposure to nitrous oxide may produce the identical condition when subclinical serum cobalamin deficiency exists (87). Nitrous oxide interferes with cobalamin activity and therefore clinically appears similar to $B_{12}$ deficiency. However, abstinence from nitrous oxide without $B_{12}$ supplements is sufficient for reversal of the myeloneuropathy (88).

In nitrous oxide–induced myeloneuropathy, axonal neuropathy and myeloneuropathy predominate (88–92). The most common clinical presentation consists of paresthesia and weakness in the limbs, sometimes producing disequilibrium. Nerve conduction studies found slowed motor and sensory conduction velocity both proximally and distally (92,93). Somatosensory evoked potentials from the tibial nerve showed prolonged latencies (92). As with other toxic neuropathies abstinence improves the neuropathy.

## ORGANOPHOSPHORUS COMPOUNDS

The primary utilization of organophosphorus (OP) compound is as pesticides. Other uses of OP agents include plasticizers, stabilizers in lubricating and hydraulic oils, flame retardants, and gasoline additives. The most common clinical presentation of OP toxicity is secondary to acetylcholinesterase inhibition of muscarinic and nicotinic receptors (94). The organophosphate-induced delayed neuropathy (OPIDN) that may occur 1 to 3 weeks following exposure (95) involves the inhibition of a different esterase, neuropathy target esterase (NTE) (96). It is important to remember that not all OP compounds inhibit NTE. OP compounds capable of NTE inhibition may produce a neuropathy but require different levels of inhibition. Usually 70% to 80% inhibition of NTE with aging is required before OPIDN develops; however, OP compounds that inhibit NTE but do not age may cause OPIDN at higher levels of NTE inhibition (90–100%). Aging refers to an intramolecular rearrangment of the phosphorylated NTE that leaves the enzyme irreversibly inhibited (97). OP agents that inhibit NTE, but do not age, have the potential to protect against the development of OPIDN if administered at low doses prior to the neuropathic OP compound. This same OP compound that provided protection by blocking the active site of NTE is capable of initiating or promoting OPIDN if administered after the neuropathic OP compound (97–100). For example, phenylmethanesulfonyl fluoride (PMSF), capable of inhibiting NTE, does not produce OPIDN when given alone (unless in high and repeated doses), but it was able to promote OPIDN when NTE was previously partially inhibited by diisopropyl phosphorofluoridate or chlorpyrifos (Fig. 2) (98). In another example, phenyl *N*-methyl *N*-benzyl carbamate inhibits NTE (>90%) without aging; OPIDN does not develop (unless in high and repeated doses). When PMSF administration followed the carbamate, clinical neuropathy developed (101). This new principle of promotion of OPIDN derived from animal studies will be important to incorporate into human exposure assessment, particularly in the farming industry where combinations of exposure to OP compounds occurs. In humans, OP compounds reported to cause OPIDN include chlorpyrifos, dichlorvos, ethyl 4-nitrophenyl phenylphosphonothionate (EPN), leptophos, methamidophos, mipafox, omethoate, parathion, tri-ortho-cresyl phosphate (TOCP), trichlorfon, and trichlornat (99).

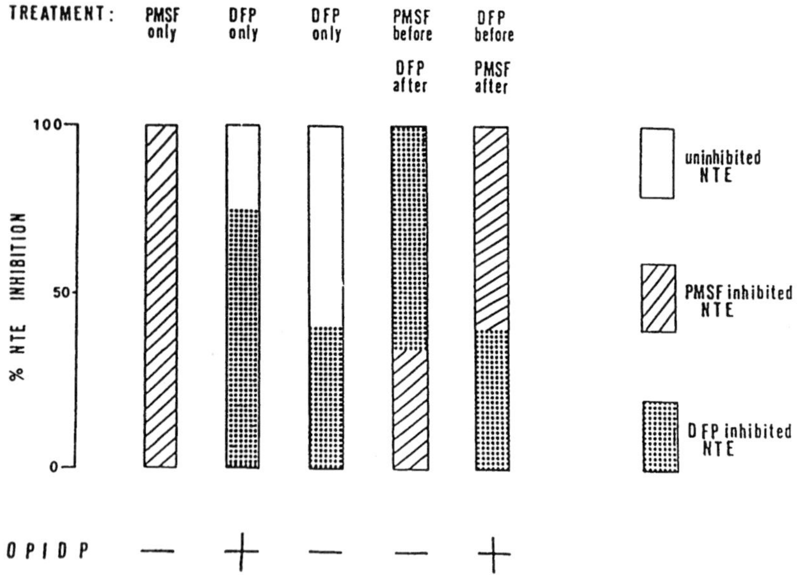


**FIG. 2.** Explicative summary of initiation, protection, and promotion of OPIDN. Relationships among dosing, NTE in inhibition, and clinical responses when diisopropyl phosphorofluoridate (DFP) and PMSF are given alone or in combination. (From ref. 98, with permission.)

Organophosphate-induced delayed neuropathy begins 1 to 3 weeks after exposure and therefore may develop after the individual is discharged from the hospital following treatment for acute cholinergic symptoms. Onset of symptoms begins with cramping in the legs that may progress to weakness, followed by similar symptoms in the arms. Sensory symptoms, if present, begin as numbness and tingling in the feet that may progress to the hands. Sensory abnormalities, if present on examination, are overshadowed by motor abnormalities. Balance is impaired when bilateral footdrop occurs (102). Even with recovery from the peripheral neuropathy, a spastic paraparesis may persist due to involvement of long tracts in the spinal cord (103).

An intermediate syndrome, OP-induced myopathy, occurs 24 to 96 hours after acute poisoning (104,105) with paralysis of the respiratory muscles. Respiratory insufficiency is accompanied by weakness in the proximal limb muscles, neck flexors, and cranial nerve palsies. An earlier case (106) in which the authors were able to examine the diaphragm showed segmental muscle fiber necrosis similar to that in animal models. In OP-induced myopathy the underlying mechanism is believed to be overstimulation of the postsynaptic muscle fiber membrane by acetylcholine overflow, leading to muscle necrosis. In contrast to OPIDN, atropine protects from OP-induced myopathy (94).

As in other toxic neuropathies, the larger and longer nerve fibers are more vulnerable (107) in a central-peripheral dying-back pattern. Even though sensory symptoms are a minor feature of OPIDN, diminished sensory potential amplitude is present early in the development of the neuropathy. Normal motor nerve conduction velocity is frequently found because large diameter fibers are not selectively affected (108).

Atropine, the standard treatment for the cholinergic symptoms, has no benefit for the neuropathy; in fact, there is no treatment for OPIDN.

## THALLIUM

Thallium is chiefly found as an impurity in pyrites. Therefore, exposure may occur from flue dust residues of zinc and lead smelters. Use of thallium-containing rodenticides was discontinued in 1965, but thallium-handling cement plants still pose a potential for exposure.

Thallium intoxication affects numerous organ systems including gastrointestinal, liver, kidney, muscle, and nerves. Numerous affected areas in the nervous system include the cranial nerves, autonomic nerves, spinal ganglia, posterior columns, anterior horn cells, and areas of cortex and basal ganglia. Painful paresthesia begins after a few days. A motor neuropathy is responsible for weakness, but reflexes are maintained until late in the course. Muscle tenderness, arthralgia, and rash follow. The hallmark of thallium intoxication is hair loss that begins after 1 to 3 weeks. Autonomic dysfunction may contribute to the alopecia and produces tachycardia, hypertension, increased salivation, and fever (109).

Nerve conduction studies are usually normal or show mild changes suggestive of axonal loss. Nerve biopsies late in the clinical course find both demyelinization and axonal destruction (110). Animal studies of the neuropathy found vacuolization of axons beneath the nodes of Ranvier. These vacuoles are filled with dilated mitochondria (111). Human nerve biopsies show axonal vacuoles (112,113). The mechanism for thallium toxicity in the nervous system is not known but the pattern is similar to other dying-back neuropathies with distal peripheral axonal disintegration and proximal fiber preservation (114).

## TRICHLOROETHYLENE

Trichloroethylene, a solvent, is primarily used as a degreasing agent in a wide range of operations from heavy construction to the manufacture of microcomputers. If a surface is to be soldered, welded, or coated, it will be made clean of oils and impurities with trichloroethylene. As with other solvents, prenarcotic symptoms, dizziness, fatigue, mental confusion, headaches, loss of coordination, and nausea occur at relatively low levels (114). In the past trichloroethylene was used as an anesthetic and to treat trigeminal neuralgia. Compared to other halogenated hydrocarbons it is a weak carcinogen (115). Trichloroethylene alters alcohol metabolism, leading to intolerance and flushing of the skin in humans. Cardiac and hepatic abnormalities occur but principally the nervous system is involved.

The etiology of the trigeminal neuropathy associated with tricholorethylene is controversial since originally it developed when trichloroethylene reacted with soda lime during anesthesia to form dichloroacetylene, a known neurotoxin with specific effects on the trigeminal nerve. Removal of the soda lime rebreathing canister during anesthesia eliminated trigeminal neuropathy (116). In spite of this controversy many reports in the literature indicate facial numbness in workers exposed to trichloroethylene. Acute exposure inside the boiler-feed tanks of a frigate resulted in the death of a worker who complained of severe headache, dizziness, and unsteadiness at the end of shift. Postmortem studies found demyelination of the fifth nerve tracts and nuclei, particularly the sensory divisions (117). It has been argued that occupational exposure frequently provided conditions that allowed for the formation of dichloroacetylene (118). Other hypotheses for the trigeminal neuropathy include reactivation of orofacial herpes simplex (119) and vascular permeability in that brain stem area (120).

Integrity of the trigeminal nerve as measured in the blink reflex, shows a dose-effect relationship with indices of trichloroethylene dose (121). Trigeminal somatosensory evoked potentials are correlated with facial numbness and exposure (122). A case report attributed trigeminal sensory loss and peripheral neuropathy to trichloroethylene exposure from a leaking overheated degreasing machine (123), but overall peripheral neuropathy is not an outcome found with trichloroethylene exposure.

## REFERENCES


1. Prineas J. Polyneuropathies of undetermined cause. *Acta Neurol Scand* 1970;46:4–72.
2. Dyck PJ, Oviatt KF, Lambert EH. Intensive evaluation of referred unclassified neuropathies yields improved diagnosis. *Ann Neurol* 1981;10:222–226.
3. Munsat TL. *Quantification of neurologic deficit.* Stoneham, MA: Butterworth, 1989.
4. Fullerton PM. Toxic chemicals and peripheral neuropathy. *Proc R Soc Med* 1969;62:201–210.
5. Bleecker ML, Lindgren KN, Ford DP. Differential contribution of current and cumulative indices of lead dose to neuropsychological performance by age. *Neurology* 1997;48:639–645.
6. Hopkins AP, Morgan-Hughes JA. The effect of local pressure in diphtheritic neuropathy. *J Neurol Neurosurg Psychiatry* 1969;32: 614–623.
7. Shimpo T, Gilliatt RW, Kennett RP, Allen PJ. Susceptibility to pressure neuropathy distal to a constricting ligature in the guinea-pig. *J Neurol Neurosurg Psychiatry* 1987;50:1625–1632.
8. Bleecker ML. *Occupational neurology and clinical neurotoxicology.* Baltimore, MD: Williams and Wilkins, 1994.
9. Chaudhry V, Rowinshy EK, Sartorius SE, Donehower RC, Cornblath DR. Peripheral neuropathy from Taxol and cisplatin combination chemotherapy: clinical and electrophysiological studies. *Ann Neurol* 1994;25:304–311.
10. Chaudhry V, Eisenberger MA, Sinibaldi VJ, Sheikh K, Griffin JW, Cornblath DR. A prospective study of suramin-induced peripheral neuropathy. *Brain* 1996;119:101–114.
11. Yarnitsky D. Quantitative sensory testing. *Muscle Nerve* 1997;20: 198–204.
12. Chado HN. The current perception threshold evaluation of sensory nerve function in pain management. *Pain Digest* 1995;5:127–134.
13. Dyck PJ, Zimmerman I, Gillen DA, Johnson D, Karnes JL, O'Brien PC. Cool, Warm, and heat-pain detection thresholds: testing methods and inferences about anatomic distribution of receptors. *Neurology* 1993;43:1500–1508.
14. LeQuesne PM. Electrophysiological investigation of toxic neuropathies in man. 6th International Congress of EMG. *Acta Neurol Scand* 1979;60:54–55.
15. Chaudhry V, Cornblath DR, Mellits ED, et al. Inter- and intra-examiner reliability of nerve conduction measurements in normal subjects. *Ann Neurol* 1991;30:841–843.
16. Dyck PJ, Litchy WJ, Lehman KA, Hokanson JL, Low PA, O'Brian PC. Variables influencing neuropathic endpoints: the Rochester Diabetic Neuropathy Study of Healthy Subjects. *Neurology* 1995;45: 1115–1121.
17. Spencer PS, Schaumburg HH. Central-peripheral distal axonopathy—the pathology of dying-back polyneuropathies. In: Zimmerman HM, ed. *Progress in neuropathology.* New York: Grune & Stratton, 1976; 253–295.
18. Korobkin R, Asbury AK, Sumner AJ, Nielsen SL. Glue-sniffing neuropathy. *Arch Neurol* 1975;219:159.
19. Spencer PS, Schaumburg HH. *Experimental and clinical neurotoxicology.* Baltimore: Williams & Wilkins, 1980.
20. Fullerton PM. Electrophysiological and histological observations on peripheral nerves in acrylamide poisoning in man. *J Neurol Neurosurg Psychiatry* 1969;32:186–192.
21. LeQuesne PM. Acrylamide. In: Spencer PS, Schaumburg HH, eds. *Experimental and clinical neurotoxicology.* Baltimore, MD: Williams & Wilkins, 1980;309–325.
22. Arezzo JC, Schaumberg HH, Petersen CA. Rapid screening for peripheral neuropathy: a field study with Optacon. *Neurology* 1983;33: 626–629.
23. EPA. *Protein adduct forming chemicals for exposure monitoring:* literature, *summary, and recommendations.* Washington, DC: USEPA 1990;134.
24. Costa LG, Manzo L. Biochemical markers of neurotoxicity: research strategies and epidemiological applications. *Toxicol Lett* 1995;77: 137–144.
25. Donofrio PD, Wilbourn AJ, Albers JW, Rogers L, Salanga V, Greenberg HS. Acute arsenic intoxication presenting as Guillain-Barré–like syndrome. *Muscle Nerve* 1987;10:114–120.
26. Feldman RG, Niles CA, Kelly-Haynes M, et al. Peripheral neuropathy in arsenic smelter workers. *Neurology* 1979;29:939–944.
27. Foa V, Colombi A, Maroni M. The speciation of the chemical forms of arsenic in the biological monitoring of exposure to inorganic arsenic. *Sci Total Environ* 1984;34:241–259.
28. Sexton GB, Gowdey CW. Relation between thiamine and arsenic toxicity. *Arch Dermatol Syph* 1963;56:634–647.
29. Beauchamp RO, Bus JS, Popp JA, Boreiko CJ, Goldberg L. A critical review of the literature on carbon disulfide toxicity. *CRC Crit Rev Toxicol* 1983;11:169–278.
30. ACGIH. *Carbon disulfide. Documentation of the threshold limit values and biological exposure markers,* 6th ed. Washington, DC: ACGIH, 1991;224–227.

31. Seppalainen A, Tolonen MT. Neurotoxicity of long-term exposure to carbon disulfide in the viscose rayon industry: a neurophysiological study. *J Scand Work Environ Health* 1974;11:145–153.
32. Chu CC, Huang CC, Chen RS, Shih TS. Polyneuropathy induced by carbon disulfide in viscose rayon workers. *Occup Environ Med* 1995; 52:404–407.
33. Vanhoorne MH, Ceulemans L, DeBacquer DA, DeSmet FP. An epidemiological study of the effects of carbon disulfide on the peripheral nerve. *Int J Occup Environ Health* 1995;1:295–302.
34. Seppalainen AM, Haltia M. Carbon disulfide. In: Spencer PS, Schaumburg HH, eds. *Experimental and clinical neurotoxicology.* Baltimore: Williams & Wilkins, 1980;356–370.
35. Teisinger J. Some mechanisms of chronic carbon disulfide poisoning. *Prac Lek* 1971;23:306.
36. Keogh JP, Pestronk A, Wertheimer D, Moreland R. An epidemic of urinary retention caused by dimethylaminopropionitrile. *JAMA* 1980; 243:746–749.
37. Kreiss K, Wegman DH, Niles CA, Siroky MB, Krane RJ, Feldman RG. Neurologic dysfunction of the bladder in workers exposed to dimethylaminopropionitrile. *JAMA* 1980;243:741–745.
38. Pestronk A, Keogh JP, Griffin JW. Dimethylaminopropionitrile. In: Spencer PS, Schaumburg HH, eds. *Experimental and clinical neurotoxicology.* Baltimore: Williams & Wilkins, 1980;422–429.
39. CDC. Occupationally related neurologic abnormalities. *MWMR* 1981; 30:365–366.
40. Pestronk A, Keogh JP, Griffin JW. Dimethylaminopropionitrile (DMAPN) intoxication: a new industrial neuropathy. *Neurology* 1979; 29:540.
41. Ohnishi A, Inoue N, Yamamoto T, et al. Ethylene oxide neuropathy in rats exposed to 250 ppm. *J Neurol Sci* 1986;74:215–221.
42. Yager JW, Hines CJ, Spear RC. Exposure to ethylene oxide at work increases sister chromatid exchanges in human peripheral lymphocytes. *Science* 1983;219:1121–1123.
43. Klees JE, Lash A, Bowler RM, Shore M, Becker CE. Neuropsychologic "impairment" in a cohort of hospital workers chronically exposed to ethylene oxide. *J Clin Toxicol* 1990;28:21–28.
44. Crystal HA, Schaumburg HH, Grober E, Fuld PA, Lipton RB. Cognitive impairment and sensory loss associated with chronic low-level ethylene oxide exposure. *Neurology* 1988;38:567–569.
45. Brashear A, Unverzagt FW, Farber MO, Bonnin JM, Garcia JGN, Grober E. Ethylene oxide neurotoxicity: a cluster of 12 nurses with peripheral and central nervous system toxicity. *Neurology* 1996;46: 992–998.
46. Kuzuhara S, Kanazawa I, Nakanishi T, Egashira T. Ethylene oxide polyneuropathy. *Neurology* 1983;33:377–380.
47. Gross JA, Haas ML, Swift TR. Ethylene oxide neurotoxicity: report of four cases and review of the literature. *Neurology* 1979;29: 978–983.
48. Finelli PF, Morgan TF, Yaar I, Granger CV. Ethylene oxide-induced polyneuropathy: a clinical and electrophysiologic study. *Arch Neurol* 1983;40:419–421.
49. Graham DG, Anthony DC, Boekelheide K, et al. Studies of the molecular pathogenesis of hexane neuropathy. II. Evidence that pyrrole derivatization of lysyl residues leads to protein cross-linking. *Toxicol Appl Pharmacol* 1982;64:415–422.
50. Passero S, Battistini N, Cioni R, et al. Toxic polyneuropathy of shoe workers in Italy. A clinical, neurophysiological and follow-up study. *Ital J Neurol* 1983;4:463.
51. Yokoyama K, Feldman RG, Sax DS, Salzsider BT, Kucera J. Relation of distribution of conduction velocities to nerve biopsy findings in *n*-hexane poisoning. *Muscle Nerve* 1990;13:314–320.
52. Huang C, Shih T, Cheng S, Chen S, Tchen P. *n*-Hexane polyneuropathy in a ball-manufacturing factory. *J Occup Med* 1991;33:139–142.
53. Pastore C, Marhuenda D, Marti J, Cardona A. Early diagnosis of *n*-hexane-caused neuropathy. *Muscle Nerve* 1994;17:981–986.
54. Barregard L, Sallsten G, Nordborg C, Gieth W. Polyneuropathy possibly caused by 30 years of low exposure to *n*-hexane. *Scand J Work Environ Health* 1991;17:205–207.
55. Altenkirch H, Mager J, Stoltenburg G, Helmbrecht. Toxic polyneuropathies after sniffing a glue thinner. *J Neurol* 1977;214:137–152.
56. Altenkirch H, Wagner HM, Stoltenburg-Didinger G, Steppat R. Potentiation of hexacarbon-neurotoxicity by methyl-ethyl-ketone (MEK) and other substances: clinical and experimental aspects. *Neurobehav Toxicol Teratol* 1982;4:623–627.
57. Allen N, Mendell JR, Billmaier DJ, Fontaine RE, O'Neill J. Toxic polyneuropathy due to methyl *n*-butyl ketone: an industrial outbreak. *Arch Neurol* 1975;32:209–218.
58. Saida K, Mendell JR, Weiss HS. Peripheral changes induced by methyl *n*-butyl ketone and potentiation by methyl ethyl ketone. *J Neuropathol Neurol* 1976;35:207–224.
59. Billmaier D, Yee HT, Craft B, et al. Peripheral neuropathy in a coated fabrics plant. *J Occup Med* 1974;16:665–671.
60. Bleecker ML, Bolla KI, Agnew J, Schwartz BS, Ford DP. Dose-related subclinical neurobehavioral effects of chronic exposure to low levels of organic solvents. *Am J Ind Med* 1991;19:715–728.
61. Cantarow A, Trumper M. *Lead poisoning.* Baltimore, MD: Williams & Wilkins, 1944.
62. Boothby JA, DeJesus PV, Rowland LP. Reversible forms of motor neuron disease; lead "neuritis." *Arch Neurol* 1974;31:18–22.
63. Buchthal F, Behse F. Electrophysiology and nerve biopsy in men exposed to lead. *Br J Ind Med* 1979;26:135–147.
64. Oh JS. Lead neuropathy: case report. *Arch Phys Med Rehabil* 1975; 56:312–317.
65. Fullerton PM. Chronic peripheral neuropathy produced by lead poisoning in guinea pigs. *J Neuropathol Exp Neurol* 1966;25: 214–236.
66. Hopkins A. Experimental lead poisoning in the baboon. *Br J Ind Med* 1970;27:130–140.
67. Ohnishi A, Schilling K, Brimijoin WS, Lambert EH, Fairbanks VF, Dyck PJ. Lead neuropathy. *J Neuropathol Exp Neurol* 1977;36: 499–518.
68. Myers RR, Powell HC, Shapiro HM, Costello ML, Lampert PW. Changes in endoneurial fluid pressure, permeability, and peripheral nerve ultrastructure in experimental lead neuropathy. *Ann Neurol* 1979;8:392–401.
69. Wu P, Kingery WS, Date ES. An EMG case report of lead neuropathy 19 years after a shotgun injury. *Muscle Nerve* 1995;18:326–329.
70. Ehle A. Lead Neuropathy and electrophysiological studies in low level lead exposure: a critical review. *Neurotoxicology* 1986;7:203–216.
71. Seppalainen AM, Hernberg S, Vesanto R. Early neurotoxic effects of occupational lead exposure: a prospective study. *Neurotoxicology* 1983;4:181–192.
72. Zi-qiang C, Qi-ing C, Chin-chin P, Jia-ying Q. Peripheral nerve conduction velocity in workers occupationally exposed to lead. *Scand J Work Environ Health* 1985;4:26–28.
73. Chia S, Chia K, Chia H, Ong C, Jeyaratnam J. Three-year follow-up of serial nerve conduction among lead-exposed workers. *Scand J Work Environ Health* 1996;22:374–380.
74. Davis JM, Svendsgaard DJ. *Nerve conduction velocity and lead:* A critical review and meta-analysis. *Advances in neurobehavioral toxicology.* Chelsea, MI: Lewis, 1990:353–376.
75. Bleecker ML, McNeil FE, Lindgren KN, Masten VL, Ford DP. Relationship between bone lead and other indices of lead exposure in smelter workers. *Toxicol Lett* 1995;80:173–174.
76. Araki S, Honma T, Ushio K. Recovery of slowed nerve conduction velocity in lead-exposed workers. *Int Arch Occup Environ Health* 1980;46:151–157.
77. Muijser H, Hoogendijk E, Hooisma J, Twisk D. Lead exposure during demolition of a steel structure coated with lead-based paints. *Scand J Work Environ Health* 1987;13:56–61.
78. Shapiro IM, Cornblath DR, Sumner AJ, et al. Neurophysiological and neuropsychological functions in mercury-exposed dentists. *Lancet* 1982;i:1147–1150.
79. Albers JW, Cavender D, Levine SP, Langolf GD. Asymptomatic sensorimotor polyneuropathy in workers exposed to elemental mercury. *Neurology* 1982;32:1168–1174.
80. Levine SP, Cavender GD, Langolf GD, Albers JW. Elemental mercury exposure: peripheral neurotoxicity. *Br J Ind Med* 1982;39: 136–139.
81. Albers JW, Kallenbach LR, Fine LJ, et al. Neurological abnormalities associated with remote occupational elemental mercury exposure. *Ann Neurol* 1988;24(5):651–659.
82. Mano S, Andreae MO. Emission of methyl bromide from biomass burning. *Science* 1994;263:1255–1258.
83. Zatuchni J, Hong K. Methyl bromide poisoning seen initially as psychosis. *Arch Neurol* 1981;38:529–530.
84. Rathus EM, Landy PJ. Methyl bromide poisoning. *Br J Ind Med* 1960;18:53–57.

85. Kantarjian AD, Shaheen AS. Methyl bromide poisoning with nervous system manifestations resembling polyneuropathy. *Neurology* 1963; 13:1054–1058.
86. Sahenk Z, Mendell JR, Couri D, Nachtman J. Polyneuropathy from inhalation of $N_2O$ cartridges through a whipped cream dispenser. *Neurology* 1978;28:485–487.
87. Kinsella LJ, Green R. "Anesthesia paresthetica": nitrous oxide-induced cobalamin deficiency. *Neurology* 1995;45:1608–1610.
88. Layzer RB, Fishman RA, Schafer JA. Neuropathy following abuse of nitrous oxide. *Neurology* 1978;28:504–506.
89. Layzer RB. Myeloneuropathy after prolonged exposure to nitrous oxide. *Lancet* 1978;2:1227–1230.
90. Gutman L, Farrell B, Crosby T, Johnson D. Nitrous oxide-induced myelopathy-neuropathy: potential for chronic misuse by dentists. *J Am Dent Assoc* 1979;98:58–59.
91. Blanco G, Peters HA. Myeloneuropathy and macrocytosis associated with nitrous oxide abuse. *Arch Neurol* 1983;40:416–418.
92. Heyer EJ, Simpson DM, Bodis-Wollner I, Diamond SP. Nitrous oxide: clinical and electrophysiologic investigation of neurologic complications. *Neurology* 1986;36:1618–1622.
93. Vishnubhakat SM, Beresford HR. Reversible myeloneuropathy of nitrous oxide abuse: serial electrophysiological studies. *Muscle Nerve* 1991;14:22–26.
94. De Bleecker JL, De Reuck JL, Willems JL. Neurological aspects of organophosphate poisoning. *Clin Neurol Neurosurg* 1992;94: 93–103.
95. Lotti M, Becker CE, Aminoff MJ. Organophosphate polyneuropathy: pathogenesis and prevention. *Neurology* 1984;34:658–662.
96. Johnson MK. The target for initiation of delayed neurotoxicity by organophosphate esters: biochemical studies and toxicological applications. *Rev Biochem Toxicol* 1982;4:141–212.
97. Lotti M, Caroldi S, Capodicasa E, Moretto A. Promotion of organophosphate induced delayed polyneuropathy by phenylmethanesulfonyl fluoride. *Toxicol Appl Pharmacol* 1991;108:234–241.
98. Pope CN, Padilla S. Potentiation of organophosphorus induced delayed neurotoxicity by phenylmethylsulfonyl fluoride. *J Toxicol Environ Health* 1990;31:261–273.
99. Lotti M. The pathogenesis of organophosphate polyneuropathy. *Crit Rev Toxicol* 1992;21:465–487.
100. Lotti M, Moretto A, Capodicasa E, Bertolazzi M, Peraica M, Scapellato ML. Interactions between neuropathy target esterase and its inhibitors and the development of polyneuropathy. *Toxicol Appl Pharmacol* 1993;122:165–171.
101. Moretto A, Bertolazzi E, Capodicasa M, et al. Phenylmethanesulfonyl fluoride elicits and intensifies the clinical expression of neuropathic insults. *Arch Toxicol* 1992;66:67–72.
102. Bidstrup PL, Bonnell JA, Beckett AG. Paralysis following poisoning by a new organic phosphorous insecticide (mipafox). *Br Med J* 1953; 1:1068–1072.
103. Morgan JP, Penovich P. Jamaica ginger paralysis. *Arch Neurol* 1978; 35:530–532.
104. Senanayake N, Karalliedde L. Neurotoxic effects of organophosphate insecticides. An intermediate syndrome. *N Engl J Med* 1987; 316:761–763.
105. Karademir M, Erturk F, Kocak R. Two cases of organophosphate poisoning with development of intermediate syndrome. *Hum Exp Toxicol* 1990;9:187.
106. De Reuck J, Colardyn F, Willems J. Fatal encephalopathy in acute poisoning with organophosphorus insecticides. A clinico-pathologic study of two cases. *Clin Neurol Neurosurg* 1979;81:247–254.
107. Spencer PS, Schaumburg HH. Pathobiology of neurotoxic axonal degeneration. In: Waxman SG, ed. *Physiology and pathobiology of axons.* New York: Raven Press, 1978;265–282.
108. Le Quesne PM. *Neurotoxic substances. Modern trends in neurology.* London: Butterworth, 1975;6:83–97.
109. Bank WJ. Thallium. In: Spencer PS, Schaumburg HH, eds. *Experimental and clinical neurotoxicology.* Baltimore: Williams & Wilkins, 1980;570–577.
110. Gastel B. Thallium poisoning: clinical conferences at the Johns Hopkins Hospital. *Johns Hopkins Med J* 1978;142:27–31.
111. Spencer PS, et al. Effects of thallium salts on neuronal mitochondria in organotypic cord-ganglia-muscle combination cultures. *J Cell Biol* 1973;58:79.
112. Bank WJ. Thallium poisoning. *Arch Neurol* 1972;26:456–464.
113. Cavanaugh JB, Fuller NH, Johnson P. The effects of thallium slats with particular reference to nervous system changes. *Q J Med* 1974; 43:293–319.
114. Lilis R, Stanescu D, Muica N, Roventa A. Chronic effects of trichloroethylene exposure. *Med Lav* 1969;60:595–601.
115. Laid RJ, Stockle G, Bolt HM, Kunz W. Vinyl chloride and trichloroethylene: comparison of alkylating effects of metabolites and induction of preneoplastic enzyme deficiencies in rat liver. *J Cancer Res Clin Oncol* 1979;94:139–147.
116. Pembleton W. Trichloroethylene anesthesia re-evaluated. *Anesth Analg* 1974;53:730–733.
117. Buxton PH, Hayward M. Polyneuritis cranialis associated with industrial trichloroethylene poisoning. *J Neurol Neurosurg Psychiatry* 1967;30:511–518.
118. Lash TL, Green LC. Letters to the editor: blink reflex measurement of effects of trichloroethylene exposure on the trigeminal nerve. *Muscle Nerve* 1993;16:217–218.
119. Cavanagh JB, Buxton PH. Trichloroethylene cranial neuropathy: Is it really a toxic neuropathy or does it activate latent herpes virus? *J Neurol Neurosurg Psychiatry* 1989;52:297–303.
120. Jacobs JM. Vascular permeability and neurotoxicity. *Environ Health Perspect* 1978;26:107–116.
121. Feldman RG, Niles C, Proctor SP, Jabre J. Blink reflex measurement of effects of trichloroethylene exposure on the trigeminal nerve. *Muscle Nerve* 1992;15:490–495.
122. Barret L, Garrel S, Daniel V. Chronic trichloroethylene intoxication: a new approach by trigeminal-evoked potentials? *Arch Environ Health* 1987;42:297–302.
123. Feldman RG, Mayer RM, Taub A. Evidence for peripheral neurotoxic effect of trichloroethylene. *Neurology* 1970;20:599–606.

*Environmental and Occupational Medicine, Third Edition,* edited by William N. Rom.
Published by Lippincott–Raven Publishers,
Philadelphia, 1998.

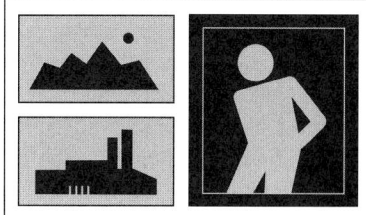

CHAPTER 48

# Human Behavioral Neurotoxicology: Workplace and Community Assessments

W. Kent Anger, Daniel Storzbach, Robert W. Amler, and O. J. Sizemore

Behavioral neurotoxicology is the science of the nontherapeutic effects of chemicals on behavior (1). Although it is a relatively new specialty in toxicology, a steadily growing body of experimental research documents the effects of chemicals on the behavior of humans studied in the laboratory (2), occupational (3), and community (4) settings, and in experimental animal research (5). This chapter focuses on research and methods to identify objective neurobehavioral deficits and psychosocial differences in people exposed to chemicals in the workplace or the community.

Human behavioral neurotoxicology in the United States began in the early 1960s as a result of the progress in behavioral pharmacology, the interest of toxicologists and government regulators who recommended or set occupational and environmental standards, and the lower Soviet exposure limits based on evidence from Pavlovian conditioning research (6–8). This field of research has now grown to encompass four objectives:

1. Detect and monitor adverse effects of exposure to neurotoxic chemicals, using noninvasive methods.
2. Identify functional nervous system impairment occurring at exposure concentrations below those associated with tissue damage.
3. Provide objective functional correlates of clinical signs and symptoms as a complement to other methods (e.g., neurologic).
4. Detect impaired behavior that could compromise safe job performance or normal development.

Human behavioral neurotoxicology research has developed along two fronts: (a) epidemiologic studies of occupational groups or community residents designed to detect the effects of chronic exposures; and (b) laboratory exposure of human volunteers to low concentrations of occupational or environmental chemicals to detect reversible effects of brief acute exposures. The 1980s and 1990s saw tremendous growth in the number and breadth of behavioral studies in the workplace (3,9), the community (4), and the laboratory (2). This chapter focuses on the epidemiologic literature to (a) describe the neurobehavioral effects of well-established neurotoxic chemicals; (b) provide an overview of human behavioral test methods, and the consensus test batteries and computerized neurobehavioral tests used in occupational and environmental research; and (c) describe procedural steps to conduct an epidemiologic study using behavioral test methods.

## NEUROTOXIC CHEMICALS

Investigations of the behavioral effects of chemical agents continue to build a base of consistent findings. This research seeks to determine whether people exposed to a given chemical or chemical mixture differ from referents not exposed to that chemical. However, the independent (exposure) variable is never measured directly over the full course of exposures. Rather, an index of perhaps one to two decades of exposures to that

W. K. Anger and O. J. Sizemore: Center for Research on Occupational and Environmental Toxicology, Oregon Health Sciences University, Portland, Oregon 97201-3098.

D. Storzbach: Veterans Medical Center, Portland, Oregon 97201.

R. W. Amler: Emory University Center School of Medicine, Agency for Toxic Substances and Disease Registry, U.S. Department of Health and Human Services, Atlanta Georgia 30333.

chemical must be estimated on the basis of employment or residence records, recollection, measures of current (rarely historical) exposures, and measures of current (blood, urine) or recent (tissue or hair sample) body burden of that chemical. This makes comparisons between studies with varying results difficult if not impossible. Nonetheless, the greatest value in this literature lies in its use of comparable or identical tests to study different populations exposed to the same chemicals. Although many of the individual studies can be criticized, the common findings that emerge, despite tests administered in different languages with slightly different protocols, despite different exposure histories, and despite methodologic errors or errors of analysis, are the more compelling for the differences. Thus, the following discussion is limited to chemicals that have been the subject of several studies (3). This is a small number of chemical agents. Further, the analysis focuses on the common methods and findings rather than attempting to identify threshold levels at which effects are first identified. This provides a basis for selecting tests relevant to a given chemical or for evaluating a reported effect of a chemical on a given test.

### Carbon Disulfide

Carbon disulfide ($CS_2$) is a classic neurotoxic solvent. At high concentrations, it produces serious central and peripheral nervous system damage, including a broad range of cognitive, motor, and sensory functions (10–15). The literature reveals abnormal performance on tests for coding, intelligence, memory, spatial relations, vigilance, coordination, and response speed that are replicated in multiple studies (3).

The pioneering research in human work-site behavioral neurotoxicology was conducted by Dr. Helena Hänninen on workers exposed to $CS_2$ in Finland. Hänninen (10,16,17) studied male workers at a viscose rayon factory who were (a) poisoned or symptomatic due to $CS_2$ exposure or (b) asymptomatic but exposed to $CS_2$ for 5 years or more, along with a matched reference group with no $CS_2$ exposure. Average monthly carbon disulfide levels in the workplace air had ranged from 130 to 30 mg/m$^3$ for 20 years, declining over that time. Statistically significant differences were found between the poisoned and unexposed referent groups in most measures involving speed and manual dexterity (Mira test, Santa Ana test), memory (Benton visual retention), coding (Digit Symbol), and other measures of higher intellectual function (Picture Completion, Block Design); smaller differences from the reference group were seen in the exposed but not poisoned workers (18). Hänninen concluded that "Carbon disulfide thus apparently affects the working capacity and sociability of exposed workers earlier than can be diagnosed by purely medical means" (10). This was the first evidence that behavioral measures could serve as early indicators of adverse effects of exposure to a workplace chemical.

More recent research on $CS_2$-exposed workers has supported this conclusion, but at exposure concentrations that may be lower. These include significantly reduced performance of exposed as compared to reference participants on color vision [100-HUE test (15)], performance speed [Bourdon-Wiersma (19,20), simple reaction time (21)], speed and dexterity [Santa Ana (19–21), finger tapping (22)], rate of visual search (Neisser test), spatial relations [Block Design (21,22)], coding [Digit Symbol (22)], other measures of intellectual function [Similarities (22)], attention and memory [Digit Span (22)], and depression [gleaned from the Rorschach personality test (19,20)]. Evidence from a prospective study of textile workers exposed to declining concentrations of $CS_2$ over 15 years suggests that even relatively low concentrations may produce or maintain adverse behavioral effects (14).

In a study of $CS_2$ exposures below 20 ppm for several years in a textile plant, Putz-Anderson and colleagues (23) found that only self-reports of minor symptoms differed between exposed and control participants tested on a battery of behavioral tests, suggesting that such symptoms may be the earliest indicators of the effects of exposure to this solvent.

### Perchloroethylene/Tetrachloroethylene

Performance differences have been reported in workers chronically exposed to perchloroethylene. Seeber (24) tested 101 dry cleaners with a mean exposure level of 30 to 35 ppm (205 mg/m$^3$), compared to 84 store workers. Performance deficits were seen on the Digit Span, Digit Symbol, d2 (vigilance), pattern vision, and Choice Reaction Time tests. More recent reports identify deficits in pattern recognition and reproduction, latency in a pattern memory task (25), color vision (26), and Simple Reaction Time (27). The data remain limited but continue to suggest the need for vigilance for possible neurotoxic effects in dry cleaners and other occupations using perchloroethylene, and even in homes above dry cleaning establishments (28).

### Styrene

Lindström and colleagues (29) in Finland initiated work-site research on styrene, finding clear differences between 98 male workers exposed to styrene during the manufacture of reinforced polyester plastic products and 43 concrete reinforcement workers who were not exposed to styrene. Deficits on Symmetry Drawing, tests of coordination (Symmetry Drawing, Mira test), and vigilance (Bourdon-Wiersma accuracy) were associated with increased urinary mandelic acid (MA) concentrations (29).

Mutti and colleagues (30,31) reported deficits, compared to matched unexposed referents, on Choice Reaction Time, Story Memory (immediate and at 30 minutes), word recall (immediate and at 30 minutes), Block Design, and Embedded Figures in workers building fiberglass silos, but not Digit Symbol, although performance was lower in the fiberglass workers. The ambient styrene exposure varied between 10 and 300 ppm, and the average MA plus phenylglyoxylic acid (PGA) value on the morning after exposure was 306 nmol/mol creatinine. These results were examined for dose-response relationships between the mean MA plus PGA levels of 75, 216, 367, and 571 and performance, revealing Block Design, immediate Story Memory, and Simple Reaction Time deficits associated with three or four doses, and similar results for at least two concentrations were found for the Story Memory at 30 minutes, Embedded Figures, and Digit Symbol.

Reports in the 1990s of workers exposed to styrene have described changes in tests of the same or highly related functions, including decrements in boat manufacturers on the Continuous Performance Test, vibration threshold (32), balance (33), Digit Span, Digit Symbol, and the Benton Visual Retention test (34); in dockyard workers on the Digit Span and Simple Reaction Time (35); and Simple Reaction Time deficits in fiberglass manufacturers (36). These findings were reported in workers exposed to styrene at or below 50 ppm or at comparably low MA or PGA levels. In addition, a number of recent studies have reported color vision deficits in styrene-exposed workers with the Lanthony D-15 or Farnsworth 100 hue test (34,37–40).

While Rebert (41) concludes that many of these reports (or their conclusions) are flawed, there is sufficient consistency in these findings to support further research on low-level styrene exposure. Overall, there is a consistent picture from the styrene research that has employed tests of memory and reaction time, which has found statistically significant differences between styrene-exposed and reference groups (3).

### Toluene

Deficits in tests of memory and attention, coding, and coordination, based on comparisons with control groups, have been reported in workers exposed to toluene (3) at concentrations between 40 and 150 ppm. Foo and colleagues (42) found significant deficits in Digit Span, Digit Symbol, Visual Reproduction, Benton visual retention, Grooved Pegboard, and Trail Making in 30 female electronics workers exposed to a mean of 88 ppm toluene when compared to co-workers with 13 ppm exposures, although these changes were not associated with years of exposure (43). Ørbæk and Nise (44) reported deficits in coding (Digit Symbol), memory (Benton visual retention), and vocabulary (Synonyms) in a study of 30 printers exposed to toluene (43 ppm in one company and 157 ppm in a second company) when compared to 72 referents in various manufacturing occupations. Iregren (45) found differences between 38 rotogravure printers (exposed daily to 50 ppm at the time of the study but to about 150 ppm in prior years) and 38 electronics workers (control data gathered earlier) on a test of Simple Reaction Time, and Cherry et al. (46,47) reported coordination (Grooved Pegboard speed) and reading deficits in 49 rubberized mat workers (exposed daily to about 100 ppm toluene but with peak exposures up to 500 ppm in prior years) as compared to 59 manual laborers not exposed to toluene. Hänninen's group (48) observed greater distractibility (Embedded Figures) and poorer performance in a test of spatial relations (Block Design) in 43 rotogravure printers exposed to a mean toluene concentration of 117 ppm as compared with offset (unexposed) printers. Thus, the Digit Symbol test of coding, tests of attention and memory (Digit Span, Benton Visual Retention), and tests of coordination (Grooved Pegboard) are seen in two of the studies in this very small body of research.

### Solvent Mixtures

Combinations of solvents such as those in motor fuels or released from hazardous waste sites typify problematic occupational and community environmental exposures. Solvent mixtures have been a dominant theme in worksite behavioral research in recent years. The primary issues have been the development of "solvent encephalopathy" in workers chronically exposed in diverse occupations, and the reversibility of the effects of chronic solvent exposure. This has been driven in part by the high workers' compensation costs associated in some European countries with disability in solvent-exposed workers, and concern that these costs could expand.

That chronic high-concentration solvent exposure or abuse can lead to neuropsychiatric disorders and deficits in neurobehavioral test performance has been well established for some time (49,50), although the existence of the phenomenon may remain controversial for some (51,52). Reports continue to surface of cognitive and motor performance deficits in workers exposed to mixed solvents (53–55), and imaging techniques have revealed evidence of increased brain atrophy in at least some solvent-exposed workers (56). Adding to the evidence, Ørbæk (57) points out that performance deficits do not progress after solvent-pensioned individuals are removed from exposure (58,59), and that there is evidence of limited reversibility, especially if the workers receive educational retraining in the affected functions (60). The huge differences in reports of encephalopathy in various countries initially troubled both the scientific and regulatory community, but Mikkelsen (61) has pointed out that the huge differences between criteria for psychiatric diagnoses and disability pensions between countries likely account for these differences.

Each of the many studies of solvent-exposed workers must be viewed as unique in the sense that no two populations could have been exposed to the same solvents or at least to the same history of exposures at similar concentrations (62). The value of this body of research lies in the identification of tests that reveal differences in many studies and are therefore sensitive to a range of solvent exposures. These results can thus serve as a guide to tests for future research aimed at detecting adverse effects of chronic solvent exposures.

Solvent research has particularly focused on cognitive measures. Performance on the Paired Associates test, drawn from the Wechsler Memory Scale (WMS), is the primary measure of learning affected by solvent exposures (18,58,63–65). Reduced performance on a widely used test from the Wechsler Adult Intelligence Scale (WAIS), the Block Design which assesses spatial relations, is also associated with reduced performance following solvent exposures (63,66–76). The Digit Symbol and the computer-implemented version of this test, the Symbol Digit, have emerged as arguably the most universally sensitive test of chemical neurotoxicity, in part because of the extensive reports of effects in solvent research (64,66–68,70–73,77–88). Tests of memory and attention that have detected group differences are the Digit Span (63–65,68,71,73–77, 80,83,89–94) and Benton Visual Retention tests (58,63,73,81,95,96), and the Bourdon-Wiersma test has been the most sensitive test of vigilance (97,98), although computerized tests of this function are recommended because they can provide a great deal more information about performance.

Tests of primarily motor performance that have frequently revealed reduced performance in solvent-exposed workers are the Santa Ana test of coordination and speed (63,68,77,91,97,98) and the Simple Reaction Time test (58,46,47,70,72,79,85,95,99–106). The Farnsworth and Lanthony tests of color vision have also revealed deficits in a number of studies of solvent-exposed workers (107–114).

### Organophosphates

Human research increasingly supports the development of permanent sequelae following acute (115–118) or chronic (119–128) organophosphate (OP) exposure. Three cross-sectional studies conducted on sizable worker populations who met clinical criteria of "poisoning" following OP pesticide exposure incidents provide consistent evidence of permanent effects. In each study, comparable behavioral tests (in some cases the same tests) were administered to detect neurotoxic effects in those workers as compared to referents, and each study reported a very similar although not identical pattern of results. Savage et al. (129) studied 100 workers (drawn from Texas and Colorado pesticide poisoning registries) aged 16 to 70 years with an incident of documented OP exposure and a physician's report of symptoms consistent with OP poisoning during the preceding 16 (Texas) to 26 (Colorado) years. The poisoning incident occurred a minimum of 3 months prior to testing. Rosenstock et al. (130) studied 36 workers aged 15 to 44 years with documented OP poisoning (criteria not specified) drawn from Leon, Nicaragua, hospital discharge records during a 3-year period ending approximately 1 year prior to testing. Steenland et al. (131) recruited 128 males, 16 years and older, reported in the California pesticide illness registry to have OP pesticide poisoning during 1982 to 1990. Each study was comprehensive in recruiting all volunteer participants from their respective selection lists. Each study selected referents matched on key participant variables (age, education), although the referents were referred by the participants themselves.

Significant differences on neurobehavioral tests between referents and exposed subjects were reported by Savage et al. (129) for 19 of 34 (56%), by Rosenstock et al. (130) for 8 of 11 (73%), and by Steenland et al. (131) for 5 of 10 (50%) of the measures they used. There is consistency in the tests that identified significant differences that emerges from very diverse backgrounds, languages, and cultures in these three studies. Deficits, compared to referent performance, emerged in complex cognitive tasks, including coding (Digit Symbol or Symbol Digit) in all three studies, and spatial relations (Block Design), attention (Digit Vigilance and Continuous Performance Test), and attention and memory (Digit Span and Benton Pattern Memory test) in two of the three studies. Response speed and coordination (Tapping) differences were found in two of three studies, and various other motor tests (Aiming, Santa Ana, Grooved Pegboard, Simple Reaction Time) were seen in at least one study but not in a second study. Recent reports by Daniell et al. (125) of orchard pesticide applicators (compared to beef slaughterhouse workers) revealed statistically significant differences on the Digit Symbol, and Stephens et al. (128) of farmers exposed to OPs in sheep dipping (compared to quarry workers) found statistically significant deficits in Symbol Digit, Simple Reaction Time, and (latency to) Syntactic Reasoning (a word classification test), directly supporting the findings in the OP-poisoned patients.

The Savage et al. (129), Rosenstock et al. (130), and Steenland et al. (131) studies suggest strongly that people who have developed clinically observable symptoms following a single, high-concentration OP exposure have deficits in attention, memory, and coordination that persist for many years. The possibility that a background of previous lower-level exposures to other pesticides provides a required substrate or is even causal is an open question.

### Lead

#### *Workers*

The neurobehavioral effects of occupational exposure to inorganic lead have been the subject of more studies than any other chemical found in the environment.

Changes have been reported in psychomotor tasks (hand steadiness, eye-hand coordination), hearing, and psychological functions (hostility, aggression, and general dysphoria) in battery manufacturers with blood lead (PbB) levels between 70 and 79 μg/dl (132). At blood lead concentrations between 30 to 70 μg/dl, significantly slower Simple Reaction Times are frequently reported (133–136), although performance deficits have also been reported on tests of Choice Reaction Time (137,138), strength [e.g., Dynamometer (139)], dexterity [e.g., the Santa Ana (136,140), Tapping (139), Purdue Pegboard (141)], sensory capabilities [e.g., auditory threshold (133)], attention and memory [e.g., Digit Span (139,140), Benton or NES test of visual memory (135,139)], and various tests of higher cognitive function [e.g., Trail Making (136,141), Logical Memory (141), Bourdon-Wiersma (vigilance), flicker fusion (136), Digit Symbol (136,141, 142), Picture Completion (141), and Block Design (140)].

Prospective studies are rare in the occupational field, but a cohort of Finnish battery workers (143) was evaluated before occupational exposure commenced (89 workers), and after 1 year (24 workers remaining), and 2 years (16 workers). The time-weighted PbB values ranged between 14 and 45 μg/dl (calculated as the average of 24 months' bimonthly PbB values). Performance on the Santa Ana, Digit Span and Block Design tests was significantly impaired in the 2 years' follow-up. Five WAIS performance scale subtests were administered to 19 Japanese foundry workers whose initial PbB concentrations were in the range of 30 to 64 μg/100 ml, and to 10 comparison workers, and performance on the Picture Completion test was significantly reduced. Over a period of 2 years, improvements in hygiene conditions reduced PbB values in some workers to a range between 26 and 59 μg/dl; Picture Completion performance no longer differed between the groups (144).

A variety of subjective symptoms have been associated with exposure to lead, although there is little consistency between the studies, perhaps due to the diverse methods for measuring the symptoms. Johnson and colleagues (134) found smelter workers (mean 56 μg/dl PbB) more depressed and hostile using the Multiple Adjective Affect Checklist compared to clinical norms. Using the Profile of Mood States test, Baker and associates (145) observed increased anger, depression, fatigue, and confusion in workers with PbB levels between 40 and 60 μg/dl. Hänninen and colleagues (140) recorded more frequent symptoms of absentmindedness, lability, and sleep disturbances in 49 lead workers (group mean PbB, 32.3 μg/dl) compared to 24 comparison participants (PbB, 11.9). Hogstedt and colleagues (135) reported significantly more symptoms of irritability, reduced libido, and depression in lead-exposed workers, compared to a referent group. In a study of lead-exposed workers in Singapore, Jeyaratnam and colleagues (136) found significantly more complaints of anxiety and depressed mood, poor concentration, and forgetfulness among lead workers whose mean PbB value was 2.35 μmol/L (48 μg/dl) than in controls. Maizlish and Parra (146) reported significant elevations of anger, depression, fatigue, and joint pain in lead-exposed smelter workers with blood lead concentrations of 15 μg/dl PbB.

### *Community Residents*

Little attention was paid to health investigations of community members prior to the 1970s because of the belief that exposure levels were safely low. However, investigations continue to demonstrate the pervasiveness of lead exposures. For example, the Agency for Toxic Substances and Disease Registry (ATSDR) (147) has determined that lead is released at more uncontrolled hazardous waste sites (59% of sites) than any other compound. Trichloroethylene (released at 53% of sites), chromium (47% of sites), benzene (46% of sites), and arsenic (45% of sites) followed lead exposure as the most frequent contaminants. Dust and soil lead derived from flaking, weathering, and chalking paint, plus airborne lead fallout and waste disposal over the years, are now recognized as the major proximate sources of potential childhood lead exposures. In communities throughout the United States that are adjacent to many hazardous waste sites on the National Priorities List, elevated blood lead levels have been found in children who played near the sites, washed their hands infrequently, and had other behavioral risk factors (148–152). Given the success of public health efforts to remove lead from gasoline, house paint, and food cans, the main source of exposure during the 1990s is existing lead-based paint in older houses. Soil and dust contaminated with lead from primary sources such as old paint act as exposure pathways to children. Because lead does not dissipate, biodegrade, or decay, the lead deposited into dust and soil is a long-term source of lead exposure. Lead exposure also continues from industrial facilities, via the effluent from plants or the clothes of workers (153).

Longitudinal investigations of young American children exposed to lead have provided revealing evidence that even very low lead levels can cause serious effects on cognitive development, intelligence, and indicators of social skill (154). Needleman and associates (155) measured neuropsychological performance in a sample of 158 first- and second-grade children. The 58 children with high lead dentine levels in their deciduous teeth scored significantly lower on tests of intelligence (Wechsler Intelligence Scale for Children–Revised), verbal and auditory processing, attention (as measured by reaction time), and classroom behavior (as assessed by teachers) than 100 children who had low dentine lead values. In a remarkable follow-up investigation of this same cohort 11 years later, Needleman's group (156) found that the associations reported earlier between lead and children's academic and cognitive functioning persisted in young adulthood. Moreover, children with the greatest lead levels were about seven times more likely to drop out of high school than those who as children had low dentine lead levels. The investigators concluded: "Exposure to lead, even in children who remain asymptomatic, may have an important and enduring effect on the success in life of such children."

Dietrich and colleagues (157) conducted a prospective study to assess the effects of fetal lead exposure on neurodevelopmental status of 3- and 6-month-old infants in Cincinnati, Ohio. The study sampled 305 mothers, fetal-placental units, and neonates (10 days and 3 months) who had PbB levels below 30 μg/dl. Infant development was measured with the Bayley Mental Developmental Index (MDI) scales at 3 and 6 months of age. Prenatal and umbilical cord PbB levels were associated with MDI deficits at both ages. Bellinger et al. (158) reported comparable findings in a prospective cohort study of children from the Boston area that assessed the association between early development and low-level prenatal and postnatal lead exposure. Infant performance on the MDI between 6 months and 24 months declined with increasing PbB levels. This association varied with children's age at exposure, degree of lead exposure, and socioeconomic status. Bellinger et al. have suggested that early postnatal PbB levels between 10 and 25 μg/dl are associated with lower MDI scores, but only among children in lower socioeconomic strata.

McMichael and colleagues (159,160) studied a cohort of 537 Australian children born to women living in a community situated near a lead smelter. Maternal PbB levels were measured antenatally, at delivery (maternal and umbilical cord), and in the children at the ages of 6, 15, and 24 months, and annually thereafter. The mean PbB concentration varied from 9 μg/dl in midpregnancy to a peak of 21 μg/dl at age 2 years (159). The PbB level was inversely related to development (McCarthy Scales of Children's Abilities; and personal, family, medical, and environmental factors) at the ages of 2 and 4 years (159,160). The persistence of these deficits in adulthood has received support (161), although there is also evidence that reductions in blood lead may be associated with limited reversibility (162). Although controversial, lead exposure has recently been linked with adolescent aggressive behavior (163).

The impact of this research was not lost on the regulatory community. In the 1970s, the U.S. Public Health Service recognized the predominance of lead as a neurotoxicant in developing infants and children. In the 1980s, the blood lead level used as an action level was reduced from 30 to 25 μg/dl (164). The importance of preventing toxic exposures was emphasized in a key report, "The Nature and Extent of Lead Poisoning in Children in the United States: A Report to Congress" (165), and in 1991 the action level was again reduced, to 10 μg/dl of blood lead (166,167).

### Manganese

The neurotoxicity of manganese in miners was established decades ago. One of the symptoms was the mask-like expression associated with parkinsonism, and there was evidence that this could progress to full-blown Parkinson's disease unless exposures were terminated (168,169). Reductions in workplace exposures largely eliminated this problem, although isolated instances (170,171) or advanced cases (172) are still reported. Recent reports have revealed adverse neurobehavioral differences in populations exposed to manganese in manufacturing operations. Motor deficits have been consistently reported, including Tapping (173–176), Simple Reaction Time (173,174,177), and measures of hand tremor or steadiness (175,177). Cognitive measures have not been employed extensively, but there is evidence of differences from controls in the Rey memory task (177), Symbol Digit, Digit Span, and an addition task (176).

### Mercury

Mercury, known since antiquity to be dangerous, continues to produce toxicity in the workplace (3) and the community (178). While some of the most serious and poignant reports concern methylmercury such as the cerebral palsy in children following consumption of fish from Japan's Minimata Bay (179,180), the research literature is dominated by the consequences of inorganic mercury exposures. The extensive research on central nervous system deficits of inorganic or elemental mercury has focused on assessments of memory and attention (e.g., Digit Span, Sternberg). In cross-sectional research on mercury-exposed workers, poorer performance has also been seen in measures of general intellectual function (e.g., Raven Progressive Matrices), coding (Digit Symbol), spatial relations (Block Design), and in personality differences (Eysenck Personality Inventory). Deficits in primarily motor test performance (e.g., Tapping, Michigan Eye-Hand Coordination, Simple Reaction Time) have also been reported, including tremor, the most frequently studied measure of mercury exposure (3).

Tests of memory and steadiness or tremor have been refined over the years, and they exemplify how growth in technology has allowed scientists to provide increasingly sensitive analyses of this sign of mercury exposure. A simple test of steadiness or tremor requires the participant to insert a pencil-like stylus into a series of increasingly smaller holes without touching the sides of the holes. More contact with the sides reflects greater unsteadiness. Williamson and colleagues (181) found a significant increase in rates of touching the sides of such a device in 12 gold-refining and fungicide workers with current urine mercury measures of less than 0.01 to 2.5 mg/L and prior-year exposures of 0.03 to 0.30 mg/L (although measures of some participants were missing) for in excess of 180 hours (to 2,532 hours among those with measures). The measure of hand steadiness correlated significantly with current urine mercury levels.

Wood and colleagues (182) first studied the finger and arm tremor spectra (amplitude of tremor by frequency) in two women exposed to mercury vapor while calibrating glass pipettes. Langolf et al. (183) recorded electromyograms (EMGs) in chloralkali workers with a mean urine mercury concentration of 0.24 mg/L, and the highest peak exposure for the past 3, 6, or 12 months was correlated with response variables. The mean time-weighted average concentration for the prior year was 0.04 $mg/m^3$, and half the participants were not actively exposed to mercury at the time of testing. The EMG was recorded while the participant was told to aim a hand-held pointer, and they evaluated the spectral characteristics of the EMG and a linear potentiometer attached to the pointer. The best correlation with increased neuromuscular tremor (from the potentiometer) was the number of peak urine mercury concentrations in excess of 0.5 mg/L. Chapman et al. (184) reports that the greatest tremor amplitude occurs in the 5- to 15-Hz range. Happily, retrospective analyses suggest that reductions in mean urine mercury are associated with reversals in tremor frequency to a more normal band width (183).

Verberk et al. (185) employed both a stylus-in-hole test and a test in which the participant was asked to balance a piezoelectric crystal (to transduce acceleration) on a fingernail for 10 seconds. In participants with a current mean urine mercury concentration of 20 μmol/mol creatinine and with an annual mean of 19 μmol/mol creatinine (from bimonthly measures over the most recent year), there was a correlation between current urine mercury and acceleration amplitude in the crystal test and with time touching the side in the stylus-in-hole test.

Roels and co-workers (186) attached an accelerometer to the back of each participants' hand and analyzed the tremor spectrum. Female ($n$ = 54) and male ($n$ = 131) workers exposed to mercury vapor were compared to controls (48 females, 114 males). Females had a mean mercury concentration of 0.037 mg/g creatinine in urine and 0.90 μg/dl in blood; males had 0.052 mg/g creatinine in urine and 1.4 μg/dl in blood. Group differences were significant for males who had the higher mercury concentrations, supporting the authors' conclusion that abnormal findings are associated with urine mercury levels in excess of 0.05 mg/g.

There is consistency in these results, regardless of the type of device. The stylus-in-hole test has the disadvantage of being crude and susceptible to intentional errors, but it has the advantage of being simple and inexpensive to implement and interpret. The other tests are more sensitive and capable of identifying subtle changes, such as greater steadiness following reduced urine mercury concentrations, but they require sophisticated hardware and software.

Measures of memory and attention are frequently used to assess central changes in mercury-exposed workers. Significantly reduced performance has been reported on the Sternberg (181,187), Paired Associates (181), Recurrent Figures (memory for shapes) (188), Logical Memory (189,190), Digit Span (189–193), Serial Digit recall (191), Rey's Complex Figures (194), and word recall (195) tests. Significant relationships have been reported between 12-month average urinary mercury (0.18 mg/L and 0.10 mg/L) and Serial Digit threshold (191), and between two measures of mercury exposure (urine mercury peaks above 0.3 mg/L and blood mercury concentrations above 75 nmol/L) and two tests of learning and memory, the Digit Span and Logical Memory (189).

Recent reports have supported these findings in dentists with lower exposures to elemental mercury (190,193), as public attention has focused on dental amalgams, which release very small amounts of mercury (196). Other deficits associated with mercury exposure in multiple studies, include Tapping (183,190,197–199), Simple Reaction Time (193,200–202), Choice Reaction Time (198,200,201), Digit Symbol (190,200,201,203,204), Raven Progressive Matrices (200,201,203–205), and Eysenck Personality Inventory (204–206).

## NEUROTOXICOLOGY ASSESSMENTS IN THE FIELD: POPULATION ASSESSMENT

An epidemiologic field study, such as those described above, is conducted to determine if a neurotoxic exposure may be responsible for an adverse health effect in a defined population. The adverse effect is inferred from the poorer performance of the exposed group. There are two approaches to assessment that have been effective in occupational and community research. The approach employed most frequently is to select a structured series of psychometric tests that assess participant symptoms and effects reported for the chemical to which the population is exposed, or select a broad range of tests of diverse functions (3). The less common approach is the clinical neuropsychological evaluation employing experienced neuropsychologists using semistructured test selection strategies, but employing clinical experience and judgment and a knowledge of neuropsychological constructs to guide the assessment process (207,208). This relatively expensive approach is described later in this chapter. Some have attempted to meld these strategies by developing broadly sensitive neuropsychological test batteries (209,210). We begin with the structured test selection approach for cross-sectional population assessments.

### Frequently Used Tests

Drawn principally from the subdisciplines of neuropsychology and experimental psychology, over 250 dif-

**TABLE 1.** *Most frequently used tests in work-site research and computerized test options*

| Function | Most frequently used test | Computerized test |
|---|---|---|
| Cognitive | | |
| General intelligence[a] | Picture Completion | Vocabulary |
| Spatial relations | Block Design | |
| Learning | Paired Associates | Serial Digit Learning |
| Attention/memory | Digit Span | Digit Span |
| Vigilance | Bourdon-Wiersma | Continuous Performance Test |
| Coding | Digit Symbol | Symbol Digit |
| Concept shifting | Trail Making | Trail Making |
| Distractibility | Embedded Figures | |
| Categorization | Figure Classification | |
| Motor | | |
| Grip strength | Dynamometer | |
| Coordination/speed | Santa Ana | Tapping |
| Response speed | Simple Reaction Time | Simple Reaction Time |
| Response speed + decision | Choice Reaction Time | Choice Reaction Time |
| Steadiness | Stylus-in-hole | Accelerometry |
| Balance | Rail balancing | Accusway platform |
| Sensory | | |
| Vision-acuity | Commercially available | |
| Vision-color | Lanthony or Farnsworth | |
| Vision-pattern | Benton | Pattern recognition |
| Audition | Audiometer | Audiometer |
| Olfaction/absolute | Commercially available | |
| Olfaction/recognition | UPSIT | |
| Tactile-vibration | Vibratron | |
| Affect/personality | | |
| Affect | Profile of Mood States | Mood Test |
| Personality | Eysenck Personality Inventory | MMPI |

[a]Should not be interpreted as a measure of intelligence independent of other tests.

ferent behavioral tests were identified in published work-site studies at the beginning of the 1990s (3). This number has continued to grow, although the development of consensus test batteries and computerized testing, discussed below, have stemmed this growth, making test selection for the nonspecialist a bit less daunting. Described next are the neurobehavioral tests used most frequently in population neurotoxicity research, and they are also used extensively in in-depth neuropsychological assessments. This is followed by a discussion of the standardized consensus neurobehavioral assessment batteries that can simplify the process of test selection for focused research.

The neurobehavioral tests employed in neurotoxicity evaluations can be divided into two categories: (a) behavioral performance tests, and (b) questionnaire-based tests of psychosocial function and personality. Performance tests measure a person's functional capability in a direct and objective manner, whereas psychosocial and personality tests address complex human factors by asking questions based on well-established questionnaire responses in clinical populations (207). Table 1 identifies the generic functions most widely assessed in work-site research, the most frequently employed tests of each function (3), and available test options from computer-implemented batteries of neurobehavioral tests aimed at neurotoxicity assessments, also described below.

Performance tests can be divided into traditional functional categories in experimental psychology—cognitive, motor, and sensory—although these are not mutually exclusive or independent categories. The judgment on categorization is based on the primary evaluative function.

### Cognitive Tests

A rich variety of cognitive tests has been employed in occupational and community health studies. Following the order in Table 1, the psychological construct of intelligence is evaluated by the integration of a variety of tests sampling multiple domains of function (211) that cannot be readily categorized. One measure of complex function drawn from intelligence scales found frequently in assessments of neurotoxic exposures (68) is the Picture Completion test, which requires the participant to name a missing part from an incomplete picture (e.g., an arm). On occasion, the entire WAIS (Information, Comprehension, Arithmetic, Similarities, Digit Span, Digit Symbol, Picture Completion, Block Design, Picture Arrangement, Object Assembly, Vocabulary) (212) or a significant subset of the WAIS has been administered to identify neurotoxic effects (213). However, measures of vocabulary are often seen as an index of preexposure intellectual capability that is unaffected by neurotoxic exposures except in cases of the most extreme overexposure, an issue discussed below.

The Block Design subtest of the WAIS assesses spatial relations. The participant is shown a design formed of red, white, or red and white squares, and is asked to construct that design using blocks that have red, white, or red and white sides (214). Acquisition or learning has often been assessed by the Paired Associates (or associates learning) test, in which a list of word pairs (e.g., bicycle–car) is read to the participant, who is then asked to recall which word was paired with one member of the pair (e.g., which was paired with bicycle) (215).

The Digit Span subtest of the WAIS is the most frequently used test of memory and attention. It consists of the presentation of sets of three to nine digits (increasing from three to nine); the participant is instructed to repeat them back to the examiner in either the same or reverse order. The longest string of digits correctly repeated both forward and backward serve as the two measures on this test (214). In the Benton visual retention test, groups of symbols (e.g., triangles, squares) are shown to participants, who are then asked to select from four similar groupings that which is identical to the initial grouping (10).

Vigilance tasks include the Bourdon-Wiersma, in which the participant is instructed to rapidly strike out sets of dots with a pencil (216). The Continuous Performance Test (CPT) requires the participant to monitor a series of letter presentations and to respond by rapidly pressing a button when they see the less frequently presented letter (84).

Coding is assessed by the Digit Symbol subtest of the WAIS. The participant is instructed to use a coding key with a set of symbols that is each associated with a digit, to draw the appropriate symbol (e.g., Æ) in a blank space that is paired with a digit (212). As noted below, the Digit Symbol samples among the widest range of neuropsychological functions of any test used in this field of research (207), and is among the most sensitive to neurotoxicants (3).

The most frequently employed test of concept shifting is the Trail Making test. The test page contains both numbers and letters, and the participant is instructed to draw a line from the number 1 to the letter A, to the number 2, to the letter B, and so on. Basically, the participant must shift between the concepts of number and letter (217). The Embedded Figures test of distractibility presents drawings of objects (e.g., a truck) with lines drawn across them. The lines make it difficult for participants with certain chemical exposures to identify the object, but normal participants are not confused (69). Categorization tests involve sorting symbols or pictures into various categories (89).

Included in the first line and rightmost column of Table 1, tests of vocabulary are sometimes used to establish similarity of intellectual ability between groups. The rationale is that vocabulary is resistant to the effects of many chemical insults to the brain, although this is speculative (218), as noted below. The Synonyms test requires the participant to select, from among several alternatives, the word most nearly synonymous with the word to be defined (207). Many vocabulary tests merely require the participant to select from a list of three or four options the best definition of a word (145).

Many of the tests described above are time-consuming. While these tests, particularly those from the WAIS, are among the foremost standardized tests of intellectual function, other tests of these functions may be found in standard texts on psychological tests (207).

### Tests of Motor Function

Tests of motor function require some sensory input in the form of a stimulus to cue the response. Unlike sensory tests that manipulate the stimulus to determine the sensitivity of the observer, motor tests emphasize the speed or accuracy of the response.

Tests of grip strength employ a dynamometer. The participant grips a handle with as much strength as possible, pulling against a spring or strain gauge to measure the strength of the pull (139). Many tests of coordination have been used in neurotoxicology research; some also involve speed. The Santa Ana consists of cylindrical pegs with a square base that are placed in square depressions arranged in rows on a board. The participant is instructed to lift, turn 180 degrees, and reinsert as many pegs as possible in 30 seconds for several trials (219). In tapping tests, the participant taps his or her finger or toe at a fixed or maximum rate, and speed of interresponse variability is evaluated (139).

To measure response speed, participants are instructed to respond as rapidly as possible, and the success of the test depends on the effectiveness with which that instruction is conveyed. In the Simple Reaction Time, the participant presses a button when a cuing stimulus is presented. Choice reaction time tests simply provide two or more potential responses and associated stimuli, requiring the participant to discriminate the onset of a stimulus and then to choose the response associated with that stimulus (58).

Finger and arm steadiness have been studied using strain gauges and accelerometers to detect movement. Movement is converted to a direct current voltage, and the voltage changes are analyzed (186). A cruder but simpler evaluation is provided by the stylus-in-hole test, which requires the participant to place a stylus shaped like a pen in a series of progressively smaller holes (1 cm to 1 mm diameter). The time touching the side of the hole, which the participant is instructed to not do, is recorded (185). Balance is measured in a complex fashion by having the participant stand on a "force" platform, which contains a large array of strain gauges to measure pressure changes (by integrating the response across the strain gauges) as the person stands on the platform, inadvertently swaying (220).

### Sensory Tests

Sensory tests have achieved increasing prominence due to their sensitivity to neurotoxic exposures (e.g., see Solvents Mixtures, above). Visual function is assessed with standardized tests of visual resolution or acuity, which have substantial normative data. These tests require the participant to distinguish gaps or spatial separations of various sizes between lines (85,221). Tests of color vision require the arrangement of buttons of different hue and saturation in an order based on their similarity in color (107–114). There are a variety of pattern discrimination tests (3), each of which requires the participant to view a pattern or figure and (a) decide if a second figure is the same or different, (b) select a similar figure, (c) draw the figure, or (d) report or describe the pattern. In some of these cases, memory is a significant factor. The tests of visual field provide flashes of light at various points in the periphery around the field of view to determine the outer boundaries of the visual field (222).

Hearing loss is evaluated by a standard audiometer to determine the absolute threshold of audibility for several pure tone frequencies. A beeping tone that is decreasing in amplitude or loudness is presented through headphones to the listener who pushes a button to indicate when he or she can no longer hear the sound of the test tone. The tone amplitude is then increased and the listener releases the button when they can hear it again. In effect, the participant tracks his or her own hearing threshold (223). Tests of speech recognition have also been employed as an objective measure of complex auditory discrimination (224).

Olfactory thresholds have been studied with the University of Pennsylvania Smell Identification Test (UPSIT) (3). Tests of tactile vibratory sensitivity include the Vibratron, which requires the participant to touch a post and report the occurrence of vibration, which is manipulated by altering the oscilation amplitude in a tracking-type procedure. Deficits on vibration tests may reflect early stages of some forms of peripheral neuropathy (225).

### Psychosocial Tests

Psychosocial tests assess such aspects of human functioning as personality, mood, attitudes, and psychiatric symptoms. Examples of these tests used in neurotoxicology research include the Neurobehavioral Evaluation System 2 Mood Test (226) and the Profile of Mood State test (227). These tests present adjectives, such as *fearful, loving,* or *disgusted,* which participants select as being either descriptive or not descriptive of their current or recent psychological state (139). These questionnaires have been useful in distinguishing between exposed and unexposed populations (3).

Personality scales are standardized psychological tests designed for the detection of abnormal personalities. The Eysenck Maudsley Personality Inventory assesses personality constructs through questions about, for example, the existence of food aversions, body sway in response to the suggestion of falling, and the length of time the respondents can hold their breath (228). The Minnesota Multiphasic Personality Inventory (MMPI) measures diverse aspects of psychosocial function, including personality characteristics and psychopathology.

Virtually all of the tests identified above can be given by technically trained individuals following procedures described later in this chapter. The analysis and interpretation of the results, on the other hand, requires the assistance of experimental or clinical psychologists or neuropsychologists who are familiar with relationships between tests and factors that may affect performance (207,229,230). The involvement of such individuals in test selection and examiner (the people who administer the tests) training is essential.

### Computerized Test Batteries

The development of computer-implemented behavioral test batteries to screen for neurotoxic effects has begun to have a major impact on epidemiologic research in this field. The computer-implemented Neurobehavioral Evaluation System (NES-2) (226,231–233) is the most extensively used test battery, and its on-screen instructions have been translated into several languages, including Chinese, Japanese, Finnish, French, and Spanish (32,54,139,226,230,234–239). The NES and other computerized neurotoxicity assessment batteries, including Behavioral Assessment and Research System (BARS) (240–242), Swedish Performance Evaluation System (SPES) (243,244), Milan Automated Neurobehavioral System (MANS) (229,245,246), Automated Cognitive Test (ACT) (247), and Automated Performance Test System (APTS) (248–250), now contain computer-implemented variants of several tests identified in Table 1 (right column).

Anger and colleagues (251) held in 1995 the first symposium exclusively focused on computer-implemented neurobehavioral testing, in this robust field of research. This symposium highlighted a number of recent developments in this field. These included a prototype of the first pen-based testing system, the NES-3 (252); computerized testing systems used primarily in primate research (253); validation efforts (254–256); and analytic issues (257). Two test batteries developed in our laboratory featured significant improvements in testing efficiency, among other benefits, described next.

Anger and colleagues (240–242) developed the Behavioral Assessment and Research System (BARS) to present behavioral tests with high-quality graphics and an extensive series of modifiable parameters (e.g., number of trials, length of intertrial intervals, type of instruction, type of stimulus). A durable response input device with nine back-lightable numbered buttons was developed to overcome the computer keyboard, which is insufficiently durable or ergonomically acceptable for behavioral testing of human subjects. BARS tests are programmed with written instructions in a series of conceptually independent and specific steps, including practice, feedback, and appropriate reinforcements or punishers (time out from the task). These we have termed "stepped" instructions (242) to distinguish them from the traditional page of instructions found in most computerized tests. Spoken instructions and non–language training methods (which we term "shaping") are also available for several BARS tests. The simplicity in instructions extends the reach of computerized neurobehavioral testing to children (241) and the less educated (242).

Also described at the 1995 symposium was the first computerized system for administering a broad range of psychosocial tests, including measures of personality, mood and other psychosocial factors, posttraumatic stress disorder, and health symptoms. This system, the Health Screening System (HSS), presents 12 tests requiring 3 hours to complete, with programmed breaks and a training module at the outset of testing. This represents an added dimension in neurotoxicology research. A broad range of psychological factors are rarely assessed in detail, yet these factors may contribute significantly to performance on neurobehavioral tests or incidents of neurotoxicity. The diverse HSS tests are administered in a common format using the same development software and the same nine-button input unit used by BARS. Common to both BARS and HSS is the capability of testing up to ten people at a time by a single technician, due to the instruction clarity and intuitive appearance of the tests (258). This is a major step in the efficiency of neurobehavioral testing.

### Consensus Neurotoxicity Assessment Batteries

The decade of the 1980s was marked by the development of standardized behavioral test batteries for worldwide use, while the 1990s has witnessed the ascendancy of computerized batteries for conducting field neurotoxicology investigations in the industrialized nations. The expense, equipment service, and educational factors may limit the use of computerized batteries in some developing countries. These batteries were developed to provide time-limited screening measures for use in epidemiologic studies of large work groups exposed to neurotoxic or putative neurotoxic chemicals.

Dr. Helena Hänninen at the Finland Institute of Occupational Health (FIOH) developed the first screening test battery for behavioral neurotoxicology during the 1960s and 1970s, although refinements continued through the 1980s (219). Using her experience and that of the handful of researchers who had employed these tests in field settings, a working group sponsored by the World Health Organization (WHO) and the National Institute for Occupational Safety and Health (NIOSH), developed the Neurobehavioral Core Test Battery (NCTB; Table 2). This

**TABLE 2.** *Functions tested and tests in the two Consensus Adult Neurobehavioral Test Batteries for neurotoxicity assessments*

| Function | NCTB tests | AENTB tests |
|---|---|---|
| Cognitive | | |
| Learning | | Serial Digit Learning[a] |
| Attention and memory | Digit Symbol | Symbol Digit (+ delayed recall)[a] |
| | Digit Span | Digit Span[a] |
| | Benton visual retention | |
| | | Raven Progressive Matrices |
| Vocabulary | | Vocabulary[a] |
| Sensory | | |
| Vision-acuity | | Visual acuity[b] |
| Vision-contrast sensitivity | | Contrast sensitivity[b] |
| Vision-color | | Lanthony |
| Tactile-vibration | | Vibractile threshold[b] |
| Motor | | |
| Response speed | Simple Reaction Time[b] | Simple Reaction Time[a] |
| Finger-speed coordination | Aiming II | Tapping[a] |
| Hand-speed coordination | Santa Ana | Santa Ana |
| Grip + fatigue | | Dynamometer |
| Psychosocial | | |
| Mood | Profile of Mood States | Mood test[a] |

[a]Fully computerized test available.
[b]Instrumented test available.

was the first consensus test battery developed for neurotoxicity assessments, and it was intended as a screening and research tool (259).

The NCTB consists of seven tests (Table 2) that were recommended by the WHO working group to screen for neurotoxic effects in work-site evaluations. NCTB tests had distinguished exposed from control groups in published work-site studies, and they could be administered in the field by technicians with minimal training using economical materials and equipment (259). Anger and colleagues (260) administered the NCTB to over 2,300 unexposed, control participants in a cross-cultural study carried out in ten countries spanning four continents. The results revealed a surprising consistency in mean performance (and performance variability) from country to country. Only the Nicaraguan sample of rural peasants with an average of 3 years of education (compared to 12 years in the other countries) displayed distinctly lower performance on most tests. Thus, the NCTB is suitable for administration to broad populations with 10 or more years of education. Since the test instructions are administered by a human examiner who may be a technician schooled to follow the NCTB Operational Guide (available from the senior author of this chapter), the NCTB can be used in developing countries, with the caveat that the participants' educational levels must be 10 or more years (260). The individual core tests remain the most widely used in neurotoxicology research (3), and NCTB has seen use as a battery of tests in several studies (92,146,261–263).

A second consensus test battery was developed in 1994 by a committee selected by the Agency for Toxic Substances and Disease Registry (ATSDR) with the express purpose of assessing populations working in or living near hazardous waste sites. The committee included members of the WHO NCTB working group from 10 years earlier (259), but a great deal more experience in work-site research had accumulated (3). Anger et al. (264) employed the same basic requirements used by the previous WHO group to select the tests that they recommended to ATSDR, although a wider range of cognitive and sensory tests were recommended to and adopted by ATSDR (Table 2). Named by ATSDR (265) the Adult Environmental Neurobehavioral Test Battery (AENTB), the AENTB has been employed in three studies of communities living near hazardous waste sites using a training manual developed for this battery (266). An analysis of the subject variables affecting the AENTB (230) and research needs for this battery (267) have been discussed.

The ATSDR did not stop with the AENTB. Concern about children living adjacent to hazardous waste sites or to businesses where they could be exposed to low-level concentrations of hazardous substances has often been voiced individually, but there was no published battery of tests to address this need. The ATSDR took the first step to fill this gap by developing a test battery to assess nervous system dysfunction in children. Named the Pediatric Environmental Neurobehavioral Test Battery (PENTB), it focuses on observational methods in very young children, adding performance measures in school-age children (268).

## Test Selection

The tests described above and referred to in the literature cited here have the attribute of successfully detecting neurotoxic effects in occupational groups when compared to referent groups, and should therefore serve as the core of tests to be used in human behavioral neurotoxicology research. The exclusive use of new or previously unused tests in epidemiologic research is risky because failure to detect group differences could be a result of test insensitivity. Using a core set of proven tests with additions to assess specific symptoms or signs in the exposed groups is a recommended strategy (259,264).

Once neurobehavioral tests are identified for a study of people exposed to neurotoxic substances, test parameters should be considered. Test duration is one of the most critical and it is often manipulated to accommodate time constraints. At the simplest level, neurobehavioral tests can be seen to consist of an instructional and practice period and the test itself (242). The instructions must be clear to the audience being tested, the practice must be sufficient to establish a common level of performance for all participants, and the test itself needs to obtain a sufficient sample of behavior to produce a reliable result. Thus, test duration is a critical factor. While some tests have a fixed duration, the duration of many tests can be adjusted to achieve the desired length of the test period. However, this can be a critical decision. Figure 1 depicts performance on the BARS Tapping test by eight volunteers (normal controls compensated for their time) in eight sessions conducted in 1 week. This is a typical result that reveals that performance often does not reach asymptote within a single test session.

It is, however, possible to establish stable performance within a single test session as shown by data from the first session (Fig. 2) of the tapping test shown in Fig. 1.

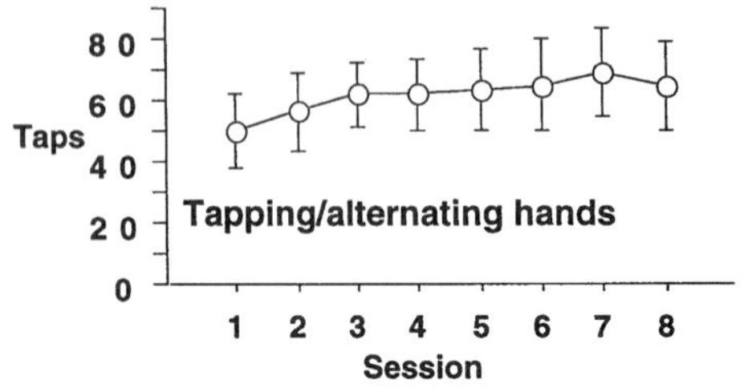


**FIG. 1.** Mean (+ 1 SD) performance by eight participants on the Tapping (alternating right/left hand index finger) test over eight sessions (in 5 days; maximum of two sessions per day).

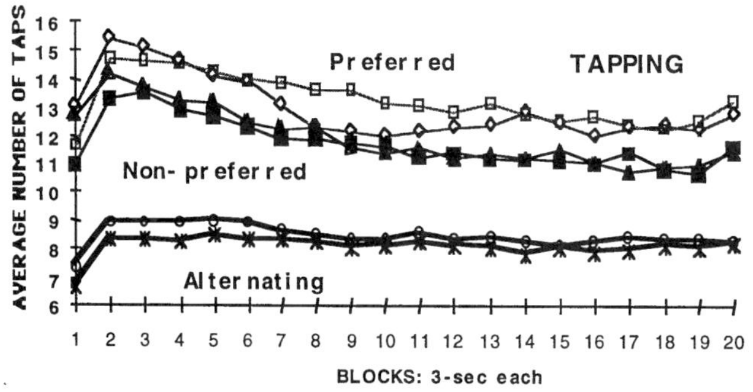


**FIG. 2.** Performance on BARS Tapping test (preferred, non-preferred hand index finger, and alternating between hands) by eight participants.

Equality among study participants in all groups may be achieved either by giving the groups the same number of trials on the test or by bringing the subjects within the groups to a common level of performance. The latter method is not practical for workplace testing, although this procedure is often used in laboratory research in which there is often more available time. Typically, a uniform number of practice trials is employed to establish adequate participant understanding. Comparisons are best made when performance is past the initial, generally steep rise of the learning curve, which could introduce significant variance into the results.

Since educational systems, cultural background, and occupational experience may vary from place to place, administration of the planned tests to a small sample (five to ten people) from the intended study population can answer questions about adequacy of instructions and practice, and test duration. A pilot study such as this is highly recommended, as it can also reveal other important factors. For example, it can generally be assumed that participants have not had significant practice on the neurobehavioral tests used in neurotoxicology research, but they may have experience on related activities. More concretely, persons with typing skills would be expected to perform well on tests of fine motor coordination, and reference participants should have had comparable experience to prevent misleading comparisons. A pilot study can answer these questions efficiently.

### From the Group to the Individual

In a small number of epidemiologic studies, historical or clinical norms have been used in lieu of testing a reference group (269). Such a procedure should be undertaken with great caution. The tests described above are well-established neuropsychological tests (207) used often in clinical evaluations, but their norms were developed with subjects (e.g., clinical patients, college students) who may not be representative of worker groups and may reflect unrecognized racial, cultural, or gender bias. The equipment or procedures used to derive the norms may have been different from those used in any given study. There are no norms for occupational or community groups, although the factors that affect performance in community groups have received some attention (229,257).

Individually the tests described above are not diagnostic tools. The problem of relating the findings from a behavioral study of groups of workers to the individuals within the groups is a vexing one. For example, how far from the reference group's mean does an individual's data have to lie before they are identified as abnormal? We have used an arbitrary convention of 1.5 or 2 standard deviations on multiple tests on which to base the recommendation to seek an in-depth neuropsychological evaluation (207,208,270), possibly combined with clinical neurologic evaluations and electrophysiologic tests (271). The neurobehavioral assessment thus serves a screening function for the individual, limiting the more expensive and time-consuming neuropsychological evaluation to those in clear need of the examination. The clinical neuropsychological examination focused on neurotoxic exposures is described next.

## CLINICAL NEUROPSYCHOLOGICAL ASSESSMENT—EVALUATING THE INDIVIDUAL

Clinical neuropsychological assessment of persons with possible neurotoxic exposure should provide clinically relevant information about the neurobehavioral functioning of the individual patient, including mood and personality. Because psychometric test batteries developed for neurotoxicologic research are constrained by time limitations and procedural rigidity, they cannot provide the information required for a comprehensive clinical neuropsychological assessment. Focused on individualized evaluation for aiding diagnosis, determining changes in individual performance, and guiding treatment, a complete clinical neuropsychological examination consists of an interview of the patient (and sometimes persons who know the patient well), behavioral observations, and a battery of psychometric tests (207). Because patterns of neuropsychological test performance associated with exposure to some neurotoxicants are beginning to be clarified and most neurologic and psychological conditions have been described in the literature, neuropsychological assessment can contribute importantly to differential diagnosis between neurotoxic disorders and neurologic or psychological conditions. Assessment can further lead to treatment recommendations such as pharmacotherapy for neuropsychiatric symptoms, training in stress coping skills, and vocational adjustments. Neuropsychological assessment should be considered to establish baseline functioning for the neurotoxicant-exposed patient with no previous neuropsychological assessment. Subsequent longitudinal assessment can then be used to measure change in function after treatment and/or termination of the exposure, or for documenting decline with continued exposure.

Desirable characteristics of a comprehensive clinical neuropsychological assessment of neurotoxic exposure have been previously described (272). The assessment should utilize standardized psychometric tests with well-defined psychometric properties and normative scores stratified or adjusted for demographic variables such as gender, age, and education. The examination should also include tests that can be used in conjunction with demographic variables such educational and vocational attainment to estimate premorbid baseline neurocognitive function (207). To aid differential diagnosis, tests both sensitive and insensitive to the neurotoxicant in question, as well as tests sensitive to other possible disorders, are needed to rule out other possible etiologies for any demonstrated deficits. Because normal human neurocognitive function changes across the life span, the assessment should be specifically designed for the developmental level of the person being assessed. Finally, the assessment battery should be sufficiently comprehensive to describe the patient's cognitive and behavioral strengths and weaknesses in enough detail to provide recommendations regarding any likely limitations on activities of daily living.

Clinical neuropsychological assessment is a complex and often subtle process that cannot be appropriately administered in rigidly predetermined fashion (207). Therefore, tests comprising specific neuropsychological evaluations vary considerably from patient to patient, depending on personal and situational variables. Nonetheless, a complete neuropsychological evaluation of neurotoxicant exposure should include tests sampling all important domains of function, including psychomotor function, language, visuospatial function, learning and memory, attention, executive function, and personality and mood. Yet because neuropsychological assessment can be a time-consuming, arduous, and expensive process, there are clear benefits to limiting the assessment as much as is feasible. Therefore, it is cost-effective to emphasize assessment of those neurocognitive functions that are most likely to be affected based on the literature. For most neurotoxicants studied to date, deficits have been most frequently and consistently demonstrated in the domains of learning and memory, attention, and psychomotor slowing (207). Some suggestions for neuropsychological assessment of neurotoxicant-exposed patients are offered below. Because child and geriatric neuropsychology are beyond the scope of the present discussion, these recommendations only address clinical neuropsychological assessment of nongeriatric adults.

Because problems with learning and memory are among the most prominent complaints of patients exposed to neurotoxicants (207), the assessment of these patients should include a thorough evaluation of memory functions. However, the psychological construct of "memory" is an amalgam of different cognitive functions. Moreover, research suggests that tests of complex learning and memory are the most sensitive to deficits of some neurotoxicants (273). For these reasons, it is important that a clinical neurospychological assessment includes tests of learning and memory that sample different modalities, different kinds of memory function, and multiple levels of complexity. A complete assessment should minimally include tests of verbal list learning, immediate and delayed verbal story recall, and at least one test of visual memory. Therefore, verbal memory measures should include tests of (a) a verbal list learning and recall, such as the Rey Auditory Verbal Learning Test (207,274) or California Verbal Learning Test (275); (b) delayed and immediate story recall, such as the Wechsler Memory Scale–Revised (WMS-R) Logical Memories (276); and (c) visual memory, such as the Continuous Visual Memory Test (277) or WMS-R Visual Reproduction (276). Brown Peterson Consonant Trigrams (207,278), a difficult verbal memory task with a concurrent secondary attentional distraction task, may be more sensitive than simpler memory tasks to neurotoxic deficits.

Attentional dysfunction is also among the most commonly reported effects of neurotoxicants. However, there are no tests that specifically measure attention in isolation (207). Moreover, attention is also highly sensitive to nonspecific organismic or situational factors, such as emotional disturbance or lack of sleep, and is almost universally affected by most causes of neurocognitive dysfunction. For these reasons, it is important that a clinical neuropsychological assessment includes multiple tests that sample performance dependent on attention. The WAIS-R forward and backward Digit Span (279), which has a large attentional component, tends to be reduced in individuals chronically exposed to solvents (280). Summated as a single scale score in the WAIS-R version, these are actually distinct but related tests, and their scores should be reported and interpreted separately (207). Other tests of attention that are rarely employed in the neurotoxicology literature are WAIS-R Arithmetic (279), in the absence of specific calculation deficits, the Attentional Capacity Test (281), and the Continuous Performance Test (282). Sentence Repetition may more closely resemble tasks encountered in day-to-day function, and therefore more accurately reflect the patient's complaints (207). For early stages of exposure or in patients for whom exposure-related deficits are questionable, test sensitivity may be particularly important. In these cases, the Paced Auditory Serial Addition Test (283) and Stroop (284) are difficult attention tasks that may be especially sensitive to neurocognitive decline.

Psychomotor slowing is also among the most commonly reported effects of neurotoxicants. Common tests of psychomotor slowing are Simple Reaction Time (207), finger tapping (285), pegboard tests (286,287), Trail Making (285), WAIS-R Digit Symbol (279), and the Symbol Digit Modalities Test (SDMT) (288). However, Trail Making, WAIS-R Digit Symbol, and SDMT are neuropsychologically complex and may also reflect complex attention (207). The similar Digit Symbol and SDMT are among the most sensitive but least specific tests of neurotoxic exposure, possibly because they reflect many different functions (289). Thus, though nonspecific, these complex tests may be an excellent index of neurocognitive decline (207).

As with attention, measures of executive function of necessity entail confounding influences of other functional domains, and executive influences can be discerned in most complex tasks. Some of the complex tasks categorized above as attention and/or complex psychomotor tasks (e.g., Trail Making, Stroop) have also been classified as tests of executive functioning. Other commonly used tests of executive function are the Wisconsin Card Sorting Test (290) and the Tower of London (291).

Although tests of language function generally appear to be insensitive to neurotoxic effects in adults, they should be included in a clinical assessment where neurotoxicity is suspected, for at least two reasons. First, they may serve as "hold" tests to estimate premorbid baseline neurocognitive functioning (based somewhat on educational and vocational attainment). However, some language tests may be more sensitive to neurotoxic effects than originally thought (218). The estimation of preexposure baseline functioning should therefore be based on a wider array of information (207). Second, specific patterns of impaired language function may be indicative of etiology other than neurotoxic exposure such as neurologically based language disorders or developmental (preexposure) learning disability. A complete assessment might reasonably include at least some of the WAIS-R verbal subtests of Information, Vocabulary, Similarities, and Comprehension (279). The Controlled Oral Word Association Test (292) and Boston Naming Test (293) are usefully included and may assist in differential diagnosis. Assessments of reading skills, such the Gates-MacGinitie Reading Tests (294) and the Boston Diagnostic Aphasia Exam Reading Comprehension (295) should also be included.

Comprehensive coverage also requires administration of tests of nonverbal cognitive function. Block Design (279), sensitive to some neurotoxicants (3) but also frequently affected by other disorders as well (e.g., dementia, stroke), should always be included. Other potentially useful nonverbal tests are WAIS-R Picture Completion and/or Picture Arrangement (279), the copy trial of the Rey-Osterreith Complex Figure test (296), the Hooper Visual Organization Test (297), and the Boston Visuospatial Quantitative Battery (295).

Because alterations in personality and mood can both affect neurocognitive test performance and also be an effect of neurotoxic exposure, the neuropsychological evaluation must assess this domain. The MMPI-2 (298), commonly used for this purpose, requires considerable time to administer and specialized training to interpret. The Symptom Checklist (SCL-90-R) (299) samples a wide range of psychiatric symptomatology, and is considerably briefer to administer. Tests of a more narrow range of symptomatology that have also been used to study neurotoxic disorders are the Beck Depression Inventory (300), Beck Anxiety Inventory (301), and the Profile of Mood States (227).

Psychometric tests inherently sample complex neuropsychological functions, and there are no purely domain-, modality-, or diagnosis-specific neuropsychological tests. Some tests, particularly those that most widely draw on multiple functional domains, are highly sensitive to generalized neurocognitive dysfunction (e.g., Digit Symbol) but may reflect a wide range of etiologies or syndromes, not purely neurotoxicity. Discerning the specific domains of dysfunction that contribute to differential diagnosis—discrimination of neurotoxicity from neurodegenerative disorders, for example—is accomplished by the analysis of relationships between multiple measures. This requires the training and experience of a clinical neuropsychologist. The value of the neuropsychological assessment is the integration of clues from performance on diverse tests and sources of information, not just psychometric testing, that contributes to accurate individual diagnosis and treatment recommendations.

## CONDUCTING THE ASSESSMENT IN THE FIELD

The decision to conduct a work-site or community assessment begins with a question to study or a hypothesis to test. An individual neuropsychological assessment, described above, can be conducted at a remote site, but the expense of this approach in testing and personnel time is prohibitive. Thus, the typical study design is a cross-sectional comparison in which a preselected battery of psychometric tests is administered to a population exposed to a neurotoxic chemical and to a comparable control or reference group. An adverse health effect is inferred if the performance of the exposed group is inferior to the performance of the reference group.

In a cross-sectional study, the appropriate reference group is chosen to be roughly equated or matched for the main factors known to affect performance on neurobehavioral tests—age, sex, and education (229,230)—and occupational factors such as work history. While the clinical neuropsychological evaluation can seek convergent information from a variety of tests and norm groups, the cross-sectional study employing a preselected battery of tests must depend on the equality of the exposed and reference group with regard to factors that affect test performance. On NCTB and AENTB tests, for example, age is a relatively minor factor below 45 years (230), although it assumes progressively increasing importance above 45 years (229) and below age 16. Gender is important primarily for motor tests involving strength (229,230). Education is an important factor when participants have fewer than 10, and especially fewer than 6, years of formal education (230), or in persons above 50 years of age with more than 10 years of education (229). Further, there is strongly suggestive data that ethnicity or cultural background can interact in complex ways with low levels of education. This is especially the case if members of different ethnic groups are educated in different educational systems. Statistical control methods such as covariance analysis cannot clarify this complexity (230).

Performance on behavioral tests may obviously be impaired by participant background. Examples are hobbies, fatigue, substance use, or occupation (e.g., historical exposures to chemicals or job activities, such as the use of vibrating tools, that can cause nerve damage). Drug use and various disease conditions that affect the nervous system can be assessed through questionnaires, although the issue of honesty and response bias must be considered. There is evidence that computerized questionnaires produce more honest responses than individually administered questionnaires (302). Criteria should be established before data are collected in order to exclude inappropriate subjects from the data analysis. If this cannot be achieved, known confounding factors must be managed by statistical analysis techniques; unknown factors are dealt with by randomization and an appropriate experimental design.

### Setting Up the Field Site

Conducting experimental research with human subjects presents difficulties in almost any setting. The ideal study is conducted in an experimental laboratory in which all equipment has been repeatedly calibrated and employed in the testing location, personnel are experienced in using the equipment with established protocols, and the setting is well controlled (e.g., noise, temperature). Mounting a study in the field compounds these difficulties by siting the study in a remote location where the study staff must deliver all the necessary services and equipment to conduct the study. This section describes the procedural factors involved in a human neurobehavioral field study [based on research with several thousand subjects by Anger and colleagues (230,260,267,303,304)].

The testing site often must be arranged to administer tests of multiple end points. For behavioral tests, a separate room is required to prevent distraction by other activities or sounds, although the use of headphones and partitions can usually accomplish this effectively in a single room if the testing is exclusively computer-administered.

If all study tests can be administered by technically competent but nonspecialized personnel (230,267), participants can be processed conveniently at one or more equivalent test stations. Unique stations, each with only a subset of the tests, are required if costly equipment or specialized expertise is needed for some tests, e.g., Anger et al. (304) used eight stations. The primary advantage of administering all tests at equivalent stations is that the participant will not be kept waiting at "backed-up" stations due to individual differences in test-taking speed.

Tests that do not require individual attention allow testing of several people by one examiner, which is cost-efficient. Computer implementation of behavioral (241) and psychological (258) tests have allowed us, with a single examiner, to administer a 4-hour battery of tests to up to ten people. Critical to the efficiency of this process was the development of simple, clear, effective written instructions (242) plus the option for spoken instructions and questionnaire tests.

### Examiner Training Program

The examiner training program must be targeted to the qualifications of the examiners. Both the NCTB and the AENTB were developed to allow technically trained individuals to administer the tests following rigorous protocols in an examiner training manual (266). The training consists of four components: (a) a review of research using the tests, to gain commitment to the study; (b) demonstration of administration procedures and technique; (c) practice by examiners on each other; and (d) practice administration to five to six naive participants. The practice with naive participants requires the bulk of the training time, and it is in this period in which the examiner trainee actually learns the skills involved in administering the tests. During this period, the trainer helps to the extent needed to avoid errors of administration, slowly fading out their active presence with each succeeding practice participant. The final administration becomes the "certification" examination, which should achieve the following criteria:

- Greet and interact with the participant with a positive, pleasant manner, yet maintain professional distance
- Demonstrate testing behaviors described in the training manual
- Read the instructions in the training manual smoothly and accurately
- Manipulate test equipment efficiently
- Record information on the data form with 100% accuracy
- Present a professional appearance throughout testing.

### Procedural Matters

Numerous procedural factors are critical to the success of any field study. The most important follow:

1. Equipment must be tested and calibrated prior to shipping to the field site, and after it is set up at the field site.
2. Because failure to maintain a study schedule can have serious consequences (inability to reschedule critical subjects, credibility in a community or work site where the field study is a major topic of conversation), backup equipment or rapid service is desirable.
3. Exposed and nonexposed participants should be intermixed or randomized with regard to the order in which they are tested, and examiners should be blind to the exposure or treatment history of persons being evaluated to avoid intentional or unintentional bias. The potential for bias may create a serious credibility issue for any study.
4. A full dress-rehearsal will identify study flow and technical problems, and assure new examiners a high comfort level, leading to a more professional and thus effective delivery of instructions on study day one.
5. There should be a site leader who is responsible for site coordination, authorized to make procedural decisions (for this they need a science background), and able to approach the process with an air of calm confidence.
6. One or more mid-study observations by the trainer is needed to determine that examiners are administering the tests properly and allow the correction of minor procedural errors (examiner drift) in the debriefing.

## CONCLUSION

There has been a continued growth of research in this field since the last edition of this text in 1992. Of the many chemicals studied in behavioral neurotoxicology, replicated findings have emerged for only a few: carbon disulfide, styrene, trichloroethylene, organophosphate pesticides, lead, manganese, and mercury. Perhaps the most interesting and worrisome development has been the growing recognition of the effects of lead in younger populations and at ever-lower concentrations (154–158), and the evidence that the neurotoxic effects in young children do not appear to reverse with time (161). Multiple solvent exposures have received the greatest amount of experimental attention. The results are compelling, but little new information has emerged on the specific solvents that present the greatest toxic potential. The most interesting research on such solvents indicates that persons placed on disability and removed from exposure do not become progressively worse; in fact, they change little at all in the succeeding 5 to 10 years (57–59).

The growth in the number of behavioral test methods has not continued its previous pace. Most encouraging, two of the test batteries have been administered in diverse international populations using different languages (226,260), holding out hope for increasing test standardization. Standardization is particularly valuable as new chemicals are studied in new populations exposed to established neurotoxicants at lower concentrations than were previously studied. Finally, the growing efficiency in testing brought about by computerized test batteries (241,258) has reduced the cost of behavioral neurotoxicology research, a critical factor in growing this field and serving working and community populations.

## ACKNOWLEDGMENTS

This work was supported by Environmental Protection Agency grants C R 822789-01-0 and 1RO1ES06475-01, and the Department of Veterans Affairs and the Portland Environmental Hazards Research Center, a joint project of the Portland Veterans Affairs Medical Center and the Center for Research on Occupational and Environmental Toxicology of the Oregon Health Sciences University to W. K. Anger; and, for R. W. Amler, funds from the Comprehensive Environmental Response, Compensation, and Liability Act trust fund through the Agency for Toxic Substances and Disease Registry (ATSDR), Public Health Service (PHS), U.S. Department of Health and Human Services (DHHS). The use of company or product names is for identification only and does not constitute endorsement by ATSDR, PHS, or DHHS. Appreciation is extended to Kelly Davis, who copied much of the recent literature for this review; Joanne Brown, who provided assistance in formatting references; and Betty Phifer, who contributed to the section on implementing field studies.

## REFERENCES

1. Dews PB. An overview of behavioral toxicology. In: Weiss B, Laties VJ, eds. *Behavioral toxicology.* New York: Plenum, 1975;439–445.
2. Dick RB. Neurobehavioral assessment of occupationally relevant solvents and chemical in humans. In: Chang LW, Dyer RS, eds. *Handbook of neurotoxicology.* New York: Marcel Dekker, 1995;217–322.
3. Anger WK. Worksite behavioral research: results, sensitive methods, test batteries and the transition from laboratory data to human health. *Neurotoxicology* 1990;11:629–720.
4. Johnson BL, Grandjean P, Amler RW. Neurobehavioral testing and hazardous chemical sites. *Neurotoxicol Teratol* 1994;16:485–487.
5. Chang LW, Dyer RS, eds. *Handbook of neurotoxicology.* New York: Marcel Dekker, 1995.
6. Armstrong RD, Leach LJ, Belluscio PR, et al. Behavioral changes in the pigeon following inhalation of mercury vapor. *Am Ind Hyg Assoc J* 1963;24:366–375.
7. Beard RR. Early development of behavioral toxicology in the U.S. In: Xintaras C, Johnson BL, de Groot I, eds. *Behavioral toxicology:* early detection of occupational hazards. DHEW publication (NIOSH) # 74-126. Washington, DC: U.S. Government Printing Office, 1974; 427–431.
8. Ekel GJ, Teichner WH. *An analysis and critique of behavioral toxicology in the USSR.* DHEW publication (NIOSH). Washington, DC: U.S. Government Printing Office, 1976;77–160.
9. Anger WK. Neurobehavioral testing of chemicals: impact on recommended standards. *Neurobehav Toxicol Teratol* 1984;6:147–153.

10. Hänninen H. Psychological picture of manifest and latent carbon disulphide poisoning. *Br J Ind Med* 1971;28:374–381.
11. Vigliani EC. Carbon disulphide poisoning in viscose rayon factories. *Br J Ind Med* 1954;11:235–244.
12. Braceland FJ. Mental symptoms following carbon disulphide absorption and intoxication. *Ann Intern Med* 1942;16:246–261.
13. Spencer PS, Schaumburg HH, eds. *Experimental and clinical neurotoxicology.* Baltimore: Williams & Wilkins, 1980.
14. Cassitto MG, Camerino D, Imbriani M, Contardi T, Masera L. Carbon disulfide and the central nervous system: a 15-year neurobehavioral surveillance of an exposed population. *Environ Res* 1993;63:252–263.
15. Vanhoorne M, De Rouck A. Epidemiological study of the systemic ophthalmological effects of carbon disulfide. *Arch Environ Health* 1996;51:181–188.
16. Hänninen H. Behavioral study of the effects of carbon disulfide. In: Xintaras C, Johnson BL, de Groot I, eds. *Behavioral toxicology:* early detection of occupational hazards. DHEW publication (NIOSH) 74-126. Washington, DC: Department of Health, Education, and Welfare, 1974;73–80.
17. Hänninen H. Psychological tests in the diagnosis of carbon disulfide poisoning. *Work Environ Health* 1966;2:16–20.
18. Hänninen H, Eskelinen L, Husman K, Nurminen M. Behavioral effects of long-term exposure to a mixture of organic solvents. *Scand J Work Environ Health* 1976;2:240–255.
19. Hänninen H, Nurminen M, Tolonen M, Martelin T. Psychological tests as indicators of excessive exposure to carbon disulfide. *Scand J Psychol* 1978;19:163–174.
20. Tolonen M, Hänninen H. Psychological tests specific to individual carbon disulfide exposure. *Scand J Psychol* 1978;19:241–245.
21. Tuttle TC, Wood GD, Grether CB. *Behavioral and neurological evaluation of workers exposed to carbon disulfide.* DHEW publication (NIOSH). Washington, DC: US Government Printing Office, 1976; 77–128.
22. Liang Y-x, Jin X-p, Lu P-q, et al. A neuropsychological study among workers exposed to low levels of carbon disulfide. In: Liang Y-X, Jiang X-Z, Wang Y-I, eds. *Occupational health bulletin.* Shanghai: Shanghai School of Public Health 1985;1:142–144.
23. Putz-Anderson V, Albright BE, Lee ST, et al. A behavioral examination of workers exposed to carbon disulfide. *Neurotoxicology* 1983;4: 67–78.
24. Seeber A. Neurobehavioral toxicity of long-term exposure to tetrachloroethylene. *Neurotoxicol Teratol* 1989;11:579–583.
25. Echeverria D, White RF. A behavioral evaluation of PCE exposure in patients and dry cleaners: a possible relationship between clinical and preclinical effects. *J Occup Environ Med* 1995;37:667–680.
26. Cavalleri A, Gobba F, Paltrinieri M, Fantuzzi G, Righi E. Perchloroethylene exposure can induce color vision loss. *Neurosci Lett* 1994;179:162–166.
27. Ferroni C, Selis L, Mutti A, Folli D, Bergamaschi E. Neurobehavioral and neuroendocrine effects of occupational exposure to perchloroethylene. *Neurotoxicology* 1992;13:243–247.
28. Schreiber JS, House S, Prohonic E, Smead G, Hudson C, Styk M. An investigation of indoor air contamination in residences above dry cleaners. *Risk Anal* 1993;13:335–344.
29. Lindström K, Härkönen H, Hernberg S. Disturbances in psychological functions of workers occupationally exposed to styrene. *Scand J Work Environ Health* 1976;3:129–139.
30. Mutti A, Mazzucchi A, Frigeri G, Falzoi M, Argini G, Franchini I. Neuropsychological investigation on styrene exposed workers. In: Gilioli R, Cassitto MG, Foa V, eds. *Advances in the biosciences, neurobehavioral methods in occupational health.* New York: Pergamon Press, 1983;46:271–281.
31. Mutti A, Mazzucchi A, Rustichelli P, Frigeri G, Arfini G, Franchini I. Exposure-effect and exposure-response relationships between occupational exposure to styrene and neuropsychological functions. *Am J Ind Med* 1984;5:275–286.
32. Tsai S-Y, Chen J-D. Neurobehavioral effects of occupational exposure to low-level styrene. *Neurotoxicol Teratol* 1996;18:463–469.
33. Möller C, Ödkvist L, Larsby B, Tham R, Ledin T, Bergholtz L. Otoneurological findings in workers exposed to styrene. *Scand J Work Environ Health* 1990;16:189–194.
34. Chia SE, Jeyaratnam J, Ong CN, Ng TP. Impairment of color vision among workers exposed to low concentrations of styrene. *Am J Ind Med* 1994;26:481–488.
35. Jégaden D, Amann D, Simon JF, Habault M, Legoux B, Galopin P. Study of the neurobehavioral toxicity of styrene at low levels of exposure. *Int Arch Occup Environ Health* 1993;64:527–531.
36. Cherry N, Gautrin D. Neurotoxic effects of styrene: further evidence. *Br J Ind Med* 1990;47:29–37.
37. Gobba F, Galassi C, Imbriani M, Ghittori S, Candela S. Acquired dyschromatopsia among styrene-exposed workers. *J Occup Med* 1991;33:761–765.
38. Campagna D, Mergler D, Huel G, Belanger S, Truchon G, Ostiguy C. Visual dysfunction among styrene-exposed workers. *Scand J Work Environ Health* 1995;21:382–90.
39. Eguchi T, Kishi R, Harabuchi I, Yuasa J, Arata Y, Katakura Y. Impaired colour discrimination among workers exposed to styrene: relevance of a urinary metabolite. *Occup Environ Med* 1995;52:534–538.
40. Fallas C, Fallas J, Maslard P. Subclinical impairment of colour vision among workers exposed to styrene. *Br J Ind Med* 1992;49:679–682.
41. Rebert CS. The neuroepidemiology of styrene: a critical review of representative literature. *Crit Rev Toxicol* 1994;24(suppl):S57–106.
42. Foo SC, Jeyaratnam J, Koh D. Chronic neurobehavioral effects of toluene. *Br J Ind Med* 1990;47:480–484.
43. Foo SC, Ngim CH, Salleh I, Jeyaratnam J. Neurobehavioral effects in occupational chemical exposure. *Environ Res* 1993;60:267–273.
44. Ørbæk P, Nise G. Neurasthenic complaints and psychometric function of toluene-exposed rotogravure printers. *Am J Ind Med* 1989;16: 67–77.
45. Iregren A. Effects on psychological test performance of workers exposed to a single solvent (toluene)—a comparison with effects of exposure to a mixture of organic solvents. *Neurobehav Toxicol Teratol 1982;*4:695–701.
46. Cherry N, Venables H, Waldron HA. Research in Britain. In: Cherry N, Waldron HA, eds. *The neuropsychological effects of solvent exposure.* Hampshire, United Kingdom: Colt Foundation, 1983:136–153.
47. Cherry N, Venables H, Waldron HA. British studies on the neuropsychological effects of solvent exposure. *Scand J Work Environ Health* 1984;10(suppl 1):10–12.
48. Hänninen H, Antti-Poika M, Savolainen P. Psychological performance, toluene exposure and alcohol consumption in rotogravure printers. *Int Arch Occup Environ Health* 1987;59:475–483.
49. Cranmer JM, Goldberg L, eds. Neurobehavioral effects solvents: proceedings of the workshop on neurobehavioral effects of solvents. *Neurotoxicology* 1986;7:1–95.
50. Hogstedt C. Has the Scandinavian solvent syndrome controversy been solved? *Scand J Work Environ Health* 1994;20:59–64.
51. Gade A, Mortensen EL, Bruhn P. "Chronic painter's syndrome." A reanalysis of psychological test data in a group of diagnosed cases, based on comparisons with matched controls. *Acta Neurol Scand* 1988;77:293–306.
52. O'Flynn RR. Do organic solvents "cause dementia"? *Int J Geriatr Psychiatry* 1988;3:5–15.
53. van Vliet C, Swaen GMH, Volovics A, et al. Neuropsychiatric disorders among solvent-exposed workers. First results from a Dutch case-control study. *Int Arch Occup Environ Health* 1990;62:127–132.
54. Spurgeon A, Gray CN, Sims J, et al. Neurobehavioral effects of long-term occupational exposure to organic solvents: two comparable studies. *Am J Ind Med* 1992;22:325–335.
55. Rasmussen K, Arlien-Søborg A, Sabroe S. Clinical neurological findings among metal degreasers exposed to chlorinated solvents. *Acta Neurol Scand* 1993;87:200–204.
56. Ellingsen DG, Bekken M, Kolsaker L, Langård S. Patients with suspected solvent-induced encephalopathy examined with cerebral computed tomography. *J Occup Med* 1993;35:155–160.
57. Ørbæk P. Solvent-induced disability and recovery after cessation of exposure. In: Chang LW, Dyer RS, eds. *Handbook of neurotoxicology.* New York: Marcel Dekker, 1995;339–354.
58. Ørbæk P, Lindgren M. Prospective clinical and psychometric investigation of patients with chronic toxic encephalopathy induced by solvents. *Scand J Work Environ Health* 1988;14:37–44.
59. Bruhn P, Arlien-S borg P, Gyldensted C, Christensen EL. Prognosis in chronic toxic encephalopathy: a two-year follow-up study in 26 house painters with occupational encephalopathy. *Acta Neurol Scand* 1981; 64:259–272.
60. Lindström K, Antti-Poika M, Tola S, Hyytiäinen A. Psychological prognosis of diagnosed chronic organic solvent intoxication. *Neurobehav Toxicol Teratol* 1982;4:581–588.

61. Mikkelsen S, Solvent encephalopathy: disability pension studies and other case studies. In: Chang LW, Dyer RS, eds. *Handbook of Neurotoxicology.* New York: Marcel Dekker, 1995;323–338.
62. Kyrklund T. The use of experimental studies to reveal suspected neurotoxic chemicals as occupational hazards: acute and chronic exposures to organic solvents. *Am J Ind Med* 1992;21:15–24.
63. Maxmilian VA, Risberg J, Prohovnik I, Rehnström S. Regional bloodflow and verbal memory after chronic exposure to organic solvents. *Brain Cogn* 1982;1:196–205.
64. Reinvang I, Borchgrevink HM, Aaserud O, et al. Neuropsychological findings in a non-clinical sample of workers exposed to solvents. *J Neurol Neurosurg Psychiatry* 1994;57:614–616.
65. Morrow LA, Robin N, Hodgson MJ. Assessment of attention and memory efficiency in persons with solvent neurotoxicity. *Neuropsychologia* 1992;30:911–922.
66. Linz DH, deGarmo PL, Morton WE, Wiens AN, Coull BM, Maricle RA. Organic solvent-induced encephalopathy in industrial painters. *J Occup Med* 1986;28:119–125.
67. Ryan CM, Morrow LA, Hodgson M. Cacosmia and neurobehavioral dysfunction associated with occupational exposure to mixtures of organic solvents. *Am J Psychiatry* 1988;145:1442–1445.
68. Eskelinen L, Luisto M, Tenkanen L, Mattei O. Neuropsychological methods in the differentiation of organic solvent intoxication from certain neurological conditions. *J Clin Exp Neuropsychol* 1986;8: 239–256.
69. Valciukas JA, Lilis R, Singer RM, Glickman L, Nicholson WJ. Neurobehavioral changes among shipyard painters exposed to solvents. *Arch Environ Health* 1985;40:47–52.
70. Elofsson S-A, Gamberale F, Hindmarsh T, et al. Exposure to organic solvents. A cross-sectional epidemiologic investigation on occupationally exposed car and industrial spray painters with special reference to the nervous system. *Scand J Work Environ Health* 1980;6: 239–273.
71. Seppäläinen AM, Lindström K, Martelin T. Neurophysiological and psychological picture of solvent poisoning. *Am J Ind Med* 1980;1: 31–42.
72. Lindström K, Wickstrom G. Psychological function changes among maintenance house painters exposed to low levels of organic solvent mixtures. *Acta Psychiatr Scand* 1983;67(suppl 303):81–89.
73. Kishi R, Harabuchi I, Katakura Y, Ikeda T. Neurobehavioral effects of chronic occupational exposure to organic solvents among Japanese industrial painters. *Environ Res* 1993;62:303–313.
74. Hänninen H, Antti-Poika M, Juntunen J. Exposure to organic solvents and neuropsychological dysfunction: a study on monozygotic twins. *Br J Ind Med* 1991;48:18–25.
75. Kilburn KH. Effects on neurobehavioral performance of chronic exposure to chemically contaminated well water. *Toxicol Ind Health* 1993;9:391–404.
76. Kilburn KH. Neurotoxic effects from residential exposure to chemicals from an oil reprocessing facility and superfund site. *Neurotoxicol Teratol* 1995;17:89–102.
77. Lindström K. Changes in psychological performances of solvent-poisoned and solvent-exposed workers. *Am J Ind Med* 1980;1: 69–84.
78. Mikkelsen S, Jorgensen M, Browne E, Gyldensted C. Mixed solvent exposure and organic brain damage. *Acta Neurol Scand* 1988; 78(suppl 118):1–143.
79. Escalona E, Yanes L, Feo O. Neurobehavioral evaluation of Venezuelan workers exposed to organic solvent mixtures. *Am J Ind Med* 1995; 27:15–27.
80. Ng TP, Ong SG, Lam WK. Neurobehavioural effects of industrial mixed solvent exposure in Chinese printing and paint workers. *Neurotoxicol Teratol* 1990;12:661–664.
81. Ng TP, Lim LC. An investigation of solvent-induced neuro-psychiatric disorders in spray painters. *Ann Acad Med Singapore* 1992;21: 797–803.
82. Kumar P, Gupta BN, Pandya KP. Behavioral studies in petrol pump workers. *Int Arch Occup Environ Health* 1988;61:35–38.
83. Fidler AT, Baker EL, Letz RE. Neurobehavioral effects of occupational exposure to organic solvents among construction workers. *Br J Ind Med* 1987;44:292–308.
84. Baker EL, Letz RE, Eisen EA, et al. Neurobehavioral effects of solvents in construction painters. *J Occup Med* 1988;30:116–123.
85. Broadwell DK, Darcey DJ, Hudnell HK, Otto DA, Boyes WK. Worksite clinical and neurobehavioral assessment of solvent-exposed microelectronics workers. *Am J Ind Med* 1995;27:677–698.
86. Zur J. Chronic solvent abuse. 1. Cognitive sequelae. *Child Care Health Dev* 1990;16:1–20.
87. Ohnishi A, Mori K, Fujishiro K, Kohriyama K, Miyata M, Murai Y. Application of neurobehavioral tests in a manufacturing automotive parts factory. *Sangyo Ika Daigaku Zasshi* 1995;17:165–172.
88. Agnew J, Schwartz BS, Bolla KI, Ford DP. Comparison of computerized and examiner-administered neurobehavioral testing techniques. *J Occup Med* 1991;33:1156–1162.
89. Gregersen P, Angels B, Nielsen TE, N rgaard B, Uldal C. Neurotoxic effects of organic solvents in exposed workers: an occupational, neuropsychological, and neurological investigation. *Am J Ind Med* 1984; 5:201–225.
90. Foo SC, Lwin S, Chia SE. Chronic neurobehavioural effects in paint formulators exposed to solvents and noise. *Ann Acad Med Singapore* 1994;23:650–654.
91. Chia SE, Ong CN, Phoon WH, Tan KT. Neurobehavioural effects on workers in a video tape manufacturing factory in Singapore. *Neurotoxicology* 1993;14:51–56.
92. Colvin M, Myers J, Nell V, Rees D, Cronje R. A cross-sectional survey of neurobehavioral effects of chronic solvent exposure on workers in a paint manufacturing plant. *Environ Res* 1993;63:122–132.
93. Milanovic L, Spilich G, Vucinic G, Knezevic S, Ribaric B. Effects of occupational exposure to organic solvents upon cognitive performance. *Neurotoxicol Teratol* 1990;12:657–660.
94. Maizlish NA, Langolf GD, Whitehead LW, Fine LJ, Albers JW, Goldberg J. Behavioural evaluation of workers exposed to mixtures of organic solvents. *Br J Ind Med* 1985;42:579–590.
95. Lindgren M, Ørbaek P, Haeger-Aronsen B. Prospective psychometric investigation of patients with organic psychosyndrome due to organic solvents. In: *Neurobehavioural methods in occupational and environmental health.* Copenhagen: World Health Organization, 1985; 125–129.
96. Lee SH. A study on the neurobehavioral effects of occupational exposure to organic solvents in Korean workers. *Environ Res* 1993;60: 227–232.
97. Singh J, Dwivedi K, Saxena VB. Disturbances in psychological functions of automobile painters. *Indian J Clin Psychol* 1987;14:43–45.
98. Lindström K. Psychological performances of workers exposed to various solvents. *Work Environ Health* 1973;10:151–155.
99. Anshelm Olson B, Gamberale F, Grönqvist B, Andersson K. Effects of solvents on reaction performance of foundry workers: a longitudinal study (translation). *Arbete Och Halsa* 1979;16:5–16.
100. Anshelm Olson B, Gamberale F, Grönqvist B. Reaction time changes among steel workers exposed to solvent vapors. *Int Arch Occup Environ Health* 1981;48:211–218.
101. Ørbæk P, Lindgren M, Olivecrona H, Hæger-Aronsen B. Computed tomography and psychometric test performance in patients with solvent induced chronic toxic encephalopathy and healthy controls. *Br J Ind Med* 1987;44:175–179.
102. Cherry N, Hutchins H, Pace T, Waldron HA. Neurobehavioral effects of repeated occupational exposure to toluene and paint solvents. *Br J Ind Med* 1985;42:291–300.
103. Anshelm Olson B. Effects of organic solvents on behavioral performance of workers in the paint industry (translation). *Arbete Och Halsa* 1982;25:1–25.
104. Anshelm Olson B. Effects of organic solvents on behavioral performance of workers in the paint industry. *Neurobehav Toxicol Teratol* 1982;4:703–708.
105. Gregersen P, Stigsby B. Reaction time of industrial workers exposed to organic solvents: relationship to degree of exposure and psychological performance. *Am J Ind Med* 1981;2:313–321.
106. Waszkowska M. Psychological evaluation of the effects of chronic occupational exposure of paint shop workers to the mixture of organic solvents. *Med Pr* 1992;43:35–39.
107. Blain L, Lagacé JP, Mergler D. Sensitivity and specificity of the lanthony desaturated D-15 panel to assess chromatic discrimination loss among solvent-exposed workers. In: *Neurobehavioural methods in occupational and environmental health.* Copenhagen: World Health Organization (Environmental Health Document 3), 1985;105–109.
108. Mergler D, Blain L. Assessing color vision loss among solvent-exposed workers. *Am J Ind Med* 1987;12:195–203.
109. Mergler D, Blain L, Lagacé J-P. Solvent related colour vision loss: an

indicator of neural damage? *Int Arch Occup Environ Health* 1987; 59:313–32.1.
110. Braun CMJ, Daigneault S, Gilbert B. Color discrimination testing reveals early printshop solvent neurotoxicity better than a neuropsychological test battery. *Arch Clin Neuropsychol* 1989;4:1–13.
111. Mergler D, Bélanger S, De Grosbois S, Vachon N. Chromal focus of acquired chromatic discrimination loss and solvent exposure among printshop workers. *Toxicology* 1988;49:341–348.
112. Zdzieszynska M. Acquired color vision disturbances as a sensitive marker of chronic exposure to petroleum derivatives. *Med Pr* 1995; 46:121–135.
113. Mergler D, Huel G, Bowler R, Frenette B. Visual dysfunction among former microelectronics assembly workers. *Arch Environ Health* 1991;46:326–334.
114. Trzcinski J, Stepien J. Disorders of color vision in employees of the Masovian refining and petrochemical industries in Píock. *Klin Oczna* 1989;91:43–44.
115. Zwiener RJ, Ginsburg CM. Organophosphate and carbamate poisoning in infants and children. *Pediatrics* 1988;81:121–126.
116. Richter ED, Chuwers P, Levy Y, et al. Health effects from exposure to organophosphate pesticides in workers and residents in Israel. *Isr J Med Sci* 1992;28:584–98.
117. Aiuto LA, Pavalakis SG, Boxer RA. Life-threatening organophosphate-induced delayed polyneuropathy in a child after accidental chlorpyrifos ingestion. *J Pediatrics* 1993;122:658–660.
118. McConnell R, Keifer M, Rosenstock L. Elevated quantitative vibrotactile threshold among workers previously poisoned with methamidophos and other organophosphate pesticides. *Am J Ind Med* 1994;25: 325–334.
119. Gershon S, Shaw FH. Psychiatric sequelae of chronic exposure to organophosphorous insecticides. *Lancet* 1961;1:1371–1374.
120. Jager KW, Roberts DV, Wilson A. Neuromuscular function in pesticide workers. *Br J Ind Med* 1970;27:273–278.
121. Korsak RJ, Sato MM. Effects of chronic organophosphate pesticide exposure on the central nervous system. *Clin Toxicol* 1977;11:83–95.
122. Duffy FH, Burchfiel JL, Bartels PH, Gaon M, Sim VM. Long-term effects of an organophosphate upon the human electroencephalogram. *Toxicol Appl Pharmacol* 1979;47:161–176.
123. Duffy FH, Burchfiel JL. Long term effects of the organophosphate sarin on EEG's in monkeys and humans. *Neurotoxicology* 1980;1: 667–689.
124. Kaloianova F, Verkhieva R, Dincheva V, et al. Epidemiological studies of the effect of organophosphate pesticides on health (abstract). *Probl Khig* 1989;14:38–75.
125. Daniell W, Barnhart S, Demers P, et al. Neuropsychological performance among agricultural pesticide applicators. *Environ Res* 1992;59: 217–228.
126. Kaplan JG, Kessler J, Rosenberg N, Pack D. Sensory neuropathy associated with Dursban (chlorpyrifos) exposure. *Neurology* 1993;43: 2193–2196.
127. Wagner SL. Chronic organophosphate exposure associated with transient hypertonia in an infant. *Pediatrics* 1994;94:94–97.
128. Stephens R, Spurgeon A, Calvert IA, et al. Neuropsychological effects of long-term exposure to organophosphates in sheep dip. *Lancet* 1995; 345:1135–1139.
129. Savage EP, Keefe TJ, Mounce LM, Heaton RK, Lewis JA, Burcar PJ. Chronic neurological sequelae of acute organophosphate pesticide poisoning. *Arch Environ Health* 1988;43:38–45.
130. Rosenstock L, Keifer M, Daniell WE, McConnell R, Claypoole K. Chronic central nervous system effects of acute organophosphate pesticide intoxication. *Lancet* 1991;338:223–227.
131. Steenland K, Jenkins B, Ames RG, O'Malley M, Chrislip D, Russo J. Chronic neurological sequelae to organophosphate pesticide poisoning. *Am J Public Health* 1994;84:731–736.
132. Repko JD, Morgan BB Jr, Nicholson J. *Behavioral effects of occupational exposure to lead.* US DHEW publication (NIOSH). Washington, DC: US Government Printing Office, 1975;75–184.
133. Repko JD, Corum CR, Jones PD, Garcia LS. *The effects of inorganic lead on behavioral and neurologic function.* DHEW publication (NIOSH). Washington, DC: US Government Printing Office, 1978; 78–128.
134. Johnson BL, Burg JR, Xintaras C, Handke JL. A neurobehavioral examination of workers from a primary nonferrous smelter. *Neurotoxicology* 1980;1:561–581.
135. Hogstedt C, Hane M, Agrell A, Bodin L. Neuropsychological test results and symptoms among workers with well-defined long-term exposure to lead. *Br J Ind Med* 1983;40:99–105.
136. Jeyaratnam J, Boey KW, Ong CN, Chia CB, Phoon WO. Neuropsychological studies on lead workers in Singapore. *Br J Ind Med* 1986; 43:626–629.
137. Stollery BT, Banks HA, Broadbent DE, Lee WR. Cognitive functioning in lead workers. *Br J Ind Med* 1989;46:698–707.
138. Stollery BT. Reaction time changes in workers exposed to lead. *Neurotoxicol Teratol* 1996;18:477–483.
139. Pasternak G, Becker CE, Lash A, Bowler R, Estrin WJ, Law D. Cross-sectional neurotoxicology study of lead-exposed cohort. *Clin Toxicol* 1989;27:37–51.
140. Haenninen H, Hernberg S, Mantere P, Vesanto R, Jalkanen M. Psychological performance of subjects with low exposure to lead. *J Occup Med* 1978;20:683–689.
141. Lindgren KN, Masten VL, Ford DP. Relation of cumulative exposure to inorganic lead and neuropsychological test performance. *Occup Environ Med* 1996;53:472–477.
142. Campara P, D'Andrea F, Micciolo R, Savonitto C, Tansella M, Zimmerman-Tansella CH. Psychological performance of workers with blood lead concentration below the current threshold limit value. *Int Arch Occup Environ Health* 1984;53:233–246.
143. Mantere P, Hänninen H, Hernberg S, Luukkonen R. A prospective follow-up study on psychological effects in workers exposed to low levels of lead. *Scand J Work Environ Health* 1984;10:43–50.
144. Yokoyama K, Araki S, Aono H. Reversibility of psychological performance in subclinical lead absorption. *Neurotoxicology* 1988;9:405–410.
145. Baker EL, Feldman RG, White RA, Harley JP, Dinse GE, Berkey CS. Occupational lead neurotoxicity: a behavioral and electrophysiological evaluation. Study design and year one results. *Br J Ind Med* 1984; 41:352–361.
146. Maizlish NA, Parra G. Neurobehavioural evaluation of Venezuelan workers exposed to inorganic lead. *Occup Environ Med* 1995;52: 408–14.
147. Agency for Toxic Substances and Disease Registry (ATSDR). *ATSDR report to Congress: 1993, 1994, 1995.* Atlanta: US Department of Health and Human Services, Public Health Service, Agency for Toxic Substances and Disease Registry, 1996.
148. Alabama Department of Public Health. *Child lead exposure study, Leeds, Alabama:* final report. Atlanta: US Department of Health and Human Services, Public Health Service, Agency for Toxic Substances and Disease Registry, September 1991.
149. Agency for Toxic Substances and Disease Registry (ATSDR). *The Silver Creek Mine Tailing Exposures Study:* final report. Atlanta: US Department of Health and Human Services, Public Health Service, Agency for Toxic Substances and Disease Registry, June 1988.
150. Agency for Toxic Substances and Disease Registry (ATSDR). *Multisite Lead and Cadmium Exposure Study with biological markers incorporated:* final report. Atlanta: US Department of Health and Human Services, Public Health Service, Agency for Toxic Substances and Disease Registry, April 1995.
151. Agency for Toxic Substances and Disease Registry (ATSDR) and City of Dallas, Department of Health and Human Services. *Biologic indicators of exposure to lead, RSR Smelter Site, Dallas, Texas.* Atlanta: US Department of Health and Human Services, Agency for Toxic Substances and Disease Registry, September 1995.
152. Colorado Department of Health. *Clear Creek/Central City Mine Waste Exposure Study, part I, Smuggler Mountain Site, Colorado:* final report. Atlanta: US Department of Health and Human Services, Public Health Service, Agency for Toxic Substances and Disease Registry, September 1992.
153. National Institute for Occupational Safety and Health (NIOSH). *Report to Congress on Workers' Home Contamination Study conducted under the Workers' Family Protection Act (29 U.S.C. 671a).* Cincinnati, OH: US Department of Health and Human Services, Public Health Service, Centers for Disease Control and Prevention, National Institute for Occupational Safety and Health, 1995.
154. Agency for Toxic Substances and Disease Registry. *The nature and extent of lead poisoning in children in the United States:* a report to Congress. Atlanta: US Department of Health and Human Services, 1988.
155. Needleman HL, Gunnoe C, Leviton A, et al. Deficits in psychologic and classroom performance of children with elevated dentine lead levels. *N Engl J Med* 1979;300:689–695.
156. Needleman HL, Schell A, Bellinger D, Leviton A, Allred EN. The

long-term effects of exposure to low doses of lead in childhood: an 11-year follow-up report. *N Engl J Med* 1990;322:83–88.
157. Dietrich KN, Krafft KM, Bornschein RL, Hammond PB, Berger O, Succop PA. Low-level fetal lead exposure effect on neurobehavioral development in early infancy. *Pediatrics* 1987;80:721–730.
158. Bellinger D, Leviton A, Waternaux C, Needleman H, Rabinowitz M. Low-level lead exposure, social class, and infant development. *Neurotoxicol Teratol* 1989;10:497–503.
159. McMichael AJ, Baghurst PA, Wigg NR, Vimpani GV, Robertson EF, Roberts RJ. Port Pirie cohort study: environmental exposure to lead and children's abilities at the age of four years. *N Engl J Med* 1988;319:468–475.
160. Wigg NR, Vimpani GV, McMichael AJ, Baghurst PA, Robertson EF, Roberts RJ. Port Pirie cohort study: childhood blood lead and neuropsychological development at age two years. *J Epidemiol Commun Health* 1988;42:213–219.
161. White RF, Diamond R, Proctor S, Morey C, Hu H. Residual cognitive deficits 50 years after lead poisoning during childhood. *Br J Ind Med* 1993;50:613–622.
162. Ruff HA, Bijur PE, Markowitz M, Ma Y-C, Rosen JF. Declining blood lead levels and cognitive changes in moderately lead-poisoned children. *JAMA* 1993;269:1641–1646.
163. Needleman HL, Riess JA, Tobin MJ, Biesectker GE, Greenhouse JB. Bone lead levels and delinquent behavior. *JAMA* 1996;275:363–369.
164. Centers for Disease Control (CDC). *Preventing lead poisoning in young Children:* a statement by the Centers for Disease Control. CDC report no. 99-2230. Atlanta: US Department of Health and Human Services, Public Health Service, Centers for Disease Control, 1985.
165. Agency for Toxic Substances and Disease Registry (ATSDR). *The nature and extent of lead poisoning in the United States:* a report to Congress. Atlanta: US Department of Health and Human Services, Agency for Toxic Substances and Disease Registry, 1988.
166. Centers for Disease Control (CDC). *Preventing lead poisoning in young children:* a statement by Centers for Disease Control. Atlanta: US Department of Public Health and Human Services, Public Health Service, Centers for Disease Control, October 1991.
167. Centers for Disease Control and Prevention (CDC). Update: blood lead levels—United States, 1991–1994. *MMWR* 1997;46(7):141–144.
168. Rodier J. Manganese poisoning in Moroccan miners. *Br J Ind Med* 1955;12:21–35.
169. Mena I, Marin O, Fuenzalida S, Cotzias GC. Chronic manganese poisoning—clinical picture and manganese turnover. *Neurology* 1967;17:128–136.
170. Hua M-S, Huang C-C. Chronic occupational exposure to manganes and neurobehavioral function. *J Clin Exp Neuropsychol* 1991;13:495-507.
171. Nelson K, Golnick J, Korn T, Angle C. Manganese encephalopathy: utility of early magnetic resonance imaging. *Br J Ind Med* 1993;50:510–513.
172. Meco G, Bonafati V, Vanacore N, Fabrizio E. Parkinsonism after chronic exposure to the fungicide maneb (manganese ethylene-bis-dithiocarbamate). *Scand J Work Environ Health* 1994;20:301–305.
173. Iregren A. Psychological test performance in foundry workers exposed to low levels of manganese. *Neurotoxicol Teratol* 1990;12:673–675.
174. Wennberg A, Iregren A, Struwe G, Cizinsky G, Haman M, Johansson L. Manganese exposure in steel smelters a health hazard to the nervous system. *Scand J Work Environ Health* 1991;17:255–262.
175. Mergler D, Huel G, Bowler R, et al. Nervous system dysfunction among workers with long-term exposure to manganese. *Environ Res* 1994;64:151–180.
176. Lucchini R, Selis L, Folli D, et al. Neurobehavioral effects of manganese in workers from a ferroalloy plant after temporary cessation of exposure. *Scand J Work Environ Health* 1995;21:143–149.
177. Roels H, Lauwerys R, Buchet J-P, et al. Epidemiological survey among workers exposed to manganese: effects on lung, central nervous system, and some biological indices. *Am J Ind Med* 1987;11:307–327.
178. Agocs MM, Etzel RA, Parrish RG, et al. Mercury exposure from interior latex paint. *N Engl J Med* 1990;323:1096–1101.
179. Mitra S. *Mercury in the ecosystem.* Lancaster, PA: Technomic, 1986.
180. Weiss B. Long ago and far away: a retrospective on the implications of Minamata. *Neurotoxicology* 1996;17:257–263.
181. Williamson AM, Teo RKC, Sanderson J. Occupational mercury exposure and its consequences for behavior. *Int Arch Occup Environ Health* 1982;50:273–286.
182. Wood RW, Weiss AB, Weiss B. Hand tremor induced by industrial exposure to inorganic mercury. *Arch Environ Health* 1973;26:249–252.
183. Langolf GD, Chaffin DB, Henderson R, Whittle HP. Evaluation of workers exposed to elemental mercury using quantitative tests of tremor and neuromuscular functions. *Am Ind Hyg Assoc J* 1978;39:976–984.
184. Chapman LJ, Sauter SL, Henning RA, Dodson VN, Reddan WG, Matthews CG. Differences in frequency of finger tremor in otherwise asymptomatic mercury workers. *Br J Ind Med* 1990;47:838–843.
185. Verberk MM, LaSalle HJA, Kemper CH. Tremor in workers with low exposure to metallic mercury. *Am Ind Hyg Assoc J* 1986;47:559–562.
186. Roels H, Gennary J-P, Lauwerys R, Buchet J-P, Malchaire J, Bernard A. Surveillance of workers exposed to mercury vapour: validation of a previously proposed biological threshold limit value for mercury concentrations in urine. *Am J Ind Med* 1985;7:45–71.
187. Smith PJ, Langolf GD. The use of Sternberg's memory-scanning paradigm in assessing effects of chemical exposure. *Hum Factors* 1981;23:701–708.
188. Uzzell BP, Oler J. Chronic low-level mercury exposure and neuropsychological functioning. *J Clin Exp Neuropsychol* 1986;8:581–593.
189. Piikivi L, Hänninen H, Martelin T, Mantere P. Psychological performance and long-term exposure to mercury vapors. *Scand J Work Environ Health* 1984;10:35–41.
190. Ngim CH, Foo SC, Boey KW. Chronic neurobehavioral effects of elemental mercury. *Br J Ind Med* 1992;49:782–790.
191. Smith PJ, Langolf GD, Goldberg J. Effects of occupational exposure to elemental mercury on short-term memory. *Br J Ind Med* 1983;40:413–419.
192. Soleno L, Urbano ML, Petrera V, Ambrosi L. Effects of low exposure to inorganic mercury on psychological effects. *Br J Ind Med* 1990;47:105–109.
193. Echeverria D, Heyer NJ, Martin MD, Naleway CA, Woods JS, Bittner AC. Behavioral effects of low-level exposure to Hgo among dentists. *Neurotoxicol Teratol* 1995;17:161–168.
194. Martinez Vazquez C, Rodriguez Saez C, Gil Fernandez M, et al. Evoked potentials and psychometric tests in the diagnosis of subclinical neurological damage in a group of workers exposed to low concentrations of mercury vapor. *An Med Interna* 1996;13:211–216.
195. Ritchie KA, MacDonald EB, Hammersley R, O'Neil JM, McGowan DA, Dale IM. A pilot study of the effect of low level exposure to mercury on the health of dental surgeons. *Occup Environ Med* 1995;52:813–817.
196. Skare I, Engqvist A. Human exposure to mercury and silver released from dental amalgam restorations. *Arch Environ Health* 1994;49:384–394.
197. Miller JM, Chaffin DB, Smith RG. Subclinical psychomotor and neuromuscular changes in workers exposed to inorganic mercury. *Am Ind Hyg Assoc J* 1975;36:725–733.
198. Liang Y-X, Sun R-K, Sun Y, Chen Z-Q, Li L-H. Psychological effects of low exposure to mercury vapor: application of a computer-administered Neurobehavioral Evaluation System. *Environ Res* 1993;60:320–327.
199. Kishi R, Doi R, Fukuchi Y, et al. Residual neurobehavioural effects associated with chronic exposure to mercury vapour. *Occup Environ Med* 1994;51:35–41.
200. Angotzi G, Cassitto MG, Camerino D, et al. Rapporti tra esposizione a mercurioe candizioni di salute in un gruppo di lavoratori addetti alla distillazione di mercurio in uno stabilimento della provincia di Siena. [Correlations between exposure to mercury and health in a group of workers at a mercury distillation plant in the province of Siena.] *Med Lav* 1980;71:463–480.
201. Angotzi G, Camerino D, Carboncini F, et al. Neurobehavioral follow-up study of mercury exposure. In: Gilioli R, Cassitto MC, Foà V, eds., *Advances in the biosciences, neurobehavioral methods in occupational health.* New York: Pergamon Press, 1983;46:247–253.
202. Kishi R, Doi R, Fukuchi Y, et al. Subjective symptoms and neurobehavioral performances of ex-mercury miners at an average of 18 years after the cessation of chronic exposure to mercury vapor. Mercury Workers Study Group. *Environ Res* 1993;62:289–302.
203. Forzi M, Cassitto MG, Gilioli R, Armeli G, Foà V. Persönlichke-its-fehlentwicklungen in arbeitern bei der elektrolytischen chlor-alkali-gewinnung. In: Deutschova E, Lukas E, eds. *Proceedings of the Sec-*

*ond International Industrial and Environmental Neurology Congress.* Prague: Univerzita Karlova, 1976;79–82 (partial translation).
204. Istoc-Bobis M, Gabor S. Psychological disfunctions in lead- and mercury-occupational exposure. *Rev Roumaine Sci Soc Serie Psychol* 1987;31:183–191.
205. Forzi M, Cassitto MG, Bulgheroni C, Foà V. Psychological measures in workers occupationally exposed to mercury vapors: a validation study. In: Horváth M, ed. *Adverse effects of environmental chemicals and psychotropic drugs.* New York: Elsevier, 1976;2:165–171.
206. Langworth S, Almkvist O, Söderman E, Wikström B-O. Effects of occupational exposure to mercury vapour on the central nervous system. *Br J Ind Med* 1992;49:545–555.
207. Lezak MD. *Neuropsychological assessment.* New York: Oxford University Press, 1995.
208. White RF. Clinical neuropsychological investigation of solvent neurotoxicity. In: Chang LW, Dyer RS, eds. *Handbook of neurotoxicology.* New York: Marcel Dekker, 1995;355–376.
209. Ryan CM, Morrow LA, Bromet EF, Parkinson DK. Assessment of neurological dysfunction in the workplace: normative data from the Pittsburgh Occupational Exposures Test battery. *J Clin Exp Neuropsychol* 1987;9:665–679.
210. Bowler RM, Thaler CD, Becker CE. California Neuropsychological Screening Battery (CNS/B I & II). *J Clin Psychol* 1986;42:946–955.
211. Kaufman AS. *Assessing adolescent and adult intelligence.* Boston: Allyn and Bacon, 1990.
212. Matarazzo JD. *Wechsler's measurement and appraisal of adult intelligence,* 5th ed. New York: Oxford University Press, 1972.
213. Grandjean P, Arnvig E, Beckmann J. Psychological dysfunctions in lead-exposed workers: relation to biological parameters of exposure. *Scand J Work Environ Health* 1978;4:295–303.
214. Mantere P, Hänninen H, Hernberg S. Subclinical neurotoxic lead effects: two-year follow-up studies with psychological test methods. *Neurobehav Toxicol Teratol* 1982;4:725–727.
215. Williamson AM, Clarke B, Edmonds C. Neurobehavioral effects of professional abalone diving. *Br J Ind Med* 1987;44:459–466.
216. Harkonen H, Lindström K, Seppäläinen AM, Asp S, Hernberg S. Exposure-response relationship between styrene exposure and central nervous functions. *Scand J Work Environ Health* 1978;4:53–59.
217. Cherry N, Venables H, Waldron HA. Description of the tests in the London School of Hygiene Test Battery. *Scand J Work Environ Health* 1984;10(suppl 1):18–19.
218. Michelsen, H, Lundber, I. Neuropsychological verbal tests may lack "hold" properties in occupational studies of neurotoxic effects. *Occup Environ Med* 1996;53:478–483.
219. Hänninen H, Lindström K. *Neurobehavioral test battery of the Institute of Occupational Health.* Helsinki: Institute of Occupational Health, 1989.
220. Bhattacharya A. Quantitative posturography as an early monitoring tool for chemical toxicity. In: Quehee S, ed. *Biological monitoring.* New York: Van Nostrand Reinhold, 1993;421–434.
221. Pifer JW, Friedlander BR, Kintz RT, Stockdale DK. Absence of toxic effects in silver reclamation workers. *Scand J Work Environ Health* 1989;15:210–221.
222. Cavalleri A, Trimarchi F, Glemi C, et al. Effects of lead on the visual system of occupationally exposed subjects. *Scand J Work Environ Health* 1982;8(suppl 1):148–151.
223. Morata TC. Study of the effects of simultaneous exposure to noise and carbon disulfide on workers' hearing. *Scand Audiol* 1989;18: 53–58.
224. Bergholtz LM, Ödqvist LM. Audiological findings in solvent exposed workers. *Acta Otolaryngol Stockh* 1984;412(suppl):109–110.
225. Arezzo JC, Schaumburg HH. The use of the Optacon as a screening device. A new technique for detecting sensory loss in individuals exposed to neurotoxins. *J Occup Med* 1980;22:461–464.
226. Letz R. The Neurobehavioral evaluation system: an international effort. In: Johnson BL, Anger WK, Durao A, Xintaras C, eds. *Advances in neurobehavioral toxicology:* applications in environmental and occupational health. Chelsea, MI: Lewis, 1990;489–495.
227. McNair DM, Lorr M, Droppleman, LF. *Manual for the profile of mood states.* San Diego, CA: Educational and Industrial Testing Services, 1981.
228. Maroni M, Bulgheroni C, Cassitto MG, Merluzzi F, Gilioli R, Foa V. A clinical, neurophysiological and behavioral study of female workers exposed to 1,1,1-trichloroethane. *Scand J Work Environ Health* 1977; 3:16–22.
229. Fittro KP, Bolla KI, Heller JR, Meyd CJ. The Milan Automated Neurobehavioral System—age, sex, and education differences. *J Occup Med* 1992;3:918–922.
230. Anger WK, Sizemore OJ, Grossmann SJ, Glasser JA, Letz R, Bowler R. Human neurobehavioral research methods: impact of subject variables. *Environ Res* 1997;73:18–41.
231. Baker EL, Letz R, Fidler AT. A computer-administered neurobehavioral evaluation system for occupational and environmental epidemiology. *J Occup Med* 1985;27:206–212.
232. Letz R, Baker EL. Computer-administered neurobehavioral testing in occupational health. *Semin Occup Med* 1986;1:197–203.
233. Letz R. Use of computerized tests batteries for quantifying neurobehavioral outcomes. *Environ Health Perspect* 1991;90:195–198.
234. Yokoyama K, Araki S, Osuga J, Karita T, Kurokawa M. Development of Japanese edition of Neurobehavioral Evaluation System (NES) and WHO Neurobehavioral Core Test Battery (NCTB): with assessment of reliability. *Sangyo Igaku* 1990;32:354–355.
235. Otto D, Skalik I, Hudnell HK, Ratcliffe J. Association of mercury exposure with neurobehavioral performance of children in Bohemia (abstract). *Neurotoxicology* 1994;15:962.
236. Maizlish N, Schenker M, Weisskopf C, Seiber J, Samuels S. A behavioral evaluation of pest control workers with short-term low-level exposure to the organophosphate Diazinon. *Am J Ind Med* 1987;12: 153–172.
237. Baker EL, Letz RE, Fidler AT, Shalat S, Plantamura D. A computer-based neurobehavioral evaluation system for occupational and environmental epidemiology: methodology and validation studies. *Neurobehav Toxicol Teratol* 1985;7:369–377.
238. Muijser H, Geuskens RBM, Hooisma J, Emmen HH, Kulig BM. Behavioral effects of exposures to organic solvents in carpet layers. *Neurotoxicol Teratol* 1996;18:455–462.
239. Bowler RM. Thaler CD, Law D. Comparison of the NES and CNS/B neuropsychological screening batteries. *Neurotoxicology* 1990;11: 451–464.
240. Anger WK, Rohlman DS, Sizemore OJ. A comparison of instruction formats for administering a computerized behavioral test. *Behav Res Methods Instrum Comput* 1994;26:209–212.
241. Anger WK, Rohlman DS, Sizemore OJ, Kovera CA, Gibertini M, Ger J. Human behavioral assessment in neurotoxicology: producing appropriate test performance with written and shaping instructions. *Neurotoxicol Teratol* 1996;18:371–379.
242. Rohlman DS, Sizemore OJ, Anger WK, Kovera CA. Computerized neurobehavioral testing: techniques for improving test instructions. *Neurotoxicol Teratol* 1996;18:407–412.
243. Gamberale F, Iregren A, Kjellberg A. Computerized performance testing in neurotoxicology: Who, what, how, and where to? The SPES Example. In: Russell RW, Flattau PE, Pope AM, eds. *Behavioral measures of neurotoxicity.* Washington, DC: National Academy Press, 1990;359–394.
244. Iregren A, Gamberale F, Kjellberg A. SPES: a psychological test system to diagnose environmental hazards. *Neurotoxicol Teratol* 1996;18: 485–491.
245. Cassitto MG, Gilioli R, Camerino D. Experiences with the Milan Automated Neurobehavioral System (MANS). *Neurotoxicol Teratol* 1989;11:571–574.
246. Camerino D; Cassitto MG. Prevalence of abnormal neurobehavioral scores in populations exposed to different industrial chemicals. *Environ Res* 1993;61:251–257.
247. Stollery BT. The Automated Cognitive Test (ACT) system. *Neurotoxicol Teratol* 1996;18:493–497.
248. Kennedy RS, Wilkes RL, Dunlap WP, Kuntz LA. Development of an automated performance test system for environmental and behavioral toxicology studies. *Percept Mot Skills* 1987;65:947–962.
249. Turnage JJ, Kennedy RS, Smith MG, Baltzley DR, Lane NE. Development of microcomputer-based mental acuity tests. *Ergonomics* 1992;35:1271–1295.
250. Turnage JJ, Kennedy RS. The development and use of a computerized human performance test battery for repeated-measures applications. *Hum Performance* 1992;5:265–301.
251. Anger WK, Otto DA, Letz R. Symposium on computerized behavioral testing of humans in neurotoxicology research: overview of the proceedings. *Neurotoxicol Teratol* 1996;18:347–350.
252. Letz R, Green RC, Woodward JL. Development of a computer-based battery designed to screen adults for neuropsychological impairment. *Neurotoxicol Teratol* 1996;18:365–370.

253. Fray PJ, Robbins TW. CANTAB battery: proposed utility in neurotoxicology. *Neurotoxicol Teratol* 1996;18:499–504.
254. Dahl R, White RF, Weihe P, et al. Feasibility and validity of three computer-assisted neurobehavioral tests in 7-year-old children. *Neurotoxicol Teratol* 1996;18:413–419.
255. Krengel M, White RF, Diamond R, Letz R, Cyrus P, Durso R. A comparison of NES2 and traditional neuropsychological tests in a neurologic sample. *Neurotoxicol Teratol* 1996;18:435–439.
256. White RF, Diamond R, Krengel M, Lindem K, Feldman RG. Validation of the NES2 in patients with neurologic patient sample. *Neurotoxicol Teratol* 1996;18:441–448.
257. Heyer NA, Bittner AC Jr, Echeverria D. Analyzing multivariate neurobehavioral outcomes in occupational studies: a comparison of approaches. *Neurotoxicol Teratol* 1996;18:401–406.
258. Kovera CA, Anger WK, Campbell KA, et al. Computer-administration of questionnaires: a health screening system (HSS) developed for veterans. *Neurotoxicol Teratol* 1996;18:511–518.
259. Johnson BL, Baker EL, El Batawi M, et al., eds. *Prevention of neurotoxic illness in working populations.* New York: John Wiley, 1987.
260. Anger WK, Cassitto MG, Liang Y-X, et al. Comparison of performance from three continents on the WHO-recommended neurobehavioral core test battery. *Environ Res* 1993;62:125–147.
261. Cassitto MG, Camerino D, Hänninen H, Anger WK. International collaboration to evaluate the WHO Neurobehavioral Core Test Battery. In: Johnson BL, Anger WK, Durao A, Xintaras C, eds. *Advances in neurobehavioral toxicology:* applications in environmental and occupational health. Chelsea, MI: Lewis, 1990;203–223.
262. Liang Y-X, Chen Z-Q, Sun R-K, Fang Y-F, Yu J-H. Application of the WHO Neurobehavioral Core Test Battery and other neurobehavioral screening methods. In: Johnson BL, Anger WK, Durao A, Xintaras C, eds. *Advances in neurobehavioral toxicology:* applications in environmental and occupational health. Chelsea, MI: Lewis, 1990; 225–243.
263. Dudek B. Adaptation of the WHO NCTB for use in Poland for detection of effects of exposure to neurotoxic agents. *Environ Res* 1993;61: 349–356.
264. Anger WK, Letz R, Chrislip DW, et al. Neurobehavioral test methods for environmental health studies of adults. *Neurotoxicol Teratol* 1994; 16:489–497.
265. Amler RW, Lybarger JA, Anger WK, Phifer BL, Chappell W, Hutchinson LJ. Adoption of an Adult Environmental Neurobehavioral Test Battery (AENTB). *Neurotoxicol Teratol* 1994;16:525–530.
266. Amler RW, Anger WK, Sizemore OJ. *Adult Environmental Neurobehavioral Test Battery (training manual).* Atlanta: US DHHS PHS, Agency for Toxic Substances an Disease Registry, 1995.
267. Anger WK, Sizemore OJ. Variables affecting performance on the ATSDR Adult Environmental Neurobehavioral Test Battery: research needs. In: Andrews JS, Frumkin H, Johnson BL, Mehlman MA, Xintaras C, Bucsela JA, eds. *Hazardous waste and public health:* International Congress on the Health Effects of Hazardous Waste. Atlanta: US DHHS PHS, Agency for Toxic Substances an Disease Registry, 1995;698–711.
268. Amler RW, Gibertini M, Lybarger JA, et al. Selective approaches to basic neurobehavioral testing of children in environmental health studies. *Neurotoxicol Teratol* 1996;18:429–434.
269. Crossen JR, Wiens AN. Wechsler Memory Scale–Revised: deficits in performance associated with neurotoxic solvent exposure. *Clin Neuropsychol* 1988;2:181–187.
270. White RF, Feldman RG. Neuropsychological assessment of toxic encephalopathy. *Am J Ind Med* 1987;395–398.
271. Albers JW. Standardized neurological testing in neurotoxicology studies. In: Johnson BL, Anger WK, Durao A, Xintaras C, eds. *Advances in neurobehavioral toxicology:* application in environmental and occupational health. Chelsea, MI: Lewis, 1990;151–164.
272. White RF, Proctor SP. Research and clinical criteria for development of neurobehavioral test batteries. *J Occup Med* 1992;34: 140–148.
273. Morrow LA, Steinhauer SR, Condray R, Hodgson M. Neuropsychological performance of journeymen painters under acute solvent exposure and exposure-free conditions. *J Int Neuropsychol Soc* 1997;3: 269–275.
274. Rey A. *L'examen clinique en psychologie.* Paris: Presses Universitaires de France, 1964.
275. Dellis D, Kramer JH, Kaplan E, Ober BA. *California Verbal Learning Test manual.* New York: Psychological Corporation, 1987.
276. Wechsler D. *Wechsler Memory Scale–Revised manual.* San Antonio, TX: Psychological Corporation, 1987.
277. Trahan DE, Larrabee GJ. *Continuous Visual Memory Test.* Odessa, FL: Psychological Assessment Research, 1988.
278. Peterson LR, Peterson MJ. Short-term retention of individual verbal items. *J Exp Psychol* 1959;58:193–198.
279. Wechsler D. *WAIS-R manual.* New York: Psychological Corporation, 1981.
280. Morrow LA, Robin N, Hodgson MJ, Kamis H. Assessment of attention and memory efficiency in persons with solvent neurotoxicity. *Neuropsychologia* 1992;30:911–922.
281. Weber AM. A new clinical measure of attention: the Attentional Capacity Test. *Neuropsychology* 1988;2;59–71.
282. Rosvold H, Mirsky A, Sarason I, et al. A continuous performance test of brain damage. *J Consult Clin Psychol* 1956;20:343–350.
283. Gronwall D, Wrightson P. Memory and information processing capacity after closed head injury. *J Neurol Neurosurg Psychiatry* 1981;44: 889–895.
284. Stroop JR. Studies of interference in serial verbal reactions. *J Exp Psychol* 1935;18:643–662.
285. Reitan RM, Wolfson D. *The Halstead-Reitan Neuropsychological Test Battery:* theory and clinical interpretation. Tucson, AZ: Neuropsychology Press, 1993.
286. Tiffin J. *Purdue Pegboard Examiner's manual.* Rosemont, IL: London House, 1968.
287. Klove H. Clinical neuropsychology. In: Forster FM, ed. *The medical clinics of North America.* New York: Saunders, 1963.
288. Smith A. *Symbol Digit Modalities Test (SDMT) manual (revised).* Los Angeles: Western Psychological Services, 1982.
289. Glosser G, Butters N, Kaplan E. Visuoperceptual processes in brain damaged patients on the Digit Symbol Substitution Test. *Int J Neuroscience* 1977;7:59–66.
290. Heaton RK. *Wisconsin Card Sorting Test (WCST).* Odessa, FL: Psychological Assessment Resources, 1981.
291. Shallice T. Specific impairments of planning. *Philos Trans R Soc Lond* 1982;198:199–209.
292. Benton AL, Hamsher Kde S. *Multilingual Aphasia Examination.* Iowa City, IA: AJA Associates, 1989.
293. Kaplan EF, Goodglass H, Weintraub S. *The Boston Naming Test,* 2nd ed. Philadelphia: Lea & Febiger, 1983.
294. MacGinitie WH. *Gates-MacGinitie Reading Tests,* 2nd ed. Boston: Houghton Mifflin, 1978.
295. Goodglass H, Kaplan E. *Boston Diagnostic Aphasia Examination (BDAE).* Odessa, FL: Psychological Assessment Resources, 1983.
296. Osterreith PA. Le test de copie d'une figure complexe. *Arch Psychol* 1944;30:206–356.
297. Hooper HE. *Hooper Visual Organization Test (VOT).* Los Angeles: Western Psychological Services, 1983.
298. Butcher JN, Dahlstrom WG, Graham JR, et al. *Manual for the Restandardized Minnesota Multiphasic Personality Inventory:* MMPI-2. Minneapolis: University of Minneapolis Press, 1989.
299. Derogatis LR. *Symptom Checklist-90-R (SCL-90-R) Administration, Scoring, and Procedures Manual.* Minneapolis: National Computer Systems, 1994.
300. Beck AT. *Beck Depression Inventory.* San Antonio, TX: Psychological Corporation, 1987.
301. Beck AT, Epstein N, Brown G, Steer RA. An inventory for measuring clinical anxiety: psychometric properties. *J Consulting Clin Psychol* 1988;56:893–897.
302. Malcolm R, Sturgis ET, Anton RF, Williams L. Computer-assisted diagnosis of alcoholism. *Comput Hum Serv* 1990;5:163–170.
303. Reif JS, Tsongas RA, Anger WK, et al. Two-stage evaluation of exposure to mercury and biomarkers of neurotoxicity at a hazardous waste site. *J Toxicol Environ Health* 1993;40:413–422.
304. Anger WK, Moody L, Burg J, et al. Neurobehavioral evaluation of soil and structural fumigators using methyl bromide and sulfuryl fluoride. *Neurotoxicology* 1986;7:137–156.

*Environmental and Occupational Medicine, Third Edition,* edited by William N. Rom.
Lippincott–Raven Publishers, Philadelphia © 1998.

# CHAPTER 49

# Occupational Heart Disease

Kenneth D. Rosenman

The effect of work on the heart is mediated by chemical and physical as well as by psychological stressors. All too often, however, clinicians and researchers tend to overlook the potential of a cardiovascular effect from work. Assessment of personal risk factors such as cigarette smoking, hypertension, and cholesterol are done routinely. Evaluation of an association between acute symptoms and the level of a patient's activity at the time of acute symptoms is also standard practice. What is typically not considered is an assessment of workplace risk factors and the location and possible exposures associated with that location where the acute symptoms of the patient have occurred.

The most dramatic consequence of this lack of attention to exposures and location is highlighted by a case report from the mid-1970s (1). A retired executive without a previous history of clinical heart disease developed an acute anterior wall myocardial infarction after exposure to paint stripper that contained methylene chloride. Methylene chloride is metabolized in the body to carbon monoxide. The patient inquired of his physician about the possible association between the exposure and his heart attack. The physician did not make any connection between the exposure and the patient's heart attack. The patient developed a second heart attack on reexposure but again no association was appreciated. During his next reexposure the patient was found dead in his basement where he had been using the methylene chloride containing product (1). Diagnostic delays recognizing the acute precipitation of cardiac disease after carbon monoxide exposure continue to be reported (2). Articles on the occupational disease burden in the United States estimate that 1% to 3% of deaths from cardiovascular disease are work related (3). Lower socioeconomic status and educational levels are associated with increased ischemic heart disease (4). This has typically been attributed to psychosocial stresses and increased personal risk factors. A recent Swedish study controlling for these factors attributed 16% of ischemic heart disease in lower socioeconomic groups to chemical exposure, particularly solvents and soldering fumes (5).

Proliferation of smooth muscle cells is an essential component of atherosclerotic plaque formation. One of the competing, although less accepted, hypotheses for smooth muscle proliferation in the endothelium is that atherosclerosis is a process that involves benign smooth muscle cell tumors of the artery wall (6). This theory was first suggested in 1973 by the Benditts (6a) as the "monoclonal hypothesis." Using plaque samples from human autopsy specimens they showed that only one glucose 6-phosphate dehydrogenase (G-6-PD) isoenzyme type was seen in plaques (single cell origin) versus both enzymes types in normal artery wall samples (polyclonal cell origin). Studies in animals have shown limited support for this hypothesis (7). If this were a valid mechanism, the number of chemicals potentially associated with occupational heart disease would markedly expand.

Table 1 summarizes the known and suspected adverse effects of work on the heart. A more detailed review of each factor follows.

## CARBON MONOXIDE

Internal combustion engines (e.g., gasoline, diesel, or propane) or any process where there is combustion of carbonaceous material (e.g., coal, oil, tobacco, or wood)

K. D. Rosenman: Department of Medicine, Michigan State University, East Lansing, Michigan 48824-1316.

**TABLE 1.** *Occupational risk factors for heart disease*

| Substance | Cardiovascular abnormalities: Acute | Cardiovascular abnormalities: Chronic |
|---|---|---|
| Arsenic | — | Cardiomyopathy<br>Hypertension?<br>Peripheral vascular disease? |
| Carbon disulfide | — | Coronary artery disease |
| Carbon monoxide | Angina<br>Claudication<br>Myocardial infarction<br>Sudden death | Coronary artery disease? |
| Cobalt | — | Cardiomyopathy |
| Cold | Angina<br>Myocardial infarction<br>Sudden death | — |
| Fibrogenic dusts | — | Cor pulmonale<br>Coronary artery disease? |
| Fluorocarbons | Arrhythmias<br>Sudden death | — |
| Heat | Angina<br>Myocardial infarction<br>Sudden death | — |
| Hydrocarbons | Arrhythmias<br>Sudden death | Coronary artery disease? |
| Lead | ECG changes<br>Myocarditis | Hypertension |
| Nitrates | Angina<br>Myocardial infarction<br>Sudden death | Coronary artery disease? |
| Noise | — | Hypertension |
| Vibration | — | Peripheral vascular disease |
| Psychological strain (high work demand + low job control) | Acute myocardial infarction<br>Sudden death | Coronary artery disease? |
| Physical inactivity | — | Coronary artery disease |

produce the odorless, colorless gas, carbon monoxide. Transportation vehicles and power plants are the major ambient air sources. Concentrations of carbon monoxide build up when a combustion engine is run inside a structure (such as a car in a garage, or a gasoline-powered pressure washer in a barn, or a propane forklift in a warehouse), when a furnace is improperly vented, or when combustion is out of control as with a fire. Low-level exposure to carbon monoxide occurs from passive cigarette smoking. Because of their metabolic breakdown in the body, exposure to dichloromethane (methylene chloride) as well as other dihalomethanes (dibromomethane, bromochloromethane, and diiodomethane) also increases body burdens of carbon monoxide.

The acute adverse health effects of carbon monoxide are based on a number of factors: a greater than 200-fold preferential binding between hemoglobin and carbon monoxide versus hemoglobin and oxygen; a 50-fold preferential binding between myoglobin and carbon monoxide versus myoglobin and oxygen; a reduction of oxygen delivery to the tissues by shifting the oxyhemoglobin curve to the left; an inhibition of mitochondrial enzymes; an impairment of oxygen diffusion into mitochondria; and an increase of platelet adhesiveness. Cardiovascular physiologic changes noted after acute exposure include decreased cardiac output, increased myocardial lactate production, and lowered threshold for ventricular fibrillation.

Clinically, carboxyhemoglobin can be measured in either arterial or venous blood. A cherry-red color of the mucous membranes may be seen on physical examination but its absence is not a reliable sign of a normal carboxyhemoglobin level. Carbon monoxide can also be measured in exhaled air and the carboxyhemoglobin level can then be estimated. With arterial blood gas measurements, the value for oxygen saturation that is not measured but calculated from the arterial oxygen content and the pH is not correct in a patient with carbon monoxide poisoning. The calculated oxygen saturation is an estimate of the hemoglobin-binding sites bound to oxygen of those available for oxygen association. In the patient with carbon monoxide poisoning the hemoglobin-binding sites available for oxygen association are reduced because of binding to carbon monoxide. This reduction in available binding sites for oxygen is not factored in when calculating the oxygen saturation. Similarly, pulse oximeters that measure functional rather than fractional arterial oxygen saturation overestimate oxygen saturation in the presence of carboxyhemoglobin.

Table 2 shows ambient air levels of exposure to carbon monoxide and the associated carboxyhemoglobin levels. Fetal carboxyhemoglobin levels are 10% to 15% higher than in the mother. Endogenous production is secondary to the normal turnover of hemoglobin and is increased with conditions causing hemolysis. Medications that induce hepatic cytochrome activity such as phenobarbital and phenytoin also increase the endogenous production. With exposure to carbon monoxide in the air, carboxyhemoglobin levels increase with increased length of exposure, and with increased physical activity, which increases pulmonary ventilation. Similarly, carboxyhemoglobin levels decrease with removal from exposure. Increased activity or the administration of oxygen speeds up the removal of carbon monoxide from the body. The relationship between the blood carboxyhemoglobin level and the carbon monoxide concentration in ambient air can be estimated by using the following equation:

$$\underset{\text{(measured in venous or arterial blood)}}{\%\ \text{Carboxyhemoglobin}} = \underset{(10{,}000\ \text{ppm} = 1\%)}{\%\ \text{carbon monoxide in air}} \times \underset{\text{(in minutes)}}{\text{Time}} \times K \qquad [1]$$

where $K = 3$ at rest, 5 for light physical work, and 11 for heavy physical work).

Carboxyhemoglobin reaches an equilibrium with constant carbon monoxide exposure. The time used in the equation cannot be greater than the time used to reach an equilibrium. At rest equilibrium is reached in approximately 8 hours; with increased activity equilibrium is reached sooner. The half-life for removal is considered to be approximately 4 to 6 hours with normal activity.

Methylene chloride is metabolized via a saturable pathway and maximum CoHgb levels after exposure are 10% to 12%.

Repeated studies have shown that low-level carbon monoxide exposure that resulted in carboxyhemoglobin levels of 2% to 4% reduced exercise tolerance and length of time to ST segment changes in individuals with angina (8). Similarly, individuals with claudication or chronic obstructive lung disease have been shown to have decreased exercise tolerance with similar low levels of carboxyhemoglobin. Levels of 6% carboxyhemoglobin have been shown to increase the frequency of multiple ventricular premature contractions after exercise but not at rest (9), although these results were not confirmed in a recent study (10). Case reports of acute myocardial infarction have been reported at carboxyhemoglobin levels as low as 10% (11,12). Patients with q wave infarcts who had carboxyhemoglobin levels ≥5% had higher levels of creatinine kinase and a higher incidence of serious arrhythmias (13).

Associated symptoms that may be reported by patients with elevated carboxyhemoglobin levels are headaches, giddiness, tinnitus at 10% CoHgb levels, nausea, and weakness at 20% CoHgb levels, and clouding of mental alertness and increased weakness at 30% CoHgb levels. At CoHgb levels of 35% or above the patient is increasingly likely to collapse and be comatose.

Although there are animal studies that suggest that carbon monoxide can increase vascular permeability with the potential to increase lipid deposition in vessel walls, increase arterial wall hypoxia, and increase platelet adhesiveness, there are relatively sparse data from epidemiologic studies to support a long-term ath-

**TABLE 2.** *Carboxyhemogloblin (COHb) at equilibrium for varying concentrations of carbon monoxide*

| Concentration of carbon monoxide (ppm) | Carboxyhemoglobin (%) | Comments |
|---|---|---|
| 0 | 0.36–0.9 (average 0.5) | Endogenous production increases with hemolysis, pregnancy, and use of phenytoin and phenobarbital |
| 9 | 1.7 | Environmental Protection Agency 8-hour standard not to be exceeded more than once/year |
| 25 | 3.5 | American Conference of Governmental Industrial Hygienists recommended 8-hour time-weighted average |
| 35 | 5.4 | Environmental Protection Agency 1-hour ceiling standard not to be exceeded more than once/year; National Institution Occupational Safety and Health recommended 10-hour time-weighted average |
| 50 | 7.36 | Occupational Safety and Health Administration allowable 8-hour time-weighted average |
| 400 | 1–10 (average: cigarette smokers 4.7, cigar smokers 2.9, pipe smokers 2.2) | Average concentration in cigarette smoke |

erosclerotic effect from carbon monoxide exposure. Within 1 year of quitting smoking the risk of coronary heart disease dramatically decreases in comparison to the risk in individuals who continue to smoke (14). The risk of cardiovascular mortality among ex-smokers who smoked less than one pack per day reverts back to that of the nonsmoker (15), although for ex-smokers who smoked more than a pack of cigarettes a day the risk of cardiovascular disease, although reduced from smokers, remains above that of nonsmokers. This increase in risk, although reduced from that of the smoker, persists for at least 20 years after cessation (16). Occupational cohort groups exposed to carbon monoxide that have been studied for heart disease include bridge and tunnel officers, firefighters, and foundry workers. Increased mortality from cardiovascular disease have been reported among all three of these groups, although the results among firefighters have not been consistent (17–19). However, when the risk after cessation of exposure has been investigated, this risk has decreased similar to the reduced risk seen with ex–cigarette smokers (19,20). Overall the evidence is not particularly convincing that carbon monoxide has a chronic effect in promoting atherosclerosis.

Another possible source of exposure to carbon monoxide is from exposure to environmental tobacco smoke. Based on measurements of urinary cotinine levels in nonsmokers who live with smokers, it is estimated that the nonsmoker is absorbing the equivalent of combustion material as if they smoked 0.1 to 1.0 cigarette per day. Levels of carbon monoxide are greater in sidestream smoke than the mainstream smoke inhaled by the smoker. Carboxyhemoglobin levels in individuals highly exposed to environmental tobacco smoke have shown an increase of 0.5% to 1.0% in carboxyhemoglobin levels. Assuming an acute adverse effort from smoking cigarettes and that there is an effect from cigarettes up to 15 years after quitting, then 32,000 to 45,000 heart disease deaths have been estimated to occur each year from exposure to environmental tobacco smoke (21).

## NITRATES

Exposures in the explosive industry to ammonium and sodium nitrate, ethylene glycol dinitrate, nitroglycerin, and dinitrotoluene have been associated with both acute and chronic heart disease. Sudden death ("Monday morning death") and headache ("powder head") have been described in workers when they are away from work for a couple of days on the weekend or on vacation. The headache has also occurred in family members with exposure to dust brought home on clothes. Workers first noted in the late 1800s that they would build up a tolerance throughout the working week to the health effects of explosives, and therefore to prevent the headache they would put a few grains of explosive powder in their hatband to maintain exposure on the weekends. Both an increase in cerebrospinal fluid pressure and blood flow in the middle cerebral artery have been correlated with the onset of the headache associated with nitroglycerine exposure (22).

Sudden death after short-term absence from exposure was first described in the 1930s. Subsequent case reports including autopsies and/or cardiac catheterization have shown coronary arteries without significant obstruction or vasospasm (not responsive to ergonovine) (23). The mechanism for myocardial infarction and/or sudden death is presumed to be rebound vasospasm from withdrawal of the nitrates.

Increased mortality from heart disease and strokes has also been reported after chronic exposure (24–27). These results are compatible with previous autopsy case reports of nonatheromatous sclerosis with hyalinization of the coronary arteries among long-term explosive workers (28).

Methemoglobinemia may occur with exposure. Also, Raynaud's phenomenon and peripheral neuropathy have been described in exposed workers.

## NOISE

Acute exposure to noise increases epinephrine levels, vascular resistance, heart rate, and blood pressure (29,30). With repeated exposure to noise there is attenuation and/or loss of the acute effect. The majority of epidemiologic studies of workers with long-term exposure to noise above either 85 or 90 db have demonstrated an increased risk of hypertension (31–33). Although less frequently, similar results of increased risk of hypertension have been reported among workers with noise-induced hearing loss (34). A nonoccupational study comparing normal-hearing children with children with congenital loss of hearing found significantly higher systolic and diastolic blood pressure in the children with normal hearing (35).

A number of studies, however, have found no association between elevated blood pressure and either duration of noise exposure or presence of hearing loss (36,37). Methodologic issues including cohort size, noise exposure measurements, age of the cohort, and control of confounding factors probably all contribute to differences in results found among studies. No controlled studies have been conducted to evaluate whether reduction of noise exposure is useful in treating hypertension.

Repeated studies have found an association between hyperlipidemia and hearing loss (38). These studies have not been able to distinguish between hyperlipidemia being a confounding risk factor for noise exposure versus a mechanistic pathway for noise's effect on the basilar membrane and/or interference with the cochlear blood supply.

## CARBON DISULFIDE

Carbon disulfide is the one workplace exposure that has clearly been associated with the development of atherosclerosis. Initially case reports in the 1940s followed by epidemiologic studies beginning in the late 1960s have consistently shown increased atherosclerosis and cardiovascular mortality among carbon disulfide–exposed workers involved in the manufacture of rayon (39,40). The mechanism appears to be mediated through an effect on lipoproteins and blood pressure (41,42). The effect appears reversible with cessation of exposure and early diagnosis; removal of symptomatic individuals has been effective in reducing atherosclerotic heart disease among exposed workers (43,44).

## HOT AND COLD

Work in temperature extremes at either end of the scale has been associated in case reports with the acute manifestations of coronary artery disease. Excess deaths from cardiovascular disease occur in winter months (45). Physiologic changes induced by hot or cold weather would exacerbate a heart problem in a person already compromised by coronary artery disease. There are no long-term epidemiologic studies among workers chronically exposed to cold environments. Limited studies of workers exposed to heat in the steel industry have not shown increased mortality in long-term heat-exposed workers (46), although there is a recent study showing an increased risk of heart disease mortality in underground potash miners exposed to heat (47).

## VIBRATION

Handheld equipment that vibrates particularly when used under cold, wet conditions causes a high incidence of Raynaud's disease. In the general medical literature, case series of Raynaud's phenomenon that evaluate treatment modalities usually include more women than men. However, in the occupational literature the prevalence of Raynaud's phenomenon has ranged from 50% to 80% among a number of different male-dominated cohorts. These include studies of chippers and grinders in foundries and shipyards, lumbermen, jackhammer operators, and miners. Among lumbermen, an association has been noted between hearing loss and Raynaud's phenomenon. The common etiology is the use of chain saws. Fish filleters, traditionally women, also have high rates of disease. Historically, individuals involved in cleaning vinyl chloride reaction kettles have had advanced changes of peripheral vascular disease, including acro-osteolysis. Exposure to arsenic among smelter workers is also associated with vasospastic disease.

Once an individual is symptomatic, even the sound of the vibrating equipment or the chain saw or vibration in the opposite hand may induce vasospasm. The primary pathologic reaction is increased peripheral resistance of the finger circulation. Chronic neuropathy with fibrosis has been reported on biopsy in patients with long-term clinical courses. An increase in blood viscosity has also been reported in patients with vibration-induced Raynaud's phenomenon.

Early diagnosis with ongoing medical surveillance and removal from exposure reduces the sequelea. Prevention of Raynaud's phenomenon requires engineering controls such as modification of production lines to eliminate the need to use vibrating hand tools and design of equipment with lower vibration levels, and work practice controls such as proper maintenance of equipment, frequent rest periods, wearing adequate clothing and gloves to keep the body and hands warm, and learning to grasp the tool as lightly as possible while still maintaining control of it.

## LUNG FUNCTION

Besides the well-known relationship between advanced lung disease and right-sided heart failure, decrements in lung function are a risk factor for mortality from atherosclerotic heart disease (48). The association has been found in both cross-sectional and longitudinal studies and among cigarette and non–cigarette smokers (49). Alternate explanations for the associations that have been put forward include (a) an hypoxic effect on the heart, (b) a spurious association secondary to preexisting heart failure, (c) a spurious association secondary to confounding by cigarette smoking, and (d) a spurious association secondary to confounding by obesity and decreased physical activity. Although one review of the literature has attributed the inverse relationship to the manner in which cigarette smoking has been controlled for in the studies, the association has also been reported among nonsmokers (48,50).

These studies generally have not considered the etiology of the pulmonary function decrements. However, a recent study of shipyard workers with asbestosis found a threefold risk of ischemic heart disease in workers with a forced expiratory volume in 1 second ($FEV_1$) or a forced vital capacity (FVC) of less than 80%, or x-ray or biopsy evidence of asbestosis (51). No increased risk was found for pleural plaques alone.

## SOLVENTS

A large number of different types of chemicals including gasoline, benzene, fluorocarbons, perchloroethylene, trichloroethylene, trichloromethane, and xylene have been associated with both arrhythmias and sudden death. Initial concern about the arrhythmogenic effect of solvents was raised by sudden deaths among teenagers abusing various commercial and household products (52).

Case reports of arrhythmias and/or sudden death from solvent exposure have been reported in industrial settings (53,54), in a dry cleaner store (55), in a hospital pathology lab (56), and among pesticide sprayers (57).

Recent epidemiologic studies of fluorocarbon exposure have not found a significant increase in arrhythmias under normal working conditions (58–61). These studies do not negate the potential toxicity of these substances in situations where exposures are particularly high such as in a confined space or after a spill or in individuals with underlying heart disease.

The fluorocarbons and hydrocarbons directly affect myocardial tissue and increase cardiac sensitivity to catecholamines (62). A dog model has been used to assess the relative cardiotoxicity of many hydrocarbons and fluorocarbons (63). Benzene, chloroform, heptane, and trichlorethylene were the most active in this experimental model. The following general conclusions can be reached based on the animal testing: (a) the threshold concentration for the initiation of an arrhythmia is independent of the duration of exposure, (b) sensitization of the myocardium to epinephrine after exposure to a halogenated hydrocarbon ceases once the hydrocarbon is eliminated from the bloodstream, (c) the arrhythmogenic effect differs among animal species, and (d) halogenated derivatives of aliphatic hydrocarbons are more active than the corresponding unsubstituted hydrocarbons (e.g., tetrachloroethane is more active than ethane). All the fluorocarbons have an arrhythmogenic effect, although at various concentrations and to different percentages of dogs. Combined exposure to noise and a fluorocarbon was more sensitizing than exposure to the fluorocarbon alone. The fact that sensitization of the myocardium to epinephrine is based on tissue levels of the chemicals suggests that arrhythmias can occur on the way home and after work and still be work related.

In addition to sensitizing the heart to the arrhythmogenic effect of an epinephrine challenge, these substances have a negative inotropic effect. There are several hypotheses on the mechanism for the arrhythmogenic effect of hydrocarbons and fluorocarbons. There is experimental evidence to indicate a role for an effect through the central nervous system, an effect through respiratory reflexes, an effect through a change in potassium levels, a direct effect on the cardiac conduction system, or an effect through adrenergic or cholinergic receptors or both. Similarly, a number of mechanisms have been suggested for the depressant effect of solvents on the heart. These mechanisms include interference with the autonomic nervous control of the heart, the availability of fuel substrate, oxygen extraction, metabolic processes for energy production or utilization, or the process of excitation-contraction coupling.

Other than carbon disulfide, mortality studies of workers chronically exposed to solvents have generally not found an increase in deaths from cardiovascular disease. A single study reported increased mortality with exposure to methylene chloride, ethanol, and phenol (64). Other studies on methylene chloride have found no increase in cardiovascular mortality.

Associated central nervous system or mucous membrane symptoms that may occur in patients who are exposed to solvents include recurrent dizziness, headaches, light-headedness, nausea, and eye or nose irritation. On physical examination, they may have reddened mucous membranes of the throat, tearing, or a runny nose. Depending on the particular solvent, abnormalities in the blood and in kidney or liver function may be found by laboratory testing. For instance, renal tubular acidosis has been described in toluene sniffers. Although not necessarily readily available, measurement of the chemical in serum, exhaled air, or as a metabolite in the urine is possible. Dysrhythmias attributable to chemical exposure can be either supraventricular or ventricular in origin and are indistinguishable from the dysrhythmias of coronary artery disease. Continuous ECG monitoring during suspected exposures with a simultaneous diary of activity can document the exposure relatedness of a dysrhythmia. Simultaneous air sampling or biologic monitoring of urine or exhaled air for the suspected substances is useful for confirming the diagnosis.

## HEAVY METALS

Arsenic and cobalt ingestion after their addition to beer have historically been found to cause outbreaks of cardiomyopathy.

Arsenic was first noted to have an effect on the heart in 1900, when a clinician described a syndrome that occurred among beer drinkers (65). Arsenic contamination of beer was traced to one supplier for breweries who had used sulfuric acid contaminated with arsenic to make invert sugar from sugar cane. Beer from 100 breweries in Northern England was affected, and thousands of cases of arsenic poisoning were reported. Fatalities from congestive heart failure were noted, although the fatality rate is unknown. The concentration of arsenic in the beer ranged from 2 to 4 ppm. Other reports of arsenic poisoning have not found congestive heart failure but rather peripheral vascular disease (66).

An increased prevalence of peripheral vascular disease has been described as a consequence of levels of arsenic of 0.8 to 1.82 ppm in drinking water in Chile and Taiwan. Normal concentrations of arsenic in drinking water are less than 0.01 ppm. Associated skin changes seen in patients with arsenic toxicity are hyperpigmentation and keratosis. In Taiwan because of gangrenous changes the clinical picture was described as "blackfoot disease." Pathologically the changes were either arteriosclerotic or thromboangiitis obliterans. Experimental studies have suggested that reduced tissues levels of zinc may contribute to the development of adverse health effects from arsenic. Long-term exposure to arsenic has been associated with hypertension (67).

Vasospastic (Raynaud's) disease has been associated with arsenic exposure among smelter workers and German vineyard workers. The problem has diminished in severity with tighter workplace exposure controls. Smelter workers' total exposure of 4 to 9 g is less than the total estimated exposure of 20 g for individuals with blackfoot disease. Among vineyard workers, inorganic arsenical pesticides, the presumed etiologic agents, are now generally not used. Organic arsenicals still in use have not been associated with similar changes.

Brewers in Canada in the 1960s began to add cobalt to beer in concentrations of 1.2 ppm to stabilize the foam. The usual concentration of cobalt previously had been 0.075 ppm. A few months after the changes in formulation cases of cardiomyopathy began to be reported in heavy beer drinkers. Case series were reported from Belgium, Nebraska, Minnesota, and Quebec with mortality rates up to 22%. The problem ceased once the cobalt was no longer added to the beer. Four cases of cobalt toxicity have been reported from the industrial setting (68). For the majority of patients with cardiomyopathy the etiology of their heart problem is considered idiopathic and it is not clear if the relatively few cases of cobalt cardiomyopathy recognized are secondary to an infrequent occurrence or to the lack of attention by the treating physician to an exposure history.

Individuals dying with cobalt cardiomyopathy have had similar autopsy findings including myocardial tissue destruction, thrombi in the heart and major arteries, polycythemia, pericardial effusions, and thyroid hyperplasia. Why an individual who drank 24 pints of beer and ingested 8 mg of cobalt had a toxic effect when as much as 150 mg of cobalt per day had been previously prescribed by physicians for anemic individuals has never been adequately explained. It has been hypothesized that a synergistic effect on enzyme metabolism of alcohol, cobalt, and a protein-poor diet was the explanation for cobalt's toxic effect at the relatively low doses found in the beer.

Electrophysiologic changes and interstitial myocarditis have been reported among children with lead poisoning from ingestion of paint chips (69). Mercury exposure has also been reported to cause electrocardiographic changes. Chelating agents have proven useful in reversing the cardiac changes associated with lead (70). The major concern, however, about lead is its effect on blood pressure. In studies of the general population, doubling of lead is associated with a rise of 1 to 2 mm Hg in systolic and a smaller rise in diastolic pressure. This effect is seen at relatively low blood levels <25 μg/dl (71). Similarly, results have been seen in occupational cohorts at these lower levels. The lack of a more dramatic effect in workers with higher blood lead levels is presumably because the effect of lead is secondary to a chronic exposure and does not correlate with higher acute blood lead levels that are found among workers in the occupational studies. It has been estimated that 24,000 fewer myocardial infarctions per year would occur if blood lead levels were reduced in half (72).

Newly identified hypertensive patients with serum creatinine concentrations exceeding 1.5 μg/dl have increased body burdens of lead as measured by an ethylenediaminetetraacetic acid (EDTA) mobilization test (measurement of urinary lead for 3 days after two 1-g intramuscular injections of EDTA given 8 to 12 hours apart) (73,74). Renal biopsies have shown interstitial disease and immunoglobulin deposition in glomeruli (75). Similarly, individuals with gout and increased serum creatinine with or without increased blood pressure have elevated body burdens of lead according to the EDTA mobilization test (76). There are no controlled studies to indicate chelation therapy is useful in this situation, but removal from continuing exposure has been recommended.

## PSYCHOSOCIAL FACTORS

In the last 15 years, multiple investigators have addressed the hypothesis put forth by Korasek that high-demand jobs with low job-decision latitude increased the risk for heart disease. In Sweden, 7% to 16% of cardiovascular disease has been estimated to be secondary to the high-strain risk of high-demand and low-control jobs (77). The reproducibility of an association has been mixed (78). However, a recent review article concluded that the weight of the evidence would suggest a causal association (79). Risk ratios up to 2.6 have been reported. The pathophysiologic mechanism may be that job strain increases a known risk factor (i.e., high blood pressure). For example, there are eight epidemiologic studies that have found an increased prevalence of hypertension in bus drivers (80). Some authors have suggested that the association between cardiovascular disease and high-demand/low-control jobs is not secondary to particular work stressors but rather secondary to confounding by socioeconomic status (81). Further work on understanding the association is needed, particularly in the area of intervention to determine if work can be modified to reverse or mitigate the association.

There have been both positive and negative studies on the effect of shiftwork and cardiovascular disease (82). Two recent studies have both reported an absence of an effect (83,84). A number of the studies have methodologic problems in controlling for selection bias on who is assigned to shift work.

## PHYSICAL INACTIVITY

Physical inactivity is a risk factor for ischemic heart disease. Studies have examined both leisure and work physical activity. A meta-analysis found a summary relative risk of death of 1.9 for coronary heart disease and evidence of a dose response among sedentary versus moderate and high activity at work (85). High leisure activity was equally protective.

## IMPAIRMENT/DISABILITY

Heart disease is a common cause for disability in the Social Security Disability Insurance (SSDI) program. The American Medical Association has published the most comprehensive guide for determining fitness to return to work and evaluating impairment (86). There are specific requirements on fitness to work that include evaluation for heart disease that have been developed for pilots by the Federal Aviation Administration and for commercial bus and truck drivers by the Department of Transportation.

Workers' compensation for heart disease is relatively rare except for firefighters and police. Psychological and/or physical stress, not chemical exposure, is the typical reason compensation is requested and awarded. Each state has its own individualized criteria to evaluate stress-related disease. Chronic stress and/or strain is usually not recognized for compensation purposes. Rather common criteria used by states include determination of whether an acute cardiac event has occurred on a day of unusual stress or strain and how an individual's stress or strain at work compares with stress or strain in their nonwork life.

Firefighters and police in many states are treated under special provisions, commonly called "heart laws," when they apply for heart-related disability. In some states, the employer must prove heart disease is not related to work; other states disallow the use of evidence of previous heart disease, and in other states, heart disease in police and firefighters is presumed to be work related and is virtually irrefutable. The provisions for police and firefighters have typically been enacted because of the perceived stress and strain of the job and not because of exposure to a particular substance such as carbon monoxide.

For individuals with cardiac disease returning to work at jobs with specific exposures, there is a presumed though not medically documented need to recommend medical restrictions. This would be particularly true for carbon monoxide where the current work standard allows a carboxyhemoglobin of 7.4%. This level is above experimental carbon monoxide exposures associated with adverse cardiac outcomes. Other restrictions to consider would be work with solvents, particularly in jobs with the potential for overexposure; work in heat or cold, particularly when associated with physical activity; and work in hot environments, such as around furnaces or ovens or in construction in the summer, because of the increased risk of the development of heat stress for individuals on cardiac medications such as diuretics or beta-blocks.

## REFERENCES


1. Stewart RD, Hake CL. Paint remover hazard. *JAMA* 1976;235:398–401.
2. Mevorach D, Heyman SN. Clinical problem solving pain in the marriage. *N Engl J Med* 1995;332:48–50.
3. Baker DB, Landrigan PH. Occupationally related disorders. *Med Clin North Am Environ Med* 1990;74:441–460.
4. Hammar N, Alfredsson L, Smedberg M, Ahlbom A. Differences in the incidence of myocardial infarction among occupational groups. *Scand J Work Environ Health* 1992;18:178–185.
5. Suadicani P, Hein HO, Gyntelberg F. Do physical and chemical working conditions explain the association of social class with ischemic heart disease? *Atherosclerosis* 1995;113:63–69.
6. Penn A. Mutational events in the etiology of atherosclerotic plaques. *Mutat Res* 1990;239:149–162.

6a. Benditt EP, Benditt JM. Evidence for a monoclonal origin of human atherosclerotic plaque. *Proc Natl Acad Sci USA* 1973;70:1753–1756.

7. Wakabayashi K. Animal studies suggesting involvement of mutagen/carcinogen exposure in atherosclerosis. *Mutat Res* 1990;239:181–187.
8. Allard EN, Bleecker ER, Chaitman BR, et al. Short-term effects of carbon monoxide exposure on the exercise performance of subjects with coronary artery disease. *N Engl J Med* 1989;321:1426–1432.
9. Sheps DS, Herbst MC, Hinderliter AL, et al. Productions of arrhythmias by elevated carboxyhemoglobin in patients with coronary artery disease. *Ann Intern Med* 1990;113:343–351.
10. Dahms TE, Younis LT, Wiens RD, Zarnegar S, Byers SL, Chaitman BR. Effects of carbon monoxide exposure in patients with documented cardiac arrhythmias. *J Am Coll Cardiol* 1993;21:442– 450.
11. Atkins EH, Baker EL. Exacerbation of coronary artery disease by occupational carbon monoxide exposure: a report of two fatalities and a review of the literature. *Am J Ind Med* 1985;7:73–79.
12. Balraj EK. Atherosclerotic coronary artery disease and "low" levels of carboxyhemoglobin; report of fatalities and discussion of pathophysiologic mechanisms of death. *J Forensic Sci* 1984;29:1150–1159.
13. Elsasser S, Mall T, Grossenbacher M, Zuber M, Perruchoud AP, Ritz R. Influence of carbon monoxide on the early course of acute myocardial infarction. *Intensive Care Med* 1995;21:716–722.
14. Ockene JK, Kuller LH, Svendsen, Meilahn E. The relationship of smoking cessation to coronary heart disease and lung cancer in the Multiple Risk Factor Intervention Trial (MRFIT). *Am J Public Health* 1990;80:954–958.
15. Rosenberg L, Kaufman DW, Helmrich ST, et. al. The risk of myocardial infarction after quitting smoking in men under 55 years of age. *N Engl J Med* 1985;313:1511–1514.
16. Omenn GS. Anderson KW, Kronmal KA, Vlietstra RT. The temporal pattern of reduction of mortality risk after smoking cessation. *Am J Prevent Med* 1990;6:251–257.
17. Koskela RS. Cardiovascular disease among foundry workers exposed to carbon monoxide. *Scand J Work Environ Health* 1994;20:286–293.
18. Guidotti TL. Occupational mortality among firefighters: assessing the association. *J Occup Environ Med* 1995;37:1348–1356.
19. Stern FB, Halperin WE, Hornung RW, Rungenburg VL, McCammon CS. Heart disease mortality among bridge and tunnel officers exposed to carbon monoxide. *Am J Epidemiol* 1988;128:1276–1288.
20. Feuer E, Rosenman KD. Mortality in police and firefighters in New Jersey. *Am J Ind Med* 1986;9:517–527.
21. Steenland K. Passive smoking and the risk of heart disease. *JAMA* 1992;267:94– 99.
22. Hannerz J, Greitz D. Cerebrospinal fluid pressure and venous pressure in "dynamite" headache and cluster headache attacks. *Headache* 1992; 32:436–438.
23. Przybojewski JZ, Heyns MH. Acute myocardial infarction due to coronary vasospasm secondary to industrial nitroglycerin withdrawal. A case report. *S Afr Med J* 1983;16:101–104.
24. Hogstedt C, Axelson O. Mortality from cardio-cerebrovascular diseases among dynamite workers—an extended case-referent study. *Ann Acad Med* 1984;13(suppl 2):399–403.
25. Levine RJ, Andjelkovich DA, Kersteter SL, et al. Heart disease in workers exposed to dinitrotoluene. *J Occup Med* 1986;28:811–816.
26. Reeve G, Bloom T, Rinsky, Smith A. Cardiovascular disease among nitroglycerin-exposed workers. *Am J Epidemiol* 1983;188:418.
27. Craig R, Gillis CR, Hole DJ, Paddle GM. Sixteen year follow-up of workers in an explosive factory. *J Soc Occup Med* 1985;35:107–110.
28. Carmichael P, Lieben J. Sudden deaths in explosive workers. *Arch Environ Health* 1963;7:50–65.

29. Cavatorta A, Falzoi M, Romanelli A, et al. Adrenal response in the pathogenesis of arterial hypertension in workers exposed to high noise levels. *J Hypertens* 1987;5:S463–S466.
30. Kristal-Boneh E, Melamed S, Harari G, Green MS. Acute and chronic effects of noise exposure on blood pressure and heart rate among industrial employees: the Cordis study. *Arch Environ Health* 1995;50: 298–304.
31. Fogari R, Zoppi A, Vanasia A, Marasi G, Villa G. Occupational noise exposure and blood pressure. *J Hypertens* 1994;12:475–479.
32. Lang T, Fouriaud C, Jacquinet-Salord MC. Length of occupational noise exposure and blood pressure. *Int Arch Occup Environ Health* 1992;63:369–372.
33. Milkovic-Kraus S. Noise-induced hearing loss and blood pressure. *Int Arch Occup Environ Health* 1990;62:259–260.
34. Talbott EO, Findlay RC, Kuller LH, et al. Noise induced hearing loss: a possible marker for high blood pressure in older noise-exposed populations. *J Occup Med* 1990;32:690–697.
35. Wu TN, Chiang HC, Huang JT, Chang PY. Comparison of blood pressure in deaf-mute children and children with normal hearing: association between noise and blood pressure. *Int Arch Occup Environ Health* 1993;65:119–123.
36. Hessel PA, Sluis-Cremer GK. Occupational noise exposure and blood pressure: longitudinal and cross-sectional observations in a group of underground miners. *Arch Environ Health* 1994;49:128–134.
37. Kent SJ, Von Gierke HE, Eng DR, Tolan GD. Analysis of the potential association between noise-induced hearing loss and cardiovascular disease in USAF air crew members. *Aviat Space Environ Med* 1986;57: 348–361.
38. Campbell KCM, Rybak L, Khardori R. Sensorineural hearing loss and dyslipidemia. *Am J Audiol* 1996;5:11–14.
39. Tiller JR, Schilling RSF, Morris JN. Occupational toxic factor in mortality from coronary heart disease. *Br Med J* 1968;4:407–411.
40. Swaen GMH, Braun C, Slangen JJM. Mortality of Dutch workers exposed to carbon disulfide. *Int Arch Occup Environ Health* 1994;66: 103–110.
41. Egeland GM, Burkhart GA, Schnorr TM, Hornung RW, Fajen JM, Lee ST. Effects of exposure to carbon disulfide on low density lipoprotein cholesterol concentration and diastolic blood pressure. *Br J Ind Med* 1992;49:287–293.
42. Vanhoorne M, De Bacquer D, De Backer G. Epidemiological study of the cardiovascular effects of carbon disulfide. *Int J Epidemiol* 1992;21: 745–752.
43. Nurminen M, Hernberg S. Effects of intervention on the cardiovascular mortality of workers exposed to carbon disulfide: a 15-year follow up. *Br J Ind Med* 1985;42:32–35.
44. Sweetnam PM, Taylor SWC, Elwood PC. Exposure to carbon disulfide and ischemic heart disease in a viscose rayon factory. *Br J Ind Med* 1987;44:220–227.
45. Lloyd EL. The role of cold in ischaemic heart disease: a review. *Public Health* 1991;105:205–215.
46. Redmond CK, Emes JJ, Mazumdar S, Magee PC, Kavron E. Mortality of steel workers employed in hot jobs. *J Environ Pathol Toxicol* 1979; 2:75–96.
47. Wild P, Moulin JJ, Ley FX, Schaffer P. Mortality from cardiovascular diseases among potash miners exposed to heat. *Epidemiology* 1995;6: 243–247.
48. Tockman MS, Pearson JD, Fleg JL, et al. Rapid decline in $FEV_1$, a new risk factor for coronary heart disease mortality. *Am J Respir Crit Care Med* 1995;151:390–398.
49. Weiss S. Pulmonary function as a phenotype physiologic marker of cardiovascular morbidity and mortality. *Chest* 1991;99:265–266.
50. Marcus EB, Curb J, Maclean C, et al. Pulmonary function as a predictor of coronary heart disease. *Am J Epidemiol* 1989;129:97–104.
51. Sanden A, Jaruhold B, Larsson S. The importance of lung function, non-malignant diseases associated with asbestos, and symptoms as predictors of ischaemic heart disease in shipyard workers exposed to asbestos. *Br J Ind Med* 1993;50:785–790.
52. Bass M. Sudden sniffing death. *JAMA* 1970;212:2075–2079.
53. Jones RD, Winter DP. Two case reports of deaths on industrial premises attributed to 1,1,1-trichloroethane. *Arch Environ Health* 1983;38:59–61.
54. Lerman Y, Winkler E, Tirosh MS, Danon Y, Almo G. Fatal accidental inhalation of bromochlorodifluoromethane. *Hum Exp Toxicol* 1991;10: 125–128.
55. Abedin Z, Cook RC, Milberg BS. Cardiac toxicity of perchloroethylene (a dry cleaning agent). *South Med J* 1980;73:1081–1083.
56. Speyer FE, Wegman DH, Raminey A. Palpitation rates associated with fluorocarbon exposure in hospital setting. *N Engl J Med* 1975;292:624–626.
57. Saiyed HN, Sadhu HG, Bhatnagar NK, Dewan A, Venkaiah K, Kashyap SK. Cardiac toxicity following short-term exposure to methomyl in sprayman and rabbits. *Hum Exp Toxicol* 1992;11:93–97.
58. Antti-Poika M, Heikkila J, Saarinen L. Cardiac arrhythmias during occupational exposure to fluorinated hydrocarbons. *Br J Ind Med* 1990; 47:138–140.
59. Edling C, Ohlson CG, Ljungkvist G, Oliv A, Soderholm B. Cardiac arrhythmia in refrigerator repairmen exposed to fluorocarbons. *Br J Ind Med* 1990;47:207–212.
60. Egeland GM, Bloom TF, Schnorr TM, Hornung RW, Suruda AJ, Wille KK. Fluorocarbon 113 exposure and cardiac dysrhythmias among aerospace workers. *Am J Ind Med* 1992;22:851–857.
61. Kaufman JD, Morgan MS, Marks ML, Greene HL, Rosenstock L. A study of the cardiac effects of bromochlorodifluoromethane (Halon 1211) exposure during exercise. *Am J Ind Med* 1992;21:223–233.
62. Zakhari S, Aviado DM. Cardiovascular toxicology of aerosol propellants, refrigerants, and related solvents. In: Van Stee EW, ed. *Cardiovascular toxicology.* New York: Raven Press, 1982;281–314.
63. Reinhardt CF, Azar A, Maxfield ME, et al. Cardiac arrhythmias and aerosol "sniffing." *Arch Environ Health* 1971;22:265–279.
64. Wilcosky TC, Simonsen NR. Solvent exposure and cardiovascular disease. *Am J Ind Med* 1991;19:569–586.
65. Reynolds ES. An account of the epidemic outbreak of arsenical poisoning occurring in beer drinkers in the north of England and midland countries in 1900. *Lancet* 1901;1:166–170.
66. Engel RR, Hopenhayn-Rich C, Receveur O, Smith AH. Vascular effects of chronic arsenic exposure: a review. *Epidemiol Rev* 1994;16:184–209.
67. Chen CJ, Hsueh YM, Lai MS, et al. Increased prevalence of hypertension and long-term arsenic exposure. *Hypertension* 1995;25:53–60.
68. Jarvis JQ, Hammond E, Meier R, Robinson C. Cobalt cardiomyopathy. *J Occup Med* 1992;34:620–626.
69. Silver W, Rodriguez-Torres R. Electrocardiographic studies in children with lead poisoning. *Pediatrics* 1968;41:1124–1127.
70. Freeman R. Reversible myocarditis due to chronic lead poisoning in childhood. *Arch Dis Child* 1965;40:389–393.
71. Hertz-Picciotto I, Croft J. Review of the relation between blood lead and blood pressure. *Epidemiol Rev* 1993;15:352–373.
72. Schwartz J. Lead, blood pressure, and cardiovascular disease in men and women. *Environ Health Perspect* 1991;91:71–75.
73. Batuman V. Lead nephropathy, gout and hypertension. *Am J Med Sci* 1993;305:241–247.
74. Batuman V, Landy E, Maesaka JK, et al. Contribution of lead to hypertension with renal impairment. *N Engl J Med* 1983;309:17–21.
75. Wedeen RP, Maesaka JK, Weiner B, et al. Occupational lead nephropathy. *Am J Med* 1975;59:630–641.
76. Batuman V, Maesaka JK, Haddad B, et al. The role of lead in gout nephropathy. *N Engl J Med* 1981;304:520–523.
77. Johnson JV, Stewart W, Hall EM, Fredlund P, Theorell T. Long-term psychosocial work environmental and cardiovascular mortality among Swedish men. *Am J Public Health* 1996;86:324–331.
78. Alterman T, Shekelle RB, Vernon SW, Burau KD. Decision latitude, psychological demand, job strain and coronary heart disease in the Western Electric Study. *Am J Epidemiol* 1994;139:620–627.
79. Schnall PL, Landsbergis PA, Baker D. Job strain and cardiovascular disease. *Annu Rev Public Health* 1994;15:381–411.
80. Winkleby MA, Ragland DR, Fisher JM, et al. Excess risk of sickness and disease in bus drivers: a review and synthesis of epidemiological studies. *Int J Epidemiol* 1988;17:255–262.
81. Albright CL, Winkleby MA, Ragland DR, Fisher J, Syme SL. Job strain and prevalence of hypertension in a biracial population of urban bus drivers. *Am J Public Health* 1992;82:984–989.
82. Harrington JM. Shiftwork and health—a critical review of the literature on working hours. *Ann Acad Med Singapore* 1994;23:699–705.
83. McNamee R, Binks K, Jones S, Faulkner D, Slovak A, Cherry NM. Shift work and mortality from ischaemic heart disease. *Occup Environ Med* 1996;53:367–373.
84. Steenland K, Fine L. Shift work shift change and risk of death from heart disease at work. *Am J Ind Med* 1996;29: 278–281.
85. Berlin JA, Colditz GA. A meta-analysis of physical activity in the prevention of coronary heart disease. *Am J Epidemiol* 1990;132:612– 628.
86. American Medical Association. *The cardiovascular system in guides to the evaluation of permanent impairment,* 4th ed. Chicago: AMA, 1993; 119–144.

*Environmental and Occupational Medicine, Third Edition,* edited by William N. Rom.
Lippincott–Raven Publishers, Philadelphia © 1998.

CHAPTER 50

# Occupational Eye Disorders

Norman A. Zabriskie and Randall J. Olson

Occupational ophthalmology is an important part of modern-day eye care. The increased significance of this ophthalmologic specialty has been driven both by a greater understanding of the ocular effects of new technology, such as video display units, and also by a greater appreciation for the ergonomic impact of such common things as refractive error and presbyopia. No longer is this a discipline solely concerned with work-related eye trauma and exposure to hazardous compounds, although certainly these aspects continue to be profoundly important. Increased awareness of the complexity of occupational eye diseases is due in part to the efforts of the International Ergophthalmology Society, which was formed in 1965. The term *ergophthalmology,* from the Greek *ergo,* indicates the relationship of the discipline to the work environment (1). The emphasis of ergophthalmology is to extend the concepts of prevention to all aspects of eye care in the workplace, from eye trauma to eye strain and from preemployment examinations to quantification of work-related vision loss (1).

The magnitude of work-related eye diseases can be estimated from two viewpoints: (a) Of all work-related accidents or illnesses, how many are eye disorders? (b) Of all eye injuries and disorders, what percentage are occupation-related? Several studies have attempted to answer the first of these questions. One study estimated that 5% to 19% of all industrial accidents were eye injuries (2). In Finland in 1973, 11.9% of all industrial accidents were ocular traumas (3). The most common insult was superficial eye injury (79.2%) followed by posttraumatic infections (5.8%), ultraviolet burns of the cornea (3.9%), eye burns (3.6%), blunt ocular trauma (2.5%), and penetrating wounds (2.4%) (3). A prospective study among 63,000 chemical industry workers found that 8.4% of all injuries reported during a 1-month period were eye injuries (4). In the same work group, a retrospective study of the previous year showed that 11.7% of all injuries were ocular (4). In terms of actual numbers, a Canadian study reported that 300 occupational eye injuries occurred per day in that country (5). Males account for the great majority of these occupational eye injuries. The male/female ratio varies from 3:1 in Australia to 20:1 in Brazil (2,6).

The percentage of eye injuries that are work related appears not to be as high as originally thought. Garrow (7) in 1923 demonstrated that 71% of all severe eye injuries requiring hospitalization were work related (7). Recent studies indicate that the percentage of eye injuries occurring at work ranges from 7.7% to 59% (8–13). Two studies in urban populations found a lower percentage of eye injuries to be work related (8% and 13%, respectively), which indicated that the inner-city population was more likely to be unemployed (14,15). Another study found 24% of ruptured globes occurred at work (16). Desai et al. (17) found that 24% of ocular injuries ending in blindness resulted from an occupational accident.

These serious work-related eye disorders are obviously a significant part of occupational medicine. And yet the above studies do not fully quantify the magnitude of the problem. Blurry vision at work, eye strain, and eye fatigue are complaints not included in published studies but frequently heard by company medical personnel. These less devastating but very common ocular problems must be included in any complete discussion of occupational eye disorders. It also must be emphasized that the majority of these disorders are preventable. The National

N. A. Zabriskie and R. J. Olson: Department of Ophthalmology, John A. Moran Eye Center, University of Utah Hospital, Salt Lake City, Utah 84132.

Society to Prevent Blindness estimates that with proper education and eye protection, 90% of eye injuries could be prevented (18).

## ASSESSMENT OF VISUAL FUNCTION

### Visual Acuity

Visual acuity is the most common measure of visual function, even though it may not be the best indicator of one's visual ability to perform a particular task. Nevertheless, it is the most important first step in evaluating visual capability. Visual acuity as we know it is synonymous with Snellen acuity (measured on the Snellen eye chart) and is a measure of central vision. This value is determined by having the individual read the smallest letter possible on a standardized eye chart at 20 feet (or 6 meters). The result is expressed as a fraction, e.g., 20/20 or 6/12. The 20/20 Snellen letter or optotype is standardized so that at 20 feet, the letter subtends an angle of 5 minutes of arc and each part or stroke of the letter subtends an angle of 1 minute of arc. The 20/20 letter measures 8.9 mm in height, and the ability to read this optotype at 20 feet is considered normal vision. However, an individual may have the ability to read the 20/20 line at 20 feet and yet have very abnormal vision, e.g., visual field defect, color deficiency, etc. When the 20/20 letters cannot be read, the smallest line that can be distinguished is recorded, such as 20/60. This indicates that the individual can read at 20 feet what a person with 20/20 vision can distinguish at 60 feet.

Near visual acuity should also be measured since it has particular occupational implications. Unfortunately, there is no standardized method of measuring near acuity. Jaeger notation is often used, which utilizes printed text of various sizes and the smallest line read is recorded as the near visual acuity, e.g., Jaeger 2. This notation is in common use, but the testing conditions are quite variable.

Many occupations have minimum acuity requirements. Commercial truck drivers and law enforcement officers for example have visual acuity requirements that often must be attested by an ophthalmic professional. The aviation industry has the most stringent minimum acuity requirements and these are set by the International Civil Aviation Organization (ICAO) (19). Listing the visual requirements for each occupation is beyond the scope of this chapter, but this information is easily obtained when needed from the particular agency in question.

### Color Vision

Many occupations require normal color discrimination. An example is the transportation industry where the ability to discern traffic lights is important for public safety. Accordingly, commercial drivers are usually required to have normal color perception. Other employers may require normal color vision in their employees depending on the task required.

The pseudoisochromatic Ishihara plates are a good example of a screening color vision test. These plates can detect even minor red-green color defects. A quantitative test, such as Farnsworth's D-15 panel, can be used to give specific information about the degree of a color vision defect. The test panel consists of 15 movable color caps and one fixed cap at the end of the panel. The object is to arrange the caps according to color. The test is quick and easily scored (20).

Both the screening Ishihara test and the quantitative D-15 panel can be administered by a technician. More detailed tests such as the Farnsworth-Munsell 100 hue or the anomaloscope require an experienced ophthalmologist for proper interpretation (20).

### Contrast Sensitivity

Contrast sensitivity is the ability to detect a pattern from a homogeneous background. The differences in luminance are distinguished without the help of sharp borders or contours. Standardized charts are available for clinical testing and are as easily administered as Snellen visual acuity. Like visual acuity, it is important to control for lighting and distance when testing with contrast sensitivity charts.

Contrast sensitivity has particular application in occupational medicine. Few occupations have minimum contrast sensitivity requirements. However, contrast sensitivity is a sensitive measure of ocular disease. Common eye diseases such as cataract and macular degeneration can reduce contrast sensitivity more than Snellen acuity. Thus visual performance at low contrast levels can be affected even though Snellen acuity may be normal. With more and more senior citizens at risk for these common eye diseases in the work force, contrast sensitivity will most likely be an increasingly important measure of visual function in the workplace.

### Visual Field

The visual field examination is an important part of any full assessment of visual function. As indicated earlier, the visual field can be markedly abnormal despite 20/20 visual acuity. Gross assessment of the visual field can be performed quickly using confrontation. In this test, the patient covers one eye while the examiner presents an object into each visual quadrant. Usually the examiner holds up one or two fingers and the patient responds with the appropriate number. The test is then repeated with the opposite eye covered. The sensitivity of this method can be increased greatly by using a red object to test for differences in color intensity in the different visual quadrants. An experienced examiner can become extremely adept at detecting even minor defects by the confrontation method.

If a defect is suspected on confrontation, visual field testing should be performed by either manual or automated perimetry. This quantifies the defect and provides a baseline for assessment of future progression. Although not available to most general occupational physicians, the instrumentation for this type of formal visual field testing is available to most ophthalmologists since it is such an integral part of modern-day eye care.

Many occupational tasks could be adversely affected by loss of visual field. The effects of visual field loss on driving ability has received particular interest. Johnson and Keltner (21) performed automated visual field screening on 10,000 volunteers. A visual field defect was found in 3.3%. The percentage increased with age and 13% of those over age 65 had a visual field defect. Half of the individuals with a visual field defect were unaware of any visual abnormality. Driving records for these 10,000 individuals were obtained and reviewed relative to visual field loss. Those with a monocular visual field defect did not show a significant difference in driving records compared to an age- and sex-matched control set of subjects with normal visual fields. However, those with visual loss in both eyes had markedly worse driving records. Both the accident rate and traffic violation conviction rate were more than twice as high as for an age- and sex- matched control group. Data such as these have made it clear that proper vision screening for a driver's license should include visual field assessment. Particularly for a commercial driver's license, a minimum visual field requirement is increasingly a part of the licensing procedure in the United States and elsewhere (22,23). Further studies on the effects of reduced visual field on task performance will no doubt lead to similar minimum field requirements in other industries.

## OCULAR FOREIGN BODY INJURIES

### Superficial

Two studies indicate that nearly 75% of all work-related eye injuries are superficial corneal injuries and foreign bodies (3,5). The majority of these heal quickly. In a study of 504 patients with corneal foreign body injuries, the median time lost from work was 4 hours, and 30% took no time off work (24). Evaluation of a suspected corneal foreign body includes instillation of fluorescein dye. This stain is taken up by damaged epithelial cells and helps to delineate the foreign body or residual abrasion. A foreign body embedded in the upper lid tarsal plate leaves a characteristic linear, vertical fluorescein staining pattern (Fig. 1). Treatment consists of foreign body removal, placement of antibiotic ointment, and patching overnight. This regimen usually results in complete healing of any corneal defect in 24 to 48 hours, depending on the initial size.

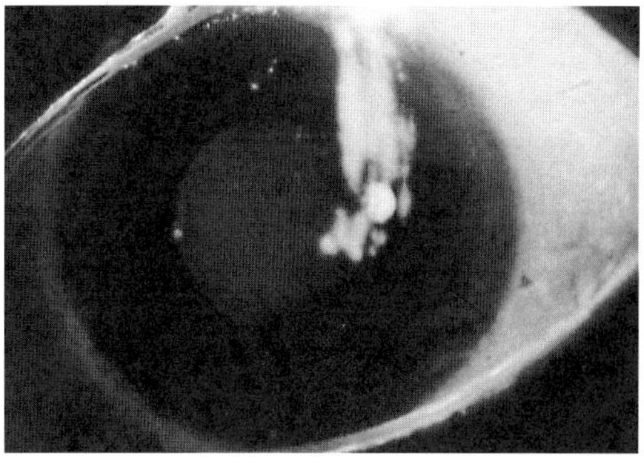

**FIG. 1.** Fluorescein staining pattern of a corneal abrasion from an embedded piece of metal in the upper tarsal plate.

The most dreaded complication of superficial eye trauma is infection. A defect in the ocular epithelial surface provides a route for bacteria and fungi to infect the avascular corneal stroma. Abrasions secondary to organic foreign bodies are thought to be particularly susceptible to posttraumatic infection. Topical antibiotic is typically used until the epithelium is completely healed in an attempt to reduce the infection rate.

Recurrent corneal erosion is another potential complication of superficial corneal injury. In this condition, the epithelium fails to firmly attach to the traumatically damaged basement membrane. During repair of the basement membrane, minor trauma, such as eye rubbing, can result in sloughing of the epithelium. This is often a painful event characterized by blurry vision and tearing. Treatment attempts to immobilize the epithelium long enough to allow firm adherence to normal reformed basement membrane. Bedtime ointment for 3 months is often required. Bandage contact lenses have proven particularly beneficial in this condition. In some cases, debridement of the epithelium and damaged basement membrane is required (25). Vision loss can occur in recurrent erosion syndrome if healing is associated with significant scarring.

### Penetrating

Penetrating ocular injuries represent 1.4% to 4% of all ocular injuries, yet they are a substantial proportion of those that result in legal blindness (Fig. 2) (3,5). In a study of 320 perforating eye injuries, paid work was the most common activity at the time of injury (27%) (26). Two other studies found the proportion of penetrating ocular injuries occurring at work to be 36% and 27% (27,28). Eighty percent or more of these injuries occurred in males. These studies indicated that the occupational groups at greatest risk for penetrating eye injuries were construction and industry. It is not surprising, therefore, that the most common perforating objects are metal frag-

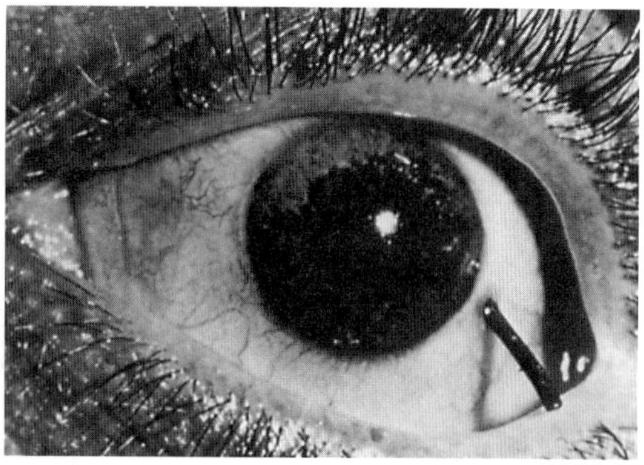

**FIG. 2.** A thorn penetrates the eye at the limbus. Penetrating injuries with organic materials often lead to endophthalmitis and loss of the eye.

ments, glass, and nails (26,29). A very important study on the epidemiology of occupational penetrating ocular trauma was published in 1992 using data from the National Eye Trauma System Registry (NETS Registry) (30). In 2,939 cases of penetrating eye trauma recorded between 1985 and 1991, 635 (22%) were work related. Projectiles were the commonest cause of injury and 97% of the injured were male. Only 6% were wearing safety eyewear at the time of injury.

At times it is obvious that the eye has been penetrated. Extruded intraocular contents can be seen outside the eye and the globe may appear flat. At other times, less dramatic signs of a penetrating injury, such as severely decreased vision, low intraocular pressure, large hyphema, or tense subconjunctival hemorrhage, may make an examiner suspicious of penetrating trauma. Any patient suspected of having a ruptured globe should be immediately referred for a full ophthalmologic examination.

There is a subgroup of individuals with penetrating eye trauma who present with relatively minor or no symptoms. These are usually caused by high-velocity metal fragments that can penetrate the eye with a self-sealing entry wound. These injuries can be surprisingly painless and vision can be well preserved, hiding the true severity of the injury. The single most important element of the patient's history is a report of pounding or grinding metal on metal. Any individual presenting with an ocular foreign body injury or reporting that something flew into their eye, who has a history of pounding metal on metal, needs a full ophthalmologic examination including a dilated retinal examination. Radiologic studies are sometimes required to rule out a metallic intraocular foreign body. These x-ray studies are particularly indicated if unexplained intraocular inflammation or cataract occurs in an individual with a history of metal-on-metal work (31).

Penetrating eye trauma usually requires surgical treatment. The integrity of the globe must be reestablished. Intraocular foreign bodies are removed at the time of surgery. Accompanying injuries such as traumatic cataract and retinal detachment are commonly seen and can be dealt with at the time of primary repair (32).

Another potential complication of a retained iron intraocular foreign body is siderosis. Siderosis is characterized by cataract and retinal toxicity, which can lead to significant vision loss. When advanced, the toxicity is irreversible. While still in the reversible stage, siderosis is associated with a rusty increase in pigmentation throughout the eye. Early siderosis also shows characteristic changes on the electroretinogram (ERG) (33,34). Treatment consists of removal of the offending foreign body. Desferrioxamine has been used successfully when removal of the iron-containing fragment has not prevented ERG changes (35).

## CHEMICAL OCULAR INJURIES

Chemical injuries constitute a relatively small proportion of industrial ocular injuries (3). However, they represent a significant percentage of severe injuries. A study in a British chemical plant showed the 1 year incidence of ocular chemical injuries among all employees to be 10%. Most of the injuries were minor, but 8 of 129 accidents resulted in time lost from work and one worker lost an eye (36). A report of 102 consecutive chemical eye injuries in India found that 6.9% of the eyes progressed to phthisis bulbi, an ophthalmic condition characterized by no light perception and loss of normal eye structure (37). Kuckelkorn et al. (38) found in a series of 131 eyes with chemical burns that 47% of eyes were left with only light perception vision and two eyes were enucleated. Also of concern is the relatively high risk of bilateral severe injury from an accidental chemical splash. In the same Indian study, 42% had bilateral injuries (37).

A multitude of chemicals have been implicated in ocular disease, but the most important are the strong acids and bases (37–39). The most common route of injury is an accidental splash of these chemicals into the eye (39). The intact corneal epithelium is resistant to pH changes in the range of pH 4 to 10. But with a pH outside of this range, the epithelium is rapidly destroyed and the substances have access to the underlying tissues. Strong acids tend to precipitate proteins (39). Although the tissue damage can be extensive, this precipitation of proteins effectively forms a buffering barrier, limiting the penetration of the acid into the eye. Strong bases, on the other hand, saponify fatty acids, which disrupts cell membranes and therefore no such barrier is created. The penetration continues and the entire anterior segment of the eye can be destroyed. Alkali chemical burns are therefore some of the most devastating of all ocular injuries.

In no other injury is immediate therapeutic intervention more critical than in the case of an ocular chemical burn. Thorough irrigation of the eye and the conjunctival fornices, preferably with isotonic saline or lactated Ringer's solution, is imperative. However, in an emergency it is better to use tap water than to search for saline solution. Any laboratory or industrial work area where potentially harmful chemicals are used should have an emergency eye wash station readily available. Irrigation should be copious and, particularly when a strong acid or alkali solution is involved, should be continued for at least 30 minutes. This may require several bags of saline IV solution delivered through a special irrigating contact lens, or extensive irrigation with an eye bath. It is critical that the eyes be open during irrigation, which usually requires topical anesthetic, a lid speculum, and/or the help of a colleague or medical personnel. There is really no need to check the pH until this extensive irrigation has been done since it should continue for 30 minutes (in the case of strong acid or base) even if the pH has returned to normal. The conjunctival fornices should be examined for particulate matter and this should be removed. Even after copious irrigation, residual solid chemicals can continue to cause extensive damage. The surrounding cutaneous structures should be cleared of particulate matter. It has been recommended that irrigation be continued during transport (40).

It has been clearly demonstrated that this type of immediate and thorough irrigation can profoundly impact the final outcome of an eye with a severe chemical injury. Unfortunately, this fact is not well appreciated in the workplace or at home. A recent study found that out of 101 patients with significant chemical or thermal (liquid metal) eye injury, only 50% received immediate irrigation (38). Yet this same study showed that those who were immediately irrigated had significantly better final visual acuity, fewer operations, and less hospitalization than those who were not irrigated. Saari et al. (41) showed beneficial effects of prolonged irrigation, 1 to 2 hours, versus conventional irrigation.

Prompt referral to an ophthalmologist is indicated after irrigation. Further ophthalmic care depends on the extent of the injury. Many people have only mild chemical or thermal superficial injury that will completely heal with time. Supportive measures such as antibiotics, cycloplegia for pain control, and patching are used during this healing process. A severe chemical injury to the eye, on the other hand, is one of the most challenging therapeutic problems in ophthalmology. The primary goals are (a) healing of the corneal epithelium and (b) reducing subsequent scarring. Lubrication, patching, and bandage contact lenses have all been used to promote epithelial healing. Antiinflammatory therapy is also indicated. Polymorphonuclear leukocytes are quickly recruited to the damaged area. These activated cells secrete lysosomal enzymes and free radicals (38). Excessive amounts of these enzymes and free radicals can lead to corneal perforation. Newer treatments include the use of 10% potassium ascorbate, which is thought to scavenge free radicals and collagenase-blocking agents such as ethylenediaminetetraacetic acid (EDTA), acetylcysteine, and l-cysteine, which are thought to slow the effects of the released lytic enzymes (42). There is also evidence that large doses of vitamin C can help prevent some damage. More work is needed in this area to improve what often is an extremely unfavorable outcome (43). An evolving method of surgical treatment is the transplantation of more normal epithelium and conjunctiva from the opposite, uninvolved or less damaged, eye.

Not all chemical injuries of the eye result in severe destructive injury. Some chemicals, even in extremely small amounts, can produce marked pharmacologic ocular dysfunction. This ocular dysfunction can indicate more threatening systemic toxicity. Parasympathomimetic agents are particularly important offenders. Many insecticides permanently poison acetyl cholinesterase. The resulting parasympathomimetic effects include small pinpoint pupils, myopia, eye injection, and headache. Agricultural workers who use these insecticides are at risk for parasympathomimetic poisoning. Again, the importance of the eye findings is their correlation with systemic toxicity.

## OCULAR INJURY FROM ELECTROMAGNETIC RADIATION

### Visible Light

Visible light has a wavelength between 400 and 700 nm. Exposure to visible light has been listed as a risk factor for cataract, pterygium, some corneal degenerations, and macular degeneration. In some professions such as fisherman, high-altitude worker, and outdoor laborer, among others, the lifetime exposure to light in the visible spectrum is high. If there were an association between light exposure and ocular injury, these workers exposed to large amounts of visible light would have an increased need for eye protection.

An important recent study among watermen on Chesapeake Bay has established just such an association (44). This population-based survey of 838 watermen showed pterygium and climatic droplet keratopathy (a corneal degeneration) to be associated with higher exposures to all the visible wavelengths. This same study showed an association between advanced macular degeneration and exposure to blue light (400 to 500 nm). There was no association between nuclear or cortical cataract and visible light exposure.

Visible-light dental curing units are also a potential ocular hazard. A Texas study looked at 11 of these visible-light curing units and concluded that no thermal hazard existed. The photochemical reaction caused by the blue light was not a hazard in normal use of the units. The maximum exposure time needed to cause damage varied with the unit used, ranging from 2.4 to 16.4 minutes per

24 hours. This time could not be achieved unless the operator focused on the source of light for an extended period of time (45).

### Ultraviolet

Ultraviolet light has a wavelength between 100 and 400 nm and is divided into three bands: UV-A (400 to 320 nm), UV-B (320 to 290 nm), and UV-C (290 to 100 nm). UV-C does not normally penetrate the earth's atmosphere. Ultraviolet exposure has been linked to various ocular disorders. The study among Chesapeake Bay fisherman looked also at the relationship of ultraviolet light exposure to eye disease. A positive association was found between UV-B exposure and cortical cataract (46). An association was not found with UV-A exposure. There was also a strong correlation between pterygium and climatic droplet keratopathy and both UV-A and UV-B exposure (47). Unlike the study of visible light, no association between UV-A or UV-B exposure and macular degeneration was found (48). An association between UV-B exposure in men, but not in women, and cortical cataract was found in another population-based study (49).

Studies have also suggested a link between intraocular melanoma and ultraviolet exposure (50,51), although, as Seddon et al. (51) point out, one must be cautious in establishing a specific causal relationship between intraocular melanoma and UV exposure. Another study evaluating any potential association of uveal melanoma and occupation showed that the odds ratio of intraocular melanoma increased in association with agriculture, fishing, and forestry (52). Whether or not this was due to UV exposure could not be assessed by the design of the study.

### Infrared

A high rate of cataract formation has been observed in glass and metal workers for over 100 years. Lydahl (53) found a greater incidence of lens changes in older glass and metal workers than in age-matched controls.

Exposure to the short-wave infrared (IR) radiation emitted from the molten glass and metal is thought to be the cause. The iris absorbs the IR radiation and is heated. This heating of the iris secondarily induces cataractous changes in the underlying lens (53). All major lens opacities, e.g., nuclear, cortical, and posterior subcapsular, are seen with increased frequency in IR-exposed workers (53). Exfoliation or splitting of the anterior lens capsule, however, is thought to be pathognomonic for IR-induced lens damage. In Lydahl's study, exfoliation of the lens capsule was seen only in the IR-exposed workers (53).

### Microwave

Microwaves vary tremendously in their biologic effects. Microwaves of frequencies greater than 10,000 MHz do not penetrate beyond the skin and cause only surface heating. Microwave frequencies less than 150 MHz penetrate the body with very little loss of energy. Therefore, the body's most sensitive organs can be affected by frequencies between 150 and 10,000 MHz. The two most sensitive organs are the testes and the eyes.

Microwaves have induced cataracts in animals. In humans, early cataracts have been associated with microwave exposure among radar facility workers. A 1977 study of 800 microwave and laser workers did not find changes in the lens or retina that could be attributed to work (54). However, a 1988 study showed an increased incidence of cataract formation in military personnel that was thought to be associated with the powerful radar equipment used (55). There have been other documented cases of cataract formation after accidental exposure to large quantities of microwave irradiation in the sensitive range (56).

### Lasers

There has been a dramatic proliferation of lasers in industry over the last 30 years. Lasers have the potential to cause significant ocular damage even at low energy levels. Laser light inadvertently focused on the macular region of the retina can immediately reduce visual acuity, at times with little recovery. There are scattered reports in the literature of industrial laser ocular injuries (57,58). It is speculated that many accidental extramacular laser burns go unreported because of lack of symptoms (57).

In the medical industry, five types of lasers are in common use. Each uses a different medium to produce the laser, and they each have different potential ocular effects (59). The neodymium:yttrium-aluminum-garnet (Nd:YAG) laser can cause a burn or tissue disruption in any ocular layer. The carbon dioxide laser causes ocular coat damage. Argon and dye lasers can produce photochemical and thermal retinal injuries. The excimer laser creates a photokeratitis. These laser effects have important therapeutic uses in the eye when directed appropriately, and important toxicity when accidentally focused on ocular structures.

The following precautions have been recommended for workers exposed to laser light (60):

1. Workers should be alerted to areas of laser use and the associated admittance restrictions.
2. Eyes should be protected using laser-safe eye protection of the appropriate wavelength and optical density.
3. Skin should be protected from aberrant and reflected laser beams.
4. Workers should be protected from inhaling fumes associated with laser use.
5. Workers should be protected from fire hazards associated with laser use.

6. Workers should be protected from electrical hazards associated with laser use.
7. Policies and procedures for laser safety should be developed within the work setting.

These recommendations were established for health care workers (60), but they can be applied to other industries that use lasers. Protective shields can prevent accidental laser damage, but even these can be destroyed at high energy levels. Another consideration is the pupillary dilation associated with low lighting. This can increase the accessibility of laser light to the retina by 16- to 25-fold (61).

### Welding Arc

Welding eye injuries are common enough to be considered as a separate category. In 1985, 21% of all ocular injury claims filed with the Workers' Compensation Board of Alberta were from welders (62). Most of these injuries were due to metallic foreign bodies, but 23% were radiation injuries.

Welding arcs emit radiation across a broad wavelength spectrum (200 to 1,400 nm) (63). UV radiation (200 to 400 nm) is absorbed by the cornea and can cause the typical keratoconjunctivitis seen in welders not wearing adequate protection (63). Some of the UV, the visible (400 to 700 nm) and the IR (700 to 1,400 nm) radiation can penetrate to the retina and potentially damage it (63). Welding arc maculopathy has been reported in welders not wearing filtering goggles (63,64). Radiation damage to the retina can occur by three mechanisms (65). Mechanical damage results when the laser power is so high that shock waves disrupt retinal tissue. Photochemical injury is caused by chronic exposure to light sources with blue and near ultraviolet components (65). Thermal injury is due to an intense, short burst of light that increases the retinal and pigment epithelial temperature by 10° to 20°C (65). Retinal burns from welding arcs have reportedly been due to thermal (63) and photochemical (65) insults.

## EYE INJURIES IN AGRICULTURE

Agricultural eye injuries are different from other occupational ocular accidents in a few important ways. A study of agricultural injuries in Ireland (66) showed that minor corneal and conjunctival abrasions were still the most common injuries, but the major source of the trauma was contact with bushes. Superficial ocular trauma such as this caused by organic material is probably at greater risk for posttraumatic infection. Prophylactic treatment with topical antibiotics until the corneal epithelium has healed is essential.

Gathering and breaking sticks and chopping wood were responsible for almost 15% of the agricultural injuries (66). Fertilizers and pesticides used by agricultural workers can cause severe chemical damage to the eye. Equipment failure, accidental spill, and spray drift are common reasons for ocular exposure to these agricultural chemicals (67).

A very important finding was that penetrating injuries were almost as frequent as nonpenetrating traumas (66). Penetrating ocular injuries in the rural setting are not only at increased risk for intraocular infection, but the offending bacteria are often quite virulent, resulting in devastating outcomes (68). Any potentially penetrating eye trauma in the rural or agricultural setting should be referred immediately for a complete ophthalmologic evaluation.

Education and the use of properly fitting safety goggles are essential components in the reduction of agricultural ocular injuries (67). In Finland between the years 1955 and 1957, 16.4% of all perforating eye injuries were due to agricultural ocular trauma (69). Twenty years later, between 1972 and 1979, the corresponding figure was unchanged at 17.5%. This was despite a decrease in the proportion of people in agriculture from 41.4% to 12.2% during the same 20-year span. This suggests that eye protection in agriculture is insufficient (69).

## PREVENTION

The various occupational eye disorders discussed thus far represent work-related accidents and harmful exposures. The cost to industry worldwide is enormous. The cost to the individual who loses an eye in an accident is incalculable. The astounding truth, however, is that essentially all of the above injuries are preventable. It is estimated that 90% of all ocular injuries are preventable (18). In all the studies reviewed in this chapter, it is striking that the overwhelming majority of the injured were not wearing eye protection, even though it was readily available to them.

An effective eye safety program in the workplace entails a combination of attitude and implementation. Firms with successful eye protection programs consistently show that all levels of the company—management and labor—must be actively involved and demonstrate a positive attitude toward safety (70,71). Performance standards and audit systems must be implemented and continuing education is essential (70). A good program is specific and well researched. One study suggested that the following issues be carefully addressed when developing an eye safety program (72):

1. What are the possibilities of eye accidents in the workplace?
2. What kind of eye accidents have occurred in the past?
3. How can the danger factors be avoided?
4. How can the choice and purchase of safety eyewear be best arranged?

5. What must the employee do to get shockproof lenses in their personal glasses?
6. How is the maintenance of safety eyewear organized?
7. What are the duties of the employers in preventing eye accidents?
8. What are the duties of the employees in preventing eye accidents?
9. What are the duties of the foremen in controlling the usage of safety eyewear?

Specific safety steps start with the identification and correction of poor vision. Uncorrected visual problems can contribute to accidents (70,71). One study suggested that more than 30% of workers have visual defects that are either inadequately corrected or uncorrected (73). This same study found that the number of accidents among workers with poor vision was three times that among workers with normal vision. Proper vision screening of all new employees can identify problems and allow for appropriate referral. Multiple visual functions should ideally be tested: Snellen visual acuity, color discrimination, and depth perception (70). Proper lighting in the workplace should be provided to maximize vision and thereby afford increased protection (71).

Safety glasses and goggles are a fundamentally important part of any eye protection plan. Safety goggles of high-impact–resistant materials are needed to prevent injury (74). In the United States, all safety eye protection must meet or exceed the American National Standard Z87.1 (70). They must be available to all workers and well maintained. Shields on the sides, top, or bottom of the glasses should be worn by any worker exposed to splashing of potentially harmful agents.

Safety eyewear, no matter how high its quality, is of no help if it is not worn. It is difficult at times to convince workers that the goggles are necessary, in part because goggles often decrease visual acuity, especially when they become dirty or worn out. Also, goggles are hot and uncomfortable, and condensation forms rapidly on the lenses. Despite these disadvantages, a properly fitted pair of safety goggles can prevent most industrial eye injuries. Since injuries are difficult to predict and most areas of the workplace carry at least some risk, it has been suggested that for maximal eye protection a 100% mandatory program requiring eye protection in all areas of the industrial workplace be adopted (70).

Glasses with the appropriate absorbency can prevent injury from electromagnetic radiation. Rooms and laboratories that house lasers must have a clear warning label on the door and appropriate goggles available to any entering personnel. Exposure to the sun's radiation can also be reduced by suitable sunglasses (75) and even to some extent by regular prescription eyewear (76). Even something as simple as wearing a brimmed hat can significantly reduce workers ocular exposure to ultraviolet radiation (77). It is reasonable for an outdoor worker to consider such precautions.

## LESS COMMON CAUSES OF OCCUPATIONAL EYE DISORDERS AND INJURIES

Compressed air injury to the eyes is particularly common among mechanics and service station attendants, usually due to a burst air hose. Thermal and blast burns to the cornea, conjunctiva, and lid may result. Foreign debris can be propelled at high speed into ocular structures. Protection can be provided by well-fitting goggles (78).

As little as 0.5 oz. of methanol can cause a blinding retinopathy and optic neuropathy. The ganglion cell layer and optic nerve are destroyed. Damage has even been reported from inhalation. No symptoms appear until 18 to 48 hours after digestion. The degree of metabolic acidosis correlates well with the amount of ocular damage. Systemic sodium bicarbonate to counteract the acidosis and ethanol to block methanol metabolism are important treatment modalities. Any visual recovery is usually appreciated within 6 days of ingestion (79). Ocular disorders have also been reported with exposure to styrene (80), hydrogen sulfide (81), and polychlorinated biphenyls (PCBs) (82).

Direct contact with a high-energy electrical source can produce total destruction of the eye. The injury results from either a thermal burn or intense ultraviolet and infrared electromagnetic injury. Electrical cataracts can occur with direct electrical flow through the eye at relatively low energy levels (83).

Adenovirus type VIII can cause a very severe infectious conjunctivitis that is often bilateral. Recovery is usually complete, but corneal opacities can occur and cause decreased visual acuity. The morbidity of this particular disease is great. And it can spread rapidly in the workplace (84). A communal towel, a shared pen, and even a doorknob can be potential vectors. A patient with adenoviral conjunctivitis seen in the company infirmary can contaminate the medical personnel and any instruments used to examine the patient. Any worker with suspected viral conjunctivitis should be sent home from work. All those coming into contact with the individual should wash their hands frequently to avoid spread. Any instrument used for examination should be segregated and sterilized. It is best that the examiner not touch the lids of such patients. A cotton-tipped applicator should instead be used.

## OCCUPATIONAL IMPLICATIONS OF REFRACTIVE ERROR

As mentioned earlier, one of the most important issues in occupational eye safety is the identification of poor visual acuity. Perhaps the most common cause of decreased vision among workers is uncorrected refractive error. Refractive error has important implications in both its uncorrected and corrected states. The common refractive states are hyperopia, myopia, astigmatism, and presbyopia. This section focuses on those states with occupational implications.

### Hyperopia, Aphakia, and Pseudophakia

Hyperopia is commonly referred to as farsightedness. In this condition, the eye does not have enough focusing power so that an object placed at infinity comes into focus behind the eye. Hyperopia is corrected with plus lenses, which add focusing power to the visual system. Accommodation, which adds focusing power to the eye, can be used to compensate for uncorrected hyperopia. Large amounts of hyperopia can be compensated by a young individual who has a large accommodative amplitude. With age, however, accommodative amplitude decreases and the existing hyperopia is now compensated only with great effort. Uncorrected hyperopia is therefore a very important cause of eye strain, especially among those 35 to 45 years old. Latent hyperopia can be uncovered with a cycloplegic refraction, in which one's accommodative power is eliminated with eye drops. This test should be done on all patients complaining of eye strain. Proper spectacle correction decreases or eliminates their need for accommodation, and thereby relieves the strain. Generally, latent hyperopes experience strain only when trying to read, which requires the greatest accommodation. Without a cycloplegic refraction, they may be mistakenly prescribed bifocals when the real problem is the uncorrected hyperopia. Proper hyperopic correction in this instance will likely make the patient more comfortable all the time, and also may postpone the need for bifocals. Again, any worker complaining of eye strain or difficulty with near work should have a cycloplegic refraction as part of their examination.

Aphakia is an important high hyperopic state. Aphakia is the absence of the natural lens of the eye. This condition is usually surgically induced with the removal of a cataractous lens. Since the natural lens provides a significant amount of the eye's focusing power, an aphakic individual requires a high plus lens for good visual acuity. Plus lenses of this power induce several visual side effects that may impede a worker's ability to perform certain tasks: (a) objects are magnified from 20% to 35%; (b) this magnification alters depth perception; (c) pincushion distortion occurs, with which, for example, doors appear to bow inward; (d) hand-eye coordination is decreased; and (e) ringed blind areas induced by the edges of the thick lenses cause objects to jump in and out of the visual field, which is referred to as the jack-in-the-box phenomenon (85).

Contact lens correction can decrease many of these side effects induced by high plus spectacle correction. The object magnification with an aphakic contact lens is 7% to 12%. However, even with good visual acuity, a contact lens–corrected aphakic eye has been shown to have decreased contrast sensitivity relative to a normal phakic eye (86). This decrease in contrast sensitivity is accentuated by glare. Successful aphakic contact lens wear depends in part on lens handling ability, an ability that can be compromised in older patients (87).

Unilateral aphakia is particularly troublesome because of the usually large refractive difference between the two eyes. This difference, called anisometropia, severely decreases stereoacuity and depth perception. One study of six unilateral aphakic patients with spectacle correction showed that none had good stereoacuity (88). The same report showed that in 27 unilateral aphakic patients with contact lens correction, 41% had good stereoacuity.

Another consideration in the aphakic patient is the increased risk of retinal exposure to ultraviolet light. The natural lens absorbs damaging ultraviolet rays, particularly between 300 and 400 nm (89). The retina is thus shielded from this potentially damaging radiation. The aphakic patient has no such shield and is thought to be at greater risk for the harmful retinal affects of UV radiation discussed earlier. Protective UV absorbing spectacles should probably be prescribed in these individuals.

Fortunately, almost all these problems with aphakia can now be alleviated with modern-day intraocular lens technology. Pseudophakia refers to an ocular state in which the natural lens has been replaced with an implant lens. This is an extremely common condition, in part because cataracts are so common. Annually, approximately 1.2 million cataracts are removed in the United States. As the work force ages, more employees will be faced with progressive visual loss due to cataract. This visual loss can be exacerbated by bright light (90). Cataract extraction and intraocular lens implantation usually provides excellent visual rehabilitation in such individuals.

An intraocular implant lens is the ideal means of optical correction following cataract extraction. The image magnification from an implant lens is on the order of 4%. This allows a majority of patients to have good stereoacuity and depth perception, even in unilateral pseudophakia (88). Newer implants have radiation-absorbing properties that protect the retina from harmful UV light. Implants are usually chosen to allow the distance to be in focus with little or no correction. Thus, most pseudophakic workers require a corrective lens for near work.

Implant lenses have truly revolutionized visual function after cataract surgery. Aphakic individuals, most of them having had their cataracts removed before the widespread use of intraocular lenses, who struggle with aphakic spectacles or contact lenses are usually good candidates for a secondary intraocular lens.

**Myopia**

Myopia, or nearsightedness, is more common than hyperopia. In myopia, the eye has too much focusing power and a distant object is focused in front of the retina. Myopia is corrected with minus, or diverging, lenses. Improper correction of myopia can also be a source of eye strain. Young people with large accommodative amplitudes often prefer to have their myopic glasses overcorrected, forcing them to accommodate to have clear vision. If lens prescribers are not fully aware of this fact, a young person may be given a diopter, or more, of excess myopic correction in their glasses. This is easily compensated in a 20-year-old. But in a 40-year-old, this forced accommodation can be very straining. Again, a cycloplegic refraction can uncover the problem, and with proper correction the eye strain can be reduced and bifocals postponed.

Surgical correction of myopia is becoming more popular among working-age individuals. This is an important option for those myopic individuals who do not meet the minimum uncorrected vision requirement for their desired profession, such as a law enforcement officer. Two forms of surgical correction are common. The first is radial keratotomy (RK). In this procedure, a diamond blade is used to make deep radial cuts in the cornea. These cuts allow the cornea to flatten, thereby reducing the myopia. The number, depth, and length of the incisions depend on the amount of myopia to be corrected. Most patients undergoing radial keratotomy do well and have good correction of their myopia. As in all surgery, there are potential complications that can compromise visual acuity (91). The most important occupational implication of RK is the weakening of the eye. This leaves the RK patient more susceptible to the effects of blunt trauma. In a worker who has had RK surgery, safety glasses are imperative.

The second form of surgical correction of myopia uses the excimer laser in a procedure called photorefractive keratectomy (PRK). The laser is used to ablate a certain amount of the central cornea, again dependent on the amount of myopia to be corrected. It is felt by many that the postoperative results are both more predictable and more stable compared to radial keratotomy. An important difference is that PRK does not weaken the eye like radial keratotomy. Excimer laser PRK is, therefore, probably the preferred procedure in anyone occupationally at risk for ocular blunt trauma. LASIK is the latest refractive procedure. It is similar to PRK, but recovery is quicker. LASIK is proving to be better for high myopia and can even correct some hyperopia. It may prove to be the most effective refractive surgery technique of those presently available.

**Presbyopia**

Presbyopia is the age-related loss of accommodative amplitude. This condition is manifested as a decreased ability to see up close. It becomes a clinical problem when one no longer has the accommodative reserve to comfortably carry out one's usual near visual tasks. This not only leads to blurry near vision, but it also is an important cause of eye strain.

An average 20-year-old has 11 diopters of accommodative amplitude. A 40-year-old has on average 6 diopters. A common rule is that to comfortably perform a visual task, half of the accommodative amplitude must be held in reserve. For example, to read at a distance of 25 cm, 4 diopters of accommodation are required. Thus, to comfortably work at this distance, 8 total diopters of accommodation must be present. An average 40-year-old has only 6 diopters, so visual tasks at 25 cm would be at the least uncomfortable, and at the most impossible due to blurry vision. In this situation, reading lenses or reading bifocals can be used to make up the accommodation deficit.

Reading bifocals need to be carefully fit to meet the worker's specific needs. Common working distances need to be discussed. Some may require correction for different distances, e.g., the desktop, the computer screen, and the normal reading position. A trifocal lens can be added to accommodate these midrange distances. Usually with careful history taking and appropriate prescribing, a pair of suitable glasses can be made.

**Contact Lenses in the Workplace**

Controversy exists regarding contact lens use in the workplace. Both hard and soft lenses are used commonly by young workers. The majority of those who wear lenses do so for cosmetic or convenience reasons. In some individuals, however, contact lenses have specific visual advantages. As mentioned earlier, spectacle correction of moderate to high hyperopes and myopes is associated with changes in image size and loss of stereoacuity. These side effects are minimized by contact lenses. Contact lenses do, however, pose specific hazards. Soft contacts especially have an affinity for particulate foreign bodies. Small particles normally removed by the tears may be trapped by a contact lens (92). Foreign bodies are more commonly trapped under a hard lens than a soft one (92). Soft lenses are known to accumulate some toxic substances, including industrial gases and fumes (93–95). UV and IR radiation can be absorbed by the contact lens. This causes heating of the contact lens, which can injure the cornea (92).

In summary, contact lenses offer no protective barrier. In fact, the need for protective eyewear is probably increased in the contact lens wearer.

**SUMMARY**

Occupational eye disorders represent a complex group of traumatic injuries, harmful exposures, uncorrected and undiagnosed ocular diseases, eye strain and fatigue, and other miscellaneous ocular complaints. These diseases constitute a significant percentage of all work-related illnesses. Many advancements have been made in the treatment of these ocular disorders; penetrating injuries can now be better repaired and new medicines and surgical techniques are available to the worker with a chemical eye injury.

Most importantly, essentially all of these disorders are more easily prevented than treated. Good, effective eye protection exists in the form of safety glasses and goggles. Even eye strain and fatigue can be prevented with the application of sound refraction principles and attention to ergonomic detail. With such preventative measures readily available, management and labor should aggressively work to decrease the number of workers affected with an occupational eye disorder.

## REFERENCES


1. Keeney AH. The progressive pathway of ergophthalmology. *Acta Ophthalmol* 1984;164(suppl):9–13.
2. Belfort R, Bonomo PP, Neustein I. Industrial eye injuries: analysis of 500 cases. *Ind Med* 1972;41:30–32.
3. Saari KM, Parvi V. Occupational eye injuries in Finland. *Acta Ophthalmol* 1984;161(suppl):17–28.
4. Jones NP, Griffith AP. Eye injuries at work: a prospective population-based survey within the chemical industry. *Eye* 1992;6:381–385.
5. Schmidt BT. Are new emphases needed in occupational vision care? *Can J Optom* 1978;69:61–67.
6. Wigglesworth EC. Occupational injuries: an exploratory analysis of successful Australian strategies. *Med J Aust* 1976;1:335–340.
7. Garrow A. A statistical inquiry into 1000 cases of eye injuries. *Br J Ophthalmol* 1923;7:65–80.
8. Cohen GR, Zaidman GW. Work-related eye injuries. *Ann Ophthalmol* 1986;18:19–21.
9. Karlson TA, Klein BEK. The incidence of acute hospital-treated eye injuries. *Arch Ophthalmol* 1986;104:1473–1476.
10. Baker RS, Wilson MR, Flowers CH, Lee DA, Wheeler NC. Demographic factors in a population-based survey of hospitalized, work-related, ocular injury. *Am J Ophthalmol* 1996;122:213–219.
11. White MF Jr, Morris R, Feist RM, Witherspoon CD, Helms HA, John GR. Eye injury: prevalence and prognosis by setting. *South Med J* 1989;82:151–158.
12. Schein OD, Hibbard PL, Shingleton BJ, et al. The spectrum and burden of ocular injury. *Ophthalmology* 1988;95:300–305.
13. Glynn RJ, Seddon JM, Berlin BM. The incidence of eye injuries in New England adults. *Arch Ophthalmol* 1988;106:785–789.
14. Zagelbaum BM, Tostanoski JR, Kerner DJ, Hersh PS. Urban eye trauma. *Ophthalmology* 1993;100:851–856.
15. Liggett PE, Pince KJ, Barlow W, Ragen M, Ryan SJ. Ocular trauma in an urban population. Review of 1132 cases. *Ophthalmology* 1990;97:581–584.
16. Dunn ES, Jaeger EA, Jeffers JB, Freitag, BA. The epidemiology of ruptured globes. *Ann Ophthalmol* 1992;24:405–410.
17. Desai P, MacEwen CJ, Baines P, Minassian DC. Incidence of cases of ocular trauma admitted to hospital and incidence of blinding outcome. *Br J Ophthalmol* 1996;80:592–596.
18. National Society to Prevent Blindness. *Eye safety is no accident* [brochure]. Schaumberg, IL: NSPB, 1990.
19. Aine E. Minimum visual requirements in different occupations in Finland. *Acta Ophthalmol* 1984;161(suppl):104–110.
20. Aarnisalo E. Testing of color vision for vocational purposes. *Acta Ophthalmol* 1984;161(suppl):135–138.
21. Johnson CA, Keltner JL. Incidence of visual field loss in 20,000 eyes and its relationship to driving performance. *Arch Ophthalmol* 1983; 101:371–375.
22. Keltner JL, Johnson CA. Visual function, driving safety, and the elderly. *Ophthalmology* 1987;94:1180–1187
23. Parisi JL, Bell RA, Yassein H. Homonymous hemianopic field defects and driving in Canada. *Can J Ophthalmol* 1991;26:252–256.
24. Alexander MM, MacLeod DA, Hall NF, Elkington AR. More than meets the eye: a study of the time lost from work by patients who incurred injuries from corneal foreign bodies. *Br J Ophthalmol* 1991;75:740–742.
25. Brodrick J, Dark A, Peace G. Fingerprint dystrophy of the cornea. *Arch Ophthalmol* 1974;92:483–489.
26. Blohmdahl S, Norell S. Perforating eye injury in the Stockholm population. *Acta Ophthalmol* 1984;62:378–390.
27. Punnonen E. Epidemiological and social aspects of perforating eye injuries. *Acta Ophthalmol* 1989;67:492–498.
28. Patel BCK, Morgan LH. Work-related penetrating eye injuries. *Acta Ophthalmol* 1991;69:377–381.
29. Neubert FR. Nail-gun and masonry nail accidents. *Br Med J* 1968;1:511.
30. Dannenberg AL, Parver LM, Brechner RJ, Khoo L. Penetrating eye injuries in the workplace. The National Eye Trauma System Registry. *Arch Ophthalmol* 1992;110:843–848.
31. Keeney AH. Intralenticular foreign bodies. *Arch Ophthalmol* 1971;86: 499–501.
32. Percival SPB. Late complications from posterior segment intraocular foreign bodies. *Br J Ophthalmol* 1972;56:462–465.
33. Apple I, Barishak YR. Histopathological changes in siderosis bulbi. *Ophthalmologica* 1978;176:205–210.
34. Declercq SS, Meredith PC, Rosenthal AR. Experimental siderosis in the rabbit. *Arch Ophthalmol* 1977;95:1051–1058.
35. Falbe-Hansen I. Treatment of ocular siderosis and haemochromatosis with desferrioxamine. *Acta Ophthalmol* 1966;44:95–99.
36. Whitehead P. Chemical burns of the eye. *Nursing Times* 1971;67: 759–762.
37. Saini JS, Sharma A. Ocular chemical burns-clinical and demographic profile. *Burns* 1993;19:67–69.
38. Kuckelkorn R, Kottek A, Schrage N, Reim M. Poor prognosis of severe chemical and thermal eye burns: the need for adequate emergency care and primary prevention. *Int Arch Occup Environ Health* 1995;67: 281–284.
39. Teir H. Toxicologic effects on the eyes at work. *Acta Ophthalmol* 1984; 161(suppl):60–65.
40. Pfister RP. Chemical corneal burns. In: Olson RJ, ed. *Common corneal problems.* Boston: Little, Brown, 1984;157–169.
41. Saari KM, Leinonen J, Aine E. Management of chemical injuries with prolonged irrigation. *Acta Ophthalmol* 1984;161(suppl):52–59.
42. Morgan SJ. Chemical burns of the eye: causes and management. *Br J Ophthalmol* 1987;71:854–857.
43. Thoft RA. Chemical and thermal injury. *Int Ophthalmol Clin* 1979; 19:243–256.
44. Taylor HR, West S, Munoz B, Rosenthal FS, Bressler SB, Bressler NM. The long term effects of visible light on the eye. *Arch Ophthalmol* 1992;110:99–104.
45. Foster CD, Satrom DK, Morris MA. Potential retinal hazards of dental visible light resin-curing units. *Biomed Sci Instrum* 1988;24:251–257.
46. Taylor HR, West SK, Rosenthal FS, et al. Effect of ultraviolet radiation on cataract formation. *N Engl J Med* 1988;319:1429–1433.
47. Taylor HR, West SK, Rosenthal FS, Munoz B, Newland HS, Emmett EA. Corneal changes associated with chronic UV irradiation. *Arch Ophthalmol* 1989;107:1481–1484.
48. West SK, Rosenthal FS, Bressler NM, et al. Exposure to sunlight and other risk factors for age-related macular degeneration. *Arch Ophthalmol* 1989;107:875–879.
49. Cruickshanks KJ, Klein EK, Klein R. Ultraviolet light exposure and lens opacities: the Beaver Dam eye study. *Am J Public Health* 1992; 82:1658–1662.
50. Tucker MA, Shields JA, Hartge P, Augsburger J, Hoover RN, Fraumeni JF. Sunlight as a risk factor for intraocular malignant melanoma. *N Engl J* Med 1985;313:789–792.
51. Seddon JM, Gradougas ES, Glynn RJ, Egan KM, Albert DM, Blitzer PH. Host factors, UV radiation, and risk of uveal melanoma- A case control study. *Arch Ophthalmol* 1990;108:1274–1280.
52. Ajani UA, Seddon JM, Hsieh C, Egan KM, Albert DM, Gradougas, ES. Occupation and risk of uveal melanoma. *Cancer* 1992;70:2891–2900.
53. Lydahl E. Infrared radiation and cataract. *Acta Ophthalmol* 1984; 166(suppl):1- 63.

54. Hathaway JA, Stern N, Soles EM, Leighton E. Ocular medical surveillance on microwave and laser workers. *J Occup Med* 1977;19:683–688.
55. Harding JJ, van Heyningen R. Beer, cigarettes and military work as risk factors for cataract. *Dev Ophthalmol* 1989;17:13–16.
56. McRee DI. Environmental aspects of microwave radiation. *Environ Health Perspect* 1972;2:41–53.
57. Boldrey EE, Little HL, Flocks M, Vassiliadis A. Retinal injury due to industrial laser burns. *Ophthalmology* 1981;88:101–107.
58. Fowler BJ. Accidental industrial laser burn of the macula. *Ann Ophthalmol* 1983;15:481–483.
59. Ben-zvi S. Laser safety: guidelines for use and maintenance. *Biomed Instrum Technol* 1989;23:360–368.
60. Technical Practices Coordinating Committee. Recommended Practices. Laser safety in the practice setting. *AORN J* 1989;50:1015, 1018–1020.
61. Goldman L, Hornby P. Personal protection from high-energy lasers. *Am Ind Hyg Assoc J* 1965;26:553–557.
62. Reesal MR, Dufresne RM, Suggett D, Alleyne BC. Welder eye injuries. *J Occup Med* 1989;31:1003–1006.
63. Romanchuk KG, Pollak V, Schneider RJ. Retinal burn from a welding arc. *Can J Ophthalmol* 1978;13:120–122.
64. Uniat L, Olk RJ, Hanish SJ. Welding arc maculopathy. *Am J Ophthalmol* 1986;102:394–395.
65. Mainster MA, Ham WT, Delori FC. Potential retinal hazards. *Ophthalmology* 1983;90:927–932.
66. Blake J. Eye injuries in agriculture. *Ir Med J* 1971;64:420–423.
67. Rettig BA, Klein DK, Sneizek JE. The incidence of hospitalizations and emergency room visits resulting from exposure to chemicals used in agriculture. *Nebr Med J* 1987;72:215–219.
68. Boldt HC, Pulido JS, Blodi CF, Folk JC, Weingeist TA. Rural endophthalmitis. *Ophthalmology* 1989;96:1722–1726.
69. Saari KM, Aine E. Eye injuries in agriculture. *Acta Ophthalmol* 1984; 161(suppl):42–51.
70. Hall E. Protective eyewear, proper care help stop injuries, blindness at work. *Occup Health Saf* 1987;56:70–71,80.
71. Parvinen A. The role of occupational health physician in protection of the eyes and vision. *Acta Ophthalmol* 1984;161 (suppl):29–33.
72. Lehtonen KE. Practical principles of the prevention of occupational eye injuries. *Acta Ophthalmol* 1984;161(suppl):38–41.
73. Liukkonen I. The role of an optician in the eye protection activities. *Acta Ophthalmol* 1984;161(suppl):34–37.
74. Keeney AH, Renaldo DP. Impact resistance of ophthalmic lenses of various strengths and the influence of frame design. *Sight Sav Rev* 1975;45:105–115.
75. Fishman GA. Ocular phototoxicity: guidelines for selecting sunglasses. *Surv Ophthalmol* 1986;31:119–124.
76. Rosenthal FS, Bakalian AE, Taylor HR. The effect of prescription eyewear on ocular exposure to ultraviolet radiation. *Am J Public Health* 1986;76:1216–1220.
77. Rosenthal FS, Phoon C, Bakalian AE, Taylor HR. The ocular dose of ultraviolet radiation to outdoor workers. *Invest Ophthalmol Vis Sci* 1988;29:649–656.
78. Hitchings R, McGill JI. Compressed air injury of the eye. *Br J Ophthalmol* 1970;86:634–635.
79. Greenseid DZ, Leopold IH. Toxic retinopathies. In: Duane D, ed. *Clinical ophthalmology.* Hagerstown, MD: Harper & Row, 1980;3:8.
80. Eguchi T, Kishi R, Harabuchi I, et al. Impaired colour discrimination among workers exposed to styrene: relevance of a urinary metabolite. *Occup Environ Med* 1995;52:534–538.
81. Kilburn KH. Case report: profound neurobehavioral deficits in an oil field worker overcome by hydrogen sulfide. *Am J Med Sci* 1993;306: 301–305.
82. Fischbein A, Rizzo JN, Solomon SJ, Wolff MS. Oculodermatological findings in workers with occupational exposure to polychlorinated biphenyls (PCBs). *Br J Ind Med* 1985;42:426–430.
83. Von Bahr G. Electrical injuries. *Ophthalmologica* 1969;158:109–117.
84. Sprague JB, Hierholzer JC, Currier RW, et al. Epidemic keratoconjunctivitis. *N Engl J Med* 1973;289:1341–1346.
85. American Academy of Ophthalmology. *Prescribing special lenses. Basic clinical and science course.* Section 3—Optics, refraction, and contact lenses. 1991;198.
86. Harper RA, Halliday BL. Glare and contrast sensitivity in contact lens corrected aphakia, epikeratophakia, and pseudophakia. *Eye* 1989;3: 562–570.
87. Graham CM, Dart JKG, Wilson-Holt NW, Buckley RJ. Prospects for contact lens wear in aphakia. *Eye* 1988;2:48–55.
88. Katsumi O, Miyanaga Y, Hirose T, Okuno H, Asaoka I. Binocular function in unilateral aphakia. *Ophthalmology* 1988;95:1088–1093.
89. Kraff MC, Sanders DR, Jampol LM, Lieberman HL. Effect of an ultraviolet-filtering intraocular lens on cystoid macular edema. *Ophthalmology* 1985;92:366–369.
90. McCaslin MF. Cataracts. *J Occup Med* 1970;12:345–347.
91. Marmer RH. Radial keratotomy complications. *Ann Ophthalmol* 1987; 19:409–411.
92. Makitie J. Contact lenses and the work environment. *Acta Ophthalmol* 1984;161(suppl):115–122.
93. Dixon WS. Contact lenses: Do they belong in the workplace? *Occup Health Saf* 1978;47:36.
94. Novak JF, Saul RW. Contact lenses in industry. *J Occup Med* 1971; 13:175–178.
95. Randolph SA, Mitchell RZ. Guidelines for contact lens use in industry. *J Occup Med* 1987;29:237–242.

## FURTHER READING

Shingleton BJ. Current concepts: eye injuries. *N Engl J Med 1991;* 325:408–413.

Taylor HR. Ultraviolet radiation and the eye: an epidemiologic study. *Trans Am Ophthalmol Soc* 1989;97:802–852.

*Environmental and Occupational Medicine, Third Edition,* edited by William N. Rom.
Lippincott–Raven Publishers, Philadelphia © 1998.

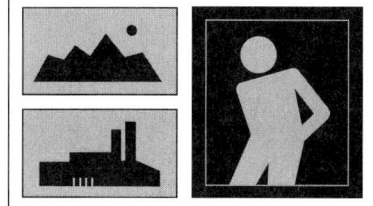

CHAPTER 51

# Occupational Infections

Kevin D. Dieckhaus and Richard A. Garibaldi

In the United States, there are over 100 infectious diseases whose reporting to state health departments may be mandated by law (1), including most infections that impact workers at their place of employment (Tables 1 to 3). Traditionally, infections acquired from animal exposure or unsanitary work environments have accounted for the majority of occupationally acquired infections. However, modernization of agrarian life and improved sanitary standards have markedly diminished the incidence of these infections. The increasingly rare reports of animal-related human infections with such organisms as *Brucella* spp., *Chlamydia psittici,* and *Coxiella burnettii* in the United States speaks to the success of animal vaccination programs and disease elimination programs in reducing the incidence of zoonotic infections. However, just as the modern work force is less likely to be exposed to infectious animals or animal products, it is increasingly likely to come into contact with the infectious diseases that affect other humans. A prime setting for this disease transmission is the hospital and other health care facilities that place health care workers (HCWs) in close proximity to patients with a wide variety of infectious illnesses. In addition, those not directly related to patient care such as clinical lab workers may be exposed to potentially infectious tissues or fluids. With the development of biomedical and research laboratory science, workers in such institutions may increasingly come into contact with infectious agents via laboratory animals, infected cell lines, or microorganisms used for the production of pharmaceutical agents or other biologic products. Finally, residents from industrialized nations are traveling more and more frequently to developing areas of the world for professional and recreational reasons. Contact with unsanitary conditions and exposures to new potential pathogens puts these travelers at risk for an entire host of new infectious agents to which they may not be immune.

## OCCUPATIONAL INFECTIONS ACQUIRED FROM HUMANS

The majority of infections acquired through occupational exposures result from exposure to patients and other infected people in a health care setting (Table 4). The health care industry of the United States employs approximately 9.7 million people (2) and consumes over $750 billion, 13.2% of the gross domestic product (3). HCWs are brought into daily, direct contact with sick patients who may be infected with potentially highly contagious agents. Fortunately, the majority of these infections are pathogenic only to the patient who has underlying conditions that compromise the body's ability to defend itself. Nevertheless, the HCW can be exposed to a wide variety of dangerous agents through direct contact with patients, inhalation, percutaneous inoculation, or fecal-oral transmission.

Hospital infection control practices are designed to minimize the possibility of transmitting an infectious agent from patient to HCW. Proper hand washing has been shown to be critically important to limit the spread of microorganisms (4,5). The most useful measure to limit cross-transmission in health care settings has been the adoption of universal precautions. Under these guidelines, any body fluid is considered to be potentially infec-

K. D. Dieckhaus: Division of Infectious Diseases, Department of Medicine, University of Connecticut Health Center, Farmington, Connecticut 06030-3212.
R. A. Garibaldi: Department of Medicine, University of Connecticut Health Center, Farmington, Connecticut 06030-3945.

**TABLE 1.** *Important bacterial diseases associated with occupational illness*

| Disease | Causative agent | Manifestations of disease | Disease-specific prevention |
|---|---|---|---|
| Anthrax | *Bacillus anthracis* | Necrotizing cutaneous lesion; pneumonia; gastroenteritis with necrotizing oropharyngeal lesions | Animal vaccine, reducing dust exposure, decontaminating imported hides |
| Brucellosis | *Brucella abortus, B. canis, B. melitensis, B. suis* | Systemic syndrome with fever, lymphadenopathy, splenomegaly, hepatomegaly, synovitis | Animal vaccine |
| Infectious diarrhea | *Campylobacter jejuni, Clostridium difficile, Escherichia coli, Salmonella enteritidis, Shigella* | Gastroenteritis | |
| Legionnaires' disease, Pontiac fever | *Legionella pneumophilia* | Pneumonia, influenza-like illness | Reservoir disinfection |
| Leptospirosis | *Leptospira interrogans* | Hepatitis, conjunctivitis, meningitis, jaundice, renal failure, myocarditis | Animal vaccination, disinfection of work areas, doxycycline for those at risk (military) |
| Lyme disease | *Borrelia burgdorferi* | Erythema migrans, meningoencephalitis, cranial neuritis, cardiac dysrhythmias, arthritis | Tick avoidance, human vaccine trials in process, no benefit to prophylactic antibiotics for tick bites |
| Tularemia | *Francisella tularensis* | Skin ulcer, fever, lymphadenopathy, conjunctivitis | Personal protective devices (gloves, eye protection), hygienic work conditions |

tious. Therefore, specific protective barriers to reduce parenteral, mucous membrane and nonintact skin contact with these fluids is required for all patients, whether or not they are considered to be infected.

Because no procedures or policies can be completely effective in preventing exposure to infection, employee health programs have been developed to provide protection to HCWs and other hospital personnel before or after an exposure has occurred. Preemployment evaluation is designed to identify workers who are susceptible to infectious agents to which they may be exposed in the health care industry. Many of these agents have vaccines available for disease prevention. Immunizations are recommended for protection against infections with such agents as influenza, hepatitis A and B, measles, rubella, and varicella. Should an HCW be inadvertently exposed to certain infectious agents, postexposure therapy may reduce the incidence or attenuate the course of the disease.

## INFECTIONS ACQUIRED BY PERCUTANEOUS INOCULATION

Infections acquired by percutaneous inoculation are among the most feared complications of working in the health care arena. A variety of organisms may be transmitted by the direct inoculation of infectious material. This usually occurs in the setting of a needlestick injury. However, other items such as medical instruments including respirators and endoscopes (6,7), laboratory equipment, and glassware (8) may become contaminated and transmit disease to a care provider or laboratory worker. Direct contact of infected blood or other tissues with conjunctiva or broken skin provides another route of percutaneous transmission.

Prevention of needlestick injuries is the single most cost-effective way to limit morbidity from agents that can be transmitted percutaneously. Hospital-based and office-based infection control programs emphasize the importance of meticulous technique when handling sharps. Gloves and eye protection should be worn when exposure to blood is anticipated. Recapping of needles should be avoided. Engineering controls such as needle sheathing devices or self-blunting needles, easy access to sharps disposal units, and proper disposal of infectious materials are important as well. Guidelines are provided by the Occupational Safety and Health Administration (9).

### Hepatitis B

Infection with hepatitis B virus (HBV) has been one of the more common of the hospital infections for which HCWs are at risk. HBV infection can cause a subacute illness characterized by anorexia, fatigue, liver tenderness, and jaundice. A small percent of patients have infections that progress to chronic active hepatitis, cirrhosis, or hepatocellular carcinoma. The treatment of chronic hepatitis B infection centers on supportive management of liver dysfunction. Administration of interferon-$\alpha$ may lessen liver injury in some patients. Prior to the widespread use of vaccine, it was estimated that up to 9,000

**TABLE 2.** *Nonbacterial diseases commonly associated with occupational illness*

| Disease | Causative agent(s) | Manifestations of disease | Disease-specific prevention |
|---|---|---|---|
| Chlamydial/Rickettsial | | | |
| Ornithosis | *Chlamydia psittici* | Pneumonia, septic abortion | Treatment of infected imported birds, environmental sanitation, avoid birthing sheep |
| Q fever | *Coxiella burnetii* | Fever, pneumonia, endocarditis, hepatitis | Personal protective gear (gloves, mask) when working with infected animals |
| Fungal | | | |
| Coccidiodomycosis | *Coccidiodes immitis* | Pneumonia, erythema nodosum | Dust reduction |
| Histoplasmosis | *Histoplasma capsulatum* | Pneumonia, granulomatous disease | Wetting soil prior to digging, respirator for dusty procedures |
| Ringworm | *Microsporum canis, M. gallinae, M. nanum, Trichophytan equinum, T. mentagrophytes, T. verrucosum* | Cutaneous infection | Avoid overcrowding, isolation of infected animals, personal protective gear when working with infected animals |
| Sporotrichosis | *Sporothrix schenckii* | Cutaneous and lymphangitic infection | Personal protective gear |
| Protozoan/Parasitic | | | |
| Echinococcosis | *Echinococcus granulosus, E. multilocularis* | Hydatid cyst disease in liver, lung, CNS | Adequate hygiene and food preparation, dog screening programs, empiric treatment of dogs |
| Schistosomiasis | *Schistosoma mansoni, S. japonicum, S. haematobium,* avian schistosome species | Dermatitis, acute febrile syndrome, portal hypertension, *S. haematobium*: hematuria | Avoidance of direct contact with infected water |
| Toxoplasmosis | *Toxoplasma gondii* | Febrile syndrome, lymphadenitis, chorioretinitis; congenital syndrome | Hygienic measures, adequate food preparation |
| Viral | | | |
| Acquired immune deficiency syndrome | Human immunodeficiency virus | Acquired immune deficiency syndrome | Postexposure antiretroviral agents |
| Hepatitis A | Hepatitis A virus | Hepatitis | Vaccine, immune globulin |
| Hepatitis B | Hepatitis B virus | Hepatitis | Vaccine, immune globulin |
| Hepatitis C | Hepatitis C virus | Hepatitis | None |
| Herpes | Herpes simplex I and II | Whitlow | None |
| Influenza | Influenza A virus | Influenza | Vaccine, Amantadine, Rimantidine |
| Measles | Measles virus | Febrile syndrome, rash | Vaccine, postexposure immunoglobulin |
| Parvovirus B19 | Parvovirus B19 | Erythema infectiosum, aplastic crisis, arthropathy, hydrops fetalis | None, pregnant women should avoid infected patients |
| Rabies | Rabies virus | Rabies | Vaccine for occupations at risk, postexposure prophylaxis with vaccine and immune globulin, animal vaccination |
| Respiratory syncytial virus | Respiratory syncytial virus | Respiratory illness | None |
| Varicella | Varicella-Zoster virus | Chickenpox, shingles | Vaccine, immune globulin |
| Other syndromes | | | |
| Animal bite | *Staphylococci, Streptococci, Pasteurella multocida, Capnocytophaga canimorsus, anaerobes* | Cellulitis, wound infection | None |
| Ectoparasites | Lice, scabies | Dermatitis | None |
| Farmer's lung | *Streptomyces rectivirgula, Aspergillus spp.,* Thermophilic *actinomyces* | Acute, subacute, or chronic pulmonary syndrome | Dust reduction |

**TABLE 3.** *Occupations and their specific infectious diseases*

| Occupation | Associated diseases |
|---|---|
| Abattoir workers, butchers, and meat handlers | Anthrax, brucellosis, cryptosporidiosis, erysipeloid, infectious diarrhea, leptospirosis, *Mycobacterium bovis,* Newcastle disease, orf, ornithosis, Q fever, *Streptococcus suis* meningitis, toxoplasmosis, tularemia, vesicular stomatitis |
| Animal handlers | |
| Animal control officer | Bite wounds, rabies |
| Cattle | Babesiosis, bovine papular stomatitis, brucellosis, cryptosporidiosis, erysipeloid, *Mycobacterium bovis,* pseudocowpox, Q fever, ringworm, vesicular stomatitis |
| Fish/crustaceans | Erysipeloid, leptospirosis, *Mycobacterium marinum,* nanophyetiasis |
| Pet shop employees | Bite wounds, *Mycobacterium marinum,* Newcastle disease, ornithosis, ringworm, toxoplasmosis |
| Poultry | Campylobacteriosis, erysipeloid, histoplasmosis, infectious diarrhea, Newcastle disease, ornithosis, ringworm |
| Sheep/goats | Brucellosis, cryptosporidiosis, echinococcosis, erysipeloid, louping-ill, orf, ornithosis, Q fever, tularemia |
| Swine | Erysipeloid, influenza, ringworm, *Streptococcus suis* meningitis |
| Veterinarians | Anthrax, bite wounds, brucellosis, cryptosporidiosis, echinococcosis, herpes simiae, leptospirosis, *Mycobacterium bovis,* Newcastle disease, orf, ornithosis, Q fever, rabies, ringworm, toxoplasmosis, tularemia, vesicular stomatitis |
| Zoo personnel | Bite wounds, herpes simiae, *Mycobacterium marinum,* ringworm, sealpox |
| Archeologists | Coccidiodomycosis |
| Construction workers | Coccidiodomycosis, histoplasmosis, tetanus |
| Day-care providers | Cytomegalovirus, hepatitis A, infectious diarrhea, upper respiratory tract infections |
| Farmers | Brucellosis, campylobacteriosis, coccidiodomycosis, cryptosporidiosis, histoplasmosis, hypersensitivity pneumonitis, orf, Q fever, ringworm, sporotrichosis, tetanus, toxoplasmosis, tularemia, vesicular stomatitis |
| Foundry workers | Acinetobacter pneumonia |
| Health care personnel | Clostridium difficile, hepatitis A, B, C, and delta, herpes simplex virus, human immunodeficiency virus, influenza, lice, measles, *Mycobacterium tuberculosis, Neisseria meningitidis,* parvovirus, respiratory syncytial virus, *Salmonella,* scabies, varicella-zoster virus |
| Hide processors | Anthrax, tularemia |
| Laboratory worker | |
| Research lab | Campylobacteriosis, filoviruses, hepatitis A, herpes simiae, influenza, leptospirosis, lymphocytic choreomeningitis, ornithosis, Q fever, rat-bite fever, ringworm, *Salmonella,* toxoplasmosis |
| Clinical microbiology lab | Brucellosis, campylobacteriosis, coccidioidomycosis, *Salmonella,* tularemia |
| Military personnel | Adenovirus, coccidioidomycosis, hepatitis A, leptospirosis, *Neisseria meningitidis,* ringworm, tetanus, upper respiratory tract infections |
| Miners | Leptospirosis, ringworm |
| Office workers | Influenza, legionellosis |
| Outdoor/rural occupation | Babesiosis, leptospirosis, Lyme disease, Q fever |
| Plant and plant product exposure | Hypersensitivity pneumonitis, sporotrichosis |
| Sewer workers | Hepatitis A, leptospirosis, tetanus |
| Sandblasters, miners, quarry workers, ceramic workers | Silicotuberculosis |

HCWs were infected with HBV annually, resulting in 125 to 190 deaths per year (10).

There are between 750,000 and 1 million HBV carriers in the United States. Approximately 80% to 90% of hepatitis B surface antigen (HBsAg) carriers are asymptomatic and unaware of their potential infectivity. Over 10,000 patients are admitted to hospitals annually with hepatitis B (11,12) and between 1% and 1.5% of all patients admitted to hospitals are asymptomatic carriers of HBV. Patients with certain risk factors have a much higher prevalence of low-grade, chronic infection, and thus can transmit the virus unknowingly to unsuspecting, susceptible HCWs. Patients who have a history of intravenous drug abuse, promiscuous homosexual activity, hemophilia, or chronic liver disease, and patients originating from Southeast Asia have a higher incidence of chronic infection. HCWs who have frequent contact with blood or blood products, such as surgical, dental, and

**TABLE 4.** *Occupational illness acquired through contact with humans*

| Type of contact | Agents | Prevention |
|---|---|---|
| Percutaneous inoculation | Hepatitis B, C, and delta, human immunodeficiency virus | Gloves, needlestick prevention programs |
| Airborne transmission | Tuberculosis, varicella-zoster virus, measles | Respiratory isolation, air filtration (for *M. tuberculosis)* |
| Respiratory droplets | Diphtheria, *Mycoplasma, Neisseria meningitidis,* rubella, respiratory syncytial virus, influenza virus, mumps, pertussis, parvovirus B19 | Respiratory isolation, respiratory droplet precautions |
| Fecal-oral transmission | Campylobacter jejuni, *Clostridium difficile, Escherichia coli, Salmonella, Shigella, Vibrio, Yersinia,* hepatitis A, rotavirus, *Giardia lamblia* | Hand washing, gloves |
| Direct contact | Varicella-zoster virus, respiratory syncytial virus (via fomites), herpes simplex virus, staphylococci, ectoparasites | Gloves, protective clothing |

hemodialysis staff, as well as clinical laboratory workers, are at risk for developing hepatitis B. As many as 30% of these hospital staff members have evidence of past infection with HBV compared to only 5% of the general population. Medical personnel are exposed to HBV through percutaneous inoculations in most instances, although contact with eyes and nonintact skin have also led to infection. The presence of HBsAg in the patient's blood indicates a high-risk exposure, although HBsAg-negative blood has occasionally also been shown to harbor infectious virus and cause infection (13). The presence of hepatitis B e-antigen has been correlated with a markedly increased risk of viral transmission. Whereas 1% to 6% of needlesticks with e-antigen negative blood result in infection, 22% to 40% of needlestick injuries involving blood positive for e-antigen result in infection (14).

A plasma-derived vaccine for hepatitis B has been available since 1982. This was replaced in the United States by a recombinant subunit vaccine in 1986. Routine preexposure vaccination is recommended for all HCWs who have regular contact with blood (11). Postexposure prophylaxis is recommended after a nonimmune HCW has been exposed to potentially infectious blood. This includes both passive protection with the administration of hepatitis B immune globulin (HBIG) and active immunization with a three-dose series of hepatitis B vaccine. HCWs who have been previously vaccinated and demonstrate protective levels of antibody to HBsAg (>10 mIU/ml) do not require postexposure prophylaxis.

### Hepatitis C

Hepatitis C virus (HCV) used to be included under the rubric "non-A, non-B hepatitis." HCV has now been characterized as a member of the flavivirus family, and a specific serologic test has been developed to identify carriers who may be infectious to others. Hepatitis C is contracted primarily through parenteral inoculation, especially blood transfusions (15). HCWs sustaining needlestick injuries from known HCV carriers have a 2.7% to 10% risk of acquiring infection (16,17). As many as 12% of source patients in needlestick incidents are positive for HCV (18). The incidence is highest in injection drug users, hemophiliacs, and hemodialysis patients. A minority of infections are acquired nonparentally by sexual contact, household exposure, or otherwise undefined exposures. Most people infected with HCV are asymptomatic and cannot pinpoint the time of their acute infection. Clinical consequences of HCV infection include acute hepatitis, life-long carrier state, chronic active hepatitis, cirrhosis, and primary hepatocellular carcinoma.

Treatment of HCV infection rests primarily on supportive therapy of chronic liver dysfunction. Interferon-α is a Food and Drug Administration (FDA)-approved treatment for chronic HCV infections and has been used with moderate success in lessening liver injury in some patients (19–23). However, these beneficial effects are generally short-lived after completion of therapy. Other investigational agents include ribavirin and interferon-β. The only known strategy to prevent nosocomial hepatitis C infection is to prevent inoculation injuries. Transfusion-associated hepatitis C has been virtually eliminated in the United States because all blood is routinely screened for antibody to HCV prior to transfusion. As yet, no vaccine is available to protect HCWs against HCV, before or after exposure. Immunoglobulin prophylaxis has been used following exposure; however, it is not recommended as a routine measure (24).

### Human Immunodeficiency Virus (HIV) (See Also Chapter 52)

Human immunodeficiency virus (HIV) is the pathogen of the acquired immune deficiency syndrome (AIDS). Over 500,000 cases of AIDS have been reported to the Centers for Disease Control and it is estimated that over 1.5 million people in the United States are infected with

HIV. The infection is transmitted to HCWs via percutaneous injuries with sharps that are contaminated with HIV-positive blood. Guidelines for postexposure prophylaxis of HIV for HCWs have recently been published (25).

### Other Percutaneously Acquired Infections

Virtually any infectious agent is capable of causing a localized infection when it is inoculated directly into the skin or comes in contact with an abrasion or open wound. Often, the inoculation results in a suppurative lesion, especially when the pathogen is a bacterium such as *Staphylococcus aureus* or a virulent gram-negative bacillus. Other agents, including fungi like *Candida albicans* or *Cryptococcus neoformans,* mycobacteria like *Mycobacterium fortuitum,* or spirochetes like *Treponema pallidum,* have been reported to cause infections associated with inoculation injuries in HCWs.

## INFECTIONS ACQUIRED BY THE AIRBORNE ROUTE

Organisms such as measles, tuberculosis, and varicella may be transmitted via aerosolation of particles from evaporated respiratory secretions called droplet nuclei (26). These are small (5 μm or less) particles that may remain suspended in the air for long periods and may be widely dispersed by air currents. Patients with infections that can be transmitted via droplet nuclei should be placed in a respiratory isolation room and caregivers should be versed in the use of appropriate personal protective respiratory equipment. Should transport be necessary, patients should wear masks to minimize dispersal of droplet nuclei. HCWs immune to measles or varicella do not require such precautions for protection against these agents.

### Measles

Measles is a highly transmittable disease caused by the rubeola virus. It is characterized by cough, coryza, fever and a maculopapular rash. It is usually considered as a disease of childhood, but with the institution of widespread immunization programs in the United States in 1963 the incidence during childhood has been dramatically reduced. A resurgence in measles cases has recently been observed in people who had received only a single dose of measles vaccine during childhood and who were subsequently exposed to wild virus during adulthood.

Patients with measles should be placed in respiratory isolation until after the fourth day of the rash, after which they are no longer considered infectious. Nonimmune contacts may be given vaccine within 3 days of contact or, if live virus is contraindicated, immunoglobulin within 6 days of contact to attenuate the clinical course of infection (27). All HCWs should be assessed for susceptibility to measles prior to employment and receive vaccine unless they were born prior to 1957 or have a history of physician-diagnosed measles, serologic evidence of prior infection, or documentation of two doses of measles vaccine after their first birthday (28).

### Mycobacterium Tuberculosis (See Also Chapter 53)

Tuberculosis remains a significant hazard to hospital personnel. Despite the widespread use of screening tests for the early identification of cases, knowledge of how the disease is spread, and availability of effective therapy, medical students and physicians are reported to have two to three times the prevalence of tuberculosis compared with nonmedical, age-matched controls. The AIDS epidemic has increased the possibility that HCWs will come in contact with active pulmonary tuberculosis. Disseminated tuberculosis is one of the opportunistic infections seen in patients with AIDS. It is often unrecognized by medical personnel at the time of the patient's admission, when transmission is likely to occur. Patients with HIV, those from highly endemic urban areas, and patients from homeless shelters or prison are at risk for having and transmitting drug-resistant strains of tuberculosis.

Patients with active pulmonary tuberculosis or laryngeal involvement may transmit infection via the respiratory route. Coughing or sneezing aerosolizes infectious particles that may remain suspended in the air on small droplet nuclei for several hours. Inhalation of these particles by a HCW may cause focal pulmonary infection that heals with a characteristic radiographic appearance. This infection may later recrudesce into pneumonia or disseminated, systemic illness. Nonpulmonary tuberculosis is generally noncommunicable to the HCW.

Infection with tuberculosis generates a cellular immune response that may be demonstrated by a positive reaction to a tuberculin skin test within 2 to 8 weeks after exposure. Hospital employees should be tested at the time of their employment and subsequently at regular intervals based on risk assessment. The use of a two-step method may increase sensitivity of skin testing for HCWs who have not had a documented negative result in the preceding 12 months (29). HCWs should also be tested after exposure to a tuberculosis patient when appropriate preventive measures were not employed. A skin test result of 10-mm induration or greater is generally considered positive for HCWs (30). HCWs with a skin test that converts to positive need to be evaluated by physical examination and chest x-ray to exclude progressive primary infection. If the x-ray reveals no pneumonia, preventive therapy with isoniazid for 6 months is recommended. Identification of active pulmonary disease necessitates treatment with two or more drugs. Antituberculous therapy is very effective in controlling active infection and decreasing the likelihood of additional respiratory transmission.

### *Varicella-Zoster Virus*

Varicella-zoster virus (VZV) is a member of the herpes virus family and is the etiologic agent of chickenpox and shingles. Chickenpox is highly infectious and is spread via airborne droplet nuclei, larger respiratory droplets (31), and direct contact with involved lesions. Systemic disease is usually seen in children and is characterized by a vesicular rash, fever, and lassitude. In adults or immunocompromised patients, the infection may reactivate, resulting in a dermatomally distributed rash—shingles. Nonimmune adults are at risk of serious complications, particularly varicella pneumonia, after acquiring primary VZV infection.

Hospital personnel should have their antibody status assessed at the time of employment. A clearly positive history of chickenpox is usually sufficient to predict protective immunity. HCWs with a negative or equivocal history should have serologic screening and be offered vaccination if negative for past infection (32). Because varicella may be transmitted during the incubation period prior to the onset of clinical illness, susceptible employees who are exposed to active cases should be placed on administrative leave from 10 to 21 days after the exposure.

## INFECTIONS ACQUIRED VIA RESPIRATORY DROPLET INHALATION

Larger aerosolized respiratory particles that may contain infectious agents are generated by coughing, sneezing, talking, and by certain respiratory procedures such as suctioning or bronchoscopy. These droplets may be propelled short distances and deposited on the hands or the nasal mucosa, conjunctiva, or mouth of a susceptible host. Agents transmitted this way include influenza virus, respiratory syncytial virus (RSV), rubella, mumps, parvovirus, diphtheria, *Mycoplasma pneumonia, Neisseria meningitis,* pertussis, and pneumonic plague. Affected patients should be placed in isolation during the period of infectivity. While working with infected patients, susceptible employees should wash their hands and wear masks, gowns, and gloves to reduce contact with these secretions, but specialized ventilation systems are not necessary (26).

### Influenza

Health care workers are at risk for influenza infection during the winter and spring months each year. Patients who are admitted with active influenza are the prime sources of virus, but visitors or hospital personnel may also introduce influenza into the institutional setting.

Influenza virus causes an acute respiratory infection with a spectrum of clinical presentations that range from a mild pharyngitis to an acute tracheobronchitis or severe pneumonia. Patients with infections sometimes require ventilatory support and intensive care. Each year, the U.S. Public Health Service directs the production of influenza vaccine against what is predicted to be the most likely serotypes of epidemic influenza A and influenza B viruses. It is recommended that hospital personnel who may be involved in the care of patients with influenza pneumonia be immunized annually (33). Unfortunately, acceptance of influenza immunizations by HCWs is quite poor. Thus, hospitals, nursing homes, and other health care settings remain susceptible to epidemic transmission of influenza A. Once an active case is introduced into these settings, prophylactic treatment of susceptible personnel and patients with amantadine or rimantidine is recommended to decrease staff absenteeism from influenza A and to reduce the morbidity and mortality in susceptible patients (33). Some studies suggest that the administration of influenza vaccine to employees is cost-effective by reducing employee absenteeism due to upper respiratory illness during the winter months (34).

### Mumps

Outbreaks of mumps in health care facilities are uncommon due to the high rate of vaccination with the measles-mumps-rubella (MMR) vaccine but have been described (35,36). Facilities that provide chronic care for adolescents and young adults appear to be at greatest risk. Immunization should be considered at the time of the pre-employment evaluation for HCWs who do not have documentation of disease or adequate immunization.

### Neisseria Meningitidis

Meningococcal meningitis is a disease that is feared by HCWs. Infection with *N. meningitidis* can run an acute fulminant course with meningitis, coma, shock, disseminated intravascular coagulation, and death within 12 to 24 hours after exposure. HCWs may come in contact with this organism as they care for patients with acute infection. The organism colonizes the nasopharynx of infected patients and may be transmitted by respiratory droplets or direct contact with respiratory secretions. Activities that increase the likelihood of exposure include suctioning, intubating, or performing mouth-to-mouth resuscitation (37). HCWs with short periods of low-risk exposure need not be prophylaxed (38). Those who are likely to have been exposed to respiratory droplets or secretions of patients with meningococcal disease should receive prophylactic therapy with rifampin (39). This eradicates early nasopharyngeal colonization and prevents active infection.

### Parvovirus B19

Human parvovirus B19 is the etiologic agent of erythema infectiosum or fifth disease; it also can cause arthropathy, aplastic anemia in patients with AIDS or sickle cell anemia, and hydrops fetalis in pregnant women. It is spread via respiratory secretions and direct contact with infected individuals. HCWs should wear gloves, gowns, and masks while working in close proximity with infected patients during the period of infectivity. Because of the small but defined risk of fetal demise associated with acute infection during pregnancy (40), some authorities recommend that pregnant HCWs not participate in the direct care of patients with aplastic crises to minimize the risk of becoming infected with parvovirus (41). Once a rash has developed, the disease is no longer transmissable and specific precautions are no longer indicated.

### Acute Respiratory Tract Diseases

There are over 100 agents that are etiologically responsible for syndromes of pharyngitis or upper respiratory tract disease. These include bacteria such as *Streptococcus pyogenes, Mycoplasma pneumoniae, Chlamydia pneumoniae,* and a host of viruses including RSV; rhinovirus; adenovirus; parainfluenza 1, 2, and 3 viruses; coxsackie A and B viruses; coronavirus; and echovirus. Most of these agents are spread by direct contact with respiratory secretions from coughing, hand contamination, or touching contaminated environmental surfaces. While participating in the care of an infected patient, particularly in outbreak situations, the HCW should be meticulous with hand washing.

Respiratory syncytial virus is a particularly common agent of bronchiolitis among young children. It is frequently transmitted to HCWs and subsequently to other patients. Adenovirus is a common cause of respiratory disease in military recruits. Use of oral live virus vaccine has reduced the incidence of adenovirus pulmonary disease in this population (42). However, this vaccine is not recommended for the general public.

### Rubella

Rubella, or German measles, usually causes a mild febrile disease with an exanthem in children. Active infection in a pregnant woman, however, may result in prematurity, congenital birth defects, or fetal death. Female HCWs of child-bearing age should be offered rubella vaccination at their preemployment evaluation if they are not immune (43). Pregnant HCWs who are nonimmune should not be involved with the direct care of patients with active rubella infection.

### Cytomegalovirus

Cytomegalovirus (CMV) is a common cause of an infectious mononucleosis-like syndrome. CMV has also been associated with the risk of congenital infection in children born to mothers who acquire infection early during pregnancy. This is an important consideration for HCWs and child-care providers in day-care centers or preschools, many of whom are of childbearing age. Asymptomatic carriers may excrete CMV viral particles in saliva, urine, stool, respiratory tract secretions, blood, and breast milk. Contact with these fluids directly or indirectly may increase the risk of acquiring acute CMV. However, epidemiologic studies have not shown evidence of significantly increased rates of CMV infection in HCWs in any of the suspected high-risk hospital settings (44). On the other hand, day-care providers and mothers of children who excrete CMV appear to be at greatest risk for acquiring the virus (45,46). Aside from meticulous attention to hand washing and proper handling of diapers, blood, and other potentially secretions or excretions, no additional precautions are currently recommended for pregnant women (47).

## INFECTIONS ACQUIRED BY INGESTION (FECAL-ORAL TRANSMISSION)

Fecal-oral transmission of a variety of agents has been reported frequently within health care settings. Other types of employment, such as providing day care or performing sanitation or sewer work, may also increase the risk for acquiring infection with these pathogens. Employees should be instructed in proper barrier precautions, especially glove use, when working with potentially infectious materials, and be meticulous about proper hand washing to reduce the transmission of these agents.

### Agents of Infectious Diarrhea

Patients are admitted to the hospital with a variety of acute diarrheal infections. Likely diarrheal pathogens include *Salmonella, Shigella,* enteroinvasive *Escherichia coli, Campylobacter jejuni, Yersinia, Vibrio, Clostridium difficile, Giardia lamblia,* and rotavirus, among others. *C. difficile* is the agent of antibiotic-associated colitis. More frequently, however, the clinical presentation of *C. difficile* infection includes only mild to moderate diarrhea. Usually, the syndrome is linked to the administration of antibiotics. However it is now well demonstrated that *C. difficile* may be transmitted from patient to patient or patient to HCW in the hospital setting (48). *C. difficile* is excreted in the feces. Some patients, particularly those receiving antibiotics, may be asymptomatic carriers. Bacteria are spread from patient to patient on the hands of hospital personnel or by contact with contaminated environmental surfaces. Symptomatic infections are treated with fluid replacement, discontinuation of the implicated antibiotic, and metronidazole or oral vancomycin. If epidemic spread in the hospital is identified, decontamination of possibly contaminated surfaces is also recommended.

Because of difficulties in maintaining adequate hygiene, outbreaks of infectious diarrhea are frequently reported in day-care centers, affecting both children and their teachers. *Giardia lamblia, Shigella, C. jejuni, Cryptosporidium,* and *C. difficile* have been implicated as epidemic infections from these settings.

### Hepatitis A

Cases of hepatitis A virus (HAV) infection among hospital personnel are not often reported. This may be because infection of hospital personnel is often asymptomatic or because adults, in general, have high levels of immunity against HAV infection. Hospital personnel are at some increased risk for acquiring hepatitis A. However, because the period of excretion of HAV in the stool is limited to the prodromal period, transmission to HCWs is uncommon. There have, however, been isolated reports of common-source contamination of hospital foods that have resulted in institutional outbreaks. When indicated, immune serum globulin provides excellent passive protection against HAV infection. An inactivated virus vaccine is now available for active immunization for those who are at high risk of acquiring hepatitis A. Groups that may benefit from vaccination include travelers to areas of the world where HAV is endemic, military personnel, day-care workers, staff of institutions for the mentally handicapped, and any HCW having contact with active cases or handling live hepatitis A virus (49).

## INFECTIONS ACQUIRED BY DIRECT CONTACT

Many organisms may be transmitted by direct contact to HCWs. Usually this involves direct contact with an active infectious lesion, body fluid, or tissue, or indirect contact with a contaminated environmental surface. Infections that may be transmitted to HCWs from an affected patient include conjunctivitis, impetigo, staphylococcal infections, ectoparasitic diseases, cutaneous diphtheria, varicella-zoster, and herpes simplex, among others. HCWs should wear appropriate barrier precautions, including gloves and protective gowns, and wash their hands if substantial contact with the patient, environmental surfaces, body fluids, or tissues is anticipated.

### Herpes Simplex Virus

Hospital personnel in critical care units are at risk of acquiring herpes simplex virus (HSV) infection by direct contact. Critically ill patients frequently develop labial herpes infections; in addition, approximately 20% of patients in intensive care units have been shown to harbor HSV in oral secretions even though they are asymptomatic. Persons involved in suctioning oropharyngeal secretions from these patients are at risk of inoculating periungual skin and developing herpetic whitlows. These lesions are painful deep vesicles that may be mistaken for a pyogenic infection. They will not respond to antibacterial agents, but oral acyclovir may induce early remission and provide symptomatic relief (50).

### Ectoparasitic Diseases

Hospital personnel or other individuals who have close bodily contact with others are at risk for certain ectoparasitic diseases such as scabies and pediculosis. Scabies, a skin infection caused by a burrowing mite, usually involves the interdigital spaces of the hands and the flexor surface of the wrists. Typically, a papular or eczematous reaction with intense itching develops 2 to 6 weeks after exposure to an infected patient. The diagnosis is confirmed by microscopic examination of tissue scrapings with 10% potassium hydroxide. An agent such as γ-benzene hexachloride (Kwell) is prescribed for treatment.

Head and pubic lice are found on patients of all socioeconomic classes. Body lice are typically seen in destitute patients who are unable to maintain even a minimal level of personal hygiene. Lice are transmitted from person to person by direct contact or by contact with clothing in which the ectoparasite can survive as long as a week. The diagnosis is confirmed by finding adult lice or nits on the hair or clothing of infested persons. As with scabies, treatment with γ-benzene hexachloride is usually effective.

## INFECTIONS ACQUIRED THROUGH CONTACT WITH ANIMALS

The vast majority of occupational infections acquired by workers who are not in the medical or scientific communities are zoonoses (Tables 5 and 6). Workers become infected because their occupation places them in direct contact with animals, their secretions, or their by-products. Whereas in years past, occupational infectious diseases were a prominent cause of workplace-related disease, extramedical occupational infections are now infrequent. The fact that brucellosis, psittacosis, and other previously common workplace-related infections are not seen very often today is a tribute to the efficacy of surveillance and animal vaccination and disease elimination programs that have reduced the incidence of these diseases in animals, and consequently in their human contacts. Occupational zoonoses of particular concern are described here based on their common modes of acquisition.

## ZOONOSES ACQUIRED BY AIRBORNE TRANSMISSION

### Chlamydia Psittici

*Chlamydia psittici,* the etiologic agent of ornithosis, generally causes an atypical pneumonia with fever, cough, headache, myalgias and other nonspecific symptoms. The organism may be found in a variety of animals including

**TABLE 5.** *Bacterial disease acquired through direct or indirect contact with animals*

| Type of contact | Disease | Animal exposure |
|---|---|---|
| Airborne transmission | Anthrax | Cattle, goats, donkeys, various other wild herbivores |
| | Brucellosis | Cattle, goats, swine, dogs |
| | Plague | Urban and domestic rats, ground squirrels, prairie dogs, rock squirrels, chipmunks, mice, bobcats, rabbits |
| | Tularemia | Rabbits, hares, rodents, beavers, squirrels, muskrats, birds |
| Direct contact with infected animal or tissue | Anthrax | Cattle, goats, donkeys, various other wild herbivores |
| | Brucellosis | Cattle, goats, swine, dogs |
| | Erysipeloid | Cattle, chickens, ducks, fish, pheasants, sheep, shellfish, swine, turkeys |
| | Fish tank granuloma | Fish, crustaceans |
| | Leptospirosis | Cattle, cats, dogs, raccoon, rats, swine |
| | *Streptococcus suis* meningitis | Pigs |
| | Tularemia | Rabbits, hares, rodents, beavers, squirrels, muskrats, birds |
| Ingestion/fecal-oral transmission | Infectious diarrhea | Cattle, cats, dogs, chickens, rodents, sheep, swine |

birds, cows, sheep, and goats. Organisms associated with psitticine birds such as turkeys and chickens appear to be the most common cause of human disease. Infected birds may be obviously sick or completely asymptomatic carriers. The disease is spread by direct contact or inhalation of aerosolized infectious particles or dust. The organism has been implicated as a cause of septicemia with spontaneous abortion in women who acquired the infection from sheep during the lambing process (51). Other occupations of particular hazard include ranchers, pet shop employees, abattoir workers, poultry farmers, and veterinarians. Treatment of active disease is with doxycycline or erythromycin. Quarantine and treatment of imported birds with doxycycline may reduce the incidence of psitticosis in some groups. Pregnant women should avoid contact with sheep during birthing or handling of the newborn lambs.

## Coxiella Burnetii

*Coxiella burnetii* is a pleomorphic coccobacillus related to the rickettsiae that cause the syndromes of Q fever (52). The most common animal reservoirs are cattle, goats, and sheep, although a large number of other animals have been shown to harbor the organism. Placenta of infected animals have large numbers of the organism. Inhalation of infectious particles is the usual mode of acquiring infection. Other routes of infection include direct contact with infected animals or ingestion of contaminated milk. Clinical laboratory-related infections have occurred.

Clinical manifestations of Q fever may include a nonspecific febrile illness, pneumonia, osteomyelitis, endocarditis, or hepatitis. Occupations that have been associ-

**TABLE 6.** *Nonbacterial diseases acquired through contact with animals*

| Type of contact | Disease | Animal exposure |
|---|---|---|
| Airborne transmission | Ornithosis (psittacosis) | Birds, poultry |
| | Q fever | Cattle, sheep, goats, rabbits, cats, many others |
| Direct contact with infected animal or tissue | Erysipeloid | Fish, whales, crabs, swine, turkeys, ducks, sheep |
| | Influenza | Pigs, horses, birds |
| | Lymphocytic choreomeningitis | Mice, hamsters |
| | Newcastle disease | Birds, especially chickens and turkeys |
| | Orf | Sheep, goats |
| | Parapoxviruses | Cattle, goats, seals, sheep |
| | Q fever | Cattle, sheep, goats, rabbits, cats, many others |
| | Rabies | Skunk, fox, raccoons, bats, cattle, monkeys, cats, horses, sheep, most mammals |
| | Ringworm | Dogs, cats, poultry, pigs, rodents, horses, cattle |
| | Vesicular stomatitis | Horses, cattle |
| Ingestion/fecal-oral transmission | Cryptosporidiosis | Cattle, sheep |
| | Echinococcosis | Dogs, sheep, goats, camels, horses |
| | Nanophyetiasis | Fish, particularly salmonids |
| | Toxoplasmosis | Cats, birds, sheep, goats, swine, cattle |
| | Q fever | Unpasteurized milk |

ated with acquisition of Q fever include farmers, dairy workers, sheep workers, abattoir workers, veterinarians, and meat handlers. Research laboratory workers using sheep may also become infected. Frequently, infection occurs without a specific animal exposure and is likely due to inhalation of the organism from a distant site. Simply working or living in a rural environment may put individuals at increased risk of inhalation-related disease.

### Newcastle Disease

Newcastle disease is caused by a paramyxovirus and is characterized by a self-limited influenza-like syndrome with conjunctivitis. It is associated with contact with birds, particularly turkeys and chickens. The organism can be acquired by direct inhalation of infectious particles or by inoculation into the conjunctiva. Imported birds are required to be quarantined prior to entry into the United States to prevent the introduction of the disease.

### Lymphocytic Choreomeningitis

Lymphocytic choreomeningitis virus (LCV) commonly infects mice, including those used in research laboratories. Rodent breeders, researchers, and laboratory technicians who work with mice or hamsters may be exposed to infectious aerosols (53). Clinically, infection presents with biphasic symptoms of fever, headache, and signs of meningitis or encephalomyelitis. Infection during pregnancy is associated with congenital complications (54). Treatment of meningitis is supportive.

## INFECTIONS ACQUIRED THROUGH DIRECT CONTACT WITH ANIMALS

### Animal Bites

Numerous organisms may be inoculated into the skin and soft tissue of workers who are bitten by animals (55). Occupations such as farmers, veterinarians, zoo personnel, research laboratory workers, and animal control officers are at particular risk of suffering a bite-related infection. In addition to the common isolates of *S. aureus,* streptococci, and/or anaerobes causing local infection at the site of inoculation, several organisms are considered uniquely related to animal exposures.

*Capnocytophaga canimorsus,* previously identified as DF-2, may be acquired through a dog bite. Clinical symptoms may range from a localized infection to overwhelming sepsis and death, particularly in people who have undergone splenectomy or who are taking corticosteroids (55).

*Pasteurella* spp. are found in a wide variety of animals. Infection has been described after bites from cats, dogs, lions, panthers, opposums, rabbits, and rats (56). The organism generally causes a cellulitic or suppurative soft tissue infection, but may cause sepsis, osteomyelitis or other systemic illness. Nonbite transmission has been described for this organism in a number of occupations requiring close contact with these animal reservoirs (57,58).

Rabies is caused by a rhabdovirus that may be found in domestic animals and livestock such dogs, cats, cattle, horses, and swine, as well as wild animals such as skunks, raccoons, foxes, coyotes, and bats. Human cases usually result from the bite of an infected animal. Because of the nearly uniform mortality of the disease and its ability to be prevented with appropriate preexposure vaccination, workers in occupations at high risk for exposure to rabies should receive preexposure vaccination. Occupations for whom immunization should be considered include rabies research or diagnostic laboratory workers, veterinarians and their staff, animal control officers, and wildlife workers (59). Postexposure guidelines include thorough cleansing of the wound, local injection of rabies immune globulin, and rabies vaccination based on risk assessment.

Rat-bite fever encompasses two clinically similar diseases caused by *Spirillium minus* and *Streptobacillus moniliformis.* Laboratory workers (60) or rodent breeders (61) who are bitten by rodents may develop local inflammation or eschar formation with or without regional lymphadenitis, relapsing fever, chills, rash, and headache beginning 1 to 4 weeks after the bite of a rat. Both organisms are susceptible to penicillin.

### Bacillus Anthracis

*Bacillus anthracis*, a gram-positive rod that is the etiologic agent of anthrax, has been the cause of much human illness throughout history. It is found in association with a variety of animals, but most commonly with larger herbivores. It may also contaminate soil in areas where these animals graze. Occupational illness is generally through direct inoculation into the skin while working with infected animals, soil, tissues or the hides of infected animals. This results in a characteristic black eschar. Outbreaks have been described in industrialized countries due to the importation of contaminated animal products, especially goat hair (62). In developing countries, large outbreaks have been described in association with agricultural animals, particularly cattle. Occasionally, inhalation of spores may cause a pulmonary illness. Animal vaccination programs, improvements in industrial dust control, and disinfection of imported animal fibers have significantly reduced the incidence of anthrax in industrialized countries.

### Brucella Spp.

Several different species of *Brucella* have been implicated in human disease, including *B. suis, B. melitensis,* and *B. abortus,* among others. Disease from these organisms is almost always derived from direct or indirect exposure to a wide variety of animals including, but not limited to, goats, sheep, camels, cattle, pigs, dogs, buffalo, and yaks. Human disease is usually contracted by direct cutaneous contact or conjunctival inoculation from an infected animal, animal tissues or placenta, or ingestion of unpasteurized milk products. Direct inhalation of infected aerosols may also produce disease. Occupations at risk for disease involve the direct handling of potentially infected animals, such as ranchers, veterinarians, abattoir workers, hunters, farmers, and butchers. Accidental conjunctival inoculation of live brucella animal vaccine strains has been described in veterinarians and ranchers. Clinical laboratory workers may become infected via inhalation of the organism during routine handling of clinical specimens (63).

Brucellosis is manifested by a wide array of clinical syndromes. Symptoms are often nonspecific with fever, rigors, malaise, anorexia, and arthralgia. Local suppurative complications including splenic and hepatic abscesses may occur. Osteoarticular complications are common and may present as sacroiliitis, osteomyelitis, tenosynovitis, arthritis, or bursitis (64). Granulomatous hepatitis, meningitis, endocarditis, pulmonary lesions, epididymitis, orchitis, and colitis may occasionally occur.

Treatment of brucellosis requires combination therapy with a tetracycline in addition to an aminoglycoside or rifampin. Animal control programs, including improved sanitary conditions for swine, cattle vaccination, and serologic testing of cattle herds with elimination of infected cattle, have significantly reduced the incidence of brucellosis in the United States.

### Francisella Tularensis

*Francisella tularensis* is a gram-negative pleomorphic bacillus that is the etiologic agent of tularemia (65). It is found in hundreds of animal species including rodents, squirrels, muskrats, voles, beavers, rabbits, hares, birds, sheep, goats, and mice. Disease transmission most commonly occurs due to direct contact with or bite from an infected animal, contact with infected animal tissues, or through the bite of an infected insect. Insect vectors vary according to geographic locale, but ticks, biting flies, and mosquitoes may transmit the organism. Other less common modes of transmission include inhalation of aerosolized particles during slaughtering of infected animals, during routine microbiologic handling, or through direct contact with contaminated water or mud. Any activity that places a worker in contact with animals entails the risk of contracting tularemia. Thus hunters, trappers, skinners, meat handlers, sheep shearers, farmers, clinical laboratory workers, and veterinarians may have occupational exposure to the organism.

Clinical disease may present as one of several syndromes and varies according to the site of inoculation. The most common presentation is an ulcer at the site of inoculation associated with local lymphadenopathy. Other syndromes include lymphadenopathy without skin lesions, an enteric illness, pneumonia, conjunctival disease, pharyngitis, and nonspecific symptoms such as fever, chills, myalgias, headache, hepatitis, splenomegaly, or diarrhea. Symptomatic patients are treated with parenteral aminoglycosides. Prevention of disease is best accomplished by limiting exposure to potentially infected animals. When exposure is unavoidable, proper barrier precautions with masks, gloves, and eye protection should be worn. Outdoor workers in endemic areas should be encouraged to wear appropriate clothing and repellents to avoid mosquito and tick bites.

### Leptospira Interrogans

Leptospirosis is caused by a number of serovariants of the spirochete *Leptospira interrogans.* Leptospires are found in a variety of animals. The organism has been recovered from rats, swine, dogs, cats, raccoons, and cattle, among a variety of other mammals. Human disease is contracted by direct exposure to an infected animal, its tissues or urine, or by indirect contact with soil or water contaminated by infected urine. Ingestion of contaminated food and inhalation of infectious aerosols have also been implicated as modes of transmission. Occupations at risk for direct inoculation include veterinarians, dairymen, abattoir workers, meat handlers, farmers, research laboratory personnel and others involved in animal husbandry. Additionally, any occupation that places workers in contact with contaminated soil or water is associated with an increased risk of acquiring the organism. Such occupations include sugar cane or rice field workers, miners, sewer workers, farmers, fishery workers, and military troops (66).

Clinical manifestations of leptospirosis are varied but usually include nonspecific constitutional symptoms, fever, headache, myalgias, and nausea. Severe illness is characterized by conjunctivitis, hepatic dysfunction with jaundice, meningitis, and renal failure (66). Treatment usually involves doxycycline (67) along with supportive care for renal and/or hepatic dysfunction. Prevention of disease centers on limiting direct contact of workers to livestock, rodents, and other animals as well as avoiding exposure to contaminated environments by providing gloves, boots, and aprons, and by disinfecting contaminated work areas. Livestock vaccination programs may also be effective in reducing the incidence of disease. Prophylactic weekly doxycycline has been proven effective for military personnel during high-risk activities (68).

### Streptococcus Suis

*Streptococcus suis* has been recognized as an agent of septicemia, pneumonia, and pyogenic meningitis in individuals who are exposed to pigs (69). The organism likely penetrates through nonintact skin, although inhalation seems possible as well. Occupations that involve contact with swine or meat handling, such as farmer, abattoir worker, butcher, and meat packer, are at risk. Prevention of disease in occupational settings may be accomplished by protective attire and protection of skin abrasions by appropriate occlusive dressings.

### Erysipelothrix Rhusiopathiae

Erysipeloid, caused by the gram-positive bacillus *Erysipelothrix rhusiopathiae,* usually causes a localized cellulitis at the site of inoculation (70). The organism may be found in a wide variety of fish and both wild and domestic animals. It is transmitted through direct contact of an infected animal with broken skin by people handling swine, turkeys, chicken, sheep, cattle, pheasants, fish, shellfish, or their tissues. Because these occupations involve direct hand contact with animal reservoirs, most occupationally related infections appear on the upper extremity. The bacterium is susceptible to many antibiotics; treatment is usually with a penicillin, fluoroquinolone, or cephalosporin. Prevention of disease centers on appropriate barrier precautions such as occlusive dressings applied over any breaks in the skin and glove use while working with animals or tissues.

### Ringworm

Ringworm is a cutaneous fungal infection that is caused by one of several fungal species. These fungi generally cause superficial dermatophytic infections of their animal host and may occasionally cause superficial skin disease in humans as well. Wild, domestic and laboratory animals have been implicated including horses, mice, monkeys, cattle, cats, dogs, poultry, and swine. Any occupation or avocation that places a worker in direct physical contact with these animals may pose a risk for development of disease. In addition, individuals are at increased risk when large numbers of people share common facilities, such as crowded workplaces or military camps. Treatment consists of topical or sometimes oral antifungal therapy.

### Parapoxviruses

Several related but antigenically different parapoxviruses may infect humans who work in close contact with animal hosts. Orf (71), or contagious ecthyma, affects those working with sheep and goats. Bovine papular stomatitis (72) and pseudocowpox, or milker's nodule, may occur after contact with cattle. Sealpox occurs in seal hunters and zoo personnel who work with seals. The pathologic lesions begin as vesicles that may progress to coalescing pustules. They usually involve the hands or upper extremities. There is no known treatment for these infections.

### Vesicular Stomatitis Virus

Vesicular stomatitis virus (VSV) is a rhabdovirus that infects a wide array of wild and domestic animals. Infection may be transmitted to humans by direct contact with the oral secretions of an infected animal host (73). The virus gains entry via nonintact skin or inoculation into the conjunctiva or oral mucosa. In animals, VSV causes a febrile illness with oral and mammary vesiculation. In humans, it generally results in an acute flu-like illness with myalgias, fever, chills, nausea, or pharyngitis for 4 to 7 days. Vesicle formation is only occasionally noted in human illness.

## ZOONOSES ACQUIRED THROUGH FECAL-ORAL TRANSMISSION

### Infectious Diarrhea

Several agents that cause infectious diarrhea in humans can be acquired through animal exposures. *C. jejuni* and *Salmonella* spp. are frequently found in the gastrointestinal tract of cattle, sheep, swine, dogs, cats, rodents, and most importantly poultry (74). Both are transmitted to human hosts by ingestion of foods derived from an infected animal or ingestion of food contaminated by the feces of an infected animal. Clinically, these agent cause acute gastroenteritis, although systemic illness has also been described. *Cryptosporidium parvum* is a coccidian protozoan whose primary animal reservoir is cattle. Direct contact with infected animal by-products or ingestion of contaminated water results in human disease. Symptoms generally include profuse diarrhea with abdominal cramping. These symptoms are usually self-limited in immunocompetent hosts, but may produce prolonged disability in the immunocompromised host.

Any occupation that places workers in direct contact with these infected animals or contaminated water or food confers a risk of acute diarrheal disease. Prevention is best accomplished by maintenance of strict hygienic standards including hand washing and appropriate protective attire. Potentially contaminated water may be boiled to remove the oocysts of *C. parvum.*

### Echinococcus Spp.

The dog tapeworms *Echinococcus multilocularis* and *E. granulosus* are intestinal parasites that are found in dogs or related species worldwide. Domestic livestock, particularly sheep, goats, camels, and horses, play a vital role in the natural life cycle of the organism. The disease may be found in people, such as shepherds, who work directly with both grazing animals and dogs. Infection in a human host is initiated by inadvertent hand-to-mouth transfer of eggs originating from the fecal material of the infected dog. Once ingested, the organisms migrate to the liver, lung, or other organ to form a cystic structure that causes symptoms related to local mass effect. Definitive therapy requires surgical removal, but mebendazole and albendazole have been used for inoperative cases. Workers should maintain good hygiene while working with the animals or preparing food. Dog screening programs or empiric treatment of dogs in hyperendemic areas may limit transmission to human hosts.

### Nanophetus Salmincola

Infection with the intestinal trematode *Nanophetus salmincola* is seen with occupational or recreational contact with freshwater fish. Infection is acquired through ingestion of raw or undercooked fish or inadvertent fecal-oral transmission after contact with an infected fish. Fish handlers, research biologists, and others who have frequent contact with fish, particularly salmonids, may develop gastrointestinal symptoms with eosinophilia as a result of infection (75). Praziquantel appears to be effective therapy (76).

### Toxoplasma Gondii

*Toxoplasma gondii* is a protozoan parasite whose definitive host is the cat and whose intermediate hosts include birds, sheep, goats, swine, cattle, and chicken, among others. Occupational infection is generally acquired through inadvertent fecal-oral contact while working with infected meat products or contact with cat feces containing viable oocysts (77). Abattoir workers, butchers, pet store personnel, cat breeders, and veterinarians are often exposed directly or indirectly to the organism. Clinical laboratory workers and pathologists may acquire infection in the health care setting through accidental self-inoculation (78).

Acute disease in the human host may be asymptomatic or may produce a nonspecific mononucleosis-like illness with fever, lymphadenopathy, and lymphocytosis. Acute infection or reactivation of latent disease in the immunocompromised patient may result in choreoretinitis or cerebritis. Women who acquire infection during pregnancy may have offspring with congenital infection (79).

Individuals who work with meat or cats should pay meticulous attention to hand washing. Women who are pregnant should be advised to avoid cat litter boxes or cats with an unknown feeding history. Litter boxes should be changed daily. Treatment of acute disease is generally not indicated in the absence of pregnancy or specific organ involvement. Pyrimethamine is given with sulfadiazine or clindamycin for severe disease.

## VECTOR-BORNE ZOONOSES

A variety of agents may be transmitted from an animal reservoir to a human host by means of an insect vector (Table 7). Occupations that place a worker in the same environment as or in direct contact with an animal reservoir may confer an increased risk of these infections. Prevention of bites from ticks, flies, and fleas with appropriate repellents and clothing while working in endemic areas limits the acquisition of these agents. Clothing should include long pants and sleeves. Inspection of the skin should be performed to identify and remove any attached ticks upon leaving the endemic area.

Lyme disease, caused by the spirochete *Borrelia burgdorferi,* is transmitted by a tick bite and may cause a characteristic rash, fever, arthralgias, arthritis, carditis, or neurologic abnormalities (80). It is common in outdoor workers in endemic areas (81). Treatment with amoxacillin or doxycycline usually is sufficient for early disease stages. A vaccine study for prevention of Lyme disease in people at high risk is currently in progress.

Viral agents such as Russian spring-summer encephalitis and Central European encephalitis are common tick-borne illnesses in Siberia and Eastern Europe that are acquired in occupations that require outdoor work. Many cases are asymptomatic. Use of a vaccine has lowered the incidence of disease in endemic areas. Louping ill is a tick-borne viral illness found in Great Britain that may cause encephalitis in those who work near its natural reservoirs such as sheep and rodents.

*Babesia microti,* an intraerythrocytic parasite, may be transmitted by a tick-bite in endemic areas. Cattle appear to be the major reservoir for this occupational illness.

*Francisella tularensis* may also be transmitted by tick bite to workers in endemic areas.

**TABLE 7.** *Diseases acquired through vector exposure*

| Disease | Vector | Reservoir |
|---|---|---|
| Babesiosis | Tick | Cattle |
| Louping-ill | Tick | Sheep, rodents |
| Lyme disease | Tick | Deer, mice |
| Plague | Fleas | Rodents, bobcats, rabbits |
| Russian spring-summer encephalitis | Tick | Rodents, birds, cattle, goats |
| Tularemia | Tick or other insect bite | Rabbits, hares, rodents, beavers, squirrels, muskrats, birds |

*Yersinia pestis,* the agent of plague, may be acquired from a flea bite in individuals who work with rodents, rabbits, and other wild animals in endemic areas. A killed vaccine is available for those who anticipate high-risk exposures.

## DISEASES ACQUIRED THROUGH CONTACT WITH ENVIRONMENT

Some occupations place individuals in contact with a variety of infectious agents found primarily in the environment (Table 8). These organisms can be free-living in the environment, but may cause disease if inhaled or inoculated into a susceptible host. Measures to control these agents focus on reducing dust and using respiratory equipment in construction, excavation, and farming occupations. Sometimes infections may occur when a uniquely sensitized worker is exposed to an airborne pathogen. An example is pneumonia due to *Acinetobacter* in foundry workers (82) or tuberculosis in those with pulmonary silicosis (83). Other infectious agents are prevented by minimizing work-related traumatic or bite-related injuries and appropriate wound management.

## AIRBORNE TRANSMISSION

### Coccidioides Immitis

*Coccidioides immitis* is a saprophytic fungus that grows in soil in the lower Sonoran life zone including the southwestern United States, Mexico, and Central and South America (84). The organism may become aerosolized and inhaled due to heavy winds, excavation, or any other activity that leads to dust formation. Occupations including military personnel, farm workers, construction workers, and archeologists in endemic areas are at increased risk of developing disease (85). When isolated in a clinical laboratory, infectious arthroconidia may become airborne and infect laboratory workers. Infection characteristically causes a nonspecific respiratory illness but may also cause erythema nodosum, a thin-walled pulmonary cavity, or disseminated disease (86). Most cases do not require specific therapy and resolve spontaneously. Patients with mild symptomatic infections are treated with azole antifungal agents; amphotericin B is prescribed for more severe illness. Dust control measures including planting vegetation, wetting soil, and use of respiratory equipment may lessen the incidence of the disease among high-risk occupations.

### Histoplasma Capsulatum

Histoplasmosis is caused by the dimorphic fungus *Histoplasma capsulatum* (87). The organism is endemic to the Midwest United States and lives in mycelial form in soil. Earth that has been enriched with the droppings of birds or bats may harbor large numbers of fungi. Disturbance of the soil through farming, excavation, or other activities aerosolizes the organism, which is then acquired by inhalation. Individuals who work with soil or are exposed to dust in endemic areas may develop active histoplasmosis. Usually this presents as a self-limited respiratory illness, although fulminant pneumonia or dissemination with sepsis, lymphadenopathy, endocarditis, ocular disease, or skin lesions may occur. Treatment of severe disease requires antifungal therapy with itraconazole or amphotericin B. Prevention of histoplasmosis centers on dust control and protective respiratory equipment. Heavily contaminated soil, such as that found in chicken coops, can be treated with a formalin solution to inactivate infectious particles prior to excavation (88).

**TABLE 8.** *Disease acquired through contact with environment*

| Disease | Source | Prevention |
|---|---|---|
| *Acinetobacter* pneumonia | Foundry workers | None |
| Coccidiodomycosis (San Joaquin Valley fever, desert fever) | Soil | Minimize dust exposure |
| Histoplasmosis | Soil enriched with bird or bat droppings | Minimize dust exposure |
| Hypersensitivity pneumonitis (Farmer's lung) | Agricultural dusts | Minimize dust exposure |
| Legionella (Legionnaire's disease, Pontiac fever) | Potable water systems, air conditioning systems, cooling towers | Reservoir disinfection |
| *Mycobacterium marinum* | Water, marine animals | Gloves |
| Silicotuberculosis | Tuberculous exposure in patients with pulmonary silicosis | None, prevention of pulmonary silicosis by dust reduction, mask, etc. |
| Sporotrichosis | Soil, plants, plant products | Gloves |
| Tetanus | Soil | Wound cleansing, vaccine, postexposure immunoglobulin |

### Legionella Pneumophilia

*Legionella pneumophilia* is a gram-negative rod that grows in environmental water and has a particular predilection for potable water reservoirs such air conditioning cooling towers, fountains, humidifiers, spas, and evaporative condensers. The organism has been implicated in two distinct diseases, Legionnaires' disease, and Pontiac fever. Most infections result in pneumonia from inhalation or aspiration of the organism. Standard treatment of pneumonia involves erythromycin in high doses. Pontiac fever is a self-limited flu-like illness without pneumonia first described in an office building with a contaminated air conditioning unit (89). It has a high attack rate (>90%) and is likely due to inhalation of bacterial antigens.

### Hypersensitivity Pneumonitis (Farmer's Lung)

Farmers, brewery workers, cotton workers, cork workers, sugar cane workers, and others who have close contact with organic fibers may develop acute pulmonary inflammation in response to inhalation of these particles (90). Often, these materials have large numbers of saprophytic organisms such as *Streptomyces rectivirgula, Aspergillus* spp. or thermophilic *actinomyces* growing in them. Although not an infection per se, inhalation of bacterial antigens and endotoxin contributes to the pulmonary inflammation (91). Lung injury may be acute, subacute, or chronic with symptoms of cough, fever, chills, myalgias, and dyspnea with diffuse or patchy pulmonary infiltrates by chest roentgenogram. Repeated exposure can lead to chronic disabling lung injury. Treatment involves corticosteroids and removal from the source of antigens. Prevention of Farmer's lung centers on limiting dust generation by heavy equipment, ventilation of work areas, and the use of masks or personal respirators.

## DIRECT INOCULATION

### Mycobacterium Marinum

Individuals who work with marine life or in an aquatic environment may be exposed to *Mycobacterium marinum* infection. These risk groups include fishermen, marine biologists, pet store employees, and zoo personnel. The organism gains entry into the host through breaks in the skin, often obtained while working in water or from being bitten or nipped by marine organisms. It then may cause a nonhealing ulcer, arthritis, lymphadenitis, suppuration, or tenosynovitis in the involved extremity (92). Use of appropriate work gloves for occupations at risk prevent these often innocuous injuries. Drug treatment usually involves multiple agents that are active against tuberculosis or trimethoprim-sulfamethoxazole.

### *Sporothrix Schenckii*

*Sporothrix schenckii* is a dimorphic fungus that may be isolated from soil, plants, or plant products. Infection has been described resulting from contact with thorned plants, sphagnum moss, hay, straw, and mining timbers. The organism enters through breaks in the skin that are usually sustained while working with these materials. Horticulturalists, gardeners, and farmers are at particularly high risk of developing disease. Infection most commonly results in nodular skin lesions that extend proximally from the site of inoculation along lymphatic channels. Dissemination may occur rarely. Therapy involves potassium iodide or itraconazole.

### *Tetanus*

Tetanus is a toxin-mediated disease caused by *Clostridium tetani* (93). The organism may be found as normal flora in the intestines of humans and animals. Spores are ubiquitous in the soil and environment, particularly in areas contaminated by animal feces. Tetanus develops after spores are inoculated into an open wound and produce a toxin that causes muscle spasm. Fortunately, the disease is preventable by immunization with tetanus toxoid. Immunization is universally recommended and provides protection for 10 years. Immunization is especially important for people who might anticipate a higher risk of traumatic work-related injury such as policemen, military personnel, or workers in contact with farm animals, soil, or sewage. Following an injury, proper wound management is imperative. Wounds should be thoroughly cleansed and debrided. For injuries sustained in potentially contaminated environments, a tetanus booster is given if more than 5 years has elapsed since the last immunization. Immune globulin is available for postexposure prophylaxis of tetanus-prone wounds or for individuals who have been inadequately immunized (94).

## LABORATORY-RELATED INFECTIONS

Personnel in biotechnology, research, and clinical laboratories may encounter a wide array of virulent pathogens. Over 4,000 cases of laboratory-acquired infection with greater than 160 different infectious agents and 168 deaths have been reported worldwide in the literature (95). Infectious agents may be classified into biosafety levels that require different combinations of laboratory techniques, safety equipment, and facilities to minimize potential exposure of laboratory personnel (96).

Clinical laboratory workers in hospitals may be exposed to any agent that causes human disease by working directly with the body fluids, tissues, and cultures of potentially highly infectious agents. Containment of potentially infectious specimens by appropriate transportation devices, work hoods, barrier precautions, and disposal systems is mandatory.

Workers in the biotechnology industry often work with bacteria of low human pathogenicity in the processes of producing enzymes, fermentation products, vaccines, and development of other biologic products. Nevertheless, repeated or high-grade exposure to many of these agents has been reported to cause human illness.

Biomedical researchers in hospitals, universities, and research institutions are at risk of acquiring infection from a variety of virulent pathogens. Active research is ongoing with such pathogens as smallpox, rabies, anthrax, Lassa fever virus, hepatitis B, and HIV, among others. Some animals used in medical research may harbor pathogens of human disease. Researchers, veterinarians, and animal handlers should be educated to recognize the signs and symptoms of infection in animals and the routes by which they may become infected. Similarly to HCWs who are caring for hospitalized patients, researchers using animals should practice meticulous universal precautions to avoid direct contact with animal body fluids. Researchers working with infected cell lines in vitro need to use appropriate protective equipment, such as laminar air flow hoods with flow vented to the outside, and outerwear, such as gloves, gowns with sleeves, masks, and goggles, to avoid direct contact or exposure to aerosols.

## INFECTIONS FROM OCCUPATION-RELATED TRAVEL

With the growth of air travel and the opening of new markets in developing countries, businesspeople from industrialized nations travel to underdeveloped countries where the threat of acquiring infectious illnesses requires specific precautions (Table 9). Pretravel medical care should be encouraged in order to identify risk factors for acquiring certain infectious diseases and implementing appropriate precautionary measures. The individual's itinerary, anticipated length of stay, and specific exposures often dictate the precautionary measures that are warranted. In addition to vaccinations and education about how to avoid infectious illnesses, this visit may be used to address such issues as personal safety, jet lag, and altitude sickness when appropriate. A detailed itinerary and exposure history is important because many people extend their travels to include recreational activities that may increase the risks for acquiring a travel-related infection. Many insurance companies in the United States do not provide medical coverage for care obtained outside the country. Therefore, clarification of the patient's medical coverage is imperative. Many companies offer medical insurance for international travelers. Space limitations preclude a full discussion of all infectious risks pertinent to the international traveler, so the reader is referred to the Centers for Diseases Control (97) for updated and itinerary-specific recommendations.

**TABLE 9.** *Infectious agents associated with international travel*

| Agent | Specific precautions |
|---|---|
| Cholera | Vaccine |
| Hepatitis A | Immune globulin, vaccine |
| Hepatitis B | Vaccine |
| Malaria (*Plasmodium* spp.) | Chemoprophylaxis |
| Measles | Vaccine |
| *Neisseria meningitidis* | Vaccine |
| Polio | Vaccine |
| Rabies | Vaccine |
| Rubella | Vaccine |
| *Salmonella typhi* | Oral live attenuated vaccine, parenteral subunit vaccine |
| Tetanus | Vaccine |
| Traveler's diarrhea | Early treatment of symptoms |
| Yellow fever | Vaccine |

### Diseases Acquired by Ingestion

Some of the most common travel-related illnesses are acquired through ingestion of contaminated food or water. To reduce the risk of travel-associated gastrointestinal illnesses, meticulous attention should be paid to food and water hygiene. Limiting fluid ingestion to bottled, carbonated, or heated, previously boiled drinks and food consumption to well-cooked or canned foods and fruit that must be peeled may reduce, but not eliminate, the risk of acquiring a pathogen. Unpasteurized dairy products, tap water, ice cubes, food from street vendors, and fresh, ground-grown leafy vegetables should be avoided (98). Most larger hotels that cater to international business people have adequately sanitized food preparation and water purification.

Traveler's diarrhea is very common during or after international travel, affecting up to 30% to 50% of visitors to developing areas (99). Most cases are caused by toxigenic strains of *E. coli.* Symptoms of diarrhea with abdominal cramping usually start within the first week of a stay in a foreign country and lasts 3 to 4 days if untreated. Although not usually life threatening, this may lead to significant morbidity or prevent the business traveler from performing his duties. Aside from meticulous food and water precautions, early self-treatment with a short course of trimethoprim-sulfamethoxazole or a fluoroquinolone, combined with loperamide, may attenuate symptoms. It is helpful for the international traveler to bring these items with them rather than attempt to find health care urgently in a foreign country.

*Salmonella typhi* or hepatitis A may also be acquired by food or water ingestion in underdeveloped countries (100,101). Specific vaccines are available for those who might anticipate exposure to these agents (101,102). Immune globulin may also be given for immediate passive protection from hepatitis A; however, the preparation is in increasingly short supply in the United States and protection lasts only 2 to 6 months.

Other agents such as amebae, cyclospora, or *cryptosporidium* may occasionally cause persistent diarrhea in a traveler. *Giardia lamblia* contaminates some public water systems of the former Soviet Union and may cause diarrhea in travelers to these areas. Cholera vaccine is no longer required for international travel due to low risk of infection in travelers, vaccine ineffectiveness, and a high rate of undesirable side effects (103).

Polio remains endemic throughout Asia and Africa. The risk to the international traveler is low, but those who will be exposed to poor food and water sanitation in these areas should be immunized.

### Diseases Acquired by Insect Vectors

Mosquito-borne transmission of infectious diseases is a common concern of travelers to tropical or subtropical climates. Minimizing exposure to mosquitoes by avoiding outdoor activities at dusk or night, wearing appropriate clothing, and using mosquito netting and insect repellents lessens the risk of acquiring yellow fever, malaria, and Japanese encephalitis while in endemic areas. Mosquito repellent containing a 30% to 35% concentration of diethyltoluamide (DEET) provides the best protection. It should be applied only to areas of exposed skin and washed off immediately after returning indoors.

Yellow fever is a mosquito-borne viral illness endemic to central Africa and South America. Those traveling to countries known to have yellow fever should be vaccinated with live-attenuated yellow fever vaccine (97,104). This vaccine is given only at approved yellow fever vaccination centers and provides protection from 10 days after vaccination up to 10 years. Some countries require that travelers provide documentation of immunization prior to entry from endemic areas.

Malaria is one of the most common concerns for travelers going to tropical or subtropical climates. It usually causes a febrile flu-like illness. Travelers from nonendemic areas who develop falciparum malaria are at risk for more severe disease, including cerebral, pulmonary, and renal failure. In addition to the usual mosquito precautions, chemoprophylaxis is indicated for most travelers to malarious areas. Depending on local drug resistance patterns and the medical history of the patient, one of several drugs such as mefloquine, chloroquine, or doxycycline may be prescribed (105). The Centers for Disease Control publishes updated, country-specific risks of malaria and local patterns of drug resistance (97). For prolonged travel to areas endemic for *Plasmodium vivax* or *P. ovale,* primaquine is given at the conclusion of the chemoprophylactic regimen in order to reduce the potential for late relapses. It is important to note that no prophylactic regimen is 100% effective in preventing malaria and that active disease may develop months after return from a malarious area.

Travelers remaining in rural areas of Southeast Asia and the Indian subcontinent for prolonged periods are at risk of acquiring Japanese encephalitis virus. Most people engaged in international business remain in urban centers or tourist centers and travel for less than 4 weeks. Thus, these travelers do not require specific immunization for the virus. For those who are at risk, a three-dose series of inactivated vaccine may be administered (106). Substantial toxicity exists with the vaccine, including local, systemic, and delayed-type hypersensitivity reactions (106,107).

### Diseases Acquired by Respiratory Transmission

Travelers may be exposed to virulent pathogens through respiratory transmission. Prior to departure, the traveler should have an updated influenza, pneumococcal, and measles-mumps-rubella (MMR) vaccines if indicated. Those going to sub-Saharan Africa, Nepal, portions of India, or Saudi Arabia should consider meningococcal vaccine if a prolonged stay or contact with crowds is anticipated (108). A major outbreak of diphtheria has been ongoing in the states of the former Soviet Union (109,110). Thus diphtheria vaccination, most often combined with tetanus immunization, must be up to date for travelers going to these areas.

### Diseases Acquired by Other Means

Depending on the specific location of travel and exposures that are anticipated, precautions may be indicated for dengue, hepatitis B or E, schistosomiasis, plague (111), or rabies (59). Tetanus vaccination should be updated prior to departure.

Travelers must be cautioned that casual sexual relations may result in infection with HIV or one of several sexually transmitted diseases. The prevalence of HIV in commercial sex workers may be extraordinarily high, with infection rates of up to 90% in some urban areas of Africa (112). In addition to syphilis and herpes simplex virus, some sexually transmitted diseases, such as chancroid, lymphogranuloma venereum, and granuloma inguinale, are unusual in the United States and may not be promptly diagnosed if imported from exposure abroad. Drug-resistant *Neisseria gonorrhoeae* may be acquired in southeast Asia or Africa.

## REFERENCES

1. Centers for Disease Control and Prevention. Mandatory reporting of infectious disease by clinicians. *MMWR* 1990;39(RR-9):1–17.
2. U.S. Department of Commerce. Statistical abstract of the United States, 1995. Washington, DC: 1995.
3. U.S. Department of Health and Human Services, Centers for Diseases Control, National Center for Health Statistics, Public Health Service. Health, United States, 1992. Hyattsville, MD: 1993.

4. Larson EL. APIC guideline for handwashing and hand antisepsis in health care settings. *Am J Infect Control* 1995;23:251–269.
5. Centers for Disease Control. Guidelines for the prevention and control of nosocomial infection, 1985. Atlanta: U.S. Department of Health and Human Services, Public Health Service, Centers for Disease Control, 1985.
6. Morris IM, Cattle DS, Smits BJ. Endoscopy and transmission of hepatitis B. *Lancet* 1975;2:1152.
7. McDonald GB, Silverstein FE. Can gastrointestinal endoscopy transmit hepatitis B to patients? *Gastrointest Endosc* 1975;22:168.
8. Lauer JL, Van Drunen NA, Washburn JW, et al. Transmission of hepatitis B virus in clinical laboratory areas. *J Infect Dis* 1979;140: 513.
9. Occupational Safety and Health Administration. Occupational exposure to bloodborne pathogens, final rule. *Fed Lett* 1991;56: 64175–64182.
10. Mast EE. Prevention of hepatitis B virus infection in health-care workers. In: Ellis RW, ed. Hepatitis B vaccines in clinical practice. New York: Marcel Dekker, 1993;295–307.
11. Centers for Disease Control. Protection against viral hepatitis. Recommendations of the Advisory Committee for Immunization Practices (ACIP). *MMWR* 1990;39(RR-2).
12. Centers for Disease Control. Hepatitis surveillance. Atlanta: U.S. Department of Health and Human Services, Public Health and Human Services, Health Service, 1989.
13. Hoofnagle JH, Seeff LB, Bales ZB, et al. The Veterans Administration Hepatitis Cooperative Study Group: type B hepatitis after transfusion with blood containing antibody to hepatitis B core antigen. *N Engl J Med* 1978;298:1379–1383.
14. Sepkowitz KA. Occupationally acquired infection in health care workers. *Ann Intern Med* 1996;125:917–928.
15. Alter HJ, Purcell RH, Shih JW. Detection of antibody to hepatitis C virus in prospectively followed transfusion recipients with acute and chronic non-A, non-B hepatitis. *N Engl J Med* 1989;321:1494–1500.
16. Kiyosawa K, Sodeyama T, Tanaka E, et al. Hepatitis C in hospital employees with needlestick injuries. *Ann Intern Med* 1991;115: 367–369.
17. Mitsui T, Iwano K, Masuko D, et al. Hepatitis C virus infection in medical personnel after needlestick accident. *Hepatology* 1992;16: 1109–1114.
18. Lanphear BP, Linneman CCJ, Cannon CG, et al. Hepatitis C virus infection in healthcare workers: risk of exposure and infection. *Infect Control Hosp Epidemiol* 1994;15:745–750.
19. Davis GL, Balart LA, Schiff ER, et al. Treatment of chronic hepatitis C with recombinant interferon alfa: a multicenter randomized, controlled trial. *N Engl J Med* 1989;321:1501–1506.
20. DiBiscegle AM, Martin P, Kassianides C, et al. Recombinant interferon alpha therapy for chronic hepatitis C: a randomized, double-blind, placebo-controlled trial. *N Engl J Med* 1989;321:1506–1510.
21. Saez-Royuela F, Porres JC, Moreno A, et al. High doses of recombinant alpha-interferon or gamma-interferon for chronic hepatitis C: a randomized, controlled trial. *Hepatology* 1991;13:327–331.
22. Makris M, Preston FE, Triger DR, et al. A randomized controlled trial of recombinant interferon-alpha in chronic hepatitis C in hemophiliacs. *Blood* 1991;78:1672–1677.
23. Viladomiu L, Genesca J, Estaban J, et al. Interferon-alpha in acute posttransfusion hepatitis C: a randomized, controlled trial. *Hepatology* 1992;15:767–769.
24. Alter MJ. Exposure to hepatitis C virus: a dilemma. *Infect Control Hosp Epidemiol* 1994;15:742–744.
25. Centers for Disease Control. Update: Provisional Public Health Service: recommendations for chemoprophylaxis after occupational exposure to HIV. *MMWR* 1996;45:468–472.
26. Garner JS. The Hospital Infection Control Practices Advisory Committee. Recommendations for isolation precautions in hospitals. *Am J Infect Control* 1996;24:32–51.
27. Benenson AS. Control of communicable diseases manual. Washington, DC: American Public Health Association, 1995.
28. Centers for Disease Control. Measles prevention: recommendations of the Immunization Practices Advisory Committed (ACIP). *MMWR* 1989;38(S-9):1–18.
29. Centers for Disease Control. Guidelines for preventing the transmission of *Mycobacterium tuberculosis* in health-care facilities. *MMWR* 1996;43(RR-13).
30. American Thoracic Society. Diagnostic standards and classification of tuberculosis. *Am Rev Respir Dis* 1990;142:725–735.
31. Williams WW. Guideline for infection control in hospital personnel. *Am J Infect Control* 1984;12:34–56.
32. Centers for Disease Control. Prevention of varicella: recommendations of the Advisory Committee on Immunization Practices (ACIP). *MMWR* 1996;45(RR-11):13–15.
33. Centers for Disease Control. Influenza prevention and control: recommendations of the Advisory Committee on Immunization Practices (ACIP). *MMWR* 1996;45(RR-5).
34. Nichol KL, Lind A, Margolis K. The effectiveness of vaccination against influenza in healthy, working adults. *N Engl J Med* 1995;333: 889–893.
35. Wharton M, Cochi SL, Hutcheson RH, Schaffner W. Mumps transmission in hospitals. *Arch Intern Med* 1990;150:47–49.
36. Fischer PR, Brunetti C, Welch V, Christenson JC. Nosocomial mumps: report of an outbreak and its control. *Am J Infect Control* 1996;24: 13–18.
37. Centers for Disease Control. Meningococcal disease—United States, 1981. *MMWR* 1981;30:113–115.
38. Artenstein MS, Ellis RE. The risk of exposure to a patient with meningococcal meningitis. *Milit Med* 1968;133:474–477.
39. Jacobson JA, Fraser DW. A simplified approach to meningococcal disease prophlylaxis. *JAMA* 1976;236:1053–1054.
40. Rodis JF, Quinn DL, Gary W, et al. Management and outcomes of pregnancies complicated by human B19 parvovirus infections: a prospective study. *Am J Obstet Gynecol* 1990;163:1168–1171.
41. Committee on Infectious Diseases, American Academy of Pediatrics. Parvovirus, erythema infectiosum, and pregnancy. *Pediatrics* 1990;85: 131–133.
42. Dudding BA, Top FHJ, Winter PE, et al. Acute respiratory disease in military trainees. The adenovirus surveillance program 1966–1971. *Am J Epidemiol* 1973;97:187–198.
43. Ewar DP, Frederick PD, Mascola L. Resurgence of congenital rubella syndrome in the 1990's. Report on missed opportunities and failed prevention policies among women of childbearing age. *JAMA* 1992;267:2616–2620.
44. Balcarek KB, Bagley R, Cloud GA, Pass RF. Cytomegalovirus among employees of a children's hospital. No evidence for increased risk associated with patient care. *JAMA* 1990;263:840–844.
45. Pass RF, Hutto C, Ricks R, Cloud GA. Increased rate of cytomegalovirus among parents of children attending day-care centers. *N Engl J Med* 1986;314:1414–1418.
46. Adler SP. Cytomegalovirus and child day care Evidence for an increased infection rate among day-care workers. *N Engl J Med* 1989; 321:1290–1296.
47. Siegel JD. Risks and exposures for the pregnant health-care worker. In: Olmstead RN, ed. Infection control and applied epidemiology. St. Louis: Mosby, 1996;22:1–8.
48. McFarland LV, Stamm WE. Review of *Clostridium difficile*-associated diseases. *Am J Infect Control* 1986;14:99–109.
49. Poland GA, Haiduven DJ. Adult immunizations in the health-care worker. In: Olmstead RN, ed. Infection control and applied epidemiology. St. Louis: Mosby, 1996;24:1–34.
50. Gill MJ, Arlette J, Tyrrel DL, Buchan MB. Herpes simplex virus infection of the hand. Clinical features and management. *Am J Med* 1988; 85:53–56.
51. Beer RJS, Bradford WP, Hart RJC. Pregnancy complicated by psittacosis acquired from sheep. *Br Med J* 1982;284:1156–1157.
52. Sawyer LA, Fishbein DB, McDade JE. Q fever: current concepts. *Rev Infect Dis* 1987;9:935–946.
53. Hinman AR, Fraser DW, Douglas RG, et al. Outbreak of lymphocytic choriomeningitis virus infection in medical center personnel. *Am J Epidemiol* 1975;101:103–110.
54. Barton LL, Budd SC, Morfitt WS. Congenital lymphocytic choreomeningitis virus infection in twins. *Pediatr Infect Dis* 1993;12: 942–946.
55. Weber DJ, Hanson AR. Infections resulting from animal bites. *Infect Dis Clin North Am* 1991;5:663–680.
56. Hubbert WT, Rosen MN. *Pasteurella multocida* infection due to animal bite. *Am J Public Health* 1970;60:1103–1108.
57. Weber DL, Wolfson JS, Swartz MN, et al. *Pasteurella multocida* infections. Report of 34 cases and review of the literature. *Medicine* 1984;63:133–154.

58. Hubbert WT, Rosen MN. *Pasteurella multocida* infection in man unrelated to animal bite. *Am J Public Health* 1970;60:1109–1117.
59. Centers for Diseases Control. Rabies prevention—1991 Recommendations of the Immunization Practices Advisory Committee (ACIP). *MMWR* 1991;40(RR-3).
60. Anderson LC, Leary SL, Manning PJ. Rat-bite fever in animal research laboratory personnel. *Lab Anim Sci* 1983;33:292–294.
61. Wilkins EGL, Millar JGB, Cockroft PM, et al. Rat-bite fever in a gerbil breeder. *J Infect* 1988;16:177–180.
62. LaForce FM. Anthrax. *Clin Infect Dis* 1994;19:1009–1014.
63. Kiel FW, Khan MY. Brucellosis among hospital employees in Saudi Arabia. *Infect Control Hosp Epidemiol* 1993;14:268–272.
64. Mousa AR, Muhtaseb SA, Almudallal DS, et al. Osteoarticular complications of brucellosis: a study of 169 cases. *Rev Infect Dis* 1987;9: 531–543.
65. Evans ME, Gregory DW, Schaffner W, McGee ZA. Tularemia: a 30-year experience with 88 cases. *Medicine* 1985;64:251–268.
66. Farr RW. Leptospirosis. *Clin Infect Dis* 1995;21:1–8.
67. McClain JB, Ballou WR, Harrison SM, Steinweg DL. Doxycycline therapy for leptospirosis. *Ann Intern Med* 1984;100:696–698.
68. Takafuji ET, Kirkpatrick JW, Miller RN, et al. An efficacy trial of doxycycline chemoprophylaxis against leptospirosis. *N Engl J Med* 1984;310:497–500.
69. Andrends JP, Zanen HC. Meningitis caused by *Streptococcus suis* in humans. *Rev Infect Dis* 1988;10:131–137.
70. Reboli AC, Farrar WE. *Erysipelothrix rhusiopathiae*: an occupational pathogen. *Clin Microbiol Rev* 1989;2:354–359.
71. Maki A, Hinsburg A, Percheson P, Marshall DG. Orf: contagious pustular dermatitis. *Can Med Assoc J* 1988;139:971–972.
72. Bowman KF, Barbery RT, Swango LJ, Schnurrenberger PR. Cutaneous form of bovine papular stomatitis in man. *JAMA* 1981;246: 2813–2818.
73. Reif JS, Webb PA, Monath TP, et al. Epizotic vesicular stomatitis virus in Colorado, 1982: infection in occupational risk groups. *Am J Trop Med Hyg* 1987;36:17–82.
74. Blaser MJ, Taylor DN, Feldman RA, Epidemiology of *Campylobacter jejuni* infections. *Epidemiol Rev* 1983;5:157–176.
75. Harrel LW, Deardorff TL. Human nanophyetiasis: transmission by handling naturally infected coho salmon (*Oncorhynchus kisutch*). *J Infect Dis* 1990;161:146–148.
76. Fritsche TR, Eastburn RL, Wiggens LH, et al. Praziquantel for treatment of human *Nanophyetus salmincola (Trogloytema salmincola)* infection. *J Infect Dis* 1989;160:896–899.
77. Teutsch SM, Juranek DD, Sulzer A, et al. Epidemic toxoplasmosis associated with infected cats. *N Engl J Med* 1979;300:695–699.
78. Neu HC. Toxoplasmosis transmitted at autopsy. *JAMA* 1967;202: 284–285.
79. Remington JS. The tragedy of toxoplasmosis. *Pediatr Infect Dis J* 1990;9:762–763.
80. Steere AC. Lyme disease. *N Engl J Med* 1989;321:586–596.
81. Schwartz BS, Goldstein MD. Lyme disease in outdoor workers: risk factors, preventive measures, and tick removal methods. *Am J Epidemiol* 1990;131:877–885.
82. Cordes LG, Brink EW, Checko PJ, et al. A cluster of *Acinetobacter* pneumonia in foundry workers. *Ann Intern Med* 1981;95:688–693.
83. Snider DE. The relationship between tuberculosis and silicosis. *Am Rev Respir Dis* 1978;118:455–460.
84. Pappagianis D. Epidemiology of coccidioidomycosis. *Curr Top Med Mycol* 1988;2:199–238.
85. Johnson WM. Occupational factors in coccidioidomycosis. *J Occup Med* 1981;23:367–374.
86. Stevens DA. Coccidioidomycosis. *N Engl J Med* 1995;332:1077–1082.
87. Wheat LJ. Histoplasmosis. *Infect Dis Clin North Am* 1988;2:841–859.
88. Bartlett PC, Weeks RJ, Ajello L. Decontamination of a *Histoplasma capsulatum*–infested bird roost in Illinois. *Arch Environ Health* 1982; 37:221–223.
89. Kaufman A, McDade J, Patton C, et al. Pontiac fever: Isolation of the etiologic agent (*Legionella pneumophilia*) and demonstration of its mode of transmission. *Am J Epidemiol* 1981;114:337–347.
90. Sharma OP. Hypersensitivity Pneumonitis. *Dis Mon* 1991;37: 411–471.
91. Castellan RM, Olenchock SA, Kinsley KB, Hankinson JL. Inhaled endotoxin and decreased spirometric values. An exposure response relation for cotton dust. *N Engl J Med* 1987;317:605–610.
92. Edelstein H. *Mycobacterium marinum* skin infection. *Arch Intern Med* 1994;154:1359–1364.
93. Bleck TP. Tetanus. *Dis Mon* 1991;37:556–603.
94. Centers for Disease Control. Diphtheria, tetanus, and pertussis: recommendations for vaccine us and other preventive measures. Recommendations of the Immunization Practices Advisory Committee (ACIP). *MMWR* 1991;40(RR-10).
95. Pike RM. Past and present hazards of working with infectious hazards. *Arch Pathol Lab Med* 1978;102:333–336.
96. Centers for Disease Control/National Institute of Health. Biosafety in microbiological and biomedical laboratories. Washington, DC: U.S. Government Printing Office, 1993.
97. Centers for Disease Control. Health information for international travel. Atlanta: U.S. Department of Health and Human Services, Public Health Service, 1996–1997.
98. Hill DR, Pearson RD. Health advice for international travel. In: Reese RE, Betts RF, eds. A practical approach to infectious disease. Boston: Little, Brown, 1995;812–845.
99. DuPont HL, Ericsson CD. Prevention and treatment of traveler's diarrhea. *N Engl J Med* 1993;328:1821–1827.
100. Steffen R, Kane MA, Shapiro CN, et al. Epidemiology and prevention of hepatitis A in travelers. *JAMA* 1994;272:885–889.
101. Ryan CA, Hargrett-Bean NT, Blake PA. *Salmonella typhi* infections in the United States, 1975–1984: increasing role of foreign travel. *Rev Infect Dis* 1989;11:1–8.
102. Woodruff BA, Pavia AT, Blake PA. A new look at typhoid vaccination. Information for the practicing physician. *JAMA* 1991;265: 756–759.
103. Centers for Disease Control. Cholera vaccine. Recommendations of the Immunization Practices Advisory Committee (ACIP). *MMWR* 1988;37:617–618, 623–624.
104. Centers for Disease Control. Yellow fever vaccine. Recommendations of the Immunization Practices Advisory Committee (ACIP). *MMWR* 1990;39(RR-6).
105. Wyler DJ. Malaria chemoprophylaxis for the traveler. *N Engl J Med* 1993;329:31–37.
106. Centers for Diseases Control. Inactivated Japanese encephalitis virus vaccine. Recommendations of the Immunization Practices Advisory Committee (ACIP). *MMWR* 1993;42(RR-1).
107. Poland JD, Cropp CB, Craven RB, Monath TP. Evaluation of the potency and safety of inactivated Japanese encephalitis vaccine in US inhabitants. *J Infect Dis* 1990;161:878–882.
108. Wolfe MS. Meningococcal meningitis vaccine for travelers. *Inf Dis Clin Pract* 1992;1:409–410.
109. Centers for Disease Control. Diphtheria outbreak epidemic—new independent states of the former Soviet Union, 1990–1994. *MMWR* 1995;44:177–81.
110. Centers for Disease Control. Diphtheria acquired by U.S. citizens in the Russian Federation and Ukraine—1994. *MMWR* 1995;44:237, 243–244.
111. Wolfe MS, Tuazon MD, Schultz R. Imported bubonic plague—District of Columbia. *MMWR* 1990;39:895.
112. von Reyn CF, Mann JM, Chin J. International travel and HIV infection. *Bull WHO* 1990;68:251–259.

*Environmental and Occupational Medicine, Third Edition,* edited by William N. Rom.
Published by Lippincott–Raven Publishers,
Philadelphia, 1998.

# CHAPTER 52

# HIV in the Workplace

Lynn G. Stansbury, James M. Schmitt, and Martin H. Markowitz

The first case of the acquired immune deficiency syndrome (AIDS) in a Westerner was work related. A Danish woman surgeon, with no risk factors other than service in a rural hospital in Zaire, died in 1976 of the signature immune collapse that we now know is caused by the human immunodeficiency virus (HIV) (1,2). However, once the transmission of AIDS was characterized—even before a specific agent was identified—the ability of people at job-related risk to alter job-related behaviors and, more recently, the use of postexposure chemoprophylaxis have greatly reduced the risk of occupational transmission of HIV.

In contrast, those aspects of personal experience not so easy to change—sexual behavior, intravenous drug use, or birth to a HIV-infected mother—continue to put large numbers of people at risk. In the United States alone, as of June 1996, between 70,000 and 80,000 new cases of AIDS and about the same number of new HIV infections were documented annually (3). While there is some suggestion that these numbers may be leveling off or indeed falling, they are 10% to 20% higher than what was predicted 5 years ago (4). Some of the surprise these numbers still generate may reflect the growing endemicity of HIV in marginalized social groups, in male homosexuals and intravenous drug users and their contacts in the United States, and therefore a certain complacency in the wider society (5). However, HIV is and will continue to be for the foreseeable future a vast and growing problem and, as such, will continue to affect people who work.

L. G. Stansbury and J. M. Schmitt: Occupational Medical Service, National Institutes of Health, Bethesda, Maryland 20892-1584.

M. H. Markowitz: Aaron Diamond AIDS Research Center, Rockefeller University, New York, New York 10024.

## BASIC SCIENCE OF HIV

### HIV: Structure and Biology

#### *Virology*

Human immunodeficiency virus is a member of the lentivirus subfamily of retroviruses. There are two distinct viruses pathologic in humans, HIV-1 and HIV-2. Both are known to cause immunodeficiency disease; however, the latter is less pathogenic and epidemiologically distinct from HIV-1. This discussion focuses on HIV-1 infection and pathogenesis. Interested readers are referred elsewhere for a complete review of HIV-2 infection (6). HIV is the virus that causes AIDS and has the distinction of being at the center of a pandemic widely distributed among the industrialized and developing nations of the world (7). Being a retrovirus, its genetic material is single-stranded RNA, and reverse transcription to DNA to successfully complete its life cycle is required (8).

The basic genomic structure of HIV-1 is typical of retroviruses, as shown in Fig. 1 (9). Two terminal long terminal repeats flank nine open reading frames for the structural proteins gag and env, the constitutive enzyme pol, the required regulatory proteins tat and rev, and the accessory regulatory proteins vif, vpr, vpu, and nef (9). The functions of the accessory regulatory proteins are reviewed elsewhere (10,11). In general, they are not required for viral replication but are important and perhaps critical determinants of degrees of viral replication and pathogenicity.

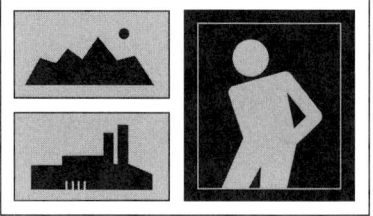

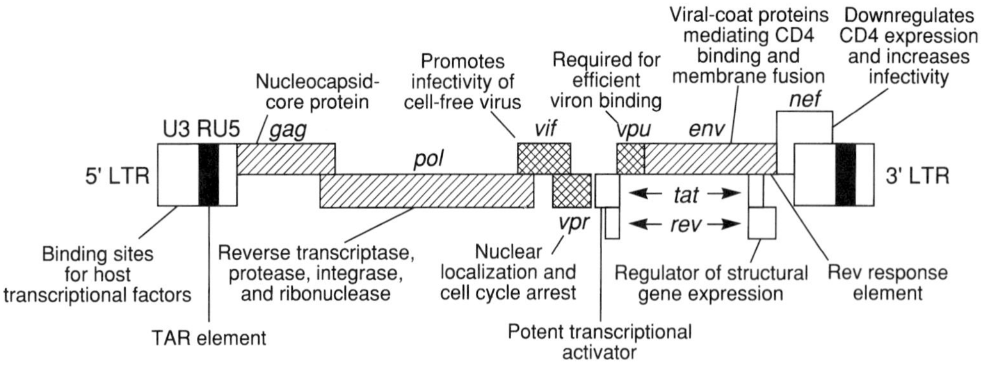


**FIG. 1.** Genomic structure of HIV-1. Each of the known genes of HIV-1 is shown, and their recognized primary functions are summarized. The 5′ and 3′ long terminal repeats (LTRs) containing regulatory sequences recognized by various host transcription factors are also depicted, and the positions of the tat and rev RNA response elements (TAR [transactivations response] element and Rev response element) are indicated. (From ref. 9.)

The virus is a 100- to 150-nm icosahedron with an inner dense core of two single strands of RNA and associated proteins and enzymes including nucleocapsid (p7), p6, p2, p1, and reverse transcriptase. The regulatory proteins vpr, nef, and vif are also packaged into the virion; however, their precise location is unknown (11). The central nucleic acid is surrounded by a capsid (p24) and matrix protein (p17). Forming the outermost surface is the viral envelope, which consists of a lipid bilayer including the env viral glycoproteins gp120 and gp41 (transmembrane anchor), in addition to host cell proteins. A schematic of the structure of the virion is shown in Fig. 2 (12).

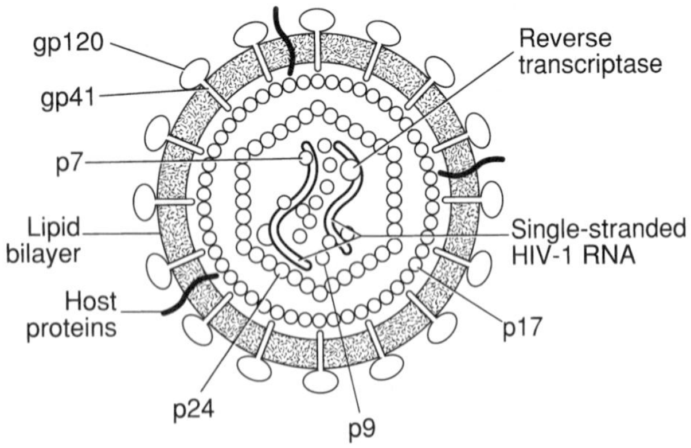


**FIG. 2.** Schematic diagram of the HIV-1 virion. The virion proteins making up the envelope (gp $120^{env}$ and gp $41^{env}$), matrix ($p17^{gag}$), capsid ($p24^{gag}$), and nucleocapsid ($7^{gag}$), and $p6^{gag}$, $p2^{gag}$, and $p1^{gag}$ are identified. In addition, the diploid RNA genome is shown associated with reverse transcriptase, and RNA-dependent DNA polymerase. (From ref. 9.)

### *Life Cycle*

The life cycle of HIV can be separated into cell entry, reverse transcription, integration, viral messenger RNA (mRNA) and protein expression, and finally virus assembly and budding (Fig. 3) (13).

It has long been clear that HIV enters cells expressing CD4 due to a high-affinity interaction between the viral gp120 and CD4 expressed on the cell surface (14). Recently a family of transmembrane proteins have been identified that serve as co-receptors for HIV entry into a CD4 expressing cell. These proteins serve as receptors for a family of inflammatory chemoattractants called chemokines (15–18). A subset, the β-chemokines, has been shown to inhibit HIV-1 replication in vitro (19). These findings, discussed below, have facilitated important insights into the pathogenesis of HIV infection.

Following entry, the viral RNA is uncoated, reverse transcribed, and degraded (20). The newly formed double-stranded DNA is ushered into the nucleus as the preintegration complex and enzymatically integrated into the host genome by the viral protein integrase (21,22). The crystal structure of the active site of this virus specific enzyme has been recently published, and is the logical next target for structure-based design of drugs to inhibit viral replication by disrupting the viral life cycle (23). Once integrated, viral DNA is referred to as provirus. Of note is that many proviruses are defective and are incapable of producing infectious particles due to the error-prone nature of reverse transcriptase, which during reverse transcription allows for multiple lethal mutations, deletions, and substitutions. Conversely, this property of the enzyme does result in enormous genetic diversity among those viruses actively replicating, allowing for escape from immunologic control and therapeutic efforts (8).

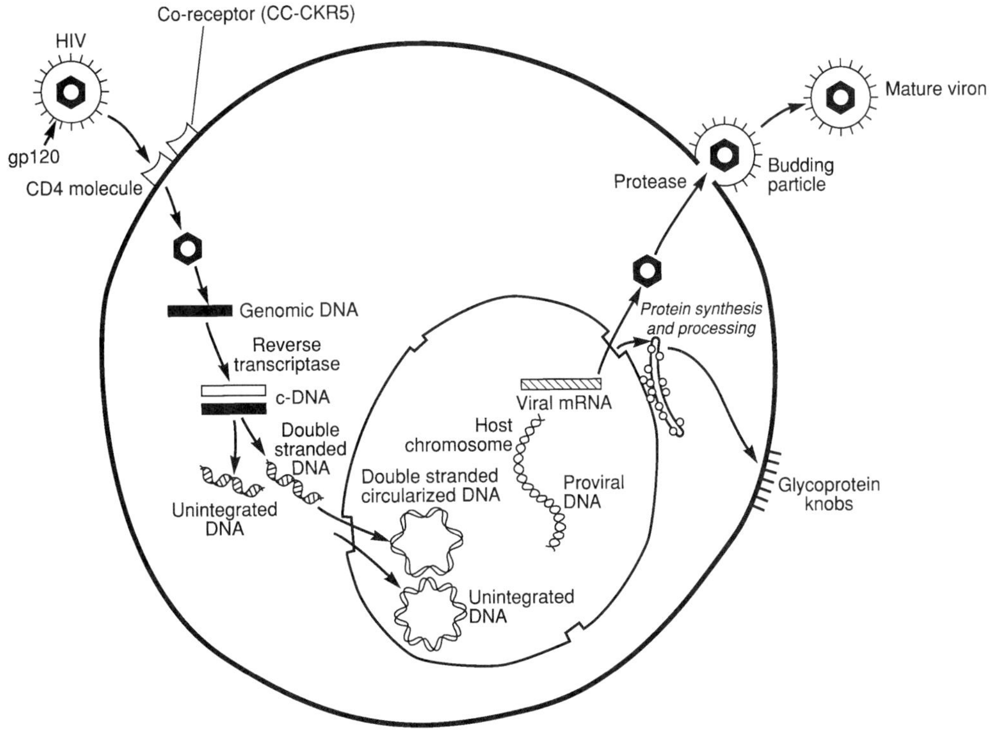


**FIG. 3.** HIV life cycle. The interaction of viral gp120 with the CD4 receptor and the co-receptor allows for the gp41-mediated membrane fusion, which enables the RNA to enter the cytoplasm. The RNA is uncoated and reverse transcribed. In association with the preintegration complex, including p17, integrase, and vpr, it is ushered into the nucleus for integration to occur. Host transcription factors allow for the expression of regulatory mRNA, which are translated and serve to upregulate the expression of the structural genes. Viral proteins are localized to the membrane, processed by the viral protease, and finally bud associated with host membrane proteins. (From ref.13.)

With cellular activation, viral specific mRNA is expressed. On expression, regulatory multiply spliced mRNA products of tat, nef, and rev are translated to proteins. The tat protein binds to the transactivation response element (TAR) and upregulates the expression of viral mRNA. The rev protein binds to the rev-response element (RRE) and is involved in the transport of viral mRNA coding for structural and enzymatic proteins from the nucleus to the cytoplasm of an activated cell (10). Once translated, these proteins are directed to the cell membrane where they undergo proteolytic cleavage by the HIV-1 protease, and associate with the viral envelope glycoproteins, gp120 and gp 41, as well as host cellular proteins as budding occurs (24). The HIV-1 protease has served as a fruitful target for antiviral therapy development (25). Inhibitors of this enzyme, saquinavir, ritonavir, and indinavir, have received rapid approval by the Food and Drug Administration and represent dramatic breakthroughs in the area of antiretroviral therapy when used in combination with established therapies such as the nucleoside inhibitors of reverse transcriptase (26).

## TRANSMISSION OF HIV

The routes of transmission and nontransmission of HIV have been well characterized (27). HIV-1 has been isolated from and transmitted by the blood of infected individuals, the semen of infected men, and the vaginal secretions and breast milk of infected women. Despite the isolation of virus from saliva, tears, and urine, there is no evidence that casual contact with these fluids can result in HIV infection.

### Sexual Transmission

Sexual transmission of HIV-1 can occur during both homosexual and heterosexual sexual practices that promote the exchange of bodily fluids including blood, semen, and vaginal fluid. The proper use of condoms can prevent HIV-1 transmission (28). Currently, sexual intercourse accounts for 75% of all HIV infections worldwide (7). The ratio of infected men to women is 3:2; however, by the year 2000 it is estimated that the ratio will be closer to 1:1, which will in turn increase the number of HIV-infected children worldwide. In North America, the

Centers for Disease Control and Prevention (CDC) has reported that the number of new HIV infections resulting from homosexual sex has dropped significantly; however, transmission via heterosexual intercourse is on the rise (29), particularly in inner city areas, where injecting drug use, crack use, and concomitant venereal infection are common (30). Interestingly, a small number of repeatedly exposed but uninfected individuals have been recently identified (31). These individuals were found to have CD4$^{+}$ T cells that were unable to be infected in vitro with viruses isolated from persons with AIDS. Subsequently, these individuals have been found to be homozygous for a nonfunctional chemokine co-receptor, CC-CKR5 (32). This is the first description of a genetic basis for resistance to HIV infection. The homozygous absence of this receptor does not have any deleterious effects, therefore, making it an interesting option in the search for therapeutic or vaccine development opportunities.

### Transmission by Blood and Blood Products

The transfer of blood by intravenous drug use remains a significant route of HIV infection. In both Western Europe and North America this route of transmission is still on the rise (7). Efforts to curb this mode of transmission have included needle exchange programs, methadone maintenance, and education. However, these efforts have for the most part met strong community opposition.

Inadvertent needlestick and other high-risk exposure does occur in the occupational setting, and postexposure prophylaxis with combination antiretroviral therapy is strongly recommended (33). Blood transfusion and/or the use of blood products does not remain a significant route of HIV infection in developed countries owing to more efficient screening of the blood supply and heat treatment of factor concentrates.

### Maternal-Infant Transmission

Maternal-infant transmission of infection perinatally is the third common route of HIV-1 transmission. Rates have varied worldwide, from 14% to 30% in the pretreatment era, the variation likely a reflection of access to good prenatal care and medical care in general (7,34). Worldwide, one-third of children born to HIV-infected mothers are infected. While in utero transmission does occur, most cases occur during parturition as the newborn traverses the birth canal or postpartum via breast-feeding. High levels of virus in the blood of mothers as well as prolonged rupture of membranes at delivery are factors associated with increased risk of transmission (35,36). A recent clinical trial, AIDS Clinical Trial group (ACTG) 076, investigated the administration of zidovudine (AZT) between weeks 14 and 34 of pregnancy and postdelivery to the infants for 6 weeks. Reduced rates of transmission, 23% to 7%, were observed in the drug-treated mother-infant pairs, when compared to those pairs receiving placebo (37). The success of AZT monotherapy in this setting is somewhat surprising as the drug when used alone has been shown to be a relatively weak antiretroviral agent (38). However, it is likely that the effect is due to both the antiviral effect in the mother and postexposure prophylaxis in the infant. More aggressive regimens including multiple antiretrovirals are currently being studied.

## DIAGNOSTIC TESTING FOR HIV INFECTION

### Screening

The diagnosis of HIV infection can be made by detecting viral markers of infection or more commonly, and perhaps more efficiently, the serologic response to the pathogen. Serologic tests for the presence of antibodies to HIV-1 have been used as an effective screening tool in evaluating the population for evidence of HIV-1 infection. In general the period between infection and the presence of HIV-specific antibodies is 4 to 12 weeks (39). There are many commercially available enzyme-linked immunosorbent assay (ELISA or EIA) kits available to detect HIV-specific antibodies with a high degree of sensitivity but limited specificity (40). These tests use either whole virus lysates or synthetic and/or recombinant HIV antigens that bind HIV-specific antibodies. Although highly sensitive when applied to the proper population, the specificity of these tests is limited by the presence of false-positive results, particularly in low-prevalence populations. False-positive tests are more commonly seen in persons with autoimmune diseases, dysproteinemias, and those exposed and sensitized to multiple foreign human leukocyte antigens (HLAs) by either transfusion or multiple pregnancies (39,41). Therefore, a repeatedly positive test requires confirmation with a more specific test before a diagnosis of HIV infection can be made with confidence.

### Confirmatory Tests

The test most commonly used to confirm a repeatedly positive ELISA is the Western blot, although immunofluorescent assays (IFA) have been developed for similar purposes. The Western blot test relies on immunoelectrophoresis and transfer to nitrocellulose paper to detect specific bands that correspond to specific HIV-related proteins: envelope (gp160/gp120, gp41), gag (p55, p24,p17), and pol (p66, p51, p31) (Table 1). These tests are read as negative, indeterminate, or positive, based on the observed banding pattern. A negative test is easiest to interpret, and reveals the absence of all bands. To interpret a positive test, the bands of major significance on a Western blot are p24, gp41, and gp120/160, and a blot is interpreted as positive by the presence of at least two of these. It is important to note that there are slightly differ-

**TABLE 1.** *Major genes and gene products of HIV-1*

| Gene | Gene products |
|---|---|
| Group-specific antigen/core (gag) | p17, p24, p55 |
| Polymerase (pol) | p31, p51, p66 |
| Envelope (env) | gp41, gp120, gp160 |

p, protein; gp, glycoprotein; numbers, approx. molecular weight (kd).
Adapted from ref. 37.

ent criteria for positive Western blots in individual laboratories. The criteria for positive interpretations are shown in Table 2. An indeterminate result may be the most difficult to interpret. A blot is indeterminate when isolated single bands are observed. Generally these occur in the gag region, either p24 or p17 (41). An indeterminate Western blot can be associated with very early HIV-1 infection or HIV-2 infection. Sixty to ninety percent of HIV-2 infected individuals test positive with EIA tests using whole-virus HIV-1 lysates. This increases to 99% using HIV-2–specific EIAs. As is the case for HIV-1, repeatedly positive HIV-2 EIAs should be followed by with a confirmatory test, usually an HIV-2–specific Western blot (42). Repeatedly indeterminate Western blots in the presence of positive EIAs should be evaluated with an HIV-specific test as detailed below. However, in a series of healthy blood donors without known risk factors for HIV infection, all indeterminate blots with either isolated positive or negative screening EIAs were false positives and not indicative of HIV infection (43). Finally, the time between documented infection with the virus and the ability to detect an immune response is variable, and may be quite prolonged in certain individuals (44). Therefore, when suspicion is high but there is no serologic evidence of HIV infection, the use of virologic markers may be employed to confirm a diagnosis of HIV infection.

**TABLE 2.** *Criteria for positive interpretation of Western blot tests*

| Organization | Criteria |
|---|---|
| ASTPHL/CDC[a] | Any 2 of p24, gp41, gp120/160[c] |
| FDA-licensed DuPont test | p24 and p31 and gp41 or gp120/160 |
| American Red Cross | 1 band from each gene-product grp: gag and pol and env |
| CRSS[b] | Bands: p24 *or* p31 + gp41 or gp120/160 |

[a]Association of State and Territorial Public Health Laboratories.
[b]Consortium for Retrovirus Serology Standardization.
[c]Distinguishing gp120 and 160 is difficult; may be interpreted as single reactant for purposes of Western blot interpretation.
Adapted from ref. 38.

### Virologic Markers

Reliable viral markers that serve both diagnostically and as indicators of disease progression have evolved quickly over the past 5 years, and have met the demands of sensitivity, specificity, and reproducibility. Older tests including the p24 antigen assay and the virologic coculture assay have been reviewed elsewhere (45).

The p24 antigen test is an enzyme immunoassay for a major viral core protein. It is commercially available and easily performed. The level of antigen is generally high during acute infection, but lacks sensitivity with the appearance of HIV-1–specific antibodies, even in end-stage patients, with detectable antigen being found in 20% to 95% (46). The addition of an acid dissociation step improves the sensitivity of the assay, yet the test may be positive in as few as 45% of known HIV-infected patients (47).

Viral isolation from peripheral blood mononuclear cells (PBMCs) is both a sensitive and specific test for the presence of HIV infection, with positive results being obtained in nearly all HIV-infected subjects (48). However, it is expensive, labor intensive, and impractical for widespread clinical use. Viral isolation from plasma is slightly less labor intensive but is also less sensitive and equally impractical (49).

The qualitative HIV-1 DNA polymerase chain reaction (PCR) assay may be diagnostic of HIV infection when used as a confirmatory test. When performed properly, DNA PCR exhibits a sensitivity and specificity of 98.7% and 100%, respectively, and can be used to diagnose HIV infection in the absence of positive serology (50,51).

The determination of levels of virion-associated HIV-1 RNA in the plasma has emerged as an ideal test to determine the level of viral activity in an HIV-infected person. It is a reliable and reproducible measurement of disease activity and as discussed below is predictive of both clinical course and response to therapy. Piatak and coworkers (52), using a competitive PCR-based assay, initially demonstrated that HIV-1 RNA can be detected in virtually all HIV-1–infected subjects and correlated well with stage of disease. The determination of HIV-1–specific viral RNA is sensitive, specific, and reproducible, regardless of the method used. Commercially available assays include the PCR-based (53) Amplicor assay developed by Roche Laboratories and the signal amplification–based assay developed by Chiron, known as the branched-chain DNA assay (bDNA) (54). Both assays are now routinely used to diagnose and guide the treatment of HIV infection. Results are expressed in copies of RNA per milliliter of plasma, and both assays in their current form have similar dynamic ranges.

## PATHOGENESIS

Credit for the discovery of HIV, previously known as human T-cell leukemia virus (HTLV-III) and lymphadenopathy-associated virus (LAV), as the cause of AIDS in 1984 is shared by the French and American groups led by Barre-Sinoussi et al. (55) and Gallo (56, 57). Early clinical observations included an early symptomatic period with flu-like symptoms not dissimilar to a viral illness like mononucleosis or cytomegalovirus (CMV) (58,59). This was followed by a clinically latent period during which there was minimal evidence of viral activity in the blood of infected persons but a gradual drop in CD4 cell count. The final stages of the disease were most readily and easily identifiable. Precipitated by unknown factors, and characterized by both clinical decline and measurable virologic activity, this phase inexorably led to profound and progressive immunodeficiency, recurrent opportunistic infections, and ultimately death. These observations were indeed limited by technology, and with improved abilities to detect viral activity, specifically plasma viral RNA, a new understanding of HIV pathogenesis has emerged.

Central to the model is the realization that following primary infection, persistently high levels of viral replication are present throughout the course of infection. It had been appreciated by 1989 that HIV-1 could be cultured from the blood of infected persons, and the levels of infectious virus were correlated with clinical status (48,49). In 1991 groups led by Daar (60) and Clark et al. (61) documented high levels of viral replication at the time of acute infection, higher than had been previously appreciated. In 1993 Piatak and co-workers (52), using a quantitative PCR technique, showed that levels of HIV RNA were quantifiable in the blood of infected persons. In addition, they documented a correlation with clinical status; that is, high levels were associated with low CD4 and clinically advanced disease. These observations were followed by reports by Pantaleo et al. (62) and Embreston et al. (63) documenting high levels of viral replication in lymphatic tissue during the period of clinical latency, previously thought to be one characterized by viral latency. Thus it became clear that viral replication was massive and ongoing during clinical latency despite relatively stable clinical profiles.

The actual dynamics of viral turnover were not appreciated until 1995, when two simultaneous reports appeared. Two groups, led by Ho (64) and Wei (65), independently discovered that the virions that were now detectable in the blood as well as the infected cells producing them were turning over at alarming rates. The minimal half-life of both plasma virus and the actively infected CD4 cell was less than 2 days. In other words, every 2 days or so half the circulating free virus and the infected CD4 cells producing this virus is the result of new infection. Thus, the notion of HIV infection being a latent infection was dispelled. It appears that clinical progression and immune dysfunction is a result of unchecked viral replication. Subsequently, Ho's group (66) has shown that, on average, $10^{10}$ virions are produced and cleared daily, with half the free virus in the plasma being replaced every 6 hours at a minimum. The consequences of this degree of viral replication is limitless genetic diversity that lends itself to drug resistance, escape from immune surveillance, and the emergence of more virulent viruses.

The specific mechanisms that link HIV-1 replication and CD4 cell destruction are yet to be clearly defined. Possible proposed mechanisms include direct viral cytopathicity as a consequence of productive infection (67), indirect CD4 cell destruction by immune surveillance of virus expressing cells (68), T-cell receptor–induced apoptosis (programmed cell death) due to HIV-related proteins such as gp120 and tat (69), or HIV-induced cytokine dysregulation (70). Independent of the precise mechanism(s) at play, antiviral regimens that result in significant reductions in viral load have recently translated into unprecedented improvements in CD4 cell counts (38,71–74) and have been associated with clinical benefit (75), suggesting an improvement in both CD4 cell number and immune function.

### Acute or Primary Infection

Regardless of the route, symptomatic acute HIV infection is characterized by a burst of viremia (60,61) associated with the onset of a nondistinct clinical syndrome suggestive of an acute viral illness. Recent studies suggest that approximately 90% of individuals are symptomatic during primary infection. The signs and symptoms include fever, fatigue, pharyngitis, weight loss, lymphadenopathy, headache, myalgia, nausea with vomiting, diarrhea, and rash (59,76,77). In addition, a clinical syndrome resembling aseptic meningitis with fever, headache, photophobia, and meningismus has been reported in as many as 10% of those newly infected.

The spontaneous reduction in plasma viremia is temporally associated with the appearance of measurable cell-mediated immune responses (78). Antibody responses appear to play a relatively minor role in the immune-mediated clearance of antigen (79). The drop in the level of plasma viremia following resolution of the peak viremia is highly predictive of clinical course. O'Brien et al. (80) obtained viral loads 12 to 36 months postseroconversion in a cohort of 165 hemophiliacs. They reported a progression rate to AIDS of 72%, 52%, 22%, and 0% in groups with plasma RNA levels of $10^5$ or more, between $10^5$ and $10^4$, between $10^3$ and $10^4$, and less than $10^3$, respectively. Similarly, Mellors and co-workers (81), following a cohort of newly infected gay and bisexual men, found a detectable plasma HIV RNA (using an assay with a lower limit of $10^4$ HIV RNA copies/ml) at the first postseroconversion visit to be the most predictive variant of the development of AIDS and CD4 cell decline. Given these observations, the paramount question is, What is the determinant of the viral set-point postinfection?

Characterization of the cellular immune response to HIV has revealed differences between individuals in the broadness of this response by studying the Vβ repertoire of the HIV-specific cytotoxic T cells (CD8 positive) (82). The T-cell receptor is composed of an α and β chain that allow for the polymorphic nature of the immune response to a wide variety of antigens. Put simply, individuals with rapid clinical progression appear to have a limited cellular immune response, as evidenced by a narrow Vβ response, as opposed to slower progressors in whom a broader degree of Vβ usage is observed (83). Thus it would appear that the clinical course of an HIV-infected subject relies on the interplay between host and viral factors that ultimately determine the degree of viral replication in an individual.

The issue of early treatment of HIV infection has come to the forefront in HIV research. Six months of zidovudine (AZT) monotherapy given to subjects with evidence of primary infection reduced the incidence of minor HIV-related conditions and resulted in slightly higher CD4 cell counts when compared to a similar group treated with placebo (84). Currently, aggressive treatment regimens such as those containing two nucleoside inhibitors of reverse transcriptase in combination with a potent protease inhibitor have resulted in excellent virologic and immunologic responses in limited numbers of newly infected subjects (77,85).

**Asymptomatic Phase**

Following the acute phase of HIV infection, the typical untreated host enters a period during which there is ongoing viral replication and CD4 cell destruction with immune compensation that is compromised over time. During this period, symptoms are minimal. The duration of this phase may be brief in rapid progressors or apparently never ending in the long-term nonprogressors. On average, the asymptomatic phase lasts for approximately 7 to 10 years, at the end of which 90% or so of those infected have developed AIDS, as defined below (86,87). It is now appreciated that during this phase a viral set point is maintained at a relatively constant level, characterized by high levels of viral production and clearance and associated with immunologic compensation (64,65). Although the determinants of this set point are unclear, host factors clearly play a role. It has recently been reported that HIV-infected persons heterozygous for the CC-CKR5 deletion progress more slowly to AIDS than those with the homozygous wild type (88).

Although the determinants of levels of viral replication in an HIV-infected host remain to be defined, the resultant steady-state level of viral replication is critical. Mellors et al. (89) reported the prognostic value of a single plasma HIV RNA measurement in a cohort of homosexual and bisexual men followed longitudinally over a period of 10 years. For example, patients with less than 4,530 RNA copies/ml plasma had a 30% rate to progression to AIDS at 10 years, whereas those with plasma HIV RNA values above 36,270 had an 80% progression rate over the same time period. The CD4 cell count, however, was far less predictive of subsequent course. From this study emerged the following conclusions: plasma HIV RNA is highly predictive of prognosis, there is a strong time-dependent prognostic relationship between plasma HIV-1 RNA and the development of AIDS and death, and reduced HIV-1 RNA levels in response to therapy are associated with improved outcomes (89).

In the not too distant past, therapeutic intervention with AZT monotherapy during this stage had been advocated based on results showing improved CD4 cell count, reduced p24 antigen levels, and a reduced rate of progression to AIDS or AIDS-related complex in patients with fewer than 500 CD4 cells/mm$^3$ treated with AZT in doses of 500 mg daily (90). However, subsequent studies failed to show a sustained benefit from early intervention with AZT monotherapy compared to deferred therapy at this stage of HIV infection (91). Given the present understanding of the dynamics of HIV replication in vivo and the limited antiviral activity of AZT monotherapy, these data became easier to understand and in some ways highlighted the need for a more aggressive approach to the treatment of HIV infection. Guidelines to therapy, once simple, have indeed become controversial (92), with some advocating multiple drug therapy guided by maximum suppression of plasma RNA levels to below detection (93). It can be argued that shutting down viral replication effectively during this phase may indeed prolong or even abrogate the progression to symptomatic HIV-1 infection.

During this phase, chronic viral replication is associated with chronic immune activation as evidenced by lymphoid hyperplasia, increased expression of cyotkines, increased expression of activation markers on both CD4 and CD8 cells, autoimmune phenomena, and hypergammaglobulinemia due to B cell activation (86,94). The consequences of chronic immune activation remain unclear. Negative effects would include the creation of more activated CD4 cells favoring expression of provirus and viral replication, as well as the elaboration of cytokines such as TNF-α and interleukins IL-2 and IL-6, which upregulate HIV replication in vitro. On the other hand, the production of soluble factors, such as chemokines and certain cytokines that inhibit viral replication, may dominate and favor clinical stability. It would appear that the factors that affect the duration of this stage would be multiple, with both viral and host factors being critical.

A good example of this interaction is the select group of patients, generally estimated at 5% to 10% of those chronically infected with HIV-1, who do not show typical signs of progression from this chronic phase to later stages. These are the nonprogressors, a group that is virologically and immunologically quite heterogeneous. In general, however, these patients have high measurable immune responses to HIV, both cell mediated and humoral, low plasma HIV RNA levels, generally below the level of detection, and in many cases unculturable virus by standard PBMC coculture methods, some with high levels of soluble cofactors that inhibit viral replication *in vitro* (95,96).

### Symptomatic Phase

Progression to symptomatic HIV infection and/or clinical AIDS is preceded by dropping CD4 cell counts and increasing levels of viral activity as measure by plasma HIV RNA. The diagnosis of AIDS is based on absolute CD4 cell levels below 200 cells/mm$^3$, or the presence of one of the conditions listed in Table 3 (97). In some patients a switch in the quality of the virus isolated from the blood is observed. A switch from a predominantly macrophage-tropic, slow growing viral population to a more rapidly replicating, T-cell tropic, syncytium-forming virus precedes the onset of AIDS (98,99). This switch has recently been found to be linked to a switch in co-receptor usage by HIV-1 to gain entry into a CD4 positive cell. At present the conditions that favor the switch are unclear, but recent findings indicate that changes in the conformation of the viral envelope emerge that favor CXCR4 or other co-receptor usage (18,100).

In addition to changes in viral tropism and replication properties, the effects of relentless viral replication in the lymphatic system result in progressive destruction of the nodal architecture and perhaps irreversible immune dysfunction. It is hypothesized that the loss of nodal architecture may result in a cytokine environment that promotes viral replication as opposed to a cytokine environment that favors inhibition of viral replication (94).

Therapeutics during this stage include combination antiviral therapy and prophylaxis for multiple opportunistic pathogens such as *Pneumocystic carinii, Mycobacterium avium* complex (MAC), cytomegalovirus, and *Candida.*

The presentation of infectious and neoplastic complications of AIDS and symptomatic HIV infection are protean and include nearly all organ systems (101). Important new developments include the identification of a herpes virus (HHV-8) that is associated with HIV-related Kaposi's sarcoma (102), suggesting a viral etiology for this AIDS-related malignancy.

The neurologic complications of HIV infection merit special attention. Neurologic manifestations of HIV infection may occur both early and late in the course of disease. Direct effects of HIV may range from a meningoencephalitis associated with primary infection to advanced dementia in the end stages of AIDS. Opportunistic infections may include infectious manifestations of toxoplasmosis, cytomegalovirus, cryptococcus, mycobacteria, or syphilis. Neoplasia, particularly primary CNS lymphoma, may also complicate HIV infection. Demyelinating diseases both centrally and peripherally have been associated with HIV infection (103). Of present concern is the possibility of the central nervous system as an untreated reservoir of viral replication. Recent advances in therapeutics have resulted in unprecedented reduction of viral activity in both blood and lymphoid tissue (85,104). A mathematical model has even been proposed addressing the possibility of eradication from an HIV-infected host (105). However, critical to this theory is the absence of an untreatable reservoir, such as

**TABLE 3.** *CDC surveillance case definition for AIDS*

| |
|---|
| Diseases diagnosed definitively without confirmation of HIV infection in patients without other causes of immunodeficiency |
| Candidiasis of the esophagus, trachea, bronchi, or lungs |
| Cryptococcosis, extrapulmonary |
| Cryptosporidiosis >1 month duration |
| Cytomegalovirus (CMV) infection of any organ except the liver, spleen, or lymph nodes |
| Herpes simplex infection, mucocutaneous (>1 month duration) or of the bronchi, lungs, or esophagus in patients (1 month duration) |
| Kaposi's sarcoma in patients <60 years old |
| Lymphoid interstitial pneumonitis (LIP) and/or pulmonary lymphoid hyperplasia (PLH) |
| *Mycobacterium avium* complex or *M. kansasii* disseminated |
| *Pneumocystis carinii* pneumonia |
| Progressive multifocal leukoencephalopathy |
| Toxoplasmosis of the brain in patients >1 month old |
| Diseases diagnosed definitively with confirmation of HIV infection |
| Multiple or recurrent pyogenic bacterial infection in patients <13 years old |
| Coccidioidomycosis, disseminated |
| Histoplasmosis, disseminated |
| Isosporiasis >1 month duration |
| Kaposi's sarcoma, any age |
| Primary CNS lymphoma, any age |
| Non-Hodgkin's lymphoma (small, noncleaved lymphoma; Burkitt or non-Burkitt type; or immunoblastic sarcoma) |
| Mycobacterial disease other than *M. tuberculosis,* disseminated |
| *M. tuberculosis,* extrapulmonary |
| *Salmonella* septicemia, recurrent CD4 cell count, <200 cells/mm$^3$ |
| Diseases diagnosed presumptively with confirmation of HIV infection |
| Candidiasis of the esophagus |
| CMV retinitis |
| Kaposi's sarcoma |
| LIP/PLH in patients <13 years old |
| Disseminated mycobacterial disease (not cultured) |
| *Pneumocystis carinii* pneumonia |
| Toxoplasmosis of the brain in patients >1 month old |
| HIV encephalopathy |
| HIV wasting syndrome |

the central nervous system. Among the available approved drugs to treat HIV infection, only zidovudine (AZT) and stavudine (D4T) effectively cross the blood-brain barrier. If indeed the central nervous system is a sanctuary, then therapeutic efforts must be directed to address this issue.

## OCCUPATIONAL RISK OF HIV

With the exception of prostitution, the occupational risk of HIV transmission is directly proportional to the risk of significant exposure to HIV-infected blood. Significant exposure to blood in the workplace is primarily percutaneous, most often in the usual medical sense of penetration of intact skin by a sharp object (106–112). However, the common occurrence of acutely broken skin in the course of military and safety/rescue operations and in some professional sports is also of concern and, theoretically at least, increases the risk of HIV transmission in these special work groups.

### Fire-Rescue/Public Safety: The Role of Education

By 1983, although a specific AIDS agent had not yet been found, transmission had been characterized epidemiologically and those results published in the scientific literature (113).

The discovery of HIV in 1984 did not significantly change the basic understanding of transmission (114), nor has it changed since (115,116), although the recent elucidation of the CCR5 receptor allele (88) may explain some of the excess transmission consistently seen in non-European racial groups (115,117–120). But at least another 5 years would pass before this information, and its backhanded reassurance, took root in the general public understanding of AIDS. The interim was a period of public hysteria about AIDS that touched all aspects of personal and social life (121).

During this period, fire-rescue/public safety workers held a special position. The nature of their work includes the routine risk of exposure to human blood and body fluids, often in highly uncontrolled situations, but their training, at least up to this time, did not emphasize infectious disease risks or prevention. Thus there were a number of widely publicized incidents resulting from police and fire/rescue personnel fears of contact with people with AIDS or people believed to have the disease for social rather than clinical reasons (122).

From the beginning of the epidemic, the CDC published and periodically updated guidelines for health care and laboratory workers to avoid high-risk exposure to the AIDS agent (110,113,123–125). In June 1988 the federal government mailed to all households in the United States a brochure discussing the transmission and prevention of HIV/AIDS (126). The National Health Interview Survey done in August of that year did document a substantial increase in respondents who understood that HIV was not acquired by casual contact (127). In 1989 additional guidelines were published by the CDC that addressed the special circumstances and risks of fire-rescue/public-safety personnel (128). In particular, these guidelines discuss the risks imposed by bloody trauma and crime scenes, violence, and sharp objects in unexpected places. To date, no seroconversions are documented to have been directly associated with fire-rescue/public-safety work.

### The Military

#### *The Role of Testing*

The association of AIDS in the public mind with despised behaviors and expensive dying put an early crimp in the public health response to the epidemic in the United States. Screening, counseling, contact notification, and early treatment and preventive measures, mainstays of the classic response to epidemics, were not possible in the social and health care economics settings of the first decade of the AIDS epidemic. Even when testing for HIV antibody became available early in 1985, though seized upon by blood banks for screening of potential donors, it was otherwise used only cautiously in other contexts and amid debate that paralyzed any focus on the HIV epidemic other than its clinically visible end stage.

Only in the U.S. military was the overpowering need to secure the health of active duty personnel coupled with sufficient social control to implement a universal testing program (129). However, unlike screening in general, which tolerates some latitude in specificity and sensitivity, the designers of the military testing did not feel that they could afford this. Although they believed that the security of its data system was a major virtue of their program, a risk of having personnel falsely labeled as HIV positive was not acceptable (130).

False negatives, particularly among new recruits, were viewed as a threat for a number of reasons. Unidentified infection potentially undermined the safety of the military's "walking blood bank." In addition, the long-term medical care of AIDS patients was not something that the military health care system could afford knowingly to take on in advance. Early experience also showed that HIV-positive individuals may not safely receive live virus vaccination (131). That, along with the increased potential for exposure to infectious diseases and less ready access to medical care when deployed overseas, meant that people infected with HIV could not be deployed overseas. Finally, from the standpoint of military readiness, nothing in the known natural history of HIV disease suggests that an individual entering service already infected with HIV will be able to provide 10 years of full duty service, the median hoped for with any recruit (132).

The strict requirements of the U.S. Army testing program have set the subsequent standard for testing in the United States. The military testing programs have provided information on evolving patterns of the HIV epidemic not available from other sources. For example, data coming out of testing of recruits first heralded the shift of the epidemic into heterosexual adolescent populations (133,134). Also, because military service tends to erase the confounding links of race to socioeconomic status (with the further link of socioeconomic status to access to medical care), it has been possible to explore aspects of racial-cultural differences in attitudes toward the epidemic, including toward risky behaviors and prevention, that cannot be approached as clearly in the civilian population (135). There are two caveats in using these data. With the proscription of openly homosexual behavior for military service, lying about this aspect of one's life—"Don't ask; don't tell"—is presently official policy. It is also likely that some degree of self-de-selection, both in terms of sexual orientation and preexisting HIV infection, are operative in the formation of the groups who ultimately constitute the military population.

### *Fitness for Duty*

Although the day-to-day activities of military personnel are largely administrative and tend to be sedentary, military readiness requires sustained physical fitness and the tacit acceptance of bloodshed. Current U.S. Army regulations use both the day-to-day realities and readiness-potential aspects of military life in setting fitness-for-duty standards for soldiers with HIV infection (136). These regulations may suggest guidelines for civilian employers deciding fitness-for-duty issues.

In general, HIV-positive military personnel may not serve overseas unless that overseas post happens to be their home (Guam, Puerto Rico, etc.), because of the vaccination and health care issues noted above. They may not serve in combat units because of the risk of bloodshed—both the risk of exposing their comrades to HIV-infected blood and the risk of those comrades having open wounds themselves if that happens. They may not enroll in educational programs that incur additional service obligations, but they may reenlist if they meet the basic fitness standards required of all Army personnel.

Once infection has progressed to the point of needing frequent medical follow-up, HIV-infected soldiers may not be assigned to areas remote from a military medical facility (for example, as a recruiter). Only when the HIV-infected soldier shows progressive clinical illness or significant immunologic deficiency are medical separation procedures begun.

To date, there have been no recognized cases of action-related transmission of HIV infection. However, the prospect of even limited military action, as in peacekeeping and humanitarian efforts, in areas of the world with high prevalence of HIV such as central Africa or Southeast Asia, may appropriately provoke concern about such transmission.

### Professional Sports

Unlike the military, professional sports present their tangle of fitness-for-duty and fear-of-transmission issues in the setting of extremely high stakes free-market economics. As in the first two occupational groups discussed, as of this writing no transmission of HIV has been clearly documented in a professional athlete as a result of the athletic activity itself. The report of seroconversion in an soccer player after he collided head-on with a player known to be HIV positive, both players suffering facial lacerations that bled copiously (137), has been contested (138), but there is no intrinsic reason why this incident could not have resulted in transmission. However, traumatic skin disruption and potential exchange of blood, routine in boxing and at least not unexpected in other sports such as basketball, football, or hockey, mean that the potential for blood-borne pathogen transmission must be addressed.

By mid-1987, the New Jersey Athletic Commission had ruled that all ring-side personnel must wear water-impervious gloves while assisting fighters (139). Later that same year, the Nevada Boxing Commission ruled that any boxer fighting in Nevada had to be tested for HIV (140).

Earvin "Magic" Johnson's announcement, in November 1991, that he had tested positive for HIV dramatized the need for a clear response to the HIV epidemic in professional sports. After Johnson's first retirement, the National Basketball Association (NBA), at the request of the NBA Players' Association, began an ongoing program to provide AIDS prevention education to all the players on all 27 NBA teams, in association with the Johns Hopkins School of Hygiene and Public Health (141). Meeting in February 1992, representatives from the NBA, the National Football League (NFL), the National Hockey League, professional baseball, the National College Athletics Association, and the National Federation of State High School Associations agreed to informally adopt the World Health Organization (WHO) Consensus Statement guidelines on AIDS and sports, first published in 1989 and revised in 1991.

These guidelines, which agree with the recommendations of the American Academy of Pediatrics (AAP) Commission on Sports Medicine and Fitness (142), do not recommend routine testing of athletes for HIV and do not recommend restricting the HIV-positive athlete from playing. They provide specific recommendations for on-field blood/body fluid management. Both the AAP and the WHO emphasize the need for education and counseling of HIV-positive athletes about transmission potential in contact sports, including encouraging transfer to a noncontact sport. The AAP, from the point of view of pediatric practice in an American legal context, strongly emphasizes confidentiality, including not disclosing the presence of a HIV-infected individual on a team unless the understanding of risk of transmission in sports contact changes with further experience.

From this base, the NFL went on to develop and implement, by July 1992, a policy on HIV/AIDS specific to professional football. In general, this policy agrees with the AAP/WHO guidelines, with two interesting differences. A specific decision was made *not* to stop play if a bloody injury occurred. This decision was based on the observations that in professional football, essentially all bloody injuries are abrasions rather than lacerations and that the equipment worn by players covers about 90% of skin surface. Both factors were felt to reduce the likelihood of significant blood contact sufficiently to obviate the need to stop play only because a bloody injury occurs. Further, official NFL policy not only emphasizes confidentiality, as per the WHO/AAP guidelines, but discourages players from disclosing their HIV status at all, given the inconsistency of interstate rulings on HIV and the lack of relevance of HIV status to a player's performance (143).

Baseball, which views itself as relatively low risk for directly occupational transmission, has tended to approach HIV issues through the employee assistance programs of individual teams, and in rookie career development "Baseball Off the Field" programs (141).

The WHO guidelines make passing reference to the possibility of risk to the health of the HIV-infected athlete by continued play. The concern that intense physical activity might accelerate progression of disease was based in part on observations of disturbances in immune markers after intense physical activity (144). For professional sports, these observations have not had much practical significance as the debility imposed by advancing AIDS precludes activity of the intensity required either to perform professionally or to produce the experimentally observed shifts (145). Furthermore, people who are HIV positive and asymptomatic have shown improvements in CD4 and associated cell counts under a program of graded physical training (146). Both asymptomatic and early symptomatic HIV-positive individuals appear to respond normally to physiometric and psychometric assessment of physical training (147). Finally, HIV-positive, asymptomatic individuals do not show neuropsychiatric impairment (148,149). In summary, there seems to be little evidence of increased risk in the continued activity of HIV-positive athletes.

Far more important than any theoretical risk of HIV transmission in sports contact, the superstar lifestyles of many professional athletes greatly increases their social—as compared with intrinsically occupational—risk of exposure, eliminates privacy if they do become infected, and magnifies concerns over occupational transmission and fitness for duty out of proportion to the actual risks involved. In addition, as well as being personally devastating to the athletes involved, the media circus that often erupts around a professional athlete's testing positive for HIV tends to distract public attention and debate from much more important aspects of transmission and prevention.

### Health Care Workers

In the early stages of the AIDS epidemic, the emotional impact on nurses, physicians, and other health care workers (HCWs), both the specter of young patients dying horribly and the association with social groups about whom many of them felt at least ambivalent, was far greater than visible risks to themselves (150,151). As transmission patterns emerged and the epidemic grew, so did concern over personal risk, sufficient, at least among house staff and medical and dental students, to affect career choices (152). It should be noted, however, that other issues, including the volume of work required by these patients and the social groups from which they came, appeared to continue to have as much to do with the distress expressed by a substantial proportion of HCWs over caring for AIDS patients as the amount of personal risk perceived (152,153).

But even as serologic testing enormously expanded the identified prevalence of HIV and at a time when the true prevalence was increasing as well, a work-related epidemic of HIV in HCWs never emerged. Overall work-related transmission of HIV to HCWs remains very low even though the pool of HCW who may encounter HIV-infected patients in the course of normal job tasks has greatly increased (154–156). There are three objective reasons for this. First, the relative risk of transmission from a single percutaneous exposure to HIV-positive blood via a contaminated hollow-core needle—the overwhelmingly most common form of significant exposure—is about 1 in 300 (157). The relative risk for laboratory workers of seroconversion after accidents handling high-titer virus cultures is considered to be in the same range, though there is less specific prospective data on this group of workers (158). This level of risk is much less than the relative risks of transmission from the most common nonoccupational exposures. In comparison, sexual transmission is estimated to range, in North American populations, from 1 in 1,000 contacts with any infected partner to 1 in 150 to 200 for receptive intercourse with a penetrating partner with AIDS. Among Thai women working as prostitutes, whose susceptibility may more closely approximate Africans working as prostitutes, risk of transmission is estimated at about 1 in 30 contacts. Transmission rates as high as 1 in 10 may occur in the presence of other sexually transmitted diseases (159). About one in three infants born to HIV-positive mothers and two in three recipients of HIV-infected blood transfusions are infected (27,160–162).

**TABLE 4.** *Factors predicting transmission of human immunodeficiency virus to health care providers after percutaneous exposure*

| Factor | Adjusted odds ratio (95% confidence level) |
|---|---|
| Deep (intramuscular) injury | 16.1 (6.1 to 44.6) |
| Visible blood on sharp device | 5.2 (1.8 to 17.7) |
| Needle used to enter blood vessel | 5.1 (1.9 to 14.8) |
| Source patient with terminal AIDS | 6.4 (2.2 to 18.9) |
| Zidovudine prophylaxis used | 0.2 (0.1 to 0.6) |

From ref. 164.

### *Risk Associated with Percutaneous Exposure*

Several factors are associated with the risk of transmission from percutaneous exposure. The quantity and depth of injection are critical (163,164). As shown in Table 4, deep intramuscular injection converts an expected transmission of about 1 in 300 to an observed transmission of about 1 in 20. Skin penetration only or surface scratches clearly convey much less risk. The quantity of infectious material involved can be estimated by degree of contamination of the device involved; visible blood or use of the device in a blood vessel clearly enhances risk of transmission. The potential infectivity of the blood itself is also important. Viral titers tend to be particularly high in individuals during the acute viral syndrome period of the disease just after infection and in the final advanced stages of the disease (48).

### *Other Exposures*

In the health care setting, exposure of nonintact skin to, especially, large quantities of blood has resulted in infection with HIV (157). Transmission via mucous membrane exposure in the health care setting is extremely rare but has occurred (165).

### *Primary Prevention*

The second reason for the low transmission rates to HCWs is that effective, simple, cheap, and familiar means of primary prevention (see Appendix A) are readily available and easily incorporated into routine health care practices (108,109,113,122–125,166–170). Although manufacturers have eagerly promoted new, safer equipment, simple changes in work practices, such as non-recapping of needles and the location and numbers of impervious containers for contaminated sharp equipment, with the overall practice of "Standard Precautions" (formerly "Universal Precautions"; see Appendix A), are the only modifications that have been proved to significantly reduce percutaneous injuries in health care settings (167–169).

### *Secondary Prevention: Decontamination of Wounds*

The effectiveness of simple methods is also true of secondary preventive measures. Povidone-iodine solution at 1/40 the concentration of commercial preparations (Betadine and others) destroys HIV completely after very brief applications (171).

Central to postexposure care is immediate scrubbing with povidone-iodine scrub or solution (or alternate standard surgical scrub solutions for iodine-sensitive individuals) for 10 minutes. Mucous membrane exposures are cleansed with a 15-minute flow of sterile normal saline.

### *Secondary Prevention: Postexposure Chemoprophylaxis*

A third reason for low transmission rates to HCW has only recently been clearly appreciated. Postexposure chemoprophylaxis for HIV was first proposed in the late 1980s based on observations in animals that zidovudine (AZT) administered shortly after exposure to HIV could suppress or eliminate viral replication (172,173). Despite the difficulty of generalizing from this work, many cen-

**TABLE 5.** *Summary protocol: multicenter trial of postexposure prophylaxis for health care providers exposed to HIV*[a]

Zidovudine dosage: 200 mg orally, three times per day
Lamivudine dosage: 150 mg orally, twice per day
Indinavir dosage: 800 mg orally, three times per day[b]
Initiation: As soon as possible after known or possible exposure to HIV, but within 72 hours
Treatment duration: 4 weeks
Toxicity monitoring
- Symptoms
- Focused physical examination
- Complete blood count
- Liver function tests
- Amylase tests
- Renal function tests
- Urinalysis

Monitoring frequency
- Every 2 weeks while receiving treatment
- At 6 weeks, 3 months, 6 months, and 12 months

HIV monitoring
- HIV antibody test at baseline, 6 months, and 12 months (required)
- HIV antibody test at 6 weeks and 3 months (optional)
- HIV antigen test, HIV polymerase chain reaction, and culture if symptoms of acute retrovirus illness occur in a seronegative health care worker

[a]Principal investigators: J. L. Gerberding (University of California–San Francisco and San Francisco General Hospital) and D. K. Henderson (Clinical Center, National Institutes of Health, Bethesda, MD). Complete study protocol is available at http://epi-center.ucsf.edu.

[b]If the source patient has experience with zidovudine and lamivudine or when the exposure is to a large volume of material with a high titer of virus.

From ref. 164.

ters attempted some form of chemoprophylaxis. The results, though generally supportive, were confounded by widely varying dosages and schedules and by low natural rates of transmission in this setting (154).

In 1989, San Francisco General Hospital (SFG) and the Warren G. Magnuson Clinical Center of the National Institutes of Health (NIH), began a collaborative, prospective trial of postexposure chemoprophylaxis of health care workers at first using AZT alone and more recently with additional agents (Table 5) (174,175). The statistical challenge of proving efficacy prospectively is daunting. A previous attempt at a prospective trial was halted (176). However, the observation that transmission of HIV infection can be reduced in a substantial proportion of cases by giving AZT to HIV-positive women in the last trimester of pregnancy followed by treatment of the child post partum (37,177) gave important support to the concept of postexposure prophylaxis (PEP).

In December 1995 the CDC published the results of case-control follow-up of HCWs after percutaneous exposure to HIV-positive blood (163). These showed a 79% reduction in the risk for HIV infection among HCWs who used AZT appropriately after percutaneous exposure to HIV-infected blood. PEP is now recommended for any significant occupational exposure to HIV-infected blood, body fluids contaminated with blood, or those body fluids known to transmit HIV (164,178). Table 6 outlines the advice provided to employees exposed to HIV at SFG, which is in accordance with the current Public Health Service recommendations.

The efficacy of chemoprophylaxis, ideally within 2 hours and no later than 5 days after exposure, is sufficiently convincing that most authorities recommend a first dose at least of AZT/3TC essentially as soon as the exposure is reported, unless there is an overriding contraindication to such action. Pregnancy is *not* considered such a contraindication. The addition of indinavir (Crixivan) in doses of 800 mg orally every 8 hours should be recommended in high-risk exposures.

### *Chemoprophylaxis in Pregnancy*

Pregnant workers are not eligible for entry into the prospective studies under way at SFG and the NIH, nor has PEP been recommended for pregnant workers in the past (179). However, pregnancy per se is not a contraindication to the use of AZT and probably not 3TC. The sum of evidence available at present suggests that, given the role of studies of HIV-positive pregnant women in supporting chemoprophylaxis and the high risk of mother-to-child perinatal transmission when primary infection occurs during pregnancy, PEP of at least those two agents should be offered to any pregnant worker exposed in a manner that would otherwise suggest the need for it.

## Funeral/Mortuary Workers

Mortuary workers share much of the same risk as both health care and rescue workers (180). HIV has been cul-

**TABLE 6.** *Advice about prophylaxis after exposure to human immunodeficiency virus at San Francisco General Hospital*

| | Attributes of the source patient | | |
|---|---|---|---|
| Attributes of the exposure | Asymptomatic, known low titer | AIDS, symptomatic infection | Preterminal AIDS, acute infection, known high titer |
| Percutaneous injuries | | | |
| Superficial injury | Offer | Recommend | Strongly encourage |
| Visible bloody device used in artery or vein | Recommend | Recommend | Strongly encourage |
| Deep intramuscular injury or actual injection | Recommend | Strongly encourage | Strongly encourage |
| Mucosal contacts | | | |
| Small volume; brief contact | Offer | Offer | Offer |
| Large volume or prolonged contact | Offer | Recommend | Recommend |
| Large volume; prolonged contact | Recommend | Recommend | Recommend |
| Cutaneous contacts | | | |
| Small volume; brief contact | Offer if obvious portal of entry | Offer if obvious portal of entry | Offer if obvious portal of entry |
| Large volume or prolonged contact | Offer (recommend if obvious portal) | Offer (recommend if obvious portal) | Offer (recommend if obvious portal) |
| Large volume and prolonged contact | Offer (recommend if obvious portal) | Offer (recommend if obvious portal) | Recommend (especially with obvious portal) |

From ref. 164.

tured from blood for up to 21 hours after death and from other tissues, including bone, brain, and viscera, for as long as 2 weeks after death in the absence of refrigeration (181,182). The risk of percutaneous exposure to blood and body fluids during autopsy and embalming procedures is obvious. Less well appreciated is the participation of these workers in the extrication and transport of bodies from out-of-hospital sites to the mortuary. Although the overall risk of transmission appears equivalent with other HCWs, it may be increased by complacency, frequent lack of knowledge about the premorbid state of the deceased, and the reliance of the funeral industry for care of work-related injuries on local contract health care providers who may not be fully aware of the risks and treatment of blood-borne pathogen exposures (183).

Although there is no overt policy in the funeral injury for recommendation of postexposure prophylaxis, these workers are covered by the Occupational Safety and Health Administration (OSHA) regulations for workers at risk for blood-borne pathogen exposure, and these regulations do recommend PEP (see Appendix B) (184). Any funeral or mortuary worker with a significant exposure to HIV-positive blood or body fluids should be offered PEP as noted above.

### Professional-to-Patient Transmission

Transmission of HIV from an infected HCW to patients in the course of normal professional practice has been documented only once, in a dental practice, although the exact process by which this happened has never been determined (185). Although the risk of HCW-to-patient transmission appears to be extremely low (186), transmission of HIV from patient to patient in a surgical practice has also occurred once (187,188). Again, the process by which this occurred is not clear, although it also appears to have been in the course of normal practice.

### Sex Workers: The International Experience

By far the greatest risk for occupational transmission of HIV worldwide is in commercial sex workers (CSWs) (189–191).

Unlike Europe and the United States, where intravenous drug use (IVDU) appears to have been the critical factor in the expansion of HIV in heterosexual populations (114,189,190), in sub-Saharan Africa and Southeast Asia the relative economic and/or social legitimization of commercial sex appears to have been the primary amplifying factor (192). Retrospective testing of serum samples from female prostitutes in Nairobi, Kenya, showed that 4% were HIV positive by 1981 and 65% by 1985 (193). The first case of AIDS in Thailand was documented in 1985 in a homosexual male, but by 1989 40% of the commercial sex workers in seven northern provinces were HIV positive; by 1991, 65%. By 1993, 12% of the general population of this region were HIV positive (194).

In sub-Saharan Africa and in India, long-distance truckers appear to be a major additional factor in the spread of HIV (195–197). In India, the prevalence of HIV seropositivity in CSWs shows a striking west-to-east pattern. Among prostitutes in Bombay, on the western coast facing Africa, the prevalence was 1.6% in 1988 and 23% by 1990 (198). In 1992, in Calcutta, on the eastern coast, HIV seropositivity among prostitutes was still only slightly above 1%, though the prevalence of other sexually transmitted diseases (STDs) was more than 80% and the use of condoms around 10% (199,200). In New Delhi, in north-central India, in 1988 the prevalence of HIV seropositivity was 1/700 and in 1990, still only 1/600, a success attributed to an active condom promotion campaign (195). Along the "AIDS highway" through central and east Africa HIV seropositivity in CSWs has reached nearly 90% (189,191–193,201).

In other parts of the world, the prevalence of HIV infection among CSWs, particularly when IVDU is not an issue, can be very low (189–191). Although recent work on the molecular biology of HIV transmission suggests that susceptibility factors (88) may have an important role in the repeated observation of higher prevalence of seropositivity in non-European racial groups, social factors that influence the use of condoms are probably more important for CSWs. The efficacy of consistent condom use in preventing HIV transmission to CSWs has been demonstrated repeatedly in prospective, community-based studies all over the world (202–206). But even with full appreciation of risk of infection, actual condom use varies greatly. There is as yet no satisfactory prophylactic totally in the control of the receptive individual: brief hopes for the chemical spermicide nonoxinol-9 were not confirmed in community-based studies (207).

Factors that support condom use include specific laws regarding commercial sex work. In Nevada there has been no transmission of HIV to a sex worker since 1987 (202,208). Commercial sex work in brothels is legal in many communities in Nevada. CSWs must be licensed and HIV negative, and condom use and regular HIV testing are mandatory; compliance has been essentially 100%. The availability or cost of condoms also have some role in utilization by CSWs (209,210), but clearly other factors are also at work. In Thailand, where commercial sex is actually illegal, the frightening rise in HIV infection in prostitutes in the late 1980s was reflected in a steady rise in seropositivity in military recruits. In 1989, the Thai Ministry of Health initiated a vigorous program to promote condom use among CSWs, including providing mass quantities of free condoms to these workers. The program appears to have greatly reduced other STD transmission and can probably be credited with slowing the epidemic of HIV. The failure to stop transmission of HIV, however, appears due to human factors: the lukewarm support of brothel keepers and clients and the relative social position of the CSWs (211,212).

Gender factors—the social position of women and homosexuals—are probably important in condom use by CSWs but also probably more complex than is allowed by most writers on the subject. Along the long-distance trucking routes of Africa and India, for example, where both male and female rural CSWs tend to be isolated and socially powerless, the request that a client use a condom is often met with violence or at least reduced payment (195,196). However, the discounting of payment for condom use (and a general preference for accepting the risk and full payment or even a payment bonus for going without) appears across cultures and genders, being noted in female CSWs in Thailand and Britain and male CSWs in Britain and Italy (213–216). Emotional factors play a role: repeat customers—"I know him: he's healthy"—are often not asked to use a condom. Probably more importantly, worldwide, CSWs of either sex do not use condoms with personal, as against professional, sexual contacts (194,217–222). This greatly increases their nonoccupational risk of infection with HIV, particularly in social groups in which IVDU is widespread, and in turn the risk of spread into the client community (190,209,221,223).

For medical and public health providers involved in the care of CSWs, a clear understanding of the social factors at work in their particular community of CSWs and the ability to provide both basic and ongoing education and social support for the use of condoms among them is central in minimizing HIV transmission (205,224). Other STDs also appear to have a significant role in promoting transmission of HIV (192,201,224–226), so measures that increase access to and utilization of STD diagnostic and treatment services may also be important in limiting transmission of HIV. Although postexposure chemoprophylaxis is now the standard of care for health care workers exposed to HIV via a considerably less efficient route than sexual intercourse, it seems highly unlikely that this modality will be extended to commercial sex workers any time in the foreseeable future.

## REFERENCES


1. Shilts R. *And the band played on.* New York: Penguin Books, 1988; 3–7.
2. Bygbjerg IC. AIDS in a Danish surgeon. *Lancet* 1983;1:925.
3. CDC. HIV/AIDS surveillance report. *National AIDS Clearinghouse* 1996;8:5.
4. Brookmeyer R. Reconstruction and future trends of the AIDS epidemic in the United States. *Science* 1991;253:37–42.
5. Brandt AM. AIDS: from public history to public policy. In: Hannaway C, Harden VA, Parascandola J, eds. *AIDS and the public debate.* Amsterdam: IOS Press, 1995;124–131.
6. Markovitz DM. Infection with the human immunodeficiency virus type 2. *Ann Intern Med* 1993;118:211–218.
7. Mertens TE, Belsey E, Stoneburner RL, et al. Global estimates and epidemiology of HIV-1 infections and AIDS: further heterogeneity in spread and impact. *AIDS* 1995;9(suppl A):s259–s272.
8. Varmus H. Retroviruses. *Science* 1988;240:1427–1435.
9. Greene WC. The molecular biology of human immunodeficiency virus type 1 infection. *N Engl J Med* 1991;324:308–317.
10. Cullen BR. Regulation of HIV gene expression. *AIDS* 1995;9(suppl A):s19–s32.
11. Subramanian RA, Cohen EA. Molecular biology of the HIV accessory proteins. *J Virol* 1994;68:6831–6835.
12. Gelderblom H. Assembly and morphology of HIV: potential effect of structure on viral function. *AIDS* 1991;5:617–638.
13. Ho DD, Pomerantz RJ, Kaplan JC. Pathogenesis of infection with human immunodeficiency virus. *N Engl J Med* 1987;317:278–286.
14. Maddon PJ, Dalgleish AG, McDougal JS, Clapham PR, Weiss RA, Axel R. The T4 gene encodes the AIDS virus receptor and is expressed in the immune system and the brain. *Cell* 1986;47:333–348.
15. Dragic T, Litwin V, Allaway GP, et al. HIV-1 entry into CD4 cells is mediated by the chemokine receptor CC-CKR-5. *Nature* 1996;381: 667–673.
16. Deng H-K, Lui R, Ellmeier W, et al. Identification of a major coreceptor for primary isolates of HIV-1. *Nature* 1996;381:661–666.
17. Bleul CC, Farzan M, Choe H, et al. The lymphocyte chemoattractant SDF-1 is a ligand for LESTR/fusin and blocks HIV-1 entry. *Nature* 1996;382:829–832.
18. Feng Y, Broder CC, Kennedy PE, Berger EA. HIV-1 entry cofactor: functional cDNA cloning of a seven-transmembrane G protein-coupled receptor. *Science* 1996;272:872–877.
19. Cocchi F, DeVico AL, Garzino-Demo A, Arya SK, Gallo RC, Lusso P. Identification of RANTES, MIP-1 alpha, and MIP-1 beta as the major HIV-suppressive factors produced by CD8- T cells. *Science* 1995;270:1811–1815.
20. Goff SP. Retroviral reverse transcriptase: synthesis, structure, and function. *J AIDS* 1990;3:817–831.
21. Bukrinsky M, Sharova N, McDonald TL, Pushkarskaya T, Tarplay G, Stevenson M. Association of integrase, matrix, and reverse transcriptase antigens of HIV-1 with viral nucleic acids following acute infection. *Proc Natl Acad Sci USA* 1993;90:6125–6129.
22. Bushman FD, Fujiwara T, Craigie R. Retroviral DNA integration directed by HIV integration protein in vitro. *Science* 1990;249: 1555–1558.
23. Dyda F, Hickman AB, Jenkins TM, Engleman A, Craigie R, Davies DR. Crystal structure of the catalytic domain of HIV-1 Integrase: similarity to other polynucleotidyl transferases. *Science* 1994;266:1981–1986.
24. Arthur LO, Bess JW Jr, Sowder RC II, et al. Cellular proteins bound to immunodeficiency viruses: implications for pathogenesis and vaccines. *Science* 1992;258:1935–1938.
25. DeBouck C. The HIV-1 protease as a therapeutic target for AIDS. *AIDS Res Hum Retroviruses* 1992;8:153–164.
26. Deeks SG, Smith M, Holodiny M, Kahn J. HIV-1 Protease Inhibitors. *JAMA* 1997;277:145–153.
27. Friedland GH, Klein RS. Transmission of the human immunodeficiency virus. *N Engl J Med* 1987;317:1125–1135.
28. Conant M, Hardy D, Sernatinger J, Spicer DW, Levy J. Condoms prevent transmission of AIDS associated retrovirus. JAMA 1986;255: 1706–1709.
29. Prevots DR, Ancelle PR, Neal JJ, Remis RS. The epidemiology of heterosexually acquired HIV infections and AIDS in western industrialized countries. *AIDS* 1994;8:S109–117.
30. Edlin BR, Irwin K, Farque S, et al. Intersecting epidemics-crack cocaine and HIV infection among inner-city young adults. *N Engl J Med* 1994;331:1422–1427.
31. Paxton WA, Martin SR, Tse D, et al. Relative resistance to HIV-1 infection of CD4 lymphocytes from persons who remain uninfected despite multiple high-risk sexual exposures. *Nature Med* 1996;2: 412–417.
32. Liu R, Paxton WA, Choe S, et al. Homozygous defect in HIV-1 coreceptor accounts for resistance of some multiply-exposed individuals to HIV-1 infection. *Cell* 1996;86:367–377.
33. CDC Update: provisional Public Health Service recommendations for chemoprophylaxis after occupational exposure to HIV. *MMWR* 1996; 44:468–472, 45:422.
34. Study EC. Risk factors for mother-to-child transmission of HIV-1. *Lancet* 1991;339:1007–1012.
35. Sperling RS, Shapiro DE, Coombs R, et al. Maternal plasma HIV-RNA and the success of zidovudine (ZDV) in the prevention of mother-child-transmission. 3rd Conf. *Retrovir Opp Infect* 1996; Abstract:LB1.
36. Landesman SH, Kalish LA, Burns DN, et al. Obstetrical factors and

the transmission of human immunodeficiency virus type 1 from mother to child. The Women and Infants Transmission Study. *N Engl J Med* 1996;334:1617–1623.
37. Connor EM, Sperling RS, Gelber R, et al. Reduction of maternal-infant transmission of human immunodeficiency virus type 1 with zidovudine treatment. *N Engl J Med* 1994;331:1173–1180.
38. Eron JJ, Benoit SL, Jemsek J, et al. Treatment with lamivudine, zidovudine, or both in HIV-positive patients with 200 to 500 CD4-cells per cubic millimeter. *N Engl J Med* 1995;333:1662–1669.
39. Burke DS. Laboratory Diagnosis of Human Immunodeficiency Infection. *Clin Lab Med* 1989;9:369–392.
40. Reesink HW, Huisman JG, Gonsalves M, et al. Evaluation of six enzyme immunoassays for antibody against HIV. *Lancet* 1986:483–486.
41. Second Consensus Conference on HIV Testing, Committee on HIV Association of State and Territorial Public Health Laboratory Directors, Atlanta, Georgia, 1987.
42. CDC. Testing for antibodies to HIV-2 in the United States. *MMWR* 1992;41:1–8.
43. Midthun K, Garrison L, Clements M, et al. Frequency of indeterminate Western blot tests in healthy adults at low risk for HIV infection. *J Infect Dis* 1990;162:1379–1382.
44. Imagawa DT, Lee MH, Wolinsky SM, et al. Human immunodeficiency virus type 1 infection in homosexual men who remain seronegative for prolonged periods. *N Engl J Med* 1989;320:1458–1462.
45. Hammer S, Crumpacker C, D'Aquila R, et al. Use of virologic assays for detection of human immunodeficiency virus in clinical trials: recommendations of the AIDS Clinical Trials Group Virology Committee. *J Clin Microbiol* 1993;31:2557–2564.
46. Allain J, Laurian Y, Paul DA, et al. Long-term evaluation of HIV antigen and antibodies to p24 and gp41 in patients with hemophilia. *N Engl J Med* 1987;317:1114–1121.
47. Bollinger RC, Kline RL, Francis HL, Moss MW, Bartlett JG, Quinn TC. Acid dissociation increases the sensitivity of p24 antigen detection in the evaluation of antiviral therapy and disease progression in asymptomatic HIV infected-persons. *J Infect Dis* 1992;165:913–916.
48. Ho DD, Moudgil T, Alam M. Quantitation of human immunodeficiency virus type 1 in the blood of infected persons. *N Engl J Med* 1989;321:1621–1625.
49. Coombs RW, Collier AC, Allain JP, et al. Plasma viremia in human immunodeficiency virus infection. *N Engl J Med* 1989;321:1626–1631.
50. Khadir A, Coutlee F, Saint-Antoine P, Olivier C, Voyer H, Kessous-Elbaz A. Clinical evaluation of Amplicor HIV-1 test for detection of human immunodeficiency virus type 1 proviral DNA in peripheral blood mononuclear cells. *J AIDS Hum Retrovirol* 1995;9:257–263.
51. Wolinsky SM, Rinaldo CR, Snisky JJ, et al. Human Immunodeficiency virus type 1 (HIV-1) infection a median of 18 months before a diagnostic western blot. *Ann Intern Med* 1989;111:961–972.
52. Piatak MJ, Saag MS, Yang LC, et al. High levels of HIV-1 in plasma during all stages of infection determined by competitive PCR. *Science* 1993;259:1749–1754.
53. Mulder J, McKinney N, Christopherson C, Sninsky J, Greenfield L, Kwok S. Rapid and simple PCR assay for quantification of HIV-1 RNA in plasma: application to acute retroviral infection. *J Clin Microbiol* 1994;32:292–300.
54. Cao Y, Ho DD, Todd J, et al. Clinical evaluation of branched DNA signal amplification for quantifying HIV type 1 in human plasma. *AIDS Res Hum Retroviruses* 1995;11:353–361.
55. Barre-Sinoussi F, Chermann JC, Rey F, et al. Isolation of a T-lymphotropic retrovirus from a patient at risk for acquired immune deficiency syndrome (AIDS). *Science* 1983;220:868–871.
56. Popovic M, Sarngadharan MG, Read E, Gallo RC. Detection, isolation, and continuous production of cytopathic retroviruses (HTLV-III) from patients with AIDS and pre-AIDS. *Science* 1984;224: 497–500.
57. Gallo RC, Salahuddin SZ, Popovic M, et al. Frequent detection and isolation of cytopathic retroviruses (HTLV-III) from patients with AIDS and at risk for AIDS. *Science* 1984;224:500–503.
58. Ho DD, Sargadharan MG, Resnick L, DiMarzo-Veronese F, Rota TR, Hirsch MS. Primary human T-lymphotropic virus type III infection. *Ann Intern Med* 1985;103:880–883.
59. Cooper DA, Gold J, MacLean P, et al. Acute AIDS retrovirus infection: definition of a clinical illness associated with seroconversion. *Lancet* 1985;i:537–540.
60. Daar ES, Moudgil T, Meyer RD, Ho DD. Transient high levels of viremia in patients with primary human immunodeficiency virus type 1 infection. *N Engl J Med* 1991;324:961–964.
61. Clark SJ, Saag MS, Decker WD, et al. High titers of cytopathic virus in plasma of patients with symptomatic primary HIV-1 infection. *N Engl J Med* 1991;324:954–960.
62. Pantaleo G, Graziosi C, Demarest JF, et al. HIV infection is active and progressive in lymphoid tissue during the clinically latent stage of disease. *Nature* 1993;362:355–358.
63. Embreston J, Zupanic M, Beneke J, et al. Analysis of human immunodeficiency virus-infected tissues by amplification and in situ hybridization reveals latent and permissive infections at single-cell resolution. *Proc Natl Acad Sci USA* 1993;90:357–361.
64. Ho DD, Neumann AU, Perelson AS, Chen W, Leonard JM, Markowitz M. Rapid turnover of plasma virions and CD4 lymphocytes in HIV-1 infection. *Nature* 1995;373:123–126.
65. Wei X, Ghosh SK, Taylor ME, et al. Viral dynamics in human immunodeficiency virus type 1 infection. *Nature* 1995;373:117–122.
66. Perelson AS, Neumann AU, Markowitz M, Leonard JM, Ho DD. HIV-1 dynamics in vivo: virion clearance rate, infected cell life span, and viral generation time. *Science* 1996;271:1582–1586.
67. Tersmette M, Schuitemaker H. Virulent AIDS strains? *AIDS* 1993;7: 1123–1125.
68. Zinkernagel RM, Hengartner H. T-cell-mediated immunopathology versus direct cytolysis by virus: implications for HIV and AIDS. *Immunol Today* 1994;15:262–268.
69. Westendorp MO, Frank R, Ochsenbauer C, et al. Sensitization of T cells to CD95-mediated apoptosis by HIV-1 Tat and gp120. *Nature* 1995;375:497–500.
70. Meyaard L, Schuitemaker H, Miedema F. T-cell dysfunction in HIV infection: anergy due to defective antigen-presenting cell function. *Immunol Today* 1993;14:161–163.
71. Danner SA, Carr A, Leonard JM, et al. A short-term study of the safety, pharmacokinetics, and efficacy of ritonavir, an inhibitor of HIV-1 protease. *N Engl J Med* 1995;333:1528–1533.
72. Markowitz M, Saag M, Powderly WG, et al. A preliminary study of ritonavir, an inhibitor of HIV-1 protease, to treat HIV-1 infection. *N Engl J Med* 1995;333:1534–1539.
73. Steigbigel RT, Berry P, Mellors J, et al. Efficacy and safety of the HIV protease inhibitor indinavir sulfate (MK639) at escalating dose. 3rd Conference on Retroviruses and Opportunistic Infections, Washington, DC 1996;146.
74. Gulick RM, Mellors J, Havlir D, et al. Potent and sustained antiretroviral activity of indinavir (IDV), zidovudine (ZDV) and lamivudine (3TC). XI International Conference on AIDS, Vancouver, British Columbia, Canada 1996;Th.B.931.
75. Cameron B, Heath-Chiozzi M, Kravcik S. Prolongation of life and prevention of AIDS in advanced HIV immunodeficiency with ritonavir. 3rd Conference on Retroviruses and Opportunistic Infections, Washington, DC 1996;LB6a.
76. Schacker T, Collier AC, Hughes J, Shea T, Corey L. Clinical and epidemiologic features of primary HIV infection. *Ann Intern Med* 1996; 125:257–264.
77. Markowitz M, Y. C, Hurley A, et al. Triple therapy with AZT,3TC, and ritonavir in 12 subjects newly infected with HIV-1, XI International Conference on AIDS, Vancouver, Canada, 1996.
78. Koup RA, Safrit JT, Cao Y, et al. Temporal association of cellular immune responses with the initial control of viremia in primary HIV-1 syndrome. *J Virol* 1994;68:4650–4655.
79. Moore JP, Cao Y, Ho DD, Koup RA. Development of the anti-gp120 antibody response during seroconversion to human immunodeficiency virus type 1. *J Virol* 1994;68:5142–5155.
80. O'Brien TR, Blattner WA, Waters D, et al. Serum HIV-1 RNA levels and time to development of AIDS in the multicenter hemophilia cohort study. *JAMA* 1996;276:105–110.
81. Mellors JW, Kingsley LA, Rinaldo Jr. CR, et al. Quantitation of HIV-1 RNA in plasma predicts outcome after seroconversion. *Ann Intern Med* 1995;122:573–579.
82. Pantaleo G, Demarest JF, Soudeyns H, et al. Major expansion of CD8-T lymphocytes with a predominant V$\beta$ usage during the primary immune response to HIV. *Nature* 1994;370:463–467.
83. Pantaleo G, Demarest JF, Schacker T, et al. The qualitative nature of the primary immune response to HIV infection is a prognosticator of disease progression independent of the initial level of plasma viremia. *Proc Natl Acad Sci USA* 1997;94:254–258.

84. Kinloch-de Lo s S, Hirschel BJ, Hoen B, et al. A controlled trial of zidovudine in primary human immunodeficiency virus infection. *N Engl J Med* 1995;333:408–413.
85. Markowitz M, Cao Y, Vesanen M, et al. Recent HIV infection treated with AZT, 3TC, and a potent protease inhibitor. 4th Conference on Retroviruses and Opportunistic Infections, Washington, DC, 1997.
86. Fauci AS. Multifactorial nature of human immunodeficiency virus disease: implications for therapy. *Science* 1993;262:1011–1018.
87. Haynes B, Pantaleo G, Fauci AS. Toward an understanding of the correlates of protective immunity to HIV infection. *Science* 1996;271: 324–327.
88. Huang Y, Paxton WA, Wolinsky SM, et al. The role of a mutant CCR5 allele in HIV-1 transmission and disease progression. *Nature Med* 1996;2(11):1240–1243.
89. Mellors JW, Rinaldo Jr. CR, Gupta P, White RM, Todd JA, Kingsley LA. Prognosis in HIV-1 infection predicted by the quantity of virus in plasma. *Science* 1996;272:1167–1170.
90. Volberding PA, Lagakos SW, Koch MA, et al. Zidovudine in asymptomatic human immunodeficiency virus infection: a controlled trial in persons with fewer than 500 CD4-positive cells per cubic millimeter. *N Engl J Med* 1990;322:941–949.
91. Concorde Committee: MRC/ANRS randomised double-blind controlled trial of immediate and deferred zidovudine in symptom-free HIV infection. *Lancet* 1994;343:871–881.
92. Carpenter CCJ, Fischl MA, Hammer SM, et al. Antiretroviral therapy for HIV infection in 1996. *JAMA* 1996;276:146–152.
93. Ho DD. Time to hit HIV early and hard (editorial). *N Engl J Med* 1995;333:450–451.
94. Fauci AS. Host factors and the pathogenesis of HIV-induced disease. *Nature* 1996;384:530–534.
95. Cao Y, Qin L, Zhang L, Safrit J, Ho DD. Virologic and immunologic characterization of long-term survivors of human immunodeficiency virus type 1 infection. *N Engl J Med* 1995;332:201–208.
96. Pantaleo G, Menzo S, Vaccarezza M, et al. Studies in subjects with long-term nonprogressive human immunodeficiency virus infection. *N Engl J Med* 1995;332:209–216.
97. CDC surveillance case definitions for acquired immunodeficiency syndrome. *MMWR* 1987;36(suppl).
98. Connor RI, Ho DD. Human immunodeficiency virus type 1 variants with increased replicative capacity develop during the asymptomatic stage before disease progression. *J Virol* 1994;68:4400–4408.
99. Connor RI, Mohri H, Cao Y, Ho DD. Increased viral burden and cytopathicity correlate temporally with CD4- T-lymphocyte decline and clinical progression in HIV-1 infected individuals. *J Virol* 1993;67: 1772–1778.
100. Doranz BJ, Rucker J, Yanjie Y, et al. A dual-tropic primary HIV-1 isolate that uses fusin and the b-chemokine receptors CKR-5, CKR-3, and CKR-2b as fusion cofactors. *Cell* 1996;85:1149–1158.
101. Connor R, Ho D, Kuritzkes D, Richman D. Human Immunodeficiency Virus. In: Richman D, Whitley R, Hayden F, eds. *Clinical virology.* New York: Churchill-Livingstone, 1997;707–754.
102. Chang Y, Cesarman E, Pessin MS, et al. Identification of herpesvirus-like DNA sequences in AIDS-associated Kaposi's sarcoma. *Science* 1994;266:1865–1869.
103. Simpson DM, Tagliati M. Neurologic manifestations of HIV infection. *Ann Intern Med* 1994;121:769–785.
104. Cavert W, Staskus K, Zupancic M, et al. Quantitative in situ hybridization measurement of HIV-1 RNA clearance kinetics from lymphoid tissue cellular compartments during triple-drug therapy. 4th Conference on Retroviruses and Opportunistic Infections, Washington, DC, 1997.
105. Perelson AS, Essunger P, Markowitz M, Ho DD. How long should treatment be given if we had an antiretroviral regimen that completely blocks HIV replication? XI International Conference on AIDS, Vancouver, British Columbia, Canada 1996;LB.930.
106. McCray E, Group TcNS. Occupational risk of the acquired immunodeficiency syndrome among health care workers. *N Engl J Med* 1986; 314:1127–1132.
107. Henderson DK, Saah A, Zak B. Risk of nosocomial infection with human T-cell lymphotropic virus type III/lymphadenopathy-associated virus in a large cohort of intensively exposed health care workers. *Ann Intern Med* 1986;104:644–647.
108. Gerberding JL, Littell C, Tarkington A, Brown A, Schecter WP. Risk of exposure of surgical personnel to patients' blood during surgery at San Francisco General Hospital. *N Engl J Med* 1990;322:1788–1793.
109. CDC. Evaluation of human T-lymphotropic virus type III/lymphadenopathy-associated virus infection in health-care personnel—United States. *MMWR* 1985;34:575–578.
110. CDC. Summary and recommendations for preventing transmission of infection with human T-lymphotropic virus type III/lymphadenopathy-associated virus in the workplace. *MMWR* 1985;34:681–685, 691–695.
111. CDC. Human immunodeficiency virus infections in health-care workers exposed to blood of infected patients. *MMWR* 1987;36:285–289.
112. Henderson DK, Fahey B, Willy M. Risk for occupational transmission of human immunodeficiency virus type 1 (HIV-1) associated with clinical exposures: a prospective evaluation. *Ann Intern Med* 1990; 113:740–746.
113. CDC. Acquired immune deficiency syndrome: precautions for clinical and laboratory staffs. *MMWR* 1982;31:577–580.
114. Curran J, Morgan W, Hardy A, Jaffe HW, Darrow WW, Dowdle WR. The epidemiology of AIDS: current status and future prospects. *Science* 1985;229:1352–1357.
115. Curran J, Jaffe H, Hardy A, Morgan WM, Selik RM, Dondero TJ. Epidemiology of HIV infection and AIDS in the United States. *Science* 1988;239:610–616.
116. Gershon R, Vlahov D, Nelson K. The risk of transmission of HIV-1 through nonpercutaneous, non-sexual modes—a review. *AIDS* 1990; 4:645–650.
117. Burke DS, Brundage JF, Herbold JR. Human immunodeficiency virus infections among civilian applicants for United States military service, October 1985 to March 1986. *N Engl J Med* 1987;317:131–136.
118. CDC. Trends in human immunodeficiency virus infection among civilian applicants for military service— United States, October 1985-December 1986. *MMWR* 1987;35:273–276.
119. Robert-Guroff M, Weiss SH, Giron JA, et al. Prevalence of antibodies to HTLV-I, -II, -II in intravenous drug abusers from an AIDS endemic region. *JAMA* 1986;255:3133–3137.
120. Chaisson RE, Moss AR, Onnishi R, Osmond D, Carlson JR. Human immunodeficiency virus infection in heterosexual intravenous drug users in San Francisco. *Am J Public Health* 1988;77:169–172.
121. Thomas E, Booth C, Riley MG. The new untouchables: anxiety over AIDS is verging on hysteria in some parts of the country. *Time* 1985; 126:24–26.
122. Fear of AIDS infects the nation. *US News World Rep* 1983;94:13.
123. CDC. Recommendations for preventing transmission of infection with human T-lymphotropic virus type III/lymphadenopathy-associated virus during invasive procedures. *MMWR* 1986;35:221–223.
124. CDC. Recommendations for prevention of HIV transmission in health-care settings. *MMWR* 1987;36(suppl 2S):1S–19S.
125. CDC. Universal precautions for prevention of transmission of human immunodeficiency virus, hepatitis B virus, and other bloodborne pathogens in health-care setting. *MMWR* 1988;37:377–382, 387–388.
126. CDC. Understanding AIDS: an information brochure being mailed to all US households. *MMWR* 1988;37:261–269.
127. CDC. HIV epidemic and AIDS: trends in knowledge—United States. *MMWR* 1989;38:353–358, 363.
128. CDC. Guidelines for prevention of human immunodeficiency virus and hepatitis B virus to health care and public safety workers. *MMWR* 1989;38:S–6.
129. Herbold JR. AIDS policy development within the Department of Defense. *Milit Med* 1986;151:623–627.
130. Damato JJ, O'Bryen BN, Fuller SA, Roberts CR, Redfield RR, Burke DS. Resolution of indeterminate HIV-1 test data using the Department of Defense HIV-1 testing program. *Lab Med* 1991;22:107–113.
131. Redfield RR, Wright DC, James WD, Jones TS, Brown C, Burke DS. Disseminated vaccinia in a military recruit with HTLV-III disease. *N Engl J Med* 1987;316:673–676.
132. Brown AA, Brundage JF, Tomlinson JP, Burke DS. The US army HIV testing program: the first decade. *Milit Med* 1996;161:117–122.
133. Tramont EC, Redfield R, Burke D, Takafuji ET, Wright C, Moore W. HTLV-111/LAV infections in the military. *Milit Med* 1987;152: 105–106.
134. Garland FC, Mayers DL, Hickey TM. Incidence of human immunodeficiency virus seroconversion in US Navy and Marine Corps personnel, 1986 through 1988. *JAMA* 1989;262:3161–3165.
135. Brown AE, Newby JH, Ray KL, Jackson JN, Burke DS. Prevention and treatment of HIV infections in minorities in the US military: a review of military research. *Milit Med* 1996;161:123–127.

136. Department of the Army. Identification, surveillance, and administration of personnel infected with human immunodeficiency virus (HIV) (revised 1994). *Army Regulation* 1988;600–110.
137. Torre D, Sampietro C, Ferraro G, Zeroli C, Speranza F. Transmission of HIV-1 via sports injury. *Lancet* 1990;335:1105.
138. Loveday C, and others. HIV and sport. *Lancet* 1990;335:1532.
139. Putting on the gloves to fight AIDS. *Newsweek* 1987;110:49.
140. Gunby P. Boxing: AIDS. *JAMA* 1988;259:1613.
141. Goldsmith MF. When sports and HIV share the bill, smart money goes on common sense. *JAMA* 1992;267:1311–1314.
142. American Academy of Pediatrics Committee on Sports Medicine and Fitness. Human immunodeficiency virus [acquired immunodeficiency syndrome (AIDS) virus] in the athletic setting. *Pediatrics* 1991;88:640–641.
143. Brown LS, Phillips RY, Brown CL, Knowlan D, Castle L, Moyer J. HIV/AIDS policies and sports: the national football league. *Med Sci Sports Exerc* 1994;26:403–407.
144. Shepherd RJ, Verde TJ, Thomas SG, Shek P. Physical activity and the immune system. *Can J Sport Sci* 1991;16:169–185.
145. Johnson RJ. HIV in athletes: What are the risks? Who can compete? *Postgrad Med* 1992;92:73–75, 79–80.
146. LaPerriere A, Fletcher MA, Antoni MH, Klimas NG, Ironson G, Schneiderman N. Aerobic exercise training in an AIDS risk group. *Int J Sports Med* 1991;12(suppl 1):S53–57.
147. Rigsby LW, Dishman RK, Jackson AW, Maclean GS, Raven PB. Effects of exercise training on men seropositive for the human immunodeficiency virus-1. *Med Sci Sports Exerc* 1992;24:6–12.
148. Levy R, Bredesen D. Controversies in HIV-related central nervous system disease: neuropsychological aspects of HIV-1 infection. In: Volberding P, Jacobson M, eds. *AIDS clinical review.* New York: Marcel Dekker, 1989;151–191.
149. Clifford D, Jacoby R, Miller J, Seyfried WZ, Glicksman M. Neuropsychometric performance of asymptomatic HIV-infected subjects. *AIDS* 1990;4:767–774.
150. American College of Physicians. Position paper: acquired immunodeficiency syndrome. *Ann Intern Med* 1986;104:575–581.
151. Stienbrook R, Lo B, Tirpack J. Ethical dilemmas in caring for patients with the acquired immunodeficiency syndrome. *Ann Intern Med* 1985;103:787–790.
152. Bernstein C, Rabkin J, Wolland H. Medical and dental students' attitudes about the AIDS epidemic. *Acad Med* 1990;65:458–460.
153. Hayward R, Shapiro M. A national study of AIDS and residency training: experiences, concerns, and consequences. *Ann Intern Med* 1991; 114:23–32.
154. Tokars JI, Marcus R, Culver DH, et al. Surveillance of HIV infection and zidovudine use among health care workers after occupational exposure to HIV-infected blood. The CDC Cooperative Needlestick Surveillance Group. *Ann Intern Med* 1993;118:913–919.
155. Ippolito G, Puro P, DeCarli G. The Italian Study Group on Occupational Risk of HIV Infection. The risk of occupational HIV infection in health care workers: Italian multicenter study. *Arch Int Med* 1993; 153:1451–1458.
156. CDC. Health-care workers with documented and possible occupationally acquired AIDS/HIV infection, by occupation, reported through March 1993, United States. *HIV/AIDS Surveillance Report* 1993 (May).
157. Henderson D. HIV in the health care setting. In: Mandell GE, Bennet JE, Dolin R, eds. *Principles and practice of infectious diseases.* New York: Churchill-Livingstone, 1995:2632–2656.
158. Weiss S, Goedert J, Gartner S. Risk of human immunodeficiency virus (HIV-1) infection among laboratory workers. *Science* 1988;239:68–71.
159. Mastro TD, Satten GA, Nopkesorn T, Sangkharomys S, Longini IM. Probability of female to male transmission of HIV-1 in Thailand. *Lancet* 1994;343:204–207.
160. Fischl M, Dickenson GM, Scott GB, Klimas N, Fletcher MA, Parks W. Evaluation of heterosexual partners, children, and household contacts of adults with AIDS. *JAMA* 1987;257:640–644.
161. Andiman WA, Modlin JF. Vertical transmission. In: Pizzo PA, Wilfert CM, eds. *Pediatric AIDS.* Baltimore: Williams and Wilkins, 1991: 140–155.
162. Ward JW, Deppe DA, Samson S. Risk of human immunodeficiency virus infection from blood donors who later developed the acquired immunodeficiency virus syndrome. *Ann Intern Med* 1987;106:61–62.
163. CDC. Case-control study of HIV seroconversion in health-care workers after percutaneous exposure to HIV-infected blood—France, United Kingdom, and United States, January 1988-August 1994. *MMWR* 1995;44:929–933.
164. Gerberding J. Prophylaxis for occupational exposure to HIV. *Ann Intern Med* 1996;125:497–501.
165. CDC. Surveillance for occupationally acquired HIV infection—United States 1981–1992. *MMWR* 1992;41:823–825.
166. Gerberding JL, Henderson DK. Design of rational infection control policies for human immunodeficiency virus infection. *J Infect Dis* 1987;156:861–864.
167. Whitby M, Stead P, Saiman J. Needlestick injury: impact of a recapping device and an associated education program. *Infect Control Hosp Epidemiol* 1991;12:220–225.
168. Beekman SE, Vlahov D, Koziol DE, McShalley ED, Schmitt JM. Temporal association between implementation of universal precautions and a sustained, progressive decrease in percutaneous exposures to blood. *Clin Infect Dis* 1994;18:562–569.
169. Haiduven D, DeMaio T, Stevens D. A five year study of needlestick injuries: significant reduction associated with communication, education, and convenient placement of sharps containers. *Infect Control Hosp Epidemiol* 1992;13:265–271.
170. Garner JS, Hospital Infection Control Practices Advisory Committee. Guideline for isolation precautions in hospitals. *Infect Control Hosp Epidemiol* 1996;17:53–80.
171. Kaplan JC, Crawford DC, Durno AG, Schooley RT. Inactivation of human immunodeficiency virus by Betadine. *Infect Control* 1987;8: 412–414.
172. Ruprecht RM, O'Brien LG, Rossoni LD, Nusinoff S. Suppression of mouse viraemia and retroviral disease by 3′-azido-3′ deoxythymidine. *Nature* 1986;323:467–469.
173. Tavares L, Roneker C, Johnston K, Lehrman SN, de Noronha F. 3′-azido-3′ deoxythymidine in feline leukemia virus-infected cats: a model of therapy and prophylaxis of AIDS. *Cancer Res* 1987;47: 3190–3194.
174. Henderson DK, Gerberding JL. Prophylactic zidovudine after occupational exposure to the human immunodeficiency virus: an interim analysis. *J Infect Dis* 1989;160:321–327.
175. Henderson DK, Beekman SE, Gerberding JL. Post-exposure antiviral chemoprophylaxis following occupational exposure to the human immunodeficiency virus. *AIDS Updates* 1990;3:1–8.
176. LaFon S, Mooney B, McMullen J, et al. A double-blind, placebo-controlled study of the safety and efficacy of Retrovir (zidovudine) as a chemoprophylactic agent in health care workers exposed to HIV. 30th Interscience Conference on Antimicrobial Agents and Chemotherapy 1990:Abstract 489.
177. CDC. Recommendation of the US Public Health Service Task Force on the use of zidovudine to reduce perinatal transmission of human immunodeficiency virus. *MMWR* 1994;43(RR-11):1–20.
178. CDC. Update: provisional Public Health Service recommendations for chemoprophylaxis after occupational exposure to HIV. *MMWR* 1996;44:468–472, 45:422.
179. Gerberding JL. Management of occupational exposures to bloodborne viruses. *N Engl J Med* 1995;322:444–451.
180. CDC. Current trends: acquired immunodeficiency syndrome (AIDS). Precautions for health care workers and allied professionals. *MMWR* 1983;32:450–451.
181. Bankowski MJ, Landay AL, Staes B, et al. Postmortem recovery of human immunodeficiency virus type 1 from plasma and mononuclear cells. Implications for occupational exposure. *Arch Pathol Lab Med* 1992;116:1124–1127.
182. Nyberg M, Suni J, Heldis M. Isolation of human immunodeficiency virus (HIV) at autopsy. *Am J Clin Pathol* 1990;94:422–425.
183. Atlantic Region/Eastern Division SCI. Occupational exposure to bloodborne pathogens. *OSHA compliance training lesson plan* 1992; Module 2:(unpublished), revised March 1992.
184. Department of Labor. Occupational exposure to bloodborne pathogens: final rule. *Fed Register* 1991;56:64175–64182.
185. Ciesielski C, Marianos D, Ou C-Y, et al. Transmission of human immunodeficiency virus in a dental practice. *Ann Intern Med* 1992; 116:798–805.
186. Lowenfels A, Wormser G. Risk of transmission of HIV from surgeon to patient. *N Engl J Med* 1991;325:888–889.
187. Chant K, Lowe D, Rubin G, et al. Patient-to-patient transmission of HIV in private surgical consulting rooms. *Lancet* 1993;342:1548–1549.

188. Ragg M. Patient-to-patient HIV transmission trial. *Lancet* 1994;344: 1695.
189. CDC. Antibody to human immunodeficiency virus in female prostitutes. *MMWR* 1987;36:157–161.
190. Padian N. Prostitute women and AIDS: epidemiology. *AIDS* 1988;2: 413–419.
191. Piot P, Kreiss JK, Ndinya-Achola JO,et al. Heterosexual transmission of AIDS. *AIDS* 1987;1:199–206.
192. Day S. Prostitute women and AIDS: anthropology. *AIDS* 1988;2: 421–428.
193. Piot P, Plummer FA, Rey M-A, et al. Retrospective sero-epidemiology of AIDS virus infection in Nairobi populations. *J Infect Dis* 1987;155: 1108–1112.
194. Kunawararak P, Beyrer C, Natpratan C, et al. The epidemiology of HIV and syphilis among male commercial sex workers in norther Thailand. *AIDS* 1995;9:517–521.
195. Singh YN. Long distance truck drivers in India: HIV infection and their possible role in disseminating HIV into rural areas. *Int J STD AIDS* 1994;5:137–138.
196. Karim Q, Karim SSA, Soldan K, Zondi M. Reducing the risk of HIV infection among South African sex workers: socioeconomic and gender barriers. *Am J Public Health* 1995;85:1521–1525.
197. Carswell JW, Lloyd G, Howells J. Prevalence of HIV-1 in East African lorry drivers. *AIDS* 1989;3:767–768.
198. Singh YN, Mlaviya AN. Experience of HIV prevention interventions among female sex workers in Delhi, India. *Int J STD AIDS* 1994;5: 56–57.
199. Das A, Jana S, Chakraborty AK, Khodakevic L, Chakraborty MS, Pal NK. Community-based survey of STD/HIV infection among commercial sex workers in Calcutta (India), Part III: clinical findings of sexually transmitted diseases. *J Commun Dis* 1994;26:192–196.
200. Pal NK, Chakraborty MS, Das A, Kodakevich L, Jana S, Chakraborty AK. Community-based survey of STD/HIV infection among commercial sex workers in Calcutta (India), Part IV: STDs and related risk factors. *J Commun Dis* 1994;26:197–202.
201. Kreiss JK, Koech D, Plummer FA, et al. AIDS virus infection in Nairobi prostitutes: spread of the epidemic to East Africa. *N Engl J Med* 1986;314:414–418.
202. Albert AE, Warner DL, Hatcher RA, Trussel J, Bennet C. Condom use among female commercial sex workers in Nevada's legal brothels. *Am J Public Health* 1995;85:1514–1520.
203. Richters J, Donovan B, Gerofi J, Watson L. Low condom breakage rate in commercial sex. *Lancet* 1988;2:1487–1488.
204. Mann J, Quinn TC, Piot P. Condom use and HIV infections among prostitutes in Zaire. *N Engl J Med* 1987;316:345.
205. Ngugi EN, Simonsen JN, Bosire M, et al. Prevention of transmission of human immunodeficiency virus in Africa: effectiveness of condom promotion and health education among prostitutes. *Lancet* 1988;2: 887.
206. Roumeliotou A, Papautsakis G, Kallinikos G, Papaevangelou G. Effectiveness of condom use in preventing HIV infection in prostitutes. *Lancet* 1988;2:1249.
207. Kreiss J, Ngugi E, holmes K, Ndinya-Achola J, Waiyaki P. Efficacy of nonoxynol-9 contraceptive sponge use in preventing heterosexual acquisition of HIV in Nairobi prostitutes. *JAMA* 1992;268: 477–482.
208. Stein ZA. More on women and the prevention of HIV infection. *Am J Public Health* 1995;85:1485–1487.
209. Fischbacher CM, Njeru JM. Impact of improved condom supply on condom use by prostitute women. *AIDS* 1994;8:856–857.
210. Limanonda B, VanGriensven GJP, Changvatana N, et al. Condom use and risk factors for HIV-1 infection among female commercial sex workers in Thailand. *Am J Public Health* 1994;84:2026–2027.
211. Mastro TD, Limpakarnjanarat K. Condom use in Thailand: How much is it slowing the HIV/AIDS epidemic? *AIDS* 1995;9:523–525.
212. Hannenberg RS, Rojanapithayakorn W, Kunasol P, Sokal DC. Impact of Thailand's HIV-control programme as indicated by the decline of STDs. *Lancet* 1994;344:243–245.
213. McKeganey NP, Finlay A, Barnard MA. The inappropriateness of psycho-social models of risk behavior for understanding HIV-related risk practices among Glasgow male prostitutes. *AIDS Care* 1992;4: 131–137.
214. Gattari P, Spizzichino L, Valenzi C, Zaccarelli M, Rezza G. Behavioral patterns and HIV infection among drug-using transvestites practicing prostitution in Rome. *AIDS Care* 1992;4:83–87.
215. Morris M, Pramvalratana A, Podhisita C, Wawer M. Determinants of condom use with commercial sex partners in Thailand. *AIDS* 1994;8: 504–515.
216. Morrison CC, Ruben SM, Wakefield D. Female street prostitution in Liverpool. *AIDS* 1994;8:1194–1195.
217. Coutinho RA, van Andel RLM, Rijsdijk TJ. Role of male prostitutes in the spread of sexually transmitted diseases and human immunodeficiency virus. *Genitourin Med* 1988;64:207–208.
218. Wirawan DN, Fajans P, Ford K. AIDS and STDs: risk behavior patterns in female sex workers in Bali, Indonesia. *AIDS Care* 1993;5: 289–303.
219. Archibald CP, Chan RKW, Wong ML, Goh A, Goh CL. Evaluation of a safe-sex intervention program among sex workers in Singapore. *Int J STD AIDS* 1994;5:268–272.
220. Wong KL, LSS, Lo YC, Lo KK. Condom use among female commercial sex workers and male clients in Hong Kong. *Int J STD AIDS* 1994;5:287–289.
221. Van den Hoek J, Coutinho RA, van Haastrecht HJA, van Zadelhoff AW, Goudsmit J. Prevalence and risk factors of HIV infections among drug users and drug-using prostitutes in Amsterdam. *AIDS* 1988;2:55–60.
222. Celentano DD, Pasakorn A, Sussman L, et al. HIV-1 infection among lower-class commercial sex workers in Chiang Mai, Thailand. *AIDS* 1994;8:533–537.
223. Aim G, DeVincenzi I, Ancelle-Park R, Brunet J-B, Catalon F. HIV infection in French prostitutes. *AIDS* 1989;3:767–768.
224. Asamoah-Adu A, Weir S, Pappoe M, Kanlisi N, Neequaye A, Lamptey P. Evaluation of a targeted AIDS prevention intervention to increase condom use in Ghana. *AIDS* 1994;8:239–246.
225. Laga MA, Alary M, Nzila N, et al. Condom promotion, STDs treatment, and declining incidence of HIV-1 infection in female Zairian sex workers. *Lancet* 1994;344:246–248.
226. Anzala OA, Nagelkerke NJD, Bwayo JJ, et al. Rapid progression to disease in African sex workers. *J Infect Dis* 1995;171:686–689.


## APPENDIX A: STANDARD PRECAUTIONS TO PREVENT TRANSMISSION

In 1985, the CDC published guidelines intended to reduce the risk of occupational transmission of blood-borne pathogens. These centered on the concept that all patients should be assumed to be infectious for HIV and other blood-borne pathogens. Initially called "Universal Precautions," these guidelines were recently renamed "Standard Precautions" with the recognition that they form the necessary basis of infection control practice but must be supplemented by additional precautions appropriate to other modes of pathogen transmission.

### Standard Precautions: Personal Protective Gear

With all patients, contact with moist body substances and surfaces should be minimized by the use of handwashing, gloves, gowns, and face shields or other eye/mouth barriers.

Hand washing: Wash skin surfaces contaminated with moist body substances (except sweat) or by potentially contaminated items immediately and thoroughly with warm water and plain soap. Antimicrobial agents are not necessary except in special, epidemic/outbreak circumstances. Wash hands after gloves are removed, even if the gloves are intact. Waterless antiseptic hand cleanser should be provided on response units where adequate conventional facilities are not available.

Barriers: Put on clean gloves just before touching blood, body fluids, secretions, excretions, or contaminated items or mucous membranes or nonintact skin. Change gloves between tasks and procedures on the same patient after contact with highly contaminated material and remove them promptly before going on to the next patient or touching noncontaminated surfaces or items. Wash hands after removing gloves.

A gown and face shield (or mask/goggles combination) should be used during procedures and patient care activities likely to generate splashes or sprays of blood or body fluids. Remove these as soon as possible and dispose of them appropriately to minimize contamination to the practitioner, other patients, and the environment.

Keep mouthpieces, resuscitation bags, or other ventilation devices available for use in areas where resuscitation is predictable.

## Standard Precautions: Disinfection, Decontamination, and Disposal

### *Needles and Sharps Disposal*

Do not recap or otherwise manipulate used needles in any way. After use, put disposable syringe/needle units, scalpel blades, and other sharp items in puncture-resistant containers for disposal. Place these containers as close as practical to use areas, including carrying smaller ones to emergency response sites such as "codes" or accident scenes. Leave reusable needles on syringe bodies and place in a puncture-resistant container for transport to the reprocessing area.

### *Cleaning and Decontaminating Blood Spills*

Promptly clean up all spills of blood and potentially infectious body fluids using an Environmental Protection Agency (EPA)-approved germicide or a 1:100 solution of household bleach.

Remove visible material with disposable or other appropriate means that will ensure against direct contact with blood and while wearing gloves and barrier clothing appropriate to Standard Precautions. Wear impervious shoe covers where there is massive contamination on floors.

Decontaminate the area with an appropriate germicide.

Remove soiled cleaning materials in plastic bags or other containers that minimize risk of secondary contamination to disposal or decontamination areas. Dispose of/process according to agency/OSHA policy. Remove soiled protective clothing *while still wearing gloves*; dispose of or contain for decontamination as appropriate.

Dispose of gloves last *and wash hands after removing gloves.*

### *Laundry*

The risk of disease transmission from blood-borne pathogens via soiled linen is negligible. Hygienic storage of clean and soiled linen are adequate and recommended. However, handle or agitate soiled linen as little as possible to minimize gross microbial contamination of the air and those handling the linen. Soiled linen should be bagged at origin. If blood-soiled, it should be transported in impervious bags. Normal hospital standard laundry cycles and cleansers are adequate and appropriate.

### *Decontamination and Laundering of Protective Clothing*

Handle contaminated protective work clothing in the same manner as linens. Those who bag, transport, or launder such clothing should wear gloves. Boots and leather goods can be decontaminated by brush-scrubbing with soap and hot water, with care to avoid splattering.

### *Infectious Waste*

Procedures for disposal of infectious waste are determined by risk of disease transmission and by local regulation. *Local regulations vary widely and must be followed.*

Infectious waste, in general, is incinerated or decontaminated and placed in a sanitary landfill. Bulk blood, suctioned fluids, excretions, and secretions may be carefully poured down a drain connected to a sanitary sewer, where local law permits this. Sanitary sewers can also be used to dispose of other infectious wastes that can be ground and flushed into the sewer, again, if permitted. Sharps containers must be placed in impervious bags for transport to appropriate—and legal—disposal locations.

## APPENDIX B: HIV POSTEXPOSURE MANAGEMENT

For any occupational exposure with potential for transmission of HIV, every effort must be made to obtain current information on the source. The interests of injured workers must take precedence over strict confidentiality. However, worker confidentiality must be protected through all phases of postinjury follow-up.

Cleanse wounds as described above (see Secondary Prevention: Decontamination of Wounds, in text above).

If the source is seronegative, offer baseline testing of exposed workers with follow-up testing 12 weeks later.

If the source is unknown, refuses testing, is known to be HIV positive, or has AIDS, counsel exposed workers about the risk of infection and evaluate them clinically and serologically for evidence of HIV infection as soon as possible. Postexposure chemoprophylaxis (PEP) is now the standard of care (see Tables 5 and 6), but medications and protocols may change. Those providing medical care to workers potentially exposed to HIV must stay well informed on Public Health Service (PHS) guidelines.

Advise exposed workers to report and seek evaluation of any acute febrile illness that occurs within 12 weeks after the exposure. (Such an illness, particularly if accompanied by rash or lymphadenopathy, may indicate HIV infection.) Retest those initially seronegative at 6, 12, and 26 weeks after exposure. During this period (particularly in the first 12 weeks after exposure, by which time most infected people will seroconvert), exposed workers should avoid donating blood and use appropriate sexual prophylaxis.

*Environmental and Occupational Medicine, Third Edition,* edited by William N. Rom.
Lippincott–Raven Publishers, Philadelphia © 1998.

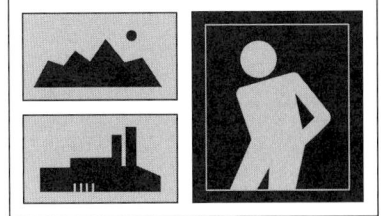

CHAPTER 53

# The Occupational Risk of Tuberculosis Care

Kent A. Sepkowitz and Neil W. Schluger

The occupational risk of tuberculosis (TB) continues to be a subject of intense debate even as the annual incidence of TB has decreased in the United States (1). Cases of both sensitive and multidrug-resistant tuberculosis (MDR-TB) (2) have spread to health care workers (HCWs). According to the Centers for Disease Control and Prevention (CDC), at least 17 workers have developed nosocomially acquired MDR-TB and several have died. Employee tuberculin skin test conversion rates from outbreak hospitals have ranged from 20% to 50% (2), indicating the presence of a large reservoir of HCWs latently infected with resistant strains.

The CDC has periodically updated its recommendations for control of nosocomial TB, most recently in 1994 (3). Three hierarchical elements compose the core of the recommendations, including administrative measures (highest priority), environmental controls, and the use of personal respiratory protective equipment. Because of the potential cost of certain aspects of these recommendations, much controversy and some reconsideration have occurred. Most notably, the type of mask considered acceptable has been broadened to include cheaper and more comfortable equipment.

Despite the concern, the many recommendations, and the reports of nosocomial spread, few scientific studies are available to point the way toward improved occupational control of TB. Early isolation of patients continues to appear to be the best means of controlling TB in hospitals. This chapter reviews historical aspects of the problem, the fundamental principles of transmission, and the various interventions promulgated to improve HCW safety.

K. A. Sepkowitz: Department of Medicine, Memorial Sloan-Kettering Cancer Center, Cornell University Medical College, New York, New York 10021.
N. W. Schluger: Division of Pulmonary and Critical Care Medicine, Chest Service, Bellevue Hospital Center, New York University Medical Center, New York, New York 10016.

## TUBERCULOSIS AS AN OCCUPATIONAL RISK

Health care workers are at increased risk for numerous occupationally acquired infections, ranging from the trivial, such as the common cold, to the serious, including measles and hepatitis B, to the potentially fatal, such as Ebola virus and human immunodeficiency virus (HIV) (4). Physicians' sense of professional duty has varied through the centuries. The debate about a physician's obligation to treat the potentially contagious was reexamined in the 1980s, in the context of the emerging HIV epidemic (5).

A consensus that care of the tuberculous represented an occupational hazard evolved in the 1950s, as a result of dozens of well-conducted prospective studies of infection and disease rates in nursing and medical students (6). Overall, HCWs were determined to have a risk about 2 to 10 times that of the general public, with the highest rates seen in nurses. This recognition led to inclusion of TB as a disease potentially covered by workers' compensation and the development of numerous federally mandated regulations designed to better protect the HCW (6).

## THE TUBERCULIN SKIN TEST: GENERAL CONSIDERATIONS

Tuberculosis is unusual among infections potentially spread to hospital and other staff in that the test used to diagnose the latent disease, the tuberculin skin test, is neither sensitive nor specific. Thus, outbreak investigations, as well as establishment of the baseline prevalence and

**TABLE 1.** *Potential causes of false-negative tuberculin skin-test reactions*

| Category | Factor |
|---|---|
| Related to person tested | Infection (viral,[a] bacterial,[b] fungal[c]) |
| | Live-virus vaccination (measles, mumps, polio) |
| | Metabolic derangements (chronic renal failure) |
| | Nutritional factors (severe protein depletion) |
| | Diseases affecting lymphoid organs (Hodgkin's disease, lymphoma, chronic lymphocytic leukemia, sarcoidosis) |
| | Drugs (corticosteroids, many other immunosuppressive agents) |
| | Age (newborns, elderly patients whose sensitivity has waned) |
| | Recent or overwhelming infection with *M. tuberculosis* |
| | Stress (surgery, burns, mental illness, graft-vs-host reactions) |
| Related to tuberculin used | Improper storage (exposure to light and heat) |
| | Improper dilutions |
| | Chemical denaturation |
| | Contamination |
| | Adsorption (partially controlled by addition of Tween 80) |
| Related to method of tuberculin administration | Injection of too little antigen |
| | Delay in administration after drawing of preparation into syringe |
| | Injection too deep |
| Related to reading of test and recording of results | Inexperienced reader |
| | Conscious or unconscious bias |
| | Error in reading |

[a]HIV, measles, mumps, chickenpox.
[b]Typhoid fever, brucellosis, typhus, leprosy, pertussis, overwhelming TB, TB pleurisy.
[c]South American blastomycosis.
From ref. 12, with permission.

incidence of a reactive test, are confounded by the intrinsic difficulty interpreting the test. Problems with the test may arise at several points: (a) administration of the test, (b) the tuberculin preparation, (c) interpretation of the test, and (d) the status of the host (employee receiving the test). Table 1 lists many of the problems with injecting and interpreting the tuberculin skin test, which are discussed in more detail below.

### The Administration of the Test

Proper technique for administration is well demonstrated on a videotape produced by the CDC ("Mantoux Tuberculin Skin Testing," available free of charge from the CDC, phone number 1-404-639-1819, order #005457; wall charts are also available, order #005564). It is important to "raise a bleb" to be confident that the subsequent result is meaningful. Although the technique is relatively simple, persons who do not administer the test frequently may become less adept at placement of a tuberculin test. Whenever possible, a test should be administered by the person with the most experience and the most recent experience, such as an employee health nurse, rather than someone, such as an attending physician, who is less likely to have performed numerous tests recently.

### The Tuberculin Preparation

In the United States, two tuberculin compounds are approved by the Food and Drug Administration (FDA) for use: Aplisol (Park-Davis, Morris Plains, NJ) and Tubersol (Connaught, Swiftwater, PA). Several recent reports have demonstrated an unacceptably high rate of false-positive responses to Aplisol, leading experts to strongly recommend use of Tubersol only (7,8). Other reports have not demonstrated a problem (9). The multidose preparation must be refrigerated. Once opened, the preparation can be used for about a month. The multipuncture tine test should not be used.

### Interpretation of the Test

Chaparas and colleagues (10) reported a disheartening study that demonstrated the potential for interpretative error, even among experts. In this study, persons with known previous TB and controls were given two tuberculin skin tests (one in each arm) on the same day, using the same lot of tuberculin preparation. Thus, potential variation in the injector, the tuberculin preparation, and the host were controlled for. The result in one arm was then interpreted by one expert, while the result in the contralateral arm was interpreted by a second expert. Analysis showed that the rate of arm-to-arm discordance was as high as 15%.

In addition, exact measurement of the induration provoked by the tuberculin skin test remains difficult. Trained staff must be able to reliably measure the area of induration and record specifics into an employee's chart. A recent French study compared measurement using the palpation technique versus the "ballpoint pen" technique

(11), in which a ballpoint pen is used to draw a line along the arm of the patient from normal skin toward the putative induration. The tip of the pen will get stuck as it hits against the base of the induration. The study found the ballpoint pen technique superior, but still found substantial intraobserver variation and cautioned that interpretation of results near the cutoff point for treatment must include an element of clinical judgment. If used, the ballpoint pen technique should include drawing toward the induration from four directions. The resulting measurement then should be expressed as a two-dimensional size (for example, 8 by 12 mm).

### The Status of the Host

Numerous conditions are associated with false-negative skin tests (Table 1) (12). Most common to clinical practice, the progressive immunodeficiency seen in persons with HIV infection may render a patient anergic (13). The utility of anergy panel testing, however, has not been proven and should not routinely be a part of occupational health evaluation (14).

Other factors may influence the likelihood of a positive response, including age and BCG-vaccination status. A study from Montreal demonstrated that childhood bacille Calmette-Guérin (BCG) vaccination was associated with a positive adult tuberculin result (15), especially when the person was given a two-step test. Such an observation is particularly pertinent in areas such as New York City, where foreign-born, BCG-vaccinated workers constitute a substantial proportion of the health care work force. In such individuals, who are skin tested every 6 to 12 months, some tuberculin "conversions" may in fact represent boosted responses to remote BCG vaccination, not new infection with *Mycobacterium tuberculosis* (MTB), further confounding interpretation of infection control interventions (16). In addition, rates of tuberculin reactivity increase with increasing age in most reported studies.

### The Two-Step Tuberculin Skin Test

A "boosted" response may occur when latently infected persons have a negative response to initial skin testing, but demonstrate a positive response to a second tuberculin test administered within 1 year of the original test (3). This boosting is thought to be due to a sluggish initial response that is more brisk after the second exposure to antigen. Such a change in skin test result may be misinterpreted as new infection due to occupational exposure, particularly if tests are given 6 months apart, rather than from skin test boosting. This response has been called a pseudoconversion (2) and may lead to inaccurate HCW tuberculin conversion rates (17).

The use of two-step testing has been shown to "reduce the likelihood that a boosted reaction is misinterpreted as a new infection" (3) and therefore is recommended by the CDC (3) for hospital employee health programs, depending on the hospital TB rate. In a two-step program, new employees are given the first skin test, and then, among those with a negative initial test, are retested 1 week later. Those reacting to the first or second test are considered tuberculin positive. Once a baseline test has been determined using a two-step approach, two-step testing need not be performed on subsequent skin tests. Previous studies have demonstrated that older age (17,18), atypical mycobacterial infections (19), and previous BCG vaccination (17,20) are associated with higher rates of skin test boosting.

Employee health programs will continue to depend on the relatively undependable tuberculin skin test for many years to come. It has been suggested that complete control of TB may await development of an improved means of identifying patients with latent infection.

## PREVALENCE OF A POSITIVE TEST

The CDC estimates that about 5% of the U.S. population is tuberculin positive, with the rate varying considerably according to age, ethnic group, and location (21). No large-scale surveys, however, have been conducted recently. In the 1970s, Reichman and O'Day (22) found that 12% of 61,000 Board of Education workers in New York City were tuberculin positive, ranging from 8% to 25% according to race (Table 2). From 1980 to 1986, over 2 million skin tests were administered to active duty U. S. Navy and Marine personnel, of whom 0.97% were positive (23). Recent reports from New York City found tuberculin reactivity rates of 7.8% among 2,011 firemen

**TABLE 2.** *Prevalence of tuberculin reactivity among various U.S. groups*

| Institution (reference) | Year | No. of persons tested | Prevalence (%) |
|---|---|---|---|
| U.S. population (21) | 1994 | U.S. population | 4 |
| New York City Board of Education (22) | 1973–1974 | 61,000 | 12 |
| U.S. Navy and U.S. Marines, active-duty personnel (23) | 1980–1986 | 2,000,000 | 0.97 |
| New Mexico Corrections Department (30) | 1986–1987 | — | 10.50 |
| New York State Department of Corrections facilities (30) | 1991 | — | 5.82 |
| New York City firefighters (24) | 1990s | 2,011 | 7.8 |
| Persons seeking social services, New York City (25) | 1990s | 651 | 41 |

**TABLE 3.** *Prevalence of tuberculin reactivity among various U.S. health care worker groups*

| Institution (reference) | Year | No. of persons tested | Prevalence (%) |
|---|---|---|---|
| Pittsburgh VAMC chronic care facility (30) | 1985–1986 | — | 28 |
| Barnes Hospital, St. Louis (all employees) (86) | 1989–1991 | 6,070 | 11.3 |
| Montreal (two hospitals) (27) | 1992–1993 | 522 | 38 |
| St. Clare's Hospital, New York City (new employees)(26) | 1993 | 313 | 40 |
| New York Hospital, New York City (all employees) (45) | 1991–1993 | 773 | 36 |
| Philadelphia (87) | 1993 | 109 | 37 |

(24) and 41% among 651 persons seeking social services (25).

The prevalence of tuberculin reactivity among HCWs is higher than that in the general population (Table 3). This may be due to the large number of HCWs in the United States who were born in TB-endemic countries or who have received BCG vaccination, as well as to the accumulation over time of occupationally transmitted infections. Studies among urban HCWs have found rates ranging from 20% to 40% (Table 3). In one study rates were higher among non-U.S. born (70%) versus U.S. born (20%), as well as among persons >40 years of age (26). In another, rates correlated with duration of employment in a hospital (27).

## INCIDENCE OF TUBERCULIN CONVERSION

### Baseline Conversion Rates

The anticipated conversion rate in non-outbreak settings is poorly defined (Table 3). A survey of 210 U.S. hospitals conducted by the Society for Healthcare Epidemiology of America (SHEA) and the CDC found 561 (0.64%) tuberculin conversions among 87,156 tests performed in HCWs in 1992 (28,28a). Rates in certain urban settings may be higher and exceed 3% annually when community rates are high, even in non-outbreak settings (29). Bowden and McDiarmid (30), reviewing results from 25 studies conducted at institutions not in the midst of outbreaks, found a range varying from less than 0.09% per year among employees in 114 hospitals in Washington State to 5.0% among correctional facility staff in Sacramento, California. Fagan and Poland (31), in a survey of medical students in the United States, found the mean annual conversion rate for all schools was 1.8% (range 0–12%).

### Conversion Rates in Outbreaks

The CDC has reported numerous outbreaks of TB in recent years, and in some the rates of tuberculin conversion among employees have been defined (range 20–50%) (2). Many recent outbreaks have occurred among the HIV infected, with spread resulting from delays in patient isolation and diagnosis. In one outbreak, exposure to an HCW with TB also constituted a significant risk (32).

Investigation of outbreaks prior to the AIDS epidemic established several important transmission principles. In Miami, inadequate ventilation resulted in recirculation of contaminated air and tuberculin conversion among 35% of 60 employees (33). Bronchoscopy of an acid-fast bacillus (AFB) smear–negative patient in San Diego resulted in tuberculin conversion among 10 of 13 present at the procedure (34). This outbreak suggests how significantly certain procedures such as bronchoscopy can amplify risk. Nasotracheal suctioning similarly can augment risk, as demonstrated by an outbreak in a Dallas emergency room where an intubated man, present for only 4 hours, spread infection to at least 16 (14%) of 112 emergency room staff (35). The impact of the unsuspected case was demonstrated by Craven et al. (36), who reported the consequences of 17 unsuspected cases of TB admitted to a teaching hospital and found a significantly higher risk for tuberculin conversion among staff exposed to an unsuspected case versus those not exposed. In Los Angeles in the early 1950s, the number of cases of TB among employees of a city hospital decreased dramatically after introduction of routine patient admission chest radiographs, further demonstrating the effect on HCW risk of the unsuspected case (37).

## PRINCIPLES OF TRANSMISSION IN AND OUT OF HOSPITALS

Little deliberate scientific study has gone into determining the principles of transmission of TB in the hospital/congregate setting or in the community. More commonly, investigation of an outbreak—an "accident of nature"—has led to a new appreciation of a principle of TB transmission, or a broadened understanding of an established tenet. Lincoln (38), reviewing the world literature of community-based outbreaks in 1964, concluded that a delay in diagnosis, overcrowding with large numbers of susceptible persons, and inadequate ventilation all contributed to outbreaks, an observation confirmed by a more recent review (39).

In the 1950s and early 1960s, the group headed by Riley (40–42) performed ground-breaking studies on transmission utilizing newly diagnosed patients with TB, a specifically fitted ventilation system, and hundreds of tuberculin-negative guinea pigs, who were placed "downwind" from the still coughing source cases. Although Riley et al. determined that a small number of source patients were responsible for a majority of the transmission to guinea pigs, they were unable to associate any specific clinical or microscopic characteristic to the "superdisseminators." All were AFB sputum smear positive, but quantification of AFB smear status was insufficient to predict who would and would not efficiently spread MTB.

Little additional information has been added since that time. Recently, a group of investigators in New York City determined that a specific strain of drug-sensitive TB, labeled the "c" strain according to its molecular fingerprinting characteristics, was responsible for a disproportionate number of cases throughout New York City (43). Further understanding of how and why this particular strain appears more likely to cause disease may lead to an understanding of the pathogen-specific characteristics that favor spread.

Most studies of hospital-based outbreaks have stressed the problems caused by a delay in diagnosis and, less commonly, by inadequate ventilation. Appreciation of the subtle presentations of TB among the HIV infected has led to a broadening of respiratory isolation policies, with a subsequent decrease in nosocomial spread of MTB. Specific measures to prevent spread in hospitals are discussed below.

## SPECIFIC HEALTH CARE WORKER GROUPS AT RISK

### Nurses

Nurses were the first HCW group documented to have increased risk of occupational TB (6). Heimbeck (44), followed by at least 30 other groups (6), documented increased rates of infection and disease among student nurses versus the general population. In key studies conducted in Oslo, Philadelphia, Montreal, Boston, and Wisconsin, 906 (86%) of 1,053 susceptible nursing students tuberculin converted, of whom 209 (20%) developed active disease (45).

At least two old studies considered relative rates of disease among occupations, and in both studies nurses had the highest rate of infection and/or disease. In a 1952 review of rates of TB among worker groups at several New York State TB sanatoria, nurses were found to have the highest rate of disease, about twice that of any other occupational group, and three times that of physicians (46). In the British Prophit Survey, which studied rates of TB among 10,000 young adults from 1935 to 1944, nurses had two to three times the rate of infection and disease compared to medical students, and 3 to 20 times that seen in controls (47).

Recent studies at hospitals with high rates of TB have found a 4% to 13% tuberculin conversion rate among nurses, significantly higher than most other occupational groups (29,48,49). Institution of CDC-recommended control measures, including early isolation of patients with suspected disease, resulted in a significant improvement of this rate.

### Pathologists

Prosector's wart (inoculation TB) is an established occupational hazard for pathologists. An additional risk for pathologists is potential spread via the aerosol route from performing autopsies on tuberculous patients (6). In one older study, discontinuation of autopsies on patients with TB resulted in a decrease in tuberculin conversions among medical students, from 81% to 4% (50).

Spread continues to occur from autopsies performed on patients not suspected to have TB. In one report, an elderly man with progressive small cell lung cancer died of respiratory failure thought due to his tumor (51), but in fact due to TB. Eight (14.5%) of 55 employees exposed at his autopsy, including several pathologists, developed tuberculin conversions and two developed active disease. More recently, Templeton and colleagues (52) have shown that patients who were not sputum smear positive (infectious) during life may transmit TB infection during autopsy.

### Laboratory Workers

In the laboratory, infection may occur via either accidental aerosolization with inhalation or inadvertent inoculation. Pike (53), reviewing the world literature, found 194 reported cases of laboratory-acquired TB, including four fatal cases, making TB the sixth most common occupationally acquired infection among laboratory workers. Collins (54) noted that most series estimated that laboratory workers had two to nine times the risk of developing TB, when compared to the general population.

### Specialists in Pulmonary Medicine

One study found that the tuberculin conversion rates of pulmonary fellows-in-training was increased compared to that of infectious disease fellows-in-training [7/62 (11%) vs. 1/42 (2.4%)] (55). Because infectious disease and pulmonary fellows-in-training presumably spend equal amounts of time with TB patients, the higher rate of tuberculin conversion was thought due to the additional risk of performing bronchoscopy, or from time spent in intensive care units. Catanzaro (34) had described similar risks.

### HIV-Positive Health Care Workers

According to the CDC, seven of the nine fatal cases of occupationally acquired MDR-TB have occurred among HIV-infected HCWs. A molecular epidemiologic study from six non-outbreak hospitals in New York City examined rates of clonal, or clustered, disease among HCWs (56). In this analysis, the HCW occupation was a significant association for clonal disease, suggesting that even without recognized outbreaks the risk for transmission persists. In addition, HIV-positive HCWs had the highest rate of clustered disease (89%). The ethical issues raised by this situation have no simple resolution. HIV-positive HCWs should decide after being made aware of the potential risk.

### Housekeeping Personnel

Several studies in the past decades have identified housekeeping personnel at higher risk for tuberculin conversion, with annual conversion rates as high as 10% (29,48). One study controlled for BCG status, country of birth, age, sex, and rates of TB disease in zip code of residence in a multivariate analysis and found that the group of employees that included housekeeping, dietary, and security personnel had a the highest rate of tuberculin conversion (29).

## INTERVENTIONS

### Treatment of a Positive Tuberculin Skin Test

The cornerstone of all TB control efforts is an active tuberculin skin test program. Once identified, tuberculin-positive persons are treated with a 6-month course of isoniazid therapy (300 mg QD), with or without pyridoxine (vitamin $B_6$, 50 mg QD). Persons with HIV infection should receive 12 months of therapy (3).

The CDC carefully has carefully defined the cutoff by size of tuberculin induration. However, all experts agree that, given the poor sensitivity and specificity of the tuberculin skin test, clinical judgment remains the most important element in the decision to initiate or not initiate preventative therapy. Table 4 shows the groups for which initiation of therapy should be considered.

**TABLE 4.** *Summary of interpretation of purified protein derivative (PPD)-tuberculin skin-test results*

1. An induration of ≥5 mm is classified as positive in:
   - persons who have human immunodeficiency virus (HIV) infection or risk factors for HIV infection but unknown HIV status
   - persons who have had recent close contact[a] with persons who have active tuberculosis (TB)
   - persons who have fibrotic chest radiographs (consistent with TB)
2. An induration of ≥10 mm is classified as positive in all persons who do not meet any of the criteria above but who have other risks factors for TB, including:

   High-risk groups
   - injecting-drug users known to be HIV seronegative
   - persons who have other medical conditions that reportedly increase the risk for progressing from latent TB infection to active TB (e.g., silicosis; gastrectomy or jejuno-ileal bypass; being ≥10% below ideal body weight; chronic renal failure with renal dialysis; diabetes mellitus; high-dose corticosteroid or other immunosuppressive therapy; some hematologic disorders, including malignancies such as leukemias and lymphomas; and other malignancies)
   - children <4 years of age

   High-prevalence groups
   - persons born in countries in Asia, Africa, the Caribbean, and Latin America that have high prevalence of TB
   - persons from medically underserved, low-income populations
   - residents of long-term-care facilities (e.g., correctional institutions and nursing homes)
   - persons from high-risk populations in their communities, as determined by local public health authorities
3. An induration of ≥15 mm is classified as positive in persons who do not meet any of the above criteria
4. Recent converters are defined on the basis of both size of induration and age of the person being tested
   - ≥10 mm increase within a 2-year period is classified as a recent conversion for persons <35 years of age
   - ≥15 mm increase within a 2-year period is classified as a recent conversion for persons ≥35 years of age
5. PPD skin-test results in health care workers (HCWs)
   - In general, the recommendations in sections 1, 2, and 3 above should be followed when interpreting skin-test results in HCWs. However, the prevalence of TB in the facility should be considered when choosing the appropriate cutoff point for defining a positive PPD reaction. In facilities where there is essentially no risk for exposure to *Mycobacterium tuberculosis* (i.e., minimal or very low risk facilities), an induration ≥15 mm may be a suitable cutoff point for HCWs who have no other risk factors. In facilities where TB patients receive care, the cutoff point for HCWs with no other risk factors may be ≥10 mm.
   - A recent conversion in an HCW should be defined generally as a ≥10 mm increase in size of induration within a 2-year period. For HCWs who work in facilities where exposure to TB is very unlikely (e.g., minimal-risk facilities), an increase of ≥15 mm within a 2-year period may be more appropriate for defining a recent conversion because of the lower positive-predictive value of the test in such groups.

[a]Recent close contact implies either household or social contact or unprotected occupational exposure similar in intensity and duration to household contact.

Adapted from ref. 88.

### The Role of BCG

The potential utility of BCG vaccination for TB control continues to be debated, more than 70 years after its introduction and with over 1,264 studies reported (57). A meta-analysis of all prospective randomized trials reported (26 of the 1,264 studies) revealed that BCG reduced the risk of TB by about 50%, a benefit extending to tuberculous meningitis, disseminated disease, and tuberculous death. A consideration of studies limited to HCWs (58) showed similar benefit.

The potential problem created by wide-scale vaccination of HCWs in low-prevalence areas is that response to vaccination predictably results in a positive tuberculin skin test. Thus, the one means of identifying TB outbreaks early—the rate of tuberculin skin test conversion—is sacrificed to a larger public health effort utilizing a 50% effective vaccine.

### The Benefit of Previous Infection

Native immunity to *M. tuberculosis,* reflected by either a previous history of disease or a positive tuberculin test, affords protection against reinfection. Some older studies go so far as to suggest that only tuberculin-positive persons work among the tuberculous (59). Exogenous reinfection has occurred among specific hosts, including the homeless (60), veterans (61), persons with AIDS (62), or those with sustained exposure, such as family members (63).

The British Prophit Survey of Young Adults demonstrated that protective immunity among the already-tuberculin positive is incomplete (47). In an analysis of baseline tuberculin-positive nurses, rates of TB disease were twice as high for nurses who worked in hospitals with TB wards than for nurses who cared for few TB patients (64). The authors conclude, "Any evidence that previously infected persons who are heavily exposed contract TB more often than infected persons not so exposed is strong evidence that the added exposure is responsible for the disease" (47).

### CDC Guidelines to Prevent Transmission in Health Care Facilities

The CDC periodically updates guidelines for prevention of the spread of TB in health care facilities (3). The 1994 guidelines were met with some criticism, particularly from areas with low rates of TB, due to the potentially onerous cost. The CDC regulations include implementation of three hierarchical levels of intervention (in order of decreasing priority):

#### *1. Isolation of Potentially Infectious Cases*

The undiagnosed case of TB has long been considered the greatest potential disseminator of disease. Appropriate placement of patients into respiratory isolation has reduced the rate of employee infection and disease in studies reported over the past 40 years (36,37,49).

The subtlety of presenting symptoms in many patients with TB, particularly those who are HIV infected, continues to complicate guidelines concerning whom to place into respiratory isolation and whom to remove. Many hospitals adopted an approach that "all patients are presumed to have TB until proven otherwise," meaning that persons with known or suspected HIV infection and fever or respiratory symptoms are placed into respiratory isolation, pending "rule-out" for TB (65). The ratio of patients placed into isolation to those who eventually are diagnosed with TB ranges from 5–10 to 1 (65–67). Attempts to develop predictive guidelines have been met with some problems (66,67). The average length of stay in isolation for patients who eventually "rule out" is about 5 days (65).

Of note, about 50% of patients with pulmonary TB are AFB smear–negative (68), meaning that many patients are removed from respiratory isolation despite having pulmonary TB. Due to the markedly reduced infectiousness of the AFB smear–negative case (69,70), this has remained a safe and effective approach.

#### *2. Engineering Controls*

Three different engineering controls are recommended to reduce the concentration of infectious droplet nuclei:

(a) Appropriate ventilation is necessary for respiratory isolation rooms. Several outbreaks from recirculation of contaminated air have been reported (33,71). Current recommendations include negative pressure ventilation with at least six air exchanges per hour for isolation rooms. More specifics are given in the guidelines (3).

(b) High-efficiency particulate (HEPA) filtration use, with placement of units into existing ducts, is suggested as an additional engineering control. To be effective, units must be serviced and cleaned regularly. At one hospital, maintenance of HEPA filtration and ultraviolet germicidal irradiation units (see below), and monitoring negative pressure flow required adding an additional full-time employee (65).

(c) Ultraviolet germicidal irradiation is suggested as an additional supplement for settings with high rates of transmission. The relatively cheap cost and evidence of benefit both in animal experiments (42) and in uncontrolled hospital-based reports (72) have led to its enthusiastic recommendation by many experts in the field (73–75).

#### *3. Personal Protective Equipment*

Even more intense controversy surrounds the recommendations for masks and respirators, or "personal protective equipment." Recently, additional equipment, such as the N-95 respirator, has been approved for use. The cheaper per unit cost and vastly improved comfort of this respirator make it more popular among workers and administrators alike. No objective evidence of the effectiveness of this or other units has been established. Indeed, rates of employee conversion had decreased long before introduction of this costly and uncomfortable intervention (76,77). Thus, the optimal mask is unknown and it is unlikely that studies can be designed to identify such equipment. Therefore, common sense must prevail, weighing need to protect against need for worker comfort and overall equipment cost.

## SUMMARY

The hope of global control of TB has been severely hampered by the emergence of the HIV epidemic. However, in the United States better control of TB once again appears possible, with a decrease in annual case-rates (1), better understanding of urban transmission (78–81), and improved survival among patients with resistant disease (82,83).

Considerable resources and attention have been given to the occupational risk of TB. Current CDC recommendations are rigorous and their implementation costly, which precipitated a contentious debate. In addition, studies clearly have shown that TB is not highly contagious (70) and that the cost to prevent a case, much less a death, is quite high (84,85).The key to all TB control efforts is an active PPD surveillance program, which allows targeted educational, environmental, and other interventions. The goal of all involved, including HCWs, federal regulatory bodies, and hospital administrators, is the same—making hospitals safe for patients and workers alike. Attempts to achieve this goal have disclosed numerous contentious and still unresolved issues.

As guidelines are promulgated and revised, it is important to remember that the risk of occupational transmission will be reduced to zero only when the diagnosis of TB can reliably be made in a matter of hours rather than weeks. Improved environmental controls can afford only tiny increments of improved safety, since patients with unsuspected disease will continue to spread disease. Also, it is unlikely that the previous guidelines were wrong. Decreases in employee tuberculin conversion rates occurred before implementation of 1994 guidelines by following basic principles of infection control: prompt identification and isolation of suspected cases and immediate institution of effective therapy. Thus it appears that guidelines dating back at least the 1930s (6) were appropriate for most hospitals; compliance with the guidelines was inadequate, not the guidelines themselves.

A safer work environment awaits new means of diagnosis, not a better mask or an increased air-exchange rate. The already complicated issue of occupationally acquired TB is only compounded by calls for a risk-free workplace. Perhaps only when a realistic premise is established—that working with the tuberculous confers an occupational risk—can rational programs to balance cost and safety and worker safety be developed.

## REFERENCES


1. Centers for Disease Control and Prevention. Tuberculosis morbidity—US, 1995. *MMWR* 1996;45:365–370.
2. Centers for Disease Control and Prevention. Nosocomial transmission of multidrug-resistant tuberculosis among HIV-infected persons—Florida and New York, 1988–1991. *MMWR* 1991;40: 585–591.
3. Centers for Disease Control and Prevention. Guidelines for preventing the transmission *Mycobacterium tuberculosis* in health-care facilities, 1994. *MMWR* 1994;43(No. RR-13):1–132.
4. Sepkowitz KA. Occupationally-acquired infections in health care workers. Part I & II. *Ann Intern Med* 1996;125:826–834, 917–928.
5. Zuger A, Miles SH. Physicians, AIDS, and occupational risk. *JAMA* 1987;258:1924–1928.
6. Sepkowitz KA. Tuberculosis and the health care worker: a historical perspective. *Ann Intern Med* 1994;120:71–79.
7. Shands JW, Boeff D, Fauerbach L, Gutekunst RR. Tuberculin testing in a tertiary hospital: product variability. *Infect Control Hosp Epidemiol* 1994;15:758–760.
8. Lamphear BP, Linnemann CC, Cannon CG. A high false positive rate of tuberculosis associated with Aplisol: an investigation among health care workers. *J Infect Dis* 1994;169:703–704.
9. Johnson JL, Nyole S, Shepardson L, Mugerwa R, Ellner JJ. Simultaneous comparison of two commercial tuberculin skin test reagents in an area with a high prevalence of tuberculosis [Letter]. *J Infect Dis* 1995;171:1066–1068.
10. Chaparas SD, Vandiviere HM, Melvin I, Koch G, Becker C. Tuberculin test. Variability with the Mantoux procedure. *Am Rev Respir Dis* 1985;132:175–177.
11. Pouchot J, Grasland A, Collet C, Coste J, Esdaile JM, Vinceneux P. Reliability of tuberculin skin test measurement. *Ann Intern Med* 1997; 126:210–214.
12. Huebner RE, Schein MF, Bass JB. The tuberculin skin test. *Clin Infect Dis* 1993;17:968–975.
13. Markowitz N, Hansen NI, Wilcosky TC, et al. Tuberculin and anergy testing in HIV-seropositive and HIV-seronegative persons. *Ann Intern Med* 1993;119:185–193.
14. Centers for Disease Control and Prevention. Anergy skin testing and preventative therapy for HIV-infected persons: revised recommendations. *MMWR* 1997;46:1–10.
15. Menzies R, Vissandjee B, Rocher I, St. Germain Y. The booster effect in two-step tuberculin testing among young adults in Montreal. *Ann Intern Med* 1994;120:190–198.
16. Horowitz H, Luciano BB, Kadel JR, Wormser GP. Tuberculin skin test conversion in hospital employees vaccinated with bacille Calmette-Guerin: recent *Mycobacterium tuberculosis* infection or booster effect. *Am J Infect Control* 1995;23:181–187.
17. Sepkowitz KA, Feldman J, Louther J, Rivera P, Villa N, DeHovitz J. Benefit of 2-step PPD testing of new employees at a New York City hospital. *Am J Infect Control* 1997;25:283–286.
18. Rosenberg T, Manfreda J, Hershfield ES. Two-step tuberculin testing in staff and residents of a nursing home. *Am Rev Respir Dis* 1993;148: 1537–1540.
19. Cauthen GM, Snider DE, Onorato IM. Boosting of tuberculin sensitivity among Southeast Asian refugees. *Am J Respir Crit Care Med* 1994;49:1597–1600.
20. Menzies R, Vissandjee B, Amyot D. Factors associated with tuberculin reactivity among the foreign-born in Montreal. *Am Rev Respir Dis* 1992;146:752–756.
21. Rosenblum LG, Castro KG, Dooley S, Morgan M. Effect of HIV infection and tuberculosis on hospitalizations and cost of care for young adults in the United States, 1985 to 1990. *Ann Intern Med* 1994;121:786–792.
22. Reichman LB, O'Day R. Tuberculosis screening in a large urban population. *Am Rev Respir Dis* 1978;117:705–712.
23. Cross ER, Hyams KC. Tuberculin skin testing in US Navy and Marine

Corps personnel and recruits, 1980–1986. *Am J Public Health* 1990; 80:435–438.
24. Prezant DJ, Kelly KJ, Karwa ML, Kavanauugh K. Self-assessment of tuberculin skin test reactions by New York City firefighters: reliability and cost-effectiveness in an occupational health care setting. *Ann Intern Med* 1996;125:280–283.
25. Schluger NW, Huberman R, Wolinsky N, Dooley R, Rom WN, Holzman RS. Tuberculosis infection and disease among persons seeking social services in New York City. *Int J Tuberc Lung Dis* 1997;1:31–37.
26. Sepkowitz KA, Fella P, Rivera P, Villa N, DeHovitz J. Prevalence of PPD positivity among new employees at a hospital in New York City. *Infect Control Hosp Epidemiol* 1995;16:344–347.
27. Schwartzman K, Loo V, Pasztor J, Menzies D. Tuberculosis infection among health care workers in Montreal. *Am J Respir Crit Care Med* 1996;154:1006–1012.
28. Fridkin SK, Manangaan L, Bolyard E, Jarvis WR. SHEA-CDC TB survey, part I: status of TB infection control programs at member hospitals, 1989–1992. *Infect Control Hosp Epidemiol* 1995;16:129–134.
28a. Fridkin SK, Manangaan L, Bolyard E, Jarvis WR. SHEA-CDC TB survey, part II: efficacy of TB infection control programs at member hospitals, 1989–1992. *Infect Control Hosp Epidemiol* 1995;16:135–140.
29. Louther J, Rivera P, Feldman J, Villa R, DeHovitz J, Sepkowitz KA. Risk for PPD conversion among health care workers at a NYC hospital. *Am J Respir Crit Care Med* 1997;156:201–205.
30. Bowden KM, McDiarmid MA. Occupationally acquired tuberculosis: what's known. *J Occup Environ Med* 1994;36:320–325.
31. Fagan MJ, Poland GA. Tuberculin skin testing in medical students: a survey of US medical schools. *Ann Intern Med* 1994;120:930–931.
32. Zaza S, Blumberg HM, Beck-Sague C, et al. Nosocomial transmission of Mycobacterium tuberculosis: role of health care workers in outbreak propagation. *J Infect Dis* 1995;172:1542–1549.
33. Ehrenkranz NJ, Kicklighter JL. Tuberculosis outbreak in a general hospital: evidence for airborne spread of infection. *Ann Intern Med* 1972;77:377–382.
34. Catanzaro A. Nosocomial tuberculosis. *Am Rev Respir Dis* 1982;125: 559–562.
35. Haley CE, McDonald RC, Rossi L, Jones WD, Haley RW, Luby JP. Tuberculosis epidemic among hospital personnel. *Infect Control Hosp Epidemiol* 1989;10:204–210.
36. Craven RB, Wenzel RP, Atuk NO. Minimizing tuberculosis risk to hospital personnel and students exposed to unsuspected disease. *Ann Intern Med* 1975;82:628–632.
37. Jacobson G, Hoyt DD, Bogen E. Tuberculosis in hospital employees as affected by an admission chest X-ray screening program. *Dis Chest* 1957;32:27–39.
38. Lincoln E. Epidemics of tuberculosis. *Adv Tuberc Res* 1965;14: 157–201.
39. Raffalli J, Sepkowitz KA, Armstrong D. Community-based outbreaks of tuberculosis. *Arch Intern Med* 1996;156:1053–1061.
40. Riley RL, Mills CC, Nyka W, et al. Aerial dissemination of pulmonary tuberculosis: a two year study of contagion in a tuberculosis ward. *Am J Hyg* 1959;70:185–196.
41. Sultan LU, Nyka W, Mills CC, O'Grady F, Wells WF, Riley RL. Tuberculosis disseminators: a study of the variability of aerial infectivity of tuberculosis patients. *Am Rev Respir Dis* 1960;82:358–369.
42. Riley RL, Mills CC, O'Grady F, Sultan LU, Wittstadt F, Shivpuri DN. Infectiousness of air from a tuberculosis ward. Ultraviolet irradiation of infected air: comparative infectiousness of different patients. *Am Rev Respir Dis* 1962;85:511–525.
43. Friedman CR, Quinn GC, Kreiswirth BN, et al. Widespread dissemination of a single drug-susceptible strain of *Mycobacterium tuberculosis. J Infect Dis* 1997;176:478–484.
44. Heimbeck J. Incidence of tuberculosis in young adult women with special reference to employment. *Br J Tubercle* 1938;32:154–166.
45. Sepkowitz KA. AIDS, tuberculosis, and the health care worker. *Clin Infect Dis* 1995;20:232–242.
46. Mikol EX, Horton R. Lincoln NS, Stokes AM. Incidence of pulmonary tuberculosis among employees of tuberculosis hospitals. *Am Rev Tuberc* 1952;66:16–27.
47. Daniels M, Ridehalgh F, Springett VH, Hall IM. *Tuberculosis in young adults:* report on the Prophit Tuberculosis Survey, *1935–1944.* London: HK Lewis, 1948.
48. Holzman RS. A comprehensive control program reduces transmission of tuberculosis (TB) to hospital staff. *Clin Infect Dis* 1995;21:733.
49. Blumberg HM, Watkins DL, Berschling JD, et al. Preventing the nosocomial transmission of tuberculosis. *Ann Intern Med* 1995;122: 658–663.
50. Meade GM. The prevention of primary tuberculous infections in medical students: the autopsy as a source of primary infection. *Am Rev Tuberc* 1948;58:675–683.
51. Kantor HS, Poblete R, Pusateri SL. Nosocomial transmission of tuberculosis from unsuspected disease. *Am J Med* 1988;84:833–838.
52. Templeton GL, Illing LA, Young L, Cave D, Stead WW, Bates JH. The risk for transmission of *Mycobacterium tuberculosis* at the bedside and during autopsy. *Ann Intern Med* 1995;122:922–925.
53. Pike RM. Laboratory-associated infections: incidence, fatalities, causes, and prevention. *Annu Rev Microbiol* 1979;33:41–66.
54. Collins HC. *Laboratory-acquired infections*, 2nd ed. London: Butterworth, 1988.
55. Malasky C, Jordan T, Potulski F, Reichman LB. Occupational tuberculosis infections among pulmonary physicians in training. *Am Rev Respir Dis* 1990;142:505–507.
56. Sepkowitz KA, Friedman C, Hafner A, et al. Tuberculosis among urban health care workers: a study utilizing restriction fragment length polymorphism typing. *Clin Infect Dis* 1995;21:1098–1101.
57. Colditz GA, Brewer TF, Berkey CS, et al. Efficacy of BCG vaccine in the prevention of tuberculosis. *JAMA* 1994;271:698–702.
58. Brewer TF, Colditz GA. Bacille Calmette-Guerin vaccination for the prevention of tuberculosis in health care workers. *Clin Infect Dis* 1995;20:136–142.
59. Stead WW. Pathogenesis of a first episode of chronic pulmonary tuberculosis in man: recrudescence of residuals of the primary infection or exogenous re-infection? *Am Rev Respir Dis* 1967;95:729–745.
60. Nardell E, McInnis B, Thomas B, Weidhaas S. Exogenous reinfection with tuberculosis in a shelter for the homeless. *N Engl J Med* 1986; 315:1570–1575.
61. Raleigh JW, Wichelhausen RH, Rado TA, Bates JH. Evidence for infection by two distinct strains of *Mycobacterium tuberculosis* in pulmonary tuberculosis: report of 9 cases. *Am Rev Respir Dis* 1975;112: 497–503.
62. Small P, Shafer RW, Hopewell P, et al. Exogenous reinfection with multidrug-resistant mycobacterium tuberculosis in patients with advanced HIV infection. *N Engl J Med* 1993;328:1137–1144.
63. Ormerod P, Skinner C. Reinfection tuberculosis: two cases in the family of a patient with drug-resistant disease. *Thorax* 1980;35:56–59.
64. Sepkowitz KA. The tuberculin skin test and the health care worker: the Prophit Survey reconsidered. *Tuberc Lung Dis* 1996;77:81–85.
65. Fella P, Rivera P, Hale M, Squires KE, Sepkowitz KA. Dramatic decrease in tuberculin conversion rates among employees at a hospital in New York City. *Am J Infect Control* 1995;23:352–356.
66. Bock NN, McGowan JE, Ahn J, Aptia J, Blumberg HM. Clinical predictors of tuberculosis as a guide for a respiratory isolation policy. *Am J Respir Crit Care Med* 1996;154:1468–1472.
67. Pegues CF, Johnson DC, Pegues DA, Spencer M, Hopkins CC. Implementation and evaluation of an algorithm for isolation of patients with suspected pulmonary tuberculosis. *Infect Control Hosp Epidemiol* 1996;17:412–418.
68. Schluger N, Rom W. Current approaches to the diagnosis of active pulmonary tuberculosis. *Am J Respir Crit Care Med* 1994;149: 264–267.
69. Grzybowski S, Barnett GD, Stylbo K. Contacts of cases of active pulmonary tuberculosis. *Bull Int Union Tuberc* 1975;50:90–106.
70. Sepkowitz KA. How contagious is tuberculosis? *Clin Infect Dis* 1996; 23:954–962.
71. Houk VN, Kent DC, Baker JH, Sorensen K, Hanzel GD. The Byrd study: in-depth analysis of a micro-outbreak of tuberculosis in a closed environment. *Arch Environ Health* 1968;16:4–6.
72. Madsen L, Carbajal J, Iseman M. Low incidence of nosocomial infection of health care workers on a tuberculosis ward equipped with ultraviolet light irradiation. *Am J Respir Crit Care Med* 1994;A855.
73. Nardell EA, Keegan J, Cheney SA, Etkind SC. Airborne infection: theoretical limits of protection achievable by building ventilation. *Am Rev Respir Dis* 1991;144:302–306.
74. Iseman MD. A leap of faith: what can we do to curtail intrainstitutional transmission of tuberculosis? *Ann Intern Med* 1992;117: 251–253.
75. Riley RL, Nardell EA. Clearing the air: the theory and application of ultraviolet air disinfection. *Am Rev Respir Dis* 1989;139:1286–1294.

76. Segal-Maurer S, Kalkut GE. Environmental control of tuberculosis: continuing controversy. *Clin Infect Dis* 1994;19:299–308.
77. Rivera P, Louther J, Mohr J, Campbell A, DeHovitz J, Sepkowitz KA. Does a cheaper mask save money? The cost of implementing a personal protection equipment program at a hospital in New York City. *Infect Control Hosp Epidemiol* 1997;18:24–27.
78. Genewein A, Telenti A, Bernasconi C, et al. Molecular approach to identifying route of transmission of tuberculosis in the community. *Lancet* 1993;342:841–844.
79. Small PM, Hopewell PC, Singh SP, et al. The epidemiology of tuberculosis in San Francisco. *N Engl J Med* 1994;330:1703–1709.
80. Alland D, Kalkut GE, Moss AR, et al. Transmission of tuberculosis in New York City: an analysis by DNA fingerprinting and conventional epidemiologic methods. *N Engl J Med* 1994;330:1710–1716.
81. Friedman CR, Stoeckle MY, Kreiswirth BN, et al. Transmission of multidrug-resistant tuberculosis in a large urban setting. *Am J Respir Crit Care Med* 1995;152:355–359.
82. Telzak EE, Sepkowitz KA, Alpert P, et al. Successful treatment of multidrug-resistant tuberculosis (MDRTB) among HIV-negative patients. *N Engl J Med* 1995;33:907–911.
83. Park MM, Davis AL, Schluger NW, Cohen H, Rom WN. Outcome of MDR-TB patients. Prolonged survival with appropriate therapy. *Am J Respir Crit Care Med* 1996;153:317–324.
84. Nettleman MD, Fredrickson M, Good NL, Hunter SA. Tuberculosis control strategies: the cost of particulate respirators. *Ann Intern Med* 1994;121:37–40.
85. Adal KA, Anglim AM, Palumbo CL, Titus MG, Coyner BJ, Farr BM. The use of high efficiency particulate air-filter respirators to protect hospital workers from tuberculosis. *N Engl J Med* 1994;331: 169–173.
86. Bailey TC, Fraser VJ, Spitznagel EL, Dunagan WC. Risk Factors for a positive tuberculin skin test among employees of an urban, Midwestern teaching hospital. *Ann Intern Med* 1995;122:580–585.
87. Rattner SL, Fleischer JA, Davidson BL. Tuberculin positivity and patient contact in healthcare workers in the urban United States. *Infect Control Hosp Epidemiol* 1996;17:369–371.
88. Centers for Disease Control. Screening for tuberculosis and tuberculosis infection in high-risk populations and the use of preventive therapy for tuberculous infection in the United States. *MMWR* 1990;39: 1–12.

*Environmental and Occupational Medicine, Third Edition,* edited by William N. Rom.
Lippincott–Raven Publishers, Philadelphia © 1998.

CHAPTER 54

# Endocrine Disruption from Environmental Toxicants

Theo Colborn

A growing body of literature has focused on the sensitivity of the embryo, fetus, and neonate to synthetic chemicals that can interfere with the natural hormones, neurotransmitters, and growth factors that control development (1). The untoward effects of endocrine disruption during these early stages of development in most instances are irreversible (2). For physicians who are trained as healers this could be quite perplexing. This, however, should not deter physicians from becoming familiar with the hazards to human development posed by commonly encountered synthetic chemicals. As physicians become knowledgeable about the effects of endocrine disruption they should begin to appreciate the value of this information as an integral part of their diagnostic procedures and prevention programs.

This chapter provides a brief overview of what is currently known about the effects of man-made chemicals that mimic or interfere with the naturally produced signaling molecules that control development. Physicians may not recognize the health decrements in infants at birth, or even in early childhood, because the effects may be expressed as loss of function or changes in behavior, which often require specialists and trained technicians to be detected (3,4). In some cases the effects may not be discovered until the individual matures. For instance, in utero exposure to the synthetic estrogen-like compound, diethylstilbestrol (DES), can lead to changes in female reproductive tracts that may not be discovered until adulthood. These effects include vaginal epithelial cell cornification, clear cell vaginal adenocarcinoma, T-shaped uteri, and other reproductive problems (2,5). On the other hand, some effects could remain undiagnosed throughout life, such as reductions in IQ and human semen quality and sperm count. However, these unrecognized effects, if allowed to become widely prevalent at the population level, could have significant impacts on a society and its survival (6).

T. Colborn: Wildlife and Contaminants Program, World Wildlife Fund, Washington, D.C. 20037-1175.

## PROFILE OF ENDOCRINE DISRUPTION

A number of widely used synthetic chemicals are known endocrine disruptors and reproductive toxicants (Table 1). As the list of chemicals grows so does the list of their mechanisms of action, regardless of the affected system (e.g., thyroid, neuroendocrine, adrenal, reproductive). The mechanisms of action of contaminants to date fall into six general categories. Contaminants can act by:

1. binding to receptors and enhancing effects as agonists;
2. blocking receptors and inhibiting effects as antagonists;
3. directly interfering with endogenous hormones;
4. indirectly interfering with endogenous hormones or other naturally produced chemical messengers;
5. altering steroidogenesis, metabolism, and excretion;
6. altering hormone receptor levels (1).

A contaminant can interfere with homeostasis in more than one way, and toxicity may in some cases depend more on timing of exposure than on dose (7). Several review papers describing the role of contaminants as disruptors in specific endocrine systems are available (8,9).

**TABLE 1.** *Chemicals in the environment reported to have reproductive and endocrine disrupting effects*

| Chemical | Reference |
|---|---|
| Pesticides | |
| Herbicides | |
| 2,4 D | 73,74 |
| 2,4,5 T | 75 |
| Alachlor | 76,77 |
| Amitrole | 78,79 |
| Atrazine | 80–82 |
| Metribuzin | 83 |
| Nitrofen | 9 |
| Trifluralin | 84 |
| Fungicides | |
| Benomyl | 85 |
| Ethylene thiourea (ETU) | 86 |
| Fenarimol | 9 |
| Hexachlorobenzene | 87–90 |
| Mancozeb | 91 |
| Maneb | 92,86 |
| Metiram | 93 |
| Tributyltin | 94,95 |
| Vinclozolin | 96 |
| Zineb | 86 |
| Ziram | 76 |
| Insecticides | |
| Aldrin | 33 |
| β-HCH | 97 |
| Carbaryl | 75 |
| Chlordane | 89,98 |
| Chlordecone | 99 |
| DDT and metabolites | 25,99,100 |
| Dicofol | 25 |
| Dieldrin | 65,89 |
| Endosulfan (α and β) | 65,101 |
| Heptachlor and H-epoxide | 89 |
| Lindane (gamma-HCH) | 102 |
| Malathion | 103,104 |
| Methomyl | 105 |
| Methoxychlor | 60,106,107 |
| Oxychlordane | 98 |
| Parathion | 108 |
| Synthetic pyrethroids | 109 |
| Toxaphene | 65 |
| Transnonachlor | 98 |
| Nematocides | |
| Aldicarb | 105 |
| DBCP | 9,76 |
| Industrial chemicals | |
| 4-OH Alkyl phenol | 99 |
| 4-OH Biphenyl | 99 |
| Benzylbutylphthalate | 99 |
| Bisphenol A | 99,39,110 |
| t-Butylhydroxyanisole | 99 |
| Cadmium | 111 |
| Dioxin | 112–114 |
| Lead | 115,116 |
| Mercury | 117 |
| PBBs | 118 |
| PCBs | 119–121 |
| 2 to 4-OH 2′,5′ Dichlorobiphenyl | 99 |
| 2,3,4 Trichlorobiphenyl | 99 |
| 4-OH Trichlorobiphenyls (2,2′,5;2′,4′,6′) | 99 |
| PCBs *(continued)* | |
| 3-OH 2′,3′,4′,5′ Tetrachlorobiphenyl | 99 |
| 4-OH 2′,3′,4′,5′ Tetrachlorobiphenyl | 99 |
| 2,2′,3,3′,6,6′ Hexachlorobiphenyl | 99 |
| Pentabromodiphenyl ether | 122 |
| Pentachlorophenol | 123 |
| Penta- to nonylphenols | 38 |
| Phthalates | 41,124–128 |
| Styrenes | 38,129,130 |

Modified from ref. 11.

One of the most compelling describes the myriad of axes where organochlorine contaminants interfere with the thyroid system and could undermine the development of the brain, intelligence, and behavior in wildlife, laboratory animals, and humans (10).

## WIDESPREAD EXPOSURE

Exposure to endocrine disrupting chemicals is far greater than most individuals realize (Table 2). Today, at least 500 measurable chemicals, and many more that have not been identified yet, are present in human tissue that were never there before the 1920s. Some of these chemicals are capable of bypassing the placental and brain barriers and the hormone binding serum proteins that protect the fetus and the mother, respectively, from excessive hormone exposure. This allows foreign chemicals to mingle in the womb with the natural chemicals that control development, to interfere with normal gene expression, and to influence the determination of the future of the embryo and fetus (1,11).

A great deal of the current knowledge about endocrine disruption evolved through research with chemicals that do not degrade readily and thus accumulate in the environment. Their persistence and their lipophilic properties together allow them to accumulate in animal and plant tissue and build up in food webs on which wildlife and humans are dependent (12,13). Exposure to endocrine-disrupting chemicals in the environment has been associated with the following effects in wildlife: abnormal thy-

**TABLE 2.** *Chronological examination of human exposure*

| | |
|---|---|
| 1929 | PCBs introduced |
| 1938 | DDT first manufactured |
| 1940–WWII | First wide scale exposure to man-made chemicals |
| 1940s–1950s | First generation exposed postnatally |
| 1950s–1970s | First generation born that was exposed in womb |
| 1970s–1990s | First generation exposed in womb reaching reproductive age |

roid function in birds (14) and fish (15); decreased fertility in birds (16), fish (17), shellfish (18), reptiles (19), and mammals (20); decreased hatching success in fish (21), birds (22), and turtles (23); loss of parental attention in birds (22); metabolic disorders in birds (22) and mammals (20); demasculinization and feminization of male fish (24), birds (25), and mammals (26); defeminization and masculinization in female fish (27), gastropods (28), and birds (25); and altered immune function in birds (29) and mammals (30). The above effects were not reported before the 1950s and are still reported today in animals in geographic regions where the presence of synthetic chemicals, such as pesticides, industrial and commercial products, and their by-products, have accumulated. The Great Lakes region, the lower Columbia River in Washington, central lakes in Florida, and the Baltic and Mediterranean Seas provide patterns of chemical contamination associated with biologic effects and health concerns (12). It is important to note that contamination in the Great Lakes region is no greater than some of the other major river drainage basins in the United States (31).

These persistent organic pollutants (POPs), designated in international conventions to reduce their production and release into the environment, include organochlorine compounds such as polychlorinated biphenyls (PCBs), dioxins, and furans. The PCBs were used most extensively as heat transfer fluids and fire retardants in electrical equipment and structural material from 1929 to 1979 when their production was banned in the United States. PCBs are a complex mixture of 209 compounds called congeners, depending on the position and number of chlorine atoms on the biphenyl rings (32). It is estimated that some of the congeners have a half-life of over 1,000 years. Dioxins and furans are not produced intentionally. Their greatest source is from incomplete combustion of material containing organochlorine chemicals, such as polyvinyl chloride (PVC), or as a by-product in the production of organochlorine pesticides.

Another group of persistent chemicals are the organochlorine pesticides such as DDT, dieldrin, lindane, mirex, chlordane, toxaphene, and hexachlorobenzene (HCB). HCB is also produced unintentionally when organochlorine compounds are burned or as a by-product in pesticide production. Commencing in the early 1970s many of these chemicals were partially regulated in the United States, Canada, the United Kingdom, Europe, and Scandinavia and as result their widespread, heavy releases into the environment were curtailed considerably. Despite this, these chemicals are found regularly in human and wildlife tissue around the world (1). The problem persists because of the reluctance of governments to completely ban their production and use, and is exacerbated because many pesticides are still used in vast amounts in the developing world.

For instance, dieldrin was restricted in the United States as an agricultural insecticide in 1974 but it was only in 1987 that its use as an insecticide (moth-proofer) in carpets and wool clothing and as a termiticide was stopped (33). Although DDT use as an agricultural chemical is banned in the United States, it can still be produced legally in the United States and is imported into and exported out of the country. Furthermore, DDT can still be used in the United States for public health reasons and emergency insect infestations in agriculture when an exemption is sought through the appropriate government agency. Almost everyone in the United States has measurable levels of DDE, a breakdown product of DDT, in his or her tissue. The global use of DDT is greater today than before its use was restricted in the United States in 1992. Recently, fresh DDT was discovered in the eggs and blood of albatrosses that feed only on the surface of the North Pacific Ocean, 500 or more miles from any land area (34). DDT and its breakdown products have a half-life of 57.5 years in orchard soils in the state of Washington and over 200 years in the Arctic (35).

It is now recognized that widespread, unavoidable exposure to endocrine disruptors occurs via global atmospheric and oceanic transport, as well as via commonly encountered plastic items that are an integral part of commerce and daily life, from the lining of canned food products (36) to dental sealants (37). Two serendipitous findings in separate laboratories studying human breast cancer cells led to the discovery that components of common plastic products can interfere with estrogen-mediated pathways by binding to the estrogen receptor. Bisphenol-A (BPA), a monomer used to make polycarbonates, and alkylphenol ethoxylates, used as plasticizers (in this case, polystyrene), were found to have an affinity for the estrogen receptor and cause breast cancer cells to proliferate *in vitro* (38,39). In addition, scientists have known since 1975 that phthalates are widely distributed in the environment (40,41). Some phthalates, extensively used in PVC products and to make plastic products flexible, also bind to the estrogen receptor. In other modes of action, phthalates induce seminiferous tubule atrophy, and reduce testis and epididymis weight, and spermatogenesis (42). It appears that as heavy-dose exposure to several organochlorine chemicals has abated somewhat because of regulation in the past 20 years, exposure to biologically active plastic components and plasticizers has increased (43).

Human adipose tissue studies in the United States reveal that although extremely high concentrations of contaminants are found less frequently in individuals, these chemicals have become more evenly dispersed throughout the population, leading to fewer individuals with no measurable concentrations in their tissue (44). This introduces a problem if one depends on mean values to judge exposure trends. Average exposure may not have declined at all, since the absence of individuals with high concentrations may be balanced by the lack of individuals with no detectable contamination.

In the Great Lakes region, birds are still adversely affected by environmental contaminants even though their fish food base is less contaminated than it was in the mid-1970s (45). This suggests that exposure levels of organochlorine chemicals are still not low enough to protect wildlife and human health and/or that perhaps the growing use of other synthetic chemicals that also behave as endocrine disruptors, but as yet unidentified by standard analytical techniques, is contributing to the problem.

## WIDESPREAD HUMAN HEALTH EFFECTS

A growing number of infant/mother cohort studies report an association between exposure to synthetic chemicals and effects in offspring and support the premise that ambient exposure is now at, or above, levels at which humans are being affected. For example, children whose mothers consumed Lake Michigan fish for at least 6 years prior to their pregnancies (1980–1981) were examined by trained psychologists shortly after birth (46). A majority of the mothers ate an average of two to three fish meals a month. Those children whose mothers carried the highest concentrations of PCBs in their umbilical cord blood fat were found at birth to have measurable neurologic decrements and at age 4 had short-term memory problems (47). At age 11, the children with the highest prenatal exposure to PCBs had a 6.2 IQ point deficit and were more than a year behind their peers in school (3). The 6.2 IQ point deficit correlated with the concentrations of PCBs in their mothers' blood, not the concentration of PCBs in their blood at age 11. Children exposed to 1.25 ppm PCBs in their mothers' fat were significantly affected (48). This is within the range of PCB concentration in human adipose tissue from around the world, suggesting that a sizable number of children born today are affected.

A more recent study evaluated neurobehavioral development of infants whose mothers ate the equivalent of 40 lb of Lake Ontario fish over their lifetime prior to their pregnancies (1991–1993). Although the study design was not identical to the Lake Michigan study, the infants in this study also exhibited some of the same neurobehavioral decrements (4). In both studies, lifetime fish consumption, not what the mother ate during pregnancy, was associated with the problems in the children. In this study, the newborns were also given additional tests in which the more highly exposed infants were found to be hyperreactive. In this case the infants did not accommodate to common disturbances such as a ringing bell. This finding is consistent with the results of a series of studies in which rats were fed a diet of Lake Ontario salmon (49). At the end of 20 days on a 30% Lake Ontario salmon diet, the rats could not cope with adverse events such as a mild shock, a reduction in the number of food pellet offerings, or a change of scenery in their cages. The same effects were measurable in rats after 60 days on a 10% Lake Ontario salmon diet. The adults in these studies were bred and the same effect was reported in their offspring (50).

Two other epidemiologic studies undertaken in the Netherlands and the United States support the findings in the Great Lakes studies that neurologic changes are measurable in infants and children at contemporary exposure levels to organochlorine chemicals. Healthy mother-infant pairs were recruited for a nationwide study in the Netherlands (1990–1992) to determine psychomotor development and immune status of the infants relative to the mothers' plasma and breast milk levels of PCBs, dioxin, and dioxin toxicity equivalents (TEQs) measured as cytochrome P-450 enzyme activity (51–53). The results of this series of studies suggest that background exposure to PCBs and dioxins can have a small adverse effect on early psychomotor development, although the effect(s) were no longer detectable by the same battery of tests as the infants approached age 2. The authors note that they are not certain how or if this will be expressed in some other manner as the children mature. Background levels of PCBs/dioxin in the infants were inversely associated with monocyte and granulocyte counts at 3 months and positively associated with T cell subpopulations at 18 months. An inverse relationship between thyroid hormone ($T_4$,$T_3$) levels and dioxin TEQs was also discovered in these infants.

A similar study was conducted in North Carolina in 1986 where again a cross section of a healthy mother-infant population was examined and an inverse relationship between PCBs and hypotonicity and hyporeflexivity was discovered within several months after birth (54). In addition, this study also revealed a reduction in both breast milk production and length of lactation, which was correlated with the amount of DDT in the mother's breast milk fat. The same team confirmed these effects in a more recent study conducted in Mexico (55).

In each of the above studies, even though the decrement in the child was statistically significant, it would not have been recognized by the infants' parents or doctors. It took skilled psychologists and technicians with a battery of developmental tools and biochemical laboratory assays to quantify the changes in the children. These children are not retarded or obviously different; nevertheless, they are not developing to their fullest potential.

Findings such as this led to the convening of a group of environmental health scientists and physicians to review the current state of knowledge concerning the loss of human potential resulting from exposure to certain synthetic chemicals and their effects on the developing brain, behavior, and the thyroid system. The group was certain that "widespread loss of this nature can change the character of human societies." (6) In their judgment, "The benefits of reduced health care costs could be substantial if exposure to endocrine-disrupting chemicals were reduced." The economic and social costs of population-wide effects of this nature are only now being taken into consideration.

## CHARACTERISTICS OF THE ENDOCRINE SYSTEM THAT LEAD TO VULNERABILITY FROM ENDOCRINE DISRUPTORS

### Exquisitely Low Concentrations of Natural Chemicals Drive the Endocrine System

It is easy to brush aside the vast amount of data about the widespread dispersal of endocrine disruptors and the extent of exposure to them because the chemicals are not visible and the effects are not readily observed. In addition, it is easy to assume that because exposure to synthetic chemicals appears to be extremely low, it is not harmful. This mind-set probably evolved as a result of the traditional toxicologic paradigm for testing chemical safety that assumed if a compound does not cause cancer or other untoward effects at high doses, the compound is safe. Under this protocol, laboratory animals were exposed to chemicals at two to six orders of magnitude higher concentrations than daily exposure levels. Effects expressed at these high doses were then used to extrapolate down to a no-effect level at which regulatory standards were established. However, recent research has demonstrated that effects resulting from high-dose testing do not reflect the extent of harm at lower doses and do not take into consideration the safety of a compound at ambient exposure. Most important, high-dose extrapolation does not consider the effects that are initiated during the critical period of in utero exposure (56).

Prenatal development takes place at extremely low concentrations in the range of $10^{-13}$ g/ml for free estradiol (57) and $10^{-12}$ g/ml for free thyroxine (58). For example, an increase of $10^{-13}$ g/ml (1/10th part per trillion g/ml) free estradiol in serum of male mouse fetuses can alter the development of their prostates (59). Their prostate glands will be heavier because of a threefold increase in androgen receptors (59) and the pups will become more aggressive (60). Aggressiveness in this case is measured as the rate of urine marking (territoriality). Male mouse pups whose mothers were given DES (0.0001, 0.001, 0.01, 1.0, and 10 μg/day) and either of two pesticides, methoxychlor and o,p′-DDT (0.1, 1.0, and 100 μg/day), also showed an increase in territorial marking behavior. Methoxychlor is a contemporary-use pesticide that has been substituted for DDT. Its metabolites are estrogenic. o,p′-DDT is a mildly estrogenic isomer found in freshly produced DDT (9). The doses used in this case were based on their binding affinity for the estrogen receptor in serum when compared with free estradiol. Prostate size and aggression increased as the lowest doses of DES increased. But after a point, the effects abated, and as the dose increased more, the prostate became smaller and atrophied and increases in aggression abated (59). An inverted U-shaped dose-response curve was produced. High-dose testing would not have detected these significant changes that occurred at ambient exposure levels.

The inverted-U response curve was also demonstrated in two other reports. Pups of pregnant rats fed 10 and 20 μg/kg/body weight of PCB 126 (one of the 209 PCB congeners) exhibited mortality, fetotoxicity, liver enzyme induction, and delayed physical maturation (61). However, pups of pregnant rats fed 2 μg/kg/body weight of PCB 126 showed none of the above effects but exhibited poorer visual discrimination and higher activity levels (62). In the above studies, it is thought that high doses caused cytotoxicity and/or shut down receptors and thus masked the less visible effects on development and functionality (57,61).

### The Sensitive Embryo, Fetus, Newborn, and Child

The early stages of development are by far the most sensitive to endocrine disruption and therefore the most vulnerable to endocrine disruptors (2). For example, a single meal of 0.064 μg/kg/body weight 2,3,7,8-TCDD (dioxin) fed to pregnant rats on day 15 of gestation altered the sexual and behavioral development of the male pups, e.g., reduction in sperm per cauda epididymis, daily sperm production, and seminiferous tubule diameter, and demasculinized behavior. (Sexual differentiation commences in the rat fetus at approximately gestation day 15.) For years, dioxin research was directed toward its probability as a carcinogen. This new, low-dose testing regime, however, has revealed that exposure to dioxin in utero can lead to permanent alteration in reproductive function and development in both males and females (63).

Females have evolved with hormone-binding proteins in their blood that protect not only the mother from excess estrogenic hormones but also her offspring. However, several of the synthetic chemicals introduced in the past 50 years show little or no affinity for the these binding proteins and therefore compete with unbound hormones for the embryo's receptors (64). Although a synthetic contaminant may be 3 or 4 orders of magnitude weaker than free estradiol that operates in the range of $10^{-12}$ g and $10^{-13}$ g, individuals can carry as much as $10^{-6}$ g/g and $10^{-9}$ g/g in body fat of a single estradiol mimic. Consideration must be given to the fact that individuals in the developed world simultaneously carry a number of chemicals that bind to the estrogen receptor and that additivity and synergy among estrogen receptor binding chemicals has been demonstrated (65). Although DES is not an environmental contaminant, it provides a model for a synthetic chemical that does not bind to serum hormone binding proteins. Most of the adverse effects of in utero exposure to DES among humans were not recognized until the secondarily exposed individuals reached adulthood. The effects reported in the DES-exposed individuals have been replayed in the laboratory mouse (2).

### Homeostatic Control by the Endocrine System Foils High-Dose Testing

The exquisite feedback mechanisms that maintain homeostasis in the endocrine system complicate the ability to assess the hazard of exposure to synthetic chemicals. The protocol of setting acceptable thresholds for contaminants does not hold for the endocrine system, which is always "up and running." The addition of an agonist to the system could give a boost and trigger an increased DNA response, while an antagonist could reduce the endogenously programmed response. As mentioned above, exposure to endocrine disruptors can lead to uploading and downloading of response tissue in developing organs with the alteration dependent on the tissue involved, and the sex and stage of development of the individual. In addition, it is impossible to predict the vulnerability of the vast number of axes and opportunities for cross-talk between and among cells, tissues, and organs involved in homeostasis. In turn, it is now recognized that one synthetic chemical can initiate a number of effects depending on the stage of development, the sex, and the sensitivity of the individual. These characteristics of the endocrine system pose severe limitations on our ability to determine the safety of synthetic chemicals, and as a consequence have led to a large number of endocrine disruptors in the environment of our homes, work places, recreation centers, and the outdoors.

## THE ROLE OF THE PHYSICIAN

The effects of endocrine disruption during development pose a challenge to the physician because they are insidious and more often expressed as a reduction in function rather than as a specific clinical disease. Because of the subtlety of this damage it is improbable that a physician could determine if a patient's intelligence, behavior, immune system, and reproductive success have been compromised. In addition, few of the known adverse health effects that can be related to endocrine disruption require registration with public health authorities, and, therefore, little is known about their actual incidence. Increases in cryptorchidism and hypospadias, testicular cancers, and reduction in sperm counts have been reported in various geographical regions of the developed world but with little consistency and accuracy. Is it possible for physicians to determine if they are being presented with more cases of cryptorchidism now than in the past? This is still a relatively rare event. How does the physician know if a suspected increase is not just chance?

Physicians should become familiar with the classes of chemicals their patients might be encountering in their service areas. For instance, in the Midwest corn belt region of the United States, herbicides and insecticides are used heavily and are routinely found in ground water, surface water, wells, and municipal drinking water supplies. Large cities that receive water from these areas are delivering herbicide-contaminated water to their citizens on a daily basis and in seasonal pulses (66). Individuals living in agricultural regions, although they may not be farming, are also vulnerable because farm chemicals are volatile and travel in air currents and move in water supplies. For example, infants conceived in the spring in the beet, wheat, and potato growing region of western Minnesota exhibited an increase in male/female sex ratio for birth anomalies (circulatory/respiratory, urogenital, and musculoskeletal/integumental) whether they were offspring of pesticide applicators or offspring of residents living in the same general region of the state (67). The rate of these anomalies in 1,000 births was 26.9 and 30.0 in the bean, wheat, and corn section of the state for the general population and farmers, respectively. The rate was 18.3 in the urban and 23.7 in the forest sections of the state. Physicians in this part of Minnesota and other agricultural regions should be alert for concurrent functional deficits in their patients and other members of their families.

Physicians treating individuals in the United States and Canada who are dependent on food resources from aquatic systems, such as gulfs and bays, rivers, and lakes, should become familiarized with the fish advisories released by state or provincial departments of health in cooperation with state and provincial departments of fish and game. These advisories are generated to warn people, especially pregnant women, females of childbearing age, youngsters, and the aged, not to eat the fish. Although these advisories are based on the risk of getting cancer, they at least signal which fish are the most contaminated and, therefore, should be excluded from human consumption.

Traditional epidemiology tends to seek the problem in the directly exposed individual, which, in the case of endocrine disruptors, would lead to a type II error (a false negative). Instead, transgenerational exposure must be taken into consideration. For example, the health of the children of those who have handled or produced synthetic chemicals should be examined (68). Current epidemiologic studies seeking the etiology of breast cancer should include a prenatal history of the cancer patients from the time of their conception as well as their parents' exposure prior to their conception. It could be futile to try to find an association between breast cancer and the current concentration of chemicals in a patient's body at the time the cancer is discovered. The damage may well have been laid down prenatally when the patient's mother was exposed to elevated levels of estrogenic compounds that programmed or uploaded the estrogen response tissue in her fetus. For example, increased birth weight is associated with the increased incidence and mortality of breast, prostatic, and testicular cancer (69–71). Since premature birth and eclampsia reduce the risk of these cancers, consideration is given in these studies to the possibility that longer-term, elevated exposure to estrogenic hormones in utero may be a factor.

It is imperative to create case histories that probe into the memory of individuals who are suffering from autoimmune problems, such as arthritis, lupus, and early diabetes. The list should include those with endometriosis, reproductive problems, any thyroid disturbances, problems socially integrating, and attention deficit hyperactivity disorder (ADHD), as well as men with breast cancer and boys with obvious developmental problems at birth (undescended testicles and hypospadias, for example). The latter, appearing at birth, provide an unequivocal connection with prenatal experience, a period of time that is still well imprinted in the mother's mind. Physicians should take advantage of the fact that pregnancy is a special period in a woman's life when she is probably more aware of her body and where she has been and what she ate than any other time in her life.

Case histories need to address the following: Where was the patient born? Where were the patient's parents throughout their lives prior to the patient's conception? What was maternal and paternal exposure prior to, and during, pregnancy? What were the patient's parents' avocations and occupations? Did they farm or garden, fish, and hunt? Did they work with electronic equipment? Were they artists? What ethnic, regional, or unusual food habits were customary in the patient's home?

The single practitioner can document an increase or unusual endocrine-driven problem that he or she might see in a practice, but there are no coordinated programs to collect and summarize the findings. Information such as this, however, could be shared during grand rounds, local medical society meetings, or during specialty meetings. Remember, it took only a conversation between a physician and a questioning mother who wondered whether the DES she took during her pregnancy induced her daughter's clear cell vaginal adenocarcinoma (CCVA) and the physician's willingness to ask the mother of his next patient with CCVA if she had taken DES, for the cause of this long-term, delayed outcome to be recognized (72). Without this communication between a physician and his patient and subsequent patients, DES might still be used during pregnancies today. Unfortunately, in the case of endocrine disruptors we are not dealing with a single pharmaceutical that is relatively easy to track and regulate. Instead, we are dealing with complex mixtures of many widely used compounds that society has become dependent on and whose interactions are totally unpredictable.

## REFERENCES


1. Colborn T, Clement C, eds. *Chemically-induced alterations in sexual and functional development:* the wildlife/human connection. Princeton, NJ: Princeton Scientific Publishing, 1992.
2. Bern HA. The fragile fetus. In: Colborn T, Clement C, eds. *Chemically-induced alterations in sexual and functional development:* the wildlife/human connection. Princeton, NJ: Princeton Scientific Publishing, 1992;9–15.
3. Jacobson JL, Jacobson SW. Intellectual impairment in children exposed to polychlorinated biphenyls in utero. *N Engl J Med* 1996; 335(11):783–789.
4. Lonky E, Reihman J, Darvill T, Mather J, Daly H. Neonatal behavioral assessment scale performance in humans influenced by maternal consumption of environmentally contaminated Lake Ontario fish. *J Great Lakes Res* 1996;22(2):198–212.
5. Rotmensch J, Frey K, Herbst AL. Effects on female offspring and mothers after exposure to diethylstilbestrol. In: Mori T, Nagasawa H, eds. *Toxicity of hormones in perinatal life.* Boca Raton, Florida: CRC Press, 1988;143–159.
6. Consensus Statement from the work session on environmental endocrine-disrupting chemicals: Neural, endocrine, and behavioral effects. *Toxicol Ind Health* 1998;14(1/2):1–8.
7. Peterson RE, Moore RW, Mably TA, Bjerke DL, Goy RW. Male reproductive system ontogeny: Effects of perinatal exposure to 2,3,7,8-Tetrachlorodibenzo-p-dioxin. In: Colborn T, Clement C, eds. *Chemically-induced alterations in sexual and functional development:* the wildlife/human connection. Princeton, NJ: Princeton Scientific Publishing, 1992;175–194.
8. Brouwer A, Morse DC, Lans MC, et al. Interactions of persistent environmental organohalogens with the thyroid hormone system: Mechanisms and possible consequences for animal and human health. *Toxicol Ind Health* 1998;14(1/2):59–84.
9. Gray, LE. Chemical-induced alterations of sexual differentiation: A review of effects in humans and rodents. In: Colborn T, Clement C, eds. *Chemically-induced alterations in sexual and functional development:* the wildlife/human connection. Princeton, NJ: Princeton Scientific Publishing, 1992;203–230.
10. Porterfield, SP. Vulnerability of the developing brain to thyroid abnormalities: Environmental insults to the thyroid system. Environ Health Perspect 1994;102(Suppl 2):125–130.
11. Colborn T, vom Saal FS, Soto AM. Developmental effects of endocrine-disrupting chemicals in wildlife and humans. *Environ Health Perspect* 1993;101:378–384.
12. Rolland R, Gilbertson M, Colborn T, eds. Environmentally induced alterations in development: A focus on wildlife. *Environ Health Perspect* 1995;103(suppl 4).
13. Colborn T, Smolen MJ. Epidemiological analysis of persistent organochlorine contaminants in cetaceans. *Rev Environ Contam Toxicol* 1996;146:91–172.
14. Moccia R, Fox GA, Britton AJ. A quantitative assessment of thyroid histopathology of herring gulls *(Larus argentatus)* from the Great Lakes and a hypothesis on the causal role of environmental contaminants. *J Wild Dis* 1986;22:60–70.
15. Moccia RD, Leatherland JF, Sonstegard RA. Quantitative interlake comparison of thyroid pathology in Great Lakes coho *(Oncorhynchus kisutch)* and chinook *(Oncorhynchus tschawytscha)* salmon. *Cancer Res* 1981;41:2200–2210.
16. Shugart GW. Frequency and distribution of polygyny in Great Lakes herring gulls in 1978. *Condor* 1980;82:426–429.
17. Leatherland JF. Endocrine and reproductive function in Great Lakes salmon. In: Colborn T, Clement C, eds. *Chemically-induced alterations in sexual and functional development:* the wildlife/human connection. Princeton, NJ: Princeton Scientific Publishing, 1992; 129–145.
18. Gibbs PE, Pascoe PL, Burt GR. Sex change in the female dog-whelk, Nucella lapillus, induced by tributyltin from antifouling paints. *J Mar Biol Assoc UK* 1988;68:715–731.
19. Guillette LJ Jr, Pickford DB, Crain DA, Rooney AA, Percival HF. Reduction in penis size and plasma testosterone concentrations in juvenile alligators living in a contaminated environment. *Gen Compar Endocrinol* 1996;101:32–42.
20. Reijnders PJH. Reproductive failure in common seals feeding on fish from polluted coastal waters. *Nature* 1986;324:456–457.
21. Mac MJ, Schwartz TR, Edsall CC. Correlating PCB effects on fish reproduction using dioxin equivalents. *Soc Environ Toxicol Chem* 1988;116(abstr).
22. Kubiak TJ, Harris HJ, Smith LM, et al. Microcontaminants and reproductive impairment of the Forster's tern on Green Bay, Lake Michigan-1983. *Arch Environ Contam Toxicol* 1989;18:706–727.
23. Bishop CA, Brooks RJ, Carey JH, Ng P, Norstrom RJ, Lean DRS. The case for a cause-effect linkage between environmental contamination and development in eggs of the common snapping turtle (Chelydra s. serpentina) from Ontario, Canada. *J Toxicol Environ Health* 1991;33: 521–547.
24. Munkittrick KR, Portt CB, Van Der Kraak GJ, Smith IR, Rokosh DA. Impact of bleached kraft mill effluent on population characteristics, liver MFO activity, and serum steroid levels of a Lake Superior white

sucker *(Catostomus commersoni)* population. *Can J Fish Aquat Sci* 1991;48:1371–1380.
25. Fry DM, Toone CK. DDT-induced feminization of gull embryos. *Science* 1981;231:922–924.
26. De Guise S, Legace A, Beland P. True hermaphroditism in a St. Lawrence beluga whale *(Delphinapterus leucas)*. *J Wild Dis* 1994; 30(2):287–290.
27. Davis WP, Bortone SA. Effects of kraft mill effluent on the sexuality of fishes: An environmental early warning? In: Colborn T, Clement C, eds. *Chemically-induced alterations in sexual and functional development:* the wildlife/human connection. Princeton, NJ: Princeton Scientific Publishing, 1992;113–127.
28. Ellis DV, Pattisina LA. Widespread neogastropod imposex: A biological indicator of global TBT contamination? *Mar Pollut Bull* 1990;21: 248–253.
29. Grasman KA, Fox GA, Scanlon PF, Ludwig JP. Organochlorine-associated immunosuppression in prefledgling caspian terns and herring gulls from the Great Lakes: An ecoepidemiological study. *Environ Health Perspect* 1996;104(suppl 4):829–842.
30. Martineau D, Legacé A, Béland P, Higgins R, Armstrong D, Shugart LR. Pathology of stranded beluga whales *(Delphinapterus leucas)* from the St. Lawrence estuary, Québec, Canada. *J Comp Pathol* 1988; 98:287–311.
31. Phillips LJ, Birchard GF. An evaluation of the potential for toxics exposure in the Great Lakes region using STORET data. *Chemosphere* 1990;20:587–598.
32. Safe S. Toxicology, structure-function relationship, and human and environmental health impacts of polychlorinated biphenyls: Progress and problems. *Environ Health Perspect* 1992;100:259–268.
33. Agency for Toxic Substances and Disease Registry (ATSDR). *Toxicological profile for aldrin/dieldrin:* draft for public comment. Washington, DC: US Dept of Health and Human Services, Public Health Service, 1992;107.
34. Jones PD, Hannah DJ, Buckland SJ, et al. Persistent synthetic chlorinated hydrocarbons in albatross tissue samples from midway atoll. *Environ Toxicol Chem* 1996;15(10):1793–1800.
35. Blus LJ, Henny CJ, Stafford CJ, Grove, RA. Persistence of DDT and metabolites in wildlife from Washington state orchards. *Arch Environ Contam Toxicol* 1987;16:467–476.
36. Brotons JA, Olea-Serrano MF, Villalobos M, Pedraza V, Olea N. Xenoestrogens released from lacquer coating in food cans. *Environ Health Perspect* 1995;103:608–612.
37. Olea N, Pulgar R, Perez P, et al. Estrogenicity of resin-based composites and sealants used in dentistry. *Environ Health Perspect* 1996; 104(3):298–305.
38. Soto A, Justica H, Wray J, Sonnenschein C. p-Nonylphenol: An estrogenic xenobiotic released from "modified polystyrene." *Environ Health Perspect* 1991;92:167–173.
39. Krishnan AV, Stathis P, Permuth SF, Tokes L, Feldman D. Bisphenol-A: An estrogenic substance is released from polycarbonate flasks during autoclaving. *Endocrinology* 1993;132:2279–2286.
40. Peakall DB. Phthalate esters: Occurrence and biological effects. *Residue Rev* 1975;54:1–41.
41. Wams TJ. Diethylhexylphthalate as an environmental contaminant: A review. *Sci Total Environ* 1987;66:1–16.
42. Heindel JJ, Gulati DK, Mounce RC, Russell SR, Lamb JC. Reproductive toxicity of three phthalic acid esters in a continuous breeding protocol. *Fundam Appl Toxicol* 1989;12:508–518.
43. Reisch, MS. Dow wants more. *Chem Eng News* 1996(November 26); 19–23.
44. Kutz FW, Carey AE. Pesticides and toxic substances in the environment. *J Arboriculture* 1986;12(4):92–95.
45. Giesy JP, Ludwig JP, Tillitt, DE. Deformities in birds of the Great Lakes region: Assigning causality. *Environ Sci Tech* 1994;28(3): 128–135.
46. Jacobson SW, Fein GG, Jacobson JL, Schwartz PM, Dowler JK. The effect of intrauterine PCB exposure on visual recognition memory. *Child Develop* 1985;56:853–860.
47. Jacobson JL, Jacobson SW. A 4-year follow-up study of children born to consumers of Lake Michigan fish. *J Great Lakes Res* 1993;19(4): 776–783.
48. Jacobson JL, Jacobson SW. Dose-response in perinatal exposure to polychlorinated biphenyls (PCBs): The Michigan and North Carolina cohort studies. *Toxicol Ind Health* 1996;12(3/4):435–445.
49. Daly HB, Hertzler DR, Sargent DM. Ingestion of environmentally contaminated Lake Ontario salmon by laboratory rats increases avoidance of unpredictable aversive nonreward and mild electric shock. *Behav Neurosci* 1989;103(6):1356–1365.
50. Daly HB. The evaluation of behavioral changes produced by consumption of environmentally contaminated fish. In: Isaacson RL, Jensen KF, eds. *The vulnerable brain and environmental risks, vol 1:* Malnutrition and hazard assessment. New York: Plenum Press, 1992; 151–171.
51. Koopman-Esseboom CM, Morse DC, Weisglas-Kuperus N, et al. Effects of dioxins and polychlorinated biphenyls on thyroid hormone status of pregnant women and their infants. *Pediatr Res* 1994;36: 468–473.
52. Koopman-Esseboom C, Weisglas-Kuperus N, de Ridder MAJ, Van der Paauw CG, Tuinstra LGMT, Sauer PJJ. Effects of polychlorinated biphenyl/dioxin exposure and feeding type on infants' mental and psychomotor development. *Pediatrics* 1996;97(5):700–706.
53. Weisglas-Kuperus N, Sas TCJ, Koopman-Esseboom C, et al. Immunologic effects of background prenatal and postnatal exposure to dioxins and polychlorinated biphenyls in Dutch infants. *Pediatr Res* 1995; 38(3):404–410.
54. Rogan WJ, Gladen BC, McKinney JD, et al. Neonatal effects of transplacental exposure to PCBs and DDE. *J Pediatr* 1986;109: 335–341.
55. Gladen BC, Rogan WJ. DDE and shortened duration of lactation in a northern Mexican town. *Am J Public Health* 1995;85(4):504–508.
56. Sheehan DM, Thayer CA, Vom Saal F. A paradigm inversion for low dose toxicity studies. Abstract for Teratology Society Meeting, Keystone, CO, March, 1996.
57. vom Saal FS, Montano MM, Wang MH. Sexual differentiation in mammals. In: Colborn T, Clement C, eds. *Chemically-induced alterations in sexual and functional development:* the wildlife/human connection. Princeton, NJ: Princeton Scientific Publishing, 1992;17–83.
58. Porterfield SP, Hendrich CE. Tissue iodothyronine levels in fetuses of control and hypothyroid rats at 13 and 16 days gestation. *Endocrinology* 1992;131:195–200.
59. vom Saal FS, Timms BG, Montano MM, et al. Prostate enlargement in mice due to fetal exposure to low doses of estradiol or diethylstilbestrol and opposite effects at high doses. *Proc Natl Acad Sci USA* 1997;94:2056–2061.
60. vom Saal FS, Nagel SC, Palanza P, et al. Estrogenic pesticides: Binding relative to estradiol in MCF-7 cells and effects of exposure during fetal life on subsequent territorial behaviour in male mice. *Toxicol Lett* 1995;77:343–350.
61. Bernhoft A, Nafstad I, Engen P, Skaare JU. Effects of pre- and postnatal exposure to 3,3′,4,4′,5-pentachlorobiphenyl on physical development, neurobehavior and xenobiotic metabolizing enzymes in rats. *Environ Toxicol Chem* 1994;13(10):1589–1597.
62. Holene E, Nafstad I, Skaare JU, Bernhoft A, Engen P, Sagvolden T. Behavioral effects of pre- and postnatal exposure to individual polychlorinated biphenyl congeners in rats. *Environ Toxicol Chem* 1995; 14(6):967–976.
63. Gray LE Jr, Ostby JS. In utero 2,3,7,8-tetrachlorodibenzo-p-dioxin (TCDD) alters reproductive morphology and function in female rat offspring. *Toxicol Appl Pharmacol* 1995;133:285–294.
64. Arnold SF, Robinson MK, Notides AC, Guillette LJ Jr, McLachlan JA. A yeast estrogen screen for examining the relative exposure of cells to natural and xenoestrogens. *Environ Health Perspect* 1996;104(5): 544–548.
65. Soto AM, Chung KL, Sonnenschein C. The pesticides endosulfan, toxaphene, and dieldrin have estrogenic effects on human estrogen-sensitive cells. *Environ Health Perspect* 1994;102(4):380–383.
66. Wiles R, Cohen B, Campbell C, Elderkin S. *Tap water blues:* herbicides in drinking water. Environmental Working Group, Physicians for Social Responsibility. Washington, DC: The Tides Foundation, 1994.
67. Garry VF, Schreinemachers D, Harkins ME, Griffith J. Pesticide appliers, biocides, and birth defects in rural Minnesota. *Environ Health Perspect* 1996;104(4):394–399.
68. Agency for Toxic Substances and Disease Registry. *Health panel summary report from expert panel workshop to evaluate the public health implications of the treatment and disposal of polychlorinated biphenyls-contaminated waste.* Bloomington, IN: Agency for Toxic Substances and Disease Registry (ATSDR), 1994(May);15,29.

69. Michels KB, Trichopoulos D, Robins JM, et al. Birthweight as a risk factor for breast cancer. *Lancet* 1996;348:1542–1546.
70. Ekbom A, Hsieh CC, Lipworth L, et al. Perinatal characteristics in relation to incidence of and mortality from prostate cancer. *Br Med J* 1996;313:337–341.
71. Akre O, Ekbom A, Hsieh CC, Trichopoulos D, Adami HO. Testicular nonseminoma and seminoma in relation to perinatal characteristics. *J Natl Cancer Inst* 1996;88(13):883–889.
72. Herbst AL, Ulfelder H, Poskanzer DC. Adenocarcinoma of the vagina: Association of maternal stilbestrol therapy with tumor appearance in young women. *N Engl J Med* 1971;284:878–881.
73. Berwick P. 2,4-Dichlorophenoxyacetic acid poisoning in man. *JAMA* 1970;214:1114–1117.
74. de Duffard AME, de Alderte MN, Duffard R. Changes in brain serotonin and 5-hydroxyindolacetic acid levels induced by 2,4- dichlorophenoxyacetic butyl ester. *Toxicology* 1990;64:265–270.
75. Amdur MO, Doull J, Klaassen CD, eds. *Casarett and Doull's toxicology, the basic science of poisons.* New York: Pergamon Press, 1991.
76. Hayes WJ, Laws ER, eds. *Handbook of pesticide toxicology.* San Diego, CA: Academic Press, 1991.
77. USEPA. *Guidance for the reregistration of pesticide products containing as the active ingredient Alachlor (090501).* Washington, DC: Office of Pesticide Programs, US Environmental Protection Agency, 1984.
78. Tjalve H. Fetal uptake and embryogenetic effects of aminotriazole in mice. *Arch Toxicol* 1974;33:41–48.
79. Jukes TH, Shaffer CB. Antithyroid effects of aminotriazole. *Science* 1960;132:296.
80. Simic B, Kniewald Z, Davies JE, Kniewald J. Reversibility of the inhibitory effect of atrazine and lindane on cytosol 15 alpha-dihydrotestosterone-receptor complex formation in rat prostate. *Bull Environ Contam Toxicol* 1991;46:92–99.
81. Babic-Gojmerac T, Kniewald Z, Kniewald J. Testosterone metabolism in neuroendocrine organs in male rats under atrazine and deethylatrazine influence. *J Steroid Biochem* 1989;33:141–146.
82. Kniewald J, Peruzovic M, Gojmerac T, Milkovic K, Kniewald Z. Indirect influence of s-atrazines on rat gonadotrophic mechanism at early postnatal period. *J Steroid Biochem* 1987;27:1095–1100.
83. Porter WP, Green SM, Debbink NL, Carlson I. Ground water pesticides: Interactive effects of low concentrations of carbamates aldicarb and methomyl and the triazine metribuzin on thyroxine and somatotropin levels in white rats. *J Toxicol Environ Health* 1993;40:15–34.
84. Couch JA. Histopathology and enlargement of the pituitary of a teleost exposed to the herbicide trifluralin. *J Fish Dis* 1984;7:157–163.
85. Hess RA, Moore BJ, Forrer J, Linder RE, Abuel-Atta AA. The fungicide benomyl (methyl 1-(butylcarbamoyl)-2- benzimidazolecarbamate) causes testicular dysfunction by inducing the sloughing of germ cells and occlusion of efferent ductules. *Fundam Appl Toxicol* 1991;17:733–745.
86. Laisi A, Tuominen R, Mannisto P, Savolainen K, Mattila J. The effect of maneb, zineb, and ethylenethiourea on the humoral activity of the pituitary-thyroid axis in rat. *Arch Toxicol Suppl* 1985;8:253–258.
87. Gocmen A, Peters HA, Cripps DJ, Bryan GT, Morris CR. Hexachlorobenzene episode in Turkey. *Biomed Environ Sci* 1989;2:36–43.
88. Smith A, Dinsdale D, Cabral J, Wright A. Goiter and wasting induced in hamsters by hexachlorobenzene. *Arch Toxicol* 1987;60:343–349.
89. Haake J, Kelley M, Keys B, Safe S. The effects of organochlorine pesticides as inducers of testosterone and benzo-a-pyrene hydroxylases. *Gen Pharmacol* 1987;18(2):165–169.
90. Arnold D, Moodie C, Charbonneau S, et al. Long-term toxicity of hexachlorobenzene in the rat and the effect of dietary vitamin A. *Food Chem Toxicol* 1985;23:779–793.
91. USEPA. *Guidance for the reregistration of pesticide products containing mancozeb as the active ingredient.* Washington, DC: Office of Pesticide Programs, US Environmental Protection Agency, 1987.
92. USEPA. *Guidance for the reregistration of pesticide products containing maneb as the active ingredient.* Washington, DC: Office of Pesticide Programs, US Environmental Protection Agency, 1988.
93. USEPA. *Guidance for the reregistration of pesticide products containing metiram as the active ingredient.* Washington, DC: Office of Pesticide Programs, US Environmental Protection Agency, 1988.
94. Huggett R, Unger MA, Siligman PF, Valkirs AO. The marine biocide tributyltin: Assessing and managing the environmental risks. *Environ Sci Technol* 1992;26(2):232–237.
95. Bryan GW, Gibbs PE, Burt GR, Hummerstone LG. The effects of tributyltin (TBT) accumulation on adult dog whelks, *Nucella lapillus: Long-term field and laboratory experiments.* J Mar Biol Assoc UK 1987;67:525–544.
96. Gray LE, Ostby JA, Kelce WR. Developmental effects of an environmental antiandrogen—the fungicide vinclozolin alters sex differentiation of the male rat. *Toxicol Appl Pharmacol* 1994;129:46–52.
97. van Velsen FL, Danse LHJC, van Leeuwen FXR, Dormans JAMA, van Logten MJ. The subchronic oral toxicity of the B-isomer of hexachlorocyclohexane in rats. *Fundam Appl Toxicol* 1986;6:697–712.
98. Cranmer JM, Cranmer MF, Goad PT. Prenatal chlordane exposure: Effects on plasma corticosterone concentrations over the life span of mice. *Environ Res* 1984;35:204–210.
99. Soto AM, Sonnenschein C, Chung KL, Fernandez MF, Olea N, Serrano FO. The E-screen assay as a tool to identify estrogens: An update on estrogenic environmental pollutants. *Environ Health Perspect* 1995;103(suppl 7):113–122.
100. Kelce W, Stone C, Laws S, Gray L, Kemppainen JA, Wilson E. Persistent DDT metabolite p,p'-DDE is a potent androgen receptor antagonist. *Nature* 1995;375:581–585.
101. ATSDR. *Toxicological profile for endosulfan, endosulfan alpha, endosulfan beta, endosulfan sulfate.* Atlanta, GA: Agency for Toxic Substances and Disease Registry, 1990.
102. Chowdhury AR, Venkatakrishna-Bhatt H, Gautam AK. Testicular changes in rats under lindane treatment. *Bull Environ Contam Toxicol* 1987;38:154–156.
103. Inbaraj RM, Haider S. Effect of malathion and endosulfan on brain acetylcholinesterase and ovarian steroidogenesis of Channa punctatus (Bloch). *Ecotoxicol Environ Safety* 1988;16:123–128.
104. Reuber MD. Carcinogenicity and toxicity of malathion and malaoxon. *Environ Res* 1985;37:119–153.
105. Porter WP, Green SM, Debbink NL, Carlson I. Ground water pesticides: Interactive effects of low-level concentrations of carbamates, aldicarb, methomyl, and the triazine metribuzin on thyroxine and somatotropin levels in white rats. *J Toxicol Environ Health* 1993;40:15–34.
106. Gray LE, Ostby J, Ferrell J, et al. A dose-response analysis of methoxychlor-induced alterations of reproductive development and function in the rat. *Fundam Appl Toxicol* 1989;12:92–108.
107. Cummings AM, Gray LE. Methoxychlor affects the decidual cell response of the uterus but not other progestational parameters in female rats. *Toxicol Appl Pharmacol* 1987;90:330–336.
108. Rattner BA, Clarke RN, Ottinger MA. Depression of plasma luteinizing hormone concentration in quail by the anticholinesterase insecticide parathion. *Comp Biochem Physiol* 1986;83C:451–453.
109. Eil C, Nisula BC. The binding properties of pyrethroids to human skin fibroblast androgen receptors and to sex hormone binding globulin. *J Steroid Biochem* 1990;35(3/4):409–414.
110. Nagel SC, vom Saal FS, Thayer KA, Dhar MG, Boechler M, Welshons WV. Relative binding affinity-serum modified access (RBA-SMA) assay predicts the relative in vivo bioactivity of the xenoestrogens bisphenol A and octylphenol. *Environ Health Perspect* 1997;105:70–76.
111. ATSDR. *Toxicological profile for cadmium.* Atlanta, GA: Agency for Toxic Substances and Disease Registry, 1991.
112. Mably TA, Bjerke DL, Moore RW, Gendron-Fitzpatrick A, Peterson RE. In utero and lactational exposure of male rats to 2,3,7,8-tetrachlorodibenzo-p-dioxin. 3. Effects on spermatogenesis and reproductive capability. *Toxicol Appl Pharmacol* 1992;114(1):118–126.
113. Mably TA, Moore RW, Peterson RE. In utero and lactational exposure of male rats to 2,3,7,8-tetrachlorodibenzo-p-dioxin. 1. Effects on androgenic status. *Toxicol Appl Pharmacol* 1992;114:97–107.
114. Mably TA, Moore RW, Goy RW, Peterson RE. In utero and lactational exposure of male rats to 2,3,7,8-tetrachlorodibenzo-p-dioxin. 2. Effects on sexual behavior and the regulation of luteinizing hormone secretion in adulthood. *Toxicol Appl Pharmacol* 1992;114:108–117.
115. ATSDR. *Toxicological profile for lead.* Atlanta, GA: Agency for Toxic Substances and Disease Registry, 1991.
116. Cullen MR, Kayne RD, Robins JM. Endocrine and reproductive dysfunction in men associated with occupational inorganic lead intoxication. *Arch Environ Health* 1984;39(6):431–440.

117. ATSDR. *Toxicological profile for mercury.* Atlanta, GA: Agency for Toxic Substances and Disease Registry, 1988.
118. Allen-Rowlands CF, Castracane VD, Hamilton MG, Seifter J. Effect of polybrominated biphenyls (PBB) on the pituitary-thyroid axis of the rat (41099). *Proc Soc Exp Bio Med* 1981;166:506–514.
119. Bush B, Bennett A, Snow J. Polychlorobiphenyl congeners, p,p'-DDE, and sperm function in humans. *Arch Environ Contam Toxicol* 1986;15: 333–341.
120. Sager DB, Shih-Schroeder W, Girard D. Effect of early postnatal exposure to polychlorinated biphenyls (PCBs) on fertility in male rats. *Bull Environ Contam Toxicol* 1987;38:946–953.
121. Dieringer CS, Lamartiniere CA, Schiller CM, Lucier GW. Altered ontogeny of hepatic steroid-metabolizing enzymes by pure polychlorinated biphenyl congeners. *Biochem Pharmacol* 1979;28:2511–2514.
122. Fowles JR, Fairbrother A, Baecher-Steppan L, Kerkvliet NI. Immunologic and endocrine effects of the flame-retardant pentabromodiphenyl ether (DE-71) in C57BL/6J mice. *Toxicology* 1994;86:49–61.
123. Choudhury H, Coleman J, DeRosa CT, Stara JF. Pentachlorophenol: Health and environmental effects profile. *Toxicol Ind Health* 1986; 2(4):483–553.
124. Treinen KA, Dodson WC, Heindel JJ. Inhibition of FSH-stimulated cAMP accumulation and progesterone production by mono(2-ethylhexyl) phthalate in rat granulosa cell cultures. *Toxicol Appl Pharmacol* 1990;106:334–340.
125. Lloyd SC, Foster PMD. Effect of mono-(2-ethylhexyl)phthalate on follicle-stimulating hormone responsiveness of cultured rat Sertoli cells. *Toxicol Appl Pharmacol* 1988;95:484–489.
126. Gray TJB, Gangolli SD. Aspects of the testicular toxicity of phthalate esters. *Environ Health Perspect* 1986;65:229–235.
127. Thysen B, Morris PL, Gatz M, Bloch E. The effect of mono(2-ethylhexyl) phthalate on sertoli cell transferrin secretion in vitro. *Toxicol Appl Pharmacol* 1990;106:154–157.
128. Laskey JW, Berman E. Steroidogenic assessment using ovary culture in cycling rats: Effects of bis(2-diethylhexyl) phthalate on ovarian steroid production. *Reprod Toxicol* 1993;7:25–33.
129. Arfini G, Mutti A, Vescovi PP, et al. Impaired dopaminergic modulation of pituitary secretion in workers occupationally exposed to styrene: Further evidence from PRL response to TRH stimulation. *J Occup Med* 1987;29(10):826–830.
130. Mutti A, Vescovi PP, Falzoi M, Arfini G, Valenti G, Franchini I. Neuroendocrine effects of styrene on occupationally exposed workers. *Scand J Work Environ Health* 1984;10:225–228.

*Environmental and Occupational Medicine, Third Edition,* edited by William N. Rom.
Lippincott–Raven Publishers, Philadelphia © 1998.

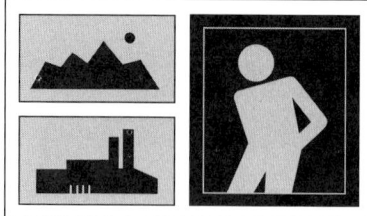

CHAPTER 55

# Hematologic Effects of Occupational Hazards

John H. Ward

The hematopoietic system is a complex organ consisting of two parts, the marrow and the blood. The bone marrow is the site of cell production, continually replacing the cellular elements of the blood, erythrocytes, neutrophils, and platelets. Production is under tight control of a group of growth factors. Neutrophils and platelets are used as they perform their physiologic functions, and erythrocytes eventually become senescent and outlive their usefulness. For successful function, the cellular elements of the blood must circulate in proper numbers and retain both their structural and physiologic integrity. Erythrocytes contain hemoglobin, which permits uptake and delivery of oxygen to tissues to sustain cellular metabolism. Erythrocytes normally survive in the circulation for 120 days while sustaining this function. Neutrophils are found in blood on their way to tissues to repel microbial invasion. Circulating platelets play a key role in hemostasis.

The production requirement of the bone marrow is a prodigious one. Daily, the marrow replaces 3 billion erythrocytes per kilogram of body weight (1). Neutrophils have a circulating half-life of only 6 hours, and 1.6 billion neutrophils per kilogram of body weight must be produced each day (2). The entire platelet population must be replaced every 9.9 days (3). Because of the need to produce large numbers of functional cells, the marrow is remarkably sensitive to any infectious, chemical, metabolic, or environmental insult that impairs DNA synthesis or disrupts the formation of the vital subcellular machinery of the erythrocytes, leukocytes, or platelets. Further, since the blood cells are marrow progeny, the peripheral blood serves as a sensitive and accurate mirror of bone marrow activity. Blood is readily available for assay via venipuncture, and examination of the blood can provide an early clue of environmentally induced illness.

J. H. Ward: Division of Hematology–Oncology, Department of Internal Medicine, University of Utah Health Sciences, Salt Lake City, Utah 84132.

## SCREENING FOR HEMATOLOGIC DISEASE

The hematopoietic system can be evaluated by means of the history and physical examination as well as with the assistance of the laboratory.

### History

The initial evaluation for possible hematologic illness must include a careful history. Symptoms usually are not specific for hematologic ailments and may give rise to symptoms in all other organ systems. Attention should be directed to the nonspecific symptoms of anemia, including weakness, malaise, and lassitude; in more severe cases, dyspnea, angina pectoris, and confusion may be found. A history of jaundice or pigmenturia may suggest a hemolytic process. The onset of infection may signal neutropenia. Thrombocytopenia may be discovered because of complaints of easy bruising, epistaxis, or petechiae. A thorough drug history, a detailed work history, and a history of exposure to any potentially toxic substances is imperative.

### Physical Examination

The physical examination may aid in focusing on the specific problem. Examination of the skin and mucous membranes may reveal pallor, suggesting anemia. Jaundice may signal hemolysis. Cyanosis may indicate a defect in oxygen transport. Abnormal bleeding or petechiae may suggest a problem with platelet number or

**TABLE 1.** *Normal adult blood values*

| Determination | Reference range: Conventional units | Reference range: SI units |
|---|---|---|
| Hematocrit | | |
| Male | 45–52% | 0.42–0.52 |
| Female | 37–48% | 0.37–0.48 |
| Hemoglobin | | |
| Male | 13–18 g/dl | 8.1–11.2 mmol/L |
| Female | 12–16 g/dl | 7.4–9.9 mmol/L |
| Leukocyte count | 4,300–10,800/mm$^3$ | 4.3–10.8 × 10$^9$/L |
| Neutrophils | 1,800–7,700/mm$^3$ | 1.8–7.7 × 10$^9$/L |
| Lymphocytes | 1,000–4,800/mm$^3$ | 1.0–4.8 × 10$^9$/L |
| Monocytes | 0–800/mm$^3$ | 0–0.8 × 10$^9$/L |
| Eosinophils | 0–450/mm$^3$ | 0–0.45 × 10$^9$/L |
| Basophils | 0–200/mm$^3$ | 0–0.2 × 10$^9$/L |
| Platelet count | 150,000–350,000/mm$^3$ | 150–350 × 10$^9$/L |
| Erythrocyte count (RBC) | 4.2–5.9 million/mm$^3$ | 4.2–5.9 × 10$^{12}$/L |
| Mean corpuscular volume (MCV) | 80–94 μm$^3$ | 80–94 fl |
| Mean corpuscular hemoglobin (MCH) | 27–32 pg/cell | 1.7–2.0 fmol |
| Mean corpuscular hemoglobin concentration | 32–36% | 0.32–0.36 |
| Reticulocyte count | 0.2–2.0% | 10–100 × 10$^9$/L |
| Serum iron | 50–150 μg/dl | 9–26.9 μmol/L |
| Iron-binding capacity | 250–410 μg/dl | 44.8–73.4 μmol |

SI, *Système International.*
Adapted from ref. 7.

function. Examination of the fundi and mucous membranes may disclose otherwise unrecognized evidence of bleeding. Particular attention should be paid to examination of lymph nodes and spleen, remembering that in 95% of normal subjects the spleen is not palpable. Physical evidence of infection may be found when neutrophil production is impaired, and bone tenderness, particularly of the sternum, should raise the possibility of leukemia.

### Examination of the Blood

To evaluate the hematopoietic system, one must examine the blood itself. Hemoglobin is measured by converting it to cyanmethemoglobin and measuring its absorbance at 540 nm (4). The hematocrit, or percentage of blood consisting of erythrocytes, can be determined by centrifugation; in automated systems, it may be calculated as the product of the mean corpuscular voiume (MCV) and red blood cell (red blood cell) count. The red blood cell count can be measured electronically, by quantitating a decrease in conductance whenever a cell interrupts the passage of current between two electrodes. The magnitude of this change in conductance parallels the MCV. After lysis of the red cells, the leukocyte and platelet counts can be similarly determined (5).

Other red blood cell indices may be calculated from the previously derived parameters (5):

*Mean corpuscular hemoglobin (MCH), pg/cell = [hemoglobin (g/dl)]/[red blood cell count (× 10$^{12/L}$)]*

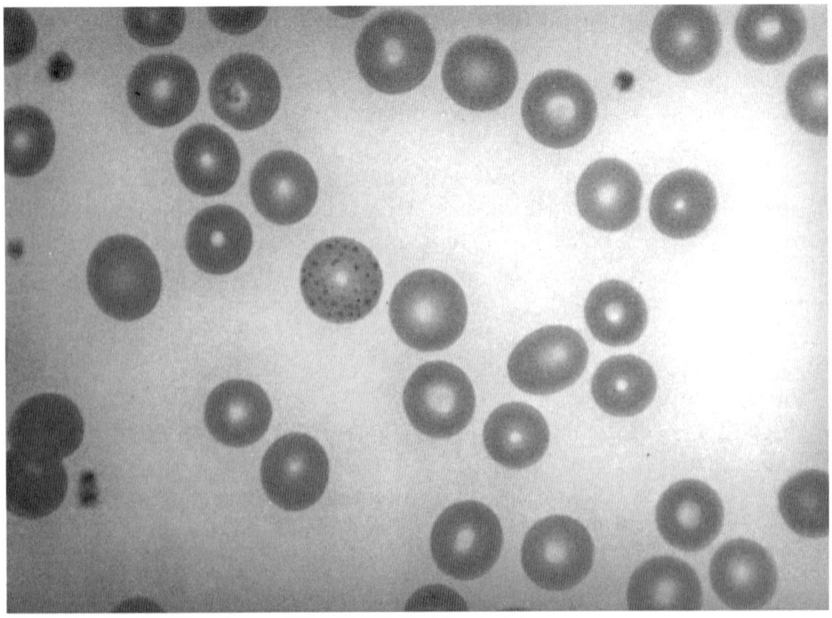

**FIG. 1.** Basophilic stippling (residual RNA inclusions in the RBCs is a finding of lead poisoning). (Courtesy of Sherri Perkins, M.D.)

*Mean corpuscular hemoglobin concentration (MCHC), % = [hemoglobin (g/dl)]/[volume packed red cells (%)]*

The red cell indices may be helpful in clarifying anemias for diagnostic purposes (6). Normal values are shown in Table 1 (7).

Examination of the peripheral blood smear is an indispensable aid in the evaluation of hematologic illness. Wright-stained smears enable the examiner to assess the accuracy of reported leukocyte and platelet counts and allow evaluation of red cell morphology and leukocyte differential count. Since the MCV is the average red blood cell size, populations of different sizes may produce a faulty impression of red blood cell size unless the smear is examined. The shape of the RBCs also is important. Damaged, fragmented cells can suggest hemolysis, and large, polychromatophilic, young red cells can indicate increased red cell production because of red cell loss or destruction. The presence of red blood cell inclusions may be the initial clue for some illnesses, as with the basophilic stippling found in lead poisoning (Fig. 1). A direct determination of the reticulocyte count may be increased if there is evidence of hyperfunctioning bone marrow, or reduced in the presence of a hypoproliferative marrow disorder. Determination of the leukocyte differential is critical in ascertaining the absolute numbers of the individual types (neutrophils, lymphocytes, monocytes, basophils, eosinophils), since the concentration of the cell type multiplied by the leukocyte count gives the absolute cell number. For some leukemias, examination of the blood smear alone may be sufficient to establish a diagnosis.

### Bone Marrow Examination

When hematologic problems are discovered, examination of bone marrow obtained safely and rapidly from the sternum or iliac crest may yield valuable additional information. Erythroid and myeloid cells at all stages of maturation can be observed and their relative numbers determined. The presence of cells foreign to the marrow (such as tumor cells) or abnormal hematopoietic cells (such as iron-laden erythroid precursors or leukemic cells) may be recognized. Chromosome studies can be done as well.

Chromosome abnormalities have become increasingly important in evaluating hematologic malignancies and will likely lead to better prognostic information, and perhaps to more specific therapies. Our understanding of oncogenes is also beginning to have clinical applications (8–11). Proto-oncogenes (cellular oncogenes) are certain genes present in normal tissues that are highly conserved and code for proteins important in key cellular functions, such as protein kinases or receptors. Correlates to cellular oncogenes, termed viral oncogenes, are found in the group of viruses called retroviruses. Such viruses may induce neoplasia in some animals and tissue culture systems. The viral oncogenes are thought to represent normal proto-oncogenes that have been incorporated into the viral genome. In certain circumstances, as in chronic myelogenous leukemia, altered proto-oncogenes likely play a role in human neoplasia. This field continues to evolve rapidly.

The Philadelphia chromosome is evident in the malignant cells of most patients with chronic myelogenous leukemia. This abnormality, due to a reciprocal translocation between chromosomes 9 and 22, has been recognized for many years using standard karyotyping. At the molecular level, this results in the translocation of the proto-oncogene c-*abl*, on chromosome 9, to a region on chromosome 22 termed the breakpoint cluster region (bcr) (12–14). This translocation yields a chimeric gene, *bcr-abl,* which encodes a very active tyrosine kinase thought to be pathogenic in chronic myelogenous leukemia.

In one form of acute leukemia, acute promyelocytic leukemia, there is a characteristic 15;17 translocation, a rearrangement of the gene that encodes the retinoic acid receptor-α. Recent information suggests that pharmacologic doses of retinoic acid can induce differentiation of malignant cells and allow many patients to achieve complete remission without the initial use of cytotoxic chemotherapy (15,16).

### Other Studies

When a bleeding disorder is present, evaluation of the platelet count, bleeding time, prothrombin time (PT), and partial thromboplastin time (PTT) usually pinpoints the locus. Prolonged bleeding time indicates a functional platelet defect or thrombocytopenia. An abnormal PT or PTT points to a disorder of the coagulation cascade. Measurement of the serum iron, total iron-binding capacity (TIBC), and serum ferritin can be used to estimate the iron stores. Levels of lactic dehydrogenase and indirect bilirubin may be elevated in the presence of hemolysis. Rapid cell turnover may be reflected by an elevated serum uric acid value.

Environmental agents can interfere with the hematopoietic system in several ways—inhibition of hemoglobin synthesis, inhibition of cell production, leukemogenesis, and increased red blood cell destruction, among others. Other agents may interact with hemoglobin, inhibiting oxygen delivery. Some agents, such as radiation and benzene, may act via more than one mechanism. Prototype causative agents are discussed in the following sections.

## INHIBITION OF HEMOGLOBIN SYNTHESIS: LEAD POISONING

### Exposure Sources

Lead poisoning results in multisystem disease. Its history as a public health problem began at least with the Roman Empire, when pottery was lead glazed and water was transported through lead-lined pipes. Lead has been used to sweeten wines, and the addition of lead to wine in the 15th and 16th centuries was a potential capital offense in Germany. Today exposure to lead from many potential sources remains a problem. In addition to lead miners, lead poisoning has been documented in "urban lead miners," people who remove lead paint from older homes (17). Lead poisoning also occurred in persons responsible for disposal of lead-containing batteries (18). While lead is not used in commercial distilling, it remains a potential toxin in the production of illicit alcohol. In one survey in the southeastern United States, 30% of the samples of moonshine contained lead concentrations greater than 1,000 g/L, and 86% of all moonshine contained detectable lead derived from distillation equipment (19). In one year alone, 50 million gallons of moonshine were confiscated in the United States, confirming the importance of this potential exposure source. One family contracted lead poisoning from the unexpected source of cocktail glasses that released lead from the applied decorations (20). Some pottery glazes also may contribute lead to foodstuffs contained in them. In another instance, lead poisoning occurred as the element was slowly released from an embedded bullet (21).

### Symptoms and Signs of Lead Poisoning

Lead poisoning most commonly presents as abdominal pain (22). It may mimic peritonitis because of its intensity and association with a rigid abdominal wall. This has been termed lead colic. Other gastrointestinal symptoms include constipation, vomiting, and anorexia. Less commonly, peripheral neuropathy involving paralysis of frequently used muscle groups is present (23). For example, a painter may experience wrist drop. Lead encephalopathy may be manifest as seizures (82%), coma or stupor (40%), or a variety of other complaints including confusion and headaches (19). Since anemia is virtually always present, pallor is frequently found. As many as 70% of patients have been reported to have the so-called lead line, a deposit of bluish lead sulfide in the gingival margin (22). Stippling of the retina was reported in Egyptian cases (23).

### Lead Poisoning and Anemia: The Basic Defect

The anemia of lead poisoning is due to the ability of lead to inhibit hemoglobin synthesis in a variety of ways (Fig. 2). For example, lead interferes with the production of the iron-protoporphyrin moiety of hemoglobin, heme, as it inhibits the action of the synthetic enzymes, δ-aminolevulinic acid (δ-ALA) synthetase, ALA dehydrase, uroporphyrinogen decarboxylase, coproporphyrinogen oxidase, and heme synthetase (24,25). Then, by-products of the disordered synthetic pathway, δ-ALA and coproporphyrin, can be found in the urine and may serve as diagnostic aids. In addition to inhibition of heme synthesis, lead poisoning is associated with a defect in the incorporation of labeled leucine into the globin protein chains of hemoglobin, indicating that globin synthesis is impaired as well (26).

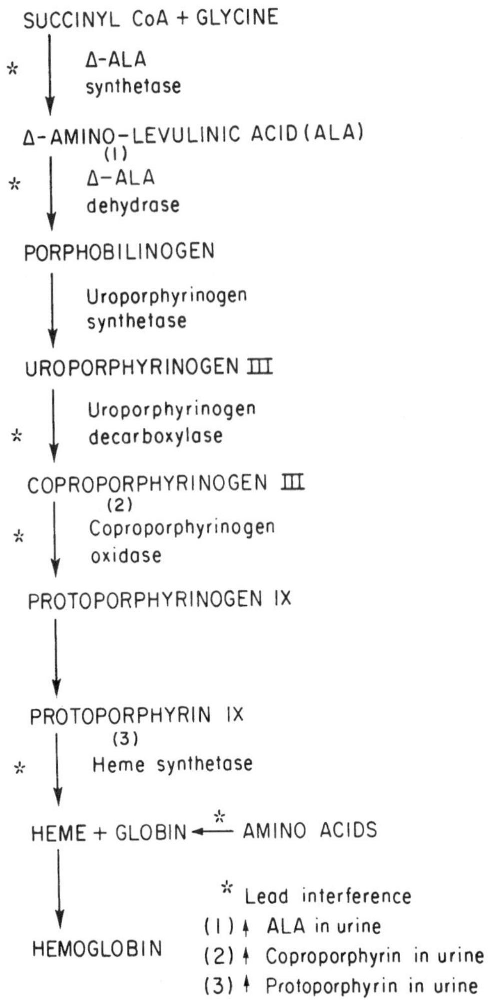


**FIG. 2.** Multiple sites of lead interference with hemoglobin synthesis.

Another prominent feature of lead poisoning is impairment of the synthesis of the enzyme, pyrimidine 5′-nucleotidase (27,28). This enzyme promotes the catabolism of RNA in immature red cells. In lead poisoning, RNA accumulates and can be seen as basophilic inclusions, or stippling, on Wright-stained blood smears (see Fig. 1). Apparently because heme synthesis is impaired, iron also accumulates during red cell maturation, and when the marrow is examined iron-laden mitochondria can be seen about the nuclear border of normoblasts, which explains the finding of ringed sideroblasts . Understanding of this constellation of findings informs the diagnosis of lead toxicity.

## LABORATORY FINDINGS IN THE ANEMIA OF LEAD POISONING

Anemia is a feature of more than 90% of cases of lead poisoning (22). Usually it is mild, with a hematocrit of 0.29 to 0.43 (mean 0.35) and a hemoglobin value of 8.1 to

12.8 g/dl (mean 10.7 g/dl) (25). In patients with lead encephalopathy, the anemia is typically worse, the hematocrit averaging between 0.20 and 0.30 (19). The red cells are mildly microcytic, with an MCV of 79 femtoliter (fl). The mean corpuscular hemoglobin concentration (MCHC) usually is slightly reduced, with an average value of 31%. Basophilic stippling of circulating red cells occurs in 70% of patients (22); on average, 1.8% of cells demonstrate stippling, which can be coarse or fine (25). The reticulocyte count is mildly elevated (mean 4.4%). Other laboratory findings include increased urinary excretion of δ-ALA, coproporphyrin III, and, to a lesser extent, uroporphyrin. Free erythrocyte protoporphyrin is increased as well. The diagnosis can be made by demonstrating elevated lead levels in blood or urine. In persons with equivocal values, an infusion of calcium ethylenediaminetetraacetic acid (CaEDTA), 1 g in 500 ml 5% dextrose in water over 6 hours, followed by a 24-hour urinary lead determination, should yield less than 0.5 mg lead. With lead toxicity the value usually is greater than 1.0 mg.

## INHIBITION OF CELL PRODUCTION: BENZENE POISONING

### Exposure Sources

Benzene is a cyclic hydrocarbon obtained by the distillation of coal tar. It also can be produced in the process of compressing the distillation products of petroleum and fuel oil. Benzene is highly volatile under ambient conditions. Industrial practices offer numerous potential sources of benzene exposure, since it is used in the manufacture of explosives and the production of cosmetics, soaps, perfumes, and drugs. Benzene also finds use in the dye industry and is employed in dry cleaning. Although clear standards for regulation of occupational benzene exposure have been put forth by the Occupational Safety and Health Administration (OSHA), it is estimated that more than 2 million workers have at least the potential for exposure to this agent. A reduction in the permissible exposure limit could likely decrease benzene-related hematopoietic problems (29). The primary route of exposure is via volatile benzene in ambient air, and concentrations well below the threshold for smell are associated with toxicity (30). Although recognized as an important occupational danger, large-scale problems may still be seen (31).

### Signs and Symptoms

Benzene toxicity may be present as an acute illness or as a chronic disease that develops after as many as 29 years' exposure (32). With acute illness, subjects may complain of headache, dizziness, and vertigo, symptoms believed to be due to the early localization of inhaled benzene in the brain.

The chronic form of the illness is related to the localization of benzene in the bone marrow. In one series of 217 Turkish shoe workers, 23.5% demonstrated some hematologic abnormality indicative of chronic benzene poisoning (33). Here the benzene seems to exert a colchicine-like effect, blocking mitosis of the marrow proliferative cells. Further, some mutagenic effects occur that probably have a role in the occasional subsequent development of leukemia. As marrow cell proliferation is inhibited, the concentration of the circulating marrow progeny decreases and symptoms appear. The red cell mass decreases, and shortness of breath and pallor develop. A reduction in the platelet count results in a bleeding diathesis, with petechiae and purpura. As the neutrophil number and supply diminish, infection may ensue, and a painful mouth (agranulocytic angina) may be seen. These symptoms of blood cell deficiency are those that most often bring patients with chronic benzene intoxication to the physician. On physical examination, the patient may be pale and exhibit petechiae and bruises. Signs of infection such as fever also may be present, and in the febrile subject a careful history is most helpful in localizing the source. In patients with compromised cardiac circulation, the development of anemia may lead to the unmasking of coronary artery insufficiency and angina. The presence of fever or angina should be considered an indication for immediate hospitalization.

### Laboratory Findings

Careful examination of the blood is a first step in investigating possible benzene toxicity. The initial examination should include measures of the hematocrit, total leukocyte count, and platelet count. A smear of blood from the fingertip should be prepared to evaluate the red cell morphology, white cell varieties, and platelet number. Patients usually present with pancytopenia, though any combination of anemia, leukopenia, or thrombocytopenia may occur (34). The anemia is usually normocytic and normochromic, although macrocytic indices of the red cell may be noted. Red cell morphology usually is normal, and polychromatophilia is not prominent. White cell morphology is normal, with a decrease in the concentration of neutrophils and a reciprocal increase in the concentration of mononuclear cells. The platelet count may be decreased. The degrees of anemia, neutropenia, and thrombocytopenia vary, but anemic symptoms are most common with hematocrit values less than 0.30. The rate of infection increases as the neutrophil count falls below $0.5 \times 10^9$/L, and often bleeding and purpura are associated with platelet counts less than $60 \times 10^9$/L. An inappropriately low reticulocyte count for the degree of anemia almost always is found and highlights the defect as a hypoplastic state. Similarly, normal values for lactic dehydrogenase (LDH) and for haptoglobin confirm that red cell destruction is not increased. Once the presumptive diagnosis of cytopenia due to hypoplastic marrow has been reached, marrow aspiration should be performed, and at the same

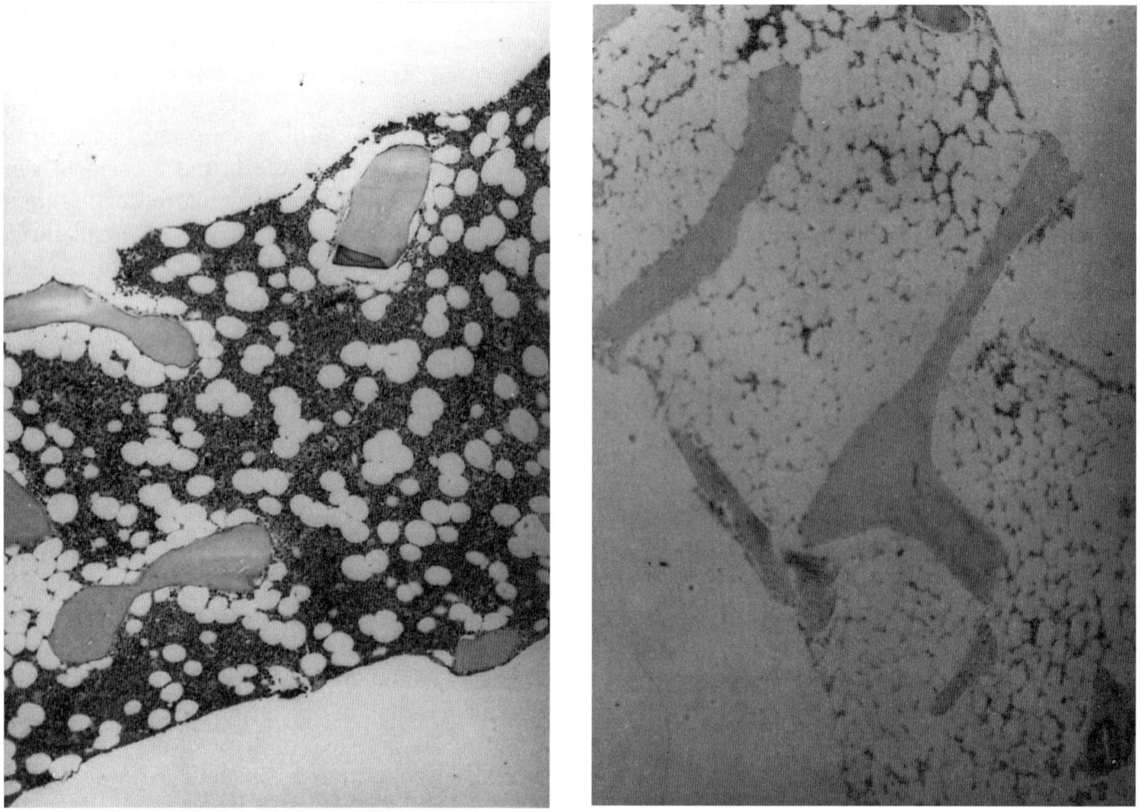

**FIG. 3.** Benzene-induced aplastic anemia. A microscopic section of the bone marrow exhibits hypocellularity *(right)*. A normal bone marrow biopsy is shown for comparison *(left)*. (Courtesy of Sherri Perkins, M.D.)

time biopsy of the bone marrow, since aspirates are relatively unreliable for assessing marrow cellularity.

Examination of the marrow aspirate ordinarily reveals a hypocellular specimen with a relative predominance of lymphocytes. In some cases, however, numerous immature forms of the red cell, neutrophil, and megakaryocyte series may be seen. Examination of sections of the bone marrow biopsy usually reveals hypocellularity (Fig. 3). Pancytopenia may occur with either normocellular or hypocellular marrow, though. In some cases, the marrow contains numerous immature forms (35). Fibrosis is not seen. Acute myelogenous leukemia may develop on the substrate of benzene-induced cytopenia, and when this occurs, it is most likely acute myeloid leukemia (36–39). Other hematologic entities including myeloma, chronic lymphocytic leukemia, hairy cell leukemia, and chronic myelogenous leukemia may be seen in workers exposed at their jobs, and the risk increases with the level of cumulative exposure (40–42).

## Management

Once the diagnosis of benzene-induced marrow injury is established, the worker should be removed from benzene exposure permanently. Such an approach is advisable even in cases of relatively mild toxicity, since patients with already damaged marrow may be more sensitive than expected when reexposed to the agent.

Principles for the management of benzene-induced cytopenia may be derived from experience with hypoplastic anemias in general. In this setting, the therapeutic approach is dictated by the degree and variety of cytopenia and the patient's reaction to it. For example, anemia sufficient to cause limitation of activity may require repeated transfusions. In patients with vascular insufficiency, particularly of the coronary vessels, transfusion therapy should be given to maintain a hematocrit value above 0.30, since at this level the physiologic compensatory mechanisms for anemia have their maximum effect. Neutrophil counts less than $0.5 \times 10^9$/L are associated with increased risk of infection.

The course of benzene-induced aplastic anemia does not appear to differ from that of other aplastic anemias. In general, the 5-year survival rate for patients with aplastic anemia is only 30%, and half of the deaths are likely to occur during the first 6 months following diagnosis. An attempt has been made to identify the subgroup of patients who are most likely to die of their disease so that aggressive treatment can be instituted. Lynch and co-workers (43) found that severe thrombocytopenia and a predominance of lymphoid cells in the marrow seem to be prominent features of patients who have the highest mortality rate. These data, however, apply to aplastic anemia patients in general, and their application to the specific instance of benzene toxicity has not been tested directly.

Bone marrow transplantation from human leukocyte antigen (HLA)-identical siblings to patients with severe aplastic anemia is very successful, though perhaps less so for patients who have received transfusions (44,45). Transplant is most successful in young persons, and because of the need for a matched sibling, this form of treatment remains applicable to only a portion of persons who have aplastic anemia. Patients who receive syngeneic bone marrow transplants require immunosuppression as well as bone marrow, suggesting that aplastic anemia is due to more than just a depletion of pluripotent stem cells (46). For those who are not candidates for marrow transplant, immunosuppression may improve survival (47). Recent evidence suggests a combination of antilymphocyte globulin, methylprednisone, and cyclosporine produces either a complete or a partial response in 65% of patients (48). High doses of cyclophosphamide given without bone marrow transplant may also prove effective (49). In severe aplastic anemia, the application of androgens seemed effective in certain patients but had no effect on mortality in general (50).

### Inhibition of Marrow Growth by Other Agents

Aplastic anemia has been reported in association with a variety of other agents, including insecticides such as lindane (benzene hexachloride) (51,52), hydrocarbon glues (53), trinitrotoluene (54), kerosene, carbon tetrachloride, and other solvents (55,56). Both transient and irreversible suppression of the bone marrow occur after exposure to ionizing radiation (57). One unusual case of aplastic anemia was reported in a runner who applied rubber cement containing a benzene impurity to foot blisters (58).

## INDUCTION OF LEUKEMIA: IONIZING RADIATION

### Exposure Sources

Ionizing radiation is that particulate or electromagnetic radiation that has sufficient energy to ionize molecules. α-Particles, β-particles, and cosmic rays (atomic nuclei) directly ionize molecules, while δ-rays and x-rays indirectly ionize molecules because they generate secondary particles that possess ionizing properties. Neutrons also possess a secondary ionizing effect. Standardized units for the measurement of ionizing radiation attempt to quantify the absorbed dose, the amount of energy transferred, and the penetrative quality of the radiation source. Attempts are being made to relate the dose to a predictable biologic result, so as to establish what risks might be encountered in occupational situations.

The knowledge that radiation and cancer were related began to accumulate soon after the discovery of x-rays. These cases were primarily skin malignancies, but evidence for the induction of leukemia by ionizing radiation also accumulated; indeed, this proved to be the malignancy most often induced. A major potential source of radiation exposure is medical workplaces. Radiologists, radiation therapists, radiation technicians, and radiopharmacists all work in an environment where they require protection from radiation. Indeed, before adequate shielding was routinely used, it is estimated that radiologists received an exposure of 100 R each year, and over a working lifetime likely 20 times that or more. This resulted in a high rate of leukemia in radiologists in the period 1930 to 1950, and a latent period of some 18 years was estimated before disease developed (59,60). Following the nuclear explosions in Japan, the incidence of leukemia began to increase 1½ years later; the peak increase in leukemia occurred 4 to 7 years later (61). Risk was directly related to proximity to the explosion.

Long-term review of atomic bomb survivors has substantiated the increased risk of leukemia, though the latency period may be longer than initial reports suggested (62). Continued analysis appears to also show an excess of patients with the myeloproliferative disorder polycythemia rubra vera (63,64). All subsets of acute nonlymphoblastic leukemia are represented, including the recently recognized acute megakaryoblastic leukemia, which is characterized by a syndrome of acute myelofibrosis. Others exposed to radiation may present with a preleukemic phase consisting of cytopenias despite a remarkably cellular bone marrow that may show evidence of disordered erythroid maturation (dyserythropoiesis), ringed sideroblasts, and variable numbers of blasts in insufficient numbers to represent leukemia. These preleukemic disorders are now called myelodysplastic syndromes and have been strictly defined in morphologic terms (65). In addition to atomic bomb survivors, military personnel who witnessed nuclear testing are also at higher risk for leukemia (66,67). Although this is controversial, the risk of acute leukemia may be slightly increased for persons living in southern Utah who are exposed to fallout from above-ground nuclear testing (68).

It is certainly possible that other bone marrow disorders would become evident with continued follow-up. The suggestion that plasma cell myeloma is now more frequent among atomic bomb survivors indicates the need for continued surveillance (69). Similar data confirmed the potential leukemogenic effect of x-rays from a study of subjects who received radiation in a variety of medical occupations (70), and a risk of leukemia is also conferred to fetuses exposed to diagnostic radiation in utero (71). In each case, radiation exposure may be limited by removing personnel from the source or by adequate shielding to prevent emitted radiation from reaching workers.

### Signs and Symptoms

Whole-body exposure to radiation in single doses results in suppression of marrow growth, and usually a single whole-body dose of 300 to 400 cGy is fatal to humans. With sublethal exposure, symptoms of acute nausea and diarrhea may occur. Cytopenias follow and can be predicted by the kinetics of the production, storage, and circulation of the various cell lines. Platelet survival time is 7 to 9 days, and petechiae or purpura may be seen following a fall of the platelet count to less than $50 \times 10^9$/L. The pallor of anemia and its symptoms of dyspnea, tachycardia, and malaise are not expected until the red cells circulating are removed after their 120-day life span, when the hematocrit value falls. Neutrophils are stored for 7 to 10 days in the marrow, so despite their short intravascular survival time, neutropenia and infection do not ordinarily occur until a week or more after exposure. The interval between exposure and development of leukemia may be 8 to 18 years. Then the presence of hematopoietic malignancy may be detected because of either abnormalities found on routine blood examination or symptoms of the cytopenias that develop as a result of the leukemia. Physical examination of symptomatic patients may reveal pallor, petechiae, purpura, and signs of infection. In asymptomatic patients the physical examination may reveal only splenomegaly and sternal tenderness.

### Laboratory Findings

Following radiation exposure, either acute or chronic leukemia may occur, with chronic myelogenous leukemia (CML) being most frequent (61). Interestingly, chronic lymphocytic leukemia was not seen as a consequence of the atomic bombs dropped on Hiroshima and Nagasaki. In a follow-up of the Japanese blasts, the specific rates of increased risk for persons who were within 1,500 m of the hypocenter were 8.1 for acute nonlymphocytic leukemia, 25.6 for CML, and 21.7 for acute lymphoblastic leukemia (61). With CML the patient may be neither anemic nor thrombocytopenic at the time of diagnosis. The leukocyte count is typically increased, to greater than $50 \times 10^9$/L, and examination of the blood film discloses neutrophils in all stages of maturation as well as an increase in the number of eosinophils and basophils (Fig. 4). Because such a blood picture is rarely seen except during CML this is a finding of considerable diagnostic importance. The diagnosis is further supported when the marrow reveals increased cellularity, predominantly of neutrophils and their precursors, and chromosome analysis discloses the presence of Philadelphia chromosome.

The concept of the Philadelphia chromosome was introduced earlier in this chapter. This reciprocal translocation between chromosomes 9 and 22 yields a fusion gene *(bcr-abl)* that encodes a protein that is an aberrant version of the normal gene product. The resultant tyrosine kinase is more active than its normal counterpart. Although the typical translocation can usually be seen on routine karyotyping, a small percentage of patients are abnormal within the breakpoint cluster region of chro-

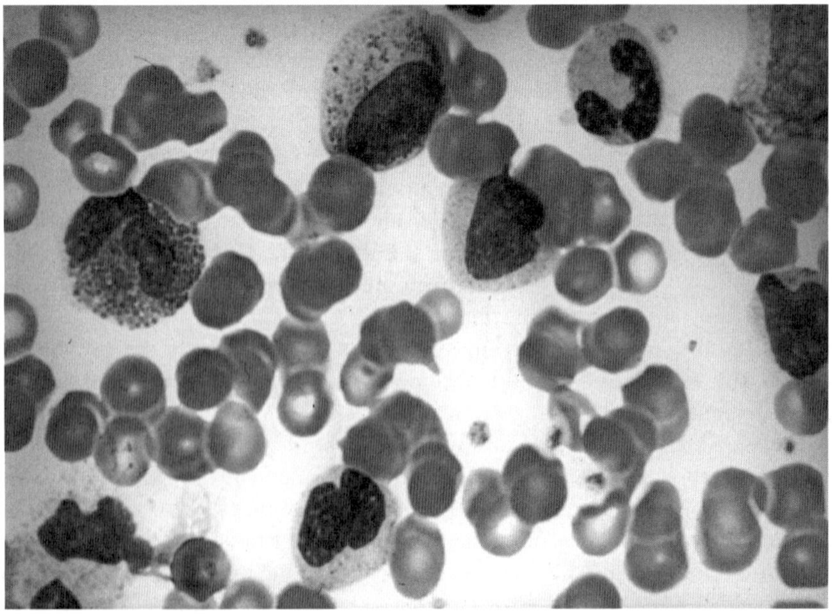

**FIG. 4.** In chronic myelocytic leukemia, the blood contains immature neutrophils in all stages of development. (Courtesy of Sherri Perkins, M.D.)

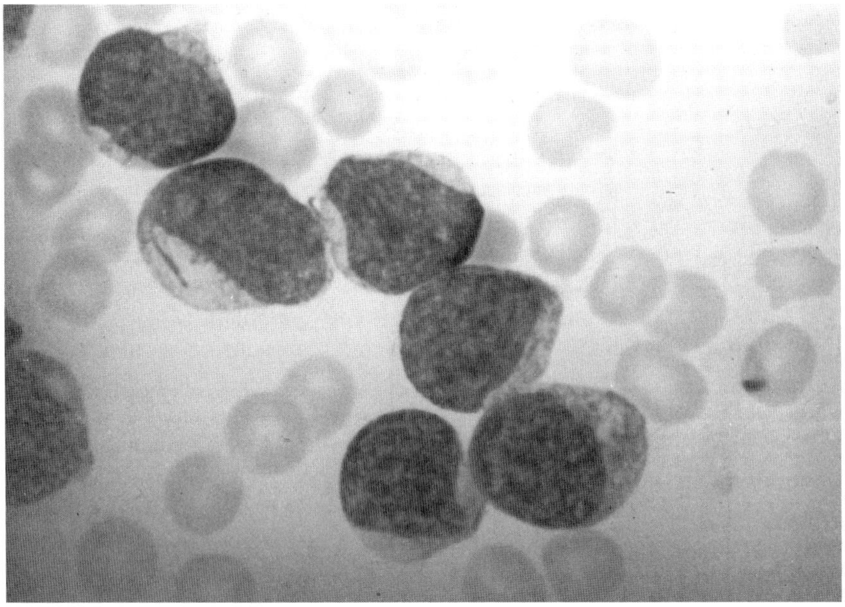

**FIG. 5.** Acute leukemia: myoblasts, one of which contains an Auer rod. (Courtesy of Sherri Perkins, M.D.)

mosome 22, which can be detected by Southern blot analysis (72). The actual size of the breakpoint within the bcr appears to correlate with the duration of the chronic phase of CML (73).

In other patients, examination of the blood may reflect the development of acute myelogenous leukemia. In this setting, anemia and thrombocytopenia are nearly universal. In half the cases, the leukocyte count is elevated; in the others, it is normal or low. Most patients have blast cells circulating at the time of diagnosis, and some of these may contain Auer rods, which appear as pinkish rods or strands that stain positive for peroxidase (Fig. 5). The marrow may be either hypocellular or hypercellular, and it almost always contains 30% blasts or more. Megakaryocytes usually are reduced in number, as are the neutrophil and red cell precursors.

### Management

With CML, survival time averages 2½ to 3 years from the date of diagnosis, and the institution of standard treatment has little effect on survival, although it may be effective in reducing the fatigue and subjective symptoms of the disease. Treatment with alkylating agents such as busulfan usually results in clinical remission of the disease, and repeated courses are given as the clinical picture dictates. In the terminal stage many patients develop an acute leukemia–like picture, and usually this predicts a survival time of 6 months or less. Some of these patients in so-called blast crisis respond to chemotherapy transiently.

Bone marrow transplantation offers the only hope of cure for CML. When used in the chronic phase of the disorder, bone marrow transplantation results in better than 50% long-term survival. If reserved until blast crisis, long-term survival is less than 20% (74–78). This approach is limited by the availability of a matched donor (usually a sibling), physiologically young patients, as older patients have increasing numbers of complications. Recently there has been success with HLA-matched unrelated donors, but the availability of such donors is low and the frequency of graft-versus-host disease high (79).

With acute myelogenous leukemia survival depends on the ability of the treatment to induce remission. For subjects who do not experience remission survival is measured in weeks. Thus far, few data have been obtained to evaluate the effect of modern chemotherapy on leukemia induced by radiation; however, survival of 2 more years may be expected for many of the patients who obtain complete remission, and some patients may experience disease-free intervals of 5 years or more.

The treatment of acute myelogenous leukemia depends on successful eradication of the malignant clone of cells from the bone marrow. Cytotoxic therapy can result in complete remission in 60% to 85% of patients. A subset of about 20% of these complete responders remain in remission for years. The use of HLA-matched allogenic bone marrow transplantation during the first remission appears to result in long-term survival for close to 50% (80–82). In carefully selected patients with similar demographic parameters, bone marrow transplantation probably offers a 20% to 30% better chance of cure than chemotherapy alone (83). As with CML, the utility of transplant is restricted by the physiologic age of the patient and the necessity for a properly matched donor.

The health and functional status of adult bone marrow transplant survivors are remarkably good, whether the transplant is used to treat aplastic anemia or leukemia (84).

## HEMOLYTIC DISEASE: ARSINE POISONING

### Exposure Sources

Arsine (arseniuretted hydrogen) is a colorless, nonirritating gas, that in high concentration possess a mild garlic odor. Arsine is generated when hydrogen and arsenic interact and when a reaction between water and a metallic arsenide occurs. In the industrial setting, the treatment of metals or ores with acid, as in the refining of metals, can lead to arsine formation. Further, the processes of galvanizing, soldering, and lead-plating have been reported to generate lethal concentrations of the gas (17). Certain fungi can generate arsine in sewage. Present regulations limit arsine exposure to 0.05 parts of gas per million parts of air as a time-weighted average for an 8-hour work shift of a standard workweek. In a 15-minute exposure period, the arsenic limit of 0.002 $mg/m^3$ has been established (85). It is estimated that the most effective measures against arsine exposure include careful monitoring of ambient air and rigid measures to prevent or limit contact of arsenic-containing materials with nascent hydrogen or acid. The magnitude of potential worker exposure to arsine is considerable, and it is estimated to be 900,000 or more. Further, since many sources of coal contain arsenic, the potential for increased worker exposure as coal is developed as an energy source is real.

### Signs and Symptoms

A history of exposure to arsenic or arsine is helpful in alerting the observer to the possibility of arsine intoxication. Inhalation of 250 ppm has been reported as instantly lethal, whereas exposures to 25 to 50 ppm for 30 minutes also have been associated with death (86). The clear minimum lethal dose in humans has not been established. Since arsine can damage red blood cells and lead to their destruction, some of the symptoms and signs are related to hemolysis. Subjects may complain of dark urine and back pain, followed by scanty urine as intravascular hemolysis occurs and the kidneys are damaged by the byproducts of red cell destruction. As anemia develops, the subject may complain of shortness of breath as well as dizziness on standing abruptly. Jaundice ensues as the liberated hemoglobin exceeds the capacity of the liver to metabolize and excrete it. Subjective symptoms include nausea, abdominal pain, and headache.

The physical examination typically reveals a pale, jaundiced patient with tachycardia and sometimes postural hypotension upon assuming the standing position. There may be fever. Examination of the skin may reveal bronzing, and the skin of the palms and soles of the feet may be thickened. Liver tenderness has been reported (86).

### Laboratory Findings

The hematologic effects of arsine poisoning are largely due to the ability of arsine to associate with the red blood cell and to induce hemolysis. Some workers have sug-

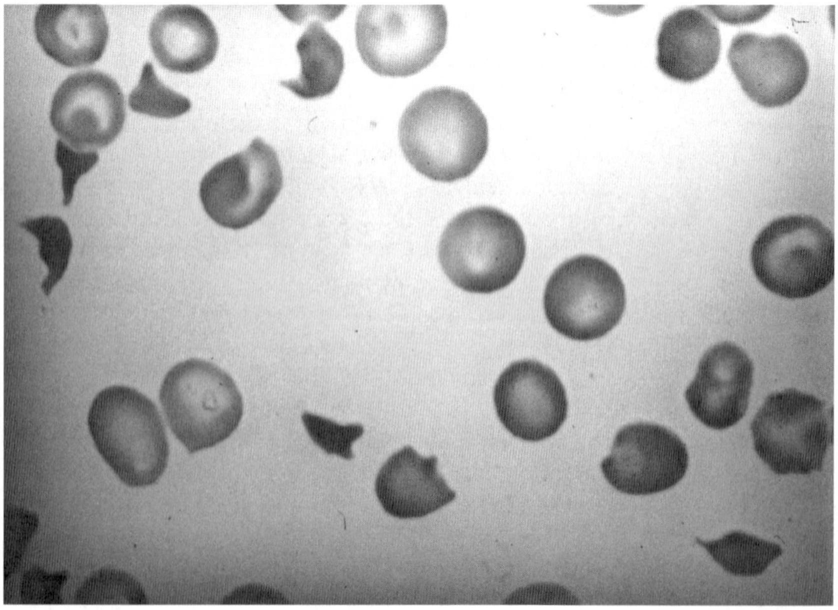

**FIG. 6.** With arsine-induced hemolysis, numerous fragmented erythrocytes can be seen. (Courtesy of Sherri Perkins, M.D.)

gested that an interaction with oxygen produces elemental arsenic, which is the ultimate hemolytic factor. Other studies suggest that arsine leads to accumulation of erythrocytic hydrogen peroxide, which is responsible for red cell destruction. Arsine may interfere with the sodium-potassium pump of the red cell, leading to osmotic cell destruction (87).

Examination of the blood reveals anemia with poikilocytes, red cell fragments, and red cell ghosts (Fig. 6). Red cell destruction appears to take place intravascularly, so hemoglobin is liberated directly into the plasma, where concentrations greater than 2 mg/ml are noted (86). Dimers of hemoglobin are excreted in the urine, so results of the test for heme are positive. Reticulocytosis usually is seen as the marrow compensates for the anemia. Further examination of the blood discloses leukocytosis, and the stained neutrophils may demonstrate toxic granules. Also, unstained leukocytes may contain greenish nuclei (88). Chemical determinations of the plasma reveal the products and by-products of hemolysis. Indirect, or unconjugated, bilirubin concentrations increase, and the values for lactic dehydrogenase rise as well. As hemoglobin binds with haptoglobin, the concentration of the latter declines, and it is frequently entirely absent. Hemopexin, a heme-binding protein, also declines. Tests for antibody to red cells are negative. If the marrow is examined, hyperplasia of the red cell precursors is observed.

The urine sediment is initially normal, but cellular elements may be recognized if tubular necrosis is present. The urine arsenic levels are elevated as high as 2 mg/L. Oliguria can occur as an early manifestation of the disease, and renal failure is likely to be the cause of death in fatally intoxicated subjects.

### Treatment

Even if subjects are removed from the source of toxic exposure, hemolysis is likely to continue and may last as long as 4 days (86). The treatment of choice for severely intoxicated subjects is exchange transfusion to remove irreversibly damaged and arsenic-bearing red cells. Alkaline diuresis is recommended to minimize precipitation of hemoglobin in the kidney. For severely oliguric patients and those with anuria, dialysis of the blood and measures to reduce a much elevated serum potassium value are advisable. Attempts to remove accumulated arsenic with chelating agents such as dimercaprol have been disappointing in preventing further hemolysis (89).

## HEMOLYTIC DISEASE RELATED TO OTHER CAUSES

Hemolytic anemia has been reported as a consequence of exposure to naphthalene, a prominent component of moth balls (90,91). This occurs most frequently in persons who are deficient in glucose-6 phosphate dehydrogenase (G6PD) and appears to be due to a naphthalene metabolite. G6PD is an enzyme in the pentose phosphate pathway, and is necessary for the reduction of nicotinamide adenine dinucleotide phosphate (NADP) to NADPH, which in turn is required for the maintenance of intracellular levels of reduced glutathione. Individuals with G6PD deficiency may develop hemolytic anemia when exposed to certain agents that produce oxidative stress, as their red cells have insufficient reducing power. G6PD deficiency affects more than 100 million people worldwide, and the potential for offending agents to cause harm is thus considerable. Twelve percent of African-American males may carry G6PD deficiency (92). A variety of pharmaceuticals, dyes, and other agents can precipitate G6PD deficiency–related hemolysis (93).

An interesting entity, termed march hemoglobinuria and characterized by hemoglobinuria, increased plasma hemoglobin, and decreased plasma haptoglobin, can occur in workers who sustain repeated bodily contact with a hard surface. It has been reported in soldiers during marches (94), karate practitioners (95), and a conga drummer (96). Interestingly, red blood cell morphology usually is normal.

Immune-related hemolytic anemia may also be seen after exposure to a variety of pharmaceuticals. Trimellitic anhydride (TMA), an agent used as a curing resin, has been associated with a syndrome characterized by immune-mediated hemolytic anemia, restrictive lung disease, fever, and dyspnea. Removal of exposure leads to resolution of the syndrome, and with current environmental controls, this syndrome is unusual (97).

## AGENTS THAT INTERFERE WITH OXYGEN DELIVERY

Oxygen delivery depends on an adequate level of hemoglobin, with the iron in the reduced (ferrous) state. The normal hemoglobin level is about 15 g/dl. When the reduced hemoglobin level exceeds 5 g/dl, cyanosis is apparent in physical examination. When heme is in the oxidized (ferric) state, the molecule is termed methemoglobin. Because of the red blood cell's effective capacity to reduce hemoglobin, less than 1% of the total hemoglobin is in the form of methemoglobin. In concentrations of 2 g/dl, methemoglobin causes cyanosis.

Acquired methemoglobinemia can occur with exposure to a variety of compounds used in the home and industry which are capable of increasing the rate of heme oxidation. Naphthalene, various dyes, and waters high in nitrates are among the long list of agents that can cause methemoglobinemia (98). Usually methemoglobinemia is simply a curiosity causing cyanosis. If high levels are present (more than 35%), symptoms of poor oxygen delivery can occur, an unusual situation in adults. The treatment is to terminate exposure to the offending agent.

If the patient is symptomatic, methylene blue can be given by vein (99). This results in nonenzymatic reduction of the methemoglobin. Methylene blue requires the pentose phosphate pathway to function, and is ineffective in patients with G6PD deficiency (100).

Sulfhemoglobinemia can cause cyanosis with a concentration as low as 0.5 g/dl. This molecule, too, is incapable of oxygen transport. It occurs when sulfur is incorporated into the porphyrin ring, resulting in a reduced oxygen affinity (101). This can occur with exposure to sulfur compounds found in the workplace and in polluted areas (98,101–103). Sulfhemoglobinemia causes marked cyanosis but few other symptoms except in rare cases (103), such as the case of two fishermen who died of sulfhemoglobinemia-related asphyxia thought to be secondary to hydrogen sulfide gas in a ship's hold containing decaying shrimp. Treatment requires removing the offending agent. Once sulfhemoglobin is formed, it remains throughout the life of the red blood cell.

Carbon monoxide reversibly binds to heme iron in the ferrous state (carboxyhemoglobin) with such a high affinity that it precludes oxygen binding. Levels of 30% can cause symptoms of headaches and dizziness. Levels of 50% can cause asphyxiation. Unlike the cyanosis caused by methemoglobin and sulfhemoglobin, carboxyhemoglobin is bright red, causing the skin to appear cherry-red. Treatment of carbon monoxide poisoning is ventilation with inspired oxygen concentration of 100%.

## REFERENCES


1. Donohue DM, Reiff RH, Hanson ML, et al. Quantitative measurement of the erythrocytic and granulocytic cells of the marrow and blood. *J Clin Invest* 1958;37:1571–1576.
2. Golde DW, Cline MJ. Production, distribution, and fate of granulocytes. In: Williams WJ, Beutler E, Erslev AJ, et al., eds. *Hematology.* New York: McGraw-Hill, 1977;699–706.
3. Harker LA, Finch CA. Thrombokinetics in man. *J Clin Invest* 1969; 48:963–974.
4. International Committee for Standardization in Haematology. Recommendations for hemoglobinometry in human blood. *Br J Haematol* 1967;13(suppl):71.
5. Williams WJ, Schneider AS. Examination of the peripheral blood. In: Williams WJ, Beutler E, Erslev AJ, et al., eds. *Hematology.* New York: McGraw-Hill, 1977;10–25.
6. Wintrobe MM. The size and hemoglobin content of the erythrocyte. *J Lab Clin Med* 1932;17:899–912.
7. Normal reference laboratory values. *N Engl J Med* 1986;314:39–49.
8. Bishop JM. Oncogenes. *Sci Am* 1982;246:80–92.
9. Cline MJ, Slamon DJ, Lipsick JS. Oncogenes: implications for the diagnosis and treatment of cancer. *Ann Intern Med* 1984;101: 223–233.
10. Friend SH, Dryja TP, Weinberg RA. Oncogenes and tumor-suppressing genes. *N Engl J Med* 1988;319:618–622.
11. Bishop JM. The molecular genetics of cancer. *Science* 1987;235: 305–310.
12. Stam K, Heisterkamp N, Grosveld G, et al. Evidence of a new chimeric bcr/c-abl mRNA in patients with chronic myelocytic leukemia and the Philadelphia chromosome. *N Engl J Med* 1985;313: 1429–1433.
13. Ben-Neriah Y, Daley GQ, Mes-Masson AM, Witte ON, Baltimore D. The chronic myelogenous leukemia-specific P210 protein is the product of the bcr/abl hybrid gene. *Science* 1986;233:212–214.
14. Kurzrock R, Gutterman JU, Talpaz M. The molecular genetics of Philadelphia chromosome-positive leukemias. *N Engl J Med* 1988; 319:990–998.
15. Warrell RP, Frankel SR, Miller WH, et al. Differentiation therapy of acute promyelocytic leukemia with tretinoin (all-trans-retinoic acid). *N Engl J Med* 1991;324:1385–1393.
16. Fenaux P, Le Deley MC, Castaigne S, et al. Effect of all trans-retinoic acid in newly diagnosed acute promyelocytic leukemia. *Blood* 1993; 82:3241–3249.
17. Feldman RG. Urban lead mining: lead intoxication among deleaders. *N Engl J Med* 1978;298:1143–1145.
18. Travers T, Rendle-Short J, Harvey CC. The Rotterdam lead poisoning outbreak. *Lancet* 1956;2:113–116.
19. Whitfeld CL, Chien LT, Whitehead JD. Lead encephalopathy in adults. *Am J Med* 1972;52:289–298.
20. Dickinson L, Reichert EL, Ho RCS, et al. Lead poisoning in a family due to cocktail glasses. *Am J Med* 1972;52:391–394.
21. Cagin CR, Diloy-Puray M, Westerman MP. Bullets, lead poisoning and thyrotoxicosis. *Ann Intern Med* 1978;89:509–511.
22. Dagg JH, Goldberg A, Lockhead A, et al. The relationship of lead poisoning to acute intermittent porphyria. *Q J Med* 1965;34: 163–175.
23. Browder AA, Joselow MM, Louria DB. The problem of lead poisoning. *Medicine (Baltimore)* 1973;52:121–139.
24. Goldberg A. Lead poisoning and haem biosynthesis. *Br J Haematol* 1972;23:521–524.
25. Griggs RC. Lead poisoning: hematologic aspects. *Prog Hematol* 1964;4:117–137.
26. Ali MAM, Quinlan A. Effect of lead on globin synthesis in vivo. *Am J Clin Pathol* 1977;67:77–79.
27. Paglia DE, Valentine WN, Dahlgren JG. Effects of low-level lead exposure on pyrimidine 5′-nucleotidase and other erythrocyte enzymes. *J Clin Invest* 1975;56:1164–1169.
28. Paglia DE, Valentine WN, Fink K. Lead poisoning: further observations on erythrocyte pyrimidine nucleotidase deficiency and intracellular accumulation of pyrimidine nucleotides. *J Clin Invest* 1977;60: 1362–1366.
29. Rinsky RA, Smith AB, Hornung R, et al. Benzene and leukemia. An epidemiologic risk assessment. *N Engl J Med* 1991;316:1044–1050.
30. Saccomanno GV, Archer E, Auerback O, et al. Histologic types of lung cancer among uranium miners. *Cancer* 1971;27:515–523.
31. Ruiz MA, Vassalo J, DeSouza C. A morphologic study of the bone marrow of neutropenic patients exposed to benzene of the metallurgical industry of Cubatao, Sao Paolo, Brazil (letter). *J Occup Med* 1991;33:83.
32. Saita G. Benzene induced hypoplastic anemias and leukemias. In: Saita G. Blood Disorders Due to Drugs and Other Agents. *Excerpta Medica* 1974;25:1.
33. Aksoy M, Dincol K, Akgun T, et al. Haematological effects of chronic benzene poisoning in 217 workers. *Br J Ind Med* 1971;28:296–302.
34. Vigliani EC, Saita G. Benzene and leukemia. *N Engl J Med* 1964; 271:872–876.
35. Aksoy M, Dincol K, Erdem S, et al. Details of blood changes in 32 patients with long-term exposure to benzene. *Br J Ind Med* 1972;29: 56–64.
36. Young NS, Maciejewski. The pathophysiology of acquired aplastic anemia. *N Engl J Med* 1997;336:1365–1372.
37. DeGowin RL. Benzene exposure and aplastic anemia followed by leukemia fifteen years later. *JAMA* 1963;185:748–751.
38. Aksoy M, Dincol K, Erdem S, et al. Acute leukemia due to chronic exposure to benzene. *Am J Med* 1972;52:160–166.
39. Aksoy M, Erdem S, Dincol K. Leukemia in shoe workers exposed chronically to benzene. *Blood* 1974;44:837–841.
40. Aksog M. Chronic lymphoid leukemia and hairy cell leukemia due to chronic exposure to benzene: report of three cases. *Br J Haematol* 1987;66:209–211.
41. Checkoway H, Wilcosky T, Wolf P, et al. Malignancies due to occupational exposure to benzene. *Haematologica* 1980;65:370–373.
42. Paci E, Buiatti E, Costantini AS, et al. Aplastic anemia, leukemia, and other cancer mortality in a cohort of shoe workers exposed to benezene. *Scand J Work Environ Health* 1989;15:313–318.
43. Lynch RE, Williams DM, Reading JC, et al. The prognosis in aplastic anemia. *Blood* 1975;45:517–528.

44. Storb R, Thomas ED, Buckner CD, et al. Marrow transplantation in thirty untransfused patients with severe aplastic anemia. *Ann Intern Med* 1980;92:30–36.
45. McGlave PB, Haake R, Miller W, Kim T, Kersey J, Ramsay NKC. Therapy of severe aplastic anemia in young adults and children with allogeneic bone marrow transplantation. *Blood* 1987;70:1325–1330.
46. Champlin RE, Feig SA, Sparkes RS, et al. Bone marrow transplantation from identical twins in the treatment of aplastic anemia: implications for the pathogenesis of the disease. *Br J Haematol* 1984;56:455–463.
47. Gluckman E, Devergie A, Poros A, Degoulet P. Results of immunosuppression in 170 cases of severe aplastic anemia. *Br J Haematol* 1982;51:541–550.
48. Frickhofen N, Kaltwasser JP, Schrezenmeier H, et al. Treatment of aplastic anemia with antilymphocyte globulin and methylprednisolone with or without cyclosporine. *N Engl J Med* 1991;324: 1299–1304.
49. Brodsky RA, Sensenbrenner LL, Jones RJ. Complete remission in severe aplastic anemia after high dose cyclophosphamide without bone marrow transplantation. *Blood* 1996;87:491–494.
50. Williams DM, Lynch RE, Cartwright GE. Drug-induced aplastic anemia. *Semin Hematol* 1973;10:195–223.
51. Loge JP. Aplastic anemia following exposure to benzene hexachloride (Lindane). *JAMA* 1965;193:110–114.
52. Sanchez-Medal L, Castanedo JP, Garcia-Rojas F. Insecticides and aplastic anemia. *N Engl J Med* 1963;269:1365–1367.
53. Powers D. Aplastic anemia secondary to glue sniffing. *N Engl J Med* 1965;273:700–702.
54. Crawford MAD. Aplastic anemia due to trinitrotoluene intoxication. *Br Med J* 1954;2:430–437.
55. Hiebel J, Gant HC, Schwartz SO, et al. Bone marrow depression following exposure to kerosene. *Am J Med Sci* 1963;246:185–191.
56. Straus B. Aplastic anemia following exposure to carbon tetrachloride. *JAMA* 1954;156:1428.
57. Champlin RE, Kastenberg WE, Gale RP. Radiation accidents and nuclear energy: medical consequences and therapy. *Ann Intern Med* 1988;109:730–744.
58. Roodman GD, Reese EP, Cardamone JM. Aplastic anemia associated with rubber cement use by a marathon runner. *Arch Intern Med* 1980;140:703–709.
59. March HC. Leukemia in radiologists in a 20-year period. *Am J Med Sci* 1950;220:282–286.
60. March HC. Leukemia in radiologists, ten years later. *Am J Med Sci* 1961;242:137–149.
61. Bull AB, Tomonaga M, Hegssel RM. Leukemia in man following exposure to ionizing radiation: a summary of the findings in Hiroshima and Nagasaki, and a comparison of the findings with other human experience. *Ann Intern Med* 1962;56:590–609.
62. Moloney WC. Radiogenic leukemia revisited. *Blood* 1987;70: 905–908.
63. Caldwell GG, Kelley DB, Heath CW Jr, Zack M. Polycythemia vera among participants of a nuclear weapons test. *JAMA* 1984;252: 662–664.
64. Weinberg JB. Sequential development of polycythemia vera and chronic myelocytic leukemia in a patient following radiation exposure from nuclear weapons testing. *Am J Med* 1989;87:121–123.
65. Bennett JM, Catovsky D, Daniel MT, et al. Proposals for the classification of the myelodysplastic syndromes. *Br J Haematol* 1982;51: 189–199.
66. Caldwell GG, Kelley DB, Heath CW Jr. Leukemia among participants in military maneuvers at a nuclear bomb test. *JAMA* 1980;244: 1575–1578.
67. Caldwell GG, Kelley D, Zack M, Falk H, Heath CW Jr. Mortality and cancer frequency among military nuclear test (smoky) participants, 1957 through 1979. *JAMA* 1983;250:620–624.
68. Stevens W, Thomas DC, Lyon JL, et al. Leukemia in Utah and radioactive fallout from the Nevada test site. *JAMA* 1990;264:585–591.
69. Shimizu Y, Schull WJ, Kato H. Cancer risk among atomic bomb survivors. *JAMA* 1990;264:601–604.
70. Seltser R, Sartwell P. The influence of occupational exposure to radiation on the mortality of American radiologists and other medical specialists. *Am J Epidemiol* 1965;81:2–22.
71. Mole RH. Antenatal irradiation and childhood cancer: causation or coincidence? *Br J Cancer* 1974;30:199–208.
72. Kurzrock R, Blick MB, Talpaz M, et al. Rearrangement in the breakpoint cluster region and the clinical course in Philadelphia-negative chronic myelogenous leukemia. *Ann Intern Med* 1986;105:673–679.
73. Mills KI, MacKenzie ED, Birnie GD. The site of the breakpoint within the bcr is a prognostic factor in Philadelphia-positive CML patients. *Blood* 1988;72:1237–1241.
74. Segel GB, Simon W, Lichtman MA. Variables influencing the timing of marrow transplantation in patients with chronic myelogenous leukemia. *Blood* 1986;68:1055–1064.
75. Thomas ED, Clift RA, Fefer A, et al. Marrow transplantation for the treatment of chronic myelogenous leukemia. *Ann Intern Med* 1986; 104:155–163.
76. Goldman JM, Apperley JF, Jones L, et al. Bone marrow transplantation for patients with chronic myeloid leukemia. *N Engl J Med* 1986; 314:202–207.
77. Goldman JM, Gale RP, Horowitz MM, et al. Bone marrow transplantation for chronic myelogenous leukemia in chronic phase. *Ann Intern Med* 1988;108:806–814.
78. Arthur CK, Apperley JF, Guo AP, Rassool F, Gao LM, Goldman JM. Cytogenetic events after bone marrow transplantation for chronic myeloid leukemia in chronic phase. *Blood* 1988;71:1179–1186.
79. Hows JM, Yin JL, March J, et al. Histocompatible unrelated volunteer donors compared with HLA nonidentical family donors in marrow transplantation for aplastic anemia and leukemia. *Blood* 1986;68: 1322–1328.
80. Appelbaum FR, Dahlberg S, Thomas ED, et al. Bone marrow transplantation or chemotherapy after remission induction for adults with nonlymphocytic leukemia. *Ann Intern Med* 1984;101:581–588.
81. Bostrom B, Brunning RD, McGlave P, et al. Bone marrow transplantation for acute nonlymphocytic leukemia in first remission: analysis of prognostic factors. *Blood* 1985;65:1191-1196.
82. Appelbaum FR, Fisher LD, Thomas ED, and the Seattle Marrow Transplant Team. Chemotherapy v marrow transplantation for adults with acute nonlymphocytic leukemia: a five-year follow-up. *Blood* 1988;72:179–184.
83. Santos GW. Marrow transplantation in acute nonlymphocytic leukemia. *Blood* 1989;74:901–908.
84. Wingard JR, Curbow B, Baker F, Piantadosi S. Health, functional status, and employment of adult survivors of bone marrow transplantation. *Ann Intern Med* 1991;114:113–118.
85. *Arsine poisoning in the workplace.* USDHEW publication (NIOSH). Washington, DC: U.S. Government Printing Office, 1979;79–142.
86. Fowler BA, Weissberg JB. Arsine poisoning. *N Engl J Med* 1974;291: 1171–1174.
87. Levinsky WJ, Smally RV, Hillyer PN, et al. Arsine hemolysis. *Arch Environ Health* 1970;20:436–440.
88. Teitelebaum DT, Kier LC. Arsine poisoning: report of five cases in the petroleum industry and a discussion of the indications for exchange transfusion and hemodialysis. *Arch Environ Health* 1969; 19:133–143.
89. Kessler CJ, Akels JC, Rhoads CP. Arsine poisoning: mode of action and treatment. *J Pharmacol Exp Ther* 1946;88:99–108.
90. Valaes T, Doxiadis SA, Fessas P. Acute hemolysis due to naphthalene ingestion. *J Pediatr* 1963;63:904–915.
91. Zinkham WH, Childs B. A defect of glutathione metabolism in erythrocytes from patients with a naphthalene-induced hemolytic anemia. *Pediatrics* 1953;22:461–471.
92. Petrakis NL, Wiesenfeld SL, Sams BJ, et al. Prevalence of sickle-cell trait and glucose-6-phospate dehydrogenase deficiency. *N Engl J Med* 1970;282:767–770.
93. Valentine WN, Paglia DE. Erythrocyte enzymopathies, hemolytic anemia, and multisystem disease: an annotated review. *Blood* 1984;64: 583–591.
94. Gilligan DR, Blumgart HL. March hemoglobinuria: studies of the clinical characteristics, blood metabolism, and mechanisms with observations on three new cases and review of the literature. *Medicine (Baltimore)* 1941;20:341–395.
95. Streeton JS. Traumatic hemoglobinuria caused by karate exercises. *Lancet* 1967;2:191–192.
96. Furie B, Penn AS. Pigment from conga drumming: hemoglobinuria and myoglobinuria. *Ann Intern Med* 1974;80:727–729.
97. Zeiss CR, Patterson R, Pruzansky JJ, et al. Trimellitic anhydride-induced airway syndromes: clinical and immunologic studies. *J Allergy Clin Immunol* 1977;60:96–103.

98. Lukens JN. Methemoglobinemia and other disorders accompanied by cyanosis. In: Lee GR, Bitchell TC, Foerster J, et al., eds. *Wintrobe's clinical hematology,* 9th ed. Philadelphia: Lea & Febiger, 1993; 1262–1271.
99. Kearney TE, Manoguerra AS, Dunford JV. Chemically induced methemoglobinemia from aniline poisoning. *West J Med* 1984;140: 282–286.
100. Rosen PJ, Johnson C, McGehee WG, et al. Failure of methylene blue treatment in toxic methemoglobinemia associated with glucose 6-phosphate dehydrogenase deficiency. *Ann Intern Med* 1971;75: 83–86.
101. Park CM, Nagel RL. Sulfhemoglobinemia: clinical and molecular aspects. *N Engl J Med* 1984;310:1579–1584.
102. Medeiros MHG, Bechara EJH, Naoum PC, et al. Oxygen toxicity and hemoglobinemia in subjects from a highly polluted town. *Arch Environ Health* 1983;38:11–16.
103. Ford R, Shkor J, Akman WV, et al. Deaths from asphyxia among fishermen. *MMWR* 1978;27:309–315.

*Environmental and Occupational Medicine,*
*Third Edition,* edited by William N. Rom.
Lippincott–Raven Publishers, Philadelphia © 1998.

# CHAPTER 56

# Toxic Liver Disorders

Jia-Sheng Wang and John D. Groopman

Normally the liver functions to maintain homeostasis by processing nutrients such as dietary amino acids, carbohydrates, lipids, and vitamins. The liver is also involved in the phagocytosis of particulate material in the splanchnic circulation, synthesis of serum proteins, formation of bile, and biliary excretion of endogenous products and xenobiotics. This organ is the major site of biotransformation and detoxification of drugs, chemicals, and circulating metabolites in the body (1,2). The liver's central role in total health status makes it vulnerable to a wide variety of environmental and occupational hepatotoxic insults.

Toxic liver disorders can be divided into three categories according to their etiology: viral hepatitis, chemical-induced injuries, and physical agent–induced lesions (3–5). Many of these disorders are difficult to clinically diagnose and treat because of the similarity of the presenting symptoms. People with acute toxic liver disorders frequently have nonspecific clinical manifestations and those suffering from chronic liver injury usually are asymptomatic until the disease progresses to its end stage. Sometimes toxic liver disorders are inferred in certain occupational settings by epidemiologic exposure studies or when regular liver function screening tests have been carried out (5). Simultaneous exposure of agents, such as viral hepatitis and/or alcohol and drug abuse, may confound the liver disorder caused by the specific occupational or environmental hepatotoxic agent (3). Further, host-susceptibility factors including genetic polymorphisms of metabolic and detoxifying enzymes complicate the direct interpretations of descriptive epidemiology studies. In the future, the application of molecular biomarkers specific for environmental or occupational hepatotoxic agent and specific biomarkers for the liver disease may help resolve some of these difficulties.

J.-S. Wang and J. D. Groopman: Department of Environmental Health Sciences, The Johns Hopkins University, Baltimore, Maryland 21205.

## INFLAMMATORY LIVER DISORDERS

Inflammatory liver disorders are the predominant cause of morbidity seen in clinical practice of hepatology since many insults to the liver can kill hepatocytes and recruit inflammatory cells to sites of tissue injury (6). These disorders are frequently chronic conditions, which may progress inexorably to cirrhosis and hepatic failure due to a lack of effective treatment protocols. The primary cause of hepatic inflammation are infections by viral hepatitis, although miliary tuberculosis, malaria, staphylococcal bacteremia, the salmonelloses, candida, and amebiasis also can cause inflammatory hepatic lesions (7). Two major causes of inflammatory liver disorders are discussed in the following subsections.

### Viral Hepatitis

Viral hepatitis is a systemic viral infection causing hepatic cell necrosis and hepatic inflammation. There are numerous characteristic clinical, biochemical, immunologic, and morphologic features of viral hepatitis in the patient (8). There are at least five known viral etiologic agents—hepatitis A virus (HAV), B virus (HBV), C virus (HCV), D virus (HDV), and E virus (HEV) (9)—each having distinctive immunoserologic characteristics and specific epidemiologic attributes. Viral hepatitis may also be caused by infections with viruses, such as yellow fever virus, Epstein-Barr virus, cytomegalovirus, four exotic viruses (Ebola, Marburg, Lassa fever, and Rift Valley fever viruses), herpes hominis, rubella, adenoviruses, and enteroviruses (10). The majority of cases presenting with viral hepatitis are due to infections with the five specific hepatitis viruses A to E. Viral hepatitis is an endemic disease in some parts of Asia and Africa, and is also commonly reported in occupational liver disease reports. Health care workers are especially at risk for HBV and HCV infections (11).

### Chronic Active Hepatitis (CAH)

Chronic active hepatitis, sometimes also called chronic aggressive hepatitis, is one of the three major forms of chronic hepatitis (12). The other two forms, chronic persistent hepatitis (CPH) and chronic lobular hepatitis (CLH), are usually clinically mild and histologically nonprogressive and therefore are considered benign. CAH, on the other hand, is frequently, but not invariably, characterized by the presence of symptoms and abnormality of liver function or histologic status that indicate a high expectation for the condition to progress to cirrhosis (12). This syndrome is a serious progressive disorder that warrants major concern for the patient. Infections with HBV, HCV, and HDV, drug-induced autoimmune reactions, and genetic metabolic disorders (13–16) are well-established causes for most cases of CAH; however, there are a number of patients with unknown nonviral diagnosis (12). Epidemiologic studies suggest that this portion of unexplained liver disorders may be due to occupational or environmental exposures to certain hepatotoxins (17,18). Although alcohol may cause CAH, its role in pathogenesis of the disease is still under active investigation (19,20).

Histopathologically, CAH is characterized as a chronic necrotizing and fibrosing hepatic disease. The general morphologic features of CAH include: (a) an exuberant portal inflammatory infiltrate that spills out of the portal tracts, (b) piecemeal necrosis, (c) bridging necrosis, and (d) progressive fibrosis extending from the portal tracts into the hepatic parenchyma, often leading to fully developed cirrhosis (6,12). The clinical presentation of CAH is highly variable and some cases are marked by the features seen in acute hepatitis, i.e., fatigue, malaise, mild fever, and jaundice. Some patients may be virtually asymptomatic, and the underlying liver disorder comes to attention only by the appearance of ascites and other manifestations of portal hypertension, when the scarring and cirrhosis are already well developed (12). Laboratory studies in almost all cases reveal elevated serum transaminase levels, prolongation of the prothrombin time, and in some instances, hyperglobulinemia and hyperbilirubinemia. The clinical course of CAH is unpredictable; some patients have rapidly progressive disease, particularly those with combined HBV-HDV infections, and they develop cirrhosis within a few years. The overall 5-year mortality for CAH is about 25% to 50%. The major causes of death are liver failure with hepatic encephalopathy, cirrhosis with massive hematemesis from esophageal varices, and, in those people who acquire the HBV or HCV early in life, hepatocellular carcinoma can develop (21,22).

There is no specific treatment available for CAH, and liver transplantation is usually not done. Therapy varies on recognized causative agents, such as treatment of chronic viral infection with antiviral and immunomodulatory agents and the withdrawal of the offending drugs. Corticosteroid therapy sometimes prevents or retards the progressive process in patients with autoimmune reactions (12).

## SEROLOGIC MARKERS FOR LIVER DISORDERS

Two major categories of serologic markers are currently used for the diagnosis of liver disorders: (a) markers for specific pathogens, such as serologic viral markers and their antibodies; and (b) markers of liver function, such as hepatic enzymes released into the blood (23). Determination of the viral markers usually reveal the cause and the stage of the disease, and measurement of the serum enzyme markers indicates the extent of hepatic injury. It is necessary to use markers from both categories and combine all the test results before making a final diagnosis.

### Serologic Markers for Viral Hepatitis

Hepatitis A virus (HAV) is a small, nonenveloped, single-stranded RNA picornavirus. A specific immunoglobulin M (IgM) antibody against HAV appears in serum at the onset of symptoms, constituting a reliable marker of acute infection. The IgM response in serum usually begins to decline in a few months and is followed by the appearance of IgG anti-HAV, which persists for years. This persistent response provides protective immunity against reinfection by all strains of HAV, and this has formed the strategy for developing a vaccine (24). In developing countries the majority of people have detectable anti-HAV in their serum by age 10 years. In developed countries seropositivity for this marker increases with age, reaching 50% by age 50 years in the United States (6).

Hepatitis B virus (HBV) is a member of the hepadnavirus family, a group of DNA-containing viruses. The genome of HBV is a partially double-stranded circular DNA molecule having 3,200 nucleotides (25). The organization of the HBV genome includes a nucleocapsid, called hepatitis B core antigen (HBcAg); an envelope glycoprotein, called hepatitis B surface antigen (HBsAg); DNA polymerase (a product of the P gene); and a protein from the X gene. HBeAg is a polypeptide virtually identical to HBcAg. HBV-infected hepatocytes are capable of synthesizing and secreting massive quantities of noninfective HBsAg, which appears in serum before the onset of symptoms and peaks during overt disease. HBsAg levels decline to undetectable amounts in 3 to 6 months following infection. HBeAg, HBV-DNA, and DNA polymerase appear in the serum soon after HBsAg and these are all markers of active viral replication (26). Persistence of HBeAg is an important clinical indicator and probably marks progression to chronic hepatitis. Anti-HBe is detectable shortly after the disappearance of HBeAg, implying that the acute infection has peaked and this phase of the disease is declining. IgM anti-HBc begins to be detectable in the serum shortly before the onset of symptoms and usually concurrent with the onset of elevated liver serum transaminases. Over several months, the IgM antibody is replaced by IgG anti-HBc, and thus an elevated level of IgM anti-HBc indicates a recent acute infection. Anti-HBs does not rise until the acute disease is over and is usually not detectable for a few weeks to several months after the disappearance of HBsAg. During this interval anti-HBc and anti-HBe are the only markers of the disease. Anti-HBs persists for many years, conferring protection and forming the basis for current vaccination strategies (8,12). Thus, the complex but well-defined pattern of these markers has been important in characterizing the progression of this infection in people.

Hepatitis C virus (HCV) is a small, enveloped, single-stranded RNA virus with continued alteration in envelope antigen expression (27). The genome codes for a single polypeptide of approximately 3,010 amino acids in one single open reading frame. This set of peptides is subsequently processed into a functional protein. HCV RNA is detectable in serum for 1 to 3 weeks after infection, coincident with elevations in serum transaminase. Circulating HCV RNA persists in many patients despite the presence of neutralizing antibodies, which indicates that the anti-HCV IgG following active infection does not confer effective protective immunity to subsequent HCV infections. This seriously hampers efforts to develop an effective HCV vaccine. Indeed, HCV has a high rate (more than 50%) of progression to chronic disease and eventual cirrhosis. Currently, HCV is the leading cause of chronic liver disease in many Western countries and Japan (6).

Hepatitis D virus (HDV) is a unique RNA virus that is replication defective, causing infection only when it is encapsulated by HBsAg. This acute coinfection occurs following exposure to both HDV and HBV (28). HDV usually infects the chronic carrier of HBV, called superinfection. HDV RNA is detectable in serum and liver just before and in the early days of acute symptomatic disease. IgM anti-HDV is the most reliable indicator of recent HDV exposure. Acute coinfection by HDV and HBV is best indicated by detection of IgM against both HDV Ag (delta antigen) and HBcAg. With chronic HDV, HBsAg is present in serum and anti-HDV persists for months or longer.

Hepatitis E virus (HEV) is an unenveloped single-stranded RNA virus that is classified as a calicivirus (29). The RNA genome is approximately 7.6 kb. A specific antigen (HEVAg) can be identified in the cytoplasm of hepatocytes during active infection. Diagnosis has been based on the detection of anti-HEV in serum (30).

**Serologic Markers for Liver Function**

The detection of elevated activity of hepatic enzymes reflecting the release of these intracellular proteins into blood is one of the most useful tools in the diagnosis of liver disease following cytotoxic injury (23). Enzyme release usually results from increased hepatocyte membrane permeability caused by the liver damage. Four groups of enzymes, based on specificity and sensitivity, have been proposed as serologic markers for different types of liver injury (31,32). The first group of enzymes are alkaline phosphatase (AP), 5′-nucleotidase (5′-NT), and γ-glutamyltranspeptidase (γ-GT). Elevated serum activities of these proteins appear to reflect cholestatic injury. In contrast, a second group of enzymes includes those that are more sensitive to cytotoxic hepatic injury. This group has been further subdivided into (a) enzymes that are somewhat nonspecific and reflect injury to extrahepatic tissue, for example, aspartate aminotransferase (AST or SGOT) and lactic dehydrogenase (LDH); (b) enzymes found mainly in the liver, for example, alanine aminotransferase (ALT or SGPT); and (c) enzymes that are almost exclusively located in the liver, for example, ornithine carbamyltransferase (OCT) and sorbitol dehydrogenase (SDH). These enzymes may be particularly useful markers of toxic injury when studying agents with unknown hepatotoxic potential. In some cases, elevated serum activity of the aminotransferases reflects injury to extrahepatic organs such as the heart, skeletal muscle, or kidney; however, elevated levels of all ALT, OCT, and SDH activities are reliable indicators of specific hepatic injury. The third and fourth groups of serum enzymes contain those that are generally only elevated with extrahepatic diseases, for example, creatine phosphokinase (CPK). In one case, there is a depressed serum activity during liver disease, with the measurement of cholinesterase (ChE).

Aspartate aminotransferase and alanine aminotransferase are probably the most frequently used serum markers of hepatic damage and both have been validated in a wide variety of clinical and experimental settings. In general, a two- to threefold elevation is seen in chronic hepatocellular injury or less severe acute injury (33,34). ALT levels of greater than 300 are uncommon in alcoholic liver injury. Thus, the pattern of transaminase elevation can be helpful in distinguishing alcoholic liver disease from other hepatotoxic injury. Alcohol selectively inhibits ALT activity, often resulting in an AST/ALT ratio of greater than 1 in alcohol-related liver disorders. In contrast, other hepatotoxin- and viral-induced hepatic injury usually results in an AST/ALT ratio of less than 1. Unfortunately for early detection situations, subclinical disease can occur despite normal serum aminotransferase. In certain cases, specific enzymes such as OCT, SDH, and LDH isoenzymes may select to improve the diagnosis probability (35,36). In summary, serum enzyme activities are valuable, but imprecise, tools for detecting liver injury. Positive results are strongly suggestive of disease, whereas negative data cannot be used to rule out liver disease.

## CHEMICALLY INDUCED LIVER DISORDERS

Human liver disorders caused by chemicals have been recognized for more than a century. Early documentation of hepatic deposition of lipids following exposure to yellow phosphorus was well described in the literature (37). Clinical cases and experimental studies on hepatic lesions produced by diverse agents, such as arsphenamine, carbon tetrachloride ($CCl_4$), trinitrotoluene (TNT), dimethylnitrosamine (DMN), chloroform, and the polychlorinated biphenyls (PCB), were reported in the first half of this century (38). At the same time the correlation between liver disorders and excessive ethanol consumption was widely recognized. Recently, liver disorders caused by adverse drug reactions have also been well studied and described.

Hepatotoxic chemicals are encountered in a variety of occupations, including painting, textile, and dye manufacturing. More than 100 chemicals have been found to be toxic to the liver in occupationally exposed workers (39). Hepatotoxic exposures can also occur in the homes when chemicals, such as cleaning agents, paints, or paint removers are inappropriately used. Environmental exposure to contaminated water, air, soil, or food, or with naturally occurring hepatotoxins, also has been demonstrated (40). Rare instances of liver disease associated with massive environmental contamination have been reported, such as cooking oil heavily contaminated with PCBs (Japan, 1968), wheat with hexachlorobenzene (Turkey, 1955 to 1957), and flour with 4,4′-diaminodiphenyl-methane (England, 1965) (41). Some industrial chemicals, despite premarket safety testing, are found to be hepatotoxic in workplace settings long after their release, due to insufficient appreciation of their toxicity or inappropriate use. Although exposures to many common hepatotoxic chemicals have been reduced through regulation and education, new chemicals are found to damage the liver. For example, the recent clinical trial for the promising drug fialuridine that was used as a therapy for chronic hepatitis was terminated in 1993 when patients suddenly died from liver failure (42).

### Classification of Chemical Hepatotoxins

Hepatotoxic chemical agents include both naturally occurring and synthetic hepatotoxins. The naturally occurring toxins include bacterial toxins, mycotoxins, mushroom toxins, and algae toxins. Among these aflatoxins, phalloidin and microcystin are potent hepatotoxins described for humans and animals (43). The synthetic hepatotoxic chemicals include therapeutic drugs, pesticides, metals, ethanol, and industrial chemicals. Among the industrial chemicals are classes of agents, such as aromatic hydrocarbons, halogenated hydrocarbons, chlorinated aromatic compounds, and nitro compounds (3,44).

Hepatotoxins have also been classified as either intrinsic or idiosyncratic based on their presumptive mechanisms of action (5). Most hepatotoxins are intrinsic toxins, that is, their hepatotoxicity is a predictable property of the substance itself, and most individuals will be affected if the dose is high. With most intrinsic toxins, called direct toxins, the substance or its metabolite directly injures the liver rather than indirectly interfering with metabolic pathways. Acute and subacute injury by such agents produce varying degrees of hepatocellular injury with necrosis and steatosis (45). A few hepatotoxins (e.g., beryllium) are idiosyncratic in that they cause liver injury that is sporadic and generally not dose related, possibly due to a hypersensitivity or immunologic-type reaction.

### Clinical Syndromes Induced by Chemical Hepatotoxins

Chemically induced liver disorders can be acute, subacute, and chronic hepatic injuries based on their clinical presentations, and specific hepatotoxins may induce both acute and chronic lesions. Pathologically, chemical liver injury manifests itself in different ways (37). Acute injury often results in an accumulation of lipids (steatosis) and the appearance of degenerative processes, leading to cell death (necrosis). The necrotic process can affect small groups of isolated parenchymal cells (focal necrosis), groups of cells located in zones (centrilobular, midzonal, or periportal necrosis), or virtually all the cells within a hepatic lobule (massive necrosis). Although acute injury may cause both necrosis and fat accumulation, it is not a consistent outcome that both features are present. Chronic injuries usually present with piecemeal and bridging necrosis, influx of chronic inflammatory cells accompanied by hepatocyte regeneration, and fibrous septum formation (6).

### Cholestatic Injury

The cholestatic lesion is an important form of liver injury (46,47) resulting in diminution or cessation of bile flow and retention of bile salts and bilirubin. The appearance of jaundice is an outstanding characteristic of the disorder. Acute cholestatic liver injury is rare, but has been reported following exposure to the chemical methylene dianiline (MDA), an aromatic amine used as an epoxy resin hardener. An epidemic of cholestatic jaundice occurred in Epping, England (so-called Epping jaundice) in 1965 after bread was made from flour contaminated with MDA (48). Similar cases were reported in workers following occupational exposure during the manufacture or handling of MDA. These clinical symptoms included abdominal pain, pruritus, fever, and jaundice. Laboratory studies showed elevated bilirubin, AP, and aminotransferase activities. A similar pattern of injury with bile stasis, portal inflammation, and variable hepatic necrosis was determined in liver biopsy samples.

Chronic cholestatic liver disorder was reported with the Spanish toxic oil syndrome associated with accidental high ingestion of denatured rapeseed oil (49). In addition to systemic illnesses, liver biopsy specimens revealed chronic biliary disease, fibrosteatosis, and chronic hepatitis. Clinical manifestations ranged from transient increases of serum aminotransferase activity to increased aminotransferase, AP, and bilirubin values for up to 30 months after exposure.

### Fatty Liver (Steatosis)

Steatosis, fatty change in the liver, was first characterized in patients suffering from alcohol-related liver disease. Steatosis is defined morphologically as greater than 5% of the hepatocytes containing fat, or quantitatively, as greater than 5 g lipid per 100 g hepatic tissue. This syndrome also occurs in other disorders, including diabetes mellitus, hypertriglyceridemias, and obesity. Some degree of steatosis is usually found accompanying acute hepatocellular necrosis; however, marked steatosis is more commonly seen in exposure to a chronic hepatotoxic agent (6).

Fatty liver associated with chemicals, as previously mentioned, was first described with yellow phosphorus poisoning, and pronounced steatosis and necrosis was found at autopsy (37). Steatosis has also been associated with occupational exposure to styrene, toluene, trichloroethane (TCE), and other aromatic compounds (50–52). Similar cases of acute massive necrosis and steatosis have been described with TNT in munitions industries, arsenical pesticide use in vintners, and the use of certain chlorinated aliphatic solvents (such as $CCl_4$, methyl chloroform, and TCE) (53). More subtle microsteatosis was described following short-term low-level exposure to dimethylformamide (DMF) in a fabric-coating factory (54). Chronic exposure to chlorinated solvents such as $CCl_4$ causes varying degrees of steatosis and hepatocellular injury. Several studies have reported steatosis in workers chronically exposed to nonchlorinated solvents, including DMF, toluene, and mixed aliphatic and aromatic solvents (53).

### Hepatoportal Sclerosis

Hepatoportal sclerosis is a rare form of noncirrhotic periportal fibrosis, that can lead to portal hypertension. This syndrome has been associated with occupational exposure to the vinyl chloride monomer in polyvinyl chloride polymerization manufacturing plants, inorganic arsenicals, and thorium compounds (5). Liver histology has shown hyperplasia of hepatocytes and sinusoidal cells, with dilatation of sinusoids and progressive subcapsular, portal, perisinusoidal, and occasionally intralobular fibrosis, which is accompanied by portal hypertension and splenomegaly.

### Fulminant Hepatic Failure and Necrosis

Fulminant hepatic failure is a severe liver disorder in which hepatic insufficiency progresses from the onset of symptoms to hepatic encephalopathy within 2 to 3 weeks, resulting in liver necrosis and liver failure (6). This disorder was reported following exposure to TNT, used extensively in munitions manufacture during World War I and II. The symptoms included jaundice, hepatomegaly, and severe liver necrosis (32). Even people who survive the acute phases of the disease often later develop postnecrotic cirrhosis or aplastic anemia. This severe liver disorder can also be induced by $CCl_4$ and chloroform after inhalation exposure in an enclosed space. Onset of symptoms developed 2 to 4 days after exposure, often accompanied by renal failure in severe cases. Those who survived the acute stages recovered in 2 to 4 weeks, but repeated subclinical exposure could induce cirrhosis (50).

As many as 10% of workers exposed over 30 work-years to TCE reportedly became jaundiced, and on autopsy subacute or massive hepatic necrosis and postnecrotic scarring were noted (50). Exposure to trichloroethylene also can result in hepatic necrosis similar to that seen with $CCl_4$. Similar findings were reported after occupational exposure in an enclosed space to an epoxy resin coating containing 2-nitropropane. In several cases, this resulted in the death, and some of the workers who recovered had persistent serum transaminase elevation (55).

### Cirrhosis

Cirrhosis is a chronic, irreversible condition where the normal lobular architecture is replaced by fibrous tissue and regenerating nodules derived from the remaining hepatocytes (6). Although cirrhosis is most commonly due to chronic viral infection and alcohol abuse, increased morbidity of cirrhosis has been noted in several studies of shipyard workers and printers who were daily exposed to a variety of organic solvents (56,57). In addition, other workers exposed to dimethylnitrosamine (DMN), TNT, TCE, various pesticides, and hydrazines have also been found to have increased rates of cirrhosis (17). Cirrhosis and other liver disorders have been reported to be more prevalent among anesthesiologists compared to other hospital personnel (58). Morticians exposed long term to formaldehyde had a greater prevalence of cirrhosis than an unexposed control population, although ethanol was a possible confounding factor (59). Increased prevalence of cirrhosis has also been found to associate with arsenic exposure, as in vineyard workers using arsenic compounds as a pesticide (60). An increased death rate for cirrhosis was also found in a retrospective cohort study of 2,567 workers in two plants where PCBs were used in the manufacture of electrical capacitors (61).

### Granulomatous Disease of the Liver

Granulomatous liver disease has been reported in occupational exposure setting where beryllium and copper are used. In beryllium injury the histopathologic appearance of the liver biopsy specimen can be indistinguishable from sarcoidosis. Berylliosis may include associated granulomas in the spleen, bone marrow, and lungs, as well as the usual granulomatous interstitial lung disease. Thirty workers who suffered from vineyard sprayer's lung were also found to have liver damage with inclusion of copper in biopsy tissue. The liver disorder included proliferation and swelling of the Kupffer cells, sarcoid like granulomas, fibrosis, micronodular cirrhosis, hepatic angiosarcomas, and idiopathic portal hypertension (62).

### Porphyria Cutanea Tarda and Related Abnormalities

A chronic hepatic disorder of porphyrin metabolism was found in 36 workers who suffered vinyl chloride–induced hepatic injury due to long-term industrial exposure. This abnormality was apparently induced by the inhibition of a number of hepatic enzymes in the porphyrin biosynthesis pathway. Porphyrinuria due to vinyl chloride exposure is rare (63). The disorder has also been described in association with methyl chloride poisoning, dioxin exposure, hexachlorobenzene and other kinds of polyhalogenated aromatic hydrocarbon induced liver injury (64). Occupational exposure to 2,4,5-trichlorophenoxy-acetic acid (2,4,5-T) and PCBs can cause porphyria (65). Following exposure to tetrachlordibenzo-p-dioxin (TCDD), porphyria cutanea tarda seems to be quite a specific disorder, producing increased urinary concentrations of uroporphyrin (66). Eleven out of 55 workers who had been exposed during the manufacture of TCDD were diagnosed and then were followed for 10 years because of liver abnormalities (67).

### Other Liver Abnormalities Reported Following Chemical Exposures

Transient increases in values of liver function tests were recorded in several cases following occupational exposure to methylene chloride (68). Increased transaminase values were found in DMF-exposed workers who had microvesicular fat and hepatocellular changes in liver biopsy specimens (69). Liver biopsy of workers manufacturing the pesticide Kepone (chlordecone) showed increased fat, numerous dense bodies, and proliferative smooth endoplasmic reticulum, as well as severe neurologic symptoms (70). A variety of jaundice and mild transient liver necrosis has been diagnosed in workers exposed to chrome during chrome plating operations (71).

Transient liver function abnormalities were also found in association with TCDD exposure. Ten percent of the Seveso (Italy) population environmentally exposed to TCDD after an industrial explosion had modest elevations of $\gamma$-GT. Separately, workers exposed to tetrachlorophenol (TCP) and TCDD had prolonged prothrombin time and elevated plasma lipid and other liver transaminase values. Mild steatosis, periportal fibrosis, activation of Kupffer cells, as well as porphyria cutanea tarda, were reported in workers who manufactured TCDD (67). In Japan and Taiwan, more than 2,000 people who ingested cooking rice oil contaminated with PCB and related compounds had abnormal liver function tests, hepatomegaly in severe cases, and electron microscopic alterations in the endoplasmic reticulum and mitochondria in biopsy samples (72–74). A variety of liver abnormalities have also been reported following occupational PCB exposure. In one study of electrical workers who had PCB levels in blood (41 to 1,319 $\mu$g/kg), 16 of 80 workers had variably increased $\gamma$-GT, AST, and ALT values and hepatomegaly (75).

Residents near a toxic waste dump with leachate-contaminated drinking water sources exhibited statistically significant differences in the liver function tests (AP and AST) and a greater prevalence of hepatomegaly compared to area residents drinking uncontaminated water (76). Increased hepatic enzyme values (especially $\gamma$-GT and ALT) were seen in human populations that consumed water from a reservoir contaminated with a heavy bloom of the toxic blue-green alga, *Microcystis aeruginosa,* compared to an adjacent population that drank water from other sources (77). Finally, an outbreak of toxic hepatitis occurred in India in 1974 with a high mortality among the exposed villagers and animals. This incident has been associated with food contamination with aflatoxin and other mycotoxins (78).

## LIVER DISORDERS INDUCED BY PHYSICAL AGENTS

Environmentally induced hyperthermia (heat stroke) can cause acute hepatic injury characterized by centrilobular necrosis and cholestasis (79). Exposure to a cumulative dose of ionizing radiation in excess of 3,000 to 6,000 rad gives rise to radiation-induced hepatitis 2 to 6 weeks later. Those who survived often subsequently develop cirrhosis with progressive fibrosis and obliteration of the central veins with centrilobular congestion. Radiation-induced hepatitis has been reported after accidental intense exposure. For example, a group of Japanese fishermen exposed to radioactivity from hydrogen bomb experiments in the Bikini Islands in 1955 had liver fibrosis and proliferation of bile canaliculi in biopsy specimens (41).

## MALIGNANT LIVER DISEASE

There are two types of human malignant liver disorders associated with occupational and environmental hepatotoxicants: hepatocellular carcinoma (HCC) and hepatic angiosarcoma (HAS). HAS, also described as endothelial cell sarcoma, is a rare malignant tumor in people and was found to be associated with chronic exposure to vinyl chloride monomer, arsenic, anabolic steroids, and Thorotrast, an obsolete scintigraphy contrast agent that contained colloidal thorium dioxide, an emitter of $\alpha$-particle ionizing radiation (80–82). Many of the reported HAS cases appeared to be workers who were exposed to vinyl chloride for many years in a few specific plants (83,84). HAS has also been diagnosed in vineyard workers and others who used arsenicals, including Fowler's solution (1% potassium arsenite), or copper as a pesticide (85). In addition, there were several case reports that long-term ingestion of arsenic-contaminated well-water could cause HAS (86).

Hepatocellular carcinoma is one of the leading causes of cancer mortality in Asia and Africa (87). In the People's Republic of China, this disease is the third leading cause of cancer mortality and accounts for at least 150,000 deaths per year with an incidence rate in some areas of the country approaching 100 cases per 100,000 per year (88). In contrast, HCC incidence in the United States is about 1.5 cases per 100,000 per year. Thus, the malignancy varies worldwide by at least 100- to 1,000-fold.

In the United States and most Western countries, excessive ethanol consumption, HBV, and/or HCV infections, and possible exposure to chlorinated hydrocarbons, have been estimated to account for as many as 75% of HCC cases (89–91). In addition, a slightly increased risk is thought to be associated with the use of oral contraceptives or androgenic-anabolic steroid hormones (6). A number of epidemiologic studies have also examined the association between occupation and risk of HCC (92,93). In Texas, an excess risk of HCC mortality has been described in certain occupations, such as oil refinery workers, plumbers, pipefitters, butchers and meat cutters, textile workers, and longshoremen (all odds ratios at least 2.0 and significant at 95%) (94). Another study reported increase risk of HCC in the chemical or petrochemical industry (95). A case-control study of HCC in New Jersey found an association with road builders, manufacturers of automobiles and plastics, workers exposed to anesthetics, gas station workers, and (even after adjustment for level of ethanol consumption ) workers in eating and drinking places (96). Studies also found increases in HCC in the highway construction industry, especially among workers who were exposed to asphalt (97), synthetic abrasive manufacture (98), and automobile workers (99). Many of these studies, however, did not adjust for other known risk factors, such as ethanol consumption, and HBV and HCV infection.

In contrast to North America, the major risk factors for HCC in Africa and Asia, including China, are chronic infection with hepatitis viruses and exposure to aflatoxins (100). Aflatoxins are mycotoxins produced by *Aspergillus flavus* and *Aspergillus parasiticus*. Aflatoxin $B_1$ ($AFB_1$) is a potent hepatocarcinogen in the diet that has been classified as a group I human carcinogen by the International Agency for Research on Cancer (IARC) (101–103). Over the past 30 years there have been extensive efforts to investigate the association between aflatoxin exposure and human HCC. Several epidemiologic studies found that increased aflatoxin ingestion corresponded to increased HCC incidence (104).

The role of HBV infection, dietary aflatoxin exposure, and other potential etiologies, such as polluted drinking water, pesticide exposure, and nitrosoamine contamination, were reviewed by Yeh et al. (105,106), who described several decades of research on the epidemiology of HCC in China. One of the most extensive investigations described was done in the Guangxi autonomous region. The staple food of people living in this region during the 1960s and 1970s was corn that was often contaminated with high levels of $AFB_1$. In the heavily contaminated areas, $AFB_1$ content in corn ranged from 53.8 to 303 ppb, while the lightly contaminated regions showed $AFB_1$ levels in grains of less than 5 ppb. After 5 to 8 years of follow-up, HCC incidence was determined for these two aflatoxin contamination regions. Those individuals who were HBsAg positive and found to have heavy aflatoxin exposure had a HCC incidence of 649.35 cases per 100,000 compared with 65.92 cases per 100,000 in aflatoxin lightly contaminated areas. Those people who were HBsAg negative and eating heavily contaminated aflatoxin diets had a HCC rate of 98.57 per 100,000 compared with zero cases detected in the light contaminated area.

Several recent studies have used newly developed molecular biomarkers for aflatoxins to study the intercorrelations between aflatoxin exposure and HBV infection and HCC. A cohort study initiated in 1986 in Shanghai collected 18,244 urine samples from healthy males between the ages of 45 and 64. In the subsequent 7 years, 50 of these individuals developed HCC. The urine samples from these cases were age- and residence-matched with 267 controls and analyzed for both aflatoxin biomarkers and HBsAg status. The data revealed a highly significant increase in the relative risk (RR = 3.4) for those HCC cases in whom urinary aflatoxins were detected. For

HBsAg positive people, the RR is 7, but for individuals with both urinary aflatoxins and positive HBsAg status, the RR is 59 (107,108). These results show a causal relationship between the presence of two specific biomarkers (aflatoxin and HBsAg) and HCC risk.

In Qidong county, Jiangsu province, China, HCC accounts for 10% of all adult deaths and both HBV and aflatoxin exposures are common (109). A prospective nested case-control study collected serum samples from 804 healthy HBsAg positive individuals (728 male, 76 female) aged 30 to 65 years in 1992. Between the years 1993 and 1995, 38 of these individuals developed HCC. The serum samples from 34 of these cases were matched by age, gender, residence, and time of sampling to 170 controls. $AFB_1$-albumin adduct levels were determined by radioimmunoassay. The relative risk for HCC cases among $AFB_1$-albumin positive individuals was 2.4 [95% confidence interval (CI) 1.2, 4.7] (110). Another nested case-control study (111) was carried out in Taiwan. A cohort of 8,068 men was followed-up for 3 years, and 27 cases of HCC were identified and matched with 120 healthy controls. Serum samples were analyzed for $AFB_1$-albumin adducts by enzyme-linked immmunosorbent assay (ELISA). The proportion of subjects with a detectable serum $AFB_1$-albumin adducts was higher for HCC cases (74%) than matched controls (66%) with an odds ratio of 1.5. There was also a statistically significant association between detectable levels of $AFB_1$-albumin adduct and HCC risk among men younger than 52 years old, showing a multivariant-adjusted odds ratio of 5.3.

The relationship between aflatoxin exposure and development of human HCC is further highlighted by the recent studies of the p53 tumor suppressor gene, the most common mutated gene detected in many human cancers (112,113). The initial results came from three independent studies of p53 mutations in HCCs occurring in populations exposed to high levels of dietary aflatoxin and showed that there were high frequencies of G→T transversions, with clustering at codon 249 (114–116). On the other hand, studies of p53 mutations in HCCs from Japan and other areas where there is little exposure to aflatoxin revealed no mutations at codon 249 (117). These studies provided the circumstantial linkage between this signature mutation of p53 and aflatoxin exposure in HCC from China and Southern Africa.

Fujimoto et al. (118) further examined HCC tissues obtained from two different areas in China: Qidong, where exposure to HBV and $AFB_1$ is high, and Beijing, where exposure to HBV is high but that of $AFB_1$ is low. They analyzed these tumors for mutations in the p53 gene and loss of heterozygosity for the p53, Rb, and APC genes. The frequencies of mutation, loss, and aberration of the p53 gene in 25 HCC specimens from Qidong were 60%, 58%, and 80%, respectively. The frequencies in nine HCC specimens from Beijing were 56%, 57%, and 78%; however, the frequency of a G to T transversion at codon 249 in HCCs from Qidong and Beijing were 52% and 0%, respectively. These data show distinct differences in the pattern of p53 mutations at codon 249 between HCCs in Qidong and Beijing and suggest that $AFB_1$ and/or other environmental carcinogens may contribute to this difference.

The observation of the codon 249 mutation in p53 with aflatoxin exposure is not limited to only China and Southern Africa. Senegal is a country where HCC incidence is one of the highest in the world and where people are exposed to high levels of aflatoxins. Fifteen HCC tissues from this country were examined for mutation at codon 249 of the p53 gene (119). Mutations at codon 249 of the p53 gene was detected in 10 of the 15 tumor tissues tested (67%). This frequency of mutation in codon 249 of the p53 gene is the highest described to date in the literature. Aguilar et al. (120) examined the role of $AFB_1$ and p53 mutations in HCCs and in normal liver samples from the United States, Thailand, and Qidong, China, where $AFB_1$ exposures are negligible, low, and high, respectively. The frequency of the AGG to AGT mutation at codon 249 paralleled the level of $AFB_1$ exposure, which further supports the hypothesis that aflatoxin has a causative and probably early role in human hepatocarcinogenesis.

Results from experimental studies have also linked aflatoxin as a causative agent in the described p53 mutations. Previous work had shown that $AFB_1$ exposure causes almost exclusively G→T transversions in bacteria (121), and that aflatoxin-epoxide can bind to the particular codon 249 of p53 in a plasmid in vitro (122). Further study (123) examined the mutagenesis of codons 247 to 250 of p53 gene by rat liver microsome-activated $AFB_1$ in human HCC HepG2 cells and found that $AFB_1$ preferentially induced the transversion of G→T in the third position of codon 249; however, $AFB_1$ also induced G→T and C→A transversions into adjacent codons, albeit at lower frequencies. Cerutti et al. (124) studied the mutability of codons 247 to 250 of p53 with $AFB_1$ in human hepatocytes using the same strategy and found that $AFB_1$ preferentially induced the transversion of G to T in the third position of codon 249, generating the same mutation, which is found in a large fraction of HCCs from regions of the world with $AFB_1$-contaminated food. These experimental results support $AFB_1$ as an etiologic factor for HCCs in $AFB_1$-contaminated areas.

## SUMMARY

The liver is a critical organ for maintaining normal homeostasis. Since virtually all internalized agents that are absorbed into the blood pass through the liver, the opportunity for acute and chronic damage to this organ is very high. The liver has an enormous capacity to recover from acute toxic injuries, and only when an overwhelming number of hepatocytes have been damaged is there a clinical manifestation. Unfortunately, once these toxic injuries begin to accumulate, many of the syndromes arising from these injuries prove to be difficult to manage and cure. While in some cases liver transplantation is the only course to survival, the very nature of many liver diseases preclude this method of therapy. This is particularly true in liver cancer, where there is 5-year survival rate of less than a 5%. In this chapter, we have attempted to highlight some of the major liver disorders, and it is clear that the high mortality rates of these disorders is due in part to a lack of sensitive and specific early detection methods. This is an urgent challenge to the developing biomarker community, and perhaps in the next decade, as our understanding of the molecular basis of these disease processes increases, we will begin to have the requisite tools necessary to make early diagnosis of liver injury practical.

## REFERENCES


1. Gumucio JJ, Chianale J. Liver cell heterogeneity and liver function. In: Arias IM, ed. *The liver:* biology and pathobiology, 2nd ed. New York: Raven Press, 1988;931–947.
2. Rappaport AM, Wanless IR. Physioanatomic consideration. In: Schiff L, Schiff ER, eds. *Diseases of the liver,* vol 1, 7th ed. Philadelphia: JB Lippincott, 1993;1–41.
3. Zimmerman HJ, Maddrey WC. Toxic and drug-induced hepatitis. In: Schiff L, Schiff ER, eds. *Diseases of the liver,* vol 1, 7th ed. Philadelphia: JB Lippincott, 1993;707–783.
4. Moslen MT. Toxic responses of the liver. In: Klaassen CD, ed. *Casarett and Doull's toxicology:* the basic science of poisons, 5th ed. New York: McGraw-Hill, 1996;403–416.
5. Redlich C, Brodkin CA. Gastrointestinal disorders: liver diseases. In: Rosenstock L, Cullen MR, eds. *Textbook of clinical occupational and environmental medicine.* Philadelphia: WB Saunders, 1994;423–436.
6. Crawford JM. The liver and the biliary tract. In: Cotran RS, Kumar V, Robbins SL, eds. *Robbins pathologic basis of disease,* 5th ed. Philadelphia: WB Saunders, 1994;831–896.
7. Samuelson J, Von Lichtenberg F. Infectious diseases. In: Cotran RS, Kumar V, Robbins SL, eds. *Robbins pathologic basis of disease,* 5th ed. Philadelphia: WB Saunders, 1994;305–377.
8. Koff RS. Viral hepatitis. In: Schiff L, Schiff ER, eds. *Diseases of the liver,* vol 1, 7th ed. Philadelphia: JB Lippincott, 1993;492–577.
9. Lau JYN, Alexander GJM, Alberti A. Viral hepatitis. *Gut* 1991; 32(suppl):47–62.
10. Schiff GM. Hepatitis caused by viruses other than hepatitis A, hepatitis B, and non-A, non-B hepatitis viruses. In: Schiff L, Schiff ER, eds. *Diseases of the liver,* vol 1, 7th ed. Philadelphia: JB Lippincott, 1993; 578–585.
11. Abb J. Prevalence of hepatitis C virus in hospital personnel. *J Med Microbiol* 1991;274:543–547.
12. Boyer JL, Reuben A. Chronic hepatitis. In: Schiff L, Schiff ER, eds. *Diseases of the liver,* vol 1, 7th ed. Philadelphia: JB Lippincott, 1993; 586–637.
13. Black M, Rabin L, Schatz N. Nitrofurantoin-induced chronic active hepatitis. *Ann Intern Med* 1980;92:62–64.
14. Babany G, Larrey D, Passayre D, Degott C, Rueff B, Benhamou J-P. Chronic active hepatitis caused by benzarone. *J Hepatol* 1987;5: 332–335.
15. Bach N, Thung SN. The histologic feature of chronic hepatitis C and autoimmune hepatitis: a comparative analysis. *Hepatology* 1992;15: 572–577.
16. Hodges JR, Millward-Sadler GN, Barbatis C, Wright R. Heterozygous MZ $\alpha_1$-antitrypsin deficiency in adults with chronic active hepatitis and cryptogenic cirrhosis. *N Engl J Med* 1981;304:557–560.
17. Dossing M, Skinhoj P. Occupational liver injury. *Int Arch Environ Health* 1985;56:1–21.
18. Guzelian PS. Hepatic injury due to environmental agents. *Clin Lab Med* 1984;4:483–488.
19. Sato H, Takase S, Takada A. Diagnosis of chronic hepatitis induced by alcohol. In: Kuriyama K, Takada A, Ishii H, eds. *Biomedical and social aspects of alcohol and alcoholism.* Amsterdam: Excerpta Medica, 1988;729–732.
20. Takase S, Takada N, Enomoto N, Yasuhara M, Takada A. Different types of chronic hepatitis in alcoholic patients: Does chronic hepatitis induced by alcohol exist? *Hepatology* 1991;13:876–881.
21. Alward WLM, McMahon BJ, Hall DB, Heyward WI, Francis DP, Bender TR. The long-term serological course of asymptomatic hepatitis B virus carriers and the development of primary hepatocellular carcinoma. *J Infect Dis* 1985;151:604–609.
22. Colombo M, Kuo G, Choo Q-L, Donnato MF, DelNino E, Tommasini MA, Prevalence of antibodies to hepatitis C virus in Italian patients with hepatocellular carcinoma. *Lancet* 1989;2:1006–1008.
23. Kaplan MM. Laboratory tests. In: Schiff L, Schiff ER, eds. *Diseases of the liver,* vol 1, 7th ed. Philadelphia: JB Lippincott, 1993;108–144.
24. Lemon SM. Inactivated hepatitis A virus vaccines. *Hepatology* 1992;15:1194–1197.
25. Lau JYN, Wright TL. Molecular virology and pathogenesis of hepatitis B. *Lancet* 1993;342:1335–1340.
26. Hoofnagle JH, Schafer DF. Serologic markers of hepatitis B virus infection. *Semin Liver Dis* 1986;6:1–10.
27. Weiland O, Schvarcz R. Hepatitis C: virology, epidemiology, clinical course, and treatment. *Scand J Gastroenterol* 1992;27:337–342.
28. Hoofnagle JH. Type D (delta) hepatitis. *JAMA* 1989;261: 1321–1325.
29. Hoofnagle JH, Di Bisceglie AM. Serologic diagnosis of acute and chronic viral hepatitis. *Semin Liver Dis* 1991;11:73–83.
30. Goldsmith R et al. Enzyme-linked immunosorbent assay for diagnosis of acute sporadic hepatitis E in Egyptian children. *Lancet* 1992;339: 328–331.
31. Plaa GL, Charbonneau M. Detection and evaluation of chemically induced liver injury. In: Hayes AW, ed. *Principles and methods of toxicology,* 3rd ed. New York: Raven Press, 1994;839–870.
32. Zimmerman HJ. *Hepatotoxicity.* New York: Appleton-Century-Crofts, 1978.
33. Wroblewski F. The clinical significance of transaminase activities of serum. *Am J Med* 1959;27:911–923.
34. Molander DW, Wroblewski F, LaDue JS. Serum glutamic oxalacetic transaminase as an index of hepatocellular injury. *J Lab Clin Med* 1955;46:831–839.
35. Reichard H. Ornithine carbamoyl transferase activity in human serum in diseases of the liver and biliary system. *J Lab Clin Med* 1961;57: 78–87.
36. Cornelius CE. Liver function tests. In: Meeks RG, Harrison SD, Bull RJ, eds. *Hepatotoxicology.* Boca Raton, FL: CRC Press, 1991; 181–213.
37. Plaa GL. Toxic responses of the liver. In: Amdur MO, Klaassen CD, Doull J, eds. *Toxicology:* the basic science of poisons. New York: Pergamon Press, 1991;334–353.
38. Reynolds ES, Moslen MT. Environmental liver injury: halogenated hydrocarbons. In: Farber E, Fisher MM, eds. *Toxic injury of the liver.* New York: Marcel Dekker, 1980;541–596.
39. Davidson SC, Leevy CM, Chamberlayne EC. *Guidelines for detection of hepatotoxicity due to drugs and chemicals.* NIH Publication. Washington, DC: U.S. Department of Health, Education and Welfare, 1979; 79–313.
40. Cotran RS, Kumar V, Robbins SL. Environmental and nutritional diseases. In: Cotran RS, Kumar V, Robbins SL, eds. *Robbins pathologic basis of disease,* 5th ed. Philadelphia: WB Saunders, 1994; 379–430.
41. Fleming LE, Beckett WS. Occupational and environmental disease of the gastrointestinal system. In: Rom WN, ed. *Environmental and occupational medicine*, 2nd ed. Boston: Little, Brown, 1992;633–647.
42. Macilwain C. NIH, FDA seeks lessons from hepatitis B drug trial deaths. *Nature* 1993;364:275.
43. Reddy CS, Hayes AW. Food-borne toxicants. In: Hayes AW, ed. *Principles and methods of toxicology,* 3rd ed. New York: Raven Press, 1994;317–360.
44. Lauwerys RR. Occupational toxicology. In: Klaassen CD, ed. *Casarett and Doull's toxicology:* the basic science of poisons, 5th ed. New York: McGraw-Hill, 1996;987–1009.
45. Holzbach T. Nonalcoholic fatty liver: structural and clinical implications. *Cleve Clin J Med* 1988;55:136–144.
46. Oelberg DG, Lester R. Cellular mechanisms of cholestasis. *Annu Rev Med* 1986;37:297–317.
47. Reichen J. Mechanisms of cholestasis. In: Travoloni N, Berk PD, eds.

*Hepatic transport and bile secretion:* physiology and pathophysiology. New York: Raven Press, 1993;665–672.
48. Kopelman H, Scheuer PJ, Williams R. The liver lesion of the Epping jaundice. *Q J Med* 1966;35:553–564.
49. Velicia R, Sanz C, Martinez-Barredo F, Sanchez-Tapias JM, Bruguera M, Rodes J. Hepatic disease in the Spanish toxic oil syndrome. *J Hepatol* 1986;3:59–65.
50. Klockars M. Solvents and the liver. In: Riihimaki V, Ulvarson U eds. *Safety and health aspects of organic solvents.* New York: Alan R. Liss, 1986;139–154.
51. Guzelian P, Mills S, Fallon HJ. Liver structure and function in print workers exposed to toluene. *J Occup Med* 1988;30:791–796.
52. Hodgson MJ, Heyl AE, Van Thiel DH. Liver disease associated with exposure to 1,1,1-trichloroethane. *Arch Intern Med* 1989;149: 1793–1798.
53. Snyder R, Andrews LS. Toxic effects of solvents and vapors. In: Klaassen CD, ed. *Casarett and Doull's toxicology:* the basic science of poisons, 5th ed. New York: McGraw-Hill, 1996;737–771.
54. Fleming LE, Shalat SL, Redlich CA. Liver injury in workers exposed to ethylformamide. *Scand J Work Environ Health* 1990;16:289–292.
55. Harrison R, Letz G, Pasternak G, Blanc P. Fulminant hepatic failure after occupational exposure to 2-nitropropane. *Ann Intern Med* 1987;107:466–468.
56. Chiazz L, Ference LD, Wolf PH. Mortality among automobile assembly workers. *J Occup Med* 1980;22:520–526.
57. Paganini-Hill A, Glazer E, Henderson BE, Ross RK. Cause-specific mortality among newspaper web pressmen. *J Occup Med* 1980;22: 542–544.
58. Edling C. Anesthetic gases as an occupational hazard-a review. *Scand J Work Environ Health* 1980;6:85–93.
59. Levine RH. Mortality of undertakers. *CHT Activities* 1982;2:3–5.
60. Hine CH, Pinto SS, Nelson KW. Medical problems associated with arsenic exposure. *J Occup Med* 1977;19:391–396.
61. Brown DP, Jones M. Mortality and industrial hygiene study of workers exposed to PCBs. *Arch Environ Health* 1981;36:120–129.
62. Pimentel JC, Menezes AP. Liver diseases in vineyard sprayers. *Gastroenterology* 1977;72:275–283.
63. Tamburro CH. Relationship of vinyl monomers and liver cancers: angiosarcoma and hepatocellular carcinoma. *Semin Liver Dis* 1984;4:158–169.
64. Doss M, Lange C-E,Veltman A. Vinyl chloride induced hepatic coproporphyrinuria with transition to chronic hepatic porphyria. *Klin Wochenschr* 1984;64:175–178.
65. Kimbrough D. Toxicity of chlorinated hydrocarbons and related compounds. *Arch Environ Health* 1972;25:125–131.
66. Webb KB, Ayres SM, Miles J, Evans RG. The diagnosis of dioxin-associated illness. *Am J Prev Med* 1986;2:103–108.
67. Pazderova-Vehlupkova J, Nemcova M, Pickova J, Jirasek L, Lukas E. The development and prognosis of chronic intoxication by tetrachlordibenzo-p-dioxin in men. *Arch Environ Health* 1981;36:5–11.
68. Cordes DH, Brown WD, Quinn KM. Chemically induced hepatitis after inhaling organic solvents. *West J Med* 1988;148:458–460.
69. Redlich CA, Beckett WS, Sparer JS, et al. Liver disease associated with occupational exposure to the solvent Dimethylformamide. *Ann Intern Med* 1988;108:680–686.
70. Cohn WH, Blanke HT, Griffith FD, Guzelian PS. Distribution and excretion of Kepone in humans. *Gastroenterology* 1976;A-8:901.
71. Pascale LR, Waldstein SS, Endbring G, Dubin A, Szanto PB. Chromium intoxication, with special reference to hepatic injury. *JAMA* 1952;149:1385–1389.
72. Higuchi K, ed. *PCB poisoning and pollution.* Tokyo: Kodansha and Academic Press, 1976.
73. Lu YC, Wong PN. Dermatological, medical and laboratory findings of patients in Taiwan and their treatments. *Am J Ind Med* 1984;5: 81–115.
74. Hsu S-T, Ma C-I, Hsu S K-H, et al. Discovery and epidemiology of PCB poisoning in Taiwan: a four-year follow-up. *Environ Health Perspect* 1985;59:5–10.
75. Maroni M, Colombi A, Arbusti G, Cantoni S, Foa V. Occupational exposure to PCBs in electrical workers. II. Health effects. *Br J Ind Med* 1981;38:55–60.
76. Meyer CR. Liver dysfunction in residents exposed to leachate from a toxic waste dump. *Environ Health Perspect* 1983;48:9–13.
77. Falconer IR, Beresford AM, Runnegar MTC. Evidence of liver damage by toxin from a bloom of the blue-green alga, *Microcystis aeruginosa. Med J Aust* 1983;1:511–514.
78. Krishnamachari KAVR, Bhat RV, Nagarajan V, Tilak TBG. Hepatitis due to aflatoxicosis. *Lancet* 1975;1(7915):1061–1063.
79. Bianchi L, Ohnacker H, Beck K, Zimmerli-Ning M. Liver damage in heatstroke and its regression. *Hum Pathol* 1972;3:237–248.
80. Creech JL, Johnson MN. Angiosarcoma of the liver in the manufacture of polyvinyl chloride. *J Occup Med* 1981;16:150–151.
81. Falk H, Thomas LB, Popper H, Ishak KG. Hepatic angiosarcoma associated with androgenic anabolic steroids. *Lancet* 1979;2:1120–1123.
82. Falk H, Caldwell GG, Ishak KG, Thomas LB, Popper H. Arsenic-related hepatic angiosarcoma. *Am J Ind Med* 1981;2:43–50.
83. Forman D, Bennett B, Stafford J, Doll R. Exposure to vinyl chloride and angiosarcoma of the liver: a report of the register of cases. *Br J Ind Med* 1985;42:750–753.
84. Falk H, Creech JL, Heath CW, Johnson MN, Key MM. Hepatic disease among workers at a vinyl chloride polymerization plant. *JAMA* 1974;230:59–63.
85. Popper H, Thomas LB, Telles NC, Falk H, Selikoff IJ. Development of hepatic angiosarcoma in man induced by vinyl chloride, Thorotrast and arsenic. *Am J Pathol* 1978;92:349–376.
86. Zaldivar R, Prunes L, Ghai GL. Arsenic dose in patients with cutaneous carcinomata and hepatic haemangioendothelioma after environmental and occupational exposure. *Arch Toxicol* 1981;47:154.
87. Okuda K, Kojiro M, Okuda H. Neoplasms of the liver. In: Schiff L, Schiff ER, eds. *Diseases of the liver,* vol 2, 7th ed. Philadelphia: JB Lippincott, 1993;1236–1296.
88. National Cancer Office of the Ministry of Public Health, P.R.C. *Studies on mortality rates of cancer in China.* Beijing: People's Publishing House, 1980.
89. Popper H. Hepatic cancers in man: quantitative perspectives. *Environ Res* 1979;19:482–494.
90. Popper H, Thomas LB. Environmental liver tumors. *Kurume Med J* 1979;26:189–204.
91. Colombo M, Kuo G, Choo QL, et al. Prevalence of antibodies to hepatitis C virus in Italian patients with hepatocellular carcinoma. *Lancet* 1989;2:1006–1008.
92. Chow WH, McLaughlin JK, Zheng W, Blot WJ, Gao YT. Occupational risks for primary liver cancer in Shanghai, China. *Am J Ind Med* 1993;24:93–100.
93. Hsueh YM, Cheng GS, Wu MM, Yu HS, Kuo TL, Chen CJ. Multiple risk factors associated with arsenic-induced skin cancer: effects of chronic liver disease and malnutritional status. *Br J Cancer* 1995;71:109–114.
94. Suarez L, Weiss NS, Martin J. Primary liver cancer death and occupation in Texas. *Am J Ind Med* 1989;15:167–175.
95. Hoover R, Fraumeni JF. Cancer mortality in the US counties with chemical industries. *Environ Res* 1975;9:196–207.
96. Stemhagen A, Slade J, Altman R, Bill J. Occupational risk factors and liver cancer: a retrospective case control study of primary liver cancer in New Jersey. *Am J Epidemiol* 1983;117:443–454.
97. Austin H, Delzell E, Grufferman S, et al. Case-control study of hepatocellular carcinoma, occupation and chemical exposures. *J Occup Med* 1987;29:665–669.
98. Wegman DH, Eisen E. Causes of death among employees of a synthetic abrasive product manufacturing company. *J Occup Med* 1981; 11:748–753.
99. Vena JE, Sultz HA, Fiedler RC, et al. Mortality of workers in an automobile engine and parts manufacturing complex. *Br J Ind Med* 1985; 42:85–93.
100. Harris CC, Sun T-T. Multifactorial etiology of human liver cancer. *Carcinogenesis* 1984;5:697–701.
101. Wogan GN. Aflatoxins as risk factors for hepatocellular carcinoma in humans. *Cancer Res* 1992;52(suppl):2114s–2118s.
102. Groopman JD, Cain LG, Kensler TW. Aflatoxin exposure in human populations and relationship to cancer. *CRC Crit Rev Toxicol* 1988;19: 113–145.
103. IARC Working Group on the Evaluation of Carcinogenic Risk to Humans. *Some naturally occurring substances:* food items and constituents, *heterocyclic aromatic amines and mycotoxins.* Lyon, France: IARC Press, 1993;245–395.
104. Groopman JD, Wang J-S, Scholl P. Molecular biomarkers for aflatoxins: from adducts to gene mutations to human liver cancer. *Can J Physiol Pharmacol* 1996;74:203–209.

105. Yeh F-S, Shen K-N. Epidemiology and early diagnosis of primary liver cancer in China. *Adv Cancer Res* 1986;47:297–329.
106. Yeh F-S, Yu MC, Mo C, Luo S, Tong MJ, Henderson BE. Hepatitis B virus, aflatoxins, and hepatocellular carcinoma in southern Guangxi, China. *Cancer Res* 1989;49:2506–2509.
107. Ross R, Yuan J-M, Yu MC, et al. Urinary aflatoxin biomarkers and risk of hepatocellular carcinoma. *Lancet* 1992;339:943–946.
108. Qian G-S, Yu MC, Ross R, et al. A follow-up study of urinary markers of aflatoxin exposure and liver cancer risk in Shanghai, P.R.C. *Cancer Epidemiol Biomarkers Prev* 1994;3:3–11.
109. Wang J-S, Qian G-S, Zarba A, et al. Temporal patterns of aflatoxin-albumin adducts in hepatitis B surface antigen-positive and antigen-negative residents of Daxin, Qidong county, People's Republic of China. *Cancer Epidemiol Biomarkers Prev* 1996;5:253–261.
110. Kuang S-Y, Fang X, Lu P-X, et al. Aflatoxin-albumin adducts and risk for hepatocellular carcinoma in residents of Qidong, People's Republic of China. *Proc Am Assoc Cancer Res* 1996;37:1714.
111. Yu M-W, Chen C-J, Wang L-W, Santella RM. Aflatoxin $B_1$ adduct level and risk of hepatocellular carcinoma. *Proc Am Assoc Cancer Res* 1995;36:1644.
112. Harris CC. Deichman Lecture—p53 tumor suppressor gene: at the crossroads of molecular carcinogenesis, molecular epidemiology and cancer risk assessment. *Toxicol Lett* 1995;82/83:1–7.
113. Harris CC. p53 tumor suppressor gene: from the basic research laboratory to the clinician abridged historical perspective. *Carcinogenesis* 1996;17:1187–1198.
114. Hsu IC, Metcalf RA, Sun T, Wesh JA, Wang NJ, Harris CC. Mutational hotspot in the p53 gene in human hepatocellular carcinomas. *Nature* 1991;350:427–428.
115. Bressac B, Kew M, Wands J, Ozturk M. Selective G to T mutations of p53 gene in hepatocellular carcinoma from Southern Africa. *Nature* 1991;350:429–431.
116. Li D, Gao Y, He L, Wang NJ, Gu J, Aberrations of p53 gene in human hepatocellular carcinoma from China. *Carcinogenesis* 1993;14: 169–173.
117. Ozturk M and collaborators, p53 mutation in hepatocellular carcinoma after aflatoxin exposure. *Lancet* 1991;338:1356–1359.
118. Fujimoto Y, Hampton LL, Wirth PJ, Wang NJ, Xie JP, Thorgeirsson SS. Alterations of tumor suppressor genes and allelic losses in human hepatocellular carcinoma in China. *Cancer Res* 1994;54:281–285.
119. Coursaget P, Depril N, Chabaud M, et al. High prevalence of mutations at codon 249 of the p53 gene in hepatocellular carcinomas from Senegal. *Br J Cancer* 1993;67:1395–1397.
120. Aguilar F, Harris CC, Sun T, Hollstein M, Cerutti P. Geographic variation of p53 mutational profile in nonmalignant human liver. *Science* 1994;264:1317–1319.
121. Foster PL, Eisenstadt E, Miller JH. Base substitution mutation induced by metabolically activated aflatoxin $B_1$. *Proc Natl Acad Sci USA* 1983;80:2695–2698.
122. Puisieux A, Lim S, Groopman JD, Ozturk M. Selective targeting of p53 gene mutational hotspots in human cancers by etiologically defined carcinogens. *Cancer Res* 1991;51:6185–6189.
123. Aguilar F, Hussain SP, Cerutti P. Aflatoxin $B_1$ induces the transversion of G→T in codon 249 of the p53 tumor suppressor gene in human hepatocytes. *Proc Natl Acad Sci USA* 1993;90:8586–8590.
124. Cerutti P, Hussain P, Pourzand C, Aguilar F. Mutagenesis of the H-ras protooncogene and the p53 tumor suppressor gene. *Cancer Res* 1994;54:1934s–1938s.

*Environmental and Occupational Medicine,*
*Third Edition,* edited by William N. Rom.
Lippincott–Raven Publishers, Philadelphia © 1998.

CHAPTER 57

# Environmental and Occupational Causes of Toxic Injury to the Kidneys and Urinary Tract

Edward T. Zawada, Jr., Fred K. Alavi, and David A. Maddox

In our environment and at the workplace there are biologic, elemental, chemical, and pharmaceutical exposures that cause acute and chronic toxicity to the kidneys and urinary tract, the renal-urinary system. Pharmacologic toxicity is often iatrogenic, results usually in acute, reversible injury, and is often easy to identify due to the rapid onset of toxicity and the prospective scrutiny of the patient. The other toxic agents are often more chronic, difficult to identify, and more inexorably destructive. This is especially true for environmental exposure to toxic agents. In industrial settings prospective surveillance programs developed for screening for injury now tend to remove the individual from exposure at the first sign of abnormal screening results, thereby minimizing the long-term risk. Nevertheless, environmental and occupational renal urinary toxic injury are still underestimated and underinvestigated. For example, in the United States nearly $7 billion is spent annually for dialysis and transplantation of patients with end-stage renal failure. The United States Renal Data System Report cites the cause of all but 7% of these patients. No occupational or environmental renal diseases, which are known causes of renal failure, appear in this report. Thus, it has been suggested that the underestimation and underinvestigation of environmental/occupational causes of renal failure is some fraction of this 7% (1).

This chapter begins with a listing of the classic syndromes of diseases of the kidneys and urinary tract, and then discusses the workup and diagnosis of toxic diseases of the renal-urinary system, emphasizing cellular and molecular mechanisms of toxicity. The laboratory methods of quantitating the toxic injury before end-stage injury are presented for the most common syndromes. Case studies from the literature or from the authors' experience are used to illustrate the clinical course of the most common toxic patterns of renal dysfunction.

E. T. Zawada, Jr., F. K. Alavi, and D. A. Maddox: Department of Internal Medicine, University of South Dakota School of Medicine; and the Royal C. Johnson Veterans Memorial Hospital, Sioux Falls, South Dakota 57105.

## SYNDROMES OF RENAL-URINARY SYSTEM DISEASES

### Hematuria

Using standard urinalysis dipsticks, hematuria can be detected as a change in color proportional to the amount of blood in the urine, with a visual scale provided for qualitative analysis of the degree of hematuria. Such bleeding is also seen as numerous red blood cells (RBCs) on microscopic examination of the urinary sediment. Urinary tract carcinogens present clinically as hematuria. These include benzidine, the aniline dyes, asbestos, arsenic, gasoline, and analgesic pharmaceuticals. Papillary necrosis occurs when a confluence of collecting ducts becomes injured and ischemic, and it eventually sloughs into the urine. There is a defect remaining in the renal parenchyma, which results in interrupted circulation and bleeding into the urinary tract. Papillary necrosis can result from prolonged exposure to salicylates, analgesic mixtures, and nonsteroidal antiinflammatory drugs (NSAIDs). The pyelographic findings in papillary necrosis include contrast dye pooling in the defect resulting from the sloughed papilla. Hydrocarbon solvents and silica exposure cause glomerulonephritis, which also causes hematuria, and red blood cell cast formation in the urinary sediment.

## Proteinuria

### *High Molecular Weight Proteinuria*

High molecular weight proteinuria (primarily reflecting albuminuria) is detected by the routine dipstick. A 24-hour urine collection can be used for quantitation, with the normal being less than 150 mg of protein excreted in a day. With glomerular injury, urinary albumin excretion can exceed 3 g/24 hours. This level of proteinuria is defined as the nephrotic range since it may result in the nephrotic syndrome. Mercury, gold, d-penicillamine, and nonsteroidal analgesics can cause the nephrotic syndrome. Spillage of large quantities of albumin into the urine results in low serum albumin. Liver metabolism is altered, resulting in hyperlipidemia, hypercholesterolemia, lipiduria, increased production of clotting factors, and a hypercoagulable state. The hypercoagulable state also results from urinary loss of coagulation system inactivators such as antithrombin III. The lipiduria is seen as fat droplets in the urine, which seem like small bubbles under high-power examination of the sediment. These droplets deflect the light, in the pattern of a Maltese cross, under polarization microscopy of the urinary sediment. The droplets may be taken up by macrophages and have the appearance of cells stuffed with fat droplets, the so-called oval fat bodies. Thus if the urinalysis screen displays any of these abnormalities or the quantitation of protein excretion illustrates that there is >3 g protein excreted per 24 hours, exposure to any of the agents listed above should be considered as a possible causative factor. These agents cause the heavy proteinuria by depositing in the glomerulus directly or complexed with an antibody (immune complex) that alters the charge barrier, allowing the negatively charged albumin to pass into Bowman's space from the capillary lumen. Whether the immune complexes directly alter the charge barrier or do so through the fixation and activation of the complement cascade is not known at the present time. Alternately, the toxin or immune complex may induce an antibody to the epithelial cells, which binds to the cell and alters the charge barrier. The analgesics may indirectly alter the charge barrier through the liberation from activated lymphocytes of permeability factors whose mechanism of action is not entirely understood.

### *Low Molecular Weight Proteinuria*

Smaller proteins in the plasma, such as $\beta_2$-microglobulin and retinol-binding protein (RBP), are normally filtered at the glomerulus and reabsorbed by the renal tubules through endocytosis. In tubular injuries there may be increased urinary appearance of these protein molecules. Lead nephropathy can result in low molecular weight proteinuria. Urinary protein electrophoresis can distinguish high molecular weight proteinuria from low molecular weight proteinuria, and thus distinguish glomerular from tubular proteinuria, either of which may cause greater than 150 mg protein excretion per 24 hours.

## Acute Renal Failure Due to Tubular Necrosis

This is the most common syndrome of "renal shutdown," which is often accompanied by oliguria and electrolyte disturbances and necessitates dialysis. It is the most common life-threatening toxicant-induced renal syndrome. Those agents which directly cause acute tubular necrosis include heavy metals (brief exposure to high doses), organic solvents, aminoglycoside antibiotics, amphotericin antifungal therapy, chemotherapy drugs (especially those with platinum), NSAIDs, and radiographic contrast agents. Poisonous snakebites and certain food toxins can also precipitate acute tubular necrosis indirectly by causing toxin-induced hemolysis or rhabdomyolysis. This syndrome is usually diagnosed by the progressive rise in serum creatinine and blood urea nitrogen daily over a 2- to 3-day period of serial measurement. Other electrolyte abnormalities usually include hyperkalemia and metabolic acidosis. The oliguria often results in fluid retention, edema, and congestive heart failure. Renal imaging in this syndrome shows normal to slightly enlarged kidneys with no dilation of the tubules. The urinary sediment may show pigmented granular casts resulting from degenerating sloughed tubular cells.

## Acute Renal Failure Due to Hemolytic-Uremic Syndrome

The pathophysiology of this syndrome involves the interplay between hematologic disturbances with resultant coagulopathy. Toxins can initiate this process by destroying red cells and producing hemolysis. The red cell fragments activate clotting, which consumes platelets in a form of a local intravascular coagulation. Microthrombi then cause renal circulatory dysfunction and renal ischemia. Acute renal failure with oliguria and electrolyte disorders ensue, requiring dialysis. After an intermediate time period of a few weeks the hemolysis often stops, the thrombocytopenia improves, and finally the renal failure resolves. The agents that have been known to produce the syndrome include bacterial toxins, elements including arsenic, cancer without therapy in which there is a hematologic disturbance, and chemotherapy agents such as mitomycin (2). Most recently Hanta virus has been associated with the syndrome.

### Acute Renal Failure Due to Acute Glomerulonephritis

The classic syndrome of acute glomerulonephritis due to streptococcal infections has now been attributed to a growing number of biologic, elemental, chemical, and pharmaceutical agents (Table 1). Originally thought to occur only due to strep throat, this form of acute renal failure is seen more commonly due to skin infections with streptococci or staphylococci. Other bacterial infections can produce the same result. As an example from the authors' experience, typhoid fever with documented evidence of infection of salmonella produced a 3-week episode of acute nephritis in a middle-aged Hispanic female, followed by complete recovery from the nephritis. More importantly viruses have now been found to cause the same pathophysiology. They would represent a more frequent exposure and thus have the likelihood of eclipsing streptococci as the most common cause of acute glomerulonephritis. The syndrome has thus now become known as postinfectious glomerulonephritis to illustrate our changing knowledge of the risk factors. The pathophysiology is summarized as the deposition of infectious fragments coupled with antibody as an immune complex, which lands in the glomerulus due to the high rate of renal blood flow. The deposited immune complex activates complement. Depending on the size of the complex, the antibody type, [i.e., immunoglobulin A (IgA) vs. IgG], the location of the deposit within the glomerular ultrastructure (subepithelial location vs. subendothelial vs. mesangial location), or other still unknown factors, there may be alterations of the charge barrier to glomerular permselectivity, cytotoxicity of the endothelial cells, lysis of the basement membrane, and chemotaxis to a varying degree. Depending on these same variables, there are differing attempts at healing: endothelial and mesangial cell proliferation, basement membrane repair or duplication, and epithelial cell proliferation. There result several histologic patterns of response: mesangial expansion, focal proliferative glomerular changes, diffuse proliferative glomerular changes, and membrano-proliferative changes that have different prognosis for recovery.

Poststreptococcal glomerulonephritis has a diffuse proliferative histologic pattern due to large aggregates of subepithelial deposits of strep antigen complexed with IgG. Complement is activated and serum complement levels are low. The syndrome is short-lived with total recovery in nearly all cases within 2 to 3 weeks. The case described above due to typhoid fever also fits this same pattern of diffuse proliferative histology, IgG complexes, low serum complement, 3-week course, and total recovery. On the other hand much more common is a nephritis that appears after an upper respiratory infection due to common viruses. A focal proliferative histology is seen with mesangial location of immune complexes involving IgA as the antibody response. This form of nephritis often has a subacute course with recurrent episodes of hematuria anamnestically occurring with subsequent upper respiratory illnesses. After 1 or 2 years the process usually subsides.

### Acute Noninfectious Glomerulonephritis

The same pathophysiology as described above for streptococci, other bacteria, and viruses has also occurred after exposure to silica. A focal or diffuse proliferative pattern has been described.

### Rapidly Progressive Glomerulonephritis (RPGN)

Inhalation of hydrocarbon solvents has been associated with a more acutely aggressive pattern of glomerulonephritis known as rapidly progressive glomerulonephritis (RPGN). The histologic pattern is described

**TABLE 1.** *Glomerular histologic patterns and mechanisms of immune injury due to environmental and occupational toxins*

| Histologic pattern | Type of immune injury | Location of immune injury | Agent |
|---|---|---|---|
| Nil lesion[a] | Lymphocyte production of permeability factors | Loss of charge barrier | NSAIDs, mercury |
| Focal proliferative nephritis | Immune complex (antibody-antigen) | Mesangium | Silica, rhinoviruses |
| Diffuse proliferative nephritis | Immune complex | Subepithelial | Streptococci, bacteria, hepatitis viruses, silica |
| Membranous nephropathy | Immune complex, may involve cryoglobulins | Subepithelial | Hepatitis viruses, gold, mercury, penicillamine |
| Membrano-proliferative nephritis | Immune complex | Subepithelial, mesangium, subendothelial | Hepatitis viruses |
| Focal sclerosis nephropathy | Immune complex | Subepithelial | HIV |
| Crescentic nephritis (RPGN) | Antiglomerular antibody | Linear along basement membrane | Solvents, mercury |

[a]Nil lesion, no lesion or normal looking light microscopy. The pathology is seen on electron microscopy of fused foot processes of glomerular epithelial cells.

as crescentic glomerular injury because the capillary walls leak large quantities of fibrin into Bowman's space, which then interacts with the epithelial cell to expand and rapidly squash normal glomerular architecture, rapidly reducing the glomerular filtration rate (GFR). The immune process is most often due to production of antiglomerular basement membrane antibody, which attaches in a continuous fashion to the entire glomerular basement membrane, presumably increasing the intensity of the inflammation and fibrin leak. A similar process of lung injury due to antiglomerular basement membrane antibody fixation to alveolar capillary basement membrane occurs with resultant pulmonary injury including hemoptysis and pulmonary hemorrhage, hypoxemia with alveolar-capillary leak, and interstitial pneumonitis. It is tempting to speculate that the inhalation leads to pulmonary basement membrane lodging of the solvent, which serves as a hapten to induce an antiglomerular basement membrane antibody that then attacks the lung and cross-reacts with renal glomerular basement membrane to attack the kidneys.

### Chronic Glomerulonephritis

Hepatitis B, C, and HIV viruses have now all been associated with acute-proceeding-to-chronic glomerulonephritis. In some cases, with any of these agents, cryoglobulin production occurs, contributing to the renal injury by serving as an immune complex. The glomerular patterns identified include membranous, membrano-proliferative, and focal sclerosing glomerulonephritis.

### Chronic Tubular Syndromes Due to Interstitial Nephritis and Fibrosis

Early tubular injury is now being monitored by the measurement of enzymuria. Of the several that have been reported in the literature, *N*-acetyl-β-D-glucosaminidase (NAG) is the most widely measured and reported. Next in the progression of injury due to short-term exposure are electrolyte abnormalities, since tubular reabsorption and secretion fine-tune blood electrolyte homeostasis. These most commonly include hyperuricemia (lead), the Fanconi syndrome of proximal tubular wasting of bicarbonate (renal tubular acidosis type II), glucose, phosphate (lead), hypernatremia due to renal water wasting or nephrogenic diabetes (lithium), and distal tubular inability to lower urinary pH below 5.5 (renal tubular acidosis type I). Global distal tubular injury that results in hyperkalemia and the inability to regenerate bicarbonate (renal tubular acidosis type IV) also occurs and, like the other types of renal tubular acidosis, manifests as a nonanion gap metabolic acidosis (NSAIDs). Urinary white blood cells or granular casts from the desquamated tubular cells and tubular proteins may also be seen on examination of the urinary sediment. Long-term exposure usually finds some of the above electrolyte abnormalities to have disappeared or to have been compensated. Azotemia (elevated serum creatinine, blood urea nitrogen) has supervened and may be quite severe. Renal imaging shows small kidneys with echogenicity due to atrophy of some portions of renal tubules and dilation of others. Renal biopsy confirms the damaged or degenerated renal tubules. There may be an interstitial infiltrate of white blood cells in earlier stages of the toxic exposure. Later, with nephron dropout, there is fibrosis replacing the damaged parenchyma. End-stage histology confirms varying amounts of atrophic tubules alternating with dilated colloid filled tubular remnants, the so-called thyroidization of the kidney.

### Acute Interstitial Nephritis

This is a rare form of acute renal failure that results from an inflammatory injury to tubules. In this form of injury the agent is likely to accumulate in the peritubular blood, and then in the interstitium between tubules. There is an inflammation, and the white cell degeneration releases lysosomal enzymes, which destroy the tubules.

**TABLE 2.** *Diagnostic tests for renal-urinary toxicity*

| |
|---|
| Urinalysis dipstick |
|   Glycosuria |
|   Hematuria |
|   Albuminuria |
|   High urinary pH |
| Urinalysis sediment examination |
|   Red blood cells |
|   Red blood cell casts |
|   Desquamated renal epithelial cells |
|   Granular casts |
| Quantitative urinary protein measurement |
|   24-hour urinary protein excretion |
|   Urinary protein electrophoresis |
| Serum electrolytes |
|   Serum sodium abnormalities (hypernatremia) |
|   Serum potassium abnormalities (hyperkalemia) |
|   Serum bicarbonate abnormalities (nonanion gap metabolic acidosis) |
|   Other blood chemistry abnormalities (low serum phosphorus, elevated serum uric acid) |
| Azotemia |
|   Elevated serum creatinine |
|   Elevated serum blood urea nitrogen (bun) |
| Urinary enzyme excretion |
|   N-acetyl-β-D-glucosaminidase |
|   Specialized tests of tubular enzymes or antigens |
| Renal imaging |
|   Renal ultrasound |
|   Intravenous pyelogram (IVP) |
| Measurements of reduced glomerular filtration |
|   24-hour urine for creatinine clearance |
|   Iothalamate clearance |
| Measurements of tubular biochemical function |
|   Urinary prostanoid excretion |
| Renal biopsy |

## DIAGNOSTIC WORKUP

Table 2 lists the screening tests needed to detect injury to the renal-urinary system from toxic exposure to biologic organisms, elements, chemicals, and pharmaceutical agents. Measurement of elevated blood or urinary or tissue concentrations of a toxic substance would be important to suggest renal-urinary toxicity. The problem is that these tests are not readily available. In addition, chronic exposure may often result in reduction of blood and urinary levels to normal values. Provocative testing may be necessary to mobilize substances from body stores. Such provocative tests are difficult to perform in that they are time-consuming, patient compliance with testing is sometimes poor, complex measuring methodology is required that is not often readily available, and interpretation is difficult due to overlap with normal individuals.

## CASE REPORTS

### Case 1

This case illustrates the use of diagnostic testing for screening for renal-urinary toxicity secondary to occupational exposure (3). Twenty-two mechanics aged 20 to 45 years actively employed in automobile garages were compared to 27 clerical male employees with an age range of 22 to 45 years. Blood lead levels were 24.3 to 62.4 μg/dl in the mechanics and 19.4 to 30.6 μg/dl in the clerical employees. Symptoms of loss of appetite, fatigue, headache, metallic taste, abdominal colic, intermittent vomiting, and insomnia appeared commonly in those with lead levels >35 μg/dl. Physical findings of lead line, tremors, and sensory and motor disturbances in the extremities were noted in eight or 36% of the mechanics. Urinary NAG levels were measured and found to be 14.8 ± 1.63 in the mechanics vs. 4.3 ± 0.57 μmol/min/g creatinine in the controls. Urinary $\beta_2$-microglobulin levels were 508 ± 55.2 in the mechanics vs. 395 ± 34.4 μg/g creatinine in the controls. There were no differences in the hemoglobin levels, serum albumin, serum creatinine, or creatinine clearance between the two groups. There was a significant correlation between NAG and blood lead level and between NAG and $\beta_2$-microglobulin results (3). This report demonstrates that enzymuria detected the influence of lead on the kidneys earlier than changes in serum creatinine or creatinine clearance, which are later and more severe consequences of loss of parenchymal structure and function.

### Case 2

At a major United States university medical center the rheumatology clinic on certain scheduled days is focused on a single common disease for management. When the rheumatoid arthritis clinic is held, patients report in the midmorning for laboratory tests and x-rays, and return in the afternoon to see their assigned physician. One afternoon the patient mix includes 16 patients receiving NSAIDs alone, 10 patients receiving auranofin (oral gold), and 15 patients receiving methotrexate. The routine laboratory tests on all patients include complete blood count (CBC) to search for leukopenia, urinalysis, serum electrolytes, blood urea nitrogen (BUN), serum creatinine (PCr), and liver function tests. Of the patients receiving auranofin, three test positive for proteinuria. In these patients the auranofin is discontinued on the basis of early renal toxicity.

### Case 3

A 16-year-old black male is brought to an inner city emergency room with delirium. The other youths who accompany him state that he has had the habit of toluene sniffing. Examination reveals his blood pressure to be 180/100 mm Hg. His respiratory rate is increased, but his lungs are clear on examination. Serum arterial blood gases reveal pH 7.30, $pCO_2$ of 32 mm Hg, and $pO_2$ of 140 mm Hg. Serum electrolytes reveal serum sodium of 140 mEq/L, potassium of 3.3 mEq/L, chloride of 110 mEq/L, and total $CO_2$ of 18 mEq/L. Urinary pH is 6. The correct diagnosis is renal tubular acidosis due to toluene renal toxicity. There is a nonanion gap metabolic acidosis.

$$\text{Anion gap} = \text{Plasma sodium} - (\text{plasma chloride} + \text{total } CO_2) \quad [1]$$

Normal is 12 ± 2.

In the above case,

$$\text{Anion gap} = 140 - (110 + 18) = 12,$$

which is normal. The low total $CO_2$ with the normal anion gap represents a nonanion gap metabolic acidosis consistent with renal tubular toxicity, i.e., renal tubular acidosis. The high urinary pH, i.e., >5.5 in the face of systemic acidosis, confirms a distal tubular inability to lower urinary pH to excrete acid.

### Case 4

A 5-year-old white boy develops nausea, anorexia, and diarrhea. Over a 3-day period these symptoms do not improve. He develops fever and bloody stools. He is seen briefly by his primary care physician, but sent to a tertiary care center because his laboratory findings show severe anemia, thrombocytopenia, hematuria, and moderately advanced azotemia. In the hospital a history of onset of symptoms 2 days after a picnic in which hamburger was cooked over an outdoor campfire was obtained. On examination he is flushed, and he has poor skin turgor. His urine output is low over the next several days. His serum BUN and creatinine rise progressively. Dialysis is initiated. After 3 weeks of dialysis and administration of blood products, his urine output improves, and his serum creatinine spontaneously declines toward normal. Dialysis is discontinued, and he is discharged to home. In the hospital stool culture was not positive for any toxins or abnormal strains of bacteria. At home his water supply was tested. The well water he was exposed to had a culture positive for *Escherichia coli* 0157:H7. This case illustrates acute renal failure due to hemolytic-uremic syndrome due to a verotoxin produced by certain strains of *E. coli,* to be described in greater detail below.

## THE MOST IMPORTANT RENAL-URINARY TOXINS

### Biologic

In the past decade the biologic agents in our environment have reemerged as preeminent causes of renal injury. The case above described the hemolytic-uremic syndrome secondary to bacterial toxic injury to the gastrointestinal tract. This hematologic disturbance followed by microthrombi-induced acute renal failure is now by far the most common cause of acute renal failure in infants and children. The usual exposure is through incompletely cooked hamburger. After a prolonged period of intensive care, the outcome is often favorable. However, there is an increased mortality rate in these patients. In our experience bowel ischemia and sepsis can be the cause of death. In addition to bacterial toxic injury, the documentation of viruses as the cause of acute and chronic glomerular renal injury is expanding each year (4). Balkan nephropathy is a disease affecting large numbers of people in Bulgaria, Romania, and Yugoslavia. The highest foci of occurrence are along the Danube or its tributaries. A variety of theories have been postulated, but the cause of this problem is as yet unproven. Hereditary factors, trace elements in excess or in deficient amounts, and mycotoxins (i.e., ochratoxin A) consumed in the cereals, poultry, and dried fruit have been suggested. Viral particles have been observed in kidney tissue of affected individuals. The latest hypothesis is therefore that a slow virus is spread to the people through rodents (5). This theory has also been investigated as a possible cause of the chronic renal failure of unknown etiology observed in inner cities of the United States (4). Besides nephropathy, there is a higher incidence of tumors of the renal urinary system in the Balkans. In summary, bacteria, bacterial toxins, viruses, and fungal toxins suggest that the most common environmental exposure as a cause of injury to the renal-urinary system is biologic. If one further considers that venom from poisonous snakes can cause hemolysis and resultant hemoglobin-induced acute tubular necrosis, it can be seen that biologic sources may now be the most important cause of serious toxicity to the excretory system.

### Elemental

#### *Lead*

Lead is one of the most important and well-documented environmental or occupational causes of renal disease. The main features of the syndrome of acute lead intoxication (plumbism) are colic and central nervous system toxicity. Clinical manifestations of chronic lead exposure include impairment of proximal tubule transport of amino acids, glucose, bicarbonate, uric acid, and phosphate, resulting in a Fanconi-type syndrome (6,7). Chronic intoxication leads to small contracted kidneys and renal failure. Light and electron microscopic examinations of rats exposed to lead demonstrate significant proximal tubular injury with frequent mitoses, interstitial fibrosis, and the formation of lead-containing intranuclear inclusion bodies (8–10). A nonanion gap metabolic acidosis occurs due to a type II or proximal renal tubular acidosis. Renal cancer has been reported due to lead intoxication. Since lead interferes with hemoglobin synthesis, anemia also occurs.

A complete review of the mechanisms responsible for lead-induced proximal tubule impairment is beyond the scope of this chapter, but the reader is referred to excellent summaries of our current knowledge (6,7). To summarize, most of the lead in the circulation is associated with the red cells, but a significant portion binds to a low molecular weight (17 kd) acidic protein, $\alpha_{2\mu}$-globulin, which is synthesized in the liver and filtered by the kidney. The proximal tubule cells probably take up this metal-protein complex by endocytosis. Within the cells this complex aggregates to form dimers, tetramers, and other higher molecular weight species, leading to the formation of the cytosolic and intranuclear inclusion bodies. The marked alterations in renal DNA, RNA, and protein synthesis caused by lead are associated with lead-induced mitosis and the formation of the lead intranuclear inclusion bodies (6,7).

Lead exposure has little or no effect on urinary excretion of albumin and other large proteins suggesting little or no significant damage to the glomerulus (11,12). In fact, in one group of lead smelter workers exposed to lead for a prolonged period (mean = 18 years), baseline GFR and the GFR after exposure to a protein meal were actually higher in the lead workers than in the control group and the age-related decline in GFR in the lead workers was actually lower (by a factor of two) than in the control group (12). Thus, at least for workers with blood levels less than 700 μg/L, as in that study (12), no significant impairment of glomerular function has been observed. One group observed a significant (50%) reduction in creatinine clearance (an indicator of GFR) in young rats maintained on lead acetate in the drinking water from weaning (and derived from females maintained on the same lead-containing drinking water throughout pregnancy and lactation) vs. the control animals (10). It is likely, however, that this reduction in GFR was the consequence of a reduction in food consumption (and hence protein intake) rather than glomerular injury since the lead-exposed rats weighed significantly less than controls by the end of the study (10).

Diagnosis of lead poisoning is made by measuring levels of lead in the blood or of measuring δ-aminolevulinic acid, a porphyrin precursor to hemoglobin. The most dependable marker for lead intoxication is measurement of urinary excretion of lead for 3 days after the patient takes two doses of 1 g of ethylenediaminetetraacetic acid (EDTA) at an interval of 8 hours. Normal people excrete less than 600 μg lead. Persons with lead intoxication excrete more than 1,000 μg of lead. Chelation therapy with EDTA and other agents has been shown to improve renal function. Classic cases of nephrotoxicity have followed inadvertent ingestion of leaded paint, especially by children who live in tenements. A recent follow-up study of 454 patients at Boston Children's Hospital who had been diagnosed with severe lead poisoning between 1923 and 1966, however, indicated that chronic nephritis was not a significant cause of death (13). Other lead hazards are present in battery manufacturing, construction and building wrecking, primary metal industries, machinery manufacturing, fabrication of metal parts, and mining. Environmental exposure can occur since lead can be ingested in moonshine whiskey contaminated with leaded solder in stills and in contaminated foods such as flour. Although gasoline contains lead, it is not a common source of lead intoxication. Air pollution and crop contamination by the products of combustion of leaded gasoline are potential sources of lead intoxication. Treatment for chronic lead intoxication by chelation has been improved in that newer, safer chelating agents such as succimer have been developed. Previously calcium EDTA, dimercaprol (BAL), or D-penicillamine were used for chelation of lead. These agents are also nephrotoxic.

### *Cadmium*

Cadmium is a highly toxic metal used in the manufacture of alloys, paints, plasters, glass, and electrical equipment. It is also used in electroplating and soldering, and is a by-product of zinc smelting. Rice contaminated with cadmium from industrial pollutants causes *itai-itai byo* (ouch-ouch disease) in Japan. Slowly progressive renal dysfunction is usual, and on rare occasions total renal failure requires dialysis or transplantation. Roels and coworkers (14) studied male workers from zinc and cadmium smelters in Belgium. The workers had been only moderately exposed to Cd, yet the indicators of nephrotoxicity were elevated, in direct degree to the level of exposure. At exposure levels that yielded urinary concentrations of Cd around 2 μg Cd/g creatinine they observed increased urinary 6-keto–prostaglandin $F_{1\alpha}$ ($PGF_{1\alpha}$) and sialic acid concentrations. When the levels reached ~4 μg Cd/g creatinine they observed the appearance of high molecular weight proteins (e.g., albumin), tubular antigens, and tubular enzymes, while at ~10 μg/g creatinine they found low molecular weight proteins such as $\beta_2$-microglobulin (14). The observed albuminuria may have been the result of a loss of glomerular polyanion charge.

Proximal tubular wasting of calcium leads to calcium deficits with osteomalacia, nephrolithiasis, and bone pain (15). Cadmium is bound by metallothionein, a low molecular weight protein (6.6 kd) that is synthesized in the liver. This complex is released into the circulation and transported to the kidney where it is freely filtered across the glomerulus, then reabsorbed by the proximal tubule with great efficiency. Cellular lysosomes rapidly degrade the complex with release of cadmium ions (6,7). Renal cell synthesis of metallothionein binds the cadmium until a finite capacity is reached. When that capacity is exceeded the free cadmium leads to vesiculation of cells with an increased number of electron-dense lysosomes. This leads to decreases in lysosomal protease activity, low molecular weight proteinuria, and calciuria. The vesiculation is thought to be associated with the induction of intracellular stress proteins, activation of calmodulin, and damage to the cytoskeleton (6,7).

### *Mercury*

Mercury is found in the environment in several forms including mercuric chloride (corrosive sublimate) and mercurous chloride (calomel), and metallic mercury. Occupational hazards are inhaled vapors in industry, mines, dental offices, and research laboratories. Metallic mercury is used today in the manufacture of mirrors, batteries, alloys, and scientific instruments.

Mercuric chloride is highly nephrotoxic (16). $Hg^{2+}$ specifically affects the $S_3$ segment of the proximal tubule (17). $Hg^{2+}$ creates blebbing and exfoliation of brush border membranes of proximal tubular cells. This leads to massive influx of calcium associated with cell death (18). In the past mercuric chloride was used as a medicinal agent in germicides, douches, antiseptics, and ointments. Exposure to these products often led to acute tubular necrosis by interfering with cellular sulfhydryl enzymes. Mercuric chloride also stimulates renal hydrogen peroxide production, leading to oxidative stress and contributing to renal dysfunction (19). Mercuric chloride was also used in the fur hat felting process and long-term exposure to mercury vapors led to central nervous system toxicity with psychosis. In addition to its effects on the proximal tubule, $HgCl_2$ induces renin release from isolated juxtaglomerular apparatus (20), and thereby can indirectly affect blood pressure and glomerular filtration.

Methyl, ethyl, and phenoxyethyl mercury are important organomercurial contaminants from industrial and agricultural sources (21). Phenyl and methoxy methyl mercuric salts are nephrotoxic (22). Methyl mercury poisoning arising from ingestion of contaminated fish by industrial effluents into Minimata Bay in Japan led to severe neurologic defects (23), and chronic methyl mercury ingestion leads to low molecular weight proteinuria and proximal tubular lysosomal and mitochondrial abnormalities. The lipid soluble organomercurial $CH_3Hg^+$ is one of the more stable organomercurials and does not induce or bind to metallothionein (7). It produces toxicity in both the $S_2$ and $S_3$ segments of the proximal tubule where it damages the mitochondria and alters the lysosomal apparatus (24). Organomercurials such as ethyl and phenyl mercurials are more rapidly broken down to yield $Hg^{2+}$, and their toxicology more closely resembles that of agents such as mercuric chloride (7).

The common use of mercury-silver amalgams for dental fillings carries the risk of constant low dose exposure to mercury for many individuals. The potential renal dysfunction that might be caused by chronic exposure to mercury released from dental amalgams has therefore received considerable attention. Nylander and co-workers (25) examined the mercury content of tissue samples collected from autopsies of eight dental staff cases and 27 controls (with fillings). Mercury levels tended to be higher in tissues obtained from the dental staff than in controls, including in the kidney (25). The kidney concentrates mercury in the tissues to a greater extent than many other tissues (26). Systemic mercury concentrations rise rapidly in rats exposed to drilling of a dental amalgam surface, rising almost instantaneously in the lung where it is absorbed, rapidly transferred to the blood, then taken up by the liver, heart, brain, and kidney over the next 24 to 72 hours (27). Mercury from dental amalgams can also be absorbed from the intestinal tract and through tissues in the mouth (28). In monkeys and ewes receiving amalgam fillings or maxillary bone implants of amalgam, organs such as the adrenal gland, pituitary, and kidneys had higher mercury levels than in untreated animals (28–30). Despite the theoretical potential for mercury nephrotoxicity from dental amalgams, there is no clear-cut evidence in humans that such a problem exists, at least for the patient. Herrström and co-workers (23) studied 48 healthy young males and examined the relationship between the number of amalgam fillings and urinary mercury concentration vs. urinary albumin excretion (as a measure of glomerular injury) and $\alpha_1$-microglobulin, kappa and lambda light chains, or *N*-acetyl-β-D-glucosaminidase excretion as indicators of tubular dysfunction. No renal dysfunction was noted. Furthermore, massive oral ingestion of mercury was found in one study to be virtually harmless (31). Bluhm and co-workers (32) studied a group of workers from a chlorine plant 19 to 36 days after exposure to elemental mercury vapor while performing maintenance work on mercury cell lines. Despite blood mercury levels of ~50 ng/ml at the onset of measurements, only 1 of 11 patients exhibited proteinuria, and that was only transitory (32). Moreover, creatinine clearance was not affected (32). The primary defects were neurologic (32).

### *Chromium*

Experimental and occupational exposure to the hexavalent chromium ion, $Cr^{6+}$, results in proximal tubular necrosis, particularly in the $S_1$ and $S_2$ segments (33). There is disruption of the brush border membrane accompanied by a decreased proximal reabsorptive capacity as evidenced by glucosuria (24,34). Vyskocil and co-workers (35) gave chromium in the drinking water to rats (potassium dichromate) for 3 to 6 months. Female rats appeared to be more sensitive than male rats and developed a mild albuminuria and mild $\beta_2$-microglobulinuria (marker of tubule dysfunction) while the male rats did not. Bonde and Vittinghus (36) examined urinary protein excretion in steel welders who are chronically exposed to chromium, nickel, and manganese. Stainless steel welders had higher creatinine-adjusted urinary chromium levels than mild steel welders, ex-welders, or never-welders (36). They observed increased urinary protein excretion in stainless as well as "mild" steel workers but ex-welders only had sustained increase in albumin excretion. These investigators therefore questioned whether welding exposure actually increased clinically significant kidney disease (36). Vyskocil and co-workers examined the renal effects of chronic (18-year) exposure to chromium and nickel in stainless steel welders (37). Despite high concentrations of chromium in the urine the workers had no significant glomerular damage as assessed by the lack of albumin and transferrin in the urine and no significant tubular dysfunction as assessed by unchanged urinary excretion of enzymes and low molecular weight proteins associated with tubular damage (37). Thus, after chronic exposure to chromium, at least as long as urinary chromium does not exceed ~65 nmol chromium/mmol creatinine, there is little or no renal damage (37). More significant exposure, however, leads to proximal tubular and glomerular dysfunction in the human as it does in the rat (33,38). Chronic interstitial nephropathy was observed in a 48-year-old man who worked as a plasma cutter (cutting process using superheated ionized gas at high speed) of stainless steel (39). The nephropathy was due to exposure of the worker to the chromium-containing smoke emitted during the process (39). The patient had a blood chromium level seven times the normal value.

### *Other Heavy Metals*

Other heavy metals that infrequently cause renal disease include bismuth, silver (in photographic developers), and copper sulfate. Uranium has been used to create an animal model of acute renal failure. Several medicinal metals such as gold, platinum, and antimony are described below.

## Chemical

### *Hydrocarbons*

A wide range of hydrocarbons, including petroleum products (gasoline, diesel fuel, and other petroleum distillates), solvents used in glue and paints (e.g., turpentine, toluene, mineral spirits), halogenated hydrocarbons (e.g., chloroform, carbon tetrachloride, pesticides), and glycols (e.g., ethylene glycol, diethylene glycol, dioxane, glycerol), can be nephrotoxic. Within the American work force, these compounds represent one of the highest probabilities for occupational exposure; many millions of workers annually work in industry involving exposure to these agents. The lipophilic characteristics of hydrocarbons allow them to readily cross the skin, gastrointestinal tract, or lungs into the circulation where with highest concentrations they accumulate in adipose tissue (40). The liver has a great capacity to remove most of the ingested hydrocarbons with its first-pass effect after absorption from the gastrointestinal tract. However, exposure to solvents and petroleum products commonly occurs via the lungs, thereby escaping the first-pass effect, yielding higher accumulations in the brain. The capacity of liver to detoxify hydrocarbons can be exceeded after oral ingestion of large quantities of the hydrocarbon (41).

In a study conducted by Steenland and co-workers (42) in patients with end-stage renal disease (ESRD), the risk associated with occupational solvent exposure [odds ratio (OR) = 1.51) was relatively low compare to phenacetin or acetaminophen (OR = 2.66). When degreasers and cleaning solvents were analyzed independently, however, the risk of developing ESRD increased (OR = 2.5), suggesting that these agents are particularly nephrotoxic (42). Acute exposure to petroleum distillates by ingestion can cause acute tubular necrosis characterized by oliguria and azotemia (43). However, exposure of male rats to inhalation of C4 and C5, common constituents of gasoline, for 21 days (gasoline vapor concentrations up to 4,437 ppm) yielded no significant clinical signs or renal lesions, suggesting that short-term exposure to gasoline vapors at the workplace or by consumers may have no significant nephrotoxicity in humans (44).

Our understanding of the specific mechanisms of hydrocarbon nephrotoxicity is limited. It appears that the mechanism by which hydrocarbons can induce renal toxicity may depend on the duration of exposure and the type of hydrocarbons (45). Acute exposure results in more direct toxicity to the renal-urinary system, whereas chronic exposure may involve immunomediated pathophysiology. The latter may occur either through damage to nephron segments and release of cellular antigens resulting in an autoimmune response (46) or through damage to the immune system, leading to impaired clearance of antigens that then accumulate and produce an inflammatory response in the glomerulus (47). In support of this theory, chronic exposure to hydrocarbons can lead to glomerulonephritis characterized by mild proteinuria, deposition of antiglomerular basement membrane antigen-antibody complex, and thickening of the glomerular basement membrane (43,47–52). Ravnskov (47) suggests that most patients with glomerulonephritis are in state of immune deficiency and that hydrocarbons and other immunotoxic environmental contaminants are perhaps primary offenders. In an earlier survey, Ravnskov et al. (53) found that 50% of patients with glomerulonephritis had been exposed to organic solvents compared to 20% of the controls, suggesting that exposure to organic solvents may frequently play a role in glomerulonephritis. In contrast, others found no significant evidence supporting the association between hydrocarbon exposure and glomerulonephritis (45,54) and Viau and co-workers (55) were unable to find a significant relationship between hydrocarbons and the occurrence of renal disease in refinery workers. The differing results may be the consequence of differences in the dose and duration of exposure and perhaps differences in preexisting medical conditions.

### *Benzidine*

Benzidine and similar aromatic amines including aniline compounds are found in most synthetic organic dyes in the United States. Numerous studies have shown an increased incidence of bladder cancer in dye workers (56). The epithelium of the urinary collecting system is exposed to many substances that are ingested, absorbed through the skin, or inhaled, and that are potential mutagens in their native form or after being transformed by the liver or intestinal microflora. Analgesic mixtures containing phenacetin were marketed prior to the mid-1970s. Such agents caused chronic tubulointerstitial nephritis and transitional cell malignancies.

### *Alcohols*

A variety of alcohols are substituted for ethanol in alcoholics unable to afford alcoholic beverages. Methanol is found in windshield washer fluid, Sterno brand portable stove fuel, and in Heat® brand gasoline deicer. It causes an anion gap metabolic acidosis since it is metabolized to formaldehyde and then formic acid. Its ingestion causes blindness and acute tubular necrosis. Ethylene glycol is ingested from antifreeze and is metabolized by alcohol dehydrogenase and other enzymes to ultimately yield oxalic acid and calcium oxalate. An anion gap metabolic acidosis occurs and acute renal failure develops in untreated individuals. The histologic examination of the kidney reveals acute tubulointerstitial nephritis and chronic fibrosis due to accumulation of calcium oxalate crystals, and these crystals appear to be responsible for most of the organ damage (57). The insoluble crystals form in the urine, the peritubular blood, and the interstitium between tubules. The resultant inflammatory reaction leads to tubular injury and death due to release of lysosomal enzymes from the white blood cells. Ethylene glycol-induced inflammatory injury to the tubules is relatively rare and is different from the noninflammatory injury seen in acute tubular necrosis. Lysol®, a household cleaner and disinfectant, is also ingested as an ethanol substitute. This practice has been seen in the Native-American population of the Northern Plains and also causes acute tubular necrosis.

### Other Nephrotoxic Agents

#### *Arsenic*

Arsenic trioxide, a by-product of copper smelting, is found in pesticides and defoliants, and as a contaminant of moonshine whiskey. Arsine ($AsH_3$), a highly toxic gas formed by the action of acid on arsenic in metal and coal processing, is more nephrotoxic than arsenic. Both arsenic and arsine cause acute tubular necrosis (58). Acute intoxication with arsine causes fulminant intravascular hemolysis. The hemoglobinopathy contributes to the nephrotoxicity.

#### *Asbestos*

Asbestos has been shown in human studies to be associated with excess mortality due to kidney cancer (59) in individuals who worked in shipyards or in the insulation industry.

#### *Silica*

Silica exposure occurs in underground mining, granite extraction, and cutting foundry operations that use sand. Exposure also occurs in the manufacture of pottery and refractory materials such as lenses and glasses. Silica produces glomerulonephritis (60). Early case reports documented albuminuria. More recently, case reports have documented proteinuria, hematuria, and azotemia. In many of these cases, a high concentration of silica was documented in renal tissue. It has been postulated that renal silica deposits may alter renal tissue protein, creating immunogenicity. Alternatively, silica may produce a lupus-like syndrome, since several affected persons had elevated titers of antinuclear antibodies (ANA). Analysis of large-scale screening studies has documented increased prevalence of ANA in silica workers.

#### *Cocaine*

Cocaine intoxication is associated with acute tubular necrosis due to tubular ischemia from the vasospasm produced by the vascular effects of the agent. There may also be muscle injury, which results in release of myoglobin, which is toxic to the tubules and produces acute tubular necrosis (61).

### Radiation

Radiation causes renal injury when the kidneys have been included in the therapeutic field of radiation for cancer. In one large study 54 patients treated with radiation developed proteinuria, severe hypertension and chronic renal failure accompanied by severe interstitial fibrosis (62). Workers exposed to nuclear power plant accidents are at risk for nephrotoxicity. Improperly handled radioactive waste will continue to be a potential environmental nephrotoxicant.

## CATALOGUE OF MISCELLANEOUS TOXINS OF THE RENAL-URINARY SYSTEM

The following discussion presents newer reports of renal-urinary injury occurrences documented in the literature:

### Copper

Acute renal failure due to ingestion of "green water" as part of a religious ritual in which the water was contaminated with copper was reported in a 37-year-old Nigerian man in California. The acute renal failure was thought to be due to massive hemolysis, which occurred acutely in this patient. The outcome was recovery of renal function and discontinuation of dialysis (63).

### Potassium Bromate

Acute renal failure in humans has been observed as has carcinogenicity (renal cell) in rodents due to potassium bromate (64). Potassium bromate is used in permanent wave hairdressing treatments and as a maturing agent for flour (64).

### Tungsten Carbide/Cobalt Alloy

Rapidly progressive glomerulonephritis due to Goodpasture's syndrome was reported in a 26-year-old man with exposure to hard metal dust. The metal was an alloy of inert tungsten carbide and cobalt, which caused the hard metal lung disease (65). The patient underwent plasmapheresis of the antiglomerular basement membrane antibodies, received steroids and immunosuppressive therapy, and recovered renal function.

### Formaldehyde

High molecular weight proteinuria and nephrotic syndrome due to membranous glomerular nephropathy has been documented in four patients exposed to formaldehyde (66). All had worked with materials that contained formaldehyde or had moved into new homes that had substantial amounts of formaldehyde in the insulation or cabinetry. In three of the four cases the patient or a family member had a history of eye or upper respiratory problems related to the formaldehyde fumes. The younger two of the four patients recovered after corticosteroid therapy. One older patient persisted with the nephrotic syndrome. One middle-aged patient required dialysis.

### Paper Printers

Renal cell cancer among paperboard printing workers was evaluated by a retrospective cohort mortality study and by a case-control study. The report concluded that the standardized incidence ratio in these workers was greater than expected and that the risk of renal cell cancer was associated with overall length of employment. It was suspected that the toxicity was due to exposure to benzidine or toluidine types of pigment (67).

## IATROGENIC PHARMACEUTICAL TOXICANTS OF THE KIDNEYS AND URINARY SYSTEM

### Aminoglycoside Antibiotics

Aminoglycoside antibiotics, which are still used as empiric therapy for patients with presumed septic shock and for gram-negative infections documented to be due to pseudomonas, cause acute tubular necrosis (mainly to the proximal convoluted tubule). It is often nonoliguric and has low mortality and excellent probability for total recovery. A milder form of tubular injury with electrolyte abnormalities such as magnesium wasting without full-blown acute renal failure has also been commonly documented. The most important risk for aminoglycoside nephrotoxicity is the period of time of sustained trough level elevations. Thus dose adjustment for reduced renal function becomes the most important way to reduce the incidence of renal failure because the kidney primarily eliminates the agent. Several strategies for administration of aminoglycosides have been developed for giving the agent to patients with reduced renal function. The first is the use of the Cockroft and Gault formula for estimating GFR.

$$\text{GFR} = [(140 - \text{Age}) \times \text{Wt (kg)}/(72 \times \text{Serum Creatinine})] \quad [2]$$

This equation applies to males. For females, the result is then multiplied by 0.85. As an example, a 68-year-old 40-kg female with a serum creatinine of 1.0 mg/dl, which appears normal, would have a GFR estimated to be:

$$\text{GFR} = [(140-68)\times 40/(72\times 1)]\times 0.85 = [(72)\times 40/(72)]\times 0.85 = 40\times 0.85 = 34$$

Since a normal GFR is approximately 100 cc/min, 34 cc/min represents a reduction of the elimination of an aminoglycoside to 33% as efficiently. Thus the interval should not be 8 hours but 8/0.33 = 24 hours. A somewhat simpler strategy has been to automatically administer aminoglycosides at 24-hour intervals for anyone over the age of 65. These measures have proved effective in reducing the risk of renal toxicity due to aminoglycosides. Within the group of agents tobramycin appears less nephrotoxic than neomycin, gentamicin, or amikacin (68), but has in the past been considerably more expensive. More recently the cost has been reduced, making it more useful.

### Platinum Chemotherapy

Platinum chemotherapy (e.g., cisplatin) also produces an early picture of electrolyte abnormalities due to acute proximal tubular injury (7). Hypomagnesemia due to renal magnesium wasting is also quite common. The hypomagnesemia in turn causes a refractory hypokalemia. In many cases the toxicity progresses to acute renal failure due to acute tubular necrosis. Hydration prior to chemotherapy and prevention of dehydration due to nausea and vomiting after the chemotherapy are ways in which renal toxicity is reduced.

### Radiocontrast Agents

Radiocontrast agents also cause tubular obstruction, renal ischemia, and acute tubular necrosis (69). The newer nonionic dyes have a reduced incidence of acute renal failure. Risks factors for contrast-induced renal toxicity include advanced age, dehydration, advanced renal insufficiency of any etiology, multiple myeloma, and diabetes. Hydration prior to contrast administration has become the standard method of reduction of risk. It has replaced complicated protocols, which had included loop diuretics or mannitol administration. The degree of hydration must be vigorous, i.e., 150 ml/hr of normal saline. For those unable to handle this volume challenge without precipitating congestive heart failure, a lower rate of 50 to 75 cc/hour is used. New angiography agents such as $CO_2$ angiography or gadolinium magnetic resonance angiography have no renal toxicity.

### Amphotericin

Amphotericin is used to treat serious fungal infections. It is not used for empiric therapy where fluconazole has now assumed its role. Amphotericin acts as a detergent, altering cell membrane permeability to small solutes. Early in its administration it causes electrolyte abnormalities due to tubular toxicity. Although magnesium wasting and hypokalemia are common, the classic sign of early amphotericin injury is a distal renal tubular acidosis due to back leak of hydrogen ions pumped into the urinary lumen. The back leak into the cells reduces the effective acid excretion. A nonanion gap metabolic acidosis with an inability to lower the urinary pH below 5.5 despite severe acidosis occurs. With progressive injury, acute tubular necrosis ensues (68).

### Nonsteroidal Antiinflammatory Agents

Nonsteroidal antiinflammatory agents (NSAIDs) cause a nil lesion glomerular toxicity that results in heavy proteinuria. Also acute interstitial nephritis with acute renal failure has been reported. This appears to be a lymphocytic acute infiltration of the kidneys. Finally, tubular dysfunction with renal tubular acidosis type IV or isolated hyperkalemia may precede acute tubular necrosis. Propionic acid subtypes and ketorolac used for pain management seem to have the highest risk. The tubular injury appears directly related to prostaglandin inhibition, which interferes with reserve renal capacity to perform normal physiologic events (70).

### Gold

Gold is used in an oral or intramuscular injection form as a disease-modifying agent for rheumatoid arthritis. It causes a membranous nephropathy with heavy proteinuria.

### Antimony

Antimony is used as an antihelminthic agent. It can cause acute tubular necrosis.

### Methotrexate

Methotrexate in high doses precipitates in the tubules as an insoluble crystal resulting in intrarenal obstruction and acute renal failure. Hydration reduces the risk of this phenomenon.

### Sulfonamides

Sulfonamides cause an acute interstitial nephritis. In this form of acute renal failure eosinophils accumulate in the renal interstitium. This is a hypersensitivity type of allergic reaction. Besides the nephritis, there is fever and eosinophilia in the peripheral blood. Discontinuation of the drug and even a short course of high-dose steroid therapy have been reported to reduce the hypersensitivity reaction. Thiazide diuretics and furosemide have a structural similarity to sulfa and have been reported to cause an acute interstitial nephritis. Oral hypoglycemic agents and some antituberculous drugs also have a sulfa-like structure and cause the same renal toxic phenomenon.

### Penicillins

Penicillins were among the first to cause an eosinophilic interstitial nephritis syndrome. At first the semisynthetic penicillins were found to cause the problem. However, in time all penicillins and some cephalosporins have been found to cause eosinophilic interstitial nephritis syndrome

### Anticonvulsants

Anticonvulsants and allopurinol also have been shown to cause eosinophilic interstitial nephritis.

### Lithium

Lithium, used for manic-depressive psychiatric illness, produces an early tubular dysfunction consisting of a nephrogenic diabetes insipidus. Polyuria, clinical dehydration, and hyponatremia are often the presenting manifestations. The renal toxicity is directly related to elevated lithium blood levels. Thiazide diuretics have been known to elevate blood levels of lithium and aggravate the risk of lithium renal toxicity. Prolonged lithium exposure can lead to chronic tubulointerstitial nephritis and mild to moderate chronic azotemia. The injury stabilizes upon discontinuation of the drug so that progression to end-stage renal disease is uncommon.

## REFERENCES


1. Wedeen RP. Renal diseases of occupational origin. *Occup Med* 1992; 7:449–463.
2. Ives HE, Daniel TO. Vascular diseases of the kidney. In: Brenner BM, Rector FC Jr, eds. *The kidney.* Philadelphia: WB Saunders, 1991; 1497–1550.
3. Kumar BD, Krishnaswamy K. Detection of occupational lead nephropathy using early renal markers. *Clin Toxicol* 1995;33(4): 331–335.
4. Rodriguez-Iturbe B. Glomerulonephritis associated with infection. In: Massry SG, Glassock RJ, eds. *Textbook of nephrology,* 3rd ed. Baltimore: Williams and Wilkins, 1995;698–710.
5. Radovanovic Z. Epidemiological evidence on Balkan nephropathy as a viral disease. *Med Hypoth* 1987;22:171–175.
6. Fowler BA. Mechanisms of kidney cell injury from metals. *Environ Health Perspect* 1992;100:57–63.
7. Conner EA and Fowler BA. Mechanisms of metal-induced nephrotoxicity. In: Hook JB, Goldstein RS, eds. *Toxicology of the kidney.* New York: Raven Press, 1993;437–457.
8. Richter GW. Evolution of cytoplasmic fibrillar bodies induced by lead in rat and mouse kidneys. *Am J Pathol* 1976;83:135–149.
9. Murakami M, Kawamura R, Nishi S, Karsunuma H. Early appearance and localization of intranuclear inclusions in the segments of renal proximal tubules of rats following ingestion of lead. *Br J Exp Pathol* 1983;64:144–155.
10. Oberley TD, Friedman AL, Moser R, Siegel FL. Effects of lead administration on developing rat kidney. II. Functional, morphologic, and immunohistochemical studies. *Toxicol Appl Pharmacol* 1995;131: 94–107.
11. Vyskocil A, Cizkova M, Tejnorova I. Effect of prenatal and postnatal exposure to lead on kidney function in male and female rats. *J Appl Toxicol* 1995;15:327–328.
12. Roels H, Lauwerys R, Konings J, et al. Renal function and hyperfiltration capacity in lead smelter workers with high bone density. *Occup Environ Med* 1994;51:505–512.
13. McDonald JA, Potter NU. Lead's lagacy? Early and late mortality of 454 lead-poisoned children. *Arch Environ Health* 1996;51:116–121.
14. Roels H, Bernard AM, Cárdenas A, et al. Markers of early renal changes induced by industrial pollutants. III. Application to workers exposed to cadmium. *Br J Ind Med* 1993;50:37–48.
15. Kazantis G, Flynn FV, Spowage JS, Trott DG. Renal tubular malfunction and pulmonary emphysema in cadmium pigment workers. *Q J Med* 1963;32:165–192.

16. Biber TUL, Mylle M, Baines AD, et al. A study by micropuncture and microdissection of acute renal damage in rats. *Am J Med* 1968;44:464.
17. Gritzka TL, Trump BF. Renal tubular lesions caused by mercuric chloride: electron microscopic observations: degeneration of the pars recta. *Am J Pathol* 1968;52:1225.
18. Kempson SA, Ellis BG, Price RG. Changes in rat renal cortex, isolated plasma membranes, and urinary enzymes following the injection of mercury chloride. *Chem Biol Interact* 1977;18:217–220.
19. Nath KA, Croatt AJ, Likely S, Behrens TW, Warden D. Renal oxidant injury and oxidant response by mercury. *Kidney Int* 1996;50:1032–1043.
20. Kozma L, Lenkey A, Varga E, Gomba SZ. Induction of renin release from isolated glomeruli by inorganic mercury (II). *Toxicol Lett* 1996; 85:49–54.
21. Wedeen RP. Heavy metals. In: Schrier RW, Gottchalk CW, eds. *Diseases of the kidney,* 4th ed. Boston: Little, Brown, 1988;1367–1376.
22. Magos L, Sparrow S, Snowden R. The comparative renal toxicology of phenylmercury and mercuric chloride. *Arch Toxicol* 1982;50:133.
23. Herrström P, Schütz A, Raihle G, Holthus N, Högstedt B, Råstam L. Dental amalgam, low-dose exposure to mercury, and urinary proteins in young Swedish men. *Arch Environ Health* 1995;50:103–107.
24. Fowler BA, Brown HW, Lucier GW, Krigman MR. The effect of chronic oral methyl mercury exposure on the lysosome system of rat kidney. Morphometric and biochemical studies. *Lab Invest* 1975;32:313–322.
25. Nylander M, Friber L, Eggleston D, Björkman L. Mercury accumulation in tissues from dental staff and controls in relation to exposure. *Swed Dent J* 1989;13:235–243.
26. Nylander M, Friberg L, Lind B. Mercury concentrations in the human brain and kidneys in relation to exposure from dental amalgam fillings. *Swed Dent J* 1987;11:179–187.
27. Cutright DE, Miller RA, Battistone GC, Millikan LJ. Systemic mercury caused by inhaling dust during high-speed amalgam grinding. *J Oral Med* 1973;28:100–104.
28. Hahn LJ, Kloiber R, Vimy MJ, Takahashi Y, Lorscheider FL. Dental "silver" tooth fillings: a source of mercury exposure revealed by whole-body image scan and tissue analysis. *FASEB J* 1989;3:2641–2646.
29. Danscher G, Hørsted-Bindsley P, Rungby J. Traces of mercury in organs from primates with amalgam fillings. *Exp Mol Pathol* 1990;52: 291–299.
30. Vimy MJ, Takahashi Y, Lorscheider FL. Maternal-fetal distribution of mercury ($^{203}Hg$) released from dental amalgam fillings. *Am J Physiol* 1990;258:R939–R945.
31. Yver L, Yeoman WB, Carter GF. Massive oral ingestion of elemental mercury without poisoning. *Lancet* 1980;1:206.
32. Bluhm RE, Breyer JA, Bobbitt RG, Welch LW, Wood AJJ, Branch RA. Elemental mercury vapour toxicity, treatment, and prognosis after acute, intensive exposure in chloralkali plant workers. Part II: hyperchloraemia and genitourinary symptoms. *Hum Exp Toxicol* 1992;11:211–215.
33. Franchini I, Mutti A, Cavatorta A, et al. Nephrotoxicity of chromium. *Contrib Nephrol* 1978;10:98–110.
34. Evan AP, Dail WG Jr. The effects of sodium chromate on the proximal tubules of the rat kidney: fine structural damage and lysozymuria. *Lab Invest* 1974;30:704–715.
35. Vyskocil A, Vlau C, Cizkova M, Truchon G. Kidney function in male and female rats chronically exposed to potassium dichromate. Kidney function in male and female rats chronically exposed to potassium dichromate. *J Appl Toxicol* 1993;13:375–376.
36. Bonde JP, Vittinghus E. Urinary excretion of proteins among metal workers. *Hum Exp Toxicol* 1996;15:1–4.
37. Vyskocil A, Smejkalova J, Tejral J, et al. Lack of renal changes in stainless steel workers exposed to chromium and nickel. *Scand J Work Environ Health* 1992;18:252–256.
38. Verschoor MA, Bragt PC, Herber RFM, Zeilhus RL, Zwennis WC. Renal function of chrome plating workers and welders. *Int Arch Occup Environ Health* 1988;60:67–70.
39. Petersen R, Mikkelsen S, Thomsen O. Chronic interstitial nephropathy after plasma cutting in stainless steel. *Occup Environ Med* 1994;51: 259–261.
40. Pedersen LM. Biological studies in human exposure to and poisoning with organic solvents. *Pharmacol Toxicol* 1987;61(suppl 3):1–38.
41. Janssen S, Van der Geest S, Meijer S, Uges DRA. Impairment of organ function after oral ingestion of refined petrol. *Intensive Care Med* 1988;14:238–240.
42. Steenland NK, Thun MJ, Ferguson CW, Port FK. Occupational and other exposures associated with male end-stage renal disease: a case/control study. *Am J Public Health* 1990;80:153–159.
43. Phillips SC, Petrone RL, Hemstreet GP III. A review of the non-neoplastic kidney effects of hydrocarbon exposure in humans. *Occup Med* 1988;3(3):495–509.
44. Halder CA, Van Gorp GS, Hatoum NS, Warne TM. Gasoline vapor exposures. Part II. Evaluation of nephrotoxicity of the major C4/C5 hydrocarbon components. *Am Ind Hyg Assoc J* 1986;47(3):173–175.
45. van der Laan G. Chronic glomerulonephritis and organic solvents. *Int Arch Occup Environ Health* 1980;47:1–8.
46. Ogawa M, Moti T, Mori Y, et al. Study on chronic renal injuries induced by carbon tetrachloride: selective inhibition of the nephrotoxicity by irradiation. *Nephron* 1992;60:68–73.
47. Ravnskov U, Possible mechanisms of hydrocarbon-associated glomerulonephritis. *Clin Nephrol* 1985;23(6):294–298.
48. Zimmerman SW, Groehler K, Beirne GJ. Hydrocarbon exposure and chronic glomerulonephritis. *Lancet* 1975;1:199–201.
49. Roy AT, Brautbar N, Lee DBN. Hydrocarbons and renal failure. *Nephron* 1991;58:385–392.
50. Daniell WE, Couser WG, Rosenstock L. Occupational solvent exposure and glomerulonephritis: a case report and review of the literature. *JAMA* 1988;259:2280–2283.
51. Lehman-McKeeman LD. Male rat-specific light hydrocarbon nephropathy, In: Hook JB, Goldstein RS, eds. *Toxicology to the kidney,* 2nd ed. New York: Raven Press, 1993, 477–494.
52. Yaqoob M, Bell GM, Stevenson A, Mason H, Percy DF. Renal impairment with chronic hydrocarbon exposure. *Q J Med* 1993;86:165–174.
53. Ravnskov U, Forsberg B, Skerfving S. Glomerulonephritis and exposure to organic solvent. *Acta Med Scand* 1979;205:575–579.
54. Asal NR, Cleveland HL, Kaufman C, et al. Hydrocarbon exposure and chronic renal disease. *Int Arch Occup Environ Health* 1996;68:229–235.
55. Viau C, Bernard A, Lauwerys R, et al. A cross-sectional survey of kidney function in refinery employees. *Am J Ind Med* 1987;11:177–187.
56. Shulte PA, Ringen K, Hemstreet GP, Ward E. Occupational cancer of the urinary tract. *Occup Med State Art Rev* 1987:2;85–107.
57. Boogaerts MA, Hammerschmidt DE, Roelant C, Verwilghen RL, Jacob HS. Mechanisms of vascular damage in gout and oxalosis: crystal induced, granulocyte mediated, endothelial injury. *Thromb Haemost* 1983;50(2):576–580.
58. Giberson A, Vaziri ND, Mirahamadi K, Rosen SM. Hemodialysis of acute arsenic intoxication with transient renal failure. *Arch Intern Med* 1976;136:1303–1304.
59. Smith AH, Sheam VI, Wood R. Asbestos and kidney cancer: the evidence supports a causal association. *Am J Ind Med* 1989;16:159–166.
60. Osoria AM, Thun MJ, Novak RF, Cura JV, Avner ED. Silica and glomerulonephritis: case report and review of the literature. *Am J Kidney Dis* 1987:9:224–230.
61. Roth D, Alarcon FJ, Fernandez JA, Preston RA, Bourgoignie JJ Acute rhabdomyolysis associated with cocaine intoxication. *N Engl J Med* 1988;319:673–677.
62. Luxton RW. Radiation nephritis: a long-term study of 54 patients. *Lancet* 1961;1:1221–1224.
63. Sontz E, Schwieger J. The "green water" syndrome: copper-induced hemolysis and subsequent renal failure as a consequence of religious ritual. *Am J Med* 1995;98:311–315.
64. Kurokawa Y, Maekawa A, Takahashi M, Hayashi Y. Toxicity and carcinogenicity of potassium bromate—a renal carcinogen. *Environ Health Perspect* 1990;87:309–335.
65. Lechleitner P, Defregger M, Lhotta K, Totsch M, Fend F. Goodpasture's syndrome: unusual presentation after exposure to hard metal dust. *Chest* 1993;103:956–957.
66. Breysse P, Couser WG, Alpers CE, Nelson K, Gaur L, Johnson RJ. Membranous nephropathy and formaldehyde exposure. *Ann Intern Med* 1994;120:396–397.
67. Sinks T, Lushniak B, Haussler BJ, et al. Renal cell cancer among paperboard printing workers. *Epidemiology* 1992;3:483–489.
68. Walker RJ, Duggin GG. Drug nephrotoxicity. *Annu Rev Pharmacol Toxicol* 1988;28:331–345.
69. Barrett BJ. Contrast nephrotoxicity. *J Am Soc Nephrol* 1994;5:125–137.
70. Murray MD, Brater DC. Renal toxicity of nonsteroidal anti-inflammatory drugs. *Annu Rev Pharmacol Toxicol* 1993;32:435–465.

*Environmental and Occupational Medicine, Third Edition,* edited by William N. Rom.
Lippincott–Raven Publishers, Philadelphia © 1998.

# CHAPTER 58

# Bladder Carcinogens

Michael D. Goldstein, Peter D. Griffin, and Paul W. Brandt-Rauf

The link between specific occupations and subsequent risk for the development of bladder cancer was first identified in 1895. L. Rehn (1), a surgeon, identified a cluster of bladder cancer cases among workers in the dyestuffs industry who were manufacturing magenta from aniline. Numerous studies since that time have investigated the epidemiology, toxicology, and clinical aspects of occupational bladder cancer.

In 1994, cancer of the urinary bladder accounted for 51,200 new cases in the United States. Approximately 10,000 deaths were recorded from bladder cancer in that same period (2). There had been a striking increase in bladder cancer in past decades reaching a peak mortality incidence in the early 1970s. Among white males in the United States the reported incidence from 1937 to 1939 was 14.1 per 100,000 person-years, and it had jumped to 21.3 per 100,000 person-years by 1971 (3). While the overall incidence of bladder cancer has increased 10% from 1973 to 1991, mortality rates for this disease have declined over the past two decades (4).

The current incidence rate of 32.3 cases per 100,000 population among white men is more than twice that found in nonwhite men but there has been a 28% increase for black men and a 34% increase for black women (5). From the early 1960s, 5-year relative survivorship has increased more than 50%. This improvement in survival rates among persons with bladder cancer may in part be due to earlier diagnosis, which may have contributed to the decline in mortality (6). Internationally, the incidence of bladder cancer varies about tenfold (7). Bladder cancer occurs most often in Western Europe and North America and least often in Eastern Europe and several areas of Asia (5).

Additional risk may be incurred by environmental exposure to bladder carcinogens. Some of this increase is attributable to occupational exposures. The percent attributable risk (PAR) of bladder cancer to occupational exposure has been estimated at 21% to 25% for males and 11% for females (8). In England and the United States it has been shown that there is a marked change in incidence rates from one part of the country to another with higher rates being recorded in urban rather than rural areas. New Jersey has the highest mortality rate for bladder cancer among white males of any state in the United States (9). It has been speculated that excess deaths in New Jersey may be related to the concentration of chemical manufacturing industries in that state.

In terms of carcinogenesis, the lower urinary tract—renal pelves, ureters, bladder, and urethra—may be considered as a unit. All of it is lined by transitional epithelium, and potentially carcinogenic substances and metabolites excreted through the kidneys directly contact this mucosa. Studies indicate that 90% to 95% of lower urinary tract tumors are in the bladder, 1% to 6% in the ureters, and 2% to 6% in the renal pelves (10). There is evidence that occupational carcinogens can act on all of the transitional epithelium, though more intense exposure may be needed to cause cancer in the renal pelves and ureters (10). In occupational carcinogenesis of the lower urinary tract, the area of the greatest concern, and hence most study, has been the bladder.

## HISTORICAL PERSPECTIVE

In the decades after 1895, when the initial cluster of three cases of bladder cancer was reported among dyestuffs workers, cases of bladder cancer associated

M. D. Goldstein and P. W. Brandt-Rauf: Division of Environmental Health Sciences, Columbia University School of Public Health, New York, New York 10032.
P. D. Griffin: Corporate Medical Consultant, Westport, Connecticut 06880.

with work in this industry were reported throughout Europe. In 1938 it was shown that feeding 2-naphthylamine to dogs induced bladder cancer (11). A significant amount of evidence suggested that certain aromatic amines could cause bladder cancer in the industrial environment, but it was not until the 1950s, and the epidemiologic investigations of Case and co-workers (12) of the chemical and rubber industries in the United Kingdom, that it was generally accepted that bladder cancer is an occupational disease. They studied 4,622 men who worked longer than 6 months in the British chemical industry. Using death certificates they uncovered 127 men who died of bladder cancer and who were exposed to 2-naphthylamine and benzidine, when in fact only three to five deaths from bladder cancer were expected. They estimated that the risk of dying of bladder cancer when exposed to these chemicals was 30 times the baseline risk. Case's group also investigated the rubber industry in the United Kingdom, where they likewise identified increased risk of developing bladder cancer (13). It was determined that 2-naphthylamine, which was known from the chemical industry study to be a potent bladder carcinogen, was a principal ingredient of an important additive, Nonox S, used extensively in the British rubber industry until 1949 (14).

## SUBSTANCES OF CONCERN

In 1955 in the United States, Melick and associates (15) showed that 4-aminobiphenyl (xenylamine), a by-product of aniline dye manufacturing used as a rubber antioxidant, is another occupational bladder carcinogen and may cause cancer of the ureters and renal pelves as well. Other compounds that are recognized or strongly suspected to be potential occupational bladder carcinogens are benzidine, benzidine-derived dyes, 3,3-dichlorobenzidine, nitrobiphenyl, 4,4-methylene-bis(2-chloroaniline) (MOCA), and 4,4-methylene dianiline (MDA) (16). Many of the hundreds of synthetic organic dyes used in the United States contain benzidine or benzidine congeners such as *o*-toluidine or *o*-dianisidine and are used to color textiles, leather, and paper. Numerous animal studies and several human studies of occupational dye users provide support for the role of these dyes in bladder carcinogenesis (17). Four dyes are of particular concern: direct black-38, direct green-1, direct red-17, and direct red-28. Long-term studies in Japanese dye stuff workers by Naito (18) demonstrated a remarkable increased risk for bladder carcinoma among 442 employees engaged in benzidine manufacture [Standard Mortality Ratio (SMR) = 63.6] and β-naphthylamine manufacture (SMR = 48.4). The average observation period was 39.4 years. The adjusted rate of urothelial carcinoma increased with the duration of exposure.

Other substances that are structurally similar to benzidine, such as 3,3-dichlorobenzidine and MDA, are also bladder carcinogens. The former is a known animal carcinogen, although occupational studies are equivocal. MDA is also a known animal carcinogen used in the production of rigid polyurethane foams, as a curing agent, and as an epoxy resin hardener. A proportionate mortality study of workers at a facility using MDA as a curing agent revealed a statistically significant threefold excess of bladder cancer. MOCA is another aromatic amine used as a curing agent for isocyanate-containing polymers. Approximately 33,000 workers are estimated to be exposed to MOCA in the United States, most in the polyurethane industry. Although it is a known animal carcinogen, MOCA has not been confirmed to be a human carcinogen owing to methodologic difficulties of study design, i.e., MOCA has been in widespread commercial use for about 30 years (short latency) and most cases have been in small plants with very few exposed workers (limited statistical power) (16).

It must also be kept in mind that cigarette smoking is probably the largest single attributable risk for the development of bladder cancer. Arylamines are found in tobacco smoke and may explain the risk association. The risk ratio for cigarette smoking and bladder cancer has been measured between 2:1 and 5:1 (19–23). Studies that have assessed the interaction between occupational exposure and cigarette smoking have usually found a synergistic relationship, sometimes additive and sometimes multiplicative (24–26).

New potential bladder carcinogens are constantly being uncovered. The benzidine congeners MDA and MOCA have already been noted. Perchloroethylene (PCE) has been implicated as a possible cause of excess mortality from bladder cancer among dry-cleaning workers (27). Occupational exposures to polycyclic aromatic hydrocarbons (PAHs) (28,29), asbestos (30), arsenic (31), and lead (32) have also been associated with increased risk of bladder cancer. The PAH link has received a good deal of attention in recent years. Several studies have focused on workers in aluminum smelting plants with exposures to coal tar pitch volatiles and found an association with increased bladder cancer risk (33,34). Investigations of other cohorts have also supported an association between PAH exposures and bladder cancer (35–37).

A National Institute for Occupational Safety and Health (NIOSH) investigation of occupational exposure to animal bladder tumorigens attempted to estimate the number of United States workers previously and currently exposed to bladder carcinogens (38). Utilizing the Registry of Toxic Effect of Chemical Substances (RTECS) and the National Occupational Exposure Survey (NOES), it was estimated that 700,000 U.S. workers were potentially exposed on a full-time (more than 4 hours per day) basis and 3.5 million on a part-time basis to 200 substances associated with animal bladder tumors. It should be noted that some animal tumorigens may not be human carcinogens and that individual risks are related to potency, duration, and intensity of the actual exposures. These numbers are helpful, however, in estimating the magnitude of potential exposures to occupational bladder carcinogens.

## EPIDEMIOLOGY

In recent years there have been many cohort and case-control studies that have associated various occupations with increased risk of bladder cancer but that have not necessarily identified the specific carcinogen involved. The following have been identified in one or another study as being at occupational risk: leather workers, kimono painters, textile workers, hairdressers and barbers, dye manufacturers, machinists, painters, aluminum smelter workers, tailors, cooks and kitchen hands, food counter workers, rubber workers, butchers, crop sprayers, glass processors, railroad workers, truck drivers, vehicle mechanics, nuclear fuel workers, petroleum workers, printers, rodenticide applicators, gas station workers, clerical workers, cable manufacturers, carpenters, chemical workers, civil engineers, purchasing agents, coal miners, electricians, metal workers, farmers, medical workers, nurserymen, photography workers, plumbers, welders, stone masons, tool and die makers, food processors, dry cleaning and laundry workers, construction industry workers, female computer manufacturers aircraft and ship officers, street vendors, and workers exposed to high power frequency electromagnetic fields (16,24,39–71). The list is remarkable for its variety and the differences in strength of association between various occupations and bladder cancer. Some of these occupations—dye, leather, hairdresser, and chemical worker—appear in numerous studies and over time continue to have a statistically significant association with bladder cancer. Other jobs such as butchering and food handling appear in only occasional studies to carry a risk, and one remains skeptical of the validity of the association.

These inconsistencies may be explained by considering how exposures differ over time and from place to place. It has been shown in the rubber industry, for example, how removal of one chemical (Nonox S) in the United Kingdom has neutralized the risk inherent in one occupation (14). It should also be noted that workers who have the same occupational title may in fact have different exposure levels in different companies or different countries. Attempts have been made to overcome this obstacle by using an exposure-to-classes-of-chemicals matrix, rather than a job title or industry affiliation matrix (72,73). New causal agents have not been uncovered in this way, however. In case-control studies a finite number of cases of bladder cancer may be divided up among many job titles, to the point where a statistically significant association may be based on very few cases. Alternatively, a real occupational risk may be diluted into an insignificant relative risk if it is classified along with groups with different exposures. Insufficient dose, insufficient duration of exposure, and analysis of cases during the latent period (which for bladder cancer can range from 2 to 48 years) (74) may also mask a real association.

Although exposure to well-documented occupational bladder carcinogens has been curtailed to a considerable extent, exposure may continue by various and different means. For example, impurities of known bladder carcinogens can be mixed in with other substances. Such is the case with the rodenticide ANTU. Workers who handled it were found to have an increased risk of developing bladder cancer, and it was discovered that 2-naphthylamine was mixed with the ANTU (25,75). The carcinogenicity of 1-naphthylamine can likewise be attributed to contamination with 2-naphthylamine. Some cutting oils and lubricants may contain aromatic amines as antioxidants or may have contained polycyclic aromatic hydrocarbons in the past. Some substances that are related to the known bladder carcinogens can be metabolized in vivo into the carcinogens. It has been shown that the benzidine-based dyes direct black-38, direct blue-6, and direct brown-95 are metabolized by bacteria in the human gut into benzidine. Workers exposed to benzidine-based dyes have been found to excrete benzidine in their urine (76). Japanese kimono painters, who have an increased risk of bladder cancer, tip brushes with these benzidine-based paints in the mouth to achieve a sharper point (46). Many of the aromatic amines are lipid soluble, and absorption can be transdermal as well as by inhalation and ingestion.

## MECHANISMS OF DISEASE

Most chemical carcinogens probably affect the urothelial cells via their presence in the urine. The metabolism of these compounds is a crucial part of the initial host response to the environmental exposure. It has been postulated that disturbances in the balance between activation and detoxification may explain the individual variations in responses to carcinogen exposures (77). The majority of chemical carcinogens require metabolic activation before they interact with cellular macromolecules and can cause cancer initiation. Defective *N*-acetyltransferase (NAT) and glutathione-S-transferase enzymes have been associated with an increased risk of developing bladder cancer (78). NAT is an enzyme involved in the metabolism of arylamines. Human populations show a genetically based polymorphism. Increased bladder cancer risk has been associated with slow acetylation by NAT in human phenotyping studies (79,80). This effect does not appear to hold for benzidine exposures. In fact, a recent National Cancer Institute study concluded that slow acetylation by NAT is not associated with an increased risk of bladder cancer in workers exposed to benzidine and may in fact actually have a protective effect (81).

Glutathione-S-transferase M1 (GSTM1) is an enzyme that metabolizes foreign compounds. The GSTM1 gene may modulate the internal dose of environmental carcinogens and thereby affect the risk of developing bladder cancer. Approximately 50% of all humans inherit two deleted copies of the GSTM1 gene. Two recent case control studies investigated GSTM1 deficiency in relation to environmental risk factors and bladder cancer. Both studies concluded that a significant proportion (between 17% and 25%) of all bladder cancer may be attributable to the at risk GSTM1 0/0 genotype (82,83).

Investigations of bladder cancer disease mechanisms have also utilized tools such as DNA adducts and oncogenes. Biochemical studies have revealed aminobiphenyl DNA adduct formation in human uroepithelial cells (84). In one particular study the concentration of ABP hemoglobin adducts was significantly higher in slow NAT acetylators (85). Another study of bladder cancer patients revealed a dose-response relationship between smoking levels and adduct levels (86). Oncogene investigations have focused primarily on the P53 and *ras* oncogenes. Point mutations in the P53 tumor suppressor gene are the most common genetic alterations in human cancers. A recent study analyzed a group of 109 bladder cancer patients for P53 nuclear overexpression (87). The researchers found associations between cigarettes smoked, dye/ink-related occupations, cooking-related occupations, and P53 nuclear overexpression. Another study, however, found no difference in the frequency and pattern of P53 mutations between bladder cancer patients with and without documented occupational exposures (88). Researchers have also looked at the *ras* oncogene in terms of an association with bladder cancer. One recent study (albeit based on small numbers) has reported an apparent association between occupational exposures (to naphthylamine and benzidine) and overexpression of the ras protein products (89).

In addition to the direct effects of the various carcinogens upon the urothelial cells, physical inflammation may be an important cofactor. Cell proliferative activity may be increased by urinary bladder infection and/or irritation caused by bladder stones (90,91). The association between cancer and inflammation, however, does appear to be stronger for squamous cell as opposed to transitional cell cancers.

## SURVEILLANCE

Research into the effectiveness of and methods for screening for occupationally related bladder cancer has expanded rapidly over the past several years. Many of these investigations have been aimed at more closely evaluating the impact of traditional screening methods utilizing tests for urinary cytology and microhematuria. Additional studies have focused on newer areas of detection technology, such as quantitative fluorescence image analysis (QFIA) and deoxyribonucleic acid (DNA) flow cytometry.

The use of urine cytologic examination to evaluate workers at occupational risk for bladder cancer has been the mainstay of screening programs to date. Recent studies have been directed at evaluating the efficacy of such screening. Ellwein (92) evaluated the value of screening asymptomatic high-risk populations using a biologically based model of bladder cancer. The analyses assumed biennial cytologic screening of voided urine, beginning at 30 years of age with 100% attendance until age 65 and 60% attendance thereafter. Based on these analyses, cytologic screening was projected to increase life expectancy by 1 to 3 years among those diagnosed and to reduce deaths from bladder cancer by more than 50%. Farrow (93) also reviewed the utility of urine cytologic screening in high-risk populations and noted that the majority of bladder tumors begin as superficial, noninvasive growths and remain so. A smaller subpopulation exhibit aggressive malignant behavior. He therefore concluded that urine cytologic examination is an effective method of detecting lethal forms of bladder cancer in early stages but that detection strategies should concentrate on the higher-grade and lethal forms of the disease and recognize and accept that a significant proportion of cases of well-differentiated nonlethal superficial tumors will go undetected.

Although urinary Papanicolaou (PAP) cytology does have a high sensitivity for dangerous, invasive bladder cancer, the slightly earlier detection of these high-grade tumors rarely alters unfavorable outcomes (94). Sensitivity to low-grade papillary tumors is low (95). A recent study evaluated the results of specific cytologic screening programs in Canada (96). In this cohort of Canadian aluminum workers, 79 cases of bladder cancer were identified between 1970 and 1986. Cases diagnosed after the screening program was introduced in 1980 were compared with those diagnosed earlier. In cases diagnosed after the screening program was introduced the proportion identified at early stages was higher and survival seemed improved, but the differences were not statistically significant.

Some studies have suggested that urinary mutagen (Ames) testing, has application as a surveillance tool for workplace hazardous exposures, though sensitivity and specificity are low (97).

Most bladder cancers, even when noninvasive, produce hematuria (98). Therefore, screening asymptomatic high-risk populations for hematuria is potentially useful as a means for early detection. In one study of 235 men, older than 50 years, from the general population who performed home dipstick testing for hematuria, 8 (3.4%) were found to have unsuspected urinary cancers diagnosed early enough to allow institution of seemingly conservative treatment (98). A British study of dipstick screening of 578 men over age 60 for hematuria revealed four previously undiagnosed cases of bladder cancer (99). The authors conclude that the introduction of less invasive methods of follow-up investigation (flexible cystoscopy and ultrasonography) makes screening for bladder cancer in the community more feasible. It should be noted that

**TABLE 1.** *Scenarios for screening programs*

| | Known carcinogen | Suspect carcinogen |
|---|---|---|
| High exposure | Cytology every 6 months, RBC test every 6 months to ensure acceptability | Cytology every 6 months, RBC test every 6 months to catch low-grade tumors |
| Low exposure | Cytology after 2 years, then every 5 years | Cytology depending on circumstances |

Educational and psychosocial support would be included in each scenario. Frequency of screening would be modified depending on the degree of exposure, carcinogenicity, and interval since first exposure.

high sensitivity is achieved only in the face of multiple screenings (100). Others have suggested that hematuria may not be a useful test for screening of occupational groups at risk of bladder cancer given the limitations of available information concerning normal urinalysis. The extremely low positive predictive value of routine screening in the general population has caused most authoritative bodies to recommend against this application as a screening tool. A recent review by the U.S. Preventative Services Task Force concluded that the routine screening of asymptomatic individuals is not justified.

Quantitative fluorescence image analysis is a technology that makes biochemical and immunochemical measurements at the molecular level in single cells using fluorescent probes (101). Normal cells contain 46 chromosomes (2C) and dividing cells up to 92 chromosomes (4C). Utilizing QFIA, the diagnosis of cancer can be made if a single unambiguous cancer cell with 5C DNA can be identified, although viruses and premalignant lesions can also yield abnormal cells with 5C DNA. QFIA screening of 504 persons within a 2-naphthylamine cohort found that DNA hyperploidy correlated with exposure duration and smoking history (101). The authors concluded that results to date indicate that QFIA measurements on voided urine cells can play an important role in occupational screening programs.

Another recently developed method for evaluating bladder tumors involves flow cytometry. This method utilizes automated cell spectrophotometry to detect increased DNA content indicative of malignant cells (102). Flow cytometry typically requires evaluation of a bladder irrigation specimen. Since this is an invasive procedure its principal role to date has been in predicting and monitoring response to therapy in patients with known bladder cancer. This method has recently been evaluated as a screening tool for bladder cancer utilizing voided urine specimens (103). This study determined that while flow cytometry of voided urine specimens may be helpful in following patients with a history of bladder cancer, it is not recommended for widespread screening (103,104).

Additional studies have examined other methods that may prove useful in screening for bladder cancer. These include the use of monoclonal antibodies specific to several known antigens associated with human bladder cancer (105), cystoscopic screening of asymptomatic high-risk cohorts (106), tumor markers such as autocrine motility factor and tumor cell collagenase-stimulating factor (107), and screening protocols employing a combination of methods (108,109). Bi et al. (110) have suggested that the use of cellular and molecular probes in combination with medical and epidemiologic screening can identify early, low-grade bladder cancer cases. A cohort of Chinese workers who had been exposed to benzidine and identified with bladder cancer underwent screening tests included PAP urinary cytology, QFIA cytology, and quantitative fluorescence to detect expression of a low-grade bladder tumor-associated antigen (p300) by exfoliated urothelial cells and elevated expression of the *neu* oncogene product (p185). P300 markers detected by the M344 monoclonal antibody had higher sensitivity and specificity that either QFIA or PAP cytology and appears to have potential as a marker to screen high-risk groups (110).

The 1989 International Conference on Bladder Cancer Screening in High-Risk Groups sponsored by NIOSH, at which many of the above noted studies were presented, produced several summary recommendations of note (111):

1. Screening for bladder cancer should be viewed as a research endeavor whose benefits for persons or the populations screened are not yet delineated.
2. Techniques for screening are evolving; it would be wise to bank serum and urine samples.
3. The natural history of bladder cancer is unclear; hence, the value to the individual of detecting superficial versus invasive lesions is unclear.

Recommended guidelines for bladder cancer screening are outlined in Table 1 (111).

## REFERENCES


1. Rehn L. Blasengeschwulste bei fuchsin Arbeitern. *Arch Klin Chir* 1895;50:588–600.
2. Boring CC, Squire TS and Tong T. Cancer Statistics, 1994. *CA* 1994; 44:7–26.
3. Devesa SS, Silverman DT. Cancer incidence and mortality trends in the U.S. 1935–1974. *J Natl Cancer Inst* 1978;60:545–571.
4. Ries LAG, Hankey BF, et al., eds. *SEER Cancer Statistics Review 1973–1990.* NIH Publication No. 93-2789. Bethesda, MD: National Cancer Institute, 1993.
5. Silverman DT, et al. Urinary bladder. In: Harras A, Edwards B, Gloeckler-Reis L, Blot W. *Cancer rates and risks,* 4th ed. 1996.
6. Hanky BF, Silverman DT. Urinary bladder. In: Miller BA, Ries LAG, Hankey BF, et al., eds. *SEER cancer statistics review* 1973–1990.

NIH Publication No. 93-2789. Bethesda, MD: National Cancer Institute, 1993.
7. Parkin DM, Muir CS, Whelan S. *Cancer incidence in five continents,* vol VI. IARC Scientific Publication No. 120. Lyon, France: World Health Organization, International Agency for Research on Cancer, 1992.
8. Silverman DT. Occupational risks of bladder cancer among white women in the United States. *Am J Epidemiol* 1990;132:453–461.
9. Schoenberg JB, Stemhagen A, Mogielnicki AP, Altman R, Abe T, Mason TJ. Case-control study of bladder cancer in New Jersey. 1. Occupational exposures in white males. *J Natl Cancer Inst* 1984;72: 973–981.
10. Schmauz R, Cole P. Epidemiology of cancer of the renal pelvis and ureter. *J Natl Cancer Inst* 1974;52:1431–1434.
11. Hueper WC, Wiley FH, Wolfe HD, Ranta KE, Leming MF, Blood FR. Experimental production of bladder tumors in dogs by administration of beta-naphthylamine. *J Ind Hyg* 1938;20:46–84.
12. Case R, Hosker M, McDonald D, Pearson J. Tumours of the urinary bladder in workmen engaged in the manufacture and use of certain dyestuff intermediates in the British chemical industry. *Br J Ind Med* 1954;11:75–104.
13. Case R, Hosker M. Tumour of the urinary bladder as an occupational disease in the rubber industry in England and Wales. *Br J Prevent Soc Med* 1954;8:39–50.
14. Nutt AR. *Toxic hazards of rubber chemicals.* London: Elsevier, 1984.
15. Melick WH, Escue HM, Naryka JJ, Mezera RA, Wheeler EP. The first reported cases of human bladder tumors due to a new carcinogen—xenylamine. *J Urol* 1955;74:760–766.
16. Schulte PA, Ringen K, Hemstreet GP, Ward E. Occupational cancer of the urinary tract. *J Occup Med* 1987;2:85–107.
17. Bulbulyan MA, Figgs LW, et.al. Cancer incidents and mortality among beta-naphthylamine and benzidine dye workers in Moscow. *Int J Epidemiol* 1995;24(2):266–275.
18. Naito S, Tanaka K, Koga H, et al. Cancer occurrence among dyestuff workers exposed to aromatic amines. *Cancer* 1995;76:1445–1452.
19. Javadpour N, ed. *Epidemiologic considerations in bladder cancer.* Baltimore: Williams & Wilkins, 1984.
20. Burch JD, Rohan TE, Howe GR, et al. Risk of bladder cancer by source and type of tobacco exposure: a case-control study. *Int J Cancer* 1989;44:622–628.
21. Schifflers E, Jamart J, Renard V. Tobacco and occupation as risk factors in bladder cancer: a case-control study in Southern Belgium. *Int J Cancer* 1987;39:287–292.
22. Howe GR, Burch JD, Miller AB, et al. Tobacco use, occupation, coffee, various nutrients and bladder cancer. *J Natl Cancer Inst* 1980;64: 701–713.
23. Siemiatycki J, Krewski D, et.al. Associations between cigarette smoking in each of twenty-one types of cancer; A multi-site case control study. *Int J Epidemiol* 1995;24(3):504–514.
24. Gonzalez CA, Lopez-Abente G, Errezola M, et al. Occupation and bladder cancer in Spain: a multicentre case-control study. *Int J Epidemiol* 1989;18:569–577.
25. Vineu P, Esteve J, Terracini B. Bladder cancer and smoking in males: types of cigarettes, age at start, effect of stopping and interaction with occupation. *Int J Cancer* 1984;34:165–170.
26. Cartwright RA. Occupational bladder cancer and cigarette smoking in West Yorkshire. *Scand J Work Environ Health* 1982;8:79–82.
27. Ruder AM, Ward EM, Brown DP, et al. Cancer mortality in female and male dry-cleaning workers. *J Occup Med* 1994;36(8):867–874.
28. Bonassi S, Merlo F, Pearce N, Puntoni R. Bladder cancer and occupational exposure to polycyclic aromatic hydrocarbons. *Int J Cancer* 1989;44:648–651.
29. Momas I, Daures JT, et al. Relative importance of risk factors in bladder carcinogenesis: some new results about Mediterranean habits. *Cancer Causes Control* 1994;5(4):326–332.
30. Bravo MP, Del Rey-Calero J, Conde M. Bladder cancer and asbestos in Spain. *Rev Epidemiol Sante Publique* 1988;36:10–14.
31. Maloney ME. Arsenic in dermatology. *Dermatol Surg* 1996;22(3): 301–304.
32. Fu H, Boffetta P. Cancer and occupational exposure to inorganic lead compound. *Occup Environ Med* 1995;52(2):73–81.
33. Ronneberg A, Andersen A. Mortality and cancer morbidity in workers from an aluminum smelter. *Occup Environ Med* 1995;52(4):250–254.
34. Tremblay C, Armstrong B, et al. Estimation of risk of developing bladder cancer among workers exposed to cold tar pitch volatiles in the primary aluminum industry. *Am J Ind Med* 1995;27(3):335–348.
35. Clavel J, Mandereau L, et al. Occupational exposure to polycyclate aromatic hydrocarbons and the risk of bladder cancer: a French case-controlled study. *Int J Epidemiol* 1994;23(6):1145–1153.
36. Hours M, Dananche B, et al. Bladder cancer and occupational exposures. *Scand J Work Environ Health* 1994;20(5):322–330.
37. Evanoff BA, Gustavsson T, et al. Mortality and incidence of cancer in a cohort of Swedish chimney sweeps: an extended follow-up study. *Br J Ind Med* 1993;50(5):450–459.
38. Ruder AM, Fine LJ, Sundin DS. National estimates of occupational exposure to animal bladder tumorigens. *J Occup Med* 1990;32: 797–805.
39. Porru S,Aulenti V, et al. Bladder cancer and occupation: a case controlled study in northern Italy. *Occup Environ Med* 1996;53(1):6–10.
40. Brown LM, Zahm SH, et al. High bladder cancer mortality in rural New England: an etiologic study. *Cancer Causes Control* 1995;6(4): 361–368.
41. Swanson GM, Burns TB. Cancer incidence among women in the work place. *J Occup Environ Med* 1995;37(3):282–287.
42. LaVecchia C, Tavani A. Epidemiologic evidence on hair dyes and the risk of cancer in humans. *Eur J Cancer Prev* 1995;4(1):31–43.
43. Skov T, Lynge E. Cancer risk and exposures to carcinogens in hair dressers. *Skin Pharmacol* 1994;7(1-2):94–100.
44. Cordier S, Clavel J, et al. Occupational risks of bladder cancer in France: a multi-center case control study. *Int J Epidemiol* 1993;22(3): 403–411.
45. Notani PN, Shah P, et al. Occupation and cancers of the lung and bladder: a case control study in Bombay. *Int J Epidemiol* 1993;22(2): 185–191.
46. Brown DP, Kaplan SD. Retrospective cohort mortality study of dry cleaners workers using perchloroethylene. *J Occup Med* 1987;29: 535–541.
47. Cole P, Hoover R, Friedell G. Occupation and cancer of the lower urinary tract. *Cancer* 1972;29:1250–1260.
48. Theriault G, DeGuire L, Cordier S. Reducing aluminum: an occupation possibly associated with bladder cancer. *CMA J* 1981;124: 419–425.
49. Theriault G, Cordier S, Tremblay C, Gergras S. Bladder cancer in the aluminum industry. *Lancet* 1984;1:947–950.
50. Smith EM, Miller E, Woolson R, Brown C. Bladder cancer risk among auto and truck mechanics and chemically related occupations. *Am J Public Health* 1985;75:881–883.
51. Davies JM, Thomas HF, Mawson D. Bladder tumors among rodent operatives handling ANTU. *Br Med J* 1982;285:927–931.
52. Wertheimer N, Leeper E. Magnetic field exposure related to cancer subtypes. *Ann NY Acad Sci* 1987;502:43–54.
53. Matnoski GM, Elliot EA. Bladder cancer epidemiology. *Epidemiol Rev* 1981;3:203–229.
54. Tola S. Occupational cancer of the urinary bladder. In: Vanio H, Sorsa M, Hemminki K, eds. *Occupational cancer and carcinogens.* Washington, DC: Hemisphere, 1981.
55. Silverman DT, Hoover RN, Albert S, Graff KM. Occupation and cancer of the lower urinary tract in Detroit. *J Natl Cancer Inst* 1983;70: 237–245.
56. Marrett LD, Hartge P, Meigs JW. Bladder cancer and occupational exposure to leather. *Br J Ind Med* 1986;43:96–100.
57. Garabrant D, Wegman D. Cancer mortality among shoe and leather workers in Massachusetts. *Am J Ind Med* 1984;5:303–314.
58. Hoar L, Hoover R. Truck driving and bladder cancer mortality in rural New England. *J Natl Cancer Inst* 1985;74:771–74.
59. Silverman DT, Hoover RN, Mason TJ, Swanson MG. Motor exhaust–related occupations and bladder cancer. *Cancer Res* 1986;46: 2113–2116.
60. Jenson OM, Wahrendorf J, Knudsen J, Sorensen BL. The Copenhagen case-referent study on bladder cancer. *Scand J Work Environ Health* 1987;13:129–134.
61. Delzell E, Monson R. Mortality among rubber workers. *Am J Ind Med* 1984;6:273–279.
62. Boyko RW, Cartwright MA, Glashan RW. Bladder cancer in dye manufacturing workers. *J Occup Med* 1985;27:799–803.
63. Meigs JW, Marrett LD, Ulrich FV, Flannery JT. Bladder tumor incidence among workers exposed to benzidine: a thirty-year follow-up. *J Natl Cancer Inst* 1986;76:1–8.

64. Obata K, Ohno Y, Aoki K. Epidemiological investigation on bladder cancer and occupations. *Hinyokika Kiyo* 1989;35:2057–2061.
65. Miyakawa M, Yoshida O. Benzidine dyes and risk of bladder cancer. *Hinyokika Kiyo* 1989;35:2049–2056.
66. Silverman DT, Levin LI, Hoover RN. Occupational risks of bladder cancer in the United States: II. Nonwhite men. *J Natl Cancer Inst* 1989;81:1480–1483.
67. Silverman DT, Levin LI, Hoover RN, Hartge P. Occupational risks of bladder cancer in the United States: I. White men. *J Natl Cancer Inst* 1989;81:1472–1480.
68. Schumacher MC, Slattery ML, West DW. Occupation and bladder cancer in Utah. *Am J Ind Med* 1989;16:89–102.
69. Steenland K, Burnett C, Osorio AM. A case-control study of bladder cancer using city directories as a source of occupational data. *Am J Epidemiol* 1987;126:247–257.
70. Armstrong BG, Tremblay CG, Cyr D, Theriault GP. Estimating the relationship between exposure to tar volatiles and the incidence of bladder cancer in aluminum smelter workers. *Scand J Work Environ Health* 1986;12:486–493.
71. Silverman DT, Hoover RN, Mason TJ, Swanson GM. Motor exhaust–related occupations and bladder cancer. *Cancer Res* 1986;46: 2113–2116.
72. Coggan D, Pannett B, Acheson ED. Use of job-exposure matrix in an occupational analysis of lung and bladder cancers on the basis of death certificates. *J Natl Cancer Inst* 1984;72:61–65.
73. Vinei SP, Magnani C. Occupation and bladder cancers in males: a case-control study. *Int J Cancer* 1985;35:599–606.
74. Schulte PA, Ringen K, Hemstreet G, et al. Risk assessment of a cohort exposed to aromatic amines. *J Occup Med* 1985;27:115–121
75. Lindstedt G, Sollenberg J. Polycyclic aromatic hydrocarbons in the occupational environment. *Scand J Work Environ Health* 1982;8:1–19.
76. *Monographs on the evaluation of the carcinogenic risk of chemicals to humans.* Lyon, France: IARC, 1982.
77. Hirvonen A. Genetic factors in individual responses to environmental exposures. *J Occup Environ Med* 1995;37(1):37–43.
78. Raunio H, et al. Diagnosis of polymorphisms in carcinogen-activating and inactivating enzymes and cancer susceptibility–a review. *Gene* 1995;159(1):113–121.
79. Hayes RB. Genetic susceptibility in occupational cancer. *Med Lav* 1995;86(3):206–213.
80. Risch A, Wallace DM, et al. Slow N-acetylation genotype is a susceptibility factor in occupational and smoking-related bladder cancer. *Hum Mol Genet* 1995;4(2):231–236.
81. Hayes RB, Ibi-W, et al. N-acetylation phenotype and genotype and risk of bladder cancer in benzidine-exposed workers. *Carcinogenesis* 1993;14(4):675–678.
82. Brockmoller J, Kerb R, et al. Glutathione S-transferase M1 and its variants AB as host factors of bladder cancer susceptibility, a case-controlled study. *Cancer Res* 1994;54(15):4103–4111.
83. Bell DA, Taylor JA, et al. Genetic risk and carcinogen exposure: a common inherited defect of the carcinogen-metabolism gene glutathione S-transferase. *J Natl Cancer Inst* 1993;85(14):1159–1164.
84. Reznikoff CA, Kao C, et al. A molecular genetic bottle of human bladder carcinogenesis. *Semin Cancer Biol* 1993;4(3):143–152.
85. Vineis P. Epidemiological models of carcinogenesis: the example of bladder cancer. *Cancer Epidemiol Biomarkers Prev* 1992;1:149–153.
86. Talaska G, Schamer M, et al. Carcinogen-DNA adducts in bladder biopsies and urothelial cells. *Cancer Lett* 1994;84(1):93–97.
87. Zhang ZF, Sarkis AS, et al. Tobacco smoking, occupation and p53 nuclear overexpression in early stage bladder cancer. *Cancer Epidemiol Biomarkers Prev* 1994;3(1):19–24.
88. Taylor JA, Li Y, et al. P53 Mutations in bladder tumors from arylamine exposed workers. *Cancer Res* 1996;56(2):294–298.
89. Novara R, Coda R, et al. Exposure to aromatic amines and ras and c-erB-2 overexpression in bladder cancer. *J Occup Environ Med* 1996; 38:390–393.
90. Burin GJ, Gibb HJ, Hill RN. Human bladder cancer: evidence for a potential irritation-induced mechanism. *Food Chem Toxicol* 1995; 33(9):785–795.
91. Shirai T, Fradet Y. The etiology of bladder cancer—are there any new clues or predictors of behavior? *Int J Urol* 1995;2(suppl 2):64–75.
92. Ellwein LB. Bladder cancer screening: lessons from a biologically based model of bladder cancer progression and therapeutic intervention. *J Occup Med* 1990;32:806–811.
93. Farrow GM. Urine cytology in the detection of bladder cancer: a critical approach. *J Occup Med* 1990;32:817–821.
94. Cole PL. Basic issues in population screening for cancer. *J Natl Cancer Inst* 1980;64:1263–1272
95. Farrow GM. Urine cytology in the detection of bladder cancer: a critical appraisal. *J Occup Med* 1990;32(9):817–821.
96. Theriault GP, Tremblay CG, Armstrong BG. Bladder cancer screening among primary aluminum production workers in Quebec. *J Occup Med* 1990;32:869–872.
97. Choi BC, Connolly JG, Zhou RH, et al. Application of urinary mutagen testing to detect workplace hazardous exposure and bladder cancer. *Mutat Res* 1995;341:207–216.
98. Messing EM, Vaillancourt A. Hematuria screening for bladder cancer. *J Occup Med* 1990;32:838–845.
99. Britton JP, Dowell AC, Whelan P. Dipstick haematuria and bladder cancer in men over 60: results of a community study. *Br Med J* 1989; 299:1010–1012.
100. Messing EM. Hematuria screening for bladder cancer. *J Occup Med* 1990;32:838–845.
101. Hemstreet GP III, Hurst RE, Bass RA, Rao JY. Quantitative fluorescence image analysis in bladder cancer screening. *J Occup Med* 1990; 32:822–828.
102. Melamed MR. Flow cytometry detection and evaluation of bladder tumors. *J Occup Med* 1990;32:829–833.
103. Deitch AD, Anderson KA, DeVere-White RW. Evaluation of DNA flow cytometry as a screening test for bladder cancer. *J Occup Med* 1990;32:898–903.
104. Hermansen DK, Badalament RA, Bretton PR, et al. Voided urine flow cytometry in screening high-risk patients for the presence of bladder cancer. *J Occup Med* 1990;32:894–897.
105. Lin CW, Kirley SD, Khaw AH, Zhang DS, Prout GR Jr. Detection of exfoliated bladder cancer cells by monoclonal antibodies to tumor-associated cell surface antigens. *J Occup Med* 1990;32:910–916.
106. Ward E, Halperin W, Thun M, et al. Screening workers exposed to 4,4′-methylenebis(2-chloroaniline) for bladder cancer by cystoscopy. *J Occup Med* 1990;32:865–868.
107. Guirguis R, Javadpour N, Sharareh S, et al. A new method for evaluation of urinary autocrine motility factor and tumor cell collagenase–stimulating factor as markers for urinary tract cancers. *J Occup Med* 1990;32:846–853.
108. Mason TJ, Vogler WJ. Bladder cancer screening at the DuPont Chambers Works: a new initiative. *J Occup Med* 1990;32:874–877.
109. Marsh GM, Callahan C, Pavlock D, Leviton LC, Talbott EO, Hemstreet G. A protocol for bladder cancer screening and medical surveillance among high-risk groups: the Drake Health Registry experience. *J Occup Med* 1990;32:881–886.
110. Bi W, Rao JY, Hemstreet GP, et al. Field molecular epidemiology: feasibility of monitoring for the malignant bladder cell phenotype in a benzidine-exposed occupational cohort. *J Occup Med* 1993;35(1): 20–27.
111. Schulte P, Halperin W, Ward E. Final discussion: Where do we go from here? *J Occup Med* 1990;32:936–945.

*Environmental and Occupational Medicine, Third Edition,* edited by William N. Rom.
Lippincott–Raven Publishers, Philadelphia © 1998.

CHAPTER 59

# Alcohol and Drug Abuse in Industry

Kent W. Peterson and Donna R. Smith

Substance abuse includes unauthorized or inappropriate use of controlled substances, alcohol, prescription drugs, and tobacco. During the past decade, increasing employer resources have been directed toward workplace substance abuse issues, as evidenced by the growth of written policies, supervisor and employee education, drug and alcohol testing, employee assistance programs, and rehabilitation efforts.

This chapter covers five areas. First, epidemiologic data on the prevalence of substance use in the United States, both in the general population and among employees, is reviewed, as well as the impact of drug and alcohol use at the workplace. Second, industry and government programs are discussed, including prevention and control measures. Third, information about major substances of abuse, including psychedelics, stimulants, opiates, and alcohol, is summarized. Fourth, substance abuse treatment and rehabilitation are presented. Fifth, workplace drug and alcohol testing programs are discussed, including types and methods of testing, as well as specimen collection, laboratory analysis, and medical review officer (MRO) functions. The chapter concludes by identifying current substance abuse testing issues and future trends.

## EPIDEMIOLOGY

### Scope of the Problem

The best information about U.S. patterns of alcohol and drug use comes from the U.S. Department of Health and Human Services (DHHS) Substance Abuse and Mental Health Services Administration (SAMHSA) National Household Survey on Drug Abuse (1). Prevalent trends from 1979 to 1995 are summarized in Tables 1 to 3. In 1995, 12.8 million Americans used one or more illicit drugs during the previous month, representing 6.1% of the population 12 years and older. Of the 17.8 million people who in 1994 used marijuana at least once during the past year, 5.7 million used it once a week or more, and 3.1 million used it daily or almost daily. In 1995, 1.4 million people reported having used cocaine in the last month. Although the prevalence of illicit drug use in 1995 has continued to decrease slightly, these figures are still high, and prevalence has remained constant among frequent cocaine users. Recidivism after rehabilitation for illicit drug abuse is high compared to those treated for alcoholism (2).

Drugs in the workplace are a concern because 74% of current illicit drug users are employed, 54.7% full-time and 19.3% part-time. Illicit drug use is higher among males than females. Among employees 18 years or older, 7.9% of males and 4.3% of females were current illicit drug users in 1994. Even more dramatic is the variation by age as shown in Table 2. Illicit drug use is heavily concentrated among those aged 18 to 34. Based on 1994 surveys, 9.3% of full-time employees aged 18 to 34 use illicit drugs, largely marijuana (8.1%) and cocaine (1.3%). This percentage of use is considerably higher than the rates of positive urine drug screens among this age group, for example, as shown in Table 4. Reasons for this gap between reported use and drug test positives include recreational users abstaining from drug use prior to scheduled drug tests, and urine dilution, substitution, or adulteration. Illicit drug use crosses all industries, being highest in food preparation, food serving, and

K. W. Peterson: Department of Environmental Medicine, New York University Medical Center, New York, New York 10016; and Occupational Health Strategies, Charlottesville, Virginia 22903-4491.
D. R. Smith: Department of Education and Training, Substance Abuse Management, Inc., Boca Raton, Florida 33431.

**TABLE 1.** *Past month illicit drug, alcohol, and tobacco use in the U.S. population ages 12 and older (percent)*

| Drug | 1979 | 1982 | 1985 | 1988 | 1990 | 1991 | 1992 | 1993 | 1994 | 1995 |
|---|---|---|---|---|---|---|---|---|---|---|
| Any illicit drug | 14.1 | — | 12.1 | 7.7 | 6.7 | 6.6 | 5.8 | 5.9 | 6.0 | 6.1 |
| Marijuana and hashish | 13.2 | 11.5 | 9.7 | 6.2 | 5.4 | 5.1 | 4.7 | 4.6 | 4.8 | 4.7 |
| Cocaine | 2.6 | 2.4 | 3.0 | 1.6 | 0.9 | 1.0 | 0.7 | 0.7 | 0.7 | 0.7 |
| Crack | — | — | — | 0.3 | 0.3 | 0.3 | 0.2 | 0.3 | 0.2 | 0.2 |
| Inhalants | — | — | 0.6 | 0.4 | 0.4 | 0.4 | 0.3 | 0.3 | 0.4 | 0.4 |
| Hallucinogens | 1.9 | 0.9 | 1.2 | 0.6 | 0.4 | 0.5 | 0.4 | 0.4 | 0.5 | 0.7 |
| PCP | — | — | — | — | — | — | 0.0 | 0.0 | 0.0 | 0.0 |
| LSD | — | — | — | — | — | — | — | — | 0.2 | 0.3 |
| Heroin | 0.1 | 0.1 | 0.1 | 0.0 | 0.0 | 0.0 | 0.0 | 0.0 | 0.1 | 0.1 |
| Nonmedical use of any | | | | | | | | | | |
| Psychotherapeutic | — | — | 3.8 | 2.1 | 1.7 | 1.9 | 1.5 | 1.5 | 1.2 | 1.2 |
| Stimulants | — | — | 1.8 | 1.2 | 0.6 | 0.4 | 0.3 | 0.5 | 0.3 | 0.4 |
| Sedatives | — | — | 0.5 | 0.2 | 0.2 | 0.2 | 0.2 | 0.2 | 0.1 | 0.2 |
| Tranquilizers | — | — | 2.2 | 1.3 | 0.6 | 1.1 | 0.8 | 0.6 | 0.5 | 0.4 |
| Analgesics | — | — | 1.4 | 0.7 | 0.9 | 0.8 | 0.9 | 0.8 | 0.7 | 0.6 |
| Any illicit drug other than marijuana | — | — | 6.1 | 3.4 | 2.7 | 3.0 | 2.4 | 2.4 | 2.3 | 2.6 |
| Alcohol | 63.2 | 56.6 | 60.2 | 54.9 | 52.6 | 52.2 | 49.0 | 50.8 | 53.9 | 52.2 |
| Binge alcohol use | — | — | 20.2 | 15.0 | 14.4 | 15.5 | 14.5 | 14.6 | 16.5 | 15.8 |
| Heavy alcohol use | — | — | 8.3 | 5.8 | 6.3 | 6.8 | 6.2 | 6.7 | 6.2 | 5.5 |
| Cigarettes | — | — | 38.7 | 35.3 | 32.6 | 33.0 | 31.9 | 29.6 | 28.6 | 28.8 |
| Smokeless tobacco | — | — | — | 3.9 | 3.9 | 3.7 | 4.0 | 3.2 | 3.3 | 3.3 |

From ref. 1.

wholesale/retail trades (17.5%, 16.3%, and 15.4%, respectively). Interestingly, the transportation industry is clustered in the middle of other industries.

The DHHS Household Survey on Drug Abuse also provides some data on alcohol use prevalence and heavy alcohol usage, a sample of which is reported in Table 3. Heavy alcohol use is defined as consuming five or more drinks per occasion on 5 or more days in the past month. Of persons 12 years or older, 52.2% reported using alcohol in the last month in 1995. This percentage remains relatively unchanged from previous years. Heavy alcohol use was reported in 1994 by 6.2% of the population over 12 years of age. Underage alcohol use continues with 2.5% of teens 12 to 17 years of age reporting heavy alcohol use, and 13.2% of 18- to 25-year-olds. Of full-time employed persons 18 years and older, 7.8% are heavy alcohol users, as are 6.7% of part-time employees. There is a significant difference between males and females in heavy alcohol use with 10.3% of males and 2.5% of females 12 years and older identified as heavy alcohol users. More than 20% of men employed full time in construction, transportation, and wholesale trade were heavy drinkers.

Other investigations of the prevalence of alcohol use by employed individuals have demonstrated variations across occupational groups. Percentages of white collar workers who are current users of alcohol are higher than blue collar workers. However, current blue collar drinkers

**TABLE 2.** *Past month use of marijuana by age, race, and sex (percent)*

| Demographic characteristics | 1979 | 1982 | 1985 | 1988 | 1990 | 1991 | 1992 | 1993 | 1994 | 1995 |
|---|---|---|---|---|---|---|---|---|---|---|
| Total | 13.2 | 11.5 | 9.7 | 6.2 | 5.4 | 5.1 | 4.7 | 4.6 | 4.8 | 4.7 |
| Age group | | | | | | | | | | |
| 12–17 | 14.2 | 9.9 | 10.2 | 5.4 | 4.4 | 3.6 | 3.4 | 4.0 | 6.0 | 8.2 |
| 18–25 | 35.6 | 27.2 | 21.7 | 15.3 | 12.7 | 12.9 | 10.9 | 11.1 | 12.1 | 12.0 |
| 26–34 | 19.7 | 19.0 | 19.0 | 12.3 | 9.5 | 7.7 | 9.3 | 7.5 | 6.9 | 6.7 |
| ≥35 | 2.9 | 3.9 | 2.6 | 1.8 | 2.4 | 2.6 | 2.0 | 2.4 | 2.3 | 1.8 |
| Race/ethnicity | | | | | | | | | | |
| White | 13.6 | 11.9 | 10.0 | 6.3 | 5.7 | 5.2 | 5.1 | 4.9 | 4.8 | 4.7 |
| Black | 11.0 | 11.5 | 9.9 | 4.7 | 5.1 | 5.5 | 3.9 | 4.2 | 5.9 | 5.9 |
| Hispanic | 11.4 | 8.6 | 6.4 | 4.9 | 3.9 | 3.6 | 3.0 | 3.9 | 4.1 | 3.9 |
| Other | 12.2 | — | 7.6 | — | — | 4.2 | 2.6 | 3.2 | 3.0 | 2.8 |
| Sex | | | | | | | | | | |
| Male | 18.1 | 16.4 | 12.6 | 8.4 | 6.8 | 6.8 | 6.4 | 6.4 | 6.7 | 6.2 |
| Female | 8.7 | 7.1 | 7.1 | 4.2 | 4.2 | 3.6 | 3.1 | 3.0 | 3.1 | 3.3 |

From ref. 1.

**TABLE 3.** *Past month "binge" alcohol use by age, race and sex (percent)*[a]

| Demographic characteristics | 1979 | 1982 | 1985 | 1988 | 1990 | 1991 | 1992 | 1993 | 1994 | 1995 |
|---|---|---|---|---|---|---|---|---|---|---|
| Total | — | — | 20.2 | 15.0 | 14.4 | 15.5 | 14.5 | 14.6 | 16.5 | 15.8 |
| Age group | | | | | | | | | | |
| 12–17 | — | — | 21.9 | 15.1 | 15.4 | 13.2 | 10.0 | 11.0 | 8.3 | 7.9 |
| 18–25 | — | — | 34.4 | 28.2 | 29.5 | 31.2 | 29.9 | 29.1 | 33.6 | 29.9 |
| 26–34 | — | — | 12.9 | 9.7 | 8.0 | 10.1 | 9.0 | 9.6 | 11.8 | 11.8 |
| ≥35 | — | — | 12.9 | 9.7 | 8.0 | 10.1 | 9.0 | 9.6 | 11.8 | 11.8 |
| Race/ethnicity | | | | | | | | | | |
| White | — | — | 21.6 | 15.8 | 14.9 | 16.2 | 15.3 | 15.6 | 17.1 | 16.6 |
| Black | — | — | 12.1 | 8.9 | 11.1 | 11.0 | 10.3 | 9.0 | 11.5 | 11.2 |
| Hispanic | — | — | 19.1 | 15.7 | 16.9 | 18.4 | 16.3 | 17.2 | 18.3 | 17.2 |
| Other | — | — | 11.1 | 13.7 | 4.7 | 9.6 | 7.6 | 6.5 | 13.0 | 9.7 |
| Sex | | | | | | | | | | |
| Male | — | — | 31.6 | 23.2 | 22.1 | 23.5 | 21.9 | 22.7 | 24.7 | 23.8 |
| Female | — | — | 9.8 | 7.5 | 7.3 | 8.3 | 7.7 | 7.3 | 8.9 | 8.5 |

[a]Note: "Binge" alcohol use is defined as drinking five or more drinks on the same occasion in at least one day in the past 30 days.
From ref. 1.

had higher daily consumption levels, alcohol dependence, and severe dependence rates than white collar workers (2). On the job use of alcohol is far more common than on the job use of illicit drugs (3). Several studies have estimated on the job use of alcohol at 5% to 8% for men and 1% to 3% for women.

### Impact of Substance Abuse in the Workplace

Illicit drug use among employees is associated with higher rates of absenteeism, accidental injury, involuntary separation, medical care usage, and health care costs. For example, in a study of U.S. Postal service applicants, those who screened positive for drugs had 66% higher absenteeism, 77% greater likelihood of being fired, 143% more employee assistance program referrals, and 26% higher medical claims over a 3.3-year period than those who screened negative (4). Even though supervisors did not know the results of employment drug tests, disciplinary action for problems of attendance, performance, and conduct was almost twice as high for those with positive tests. In a study of Georgia Power employees, hours of absenteeism for those testing positive for drugs was 165, compared to 91 for those treated for drug abuse, 73 for those treated for alcohol, and 41 for the average worker (5). Annual general medical benefit costs were $1,314 for those testing positive for drugs, $1,347 for those treated for drugs, and $842 for those treated for alcohol, in contrast to $590 for the average worker.

**TABLE 4.** *Percent of laboratory specimens testing positive*

| Drug category | 1996 | 1995 | 1994 | 1993 |
|---|---|---|---|---|
| Marijuana | 3.6% | 3.7% | 3.5% | 3.4% |
| Cocaine | 1.0% | 1.4% | 1.8% | 2.4% |
| Benzodiazepine | 0.5% | 0.5% | 0.8% | 1.1% |
| Opiates | 0.4% | 0.5% | 0.5% | 0.8% |
| Barbiturates | 0.2% | 0.3% | 0.3% | 0.4% |

From ref. 37.

Workplace productivity losses from alcohol abuse are estimated at $33 billion. Alcohol abuse and workplace accidents are highly correlated. The five states with the highest alcohol consumption rates have 3.3% higher average workers' compensation costs (6). The majority of studies evaluating the effects of alcohol on work performance have demonstrated that alcohol does disrupt performance. Tracking, visual vigilance, divided attention, postural stability, and cancellation tasks are particularly affected by alcohol. Memory, judgment, and other cognitive tasks are also affected, but with greater variability in individuals. Visual, coordination, and fine motor performance is impaired at low blood alcohol levels, e.g., 0.02% blood alcohol concentration (BAC). There is evidence that alcohol hangover effects can degrade task performance. Even though studies indicate that the extent of impairment is also related to age and experience with the task, degradation in task performance was measured 4 to 8 hours after reaching peak blood alcohol levels.

There is clear evidence that alcohol abuse is linked to both workplace absenteeism and accidents. Heavy alcohol users are generally absent two to three times more often than nonusers (7). In fatal transportation accident investigations, body fluid analysis for alcohol has shown positive findings in 9% to 15% (8). Investigations of fatal accidents in other industries have also found 11% to 13% with positive BACs (≥0.02%) (9). The negative impact of alcohol abuse on other work-related issues, such as employee turnover, job satisfaction, disciplinary actions, and medical benefit usage, is also supportable, though largely through observation/field study data.

## INDUSTRY RESPONSE

### Education, Awareness, and Training

In response to the potential impacts of substance abuse on productivity, performance, and people, employers began in the 1970s to develop and implement education and awareness programs for both labor and management employees to emphasize the dangers of substance abuse in the workplace. These programs were aimed at helping supervisors recognize the signs and symptoms of substance abuse, providing employees with drug and alcohol information to deter abuse, and encouraging those with substance abuse problems to seek help (10). These education efforts were often linked to workplace safety programs, employee health and wellness programs, and to initiatives in the human resources area of the corporate structure.

### Employee Assistance Programs

The 1970s also saw growth in employee assistance programs (EAPs) in large corporations. Early EAPs, which began after World War II, were focused on substance abuse problem identification and intervention (11). In later years, EAPs became much broader based, addressing employee mental health, marital, and financial problems that impact their ability to function effectively in the workplace. Education and awareness activities are central functions of the EAP model. Confidentiality and access to treatment are essential components. EAPs, in many ways, serve as the employee's information and referral source for personal and family problems.

In the early stages of EAP development, many programs were staffed by recovering substance abusers. The programs often used 12-step (Alcoholics Anonymous) models for monitoring and supporting employees after return to work following treatment for substance abuse problems. As EAPs have matured, they have less of a counseling and treatment flavor, and more emphasis on assessment, referral, and case management. Many employers have outsourced their EAPs, and employees use community-based organizations for information, assessment, and treatment referral (12).

Beginning in the 1990s, emphasis has been placed on increasing employee access to EAPs (13). As employers began to craft specific policies addressing substance abuse in the workplace, impose sanctions against employees who violate these policies, and enforce these policies with drug and alcohol testing programs, having an EAP became a crucial issue in employee acceptance of the new substance abuse prevention and control initiatives. Recent data from the U.S. Department of Labor and the American Management Association indicate that 75% to 80% of large employers in the United States provide some form of EAP access for their employees.

### Peer Programs

Coinciding with the development and implementation of EAPs was a peer counseling movement. Labor unions, in particular, were heavily involved in developing peer programs for the workplace. The idea behind peer programs was to encourage substance abusers to seek help through the advice and counsel of their peers and to ensure confidentiality and job security for those who voluntarily sought help. A key component of peer programs was intensive mentoring and monitoring of employees after return to work. The peer program model has been especially successful in the transportation and manufacturing industries where labor groups and management have cooperated in funding and publicizing the programs. Peer programs traditionally rely on the use of recovering alcoholics and addicts as peer counselors and mentors for aftercare support and monitoring. Peer programs such as Operation Red Block in the railroad industry, and AFL/CIO programs in manufacturing demonstrate greater success in workplace interventions and follow-up abstinence than do traditional EAP models.

### Substance Abuse Policies and Sanctions

Today, most large and medium-size companies have written substance abuse policies (14), in large part due to requirements placed on employers by the Drug-Free Workplace Act of 1988, the Department of Transportation Drug and Alcohol Rules, and other federal legislative or regulatory initiatives (15,16). Beginning in 1990, companies that do business (grants or contracts) with the federal government, that are regulated by the Departments of Transportation, Energy, and Defense, or that are licensed or certified by the U.S. government must have written policies that specifically address illicit drugs. Along with the requirement for written policies come sanctions against employees who violate them, and employers' responsibility to enforce the policies and sanctions.

In many cases, the development and implementation of a substance abuse policy are functions shared by the corporate medical staff and human resources or safety personnel (17,18). While earlier employer policies may have been limited to the issue of illicit drugs, today companies are beginning to incorporate alcohol use and abuse into these policies. Policies on alcohol use were traditionally limited to prohibitions of alcohol intoxication or being under the influence of alcohol. Now, employers are addressing alcohol testing in the workplace, use of alcohol proximate to being on duty, and accident or injury investigations that include detecting alcohol misuse.

The 1988 Americans with Disabilities Act (ADA) also impacts substance abuse policies, employee sanctions, and workplace alcohol and drug abuse prevention and control programs. Although the ADA identifies both alcoholism and drug addiction as disabilities entitling job applicants and employees to reasonable accommodation and nondiscrimination of their disabilities, current illicit drug users and those who misuse alcohol in violation of company policy are not protected. Someone who is currently using illicit drugs, or uses alcohol while on duty, cannot claim a disability and thus avoid discipline or sanctions under the employer's policy. Employee drug and alcohol testing are both permitted under the provisions of the ADA. Recovering addicts and alcoholics can be held to the same standards of conduct relative to alcohol and drug use as all other employees.

### Deterrent and Detection Programs

In addition to written substance abuse policies, education and training programs, and EAPs, many employers include specific programs to deter and detect drug and alcohol abuse in their workplaces. Deterrence programs are prevention-oriented, aimed at sending a powerful message that substance abuse will not be tolerated. Detection programs are intervention actions aimed at enforcement of the company policy.

Deterrence programs include employee testing, EAP incentive programs, and employee education activities. Detection programs include employee testing, workplace searches, and security and surveillance measures. Many drug-free workplace programs include elements of both deterrence and detection.

## GOVERNMENTAL RESPONSE

### Federal Level

In 1986, President Reagan focused the nation's attention on workplace substance abuse by issuing Executive Order 12564, which required all 135 federal agencies of the executive branch of government to adopt drug-free workplace policies and programs. U.S. policy was in the midst of the war on drugs, which by all indicators was being lost (19). In issuing the order that would require testing for drugs of abuse of over 1.5 million federal workers in safety/security-related positions, the president stated, "The federal government as the largest employer in the nation can and should lead the way in establishing drug-free workplaces" (20). The executive order and supporting federal legislation charged the U.S. Department of Health and Human Services with the responsibilities of (a) guiding the federal agencies through the process of developing substance abuse policies and programs, (b) developing guidelines for employee testing programs, and (c) establishing a federal certification program for laboratories that would engage in drugs of abuse testing. These emerged as Mandatory Guidelines for Federal Workplace testing Programs, first released in April 1988, and later updated in June 1994 (21).

Shortly thereafter, the Drug-Free Workplace Act of 1988 required all companies and individuals who are awarded federal grants or contracts to establish drug-free workplace policies and programs as a condition of receiving federal funds. Although the Drug-Free Workplace Act stopped short of requiring drug or alcohol testing of employees or contractors, it did address prohibitions of illicit drug use, possession, traffic, and sale at the work site.

The Department of Transportation (DOT) and the Nuclear Regulatory Commission (NRC) issued regulations in 1988 and 1989 that mandated drug-free workplace programs in private and public sector companies that they regulate (22,23). Although both the DOT and the NRC rules require drug testing of employees, the two programs have a different emphasis. The DOT rules focus clearly on a deterrent model of addressing illicit drug use; the NRC rule is a fitness for duty program that aims to deter and detect all forms of substance misuse or abuse including alcohol, prescription drugs, and illicit controlled substances.

These safety-based initiatives were both presented as federal strategies to protect the American public from the dangers of substance abuse by workers in the commercial transportation and nuclear power industries. The DOT rules were issued, in large part, in response to a fatal Amtrak/Conrail train wreck in early 1987 in which nine people died and scores were injured. The crash investigators concluded that (a) the wreck was caused by human error due to drug use by train employees, and (b) on-the-job alcohol and drug use in the railroad industry was endemic and epidemic. The NRC rule required comprehensive alcohol and drug testing of employees at nuclear power sites as a way of ensuring that employees who had access to sensitive and critical areas of nuclear power operations were drug-free. The DOT rules did not address alcohol abuse or alcohol testing of transportation employees, beyond the investigative role of testing in fatal accidents.

In 1991, after another rail accident, this time on a metropolitan mass transit subway system, congress passed the Omnibus Transportation Employee Testing Act, mandating by federal law drug and alcohol testing of over seven million employees in the aviation, rail, highway (commercial trucks and buses), and mass transit transportation industries (24). The operator of the subway train in the New York City fatal crash was determined to be under the influence of alcohol at the time of the wreck. Drug tests were not done on the train operator. The 1988 DOT drug testing rules applied only to interstate transportation. Thus, school bus drivers, intrastate truck drivers, city and county transit systems, and other non–federally regulated transportation operations were not subject to the DOT rules. The Omnibus Act expanded the coverage of the drug rules and imposed requirements for workplace alcohol use policies and alcohol testing on transportation employers.

Since the mid-1990s, several states have enacted drug-free workplace legislation (25). Most of these statutes provide incentives to employers to adopt drug-free workplace policies and programs, including employee testing. Florida and other state initiatives provide employer credits or discounts on workers' compensation premiums or fund payments in exchange for drug-free workplace programs that include sanctions against illicit drug use, applicant and employee testing programs, and drug abuse awareness education and training. In March 1997, the Florida Supreme Court invalidated the part of the act that presumes that drugs or alcohol caused the injury if the postaccident test result is positive (26). The federal and state initiatives in workplace substance abuse prevention and control have sparked interest in the commercial insurance industry to offer incentive programs to employers in the form of discounts on liability, medical benefits, and other insurance premiums when drug-free workplace policies and programs are in place.

## SUBSTANCE ABUSE PREVENTION AND CONTROL

### Prevention Strategies

Many workplaces approach substance abuse prevention in the same way they seek to prevent other potential workplace hazards and problems—through education and training. Along with mandatory training programs in workplace safety, sexual harassment, and workplace violence, most supervisory personnel in today's work force receive specific education in substance abuse prevention and identification. Many progressive companies provide drug and alcohol education and awareness materials and programs for employees that seek to expand their knowledge of substance abuse for application to their own families and friends. Some corporate wellness programs have a substance abuse awareness component.

Applicant validation programs seek to identify, through personnel screening and drug testing, applicants who have a substance abuse problem before they enter the work force. While these efforts are not totally effective in eliminating substance abusers from the work force, they often send a message to job applicants that drug and alcohol abuse is not compatible with employment.

Employer substance abuse policies and the sanctions imposed for violations of the policy serve to foster prevention and deterrence. They reinforce employees' decisions to be drug-free, and encourage abusers to get help if they want to retain their employment.

### Control Strategies

Substance abuse control is an important element of risk management. Most companies today use drug and alcohol abuse control strategies to reinforce and supplement their prevention efforts. Last-chance agreements or posttreatment contracts with employees who have had substance abuse problems in the workplace are used to motivate employees to enter treatment and to monitor their progress and recovery after rehabilitation. Although many in the EAP or addiction medicine disciplines have viewed last-chance agreements and posttreatment contracts to be punitive, the current trend is to view these measures as helpful in relapse prevention and aftercare motivation. Drug and alcohol testing programs are also examples of tools that serve both a prevention and a control objective. When workplace testing is a part of the company culture, employees have a perceived risk of being identified if they continue to use drugs or misuse alcohol.

Work sites reflect the influences of the communities in which they are located and the people who work there. Thus, work sites can become locations for dealing drugs, making illicit drug contacts, and fostering alcohol abuse. Searches, surveillance efforts, and other drug enforcement measures are sometimes needed to eradicate illegal activity that supports substance abuse.

## ILLICIT DRUG USE

Drugs of abuse are any substances taken through any route of administration that alter the mood, the level of perception, or brain functioning (27). There are several classification schemes for drugs of abuse, some using pharmacologic properties, others using addictive potential, and others based on clinical effects. The Federal Drug Enforcement Agency (DEA) categorizes drugs of abuse in a series of schedules based on the degree of medical usefulness and the abuse potential of the drug. These DEA schedules are labeled I to V, with schedule I substances identified as having no accepted medical use and high abuse potential, and schedules II to V drugs as having accepted medical uses and decreasing abuse potential through schedule V. Table 5 summarizes the DEA drug schedules and lists some examples. Seymour and Smith (28) classify drugs of abuse in four basic categories: opiates, stimulants, psychedelics, and sedative-hypnotics. The *Diagnostic and Statistical Manual of Mental Disorders* (DSM-IV) classifies psychoactive substance use disorders in ten basic categories: alcohol, amphetamines, cannabis, cocaine, hallucinogens, inhalants, nicotine, opiates, phencyclidine, and sedative-hypnotics.

The following discussion focuses on three classes of drugs—psychedelics, stimulants, and opiates—with particular emphasis on the specific drugs that are more frequently tested for and identified in workplace substance abuse prevention and control programs.

**TABLE 5.** *Drug Enforcement Agency (DEA) drug schedules with examples*

| |
|---|
| Schedule I (No accepted medical use; high abuse potential) |
| Heroin |
| Hallucinogens |
| Marijuana |
| Methaqualone (Quaalude) |
| Schedule II |
| Opium or morphine |
| Codeine |
| Synthetic opiates [e.g., meperidine (Demerol)] |
| Selected barbiturates [e.g., secobarbital (Seconal)] |
| Amphetamines, methylphenidate (Ritalin), and phenmetrazine (Preludin) |
| Gluthimide (Doriden) |
| PCP |
| Schedule III |
| Aspirin with codeine |
| Paregoric |
| Methyprylon (Noludar) |
| Schedule IV |
| Chloral hydrate (Noctac) |
| Ethchlorvynol (Placidyl) |
| Flurazepam (Dalmane) |
| Pentazocine (Talwin) |
| Chlordiazepoxide (Librium) |
| Propoxyphene (Darvon) |
| Diethylpropion (Tenuate) |
| Schedule V (Accepted medical use; low abuse potential) |
| Narcotic-atropine mixtures (Lomotil) |
| Codeine mixtures (200 mg per 100 ml) |

## Psychedelics

This term is generally applied to drugs that are ingested or inoculated to achieve an altered state of consciousness. Drugs in this category are also called hallucinogens because they may produce sensory enhancements, illusions, or more rarely, hallucinations. Examples of psychedelic drugs include: LSD, psilocybin, mescaline, δ-9-tetrahydrocannabinol (THC) (in marijuana or hashish), phencyclidine (PCP), methylene dioxy amphetamine (MDA), methylene dioxy methamphetamine (MDMA) (ecstasy), and other "designer drugs." These drugs are usually orally ingested, smoked, or snorted. The duration of the intoxicating effects of psychedelic substances ranges from less than 1 hour to up to 12 hours after administration. Most psychedelic substances have clinically relevant actions between 2 and 8 hours. Effects of these drugs include increased awareness of sensory input, subjective feeling of enhanced mental activity, altered body images, distorted perception of ordinary environmental stimuli, and marked introspection. Physiologically, the intoxicated individual usually exhibits dilated pupils, flushed complexion, fine tremors, increased blood pressure, elevated blood sugar, and increased body temperature. With THC use, both blood pressure and body temperature may be slightly decreased.

### *Marijuana*

δ-9-Tetrahydrocannabinol (THC) originates with the cannabis sativa plant. The less potent form of THC comes from marijuana or the dried plant leaves, while more potent THC is found in hashish, the resins of the plant flowers. THC is used by smoking or eating the marijuana product. An average marijuana cigarette contains 2.5 to 6.0 mg of THC, although not all of the drug is absorbed through smoking. Intoxication from smoking generally lasts 2 to 3 hours, while a longer high is achieved from oral ingestion (usually in a high-fat content food such as brownies, pizza, or cookies) with the intoxicating effects peaking at 2 to 3 hours after eating but lasting up to 8 hours.

One of the greatest dangers associated with THC use is accidents as a consequence of decreased judgment, impaired time and distance estimates, and impaired motor performance. Impairment of cognitive and motor functioning can be demonstrated up to 24 hours after use (29).

In recent surveys of employees, as many as 33% report that they know co-workers who use illicit drugs. Marijuana use is the most prevalent usage reported in these surveys. Although the majority of employed individuals who admit to current use of marijuana state that they don t use it while on duty, 20% of employed marijuana users acknowledge absenteeism or poor job performance related to their marijuana use. While the research data about the intoxicating effects of marijuana on task performance have produced some conflicting results and conclusions, the negative impact of marijuana use on certain psychomotor and cognitive functions is well documented. Disturbances and disruption of immediate recall functions, time orientation, event sequencing, and visual orientation in three-dimensional space are associated with marijuana use. Routine repetitive tasks may not be affected by marijuana use; however, work requiring cognitive integration is adversely impacted. The impact of marijuana on task functioning is not limited to the period of acute intoxication. Skill impairment is measurable after a single dose for more than 8 to 10 hours, long after the individual has lost awareness of feeling high. In studies involving very complex cognitive-psychomotor interactions, some degree of functional impairment has been shown 24 hours after smoking marijuana.

### *Other Psychedelics*

Other psychedelic drugs are more certain to produce illusions and hallucinations (usually visual) than THC. LSD and PCP are synthetic drugs, while psilocybin (mushrooms) and mescaline (cacti) are plant products. LSD is one of the most potent of the hallucinogens. Usual street doses of this drug range from 50 to 100 pg, although the upper range may be as high as 300 pg. LSD is sold as a powder, solution, or pill. The liquid is colorless, odorless, and tasteless, and is often dissolved on colorful blotter paper and offered as stickers that are attractive to adolescents. The most common hallucinogen use problems are panic reactions, flashbacks, and toxic reactions.

Phencyclidine (PCP) is a synthetic substance first produced as a general anesthetic for both humans and animals. PCP produces a dissociative state in which the subject does not experience pain, but is not in a coma state. However, the postoperative agitation and hallucinations occurring in human subjects resulted in its withdrawal from medical use. PCP can be smoked, eaten, or injected intravenously. It is frequently sprayed or added to other drugs such as marijuana. Normal doses range from 1 to 10 mg; however, PCP-laced marijuana cigarettes often contain 12 to 25 mg of PCP powder. In a state of confusion and agitation produced by PCP, users may harm themselves through accidents, physical violence, and apparent suicide attempts.

While most employed individuals who admit to hallucinogen abuse state that their use is confined to nonduty periods, the possibility of flashback or other sensory perceptual disturbances outside the periods of intoxication present potential dangers in the work environment. Hallucinogen abusers tend to be risk takers and thrill seekers, and often exhibit underlying personality disorders. The unpredictability of the hallucinogen abuser represents the greatest danger to co-workers and others around him/her. Because hallucinogenic drugs can induce a temporary psychotic state (i.e., the user's perceptions of reality are altered), an episode of hallucinogen use in the workplace is always a potential crisis requiring immediate medical and security attention.

## Stimulants

Stimulants, including amphetamines and cocaine share the ability to stimulate the central nervous system. Stimulants affect the central nervous system by causing the release of neurotransmitters from nerve cells. Some stimulants also mimic the functions of transmitters through a direct effect on the nerve cells themselves. Stimulants include cocaine, amphetamine, and methamphetamine.

### *Cocaine*

Cocaine is sold as a powder, and either injected intravenously or snorted intranasally. The average dose used by the nontolerant user is 20 to 100 mg. Cocaine powder is often free based for smoking. Free-base cocaine is produced by adding a strong base to the cocaine solution, heating it, and then extracting the alkaline free-base precipitate (29). The crystallized form of cocaine, known as rock or crack, has a relatively low melting point and is readily soluble in water, and thus has led to widespread usage as an easily smokable form. The onset of euphoria is more intense and rapid when cocaine is smoked. Cocaine produces a quick, short high (5–30 minutes), with most of the psychoactive effects gone within 1 to 2 hours. Stimulants cause euphoria, decrease fatigue, increase feelings of sexuality, decrease appetite, increase energy, and interfere with normal sleep patterns. Impaired judgment and psychological changes are also common. Physical effects include tremors, tachycardia and arrhythmias, dilated pupils, and increased body temperature and blood pressure. Chronic stimulant abuse may produce psychoses characterized by paranoia, hallucinations, and aggressive behavior.

As a powerful stimulant, cocaine is frequently attractive to workers who feel pressure to achieve, produce under stressful conditions, and work long and arduous hours. The initial effects of cocaine—increased alertness, accelerated thinking, hyperenergized state, and feelings of competence and power—are conducive to making employees think and feel that they are more productive. Even in small amounts, cocaine does impair judgment and decision making. Perhaps the greater danger associated with cocaine use in the workplace is the speed with which users develop dose tolerance and addiction. Since it takes more and more cocaine to repeat the euphoric experiences and sensations of power, the individual is forced to increase both the frequency and amount of use. The cocaine user who initially limits his/her use to off-duty periods is soon having to use on the job to avoid the depression, agitation, and paranoia associated with coming down from a cocaine high. With increased use and addiction, the lows of the cocaine cycle become as disabling as the highs of intoxication. Because cocaine addiction requires more and more of the drug, the expense of a cocaine habit can be financially ruinous. This often leads to other workplace problems such as theft and trafficking to support the addiction.

### *Amphetamine and Methamphetamine*

Amphetamine and methamphetamine are sympathomimetic drugs. Both substances are available as therapeutic drugs. Both are also manufactured illicitly. Methamphetamine is generally produced in clandestine laboratories, and sold in the crystalline form as crystal meth or "ice." Amphetamine is ingested orally as pills or capsules, or injected intravenously. Crystal meth is snorted or injected, while ice is volatized and smoked. The stimulant effects of amphetamine and methamphetamine generally last longer than those of cocaine. The toxicologic and pharmacologic effects are similar to cocaine. Tolerance to these drugs builds rapidly. It is not uncommon for IV intravenous amphetamine users to inject 70 to 100 mg in a single dose.

The use of illicit amphetamine and methamphetamine is not as common in the workplace as either marijuana or cocaine. However, stimulant abuse is particularly dangerous in the workplace. Amphetamine abusers who work when under the influence of the drugs often ignore safety precautions, take inappropriate risks, and demonstrate impaired cognitive-psychomotor interactions. Equally as dangerous are amphetamine abusers who work during periods of "crashing" after a "speeding binge." These abusers are often sleep deprived, irritable, and anxious; they exhibit decreased attention spans, and are unable to process new cognitive data.

### Opiates

The major opiates include natural substances (e.g., opium, morphine, codeine), semisynthetic drugs produced from basic poppy plant products (e.g., heroin, hydromorphone, oxycodone), and synthetic analgesic drugs (e.g., propoxyphene, meperidine). The opiates all produce analgesia, drowsiness, changes in mood, and clouding of mental functioning (in higher doses). Opiates when used as drugs of abuse are taken orally, intravenously, intranasally, or are smoked (opium, heroin). IV ingestion is the most reinforcing. The immediate effects of heroin use include a warm "rush" feeling, followed by a floating intoxicating feeling. The respiratory rate is decreased, and pupils are pinpoint. Recent research on the pharmacology of opiates has led to the identification of subtypes of opiate receptors in the central nervous system (CNS). There is evidence that the major reinforcing properties of opiates may be the result of changes in the types of receptors. Heroin has, by far, the greatest potential for abuse, and is not used therapeutically in the United States. Morphine and codeine addiction or abuse are relatively rare. It is estimated that less than 1% of the U.S. adult population uses opiates without medical supervision. Morphine abuse or addiction is most commonly associated with attempts for relief from chronic pain. Opiate abusers, particularly those using "street drugs," often present for medical care as a consequence of overdoses, toxicity to adulterants used in opiate mixtures, or complications from intravenous ingestion.

Heroin abuse has generally been associated with the unemployed. However, recent epidemiologic data show that its popularity with young, urban, skilled and professional workers is on the rise. Heroin is readily available in metropolitan areas, is cheap in comparison to other drugs, and is now sold in a processed smokable form that makes it attractive to users who avoided heroin because of the fear of IV administration. Narcotics users present dangers in the workplace because of the psychomotor retardation, confused mental state, and sensory disturbances that are associated with heroin intoxication. The long-term effects of chronic heroin use manifest themselves in physical complications associated with addiction, such as malnutrition, chronic fatigue, immune system deficiencies, etc. Narcotics abuse by workers who operate machinery, vehicles, or other equipment is particularly dangerous because of the potential for accidents and injury to themselves, co-workers, or others in close proximity to the impaired worker.

## ALCOHOL ABUSE AND ALCOHOLISM

### Alcohol Abuse and Alcohol Dependence

There are many definitions of alcohol abuse, alcohol dependence, alcoholism, and alcohol misuse. The DSM-IV (30) distinguishes between alcohol abuse and alcohol dependence. Alcohol abuse is characterized as a maladaptive pattern on alcohol use leading to clinically significant impairment or distress as manifested by one or more of the following, occurring at any time in the same 12-month period: (a) recurrent alcohol use resulting in a failure to fulfill major role obligations at work, school, or home; (b) recurrent alcohol use in situations in which it is physically hazardous; (c) recurrent alcohol related legal problems; and (d) continued alcohol use despite having persistent or recurrent social or interpersonal problems caused or exacerbated by the effects of alcohol. Alcohol dependence is characterized as a maladaptive pattern of alcohol use leading to clinically significant impairment or distress, as manifested by at least three of the following occurring at any time in the same 12-month period: (a) tolerance, (b) withdrawal, (c) alcohol consumed in larger amounts or over a longer period than was intended, and (d) persistent desire or unsuccessful efforts to cut down or control alcohol use.

There is general agreement that alcoholism or alcohol dependence is a pathologic state characterized by a compulsive desire for alcohol, loss of control when exposed to alcohol, and continued use of alcohol in spite of adverse consequences.

Most occupational medicine practitioners see more workers as patients due to the effects of alcohol abuse and alcoholism than as a result of illicit drug abuse or addiction. While the extreme physiologic and clinical signs of chronic alcoholism such as delirium tremors, withdrawal seizures, hallucinosis, or jaundice are not commonly seen in the workplace occupational health setting, the physical and mental complications and disease processes associated with alcoholism are frequently encountered. Gastrointestinal disorders, cardiac dysfunction, malnutrition, neuropathy, and other commonly associated disease processes are manifested in the working population. A thorough alcohol use history is an essential ingredient in assessing many chronic disorders that bring workers to occupational medicine facilities.

It is generally safe to assume that if an employee exhibits work-related problems (absenteeism, poor performance, disciplinary actions, etc.) due to alcohol abuse, he/she also manifests alcohol-related problems in other areas of his/her life, e.g., family, marriage, health, and financial. The most striking feature of the psychological and physical dependence on alcohol is the continuance of drinking behavior despite known adverse consequences to one's health, relationships, and employment. Unfortunately, by the time alcohol-related problems are identified by supervisors or co-workers, the employee is well down the path of alcohol dependence. Losing control of one's drinking to the extent that it is identified at work is usually far into the disease process.

### Alcohol Abuse and Misuse

In the workplace, the concern about alcohol abuse and misuse focuses on the impact of alcohol use on task performance and safety. Many workplace substance abuse policies address alcohol use in terms of prohibiting employees from being "under the influence," impaired, or intoxicated. Legally, these terms were often defined using drunk driving enforcement standards for driving while intoxicated (DWI) or driving under the influence (DUI), generally 0.08% or 0.10% BAC. However, recent research data from studies designed to approximate workplace conditions demonstrate that much lower alcohol levels adversely impact individuals' abilities to perform cognitive and psychomotor skills used in most job functions. Even at levels as low as 0.02% BAC, workers exhibit evidence of impairment in alertness, judgment, cognitive skills, decision making, divided attention task accomplishment, short-term memory, and motor coordination. The more complicated the task, or the greater the need for spontaneous judgments or alterations in procedures, the more significant the impairment at low levels of alcohol concentration.

Principally as a result of federal regulations, the standard for defining alcohol impairment in the workplace has gradually evolved to 0.04% BAC or 0.04 breath alcohol concentration (BrAC). For all safety-sensitive occupations in the transportation industries (pilots, truck drivers, railroad engineers, mechanics, etc.) 0.04% BAC/BrAC is the per se level for determining that an individual is unfit to perform safety-sensitive functions. In adopting the 0.04% BAC/BrAC alcohol misuse standard, the DOT went one step further in addressing the potential adverse impacts of even lower alcohol concentrations on task performance and public safety. If a transportation employee is tested for breath alcohol and has an alcohol concentration of 0.02 or greater, even though he/she may exhibit no signs of impairment or intoxication, the employee cannot continue to perform safety-sensitive duties and must be removed from such duties for at least 8 hours.

### Hangovers, Tolerance, and Withdrawal

In addition to the dangers associated with impairment from breath alcohol concentrations as low as 0.02, worker performance and safety are often impacted by other aspects of alcohol misuse and abuse. Hangovers, the physical and psychological impact of excessive alcohol intake experienced after the body has detoxified the ethanol, also affect employee productivity and performance. The manifestations of a hangover include nausea, irritability, hypersensitivity to light, noise, and temperature, sluggish psychomotor responses, memory and cognitive disturbances, tremors, and generalized feelings of malaise. Some estimates of absenteeism and lateness due to hangovers are as high as 40% of all time and attendance problems. Research data show that impairment in cognitive and motor functioning is associated with the alcohol hangover syndrome. In part due to the adverse impact of alcohol hangovers on worker performance, the DOT alcohol misuse rules include a preduty alcohol abstinence period ranging from 4 to 8 hours for safety-sensitive occupations.

Alcohol tolerance and withdrawal symptoms are generally associated with alcohol dependence or alcoholism. Alcoholics develop a tolerance for alcohol that requires higher and higher blood alcohol concentrations for them to feel the desired effects of alcohol consumption. It is not unusual for alcoholic workers to consume large quantities of alcohol (e.g., a fifth per day) and appear to function normally. In many cases, alcoholics become quite adept at hiding or compensating for the usual signs or symptoms associated with intoxication. As the disease of alcoholism progresses, the probability of alcohol withdrawal symptoms occurring when the blood alcohol concentration declines or reaches 0.00% increases. The physiologic dependence creates tremors, mental confusion, gastric distress, and ultimately seizures and hallucinations. The dangers associated with alcohol withdrawal in the work environment are obvious, and the fear and pain of withdrawal for the alcohol dependent employee are usually what motivates him/her to risk on-duty alcohol use.

## SUBSTANCE ABUSE TREATMENT AND REHABILITATION

### Workplace Interventions

The workplace is in many aspects an ideal place for intervention, motivation for treatment, and rehabilitation of substance abusers. Denial of a problem with substance abuse is the most powerful obstacle to treatment and recovery. When the employee is confronted with work-related substance abuse problems, he/she is forced to make a hard choice: get help and get sober, or risk losing a job. The job usually represents being able to continue to get drugs and/or alcohol. Workplace interventions and referrals for treatment should be focused on facts of the employee's performance, time and attendance, conduct, and productivity.

Alcoholism and drug addiction are treatable diseases. Employees can and do make successful recoveries from addiction. It is in the employer's best interest to identify substance-abuse–related problems early, refer the employee for assessment and appropriate treatment, and return him/her to duty as a functional, recovering individual. Once the employer has invested hiring, training, salary, and benefits costs in an employee, it is far more cost-effective to rehabilitate that employee and have him/her return to work than it is to find a new employee who will require training and time before being fully productive. Early identification of and intervention with substance abusers is crucial. The old adage that substance abusers must hit bottom before treatment is successful is not supported by treatment outcome data. Of much greater importance in determining the probability of successful rehabilitation are the structure and expectations provided to the employee and the attention to aftercare and posttreatment monitoring and support after return to work.

The data available on the effectiveness of EAPs are largely inconclusive. Most studies of EAP effectiveness use job performance outcomes as criterion measures. Absenteeism, accidents, grievances, disciplinary actions, and sick time usage are variables on which improvements are shown when compared posttreatment to pretreatment (31). The role of the EAP in posttreatment follow-up may be a critical element in effecting relapse and treatment recidivism. At least one study has found that employees who participated in intensive closely monitored follow-up programs had fewer hospitalizations and reduced alcohol- or drug-related health benefit claims than the control group who received no special EAP follow-up services (32). The intensive follow-up services group showed significant reductions in alcohol and other drug abuse disability, alcohol and other drug abuse treatment costs, and relapse hospitalizations for alcohol or other drug abuse.

### Treatment Options and Placement Criteria

In this era of managed care, capitated fees, and multiple-level benefit plans, many employees do not have adequate insurance coverage for substance abuse and other mental health treatment. In-patient treatment programs are reserved for those whose diagnostic assessment clearly meets the criteria for hospital-based care outlined by the American Society for Addiction Medicine (ASAM) (33). However, a wide variety of outpatient programs designed to treat substance abusers and their family members are available. Night and partial-day residential rehabilitation programs present innovative approaches to rehabilitation while maintaining the individual in the work environment. Twelve-step and other support group approaches have expanded beyond the traditional Alcoholics Anonymous (AA) and Narcotics Anonymous (NA) models. Some labor unions sponsor treatment programs, and there are specialized programs for specific occupational or professional groups and support group models that are not based on the spiritual component of healing and recovery for which AA and NA are noted. The key components to successful treatment of substance abusing employees are (a) selecting the best available treatment program; (b) intervening sooner rather than later; and (c) developing a structured, individualized aftercare program coordinated with the work environment.

The impact of level of care for alcohol and drug abuse problems is another issue bearing on treatment success and recidivism. With the growth in managed care and health maintenance organizations, access to inpatient or residential care has become restricted. There is at least one study that indicates that employees who had short-term inpatient treatment followed by AA participation were more successful in maintaining sobriety over a 2-year follow-up period than were employees who had no inpatient treatment and were participating only in AA. The study draws the conclusion that inpatient treatment is as cost-effective as self-help modalities because of higher relapse rates among those who had only self-help modalities of treatment (34). The treatment outcome studies comparing outpatient treatment with either inpatient or self-help groups have not been definitive in attributing success or failure to the level of care. When compared to other chronic medical disorders, and not viewed as acute problems, alcohol and other drug abuse treatment produces as much improvement in work-related performance measures as are achieved for other long-term, progressive illnesses (35).

## WORKPLACE DRUG AND ALCOHOL TESTING PROGRAMS

Employee drug testing has grown dramatically during the last decade. In 1980, drug testing was confined to the military, nuclear power industry, and a few other employers. Now, almost every Fortune 500 company prohibits illegal drug use on or off the job and requires preemployment drug tests. Approximately 10 million Americans are subject to federal drug testing requirements.

The extraordinary growth of drug testing is due to many factors. Most essential was the technological breakthrough of simple, inexpensive immunoassay urine screening tests in the 1960s. But sensitive immunoassay tests produce many false positives due to cross-reactivity with other substances. Testing using this method alone adversely affected some of those tested, with consequent litigation. A two-test standard has evolved, with a more specific test—gas chromatography/mass spectrometry (GC/MS)—used to confirm positive screening test results. GC/MS has become the "gold standard" for forensic drug testing and is required in all federally mandated programs.

### Types of Drug Testing

There are six major situations in which drug testing is performed at the work site.

#### *Preemployment/Preplacement*

This is the most prevalent form of drug testing. For federal employees, it is limited to those in safety-sensitive positions and all military personnel. But many private employers require preemployment drug tests of all those entering the workplace. Preplacement testing can include employees who are transferred and/or promoted to covered positions and those who are returning to work after extended absences. Although the Americans with Disabilities Act (ADA) prohibits preoffer preemployment medical examinations, it specifically allows drug testing before or after a job offer is made.

### *Periodic*

Employers may require drug testing as part of fitness-for-duty or other examinations. Because these exams are scheduled in advance, recreational users can abstain from drug use prior to testing and positive rates tend to be low. Scheduled drug tests are not included in the most recently proposed DOT regulations.

### *Postaccident/Incident*

Testing may be required after an accident, incident, and/or safety violation. Each employer must define specific conditions under which postaccident testing is required. The DOT regulations define conditions that trigger postaccident testing. Postaccident specimens must be collected quickly, often after-hours and away from the usual collection site. In anticipation of this, the employer should explore available collection options. Proper urine collection, chain-of-custody techniques, and consent procedures must be observed in the emergency department or other clinical setting. A number of employers have been successful in invoking the "voluntary intoxication defense" in order to avoid paying workers' compensation claims for injuries when the employee tested positive (36).

### *Reasonable Cause/Reasonable Suspicion*

This testing is performed when there is reason to believe that the employee has used drugs in violation of company policy or agency rules. A supervisor must document the behavior and usually obtain the approval of a second supervisor prior to testing. Indications for testing can include unsafe practices, violating operating rules, changes in personality, or aberrant behavior.

### *Return to Duty and Follow-Up*

An employee who has refused or previously failed a drug test may be required to provide drug-free urine before returning to work. Frequently, employees completing a rehabilitation program are subject to unannounced follow-up testing for 6 months to 5 years. Department of Transportation rules require a minimum of six follow-up tests in the first 12 months after returning to duty following treatment.

### *Random*

Unannounced random drug testing provides the highest deterrent against drug use. Usually, names of employees in specific safety-sensitive jobs (e.g., pilots, drivers, or security personnel) are included in a pool, from which individuals are selected based on randomly generated numbers. Tests are conducted on short notice, e.g., within 1 to 3 hours. To maintain the deterrent effect, employees who have already tested negative remain within the pool and subject to retesting. It is crucial that information about the dates of random testing, locations, and employees to be tested be kept confidential.

Random testing also raises the greatest threat among rank-and-file employees and concerns of civil libertarians about the invasion of individual privacy and possible unreasonable search and seizure. Proposed random testing among private companies of all employees regardless of job category has led to employee relations concerns and legal challenges. Employers are urged to adopt policies that are reasonable as well as legally defensible, that recognize that the vast majority of employees are not illicit drug users, and that presume innocence rather than guilt.

## Drug Testing Practices

Currently, two divergent worlds of drug testing exist. In the unregulated private sector, a wide spectrum of approaches is found. For example, urine may be tested for 2 to 20 different drugs; custody and control forms may include the employee's name and list prescription drugs taken within the last 2 weeks. Urine may be analyzed at any laboratory; laboratory cutoff levels may be specified by the employer; and results may go directly to the employer, without physician review. Because of concerns about the quality and appropriateness of some company drug testing programs, Congress is considering legislation that would establish a federal standard for all workplace drug testing in the United States.

The other world of drug testing is prescribed by detailed government regulations from the DHHS, Departments of Transportation, Energy, and Defense, and other agencies. DOT regulations are particularly important, because they currently affect over 8 million Americans in six commercial transportation industries: trucking, aviation, mass transit, marine, pipelines, and railroads. Federal regulations contain detailed procedures for urine collection, completion of custody and control forms, analysis by laboratories certified by DHHS Substance Abuse and Mental Health Services Administration (SAMHSA) for only five specified illicit drugs or drug categories (amphetamines, cocaine, marijuana, opiates, and PCP), and mandatory reporting of all results to a medical review officer (MRO) for review and interpretation before reporting to the employer.

The DHHS-DOT regulations have clearly emerged as the gold standard of practice. The remainder of this chapter summarizes these detailed federal drug testing procedures. Those conducting urine collection and medical review are urged to carefully review federal regulations and participate in training offered by federal agencies or by professional societies such as the American College of Occupational and Environmental Medicine (ACOEM) or ASAM.

Drug testing can be broken down into three steps: (a) collection of the specimen and completion of custody and control forms; (b) laboratory analysis for screening and confirmation of positive tests; and (c) review, verification, and reporting to the employer of test results.

### Laboratory Analysis

The cutoff levels issued by DHHS for both screening and confirmation tests are shown on Table 6. The screening level for marijuana of 50 ng/ml represents a variety of metabolites; the confirmation cutoff level of 15 ng/ml represents one specific metabolite (11-nor-δ-9-tetrahydrocannabinol-9-carboxylic acid). The cocaine screening level of 300 ng/ml is also for various metabolites, whereas the confirmation cutoff level of 150 ng/ml is for benzoylecgonine. For opiates and PCP, the respective screening and confirmation levels are identical. The screening level for amphetamines is 1000 ng/ml, with confirmation cutoff levels of 500 ng/ml each for amphetamine and methamphetamine.

With the increasing amount of workplace drug testing, commercial laboratories have compiled data on urine drug test positives. One laboratory that has compiled data on over 24 million employee drug tests beginning in 1987 reported an overall positive rate of 5.1% in 1996. This represents a decline of almost 68% from 1987, when the positive rate was 18% (32). Laboratory positive test data continue to show that the majority of positive tests detect marijuana (54.4%). Cocaine is detected in 22.5% of the positive specimens, and opiates (including heroin) are found in 8.5% of the positive tests (37). Drug testing positive test data is shown at Table 4. These data should not be interpreted as prevalence of employee drug use. The testing data show only those applicants and employees who tested positive. Because of the short detection windows for identifying drug use by urinalysis, many drug users are not identified by workplace urine tests.

**TABLE 6.** *Department of Health and Human Services (DHHS) cuttoff levels for drugs of abuse*

| Drugs | Initial (screening) ng/ml | Confirmatory (GC/MS) |
|---|---|---|
| Marijuana metabolites | 50 | 15[a] |
| Cocaine metabolites | 300 | 150[b] |
| Opiate metabolites | 300 | |
| Morphine | | 300 |
| Codeine | | 300 |
| Phencyclidine | 25 | 25 |
| Amphetamines | 1,000 | |
| Amphetamine | | 500 |
| Methamphetamine | | 500 |

[a]As δ-9-tetrahydrocannabinol-9-carboxylic acid.
[b]As benzoylecgonine.
From ref. 38.

### Review of Test Results by a Medical Review Officer (MRO)

The medical review officer (MRO) designation and role emerged from federal regulations, which referenced a "medical review official." For example, the DHHS mandatory guidelines governing drug testing under the federal Drug Free Workplace Program described the MRO as "a licensed physician with knowledge of substance abuse disorders" (38).

By receiving, reviewing, interpreting, verifying, and reporting drug test results, the MRO plays a vital role in protecting individuals from being inappropriately labeled as drug users, with adverse consequences. Approximately 7,000 MROs have received 2-day training from organizations such as the ACOEM, ASAM, Federal Aviation Administration, DOT, and others. MRO manuals have been published by NIDA, DOT, professional societies, and experienced MROs (39–42).

Many prescription and OTC drugs can cause positive tests. Verification of legitimate medical explanations for positive tests often requires clinical judgment. For example, tetrahydrocannabinol, the active ingredient of marijuana, is used as an antinausea agent for cancer patients under the prescription name Marinol. Although inhalation of sidestream marijuana smoke is offered as an explanation for a positive test, toxicology studies have not confirmed this as a feasible explanation. Cocaine is used in ENT, ophthalmology, and surgical procedures, such as injection of TAC (tetracaine, adrenaline, and cocaine) for suturing skin lacerations. Because L-methamphetamine, found in Vick's inhaler, can cause a positive test, the MRO should request D- and L-isomer isolation on methamphetamine positive specimens. Ingestion of poppy seeds can cause an opiate-positive test. The federal regulations specify that verification of an opiate test as positive requires clinical evidence of unauthorized opiate use, or the detection of the heroin metabolite monoacetyl-morphine (6-MAM). Clinical evidence includes a positive medical history, physical findings, or the donor's admission of illicit use. Medical review officers must often determine whether quantitative levels are compatible with legitimate prescription drug use.

### DOT Forensic and Evidential Procedures for Breath and Saliva Alcohol Testing

In the Omnibus Transportation Employee Testing Act of 1991, Congress mandated testing for misuse of alcohol as well as controlled substances in preemployment, random, reasonable suspicion, postaccident, and posttreatment testing in most transportation sectors. It also provided legislative authority for drug and alcohol testing for mass transit vehicle operators, controllers, and maintenance workers. The February 15, 1994 final rules require those subject to urine drug testing to also undergo alcohol breath testing (43). In effect, these regulations broaden the previous deterrent program into a fitness-for-duty program. Individuals in qualified safety-sensitive positions cannot work (a) with breath alcohol concentrations of 0.04 or greater, (b) while their behavior or appearance indicates intoxication or impairment, (c) while using alcohol, or (d) within 4 to 8 hours after using alcohol. Employees involved in an accident cannot use alcohol until they have been tested or 8 hours have passed.

The consequences of alcohol concentration of 0.04 or greater include immediate removal from safety-sensitive duty. Return to work is permitted only after evaluation and rehabilitation, if indicated, as well as return-to-work and follow-up testing. The regulations also call for immediate removal from safety sensitive duty if the alcohol concentration is between 0.02 and 0.04 for 8 to 24 hours or until the tested alcohol concentration falls below 0.02. While cumbersome to implement, this two-tier consequence provision underscores the DOT's concern that even low levels of alcohol are inconsistent with safety.

The alcohol testing rules affect approximately 7.5 million people, including intrastate vehicle operators who hold a commercial drivers' license. Although DOT rules do not permit or authorize blood alcohol testing, many employers, law enforcement agencies, and clinical settings use blood alcohol methodology for measuring alcohol concentration.

## CURRENT SUBSTANCE ABUSE TESTING ISSUES

### *Individual Privacy versus Public Health and Safety*

Drug testing programs must balance carefully the individual right to privacy and personal freedom versus public health and safety needs. The federal drug testing regulations seek to protect the individual against false accusation of illicit drug use and, in the collection process, to balance the right to privacy against unreasonable search and seizure. For this reason, directly witnessed specimen collection is permitted only in instances of likely specimen adulteration or substitution. Drug testing is also restricted to those in safety sensitive job positions. Although private sector drug testing is not restricted to those in safety sensitive positions, health professionals are urged to be sensitive to privacy issues, to recognize that the vast majority of those tested are not illicit drug users, and to assure each individual confidentiality and respect.

### *MRO Credentialing*

Because of concerns about quality of MRO services, federal officials urged establishment of voluntary MRO credentialing and certification within the private sectors. Although, MRO certification is not required by current federal regulations, physicians seeking to demonstrate their competence in a competitive marketplace and a litigious environment have shown strong interest in MRO credentialing. The Medical Review Officer Certification Council (MROCC) was established in 1992 by ACOEM and has been joined by the American Medical Association, the American Academy of Family Practice, the College of American Pathologists, the American Society of Clinical Toxicologists, and other medical specialty societies. MROCC eligibility requires at least 12 hours of approved MRO training, followed by a rigorous certifying examination. To date more than 1,000 physicians have been certified by MROCC (39). Certificates are valid for 5 years.

## CONCLUSION

Attention to workplace substance abuse prevention, control, and rehabilitation has increased markedly in the past 20 years. In part this is a reflection of American society as a whole. U.S. public policy and governmental intervention have been unable to impact the destruction (individual and collective) caused by illicit drugs through interdiction efforts aimed at eradicating the supply of drugs. The focus on demand reduction, decreasing Americans desire for illicit substances, has included the workplace as a target for those efforts. While education and awareness initiatives have met with some measured success in changing people's attitudes about illicit drugs, other strategies for deference and intervention are needed to modify behavior.

As American companies struggle to compete in a global economy, worker productivity and quality performance become even more important. As the total costs of economic losses attributable to drug and alcohol abuse continue to mount, corporate America is sending a message that substance abuse in the workplace will not be tolerated. Today, close to 85% of companies employing more than 250 people require their job applicants to pass a drug test before they are hired. Seven million workers in transportation occupations are subject to random drug and alcohol tests wherever they work. The North American Free Trade Agreement (NAFTA) included requirements for Canadian and Mexican employers transporting goods into the United States to implement alcohol and drug prevention and control programs. Companies are reexamining the role of alcohol in their workplaces. Worker opinion polls reflect diminishing tolerance for alcohol and drug use in the workplace.

Are there any indications that drug-free workplace programs are effective prevention or intervention strategies? Anecdotally—yes; solid research data—not yet. If the experiences of the U.S. military in implementing policies, sanctions, treatment programs, and drug and alcohol testing can be replicated, then success may be measurable in other workplaces. A decade of substance abuse prevention and control policies and programs for Department of Defense uniformed personnel resulted in a reduction in the prevalence of illicit drug use from almost 25% to less than 5%. Likewise, initiatives to alter a corporate culture in the military services that condoned and often fostered alcohol abuse have significantly reduced alcohol-related accidents, crime, and hospital admissions.

Alcohol and drug abuse often reflect dissatisfaction with one's life, be it personal or at work. Employers must seek ways to foster healthier work environments, filled with challenge, support, creativity, and human concern. Addressing these issues will help solve the drug problem our society faces.

## REFERENCES


1. U.S. Department of Health and Human Services. *National household survey on drug abuse.* Rockville, MD: Substance Abuse and Mental Health Services Administration, 1979–1995.
2. Parker DA, Harford TC. The epidemiology of alcohol consumption and dependence across occupations in the United States. *Alcohol Health Res World* 1992;16:97–105.
3. National Research Council/Institute of Medicine, Normand J, Lempert R, O'Brien C, et al., eds. *Under the influence? Drugs and the American workforce.* Washington, DC: National Academy Press, 1994;65–99.
4. Zwerling C, Ryan J, Orav EJ. The efficacy of preemployment drug screening for marijuana and cocaine in predicting employment outcome. *JAMA* 1990;264:2639–2643.
5. Sheridan JR, Winkler H. An evaluation of drug testing in the workplace. In: Gust SW, Walsh JM, eds. *Drugs in the workplace:* research and evaluation data. NIDA Research Monograph 91. Washington, DC: U.S. Department of Health and Human Services;Alcohol, Drug Abuse, and Mental Health Administration, National Institute on Drug Abuse, 1989;195–216.
6. Durbin DL. Alcohol consumption and workplace accidents. *NCCI Dig* 1991;6(4):36–63.
7. Rosenbaum AL, Lehman WEK, Olson KE, Holcom ML. *Prevalence of substance use and its association with performance among municipal workers in a Southwestern City.* Fort Worth, TX: Institute of Behavioral Research, 1992.
8. Transportation Research Board. *Alcohol and other drugs in transportation:* research needs for the next decade. Washington, DC: National Research Council, National Academy Press, 1993.
9. Alleyne BC, Stuart P, Copes R, et al. Alcohol and other drug use in occupational fatalities. *J Occup Med* 1991;33:496–500.
10. Roman PM, Blum TC. Formal intervention in employee health: comparisons of the nature and structure of employee assistance programs and health promotion programs. *Soc Sci Med* 1988;26:503–514.
11. Stockman LV. Employee assistance programs. In: Swotinsky RB, ed. *The medical review officer's guide to drug testing.* New York: Van Nostrand Reinhold, 1992;141–162.
12. Roman PM. Growth and transformation in workplace alcoholism programming. In: Galanter M, ed. *Recent developments in alcoholism,* vol. 6. New York: Plenum Press, 1988;131–158.
13. Blum TC, Martin JK, Roman PM. EAP prevalence, components and utilization. *J Employ Assist Res* 1992;1(l):209–229.
14. American Management Association. *Workplace drug testing and Drug abuse policies survey.* New York: AMA, 1995.
15. Public Law 100-690, title V, subtitle D, Drug Free Workplace Act: 1988.
16. U.S. Department of Transportation. Final rules for alcohol misuse prevention programs and controlled substances testing programs. *Federal Register* 1994;59(31):7302–7611.
17. Peterson K. Employee drug screening: issues to be resolved in implementing a program. *Clin Chem* 1987;33(11):54B–60B.
18. ACOEM. ACOEM committee report: drug screening in the workplace: ethical guidelines. *J Occup Med* 1991:33(5):651–652.
19. Shannon E. A losing battle: despite billions of dollars and more than a million arrests, the war on drugs has barely dented addiction or violent crime. *Time* 1990(December 3);44–48.
20. Executive Order 12564: Drug-free federal workplace. *Federal Register* 1986;51(180):32889–32893.
21. Substance Abuse and Mental Health Services Administration, DHHS. Mandatory guidelines for federal workplace drug testing programs. *Federal Register* 1994;59(110):29908–29931.
22. U. S. Department of Transportation. Final rules: anti-drug and controlled substances testing programs. *Federal Register* 1988;53(224): 47024–47177.
23. U. S. Nuclear Regulatory Commission. Fitness for duty programs: final rule. *Federal Register* 1989;54(108):24468–24508.
24. Public Law 102-143, Title V—Omnibus Transportation Employee Testing Act, October 28, 1991.
25. DeBernardo M, Delogu N. *Guide to state and federal drug testing laws.* Washington, DC: Institute for a Drug Free Workplace, 1996.
26. Recchi America Inc. vs Astley Hall: Court rejects part of Florida's drug-free workplace act. In: Swotinsky RB, ed. *MRO update.* Arlington Heights, IL: American College of Occupational and Environmental Medicine, 1997;2–3.
27. Shuckit N. Drug classes and problems. *Drug Abuse Alcohol Newsletter* 1988;17(1):1–4.
28. Seymour RB, Smith DE. Identifying and responding to drug abuse in the workplace. *J Psychoactive Drugs* 1990;22(4):383–405.
29. Shuckit MA. *Drugs and alcohol abuse:* a chemical guide to diagnosis and treatment. New York: Plenum Press, 1990;158–160.
30. American Psychiatric Association. Diagnostic criteria. In: *Diagnostic and statistical manual of mental disorders,* 4th ed. Washington, DC: AMA, 1994;175–272.
31. Kurtz NR, Boogins D, Howard WC. Measuring the success of occupational alcoholism programs. *J Stud Alcohol* 1984;45:3–45.
32. Foote A, Erfurt JC. Effects of EAP follow-up on prevention of relapse among substance abuse clients. *J Stud Alcohol* 1991;52:241–248.
33. American Society of Addiction Medicine. *Patient placement criteria for the treatment of psychoactive substance use disorders.* Washington, DC: American Society of Addiction Medicine, 1991.
34. Walsh DC, et al. A randomized trial of treatment options for alcohol abusing workers. *N Engl J Med* 1991;325:775–782.
35. McLellan AT, Metzger D, Allerman AI, Cornish J, Urschel H. How effective is substance abuse treatment? In: O'Brien CP, Goffe J, eds. *Advances in understanding the addictive states.* New York: Raven Press, 1992;202–231.
36. Judge WJ. *Outside the circle:* the impact of drug testing on workers' compensation. Washington, DC: Tort and Insurance Practice Section, American Bar Association, 1991.
37. Smith Kline Beecham Clinical Laboratories, College Park, PA, January 1997.
38. Substance Abuse and Mental Health Services Administration, DHHS. Mandatory guidelines for federal workplace drug testing programs. *Federal Register* 1994;59(110):29924.
39. Department of Health and Human Services. *Medical review officer manual:* a guide to evaluating urine drug analysis. Washington, DC: US Department of Health and Human Services, National Institute on Drug Abuse, 1997.
40. *Medical review officer guide.* Washington, DC: U.S. Department of Transportation, Office of the Secretary, 1990.
41. Peterson KW, et al. *Medical review officer information handbook.* Arlington Heights, IL: American College of Occupational and Environmental Medicine, 1977.
42. Swotinsky R. *The medical review officer's guide to drug testing.* New York: Van Nostrand Reinhold, 1992.
43. Department of Transportation. Drug and alcohol testing programs: final rules. *Federal Register* 1994;59:7302–7625.

*Environmental and Occupational Medicine, Third Edition*, edited by William N. Rom.
Lippincott–Raven Publishers, Philadelphia © 1998.

# CHAPTER 60

# Psychiatric Syndromes Common to the Workplace

Robert C. Larsen

Given the incidence of mental disorders in the general population, it is not unexpected that behavioral problems frequently manifest themselves in the work environment. According to a World Health Organization study, five of the ten leading causes of disability in 1990 worldwide involve psychiatric conditions, i.e., unipolar depression, alcoholism, bipolar disorder, schizophrenia, and obsessive-compulsive disorder. By the year 2020 unipolar depression will be second to ischemic heart disease as the major cause of disability (1). Certain psychiatric conditions would present irrespective of the work setting. However, even with a preexisting condition, such as bipolar disorder, the influence of external factors can exacerbate the illness. Shift work in such a vulnerable individual might well bring on a manic episode. Trauma increasingly associated with workplace violence is recognized as responsible for homicide as the second leading cause of occupational fatalities (2). Survivors of workplace violence may develop new cases of posttraumatic stress disorder. Even where the work site is passive to the expression of individual psychopathology, it may be affected by the actions of a troubled employee. Furthermore, as the nature of work evolves and the pace of change accelerates, psychiatric syndromes can be expected to be more prevalent in the modern work environment. Rather than hernias and low back syndromes of the physical labor-intense workplace, today's service-based employment setting will commonly find psychiatric injuries occurring. It is thus prudent that the occupational health professional have a good appreciation of the range of psychiatric conditions that are frequently encountered at work.

Occupational psychiatry brings together the fields of occupational medicine and psychiatry (3). Here attention is given to disturbances of thought, mood, behavior, perception, and interpersonal interchange at work. Given the nature of psychiatric disorders, the professional addressing such presentations must be aware not only of the individual's symptoms but also the impact on the work group as well as the larger organization. This chapter focuses on the individual employee who presents with psychiatric symptoms in the work setting. Occupational psychiatrists, industrial psychologists, and social scientists also address the broader organizational dynamics and psychosocial factors with which the concept of health promotion is firmly associated. These factors are not covered here; the interested reader is referred elsewhere for a discussion of the impact of these factors on the work orgaization in U.S. companies (4,5).

## WHEN TO OBTAIN A PSYCHIATRIC CONSULT

The occupational health practitioner must be capable of recognizing and intervening in a wide range of work-related health problems. There are instances where psychiatric consultation is advisable. These include clarification of diagnosis, treatment planning, fitness for duty assessment, disability evaluation, threat assessment, adjustment of pharmacotherapy, psychotherapy, and psychometric testing (Table 1).

The occupational medicine clinician makes use of mental health practitioners to establish parameters of

R. C. Larsen: Department of Psychiatry, Center for Occupational Psychiatry, University of California, San Francisco, San Francisco, California 94104.

**TABLE 1.** *Reasons for psychiatric consultation*

| |
|---|
| Diagnostic clarification |
| Treatment planning |
| Fitness for duty assessment |
| Disability evaluation |
| Threat assessment |
| Pharmacotherapy adjustment |
| Psychotherapy |
| Psychometric testing |

**TABLE 2.** *Common triggers for psychiatric consultation*

| |
|---|
| Erratic behavior |
| Mood instability |
| Recognizable life-threatening trauma |
| Potential dangerousness |
| History of head trauma |
| Pattern of conflict with co-workers, supervisors, or clients |
| Unexplained change in productivity |

treatment and case management in employees with mental disorders. Erratic behavior, mood instability, exposure to life-threatening trauma, concern about dangerousness, or a history of head injury are all examples of situations in which psychiatric consultation is indicated (Table 2).

One role of the occupational physician or nurse is to recognize the need for such consultations. The clinician may oversee aspects of treatment especially when the pharmacotherapy regimen is well established. Counseling that is more involved than coaching should best be left to a competent psychologist or psychiatrist. The occupational health clinician frequently assumes administrative and case management functions where psychiatric issues are present. Thus, such professionals should have a reasonable familiarity with psychiatric conditions common to the work force. Case histories are presented here to illustrate the complexities of issues faced by the occupational physician addressing psychiatric issues among employees. (Confidentiality has been preserved in all case histories with employees' names and characteristics having been altered.)

## COMMON PSYCHIATRIC DISORDERS IN THE WORKING POPULATION

### Adjustment Disorders

Perhaps most common among the emotional problems that working people experience are the mild reactions to recognizable psychosocial stressors termed adjustment disorders. These time-limited conditions come forth in response to external stressors. Mergers, downsizing, performance plans, and prolonged supervisor-supervisee conflict can precipitate anxiety, depression, and psychophysiologic symptoms.

#### *Case History: Combined Job and Personal Stressors*

Mr. Smith, a 39-year-old manager for an insurance company, presents for the first time to the company medical department complaining of headaches and cervical pain. The only history of trauma involves a motor vehicle accident in the course of his regular duties 2 months previously. The manager has not sought out medical attention to this point in time. He indicates that he has continued to work long hours and does not feel he has had the opportunity to take time off from his busy schedule. Mr. Smith has found himself irritable both at work and at home. His sleep is regularly interrupted due to physical pain. He admits that he has been having problems in his personal life; he and his wife have been in counseling for the last 6 months. He is perplexed by whether his physical discomfort, which began within days of the accident, relates to the vehicular accident, to job stress he is experiencing in trying to prove himself to a new vice president, or to the problems in his personal life. He does not wish to take time off work. He has not felt comfortable in discussing in the couples counseling with his wife issues he feels are peripheral to his marriage.

This case of a relatively high functioning management employee points out the complexity of issues that can present themselves to the occupational physician. Mr. Smith is someone with a history of a legitimate physical injury associated with employment, and psychosocial stressors associated with both employment and personal concerns.

When symptoms do not come forth to the degree that warrant recognition as a psychological syndrome, the employee may still be viewed as upset in relation to these same types and severity of work-related stressors. In these situations the employee might best be conceptualized as struggling with either an occupational problem, or a nonclinical, expectable, and normal human response, such as grief in response to a death in the family, i.e., a nonpathologic state of distress. The majority of employees exposed to downsizing, reorganization, or discipline at work do not develop a psychiatric problem, but some do.

### Mood Disorders

It is well recognized that there are multifactorial causes for mood disorders. Biologic predisposition, psychodynamic underpinnings, social factors, and environmental precipitants can all lead to the development of a clinical depression. Typically these disorders are more chronic or more severe when compared to the milder adjustment disorders. *Dysthymic disorder* is neurotic depression with symptoms such as dysphoria, low self-esteem, indecision, and fatigue present over a period of 2 years or more. This type of depressive disorder often arises in persons with histories of loss, deprivation, and disappointment. *Major depression* is characterized by more extensive and severe symptoms impacting on the individual's functional ability. Disturbances of appetite, sleep, and cognition can be profound and accompanied by markedly reduced interest in and pleasure associated with normal activities. Severe cases result in social withdrawal, pseudodementia, and suicidal ideation.

#### *Case History: The Beaten-Down Employee*

Mr. Jones, a 41-year-old security manager for a major bank, presents to the company personnel department 6 months after having taken a personal leave of absence. The employee gives a history of having worked under the direction of a regional manager who repeatedly undermined his efforts. He describes functioning under significant staff cutbacks following a company reorganization. He reports putting in long hours, sometimes being expected to work at night and on weekends for weeks at end. Not only did Mr. Jones receive no additional compensation for the extra hours demanded of him by his supervisor, but he was expected to be available on a 24-hour basis except when on vacation. Although he had been with the bank for less than 1 year at the time that he went on leave, he had been in a similar position with another financial institution for a decade. While on his leave he applied for job positions elsewhere. He reluctantly listed his regional manager as a reference. A potential employer disclosed to Mr. Jones that he was not given a job position when his supervisor indicated that the employee had a "nervous breakdown" resulting in the need for the leave from work. In fact, Mr. Jones had entered outpatient psychiatric care and was being treated with an antidepressant, though he assumed that this was confidential information. He had never given consent to his supervisor to report to others about this matter. Mr. Jones now discloses that he has found himself struggling with suicidal thoughts. The situation has escalated as his permit to carry a handgun in the course of his security duties is in jeopardy. He is now approaching the personnel department feeling both angry and hopeless.

This case, which was later referred by the personnel department for medical evaluation, involves an employee clearly suffering from a mood disorder for which psychiatric treatment services are already in place. It is further complicated by legal, corporate policy, and ethical issues.

Although less common than unipolar depressions, *bipolar disorder*, in which episodes of mania are evident, can be very disruptive to the work site. During manic episodes, pressured speech, racing thoughts, agitation, distractibility, grandiosity, and euphoria may be apparent to others observing the person so affected. While the depressed employee may elicit concern from co-workers, the employee beset with mania causes others to be frightened, worried, or angry. An individual with vacillating moods that do not reach the level of mania is noted to experience hypomanic episodes and would be diagnosed with *cyclothymic disorder*. Pharmacotherapy for cyclical mood disorders is a mainstay of treatment, including lithium, neuroleptics, anticonvulsants, and antidepressants (6).

### Anxiety Disorders

Perhaps as prevalent if not more so than the mood disorders in the general population are the anxiety disorders (7). *Panic disorder* is a condition distinguished by recurrent episodes of intense fear involving palpitations, shortness of breath, chest pain, trembling, and a sense of dread. Panic attack is the current term for what in the past would have been referred to as an anxiety attack. Panic disorder may occur in conjunction with symptoms of agoraphobia in which the individual fears venturing out, being in crowded situations, or traveling. While there is evidence for panic disorder having a biologic cause, external stressors may precipitate panic attacks in an individual vulnerable to acute anxiety.

#### *Case History: Full Duty or No Duty*

Ms. Frank, a 29-year-old sheriff's deputy, presents to her family physician reporting circumscribed episodes of shortness of breath and tachycardia while working in a jail. No precipitant is apparent other than that she was transferred to the jail setting within the prior week. A physical examination is within normal limits, except that the patient appeared quite anxious. During the course of the clinical interview Ms. Frank's anxious affect gradually recedes. The record notes a similar set of symptoms that followed an inmate assault 3 years ago that resulted in significant orthopedic injuries necessitating hospitalization. When Ms. Frank attempted to return to work within 1 month of the assault, she experienced panic symptoms and avoidant behavior in the jail setting. At the treating doctor's recommendation following the assault, brief psychiatric treatment was implemented. At the recommendation of the treating psychiatrist at that time, an alternative assignment was found wherein the deputy functioned as a bailiff in the county court system. Her symptoms remitted and she continued working on a full-time basis.

Now, with his patient's permission, the family physician contacts the personnel manager for the sheriff's department only to learn that deputies cannot be "coddled" and no limited duty assignment is possible. The manager indicates that the jail to which the deputy was recently assigned is a new facility and has a lower inmate-to-deputy ratio than the old institution.

This case of an individual with clear symptoms of acute anxiety associated with her duties in law enforcement involves clinical issues that have administrative implications for the affected individual. The physician can address the patient's symptoms or impairment associated with the current duties, but the employee may also need professional assistance from her union representative or from legal counsel.

## Stress Disorders

*Posttraumatic stress disorder* (PTSD) was first described in the *Diagnostic and Statistical Manual of Mental Disorders,* 3rd edition (DSM-III), published in 1980. However, the concept of a psychological response to severe trauma has been described in the clinical literature for over a century, typically in reports involving soldiers and disaster victims (8). According to DSM-IV, the individual with PTSD responds to life-threatening trauma by experiencing fear, helplessness, or horror. Persistent reexperiencing comes forth in recurrent intrusive recollections and frightening dreams. This is accompanied by avoidant behavior for activities, places, and persons reminiscent of the trauma. Sleep disturbance, irritability, hypervigilance and startle reactions are common. *Acute stress disorder* can be diagnosed 2 days and for up to 1 month after a recognizable trauma, whereas PTSD is diagnosed after 1 month following the same type of event.

**TABLE 3.** *Events that may precipitate posttraumatic stress disorder*

| |
|---|
| Sexual assault |
| Physical attack |
| Robbery |
| Mugging |
| Hostage situations |
| Disasters |
| Severe automobile accident |

From. ref. 9.

Not uncommonly individuals with PTSD symptoms respond to a number of stressors that have a cumulative effect. Early intervention and workplace accommodation may allow for individuals so affected by recognizable traumas to work through certain consequences of traumatic exposure and return to a more functional status (Table 3).

Intervention for employees experiencing PTSD is described below. Other anxiety disorders that can present in the working population include specific phobias, social phobias, and obsessive-compulsive disorders. It should be recognized that individuals meeting the criteria for the diagnosis of an anxiety disorder not uncommonly present with depressive symptoms as well.

### *Case History: Posttraumatic Stress*

Mr. Jeffers is a battalion chief and 20-year veteran of a municipal fire department who is referred by his departmental physician for a fitness for duty evaluation. Mr. Jeffers has been noted recently to act uncharacteristically. He has been avoiding going out to major alarm fires, or arriving at the scene much later than is required of him in his management role. He is expected to coordinate fire units at such major events. He reluctantly discloses that he has found himself experiencing profound fearfulness at the prospect of being at the site of a major blaze and having to make decisions. He has been experiencing intrusive recollections of other fires including one that took place 2 months earlier in which he witnessed one of the firefighters in his command die. His sleep is disturbed and regularly interrupted by disturbing dreams involving disaster scenes. He has found himself procrastinating, having difficulty concentrating, and being more irritable both at work and at home. He describes a lengthy career in which he has been exposed to numerous disasters involving fires, earthquakes, and motor vehicle accidents. He reports that he can no longer enjoy attending departmental barbecues; he finds the mere smell of cooking meat repulsive, as it seems to be associated with memories of charred victims. He emphasizes his desire to remain a productive member of his department, yet finds himself terrified of the prospect that decisions that he will make may result in untoward effects for others.

## Substance Abuse

Substance abuse or chemical dependency should be considered early in the differential diagnosis of the employee presenting with erratic behavior, mood instability, and interpersonal conflict at work. Work cultures can reinforce alcoholic behavior through the emphasis on entertaining clients or socializing with co-workers after hours. The professions of health care and law enforcement can expose the vulnerable worker to pharmaceuticals and illicit substances, respectively. At the point that tolerance, craving, and withdrawal are present the individual so affected by alcohol, prescription medication, or illicit drugs has developed features of chemical dependency, a step on the continuum beyond abuse. Not uncommonly employees with substance abuse problems have other axis I psychiatric conditions such as depression or anxiety, an axis II personality disorder, and/or an axis III medical condition such as a chronic pain syndrome.

### *Case History: In Need of Intervention*

Mr. Reed, a successful 32-year-old account representative for a major microelectronics manufacturer, is referred by management to his company's employee assistance program for consultation. He is aware that the purpose of the consultation is to determine his fitness for duty given certain incidents that have troubled his sales manager. Over the course of the prior 6 months Mr. Reed has been late to a number of important meetings and has lost a couple of major accounts. Most recently he fell down some stairs at a trade show resulting in his injuring his leg. Other co-workers have expressed some concern about the number of drinks he had at a company-sponsored reception on that occasion. In the course of the consultation Mr. Reed admits that his drinking has increased over time, though he does not see it as worrisome as he has never had a blackout or been charged with driving under the influence. When asked about the use of illicit substances he admits to having made repeated use of amphetamines but denies that it has ever represented a problem for him. Reluctantly he agrees to enter a chemical dependency treatment program when the alternative he is faced with is severance of his employment with the company based on his having failed the current performance plan.

Clinicians working with management need to be attuned to the warning signs of substance abuse to minimize the chances of serious deleterious consequences to the employee and the work site.

### Somatoform Disorders

Just as physicians in hospital and clinical settings must be mindful of hysterical presentations, so too must the occupational medicine clinician be attentive to the occurrence of somatoform disorders in the population of workers with claims of physical injury and disability. Nonanatomic neurologic complaints (those that do not coincide with known neurologic pathways), diffuse pain, and dramatic complaints are characteristic of these psychosomatic illnesses. Rather than the somatisizing patient improving with the passage of time following a physical injury, a progressive deterioration to a passive, dependent status takes place. Objective findings in the physical examination and within the diagnostic studies performed are typically within normal limits and unimpressive. Yet the worker so afflicted with psychogenic pain or some other variant of a somatoform disorder continues to seek out consultation and treatment despite the lack of evidence supportive of a biologically based disease process. There may or may not be an accompanying affective component. Physicians at times note that such patients present with minimal emotional distress associated with the chronicity of their complaints, i.e., "la belle indifference." These hysterical reactions have long been recognized and described as distinct from, though at times coexisting with, hysterical personality (10).

*Somatization disorder* is a somatoform diagnosis made when there is a lengthy history of physical complaints dating back to early adulthood resulting in treatment and/or functional impairment, yet investigation cannot identify a medical condition that can account for the subjective complaints. A *conversion disorder* should be considered when deficits involving voluntary motor or sensory functions cannot be explained by a physical disorder and where psychological factors are considered operative as evidenced by conflict and external stressors. *Hypochondriasis* involves a preoccupation or conviction that one is beset with a serious illness despite medical evidence to the contrary. Individuals with hypochondriacal predispositions often have a naive notion of how their bodies function. They tend to misinterpret the bodily cues or symptoms perceived. *Pain disorder* is the current terminology for what in the past had been labeled as psychogenic or somatoform pain. In general, unconscious processes are causally related to the unexplained physical complaints in persons with somatoform disorders. There may be a steadfast denial of any possible psychological problem and psychotherapy often achieves disappointing results.

#### *Case History: Prolonged Disability, Physical versus Psychiatric*

Mr. Adams is a 45-year-old married man who presents for psychiatric assessment of his situation 2 years after a documented fall at work. He stumbled down a flight of stairs at the restaurant where he was employed as a dishwasher. Extensive medical evaluation has been performed by neurologists, orthopedists, physical medicine specialists, and neuropsychologists. Magnetic resonance imaging (MRI) scans of the head and neck, bone scans, EEGs, and extensive neuropsychological testing have been performed. The employee has not returned to work and describes an existence wherein he can take on little if any normal activities. He complains of "total body pain." There is a dramatic quality to his complaints and he implores the evaluating physician to somehow find the cause and alleviate his discomfort. The voluminous medical file repeatedly makes reference to an absence of objective findings of neurologic dysfunction. Neuropsychological testing was interpreted as consistent with a postconcussive head syndrome with an associated disturbance of cognition, mood, and behavior. The treating neurologist has diagnosed the patient as having a posttraumatic head syndrome that precludes his returning to work as a dishwasher. Interestingly, none of the evaluating or treating clinicians have requested a copy of the initial hospital record containing the emergency room report from the date of injury. While the employee gives a history of loss of consciousness, that is not corroborated by the initial emergency room record. Furthermore, Mr. Adams is noted to complain at that time of "total body pain" while still in the emergency facility. His "memory problem" is now so severe that he cannot recall his date of birth or his age. At the same time he is completely fluent in his native language.

A further review of records from the hospital at which he presented on an emergency basis 2 years ago includes a number of contacts that predate the workplace injury. The employee had presented on a number of occasions with complaints of chest pain, gastrointestinal difficulties, back pain, and various other maladies, though none of these had been found to have an organic basis. The record makes frequent reference on these occasions to functional overlay, anxiety, and hysteria. The employee had never previously filed a workers' compensation claim nor had he ever put forth a litigated claim of any sort in the past.

This case points out the importance of obtaining sources of information other than the patient when considering complaints that appear to have a somatoform quality. A patient such as Mr. Adams can end up receiving extensive medical services to the point that he is at risk for an iatrogenic complication. It can be difficult for physicians to curtail further examination in an individual who so vehemently wishes to pursue the source of the serious physical problem that he is convinced must be present.

Somewhat distinct from the somatoform disorders are the factitious disorders. While the unconscious is again involved in the development of physical complaints, these presentations also incorporate conscious, willful behavior that perpetuates the symptoms. The drive in these cases is to achieve and maintain the sick role. What differentiates factitious disorders from malingering is the willingness to undergo invasive medical procedures and even surgery. A unifying theme to these somatoform disorders, factitious disorders, and cases of conscious malingering is the element of symptom exaggeration or embellishment that goes beyond what is expected given the history of the injurious event, the physical examination, and the diagnostic test results. Psychometric testing often detects this element of exaggeration as well as hypochondriacal and hysterical features in cases of somatoform or factitious disorders. Once a diagnosis has been established of a somatoform or factitious disorder, minimizing the potential harm that can come from unnecessary testing and medical treatment should be a guiding principle of case management. There have been instances of mass psychogenic illness where multiple employees have developed an unexplained panoply of symptoms that has the appearance of an epidemic. Brodsky (11) has emphasized the contribution made by social systems, attorneys, and physicians to outbreaks of hysterical illness in a variety of work settings.

### Personality Disorders

When personality characteristics become maladaptive and result in a pattern of dysfunction at work or socially, a *personality disorder* should be considered. The diagnosis of a personality disorder is listed on axis II of the multiaxial assessment used in psychiatry. Disturbances of personality are thus differentiated from axis I conditions such as the mood, anxiety, and somatoform disorders. Personality disorders are manifest by an enduring pattern of inflexibility in cognition, affect, interpersonal interchange, or impulse control. The current diagnostic nomenclature identifies ten specific personality disorders grouped into three clusters (Table 4).

**TABLE 4.** *Personality disorders, DSM-VI clusters*

| |
|---|
| Cluster A |
| Paranoid, schizoid, schizotypal |
| Cluster B |
| Antisocial, borderline, histrionic, narcissistic |
| Cluster C |
| Avoidant, dependent, obsessive-compulsive |

From. ref. 12.

#### *Case History: Damned If You Do, Damned If You Don't*

Ms. Hall is a 45-year-old lower-level administrator for a transit company, referred for psychiatric consultation by the attorney representing her in multiple legal claims against the employer. Ms. Hall complains of depression and resentment related to what she perceives to be both racial and sexual discrimination. Following 6 months' employment in a job position as an assistant program director, she has been demoted. The reasons cited in the personnel file include poor organizational skills and conflict with both managers and subordinates. The employee had repeatedly complained about not having been promoted in her first 5 years with the company. The employer reluctantly granted the promotion to assistant director, indicating certain goals would have to be attained within the first 6 months. The personnel file further includes documentation of Ms. Hall's not having met these goals. In fact, a department that had previously been quite stable is noted to have undergone a dramatic attrition rate, with many long-term employees either leaving the company or requesting a transfer. Rather than viewing herself as responsible for the problem, Ms. Hall insists that she was removed from the position because of being "too progressive." Psychological testing is positive for symptoms of depression, passive-aggressive personality features, profound mistrust, and intellectual abilities falling within the low-average range of adult intelligence. Ms. Hall vehemently denies that her having other obligations including responsibility for two severely ill parents has in any way contributed to her "anxiety."

Perhaps there is little the employer could have done to have avoided the conflict that developed in this situation. It has now taken on not only clinical manifestations for the employee but organizational problems at the work site as well as legal complications.

### Psychotic Disorders

The occupational physician at times is confronted with assessing an employee with idiosyncratic thoughts and odd behaviors. While it would be somewhat unusual for a work environment to cause a psychotic illness, individuals vulnerable to the development of delusions, hallucinations, and eccentric behavior do at times present a challenge to management and occupational medicine. Referral to a psychiatrist to establish an accurate diagnosis and treatment plan is essential. Schizophrenia, schizoaffective disorder, and delusional disorder are severe diagnoses that, while uncommon in the work population, can be quite notable when present. Dementias and amnestic disorders can result from closed head trauma or chemical exposure such as to heavy metal vapors. A thorough history of the traumatic incident or exposure and corroboration of the trauma/exposure should be obtained. Serial neuropsychological testing can be helpful in determining whether the cognitive dysfunction is exaggerated, progressive, or stabilizing.

## SPECIAL SITUATIONS

Certain circumstances involving behavioral issues have implications that are so profound for the workplace that they warrant particular attention. Violence, the threat of violence, and harassment can have serious consequences for victims of such aggressive acts. The employee plagued by fear and mistrust as the result of workplace aggression may seek out clinical services through various means. The occupational physician may be faced with making a referral for psychiatric evaluation and/or treatment. These cases may assume additional complexity due to other sources of psychological trauma, concurrent nonindustrial stressors, administrative/personnel issues, and legal concerns. Proper disposition can not only address the needs of the individual employee but maintain morale in the work group while helping to dispel concerns about safety in the employment setting.

### Threat Assessment

Situations arise from time to time where a particular worker comes to be seen as a potential threat to others at work. Aggressive behavior may be verbal and overtly stated. A threat may be directed toward a single individual or to a particular group, or be nonspecific and vaguely intended. Threats can also be communicated in writing, by telephone, or via computers. The message may come from an anonymous source. The alleged threat may be witnessed or not. When concern arises about the potential for a particular employee to become a danger to others or to the company's physical plant, a comprehensive threat assessment should be done. Wherever possible this type of fitness for duty examination of an individual with the potential to act out in a destructive manner should be performed by a clinician with expertise in identifying risk factors for violence (Table 5).

**TABLE 5.** *Factors contributing to workplace violence*

| |
|---|
| Antisocial personality |
| Paranoid personality |
| Alcohol and drug abuse |
| Job loss |
| Desire for retaliation |

From ref. 13.

Psychiatric consultants utilize protocols for assessing the seriousness of a threat or an individual's potential to become violent (14). The information developed can then allow employer representatives to take appropriate administrative steps by restricting the employee's access to the work site and intended victims.

### Trauma Intervention

When an incident has occurred that can be expected to have psychologically traumatic effects on employees, early intervention is advised. Bank robberies, plant explosions, natural disasters, and other workplace events that represent a recognizable threat to physical integrity can leave employees vulnerable to an acute stress syndrome or some other reactive emotional condition. Where multiple employees are exposed management should consider an educational/clinical intervention by a skilled clinician familiar with working with victims of trauma. *Critical incident stress debriefing* is a method of educating employees about the aftereffects of a serious trauma. The group format at the work site allows for a sharing of the common experience. It serves as an acknowledgment that management recognizes that the incident was unusual and disturbing. Furthermore, individuals who are symptomatic can be encouraged to obtain treatment (15–17).

In addition to employee education and psychiatric treatment, attention to security measures and plant safety may be necessary. Guidelines for treatment of workers diagnosed with PTSD have been developed by the Industrial Medical Council of the State of California. These guidelines emphasize early intervention, workplace accommodation, and nonclinical measures aside from psychotherapy and pharmacotherapy (18). For example, transferring a bank teller who had been robbed to a position removed from the teller line may allow for that individual to return to work much sooner than if only full teller duties are made available. Similarly, a bus driver who has been the victim of an assault may feel empowered and less vulnerable by taking a self-defense course, again allowing for a resumption of work duties. Even when administrative issues are properly addressed legal issues are frequently associated with PTSD cases resulting in the need for forensic evaluation (19,20).

### Harassment and Bullying

Harassment or intimidation, like threats of violence, can be overt or implied. The underlying dynamics can center around race, gender, age, or lifestyle. Harassment by definition involves power used abusively. Subtle forms of sexual harassment can involve the implied quid pro quo of a desired job promotion in exchange for the harasser achieving a nonprofessional social relationship. While companies can develop policy to prohibit harassment, it still arises. Investigation of allegations of harassment often requires involvement by management, legal council, and clinicians. Attention to confidentiality is crucial. Litigation can involve workers' compensation, civil tort, and criminal arenas. Such cases can be highly charged emotionally, and potential bias on the part of the psychiatric examiner needs to be considered (21). It should also be recognized that interpersonal conflict is determined in part by culture. For example, what is acceptable behavior in a work site in a rural location may be considered quite offensive in an urban office setting. Other cultures do not recognize the concept of harassment in quite the manner acknowledged in the United States. In Japan, rather than harassment, the concept of "bullying," where the individual is forced to conform to the norm of the work group, is a common phenomenon (22).

## PREVENTION OF AND INTERVENTION IN WORKPLACE CONFLICT

While predicting when and by whom interpersonal conflict will develop is difficult, planning for its occurrence should be a component of a company's health and safety management. The concept of early intervention for PTSD, addressed above, also applies to the broader concept of stress prevention and conflict management. Psychiatric injury claims can follow from an initial physical injury, as a response to a recognizable psychologically traumatic event, or from cumulative work stressors. Interpersonal conflict is frequently a manifestation of a psychiatric condition and comes forth as the troubled employee becomes dysfunctional in the workplace in interactions with co-workers or clients. A structure of preventative measures should result in appropriate case disposition, thus reducing the costs of mental disorders to both the individual employee and the work organization (Table 6).

**TABLE 6.** *Psychiatric injury claims: preventative measures*

| |
|---|
| Employee education |
| Supervisor training |
| Employee assistance programs |
| Early intervention |
| Mediation services |
| Outpatient mental health benefit |
| Comprehensive psychiatric exam |
| Claims review |
| Standardized personnel policy |
| Executive consultation |

From ref. 23.

Employee education is a low-cost method of involving the individual in health promotion. Instructing managers in the warning signs of behavioral problems and appropriate means of discipline should be part of supervisor training. Employee assistance programs (EAPs) can be internal to the work organization or services provided by external mental health groups. They can serve a central function in education, evaluation, short-term therapy, and referral (24). Proper coordination between the company's EAP program, the human resources/personnel department, and the occupational physician can allow for early intervention when supervisor/supervisee, peer/peer, or other interpersonal conflict arises in the work environment. Clinical intervention soon after a critical incident is crucial. Resolving conflict through mediation services can be considered when management efforts have failed. The goal here is to maintain productivity of the work group while reducing the chance of litigation and disability.

Outpatient mental health services can encourage an employee with emotional or behavioral problems, irrespective of the cause, to obtain appropriate treatment. When claims are filed comprehensive psychiatric examination allows for administrative and benefits decisions to be made in a timely manner (25). Risk factors within the organization can be identified via a claims review of workers' compensation or long-term disability psychiatric claims. Standardized personnel policy governing performance reviews and disciplinary action should assure the presence of lawful, nondiscriminatory personnel actions. This component of the structure is intended to allow adequate documentation of proper procedure to defend against nonmeritorious claims. Management can benefit from executive consultation on a variety of issues such as corporate strategy, intergroup rivalry, and successor planning (26). The company that addresses the inevitable conflict that arises in the workplace through a comprehensive structure of policy and services will be better able to address the needs of the individual, the work group, and the larger corporation. Corporations in the 21st century must plan for change and conflict. Organizations that do so will grow and adapt. The occupational medicine specialist will also need to change and adapt by understanding more about mental health problems of employees, work-related stressors, and intervention strategies. The physician accepting this challenge will be better able to provide clinical, administrative, and consulting services to work organizations.

## REFERENCES


1. Murray CJ, Lopez AD, eds. *The global burden of disease:* a comprehensive assessment of mortality and disability from diseases, *injuries and risk factors in 1990 and projected to 2020.* Cambridge, MA: Harvard University Press, 1996.
2. Toscano G, Weber W. Patterns of fatal workplace assaults differ from those of non-fatal ones. In: *Fatal workplace injuries in 1993:* a collection of data and analysis [Bureau of Labor Statistics Report No. 891.] Washington, DC: US Department of Labor, Bureau of Labor Statistics, 1995;43–50.
3. Committee on Psychiatry in Industry, Group for Advancement of Psychiatry. *Introduction to occupational psychiatry.* Washington, DC: American Psychiatric Press, 1994;vii–xiv.
4. Sperry L. Organizational dynamics. In: *Corporate therapy and consulting.* New York: Brunner Mazel, 1996;30–68.
5. Sperry L. Understanding organizations: a primer for occupational medicine physicians. In: Farid A, Brodsky C, eds. *Psychosocial and corporate issues in occupational dysfunctions. Occupational medicine:* state of the art reviews. Philadelphia: Hanley and Belfus, 1996;651–661.
6. Hirshfield RMA. Guidelines for the long-term treatment of depression. *J Clin Psychiatry* 1994;55:61–69.
7. Kessler RC, McGonagle KA, Zhao S, et al. Lifetime and 12 month prevalence of DSM-III-R psychiatric disorders in the United States. *Arch Gen Psychiatry* 1994;51:8–19.
8. Davidson JRT. Posttraumatic stress disorder and acute stress disorder. In: Kaplan HI, Sadock BJ, eds. *Comprehensive textbook of psychiatry,* 6th ed. Baltimore: Williams and Wilkins, 1995;1227–1236.
9. American Psychiatric Association. *Diagnostic and Statistical Manual of Mental Disorders,* 4th ed. Washington, DC: American Psychiatric Press, 1994;424–429.
10. Chodoff P, Lyons H. Hysteria, the hysterical personality and "hysterical" conversion. *Am J Psychiatry* 1958;114:734–740.
11. Brodsky CM, The psychiatric epidemic in the American workplace. In: Larsen RC, Felton JS, eds. *Psychiatric injury in the workplace. Occupational medicine:* state of the art reviews. Philadelphia: Hanley and Belfus, 1988;653–662.
12. American Psychiatric Association. *Diagnostic and statistical manual of mental disorders,* 4th edition. Washington, DC: American Psychiatric Press, 1994;629–673.
13. Warshaw LJ, Messite J. Workplace violence: preventive and interventive strategies. *J Occup Environ Med* 1996;38:993–1006.
14. Resnick PJ, Kausch O. Violence in the workplace: role of the consultant. *Consult Psychol J* 1995;47:213–222.
15. White SG, Hatcher C. Violence and trauma response. In: Larsen RC, Felton JS, eds. *Psychiatric injury in the workplace. Occupational medicine:* state of the art reviews. Philadelphia: Hanley and Belfus, 1988; 677–694.
16. Mitchell JT. Development and functions of a critical incident stress debriefing team. *J Emerg Med Serv* 1988;13:43–46.
17. Mitchell, JT. History, status and future of critical incident stress debriefing. *J Emerg Med Serv* 1988;13:49–52.
18. Industrial Medical Council of California. *Treatment guideline for posttraumatic stress disorder.* Sacramento, CA: Department of Industrial Relations, State of California, 1996.
19. Stone AA. Post-traumatic stress disorder and the law: critical review of the new frontier. *Bull Am Acad Psychiatry Law* 1993;21:23–36.
20. Simon RI. *Posttraumatic stress disorder in litigation:* guidelines for forensic assessment. Washington, DC: American Psychiatric Press, 1995.
21. Simon RI. The credible forensic psychiatric evaluation in sexual harassment litigation. *Psychiatr Ann* 1996;26:139–148.
22. Shima S, Arai M, Fujita O. Bullying and harassment at the job place in Japan. Presented at the Group for the Advancement of Psychiatry, White Plains, New York, April 1995.
23. Larsen RC. Workers' compensation stress claims: workplace causes and prevention. *Psychiatr Ann* 1995;25:234–237.
24. Lawton B. The EAP and workplace psychiatric injury. In: Larsen RC, Felton JS, eds. *Psychiatric injury in the workplace. Occupational medicine:* state of the art reviews. Philadelphia: Hanley and Belfus, 1988; 645–706.
25. Grant B, Robbins DB. Disability, workers' compensation and fitness for duty. In: Kahn J, ed. *Mental health in the workplace.* New York: Van Nostrand Reinhold, 1993;83–105.
26. Morrison D. Psychiatric consultation to management. *Psychiatr Ann* 1978;12:47–57.

*Environmental and Occupational Medicine, Third Edition,* edited by William N. Rom.
Lippincott–Raven Publishers, Philadelphia © 1998.

CHAPTER 61

# Multiple Chemical Sensitivity

Alan M. Ducatman

The previous edition of this text did not have a chapter on multiple chemical sensitivity (MCS), thus avoiding controversy in the face of inconclusive research. Now this ubiquitous and problematic condition in occupational health practice can no longer be ignored. It is uncertain, however, that future generations will use this term or consider the present treatment of this condition wise.

Everything about MCS engenders controversy except for the suffering it causes, which clinicians need to address. The isolation, frustration, and marginalization of MCS patients is widely acknowledged by clinicians. The physiologic mechanisms in MCS that lead to these social outcomes are unclear. The various hypotheses invoked to explain the phenomenon of MCS have their supporters and detractors, resulting in a polarized MCS community of patients, advocates, and clinicians. This chapter reviews what we know about MCS and what has been hypothesized, discusses when absence of confirmatory data for a hypothesis amounts to absence of causation, addresses what helps clinically and what appears to be unhelpful, and speculates about what might be useful in the future. The views of professional societies that are concerned with MCS phenomenon are discussed, along with whether new research results should alter these societies' official positions. The utility of MCS as a concept for patients, physicians, researchers, and policy makers, in that order of importance, is discussed. It is the editor's wisdom that this chapter should be written by a relative nonparticipant in the MCS wars, whose status will undoubtedly change upon publication. The history of MCS suggests that not all readers will be fully pleased by the effort, and that definitions, hypotheses, and arguments will continue to change after publication of this text.

Yet the suffering will remain. Determining which interventions are beneficial and which are not is among the most critical evidence-based needs in the field of MCS. To date, opinions outweigh evidence.

A. M. Ducatman: Department of Community Medicine, Institute of Occupational and Environmental Health, West Virginia University School of Medicine, Morgantown, West Virginia 26506-9190.

## DEFINITION AND DIAGNOSTIC CRITERIA

Cullen (1) defined MCS as "an acquired disorder characterized by recurrent symptoms, referable to multiple organ systems, occurring in response to demonstrable exposure to many chemically unrelated compounds at doses far below those established in the general population to cause harmful effects. No single widely accepted test of physiologic function can be shown to correlate with symptoms."

Using this definition, seven major diagnostic features were distinguished (1):

1. The disorder is acquired in relation to some documentable environmental exposure(s), insult(s), or illness(s).
2. Symptoms involve more than one organ system.
3. Symptoms recur and abate in response to predictable stimuli.
4. Symptoms are elicited by exposures to chemicals of diverse structural classes and toxicologic modes of action.
5. Symptoms are elicited by exposures that are demonstrable (albeit of low level).
6. Exposures that elicit symptoms must be very low, many standard deviations below average exposures known to cause adverse human responses.
7. No single widely available test of organ system function can explain symptoms.

These criteria were useful in that they described a growing subset of patients whose problems set the tone for subsequent descriptions and investigations. An essential shorthand developed for describing a complex type of patient. The willingness of skilled researchers to consider the population increased. The criteria also contained within them important limitations and, in hindsight, an unfortunate choice of terms. The word *sensitivity* suggests to clinicians an immunologic process, and the assumption by both research and clinical communities was that immunologic derangements were the issue to address. This assumption, implicit in the term *multiple chemical sensitivity*, may have spurred the controversy.

Other diagnostic criteria have been proposed (2,3). The least proscriptive case definition comes from the National Research Council (2), which suggested that symptoms need occur in more than one organ system, be elicited by low level exposures, and wane in the absence of exposure. There are problems with this definition. On the one hand, environmental asthma with rhinitis might inappropriately be termed MCS under this definition. On the other hand, the concept that symptoms wane in the absence of exposure has communication utility but limited toxicologic meaning, as minute exposures are ubiquitous and unavoidable, and MCS patients most often have large number of inciting substances whose ambient presence cannot be reliably predicted or measured. Ashford and Miller (4) have defined MCS in operational terms. The MCS patient is identified by improvements following removal from suspected offending agents and by problems following subsequent rechallenge under strictly controlled environmental conditions. This definition holds promise for research, although the nature of the challenge, the evident need for careful blinding of both subjects and researchers (and the difficulty of so doing), and a definition of a positive outcome need clarification. One hopes that repeatable tests and objective outcome measures can eventually be proposed. Rest's (5) definition of MCS requires a change in health status including a stereotypic set of reported symptoms referable to three or more organs, and the exclusion of other health conditions. This definition is useful because it implies no particular etiologic hypothesis, does not rely on presently unachievable test methods, and does not require confirmation of exposure. Wide clinical acceptance of the Rest definition would have decreased but not eliminated the controversy engendered by the MCS diagnosis. Scientific controversy would be further reduced by elimination of references to exposure, at any dose, but such proposals infuriate MCS interest groups. Suggestions that the MCS phenomenon be relabeled with a purely descriptive name such as multiorgan dysesthesia have met with resistance.

One such definition was proposed by Simon (6): "MCS can be most clearly defined in terms of beliefs and behaviors. Patients with MCS believe that their symptoms result from low-level exposure." This definition is technically accurate because it eliminates neither psychologic nor physiologic etiologies. It is also unlikely to gain wide acceptance in the MCS advocacy community because it features and favors the possibility of a psychologic explanation. The importance of these definitions and the concept of MCS is apparent to clinicians. Low-level exposures are ubiquitous, whether perceived or not. Perceptions of low-level exposures are also very common.

## HISTORIC ANTECEDENTS

Multiple chemical sensitivity descends most directly from Theron Randolph's (7) concepts of chemical sensitivity. The description of chemical sensitivity resembles Cullen's subsequent MCS criteria in several ways. According to Randolph chemical sensitivity was:

- an acquired disorder
- an outcome that often follows an acute chemical exposure.
- accompanied by symptoms that occur following low-level exposures to chemicals
- an adaptation phenomenon that results in the masking of symptoms (at least initially); patients who are chronically ill during chronic exposure to chemicals go through a withdrawal period when removed from exposure, and they subsequently become acutely reactive to chemical challenge
- a spreading phenomenon; patients become sensitive to an increasing number of chemicals.

Treatments proposed by Randolph (7) and clinical adherents included sauna therapy, vitamin and mineral supplementation, and sublingual or intradermal administration of chemicals for both diagnoses and treatment. Randolph's hypothesis gave rise to a movement often called "clinical ecology," which relied heavily on provocation diagnoses (often of subjective feelings) and provocation-neutralization treatments. This approach is now widely discredited for a variety of reasons, including consistent inability to stand up to truly blind provocation testing. The clinical ecology movement engendered a host of descriptions for what later became the MCS phenomenon including environmental illness, cerebral allergy, environmental maladaptation syndrome, ecologic illness, immune dysregulation, total allergy syndrome, universal allergy, 20th century disease, and chemical AIDS. Some of these terms persist and most contain some concept of immunologic derangement, an etiologic concept now considered relatively unlikely as an explanation for MCS. In the early 1980s, it was possible to see patients from clinical ecology clinics (mostly but not exclusively in the Midwest) who had been patch tested to skin irritants, placed on extremely restricted diets with specialty food and supplement items purchased from their clinician, treated for *Candida* infection over a long period, and given a wide range of nonstandard medical remedies. Clinicians and scientists concur that it is unreasonable to criticize present MCS clinical practices and scientific hypotheses related to MCS because of the historical background in clinical ecology. Of importance, however, the same treatment strategies persist and patients receiving them are encountered quite commonly in referral clinics.

Historical antecedents also precede the clinical ecology movement. A common assumption, that nonspecific complaints began in the late 20th century with the introduction of synthetic chemistry to industry and consumer goods, lacks historical perspective. The neurasthenia diagnosis of the 19th century generally attributed to Glenard (8) but actually around since the end of the Civil War (9), also attempted to explain generalized, non–organ-specific symptoms. Neurasthenia appears to have become an even more common middle-class diagnosis during the 19th century than MCS today. By the turn of the century, more than 1,000 articles and numerous books had appeared concerning Glenard's disease (10). Many authorities eventually considered the syndrome to be due to autointoxication. Autointoxication was hypothesized to be the production of internal toxins at a rate faster than the detoxification mechanism of the liver and kidneys. It shared with MCS a primarily middle class, female sex, Caucasian race population background, as well as symptoms of "dopiness," headaches, abdominal discomfort, and decreased appetite (not necessarily accompanied by weight loss). For neurasthenia then and for MCS now, there is a contrast with the usual population demographics of somatization disorder, which is more common in disadvantaged socioeconomic groups. Neurasthenia and MCS clearly started as middle-class afflictions. Marcel Proust (1871–1922) was a famous neurasthenia-type sufferer. His affliction was as modern as his prose. Proust is said to have lived the last years of his life in a cork-lined bedroom and instructed visitors not to wear perfume.

In the 1930s, Selye proposed that similar nonspecific symptoms might be a general adaptation syndrome related to stress (10). His writings are being reevaluated in a neuroendocrine context by those who believe that olfactory sensations may cue some individuals to cope less successfully. In the 1950s, the allergic tension-fatigue syndrome was considered to cause dysfunctional behavior patterns, uniting Selye's concepts of stress with growing appreciation of immunologic responses such as allergy. Two other syndromes, chronic brucellosis and chronic hypoglycemia, were also invoked to explain multisystem complaints during the 1950s and subsequently. Some aspects of the hypoglycemia hypothesis are still held in Japan (11), but used to explain a much narrower range of behavioral symptoms restricted to judgment deficits and poor performance.

Clinical ecology relied heavily on neutralization concepts, but was not the first or most prominent movement to do so. Similarities in the belief systems of clinical ecologists today and homeopaths of two centuries ago have been inadequately discussed, as have reasons why such belief systems might persist in the absence of evidence. Other echoes of clinical ecology and still earlier concepts can recur in modern MCS discussions. Ashford and Miller (4) regard adaptation as habituation or tolerance with repeated exposures that result in a masking of symptoms. Withdrawal symptoms occur when exposure is discontinued. The adaptation is considered to obscure the effects of a specific exposure in the already-sensitized individual, and chemical exposures may adversely impact adaptation mechanisms. These concepts hark directly back to Randolph. The suggested treatment relies on a reversal of adaptation that parallels the diagnostic approach. Physicians are advised to "de-adapt" the patient with options including an environmental unit as well as judicious avoidance (4). Avoidance is the most prominent surviving clinical ecology recommendation in the MCS armamentarium, and the hardest to quantify. Depending on clinician and patient, it can be a useful coping strategy or a socially devastating prescription.

## CURRENT OVERLAP SYNDROMES

Several other syndromes resemble MCS, including chronic fibromyalgia, chronic candidiasis-hypersensitivity syndrome, chronic Epstein-Barr virus syndrome (now considered to be a relatively less likely cause of chronic fatigue), chronic fatigue syndrome, and chronic food sensitivity. In Sweden, symptoms resembling those of North American MCS patients are commonly ascribed to exposure to electromagnetic fields (12). There are several differences between the overlap syndromes and MCS. The essential difference is that MCS patients necessarily attribute initial causation and subsequent symptoms to chemical exposure, triggered following olfactory or occasionally visual cues. Besides the less certain reference to environmental olfactory-perceptible exposure, the other overlap syndromes are in some way more specific. They may rely on a specific if controversial laboratory test (as in Epstein-Barr virus syndrome), a stereotypic set of reproducible if subjective clinical findings (chronic fibromyalgia), or a sina qua non complaint (chronic fatigue). Nevertheless, MCS patients commonly carry several of the overlap diagnoses from one or more of their providers. As in the days of clinical ecology, many have been treated chronically for yeast infection. A prominent MCS clinician has pointed out that many patients carrying the more common fibromyalgia label might actually have MCS or chronic fatigue syndrome (13).

Similarities of MCS, chronic fatigue, and fibromyalgia include mean age (41 to 44), gender (60% to 90% female), unmarried status (for MCS and fibromyalgia), and relatively high educational attainment (mean 14.7 to 14.9 years in clinical series). Shared complaints include myalgia, arthralgia, fatigue, sleep disturbance, confusion or similar thought problem, and headache (14). An important point for an occupational health readership is the very low degree of current employment in all three groups, usually under 20% for MCS patients. It is reasonable to investigate whether the specific diagnosis for the overlap syndromes in local populations might vary substantially in small area analyses.

Research regarding the overlap syndromes has been potentially instructive for MCS; the concept of overlap stems from similarity of symptoms and frequency of shared diagnoses. Where overlap syndromes have proposed specific causes or outcomes, well-designed studies can be devised to test the proposed relationship. A randomized, double-blind trial of nystatin therapy did not reduce systemic or psychologic symptoms of women with presumed chronic candidiasis-hypersensitivity syndrome, compared to placebo (15). An accompanying editorial pointed out the disconnection between the opinions of leading scientists and those of the public, noting that 775,000 copies of the book *The Yeast Connection* had already been sold (16). This editorial touched upon the generalized limitation of any well-designed study of an alleged phenomenon that leads to a negative outcome; it is only a beginning point for the evaluation of the presence or absence of a hypothesized etiologic relationship. This problem certainly exists in the interpretation of MCS literature.

A similarly robust double-blind study design was used to evaluate the clinical hypothesis that respiratory and CNS outcomes of food allergy can be identified by intradermal injection of extracts of the offending allergens, which are used to reproduce symptoms. The similarity of this technique to diagnostic processes of clinical ecology and neutralization treatments concepts of MCS is noteworthy. It was found that when symptom provocation was evaluated under true double-blind conditions, provocation testing and the use of treatments based on neutralizing doses were unrelated to symptoms and outcomes (17). The accompanying editorial emphasized that food allergies are very real and referable to specific organs and outcomes. Generalized psychologic reactions, on the other hand, need to be addressed through truly blind challenges or else patient and caregiver alike risk self-deception (18).

## EPIDEMIOLOGY

Several case series show the treated MCS population to be 70% to 88% female (19). A clinical sample of 705 sequential patients at an academic center found that 27/224 women and 12/471 men met the clinic's clinical criteria for MCS diagnosis (a few patients could not participate) (20). The authors noted that symptomatic reactivity was also high among asthma patients, although not so high as among MCS patients. Women responded to a significantly greater number of substances overall, independent of the MCS diagnosis. Other common clinic-based demographic factors in several case series are enormous preponderance of Caucasian race and a plurality of the college educated. While clinic-based studies may overestimate the degree of unemployment in the MCS population, as high as 85% in some case series (21), unemployment is clearly very common.

No reliable estimate of population prevalence or incidence can be presented. The descriptive epidemiology has been based on case series. Nonrepresentative clinic samples are a particular concern in academic clinics, due to their referral nature. A nonrandom survey of 122 clinicians, heavily linked to academic centers, revealed that 71% had made a diagnosis of MCS (22).

Some population data exist concerning odor perception. A required classroom questionnaire of 543 college students identified 66% who reported illness following exposure to one of the following substances: pesticides, automobile exhaust, paint, new carpet, and perfume. Fifteen percent reported sickness after smelling at least four of these (23). This demonstrated that reactions to odors are common, but it leaves open the question of how common are subsequent decompensatory episodes. One of the physiologic hypotheses for MCS relates to olfactory disturbances. Olfactory disturbance is not at all unique to the MCS setting. Olfactory disturbance is also said to be common in exposed workers (24–26). Asthma patients also share with MCS patients a perception that odors make them worse. A random telephone survey of 1,446 households in rural North Carolina defined the chemically sensitive as individuals who admitted that chemical odors made them sick. Approximately one-third of respondents were said to suffer chemical sensitivity after interviewer prompting that potential irritating agents included perfume, pesticides, fresh paint, environmental cigarette smoke, new carpets, and car exhaust (27). Again, the definition of illness was unclear. Perception that odors are unpleasant to participants is indistinguishable in this study design from the decompensation and adverse social consequences experienced by MCS patients. The North Carolina survey researchers did find an intriguing increased disability among those who fit their odor dislike definition of chemical sensitivity, but did not clarify if disability preceded odor intolerance or was attributed to odor intolerance in the survey population, nor whether demographic factors related to the disability or intermediate outcome of odor intolerance. If a purpose of the survey had been to better understand the MCS phenomenon, use of the more complete questionnaire validated by Kipen and colleagues (20) would have been helpful.

Populations at risk because of exposure characteristics have been suggested to include industrial workers, sick building occupants, inhabitants of contaminated communities, and individuals (28). These clinical risk factors are inclusive, and should not be confused with epidemiologic concepts of excess risk. No reliable etiologic studies have been done concerning risk factors. Creation of such studies will be challenging given the variability of case definition and the absence of physiologic correlates, and the potential social incentives (and disincentives) pertaining to sufferers, clinicians, and insurers.

Prospective designs are needed but may be unaffordable. If population concepts of MCS are to advance, the relatively protective factors of blue collar work, low socioeconomic class, and possibly actual exposure to toxic chemicals will have to be explained. The explanation will need to relate epidemiologic findings to physiologic characteristics, presumably in terms acceptable to scientists and clinicians. Case series have both suggested and refuted high rates of preexisting psychiatric disorders (19,29). This remains a point of heated disagreement. The best-designed studies suggest excess premorbid somatization, even in comparison to a control population at high risk (low back pain patients receiving compensation) (30), but wide agreement has not been reached. Broad coverage of symptom surveys is unwarranted here, as poor study design and conflicting evidence still characterize a field dominated by subjective complaint epidemiology. In short, inadequate population data concerning premorbid risk factors exist to date despite copious publication.

Important population issues that have not been addressed include the incidence/prevalence of those meeting some standard case definition, demographic variability including geographic and socioeconomic status factors, longitudinal studies that can address premorbid conditions and potential risk factors, useful (or useless) therapies for some of the more common symptoms, as well as natural history for subsequent coded diagnoses, mortality, and socioeconomic outcomes. Small area studies for comparison of MCS diagnoses and practices would be helpful, but do not yet exist.

Population cognitive research is also indicated in the MCS population. By definition, MCS patients are selected for resistance to psychologic interpretations for their neuropsychologic outcomes such as confusion, memory loss, and lethargy. Much of the case series literature focuses on coexisting DSM diagnoses. In contrast, designed epidemiologic studies have less predictably shown that MCS patients have intercurrent psychiatric diagnoses. The issue is complicated by the ubiquitous symptoms of intermittent and sometimes permanent psychologic deficits in the MCS population, a clear complaint-based clinical outcome whose cause is in dispute in population surveys. Similar populations in Scandinavia, whose behavioral patterns are often attributed to electric fields rather than chemicals, have been willing to receive psychologic testing and (apparently successful) intervention, so long as it was packaged in the context of research (12).

Clinical population observations that have not been addressed by either case-control or longitudinal methodology include the prevalence of earlier abdominal and gynecologic surgery in MCS patients, and the likelihood that initial clinician visits by MCS patients will be made accompanied by a significant other or patient advocate. These descriptive statistics, if available, could be compared to similar findings in other conditions. The effect of the Internet and other means of communication upon the prevalence of MCS would also be important population information, but difficult to obtain. Among 112 patients who reported MCS symptoms following well-documented exposures to either organophosphate or carbamate pesticides, or else to building remodeling activities, Miller and Mitzel (21) noted that nearly 25% also reported subsequent sensitivity to watching television. This suggests more North American similarity to the Scandinavian experience (12) than is commonly discussed. Miller and Mitzel hypothesized that such reports were not independent phenomena, and may have resulted from communication among patients. Their conclusion was that such reports are fertile grounds for cognitive research.

An interesting aspect of MCS and the overlap syndromes is a perception that they are less commonly diagnosed in developing countries, despite plentiful encounters with chemicals in poorly controlled industry and in daily life. The possible reasons for the perceived difference (if real) include absence of clinical acumen (in either developed or developing countries), differences in reporting, differences in social interpretation of symptoms by patients or clinicians, and true differences in epidemiology between developed and developing countries.

## ETIOLOGIC HYPOTHESES AND RESULTS OF STUDIES

Etiologic hypotheses by clinical ecologists about MCS centered, initially, on the immune system first and then on opposing psychological explanations. Clinical ecologists proposed that MCS related to either the total environmental load of all toxic stressors or the patient's adaptation to toxic stressors. As most MCS patients have relatively low ongoing exposures, scientific hypotheses centered upon immunology and psychology. What else could explain idiosyncratic, dose-independent production of dramatic reversible symptoms not explicable by easily measured physiologic changes? Furthermore, sensitivity is immunology to most doctors and in the eyes of toxicologists.

For a while, there appeared to be support for immunologic changes in MCS populations. Batteries including multiple immunologic parameters with low thresholds for abnormalities were reported to be abnormal in MCS sufferers, even in comparison to control populations. A literature including some peer review publications concerning MCS immunologic abnormalities sprang from these unconventional applications of immunologic testing, but it was clear that the tests had not been performed blindly and compared to matched blind controls. Furthermore, the substantial normal variability and age-dependence of the measures and their ratios (31) were rarely accounted. Researchers in Washington State replicated the battery of immunologic tests on 41 MCS patients from a single practitioner (30). The immunologic battery duplicated the practice of the same laboratory that had participated earlier in nonblind peer review publication. Blinded specimens were sent to this laboratory along with control specimens from a population suffering from back pain. The key to the study design was the addition of the blinded control population for comparison of laboratory outcomes. The choice of back pain patients as the control group was excellent. Back pain patients face social stressors, but they are not hypothesized to have immunologic deficits as a cause of their condition. The study found that control patients were as likely or more likely to have reported immunologic abnormalities, including anti–smooth muscle, anti–parietal cell, anti–brush border, antimitochondrial, and antinuclear antibodies (30). The finding of 63% of cases and 68% controls with autoimmune antibodies will remind clinician readers of the profoundly unacceptable laboratory interpretations that accompanied MCS patient care and MCS research at the advent of the 1990s. (While the research is now much better, MCS patients still may come to the office with unconventional, seldom repeatable, probably meaningless immunologic results.)

Reactions of the medical community were then and have remained predictable. A mainstream perspective, outside of a few centers and clinical ecology clinics, holds that hypersensitivity of MCS patients is not based on reproducible immunologic findings. Causes of MCS or MCS-like symptoms have been attributed to depression (29), somatoform disorder (32,33), posttraumatic stress (e.g., to sexual abuse) (34), psychosis (33), anxiety disorder (33), panic disorder (29,35,36), personality disorder (33), obsessive or paranoid personality (37), and conditioned response (38). Physiologic proposals include abnormal red cell glycolytic energy metabolism, suspected abnormalities of heme synthesis such as porphyria, labile autonomic function with cognitive sequelae (39), and a never quite disappearing variety of proposed autoimmune abnormalities including both high and low helper/suppressor ratios (40). Abnormal neuropeptide mediator release or abnormal hypothalamic control form another class of hypotheses. These are plausible, and await their first well-designed experiments. Gots (41) has pointed out that current understanding of pathophysiology connects the multiorgan system complaints of MCS patients to a toxicodynamic process only through behavioral mechanisms, of whatever cause. Labile autonomic function might be considered a physiologic factor that affects emotions, or the reverse depending on circumstance and preference. This pertains more clearly to theories of limbic kindling, as exploration of the neurophysiology of the multiple system responder still fails to distinguish between classical conditioning and organic disease (41).

CNS changes following perception of stimuli are real and will be demonstrated. Whether the cause is conditioned and whether the process is toxicologic will be disputed. The difficulty of making this distinction can be seen in a nicely designed experiment pertaining to patients with electrical hypersensitivity. Ten patients complaining of electrical hypersensitivity and matched controls were exposed to amplitude-modulated light, between 20 and 75 flashes per second. Visual evoked potentials were measured and found to be phase-locked to the oscillations, as expected. The visual evoked potential amplitudes were higher in electrical sensitivity patients than controls at all frequencies (42). This study of a syndrome related by outcome to MCS provides a Rorschach test for our personal prejudices about mind-body phenomena. Does the result show a baseline physiologic or a psychologic difference in response between populations? The authors stressed that hyperreactive nervous systems of case subjects may or may not explain their subjective symptoms or the reported association to electrical fields. Studies using sophisticated neuroimaging or other technologies will face similar philosophical hurdles of interpretation. As we are able to clearly visualize the chemical changes of the depressed or frightened brain, are we then seeing physiologic change, psychologic change, or both, and is the cause intrinsic to the brain or due to external environmental factors? What experimental protocol will allow us to tease these issues apart?

There is already ample evidence that psychologic stress in normal humans causes measurable and eventually irreversible physiologic change. The relationship of chronic anger to heart disease provides one example. Far from the MCS battlefront, research is now under way to determine if prayer and meditation can be regarded as important preventive or mitigating factors for outcomes ranging from heart disease to chronic pain. Not surprisingly, this mind-body research is also interpreted in quite polarized ways (43,44), ranging from praise for cutting-edge innovation to judgments of junk science. If perceptions of stress cause harm, and meditation or prayer are hypothesized to be associated with positive outcomes, then the mind-body dualism requiring that MCS suffering be due to emotions or to physiology may not be clinically important. (The related question concerning whether the causes are external or internal to the patient may be easier to address, but only so long as we consider stress reactions as solely internal or solely external force.). Furthermore, a perception is growing that diagnoses that separate the mind and body, such as somatization disorder, are overly simplistic and show an absence of care for the patient (45). In a more complex biopsychosocial model of disease (46), perceptions about mind-body dualism change rapidly. Nevertheless, concepts of causation (whether psychological, physiologic, or biopsychosocial) remain central to social application of insurance and responsibility for payments. It is likely that monetary linkages to causation will remain central to insurance systems such as workers' compensation as well as to tort law. The question concerning intrinsic versus extrinsic cause remains fundamental to our socioeconomic system of just compensation, even as the biopsychosocial model overtakes dualism in our concept of physiology. Future maturation of physiologic understanding and increased compassion hold unpredictable impact for future application of insurance and tort transfers of wealth. The need to distinguish between intrinsic and extrinsic factors will not disappear until the social setting changes dramatically, despite more sophisticated biopsychosocial concepts.

Scientific data demonstrate repeated linkages between emotional patterns such as bereavement or depression and immunologic parameters such as natural killer (NK) cell activity, T-helper/suppressor ratios, and B antibody titers, as well as with endocrinologic parameters such as circulating glucocorticoids (47). These linkages suggest the very high degree of difficulty in the leap from asserting to proving that the chemical exposure itself is externally responsible for independently verifiable physiologic change, when evidence of organ damage is absent. Furthermore, immunologic conditioned-response to perceived stress has been demonstrated for a decade (48). Similar observations abound for neurologic measures. The normal human EEG changes in response to odors (49). Most studies purporting to evaluate presence/absence of behavior-caused or behavior-free neurohumoral or neuroendocrine changes in MCS patients are of completely inadequate design in the context of what is already known about this topic. In a biopsychosocial model of MCS, the definition of MCS could refer to the perception of exposure rather than exposure. For reasons that may relate to insurance, indemnity, and self-image, the MCS advocacy community is not ready for this step.

## DESIGNED TRIALS POTENTIALLY RELATED TO ETIOLOGY

A double-blind chamber controlled challenge to substances identified by consenting MCS patients as inciting reactions, and to sham substances, was conducted at the Allergy Respiratory Institute of Colorado from 1985 to 1988 (50). All exposures were accompanied by a patient-tolerated odor masking agent such as cinnamon. All exposures were below the threshold limit value (TLV®). Active agents included formaldehyde, natural gas, cleaners, and several solvents. For the 145 challenges to 20 patients, response sensitivity was 33%; response specificity was 65%; response efficiency was 52%. The authors concluded that MCS patients could not differentiate active agents from controls. Given present controversies of context, presentation of economic support and institutional review board information would be important for those who attempt to validate this finding or undertake similar research in future. A conclusion that might be drawn from challenge data to date is that MCS patients do not experience their symptoms following exposures that lack sensory-environmental cues. Present evidence suggests that chemical exposure without perceived odor or other sensory confirmation of exposure might not incite the syndrome.

Designed provocative challenges of MCS patients have occurred in several settings. In a study that does have a clear positive statement about institutional review, Leznoff (51) exposed patients to self-identified stressors ranging from hairspray to the Yellow Pages. Challenges reproduced symptoms predictably, including tachycardia, tremor, and pallor in some cases. Declines in $CO_2$ were noted, without change in $SaO_2$ or flow volume curves. The author concluded that hyperventilation was the condition most consistent with the data and hypothesized that the cause was anxiety reaction. Support for a broad anxiety etiology, as opposed to specific olfactory limbic stimulation, came from patients who reacted to odorless (but tactile-perceptible) stimulants.

In a smaller and more invasive study that also had a clear institutional review, Binkley and Kutcher (52) exposed five MCS patients to single-blind intravenous infusions of normal saline placebo or sodium lactate. Patients selected for study did not have major psychiatric diagnoses, in keeping with the relative absence of major psychiatric diagnoses in most MCS populations. Subjects completed acute panic inventories during the procedure; five of five experienced a panic-like state during lactate infusion. Nonlactate infusion and non-MCS control groups were not used, a potential design weakness. The authors provide references concerning the utility of the lactate infusion in the diagnosis of panic attacks. This study warrants double-blind repetition in a larger population with appropriate population and infusion controls. The authors did not discuss that their data indirectly address and do not support (but cannot rule out) hypotheses such as abnormal glycolytic energy metabolism, which would affect oxygen carrying capacity of red cells. In an earlier study of 18 matched cases and controls, olfactory thresholds were not different in MCS patients, but MCS patients had higher nasal resistance, respiratory rates, and depression inventories (53). The higher respiratory rate is also consistent with but not proof of an anxiety-hyperventilation hypothesis.

## IMPACT OF COMMUNITY ACTIVISM

The history of community activism to combat environmental evils goes back a long way, and includes efforts to provide cleaner heating fuels in urban areas, better housing in ghettos, and unadulterated food. The MCS community and its antecedent clinical ecology movement have been similarly engaged. Furthermore, apparently low employment rates among a relatively well-educated population suggest favorable conditions for advocacy.

There are numerous support groups, patient advocacy groups, and clinician advocacy groups, such as the Human Action Ecology League, the Environmental Illness Society of Canada, the American Academy of Environmental Medicine, and MCS Referral and Resources, as well as patient support newsletters. Patient contributors describe themselves as "universal reactors," "chemies," or "canaries" (54). By 1988, the psychologist leader of an MCS support group could testify before a state senate that she was part of a larger group of 2,000 individuals in Maryland alone. MCS patients and clinicians (including former clinical ecologists) frequently appear in numbers at state and federal proceedings relating to their clinical and economic interests. These are typically American aspects of advocacy, and it is not surprising that advocacy accompanies a controversial diagnosis affecting a patient population with strong needs for institutional and governmental support. The Association of Trial Lawyers of America established a clearinghouse on legal aspects of ecologic illness in 1989. More recently, counterorganizations have appeared with an oppositional mission to debunk MCS practice.

The advent of Internet communication has facilitated a full flowering support group strategy. There are recruitment functions for new patients, who are given their Internet diagnosis once inquiries are made. Thought-provoking communications with or from patients appear routinely. There are what amount to advertisements for new recruits featuring possible symptoms such as "tired and sleepy 30 minutes after eating," "hyper after meals or a birthday party," "recurrent urinary problems," and "depression" among symptoms of environmental illness. Interpersonal support functions are strongly represented. An interesting Internet trend is the rapid identification of what amounts to an enemies list, with personal and professional attacks on authors of contradictory opinions. Communication from patients and clinicians about legal or public relations battles and victories, and information concerning how on-line communicants may join in productively are also featured. This trend is probably not unique to MCS.

An ongoing and problematic aspect of community activism has been the history of identifying problem environments and environmental causation based on inadequate data. At the local level, MCS clinicians and building managers may make competing assumptions about environments, often school environments with children as pawns in political battles. These assumptions may rely on inadequate environmental data for either side to determine if there is a problem other than symptom complaints of one or several individuals. Sometimes the controversy reaches the headlines. The article by Simon and colleagues (30) debunking immunologic diagnoses of MCS (described in the section Etiologic Hypotheses) followed months of major newspaper headlines concerning alleged environmental problems and population outcomes at the work site of a local employer, diagnosed by a single practitioner and relying on the laboratory whose tests were subsequently found to have little value in the context used. The newspaper publishing the articles gave little evidence that it was aware that its story was based on unconventional uses of diagnostic data, or that it cared that a well-designed study of this or another population from the same clinician could be predicted to debunk some of its headlines. (Simon and colleagues studied another population from the same clinician.) It is unclear if residents of the community have been told in equally bold terms of the significance of subsequent research.

Fear of retribution following publication of studies or expression of opinions that disagree with those of special interest groups is a societal problem of intolerance that MCS has not escaped. The best-known attack was on Simon and colleagues following their well-designed blinded study of immunologic parameters in MCS patients. Attacks on their conduct and research led to a long inquiry process within their institutions, state medical board, and the federal Office of Research Integrity before they were exonerated. A recounting of the deliberate and unwarranted personal interference with the authors lives is understated in their subsequent editorial about the experience (55). Every author who evaluates or discusses MCS must consider the possibility of personal hardship, including potential attacks by colleagues or advocacy groups. Nor are attacks limited to one side.

A recent news exposé on a major network program revealed potentially problematic aspects of MCS practice to the public, but it also provided a substantial dose of innuendo, entrapment, and sloppy vocabulary in the eyes of MCS patients and practitioners. In the news-entertainment forum, there is little room for rebuttal or scientific discussion. MCS advocates presented their countercharges in court and on the Internet. Legal charges against the producers of the news program were investigated by the Maryland attorney general and dropped.

MCS controversies highlight tensions between professional standards and advocacy perceptions, with a subtext of scientific values and potential harm to patients versus self-determination of individuals in a free society. A recent Internet inquiry from a physician concerned a search for the evidence basis of oxygen therapy in MCS. The advocacy response was related to but slightly off the mark from the scientific inquiry: "Our paper on Recognition of MCS lists one court case involving oxygen treatments." A case citation is given, "in which the plaintiffs won the right to receive oxygen treatments for MCS by successfully appealing to the Superior Court of Alameda

County that overturned the prior ruling of an administrative law judge."

Public discussion about diagnosis and care of MCS patients typically speeds by scientific evidence and dwells on familiar aspects of public conflict in our society: personal rights, personal interests of patients, potential conflicts of interest of investigators, legal victories and losses, and how to obtain or avoid paying for desired goods, services, and indemnity support. Inflexible advocacy positions present major impediments for thoughtful researchers seeking an evidence basis for MCS.

## POSITIONS OF PROFESSIONAL SOCIETIES

The American Academy of Allergy was the first professional society to deem the phenomenon of MCS worthy of a position paper. The academy labeled the clinical ecology movement "unproved and experimental" (56). The California Medical Association considered clinical ecology concepts to be inadequately supported by the medical literature (57).

The American College of Physicians took its position in 1989 (58). It acknowledged Cullen's work and the MCS definition, but it did not distinguish the clinical ecology movement from the later MCS phenomenon. The position paper evaluated provocation neutralization testing, immunologic test outcomes, and associated treatment including avoidance therapy. The American College of Physicians concluded, "Review of the clinical ecology movement provides inadequate support for the beliefs and practices of clinical ecology. The existence of an environmental illness as presented in clinical ecology theory must be questioned because of the lack of a clinical definition. Diagnoses and treatments involve procedures of no proven efficacy." The American College paper also pointed out that the practice of environmental medicine cannot be considered harmless. Severe restraints are placed on patients lives, and in many cases invalidism is reinforced as patients develop increasingly iatrogenic disability. Treatment frequently creates a severe financial burden for patients and health insurers. The position paper was authored primarily by Dr. Abba Terr, who has also editorialized against the MCS diagnosis and clinical practice in other settings. Most of the criticisms in the editorial were directed against provocation-neutralization testing and neutralizing therapy. Fortunately, these practices were already becoming less common in the MCS research community be the time the editorial appeared. The inclusion of the term *environmental medicine* for opprobrium was distinctly unfortunate. The American College confused a laudable mainstream interdisciplinary trend, the consideration of preventable causes of environmental illness ranging from lead poisoning to ozone depletion, with the MCS controversy.

The American Medical Association (AMA) published a council report on MCS in 1992 (59). It pointed out that clinical ecology and MCS need not be synonymous, but chose to treat them as one issue. The AMA concurred with the universal wisdom that "there are no well-controlled studies establishing a clear mechanism of cause," and pointed out that "[no] confirmation of the efficacy of the diagnostic and therapeutic modalities existed." The AMA recommended that the burden of proof for support of new tests or treatments must be by controlled peer review trials and that the responsibility is on the shoulders of those who use them. This position is not substantially different from those expressed by other organizations.

The American College of Occupational and Environmental Medicine (ACOEM) first stated its position in 1991 (60). It characterized MCS as a "poorly defined entity" and concluded that the existence of a multiple chemical hypersensitivity syndrome is an unproven hypothesis, that current treatment methods represent an experimental methodology, and that scientific research was needed, and the college further admonished that such research should adhere to established principles of scientific inquiry. A 1993 addendum to the position noted that the impact of some experimental treatment modalities on lifestyle and productivity may be significant. ACOEM offered specific guidelines for conduct and goals of research based on this observation. Paraphrasing from their document:

- A clear case definition with established diagnostic criteria is needed. Investigators should specify criteria for inclusion/exclusion and adhere to the case definition.
- The case definition must distinguish between MCS and other medical conditions including allergy, skin conditions, chronic fatigue, and toxic or neurologic conditions.
- Demographic data of the affected population are needed.
- The efficacy, side effects, and long-term outcomes of treatment modalities must be examined (ACOEM characterized this as the most important research need).
- Hypothesized pathophysiologic and psychologic mechanisms leading to the development of MCS should be investigated.

ACOEM reiterated the need for peer review. It further cautioned investigators that MCS research is not synonymous with indoor air quality (IAQ) investigations, and suggested MCS considerations incorporated into IAQ research would only confuse the IAQ investigative process. It should be noted that the revised position was written before the advent of survey research on Persian Gulf war veterans, and may now require further consideration concerning areas of potential avoidable confusion in clinic and research settings.

An International Labor Office–sponsored panel prepared a preliminary document in 1996 about MCS under the aegis of the International Programme on Chemical Safety. The panel recommended that the term *multiple chemical sensitivity* be changed because it suggested an unsupported judgment about causation. An alternative *term—idiopathic environmental intolerances*—was proposed in draft. The panel noted that the relationship between exposures and symptoms is unknown, and that there are no validated criteria for diagnosis. Other than a proposed name change, this recommendation is merely a rearticulation of the caveats in earlier discussions and should not have been seen as controversial. Those interested in the politics of MCS should read subsequent Internet discussions, personal accusations, and organizational conspiracy discussions. The proposed name change will not become an official recommendation, in all likelihood, and international groups will likely be more cautious in the future before treading on this primarily North American turf.

Among official positions, ACOEM (60) has drawn the clearest distinction between the clinical ecology practitioner and the research needs related to more modern concepts of MCS. The initial position used the term *multiple chemical hypersensitivity syndrome,* suggesting that skepticism was directed at an immunologic hypothesis. In the addendum focusing on research needs, the broader MCS term was used. ACOEM has also recognized the gradual assumption by MCS practitioners that indoor air problems are a primary etiologic cause of the MCS phenomenon, and addresses the corresponding confusion of building engineering consensus about indoor air quality in habitable buildings with MCS outcomes.

Among official positions, the AMA and ACOEM clearly designate that they are dealing with MCS as a syndrome as well as with clinical ecologists as practitioners. ACOEM alone addresses an industrial hygiene public health issue. All official positions uniformly state that the burden of proof for clinical practices, including diagnosis and treatment, has not been met.

## CLINICAL PRESENTATION OF MCS PATIENTS

By definition, MCS patients present with symptoms out of proportion to physical findings. In other ways, MCS patients differ remarkably from one another, far more than patients with other syndromes of unknown cause, such as sarcoidosis or most headaches. First, MCS patients have different triggers, especially at the onset of their presentation. Patients may report their first negative experiences with substantial or insubstantial exposure to transportation fuels, batch chemicals of numerous unrelated classes, pesticide applications, fertilizer applications, paints and varnishes, "sick" buildings, products of incomplete combustion, and cleaners. Many patients also describe intolerance to tap water, prescription and over-the-counter pharmaceuticals other than herbal remedies, and a variety of foods. This list is incomplete. Its variability is not surprising in either a physiologic or a psychological model of causation. After all, hundreds of different agents cause occupational asthma, and asthma alone has many presentations. Many stressors can lead to anxiety, depression, and feelings of hopelessness, in the presence or absence of MCS.

Symptoms and especially chief complaints also vary dramatically among MCS patients. Many have intermittent memory deficits, sparing the part of the brain that recalls exposures. Patients may be most concerned about light-headedness, intermittent or permanent memory loss or orientation difficulties, sudden losses of alertness or even consciousness, chronic fatigue (both lethargy and somnolence), muscle aches, muscle twitches, rashes, tremor, paresthesia, incoordination, breathlessness (without clinical detection of reversible airway obstruction), intermittent weakness or even paralysis of specific parts of the body or the entire body, headache, gastrointestinal pain or other gastrointestinal discomfort, and panic (1,61). Of these complaints, rashes and specific areas of weakness should be amenable to external validation. The concept that MCS patients feel well between exposures or between episodes need not be true. Many MCS patients feel bad all the time, and worse during episodes.

Common distinguishing presentations of many long-term MCS patients include a desire for separate access to the clinician, away from other patients who may wear perfume or use scented soap, and away from hospital materials (such as antiseptics and cleaning materials). More recent sufferers are less likely to request separate access. A few will be wearing respirators. Over time, MCS patients have improved their choice of respirators so that most respirator wearers now use the correct filters for routine chemical filtration. This is too bad, as previous paper respirator use was less isolating, and there has been no difference in perceived efficacy.

Many MCS patients are accompanied to the clinician by a significant other. The clinician should attempt to take the history from the patient, but the social dynamic between the patient and the significant others also provides information. It is likely that the social disruption associated with the syndrome fosters relationships with solicitous others, but that relationships with those who are not solicitous may end. It is possible, however, that solicitousness and acquiescence of family and friends is a part of the syndrome. Designing studies to address this clinical perception would be difficult.

MCS patients are also not cut from a cookie cutter in their self-perception and in their approach to cosmetics or even perfumes. Some MCS patients wear lipstick and eye shadow. A few have discovered that only specific perfumes and deodorants bother them. Some work on their cars, noting for example that grease does not bother them but cleanup solvents are a problem. MCS patients are a substantially labile population group, but some MCS patients remain composed and respond in a straightforward manner throughout their evaluation. Many express insight and concern that their symptoms may sound crazy, and most but not all are sure that there is no important psychological context for their experiences. Over time, male and even occasional blue-collar MCS patients have become more common, although they are still not the norm. Over time, it is very likely that MCS will follow the trajectory of historical antecedent diagnoses and find a home in the lower socioeconomic classes.

The physical examination is generally normal. Serious abnormalities have other diagnostic categories. These abnormalities may not preclude the MCS diagnosis, but they most often take precedence in the clinical assessment. It is therefore not surprising that MCS patients have normal findings.

Experienced MCS patients become aware that traditional clinicians often do little to reverse the course of their disease. Many but not all have sought nontraditional forms of therapy. This should be recognized as a potential danger point for patients, on several levels. Patients seek multiple providers and many have encounters with expensive therapies including unusual diet, sauna, special habitations, and unusual and even dangerous remedies such as chelation, supplements, and herbs. These therapies are often not covered by insurance, and thus patients face the economic consequences. To put this in perspective, adverse economic outcomes of health care provision are neither exclusively nor largely the domain of nontraditional providers.

Patient presentations also warrant discussion in a public health and population context. School superintendents or employers may receive letters about responsibility and liability from MCS clinicians, letters that often originate far from the patient's school or workplace. The contents of these letters are sometimes quite threatening, and recipients may be shocked into action and seek advice of public health departments or clinicians with environmental expertise. From a public health perspective, the problem that can be addressed is most often a potentially "sick" building. The building itself should not be confused with the symptoms. Building evaluation is critical, based on common engineering and industrial hygiene principles.

A central clinical assessment need for patients going to nontraditional providers is the degree of and further increase in social isolation. It is not possible to say if withdrawal from one's social life is an outcome of nontraditional care, or only a consequence of the same symptom complex that drives patients to seek unsubstantiated therapies. No good studies exist on this topic.

## EVALUATION AND TREATMENT

It is easier to discuss what does not work, what is not evidence-based, and what is socially isolating and potentially harmful than it is to recommend what is helpful. The best results are obtained by clinicians who exhibit a strong sense of compassion and a willingness to spend time to build a clinical bond, and who have a healthy sense of the harm they can do if they try to do more than gently challenge the patient to improve. Evaluation should be directed to ruling out other diagnoses. This is usually simple, unless previous inappropriate testing requires more extensive follow-up.

The diagnosis is made by history and ruling out other diagnoses. In the hands of a skilled clinician, little testing should be necessary. Potentially useful additions to the physical examination include Schirmer's test for dry eyes, evaluation of postural blood pressure changes, and voluntary hyperventilation in the event that symptoms are reproduced. More difficult decisions are faced when patients provide histories that might be descriptions of asthma or other reversible airway disorder, or neurologic conditions that might just be epilepsy or other organic brain diagnosis. The pulmonary function test with selective β-adrenergic stimulation (if indicated by obstruction) is a standard procedure in the initial workup of environmental asthma. It is diagnostically valuable in patients who appear to meet criteria for MCS but might also have asthma. The clinician should be prepared for inadequate test results, however, due to poor repeatability of flow volume curves by MCS patients who have not established trust. Poor repeatability of spirometry has its own diagnostic value in the MCS setting, but excessive challenges to patient trust may decrease the success of other interventions that rely on a strong sense of therapeutic bonding. A more dramatic outcome is hyperventilation or other anxiety manifestations during such tests as computed tomography (CT), magnetic resonance imaging (MRI), pulmonary function testing, and especially methacholine challenge. In addition to hyperventilation, sudden paralyses or apparent diminishment of consciousness, or other similar reversible reactions during testing can be manifested. These responses provide useful information about the patient's reaction to stress, but they are obtained at a potential risk to the establishment of a positive partnership. Clinical information can be gained, but the goal should be progress toward increased coping and decreasing symptoms.

When patients receive unconventional test results or unconventional interpretations of test results likely to increase stress, it is helpful and it can be cost-effective to repeat the test on behalf of the patient. This is a part of the treatment. Individuals suffering from MCS deserve to know that their levels of certain chemicals are indeed within population norms (and usually unrelated to distant inciting exposure). They may benefit from seeing proof that their immune system is not abnormal. Physicians may repeat unconventional tests with high-quality conventional laboratories, lest a patient believe in a nonexistent problem. Alternatively, repeat testing may confirm a real immunologic deficiency (a rare occurrence but a theoretical possibility that should not be overlooked). Helpful tests in this setting are discussed by Salvaggio and Terr (62). It should be noted, however, that extensive testing is required only when findings indicate or when there is a preexisting belief in abnormal values. Another consideration is whether to repeat tests, such as single photon emission computed tomography (SPECT) scan, for which normal expectations are not established. Probably positron emission tomography (PET) scan studies of case and control populations (with blind interpretations by investigators) are needed before this kind of imaging warrants consideration. In general, exhaustive radiographic and laboratory testing is not helpful and should be used only to rule out diseases requiring specific therapy (63).

It is very important to understand what therapies a patient is receiving before initiating new ones. Patients often do not provide complete lists initially. At the time of evaluation, questions should be posed about the following: sauna or chelation to eliminate chemicals and boost the immune system; vitamins, including some still unknown to science; sublingual or other similar desensitization schemes; other detoxifications (pellets for reversal of anthrax toxicity are an Internet favorite); oxygen therapy; and elimination or rotation diets, which are controversial in MCS as they are in other aspects of health care. Oxygen therapy proposals have not been justified by any clinical study, legal precedents notwithstanding. These therapies are at best not evidence-based. Some are harmful. It is important to understand the patient's experiences, including specific unsubstantiated therapeutic activities that the patient is willing to give up.

Prudent avoidance of the patient's particular stressors sounds reasonable, especially for patients with very specific symptom inducers. Prudent avoidance may also lead to increasing social withdrawal, including loss of contact with family, social supports, community, and employment (with associated loss of income). Psychiatric evaluation and psychologic counseling are tempting at the first nonphysiologic symptoms or when a social withdrawal cascade commences, but most MCS patients will not tolerate special psychologic approaches and will seek other providers if such suggestion is made. Psychological referral removes the patient from the office and solves the clinician's problem, but not always the patient's! Many MCS patients are shunted among (or seek) numerous clinicians. In one case series of 112 patients, 40% had consulted ten or more practitioners (21). Rather than simply refer elsewhere, the clinician can help the patient by evaluating present social function, and helping the patient cope with problems in small steps.

Patients should be encouraged to stick with their primary care physicians whenever feasible. Equally important, primary care physicians should be encouraged by consulting physicians to stick with their patients. The risk of social isolation and other harm appears to increase when this caring bond is broken. Rapport can be developed by honest admission that the causes of MCS are uncertain, and that the syndrome has important psychosocial consequences whether or not they are its cause. Rapport can be increased over time by gentle and consistent strategies that emphasize increased coping over time.

The ongoing relationship with a primary care provider does more than just protect the MCS patient from physiologically detrimental and socially isolating practices. Rapport with a health care provider is essential in any chronic disease status, and MCS qualifies whatever its cause. A primary care provider can address beneficial coping strategies and the need for exercise and social intercourse as competently as mental health professionals. While some authorities also recommend psychiatric consultation (6,62), only a minority of MCS patients comply. A regular appointment schedule with the primary care provider, independent of the need for triggering events, is important. Small and achievable goal increments, frequent encouragement, and compassion are not high tech, although they are certainly time-consuming. They are nevertheless the most successful care that MCS patients receive. Unfortunately, insurance plans generally do not cover additional frequent contact with social workers and wellness counselors.

Particularly successful strategies include emphasis that the condition has never been reported to be fatal or to cause ongoing damage to any organ system, and the gentle persuasion that patients who can focus on goals and positive outcomes do much better. Some clinicians have reported anecdotal success with masking odors (such as cinnamon) coupled with relaxation techniques. These are hopeful reports, and any evidence that these techniques work for less committed clinicians would be most welcome.

Finally the role of MCS patients' cultural views of the environment also warrants assessment (64) at both the experimental and clinical level. Understanding the belief system of the patient is critical to understanding MCS in its long-standing yet ever changing cultural context.

## DISCUSSION

Professional societies should update their recommendations concerning MCS to reflect the results of recent studies. Many MCS hypotheses have now been examined, and there are few known, extrinsic causes of MCS supported by research. Immunologic abnormality now appears to be a less plausible cause. Neuroendocrine changes are still plausible, but the understanding of normal hormonal variation in response to stress has advanced. Case reports (65,66) and case series (67) and small designed trials (51,52) have revealed a probable role of conditioned response. The role of stimulus conditioning for functions as physiologic as a cell response (68) should give pause to those who favor exclusively psychological or physiologic explanations. Findings from the Monell Chemical Senses Center, our leading odor research center, demonstrated that cognitive factors probably modulate odor perception in individuals who exhibit extreme sensitivity and do not adapt (69). Stress is real. Conditioned response is real.

Conditioned response to odor is where the best research on MCS is now taking place.

The MCS concept has always faced a number of important shortcomings, including a definition that precludes important clinical findings, and the belief of patient advocacy groups that physiologic explanations and specific etiologic causation must be supported. MCS has been an improvement over clinical ecology for research purposes, but clinical behavior remains unacceptable and little changed in many cases from the clinical ecology days.

How did a profession devoted to public health find its way into this acrimonious debate? On a grand scale, we can discuss mind-body dualism and the limitations of dualistic thinking when we know that emotional stressors are real, and that they have real physiologic consequences. That discussion is illuminating, but it does not adequately explain the anger, the personal attacks on researchers, and the need to discount and even attack the motivation for scientific investigation. It also does not address the unacceptable disdain expressed for the real suffering encountered. The acrimony is not explained by normal differences in scientific interpretation because it involves societal values, compensation indemnity for individuals who either cannot or will not cope, and the need of sufferers for social support versus the desire of potential sources of support to avoid investment in unproductive lifestyles. At its heart, the MCS debate is about social values and money.

Insurance has been inadequately discussed in the scientific community, but it is central to understanding MCS. The future diagnosis and treatment of MCS is more closely linked to insurance requirements than to scientific study. Advocacy groups understand this intuitively and they protest research that might lead to policy or policy decisions that threaten support systems. As with other illnesses of uncertain etiology, the prevalence of MCS varies depending on social support. This has already happened with chronic fibromyalgia in Canada, with the diagnosis of carpal tunnel syndrome in states that do not cover it for workers' compensation, and with low back pain in many countries, where it is treated differently than in the United States. The need for social research is great, especially on the impact of insurance coverage.

Finally, it is important to reiterate that whatever the cause of the syndrome and whatever the social controversy, MCS patients deserve competent and compassionate evaluation and treatment.

## REFERENCES


1. Cullen MR. The worker with multiple chemical sensitivities: an overview. *Occup Med State Art Rev* 1987;2:655–661.
2. National Research Council. *Multiple chemical sensitivities:* addendum to biologic markers in toxicology. Washington, DC: National Academy Press, 1992.
3. Nethercott JR, Davidoff LL, Curbow B, Abbey H. Multiple chemical sensitivities syndrome: toward a working case definition. *Arch Environ Health* 1993;48:19–26.
4. Ashford NA, Miller CS. Multiple chemical sensitivity. *Health Environ Dig* 1993;6:1–4.
5. Rest KM. Advancing the understanding of multiple chemical sensitivities (MCS): overview and recommendations from an AOEC workshop. *Toxicol Ind Health* 1992;8:1–13.
6. Simon GE. Psychiatric treatments in multiple chemical sensitivity. *Toxicol Ind Health* 1992;8:67–72.
7. Randolph TG. *Human ecology and susceptibility to the chemical environment.* Springfield, IL: Charles Thomas, 1962.
8. Glenard F. Neurasthenie et enteroptose. *Semaine Medicale* 1886;6: 211–212.
9. Beard GM. Neurasthenia, or nervous exhaustion. *Boston Med Surg J* 1869;3(new series):217–221.
10. Gots RE. Medical hypothesis and medical practice: autointoxication and multiple chemical sensitivities. *Regul Toxicol Pharmacol* 1993;18: 2–12.
11. Mogi T, Wada Y, Hirosawa I, Sasaki M, Koizami M. Epidemiological study on hypoglycemia endemic to female nurses and other workers. *Ind Health* 1996;34:335–346.
12. Andersson B, Berg M, Arnetz BB, Melin L, Langlet I, Liden S. A cognitive-behavioral treatment of patients suffering from electric hypersensitivity. *J Occup Environ Med* 1996;38:752–758.
13. Ziem G. Chronic fatigue, fibromyalgia, and chemical sensitivity: overlapping disorders [letter]. *Arch Intern Med* 1995;155:1913.
14. Buchwald D, Garrity D. Comparison of patients with chronic fatigue syndrome: similarities and differences. *Rheum Dis Clin North Am* 1996;22:219–243.
15. Dismukes WE, Wade JS, Lee JY, Dockery BK, Hain JD. A randomized double-blind trial of nystatin therapy for the candidiasis hypersensitivity syndrome. *N Engl J Med* 1990;323:1717–1723.
16. Bennett JE. Searching for the yeast connection (editorial). *N Engl J Med* 1990;323:1766–1767.
17. Jewett DL, Fein G, Greenberg MH. A double-blind study of symptom provocation to determine food sensitivity. *N Engl J Med* 1990;323: 429–433.
18. Ferguson A. Food sensitivity or self deception? (editorial). *N Engl J Med* 1990;323:476–478.
19. Sparks PJ, Daniell W, Black DW, et al. Multiple chemical sensitivity syndrome: a clinical perspective. I. Case definition; theories of pathogenesis, and research needs. *J Occup Environ Med* 1994;36:718–730.
20. Kipen HM, Hallman W, Kelly-McNeil K, Kriedler N. Measuring chemical sensitivity prevalence: a questionnaire for population studies. *Am J Public Health* 1995;85:574–577.
21. Miller CS, Mitzel HC. Chemical sensitivity attributed to pesticide exposure versus remodeling. *Arch Environ Health* 1995;50:119–129.
22. Rest KM. A survey of AOEC physician practices and attitudes regarding multiple chemical sensitivity. *Toxicol Ind Health* 1992;8:51–65.
23. Bell IR, Schwartz GE, Peterson JM, Amend D. Self-reported illness from chemical odors in young adults without clinical syndromes or occupational exposures. *Arch Environ Health* 1993;48:6–13.
24. Henkin RI, Schecter PJ, Hoye R, Mattern CF. Idiopathic hypogeusia with dysgeusia, dyposmia, and dysosmia. *JAMA* 1971;217:434–40.
25. Schwartz BS, Doty RL, Monroe C, Frye R, Barker S. Olfactory function in chemical workers exposed to acrylate and methacrylate vapors. *Am J Public Health* 1989;79:613–8.
26. Schwartz BS, Ford DP, Bolla KI, Agnew J, Rothman N, Bleecker ML. Solvent-associated decrements in olfactory function in paint manufacturing workers. *Am J Ind Med* 1990;18:697–706.
27. Meggs WJ, Dunn KA, Bloch RM, Goodman PE, Davidoff AL. Prevalence and nature of allergy and chemical sensitivity in the general population. *Arch Environ Health* 1996;51:275–282.
28. Miller CS. White paper: chemical sensitivity: history and phenomenology. *Toxicol Ind Health* 1994;253–276.
29. Sparks PJ, Simon GE, Katon WJ, Altman LC, Ayars GH, Johnson RL. An outbreak of illness among aerospace workers. *West J Med* 1990:15; 28–33.
30. Simon G, Daniell W, Stockbridge H, Claypool K, Rosenstock L. Immunologic, psychological, and neuropsychological factors in multiple chemical sensitivity: a controlled study. *Ann Intern Med* 1993; 119:97–103.
31. Lifson JD, Finch SL, Sasaki DT, Engleman EG. Variables affecting T-

lymphocyte subsets in a volunteer blood donor population. *Clin Immunol Immunopathol* 1985;36:151–160.
32. Stewart DE, Raskin J. Psychiatric assessment of patients with 20th-century disease (total allergy syndrome). *Can Med Assoc J* 1985;133: 1001–1006.
33. Barsky AJ, Borus JF. Somatization and medicalization in the era of managed care. *JAMA* 1995;274:1931–1934.
34. Staudenmeyer H, Selner ME, Selner JC. Adult sequelae of childhood abuse presenting as environmental illness. *Ann Allergy* 1993;71: 538–546.
35. Dager SR, Holland JP, Cowley DS, Dunner DL. Panic disorder precipitated by exposure to organic solvents in the workplace. *Am J Psychiatr* 1987;144:1056–1058.
36. Kurt TL. Multiple chemical sensitivities—a syndrome of pseudotoxicity manifest as exposure perceived symptoms. *Clin Toxicol* 1995;33: 101–105.
37. Rosenberg SJ, Freedman MR, Schmaling KB, Rose C. Personality styles and environmental illness. *J Occup Environ Med* 1990;32: 678–681.
38. Arnetz BB, Berg M, Andersen I, Lundeberg T, Haker E. A nonconventional approach to the treatment of environmental illness. *J Occup Environ Med* 1995;37:838–844.
39. Bell I, Schwartz GE, Bootzin RR, Wyatt JK. Time-dependent sensitization of heart rate and blood pressure over multiple laboratory sessions in elderly individuals with chemical odor intolerance. *Arch Environ Health* 1997;52:6–17.
40. Vojdani A, Ghomeum M, Brautbar N. Immune alteration associated with exposure to toxic chemicals. *Toxicol Ind Health* 1992;8:239–254.
41. Gots RE. Multiple chemical sensitivities: distinguishing between psychogenic and toxicodynamic. *Regul Toxicol Pharmacol* 1996;24: S8–S15.
42. Sandstrom M, Lyskov E, Berglund A, Medvedev S, Hansson K. Neurophysiological effects in patients with perceived electrical hypersensitivity. *J Occup Environ Med* 1997;39:15–22.
43. Roush W. Herbert Benson: mind-body maverick pushes the envelope (research news). *Science* 1997;276:357–359.
44. Tessman I, Tessman J. Mind and body (Book review of *Timeless Healing* by Herbert Benson). *Science* 1997;276:369–370.
45. McWhinney IR, Epstein RM, Freeman TR. Rethinking somatization (editorial). *Ann Intern Med* 1997;126:747–750.
46. Engel GL. The clinical application of the biopsychosocial model. *Am J Psychiatry* 1980;137:535–44.
47. Ader R, Cohen N, Felten D. Psychoneuroimmunology: interactions between the nervous system and the immune system. *Lancet* 1995;345:99–103.
48. Lysle DT, Cunnick JE, Fowler H, Rabin B. Pavlovian conditioning of shock-induced suppression of lymphocyte reactivity: acquisition, extinction, and preexposure effects. *Life Sci* 1988;42:2185–94.
49. Lorig TS, Schwarts GE. Brain and odor: I. Alteration of human EEG by odor administration. *Psychobiology* 1988;16:281–284.
50. Staudenmeyer H, Selner JC, Buhr MP. Double blind provocation chamber challenges in 20 patients presenting with multiple chemical sensitivity. *Regul Toxicol Pharmacol* 1993;18:44–53.
51. Leznoff A. Provocative challenges in patients with multiple chemical sensitivity. *J Allergy Clin Immunol* 1997;99:438–442.
52. Binkley KE, Kutcher S. Panic response to sodium lactate infusion in patients with multiple chemical sensitivity. *J Allergy Clin Immunol* 1997;99:570–574.
53. Doty RL, Deems DA, Frye RE, Pelberg R, Shapiro A. Olfactory sensitivity, nasal resistance, and autonomic function in patients with multiple chemical sensitivities. *Arch Otolaryngol Head Neck Surg* 1988;114: 1422–1427.
54. Twombly R. MCS: a sensitive issue (focus article). *Environ Health Perspect* 1994;102:746–750.
55. Deyo RA, Psaty BM, Simon G, Wagner EH, Omenn GS. The messenger under attack—intimidation of researchers by special interest groups. *N Engl J Med* 1997;336:1176–1180.
56. American College of Allergy and Immunology. Executive Committee of the American College of Allergy and Immunology. Position statements—clinical ecology. *Allergy Clin Immunol* 1986;78:269–271.
57. California Medical Association Scientific Board Task Force on Clinical Ecology. Clinical ecology: a critical appraisal. *West J Med* 1986;144: 239–245.
58. American College of Physicians. Position paper: clinical ecology. *Ann Intern Med* 1989;111:168–178.
59. Council on Scientific Affairs, American Medical Association. Clinical ecology. *JAMA* 1992;268:3465–3467.
60. American College of Occupational and Environmental Medicine. ACOEM Statement on multiple chemical hypersensitivity syndrome, multiple chemical sensitivities, environmental tobacco smoke, and indoor air quality. Multiple Chemical hypersensitivity syndrome, May 2, 1991. Multiple Chemical Sensitivities (Addendum, 1993). (Available from the college.)
61. Mooser SB. The epidemiology of multiple chemical sensitivities (MCS). In: Cullen MR, ed. *Workers with multiple chemical sensitivities. Occupational medicine:* state of the art reviews. Philadelphia: Hanley and Belfus, 1987;2:663–668.
62. Salvaggio JE, Terr AI. Multiple chemical sensitivity multiorgan dysesthesia, multiple somatoform complex, and multiple confusion: problems in diagnosing the patient presenting with unexplained multisystemic symptoms. *Crit Rev Toxicol* 1996;26:617–631.
63. Weaver VM. Medical management of the multiple chemical sensitivity patient. *Regul Toxicol Pharmacol* 1996;24:S111–115.
64. Abbey SE, Garfinkel PE. Neurasthenia and chronic fatigue syndrome: the role of culture in making the diagnosis. *Am J Psychiatr* 1991;148: 1638–1646.
65. Bolla-Wilson KB, Wilson RJ, Bleeker ML. Conditioning of physical symptoms after neurotoxic exposure. *J Occup Environ Med* 1988;30: 684–685.
66. Shusterman D, Balmes J, Cone J. Behavioral sensitization to irritants/odorants after acute exposures. *J Occup Environ Med* 1989;30: 565–567.
67. Black DW, Rathe A, Goldstein R. Environmental illness: a controlled study of 26 subjects with 20th Century Disease. *JAMA* 1990;264: 3166–3170.
68. MacQueen G, Marshall J, Perdue M, Siegel S, Bienenstock J. Pavlovian conditioning of rat musocal mast cells to secrete rate most cell protease II. *Science* 1989;243:83–85.
69. Dalton P. Odor perception and beliefs about risk. *Chem Senses* 1996; 21:447–458.

*Environmental and Occupational Medicine, Third Edition,* edited by William N. Rom.
Published by Lippincott–Raven Publishers, Philadelphia, 1998.

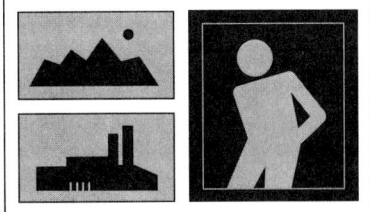

# CHAPTER 62

# Psychological Job Stress

Joseph J. Hurrell, Jr., and Lawrence R. Murphy

As made evident in recent discussions of health care reform in the United States, costs associated with chronic diseases represent a massive drain on the U.S. economy. Nowhere are the rising costs of work-related chronic ill health more evident than in the area of occupational stress. California workers' compensation data, for example, show a rapid increase beginning in 1981 in the rate for mental problems, whereas compensation rates for all other types of claims continued a modest decline (1). Similarly, a study by the Northwestern National Life Insurance Company found that the percentage of stress-related disability claims managed by the company rose from 6% in 1982 to fully 13% in 1990 (2). Disability due to job stress alone, without evidence of any physical injury or illness, is now a compensable condition in about one-half of the states (3).

Despite increased recognition by the legal, medical, and insurance communities, for many workers (even those in the scientific community) stress remains a complex and nebulous construct implying numerous events and processes. In the hope of reducing some of this ambiguity, this chapter provides an integrative review of the occupational stress literature. A history of the job stress concept is provided first, followed by a model of occupational stress-health relationships. Stress reduction methods are then described, and research needs and future directions are discussed.

J. J. Hurrell, Jr.: Division of Surveillance, Hazard Evaluations, and Field Studies, National Institute for Occupational Safety and Health, Cincinnati, Ohio 45226.

L. R. Murphy: Applied Psychology and Ergonomics Branch, National Institute for Occupational Safety and Health, Centers for Disease Control and Prevention, U. S. Public Health Service, Cincinnati, Ohio 45226.

## A BRIEF HISTORY OF JOB STRESS

Occupational stress, as a field of inquiry examining job conditions and their health and performance consequences, is a relatively new research domain that crystallized in the early 1970s. Its conceptual roots can be traced to the animal research of Hans Selye (4) and to Walter Cannon's (5) work on the physiologic concomitants of emotion. In the early 1930s, Hans Selye discovered that a wide variety of noxious stimuli (which he later referred to as stressors), such as exposure to temperature extremes, physical injury, and injection of toxic substances, evoked identical patterns of physiologic changes in laboratory animals. In each case, the cortex of the adrenal gland became enlarged, the thymus and other lymphatic structures became involuted, and deep-bleeding ulcers developed in the stomach and intestines. These effects were "nonspecific"; that is, they occurred regardless of the particular stressor and were superimposed on any specific effects associated with the individual agents. Some years later, Selye (6) described this somatic response as the general adaptation syndrome (GAS) and defined stress as the nonspecific response of the body to any demand. His mention of "nervous stimuli" among the stressor agents capable of eliciting the GAS had an energizing effect on investigators working in the field of psychosomatic medicine. Earlier Cannon (5) had laid the groundwork for an understanding of how emotions affect physiologic functions and disease states in his description of the "fight-or-flight" response. This response, elicited by potentially dangerous situations, involved elevated heart rate and blood pressure, redistribution of blood flow to the brain and major muscle groups and away from distal body parts, and a decrease in vegetative functions. Perhaps equally important, Cannon (7) advanced the concept of physiologic homeostasis, and developed an engineering concept of stress and strain (i.e., stress as the inputs, strain the response). In particular, Cannon proposed the notion of critical stress levels that were capable of producing strain in the homeostatic mechanisms. Although he used the term somewhat casually, Cannon, like Selye, conceived of stress as involving physical as well as emotional stimuli (8).

In the 1960s and 1970s. Richard Lazarus and his colleagues (9) added immensely to the study of stress by describing in specific terms how an organism's perceptions or appraisals of objective events determine its health valence. Cognitive appraisal was described by Lazarus as an intrapsychic process that translates objective events into stressful experiences. The importance of this formulation lies in its recognition that subjective factors can play a much larger role in the experience of stress than objective events. Indeed, any given objective event can at once be perceived positively by one person and negatively by another (i.e., "One person's meat is another person's poison").

The study of occupational stress was given impetus in the early 1970s by the establishment of the National Institute for Occupational Safety and Health (NIOSH) under Public Law 91-596 (10). The stated goal of this agency is to ensure safe and healthful working conditions for America's working men and women. NIOSH is the principal federal agency in the United States engaged in research aimed at the recognition and control of job-related hazards. The importance of behavioral and motivational factors was clearly acknowledged in certain research provisions of the Occupational Safety and Health (OSHA) Act. For example, sections 20(a)(1) and 20(a)(4) of the OSHA act (10) explicitly directed NIOSH to include psychological, behavioral, and motivational factors in research on problems of worker safety and health, and in developing remedial approaches for offsetting such problems. Job-related hazards were interpreted broadly to include conditions of a psychological nature—undue task demands, work conditions, or work regimens that, apart from or combined with exposure to physical and chemical hazards, may degrade workers' physical or mental health (11). Since its inception, NIOSH has sponsored and conducted a large number of research studies, which have helped shape the course of job stress research in the United States. In 1988, NIOSH proposed a national strategy for prevention of work-related psychological disorders (12). Key elements in this prevention strategy include abatement of known job (environmental) risk factors, research to improve understanding of these risk factors, surveillance to detect and track risk factors, education and training to facilitate recognition of risk factors and their control, and improved mental health services. Most recently, NIOSH has identified the "organization of work," which includes work-related psychosocial stressors as one of 21 national occupational safety and health research priorities (13).

## A MODEL OF JOB STRESS AND HEALTH

Over the past 25 years a paradigm of stress was developed by researchers at NIOSH to guide efforts at examining the relationship between working conditions and health consequences (Fig. 1). This model builds on frameworks proposed by Caplan and coworkers (14), Cooper and Marshall (15), and Levi (16). In the model, job stress

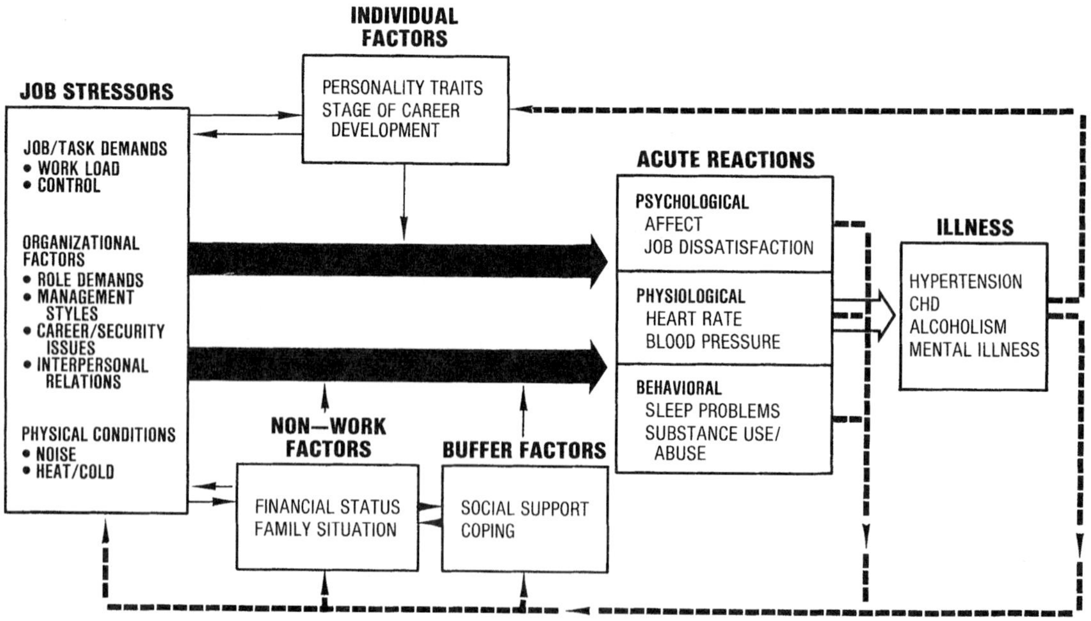


**FIG. 1.** Model of job stress and health.

is viewed as a situation in which a working condition (stressor) or combination of working conditions interacts with individual worker characteristics and results in an acute disruption of psychological or physiologic homeostasis. These acute reactions or disruptions, if prolonged, are thought to lead to a variety of illnesses. As Fig. 1 shows, the most studied of these job stress-related illnesses have been hypertension, coronary heart disease, alcoholism, and mental disorders. Evidence is also accumulating that seems to suggest that job stressors are linked to risk of workplace violence (17).

### Job Stressors and Their Consequences

Unlike physical and chemical hazards, psychosocial stressors (i.e., those embedded in the psychological or social environment) respect no occupational boundaries. The potential for exposure to this class of health risks is ubiquitous, and many psychosocial factors have been identified as potentially hazardous. The most firmly established risk factors, in terms of quantity and convergence of evidence, are discussed below (18–20).

In general, job stressors fall into three broad categories: job/task demands, organizational factors, and physical conditions. Examples of common stressors in each category are described in the following sections.

#### *Job or Task Demands*

Work load is a feature of occupations that is easily recognized as stressful, and has received substantial empirical attention. Working excessive hours or performing more than one job, for example, has been associated with coronary heart disease (CHD) morbidity and mortality (21). Studies showing a relationship between work load and serum cholesterol levels also suggest a CHD-work load relationship (22,23).

Karasek (24) postulated that the amount of work does not seem to be as critical to worker health as the interaction of work load with the amount of control or discretion the worker has over the work and related work processes (referred to as "decision latitude").

Karasek and colleagues (24–26) combined a database containing information on worker self-reports of job conditions with national health databases to examine the relationship between work load, work pace, and degree of decision latitude. Their findings indicate that workers who experienced both a heavier psychological work load and lower decision latitude (termed job strain), were at greater risk for coronary heart disease, had higher blood pressure, and smoked more than workers in jobs without these characteristics. Recent reviews of the growing body of cardiovascular job strain research have concluded that the combination of low decision latitude and high psychological demands is a risk factor for cardiovascular mortality in a majority of studies (27,28). Indeed, the concept that worker control or discretion over working conditions is integral to health has become almost ubiquitous in the occupational stress area (29). The theoretic bases and mechanisms of the effects of control on health, however, are not clear.

Shift work is another job demand associated with health and safety consequences. There is converging evidence that working a shift other than the first shift (e.g., 7:00 A.M. to 3:00 P.M.), and rotating shift schedules in particular, are associated with sleep disorders, gastrointestinal disorders, emotional disturbances, and increased risk of occupational injury (30,31). The primary mechanism responsible for these effects appears to be disruption of biologic rhythms resulting in physiologic and biochemical disturbances (31). Shift work also has behavioral effects on health, including altered sleep patterns and eating habits, and increased alcohol and tobacco use (31).

#### *Organizational Factors*

Many studies have examined the psychological and physical effects of role relationships in work organizations. One of the first of these investigations was conducted in the early 1960s by Robert Kahn and his colleagues at the Institute for Social Research, University of Michigan. Kahn's group (32) found that men who experienced role ambiguity (i.e., lack of clarity about objectives associated with the work role, expectations concerning the work role, and the scope and responsibilities of the job) experienced low self-confidence, high job-related tension, and low job satisfaction. Likewise, workers who experienced role conflict (i.e., conflicting lob demands) have been found to experience more job-related tension and less job satisfaction (32,33). Other studies not only confirmed the association between role ambiguity or conflict and affective reactions, but have also suggested that role stressors are correlated as well to absenteeism and poor job performance (34—36). Finally, role ambiguity and conflict have been related to physiologic responses, including increased heart rate and blood pressure (22,36).

Various management styles, including tolerance of little or no worker participation in decision making, lack of effective consultation, and excessive restrictions on worker behavior, also have been viewed as stressful (37). Of these style characteristics, exclusion from decision making has received the most research attention. Early field studies demonstrated that greater participation in decision making led to greater job satisfaction, lower turnover, better supervisor-subordinate relationships, and greater productivity (38,39). In a nationally representative sample of 1,500 workers, nonparticipation at work also was found to be significantly related not only to low self-esteem and low job satisfaction but to overall poor physical health, excessive drinking, depressed mood, and absenteeism (40). More recently, Jackson (41) found the increasing worker participation in a broad range of work-related decisions can substantially reduce work-related emotional strain.

Factors related to career development also have been linked to health consequences. These factors include overpromotion, underpromotion, status incongruence, lack of job security and fear of task redundancy, job obsolescence, and early retirement (37). One of the most potent of these stressors appears to be ambiguity about job future. For instance, uncertainty about continued employment has been found to be related to low job satisfaction, low life satisfaction, low self-esteem, excessive drinking, and overall poor physical health (39,42).

Poor relationships with colleagues, supervisors, and subordinates at work have been identified as sources of job stress (37,43). For example, the most common sources of stress for a sample of 5,000 managers included inadequate support by supervisors, ineffective performance by supervisors, and conflict and ambiguity about job expectations (44).

The association of organizational culture/climate with worker stress is not at issue as much as the mechanism through which it exerts effects (45). Some researchers suggest that culture/climate moderates the effects of job stressors on worker well-being (46), while other authors reverse the causal sequence, proposing that culture/climate factors influence the job stressors, which in turn affects well-being. Still other authors propose a direct relationship between climate/culture and perceived stress (47). Also, there is some disagreement on how to dimensionalize organizational culture/climate characteristics. Despite these theoretical differences, however, there appears to be an important link between culture/climate factors and worker well-being, and thus a significant role for these factors in future stress research.

### *Physical Conditions*

Adverse environmental conditions serve to exacerbate the overall job demands placed on employees, thus lowering worker tolerance to other stressors and decreasing worker motivation. Environmental conditions, including excessive noise, heat or cold, poor ventilation, inadequate lighting, and ergonomic design deficiencies have been linked to employee physical and psychological health complaints, as well as to attitude and behavior problems (14, 15). For example, outbreaks of mass psychogenic illness typically occur in workplaces that employees regard as physically uncomfortable (48). Evidence is also accruing that psychological job stressors produce increments in muscle tension that may exacerbate muscle loads and symptoms resulting from physical task demands (49).

## Moderating Factors

A number of personal and situational characteristics can alter or modify the way individual workers exposed to a work environment perceive or react to it. These variables, known as "moderators," are depicted in Fig. 1, in the blocks labeled Individual Factors, Nonwork Factors, and Buffer Factors. These factors are discussed separately below.

### *Individual Factors*

The most widely discussed personal characteristic related to stress at work has been the coronary artery disease–prone type A behavior pattern. Type A behavior is characterized by intense striving for achievement, competitiveness, time urgency, excessive drive, and overcommitment to vocation or profession. While investigators in the past have reported the type A pattern to be independently associated with coronary artery disease (50), more recent studies have suggested that the variables of hostility, cynicism, anger, irritability, and suspicion may be the primary pathogenic component of type A found to be significant in earlier investigations (51). Similarly, while earlier investigations suggested an interaction between certain job stressors and type A characteristics that may lead to heart disease (52), overall the evidence that people with type A are more adversely affected by various job stressors is limited (53).

The hardy personality style and an internal locus of control are also thought to mediate the stressor-illness relationship. Hardy persons are believed to possess various beliefs and tendencies that are useful in coping with stressors (54), such as optimistic appraisals of events and decisive actions in coping (55). In both a retrospective and prospective study of executives, hardy persons were found to report less illness in the presence of stressors (55). Persons with an internal locus of control (i.e., a general belief that events in life are controlled by their actions) also have shown a consistent tendency to report better health than those who believe that life events are beyond their control (56).

Stage of career development, though little studied, may also moderate the stressor-illness relationship. For example, work experience (i.e., job tenure) seems to moderate worker responses to negative events at work (57). Indeed, a recent study of more than 6,000 postal workers (58) found that, for persons in the middle stage of their careers, job stressors lose potency in affecting physical health but stressful events outside the job domain become increasingly deleterious to health.

## Extraoccupational Factors

Workers clearly do not leave their family and personal problems behind when they go to work, nor do they forget job problems on returning home. Nearly all models of job stress acknowledge extraoccupational factors and their potential interaction with work in affecting health outcomes. Few studies, however, have attempted to examine the respective health effects of job and extraorganizational stressors (59). While some investigators, e.g., Hurrell (60), have incorporated generic stressful life events scales into job stress surveys, these scales provide only crude indications of social, familial, and financial stressors. It is clear that in future studies more attention needs to be paid to nonwork factors. Interpersonal, marital, financial, and child-rearing stressors can exacerbate existing job stressors to promote acute stress reactions (59,61). Alternatively, the absence of extraorganizational problems may make stressful job situations more tolerable (i.e., less stressful) and may impede the development of stress reactions.

## Buffer Factors

### *Social Support*

Stress researchers have sought to identify factors, generally referred to as "buffer factors," that reduce or eliminate the effects of job stressors. One of the most extensively studied buffer factors has been the degree of social support an individual worker receives from work and nonwork sources. To date, however, evidence for a buffering effect of social support has been mixed. While a number of studies (5,62) have found that social support buffers the relationship between a variety of job stressors and psychological symptoms, other investigations (63,64) have found no such buffering effect. At least in part, these disparate results appear to be the result of differences among investigators in conceptualizing and measuring support. Wethington and Kessler (65), for example, have shown that measures of perceived support fare better than measures of received support in predicting adjustment to stressful situations.

### *Coping*

Another potential buffering factor is coping. The literature on coping is voluminous, but until recently little of this knowledge has been incorporated into studies of occupational stress and health. Lazarus and colleagues (66,67) proposed that coping is not a stable trait or disposition but rather a transactional process that is modified continually by experience within and between stressful episodes. Further, a specific coping strategy that alleviates stress in one situation may not alleviate stress, or may actually increase perceived stress, in other situations (66).

Pearlin and Schooler (68) believe the coping responses that people use are a function of the social and psychological resources at their disposal. Social supports and psychological resources, like mastery and self-esteem, are what people draw upon in developing coping strategies. Research has shown that these resources vary by educational level and income (68). Persons who are better educated and more affluent possess more resources and a wider range of coping alternatives (68). The authors concluded that no single coping response was uniformly protective across nonwork and work situations but that having a large and varied coping repertoire was effective in reducing stressor-strain relationships. Particularly important was Pearlin and Schooler's finding that, while various coping responses were effective in the areas of marriage, child rearing, and household finances, coping was strikingly ineffective when applied to occupational problems. The authors suggested that the resistance of occupational stress to coping may be due to the impersonal nature of work and the lack of worker control over this class of stressors (i.e., little support is available across a wide variety of jobs).

Evidence from other recent studies suggests that some coping behaviors may actually increase stress. Parasuraman and Cleek (69) examined adaptive and maladaptive coping responses used in work settings. They found that adaptive coping responses (e.g., prioritizing assignments) had no buffering effects on perceived stress or job satisfaction but were associated with higher trait anxiety. Maladaptive coping (e.g., working harder, but making more mistakes) was associated with perceived stress. The authors concluded that avoiding maladaptive coping strategies was the most efficient stress reduction strategy.

From such research it is clear that coping responses can increase, decrease, or have no effect on stressor-health relationships. Those that increase or decrease stress reactions need to be factored into job stress assessment instruments to improve ecologic validity, (i.e., to "fine tune" descriptions of stressor-health relationships). Furthermore, future research would benefit from a clear delineation of the various types of coping strategies and their relative effectiveness across work and nonwork situations. In this regard, Latack and Havlovic (70) proposed an evaluative framework that cross-classifies coping responses according to the *focus* of coping (problem-focused or emotion-focused) and the *method* of coping (cognitive or behavioral). Cognitive methods of coping are subdivided according to whether the method involves attempts to *control* the stressor or *escape* from the stressor. Behavioral methods are divided into four dimensions—*control*, *escape*, *social*, and *solitary*—that are not mutually exclusive. When the focus and methods of coping are better delineated in future research, we will be in a better position to predict the effects of coping on stressor-health relationships.

### *Lifestyle Factors*

The 1980s witnessed a surge of interest in lifestyle factors related to individual health and well-being. Generally discussed under the rubric "health promotion," lifestyle factors include physical fitness and exercise, smoking cessation, sound nutrition habits, and stress management. Such factors clearly have the potential for buffering the health effects of job stressors. Two publications by the U.S. Department of Health and Human Services, *Healthy*

*People* (71) and *Promoting Health/Preventing Disease: Objectives for the Nation* (72), served to stimulate interest in lifestyle. Another impetus for this interest is the relationship between lifestyle factors and soaring health care costs that was recognized during the decade of the 1980s.

The workplace was viewed as an ideal site for programmatic efforts to promote employee health (73). Worksite health promotion programs dealing with physical fitness, smoking cessation, hypertension screening and control, nutrition, and stress management were implemented in numerous organizations during the 1980s. Although early efforts at program evaluation were not scientifically sophisticated [see Fielding (74) for a review], more recent studies have used a stronger methodologic design and increasingly are demonstrating the cost-effectiveness of these programs, especially those that emphasize physical fitness (75). A recent set of reviews of all the major health promotion areas uniformly recommended the use of stronger experimental designs in this research as well as the development and application of theoretical models to guide study design and evaluation (76).

## JOB STRESS REDUCTION

Despite the complexities in job stress research, the merits of both individual-oriented stress management and, to a lesser extent, work-oriented approaches to reduce stress have been explored. Given the conceptual framework that emphasizes the subjective element of stress, it is not surprising to find that most stress reduction studies in the literature have focused on changing individual workers rather than the organization and have used individual-oriented measures (e.g., self-reported anxiety) to evaluate program success. Such studies have supported the efficacy of stress-management training in reducing psychophysiologic and self-report signs of stress (77).

A recent review of this literature indicates that stress management interventions use a variety of training techniques and evaluated effects on a range of health outcomes (78). The effectiveness of stress management interventions varied according to the type of outcome measured. Cognitive-behavioral skills training was effective in reducing psychological symptoms of stress, while muscle relaxation training has its main effects on physiologic indicators (i.e., muscle activity). Combinations of techniques, especially muscle relaxation plus cognitive-behavioral skills training, were the most common type of stress management intervention, and generally were the most effective across all types of outcome measures (i.e., psychological, physiologic, and behavioral). However, none of the stress management interventions was consistently effective in producing effects on job/organization-relevant outcomes, such as productivity, absenteeism, or job satisfaction. This is not surprising since these interventions focused on changing the individual worker, not the job-related sources of stress.

In contrast to the growing number of stress management interventions, efforts to reduce or eliminate the sources of stress at work remain sparse (79). Reasons for this discrepancy seem straightforward: Individual-oriented strategies are easy to implement, can be evaluated in the short term, do not require disruptions in production schedules or organizational structure, and fit nicely with management's view of stress as an individual problem rather than an organizational one (80). Individual strategies also are compatible with the expanding interest of employers in health promotion and disease prevention programs that focus exclusively on individual lifestyle and behavior changes to improve health. In contrast, organizational change approaches require an assessment of the work conditions that generate stress and a knowledge of the dynamics of change processes in organizations, e.g., Alderfer's (81). These change strategies can be expensive and disruptive, and may makes them less appealing to management. Nevertheless, job redesign and organizational change approaches are the most desirable type of intervention because they focus on reducing or eliminating the sources of the problem, not just the symptoms.

Organizational strategies that could prevent or reduce stress include (1) job redesign, (2) quality circles (which bring bench-level workers into the decision-making process), (3) worker representation on health and safety committees, (4) extensive training programs for workers whose jobs are being revised owing to the introduction of new technology, (5) more open communication channels within an organization, and (6) development of clear job descriptions. These types of interventions, however, have not been subjected to rigorous scientific evaluation. Evaluation schemes for such interventions should include cost-benefit analyses in addition to assessments of worker satisfaction, job stressors, performance, absenteeism, and health status. A recent job redesign study (82) involving the enlargement of the scope and responsibility of jobs, however, clearly suggests that it is possible to gain benefits through redesign without incurring excess costs.

It is important to recognize that universal solutions to problems of work stress are not likely to be successful because, more often than not, stress problems require solutions that are specific to each organization. The intervention process, on the other hand, may be both generic and effective. For example, Murphy and Hurrell (83) designed an intervention that involved combined individual stress management and job redesign-organizational change approaches for reducing employee stress. Briefly, a stress reduction committee was formed with representatives from each unit of the organization. The committee acquired the services of the present authors, who recommended a two-pronged approach. First, stress management workshops were held to educate employees about the nature, sources, and consequences of work and nonwork stress, and elicit feedback from employees regarding job stressors in the organization. Second, based on the employee feedback obtained during the workshops, a survey designed to identify sources of organizational stress was administered to all employees. The job, task, and organizational stressors identified in the employee survey then were reviewed by the committee and prioritized according to their importance to employee health and well-being and their amenability to primary prevention efforts. Organizational changes to eliminate or reduce the highest-priority stressors then were formulated and presented to management, with recommendations for implementation and repeated evaluation at annual intervals. Although no organizational changes were implemented as a result of this effort, the process and methods developed under it warrant further research attention.

## FUTURE DIRECTIONS

### Job Stress and the Immune System

Despite the amount of data linking stressful job conditions to poor health, surprisingly little is known about the actual physiologic mechanisms that underlie the relationships between stress and disease. Evidence is accumulating that immune system responses may mediate some of these relationships. A large number of animal studies, for example, have demonstrated that experimentally induced stress increases both susceptibility to a variety of infectious agents and the incidence and rate of growth of certain tumors (84). Although they are fewer, human studies have shown that psychosocial factors, including stressful life events, are related to diseases that are under immune system regulation (85). Other animal and human research findings provide more direct evidence that stress can affect immune competence (i.e., the ability of an organism's immune system to defend against challenge). For example, stress has been linked to changes in levels of circulating antibodies, lymphocyte cytotoxicity, and lymphocyte proliferation (86). Even commonplace stressors, such as academic demand, marital separation, divorce, and bereavement, have been shown to produce changes in measures of immune competence (86). While there is yet only limited research evidence, there is every reason to believe that stressful elements of the work environment also may elicit changes in immune competence and so influence health status.

Technologic developments in the quantification of immune competence, as well as better understanding of the connection of nervous and immune systems, are beginning to make possible studies of job stress and immune competence.

### Economic Trends and Work Force Changes

Emerging trends in the economy, technology, and demographic characteristics of the work force may increase the risk for psychological disorders (87). The U.S. economy is no longer dominated by manufacturing, and an ever-increasing number of workers are employed in service-producing industries. This sector of the economy is projected to account for nearly 94% of all newly created jobs between 1990 and 2005, with its share of all jobs expected to rise from 69% in 1990 to 73% in 2005 (88). This change has a dramatic impact on the kinds of jobs that are available, the type of worker employed, and the characteristics of the workplace. Of particular concern is the fact that workers in service industry jobs are at increased risk for psychological disorders (89).

Against this backdrop, the face of the U.S. national work force has changed, with the fastest growing segments of the working population being women, ethnic minorities, and older workers, with the median age of the labor force expected to rise from 36.6 years in 1990 to 40.6 years in 2005 (88). Despite these radical changes in the makeup of the work force and the availability of new research findings, sufficient data still do not exist on the particular stressors experienced by female, ethnic minority, and aging workers who will make up a large percentage of the work force in the years to come. One fact, however, is abundantly clear. As a result of changes in employee demographics, and particularly because of the increasing numbers of women in the work force, balancing the demands of work and family has become a major challenge for many working adults (90). Although occupying multiple roles may have psychological benefits, there is increasing evidence that there are both individual and organizational costs associated with, for example, simultaneously occupying the roles of worker, spouse, and caregiver (91).

Corporate closing and downsizing in the United States have been occurring at an unprecedented rate since the mid-1980s. It is estimated that 9 million workers were permanently and involuntarily separated from their jobs between January 1991 and December 1993 (92). As research literature from the 1930s to the present has documented the psychological and social cost of job loss for the unemployed person, for individual members of the person's family, and for the family as a whole (93), this trend represents a serious concern for occupational health professionals. There is also growing evidence that downsizing efforts may have a profound effect on survivors within an organization, increasing their role ambiguity, conflict, and workload (93).

### Surveillance of Psychological Disorders

Surveillance of psychosocial job risk factors and psychological disorders presents unique problems that have not been encountered in traditional occupational safety and health surveillance. For example, psychological disorders do not fit the infectious disease model in that there is no single agent that leads to a particular disease. Rather, the work environment contains a variety of risk factors or hazards that interact with characteristics of the individual to produce health outcomes. Kasl (94) described these problems and concluded that current surveillance systems are inadequate for assessing job risk factors and psychological disorders.

### Controlling Organizational Stress

Emerging changes in the work environment (e.g., downsizing/reorganization, flexiplace arrangements (as necessary), total quality management) and changes in work force demographics (e.g., cultural diversity) signal that job stress will increase or at least continue to be a problem in the near future. Increasingly, companies will seek effective interventions to reduce employee stress, lower health care costs, and improve productivity.

To maximize their effectiveness, stress interventions will need to become more comprehensive and attend to the prevalent stressors in the work environment in order to produce significant effects on job/organizational outcomes. Teaching workers stress management skills is necessary and serves a useful purpose, but it deals with only part of the problem. The workplace is the source of powerful stressors that can be targeted for change. A few studies have documented the health-enhancing effects of implementing flexible work schedules, increasing worker participation in decision making, and increasing worker autonomy. Ideally, comprehensive interventions should include attention to both individual- and organization-level factors.

Increasing worker participation and involvement in stress interventions will shift some of the emphasis to the process, without ignoring either the content or outcomes of training (77,95).

Stress intervention studies need to be designed and evaluated within the context of a well-defined conceptual/theoretical model. A conceptual model is useful for defining the stressors, the short- and long-term consequences of stress, key intervening variables, and the nature of relationships among stressors, outcomes, and intervening variables. Once a model is specified, it serves to guide the choice of stressors to measure the targeting of intervention strategies and decisions on how to implement the intervention and evaluate its effectiveness. A number of authors have proposed conceptual models for stress intervention, but the models remain underutilized by researchers and practitioners (96,97). Ideas for controlling job stress through collaboration among employee assistance and human resource management departments also have been offered.

Although company goals of profitability and competitiveness are often assumed to be in opposition to worker goals of well-being and job satisfaction, recent research at NIOSH is challenging this assumption. This new research attempts to identify job and organizational characteristics that promote both productivity and employee health and well-being (98). The research is being performed collaboratively with industry and will operationalize the key characteristics of a healthy work organization by linking organizational factors with objective outcome measures (i.e., measures of employee health and performance). Based on these results, a healthy work organization profile will be formulated and used to design and evaluate pilot studies of selected companies.

### Methodologic Needs

Researchers need to address several methodologic problems associated with occupational stress research. Particularly important are (1) increased use of prospective and follow-up research designs of psychological outcomes, (2) development of more standardized methods for assessing psychosocial risk factors on the job, (3) greater adherence to the use of standard psychometric instruments in assessing psychological outcomes, (4) more extensive use of collateral measures of working conditions (e.g., assessments by co-workers, managers, objective measurements) as well as indicators of psychological health effects (e.g., self-reports, medical and personnel records, psychophysiologic measures, performance, attendance, supervisory and peer evaluations), (5) increased efforts to ensure that the findings of particular studies will have general application or external validity (e.g., the use of multiple work sites or industries), and (6) increased use of advanced statistical methods such as structural analysis to improve the understanding of causal mechanisms and pathways.

In addition, researchers need to explore methods that could supplement self-report approaches. Karasek's (99) work, which supplements self-report data on job stressors with objective health data, is an example of the effective use of supplementary methods. A related, but more global, method was used by Shaw and Riskind (100) and by Murphy (101); the work environment for many different jobs was characterized via job analysis, and the resulting standardized job dimension scores were used as predictors of health outcomes. The method involves merging job analysis data with cardiovascular and psychological health outcome data derived from questionnaire surveys, organizational records, or death certificates. Occupational title is used as the common (i.e., merging or linking) variable. Results from two studies using this method indicated increased risk of cardiovascular diseases for workers whose jobs required much vigilance and involved great responsibility.

## CONCLUSION

This chapter has described a growing knowledge base on occupational stress and health. Although the area is complex and much additional research is needed, it is clear that organizations cannot afford to ignore the human and organizational costs of stress. It seems likely that stress at work will increase over the next decade, owing to the continued introduction of new technological developments in the work environment, new management principles (e.g., total quality management), downsizing/reorganization, and changes in work force demographics. All of these factors will require workers and organizations to change and adapt, thereby increasing perceptions of stress. Progressive companies will equip themselves to better understand work stress and how to manage its health and productivity consequences, which should result in reduced health care costs and improved productivity, and will assist companies in remaining competitive in an increasingly global economy. One mechanism for meeting this challenge is improved collaboration among company departments, bringing expertise from different disciplines to bear on the problem of stress and the design of stress interventions. The most successful interventions will be those that jointly meet the company goals of profitability and competitiveness, and the employee goals of job satisfaction and mental and physical health.

## REFERENCES


1. California Worker's Compensation Institute. *Mental stress claims in California workers' compensation—incidence costs and trends.* San Francisco: California Workers Compensation Institute, 1990.
2. Northwestern National Life Insurance Company. *Employee burnout:* America's newest epidemic. Minneapolis, MN: Northwestern National Life Insurance, 1991.
3. Elisburg D. Workers' compensation issues for psychologists: the workers point of view. In: Murphy LR, Hurrell JJ, Sauter S, Keita G, eds. *Job stress interventions.* Washington, DC: American Psychological Association, 1995;369–381.
4. Selye H. A syndrome produced by diverse noxious agents. *Nature* 1936; 138:32.
5. Cannon WB. *Bodily changes in pain, hunger, fear, and rage.* Boston: CT Branford, 1929.
6. Selye H. The general adaptation syndrome and diseases of adaptation. *J Clin Endocrinol* 1946;6:217–230.
7. Cannon WB. Stresses and strains of homeostasis. *Am J Med Sci* 1935; 189:1–14.
8. Mason JW. A historical view of the stress field: Part I. *J Human Stress* 1975;1:6–12.
9. Lazarus RS, Folkman S. *Stress appraisal and coping.* New York: Springer-Verlag, 1984.
10. Occupational Safety and Health Act (1970). Pub. L 91-596, Star 2193.
11. Cohen A, Margolis B. Initial psychological research related to the Occupational Safety and Health Act of 1970. *Am Psychol* 1973;28: 600–606.
12. Sauter S, Murphy LR, Hurrell JJ Jr. Prevention of work-related psychological disorders: a national strategy proposed by the National Institute for Occupational Safety and Health. *Am Psychol* 1990;45: 1146–1158.
13. Rosenstock, L. Work organization at the National Institute for Occupational Safety and Health. *J Occup Health Psychol* 1997;2:7–10.
14. Caplan RD, Cobb S, French JRP Jr, Min Harrison R, Pinneau SR. *Job demands and worker health.* NIOSH publication 75-160. Washington, DC: DHEW, 1975.
15. Cooper CL, Marshall J. Occupational sources of stress: a review of the literature relating to coronary heart disease and mental ill health. *J Occup Psychol* 1976;49:11–28.
16. Levi L, ed. *Society, stress, and disease.* London: Oxford University Press, 1971.
17. Vandenbos GR, Bulato EQ. *Violence on the job.* Washington DC: American Psychological Association, 1996.
18. Quick JC, Quick JD, Nelson DL, Hurrell JJ Jr. *Preventive stress management in organizations.* Washington, DC: American Psychological Association, 1997.
19. Hurrell JJ Jr, Murphy LR. An overview of psychological job stress. In: Rom WN, ed. *Environmental and occupational medicine,* 2nd ed. Boston: Little, Brown, 1992;675–648.
20. Holt RR. Occupational stress. In: Goldberger L, Breznitz S, eds. *Handbook of stress,* 2nd ed. New York: Free Press, 1993;342–367.
21. Kasl S. The influence of the work environment on cardiovascular health: a historical, conceptual, and methodological perspective. *J Occup Health Psychol* 1996;1:42–56.
22. French JRP Jr, Caplan RD. Organizational stress and individual strain. In: Manow AJ, ed. *The failure of success.* New York: AMACOM, 1972;30–66.
23. Friedman MD, Rosenmann RD, Carroll V. Changes in serum cholesterol and blood clotting time in men subject to cyclic variation of occupational stress. *Circulation* 1958;17:852–861.
24. Karasek RA. Job demands, decision latitude, and mental strain: implications for job redesign. *Admin Sci Q* 1979;24:285–307.
25. Karasek RA, Schwartz J, Theorell T. *Job characteristics, occupation, and coronary heart disease.* (Final report on Contract No. R-01-0H00906.) Cincinnati, OH: NIOSH, 1982.
26. Karasek RA, Theorell T, Schwartz JE, Schnall PL, Pieper CF, Michela JL. Job characteristics in relation to the prevalence of myocardial infarction in the U.S. Health Examination Survey (HES) and the Health and Nutrition Examination Survey (HANES). *Am J Public Health* 1988;78:682–684.
27. Schnall PL, Landsbergis PA. Job strain and cardiovascular disease. *Annu Rev Public Health* 1994;15:381–411.
28. Kristensen TS. The demands–control–support model: methodological challenges for future research. *Stress Med* 1995;11:17–26.
29. Sauter S, Hurrell JJ Jr, Cooper CL. *Job control and worker health.* Chichester: John Wiley, 1990.
30. Scott AJ, ed. *Occupational medicine:* state of the art reviews. Philadelphia: Hanley & Belfus, 1990;5.
31. Scott AJ, Landow JL. Shiftwork: effects on sleep and health with recommendations for medical surveillance and screening. In: Scott AJ, ed. *Occupational medicine: state of the art reviews.* Philadelphia: Hanley & Belfus, 1990;5.
32. Kahn RL, Wolfe DM, Quinn RP, Snoek JD, Rosenthal RA. *Organizational stress:* studies in role conflict and ambiguity. New York: John Wiley, 1964.
33. Bacharach SB, Bamberger P, Conley S. Work-home conflict among nurses and engineers: mediating the impact of role stress on burnout and satisfaction. *J Org Behav* 1991;12:40–53.
34. Jackson S, Schuler R. A metaanalysis and conceptual critique of research on role ambiguity and role conflict in work settings. *Org Behav Hum Decision* 1985;36:16–28.
35. Caplan RD, Jones K. Effects of work load, role ambiguity and type A personality on anxiety, depression, and heart rate. *J Appl Psychol* 1975;60:713–719.
36. Ivancevich JM, Matteson MI, Preston C. Occupational stress, type A behavior and physical well-being. *Acad Manag J* 1982;25:373–391.
37. Beehr IA, Newman JE. Job stress, employee health, and organizational effectiveness: a facet analysis, model, and literature review. *Personnel Psychol* 1978;31:665–699.
38. Coch L, French JRP Jr. Overcoming resistance to change. *Hum Relat* 1948;1:1–21.
39. French JRP Jr, Israel J, Aas D. An experiment in participation in a Norwegian factory. *Hum Relat* 1960;13:3–19.
40. Margolis B, Kroes W, Quinn RP. Job stress: an unlisted occupational hazard. *J Occup Med* 1974;16:659–661.
41. Jackson SE. Participation in decision making as a strategy for reducing job-related strain. *J Appl Psychol* 1983:68:3–19.
42. Roskies E, Louis-Guerin C. Job insecurity in managers: antecedents and consequences. *J Org Behav* 1990;11:345–359.
43. Davidson MI, Cooper CL. A model of occupational stress. *J Occup Med* 1981;23:564–50.
44. Pearse R. *What managers think about their managerial careers.* New York: AMACOM, 1977.

45. Sauter SL, Murphy LR, eds. *Organizational risk factors for job stress.* Washington, DC: American Psychological Association, 1995.
46. Jones B, Flynn DM, Kelloway EK. Perception of support from the organization in relation to work stress, satisfaction, and commitment. In: Sauter SL, Murphy LR, eds. *Organizational risk factors for job stress.* Washington, DC: American Psychological Association, 1995; 41–52.
47. Michela JL, Lukaszewski MP, Allegrante JP. Defining and measuring hostile environment: development of the hostile environment inventory. In: Sauter SL, Murphy LR, eds. *Organizational risk factors for job stress.* Washington, DC: American Psychological Association, 1995;61–80.
48. Colligan MI, Murphy LR. Mass psychogenic illness in organizations: an overview. *J Occup Psychol* 1979;52:77–90.
49. Sauter SL, Swanson NG. An ecological model of musculoskeletal disorders in office work. In: Moon S, Sauter SL, eds. *Psychological aspects of musculoskeletal disorders in office workers.* London: Taylor & Francis, 1996;3–21.
50. Cooper T, Detre T, Weiss SM, et al. Coronary-prone behavior and coronary heart disease: a critical review. *Circulation* 1981;63:1200–1215.
51. Goldstein MG, Niaura R. Psychological factors affecting physical conditions: cardiovascular disease literature review. *Psychosomatics* 1992;33:134–155.
52. Ivancevich JM, Matteson MT. A type A person-work environment interaction model for examining occupational stress consequences. *Hum Relat* 1984;37:491–513.
53. Parkes KR. Individual differences and work stress: personality characteristics as moderators. In: Levi L, LaFerla F, eds. *A healthier work environment.* Copenhagen: World Health Organization, 1993;122–142.
54. Kobasa SC, Maddi SR, Courington S. Personality and constitution as mediators in the stress-illness relationship. *J Health Soc Behav* 1981; 22:368–378.
55. Ouelette SC. Inquiries into hardiness. In: Goldberger L, Breznitz S, eds. *Handbook of stress.* New York: Free Press, 1993;77–100.
56. Hurrell JJ, Murphy LR. Locus of control, job demands and health. In: Cooper R, Payne R, eds. *Personality and stress:* individual differences in the stress process. Chichester: John Wiley, 1991;133–150.
57. Wanous JP. Effects of a realistic job preview on job acceptance, job attitudes, and job survival. *J Appl Psychol* 1973;58:327–332.
58. Hurrell JJ Jr, McLaney A, Murphy LR. The middle years: career stage differences. *Prev Hum Serv* 1990;8:179–203.
59. Bhagat P, McQuaid SJ, Lindholm H, Segovis J. Total life stress: a multimethod validation of the construct and its effects on organizationally valued outcomes and withdrawal behaviors. *J Appl Psychol* 1985;70: 202–214.
60. Hurrell JJ Jr. Machine-paced work and the type A behaviour pattern. *J Occur Psychol* 1985;58:15–25.
61. Barling J, MacEwan KE. Linking work experiences to facets of marital functioning. *J Org Behav* 1992;13:673–683.
62. LaRocco JM, House JS, French JRP Jr. Social support, occupational stress, and health. *J Health Soc Behav* 1980;21:202–208.
63. Blau G. An empirical investigation of job stress, social support, service length and job strain. *Org Behav Hum Perform* 1981;27:279–302.
64. Ganster DC, Fusilier MR, Mays BT. Role of social support in the experience of stress at work. *J Appl Psychol* 1986;1:102–110.
65. Wethington E, Kessler R. Perceived support, received support, and adjustment to stressful life events. *J Health Soc Behav* 1986;27:78–89.
66. Cohen F, Lazarus RS. Coping with the stresses of illness. In: Stone GC, Cohen F, Adler NE, eds. *Health psychology—a handbook.* San Francisco: Jossey-Bass, 1979;217–254.
67. Folkman S, Lazarus RS. An analysis of coping in a middle-aged community sample. *J Health Soc Behav* 1980;21:219–239.
68. Pearlin LI, Schooler C. The structure of coping. *J Health Soc Behav* 1978;19:2–21.
69. Parasuraman S, Cleek MA. Coping behaviors and managers' affective reactions to role stressors. *J Vocat Behav* 1984;24:179–193.
70. Latack JC, Havlovic SJ. Coping with job stress: a conceptual evaluation framework for coping measures. *J Org Behav* 1992;13:479–508.
71. Department of Health and Human Services. *Healthy people, the Surgeon General's report on health promotion and disease prevention.* PHS publication 79-55071. Washington, DC: Department of Health and Human Services, 1979.
72. Department of Health and Human Services. *Promoting health/preventing disease:* objectives for the nation. Washington, DC: Department of Health and Human Services, 1980.
73. Parkinson R. *Managing health promotion in the work-place:* guidelines for implementations and evaluation. Palo Alto, CA: Mayfield, 1982.
74. Fielding JE. The challenges of work-place health promotion. In: Weiss SM, Fielding JE, Baun WB, eds. *Health at work.* Hillsdale, NJ: Erlbaum, 1990;13–28.
75. Bertera RL. The effects of workplace health promotion on absenteeism and employment costs in a large industrial population. *Am J Public Health* 1990;80:1101–1105.
76. Wilson MG. A comprehensive review of the effects of worksite health promotion on health-related outcomes: an update. *Am J Health Promot* 1996;11:107–157.
77. Murphy LR. Managing job stress: an employee assistance/human resource management partnership. *Personnel Rev* 1995;24:41–50.
78. Murphy LR. Stress management in work settings: a critical review of the research literature. *Am J Health Promot* 1996;11:112–135.
79. Murphy LR. Workplace interventions for stress reduction and prevention. In: Cooper CL, Payne P, eds. *Causes, coping and consequences of stress at work.* Chichester: John Wiley, 1989;301–342.
80. Neale MS, Singer JA, Schwartz GE, Schwartz J. *Conflicting perspectives on stress reduction in occupational settings:* a systems approach to their resolution. Department of Health and Human Services publication 82-1058. Cincinnati, OH: NIOSH, 1982.
81. Alderfer CP. Change processes in organizations. In: Dunnette MD, ed. *Handbook of industrial and organizational psychology.* Chicago: Rand McNally, 1976;1591–1638.
82. Campion MA, McClelland CL. Interdisciplinary examination of the costs and benefits of enlarged jobs: a job design quasi-experiment. *J Appl Psychol* 1991;6:186–198.
83. Murphy LR, Hurrell JJ Jr. Stress management in the process of occupational stress reduction. *J Manag Psychol* 1987;2:18–23.
84. Borysenko M, Borysenko J. Stress, behavior, and immunity: animal models and mediating mechanisms. *Gen Hosp Psychiatr* 1982;4: 59–67.
85. Jemmon JB, Locke SE. Psychosocial factors, immunologic mediation and human susceptibility to infectious diseases: How much do we know? *Psychol Bull* 1984;95:8–108.
86. Baker GHB. Psychological factors and immunity. *J Psychosom Res* 1987;31:1–10.
87. Keita GP, Hurrell JJ Jr, eds. *Job stress in a changing workforce.* Washington DC: American Psychological Association, 1994.
88. U.S. Department of Labor Women's Bureau. *Women workers outlook to 2005.* Washington DC: U.S. Department of Labor, 1992.
89. Landy FJ. Work design and stress. In: Keita GP, Sauter SL, eds. *Work and well-being:* an agenda for the 1990s. Washington, DC: American Psychological Association, 1992;119–158.
90. Williams KJ, Alliger GM. Role stressors, mood spillover, and perceptions of work family conflict in employed parents. *Acad Manag J* 1994;37:837–868.
91. Greenhaus JH, Parasuraman S. A work-nonwork interactive perspective of stress and its consequences. *J Org Behav Manag* 1986;8: 37–55.
92. Walsh DP, Dillon H. Where the workers are: a state by state guide to occupations. *Occup Outlook Q* 1994(Fall);10–23.
93. Noer DM. *Healing the wounds:* overcoming the trauma of layoffs and revitalizing *the downsized organization.* San Francisco: Jossey-Bass, 1993.
94. Kasl SV. Surveillance of psychological disorders in the workplace. In: Keita GP, Sauter SL, eds. *Work and well-being: an agenda for the 1990s.* Washington, DC: American Psychological Association, 1992; 73–95.
95. Hurrell JJ Jr, Murphy LR. Occupational stress intervention. *Am J Ind Med* 1996;29:338–341.
96. Stoner CR, Fry FL. Developing a corporate policy for managing stress. *Personnel* 1983(May/June);66–76.
97. Heaney CA, van Ryn M. Broadening the scope of worksite stress programs: a guiding framework. *Am J Health Promot* 1990;4:413–420.
98. Sauter SL, Lim SY, Murphy LR. *Organizational health:* a new paradigm for occupational stress research at NIOSH. *Jpn J Occup Mental Health* 1996;4:248–254.
99. Karasek RA, Theorell T. *Healthy work.* New York: Basic Books, 1990.
100. Shaw JB, Riskind JH. Predicting lob stress using data from the Position Analysis Questionnaire. *J Appl Psychol* 1983;68:253–261.
101. Murphy L. Job dimensions associated with severe disability due to cardiovascular disease. *J Clin Epidemiol* 1991;44:155–166.

*Environmental and Occupational Medicine,*
*Third Edition,* edited by William N. Rom.
Lippincott–Raven Publishers, Philadelphia © 1998.

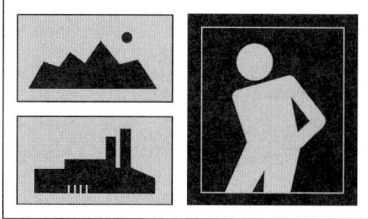

CHAPTER 63

# Epidemiology of Occupational Injury

Mary-Louise Skovron

Occupational injury is a major cause of death and disability among working people in the United States. Occupational musculoskeletal injuries and severe traumatic injuries have been ranked second and fourth, respectively, as causes of work-related disability and death (1). In 1991 there were 2.8 million on-the-job injuries resulting in restricted activity or lost work time. These resulted in approximately 60 million person-days of restricted activity or lost work time. The total cost of occupational injuries in that year was estimated at $63.3 billion (2). The National Safety Council (NSC) estimates that there were approximately 10,600 work-related deaths in 1988, a death rate of 9 per 100,000 workers. The average cost per death was $550,000 (3). Indirect costs were estimated to be $145 billion plus another $26 billion for occupational diseases (3).

Occupational injury as defined under the record-keeping requirements of the Occupational Safety and Health Administration (OSHA) (1970, revised 1978) is any injury, such as a cut, fracture, sprain, amputation, that results from a work accident or from an exposure involving a single incident in the work environment. Reportable injuries involve one of the following: loss of consciousness, restriction of work or motion, transfer to another job, or medical treatment other than first aid. Disabling (lost workday) injuries involve days away from work or days of restricted work activity. Fatal occupational injuries are work-related accidents resulting in death, regardless of the time between injury and death. This chapter focuses on the epidemiology of occupational injury in the United States, as defined above.

M-L. Skovron: Genentech Inc., Medical Affairs/Epidemiology, San Francisco, California 94080; and New York University Medical Center, New York, New York 10016.

## FATAL OCCUPATIONAL INJURIES

Information on the frequency, distribution, and causes of occupational injuries is available from a variety of sources, each developed for different purposes, using different capture methods, definitions, and covered populations (4). These include the Bureau of Labor Statistics (BLS), which compiles information from a sample of some 280,000 private establishments that have at least 11 employees; the NSC, employing multiple sources, including the National Center for Health Statistics, state health departments, and state industrial commissions; and the National Traumatic Occupational Fatality (NTOF) surveillance system implemented by the National Institute for Occupational Safety and Health (NIOSH), which relies on death certificate data and is a source of information for deaths beginning in 1980. In addition, the NIOSH Fatal Accident Circumstances and Epidemiology (FACE) project, which compiles information on electrocutions and fatal falls, and the Department of Transportation Fatal Accident Reporting System (FARS) provide data on certain types of fatal on-the-job injuries. OSHA files of reported fatalities in regulated states are also useful, but exclude miners, truckers in interstate commerce, aircraft flight crews, seamen, railroad workers, and all public employees.

Information on the numbers of workers at risk, necessary for computing fatality rates, may be based on reports of hours worked by employees in covered industries (BLS, NSC) or on data from the Bureau of the Census (NTOF). The variety of sources of information, industries and establishment sizes covered, definitions of fatal occupational injuries, and sources of denominator data lead to substantial variations in estimates of the frequency of deaths derived from the different sources. For example, there were 13,000 work-related deaths among 96.8 million workers in 1980, a rate of 13 per 100,000, while the BLS reported 41 deaths in 61.7 million covered workers (7 per 100,000) (5). For the same year, the NTOF estimate was 7,700 deaths, a rate of 9.1 per 100,000 (6). Among the sources of information on work-related deaths, Stout and Bell (7) have concluded that death certificates provide the best single source for identifying occupational injuries and that these, on average, captured only 36% of deaths in the studies reviewed.

The NSC, which has compiled fatality data for the better part of this century, reports a long-term decline in occupational fatality rates, from 37 per 100,000 in 1933 to 9 per 100,000 in 1988 (2).

**TABLE 1.** *Occupational fatality rates by major industrial group, United States (6)*

| | Number of deaths | Average annual rate[a] |
|---|---|---|
| Agriculture, forestry, fishing | 5,264 | 20.30 |
| Mining | 1,974 | 28.08 |
| Construction | 7,482 | 25.13 |
| Manufacturing | 4,917 | 3.58 |
| Transportation | 7,686 | 23.44 |
| Wholesale trade | 738 | 1.96 |
| Retail trade | 3,090 | 2.78 |
| Finance/insurance/real estate | 474 | 1.19 |
| Service | 3,518 | 2.56 |
| Public administration | 2,255 | 6.41 |
| Total | 45,089 | 7.54 |

[a]Deaths per 100,000 workers per year.

## Occupational Risk Factors

Despite discrepancies in absolute fatality rate estimates, the principal sources (NTOF, NSC, BLS) yield similar rankings of the different covered industrial sectors by fatality rates (5,8). For the period 1980 through 1986, NTOF data (Table 1) indicate that the highest annual fatality rates were in mining (28.1 per 100,000); construction (25.1 per 100,000); transportation, communication, and public utilities (23.4 per 100,000); and agriculture, forestry, and fishing (20.3 per 100,000) (9). In an analysis of OSHA fatality cases for the period 1977 through 1986, fatality rates within industry sectors were inversely related to establishment size (10).

Among all causes, motor vehicle accidents are most important, accounting for more than 20% of occupational fatalities, and the leading cause in all industrial sectors except construction, where the leading cause is falls (8) (Table 2). Approximately two-thirds of occupational motor vehicle deaths involve occupants of the vehicles (11,12). Reports of the high proportion of fatal occupational injuries occurring in motor vehicles have led to a call for installation of seat belts and air bags in such vehicles and for enforcement of their use.

Several recent studies focused on fatality patterns in specific industries, urging regulatory changes to reduce fatalities. Karlson and Noren (13) in Wisconsin, and Goodman and co-workers (14) in Georgia documented that fatal farm tractor injury rates for males generally increase with age and that one-half to three-quarters of such deaths are attributable to rollovers. The high rate of fatal injuries in males, and the preponderance of tractor rollover fatalities among them, has also been documented by Erlich and colleagues (15) in Australia. Rivara (16), studying several national data sources, indicated that tractor accidents are responsible for 26% of fatal farm injuries in children and adolescents. These findings were reinforced by a recent study of NTOF data, which found that 69% of farm fatalities involved tractors, 52% of which were rollovers (17). These reports urged the adoption of mandatory protection features such as roll bars or reinforced protective cabs, noting that, while they have long been available, they have not been widely applied on a voluntary basis.

Examining fatal injury rates in bituminous coal mining, Weeks and Fox (18) pointed out that a decline in mortality rates followed the passage of the Coal Mine Safety and Health Act in 1969. The declining trend in fatality rates that had been observed during the 1970s, however, appeared to reverse in underground coal mining operations toward the end of the decade, consistent with the investigators' hypothesis that reductions in agency enforcement personnel and relaxation of enforcement policies after 1978 would be reflected in mortality rates. A return to the more rigorous policies of the early 1970s was urged.

A high proportion of fatal injuries in construction workers are transportation injuries (19). A study of fatalities from trench cave-ins in the construction industry reported that 94% of deaths occurred in companies that had previously been cited by OSHA for safety violations. Sewer line construction firms were responsible for 33% of deaths in trench cave-ins. Firms with fewer than 11 employees presented the highest standardized mortality ratios (SMRs) for cave-ins (19). The authors called for a revision of OSHA standards for trenches, to mandate long-known measures for preventing cave-ins.

**TABLE 2.** *Leading causes of death in highest-risk industrial groups (8)*

| Industrial group | Cause | Fatality rate[a] | Percent of deaths |
|---|---|---|---|
| Mining | Struck by falling | 4.48 | 21 |
| | Motor vehicle | 4.05 | 16 |
| Construction | Fall | 6.51 | 26 |
| | Electrocution | 3.91 | 16 |
| Agriculture/ forestry/fishery | Machinery | 7.14 | 35 |
| | Motor vehicle | 3.04 | 15 |
| Transportation | Motor vehicle | 11.42 | 49 |
| | Air transport | 1.92 | 8 |

[a]Fatalities per 100,000 workers per year.

### Individual Risk Factors

Bell and colleagues (6) have reported, based on NTOF data for 1980 to 1985, that age-specific worker death rates are relatively constant until age 65, when they increase sharply, although the relatively small numbers of workers over age 65 leads to some instability in their occupational fatality rates. The risk of occupational fatality is substantially higher for men (11.1 per 100,000) than women (0.9 per 100,000). The distribution of causes of death by gender is quite different: homicides account for 39% of women's deaths and 11% of men's. In the same report, black and other non-Caucasian workers had higher death rates than whites—7.7 and 7.6 versus 6.5 per 100,000.

The indication from two state-based studies that a high proportion of occupational fatalities in women were murders (11,20) led to an analysis of NTOF data from 1980 to 1985 on female homicides. The highest-risk industrial category was retail trade with a rate (8.7 per million) approximately twice the rate for all industries combined (4.5 per million). Sixty-four percent of deaths were from gunshots and 19% from stabbings and slashings. Seventy-five percent of the women worked in food stores or eating and drinking establishments (21). In light of information that approximately 50% of confirmed workplace homicides in a subset of counties occurred during robberies, antirobbery safety regulations have been urged. Indeed, in at least one national convenience store chain, robbery-prevention programs have already been implemented.

Alcohol ingestion has been implicated as a cause of occupational fatalities. Descriptive studies have reported detectable blood alcohol levels in 4% to 11% of fatally injured workers (11,22,23). Among seamen it has been reported that alcohol contributed to at least one-half the fatalities (24).

## DISABLING OCCUPATIONAL INJURIES

Information on the frequency, distribution, and causes of disabling occupational injuries is less readily available than fatality data. The BLS, in addition to its annual survey, maintains the Supplementary Data System (SDS), with descriptive information on workers' compensation claims in OSHA-regulated states. This information covers fewer than 30 states and excludes public sector employees and certain other industrial groups. The NSC publishes information based on firms that participate in its occupational safety and health awards program but states explicitly that these firms cannot be construed as being representative of their industries. An additional database, the National Electronic Injury Surveillance System (NEISS) of the Consumer Product Safety Commission covers only injuries treated at emergency rooms but focuses on product-related injuries.

**TABLE 3.** *Disabling injuries by major industrial group (25)*

| Industrial group | Disabling injuries 1988 | Injury rates 1987 |
|---|---|---|
| Agriculture, forestry, fishing | 140,000 | 5.7 |
| Mining | 30,000 | 4.9 |
| Construction | 210,000 | 6.8 |
| Manufacturing | 350,000 | 5.3 |
| Transportation or utilities | 140,000 | 4.9 |
| Trade | 320,000 | 3.4 |
| Services | 330,000 | 2.7 |
| Governmental | 200,000 | — |
| Total | 1,800,000 | 3.6[a] |

[a]Private sector only.

Bureau of Labor Statistics data indicate that occupational injuries accounted for 93% of compensation cases closed in 1985. Sprains and strains, the most common injury, accounted for 45% of all cases, followed by fractures (12%); cuts, lacerations, and punctures (11%); and contusions, crushes, and bruises (10%) (25). Table 3 shows estimated rates of disabling injuries by major industrial groups in the private sector for 1987. The highest rates occurred in construction (6.8 per 100), agriculture (5.7 per 100), and manufacturing (5.3 per 100). Data from the BLS SDS indicate that "overexertion" injuries were the most common type of injury in 18 states in 1983, accounting for 28% of the total. "Struck by or against" injuries ranked next, accounting for 26%, and falls ranked third (16%). These were the three most common types of injury in each industrial group (25) (Table 4). Available United States data are evidence of a long-term decline in disabling injury rates in the construction and mining industries, which, however, appeared to be reversing in the late 1970s. In the manufacturing industry, the general trend toward declining rates appears to have reversed early in the same decade. This time pattern appeared to hold for all types of injuries (26).

**TABLE 4.** *Leading types of disabling work injury for high-risk industrial sectors (25)*

| Industrial sector | Type of accident | Percent of injuries in sector |
|---|---|---|
| Construction | Struck by or against | 29 |
| | Overexertion | 24 |
| | Falls | 21 |
| Agriculture, forestry, fishing | Struck by or against | 32 |
| | Overexertion | 22 |
| | Falls | 18 |
| Manufacturing | Overexertion | 29 |
| | Struck by or against | 27 |
| | Falls | 12 |

### Occupational Back Injuries

Occupational back injuries are the single most common nonfatal occupational injury in the United States. Occurring at the rate of 3.5 per 100 workers, back injuries accounted for 22% of lost-work injuries in 1988 (2) and 32% of workers' compensation costs in 1985 to 1987. The average indemnity compensation in 1985 was $5,193 and the average medical payment $2,358 (27).

The overwhelming majority of back injuries are classified as sprains and strains, and a pathoanatomic explanation is found in fewer than 15% of cases (27). Back injury episodes are largely self-limited; 75% of injured workers return to work within a month and 90% within 2 months. Approximately 5% of back-injured workers become chronically disabled, remaining out of work 6 months or longer (28). Although chronicity is infrequent, recurrence is common; some 50% of patients experience subsequent episodes. In fact, in several studies the most powerful individual predictor of a work-related back injury is a history of back pain (29–31).

#### *Occupational Risk Factors*

Occupational risk factors for back injury include manual materials handling, particularly heavy lifting (29,31–38) and lifting while twisting (39), and static postures (40,41). The mechanical load on the spine resulting from heavy lifting can be reduced by optimizing work technique and redesigning the workplace (42). Physiologic work load, as indicated by energy expenditure during studied tasks, can also be reduced by task redesign. When tasks are not amenable to redesign, such as patient lifting by nurses, reducing the speed of lifting is an important mitigating factor in work load (43).

Occupational groups exposed to whole-body vibration, such as tractor, truck, and bus drivers, are also at increased risk of back injuries, particularly disk herniation (44–47). Falls are cited as the cause of about 10% of occupational back injuries (48,49).

#### *Individual Risk Factors*

Peak onset of occupational back injury occurs in the third decade of life, in the first years of employment in the job (50). Disabling occupational back injury occurs more frequently in men (51); this is most probably due to the preponderance of males in occupations that require heavy lifting. Back injury rates in nursing occupations, in which women predominate, are among the highest in any occupation (40). Height, weight, isometric trunk strength, dynamic strength, endurance, and spinal flexibility have all been implicated as possible risk factors; however, there is not consistently convincing evidence for any (32,51–60).

Among lifestyles factors, smoking has repeatedly been associated with back injury—specifically with herniated disk (31,47,59). Reported associations of alcohol consumption and back pain have been confined to studies of chronic back–disabled patients (61); this factor requires further examination in prospective studies.

#### *Psychosocial Factors*

Psychosocial factors have been associated with reporting of occupational back pain (30,48,62–66). The relative importance of these psychosocial factors and physical demands of work were not analyzed in these studies, and the question requires further investigation. A controlled trial of an educational program to prevent low back injuries found no long-term benefit in reducing the rate of low back injury, the time off from work, or median cost (67).

A relationship between socioeconomic factors, such as divorced or widowed marital status, and education and availability of wage replacement has also been suggested but not consistently demonstrated (35,68–70).

### Injury Patterns in Selected Occupational Groups

While considerable attention has been given to the epidemiology of back injuries, the epidemiology of other types of disabling occupational injuries has been studied less thoroughly. Reports of injury patterns in specific occupational groups are summarized below for selected occupations.

#### *Firefighters*

Approximately 60% of firefighter injuries occur while fighting fires. Of these, two thirds are the results of burns, falls, and smoke inhalation (71).

In a case-control study, 75 injuries on the fireground were identified among approximately 1,200 firefighters in 1986, an incidence rate of 6.2 per 100; 39% were burns, another 39% falls, 15% smoke inhalations, and 7% a combination of falls and burns. Risk factors for burns included basement origin of the fire, injury on duty in the preceding 12 months, and firefighter training outside the department. Nozzle operators, engine officers, and forcible-entry firefighters were at highest risk of burns. Firefighters in truck companies were at increased risk of falls. Injury risk overall was not associated with age or years of experience (72).

#### *Law Enforcement Personnel*

In a study of traumatic injuries to law enforcement personnel in California, there were 1,901 paid workers compensation claims among 7,787 permanent employees in 1982 (24.4 per 100). The highest injury rates were in deputies (30 per 100) and for both males and females in the age range 30 to 34 years. In a sample of cases, altercations (26%), being struck by or striking a foreign object (20%), and overexertion (19%) were the leading causes of injury. The most common injuries were to the hand and wrist (23%), followed by back (16%) and knee (10%) injuries (73).

### *Agricultural Workers*

In addition to the high rate of fatal injuries described above, agricultural workers are at high risk of disabling injuries. In a study of dairy farm workers in New York State, Pratt et al. (74) found, in monthly telephone interviews conducted over a 2-year period, an injury event rate of 166/1,000 person-years. In this study, 30% of reported injuries did not result in restricted activity. In eastern Ontario, Brison and Pickett (75) found, based on personal interviews, a self-reported injury incidence rate of 7 per 100 person-years. Zhou and Roseman (76) found, using mailed questionnaires, a similar rate in Alabama farmers; 7.8 per 100 farmers were injured per year. Some farm workers experience more than one injury in a given year; in this study, the annual event rate, 9.9/100, was also reported. The respondents sought medical attention for 90% of the injuries. In both these studies, injuries were counted if they resulted in restricted activity or seeking medical attention. Further, they relied on longer recall than Pratt and colleagues. It has been estimated that 1-month recall yields a reported injury rate 36% higher than 1-year recall (77). In a population-based study in Wisconsin, Nordstrom and colleagues (78) reported that 1 in 31 (3.2/100 persons/year) farm workers sought medical care for a farm-work–related injury annually, and that injury rates were highest among dairy farm workers and among adult males. This incidence rate is lower than reported in other studies, partly because it only counted injuries for which medical care was sought and partly because the source of information was medical care records rather than self-report, which is subject to recall problems. A large proportion of the injuries reported in these and other studies are machine related, but injuries from animals on dairy and beef farms are also important (74–76,78–80).

### *Manufacturing Workers*

Manufacturing industry workers, in addition to being at risk for sprains and strains (principally of the back), are the group at highest risk of amputations. It has been reported that in 1977 60% of all amputations occurred in manufacturing, where only 30% of workers were employed (81). Olson and Gerberich (82), reporting a special study of manufacturing workers in Minnesota, indicated that 94% of amputated parts were fingers. Sorock and colleagues (83) report that persons working with machines or maintaining them in factories are at highest risk of hospitalization for finger amputations.

## COMMENT

Our knowledge of the epidemiology of fatal injuries is based largely on surveillance data, whose completeness and validity have been questioned. The focus of attention on the prevention of occupational injuries by NIOSH in the mid-1980s (1) has led to an increase in analytic research on risk factors for occupational injury, several of which have been highlighted here. It is hoped that within 10 years our understanding of the causes of fatal and nonfatal occupational injuries will have improved accordingly. The relative importance of individual risk factors for occupational injury to the back, the most often injured part of the body, remain to be clarified, although its epidemiology has been under study for at least three decades. Recent attention to occupational injury of agricultural workers has begun to illuminate the seriousness of the risk to farm workers. Finally, the epidemiology of other types of disabling occupational injury and of injuries to specific occupational groups needs continued elaboration.

## REFERENCES


1. Millar JD. Leading work-related diseases and injuries. *Scand J Work Environ Health* 1988;14(suppl 1):5–6.
2. *Accident facts, 1992, and work injury and illness rates.* Chicago: National Safety Council, 1992.
3. Leigh JP, Markowitz SB, Faks M, Shin C, Landrigan PJ. Occupational injury and illness in the United States. Estimates of costs, morbidity, and mortality. *Arch Intern Med* 1997;157:1557–1568.
4. Rubens AJ, Oleckno WA, Papaeliou L. Establishing guidelines for the identification of occupational injuries: a systematic appraisal. *J Occup Environ Med* 1995;37:151–159.
5. Kraus JF. Fatal and nonfatal injuries in occupational settings: a review. *Annu Rev Public Health* 1985;6:403–418.
6. Bell CA, Stout NA, Bender TR, Conroy CS, Crouse WE, Myers JR. Fatal occupational injuries in the United States, 1980 through 1985. *JAMA* 1990;263:3047–3050.
7. Stout N, Bell C. Effectiveness of source documents for identifying fatal occupational injuries: a synthesis of studies. *Am J Public Health* 1991; 81:725–728.
8. Stout-Wiegand N. Fatal occupational injuries in US industries, 1984: comparison of two national surveillance systems. *Am J Public Health* 1988;78:1215–1217.
9. Panel on Occupational Injury. *Prevention of occupational injury.* CDC-NIOSH Third National Injury Control Conference, 1991.
10. Mendeloff JM, Kagey BT. Using occupational safety and health administration accident investigations to study patterns in work fatalities. *J Occup Med* 1990;32:1117–1123.
11. Baker SP, Samkoff JS, Fisher RS, Van Buren CB. Fatal occupational injuries. *JAMA* 1982;248:692–697.
12. Loomis DP. Occupation, industry, and fatal motor vehicle crashes in 20 states, 1986–1987. *Am J Public Health* 1991;81:733–735.
13. Karlson T, Noren J. Farm tractor fatalities: the failure of voluntary safety standards. *Am J Public Health* 1979;69:146–149.
14. Goodman RA, Smith JD, Sikes RK, Rogers DL, Mickey JL. Fatalities associated with farm tractor injuries: an epidemiologic study. *Public Health Rep* 1985;100:329–333.
15. Erlich SM, Driscoll TR, Harrison JE, Frommer MS, Leigh J. Work-related agricultural fatalities in Australia, 1982–1984. *Scand J Work Environ Health* 1993;19:162–167.
16. Rivara FP. Fatal and nonfatal farm injuries to children and adolescents in the United States. *Pediatrics* 1985;76:567–573.
17. Etherton JR, Myers JR, Jensen RC, Russell JC, Braddee RW. Agricultural machine-related deaths. *Am J Public Health* 1991;81:766–768.
18. Weeks JL, Fox M. Fatality rates and regulatory policies in bituminous

coal mining, United States, 1959–1981. *Am J Public Health* 1983;73: 1278–1280.
19. Suruda A, Smith G, Baker SP. Deaths from trench cave-in in the construction industry. *J Occup Med* 1988;30:552–555.
20. Davis H, Honchar PA, Suarez L. Fatal occupational injuries of women, Texas 1975–84. *Am J Public Health* 1987;77:1524–1527.
21. Bell CA. Female homicides in United States workplaces, 1980–1985. *Am J Public Health* 1991;81:729–732.
22. Sanderson L, Smith GS. Alcohol and residential, recreational, and occupational injuries: a review of the epidemiologic evidence. *Annu Rev Public Health* 1988;9:99–121.
23. Parkinson DK, Gauss WF, Perper JA, Elliott SA. Traumatic workplace deaths in Allegheny County, Pennsylvania 1983 and 1984. *J Occup Med* 1986;28:100–102.
24. Arner O. The role of alcohol in fatal accidents among seamen. *Br J Addict* 1973;68:185–189.
25. *Accident facts 1989.* Chicago: National Safety Council, 1990.
26. Robinson JC. The rising long-term trend in occupational injury rates. *Am J Public Health* 1988;78:276–281.
27. Nachemson AL. The lumbar spine: an orthopaedic challenge. *Spine* 1976;1:59–71.
28. Spitzer WO, LeBlanc FE, DuPuis M, et al. Scientific approach to the assessment and management of activity-related spinal disorders; Report of the Quebec Task Force on Spinal Disorders. *Spine* 1987; 12(suppl 1):S1–S59.
29. Biering-Sorensen F. A prospective study of low back pain in a general population. III. Medical service-work consequence. *Scand J Rehabil Med* 1983;15:89–96.
30. Bigos SJ, Battie MC, Spengler DM, et al. A prospective study of work perceptions and psychosocial factors affecting the report of back injury. *Spine* 1991;16:1–6.
31. Skovron ML, Nordin M, Sterling RC, Mulvihill MN. Patient care and low back injury in nursing personnel. *Hum Factors* 1986;4:855–862.
32. Chaffin DB, Park KS. A longitudinal study of low back pain as associated with occupational weight lifting factors. *Am Ind Hyg Assoc J* 1973;34:513–524.
33. Damkot DK, Pope MH, Lord J, Frymoyer JW. The relationship between work history, work environment and low back pain in men. *Spine* 1984;9:395–399.
34. Frymoyer JW, Pope MH, Clements JH. Risk factors in low back pain. *J Bone Joint Surg* 1983;65:213–218.
35. Gyntelberg F. One-year incidence of low back pain among male residents of Copenhagen aged 40–59. *Dan Med Bull* 1974;21:30–36.
36. Magora A. Investigation of the relation of low back pain and occupation. III. Physical requirements: sitting, standing, and weightlifting. *Ind Med Surg* 1972;41:5.
37. Riihimaki H. Back pain and heavy physical work: a comparative study of concrete reinforcement workers and maintenance house painters. *Br J Ind Med* 1985;42:226–232.
38. Venning PJ, Walter SD, Stitt LW. Personal and job-related factors as determinants of incidence of back injuries among nursing personnel. *J Occup Med* 1987;29:820–825.
39. Kelsey JL, Githens PB, White AA, et al. An epidemiologic study of lifting and twisting on the job and risk of acute prolapsed lumbar intervertebral disk. *J Orthop Res* 1984;2:61–66.
40. Klein BP, Jensen RC, Sanderson LM. Assessment of workers' compensation claims for back strains/sprains. *J Occup Med* 1984;26: 443–448.
41. Kelsey JL, Golden AL. Occupational and workplace factors. *Occup Med* 1988;3:7–16.
42. Hultman G, Nordin M, Ortengren R. The influence of a preventive educational program on trunk flexion in janitors. *Appl Ergonometr* 1984;15:127.
43. Nordin M, Ortengren R, Andersson GBJ. Measurement of trunk movement during work. *Spine* 1984;9:465.
44. Gruber GJ. *Relationships between whole-body vibration and morbidity patterns among interstate truck drivers.* NIOSH publication 77–168. Washington, DC: National Institute of Occupational Safety and Health, 1976.
45. Gruber GJ. *Relationships between whole-body vibration and morbidity patterns among motor coach operators.* NIOSH publication 75–104. Washington, DC: National Institute of Occupational Safety and Health, 1974.
46. Kelsey JL, Hardy RJ. Driving of motor vehicles as a risk factor for acute herniated lumbar intervertebral disc. *Am J Epidemiol* 1975; 102:63–73.
47. Kelsey JL, Githens PB, O'Connor T, et al. Acute prolapsed lumbar intervertebral disc: an epidemiologic study with special reference to driving automobiles and cigarette smoking. *Spine* 1984;9:608.
48. Bigos SJ, Spengler DM, Martin NA, et al. Back injuries in industry: a retrospective study. II. Injury factors. *Spine* 1986;116:246–251.
49. Snook SH, Campanelli RA, Hart JW. A study of three preventive approaches to low back injury. *J Occup Med* 1978;20:478–481.
50. Bigos SJ, Spengler DM, Martin NA, Zeh J, Fisher L, Nachemson A. Back injuries in industry: a retrospective study. III. Employee-related factors. *Spine* 1986;11:252–255.
51. Snook SH. Low back pain in industry. In: White AA, Gordon SL, eds. *AAOS symposium on low back pain.* St. Louis: CV Mosby; 1982.
52. Keyserling WM, Herrin GD, Chaffin DG. Isometric strength testing as a means of controlling medical incidents on strenuous jobs. *J Occup Med* 1980;22:332.
53. Battie MC, Bigos SJ, Fisher LD, Hansson TH, Jones ME, Wortley MD. Isometric lifting strength as a predictor of industrial back pain. *Spine* 1989;14:851.
54. Troup JDG, Foreman TK, Baxter CE, Brown D. The perception of back pain and the role of psychophysical testing of lifting capacity. *Spine* 1987;12:645.
55. Himmelstein JS, Andersson GBJ. Low back pain: risk evaluation and preplacement screening. State of the art reviews. *Occup Med* 1988;3: 255–69.
56. Battie MC, Bigos SJ, Fisher LD, et al. The role of spinal flexibility in back pain complaints within industry: a prospective study. *Spine* 1990; 15:768–773.
57. Biering-Sorensen F. Physical measurements as risk indicators of low-back trouble over a 1-year period. *Spine* 1984;9:106–119.
58. Cady LS, Bischoff DP, O'Connell ER. Strength and fitness and subsequent back injury in firefighters. *J Occup Med* 1979;21:269–272.
59. Battie MC, Bigos SJ, Fisher LD, et al. A prospective study of the role of cardiovascular risk factors and fitness in industrial back complaints. *Spine* 1989;14:141.
60. Magnusson M, Granqvist M, Jonson R, et al. The loads on the lumbar spine during work at an assembly line. The risks for fatigue injuries of vertebral bodies. *Spine* 1990;15:774–779.
61. Sandstrom J, Andersson GBJ, Wallerstedt S. The role of alcohol abuse in working disability in patients with low back pain. *Scand J Rehabil Med* 1984;16:147–149.
62. Love A, Peck C. The MMPI and psychological factors in chronic low back pain: a review. *Pain* 1987;28:1–12.
63. Sandstrom J, Esbjornsson E. Return to work after rehabilitation. The significance of the patient's own prediction. *Scand J Rehabil Med* 1986;18:29–33.
64. Waddell G, Main CJ, Morris EW, DiPaola M, Gray ICM. Chronic low-back pain, psychologic distress, and illness behavior. *Spine* 1984;9: 209–213.
65. Craufurd DIO, Creed F, Jayson MIV. Life events and psychological disturbance in patients with low-back pain. *Spine* 1990;15:490–494.
66. Turner RS, Leiding WC. Correlation of the MMPI with lumbosacral spine fusion results. *Spine* 1985;10:932–936.
67. Daltrov LH, Iversen MD, Larson MG, et al. A controlled trial of an educational program to prevent low back injuries. *N Engl J Med* 1997;337:322–328.
68. Simons GR, Mirabile MP. An analysis and interpretation of industrial medical data with concentration on back problems. *J Occup Med* 1972; 14:227–231.
69. Walsh NE, Dimitri D. Financial compensation and recovery from low back pain. *Occup Med* 1988;3:109–122.
70. Hammonds W, Brena SF, Unikel IP. Compensation for work-related injuries and rehabilitation of patients with chronic pain. *South Med J* 1978;71:664–666.
71. Karter MJ, LeBlanc PR, Washburn AE. U.S. firefighter injuries 1986. *Fire Command* 1987(November);35–44.
72. Heineman EF, Shy CM, Checkoway H. Injuries on the fireground: risk factors for traumatic injuries among professional firefighters. *Am J Ind Med* 1989;15:267–282.
73. Sullivan CSB, Shimizu KT. Epidemiological studies of work-related injuries among law enforcement personnel. *J Soc Occup Med* 1988;38: 33–40.
74. Pratt DS, Marcel LH, Darrow D, Stallones L, May JJ, Jenkins P. The

dangers of dairy farming: the injury experience of 600 workers followed for two years. *Am J Ind Med* 1992;21:637–650
75. Brison RJ, Pickett CWL. Non-fatal farm injuries on 117 Eastern Ontario beef and dairy farms: a one-year study. *Am J Ind Med* 1992;21:623–636.
76. Zhou C, Roseman JM. Agricultural injuries among a population-based sample of farm operators in Alabama. *Am J Ind Med* 1994;25:385–402.
77. Zwerling C, Sprince NL, Wallace RB, Davis CS, Whitten PS, Heerings SG. Effect of recall on the reporting of occupational injuries among older workers in the Health and Retirement Study. *Am J Ind Med* 1995;28:583–590.
78. Nordstrom DL, Layde PM, Olson KA, Stueland D, Brand L, Follen MA. Incidence of farm-work-related acute injury in a defined population. *Am J Ind Med* 1995;28:551–564.
79. Simpson SG. Farm machine injuries. *J Trauma* 1984;24:150–152.
80. Beatty ME, Zook EG, Russell RC, Kinkead LR. Grain auger injuries: the replacement of the corn picker injury? *Plast Reconstr Surg* 1982;69:96–102.
81. McCaffrey DP. Work-related amputations by type and prevalence. *Monthly Labor Rev* 1982;35–41.
82. Olson DK, Gerberich SG. Traumatic amputations in the workplace. *J Occup Med* 1986;28:480–485.
83. Sorock GS, Smith E, Hall N. Hospitalized occupational finger amputations, New Jersy, 1985 and 1986. *Am J Ind Med* 1993;23:439–447.

*Environmental and Occupational Medicine, Third Edition,* edited by William N. Rom.
Published by Lippincott–Raven Publishers, Philadelphia, 1998.

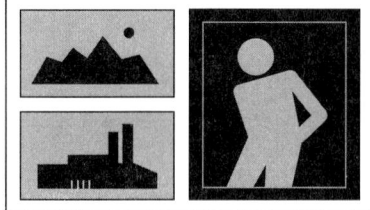

CHAPTER 64

# Occupational Safety and Human Factors

Hongwei Hsiao and William E. Halperin

Occupational injuries pose a continuing major threat to the health and well-being of American workers. They account for a significant amount of human suffering, loss of productivity, and economic burden to employers. The Bureau of Labor Statistics estimated 6.3 million nonfatal injuries occurred in U.S. workplaces in 1992 (1). The leading causes of these injuries were overexertion, contact with objects or equipment, and falls. In addition, according to the National Traumatic Occupational Fatalities (NTOF) surveillance system, more than 77,000 workers died as a result of work-related injuries during the period 1980 through 1992. This means that an average of 16 workers died each day from a traumatic injury (2). The leading causes of death were motor vehicles, machines, homicide, worker falls, electrocution, and workers being struck by objects. The injuries and fatalities affect different segments of the working population and all industrial settings. The total costs (direct and indirect) of work-related injuries and fatalities to U.S. industries and societies are estimated to be as high as $121 billion per year (3).

Occupational injuries often result when forces, stresses, or conditions imposed by work exceed levels that workers can physically tolerate or when the workplace creates conditions to which workers cannot effectively adapt or respond, either physically or cognitively. Most of the injury-producing incidents have multiple causes. Research on injury causes indicates that human performance was an important factor in about 80% of the injury incidents (4). Further research evidence suggests that these human-performance problems are often induced by poorly designed equipment, work environments, and ineffective training (5). Increased understanding of human factors will contribute to the design of new and improved systems and controls, work practices, and personal protective equipment to protect workers from injury.

The term *human factors* has multiple meanings. It refers to the elements that influence a person's ability to effectively use systems or equipment to accomplish their functions. The primary human factor elements are systems or equipment, tasks, environments, and humans themselves (6). Human factors, as a discipline, is a field that studies and applies information about human abilities, limitations, and other characteristics to the design of tools, machines, systems, tasks, jobs, and environments for safe, comfortable, and effective human use (7).

The primary emphasis of this chapter is the prevention of traumatic injuries in the workplace through human-factors intervention. Typical examples of occupational traumatic injuries include the following: A road-roller operator was found unresponsive in a ditch after his road-roller went out of control and struck a tar truck on the road. A construction worker fell from his ladder on concrete and injured his feet when the ladder slipped out from under him. A roofer, carrying a bucket of hot asphalt, tripped and spilled hot asphalt on his face and had second-degree burns to his face and wrist. A construction worker fell off a bulldozer at work, resulting in contusions and fractures to the tibia and fibula. A self-employed person suffered right inguinal hernia when lifting hay bales at a farm. A construction worker suffered an acute strain of the right shoulder and arm when lifting 200 lb of oak wood (8). A firefighter experienced heat stroke due to heavy physical work and the hot environment of a burning forest (9). The sudden roof collapse of

H. Hsiao and W. E. Halperin: Division of Safety Research, National Institute for Occupational Safety and Health, Morgantown, West Virginia 26505-2888.

a burning auto parts store claimed the lives of two firefighters (10).

There are six major areas of specialization of human factors that are most related to the development of programs for reducing occupational traumatic injuries. Applications of these disciplines are presented in the sections that follow. In addition, a public health approach for injury prevention and control is discussed. *Sensory performance* is concerned with human sensory capabilities (e.g., visual acuity, hearing ability, sensitivity) and the impact of environmental factors (e.g., lighting, noise) on human sensory systems. Sensory performance data provide important information for designing displays, guarding systems, vehicle operation controls, and communication methods to minimize the likelihood of injury incidents. *Information processing* is concerned with human mental or cognitive capabilities for storing and processing information and for making decisions. The information is important for designing an adequate work environment, equipment, and jobs that are compatible with human expectations to minimize the possibility of error. *Anthropometry* is concerned with physical measures of a person's size, form, and functional capacities. In occupational-injury prevention applications, anthropometry measurements are used to evaluate the physical interaction of workers with tasks, tools, machines, vehicles, and personal protective equipment. *Biomechanics* is concerned with the application of mechanics to living creatures (11). It uses laws of physics and engineering concepts to describe mechanical properties of human tissue, motion undergone by the various body segments, and the force acting on body parts during normal daily activities (12) (see Chapter 109). *Work physiology* is concerned with the responses of the cardiovascular, pulmonary, and musculoskeletal systems to the metabolic demands of work. Both occasional and regular physiologic overloading may represent health hazards that could lead to injury incidents in many occupational settings. *Safety management* is concerned with training, age, experience, perception of risks, motivation, and employee participation in minimizing the likelihood of occupational injuries.

## SENSORY PERFORMANCE

During human-machine interactions, several human information processing steps are involved. Information processing begins with the detection of some environmental event through human sensory systems. The information is then stored in memory and intellectual processing is performed. Actions such as movements and controls follow. During the phase of detection, some events are so noticeable that immediate detection is easily assured (e.g., identifying a broken tea pot). However, the difficulty of successful detection increases when it is necessary to detect events that are near the threshold of perception (e.g., recognizing signs in the dark). Three sensory issues most related to the development of programs for reducing occupational traumatic injuries are visual interface, voice communication, and proprioception interaction.

### Visual Interface

At the human-machine interface, most information is input through visual displays. Examples would include the ability to detect differences in the position of two controls, to recognize the presence of an object in the visual field, to distinguish between two objects close in space, and so forth. Therefore, a basic understanding of the visual-interface process is necessary. Human visibility is affected by many factors. There are at least four critical factors that must be considered in designing visual tasks. They are size of critical detail, brightness, contrast, and time available for seeing (13). In addition to the four critical factors, glare is frequently a concern of job safety (14,15). Glare causes light to scatter within the eye, causing an overall veiling brightness that reduces contrast (16).

The size of critical detail is defined as the smallest dimension or gap that must be seen for recognition. It is typically expressed in visual angles, which are the angles subtended at the eye by the viewed object. Usually, this is given in minutes of arc, as computed by the following formula: visual angle (min) = $(57.3 \times 60) \times L/D$, where $L$ is the size of the object measured perpendicular to the line of sight, and $D$ is the distance from the eye to the object. The 57.3 and 60 in the formula are constants for angles less than 600 minutes (17). For example, if a child has a body height of 120 cm, then the visual angle of the child to be seen at a distance of 300 m is $57.3 \times 60 \times 120/30{,}000 = 13.75$ minutes. Under ideal lighting and high-contrast conditions, a person with 20/20 vision can identify targets (i.e., 50% probability of detection) with critical detail size of 1 minute. For a 95% probability of accurate identification of targets, 2 minutes of critical detail size would be required (13). It is usually recommended that the visual angle for electronic displays be at least 15 minutes of arc under good viewing conditions and at least 21 minutes of arc under degraded viewing environments (18).

The brightness ($B$; unit: foot-Lambert) is defined as light reflected by a surface. $B = R \times E$, where $R$ is the percent reflection of a surface, and $E$ is the illumination, which is defined as the amount of light falling on a surface. One foot-Lambert (ft-L) is the brightness of a surface (100% reflectance) illuminated by 1 ft-candle light ($E$ or illumination). The illumination $E = I/D^2$, where $I$ is the intensity (amount of energy radiated by a source; unit: candles) and $D$ is the distance from the source. One foot-candle (ft-C) of illumination is the amount of light on a surface located 1 foot from a 1 candle source.

Contrast *(C)* is the comparison of the brightness of the target ($B_t$) to that of background ($B_g$). Cobb and Moss (19) suggest the formula $C(\%) = 100 \times (B_g - B_t)/B_g$, which covers a range of 0% to 100% contrast (19). The time available for seeing is referred to as the time allowed to view the object. The exposure times experienced in normal work activities are usually above those needed for this to be a problem (above 200 to 300 milliseconds at normal daylight levels of illumination). The relationship among size, brightness, and contrast is described in Fig. 1 (19). The vertical axis indicates the minimum separable acuity as a function of luminance (contrast ratio and brightness) in the horizontal axis at the 300-millisecond reading time.

Here is an example in a manufacturing environment. A broadcast sheet has letters of 0.011" stroke width and has illumination of 11 ft-C. The contrast is about 90%, black letters on white background; the white background has reflectance of 90%. What is the maximum acceptable reading distance at the area where this sheet is read? The brightness $B = ER = 11 \times 0.9 = 9.9$ ft-L. The contrast $C =$ 90%. The 95% threshold visual angle is found to be 1.8 minutes using Cobb and Moss curves (Fig. 1). Therefore, the maximum reading distance $D$ is $57.3 \times 60 \times 0.011"/1.8 = 21"$. This means that a person with good reading acuity (20/20) needs to get quite close to the sheet to read it. It is not unusual to find persons with 20/40 reading vision (probably age 45 or older). For them, the reading distance must be half of the 21 inches or 10.5 inches, which is a big challenge to them because people at this age cannot easily focus on a target 10.5" away (16). Therefore, it is recommended that the letters be enlarged at least two to three times.

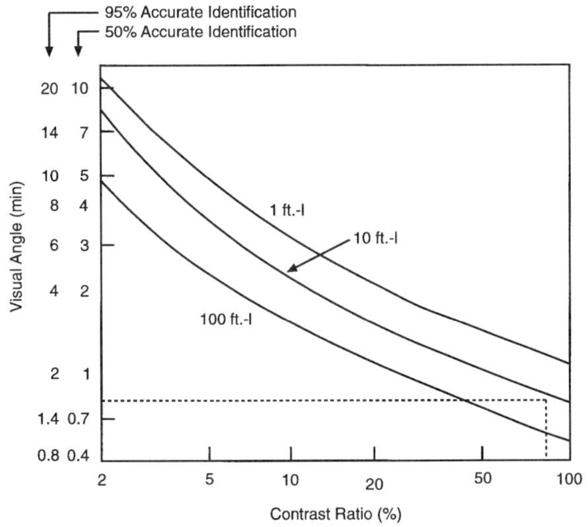


**FIG. 1.** Minimum separable acuity as a function of luminance at the 0.3-second reading time (19).

**Voice Communication**

In many occupations, the performance of people depends heavily on voice communication. An example is the job of overhead crane operator. The speaker and the listener may not be near enough for face-to-face communication, and may need to shout or use a speech transmission device. Verbal miscommunication is quite possible, and can result in dangerous conditions for ground crew, materials handlers, and hook crew. To address safety and performance concerns, a system or job that involves voice communication must be designed with speech content that will be audible, distinguishable, and properly understood (20).

Voice is a form of physical sound wave. A physical sound wave is described in terms of its frequency and intensity. Frequency is defined as the number of cycles of pressure change occurring in 1 second. If the sound pressure changes from positive to negative and back to positive 1,000 times a second, the frequency is 1,000 cycles per second or 1,000 hertz (Hz). Intensity is defined in terms of how large the sound pressure changes are. The range of sound intensities is so large that a special number scale has been developed to measure it. It is measured in decibels (dB). Sound intensity (dB) $= 10 \log(p/p_0)^2$, where $p$ = pressure measured and $p_0$ = reference pressure = 0.0002 dyn/cm$^2$. $p_0$ is the average threshold for perceiving a 1,000-Hz tone. The human ear has a frequency range of 20 to 20,000 Hz, although most persons are most sensitive to a much smaller range of sounds. Most speech sounds are between about 200 and 4,000 Hz and in the range of 60 and 75 dB at a distance of 1 m. We typically are able to manage 1 to 130 dB without harm. However, extended exposure to high sound-pressure levels (over 100 dB) may result in permanent damage to the ear.

A definition that is useful in understanding voice communication is the signal-to-noise ratio (S/N ratio). It is a measure of the relative sound intensity of speech to background noise. To compute the S/N ratio, subtract the number of decibels in a noise source from the number of decibels in the speech signal. For example, if the average intensity of speech is 75 dB and the average intensity of the noise in which the speech is spoken is 70 dB, we have an S/N ratio of +5 dB (20). At S/N = 0 dB, certain individual consonants are confused. At S/N = +12 dB, all the consonants are readily distinguished. For satisfactory communication of most voice messages in noise, the speech level should exceed the noise level by at least 6 dB (21,22).

There are other safety concerns that should be considered for designing systems requiring voice communication. When noise levels are high (80 dB or more) or when speech levels are high (85 dB or more) ear plugs will usually improve speech intelligibility in face-to-face communication (23). Noise-canceling microphones would also be helpful for improving voice communication. In addition, the use of a limited set size of the vocabulary that both the talker and listener know thoroughly has some advantages. The difference between very small (two-word) and moderate size (1,000-word) vocabularies can change by 18 dB the signal-to-noise ratio required for a given level of intelligibility. Furthermore, familiar, frequently used, and longer words will be more correctly identified than less familiar and short words. Both familiarity and length factors can change by 10 to 15 dB the signal-to-noise ratio required for a given level of intelligibility. Finally, a designer may want to have users use the International Word-Spelling Alphabet when individual characters are to be communicated verbally in noisy environments (20).

### Proprioception Interaction

The proprioception interaction refers to the perception of a person's movement and to the sensation of his or her limb positions in space. Two sensory systems play the most important role in proprioception. The vestibular system in the ear concerns itself with maintaining the body's posture and equilibrium. The kinesthetic system, which consists of sensors in the muscles and tendons, indicates the relative positions of the limbs and of different parts of the body (24–26). The proprioception interaction is important for notifying persons about the activities of their bodies without them having to actively monitor every part of it, for example, watching their hands while operating a control above their heads, or looking at their feet while walking. Many daily job activities include proprioception to a greater or lesser extent; this sense controls fine-motor activities, multilimb coordination, direction discrimination, reaction time, speed of arm movement, motor adjustment for controlling moving objects, manual dexterity, finger dexterity, aiming (speed and accuracy of placement), and arm-hand steadiness, to name a few activities (27–29).

The proprioception interaction has significant impact on fall injury prevention—a leading national occupational concern. The demands on workers postural stability to avoid falls are increased when the work surface is elevated, and under conditions such as uneven and narrow walking surfaces, slippery surfaces, unbalanced loads, or destabilizing effect of the wind. For maintenance of postural stability, especially while performing elevated activities, an integrated coordination of the proprioceptive and visual systems is essential. Normally, any external force placed on the body or displacement in the body's position will be quickly detected, and compensating reactions will be evoked, such as swaying or a change in posture; or if more serious, by staggering and sweeping of the arms. If correcting mechanisms fail to respond properly to a displacing force, a fall will occur. Such failures may be increased by fatigue, lack of lift/carry strength, or other factors. In fact, an investigation of 600 scaffold-related falls by Helander (30) revealed that approximately 60% of the falls were caused by a loss of balance that was primarily the result of a combination of human performance problems such as worker techniques and exertion level, as well as environmental factors such as work-surface condition and lighting.

## INFORMATION PROCESSING

In human-machine interaction, information processing takes place after sensory systems receive signals. Human information processing has identifiable limitations in several different aspects: absolute judgment, relative judgment, choice reaction (decision), single-channel limitation, memory, and perception.

### Absolute Judgment

Absolute judgment is the ability to accurately judge the level of a stimulus without a comparison stimulus. An example is that of an inspector of fruit quality who must categorize a given specimen into one of several size levels (e.g., small, medium, large, jumbo). Human ability to make judgments on a single sensory dimension is severely limited, if errors in judgment are to be less than 5%. This limit varies somewhat from one sensory continuum to another. It is less than four levels for saltiness of taste, about three to five levels for brightness, loudness, and vibration amplitude, about five to seven levels for length of a line, about four to five levels for pure tone frequency, and about 12 to 13 level for colors (hue) (16). While the limits of absolute judgment are severe, humans are readily able to recognize some stimuli in the environment by a combination of two or more stimulus dimensions, rather than by levels along a single dimension; for example, it is possible to recognize a person based on the weight and hair color (orthogonal dimensions) or based on the weight plus body height (correlated dimensions). Studies on human performance in absolute judgment of multidimensional auditory stimuli found that as each successive orthogonal dimension was added, subjects showed a continuous gain in total information transmitted but a loss of information transmitted per dimension (31). Studies also showed that the information loss per dimension for correlated dimensions is much less than that of orthogonal dimensions (32).

The knowledge of absolute judgment has important implications in safety. Human ability to make absolute judgments is limited to 7 ± 2 stimulus categories. Therefore, system displays and machine controls should be designed in a way that does not require operators to discern too many stimulus levels. When absolute security is required or minimal information loss is allowed, it is good to choose redundant coding (high correlation dimensions) so that two or more physical dimensions represent only one dimension of information. For example, control knobs with both shape and texture codings have been found to be useful in preventing actuation of the wrong control.

### Relative Judgment

Relative judgment is the ability to detect a difference between two or more stimuli. Assuming that $I$ is the intensity of the smaller stimulus and $DI$ is the difference between the smaller and larger stimulus, then Weber's law indicates that $(DI_{critical})/I$ = constant (16). The actual value of the constant varies with the senses; for example, 2% for brightness, 5% for length, 7% for time periods, 7% for weight, 7% for speed, and 25% for saltiness. A constant of 7% is often used as a rough guess. However, Weber's law does not apply to hearing (loudness of frequency).

### Choice Reaction

The safety application in choice reaction is the reaction time (RT) limitations. With a single and simple stimulus, human reaction time is 150 to 200 milliseconds if warning occurs about 1 second before the stimulus. The eye, brain, nerves, and muscles take about 10 to 30, 90, 20, and 30 milliseconds to react respectively. Choice reaction time increases with the number of alternatives, more specifically with the amount of information that has to be processed. If alternatives are equally likely, the amount of information $(H)$ can be expressed as $\log_2 (n)$ bits, where $n$ is the number of alternatives. Hick's law predicts average reaction time to be $RT = a + b \times H$. For stimulus lights with response buttons cases, the formula is $RT = 150 + 100 \times H$. The intercept $a$ is affected by the intensity of a stimulus, warning period and duration, and individual age. In addition, some senses (touch/vibration, hearing, vision) are faster than others (heat, smell). The slope $b$ is mainly affected by the stimulus-response compatibility. This is a very important concept in the design of human-machine interfaces (e.g., if the machine action is to go to the right, the operator should move the control to the right). Learning also affects the slope $b$. After sufficient practice (thousands of trials) $b$ can be nearly zero (33). In addition, $b$ increases with age.

The choice reaction time is an important component of real-world tasks and occupational safety concerns (34). In industrial assembly, the part may be delivered out of the chute upside down or right side up. The alternatives then become $n = 2$ instead of $n = 1$. In operating a construction vehicle following a co-worker's hand signal, the direction controls could be $n = 4$ or more. In the job design, several points can be considered to avoid or reduce choice reaction time. Since the amount of information $H = \log_2 (n)$, reducing the number of things that can happen reduces the choice reaction time; for example, the chute can be redesigned so that it always delivers the part right side up. In this case, $n = 1$ and $H = 0$, no information is processed and reaction time is minimum. Using strong stimuli and a short predictable warning period is also helpful in reducing reaction time. In addition, operating controls should be designed with high stimulus-response compatibility. Certainly, using a very experienced operator will help, too.

### Single-Channel Limitation

Humans can only pay attention to one task at a time. What often appears to be simultaneous performance of two or more tasks is actually "time sharing." For examples, some drivers use cellular phones or read maps while driving, and safety guards at big construction sites appear to guide several dirt trucks simultaneously. It is desirable to leave as much spare mental capacity as possible to deal with emergency loads (35). In the design of control systems or equipment, human channel limitation must be well considered. The controls should be designed with high stimulus-response compatibility. Shape coding, texture, and color can be used to avoid excess time in searching for controls or operating the wrong controls. Consistency of control locations (i.e., functional grouping) is also helpful to ease identification and thus reduce mental work loads. In addition, measures should be implemented to avoid accidental activation (e.g., the parking gear must be on in order to start a car engine).

### Memory

Memory is an important step in the human information process. The human central cognitive processes such as perception, intellect, and movement control all require memory to function properly. Of occupational injury prevention concern, a safety professional should be aware of at least three types of memory: sensory memory, short-term memory, and long-term memory.

The persistence of a stimulus that takes place in the sense itself, not in the brain, is defined as sensory memory. Although there do not seem to be many design-related issues associated with sensory memory, it is important for safety professionals to be aware of its existence and to make full use of its capacities when needed. In the case of vision, an image usually persists for about $^1/_4$ to 2 seconds. The duration of visual sensory memory can be lengthened by optimizing the stimulus-background contrast. The auditory sensory memory appears to last for $^1/_4$ to 5 seconds. The touch sensory memory lasts for about 0.8 seconds. Difficulties with sensory memory would likely show up as an increase in errors. If a typist or key operator were typing codes, say seven-character codes such as BKVRTSC, we would expect that there would be more errors in the rightmost positions and fewer in the left positions, and most errors would tend to occur in the fifth position.

Short-term memory (STM) is referred to as the correct recall or appropriate performance immediately or shortly after the presentation of the material. People use STM to hold information temporarily, usually for a few seconds. Information stored in STM appears to come from both external (through the senses by way of perceptual process) and internal (results of reasoning, problem-solving, or decision-making) sources. STM has a capacity of 7 ± 2 items (sometimes referred to as chunks of information). Safety engineers or system designers should particularly keep in mind problems associated with STM, such as limited capacity (six or fewer units), relatively short duration (usually less than 20 seconds), and the requirement of continued rehearsals without interference to maintain information. During the rehearsal of a code or information, other intellectual activities cannot take place; the most likely mistakes are those related to the rehearsal sensory features. If longer strings of characters (codes) must be used, they should be divided into groups of three or four to help the rehearsal (example: telephone number 202-499-1089 instead of 2024991089). Organized patterns can also help to reduce the load on the STM. For example, the statement "TFH TDH OIH OEX TEG" is considered to be 5 or 15 chunks of information. The statement "THE FOX HIT THE DOG," however, is a one- to two-chunk piece of information.

Long-term memory (LTM) is referred to as the ability to respond to a stimulus, recite a list, remember an association, and so on, after a long period of time following the material and presentation. Its slow rate of decay and great amount of remembered material distinguish it from STM. LTM relies heavily on organization to build and maintain content. Although memories are not always accessible, the evidence is unclear as to whether these memories are lost. It is desirable to reduce the number of times people need to recall information or instructions, and increase the number of opportunities to recognize one or more available alternatives. By doing this, the amount of forgetting is reduced. A practical application is that manual-selection method is better than command-input method for most personal computer users. In addition, reduction and elaboration are typical ways to help humans remember events. Reductions frequently take the form of acronyms. An example is to name the five Great Lakes: HOMES (Huron, Ontario, Michigan, Erie, Superior). Elaboration is to add information to make the material easier to remember. An example is that a person beginning to study music may be told by the teacher to learn the lines of treble clef E, G, B, D, and F. The teacher helps the student remember these letters by thinking of the sentence "Every Good Boy Does Fine." In summary, people are not expected to perform functions that put an unreasonable demand on human memory. Cues to assist human memory should be everywhere. The memory of users can be improved through the design of good facilitators, that is, providing training, instructions, and performance aids that make full use of the mnemonic concept.

### Perception

Perception may involve any sense, including hearing, tasting, smelling, or feeling. A person's perception cannot be observed directly and is usually inferred from observations of performance. Perception involves the interaction of information available through our senses and the accumulated knowledge stored in memory. Perceptual skill may be defined as developing ways of quickly and efficiently combining new experience with old. This explains why a younger child sometimes ignores information that older children and adults recognize quite effortlessly, such as the danger of crossing a street when a car is coming, or of playing with a candle's flame. A human factors engineer can help users to develop perceptual skills by designing the system with operation rules that are easy to understand and consistent. In addition, the human factors engineer can provide users with training to build the necessary schema. An example is that software with similar operational structures is beneficial to the users. Another issue is to recognize illusions and human errors. Although people are usually quite good in judging shape, size, and distance, we may be fooled by illusions. Illusions are the results of errors in the perceptual process. It may be produced when we make assumptions about "how things usually are" that causes us to distort or misunderstand the information we actually receive. Many injuries are no doubt contributed to by illusions (36,37). An example is the side-mirror image problem in causing automobile crashes. The cars are actually closer to you than what you see on the mirror.

## ANTHROPOMETRY

Anthropometry is the empirical science that defines physical measures of a person's size, form, and functional capacities. Anthropometry measurements are used to evaluate the interaction of workers with tasks, tools, machines, vehicles, and personal protective equipment. These data contribute to the design (e.g., sizing, functionality, safety, and comfort) of tools, vehicles, protective clothing, fall-protection devices, and other equipment. For example, anthropometry helps specify clearances separating the body from hazards such as surrounding equipment. It also helps human factors specialists describe spatial locations of the eyes so as to determine what can be seen and thereby identify obstructions that limit vision and cause mistakes (38). Designs that are incompatible with normal anthropometric measurements of a work force could result in undesired incidents. The misfit of a heavy-vehicle operation cockpit to the worker could produce blind spots that limit normal operation. It could also lead to a vehicle overturn or run-

**TABLE 1.** *Population stature data (in centimeters) (44)*

| Sample | Date | No. of subjects | Age | Mean | SD | 5th percentile | 95th percentile |
|---|---|---|---|---|---|---|---|
| Females | | | | | | | |
| U.S. Air Force | 1968 | 1,905 | 18–56 | 162.1 | 6.0 | 152.4 | 172.1 |
| U.S. civilians | 1974 | 8,411 | 18–74 | 161.5 | 6.4 | 151.1 | 172.2 |
| Japanese civilians | 1968 | 1,622 | 25–39 | 153.2 | 4.8 | 145.3 | 161.1 |
| Males | | | | | | | |
| U.S. Air Force | 1967 | 2,420 | 21–50 | 177.3 | 6.2 | 167.2 | 187.7 |
| U.S. civilians | 1974 | 5,260 | 18–74 | 175.3 | 7.1 | 163.6 | 186.9 |
| Japanese civilians | 1968 | 1,870 | 25–39 | 165.3 | 5.8 | 155.8 | 174.8 |

over of co-workers. A misfit of a respirator to workers could result in serious health effects in firefighting, hazardous waste cleanup, and other workplace conditions due to exposure to dangerous gases. Inadequate crew station geometry was found to be a contributor to some crew members injuries during ejection from aircraft (39). Inadequate height and step clearance for heavy-vehicle access systems also has been identified as a common cause of falls among vehicle operators (40,41). The appropriateness and limitations of children and older workers operating various machinery is also a concern to the safety community due to potential anthropometry misfits of design to the populations (42). Thus, a design process that involves the characterization of body size must consider the large variation in dimensions from person to person and from population to population. Consequently, statistical methods are used to analyze body dimensions and the results are typically reported as means and standard deviations for various body segments (43). Extensive tables of these statistics are available in reference texts (43–46). Table 1 presents an example of summary of population stature data for anthropometry applications. By assuming that human sizing data follow the normal distribution, statistical procedures are used to compute dimensions for various percentiles of the population of interest. The following equation can be used to estimate dimensions for different percentiles of the population:

$$E_p = X + (Z_p * S)$$

where $E_p$ is the estimated dimension of the $p$th percentile,

$X$ is the population mean,

$Z_p$ is a coefficient whose value varies with $p$ (some selected values of $Z$ for frequently used population percentiles are presented in Table 2), and

$S$ is the population standard deviation.

An example of the use of this equation is to compute the stature of the 1st percentile Japanese female and the 99th percentile U.S. male. The mean and standard deviation of the stature of Japanese females are $X = 153.2$ and $S = 4.8$ (see Table 1). The $Z_1$ value is −2.33 (see Table 2). Therefore, the stature of the 1st percentile Japanese female is $E_1 = 153.2 - (2.33 * 4.8) = 142.0$ cm. Similarly, the 99th percentile U.S. male stature is $E_{99} = 177.3 + (2.33 * 6.2) = 191.7$ cm.

### Anthropometric Procedures for Design Decisions

The above example demonstrates a basic statistical concept to obtain the dimensions for different percentiles of the population. In the occupational safety applications, a six-step procedure is typically used for design decisions (45,47): (1) determine the body dimension that is of essential importance (e.g., stature, shoulder height, hand width, etc.), (2) determine the population to be considered (e.g., sex, age, ethnic background, occupation etc.), (3) select the percentage of the population to be accommodated (e.g., safety, cost-benefit), (4) obtain the necessary reference materials to determine the appropriate descriptive statistics (a user may need to collect his or her own data), (5) compute the specific dimensions, and (6) adjust as necessary for clothing and other equipment (47,48).

An example is to specify the height for a doorway to avoid unintentional head injuries in manufacturing plants. The solution can be drawn by following the above-mentioned six steps. The essential dimension is stature. The population to be considered is U.S. civilians. The percentage of the population to be accommodated is 99.9% of the male population for the safety concerns (this will cover almost all females). The reference materials $X$ (mean stature) is 175.3 cm and $S$ (standard deviation) is 7.1 cm (44). The $Z$ value is $Z_{99.9} = 3.09$ and the $\text{Stature}_{99.9}$ is $175.3 + (3.09 * 7.1) = 197.2$ cm (see Tables 1 and 2). We need to adjust the height for

**TABLE 2.** *Some selected values of Z for frequently used population percentiles*

| Percentile (*p*) | $Z_p$ | Percentile (*p*) | $Z_p$ |
|---|---|---|---|
| 0.1 | -3.09 | 99.9 | 3.09 |
| 1 | -2.33 | 99 | 2.33 |
| 5 | -1.64 | 95 | 1.64 |
| 10 | -1.28 | 90 | 1.28 |
| 25 | -0.67 | 75 | 0.67 |
| 50 | 0.0 | — | — |

**TABLE 3.** *Popliteal height, sitting[a] (in centimeters) (46)*

| Percentile | 5th | 40th | 50th | 60th | 95th |
|---|---|---|---|---|---|
| Female | 35.6 | 39.1 | 39.9 | 40.6 | 44.5 |
| Male | 39.3 | 43.2 | 43.9 | 44.7 | 49.0 |

[a]Data for adults between 18 and 79 years of age.

shoes (2.5 cm) and headgear (5.0 cm) (47). Therefore, the desired opening is 197.2 + 2.5 + 5.0 = 204.7 cm.

### Design Decisions for Composite Populations

Work forces throughout the world are made up of several groups—men and women, young and old, black and white, etc. A single anthropometric data set is not appropriate for designing equipment for such work forces. However, a range of homogeneous data sets for different populations could be combined according to the mix in a particular work force to give estimates of the statistical distributions of relevant dimensions. For example, to determine the optimal range of seat height of construction vehicles for safety and effective operations, given that 85% of construction vehicle operators are males and 15% are females, the following steps can be used to synthesize the composite distribution of the two groups:

(1) We determine the essential dimension and the available group data. The popliteal height (sitting) is the essential measurement for determining the seat height. The data are available from Panero and Zelnik (46) (Table 3). (2) We then plot the male and female distributions on normal probability paper using the five points (Table 3) for each distribution and draw the best-fitting line between them (Fig. 2). (3) To determine the distribution for the composite population, we need but two points. We know that 85% of the population is male and that the 50th percentile value for male for popliteal height is 43.9 cm (Table 3). Therefore, 42.5% (i.e., 0.85 × 50%) of the composite population are males with popliteal height that equals or is less than 43.9 cm. Next, if our population consisted of only females, approximately 92% of all females have popliteal height that equals or is less than 43.9 cm. This can be found by looking at the distribution for females that we plotted on the normal probability paper (Fig. 2). Therefore, in terms of the composite population, 13.8% (i.e., 0.15 × 92%) of them are females with popliteal height that equals or is less than 43.9 cm. By adding the two numbers (42.5% + 13.8% = 56.3%), we know that 56.3% of the composite population has popliteal height equal to or less than 43.9 cm. (4) We need one more point. We know that for females, the 50th percentile is 39.9 cm. Therefore, in terms of the composite population, 7.5% (i.e., 0.15 × 50%) of them are females with popliteal height that equals or is less than 39.9 cm. And approximately 7.5% of males have popliteal height equal to or less than 39.9 cm from the distribution for males that we plotted on the normal probability paper (Fig. 2). Therefore, 6.4% (i.e., 0.85 × 7.5%) of the composite population are males with popliteal height that equals to or is less than 39.9 cm. By adding the two numbers (7.5% + 6.4% = 13.9%), we know that 13.9% of the composite population has popliteal height equal or less than 39.9 cm. (5) We plot a straight line through the two points identified in steps 3 and 4. The 5th, 50th, and 95th percentile values for our composite population are 38.1, 43.4, and 48.7, respectively. The suggested range of seat height of construction vehicles is 38.1 to 48.7 cm. This is a very valuable tool and can be used with two or more groups. In some cases, the distribution of a combined

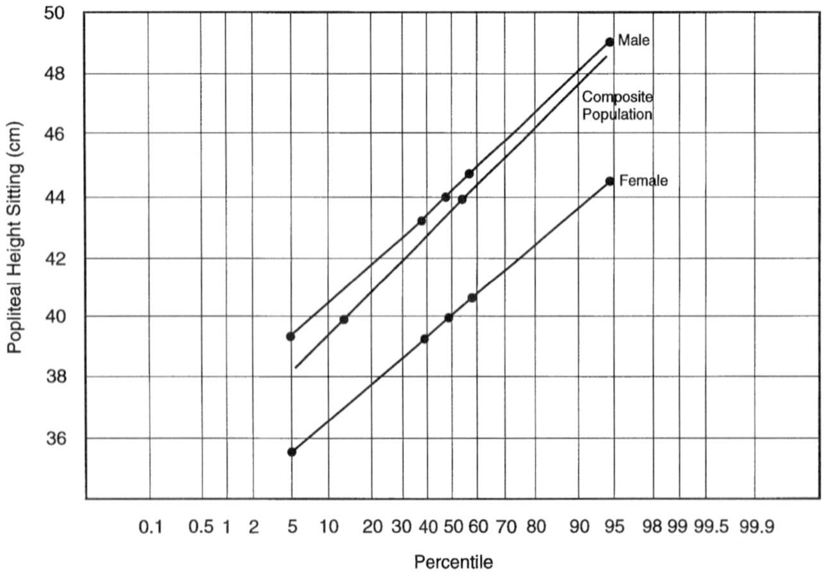


**FIG. 2.** Normal probability graph of two composite populations.

population is not normal. The distribution plots on the normal probability paper will not be a straight line. The curve can be drawn through a 5- or 10-point calculation by repeating steps 3 and 4. Computer programs can be used to calculate anthropometric data for groups of mixed populations (49).

**Design Decisions for Complex Systems**

In many occupational practices, body size accommodation is not a single-parameter question. Construction vehicles are an example. Adequate reach to controls, body clearances to enter and exit the cab, overhead clearance, and vision to internal and external environments all are functions of the operator's body size and position in the cockpit. While some measurements (most are simple clearance dimensions) can be dealt with in terms of minimum and maximum values of the population (such as the example in the section Anthropometric Procedures for Design Decisions, above), some measurements must be considered in varying combinations. Some people have long limbs and some have long torsos. Percentiles are only relevant for one dimension at a time (univariate). While a 5th-percentile stature value can be accurately located, that value tells us little or nothing about variability of other body dimensions of individuals with 5th percentile stature. For example, it is common for people to assume that the 5th percentile for both stature and weight represents a 5th percentile person. In fact a 1967 survey indicated that only 1.3% of subjects were smaller than the 5th percentile for both stature and weight measurements, while 9% were smaller for one or the other (50,51). The problem is compounded with each additional measurement used to specify the size of an individual. A multivariate accommodation approach is more adequate to address the multidegree anthropometry concerns for designing complex systems. In this way, the percentage level is accommodated, by taking into account both the size variance and proportional variability. Not only individuals who are uniformly large or small, but those whose measurements are combined (e.g., small torsos with long legs, or vice versa) will be accommodated (52).

For example, the thumb-tip reach and shoulder-height sitting are important dimensions for crane operators in locating controls. Imagine two individuals with equally short arms but different shoulder-height sitting values. Their ability to reach down to a control on a side panel or to an overhead control will differ considerably. How do we determine that a desired percentage of the population is covered in the crane cockpit design? Using the mean value for both thumb-tip reach and shoulder-height sitting as a starting point *(X)*, we draw the 90% ellipse in Fig. 3. The ellipse passes points 1 and 2, which are similar to the 5th and 95th percentile concept. They represent crane operators who are small or large for both values. The ellipse in Fig. 3 also passes the points representing a tall-shoulder, short-limb person (point 3) and a short-shoulder, long-limb person (point 4), who are just as likely to occur in the population as any other individual along the perimeter of the circle. The multivariate accommodation approach would select at least four representative points to describe size variability (51).

In the design of many workstations or systems, more than two variables are needed to ensure the proper

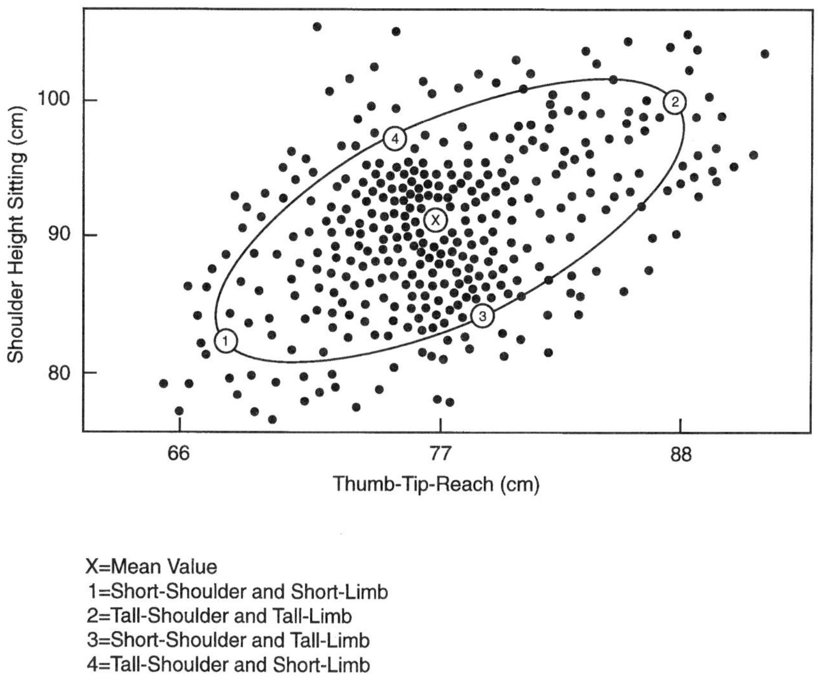


**FIG. 3.** A concept of 90% accommodation model involving thumb-tip reach and shoulder-height sitting bivariate.

accommodation of individuals and their equipment. As each additional measurement is added to the design, an additional level of complexity is added to the analysis. Clearly the problem becomes unworkable very quickly. Fortunately, for most workstation designs the total number of relevant measures can be reduced to two or three critical factors. This means that a bivariate circle or trivariate sphere can be used to define population limits and identify the representative points/cases. The results can be graphically demonstrated. Computerized human model programs are becoming commercially available for determining representative cases and reducing the accommodation problems.

## WORK PHYSIOLOGY

Work physiology is concerned with the responses of the cardiovascular, pulmonary, and musculoskeletal systems to the metabolic demands of work. Both occasional and regular physiology overloading may represent health hazards that could lead to injury incidents in many occupational settings. Best known are the ill effects of acute exposure, e.g., fainting, heat exhaustion, heat stroke, hypothermia, fatigue, increase of blood pressure, and increased risk of mortality from digestive disease (53–55). The body's core temperature must be kept to within quite narrow limits. A temperature increase of about 5°C is likely to lead to death, as is a reduction by 3 to 4°C. Small departures from this critical band can lead to decrements in both motor and cognitive performance. Studies indicate that heat affects human attention performance (56), grip strength, manual dexterity, tracking ability (57), and cognitive performance (57). Cold can affect human tactile sensitivity, tracking, reaction time, complex behaviors (58), grip strength (59), cognitive performance (60,61), and manual dexterity (59). These results have significant applications to various industries, for example, waste abatement, construction, agriculture, and food process industries, to name a few.

In handling daily occupational work, a person must be capable of performing without excessive strain or fatigue. A metabolic energy expenditure rate and heart rate are the physiologic measurements that have been suggested most often in the literature for determining the maximum task intensity that can be continuously performed without accumulating an excessive amount of physical fatigue (62). By relating the energy expended in a job to the aerobic power of the individuals for endurance effort, an objective assessment can be made of the work capacity of the worker for carrying out a particular job without undue fatigue (63). Metabolic energy expenditure has been used to evaluate alternate work methods (64), to establish duration and frequency of rest breaks, and to determine heat stress during excess temperature and humidity conditions (62). Several researchers have recommended 33% of the maximum aerobic power of a normal healthy person as the maximum energy expenditure rate that should be expended for an 8-hour workday (65). Generally, 16 kcal/min is taken as the maximum aerobic power of a normal healthy young male for a highly dynamic job. A physical work capacity limit of 5.3 kcal/min (males) or 3.5 kcal/min (females) is recommended for an 8-hour continuous workday (66). It is also recommended that the energy expenditure rate not exceed 9 kcal (males) or 6.5 kcal (females) per minute for occasional lifting tasks lasting 1 hour or less. Older workers require a much smaller physical work capacity limit. Body weight and physical fitness also impact a person's work capacity limit.

## SAFETY MANAGEMENT

Safety management has been frequently considered in developing occupational injury prevention programs. Three related subjects are discussed in this section: personality and training, age and experience, and employee participation.

### Personality and Training

It is suspected that some individuals might have personality traits that are more likely to lead to injury incidents. Accident proneness, extroversion, aggression, and risk-taking behavior are among those traits frequently discussed in the literature. Some studies showed that a small minority of workers had more accidents than others (67). However, their reports were careful to emphasize that the statistical analysis of accident records is an analysis only of what happened, not of why or how it happened. Other studies argued that accident proneness is not a permanent entity (68) and is often task-specific and generally too small to justify using selection of workers as a way of reducing accident (69). Studies also demonstrate links of high aggression or extroversion scores to severity rates of accidents (71–73). However, very little statistical evidence has been advanced to link aggressiveness or extroversion per se with accidents (25). Risk taking is the extent to which an individual performs an action that he or she has previously judged to be dangerous and to have some degree of hazard. A study on drivers' anticipated ability to drive through a progressively narrowing gap compared with their actual performance indicated that experienced drivers took less risk than inexperienced drivers (74). This result possibly means that appropriate training may result in less risk-taking behavior. However, Winsemius' (75) study on worker behavior during punch-machine operation indicated that training alone is unlikely to reduce unsafe behavior. Unless the negative-reinforcing aspects have been sufficiently incorporated into the training repertoire (such as depiction of severe hand-injury scenes), workers will bypass safe operations. The unsafe behavior is then likely to become positively reinforced as soon as the training period ends (25). From a human-machine interface-design standpoint, a machine or system should be designed with the consideration of a second-layer protection so that risk-taking behavior will be discouraged and human performance error will be corrected (e.g., a machine will stop if a foreign object is presented in certain areas or a machine cannot be operated if a safety guard is removed).

### Age and Experience

Age is one of the most frequently considered factors in accident and injury prevention research, but it is a factor confounded by the effects of experience, the task, and even by the effects of the accidents themselves, resulting in a tendency to leave the employment. Although the effects of experience and training cannot be excluded from age effects, studies matching age groups for their level of experience indicate that younger workers are more likely to have accidents (76,77). However, studies also suggest that older persons may have a significant amount of attention failure that may lead to accidents (78). Older people are less well tolerated to the tasks that require heavy perceptual demands, particularly accompanied by speed (79).

### Employee Participation

Personality, age, experience, hazard exposure, and many other factors may contribute to cause an individual to be more liable to have an accident at some times than at others. It is reasonable to assume that each person has a range of behavior, any part of which may be safe or unsafe depending on the type of hazards or environments to which the person is exposed (80). A safety problem is more likely to be a fault of the current man-machine system with all of its complexities, rather than only of the worker. Safety management's goal is to assure that all the human factors are considered at the system-design stage and safety quality is maintained at all times. It is believed that the cognition and motives of workplace participants are central to the detection, appraisal, and amelioration of workplace safety problems. Good safety management would include the involvement of employees at all levels in perceiving and responding to safety-related events. The establishment of positive safety climates, comprehensive safety programs, and increased objectivity in reporting accidents is critical in injury prevention (81). In addition, aggressive efforts to promote open and two-way communications between labor and management on safety matters are needed. A relation-oriented supervisory style is more effective than a task-oriented supervisory style when dealing with safety issues (82). Participation in safety programs promotes increased employee sensitivity, a feeling of influence, and recognition of company safety goals.

## INJURY PREVENTION AND CONTROLS

Approaches for reducing occupational injuries in the work force can be divided into three categories: (a) Primary prevention, the most efficient and cost-effective way, includes engineering controls (premarket testing, substitution, and redesign), administrative controls, and the use of personal protective devices. (b) Secondary prevention involves biomonitoring of workers exposures to hazardous substances, energy, and environment. It also includes preplacement screening to prevent assignment of particularly susceptible individuals (e.g., those incapable of performing the tasks or sustaining the stresses imposed by the tasks). (c) Tertiary prevention such as rehabilitation and compensation are usually costly and in many cases cannot reverse the consequence of injuries. This chapter focuses on primary prevention. (Table 4 shows the cascade of prevention.)

### Public Health Model

Most workplace injury incidents occur as a result of separate cause-effect sequences, each influenced by multiple factors or stressors. Each set of risk factors represents an area in need of scientific study in the multidisciplinary effort to mitigate occupational injuries. Six major areas of human factors that are most related to traumatic injury prevention have been described in the previous sections. Table 5 shows a public health model for occupational injury prevention. Surveillance has a role in problem identification, problem confirma-

**TABLE 4.** *Cascade of prevention*

| |
|---|
| Engineering controls (premarket testing, substitution, redesign) |
| Administrative controls (training, written policies, safety work practices) |
| Use of personal protective devices (e.g., respirator, protective clothing) |
| Biomonitoring (e.g., body temperature monitoring to prevent heat stress) |
| Screening (e.g., preplacement tests) |
| Clinical diagnosis |
| Rehabilitation |
| Compensation |

**TABLE 5.** *Public health model in practice for injury prevention*

| Function | Surveillance | Epidemiology | Engineering | Information dissemination |
|---|---|---|---|---|
| Problem prediction | | | × | |
| Problem identification | × | | | |
| Problem confirmation | × | × | × | |
| Etiology identification | | × | × | |
| Design intervention | | | × | |
| Field test of intervention | | × | × | |
| Implementation | | | | × |
| Evaluation | × | × | × | × |

tion, and evaluation; epidemiology may be used to identify etiologies, to confirm the existence of problems, and to perform field tests of interventions and evaluation. Engineering is typically involved in problem prediction and confirmation, etiology identification, design of interventions, field tests of interventions, and evaluation. Injury prevention and control technologies and strategies will then be disseminated to the public through health and injury communication systems. In other words, the model uses an interdisciplinary approach for injury prevention. The approach uses injury surveillance systems to identify target occupations as well as factors that may increase the risk of work-related injury. Targeted occupations are investigated for the prevalence of safety hazards by epidemiologists and engineers to identify the critical elements that contribute to the traumatic injury incidents, near-miss incidents, or stressful tasks of the occupations. Engineers then work together with partners to identify and evaluate task characteristics, perform computerized simulations, conduct laboratory and field studies, develop engineering control strategies, introduce new designs, and evaluate the efficacy of the new systems.

### Human Factors Principles

In formulating actions of primary prevention to control occupational injuries, consideration must be given to the risk factors associate with the task, the working environment, the machine/system, and the worker, simultaneously. In general, a three-tiered injury control program can be used. Engineering controls include removing the hazard, improving job and tool design, and modifying workplaces. Administrative controls change work practices or organizational and management policies. The use of personal protective equipment can serve as the last line of protection. The above-mentioned six major sections have outlined the general human factors principles and applications for traumatic injury prevention. More applications of these principles to different occupational settings can be found in the relevant literature, for example human factors in construction (83), human factors in agriculture (84), and ergonomics for meat packing (85).

### Future Protective Technologies

Although interventions are available to reduce workplace injury, many techniques still lack rigorous testing and validation. Major efforts must be made to more thoroughly study occupational-injury incidents, to expand the field of human factors study, and ultimately to reduce the suffering of our work force. Among suggested research efforts are (a) developing advanced remote-monitoring methods for hazard-exposure assessments; (b) establishing computerized anthropometry research and national anthropometry databases for improving the fit of workplace systems to workers; (c) evaluating synergistic effects among biomechanical, environmental, physiologic, and psychological factors upon industrial workers; (d) studying fall-injury characteristics, risk factors of occupational falls, and fall-exposure assessment methods, as well as developing new fall-prevention technologies, and (e) evaluating the human-equipment interface to improve the safety and performance of existing tools, machines, and safety devices. Furthermore, new technologies should be pursued to more effectively develop and evaluate interventions. Among the technologies are human-equipment interface models (e.g., virtual human models, finite element models, dynamic simulation models), reverse engineering tools (e.g., 3-D laser scanning systems and engineering drawing software), virtual reality simulation, and instrumented manikins (to study body-property behavior, such as impact-energy transfer from equipment onto the human body).

## SUMMARY

Occupational injuries often occur when forces, stresses, or conditions imposed by work exceed levels that workers can physically tolerate or when the workplace creates conditions to which workers cannot effectively adapt or respond, either physically or cognitively. Human factors is the applications of knowledge of human sensory performance, information processing, anthropometry, biomechanics, work physiology, and safety management to the design of work, to prevent injury and increase work performance. Increased understanding of human factors will contribute to the improvement of systems and controls, work practices, and personal protective equipment to protect workers from injury. This chapter addressed the theories, principles, and applications of six major areas of human factors that are most related to occupational traumatic injury prevention. In general, a three-tiered injury control approach can be used in a safety program. Engineering controls include removing the hazard, improving job and tool design, and modifying workplaces. Administrative controls change work practices or organizational and management policies. The use of personal protective equipment can serve as the last line of protection. Finally, while interventions are available to reduce workplace injury, many techniques still need to be improved and have to be rigorously tested and validated. Continual research using state-of-the-art scientific methods is needed to expand the underdeveloped human factors field, and to reduce the suffering of our work force.

## REFERENCES


1. U.S. Department of Labor. *Occupational injuries and illnesses:* counts, *rates, and characteristics.* Bulletin 2455. Washington, DC: Bureau of Labor Statistics, 1995.
2. NIOSH. *Fatal injuries to workers in the United States, 1980–1989:* a decade of surveillance. Washington, DC: National Institute for Occupational Safety and Health, 1993.
3. NIOSH. *National occupational research agenda.* Washington, DC: National Institute for Occupational Safety and Health, 1996.
4. Shaw BE, Sanders MS. Research to determine the frequency and cause of injury accidents in underground mining. Proceedings of the Human Factors Society 31st Annual Meeting, New York, 1987;2:926–930.
5. Pittsburgh Research Center. *Briefing document for human factors research program.* Washington, DC: U.S. Department of Energy, 1996.
6. Duncan JR. *Human factors concepts:* an overview. St. Joseph, MI: American Society of Agricultural Engineers, 1991.
7. Chapanis A. Some reflections on progress. *Proceedings of the Human Factors Society 29th annual meeting.* Santa Monica, CA: Human Factors Society, 1985.
8. NEISS. *National electronic injury surveillance system.* Washington, DC: U.S. Consumer Products Safety Commission, 1996.
9. NIOSH. *Hazard evaluation and technical assistance report:* international association of fire fighters, *Sedgwick County, Kansas.* Report No. HETA 90-395-2121. Morgantown, WV: National Institute for Occupational Safety and Health, 1990.
10. NIOSH. *Unpublished injury investigation report.* Morgantown, WV: Division of Safety Research, National Institute for Occupational Safety and Health, 1996.
11. North K, Stapleton C, Vogt C. *Ergonomics glossary.* Published for the Bureau of Information and Coordination of Community Ergonomics Action of the European Coal and Steel community. Utrecht/Antwerp: Bohn, Scheltema & Holkema, 1982.
12. Frankel VH, Nordin M. *Basic biomechanics of the skeletal system.* Philadelphia: Lea & Febiger, 1980.
13. Grether WF, Baker CA. Visual Presentation of Information. In: VanCott HP, Kinkade RG, eds. *Human engineering guide to equip design,* rev. ed. Washington, DC: U.S. Government Printing Office, 1972.
14. Stelmakowich A. Good indoor lighting provides a safer workplace. *Canadian Occupational Health and Safety News* 1986;9(6):4–5.
15. Nakagawara VB. Glare vision testing: applications in occupational health and safety programs. *Professional Safety* 1990;35(11):25–27.
16. Langolf G. Visual Information, Occupational Ergonomics, Engineering Summer Conferences, University of Michigan, June 11–15, 1984.
17. Graham CH. *Vision and visual perception.* New York: John Wiley, 1965.
18. Buckler AT. A review of the literature on the legibility of alphanumerics on electronic displays. ADA 040625; 1977. (Cited by Bailey RW. *Human performance engineering:* a guide for system designers. Englewood Cliffs, New Jersey: Prentice-Hall, 1982.)
19. Cobb PW, Moss FK. The four variables in the visual threshold, Franklin Institute Journal, 205; 1928. In: Van Cott HP, Kinkade RG, eds. *Human engineering guide to equipment design,* rev. ed. Washington, DC: U.S. Government Printing Office, 1972.
20. Bailey RW. *Human performance engineering:* a guide for system designers. Englewood Cliffs, New Jersey: Prentice-Hall; 1982.
21. Miller GA, Nicely PE. An analysis of perceptual confusions among some English consonants. *J Acoust Soc Am* 1955;27(2):338–352.
22. Kryter KD. Speech communication. In: VanCott HP, Kinkade RG, eds. *Human engineering guide to equipment design,* rev. ed. Washington, DC: U.S. Government Printing Office, 1972.
23. Chapanis A. *Man-machine engineering.* Monterey, CA: Brooks/Cole, 1965.
24. Reason JT, Brand JJ. *Motion sickness.* London: Academic Press, 1975.
25. Oborne DJ. *Ergonomics at work.* New York: John Wiley, 1982.
26. Sidebotham PD. Balance thru the ages of man. *J Laryngol Otolaryngol* 1988;102:203–208.
27. Fleishman EA. Human abilities and the acquisition of skill. In: Bilodeau EA, ed. *Acquisition of skill.* New York: Academic Press, 1966.
28. Dickinson J. *Proprioceptive control of human movement.* London: Lepus, 1974.
29. Ilmarinen R, Harjula R. Meat-cutters work-cold and physiologically strenuous. *Tyoe Ja Ihminen* 1987;4:366–387(English abstr).
30. Helander MG. Safety hazards and motivation for safe work in the construction industry. *Int J Ind Ergonom* 1991;8:2O5–223.
31. Pollack I and Ficks L. Information of multidimensional auditory displays. *J Acoust Soc Am* 1954;26:155–158.
32. Eriksen CW, Hake HN. Absolute judgments as a function of stimulus range and number of stimulus and response categories. *J Exp Psychol* 1955;49:323–332.
33. Welford A. *Fundamentals of skill.* London: Methuen, 1968.
34. Kantowitz BH. *Heavy vehicle driver workload assessment:* lessons from aviation. Proceedings of the Human Factors Society 36th Annual Meeting. Santa Monica, CA: Human Factors Society, 1992;2: 1113–1117.
35. Goldstein IL, Dorfman PW. Speed and load stress as determinants of performance in a time sharing task. *Hum Factors* 1978;20(5):603–609.
36. Cheung B, Money K, Wright H, Bateman W. Spatial disorientation-implicated accidents in canadian forces, 1982–92. *Aviat Space Environ Med* 1995;66(6):579–585.
37. Feggetter AJ. A method for investigating human factor aspects of aircraft accidents and incidents. *Ergonomics* 1982;25(1):1065–1075.
38. Roebuck JA. *Anthropometric methods:* designing to fit the human body. Santa Monica, CA: Human Factors and Ergonomics Society, 1993.
39. Rice EV, Ninow EH. Man-machine interface: a study of injuries incurred during ejection from U.S. navy aircraft. *Aerospace Med* 1973; 44(1):87–89.
40. Albin TJ, Adams WP. *Slip-and-fall accidents during equipment maintenance in the surface mining industry.* Information Circular. No. 9249. Washington, DC: U.S. Bureau of Mines, 1990.
41. Couch DB, Fraser TM. Access systems of heavy construction vehicles: parameters, problems and pointers. *Appl Ergonom* 1981;12(2):103–110.
42. Buttoms DJ, Butterworth DJ. Foot reach under guard rails on agricultural machinery. *Appl Ergonom* 1990;21(3):179–186.
43. Roebuck JA, Kroemer KHE, Thomson WG. *Engineering anthropometry methods.* New York: Wiley-Interscience, 1975.
44. NASA. *Anthropometric source book. Volume 1:* anthropometry for designers. Publication 1024. Washington, DC: National Aeronautics and Space Administration, 1978.
45. Pheasant S. *Bodyspace—anthropometry, ergonomics, and design.* London: Tayler & Francis, 1986.
46. Panero J, Zelnik M. *Human dimension and interior space.* London: Architectural Press, 1979.
47. Hertzberg HTE. Engineering anthropology. In: Van Cott HP, Kincade RG, eds. *Human engineering guide to equipment design,* rev. ed. Washington, DC: U.S. Government Printing Office, 1972.
48. Das B, Grady RM. Industrial workplace layout and engineering anthropology. In: Kvalseth TO, ed. *Ergonomics of workstation design.* London: Butterworths, 1983.
49. Worksafe Australia. *Worksafe Australia anthropometric database.* Sydney, Australia: Worksafe Australia, 1994.
50. Kennedy KW. *A collection of United States Air Force anthropometry.* Technical report AAMRL-TR-85-062. Wright-Patterson Air Force Base, Ohio: Armstrong Aerospace Medical Research Laboratory, 1986.

51. Zehner GF, Merndl RS, Hudson JA. *A multivariate anthropometric method for crew station design:* abridged (U). Technical Report AL-TR-1992-0164. Wright-Patterson Air Force Base, Ohio: Air Force Materiel Command, 1993.
52. Bittner AC, Wherry RJ, Glenn FA. *CADRE:* a family of manikins for workstation design. Technical Report 2100.07B. Warminster, PA: Man-Machine Integration Center, Naval air Development Center, 1986.
53. Rodahl K. *The physiology of work.* New York: Taylor & Francis, 1989.
54. Knochel JP, Beisel WR, Herndon EG, Gerard ES, Barry KG. The renal, cardiovascular, hematologic, and serum electrolyte abnormalities of heat stroke. *Am J Med* 1961;299–309.
55. Khogali M, Hales JRS. *Heat stroke and temperature regulation.* New York: Academic Press, 1983.
56. Hancock PA, Vercruyssen M. Limits of behavioral efficiency for workers in heat stress. *Int J Ind Ergonom* 1988;3(2):149–158.
57. Ramsey JD. Task performance in heat: a review. *Ergonomics* 1995; 38(1):154–165.
58. Enander A. Performance and sensory aspects of work in cold environments: a review. *Ergonomics* 1984;27(4):365–378.
59. Giesbrecht GG, Bristow GK. Decrement in manual arm performance during whole body cooling. *Aviat Space Environ Med* 1992;63(12): 1077–1081.
60. Thomas JR, Ahlers ST, House JF, Schrot J. Repeated exposure to moderate cold impairs matching-to-sample performance. *Aviat Space Environ Med* 1989;60(11):1063–1067.
61. Enander A. Effects of moderate cold on performance of psychomotor and cognitive tasks. *Ergonomics* 1987;30(10):1431–1445.
62. Astrand PO, Rodahl K. *Textbook of work physiology.* New York: McGraw-Hill, 1986.
63. Karger D, Hancock W. *Advanced work measurement.* New York: Industrial Press, 1982.
64. Speckman KL, Allan AE, Sawka MN, Young AJ, Muza SR, Pandolf KB. Perspectives in microclimate cooling involving protective clothing in hot environments. *Int J Ind Ergonom* 1988;3(2):121–147.
65. Kamon E, Ayoub M. Ergonomics guide to assessment of physical work capacity. *Am Ind Hyg Assoc J* 1976;37:1–9.
66. Chaffin DB. *Some effects of physical exertion.* Ann Arbor, Michigan: Department of Industrial and Operations Engineering, University of Michigan, 1972.
67. Greenwood M, Woods HM, Yule Gu. A report on the incidence of industrial accidents upon individuals with special reference to multiple accidents. Industrial Health Research Board Report No. 4. In: Haddon W, Suchman EA, Flein D, eds. *Accident research (1964).* New York: Harper, 1919.
68. Ganguly ON, Bhattacharya SK. Is accident proneness a myth or reality? *Ind Safety Chronicle* 1972;4(1):11–15.
69. Hale AR, Glendon AI. *Individual differences and selection. Individual behavior in the control of danger.* Industrial Safety Series 2. Amsterdam, Holland: Elsevier, 1987;309–339.
70. Shaw L, Sichel HS. *Accident proneness:* research in the occurrence, *causation, and prevention of road accidents.* Oxford: Pergamon, 1971.
71. Fine BJ. Introversion, extroversion and motor driver behavior. *Percept Motor Skill* 1963;12:95–100.
72. Wrogg SG. The role of emotions in industrial accidents. *Arch Environ Health* 1961;3:519.
73. Suchman EA. Cultural and social factors in accident occurrence and control. *J Occup Med* 1965;7:487.
74. Cohen J, Dearnaley EJ, Hansel CEM. The risk taken in driving under the influence of alcohol. *Br Med J* 1958;1:1438–1442.
75. Winsemius W. Some ergonomic aspects of safety. *Ergonomics* 1965;8: 151–162.
76. Van Zelst RH. The effects of age and experience upon accident rate. *J Appl Psychol* 1954;38:313–317.
77. Hale AR, Hale M. *A review of the industrial accident research literature.* Committee on Safety and Health at Work Paper. London: HMSO, 1972.
78. Block JR. A measurement of attention. *Environ Control Safety Manag* 1970;140:16–18.
79. Murrel KFH. Industrial aspects of aging. *Ergonomics* 1962;5:147–153.
80. Reason JT. *Man in motion:* the psychology of travel. London: Weidenfeld and Nicolson, 1974.
81. DeJoy DM. An attributional model of the safety management process in industry. Proceedings of the Annual International Industrial Ergonomics and Safety Conference, Denver, CO, 1992;161–168.
82. Forsgren RA. Developing employee psychological advantage through safety management. *Environ Control Safety Manag* 1970;140:26–30.
83. Hsiao H, Stanevich R. Injuries and ergonomic applications in construction. In: Bhattacharya A, McGlothlin JD, eds. *Occupational ergonomics.* New York: Marcel Dekker, 1996.
84. ASAE. *Human Factors.* St. Joseph, MI: American Society of Agricultural Engineers, 1991.
85. U.S. Department of Labor. *Ergonomics program management guidelines for meatpacking plants.* OSHA publication 3123. Washington, DC: U.S. Department of Labor, 1990.

*Environmental and Occupational Medicine,*
*Third Edition,* edited by William N. Rom.
Lippincott–Raven Publishers, Philadelphia © 1998.

CHAPTER 65

# Work-Related Musculoskeletal Disorders Excluding Back Pain

Margareta Nordin and Carl Zetterberg

Musculoskeletal impairments impact significantly on the population, the health care utilization, and the cost for society (1–3). It has been estimated that approximately 10% of the population is affected by some musculoskeletal injury or diseases yearly (4). In 1988 the Academy of Orthopedic Surgeons reported 29.9 million incidents in the United States. By age group the musculoskeletal impairments are most prevalent in the working age group. These impairments ranked first in frequency visits to physicians, second in frequency of hospital utilization, third for acute conditions, and fourth among reasons for surgical procedures. The total cost for the United States was estimated to be $65 billion (5).

The workplace is a significant source of occupational injury, occupational illness, and related disability (4). There were an estimated 1.8 million disabling work injuries in the United States in 1990; 10,500 resulted in fatalities and 60,000 in permanent disability. Musculoskeletal injuries and disorders are the leading category of work-related diseases and injuries in the United States that result in work loss. The data are derived from the Supplemental Data System (SDS), a federal-state cooperative program administered by the Bureau of Labor Statistics. The SDS compiles occupational injuries and illnesses data from workers' compensation records in 24 states (4). The data show the large impact of occupationally related musculoskeletal ailments in the working population in the United States. These data also indicate the importance of prevention and early care requirement of occupational musculoskeletal events and the importance of primary prevention and prevention of disability.

Occupational musculoskeletal ailments encompass acute and chronic injuries. They include injuries and illnesses to muscles, tendons, ligaments, nerves, cartilage, and bone. The term *injury* or *illness,* therefore, would include sprains, strains, inflammation, and irritations. Impairments in which skin, ligament, tendon, or bone is broken or dislocated owing to a transfer of high energy are defined as traumatic injuries and are not covered in this chapter. For comparative purposes, the national available data of work-related fractures, laceration, and amputations are displayed in Table 1.

Sprains and strains were the most frequent type of injury and accounted for 43% of cases involving work loss. The second and third most common injuries were cut, laceration, and puncture (11.6%) and fractures (9.6%), respectively. Type of accident exposure is presented in Table 2. More than two-thirds of the injuries and disorders in the musculoskeletal system are reported as overexertion (31.2%), being struck by or against another object (23.6%), or falling (17%).

Finally, these injuries and disorders are the leading cause of disability in individuals in their working years. Persons with musculoskeletal conditions have higher rates of work disability than those with other chronic conditions (6). Low back sprains and strains are by far the most frequent problem. The proposed National Strategy for the Prevention of Leading Work-Related Diseases and Injuries includes the following four elements:

M. Nordin: Occupational and Industrial Orthopaedic Center, Hospital for Joint Diseases; Program of Ergonomics and Biomechanics; and Department of Environmental Medicine, New York University Medical Center, New York, New York 10014.

C. Zetterberg: Department of Orthopaedics, School of Medicine, University of Goteborg, Sahlgren Hospital, 45 Goteborg, Sweden.

**TABLE 1.** *Occupational musculoskeletal injury and illness, type of injury in percent of distribution of cases involving work loss by gender: all reported injuries and illnesses in 24 states*

| Type of injury | Total (%) | Male (%) | Female (%) |
|---|---|---|---|
| Dislocation | 2.0 | 2.1 | 1.7 |
| Fracture | 9.6 | 10.5 | 7.4 |
| Inflammation or irritation of joints, tendons, or muscles | 1.1 | 0.7 | 2.2 |
| Sprain and strain | 43.0 | 40.9 | 48.2 |
| Amputation | 0.6 | 0.7 | 0.2 |
| Contusion, crushing, bruise | 9.2 | 8.8 | 10.0 |
| Cut, laceration, puncture | 11.6 | 13.3 | 7.5 |
| Scratch, abrasion | 2.5 | 3.0 | 1.2 |
| Multiple injuries | 2.9 | 3.0 | 2.9 |
| All other | 17.5 | 16.9 | 18.7 |
| Total | 100.0 | 100.0 | 100.0 |

Data from ref. 48.

1. *Environmental hazards.* Hazards to the musculoskeletal system associated with work are called workplace traumatogens. A traumatogen is a source of biomechanical stress stemming from job demands that exceed the worker's strength or endurance, such as heavy lifting or repetitive, forceful manual twisting. Traumatogens can be measured by determining the frequency, magnitude, duration, and direction of forces required in relation to body posture and external load.
2. *Human biologic factors.* These factors include the anthropometric or innate attributes that influence a worker's capacity for safely performing the job. Examples include the worker's physical size, strength, range of motion, work endurance, and the integrity of the musculoskeletal system. These factors partly account for variability in performance. The capability of the population, the capacities as defined by physical attributes, and the health and safety of the worker are compromised. Aging with accompanying tissue degeneration increases the risk of injury by lowering the harmful threshold of the job demand.

**TABLE 2.** *Occupational musculoskeletal disorders in percent by type of accident or exposure of cases involving work loss*

| Type of accident | Percent |
|---|---|
| Overexertion | 31.2 |
| Struck by or against | 23.6 |
| Falls | 17.0 |
| Bodily reaction | 7.3 |
| Caught in, under, between | 5.7 |
| Contact with radiation, caustics | 3.3 |
| Motor vehicle | 3.0 |
| All other | 8.9 |
| Total | 100.0 |

Data from ref. 48.

3. *Behavior factors and healthy lifestyles.* These elements are acquired behaviors or personal habits that affect the worker's risks of incurring musculoskeletal strain or injury. Such behavioral factors may include insufficient sleep or recovery from an exertion, perception of the job as being excessively demanding or hazardous, job dissatisfaction, and mental lapses due to the distraction. Lifestyle factors include obesity and physical unfitness, unhealthy diet, substance abuse, or outside work. Recent studies also have focused on some distress factors and beliefs that are predictive of delayed recovery and/or permanent disability. Recent studies also have pointed to physical activity at leisure time as a common cause of sprain and strains significantly affecting the exposure of physical load (mechanical stressors).
4. *Inadequacies in the existing health care and ancillary system.* Recent studies point to the importance of increased awareness of the psychosocial (workers' perception) work environment, managerial style, and management-union collaboration in reducing the disability of occupational musculoskeletal injuries and disorders. These elements include provision of early state-of-the-art care for the injured worker, long-term goals for prevention of injury and accidents, and education of management and the work force. Elements of particular importance include the lack of medical knowledge; inappropriate training for health care personnel in the causes, diagnosis, and treatment of musculoskeletal problems that result from biomechanical strain and hazards; delayed care due to improper referral; and misdirected case management. Recent studies have shown that ergonomic workplace factors are of importance, even more than medical factors, in long-term disability cases (7,8). Management and unions need special health and safety training in recognizing physical traumatogens and in understanding the role of biologic factors,

behavioral factors, and the hurdles to returning to work after a musculoskeletal injury. Organizations and industries that have implemented early care program are displaying lower disability costs and thereby indemnity costs (9).

This chapter focuses on the occupational musculoskeletal ailments with cumulative load exposure characteristics, i.e., osteoarthritis and cumulative trauma disorders, excluding low back pain.

## BRIEF OVERVIEW OF PHYSIOLOGIC PROPERTIES OF MUSCULOSKELETAL TISSUE

Musculoskeletal tissue responds to mechanical stress (10). With no mechanical stress, tissue will atrophy. With too much mechanical stress, tissue will be damaged. Thus it is fundamentally important to determine what is an adequate level of mechanical stress. The end point of prolonged bed rest or paralysis involves no or almost no mechanical stress. A broken bone or a ligament rupture indicates excessive stress. Most occupationally related musculoskeletal ailments occur owing to a level of stress somewhere in between these two extremes. A load event or several minor load events have been sustained by the individual, but the health care provider cannot pinpoint the structure that is causing pain. Determining level of stress is a valid approach if biomechanical, physiologic, medical, and psychological factors are understood. This section give a brief overview of the musculoskeletal tissues and factors contributing to depleting or invigorating the tissues.

### Bone Tissue

Two types of bone tissue form the skeleton: compact (cortical) and cancellous (trabecular) bone tissue. Compact bone can withstand tensile, bending, and sheer forces better than cancellous bone, by a ratio of approximately 5:1. Cancellous bone is subjected mainly to compressive forces and is found in the ends of long bones, the pelvis, and vertebrae. Compact bone gives the skeleton its strength and cancellous bone acts as a shock absorber. Bone tissue has the capacity to remodel over time. Bone strength peaks and the bone mass are at maximum density between 20 and 40 years of age; thereafter, an age-related loss of bone mass occurs and thereby also a decrease in bone strength. This age-related bone loss has never been shown to be reversible. The rate of bone loss is faster in women than men. Menopause (loss of estrogens) has some negative influence but is not the only cause. The rate of the bone loss may be altered by treatment or by a change of lifestyle. Factors that help prevent bone loss are physical activity, load bearing, estrogens, anabolic steroids, bisphosphonate, adequate calcium intake, vitamin D, and sunlight. Factors that contribute to bone loss are inactivity, disuse, immobilization, smoking, gastric resection, aging, and long-term use of drugs such as corticosteroids, heparin, and phenytoin.

### Articular Cartilage and Fibrocartilaginous Structures

Articular cartilage in diarthrodial joints is aneural, avascular, and without lymphatic supply. Nutrients are diffused through the matrix. Diffusion depends on joint motion and compressive loads. Adult articular cartilage varies in thickness from 2 to 4 mm. The cartilage is built up by water, collagen (type II), proteoglycans, glycoproteins, and cells that are unevenly distributed. This process creates the unique weight-bearing and lubrication capabilities of the cartilage. Damage to articular cartilage can disrupt the normal load-carrying ability of the tissue and thus the normal lubrication process operating in the joint. Insufficient lubrication may be a primary factor in the etiology of osteoarthritis.

Menisci are disk-shaped, fibrocartilaginous structures in some joints (e.g., tibiofemoral and acromioclavicular joints). The function of a meniscus is to distribute the load evenly over the joint surface. There are fibrocartilaginous structures in the ulnocarpal joint and also in the flexor tendon sheaths.

Joint motion is crucial for the well-being of cartilage tissue. Immobilization, long-term use of corticosteroids, long-term exposure to vibration, peak loads (impact), joint instability, and joint incongruity have deleterious effects on cartilage and fibrocartilaginous tissues.

### Muscle

The muscle tissue is the motor, or source of mechanical tension, that produces movement and torque. The natural pattern of movement of the human muscles is dynamic muscle contractions of short duration followed by relaxation. Muscle contraction derives energy from aerobic or anaerobic sources. The anaerobic threshold decreases with age. The duration and the intensity of the muscle contraction, particularly the resting or recovery period, determine the utilization of the muscle. Muscle contraction can exceed 20% to 30% of maximal voluntary contraction level only for short periods before muscle fatigue develops. Muscle work exceeding the anaerobic threshold leads to the accumulation of metabolites and lactate. Occupational demands seldom require periods of long muscle recruitment above 5% to 10% of the maximum voluntary contraction. However, certain occupations are at high risk for muscle injury due to highly repetitive work cycles or to maintaining positions for long durations.

Factors that increase muscle tissue are physical activity and exercise, and perhaps stretching. Factors that harm muscle tissue are inactivity, disuse, immobilization, aging, nutritional deficiencies (lack of protein intake), prolonged static loading, long-term repetitive loading, and vibration exposure (whole-body or segmental vibration).

### Connective Tissues: Ligaments, Tendons, and Joint Capsules

Tendons are dense, regularly arranged collagenous structures that connect muscle to bone. The collagen fibers insert directly into the bone. The tensile strength of a tendon is high. Tendons are mostly surrounded by more or less well developed tendon sheaths, some of which are synovial tendon sheaths, as in the flexor tendons of the wrist and the hand. Tendons are particularly sensitive to repetitive, monotonous load.

Ligaments are passive stabilizing structures that are found around joints (e.g., collateral ligaments) or within joints (e.g., cruciate ligaments). Joint capsules are connective tissue structures around joints. Connective tissues are strengthened by joint motion, physical activity, and perhaps stretching. Injury, immobilization, long-term use of corticosteroids, and aging weaken connective tissue.

## DISEASE STATES

Occupational musculoskeletal ailments can be specific or nonspecific (3,11). It therefore is characteristic for an employee or a worker to suffer from any of these disorders without presenting pathologic structure changes that would easily facilitate a differential diagnosis. The causes are multifactorial, having physical and psychosocial components, especially for chronic disorders (3,12). Table 3 lists components that affect the outcome of occupational respiratory diseases and musculoskeletal impairments (excluding fractures and soft-tissue ruptures). This comparison serves to illustrate the differences between the two leading occupational disorders, which can help in the formulation of a model for occupational musculoskeletal disorders. The most important link to such modeling is the exposure leading to a cause-effect relationship. Indeed, so many factors affect the outcome of functional musculoskeletal work capacity that a good model is still sought. The medical model suggested by Wood (13) implies that an individual plus a disease leads to an interaction resulting in an illness. This model has been abandoned for occupational musculoskeletal injuries and disorders involving nonspecific symptomatology. A more comprehensive model is currently popular—the biopsychosocial model proposed by Wadell (14) and Johansson (15). This chapter focuses on cumulative exposure of load and therefore describes the two most common conditions, i.e., osteoarthritis and cumulative trauma disorders in the upper extremity.

### Occupational Osteoarthritis

Osteoarthritis (OA) affects 12% of adults in the United States. Primary OA has a multifactorial background (16). Secondary OA is caused by previous known trauma (e.g., fracture, surgery, instability) or disease (e.g., hip dysplasia, osteochondritis, Perthes disease) manifestation. Individual risk factors associated with OA are age, gender, ethnic and racial background, genetic predisposition, and obesity (17).

The possibility that primary OA can be caused by prolonged occupational loading cannot be ruled out (18,19). Occupational factors that may be associated are repetitive physical activity, whole-body and segmental vibration, and occupational trauma leading to abnormal joint mechanics. Peyron's (16) review of epidemiologic studies of OA extensively cites studies that link mechanical loading and repetitive movement to primary OA. Involvement of the small joints of the hands of cotton pickers and weavers, of elbow and knee joints of coal miners, and of the metatarsophalangeal joints of ballet dancers points to occupational or repeated physical loading as an important risk factor.

**TABLE 3.** *Comparison of certain components related to outcome of work-related musculoskeletal disorders and occupational respiratory diseases*

| Variable | Musculoskeletal | Respiratory |
|---|---|---|
| Prevalence | Very high to epidemic | High |
| Incidence | Very high to epidemic | High |
| Exposure | Physical/mechanical load | Specific agent |
| Measurement of exposure | Very difficult to not possible | Easy to difficult |
| Cause | Indirect evidence, multifactorial | Direct evidence, unifactorial |
| Triggering factors | Occupational or nonoccupational environments | Occupational environment |
| Weight of one factor[a] | Variable but low | Pathognomonic |
| Pathology | Nonspecific | Characteristic |
| Functional assessment | Parameters need validation | Parameters based on physiology |
| Functional capacity | Poorly related to body size | Related to body size |
| Natural evolution | Limited and no mortality | Progressive and possibly lethal |
| Treatment | Functional training | Medical therapy and removal of exposure |
| Rehabilitation | Aim is return to previous occupation | Return to inoffensive milieu |
| Effect of latency | Allowance for psychological overlay | Deterioration of pulmonary function |
| Critical time interval | Undue delay in promoting activity | Undue delay in removing exposure |

[a]Weight of one casual factor.

High peak loading and shear stress may be a cause-effect relationship in the development of primary OA (20). The cause is thought to be overload of the subchondral bone of the joint, where the main stress is absorbed, and microfractures occur, leading progressively to increased stiffness. The relative energy absorption within the subchondral bone is thus decreased, and the risk for cartilage damage increases. Long-term prospective in vivo studies are needed to confirm the relationship. Primary OA in the lower extremity can lead to disability or job/career change. The prevalence of OA in the hip and the knee, radiographically defined as the lower height of the cartilage, is about 2% and 3%, respectively (19).

Vingard et al. (21–23) in Sweden found an increase in symptomatology leading to hospitalization caused by hip OA in men with jobs that had increased physical demands. These jobs included farmer, construction worker, firefighter, and food-processing worker [relative risk (RR) 2.5–3.8, 95% confidence interval (CI) 1.3–3.9]. When the individual engaged in a job requiring heavy physical work or in sports activity, or was obese, the relative risk increased two- to threefold. These findings imply that cumulative physical load exposure may lead to OA or at least worsen the condition. Although certain limitations are present in the above study, it confirms the findings by Axmacher and Lindberg (24) and Croft et al. (25). These two studies focused on farmers. Similar findings have been demonstrated for the knee joint. A moderately increased risk for knee OA has been shown in physically demanding work (26,27); however, some sports activity and being overweight seem to increase the risk of knee OA more than any given occupation.

A consensus symposium (19) on the etiology of OA concluded that unfavorable load bearing and repeated minor trauma may contribute to OA. This conclusion is in agreement with current biomechanical and epidemiologic hypotheses. Static load, repeated trauma over long periods, and an unnatural use of joints are likely to contribute to or exacerbate OA. Farmers and professional ballet dancers have a much higher frequency of OA, as do professional soccer players (19,25,28).

### Cumulative Trauma Disorders

Cumulative trauma disorders (CTD) or disorders associated with repeated trauma are likely to lead to musculoskeletal problems in the upper extremity (29). This definition is hardly exclusive; for instance, some repeated trauma can be acoustic and some CTDs are related to low back pain. The Bureau of Labor Statistics from 1982 to 1992 found an 800% increase in all reported cumulative trauma disorders. This increase has led to efforts by the Occupational Safety and Health Administration (OSHA) and the American National Standards Institute (ANSI) to initiate efforts to develop standards and guidelines that address the problem. The consensus reached by the ANSI Z-365 committee, which included scientists, representatives of industry and labor, and clinicians, offers recommendations for prevention. The committee formulated recommendations for surveillance factors, job analysis and design, medical management and training.

A precise epidemiologic model for CTD is lacking; however, there is a consensus that the development of CTD is a process with multifactorial causes rather than a single stimulus (30). The outcome of these stimuli may lead to a disorder. The onset of CTD may occur during work; the nomenclature itself implies a cumulative effect of physical load exposure over time. Symptom severity seems to be modified by work-organizational factors, i.e., cognitive demands and employee autonomy. The current epidemiologic models are predominantly biomechanical and inherently difficult to generalize because of the wide variation in interpreting the results of exposure measurements. The occupational risk factors for CTD are repetitive movements of a given body segment, prolonged duration of static muscle work, repetitive dynamic muscle work, and prolonged recovery time of the work environment such as exposure to vibration and cold. Definitions of rates of repetition, duration of a task, and rest periods for recovery are not uniform, which creates appreciable methodologic problems in the measurement of exposure. Despite these problems, high exposure to mechanical stressors seems to outweigh individual and work-organizational factors. Brogmus and Marko (31) found an increase in work-related repeated trauma to the upper extremity of approximately 5% from 1983 to 1993 using data of the Liberty Mutual Insurance Company. Opposite findings occurred in Sweden; a dramatic decrease in reported work injuries and diseases due to a change in legislation was reported in 1992. Figure 1 depicts the proportion of social security–approved illnesses and injuries from 1980 to 1995. The data includes musculoskeletal work-related injuries and disorders which encompass approximately 50% of all cases.

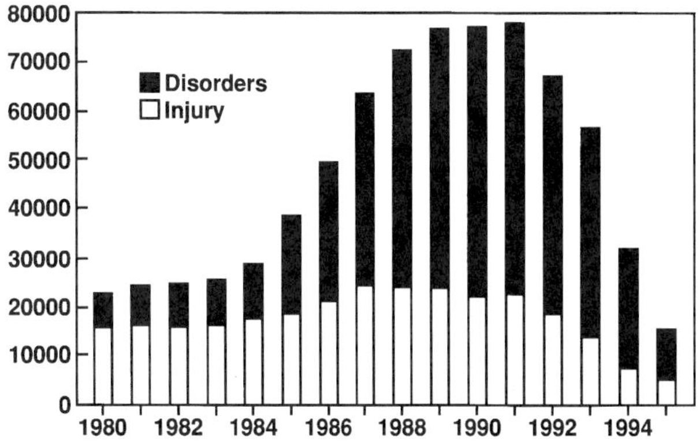


**FIG. 1.** Work-related injuries and disorders, 1980–1995 in Sweden. Only approved injuries and disorders through the social security system are shown. (Adapted from the Swedish Social Security System, SOU 1996:113.)

It is believed that hand and wrist disorders account for the majority of CTDs in the upper extremity. The food industry has the highest rate of hand, wrist, and forearm disorders: oyster, crab, and clam packing (RR 14.8, 95% CI 11.2–19.5), and meat and poultry dealers (RR 13.8, 95% CI 11.6–16.4) (32). High rates are found as well in serial production workers, textile industry workers, fine electrical and mechanical production workers, and office workers (33–37). Kuorinka and Forcier (30) have published a summary of CTD epidemiology studies available up to 1994.

Cumulative trauma disorder serves mainly as a descriptor for soft-tissue disorders and is an umbrella term for the many specific diagnoses encountered. Table 4 groups the disorders as related to tendon, nerve, joint, muscle, circulatory, and bursa.

Perhaps the most challenging task for the health care provider is to decide whether the symptomatology is work related (38,39). For example, epicondylitis traditionally has been considered as a work injury; however, good epidemiologic studies are lacking. Only one study (40) showed that 30% of the reported cases of lateral epicondylitis were work related, in this study work in an aircraft industry. The second challenge is to determine criteria for the safe return to work after treatment of the injury. The third challenge is to prevent recurrence. Medical management of CTD of the upper extremity and neck follow current practice and scientific knowledge. The literature documents little specific occupational medical management of CTD of the upper extremity and neck. Management of CTD includes a detailed interview of the job tasks, which is essential to understand the work relatedness. The history must include information on prior and current occupations, which is important in determining if the reported risk factor accords with the patient's symptomatology. Factors helpful in this determination are consistent exposure to repetitive tasks, awkward posture, high force exertion, long exertion time, and the use of handheld vibrating tools. Differential diagnosis is facilitated by the use of a standardized clinical examination of the symptoms, and a standardized assessment of such factors as onset of symptoms; quality and intensity of symptoms; site of onset; exposure to vibration; evolution, exacerbation, and relieving factors; the effect of recreational activities; and prior treatments. Finally, an understanding of psychosocial factors influencing and modifying pain behavior is essential (15,41).

Bonzani et al. (42) suggest three levels of evaluations: clinical, ergonomic, and psychosocial (Table 5). In an outcome study of 50 employees this classification could predict return to work. With this rating the authors found that subjective pain, tenderness, weakness, and sensory loss described by the patient were consistent with the clinical examination and the history of injury, and the patient responded to treatment in a predictable way. The ergonomic classification did not independently determine a patient's ability to resume work. The authors concluded that any rating higher than minor psychosocial issues was the main hurdle to returning a patient to work. Although this is one of the few outcome studies and needs further validation, the study underlines the importance of the use of the biopsychosocial model.

There is a significant association ($p < 0.01–0.02$) between symptoms and signs from the neck and upper extremity, and perceived stress at work (36). A poor psychosocial work environment combined with a high level

**TABLE 4.** *Examples of diagnosis commonly considered as work-related cumulative trauma disorders*

| Type | Disorders |
|---|---|
| Tendon-related disorders | Tendinitis/peritendinitis/tenosynovitis<br>Epicondylitis<br>De Quervain's<br>Trigger finger<br>Ganglion cyst |
| Nerve-related disorders | Carpal tunnel syndrome<br>Cubital tunnel syndrome<br>Guyon canal syndrome<br>Pronator teres syndrome<br>Radial tunnel syndrome<br>Thoracic outlet syndrome<br>Cervical syndrome (radiculopathy)<br>Digital neuritis |
| Joint-related disorders | Osteoarthritis predominantly hip and knee |
| Muscle-related disorders | Tension neck syndrome<br>Muscle sprain and strain<br>Myalgia and myositis |
| Circulatory-related disorders | Hypothenar hammer syndrome<br>Raynaud's syndrome |
| Bursa-related disorders | Bursitis of most joints |

Adapted from ref 30.

**TABLE 5.** *Suggested evaluation for upper extremity cumulative trauma disorders*

| |
|---|
| Clinical issues |
| *Objective findings:* swelling, joint or tendon crepitation, limited joint motion, abnormal radiographic or electromyographic findings |
| *Reasonable subjective findings:* pain, tenderness, sensory loss or weakness appropriate and consistent with the injury and the history |
| *Unreasonable subjective findings:* diffuse, vague unreproducible pain and tenderness not corresponding to anatomic distribution or inconsistent with history of injury |
| Ergonomic issues |
| *Minor issues:* correctable workstation problems or minor ergonomic instruction |
| *Moderate issues:* high repetition, high force or abnormal position that are correctable |
| *Major issues:* high repetition, high force or abnormal positions that are not correctable |
| Psychosocial issues |
| *Minor psychosocial issues:* usually administrative issues such as providing temporary modified duty or minor conflicts with the supervisor |
| *Moderate psychosocial issues:* job frustration, job stress, management insensitivity, or employee anger that is treatable |
| *Major psychosocial issues:* long standing unresolved frustration, anger, job stress plus degree of depression that are difficult to treat |

Adapted from ref. 42.

of physical demands increases the prevalence of neck pain by a factor of 2, as compared with the presence of either variable alone. CTD in the upper extremity, including unspecific symptomatology, requires a multidisciplinary approach to the evaluation of the patient and the workplace (43). The patient is evaluated by the health care provider in charge and the workplace by an ergonomist. The provider and ergonomist must communicate with each other.

Most CTDs fall in the category of nerve entrapment or soft-tissue inflammation. The recommended treatment in the early stage is rest of the affected area; however, few outcome studies or randomized controlled trials suggest that any form of treatment is superior in the early stage of CTD. The natural history of these different disorders is virtually unknown, which creates a dilemma for the treating physician and the patient. Therefore, until this knowledge is available, patients with symptomatology of the upper extremity or neck, occupationally related or not, are treated similarly.

A recently published reference book for prevention of work-related musculoskeletal disorders of the upper extremities and the neck provides evidence for the ergonomic intervention in primary prevention (30). These interventions need further evaluation if used as clinical tools to reduce symptomatology and to enhance the rate of return to work. Simple work modifications can alter the components of exposure, such as loads, repetition, recovery time, posture, and so forth. The involved health care provider should incorporate ergonomic knowledge in the treatment team to enhance the success of treatment for CTD (44,45).

We are strong proponents of early screening to prevent chronic pain and disability. For example, nonspecific hand and wrist pain are the most common problems. They are followed by tendinitis, ganglion, cyst, and carpal tunnel syndrome (CTS) (33). Rempel and Punnett (46) state, "In their early stages, these disorders may be manifested by nonspecific symptoms without signs and laboratory findings." Specific disorders usually do not occur in isolation. They are preceded by high rates of nonspecific symptoms and tendinitis and seem to track each other in high-risk workplaces. Of utmost importance in preventing disability are early screening, ergonomic intervention, early care, and follow-up (36,47). Epidemiologic surveillance systems are not solely of academic interest. They are necessary and essential for industry in planning intervention, maintaining a healthy work force, and cost saving.

### Patient Assessment

Placement examination should include questions about pain, weakness, and stiffness of the neck, spine, and extremities.

### Medical History

The history should include questions about injuries or diseases causing loss of function for longer than a week and previous surgery to the spine or the extremities. Hospital records should be requested. Additional historical details should include the circumstance of the injury, treatment, and results. A detailed interview of work tasks is important, as is determining what exacerbates the symptoms and what relieves the symptoms.

### Physical Examination

The physical examination is the most important tool for establishing a good doctor-patient relationship. The examination should be thorough but can be limited to the areas of medical interest. In the case of a traumatic injury to the neck, back, and extremities (especially one caused by external load), the whole region should be examined, not only the site of damage, and a neurovascular assessment (e.g., motor, sensory, and circulatory function distally in the extremities) should be done.

### Symptoms and Duration

When evaluating disabilities in a patient with a musculoskeletal impairment, the degree and duration of symptoms may have greater occupational importance than the specific underlying diagnosis itself. The clinical evaluation of musculoskeletal impairment places the patient into one of four groups, depending on the degree of symptoms:

- Completely asymptomatic: No restriction of activity.
- Symptoms associated with strenuous activity rather than with activities of daily living (ADL): Certain activities may be limited because they may initiate or exacerbate pain. These activities may be occupational or nonoccupational.
- Symptoms while undertaking ADL: Light duty or workplace modification may be necessary. Light duty should be time-limited and the condition reevaluated.
- Symptoms at rest: Limited ADL and restricted work or no work ability.

The duration of symptoms is important for future work ability. The longer the duration of the symptoms, the less the ability to work. A longer than anticipated duration of symptoms challenges the clinical examiner to ask the following questions:

1. Has the patient received the appropriate clinical evaluation, diagnosis, and treatment?
2. Are there other underlying medical, psychological, social, or legal hurdles for return to normal lifestyle and work?

### Radiographic Examinations

Radiographic studies, essential in many cases, are never a substitute for the history and physical examination. Radiographs, computed tomography (CT), and magnetic resonance imaging (MRI) of any part of the body can be done when indicated for an unknown or newly discovered abnormality. In case of fracture, dislocation, or fusion, hospital records, medical history, and clinical findings should provide sufficient information for proper placement.

### Diagnostic Tests

Laboratory blood tests in relation to musculoskeletal pain should be performed according to diagnostic requirements. Blood tests are usually normal in occupational musculoskeletal disorders. The possibility of systemic disease should be investigated if a musculoskeletal disorder has an unusual arthritic, neurologic, or myogenic presentation. In such cases, it may be necessary to consult specialists in different fields for further evaluation.

Neurophysiologic examinations such as clinic electromyography, nerve conduction velocity, and other diagnostics can be used to diagnose nerve entrapment or neuropathy. These examinations require good skills because the interpretation is subjective and specificity is poor; nevertheless, they are essential for confirming entrapment neuropathies common in occupational settings.

Arthroscopy is a diagnostic tool for evaluation traumatic or arthritic joint changes, although MRI is about to replace investigational arthroscopy. Biopsy of the muscle, nerve, or synovial tissue rarely is performed for occupational disorders, but it remains essential for unexplained myopathy, arthritis, or neurologic disease. However, these diagnostic tools do not predict work performance.

### Assessment of Work

The key to rehabilitation and successful placement of the worker is understanding his or her physiologic, physical, and mental capacities after the injury and to be certain that they meet the demands of the workplace. To make this assessment, it is necessary to be familiar with the demands of the workplace—the motions, strength, and endurance needed to perform the tasks and what loads are imposed on the musculoskeletal system. Answers to these questions, combined with knowledge of the patient's capabilities, allow proper decision making. The workplace may be modified to match the capabilities of the worker. A basic ergonomic principle is that the work load should be distributed in an optimal manner for the task required. Working conditions of special relevance to the musculoskeletal system are vibration, including driving, handling manual materials, constrained or long-sustained body position, awkward posture, impact loads, and repetitive motions.

## CONCLUSION

Injuries to the musculoskeletal system are the most important cause of work-related morbidity and disability in the United States. Occupational musculoskeletal impairment may occur acutely or may develop slowly over time. Cumulative trauma disorders of the upper extremities and osteoarthritis develop slowly. A goal for industry must be to prevent long-term morbidity and permanent disability and to become more proactive rather than reactive. This can be done through a multidisciplinary approach involving, in addition to the health care team, contributions of management, union, technical, epidemiological, and ergonomic experts with additional scientific expertise. The employee and the workplace and task must be evaluated carefully. Strategies must be implemented to deal with case management, return to work, adaptation of the work task, reinforcement of safety rules, continuing education and training, and long-term prevention. Only with such a multidisciplinary approach can we expect to reduce the prevalence, incidence, morbidity, disability, and costs of occupational musculoskeletal disorders.

## REFERENCES


1. Anderson JAD. Rheumatism in industry: a review. *Br J Ind Med* 1971; 28:103–121.
2. Cullen MR, Cherniack MG, Rosenstock L. Occupational medicine. Medical progress. *N Engl J Med* 1990;322:594–601.
3. Nordin M, Andersson GBJ, Pope MH. *Musculoskeletal disorders in the workplace. Principles and practice.* Philadelphia: Mosby, 1997.
4. Praemer A, Furner S, Rice DP. *Musculoskeletal conditions in the United States.* Park Ridge, IL: American Academy of Orthopaedic Surgeons, 1992.
5. Grazier KL, Holbrook TL, Kelsey JL, et al. *The frequency of occurrence, impact, and cost of musculoskeletal conditions in the United States.* Park Ridge, IL: American Academy of Orthopaedic Surgeons, 1984.
6. Rossman SB, Miller TR, Douglass JB. *The costs of occupational traumatic and cumulative injuries.* Cincinnati, OH: National Institute for Occupational Safety and Health, 1991.
7. Henessey JC, Muller LS. Work efforts of disabled-workers beneficiaries: preliminary findings from the new beneficiary back to work. *Soc Sec Bull* 1994;3:42–51.
8. Henessey JC, Muller LS. The effect of vocational rehabilitation and work incentives on helping the disabled-worker beneficiary back to work. *Soc Sec Bull* 1995;30:1–24.
9. Wiesel SW, Boden SD, Feffer HL. A quality-based protocol for management of musculoskeletal injuries: a ten year prospective outcome. *Clin Orthop* 1994;301:164–176.
10. Nordin M, Fankel V. *Basic biomechanics of the skeletal system.* Philadelphia: Lea & Febiger, 1989.
11. Cunningham LS, Kelsey JL. Epidemiology of musculoskeletal impairments and associated disability. *Am J Publ Health* 1984;74:594–601.
12. Bergenudd H. *Talent, occupation and locomotor discomfort.* Thesis, Department of Orthopaedics, Malmo General Hospital Lund University, S-21401 Malmo, Sweden, 1989.
13. Wood PHN. The basis of rheumatological practice, including nomenclature and classification. In: Scott JT, ed. *Coperman's textbook of the rheumatic diseases,* 6th ed. London: Churchill Livingstone, 1986; 59–142.
14. Wadell G. Biopsychosocial analysis of low back pain. In: Nordin M, Vischer TL, eds. *Common low back pain prevention of chronicity. Baillieres Clin Rheumatol* 1992;6:523–558.
15. Johansson J. *Psychosocial factors at work and their relation to musculoskeletal symptoms.* Doctoral thesis, Department of Psychology, Goteborg University, Goteborg, Sweden, 1994.
16. Peyron JG. Osteoarthritis: the epidemiology viewpoint. *Clin Orthop* 1986;213:13–19.
17. Inerot S, Heinegard D, Audell L, et al. Articular cartilage proteoglycans in aging and osteoarthritis. *Biochem J* 1978;169:143–156.
18. Moskowitz RW, Howell PS, Goldberg VM, et al. *Osteoarthritis. Diagnosis and management.* Philadelphia: WB Sanders, 1984.
19. Nilsson BE. The Tore Nilson symposium on the etiology of degenerative joint diseases. *Acta Orthop Scand Suppl* 1993;64:54–61.
20. Freeman MAR. *Adult articular cartilage.* New York: Grune & Stratton, 1973.
21. Vingard E, Alfredsson L, Goldie I, et al. Sports and osteoarthrosis of the hip. *Am J Sports Med* 1993;21:195–200.
22. Vingard E, Alfredsson L, Hogstedt C. Disability pensions due to musculoskeletal disorders among men in heavy occupations. *Scand J Soc Med* 1992;20:31–36.
23. Vingard E, Alfredsson L, Goldie I, et al. Sports and osteoarthrosis of the hip. *Am J Sports Med* 1993;21:195–200.
24. Axmacher B, Lindberg H. Coxarthrosis in farmers. *Clin Orthop* 1993; 287:82–86.
25. Croft P, Coggon D, Cruddas U, et al. Osteoarthritis of the hip: an occupational diseases in farmers. *Br J Med* 1992;304:1269–1272.
26. Felson D. Occupational physical demands, knee bending and osteo arthritis: results from the Framingham study. *J Rheumatol* 1991;18: 1587–1592.
27. Kohatsu N, Schurman D. Risk factors for the development of osteoarthritis of the knee. *Clin Orthop* 1990;261:242–246.
28. Andersson S, Nilsson B, Hessel T, et al. Degenerative joint diseases in ballet dancers. *Clin Orthop* 1989;238:233–236.
29. Putz-Anderson V. *Cumulative trauma disorders. a manual for musculoskeletal diseases of the upper limbs.* London: Taylor & Francis, 1988.
30. Kuorinka I, Forcier L. *Work-related musculoskeletal disorders:* WMSDs. *A reference book for prevention.* London: Taylor & Francis, 1995;323–348.
31. Brogmus GE, Marko R. The proportion of cumulative trauma disorders of the upper extremities in U.S. industry. Proceedings of the Human Factors Society 36th Annual Meeting, San Francisco, 1992;997–1001.
32. Franklin GM, Haug J, Heyer N, et al. Occupational carpal tunnel syndrome in Washington State 1984–1988. *Am J Public Health* 1991;81: 741–746.
33. Luopajarvi R, Kuorinka I, Virolainen M, et al. Prevalence of tenosynovitis and other injuries of the upper extremities in repetitive work. *Scand J Work Environ Health* 1979;5:48–55.
34. Silverstein BA, Fine LJ, Armstrong TJ. Occupational factors and carpal tunnel syndrome. *Am J Ind Med* 1987;11:343–358.
35. Stock SR. Workplace ergonomic factors and the development of musculoskeletal disorders of the neck and upper limbs: a meta-analysis. *Am J Ind Med* 1991;19:87–107.
36. Zetterberg C, Forsberg A, Hansson E, et al. Neck and upper extremity problems in car assembly workers. A comparison of subjective complaints, work satisfaction, physical examination and gender. *Int J Ind Ergonom,* in press.
37. Magnusson M, Pope M. Epidemiology of neck and upper extremity. In: Nordin M, Andersson GBJ, Pope MH, eds. *Musculoskeletal disorders in the workplace. principles and practice.* Philadelphia: Mosby, 1997; 328–335.
38. Fine LJ, Silverstein BA, Armstrong TJ, et al. Detection of cumulative trauma disorders of the upper extremity in the workplace. *J Occup Med* 1986;28:674–678.
39. Young VL, Seaton MK, Freely CA, et al. Detecting cumulative trauma disorders in workers performing repetitive tasks. *Am J Ind Med* 1995; 27:419–431.
40. Dimberg L. The prevalence and causation of tennis elbow (lateral humeral epicondylitis) in a population of workers in an engineering industry. *Ergonomics* 1987;30:573–580.
41. Weiser P. Psychosocial aspects of occupational musculoskeletal disorders. In: Nordin M, Andersson GBJ, Pope MH, eds. *Musculoskeletal disorders in the workplace. Principles and practice.* Philadelphia: Mosby, 1997;51–61.
42. Bonzani P, Mangieri M, Keelan B, et al. Factors prolonging disability in work-related cumulative trauma disorders. *J Hand Surg,* 1997;22(1): 30–34.
43. Keyserling WM, Stetson DS, Silverstein BA, et al. A checklist for evaluating ergonomic risk factors associated with upper extremity cumulative trauma disorder. *Ergonomics* 1993;36:807–831.
44. Armstrong TJ. Workplace adaption. In: Nordin M, Andersson GBJ, Pope MH, eds. *Musculoskeletal disorders in the workplace. Principles and practice.* Philadelphia: Mosby, 1997;411–419.
45. Radwin RG, Scoungyeon O, Carson-Oakes C. Biomechanical aspect of hand tools. In: Nordin M, Andersson GBJ, Pope MH, eds. *Musculoskeletal disorders in the workplace. Principles and practice.* Philadelphia: Mosby, 1997;467–479.
46. Rempel D, Punnett L. Epidemiology of wrist and hand disorders. In: Nordin M, Andersson GBJ, Pope MH, eds. *Musculoskeletal disorders in the workplace. Principles and practice.* Philadelphia: Mosby, 1997; 421–430.
47. Moore JS, Garg A. Upper extremity disorders in a pork processing plant: relationship between job risk factors and morbidity. *Am Ind Hyg Assoc J* 1994;55:703–715.
48. Bureau of Labor Statistics. *Supplemental data system.* Announcement 90-1. Washington, DC: U.S. Department of Labor, 1990(May).

*Environmental and Occupational Medicine, Third Edition,* edited by William N. Rom.
Lippincott–Raven Publishers, Philadelphia © 1998.

# CHAPTER 66

# Nonspecific Low Back Pain

Margareta Nordin, Sherri R. Weiser, Jan Willem van Doorn, and Rudi Hiebert

Low back pain can be characterized as specific or nonspecific. Specific low back pain entails all diagnoses that can be linked to a disorder, disease, infection, injury, trauma, or structural deformity. A potential causal relationship can be found between the diagnosis and the pain. For example, a herniated disk in the lumbar spine may compress a nerve root, thereby producing pain in the lumbar spine and sometimes in the leg (1). A tumor can generate a structural deformity and impact on the spinal canal, resulting in back pain (2). These conditions are rare and can be diagnosed early from "red flag" symptoms (Table 1) (3,4). This chapter focus on benign low back pain, which constitutes approximately 80% of all low back pain, work related or not.

## NATURAL HISTORY OF NONSPECIFIC LOW BACK PAIN

Most adults experience nonspecific low back pain (NSLBP). It is called nonspecific because no specific cause can be found to account for the patient's perceived pain. NSLBP encompasses many vague diagnostic terms such as lumbago, myofascial syndromes, muscle spasms, mechanical low back pain, back sprain, back strain, and other less traditional terms.

M. Nordin: Occupational and Industrial Orthopaedic Center, Hospital for Joint Diseases; Program of Ergonomics and Biomechanics; and Department of Environmental Medicine, New York University Medical Center, New York, New York 10014.

S. R. Weiser: Psychological Services, Occupational and Industrial Orthopaedic Center, Hospital for Joint Diseases, New York, New York 10016.

J. W. van Doorn: Business Development, Occupational and Industrial Orthopaedic and Spine Center, Hospital for Joint Diseases, New York, New York 10016.

R. Hiebert: Department of Orthopaedics, New York University Medical Center; and Musculoskeletal Epidemiology Unit, Hospital for Joint Diseases, New York, New York 10016.

Since the cause is unknown and the course and treatment is similar for all these diagnoses, the more accurate term is NSLBP (5). It is described as pain in the lumbar region that may or may not radiate down one or both thighs. It is usually exacerbated by motion of the trunk, particularly flexion in combination with rotation. NSLBP represents approximately 80% of all reported cases in patients 25 to 55 years of age (6). Table 2 displays the symptoms, signs, and expected recovery rate for NSLBP and nerve root pain (sciatica).

Extensive research has shown that the prognosis for NSLBP is good. The prognosis is based on the natural history of low back pain. Up to 90% of all patients presenting to a health care provider with NSLBP recover within 4 weeks and 96% recover between 4 and 12 weeks (3,5). Here, recovery means the resumption of normal activities, including work. If residual pain exists, it does not limit function. Approximately 4% of all patients with an initial diagnosis of NSLBP remain disabled after 12 weeks (5,7). Studies have also shown that the natural history of sciatica is good; however, recovery is slower than for NSLBP (8,9). Sciatica lifetime prevalence is estimated to be 1% to 3% in the general population (10). If pain persists or progresses, the patient has the option of surgery. Approximately 60% have complete relief of their symptoms if surgery is performed (11). This chapter does not address specific nerve root pain from the lumbar spine.

## DEFINITIONS OF ACUTE, SUBACUTE, AT-RISK, CHRONIC, AND RECURRENT NONSPECIFIC LOW BACK PAIN

The following definitions are used:

*Acute NSLBP* is impairment lasting 7 days or less (5).
*Subacute NSLBP* is impairment lasting 1 to 4 weeks (3).

**TABLE 1.** *Red flags for potentially serious conditions at initial evaluation of patient seeking treatment for low back pain (from medical history and clinical examination at first visit)*

| Red flags for possible serious spinal pathology | Red flags for possible cauda equina syndrome or widespread neurologic disorders | Inflammatory disorders |
|---|---|---|
| Age of onset less than 20 or greater than 55 years | Difficulty with micturition | Gradual onset before age of 40 |
| Violent trauma; e.g. fall from height or motor vehicle | Loss of anal sphincter tone or fecal incontinence | Marked morning stiffness |
| Constant progressive nonmechanical pain | Saddle anesthesia about the anus, perineum, or genitals | Persisting limitation of spinal movements in all directions |
| Thoracic pain | Widespread (>1 nerve root) or progressive motor weakness in the leg(s) or gait disturbances | Peripheral joint involvement |
| Past medical history of carcinoma | Sensory level | Iritis, skin rashes (psoriasis), colitis, urethral discharge |
| Systemic steroids | | Family history |
| Drug abuse, HIV | | |
| Systemically unwell | | |
| Rapid weight loss | | |
| Persisting severe restriction of lumbar flexion | | |
| Widespread neurology | | |
| Structural deformity | | |

Adapted from refs. 3,4.

*At-risk NSLBP* is impairment lasting between 4 and 12 weeks (12,13).

*Chronic low back pain* is impairment lasting longer than 12 weeks and up to 6 months (5).

*Chronic pain syndrome* is impairment and disability lasting longer than 6 months (14).

The prognosis for acute and subacute NSLBP is excellent. The term *at-risk* is used for patients who do not recover within 4 weeks (15) They are at risk for delayed recovery and prolonged disability. Their prognosis is unknown. Chronic NSLBP, however, has a progressively worse prognosis. At 6 months after the onset of pain, the likelihood of a patient ever resuming normal activities is 40% to 55%. At 2 years it is almost nil (16–19).

There is no consensual definition of *recurrent NSLBP.* Estimates of recurrencies vary from 8.9% to 44% depending on social system, culture, and type of work. These variations are also influenced by the lack of a uniform definition.

## EPIDEMIOLOGY OF LOW BACK PAIN

Differences in terminology used to describe and classify back pain result in variable estimates of frequency and cost (20,21). The following statistics include all forms of low back pain, not just NSLBP.

Estimates of prevalence vary considerably, depending on the data source and the definitions used. Praemer et al. (22), using data from the National Health Interview Survey, found that the cumulative lifetime prevalence of low back pain lasting at least 2 weeks was 16% for individuals between 25 and 74 years. Other authors found that 50% of adults have reported experiencing any low back pain at some point in their life (23). Approximately 10% of individuals report having had back pain within the last year, and 6.8% report having back pain at any one point in time (24,25). Extrapolating to the present, these figures suggest that approximately 17 million individuals have back pain at one point in time.

Back pain results in significant use of health care resources. Back pain is the second most frequently

**TABLE 2.** *Diagnostic triage for patients with nonspecific low back pain (NSLBP) and nerve root pain (sciatica)*

| Nonspecific low back pain (NSLBP) | Lumbar nerve root pain (sciatica) |
|---|---|
| Presentation between age 20 and 55 | Unilateral leg pain worse than low back pain |
| Lumbosacral region, buttocks and thighs | Pain generally radiates to foot or toes |
| Pain mechanical in nature | Numbness and paresthesia in dermatomal distribution |
| Varies with physical activity | Nerve root irritation signs |
| Varies with time | Reduced straight leg raising test (SLR), which reproduces leg pain |
| Patient medically well | Motor, sensory or reflex change |
| Prognosis good | Limited to one nerve root |
| 90% recover from acute NSLBP within 6 weeks | Prognosis reasonable |
| | 50% recover from acute onset of pain within 6 weeks |

Adapted from refs. 3,4.

reported reason for making a physician visit (26). One study found that 85% of back pain sufferers sought medical care, resulting in approximately 13 million physician visits (25). On average, patients visit medical doctors 2.8 times for each episode. This number is higher for chiropractors. Surgeries are performed in 12% of all low back pain cases (25). Some experts estimate that back pain results in as much as $50 billion per year in direct and indirect costs. Low back pain lasting longer than 3 months is disproportionately expensive to treat and compensate (20,26a).

A variety of individual characteristics have been investigated as risk factors for the onset of back pain (6,27,28). The peak incidence of low back pain occurs in the early 20s with a gradual decline thereafter. The prevalence of low back pain gradually increases with age, reflecting a cumulative effect as new cases develop (25). A low back pain episode is likely to be more severe and result in greater disability as one gets older. At age of 60 severity levels off for men but continues to increase for women. The prevalence rate of low back pain in the general population is similar for men and women (25).

## OCCUPATIONAL LOW BACK PAIN

The most recent analysis used nationally representative data from the 1988 National Health Interview Survey (29). The study found that 17.6% of respondents reported back pain symptoms lasting longer than 1 week during the past year. This percentage represents an estimated total of 22.4 million cases, resulting in an estimated 149.1 million lost workdays for the entire work force because of low back pain.

The back represents the single most common claim for compensation. One-quarter of all workers' compensation cases are for back pain, and approximately one-third of workers' compensation costs are for back pain. The direct cost of back pain in 1979 was $1 billion (29). Some authors estimated that the total direct and indirect cost of work-related back pain was as much as $50 billion in 1990 (10).

Studies have investigated the role of the physical demands of work as predictors of acute episodes of occupational low back problems. These studies show that work requirements, such as heavy lifting, frequent or prolonged forward flexion or torso twisting, prolonged standing or sitting, repetitive tasks, and exposure to whole-body vibration are associated with an increased risk of an acute episode of low back pain (30,31). Risk for injury increases as the amount of weight an individual is required to move nears or matches his or her lifting capacity (32).

The physical demands of work are also thought to be associated with the duration of pain and the risk of subsequent disability. Among male workers, construction laborers, carpenters, and agricultural workers/tractor equipment operators had the highest rates of work-related back pain (22%) (29). Among female workers, nursing aides, licensed or practical nurses, and maids had the highest rates of back pain (18%, 16%, and 15%, respectively) (29). One study found that blue-collar workers were more likely to exhibit sciatica than white-collar workers and stayed away from work longer (33).

In a recent study, exposure to whole-body vibration resulted in a threefold risk of delayed recovery (15). The same study assessed patients within 7 days of an on-the-job injury and found that altered gait (inability to perform heel or toe walk) and high self-reported perceived disability increased the odds of remaining out of work for 1 month, by 2.5 and 3 times, respectively. A retrospective study found that patients who received a specific diagnosis within 7 days of a lost work episode were 4.9 times more likely to be out of work at 6 months. Age was also important, with those individuals over 55 years of age being 4.7 times more likely to be out of work at 6 months. The combined affect of age and diagnosis yielded a tenfold risk for chronicity (1). Other studies indicate a trend for women to be twice as likely to remain out of work for 6 months. In the occupational setting, however, women experience less back pain–related absence than men. This may reflect the disproportionate employment of men in high-risk jobs.

Work stress may affect NSLBP complaints through the stress-response model, indirectly through work organization, or more likely, by the interaction of the two (34). Work satisfaction has been negatively related to reports of NSLBP and a tendency to blame the workplace for injury (35–37). Work stress conceptualized as high work pace, low decision latitude, lack of control, and/or perceived physical demands has been positively related to musculoskeletal complaints and the development of chronic NSLBP (38–44). Most reports link social support at work to decreased symptoms (44–46). Patients undergoing litigation as a result of back injury or receiving workers' compensation have poorer outcomes than others in many studies (47,48). Recent investigations suggest that this relationship does not hold true for high level or prestigious jobs or workers' compensation patients with a positive outlook and who receive proper care (49,50).

When treating occupational injuries, attention should be paid to specific risk factors regarding the worker and the work environment, in addition to nonwork factors. A comprehensive program that addresses organizational issues as well as individual risk factors has proven effective in reducing workplace injuries (51). A recent study found that blue-collar workers placed on restricted duty were not likely to ever return to their previous work (52). This suggests that for jobs with heavy work loads, restricted duty should be limited to 2 to 3 weeks.

**TABLE 3.** *Health care utilization by care professionals*

| Specialty | Percent |
|---|---|
| General practitioner | 58.6 |
| Orthopedist | 36.9 |
| Chiropractor | 30.8 |
| Osteopath | 13.8 |
| Internist | 7.6 |
| Hematologist | 2.5 |

Adapted from ref. 25.

In 1994 a group of low back pain experts convened to develop evidence-based guidelines for the treatment of acute low back pain. The result was the U.S. Agency for Health Care Policy and Research (AHCPR) guidelines (3). Around the time another task force including some of the same experts was writing "Back Pain in the Workplace: Management of Disability in Nonspecific Conditions" (47). This task force had a different focus. It went beyond the care of the patient and dealt with the sociocultural influences specific to occupational pain, with an emphasis on preventing disability. The main recommendation of this panel was that NSLBP should be reclassified as an activity-intolerance problem and not a medical one. The implications of this statement are meant to alter our perspective of workers' compensation and severely restrict the assignment of disability status. The guidelines outline the policy changes that are necessary to support this recommendation.

## HEALTH CARE UTILIZATION IN TREATMENT OF PATIENTS WITH NONSPECIFIC LOW BACK PAIN

Most of the published health care utilization data are from the 1970s. The National Health and Nutrition Examination Survey from 1976 to 1980 (NHANES II) described the use of health professionals by NSLBP sufferers (Table 3) (25). Overall, 84% had seen a health care professional, 30.9% had been hospitalized, and 11.6% had undergone surgery.

Other data provided by the 1976 National Health Interview Survey (NHIS) showed an average of 2.8 physician visits per NSLBP sufferer (53). Fifty percent were admitted to a hospital and 22% underwent surgery. Bed rest was taken by 8.3% of the NSLBP sufferers.

In 1992 to 1993, a study was performed in North Carolina to analyze the differences in care provided by various health care professionals, including an HMO practice (54). Table 4 shows all statistically significant differences ($p < 0.05$).

## OUTCOME OF PATIENT EDUCATION PROGRAMS

Patient education and training programs are frequently proposed as a means of reducing morbidity associated with NSLBP. However, there is little evidence to attest to the efficacy of these programs. To date no educational intervention, on its own, has demonstrated a decrease in the frequency, severity, duration, cost, or risk associated with NSLBP. These educational interventions range from simple pamphlets to complex educational programs based on health education theory. The most common educational program is the back school. The back school is a formal series of educational lectures and practical applications lasting about four to six sessions (55,56).

One study found that healthy individuals who volunteered for back school made fewer visits to medical doctors for low back pain during a subsequent 6-month period as compared to a matched comparison group. The frequency and severity of new back pain episodes, drug intake, and time lost from work were not different between the two groups, however (57).

Education programs and counseling can help to reduce barriers to the adoption of new behaviors, improve short-term compliance with treatment recommendations, and improve patient satisfaction with care. One study found that back education class students had views about back pain that were more congruent with the instructor's after the class than before (58). Another study found that patients who received counseling were more likely to keep their follow-up appointments than those who did not (59). Cherkin et al. (60) showed that patient satisfaction with care improved when the health care provider imparted information about treatment. In a large Health

**TABLE 4.** *Significant differences in care provided by various health care professionals*

| Provider | Mean no. of visits to this provider | Mean no. of visits to any provider | X-ray (% of patients) | CT or MRI (% of patients) | Mean no. of medications | Hospitalization (% of patients) | Median cost per episode ($) |
|---|---|---|---|---|---|---|---|
| Primary care physician (urban) | 1.9 | 4.4 | 26 | 9 | 3.3 | 3 | 169 |
| Primary care physician (rural) | 2.0 | 4.6 | 32 | 11 | 3.7 | 4 | 214 |
| HMO provider | 1.9 | 3.1 | 19 | 6 | 3.3 | 1 | 184 |
| Orthopedist | 2.2 | 5.5 | 72 | 17 | 3.6 | 6 | 383 |
| Chiropractor (urban) | 13.2 | 15.0 | 67 | 8 | 2.4 | 2 | 545 |
| Chiropractor (rural) | 9.0 | 10.1 | 68 | 7 | 2.1 | 3 | 348 |

Adapted from ref. 54.

Maintenance Organization 293 patients with benign low back pain were randomized to one of three groups: (a) the usual care was provided; (b) an educational booklet was distributed; and (c) a 15-minute session with a clinic nurse was provided, combined with the educational booklet and follow-up telephone calls. The booklet was developed by the authors for the study. It discusses (in lay language) current knowledge of what causes back pain, available treatment, and prognosis. The pamphlet stresses the importance of returning to normal physical activity quickly as a treatment for low back pain, and the value of regular exercise in preventing and minimizing the severity of low back pain episodes. Six female nurses with 20 years of clinic experience conducted the patient education sessions. The nurses received 9 hours of training specifically for the study. The patient-education session occurred immediately after the patient's physical examination by the doctor. During the education session, the nurse reviewed the material discussed in the booklet, emphasized the benign nature of back pain, and helped establish physical activity goals (walking, swimming, etc.). The nurse also reassured the patient that, even though physical activity may increase back pain momentarily, consistent, progressive, and moderate activity helps improve recovery. The nurse telephoned the patient 1 to 3 days later to answer questions, reassure the patient, and to encourage the patient to meet exercise goals. The results indicated greater patient satisfaction and exercise participation but no effect on worry and fundamental status on health care utilization.

While education programs may influence some health behaviors, the generation of new behaviors depends on environmental factors that support or discourage them. For example, poor ergonomic designs in the workplace may make it impossible to comply with biomechanical recommendations. Successful education programs should be highly specific and take into account environmental contingencies. Education programs, regardless of how extensive they are, have not yet demonstrated an impact on broad measures of back pain morbidity. They appear to be one component in the successful management of NSLBP.

## OUTCOME OF HEALTH CARE PROVIDERS EDUCATION PROGRAM

The AHCPR guidelines for the treatment of acute low back pain propose a standard clinical assessment for all patients (3). Wiesel et al. (61) found a decrease in the prevalence of low back pain, lost work days, and medical and compensation costs when such a procedure was implemented in a 2-year period.

Education programs for physicians are necessary to change clinical practice. However, little information on successful education programs for physicians is available. Geyman and Gordon (62) proposed that in order to change practice new knowledge must be accepted as valid and useful, and that judged benefits must outweigh obstacles to change. In a study of 83 primary health care physicians taught to do three new procedures, a significant retention of knowledge was found. However, this resulted in only some change in practice for two of the three procedures. The authors conclude that factors such as habit, economic disincentives, practice pressures, and skepticism may have been at play.

Ashbaugh and McKean (63) performed a medical records audit in a department of surgery and found that 94% of deficiencies in care were performance based rather than knowledge based. The authors concluded that training should be performance based, utilizing hands-on demonstrations.

An educational program to train industry-based physicians in a new low back pain assessment procedure based on the AHCPR guidelines was recently developed and evaluated (64). Physicians were instructed in a standard clinical evaluation including the completion of standard medical forms. They were also asked to categorize patients based on a clinical classification system proposed by the Quebec Task Force (5). The education program included group and individual sessions stressing performance-based training, followed by an extensive period of follow-up at the work place. Little change in clinical practice occurred with the training program alone. Significant change in physician compliance was achieved after an administrative mandate was given to the physicians. These findings point to the importance of economic incentives in changing practice and the multidetermined nature of behavior change.

## OUTCOMES OF EARLY CARE IN PATIENT POPULATIONS

Work-related and non–work-related NSLBP are the cause for up to a third of the visits to primary care physicians, chiropractors, and physical therapists. The information and treatment that the patient receives at the first contact with a health care provider is crucial in determining recovery. Several studies have pointed to the importance of a careful medical evaluation that focuses on the detection of potentially serious spinal pathology or other nonspinal pathology. Once those conditions are ruled out, a course of treatment must be discussed with the patient. In the absence of red flags, the patient should be informed that imaging is not helpful during the first 4 weeks, that recovery is most likely with noninvasive benign treatment or no treatment, and full recovery is likely (3). The health care provider should offer the following advice for patients with NSLBP:

- Over-the-counter (OTC) drugs such as nonsteroidal antiinflammatory drugs (NSAIDs) and acetaminophen are considered safe and effective for most patients. The type of drug selected should be based on comorbidity, side effects, cost, and patient and provider preference (65–67).

- Leisure and work activities should be resumed as soon as possible. Low-stress aerobic activities can safely be done within the first 2 weeks of symptoms (68). Bed rest longer than 2 days can have deleterious effects (69,70).
- Spinal manipulation can also be helpful for patients with acute NSLBP during the first month. If no improvement has occurred within this time, the manipulation should be discontinued and the patient should be reevaluated (71,72).
- Temporary symptomatic relief from heat and cold has been reported in the literature. However, no long-lasting effect can be expected. Nonetheless, teaching the patient the self-application of these techniques is an option (65,73).

No other treatments during the first 4 weeks of acute NSLBP have scientifically strongly supported benefits (3,13). Taken together, these findings point to strong evidence for early activation, OTC medications, limited manipulation, and early return to normal activity. If the patient does not improve in the 4-week period, a multidisciplinary evaluation including a back specialist, a psychologist, and a physical therapist is recommended (3,13). At this stage multidisciplinary treatment offers the best chance of preventing disability and returning the patient to normal activities.

## NONPHYSICAL FACTORS ASSOCIATED WITH OUTCOME OF TREATMENT

A recent accumulation of evidence suggests that a biopsychosocial model is more useful in understanding NSLBP than a purely physical or medical approach (74). Nonphysical factors have been associated with the outcome of NSLBP in the acute, subacute, and chronic phases and have been particularly important in determining occupational status (75). Psychosocial factors include attributes of the individual, the work environment, and the sociocultural environment. This section summarizes the nonphysical factors that influence NSLBP.

Cognition refers to beliefs about illness and mental coping strategies. Acute and chronic patients' accurate beliefs about low back pain have been associated with better functional outcomes than inaccurate beliefs (76,77). It has also been found that patients who believed that daily life and work activities would hurt their backs had poor outcomes (74). Patients' beliefs in their ability to return to work predicted work status 4 years hence (78). Cognitive coping, defined as attempts to render pain more tolerable, has been associated with pain perception and functional outcome. Attempts to overcome pain and perceived control are associated with good outcomes while catastrophizing (imagining the worst) is associated with poor outcome (79–82).

Affect, though associated with cognition, has been shown to be important in the course of NSLBP in its own right. A body of research has found that psychological distress (e.g., depression, anxiety, hysteria, somatization) is associated with poor outcome at all stages of NSLBP (35,49,83–86). Distress measured in the early stage of injury has been found to predict future disability (87,88). Pain-specific anxiety was more predictive of chronic pain symptoms than general anxiety.

There is no evidence that personality predisposes a patient to developing chronic NSLBP. However, certain aspects of personality or traits appear to be associated with outcome. Premorbid pessimism measured after injury was linked to failure to return to work, while the trait of "cooperativeness" was associated with good outcome (49). Type A personality traits, particularly speed and hard-driving competitiveness, were associated with a high level of musculoskeletal complaints (89). A history of premorbid clinical depression and alcohol abuse was found in over half of the injured workers in one study (85).

Illness behaviors such as grimacing, bracing, guarding, groaning, limping, overreacting, and periods of inactivity are physical or verbal attempts to communicate suffering and disability (18,19,90). In the acute stage such behaviors may be warranted to seek help and avoid further injury. However, in chronic patients these behaviors have no therapeutic value and undermine the patients' ability to return to normal activities (91). Pain behaviors and reports of perceived disability in early injury have been found to be predictive of future work status (13,92). One study predicted surgical outcome of spinal fusion patients at 2 years postsurgery on the basis of behavioral signs and the patients' diagrams of pain patterns (93).

Extrinsic factors may affect NSLBP. The family system may be a strong influence on the development of disability. One study found over half of the disabled patients they studied had a disabled relative (94). Finally, the influence of health care professionals can be powerful. Information that is vague, incomplete, or inaccurate can have deleterious effects. A medical care delivery plan that utilizes quality-based management systems has been shown to have good outcomes (61) .

## GUIDELINES FOR EARLY CARE

Guidelines for the treatment of low back pain have been developed to improve patient care and lower costs. The Quebec Task Force on Spinal Disorders (QTFSD) was an early attempt to develop guidelines from quality-based scientific evidence (5). Their findings emphasized the positive natural history of low back pain, early resumption of activities and return to work, the need for minimal treatment early in care, the need to study non-

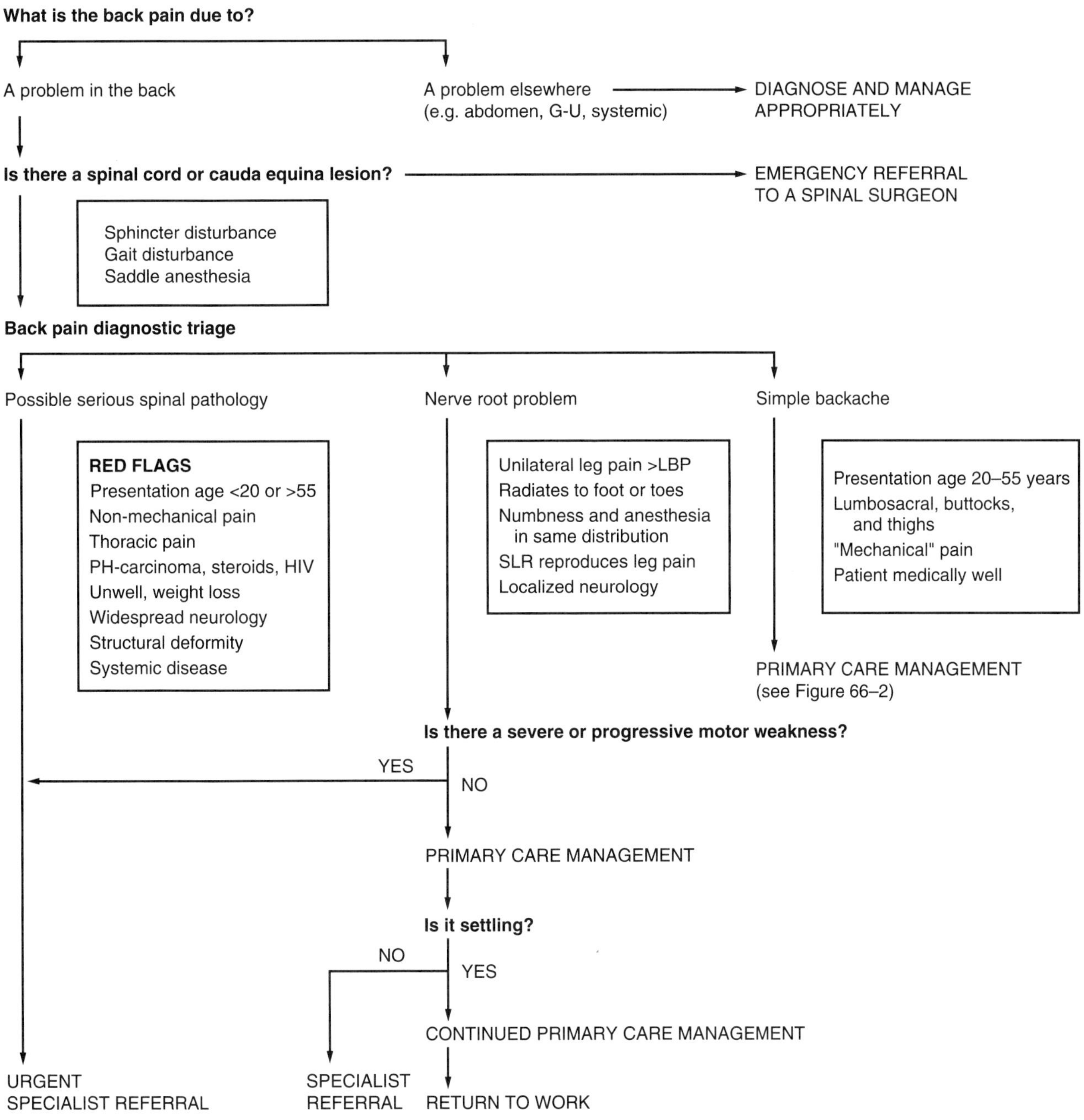


**FIG. 1.** Diagnostic triage flowchart of a patient presenting with low back pain with or without leg pain. (Adapted from refs. 3,4.)

physical factors associated with chronicity, and the importance of a standard medical assessment. The panel proposed a standard medical evaluation form and an algorithm for treatment that has subsequently been modified by other expert panels.

In 1994 a multidisciplinary panel comprised of international experts was mandated by the AHCPR to produce up-to-date guidelines for acute low back pain based on the recommendations of the Quebec Task Force (3). Using stringent methodologic criteria, the panel reviewed all existing well-designed studies and produced a summary of their findings. They devised a rating system to indicate the amount of scientific evidence that exists to support each of their conclusions. A major thrust of this effort was to shift attention away from treating pain and toward improving activity intolerance.

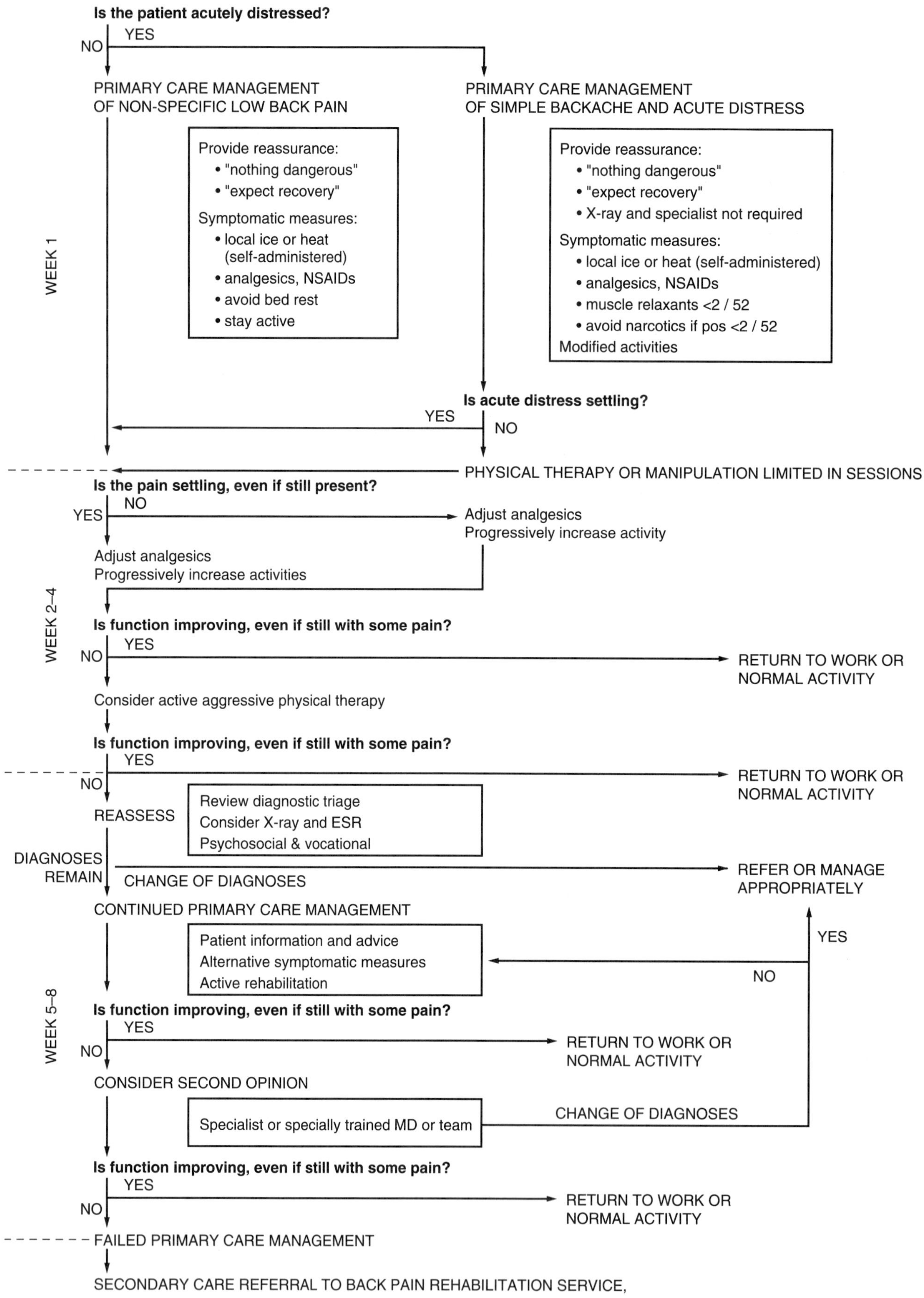


**FIG. 2.** Management of nonspecific low back pain. (Adapted from refs. 3,4.)

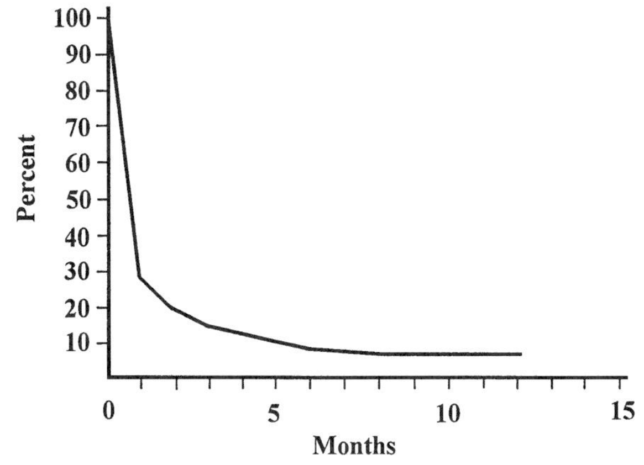


**FIG. 3.** Return to function in patients with nonspecific low back pain.

**TABLE 6.** *Risk factors for chronicity and disability in nonspecific low back pain*

| |
|---|
| Previous history of low back pain[a] |
| Total work loss (due to low back pain) in past 12 months |
| Radiating leg pain |
| Reduced straight leg raising[a] |
| Signs of nerve root involvement[a] |
| Reduced trunk muscle strength and endurance |
| Poor physical fitness |
| Self-rated health poor |
| Heavy smoking |
| Psychological distress and depressive symptoms[a] |
| Disproportionate illness behavior[a] |
| Low job satisfaction |
| Personal problems—alcohol, marital, financial |
| Adversarial medicolegal proceedings |

[a]Strong scientific evidence for delayed recovery and return to work within 4 weeks of onset of nonspecific low back pain.
Adapted from ref. 4.

Ways of identifying "red flags" that signal serious spinal conditions such as fracture, tumor, infection, or caudal equine syndrome were identified. The guidelines recommended against special studies in the absence of red flags and outlined a focused medical history and physical examination that provides the necessary information. Five algorithms are provided and include the initial evaluation of acute low back pain, the treatment of acute low back problems on initial and follow-up visits, evaluation of the slow-to-recover patient (symptoms >4 weeks), surgical considerations for patients with persistent sciatica, and further management of acute low back problems (Figs. 1 and 2).

The Clinical Guidelines for the Management of Acute Low Back Pain supported by the Royal College of Practitioners in Great Britain provides an update of the AHCPR and the "Back Pain in the Work Place" guidelines incorporating articles published as recently as April 1996 (4). New findings include even stronger support for early resumption of normal activities and greater emphasis on psychosocial factors and risk factors for chronicity (Fig. 3). The latter two findings are shown in Tables 5 and 6.

**TABLE 5.** *Biopsychosocial assessment*

| | | |
|---|---|---|
| Biomedical | | |
| | Review diagnostic triage | |
| | | Nerve root problem |
| | | Serious spinal pathology |
| | Erythrocyte sedimentation rate and plain x-ray | |
| Psychological | | |
| | Attitudes and beliefs about back pain | |
| | | Fear avoidance beliefs about activity and work |
| | | Personal responsibility for pain and rehabilitation |
| | Psychological distress and depressive symptoms | |
| | Illness behavior | |
| Social | | |
| | Family | |
| | | Attitudes and beliefs about the problem |
| | | Reinforcement of disability behavior |
| | Work | |
| | | Physical demands of job |
| | | Job satisfaction |
| | | Other health problems causing time off or job loss |
| | Nonhealth problems causing time off or job loss | |

From ref. 4.

## SUMMARY

Nonspecific low back pain (NSLBP) is a common complaint among adults. Although the prognosis is excellent, NSLBP results in significant use of health care resources as patients seek to relieve pain and distress. This chapter defines the phases of NSLBP and describes factors associated with its onset and progression. Treatment outcomes and guidelines for care are also addressed. It is purported that a greater understanding of NSLBP and its influences will lead to quality care and a reduction in costs and suffering.

## ACKNOWLEDGMENT

This chapter was supported in part by Strategic Management Technology (SMT).

## REFERENCES

1. Spangfort EV. The lumbar disc herniation. *Acta Orthop Scand* 1972; 142:1–95.
2. Deyo RA, Diehl AK. Cancer as a cause of back pain: frequency, clinical presentation, and diagnostic strategies. *J Gen Intern Med* 1988; 3: 230–238.
3. Bigos S, Bowyer O, Braen G, et al. *Acute low back problems in adults. Clinical practice guidelines.* AHCPR Publication No 95-0643. Washington, DC: U.S. Department of Health and Human Services, Public Health Service, Agency for Health Care Policy and Research, 1994.
4. Waddell G, Feder G, McIntosh A, et al. *Low back pain evidence review.* London: Royal College of General Practitioners, 1996;1–35.

5. Spitzer WO, LeBlanc FE, Dupuis M, et al. Scientific approach to the assessment and management of activity related spinal disorders: A monograph for clinicians. Report of the Quebec Task Force on Spinal Disorders. *Spine* 1987;12:S1–S59.
6. Kelsey JL, Mundt DJ, Golden AL. Epidemiology of low back pain. In: Jayson MIV, Dixon AJ, eds. *The lumbar spin and back pain,* 4th ed. London: Churchill Livingstone, 1992;537–550.
7. Abenhaim L, Rossignol M, Gobeille D, et al. The prognostic consequences in the making of the initial medical diagnosis of work-related back injuries. *Spine* 1995;20:791–795.
8. Weber H. Lumbar disc herniation: A controlled prospective study with ten years of observation. *Spine* 1983;8:131–140.
9. Riihimaki H, Wickstrom G, Hanninnen K, et al. Predictors of sciatica pain among concrete reinforcement workers and house painters: A five-year follow up. *Scand J Work Environ Health* 1989;15:415–423.
10. Frymoyer JW, Cats-Baril WL. An overview of the incidences and costs of low back pain (review). *Orthop Clin North Am* 1991;22:263–271.
11. Hanley E. Surgical outcomes for herniated lumbar discs. In: Weinstein JN, Gordon SL, eds. *Low back pain. a scientific and clinical overview.* Rosemont, IL: American Academy of Orthopaedic Surgeons (AAOS), 1996;113–124.
12. van Doorn JWC. Low back disability among self-employed dentists, veterinarians, physicians and physical therapists in the Netherlands. A retrospective study over a 13-year period (N = 1, 119) and an early intervention program with 1-year follow-up (N = 134). *Acta Orthop Scand* 1995;263:1–66.
13. Nordin M, Andersson GBJ, Pope MH. *Musculoskeletal disorders at work:* principles and practice. Philadelphia: Mosby Yearbook, 1997; 253–316.
14. Merskey H, Bogduk N. *Classification of chronic pain:* descriptions of chronic pain syndromes and definitions of terms. International Association of Pain. Seattle, WA: IASP Press, 1994.
15. Nordin M, Skovron ML, Heibert R, et al. Early predictors of delayed return to work in patients with low back pain. *J Musculoskel Pain* 1997;5:5–27.
16. McGill CM. Industrial back problems: A control program. *J Occup Med* 1968;10:174–178.
17. Nachemson A. Work for all: for those with low back pain as well. *Clin Orthop* 1983;179:77–85.
18. Waddell G. Understanding the patient with back pain. In: Jayson M, ed. *The lumbar spine and back pain,* 4th ed. Edinburgh: Churchill Livingstone, 1992;469–485.
19. Waddel G. A new clinical model for the treatment of low-back pain. *Spine* 1987;12:632–644.
20. Andersson GBJ, Pope MH, Frymoyer JW, et al. Epidemiology and cost. In: Pope MH, Andersson JGB, Chaffin BD, Frymoyer JW, eds. *Occupational low back pain:* assessment, *treatment and prevention.* St. Lous: Mosby-Year Book, 1991;95–116.
21. Frymoyer JW, Andersson GBJ. Clinical Classification. In: Pope MH, Andersson JGB, Chaffin BD, Frymoyer JW, eds. *Occupational low back pain:* assessment, *treatment and prevention.* St. Lous: Mosby-Year Book, 1991;44–70.
22. Praemer A, Furner S, Rice DP. *Musculoskeletal conditions in the United States.* Park Ridge, IL: American Academy of Orthopaedic Surgeons (AAOS), 1992;3–19.
23. Frymoyer JW, Pope MH, Costanza MC. Epidemiologic studies of low back pain. *Spine* 1980;5:419–425.
24. Andersson GBJ. The epidemiology of spinal disorders. In: Frymoyer JW, ed. *The adult spine:* principles and practice. Philadelphia: Lippincott-Raven, 1997;93–142.
25. Deyo RA, Tsui-Wu Y-J. Descriptive epidemiology of low back pain and its related medical care in the United States. *Spine* 1987;14:501–506.
26. Cypress BK. Characteristics of physician visits for back symptoms: a national perspective. *Am J Public Health* 1983;73:389–395.
26a. Spengler DM, Bigos SJ, Martin NA. Back injuries in industry: a retrospective study. I. Overview and cost analysis. *Spine* 1986;11:241–245.
27. Kelsey JL. Idiopathic low back pain: magnitude of the problem. In: White AA, Gordon SL, eda. *American Academy of Orthopaedic Surgeons Symposium on idiopathic low back pain.* St Louis: CV Mosby, 1992;5–8.
28. Skovron ML. Epidemiology of low back pain. In: Nordin MN, Vischer TL, eds. *Bailliere's clinical rheumatology practice and research, common low back pain:* prevention of chronicity. London: Bailliere, Tindall, 1992;559–574.
29. Guo HR, Tanaka S, Cameron LL, et al. Back pain among workers in the United States: national estimates and workers at high risk. *Am J Ind Med* 1995;28:591–602.
30. Frymoyer JW, Pope MH, Clements JH, et al. Risk factors in low back pain. An epidemiological survey. *J Bone Joint Surg* 1983;65:213–218.
31. Punnett L, Fine LJ, Keyserling WM, et al. Back disorders and nonneutral trunk postures of automobile assembly workers. *Scand J Work Environ Health* 1991;17:337–346.
32. Keyserling WM, Herrin GD, Chaffin DB. Isometric strength testing as a means of controlling medical incidents on strenuous jobs. *J Occup Med* 1980;22:332–336.
33. Andersson GBJ, Svensson HO, Oden A. The intensity of work recovery in low back pain. *Spine* 1983;8:880–884.
34. Bongers PM, de Winter CR, Kompier MA, et al. Psychosocial factors at work and musculoskeletal diseases. *Scand J Work Environ Health* 1993;19:297–312.
35. Bigos S, Battie M, Spengler D. A prospective study of work perceptions and psychosocial factors affecting the report of back injury. *Spine* 1991;16:1–6.
36. Linton SJ, Warg LE. Attributions (beliefs) and job satisfaction associated with back pain in an industrial setting. *Percept Motor Skills* 1993; 76:51–61.
37. Ready AE, Boreskie SI, Law SA, et al. Fitness and lifestyle parameters fail to predict back injury in nurses. *Can J Appl Phys* 1993;18:80–90.
38. Houtman IL, Bongers PM, Smulders PG. Psychosocial stressors at work and musculoskeletal problems. *Scand J Work Environ Health* 1994;20:139–145.
39. Lehto TU, Helenius HY, Alaranta HT. Musculoskeletal symptoms of dentists assessed by a multidisciplinary approach. *Community Dent Oral Epidemiol* 1991;91:38–44.
40. Eskelinen L, Toikkanen J, Tuomi K, et al. Work-related stress symptoms of aging employees in municipal occupations. *Scand J Work Environ Health* 1991;17:87–93.
41. Pickett CW, Lees RE. A cross-sectional study of health complaints among 79 data entry operators using video display terminals. *J Soc Occup Med* 1991;41:113–116.
42. Lancourt J, Kettelbut M. Predicting RTW for lower back patients receiving worker's compensation. *Spine* 1992;17:629–640.
43. Feuerstein M, Thebarge RW. Perceptions of disability and occupational stress as discriminators of work disability in patients with chronic pain. *J Occup Rehabil* 1991;1:185–195.
44. Skov T, Borg V, Orhede E. Psychosocial and physical risk factors for musculoskeletal disorders of the neck, shoulder and lower back in salespeople. *Occup Environ Med* 1996;53:352–356.
45. Leino P, Lyyra A. The effects of mental stress and social support on the development of musculoskeletal morbidity in the engineering industry. In: Sakurai H, Okazaki T, Kazuyuki O, eds. *Occupational epidemiology.* Amsterdam: Elsevier Science, 1990;267–272.
46. Leino P, Hanninen V. Psychosocial factors and work in relation to back and limb disorders. *Scand J Work Environ Health* 1995;21:134–142.
47. Fordyce W, ed. *Back pain in the workplace:* management of disability in nonspecific conditions. Task Force on Pain in the Workplace. Seattle, WA: International Association for the Study of Pain (IASP) Press, 1995;25–42.
48. Cats-Baril W, Frymoyer J. Identifying patients at risk of becoming disabled because of low back pain. The Vermont Rehabilitation Engineering Center Predictive Model. *Spine* 1991;16:1168–1172.
49. Barnes D, Smith D, Gatchel R, et al. Psycho socioeconomic predictors of treatment success/failure in chronic low-back pain patients. *Spine* 1988;14:427–430.
50. Burns JW, Sherman ML, Devine J. Association between workers' compensation and outcome following multi-disciplinary treatment for chronic pain roles of mediators and moderators. *Clin J Pain* 1995;11: 94–102.
51. Steffy BD, Jones JW, Murphy LR, et al. A demonstration of the impact of stress abatement programs on reducing employees accidents and their costs. *Am J Health Promotion* 1988;fall:25–32.
52. Skovron MLS, Hiebert R, Crane M, Nordin M. Work restrictions and outcome of nonspecific low back pain. *Spine,* in press.
53. Kramer JS, Yelin EH, Epstein WV. Social and economic impacts of four musculoskeletal conditions. A study using national community-based data. *Ann Arthritis Rheum* 1983;26:901–907.
54. Carey TS, Garrett J, Jackman A, et al. The outcomes and costs of care for acute low back pain among patients seen by primary care practitioners, chiropractors and orthopedic surgeons. *N Engl J Med* 1995; 333:913–917.

55. Battie MC, Nordin M. Rehabilitation, education, and training. In: Weisel SW, Weinstein DO, Herkowitz HN, et al., eds. *The lumbar spine,* 2nd ed. Philadelphia: WB Saunders, 1996;989–997.
56. Nordin M, Weiser S, Halpern M. Education in the prevention and treatment of low back disorders. In: Frymoyer JW, ed. *The adult spine:* principles and practice. Philadelphia: Lippincott-Raven, 1997;209–222.
57. Weber M, Cedraschi C, Roux E, et al. A prospective controlled study of low back school in the general population. *Spine* 1996;35:178–183.
58. Cedraschi C, Reust P, Lorenzi-Cioldi F, et al. The gap between back pain patients' prior knowledge and scientific knowledge and its evolution after a back school teaching programme: a quantitative evaluation. *Patient Educ Counsel* 1996;27:235–246.
59. Jones SL, Jones PK, Katz J. Compliance for low-back pain patients in the emergency department. A randomized trial. *Spine* 1988;13: 553–556.
60. Cherkin DC, Deyo RA, Street JH, et al. Pitfalls of patient education: Limited success of a program for back pain primary care. *Spine* 1996; 21:345–355.
61. Wiesel M, Boden SD, Feffer HL. A quality-based protocol for management of musculoskeletal injuries a ten-year prospective outcome study. *Clin Orthop Rel Res* 1994;301:164–176.
62. Geyman JP, Gordon MJ. Learning outcomes and practice changes after a postgraduate course in orthopedics. *J Fam Pract* 1982;15: 131–136.
63. Ashbaugh DG, McKean RS. Continuing medical education: The philosophy and use of audit. *JAMA* 1976;236:1475–1488.
64. Harwood KJ, Nordin M, Hiebert R, et al. Low back pain assessment training of industry-based physicians. *J Rehabil Res Dev* 1997;34: 371–382.
65. Postacchini F, Facchini M, Palieri P. Efficacy of various forms of conservative treatment in low back pain. A comparative study. *Neuro-Orthopaedics* 1988;6:28–35.
66. Amlie E, Weber H, Holme I. Treatment of acute low-back pain with piroxicam: results of a double-blind placebo-controlled trial. *Spine* 1987;12:473–476.
67. Berry H, Bloom B, Hamilton EBD, et al. Naproxen sodium, diflunisal, and placebo in the treatment of chronic back pain. *Ann Rheum Dis* 1982;41:129–132.
68. Campello M, Nordin M, Weiser S. Physical exercise and low back pain: A review. *Scand J Med Sci Sports* 1996;6:63–72.
69. Deyo RA, Diehl AK. How many days of bed rest for acute low back pain? A randomized clinical trial. *N Engl J Med* 1986;315: 1064–1070.
70. Malmivaara A, Hakkinen U, Aro H, et al. The treatment of acute low back pain: bed rest, exercises or ordinary activity? *N Engl J Med* 1995; 332:351–355.
71. Hadler NM, Curtis P, Gillings DB, et al. A benefit of spinal manipulation as adjunctive therapy for acute low-back pain: a stratified controlled trial. *Spine* 1987;12:703–706.
72. Shkelle PG, Adams AH, Chassin MR, et al. Spinal manipulation for low-back pain. *Ann Intern Med* 1992;117:590–598.
73. Waterworth RF, Hunter IA. An open study of diflunisal conservative and manipulative therapy in the management of acute mechanical low back pain. *N Z Med J* 1985;22:372–375.
74. Waddell G. Biopsychosocial analysis of low back pain. In: Nordin M, Vischer TL, eds. *Common low back pain:* prevention of chronicity. London: Bailliere, Tindall, 1992;523–556.
75. Weiser S. Psychosocial aspects of occupational musculoskeletal disorders. In: Nordin M, Andersson G, Pope MH, eds. *Musculoskeletal Disorders at work:* principles and practice. Philadelphia: Mosby, 1997;51–61.
76. Keefe FJ, Crisson J, Urban BJ, et al. Analyzing chronic low back pain: the relative contribution of pain coping strategies. *Pain* 1990;40:293–301.
77. Lacroix JM, Powell J, Lloyd GJ, et al. Low back pain. Factors of value in predicting outcome. *Spine* 1990;15:495–499.
78. Sandstrom J, Esbjornsson E. Return to work after rehabilitation. The significance of the patient's own prediction. *Scand J Rehabil* 1986; 18:29.
79. Turner J, Clancy S. Strategies for coping with chronic low back pain: Relationship to pain and disability. *Pain* 1986;24:355–364.
80. Turner J, Clancy S, Vialiano PP. Relationships of stress, appraisal and coping to chronic low back pain. *Behav Res Ther* 1987;25:281–288.
81. Spinhoven P, Linssen ACG. Behavorial treatment of chronic low back pain. I. Relation of copying strategy use to outcome. *Pain* 1991;45: 29–34.
82. Linton SJ, Althoff B, Melin L, et al. Psychological factors related to health, back pain and dysfunction. *J Occup Rehabil* 1994;4:3–10.
83. Deyo RA, Tsui-Wu Y-J. Functional disability due to back pain. *Ann Arthritis Rheumatol* 1987;30:1247–1253.
84. Polatin PB, Gatchel RJ, Barnes D, et al. A psychosociomedical prediction model of response to treatment by chronically disables workers with low-back pain. *Spine* 1989;14:956–961.
85. Lustman PJ, Velozo CA, Eubanks B, et al. Prior psychiatric problems in rehabilitation clients with work-related injuries. *J Occup Rehabil* 1991; 1:227–233.
86. Feyer AM, Williamson A, Mandryk de Silva I, et al. Role of psychosocial factors in work-related low back pain. *Scand J Work Environ Health* 1992;18:387–375.
87. Leino P, Magni G. Depressive and distress symptoms as predictors of low back pain, neck shoulder pain and other musculoskeletal morbidity: a 10-year follow-up of metal industry employees. *Pain* 1993;53: 89–94.
88. Main C, Watson P. What harm-pain behavior? Psychological and physical factors in the development of chronicity. *Hosp Joint Dis Bull* 1996; 55:213–216.
89. Flodmark B, Aase G. Musculoskeletal symptoms and type A behavior in blue collar workers. *Br J Ind Med* 1992;49:683–687.
90. Keefe F, Block A. Development of an observation method for assessing pain behavior in chronic low back pain patients. *Behav Ther* 1982;13: 363–375.
91. Zarkowska E, Philips HC. Recent onset vs persistent pain: evidence for distinction. *Pain* 1986;25:365–372.
92. Ohlund C, Lindstrom I, Areskoug B. Pain behavior in industrial subacute low back pain. Part I. Reliability, concurrent and predictive validity of pain behavior assessments. *Pain* 1994;58:201–209.
93. Greenough CG, Taylor LJ, Fraser RD. Anterior lumbar fusion: A comparison of noncompensation patients with compensation patients. *Clin Orthop Rel Res* 1994;300:30–37.
94. Stutts JT, Kasden M. Disability: A new psychological perspective. *J Occup Med* 1993;35:355–364.

*Environmental and Occupational Medicine, Third Edition,* edited by William N. Rom.
Published by Lippincott–Raven Publishers, Philadelphia, 1998.

CHAPTER 67

# Work-Related Disorders of the Neck and Upper Extremity

Lawrence J. Fine and Barbara A. Silverstein

The carpal tunnel syndrome (CTS) (1,2) is the best known of the common work-related disorders of the upper extremity. Other examples of these disorders that may be related to work include de Quervain's disease (3), epicondylitis (4), rotator (or rotor) cuff tendinitis (mainly supraspinatus) (5), and tension neck syndrome (6). This family of disorders may involve muscles (tension neck syndrome), tendons (supraspinatus tendinitis), joints (degenerative joint disease) (7), nerves (CTS), or blood vessels (hand arm vibration syndrome, or Raynaud's phenomenon of occupational origin) (8).

## MAGNITUDE AND COST OF THE PROBLEM

The largest data sources about the magnitude and the cost of this group of work-related musculoskeletal disorders is from the Bureau of Labor Statistics (BLS) Annual Survey of Occupational Injuries and Illnesses and from workers' compensation (WC) data sources. The Survey of Occupational Injuries and Illnesses is a federal/state program in which employer reports are collected from about 250,000 private industry establishments. The survey excludes the self-employed, farms with fewer than 11 employers, private households, and employees in all governmental agencies. The survey provides estimates of workplace injuries and illnesses based on records kept by private employers during the year (9). The survey is confidential and this may promote an accurate recording by the employer. A worker's or employer's decision to report may be influenced by personal, cultural, administrative, peer pressure, or economic factors (10). The accuracy of the survey depends on the interplay of these complex factors.

Each episode is classified into an illness or an injury. Illnesses or injuries that result in days away from work are classified on several factors: (a) the causal events or exposures such as falls or overexertion, (b) the nature of injury or illness such as sprains or strains or CTS, and (c) the source of injury or illness such as machinery or worker motion or position. Some of these categories likely represent illnesses and injuries due to physical stressors at work such as repetitive movements of the hands or lifting of objects. The BLS has two estimates for disorders or diseases and injuries related to repetitive job tasks. The first is disorders or diseases associated with repeated trauma, which are defined as illnesses due to repeated motion, vibration, or pressure such as CTS, noise-induced hearing loss, or tendinitis. This estimate includes cases involving lost time and those that only involve restriction of normal work activities or medical treatment but no lost time. For these disorders the BLS Annual Survey of Occupational Injuries and Illnesses reported that incidence rate of occupational illnesses and disorders associated with repeated trauma was 3.7 cases per 1,000 full-time workers in the private sector in 1995. There has been a steady increase from 1982, when the rate was 0.4 per 1,000, to 1994. In 1995 there were 308,000 workplace illnesses associated with repeated trauma, a decrease of 7% from 1994. Interestingly, in the

L. J. Fine: Division of Surveillance, Hazard Evaluations, and Field Studies, National Institute for Occupational Safety and Health, Centers for Disease Control and Prevention, Cincinnati, Ohio 45226–1998.
B. A. Silverstein: Safety and Health Assessment and Research for Prevention, Department of Labor and Industries, Olympia, Washington 98505.

same time period the rate for skin disorders has been more stable, from 0.67 in 1982 to 0.79 in 1995. While no precise information on the location of these illnesses by body part is available, limited analysis of the BLS data suggests that the most common site of these disorders and illnesses is the upper extremity followed by the lower extremity, since low back pain in the BLS system is usually recorded as an injury rather than a disorder or illness.

The second estimate, for disorders and injuries is derived only from cases that involve days away from work, is also based on the BLS Annual Survey of Occupational Injuries and Illnesses. All disorders and injuries involving lost time identified in the annual survey are classified based on the following question: What was the employee doing just before the incident occurred? Cases are classified as resulting from repetitive motion if they involve a bodily motion such as typing or key entry, repetitive use of tools, or repeated grasping of objects other than tools. Repetitive motion is one of the many narrowly defined categories that trained survey coders record based on the employer's response to the question about what the employee was doing prior to the injury or illness. Another event category that seems to be very relevant to estimating the number of work-related musculoskeletal disorders is overexertion, as in maneuvering especially heavy or bulky objects, such as health care patients or cartons of soft drinks. In 1994 the BLS survey reported about 92,000 (4% of the total of about 2,236,000) cases of disorders and injuries with lost time caused by repetitive motion primarily in the upper extremities (shoulder, hand, and wrist). This compared to 373,000 (17%) back cases caused by overexertion in lifting, pulling, pushing, and other activities. Overexertion of all types also caused 106,000 (5%) cases in the upper extremities. Of the wrist cases (110,232), 46% were due to repetitive motion. The annual survey also collects information on the nature of these lost-time cases. Out of total of about 2,240,000 cases in 1994, 38,000 were due to CTS. The annual survey also collects data on days away from work. For back pain cases the median is 6 days, and for carpal tunnel cases, 30 days. While these numbers do suggest that back injuries due to lifting and other manual handling activities are a larger problem than upper extremity disorders, upper extremities disorders and injuries due to overexertion or repetitive motion are approximately half as large as a problem.

From the workers' compensation data there is more information about the prevalence of CTS. In a medical-record–based study of the workers' compensation record study in the State of Washington, the rate of occupational CTS was 17 claims per 10,000 full-time workers during 1984 to 1988 (11). About a quarter of these claims also indicated that a CTS surgery had been done. More recent data from the Washington State Fund Workers' Compensation data (Fig. 1) indicate a 1993 incidence rate of 31.7 per 10,000 for CTS, 14.7 per 10,000 for epicondylitis, and 13.7 per 10,000 for rotator cuff syndrome (12). As indicated by the Washington State data, while varying by specific occupation, these disorders are probably overall less common than CTS. Besides noncontact ball sports (545 per 10,000 for epicondylitis and 1,417 per 10,000 for rotator cuff), the Washington industrial class (WIC) with the highest rate of epicondylitis was wallboard installation (105 per 10,000, 9.2 times the rate as overall industry), and for rotator cuff syndrome tree topping and pruning had the highest rate (149 per 10,000, 11.4 times the overall industry rate). In 1988, the Occupational Health Supplement to the annual National Health Interview Survey (NHIS) included questions on self-reported

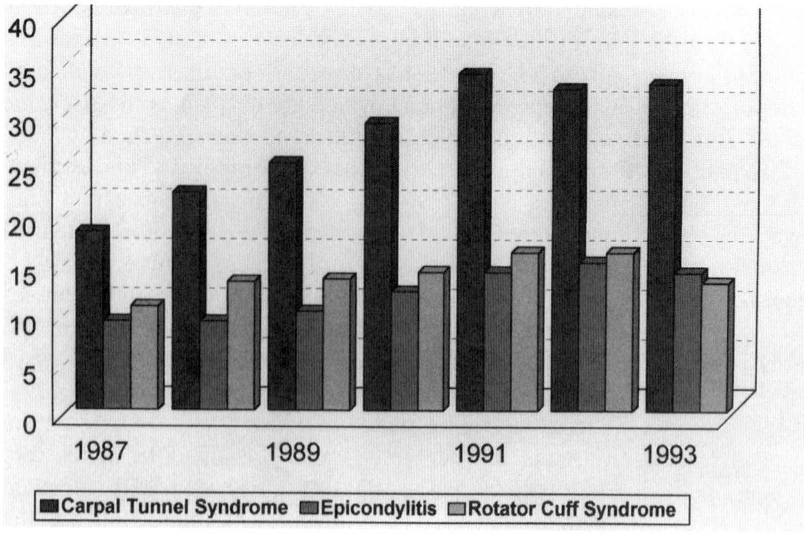


**FIG. 1.** Incidence rates of specific upper extremity conditions per 10,000 full-time equivalent workers. Washington State Fund, 1987–1993. Includes both lost time and medically accepted workers' compensation claims.

nonoccupational and occupational CTS and "prolonged" hand discomfort (20 days or more, or 7 or more consecutive days in the past 12 months). Approximately 8% of the active workers in the NHIS survey reported prolonged hand discomfort, and about 0.5% reported CTS that had been diagnosed by a medical person (13). Twenty percent of the workers with CTS had missed work as a result of their condition, compared to 6% of those with prolonged hand discomfort. Epidemiologic studies of workers in specific high-risk industries typically find that CTS cases consist of only a minority of all of the cases of upper extremity disorders noted in the surveys (14,15). From a national perspective, while the precise prevalence of work-related musculoskeletal disorders of the upper extremity is unknown, these disorders are among the most common occupational disorders, although possibly not as common as work-related low back disorders. Typical prevalence rates for CTS in workplaces with an average level of risk should be less than 1%.

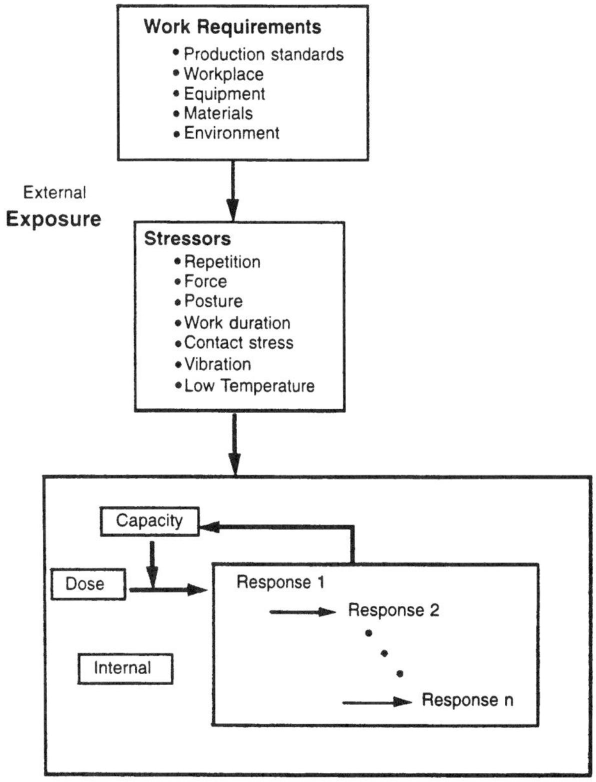


**FIG. 2.** Schematic representation of pathophysiology of work-related disorders of the upper extremity and neck. (Adapted with permission from ref. 10.)

## PATHOPHYSIOLOGY AND WORK EXPOSURES

Clinical, laboratory, and epidemiologic studies all have contributed to the current understanding of the pathophysiology of work-related musculoskeletal disorders of the upper extremity and neck. In these disorders work and nonwork factors can be important. The pathophysiologic mechanisms may also be similar both in cases where occupational exposure is important and in those where it is not important.

A model has been developed to incorporate both physical and psychosocial factors in the development of work-related musculoskeletal disorders (Fig. 2) (16). Exposures may be either physical work factors or psychosocial factors. Exposure to work factors results in a specific level of force or other disturbance on specific tissues of the upper extremity. This is called the dose. The tissue response to a specific dose is moderated by the tissue resistance to change—the capacity. Capacity could be either physiologically defined, such as strength of a specific tendon, or psychologically defined, such as the level of self-esteem. The internal changes or effects resulting from a specific dose may occur in a tendon or in the muscles of the forearm. We first discuss the physical work factors and then the proposed pathophysiology of these exposures.

Several occupational factors are important in the etiology of these disorders: repetitive motions, forceful motions, localized mechanical or contact stresses, static or awkward postures, and local vibration (Fig. 2).

Repetitive motions of the hands, wrists, shoulders, and neck commonly occur in the workplace. A data entry operator may perform 20,000 keystrokes per hour, a worker in a meat-processing plant may perform 12,000 cuts with a knife per day, and a worker on an assembly line may elevate the right shoulder above the level of the acromion 7,500 times per day. These repetitive motions in an individual may eventually exceed the ability to recover from this level of physical stress, especially if forceful contractions of muscles are involved in the repetitive motions.

For CTS, a proposed model has been suggested related to repetitive forceful hand tasks. Forceful contraction of the flexor tendons of fingers can increase the pressure in the carpal tunnel to moderately elevated levels (17). This increased pressure, if chronic, may limit microvascular flow in the median nerve, which in turn leads to tissue swelling and epineural edema. Eventually after several years epineurial fibrosis may result. Histologic studies of flexor tendon sheaths sampled during carpal tunnel surgery support the above model because vascular changes consistent with ischemia and tissue edema are commonly observed. Inflammation is usually not found (17). In lateral epicondylitis (tennis elbow) forceful and repetitive hand and wrist movements such as wrist extension and pronation are associated with the onset of the syndrome. These activities occur in sports, work, or performing arts activities (18). Similarly to CTS acute inflammation is not a histologic hallmark; rather, the pattern has been called angiofibrolastic tendinosis and is likely the result of a degenerative and avascular process. The insertion of extensor carpi radialis brevis is the most common location of this process in lateral epicondylitis. The precise steps in the development of angiofibrolastic tendinosis are not known, but have been described as the result of microruptures of the tendon or intermittent ischemic process from repetitive forceful activity. Middle-aged workers are likely at the greatest risk (18). The pathophysiology of CTS and lateral epicondylitis therefore may have a common element of forceful repetitive activity triggering a chronic process in which disturbances in microvascular system lead to an ineffective or even harmful repair process or tissue response (Fig. 2). While much remains to be learned about the role of forceful repetitive work and the pathophysiologic changes that result from these activities, plausible models have been developed for CTS and epicondylitis.

De Quervain's disease and other tenosynovitis of the hand, wrist, and forearm have been associated for decades with repetitive and forceful hand activities as one of the possible causal factors (19). De Quervain's disease is the entrapment of the tendons of the extensor pollicis brevis and abductor pollicis longus. Other similar conditions are trigger thumb and triggering of the middle and ring fingers. These are characterized by pain with motion of the affected tendon. Despite the fact that the tendon and its sheath may be swollen and tender, the histopathology shows peritendinous fibrosis without inflammation, and fibrocartilaginous metaplasia of the tendon sheath tissue. The role of inflammation early in the process is not clear (20). As with CTS or epicondylitis, acute classical inflammation does not seem a critical pathophysiologic component of the clinical condition, at least once it becomes chronic. Despite the observations that too much forceful and repetitive activity contributes to CTS and epicondylitis, the response of the tendons and the muscles to repetitive activity is likely that of a U-shaped curve. Too little and too much activity may be harmful, but intermediate levels of activity are probably beneficial. The studies of tendon and muscle physiology suggest that certain amounts of activity maintain the normal state of these tissues and lead to adaptive changes. These tissues have the definite ability to repair significant amounts of damage from some overuse. The poorly understood issue is when the overuse exceeds the ability of the tissue to repair the damage or triggers a qualitatively more harmful type of damage (20).

An important, but inadequately investigated, question is whether the repetitive stresses to the joints of upper limbs that occur in some occupations lead to the accelerated development of localized osteoarthrosis (LOA). Since LOA is not a specific disease but the final common pathway of biomechanical and pathologic changes in cartilage, subchondral bone, and bone-surrounding joints, prolonged and very repetitive and forceful stresses may accelerate its development (7,19,21).

In addition to repetitive and forceful motions, three other exposure variables that influence the development of work-related musculoskeletal disorders are external mechanical or contact stress, work performed in awkward or static postures, and segmental (localized) vibration. The use of poor-fitting gloves and exposure to cold temperatures increase hand-force requirements because of decreased sensory feedback to the fingers and due to working against the glove in order to grip tightly.

Mechanical or contact stress to nerves or other soft tissues can occur when they come into contact with structures harder than themselves, particularly external hard or sharp objects. These stresses can lead to nerve compression (3). Examples include (a) a digital neuritis associated with the edge of scissors handles or bowling ball holes coming into forceful contact with the sides of the fingers or thumb, and (b) cubital tunnel syndrome in a microscopist who must position the elbow on a hard surface for long periods. Short-handled tools that dig into the base of the palm exert as much force on the hand, particularly the superficial branches of the median nerve, as the hand does on the tool. Squeezing wire cutters with a handle pressing into the palm of the hand will be more physically stressful than resting the palm on the edge of a sharp work surface.

Work performed in awkward or static postures is another important influence on the development of work-related musculoskeletal disorders. Posture plays an important role in rotator cuff tendinitis of the shoulder. The level of mechanical stress produced by a muscle contraction varies with the posture of a joint. For example, it is believed that contraction of the finger flexors is more stressful if the wrist is flexed. Work with the arm elevated more than 60 degrees from the trunk is more stressful for the supraspinatus than work performed with the arm at the trunk. As the arm is raised or abducted the supraspinatus tendon becomes in contact with the undersurface of the acromion. They are in closest proximity between 60 and 120 degrees of arm elevation (19). The precise pathophysiology of work-related rotator cuff tendinitis is unknown. However, the role of overhead work, particularly of a static nature or very forceful exertions like those in activities such as swimming, is likely a crucial event (22,23). Impingement seems important. One suggested histologic pattern is a reversible inflammatory infiltrate, with increased vascularity and edema within the rotator cuff tendons, especially the supraspinatus tendon. This process, if it becomes chronic, has been postulated as leading to degenerative changes in the tendons. This chronic process may not produce enough pain to severely limit movement; however, eventually enough degeneration occurs that a minor trauma causes or seems to cause a partial rotator cuff tear. Since these tears are more common in older individuals regardless of their occupation, aging itself also increases the risk of rotator cuff tears (23). When evaluating individual cases, separating out the roles of work and age may be difficult.

Exposure to segmental or localized vibration from power tool use is another risk factor. Segmental vibration is not only a cause of hand-arm vibration syndrome but also may increase the risk of CTS (24). Segmental vibration is transmitted to the upper extremity from impact tools, power tools, and bench-mounted buffers and grinders. The mechanism by which localized vibration from power tools contribute to the development of work-related Raynaud's phenomenon and changes in digital nerves of the fingers is not clear. Nevertheless, it has been associated with several types of power tools, such as chain saws, rock drillers, chipping hammers, and grinding tools (25).

The adverse chronic effect of repetition and other risk factors on muscles is not as well understood as on tendons. Chronic or intermittent pain from muscles may be important in several disorders including tension neck syndrome (scapulocostal syndrome) and overuse injuries in musicians (26,27). These syndromes are often characterized by diffuse tenderness over the muscle, rather than the tendon origin, and activity limitation. While discomfort of all types in the upper extremity is common among office workers, symptoms that are severe enough to cause work limitation or days away from work are less common. For example, in a study of newspaper personnel, 40% of the employees reported at least moderate discomfort in the neck or upper extremity, while 13% reported seeing a health care provider for their complaint, 6% reported missing at least one workday because of their complaints, and 3% reported being assigned to a different job for one or more workdays because of their symptoms (28). The pathophysiology is unknown for the limited number of severe cases; however, a number of mechanisms have been proposed, including chronic inflammation (18). Two types of muscle activity may be important in work-related disorders: low-force, prolonged muscle contractions [moderate neck flexion while working on a video display terminal (VDT) for many hours without rest breaks]; and infrequent or frequent high-force muscle contractions (intermittent use of heavy tools in overhead work). Sustained static contractions can lead to increases in intramuscular pressure, which in turn may impair blood flow to cells within the muscle.

Motor nerve control of the working muscle may be important in sustained static contractions since even if the relative load on the muscle as a whole is low, the active part of the muscle can be working close to its maximal capacity. Thus, small areas of large muscles such as the trapezius may have disturbances in microcirculation that might contribute to or cause the development of muscle damage (red ragged fibers), reduce strength, higher levels of fatigue, sensitization of pain receptors in the muscle, and pain at rest (3,10). High levels of tension (strong contractions) can lead to muscle fiber Z-line rupture, muscle pain, and large, delayed increases in serum creatine kinase. These changes are reversible and can be completely repaired, often leading the muscle to be stronger. It is hypothesized that if damage occurs daily due to work activity, the muscle may not be able to repair the damage as fast as it occurs, leading to chronic muscle damage or dysfunction. The mechanism of this damage at the cellular level is not understood (10). Work activities that lead to sustained relative low-level muscle activity or higher-level muscular contractions may be a causal factor in some work-related musculoskeletal disorders. It is not clear whether models that have been developed from studies of blue-collar workers are readily applicable to the office setting, where the relative importance of physical and work organization or psychosocial factors may differ substantially.

In addition to occupational risk factors or exposures such as repetitive work, personal risk factors may influence the development of these work-related disorders. Some occupational factors such as forceful repetitive activities and the wrist extension that occurs in some recreational activities can cause the development of similar disorders. One of the differences between occupational and recreational exposures is control over the duration of exposure. Personal risk factors, such as age, gender, obesity, peak muscle strength, and the size of the carpal tunnel, may contribute to the development of some work-related disorders. For two specific disorders—rotator cuff tendinitis and epicondylitis—two important nonwork factors are age and nonoccupational repetitive or forceful activities such as tennis, performing arts, or baseball pitching (23). The nonoccupational factors for CTS that have been most thoroughly studied include coexisting medical conditions such as rheumatoid arthritis, diabetes mellitus, pregnancy, and acute trauma especially after Colles' fracture (29). Four additional possible nonoccupational risk factors are carpal tunnel size or shape, age, obesity, and gender. The evidence is stronger for age, obesity, and gender. For CTS, there is an increasing risk with age up to approximately 50 (30). In both men and women the risk for occupationally related CTS may occur earlier (10).

While most clinical- or community-based studies report a female-to-male ratio of about 3:1, studies from workplaces do not consistently report a higher risk for women in those jobs in which the proportion of men and women is approximately equal. In a study of occupational CTS in Washington State based on the workers' compensation system, female/male gender ratio was 1.2:1 (10). In one analysis of a large interview study, the following were statistically significant predictors of a medical history of CTS: bending-twisting wrist at work [odds ratio (OR) 5.9], use of a vibration tool (OR 1.85), female gender (OR 2.44), obesity (OR 2.07), cigarette use (OR 1.58), and higher income (OR 1.54). In this survey based on small numbers, nonwhite participants had a lower rate of CTS (30). Carpal canal size, both small and large, has been proposed as a risk factor based on a limited evidence (14). There is also some evidence that cigarette smoking is associated with a high rate of CTS. Few if any personal factors are strong predictors of susceptibility to work-related disorders of the upper extremity. Multiple factors are related to the development of CTS; where the exposures to forceful and repetitive work are substantial, there is strong evidence of a definite role for occupational exposures. From a community perspective, nonoccupational factors are also important.

In addition to the physical factors, psychosocial factors may be important in both the initial development of work-related musculoskeletal disorders and the subsequent long-term disability that sometimes occurs. Few studies have rigorously investigated both the psychosocial and physical factors, and their combined effects (28,31). Psychosocial factors are broadly defined; as they relate to musculoskeletal disorders, they may range from personality factors (psychological) to the way in which work is organized (social). The psychosocial factors that seem most likely to be related to musculoskeletal disorders are monotonous work, perceived high work load, time pressure, and low control and social support (32). The effects of psychosocial factors may be indirect by altering muscle tension or other physiologic processes (Fig. 3) (32). In a similar manner, psychosocial factors may influence, through physiologic mechanisms, the perception of pain. Psychosocial factors, including psychological factors, may be particularly important in determining if specific musculoskeletal disorders will evolve into chronic pain syndromes (33). In a study of the industry newspaper, the National Institute for Occupational Safety and Health (NIOSH) suggested three possible explanations for this association: (a) psychosocial demands and job stress may increase muscle tension, which may exacerbate task-related biomechanical strain; (b) psychosocial demands may affect an individual's perception and willingness to report symptoms, and affect perceptions of their cause; (c) a causal relationship exists between psychosocial and physical workload demands (28). This model is most applicable to office workers (34). Psychosocial factors appear overall to be more important in disorders of the neck/shoulder muscles than in tendon-related disorders of the forearm and the hand.

In addition to the model shown in Fig. 3, studies that have addressed psychosocial factors have often used the demand-control-support model originally introduced by Karasek and Theorell (35). In this model, high levels of psychological job demand, in an occupational setting where the worker has little ability to decide what to do and how to do a particular job task and little opportunity to use or develop job skills, may contribute to the development of work-related musculoskeletal disorders. These adverse effects are hypothesized to occur more frequently in a work environment where there is little social support from co-workers or supervisors. Similarly, nonoccupational psychosocial factors could also be important. Social and economic factors may contribute to long disability. For example, Cheadle et al. (36) used workers' compensation data to identify predictors of disability of greater than 2 months' duration. They found that female gender, age older than 45, low paying work, employment in small companies, and residing in counties with high unemployment were factors associated with an elevated risk of disability (36). Further studies are needed to better understand the complex interrelationships between physical and psychosocial occupational factors. However, where the level of exposure to several physical factors is high, the role of psychosocial factors may not be important in the initial development of these work-related musculoskeletal disorders.

In summary, excessive repetitive and forceful motions, high levels of mechanical stress, work in static or awkward postures, and the use of vibrating power tools singularly or more frequently in combination likely cause a

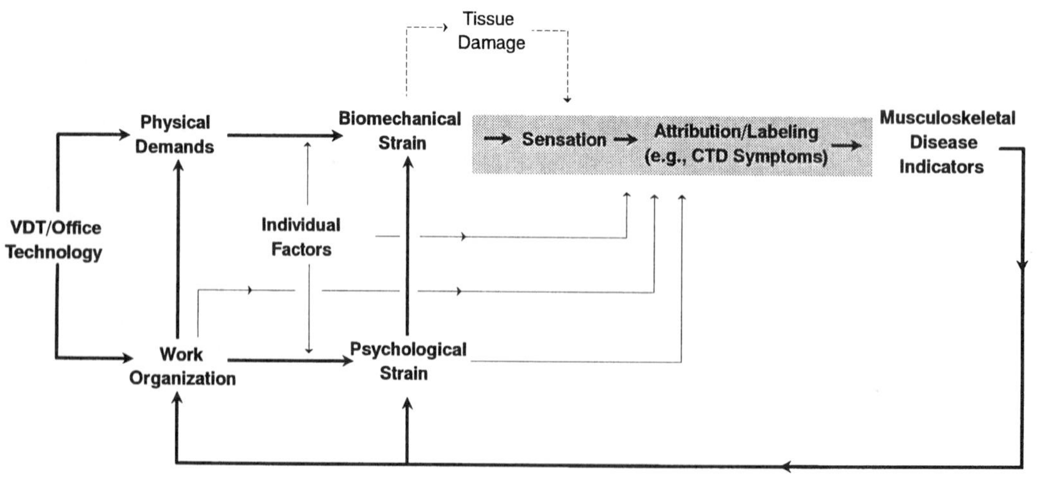


**FIG. 3.** An ecological model of musculoskeletal disorders in VDT work. (From ref. 43.)

variety of tissue responses such as increased pressure in the carpal tunnel. These tissue responses in turn contribute to the development of CTS, epicondylitis, and rotator cuff tendinitis. All of these syndromes also have been associated with one or more nonoccupational factors that also influence the magnitude of the risk with occupational exposure. Precise dose-response relationships have not been developed for the occupational risk factors. The precise role of the occupational and nonoccupational psychosocial factors needs to be further elucidated. The current level of knowledge about high exposure to physical occupational factors is incomplete, but it nevertheless guides both treatment and preventive strategies. When the exposure to several physical factors is high, then the risk of these disorders is substantially increased. The frequency, intensity, and duration of exposure are important parameters to consider in assessing the risk of musculoskeletal disorders. When the level of exposure to physical factors is more moderate, the overall level of risk may appear to be more dependent on the combination of personal attributes and physical and psychosocial factors.

## DIAGNOSIS

Work-related disorders of the neck and upper extremity have a diverse set of symptoms and physical findings. The evaluation of a patient for a suspected work-related disorder should have two major components: history of the present illness and physical examination of the upper extremity and the neck (1). The history of the present illness should fully characterize the symptoms by determining the location, radiation exposure, duration, evolution, and exacerbating factors. Employees' description of their work activities is useful. They should describe the nature of their specific work tasks by risk factors (forceful exertions, repetitive activities, and other adverse exposure). For example, a worker who for 8 hours a day uses a vibrating hand tool during a repetitive task that is repeated every 30 seconds may be at high risk for CTS. Similarly, a repetitive job that requires the arms to be elevated overhead during most of the work shift may increase the risk of a rotator cuff tendinitis. Because specific job tasks can vary within even a high-risk occupation, a careful history of specific job tasks is important. An important clue is the evidence of a lack of variety in motion/force patterns.

When a worker who has been performing the same job for a considerable time develops a disorder, the history should be directed not only at the chronic stable exposures but also at the acute factors. For example, if the worker uses a power screw driver, perhaps the symptoms started with screws from a bad batch that required more force to properly insert. Another common acute risk factor is overtime, either by lengthening the normal workday or by decreasing the number of days off that provide an opportunity for recovery from fatigue and occult injury.

Description of work tasks may not be accurate in some cases despite the conscientious efforts of the employee and careful interviewing by the physician. Direct observation or review of videotapes of the work process provides the most accurate description of the risk factors associated with specific job tasks. In addition to visiting the workplace, written descriptions of job tasks based on industrial engineering data and the results of ergonomic job analyses are additional ways of gathering information on exposure. While direct observation of the work is often required to determine with precision the level of risk-factor exposure in specific job tasks, descriptions by workers may identify many high-risk exposures with sufficient accuracy for a correct diagnosis.

Also to be considered from the history are possible precipitating factors such as changes in work pace or duration (e.g., longer or more frequent overtime). Determining predisposing medical conditions, such as prior injuries to the symptomatic area, is also important. Nonoccupational exposure to risk factors can be a potential confounding influence and should be elicited during the history interview. For nonoccupational activities to be significant causal factors, they should be similar in intensity and frequency to the known occupational exposures.

Surveillance and epidemiologic studies have identified several industries and occupations associated with risks of CTS or other work-related musculoskeletal disorders. This information can be useful in the diagnostic process by alerting physicians to the industries and occupations where adverse exposures are more common. A few illustrative industries or occupations are listed in Table 1.

Clinical experience, surveillance, and epidemiologic research suggest that many jobs with substantial exposure may adversely affect closely related muscles, tendons, or joints at the same time. As a result, workers in these high-risk jobs may present with one of several disorders such as CTS or de Quervain's disease.

In addition to the history, the physical examination can contribute useful information. An examination of the upper extremity typically involves inspection, palpation, assessment of the range of motion, evaluation of peripheral nerve function, and applicable provocative maneuvers of the upper extremity. One of the main objectives of the history and physical is to determine the precise structures in the upper extremity that are the anatomical source of the symptoms. Numbness and paresthesias often result from peripheral nerve compression. Increased pain on resisted movements such as resisted wrist extension often involves inflammation of a tendon such as the extensor carpi radialis brevis (tennis elbow). In some cases it is not possible to determine the precise source of the pain in the upper extremity, while in other cases it should be possible to determine the specific disorder, such as CTS or cubital tunnel syndrome. Cubital tunnel syndrome involves compression of the ulnar nerve out or near the medial side of the elbow. Symptoms are

**TABLE 1.** *Illustrative examples of industries and occupations with high-risk job tasks*

| Industries/occupations | Disorders |
|---|---|
| Seafood packing | Carpal tunnel syndrome (CTS) |
| Carpentry | CTS |
| Metal platers | CTS |
| Invasive cardiologists (removal of intraaortic balloon) | CTS |
| Dentists | Cervical spondylosis/degenerative changes |
| Rockblaster | Shoulder tendinitis |
| Data entry operators | Tension neck syndrome |
| Instrumental musicians | Focal dystonias and other conditions (overuse syndromes) |
| Knit underwear mills | Variety of conditions associated with repetitive motion |
| Men's and boys suits and coats | Variety of conditions associated with repetitive motion |
| Meat packing plants | Variety of conditions associated with repetitive motion |
| Poultry slaughtering and processing | Variety of conditions |
| Motor vehicles and car bodies | Variety of conditions |
| Household laundry equipment | Variety of conditions |
| Sausages and other prepared meats | Variety of conditions |
| Automotive stampings | Variety of conditions |
| Motorcycles, bicycles, and parts | Variety of conditions |

numbness and paresthesias in the small and ring finger, with abnormalities on electrodiagnostic studies of the ulnar nerve.

The severity of these disorders ranges from very mild with no significant impairment of the ability to work to severe. The physical examination is an important part of the patient evaluation with work-related musculoskeletal disorders. In addition to the disorders with specific physical findings on physical examination, workers in certain occupations (for example, keyboard operators, musicians, and newspaper reporters) often have an elevated rate of complaints of pain in the upper extremity or neck. These symptoms are similar to low back pain because a specific anatomic source of this pain often cannot readily be identified on clinical evaluation. As discussed earlier, many of these are hypothesized as involving muscle abnormalities. As with low back pain, these symptoms are common, often intermittent in nature, and sometimes lead to substantial disability and impairment (26–28).

A number of state workers' compensation programs have developed guidelines for the diagnosis and treatment of occupational CTS. For example, Washington State requires electrodiagnostic testing only when (a) the attending physician's diagnosis is occupational CTS, but the clinical criteria (appropriate neurologic symptoms and/or signs) are not met; (b) the patient has been on sick leave for CTS for more than 2 weeks and the clinical criteria are met; (c) carpal tunnel decompression surgery is requested. The diagnosis of a work-related musculoskeletal disorder is based on a three-step process. First is the determination of whether the patient has a specific disorder such as flexor tendinitis of the forearm. This is usually based on the history and physical examination. Particularly for distal neuropathies such as CTS, there is the unusual possibility of a entrapment of the nerve at two different levels such as at the wrist and cervical region. Second, there should be evidence, from direct or videotape observation of the workplace or from a detailed occupational history, of substantial exposure to specific occupational risk factors. Some employers, to facilitate return-to-work evaluations, now provide physicians with a videotape of the job that the worker normally performs. These may be useful for determining the level of exposure. Analysis of health surveillance data, such as Occupational Safety and Health Administration (OSHA) logs or workers' compensation records from the specific workplace, may be particularly helpful in confirming that a specific job is associated with an elevated risk of a work-related musculoskeletal disorder. Third, possible nonoccupational causes should be considered as possible primary causal factors or as extenuating factors based on the history and physical examination. Review and analysis of the surveillance and epidemiologic studies of similar work may provide information on the relative contribution of occupational factors compared to nonoccupational factors in the causation of a specific work-related musculoskeletal disorder in the patient's occupation and industry. With the exception of the use of electrodiagnostic tests for abnormalities in nerve conduction, elaborate diagnostic or laboratory studies are often not necessary unless there is a history of past trauma or clinical evidence suggestive of underlying systemic disease.

The most difficult part of the diagnosis of work-related musculoskeletal disorder is to determine the relative contribution of occupational factors to the etiology of the disorder. Table 2 gives an example of guidance for work-relatedness determination for CTS (35). As with other diagnostic evaluation of work-relatedness, the critical question is whether the exposure has been of sufficient intensity, frequency, and duration. Because intense periods of high exposure as short as weeks in duration can

**TABLE 2.** *Work-relatedness guideline for carpal tunnel syndrome.*

Any activity requiring extensive or continuous use of the hands in work is an appropriate exposure. In general, one of the following work conditions should be occurring on a regular basis:

1. Repetitive hand use, especially for prolonged periods (e.g., keyboard users), against force (e.g., meat cutters) or with awkward hand positions (e.g., grocery checkers) with repeated wrist flexion, extension, or deviation as well as forearm rotation, or with constant firm gripping.
2. The presence of regular, strong, vibrations (e.g., jack hammer, chain saw).
3. Regular or intermittent pressure on the wrist. (Note: acute CTS may be associated with acute trauma, e.g., fracture, crush injury of the wrist, etc.).

The types of jobs that are most frequently mentioned include meat cutting; seafood, fruit, or meat processing or canning; carpentry; roofing; dry walling; boat building; book binding; wood products work; dental hygienist; and intensive word processing.

From ref. 42.

rarely cause CTS or more commonly other work-related musculoskeletal disorders, attention should be directed at estimating the intensity and frequency of exposure. It is not uncommon for exposure to occur to multiple risk factors at the same time, such as repetitive and forceful exertions of the hands or shoulder abduction and exposure to vibration from hand tools. Unfortunately, there are no simple rules of how to assess whether exposure has been of sufficient intensity and frequency to cause a disorder. For example in one study of possible CTS cases referred for independent medical examinations, 60% were judged to be work-related CTS (35). This was based on using typical workers' compensation criteria and a standardized approach to assessing exposure using videotape or on-site inspection. Age, gender, duration of exposure, associated medical conditions, gynecologic conditions, and whether the CTS was unilateral or bilateral were not associated with work-relatedness. Fifteen percent of the cases did not have CTS but were found to have a different work-related disorders of the upper limb, such as localized muscle fatigue/myalgias, while an additional 21% had non–work-related disorders. This study demonstrates the absence of precise rules for determining work-relatedness, the need for thorough diagnostic evaluation to identify the specific disorder, and the need to assess exposure as carefully as possible.

## TREATMENT AND PROGNOSIS

The goals of treatment are elimination or reduction in symptoms and impairment, and returning the employee to work under conditions that will protect his or her health. These goals can be most easily achieved by early and conservative treatment. Treatment of work-related musculoskeletal disorders early in the course has several advantages. The treatment is less difficult and costly. Surgical procedures can be avoided, periods of absence from work or stressful exposures will be shorter, and the effectiveness of treatment is greater (37). The treatment is usually directed at two goals: to assist in the repair of any tissue damage and to reduce nerve compression. Symptomatic relief is provided by (1) the use of anti-inflammatory medications, more for their analgesic than their inflammatory properties; (2) reduced activity (sometimes facilitated by splints); and (3) application of heat or cold. Physical therapy techniques are helpful to assist in symptom relief, to ensure normal joint motion (stretching), and to recondition muscles after periods of rest or reduced use. If these more conservative measures fail to reduce symptoms and impairment for some conditions such as CTS, steroid injections or surgical treatments can be helpful. Surgery, for CTS or epicondylitis, may be ineffective if the worker is returned to his/her old job without an effort to reduce the occupational exposures that were present. Nevertheless, most individuals should be able to return to their work after CTS surgery with careful follow-up. Since only a few scientifically valid studies have evaluated the long-term effectiveness of the treatment of the work-related musculoskeletal disorders of the limb and neck, an empirical approach is indicated (38).

One needs to identify the work and nonwork activities that are the most stressful to the involved regions of the upper extremity and then to reduce these activities. Prolonged complete rest is rarely indicated. Generally within a week or two some level of activity is useful. Activity, for example, promotes tendon healing in epicondylitis. Rest of the symptomatic part of the upper extremity can be achieved by reducing or eliminating worker exposure to the known risk factors. In addition to engineering changes, restricted duty, job rotation, or temporary transfer may be effective. For job transfer or rotation to be effective, the new job duties have to result in a net reduction in the level of exposure. Conducting an evaluation of the new duties to determine if a reduction in exposure will occur is often necessary. One of the benefits of identifying ways to reduce the level of exposure for injured workers is that these same changes, if widely used, may prevent uninjured workers from developing problems or allow workers with minimal problems to continue to work. The magnitude of reduction in exposure required to facilitate recovery is often not known. In general, the more severe the disorder, the greater the reduction in magnitude and duration that will probably be required. One of the principal reasons to encourage early reporting of symptoms is the belief that earlier treatment requires less prolonged or drastic reduction in the level of activity or exposure. Because of its adverse consequences, complete removal from the work environment should be used only in severe cases or when less drastic measures have failed.

The recognition that comprehensive approaches that directly address all facets of the patient's situation may be more effective in returning the patient to work and reducing future impairment has led to the rapid development of comprehensive programs that ideally address the physical reconditioning of the worker, the psychosocial factors, and workplace factors such as ongoing exposure (38,39). Some researchers have developed models for rehabilitation of severe upper extremity cases based on the rehabilitation of low back pain and cardiac surgery (38).

## PREVENTIVE STRATEGY

Preventive strategy, largely experience-based, has not been comprehensively evaluated by scientific studies. However, a number of interventions have been studied (40). The principles outlined below must be adapted to fit the specific characteristics of each working environment. They should be viewed as only a guide, requiring ongoing scientific evaluation rather than a detailed blueprint.

Three standard preventive strategies might be considered: (a) a reduction of the exposure to suspected occupational risk factors such as vibrating hand tools, (b) a conditioning process that increases the tolerance of workers to the suspected occupational risk factors, or (c) development of a replacement process that is highly predictive and reliable in identifying those persons at usually high risk of developing an upper extremity disorder (1). Development of a replacement process is the least desirable of these strategies because (a) there are no scientifically valid screening procedures to identify those persons at high risk of developing CTS; and (b) this shifts the cost of reducing the incidence of symptoms to the workers, who are denied employment or placement, and increases the cost of the hiring and replacement processes (41).

For those persons in forceful action or repetitive-action jobs, the second approach, creating a period of time during which workers can gradually adapt their muscles and tendons to the new demands on them, could be useful. Training of new workers in the most efficient and least stressful way of performing their jobs may be useful, provided that the work tasks can be done in alternate ways, which are both less stressful and at least as fast. Similarly, workers with symptoms may, with training, be able to adapt an equally efficient, but less stressful, work method. Training activities have not been evaluated specifically. Several employers, perceiving long-term benefits in the "phasing-in" period, have established transitional or training areas where employees may work at a reduced pace for a limited time.

The standard preventive approach, which is directed at control of occupational factors, has the most promise. This approach often requires changes in the workstation, work process, or use of tools. Sometimes administrative changes, such as work restrictions, the use of personal protective equipment (for example, palm pads), or job rotation, are useful alternatives. Job rotation of work requiring different types of motions of the upper extremity, however, may simply expose a larger number of workers to a considerable degree of risk.

The first step required for instituting changes in workstations or work processes to reduce exposure is to analyze the specific characteristics of suspected high-risk jobs. While the job reviewed may be conducted by an industrial engineer or occupational health professional with training in ergonomics, the involvement of those persons most knowledgeable about the job is important. Experience has shown that not only can operators and supervisors with limited training successfully identify many of the hazardous aspects of a specific job, but also specific solutions may not be effective or accepted without their involvement in the job review and the development of solutions.

## REFERENCES


1. Fine LJ, Silverstein BA. Work-related disorders of the neck and upper extremity. In: Levy BS, Wegman DH, eds. *Occupational health: recognizing and preventing work-related disease,* 3rd ed. Boston: Little, Brown, 1995;358–365.
2. Phalen G. The carpal tunnel syndrome. Clinical evaluation of 598 hands. *Clin Orthop* 1972;83:29.
3. Finkelstein H. Stenosing tendovaginitis at the radial styloid process. *J Bone Joint Surg [Am]* 1930;12:509–540.
4. Kurppa K, et al. Incidence of tenosynovitis or peritendinitis and epicondylitis in a meat-processing factory. *Scand J Work Environ Health* 1991;17:32–37.
5. Bland D, et al. The painful shoulder. *Semin Arthritis Rheum* 1977;7(1): 21–47.
6. Waris P. Epidemiologic screening of occupational neck and upper limb disorders. *Scand J Work Environ Health* 1979;5(suppl 3):25.
7. Halder N, Gillings DB, Imbus HR, et al. Hand structure and function in an industrial setting. *Arthritis Rheum* 1978;21:210–220.
8. Cargile CH. Raynaud's disease in stonecutters using pneumatic tools. *JAMA* 1915;64:582.
9. Bureau of Labor Statistics, U.S. Department of Labor. *Workplace injuries and illnesses in 1996.* Olympia, Washington: USDL, December 1997.
10. Armstrong TJ, Buckle P, Fine LJ, et al. A conceptual model for work-related neck and upper-limb musculoskeletal disorders. *Scand J Work Environ Health* 1993;19:73–84.
11. Franklin GM, Haug J, Heyer N, Checkoway H. Occupational carpal tunnel syndrome in Washington State, 1984–1988. *Am J Public Health* 1991;81:741–746.
12. Washington State Department of Labor and Industries. *SHARP upper limb disorders in Washington State. Analysis of the state fund workers' compensation data, 1987–1993.* Technical Report 2-97. Olympia, Washington: USDL, 1997.
13. Tanaka S, Wild DK, Seligman PJ, et al. The US prevalence of self-reported carpal tunnel syndrome:1988 National Health Interview Survey data. *Am J Public Health* 1994;84:1846–1848.
14. Moore JS. Carpal tunnel syndrome. *Occup Med* 1992;7(4):741–763.
15. Hagberg M, Silverstein B. Work-related musculoskeletal disorders (WMSDS). In: Kuorinka K, Forcier M, eds. *A reference book for prevention.* Montreal: Taylor & Francis, 1995.
16. Armstrong TJ, Latko WA. Physical stressors: their characterization,

assessment, and relationship with physical work requirements. In: Gordon SL, Blair SJ, Fine LJ, eds. Rosemont, IL: American Academy of Orthopaedic Surgeons, 1995;87–98.
17. Rempel D. Musculoskeletal loading and carpal tunnel pressure in repetitive motion disorders of the upper extremity. In: Gordon SL, Blair SJ, Fine LJ, eds. Rosemont, IL: American Academy of Orthopaedic Surgeons, 1995;123–132.
18. Nirschl RP. Tennis elbow tendinosis: pathoanatomy, nonsurgical and surgical management. In: Gordon SL, Blair SJ, Fine LJ, eds. Rosemont, IL: American Academy of Orthopaedic Surgeons, 1995;467–478.
19. Amadio PC, De Quervain's Disease and Tenosynovitis. In: Gordon SL, Blair SJ, Fine LJ, eds. Rosemont, IL: American Academy of Orthopaedic Surgeons, 1995;435–448.
20. Hart DA, Frank CB, Bray RC. Inflammatory processes in repetitive motion and overuse syndromes: potential role of neurogenic mechanisms in tendons and ligaments. In: Gordon SL, Blair SJ, Fine LJ, eds. Rosemont, IL: American Academy of Orthopaedic Surgeons, 1995; 247–262.
21. Mintz G, Farga A. Severe osteoarthritis of the elbow in foundry workers An occupational hazard. *Arch Environ Health* 1973;27:78–80.
22. Andersson GBJ. Epidemiology of occupational neck and shoulder disorders. In: Gordon SL, Blair SJ, Fine LJ, eds. Rosemont, IL: American Academy of Orthopaedic Surgeons, 1995;31–42.
23. Levitz CL, Iannotti JP. Overuse injuries of the shoulder. In: Gordon SL, Blair SJ, Fine LJ, eds. Rosemont, IL: American Academy of Orthopaedic Surgeons, 1995;493–506.
24. Hagberg M, Morgenstern H, Kelsh M. Impact of occupations and job tasks on the prevalence of carpal tunnel syndrome. *Scand J Work Environ Health* 1992;18:337–345.
25. Hagberg M, Nystrom A, Zetterlund B. Recovery from symptoms after carpal tunnel syndrome surgery in males in relation to vibration exposure. *J Hand Surg* [Am] 1991;16:66–71.
26. Lockwood AH. Medical problems of musicians. *N Engl J Med* 1989; 320(4):221–227.
27. Lambert CM. Hand and upper limb problems of instrumental musicians. *Br J Rheumatol* 1992;31:572–573.
28. Bernard B, Sauter S, Fine L, et al. Job task and psychosocial risk factors for work-related musculoskeletal disorder among newspaper employees. *Scand J Work Environ Health* 1994;20:417–426.
29. Stevens JC. Conditions associated with carpal tunnel syndrome. *Mayo Clin Proc* 1992;67:541–548.
30. Tanaka S, Wild DK, Cameron LL, Freund E Jr. Association of occupational and non-occupational risk factors with the prevalence of self-reported carpal tunnel syndrome in a national survey of the working population. *Am J Ind Med* 1997;32(5):550–556.
31. Theorell T, Harms-Ringdahl K, Ahlberg-Hulten G, Westin B. Psychosocial job factors and symptoms from the locomotor system- a multi-causal analysis. *Scand J Rehabil Med* 1991;23:165–173.
32. Bongers PM, de Winter CR, Kompier MA, et al. Psychosocial factors at work and musculoskeletal disease. *Scand J Work Environ Health* 1993; 19:297–312.
33. Sauter SL, Swanson NG. The relationship between workplace psychosocial factors and musculoskeletal disorders in office work: suggested mechanisms and evidence. In: Gordon SL, Blair SJ, Fine LJ, eds. Rosemont, IL: American Academy of Orthopaedic Surgeons, 1995.
34. Moore JS. Clinical determination of work-relatedness in carpal tunnel syndrome. *J Occup Rehabil* 1991;1:145–158.
35. Karasek RA, Theorell T. *Healthy work.* New York: Basic Books, 1990.
36. Cheadle A, Franklin G, Wolfhagen C, et al. Factors influencing the duration of work-related disability: a population-based study of Washington State workers compensation. *Am J Public Health* 1994;84(2): 190–196.
37. Rempel DM, Harrison RJ, Barnhardt S. Work-related cumulative trauma disorders of the upper extremity. *JAMA* 1992;267:838–842.
38. Pransky G, Himmelstein J. Overview of complete patient management in upper extremity repetitive motion disorders. In: Gordon SL, Blair SJ, Fine LJ, eds. Rosemont, IL: American Academy of Orthopaedic Surgeons, 1995.
39. Feurstein M. A multi-disciplinary approach to the prevention, evaluation and management of work disability. *J Occup Rehabil* 1991;1:5–12.
40. NIOSH. *Elements of ergonomics programs:* a primer based on workplace evaluations of musculoskeletal disorders. DHHS (NIOSH) Publication 97-117. Cincinnati OH: U.S. Department of Health and Human Services, Public Health Service, Centers for Disease Control and Prevention, National Institute for Occupational Safety and Health, 1997.
41. Werner RA, Franzblau A, Albers JW, Buchele H, Armstrong TJ. Use of screening nerve conduction studies for predicting future carpal tunnel syndrome. *Occup Environ Med* 1997;54(2):96–100.
42. State of Washington Department of Labor and Industries. *Attending physician's handbook,* rev. ed. Olympia, Washington: State of Washington Department of Labor and Industries, 1996.
43. Sauter S, Swanson N. An ecological model of musculoskeletal disorders in office work. In: Moon S, Sauter S, eds. Beyond biomechanics-psychosocial aspects of musculoskeletal disorders in office work. London: Taylor & Francis, 1996;3–23.

# SECTION II

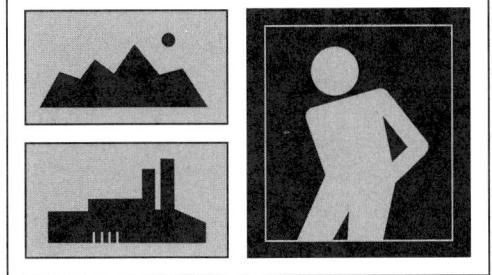

## Environmental and Occupational Exposures

*Environmental and Occupational Medicine, Third Edition*, edited by William N. Rom.
Lippincott–Raven Publishers, Philadelphia © 1998.

CHAPTER 68

# Occupational and Environmental Exposure to Lead

Alf Fischbein

You will see by it, that the opinion of this mischievous effect from lead is at least 60 years old; and you will observe with concern how long a useful truth may be known and exist, before it is generally receiv'd and practis'd on.

—Benjamin Franklin (1786)

Practically all industrial lead poisoning is due to the inhalation of dust and fume; and if you stop their inhalation, you will stop the poisoning.

—Sir Thomas Legge (1934)

## HISTORY

Lead is one of the ancient metals, produced by humans and used as early as 6,000 years ago in Asia Minor. Both its use and toxic effects can be traced to the cradle of human civilization (1,2). The numerous applications of lead throughout the ages have been as varied as the human mind can envision. To mention a few examples, the Egyptians used leaden tools and vessels, and a leaden statuette in the British Museum in London gives testimony to the fact that lead was also used by the Egyptians in the arts and crafts around 3500 B.C. The Israelites made the candelabrum in the Second Temple of an alloy containing lead (3); in the Hanging Gardens of Babylon plants were kept in leaden pots to retain moisture, while the Romans drank sapa, wines, and ciders sweetened and preserved with lead (4). The habit of drinking such beverages was prevalent among the Roman aristocracy and, according to some historians, might have been an important contributing factor to the fall of the Roman Empire (5).

Although lead may have had a major impact on society as early as two millennia ago, it is only during the past two decades that drastic measures have been taken in many industrialized countries to minimize human exposure to lead. In this respect, the United States has been in the vanguard in controlling both occupational and environmental lead exposure.

Some of the toxic effects of lead were probably known to both the Greeks and the Romans. Hippocrates (circa 370 B.C.) describes a severe attack of abdominal pain (possibly "lead colic") in a man who extracted metals, while Nicander, in the second century B.C., noted an association between exposure to lead and symptoms such as pallor, constipation, colic, and paralysis. Pliny (79 A.D.) mentions that lead-based paint was used on ships and that lead poisoning occurred among shipbuilders in his time.

The numerous epidemics of lead poisoning that occurred in the Middle Ages throughout Europe are of great historic and epidemiologic interest. The ancient Roman practice of improving the taste of poor vintages with additives containing lead was common during the Middle Ages. The many episodes of lead poisoning that occurred during this period were in fact the result of this practice. This was primarily discovered by Eberhard Gockel, an alert physician in the German city of Ulm, who realized that the severe clinical symptoms known as colica Pictonum (the colic of Poitou) that occurred among monks in monasteries in Ulm were caused by drinking wines treated with lead oxide (litharge). His

A. Fischbein: Department of Life Sciences, Division of Environmental and Occupational Health, Bar-Ilan University, Ramat-Gan 52900; and Department of Research and Development for Occupational and Environmental Health, Sanz Medical Center–Laniado Hospital, Netanya 42150, Israel.

findings were published in 1697 (4,6). Poitou was the region in France where the habit of adding lead to wines was so prevalent that the colic of Poitou was synonymous with lead colic.

Moreover, another probable cause of intoxication was drinking acidic beverages that had either been stored in lead-glazed earthenware or been contaminated with lead during manufacturing. Thus, Sir George Baker, in his classic description of the Devonshire colic in 1767, traced the disease to cider that had been contaminated with lead. Subsequently, in this episode, other lead-induced clinical effects (e.g., gout) were also associated with exposure (2).

In 1839 Tanquerel des Planches published a famous study of 1,217 cases of lead poisoning, and his clinical observations contributed much to our current knowledge of the clinical signs and symptoms of this occupational disease, including effects on the central nervous system. He realized that most cases of occupational lead poisoning were caused by inhalation of lead dust and fumes. He also suggested an association between lead exposure and renal disease. In Great Britain, great efforts to control occupational lead poisoning were introduced during the last decade of the 19th century. The pioneering work by Sir Thomas Legge, the first medical inspector of factories, resulted in strict legislation, including declaring lead poisoning a notifiable disease, in 1899.

The adverse clinical effects of lead were not confined to the European continent but occurred in colonial America as well. Symptoms of lead colic were caused by drinking rum distilled in leaden vessels, and in 1723 legislation was passed in Massachusetts "preventing abuses in distilling of rum and other strong liquors with leaden heads or pipes" (7). Serious concern over occupational lead poisoning in the United States began in 1910, with the investigations of several lead-related industries by Alice Hamilton (8), a pioneer in the field of American occupational medicine. Detailed studies of the clinical and biochemical aspects of lead poisoning were conducted during subsequent decades (9,10).

Since lead does not serve any biologic function in the body, its presence has always been taken as a sign of environmental pollution. Despite its known toxic effects and long history of lead-associated diseases, there is evidence that compounds of this metal were used for medicinal purposes, especially during the 18th century in France (11). The surgeon Thomas Goulard (circa 1784), a member of the famous medical faculty in Montpellier, used extract of Saturn (a concoction of lead monoxide in wine vinegar) externally to treat a number of conditions: inflammations, sprains, joint stiffness, ligament injuries, and gunshot wounds. Although Goulard did not recommend internal administration of lead, other medical authorities in the 18th and 19th centuries advocated taking lead acetate per os for epilepsy. It is interesting to note that these physicians were indeed aware of the "side effects" of such treatment, which included abdominal cramps (lead colic).

Although some sources of environmental lead pollution prevalent in modern society are different from those of the Middle Ages, many of the symptoms associated with excessive lead exposure remained consistent over time. Control of lead exposure achieved by legislation and modern technology has undoubtedly made acute lead poisoning a much rarer disease; however, certain neurologic and gastrointestinal symptoms, known for centuries to be lead related, are still common symptoms causing persons exposed to lead to seek medical attention.

## CHEMISTRY OF LEAD

Lead (Pb), a bluish gray metal, is distributed in the earth's crust in a large number of minerals. The most important of these, in terms of extraction of lead, is galena (PbS), which consists of 85% lead metal. Two other significant lead minerals are cerussite ($PbCO_3$) and anglesite ($PbSO_4$). Galena is usually accompanied by sulfides of silver, antimony, copper, bismuth, and tin. Lead is also found combined with zinc in sphalerite. Lead is a member of group IVB in the periodic table and has a melting point of 327°C. It has two oxidation states, Pb(II) and PB(IV) in addition to its elemental stage Pb(0). The metal is extracted from the ore by concentration of the sulfide, heating (roasting), and reduction. The metal then undergoes refining to remove other metal constituents in the ore (12).

Because of its widespread use, lead and some of its chemical compounds are nearly ubiquitous in the human environment and can be found in plants, oceans, rivers, drinking water, soil, and in various food items. Lead is also present in the air and attaches to dust particles. Consequently, the possibility of human exposure to some form of lead is great. It can be said that the presence of lead in blood and other body fluids serves as an indicator of industrial development and activities; its presence always reflects environmental pollution, whether it originates from the general or occupational environment (13).

During the past two decades much concern has been voiced over the potential health consequences of exposure to lead in both occupational and general environments. During this period several investigators have examined the effects of environmental lead exposure, particularly among infants and young children, who are most sensitive to the effects of lead in society. Through these studies it has become increasingly clear that adverse health effects are seen at levels of exposure that during previous decades were considered safe (14). Of greater concern is the fact that the levels of environmental exposure at which adverse health effects can be detected have become progressively lower and the magnitude of the lead-related public health risk to children may be greater than was hitherto estimated. Major efforts to reduce exposure to lead have been made or are in progress in many industrialized countries.

## USES AND OCCUPATIONAL SOURCES OF EXPOSURE

Lead is the most widely used nonferrous metal, and its use and the use of lead compounds still play an important role in modern industry. There has been a marked increase in its use since the 1950s. Despite widely applied restrictions on major uses of lead (e.g., gasoline additives, paints, and cans), the current annual worldwide production is approximately 5.4 million tons, 23% of which is produced in the United States. Sixty percent of lead is used for the manufacturing of batteries (automobile batteries, in particular), while the remainder is required for the production of pigments, solder, plastics, cable sheathing, ammunition, and a variety of other extruded products.

Expanding uses in the future are predicted for automobile storage batteries and products in the electronics industry (15,16). Lead, as an organic compound, is added to gasoline to raise the octane rating and serve as a scavenger of free radicals (antiknock agent); this use is declining following the introduction of lead-free gasoline. The use of lead in paints has also decreased considerably during the past decade, principally because of legislation in various countries controlling the use of leaded paint, and the subsequent widespread use of water-based latex paints. Latex paints are not necessarily metal free, and may contain other metals, such as mercury, as antimold ingredients (17). Risk for hazardous exposure to lead exists in a wide range of industrial settings, and at least 120 different occupations and job titles are associated with potential risk for exposure (18).

There are some major industrial settings and paraoccupational activities that may be of special practical interest for occupational and family physicians, in terms of identifying persons at highest risk for overexposure to lead.

Primary and secondary lead smelting and refinement are associated with considerable exposure (19,20). While primary smelting involves the extraction of the metal from lead-containing minerals by various processes (including roasting at 600°C), the secondary lead-smelting plants recycle lead from scrap metal, the majority of which is lead storage batteries. Other heavy elements, including cadmium and arsenic, are frequent co-toxicants in these industries. Although the manufacture of lead paint pigments has decreased, there has been a concomitant increase in the production of storage batteries. In fact, the battery-manufacturing industry is currently one of the largest single users of lead in the United States and thus, a frequently encountered source of occupational lead exposure.

It should be emphasized that most solid metallic lead products are considered relatively safe in normal use and are seldom thought of as posing a significant health hazard. However, when various modes of treatments, such as heating, grinding, spraying, or burning, are applied to the metal surface, the danger becomes greater. When heat is applied to the surface, lead fumes are generated. Lead oxides are formed on cooling of the fumes in the air. Oxides and suboxides are biologically active forms of lead that are readily inhaled and absorbed. Therefore, workers engaged in such operations as structural, bridge, and ornamental iron work are at increased risk of lead absorption. Despite the decline in the use of leaded paint on interior surfaces, red lead ($Pb_3O_4$) remains indispensable as a weather-resistant coating for metals. The use of red lead as a protective agent for ships, bridges, railways, and various other iron and steel structures is essential even today and of great economic significance. Workers engaged in the demolition of ships, which often have been covered with several layers of lead paint, are at risk for occupational exposure to extremely high air lead levels as they cut or burn through the painted metal. Similar operations occur in shipbuilding and ship repair as well. Lead is an effective protection against high-energy radiation and a principal constituent of shielding materials against radiation, including x-rays. Lead bonding and burning are common practices in the construction and maintenance of nuclear-powered ships and reactors. The modernization and restoration of older parts of inner cities in the United States and Europe often require the demolition of buildings and the dismantling of elevated railways that have fallen into disuse. Flame cutting with oxyacetylene-propane torches through such lead-painted steel structures is still a common source of occupational lead poisoning and poses a complex industrial hygiene and occupational health problem (21–25).

Other common potentially hazardous industries include small workshops with low standards of hygiene and inadequate medical surveillance, such as automobile radiator repair and scrap metal–smelting shops, as well as pewter and leaded pane manufacturing (26).

Some employees in the manufacturing of polyvinyl chloride–based plastics work with lead-containing stabilizers, including dibasic lead phthalate, lead chlorosilicate, and basic lead carbonates, all of which can produce dust when agitated. Lead stabilizers account for approximately 60% of all stabilizer consumption and are used especially in plastic compounds requiring heat stability and tensile strength, as in electrical insulation. Cable and wire manufacturing and splicing of cables, are other examples in which there is risk for occupational lead exposure, although the replacement of powdered stabilizers with pellet-formed stabilizers has been beneficial in reducing this risk for cable manufacturing workers (27,28).

The production of tin cans with lead-based solder is another known source of potential lead exposure. Automation and modern soldering techniques have much improved the work environment in this industry, and heavily exposed workers from this sector are rarely encountered. However, the lead-containing seam on the can has been suggested as a significant source of lead for consumers of canned food. The printing industry was long associated with risk for lead poisoning, but is today a less significant source because of the prevalence of computerized and other "cold type" printing techniques.

Firearms instructors working in poorly ventilated indoor firing ranges are at risk of absorbing considerable amounts of lead by inhalation of lead fumes and dust generated by the firing of a gun. Although the risk is greatest for those employed on a full-time basis at a firing range, increased lead absorption has also been documented among more occasional users of shooting galleries. The use of jacketed or nylon-clad ammunitions, coupled with effective ventilation, has been essential in minimizing health hazards from this type of exposure (29–32).

Other common occupations that entail the use of lead include the making of lead-glazed pottery and crystal glass. Lead hazards extend to hobbyists and their families when stained glass and pottery are made in the home environment or in studios located near the domicile (33).

In the home environment, removing lead paint can pose a great danger unless strict protective hygiene measures are taken. Nevertheless, it is common that certain professional activities are done by persons who lack specific skills, and "do-it-yourself" work is common practice among homeowners. Refurbishing interior surfaces of old houses can require removal of lead-containing paint with the assistance of either heat guns or mechanical stripping devices. Unaware of the potential health hazard that this work may pose, lay persons so engaged have also suffered lead poisoning.

## AMBIENT ENVIRONMENTAL LEAD POLLUTION

Although atmospheric lead originates from a number of industrial sources, leaded gasoline is a principal source of general environmental lead pollution (34). Tetraethyl lead was introduced as an antiknock agent in gasoline in the 1920s and has played an increasingly important role as a pollutant of the general atmosphere since. During combustion, lead alkyls decompose into lead oxides, which react with halogen scavengers also present as additives to gasoline, to produce lead halides, i.e., chlorinated and brominated compounds. These compounds are further broken down to lead carbonate, oxycarbonate, and oxides. A certain amount of organic lead is emitted in exhaust fumes in these forms.

It is estimated that 90% of the atmospheric lead originates from automobile exhaust and the increase in environmental lead concentrations observed between the 1930s and 1960s was associated mainly with emissions from leaded gasoline (35). The introduction of lead-free gasoline in the United States has contributed to a considerable decrease in air lead levels in many areas.

Although automobile traffic and consumption of leaded gasoline have been associated with lead concentrations in surface soils, it has also been demonstrated that lead in soil can occur from weathering of lead-based exterior paint, and this should be considered as a potential source of lead exposure in some locations (36,37).

Industrial emissions are also important sources in specific locales. The magnitude of the lead pollution problem in the general environment of industrialized countries is illustrated by a study in 1980 examining populations in remote mountainous areas in East Asia. The investigators reported average blood lead levels in children of approximately 3 μg/dl, substantially less than the median blood lead concentration of 13 μg/dl reported for the entire U.S. population at that time. Thus, the considerably higher blood levels in industrial populations reflect widespread environmental lead pollution, and levels considered normal, even nowadays, in an industrial society are greatly increased above the natural lead concentration in the biosphere, which is estimated to be associated with blood lead levels of 0.06 to 0.12 μg/dl (38–40).

Data from the second National Health and Nutrition Examination Survey (NHANES) indicated a decline in the geometric mean blood lead level of the U.S. population during the period 1976 through 1980, from 15.8 to 12.8 μg/dl. The decreases were found in all ages and races, and in both sexes. It has been suggested that the reduced use of leaded gasoline was a most important factor for lowering the blood lead levels in the U.S. general population (41,42). Similar data from other countries further demonstrated the beneficial effect on blood lead levels in the population subsequent to the institution of environmental controls (43,44).

A further substantial decline in blood lead levels in the entire United States population was demonstrated during the period 1988 to 1991 in a subsequent national survey (NHANES) that found a geometric mean concentration of 2.8 μg/dl. Removal of lead from gasoline and soldered cans were the most likely reasons for the observed decline. The efforts to control these sources of lead pollution must be considered a major achievement in public health (45,46). Substantial decreases in mean blood lead levels in children have also been reported from Sweden between 1978 and 1994 with a decline from 6.0 to 2.5 μg/dl, also primarily ascribed to the discontinuation of leaded gasoline (47). In a global perspective, however, in countries where lead pollution has not yet been given proper attention, lead poisoning may be a serious public health issue of growing dimensions (48).

## LEAD INTAKE AND ABSORPTION

In occupational and environmental settings, xenobiotic agents essentially enter the human body by three modes—inhalation of contaminated air; ingestion of food, beverages, or nonfood items; and absorption through the skin. The most important route of entry into the human organism for lead and its compounds is via the respiratory tract. The respiratory uptake of lead is a function of respiratory rate; particle size, shape, and charge; and the degree of solubility in body fluids. The mass median diameter of atmospheric lead particles is often within the range at which significant deposition and retention in the respiratory tract occur. It is estimated that the deposition rate of airborne lead is approximately 40% in adult humans (49). The range given by different authors varies between 30% and 85%. Most of the lead deposited in the respiratory tract is readily absorbed into the bloodstream, especially if particles are small enough for optimal deposition in the alveoli. Data about deposition and absorption of lead by children are less certain, because of their respiratory physiology; children inhale a greater volume of air in relation to body mass than adults. It has been suggested that the rate of deposition of lead in children is considerably greater than in adults (50).

In contrast to the relatively high rate of respiratory deposition and absorption of lead, gastrointestinal absorption of lead in adults is much lower. The rate has been estimated at approximately 10% to 15% from normal diets (51). The degree of absorption is influenced by several factors and can be increased considerably by fasting or by a diet deficient in calcium, iron, phosphorus, or zinc (52). Moreover, gastrointestinal absorption of lead is much greater in infants and children than in adults and is estimated to be around 50% (53). Thus, if both consume a diet with a given lead content, children are at higher exposure risk than adults. There is evidence that food is becoming less important as a source of lead (54). Despite the relatively insignificant gastrointestinal absorption rate of lead in adults, care must be taken to minimize intake via this route in certain occupational settings where there may be particularly great risk, for example in lead-contaminated lunchrooms and smoking areas. Absorption of lead from cigarette smoking, especially in a lead-contaminated work environment, can add significantly to the individual's total intake of the metal. Cigarette smoking is also a source of lead exposure both for the smoker and for others living in the household (55).

As mentioned, the particle size of a given lead compound and its solubility in body fluids are two important determinants of toxicity. The awareness of this fact may be significant for assessment of risk associated with various occupational exposures. For example, the rate of pulmonary absorption of lead sulfide (galena), the principal ore in the Missouri lead mines, is limited, whereas the lead mines in Utah contain ore that is principally lead sulfate and lead carbonate. These compounds are more readily soluble in body fluids and constitute a far greater hazard to workers. Similarly, airborne oxides of lead in fumes of molten lead are readily soluble in weak acids and expose unprotected workers to high risk of lead absorption. Risk of absorption of inorganic lead compounds via the skin is insignificant, except for absorption of lead acetate through damaged skin. Organometallic compounds, however, are lipid soluble and organic lead compounds, such as tetraethyl and tetramethyl lead, are easily absorbed via the skin. Therefore, they pose a different and more complex industrial hygiene problem than in work that involves inorganic lead compounds.

## DISTRIBUTION OF LEAD IN THE BODY

Absorption of lead via the respiratory tract is the most significant route of entry into the human organism. There is fairly rapid and direct uptake of lead into the bloodstream, and the toxic metal has easy access to sensitive target organs. Inorganic lead does not undergo any metabolic transformation, digestion in the intestines, or detoxification in the liver.

Because of the long biologic half-life of lead, a certain body burden accumulates over time. Several mathematical models of the pharmacokinetic characteristics of lead have been proposed. In one, the total body burden of lead is divided as follows: (1) a rapidly exchangeable pool in blood and soft tissues, (2) an intermediate pool of exchangeable lead in skin and muscles, and (3) a more stable pool in the skeleton. The third pool contains two subdivisions: an intermediate exchangeable pool in the marrow in the trabecular portion of the bone, and a more slowly exchangeable pool in the dense bone, including dentine (56).

In another proposed multicompartment model, consideration is given to the diffusion of lead into bone as well as to interactions between lead in plasma and erythrocytes. Division of the blood lead compartment into four subdivisions has been proposed: diffusible lead in plasma, protein-bound lead in plasma, and two erythrocyte pools (57).

The total burden of lead is distributed throughout the organism, and the biologic activity of lead varies among the compartments. The rapidly exchangeable portion of lead in the blood is the most biologically active part of the total body burden. However, this pool constitutes only about 2% of the total body burden. In blood, 99% of the metal is bound to erythrocytes (58) and only a small portion is present in plasma. The albumin-bound fractions of lead in plasma and in extracellular fluid are the main vehicles by which lead reaches the various organs of the body. Although lead in plasma may be the most direct indicator of current exposure and internal dose, measurement of lead concentration in whole blood remains the most accessible and widely used laboratory indicator for assessing exposure and absorption of lead into the body. The blood lead concentration also defines the risk of toxicity fairly accurately (59). At constant exposure, an equilibrium is established between the blood and the tissues. Lead is cleared relatively fast from the blood, in comparison with other body segments. It has been suggested that 50% of the lead absorbed under steady-state conditions is excreted rapidly and that the half-life of this portion is approximately 3 weeks (56,60). The blood lead concentration is representative only of the amount of lead recently absorbed into the body. Under exposure conditions associated with abrupt increases or declines in blood lead concentrations, the steady-state situation is difficult to predict but is a function of duration and intensity of exposure as well as of the total body burden. As mentioned, the blood lead concentration is not a reliable index of the total body burden of lead accumulated over a prolonged period.

Recently, attempts have been made to develop new methods for measuring an integrated index of cumulative exposure and absorption of lead into the body (i.e., to find a way to quantify the body burden of lead that has accumulated from lifelong environmental exposure). A great need exists for the development of more accurate means of assessing the total body burden of lead, in order to optimize evaluations of dose-response relationships in epidemiologic studies.

Noninvasive x-ray fluorescence (XRF) techniques are under evaluation as potentially safe and accurate means of in vivo assessment of cumulative absorption from past lead exposure. XRF, which involves the stimulation of characteristic x-ray emission from lead with a beam of photons, has been applied, with various methodologic approaches and modifications, by several investigators (61–66). The XRF methods are emerging as a promising new tool for assessing cumulative exposure in high-risk populations; improvements in the relatively poor sensitivity of XRF are expected to make these methods more useful in evaluating low-level community exposure as well (67,68). Whereas, initially, only limited extrapolations could be made from XRF measurements because of the complex composition and turnover rates of skeletal lead compartments, a more recent investigation has demonstrated that the technique can be useful in quantifying bone lead in occupationally exposed workers in relation to duration of employment, a time-integrated blood lead index, and employment status (active or retired). This technique can also be used for calculation of the biologic half-life of lead, estimated from examinations to be 5.2 years in the active workers (69,70).

## BIOCHEMICAL ASPECTS OF LEAD TOXICITY

Although lead is considered a toxic metal that affects many organ systems and functions in humans, there are certain biochemical mechanisms that correspond with abnormalities in diagnostic biologic response tests and with lead-induced clinical symptoms. The following description emphasizes such mechanisms (71,72).

The major biochemical effects of lead can be broadly classified into three groups. Lead is an electropositive metal with high affinity for the negatively charged sulfhydryl groups. This is manifested, in several organs, by the inhibition of sulfhydryl-dependent enzymes. Inhibition of δ-aminolevulinic acid dehydratase (ALA-D) and ferrochelatase, two enzymes in the biosynthetic pathway of heme, has been utilized in the development of some fundamental diagnostic tests. Divalent lead is similar in many aspects to calcium and acts competitively with this element in several biologic systems, such as mitochondrial respiration and various nerve functions. The similarities between calcium and lead partially explain why both elements are interchangeable in bone and why more than 90% of the total body burden of lead is stored in the skeleton. Lead also affects nucleic acids, both deoxyribonucleic acid (DNA) and ribonucleic acid (RNA), by mechanisms that are not yet fully known, but that, likewise, may be related to the divalence of the lead ion. The effect on nucleic acids may have important biologic implications (73). Some studies have reported increased rates of chromosome aberrations (74–76), but other investigators did not identify such changes (77,78). Increased frequency of sister-chromatid exchanges (SCE) and abnormal excretion of DNA-derived β-amino-isobutyric acid has been reported among lead-exposed workers (79,80).

Lead has also been shown to inhibit erythrocytic pyrimidine-5′-nucleotidase (P5N), in both children and adults exposed to lead, which results in the accumulation of nucleotides in erythrocytes affecting the stability of the cell membrane (81,82). This and other interactions with cell membranes, such as interference with $Na^+/K^+$ adenosine triphosphatase (ATPase) activity (83), $Na^+/K^+$ pump, and $Na^+/K^+$ cotransport system (84), have been suggested as the biochemical basis for a variety of lead-related effects, including shortened erythrocyte survival time and hemolysis, renal toxicity, and hypertension.

Lead has also been shown to exert complex effects on the immune system affecting both humoral and cell-mediated immune responses. The exact mechanism of action has not yet been clarified. It may be associated with the high affinity of lead for surface receptors, thereby interfering with antigen processing (85,86).

Although there is evidence that some inorganic lead compounds, such as lead acetate, lead subacetate, and lead phosphate are carcinogenic in experimental animals (87,88), there is no conclusive epidemiologic evidence that lead is carcinogenic in humans. An association between heavy occupational exposure to lead and stomach cancer, lung cancer, and bladder cancer has been suggested in a meta-analysis study of published data. Relative risk for kidney cancer was also high but did not reach statistical significance (89,90). In this context, case reports of renal cancer in workers with lead-associated neuropathy are of interest and concern (91–93).

## Lead and Heme Synthesis

One of the most important mechanisms of lead toxicity is its effect on various enzymes in the heme biosynthetic pathway (Fig. 1). The hematopoietic system is considered one of the critical organs in lead poisoning. The interference by lead in heme synthesis, discussed below in greater detail, constitutes an essential component of the clinical and biochemical features of lead poisoning. Some fundamental diagnostic blood tests aimed at detecting early, subclinical alterations have their biochemical correlates in lead-related toxicity on heme synthesis.

One biologic response test, namely measurement of blood zinc protoporphyrin (ZPP), is a practical diagnostic test that can be performed in occupational health and community surveys at the site of examination. When utilizing a portable instrument for use as a primary screening test, it is possible to rapidly examine a large number of individuals, e.g., workers and children (94–96).

The two target sites in the biosynthetic pathway of heme in which the effect of lead is of the most clinical interest are the sites of activity of ALA-D and ferrochelatase, both of which are inhibited by lead. In addition, a stimulatory effect on δ-aminolevulinic acid synthetase (ALA-S), which is the rate-limiting step in the biosynthesis of heme, has also been demonstrated. Lead-induced effects on heme synthesis are not limited to the hematopoietic system but are manifested in other organs as well (97).

ALA-D is a most sensitive indicator of both acute and chronic effects of lead, and its activity decreases with rising blood lead levels (98,99). The lowest currently observable blood level for effects in children is about 10 μg/dl (100). Inhibition of ALA-D may therefore occur among individuals of the general population at blood lead levels that previously were not regarded as cause for much concern. It was not considered feasible to use the degree of ALA-D inhibition as a practical screening parameter in industrial settings because of its high level of sensitivity to lead and the uncertainty about the health implications of inhibited ALA-D activity. Since adverse effects (e.g., including neurobehavioral abnormalities and impairment in the metabolism of 1,25-dihydroxyvitamin D in children) have been detected at blood lead concentrations of approximately 10 μg/dl (101), determination of ALA-D may emerge again as a future sensitive

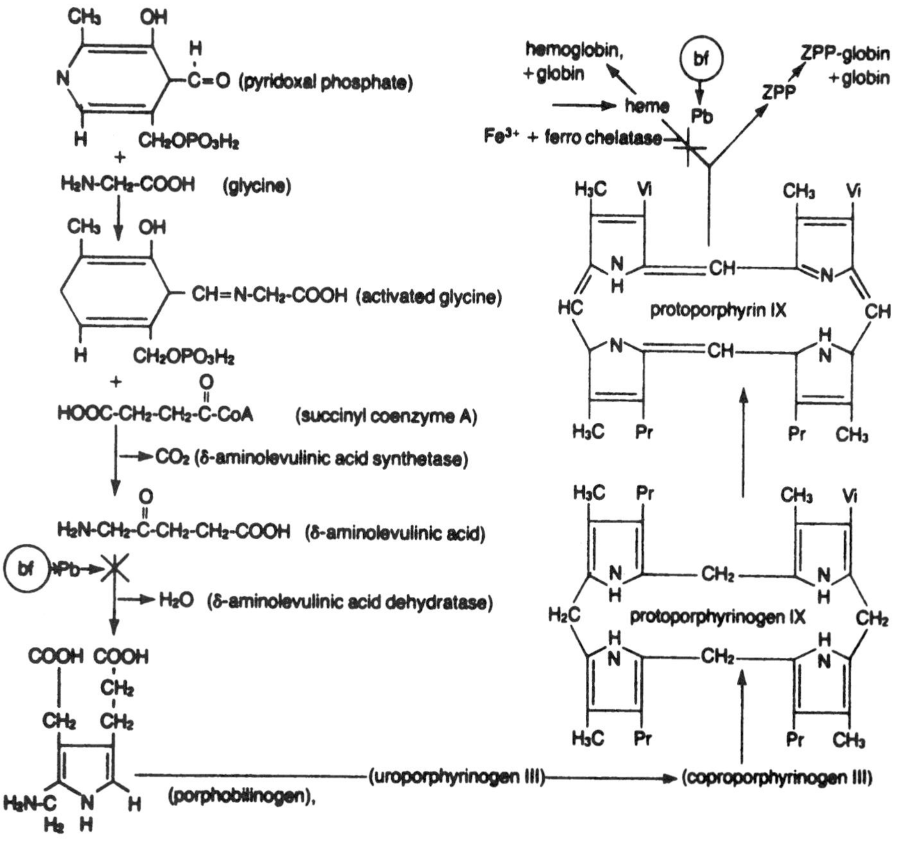


FIG. 1. Biosynthetic pathway of heme. (Courtesy of Dr. Shigeru Sassa, Rockefeller University, New York, NY.)

indicator (5) of early lead toxicity. The existence of different ALA-D alleles may determine individuals' susceptibility to the toxic effects of lead (102). The uncertainty whether a threshold exists for ALA-D inhibition is of great public health concern (103). The inhibition causes accumulation of ALA in both blood and urine; these parameters have also proven useful for evaluation of effects of lead in exposed individuals (104,105).

The enzyme ferrochelatase acts toward the completion of the biosynthetic pathway of heme. The function of ferrochelatase is to insert an iron atom into protoporphyrin IX. Lead inhibits ferrochelatase activity and therefore prevents incorporation of iron into hemoglobin. This interference results in accumulation of protoporphyrin in erythrocyte precursors in the bone marrow (106), known as free erythrocyte protoporphyrin (FEP), which can be extracted from the red blood cells quantitatively by various micro-methods. In 1974 it was demonstrated that the FEP in lead-poisoned subjects does not appear as free in the erythrocyte, but exists as a metal chelate, as zinc protoporphyrin (ZPP). The ZPP is bound to the globin moiety of the hemoglobin molecule; the hemoglobin of persons affected by lead contains higher concentrations of ZPP (94). Although the measurement of FEP in erythrocytes requires laboratory-based techniques, the discovery of ZPP in erythrocytes resulted in the development of a diagnostic biologic response test for lead toxicity. A simple, practical technique for measuring ZPP that utilizes a portable instrument, a hematofluorometer, has proven very useful for screening of large industrial and community populations (107–109). Since ZPP remains in the erythrocyte for the 120-day life span of the cell, measurement of ZPP is an indicator of a lead-related effect averaged over a 3-month period (110).

Elevated levels of ZPP are also caused by iron deficiency anemia, a condition that is often present in populations of children at high risk for lead poisoning. Iron deficiency must therefore be considered an important confounding factor in interpreting ZPP test results. Experimental studies have clarified the interaction of ZPP with both iron metabolism and other enzymes acting in the synthesis and degradation of heme (111,112). Although anemia is a characteristic clinical entity of the more advanced stages of lead poisoning, it can be explained only partly by impaired synthesis of heme. Lead-related anemia is characteristically normocytic and normochromic and can in most instances be distinguished from iron deficiency anemia, which is microcytic and hypochromic. The serum iron level is often normal or even elevated in lead poisoning. Shortened red cell survival, hemolysis, and abnormalities in erythrocyte membrane stability contribute to the low hemoglobin levels sometimes found in lead-poisoned patients (83,84).

Basophilic stippling of red blood cells, which reflects the aggregation of ribosomes, was once considered a classical sign of lead poisoning. This phenomenon, however, occurs in many other conditions and should be considered a nonspecific finding (113). Its presence does support the diagnosis, if other laboratory and clinical findings are indicative of lead poisoning.

## HEALTH EFFECTS OF LEAD

Lead poisoning is primarily a chronic disease caused by the gradual accumulation of a significant body burden of lead. The time from onset of exposure to the development of clinically observable disease depends much on the intensity of exposure. For instance, at well-controlled and low occupational exposure levels, months or even years of exposure may elapse before clinical symptoms appear. In contrast, at higher and more hazardous levels of exposure, generated, for example, by workers flame cutting lead-painted metal structures without the use of adequate respiratory protection, accumulation of toxic blood lead levels associated with clinical symptoms may appear much more rapidly, within days or weeks (21–25).

The toxic effects of lead in humans ought to be viewed as a broad spectrum of laboratory and clinical manifestations, ranging from subtle, subclinical biochemical abnormalities to severe clinical emergencies. The subclinical end of the spectrum, which by definition means absence of clinical symptoms, is the beginning point of a continuum with potential for progression to obvious adverse effects, from inhibition of enzymes and biochemical aberrations gradually developing to a stage characterized by symptoms of lead poisoning. Since various enzymatic alterations in the biosynthetic pathway of heme (ALA-D) or accumulation of enzyme substrates (FEP, ZPP, ALA) can be measured, the opportunity exists to identify effects of hazardous conditions at a relatively early stage and to prevent overt clinical lead poisoning.

Lead toxicity can manifest itself clinically in several organs (114). Although the exact mechanisms by which lead disrupts the function of sensitive organ systems, such as the central nervous system and the kidneys, are not yet completely understood, the interference by lead in the heme biosynthetic pathway can provide explanations for many clinical manifestations of lead poisoning and not solely those that are expressed as dysfunction in the hematopoietic system. Much recently acquired scientific information has shed new light on the significance of subtle clinical effects that are associated with low-level exposure to lead, both in the context of occupational and ambient environmental exposures (115,116). Since potential effects of low-level exposures are of greatest public health concern, emphasis is given in the following discussion to such effects.

### Nervous System

Both the central and the peripheral nervous systems are target organs for lead toxicity. In the most severe form of poisoning, rarely encountered nowadays in industrial settings, profound disturbances of the central nervous system are prominent, including convulsions, delirium, and coma. More frequently, however, at moderate or low occupational exposure levels, symptoms related to the nervous system are more subtle and nonspecific. These symptoms are not always readily associated with lead poisoning unless the examining physician is aware of the potential exposure source and takes a careful occupational history. Symptoms include headache, dizziness, sleep disturbances, memory deficit, and changes in personality such as increased irritability. The neurologic manifestations of lead toxicity range from subtle, nonspecific complaints to severe encephalopathy, the most serious clinical manifestation of lead poisoning. Although very rare, acute encephalopathy, is occasionally encountered in children following acute, heavy, often accidental intake of lead. The condition is therefore an important consideration as a differential diagnosis in a child presenting with signs of acute encephalopathy. Careful review of parental occupational and environmental history is of utmost importance in such cases.

As will be discussed in greater detail below, children's nervous system is more sensitive to lead toxicity than that of adults. It is widely recognized that excessive lead exposure is causally related to a wide range of developmental and behavioral dysfunctions in children (117–119).

Adult workers exposed to lead are also at risk for nervous system dysfunction, despite recent efforts to limit excessive exposure to lead at the workplace. The nonspecific central nervous system (CNS) symptoms, referred to above, are indicative of early stage CNS dysfunction with potential for developing into irreversible disease (27,120).

Evidence exists of abnormalities in a wide spectrum of neuropsychological tests applied to lead-exposed workers. Some abnormalities are consistent with the diagnosis of organic mental syndrome. Impaired performance on psychological tests has been associated with elevated levels of blood lead and ZPP concentrations (121–124). In most studies, however, measures of cumulative exposure to lead have not been available, limiting the conclusions that can be drawn regarding an association between cumulative lead exposure and adverse effects in neurobehavioural tests in adults (125). Decreased nerve conduction velocity has likewise been demonstrated in several groups of lead-exposed workers, and the literature on this subject is voluminous (34,100,126). Decreased nerve conduction velocities have been recorded by some at blood lead concentrations around 40 μg/dl (127), while others have failed to demonstrate differences between lead-exposed and control groups (128). There is a fairly good consensus that measurement of this parameter appears to be useful in documenting early changes in peripheral nerve function, which occasionally are reversible (129,130); measurement of nerve conduction velocity can be useful in documenting early, reversible changes in peripheral nerve function. Nerve conduction parameters have been reported to be more highly correlated with a calculated index for cumulative blood-years (considering both duration of exposure and blood lead concentrations) than with current blood lead levels (131). The once characteristic peripheral neurologic deficit, motor paralysis, i.e., wrist drop or foot drop, is rarely diagnosed among workers in modern industry because of improvements in environmental exposure control and enforcement of government regulations.

Several mechanisms by which lead may act on the nervous system have been proposed. Interference with neurotransmitter systems associated with behavioral disturbances, has been described in experimental animal studies (132). Hyperactivity as a manifestation of increased lead absorption in children may be a clinical correlate to the experimental findings (133).

Moreover, lead affects brain mitochondrial respiration and adenosine diphosphate (ADP) phosphorylation *in vitro* (134) and acts on newly formed neuronal components in the hippocampus, resulting in abnormal cerebral development and behavioral alterations (135). Lead has been localized in the endoneurial space of the peroneal nerve and in the myelin sheath by electron microscopic autoradiography (136).

### Effect of Lead on the Kidneys and Cardiovascular System

The kidneys constitute the main route of excretion of lead, although the gastrointestinal tract also plays an important role. There is a great individual variability in the excretory capacity of lead; the excretion involves glomerular filtration as well as transport across the tubular cells. Lead in the glomerular ultrafiltrate is also absorbed by the tubules. Besides serving as an important excretory route for lead, renal tissue is one of the soft tissues with the highest concentrations of lead (137); it is also a source of ALA production.

Lead nephropathy, during the acute phase of poisoning, includes proximal tubule damage and dysfunction with ultrastructural changes, consisting of intranuclear inclusion bodies in the proximal tubular epithelial cells and changes in cell organelles, particularly mitochondria (116,138). Renal tubular dysfunction occasionally occurs in severe childhood lead poisoning and is characterized by aminoaciduria, glucosuria, and hyperphosphaturia (i.e., Fanconi's syndrome) (139).

Whereas tubular dysfunction is considered early damage and potentially reversible with treatment (138), prolonged exposure to lead may result in progressive renal disease characterized by diffuse interstitial fibrosis and renal failure. Epidemiologic and histopathologic studies have indicated increased mortality rate among adults due to chronic lead failure related to overexposure to lead during childhood (140).

Renal dysfunction resulting from occupational exposure to lead has also been reported, manifested by nephrosclerosis with severe progressive renal insufficiency and interstitial fibrosis. Renal arterial and arteriolar vasoconstriction, which tend to occur during acute episodes of lead poisoning, are considered significant causal factors (141).

Although the adult form of acute lead nephropathy has been well described, the sequential development from the presence of proximal renal tubular damage and intranuclear inclusion bodies to interstitial fibrosis and renal insufficiency has been more difficult to demonstrate in humans (116,142). Glomerular changes and arterial damage occur in more severe cases of lead nephropathy. Associations between biochemical abnormalities in heme synthesis and kidney function tests have been reported (143), but no certain dose-response relationship has been established. The chronic renal disease observed in lead workers is usually associated with long-standing elevated blood lead concentrations (60–80 μg/dl) (141,144). Nevertheless, renal dysfunction may occur among workers at relatively low levels of exposures. Such dysfunction, which is of tubular origin, is more subtle, but is detectable by measuring the excretion of a renal tubular enzymes such as *N*-acetyl-β-D-glucosaminidase (NAG), a sensitive parameter of early tubular dysfunction (145,146). Early renal changes including alterations in renal hemodynamics, i.e., hyperfiltration state, may be related to moderate lead exposure (147,148).

*Saturnine gout* is a term used to describe a relationship between excessive lead absorption and gout nephropathy. Some patients with gout nephropathy exhibit an elevated body burden of lead as measured by the calcium ethylenediaminotetraacetic acid (CaEDTA) mobilization test, indicating that lead may be causally related to the development of gout nephropathy (149,150).

A possible association between exposure to lead and hypertension is currently a matter of much public health concern. Following an early clinical investigation in 1935 suggesting a relationship between lead exposure and hypertension (151), a number of mortality studies of lead-exposed workers have demonstrated increased risk of cerebrovascular disease, chronic renal disease, and hypertensive diseases, although the latter category was ill-defined in some studies (152–154). A fairly good consensus emerges from mortality studies of occupationally exposed persons (155) regarding excess risk for diseases of the cardiovascular system, although dose-response patterns do not always emerge; confounding factors are sometimes not accounted for (90). Cross-sectional population-based studies also suggest a relationship between hypertension and levels of blood lead that are present in the general population (156). The interaction between lead, other trace metals, and nutrients may act as a link between the observed relationship (157).

Lead-related stimulatory effects on synthesis and release of renin after brief exposure to moderate concentrations of lead have been proposed as underlying mechanisms. Moreover, lead affects the renin-angiotensin system and acts on sympathetic junctions and increases the responsiveness to stimulation of $\alpha_2$-adrenoreceptors and of cardiac vascular β-adrenergic and dopaminergic receptors (158,159). Associations have been demonstrated among lead-exposed workers between their blood lead levels and plasma concentrations of renin activity, levels of blood angiotensin I, angiotensin-converting enzyme (ACE), and aldosterone (160).

### Gastrointestinal Tract

Gastrointestinal disturbances are frequent complaints in persons with increased lead absorption. Like symptoms related to the nervous system, the severity of gastrointestinal symptoms also span a wide range. At moderately elevated blood lead concentrations, many of the symptoms are nonspecific and may consist of epigastric discomfort, nausea, anorexia, weight loss, and dyspepsia. At high blood lead concentrations, usually exceeding 80 μg/dl, these nonspecific symptoms can become accompanied by severe, intermittent abdominal cramps known as lead colic (20,161,162). The pain associated with lead colic is usually very severe. This symptom complex is typically associated with constipation of several days' duration. During a severe attack of colic, the patient's blood pressure is frequently elevated, and there is concomitant bradycardia. The origin of lead colic is uncertain, but the direct action of lead on visceral smooth muscle tone and vagal irritation associated with intestinal ischemia has been suggested as underlying pathology.

### Joint Pain

Arthralgia, often associated with muscle aches and pain, is a frequent symptom of lead poisoning. Although generally connected with chronic poisoning, joint pain is not infrequently reported by workers following exposure of rather brief duration, e.g., a few weeks, exhibiting moderately elevated blood lead concentrations. Arthralgia often prompts the experienced lead worker to seek medical attention, since it tends to indicate that the blood lead concentration is on the rise.

### Effects of Lead on Reproduction

During the past decades, increased attention has been focused on potentially adverse effects on human reproductive function caused by occupational and environmental exposures. The concern over such effects has been emphasized in the promulgation of occupational health and safety standards on exposure limits for inorganic lead (163,164).

Toxic effects of lead on reproductive organs have been well documented in both male and female laboratory animals. Lead has been found to cause a dose-related decrease in the conversion of $^{14}C$-lactate to carbon dioxide in studies of energy metabolism of isolated male rat spermatocytes, whereas studies on cultured Sertoli cells have demonstrated an increase in lactate production and a decrease in the conversion of $^{14}C$ glucose to $^{14}CO_2$ (165). Because of the high metabolic activity associated with spermatogenesis and the low concentrations of certain glycolytic enzymes in spermatocytes and spermatids, the testis may be particularly vulnerable to lead and other xenobiotic substances that interfere with energy metabolism (166).

In female animals, failure of blastocyte implantation was noted following administration of lead compounds at various stages of pregnancy. Since treatment with progesterone and estradiol brought about normal implantation, it was suggested that the inhibition of implantation by lead is due principally to its action on the hormone balance of the mother (167,168). Moreover, the ability of cultured mouse blastocytes to attach and spread was shown to be adversely affected by the presence of lead in the medium, in a dose-related manner (169). Other investigators found changes in morphology and implantation in young fetuses of mice exposed to lead during gestation, suggesting that these resulted from increased rate of chromosome aberrations in the maternal bone marrow cells (170).

In humans, lead-induced effects on reproductive function are less clearly defined. Although documentation of lead as a human teratogen is sparse, it is considered to act as such. An increased number of miscarriages, abortions, and stillbirths appear to have been related to high lead exposures of pregnant women. Lead crosses the placental barrier and can easily reach the fetus (171,172). Premature membrane rupture and preterm delivery have been associated with high lead content of fetal membranes (173). There are few data to permit assessment of the extent to which maternal exposures at currently prevailing exposure levels in a well-controlled, modern industry are associated with spontaneous abortion. At moderately elevated exposure levels, this risk is likely to be significant (174).

Other reproductive effects associated with excessive exposure to lead have been reported both among males and females. Early epidemiologic studies demonstrated both a reduction of the number of offspring in families of workers occupationally exposed to lead (175) and an increase of the miscarriage rate for women whose husbands were exposed to lead (176). More recent evidence suggests that paternal occupational exposure to lead is an important factor in causing reproductive dysfunction and adverse reproductive outcome, including spontaneous abortion (177).

Adverse effects on semen quality by occupational exposure to lead have been documented in several studies. One early study reported a dose-related decrease in sperm quality, including density, motility, and particularly morphology (178). The noted abnormalities were thought to have reflected a direct effect by lead on the gonads; no abnormalities were recorded in the gonadotropins and androgens. These findings were corroborated by a study that compared lead-exposed battery workers with nonexposed cement workers. Although no differences in hormone levels were found, the battery workers had lower sperm density than the comparison group (179). Another investigation, however, demonstrated both an impairment of the regulation of luteinizing hormone secretion and a direct effect on the testis manifested by oligozoospermia and peritubular fibrosis (180).

The potential reversibility of lead-induced effects on male reproductive function is suggested by a case report of a lead-poisoned firearms instructor who, following chelation therapy, was monitored over a 3-year period with semen quality parameters and biologic indices of lead exposure. A gradual decline in blood lead and ZPP levels was associated with improvement of sperm density and morphology; he fathered a healthy child when his blood lead level had declined to within the acceptable range (181). Partial improvement in semen quality following chelation therapy of male workers heavily exposed to lead has been reported by others (182). Dysfunction of the prostate and seminal vesicles affecting sperm motility has been observed in battery workers at relatively low blood lead concentrations (183).

Reversible lead-induced infertility has also been reported in experimental animals (184). Lead administered orally to rats caused damage to the seminiferous tubule epithelium, decreased sperm motility, and infertility in males. A subsequent report, however, failed to demonstrate changes in the morphology of rat seminiferous tubules examined by light and electron microscopy (185). An *in vitro* model of toxicity testing, in which x-ray microchemical analysis was used to localize lead in sperm cell organelles, found accumulation of the metal in the sperm head, the site in which ultramorphologic abnormalities were most prominent (186). Further epidemiologic and clinical studies are necessary to evaluate whether high levels of lead in semen may play a teratogenic role or adversely affect nucleic acids in offspring (187). Adverse effects on semen continue to be reported (188,189).

### Lead Poisoning in Children

Childhood lead poisoning is considered a major public health problem in the United States and in many countries worldwide. Data from U.S. nationwide screening programs conducted in the 1970s demonstrated that 5%

to 10% of preschool children aged 1 to 6 years residing in high-risk areas with deteriorating urban housing were exposed to hazardous levels of lead and exhibited evidence of undue lead absorption. In some cities the prevalence was close to 20%!

It was estimated that 3.9% of North American children younger than 5 years had blood lead levels of 30 μg/dl or higher and that a total of 675,000 preschool children had elevated blood lead levels (190). Subsequently, the U.S. Centers for Disease Control and Prevention lowered the definition of an elevated blood lead level from 30 to 25 μg/dl, whereas lead toxicity was considered present when the elevated blood lead concentration was accompanied by an erythrocyte protoporphyrin (EP) level of 35 μg/dl (191). An estimate published in 1988 by the Agency for Toxic Substances and Disease Registry put the number of preschool children at risk for lead toxicity at more than 5 million (192), i.e., 17.2% of preschool children.

Although there are several potential sources of lead in the child's environment, ingestion of chips or flakes of lead-based paint, which have a sweet taste, are the most important sources, resulting in acute overexposure and intoxication (193–195).

Children, however, are considered society's critical receptors for hazardous effects of ambient environmental lead pollution caused by industrial emissions and automobile exhausts (15,196). Children are more susceptible to the toxic effects of lead than adults; insufficient intake of iron, calcium, and vitamin D among some disadvantaged groups may further increase these effects (197,198). Children living in the vicinity of lead-emitting factories and children whose parents or close relatives work in industrial facilities where lead exposure occur are other populations that are at risk for increased lead absorption (199–203).

The great concern and enormous efforts now under way in many countries to control environmental lead exposure have been spurred in particular by investigations that have demonstrated abnormal neurologic development in children as a result of increased lead absorption from sources in the ambient environment, either during the fetal stage or during early childhood development (204). The blood lead levels associated with such effects are much lower than those traditionally related to (acute) childhood lead poisoning resulting from specific sources of exposure such as ingestion of lead paint chips. Children with blood lead levels associated with neurologic abnormalities have no history of clinical lead poisoning, a condition that long has been considered a cause of abnormal neurologic development. The main reason for the great concern over the public health implications of lead pollution is that several investigations have provided evidence that damage to the nervous system occur in children at blood lead levels that until the past decade were widely considered normal or safe for the general population. Such impairments include adverse effects on intellectual development, behavioral abnormalities, and learning difficulties resulting in poor school performance (205,206).

It has become increasingly clear that adverse, often subtle, neuropsychological effects can be demonstrated at levels of lead exposure that are very prevalent in modern Western society (207–210).

Of even greater concern is the observation that the degree of lead absorption at which such adverse effects can be detected appears to become progressively lower and that the health implications of blood lead concentrations that are nowadays frequently found in young children may be significant (211). Evidence is accumulating from long-term prospective studies that the magnitude of this particular public health risk to children may be greater than was hitherto estimated (212–216). A link between elevated body burden of lead and antisocial and delinquent behavior has also been reported (217).

The exposure to lead of the child begins *in utero* and the evaluation of the individual's entire exposure situation should include the fetus and its exposure via the pregnant mother (218,219).

Because of the evidence that adverse health effects are detected at progressively lower blood lead levels (191), the U.S. federal definition of lead toxicity and the blood lead level at which intervention is recommended is currently set at 10 μg/dl (220). Moreover, it is recommended that the goal of all lead poisoning prevention activities should be to reduce children's blood levels below 10 μg/dl, since the no-effect level may be below this blood level. If a significant number of children in a community exhibit blood lead levels ≥10 μg/dl, communitywide primary prevention activities should be instituted. Intervention for individual children should begin at blood lead concentrations of 15 μg/dl. Children with blood lead levels ≥20 μg/dl need complete medical evaluations.

## INDICATORS OF EXPOSURE AND EFFECTS—EXAMINATIONS OF LEAD-EXPOSED WORKERS

Several laboratory tests are available for evaluating the degree of lead absorption and related health effects. In the United States, the federal Occupational Safety and Health Administration (OSHA) of the Department of Labor promulgated legislation (lead standard) in 1978 that prescribes requirements for environmental and biologic monitoring in lead-related industries (163,164,221). Although the following discussion addresses application of diagnostic tests primarily related to the U.S. regulations, the reader must consider adherence to legislative issues in respective countries.

At present, measurement of blood lead concentration is the best available indicator of current lead absorption or dose; blood lead measurement is, in fact, the mainstay of biologic monitoring worldwide. The biologic response tests such as ZPP, FEP, and ALA-D are useful in assessing lead-related biochemical effects of occupationally exposed workers or in locations where the availability of blood lead determinations may be limited. Determinations of ZPP and FEP are recommended for screening purposes. The ZPP test can be performed at the field examination site with a portable instrument, a hematofluorometer, which has much practical value. Elevated ZPP concentrations must be confirmed and correlated with the blood lead level, which is a more specific indicator of actual lead absorption. Information about lead absorption is important, and periodic measurements of blood lead levels are the cornerstone in the biologic monitoring of workers employed at a workplace where there is potential for excessive exposure to lead.

Several attempts have been made over the years to relate blood lead levels to abnormalities in biologic response tests and to adverse health effects (222–224). Tables 1 and 2 summarize the current concepts of the relationship between blood lead levels and lead-induced abnormalities as lowest-observed-effect levels (100). The information presented in the tables should be considered approximate and not as a definitive representation of no-effect levels. It is not possible to determine a precise blood lead concentration below which symptoms never occur or a blood lead level at which symptoms are always present. Individual susceptibility must be considered in this context.

Another point to consider is the relationship between blood lead concentrations and air lead levels. Despite difficulties of establishing an exact relationship, OSHA has set a final permissible exposure limit of 50 μg/m³ averaged over 8 hours. It is estimated that this exposure level will achieve the goal of maintaining the blood lead level below 40 μg/dl in the great majority of workers. This blood lead concentration constitutes the current biologic standard for exposure to inorganic lead in the United States. Control of atmospheric lead exposure must be achieved by adequate engineering design and procedure. This is unquestionably the best method for effective, reliable control of the workplace atmosphere; acting on the emission source to eliminate or reduce exposure should be the general goal.

Biologic monitoring and medical surveillance programs must be instituted at a workplace where risk of excessive lead exposure is suspected; this is defined as a location where the concentration of lead in air is 30 μg/m³ or higher for more than 30 days per year. The final standard of OSHA and a review contains the details of such programs, and only a few pertinent general rules are discussed here (163,164,221). The frequency of blood lead and ZPP monitoring is determined by the duration of the exposure and its intensity. Sampling every 6 months is required in occupational settings where the risk for clinical intoxication is relatively low, i.e., when repeated blood lead measurements have documented levels below 40 μg/dl.

**TABLE 1.** *Summary of lowest-observed-effect levels for key lead-induced health effects in adults*

| Lowest-observed-effect level (PbB) (μg/dl) | Heme synthesis and hematologic effects | Neurologic effects | Effects on the kidney | Reproductive function effects | Cardiovascular effects |
|---|---|---|---|---|---|
| 100–120 | | Encephalopathic signs and symptoms | Chronic nephropathy | | |
| 80 | Frank anemia | | ↓ | | |
| 60 | | ↑ | | | |
| 50 | Reduced hemoglobin production | Overt subencephalopathic neurologic symptoms ↓ | | | |
| 40 | Increased urinary ALA and elevated coproporphyrins | Peripheral nerve dysfunction (slowed nerve conduction) | | | |
| 30 | | ↓ | | Female reproductive effects<br>Altered testicular function ↓ | Elevated blood pressure (white males, aged 40–59) ↓ |
| 25–30 | Erythrocyte protoporphyrin (EP) elevation in males | | | | |
| 15–20 | Erythrocyte protoporphyrin (EP) elevation in females | | | | |
| <10 | ALA-D inhibition | | | | ? |

PbB, blood lead concentrations.
From ref. 100.

**TABLE 2.** *Summary of lowest-observed-effect levels for key lead-induced health effects in children*

| Lowest-observed-effect level (PbB) (μg/dl) | Heme synthesis and hematologic effects | Neurologic and related effects | Renal system effects | Gastrointestinal effects |
|---|---|---|---|---|
| 80–100 | | Encephalopathic signs and symptoms | Chronic nephropathy (aminoaciduria, etc.) | Colic and other overt gastrointestinal symptoms ↓ |
| 70 | Frank anemia | | | |
| 60 | ↓ | Peripheral neuropathies | | |
| 50 | ? | ↓ ? | | |
| 40 | Reduced hemoglobin synthesis<br>Elevated coproporphyrin<br>Increased urinary ALA | Peripheral nerve dysfunction (slowed NCVs)<br>CNS cognitive effects (IQ deficits, etc.) | | |
| 30 | | ? | Vitamin D metabolism interference | |
| 15 | Erythrocyte protoporphyrin elevation | Altered CNS electrophysiologic responses | ↓ | |
| 10 | ALA-D inhibition<br>Py-5-N activity inhibition ↓ ? | MDI deficits, reduced gestational age and birth weight (prenatal exposure) ↓ ? | ? | |

PbB, blood lead concentrations.
Py-5-N, pyrimidine-5′-nucleotidase.
From ref. 100.

If an employee is found to have a blood lead concentration above 40 μg/dl, but below mandatory levels indicating medical removal from work, sampling for lead and ZPP levels should be repeated at least every 2 months. At extremely high levels of exposure, retesting may be required at more frequent intervals. If an employee has one blood lead concentration ≥60 μg/dl, or several blood tests averaging ≥50 μg/dl over a six-month time period, removal from the workplace is mandatory; blood lead measurements should be repeated every month. The worker may return to work only when two consecutive blood tests are at 40 μg/dl or below. Any blood level requiring removal from work must be confirmed with a second test within two weeks. However, in case of severe lead poisoning accompanied by markedly elevated levels, samplings may be required more frequently, as determined by the examining physician. In addition to laboratory tests, medical surveillance must include, over and above preemployment examination, a thorough physical examination with review of medical and occupational histories and symptoms as well as supplementary blood tests such as ZPP, complete blood count, and examination of peripheral blood smear, serum creatinine, blood urea nitrogen, routine urinalysis, and perhaps other tests indicated by the medical evaluation or the nature of work. Semen analysis or pregnancy test can be requested by the employee. Determinations of other heme enzymes and metabolites, such as ALA-D, urinary ALA, and urinary lead concentration, can be included in individual cases. The mainstays of monitoring tests, however, are the blood lead and ZPP determinations. A blood lead level exceeding 40 μg/dl and a ZPP level exceeding 50 μg/dl (70 μmol/mol heme) in an adult male should draw immediate attention to lead overexposure and should prompt investigation of the work environment. Although 40 μg/dl has been established as a maximum permissible blood lead level, it is recommended that for workers, especially those who plan to have children, the level be below 30 μg/dl.

Heavy metal registries have been established in some states (e.g., New York, California) that require reporting of abnormal blood or urine levels of lead. The current reportable blood lead concentration is 25 μg/dl. This system has the potential for securing optimal follow-up of the worker's medical condition, the work environment, and the worker's immediate family members, particularly children, who may be at risk for excessive paraoccupational lead exposure in the home. The reader is reminded that the blood lead and ZPP levels mentioned above apply only to the work environment and that the alert blood lead level for children in the community is 10 μg/dl.

The different biologic and medical representations of blood lead and ZPP should be kept in mind: The blood lead level reflects current or relatively recent exposure, whereas the ZPP represents a metabolic effect on the erythroid cells in the bone marrow. Brief significant lead exposure raises the blood lead level and is followed by an increase in ZPP. When exposure ceases, blood lead declines more rapidly than ZPP. Although individual variations in susceptibility and exposure must be considered (225,226), the administration of both tests provides sufficient information to adequately characterize both the degree of exposure (absorption) and the biologic response (effect) (20,27,227).

The laboratory tests most frequently used for the diagnosis of lead poisoning outlined above are only one aspect of the diagnostic process. The clinical symptoms previously discussed are an important constituent of clinical intoxication and should always be explored. Many of the neurologic and gastrointestinal symptoms are nonspecific, and unless the examining physician is aware of the potential source of lead exposure the diagnosis may easily be overlooked (228).

In general, physical examination may detect few signs of lead poisoning. Pallor is sometimes present in patients with anemia. Thorough examination of motor strength may reveal weakness of the extensor muscles of the wrist and fingers, particularly of the hand used more actively. Overt wrist drop, described in the past among workers with chronic lead intoxication associated with long-standing elevated blood lead levels, is rarely seen nowadays in industrialized countries that have adequate industrial hygiene practices in operation but do occur in poor working conditions. Palsies may affect other muscle groups, but the extensors of the wrist and fingers and the extensors of the foot and toes are those most frequently involved. In contrast to the neuropathy associated with exposure to arsenic, neurosensory symptoms are not typical of lead poisoning. Burton's gum lead line, one of the classic signs of lead poisoning, is rarely seen at the present time in clinical practice. Typically, the line is a bluish stippling along the lower incisors. It consists of lead sulfide, which originates from the reaction between absorbed lead and hydrogen sulfide produced by bacterial decomposition of protein material between the teeth. Improved environmental control in industry and modern preventive dental hygienic care have reduced the frequency of this physical sign; its presence strongly supports the diagnosis.

With improved exposure control of the work environment, today's occupational lead poisoning is mostly characterized by subtle, nonspecific neurologic and gastrointestinal symptoms, and the diagnosis is usually made following evaluation of the laboratory test results in conjunction with clinical evaluation.

### Lead and Nutrition

The absorption of lead from the gastrointestinal tract and the toxicity of the absorbed metal are much influenced by the nutritional status of the individual; there is evidence that deficiency in some nutrients exacerbates the toxic effects of lead (229). Lead absorption is known to be influenced by dietary intake of calcium, phosphorus, iron, vitamin D, and fat. For example, a diet low in calcium and iron tends to increase lead absorption and exacerbate the toxic effect, while a high-fat diet increases lead deposition in several tissues. Vitamin C and thiamine, as well as thiamine in combination with zinc or vitamin E, have been demonstrated to counteract some of the toxic effects of lead in experimental studies (230–232).

Since milk contains high concentrations of calcium, phosphorus, zinc, and protein, it has been traditionally promoted as a dietary supplement that has protective effects against lead poisoning. It was common practice, and still is in many circles, for lead-exposed workers to add extra milk to their daily diet. In earlier decades, administration of milk was particularly common in cases of acute lead poisoning. It was also thought that lead accompanies calcium into the skeleton and that the biologically active form of lead in the soft tissues would be deposited more rapidly in the bones, thereby avoiding significant biologic effects. Experimental studies, however, have demonstrated that lactose increases intestinal absorption of lead; the interaction between lead and calcium is very complex. Experimental animal studies have demonstrated that when lead is ingested with a calcium-deficient diet it inhibits intestinal calcium absorption, but with adequate calcium in the diet the intestinal calcium absorption was not diminished (233). The issue of additional milk intake as a protection against lead poisoning is complex but has very strong roots in many working groups (234). It is obvious, however, that preventive measures against occupational lead poisoning must rely on adequate industrial hygiene practices in the work environment, and not on dietary factors such as additional intake of milk.

## TREATMENT

When lead poisoning has been diagnosed in a worker, the first course of action is to discontinue exposure, which often is the only required treatment. The medical treatment for lead poisoning has taken many curious forms throughout history (235), but administration of chelating agents is currently the treatment of choice.

Whether discontinuation of exposure is sufficient or whether chelation therapy should be administered depends on the degree of blood lead elevation, severity of clinical symptoms, biochemical and hematologic disturbances, and type of exposure. All these factors must be taken into consideration in determining the necessity for chelation therapy. No specific blood lead concentration can be designated above which treatment with a chelating agent is always indicated. In most cases, however, it is well above 80 μg/dl, a level frequently associated with more severe symptoms. When it is necessary to treat with a chelating agent, CaEDTA is often the drug of choice. The use of dimercaprol (BAL) and penicillamine is on the decline today (236).

CaEDTA is administered in either acute symptomatic lead poisoning or, during the course of chronic lead poisoning, in cases of acute exacerbations, manifested by severe neurologic and gastrointestinal symptoms or rapid rise of the blood lead level. These are the two principal circumstances in which chelation therapy is often indicated.

Administration of chelation therapy should always be done after cessation of lead exposure and under careful medical supervision in a hospital. As mentioned, it is mandatory that the patient not be exposed to lead during the treatment for a few weeks following treatment.

Therapeutic daily doses up to 50 mg/kg, a maximum rate of administration of 20 mg per minute, and a total course of therapy restricted to 5 days is a typical treatment protocol. The medication is given intravenously in a dose of 1 g in 250 ml 5% dextrose in water as a slow infusion over 1 hour, two times a day for 5 days. In addition, 24-hour urine collections should be done to measure the amount of lead excreted during the therapy. The amount excreted during the initial 48 hours is the most informative reflection of the severity of the pretreatment situation, in terms of the amount of lead that is released from various tissue stores. Alertness should be maintained for possible occurrence of cardiac arrhythmias and for evidence of renal damage (i.e., acute tubule necrosis), potential side effects of the treatment. Daily routine urine analyses should therefore be performed.

Because of mobilization of lead from various tissue stores, the effectiveness of the treatment as a means of lowering the initially high blood lead level can only be examined approximately 5 to 7 days after the treatment course, when a blood sample should be drawn for lead analysis. If a second course is indicated, it should not be started until after a recovery period of 7 to 10 days.

The administration of CaEDTA as the so-called EDTA-mobilization test, or provocative chelation test, to obtain an estimate of the total body burden of lead is a matter of continuous debate. It has been recommended for both adults and children in cases of mild symptoms or with borderline blood lead levels, to determine whether chelation therapy is indicated. A positive result after the administration of up to 2 g CaEDTA is 600 μg lead in a 24-hour urine collection. From long clinical experience, it appears that the administration of the test is rarely indicated and that its use is declining. Recent experimental evidence that lead from bone and other soft tissues is redistributed into the central nervous system following the mobilization test has raised concern over its safety and casts doubt on its future use (237–239).

The therapeutic handling of pediatric cases is more complex. CaEDTA and BAL are often given in combination and administered intramuscularly. In general, treatment begins with an injection of BAL only, and every 4 hours thereafter BAL and CaEDTA are given simultaneously at separate intramuscular sites. The usual doses are 4 mg/kg BAL and 12.5 mg/kg CaEDTA, and a normal course is 5 days. For detailed information on treatment of children, a standard pediatrics text should be consulted.

An oral chelating agent is currently in use, 2,3-dimercaptosuccinic acid (DMSA), which has proven to be an effective antidote for lead poisoning. DMSA may be superior to CaEDTA in enhancing excretion of lead from those stores in the body that are most directly relevant to the adverse health effects of lead (240). The drug does not appear to influence the release of essential minerals such as zinc and iron from the body (241,242). Another therapeutic approach to the management of lead poisoning has been introduced utilizing S-adenosyl-L-methionine as an agent that appears to rectify biochemical abnormalities of lead poisoning on the basis of making glutathione available (243). Although the chelating agents are useful and have dramatically lowered the mortality from lead encephalopathy, especially in children, the most crucial aspect of therapy must be prompt termination of undue lead exposure, whether in the occupational or the ambient environment. Increased awareness of occupational lead poisoning, combined with case-finding efforts, has improved diagnostic laboratory methods applied in clinical field surveys, and enforcement of government regulations has enabled some countries to effectively control this preventable occupational disease (244). However, occupational lead poisoning is still a disease to be reckoned with in the United States (245–248). Major efforts continue to end the chapter of pediatric lead poisoning in the United States, and implementation of public health measures, particularly the introduction of unleaded gasoline, have proven successful (15,45,46,249).

## CASE STUDY 1

The patient, a 52-year-old iron worker, sought our attention with the chief complaint of crampy abdominal pain and vomiting during the preceding few days. The pain was severe, intermittent, and was concentrated in the periumbilical area. The patient stayed bedridden, and found he could ease the pain by assuming the fetal position. The patient also complained of extreme fatigue, dizziness, sleep disturbances, and diffuse aches and pains in joints and muscles. He reported recent loss of appetite and weight loss.

The patient, a demolition worker, had participated in the demolition of an old elevated railway line in New York City during the 4 months prior to seeking medical attention. He had used an oxyacetylene-propane torch to cut through the steel and iron structures, which were coated with lead-based paint. He had not used a respirator. His medical history included a femoral-femoral bypass operation in 1976. He had reported a previous lead poisoning incident in 1974 as a result of demolition work on another elevated railway line in the New York metropolitan area.

Laboratory workup revealed a blood lead concentration of 183 μg/dl; the blood ZPP value was 350 μg/dl, and hemoglobin 12.1 mg/dl. The patient was hospitalized and treated with calcium disodium EDTA (Versenate), 1 g twice daily for 5 days. Symptoms were relieved after a few days of treatment. The crampy, abdominal pain disappeared, and his appetite improved. The course of treatment was uneventful, and 10 days after the last treatment, the blood level was 50 μg/dl.

The patient was followed as an outpatient. Two weeks after his discharge from the hospital, he noted the return of some abdominal symptoms. His blood lead concentration at that time was 89 μg/dl. The patient was readmitted to the hospital and given a second course of chelation therapy, which he tolerated well. A 3-month follow-up revealed normalization of the blood lead level. His symptoms had disappeared, and he returned to a job that did not directly expose him to lead.

### Comment

The patient, who presented with severe gastrointestinal and neurologic symptoms of lead poisoning, had performed a job known to be associated with exposure to very high concentrations of lead. The application of an oxyacetylene-propane torch to a surface covered with red lead paint generates lead oxide fumes, which are readily inhaled by workers unless they wear proper respirators. For this type of work, a positive-pressure air-supplied respirator is usually required. The patient had been working for a 3-month period without any protection and gradually had absorbed large amounts of lead. The crampy abdominal pain, which is typical of lead colic, began abruptly one day when he was working, and was associated with constipation and vomiting. The severe symptoms and high blood lead level necessitated immediate chelation therapy. At a blood lead level of 183 μg/dl, there is risk of acute encephalopathy. Although the first course of chelation therapy lowered his blood lead level considerably, there was a second increase a few weeks later. This increase, or rebound effect, was also associated with the return of some abdominal symptoms and required a second course of chelation therapy. It is recommended that the patient have a rest period of 1 to 2 weeks between courses of chelation therapy. It should also be noted that the patient had lead poisoning 4 years prior to this incident and that an adequate respirator was not used at that particular job site. With prompt discontinuation of lead exposure and with treatment, his symptoms disappeared and the metabolic disturbances were normalized.

## CASE STUDY 2

A 42-year-old man sought medical attention because of unusual fatigue, malaise, diffuse joint and muscle pain, and abdominal discomfort. There was no history of crampy abdominal pain or constipation, but he had noticed a weight loss of 5 kg during the preceding 2 months. One year prior to this, he had bought a house that had been built in the 1840s, and 4 months prior to his seeking medical attention, he had acquired a heat gun and had begun removing old interior paint from walls and from woodwork around the doors and windows. He had noticed fumes and dust during this process and therefore used a simple paper surgical mask as respiratory protection. When he was first examined, his blood lead concentration was 98 μg/dl and his ZPP level was 220 μg/dl. There was no anemia, but urinary excretion levels of ALA and coproporphyrins were markedly elevated, 24.8 μg/ml and 4.58 nmol/L, respectively. Because of the severity of symptoms and elevated blood lead levels, the patient was admitted to the hospital and treated with calcium disodium EDTA (Versenate), 1 g twice daily for 3 days. Because of the appearance of microscopic hematuria, the chelation therapy was discontinued on the third day. During the course of therapy, 12 mg of lead was excreted. Ten days posttreatment his blood lead level had declined to 63 μg/dl, while the ZPP level was unchanged at 220 μg/dl. Urine ALA had decreased to 3.54 μg/ml. The patient's symptoms disappeared rapidly, and he noted a weight gain of 2.5 kg. One month later, the blood lead level was reduced to 54 μg/dl (250).

### Comment

Although the source of undue exposure might seem unusual, this case illustrates several points of clinical interest. The presenting symptoms were nonspecific and included fatigue, malaise, aches and pains in the muscles and joints, abdominal discomfort, and slight weight loss. None of the symptoms is specific for lead poisoning; neither lead colic nor constipation was present. However, in conjunction with a history of significant exposure to lead, a higher degree of specificity can be ascribed to such vague symptoms. The importance of obtaining a detailed occupational history is illustrated by the fact that the patient's regular occupation was not associated with any lead hazard, while his hobby or work at home was.

The chelation therapy was uneventful in this case, except for the appearance of microscopic hematuria. This emphasizes the need to carefully monitor patients who undergo chelation therapy and to perform daily urine analysis. The blood lead level fell rapidly and was within an acceptable range 10 days after treatment. The erythrocyte protoporphyrin level, however, remained elevated. This was expected, since the porphyrin concentration indicates a more chronic effect on the erythroid cells in the bone marrow. Several months elapsed before both blood lead and ZPP were completely normal, illustrating that the patient had accumulated a considerable body burden of lead from this work. The central nervous system symptoms and gastrointestinal symptoms are usually nonspecific and vague in lead poisoning. Awareness by the physician of a potential exposure source is essential in reaching a correct diagnosis. By taking a detailed, thorough occupational history, which must probe for exposure associated with hobbies and part-time occupations, the physician is more likely to succeed in identifying the work-related illness.

## CASE STUDY 3

The patient was a 35-year-old woman who sought our medical attention because of her awareness through the press of an unusual case of lead poisoning in an art conservator and because she had noted a change in the labeling on one of the products she had used for a long time in her work as a potter. The medical history was noncontributory. No specific gastrointestinal symptoms were reported, but fatigue was a prominent symptom. The patient associated this symptom with her long work hours. She reported no sleep disturbances but had experienced slight dizziness.

The findings of the physical examination were normal. The neurologic examination was normal, with no obvious weakness of the extensor muscles. A complete blood count was also normal. The patient was an artist and had been working as a potter for 17 years. She reported using an air brush when applying glazes containing fritted lead on ceramic tiles. On pottery, she routinely used nonfritted lead glazes, which she mixed herself with kaolin (clay). She devoted approximately 20 hours per week to the tile work, and described an air mist when applying the glaze. She used an OSHA-approved respirator as protection against airborne contaminants. Her studio was approximately 600 square feet and occupied half the surface of a floor in a loft. The other half served as the family's living quarters. The studio was separated from the apartment by a corridor and an opening with a plastic curtain. Of particular concern was the fact that the patient's 5-year-old daughter was often present in the studio while the mother was working, especially during a 5-month period preceding the mother's medical examination. She used to touch the glaze and to paint her own pottery and wore only a paper face mask. The daughter did not report any symptoms, such as malaise, headache, or abdominal cramps. There were no noted behavioral changes and she was functioning well in kindergarten. A routine pediatric evaluation 4 months prior to this presentation was normal.

Her examination at this time revealed normal physical and neurologic findings. A complete blood count did not reveal any abnormalities. The laboratory findings demonstrated that both the artist and her daughter manifested significantly elevated blood lead concentrations at the initial examination [48 μg/dl (2.32 μmol/L) and 54 μg/dl (2.61 μmol/L), respectively]. The EP levels were also elevated. The patient stopped using the compounds that were most likely associated with the excessive lead exposure. Six weeks later, improvements were noted in the blood lead concentrations. Almost 2 years later, despite continued work with extreme precautions and the phasing out of all lead compounds, the artist's blood lead concentration was still slightly elevated at 23 μg/dl (1.11μmol/L), which is higher than the levels of persons who have no history of a specific source of occupational lead exposure (251).

### Comment

This report describes an experienced artist-potter, who, although she used principally fritted lead glazes (but sometimes nonfritted ones), had an elevated blood lead level and other abnormal biochemical signs of lead intoxication. Although the artist took rigorous protective measures, the blood lead concentrations remained slightly elevated for a long time after the original exposure was discontinued. It is possible that low-level exposure to lead occurred during some period of this time, but the impact of several years' exposure may have also contributed to the slightly elevated blood lead levels. Of additional interest and concern was the finding of increased lead absorption in the artist's 5-year-old daughter, who was often present in the studio when work was in progress. The child, on occasions, also performed her own work, handling lead frits and painting pottery items, and she was at risk for both indirect (bystander's) and direct occupational exposure. She manifested an elevated blood lead concentration and abnormal protoporphyrin level.

This case report illustrates that artists who make pottery may handle potentially harmful substances against which industrial hygiene protective measures are necessary. The awareness of such risk, in this case by an individual artist, made early detection of adverse lead-related effects possible. This was particularly important because the artist's child was also exposed to lead. Special precautions must also be taken to prevent small children from being exposed to hazardous materials in the artist's environment. Prolonged exposure under these conditions could have resulted in serious adverse health effects for the child. Information about the contents of materials and their potential health effects ought to be more widely disseminated among artists working with pottery and ceramics. Their work area should be considered as an industrial environment that should be separated from living quarters.

## CASE STUDY 4

A 41-year-old man presented with nonspecific neurologic symptoms including dizziness, headache, irritability, and sleeplessness of 3 months' duration. In addition to these symptoms there was a history of infertility. He had fathered one child in a previous marriage 14 years prior to the examination. No diagnosis had been obtained for either the patient or his wife explaining the infertility. The patient had previously worked for 2 years as a firearms instructor, primarily at an indoor firing range. He was also in charge of cleaning and maintenance of the facility. The ventilation system of the range was reported to have intermittent malfunctions. No air measurements were available. The blood lead concentration was 88 μg/dl (4.25 μmol/L) and the blood ZPP level was 355 μg/dl—both values indicative of lead poisoning. The patient underwent chelation therapy with dimercaptosuccinic acid according to a clinical research protocol. Semen quality was evaluated prior to and after chelation therapy and during the subsequent 3-year period. After an initial sperm count of 10 million, a dramatic increase was noted, and by the time the blood lead concentration had decreased to approximately 30 μg/dl the patient's wife conceived (181).

### Comment

There are inconclusive results in the literature regarding lead-related effects on male reproductive function. This case illustrates the importance of maintaining prospective observation of lead-exposed persons which can clarify the relation between increased lead absorption and male reproductive function. The infertility problem coincided with the patient's starting work as a firearms instructor, a potentially lead-related occupation. The improvement in semen quality paralleled the decrease in blood lead and ZPP concentrations; the most significant improvements were in sperm density and total sperm count. The case further illustrates that lead-induced infertility can be reversible.

## ORGANIC LEAD COMPOUNDS

Tetraethyl lead was introduced commercially in 1923 and has been used since the 1960s as a supplementary antiknock agent in gasoline. During combustion in the engine, the compound is broken down to inorganic lead compounds such as carbonates, oxycarbonates, and oxides, which constitute most important sources of lead pollution in the general environment. However, some organic lead may also be present in automobile exhaust fumes if the compound has not undergone combustion. The organic lead compounds are colorless liquids that are insoluble in water but soluble in organic solvents. Exposure to these compounds occurs principally during synthesis, transport, and mixing with gasoline. Tetraethyl lead is normally added to gasoline together with other organic halogen compounds such as ethylene dibromide, the latter acting as a scavenger for the removal of lead after combustion. Current world production is estimated to be 300,000 tons per year.

The toxicity of organic lead compounds was recognized soon after they were first employed, and in the 1920s several cases of severe poisoning were described (252). Stricter industrial hygiene regulations were introduced in 1926, and a considerable reduction in the number of cases with clinical intoxication followed.

The toxicity of organic lead differs markedly from that of inorganic lead compounds. Tetraethyl lead is fat soluble and easily absorbed through the skin; in contrast to the inorganic lead compounds, the organic lead substances can cause lead poisoning by absorption through the skin. It should be noted that penetration of the skin usually occurs without causing local injury. Inhalation of vapor is another important route of entry into the body for organic lead compounds. Tetraethyl lead is converted to triethyl lead in the liver, and triethyl lead is the active toxic derivative (253).

Because of the solubility of organic lead in fat, accumulation occurs in the central nervous system, and symptoms of intoxication are referable primarily to this organ system. One of the early symptoms is insomnia, and it can be accompanied by headache, anxiety, restlessness, and excitation of the nervous system. In more severe cases, encephalopathy occurs with a variety of symptoms, including hallucinations, convulsions, and acute psychosis. The gastrointestinal symptoms are usually mild and include abdominal discomfort and anorexia, but the abdominal cramps (colic), so typical of inorganic lead poisoning, usually do not occur. Muscle, hepatic, and renal damage has also been observed in cases of organic lead poisoning from gasoline sniffing (254,255). A history of exposure to organic lead compounds and subsequent development of encephalopathy suggest the diagnosis. The blood lead level is slightly elevated, but the degree of elevation usually does not correspond to the severity of clinical symptoms. Erythrocyte protoporphyrin, urine aminolevulinic acid, and urine coproporphyrin levels may remain within normal range. A high level of lead in urine supports the diagnosis.

Removal from exposure and supportive treatment should be undertaken immediately, but the use of chelating agents is of doubtful value. Strict industrial hygiene measures, including personal protective equipment such as impervious clothing and goggles, is mandatory. The significance of exposure among garage employees and service station attendants is unresolved. The introduction of unleaded gasoline has lowered urban air levels of organic lead in the United States, but in countries where the number of automobiles is steadily increasing and the use of unleaded gasoline is not yet initiated, lead levels are rising. Experimental studies have demonstrated a carcinogenic effect for certain organic lead compounds (256,257). The Department of Labor standard is 0.075 $mg/m^3$ for tetraethyl lead as an 8-hour time-weighted average (TWA).

## REFERENCES


1. Nriago JO. *Lead and lead poisoning in antiquity.* New York: Wiley Interscience, 1983.
2. Wedeen RP. *Poison in the pot. The legacy of lead.* Carbondale and Edwardsville, IL: Southern Illinois University Press, 1984.
3. *The Babylonian Talmud.* In: Epstein I, ed. *Tractate: Rosh Hashana.* London: The Soncino Press, 1978;24-B.
4. Eisinger J. Lead and wine. Eberhard Gockel and the colica Pictonum. *Med Hist* 1982;26:279–302.
5. Gilfillan SC. Lead poisoning and the fall of Rome. *J Occup Med* 1965;7:53–60.
6. Gockel E. De vini acidi per acetum lithargyri cum maximo bibentium damno dulcificatione. *Ephemerides* (Misc. Curiosa) 1697; Ann. 4, Obs. 30:77–85. (Cited by Eisinger, ref. 4.)
7. McCord CP. Lead and lead poisoning in early America: Benjamin Franklin and lead poisoning. *Ind Med Surg* 1953;22:394.
8. Hamilton A. *Exploring the dangerous trades.* Boston: Little, Brown, 1943.
9. Aub JC, Fairhall LT, Minot AS, Reznikoff P. Lead poisoning. *Medicine* 1925;4:1–250.
10. Corn J. Historical perspective to a current controversy on the clinical spectrum of plumbism. *MMFQ Health Society* 1975;Winter:93–114.
11. Marks G, Beatty WK. *The precious metals of medicine.* New York: Scribners, 1975;118–127.
12. Fergusson JE. *The heavy elements:* chemistry, *environmental impact and health effects.* Oxford: Pergamon Press, 1990.
13. Patterson CC. Contaminated and natural lead environments of man. *Arch Environ Health* 1965;11:344–360.
14. Rutter M, Russel Jones R, eds. *Lead versus health.* Chichester: John Wiley, 1983.
15. Silbergeld EK. The international dimensions of lead exposure. *Int J Occup Environ Health* 1995;1:336–348.
16. Organization for Economic Cooperation and Development. *Risk reduction.* Monograph No. 1: lead. Paris, France: OECD Environment Directorate, 1993.
17. Agocs MM, Etzel RA, Parrish G, et al. Mercury exposure from interior latex paint. *N Engl J Med* 1990;323:1096–1101.
18. Committee on Lead in the Human Environment. *Lead in the human environment.* Washington, DC: Environmental Studies Board, Commission on Natural Resources, National Research Council, National Academy of Sciences, 1980.
19. Baker EL, Landrigan PJ, Barbour AG, et al. Occupational lead poisoning in the United States: clinical and biochemical findings related to blood lead levels. *Br J Ind Med* 1979;36:314–322.
20. Lilis R, Fischbein A, Eisinger J, et al. Prevalence of lead disease among secondary lead smelter workers and biological indicators of lead exposure. *Environ Res* 1977;14:255–285.
21. Fischbein A, Daum SM, Davidow B, et al. Lead hazard among ironworkers dismantling lead-painted elevated subway line in New York City. *NY State J Med* 1978;78:1250–1259.
22. Spee TS, Zwennis WCM. Lead exposure during demolition of a steel structure coated with lead-based paints. I. Environmental and biological monitoring. *Scand J Work Environ Health* 1987;13:52–55.
23. Muijser H, Hoogendijk EMG, Hooisma J, Twisk DAM. Lead exposure during demolition of a steel structure coated with lead-based paints. II. Reversible changes in the conduction velocity of the motor nerves in transiently exposed workers. *Scand J Work Environ Health* 1987;13:56–61.
24. Fischbein A, Leeds M, Solomon S. Lead exposure among ironworkers in New York City: a continuing occupational hazard in the 1980s. *NY State J Med* 1984;84:445–448.
25. Marino PE, Franzblau A, Lilis R, Landrigan P. Acute lead poisoning in construction workers: the failure of current protective standards. *Arch Environ Health* 1989;44:140–145.
26. Goldman RH. Lead poisoning in automobile radiator mechanics. *N Engl J Med* 1987;317:214–218.
27. Fischbein A, Thornton JD, Blumberg WE, et al. Health status of cable splicers with low-level exposure to lead: results of a clinical survey. *Am J Public Health* 1980;70:697–700.
28. Fischbein A, Thornton JD, Berube L, Villa F, Selikoff IJ. Lead exposure reduction in workers using stabilizers in PVC manufacture: effects of a new encapsulated stabilizer. *Am Ind Hyg Assoc J* 1982;43:652–655.
29. Fischbein A, Rice C, Sarkozi L, et al. Exposure to lead in firing ranges. *JAMA* 1979;241:1141–1144.
30. Novotny T, Cook M, Hughes J, Lee SA. Lead exposure in a firing range. *Am J Public Health* 1987;77:1225–1226.
31. Valway SE, Martyny JW, Miller JR, Cook M, Mangione EJ. Lead absorption in indoor firing range users. *Am J Public Health* 1989;79:1029–1032.
32. Ozonoff D. Lead on the range. Commentary. *Lancet* 1994;343:6–7.
33. McCann M, Barazani G, eds. *Health hazards in the arts and crafts.* Washington, DC: Society for Occupational and Environmental Health, 1980.
34. Environmental Protection Agency. *Air quality criteria for lead.* EPA publication 600/8-83/028dF. Research Triangle Park, NC: U.S. Environmental Protection Agency; 1986.
35. Murozumi M, Chow TJ, Patterson CC. Chemical concentrations of pollutant lead aerosols, terrestrial dusts and sea salt in Greenland and Antarctic snow strata. *Geochim Cosmochim Acta* 1969;33:1247–1294.
36. Yaffe Y, Flessel CP, Weselowski JJ, et al. Identification of lead sources in California children using the stable isotope ratio technique. *Arch Environ Health* 1983;38:227–245.
37. Elhelu MA, Caldwell DT, Hirpassa WD. Lead in inner-city soil and its possible contribution to children's blood lead. *Arch Environ Health* 1995;50:2:165–169.
38. Piomelli S, Corash L, Corash MB, et al. Blood lead concentrations in a remote Himalayan population. *Science* 1980;210:1135–1137.
39. Settle DM, Patterson CC. Lead in albacore: guide to lead pollution in Americans. *Science* 1980;207:1167–1176.
40. Flegal AR, Smith DR. Lead levels in preindustrial humans (letter). *N Engl J Med* 1992;326:1293–1294.
41. National Center for Health Statistics, and Center for Environmental Health (CDC). Blood lead levels in the U.S. population. *MMWR* 1982; 31:132–134.
42. Annest JL, Pirkle JL, Makric D, Neese JW, Bayse DD, Kovac MG. Chronological trend in blood lead levels between 1976 and 1980. *N Engl J Med* 1983;308:1373–1377.
43. Schutz A, Attewell R, Skerfving S. Decreasing blood lead in Swedish children, 1978–1988. *Arch Environ Health* 1989;44:391–394.
44. Ducoffre G, Claeys F, Bruaux P. Lowering time trend of blood lead levels in Belgium since 1978. *Environ Res* 1990;51:25–34.
45. Brody DJ, Pirkle J, Kramer RA, Flegal KM, Matte TD, Gunter E, Paschal DE. Blood lead levels in the US population. Phase 1 of the Third National Health and Nutrition Examination Survey (NHANES III, 1988-1991). *JAMA* 1994;272(4):277–283.
46. Pirkle J, Brody DJ, Gunter E, et al. The decline in blood lead levels in the United. The National Health and Nutrition Examination Surveys (NHANES). *JAMA* 1994;272(4):284–291.
47. Strömberg D, Schütz A, Skerfving S. Substantial decrease of blood lead in Swedish children, 1978–1994, associated with petrol lead. *Occup Environ Med* 1995;11:764–769.
48. Nriago JO, Blankson ML, Ocran K. Childhood lead poisoning in Africa: a growing public health problem. *Sci Tot Environ* 1996;181:93–100.
49. Rabinowitz M, Wetherill GW, Kopple JD. Magnitude of lead intake from respiration by normal man. *J Lab Clin Med* 1977;90:238–248.
50. James AC. Lung deposition of sub-micron aerosols calculated as a function of age and breathing rate. In: National Radiological Protection Board. *Annual research and development report.* Harwell, United Kingdom: National Radiological Protection Board, Atomic Energy Research Establishment, 1978:71–75.
51. Rabinowitz MB, Kopple JD, Wetherill GW. Effect of food intake and fasting on gastrointestinal lead absorption in humans. *Am J Clin Nutr* 1980;33:1784–1788.
52. Chisolm JJ Jr. Dose-effect relationship for lead in young children: evidence in children for interactions among lead, zinc and iron. In: Lynam DR, Piantanida LG, Cole JF, eds. *Environmental lead:* proceedings of the Second International Symposium on Environmental Lead Research. New York: Academic Press, 1981:1–7.
53. Ziegler EE, Edwards BB, Jensen RL, Mahaffey KR, Fomon SJ. Absorption and retention of lead by infants. *Pediatr Res* 1978;12:29–34.
54. Elwood PC. The source of lead in blood: a critical review. *Sci Total Environ* 1986;52:1–23.
55. Willers S, Schütz A, Attewell R, Skerfving S. Relation between lead and cadmium in blood and the involuntary smoking of children. *Scand J Work Environ Health* 1988;14:385–389.

56. Rabinowitz MB, Wetherill GW, Kopple JD. Kinetic analysis of lead metabolism in healthy humans. *J Clin Invest* 1976;58:260–270.
57. Marcus AH. Multicompartment kinetic models for lead: III. Lead in blood plasma and erythrocytes. *Environ Res* 1985;36:473–489.
58. DeSilva PE. Determination of lead in plasma and studies of its relationship to lead in erythrocytes. *Br J Ind Med* 1981;38:209–217.
59. Mushak P. New directions in the toxicokinetics of human lead exposure. *Neurotoxicology* 1993;14:29.
60. Heard MJ, Chamberlain AC. Uptake of lead by human skeleton and comparative metabolism of lead and alkaline earth elements. *Health Phys* 1984;47:857–865.
61. Ahlgren L, Liden K, Mattsson S, Tejning S. X-ray fluorescence analysis of lead in human skeleton in-vivo. *Scand J Work Environ Health* 1976;2:82–86.
62. Ahlgren L, Mattsson S. An x-ray fluorescence technique for in vivo determination of lead concentrations in a bone matrix. *Phys Med Biol* 1979;24:136–145.
63. Wielopolski L, Rosen JF, Slatkin DN, Vartsky D, Ellis KJ, Cohn SH. Non-invasive x-ray fluorescence analysis of lead in the human tibia. *Med Phys* 1983;10:248–251.
64. Somervaille LJ, Chettle DR, Scott MC, et al. In vivo tibia lead measurements as an index of cumulative exposure in occupationally exposed subjects. *Br J Ind Med* 1988;45:174–181.
65. Rosen JF, Markowitz ME, Bijur PE, et al. L-line x-ray fluorescence of cortical bone lead compared with CaNa2 EDTA test in lead-toxic children: public health implications. *Proc Natl Acad Sci USA* 1989;86: 685–689.
66. Wedeen RD. In vivo tibial XRF measurement of bone lead [editorial]. *Arch Environ Health* 1990;45:69–71.
67. Sokas RK, Besarab A, Mcdiarmid MA, Shapiro IM, Bloch P. Sensitivity of in vivo x-ray fluorescence determination of skeletal lead stores. *Arch Environ Health* 1990;45:268–272.
68. Hu H, Milder FL, Burger DE. X-ray fluorescence measurements of lead burden in subjects with low-level community lead exposure. *Arch Environ Health* 1990;45:335–341.
69. Schütz A, Skerfving S, Christoffersson JO, Ahlgren L. Lead in vertebral bone biopsies from active and retired lead workers. *Arch Environ Health* 1987;42:340–346.
70. Borjesson J, Gerhardsson L, Schütz A, Mattssom S, Skerfving S, Österberg K. In vivo measurements of lead in fingerbone in active and retired lead smelterers. *Int Arch Occup Environ Health* 1997;69: 97–105.
71. Singhal RL, Thomas JA, eds. *Lead toxicity.* Baltimore: Urban & Schwarzenberg, 1980.
72. Eisinger J. Biochemistry and measurement of environmental lead intoxication. *Q Rev Biophys* 1978;11:439–466.
73. Granick JL, Sassa S, Kappas A. Lead intoxication. *Adv Clin Chem* 1978;20:288–339.
74. Forni A, Camiaghi G, Sechi GC. Initial occupational exposure to lead: chromosome and biochemical findings. *Arch Environ Health* 1976; 31:73–78.
75. Forni A, Sciame A, Bertazzi PA, Alessio L. Chromosome and biochemical studies in women occupationally exposed to lead. *Arch Environ Health* 1980;35:139–146.
76. Nordenson I, Beckman G, Beckman L, Nordström S. Occupational and environmental risks in and around a smelter in northern Sweden: IV. Chromosomal aberrations in workers exposed to lead. *Hereditas* 1978;88:263–267.
77. Bauchinger M, Dresp J, Schmid E, Englert N, Krause C. Chromosome analyses of children after ecological lead exposure. *Mutat Res* 1977; 56:75–79.
78. Maki-Paakkanen J, Sorsa M, Vainio H. Chromosome aberrations and sister chromatid exchanges in lead-exposed workers. *Hereditas* 1981; 94:269–275.
79. Huang XP, Feng ZY, Zhai WL, Xu JH. Chromosomal aberrations and sister chromatid exchanges in workers exposed to lead. *Biomed Environ Sci* 1988;1:382–387.
80. Farkas W, Fischbein A, Solomon S, Buschman F, Borek E, Sharma OK. Elevated urinary excretion of β-aminoisobutyric acid and exposure to inorganic lead. *Arch Environ Health* 1987;42:96–99.
81. Angle CR, McIntire MS, Swanson MS, Stohs SJ. Erythrocyte nucleotides in children—increased blood lead and cytidine triphosphate. *Pediatrics* 1982;16:331–334.
82. Sakai T, Araki T, Ushio K. Accumulation of erythrocyte nucleotides and their pattern in lead workers. *Arch Environ Health* 1990;45: 273–277.
83. Hernberg S, Vihko V, Hassan J. Red cell membrane ATPases in workers exposed to inorganic lead. *Arch Environ Health* 1967;14:319–324.
84. Hajem S, Moreau T, Hannaert P, et al. Influence of environmental lead on membrane transport in a French urban male population. *Environ Res* 1990;53:105–118.
85. Fischbein A, Tsang P, Luo JCJ, Roboz JP, Jiang JD, Bekesi JG. Phenotypic aberrations of CD3+ and CD4+ cells and functional impairments of lymphocytes at low-level exposure to lead. *Clin Immunol Immunopathol* 1993;66:163–169.
86. Pyatt DW, Zheng JH, Stillman WS, Irons RD. Inorganic lead activates NF-kappa B in primary human CD4+ T lymphocytes. *Biochem Biophys Res Commun* 1996;227:380–385.
87. Boyland E, Dukes CE, Grover PL, Mitchley BCV. The induction of renal tumors by feeding lead acetate to rats. *Br J Cancer* 1962;16: 283–288.
88. Koller LO, Kerkvliet NI, Exon JH. Neoplasia induced in male rats fed lead acetate, ethylurea, and sodium nitrite. *Toxicol Pathol* 1985;13: 50–57.
89. Fu H, Bofetta P. Cancer and occupational exposure to inorganic lead compounds: a meta-analysis of published data. *Occup Environ Med* 1995;52:73–81.
90. Gerhardsson L, Hagmar L, Rylander L, Skerfving S. Mortality and cancer incidence among secondary lead smelters. *Occup Environ Med* 1995;52:667–672.
91. Cooper WC, Wong O, Kheifets L. Mortality among employees of lead battery plants and lead-producing plants 1947–1980. *Scand J Work Environ Health* 1985;11:331–345.
92. Lilis R. Long-term occupational lead exposure, chronic nephropathy, and renal cancer: a case report. *Am J Ind Med* 1981;2:293–297.
93. Baker EL, Goyer RA, Fowler RA, et al. Occupational lead exposure, nephropathy and renal cancer. *Am J Ind Med* 1980;1:139–148.
94. Lamola AA, Yamane T. Zinc protoporphyrin in the erythrocytes of patients with lead intoxication and iron deficiency anemia. *Science* 1974;186:936–938.
95. Wang YL, Lu PK, Chen ZQ, et al. Effects of occupational lead exposure. *Scand J Work Environ Health* 1985;11(suppl):20–25.
96. Wildt K, Berlin M, Isberg PE. Monitoring of zinc protoporphyrin levels in blood following occupational lead exposure. *Am J Ind Med* 1987;12:385–398.
97. Silbergeld EK, Hruska RE, Bradley D, Lamon JM, Frykholm BC.Neurotoxic aspects of porphyrinopathies: lead and succinylacetone. *Environ Res* 1982;29:459–471.
98. Granick JL, Sassa S, Granick S, et al. Studies in lead poisoning: II. Correlation between the ratio of activated to inactivated δ-aminolevulinic acid dehydratase of whole blood and the blood lead level. *Biochem Med* 1973;8:149–159.
99. Tola S, Hernberg S, Asp S, Nikkanen J. Parameters indicative of absorption and biological effect in new lead exposure. *Br J Ind Med* 1973;30:134–141.
100. ATSDR. *Toxicological profile for lead.* ATSDR publication TP-88/17. Updated version 1997. Draft toxicological profile for lead, August 1997. Atlanta, GA: U.S. Department of Health & Human Services, Public Health Service, Agency for Toxic Substances and Disease Registry, 1997.
101. Rosen JF. Metabolic abnormalities in lead toxic children: public health implications. *Bull NY Acad Med* 1989;65:1067–1083.
102. Wetmur JG, Bishop DF, Cantelmo C, Desnick RJ. Human δ-5-aminolevulinate dehydratase: nucleotide sequence of a full-length cDNA clone. *Proc Natl Acad Sci USA* 1986;83:7703–7707.
103. Chisholm JJ, Thomas DJ, Hamill TG. Erythrocyte porphobilinogen synthase activity as an indicator of lead exposure to children. *Clin Chem* 1985;31:601–605.
104. Haeger-Aronsen B. Studies on urinary excretion of δ-5-aminolevulinic acid and other haem precursors in lead workers and lead-intoxicated rabbits. *Scand J Clin Lab Invest* 1960;12(suppl 47):1–128.
105. Meredith PA, Moore MR, Campbell BC, Thompson GG, Goldberg A. δ-Aminolaevulinic acid metabolism in normal and lead-exposed humans. *Toxicology* 1978;9:1–9.
106. Sassa S, Granick JL, Granick S, et al. Studies in lead poisoning: I. Microanalysis of erythrocyte protoporphyrin levels by spectrophotometry in the detection of chronic lead intoxication in the subclinical range. *Biochem Med* 1973;8:135–148.

107. Blumberg WE, Eisinger J, Lamola AA, et al. The hematofluorometer. *Clin Chem* 1977;23:270–274.
108. Blumberg WE, Eisinger J, Lamola AA, Zuckerman DM. Zinc protoporphyrin level in blood determined by a portable hematofluorometer: a screening device for lead poisoning. *J Lab Clin Med* 1977;89: 712–723.
109. Eisinger JE, Blumberg WE, Fischbein A, et al. Zinc protoporphyrin in blood as a biological indicator of chronic lead intoxication. *J Environ Pathol Toxicol* 1978;1:897–910.
110. Lamola AA, Piomelli S, Pho-Fitzpatrick MB, Yamane T, Harber LC. Erythropoietic protoporphyria and lead intoxication: the molecular basis for difference in cutaneous photosensitivity: II. Different binding of erythrocyte protoporphyrin to hemoglobin. *J Clin Invest* 1975; 56:1528–1535.
111. Labbe RF, Rettmer RL, Shah AG, Turnlund JR. Zinc protoporphyrin. Past, present and future. *Ann NY Acad Sci* 1987;514:7–14.
112. Matsura Y, Fukuda T, Yoshida T, Kuroiwa Y. Inhibitory effect of zinc protoporphyrin on the induction of heme oxygenase and the associated decrease in cytochrome P-450 content in rats. *Toxicology* 1988; 50:169–180.
113. Cheson BD, Rom WN, Webber RC. Basophilic stippling of red blood cells—nonspecific finding of multiple etiology. *Am J Ind Med* 1984; 5:327–334.
114. Cullen MR, Robins JM, Eskenazi B. Adult inorganic lead intoxication: presentation of 31 new cases and a review of recent advances in the literature. *Medicine* 1983;62:221–247.
115. Lippmann M. Lead and human health: background and recent findings. *Environ Res* 1990;51:1–24.
116. Goyer RA. Lead toxicity: current concerns. *Environ Health Perspect* 1993;100:177–187.
117. Bryce-Smith D, Mathews Y, Stephens R. Mental health effects of lead on children. *Ambio* 1978;7:192.
118. Needleman HL, Gunnoe C, Leviton A, et al. Deficits in psychologic and classroom performance of children with elevated dentine lead levels. *N Engl J Med* 1979;300:689–695.
119. Bellinger D, Leviton A, Allred E, Rabinowitz M. Pre and post natal lead exposure and behavior problems in school-aged children. *Environ Res* 1994;66:12–30.
120. Hänninen H, Mantere P, Hernberg S, Seppäläinen AM, Kock B. Subjective symptoms to low-level exposure to lead. *Neurotoxicology* 1979;1:333–347.
121. Valciukas JA, Lilis R, Eisinger J, et al. Behavioral indicators of lead neurotoxicology: results of a clinical field survey. *Int Arch Occup Environ Health* 1978;41:217–236.
122. Johnson BL, Burg JR, Xintaras C, et al. A neurobehavioral examination of workers from a primary nonferrous smelter. *Neurotoxicology* 1980;1:561–581.
123. Hogstedt C, Hane M, Agrell A, Bodin L. Neuropsychological test results and symptoms among workers with well-defined long-term exposure to lead. *Br J Ind Med* 1983;40:99–105.
124. Stollery BT, Banks HA, Broadbent DE, Lee WR. Cognitive functioning in lead workers. *Br J Ind Med* 1989;46:698–707.
125. Balbus-Kornfeld JM, Stewart W, Bolla KI, Schwartz BS. Cumulative exposure to inorganic lead and neurobehavioural test performance in adults: an epidemiological review. *Occup Environ Med* 1995;52:2–12.
126. Arake S, Honma T. Relationships between lead absorption and peripheral nerve conduction velocities in lead workers. *Scand J Work Environ Health* 1976;4:225–231.
127. Seppäläinen AM, Hernberg S, Vesanto R, Kock B. Early neurotoxic effects of occupational lead exposure: a prospective study. *Neurotoxicology* 1983;4:181–192.
128. Spivey GH, Baloh RW, Brown CP, et al. Subclinical effects of chronic increased lead absorption—a prospective study: III. Neurologic findings at follow-up examination. *J Occup Med* 1980;22:607–612.
129. Seppäläinen AM, Tola S, Hernberg S, et al. Subclinical neuropathy at "safe" levels of lead exposure. *Arch Environ Health* 1975;30:180–183.
130. Araki S, Honma T, Yanagihara S, Ushio K. Recovery of slowed nerve conduction velocity in lead-exposed workers. *Int Arch Occup Environ Health* 1980;46:151–157.
131. Chia SE, Chia HP, Ong CN, Jeyaratnam J. Cumulative blood lead levels and nerve conduction parameters. *Occup Med* 1996;46:59–64.
132. Silbergeld EK, Hruska RE. Neurochemical investigations of low level exposure. In: Needleman HL, ed. *Low level lead exposure:* clinical implications of current research. New York: Raven Press, 1980;135–157.
133. David O, Clark J, Voeller K. Lead and hyperactivity. *Lancet* 1972;2: 900–903.
134. Dumas P, Gueldry D, Loireau A, Chomard P, Buthieau AM, Autissier N. Effects of lead poisoning on properties of brain mitochondria in young rats. *C R Soc Biol* 1985;179:175–183.
135. Slomianka L, Rungby J, West MJ, Danscher G, Andersen AH. Dose-dependent bimodal effect of low-level lead exposure on the developing hippocampal region of the rat: a volumetric study. *Neurotoxicology* 1989;10:177–190.
136. Windebank AJ, Dyck PJ. Localization of lead in rat peripheral nerve by electron microscopy. *Ann Neurol* 1985;18:197–201.
137. Brune D, Nordberg GF, Wester PO. Distribution of 23 elements in the kidney, liver and lung of workers from a smelter and refinery in North Sweden exposed to a number of elements and of a control group. *Sci Tot Environ* 1980;16:13–35.
138. Goyer RA. Renal changes associated with lead exposure. In: Mahaffey KR, ed. *Dietary and environmental lead:* human health effects. Amsterdam: Elsevier Science Publishers, 1985.
139. Chisolm JJ Jr. Aminoaciduria as a manifestation of renal tubular injury in lead intoxication and a comparison with patterns of aminoaciduria seen in other diseases. *J Pediatr* 1962;60:1–17.
140. Henderson DA. The etiology of chronic nephritis in Queensland. *Med J Aust* 1958;1:377–386.
141. Lilis R, Gavrilescu N, Nestorescu B, Dumitriu C, Roventa A. Nephropathy in chronic lead poisoning. *Br J Ind Med* 1968;25: 196–202.
142. Cramer L, Goyer RA, Jagenburg R, Marion H. Renal ultrastructure, renal function, and parameters of lead toxicity in workers with different periods of lead exposure. *Br J Ind Med* 1974;31:113–127.
143. Lilis R, Valciukas J, Fischbein A, Andrews G, Blumberg WE, Selikoff IJ. Renal function impairment in secondary lead smelter workers: correlations with zinc portoporphyrin and blood lead levels. *J Environ Pathol Toxicol* 1979;2:1447–1474.
144. Buchet JP, Roels H, Bernard A, Lauwerys R. Assessment of renal function of workers exposed to inorganic lead, cadmium or mercury vapor. *J Occup Med* 1980;22:741–752.
145. Meyer BR, Fischbein A, Rosenman K., Lerman Y, Drayer DE, Reidenberg M. Increased urinary enzyme excretion in workers exposed to nephrotoxic chemicals. *Am J Med* 1984;76:989–998.
146. Verschoor M, Wibowo A, Herber R, van Hemmen H, Zielhuis R. Influence of occupational low-level lead exposure on renal parameters. *Am J Ind Med* 1987;12:341–351.
147. Cardenas A, Roels H, Bernard AM, et al. Markers of early renal changes induced by industrial pollutants. II. Application to workers exposed to lead. *Br J Ind Med* 1993;50:28–36.
148. Roels H, Lauwerys R, Konings J, et al. Renal function and hyperfiltration capacity in lead smelter workers with high bone lead. *Occup Environ Med* 1994;51:505–512.
149. Batuman V, Maesaka JK, Haddad B, Tepper E, Wedeen RP. The role of lead in gout nephropathy. *N Engl J Med* 1981;304:520–523.
150. Wedeen R. Lead nephrotoxicity. In: Porter G, ed. *Nephrotoxic mechanisms of drugs and environmental toxins.* New York: Plenum Press, 1982.
151. Vigdortchik NA. Lead intoxication in the etiology of hypertonia. *J Ind Hyg* 1935;17:1–6.
152. Cooper WC, Gaffey WR. Mortality of lead workers. *J Occup Med* 1975;17:100–107.
153. Malcolm D, Barnett HAR. A mortality study of lead workers 1925–76. *Br J Ind Med* 1982;39:404–410.
154. Fanning D. A mortality study of lead workers, 1926–1985. *Arch Environ Health* 1988;43:247–251.
155. Kristensen TS. Cardiovascular diseases in the work environment. A critical review of the epidemiologic literature on chemical factors. *Scand J Work Environ Health* 1989;15:245–264.
156. Pocock SJ, Shaper AG, Ashby D, Delves T, Whitehead TP. Blood lead concentration, blood pressure, and renal function. *Br Med J* 1984;289: 872–874.
157. Harlan R, Landis JR, Schmouder RL, Goldstein NG, Harlan LC. Blood lead and blood pressure. Relationship in the adolescent and adult US population. *JAMA* 1985;253:530–534.
158. Boscolo P, Carmignani M. Neurohumoral blood pressure regulation in lead exposure. *Environ Health Perspect* 1988;78:101–106.
159. Schwartz J. Lead, blood pressure, and cardiovascular disease in men and women. *Environ Health Perspect* 1991;91:71–76.

160. Campbell BC, Meredith PA, Scott JJ. Lead exposure and changes in the renin-angiotensin-aldosterone system in man. *Toxicol Lett* 1985; 25:25–32.
161. Janin Y, Couinaud C, Stone A, Wise L. The lead-induced colic: syndrome in lead intoxication. *Surg Ann* 1985;17:287–307.
162. Fischbein A, Thornton JC, Lilis R, Valciukas JA, Bernstein J, Selikoff IJ. Zinc protoporphyrin, blood lead and clinical symptoms in two occupational groups with low-level exposure to lead. *Am J Ind Med* 1980;1:383–390.
163. Occupational exposure to lead: final standard. *Federal Register* 1981; 43(220):52952–53014, (225):54353–54616; 46(238):60758–60776.
164. Occupational Safety and Health Administration (OSHA), 1985. OSHA Occupational Standards. Permissable exposure limits. *Lead* 29 CFR §1910.1025.
165. Batsarseh LI, Welsh MJ, Brabec MJ. Effects of lead acetate on Sertoli cell lactate production and protein synthesis *in vitro*. *Cell Biol Toxicol* 1986;2:285–292.
166. Gray TJB. Application of *in vitro* systems in male reproductive toxicology. In: Lamb JC IV, Foster PMD, eds. *Physiology and toxicology of male reproduction.* London: Academic Press, 1987;225–256.
167. Jacquet P. Early embryonic development in lead intoxicated mice. *Arch Pathol Lab Med* 1977;101:641–643.
168. Wide M, Nilsson BO. Interference of lead with implantation in the mouse. A study of the surface ultrastructure of blastocytes and endometrium. *Teratology* 1979;20:101–114.
169. Wide M. Effect of inorganic lead on the mouse blastocyte *in vitro*. *Teratology* 1978;17:165–170.
170. Nayak BN, Ray M, Persaud TV, Nigli M. Relationship of embryotoxicity to genotoxicity of lead nitrate in mice. *Exp Pathol* 1989;36: 65–73.
171. Barltrop D. Transfer of lead to the human foetus. In: Barltrop D, Burland WL, eds. *Mineral metabolism in pediatrics.* Philadelphia: FA Davis, 1969;135–151.
172. Rabinowitz MB, Needleman HL. Temporal trends in the lead concentrations of umbilical cord blood. *Science* 1982;216:1429–1431.
173. Fahim MS, Fahim Z, Hall DG. Effects of subtoxic lead levels on pregnant women in the state of Missouri. *Res Commun Chem Pathol Pharmacol* 1976;13:309–331.
174. Sallmén M, Anttila A, Lindbohm ML, Kyyronen P, Taskinen H Hemminki K. Time to pregnancy among women occupationally exposed to lead. *J Occup Environ Med* 1995;37:931–934.
175. Chyzzer A. Des intoxications par le plomb se presentant dans le ceramique en Hongrie. *Chir Presse* 1908;44:906.
176. Rom WN. Effects of lead on the female and reproduction: a review. *Mt Sinai J Med* 1976;43:542–552.
177. Anttila A, Sallmén M. Effects of parental occupational exposure to lead and other metals on spontaneous abortion. *J Occup Environ Med* 1995;37:915–921.
178. Lancranjan J, Popescu HJ, Gavanescu O, Klepsch I, Serbanescu M.Reproductive ability of workmen occupationally exposed to lead. Arch. *Environ Health* 1975;30:396–401.
179. Assennato G, Paci C, Baser ME, et al. Sperm count suppression without endocrine dysfunction in lead-exposed men. *Arch Environ Health* 1987;42:124–127.
180. Braunstein GD, Dahlgren J, Loriaux DL. Hypogonadism in chronically lead-poisoned men. *Infertility* 1978;1:33–51.
181. Fisher-Fischbein J, Fischbein A, Melnick HD, Bardin CW. Correlation between biochemical indicators of lead exposure and semen quality in a lead-poisoned firearms instructor. *JAMA* 1987;257: 803–805.
182. Cullen MR, Kayne RD, Robins JM. Endocrine and reproductive dysfunction in men associated with occupational inorganic lead intoxication. *Arch Environ Health* 1984;39:431–440.
183. Wildt K, Eliasson R, Berlin M. Effects of occupational exposure to lead on sperm and semen. In: Clarkson TW, Nordberg CF, Sager PR, eds. *Reproductive and developmental toxicity of metals.* New York: Plenum Press, 1983;279–300.
184. Puhac I, Hrgovic N, Stankovic M. Laboratory investigation on the possibility of employing lead compounds as raticides by decreasing the reproductive capacity of rats. *Acta Vet* 1963;13:3–9.
185. Boscolo P, Carmignani M, Sacchettoni-Logroscino G, Rannelletti FO, Artese L, Preziosi P. Ultrastructure of the testis in rats with blood hypertension induced by long-term lead exposure. *Toxicol Lett* 1988; 41:129–137.
186. Fisher-Fischbein J, Bartoov B, Michaeli M, Heger-Maslansky B, Langsam J, Fischbein A. An *in vitro* model for the investigation of reproductive toxicity of chemical hazards in the male—I. metals: lead and copper. *Book of Abstracts 25th International Congress of Occupational Health,* Stockholm, September 15–20, 1996.
187. Thomas JA, Brogan WC III. Some actions of lead on the sperm and on the male reproductive system. *Am J Ind Med* 1983;4:127–134.
188. Xuezhi J, Youxin L, Yilan W. Studies of lead exposure on reproductive system: a review of work in China. *Biomed Environ Sci* 1992;5: 266–275.
189. Lerda D. Study of sperm characteristics in persons occupationally exposed to lead. *Am J Ind Med* 1992;22:567–571.
190. Mahaffey KR, Annest JL, Roberts J, Murphy RS. National estimates of blood lead levels: United States, 1976–1980. *N Engl J Med* 1982; 307:573–579.
191. Centers for Disease Control. *Preventing lead poisoning in young children.* Centers for Disease Control publication 99-2230. Atlanta, GA: U.S. Department of Health and Human Services, 1985.
192. Department of Health and Human Services. *The nature and extent of lead poisoning in children in the United States:* a report to Congress. Atlanta, GA: U.S. Department of Health and Human Services, 1988.
193. Lin-Fu JS. Lead poisoning and undue lead exposure in children: history and current status. In: Needleman HL, ed. *Low-level lead exposure:* the clinical implications of current research. New York: Raven, 1980.
194. Bornschein RL, Succop P, Krafft KM, Clark CS, Peace B, Hammond PB. Exterior surface dust lead, interior house dust lead and childhood lead exposure in an urban environment. In: Hemphil DD, eds. *Trace substances in environmental health.* Columbia, MO: University of Missouri, 1986;20:322–332.
195. Schwartz J, Levin R. The risk of lead toxicity in homes with lead paint hazard. *Environ Res* 1991;54:1–7.
196. Mauss EA. Childhood lead poisoning prevention: the tortuous trail from human health impact assessment to effective environmental policy. *Environ Impact Assess Rev* 1994;14:403–423.
197. Mahaffey KR, Gartside PS, Glueck CJ. Blood lead levels and dietary calcium intake in 1- to 11-year-old children: the Second National Health and Nutrition Examination Survey, 1976–1980. *Pediatrics* 1986;78:257–262.
198. Sorrell M, Rosen JF, Roginsky M. Interactions of lead, calcium, vitamin-D, and nutrition in lead-burdened children. *Arch Environ Health* 1977;32:160–164.
199. Delcourt JL, Hamrick HJ, O'Tauma LA, et al. Increased lead burden in children of battery workers: asymptomatic exposure resulting from contaminated work clothing. *Pediatrics* 1978;62:563–566.
200. Kaye WE, Novotny TE, Tucker M. New ceramics-related industry implicated in elevated blood lead levels in children. *Arch Environ Health* 1987;42:161–164.
201. Garrettson LK. Childhood lead poisoning in radiator mechanics' children. *Vet Hum Toxicol* 1988;30:112.
202. Wang JD, Shy WY, Chen JS, Yang KH. Parental occupational lead exposure and lead concentration of newborn cord blood. *Am J Ind Med* 1989;15:111–115.
203. Moore RS, Ducatman AM, Jozwiak JA. Home on the range: childhood lead exposure due to family occupation. Arch Pediatr Adolesc Med 1995;149:1276–1277.
204. McMichael AJ, Baghurst PA, Vimpani GV, Wigg NR, Robertson EF, Tong S. Tooth lead levels and IQ in school-age children: the Port Pirie Cohort Study. *Am J Epidemiol* 1994;140:489–499.
205. Needleman HL, Shapiro IM. Dentine lead in asymptomatic Philadelphia school children: subclinical exposure in high- and low-risk groups. *Environ Health Perspect* 1974;7:27–31.
206. de la Burde B, Choate MS Jr. Early asymptomatic lead exposure and development at school age. *J Pediatr* 1975;87:638–642.
207. Yule Q, Lansdown R, Millar IB, Urbanowicz MA. The relationship between blood lead concentrations, intelligence and attainment in a school population: a pilot study. *Dev Med Child Neurol* 1981;23: 567–576.
208. Fulton M, Raab G, Thomson G, Laxen D, Hunter R, Hepburn W. Influence of blood lead on the ability and attainment of children in Edinburgh. *Lancet* 1987;1:1221–1226.
209. Ernhart CB, Greene T. Low-level lead exposure in the prenatal and early preschool periods: language development. *Arch Environ Health* 1990;45:342–354.
210. Needleman HL, Schell A, Bellinger D, Leviton A, Allred EN. The

long- term effects of exposure to low doses of lead in childhood. An 11-year follow-up report. *N Engl J Med* 1990;322:83–88.
211. Paulozzi LJ, Shapp J, Drawbaugh RE, Carney JK. Prevalence of lead poisoning among two-year-old children in Vermont. *Pediatrics* 1995; 96:78–81.
212. Bellinger DC, Leviton A, Waternaux C, Rabinowitz M. Longitudinal analysis of prenatal and postnatal lead exposure and early cognitive development. *N Engl J Med* 1987;316:1037–1043.
213. Davis MJ, Svensgaard DJ. Lead and child development. *Nature* 1987; 329:297–300.
214. Dietrich KN, Krafft KM, Bornschein RL. Low-level fetal exposure effect on neurobehavioral development in early infancy. *Pediatrics* 1987;5:721–730.
215. McMichael AJ, Baghurst PA, Wigg NR, Vimpani GV, Robertson EF, Roberts RJ. Port Pirie cohort study: environmental exposure to lead and children's abilities at the age of 4 years. *N Engl J Med* 1988; 319:468–475.
216. Needleman HL, Gatsonis CA. Low-level lead exposure and the IQ of children. *JAMA* 1990;263:673–678.
217. Needleman H, Riess JA, Tobin MJ, Biesecker GE, Greenhouse JB. Bone lead levels and delinquent behavior. *JAMA* 1996;275:363–369.
218. Needleman H, Rabinowitz M, Leviton A, Linn S, Schoenbaum S. The relationship between prenatal exposure to lead and congenital anomalies. *JAMA* 1984;251:2956–2959.
219. Ernhart CB, Wolf AW, Kennard MJ, Erhard P, Filipovich HF, Sokol RJ. Intrauterine exposure to low levels of lead: the status of the neonate. *Arch Environ Health* 1986;41:287–291.
220. Centers for Disease Control. *Guidelines for the prevention of lead poisoning in children.* Atlanta, Georgia: U.S. Public Health Service, 1991.
221. Rempel D. The lead-exposed worker. *JAMA* 1989;262:532–534.
222. Zielhuis RL. Dose-response relationships for inorganic lead. I. Biochemical and haematological responses. *Int Arch Occup Health* 1975; 35:1–18.
223. Zielhuis RL. Dose-response relationships for inorganic lead. II. Subjective and functional responses-, chronic sequelae-, no-response levels. *Int Arch Occup Health* 1975;35:19–35.
224. Zielhuis RL. Second international workshop on permissible levels for occupational exposure to inorganic lead. *Int Arch Occup Environ Health* 1977;39:59–72.
225. Verschoor M, Herber R, Zielhuis R, Wibowo A. Zinc protoporphyrin as an indicator of lead exposure: precision of zinc protoporphyrin measurements. *Int Arch Occup Environ Health* 1987;59:613–621.
226. Grandjean P, Jørgensen PJ, Viskum S. Temporal and interindividual variation in erythrocyte zinc-protoporphyrin in lead- exposed workers. *Br J Ind Med* 1991;48:254–257.
227. Fischbein A. Zinc protoporphyrin in lead poisoning. *Lab Manag* 1981; 19:25–33.
228. Ibels LS. Lead intoxication. *Med Toxicol* 1986;1:387–410.
229. Mahaffey KR, Michaelson IA. The interaction between lead and nutrition. In: Needleman HL, ed. *Low-level lead exposure:* the clinical implications of current research. New York: Raven, 1980;159–200.
230. Dhawan M, Kachru DN, Tandon SK. Influence of thiamine and ascorbic acid supplementation on the antidotal efficacy of thiol chelators in experimental lead intoxication. *Arch Toxicol* 1988;62:301–304.
231. Flora SJ, Singh S, Tandon SK. Thiamine and zinc in prevention or therapy of lead intoxication. *J Int Med Res* 1989;17:68–75.
233. Fullmer CS, Rosen JF. Effect of dietary calcium and lead status on intestinal calcium absorption. *Environ Res* 1991;51:91–99.
234. Busnell PJ, DeLuca JF. Lactose facilitates the intestinal absorption of lead in weanling rats. *Science* 1981;211:61–63.
235. Greenberg M. *150 years in the treatment and prevention of lead poisoning by medical means—a historical review.* Report of Her Majesty's Factory Inspectorate. London: Her Majesty's Stationery Office, 1983;30–32.
236. Lilis R, Fischbein A. Chelation therapy in workers exposed to lead: a critical review. *JAMA* 1976;235:2823–2824.
237. Cory-Slechta DA, Weiss B, Cox C. Mobilization and redistribution of lead over the course of CaEDTA chelation therapy. *J Pharmacol Exp Ther* 1987;243:804–813.
238. Chisolm JJ Jr. Mobilization of lead by calcium disodium edetate. *Am J Dis Child* 1987;141:1256–1257.
239. Weinberger HL, Post EM, Schneider T, et al. An analysis of 248 initial mobilization tests performed on an ambulatory basis. *Am J Dis Child* 1987;141:1266–1270.
240. Lee BK, Schwartz B, Stewart W, Ahn KD. Provocative chelation with DMSA and EDTA:evidence for differential access to lead storage. *Occup Environ Med* 1995;52:13–19.
241. Graziano JH, Siris ES, LoIacono N, Silverberg SJ, Turgeon L. 2,3-Dimercaptosuccinic acid as an antidote for lead intoxication. *Clin Pharmacol Ther* 1985;37:431–438.
242. Graziano JH, LoIacono NJ, Meyer P. Dose-response study of oral 2,3-dimercaptosuccinic acid in children with elevated blood lead concentrations. *J Pediatr* 1988;113:751–757.
243. Paredes SR, Juknat de Geralnik AA, Batlle AM, Conti HA. Beneficial effect of S-adenosyl-L-methionine in lead intoxication. Another approach to clinical therapy. *Int J Biochem* 1985;17:625–629.
244. Hernberg S, Tola S. The battle against occupational lead poisoning in Finland: experiences during the 15-year period 1964–1978. *Scand J Work Environ Health* 1979;5:336–344.
245. Rudolph L, Sharp DS, Samuels S, Perkins C, Rosenberg J. Environmental and biological monitoring for lead exposure in California workplaces. *Am J Public Health* 1990;80:921–925.
246. Maizlish N, Rudolph L, Sutton P, Jones JR, Kizer KW. Elevated blood lead in California adults, 1987: results of a statewide surveillance program based on laboratory reports. *Am J Public Health* 1990;80: 931–934.
247. Silbergeld EK, Landrigan PJ, Froines JR, Pfeffer RM. The occupational lead standard: a goal unachieved, a process in need of repair. *New Solutions* 1991;3:18–28.
248. Chao KY, Wang JD. Increased lead absorption caused by working next to a lead recycling factory. *Am J Ind Med* 1994;26:229–235.
249. Needleman HL. Childhood lead poisoning: a disease for the history texts. *Am J Public Health* 1991;81:685–686.
250. Fischbein A, Anderson KE, Sassa S, et al. Lead poisoning from "do-it- yourself" heat guns for removing lead-based paint: report of two cases. *Environ Res* 1981;24:425–431.
251. Fischbein A, Sassa S, Butts G, Kaul B. Increased lead absorption in a potter and her family members. *NY State J Med* 1991;91:317–319.
252. Kehoe RA. Tetra-ethyl lead poisoning: clinical analysis of a series of nonfatal cases. *JAMA* 1925:85:108–110.
253. Cremer JE. Biochemical studies in the toxicity of tetraethyl lead and other organolead compounds. *Br J Ind Med* 1959:16:191–199.
254. Robinson RO. Tetraethyl lead poisoning from gasoline sniffing. *JAMA* 1978:240;1373–1374.
255. Hansen KS, Sharp FR. Gasoline sniffing, lead poisoning and myoclonus. *JAMA* 1978;240:1375–1376.
256. Epstein SS, Mantel N. Carcinogenicity of tetraethyl lead. *Experientia* 1968;24:580–581.
257. Odenbro A, Kihlstrom JE. Frequency of pregnancy and ova implantation in triethyl lead-treated mice. *Toxicol Appl Pharmacol* 1977;39: 359–363.

*Environmental and Occupational Medicine, Third Edition,* edited by William N. Rom.
Lippincott–Raven Publishers, Philadelphia © 1998.

# CHAPTER 69

# Mercury

Hugh L. Evans

## OCCURRENCE OF MERCURY IN THE ENVIRONMENT

Mercury (Hg) is a metal, and a natural component of the ocean and earth's crust. Compared to other elements, Hg is not a major component of the biosphere. The weather and human industry release Hg into the air and water, resulting in its redistribution and increasing the risk of human exposure (1,2). Everyone is exposed to Hg at some level, but any avoidable exposure to Hg is undesirable because Hg is not essential to any bodily functions.

When Hg becomes concentrated in the air, water, or foods as a result of human activity, it is considered to be a pollutant. Modern techniques can detect Hg in parts per billion (ppb) concentrations in the air or water (see Indices of Exposure, below). Mankind has used mercury since history began, most recently as a germicide and preservative, (e.g., in eye drops), for production of paper pulp, in chemical processes such as alkaline-chlorine plants, and in the manufacturing of vinyl. Hg is released from burning of fossil fuels and waste materials. Monitoring of environmental contamination may employ chemical analyses of sentinel animals or plant species that accumulate Hg from air or water, as well as specimens taken directly from humans. These monitoring strategies are discussed below.

Mercury exists in three forms: elemental (a liquid commonly known as quicksilver), inorganic mercury compounds, and organic compounds. Although all forms of Hg are toxic, the specific form of Hg influences how Hg moves through the environment and within the body. Both elemental and organic mercury are volatile and absorption by inhalation is significant. The GI tract accounts for the most significant absorption of inorganic Hg salts, and for nonoccupational exposures to organic Hg via the ingestion of foods.

H. L. Evans: Nelson Institute, New York University Medical Center, New York, New York 10016.

The toxicity of Hg compounds is the result of their affinity for sulfur and sulfhydryl groups; this affinity facilitates Hg binding with proteins, which in turn results in cytotoxicity. Alkylmercurials, the most toxic form of Hg (1), have a high absorbance from the GI tract and a slow rate of elimination from the body. These properties cause alkylmercurials to accumulate in both soft and hard tissue with continued exposure, even if the daily exposure is rather low (1,3). Details of the uptake, binding, distribution, and metabolism of Hg have been well described (1,4).

## POPULATIONS AT RISK FOR MERCURY EXPOSURE

Occupational exposure represents a significant portion of Hg poisoning cases. Miners extracting gold from Hg, or extracting Hg ore (mercuric sulfide, cinnabar, is the most prevalent form) provided early cases of occupational poisoning (5). Exposure is mostly by inhalation. Respiratory problems dominate the effects of short-term inhalation exposures. Longer-term exposures bring on signs of nervous system disorders (see Indices of Effects, below). Miners may have neurobehavioral deficits that persist for more than 10 years after the end of exposure (6).

The dental profession conveys higher risk of Hg poisoning because mercury-silver amalgams have been extensively used to fill dental caries. Exposure is by inhalation and dermal routes. Procedures for handling Hg in dentistry have improved along with increasing awareness of the health hazards of low-level exposure to Hg, and Hg amalgams are now used in only half of the dental

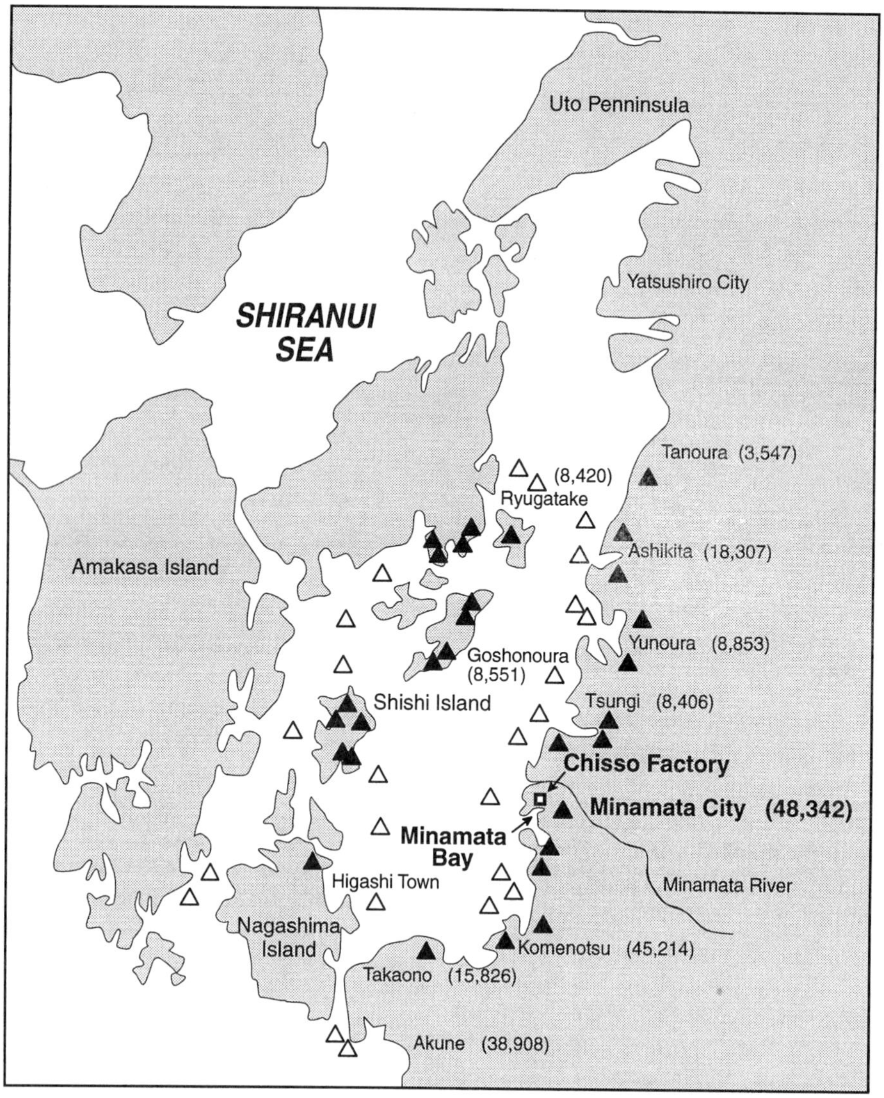


**FIG. 1.** Intoxicated cats discovered (▲) and fish found floating (△) provided early evidence of contamination of the Minamata environment by mercury. Numbers in parentheses refer to population. (Redrawn with permission from ref. 18.)

restorations of Americans. Dental personnel may have higher levels of Hg in their bodies (7,8) and may have higher incidence of nervous system impairment than employees of similar socioeconomic status who do not work with Hg (9,10). Female dental assistants whose work involved substantial use of Hg amalgams and who practiced "poor mercury hygiene" were less fertile than others who used less Hg in their work (11). Oddly, the women who used small amounts of amalgam in their work were more fertile than the control group who worked in dental offices that did not use amalgams. These results illustrate that more research is needed before we can fully understand the effects of low-level exposure to Hg.

Hg is also used in the calibration of glass, in fluorescent lamps, and in thermometers and electrical switches. Workers who had used elemental Hg to calibrate glassware illustrate the onset and recovery from Hg-induced tremor (12,13). Other current industrial uses are in paper pulp processing and in alkaline-chlorine factories (14). Clinical descriptions of these and other categories of occupational Hg poisoning of historical interest were described in the classic reference *Hunter's Diseases of Occupations* (5).

### Mercury in the Food Chain

Ingestion of Hg in food is responsible for the largest number of nonoccupational exposures. Hg is taken up by terrestrial and aquatic plants, which become food for humans and other animals. Inorganic Hg is converted to the more toxic organomercurial compounds, primarily by methylation by anaerobic microorganisms in the sedimentary layers of seas and lakes. As larger animal species feed on the plants or smaller animals, the content of Hg in the tissues becomes concentrated, reaching its highest levels in large fish such as tuna, and other predators at the top of the food chain. The major portion of Hg in fish is methylmercury (15). The risk from heavy consumption of these fish has caused public authorities to regulate the marketing of seafood having >1 part per million (ppm) Hg. Some seafoods contain significant amounts of selenium (7,16). Experiments indicate that selenium binds some of the Hg and thus reduces the toxicity that would occur with a given concentration of Hg without selenium.

The most profound examples of people poisoned by environmental Hg were in Iraq, where thousands of people were poisoned after making bread from seed grain that had been treated with methylmercury as a fungicide (17) and in Minamata, Japan (18,19) (Fig. 1). The Japanese episode illustrated the conversion of inorganic Hg to the more toxic organic forms, by aquatic organisms. Hg was discharged from a factory that used mercuric chloride in the manufacture of vinyl chloride. The effluent from the factory drained into a bay (see Fig. 1). Seafood was a principal part of the diet of the local people. The complex path of the runoff of inorganic Hg pollution from land to sea, its conversion to the highly toxic methylmercury, accumulation in the food chain, and finally the delayed manifestations of neurotoxicity among people made it difficult to trace the cause. The tragedies in Iraq and Japan also illustrated the fetus's higher vulnerability to Hg, with the most severe cases becoming apparent at birth but others displaying more subtle deficits later in the developmental process (18–20) (Fig. 2).

Attention has now shifted to children of fish-eating populations. Residents on islands (Seychelles, Faroes) where sea fish are the main component of the diet have slightly higher concentrations of Hg in their blood and hair than do other populations. These studies showed that mothers can transmit Hg to their fetus through their blood supply, and to their infant through maternal milk (21,22). Clear evidence of toxic effects is being sought for these relatively low exposures (22,23).

### Mercury Exposure from Dental Amalgams

Metallic Hg accounts for about 50% of the material in most dental fillings, and small amounts of Hg vapor are released from fillings. The World Health Organization recently concluded that Hg-silver amalgams, used in dentistry for about 150 years, offer several advantages over alternative materials for dental restorations; they provide a desirably hard surface, and are inexpensive and long-lasting. Most dentists believe that amalgams present the patient with no more health risk than that associated with alternative materials (24). However, people with Hg amalgams exhale increased levels of Hg after brushing teeth or chewing gum (25) and have higher levels of Hg in their blood or maternal milk than persons with few fillings (26). Hg from amalgams may be absorbed into the body through the buccal mucosa, the lung or the digestive tract (27,28). Hg appears in the nervous system and kidney of laboratory animals after they were given dental amalgams (27). These data demonstrate the uptake of Hg from amalgams into the body, but do not indicate whether the amount of Hg absorbed from amalgams contributes to health impairment.

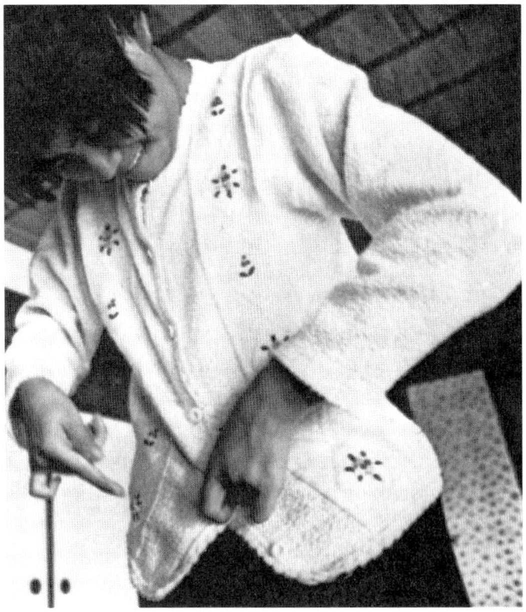

**FIG. 2.** Minamata victim: severe ataxia of upper limb displayed by buttoning. (From Putnam JJ. Quicksilver and slow death. *National Geographic* 1972;142:507.)

Long-term exposure to Hg from dental amalgams can be quantified by the number of amalgam surfaces in the mouth. The level of Hg in the urine represents primarily recent exposure, but urinary Hg levels may be proportional to the number of amalgams (7,29). Hg content of the blood and urine of adults with amalgam restorations is quite low (30,31), but Hg is known to accumulate in the kidney and nervous system, where it is less easily measured. Thus, there has been considerable speculation that accumulated Hg from dental amalgams may contribute to health problems (see Questions about Chelation Therapies, below).

There is little solid evidence of deleterious health effects that can be traced unambiguously to amalgam. The largest body of research on health effects of amalgams has been done in Sweden. Large epidemiologic studies of adults found no significant impairment of renal or immune systems related to amalgams (32–34). One study reported no relationship between amalgams and children's allergic problems (35). However, there is sufficient concern about Hg from amalgams affecting the more vulnerable, juvenile population to cause the National Institute of Dental Research to begin prospective clinical trials, the strongest experimental design for identifying health hazards from amalgams. At present, the large-scale replacement of an individual's amalgam fillings with nonmetallic materials seems unjustified because the drilling releases Hg and thus worsens the patient's exposure.

Occult religions and alternative medical practices lead to some Hg poisonings. Santeria, a quasi-religious practice that has been transplanted to the United States from the Caribbean islands (36), employs elemental Hg in potions that are thought capable of banishing evil forces from a person or their home. It is not surprising that exuberant use of such potions may result in accidental poisoning, but the extent of poisoning attributable to folk remedies is not known.

## INDICES OF EXPOSURE

### Air, Water, and Industrial Hygiene Control

Exposures to Hg in the workplace have become lower, and fewer cases of Hg poisoning are reported after governmental regulation of many organo-Hg compounds. The time-weighted average limit in the United States is 0.01 mg/m$^3$ for alkyl Hg compounds and 0.05 mg/m$^3$ for other Hg compounds (37). Exposure to Hg in the ambient air can be documented with personal monitoring devices (38).

Indices of human body burden are obtained by Hg content of hair, blood, and urine (2,39). Most cases of Hg toxicity are associated with detectable Hg in the urine. Exposure to metallic Hg vapor and inorganic Hg can be monitored in urinary Hg concentration, after adjustment for creatinine content (14). Concern should be triggered by biologic exposure Hg index values of >35 μg/g creatinine in urine (37). Exposure to methyl Hg is best indicated by the concentration of Hg in whole blood, where it is sequestered in the red cells. Blood Hg concentration is a better index of recent exposure to methylmercury than is urinary Hg. The elimination of Hg from blood and urine is much more rapid than from the whole body. Thus, blood and urine Hg concentrations are most influenced by recent exposures (e.g., within a week) and provide less evidence of past exposures (40).

A more extended chronology of past exposure to methyl Hg can be determined from the analysis of the concentration gradient of Hg along a strand of hair (41,42). Analysis of Hg in maternal hair may provide good evidence of fetal exposure during the various gestational stages. Hair and fingernails are useful indicator media for two reasons: these tissues are composed mostly of keratin, a protein that is formed from many sulfhydryl groups that can bind Hg during the growth process, and because cells of hair and nails survive for a relatively long time. However, care is required to avoid contamination of hair and nails with Hg external to the body, e.g., in dusts and cosmetic products.

Biologic specimens can be analyzed for total Hg content by atomic absorption methods. Cold vapor atomic absorption spectrometry is the most commonly used method to measure Hg in biologic samples (7,43). Digestion of the specimen may be required to liberate ionic Hg from the chemical matrix in which Hg is bound (1). Total mercury may be further analyzed into its organic and inorganic components, if gas chromatography is combined with the atomic absorption method (44). Other methods and their suitability, depending on the expected concentration of Hg in the specimen and the matrix in which Hg has been found, have been reviewed frequently (1).

### Biomarkers

Many new methods are being assessed for their ability to detect molecular or cellular changes that can be shown to indicate exposure to, or effects of, toxicants including Hg (45). Of particular relevance for Hg is the suggestion that evidence of nervous system damage caused by Hg may be seen in the peripheral blood, in the form of autoantibodies produced in response to fragments of damaged nervous system cells (46). *N*-acetyl-β-D-glucosaminidase (NAG) is one of a number of possible markers of renal changes in Hg-exposed workers (32,47,48). Elevation of urinary porphyrins, one of the earliest indices of chronic exposure to Hg in lab experiments (49), was also observed in dentists (9,50). Traditional indices of Hg effects, involving measures of behavioral and physiologic processes, are described below.

## INDICES OF EFFECTS

The kidney appears to be the critical organ for exposure to inorganic salts. The earliest change is proteinuria. Hg in all forms accumulates in the kidney and affects tubular and glomerular functions (49). Recovery of Hg-induced renal impairment is possible if the damage is not too great. Renal effects have been reported with chronic high-level occupational exposure to Hg vapor (32), in workers with intermittent exposure to Hg vapor (47), and in patients having dental amalgams (51). However, a later study found no association between amalgams and renal problems (25).

Neurotoxicity is the dominant feature of many Hg toxicity cases (1,52). Although steps have been taken to reduce exposures to Hg, improvements in testing have documented subtle neurobehavioral effects from low exposures that previously had been considered safe.

Occupational exposure to elemental Hg vapor has deleterious effects on visual-motor performance of adults (10,53). Two adolescents accidentally exposed to Hg vapor exhibited long-lasting deficits (54). Tremor (Fig. 3) was a consequence of substantial occupational exposure to Hg vapors (12,13), but was not significant in workers whose exposure was lower and intermittent (47). Studies of people have generally been confirmed by experiments with laboratory animals (19). Studies with animals are necessary to observe the effects of Hg without the influence of potentially confounding variables and to examine in detail the cellular effects of Hg on organs (45,55).

Emotional changes are probably the most commonly reported psychological symptom at a low level of chemical exposure. Affective changes, sometimes referred to as "erethism," have been frequently reported in Hg-exposed people. These changes begin with mild disorders such as anxiety and timidity. In more severe cases, there are personality changes, socially inappropriate behaviors, and performance deficits (9,50,56).

One of the most consistent findings in adults exposed to Hg vapor is slowed sensory nerve conduction velocity (1). Paresthesia, hypothesia, and tremor are commonly part of the clinical picture of Hg poisoning. Constriction of the visual field and other visual impairments are the result of damage to the central nervous system (57).

The toxicity of Hg is particularly severe during the earliest stages of prenatal and postnatal development. Cell migration and differentiation are easily disrupted by exogenous chemicals. The toxicity of Hg is also important at the end of the life span, when a critical body burden is attained after years of gradual accumulation of chemicals, and when the nervous system's reserve capacity has been diminished by cumulative loss of cells. The Japanese and Iraqi tragedies illustrates the special vulnerability at the early and late stages of the life span (18–20).

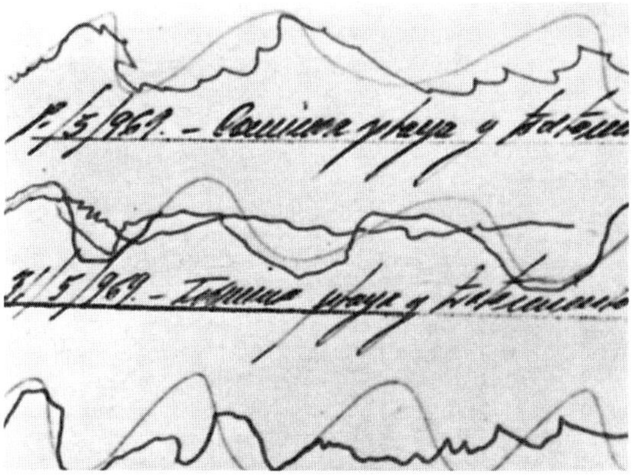

**FIG. 3.** Example of tremor affecting hands: "follow the line" test. (From Putnam JJ. Quicksilver and slow death. *National Geographic* 1972;142:507.)

Hg compounds are not carcinogenic in humans (1,58). Although evidence that Hg can affect the human immune system is sketchy, effects in animals justify further studies (1,46,59). A problem is that these effects appear to be quite variable. Hg has been associated with autoimmune diseases of the kidney and scleroderma (59). Intestinal bacteria may become resistant to Hg, and this resistance may be linked to resistance to antibiotic medication (27).

## CELLULAR AND MOLECULAR MECHANISMS

The metabolism of Hg compounds has been reviewed by Goyer (52). The molecular mechanisms of Hg toxicity have been reviewed by Clarkson (4) in terms of "molecular mimicry," in which the methylmercury cation reacts with the amino acid cysteine to form a compound that mimics the amino acid methionine and thus gains entry into the cell on the amino acid carrier. Toxicity results when Hg does not mimic essential ions and molecules in every circumstance. Additional molecular mechanisms have been reviewed by Atchison and Spitsbergen (60).

Many reports have demonstrated that Hg compounds, particularly methylmercury, damage neurons. A current question is whether the effects of Hg can be more clearly understood with reference to the role of glial cells in the brain's defense and the repair processes. Two type of glia, microglia and astroglia, may serve as filters, defending against of metals entering the brain. Glia also contribute to the repair of damaged neurons. The astroglial cells are affected in early stages of Hg neurotoxicity (46). However, the question is whether the defense and repair processes may, in some cases, occur at the expense of surviving cellular processes, and thus worsen rather than restore Hg-induced impairment (45,61).

## CHELATION THERAPY

Chelating agents have been used clinically as an antidote for severe toxicity of Hg (62,63). However, there is limited evidence of the safety and efficiency of chelating drugs to warrant their use for extended durations, for less severe cases, or for prophylactic treatment (63). Most studies have evaluated chelation outcome in terms of the metal's concentration in blood and other exposure indices (64); there is less evidence to indicate that chelation restores impaired function in the renal or nervous system toxicity of Hg (31).

Many of the neurobehavioral sequelae of Hg poisoning appear to be irreversible, and the severity of neurotoxicity is influenced by the duration of exposure as well as the magnitude of exposure (3). Thus, chelation or rehabilitation therapies may be useful only if administered in the early stages of intoxication, before irreversible changes occur. Numerous clinical case reports tell of apparently irreversible neurotoxicity of Hg that survives brief chelation treatment (64).

The most promising chelators are the dimercaprol derivatives, meso-2,3,-dimercaptsuccinic acid (DMSA, succimer) and dimercaptopropanesulfonate (DMPS, Dimaval). DMSA and DMPS have advantages over chelating agents used previously for the treatment of Hg toxicity, e.g., BAL (British anti-Lewisite, dimercaprol), EDTA (ethylenediaminetetraacetic acid), and D-penicillamine. DMSA and DMPS are water-soluble derivatives of BAL and thus may be administered orally; they are less toxic than most other chelators, and are effective in reducing metal concentrations in experimental studies (65), and in reports of clinical efficacy (52,62). It is not yet clear whether DMPS or DMSA may be the more effective. More evidence is needed to determine if chelators are capable of reversing the toxic effects of metals in the brain and kidney.

### Questions about Chelation Therapies

Several aspects of chelation therapy may pose risks to the patient. Chelation may cause redistribution of the metal, resulting in renewed exposure as a result of the liberation of bound metal. Chelation, during ongoing exposure, may enhance the absorption of Hg (66). Although chelation seems appropriate for the victim of severe poisoning, it is not clear whether chelation is appropriate for patients having less severe intoxication. The most questionable practice is administering chelation for "detoxification therapy," for patients who complain of subtle problems that are nonspecific, and for which no apparent cause has been identified. Some physicians, aware that Hg from amalgams may enter the body by absorption through the buccal mucosa, via the lung and digestive tract, refer to an allergic-toxic syndrome attributable to the accumulation of Hg and other metals in the body. They are administering chelators to people whose complaints include signs and symptoms that could be attributed to Hg (31). There is no solid scientific evidence to support such chelation therapy.

In "diagnostic chelation," administration of the chelator may be useful in revealing evidence of a significant body burden after Hg can no longer be detected in urine or blood (50,67). However, it is not yet clear how useful diagnostic chelation may be (31) or whether its benefits exceed its risks.

## ACKNOWLEDGMENTS

This work is supported by an Environmental Health Sciences Center grant (ES-00260). Dr. Stephen A. Daniel provided helpful comments on the preliminary draft.

## REFERENCES


1. ATSDR (Agency for Toxic Substances and Disease Registry). *Toxicological profile for mercury (update)*. Atlanta, GA: U.S. Public Health Service, 1994.
2. WHO (World Health Organization). *Inorganic mercury.* Environmental Health Criteria 118. Geneva, Switzerland: World Health Organization, 1991.
3. Evans HL, Garman RH, Weiss B. Methylmercury: exposure duration and regional distribution as determinants of neurotoxicity in nonhuman primates. *Toxicol Appl Pharmacol* 1977;41:15–33.
4. Clarkson TW. Molecular and ionic mimicry of toxic metals. *Annu Rev Pharmacol Toxicol* 1993;33:545–571.
5. Raffle PAB, Adams PH, Baxter PJ, Lee WR. *Hunter's diseases of occupations,* 8th ed. London: Boston E. Arnold, 1994.
6. Kishi R, Doi R, Fukuchi Y, Satoh H, et al. Residual neurobehavioral effects associated with chronic exposure to mercury vapour. *Occup Environ Med* 1994:51:35–41.
7. Akesson I, Schutz A, Attewell R, et al. Status of mercury and selenium in dental personnel: impact of amalgam work and own fillings. *Arch Environ Health* 1991;46(2):102–109.
8. Chang SB, Siew C, Gruninger SE. Factors affecting blood mercury concentrations in practicing dentists. *J Dent Res* 1992;71(1):66–74.
9. Echeverria D, Heyer NJ, Martin MD, Naleway CA, Woods JS, Bittner AC Jr. Behavioral effects of low-level exposure to Hg° among dentists. *Neurotoxicol Teratol* 1995;17:161–168.
10. Ngim, CH, Foo SC, Boey KW, Jeyaratnam J. Chronic neurobehavioural effects of elemental mercury in dentists. *Br J Ind Med* 1992;49:782–790.
11. Rowland AS, Baird DD, Weinberg CR, et al. The effect of occupational exposure to mercury vapour on the fertility of female dental assistants. *Occup Environ Med* 1994;51:28–34.
12. Roels H, Abdeladim S, Braun M, et al. Detection of hand tremor in workers exposed to mercury vapor: a comparative study of three methods. *Environ Res* 1989;49:152–165.
13. Wood RW, Weiss AB, Weiss B. Hand tremor induced by industrial exposure to inorganic mercury. *Arch Environ Health* 1973;26:249–252.
14. Langworth S, Elinder C-G, Göthe C-J, Vesterberg O. Biological monitoring of environmental and occupational exposure to mercury. *Int Arch Occup Environ Health* 1991;63:161–167.
15. Clarkson TW. Environmental contaminants in the food chain. *Am J Clin Nutr* 1995;682S–686S.
16. Grandjean P, Weihe P, Needham LL, et al. Relation of a seafood diet to mercury, selenium, arsenic, and polychlorinated biphenyl and other organochlorine concentrations in human milk. *Environ Res* 1995;71:29–38.
17. Bakir F, Damlugi SF, Amin-Zaki L, et al. Methylmercury poisoning in Iraq. *Science* 1973;181:230–241.
18. Harada M. Minamata disease: methylmercury poisoning in Japan caused by environmental pollution. *Crit Rev Toxicol* 1995;25:1–24.
19. Watanabe C, Satoh H. Evolution of our understanding of methylmercury as a health threat. *Environ Health Perspect* 1996;104:367–379.
20. Amin-Zaki L, Majeed MA, Clarkson TW, Greenwood MR. Methylmercury poisoning in Iraqi children: clinical observations over two years. *Br Med J* 1978;1:613–616.
21. Grandjean P, Weihe P, Nielsen JB. Methylmercury: significance of intrauterine and postnatal exposures. *Clin Chem* 1994;40:1395–1400.
22. Grandjean P, Weihe P, White RF. Milestone development in infants exposed to methylmercury from human milk. *Neurotoxicology* 1995;16:27–34.
23. Marsh DO, Clarkson TW, Myers GJ, et al. The Seychelles study of fetal methylmercury exposure and child development: introduction. *NeuroTox* 1995;16:583–596.
24. WHO (World Health Organization). *WHO/FDI draft consensus statement on dental amalgam.* Geneva, Switzerland: WHO, 1995.
25. Barregård L, Sällsten G, Järvholm B. People with high mercury uptake from their own dental amalgam fillings. *Occup Environ Med* 1995;52:124–128.
26. Oskarrson A, Schultz A, Skerfving S, et al. Total and inorganic mercury in breast milk in relation to fish consumption and amalgam in lactating women. *Arch Environ Health* 1996;51:234–241.
27. Lorscheider FL, Vimy MJ, Summers AO, Zwiers H. The dental amalgam mercury controversy—inorganic mercury and the CNS; genetic linkage of mercury and antibiotic resistances in intestinal bacteria. *Toxicology* 1995;97:19–22.
28. Nylander M, Friberg L, Lind B. Mercury concentrations in the human brain and kidneys in relation to exposure from dental amalgam fillings. *Swed Dent J* 1987;11:179–187.
29. Jokstad A, Thomassen Y, Bye E, et al. Dental amalgam and mercury. *Pharmacol Toxicol (Copenhagen)* 1992;70(4):308–313.

30. Halbach S. Amalgam tooth fillings and man's mercury burden. *Hum Exp Toxicol* 1994;13(7):496–501.
31. Sandborgh Englund G, Dahlqvist R, Lindelöf B, Söderman E. DMSA administration to patients with alleged mercury poisoning from dental amalgams: a placebo-controlled study. *J Dent Res* 1994;73(3): 620–628.
32. Ellingsen DG, Barregår L, Gaarder PI, Hultberg B, Kjuus H. Assessment of renal dysfunction in workers previously exposed to mercury vapor at a chloralkali plant. *Br J Ind Med* 1993;50:881–887.
33. Herrström P, Holmen A, Karlsson A, Raihle G, Schutz A, Högstedt B. Immune factors, dental amalgam, and low-dose exposure to mercury in Swedish adolescents. *Arch Environ Health* 1994;49:160–164.
34. Herrström P, Schutz A, Raihle G, Holthuis N, Högstedt B, Rastam L. Dental amalgam, low-dose exposure to mercury, and urinary proteins in young Swedish men. *Arch Environ Health* 1995;50:103–107.
35. Herrström P, Högstedt B. Dental restorative materials and the prevalence of eczema, allergic rhino-conjunctivitis, and asthma in school children. Dental amalgam and allergy in school children. *Scand J Prim Health Care* 1994;12:3–8.
36. Wendroff AP. Magico-religious exposure. *Environ Health Perspect* 1997;105:266.
37. American Conference of Industrial Hygienists (ACGIH). *Threshold limit values for chemical substances and physical agents and biological exposure indices.* Cincinnati, OH: ACGIH, 1996.
38. McCammon CS, Edwards, SL, Hull RD, Woodfin WJ. A comparison of four personal sampling methods for the determination of mercury vapor. *Am Ind Hyg Assoc J* 1980;41:528–531.
39. Vesterberg O. Automatic method for quantitation of mercury in blood, plasma and urine. *J Biochem Biophys Methods* 1991;23(3):227–236.
40. Barregård L. Biological monitoring of exposure to mercury vapor. *Scand J Work Environ Health* 1995;19(suppl 1):45–49.
41. Cox C, Clarkson TW, Marsh DO, et al. Dose-response analysis of infants prenatally exposed to methyl mercury: an application of a single compartment model to singe-strand hair analysis. *Environ Res* 1989;49:318–332.
42. Katz SA, Katz RB. Use of hair analysis for evaluating mercury intoxication of the human body: a review. *J Appl Toxicol* 1992;12:79–84.
43. Sharma DC, Davis PS. Direct determination of mercury in blood by use of sodium borohydride reduction and atomic absorption spectrophotometry. *Clin Chem* 1984;25:769–772.
44. Greenwood MR, Dhahir P, Clarkson TW. Epidemiological experience with the Magos' Reagents in the determination of different forms of mercury in biological samples by flameless atomic absorption. *J Anal Toxicol* 1977;1:265–269.
45. Evans HL. Markers of neurotoxicity: from behavior to autoantibodies against brain proteins. *Clin Chem* 1995;41(12):1874–1881.
46. El-Fawal HAN, Gong ZL, Evans HL. Exposure to methyl mercury results in serum autoantibodies to neurotypic and gliotypic proteins. *Neurotoxicology* 1996;17:267–276.
47. Boogaard PJ, Journee HL, Van Sittert NJ. Effects of exposure to elemental mercury on the nervous system and the kidneys of workers producing natural gas. *Arch Env Health* 1996;51:108–115.
48. Cárdenas A, Roels H, Bernard AM, et al. Markers of early renal changes induced by industrial pollutants. I Application to workers exposed to mercury vapour. *Br J Ind Med* 1993;50:17–27.
49. Woods JS, Bowers MA, Davis HA. Urinary porphyrin profiles as biomarkers of trace exposure and toxicity: studies on urinary porphyrin excretion patterns in rats during prolonged exposure to methyl mercury. *Toxicol Appl Pharmacol* 1991;110:464–476.
50. Gonzalez-Ramirez D, Maiorino RM, Zuniga-Charles M, et al. Sodium 2,3-dimercaptopropane-1-sulfonate challenge test for mercury in humans: II. Urinary mercury, porphyrins and neurobehavioral changes of dental workers in Monterry, Mexico. *J Pharmacol Exp Ther* 1995; 272:264–274.
51. Anneroth G, Ericson T, Johansson I, et al. Comprehensive medical examination of a group of patients with alleged adverse effects from dental amalgams. *Acta Odontol Scand* 1992;50(2):101–111.
52. Goyer RA. Toxic effects of metals. In: Klaasen CD, Amdur MO, Doull J, eds. *Casarett and Doull's toxicology,* 5th ed. New York: McGraw-Hill, 1996;691–736.
53. Liang Y-X, Sun R-K, Sun Y, Chen Z-Q, Li L-H. Psychological effects of low exposure to mercury vapor: Application of a computer-administered neurobehavioral evaluation system. *Environ Res* 1993;60: 320–327.
54. Yeates KO, Mortensen ME. Acute and chronic neuropsychological consequences of mercury vapor poisoning in two early adolescents. *J Clin Exp Neuropsychol* 1994;16:209–222.
55. Evans HL. Nonhuman primates in behavioral toxicology: issues of validity, ethics and public health. *Neurotox Teratol* 1990;12:531–536.
56. Soleo L, Ubrando ML, Petrera V, Ambrosi L. Effects of low exposure to inorganic mercury on psychological performance. *Br J Ind Med* 1990; 47:105–109.
57. Evans HL, Laties VG, Weiss B. Behavioral effects of mercury and methylmercury. *Fed Proc* 1975;34:1858–1867.
58. Klein CB, Kargacin B, Su L, Cosentino S, Snow ET, Costa M. Metal mutagenesis in transgenic Chinese hamster cell lines. *Environ Health Perspect* 1994;102(suppl 3):63–67.
59. Bigazzi PE, Autoimmunity and heavy metals. *Lupus* 1994;3:449–453.
60. Atchison WD, Spitsbergen JM. The neuromuscular junction as a target for toxicity. In: Chang LW, ed. *Principles of neurotoxicity.* New York: Marcel Dekker, 1994;265–308.
61. Aschner M, Kimelberg HK. Metallothioneins and physiological and pathological consequences of methylmercury accumulation in astrocytes. In: Aschner M, Kimelberg HK, eds. *The role of glia in neurotoxicity,* Boca Raton, FL: CRC Press, 1996;201–220.
62. Aposhian HV, Maiorino RM, Gonzalez-Ramirez D, et al. Mobilization of heavy metals by newer, therapeutically useful chelating agents. *Toxicology* 1995;97(1-3):23–38.
63. Goyer RA, Cherian MG, Jones MM, Reigart JR. Role of chelating agents for prevention, intervention, and treatment of exposure to toxic metals. *Environ Health Perspect* 1995;103:1048–1052.
64. Bluhm RE, Bobbitt RG, Welch LW, et al. Elemental mercury vapour toxicity, treatment, and prognosis after acute, intensive exposure in chloralkali plant workers. 1. History, neuropsychological findings and chelator effects. *Hum Exp Toxicol* 1992;11:201–210.
65. Aposhian MM, Maiorino RM, Xu Z, Aposhian HV. Sodium 2,3-dimercapto-1-propanesulfonate (DMPS) treatment does not redistribute lead or mercury to the brain of rat. *Toxicology* 1996;109(1):49–55
66. Ewan KBR, Pamphlett R. Increased inorganic mercury in spinal motor neurons following chelating agents *Toxicology* 1996;17(2):343–350.
67. Maiorino RM, Gonzalez-Ramirez D, Zuniga-Charles M, et al. Sodium 2,3-dimercaptopropane-1-sulfonate challenge test for mercury in humans. III. Urinary mercury after exposure to mercurous chloride. *J Pharmacol Exp Ther* 1996;277:938–944.

*Environmental and Occupational Medicine, Third Edition,* edited by William N. Rom.
Lippincott–Raven Publishers, Philadelphia © 1998.

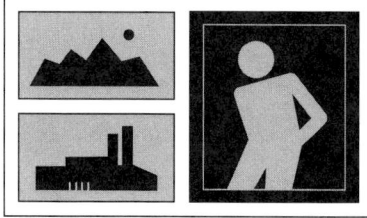

# CHAPTER 70

# Cadmium

Anthony J. Newman-Taylor

Cadmium is one of the "new" metals, first isolated by the German metallurgist Strohineyer in 1817. It serves no essential function in humans but is toxic, causing acute injury to the lungs and chronic disease of the lungs and kidneys.

Cadmium occurs in nature principally with zinc, but also with lead. It is recovered as a by-product during the smelting of zinc, and to a lesser extent of lead. World production of cadmium in 1985 was 18,660 metric tons. Its important uses are electroplating (about half); the production of cadmium alloys (such as copper cadmium and nickel cadmium), brazing solders (such as silver cadmium), and nickel cadmium batteries; the manufacture of cadmium pigments; and as a plastics stabilizer. The most important environmental source of inhaled cadmium is tobacco smoke. Each cigarette on average contains 2 μg cadmium, of which 100% may be inhaled. The concentration of cadmium is higher in livers of men who smoke than those who do not and is also higher in emphysematous than normal lungs.

## METABOLISM

Cadmium is stored in the body principally in the liver and kidneys. Nordberg and co-workers (1) estimated that cadmium in liver constituted some 14% to 18% and in the two kidneys between 50% and 56% of the total body burden.

Using these estimates Franklin and colleagues (2), from their results of neutron activation measurements of liver and kidney cadmium, estimated the mean body burden of cadmium in a population without occupational exposure to be 1.65 mg in nonsmokers and 11.34 mg in smokers, corresponding to an increase in body burden between 0.03 and 0.4 mg cadmium per pack-year.

Cadmium is transported from its site of absorption (lungs or gut) to the liver, where it induces the synthesis of metallothionein, a zinc storage protein with a high proportion of sulfur containing amino acids, which enables it to bind heavy metals. Each metallothionein molecule binds seven divalent cations, usually zinc or copper, but also cadmium, mercury, and other metals. The cadmium-metallothionein complex is released from the liver and transported in the blood to the kidneys, where it may dissociate within the tubule cells. The free metal induces intracellular synthesis of metallothionein, which binds free intracellular cadmium, providing, until the binding protein is saturated, protection against the cellular toxicity of cadmium. The biologic half-life of cadmium has been estimated to be between 10 and 30 years in kidney and between 4.7 and 9.7 years in liver (3). The half-life in both organs, particularly the kidneys, is markedly reduced with the onset of renal toxicity when tubule loss of cadmium is increased.

## ADVERSE HEALTH EFFECTS

### Acute Effects on the Lungs

Cadmium fume when inhaled in sufficient concentration is toxic to the epithelial and endothelial cells of the alveoli and causes acute pulmonary edema. Compared to the metals with which it is found, such as zinc, and with which it is alloyed, such as copper, the boiling point of cadmium (765°C) is low and its vapor pressure

A. J. Newman-Taylor: Department of Occupational and Environmental Medicine, Royal Brompton Hospital, London SW3 6NP, England.

high. Cadmium fume is therefore generated in potentially toxic concentrations in cadmium alloy production, during oxyacetylene cutting of cadmium-coated steel and rivets and in the smelting, melting, and refining of metals that contain cadmium, which is particularly hazardous when its presence is unsuspected.

Cadmium fume is insoluble, the effects on the lungs delayed, and the toxicity unrecognized by those exposed, who therefore accumulate it in increasing dose. Symptoms develop some 4 to 10 hours after onset of exposure. They are predominantly respiratory—shortness of breath, chest tightness, and cough that can be associated with flulike symptoms of chills, fever, and muscle pains—similar to those of metal fume fever. When exposure is sufficiently intense, evidence of pulmonary edema develops within 1 or 2 days, which is fatal in the more severely affected victims. The dose sufficient to cause pulmonary edema is not known. In one fatal case the average airborne concentration was estimated to be 8.6 $mg/m^3$ during 5 hours, or approximately an 8-hour time-weighted average (TWA) of 5 $mg/m^3$ (1,4). This estimate was based on cadmium content of lungs at postmortem examination, which may have been greater than the quantity necessary to cause death, and the atmospheric concentration necessary to cause pulmonary edema may therefore be considerably less.

## Chronic Effects

The focus of research into the chronic effects of cadmium, encountered both at work and in the general environment, has principally addressed the nature and severity of the effects of cadmium on the kidneys, in particular tubule function. The results of recent studies, however, suggest that exposure to cadmium, at least to inhaled cadmium fume, has more important effects on the lungs, causing respiratory disability and shortening of life. Estimates of cumulative exposure and of body burden by neutron activation analysis have also allowed assessment of exposure-response relationships both for lungs and kidneys.

### *Lungs*

Surveys of work forces exposed to cadmium published in the 1950s suggested that long-term occupational exposure to cadmium could cause emphysema (5,6); however, cigarette smoking was not taken into account and the results of subsequent investigations did not support these early conclusions. In 1982 Parkes (4) concluded, quite properly on the basis of the evidence then available, that there was little or no evidence to suggest that cadmium caused emphysema. However, confidence in the ability of the studies at that time to identify emphysema is severely limited by important methodologic problems, which include the small numbers studied, the absence of an appropriate comparison population, inclusion of currently employed workers only, failure to measure gas transfer, and the paucity of information about cadmium exposure.

A study of the mortality rates of cadmium workers in the United Kingdom reported in 1983 found that those who had experienced "ever high" exposure (which included those exposed to cadmium fume) had an increased rate of mortality from "bronchitis" (7). As compared to the expected mortality, the standardized mortality ratio from "bronchitis," in this group was 434 [95% confidence interval (CI) 224–758]. No associated increase in mortality from lung cancer or cardiovascular disease was observed, suggesting that the increase was unlikely to be the consequence of unusually high rates of tobacco consumption by persons exposed to cadmium. An update of this study, which included deaths occurring during a further 5-year period, confirmed the exposure-related excess mortality from "bronchitis"(8), with an associated excess of deaths from lung cancer. A subsequent study of copper cadmium alloy producers showed a marked excess of deaths from chronic nonmalignant respiratory disease related to cadmium exposure (9). Cumulative exposure to cadmium was categorized into three groups: <1,600, 1,600 to 4,799, >4,800 $y^2 \cdot \mu g^{-3}$. The risk of dying from chronic, nonmalignant, respiratory disease in the two higher exposure categories relative to a risk of 1 in the lowest exposure group was 4.54 (95% CI 1.96–10.51) in the medium exposure group and 4.74 (95% CI 1.81–12.43) in the highest exposure group.

Davison and colleagues (10) reported in 1988 their findings in the work force of a factory that had manufactured copper cadmium alloy since 1926. They saw all but two of the 103 men still alive and living in the United Kingdom who had ever worked in copper cadmium alloy production and compared lung function test results with those in a referent population that had been employed in the same factory complex in similar work but had never been exposed to cadmium. In addition, they made use of past measurements of airborne cadmium and knowledge of changes in production techniques, ventilation, and levels of production to determine cumulative cadmium exposure for each worker. They found that in comparison to their referents the cadmium work force had evidence of air flow limitation, hyperinflated lungs, and reduced gas transfer (Table 1), a pattern of functional abnormalities consistent with the changes characteristic of emphysema. These differences were very unlikely to be due to tobacco smoking, which was remarkably similar in the cadmium workers and their referents.

To assess whether the reductions observed in lung function were likely to be the cause of important respiratory disability, the number of cadmium workers and of referents whose results were 1.96 SD or more below pre-

**TABLE 1.** *Lung function, expressed as observed in cadmium workers minus expected from referent workers' regression equations (O−E)*

| Parameter | Workers (no.) | Mean (O−E) |
|---|---|---|
| $FEV_1$ (ml) | 97[a] | −194[d] |
| FVC (ml) | 97[a] | −27 |
| $FEV_1$/FVC % | 97[a] | −6.5[c] |
| $D_LCO$ | 75[b] | −0.81[c] |
| Radiographic TLC (ml) | 75[b] | +461[c] |
| RV (ml) | 75[b] | +402[d] |
| RV/TLC % | 75[b] | +2.9[d] |

[a]Includes those seen at factory and at home.
[b]Includes only those seen at factory.
[c]$p < 0.001$.
[d]$p < 0.05$.
From ref. 10.

dicted (11) were compared. Forced expiratory volume in 1 second ($FEV_1$) and the $FEV_1$/forced vital capacity (FVC) ratio, or both, were 1.96 SD or more below predicted in 33% of cadmium workers and 17% of referents; the carbon monoxide diffusing capacity of the lungs ($DL_{CO}$) or gas transfer coefficient (KCO), or both, were 1.96 SD or more below predicted in 19% of cadmium workers and in 3% of referents. $FEV_1$/FVC ratio was, on average, 30% below predicted values in the cadmium workers, whose $D_LCO$ or KCO was 1.96 SD below predicted. Regression analysis identified a significant relationship between the reduction in $FEV_1$, $FEV_1$/FVC ratio, $D_LCO$, and KCO, and both estimated cumulative cadmium exposure in years per microgram per meter cubed, and liver cadmium in parts per million (ppm) (Table 2). The consistency of the findings in this study, with the results of the mortality study of Kazantzis and colleagues (7,8) and of Sorahan (9) provided powerful support for the hypothesis that cadmium fume, at least when inhaled in the concentrations experienced by the men working in this factory up to the 1950s, caused chronic lung damage consistent with emphysema. Additional support comes from experimental studies in animals, which have shown that cadmium, usually soluble cadmium chloride ($CdCl_2$) instilled intratracheally, causes chronic irreversible damage to the lungs.

Niewohner and Hoidal (12) reported that intratracheal instillation of cadmium chloride to hamsters, in sufficient concentration to provoke acute lung injury, caused the functional and pathologic changes of lung fibrosis with areas of air space dilatation. However, administration by mouth of β-aminopropionitrile fumarate (BAPN) (which inhibits cross-linking of collagen and elastin by inhibiting lysyl oxidase) simultaneously with cadmium chloride inhalation was associated with the functional and pathologic changes of panlobular emphysema without fibrosis. The authors suggested that cadmium chloride caused alveolar wall destruction, possibly via endogenous proteases, and that subsequent reparative connective tissue synthesis prevented further air space enlargement and contributed to the functional evidence of stiffened lungs. Inhibition of collagen and elastin synthesis by BAPN permitted further alveolar wall destruction and bulla formation. Snider and colleagues (13), in a different series of experiments, also in hamsters, showed that cadmium chloride solution instilled into the trachea in sufficient concentration to cause pneumonia induced focal air space enlargement in alveoli adjacent to areas of focal fibrosis (13). They also found that young adult hamsters that developed these changes following cadmium chloride inhalation did not lose lung elastin, which had been radiolabeled in neonatal life. They suggested that cadmium did not cause elastin degradation, as Niewohner and Hoidal proposed, but that fibrosis and air space distention were caused by traction from adjacent areas of fibrosis.

These and other animal experiments have shown that soluble cadmium salts, inhaled in concentrations sufficient to cause pulmonary edema and pneumonia, cause irreversible lung damage, of which air space enlargement is a component. How reliable a model this is for long-term exposure to insoluble cadmium fume is not clear, but the results of animal studies are at least consistent with inhaled cadmium having the capacity to cause chronic lung damage. Chambers et al. (14) have also shown that cadmium chloride selectively inhibits the production of procollagen, but not noncollagen synthesis, in a dose-dependent fashion in fetal rat and human fetal fibroblast cell lines.

**TABLE 2.** *Mean (O−E) and regression analysis for $FEV_1$, $FEV_1$/FCV%, $D_LCO$, and KCO in three exposed groups according to liver cadmium*

| Liver cadmium (ppm) | Workers (no.) | $FEV_1$ (ml) | $FEV_1$/FVC(%) | $D_LCO$ | KCO |
|---|---|---|---|---|---|
| >25 | 24 | −146 | −8.7 | −1.4 | −0.40 |
| 12.5–25 | 23 | −120 | −6.7 | −0.7 | −0.21 |
| <12.5 | 28 | −76 | −3.7 | −0.4 | −0.14 |
| Regression analysis ($\log_c$ liver cadmium) | | | | | |
| Slope | | −59 | −1.36 | −0.38[a] | −0.08[a] |
| Intercept | | 49[a] | −2.5 | 0.21 | −0.03 |

[a]$p < 0.05$.
From ref. 10.

### *Kidneys*

The kidneys, with the liver, are the principal organs of cadmium accumulation in the body. Damage to tubule cells occurs at a critical concentration of intracellular cadmium when the capacity of metallothionein synthesized within the cell for cadmium is exceeded; the critical concentration is therefore related not to the total amount of cadmium within tubule cells but to the concentration at which free cadmium, which is nephrotoxic, begins to accumulate. This concentration may depend not only on total intracellular cadmium but on other factors as well, such as aging, that determine the capacity of renal tubule cells to synthesize metallothionein.

The principal effect of cadmium on renal function is to cause tubule proteinuria. Increased $\beta_2$-microglobulin has been used as a sensitive indicator of renal tubule damage in cadmium work forces, but it is degraded in acid urine (pH 5.5), and retinol-binding protein (RBP) has been suggested as a more reliable indicator (15). Increased excretion of $\beta_2$-microglobulin and retinol-binding protein may be accompanied by other evidence of tubule damage, such as increased excretion of amino acids, glucose, and phosphate.

The study described above, which provided evidence for a marked excess in cadmium workers of functional abnormalities consistent with emphysema, also examined differences in renal function between the cadmium work force and their referent population (14). They reported significant increases in urinary excretion of the tubular proteins $\beta_2$-microglobulin, retinol-binding protein, and the brush border enzymes *N*-acetyl-glucosaminidase (NAG), alkaline phosphatase, and $\gamma$-glutamyl transferase, and a significant decrease in renal absorption of calcium urate and phosphate. In addition, measures of glomerular filtration rate (GFR)—serum creatinine and $\beta_2$-microglobulin and creatinine clearance—were significantly reduced in the cadmium-exposed group. The great majority of the variables that were found to be different in the cadmium work force and in their referents were significantly correlated with the log of cumulative cadmium exposure index and the log of liver cadmium, supporting the relationship of these abnormalities to cadmium uptake. Roels and colleagues (16) have investigated the progression of renal abnormalities in the absence of continuing exposure. They followed 23 workers removed from exposure because of increased urinary excretion of $\beta_2$-microglobulin or retinol-binding protein, or both. During the 5-year period of follow-up, serum creatinine and $\beta_2$-microglobulin increased, indicating progressive reduction in GFR. On average, GFR decreased some five times more rapidly than the expected age-related decline. In addition, serum alkaline phosphatase increased during this period, reflecting an interference by cadmium with bone metabolism. These results suggest that accumulation of cadmium in the kidneys sufficient to cause increased urinary tubule protein excretion is also sufficient to accelerate the reduction in GFR and that tubule proteinuria should therefore be considered an adverse health effect.

### Exposure-Response Relationships

Although both the respiratory and renal consequences of chronic cadmium exposure have been shown to be related to cumulative cadmium exposure, the nature of the exposure-response relationships for the two organs is different in important respects. In their study of the chronic effects of cadmium on the lung, Davison's group (10) examined the relationship between estimated cumulative cadmium exposure and KCO in 35 workers employed 5 years or longer (chosen as men who had experienced a significant duration, as well as, in some cases, intensity of exposure). The data were consistent with a linear relationship: the slope of KCO deficit of 0.067 ($mmol \cdot min^{-1} \cdot kPa^{-1} 0.1^{-1}$) per 1,000 year per $\mu g/m^3$ with no evidence for a threshold (Fig. 1). This analysis assumed the accuracy of the estimates of intensity of exposure and that intensity and duration of exposure were equivalent in their effects on lung function. Support for the validity of the estimates of intensity of exposure was provided by the close relationship between log cumulative cadmium exposure and log liver cadmium, estimated by neutron activation analysis (15). From this analysis exposure to 2,000 yr/$\mu g/m^{-3}$ (40 years' exposure to the current occupational exposure limit of 50 $\mu g/m^3$) would, on average, cause a deficit of 0.14 $mmol \cdot min^{-1} \cdot kPa^{-1} 0.1^{-1}$ with 95% confidence limits of between 0.05 and 0.3 $mmol \cdot min^{-1} \cdot kPa^{-1} 0.1^{-1}$ (i.e., significantly different from no effect).

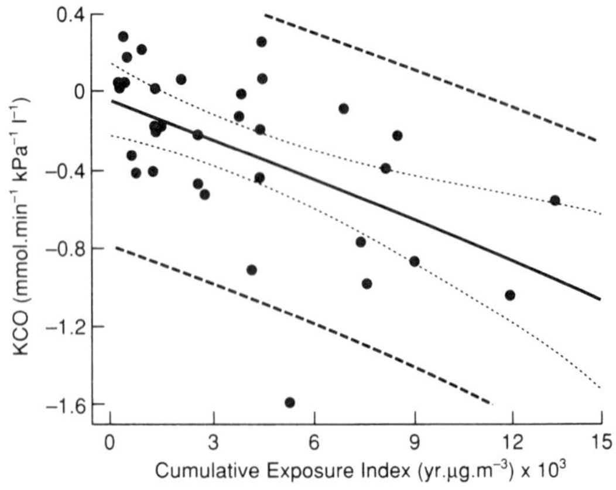


**FIG. 1.** Regression line of KCO against estimated cumulative exposure index for cadmium workers with 95% confidence limits for regression line *(dots)* and for individual values *(dashes)*. (From ref. 10.)

The pattern of the exposure-response relationship for cadmium on renal function is different. Whereas the observed deficit in KCO was consistent with a linear relationship without a threshold, the abnormalities in renal function reported by Mason and colleagues (15) were consistent with the two-phase ("broken stick") model, there being inflection points for the urinary excretion of $\beta_2$-microglobulin, retinol-binding protein, total protein, and albumin of about 1,100 y · μg/m³, with lower confidence limits between 500 and 7,000 year per μg/m³ (15). A similar two-phase model was observed using liver cadmium (Fig. 2). These observations are consistent with the results of others that use similar methods of investigation. Ellis and co-workers (3), using a logistic regression model with $\beta_2$-microglobulin as the response variable, predicted 59% renal dysfunction at 1,100 year per μg/m³ and suggested abnormal renal function developed between 400 and 550 year per μg/m³ (3). Jarup and Elinder (17) found a relationship between urinary $\beta_2$-microglobulin and cadmium excretion in a study of 561 cadmium-exposed battery workers. The prevalence of tubular proteinuria (defined as urine concentration of 34 μg $\beta_2$-microglobulin/n.mol creatinine) was 0.8% in those excreting less than 1 n.mol cadmium/n.mol creatinine and 46% in those with a mean urinary cadmium of 15n.mol cadmium/n.mol creatinine. The relationship of tubular proteinuria to urinary cadmium excretion was age dependent: a 10% prevalence of tubular proteinuria occurred at urine cadmium concentration of 1.5 n.mol/m.mol creatinine in those aged more than 60 years and at 5 n.mol cadmium/m.mol creatinine in those aged less than 60 years.

This pattern of exposure-response relationships for renal damage in humans is consistent with the results of animal studies, which have shown that raised intracellular cadmium concentrations in the kidneys induce metallothionein production and that free intracellular cadmium, which interferes with normal cellular metabolism, occurs only when the concentration of intracellular cadmium exceeds the capacity of the renal cell to synthesize metallothionein. This model implies a threshold before significant change in renal function, which occurs when the concentration in tubule cells is sufficient for non–metallothionein-bound cadmium to accumulate. The study of Mason and colleagues (15) suggested that to prevent intracellular cadmium from reaching this concentration, cumulative exposure to airborne cadmium should not exceed 1,100 year per μg/m³, the equivalent of 22 years' exposure to 50 μg/m³, the current occupational exposure limit in many countries.

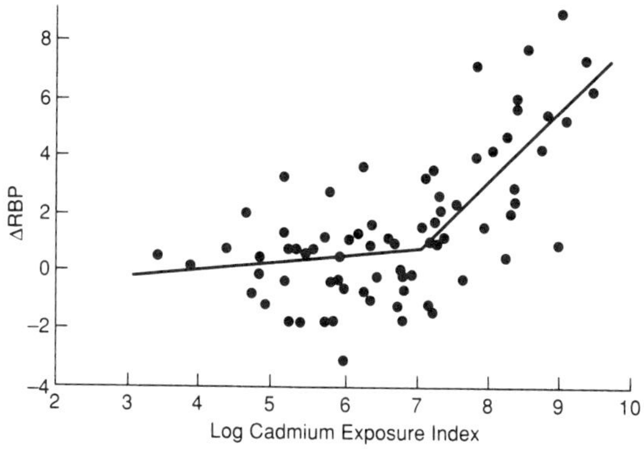


**FIG. 2.** Two-phase linear regression plot of matched pair differences of urinary retinol-binding protein (RBP) versus cumulative exposure index. (From ref. 22.)

### Carcinogenicity

Although it has been suggested that cadmium causes cancer, the evidence is weaker than that for other metals, such as arsenic, chromium, and nickel. Doll (18) has pointed out that the conclusion of an International Workshop on the Carcinogenicity of Metals (1981), which he chaired, erred in concluding that exposure to cadmium had contributed to the development of prostate cancer by including the original hypotheses-forming data in the subsequent analysis of the hypothesis-testing data (Table 3). When the original United Kingdom data are excluded, 10 cases were identified, as compared to 5.1 expected, a less than significant observation. This was confirmed by the subsequent analysis of prostate cancer rates in all men who were occupationally exposed to cadmium in England, which identified 31 deaths from prostate cancers as compared to an expected 30.9. Doll subsequently concluded that cadmium should "not now be regarded as a human carcinogen" (18).

Since that workshop mortality rates from cancer have been investigated in several cohort studies of populations occupationally exposed to cadmium in the manufacture of nickel cadmium batteries and of copper cadmium alloy and cadmium smelting. Kazantzis et al. (8) in the 5-year update of their mortality study of cadmium workers in United Kingdom found an excess of lung cancer [standardized mortality ratio (SMR) 1.30, 95% CI 1.07–1.57] which like "bronchitis" was related to estimated intensity of exposure, but no excess of prostatic cancer. In a study of cadmium smelter workers in the United States, Stayner et al. (19) found an exposure related excess of lung cancer in the entire cohort (SMR 149, 95% CI 95–222). The

**TABLE 3.** *Prostate cancer in cadmium workers: evidence available in 1981*

| Country | Observed (no.) | Expected (no.) | Characteristic |
|---|---|---|---|
| Great Britain | 4 | 0.6 | Cases |
| United States | 4 | 1.2 | Deaths |
| Sweden (1) | 2 | 1.2 | Cases |
| Sweden (2) | 4 | 2.7 | Cases |
| All countries | 14 | 5.6 | |

From ref. 18.

excess was greatest in workers with the highest estimated cadmium exposure (SMR 272, 95% CI 123–513) and in workers 20 or more years from first exposure (SMR 161, 95% CI 100–248). Similarly in a cohort study of 4,393 men employed in a zinc lead cadmium smelter Ades and Kazantzis (20) observed an excess of lung cancer (SMR 124.5, 95% CI 107–144) in men employed more than 20 years. However, the increased risk associated with increasing duration of exposure was not accounted for by exposure to cadmium, suggesting it might be due to a contaminant, such as arsenic.

In his study of 3,025 nickel cadmium battery workers Sorahan (21) observed an excess of lung cancer (SMR 1.30, 95% CI 1.07–1.57). A possible association between duration of exposure was observed in the high- or moderate-exposure group for those first employed between 1923 and 1946, but not for those first employed between 1947 and 1975. However, in a study of copper cadmium alloy workers heavily exposed to cadmium fume, Sorahan et al. (9) found no excess of lung cancer (SMR 101, 95% CI 60–159), and no evidence of an exposure response gradient.

The results of these studies remain difficult to interpret with confidence. The two studies of smelters showed an excess in mortality from lung cancer, which was more clearly associated with cadmium exposure in the Stayner than in the Ades and Kazantzis study. However both were potentially confounded by concurrent exposure to carcinogenic contaminants, particularly arsenic. The Sorahan study of nickel cadmium battery workers showed only a moderate excess of lung cancer with inconsistent relationships to cadmium exposure, which was potentially confounded by exposure to nickel. The copper cadmium alloy producers, who probably experienced the highest exposures to cadmium, showed a marked exposure-related excess mortality from chronic nonmalignant respiratory disease, but no excess from lung cancer. The evidence for cadmium as a human carcinogen remains unproven.

## REFERENCES


1. Nordberg GF, Kjellstrom T, Nordberg M. Cadmium and health. In: Friberg K, Elinder CG, Kjellstrom T, Nordberg GF, eds. Boca Raton, FL: CRC Press, 1985;103–178.
2. Franklin D, Guthrie C, Chettle D, et al. In vivo neutron activation analysis of organ cadmium burdens. Referent levels in liver and kidney and the impact of smoking. In: Shrauzer G, ed. *Biological trace element research.* Humana Press, 1990;401–406.
3. Ellis K, Cohn S, Smith T. Cadmium inhalation exposure estimates: their significance with respect to kidney and liver cadmium burden. *J Toxicol Environ Health* 1985;15:173–187.
4. Parkes W. *Occupational lung disorders,* 2nd ed. London: Butterworth, 1982.
5. Bonnell J. Emphysema and proteinuria in men casting copper-cadmium alloys. *Br J Ind Med* 1955;12:181–195.
6. Bonnell J, Kazantzis G, King E. A follow-up study of men exposed to cadmium oxide fume. *Br J Ind Med* 1959;16:135–147.
7. Armstrong B, Kazantzis G. The mortality of cadmium workers. *Lancet* 1983;1:1425–1427.
8. Kazantzis G, Lam TH, Sullman KR. Mortality of cadmium exposed workers. A five year update. *Scand J Work Environ Health* 1988; 14:220–223.
9. Sorahan T, Lister A, Gilthorpe MS, Harrington JM. Mortality of copper cadmium alloy workers with special reference to lung cancer and non malignant diseases of the respiratory system. *Occup Environ Med* 1995;52:804–812.
10. Davison A, Fayers P, Newman-Taylor A, et al. Cadmium fume inhalation and emphysema. *Lancet* 1988;1:663–667.
11. Cotes J. *Lung function,* 4th ed. Oxford: Blackwell, 1979.
12. Niewohner D, Hoidal J. Lung fibrosis and emphysema: divergent responses to a common injury? *Science* 1982;217:359–360.
13. Snider G, Lucey E, Faris B, Jung-Legg Y, Stone P, Franzblau C. Cadmium chloride induced air space enlargement with interstitial pulmonary fibrosis is not associated with destruction of lung elastin. *Am Rev Respir Dis* 1988;137:918–923.
14. Chambers RC, McAnulty RJ, Shock A, Campa JS, Newman Taylor AJ, Laurent GJ. Cadmium selectively inhibits fibroblast procollagen production and proliferation. *Am J Physiol (Lung Cell Mol Physiol)* 1994; 267:L300–L308.
15. Mason HJ, Chettle AL, Gompertz DR, Davison AG, Fayers PM, Newman Taylor AJ. The use of multiple parameters to characterize cadmium induced renal dysfunction resulting from occupational exposure. *Environ Res* 1994;65:22–41.
16. Roels H, Lauwerys P, Buchet J, Bernard A, Vos A, Over-Steyns M. Health significance of cadmium induced renal dysfunction: a 5-year follow-up. *Br J Ind Med* 1989;46:755–764.
17. Jarup L, Elinder CG. Dose-response relationships between urinary cadmium and tubular proteinuria in cadmium exposed workers. *Am J Ind Med* 1994;26:759-769.
18. Doll R. Occupational cancer: problems in interpreting human evidence. *Ann Occup Hyg* 1984;28:291–305.
19. Stayner L, Smith R, Thun M, Schnorr T, Lemen R. A dose response analysis and quantitative assessment of lung cancer risk and occupational cadmium exposure. *Ann Epidemiol* 1992;2:177–194.
20. Ades AE, Kazantzis G. Lung cancer in a non ferrous smelter: the role of cadmium. *Br J Ind Med* 1988;45:435–442.
21. Sorahan T. Mortality from lung cancer among cohort of mixed cadmium battery workers: 1946–1984. *Br J Ind Med* 1987;44:803–809.
22. Mason M, Davison A, Wright A, et al. Relations between liver cadmium, cumulative exposure and renal function in cadmium alloy workers. *Br J Ind Med* 1988;45:793–802.

*Environmental and Occupational Medicine, Third Edition,* edited by William N. Rom.
Lippincott–Raven Publishers, Philadelphia © 1998.

# CHAPTER 71

# Arsenic

Toby G. Rossman

Arsenic, a naturally occurring element in the earth's crust, is a metalloid belonging to the group V elements in the periodic table. Pure arsenic is a gray-colored metal, but arsenic in the environment is found in compounds with other elements such as oxygen, chlorine, and sulfur. Humans are exposed to arsenic compounds coming from both natural and man-made sources. Natural sources include volcanic eruptions and the leaching of arsenic from rocks and soil into drinking water. Arsenic compounds are used in wood preservation (chromated copper arsenate), insecticides, herbicides (as weed killers for railroad and telephone posts and as Agent Blue used by U.S. troops in Vietnam), desiccants to facilitate mechanical cotton harvest, algicides, in glass manufacturing, and nonferrous alloys (1–6). For example, calcium arsenate is used as an insecticide on cotton, as an herbicide for treating turf and lawns to control weeds, and as a pesticide on fruits and vegetables. Metallic arsenic is used as an alloying agent to harden lead shot and to improve the toughness and corrosion resistance of copper. Sodium arsenate is used in ant killers and in animal dips as an insecticide. Arsenic, arsenic trioxide, lead arsenate, and potassium arsenite were used in medicines, but today arsenic compounds are restricted to mostly veterinary medicine, although they still can be found in Chinese and Indian folk medicine. Arsenic and arsenic trioxide are also used in the manufacture of low-melting glasses. A new source of human exposure to arsenic may occur as a result of the discovery that crystals made of gallium arsenide (GaAs) are better superconductors than those made of silicon (7,8). Gallium arsenide crystals are now being used in semiconductors, integrated circuits, diodes, infrared detectors, and laser technology. In addition, the very toxic gas arsine ($AsH_3$) is used to make gallium arsenide. A partial list of occupations in which exposure may occur appears in Table 1.

T. G. Rossman: Nelson Institute of Environmental Medicine and Kaplan Comprehensive Cancer Center, New York University Medical Center, New York, New York 10016.

## CHRONIC HUMAN EXPOSURE

Although acute toxicity, particularly as a result of exposure to arsines, is still of concern, the major human problem today is that of chronic low-level exposure to potentially carcinogenic arsenic species. In humans, the major routes of arsenic uptake are via ingestion of food and water and via inhalation of polluted air by the lung and to a much lesser extent via dermal absorption (9). Contamination of air, water, and food by natural and man-made arsenic compounds occurs throughout the world. Drinking water may be contaminated with arsenic from arsenical pesticides, natural mineral deposits, or improperly disposed arsenical chemicals (e.g., in Superfund sites). Elevated arsenic levels in drinking water occur in Taiwan, India, New Zealand, Argentina, Chile, California, Mexico, Oregon, and Alaska. Although arsenic compounds can accumulate in the soil (10), bioaccumulation of arsenic in food does not appear to reach levels dangerous to human health (4). Elevated levels of arsenic in soil (due either to natural or man-made contamination) may lead to exposure from ingesting soil. This is of particular concern for small children who swallow bits of soil while playing. Air emissions from pesticide manufacturing facilities, smelters, cotton gins, glass manufacturing operations, tobacco smoke, and burning of fossil fuels that contain arsenic are the major sources of inhaled arsenic. Persons who handle wood treated with chromated copper arsenate (e.g., in making decks) may

**TABLE 1.** *Occupations involving exposure to arsenic compounds*

| |
|---|
| Alloy manufacturing |
| Aniline color manufacturing |
| Brass and bronze manufacturing |
| Carpentry |
| Ceramics manufacturing |
| Computer chip manufacturing |
| Drug manufacturing |
| Enameling |
| Fireworks manufacturing |
| Gold refining |
| Herbicide manufacturing and spraying |
| Hide preserving |
| Insecticide manufacturing and spraying |
| Lead shot manufacturing |
| Leather working |
| Paint manufacturing |
| Painting |
| Petroleum refining |
| Pigment manufacturing |
| Printing |
| Rodenticide manufacturing |
| Silver refining |
| Smelters (lead, copper) |
| Taxidermy |
| Textile printing |
| Tree sprayers |

be exposed to arsenic in the absence of adequate safety precautions, and inhalation of the combustion fumes from such wood caused severe arsenic poisoning in Wisconsin (11). Arsenic compounds are used to promote the growth of swine and poultry, and it has been argued that arsenic may be an essential element for humans, although no specific role for arsenic has been identified (12).

Approximately 95% of soluble trivalent arsenic compounds are absorbed from the GI tract (1). The half-life of arsenic in humans is about 10 hours (1). Although seafood is especially high in arsenic content, the form of arsenic in seafood is the less toxic arsenobetaine, which is excreted in the urine without metabolism (13). After absorption through the lungs or the GI tract, arsenic is transported in the blood to other parts of the body and distributed to the kidney, liver, spleen, skin, hair, and nails in that order (14). Arsenic in humans tends to accumulate in hair and nails, followed by skin and lungs. Approximately 70% of arsenic is excreted, mainly in urine, and recent arsenic intoxication is usually assessed by determining urinary arsenic content, whereas longer-term exposure can be detected by measuring hair and nails.

## SYMPTOMS OF ARSENIC TOXICITY

Arsine ($AsH_3$) and As(III) halogenides are more toxic than other arsenic compounds (15). Arsine intoxication in the past has occurred most often in the metal refining industry, although its newer use in semiconductor manufacture may present new problems. Within an hour after exposure, patients present with nausea, headache, signs of shock, anemia, hemoglobinurea, and coppery skin pigmentation, possibly due to methemoglobin. Arsine causes massive hemolysis that may persist for several days. As a result of the rapid hemolysis, jaundice and hemoglobinuria occur. Arsine exposure produces electrocardiograph manifestations including high, peaked T-waves, conduction disturbances, various degrees of heart block, and asystole. These effects are thought to be related in part to hyperkalemia resulting from the hemolysis. In some cases death results from cardiac failure, although more often it is caused by renal failure as the resulting arsenic acid damages the kidneys. Arsine may also directly affect the myocardium, causing a greater magnitude of cardiac failure than would be expected from the degree of anemia.

Acute symptoms of poisoning with other arsenic compounds are usually seen in humans who have ingested contaminated food or drink. The fatal human dose for ingested arsenic trioxide is 70 to 180 mg (1). Acute symptoms are characterized by profound gastrointestinal inflammation, sometimes with hemorrhage, and can include constriction of the throat followed by dysphagia, gastric pain, vomiting, diarrhea, dehydration, leg cramps, irregular pulse, shock, stupor, paralysis, and coma (1–3). Electrocardiograph changes are characterized by T-wave inversion and persistent prolongation of the Q-T interval (14). In survivors, exfoliative dermatitis, peripheral neuritis, cardiac abnormalities, and reversible anemia and leukopenia may develop. Arsenic compounds can also cause contact dermatitis and hepatotoxic effects. Around 1900 in Manchester, England, arsenic-contaminated beer caused by contaminated sugar resulted in 6,000 poisonings and approximately 71 deaths. Most of the patients presented with anorexia, brown pigmentation, peripheral neuritis characterized by muscular weakness, pain and paresthesis of the extremities, hepatic lesions, localized edema, and fatty degeneration of the heart (14). Transverse white lines across the nails (Mees' lines) often appear weeks after an episode of acute poisoning.

Chronic arsenic intoxication can have a varied clinical picture. Poisoning via inhalation tends to occur in three phases: Initially, there is weakness, loss of appetite, nausea, and diarrhea. The second phase is characterized by conjunctivitis, inflammation of the mucous membranes of the nose, larynx, and respiratory passages, mild tracheobronchitis, skin lesions, and sometimes perforation of the nasal septum at high levels of exposure. The final phase includes peripheral neuritis and sometimes anemia, and leukopenia. An increased incidence of Raynaud's disease at 0.05 to 0.5 $mg/m^2$ airborne arsenic has been reported (3). Clinical evidence of peripheral neuropathy (both of sensory and motor neurons) occurs frequently after chronic inhalation of arsenic, and more sporadically with chronic ingestion. In contrast to ingested arsenic (see below), hyperkeratosis and hyperpigmentation are not commonly seen in workers exposed primarily by inhalation.

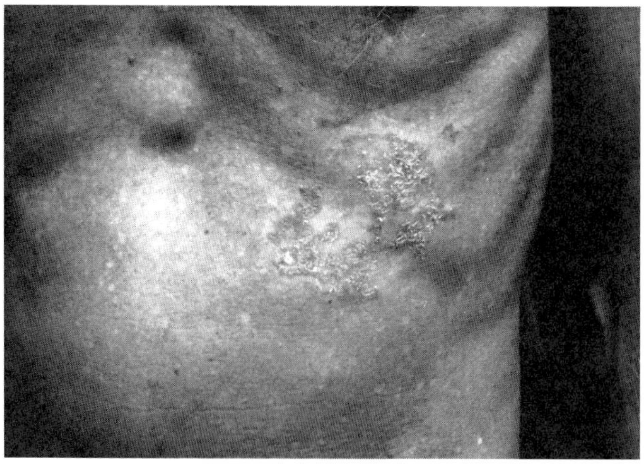

**FIG. 1.** Typical arsenical skin lesions of melanosis, depigmentation, and Bowen's disease on the trunk. (From ref. 76.) *See color plate facing page 1016.*

Early skin manifestations of chronic arsenic ingestion resemble Raynaud's syndrome (4). After many years of exposure, two of the more characteristic effects of arsenic ingestion are areas of hyperpigmentation interspersed with smaller areas of hypopigmentation (raindrop appearance) on the trunk and neck (Fig. 1) and hyperkeratosis of palms and soles characterized by small corn-like elevations and diffuse keratosis (Fig. 2). Hyperkeratotic areas may be precursors of malignant lesions. Arsenic ingestion also affects the cardiovascular system, altering myocardial depolarization and causing cardiac arrhythmias. Long-term, low-level ingestion of arsenic-contaminated water in Taiwan and Mexico leads to Blackfoot disease, a progressive loss of circulation in hands and feet, ultimately resulting in necrosis and gangrene. Drinking arsenic-contaminated water in Chile is associated with increased incidence of Raynaud's disease and thickening of small and medium-sized arteries throughout the body in children who were autopsied (3).

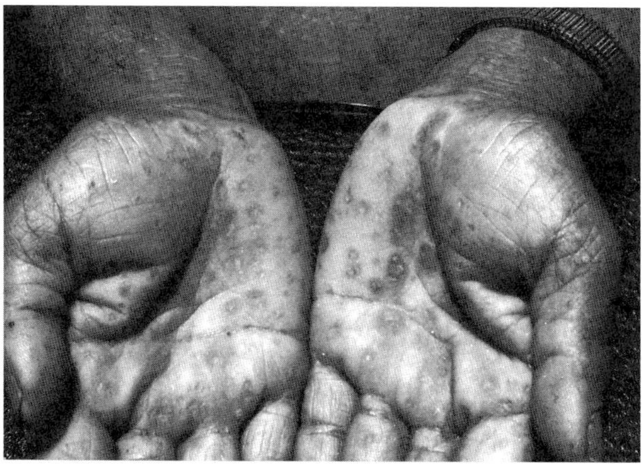

**FIG. 2.** Typical arsenical palmar hyperkeratosis. (From ref. 76.)

**TABLE 2.** *Clinical features among 13 patients[a] in West Bengal drinking arsenic-contaminated water*

| Clinical feature | Number of patients |
|---|---|
| Pigmentation | 13 |
| Anemia | 13 |
| Hepatomegaly (2–4 cm) | 13 |
| Abdominal pain | 10 |
| Tingling and numbness of hands and feet | 10 |
| Thickening of palms and soles | 10 |
| Splenomegaly (3–7 cm) | 5 |
| Anorexia | 4 |
| Nausea | 3 |
| Vomiting | 3 |
| Heartburn | 2 |
| Weakness of limbs | 2 |
| Diarrhea | 1 |
| Ascites | 1 |

[a]Patients were selected for pigmentation changes. Data taken from ref. 17.

An association between chronic arsenic ingestion and hypertension has also been seen. Gastrointestinal symptoms are less severe than in acute poisoning. Several studies have reported swollen and tender livers and sometimes elevated levels of hepatic enzymes in the blood of individuals chronically exposed. There is little evidence of renal damage or hematologic effects from chronic exposure to arsenic. Polyneuritis and motor paralysis, primarily of the fingers and toes, may occur as the sole symptoms of arsenic intoxication (4).

A recent health crisis has arisen in West Bengal, India, where high levels of arsenic have leached from natural underground sources into wells. More than 1 million people are drinking arsenic-contaminated water, and 200,000 already show skin lesions (16). The clinical features of 13 patients from this area who exhibited signs of chronic arsenical dermatosis (17) are shown in Table 2. Enlargement of the liver was seen in 92.5% of those who drank the contaminated water, but in only 6.25% of controls. Biopsy of liver samples from these patients revealed various degrees of fibrosis and expansion of the portal zone that resembled noncirrhotic portal fibrosis.

## METABOLISM OF ARSENIC COMPOUNDS

A major detoxification pathway for inorganic arsenic compounds in vivo is via methylation followed by excretion in the urine (11,18–20). Approximately 50% of excreted arsenic in human urine is dimethylarsinate and 25% is monomethylated, the remainder being inorganic (21). Reduction of arsenate to arsenite is necessary before methylation can occur, and this reaction requires glutathione (GSH) (19,22). Although arsenate reductase activity has been measured in the mammalian liver cytosol, the enzyme responsible has not been isolated or characterized.

The reduction of arsenate by GSH can also take place nonenzymatically and can proceed further to produce the arsenite-GSH conjugate $As(GS)_3$ (23), although this compound has not been detected in mammalian cells. Instead, arsenite appears to form a ternary complex with GSH and a macromolecule, possible hemoglobin in erythrocytes (24). In other cells, proteins other than hemoglobin would be expected to play a similar role. For example, in arsenite-treated Chinese hamster V79 (lung fibroblast) cells, all intracellular arsenite appears to be bound to macromolecules, probably proteins (25).

Arsenic methylation occurs primarily in the liver and to a much lesser extent in the kidney and lung (26,27). The methyl group from S-adenosyl methionine (SAM) is transferred to arsenite to form monomethylarsonic acid [MMAA(V)], which is then reduced (probably by GSH) to monomethylarsonous acid [MMAA(III)]. A second methylation (again via SAM) then forms dimethlyarsinic acid [DMAA(V)] (18,28):

$$AsO_3^{3-} + SAM \rightarrow AsO_3CH_3^{2-} \quad [1]$$
(methylarsonic acid)

$$AsO_3CH_3^{2-} + GSH \rightarrow AsO_2CH_3^{2-} \quad [2]$$
(methylarsonous acid)

$$AsO_2CH_3^{2-} + SAM \rightarrow AsO_2(CH_3)_2^{1-} \quad [3]$$
(dimethlyarsinic acid)

Depletion of GSH has been shown to block arsenic methylation and to increase the toxicity of arsenite (29). Recently, evidence has been found of a possible human genetic polymorphism in the control of arsenite methyltransferase activity (30). Differences in the rates of methylation may also partly explain why humans are more sensitive to arsenic than other species (such as rats) (20,31).

Cells other than liver appear to protect themselves against arsenic toxicity via active extrusion of arsenic from the cell, thus lowering its intracellular concentration to subtoxic levels. Bacteria have genes that express energy-dependent pumps to extrude arsenic compounds (32). The plasmid-encoded *arsA* and *arsB* gene products in *Escherichia coli* form a membrane-bound adenosine triphosphate (ATP)-coupled pump with structural and functional similarities to mammalian P-glycoprotein, the multidrug-resistant (MDR) gene product. Mammalian cells also appear to protect themselves from arsenic compounds by pumping arsenic out of the cell. SA7, an arsenite-resistant subline of CHO (Chinese hamster ovary) cells accumulated less arsenic compared to its wild-type parental cell line and had elevated levels of GSH and GSH transferase (33), the enzyme that forms GSH conjugates with toxicants. This suggests that the substrate of the efflux pump is an arsenic-GSH conjugate. However, two arsenite-resistant Chinese hamster V79 (lung fibroblast) sublines show faster efflux of arsenite (23), but do not have elevated levels of GSH or GSH S-transferase. Arsenic efflux in these cells is energy dependent and may require GSH. Biliary excretion of arsenate also requires GSH (34). Analysis of the extrusion products from V79 cells given arsenate or arsenite showed only arsenite, and not $As(GS)_3$. Similar results were seen with BALB/3T3 cells, a line of mouse fibroblasts (22). This indicates that intracellular reduction of arsenate to arsenite occurs, and that arsenite is transported as an unconjugated species, although a transient GSH conjugate cannot be ruled out.

While methylated arsenic products were not detected in arsenite-exposed BALB/3T3 cells or in V79 fibroblast cells or their medium, DMAA appeared in the medium of arsenite-treated rat hepatocytes (35), as expected if liver is the main site of arsenic methylation.

## EFFECTS OF ARSENITE ON GENE EXPRESSION

Arsenite has been shown to increase expression of the MDR gene, which codes for P-glycoprotein (36), although there is no evidence that P-glycoprotein is responsible for pumping arsenite out of cells. Arsenite also induces the MDR-associated protein (MRP) (37). This protein is responsible for pumping GSH conjugates out of cells, and may play a role in efflux of arsenite under some conditions.

Metallothionein (MT), a small metal-binding protein, was induced in the liver of rats fed arsenite (38). A cDNA subtraction library was made between RNA from HeLa cells growing for 24 hours in the presence and absence of 5 μM sodium arsenite. This led to the identification of metallothionein II and ferritin H chain as arsenite-inducible genes in human cells (39). Metallothionein I expression protects V79 cells against arsenite toxicity (40). A number of investigators have suggested that a major role of MT is to protect against electrophilic agents such as free radicals and reactive metabolites (see discussion in ref. 40). Many of the physical and chemical agents that induce metallothionein also give rise to oxidative stress. That arsenite induces metallothionein and that metallothionein can protect cells from arsenite argue for the importance of oxygen free radicals in arsenite toxicity. In the case of fibroblasts and other cells that do not appear to methylate arsenic (22,25) and thus cannot generate DMAA peroxy radical, the most likely involvement of oxygen would be via depletion of GSH after arsenite treatment, or perhaps via reaction with lipoic acid, which is also an antioxidant.

The exposure of cells to temperatures higher than those they are usually accustomed to results in thermoresistance and the expression of the so-called heat shock proteins (HSPs). Hsp genes are also activated by stimuli seemingly unrelated to heat, including arsenite (41). It has been suggested that all of the inducers of HSPs are agents that can cause the denaturation of cellular proteins (in the case of arsenite, by reacting with vicinal thiols).

Arsenite induces thermoresistance in V79 cells (42,43). Heat and arsenite induce cross-tolerance to each other in hepatoma cells (44) but not in V79 cells, where heat failed to induce arsenite tolerance (43).

Another arsenite-inducible protein has been identified as heme oxygenase (HO) (45), a protein that is also inducible by near UV, cadmium chloride, and hydrogen peroxide, but not very well by heat shock. HO is also thought to protect against oxidant damage. HO cleaves the heme tetrapyrrole ring in cellular hemoproteins involved in redox reactions, causing cellular redox potential to shift toward reduction. The enzymatic product of HO, biliverdin, is then converted to bilirubin, which is also an antioxidant (46). Induction of HO is responsive to cellular levels of GSH, and its induction by arsenite was blocked by antioxidants (47). An arsenite-resistant variant of a human lung adenocarcinoma cell line has elevated levels of heme oxygenase (48), and arsenite resistance in these cells could be blocked by tin-protoporphyrin, an inhibitor of heme oxygenase. Wild type cells, but not the arsenite-resistant variant, showed increased oxidant content after exposure to arsenite for 24 hours, thus supporting the role of oxidants in arsenite toxicity and the protective role of heme oxygenase.

Expression of the proto-oncogenes c-*fos* and c-*myc* (but not of *erbB* or c-*H-ras*) were also induced by arsenite treatment (49,50). Treatment of primary human keratinocytes in culture with arsenite induced a unique cytokine profile that included transforming growth factor-α and granulocyte-macrophage colony stimulating factor. These same cytokines were seen in arsenite-treated Ha-ras transgenic mice, a model for skin cancer (51). Arsenite induces phase 2 enzymes (the so-called electrophile counterattack) in the liver (52). Induction of these enzymes appears to be mediated by enhancer elements that contain AP-1-like sites. AP-1 is composed of the Jun and Fos proteins, both of which are induced by oxidants, as is their DNA-binding activity. Arsenite can also enhance the mitogenic effect of suboptimal serum concentrations on quiescent C3H10T$^{1/2}$ cells (53), possibly via induction of c-Fos and/or HSP70.

Some of the effects of arsenite on gene expression might be mediated by changes in protein phosphorylation. Arsenite has been shown to mimic tumor necrosis factor in inhibiting specific patterns of protein phosphorylation, probably via inactivation of protein phosphatase 2A (PP2A) (54). The induction of HSP28 is associated with such hyperphosphorylation of the protein, which can be caused by arsenite treatment (55). The p34 subunit of RPA, a DNA binding protein needed for DNA repair, is also modulated by PP2A (56), which may help to explain some of the effects of arsenite on DNA repair (see below). The tumor suppressor p53 is also modulated by reversible phosphorylation (57), which may help to explain the effects of arsenite on gene amplification described below.

Both prokaryotic and some eukaryotic cells develop tolerance when exposed to arsenic compounds. The inducible tolerance requires de novo mRNA and protein synthesis, and differs from the heat shock and metallothionein response (43). Although, as mentioned above, arsenite induces metallothionein, which is somewhat protective against arsenite, the amount of protection afforded by metallothionein is much less than that afforded by induction of arsenite tolerance by arsenite (40,43). A number of different human cell lines (including normal diploid fibroblasts from three individuals, meduloblastoma cells, SV40-transformed keratinocytes, and HeLa cells) fail to elicit a tolerance response when exposed to low concentrations of arsenite (58). All human cells tested (especially keratinocytes) are more sensitive to arsenite than are rodent cells, suggesting that failure to elicit tolerance in human cells may play a role in their greater sensitivity. This difference between human and rodent cells may underlie the different carcinogenic effects of arsenic compounds in humans, where arsenic is carcinogenic, and rodents, where it is generally not.

## BIOCHEMICAL MECHANISMS OF ARSENIC TOXICITY

Arsenite [As(III)] is more toxic in vivo and in cell culture than arsenate [As(V)] probably due at least in part to different rates of cellular uptake (22,25,35). Because arsenate is similar in structure to inorganic phosphate, it can compete with phosphate in many biochemical reactions. On a cellular level (particularly in hepatocytes), arsenate inhibits metabolic reactions in mitochondrial oxidative phosphorylation by substituting for inorganic phosphate. This results in the formation of an unstable arsenate ester that spontaneously decomposes. This arsenolysis reaction has the effect of uncoupling ATP synthesis in oxidative phosphorylation and also in glycolysis in the reaction catalyzed by glyceraldehyde 3-phosphate dehydrogenase (11). Exposure of rodents to arsenate results in hepatic mitochondrial damage (14).

Arsenite ($As^{+3}$) does not compete with phosphate, but instead tends to bind to vicinal thiol groups. Because of the risk from the chemical warfare agent Lewisite (chlorvinyldichloroarsine) during World War II, a great deal of research was conducted at that time on the arsenite-thiol interaction. It was found that some enzymes reacted with Lewisite by forming a ring involving arsenic and two thiol groups. A search for dithiol compounds that could displace arsenite from these enzymes led to the discovery of British anti-Lewisite (BAL) and the natural dithiol compound lipoic acid, a cofactor of the pyruvate dehydrogenase (PDH) multienzyme complex (4,11). PDH multienzyme complex plays an important role in controlling the supply of $C_2$ fragments to the mitochondria via production of acetyl-coenzyme A (CoA). Like Lewisite, arsenite exerts toxic effects by reacting with vicinal thiols in the cell. These thiols can exist on adjacent carbon atoms, as in lipoic acid, or on proteins where two cysteine residues act as vicinal thiols by coming into close proximity through the folding of the protein molecule. Other targets for arsenite in mammalian cells may include thiolase, glutathione reductase, DNA ligase, and glucocorticoid receptors (which have vicinal thiol groups) (9,59). Arsenite also inhibits ubiquitin-dependent proteolysis, a process that degrades abnormal proteins and controls the levels of others (60) resulting in upregulation of the levels of proteins that would otherwise be degraded. Compounds that contain vicinal thiol groups can also be used in chelation therapy for treating arsenic intoxication. BAL was used for this purpose in the past, but is now being replaced by the newer compounds meso-2,3-dimercaptosuccinic acid (DMSA) and 2,3-dimercapto-1-propanesulfonic acid (DMPS) (61).

## CARCINOGENICITY OF ARSENIC

Chronic arsenic exposure has become of more concern than acute exposure mainly because of its carcinogenic effects. Inorganic arsenic was one of the earliest identified human carcinogens. Medical treatment with inorganic arsenic compounds (mostly Fowler's solution, which contained 1% potassium arsenite and was used to treat chronic skin conditions such as psoriasis and eczema) was once common. Such patients were found to have an excess of skin cancers, a finding that has led to almost complete elimination of arsenic in human medicine. The major epidemiologic evidence linking cancers with exposure to arsenic is shown in Table 3. The increase in cancer risk observed in epidemiologic studies is attributed mainly to the presence of inorganic trivalent arsenic (62,63). There is little dispute that exposure to arsenic is associated with human skin and lung cancers. The strongest epidemiologic association between arsenic ingestion and an internal cancer is for the bladder (64), followed by kidney and liver (65). An almost tenfold increase in the incidence of lung cancer was found in copper smelter workers most heavily exposed to arsenic. Other smelter worker populations have consistent increases in lung cancer incidence, as well as increases of about 20% in the incidence of gastrointestinal cancer and of 30% for renal cancer and hematolymphatic malignancies.

With regard to the histologic type of lung cancer, a significant, relative excess of adenocarcinomas and a slight excess of oat cell cancers were seen among smelter workers. The skin tumors associated with arsenic exposure differ from sunlight-induced skin tumors in a number of ways. One often sees a gross dysplagia appearing as red, scaling lesions known as Bowen's disease. Some evidence suggests that Bowen's disease may be a marker for internal malignancy. Skin cancers often develop in regions of the body not associated with UV exposure, such as the trunk, palms of the hand, and soles of the feet. Whereas in UV-induced cancers basal cell carcinoma is more frequent than squamous cell carcinoma, the reverse is true for skin tumors associated with arsenic exposure.

Arsenic exposure appears to act synergistically with other carcinogens. For those occupationally exposed to arsenic via inhalation, a synergism with tobacco use in the causation of lung cancer is seen (66). This is also true for those exposed via drinking water (67). It is also thought that lung cancer risk in miners exposed to radon gas may be enhanced by the presence of arsenic as well. The overall prevalence of skin cancers among those drinking arsenic-contaminated water may also be affected by nutritional status and liver dysfunction due to hepatitis B infection (67).

There is no good animal model for arsenic tumorigenesis, although transgenic strains of mice hold some promise (51). Because of this, arsenic compounds are the only compounds that the International Agency for Research on Cancer considers to have sufficient evidence for human carcinogenicity, but inadequate evidence for animal carcinogenicity (62).

**TABLE 3.** *Epidemiologic evidence that arsenic is a human carcinogen*

| Exposed group | Major exposure route | Increased cancer risk |
|---|---|---|
| Smelter workers | Inhalation | Lung (possibly bladder, liver, large intestine, stomach, brain, skin, and hematolymphatic) |
| Sheep dip manufacturing workers | Inhalation | Lung |
| Arsenical pesticide manufacturing workers | | Lung |
| Populations residing near arsenical pesticide plant | Inhalation | Lung |
| Arsenical pesticide applicators | Inhalation | Lung |
| Populations with high arsenic in drinking water | Ingestion | Skin |
| Chile | | |
| Argentina | | |
| Mexico | | |
| Taiwan | | |
| Follow-up studies on Taiwan group | Ingestion | Skin, bladder, lung, liver, kidney, colon, nasal cavity, prostate |
| Patients treated with arsenic-containing medicinals | Cutaneous | Skin |

Data taken from refs. 62, 65–67.

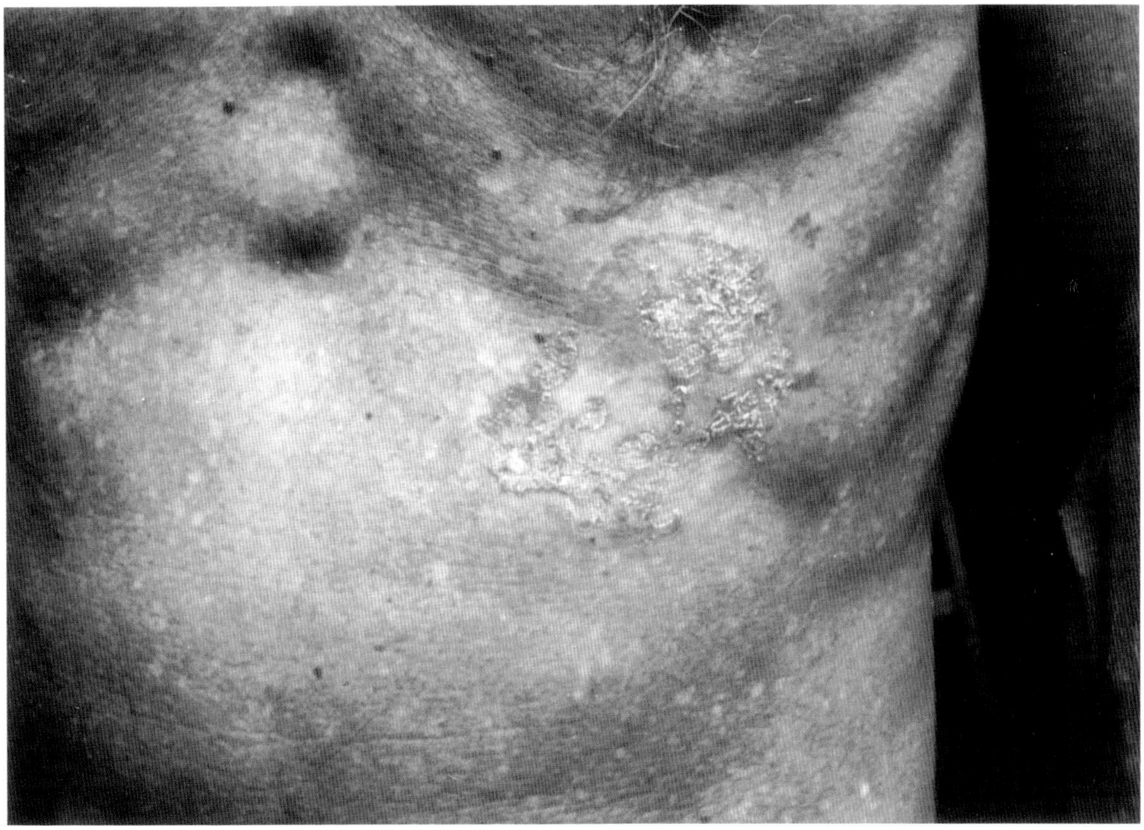

**COLOR PLATE 71–1.** Typical arsenical skin lesions of melanosis, depigmentation, and Bowen's disease on the trunk. (From ref. 76.)

## GENETIC TOXICOLOGY

Unlike many other carcinogens, arsenite is not mutagenic in bacterial or mammalian cell assays that measure mutation at single gene loci (68). Although not a mutagen, arsenite does affect the mutagenicity of other carcinogens, probably via effects on DNA repair. Arsenite enhances the mutagenicity of UV light in *E. coli* and the mutagenicity or clastogenicity of a wide variety of carcinogens in mammalian cells (69). Arsenite inhibits the completion of DNA excision repair, probably by inhibiting DNA ligase II, the last step in the excision repair pathway (59). Arsenite also potentiates the cytotoxic effect of UV in normal human fibroblasts by inhibiting excision of pyrimidine dimers, but has no effect on UV-induced cytotoxicity in cells from xeroderma pigmentosum patients who lack nucleotide excision repair (70).

In spite of its lack of mutagenicity, arsenite can induce transformation to a more malignant phenotype in a number of systems (reviewed in 68,69). Arsenite caused cell transformation and cytogenetic damage in Syrian hamster embryo cells and in 10T1/2 mouse embryo cells. Arsenite also induces neoplastic transformation in BALB/3T3 mouse embryo cells. The transformed cells gave rise to sarcomas after subcutaneous injection into athymic mice. Arsenite also enhanced cellular transformation by bovine papillomavirus and caused anchorage-independent growth (a marker of transformation) but no focus formation or immortality in diploid human fibroblasts.

One must not conclude, however, that arsenite is a nongenotoxic carcinogen (68,69). There is ample demonstration from a number of laboratories that arsenite induces both sister-chromatid exchanges (SCEs) and chromosome aberrations. Although arsenite does not damage DNA directly, DNA-protein cross-links have been detected in arsenite-treated cells. Micronuclei (markers of chromosome damage) are found in the bone marrow of mice treated with arsenite (63). Arsenite induced amplification of the *dhfr* gene in cells.

When the methylated metabolite DMAA is given to animals, lung-specific DNA damage is seen. This damage is caused by the DMAA peroxy radical, which can also induce DNA strand breaks and DNA-protein cross-links in cultured cells (71). While humans exposed to inorganic arsenic could probably never accumulate large amounts of DMAA (or its peroxy radical), free radical damage may account for some of arsenite's genotoxic effects, either via DMAA peroxy radical or via oxygen free radicals resulting from GSH or lipoic acid depletion. Toxicity and genotoxicity of a number of metals does involve oxygen radicals (68). The addition of superoxide dismutase, catalase, or vitamin E to the culture medium protects cells from arsenic toxicity (72,73).

Genetic toxicology end points have been used as biomarkers of human arsenic exposure. Individuals drinking arsenic-contaminated water in Argentina for a period of at least 20 years showed a significant elevation in lymphocyte SCE levels (74). Exfoliated bladder epithelial cells of individuals drinking arsenic-contaminated well water in Nevada had elevated micronuclei levels. The bladder cell micronucleus assay has been suggested to be the most appropriate biologic marker of arsenic genotoxicity (75).

The mechanisms by which arsenic compounds cause human cancers are not known (69). No changes in the expression of specific oncogenes or tumor suppressor genes have been demonstrated in arsenic-induced cancer cells. In transgenic mice expressing the *Ha-ras* oncogene, arsenite increased the numbers of papillomas induced by the tumor promoter phorbol ester (51). Thus, arsenite might be considered a co-promoter or a tumor enhancer. The clastogenic (chromosome breaking) effects of arsenite would be more likely to result in the loss of tumor suppressor functions (e.g., by deletion) than in altered oncogene function by point mutation. It is also likely that arsenite's ability to alter gene expression and to cause gene amplification may play an important role in its carcinogenic action.

## REFERENCES


1. Leonard A. Arsenic. In: Merian E, ed. *Metals and their compounds in the environment.* New York: Verlagsgesellschaft, 1991;751–774.
2. Landrigan PJ. Arsenic In: Rom WN, ed. *Environmental and occupational medicine,* 2nd ed. Boston, MA: Little, Brown, 1992;773–779.
3. Garcia-Vargas GG, Cebrián ME. Health effects of arsenic. In: Wang LW, ed. *Toxicology of metals.* Boca Raton, FL: CRC Press, 1996; 423–438.
4. Bencko V. Arsenic. In: Fishbein L, Furst A, Mchlman MA, eds. *Advances in modern environmental toxicology, vol 11:* Genotoxic and carcinogenic metals: *environmental and occupational occurrence and exposure.* Princeton, NJ: Princeton Scientific, 1987;1–30.
5. Squibb KS, Fowler BA. The toxicity of arsenic and its compounds. In: Fowler BA, ed. *Biological and environmental effects of arsenic.* Amsterdam: Elsevier, 1983;233.
6. Pinto SS, Nelson KW. Arsenic toxicology and industrial exposure. *Annu Rev Pharmacol Toxicol* 1976;16:95.1.
7. Carter D, Bellamy WTY. Toxicology of the group III-V intermetallic semiconductor, gallium arsenide. In: Clarkson TW, Friberg L, Nordberg GF, Sager PR, eds. *Biological monitoring of toxic metals.* New York: Plenum Press, 1988;455–468.
8. Flora SJS. Alterations in some hepatic biochemical variables following repeated gallium arsenide administration in rats. *Int Hepatol Commun* 1996;5:2.
9. Aposhian HV, Aposhian MM. New developments in arsenic toxicity. *J Am Coll Toxicol* 1989;8:1273–1281.
10. Tamaki S, Frankenberger WT Jr. Environmental biochemistry of arsenic. *Rev Environ Contamin Toxicol* 1992;124:79–110.
11. Aposhian HV. Biochemical toxicology of arsenic. *Rev Biochem Toxicol* 1989;10:265–299.
12. Uthus EO, Nielsen FH. Determination of the possible requirement and reference dose levels for arsenic in humans. *Scand J Work Environ Health* 1993;19:137–138.
13. Vahter M, Marafante E, Dencker L. Metabolism of arsenobetaine in mice, rats and rabbits. *Sci Total Environ* 1983;30:197.
14. Fowler BA. Toxicology of environmental arsenic In: Goyer GA, Mehlman MA, eds. *Toxicology of trace elements.* New York: John Wiley, 1977;79–122.
15. Klimecki WT, Carter DE. Arsine toxicity: chemical implications and mechanistic implications. *J Toxicol Environ Health* 1995;46:399–409.
16. Bagla P, Kaiser J. India's spreading health crisis draws global arsenic experts. *Science* 1996;274:174–175.
17. Mazumder DNG, Chakraborty AK, Ghose A, Gupta JD. Chronic arsenic toxicity from drinking tubewell water in rural West Bengal. *Bull World Health Org* 1988;66:499–506.
18. Aposhian HV. Enzymatic methylation of arsenic species and other new

approaches to arsenic toxicity. *Annu Rev Pharmacol Toxicol* 1997; 37:397–419.
19. Styblo M, Delnomdedieu M, Thomas DJ. Biological mechanisms and toxicological consequences of the methylation of arsenic. In: Goyer RA, Cherian, G, eds. *Toxicology of metals biochemical aspects.* New York: Springer-Verlag, 1995;407–433.
20. Vahter M. Metabolism of arsenic. In: Fowler BA, ed. *Biological and environmental effects of arsenic.* Amsterdam: Elsevier, 1983;171–198.
21. Buchet JP, Lauwerys R, Roels H. Comparison of the urinary excretion of arsenic metabolites after a single dose of sodium arsenite, monomethylarsonate or dimethylarsinate in man. *Int Arch Occup Environ Health* 1981;48:71–79.
22. Bertolero F, Pozzi G, Sabbioni E, Saffiotti U. Cellular uptake and metabolic reduction of pentavalent to trivalent arsenic as determinants of cytotoxicity and morphological transformation. *Carcinogenesis* 1987; 8:803–808.
23. Delnomdedieu M, Basti MM, Otvos JD, Thomas DJ. Reduction and binding of arsenate and dimethylarsinate by glutathione: a magnetic resonance study. *Chem Biol Interact* 1994;90:139–155.
24. Delnomdedieu M, Basti MM, Styblo M, Otvos JD, Thomas DJ. Complexation of arsenic species in rabbit erythrocytes. *Chem Res Toxicol* 1994;7:621–627.
25. Wang Z, Dey S, Rosen BP, Rossman TG. Efflux mediated resistance to arsenicals in arsenic resistant and -hypersensitive Chinese hamster cells. *Toxicol Appl Pharmacol* 1996;137:112–119.
26. Georis B, Cardenas A, Buchet JP, Lauwerys R. Inorganic arsenic methylation by rat tissue slices. *Toxicology* 1990;63:73–84.
27. Marafante E, Vahter M, Envoi J. The role of the methylation in the detoxication of arsenate in the rabbit. *Chem Biol Interact* 1985;56: 225–238.
28. Scott N, Hatlelid KM, MacKenzie NE, Carter DE. Reactions of arsenic (III) and arsenic (V) species with glutathione. *Chem Res Toxicol* 1993;6:102–106.
29. Huang H, Huang CF, Wu DR, Jinn CM, Jan KY. Glutathione as a cellular defense against arsenite toxicity in cultured Chinese hamster ovary cells. *Toxicology* 1993;79:195–204.
30. Vega L, Gonseblatt ME, Ostrosky-Wegman P. Aneugenic effect of sodium arsenite on human lymphocytes in vitro: an individual susceptibility effect detected. *Mutat Res* 1995;334:365–373.
31. Aposhian HV. Arsenic toxicology: does methylation of arsenic species have an evolutionary significance? *Metal Ions Biol Med* 1996;4: 399–401.
32. Rosen BP. Resistance mechanisms to arsenicals and antimonials. *Rev Clin Basic Pharmacol* 1995;6:251–263.
33. Lo JF, Wang HF, Tam MF, Lee TC. Glutathione S-transferase in an arsenic-resistant Chinese hamster ovary cell line. *Biochem J* 1992;288: 977–981.
34. Gyurasics A, Varga F, Gregus Z. Glutathione-dependent biliary excretion of arsenic. *Biochem Pharmacol* 1991;42:465–468.
35. Lerman SA, Clarkson TW, Gerson RJ. Arsenic uptake and metabolism by liver cells is dependent on arsenic oxidation state. *Chem Biol Interact* 1983;45:401–406.
36. Chin KV, Tanaka S, Darlington G, Pastan I, Gottesman MM. Heat shock and arsenite increase expression of the multidrug resistance (MDR1) gene in human renal carcinoma cells. *J Biol Chem* 1990;265: 221–226.
37. Ishikawa T, Bao JJ, Yamane Y. Coordinated induction of MRP/GS/X pump and g-glutamylcysteine synthetase by heavy metals in human leukemia cells. *J Biol Chem* 1996;271:14981–14988.
38. Albores A, Koropatnick J, Cherian MG, Zelazowski AJ. Arsenic induces and enhances rat hepatic metallothionein production in vivo. *Chem Biol Interact* 1992;85:127–140.
39. Guzzo A, Karatzios C, Diorio C, DuBow MS. Metallothionein-II and ferritin H mRNA levels are increased in arsenite-exposed HeLa cells. *Biochem Biophys Res Commun* 1994;205:590–595.
40. Goncharova EI, Rossman TG. The antimutagenic effects of metallothionein may involve free radical scavenging. In: Sarkar B, ed. *Genetic response to metals.* New York: Marcel Dekker, 1995;87–100.
41. Deaton MA, Bowman PD, Jones GP, Powanda MC. Stress protein synthesis in human keratinocytes treated with sodium arsenite, phenyldichloroarsine and nitrogen mustard. *Fundam Appl Toxicol* 1990;14:471–476.
42. Hatayama T, Kano E, Taniguchi Y, Nitta K. Role of heat-shock proteins in the induction of thermotolerance in Chinese hamster V79 cells by heat and chemical agents. *Int J Hyperthermia* 1991;1:61–74.
43. Wang Z, Hou G, Rossman TG. Induction of arsenite tolerance and thermotolerance by arsenite occur by different mechanisms. *Environ Health Perspect* 1994;102:97–100.
44. van Rijn J, van den Berg J, Wiegant FA, van Wijk R. Sensitization to x-rays by sodium arsenite or heat in normal cells and in cells with an induced tolerance for heat and arsenite. *Radiat Environ Biophys* 1995; 34:169–175.
45. Keyse SM, Tyrrell RM. Heme oxygenase is the major 32-kDa stress protein induced in human skin fibroblasts by UVA radiation, hydrogen peroxide, and sodium arsenite. *Proc Natl Acad Sci USA* 1989;85: 99–103.
46. Stocker RY, Yamamoto Y, McDonagh AF, Glazer, AN, Ames BN. Bilirubin is an antioxidant of possible physiological importance. *Science* 1987;235:1043–1046.
47. Lee T-C, Ho I-C. Modulation of cellular antioxidant defense activities by sodium arsenite in human fibroblasts. *Arch Toxicol* 1995;69: 498–504.
48. Lee T-C, Ho I-C. Expression of heme oxygenase in arsenic-resistant human lung adenocarcinoma cells. *Cancer Res* 1994;54:1660–1664.
49. Gubits RM. c-*fos* mRNA levels are increased by the cellular stressors, heat shock and sodium arsenite. *Oncogene* 1988;3:163–168.
50. Li J-H, Billing PC, Kennedy AR. Induction of oncogene expression by sodium arsenite in C3H/10T1/2 cells: inhibition of c-*myc* expression by the Bowman-Birk protease inhibitor. *Cancer J* 1992;5:354–358.
51. Luster MI, Wilmer JL, Germolec DR, Spalding J, et al. Role of keratinocyte-derived cytokines in chemical toxicity. *Toxicol Lett* 1995;82-83:471–476.
52. Prestera T, Zhang Y, Spencer SR, Wilczak CA, Talaly P. The electrophile counterattack response: protection against neoplasia and toxicity. *Adv Enzyme Regul* 1993;33:281–296.
53. Kullik I, Story G. Transcriptional regulators of the oxidative stress response in prokaryotes and eukaryotes. *Redox Rep* 1994;1:23–29.
54. Guy GR, Cairns J, Ng SB, Tan YH. Inactivation of a redox-sensitive protein phosphatase during the early events of tumor necrosis factor/interleukin-1 signal transduction. *J Biol Chem* 1993;268: 2141–2148.
55. Huang RN, Ho IC, Yih LH, Lee TC. Sodium arsenite induces chromosome endoreduplication and inhibits protein phosphatase activity in human fibroblasts. *Environ Mol Mutagen* 1995;25:188–196.
56. Ariza RR, Keyse SM, Moggs JG, Wood RD. Reversible protein phosphorylation modulates nucleotide excision repair of damaged DNA by human cell extracts. *Nucleic Acids Res* 1996;24:433–440.
57. Zhang W, McClain C, Gau JP, Guo XY, Deisseroth AB. Hyperphosphorylation of p53 by okadaic acid attenuates its transcriptional activation function. *Cancer Res* 1994;54:4448–4453.
58. Rossman TG, Goncharova EI, Rajah T, Wang Z. Human cells lack the inducible tolerance to arsenite seen in Chinese hamster cells. *Mutat Res* 1997;386:307–314.
59. Li J-H, Rossman TG. Inhibition of DNA ligase activity by arsenite: a possible mechanism of its comutagenesis. *Mol Toxicol* 1989;2:1–9.
60. Klemperer NS, Pickartt CM. Arsenite inhibits two steps in the ubiquitin-dependent proteolytic pathway. *J Biol Chem* 1989;264: 19245–19252.
61. Aposhian HV, Maiorion RM, Gonzales-Ramirez D, Zuniga-Charles M, Xu Z. Mobilization of heavy metals by newer, therapeutically useful chelating agents. *Toxicology* 1995;97:23–38.
62. IARC (International Agency for Research on Cancer). *IARC monographs on the evaluation of carcinogenic risk of chemicals to man, vol 23. Some metals and metallic compounds.* Lyon, France: World Health Organization, 1980.
63. Tinwell H, Stephens SC, Ashby J. Arsenite as the probable active species in the human carcinogenicity of arsenic: mouse micronucleus assays on Na and K arsenite, orpiment, and Fowler's solution. *Environ Health Perspect* 1991;95:205–210.
64. Smith AH, Hopenhayn-Rich C, Bates MN, et al. Cancer risk from arsenic in drinking water. *Environ Health Perspect* 1992;97:259–267.
65. Bates MN, Smith AH, Hopenhayn-Rich C. Arsenic ingestion and internal cancers: a review. *Am J Epidemiol* 1992;135:462–476.
66. Hertz-Piccotto I, Smith AH, Holzman D, Lipsett M, Alexeeff G. Synergism between occupational arsenic exposure and smoking in the induction of lung cancer. *Epidemiology* 1992;3:23–31.
67. Choiu H-Y, Hsueh Y-M, Liaw S-F, et al. Incidence of internal cancers and ingested inorganic arsenic: a seven-year follow-up study in Taiwan. *Cancer Res* 1995;55:1296–1300.
68. Rossman TG. Metal mutagenesis. In: Goyer RA, Cherian MG, eds.

*Toxicology of metals—biochemical aspects.* New York: Springer-Verlag, 1994;374–405.
69. Wang Z, Rossman TG. The carcinogenicity of arsenic. In: Chang LW, ed. *Toxicology of metals.* Boca Raton, FL: CRC Press, 1996;219–227.
70. Okui T, Fujiwara Y. Inhibition of human excision DNA repair by inorganic arsenic and the comutagenic effect in V79 Chinese hamster cells. *Mutat Res* 1986;172:69–76.
71. Tezuka M, Hanioka K-I, Yamanaka K, Okada S. Gene damage induced in human alveolar type II (L-1232) cells by exposure to dimethylarsinic acid. *Biochem Biophys Res Commun* 1993;191:1178–1183.
72. Wang TS, Huang H. Active oxygen species are involved in the induction of micronuclei by arsenite in XRS-5 cells. *Mutagenesis* 1994;9:253–257.
73. Lee TC, Ho IC. Differential cytotoxic effects of arsenic on human and animal cells. *Environ Health Perspect* 1994;3:101–105.
74. Lerda D. Sister-chromatid exchange (SCE) among individuals chronically exposed to arsenic in drinking water. *Mutat Res* 1994;312:111–120.
75. Warner ML, Moore LE, Smith MT, et al. Increased micronuclei in exfoliated bladder cells of individuals who chronically ingest arsenic-contaminated water in Nevada. *Cancer Epidemiol Biomarkers Prevent* 1994;3:583–590.
76. Hotta N. Clinical aspects of arsenic poisoning due to environmental and occupational pollution in and around a small refining spot. *Jpn J Constitutional Med* 1989;53:49–70.

*Environmental and Occupational Medicine, Third Edition,* edited by William N. Rom.
Lippincott–Raven Publishers, Philadelphia © 1998.

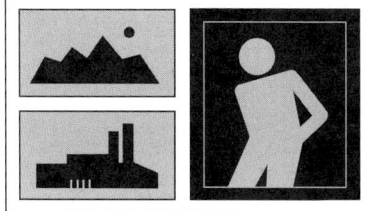

# CHAPTER 72

# Beryllium Disease

Lisa A. Maier and Lee S. Newman

Beryllium is an excellent material for high technologic applications, but it produces a number of insidious adverse health effects. It is the fourth lightest element (atomic weight = 9.02), has a low density (1.85 g/cm$^3$), high melting point, high tensile strength, and is corrosion resistant. Found in over 45 minerals, including some gemstones, beryllium is present at very low levels in soil and air in most urban centers. Exposure to beryllium occurs during the extraction of the mineral from its ores, beryl and bertrandite, and processing of beryllium into metal alloys and ceramic products. As indicated in Table 1, further exposure occurs during secondary machining and processing of the beryllium alloys and ceramic products in other industries, including electronics, aerospace, tool and die, nuclear weapons manufacturing, and dental prosthesis manufacturing. Historically, beryllium was used in the fluorescent light industry, although this practice was discontinued in the 1950s upon recognition of its health hazards. Exposure to beryllium can induce delayed-type hypersensitivity, and dermatologic, pulmonary, and systemic disease, including the granulomatous condition chronic beryllium disease (CBD) (Table 2). This chapter summarizes our present state of knowledge based on the epidemiologic workplace studies, basic research on the role of the immune response to beryllium, and clinical research on the diseases that ensue, and addresses the recent developments in CBD detection and diagnosis. The chapter emphasizes CBD, since this is now the most common form of beryllium toxicity, continuing to occur in 2% to 16% of exposed workers.

L. A. Maier: Department of Medicine, Division of Pulmonary and Critical Care Medicine, University of Colorado Health Sciences Center; and Division of Environmental and Occupational Health Sciences, National Jewish Medical and Research Center, Denver, Colorado 80207.

L. S. Newman: Department of Preventive Medicine and Biometrics, University of Colorado Health Sciences Center; and Division of Environmental and Health Sciences, National Jewish Medical and Research Center, Denver, Colorado 80206.

## HISTORICAL PERSPECTIVE

Although the element beryllium, originally named "glucinium," was first discovered in the late 1700s, its toxicity was not appreciated until the early part of this century, when the industrial processing of beryllium began in earnest. In the 1930s, reports of lung and skin diseases in workers in beryllium industries began surfacing in the European medical literature (1) and in Russia (2,3). In the early 1940s, Van Ordstrand and his colleagues (4) described beryllium workers with an acute chemical pneumonitis or bronchiolitis in the United States, although these abnormalities were misattributed initially to other chemicals in the manufacturing process. The link between beryllium and granulomatous lung disease was forged in this country when an outbreak of sarcoidosis was described in fluorescent lamp industry workers in Salem, Massachusetts by Harriet Hardy and Irving Tabershaw (5). In addition to the reports of chronic disease associated with beryllium industry workers, disease was discovered in individuals living in areas surrounding beryllium industries and among household contacts of beryllium industry workers (6–9).

Early epidemiologic and exposure assessments led Sterner and Eisenbud (7) to observe that CBD occurred at both high and low levels of exposure, without a clear association between magnitude of exposure and disease incidence. They hypothesized that beryllium-related diseases were immunologically mediated, resulting from a specific response to the antigen beryllium—quite an

**TABLE 1.** *Industries and occupations with potential beryllium exposure*

| |
|---|
| Aerospace |
| Automotive parts |
| Ceramics |
| Computers |
| Dental supplies and prosthesis manufacture |
| Electronics |
| Foundries |
| Glass manufacture |
| Nuclear reactor manufacture |
| Nuclear weapons production |
| Refractories |
| Smelters |
| Telecommunications |
| Tool and die |
| Welding |

**TABLE 2.** *Principal human health effects of beryllium exposure*

| Target organ | Disorder |
|---|---|
| Skin | Contact dermatitis |
| | Subcutaneous granulomatous nodules |
| | Ulceration |
| | Delayed wound healing |
| Eyes | Conjunctivitis |
| | Corneal ulceration, edema |
| Oral cavity | Gingivitis |
| | Salivary gland stones[a] |
| Respiratory tract | Rhinitis |
| | Nasal septal perforation |
| | Tracheitis |
| | Bronchitis |
| | Bronchiolitis |
| | Acute pneumonitis |
| | Chronic beryllium disease (CBD) (granulomatous interstitial pneumonitis with or without systemic involvement) |
| | Lung cancer |
| | Pulmonary hypertension[a], cor pulmonale[a] |
| | Pneumothorax[a] |
| Lymphatic/ hematologic | Hilar and mediastinal lymphadenopathy[a] |
| | Beryllium sensitization (delayed-type hypersensitivity, cell-mediated antigenic response to beryllium) |
| | Polyclonal gammopathy[a] |
| | Leukopenia, lymphopenia[a] |
| | Polycythemia[a] |
| Heart | Cardiomyopathy |
| | Conduction system abnormalities due to infiltration of granulomas[a] |
| Gastrointestinal | Granulomatous hepatitis and splenic infiltration[a] |
| Kidney | Nephrolithiasis[a] |
| | Hypercalcemia, hypercalcuria[a] |
| Rheumatologic | Hyperuricemia |
| Central nervous system | Granulomas, producing seizures[a] |

[a]Occurs in association with chronic beryllium disease.

advanced idea considering the limited understanding of immunology in the 1940s and 1950s. Knowing that beryllium can be retained in the lungs for many years after last exposure, Sterner and Eisenbud speculated that an individual could become immunologically sensitized to beryllium long after stopping work, which helped explain the latency of disease development noted in some cases. Much of our current understanding of the immunopathogenesis of CBD supports Sterner and Eisenbud's rudimentary theories and will be discussed in more detail below.

A beryllium exposure standard was introduced in 1949 by the Atomic Energy Commission, setting occupational exposures at a permissible exposure limit of 2 $\mu g/m^3$ for an 8-hour time-weighted average, and a peak level of 25 $\mu g/m^3$. The occupational standard was proposed after a discussion in the back of a taxicab based on existing standards for other toxic metals and on conjecture, without significant direct data on beryllium dose-response relations (10). Based on a study of neighborhood cases surrounding one beryllium plant, the environmental standard for air around factories was set at 0.01 $\mu g/m^3$ averaged over a 30-day period. As a result of these standards, some industrial controls were implemented in the late 1940s and early 1950s, leading to a reduction in the levels emitted by most industries. The U.S. Beryllium Case Registry was established at the Massachusetts General Hospital in 1952, to catalog cross-sectional and long-term information on patients with acute and chronic beryllium disease. Until the 1980s, most clinical knowledge about beryllium-related lung disease had stemmed from the study of the cases in this registry, including pathology, disease latency, progression of acute to chronic disease, and exposure information (11–14). Fortunately, after implementation of the exposure standard, acute cases of beryllium lung disease largely ceased, and the occurrence of neighborhood and household contact cases of CBD diminished. In 1978, the disease registry was moved to Cincinnati, at the National Institute of Occupational Safety and Health, but became inactive. As of 1987, over 900 cases of beryllium-related lung disease had been recorded (15), including 76 new cases since 1966, a number of which developed the disease after the implementation of the 2 $\mu g/m^3$ standard. The registry's case breakdown includes approximately 212 acute cases, 648 chronic cases, and 44 cases of disease that progressed form acute pneumonitis to CBD. Most new cases are not reported to the registry. While the reduction of beryllium levels in the workplace may have reduced the incidence of acute disease, CBD continues to occur (16–28). A case of acute berylliosis in a dental laboratory technician, whose exposure entailed grinding a beryllium alloy for 4 to 6 hours a day for 3 months, was reported in 1984 (29). Adherence to the existing standard does not afford full protection from CBD (19,28,30,31).

## TOXICOLOGY AND EXPOSURE

The number of workers with potential beryllium exposure in the United States is not known, although some estimates indicate that up to 800,000 individuals in this country have been exposed to beryllium at some time (19,32). Disease rates for CBD have been estimated at 2% to 16% of exposed workers, depending on the group studied (15,21,25,26,28,33,34). Beryllium targets primarily the lung, lymph nodes, and skin, either by direct toxicity or by its impact on the immune system, or both. Skin lesions, including granuloma formation and ulceration, occur following direct injection of beryllium into the skin. Cutaneous contact with beryllium salts can induce contact dermatitis. Inhalation of fumes and respirable dusts of beryllium salts, metal or oxides, or of beryllium-containing metal alloys results in beryllium-related respiratory diseases. Although the definitive study has not been published, exposure to the ore in the form of either beryl or bertrandite has not been shown to cause disease. However, beryllium ore workers have developed sensitization to beryllium (29). Once inhaled, the beryllium particles obey general principles of particle deposition in the lung. Most likely the chemical properties of the inhaled beryllium particle influences its toxicity. The solubility, particle size, and the form of beryllium inhaled influence the development of an immune response and disease (35). For example, beryllium oxide produced at a lower temperatures has been shown to be less immunogenic than that formed at a higher temperatures. Most of the beryllium inhaled is cleared by the lung's mucociliary escalator and airway macrophages. Some of the remaining beryllium is moved to the regional lymph nodes and pulmonary interstitium, remaining in the lung for many years after the last exposure. Beryllium is poorly absorbed through the gastrointestinal tract, making this a less likely route of exposure, but may it be distributed in the liver, kidney, and bone. Elimination occurs primarily through urine.

Certain beryllium industrial processes and job tasks increase the risk of developing an immune response to beryllium and disease. For example, machinists in both the ceramics and nuclear weapons manufacture have been found to have an increased risk of developing sensitization (25,26,28). The exact exposure-response relationship for CBD, while still unclear, does not appear to be strictly linear. However, both dose and duration of beryllium exposure have been associated with increased risk of sensitization and disease in some studies. Clearly, this is most evident with acute pneumonitis, which occurs only at high exposures (5), in the 25 $\mu g/m^3$ range or greater (36). On the other hand, CBD also develops in workers with seemingly minimal exposures, including security guards and secretaries (25,26,37–39) and after as short a duration as 4 months (33). Thus, it appears that beryllium's effects may be dose dependent, but that other factors modify the impact of beryllium exposure. In one study, tobacco smoking was found to reduce the risk of sensitization, raising the question of a protective effect from smoking (28). Genetic susceptibility to beryllium may also contribute to disease risk, as discussed below.

## IMMUNOPATHOGENESIS AND DISEASE SUSCEPTIBILITY

Many of the questions raised by beryllium's unconventional dose-response relationship promoted research in animals and in humans on the immunologic effects of beryllium. Inhalation or tracheal instillation of various beryllium moieties produces lung injury ranging from an acute chemical pneumonitis to a mononuclear cellular infiltration and formation of granulomas and/or fibrosis in rats, mice, guinea pigs, dogs, and nonhuman primates (40–49). In some of the more meticulous animal exposure studies, Haley and colleagues (43,44) challenged beagle dogs with various forms of beryllium oxide particulate and evaluated the pathologic and immune response longitudinally. Over 1 year, the dogs developed granulomas, fibrosis, and lymphocytic infiltrates in their lungs. A lymphocytic T-helper–predominant alveolitis was observed, along with an *in vitro* lymphocyte proliferative response to beryllium. Studies using T-cell lines from the beagle lung indicated a beryllium-specific immune response (44). The dog model has one significant limitation: unlike in human disease, the pathologic and immunologic response in the dog appears to resolve spontaneously. Mice and nonhuman primates mount a lymphocyte-predominant granulomatous response similar to the dog. In one mouse model, in vivo lymphocyte proliferation was demonstrated in granulomas, around blood vessels, and in areas of white blood cell aggregation (49). Although the response in the study cannot be proven to be beryllium specific, it parallels the lymphoproliferative response to beryllium that is seen in humans. Mouse and guinea pig strains that differ only in their major histocompatibility complex (MHC) loci mount varying immune responses to beryllium, suggesting genetic control (40,41,47). Cumulatively, these animal models support a beryllium-specific cell-mediated immune response with pathologic responses similar to those seen in humans that can be modified by both beryllium exposure and genetics.

Numerous lines of evidence in humans suggest that beryllium induces an antigen-specific cellular immune response. As early as 1951, Curtis (50) showed that individuals with CBD developed a cutaneous delayed-type hypersensitivity when skin patch tested with beryllium salts. Some even develop a granulomatous response at the skin patch test site weeks later (50,51). Numerous *in vitro* studies have confirmed the role of cellular immunity in

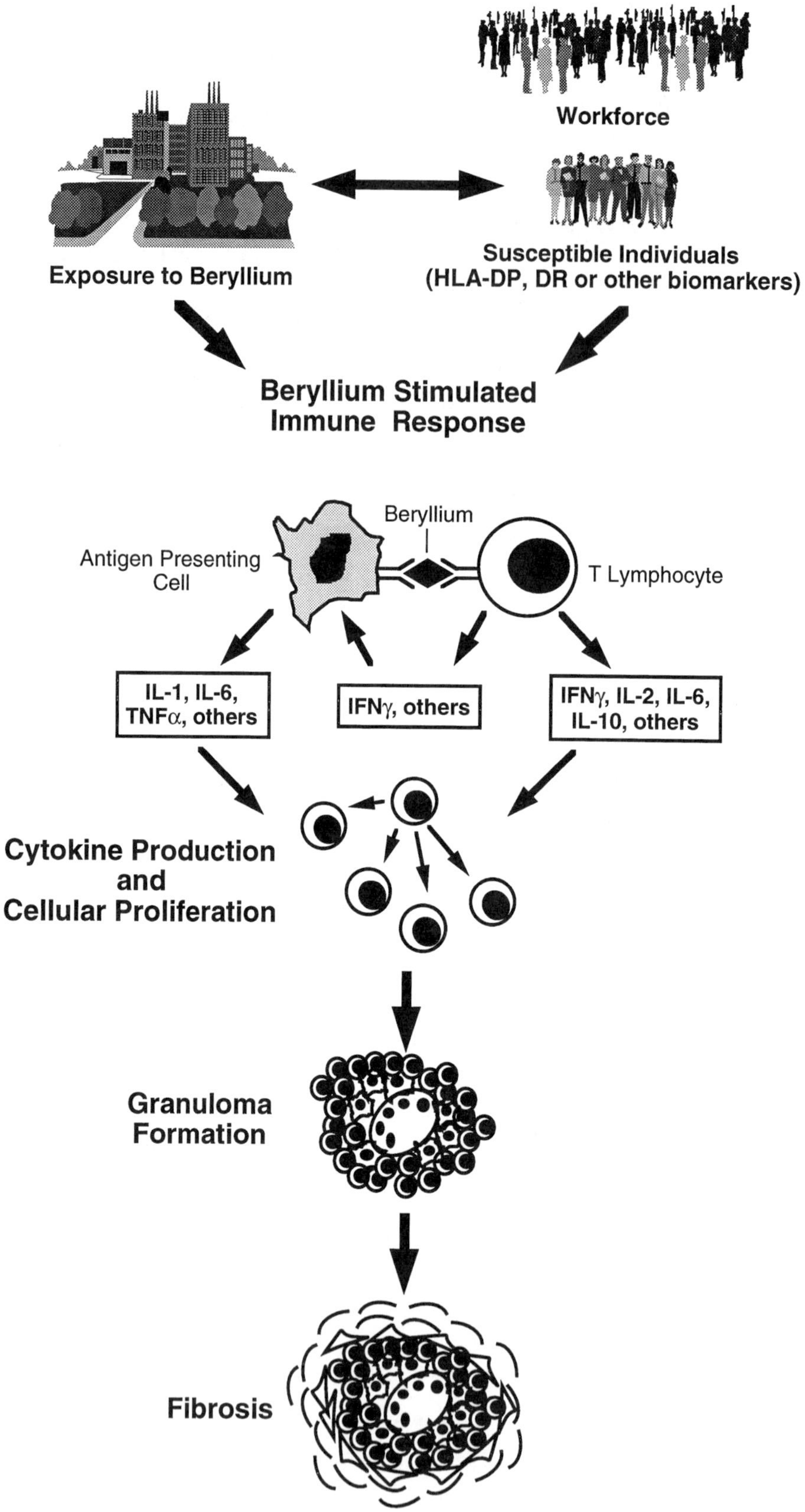

Workforce
Exposure to Beryllium
Susceptible Individuals
(HLA-DP, DR or other biomarkers)
Beryllium Stimulated
Immune Response
Beryllium
Antigen Presenting
Cell
T Lymphocyte
IL-1, IL-6,
TNFα, others
IFNγ, others
IFNγ, IL-2, IL-6,
IL-10, others
Cytokine Production
and
Cellular Proliferation
Granuloma
Formation
Fibrosis

CBD. When peripheral blood or bronchoalveolar lavage (BAL) cells are cultured in the presence of beryllium salts, those lymphocytes that possess memory for beryllium proliferate (16,17,20,21,23,24,52–55). These observations form the basis for the beryllium lymphocyte proliferation test (BeLPT), which is now widely used to detect beryllium sensitization and disease (17,20–26, 55,56). This test has been found to discriminate CBD from other granulomatous diseases; BAL cells from CBD cases show a marked proliferative response to beryllium salts while those from other granulomatous diseases, such as sarcoidosis, do not (16,20,56). When peripheral blood BeLPT was evaluated as a potential screening tool in the 1980s, Kreiss, Newman, and colleagues (21,22,24–26, 28,55) showed that this immune biomarker enhances early detection of CBD in many industries. In these studies, some individuals were found to be sensitized to beryllium, as indicated by a positive response in the BeLPT and initiation of the cellular immune response, without evidence of pulmonary disease (21,25,26,28,55,28). Some of these individuals have since developed granulomatous disease within a short follow-up period, indicating that sensitization precedes the inflammatory response in the lung and is a step in the progression from exposure to disease (25,37,39). The BeLPT and its utility in disease surveillance are discussed in more depth below. The BeLPT is performed on peripheral blood mononuclear cells (PBMCs, $2 \times 10^5$ cells/well) or BAL cells ($10^5$ cells/well) in flat-bottom 96-well microtiter plates cultured for 3, 5, and 7 days in the presence of $10^{-4}$, $10^{-5}$, and $10^{-6}$ M beryllium sulfate. Tritiated thymidine is added for the last 24 hours of incubation and the stimulation index (SI) is calculated as the highest uptake compared to incubation of unstimulated cells for any concentration of beryllium sulfate on any day of harvest. An SI of approximately 2 to 3 is considered positive, depending on laboratory specific cutoff valves that are based on testing of normal subjects' cells. Two or more elevated SI values define a positive test (37,55).

Saltini and co-workers (23,57) showed that the cellular immune response to beryllium requires class II MHC for presentation of antigen to the T cells and for proliferation of the memory T cells. Beryllium-reactive T-cell clones probably recognize the antigen via their antigen receptor. This notion is supported by the finding of a limited subset of T-cell receptors in the lungs compared to the blood of patients with CBD (38,58,59). Beryllium is likely acting in conjunction with a hapten (i.e., peptide), although the exact form of the antigen is unclear at this time. Following antigen presentation and recognition, immune effector cells become activated (52). Key inflammatory cytokines are produced, including tumor necrosis factor-α (TNF-α), interleukin-6 (IL-6) (60), IL-2, and γ-interferon (INFγ) (61,62). These cytokines enhance the inflammatory and immune response of the lymphocytes, macrophage, and other cells within the lung, while regulating the development of granulomas and the immune response in CBD (Fig. 1), thus acting in a self-propagating manner that amplifies the inflammatory response in the target organ. In CBD, the beryllium-reactive cells and immune response are largely compartmentalized to the lung (27). Other cells found at sites of granuloma formation may help limit the magnitude of this runaway pulmonary immune response. For example, mast cells found in the circumference of CBD granulomas produce fibrogenic growth factors, such as basic fibroblast growth factor (bFGF), that may help promote the formation of a fibrotic capsule surrounding the granuloma (63).

The progression from exposure to disease in CBD may hinge partly on an individual's genetic susceptibility. The finding of familial cases of CBD in identical twins (64) and in parents and children (37,38) suggests a genetic predisposition to CBD. Most striking are the results of a study by Richeldi et al. (65,66), which found an increased usage of MHC human leukocyte antigen (HLA) DPb1 with a glutamic acid residue at position 69 in patients with disease compared with exposed individuals. Other allelic differences may be found in the HLA-DR loci in individuals with CBD (67). Since HLA class II molecules are involved in the presentation of most antigens to the T-cell antigen receptor, it is hypothesized that genetic differences in the HLA may dictate the ability of a person's cells to mount an immune response to beryllium. It is unlikely that these genetic markers will be clinically useful, since a large percentage of the general population has the same allelic substitution (66). Regardless of an individual's genetics, beryllium disease does not occur unless that person has been exposed to beryllium.

**FIG. 1.** Immunopathogenesis of chronic beryllium disease. Individuals in the work force who are exposed to beryllium and who may have genetic markers of beryllium susceptibility mount a beryllium-stimulated immune response upon exposure. Within the target organ, such as the lung, beryllium is taken up by antigen-presenting cells and processed. The antigenic moiety is packaged with class II MHC molecules and transported to the surface of the cell. The MHC and antigenic material are recognized by T lymphocytes through their T cell antigen-receptor complex. This triggers the T lymphocyte to produce key cytokines that help promote T-cell proliferation and inflammatory cell recruitment. Cytokines activate other immune effector cells, such as macrophages. These cells, in turn, produce other key proinflammatory cytokines and growth factors that promote amplification of the inflammatory response in the target organ. The consequence is the accumulation of differentiated cells that constitute the typical noncaseating granuloma. Over time, areas of fibrosis form surrounding the granuloma.

## CLINICAL DISEASE

Depending on the amount, form, and route of exposure to beryllium, various diseases may result, ranging from acute to chronic lung disease, dermatologic disease, or cancer. As the respiratory diseases are most common, they are the focus of this section.

### Respiratory Manifestations

Beryllium-related pulmonary manifestations exist on a continuum from acute inhalational injury to acute pneumonitis to beryllium sensitization and the chronic indolent form of CBD. In fact, a number of early acute beryllium disease survivors eventually developed the chronic form of the disease (11,68,69).

#### *Acute Disease*

Exposure to elevated concentrations of beryllium can result in inflammation of the upper and lower respiratory tract and airways, bronchiolitis, pulmonary edema, and chemical pneumonitis (11,68,69). The manifestations of acute beryllium disease are not specific and may mimic many other inhalational injuries. The upper airway manifestations include beryllium nasopharyngitis and tracheobronchitis. The former may present with irritation of the nares and pharynx, epistaxis, a complaint of a metallic taste, or may mimic a viral upper respiratory infection (11,69). On examination, there is significant nasopharyngeal edema, hyperemia, and small areas of bleeding, and if left untreated can lead to fissures, ulcerations, and nasal perforation. Tracheobronchitis may occur rapidly or gradually, and often occurs concomitantly with chemical pneumonitis. Nonproductive cough, shortness of breath, substernal chest discomfort, and chest burning or tightness characterize this disorder. Examination reveals some similar features to the nasopharyngitis, including airway hyperemia, as well as rales or rhonchi on auscultation of the chest. Radiographic evaluation may reveal increased bronchovascular markings. Therapy is mainly supportive for acute upper airway disease and should include removal from exposure.

The symptoms of acute chemical pneumonitis are similar to those of the tracheobronchitis with cough, occasionally productive of blood-tinged sputum, chest pain or a burning sensation, and dyspnea on exertion, which may progress to dyspnea at rest. Systemic symptoms are frequently present including malaise, anorexia, and low-grade fever. In acute chemical pneumonitis, individuals usually appear quite ill, may be cyanotic, tachycardic, or tachypnic, and have rales noted on examination of the lungs. Hypoxemia may be present on arterial blood gas and low lung volumes on pulmonary function testing. The chest radiograph may be normal or may reveal diffuse bilateral alveolar infiltrates or severe bilateral pulmonary edema. Radiographic abnormalities usually develop within a few weeks of the onset of symptoms (11,69). There are no specific diagnostic criteria or laboratory evaluations available for the acute disease. The history of beryllium exposure with a compatible clinical picture are the principal means of establishing the diagnosis. Pathologically, a nongranulomatous pneumonitis is observed with nonspecific inflammatory infiltrates composed of neutrophils and lymphocytes, bronchiolitis, and intraalveolar edema.

The primary therapeutic intervention is removal from exposure. Corticosteroids, oxygen, bed rest, and even ventilatory support, if needed, are part of an appropriate treatment regimen. The signs and symptoms of the acute chemical pneumonitis may resolve within several weeks to several months. In its most severe form, this acute disease may be fatal. Approximately 17% of the acute cases in the registry progressed to CBD (68). It is unclear whether return to work and further beryllium exposure is safe for individuals who have experienced the acute pneumonitis.

#### *Beryllium Sensitization*

The use of the blood BeLPT has defined a population of exposed workers who develop a cell-mediated, antigen-driven immune response to beryllium, but in whom there are none of the pathologic or clinical features of CBD. These individuals are asymptomatic and have normal pulmonary function, exercise tolerance, chest radiographs, and lung biopsies. Although their blood BeLPT is abnormal, they have not yet developed a clinically detectable inflammatory process in the lung. The rate of beryllium sensitization without disease in a few published studies has ranged from 1% to 2% (25,26,28). A subset of these individuals eventually develop CBD (28,37,39). Thus, sensitized individuals should remain under close medical supervision and be reexamined at intervals for signs of clinical progression. The risk factors for progression from sensitization to CBD are unclear at this time, and will require long-term follow-up of the sensitized population. In some individuals who have borderline or normal blood BeLPT, sensitization can be confirmed using beryllium sulfate patch testing (51). As discussed below, serum neopterin levels may help distinguish between sensitization and granulomatous inflammation (70).

#### *Chronic Beryllium Disease*

##### *Signs and Symptoms*

Unlike acute beryllium disease, CBD can develop many years after exposure has ceased, and typically has an indolent course and insidious onset of symptoms. Occasionally disease occurs after a bout of acute beryllium disease or after a stressor such as surgery or pregnancy (11,68,69). On average, CBD develops 6 to 10 years after exposure has ceased, but has been reported to occur with a latency greater than 30 years and as early as 4 months after initial exposure. As the lung is the most commonly affected organ, nonspecific respiratory and systemic symptoms are characteristic of CBD. Most individuals with CBD present with some combination of fatigue, nonproductive cough, gradually progressive shortness of breath, and chest pain (11,68,69). Anorexia, weight loss, fevers, night sweats, and arthralgias are fairly common. Other organs besides the lung can be involved, with signs and symptoms related to liver or myocardial involvement, hypercalcemia, or nephrolithiasis. Dry bibasilar rales, cyanosis, clubbing, lymphadenopathy, and skin changes may be present on examination, with other findings depending on the severity of the disease. Hepatomegaly and/or hepatic enzyme elevations are found in approximately 10% of cases (11,68). Depending on the severity of the disease, symptoms of pulmonary hypertension, cor pulmonale, or respiratory failure may be present. In less severe disease, an abnormal chest radiograph may be the presenting feature. With increasing use of blood BeLPT screening in industry, subclinical cases of CBD are detected that are asymptomatic and have normal chest radiographs and pulmonary function, but that usually have abnormal gas exchange with exercise.

*Pulmonary Physiology*

The pulmonary function abnormalities noted in CBD are typical of many interstitial lung diseases. A restrictive pattern of decreased lung volumes occurs in advanced disease; however, normal volumes with a mild obstructive pattern are more commonly found early in CBD (12,71). Mixed obstruction and restriction may also be observed (12,13). The diffusing capacity for carbon monoxide ($DL_{CO}$) is insensitive, becoming abnormal only in more advanced disease (71). Exercise tolerance testing is the most sensitive indicator of physiologic impairment in CBD, revealing defects in pulmonary physiology even when the lung volumes, spirometry, and $DL_{CO}$ are normal (71). The most common abnormalities noted on exercise testing include reduced exercise tolerance, decreased oxygen consumption $\dot{V}O_2$), an abnormal fall in oxygen levels, widening alveolar-arterial gradient, and ventilatory limitations to exercise. Some individuals with documented CBD may have normal exercise physiology. Because alterations in exercise physiology become apparent before pulmonary function testing abnormalities do, it is a better tool to evaluate and follow gas exchange abnormalities early in the disease process.

*Imaging/Radiographic Findings*

Classical chest radiographic manifestations of CBD include bilateral middle to upper lobe predominant reticulonodular infiltrates, with mild hilar lymphadenopathy. The interstitial opacities are typically characterized as small "p" or "q" in the International Labor Organization (ILO) classification scheme (72). Chest x-ray abnormalities range in severity from normal to widespread bilateral interstitial fibrosis and honeycombing in any lung field. The large hilar nodes seen commonly in sarcoidosis are seen infrequently in CBD, although adenopathy is present on chest x-ray in approximately one-third of cases (18,73–76). Pleural abnormalities may be noted in a minority of patients, most often adjacent to areas of greatest parenchymal involvement (13). Over time, a reduction in lung volumes becomes apparent and small nodules coalesce to form larger nodular opacities (Fig. 2*A*). The chest radiograph is an insensitive screening tool (26). Disease is usually physiologically and symptomatically evident by the time the x-ray appears abnormal (21,22). Thin-section computed tomography (CT) is more sensitive than the plain radiograph (76). In one study of biopsy proven CBD, abnormalities were noted in 10/13 of the patients with normal chest radiographs and 89% of the 28 patients studied (76). The most common CT abnormalities are nodules, thickened septal lines, ground glass opacification, hilar adenopathy, and bronchial wall thickening, even in nonsmokers (Fig. 2*B*) (76,77). None of these findings is specific for CBD, but when taken in concert with specific tests like the blood BeLPT, can confirm the diagnosis.

*Bronchoalveolar Lavage*

Suspected CBD is one of the few clinical indications for BAL in the evaluation of interstitial lung diseases. BAL cells reveal an increased number of white cells with a lymphocyte predominance (16,20,22,23). The lymphocytes are principally $CD4^+$ T cells, similar to those found in sarcoidosis and in some cases of hypersensitivity pneumonitis (78). Tobacco smoke affects BAL cell function and results in an increase in the macrophage percentage, complicating the interpretation of BAL cell count and differential. The extent of BAL cellularity, lymphocytosis, and BeLPT response correlates with disease severity (27), suggesting that the magnitude of the inflammatory and antigenic response in the lung may help predict disease progression or response to therapy.

*Laboratory Abnormalities*

Besides the BeLPT and BAL findings, a number of less specific laboratory abnormalities are noted in some cases of CBD. These include hyperuricemia (79), nonspecific elevation of serum immunoglobulins (80), hypercalcemia, hypercalciuria, and abnormal hepatic enzymes (11,69). Despite the finding of increased uric acid in 40% of one patient group, gout has not been noted commonly. Despite the progressive pulmonary disease noted in some patients, polycythemia and ECG changes are uncommon (11,68). Elevated serum angiotensin converting enzyme (sACE) levels are found in some CBD patients, but levels are lower than in other granulomatous disease, such as sarcoidosis (81,82). Elevated sACE levels correlate modestly with some markers

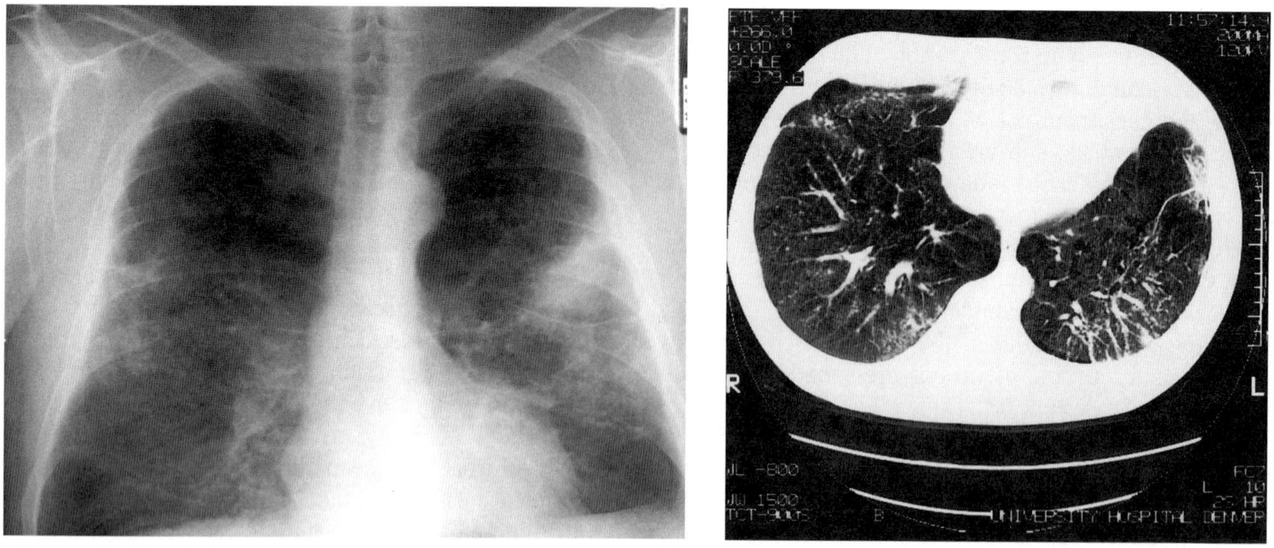


A B

**FIG. 2. A:** Posteroanterior chest radiograph of a patient with advanced chronic beryllium disease, following past exposure to beryllium oxide ceramic dust. Radiograph illustrates diffuse nodular opacities, formation on conglomerate masses with adjacent areas of emphysema, subpleural thickening, reticular lines and honeycombing, and bilateral hilar adenopathy. **B:** Thin-section computed tomography scan illustrates nodular opacities, bronchial wall thickening, diffuse ground glass opacification, and septal lines. Also observed are small areas of emphysema adjacent to areas of fibrotic/granulomatous scar.

of disease severity (81,82), although this test has shown little practical utility in CBD diagnosis or prognostication. sACE should not be used to differentiate CBD from sarcoidosis. A recent study of serum neopterin in beryllium sensitization and CBD suggests that this surrogate marker of γ-interferon production may help to distinguish between those individuals who are beryllium sensitized without disease and those with granulomatous involvement (CBD) (70).

*Pathology*

The noncaseating granuloma is the hallmark feature of CBD and of some beryllium-related skin lesions, but is histologically indistinguishable from the granulomas found in sarcoidosis. Other pathologic abnormalities commonly found include a mononuclear cell interstitial infiltrate and varying degrees of fibrosis (11,14,68,83). In a review of the pathology from the registry, over 50% of the

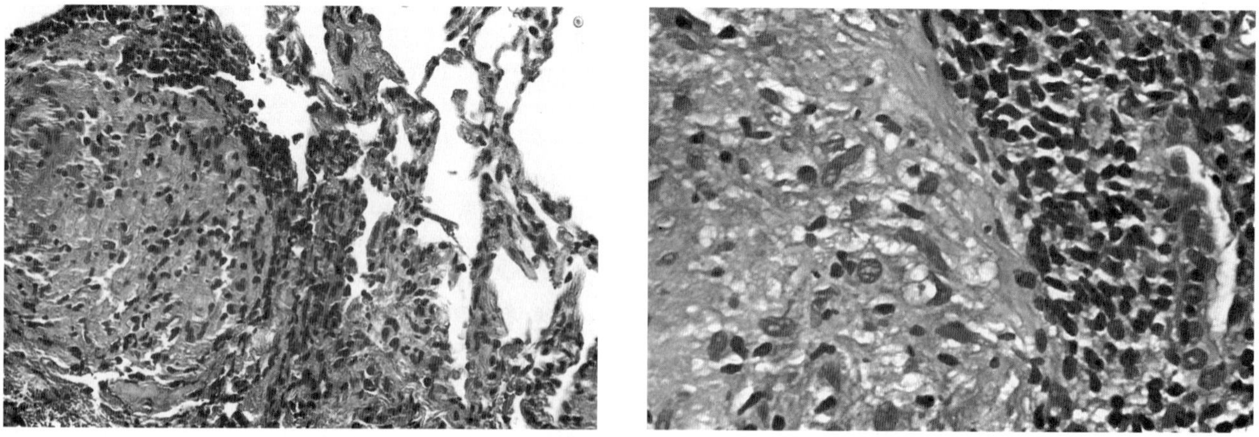

A B

**FIG. 3. A:** Low-power photomicrograph of a transbronchial lung biopsy from a patient with chronic beryllium disease illustrates a typical noncaseating granuloma composed of epithelioid cells, lymphocytes, macrophages, and a dense circumference of lymphocytes and collagen. Notably, areas adjacent to the granuloma also illustrate thickening of the alveolar septa and mononuclear cell infiltration. **B:** High-power photomicrograph shows the deposition of fibrosis and lymphocytes at the circumference of a granuloma. (Photomicrographs prepared by Dr. Yoshikazu Inoue.)

130 cases reviewed had poorly formed or no granulomas present (14). Thus, the absence of granulomas on either transbronchial biopsy or thoracoscopic lung biopsy does not fully exclude CBD. The noncaseating granuloma usually contains epithelioid cells of monocyte lineage, multinucleated giant cells, and lymphocytes that are predominantly $CD4^+$ T cells. Other immune effector cells, such as B cells, mast cells, and fibroblasts are also present (Fig. 3). The granulomas accumulate primarily in the pulmonary interstitium and bronchial submucosa, often tracking along the bronchovascular bundle, occasionally in regional lymph nodes, and rarely in the liver, abdominal, and cervical lymph nodes (84).

### *Diagnostic Evaluation*

From the 1950s to the 1970s, diagnostic criteria for CBD were based on the presence of four of the following six criteria, including one of the first two: (1) a history of beryllium exposure, (2) elevated beryllium levels in tissue, (3) characteristic chest radiographic abnormalities, (4) a restrictive and/or obstructive physiology or diffusing capacity defect, (5) pathology consistent with CBD, or (6) a clinical course consistent with a chronic respiratory disorder (13). As indicated above, the clinical features, radiographic manifestations, physiologic abnormalities, and pathologic changes present in CBD are not specific or diagnostic for this interstitial lung disease. In addition, the measure of beryllium in tissue does not establish disease and is fraught with numerous technical and interpretive problems. The implications are the same for the measurement of beryllium in the urine: it is subject to sampling and measurement error and reflects exposure, not disease. The use of these six U.S. Beryllium Case Registry criteria underestimated CBD, by definition, missing those individuals with early-stage disease. In addition, distinguishing CBD from other forms of granulomatous lung disease such as sarcoidosis or hypersensitivity pneumonitis was difficult because of the lack of tests to lend specificity to the diagnosis.

In the 1980s, the introduction of transbronchial biopsy, bronchoalveolar lavage, and the blood and lavage BeLPT improved our ability to make a more specific, accurate diagnosis of CBD. The current diagnostic algorithm is shown in Fig. 4. The diagnosis of CBD is now established by demonstrating a beryllium-specific immune response, using the blood or lavage BeLPT or beryllium salt patch test plus pathologic changes consistent with CBD (22,51, 55) (Table 3). The implications of this diagnostic schema are significant. First, while a history of beryllium exposure is helpful, its documentation is no longer essential to establish a diagnosis of CBD, since the BeLPT has been

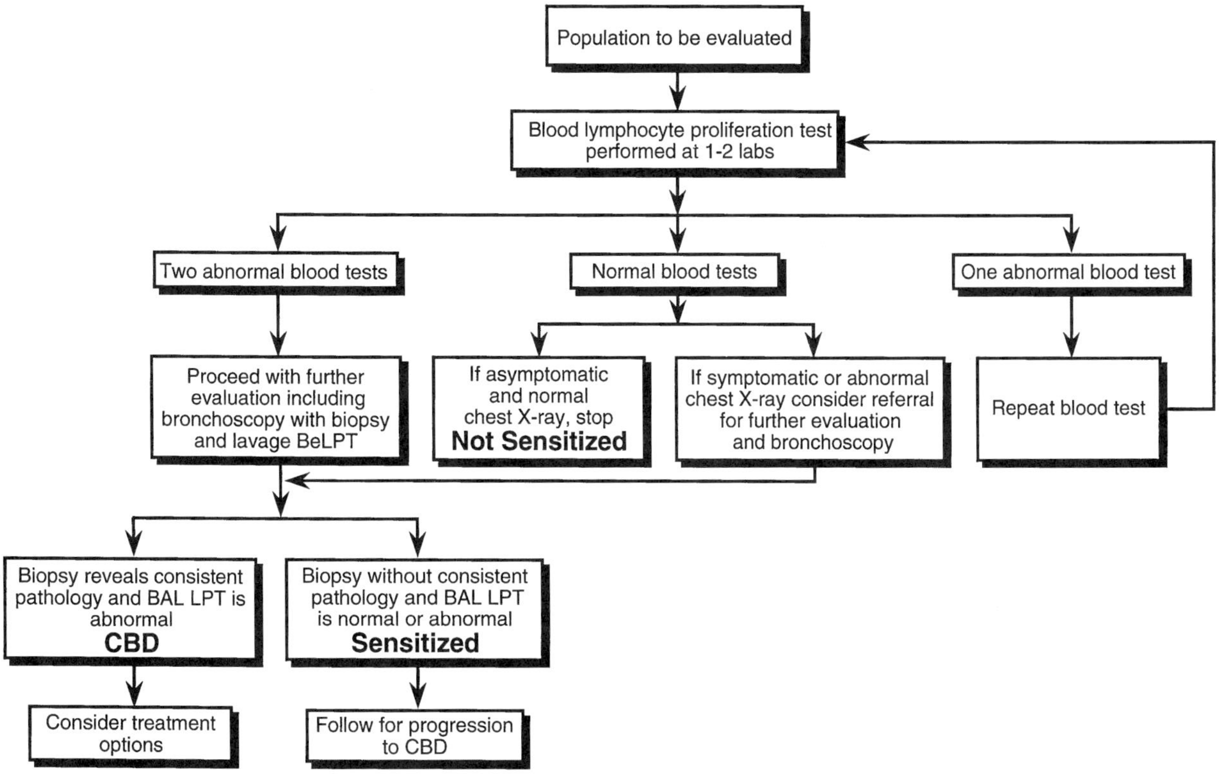


**FIG. 4.** Outline of recommended patient algorithm for evaluation of suspected chronic beryllium disease. This algorithm relies on the demonstration of an immunologic response to beryllium and findings on chest x-ray.

**TABLE 3.** *Diagnostic criteria for beryllium lung disease and sensitization*

- Beryllium sensitization
  - Beryllium-specific immune response, usually indicated by
    - an abnormal blood BeLPT
    - or positive skin patch test using beryllium salts
- Beryllium lung disease
  - Beryllium-specific immune response, usually indicated by
    - an abnormal blood BeLPT
    - abnormal BAL BeLPT
    - or positive skin patch test using beryllium salts
  - Histopathology on biopsy or radiographic alterations consistent with beryllium lung disease
  - Clinical findings, if present, may include any of the following
    - pulmonary signs or symptoms
    - compatible abnormalities on chest radiograph or chest CT scan
    - altered pulmonary physiology, demonstrated by a restrictive and/or obstructive pattern on pulmonary function testing, reduced diffusing capacity, abnormal gas exchange, ventilatory impairment on exercise testing

shown to be highly specific (22,85). This is especially important given that seemingly trivial exposures to beryllium can cause significant disease. By using an immunologic criterion, patients who have little apparent history of beryllium exposure can be detected, as illustrated by a recent report of CBD in the spouse of a beryllium production worker (86). Second, individuals may now be diagnosed with CBD at its early stages, sometimes prior to the appearance of clinical signs, symptoms, or radiographic or physiologic abnormalities. Early detection may improve disease prognosis. Third, the immunologic tests help distinguish CBD from other interstitial lung disorders, correcting misdiagnoses and directing appropriate therapeutic interventions. Like all immunologic assays and most diagnostic tests, false-negative and false-positive results occur. For example the results of the BAL and the BAL BeLPT may be affected by smoking tobacco, and the test is not 100% sensitive (24,85). In cases in which the blood and BAL BeLPT are equivocal or thought to be falsely negative, beryllium patch testing can be used safely to confirm the diagnosis (51,87,88). We recommend patch testing in those cases with a high suspicion of disease and a nondiagnostic blood or BAL BeLPT.

Occasionally, an individual may be found to have abnormal blood BeLPTs, an abnormal BAL BeLPT, and BAL lymphocytosis, but nondiagnostic lung biopsies. Although transbronchial biopsy has improved our diagnostic capabilities, it provides only small samples of lung tissue for review and thus is prone to sampling error. In such instances, repeat biopsy may be required. In some of these cases in which there is a high clinical and immunologic suspicion of disease, pathology may not be necessary for diagnosis. Similarly, when an individual has an abnormal chest x-ray or an abnormal thin-section CT and has repeatedly abnormal blood BeLPTs but is unable to undergo bronchoscopy, the diagnosis should be based on the clinical findings and two or more positive blood BeLPTs. The blood BeLPT confirms the beryllium-specific immune response, while the radiographic abnormalities confirm that there are underlying pathologic derangements.

### *Natural History*

The clinical course of CBD is quite variable. While some individuals remain stable clinically for many years, most experience a gradual worsening of symptoms and physiologic dysfunction. Another subset of patients suffers a rapidly progressive debilitating course, ultimately developing respiratory failure within a few years of diagnosis. Mortality rates range from 5% to 38% and may be related to type of exposure (37,39,89). In general, CBD worsens if not treated. A small number of cases may show spontaneously improved chest radiographic infiltrates or gas exchange after reduction or cessation of exposure (90,91). Removal from exposure and medical treatment are recommended, although the long-term impact of these interventions is unknown. The detection of CBD at a subclinical stage may improve our ability to intervene early and change the natural history of disease. A large longitudinal study currently in progress will address this issue (39).

### *Treatment and Follow-Up*

Primary prevention is superior to medical treatment of CBD. Unfortunately for current cases, there is no cure for CBD. The goals of treatment are to reduce morbidity and mortality by inhibiting inflammation and slowing disease progression. Removal from exposure is recommended. Corticosteroids are the first-line therapy for CBD, although they have never been tested conclusively in a randomized fashion or against a control population. Clinical case series have shown the efficacy of corticosteroids in reducing symptoms of CBD and improving lung function (13,92–104). It is not known if corticosteroid treatment changes the course of subclinical CBD. Before initiating corticosteroid therapy, a baseline evaluation should be performed consisting of chest radiograph, thin-section CT, complete pulmonary function tests including lung volumes, spirometry, and $DL_{CO}$, and exercise testing, ideally with arterial blood gas measurements. Indications for treatment include (1) severe symptoms, such as debilitating cough; (2) abnormal gas exchange, diminished exercise tolerance, or abnormal pulmonary physiology; (3) progressive decline in these tests of impairment; or (4) evidence of pulmonary hypertension or cor pulmonale. Initial therapy should be similar to that used in sarcoidosis: oral prednisone (or an equivalent) at a dose of approximately 0.5 to 0.6 mg/kg ideal body weight either daily or on alternate days. After 3 to 6 months, the response to therapy should be reassessed objectively and the prednisone dose tapered gradually to the minimum dose required to maintain objective and symptomatic improvement. Therapy is usually continued lifelong, because disease relapses occur after steroid withdrawal (11,68,69). If corticosteroid therapy is not initiated (e.g., in subclinical cases of CBD), follow-up examination and objective testing should be performed on a yearly basis to monitor for disease progression. Because of the need for lifelong treatment, patients should be informed of the long-term side effects of corticosteroids and be monitored and treated for consequences such as hypertension, hyperglycemia, osteoporosis, and cataracts.

In addition to steroid therapy, more severe cases may require additional supportive measures. Supplemental oxygen should be prescribed as needed to improve hypoxemia and treat pulmonary hypertension or cor pulmonale. Diuretics may be necessary to treat significant right heart failure. Symptomatic obstructive physiology and cough may respond to inhaled bronchodilators and inhaled steroids. As in other chronic illnesses, regular immunizations should be administered to prevent influenza and pneumococcal infections. Antibiotics may be needed to treat bouts of infection. In those patients who fail to respond to corticosteroids or who experience severe side effects, other immunosuppressive agents may prove efficacious. For example, as in sarcoidosis, preliminary data suggest that low-dose methotrexate (5–15 mg orally per week) has a steroid-sparing effect in CBD. Patients who are beryllium sensitized without granulomatous disease should be followed for evidence of CBD every 1 to 2 years, because of the risk of progression to disease.

### Dermatologic Manifestations

Beryllium can induce a number of dermatologic conditions, development of which may depend on the form of beryllium and magnitude of exposure. Contact dermatitis can occur on exposed areas of skin. It generally resolves with cessation of exposure. This skin lesion may occur as a result of contact irritation or a sensitization to beryllium (11,69). If the contact dermatitis involves the face, conjunctivitis, periorbital edema, and upper respiratory tract involvement may occur concomitantly (11,69). Recently, the use of beryllium-containing dental prostheses have been shown to cause the equivalent of oral contact dermatitis in two cases, and hand lesions in an individual making the oral prosthesis (87,88). Positive patch testing of these individuals indicated beryllium sensitization. Oral signs include chronic gingivitis and bleeding in the areas adjacent to beryllium-containing dental crowns and bridges. Ulceration or granulomatous nodular skin lesions may occur after accidental inoculation of the skin with splinters of beryllium metal, oxide, or crystal. The lesion will persist until the beryllium material is excised and the lesion is extensively debrided. The nodular granulomatous skin lesions may be confused with common warts and can occur without obvious skin inoculation in individuals who commonly handle beryllium and in patients with CBD.

### Carcinogenesis

Animal studies have shown that beryllium can induce cancer in many different species, with some species variability, depending on the mode of administration (46,48,49,105,106). Early studies showed that intravenous injection of beryllium induced osteogenic tumors in rabbits (107). Rats develop lung cancer after inhalational administration (46,49,108,109). The histological tumor types produced have varied from adenocarcinoma in some studies to predominantly bronchoalveolar cell carcinoma in others (49).

A number of large epidemiologic studies have shown an increased risk of lung cancer among beryllium-exposed workers and among workers with acute beryllium disease, with standardized mortality ratios (SMRs) of 1.37 to 1.97 for the production workers and 3.14 for those with acute beryllium disease (110–114). These studies have been criticized by some on methodologic grounds, such as failing to account for confounding exposures, primarily tobacco smoke (115). More recent studies have confirmed the association between beryllium and lung cancer in humans (116,117). In one study of Beryllium Case Registry cases, an increased risk of lung cancer was found in those individuals with acute and chronic beryllium disease (overall SMR = 2.00) (116). Those with acute disease had a higher risk (SMR = 2.32) compared to those with CBD (SMR = 1.57), suggesting a possible dose-response effect (116). An increased risk of lung cancer was observed in a separate study of beryllium-exposed workers, after adjusting for smoking (117). In that study, the risk to the beryllium-exposed population was less than for those beryllium lung disease (SMR = 1.26) (117). The preponderance of data support the conclusion that beryllium is a human carcinogen, especially in those with patients with beryllium-related lung disease. The International Agency for Research on Cancer (IARC) has reclassified beryllium as a class 1 human carcinogen (105,106).

## SURVEILLANCE

Advances in immunology and the beryllium epidemiologic studies of the 1980s and 1990s have helped revolutionize the approach to beryllium disease screening and surveillance. As it may not be possible to completely eliminate exposure, major beryllium users now conduct medical screening to help identify individuals at early stages of disease and those who are sensitized and at increased risk of developing CBD. Historically, screening for CBD included annual physical examination, spirometry, and chest radiography, and in some cases diffusing capacity, all of which are insensitive and nonspecific (21,71). The advent of the blood BeLPT has made disease screening in the beryllium industry a much more specific and sensitive endeavor (21,25,26,28,55). The blood BeLPT has high positive predictive value and is more sensitive than clinical evaluation, spirometry, or chest radiography (25,26, 28,55). Chest x-rays capture a small number of additional cases that may be missed by the blood BeLPT (25,26,55). The blood test identifies approximately 70% to 94% of cases (24–26,28,55,118).

Figure 5 outlines our current recommendations in conducting beryllium disease screening and suggests how to link screening to surveillance. Beryllium-exposed workers should undergo periodic testing approximately every 1 to 3 years, preferably scheduled on the basis of whether they work in high- versus low-risk areas. Such high-risk areas are identified by analyzing the frequency of disease or sensitization, by job task, title, building, etc. For example, machinists may warrant yearly or alternate-year testing, while secretaries might be tested every 3 years. In addition to discovering new cases of disease and sensitization, such periodic screening can help identify high-risk processes in manufacturing areas, leading to institution of better engineering controls.

## PREVENTION

While the current Occupational Safety and Health Administration (OSHA) standard appears sufficient to prevent most cases of acute beryllium disease, adherence to the standard does not prevent CBD. Early studies suggested that some neighborhood cases developed disease with ambient air levels as low as 0.01 μg/m$^3$ (6,7). Case series in Japan have documented cases of CBD that occurred below the 2 μg/m$^3$ threshold limit value (TLV) (119–122), consistent with recent cases that have

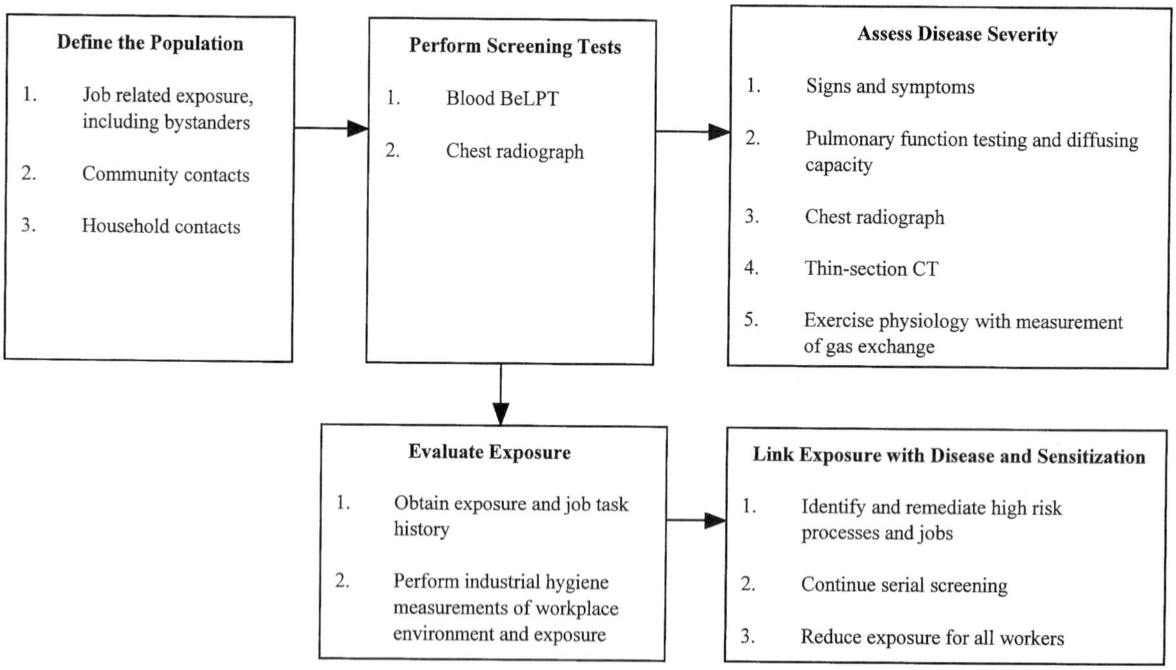


**FIG. 5.** Approach to beryllium disease medical screening and surveillance. The key elements in any workplace beryllium screening and surveillance program involve defining the population at risk; performing appropriate screening tests to identify those individuals who are most likely to be either beryllium sensitized or diseased; establishing a definitive diagnosis and assessing the severity of disease in individuals identified as having this condition. Parallel activities to evaluate exposure and to link information concerning exposure with information regarding the sensitized work force form the cornerstones of medical surveillance and can contribute to disease prevention. If the blood BeLPT test is abnormal, we recommend a second confirmatory test prior to further evaluation. Chest radiographs have been shown to identify a small number of cases missed by blood BeLPT.

occurred in nonoccupationally exposed individuals (27,48,76) and among occupationally exposed secretaries and security guards (25,26). Recent epidemiologic studies have reported the development of CBD cases at levels that were probably below the current standard (19,28, 123). Using historical industrial hygiene data, Kreiss and colleagues (28) showed that many workers in a modern beryllium ceramics plant developed sensitization and disease with median air concentrations below 2 $\mu g/m^3$. This study was unable to exclude the theoretical possibility that these individuals actually experienced higher levels of exposure since no worker is continually monitored. Nonetheless, these studies raise significant concerns about the ability of the current standard to protect workers from developing disease. Apparent adherence to the 2 $\mu g/m^3$ limit is not sufficiently protective. The threshold limit below which no cases of CBD occur is unknown, although the number of CBD cases can be decreased by improving industrial hygiene measures and reducing exposure to as low as reasonably achievable (ALARA). The best hope for prevention is to substitute safer materials, limit the number of beryllium-exposed workers, introduce tighter industrial hygiene controls, and conduct screening for early detection of individuals with sensitization or disease. Workers should be better informed of the beryllium-related health hazards through workplace education programs.

## REFERENCES


1. Weber H, Engelhardt WE. Anwendung bei der Untersuchungen von Stauben aus der Berylliumgewinnung. *Zentralbl Gewerbehyg Unfallverhuet* 1933;10:41.
2. Gelman I. Poisoning by vapors of beryllium oxyfluoride. *J Ind Hyg Toxicol* 1936;18:371–399.
3. Berkovits M, Izrael B. Changes in the lungs by beryllium oxyfluoride poisoning. *Klin Med* 1940;18:117–122.
4. Van Ordstrand HS, Hughes R, DeNardi JM, Carmody MG. Beryllium poisoning. *JAMA* 1945;129:1084–1090.
5. Hardy HL, Tabershaw IR. Delayed chemical pneumonitis in workers exposed to beryllium compounds. *J Ind Hyg Toxicol* 1946;28:197–211.
6. Eisenbud M, Wanta RC, Dustan C, Steadman LT, Harris WB, Wolf BS. Non-occupational berylliosis. *J Ind Hyg Toxicol* 1949;31:281–294.
7. Sterner JH, Eisenbud M. Epidemiology of beryllium intoxication. *Arch Ind Hyg Occup Med* 1951;4:123–151.
8. Lieben J, Metzner F. Epidemiological findings associated with beryllium extraction. *Am Ind Hyg Assoc J* 1959;20:494–499.
9. Sussman VH, Lieben J, Cleland JG. An air pollution study of a community surrounding a beryllium plant. *Am Ind Hyg Assoc J* 1959;20: 504–508.
10. Eisenbud M. Origins of the standard for control of beryllium disease (1947–1949). *Environ Res* 1982;27:79–88.
11. Tepper LB, Hardy HL, Chamberlin RI. Toxicity of beryllium compounds. In: Browning E, ed. *Elsevier monographs on toxic agents.* New York: Elsevier, 1961:1–190.
12. Andrews JL, Kazemi H, Hardy H. Patterns of lung dysfunction in chronic beryllium disease. *Am Rev Respir Dis* 1969;100:791–800.
13. Stoeckle JD, Hardy HL, Weber AL. Chronic beryllium disease: long-term follow-up of sixty cases and selective review of the literature. *Am J Med* 1969;46:545–561.
14. Freiman DG, Hardy HL. Beryllium disease: the relation of pulmonary pathology to clinical course and prognosis based on a study of 130 cases from the U.S. Beryllium Case Registry. *Hum Pathol* 1970;1: 25–44.
15. Kriebel D, Brain JD, Sprince NL, Kazemi H. The pulmonary toxicity of beryllium. *Am Rev Respir Dis* 1988;137:464–473.
16. Epstein PE, Dauber JH, Rossman MD, Daniele RP. Bronchoalveolar lavage in a patient with chronic berylliosis: evidence for hypersensitivity pneumonitis. *Ann Intern Med* 1982;97:213–216.
17. Bargon J, Kronenberger H, Bergmann L, Buhl R, Meier-Sydow J, Mitrou P. Lymphocyte transformation test in a group of foundry workers exposed to beryllium and non-exposed controls. *Eur J Respir Dis* 1986;69(suppl 136):211–215.
18. Aronchick JM, Rossman MD, Miller WT. Chronic beryllium disease: diagnosis, radiographic findings, and correlation with pulmonary function tests. *Radiology* 1987;163:677–682.
19. Cullen MR, Kominsky JR, Rossman MD, et al. Chronic beryllium disease in a precious metal refinery: clinical, epidemiologic, and immunologic evidence for continuing risk from exposure to low level beryllium fume. *Am Rev Respir Dis* 1987;135:201–208.
20. Rossman MD, Kern JA, Elias JA, et al. Proliferative response of bronchoalveolar lymphocytes to beryllium: a test for chronic beryllium disease. *Ann Intern Med* 1988;108:687–693.
21. Kreiss K, Newman LS, Mroz MM, Campbell PA. Screening blood test identifies subclinical beryllium disease. *J Occup Med* 1989;31: 603–608.
22. Newman LS, Kreiss K, King TE Jr, Seay S, Campbell PA. Pathologic and immunologic alterations in early stages of beryllium disease: re-examination of disease definition and natural history. *Am Rev Respir Dis* 1989;139:1479–1486.
23. Saltini C, Winestock K, Kirby M, Pinkston P, Crystal RG. Maintenance of alveolitis in patients with chronic beryllium disease by beryllium-specific helper T cells. *N Engl J Med* 1989;320:1103–1109.
24. Mroz MM, Kreiss K, Lezotte DC, Campbell PA, Newman LS. Re-examination of the blood lymphocyte transformation test in the diagnosis of chronic beryllium disease. *J Allergy Clin Immunol* 1991;88: 54–60.
25. Kreiss K, Mroz MM, Zhen B, Martyny J, Newman LS. Epidemiology of beryllium sensitization and disease in nuclear workers. *Am Rev Respir Dis* 1993;148:985–991.
26. Kreiss K, Wasserman S, Mroz MM, Newman LS. Beryllium disease screening in the ceramics industry: blood test performance and exposure-disease relations. *J Occup Med* 1993;35:267–274.
27. Newman LS, Bobka C, Schumacher B, et al. Compartmentalized immune response reflects clinical severity of beryllium disease. *Am J Respir Crit Care Med* 1994;150:135–142.
28. Kreiss K, Mroz MM, Newman LS, Martyny J, Zhen B. Machining risk of beryllium disease and sensitization with median exposures below 2 $mg/m^3$. *Am J Ind Med* 1996;30:16–25.
29. Rom WN, Lockey JE, Bang KM. Reversible beryllium sensitization in a prospective study of beryllium workers. *Arch Environ Health* 1983;38:302–307.
30. Izumi T, Kobara Y, Inuis S, et al. The first seven cases of chronic beryllium disease in ceramic factory workers in Japan. *Ann NY Acad Sci* 1976;278:636–653.
31. Shima S, Watanabe K, Tachikawa S. Experimental study an oral administration of beryllium compounds. *Rodo Kagaku* 1983;59:463–473.
32. Jameson CW. Introduction to the conference on beryllium-related diseases. *Environ Health Perspect* 1996;104:935–936.
33. Eisenbud M, Lisson J. Epidemiological aspects of beryllium-induced non-malignant lung disease: a 30-year update. *J Occup Med* 1983;25: 196–202.
34. Kriebel D, Sprince NL, Eisen EA, Greaves IA, Feldman HA, Greene RE. Beryllium exposure and pulmonary functions: a cross-sectional study of beryllium workers. *Br J Ind Med* 1988;45:167–173.
35. Reeves AL, Preuss OP. Immunotoxicity of beryllium. In: Dean JH, Luster MI, Munson AE, Amos H, eds. *Immunotoxicology and immunopharmacology.* New York: Raven Press, 1985:441–456.
36. Shima S. Hygienic control of beryllium. *Rodo Kagaku* 1971;26:36–46.
37. Newman LS. Significance of the blood beryllium lymphocyte proliferation test (BeLPT). *Environ Health Perspect* 1996;104:953–956.
38. Newman LS. Immunology, genetics, and epidemiology of beryllium disease. *Chest* 1996;109:40S–43S.
39. Newman LS, Lloyd J, Daniloff E. The natural history of beryllium sensitization and chronic beryllium disease. *Environ Health Perspect* 1996;104:937–943.
40. Barna BP, Deodhar SD, Chiang T, Gautam S, Edinger M. Experimental beryllium-induced lung disease: I. Differences in immunologic response to beryllium compounds in strains 2 and 13 guinea pigs. *Int Arch Allergy Appl Immunol* 1984;73:42–48.
41. Barna BP, Deodhar SD, Gautam S, Edinger M, Chiang T, McMahon

JT. Experimental beryllium-induced lung disease: II. Analyses of bronchial lavage cells in strains 2 and 13 guinea pigs. *Int Arch Allergy Appl Immunol* 1984;73:49–55.
42. Votto JJ, Barton RW, Gionfriddo MA, Cole SR, McCormick JR, Thrall RS. A model of pulmonary granulomatous induced by beryllium sulfate in the rat. *Sarcoidosis* 1987;4:71–76.
43. Haley PJ, Finch GL, Mewhinney JA, et al. A canine model of beryllium-induced granulomatous lung disease. *Lab Invest* 1989;61:219–227.
44. Haley PJ, Finch GL, Hoover MD, Muggenburg BA, Johnson NF. Immunologic specificity of lymphocyte cell lines from dogs exposed to BO. In: Thomassen DG, Shyr LJ, Bechtold WE, Bradley PL, eds. *Inhalation toxicology research institute annual report 1989–1990,* LMF-129. Springfield: National Technical Information Service, 1990; 236–239.
45. Haley PJ. Mechanisms of granulomatous lung disease from inhaled beryllium: the role of antigenicity in granuloma formation. *Toxicol Pathol* 1991;19:514–525.
46. Reeves AL. Experimental pathology. In: Rossman MD, Preuss OP, Powers MB, eds. *Beryllium:* biomedical and environmental aspects. Baltimore: Williams and Wilkins, 1991;59–76.
47. Huang H, Meyer KC, Kubai L, Auerbach R. An immune model of beryllium-induced pulmonary granulomata in mice: histopathology, immune reactivity, and flow-cytometric analysis of bronchoalveolar lavage-derived cells. *Lab Invest* 1992;67:138–146.
48. Newman LS. Beryllium lung disease: the role of cell-mediated immunity in pathogenesis. In: Dean JH, Luster MI, Munson AE, Kimber I, eds. *Immunotoxicology and immunopharmacology.* New York: Raven Press, 1994;377–393.
49. Finch GL, Hoover MD, Hahn FF, et al. Animal models of beryllium-induced lung disease. *Environ Health Perspect* 1996;104:973–979.
50. Curtis GH. Cutaneous hypersensitivity due to beryllium: a study of thirteen cases. *Arch Dermatol Syph* 1951;64:470–482.
51. Bobka CA, Stewart LA, Engelken GJ, Golitz LE, Newman LS. Comparison of in vivo and *in vitro* measures of beryllium sensitization. *J Occup Environ Med* 1997;39:540–547.
52. Hanifin JM, Epstein WL, Cline MJ. In vitro studies of granulomatous hypersensitivity to beryllium. *J Invest Dermatol* 1970;55:284–288.
53. Williams WR, Jones Williams W. Comparison of lymphocyte transformation and macrophage migration inhibition tests in the detection of beryllium hypersensitivity. *J Clin Pathol* 1982;35:684–687.
54. Williams WR, Jones Williams WJ. Development of beryllium lymphocyte transformation tests in chronic beryllium disease. *Int Arch Allergy Appl Immunol* 1982;67:175–180.
55. Kreiss K, Miller F, Newman LS, Ojo-Amaize EA, Rossman MD, Saltini C. Chronic beryllium disease: from the workplace to cellular immunology, molecular immunogenetics, and back. *Clin Immunol Immunopathol* 1994;71:123–129.
56. Rossman MD. Chronic beryllium disease. In: Daniele RP, ed. *Immunology and immunologic diseases of the lung.* Boston: Blackwell Scientific, 1988;351–359.
57. Saltini C, Kirby M, Trapnell BC, Tamura N, Crystal RB. Biased accumulation of T lymphocytes with "memory"-type CD45 leukocyte common antigen gene expression on the epithelial surface of the human lung. *J Exp Med* 1990;171:1123–1140.
58. Rossman MD, Yan H-C, R.K. M, Williams WV, Weiner DB. Chronic beryllium disease: an immune response by restricted subfamilies of T cells. *Am Rev Respir Dis* 1992;145:A415.
59. Comment CE, Kotzin BL, Schumacher BA, Newman LS. Preferential use of T cell antigen receptors in beryllium disease. *Am J Respir Crit Care Med* 1994;149:A264.
60. Bost TW, Riches DWH, Schumacher B, et al. Alveolar macrophages from patients with beryllium disease and sarcoidosis express increased levels of mRNA for TNF-a and IL-6 but not IL-1b. *Am J Respir Cell Mol Biol* 1994;10:506–513.
61. Tinkle SS, Schwitters PW, Newman LS. Cytokine production by bronchoalveolar lavage cells in chronic beryllium disease. *Environ Health Perspect* 1996;104:969–971.
62. Tinkle SS, Kittle LA, Schumacher BA, Newman LS. Beryllium induces IL-2 and IFN-g, not IL-4 in berylliosis. *J Immunol* 1997;158:518–526.
63. Inoue Y, King TE Jr, Tinkle SS, Dockstader K, Newman LS. Human mast cell basic fibroblast growth factor in pulmonary fibrotic disorders. *Am J Pathol* 1996;149:2037–2054.
64. McConnochie K, Williams WR, Kilpatrick GS, Jones Williams W. Chronic beryllium disease in identical twins. *Br J Dis Chest* 1988;82:431–435.
65. Newman LS. To $Be^{2+}$ or not to $Be^{2+}$: relating immunogenetics to occupational exposure. *Science* 1993;262:197–198.
66. Richeldi L, Sorrentino R, Saltini C. HLA-DPb1 glutamate 69: a genetic marker of beryllium disease. *Science* 1993;262:242–244.
67. Stubbs J, Argyris E, Lee CW, Monos D, Rossmann MD. Genetic markers in beryllium hypersensitivity. *Chest* 1996;109:45S.
68. Hardy HL. Beryllium poisoning: lessons in control of man-made disease. *N Engl J Med* 1965;273:1188–1199.
69. Finkel AJ, Hamilton A, Hardy HL. Beryllium. In: Finkel AJ, ed. *Hamilton & Hardy's industrial toxicology.* Boston: John Wright, 1983;26–36.
70. Harris J, Bucher Bartelson B, Barker E, Balkissoon R, Kreiss K, Newman LS. Serum neopterin in chronic beryllium disease. *Am J Ind Med* 1997;32:21–26.
71. Pappas GP, Newman LS. Early pulmonary physiologic abnormalities in beryllium disease. *Am Rev Respir Dis* 1993;148:661–666.
72. International Labour Organization. *Guidelines for the use of ILO international classification of radiographs of pneumoconioses.* Occupational Safety and Health Series, No. 22 [REV]. Geneva, Switzerland: International Labour Office, 1980.
73. Wilson SA. Delayed chemical pneumonitis or diffuse granulomatosis of the lung due to beryllium. *Radiology* 1948;50:770–779.
74. Robert AG. A consideration of the roentgen diagnosis of chronic pulmonary granulomatosis of beryllium workers. *AJR* 1950;63:467–487.
75. Weber AL, Stoeckle JD, Hardy HL. Roentgenologic patterns in long-standing beryllium disease: report of eight cases. *AJR* 1965;93:879–890.
76. Newman LS, Buschman DL, Newell JD, Jr., Lynch DA. Beryllium disease: assessment with CT. *Radiology* 1994;190:835–840.
77. Harris KM, McConnochie K, Adams H. The computed tomographic appearances in chronic berylliosis. *Clin Radiol* 1993;47:26–31.
78. Newman LS. Beryllium disease and sarcoidosis: clinical and laboratory links. *Sarcoidosis* 1995;12:7–19.
79. Kelley WN, Goldfinger SE, Hardy HL. Hyperuricemia in chronic beryllium disease. *Ann Intern Med* 1969;70:977–983.
80. Deodhar SD, Barna B, Van Ordstrand HS. A study of the immunologic aspects of chronic berylliosis. *Chest* 1973;63:309–313.
81. Sprince NL, Kazemi H, Fanburg BL. Serium angiotensin 1-converting enzyme in chronic beryllium disease. In: Jones Williams W, Davies BH, eds. *Sarcoidosis and other granulomatosis diseases.* Cardiff, Wales: Alpha Omega, 1980;287–300.
82. Newman LS, Orton R, Kreiss K. Serum angiotensin converting enzyme activity in chronic beryllium disease. *Am Rev Respir Dis* 1992;146:39–42.
83. Dutra FR. The pneumonitis and granulomatosis peculiar to beryllium workers. *Am J Pathol* 1948;24:1137–1165.
84. Jones-Williams W. United Kingdom Beryllium Registry: mortality and autopsy study. *Environ Health Perspect* 1996;104:949–951.
85. Stokes RF, Rossman MD. Blood cell proliferation response to beryllium: analysis by receiver-operating characteristics. *J Occup Med* 1991;33:23–28.
86. Newman LS. *Case reports in environmental medicine:* beryllium toxicity. Washington, DC: U.S. Public Health Service, Agency for Toxic Substances and Disease Registry, 1992;1–19.
87. Vilaplana J, Romaguera C, Grimalt F. Occupational and non-occupational allergic contact dermatitis from beryllium. *Contact Dermatitis* 1992;26:295–298.
88. Haberman AL, Pratt M, Storrs FJ. Contact dermatitis from beryllium in dental alloys. *Contact Dermatitis* 1993;28:157–162.
89. Peyton MF, Worcester J. Exposure data and epidemiology of the beryllium case registry 1958. *AMA Arch Ind Health* 1959;19:94–99.
90. Sprince NL, Kanarek DJ, Weber AL, Chamberlin RI, Kazemi H. Reversible respiratory disease in beryllium workers. *Am Rev Respir Dis* 1978;117:1011–1017.
91. Nishikawa S, Hirata T, Kitaichi M, Izumi T. Three years prospective study of mantoux reactions in factor workers exposed to beryllium oxide. In: Jones Williams W, Davies BH, eds. *Sarcoidosis and other granulomatous diseases.* Cardiff, Wales: Alpha Omega, 1980; 722–727.
92. Kennedy BJ, Pare JAP, Pump KK, Standford RL. The effect of adrenocorticotropic hormone (ACTH) on beryllium granulomatosis. *Can Med Assoc J* 1950;62:426–428.

93. Thorn GW, et al. The clinical usefulness of ACTH and cortisone. *N Engl J Med* 1950;242:865–872.
94. DeNardi JM. Chronic pulmonary interstitial granulomatosis: preliminary report on two patients treated with ACTH. *Arch Ind Hyg Occup Med* 1951;3:543–546.
95. Hardy HL, et al. General discussion on the treatment of chronic beryllium poisoning with ACTH and cortisone. *Arch Ind Hyg Occup Med* 1951;3:629–630.
96. Kennedy BJ, et al. Effect of adrenocorticotropic hormone (ACTH) on beryllium granulomatosis and silicosis. *Am J Med* 1951;10:134–155.
97. Wright GW. Interpretation of results of ACTH and cortisone therapy in chronic beryllium poisoning. *Arch Ind Hyg Occup Med* 1951;3: 617–621.
98. Hardy HL. Epidemiology, clinical character, and treatment of beryllium poisoning. *Arch Ind Health* 1955;11:273.
99. DeNardi JM. Long-term experience with beryllium disease. *Arch Ind Health* 1959;19:104–109.
100. Gaensler EA, Verstraeten JM, Weil WB, et al. Respiratory pathophysiology in chronic beryllium disease: review of 30 cases with some observations after long term steroid therapy. *Arch Ind Health* 1959;19: 132–145.
101. Hall TC, Wood CH, Stoeckle JD, Tepper LB. Case data from the beryllium registry. *Arch Ind Health* 1959;19:18–21.
102. Kline EM, Moir TW. Long-term experience with beryllium disease. *Arch Ind Health* 1959;19:104–109.
103. Seeler AO. Treatment of chronic beryllium poisoning. *Arch Ind Health* 1959;19:164–168.
104. DaHoli JA, Lieben J, Bisbing J. Chronic beryllium disease: a follow-up study. *J Occup Med* 1964;6:189–194.
105. International Agency for Research on Cancer (IARC). *Monographs on the evaluation of the carcinogenic risk of chemicals to humans, vol 23. Some metals and metallic compounds.* Lyon, France: IARC, 1980; 139–142, 205–323.
106. Meeting of the IARC working group on beryllium, cadmium, mercury, and exposures in the glass manufacturing industry. *Scand J Work Environ Health* 1993;19:360–363.
107. Gardner LU, Heslington HF. Osteosarcoma from intravenous beryllium compounds in rabbits. *Fed Proc* 1946;5:221.
108. Vorwald AJ, Reeves AL. Pathologic changes induced by beryllium compounds. *Arch Ind Health* 1959;19:190–199.
109. Vorwald AJ, Reeves AL, Urban EJ. Experimental beryllium toxicology. In: Stokinger HE, ed. *Beryllium:* its industrial hygiene aspects. New York: Academic Press, 1966;201–234.
110. Mancuso TF, El-Attar AA. Epidemiologic study of the beryllium industry. Cohort methodology and mortality studies. *J Occup Med* 1969;11:424–434.
111. Mancuso TF. Occupational lung cancer among beryllium workers. In: Lemen R, Dement J, eds. *Dust and diseases.* Forest Park, IL: Pathotox, 1979;463–472.
112. Infante PF, Wagoner JK, Sprince NL. Mortality patterns from lung cancer and non-neoplastic respiratory disease among white males in the Beryllium Case Registry. *Environ Res* 1980;21:35–43.
113. Mancuso TF. Mortality study of beryllium industry workers' occupational lung cancer. *Environ Res* 1980;21:48–55.
114. Wagoner JK, Infante PF, Bayliss DL. Beryllium: an etiologic agent in the induction of lung cancer, non-neoplastic respiratory disease, and heart disease among industrially exposed workers. *Environ Res* 1980; 21:15–34.
115. MacMahon B. The epidemiological evidence on the carcinogenicity of beryllium in humans. *J Occup Med* 1994;36:15–24.
116. Steenland K, Ward E. Lung cancer incidence among patients with beryllium disease: a cohort mortality study. *J Natl Cancer Inst* 1991; 83:1380–1385.
117. Ward E, Okun A, Ruder A, Fingerhut M, Steenland K. A mortality study of workers at seven beryllium processing plants. *Am J Ind Med* 1992;22:885–904.
118. Rossman M, D. Differential diagnosis of chronic beryllium disease. In: Rossman MD, Preuss OP, Powers MB, eds. *Beryllium:* biomedical and environmental aspects. Baltimore: Williams & Wilkins, 1991;167–175.
119. Shima S. Recommendations for the preventive management of chronic beryllium disorders. *Rodo Eisei* 1974;8:18–24.
120. Shima S. Proposal for the management and prevention of chronic beryllium lesions. *Rodo Eisei* 1974;8:12–24.
121. Izumi T, Nishikawa S. Chronic beryllium lung in Japan. *Nikkyorin* 1976;35:805–813.
122. Shima S, Taniwaki H, Tachikawa S, et al. Diagnostic value of lymphocyte transformation and macrophage migration inhibition tests in chronic beryllium disease. *J Sci Labour* 1987;63:77–84.
123. Cotes JE, Gilson JC, McKerrow CB, Oldham PD. A long-term follow-up of workers exposed to beryllium. *Br J Ind Med* 1983;40:13–21.

*Environmental and Occupational Medicine, Third Edition,* edited by William N. Rom.
Lippincott–Raven Publishers, Philadelphia © 1998.

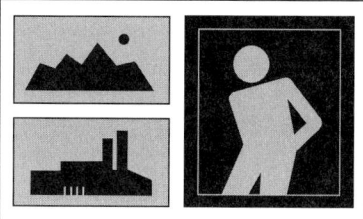

CHAPTER 73

# Hard Metal Disease

Dominique F. Lison

Hard metal (also called cemented carbide) is a composite material consisting of metallic carbide particles cemented in a matrix of cobalt metal, which is especially used for the manufacture of cutting and drilling tools for metals, rocks, and other hard materials. Workers exposed to hard metal dust are at risk of developing respiratory diseases affecting the upper respiratory tract, the bronchial tree, and the lung parenchyma. As already noted by Balmes (1), the term *hard metal disease* is somewhat confusing because, depending on the author considered, it may cover different types of parenchymal disorders, with apparently distinct clinical and pathologic presentations. Moreover, for some authors, airway manifestations are also included under the same term (2,3). The distinction may even be more complicated when, in some instances, parenchymal and airway manifestations are associated in the same patient (4). The use of the term *hard metal disease* should therefore be restricted to parenchymal manifestations occurring in hard metal workers.

## INDUSTRIAL PROCESS

Hard metal was first introduced in Germany where a powder metallurgy process called sintering was developed in the 1920s. Hard metal usually consists of more than 80% tungsten carbide particles and cobalt metal (often less than 10% but it may be as high as 25%, according to the desired applications). The usual metallurgic process includes different steps: tungsten metal powder is first reacted at 1,500°C with carbon black under an atmosphere of hydrogen to form tungsten carbide. Cobalt metal is then added to the carbide powder together with paraffin to provide cohesiveness, and organic solvents such as acetone and *n*-hexane may also be included for mixing but are removed by a drying process at a latter stage. In some cases, nickel metal or carbides of niobium, titanium, molybdenum, chromium, tantalum, or vanadium may also be added in small proportions. The material is then shaped, presintered, and deparaffinized at 500° to 800°C before grinding into its final form. Finally, it is sintered progressively (up to 1,500°C) and the product is finished by sand or shot blasting, brazing, and final grinding with diamond or carborundum wheels.

Hard metal possesses extraordinary properties of hardness (about 90% that of diamond) that, unlike other metals, increase with temperature. This characteristic is used for the manufacturing of hard metal–tipped tools such as saws, cutters, drilling bits, and other special devices such as grinding wheels, moulds, and extrusion and tunneling tools. Hard metals are also used for the nose cones of armor-piercing ammunitions and for armor plating. High-speed dental drills are made from hard metals as well. Flame plating of certain components with hard metal protects from wear; manufacturing of tire studs and some ball-point pens are other applications (1,3,5). Potential sources of exposure to hard metal dust include the manufacturing and the use of cemented carbide materials and tools.

## EPIDEMIOLOGY

The association between parenchymal lung disease and hard metal exposure was first recognized in Germany (6). Subsequently, other cases of parenchymal disease in hard metal workers were reported in Britain (7), the United States (8,9), Sweden (10), Japan (11), France (12), South Africa (13), Finland (14), and Italy (15). These descriptions were limited to case reports and/or retrospective studies initiated after the recognition of one or a few

D.F. Lison: Industrial Toxicology and Occupational Medicine Unit, Catholic University of Louvain, Brussels 1200, Belgium.

cases in a given factory. In most reports, little information is available on the intensity of exposure, and dose-response relationships are often not clearly documented.

There is only a limited number of studies designed to assess the prevalence of interstitial disorders among hard metal workers but the comparison of their results is often hampered by the use of different criteria for detecting interstitial lung disease (radiologic and/or functional). Sprince et al. (16) examined a total of 290 subjects from two different hard metal production plants. The selection of the study population, which represented 20% of the total work force, was purposely directed toward prolonged employment and high cobalt air concentrations, but there was no control group. Among the 150 subjects examined in the first plant, nine (6%) displayed radiologic and/or functional signs of parenchymal disease. Two workers from the second plant (1.4%) had interstitial infiltrates. In four of the nine workers who had been employed in the first plant, previous employment in coal mines or foundries might have contributed to radiologic abnormalities. Obstructive defects [decreased peak expiratory flow rate and forced expiratory volume in 1 second ($FEV_1$)] correlating with the length of exposure to hard metals were also detected. In a second study carried out on a population of 1,039 hard metal workers (17), the same authors found interstitial lung disease (ILD), defined on the basis of chest x-ray or pulmonary function testing, in 0.7% of the workers. In view of the absence of control groups, however, it is difficult to formally attribute these manifestations to hard metal exposure, and the changes observed may only represent the natural prevalence of ILD.

In a Japanese study (18), 319 hard metal workers were followed-up during a period of 5 years. The authors did not find any case of parenchymal disease attributed to hard metal exposure on the basis of x-rays studies. In contrast, 18 cases of bronchial asthma were diagnosed (5.6%). Later, the same team evaluated a cohort of 700 workers between 1981 and 1990 (11), and found four cases of radiographic interstitial fibrosis. No definite restrictive pulmonary function impairment could be evidenced. In contrast, nine cases of asthma were detected. In a cross-sectional survey carried out in three French factories, a total sample of 433 workers exposed to hard metal dust was compared with a group of 88 control subjects (19,20). Symptoms of chronic bronchitis (chronic cough and sputum) were more frequently reported in exposed workers than in controls, independently of smoking habits. No difference in spirometric measurements was found between controls and exposed subjects. Carbon monoxide transfer tests were also lower in exposed subjects than in controls. Slight abnormalities of chest radiographs suggestive of parenchymal disease [including International Labor Organization (ILO) scores of 0/1] were more prevalent in exposed subjects than in controls (12.8% vs 1.9%), this difference also being observed after correction for smoking habits. A cross-sectional study of Canadian saw filers found a reduction in lung capacity [$FEV_1$ and forced vital capacity (FVC)] associated with wet grinding of hard metal tools. Although a significant exposure-response relationship was found, the values for lung function were generally in the clinically normal range (21).

Although there are many more workers exposed to cobalt alone than to hard metals (in the United States about 30 times more), only rare cases of interstitial disease have been reported in workers exposed to cobalt alone (22,23). Parenchymal lung disease seems to be absent when exposure is to cobalt alone (metal, salts, or oxides; Table 1) even at high airborne concentrations

**TABLE 1.** *Exposure levels and prevalence of interstitial lung disease (ILD) in workers exposed to cobalt-containing particles*

| | Cobalt air[a] (μg/m$^3$) | Exposure duration (years) | % ILD |
|---|---|---|---|
| Hard metals | | | |
| Fairhall et al. 1947 (8) | 140–1400 | — | 2 |
| Bech et al. 1962 (7) | 18 | 0.1–20 | 2.4 |
| Sprince et al. 1984 (A) (16) | 2–438 | 25 | 6 |
| Sprince et al. 1984 (B) (16) | 3–1,480 | 17.3 | 1.4 |
| Sprince et al. 1988 (17) | 48 | 7 | 0.7 |
| Kusaka et al. 1986 (58) | 3–1,292 | — | 0 |
| Meyer-Bisch et al. 1989 (20) | 30–272 | 14 | 12.9 |
| Diamond | | | |
| Demedts et al. 1984 (44) | <45 | — | 1 |
| Nemery et al. 1992 (48) | 0.2–42.8 | — | 0 |
| Gennart et al. 1990 (66) | 15.2–135.5 | 6 | 0 |
| Cobalt | | | |
| Roto 1980 (50) | 10–100 | — | 0 |
| Morgan 1983 (67) | 200 | 10.7 | 0 |
| Raffn et al. 1988 (51) | (77 μg/L)[b] | 11 | 0 |
| Swennen et al. 1993 (24) | 125 | 8 | 0 |

[a]Mean or range.
[b]Measured in urine.
Reprinted with permission from ref. 68.

(24). This indicates that the simultaneous inhalation of other compounds, e.g., tungsten carbide, seems to be a necessary condition to induce an alveolitis that may lead to fibrosis. This hypothesis has recently been substantiated by experimental data (25–28).

## CLINICAL PRESENTATION

Although most clinical manifestations of hard metal disease are characterized by the presence of some degree of interstitial fibrosis and restrictive respiratory impairment, a large spectrum of responses with varying presentations and natural histories has been reported. In the acute or subacute form, after periods of exposure varying from some months to several years, the worker may rapidly develop fever, cough, and dyspnea during exercise. Chest x-rays may be almost normal or show wedge-shaped or ground-glass reticulonodular opacities. The symptoms may improve after removal from exposure but may recur when the subject returns to work. In other cases, the clinical picture is more insidious and progressive: the subject develops cough, labored breathing, and tachypnea; clubbing and a substantial weight loss can also be noted. Mid-to-late inspiratory crackles are often the first physical signs. Chest radiographs reveal linear striations and diffuse reticulonodular opacities. Lung function tests demonstrate a nonspecific pattern of reduced lung volumes, impaired diffusing capacity, and increased static elastic recoil. In the final stages, cor pulmonale and cardiorespiratory failure lead to death.

Taking a careful occupational history is essential for orienting the diagnosis of hard metal disease. Ruokonen et al. (29) reported the case of a young tool grinder whose occupational etiology was not timely recognized, which rapidly led to fatal outcome after further exposure. After 4 years in hard metal tool grinding, this patient started experiencing a dry cough and shortness of breath during exercise. At that stage, investigations did not reveal any cause for these symptoms and since no relation was made with occupational exposure, the patient continued to work. Several months later, he developed clinically apparent alveolitis, which proved unresponsive to corticosteroid treatment and rapidly led to irreversible pulmonary failure. The occupational cause of his disease was not recognized until lung biopsy showed typical findings of hard metal disease with interstitial fibrosis and alveolar infiltration by multinucleated giant cells (see below). The state of the patient deteriorated and necessitated a bilateral lung transplantation, but he died of pneumonia 5 months later. This case emphasizes the fact that, although invasive procedures are often useful to confirm the diagnosis, taking a detailed occupational history is of primordial importance not only for orienting the diagnosis and to take appropriate therapeutic measures. Cessation of exposure represents the first essential therapeutic measure. However, resolution may not always occur after cessation of exposure, especially in those patients with the "mural" form of the disease. There is no specific pharmacologic treatment for hard metal disease. Corticosteroids given in doses recommended in the treatment of other forms of nonspecific lung fibrosis (40–60 mg prednisone daily) may have some beneficial effect (1,10,30). A beneficial effect of cyclophosphamide (25 mg twice daily) given during 1 year has been reported in a young female patient with hard metal disease who was subsequently able to carry a full-term pregnancy with delivery by Caesarean section (1,31).

## PATHOLOGY AND MINERALOGIC ANALYSES

The pathologic descriptions of hard metal disease vary between desquamative pneumonia and overt mural fibrosis.

Alveolitis is morphologically characterized by the presence of numerous desquamated cells occupying alveolar spaces, while alveolar walls are only slightly affected by fibrosis (desquamative pneumonitis). These changes are usually distributed uniformly in the lungs. Lesions of diffuse fibrotic pattern correspond to thickened alveolar walls and few intraalveolar cells; perivascular and peribronchial fibrosis are usually present (mural form). The transition from alveolitis to permanent fibrosis is probably gradual, these two conditions being conceivably the extremes of a continuous process in which varying degrees of alveolitis and fibrosis may be observed according to the duration and severity of exposure as well as undetermined factors of individual susceptibility.

The diversity of histologic patterns of hard metal disease has also been pointed out by Rüttner et al. (32), who reviewed a series of lung biopsy or necropsy specimens from hard metal grinders. The pathologic appearances included mixed dust nodular pneumoconiosis, diffuse interstitial lung fibrosis, as well as foreign body and sarcoid-like granulomatous changes. However, an almost constant finding in all the reports was the presence, in biopsy specimens or bronchoalveolar lavage (BAL) fluid, of bizarre, cannibalistic giant multinucleated cells that are considered as a typical feature of hard metal disease. It has even been suggested that, in the absence of evidence for a viral, fungal, or mycobacterial infection, giant multinucleated cells are almost pathognomonic of hard metal disease and should stimulate an investigation on occupational exposure (33).

The mineralogic analysis of biopsy or BAL material may represent a useful approach to confirm exposure to a given particle, but the presence of a particle is not a sufficient proof of a causal relationship with the pulmonary disease. Measurement of cobalt content in BAL and/or lung tissue specimen from hard metal disease patients has yielded variable results. Most reported chemical analyses of tissues from patients with hard metal disease have demonstrated tungsten and/or tantalum- and titanium-containing particles but no or insignificant cobalt accumulation. The lower retention of cobalt has been attributed to its high solubility in biologic liquids (3). There are, however, a few reports indicating high cobalt concentrations in the tissues from hard metal disease patients. Some of these discrepancies might be explained by different latent periods between last exposure and the time when tissue or BAL was obtained for analysis. The determination of cobalt, tungsten, and tantalum in the lung but also in blood, urine, pubic hairs, and toe nails can also be used as indicators of chronic exposure to hard metal dusts (34,35).

## PATHOGENESIS

At least three different, although not mutually exclusive, hypotheses on the pathogenesis of hard metal disease have been suggested.

As in many occupational lung diseases, the great majority of hard metal workers remain unaffected, whereas only a small percentage (less than 5%; Table 1) develop interstitial disease. Several investigators have therefore suggested that the parenchymal manifestations encountered in hard metal workers may be of allergic nature and should be recognized as a form of hypersensitivity lung disease (extrinsic allergic alveolitis, EAA). This view is partly supported by different elements suggesting an allergic nature of these manifestations including the well-known sensitizing properties of cobalt (7,18); reduced helper/suppressor T cell ratios in BAL cells, which could be compatible with EAA (36); some isolated reports of positive lymphocyte transformation tests in the presence of cobalt (11); and a possible familial factor of susceptibility/hypersensitivity based on anecdotal reports (37). However, the clinical similarity between hard metal disease and EAA is incomplete and specific precipitins have never been demonstrated either in hard metal disease patients or in exposed workers. Therefore, although the possible role of allergic factors in certain forms of hard metal disease should not be overlooked, essential arguments are still lacking to confirm this hypothesis.

In addition to clinicoepidemiologic data, there is now good experimental evidence that the biologic reactivity, and in particular the lung toxicity, of cobalt metal particles is greatly increased when these particles are mixed, as in hard metal with a metallic carbide (25–28). Physicochemical investigations have shown that the unique toxicity of hard metal particles (as compared to cobalt metal alone) is due to the production of reactive oxygen species (ROSs) resulting from the interaction between cobalt metal and carbide particles (Fig. 1). The precise mechanism of this interaction is the following:

- Cobalt metal is thermodynamically able to reduce ambient oxygen but, due to the surface characteristics of the Co particles, the rate of this reaction is very low.
- Tungsten carbide is an inert material unable to react with oxygen by itself, but it is a fairly good electron conductor and possesses unique surface properties that are used in numerous catalysis processes (e.g., to replace platinum in combustion systems and petroleum chemistry).
- When both particles are associated, electrons provided by cobalt metal are easily transferred to the surface of carbide particles where reduction of oxygen can occur at a greatly increased rate and reactive oxygen species are produced in increased amounts (28).

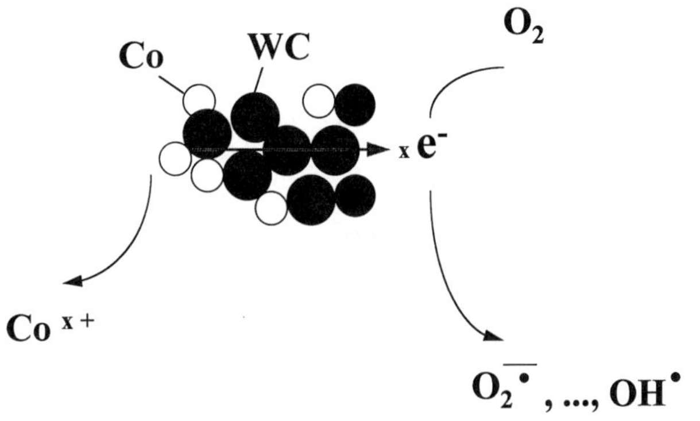


**FIG. 1.** Proposed mechanism of oxygen reduction by a mixture of cobalt (Co) and tungsten carbide (WC) particles. When both particles are in close contact, electrons ($e^-$) provided by cobalt metal and transferred to the surface of tungsten carbide particles can reduce oxygen and generate ROS; cobalt is oxidized and passes in solution ($Co^{x+}$). (Reprinted with permission from ref. 28.)

This finding might offer an attractive explanation for the fact that only a small proportion of workers exposed to hard metal dust develop an interstitial disease. It may indeed be speculated that individuals with lower antioxidant defense capacities (nutritional, constitutional) are more susceptible to the toxic effect of ROS produced by inhaled hard metal particles. Moreover, this mechanism may also contribute to explain the fact that interstitial lung diseases have rarely, if ever, been reported in workers exposed to cobalt alone even at very high airborne levels, e.g., in cobalt refineries (24).

The production of ROS by hard metal particles may also provide a basis to interpret the increased risk of lung cancer observed in hard metal (38) but not in cobalt refinery workers (39). ROSs have been demonstrated to produce significant genotoxic damage leading to the development of cancer. This hypothesis has recently been substantiated by *in vitro* data indicating a greater production of DNA single-strand breaks in human cells incubated with hard metal powders than in those treated with cobalt metal alone (unpublished results, Anard D., et al.).

It has also been suggested that tungsten oxide whiskers, which may be formed during the preparation of tungsten carbide, may play a role in the pathogenesis of the parenchymal disease (40,41). It has been shown that these fibers produce hydroxyl radicals *in vitro* and are cytotoxic at relatively high doses (42). While the possible pathogenic role of these fibers should not be ignored, it is surprising that similar fibers have never been observed in pathologic samples from hard metal disease patients.

An apparently greater prevalence of respiratory manifestations has been noted in workers who perform wet grinding as compared to those who perform dry grinding with hard metal tools (10,21). This finding has been interpreted as an exacerbating effect of certain types of coolants, which allow the dissolution of high concentrations of ionic cobalt, but it may also represent a simple additive effect due to the inhalation of metal working fluid aerosols (machine operator's lung), irrespective of its cobalt content (43).

## DIAMOND POLISHERS

Several cases of interstitial lung diseases have been described among diamond polishers (about 1% of the total work force) after the introduction of new high-speed grinding tools with a polishing surface of micro-diamonds cemented in very fine cobalt powder (44–47). No tungsten carbide was found either in the dust generated by this process or in BAL or lung tissue from patients. The clinical presentation and the pathologic findings described in diamond polishers with interstitial lung disease were essentially identical to those of hard metal disease, i.e., a fibrosing alveolitis (subacute and chronic forms) characterized by severe restrictive defects and markedly decreased diffusing capacity as well as the presence of large multinucleated cells into alveoli. These pulmonary manifestations tended to improve with cessation or reduction of exposure to cobalt disks. Corticosteroids were sometimes beneficial, especially in subacute forms of the disease. Following the discovery of this series of patients with pulmonary disease, a cross-sectional survey was performed to compare lung function tests in diamond polishers and controls (48). Spirometry showed that indices of ventilatory function (FVC and $FEV_1$) were significantly reduced in the group with the highest exposure to cobalt, but no correlation between functional impairment and years of utilization of cobalt disks could be found. Since these manifestations in diamond polishers occurred in the absence of tungsten carbide, these findings have contributed to support the view that cobalt alone was the offending compound responsible for hard metal disease, and the term *cobalt pneumopathy* was suggested as a substitute for *hard metal disease* (45,49). The exact pathogenic mechanism of this disease is still largely unsettled.

## ASTHMA

Exposure to cobaltous salts (50–52), or cobalt metal either alone or in association with other metals [i.e., hard metals (4,18,53,54) and dusts released from diamond polishing activities (55,56)] may cause typical bronchial asthma in a small proportion of workers (usually less than 5%). In some cases, in which specific immunoglobulin E (IgE) antibodies against a complex of cobalt with albumin could be identified, a type I allergic reaction has been suspected (54,57). For the remaining patients, the mechanism of cobalt-induced asthmatic reaction still remains to be elucidated (IgG-mediated, direct biochemical or irritant action). A specific inhalation challenge test with a cobalt salt (18,50,54,58,59), hard metal powder (4), or cobalt metal powder (55) may be positive. In a Japanese study (11), all patients who underwent a specific bronchial provocation test responded positively with immediate, late, or dual asthmatic reactions in approximately equal proportions. Positive (54,55) and negative (50) responses have been reported in nonspecific bronchial hyperreactivity tests (histamine or methacholine). A positive lymphocyte transformation test with cobalt has also been described in hard metal asthma, suggesting a role for cellular immunity (11,60). Cross-respiratory sensitization between nickel and cobalt has also been reported (11,61). Overall, there is therefore strong evidence that cobalt itself may cause the development of occupational asthma. However, insufficient data are available to assess whether the prevalence of asthma is higher in workers exposed to hard metal dust than in those exposed to cobalt only.

As usual in this type of disease, when an affected worker is removed from cobalt exposure, her/his asthma tends to diminish or disappear, but it may recur when exposure resumes (4,11,50). Prolonged exposure to cobalt-containing dust may also favor the development of a moderate obstructive syndrome, possibly through a nonspecific irritation (12,18).

## EXPOSURE ASSESSMENT

Exposure levels and prevalences of interstitial lung disease in hard metal workers are illustrated in Table 1. Overall, it may be concluded, however, that insufficient data are available to document dose-effect and/or dose-response relationships.

The characterization of exposure in hard metal industry has been limited to the assessment of the external and internal doses of cobalt, which is only one component of the toxic entity. Urinary excretion and blood or serum concentration of cobalt have been proposed as biologic indicators of exposure. Studying ten groups of hard metal workers (airborne cobalt concentration: 28 to 367 $\mu g/m^3$), Ichikawa et al. (62) found a good correlation between cobalt concentration in blood and cobalt in air on the basis of the mean values observed in the different groups. In a survey involving similar groups of workers (airborne cobalt concentration: 120 to 284 $\mu g/m^3$), Pellet et al. (63) have suggested that the difference between end-of-shift and beginning-of-shift urinary cobalt concentration reflected the day exposure. The concentration in urine on Friday evening was indicative of the cumulative exposure during the week, and the level of cobalt in urine collected on Monday morning mainly reflected long-term exposure. In another group of hard metal workers exposed to cobalt airborne concentrations below 100 μg/m$^3$, it has been shown that urinary cobalt concentration increased as the workweek progressed (64).

In a study in diamond polishers using cobalt-containing disks, the measurement of urine cobalt concentration, when considered on a workshop basis, was found to reflect the level of exposure to the metal (below 50 mg/m$^3$) (48). The relationships between environmental and biologic (blood and urine) parameters of exposure to different chemical forms of cobalt has been examined in a cross-sectional study in workers exposed to cobalt metal, oxides, and salts and to a mixture of cobalt and tungsten carbide (65). The main conclusion was that although biologic monitoring of workers exposed to cobalt oxides revealed increased blood and urine levels comparatively with nonexposed subjects, these parameters poorly reflected the recent exposure level. In contrast, when exposure was to soluble cobalt compounds (metal, salts, and hard metals), the measurement of urine and/or blood cobalt at the end of the workweek could be recommended for the monitoring of workers. It was calculated that an 8-hour exposure to 20 μg/m$^3$ [current recommended American Conference of Governmental Industrial Hygienists (ACGIH) threshold limit value time-weighted average (TLV-TWA)] of a soluble form of cobalt would lead to an average urinary concentration of about 20 μg of cobalt/g creatinine (postshift urine sample collected at the end of the workweek). The ACGIH (1995–96) has adopted as a biologic exposure index 15 μg cobalt/L urine (end of shift at the end of a workweek), irrespective of the conditions of exposure, e.g., association with metallic carbide or not, soluble or insoluble cobalt salt.

## REFERENCES


1. Balmes JR. Respiratory effects of hard metal dust exposure. *State Art Rev Occup Med* 1987;2:327–344.
2. Hartmann A, Wüthrich B, Bolognini G. Berufsbedingte Lungenkrankheiten bei der Hartmetallproduktion und -bearbeitung. Ein allergisches Geschehen? *Schweiz Med Wochenschr* 1982;112:1137–1141.
3. Cugell DW. The hard metal diseases. *Clin Chest Med* 1992;13:269–279.
4. Davison AG, Haslam PL, Corrin B, et al. Interstitial lung disease and asthma in hard-metal workers: bronchoalveolar lavage, ultrastructural, and analytical findings and results of bronchial provocation tests. *Thorax* 1983;38:119–128.
5. Donaldson JD, Clark SJ, Grimes SM. *Cobalt in medicine, agriculture and the environment.* The monograph series. London: Cobalt Development Institute, 1986.
6. Jobs H, Ballhausen C. The medical and technical points of view of metal ceramics as a source of dust. *Vertravensarzt Krankkasse* 1940;8:142–148.
7. Bech A, Kipling M, Heather J. Hard metal disease. *Br J Ind Med* 1962;19:239–252.
8. Fairhall LT, Castberg HT, Carrozzo NJ, Brinton HP. Industrial hygiene aspects of the cemented tungsten carbide industry. *J Occup Med* 1947;4:371–379.
9. Miller CW, Davis MW, Goldman A, Wyatt JP. Pneumoconiosis in the tungsten carbide tool industry. *Arch Ind Hyg Occup Med* 1953;8:453–465.
10. Sjögren I, Hillerdal G, Anderson A, Zetterström O. Hard metal lung disease: importance of cobalt in coolants. *Thorax* 1980;35:653–659.
11. Kusaka Y, Fujimora N, Morimoto K. Hard metal disease: epidemiology and pathogenesis. In: Kobayashi S, Bellanti JA, eds. *Advances in asthmology.* Amsterdam: Elsevier Science, 1990;271–276.
12. Tolot F, Girard R, Dorsit G, Tabourin G, Galy P, Bourret J. Manifestations pulmonaires des "métaux durs": troubles irritatifs et fibrose (Enquête et observations cliniques). *Arch Mal Prof Med Travail Securite Sociale* 1970;31:453–470.
13. Sluis-Cremer GK, Glyn Thomas R, Solomon A. Hard-metal lung disease. A report of 4 cases. *S Afr Med J* 1987;71:598–600.
14. Anttila S, Sutinen S, Paananen M, et al. Hard metal lung disease: a clinical, histological, ultrastructural and X-ray microanalytical study. *Eur Respir J* 1986;69:83–94.
15. Rizzato G, Lo Cicero S, Barberis M, Torre M, Pietra R, Sabbioni E. Trace of metal exposure in hard metal lung disease. *Chest* 1986;89:101–106.
16. Sprince N, Chamberlin R, Hales C, Weber A, Kazemi H. Respiratory disease in tungsten carbide production workers. *Chest* 1984;86:549–556.
17. Sprince NL, Oliver LC, Eisen EA, Greene RE, Chamberlin RI. Cobalt exposure and lung disease in tungsten carbide production. *Am Rev Respir Dis* 1988;138:1220–1226.
18. Kusaka Y, Ichikawa Y, Shirakawa T, Goto S. Effects of hard metal dust on ventilatory function. *Br J Ind Med* 1986;43:486–489.
19. Meyer-Bisch C, Pham QT, Mur JM, et al. Risque pulmonaire lié àl'exposition aux poussières de métaux durs. *INRS Cahiers Notes Documentaires* 1986;124:319–330.
20. Meyer-Bisch C, Pham Q, Mur JM, Massin N, Moulin JJ, Teculescu D. Respiratory hazards in hard metal workers: a cross sectional study. *Br J Ind Med* 1989;46:302–309.
21. Kennedy SM, Chan-Yeung M, Marion S, Lea J, Teschke K. Maintenance of stellite and tungsten carbide saw tips: respiratory health and exposure-response evaluations. *Occup Environ Med* 1995;52:185–191.
22. Kochetkova TA. On the question of the effect of cobalt powders. *Gig Tr Prof Zabol* 1960;4:34–38.
23. Reinl W, Schnellbächer F, Rahm G. Lungenfibrosen und entzündliche Lungenerkrankungen nach Einwirkung von Kobaltkontaktmasse. *Zbl Arbeitsmed Arbeitsschutz Prophy* 1979;29:318–325.
24. Swennen B, Buchet JP, Stanescu D, Lison D, Lauwerys R. Epidemiologic survey on workers exposed to cobalt oxides, cobalt salts and cobalt metal. *Br J Ind Med* 1993;50:835–842.
25. Lasfargues G, Lison D, Maldague P, Lauwerys R. Comparative study of the acute lung toxicity of pure cobalt powder and cobalt-tungsten carbide mixture in the rat. *Toxicol Appl Pharmacol* 1992;112:41–50.
26. Lasfargues G, Lison D, Lardot C, Delos M, Lauwerys R. Comparative study in the rat of the long term pulmonary responses to pure cobalt metal and hard metal powder. *Environ Res* 1996;69:108–121.
27. Lison D, Lauwerys R. In vitro cytotoxic effects of cobalt containing dusts on mouse peritoneal and rat alveolar macrophages. *Environ Res* 1990;52:187–198.
28. Lison D, Carbonnelle P, Mollo L, Lauwerys R, Fubini B. Physicochemical mechanism of the interaction between cobalt metal and carbide particles to generate toxic activated oxygen species. *Chem Res Toxicol* 1995;8:600–606.
29. Ruokonen E-L, Linnainmaa M, Seuri M, Juhakoski P, Söderström K-O. A fatal case of hard-metal disease. *Scand J Work Environ Health* 1996;22:62–65.
30. Cugell D, Morgan W, Perkins D, Rubin A. Respiratory effects of cobalt. *Arch Intern Med* 1990;150:177–183.
31. Ratto D, Balmes J, Boylen T, Sharma OP. Pregnancy in a woman with severe pulmonary fibrosis secondary to hard metal disease. *Chest* 1988;93:663–665.
32. Rüttner J, Spycher M, Stolkin I. Inorganic particulates in pneumoconiotic lungs of hard metal grinders. *Br J Ind Med* 1987;44:657–660.
33. Ohori NP, Sciurba FC, Owens GR, et al. Giant-cell interstitial pneumonia and hard metal pneumoconiosis. A clinico-pathological study of 4 cases and review of the literature. *Am J Surg Pathol* 1989;13:581–587.
34. Nicolaou G, Pietra R, Sabbioni E, Mosconi G, Cassina G, Seghizzi P. Multielement determination of metals in biological specimens of hard metal workers: a study carried out by neutron activation analysis. *J Trace Elem Electrolytes Health Dis* 1987;1:73–77.
35. Della Tore F, Cassani M, Segale M, Scarpazza G, Pietra R, Sabbioni E. Trace metal lung disease: A new fatal case of hard metal pneumoconiosis. *Respir* 1990;57:248–253.

36. Mosconi G, Zanelli R, Migliori M, et al. Study of lung reactions in six asymptomatic workers occupationally exposed to hard metal dusts. *Med Lav* 1991;82:131–136.
37. Moschinski G, Jurisch A, Reinl W. Pulmonary changes in sintered hard metal workers. *Arch Gewerbepath Gewerbehyg* 1959;16:697–720.
38. Lasfargues G, Wild P, Moulin JJ, et al. Lung cancer mortality in a French cohort of hard metal workers. *Am J Ind Med* 1994;26:585–596.
39. Moulin JJ, Wild P, Mur JM, Fournier-Betz M, Mercier-Gallay M. A mortality study of cobalt production workers: an extension of the follow-up. *Am J Ind Med* 1993;23:281–288.
40. Sahle W. Possible role of tungsten oxide whiskers in hard-metal pneumoconiosis. *Chest* 1992;102:1310.
41. Sahle W, Lazslo I, Krantz S, Christensson B. Airborne tungsten oxide whiskers in a hard metal industry. Preliminary findings. *Ann Occup Hyg* 1994;38:37–44.
42. Leanderson P, Sahle W. Formation of hydroxyl radicals and toxicity of tungsten oxide fibres. *Toxicol In Vitro* 1995;9:175–184.
43. Bernstein DI, Lummus ZL, Santilli G, Siskosky J, Bernstein L. Machine operator's lung. A hypersensitivity pneumonitis disorder associated with exposure to metalworking fluid aerosols. *Chest* 1995;108: 636–641.
44. Demedts M, Gheysens B, Nagels J, et al. Case reports: cobalt lung in diamond polishers. *Am Rev Respir Dis* 1984;130:130–135.
45. Lahaye D, Demedts M, van den Oever R, Roosels D. Lung diseases among diamond polishers due to cobalt? *Lancet* 1984;i:156–157.
46. Van den Eeckhout A, Varbeken E, Demedts M. La pathologie pulmonaire due au cobalt et aux métaux durs. *Rev Mal Respir* 1988;5: 201–207.
47. Van den Oever R, Roosels D, Douwen M, Vanderkeel J, Lahaye D. Exposure of diamond polishers to cobalt. *Ann Occup Hyg* 1990;34: 609–614.
48. Nemery B, Casier P, Roosels D, Lahaye D, Demedts M. Survey of cobalt exposure and respiratory health in diamond polishers. *Am Rev Respir Dis* 1992;145:610–616.
49. Demedts M, Ceuppens JL. Respiratory diseases from hard metal or cobalt exposure. Solving the enigma. *Chest* 1989;95:2–3.
50. Roto P. Asthma, symptoms of chronic bronchitis and ventilatory capacity among cobalt and zinc production workers. *Scand J Work Environ Health* 1980;6:1–49.
51. Raffn E, Mikkelsen S, Altman DG, Christensen JM, Groth S. Health effects due to occupational exposure to cobalt blue dye among plate painters in a porcelain factory in Denmark. *Scand J Work Environ Health* 1988;14:378–384.
52. Pillière F, Garnier R, Rousselin X, Dimermen S, Rosenberg N, Efthymiou ML. Asthme aux sels de cobalt. A propos d'un cas dû au résinate de cobalt. *Arch Mal Prof* 1990;51:413–417.
53. Kusaka Y. Hard metal asthma: a case of allergic bronchial asthma and contact dermatitis due to metallic cobalt. *Nippon Kyobu Shikkon Gakkai Zasshi* 1983;21:582–586.
54. Shirakawa T, Kusaka Y, Fujimura N, Goto S, Kato M, Heki S. Occupational asthma from cobalt sensitivity in workers exposed to hard metal dust. *Chest* 1989;95:29–37.
55. Gheysens B, Auwerx J, Van den Eeckhout A, Demedts M. Cobalt-induced bronchial asthma in diamond polishers. *Chest* 1985;88: 740–744.
56. Van Cutsem E, Ceuppens J, Lacquet L, Demedts M. Combined asthma and alveolitis induced by cobalt in a diamond polisher. *Eur J Respir Dis* 1987;70:54–61.
57. Shirakawa T, Kusaka Y, Fujimura N, Goto S, Morimoto K. The existence of specific antibodies to cobalt in hard metal asthma. *Clin Allergy* 1988;18:451–460.
58. Kusaka Y, Yokoyama K, Sera Y, Yamamoto S, Sone S, Kyono H. Respiratory diseases in hard metal workers: an occupational hygiene study in a factory. *Br J Ind Med* 1986;43:474–485.
59. Pisati G, Bernabeo F, Cirla AM. Utilizzo di un test di broncostimolazione specifica verso cobalto nella diagnosi dell'asma da metalli duri. *Med Lav* 1986;77:538–546.
60. Kusaka Y, Nakano Y, Shirakawa T. Lymphocyte transformation with cobalt in hard metal asthma. *Ind Health* 1989;27:155–163.
61. Shirakawa T, Kusaka Y, Fujimura N, Kato M, Heki S, Morimoto K. Hard metal asthma: cross immunological and respiratory reactivity between cobalt and nickel? *Thorax* 1990;45:267–271.
62. Ichikawa Y, Kusaka Y, Goto S. Biological monitoring of cobalt exposure, based on cobalt concentrations in blood and urine. *Int Arch Occup Environ Health* 1985;55:269–276.
63. Pellet F, Perdrix A, Vincent M, et al. Dosage biologique du cobalt urinaire. Intérêt en médecine du travail dans la surveillance des expositions aux carbures métalliques frittés. *Arch Mal Prof* 1984;45:81.
64. Scansetti G, Lamon S, Talarico S, et al. Urinary cobalt as a measure of exposure in the hard metal industry. *Int Arch Occup Environ Health* 1985;57:19–26.
65. Lison D, Buchet J-P, Swennen B, Molders J, Lauwerys R. Biological monitoring of workers exposed to cobalt metal, salt, oxide and hard metal dust. *Occup Environ Med* 1994;51:447–450.
66. Gennart J-P, Lauwerys R. Ventilatory function of workers exposed to cobalt and diamond containing dust. *Int Arch Occup Environ Health* 1990;62:333–336.
67. Morgan L. A study into the health and mortality of men exposed to cobalt and oxides. *J Soc Occup Med* 1983;33:181–186.
68. Lison D. Human toxicity of cobalt-containing dust and experimental studies on the mechanism of interstitial lung disease (hard metal disease). *Crit Rev Toxicol* 1996;26:585–616.

*Environmental and Occupational Medicine, Third Edition,* edited by William N. Rom.
Lippincott–Raven Publishers, Philadelphia © 1998.

# CHAPTER 74

# Chromium Compounds

Mitchell D. Cohen and Max Costa

## INDUSTRIAL APPLICATIONS

Chromium (Cr) is a first-series transition element from group VIB. Its earliest uses were in the production of pigments and dye mordants and for leather tanning. With industrialization, Cr was employed more for refractory processes and in alloy formation. On average, 10 million tons of chromite is consumed globally every year, making it the most commonly used Cr mineral (1). The majority of Cr is used in metallurgic applications, the remainder for refractory or chemical applications. When mixed with steel or wrought iron, Cr increases its hardness and enhances its resistance to corrosion and oxidation (i.e., stainless steel). The high melting point (2,040°C) and acid/base resistance of chromite make it ideal for refractory use, as for making mortars and castables and joining furnace bricks. Chemical applications of Cr agents, in addition to pigments, dyeing, and leather tanning, are in wood preservatives, agricultural antifungicides, antifreeze, antialgae agents, porcelain and glassmaking, photoengraving and blueprint development, the production of high-fidelity magnetic audio tapes, and tattooing. Most Cr compounds exist in the hexavalent [Cr(VI)] or trivalent [Cr(III)] oxidation state, but other oxidation states are utilized. For example, divalent (chromous chloride, $CrCl_2$) and tetravalent [chromium (IV) oxide, $CrO_2$] agents are used in chromizing processes and the manufacture of magnetic audio tapes, respectively. The trivalent or hexavalent nature of each compound affects its toxic effects—at the cellular level and ultimately on the general health of workers exposed to Cr with hexavalent Cr generally being in the order of 1000× more toxic than trivalent Cr.

M. D. Cohen: Department of Environmental Medicine, New York University Medical Center, Tuxedo, New York 10987.
M. Costa: Department of Environmental Medicine; and Department of Pharmacology, New York University Medical Center, New York, New York 10016.

## ENVIRONMENTAL EXPOSURE

The metallurgy industry is the primary user of Cr ores and also the dominant source of anthropogenic Cr emissions into the atmosphere. These emissions are almost exclusively in the form of ferrochrome particles, the total amount released depending on the technology employed (i.e., open hearth versus electric arc type furnaces). Emission control devices such as Venturi scrubbers and bag filters appreciably decrease the amounts of Cr released. Refractory processing, the second largest source of ambient Cr, produced almost 10% of the total emissions in the United States (2). Almost all Cr compounds used for chemical applications are derived from parental sodium chromite or sodium dichromate. The latter is obtained by smelting, roasting, and extracting Cr ores; atmospheric releases from these processes never exceed 0.5% of the annual total. Other sources of atmospheric Cr come from engine combustion of coal (1–100 μg Cr/g) or crude oil (5–730 ng Cr/g), the manufacture of cement (1.6 g Cr/ton), refuse (1–15 g Cr/ton) and sewer sludge (10 μg Cr/ton) incineration, and the wearing away of asbestos brake linings (3).

Typical atmospheric concentrations of Cr are, on average, 0.2 to 1.0 ng Cr/$m^3$ in remote continental regions, 1 to 10 ng Cr/$m^3$ for rural and semirural areas, and 13 to 30 ng Cr/$m^3$ in urban areas. In Cr-using industries, indoor levels have been measured at 10 to 50 μg Cr/$m^3$ (in tanning shops) to 1,220 μg Cr/$m^3$ (in steel mills) (4). Permissible exposure limits to chromates of 0.1 mg Cr/$m^3$ in a typical 40-hour workweek have been established by the

Occupational Safety and Health Administration (OSHA) (5). Differences due to oxidation states led to the establishment of two thresholds: 0.5 mg Cr/m$^3$ for Cr metal, divalent, and trivalent compounds, and 0.05 mg Cr/m$^3$ for insoluble chromates, chromite production dust, and soluble hexavalent compounds.

Contamination of water by the settling of fly ash particles, direct deposition from chromium-containing industrial sewage, or leaching from topsoil and rocks are other means by which Cr is introduced into the environment. The latter represents the most important natural source of Cr entry into water. On average, the continental crust contains 125 mg Cr/kg, and approximately 200,000 tons of Cr are released annually due to weathering processes (6). In general, most of the Cr released by natural processes is in the trivalent state. Rainwater Cr content averages <1 µg Cr/L globally, but in certain urban settings, anthropogenic contributions raise the levels >5 µg Cr/L. Industrial wastewaters can contain total amounts of Cr ranging from 0.005 to 525 mg Cr/L, with levels of hexavalent Cr averaging 0.004 to 335 mg Cr/L. On-site chemical adsorbents and filtration systems aid in the removal of much Cr from these effluents, while underground aquifers provide for natural continuous filtration of groundwater. Drinking water standards have been set at 100 µg/L or 100 parts per billion (ppb) total by the USEPA (7,8).

## CHROMIUM TRANSPORT, DISTRIBUTION, AND EXCRETION

While dermal contact provides one of the most likely means for Cr exposure, ingestion and inhalation of Cr particles are the major routes for the introduction of relatively large quantities of Cr into the body. Oral intake of water-soluble hexavalent Cr also results in a wide range of variability in absorption in humans (1–24%). Some of this hexavalent Cr is reduced to the trivalent form by gastric juices, but a substantial amount remains absorbable as Cr(VI). Uptake of trivalent Cr from the intestines is slow; the hexavalent Cr that avoids gastric reduction is absorbed there. Absorbed hexavalent Cr ions are transported via the portal vein to the liver (entering erythrocytes en route) or they are rapidly taken up by liver cells along with other absorbed materials (9).

Inhalation is the route of exposure most responsible for the associated risks from Cr exposure in occupational settings, but inhalation alone does not ensure that a given Cr particle can impart a toxic effect. Nonspecific defense mechanisms against inhaled particles and several hexavalent Cr-reducing processes can lower the potential toxic impact of any exposure. Pulmonary macrophages rapidly phagocytose hexavalent particles and reduce them within cytoplasmic phagosomes. Macrophage reduction thereby results in irreversible sequestering of Cr, since these cells have very long life spans (10). These Cr-bearing macrophages are then expectorated or swallowed, thus decreasing the chance of systemic Cr uptake. Within the bronchial tree, epithelium lining fluids directly reduce hexavalent to trivalent Cr. This second line of defense lowers the amount of inhaled hexavalent Cr that is able to enter the bloodstream through the alveoli (11).

The oxidation state of Cr is the determining factor in its mode of transport in the bloodstream. Physiologic amounts of trivalent Cr are bound to the β-globulin fraction of serum proteins or by other metal-transporting proteins such as transferrin (12,13). At high concentrations, trivalent Cr binds to serum albumin or $\alpha_1$- or $\alpha_2$-globulin. Although the trivalent form is transported via the serum, unlike the hexavalent form it cannot penetrate red blood cells. Hexavalent Cr crosses erythrocyte membranes and binds the globulin portion of hemoglobin following oxidation of the heme group (12,14).

Whole-body distribution studies indicate that the liver, spleen, kidney, and testes accumulate the majority of Cr after exposure. Other organs such as the heart, pancreas, lung, and brain take up and retain less. The subcellular distribution of Cr in the liver and kidneys results in 45% to 50% of the total cell burden locating to the nuclear fraction, with lesser amounts retained by cytoplasmic, mitochondrial, and microsomal fractions (14).

While trivalent Cr ions are cleared from the blood, hexavalent ions are retained much longer owing to internalization by red and white cells. Besides the blood, the various target organs also display different rates of clearance for each metal species. Therefore, no true equilibrium between tissue stores and circulating Cr levels can accurately be established. This makes the biologic monitoring of Cr exposure by measuring blood burdens less valuable.

Following clearance from the blood, Cr is excreted principally in the urine. Secondary excretion of small amounts of ingested metal and expectorated particles occurs via bile and feces. A minor route of excretion is through the skin and via sweat. Because the Cr found in urine is likely to have been derived from the dialyzable fraction of serum, reabsorption along the renal tubules following glomerular filtration presents another route by which circulating levels of Cr might remain elevated following acute exposure.

## CELLULAR UPTAKE AND METABOLISM

The overwhelming majority of the biologic effects following Cr exposure are due to the parental hexavalent Cr species rather than the trivalent form. It has been recognized for some time that while cells are relatively impermeable to the latter, the hexavalent form readily enters cells. These compounds exist predominantly as chromates at physiologic pH and assume tetrahedral structures similar to other physiologic anions like $PO_4^{2-}$ and $SO_4^{2-}$. Conversely, trivalent ions exist exclusively as octahedral complexes for which distinct cellular uptake mechanisms do not exist (15,16). The presence of intracellular reduced glutathione (GSH) is also necessary for the continuous uptake of hexavalent Cr via nonselective anion channels. By reducing the intracellular hexavalent Cr to the trivalent form, a concentration gradient may be maintained that allows for a steady-state influx of ions.

Although trivalent Cr does not enter cells well, the presence of numerous cation-binding sites in the cell membrane allows it to accumulate on the cell surface (17). The biologic ramifications from this effect are not clear, although interference with the binding of positively charged essential agents cannot be excluded as a mechanism of toxicity. Additionally, particulate trivalent Cr compounds may be taken up into cells by endocytotic processes (18); phagocytes treated with trivalent Cr do display genotoxic damage similar to that observed when hexavalent Cr is employed (19).

Following entry into the cytoplasm, hexavalent Cr is reduced or undergoes ligand displacement reactions (9,16,20,21). The sulfhydryl-bearing glutathione tripeptide and the nicotinamide enzymatic cofactors, reduced nicotinamide adenine dinucleotide (NADH) and reduced nicotinamide adenine dinucleotide phosphate (NADPH), readily react with hexavalent Cr (22,23). However, oxygen and hydrogen peroxide as well as thiol moieties on cysteine and proteins also act as redox participants (24,25). Because of their negative nature, the chromates ($CrO_4^{2-}$) are not directly reactive with deoxyribonucleic acid (DNA). The products of reduction—penta-, tetra-, and trivalent Cr, activated oxygen (hydroxyl radical, singlet oxygen, superoxide anion) and sulfur (thiol radicals)—rather than hexavalent Cr proper, are the ultimate genotoxins.

Microsomal and nuclear membrane phase I enzymes, like cytochrome P-450, have also been shown to enhance the toxicity of hexavalent Cr by increasing the production of intermediate oxidation state pentavalent and tetravalent forms (26). Mitochondrial reduction of hexavalent Cr may also occur. Reactions with electron transport chain complexes I and II (both of which contain Fe-S/flavin centers) and the ferricytochrome c:$O_2$ oxido-reductase complex (which bears heme and copper moieties) actively reduce hexavalent Cr (27,28). In addition to the impact on cellular respiration and the production of adenosine triphosphate (ATP) and guanosine triphosphate (GTP), the interactions of the products of hexavalent Cr reduction with mitochondrial DNA cannot be overlooked.

Whereas extracellular reduction of hexavalent Cr by ascorbate or free reduced glutathione serves as a detoxification mechanism, intracellular reduction of the hexavalent form is the critical event for the ultimate expression of potential cytotoxicity or genotoxicity. One possible mechanism for Cr genotoxicity suggests that the genotoxins generated in the cytoplasm are long-lived species that avoid cytoplasmic chelation and migrate (possibly as coordinate complexes) into the nucleus to damage DNA (19). However, the redox-generated oxygen and sulfur radicals, as well as pentavalent and hexavalent ions, are notoriously short-lived. Still, these Cr intermediates can be stabilized by complexing with select proteins or cellular ligands (29).

An alternative mechanism suggests that if cellular levels of hexavalent Cr surpass the capacity of the cytoplasmic reductants, then it might migrate directly to the nucleus and be reduced in situ without cytoplasmic modifications (9). This would then allow for generation of the reactive Cr intermediates as well as the oxygen and sulfur radicals within a short distance of the DNA. The case for both mechanisms in the induction of cancers has been demonstrated in mammalian cells with variable reductant capacities (i.e., skeletal muscle), or in cell lines where the defensive reductants have been overwhelmed (i.e., lung; see ref. 9).

**Interactions with DNA and RNA**

The ultimate form of cellular Cr, trivalent Cr, binds readily to ring nitrogen donor sites on purine nucleosides to yield bidentate structures (30). Additional linkages to the ribose oxygen atoms may give rise to even more complex structures. When phosphate groups are present, the major binding reactions occur first at the outermost phosphate moiety and subsequently with the neighboring phosphate oxygen(s) (31). Under aqueous conditions, hydroxo groups are slowly exchanged with the ligands of the parent compound in the process of olation. These olated complexes can then form long, continuous chains of metal (cross-linked through ether type of linkage following the loss of a water molecule), which can then react with nucleotides at distant sites along the DNA chain. Conversely, Cr can also react directly with nucleotides first and then undergo olation. In both scenarios, Cr-linked nucleotide complexes are formed, which may give rise to DNA-DNA intra- and interstrand cross-links (for review see ref. 32).

The magnitude and preference of trivalent Cr binding to DNA follows the order G > A > C > T among nucleic acids and nucleosides (33). The increased presence of ring carbonyl groups accounts for the differences in preference among the purines. On intact DNA, while trivalent Cr binding increases in proportion with the total (G + C) content, the major binding occurs principally via the phosphate backbone (30,31).

In addition to the formation of the DNA-DNA cross-links, trivalent Cr binding *in vitro* also results in increased resistance of DNA to hydrolysis, altered DNA perceptibility, and increased thermal denaturation [lowered melting temperature ($T_m$)] (34). While trivalent Cr induces DNA instability, it has the opposite effect with ribonucleic acid (RNA). This is due to the increased (G + C) content of RNA as compared with DNA, and the resulting linkage of neighboring guanyl sites giving rise to more compact, thermally stable structures.

The binding of Cr to DNA also impacts on the enzymology of DNA replication. The trivalent Cr-bound DNA contains novel secondary and tertiary structures that alter DNA polymerase processivity (35) or affect the recognition of bases, thereby resulting in misincorporation (36). Error repair functions are similarly inhibited, so that the trivalent Cr-induced introduction of an erroneous base into a replicated strand has little chance of being proofread, excised, and replaced. The hexavalent ions can also decrease DNA polymerase replication and fidelity (36–38), but the mechanisms are due to a different form of enzymatic competitive inhibition. Unlike trivalent Cr ions, which complex with nucleotides to form altered substrates that inhibit polymerase activity (39), the hexavalent ions are more likely to directly bind to the thiol groups along the enzyme proper or impart oxidative damage to the enzyme giving rise to the observed inhibition (40,41).

Besides affecting DNA synthesis directly, hexavalent Cr can lower nucleotide levels within cells (42,43) by altering membrane receptors involved in nucleoside uptake (i.e., nucleoside permeases) or their uptake by facilitated diffusion. The possibility of nucleotide seepage following hexavalent Cr-induced membrane oxidative perforations has been shown to be unlikely; however, inhibition of nucleotide conversion enzymes such as nucleoside diphosphokinases by trivalent ions also give rise to decreased cellular nucleotide pools (44). While trivalent ions inhibit this particular system for nucleotide pool maintenance, they have no effect on membrane permeability or related means of nucleoside uptake. This indicates that Cr compounds, in either their parental or ultimate intracellular forms, can exhibit dual toxicities at different cell target sites, resulting in nucleotide pool imbalances.

### Chromosomal Effects

Studies of trivalent and hexavalent Cr compounds in vivo reveal that hexavalent Cr is the active clastogen in intact cells, whereas the trivalent form, which is avidly reactive with both DNA and nucleic acids *in vitro*, is not effective owing to poor cellular uptake. Hexavalent Cr has been shown to induce sister-chromatid exchanges, chromosome aberrations, DNA strand breaks, formation of alkali-sensitive sites, and intrastrand DNA-DNA and DNA-protein cross-links (17,43,45–48). The most common chromosome aberrations appear as chromatid gaps and breaks, with less frequent isochromatid breaks or chromatid exchanges.

In addition to direct damage to cellular DNA, hexavalent Cr ions also alter the cell cycle (49). Mitotic delays and the inability to induce metaphase are common. Often there is aberrant cell division with a resultant increase in the frequency of cells containing dislocated metaphase chromosomes, an absence of spindles, or malformed spindles visualized as chromatin spots (50). The consequence of these defects is aneuploidy (daughter cells with chromosome imbalances).

The cell cycle is preferentially susceptible to hexavalent Cr-induced DNA damage during the S phase (51), the period in which DNA unfolds to permit replication. Unlike some other metals (i.e., nickel) which selectively damage heterochromatin, Cr does not have any preference for euchromatin or heterochromatin (52). Rather, Cr induces chromosome damage randomly.

Although hexavalent Cr itself is a powerful oxidant, it is the penta- and tetravalent intermediates that act on and cleave intact DNA. The free ions cannot act alone but apparently must be complexed with reduced glutathione during the redox reactions in order to be active (53). In addition to glutathione, microsomal enzymes and ribonucleotides are agents that can reduce hexavalent Cr in cells (54).

### Chromatin Damage

Mammalian hosts or intact cells treated with chromate, or isolated cell nuclei exposed to trivalent Cr, have an increased incidence of DNA-protein cross-links (55–59). Formation of these lesions is time- and dose-dependent (60). Under conditions *in vitro,* maximal doses for induction of the complexes can be achieved (i.e., via saturation of Cr-binding sites on protein, DNA, or both); the biologic relevance of these findings to circumstances *in vivo* is unclear, since the saturating doses used are lethal to most living organisms.

The predominant proteins that are cross-linked to DNA include the nuclear proteins such as lamins A, B, and C, several cytokeratins, and actin (57,61). Among these, actin seems to be most readily cross-linked to DNA, with complexing occurring at sublethal concentrations of hexavalent or trivalent Cr (57,60). The differences in cross-linking potentials among these and numerous other nuclear proteins demonstrate the dependence on the primary structure of the protein(s), their proximity to the DNA, the accessibility to the Cr ions, the chromatin conformation, and the DNA "strandedness" in the formation of this lesion.

### Mutation Induction

Overall, almost all hexavalent Cr compounds assayed in prokaryotic and eukaryotic systems are mutagenic. In several prokaryotes, hexavalent Cr can induce either reversions or forward mutations through base pair substitutions or frameshift mutations (43,46,62). Whether or not error-prone repair is required for Cr-induced base pair errors or mutations is not certain. Some studies using tryptophan or histidine auxotrophs that bear or lack certain types of repair mechanisms suggest that Cr-induced lesions are repaired principally through complex recombinational postreplication pathways (63). Other studies imply that chromates directly modify DNA and give rise to base pair errors despite any particular repair process (62).

Compared with the prokaryotic models, mutation studies with eukaryotic cells show similar trends with regard to the mutagenic potencies of hexavalent Cr ions as compared with those of trivalent ions (17,48,57,64). The induction of gene mutations in cultured cell lines such as the Chinese hamster lung (V79) or ovary (CHO) cells have been well documented. Endpoints, including resistance to ouabain, 6-thioguanine, 8-azaguanine, and trifluorothymidine, have all been used to demonstrate the mutagenic potential of many hexavalent Cr agents (65). Far fewer studies, such as the mouse spot test (66), have been used to detect mutagenicity *in vivo* by monitoring somatic mutations in the progeny from chromate-treated dams. The use of mammalian mutation assays also demonstrates that trivalent Cr compounds are not active in inducing mutations (17,39,46).

## HEALTH HAZARDS

### General Overview

Overall, trivalent Cr compounds have a relatively low order of toxicity as compared with hexavalent agents, owing to the low permeability in intact cells and a smaller redox potential ($E° = -0.41V$) than the strongly oxidizing hexavalent forms ($E° = +1.41V$; $+3e^-$). The most common lesion of acute Cr toxicity in occupational settings is chromate-induced ulcerations. Inhalation of chromate-bearing dusts or mists results in irritation or ulceration of nasal mucosae and possible septal perforation. Other acute responses to hexavalent Cr intoxication include gastric distress, olfactory sense impairment, and yellowing of the teeth and tongue. Contact dermatitis (dermal toxicosis) is the most widely encountered clinical manifestation from an acute overexposure to trivalent or hexavalent Cr. Although ulceration is due exclusively to hexavalent Cr ions (i.e., $CrO_4^{2-}$), breaks in the skin at the contact site allow much more of either Cr form to enter the body. The increased influx can result in renal chromate toxicosis, liver failure, and death.

The seriously detrimental effects of hexavalent Cr are primarily the result of chronic low-level exposure. Increased incidence of gingivitis and periodontitis are common, as is ocular damage, including eye lesions, conjunctivitis, and keratitis. Major health problems can arise from long-term inhalation of Cr particles or solubilized Cr in mists or dusts. Apart from the carcinogenic potential, prolonged exposure can result in chronic bronchitis, rhinitis, or sinusitis or the formation of nasal mucosal polyps. In addition to being immunosuppressive, Cr compounds can also induce acute chemical pneumonitis. Besides the lungs and intestinal tract, the liver and kidney are often target organs for chromate toxicity. Interestingly, the kidneys appear to be the most sensitive target organ to the toxic effects of trivalent Cr exposure.

### Immunotoxicologic Effects

Allergic contact dermatitis due to Cr is most commonly observed during occupational contact with low to moderate levels of chromates (67). This hypersensitivity usually occurs in the presence of other metal allergens (i.e., nickel and cobalt); however, the coexisting hypersensitivities are not due to immunologic cross-reactivities, but rather to concomitant host sensitization (68,69). That allergic contact dermatitis due to Cr exposure occurs in exposed hosts is peculiar in that some factors about Cr—the lack of universal contact sensitivity in light of widespread environmental Cr distribution, the relatively weak allergenic potency of Cr proper, variations in skin penetrability by different Cr compounds of the same and different valences, and the long time of exposure required for clinical manifestation—need to be overcome for the adverse reaction to take place. Although the concentrations of Cr necessary for sensitization are often only slightly higher than the physiologic blood levels, Cr at very low or very high concentrations, or under conditions of repeated exposures, can readily induce conditions of immunologic unresponsiveness (67,70). The penetration of hexavalent Cr through the epidermis is inversely concentration dependent (71); however, once under the dermal layers, the reduction of hexavalent Cr to its trivalent state yields the ultimate $Cr^{3+}$-protein conjugate hapten. Precisely which protein is conjugated is uncertain, but serum albumin, heparin, and glycosaminoglycans have been suggested as potential allergens (72), although questions about the importance of the conjugate protein specificity remain.

Exposed hosts that display Cr-dependent allergic contact dermatitis tend to have increased levels of serum immunoglobulins M and A (IgM and IgA) antibodies, increased Cr-induced lymphocyte transformation and proliferation, increased formation of immediate (E) rosettes, and decreased suppressor index values reflective of changes in the relative numbers of $CD4^+$-$T_H$ and $CD8^+$-$T_S$ lymphocytes (73,74). A reduction in the activity of $T_S$ cells (either through decreases in absolute numbers or Cr-mediated changes in functionality) is thought to be responsible for increases in circulating antibodies and in levels of circulating immune complexes (75). The Cr-induced lymphocyte proliferation was found to be monocyte–dependent (74); it is unclear whether monocytes/macrophages themselves, or even inflammatory polymorphonuclear leukocytes, are affected by Cr in ways that might contribute to the onset/development of the allergic response.

As inhalation of Cr is the most common route for Cr intake in industrial settings, many studies have examined the impact of Cr compounds on the functionality of cells essential to maintaining lung immunocompetence, i.e., lung macrophages. Morphologically, macrophages recovered from the lungs of experimental animals following inhalation of either hexavalent or trivalent Cr compounds display increased numbers of Cr-filled cytoplasmic inclusions, enlarged lysosomes, surface smoothing, and a decreased number of membrane blebs for cell target contact and cell mobility (76,77). Functionally, the macrophages display reductions in (a) phagocytic activity, (b) rates of oxygen consumption following stimulation with zymosan, and (c) production of reactive oxygen intermediates used for target cell killing (76,78,79). The majority of the effects of Cr on macrophage structure and function have also been reproduced *in vitro* in alveolar macrophages from a variety of hosts. However, unlike in the *in vivo* studies, trivalent Cr compounds are mainly ineffective; this lack of effect is most likely due to the differences in mechanisms of hexavalent and trivalent Cr entry into cells.

While the macrophage appears to be a primary target of Cr toxicity, immunotoxic effects are also observed in lymphocytes. At the molecular level, lymphocytes exposed to hexavalent Cr *in vivo* or *in vitro* display increased incidences of chromosomal aberrations (80,81) (including DNA strand-breaks, gaps, and interchanges) and increased levels of DNA-protein complex formation (82,83). The implications from these defects are not certain, but it has been suggested that the genetic alterations/damage to DNA integrity might result in changes in lymphocyte proliferation *in vivo* or under experimental conditions.

At the immunologic level, lymphocytes recovered from Cr-exposed hosts display altered mitogenic responsiveness (84,85). At low concentrations, soluble hexavalent Cr was slightly stimulatory, though the same compound became inhibitory with increasing concentrations; soluble trivalent Cr was ineffective at all doses tested. An *in vitro* study using rat splenocytes in mixed lymphocyte cultures or in combination with B- or T-cell–specific mitogens again demonstrated a very narrow concentration-dependent biphasic (stimulatory/inhibitory) effect with hexavalent Cr (86). However, in peripheral blood lymphocytes from Cr-exposed rats, mitogenic responsiveness was enhanced overall, with even greater responsiveness when exogenous Cr was added. The basis for the discrepancies between the *in vitro* and *in vivo* studies may be (1) that Cr added to naive splenocyte cultures reacted with cell surface proteins (i.e., surface mitogen receptors) to block the proliferative effect, while (2) extended periods of *in vivo* exposure to Cr may have resulted in host sensitization and, ultimately, selection of lymphocyte populations that proliferate in the presence of Cr ions or Cr-conjugated protein haptens (as occurs during allergic contact dermatitis).

Other Cr-induced alterations in macrophages and lymphocytes include changes in the production/release of cellular proteins required for proper immune cell function and for induction of cellular activation critical for the normal immune response. These changes include decreases in (a) the levels of circulating antibody in response to viral antigens (87); (b) formation of interferons in response to viruses or antigenic stimulation (88,89); and (c) production of interleukin-2 (85,90), the cytokine required for B-lymphocyte proliferation and differentiation during the onset of humoral immunity. These Cr-induced disturbances in immune cell intercommunications likely serve as the basis for the attenuation of cell and humoral immunity observed *in vivo*, and for the subsequent increases in the incidence/severity of infectious diseases and, possibly, cancers manifested in animals and humans exposed to Cr compounds over extended periods of time.

## CANCER IN HUMANS AND ANIMALS

By far the major health hazard due of long-term Cr exposure is the increased risk of lung/sinonasal and gastrointestinal tract (esophageal, stomach, intestinal, and pancreatic) cancers (91–93). Extensive reviews of Cr carcinogenicity have been published by several government and international organizations, as well as by individual investigators (94–102). Such studies provided epidemiologic evidence for the carcinogenicity of Cr and demonstrated in animal models that there was a direct association between selective Cr(VI) exposure and tumor formation. These studies also demonstrated the relevance of oxidation state, Cr solubility, and route of exposure as critical parameters in assessing carcinogenic potentials for Cr compounds.

### Chromium Carcinogenicity in Animal Models

Many of the earliest attempts to determine which species of Cr compounds were the causative agents for occupationally–related cancers utilized inhalation or parenteral exposures with metallic Cr, chromite ore, or several commonly–utilized Cr compounds (96,97,103–105). While a majority of studies yielded negative or equivocal results, several showed that Cr(VI) agents were often carcinogenic in test animals. Conversely, oral exposure to Cr compounds has not been shown to give rise to enhanced tumor formation in test animals when compared with vehicle controls (106,107).

Although the corresponding linkage of route of exposure to sites of Cr-induced tumor formation is remarkably similar between humans and mice/rats, this susceptibility to tumor induction varies widely among the commonly–used animal models. For example, mice and rats exposed to atmospheres or intratracheal implants containing chromates of varying solubilities displayed a greater incidence of lung squamous metaplasias, adenomas, and/or adenocarcinomas, than did controls (108–111); on the other hand, rabbits, hamsters, or guinea pigs exposed to these agents failed to develop tumors (112).

Cancers have been induced in mice and rats primarily following implantation of less soluble chromate compounds. In no cases, using intratracheal, -bronchial, muscular, -peritoneal, -venous, or -femoral implantation, have metallic or trivalent Cr compounds caused an increased incidence of tumors (99,105,109,113,114). Subcutaneous implantation of strontium, calcium, or lead chromates (but not barium chromate) resulted in spindle-cell sarcoma, rhabdomyosarcoma, or fibrosarcoma formation at the injection site (103,115). Intramuscular injections of several forms of these poorly soluble chromates also caused tumor formation (103,104,116,117). Implantation studies with highly water-soluble sodium dichromate or chromate failed to demonstrate a similar rise in formation of in-site tumors (104,108).

Direct inhalation or intratracheal, intrapleural, or intrabronchial instillation of hexavalent Cr compounds are by far the most common routes of exposure that give rise to tumor formation in animal models. The preponderance of data indicates that neither metallic nor trivalent Cr compounds give rise to lung tumors. Using direct inhalation studies, mice and rats chronically exposed to sodium dichromate aerosols, calcium chromate dusts, or chromic acid mists developed lung adenomas and carcinomas (110,111,118,119), although the incidences were not statistically significant. In mice, instillation of zinc chromate resulted in the formation of benign adenomas, but at a rate no greater than observed in vehicle controls (113,120). With rats, too, instillation of calcium chromate resulted in a greater formation of benign adenomas than adenocarcinomas, but this incidence was not significantly higher than observed in controls.

To better examine carcinogenicity in the lungs, using a method of intrabronchial implantation in which a selected zone of bronchial epithelium was subject to exposure for continuous periods, it was shown that many Cr compounds, including several trivalent species, gave rise to squamous metaplasias. However, only hexavalent agents caused significant increases in the incidences of metaplasia and carcinomas (108,109,121). When this protocol was used for introducing condensed Cr-bearing welding and thermal spraying fumes, a greater incidence of distal benign cancers (i.e., lymphomas, skin, intestine, central nervous system, thyroid, and pituitary), but oddly, not lung cancers, was obtained (122).

### Chromium Carcinogenicity in Humans

The greatest levels of human exposures to Cr(VI) occur primarily during chromate production, welding processes, chrome pigment manufacture, chrome plating, and spray painting. Exposures to other valence forms of Cr occur primarily during mining, ferrochromium and steel production, and during the cutting and grinding of Cr alloys. The results of the major epidemiologic studies of cancer formation in workers exposed to Cr during chromate production, production of Cr pigment, electroplating, the production of ferrochromium alloys, and other incidental industrial and environmental exposures have recently been reviewed (92,93) and are summarized in Table 1.

Occupational exposure to chromates has been shown to be associated with high Cr concentrations in lung tissue. While the Cr concentration in lung tissue serves as a major criterion in establishing a causal connection between occupational exposure to certain Cr compounds and development of bronchial carcinoma (123,124), the Cr content of the tumor tissue itself is not a useful criterion in this respect since it is not known whether or not the tumors store the metal during their progression. The Cr content of lung generally increases in direct relation with the duration of exposure. Most often, the concentration of Cr in the upper lobes is significantly higher than that in the lower lobes, suggesting regional differences either in clearance from, or deposition in, the lung. It has become apparent that the inhaled metal can remain in the lungs long after exposure to chromate had ceased.

The type of cancer that develops in humans following Cr exposure has been shown to vary with the type of Cr and duration of exposure. In studies where the incidence of Cr-related lung cancer was shown to be 16 times higher in exposed workers than in the general population, the predominant cancers were squamous cell and small cell carcinomas (125). Those patients who presented with small cell carcinomas were found to have been primarily engaged in the second phase of chromate production, during which they were heavily exposed to Cr(VI) dusts. The patients who primarily developed squamous cell carcinomas were found to have worked in the second, third, and fourth stages of production, all of which involve exposures to increasingly refined Cr(VI) products and increasingly lower levels of Cr(III)-bearing dusts. With regard to the duration of employment as a contributing factor to cancer development, in those Cr workers suffering from small cell carcinoma, the length of employment was significantly shorter than for those workers with squamous cell cancer. It follows then that as a function of total exposure, when the exposure to Cr agents was heavy, the major type of lung cancer that evolved was of the small cell type.

An analysis of the correlation between cancer incidence and one of several other factors, such as duration of employment in Cr industry, worker age at the beginning of employment, and estimations of the degree of chromate exposure, determined that the duration of employment/exposure was the major dependent factor in the onset of lung cancer and subsequent death (126–128). In support of this correlate, other studies have shown that modifications in plant/work environments have been associated with appreciable reductions in the overall increased risk from Cr-related lung cancer, primarily bronchogenic carcinomas (127,129).

**TABLE 1.** *Epidemiologic studies of chromium-induced cancers*[a]

| Exposed group | Site of cancer formation |
|---|---|
| Chromate-producing industries | |
| United States | Respiratory system, digestive system, oral cavity |
| United Kingdom | Lungs, nasal cavity |
| Germany | Lungs, stomach |
| Japan | Respiratory system, stomach |
| France | Lungs, stomach, brain, leukemia |
| Italy | Lungs, larynx, pleura |
| Chromate pigment ($ZnCrO_4$ and/or $PbCrO_4$) production | |
| Norway | Lungs, digestive system, nasal cavity |
| United Kingdom | Lungs |
| France | Lungs |
| Germany and Holland | Lungs |
| United States | Lungs, stomach, pancreas |
| Chrome plating industries | |
| United Kingdom | Lungs, nasal cavity, stomach, genitals |
| Japan | Lungs |
| United States | |
| Diecasting and Ni/Cr plant | Lungs |
| Electroplaters | Lungs, brain, Hodgkin's lymphoma |
| Italy (hard and bright) | Lungs, nasal cavity |
| Ferrochromium industries | |
| Soviet Union | Lungs, esophagus |
| Sweden | Lungs |
| France | Lungs, stomach, prostate, brain |
| Norway—ferrochromium/ferrosilicon plant | Lungs, kidney, prostate/stomach, kidney |
| Incidental Cr exposure | |
| Japanese workers handling Cr | Lungs |
| United States | |
| Aircraft production: spray painting/electroplating | Respiratory system |
| Ni/Cr foundries | Lungs |
| Icelandic masons | Respiratory system |
| Nordic hospital-based case control study | Nasal and paranasal sinuses |
| Canadian gold miners | Stomach |
| West German welders | Bladder, brain, genitals, thyroid, esophagus |
| Italian tannery workers | Bladder, lungs, pancreas, kidney, leukemia/lymphoma |
| Environmental exposure | |
| Swedish FeCr smelters | Lungs |
| New Jersey chromite ore sites | Lungs |
| German Ruhr district | Lungs |
| Massachusetts contaminated groundwater | Leukemia |

[a]See refs. 92 and 93 for specific reference(s) to each reported exposure group.

A greater frequency of cancers of the upper respiratory tract and oral cavity has also been reported in chromate-producing industry employees. The cancer most often involves the buccal cavity, pharynx, and esophagus. An analysis of the occurrence of nasal and sinonasal cancers with respect to various occupational exposures has shown a positive association between these cancers and exposure to Cr in welding and soldering iron fumes, Cr contaminants in hardwood, mixed wood, and softwood dusts, as well as to Cr during primary Cr production, Cr pigment production, and in chrome alloy plating (127,130,131).

Apart from cancers other than those of the lungs and sinonasal cavity, as well as the gastrointestinal tract (126,132), until recently no consistent pattern of cancer risk at other organ sites has been demonstrated in workers exposed to Cr. However, in the past decade, epidemiologic studies have demonstrated a correlation between exposure to Cr(VI) agents and an increased incidence of cancers of the prostate, stomach, bladder, brain, pancreas, kidney, genitals, and white blood cells (Table 1).

Nonoccupational sources of Cr exposure include food, air, and water; however, the levels of metal are several orders of magnitude lower than those encountered in occupational situations. In epidemiologic studies examining the relationship between non–worker-environmental exposure to Cr and mortality from lung cancer and other diseases, no significant increases in either noncarcinogenic or carcinogenic health hazards were observed, regardless of acute or chronic exposure to Cr-tainted soils and water, nor from fumes emitted from nearby smelting plants (133–135).

## REFERENCES


1. Nriagu JO. Production and uses of chromium. In: Nriagu JO, Nieboer E, eds. *Chromium in the natural and human environments.* New York: John Wiley, 1988;81–103.
2. *National emissions inventory of sources and emissions of chromium.* GCA publication (PB) 230-34. Springfield, VA: U.S. National Technical Information Service, 1973.
3. Pacyna JM. Sources of air pollution. In: Pickett EE, ed. *Atmospheric pollution.* Washington, DC: Hemisphere, 1988;33–52.
4. Nriagu JO, Pacyna JM, Milford JB, Davidson CJ. Distribution and characteristic features of chromium in the atmosphere. In: Nriagu JO, Nieboer E, eds. *Chromium in the natural and human environments.* New York: John Wiley, 1988;125–172.
5. Department of Health, Education, and Welfare. *Criteria for a recommended standard:* occupational exposure to chromium (VI). DHEW publication (NIOSH) 75-129. Washington, DC: U.S. Government Printing Office, 1980.
6. Handa BK. Occurrence and distribution of chromium in natural waters of India. In: Nriagu JO, Nieboer E, eds. *Chromium in the natural and human environments.* New York: John Wiley, 1988;189–214.
7. Environmental Protection Agency. *National interim primary drinking water regulations.* EPA publication 570/9—76/003. Washington, DC: U.S. Government Printing Office, 1976.
8. *Guidelines for Canadian drinking water quality.* Ottawa: Canadian Government Printing Office, 1979.
9. DeFlora S, Wetterhahn KE. Mechanisms of chromium metabolism and genotoxicity. *Life Chem Rep* 1989;7:169–244.
10. Hunninghake GW, Gadek JE, Szapiel SV, et al. The human alveolar macrophage. *Methods Cell Biol* 1980;21A:95–101.
11. Petrilli FL, Rossi GA, Camoirano A, et al. Metabolic reduction of chromium by alveolar macrophages and its relationship to cigarette smoke. *J Clin Invest* 1986;77:1917–1924.
12. Gray SJ, Sterling K. Tagging of red cells and plasma proteins with radioactive chromium. *J Clin Invest* 1950;29:1604–1613.
13. Harris DC. Different metal-binding properties of the two sites of human transferrin. *Biochemistry* 1977;16:560–564.
14. Saner G. Chromium in nutrition and disease. In: Albanese AA, Kritchnevsky D, eds. *Current topics in nutrition and disease.* New York: Alan R. Liss, 1980;2:26–29.
15. Arslan P, Beltrame M, Tomasi A. Intracellular chromium reduction. *Biochim Biophys Acta* 1987;931:10–15.
16. Jennette KW. The role of metals in carcinogenesis: biochemistry and metabolism. *Environ Health Perspect* 1981;40:223–252.
17. Levis AG, Majone F. Cytoxic and clastogenic effects of soluble and insoluble compounds containing hexavalent and trivalent chromium. *Br J Cancer* 1981;44:219–236.
18. Elias Z, Schneider O, Aubry F, Daniere MC, Poirot O. Sister chromatid exchanges in Chinese hamster V79 cells treated with the trivalent chromium compound chromic chloride and chromic oxide. *Carcinogenesis* 1983;4:605–611.
19. Anderson O. Effects of coal combustion products and metal compounds on sister chromatid exchange (SCE) in a macrophage-like cell line. *Environ Health Perspect* 1983;47:239–253.
20. Jennette KW. Microsomal reduction of the carcinogen chromate produces chromium (V). *J Am Chem Soc* 1982;104:874–875.
21. Standeven AM, Wetterhahn KE. Chromium(VI) toxicity: uptake, reduction, and DNA damage. *J Am Coll Toxicol* 1989;8:1275–1283.
22. Connett PH, Wetterhahn KE. Metabolism of the carcinogen chromate by cellular constituents. *Structure Bond* 1983;54:93–124.
23. Wiegand HJ, Ottenwalder H, Bolt HM. The reduction of chromium(VI) to chromium(III) by glutathione: an intracellular redox pathway in the metabolism of the carcinogen chromate. *Toxicology* 1984;33:341–348.
24. Kawanishi S, Inoue S, Sano S. Mechanism of DNA cleavage induced by sodium chromate(VI) in the presence of hydrogen peroxide. *J Biol Chem* 1986;261:5952–5958.
25. Shi X, Dalal NS. On the hydroxyl radical formation in the reaction between hydrogen peroxide and biologically generated chromium(V) species. *Arch Biochem Biophys* 1990;277:342–350.
26. Garcia JD, Jennette KW. Electron transport cytochrome $P_{450}$ system is involved in the microsomal metabolism of the carcinogen chromate. *J Inorg Biochem* 1981;14:281–295.
27. Rossi SC, Gorman N, Wetterhahn KE. Mitochondrial reduction of the carcinogen chromate: formation of chromium(V). *Chem Res Toxicol* 1988;1:101–107.
28. Rossi SC, Wetterhahn KE. Chromium(V) is produced upon reduction of chromate by mitchondrial electron transport chain complexes. *Carcinogenesis* 1989;10:913–920.
29. Goodgame DML, Joy AM. Relatively long-lived chromium(V) species are produced by the action of glutathione on carcinogenic chromium(VI). *J Inorg Biochem* 1986;26:219–224.
30. Martin RB, Mariam YH. Interactions between metal ions and nucleic bases, nucleosides, and nucleotides in solution. In: Sigel H, ed. *Metal ions in biological systems.* New York: Marcel Dekker; 1979:8:57–124.
31. Wolf T, Kasemann R, Ottenwalder H. Molecular interaction of different chromium species with nucleotides and nucleic acids. *Carcinogenesis* 1989;10:655–659.
32. Cohen M, Latta D, Coogan T, Costa M. The reactions of metal with nucleic acids. In: Foulkes E, ed. *Biological effects of heavy metals.* Boca Raton, FL: CRC Press; 1990:19–75.
33. Tsapakos MJ, Wetterhahn KE. The interaction of chromium with nucleic acids. *Chem Biol Interact* 1983;46:265–277.
34. Tamino G, Peretta L, Levis AG. Effects of trivalent and hexavalent chromium on the physicochemical properties of mammalian cell nucleic acids and synthetic polynucleotides. *Chem Biol Interact* 1981; 36:309–319.
35. Snow ET, Xu LS. Effects of chromium(III) on DNA replication in vitro. *Biol Trace Elem Res* 1989;21:61–71.
36. Tkeshelashvilli LK, Shearman CW, Zakour RA, Koplitz RM, Loeb LA. Effects of arsenic, selenium, and chromium on the fidelity of DNA synthesis. *Cancer Res* 1980;40:2455–460.
37. Sirover MA, Loeb LA. Metal-induced infidelity during DNA synthesis. *Proc Natl Acad Sci USA* 1976;73:2331–2335.
38. Zakour RA, Kunkel TA, Loeb LA. Metal-induced infidelity of DNA synthesis. *Environ Health Perspect* 1981;40:197–206.
39. Beyersmann D, Koster A. On the role of trivalent chromium in chromium genotoxicity. *Toxicol Environ Chem* 1987;14:11–22.
40. Nishio A, Uyeki EM. Inhibition of DNA synthesis by chromium compounds. *J Toxicol Environ Health* 1985;15:237–244.
41. Uyeki EM, Nishio A. Antiproliferative and genotoxic effects of chromium on cultured mammalian cells. *J Toxicol Environ Health* 1983;11:227–235.
42. Bianchi V. Nucleotide pool unbalance induced in cultured cells by treatment with different chemicals. *Toxicology* 1982;25:13–18.
43. Levis AG, Bianchi V. Mutagenic and cytogenetic effects of chromium compounds. In: Langard S, ed. *Biological and environmental aspects of chromium.* Amsterdam: Elsevier, 1982;171–208.
44. Bianchi V, Debetto P, Zantedeschi A, Levis AG. Effects of hexavalent chromium on the adenylate pools of hamster fibroblasts. *Toxicology* 1982;25:19–30.
45. Bianchi V, Dal Toso R, Debetto P, et al. Mechanisms of chromium toxicity in mammalian cell cultures. *Toxicology* 1980;17:219–24.
46. Nakamuro K, Yoshikawa K, Sayato Y, Kurata H. Comparative studies of chromosomal aberration and mutagenicity of trivalent and hexavalent chromium. *Mutat Res* 1978;58:175–181.
47. Newbold RF, Amos J, Connell SR. The cytotoxic, mutagenic, and clastogenic effects of chromium-containing compounds on mammalian cells in culture. *Mutat Res* 1979;67:55–63.
48. Venitt S. Genetic toxicology of chromium and nickel compounds. In: Stern R, Berlin A, Jarvisalo J, Fletcher A, eds. *Health hazards and biological effects of welding fumes and gases.* Amsterdam: Elsevier, 1986;249–266.
49. Jakobsen K, Bakke O, Ostgaard K, White LR, Eik-Nes KB. Effects of potassium dichromate on the cell cycle of an established human cell line. *Toxicology* 1982;24:281–292.
50. Nijs M, Kirsch-Volders M. Induction of spindle inhibition and abnormal mitotic figures by Cr(II), Cr(III), and Cr(VI) ions. *Mutagenesis* 1986;1:247–252.
51. Sugiyama M, Patierno SR, Cantoni O, Costa M. Characterization of DNA lesions induced by calcium chromate in synchronous and asynchronous cultured mammalian cells. *Mol Pharmacol* 1987;29:606–613.
52. Sen P, Conway K, Costa M. Comparison of the localization of chromosome damage induced by calcium chromate and nickel compounds. *Cancer Res* 1987;47:2142–2147.
53. Kortenkamp A, Ozolins Z, Beyersman D, O'Brien P. Generation of PM2 DNA breaks in the course of reduction of chromium(VI) by glutathione. *Mutat Res* 1989;216:19–26.

54. Goodgame DML, Hayman PB, Hathway DE. Carcinogenic chromium(VI) forms chromium(V) with ribonucleotides but not with deoxyribonucleotides. *Polyhedron* 1982;1:497–499.
55. Cupo DY, Wetterhahn KE. Binding of chromium to chromatin and DNA from liver and kidney of rats treated with sodium dichromate and chromium chloride in vivo. *Cancer Res* 1985;45:1146–1151.
56. Fornace AJ, Seres DJ, Lechner JF, Harris CC. DNA-protein cross-linking by chromium salts. *Chem Biol Interact* 1981;36:345–354.
57. Miller CA, Costa M. Characterization of DNA-protein complexes induced in intact cells by the carcinogen chromate. *Mol Carcinogen* 1988;1:125–133.
58. Tsapakos MJ, Hampton TH, Wetterhahn-Jenette K. The carcinogen chromate induces DNA cross-links in rat liver and kidney. *J Biol Chem* 1981;256:3623–3626.
59. Wedrychowski A, Schmidt WN, Hnilica LS. DNA-protein cross-linking by heavy metals in Novikoff hepatoma. *Arch Biochem Biophys* 1986;251:397–402.
60. Cohen MD, Miller CA, Xu LS, Snow ET, Costa M. A blotting method for monitoring the formation of chemically induced DNA-protein complexes. *Anal Biochem* 1990;186:1–7.
61. Wedrychowski A, Ward SW, Schmidt WN, Hnilica LS. Chromium-induced cross-linking of nuclear proteins and DNA. *J Biol Chem* 1985;260:7150–7155.
62. Venitt S, Levy LS. Mutagenicity of chromates in bacteria and relevance to chromate carcinogenesis. *Nature* 1974;250:493–495.
63. Kanematsu N, Hara M, Kada T. Rec assay and mutagenicity studies on metal compounds. *Mutat Res* 1980;77:109–116.
64. Langerwerf JS, Bakkeren HA, Jongen WM. A comparison of the mutagenicity of soluble trivalent chromium compounds with that of potassium chromate. *Ecotoxicol Environ Safety* 1985;9:92–100.
65. Rainaldi G, Colella CM, Piras A, Mariani T. Thioguanine resistance, ouabain resistance, and sister chromatid exchanges in V79/AP4 Chinese hamster cells treated with potassium dichromate. *Chem Biol Interact* 1982;42:45–51.
66. Knudsen I. The mammalian spot test and its use for the testing of potential carcinogenicity of welding fume particles. *Acta Pharmacol Toxicol* 1980;47:66–70.
67. Polak L, Turk JL, Frey JR. Studies on contact hypersensitivity to chromium compounds. *Prog Allergy* 1973;17:145–226.
68. Polak L. Immunology of chromium. In: Burrows D, ed. *Chromium metabolism and toxicity.* Boca Raton, FL: CRC Press, 1983;51–136.
69. Van Everdingen JE, Van Joost T. Hypersensitivity for nickel, chromium and cobalt; a continuous problem. *Ned T Geneesk* 1982;126: 1088–1092.
70. Vreeburg KJ, De Groot K, Von Blomberg BM, Scheper RJ. Induction of immunological tolerance by oral administration of nickel and chromium. *J Dent Res* 1984;63:124–128.
71. Spruit D, van Neer FC. Penetration rate of Cr(III) and Cr(VI). *Dermatologica* 1966;132:179–182.
72. Rytter M, Haustein UF. Hapten conjugation in the leukocyte migration inhibition test in allergic contact eczema. *Br J Dermatol* 1982; 106:161–168.
73. Janeckova V, Znojemska S, Korcakova L, Wagnerova M, Kalensky J, Svobodova J. The immune profile of contact allergy patients. *J Hyg Epidemiol Microbiol Immunol* 1989;33:121–127.
74. Al-Tawil NG, Marcusson JA, Moller E. HLA-class II restriction of the proliferative T-lymphocyte responses to nickel, cobalt, and chromium compounds. *Tissue Antigens* 1985;25:163–172.
75. Picardo M, Santucci B, Pastore R, Valesini G, Verducchi D, Bravi D. Immune complexes in patients with contact dermatitis. *Dermatologica* 1986;172:52–53.
76. Johansson A, Wiernik A, Jarstrand J, Camner P. Rabbit alveolar macrophages after inhalation of hexa- and trivalent chromium. *Environ Res* 1986;39:372–385.
77. Johansson A, Robertson B, Curstedt C, Camner P. Alveolar macrophage abnormalities in rabbits exposed to low concentrations of trivalent chromium. *Environ Res* 1987;44:279–293.
78. Galvin JB, Oberg SG. Toxicity of hexavalent chromium to the alveolar macrophage in vivo and in vitro. *Environ Res* 1984;33:7–16.
79. Glaser U, Hochrainer D, Kloppel H, Kuhnen H. Low level chromium(VI) inhalation effects on alveolar macrophages and immune functions in Wistar rats. *Arch Toxicol* 1985;57:250–256.
80. Elias Z, Mur JM, Pierre F, et al. Chromosome aberrations in peripheral blood lymphocytes of welders and characterization of their exposure by biological sample analysis. *J Occup Med* 1989;31:477–482.
81. Gao M, Binks SP, Chipman JK, Levy LS, Braithwaite RA, Brown SS. Induction of DNA strand breaks in peripheral lymphocytes by soluble chromium compounds. *Hum Exp Toxicol* 1992;11:77–82.
82. Coogan TP, Motz J, Snyder CA, Squibb KS, Costa M. Differential DNA-protein crosslinking in lymphocytes and liver following chronic drinking water exposure of rats to potassium chromate. *Toxicol Appl Pharmacol* 1991;109:60–72.
83. Toniolo P, Zhitkovich A, Costa M. Development and utilization of a new simple assay for DNA-protein crosslinks as a biomarker of exposure to welding fumes. *Int Arch Occup Environ Health* 1993; 65(suppl 1):S87–89.
84. Borella P, Manni S, Giardino A. Cadmium, nickel, chromium, and lead accumulate in human lymphocytes and interfere with PHA-induced proliferation. *J Trace Elem Electrolytes Health Dis* 1990; 4:87–95.
85. Kucharz EJ, Sierakowski SJ. Immunotoxicity of chromium compounds: effect of sodium dichromate on the T-cell activation in vitro. *Arh Hig Rada Toksikol* 1987;38:239–243.
86. Snyder CA. Immune function assays as indicators of chromate exposure. *Environ Health Perspect* 1991;92:83–86.
87. Figoni RA, Treagan L. Inhibitory effect of nickel and chromium upon antibody response of rats to immunization with T-1 phage. *Res Commun Chem Pathol Pharmacol* 1975;11:335–338.
88. Hahon N, Booth JA. Effect of chromium and manganese particles on the interferon system. *J Interferon Res* 1984;4:17–27.
89. Christensen MM, Ernst E, Ellerman-Eriksen S. Cytotoxic effects of hexavalent chromium in cultured mouse macrophages. *Arch Toxicol* 1992;66:347–353.
90. Treagan L. Metals and the immune response, a review. *Res Commun Chem Pathol Pharmacol* 1975;12:189–214.
91. Yassi A, Nieboer E. Carcinogenicity of chromium compounds. In: Nriagu JO, Nieboer E, eds. *Chromium in the natural and human environments.* New York: John Wiley, 1988;443–495.
92. Cohen, MD, Kargacin, B, Klein, CB, Costa, M. Mechanisms of chromium carcinogenicity and toxicity. *CRC Crit Rev Toxicol* 1993; 23:255–281.
93. Costa, M. Toxicity and carcinogenicity of Cr(VI) in animal models and humans. *CRC Crit Rev Toxicol* 1997;27:431–442.
94. Hayes RB. Cancer and occupational exposure to chromium chemicals. *Rev Cancer Epidemiol* 1980;1:293–333.
95. Chromium and Inorganic Chromium Compounds. *IARC Monogr Eval Carcinog Risk Chem Man* 1973;2:100–125.
96. World Health Organization. *IARC monographs on the evaluation of the carcinogenic risk of chemicals to humans:* some metals and metallic compounds. *Chromium and chromium compounds,* vol 23. Lyon, France: International Agency for Research on Cancer, 1980;205–323.
97. World Health Organization. *IARC monographs on the evaluation of the carcinogenic risk of chemicals to humans:* chromium, *nickel, and welding,* vol 49. Lyon, France: International Agency for Research on Cancer, 1990;49–256.
98. Norseth T. The carcinogenicity of chromium. *Environ Health Perspect* 1981;40:121–130.
99. Sunderman FW. Recent advances in metal carcinogenesis. *Ann Clin Lab Sci* 1984;14:93–122.
100. Agency for Toxic Substances and Diseases. *Toxicological profile for chromium.* Atlanta: Agency for Toxic Substances and Diseases, 1991.
101. *Chromium, environmental health criteria,* no. 61. Geneva: World Health Organization, 1988.
102. Leonard A, Lauwerys RR. Carcinogenicity and mutagenicity of chromium. *Mutat Res* 1980;76:227–239.
103. Payne WW. Production of cancers in mice and rats by chromium compounds. *Arch Ind Health* 1960;21:530–535.
104. Hueper WC, Payne WW. Experimental cancers in rats produced by chromium compounds and their significance to industry and public health. *Arch Environ Health* 1962;5:445–462.
105. Hueper WC. Experimental studies in metal carcinogenesis; VII. Tissue reactions to parenterally introduced powdered metallic chromium and chromite ore. *J Natl Cancer Inst* 1955;16:447–469.
106. Schroeder HA, Balassa JJ, Vinton WH. Chromium, lead, cadmium, nickel, and titanium in mice: effect on mortality, tumors, and tissue levels. *J Nutr* 1964;83:239–250.

107. Schroeder HA. Balassa JJ, Vinton WH. Chromium, cadmium, and lead in rats: effects on lifespan, tumors, and tissue levels. *J Nutr* 1965; 86:51–66.
108. Levy LS, Venitt S. Carcinogenicity and mutagenicity of chromium compounds: the association between bronchial metaplasia and neoplasia. *Carcinogenesis* 1986;7:831–835.
109. Levy LS, Martin PA, Bidstrup PL. Investigation of the potential carcinogenicity of a range of chromium-containing materials on rat lung. *Br J Ind Med* 1986;43:243–256.
110. Glaser U, Hochrainer D, Kloppel H, Oldiges H. Carcinogenicity of sodium dichromate and chromium(VI/III) oxide aerosols inhaled by male Wistar rats. *Toxicology* 1986;42:219–232.
111. Nettesheim P, Hanna MG, Doherty DG, Newell RF, Hellman A. Effect of calcium chromate dust, influenza virus, and 100 R whole-body X-irradiation on lung tumor incidence in mice. *J Natl Cancer Inst* 1971;47:1129–1144.
112. Steffe CH, Baetjer AM. Histopathologic effects of chromate chemicals. Report of studies in rabbits, guinea pigs, rats, and mice. *Arch Environ Health* 1965;11:66–75.
113. Shimkin MB, Stoner GD, Theiss JC. Lung tumor response in mice to metals and metal salts. *Adv Exp Med Biol* 1977;91:85–91.
114. Sunderman FW. A review of the carcinogenicities of nickel, chromium, and arsenic compounds in man and animals. *Prev Med* 1976;5:279–294.
115. Maltoni C, Morisi L, Chieco P. Experimental approach to the assessment of the carcinogenic risk of industrial inorganic pigments. *Adv Mod Environ Toxicol* 1982;2:77–92.
116. Furst A, Schlauder M, Sasmore DP. Tumorigenic activity of lead chromate. *Cancer Res* 1976;36:1779–1783.
117. Roe FJ, Carter RL. Chromium carcinogenesis: calcium chromate as a potent carcinogen for the subcutaneous tissues of the rat. *Br J Cancer* 1969;23:172–176.
118. Adachi S, Yoshimura H, Katayama H, Takemoto K. Effects of chromic acid mist in electroplating to ICR female mice. *Jpn J Ind Health* 1986;28:283–287.
119. Adachi S. Effects of chromium compounds on the respiratory system. Part 5. Long-term inhalation of chromic acid mist in electroplating by C57Bl6 female mice and recapitulation on our experimental studies. *Jpn J Ind Health* 1987;29:17–33, 1987.
120. Baetjer AM, Lowney JF, Steffee H, Budacz V. Effect of chromium on incidence of lung tumors in mice and rats. *Arch Ind Health* 1959;20: 124–135.
121. Laskin S, Kuschner M, Drew RT. Studies in pulmonary carcinogenesis. In: Hanna, MG, Nettesheim P, Gilbert RJ, eds. *Inhalation carcinogenesis.* US Atomic Energy Commission Symposium Series No. 18. Oak Ridge, TN: U.S. Atomic Energy Commission Division of Technical Information Extension, 1970;21–351.
122. Berg NO, Berlin M, Bohgard M, Rudell B, Schutz A, Warvinge K. Bronchocarcinogenic properties of welding and thermal spraying fumes containing chromium in the rat. *Am J Ind Med* 1987;11:39–54.
123. Tsuneta Y, Mikami H, Kimura K, Abe S, Osaki Y, Murao M, The concentration of chromium in the tissues of the respiratory tract among chromate workers with lung cancer. *Haigan* 1978;18:341–348.
124. Turhan U, Hain C, Wollburg C, Szadkowski D. Chromium and nickel content of human lungs -occupational medical aspects. In: Stalder K, ed. *Verhandlungen der Deutschen Gesellschaft fur Arbeitsmedizin.* Stuttgart: Gentner Verlag, 1983;477–480.
125. Abe S, Osaki Y, Kimura K, Tsuneta Y, Mikami H, Murao M. Chromate lung cancer with special reference to its cell type and relation to the manufacturing process. *Cancer* 1982;49:783–787.
126. Taylor FH. The relationship of mortality and duration of employment as reflected by a cohort of chromate workers. *Am J Public Health* 1966;56:218–229.
127. Alderson MR, Rattan NS, Bidstrup L. Health of workmen in the chromate-producing industry in Britain. *Br J Ind Med* 1981;38:117–124.
128. Hayes RB, Sheffet A, Spirtas R. Cancer mortality among a cohort of chromium pigment workers. *Am J Ind Med* 1989;16:127–133.
129. Hill WH, Ferguson WS. Statistical analysis of epidemiological data from a chromium chemical manufacturing plant. *J Occup Med* 1979; 21:103–106.
130. Långard S, Norseth T. A cohort study of bronchial carcinomas in workers producing chromate pigments. *Br J Ind Med* 1975;32:62–65.
131. Hernberg S, Westerholm P, Schultz-Larsen K. et al. Nasal and sinonasal cancer. Connection with occupational exposures in Denmark, Finland, and Sweden. *Scand J Work Environ Health* 1983;9:315–326.
132. Långard S, Norseth T. Cancer in the gastrointestinal tract in chromate pigment workers. *Arch Hyg Rada Toksikol* 1979;30:301–304.
133. Axellson G, Rylander R. Environmental chromium dust and lung cancer mortality. *Environ Res* 1980;23:469–476.
134. Paustenbach DJ, Meyer DM, Sheehan PJ, Lau V. An assessment and quantitative uncertainty analysis of the health risks to workers exposed to chromium-contaminated soils. *Toxicol Ind Health* 1991;7: 159–196.
135. Sheehan PJ, Meyer DM, Sauer MM, Paustenbach DJ. Assessment of the human health risks posed by exposure to chromium-contaminated soils. *J Toxicol Environ Health* 1991;32:161–201.

*Environmental and Occupational Medicine, Third Edition*, edited by William N. Rom.
Lippincott–Raven Publishers, Philadelphia © 1998.

CHAPTER 75

# Nickel Toxicity and Carcinogenesis

Elizabeth T. Snow and Max Costa

## USES AND EXPOSURE

Nickel is a commonly used, silvery white, magnetic metal that occurs naturally in the earth's crust. Alloys and compounds of nickel can provoke adverse health effects, including allergic reactions and cancer of the lungs, oral cavity, and larynx. Nickel and its compounds can be detected in all parts of the environment. Metallic nickel and nickel compounds for industrial uses come from mined ores and via recycling of nickel in scrap metal. Nickel and its compounds are used in steels and other alloys, electroplating, ceramics, permanent magnets, batteries, and fuel cells. Nickel compounds are used in chemical production, and powdered (Raney) nickel is used as a catalyst, especially in food production. Table 1 lists common uses for nickel and its compounds and jobs associated with potential exposure. Nickel-containing waste products are disposed of by landspreading, landfilling, incineration, and ocean dumping.

Nickel carbonyl, $Ni(CO)_4$, is lipid soluble and can readily cross biologic membranes without decomposing. It is the most toxic form of nickel, but because of its short half-life and limited use it is not an environmental contaminant. Nickel carbonyl is extremely reactive and produces acute effects different from those of other nickel compounds. The toxicology of this compound has recently been reviewed by Shi (1). Nickel carbonyl is produced by reacting elemental nickel with carbon monoxide and forms the basis of the Mond process for refining nickel. It has a half-life of 100 seconds and when heated decomposes to produce finely divided nickel powder, which may be used in "gas plating" of objects with nickel. Nickel carbonyl is routinely used in only two places in the Western world (2).

The general population is exposed to nickel in many forms: in the air, in food and drinking water, and in many consumer products. An in-depth overview of nickel exposure and toxicology is provided in a recent volume edited by Nieboer and Nriagu (3). Nickel allergy in the form of contact dermatitis is the most common adverse effect arising from nickel exposure (4,5), and 2% to 11% of the population may be sensitive to nickel, with females exhibiting more prevalent sensitivity than males (4). Segments of the population exposed to higher levels of nickel that are more likely to experience adverse affects include people whose diet contains foods naturally rich in nickel (e.g., urease-rich plants, cocoa, nuts), those who work at or live in the vicinity of nickel-processing facilities or those who are exposed occupationally to nickel, and those who smoke tobacco. It is estimated that approximately 2% of the work force in the nickel-producing and -using industries may be exposed to airborne nickel at concentrations at or near levels of 0.1 to 1 mg/m$^3$. The National Institute of Occupational Safety and Health (NIOSH) has estimated that 250,000 workers in the United States may be occupationally exposed to nickel and its compounds.

## EPIDEMIOLOGY

Costa (6) has recently reviewed the metabolism and toxicology of nickel and nickel compounds, and Coogan et al. (7) have reviewed nickel epidemiology and toxicology in a more extensive fashion. Nickel is an essential nutrient in animals, and nickel deficiency produces specific symptoms (8). Nickel-containing proteins and

E. T. Snow: Department of Environmental Medicine, New York University Medical Center, Tuxedo, New York 10987.
M. Costa: Department of Environmental Medicine; and Department of Pharmacology, New York University Medical Center, New York, New York 10016.

**TABLE 1.** *Common uses and exposure to nickel and its compounds*

| Substance | Uses/sources | Jobs | Possible health problems |
|---|---|---|---|
| Nickel metals and alloys | | | |
| Nickel ores and raw compounds | Nickel refineries and production plants | Refinery workers, production workers | Nasal and lung cancer, contact dermatitis, allergies |
| Powdered nickel | Chemical catalyst | Oil hydrogenators, chemical workers | Immunosuppression, nasal toxicity |
| Stainless steel (also contains chromium) | Construction, machine parts, household items | Welders, steel workers, bench mechanics, home makers, shipfitters | Contact dermatitis, allergies, asthma |
| Other alloys | Coins, magnets, spark plugs, household, surgical utensils appliances | Magnet makers, production workers, medical workers and patients | Contact dermatitis, allergies, asthma, implant-associated lymphomas |
| Nickel compounds | | | |
| Crystalline nickel subsulfide, nickel oxide | Nickel refineries | Refinery workers | Nasal and lung cancer |
| Nickel sulfate | Electroplating | Production workers | Dermatitis, nasal cancer, allergies |
| Nickel hydroxide | Nickel-cadmium batteries | Production workers | Dermatitis, allergies |
| Nickel carbonate | Electronic components | Production workers | Dermatitis, allergies |
| Nickel carbonyl | Gas plating, Mond process nickel refining | Production workers | Pulmonary insufficiency, immune dysfunction, kidney damage |
| Other/complex sources | Waste incineration, gasoline, diesel fuel, tobacco, paints | Waste handlers, fuel handlers, smokers, painters | Allergies, immune dysfunction, dermatitis |

enzymes have been identified in both plants and bacteria (9), but it has never been proven essential to humans. Dietary nickel provides 83% to 94% of the total body burden of nickel in the general population, and most of the daily intake by this route is excreted in the feces, with a small amount (approximately 1% to 5%) of absorption and subsequent excretion in urine. A small amount of absorbed nickel is also deposited in the hair, and normal persons excrete significant amounts of nickel in their sweat; however, most absorbed nickel, regardless of the route of exposure, is excreted in the urine.

## SYSTEMIC TOXICITY

Nickel-induced toxicity depends on the route of exposure and the solubility of the nickel compound. The major route of toxic nickel exposure is via pulmonary absorption. Gastrointestinal and dermal absorption of nickel compounds is significantly less important, although dermal exposure can lead to nickel sensitivity and contact dermatitis. Iatrogenic exposure can also occur due to surgical or dental implants and hemodialysis (4,10). Soluble nickel ions can be absorbed directly and insoluble or relatively insoluble nickel compounds can be phagocytosed (11). Phagocytosis of relatively insoluble nickel compounds such as $Ni_3S_2$ and NiO may play an important role in the pulmonary toxicity and carcinogenicity of nickel.

Kidney and lung are the primary organs for the accumulation of nickel. Absorbed nickel can also be measured in the blood, where it is mostly protein bound. Occupational and therapeutic exposure to a variety of compounds can alter the distribution of lipophilic nickel compounds such as $Ni(CO)_4$ (nickel carbonyl) (12). A number of chelating agents have been assessed for their ability to prevent the systemic toxicity associated with nickel exposure (13,14), including diethyldithiocarbamate (DDC), a metabolite of disulfiram (Antabuse). Although DDC is the agent of choice for acute nickel carbonyl poisoning, it should be noted that while the drug decreased the amount of nickel in the heart and lungs of $Ni(CO)_4$-treated rats and mice, it greatly increased the amount of nickel retained in the brain, suggesting the cautious use of DDC in patients with increased risk of nickel exposure, as well as the cautious use of complexing agents and chelators in acute nickel toxicity (15,16). It has been suggested that d-penicillamine be considered as an alternative chelating agent (17).

Nickel has both embryotoxic and teratogenic effects in animals. It can directly affect the developing embryo or fetus and indirectly alters the maternal hormone balance by inducing hyperglycemia (18–20). Maternal exposure can result in decreased implantation frequency, increased early and late resorption, and increased frequency of stillborn fetuses (19). Exposure to nickel during organogenesis can also result in a variety of teratogenic effects, such as exencephaly, eye malformations, and skeletal abnormalities (19,21,22). Although nickel crosses the human placenta and relatively high levels of nickel have been found in human fetuses, neonates, and stillbirths (21), nickel teratotoxicity in humans has not been established.

Nickel is hepatotoxic in animals and has been shown to effect renal function in humans. It binds to the anionic glycosaminoglycan sites of the glomerular basement membrane (23,24). Ionic blocking of these sites leads to the loss of selectivity in the filtration of albumin (23) and may explain the proteinuria associated with nickel exposure.

Low concentrations of exogenous nickel chloride have been shown to induce coronary vasoconstriction in isolated perfused rat hearts (25) and to alter the sodium conductance. Hypernickelemia has been reported in patients with acute stroke, myocardial infarction, unstable angina pectoris (26), and following extensive burn injuries, and it may be the cause of coronary vasoconstriction and myocardial injury associated with burn shock (27). Nickel contamination of intravenous fluids may also be a potential source of toxic exposure to nickel and the increase in coronary artery resistance associated with nickel may be hazardous to patients with acute myocardial infarction (28).

Inhalation is the major route of exposure to nickel compounds. Although the carcinogenic effects of nickel exposure are of most concern, other pulmonary lesions, including epithelial dysplasia and hyperplastic or polypoid rhinitis (2,29), have been described. Evidence for nickel-induced cancer of the lungs and nasal passages among exposed workers in the nickel refinery and processing industries is well documented (21). Inhalation exposure is also associated with asthma and increased susceptibility to pulmonary infections, as well as serious nasal injury such as septal perforation, chronic rhinitis, sinusitis, and anosmia (loss of the ability to smell). A number of different industrial processes have been associated with nickel carcinogenesis, especially nickel matte refining and electrolytic refining. Both occupations are associated with increased risks of nasal sinus cancer and lung cancer as well as lesser but still significant risks of laryngeal, prostate, and kidney cancer (30,31). Although changes in procedure since 1924, especially the use of gauze masks and respirators, have dramatically reduced the cancer incidence in nickel industry workers, nickel matte refining had been associated with exposure to high concentrations of dusts of nickel subsulfide and nickel oxide as well as other nickel compounds and electrolytic workers were exposed to aerosols of nickel sulfate and nickel chloride. Even after exposure to nickel dusts is discontinued, risk for nickel-induced lung and nasal cancer persists (32,33). Although it is difficult to assess exposure to specific nickel compounds in a nickel refinery, workers with high exposure to soluble nickel salts have demonstrated elevation in nasal and lung cancers (32,33). Exposure to insoluble nickel compounds cannot be ruled out. However, nasal cancers are rare and standardized mortality ratio (SMR) values show a 50-fold increase in exposed populations relative to controls.

The effect of nickel exposure on the immune system is twofold. Nickel exposure can elicit an immune response resulting in contact dermatitis or asthma (5). It is also immunotoxic, altering both the T-cell–mediated immune response and natural killer (NK) cell activity (34–37). Nickel is one of the most common causes of allergic contact dermatitis, and this type of contact dermatitis is particularly common among women (4,5,38). Nonoccupational exposure to nickel resulting in contact dermatitis has occurred from jewelry, white gold, metal clothing fasteners, wristwatches, and dental prostheses (4,5). Allergy to nickel in dental prostheses has resulted in stomatitis (39), indicating a need to determine nickel sensitivity before an alloy is used. Nickel-induced contact dermatitis represents a cellular hypersensitivity response involving antigen recognition by lymphocytes and macrophage-like cells (37,40). In addition to contact dermatitis, occupational asthma has been reported in nickel-sensitive workers (2,41). There is evidence that an immunoglobulin E (IgE) type I immunopathogenic mechanism is involved in this response.

Nickel, especially carcinogenic $Ni_3S_2$, also elicits a strong oxidative burst response in pulmonary macrophages. This response is similar to that caused by the tumor promoter phorbol 12-tetradecanoate 13-acetate (TPA) and may be an important component in both the toxicology and carcinogenesis of nickel compounds (42,43).

Nickel carbonyl is a potent toxin and produces immediate but nonspecific distress, such as coughing, dyspnea, tachycardia, cyanosis, headache, dizziness, and profound weakness (1). These symptoms may disappear after the patient is exposed to fresh air, but serious respiratory or adrenal, hepatic, and renal damage may develop hours or days later. Death may occur as the result of pneumonia, cerebral hemorrhage, or acute edema. Patients who recover from acute nickel carbonyl poisoning often develop chronic respiratory insufficiency. The severity of exposure to nickel carbonyl may be estimated from the nickel concentration in a spot urine sample collected shortly after exposure. A nickel concentration of 5 μg/dl is considered the upper boundary of normal; higher concentrations should be considered evidence of acute poisoning. Exposure to respirable nickel particulates has also been demonstrated to induce adult respiratory distress syndrome and can be fatal (44). Rapid treatment with DDC has been shown to be effective in preventing serious pneumonitis, but, as noted above, this compound is a metabolite of Antabuse, and caution should be taken to prevent complications due to concurrent alcohol consumption.

## PERMISSIBLE EXPOSURE LIMITS

The Occupational Safety and Health Administration (OSHA) permissible exposure limit for nickel and nickel compounds in the workplace (excluding nickel carbonyl) is an 8-hour time-weighted average ($TWA_8$) of 1 $mg/m^3$ (45). Comparable values from other countries range from

0.005 to 1 mg/m³. The permissible 40-hour TWA exposure for nickel carbonyl in the United States is 7 μg/m³.

## MEDICAL SURVEILLANCE

Biologic monitoring is currently available primarily in occupational settings. Nickel content can be determined in urine, serum, hair, and oral mucosa. Several methods are available for quantitation of nickel in tissue samples, the most common ones being flame or electrothermal atomic absorption spectrophotometry. Nickel is normally present in biologic samples at very low levels (0.3 to 1.1 μg/L in serum and 2.0 to 6.0 μg/L in urine) (46,47); however, dose-dependent increases in serum nickel levels have been observed after exposures to concentrations in excess of 10 μg/m³. A similar increase in urine nickel levels (with background levels in the range of 2.0 to 1.5 μg/g creatinine) (46–49) has also been observed.

## MECHANISMS OF TOXICITY AND CARCINOGENESIS

### Molecular Toxicology

The biologic and toxicologic impact of inorganic nickel in the body is believed to be due to the intracellular absorption of soluble nickel ($Ni^{2+}$), but the irritant effect of the intracellular particles cannot be ruled out. Studies of absorption of deposited particles have shown that the solubility of nickel compounds is the principal determinant of the rate and extent of absorption, distribution, and clearance of the metal. Once nickel compounds have entered the cell their transforming potential may depend only on the available concentration of the nickel ions and be independent of the original material (50,51). Insoluble nickel compounds such as $Ni_3S_2$, may be phagocytosed by various cell types (52,53). Crystalline structure, particle size, and negative surface charge are all factors in the phagocytic activity (52,54). Figure 1 is a cartoon illustrating the salient features believed to be important in nickel carcinogenesis. The ability of various nickel compounds to be taken up by cells is directly related to their ability to elevate cellular nickel levels. The phagocytosed crystalline NiS is accumulated in cytoplasmic vacuoles around the periphery of the nucleus, where they are gradually acidified and the nickel dissolved, releasing the $Ni^{2+}$ ions to the periphery of the nucleus, where they can preferentially interact with heterochromatic regions of the chromatin and DNA, forming DNA-protein complexes and, to a lesser extent, DNA strand breaks. Carcinogenesis may result from DNA or chromosome damage or from altered DNA replication due to the nickel ions, or it may result from nickel-induced alterations in DNA-protein interactions.

Recent data suggest that one of the primary effects of nickel is on DNA methylation and the structure of chromatin, often leading to the transcriptional inactivation of affected genes (52,55). The initial effect appears to be that of demethylation followed by hypermethylation and inactivation of DNA sequences adjacent to regions of constitutive heterochromatin. This can lead to the transcriptional inactivation of critical tumor suppressor or senescence genes (55, 56). Figure 2 is a cartoon illustrating how nickel-induced chromatin condensation can cause de novo DNA methylation and subsequent inactivation of tumor suppressor genes. Nickel may also induce oxidative damage to DNA by redox cycling promoted by interaction with protein histidine residues (52,57–59). Oxidation of heterochromatic regions of chromatin predominates, presumably due to the preferential binding of nickel to the nuclear matrix (43).

Exposure to water-soluble salts of nickel is characterized by rapid excretion of nickel (with a half-life of

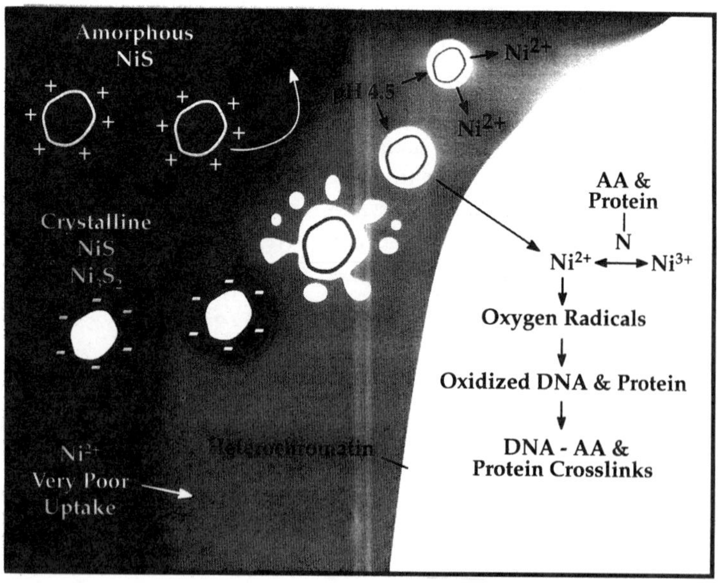


**FIG. 1.** Illustration of the selective phagocytosis and cytoplasmic dissolution of $Ni^{2+}$ ions adjacent to the nucleus and reactive upon entry into the nucleus.

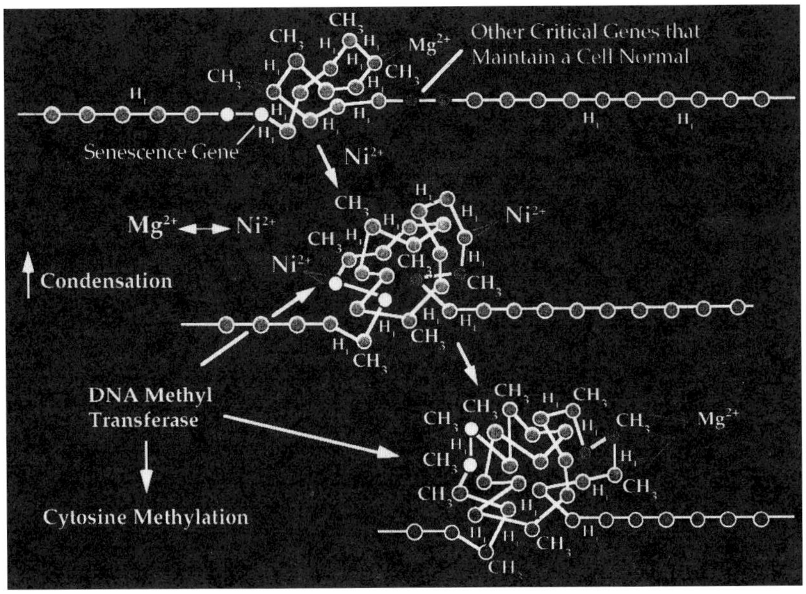


**FIG. 2.** Gene silencing model in which nickel-induced increases in heterochromatin condensation and hypermethylation of DNA may cause inherited inactivation of critical tumor suppressor or senescence genes. Cancer-relevant genes, such as tumor suppressors *(black squares)* and senescence genes *(black triangles)* may become incorporated into heterochromatin that is seeded by nickel-induced DNA condensation *(middle panel)* and stabilized by subsequent DNA methylation *(bottom panel).*

approximately 1 day) compared to exposure to solid intermediates such as nickel oxides and sulfides (with an estimated biologic half-life of up to 3 years). Soluble nickel particles deposited in the alveoli may be cleared rapidly, whereas crystalline nickel solids are less susceptible to inactivation and clearance (60). The availability of Ni to tissues and the biologic consequences of intracellular accumulation are much greater for insoluble crystalline compounds than for amorphous nickel solids.

The toxicity of nickel may be associated with its interactions with other essential metal cations. Many of the toxic and carcinogenic effects of nickel can be antagonized by magnesium ions. Much of the known toxicity of nickel may be rationalized by its interference with normal and physiologic roles, principally of magnesium, but also zinc, calcium, and manganese (61). Interactions with various other cations may potentiate or alleviate various symptoms of nickel toxicity.

### Carcinogenesis

Nickel compounds such as $Ni_3S_2$, crystalline NiS, and Ni(CO) are highly carcinogenic for rats and mice (62,63). Inhalation exposure to $Ni_3S_2$ in rats causes hyperplasia, metaplasia, adenomas, and adenocarcinomas equally in males and females. These preneoplastic changes and tumors were noted in both bronchiolar and alveolar regions. Nickel salts are not tumorigenic following ingestion; however, intramuscular injection of particulate nickel compounds induced tumors at the site of injection. Nickel is targeted to the lung not only by direct inhalation exposure but also by parenteral injection of soluble $NiCl_2$ (64). With daily injections of $NiCl_2$ into male Fischer rats, the lungs are the primary target and toxicity is severe, including hyperplasia, cellular atypia, and frequent mitoses. The resulting lesions mimic exposure by inhalation or intratracheal instillation of nickel. Water-soluble nickel compounds such as $NiCl_2$ and $NiSO_4$ were not carcinogenic in experimental animals regardless of the mode of administration. However, exposure to soluble nickel compounds has recently been associated with increased risk for human cancer, although it is difficult in such epidemiologic studies to ascertain that the people were not also exposed to water-insoluble nickel compounds as well (i.e., $Ni_3S_2$) (65,66). Tumorigenesis correlates strongly with the production of erythropoiesis by particulate nickel compounds and with phagocytic index and nickel mass fraction of the compound (67).

Both soluble and particulate forms of nickel promote morphologic cell transformation *in vitro* (67,68). Morphologic transformation of Syrian hamster embryo cells by nickel compounds depends on the uptake and long-term sequestering of these compounds in phagocytic vacuoles and the subsequent slow release of the active $Ni^{2+}$ ions inside the cell (see Fig. 1) (69).

In contrast to their carcinogenic potential, nickel compounds are only weakly mutagenic *in vitro* (70–73). Nickel is usually toxic but not mutagenic in prokaryotic assays; however, a number of studies indicate that some nickel salts may be positive in some mammalian assays (71,72). Inactivation of a bacterial gene *(gpt)* that is stably integrated into the G12 *hprt⁻* V79 cell line is strongly promoted by insoluble nickel salts such as $Ni_3S_2$. Analysis of the *gpt⁻* colonies induced by nickel shows that transcription of the *gpt* gene is inactivated by hypermethylation of the gene (55). Nickel salts have since been shown to cause the transcriptional inactivation of other cellular genes (52,57). This is now believed to be a critical process by which nickel induces cellular transformation and carcinogenesis (74).

The production of chromosome aberrations by nickel compounds has also been studied (52,75–77). Nickel is both mitostatic and clastogenic. Sister-chromatid exchange (SCE) is usually seen at doses below those that cause chromosome aberrations. Nickel salts have been shown to produce chromosome aberrations in mammalian cells both *in vivo* and *in vitro*. Nickel, together with a second agent, often gives a cooperative or synergistic response, although the metal ion by itself may be negative (78). This has also been observed in bacterial mutagenesis assays (79). Synergistic enhancement of cell transformation of Syrian hamster cells was seen with combined treatments of $NiSO_4$ and benzo[*a*]pyrene (80). These effects may be due to nickel-induced inhibition of DNA replication (81–84) or processing of DNA lesions (85–91). Combined exposure to nickel plus other metal salts can also lead to a less than additive induction of SCEs, suggesting that chromosomal damage may be poor measure of exposure in industrial settings where exposures to complex mixtures predominate (92).

Nickel preferentially damages heterochromatic regions of chromatin (6,77,93,94), and transformation of Chinese hamster embryo cells is often accompanied by inactivation of a senescence gene on the X chromosome (i.e., short arm) by DNA methylation in the transformed cells (56). $Ni^{2+}$ targets the X chromosome since it has a high concentration of heterochromatin and deletions of the heterochromatic long arm of the X chromosome are commonly observed in male transformed Chinese hamster cells (77). NiS also induced a large number of chromatid exchanges and dicentrics and a pronounced decondensation of the heterochromatic long arm of the X chromosome in CHO cells (52). $NiCl_2$ produced a much lower incidence of dicentrics and had less significant effects on the long arm of the X, unless the $NiCl_2$ was complexed with albumin and encapsulated into liposomes so that it also was taken up by the cells via phagocytosis, indicating that the specific interactions of nickel ions with heterochromatin depend on the mechanism of exposure and uptake (95). Prolonged exposure to $NiCl_2$ can also produce substantial damage in heterochromatin regions (95). The effect of magnesium in counteracting nickel toxicity is more pronounced in heterochromatin than in euchromatin (96).

## REFERENCES


1. Shi Z. Nickel carbonyl: toxicity and human health. *Sci Total Environ* 1994;148(2-3):293–298.
2. Morgan L, Usher V. Health problems associated with nickel refining and use. *Ann Occup Hyg* 1994;38(2):189–198.
3. Nieboer E, Nriagu JO. Nickel and human health: current perspectives. In: Nriagu JO, ed. *Advances in environmental science and technology,* vol 25. New York: John Wiley, 1992;680.
4. Menne T. Quantitative aspects of nickel dermatitis. Sensitization and eliciting threshold concentrations (review). *Sci Total Environ* 1994;148(2-3): 275–281.
5. Sosroseno W. The immunology of nickel-induced allergic contact dermatitis. *Asian Pacific J Allergy Immunol* 1995;13(2):173–181.
6. Costa M. Mechanisms of Nickel Genotoxicity and Carcinogenicity. In: Chang LW, ed. *Toxicology of metals.* New York: CRC Lewis, 1996; 245–252.
7. Coogan TP, Latta DM, Snow ET, Costa M. Toxicity and carcinogenicity of nickel compounds. *CRC Crit Rev Toxicol* 1989;19(4):341–384.
8. Anke M, Groppel B, Kronemann H, Grun M. Nickel-An essential element. In: Sunderman FW Jr, ed. *Nickel in the human environment.* Lyon, France: IARC Scientific, 1984;339.
9. Walsch CT, Orme-Johnson WH. Nickel enzymes. *Biochemistry* 1987; 26:4901.
10. Grandjean P. Human exposure to nickel. In: Sunderman FW Jr, ed. *Nickel in the human environment.* Publication No. 53. Lyon, France: IARC Scientific, 1984;469–485.
11. Costa M, Mollenhauer HH. Phagocytosis of nickel subsulfide particles during the early stages of neoplastic transformation in tissue culture. *Cancer Res* 1980;40:2688.
12. Baselt RC, Hanson VW. Efficacy of orally-administered chelating agents for nickel carbonyl toxicity in rats. *Res Commun Chem Pathol Pharmacol* 1982;38:113.
13. Athar M, Misra M, Srivastava RC. Evaluation of chelating drugs on the toxicity, excretion, and distribution of nickel in poisoned rats. *Fundam Appl Toxicol* 1987;9:26.
14. Tandon SK, Singh S, Jain VK, Prasad S. Chelation in metal intoxication. Effect of structurally different chelating agents in treatment of nickel intoxication in rat. *Fundam Appl Toxicol* 1996;31(2):141–148.
15. Kristenson H. How to get the best out of antabuse. *Alcohol Alcohol* 1995;30(6):775–783.
16. Nielsen G, Andersen O. Effect of tetraethylthiuramdisulphide and diethyl-dithiocarbamate on nickel toxicokinetics in mice. *Pharmacol Toxicol* 1994;75(5):285–293.
17. Sunderman FW Jr. Nickel. In: Seiler HG, Sigel H, Sigel A, eds. *Handbook on toxicity of inorganic compounds.* New York: Marcel Dekker, 1988;453–468.
18. Domingo J. Metal-induced developmental toxicity in mammals: a review. *J Toxicol Environ Health* 1994;42(2):123–141.
19. Sunderman FW Jr, Reid MC, Shen SK, Kevorkian CB. Embryotoxicity and teratogenicity of nickel compounds. In: Clarkson TW, Nordberg GF, Sayer PP, eds. *Reproductive and developmental toxicity of metals.* New York: Plenum, 1983;399.
20. Diwan B, Kasprzak K, Rice J. Transplacental carcinogenic effects of nickel(II) acetate in the renal cortex, renal pelvis and adenohypophysis in F344/NCr rats. *Carcinogenesis* 1992;13(8):1351–1357.
21. U.S. Environmental Protection Agency. *Health assessment document for nickel and nickel compounds.* Washington, DC: USEPA, 1986.
22. Berman E, Rehnberg B. *Fetotoxic effects of nickel in drinking water in mice.* Washington, DC: U.S. Environmental Protection Agency, 1983.
23. Templeton DM. Nickel at the renal glomerulus: molecular and cellular interactions. In: Nieboer E, Nriagu JO, eds. *Nickel and human health:* current perspectives. New York: John Wiley, 1992;135–170.
24. Tabata M, Sarkar B. Specific nickel(II)-transfer process between the native sequence peptide representing the nickel(II)-transport site of human serum albumin and L-histidine. *J Inorg Biochem* 1992;45(2): 93–104.
25. Edoute Y, Vanhoutte PM, Rubanyi GM. Mechanisms of nickel-induced coronary vasoconstriction in isolated perfused rat hearts. In: Nieboer E, Nriagu JO, eds. *Nickel and human health:* current perspectives. New York: John Wiley, 1992;587–602.
26. Leach CN Jr, Linden JV, Hopfer SM, Crisostomo MC, Sunderman FW Jr. Nickel concentrations in serum of patients with acute myocardial infarction or unstable angina pectoris. *Clin Chem* 1985;31:556.
27. Rubanyi G, Szabo K, Balogh I, Bakos M, Gergely A, Kovach AGB. Endogenous nickel release as a possible cause of coronary vasoconstriction and myocardial injury in acute burn of rats. *Circ Shock* 1983;10:361.
28. Sunderman FW Jr. Potential toxicity from nickel contamination of intravenous fluids. *Ann Clin Lab Sci* 1983;13:1–4.
29. Boysen M, Solberg LA, Torjussen W, Poppe S, Hgetveit AC. Histological changes, rhinoscopical findings and nickel concentration in plasma and urine in retired nickel workers. *Acta Otolaryngol (Stockh)* 1984;97: 105.
30. Kaldor J, Peto J, Easton D, Doll R, Herman L, Morgan L. Models for respiratory cancer in nickel refinery workers. *J Natl Cancer Inst* 1986; 77:841.
31. Coultas D, Samet J. Occupational lung cancer. *Clin Chest Med* 1992;13 (2):341–354.
32. Muir D, Jadon N, Julian J, Roberts R. Cancer of the respiratory tract in

nickel sinter plant workers: effect of removal from sinter plant exposure. *Occup Environ Med* 1994;51(1):19–22.
33. Andersen A. Recent follow-up of nickel refinery workers in Norway and respiratory cancer. In: Nieboer E, Nriagu JO, eds. *Nickel and human health:* current perspectives. New York: John Wiley, 1992;621–627.
34. Zeromski J, Jezewska E, Sikora J, Kasprzak K. The effect of nickel compounds on immunophenotype and natural killer cell function of normal human lymphocytes. *Toxicology* 1995;97:39–48.
35. Smialowicz RJ, Rogers RR, Rowe DG, Riddle MM, Luebke RW. The effects of nickel on immune function in the rat. *Toxicology* 1987;44: 271–281.
36. Haley PJ, Bice DE, Muggenburg BA, Hahn FF, Benjamin SA. Immunopathologic effects of nickel subsulfide on the primate pulmonary immune system. *Toxicol Appl Pharmacol* 1987;88:1–12.
37. Zeromski J, Jezewska E. Functional alterations of human blood monocytes after exposure to various nickel compounds *in vitro*: an effect on the production of hydrogen peroxide. *Immunol Lett* 1995;45(1-2):117–121.
38. Bour H, Nicolas JF, Garrigue JL, Demidem A, Schmitt D. Establishment of nickel-specific T cell lines from patients with allergic contact dermatitis: comparison of different protocols. *Clin Immunol Immunopathol* 1994;73(1):142–145.
39. Fernandez J, Vernon C, Hildebrand H, Martin P. Nickel allergy to dental prostheses. *Contact Dermatitis* 1986;14:312.
40. Merritt K. Rodrigo JJ. Immune response to synthetic materials—sensitization of patients receiving orthopaedic implants. *Clin Orthop* 1996; (326):71–79.
41. Malo JL, Cartier A, Gagnon G, Evans S, Dolovich J. Isolated late asthmatic reactions due to nickel sulfate without antibodies to nickel. *Clin Allergy* 1985;15:95–99.
42. Zhong Z, Troll W, Koenig K, Frenkel K. Carcinogenic sulfide salts of nickel and cadmium induce $H_2O_2$ formation by human polymorphonuclear leukocytes. *Cancer Res* 1990;50:7564–7570.
43. Huang X, Zhuang ZX, Frenkel K, Klein CB, Costa M. The role of nickel and nickel-mediated reactive oxygen species in the mechanism of nickel carcinogenesis. *Environ Health Perspect* 1994;102(suppl 3):281–284.
44. Rendall R, Phillips J, Renton K. Death following exposure to fine particulate nickel from a metal arc process. *Ann Occup Hyg* 1994;38:921.
45. OSHA. *Occupational standards permissible exposure limits.* Washington, DC: Occupational Safety and Health Administration, 1985.
46. Templeton D, Sunderman FJ, Herber R. Tentative reference values for nickel concentrations in human serum, plasma, blood, and urine: evaluation according to the TRACY protocol. *Sci Total Environ* 1994;148 (2-3):243–251.
47. Christensen J. Human exposure to toxic metals: factors influencing interpretation of biomonitoring results. *Sci Total Environ* 1995;166: 89–135.
48. Sunderman FJ Jr. Biological monitoring of nickel in humans. *Scand J Work Environ Health* 1993;19(suppl 1):34–38.
49. Tsai PJ, Vincent JH, Wahl G, Maldonado G. Occupational exposure to inhalable and total aerosol in the primary nickel production industry. *Occup Environ Med* 1996;53(2):793–799.
50. Hansen K, Stern RM. Toxicity and transformation of nickel compounds *in vitro*. In: Sunderman FW Jr, ed. *Nickel in the human environment.* Lyon, France: IARC Scientific, 1984;193–200.
51. Costa M, Simmons-Hansen J, Bedrossian CWM, Bonura J, Caprioli RM. Phagocytosis, cellular distribution, and carcinogenic activity of particulate nickel compounds in tissue culture. *Cancer Res* 1981;41:2868.
52. Costa M, Salnikow K, Cosentino S, Klein C, Huang X, Zhuang Z. Molecular mechanisms of nickel carcinogenesis. *Environ Health Perspect* 1994;102(suppl 3):127–130.
53. Costa M, Heck JD, Robison H. Selective phagocytosis of crystalline metal sulfide particles and DNA strand breaks as a mechanism for the induction of cellular transformation. *Cancer Res* 1982;42:2757–2763.
54. Costa M, Abbracchio MP, Simmons-Hansen J. Factors influencing the phagocytosis, neoplastic transformation and cytotoxicity of particulate nickel compounds in tissue culture systems. *Toxicol Appl Pharmacol* 1981;60:313–323.
55. Lee Y, Klein C, Kargacin B, et al. Carcinogenic nickel silences gene expression by chromatin condensation and DNA methylation: a new model for epigenetic carcinogens. *Mol Cell Biol* 1995;15:2547–2557.
56. Klein CB, Conway K, Wang XW, et al. Senescence of nickel-transformed cells by an X chromosome: possible epigenetic control. *Science* 1991;251:796–799.
57. Salnikow K, Gao M, Voitkun V, Huang X, Costa M. Altered oxidative stress responses in nickel-resistant mammalian cells. *Cancer Res* 1994;54:6407–6412.
58. Stohs S, Bagchi D. Oxidative mechanisms in the toxicity of metal ions. *Free Radic Biol Med* 1995;18(2):321–336.
59. Kasprzak K. Possible role of oxidative damage in metal-induced carcinogenesis. *Cancer Invest* 1995;13(4):411–430.
60. USEPA. *Health effects document on nickel.* Ontario: Ontario Ministry of Labour, 1986;32.
61. Nieboer E, Maxwell RI, Stafford AR. Chemical and biological reactivity of insoluble nickel compounds and the bioinorganic chemistry of nickel. In: Sunderman FW Jr, ed. *Nickel in the human environment.* Lyon, France: IARC Scientific, 1984:439.
62. Dunnick J, Elwell M, Radovsky A, et al. Comparative carcinogenic effects of nickel subsulfide, nickel oxide, or nickel sulfate hexahydrate chronic exposures in the lung. *Cancer Res* 1995;55(22):5251–5256.
63. Benson J, Cheng Y, Eidson A, Hahn F, Henderson R, Pickrell J. Pulmonary toxicity of nickel subsulfide in F344/N rats exposed for 1-22 days. *Toxicology* 1995;103(1):9–22.
64. Sunderman FW Jr, Hopfer SM, Lin S-M, et al. Toxicity to aveolar macrophages in rats following parenteral injection of nickel chloride. *Toxicol Appl Pharmacol* 1989;100:107–118.
65. Vyskocil A, Senft V, Viau C, Cizkova M, Kohout J. Biochemical renal changes in workers exposed to soluble nickel compounds. *Hum Exp Toxicol* 1994;13(4):257–261.
66. Andersen A, Berge SR, Engeland A, Norseth T. Exposure to nickel compounds and smoking in relation to incidence of lung and nasal cancer among nickel refinery workers. *Occup Environ Med* 1996;53(10): 708–713.
67. Costa M, Heck JD. Perspectives on the mechanism of nickel carcinogenesis. In: Eichorn GL, Marzilli L, eds. *Advances in inorganic biochemistry.* New York: Elsevier Science, 1984;285–309.
68. Hansen K, Stern RM. In vitro toxicity and transformation potentcy of nickel compounds. *Environ Health Perspect* 1983;51:223–226.
69. Costa M, Heck JD. Metal ion carcinogenesis: mechanistic aspects. In: Sigel H, ed. *Metal ions in biological systems.* New York: Marcel Dekker, 1986;259–278.
70. Arrouijal FZ, Hildebrand HF, Vophi H, Marzin D. Genotoxic activity of nickel subsulphide a-$Ni_3S_2$. *Mutagenesis* 1990;5(6):583–589.
71. Fletcher G, Rossetto,F, Turnbull J, Nieboer E. Toxicity, uptake, and mutagenicity of particulate and soluble nickel compounds. *Environ Health Perspect* 1994;102(suppl 3):69–79.
72. Kargacin B, Klein CB, Costa M. Mutagenic responses of nickel oxides and nickel sulfides in Chinese hamster V79 cell lines at the xanthine-guanine phosphoribosyl transferase locus. *Mutat Res* 1993;300:63–72.
73. Snow ET. Metal carcinogenesis: mechanistic implications. *Pharmacol Ther* 1992;53:31–65.
74. Costa M. Model for the epigenetic mechanism of action of nongenotoxic carcinogens. *Am J Clin Nutr* 1995;61(suppl 3):666S–669S.
75. Nishimura M, Umeda M. Induction of chromosomal aberrations in cultured mammalian cells by nickel compounds. *Mutat Res* 1979;68: 337–349.
76. Sunderman FW Jr, Hopfer SM, Nichols WW, et al. Chromosomal abnormalities and gene amplification in renal cancers induced in rats by nickel subsulfide. *Ann Clin Lab Sci* 1990;20(1):60–72.
77. Conway K, Costa M. Nonrandom chromosomal alterations in nickel-transformed Chinese hamster embryo cells. *Cancer Res* 1989;49: 6032–6038.
78. Christie NT. The synergistic interaction of Ni(II) with DNA damaging agents. *Toxicol Environ Chem* 1989;22:51–59.
79. Dubins JS, Lavelle JM. Nickel(II) genotoxicity: potentiation of mutagenesis of simple alkylating agents. *Mutat Res* 1986;162:187–199.
80. Anwer J, Mehrotra NK. Effect of simultaneous exposure of nickel chloride and benzo(a)pyrene on developing chick embryos. *Drug Chem Toxicol* 1986;9(2):171–183.
81. Snow ET, Xu L-S, Kinney PL. Effects of nickel ions on polymerase activity and fidelity during DNA replication *in vitro*. *Chem Biol Interact* 1993;88:155–173.
82. Chin YE, Snow ET, Cohen MD, Christie NT. The effect of divalent nickel ($Ni^{2+}$) on *in vitro* DNA replication by DNA polymerase alpha. *Cancer Res* 1994;54(9):2337–2341.
83. Sirover MA, Loeb LA. On the fidelity of DNA replication: effect of metal activators during synthesis with avian myeloblastosis virus DNA polymerase. *J Biol Chem* 1977;252:3605–3610.
84. Conway K, Sen P. Costa M. Antagonistic effect of magnesium chloride

on the nickel chloride-induced inhibition of DNA replication in Chinese hamster ovary cells. *J Biochem Toxicol* 1986;1(2):11–26.
85. Hartwig A, Mullenders LHF, Schlepegrell R, Krueger I, Beyersmann D. Interaction of nickel(II) with DNA repair processes—inhibition of the incision step in nucleotide excision repair. *Metal Ions Biol Med* 1994; 3:235–240.
86. Snyder RD. Effects of metal treatment on DNA repair in polyamine-depleted HeLa cells with special reference to nickel. *Environ Health Perspect* 1994;102(suppl 3):51–55.
87. Au W, Heo M, Chiewchanwit T. Toxicological interactions between nickel and radiation on chromosome damage and repair. *Environ Health Perspect* 1994;102(suppl 9):73–77.
88. Hartwig A, Kruger I, Beyersmann D. Mechanisms in nickel genotoxicity: the significance of interactions with DNA repair. *Toxicol Lett* 1994; 72(1-3):353–358.
89. Beyersmann D. Interactions in metal carcinogenicity. *Toxicol Lett* 1994; 72(1-3):333–338.
90. Lee-Chen S, Wang M, Yu C, Wu D, Jan K. Nickel chloride inhibits the DNA repair of UV-treated but not methyl methanesulfonate-treated Chinese hamster ovary cells. *Biol Trace Element Res* 1993;37(1): 39–50.
91. Zhuang ZX, Shen Y, Shen HM, Ng V, Ong CN. DNA strand breaks and poly (ADP-ribose) polymerase activation induced by crystalline nickel subsulfide in MRC-5 lung fibroblast cells. *Hum Exp Toxicol* 1996;15 (11):891–897.
92. Katsifis S, Kinney P, Hosselet S, Burns F, Christie N. Interaction of nickel with mutagens in the induction of sister chromatid exchanges in human lymphocytes. *Mutat Res* 1996;359(1):7–15.
93. Littlefield N, Hass B. Damage to DNA by cadmium or nickel in the presence of ascorbate. *Ann Clin Lab Sci* 1995;25(6):485–492.
94. Sen P, Conway K, Costa M. Comparison of the localization of chromosome damage induced by calcium chromate and nickel compounds. *Cancer Res* 1987;47:2142–2147.
95. Sen P, Costa M. Pathway of nickel uptake influences its interaction with heterochromatic DNA. *Toxicol Appl Pharmacol* 1986;84:278–285.
96. Conway K, Wang X-W, Xu L-S, Costa M. Effect of magnesium on nickel-induced genotoxicity and cell transformation. *Carcinogenesis* 1987;8(8):1115–1121.

*Environmental and Occupational Medicine, Third Edition,* edited by William N. Rom.
Lippincott–Raven Publishers, Philadelphia © 1998.

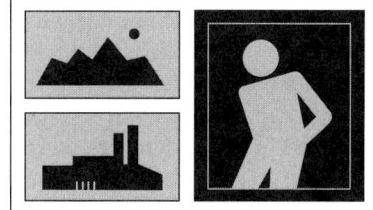

# CHAPTER 76

# Pulmonary and Neurologic Effects of Aluminum

Kaye H. Kilburn

Aluminum, atomic number 13 and atomic weight 26.98, 3b in the periodic table, is the most abundant metal in the earth's crust (8%), where it is always found combined (1,2). Bauxite is the principal ore and may contain up to 55% aluminum as the hydrated aluminum oxides gibbsite and boehmite. Commercial deposits are found in Australia, Guyana, France, Brazil, Hungary, Venezuela, and the Gulf Coast of the United States. Large-scale aluminum production began during World War II. The world's production currently exceeds 19.5 million metric tons per year.

## PRODUCTION

Bauxite is converted to alumina ($Al_2O_3{\cdot}H_2O$) by the Bayer process, in which caustic soda (sodium hydroxide) is autoclaved with bauxite at temperatures from 200° to 1,200°C. This hydrate is crystallized and calcined in a kiln. Both the autoclave and the kiln require insulation, which in the past contained asbestos.

Alumina is reduced to aluminum by an electrolytic process using carbon electrodes and cryolite, aluminum fluoride, as flux. The Hall-Heroult process invented in 1886 operates either with prebaked carbon anodes or with continuously produced coal and petroleum tar pitch electrodes—Soderberg cells. The Soderberg process is dirtier because of the boiling off of volatile polyaromatics and release of sulfur dioxide and aliphatic and aromatic compounds. Usually the electrolytic cell or pot has a gas-collection hood and with the Soderberg process a burner to ignite the volatile gases. The remainder is piped to a cleaning plant. Electrolytic reduction of aluminum requires 150,000 A and consumes 13.2 to 17.6 kW/kg. This large electric power requirement explains the location of aluminum smelters adjoining abundant hydroelectric power sources such as the Columbia River, the St. Lawrence River, the Tennessee Valley, and even in Keflavik, Iceland. There are 32 aluminum smelters in the United States (2). In Australia energy comes from abundant strip mined coal, although in New Zealand it is hydroelectric.

## ADVERSE HUMAN HEALTH EFFECTS

Recovery of bauxite, production of alumina, and refining of aluminum cause adverse health effects. The toxicants vary from silica and aluminum silicates in bauxite mining, which is usually from open pits, to the caustic soda, heat, and noise during alumina production. The recommended maximum allowable concentration of alumina in the workplace is $50 \times 10^6$ particles per cubic foot of air. However, the focus for health problems is the electrolytic cell or pot in the "potroom." Here, hydrogen fluoride, fluorine, particles of fluoride salts, alumina, pitch and tars, carbon monoxide, sulfur dioxide, metallic aluminum, and its oxides are found in abundance. Release peaks when the frozen flux and alumina are broken to charge the cell or to extract the aluminum. When prebaked electrodes are used, release of pitch products is largely confined to the anode production area (3). In the

K. H. Kilburn: Department of Internal Medicine, University of Southern California School of Medicine, Los Angeles, California 90033.

Soderberg process, more gases and fumes are released because the carbon paste or pitch is dropped into a steel casing and baked in the pot. Particles and gases escape as molten aluminum is tapped from both types of pot, alumina is added after breaking the crust, and anodes are changed. Using cryolite as flux enables electrolysis to proceed at lower temperatures, around 1,000°C (3). As the aluminum proceeds into the casting or rolling plants, fumes are released from the combustion of lubricating greases and from chlorine, which is used to clean the casting furnaces.

Health effects are adverse for several organs: lung—potroom asthma, chronic lung disease, pulmonary fibrosis, cancer (4,5); skin—telangiectasis; heart—coronary artery disease (6); and central nervous system. Perhaps the most important effects are the neurobehavioral changes, so-called potroom palsy (7), tremors, movement defects, and alterations in memory and concentration (thus, cerebral and cerebellar dysfunction) (8).

## PHYSIOLOGY AND TOXICOLOGY

Investigation of the physiologic activity of aluminum is hampered by the lack of a radioisotope, so its similarity to other metals, particularly scandium, gallium, beryllium, titanium, and zirconium, must be utilized (9). Daily human intake is 1 to 20 mg/day, and 1 g or more may be ingested as aluminum hydroxide in antacids. The body content is not known but is estimated to be 30 to 50 mg, half in the skeleton and a quarter in the lungs. The rate of excretion in the urine is estimated to be 20 to 50 μg per day, which equals intestinal absorption. Administration of 2.29 g aluminum hydroxide raised excretion from 16 to 300 μg/day.

Aluminum salts are highly insoluble at neutral pH, but solubility increases as pH decreases. Acidifying fertilizers and acid rain have increased aluminum levels in rivers and lakes. This increase, rather than decreased pH, may be responsible for gill damage and the death of young fish, and birds may be fatally intoxicated. Aluminum is toxic for plants and limits growth, probably by binding and preventing uptake of phosphate by the roots. For more details see Ganrot's (9) 1986 review.

The normal human lung contains about 25 ± 1.8 μg aluminum per gram of wet tissue (10). Aluminum in human serum, blood, urine, and tissue can be analyzed by electrothermal (flameless) atomic absorption spectrometry and neutron activation analysis (11—14). Aluminum concentrations in healthy volunteers were 2.0 ± 0.4 μg/L in serum and 12.1 ± 1.5 μg/L in whole blood. In aluminum powder workers and aluminum welders, urine aluminum levels reflect exposure better than blood aluminum concentrations (14). Bone concentrations were 8.2 ± 5.8 μg/g of fresh tissue in hemodialysis patients without osteomalacia, compared to 51 ± 20 μg/g for chronic dialysis patients with osteomalacia (11). Electron microbeam or energy-dispersive analysis can identify aluminum in tissues (10).

## POTROOM ASTHMA

The observation that potroom exposure in the aluminum refinery produces respiratory symptoms is attributed to Frostad (15) in 1936. Asthma accompanied by leukocytosis was more frequent among factory workers than in the general population. In 1960 Midttun (16) described cough, bronchitis, and fibrotic changes in the lungs of Canadian aluminum workers and reported 33 cases of bronchitis or asthma in potroom workers registered in Norway from 1955 to 1957. These workers also complained of nausea, headaches, and irritation of the conjunctiva and respiratory passages, but their most troublesome complaint was cough, which awakened them at 2:00 or 3:00 A.M. with orthopnea, dyspnea, and bubbling in the chest. Asthma and leukocytosis with eosinophilia during attacks suggested an allergic response due to fluorine or aluminum fluoride salts.

Potroom asthma is a problem in Norway, Holland, Yugoslavia, France, New Zealand, Australia, and Canada (17), but reports from the United States are lacking. Labor turnover is high—annual rates are 20% to 36% (17). In New Zealand 44% of potroom workers left in the first year (4), and in Australia 71% left within 3 years (17). Some of these workers became asymptomatic after leaving, but others continued to suffer dyspnea, wheeze, and chest tightness (18), which usually responded promptly to inhaled aerosol bronchodilators. Use of masks reduced asthma symptoms, and airstream helmets substantially reduced the numbers of workers who had to be transferred from the potroom in a Norwegian study (19). Atopy was seldom found, but family history of asthma was common (20). Skin test results have seldom been positive, even when 2% sodium fluoride was used for testing, and immunoglobulin E (IgE) levels are usually normal (4).

High workplace fluoride levels and excess urinary fluoride excretion are associated with decreases in the forced expiratory volume in 1 second ($FEV_1$) across a work shift. Precipitating events include increased dust levels following dry scrubbing, anode cleaning, pot startup, carbon or pitch cleaning, and cleaning up after batch mill breakdowns (4). The prevalence of potroom asthma varied from none to 39% in 13 recent reports (14). The high figure was from a 1983 Canadian study (21), and the low one from Norway in 1975 (22). Typically, workers had wheezing, tightness in the chest, shortness of breath, and cough with increased variability or reductions in $FEV_1$ (23), although some studies showed only persistent bronchial hyperreactivity. One longitudinal study found that men who had left had more chest tightness and a lower forced expiratory flow after 50% of vital capacity had been expelled ($FEF_{50}$) than those who stayed (24). No study of the aluminum industry has enrolled and followed a cohort to document changes in lung function and symptoms (4). Not only would such a study take 30 to 40 years, but excessive annual worker turnover makes it impossible. Six studies have followed 40 to 1,729 workers for intervals up to 11 years (4). Excessive yearly reductions in $FEV_1$ in three groups were related to both smoking and aluminum exposure, whereas in two the decrements were no greater than for control subjects (25,26). However, non-potroom workers from the same refinery were the controls, and comparison of both groups to external controls showed a greater than expected interval reduction (27,28). Most recently, $FEV_1$ and midflows were lower in potroom workers than in controls, but the differences were not statistically significant (24). In another study rapid decline in $FEV_1$ was localized to the prebaked anode plant (3).

Chest tightness, wheezing, shortness of breath often with nocturnal orthopnea, and dyspnea identified potroom asthma more than 50 years ago. When pulmonary function was evaluated, flow rates were reduced, and increased nonspecific bronchial reactivity to methacholine was seen in one study (18), though not in another (29). In addition, residual volume was increased, and diffusing capacity was decreased as a result of the airways obstruction (29). In one plant where the carbon (electrode) plant was separate from the potroom, electrode workers had greater reductions in $FEV_1$ and forced vital capacity (FVC) than potroom workers (3). In another, after only 4 months' exposure to aluminum, fluoride, and sulfate, nocturnal wheezing, breathlessness, and reversible airways obstruction were found with increased methacholine sensitivity (17 of 19 workers suffered air flow obstruction after inhaling 0.1% methacholine) (18). Bronchoalveolar lavage (BAL) fluid from potroom workers contained more fibronectin, albumin, and hyaluronate and less angiotensin-converting enzyme than fluid from unexposed men (30). In another study, asthma and alveolar macrophages in BAL fluid were least in controls, greater in administrators, and greatest in potroom workers (31).

Workers from a U.S. aluminum refinery and foundry that had closed its Soderberg cell potrooms 3 years earlier had statistically significantly more wheezing and asthma than did regional controls (32). Irregular opacities in the lung fields, indistinguishable from those of asbestosis, were found in 23% of these workers. In addition, never smokers and current smokers had lower expiratory flows than controls. A cross-shift study of 57 workers showed that midexpiratory flows ($FEF_{25-75}$) decreased more than 15% in 35% of them after they were exposed to melting and casting (recycling) of scrap aluminum.

## CHRONIC LUNG DISEASE

Eleven cross-sectional studies of chronic lung disease (CLD) in aluminum workers (4) showed variable results. Some found no difference in chronic bronchitis prevalence or in $FEV_1$ between workers and controls; others showed chronic airways obstruction, more wheeze, and increased airways resistance, which were related to accumulated exposure. As with potroom asthma the prevalences of CLD as defined by medical examination, symptoms, and spirometric evidence of impairment varied widely, from 4% to 33% (4). The survivor status of potroom workers due to high turnover was underscored in a 1972 study from Massena, New York, where 5 to 7 years after the initial examination only 66 of 231 workers could be located for examination (33). Compared to fabrication workers, they showed no health differences, skin changes, or bony fluorosis on radiography, while many Niagara Falls potroom workers had fluorosis. The prevalence of CLD was 4.9% in aluminum workers and 5.3% in skilled laborers, but aluminum workers with heavy fluoride exposure had lower $FEV_1$ and FVC than those with light or moderate exposure (33). Current workers measured below former workers and newly hired ones (34). A study of 5,406 men in one cohort and 485 in a second group, beginning about 1950, showed that the mortality rate from respiratory disease for men with 21 or more years' exposure was twice that of men who were never exposed to tars (35).

## PULMONARY FIBROSIS

Goralewski (36) found chest radiographic abnormalities of fibrosis in 26% of German aluminum powder workers in 1947. Later, in England, Mitchell et al. (37) reported similar changes in 6 of 29 workers. Neither the German nor the English workers were exposed to asbestos insulation. A ball mill worker developed progressive fibrosis and a progressive encephalopathy after 13.5 years and died of bronchopneumonia. Aluminum levels in his brain and lung were 20 times normal (7). It was thought that mineral oil used as a coating for the powder caused pulmonary fibrosis, as powder workers who used stearic acid had no fibrosis (8). Animal experiments showed no such differences, however, so the fibrosis was attributed to aluminum powder (38). Since 1960, fibrosis or granuloma has rarely been attributed to aluminum dust. A long-time aluminum polisher developed upper lobe fibrosis with high aluminum content and a carcinoma (39). Aluminum oxide fibers were considered the cause of fibrosis in one man (40). Another worker exposed to aluminum and aluminum silicates had sarcoid disease, but he had also been exposed to cobalt, vanadium, manganese, palladium, and silica (41). A shipboard aluminum welder who worked in confined spaces had dense diffuse interstitial fibrosis and alveolar filling with macrophages that were rich in aluminum (42). None of these reports mentioned ferruginous bodies or examination for asbestos fibers, despite the fact that arc welders, particularly on ships, are exposed to much asbestos.

Initial reports of exposure to alumina abrasives corundum 50 years ago by Shaver and Riddell (43) found x-ray changes in 35 of 344 furnace workers and probable changes in another 13. The abrasives were manufactured from bauxite using furnaces that produced temperatures of 2,000°C by electric arcs using carbon electrodes. When the tops of the pots were opened, dense fumes contaminated the working areas with alumina and silica as they passed to the roof. The affected workers were dyspneic, had attacks of extreme breathlessness, and produced white frothy sputum. As the disease advanced they suffered discomfort or pain from chest tightness. Pneumothorax was frequent, and seven workers died. Chest radiographs showed bilateral lacy shadows, blebs, and bullae, with widening of the mediastinum and distortion of the diaphragms. Cigarette smoking histories were not provided. In three of four autopsies, lung ash was 25% to 30% silica, so that 1.5% to 3% of the lungs' dry weight was silica. Subsequently, 46 patients were followed for fibrosis and elevated diaphragms, bullae, and pneumothorax. Ten died (44). Lungs of six patients had a gunmetal color, with many emphysematous vesicles or bullae, pleural thickening, and adhesions, particularly in the upper lobes, normal lymph nodes, and consistently diffuse fibrosis with obliterative endarteritis and variable amounts of black pigment (45). Chemical analysis showed that 21% to 31% of the lung ash was silica and 26% to 40% alumina, concentrations that matched those in the furnace fumes. There were no hallmarks of the silicotic reaction, even considering the polymorphism of experimental silicotic fibrosis. No analyses were done for asbestos fibers or ferruginous bodies.

Almost 40 years later, 1,142 men working at an Arkansas bauxite refinery and alumina products plant showed decreased $FEV_1$ related to increased duration of employment and to cumulative dust exposure. Smokers suffered greater impairment of function than those who had never smoked, although available data were insufficient to make a discrete separation (46). Later, analysis of 788 men from this same facility showed irregular opacities in about 4% of the nonsmokers and 11% to 12% of the smokers (47). Although the mechanism of alumina-induced lung disease is unclear, Dinman (48) suggested that pulmonary fibrosis was associated with surface area and catalytic activity of various aluminas, particularly low-temperature transition forms, and was critical of animal work in which massive quantities of alumina were given intratracheally. Gibbsite and boehmite, as principal ores, and corundum, the abrasive product, may trigger fibrotic reactions. However, no mention was made of asbestos or of a modified silicosis produced by alumina silicates. Four alumina dust workers showed some fibrosis on bronchoscopic lung biopsies, but only one had slight irregular opacities on chest radiography (49). The biopsy from the man with the abnormal radiograph showed 1,080 ppm (μg/g) of aluminum by neutron activation analysis.

In Australia, 32 subjects exposed to artificial aluminum silicate had minimal abnormalities, so the authors retracted their report of adverse effects associated with cat litter material (50). Nine workers were identified by chest radiographs to have a profusion of irregular opacities greater than 0/1 among 1,000 making aluminum oxide abrasive grinding wheels and aluminum oxide–tipped tools. Lung biopsy of three of them showed silica and aluminum, with asbestos fiber counts between 0.4 and $1.3 \times 10^6$ per gram of dry lung tissue (51).

## LUNG CANCER

Lung cancer mortality has been reported in three studies from the United States, two from Quebec (including the one just described), two from Norway, and one from France (4). Six studies showed a relative risk, expressed as standardized mortality rate (SMR), of over 100, and in four it was 125 or greater, the highest being 180. The two cohorts that yielded positive data, one from Quebec by Gibbs (35) and the other from Norway by Andersen et al. (52), did not include data on cigarette smoking; however, Gibbs and Horowitz (53) showed later that the lung cancers were disproportionately frequent in the exposed group. Malignant neoplasms of lung and bladder were correlated with a tar-years index and with years of aluminum production (35).

Analysis of 382 death certificates (400 deaths) from aluminum reduction plant workers in Washington State from 1946 to 1962 showed that the SMR for lung cancer was 117, for pancreatic cancer 180, for lymphatic and hematopoietic cancers 184, and for benign brain tumors 391. Pulmonary emphysema had an SMR of 204, compared to the entire state population, despite an overall SMR of 86 (54). After analyzing these data for the International Agency for Research on Cancers, Simonato (55) concluded that workers in plants that use the Soderberg process have an increased lung cancer risk expressed by the tar-years index but that more data were needed on lymphatic and hematopoietic cancer. Data on 3,954 deaths in 21,829 workers from 14 reduction plants showed excess rates of pancreatic cancers in potroom workers and of hemolymphatic and lung cancers in baked-carbon anode workers. Also, there was an excess of pulmonary emphysema deaths (56). In French aluminum workers (57), 49.1% of whose smoking status was known, differences in mortality were not explained by smoking but length of exposure covaried with duration of smoking. Follow-up of these cohorts, especially those of Andersen (52) and of Gibbs (35,53), should determine risks for lung and other cancers in the next decade.

## ANIMAL EXPERIMENTS

Hydrated alumina in rat lungs produced reticulin nodules followed by dense collagen fibrosis. Aluminum phosphate was much less fibrogenic, but condensed fume from the corundum furnace at doses equivalent to alumina resulted in high animal mortality. Smaller doses of half alumina and half silica produced fibrosis, an exudative reaction, and death (58). When powdered metallic aluminum was injected intratracheally and the controls received quartz dust, both developed fibrosis. Addition of 5% quartz to aluminum also produced more extensive fibrosis than aluminum alone (59). It was concluded that in rats, lesions from aluminum resembled those due to quartz with a similar time course to develop the lesions (60). Rats exposed to saffil alumina fibers showed no fibrosis, in contrast to those exposed to chrysotile asbestos, which showed diffuse fibrosis. They did show increased alveolar epithelialization, but no increase in tumor prevalence (61). Intratracheal introduction of large doses (100 mg) of aluminum powder produced small focal pulmonary fibrosis in rats but not in hamsters. Fibrosis occurred around respiratory bronchioles and alveolar ducts, and masses of aluminum particles were in the macrophages of the alveolar ducts and respiratory bronchioles. Alveolar proteinosis developed in some animals (62). Responses were similar to intratracheal injection of 100 mg stamped aluminum powders coated with stearine (50% stearic and 50% palmitic acid), mineral oil, and no lubricant; all three produced rapid and extensive fibrosis, as compared to granular aluminum, which caused minimal fibrosis (44). Thus, this model showed neither a protective effect for stearine nor a cofibrogenic effect of mineral oil, and stamped aluminum powder promoted fibrosis.

## FLUORIDE

Fluoride in fumes has figured in aluminum smelter problems since the introduction of the Hall-Heroult process. Fluorides released from refineries have caused fluorosis in dairy cattle downwind in upstate New York and Washington State, affecting teeth and bones so that cows, and especially calves, could neither eat nor move (63). This led in the late 1960s to hooding of pots to recover fluorides. A survey of Native American children downwind of the aluminum smelter on Cornwall Island in the St. Lawrence River showed increased pulmonary closing volumes, which correlated with fluoride levels in spot samples of urine, and fluorides were blamed (64). Similarly, increased levels of fluoride have been measured in the urine of cryolite production workers (65). Increased rates of bone cancers, in addition to dental changes, found in rats exposed to high levels of sodium fluoride raise additional concern. In a Norwegian refinery that utilized fluoride recovery onto alumina, there was an association between increased dust exposure and wheezing in potroom workers (66). Acute respiratory symptoms and reduced pulmonary function tests were related to levels of fluoride exposure in smokers, but not in nonsmokers, in a Quebec aluminum smelter (21).

## ALUMINUM POWDER TREATMENT OF SILICOSIS

In the 1940s, based on demonstration *in vitro* that aluminum powder decreased the solubility of silica, and thus formation of silicic acid, aluminum powder particles smaller than 5 μm diameter were administered to silicotic miners in Canada, the United States, and Great Britain. Interim reports from Ontario's Porcupine Gold Mines claimed 19 of 34 miners had less chest pain, cough, shortness of breath, and fatigue and that pulmonary function test results of 12 improved (67). Later, 24 of 49 U.S. miners claimed that benefit from aluminum and a hydrated form ($ALO_3$-$H_2O$) was as effective as that from metallic powder (68). However, a controlled study of 120 silicotic miners, half of whom received metallic aluminum dust and half carbon powder for 15 minutes per day, three times per week for 4 years, found no regression of radiographic abnormalities and no improvement in pulmonary function at rest, during exercise, or during maximal voluntary ventilation (69). There were no objective benefits from inhalation of aluminum dust. In fact, a 1990 follow-up study of miners in Ontario treated with McIntyre powder showed no apparent adverse effects but insufficient evidence of benefit (70).

## HEART DISEASE

Aluminum smelter (potroom) workers in Quebec showed an increased prevalence of coronary artery disease, which was not attributable to smoking, high blood pressure, hyperglycemia, high serum cholesterol, or obesity when compared to referents using a case-control study design (71). Because telangiectasis of the skin was associated with electrocardiographic abnormalities in these workers, they were examined for an association with coronary artery disease, but none was found (5).

## NEUROBEHAVIORAL ABNORMALITIES

Rapidly progressive encephalopathy was associated with years of aluminum ball mill exposure in a worker who at death also had nodular pulmonary fibrosis. Encephalopathy was attributed to increased aluminum because lung and brain levels were 20 times higher than normal (7). Despite this seminal observation, further consideration of aluminum encephalopathy evolved from studies of neurobehavioral complications of dialysis for renal insufficiency rather than from observations of occupational exposure. Thus, in the early 1970s, a severe encephalopathy with dementia, speech disorders, movement disability, and death was reported in dialysis patients who were receiving aluminum-containing phosphate-binding gels to control serum phosphorus levels (13). Progressive stuttering, memory impairment, dyspraxia of speech and then of motion, and myoclonus or fits with fatal dementia defined this disorder (72,73). Dementia, speech impairment, myoclonic seizures, and psychiatric abnormalities had occurred in more than 50% of 42 patients reviewed in 1978 (74). Alfrey and colleagues (75) measured aluminum levels of 25 ppm in gray matter of brains from encephalopathic patients compared to 6.5 ppm in uremic patients who died of other causes and 2.2 ppm in control subjects. In another study, serum aluminum levels were 35 ± 3.7 μg/L in normal subjects, 109 ± 10.6 μg/L in 47 long-term hemodialysis patients, and 369 ± 51.6 μg/L in 10 patients who had dialysis dementia (12). In children with azotemia and severe osteomalacia, aluminum hydroxide given in a phosphate binder increased the serum level of aluminum and caused intoxication without renal dialysis (76). A higher incidence of dialysis encephalopathy occurred in dialysis centers that had a high aluminum level in their tap water (77). Others observed deficient performance of digit symbol, block design, and picture arrangement from the Wechsler Adult Intelligence Scale in patients with chronic renal failure but without encephalopathy (78).

When aging human subjects were studied, those with high serum aluminum levels (504 μg/ml vs 387 μg/ml in the low-aluminum group) had impaired performance of digit symbol, serial sevens, critical flicker frequency, and Trails B, although performances on digit span, Trails A, and block design tests were not impaired (79). As the excess aluminum syndrome became understood, anemia was correlated with reduced activity of dihydropteridin reductase (DHPR), a red blood cell enzyme (80). DHPR is also present in the brain in high concentrations, where it is needed to produce tetrahydrobiopterin, tyrosine, and neurotransmitters. Aluminum neurotoxicity was associated with deficiency of DHPR in the brain (81). Aluminum may have a role in the metastatic calcification of chronic renal failure because it initiates the precipitation of calcium apatite. High serum and tissue concentrations of aluminum may be toxic to the heart by inhibiting enzymes for adenosine triphosphate (ATP) and magnesium (82). This observation may account for episodes of fatal pulmonary edema in otherwise stable patients undergoing renal dialysis. There is an inverse relationship between erythrocyte (DHPR) activity and aluminum concentrations in patients with differing serum aluminum concentrations (83).

Patients undergoing dialysis with elevated aluminum levels without overt aluminum toxicity had abnormal visual evoked potentials in recognition of flash and pattern and decreased ability to pronounce words, to do the digit symbol test, to perform the nine-choice reaction time, and to memorize 36 nouns presented serially (84). In patients being dialyzed the prevalence of muscle weakness, bone pain, fractures, and dementia was correlated with years on dialysis, or years of oral aluminum gel therapy or both (85). Reduction of serum aluminum by administering desferrioxamine (a chelating agent), renal transplantation, or reverse osmosis to lower aluminum in dialysis water have reversed the dialysis dementia syndrome (86). An exponential relationship between aluminum level in the water supply used to prepare dialysate and time until death from dialysis dementia supports this relationship (77).

Transferrin or desferrioxamine reduces the blood levels of aluminum and increases erythrocyte DHPR (87). A geographic relationship has been found between Alzheimer's disease and aluminum in drinking water in 88 districts in England and Wales (88). The risk for Alzheimer's disease was 1.5 times higher where the mean aluminum concentration of water exceeded 0.11 mg/L than in districts where concentrations were less than 0.1 mg/L. It was suggested that aluminum is more bioavailable in drinking water than when it is ingested in other forms (77).

## ALUMINUM AND ALZHEIMER'S DISEASE

The above observations have stimulated speculation concerning aluminum and Alzheimer's disease. The important metabolic characteristics of aluminum are low rate of intestinal absorption, rapid urinary excretion, and slow tissue uptake, mainly into the skeleton and reticuloendothelial cells (9,89). Intracellular aluminum is found first in the lysosomes; then it slowly accumulates in the nucleus and chromosomes. Long-lived cells such as neurons and bone may be most affected by this accumulation. It is proposed by Birchall and Chappell (89) that there is an extremely low aluminum flux in cells and across the blood-brain barrier, so that the neurons, which are long-lived, accumulate toxic levels of aluminum, while short-lived cells do not. Because aluminum is neurotoxic, brain metabolism is easily affected by three- to tenfold increases in concentration, and the assumption is that aluminum taken up by the brain cannot be eliminated, and therefore accumulates. There is speculation that specific neurologic diseases that resemble accelerated aging, like Alzheimer's disease, may be related to excess levels of aluminum in the brain (9,89).

## NEUROBEHAVIORAL ABNORMALITIES FROM WORKPLACE EXPOSURE

Almost 30 years after the seminal report (8), a progressive neurologic disorder was observed in three male potroom workers after 12 years in a large aluminum production plant in the United States (7). They complained of difficulty with balance, frequent stumbling, impaired memory, trouble concentrating, and unsteadiness of the hands. They walked with a wide-based gait, and had intention tremors and dysdiadochokinesia. These changes resembled those of dialysis encephalopathy and suggested aluminum intoxication (7). Neurologic evaluation of eight of 25 patients from the same plant showed that seven had intention tremors of hands, legs, and head and poor balance when standing or walking. Studies of 261 Ontario miners treated with finely ground aluminum and aluminum oxide (McIntyre powder) between 1944 and 1979 showed they performed less well on cognitive examinations than did 346 unexposed miners and had a higher proportion of scores in the impaired range; also, the number of scores in the impaired range increased with duration of exposure (70).

Contamination of aluminum with lithium was suggested as a mechanism for encephalopathy because psychotic patients treated with lithium salts exhibit tremors (90), either early or after several years (91). Lithium may be a neurotoxin alone, as suggested by the observation that volunteers given lithium carbonate in doses of 1,225 ± 300 mg per day for 7 days when tested in the company of distracters made more errors recalling words than when they received a placebo (92). Although lithium and aluminum may act similarly, more studies are needed to determine whether lithium contamination contributes to occupational aluminum toxicity.

## ALUMINUM RECYCLING WORKERS

In the United States more than 50% of the aluminum used for new products is recycled. Unfortunately, cans and building siding are coated with polyvinyl chloride and other plastics; also, automobile engines are melted whole with lubricating oil, and polyvinyl coated wiring harnesses and other metals are not removed before melting. Manganese, fluorides, and chlorine are added as flux during remelting. Workers described a sweet irritating odor and much black greasy dust, headache, shortness of breath, chest burning, decreased memory, and loss of balance.

Cross-sectional comparisons of 41 remelt workers to 32 local and to 66 regional referents showed workers had statistically significantly slower simple reaction time by 77 milliseconds and choice reaction times by 137 milliseconds, balance measured as sway speed was faster by 0.32 cm/s with eyes closed, and color discrimination was poorer (93). Culture Fair IQ scores were 8.3 units lower, e.g., Trails A was 10 seconds longer, Trails B was 50 seconds longer, peg placement took 9 seconds longer, and profile of mood states scores were fourfold higher after adjusting for age, bias, or confounding factors. Workers had significantly more neurobehavioral, rheumatic, and respiratory symptoms than referents. Although in remelting exposure the effects of aluminum, fluorine, chlorine, manganese, and vinyl chloride monomer could not be separated, the process is neurotoxic. Adverse health effects from aluminum remelting call for enclosed processing and other engineering controls to prevent the electrolytic refining of aluminum from causing potroom asthma. The problem of protecting workers is made more difficult as many remelting operations have replaced a few large bauxite reduction plants.

## REFERENCES


1. Dinman BD. Aluminum alloys and compounds. In: Parmeggiani L, ed. *ILO encyclopedia of occupational health and safety,* 3rd ed. Geneva: International Labour Organization, 1983;132–135.
2. Sansonetti SJ. Aluminum. In: Considine DM, ed. *Van Nostrand's scientific encyclopedia,* 6th ed. New York: Van Nostrand Reinhold, 1983; 104–112.
3. Hensley MJ, Wodlarczyk J, Field G, Dobson AJ. Lung function in an aluminum smelter: cross-sectional analysis. *Am Rev Respir Dis* 1990; 141:A82.
4. Abramson MJ, Wlodarczyk JH, Saunders NA, Hensley MJ. Does aluminum smelting cause lung disease? *Am Rev Respir Dis* 1989;139: 1042–1057.
5. Morgan WKC, Dinman BD. Pulmonary effects of aluminum. In: Gitelman HJ, ed. *Aluminum and health:* a critical review. New York: Marcel Dekker, 1988;203–234.
6. Rossignol M, Theriault G. Skin telangiectases and ischaemic disorders in primary aluminum production workers. *Br J Ind Med* 1988;45:198–200.
7. Longstreth WT Jr, Rosenstock L, Heyer NJ. Potroom palsy? Neurologic disorder in three aluminum smelter workers. *Arch Intern Med* 1985; 145:1972–1975.
8. McLaughlin AIG, Kazantzis G, King E, Teare D, Porter RJ, Owen RJ. Pulmonary fibrosis and encephalopathy associated with the inhalation of aluminum dust. *Br J Ind Med* 1962;19:253–263.
9. Ganrot PO. Metabolism and possible health effects of aluminum. *Environ Health Perspect* 1986;65:363–441.
10. Guidotti TL. Pulmonary aluminosis—a review. *Bull Soc Pharmacol Environ Pathol* 1975;111:16–18.
11. D'Haese PC, Van De Vyver FL, De Wolff FA, DeBroe ME. Measurement of aluminum in serum, blood, urine and tissues of chronic hemodialyzed patients by use of electrothermal atomic absorption spectrometry. *Clin Chem* 1985;31:24–29.
12. McKinney TD, Basinger M, Dawson E, Jones MM. Serum aluminum levels in dialysis dementia. *Nephron* 1982;32:53–56.
13. Berlyne GM, Pest D, Ben-Ari J, et al. Hyperaluminumaemia from aluminum lesions in renal failure. *Lancet* 1970;2:494–496.
14. Sjogren B, Lundberg I, Lidums V. Aluminum in blood and urine of industrially exposed workers. *Br J Ind Med* 1983;40:301–304.
15. Frostad EW. Fluoride intoxication in Norwegian aluminum plant workers. *Tidsskr Nor Laegeforen* 1936;56:179–182.
16. Midttun O. Bronchial asthma in the aluminum industry. *Acta Allergol* 1960;15:208–221.
17. Smith MM. The respiratory condition of potroom workers: the Australian experience. In: Hughes JP, ed. *Health protection in primary aluminum production.* London: International Primary Aluminum Institute, 1977;79–86.
18. O'Donnell TV, Welford B, Coleman ED. Potroom asthma: New Zealand experience and follow-up. *Am J Ind Med* 1989;15:43–49.
19. Johannessen H. The respiratory condition of potroom workers: the Norwegian experience. In: Hughes JP, ed. *Health protection in primary aluminum production.* London: International Primary Aluminum Institute, 1977;87–90.
20. Simonsson BG, Sjoberg A, Rolf C, Haeger-Aronsen B. Acute and long-term airway hyperreactivity in aluminum salt-exposed workers with nocturnal asthma. *Eur J Respir Dis* 1985;66:105–118.
21. Durand P, Martin RR, Becklake MR. Acute respiratory changes in aluminum potroom workers. *Scand J Work Environ Health* 1983;9:71.
22. Jahr J, Wannag A. A study of working conditions in the potrooms at the Alnor Aluminum Norway Ltd. Karmoy smelter. *Alum Helsentv* 1972: 19–75.
23. Field GB. Pulmonary function in aluminum smelters. *Thorax* 1984;39: 743–751.
24. Wergeland E, Lund E, Waage JE. Respiratory dysfunction after potroom asthma. *Am J Ind Med* 1987;11:627–636.
25. Chan-Yeung M, Wong R, Maclean L, et al. Epidemiologic health study of workers in an aluminum smelter in British Columbia. *Am Rev Respir Dis* 1983;127:465–469.
26. Field GB, Milne J. Occupational asthma in aluminum smelters. *Aust NZ J Med* 1975;5:475.

27. Chan-Yeung M, Enarson DA, MacLean L, Irving D. Longitudinal study of workers in an aluminum smelter. *Arch Environ Health* 1989;44:134–139.
28. Kilburn KH. Re-examination of longitudinal studies of workers. *Arch Environ Health* 1989;44:132–133.
29. Tornling G, Eklund A, Larsson K, et al. Airway obstruction and reduced diffusion capacity in Swedish aluminum potroom workers. Abstracts of Communications, VIIth International Pneumoconioses Conference, Pittsburgh, 1988.
30. Eklund A, Arns R, Blaschke E, et al. Characteristics of alveolar cells and soluble components in bronchoalveolar lavage fluid from nonsmoking aluminum potroom workers. *Br J Ind Med* 1989;46:782–786.
31. Nilsen AM, Mylius EA, Gullvag BM. Alveolar macrophages from expectorates as indicators of pulmonary irritation in primary aluminum reduction plant workers. *Am J Ind Med* 1987;12:101–112.
32. Kilburn KH, Warshaw RH. Occupational asthma and airways dysfunction in aluminum workers. *Am Rev Respir Dis* 1990;141:A79.
33. Kaltreider NL, Elder MJ, Cralley LV, Colwell MO. Health survey of aluminum workers with special reference to fluoride exposure. *J Occup Med* 1972;14:531–541.
34. Discher DP, Breitenstein BD. Prevalence of chronic pulmonary disease in aluminum potroom workers. *J Occup Med* 1976;18:379–386.
35. Gibbs GW. Mortality of aluminum reduction plant workers, 1950 through 1977. *J Occup Med* 1985;27:761–770.
36. Goralewski G. Die Aluminiumlunge: Eine neue Gewerbeerkrankung. *Z Gesamte Inn Med* 1947;2:665–673.
37. Mitchell J, Manning GB, Molyneux M, Lane RE. Pulmonary fibrosis in workers exposed to finely powdered aluminum. *Br J Ind Med* 1961; 18:10–20.
38. Corrin B. Aluminum pneumoconiosis II: effect on the rat lung of intratracheal injections of stamped aluminum powders containing different lubricating agents and of granular aluminum powder. *Br J Ind Med* 1963;20:268–276.
39. DeVuyst P, Dumortier P, Rickaert F, Van de Weyer R, Lenclud C, Yernault JC. Occupational lung fibrosis in an aluminum polisher. *Eur J Respir Dis* 1986;68:131–140.
40. Gilks B, Churg A. Aluminum-induced pulmonary fibrosis: Do fibers play a role? *Am Rev Respir Dis* 1987;136:176–179.
41. DeVuyst P, Dumortier P, Schandene L, Esteane M, Verhest A, Yernault JC. Sarcoid-like lung granuloma induced by aluminum dusts. *Am Rev Respir Dis* 1987;135:493–497.
42. Vallyathan V, Bergeron WN, Robichaux PA, Craighead JE. Pulmonary fibrosis in an aluminum arc welder. *Chest* 1982;81:372–374.
43. Shaver CG, Riddell AR. Lung changes associated with the manufacture of alumina abrasives. *J Ind Hyg Toxicol* 1947;29:145–157.
44. Shaver C. Pulmonary changes encountered in employees engaged in the manufacture of alumina abrasives. *Occup Med* 1948;5:718–728.
45. Wyatt JP, Riddell ACR. The morphology of bauxite-fume pneumoconiosis. *Am J Pathol* 1949;25:447–465.
46. Townsend MC, Enterline PHE, Sussman NB, Bonney TB, Rippey LL. Pulmonary function in relation to total dust exposure at a bauxite refinery and alumina-based chemical products plant. *Am Rev Respir Dis* 1985;132:1174–1180.
47. Townsend MC, Sussman NB, Enterline PE, Morgan WKC, Belk HD, Dinman BD. Radiographic abnormalities in relation to total dust exposure at a bauxite refinery and alumina-based chemical products plant. *Am Rev Respir Dis* 1988;138:90–95.
48. Dinman BD. Alumina-related pulmonary disease. *J Occup Med* 1988; 30:328–335.
49. Gaffuri E, Donna A, Pietra R. Pulmonary changes and aluminum levels following inhalation of alumina dust: a study on four exposed workers. *Med Lav* 1985;76:222–227.
50. Musk AW, Beck BD, Greville HW, Brain JD, Bohannon DE. Pulmonary disease from exposure to an artificial aluminum silicate: further observations. *Br J Ind Med* 1988;45:246–250.
51. Jederlinic PJ, Abraham JL, Churg A, Himmelstein JS, Epler GR, Gaensler EA. Aluminum oxide workers: investigation of nine workers with pathology and microanalysis in three cases. *Am Rev Respir Dis* 1990;142:1179–1184.
52. Andersen A, Dahlberg BE, Magnus K, Wannag A. Risk of cancer in the Norwegian aluminum industry. *Int J Cancer* 1982;29:295–298.
53. Gibbs GW, Horowitz I. Lung cancer mortality in aluminum reduction plant workers. *J Occup Med* 1979;21:347–353.
54. Milham S Jr. Mortality in aluminum reduction plant workers. *J Occup Med* 1979;21:475–480.
55. Simonato L. Carcinogenic risk in the aluminum production industry: an epidemiological overview. *Med Lav* 1981;72:266–276.
56. Rockette HE, Arena VC. Mortality studies of aluminum reduction plant workers: potroom and carbon department. *J Occup Med* 1983;25: 549–557.
57. Mur JM, Moulin J, Mayer-Bisch C, Colon JP, Loulerque J. Mortality of aluminum reduction plant workers in France. *Int J Epidemiol* 1987; 16:257–264.
58. King EJ, Harrison CV, Mohanty GP, Nagelschmidt G. The effect of various forms of alumina on the lungs of rats. *J Pathol Bacteriol* 1955; 69:81–93.
59. King EJ, Harrison CV, Mohanty GP, Yoganathan M. The effect of aluminum and of aluminum containing 5 percent of quartz in the lungs of rats. *J Pathol Bacteriol* 1958;75:429–434.
60. Stacy BD, King EJ, Harrison CV, Nagelschmidt G, Nelson S. Tissue changes in rats' lungs caused by hydroxides, oxides and phosphates of aluminum and iron. *J Pathol Bacteriol* 1959;77:417–426.
61. Pigott GH, Gaskell BA, Ishmael J. Effects of long term inhalation of alumina fibres in rats. *Br J Exp Pathol* 1981;62:323–331.
62. Gross P, Harley RA Jr, DeTreville RTP. Pulmonary reaction to metallic aluminum powders. *Arch Environ Health* 1973;26:227–234.
63. Crissman JW, Maylin GA, Krook L. New York State and U.S. federal fluoride pollution standards do not protect cattle health. *Cornell Vet* 1980;70:183–192.
64. Ernst P, Thomas D, Becklake MR. Respiratory survey of North American Indian children living in proximity to an aluminum smelter. *Am Rev Respir Dis* 1986;133:307–312.
65. Grandjean P, Horder M, Thomassen Y. Fluoride, aluminum and phosphate kinetics in cryolite workers. *J Occup Med* 1990;32:58–63.
66. Lie A, Edward W. The influence of fluoride recovery alumina and the work environment and health of aluminum pot room workers. *Med Lav* 1981;4:313–317.
67. Crombie DW, Blaidell JL, MacPherson G. The treatment of silicosis by aluminum powders. *Can Med Assoc J* 1944;50:318–328.
68. Bamberger PJ. Aluminum therapy in silicosis. *Ind Med* 1945;14:470–77.
69. Kennedy MCS. Aluminum powder inhalations in the treatment of silicosis of pottery workers and pneumoconiosis of coal miners. *Br J Ind Med* 1956;13:85–101.
70. Rifat SL, Eastwood MR, McLachlan DRC, Cory PN. Effect of exposure of miners to aluminum powder. *Lancet* 1990;2:1162–1165.
71. Theriault GP, Tremblay CG, Armstrong BG. Risk of ischemic heart disease among primary aluminum production workers. *Am J Ind Med* 1988;13:659–666.
72. Alfrey AC, Mishell JM, Burks J, et al. Syndrome of dyspraxia and multifocal seizures associated with chronic hemodialysis. *Trans Am Soc Artif Int Organs* 1972;18:257–261.
73. Mahurkar SD, Salta R, Smith EC, Dhar SK, Meyers L, Dunea G. Dialysis dementia. *Lancet* 1973;1:1412–1415.
74. Lederman RJ, Henry CE. Progressive dialysis encephalopathy. *Ann Neurol* 1978;4:199–204.
75. Alfrey AC, LeGendre GR, Kaehny WD. The dialysis encephalopathy syndrome. *N Engl J Med* 1976;294:184–188.
76. Andreoli SP, Bergstein JM, Sherrard DJ. Aluminum intoxication from aluminum containing phosphate binders in children with azotemia not undergoing dialysis. *N Engl J Med* 1984;310:1079–1084.
77. Davidson AM, Oli H, Walker GS, Lewins AM. Water supply aluminum concentration dialysis dementia and effect of reverse-osmosis water treatment. *Lancet* 1982;2:785–787.
78. English A, Savage RD, Britton PG, Ward MK, Kerr DNS. Intellectual impairment in chronic renal failure. *Br Med J* 1978;1:888–890.
79. Bowdler NC, Beasley DS, Fritze EC, et al. Behavioral effects of aluminum ingestion on animal and human subjects. *Pharmacol Biochem Behav* 1979;10:505–512.
80. Elliott HL, MacDougall AL, Fell GS. Aluminum toxicity syndrome. *Lancet* 1978;1:1203.
81. Leeming RJ, Blair JA. Dialysis dementia, aluminum and tetrahydrobiopterin metabolism. *Lancet* 1979;1:556.
82. Wills MR, Savory J. Aluminum poisoning: dialysis encephalopathy, osteomalacia and anaemia. *Lancet* 1983;2:29–33
83. Altmann P, Al-Salihi F, Butter K, et al. Serum aluminum levels and erythrocyte dihydropteridine reductase activity in patients on hemodialysis. *N Engl J Med* 1987;317:80–84.
84. Altmann P, Hamon C, Blair J, Dhanesha U, Cunningham J, Marsh F. Disturbance of cerebral function by aluminum haemodialysis patients without overt aluminum toxicity. *Lancet* 1989;2:7–12.

85. Brem AS, DiMario C, Levy DL. Perceived aluminum-related disease in dialysis population. *Arch Intern Med* 1989;149:2541–2544.
86. Sideman S, Manor D. The dialysis dementia syndrome and aluminum intoxication. *Nephron* 1982;31:1–10.
87. Aluminum and Alzheimer's disease. *Lancet* 1989;1:82–83.
88. Martyn CN, Osmond C, Edwardson JA, Barker DJP, Harris EC, Lacey RF. Geographical relation between Alzheimer's disease and aluminum in drinking water. *Lancet* 1989;1:59–62.
89. Birchall JD, Chappell JS. Aluminum, chemical physiology and Alzheimer's disease. *Lancet* 1988;2:1008–1010.
90. Cohen WJ, Cohen NH. Lithium carbonate, haloperidol and irreversible brain damage. *JAMA* 1974;230:1283–1287.
91. Donaldson IM, Cunningham J. Persisting neurologic sequelae of lithium carbonate therapy. *Arch Neurol* 1983;40:747–751.
92. Weingartner H, Rudorfer MV, Linnoila M. Cognitive effects of lithium treatment in normal volunteers. *Psycholpharmacology* 1985;69:472–474.
93. Neurobehavioral impairment and symptoms associated with aluminum remelting. *Arch Environ Health* 1998;53.

*Environmental and Occupational Medicine, Third Edition,* edited by William N. Rom.
Lippincott–Raven Publishers, Philadelphia © 1998.

# CHAPTER 77

# Metal Compounds and Rare Earths

Emily F. Madden

This chapter presents the hazards of 14 elements that are less recognized and not used extensively in industry.

## ANTIMONY

### Uses and Exposures

Antimony (Sb) is a crystalline silver-white metal and it occurs in tri- and pentavalent compounds. It is sometimes found native, but more frequently it is associated with sulfur as stibnite, and it occurs in ores associated with arsenic. Sb is a common constituent of metal alloys with copper and lead, and stibine gas is formed when these alloys are treated with acid. When antimony is heated, it releases toxic stibine fumes and stibine oxide ($Sb_2O_3$). Antimony is a poor conductor of electricity and heat, but is finding use in semiconductor technology for making infrared detectors, diodes, and Hall-effect devices. Sb is used in batteries, antifriction alloys, type metal, solders, paints, ceramics, glass, pottery, small arms, and tracer bullets, and in the manufacture of flame-proofing compounds.

Medical uses have been found for Sb compounds in tropical antihelminthic (schistosomiasis) and antiprotozoic (leishmaniasis) drugs. Trivalent Sb compounds are highly toxic, more so than the pentavalent Sb compounds, and hence their use is widely banned. Sb toxicity is usually encountered in the medical use of Sb compounds and in occupational exposures in the mining and extraction industries.

### Health Hazards

Antimony belongs in the same periodic group as arsenic, and since both elements share many characteristics, numerous industrial outbreaks and health effects were attributed to arsenic rather than antimony exposure. In 1953, Renes (1) reported the health effects of an antimony smelter with minimal arsenic exposure where the average working zone air concentrations of Sb ranged from 4.7 to 10.2 mg/m$^3$. The most common symptoms of local toxicity include dermatitis, mucous membrane irritation of the nose, throat, and mouth, and pneumoconiosis. White et al. (2) describe the occurrence of antimony spots, the pigmented follicular pustules on the skin of workers exposed to antimony dust and antimony trioxide fumes. These eruptions of the sweaty, hairy friction areas of the skin are transient, and they clear up with reduced exposure to Sb compounds. Symptoms of heavier exposure to antimony trioxide and Sb dusts include coughing, headaches, nausea, vomiting, diarrhea, stomach cramps, anorexia, dyspnea, and the inability to smell.

Antimony pneumoconiosis has been described of workers exposed to Sb dusts and fumes. This condition is marked by a fine reticulonodular infiltrate near the hilum. Pathologic studies revealed particle-laden macrophages, but no occurrence of fibrosis or affected pulmonary function in any of the cases observed (3).

The therapeutic use of antimony compounds for schistosomiasis produces electrocardiographic (ECG) abnormalities, mostly T-wave changes and QT interval prolongation, and has caused sudden death in some patients. Brieger et al. (4) describe an epidemic of sudden death and ECG abnormalities in workers exposed to antimony trisulfide. When exposure to antimony trisulfide was ceased, the ECG abnormalities persisted for some workers but no further deaths occurred. The exact mechanisms of myocardial injury by Sb compounds are not fully understood. A recent study by Tirmenstein and co-workers (5) suggests that potassium antimonyl tartrate may

E. F. Madden: Department of Toxicology, University of Maryland School of Medicine, Baltimore, Maryland 21227.

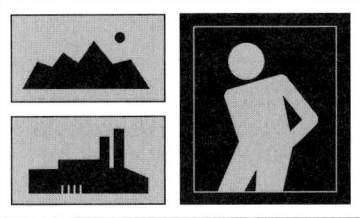

induce lipid peroxidation in cultured cardiac myocytes, and it may interact with thiol-containing molecules, contributing to cell death.

Antimony can have adverse hematologic effects, since trivalent Sb is known to bind mainly to erythrocytes, accounting for its slow elimination from the body. Case reports of hematologic effects in humans involve oral ingestion of antimony-containing therapeutic agents. Harris (6) reported a case where one patient developed hemolytic anemia following repeated injections of faudin (stibophen), an antimony-containing drug formerly used for schistosomiasis. The odorless toxic gas stibine ($SbH_3$) is known to be a potent hemolytic agent, and is associated with the formation of Heinz bodies in red blood cells. Exposure to stibine gas can produce hemolytic crisis followed by acute tubule necrosis and death.

Animal studies have shown that antimony may cause lung cancer (and heart and lung disease) in rodents. A mortality study by Schnorr and co-workers (7) of 1,014 workers at a Texas antimony smelter between 1937 and 1971 revealed an elevated mortality rate with increasing duration of employment. However, their conclusions may be limited by possible confounders and lack of appropriate referent groups.

Most mattress materials contain antimony, arsenic, and phosphorus compounds as fire-retardant additives. It has been hypothesized that microbial generation of toxic gases from antimony, arsenic, and phosphorus may be the primary cause of sudden infant death syndrome (SIDS) (8). Mattress materials in areas affected by the warmth and perspiration of the sleeping infant were found to be infected by the fungus *Scopulariopsis brevicaulis,* which is thought to be capable of generating toxic phosphines, arsines, and stibines from these materials. These gases may possibly cause anticholinesterase poisoning and cardiac failure in infants, but other contributing factors may include the prone sleeping position of the infant and overwrapping (9). Chemical and instrumental analysis of exposed test papers to these exact conditions by Warnock and coworkers (8) do not support the hypothesis that these toxic gases are actually generated and cause SIDS. But Richardson (9) has noted that in England and Wales the progressive rise in SIDS between 1951 and 1988 seems to be related to the increased use of phosphorus, antimony, and arsenic compounds as fire retardant additives in cot mattresses.

### Permissible Exposure Limit

The current Occupational Safety and Health Administration (OSHA) permissible exposure limit (PEL) for antimony metal or powder is 0.5 mg/m$^3$ for an 8-hour time-weighted average (TWA). The OSHA PEL for stibine gas is 0.5 mg/m$^3$ (0.1 ppm) for an 8-hour TWA.

## COPPER

### Uses and Exposures

Copper (Cu) is a reddish brown metal with a bright metallic luster. It is malleable, ductile, and a good conductor of electricity and heat. A member of group IB metals, copper forms either cuprous (I) or cupric (II) compounds. Metallic copper is resistant to corrosion and cannot be attacked by water, air, or nonoxidizing acids. Copper is occasionally found native, but it is found in many minerals such cuprite, malachite, azurite, chalcopyrite, and bornite. Large copper ore deposits are found in Canada, the United States, Chile, Peru, and the Congo (formerly Zaire). The important copper ores are the sulfides, carbonates, and the oxides, and from these ores copper is isolated by smelting, leaching, and electrolysis. The electrical industry is one of the greatest consumers of copper. Large quantities of copper are used in metallic items such as wire, rods, sheets, tubing, piping, roofing materials, and cooking utensils. All United States coins are made of copper alloys, and gun metals also contain copper. Copper compounds are used as pigments, fungicides, insecticides, and as algicides in water purification. The copper compound in Fehling's solution is manipulated in analytical chemistry tests for monitoring sugar levels in biologic samples. Copper is also used in chemical reagents, in pharmaceuticals, in intrauterine contraceptives, and in electroplating. Cupric oxide (black copper oxide) has many applications in batteries, electrodes, paints, ceramic colorants, and artificial gems. Cupric tungstate (VI) and cuprous selenide are used in the manufacture of semiconductors.

### Health Hazards

Copper is an essential trace element, and illness can occur when the diet is deficient or excessive in copper. The main route of exposure is ingestion, but inhalation of copper dusts and fumes can occur in industrial settings. The workers at risk include battery makers, asphalt makers, welders, solderers, gem colorers, and fungicide and insecticide manufacturers. Exposure to dust or fumes can irritate the eyes, nose, throat, and skin. Eye contact with fine copper particles in dust may lead to severe irritation, and possible damage and blindness. Penetration of the eye with elemental or copper alloy particles is referred to as chalcosis. It is marked by a brownish or greenish-brown discoloration of the lens, cornea, or iris. Copper salts can cause irritation, conjunctivitis, and eyelid edema (10). The formation of granulomas, along with the proliferation of fibroblasts, can lead to retinal detachment, and severe reactions can result in opacification (11).

Repeated exposure to copper fumes or dust may cause metal fume fever, a flu-like illness with symptoms of fever, chills, aches, a metallic taste, malaise, chest tightness, and cough. The symptoms may be delayed for several hours after exposure and may subside by the end of the workweek. The symptoms usually return upon reexposure to copper fumes after the weekend. This illness is believed to result from an immune response, and all the symptoms subside following removal from the source of copper exposure (12).

A disease called vineyard sprayer's lung was described in 1969 in Portuguese vineyard workers who sprayed grapevines with a solution of 1% to 2% copper sulfate neutralized by lime (13). These exposed workers developed interstitial pulmonary disease, which included the formation of histiocytic granulomas and nodular fibrohyaline scars containing small amounts of copper. Pulmonary fibrosis occurred among some workers, and a high incidence of alveolar cell carcinoma was noted. Liver damage was observed, and biopsies revealed fibrosis, angiosarcoma, micronodular cirrhosis, and portal hypertension (14). A study of Japanese copper smelters found an increased incidence of lung cancer types, including adenocarcinoma (15). With the exception of the various lung cancers and the incidence of liver angiosarcoma seen in vineyard workers, no evidence of other cancer types has been reported. No teratogenic effects have been reported in humans thus far, but a study in which high levels of copper were given to pregnant mice resulted in increased mortality and severe central nervous system malformations (16).

Renal abnormalities have been noted following copper sulfate ingestion. Symptoms include hematuria, elevated blood nitrogen (BUN), and oliguria. Acute tubular necrosis is often observed from urinalysis and renal biopsy (17). Suicidal copper sulfate ingestion is common in India, and the initial symptoms are nausea, vomiting, and a greenish-blue discoloration of the membranes, followed by hemorrhagic gastritis, diarrhea, and hemolytic anemia by 48 hours.

Copper toxicity has been presumed to involve catalytic hydroxyl radical formation from hydrogen peroxide and $Cu^{1+}$ ions. Excess hydroxyl radicals lead to further free radical damage to vital cellular macromolecules. Gunther et al. (18) found that a variety of copper chelators inhibited the formation of carbon-centered radical adducts, including the drugs penicillamine and triethylenetetramine, which are ordinarily used to treat Wilson's disease.

Wilson's disease is a hereditary copper metabolism disorder resulting in elevated copper levels. High copper levels lead to liver injury in humans, and a similar effect is seen in Bedlington terriers with copper toxicosis. Mental subnormality and lack of urinary catecholamine excretion is also associated with Wilson's disease. The mechanism of liver injury by copper is poorly understood, but a study by Sokol and co-workers (19) suggests that oxidant or free radical damage to hepatic mitochondria is involved in copper toxicity. The recent discovery that the gene for Wilson's disease encodes a copper-transporting adenosine triphosphatase (ATPase) may greatly improve our understanding of the pathophysiology of this disorder and of copper metabolism in humans (20).

### Permissible Exposure Limit

The OSHA PEL for copper dusts and mists is 1.0 mg/m$^3$ for an 8-hour TWA. For copper fumes the PEL is 0.1 mg/m$^3$ TWA.

## FLUORIDE

### Uses and Exposures

Fluorine is the most electronegative and reactive of all elements. It is a pale yellow, corrosive gas that reacts with most inorganic and organic substances. Fluorine-containing ores include fluorspar, fluorapatite, cryolite, and fluorite. Fluorspar ($CaF_2$) is the primary commercial source of fluorine found in the United States and Mexico. Most inorganic fluorides are prepared by the reaction of hydrofluoric acid with oxides, carbonates, hydroxides, chlorides, and metals. Production of hydrogen fluoride comes from the reaction of $CaF_2$ with sulfuric acid, and accounts for 65% of U.S. consumption of fluorspar. Hydrogen fluoride is used in the manufacture of aluminum fluoride, synthetic cryolite, fluoropolymers, and the chlorofluorocarbons used as refrigerants, solvents, and aerosols. Other applications for hydrogen fluoride include stainless steel pickling, inorganic fluoride production, uranium enrichment, and fluorine production. The steel industry employs large amounts of fluorspar, and it is added to slag to make it more reactive. Ceramic, brick, cement, glass fiber, aluminum, and foundry industries also utilize fluorspar ore. The reaction of fluorides with hydroxyapatite (found in tooth enamel) form acid-resistant and less soluble compounds. Fluorides, therefore, are added to public drinking water and toothpaste products to reduce dental caries. Metal fluorides are used in chemical vapor deposition, in ion implantation, for semiconductors, and as unreactive dielectrics. Fluorinated steroids, drugs, and anesthetics have medical applications due to their stability. The most common route of exposure is inhalation of fluoride compounds at steel, foundry, pesticide, aluminum, glass, and nuclear power industries. Ingestion is another route of exposure, with the consumption of high fluoride-contaminated water being the most common.

### Health Hazards

Acute exposure to inorganic fluoride compounds can result in severe irritation to the eyes, nose, and mucous membranes. Dermatitis and skin rashes are common after exposure. Severe skin burns from hydrofluoric acid are persistent, often necrotic, slow healing, and can lead to systemic fluoride toxicity from absorption at the burn site (21). Acute symptoms of severe nausea, vomiting, abdominal burning, diarrhea, and anorexia are associated with most fluoride compounds, and may be due to the formation of hydrofluoric acid in the stomach after ingestion (22). Accidental and suicidal ingestion of soluble fluoride compounds is a common route of acute exposure. A mass poisoning involving 263 victims at the Oregon State Hospital occurred when NaF roach powder was mistakenly added to scrambled eggs (23). Besides the acute symptoms mentioned above, some victims exhibited pallor, a shallow pulse and respiration, wet cold skin, cyanosis, mydriasis, and coma. The most common cause of death following acute fluoride poisoning is cardiovascular collapse (23). Hypotension and circulatory shock may occur from fluid loss due to excess vomiting and diarrhea, from intragastric bleeding, and possibly from central vasomotor depression and vascular smooth muscle depression.

Acute fluoride poisoning can also lead to severe hypocalcemia in which both total and ionic calcium in the plasma is reduced, and hypomagnesemia has also been observed (21). Hypocalcemic tetany may later occur, involving painful involuntary muscle contractions initially of the distal extremities. Fluoride-induced hypocalcemia may be the result of fluoride ion precipitation of calcium to form insoluble $CaF_2$, or it can result from the deposition in the bone of newly formed fluorapatite that can act as a nucleation catalyst for further calcification, hence reducing calcium plasma levels (24). The exact mechanisms responsible for fluoride-induced hypocalcemia is still uncertain.

Fluoride compounds may possibly cause toxic nephritis (22). Past studies indicate several halogenated anesthetics can induce a urinary concentrating defect, partly due to fluoride toxicity in the collecting duct cells. Cittanova and co-workers (25) investigated the effects of fluoride ion in human kidney cells. They exposed cultures of human duct cells to increasing concentrations of fluoride ion and assessed toxicity based on several established end points. Their results suggest that the mitochondrion is a target of fluoride toxicity, and its alteration is partly responsible for sodium and water disturbances observed in fluoride-exposed patients (25).

The use of fluorides in public drinking water to prevent dental caries is a widespread public health measure that has dramatically reduced dental caries in the young. Prolonged ingestion of drinking water with excess fluoride is the common cause of endemic fluorosis, especially in many developing countries.

Inhalation of fluoride particles at the workplace is a common route of exposure, and the fate of these particles depends on their size and solubility. Insoluble fluoride particles can accumulate in the lungs, and interstitial fibrosis and pneumoconiosis with dyspnea and wheezing are sometimes observed. Chest x-rays may show irregular opacities and reticulation distributed through out the lungs (22). In fact, the very first cases of pneumoconiosis in cryolite miners were originally described as silicosis. But this disease should be regarded as nonspecific pneumoconiosis, since the evidence available shows the fibrotic changes may be related to other components of cryolite ore, such as aluminum, which is known to cause fibrosis in the lungs (22).

Chronic fluorine poisoning results in a condition called fluorosis, and the toxic manifestations can take three forms: clinical, skeletal, and dental (26). The clinical (nonskeletal) phase is marked by symptoms of back stiffness, vague joint pains, synovitis, nausea, dyspepsia, anorexia, headache, and vertigo. The occurrence of dental fluorosis, a manifestation of chronic fluoride toxicity on the amleoblasts, can result from the consumption of fluoride-contaminated water, or from exposure to fluoride-containing dusts in the mining of cryolite and fluorspar ores (22,26). The teeth are often mottled in this disease. Bony or skeletal fluorosis often occurs with dental fluorosis. Skeletal fluorosis is seen after chronic fluoride exposure, and the common symptoms include nocturnal back pain, restricted trunk rotation, and slight enlargement of the trabeculae in the lumbar spine. Sclerosis of the bones is caused by the fixation of calcium by fluorine, and the vertebrae, pelvis, and ribs exhibit exostosis and osteophyte formation. There is also increased thickness of the long bones and calcification of the ligaments (22). Past research indicates that the manifestations of fluorosis are irreversible, but there is recent evidence that this may no longer be the case. Gupta and co-workers (26) conducted a study to examine the effect of a combination of calcium, vitamin $D_3$, and ascorbic acid supplementation in fluorosis-affected children. They found a significant improvement in dental, clinical, and skeletal fluorosis along with the relevant biochemical parameters in the affected children. This evidence indicates that fluorosis can be reversed by simple medical treatment.

Chronic inhalation of fluoride compounds may pose a risk for lung cancer. de Villiers and Windish (27) report excess cancer risks for a number of fluorspar miners exposed to fluoride compounds on a daily basis. But the excess cancer risks they discovered may not be directly related to fluoride exposure since these miners were also exposed to radon, a radioactive gas normally encountered in the mining industry. More studies are needed to determine the cancer risk for fluorspar miners and for other workers chronically exposed to fluoride compounds.

Fluorosis may have adverse effects on the reproductive systems of animals and humans. Kumar and Susheela (28) found that chronic fluoride toxicity in rabbits can result in defects to the spermatid and epididymal spermatozoa, thus causing infertility. It has also been observed that male patients with skeletal fluorosis had significantly reduced serum testosterone levels than their normal counterparts (29). Decreased fertility rates from chronic fluoride toxicity has been shown for most mammals studied so far. A recent survey by Freni (30) showed a possible relationship of decreased annual fertility rates of women with exposure to high fluoride levels in drinking water in several regions of the United States. The exact effects of fluoride compounds on the reproductive systems of animals and humans require further investigation.

Fluoride toxicity may also impair certain endocrine functions. For example, Trivedi and co-workers (31) found patients with endemic fluorosis exhibited glucose tolerance abnormalities. But these effects are reversible upon removal from excess fluoride exposure. The exact mechanism of fluoride toxicity on glucose tolerance and insulin secretion is unknown.

### Permissible Exposure Limit

The OSHA PEL for sodium fluoride (as fluorine) and other inorganic solid fluorides is 2.5 $mg/m^3$ for an 8-hour TWA exposure.

### Medical Surveillance

Analysis of urinary fluoride levels can be performed to determine the extent of fluoride exposure. Annual full-sized chest x-rays should be done for workers and miners exposed to fluoride dusts, and bone biopsy to determine the onset of skeletal fluorosis from chronic exposure (22). The recent studies that have shown that fluoride may have reproductive effects prompt careful medical surveillance of the fertility and reproductive health of male and female workers exposed to fluoride compounds.

## MANGANESE

### Uses and Exposures

Manganese (Mn) is a reddish-gray or silvery soft metal and a member of group VII elements of the periodic table. Manganese minerals are widely distributed, and ores containing manganese include pyrolusite, braunite, manganite, hauserite, manganesespat, tephroite, and rhodochrosite. Large quantities of manganese nodules found on the floor of the oceans may become an important source since these nodules contain about 24% manganese. Most manganese is obtained from ores found in Australia, Russia, India, and Brazil. Manganese is used to form many important alloys. In steel, manganese improves rolling and forging qualities, hardness, strength, and wear resistance. Manganese, with aluminum, antimony, and small amounts of copper, can form a highly ferromagnetic alloy. Manganese metal is reactive chemically and decomposes cold water slowly. Many steel and iron manufacturing processes need the addition of manganese to molten iron to reduce its iron oxide content by the formation of manganese oxide. Manganese compounds are used in the manufacture of dry cell batteries, and in paints, bleaching agents, and disinfectants. Manganese is also used as a colorizer and coloring agent in the manufacture of glass and ceramics. Manganese dioxide is used in the preparation of oxygen and chlorine, and in drying black paints. Permanganate is a powerful oxidizing agent and is employed in quantitative chemical analysis and in medicine. Manganese is an essential trace element, and is required for the activity of the enzymes mitochondrial superoxide dismutase, galactosyl transferase, and glutamate synthetase.

### Health Hazards

Inhalation of dusts, mists, and fumes is the primary route of occupational exposure for welders and industrial workers. Acute exposure may produce flu-like symptoms, an illness referred to as metal fume fever or manganese pneumonitis (32). A similar response is also observed of acute copper fume exposure (32). Manganese pneumonitis is more severe and may require antibiotics and bronchodilator therapy. In addition, the patient may be at extra risk of developing hyperactive airways disease and chronic pulmonary disease (33).

Chronic inhalation of manganese dioxide compounds for at least 2 years is known to cause severe neurologic disorders. It usually takes up to several months for symptoms to develop, and victims of chronic exposure tend to recover very slowly. The progression of this illness can occur in three stages (34). The first stage is marked by nonspecific symptoms of apathy, anorexia, asthenia, headaches, hypersomnia, spasms, arthalgias, weakness of the legs, and irritability. The second stage of the illness consists of psychomotor and psychic disturbances, including dysarthria, excess salivation, and difficulty in walking. The third stage is noted by a Parkinson-like syndrome with its associated symptoms. Early detection of the symptoms is crucial, because once the neurotoxic effects from manganese exposure are clinically manifested, the damage to the CNS is irreversible. More investigations are needed to detect the early signs of manganese toxicity by use of behavioral and psychological tests of exposed industrial workers (35).

The neurologic symptoms and the pathologic damage in the basal ganglia of the brain makes manganese neurotoxicity analogous to Parkinson's disease. Defazio and co-workers (36) examined the neuronal target of manganese toxicity by adding $MnCl_2$ to dissociated mesencephalic-striatal cell cultures isolated from rat embryo. Their results suggest that striatal neurons, rather than mesencephalic DA neurons, are the target of Mn toxicity.

The organic manganese compound methylcyclopentadienyl manganese tricarbonyl (MMT) was formerly used as a antiknock agent in unleaded gasoline. An animal study of dermal absorption of MMT has shown it to be very toxic, though no human toxicity has been reported (37). Inhalation exposure to MMT is very low since the agent has a low vapor pressure, and its use has been curtailed due to its interference with catalytic pollution controls.

### Permissible Exposure Limits

The OSHA PEL for manganese and its compounds (fumes) is 1 mg/m$^3$ for an 8-hour TWA, the short-term exposure limit (STEL) is 3 mg/m$^3$, and the ceiling value (CL) is 5 mg/m$^3$. The OSHA PEL for MMT is 0.1 mg/m$^3$ for an 8-hour TWA (skin), and its STEL is 5 mg/m$^3$.

### Medical Surveillance

During periods of possible Mn exposures, industrial workers and miners should receive examinations periodically to detect any changes of behavior, speech, and emotional state. Workers suspected of chronic exposure should have a complete neuropsychological evaluation, and the testing should be based on preexisting neuropsychological tests done before employment. Examination of respiratory problems is extremely important, and workers with respiratory infections should be removed from the source of Mn exposure.

## MOLYBDENUM

### Uses and Exposures

Molybdenum (Mo) metal is silvery white, very hard, but is softer and more ductile than tungsten. Molybdenum is obtained principally from molybdenite, and to lesser extent from wulfenite and powellite ores. Molybdenum can also be recovered as a by-product of tungsten and copper mining operations. Molybdenum rarely occurs in its native state. It is an essential trace element for humans and animals, and its metabolism is related to copper and sulfur metabolism. The major use of molybdenum is as a steel alloy and its utilized in the arms industry, the automobile industry, and in aeronautical engineering. The metal is used in nuclear energy applications, for missile and aircraft parts, and is a valuable catalyst in the refining of petroleum. Mo is a essential trace element in plant nutrition and is necessary for nitrogen fixation by legumes. Some lands can become barren for lack of this element in the soil, and therefore molybdenum is added to fertilizers to stimulate plant growth. Shell fish tend to have high concentrations of molybdenum, since plankton tend to concentrate molybdenum 25 times that of seawater concentrations. The average daily human uptake in food is approximately 350 μg, and Mo is ubiquitous in food products.

### Health Hazards

Chronic molybdenum poisoning due to high Mo content in foliage and in pastures have been observed in cattle and sheep and is known as molybdenosis or "teart." Symptoms include anemia, gastrointestinal disturbances, growth retardation, diarrhea, impaired reproduction, and bone and joint deformities (38). Low copper concentrations contribute to these symptoms, and when copper is added to the diet the symptoms disappear. Copper prevents the accumulation of Mo in the liver, and can antagonize Mo absorption from food. The antagonism of copper and molybdenum in the diet may depend on sulfate, and it has been suggested that sulfate may displace molybdate in the body (38). Molybdenum also has complex metabolic interactions with iron. It has been found that molybdenum may increase the response to iron in iron-deficiency anemias (39).

Molybdenum can have teratogenic effects in mammals. It has been found that water levels greater than 0.25 mg/L can disrupt embryogenesis producing increased mortality, and it can interfere with skeletal ossification in utero (40).

A few cases of pneumoconiosis have been reported among workers exposed to metallic molybdenum and molybdenum trioxide. Risk of exposure may exist in the high-temperature productions of molybdenum compounds. For example, molybdenum trioxide sublimes at 800°C, and has been shown to be irritating to the mucous membranes of animals. Soluble molybdenum compounds and fumes are more toxic than the insoluble disulfide, oxide, and halide compounds. Increased blood uric levels and gout-like symptoms have been reported among exposed workers in a copper-molybdenum plant, and anorexia, joint-muscle pains, and fatigue have been reported in Russian miners exposed to molybdenum compounds (41).

There is some uncertainty concerning the carcinogenicity of Mo compounds. Molybdenum is thought to act in cancer prevention because it has been observed that the absence of molybdenum in human and animal diets correlated with the increase of gastric and esophageal cancers due to other etiologic agents present in food (42). Molybdenum is thought to inactivate the P-450–dependent monooxygenase system. P-450 can bioactivate numerous carcinogens, including the benzopyrenes and polycyclic mycotoxins found in the diet (43). But other studies have shown that repeated exposures of experimental animals to molybdenum trioxide ($MoO_3$) solutions can give rise to increased numbers of lung tumors (44). Further studies are needed to determine the exact mechanisms of molybdenum toxicity in carcinogenesis and its role as a possible anticarcinogen in the diet.

### Permissible Exposure Limit

The OSHA PEL for soluble Mo compounds is 5 mg/m$^3$ for an 8-hour TWA, and for insoluble Mo compounds the PEL is 10 mg/m$^3$ (total dust) for an 8-hour TWA. The respirable fraction is 5 mg/m$^3$.

## OSMIUM

### Uses and Exposures

Osmium (Os) is a lustrous, bluish-white, extremely hard, dense, and brittle metal. It is a member of group VIII elements of the periodic table along with the metal platinum, and is commonly referred to as a platinoid. Platinoids are of high commercial value because of their resistance to many corrosive agents. Osmium is found in iridosule and in platinum-bearing river sands of the Urals, North America, and South America. Osmium metal is difficult to fabricate, and the powered or spongy forms slowly gives off toxic osmium tetroxide which is a strong oxidizing agent and has a unpleasant smell. Osmium can also be obtained as a by-product of copper and nickel refining. Osmium metal is almost entirely used to produce hard metal alloys with other metals of the platinoid group for use in fountain pen tips, instrument pivots, electrical contacts, phonograph needles, and watch bearings. Osmium tetroxide had been used to detect fingerprints but was discontinued due to contact dermatitis. Osmium is used as a catalysts for steroid synthesis, and as a fixing agent for electron microscopy.

### Health Hazards

Osmium itself is not highly toxic, but when heated it gives off a pungent, poisonous fume of osmium tetroxide ($OsO_4$). The principal toxic effects of osmium tetroxide exposure are ocular disturbances and an asthmatic condition caused by severe irritation to the mucous membranes (45). Symptoms of $OsO_4$ vapor inhalation include frontal headaches, severe irritation of the nose, throat, and bronchi, and the occurrence of coryza, cough, and chest tightness (45). In one study, corneal ulcerations and bronchopneumonia were observed in experimental rabbits exposed to high levels of osmium tetroxide vapor within 24 to 96 hours (46). $OsO_4$ is a very strong irritant to the eyes, and initial symptoms of acute exposure are excessive tearing, a feeling of grittiness in the eyes, and the vision of halos around lights. Long-term effects include corneal ulcerations and opacification, and some cases of irreversible blindness have been reported (46). The aqueous solutions and the solid oxide forms both yield significant amounts of $OsO_4$ vapor, and eventually it can be reduced to nontoxic osmium dioxide (47). Skin contact with $OsO_4$ may cause dermatitis and ulcerations of the skin; thus, as stated above, its use as a fingerprinting agent was discontinued.

Renal effects from $OsO_4$ exposure have been reported in humans, and clinical signs include transient hematuria, pyuria, and proteinuria. Renal tubule degeneration have been shown for experimental animals exposed to various levels of $OsO_4$ (48). More studies are needed to assess the mechanisms of osmium tetroxide toxicity to the kidneys, and the development of urinary biomarkers of exposure is necessary to monitor the early signs of hepatic toxicity.

### Permissible Exposure Limits

The OSHA PEL for osmium tetroxide is 0.0016 mg/m$^3$ (0.0002 ppm) for an 8-hour TWA exposure, and the STEL is 0.0006 ppm (Os).

## PHOSPHORUS

### Uses and Exposures

Phosphorus (P) exists in four or more allotropic forms, including white (or yellow) phosphorus; red phosphorus; black (or violet) phosphorus; and ordinary phosphorus, which is a waxy white solid, and when pure it is colorless and transparent. Phosphorus toxicity is manifested by its various forms, including elemental phosphorus, phosphoric acid, the chloro and sulfide compounds, phosphine gas, and the metal sulfides. Phosphorus does not occur free in nature; it is widely distributed in combination with other minerals. An important source of the element is phosphate rock, which contains the mineral apatite, an impure tricalcium phosphate. Large deposits are found in Florida, Tennessee, Utah, Russia, and Morocco. Red phosphorus is insoluble, nonabsorbable, nonvolatile, and fairly stable. It is used in the manufacture of safety matches, pyrotechnics, pesticides, incendiary shells, smoke bombs, and tracer bullets. White or yellow phosphorus is typically pale yellow, and when exposed to light or heat of 250°C it is converted to red phosphorus. White phosphorus can be made by several methods. One common method is the heating of tricalcium phosphate in the presence of carbon and silica in an electric or fuel-fired furnace, and collecting the vapors formed containing elementary phosphorus. White phosphorus should be kept under water since its dangerously reactive in air, and should be handled with forceps. Due to its reactivity, white phosphorus is used in munitions, pyrotechnics, explosives, smoke bombs, and other incendiaries. Phosphorus compounds are used extensively in industry. For example, phosphoric acid is employed in the manufacture of phosphate salts, detergents, fertilizers, soft drinks, pickling, for rust proofing of metals, and as acid catalysts. Calcium phosphate is found in fine chinaware, and is used to produce monocalcium phosphate used in baking powder. Trisodium phosphate is important as a cleaning agent and water softener, and for preventing the corrosion of pipes and boiler tubes. Ultrapure phosphorus is employed in the manufacture of semiconductors and for electroluminescent coatings.

### Health Hazards

Due to the variety of compounds and allotropic forms in which phosphorus exists, and also in gas, solid, and liquid phases, exposure can occur by several routes (inhalation, ocular, oral, dermal, parenteral) in the workplace. White phosphorus is a general protoplasmic poison. White phosphorus can cause serious burns that can be deep and extremely painful, with vesiculation and necrosis. Upon contact, white phosphorus can continue to burn on the skin in the presence of air until all phosphorus is consumed, or until there is the deprivation of oxygen. Healing of phosphorus burns is often slow and poor, and liver and kidney failure may occur from phosphorus absorption at the burn site (49). Burns should be treated quickly by washing with a 5% sodium bicarbonate and 1% copper sulfate solution prior to the removal of any embedded phosphorus particles. For serious burns, the patient should have serum electrolytes, phosphorus, and calcium measurements taken, and receive ECG monitoring (50).

Chronic exposure to white phosphorus may result in the condition called phossy jaw. It is the result of oral absorption of small amounts of phosphorus over long periods of time through the enamel. The disease is marked by a necrosis of the jaw, mainly periostitis, with suppuration, ulceration, and swelling of the mandible. Poor dental hygiene may contribute to this condition, and phossy jaw is reported today mostly in developing countries (51).

Phosphoric acid exposure usually occurs via inhalation. The mist is an irritant to the eyes, respiratory tract, skin, and mucous membranes. It may cause cough, tearing, and blepharospasm, and the symptoms are greater the higher the concentration of exposure. As of yet, there is no evidence that systemic phosphorus poisoning may occur from acute exposure to phosphoric acid (52). Skin contact with tetraphosphorus trisulfide can cause contact dermatitis, and phosphorus pentasulfide is an irritant to the eyes, skin, and respiratory tract.

The chloro compounds of phosphorus, which includes phosphorus trichloride and pentachloride, can produce fumes and vapors causing toxicity upon inhalation exposure. The toxic effects are primarily on the skin, mucous membranes, and the respiratory tract. The characteristic symptoms include conjunctival irritation with lacrimation and photophobia, throat pain, cough, rhinitis, and dyspnea followed by respiratory symptoms ranging from mild bronchial spasms to severe respiratory distress and pulmonary edema (53). Wason et al. (54) reported the exposure of 450 workers to a phosphorus trichloride spill, and they were evaluated in local hospitals. The most common symptoms noted were eye irritation, nausea, vomiting, subjective wheezing, lacrimation, and dyspnea, in decreasing order of severity. Pulmonary function tests also revealed changes in large and small airway resistance correlating with the distance from the spill and the duration of exposure. Chronic exposure to chloro compounds of phosphorus can lead to the development of chronic chemical bronchitis. Damage to the bone tissue may result, and these compounds are capable of penetrating the enamel and acting on the periosteum causing erosion. In an animal study to assess chronic exposure to phosphorus oxychloride, trichloride, and pentachloride, morphologic changes were found in the bone, kidney, liver, and the lungs (53). Pathology of the respiratory tract included desquamative rhinitis, tracheitis, and bronchitis, and after cessation of exposure for a number of months these symptoms still persisted (53).

Phosphine poisoning is another source of phosphorus toxicity. It is a systemic poison that causes depression of the nervous system, liver damage, pulmonary irritation, and clinical symptoms include nausea, vomiting, headache, ataxia, convulsions, and possibly coma. Acute phosphine intoxication may result in delayed pulmonary edema, and workers should be monitored after exposure for up to 48 hours.

### Permissible Exposure Limit

The OSHA PELs for phosphorus compounds are the following: white phosphorus, 0.1 $mg/m^3$; phosphoric acid, 1.0 $mg/m^3$; phosphorus oxychloride, 0.1 ppm; phosphorus pentachloride and pentasulfide, 1.0 $mg/m^3$; phosphorus trichloride, 1.5 $mg/m^3$ and a STEL of 3.0 $mg/m^3$; and phosphine, 0.4 $mg/m^3$ (0.3 ppm) for an 8-hour TWA exposure.

### Medical Surveillance

Workers exposed to white phosphorus should have physical examinations to determine medical and dental health status. Poor dental hygiene may increase the risk of phosphorus toxicity and phossy jaw. White phosphorus burns should be treated quickly to prevent systemic phosphorus toxicity. A recent study by Hu (55) showed medical treatment with an iv drip of calcium gluconate can accelerate the elimination of plasma phosphorus and prevent systemic phosphorus poisoning after major burns (55). Workers exposed to phosphorus chloro compounds, phosphorus sulfides, and phosphoric acid should receive preemployment and routine examinations to assess liver and pulmonary function and overall health status.

## SELENIUM

### Uses and Exposures

Selenium (Se) belongs to subgroup VIa of the periodic table, and has both metallic and nonmetallic properties. It is also a member of the sulfur family and resembles sulfur in its various forms. Selenium exists in several allotropic forms, and three are generally recognized. Selenium can be prepared with either an amorphous or crystalline structure. The color of amorphous selenium is either red in powder form, or black in vitreous form. Naturally occurring selenium contains six stable isotopes, and 15 other isotopes have been recognized. Selenium is found in a few rare minerals such as crooksite and clausthalite. In past years, selenium has been obtained from flue dusts remaining from the processing of copper sulfide ores, but the anode metal produced from electrolytic copper refineries now provide most of the selenium used in industry. Selenium exhibits both photovoltaic and photoconductive properties making the metal vital in the production of photocells, in exposure meters for photographic use, and in solar cells.

Selenium can convert alternating current electricity to direct current, and it is used in rectifiers. Selenium is used in xerography, in the glass industry to decolorize glass, as a photographic toner, and as an additive to stainless steel. It is also employed as a vulcanizing agent in rubber, and is used in fungicides and some medications. Elemental selenium is said to be basically nontoxic, and is considered an essential trace element. Selenium is found in many food stuffs, such as seafood (especially shrimp), meat, milk products, and grains.

### Health Hazards

Elemental selenium has low toxicity; however, hydrogen selenide and other selenium compounds are extremely toxic. Hydrogen selenide is either a by-product of the reaction of acid and water with metal selenides, or of hydrogen gas reacting with soluble selenium compounds. It is more toxic than hydrogen sulfide, but hydrogen selenide is readily converted to elemental selenium on moist surfaces of the mucous membranes and lungs. Acute airborne exposure can irritate the eyes and mucous membranes, and trigger coughs, sneezes, chest tightness, and dyspnea (56). Delayed pulmonary edema may occur 6 to 8 hours after acute exposure, and one death of a factory worker has been reported (57). Other symptoms may include nausea, vomiting, dizziness, fatigue, and garlic odor on the breath. Garlic breath is the most characteristic sign of acute Se intoxication (acute selenosis), and it is due to pulmonary excretion of volatile Se metabolites (58). The sweat may also be garlic scented.

Airborne dusts of selenium dioxide are also irritating to the eyes, nose, and throat, and acute inhalation may cause pulmonary edema. Chronic exposure may produce a pink discoloration of the eyelids, a condition called "rose eyes," and may include conjunctivitis and sensitization to any contact with selenium dioxide (59,60). It is also a strong vesicant, and may cause severe burns upon skin contact. Another condition, known as "rose cold," with symptoms of cough, sore throat, bronchitis, and coryza, can occur from exposure to dimethylselenide, and chronic exposure may lead to granulomatous respiratory disease (59,60).

Diskin et al. (60) describe the 50-year employment of a worker in a selenium refinery who exhibited the development of reddish-orange hair and fingernails, plus high Se concentrations in the lungs, hair, and nails at the autopsy. Mihajlovic (58) reports the clinical signs of chronic selenosis in horses, cattle, and swine, which include loss of hair, emaciation, hoof lesions, and lameness. In advanced cases, liver cirrhosis, atrophy of the heart, and anemia occur. The earliest written report of selenium poisoning is thought to be the detailed description by Marco Polo of a necrotic hoof disease of horses that occurred in China in the 13th century (58). Excessive ingestion of plants naturally containing selenium compounds has long been known to cause Se poisoning and teratogenic effects in animals (61,62).

Human epidemiologic evidence has suggested that selenium may be an anticarcinogen (63). The observation that the oxidation of glutathione by selenite produced superoxides opened a new area for selenium research. Spallholz (63) proposes that selenium compounds are toxic owing to their prooxidant catalytic activity, and carcinostasis appears directly correlated to selenium toxicity at supranutritional Se levels in animals. In other animal studies, selenium has been shown to be carcinogenic. The risk of cancer from selenium exposure is still a topic of debate (64).

### Permissible Exposure Limits

The OSHA PEL for elemental selenium and selenium alloys is 0.2 mg/m$^3$ for an 8-hour time exposure, and for gaseous hydrogen selenide it is 0.2 mg/m$^3$ (0.05 ppm). Gaseous selenium hexafluoride has an OSHA PEL of 0.4 mg/m$^3$ (0.05 ppm) for an 8-hour TWA.

## SILVER

### Uses and Exposures

Pure silver has a brilliant white metallic luster; it is a little harder than gold, and is very ductile and malleable. Pure silver has the highest thermal and electrical conductivity of all the metals, and possesses the lowest contact resistance. In pure air and water it is stable, but it tarnishes when exposed to ozone, hydrogen sulfide, or air containing sulfur. Alloys of silver are very important, and sterling silver is used for jewelry and silverware. Silver is utilized in photographic films with about 30% of U.S. industrial consumption going into this application. Silver has applications in dental alloys, in making solder and brazing alloys, in electrical contacts, and in high-capacity silver-cadmium and silver-zinc batteries. Silver is used in mirror production, and can be deposited on glass or metals by chemical deposition, electrodeposition, and by evaporation. The powerful explosive silver fulminate is sometimes formed during the silvering process, and silver iodide is used in seeding clouds to produce rain. Silver nitrate, also known as lunar caustic, is used extensively in photography. Silver is also used for its germicidal effects.

### Health Hazards

Occupational exposure to silver and its compounds is mainly through airborne dust, metal fumes, and mists of solutions containing silver compounds. Acute exposures to silver nitrate dusts and solutions are irritating to the skin, mucous membranes, the eyes, and the gastrointestinal tract. The tissues can become pigmented with local deposits of insoluble silver-protein complexes in elastic fibers resulting in the condition "argyria." The eyes, mucous membranes, and skin may become pigmented, and deposits in the cornea may permanently impair the vision (65). Oral doses of silver nitrate produce severe gastrointestinal irritation due to its caustic action, and the major route of exposure of silver compounds is via the gastrointestinal tract (65).

Chronic inhalation or ingestion of soluble silver compounds leads to the accumulation of silver in the body since very little silver is excreted over time (66). Complexes of silver and serum albumin can accumulate in the liver from which only a fractional amount is excreted. Chronic occupational exposure may result in the condition of industrial argyria (67), in which the skin shows widespread slate-gray pigmentations, and the skin may become black with a metallic luster (66). The eyes may become affected to such a point that the lens and vision are disturbed. The respiratory tract may also be affected in some cases (65). Exposed persons may become permanently disfigured by industrial argyria (66). Soluble silver compounds have been found to cause kidney damage in animals. A study of exposed workers producing precious-metal powder showed a decrease in creatinine clearance, but these findings may have been confounded by the effects of cadmium present in the production process (65).

Applying silver sulfadiazine to extensive burn wounds may present considerable silver concentrations in the systemic circulation and may have possible effects on delayed wound healing (68).

### Permissible Exposure Limits

The OSHA PEL is 0.01 mg/m$^3$ TWA for silver metal, dust, and fumes and for soluble silver compounds. These low exposure limits for soluble silver compounds are for the prevention of argyria.

## TELLURIUM

### Uses and Exposures

Tellurium (Te) is a silvery-white, lustrous metal that is quite brittle and can be easily pulverized. Crystalline tellurium has a silvery-white appearance, and amorphous tellurium is a black powder obtained by precipitating tellurium from a solution of telluric or tellurous acid. Tellurium is a p-type semiconductor, and its conductivity is increased when exposed to light. Tellurium is occasionally found native, but more often it is found in calaverite and with other metals. It can be recovered from anode muds that are produced during the electrolytic refining of blister copper, and from the refining and smelting of other metals such as lead and bismuth. Tellurium is used as an alloy with iron and steel to improve strength and hardness, and its addition to lead can decrease the corrosive action of sulfuric acid. It is employed as a vulcanizing agent in rubber, and is utilized in ceramic, glass, and coin productions. Tellurium is a basic ingredient in blasting caps, and is added to cast iron for chill control. Bismuth telluride is widely used in thermoelectric devices. Metal tellurides and organic tellurium compounds are also used in bactericides, drugs, photographic chemicals, plating and etching solutions, and in water treatment reagents. Dairy products, nuts, condiments, and fish have high concentrations of tellurium, and some plants, such as garlic, can accumulate tellurium from the soil. Potassium tellurate has been used as an agent to reduce sweating.

### Health Hazards

The common route of exposure to Te compounds is the inhalation of dusts, vapors, and gases. Toxicity can be produced by elemental tellurium, by the gases hydrogen telluride, tellurium hexafluoride, tellurium dioxide, and by the acid forms. Tellurium vapors and dusts are respiratory irritants. Elemental tellurium has a lower toxicity, and it is converted in the body to dimethyl telluride, which imparts a garlic-like odor to the breath and sweat (69). Foundry workers exposed to as little as 0.01 mg/m$^3$ in the air can develop tellurium breath, and experience such symptoms as nausea, anorexia, depression, itchy skin, and a metallic taste (69).

Hydrogen telluride and tellurium dioxide have a similar toxicity to that of selenium dioxide and hydrogen selenide. Acute inhalation of vapors can produce irritation of the respiratory tract, and may lead to the development of bronchitis and pneumonia. Other symptoms include headaches, malaise, eye irritation, weakness, decreased sweating, dry throat, scaly and itchy skin lesions, a metallic taste, and cardiac symptoms (69). Acute exposure to tellurium hexafluoride vapors cause severe respiratory irritation and delayed pulmonary edema, and systemic toxicity may affect the skin causing blue discolorations in the webs of the fingers (70). Clinical toxicity can also be manifested by peripheral and central neurotoxicity, and liver and kidney damage has also been observed.

A number of animal studies suggest that tellurium may cause neuropathy (71). A recent a study by Larner (72) suggests a possible role for tellurium in the pathogenesis of Alzheimer's disease. Tellurium has been reported to produce cognitive impairment and cerebral lipofuscinosis in experimental rats. These changes are similar to those seen in Kuf's disease, a condition that shares many clinical features with Alzheimer's disease. Tellurium can damage mitochondria and decrease cell metabolism, and these effects may be relevant to the pathogenesis of the disease (72). The deficiency of selenium, which can act as a physiologic antagonist to tellurium, may play an important factor in tellurium toxicity and the pathogenesis of

Alzheimer's disease (72). Animal studies indicate tellurium to have reproductive effects, and it is a teratogen at high levels. In some studies, it has been observed to cause testicular effects in rats (73). So far, no reports of these effects were reported for exposed industrial workers, and such studies are needed to assess the possibility.

### Permissible Exposure Limits

The OSHA PEL for tellurium and its compounds (dusts or fumes) is 0.1 mg/m$^3$ for an 8-hour TWA. For tellurium hexafluoride the OSHA PEL is 0.2 mg/m$^3$.

## THALLIUM

### Uses and Exposures

Thallium (Tl) is a very soft, malleable, bluish-white metal, and it is found in crooksite, lorandite, and hutchinsonite. It is also obtained from the smelting of lead and zinc ores, and can be recovered from the roasting of pyrite ores. Twenty-five isotopic forms of thallium exist with atomic masses ranging from 184 to 210, and natural thallium is a mixture of two isotopes. Thallium is used in the production of semiconductors, photoelectric equipment, optical lenses, and low-temperature thermometers. Thallium oxide has been used to produce glasses with a high index of refraction. Thallium sulfate, an odorless and tasteless compound, was widely used as a rodenticide and a insecticide in the United States, but has been prohibited since 1975 due to its high toxicity. Thallium has been used medicinally to treat scalp ringworm and other skin infections, and also as a depilatory for excess hair removal. Isotope Tl-201 is used for cardiac scanning and the diagnosis of cardiac ischemia (74). Medical use has been very limited due to the high toxicity of thallium over its therapeutic benefits.

### Health Hazards

Thallium is the most toxic of the heavy metals and the lethal oral dose ranges from 0.5 to 1.0 g for thallium salts (75). Because thallium and potassium have the same charge and similar ionic radii, thallium follows potassium distribution pathways and alters a number of $K^+$-dependent processes. The possible toxic mechanisms of thallium may include ligand formation with protein sulfhydryl groups, inhibition of cellular respiration, interaction with riboflavin-based cofactors, and the disruption of calcium homeostasis (76).

The more water-soluble salts, such as thallium sulfate, acetate, and carbonate, have the highest toxicity, and most cases of thallium toxicity occur after oral ingestion either by accident or suicidal intent. Gastrointestinal absorption is rapid and thallium can appear in the urine in 1 hour (77). The elimination half-life is between 1.7 and 30 days depending on the time of and the duration of ingestion. Thallium may act as a cumulative poison due to its long terminal elimination half-life (74). Because thallium salts are colorless, tasteless, and odorless, it has been used in poisonings and murders. Its sale is highly regulated in some countries; for example, in Britain the sale of thallium salts is strictly licensed (74).

Severe toxicity has been reported after inhalation of thallium contaminated dusts from pyrite burners and from zinc and lead smelting. Thallium toxicity has also been reported in the manufacture of cadmium after dermal absorption through protective rubber gloves (74). The principal clinical features of thallotoxicosis are gastroenteritis, peripheral neuropathy, and alopecia (76). Long-term effects may include fatigue, weakness, insomnia, poor appetite, mood changes, irritability, a metallic taste in the mouth, and pains in the arms and legs.

With acute intoxication, there may be a direct effect of thallium on both the sinus node and on cardiac muscle contractility, leading to hypotension and bradycardia (78). Hypertension can soon follow, possibly due to degeneration of the vagus nerve.

Nervous system symptoms can occur including painful peripheral neuropathies. Nerve damage is indicated by signs of numbness and dysesthesias in the arms and legs (79). Nerve damage is wallerian degeneration followed by demyelinization, a progression very similar to that in Guillain-Barré syndrome (80). Tremors, abnormal muscle jerking, loss of vision, and permanent brain damage can occur.

Gastrointestinal symptoms may include abdominal pains, bloody diarrhea, and sometimes refractory constipation. Diffuse alopecia occurs 3 to 4 weeks after ingestion if the patient survives. A dark pigmentation at the base of the hair shaft may be diagnostic of thallium exposure before the onset of alopecia (81). The hair loss may be due to disruption of energy metabolism rather than protein synthesis inhibition (82).

High concentrations of thallium in waters near the tailings of lead and zinc mines can pose an environmental concern. The thallium taken up in algae and moss are eaten by fish; thus, it may accumulate and pose a possible risk of toxicity to consumers of fish (83).

### Permissible Exposure Limits

The OSHA PEL for soluble thallium compounds is 0.1 mg/m$^3$ for an 8-hour TWA (skin).

### Medical Surveillance

The diagnosis of thallium poisoning is confirmed by the presence of elevated Tl levels in the urine or other biologic samples. Treatment with prussian blue (potassium ferrichexacyanoferrate) or with activated charcoal interrupts the enterohepatic cycling of the metal and enhance fecal elimination of Tl (76). Forced diuresis with potassium chloride loading increases renal clearance of Tl, but this treatment should be used cautiously since cardiovascular and neurologic symptoms may be exacerbated. Other supportive measures may be necessary since potassium loading is not a specific antidote for Tl intoxication (76). Other treatments include the use of dithiocarb and dithizone, but these lipophilic chelators may distribute to the CNS and may cause more neurologic damage. Potassium loading and forced diuresis combined with hemodialysis is the most effective treatment for Tl toxicity (84).

## TIN

### Uses and Exposures

Tin (Sn) is a silver-white metal; it is malleable and slightly ductile, and has a highly crystalline structure. When tin is cooled below 13.2°C, it is converted to another allotropic form called gray tin. This transformation is the "tin pest," and it may be affected by impurities such as aluminum and zinc and can be prevented by small additions of bismuth or antimony. There are very few commercial uses for gray tin. Tin is found mainly in cassiterite ($SnO_2$) and most of the world's supply comes from Bolivia, Indonesia, Malaya, the Congo, Thailand, and Nigeria. Tin is obtained by reducing the ore with coal in a reverberatory furnace. Tin is composed of nine stable isotopes, and 18 unstable isotopes are known to exist. Tin is used in tin plating of other metals since tin can take on a high polish and prevent corrosion. Alloys of tin are industrially very important, and these alloys include bronze, pewter, soft solder, gun metal, bell metal, fusible metal, type metal, and die casting alloy. Stannous chloride and inorganic tin compounds are used in the manufacture of toothpaste, ceramics, porcelain, enamel, drill glass, and ink. Stannous chloride is also employed as a reducing agent and as a mordant in calico printing. Tin salts sprayed onto glass are used to produce electrically conductive coatings, and these have been used for panel lighting and for frost-free windshields. Organotin compounds, including dibutyl and tributyl tin oxides, are used as catalysts and stabilizers in rubber and polymer productions, and dioctyl tin is a stabilizer in polyvinyl chloride film productions. Triphenyl tin is used in bactericides, sanitizing agents, fungicides, and in wood preservatives. The trialkyl and triaryl tin compounds are used as biocides, and must be handled carefully.

### Health Hazards

Tin salts are irritants to the eyes, skin, and mucous membranes, especially dusts or mists of acidic and basic tin salts. Organic tin compounds can cause skin burns that itch, especially tributyl and dibutyl oxides. Skin burns may heal if there are no secondary infections. Extended skin contact with organic tin compounds can cause erythematous dermatitis, but healing can occur quickly if contact is ceased.

Alkyl and aromatic tin compounds are highly potent neurotoxins. Trialkyl compounds, such as triethyltin, can cause encephalopathy and cerebral edema. Toxicity of alkyl compounds decreases as the number of carbon atoms in the chain increases. Prull and Rompel (85) report that excessive industrial exposures to triethyl tin produced symptoms of headaches, visual defects, nausea, and EEG changes that were slowly reversed. The trialkyl tin compounds are the most toxic of the organotins. Experimental exposures to triethyl tin was found to produce depression and cerebral edema. Tributyl tin has been shown to cause immunosuppression, weight loss, and anemia in experimental animals. Due to the toxic effects of tributyl tin, it is used as a biocide in exterior paints only, not in interior paints (86). Chronic inhalation of inorganic tin in the form of dusts or fumes can lead to a benign pneumoconiosis called stannosis (87). Inhalation of tin oxides in molten metal refining can lead to this condition. Progressive changes in chest radiographs parallel the duration and intensity of inorganic tin exposures (87). Stannosis can be readily diagnosed at its early stages by chest radiography because the inhaled tin particles are quite radiopaque and very easily seen. The changes observed with stannosis do not seem to involve any fibrosis or pulmonary function impairment (87).

Tin toxicity may involve the inhibition of certain key enzymes. It is suggested that tin may inhibit the hydrolysis of adenosine triphosphate and uncouple oxidation phosphorylation in the mitochondria (88). Tin may also inhibit enzymes acid phosphatase and hepatic succinate dehydrogenase. Tin can interfere with heme formation by the competitive antagonism with iron, zinc, and copper (89).

### Permissible Exposure Limits

The OSHA PEL for organic tin compounds is 0.1 $mg/m^3$ for an 8-hour TWA exposure, and the OSHA PEL for inorganic tin compounds (flake, metal, powder, except oxides) is 2 $mg/m^3$ TWA.

Examinations of workers exposed to organotin compounds should focus on the nervous system, the eyes, and the skin for any burns. Laboratory testing of hematologic, hepatic, and renal functions can be performed. Experimental animal studies for several therapies of tin intoxication have been performed, and dimercaprol and steroid therapy have shown great promise (90).

## URANIUM

### Uses and Exposures

Uranium (U) is a heavy metal, silvery-white in color, a little softer than steel, malleable, ductile, and widely distributed over the earth. Now considered to be more plentiful than cadmium, mercury, or silver, it is found to occur in numerous minerals such as pitchblende, carnotite, and uraninite. Uranium is pyrophoric when in a fine powder or chipform, and when exposed to air it slowly oxidizes. Uranium has known 15 isotopes, all of which are radioactive. Naturally occurring uranium contains primarily 99.28% of U-238 isotope, and 0.72% of U-235 isotope (92). Uranium is of great importance as a reactor fuel for nuclear reactors, since U-235 isotope can undergo nuclear fission with slow neutron bombardment and produce significant energy. Depleted uranium (DU), a highly dense by-product of U-235 enrichment process, has many applications, including its use as penetrators in cannon rounds, as radiation shielding material, and as counterweights for aircraft control surfaces. Inhalation is the most common mode of occupational exposure, although uranium may be absorbed through the skin or ingested. Acute renal failure is the better-known disorder resulting from acute intoxication with soluble uranium compounds, and radiotoxicity of lung tissue can result from inhalation of insoluble uranium particles (91).

The last 50 years have seen enormous expansion in the mining and processing of uranium ore. Common mining methods of uranium ore include open-pit mining, underground mining, and *in situ* leach mining. After mining, the ore is crushed and ground up, and treated with acid (leaching) to dissolve the uranium minerals. Then it is recovered from solution and heat-dried. The end product is known as yellowcake (U3O8), an uranium ore concentrate containing 70% to 90% by weight of uranium oxides (92). U3O8 is then converted into the gas uranium hexafluoride (UF6), which enables it to undergo U-235 enrichment process for use as nuclear fuel. Enrichment of UF6 can be conducted by gaseous diffusion, gas centrifuge, and laser isotope methods. Enriched UF6 is then converted into uranium dioxide ($UO_2$), which is formed into fuel pellets, placed inside thin metal tubes, and assembled into fuel rods for the core of the nuclear reactor. Depleted uranium by-product is stored as UF6 and requires highly controlled storage conditions since it is a corrosive material when moist, and radioactivity may increase with time as decay products form (91). Due to its great abundance at low cost, the military has found important uses for DU, especially its use in penetrators and armor-piercing munitions.

### Health Hazards

Uranium is radioactive, but not strongly radioactive; the radiation emitted during its decay is mostly alpha particles, though gamma rays, beta particles, and neutrons are also emitted (91). More radioactive elements encountered in uranium mining are radium and radon gas in the ore, especially if the ore is high grade. Gamma radiation comes mostly from radium, and radon gas decays into solid radon daughters polonium-218 and polonium-214, which are significantly alpha-radioactive. Inhalation of dusts and aerosol particles during the mining process is the main route of exposure to these isotopes. Solid radon daughters can deposit on the bronchial airways, and as the airway lining is only 40 μm thick, the alpha particles emitted can give up energy to nearby cells, causing genetic damage and the induction of lung cancer (93). Relative risks of lung cancer in U.S. uranium miners were estimated by Hornung and Meinhardt (93) through the use of the Cox proportional hazards model. Their results indicated that the exposure-response relationship was a slightly convex curve, predicting excess relative risks between 0.9 and 1.4 per 100 working level months (WLM) in the lower cumulative exposure range (94).

Studies of the chemical toxicity of uranium found the kidney to be the most sensitive organ to uranium exposure.

The uranyl ion is rapidly absorbed from the gastrointestinal tract where 60% is carried as a soluble bicarbonate complex, and can produce systemic toxicity in the form of acute renal damage and renal failure. Renal toxicity is believed to be brought about by filtration through the glomerulus of the uranyl-bicarbonate complex, reabsorption by the proximal tubule, and liberation of uranyl ions with subsequent damage to the tubular cells (94). This damage may reduce renal proximal tubular reabsorption of glucose, sodium, amino acids, and low molecular weight proteins. A study of uranium mill workers by Thun et al. (95) suggests that workers' long-term low-level exposure to yellowcake (U3O8) is associated with $\beta_2$-microglobulinuria and aminoaciduria, indicating reduced renal tubular reabsorption.

Depleted uranium (DU) in armor-piercing munitions was first used in combat in the Persian Gulf War. When DU munition hits its intended target, there is the release of micrometer-size uranium oxide particles upon burning of DU metal, along with the generation of DU shrapnel and dust upon impact. Long-term clinical studies are now under way to assess the toxicologic impact of exposures to embedded DU shrapnel of injured U.S. personnel.

### Permissible Exposure Limits

The OSHA PEL for soluble uranium compounds is 0.05 mg(U)/m$^3$ for an 8-hour TWA, and for insoluble uranium compounds it is 0.2 mg(U)/m$^3$.

## VANADIUM

### Uses and Exposures

Vanadium (V) is a bright white metal; it is soft and ductile, and it has good corrosion resistance to alkalis, hydrochloric and sulfuric acid, and saltwater. Vanadium has good structural strength, and it is useful in nuclear applications since it has a low fission neutron cross section. Natural vanadium is mostly a mixture of two isotopes, V-51 isotope (99.76%) and V-50 isotope (0.24%), and V-50 isotope is found to be slightly radioactive. Vanadium is found in carnotite, vanadinite, patronite, and roscoelite minerals. It is also found in certain iron ores, in phosphate rock, and in some crude fuel oils in various organic forms. Much of the vanadium being produced is formed by calcium reduction of vanadium pentaoxide ($V_2O_5$) in a pressure vessel. About 80% of vanadium produced is employed as a steel additive known as ferrovanadium. Vanadium is used in producing rust-resistant and high-speed tool steels, and is an important carbide stabilizer in making steels. Vanadium foil is utilized as a bonding agent in cladding titanium to steel. Vanadium pentoxide is used in ceramics, as a catalyst in the production of ethylene-propylene synthetic rubber, in dye mordants, in paint and varnish drying, in glass and ink manufacture, and in photographic chemicals. Vanadium is also used to produce superconductive magnets with a field of 175,000 gauss.

### Health Hazards

Vanadium compounds act mainly as conjunctivae and respiratory tract irritants. Acute local effects of exposure to vanadium-containing dusts include sneezing, rhinitis, sore throat, dry or persistent cough, and chest pains. Bronchitis and asthma may occur in workers exposed to vanadium compounds (96). Symptoms of acute exposure can disappear after immediate removal from exposure to vanadium compounds, but a dry or productive cough may persist for several weeks. A sensitization response can occur upon repeated acute exposure to vanadium-containing dusts (96). The metabolism of sulfur-containing amino acids may be affected by vanadium compounds, and workers exposed to vanadium compounds have shown decreased cysteine content in their fingernails. Vanadium may be part of the normal control of the sodium-potassium ATPase pumps in heart muscle, and vanadium may have positive and negative ionotropic action affecting the force of contractility of the atrial and ventricular myocardium (97). Other symptoms linked to industrial vanadium exposure include gastrointestinal distress, vomiting, nausea, nervous depression, and kidney damage.

It is well established that circulating levels of vanadate ($V^{5+}$) and vanadyl ($V^{4+}$) are reproductive and developmental toxicants in mammals. Decreased fertility and increased embryolethality, fetotoxicity, and teratogenicity have been reported to occur in rats, hamsters, and mice following vanadium compound exposure (98). Domingo and co-workers (99) studied the efficacy of tiron to ameliorate the developmental effects of vanadate in experimental mice. They found a decrease of reabsorbed fetuses, an increase of mean fetal weight, and a reduction of skeletal deformities when metavanadate-exposed pregnant mice were treated with the tiron chelator. The protective activity of tiron may be due to decreased vanadium levels in the embryos when tiron chelates metavanadate before it crosses the placental barrier.

In recent years, pharmacologic interest in vanadium compounds has increased. There is a medical role for vanadium as a chemotherapeutic agent since vanadium is used for chemoprotection against cancers in experimental animals (100). Sakurai (100) studied both the toxic and beneficial effects of vanadium distribution in rats, and discovered that incubation of DNA with vanadyl ion and hydrogen peroxide led to intense DNA cleavage.

### Permissible Exposure Limit

The OSHA PEL for respirable dust and fume is 0.05 mg ($V_2O_5$)/$m^3$ for an 8-hour TWA exposure.

## REFERENCES


1. Renes LE. Antimony poisoning in industry. *Arch Ind Hyg Occup Med* 1953;7:99.
2. White GP Jr, Mathias CG, Davin JS. Dermatitis in workers exposed to antimony in a melting process. *J Occup Med* 1993;35:329–395.
3. Gross P, Westrick ML, Brown THU, et al. Toxicological study of calcium halophosphate phosphors and antimony trioxide: II. Pulmonary studies. *Arch Ind Health* 1955;11;473–478.
4. Brieger H, Semisch CW, Stasneg J, et al. Industrial antimony poisoning. *Ind Med Surg* 1954;23:521–523.
5. Tirmenstein Ma, Plews PI, Walker CV, et al. Antimony-induced oxidative stress and toxicity in cultured cardiac myocytes. *Toxicol Appl Pharmacol* 1995;130:41–47.
6. Harris JW. Studies on the mechanisms of drug-induced hemolytic anemia. *J Lab Clin Med* 1956;47:760–775.
7. Schnorr TM, Steenland K, Thun MJ, Rinsky RA. Mortality in a cohort of antimony smelter workers. *Am J Ind Med* 1995;27(5):759–770.
8. Warnock DW, Delves HT, Campell CK, et al. Toxic gas generation from plastic mattresses and sudden infant death syndrome. *Lancet* 1995;346 (8989):1560–1520.
9. Richardson BA. Sudden infant death syndrome: a possible primary cause. *J Forensic Sci Soc* 1994;34(3):199–204.
10. Cohen SR. A review of the health hazards from copper exposure. *J Occup Med* 1974;16:621–624.
11. Kagorski Z. Comparative studies in chronic ocular chelosis. *Klin Oczna* 1987;91:73–74.
12. Andrews AC, Lyons TD. Binding of histamine and antihistamine to bovine serum albumin by mediation with Cu (II). *Science* 1957;126:561.
13. Pimentel JC, Marques F. Vineyard sprayer's lung. *Thorax* 1969;24: 415.
14. Pimentel JC, Manzes AP. Liver granulomas containing copper in vineyard sprayer's lung. *Am Rev Respir Dis* 1975;111:189–195.
15. Tokudome S. Histologic types of lung cancer among male Japanese copper smelter workers. *Am J Ind Med* 1988;14:137–143.
16. Agarqal K, Sharma A, Talukder G. Effects of copper on mammalian cell components. *Chem Biol Interact* 1989;69:1–16.
17. Chuttani HK, Gupta PS, Gulati S, Gupta DN. Acute copper sulfate poisoning. *Am J Med* 1965;39:849–854.
18. Gunther MR, Hanna PM, Mason RP, Cohen MS. Hydroxyl radical formation from cuprous ion and hydrogen peroxide: a spin-trapping study. *Arch Biochem Biophys* 1995;316:515–522.
19. Sokol RJ, Twedt D, McKim JM Jr, et al. Oxidant injury to hepatic mitochondria in patients with Wilson's disease and Bedlington terriers with copper toxicosis. *Gastroenterology* 1994;107(6):1788–1798.
20. Schilsky ML. Wilson disease: genetic basis of copper toxicity and natural history. *Semin Liver Dis* 1996;16:83–95.
21. Tepperman PB. Fatality due to acute systemic fluoride poisoning following a hydrofluoric acid skin burn. *J Occup Med* 1980;22:691–692.

22. Grandjean P. Occupational fluorosis through 50 years: clinical and epidemiological experiences. *Am J Ind Med* 1982;3:227–236.
23. Lidbeck WL, Hill IB, Beeman JA. Acute sodium fluoride poisoning. *JAMA* 1943;121:826–827.
24. Simpson E, Rao LGS, Evans RM, et al. Calcium metabolism in a fatal case of sodium fluoride poisoning. *Ann Clin Biochem* 1980;17:10–14.
25. Cittanova ML, Lelongt B, Verpont MC, et al. Fluoride ion toxicity in human kidney collecting duct cells. *Anesthesiology* 1996;84:428–435.
26. Gupta SK, Gupta RC, Seth AK, Gupta A. Reversal of fluorosis in children. *Acta Paediatr Jpn* 1996;38:513–519.
27. de Villiers AJ, Windish JP. Lung cancer in a fluorspar mining community. *Br J Ind Med* 1964;21:94–109.
28. Kumar A, Susheela AK. Ultrastructural studies of spermiogenesis in rabbit exposed to chronic fluoride toxicity. *Int J Fertil Menopausal Stud* 1993;39:164–171.
29. Susheela AK, Jethanandani P. Circulating testosterone levels in skeletal fluorosis patients. *J Toxicol Clin Toxicol* 1996;34:183–189.
30. Freni SC. Exposure to high fluoride concentrations in drinking water is associated with decreased birth rates. *J Toxicol Environ Health* 1994; 42:109–121.
31. Trivedi N, Mithal A, Gupta SK, Godbole MM. Reversible impairment of glucose tolerance in patients with endemic fluorosis. Fluoride Collaborative Study Group. *Diabetologia* 1993;36:826–828.
32. Piscator M. Health hazards from inhalation of metal fumes. *Environ Res* 1976;11:268–270.
33. Brooks SM, Weiss MA, Bernstein IL. Reactive airways dysfunction syndrome (RADS). Persistent asthma syndrome after high level irritant exposures. *Chest* 1985;88:376–384.
34. Saric M, Markicevic A, Hrustic O. Occupational exposure to manganese. *Br J Ind Med* 1977;34:114–118.
35. Iregren A. Using psychological tests for the early detection of neurotoxic effects of low level manganese exposure [review]. *Neurotoxicology* 1994;15:671–677.
36. Defazio G, Soleo L, Zefferino R, Livrea P. Manganese toxicity in serumless dissociated mesencephalic and striatal primary culture. *Brain Res Bull* 1996;40:257–262.
37. Hinderer RK. Toxicity studies of methylcyclopentadienyl manganese tricarbonyl (MMT). *Am Ind Hyg Assoc J* 1979;40:164–167.
38. Bremner I. The toxicity of cadmium, zinc, and molybdenum and their effects on copper metabolism. *Proc Nutr Soc* 1979;38:235–242.
39. Seelig M. Copper-molybdenum in iron deficiency and storage disease. *Am J Clin Nutr* 1973;26:657–672.
40. Nadeenko VG, Lenchenko VG, Genkina SB, et al. New data for the standardization of tungsten and molybdenum in their separate and simultaneous presence in water bodies. *Farmakol Toskikol* 1978;41:620–623.
41. Lener J, Bibr B. Effects of molybdenum on the organism. *J Hyg Epidemiol Microbiol Immunol* 1984;29:405–419.
42. Barch DH. Esophageal cancer and microelements. *J Am Coll Nutr* 1989; 8:99–107.
43. Wei HJ, Luo XM, Yang XP. Effect of molybdenum and tungsten on mammary carcinogenesis in Sprague-Dawley (SD) rats. *Chin Cancer J* 1987;9:204–207.
44. Stoner GD, Skimkin MB, Troxell MC. Test for carcinogenicity of metallic compounds by the pulmonary tumor response in strain A mice. *Cancer Res* 1976;36:1744–1747.
45. McLaughin AIG, Milton R, Perry KMA. Toxic manifestations of osmium tetroxide. *Br J Ind Med* 1946;3:138.
46. Wald P, Becker C. Toxic gases used in the microelectronics industry. *Occup Med* 1986;1:105–117.
47. Smith IC, Carson BL, Ferguson TL. Osmium: an appraisal of environmental exposure. *Environ Health Perspect* 1974;8:201–213.
48. Hygienic Guides Committee. Osmium and its compounds. *Am Ind Hyg Assoc J* 1968;29;621–623.
49. Ben-Hur N. Phosphorus burns. *Prog Surg* 1978;16:180–181.
50. Kaufman T, Ullman Y, Har Shai Y. Phosphorus burns: a practical approach to local treatment. *J Burn Care Rehabil* 1988;9:474–475.
51. Teng HQ. Health conditions and the development of mandibular injuries in workers at yellow phosphorus factory. *Chung Hua Kua Ching* 1987;23:242–243.
52. Lewis RJ Sr, Sweet DV, eds. Registry of toxic effects of chemical substances (RTECS). DHHS(NIOSH) pub no. 84. Washington, DC: Department of Health and Human Services, 1984;101–106.
53. Roshchin AV, Molodkina NN. Chlorocompounds of phosphorus as industrial hazards. *J Hyg Epidemiol Microbiol Immunol* 1977;21:387–394.
54. Wason S, Gomolin I, Gross P, Mairam S, Lovejoy FH Jr. Phosphorus trichloride toxicity: preliminary report. *Am J Med* 1984;77:1039–1042.
55. Hu AJ. Intravenous drop of calcium gluconate for phosphorus burns. *Chin J Surg* 1993;31:421–424.
56. Glover JR. Selenium and its industrial toxicity. *Ind Med* 1970;30: 50–54.
57. Schellman B, Raithel H, Schaller K. Acute fatal selenium poisoning. Toxicological and occupational medicine aspects. *Arch Toxicol* 1986; 41:354–358.
58. Mihajlovic M. Selenium toxicity in domestic animals. [Serbo-Croatian (Cyrillic)]. Glas Srp Akad Nauka [Med] 1992;42:131–144.
59. Hunter D. *The diseases of occupations,* 5th ed. Boston: Little, Brown, 1975.
60. Diskin DJ, Tomasso CL, Alper JC, et al. Long term selenium exposure. *Arch Intern Med* 1979;139:824–826.
61. National Research Council. *Selenium.* Washington, DC: National Academy of Sciences, 1976.
62. Whanger P, Vendeland S, Park YC, Xia Y. Metabolism of subtoxic levels of selenium in animals and humans [review]. *Ann Clin Lab Sci* 1996;26:99–113.
63. Spallholz JE. On the nature of selenium toxicity and carcinostatic activity [review]. *Free Radic Biol Med* 1994;17:45–64.
64. Shapiro JR. Selenium and carcinogenesis: a review. *Ann NY Acad Sci* 1972;192:215.
65. Stein R, Bourne W, Liesgant TJ. Silver nitrate injury to the cornea. *Can J Ophthalmol* 1987;22:279–281.
66. Weir FW. Health hazard from occupational exposure to metallic copper and silver dust. *Am Ind Hyg Assoc J* 1979;40:245–247.
67. Rosenman KD, Moss A, Kon S. Argyria: clinical implications of exposure to silver nitrate and silver oxide. *J Occup Med* 1979;21:430–435.
68. Hollinger MA. Toxicological aspects of topical silver pharmaceuticals. *Crit Rev Toxicol* 1996;26:255–260.
69. Blackadder ES, Manderson WG. Occupational absorption of tellurium: a report of two cases. *Br J Ind Med* 1975;32:59–61.
70. Muller R, Xeichieche W, Staffen H, Schaller K. Tellurium intoxication. *Klin Woshenschr* 1989; 67:1102–1105.
71. Walbran BB, Robins E. Effects of central nervous system accumulation of tellurium on behavior in rats. *Pharmacol Biochem Behav* 1978;9: 297–300.
72. Larner AJ. Alzheimer's disease, Kuf's disease, tellurium and selenium. *Med Hypoth* 1996;47:73–75.
73. Perez D Dregoria R, Miller R. Teratogenicity of tellurium dioxide: prenatal assessment. *Teratology* 1987;37:367–376.
74. Moore D, House I, Dixon A. Thallium poisoning. Diagnosis may be elusive but alopecia is the clue [clinical conference]. *Br Med J* 1993; 306:1527–1529.
75. Gettler A, Weiss L. Thallium poisoning: III. Clinical toxicology of thallium. *Am J Clin Pathol* 1943;13:422–426.
76. Mulkey JP, Oehme FW. A review of thallium toxicity. *Vet Hum Toxicol* 1993;35:445–453.
77. Lund A. Distribution of thallium in the organism and its elimination. *Toxicol Acta Pharmacol (Copenh)* 1956;12:251.
78. Lameijer W, Van Zweiter PA. Acute cardiovascular toxicity of thallium (I) ions. *Arch Toxicol* 1976;35:49–61.
79. Bark WJ, Pleasure DE, Suzuki MN, et al. Thallium poisoning. *Arch Neurol* 1972;26:456–464.
80. Cavanagh JB, Gregson M. Some effects of a thallium salt on the proliferation of hair follicles. *J Pathol* 1978;125:179–191.
81. Feldman J, Levisohn DR. Acute alopecia: clue to thallium toxicity. *Pediatr Dermatol* 1993;10:29–31.
82. Cavanagh JB, Fuller NH, Johnson HRM, et al. The effects of thallium salts, with particular reference to the nervous system changes. *Q J Med* 1974;43:293–319.
83. Zitko V. Toxicity and pollution potential of thallium. *Sci Total Environ* 1975;4:185–192.
84. Nogu S, Mas A, Pares A, et al. Acute thallium poisoning: an evaluation of different forms of treatment. *J Toxicol* 1982;19:1015–1023.
85. Prull G, Rompel K. EEG changes in acute poisoning with organic tin compounds. *Electroencephalogr Clin Neurophysiol* 1970;29:215.
86. *Criteria for a recommended standard:* occupational exposure to organotin compounds. Washington, DC: U.S. Government Printing Office, 1977.
87. Cremer G, Thomas R, Goldstein B, Solomon A. Stannosis. A report of two cases. *So Afr Med J* 1989;75:124–126.

88. WHO. *Environmental health criteria 15. Tin and organotin compounds: a preliminary review.* Geneva: World Health Organization, 1980.
89. Schafer S, Femfert V. Tin—a toxic heavy metal? A review of the literature. *Reg Toxicol Pharmacol* 1984;4:57–69.
90. Studer RK, Siegal BA, Morgan J, Potcher E. Dexamethasone therapy of triethyl tin-induced cerebral edema. *Exp Neurol* 1973;38: 367–376.
91. Weigel F. Uranium and uranium compounds. In: Mark HF, Othmer DF, Overberger CG, Seaborg GT, eds. *Encyclopedia of chemical technology.* New York: John Wiley, 1983; 23:502–547.
92. Edwards CR. Uranium extraction process alternatives. *CIM Bull* 1992; 85:112–136.
93. Hornung RW, Meinhardt TJ. Quantitative risk assessment of lung cancer in U.S. uranium miners. *Health Phys* 1987;52:417–430.
94. Legget RW. The behavior and chemical toxicity of U in the kidney: a reassessment. *Health Phys* 1989;57:365–383.
95. Thun MJ, Baker DB, Steenland K, Smith AB, Halperin W, Berl T. Renal toxicity in uranium mine workers. *Scand J Work Environ Health* 1985;11:83–90.
96. Musk AW, Tees J. Asthma caused by occupational exposure to vanadium compounds. *Med J Aust* 1982;1:183–184.
97. Borchard UM, Fox AAL, Greeff K, et al. Negative and positive ionotropic action of vanadate on atrial and ventricular myocardium. *Nature* 1979;279:339–341.
98. Domingo JL. Vanadiun: a review of the reproductive and developmental toxicity. *Reprod Toxicol* 1996;10:175–182.
99. Domingo JL, Bosque MA, Luna M, Corbella J. Prevention by tiron (sodium 4,5-dihydroxybenzene-1,3-disulfonate) of vanadate-induced developmental toxicity in mice. *Tetratology* 1993;48:133–138.
100. Sakurai H. Vanadium distribution in rats and DNA cleavage by vanadyl complex: implication for vanadium toxicity and biological effects. *Environ Health Perspect* 1994;3:35–36.

*Environmental and Occupational Medicine, Third Edition,* edited by William N. Rom.
Lippincott–Raven Publishers, Philadelphia © 1998.

CHAPTER 78

# Organic Solvents

Fredric Gerr and Richard Letz

Solvents are simple organic substances that are (a) liquid at room temperature and under standard atmospheric conditions, (b) relatively nonreactive, and (c) able to dissolve a wide range of organic compounds (i.e., lipophilic). Most solvents are quite volatile. While exceptions to this definition can be found, it is applicable to the majority of solvents used in industry.

Solvents may be used for the selective dissolution of one substance from a mixture (i.e., chemical extraction), for reduction of the viscosity of another substance, or as feedstock for the production of synthetics. Some solvents, such as certain alcohols as well as gasoline and other aliphatic compounds, are used as fuels. A great variety of organic solvents are currently in use in industry. Commonly used organic solvents include the aliphatic, cyclic, aromatic, halogenated, ketone, aldehyde, alcohol, and ether classes. The general structural formulas for these organic solvent classes are depicted in Fig. 1.

Approximately 49 million tons of organic solvents were produced in the United States in 1984 (1). Solvents are constituents of, or are required in the production of, a wide variety of products, including paints, varnishes and other coatings, paint removers, fuels, glues, dyes and printing inks, degreasers and dry cleaning agents, plastics, agricultural products, and pharmaceuticals (2).

Solvents affect the nervous system, liver, kidneys, and skin. Several are known human carcinogens; others are animal carcinogens suspected of possessing carcinogenic activity in humans. The acute neurologic effects are related to the anesthetic property of solvents, manifesting as transient symptoms such as dizziness and light-headedness. A chronic, irreversible solvent syndrome that can include loss of intellectual function has been described. Solvents have a wide range of potency for the induction of liver disease. Classically, the halogenated hydrocarbons are capable of inducing fatty changes and cirrhosis. The renal toxicity of solvents includes both acute tubule necrosis and glomerulonephritis. Contact dermatitis can occur in the setting of solvent exposure and is due to defatting of skin that has been in contact with organic solvents. Selected solvents have been related to cancer of the hematopoietic system and the lungs.

## EXPOSURE

The U.S. National Institute for Occupational Safety and Health (NIOSH) (1) estimated that 9.8 million workers were exposed occupationally to solvents in the United States in 1974. Because solvents are found in a wide range of products and processes, many workers are at risk of exposure. Solvent exposure is common among painters and others involved in surface coating or finishing, degreasers, printers, dry cleaners, petrochemical and refinery workers, and fiberglass laminators. In Western Europe in 1980, 43% of all organic solvents were used in paint and other surface coatings, 10% for metal cleaning, 8.1% in household products, 6.7% in adhesives, 6.1% in pharmaceutical manufacturing, 3.9% for dry cleaning, and 20% for other uses (3). Aliphatic and aromatic hydrocarbons accounted for approximately half of all solvents used in Western Europe in 1980 (3). A detailed evaluation of organic solvent use in Denmark found that 93 different solvents were used in

F. Gerr: Division of Environmental and Occupational Health, Rollins School of Public Health, Emory University, Atlanta, Georgia 30322.
R. Letz: Department of Behavioral Science and Health Education, Rollins School of Public Health, Emory University, Atlanta, Georgia 30322.

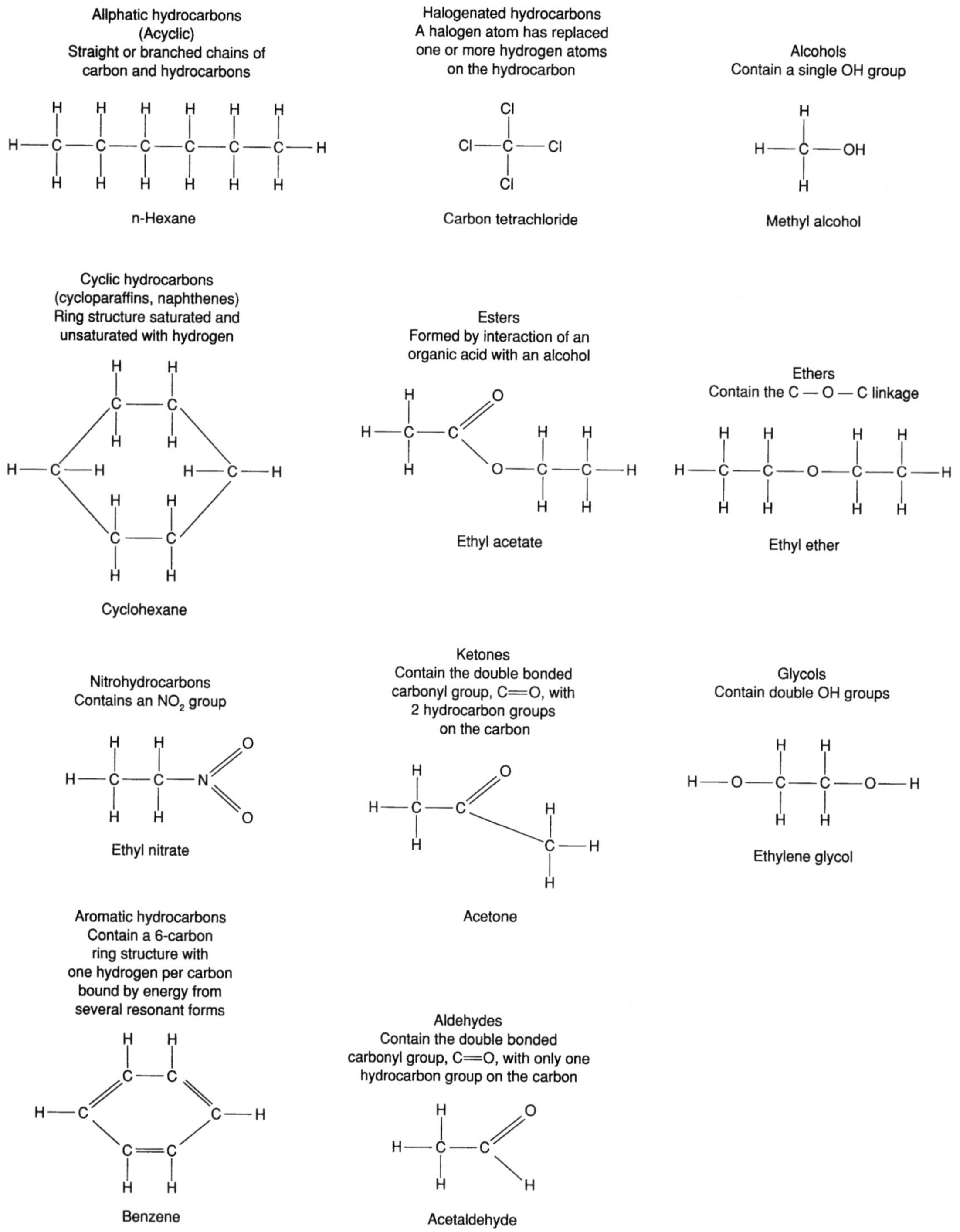


**FIG. 1.** Classes of organic solvents. (Modified from ref. 180.)

industry, most commonly ethanol, gasoline, toluene, isopropanol, and acetone (4). In a related study, the highest exposures in Denmark were found to occur in the printing and chemical industries (5). It is important to note that many workers are at risk for solvent exposure, not just those in trades with known widespread exposure. For example, an automobile mechanic may be exposed intermittently to solvents if the work requires cleaning parts in a solvent bath, a common procedure in mechanical repair.

Most occupational solvent exposure is to solvent mixtures. Indeed, many solvents are provided as mixtures—paints, thinners, mineral spirits, kerosene, jet fuel, gasoline, and white spirit, the common name for a solvent mixture composed of aliphatics and aromatics. The frequent use of solvents is problematic when estimating solvent exposure or attempting to establish permissible limits.

Some authors distinguish two types of work activities, application and process, in occupational exposure to solvents (6). Application work involves the creation of an open surface from which solvents evaporate. It is usually associated with intermittent high-level exposure. Painting and degreasing are examples. Solvent exposure in these settings can be highly variable and is related to both the work setting and ventilation (7), work in confined spaces producing especially high and potentially acutely dangerous levels. Process work is often found in the petrochemical and pharmaceutical industries, where solvents typically are enclosed to reduce occupational exposure and prevent loss of product. In these settings solvent exposure occurs during leaks or other failures of the enclosure system, product transfer, or maintenance and repair.

Estimation of occupational exposure to solvents is problematic because (a) large variations in individual exposure can occur during the workday, with periods of high exposure interspersed with periods of low exposure (7); (b) much variability of exposure can exist between individuals, even those performing the same tasks (8–10); (c) there is potential for multiple routes of entry; (d) personal protective equipment may be used; and (e) solvents are commonly used mixtures. Several methods are available for estimating occupational exposure to solvents, including environmental monitoring, biologic monitoring, and semiquantitative retrospective exposure estimation. The choice of methods depends on the exposure situation and the goals of the exposure assessment activities.

### Ambient or Environmental Monitoring

Environmental monitoring involves measuring the concentration of solvent vapor in ambient air available for respiratory uptake by workers. Both direct reading and sampling methods are available. Direct reading equipment includes indicator tubes, portable gas chromatographs, and portable infrared analyzers, among others. This method of assessing exposure is most useful when the composition of the airborne solvent contaminants is well known. Sampling methods include the use of grab samples, collection of time-weighted average samples, use of solid adsorbents, and diffusion badges. Environmental measures of exposure can be obtained from fixed locations at the work site and are called area samples. Alternatively, breathing zone samples can be obtained by requiring the worker to wear a portable device that samples air near the nose and mouth. Breathing zone samples are considered more representative of individual exposure than area samples. Environmental monitoring can be performed for virtually any solvent in air.

Solvent uptake depends on several factors in addition to the concentration of solvent in air, including both dermal uptake and work load (see Toxicokinetics, below). A disadvantage of using environmental monitoring as the sole index of exposure is that the contribution of these other factors to solvent uptake is not measured, and therefore the actual dose may be poorly estimated.

### Biologic Monitoring

Biologic monitoring is the evaluation of the internal exposure of the organism to a chemical agent (i.e., the internal dose) by a biologic method (11). "In practice, this means measuring the substance itself or its metabolites in various biologic media like blood, urine, expired air, hair, adipose tissue, etc." (11). Biologic monitoring methods have been described for a variety of industrial solvents, including benzene, toluene, xylene, styrene, trichloroethylene, tetrachloroethylene, 1,1,1-trichloroethane, and dimethylformamide (12,13). The advantages of biologic monitoring are that (a) it accounts for all routes of absorption, (b) nonoccupational exposures are also assessed, and (c) individual differences in the rate of uptake due to either use of personal protection or differential uptake secondary to work load or other factors are accounted for (11). The disadvantages of biologic monitoring include (a) the need to obtain biologic media from workers, (b) limited understanding of the association between biologic exposure measures and worker health, and (c) the limited number of solvents for which biologic measures are available.

### Estimation of Solvent Exposure from Questionnaire Data

In epidemiologic study of the health effects of solvent exposure, it is often the case that neither environmental nor biologic exposure information is available. Frequently, exposure has occurred to a variety of solvents under variable conditions of exposure. Furthermore, measures of current exposure, environmental or biologic, may not represent past or cumulative exposure. In this circumstance the duration of exposure is often used by investigators as a substitute for actual total exposure. Typically, this variable is closely correlated with age, and it may be a confounder in exposure-effect analyses. Recent attempts have been made to develop a solvent exposure index for painters that utilizes information obtained by questionnaire in combination with a weighting scheme for factors that modify individual exposure, including respirator use, method of paint application, and ventilation (14,15).

### The Solvent Mixture Problem

With the exception of styrene, it is common for workers to be exposed to mixtures of solvents. This fact adds another level of complexity to the assessment of solvent exposure, as different solvents have different toxic potency. In an attempt to develop classification schemes for mixed solvent exposure that are more accurate than simple solvent-years, some authors have utilized a summary measure called the hygienic effect. The hygienic effect is the sum, for all solvents present in a mixture, of the actual exposure to each solvent divided by its maximum permissible exposure. The assumption underlying this index is that the health effect at the maximal permissible exposure level is equivalent for all solvents and that no synergy of effect occurs. Ikeda (16) has reviewed the literature to determine possible interactive effects of multiple simultaneous chemical exposures. He concluded that the assumption of "additive effects in the case of chemicals that share similar action in toxicity" was more accurate than were assumptions of independent action, potentiation, or antagonism, a conclusion that tends to support the hygienic effect concept.

## TOXICOKINETICS

### Uptake

Inhalation and percutaneous absorption of solvents are the two routes of entry relevant to occupational medicine. Respiratory uptake of solvents depends on solvent concentration in inhaled air, the blood-air partition coefficient, alveolar ventilation, pulmonary perfusion, and the duration of exposure (17,18). Because both alveolar ventilation and pulmonary perfusion are functions of physical exertion or work load, manual labor can cause substantial variation in solvent absorption (10,19,20). Pulmonary uptake occurs via simple diffusion.

Dermal uptake is important only when liquid solvent is in contact with skin, and it may be the predominant route of entry for solvents of low vapor pressure such as the glycol ethers (21). It is dependent on the surface area of the skin in contact with solvent, skin thickness and physical characteristics (cuts, abrasions, disease), and the duration of contact (22,23). Percutaneous absorption of solvent vapor is negligible (24).

### Distribution and Transformation

The distribution of unchanged solvent in the body is a function the solvent's differential affinity for various target tissues (24), usually a function of the lipid content and vascularity of the tissue or organ. Metabolism of solvents occurs mainly in the liver and is typically mediated by the cytochrome P-450 mixed-function oxidase system. A water-soluble conjugate is produced that is subsequently excreted in the urine or bile. Biotransformation usually results in a biologically less active metabolite; however, it can produce a metabolite of greater toxicity than the parent compound, as in the case of metabolism of *n*-hexane and methyl-*n*-butyl ketone (MnBk) to 2,5-hexanedione, a peripheral neurotoxicant (see Peripheral Nervous System, below).

A great deal of recent research activity has concentrated on the development of pharmacokinetic models of solvent exposure (24,25). In these models, the body is represented as a set of compartments, and the interactions between compartments are described with differential equations. Such models may be useful for predicting the concentrations of solvents in various body tissues, and they also allow more precise estimation of dose-effect relationships. Models of increasing complexity are required when exposure to solvent mixtures is considered, when sources of variability such as work load, body build, liver function, and renal function are considered (8,9), when chronic toxicity is the outcome of interest and tissue repair processes mitigate the toxic effect of the solvent, or when bioactivation or repair mechanisms can become saturated. Pharmacokinetic models require extensive validation prior to acceptance.

### Excretion

Solvents are eliminated by exhalation of the unchanged parent compound or by urinary and biliary excretion of either the unchanged parent compound or its metabolites (1,24).

## WORKER PROTECTION

A hierarchical approach is recommended for the reduction of workers' exposure to solvents (1,26). The initial step is to substitute less toxic solvents for more toxic ones. Substitution of toluene for the carcinogen benzene and of methylisobutyl ketone for the neurotoxicant MnBk are examples of this approach. In addition, changes in use in the paint industry from solvent-based paints to both water-based paints and solventless powder coatings represents substitution or elimination of potential solvent exposure.

In addition to the substitution of safer solvents for more toxic ones, effective ventilation and enclosure of solvent-based processes is useful for reduction of solvent exposure. The spray booth found in many spray-finishing facilities represents such a mechanism, both to isolate the spray-finishing process from uninvolved workers and to establish an environment in which air flow directs solvent vapors away from the breathing zone of the involved worker.

Respirators, either air-supply or air-purifying, are the least effective means of reducing workers' exposure to solvents. In addition, their use requires a comprehensive respirator program, including worker education, evaluation of worker fitness for use, fit testing, and regular maintenance.

Because some solvents are readily absorbed through the skin, an effective worker protection program must include measures to prevent skin contact. Gloves are often used and can be effective. However, many are permeable to a variety of solvents, so gloves must be selected carefully. Barrier creams, the least effective method of reducing percutaneous absorption of solvents, are not recommended (26). In addition to gloves, reduction of percutaneous exposure includes washing areas of skin contact with soap and water and removing solvent-contaminated clothing to prevent prolonged skin contact.

## EFFECTS ON THE NERVOUS SYSTEM

Neurotoxicity induced by exposure to organic solvents has emerged as one of the most important issues in occupational health (27,28). Substantial concern stems from the essential life functions performed by the nervous system as well as the fact that damage to it may be irreversible. Although much work has been done, substantial uncertainty still exists, particularly with regard to the effects on the central nervous system of long-term, low-level exposure to solvents.

Solvents can cause depressant intoxication following acute exposure, which appears to be related to physical or chemical interactions with membranes or neurotransmitters. Long-term heavy exposure to solvents may also cause persistent, potentially irreversible impairment in cognitive function and affect, which may be associated with structural changes in neural tissue (1).

Solvents may exert their primary effect on the central nervous system (CNS), the peripheral nervous system (PNS), or both. CNS effects are typically investigated with behavioral tests or electrophysiologic evaluations. Information about the effects of occupational solvent exposure on the PNS has come from studies that utilize clinical evaluation, electrophysiologic examination, and histopathologic examination of biopsy specimens. The effects of occupational solvent exposure on the PNS are more clearly defined and easier to identify than those of the CNS, owing to the relative simplicity of both the structure and function of the PNS.

### Peripheral Nervous System

Widespread agreement exists that the solvents *n*-hexane, MnBK, and carbon disulfide cause in humans peripheral neuropathy of the distal axonal type. Other solvents suspected of having peripheral nerve effects include styrene and tetrachloroethylene (29). In this section discussion is restricted to the peripheral nerve disorder induced by the hexacarbons *n*-hexane and MnBK. An excellent review of hexacarbon-induced peripheral neuropathy is provided by Schaumburg and co-workers (30).

The hexacarbon solvents *n*-hexane and MnBK have been used mainly in thinners, glues, paints, and specialized printing materials (31). The occupational toxicity of the hexacarbons was first recognized in the 1960s when an outbreak of peripheral neuropathy occurred in a shoe factory in Japan (32). Hexacarbon-induced peripheral neuropathy was first reported in the United States in the 1970s (33,34). Occupational disease has usually occurred among workers who use glues containing hexacarbons (35). Nonoccupational cases are mostly restricted to the deliberate inhalational abuse of glues (36).

Exposure to *n*-hexane and MnBK cause changes in peripheral nerves characterized initially by axonal swelling and focal demyelination in the distal regions of the longer, larger axons. With progression, degeneration of the entire axon occurs distal to the site of axonal swelling (30,37,38).

Both *n*-hexane and MnBK share a common metabolite, 2,5-hexanedione, universally believed to be the peripheral neurotoxicant responsible for hexacarbon-induced peripheral neuropathy. This substance has been shown in animals to produce in peripheral nerves pathologic changes that are virtually identical to those caused by administration of *n*-hexane and MnBK (39).

In the occupational setting the onset of symptoms is usually gradual. Deliberate inhalational abuse is associated with a more rapid onset of signs and symptoms and can lead to disabling disease within 2 months (30). The initial complaint is usually symmetric numbness of the fingers and toes. Loss of cutaneous sensibility to light touch, vibration, pin prick, and temperature are present on physical examination, as are proprioceptive abnormalities and loss of the Achilles tendon reflex. Severe disease can include motor weakness and atrophy (30,40).

Routine clinical laboratory test results are normal in patients with hexacarbon-induced peripheral neuropathy. Electrophysiologic evaluation discovers symmetric distal electromyographic abnormalities consistent with denervation as well as mild to moderate slowing of both motor and sensory nerve conduction velocity (41).

A characteristic feature of hexacarbon-induced peripheral neuropathy is the tendency for the disease to progress for up to 4 months following cessation of exposure (30). There are no specific treatments, and the degree of recovery is proportional to the severity of disease. Hexacarbon-induced peripheral neuropathy is indistinguishable from other toxic and metabolic neuropathies, so a careful occupational and social history is required to identify the causal agent.

### Central Nervous System

A great deal of controversy exists regarding the toxic effects of solvents on the CNS. Much of the controversy is probably attributable to the use of confusing terminology and inconsistent diagnostic criteria to describe CNS impairment. Fortunately, some movement toward standardization of terminology used to describe the effects of solvents on the CNS has been made by the World Health Organization (WHO) and others (17,42). The first basic distinction in the classification scheme proposed by the WHO (17) is acute versus chronic. Acute effects are graded as mild (acute intoxication) or severe (acute toxic encephalopathy). Chronic effects were classified as mild, consisting mainly of affective changes and loss of concentration (organic affective syndrome); moderate, with some impairment of neurobehavioral functioning (mild chronic toxic encephalopathy); or severe, with significant loss of intellectual function (severe chronic toxic encephalopathy) (17). A second classification scheme is similar, except that specific names for the classifications are avoided (type 1, 2, and 3 are used instead) and the mild chronic condition is subdivided into those having primarily affective or primarily cognitive dysfunction (42).

### *Acute Effects*

The depressant effects of solvents are well recognized; some solvents have been used as general anesthetics. The ability of solvents to produce narcotic effects constitutes their main acute health hazard (43). Acute effects of exposure to solvents are pharmacologic and their intensity is generally proportional to their concentration in the brain. There may be initial euphoria and disinhibition. Higher intensity exposure may result in prenarcosis symptoms such as dizziness, nausea and vomiting, incoordination, paresthesia, increased salivation, and tachycardia. The symptoms are generally transient, disappearing quickly after exposure is terminated. Overexposure can lead to seizures, coma, and death in severe cases. The likely mechanism is anoxia following depression of central control of respiration.

Severe cases of overexposure to solvents are not common under normal working conditions. Statistical reviews are available of industrial solvent poisonings in the United Kingdom. Poisoning by simple chlorinated solvents (44) appears more common than by aromatic solvents (45), and younger workers appear to be at greater risk than older ones. About half of all reported cases (loss of more than 3 days' work) resulted in loss of consciousness, and fewer than 5% were fatal. There have been numerous case reports of accidental poisoning to a variety of alcohols, acetates, and ketone solvents, but such cases are rare, perhaps owing to the respiratory irritant qualities of these solvents (43).

Some cases of acute industrial poisoning may be the result of volatile substance abuse (VSA), but the frequency of VSA among solvent-exposed workers is unknown and presumed to be low. The overwhelming majority of VSA cases are teenagers abusing solvents recreationally (46). Adhesives are the most abused products, and toluene is the solvent detected most frequently in blood (47). Voluntary inhalation of gasoline carries additional hazard, since it may contain tetraethyl lead and *n*-hexane.

Subclinical effects of acute exposure to solvents in humans can be studied in the laboratory under experimental control. It is not ethical to expose humans to agents or concentrations that are expected to produce severe or lasting effects, so this type of study yields information only on mild, transitory effects. Typically, healthy volunteers are exposed for a few hours in chambers to well-controlled concentrations of solvent at or below the occupational permissible exposure limit. At least 50 experimental studies of effects in humans of acute exposure to solvents have been published and are briefly reviewed by Gamberale (48) and Iregren (49). The most-studied solvents have been toluene, xylene, styrene, trichloroethylene, perchloroethylene, and methylene chloride. These studies have typically shown, at most, subtle effects of short-term exposure at the current exposure limit values (50). The acute effects of most solvents are narcotic; thus, performance decrements on tests of attention and reaction time have been reported most often (51). In addition to cognitive tests, quantitative measurement of postural stability may be a sensitive outcome for assessment of acute effects of solvents on the nervous system (52,53).

The reader should be aware of some limitations in interpreting the results of experimental studies of solvent exposure. The decrements observed in performance of cognitive tests may not always be directly attributable to dysfunction of the neural systems underlying performance on these tests; rather, similar performance decrements may be observed when the primary effect of exposure is eye irritation or headache. Also, solvent exposure during these experimental studies typically lasts a few hours and occurs at intervals of several days. On the other hand, the usual exposure situation of workers may involve daily exposure, and neurobehavioral effects may result from cumulative exposure to some solvents over days or weeks. Information on extrapolation from effects of short-term exposure to those from chronic exposure or from subtle to more severe effects is lacking. Gamberale (54) provides an excellent discussion of the critical issues involved in the study of acute effects of solvent exposure.

### *Chronic Effects*

The nonspecific effects of long-term exposure to solvents range from a general negative affective state, to a subtle reduction in functional reserve capacity to perform well when fatigued or in a distracting environment, to mild slowing of psychomotor performance, to memory disturbance, and finally to severe intellectual deficits (55). The most severe condition, which has been called psychoorganic syndrome, presenile dementia, and severe chronic toxic encephalopathy, is also the most controversial. Although the existence of chronic solvent encephalopathy has been questioned (56), experts now generally agree that it occurs but do not agree on its prevalence (57,58). It has been reported most often in Scandinavia, where it is a compensable occupational illness. In Scandinavian countries it has been diagnosed more commonly in Denmark than elsewhere. The extent to which these differences reflect differences in diagnostic criteria, past exposure, or other host factors is unknown.

A great number of epidemiologic investigations of CNS outcomes among various solvent-exposed groups have been conducted. Several international conferences have been held (17,42,59), and one critical review from a conservative perspective has been published (56). It is beyond the scope of this chapter to review all these studies. Rather, an orientation to the available literature and a discussion of the relevant issues are provided.

The epidemiologic studies have been either registry-based studies of neuropsychiatric disability or cross-sectional studies comparing exposed and unexposed groups for differences in prevalence of symptoms, neurobehavioral performance level, or prevalence of abnormality on neurologic or neurobehavioral tests. The results have been almost as heterogeneous as the exposures and the methods used to assess outcome. The reader is referred to a sample of well-conducted epidemiologic studies of multiple neurologic outcomes among solvent-exposed workers (15,60–63).

*Neuropsychiatric Disability*

A number of studies based on pension or disability registries in relation to solvent exposure have been published (64–70). In general, risk of disability award on the basis of neuropsychiatric illness was found to be elevated about twofold among solvent-exposed groups such as painters and floor layers relative to comparison groups such as carpenters and electricians, although there have been some exceptions to this trend (71). In addition to registry based studies, case-control studies of the association between occupational solvent exposure and (a) psychiatric disorders requiring hospitalization (72), (b) medical disability retirement resulting from chronic neurologic and psychiatric disease (73), and (c) organic brain damage (74) have been published. Only in the study of organic brain damage was a significant association with solvent exposure observed (74). Interestingly, an interaction with alcohol consumption was observed, suggesting that alcohol consumption may modify (increase) the adverse effect of occupational solvent exposure on the central nervous system.

*Symptoms*

The rates of reporting of some symptoms were elevated above the rate reported by comparison groups in the vast majority of published epidemiologic studies of solvent-exposed workers. Those symptoms most often elevated were fatigue, irritability, depression, headaches, poor concentration, and forgetfulness. Terms such as neurasthenic syndrome and organic affective syndrome have been used to label this constellation of symptoms among solvent-exposed workers. One commonly used, brief questionnaire specifically designed for administration to solvent-exposed workers is the Swedish Questionnaire 16 (Q16) (75). Persistent expression of these symptoms has led some investigators to speak of personality changes or personality disturbances, which have been assessed with standardized personality tests (76).

*Neurobehavioral Tests*

Tests of neurobehavioral function are aimed at noninvasively assessing the functional integrity of the CNS. Many standardized neurobehavioral tests have been used to assess CNS function in solvent-exposed workers. Because of the complexity of the human nervous system and the attendant wide range of functions that can potentially be affected, sets, or batteries, of tests are usually administered to the subjects in these studies. It is generally accepted that the tests administered should sample from the perceptual, motor, psychomotor, learning-memory, attentional, and affective functional domains.

In the last 15 years at least 16 epidemiologic studies of painters (car, industrial, construction, and combinations of the three) and four studies of paint-manufacturing workers exposed to mixed solvents have been published. At least 11 studies of fiberglass fabrication workers exposed almost exclusively to styrene and at least four studies of printers exposed primarily to toluene have been published. Many other epidemiologic studies of heterogeneous groups of solvent-exposed workers have been reported. Neurobehavioral performance was reported to be poorer in the solvent-exposed groups than in the referent groups in most of these studies (63,77–80).

The findings are far from consistent, however. Some studies have failed to observe differences in neurobehavioral performance level between solvent-exposed and referent groups (81–84), and even when differences between exposure groups were observed, the pattern of differences was often inconsistent across studies of presumably similar occupational groups. Different tests were administered in different studies, and tests intended to measure the same functions, or even those bearing the same name, were sometimes quite different in practice. Also, it should be noted that decrements in performance on neurobehavioral tests are nonspecific; performance is affected by a number of factors not related to exposure (e.g., age, education, native intellectual ability, and the motivation of the subject). Furthermore, the functional significance of performance differences between exposure groups (e.g., a mean difference in reaction time of 20 milliseconds) is not always apparent. Dose-response relationships have not been observed in many investigations, probably owing to imprecise estimation of exposure to the neurotoxic agents.

*Other Tests*

Testing of three sensory systems—olfactory, auditory, and visual—that may be early targets for solvent toxicity have received attention recently. Although a Swedish study failed to show differences in smell identification between painters and referents (85), Schwartz and colleagues (86) observed decrements in smell identification among nonsmoker paint-manufacturing workers. Loss of hearing has been associated with occupational exposure to solvents. In one study of self-reported hearing difficulty, a significant association was observed with self-reported occupational solvent exposure (87). Authors of another study, in which audiometry was performed to characterize auditory function, observed a strong effect of solvent exposure on hearing. In addition, a statistically significant interaction between solvent exposure and noise exposure was observed. Several reviews of the animal and human evidence in support of this hypothesis are available (88–90). Deficits in performance of a simple color vision test have been reported among several solvent-exposed groups (91–94); however, these results have not been replicated in other investigations (95–97). Changes in visual constrast sensitivity have also been reported for solvent-exposed microelectronics workers (98) and a series of solvent-exposed patients (99).

Quantitative measurement of postural stability, or posturography, has been employed as an index of highly integrated CNS and PNS activity and findings have differed for solvent-exposed and referent groups (100–102).

Electrophysiologic outcomes such as electroencephalography and evoked potentials have been shown to differ on a group basis between solvent-exposed and referent groups (60,100,103). These methods are objective, but the findings are nonspecific and their relevance to health is usually unknown. Studies employing neurophysiologic outcomes are reviewed by Seppäläinen (38). Another physiologic measure, regional cerebral blood flow, has been shown to differ between chronic toxic encephalopathy patients and referents in one study (104), but not in another (105).

Computed tomography (CT) has been used as an index of cerebral atrophy among solvent-exposed workers and patients, but the results of such studies have been mixed (15,60,84,106,107). In addition to CT methods, several papers have been published in which single photon emission computed tomography (SPECT) was performed on solvent exposed subjects (108–110). Unfortunately, these studies are of poor methodologic quality, which severely limits inferences that can be made from them.

### Issues in Research on the CNS Effects of Solvents

The literature on the CNS effects of solvents contains many inconsistencies and, therefore, is hard to interpret. The early studies have been severely criticized on methodologic grounds, and some have concluded that they are not convincing evidence of a significant decline in CNS function due to occupational exposure to organic solvents (56,111).

This confusing state of affairs is perhaps not surprising (15). First, most of the published studies were cross-sectional, and affected persons might have left the trade. If such survivor effects were operative, the likelihood of observing true differences in neurobehavioral performance between exposure groups would have been diminished (i.e., the results would have been biased toward the null). Also, in studies sampling cross sections of currently working groups, it is not possible to distinguish relatively acute effects from chronic effects. In many studies the referent group may not have been comparable to the exposed group, particularly with respect to native intellectual abilities. In most cases this confounding would have resulted in misattributing observed differences on neurobehavioral outcomes to solvent exposure—a false-positive study result.

Another potential confounder that has been considered in many studies of solvent-exposed workers is drinking alcohol. The proportion of solvent-exposed workers who were alcoholics or heavy drinkers has been greater than referent groups in many epidemiologic studies, but not in all. Alcoholics are routinely excluded from participation or data analyses in studies of solvent-exposed workers. Self-reported level of drinking has rarely been a significant predictor of neurobehavioral performance of workers. Poorer performance among heavy drinkers than light drinkers has been reported in a few studies (112), but better performance among heavy drinkers has also been reported (113). Finally, alcohol may not be a confounder, but rather it may interact with solvent exposure in producing neurotoxicity. Whether the effect on solvent neurotoxicity of drinking alcohol is potentiating, protective, or nil awaits further research.

Many of the studies of chronic effects of solvent exposure, particularly those not reporting effects, may not have included in the exposed group enough subjects with sufficiently intense exposure to produce substantial damage to the nervous system (15). This argument requires the assumption of an effective threshold of cumulative exposure, which many experts have estimated informally to be about 10 years of relatively heavy exposure. Mikkelsen and colleagues (15) have operationalized this concept and estimated that there may be little risk of organic brain damage with less than 13 years' exposure to the equivalent of a time-weighted average of 40 ppm of white spirit. Even without assuming a threshold, heterogeneity of exposure within exposure groups would tend to bias results toward the null in epidemiologic studies that compare the level of neurobehavioral performance between exposure groups.

Exposure-response analyses, when performed, have generally used years in the trade as an index of chronic exposure. Use of this variable in regression models with another well-correlated variable, age, would yield unstable estimates of both effects. Further, years in the trade may be poorly correlated with semiquantitative exposure measures (14,15), and its validity as a surrogate for exposure to the (unknown) neurotoxic agents in mixed solvents is unknown. However, even while recognizing the considerable limitations of virtually all of the epidemiologic studies performed to date, the large number of positive findings suggests that long-term exposure to organic solvents affects the CNS. The relevant (and currently unanswered) questions are, Which are the toxic agents? and At what exposure levels?

Fortunately, the average quality of epidemiologic studies is increasing. Attempts to standardize neurobehavioral test batteries are proceeding. For example, the WHO has proposed a core test battery to be used in all epidemiologic investigations of workers exposed to neurotoxic agents (114), and studies employing it on solvent-exposed workers are beginning to appear (115). Also, the increasing use of computerized neurobehavioral tests may help standardize results (51). Blinding, at least on the interviewer's side, is now often employed to minimize observer bias and is unnecessary when a computer is administering the tests. The problem remains of study participants not being blind to their exposure, which can result in differences in motivation between groups, or even conscious manipulation of results by some persons. In our current state of ignorance of which solvents are likely to affect which functions, multiple tests will continue to be employed, and, consequently, the problems that arise from multiple statistical comparisons will need to be resolved.

Clearly, prospective studies of solvent-exposed workers are needed. Preexposure baseline values, adequate exposure monitoring, and appropriate selection of referents is required. Paradoxically, in the settings in which such studies are most feasible (large companies, Scandinavia), exposure to solvents is now generally well controlled. At least one such prospective study of painters apprentices has begun (116).

Although no long-term follow-up data from prospective studies of workers newly hired into jobs with solvent exposure have been published, there have been a few follow-up studies in Scandinavia of patients diagnosed as having chronic toxic encephalopathy. These studies have indicated that this condition is persistent in most cases even after exposure has stopped, but it does not appear to be rapidly progressive. Among 32 such patients in Sweden followed an average 4 years after diagnosis, findings at follow-up were very similar to those at their initial evaluations for physical examination and neurobehavioral performance (117), CT (107), peripheral nerve conduction measures (118), and regional blood flow (104). In a recent multicenter long-term follow-up study of another 111 solvent-exposed workers in Sweden (119), the workers who showed neurobehavioral impairment at the initial examination also showed persistence of effects after removal from exposure for at least 5 years, but rapid progression of impairment was not evident. There was evidence that removal from exposure led to symptomatic improvement in workers who had symptoms but no signs of impaired intellectual function. Finally, a Danish study has observed continued elevated reporting of symptoms of impaired memory and concentration in a group of more than 50 solvent-exposed workers at 5- and 10-year follow-up (120).

## EFFECTS OF SOLVENTS ON THE KIDNEYS

### Immediate Effects: Acute Tubule Necrosis

Acute tubule necrosis (ATN) is a potentially life-threatening renal disorder characterized by azotemia and oliguria. It is one cause of acute renal failure. Short-term, high-level exposure to selected solvents is universally accepted as a cause of ATN (121). Solvents that have been described as causing ATN include the halogenated hydrocarbons (especially carbon tetrachloride), petroleum distillates, ethylene glycol, ethylene glycol ethers, diethylene glycol, dioxane, and toluene (122,123). ATN has been reported to follow both intentional inhalational exposure (volatile substance abuse) and unintentional occupational inhalational exposure. In addition, ATN has been described following dermal exposure (i.e., hand washing) to diesel fuel (124). The mechanism of solvent-induced tubule damage is poorly understood (123). Solvent-induced ATN is not associated with glomerular disease.

When it occurs, ATN shortly follows solvent exposure, so the association with exposure is usually easy to establish. No studies are available in which the risk of solvent-associated ATN is estimated. Some authors have concluded that the risk of ATN associated with solvent exposure is low because few reports of solvent-induced acute renal failure are available despite the widespread use of solvents (125). Although in the past ATN was universally fatal, recovery is common now that renal dialysis is readily available. After the initial tubule changes associated with ATN have occurred, tubules regenerate in approximately 3 weeks. While complete recovery is possible, renal insufficiency may persist.

### Long-Term Effects

#### *Glomerulonephritis*

Glomerulonephritis is a disorder characterized by, either individually or in combination, hematuria, proteinuria, reduced glomerular filtration rate, and hypertension. It is caused by alterations in the structure and functional integrity of the glomerulus (126). Glomerulonephritis is the most commonly cited renal disease following long-term exposure to solvents (122).

Several comprehensive reviews of the literature relating solvent exposure to glomerulonephritis are currently available (122–124,127). All include a discussion of the many case reports of individual patients or series of patients with glomerular disease who have a history of exposure to solvents. Agreement exists that the results of these case series, while indicating the need for additional research, are not conclusive. In addition, they review the epidemiologic literature examining the association between glomerulonephritis and solvent exposure. Virtually all of the epidemiologic studies of the relationship between overt glomerulonephritis and solvent exposure have used a case-control design. One cross-sectional study of relevance to this issue examined both serum antiglomerular basement membrane and laminin antibody levels in relation to occupational solvent exposure (128).

The first comprehensive review included an evaluation of six studies in which a case-control design was used to determine whether glomerular disease was associated with solvent exposure (127). In five of the six studies reviewed, a significantly larger proportion of subjects with disease were exposed to solvents than were referents. In one study no association was found; however, several weaknesses in design that had the potential to bias the results of these studies have been noted (127): (a) inappropriate controls were used in three of the five positive studies, (b) blinding was a concern in four, (c) recall bias was either possibly or probably present in all, and (d) measures of exposure were either poorly defined or not explained in all. One study was judged to be of substantially higher quality than the others; an odds ratio of 3.9 for the relationship between solvent exposure and glomerulonephritis was observed in this study (129). Churchill and colleagues (127) concluded that additional studies were needed to clarify the relationship between solvents and glomerular disease.

Subsequent reviews (122–124) have included studies more recent than those included by Churchill's group (127), and the authors of all subsequent reviews also described the limitations in study design that were identified by them (127). The conclusions of the reviewers have varied, with two suggesting that the consistency with which solvent exposure has been associated with glomerular disease indicated a likely basis for concluding that a true association exists (123,124), while one suggested that the findings that relate solvent exposure to glomerular disease are inconclusive (122).

The most carefully performed case-control studies of the relationship between glomerular disease and exposure to organic solvents (129–133) controlled the above-mentioned sources of bias by (a) requiring that all cases be confirmed by biopsy, (b) using appropriate control groups, and (c) ensuring that interviewers were blinded to disease status of the subject (except refs. 130,132,133). In addition, semiquantitative measures of exposure based on interview information obtained from subjects were incorporated into three studies (131–133). Of these five studies, a significant association between solvent exposure and glomerular disease was observed in three (129,131,133). In the one cross-sectional study of circulating antibodies considered to be potential preclinical indicators of glomerulonephritis, significant associations were observed between these indicators and occupational exposure to hydrocarbons and mixed solvents.

In summary, the body of research relating solvent exposure to glomerulonephritis is suggestive of an association, although not unequivocally. However, several well-performed case-referent studies have found significantly elevated odds ratios for exposure to solvents. Others have not, although their statistical power was limited. No cohort studies of glomerular disease among solvent-exposed subjects have been published to date. Given the low incidence of the outcome, such a study would be logistically difficult and require that a huge number of subjects be followed in order for it to have adequate power to detect even a relatively large effect (127).

### *Tubule and Glomerular Dysfunction*

Several cross-sectional studies of urinary excretion of proteins and cells in subjects occupationally exposed to organic solvents have been performed. The aim of these studies was to detect renal tubule and glomerular dysfunction at an early or subclinical stage. Outcomes of interest have included not only conventional clinical measures of renal function such as proteinuria, albuminuria, and the presence of cells in urine but also novel measures of renal function, such as excretion of low molecular weight enzymes and proteins, including *N*-acetylglucosaminidase, retinol-binding protein, and $\beta_2$-microglobulin. The results of such studies have been mixed, showing both mild tubule dysfunction (134–139) and glomerular effects (138–140). Studies in which no effect was found on a variety of measures of renal function have also been reported (141–143). In summary, some inconsistency exists regarding the effects of solvents on measures of renal function among working populations exposed to solvents. However, currently, a preponderance of research findings suggest that mild tubular and glomerular effects of unknown clinical significance are detectable in solvent-exposed workers.

One study that does not fit the classification scheme used above was a case-control study of occupational and other exposures associated with end-stage renal disease in men (144). The authors observed statistically significant elevations in odds for all solvents and solvents used as cleaning agents or degreasers. However, no increase was observed for subjects who worked with solvents used in paints and glues and solvents used in other processes.

### *Summary of Renal Effects*

Solvents are widely recognized as one of the causes of ATN, and hence acute renal failure. In addition, the results of several case-control studies of glomerulonephritis suggest that solvent exposure is associated with that disorder as well. The results of cross-sectional studies indicate that mild tubule and glomerular effects can be observed among solvent-exposed groups. Finally, in one case-control study a statistically significant association was observed between solvent exposure and end-stage renal disease.

## EFFECTS ON THE LIVER

### Halogenated Hydrocarbons

Carbon tetrachloride, tetrachlorethane, and chloroform are well-known hepatotoxins, acutely causing hepatic necrosis and steatosis (145–147). In addition, hepatic cirrhosis has been observed following long-term exposure to carbon tetrachloride (145). Use of these substances has diminished over the past several decades, in large part because of their recognized hepatotoxicity and the availability of less toxic substitutes.

Evidence on human exposure to other halogenated hydrocarbon solvents such as methylene chloride, trichloroethylene, and 1,1,1-trichloroethane suggests that they are substantially less hepatotoxic than carbon tetrachloride and chloroform (148,149). A relative paucity of data from carefully performed epidemiologic studies of exposed workers necessitates guarded conclusions, however. Case reports of diffuse liver disease, including hepatic necrosis and steatosis in workers exposed to 1,1,1-trichloroethane (150) and hepatic necrosis with fibrosis in solvent abusers heavily exposed to trichloroethylene (151), suggest that these chlorinated hydrocarbon solvents have hepatotoxic potential.

### Nonhalogenated Hydrocarbons

Few or no hepatotoxic effects have been observed in well-performed cross-sectional epidemiologic studies of subjects exposed to nonhalogenated solvents, including both aliphatics (kerosene, *n*-hexane, and others) and aromatics (xylene, toluene, styrene, and others). These studies have utilized conventional noninvasive laboratory methods, such as measurement of serum hepatocellular enzymes, including aspartate aminotransferase (AST) and alanine aminotransferase (ALT), to identify the potential hepatotoxic effects.

Lundberg and Hakansson (152) studied serum hepatic enzyme activity in 47 paint industry workers exposed to a mixture of solvents, of which xylene and toluene were the most common. No significant differences were found between the solvent-exposed workers and unexposed age-matched referents. Pedersen and Rasmussen (153) compared 122 subjects with suspected solvent poisoning to 64 solvent-exposed subjects without poisoning as well as 91 unexposed referents. The exposed subjects had been exposed to many solvents, the most common being turpentine, toluene, and xylene. Some use of chlorinated solvents was reported. No differences were found in serum ALT, the only measure of liver function performed in this group. Ørbaek and colleagues (61) performed a comprehensive study of 50 male workers exposed to solvents in the paint industry and a comparison group matched for age and education level. Paint industry subjects had been exposed to nonhalogenated aliphatic and aromatic hydrocarbon solvents. The mean serum AST level was significantly decreased, and mean serum lactic acid dehydrogenase (LDH) was significantly increased in the exposed group. Mean serum ALT, alkaline phosphatase (AP), and γ-glutamyl-transpeptadase (GGTP) were not significantly different. A similar study performed by Hane and co-workers (154) demonstrated no differences in serum AST or ALT between solvent-exposed painters and age-matched comparison subjects. Elofsson and colleagues (60) compared AP, ALT, AST, and serum bilirubin levels of 80 spray painters exposed to a mixture of solvents with the levels of an unexposed comparison group. The most common toxicant was toluene, but exposure to xylene, trichloroethylene, and white spirits also occurred frequently. Serum AP was found to be significantly elevated in the solvent-exposed subjects. No significant differences were found for serum AST, ALT, or bilirubin.

Outbreaks of liver disease in the occupational setting, such as the observation of liver disease due to dimethylformamide at a coated-fabric factory in the United States (155) as well as in Taiwan (156) and the case report of two workers with fulminant hepatic failure following exposure to 2-nitropropane (157), indicate that selected nonhalogenated hydrocarbon substances are capable of inducing acute and chronic liver disease in exposed populations. These outbreaks underscore the need to identify solvents that can induce hepatic disorders before they are made available for widespread use.

### New Markers of Hepatic Effects

Some studies of the hepatic effects of solvent exposure have included assessment of antipyrine metabolism (158,159), ultrasonographic assessment of hepatic echogenicity (160), and measurement of serum bile acid concentration (161–163) as measures of liver function. Proponents of these methods suggest that they are more sensitive indicators of hepatotoxicity than conventional measures of serum levels of hepatocellular enzymes. Døssing and co-workers (158) found significant differences in antipyrene metabolism between jet fuel—exposed subjects and two comparison groups. In a recent study of workers exposed to perchloroethylene, diffuse changes in hepatic parenchymal echogenicity on ultrasound was associated with exposure while serum transaminase levels were not, suggesting that subtle effects associated with this exposure may not be detectable with conventional serologic measures of hepatic injury. Franco and associates (162) found significant elevations of serum bile acids in subjects exposed to mixed solvents as compared with unexposed referents. Edling and Tagesson (161) found elevated serum bile acids in styrene-exposed workers, and Driscoll et al. (163) observed elevated serum bile acids in two solvent exposed groups, one of which was exposed only to trichloroethylene and the other exposed to a solvent mixture that included carbon tetrachloride. The correspondence between these measures and the presence or subsequent development of hepatic disease has not been evaluated, however. At this time it is not known whether these measures are markers of exposure or actual measures of hepatotoxic effect. However, the consistency of observed effect is noteworthy and should be followed by research to determine the long-term relevance of these newer measures of hepatic structure and function.

### Summary of Hepatic Effects

Carbon tetrachloride and chloroform are well-recognized hepatotoxins. Other chlorinated hydrocarbon solvents such as trichloroethylene and 1,1,1-trichloroethane may also be hepatotoxic, although they appear to be less potent. At this time the evidence for hepatotoxicity of these chlorinated hydrocarbon solvents in humans is limited to case studies of exposed workers and a few studies using relatively new methods of detecting hepatic effects. Evidence from high-quality epidemiologic studies incorporating appropriate comparison groups indicates that the commonly used nonhalogenated hydrocarbon solvents, including both aliphatic and aromatic compounds, have few, if any, measurable effects on conventional measures of hepatic injury (i.e., serum transaminase and bilirubin levels). Additional research is required to validate the newer methods that are being used to detect hepatic effects of solvent exposure.

## OTHER EFFECTS

### Dermal Effects

Because of their ability to dissolve grease and fat, cutaneous exposure to solvents can deplete intact skin of lipids that are physiologically necessary for its functional integrity. This property of solvents results in an irritant contact dermatitis characterized by dryness, scaling, and fissuring of the skin, especially of the hands, in workers who have frequent dermal contact with solvents (164,165). This occurs either because the work requires manual handling of materials wet with solvents, as in the case of manual cleaning and degreasing, or in settings where solvents are used to wash the hands to remove glues, plastics, or other materials from the skin. These effects, which can be severe and require aggressive treatment with topical steroids, are reversible upon cessation of skin contact and are best prevented by avoiding direct skin contact with solvents.

#### *Mucous Membrane Irritation*

Solvents can be irritating to all mucous membranes. This results in irritation of the eyes, nose, and respiratory tract for workers exposed unprotected to solvent vapor. Airways irritation resulting in both bronchial and tracheal irritation have been described among solvent-exposed groups (166).

### Reproductive Effects

Few epidemiologic studies are available in which reproductive physiology or outcome is assessed in solvent-exposed workers; however, limited epidemiologic evidence available does suggest that adverse reproductive effects can occur in both male and female solvent-exposed workers (167). Occupational exposure to both carbon disulfide and benzene has been associated with menstrual abnormalities (168,169), and exposure to ethylene oxide has been associated with spontaneous abortion (170). Male shipyard painters exposed to glycol ethers have recently been shown to have lower sperm counts than unexposed referents (171). While many animal studies of reproductive effects of solvents are available, additional research is needed to clarify further the adverse reproductive effects in humans of occupational exposure to solvents.

### Carcinogenicity

The organic solvents benzene and the chloromethyl ethers, bis-chloromethyl ether (BCME) and technical-grade chloromethyl methyl ether (CMME), are well-established human carcinogens. Benzene is classified by the International Agency for Research on Cancer (IARC) as a group 1 carcinogen. It causes leukemia and other malignant hematopoietic disorders in humans. BCME is also classified by IARC as a group 1 carcinogen and is known to cause small cell carcinoma of the lung. It is used as an alkylating agent and solvent during the manufacture of polymers, ion-exchange resins, and waterproof coatings. Technical-grade CMME contains 1% to 7% BCME. Epidemiologic studies demonstrating excess small cell lung cancer in working populations exposed to BCME have come from the United States, the Federal Republic of Germany, and Japan (172).

The IARC has classified the solvent epichlorohydrin as "probably carcinogenic to humans" (group 2A), noting that the human evidence of carcinogenicity was inadequate at the time of evaluation but that evidence to declare it carcinogenic to animals was sufficient (172). Epichlorohydrin has been used in varnish, paint, and nail polish (31).

The halogenated hydrocarbons have been shown to be carcinogenic in animal systems (173); however, convincing human evidence is not available at this time. Reports of increased cancer of selected sites are available for many solvent-exposed cohorts: urologic malignancies and multiple myeloma in painters in New Zealand (174); esophageal and cervical cancers in dry cleaners (175); cancers of the lymphatic and hematopoietic system, colorectal cancer, and pancreatic cancer in commercial pressmen (176); lymphatic leukemia in rubber industry workers exposed to carbon tetrachloride and carbon disulfide (177); and primary liver cancer in solvent-exposed workers (178,179).

## CLINICAL EVALUATION

The goals of the clinical evaluation of solvent-exposed patients are to ascertain the presence of health effects attributable to solvent exposure, determine whether preexisting or underlying disease complicates the approach to the patient, and provide guidance on exposure reduction and periodic surveillance.

The evaluation of the symptomatic patient always begins with a review of presenting complaints. When a solvent-exposed worker presents for reasons other than current symptoms, such as periodic surveillance examination, a review of neurologic and dermatologic symptoms should be performed. Symptoms temporally related to exposure are a function of the anesthetic property of solvents. Specifically, dizziness, light-headedness, impaired concentration, and headache that have a temporal relationship to solvent exposure are likely the result of the acute CNS effects. In addition, unusual tiredness, sleep disturbance, appetite disturbance, mood changes, and other vegetative signs may also be related to solvent exposure, although in the absence of a close temporal association these very nonspecific symptoms may be difficult to attribute to solvent exposure in an individual case. Symptoms of dry, cracked, or itchy skin, especially of the hands, should be sought. In addition to symptoms of neurologic and dermatologic effects, symptoms of mucous membrane irritation manifesting as discomfort of the eyes, nose, and throat, should be elicited explicitly.

Review of past diagnoses or symptoms of neurologic, renal, hepatic, and dermatologic disease is required. The association between occupational solvent exposure and diagnosable conditions such as glomerulonephritis, contact dermatitis, cognitive impairment, and peripheral neuropathy may have been overlooked by other clinicians. In addition, the presence of such conditions, even if they are unrelated to current solvent exposure, may warrant more frequent medical surveillance or more aggressive exposure reduction for individual patients. The use of alcohol or medications that can affect the target organ systems of solvents must be ascertained, especially in light of increasing research evidence that toxicologically important interactions between these agents and solvents may occur.

The occupational circumstances under which the solvent exposure occurred must be elicited from the patient. Clearly, this requires knowledge not only of the job title but of daily occupational activities and the setting in which solvent exposure occurs. Exposure from the activities of co-workers should not be overlooked. An assessment of ventilation should be made, if possible. Inquiries about enclosure of solvent-related processes, use of hoods or other specialized ventilation, and specialty equipment such as spray booths should be made. The specific constituents of the solvent-containing materials used must be ascertained. This may necessitate requests for material safety data sheets (MSDS) from employers, suppliers, or manufacturers. Use and type of personal protective devices should be determined, and an assessment of the effectiveness of the program evaluated, if possible. Specific inquiry about the extent of skin contact and measures taken to prevent its occurrence should be made. The occupational history should include a general assessment of the hygienic conditions of the occupational setting, including the availability of separate washing, changing, and eating facilities.

A complete physical examination, with emphasis on the skin and the nervous system, should be performed. The skin, especially of the hands, should be inspected for redness, drying, cracking, or fissuring. A mental status examination that includes evaluation of alertness, orientation, cognition, and short-term memory should be performed. Evaluation of peripheral nerve function by assessing proprioception, deep tendon reflexes, motor strength, postural stability (Romberg test), and cutaneous sensibility to vibration, light touch, and pin prick should always be included in the evaluation. Clinical assessment of liver size and tenderness should be performed as it can be done quickly, although the clinician must recognize that it is not very sensitive.

Routine laboratory evaluation should be guided, in part, by the known toxicity of the solvents. For example, liver function tests are more likely to be of value in patients exposed to halogenated hydrocarbon solvents than in those exposed to nonhalogenated solvents. The consumption of alcohol must be considered when interpreting liver function test results. Routine urinalysis and measures of renal function (blood urea nitrogen and serum creatinine) are also reasonable for inclusion in the laboratory evaluation of solvent-exposed workers, although, again, their utility is limited by modest test sensitivity for early renal changes. The choice of additional tests must be guided by the clinical presentation of the patient. Those with complaints of persistent mood alteration or cognitive dysfunction, including memory loss, should be referred to a clinical neuropsychologist for evaluation, and a complete dementia workup should be considered. Those with persistent neuritic complaints, such as numbness, tingling, weakness, or pain, should be referred for neurologic consultation or electrophysiologic evaluation of peripheral nerve function (nerve conduction measurement and electromyography).

The health effects of exposure to organic solvents are nonspecific. Currently it is not known what proportion of neurologic, hepatic, renal, and dermatologic disease in exposed populations is attributable to solvents. Furthermore, the marked variety of exposures precludes sweeping generalization. Prior to making a diagnosis of solvent-related disease, other causes must be sought and their contribution to the current problem assessed. Organic brain syndrome secondary to solvent exposure is a diagnosis of exclusion. Substantial difficulties in estimating attribution of end-organ disease (e.g., peripheral neuropathy) due to solvent exposure occur when other disorders (e.g., diabetes) present at the same time could cause the same outcome.

Evaluation of the solvent-exposed worker provides an opportunity to address the exposure situation for the purpose of reducing exposures and preventing additional health effects for both the patient and co-workers. Unfortunately, access to the workplace may be limited, and often neither ambient nor biologic measures of exposure are available to allow quantification of the magnitude of exposure. In addition, patient confidentiality requirements may make workplace intervention difficult or impossible. Regardless, when the results of clinical evaluation suggest that biologically meaningful exposure is occurring, the clinician is obligated to explore avenues of exposure reduction within the confines of protection of patient confidentiality.

Much remains unknown about the rational approach to the solvent-exposed worker. Additional research is needed to clarify the clinical syndromes caused by solvent exposure, to provide guidance for treatment, and to attribute nonspecific outcomes to solvent exposure.

## SUMMARY

Exposure to a wide variety of organic solvents with a broad range of toxic effects is common in modern industry. Exposure to solvent mixtures is more common than exposure to pure substances. Solvents affect the nervous system, kidneys, liver, skin, and mucous membranes. Many of the health effects are controversial, including the existence and nature of chronic solvent effects on the CNS, the relationship between solvents and chronic renal disease, the hepatotoxicity of certain halogenated hydrocarbon solvents, and the human carcinogenicity of certain solvents. These areas of controversy exist, in part, because of the difficulties associated with epidemiologic research is this area of occupational toxicology. Specifically, retrospective ascertainment of exposure to solvents is especially difficult and can result in substantial misclassification. The definitions of health outcomes, especially chronic neurologic outcomes, are controversial. Virtually all solvent-related health outcomes are nonspecific, and the contribution of extraoccupational factors continues to be an area of concern. The effect of alcohol consumption on neurobehavioral outcomes is an especially good example of this problem. Furthermore, the use of so-called subclinical measures of neurologic, renal, and hepatic organ system effects has led to disagreement regarding the relationship between study results and the eventual development of disease or dysfunction. Finally, considerable additional research is needed to address the question of human carcinogenesis for those solvents that are known to cause cancer in animal systems.

The clinical evaluation of solvent-exposed workers is also complicated by difficulties of ascertainment of exposure, the nonspecific nature of the effects, poorly defined health outcomes, presence of other diseases, use of alcohol and medications, and attribution of effect to exposure. Little guidance is available for medical surveillance of solvent-exposed workers.

Regardless of the current controversies concerning the health effects of solvent exposure, overwhelming evidence is available for the existence of certain neurologic, hepatic, renal, and dermatologic health effects. Efforts to eliminate exposure by substituting safer solvents or by using solventless systems should continue. From the public health and preventive medicine perspective, reduction of occupational exposure to solvents will invariably reduce the burden of adverse health effects resulting from these agents, and should be pursued aggressively.

## REFERENCES

1. *Organic solvent neurotoxicity.* DHHS publication (NIOSH) 87—104. Cincinnati, OH: U.S. Department of Health and Human Services, 1987;1–39.
2. *Neurotoxicity:* identifying and controlling poisons of the nervous system. Washington, DC: U.S. Congress Office of Technology Assessment; 1990;267–311.
3. Parker SE. Use and abuse of volatile substances in industry. *Hum Toxicol* 1989;8:271–275.
4. Seedorff L, Olsen E. Exposure to organic solvents-I. A survey on the use of solvents. *Ann Occup Hyg* 1990;34:371–378.
5. Olsen E, Seedorff L. Exposure to organic solvents-II. An exposure epidemiology study. *Ann Occup Hyg* 1990;34:379–389.
6. Kalliokoski P. Solvent containing processes and work practices: environmental observations. In: Riihimäki V, Ulfvarson U, eds. *Safety and health aspects of organic solvents.* New York: Alan R. Liss, 1986; 21–30.
7. Baker EL, Smith TJ. Evaluation of exposure to organic solvents. In: Harrington JM, ed. *Recent advances in occupational health.* Edinburgh: Churchill Livingstone, 1984;89–105.
8. Droz PO, Wu MM, Cumberland WG, Berode M. Variability in biological monitoring of solvent exposure. I. Development of a population physiological model. *Br J Ind Med* 1989;46:447–460.
9. Droz PO, Wu MM, Cumberland WG. Variability in biological monitoring of organic solvent exposure. II. Application of a population physiological model. *Br J Ind Med* 1989;46:547–558.
10. Opdam JJG. Intra- and interindividual variability in the kinetics of a poorly and highly metabolising solvent. *Br J Ind Med* 1989;46: 831–845.
11. Lauwerys RR. Objectives of biological monitoring in occupational health practice. In: Aitio A, Riihimäki V, Vainio H, eds. *Biological monitoring and surveillance of workers exposed to chemicals.* Washington, DC: Hemisphere, 1984;3–6.
12. Aitio A, Riihimäki V, Vainio H, eds. *Biological monitoring and sur-*

veillance of workers exposed to chemicals.* Washington, DC: Hemisphere, 1984.
13. Lauwerys RR. *Industrial chemical exposure:* guidelines for biological monitoring. Davis, CA: Biomedical, 1983.
14. Fidler AT, Baker EL, Letz R. Estimation of long-term exposure to mixed solvents from questionnaire data: a tool for epidemiological investigations. *Br J Ind Med* 1987;44:133–141.
15. Mikkelsen S, J ørgensen M, Browne E, Gyldensted C. Mixed solvent exposure and organic brain damage: a study of painters. *Acta Neurol Scand* 1988;78(suppl 118):1–143.
16. Ikeda M. Multiple exposure to chemicals. *Reg Toxicol Pharmacol* 1988; 8:414–421.
17. *Organic solvents and the central nervous system.* Copenhagen: World Health Organization European Office, 1985.
18. Åstrand I. Uptake of solvents in the blood and tissues of man: a review. *Scand J Work Environ Health* 1975;1:199–218.
19. Cohr K-H. Uptake and distribution of common industrial solvents. In: Riihimäki V, Ulfvarson U, eds. *Safety and health aspects of organic solvents.* New York: Alan R. Liss, 1986;45–60.
20. Åstrand I. Work load and uptake of solvents in tissues of man. In: England A, Ringen K, Mehlman MA, eds. *Occupational health hazards of solvents.* Princeton, NJ: Princeton Scientific, 1986;2:141–152.
21. Angerer J, Lichterbeck E, Bergerow J, Jekel S, Lehnert G. Occupational chronic exposure to organic solvents. XIII. Glycolether exposure during the production of varnishes. *Int Arch Occup Environ Health* 1990;62:123–126.
22. Riihimäki V, Pfaffli P. Percutaneous absorption of solvent vapors in man. *Scand J Work Environ Health* 1978;4:73–85.
23. Bird M. Industrial solvents: some factors affecting their passage into and through the skin. *Ann Occup Hyg* 1981;24:235–244.
24. Sato A, Nakajima T. Pharmacokinetics of organic solvent vapors in relation to their toxicity. *Scand J Work Environ Health* 1987;13:81–93.
25. Fiserova-Bergerova V. Toxicokinetics of organic solvents. *Scand J Work Environ Health* 1985;11(suppl 1):7–21.
26. McFee DR, Zavon P. Solvents. In: Plog BA, ed. *Fundamentals of industrial hygiene,* 3rd ed. Chicago: National Safety Council, 1988; 95–121.
27. Baker EL. Organic solvent neurotoxicity. *Annu Rev Public Health* 1988;9:223–232.
28. Leading work-related disease and injuries—United States. *MMWR* 1983;32:24–26.
29. Spencer PS, Schaumburg HH. Organic solvent neurotoxicity: facts and research needs. *Scand J Work Environ Health* 1985;11:53–60.
30. Schaumburg HH, Spencer PS, Thomas PK. Toxic neuropathy: occupational, biological and environmental agents. In: Schaumburg HH, Spencer PS, Thomas PK, eds. *Disorders of peripheral nerves.* Philadelphia: F.A. Davis, 1983;131–155.
31. Gosselin RE, Smith RP, Hodge HC. *Clinical toxicology of commercial products.* Baltimore: Williams & Wilkins, 1984.
32. Iida M, Yamamura Y, Sobue I. Electromyographic findings and conduction velocity on *n*-hexane polyneuropathy. *Electromyogr Clin Neurophysiol* 1969;9:247.
33. Billmaier D, Yee HT, Allen N, et al. Peripheral neuropathy in a coated fabrics plant. *J Occup Med* 1974;16:665.
34. Allen N, Mendell JR, Billmaier D, Fontaine R, O'Neill J Jr. Toxic polyneuropathy due to methyl *n*-butyl ketone. *Arch Neurol* 1975;32:209.
35. Cianchetti C, Abbritti G, Petriconi G, Siracusa A, Curradi F. Toxic polyneuropathy of shoe industry workers: a study of 122 cases. *J Neurol Neurosurg Psychiatry* 1976;39:1151.
36. Korobkin R, Asbury AK, Sumner AJ, Nielsen SL. Glue-sniffing neuropathy. *Arch Neurol* 1975;32:158.
37. Thomas PK. The peripheral nervous system as a target for toxic substances. In: Spencer PS, Schaumburg HH, eds. *Experimental and clinical neurotoxicology.* Baltimore: Williams & Wilkins, 1980;35–47.
38. Seppäläinen AM. Neurophysiological approaches to the detection of early neurotoxicity in humans. *CRC Crit Rev Toxicol* 1988;18: 245–298.
39. Andrews LS, Snyder R. Toxic effects of solvents and vapors. In: Klaassen CD, Amdur MO, Doull J, eds. *Cassarett and Doull's toxicology:* the basic science of poisons. 3rd ed. New York: Macmillan, 1986; 636–668.
40. Buiatti E, Cecchini S, Ronchi O, Dolara P, Bulgarelli G. Relationship between clinical and electromyographic findings and exposure to solvents in shoe and leather workers. *Br J Ind Med* 1978;35:168–173.
41. Mutti A, Ferri F, Lommi G, et al. *n*-hexane induced changes in nerve conduction velocities and somatosensory evoked potentials. *Int Arch Occup Environ Health* 1982;51:45–54.
42. Cranmer JM, Goldberg L. Proceedings of the workshop on the neurobehavioral effects of solvents. *Neurotoxicology* 1986;7:1–123.
43. Laine A, Riihimäki V. Acute solvent intoxication. In: Riihimäki V, Ulfvarson U, eds. *Safety and health aspects of organic solvents.* New York: Alan R. Liss, 1986;123–131.
44. McCarthy TB, Jones RD. Industrial gassing poisonings due to trichlorethylene, perchlorethylene, and 1-1-1 trichlorethane, 1961–1980. *Br J Ind Med* 1983;40:450–455.
45. Bakinson MA, Jones RD. Gassings due to methylene chloride, xylene, toluene, and styrene reported to Her Majesty's Factory Inspectorate 1961–1980. *Br J Ind Med* 1985;42:184–190.
46. Ramsey J, Anderson HR, Bloor K, Flanagan RJ. An introduction to the practice, prevalence and chemical toxicology of volatile substance abuse. *Hum Toxicol* 1989;8:261–269.
47. Meredith TJ, Ruprah M, Liddle A, Flanagan RJ. Diagnosis and treatment of acute poisoning with volatile substances. *Hum Toxicol* 1989; 8:277–286.
48. Gamberale F. Application of psychometric techniques in the assessment of solvent toxicity. In: Riihimäki V, Ulfvarson U, eds. *Safety and health aspects of organic solvents.* New York: Alan R. Liss, 1986; 203–224.
49. Iregren A. Effects on human performance from acute and chronic exposure to organic solvents: a short review. *Toxicology* 1988;49: 349–358.
50. Dick RB. Short duration exposures to organic solvents: the relationship between neurobehavioral test results and other indicators. *Neurotoxicol Teratol* 1988;10:39–50.
51. Anger WK. Worksite behavioral research: results, sensitive methods, test batteries and the transition from laboratory data to human health. *Neurotoxicology* 1990;11:629–720.
52. Savolainen K, Riihimäki V, Laine A. Biphasic effects of inhaled solvents on human equilibrium. *Acta Pharmacol Toxicol* 1982;51:237–242.
53. Dick RB, Bhattacharya A, Shukla R. Use of a computerized postural sway measurement system for neurobehavioral toxicology. *Neurotoxicol Teratol* 1990;12:1–6.
54. Gamberale F. Critical issues in the study of the acute effects of solvent exposure. *Neurotoxicol Teratol* 1989;11:565–570.
55. Hänninen H. Neurobehavioral assessment of long-term solvent effects on man. In: Riihimäki V, Ulfvarson U, eds. *Safety and health aspects of organic solvents.* New York: Alan R. Liss, 1986;225–236.
56. Grasso P, Sharratt M, Davies DM, Irvine D. Neurophysiological and psychological disorders and occupational exposure to organic solvents. *Food Chem Toxicol* 1984;10:819–852.
57. *Organic solvents and the nervous system:* report of a conference. Copenhagen: CEC/Danish Ministry of the Environment, 1991.
58. Hogstedt C. Has the Scandinavian solvent syndrome controversy been solved? *Scand J Work Environ Health* 1994;20:59-64.
59. Lundberg P. International conference on organic solvent toxicity. *Scand J Work Environ Health* 1985;11(suppl 1):1–103.
60. Elofsson SA, Gamberale F, Hindmarsh T, et al. Exposure to organic solvents: a cross-sectional epidemiologic investigation on occupationally exposed car and industrial spray painters with special reference to the nervous system. *Scand J Work Environ Health* 1980;6:239–273.
61. Ørbaek P, Risberg J, Rosén I, et al. Effects of long-term exposure to solvents in the paint industry. *Scand J Work Environ Health* 1985; 11(suppl 2):1–28.
62. Baker EL, Letz R, Eisen EA, et al. Neurobehavioral effects of solvents in construction painters. *J Occup Med* 1988;30:116–123.
63. Spurgeon A, Gray CN, Sims J, et al. Neurobehavioral effects of long-term occupational exposure to organic solvents: two comparable studies. *Am J Ind Med* 1992;22:325-335.
64. Axelson O, Hane M, Hogstedt C. A case-referent study on neuropsychiatric disorders among workers exposed to solvents. *Scand J Work Environ Health* 1976;2:14–20.
65. Mikkelsen S. A cohort study of disability pension and death among painters with special regard to disabling presenile dementia as an occupational disease. *Scand J Soc Med* 1980;16:34–43.
66. Lindström K, Riihimäki H, Hänninen K. Occupational solvent exposure and neuropsychiatric disorders. *Scand J Work Environ Health* 1984;10:321–323.
67. Gubéran E, Usel M, Raymond L, Tissot R, Sweetnam PM. Disability,

mortality, and incidence of cancer among Geneva painters and electricians: a historical prospective study. *Br J Ind Med* 1989;46:16–23.
68. van Vliet C, Swaen GMH, Volovics A, et al. Exposure-outcome relationships between organic solvent exposure and neuropsychiatric disorders: results from a Dutch case-control study. *Am J Ind Med* 1989;16:707–718.
69. Brackbill RM, Maizlish NA, Fischbach T. Risk of neuropsychiatric disability among painters in the United States. *Scand J Work Environ Health* 1990;16:182–188.
70. Riise T, Kyvik KR, Moen B. A cohort study of disability pensioning among Norwegian painters, construction workers, and workers in food processing. *Epidemiology* 1995;6:132–136.
71. Cherry N, Waldron HA. The prevalence of psychiatric morbidity in solvent workers in Britain. *Int J Epidemiol* 1984;13:197–200.
72. Labreche FP, Cherry NM, McDonald JC. Psychiatric disorders and occupational exposure to solvents. *Br J Ind Med* 1992;49:820–825.
73. Nelson NA, Robins TG, White RF, Garrison RP. A case-control study of chronic neuropsychiatric disease and organic solvent exposure in automobile assembly plant workers. *Occup Environ Med* 1994;51: 302–307.
74. Cherry NM, Labreche FP, McDonald JC. Organic brain damage and occupational solvent exposure. *Br J Ind Med* 1992;49:776–781.
75. Hogstedt C, Andersson K, Hane M. A questionnaire approach to the monitoring of early disturbances in central nervous functions. In: Aitio A, Riihimäki V, Vainio H, eds. *Biological monitoring and surveillance of workers exposed to chemicals.* New York: Hemisphere, 1984;275–287.
76. Morrow LA, Ryan CM, Hodgson MJ, Robin N. Alterations in cognitive and psychological functioning after organic solvent exposure. *J Occup Med* 1990;32:444–450.
77. Rasmussen K, Arlien-Soborg P, Sabroe S. Clinical neurological findings among metal degreasers exposed to chlorinated solvents. *Acta Neurol Scand* 1993;87:200–204.
78. White RF, Proctor SP, Echeverria D, Schweikert J, Feldman RG. Neurobehavioral effects of acute and chronic mixed-solvent exposure in the screen printing industry. *Am J Ind Med* 1995;28:221–231.
79. Daniell W, Stebbins A, O'Donnell J, Horstman SW, Rosenstock L. Neuropsychological performance and solvent exposure among car body repair shop workers. *Br J Ind Med* 1993;50:368–377.
80. Hänninen H, Antti-Poika M, Juntunen J, Koskenvuo M. Exposure to organic solvents and neuropsychological dysfunction: a study on monozygotic twins. *Br J Ind Med* 1991;48:18–25.
81. Spurgeon A, Glass DC, Calvert IA, Cunningham-Hill M, Harrington JM. Investigation of dose related neurobehavioural effects in paintmakers exposed to low levels of solvents. *Occup Environ Med* 1994; 51:626–630.
82. White RF, Robins TG, Proctor S, Echeverria D, Rocskay AS. Neuropsychological effects of exposure to naphtha among automotive workers. *Occup Environ Med* 1994;51:102–112.
83. Hooisma J, Hänninen H, Emmen HH, Kulig BM. Behavioral effects of exposure to organic solvents in Dutch painters. *Neurotoxicol Teratol* 1993;15:397–406.
84. Triebig G, Barocka A, Erbguth F, et al. Neurotoxicity of solvent mixtures in spray painters. II. Neurologic, psychiatric, psychological, and neuroradiologic findings. *Int Arch Occup Environ Health* 1992;64: 361–372.
85. Sandmark B, Broms I, Löfgren L, Ohlson C. Olfactory function in painters exposed to organic solvents. *Scand J Work Environ Health* 1989;15:60–63.
86. Schwartz BS, Ford DP, Bolla KI, et al. Solvent-associated decrements in olfactory function in paint manufacturing workers. *Am J Ind Med* 1990;18:697–706.
87. Jacobsen P, Hein HO, Suadicani P, Parving A, Gyntelberg F. Mixed solvent exposure and hearing impairment: an epidemiological study of 3284 men. The Copenhagen male study. *Occup Med* 1993;43: 180–184.
88. Morata TC, Nylen P, Johnson AC, Dunn DE. Auditory and vestibular functions after single or combined exposure to toluene: a review. *Arch Toxicol* 1995;69:431–443.
89. Morata TC, Dunn DE, Sieber WK. Occupational exposure to noise and ototoxic organic solvents. *Arch Environ Health* 1994;49: 359–365.
90. Johnson AC, Nylen PR. Effects of industrial solvents on hearing. *Occup Med* 1995;10:623–640.
91. Riatta C, Teir H, Tolonen M, et al. Impaired color discrimination among viscose rayon workers exposed to carbon disulfide. *J Occup Med* 1981;23:189–192.
92. Mergler D, Blain L. Assessing color vision loss among solvent-exposed workers. *Am J Ind Med* 1987;12:195–203.
93. Mergler D, Belanger S, De Grosbois S, Vachon N. Chromal focus of acquired chromatic discrimination loss and solvent exposure among printshop workers. *Toxicology* 1988;49:341–348.
94. Mergler D, Bowler R, Cone J. Colour vision loss among disabled workers with neuropsychological impairment. *Neurotoxicol Teratol* 1990;12:669–672.
95. Ruijten MW, Salle HJ, Verberk MM, Muijser H. Special nerve functions and colour discrimination in workers with long term low level exposure to carbon disulphide. *Br J Ind Med* 1990;47:589–595.
96. Baird B, Camp J, Daniell W, Antonelli J. Solvents and color discrimination ability. Nonreplication of previous findings. *J Occup Med* 1994; 36:747–751.
97. Nakatsuka H, Watanabe T, Takeuchi Y, et al. Absence of blue-yellow color vision loss among workers exposed to toluene or tetrachloroethylene, mostly at levels below occupational exposure limits. *Int Arch Occup Environ Health* 1992;64:113–117.
98. Frenette B, Mergler D, Bowler R. Contrast-sensitivity loss in a group of former microelectronics workers with normal visual acuity. *Optom Vis Sci* 1991;68:556–560.
99. Donoghue AM, Dryson EW, Wynn-Williams G. Contrast sensitivity in organic-solvent-induced chronic toxic encephalopathy. *J Occup Environ Med* 1995;37:1357–1363.
100. Antti-Poika M, Ojala M, Matikainen E, Vaheri E, Juntunen J. Occupational exposure to solvents and cerebellar, brainstem and vestibular functions. *Int Arch Occup Environ Health* 1989;61:397–401.
101. Ledin T, Ødkvist L, Möller C. Posturography findings in workers exposed to industrial solvents. *Acta Otolaryngol (Stockh)* 1989;107: 357–361.
102. Möller C, Ødkvist L, Larsby B, et al. Otoneurological findings in workers exposed to styrene. *Scand J Work Environ Health* 1990;16: 189–194.
103. Ørbaek P, Rosén I, Svensson K. Power spectrum analysis of EEG at diagnosis and follow-up of patients with solvent-induced chronic toxic encephalopathy. *Br J Ind Med* 1988;45:476–482.
104. Hagstadius S, Ørbaek P, Risberg J, Lindgren M. Regional cerebral blood flow at the time of diagnosis of chronic toxic encephalopathy induced by organic solvent exposure and after the cessation of exposure. *Scand J Work Environ Health* 1989;15:130–135.
105. Deschamps D, Garnier R, Lille F, et al. Evoked potentials and cerebral blood flow in solvent induced psycho-organic syndrome. *Br J Ind Med* 1993;50:325–330.
106. Juntunen J, Matikainen E, Antti-Poika M, Suoranta H, Valle M. Nervous system effects of long-term occupational exposure to toluene. *Acta Neurol Scand* 1985;72:512–517.
107. Ørbaek P, Lindgren M, Olivecrona H, Haeger-Aronsen B. Computed tomography and psychometric test performances in patients with solvent induced chronic toxic encephalopathy and healthy controls. *Br J Ind Med* 1987;44:175–179.
108. Callender TJ, Morrow L, Subramanian K, Duhon D, Ristovv M. Three-dimensional brain metabolic imaging in patients with toxic encephalopathy. *Environ Res* 1993;60:295–319.
109. Heuser G, Mena I, Alamos F. NeuroSPECT findings in patients exposed to neurotoxic chemicals. *Toxicol Ind Health* 1994;10:561–571.
110. Fincher CE, Chang TS, Harrell EH, et al. Comparison of single photon emission computed tomography findings in cases of healthy adults and solvent-exposed adults. *Am J Ind Med* 1997;31:4–14.
111. Errebo-Knudsen EO, Olsen F. Organic solvents and presenile dementia (the painters' syndrome). A critical review of the Danish literature. *Sci Tot Environ* 1986;48:45–67.
112. Ørbaek P, Nise G. Neurasthenic complaints and psychometric function of toluene-exposed rotogravure printers. *Am J Ind Med* 1989;16:67–77.
113. Hänninen H, Antti-Poika M, Savolainen P. Psychological performance, toluene exposure and alcohol consumption in rotogravure printers. *Int Arch Occup Environ Health* 1987;59:475–483.
114. Johnson BL, ed. *Prevention of neurotoxic illness in working populations.* New York: John Wiley, 1987.
115. Bleecker ML, Bolla K, Agnew J, Schwartz BS, Ford DP. Dose-related subclinical neurobehavioral effects of chronic exposure to low levels of organic solvents. *Am J Ind Med* 1991;19;715–728.
116. Williamson AM, Winder C. A prospective cohort study of the chronic effects of solvent exposure. *Environ Res* 1993;62:256–271.

117. Ørbaek P, Lindgren M. Prospective clinical and psychometric investigation of patients with chronic toxic encephalopathy induced by solvents. *Scand J Work Environ Health* 1988;14:37–44.
118. Ørbaek P, Rosén I, Svensson K. Electroneurographic findings in patients with solvent-induced central nervous system dysfunction. *Br J Ind Med* 1988;45:409–414.
119. Edling C, Ekberg K, Ahlborg G Jr, et al. Long-term follow-up of workers exposed to solvents. *Br J Ind Med* 1990;47:75–82.
120. Gregersen P. Neurotoxic effects of organic solvents in exposed workers: two controlled follow-up studies after 5.5 and 10.6 years. *Am J Ind Med* 1988;14:681–701.
121. Schrier RW, Conger JD. Acute renal failure: pathogenesis, diagnosis, and management. In: Schrier RW, ed. *Renal and electrolyte disorders,* 2nd ed. Boston: Little, Brown, 1980;375–408.
122. Phillips SC, Petrone RL, Hemstreet GP. A review of the nonneoplastic kidney effects of hydrocarbon exposure in humans. *Occup Med* 1988;3:495–509.
123. Lauwerys RR, Bernard A, Viau C, Buchet JP. Kidney disorders and hematotoxicity from organic solvent exposure. *Scand J Work Environ Health* 1985;11:83–90.
124. Nelson NA, Robins TG, Port FK. Solvent nephrotoxicity in humans and experimental animals. *Am J Nephrol* 1990;10:10–20.
125. Barrientos A, Ortuno MT, Morales JM, Martinez T, Rodicio JL. Acute renal failure after use of diesel fuel as shampoo. *Arch Intern Med* 1977;137:1217.
126. Glassock RJ, Brenner BM. The major glomerulopathies. In: Braunwald E, Isselbacher KJ, Petersdorf RG, Wilson JD, Martin JB, Fauci AS, eds. *Harrison's principals of internal medicine,* 11th ed. New York: McGraw-Hill, 1987;1173–1183.
127. Churchill DN, Fine A, Gault MH. Association between hydrocarbon exposure and glomerulonephritis. An appraisal of the evidence. *Nephron* 1983;33:169–172.
128. Stevenson A, Yaqoob M, Mason H, Pai P, Bell GM. Biochemical markers of basement membrane disturbances and occupational exposure to hydrocarbons and mixed solvents. *Q J Med* 1995;88:23–28.
129. Ravnskov U, Forsberg B, Skerfving S. Glomerulonephritis and exposure to organic solvents: a case-control study. *Acta Med Scand* 1979; 205:575–579.
130. van der Laan G. Chronic glomerulonephritis and organic solvents: a case-control study. *Int Arch Occup Environ Health* 1980;47:1–8.
131. Bell GM, Gordon ACH, Lee P, et al. Proliferative glomerulonephritis and exposure to organic solvents. *Nephron* 1985;40:161–165.
132. Harrington JM, Whitby H, Gray CN, et al. Renal disease and occupational exposure to organic solvents: a case referent approach. *Br J Ind Med* 1989;46:643–650.
133. Porro A, Lomonte C, Coratelli P, et al. Chronic glomerulonephritis and exposure to solvents: a case-referent study. *Br J Ind Med* 1992;49: 738–742.
134. Franchini L, Cavatorta A, Falzoi M, et al. Early indicators of renal damage in workers exposed to organic solvents. *Int Arch Occup Environ Health* 1983;52:1–9.
135. Viau C, Bernard A, Lauwerys R, et al. A cross-sectional survey of kidney function in refinery employees. *Am J Ind Med* 1987;11:177–187.
136. Meyer BR, Rosenman K, Lerman Y, et al. Increased urinary enzyme excretion in workers exposed to nephrotoxic chemicals. *Am J Med* 1984;76:989–998.
137. Mutti A, Lucertini S, Falzoi M. Organic solvents and chronic glomerulonephritis: a cross-sectional study with negative findings for aliphatic and alicyclic C5–C7 hydrocarbons. *Appl Toxicol* 1981;1:224.
138. Hotz P, Pilliod J, Söderstrom D, et al. Relation between renal function tests and a retrospective organic solvent exposure score. *Br J Ind Med* 1989;46:815–819.
139. Mutti A, Alinovi R, Bergamaschi E, et al. Nephropathies and exposure to perchloroethylene in dry-cleaners. *Lancet* 1992;340:189–193.
140. Askergren A. Organic solvents and kidney function. In: Englund A, Ringen K, Mehlman MA, eds. *Occupational health hazards of solvents.* Princeton, NJ: Princeton Scientific, 1986;157–172.
141. Krusell L, Kraemmer Nielsen H, Baelum J, et al. Renal effects of chronic exposure to organic solvents. *Acta Med Scand* 1985;218: 323–327.
142. Vyskocil A, Emminger S, Malir F, et al. Lack of nephrotoxicity of styrene at current TLV level (50 ppm). *Int Arch Occup Environ Health* 1989;61:409–411.
143. Solet D, Robins TG. Renal function in dry cleaning workers exposed to perchloroethylene. *Am J Ind Med* 1991;20:601–614.
144. Steenland NK, Thun MJ, Ferguson CW, Port FK. Occupational and other exposures associated with male end-stage renal disease: a case/control study. *Am J Public Health* 1990;80:153–157.
145. Zimmerman HJ, Ishak KG. Hepatic injury due to drugs and toxins. In: MacSween RNM, Anthony PP, Scheuer PJ, eds. *Pathology of the liver,* 2nd ed. Edinburgh: Churchill Livingstone, 1987;503–573.
146. Gurney R. Tetrachlorethane intoxication: early recognition of liver damage, and means of prevention. *Gastroenterology* 1943;1:1112–1116.
147. McDermott WV, Hardy H. Cirrhosis of the liver following chronic exposure to carbon tetrachloride. *J Occup Med* 1963;5:249–251.
148. Kramer CG, Ott MG, Fulkerson JE, Hicks N, Imbus HR. Health of workers exposed to 1,1,1,-trichloroethylene: a matched-pair study. *Arch Environ Health* 1978;331–342.
149. Soden KJ. An evaluation of chronic methylene chloride exposure. *J Occup Med* 1993;35:282–286.
150. Hodgson M, Heyl AE, Van Thiel DH. Liver disease associated with exposure to 1,1,1-trichloroethane. *Arch Intern Med* 1989;149: 1793–1798.
151. Baerg RD, Kimberg DV. Centrilobular hepatic necrosis and acute renal failure in solvent sniffers. *Ann Intern Med* 1970;73:713–720.
152. Lundberg I, Hakansson M. Normal serum activities of liver enzymes in Swedish paint industry workers with heavy exposure to organic solvents. *Br J Ind Med* 1985;42:596–600.
153. Pedersen LM, Rasmussen JM. The haematological and biochemical pattern in occupational organic solvent poisoning and exposure. *Int Arch Occup Environ Health* 1982;51:113–126.
154. Hane M, Axelson O, Blume J, et al. Psychological function changes among house painters. *Scand J Work Environ Health* 1977;3:91–99.
155. Redlich CA, Beckett WS, Sparer J, et al. Liver disease associated with occupational exposure to the solvent dimethylformamide. *Ann Intern Med* 1988;108:680–686.
156. Wang JD, Lai MY, Chen JS, et al. Dimethylformamide-induced liver damage among synthetic leather workers. *Arch Environ Health* 1991; 46:161–166.
157. Harrison R, Letz G, Pasternak G, Blanc P. Fulminant hepatic failure after occupational exposure to 2-nitropropane. *Ann Intern Med* 1987; 107:466–468.
158. Døssing M. Changes in hepatic microsomal enzyme function in workers exposed to mixtures of chemicals. *Clin Pharmacol Ther* 1982;32: 340–346.
159. Døssing M, Loft S, Schroeder E. Jet fuel and liver function. *Scand J Work Environ Health* 1985;11:433–437.
160. Brodkin CA, Daniell W, Checkoway H, et al. Hepatic ultrasonic changes in workers exposed to perchloroethylene. *Occup Environ Med* 1995;52:679–685.
161. Edling C, Tagesson C. Raised serum bile acid concentrations after occupational exposure to styrene: a possible sign of hepatotoxicity? *Br J Ind Med* 1984;41:257–259.
162. Franco G, Fonte R, Tempini G, Candura F. Serum bile acid concentrations as a liver function test in workers occupationally exposed to organic solvents. *Int Arch Occup Environ Health* 1986;58:157–164.
163. Driscoll TR, Hamdan HH, Wang G, Wright PF, Stacey NH. Concentrations of individual serum or plasma bile acids in workers exposed to chlorinated aliphatic hydrocarbons. *Br J Ind Med* 1992;49:700–705.
164. Mathias CGT. Contact dermatitis from use or misuse of soaps, detergents, and cleansers in the workplace. *Occup Med State Art Rev* 1986; 1:205–228.
165. Andersen KE. Solvent dermatitis. In: Riihimäki V, Ulf–Varson U, eds. *Safety and health aspects of organic solvents.* New York: Alan R. Liss, 1986;133–138.
166. Lorimer WV, Lilis R, Nicholson WJ, et al. Clinical studies of styrene workers: initial findings. *Environ Health Perspect* 1976;17:171–181.
167. *Reproductive hazards in the workplace.* Washington, DC: U.S. Government Printing Office, 1985.
168. Cai SX, Boa YS. Placental transfer, secretion into mother's milk, and the effects on maternal function of female viscose rayon workers. *Ind Health* 1981;19:15–29.
169. Hunt VR. *Work and the health of women.* Boca Raton, FL: CRC Press, 1979.
170. Hemminki K, Mutagen P, Saloniemi I, Niemi ML, Vaino N. Spontaneous abortions in hospital staff engaged in sterilizing instruments with chemical agents. *Br Med J* 1982;285:1461–1463.
171. Welch LH, Schrader SM, Turner TW, Cullen MR. Effects of exposure to ethylene glycol ethers on shipyard painters: II. Male reproduction. *Am J Ind Med* 1988;14:509–526.

172. *The toxicology of chemicals:* carcinogenicity. Luxembourg: Commission of the European Communities, 1989;1.
173. Decouflé P. Occupation. In: Schottenfeld D, Fraumeni JF Jr, eds. *Cancer epidemiology and prevention.* Philadelphia: WB Saunders, 1982; 318–335.
174. Bethwaite PB, Pearce N, Fraser J. Cancer risks in painters: study based on the New Zealand Cancer Registry. *Br J Ind Med* 1990;47:742–746.
175. Blair A, Stewart PA, Tolbert PE, Grauman D. Cancer and other causes of death among a cohort of dry cleaners. *Br J Ind Med* 1990;47:162–168.
176. Zoloth SR, Michaels DM, Villalbi JR, Lacher M. Patterns of mortality among commercial pressmen. *J Natl Cancer Inst* 1986;76:1047–1051.
177. Wilcosky TC, Checkoway H, Marshall EG, Tyroler HA. Cancer mortality and solvent exposure in the rubber industry. *Am Ind Hyg Assoc J* 1990;45:809–811.
178. Hernberg S, Korkala ML, Asikainen U, Riala R. Primary liver cancer and exposure to solvents. *Scand J Work Environ Health* 1984;54: 147–153.
179. Hernberg S, Kauppinen T, Riala R, Korkala ML, Asikainen U. Increased risk for primary liver cancer among women exposed to solvents. *Scand J Work Environ Health* 1988;14:356–365.
180. Alliance of American Insurers. *Handbook of organic industrial solvents,* 6th ed. 1987.

*Environmental and Occupational Medicine, Third Edition,* edited by William N. Rom.
Lippincott–Raven Publishers, Philadelphia © 1998.

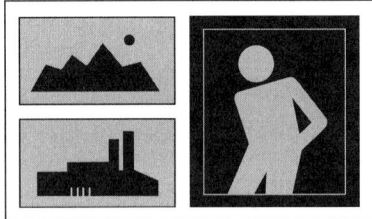

# CHAPTER 79

# Benzene

Philip J. Landrigan and William J. Nicholson

Benzene ($C_6H_6$) is the simplest and the prototypical aromatic hydrocarbon. It is a known cause of aplastic anemia, leukemia, and lymphoma. It is among the most widely used of all organic chemicals and has the highest production volume of all known human carcinogens (1). Historically, benzene was produced as a by-product of coal gasification and coke production. Today, however, it is produced principally by the petrochemical and petroleum-refining industries, and these sources are responsible for 98% of the total United States production (2). An estimated 2 million American workers have potential occupational exposure to benzene (3).

Benzene is a clear, colorless, noncorrosive, highly flammable liquid with a strong and rather pleasant odor. Its low boiling point and high vapor pressure cause rapid evaporation under ordinary atmospheric conditions; the resulting vapors are nearly three times heavier than air (4).

## HUMAN EXPOSURE

Benzene is used as a solvent, a degreasing agent, and as a fundamental building block in many processes in the synthetic chemical industry (1). Occupational exposure occurs in the chemical, printing, rubber, paint, and petroleum industries (2). Particularly heavy exposure occurs in maintenance, clean-up, product sampling, and petroleum bulk transfer operations. Although benzene's use has declined in recent years in the United States and in other industrially developed nations, data from developing countries suggest that exposures there are widespread (5), especially in artisan work, shoe manufacture, small chemical industries, and work involving children (6).

Environmental exposure to benzene is extensive, because benzene is a constituent of both inhaled and environmental tobacco smoke. Also benzene constitutes 1% to 2% of American unleaded gasoline by weight, and 3% to 5% of European gasoline; exposure occurs during the pumping and handling of gasoline (7).

Occupational absorption of benzene occurs predominantly through inhalation of benzene vapor (1,3). Experimental studies indicate that approximately 50% of inhaled benzene is absorbed into the body and the remainder is exhaled (8). Ingested liquid benzene is rapidly absorbed through the gastrointestinal mucosa.

Benzene can also be absorbed through the skin (1). Dermal absorption is substantially enhanced when the skin is cracked, blistered, or abraded, as occurs in rubber workers engaged in tire building. It is estimated that a rubber worker who produces 150 tires a day using benzene-containing rubber solvent could absorb 6 mg of benzene through the skin; this compares with an estimated 14 mg absorbed by inhalation per 8-hour day in an atmosphere containing 1 ppm benzene vapor (2).

### Metabolism and Mechanisms of Injury

Benzene is rapidly metabolized, principally in the liver. Its metabolic products are excreted, mainly as water-soluble metabolites in urine, within 48 hours of absorption. The oxidative products of benzene include phenol, catechol, quinol, hydroxyquinol, and muconic acid (8).

Metabolism of benzene is required for toxicity (9). This metabolism occurs principally in the liver via the cytochrome P-450 and mixed-function oxidase systems

P. J. Landrigan: Department of Community and Preventive Medicine, Mt. Sinai School of Medicine, New York, New York 10029.
W. J. Nicholson: Division of Environmental and Occupational Medicine, Department of Community and Preventive Medicine, Mt. Sinai School of Medicine, New York, New York 10022.

(10,11). Production of benzene metabolites in the liver is followed by their transport to the bone marrow and other organs. Substantial evidence indicates that benzene per se is not myelotoxic, and that its toxicity is due to several of its metabolic products, particularly benzoquinone and muconaldehyde (12,13). These compounds have the ability to react with DNA to form adducts (9). Benzene metabolism is quantitatively different at different dose levels, and at low doses a relatively higher proportion of benzene is converted to hydroquinones and other more highly toxic metabolites than at higher doses; this finding suggests that linear extrapolation of risk from high-dose studies may underestimate the true risk of low-level benzene exposure (13).

Benzene itself is not mutagenic. However, various of its products are mutagenic in bacterial species (14). Presumably, these active products such as the quinones are involved in the causation of the chromosome damage, with increased numbers of strand breaks, hyperploidy, and deletions observed in humans and animal species exposed to benzene (9,15). It is hypothesized that these chromosomal aberrations induced by benzene may lead to inactivation of p53 or other tumor suppressor genes, and that these genomic events are involved in leukemogenesis (16). Recently, an association has been suggested between benzene exposure and deletion of the long arm of chromosome 5; this 5q-deletion is linked to myelodysplastic syndrome, a preleukemic condition, and the deletion is hypothesized to result in inactivation of a leukemia tumor suppressor gene, possibly the gene encoding purα, located at 5q31; the purα protein is involved in cell cycle control of DNA replication (17).

### Exposure Monitoring

Occupational exposure to benzene is assessed principally through personal (breathing zone) air sampling (2). Measurement of the blood benzene level has traditionally been considered to be insensitive for occupational exposure monitoring; however, recent studies with new high-resolution gas chromatographic techniques suggest that blood sampling may be a useful indicator of current benzene exposure (18). Timing is very important in the determination of the blood level of benzene because of the short half-life of the compound in blood. Measurement of benzene in exhaled breath is another sensitive means of assessing exposure. Approximately 50% of benzene is exhaled unmetabolized; this measurement also is very time dependent (18).

Urinary phenol determination is a good biologic marker of recent industrial benzene exposure (16). Recent studies in China and Japan indicate that there is a close quantitative relation between level of benzene vapor in workroom air and urine phenol level (19). By contrast, urinary markers are not useful as indicators of low-level benzene exposure in the general environment (20).

The principal screening tool for clinical assessment of benzene toxicity is the complete blood count (CBC), including a platelet count and a white cell differential count as well as a red blood cell count, hemoglobin, hematocrit, and red blood cell indices (1,2). These hematologic indices do not appear to be sufficiently sensitive to detect toxic changes in workers whose exposures are within current exposure standards. However, at high levels of exposure, benzene is associated with significant decreases in white and red cell counts as well as in hemoglobin levels. Therefore, periodic hematologic testing of benzene workers may be useful to detect those who are exposed to higher-than-average ambient levels. Also, it is at least theoretically possible that periodic biologic monitoring of workers exposed to benzene may detect any who are unusually sensitive, although such sensitivity has not been well documented.

Chromosome aberrations have been seen in several studies of workers exposed to benzene, even at low levels (21). These changes consist of chromatid deletions and gaps (22) as well as increased numbers of strand breaks and micronuclei (15). The utility of these cytogenetic abnormalities as quantitative screening tests for benzene exposure and toxicity is not yet established and will require prospective epidemiologic follow-up of exposed groups (15).

An important unmet need in benzene toxicology is for a stable biologic marker of exposure. There is need for a marker that better reflects cumulative exposure over time than the measurement of evanescent levels of benzene in exhaled breath or blood or the measurement of relatively rapidly excreted phenol in urine.

## TOXICITY

### Immediate Effects

Central nervous system toxicity is the most important aspect of acute high-dose exposure to benzene. Like many solvents, benzene is readily soluble in lipids and rapidly crosses the blood-brain barrier to enter the central nervous system. Low-level neurologic exposure causes headache and nausea, whereas higher levels cause alteration of consciousness progressing to coma and respiratory arrest (1,4). Acute benzene exposure is toxic to the liver and kidneys; elevations in the serum creatinine level as well as in liver function enzymes and serum bilirubin can result (1). Benzene is toxic to the skin. Direct contact may cause erythema and blistering (4). Long-term direct contact removes lipids from the skin tissue and may result in the development of a dry, scaly dermatitis. Benzene is poorly absorbed through intact skin but is readily absorbed through cracked, dry, or fissured skin (2). Immediate effects of ingestion of liquid benzene are local irritation of the mouth, throat, esophagus, and stomach. Subsequent absorption of ingested benzene into the blood leads to the signs and symptoms of systemic intoxication (4). High concentrations of benzene vapor are irritating to the mucous membranes of the eyes, nose, and respiratory tract (4).

### Long-Term Effects

Aplastic anemia is the classic cause of death in chronic benzene poisoning (1), and the association between benzene exposure and bone marrow suppression has been recognized since 1897 (23).

Leukemia in workers exposed occupationally to benzene was first recognized in the 1920s (24). Additional case reports and case series published from the 1920s to the 1960s repeatedly noted the association between leukemia and exposure to benzene (24–26). All types of leukemia are observed in reports of workers exposed to benzene. Myeloid and myelomonocytic leukemias are the cell types most commonly seen, but also acute and chronic lymphocytic leukemia are encountered (1,9,27,28). Additionally, benzene exposure has been linked in clinical and epidemiologic studies to lymphoma, including non-Hodgkin's lymphoma and multiple myeloma (29,30).

To evaluate systematically the association between benzene and leukemia, the National Institute for Occupational Safety and Health (NIOSH) undertook a series of epidemiologic studies beginning in the 1970s. The studies employed a retrospective cohort design. They examined a population of 1,165 rubber workers occupationally exposed to benzene at two plants in Ohio that produced thin sheets of latex rubber called Pliofilm. Benzene was the only hematotoxic substance in these factories (31,32).

Initial analyses of mortality in this population were primarily qualitative, and they showed a significantly increased rate of deaths from leukemia in workers exposed to benzene (31) as well as a particularly striking increase in leukemia mortality among workers employed for 5 or more years (32). Then, in the most recent study in this series, an extensive effort was made to examine quantitatively the dose-response relationship between benzene and leukemia; to this end, a cumulative exposure index (ppm-years) was calculated for each worker (29). Exposure indices were based on extensive air-sampling data and were derived from a job-exposure matrix. Nine deaths from leukemia were observed, versus 2.9 expected. The overall standardized mortality ratio (SMR) for leukemia in the population was 337. A strongly positive trend in leukemia mortality was observed with increasing cumulative exposure to benzene (30). In workers with less than 40 ppm-years of cumulative exposure the SMR was 108, a value not significantly different from background mortality; 40 ppm-years of cumulative exposure corresponds to a working lifetime (40 years) of exposure at an exposure level of 1 ppm. By contrast, in workers with 400 or more ppm-years (corresponding to 40 years exposure at 10 ppm) the SMR was 6,637 (Table 1).

An additional finding in the NIOSH studies of workers exposed to benzene was that there were four deaths from multiple myeloma, as compared to 1.0 expected (SMR 409) (29). This observation, coupled with the observation of lymphomas in other populations exposed to benzene as well as in animal studies, further supports the conclusion that benzene can cause lymphomas and lymphocytic leukemias, in addition to myelomonocytic leukemias (29).

The NIOSH findings on benzene and leukemia are corroborated by data from an ongoing epidemiologic study conducted by the Dow Chemical Company (33) and by an industrywide study of American chemical workers (27). They are corroborated further by studies of workers exposed to benzene in China (34).

Benzene-induced leukemia may develop in some cases in persons who previously have had aplastic anemia. In other cases, however, no preceding aplastic anemia is seen; thus aplastic anemia does not appear to be a necessary precursor to benzene-induced leukemia.

Three major animal studies have found that the benzene is capable of causing leukemia or other forms of cancer in experimental animals (35–37).

### Prevention

The toxic effects of benzene are best prevented by replacing it with less toxic compounds and thus eliminating exposure (2). There are many solvents safer than benzene. Where benzene cannot readily be replaced, for example in the synthetic chemical industry where it is used widely as a basic chemical building block, it is

**TABLE 1.** *Benzene mortality among rubber workers by cumulative exposure to benzene*

| Cumulative exposure (ppm) | $TWA_8$ equivalent[a] | Deaths observed | SMR | Confidence interval |
|---|---|---|---|---|
| 0.001–40 | <1 | 2 | 109 | 12–394 |
| 40–200 | 1–5 | 2 | 322 | 36–1,165 |
| 200–400 | 5–10 | 2 | 1,186 | 133–4,285 |
| >400 | >10 | 3 | 6,637 | 1,334–19,393 |
| TOTAL | — | 9 | 337 | 154–641 |

[a]Exposure that over a working lifetime (40 years) would result in this exposure.
Adapted from ref. 30.

essential that processes be enclosed to the extent possible and that leaks and spills be vented away from workers. The greatest risk of exposure in modern chemical factories is for maintenance and cleanup workers. Also there may be substantial risk to workers engaged in process sampling, laboratory analysis of process samples, and bulk transfer operations (2,3). Protective efforts should therefore be targeted at those specific job operations.

## CASE STUDY: BENZENE AND LEUKEMIA

Although an association between benzene and leukemia was first suggested in the 1920s (24), the regulatory history of benzene has been turbulent and protracted. Particular controversy has surrounded efforts to regulate occupational exposure to relatively low levels of benzene. Review of this history affords insights into the interaction between science and regulatory policy in occupational medicine.

In 1978, in an effort to reduce occupational exposure to benzene, the Occupational Safety and Health Administration (OSHA) promulgated an occupational exposure standard reducing permissible worker exposures tenfold, from the previously acceptable 8-hour time-weighted average ($TWA_8$) standard of 10 ppm to a new standard level of 1 ppm (38). This action was based on information from case reports and from the first generation of NIOSH epidemiologic studies (31).

These early epidemiologic studies showed that occupational exposure to benzene was statistically associated with excess numbers of deaths from leukemia (30,31). Seven leukemia deaths occurred in the NIOSH study population, as compared to 1.25 expected (SMR 560; $p$ <0.001) (31). When these observed leukemia deaths were examined by duration of employment, it was found that workers with less than 5 years' employment had two deaths versus 1.0 expected (SMR 2.0). By contrast, workers with 5 or more years' employment had five leukemia deaths versus 0.23 expected (SMR 2,100) (32). This result supported the notion that there is an increased risk of death from leukemia with increasing cumulative exposure to benzene. By themselves, however, these data provided no quantitative information on risk of leukemia at specific levels of airborne exposure.

The 1978 OSHA standard was challenged by the petrochemical industry. The case went before the U.S. Supreme Court, which on July 2, 1980 invalidated the proposed standard (39). The Court ruled that OSHA had failed to provide substantial evidence of the need for regulation, in that it had not quantified a "significant risk of material health impairment" at the previous level of 10 ppm and had not established that a new standard would achieve "a substantial reduction in significant risk." As a result of this decision, workers in the United States were legally allowed to continue to be exposed to benzene at levels up to 10 ppm.

The Supreme Court benzene decision has had profound implications for government regulatory policy. As a consequence of this decision, it became mandatory for government agencies to develop quantitative information on risks to human health before setting a standard. Although qualitative evidence was available in 1980 showing that the new 1 ppm standard would reduce the risk of benzene-induced leukemia, the actual risk reduction, that is, the number of lives that would be saved by imposing the lower exposure level, could not at that time be precisely quantified. Thus application of the new standard was blocked for many a decade.

The implications of the Supreme Court ruling were discussed by Justice Thurgood Marshall in his dissenting opinion: "The critical problem in cases like the ones at bar is scientific uncertainty.... The risk issue has hardly been shown to be insignificant, indeed future research may reveal the risk is in fact considerable. But the existing evidence may frequently be inadequate to enable the Secretary [of Labor] to make the threshold finding of significance that the court requires today.... Such an approach would place the burden of medical uncertainty squarely on the shoulders of the American worker, the intended beneficiary of the Occupational Safety and Health Act" (38).

Subsequent to the Supreme Court decision, several quantitative assessments of the risk of benzene-induced leukemia were undertaken. The International Agency for Research on Cancer (IARC) projected that a minimum excess of 140 to 170 leukemia deaths would occur per 1,000 workers exposed during a working lifetime to 100 ppm of benzene; this determination extrapolates to 14 excess deaths per 1,000 workers as a low estimate and 17 as a high estimate for lifetime exposure at 10 ppm (40). Also, the NIOSH investigators updated their mortality study (29). By merging industrial hygiene data with personnel records, cumulative benzene exposures (ppm-years) were calculated for each member of the work force. This approach provided a more directly quantitative index of exposure than analysis of length of employment and demonstrated a strong dose-response relationship (see Table 1). The Environmental Protection Agency (EPA) also conducted a quantitative risk assessment and documented increased risk of leukemia at low levels of benzene exposure (41).

On the basis of these new highly quantitative data showing an increased risk of leukemia at low levels of exposure to benzene, OSHA reissued a 1 ppm standard for occupational exposure to benzene in December 1987 (2). That standard is in force today.

To assess the damage that resulted from this 9-year delay in federal regulation of benzene, an epidemiologic analysis has been conducted (37). Data on numbers of persons exposed to benzene in seven occupational categories were merged with dose-response data from three epidemiologic studies. It was then calculated that between 30 and 490 excess leukemia deaths will ultimately result from occupational exposures to benzene greater than 1 ppm that occurred between 1978 and 1987. Deaths from aplastic anemia and lymphoma likely will add to this total (38).

These findings confirm the risk of regulatory delay. They suggest that the courts, in reviewing public health regulations, must beware of cost-benefit arguments and be open to the possibility of accepting strong evidence of health risk even when quantitative data are incomplete.

## REFERENCES


1. Goldstein BD, Witz G. Benzene. In: Lippmann M, ed. *Environmental toxicants:* human exposures and their health effects. New York: Van Nostrand Reinhold, 1992.
2. Occupational exposure to benzene: proposed rule and notice of hearing. 50 *Federal Register* 50512–50586.
3. NIOSH. *Revised recommendation for an occupational exposure standard for benzene.* DHEW publication (NIOSH) 76-76-137-a. Cincinnati, OH: National Institute for Occupational Safety and Health, 1976.
4. Gerarde HW. *Toxicology and biochemistry of aromatic hydrocarbons.* Amsterdam: Elsevier, 1960;98–105.
5. Nordlinder R. Exposure to benzene at different work places. In: Irmbriani M, Ghittori S, Pezzagno G, Capodaglio E, eds. *Update on benzene. Advances in occupational medicine and rehabilitation,* vol 1. 1995;1–8..
6. Dosemeci M, Li GL, Hayes RB, et al. Cohort study among workers exposed to benzene in China: II. Exposure assessment. *Am J Ind Med* 1994;26:401–411.
7. Wallace L. Environmental exposure to benzene: an update. *Environ Health Perspect* 1996;104(suppl 6):1129–1136.
8. Snyder R, Hedli CC. An overview of benzene metabolism. *Environ Health Perspect* 1996;104(suppl 6):1165–1171.
9. Kalf GF. Recent advances in the metabolism and toxicity of benzene. *CRC Crit Rev Toxicol* 1987;18:141–159.
10. Synder R, Witz G, Goldstein BD. The toxicity of benzene. *Environ Health Perspect* 1993;100:293–306.
11. Snyder R, Dimitriadis E, Guy R, et al. Studies on the mechanism of benzene toxicity. *Environ Health Perspect* 1989;82:31–35.
12. Witz G, Latriano L, Goldstein BD. Metabolism and toxicity of trans, trans-muconaldehyde, an open-ring microsomal metabolite of benzene. *Environ Health Perspect* 1989;82:9–22.
13. Henderson RF. Species differences in the metabolism of benzene. *Environ Health Perspect* 1996;104(suppl 6):1173–1175.
14. Glatt H, Padykula R, Berchtold GA, et al. Multiple activation pathways of benzene leading to products with varying genotoxic characteristics. *Environ Health Perspect* 1989;82:81–89.
15. Forni A. Benzene induced chromosome aberrations: a follow-up study. *Environ Health Perspect* 1996;104(suppl 6):1309–1317.
16. Irons RD, Stillman WS. The process of leukemogenesis. *Environ Health Perspect* 1996;104(suppl 6):1239–1246.
17. Lezon-Geyda KA, Najfeld V, Johnson EM. The PUR-A gene, encoding the single-stranded DNA-binding protein pur-, as a marker for 5z31 alterations in myeloproliferative disorders, a potential early step in induction of AML. *FASEB J* 1997;11:A100.
18. Brugnone F, Perbellini L, Faccini GB, et al. Benzene in the blood and breath of normal people and occupationally exposed workers. *Am J Ind Med* 1989;16:385–399.
19. Inoue O, Seidi K, Kasahara M, et al. Quantitative relation of urinary phenol levels to breathzone benzene concentrations: a factory survey. *Br J Ind Med* 1988;45:487–492.
20. Ong CN, Kok PW, Ong HY, et al. Biomarkers of exposure to low concentrations of benzene. A field assessment. *Occup Environ Med* 1996; 53:328–333.
21. Tice RR, Costa DL, Drew RT. Cytogenetic effects of inhaled benzene in murine bone marrow: induction of sister chromatid exchanges, chromosomal aberrations, and cellular proliferation inhibition in DBA/2 mice. *Proc Natl Acad Sci* USA 1980;77:2148–2152.
22. Yardley-Jones A, Anderson D, Jenkinson PC, Lovell DP, Blowers SD, Davies MJ. Genotoxic effects in peripheral blood and urine of workers exposed to low level benzene. *Br J Ind Med* 1988;45:694–700.
23. Santesson CG. Uber chronische Vergiftungen mit Steinkohlenteerbenzin: vier Todesfalle. *Arch Hyg Berlin* 1897;31:336–349.
24. Delore P, Borgomano C. Leucemie aigue au cours de l'intoxication benzenique: Sur l'origine toxique de certaines leucemies aigues et leurs relations avec les anemies graves. *J Med Lyon* 1928;9:227–233.
25. Aksoy M, Erdem S, DinCol G. Leukemia in shoe workers exposed chronically to benzene. *Blood* 1974;44:837–841.
26. Vigliani EC, Saita G. Benzene and leukemia. *N Engl J Med* 1964;271: 872–876.
27. Wong O. An industrywide mortality study of chemical workers occupationally exposed to benzene. I. General results. II. Dose-response analyses. *Br J Ind Med* 1987;44:365–381;382–395.
28. Savitz DA, Andrews KW. Review of epidemiologic evidence on benzene and lymphatic and hematopoietic cancers. *Am J Ind Med* 1997;31: 287–295.
29. Young N. Benzene and lymphoma. *Am J Ind Med* 1989;15:495–498.
30. Rinsky RA, Smith JB, Hornung R, Filloon TG, Young RJ, Landrigan PJ. Benzene and leukemia—an epidemiologic risk assessment. *N Engl J Med* 1987;316:1044–1050.
31. Infante PF, Rinsky RA, Wagoner JK, Young RJ. Leukemia in benzene workers. *Lancet* 1977;2:76–78.
32. Rinsky RA, Young RJ, Smith JB. Leukemia in benzene workers. *Am J Ind Med* 1981;2:217–245.
33. Ott GM, Townsend JC, Fishbeck WA, Langner RA. Mortality among individuals occupationally exposed to benzene. *Arch Environ Health* 1978;33:3–10.
34. Travis LB, Li C-Y, Zhang Z-N, et al. Hematopoietic malignancies and related disorders among benzene-exposed workers in China. *Leukemia Lymphoma* 1994;14:91–102.
35. Snyder CA, Goldstein BD, Sellumar AR, Bromberg I, Laskin S, Albert RE. The inhalation toxicology of benzene: incidence of hematopoietic neoplasms and hematoxicity in AKR/J and C57DBL/6J mice. *Toxicol Appl Pharmacol* 1980;54:323–331.
36. Maltoni C, Conti B, Cotti G. Benzene: a multipotential carcinogen: results of long-term bioassays performed at the Bologna Institute of Oncology. *Am J Ind Med* 1983;4:589–630.
37. National Toxicology Program. *Technical report on the toxicology and carcinogenesis studies of benzene in F344/N rats and B6C3F, mice (gavage studies).* NIH publication 86-2545. Research Triangle Park, NC: NTP, 1986.
38. Nicholson WJ, Landrigan PJ. Quantitative assessment of lives lost due to delay in the regulation of occupational exposure to benzene. *Environ Health Perspect* 1989;82:685–688.
39. Industrial Union Department vs. American Petroleum Institute. *US Reports* 1980(July 2);448, 607.
40. *Evaluation of the carcinogenic risk of chemicals to humans:* some industrial chemicals and dyestuffs. Lyon, France: International Agency for Research on Cancer, 1982;93–148.
41. Albert RE. *Carcinogen assessment group's final report on population risk to ambient benzene exposures.* EPA Publication 450/5-890-004. Research Triangle Park, NC: United States Environmental Protection Agency, 1979.

*Environmental and Occupational Medicine, Third Edition*, edited by William N. Rom.
Lippincott–Raven Publishers, Philadelphia © 1998.

# CHAPTER 80

# Formaldehyde

Dean B. Baker

Formaldehyde is a highly reactive chemical that is ubiquitous in the natural environment and widely used in occupational and environmental settings. It is present in many consumer products. It is also an endogenous chemical found in living cells, where small quantities derive from the metabolism of amino acids, and its metabolites are in equilibrium with the labile methyl group pool.

The health effects of formaldehyde are controversial and have been the subject of a large amount of research (1,2). Formaldehyde causes mucous membrane and upper respiratory tract irritation at relatively low exposure. Inhalation at high concentrations can cause reversible bronchoconstriction; however, allergic sensitization does not appear to play a substantial role in formaldehyde-associated pulmonary effects (3–5). Formaldehyde off-gassing from building materials and furnishings has been cited as a contributing cause of indoor air quality problems.

Formaldehyde is a proven animal carcinogen (6,7), but the findings of epidemiologic studies have been equivocal, so its carcinogenicity in humans remains uncertain (1,8–11). The strongest evidence of human cancer risk is for cancer of the nasopharynx, with weaker evidence for nasal cancer (1,9). Formaldehyde is considered a probable human carcinogen by the International Agency for Research on Cancer (IARC) and United States governmental agencies (12–14).

## CHEMICAL AND PHYSICAL PROPERTIES

Formaldehyde (HCOH) is a flammable, colorless gas with a pungent odor at room temperature and atmospheric pressure. It is the simplest of the aldehydes, consisting of a single carbonyl group flanked by two hydrogen atoms. Formaldehyde has a relative molecular mass of 30.03, boiling point of −21°C, and melting point of −92°C (1). For conversion of units, 1 ppm = 1.23 mg/m$^3$ at normal temperature and pressure.

Formaldehyde is soluble in water, ethanol, and diethyl ether. Formaldehyde-alcohol solutions are stable, as is the gaseous form of the compound in the absence of water. It is incompatible with acids, alkalis, oxidizers, phenols, and urea (15–17). Formaldehyde reacts explosively with peroxide, nitrogen oxide, and performic acid. It can also react with hydrogen chloride and other inorganic chlorides to form bis-(chloromethyl) ether, a potent carcinogen (15–17).

## PRODUCTION AND USE

Formaldehyde is produced by the oxidation of methanol, most commonly using the metal oxide catalyst and silver catalyst processes (15,17). Approximately 12 million metric tons were manufactured worldwide in 1992 (1). The United States is the leading manufacturer, with a reported annual production of more than 3.5 million metric tons (18,19). Other leading producers include Japan, Germany, China, and Sweden. Formaldehyde is most commonly available as formalin, a 30% to 50% by weight aqueous solution. It is also marketed in a solid form as trioxane $(CH_2O)_3$ or its polymer, paraformaldehyde (1).

Formaldehyde is used mainly in the production of urea, phenol, melamine, and acetal resins, which account for approximately 70% of the formaldehyde produced (18). These resins are used as adhesives and impregnating resins in the manufacture of wood-based products, such

D. B. Baker: Department of Medicine, Center for Occupational and Environmental Health, University of California, Irvine, Irvine, California 92612.

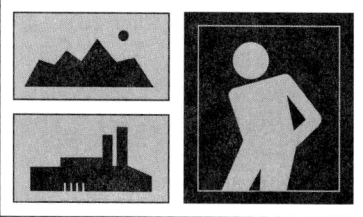

as particleboard, plywood fiberboard, and furniture. They are also used as raw materials in the production of surface coatings and controlled-release nitrogen fertilizers. Other applications include paper treating and coating, molding, and foams for insulating materials. Resins also act as binders for foundry sand, abrasive paper, and brake linings. Approximately 20% of formaldehyde is used in the production of chemical intermediates, including acetylenic chemicals and methylene diisocynate.

Formaldehyde is used in aqueous solution (formalin) for the disinfection of hospital wards and acts as an antimicrobial agent in a variety of cosmetic products, such as makeup, nail products, lotions, hair products, shampoos, deodorants, and soaps. It is used as a tissue preservative and disinfectant in embalming fluids.

## EXPOSURE

### Occupational Exposures

Several million people are occupationally exposed to formaldehyde in industrialized countries alone. According to the National Occupational Exposure Survey covering the years 1981 to 1983, approximately 1.5 million workers in the United States were exposed all or part of the time (20). More than 50,000 workers in each of the following industries had some formaldehyde exposure: manufacture of chemicals and allied products, furniture and fixtures, paper and allied products, printing and publishing, apparel and allied products, health services, machinery, transport equipment, personal services, and business services.

The main pathway of exposure in occupational settings is inhalation of formaldehyde gas, which arises as a vapor from formalin or from decomposition of polymer resins. When powdered resins are used, inhalation of formaldehyde-containing particulates may occur (21). In addition, formaldehyde-based resins may also become airborne when attached to wood dust or other carrier agents (22). Dermal exposure may also occur if liquid resins or formalin solutions come into contact with the skin.

The highest continuous exposures have been measured in particleboard mills, during the varnishing of furniture (23,24) and wooden floors (25), in foundries, and during the finishing of textiles (26,27). Somewhat lower exposures occur in plywood mills and in embalming areas of mortuaries. Short-term high exposures can occur during disinfection in hospitals and food processing plants, as well as in some agriculture operations and during firefighting. In general occupational exposures have decreased over time because of the development of resins that release less formaldehyde (1). Many occupations with formaldehyde exposure have concurrent exposures to other substances (1,28) (Table 1).

### Environmental Exposures

#### *Ambient Air*

While formaldehyde occurs naturally in ambient air, levels in remote areas are generally <1 μg/m$^3$ [0.8 parts per billion (ppb)]. Hence, most of the formaldehyde found in populated regions may be attributed to anthropogenic sources. Urban environments have variable outdoor air concentrations of formaldehyde, which are highly dependent on local conditions and range between 1 and 20 μg/m$^3$ (0.8 to 16 ppb) (2,29–31). Ambient urban air levels up to 100 μg/m$^3$ (81 ppb) have been found during periods of heavy traffic or severe inversions (2,29,30).

Stationary sources, such as incinerators and home fires, as well as mobile sources, including internal combustion, diesel, and jet engines, release formaldehyde into the environment. Vehicular emissions are a major source of formaldehyde in outdoor urban air (2,32). Emitted hydrocarbons from these sources can also produce formaldehyde through secondary photochemical reactions.

**TABLE 1.** *Formaldehyde exposures by occupational group*

| Group | Formaldehyde source: Vapor/gas | Formaldehyde source: Particle | Other exposures |
|---|---|---|---|
| Anatomists and pathologists | Formalin | | Other preservatives, xylene, toluene, chloroform, methyl methacrylate |
| Embalmers | Formalin | Paraformaldehyde dust | Solvents in disinfectant sprays, methanol, phenolic solutions |
| Wood and paper industries | Polymer decomposition | Polymer dust | Wood dust, pesticides, other preservatives |
| Textiles | Polymer decomposition | Polymer dust | Cotton dust, oil mists |
| Plastics production | Formalin, polymer decomposition | Polymer dust | Other raw materials |
| Chemical production | Formalin, polymer decomposition | Polymer dust | Other raw materials |

Adapted from ref. 28.

### *Residential Indoor Air*

It is estimated that more than 11 million people in the United States have potential exposure to formaldehyde in their homes because of off-gassing from building materials or other indoor sources (33). Indoor air levels are determined by the formaldehyde sources present, age of the source materials, ventilation, humidity, and temperature. Formaldehyde concentrations found indoors are usually higher than those found outdoors. For most individuals, the home is the primary source of formaldehyde exposure (34).

Common sources of indoor formaldehyde include release from structural materials, furnishings, insulation, clothing, and cosmetics (35,36). Tobacco smoking and wood burning also generate formaldehyde. Formaldehyde in mobile homes, due to off-gassing of particleboard, has been studied since the 1970s (37,38). Levels decrease as the formaldehyde-based resins age, with a half-life of 4 to 5 years (31). Due to standards established in the 1980s for mobile home building materials and to voluntary reductions adopted by manufacturers, mean formaldehyde levels in mobile homes have dropped from 0.4 ppm in the 1980s to 0.1 ppm or less today (37–40).

### *Consumer Products*

Cigarette smoke from one cigarette may contain from a few micrograms to several milligrams of formaldehyde. A pack-a-day smoker may inhale 0.4 to 2.0 mg formaldehyde (2,41). Consumers may be exposed to formaldehyde, formalin, and paraformaldehyde through the use of cosmetic products. Ingredient labels of cosmetics and toiletries rarely list formaldehyde itself as a component of the product. However, formaldehyde may be released from several preservatives or be present as an impurity. Typically, the concentration of a preservative in a commercial product is 0.1% to 0.2%. Concentrations of formaldehyde are thus even lower. However, even minute concentrations may induce allergic contact dermatitis among sensitized individuals.

Foods naturally contain small amounts of formaldehyde, but they may also be contaminated through fumigation, cooking, or release from formaldehyde resin–based cooking utensils or tableware (2). Formaldehyde has also been used as a bacteriostatic in cheeses and other foods (42).

## INDICATORS OF EXPOSURE

Formaldehyde exposure is usually monitored by measuring the concentration of formaldehyde gas in the air. Area air or personal samples may be taken. Most air measurements of formaldehyde were intended for use in occupational environments. Therefore, caution is required when these methods are used in nonoccupational settings, which usually have substantially lower levels of formaldehyde (43,44). In recent years, passive monitors have been developed to monitor workplace exposure. Methodologies for compliance monitoring of formaldehyde, specified by the Occupational Safety and Health Administration (OSHA) or the National Institute for Occupational Safety and Health (NIOSH), refer to passive badges as alternative sampling techniques to those specified in the OSHA or NIOSH method. Other countries have also accepted the use of passive monitors for exposure monitoring (45).

Biologic monitoring of formaldehyde exposure is not considered feasible. Because formaldehyde is rapidly metabolized, no increase in blood concentration is detectable even moments after exposure (46–49). Urinary excretion of formic acid has been suggested as a possible biologic monitoring method. To test this theory, the urine of veterinary medical students exposed to low concentrations of formaldehyde was analyzed over a period of 3 weeks. Although levels varied within and between subjects, no significant changes in concentration were detected, so it was concluded that formic acid in urine is not a feasible monitoring technique (50).

At present, no techniques are available for reliable measurement of formaldehyde in tissue or for detection of formaldehyde adducts formed with macromolecules. In a small study examining the presence of DNA-protein cross-links (DPX) in white blood cells taken from 12 exposed workers and eight controls, a significant difference was found in the amount of DPX among exposed versus unexposed. This suggests that DPX may be used as a biologic marker for monitoring formaldehyde exposure (51). However, findings of this study have been challenged (48). A study examining methods to measure hydroxylmethyl adducts in DNA as an indicator of formaldehyde exposure concluded that this approach was not feasible (52).

## ABSORPTION AND BIOTRANSFORMATION

Because formaldehyde has a high aqueous solubility, the upper respiratory tract is its principal site of deposition with inhalation exposure (53). Essentially all inhaled formaldehyde will deposit in the nasal and nasopharyngeal mucosa during nasal breathing. Experimental studies in animals indicate that any formaldehyde that penetrates the nasal cavity or upper airways will be deposited in the lower airways (54,55).

There are two major protective mechanisms in the nasal passages—mucous clearance and glutathione (GSH)-dependent detoxification (56,57). Formaldehyde reacts with the proteins and polysaccharides of the mucous layer, reducing the concentration of formaldehyde to which epithelial cells are exposed. Also there is constant mucus removal by ciliary motion, which tends to limit the extent and severity of formaldehyde cytotoxicity. However, when the inhaled dose of formaldehyde reaches a sufficient level, formaldehyde produces inhibition of mucociliary function and a decrease in mucus flow.

Once in the cell, formaldehyde may react with nucleic acids or proteins, or be metabolized to formic acid. It is metabolized by incorporation into the labile methyl group pool via tetrahydrofolate-dependent pathways. In addition, formaldehyde reacts with GSH, and further biotransformation is mediated by formaldehyde dehydrogenase to produce the thiol ester of formic acid, S-formylglutathione, which yields free GSH and formic acid. The latter is subsequently degraded to $CO_2$ and exhaled, incorporated into the labile methyl group, or excreted in the urine.

The metabolic pathway involving GSH and formaldehyde dehydrogenase is an important defense mechanism because this pathway tends to inhibit the covalent reaction of formaldehyde with nucleic acids. Depletion of GSH diminished the capacity of the respiratory mucosa to protect itself from the formation of DPX after administration of formaldehyde (58). At concentrations that exceed the endogenous protective mechanisms, formaldehyde can produce higher concentrations of DPX per unit of time, as well a greater cellular toxicity and enhanced cell proliferation.

Formaldehyde or its metabolites may also penetrate human skin (59).

## HEALTH EFFECTS

Because inhaled formaldehyde is completely absorbed and metabolized in the upper respiratory tract except with very high exposure, in which case some may reach the lower respiratory tract, it is unlikely to produce systemic toxicity, including carcinogenicity, in organs distant from the site of absorption. Thus, most health effects associated with formaldehyde occur in the mucosa of the eyes and upper respiratory tract, and the skin. Gastrointestinal and systematic toxicity have been reported in cases of ingested formalin.

### Mucosa and Respiratory Tract

#### *Irritation*

Formaldehyde is a known irritant of the eyes and upper respiratory tract. The threshold for eye, nose, and throat irritation in most people is 0.5 to 1.0 ppm (60,61), although eye and respiratory irritation have been reported by some persons with exposure to formaldehyde concentrations as low as 0.1 ppm (1). Controlled human exposure studies indicated that the no-observable-effect level for symptoms of eye and respiratory irritation is 0.4 ppm, with definitive reports of symptoms at ≥0.8 ppm (62). With increasing concentrations of formaldehyde, the proportion of persons reporting eye irritation and the severity of the irritation increased (63). A short-term tolerance usually develops to low doses but is lost if exposure is resumed after a 1- to 2-hour interruption.

Wilhelmsson and Holmström (64) studied workers with occupational exposure to formaldehyde and a reference group to investigate the mechanism of formaldehyde-associated upper airway discomfort. They concluded that formaldehyde can induce an immunoglobulin E (IgE)-mediated reaction in the nose in rare instances, but in most cases the nasal symptoms are due to varying sensitivity to irritation among the population.

#### *Nasal Epithelial Damage*

Histopathologic effects and cytogenic changes in the nasal mucosa have been reported among persons with occupational or residential exposure to formaldehyde. Exposure to formaldehyde appeared to be associated with increased prevalence of squamous metaplasia, based on cell smears or biopsy samples, among persons living in urea-formaldehyde foam-insulated homes (65) and workers in phenol-formaldehyde plants (66), particleboard plants (67), and resin manufacturing plants or furniture factories (68); but there was no consistent association with formaldehyde exposure concentrations or duration (1). Higher frequencies of micronucleated nasal respiratory cells and squamous metaplasia were seen among exposed workers compared to control workers in a warehouse area of a plywood factory (69). Increased micronuclei were seen in buccal cells, but not nasal cells in mortuary science students exposed to embalming fluid containing formaldehyde following a 90-day embalming class (70).

That formaldehyde causes epithelial damage has been confirmed in animal studies. Exposure to airborne formaldehyde produced purulent rhinitis, epithelial dysplasia, squamous metaplasia and hyperplasia, and squamous cell carcinoma of the nasal cavity in Fischer 344 rats (56). In other animal inhalation studies, it was found that epithelial dysplasia preceded the appearance of squamous metaplasia (71). The frequency and severity of squamous metaplasia and rhinitis increased in a time- and dose-dependent manner during 24 months of exposure. After daily exposure to formaldehyde was discontinued, the incidence of squamous metaplasia and rhinitis decreased, indicating reversibility of cellular damage.

#### *Pulmonary Effects*

Acute changes in pulmonary function with formaldehyde exposure have been studied using controlled exposure studies and cross-sectional occupational studies. The findings are not completely consistent, but the studies generally indicate that formaldehyde does not cause significant bronchoconstriction or airway hyperresponsiveness at exposure levels below about 3 ppm. Reversible bronchoconstriction can occur following high exposure to formaldehyde (>5 ppm). There have been case reports of asthma in individuals exposed to formaldehyde (3,72–76).

In controlled exposure studies, exposures up to 3 ppm formaldehyde caused upper respiratory tract irritation, but no bronchoconstriction. Pulmonary function was not significantly altered in healthy nonsmokers and asthmatic subjects exposed to 2 ppm for 40 minutes (77), in hospital laboratory workers exposed to 2 ppm for 40 minutes (78), in nonsmokers exposed to 2 ppm while exercising (61), or in nonsmokers exposed to 3 ppm (61).

Some studies of workers with exposures in the range of 0.02 to 5.0 ppm formaldehyde have found symptoms of bronchoconstriction and reversible reductions in pulmonary function measures [e.g., forced expiratory volume in 1 second ($FEV_1$)] including particleboard and plywood workers (63), urea-formaldehyde resin producers, embalmers, and anatomy and histology workers (1,79). A study of students exposed to 0.5 to 0.9 ppm formaldehyde while dissecting cadavers 3 hours per week found increasing irritant symptoms to eyes, nose, and throat over the course of a laboratory session. Peak expiratory flow rate declined significantly over a 10-week course, but returned to normal after the course ended (80). An earlier study of medical students exposed to formaldehyde, however, provided no evidence of reduced pulmonary function (81). Other occupational studies also did not find effects on pulmonary function associated with lower exposures to formaldehyde.

One explanation for the inconsistency is that some occupational groups may be exposed intermittently to high concentrations of formaldehyde, which is not reflected in the time-weighted exposure measurements. Another explanation is that in some workplaces formaldehyde may be adsorbed to fine particles and then transported to the lower respiratory tract, causing the airways effect (82). Also, several occupational groups are exposed to other irritating substances that may contribute to the pulmonary effects.

Lower respiratory tract effects have been reported in particular circumstances. For example, chemical pneumonitis and pulmonary edema have been reported after very high levels of exposures. Inhalation of paraformaldehyde particles may penetrate more deeply into the lungs than inhalation of formaldehyde vapors, resulting in pulmonary irritation (83).

### *Role of Allergic Sensitization*

There has been substantial discussion about whether formaldehyde can cause immunologically mediated respiratory disease (3–5,84,85). This issue is relevant because some individuals report experiencing lower respiratory tract symptoms at formaldehyde concentrations that are too low to be consistent with irritation.

Formaldehyde exposure is capable of causing antibody-mediated hypersensitivity. IgE, IgG, and IgM antibodies to formaldehyde-hemolytic red blood cell membrane protein and formaldehyde-human serum albumin conjugates have been identified in persons who received intravenous formaldehyde during dialysis (86–89). Nevertheless, studies that have measured formaldehyde-specific antibodies in the sera of occupationally and environmentally exposed persons have found that only a small proportion of exposed individuals develop specific IgE or IgG (4,5,84,85). Furthermore, among these groups, specific antibodies did not correlate with symptoms. For example, Patterson et al. (89) found that IgG antibody against formaldehyde-human serum albumin (F-HSA) could be identified in some persons, but there was no correlation between the presence of IgG antibodies to F-HSA and gaseous formaldehyde exposure, or symptoms from formaldehyde exposure. Dykewicz et al. (90) performed environmental assessments, respiratory challenges, and immunologic testing on 55 volunteers, 34 with reported occupational exposure to formaldehyde. Although antibodies to F-HSA were found in some subjects, there was no relation between the presence of IgE or IgG to F-HSA and a history of formaldehyde exposure or a history of respiratory symptoms from gaseous formaldehyde exposure. Pross et al. (91) conducted immunologic studies on persons with potential exposure to formaldehyde from urea-foam formaldehyde insulated homes and also concluded that there was no evidence that exposure to gaseous formaldehyde can induce a specific immune response. Wantke et al. (92) did report that the presence of formaldehyde-specific IgE correlated with measured formaldehyde in schoolchildren; however, elevated IgE levels to formaldehyde did not correlate with symptoms. In animal studies, formaldehyde displayed no significant potential to influence serum IgE levels in the mouse IgE test (4). An investigation by Potter and Wederbrand (93) also found that formaldehyde did not influence the serum concentration of IgE in mice. The general conclusion has been that exposure to gaseous formaldehyde rarely if ever causes immunologically mediated respiratory disease (3–5).

### *Chronic Pulmonary Effects*

Findings of studies on the long-term effects of formaldehyde exposure on pulmonary function have been inconsistent (82). Studies using pulmonary function tests performed on a variety of groups with occupational exposure have generally found that formaldehyde does not induce chronic decrement in lung function (1,94), although some studies have found evidence of chronic airway obstruction in workers who handle phenol formaldehyde resins (95). Several mortality studies in industries with formaldehyde exposure have not generally shown increased risk for noncancerous respiratory causes (1,96,97).

## Dermatitis

Formaldehyde is an acute skin irritant and an important cause of occupational allergic contact dermatitis (4,98–100). Formaldehyde induces cell-mediated hypersensitivity, which results in allergic contact dermatitis. Experimental studies using the guinea pig test methods and the local lymph node assay demonstrated the contact-sensitizing potential of formaldehyde (4). In a study of persons with positive patch tests to formaldehyde, only two of 15 persons demonstrated formaldehyde-specific serum IgE and these two persons had no clinical signs of atopy, indicating that specific IgE antibodies are not involved in the pathogenesis of contact sensitivity to formaldehyde in either nonatopic or atopic persons (101).

Other than occupational exposures, the most common sources of exposure include cosmetics, skin and hair products, and permanent press textiles. In the past, contact dermatitis caused by formaldehyde-based textile resins was common. Introduction of formaldehyde resins that release little or no formaldehyde has brought about a substantial reduction in the incidence of dermatitis from permanent press clothing. People who are allergic or sensitive to formaldehyde-based textile resins in permanent press clothing may react to the resin, to formaldehyde, or to the monomers themselves. Individuals who are hypersensitive to formaldehyde resins are often not allergic to formaldehyde itself. For example, people who are affected by permanent press clothing may actually be allergic to a fabric finish that contains a formaldehyde resin. Because these individuals do not have positive patch test reactions to formaldehyde, formaldehyde alone cannot be reliably used for screening. Instead, resins should be tested as well. Although fabric tests are often negative, they should also be conducted in order to rule out dye allergy (102).

## Carcinogenicity

The question of whether formaldehyde causes cancer in humans has been the subject of considerable controversy since it was reported that exposure to high concentrations of formaldehyde gas produced squamous cell carcinomas in the nasal cavities of rats (6,7).

There have been three main bodies of research pertaining to the carcinogenic effects of formaldehyde. First, animal and *in vitro* experimental research demonstrated that formaldehyde is an animal carcinogen and directly genotoxic in a variety of experimental systems (1). It was found that formaldehyde exhibits a sublinear dose-response for animal carcinogenicity with little or no effect at low exposure levels (1,56,103). Tumors appear to occur only in tissues with direct contact to high concentrations of formaldehyde (56). These findings then motivated a large number of epidemiologic studies. The epidemiologic findings provided inconsistent evidence of cancer risk, which then led to a series of studies examining mechanisms for formaldehyde carcinogenicity in order to refine estimates of potential cancer risk in humans. These latter studies used animal and *in vitro* experiments, as well as computer models, to analyze tissue dosimetry and cellular responses at different formaldehyde exposures.

### *Epidemiologic Studies*

The relationship between formaldehyde exposure and cancer has been investigated in more than 25 cohort studies of professional groups and industrial workers. Case-control studies have investigated formaldehyde exposure related to various tumor types, including nasal cavities, nasopharynx, and lung. Reviews have summarized the epidemiologic data (1,8,9,11).

#### *Professional Workers*

Professional groups such as pathologists, anatomists, embalmers, and funeral directors have been studied because they are exposed to formalin as a tissue preservative. The cohorts were identified from occupational associations or lists of professional licensees. These studies include a cohort mortality study of pathologists and medical laboratory technicians in the United Kingdom (104–106); cohort mortality studies of pathologists (107) and anatomists in the United States (108); proportionate mortality studies of embalmers in New York State (97), California (109), and the United States excluding New York and California (110); and a cohort mortality study of embalmers in Ontario (111).

The findings were summarized by Blair et al. (8) in a meta-analysis. Among professionals, significant excess mortality occurred for leukemia [cumulative relative risk (CRR) = 1.6], brain cancer (CRR = 1.5), and colon cancer (CRR = 1.3). There were fewer deaths than expected due to lung cancer, with a significant deficit (CRR = 0.3) among anatomists and pathologists. Similar findings were reported in the meta-analysis by Partanen (9), as summarized in Table 2. This pattern of cancer deaths was quite different from that observed among the industrial worker cohorts, which did not have excess risk of leukemia, brain cancer, or colon cancer. There were too few expected deaths from nasal cancer or nasopharyngeal cancer to draw meaningful inferences in these studies, although one of the larger studies observed a nonsignificant increase in nasopharyngeal cancer risk (110).

Concerns have been raised about the studies of professionals. First, data on formaldehyde exposure were not available. In many instances, it was not even possible to

**TABLE 2.** *Aggregated relative risks for respiratory cancers associated with occupational formaldehyde exposure*

| | Level or duration of exposure to formaldehyde | | | | | |
|---|---|---|---|---|---|---|
| | Any | | Low/medium | | Substantial | |
| Site | O/E | RR (95% CI) | O/E | RR (95% CI) | O/E | RR (95% CI) |
| Nose and nasal sinuses | 93/78 | 1.1 (0.8–1.5) | 33/30 | 1.1 (0.7–1.8) | 36/21 | 1.7 (1.0–2.8) |
| Nasopharynx | 36/21 | 2.0 (1.4–2.9) | 23/16 | 1.6 (1.0–2.7) | 11/4 | 2.7 (1.4–5.6) |
| Lung | | | | | | |
| Industrial workers | 833/752 | 1.1 (1.0–1.2) | 518/425 | 1.2 (1.1–1.3) | 233/216 | 1.1 (1.0–1.2) |
| Medical professions (e.g., anatomists, pathologists) | 54/160 | 0.3 (0.3–0.4) | | | | |
| Nonmedical professions (e.g., embalmers, undertakers) | 474/486 | 1.0 (0.9–1.1) | | | | |

O/E, aggregated number of observed and expected in all studies; RR, relative risk; 95% CI, 95% confidence interval of the relative risk. The data were aggregated using a log-Gaussian, fixed-effect model for risk ratios.

Adapted from refs 1 and 9.

analyze risk by duration of employment. Second, data were not generally available to adjust for tobacco use or potentially confounding occupational exposures, such as solvents and other chemicals used by embalmers and in anatomy laboratories. Third, many of the studies used external population comparisons, which introduced the possibility of diagnostic bias or confounding due to differences in socioeconomic status between the professional groups and the referent populations. Blair et al. (8), as well as others (1), have concluded that the excess risk for leukemia, brain cancer, and colon cancer seen in professional workers was not due to formaldehyde.

### *Industrial Workers*

The cohort studies of industrial workers are important because some of them were large and had quantitative estimates of formaldehyde exposure. The principal studies were a National Cancer Institute study of U.S. industrial workers (96,112) and a study of British industrial workers (113,114) exposed to formaldehyde.

The National Cancer Institute study included more than 25,000 workers in ten facilities producing a variety of products such as formaldehyde, formaldehyde resins and molding compounds, laminates, photographic film, and plywood (96,112). Formaldehyde exposures were estimated based on the combination of job, department, plant, and calendar-year linked with results of plant visits, job descriptions, process descriptions, work processes, and current and historical monitoring data. Only 4% of the cohort was estimated to have formaldehyde exposures above 2.0 ppm. The cohort was followed for mortality. Blair et al. (112) observed no excess of nasal cancer (2 versus 2.2 expected), but did identify an excess of nasopharyngeal cancers (6 versus 2.2) among exposed workers with a suggestive exposure-response relationship. The study found a small excess risk of lung cancer for some groups of workers exposed to formaldehyde, but there was no clear exposure-response gradient using several measures of exposure. This study has been subjected to several reanalyses by different investigators regarding the apparent excess lung cancer risk (cited in ref. 10).

The other major study of industrial workers was based on about 14,000 British workers from six facilities producing formaldehyde, formaldehyde resins, adhesives, paraform, and alcoforms (113,114). Estimates of formaldehyde exposure were made for each job. Twenty-five percent of the cohort were unexposed, while 35% were in the highest exposure category (>2.0 ppm). The cohort was followed for mortality and for cancer incidence using a national cancer registry. One death occurred from nasal cancer (1.7 expected) and none from nasopharyngeal cancer (1.3 expected). The relative risk [standardized mortality ratio (SMR)] for lung cancer among workers first employed before 1965 was 1.2 [95% confidence interval (CI) 1.1–1.4], but there was no apparent trend with estimates of cumulative exposure. The investigators felt that the excess lung cancer risk was consistent with confounding effects of cigarette smoking.

Mortality was also studied among workers in a resin manufacturing plant in Italy (115,116), the abrasives industry in Sweden (117), garment manufacturing plants in the United States (118), and an iron foundry in the United States (119). These studies did not find significant lung cancer mortality risk associated with formaldehyde exposure and they were too small to meaningfully evaluate risk for sinonasal or nasopharyngeal cancer.

### ***Case-Control Studies***

Several case-control studies have evaluated cancer risk associated with formaldehyde exposure. The most pertinent are those related to cancers of the nasal cavity, nasopharynx, and lung because of findings in the animal studies and cohort studies. Four studies accounted for most of the exposed cases and therefore contributed most to the meta-analyses (8,9).

Olsen et al. (120) studied cases with cancer of the sinonasal cavities and nasopharynx reported to a cancer registry in Denmark, using controls with cancers of other sites. Exposure histories were assessed by industrial hygienists. Because of concern about confounding due to wood dust exposure, a reanalysis was performed in which squamous cell carcinoma and adenocarcinoma of the sinonasal cavities were examined separately. A nonsignificant increased risk of squamous cell carcinoma was observed for persons who had been exposed to formaldehyde, adjusted for wood dust exposure [odds ratio (OR) = 2.0; 95% CI = 0.7–5.9] (121).

Hayes et al. (122) conducted a case-control study of cancer of the nasal cavities and paranasal sinuses in the Netherlands using medical records from major medical institutions, with age-matched population controls. Work and exposure histories were obtained from the subjects or next-of-kin and evaluated by industrial hygienists for formaldehyde exposure. An excess was found for adenocarcinoma associated with wood dust exposure. Therefore, a separate analysis was done for squamous cell cancer, which found significantly increased risk associated with formaldehyde exposure alone. Concerns were raised about this study because of differences in use of next of kin for information and due to incomplete agreement on exposure rankings by two independent industrial hygienists (11); however, it was noted that significant associations were observed using either exposure rating (1).

Roush et al. (123) conducted a population-based case-control study of sinonasal or nasopharyngeal cancer mortality using a tumor registry in Connecticut. Controls were randomly selected from state death certificates. Occupations of subjects were identified from the death certificates and city directories, and coded by an industrial hygienist. Relative risks for sinonasal cancer and for nasopharyngeal cancer were increased among subjects who had probably been exposed to high levels of formaldehyde at some point 20 or more years before death.

Vaughan et al. (124,125) examined both occupational and residential exposure to formaldehyde in a population-based case-control study in Washington State. Occupational exposure was assessed based on interviews with subjects or next-of-kin using a job-exposure linkage system. Increased relative risks for nasopharyngeal cancer were associated with occupational formaldehyde exposure and with a residential history of living in a mobile home or in a home with formaldehyde-containing insulation and plywood or particleboard. Sinonasal cancer was associated with a nonsignificantly decreased risk with occupational formaldehyde exposure; mixed associations were found for residential formaldehyde exposure.

Other case-control studies also examined the association between formaldehyde exposure and either sinonasal or nasopharyngeal cancer. Some studies reported increased risk for nasal cancer, while others did not find excess risk (1,8,9,126).

### *Cancer Risk by Site*

Considered as a whole, the epidemiologic studies suggest that formaldehyde is most likely to have a causal relationship with nasopharyngeal cancer and, to a lesser extent, with sinonasal cancer. Excess risk for nasopharyngeal cancer was reported in a number of studies, including a few cohort studies and several case-control studies. While the power of individual studies has been limited, the meta-analyses found a significant increase in risk (8,9). Suggestive dose-response relationships were found among three studies with exposure data—a cohort (96,127) and two case-control (123,124) studies.

The evidence supporting a relationship between formaldehyde and sinonasal cancer is less clear. The cohort studies did not suggest any increased risk, although these studies were limited by a small number of expected cases. Findings of the case-controls studies were inconsistent. In several studies, confounding wood dust exposure was a problem, but some studies addressed this problem by focusing on squamous cell carcinoma and adjusting for wood dust exposure, and still found increased risk.

The overall findings indicate that excess lung cancer risk is unlikely. The significant deficits of lung cancer among anatomists and pathologists were most likely due to lower prevalences of smoking in those health professions. No excesses of lung cancer were found among embalmers, a group in which the prevalence of smoking is similar to that of the general population (128). The larger studies of industrial workers found small excesses in lung cancer. However, the risk of lung cancer did not increase with duration of employment or level of exposure; in fact, there was a slight inverse exposure-response gradient. In the multiple plant studies in the United States and United Kingdom, excess mortality from lung cancer was largely confined to workers involved in the production of resins and molding compounds, which suggests that there may be increased lung cancer risk in these types of facilities, but it is not likely due to formaldehyde per se (112).

The findings of the epidemiologic studies have been reviewed by IARC (1) and combined in meta-analyses by Blair et al. (8) and Partanen (9). The aggregated relative risks for respiratory cancers calculated in the meta-analysis by Partanen are shown in Table 2.

### *Cancer Mechanisms*

Possible mechanisms for formaldehyde carcinogenicity have been discussed (56,103,129). The current understanding is that formaldehyde is a direct-acting, genotoxic carcinogen that exhibits sublinear dose-responses for DNA reactivity, enhancement of cell proliferation, and carcinogenicity (56). Formaldehyde can cause DNA-protein cross-links, DNA-DNA cross-links, point mutations, and single- and double-strand DNA breaks, which result in cytogenetic damage (70). Conversion of the initial DNA damage into chromosome aberrations and micronuclei appears to be facilitated by increases in cell proliferation and formaldehyde inhibition of DNA repair (56,70,130). The sublinear dose-response relationship presumably derives from the endogenous protective mechanisms in the nasal passages (56–58).

*DNA Reactivity*

A focus of research on DNA reactivity has been on the ability of formaldehyde to form DPX (131–134) (Fig. 1). DPXs induced by formaldehyde exposure were measured in the nasal mucosa of the upper respiratory tract of exposed animals. The formation of DPX was a sublinear function of formaldehyde concentration in inhaled air (131). There was no detectable accumulation of DPX during repeated exposures (133). Studies of the repair of DPXs caused by formaldehyde showed that they are removed from cells with a half-life of 2 to 3 hours (135). These findings suggest that formation of DPX must be accompanied by cell proliferation or inhibition of DNA repair mechanisms in order to induce carcinogenesis.

In comparing species, the concentrations of cross-links in the turbinates and anterior nasal mucosa were significant lower in monkeys than in rats (132). Cross-links were formed in the nasopharynx of monkeys, but they were not detected in the sinus, proximal lung or bone marrow. These findings suggest that differences between the species may be due to differences in nasal cavity deposition and in the elimination of absorbed formaldehyde (132,134).

Although DPXs are considered to play a role in formaldehyde carcinogenesis, other mechanisms may also be involved, as suggested by reports that formaldehyde exposure potentiated the tumor rate when administered in combination with known carcinogens such as *N*-nitrosodimethylamine (1,136).

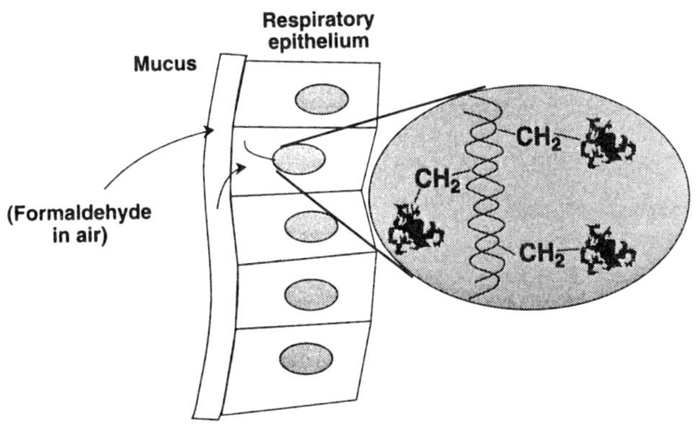


**FIG. 1.** Relationship between formaldehyde in inhaled air and the formation of DNA-protein cross-links by formaldehyde residues. (From ref. 103.)

*Role of Cell Proliferation*

Monticello et al. (33,137–139) studied the correlation of cell proliferation indices with sites of formaldehyde-induced squamous cell carcinoma in rats. They found that formaldehyde induced squamous cell carcinoma in a nonlinear fashion with no observed effect at an exposure of 2 ppm. There was a good spatial correlation between a cell population-weighted index of cell proliferation and regional tumor incidence. The dose-response curve for cell proliferation also correlated well with nasal epithelial lesions and other biologic effects, such as inhibition of mucociliary function (137). The basis for disturbances in cell proliferation have not yet been determined but may involve direct reaction of formaldehyde with DNA or other macromolecules, growth factors, mutations in growth regulatory genes, or an imbalance between cell proliferation and cell loss (33). Point mutations in the p53 gene have been demonstrated in formaldehyde-induced nasal squamous cell carcinoma in the rat. These data support the concept that mucosal regeneration associated with toxic concentrations of formaldehyde enhances neoplastic development in the nasal cavity.

A critical issue in evaluating the mechanism of carcinogenesis is whether exposure to low concentrations of formaldehyde enhances cell proliferation (1). However, the evidence has been inconclusive. One study reported that subacute exposure to low concentration of formaldehyde (1 ppm, 6 hours a day for 3 days) induced a small, transient increase in nasal epithelial cell turnover in Wistar rats (140), but this finding was not confirmed in later studies (1,141), and investigators did not detect an increase in cell turnover in the nasal epithelium of Fischer 344 rats (1). Cell replication was observed in rats with higher exposure (3 ppm, 6 hours a day for 3 days). In evaluating the relative importance of concentration and total dose, investigators have concluded that concentration, not total dose, is the primary determinant of the cytotoxicity of formaldehyde.

It is difficult to relate findings of the animal studies to the findings of the epidemiologic studies because virtually none of the epidemiologic studies had information on peak exposures. What information does exist suggests that formaldehyde exposures are not generally high enough to cause epithelial damage and cellular proliferation in most occupational or residential settings.

## Systematic Effects

### *Effects of Ingestion*

Toxic effects following ingestion of formaldehyde have been confirmed by reports of a number of deaths attributed to this type of exposure. Ingestion of large amounts of formaldehyde has been known to cause severe corrosive damage to the esophagus and stomach. Ingestion of formalin may cause corrosive gastritis with associated nausea, vomiting, pain, and bleeding. Ingestion of concentrated formaldehyde solutions can result in necrosis and ulceration of the stomach and intestine (142). Metabolic acidosis can develop following ingestion due to the metabolism of formaldehyde to formic acid.

### *Reproductive and Developmental Toxicity*

The reproductive and developmental toxicity of formaldehyde has been reviewed (1,2). In animal experimental systems, formaldehyde did not exert adverse effects on reproduction or fetal development whether administered by inhalation, ingestion, or skin exposure to various rodent species. In humans, studies among hospital staff and nurses in Finland using record linkage and case-control designs found no consistent associations with spontaneous abortion or congenital malformations (143,144). A small increase in spontaneous abortion was observed in one study (OR = 3.5, 95% confidence interval, 1.1–11), but most of the cases and controls that had been exposed to formalin were also exposed to xylene (145).

### *Neurologic Effects*

Neurobehavioral effects, including impaired memory, equilibrium, and dexterity, have been reported among histology technicians (146). However, because of rapid metabolism and no documented increases in blood concentration following exposure, it is unlikely that formaldehyde would reach the brain to cause direct central nervous system effects.

## REGULATIONS

In the United States, occupational exposure to formaldehyde is regulated under an OSHA standard that specifies exposure limits and monitoring, respiratory and hygiene protection, medical surveillance, medical removal, and worker training (13). The permissible exposure limit (PEL) is 0.75 ppm as an 8-hour time-weighted average, the action level is 0.5 ppm as an 8-hour time-weighted average, and the short-term exposure limit (STEL) is 2 ppm over 15 minutes.

Medical surveillance is mandated for all workers exposed at or above the action level or STEL, as well as for workers who experience symptoms or signs consistent with formaldehyde overexposure. The examinations should be performed prior to exposure, annually in those who will use respirators, and at the discretion of the physician. The examination must include a questionnaire about occupational exposures, smoking, and medical history, focusing on evidence of eye, nose, or throat irritation; upper or lower respiratory problems; chronic airways problems or hyperreactive airway disease; or allergic skin conditions or dermatitis. Medical examinations are given if the physician feels the worker may be at increased risk from formaldehyde exposure and annually to those who use respirators. Workers who use respirators should have baseline and annual pulmonary function tests. The surveillance provisions of this regulation may be used as a guideline for the clinical evaluation of any person with potential formaldehyde exposure.

The U.S. Environmental Protection Agency (EPA) has declared formaldehyde a hazardous air pollutant, water pollutant, waste constituent, and inert ingredient of pesticide products. The EPA regulates formaldehyde under the Clean Air Act (CAA); Comprehensive Environmental Response, Compensation, and Liability Act (CERCLA); Food, Drug, and Cosmetic Act (FD&CA); Resource Conservation and Recovery Act (RCRA); Superfund Amendments and Reauthorization Act (SARA); and Toxic Substances Control Act (TSCA). Under CWA, the EPA established a reportable quantity (RQ) of 1,000 pounds; under CERCLA, the EPA lowered the RQ to 100 pounds. The EPA also requires that safety and health studies be submitted by manufacturers in relation to exposure to urea-formaldehyde resins. Formaldehyde is regulated as an indirect food additive under TSCA. Under SARA, the EPA established general threshold amounts and a threshold planning quantity. Carcinogen risk estimates by the EPA have been revised over time to reflect the sublinear, rather than linear, dose-response of formaldehyde on cell proliferation and animal carcinogenicity (14).

Under the authority of the Federal Hazardous Substances Act (FHSA), the Consumer Products Safety Commission (CPSC) requires household products containing 1% or more of formaldehyde to be labeled with a warning that formaldehyde is a strong sensitizer. CPSC also banned the use of urea-formaldehyde foam insulation in residences and schools, acting under the authority of the Consumer Product Safety Act (CPSA), but a U.S. Court of Appeals later ruled that the ban be vacated. After studying the bioavailability and dermal penetration of formaldehyde from textiles, CPSC did not find that formaldehyde from this source penetrated intact skin; consequently, no action based on carcinogenic risk was taken regarding the use of formaldehyde in the textile industry.

## ACKNOWLEDGMENTS

The assistance of Ms. Stacey Kojaku is gratefully acknowledged. Ms. Irma Nicola obtained many of the cited articles.

## REFERENCES

1. International Agency for Research on Cancer. *IARC monographs on the evaluation of carcinogenic risks to humans, vol 62. Formaldehyde.* Lyon, France: IARC, 1995;217–375.

2. World Health Organization. *Formaldehyde* (Environmental Health Criteria 89). Geneva: International Programme on Chemical Safety, 1989.
3. Smedley J. Is formaldehyde an important cause of allergic respiratory disease? (editorial). *Clin Exp Allergy* 1996;26:247–249.
4. Hilton J, Dearman RJ, Basketter DA, Scholes EW, Kimber I. Experimental assessment of the sensitizing properties of formaldehyde. *Food Chem Toxicol* 1996;34:571–578.
5. Grammer LC, Harris KE, Cugell DW, Patterson R. Evaluation of a worker with possible formaldehyde-induced asthma. *J Allergy Clin Immunol* 1993;92(Pt 1):29–33.
6. Albert RE, Sellakumar AR, Laskin S, Kuschner M, Nelson A, Snyder CA. Nasal cancer in the rat induced by gaseous formaldehyde and hydrogen chloride. *J Natl Cancer Inst* 1982;68:597–603.
7. Kerns WD, Pavkov KL, Donofrio DJ, Gralia EJ, Swenberg JA. Carcinogenicity of formaldehyde in rats and mice after long-term inhalation exposure. *Cancer Res* 1983;43:4382–4392.
8. Blair A, Saracci R, Stewart PA, Hayes RB, Shy C. Epidemiologic evidence on the relationship between formaldehyde exposure and cancer. *Scand J Work Environ Health* 1990;16:381–393.
9. Partanen T. Formaldehyde exposure and respiratory cancer—a meta-analysis of the epidemiologic evidence. *Scand J Work Environ Health* 1993;19:8–15.
10. Callas PW, Pastides H, Hosmer DW Jr. Lung cancer mortality among workers in formaldehyde industries (editorial). *J Occup Environ Med* 1996;38:747–748.
11. McLaughlin JK. Formaldehyde and cancer: a critical review. *Int Arch Occup Environ Health* 1994;66(5):295–301.
12. National Institute for Occupational Safety and Health. *Evaluation of the National Cancer Institute epidemiologic and industrial hygiene studies of the formaldehyde industry.* Cincinnati: DHEW (NIOSH), 1986(June 19).
13. Occupational Safety and Health Administration. *Occupational Safety and Health standard for formaldehyde.* 29 CFR Section 1910.1048.
14. Environmental Protection Agency. *Formaldehyde risk assessment update final draft.* Washington, DC: Office of Toxic Substances, Environmental Protection Agency, 1991.
15. Gerberich HR, Seaman GC. Formaldehyde. In: Kroschwitz JI, Howe-Grant M, eds. *Kirk-Othmer encyclopedia of chemical technology,* 4th ed, vol 11. New York: John Wiley, 1994;929–951.
16. International Agency for Research on Cancer. *IARC monographs on the evaluation of the carcinogenic risk of chemicals to humans. Vol 29. Some industrial chemicals and dyestuffs.* Lyon, France: IARC, 1982; 345–389.
17. Reuss G, Disteldorf W, Grundler O, Hilt A. Formaldehyde. In: Gerhart W, Yamamoto YS, Elvers B, Rounsaville JF, Schulz G, eds. *Ullmann's encyclopedia of industrial chemistry,* 5th ed., rev., vol A11. New York: VCH Publishers, 1988;619–651.
18. Formaldehyde. *Chemical Week* 1996;158(8):26.
19. *Directory of chemical producers.* Menlo Park (CA): SRI International, 1985;617.
20. National Institute of Occupational Safety and Health. *National occupational exposure survey 1981–83.* Cincinnati: NIOSH, 1990.
21. Stewart PA, Cubit DA, Blair A. Formaldehyde levels in seven industries. *Appl Ind Hyg* 1987;2:231–236.
22. Kauppinen T. Occupational exposure to chemical agents in the plywood industry. *Ann Occup Hyg* 1986;30:19–29.
23. Priha E, Riipinen H, Korhonen K. Exposure to formaldehyde and solvents in Finnish furniture factories in 1975–1984. *Ann Occup Hyg* 1986;30:289–294.
24. Alexandersson R, Hedenstierna G. Respiratory hazards associated with exposure to formaldehyde and solvents in acid-curing paints. *Arch Environ Health* 1988;43:222–227.
25. Riala RE, Riihimäki HA. Solvent and formaldehyde exposure in parquet and carpet work. *Appl Occup Environ Hyg* 1991;6:301–308.
26. Cooke TF, Weigmann L. The chemistry of formaldehyde release from durable-press fabrics. *Text Chem Colorist* 1982;14:25.
27. Elliott LJ, Stayner LT, Blade LM, Halperin W, Keenlyside R. *Formaldehyde exposure characterization in garment manufacturing plants:* a composite summary of three in-depth industrial hygiene surveys. Cincinnati: Department of Health and Human Services, Public Health Service, Centers for Disease Control, National Institute for Occupational Safety and Health, 1987.
28. Higginson J, Jenson OM, Kinley L, et al. Epidemiology of chronic occupational exposure to formaldehyde: report of the ad hoc panel on health aspects of formaldehyde. *Toxicol Ind Health* 1988;4:77–90.
29. National Research Council. *Formaldehyde:* an assessment of its health effects. Washington, DC: National Academy Press, 1980.
30. National Research Council. Health effects of formaldehyde. In: *Formaldehyde and other aldehydes.* Washington, DC: National Academy Press, 1981;175–220,306–340.
31. Preuss PW, Dailey RL, Lehman ES. Exposure to formaldehyde. In: Turoski V, ed. *Advances in chemistry series. Vol 210. Formaldehyde. Analytical chemistry and toxicology.* Washington, DC: American Chemical Society, 1985;247–259.
32. Vaught C. *Locating and estimating air emissions from sources of formaldehyde (revised).* Report No. EPA-450/4-91-012; US NTIS PB91-181842. Research Triangle Park (NC): Environmental Protection Agency, 1991.
33. Monticello TM, Swenberg JA, Gross EA, et al. Correlation of regional and nonlinear formaldehyde-induced nasal cancer with proliferating populations of cells. *Cancer Res* 1996;56:1012–1022.
34. Songco G, Fahey PJ. Indoor and outdoor air pollutants and health. *Compr Ther* 1987;13:41–48.
35. Gupta KC, Ulsamer AG, Preuso PW. Formaldehyde in indoor air. Sources and toxicity. *Environ Int* 1982;8:349–354.
36. Pickrell JA, Griffs LC, Mokler BV, Vanapilly GM, Hobbs CH. Release of formaldehyde from various consumer products. *Environ Sci Technol* 1983;17:753–764.
37. Gammage RG, Travis CC. Formaldehyde exposure and risk in mobile homes. In: Paustenbach DJ, ed. *The risk assessment of environmental and human health hazards:* a textbook of case studies. New York: John Wiley, 1989:601–611.
38. Sexton K, Petreas MX, Liu KS. Formaldehyde exposures inside mobile homes. *Environ Sci Technol* 1989;23:985–988.
39. Gylseth B, Digernes V. *The European development of regulations and standards for formaldehyde in air and in wood composite boards. Proceedings of the Pacific Rim Bio-based Composites Symposium;* 1992 November 9–13. Rotorua, New Zealand: Forest Products Research Institute, 1992:199–206.
40. Lehmann WF, Roffael E. International guidelines and regulations for formaldehyde emissions. In: *Proceedings of the 26th Washington State University International Particleboard/Composite Material Symposium.* Pullman, WA: Washington State University, 1992;124–150.
41. International Agency for Research on Cancer. *IARC monographs on the evaluation of the carcinogenic risk of chemicals to humans. Vol 38. Tobacco smoking.* Lyon, France: IARC, 1986;96.
42. Restani P, Restelli AR, Galli CL. Formaldehyde and hexamethylenetetramine as food additives: chemical interactions and toxicology. *Food Addit Contam* 1992;9:597–605.
43. Indoor pollutants/Committee on Indoor Pollutants. National Research Council. Washington, DC: National Academy of Sciences, 1981.
44. National Institute for Occupational Safety and Health. Problems with the performance of passive monitors for formaldehyde. *MMWR* 1983; 32:615–621.
45. Pristas R. Passive badges for compliance monitoring internationally. *Am Ind Hyg Assoc J* 1994;55:841–844.
46. Heck Hd'A, Casanova-Schmitz M, Dodd PB, Schachter EN, Witek T, Tosun T. Formaldehyde ($CH_2O$) concentrations in the blood of humans and Fischer 344 rats exposed to $CH_2O$ under controlled conditions. *Am Ind Hyg Assoc J* 1985;46:1–3.
47. Heck Hd'A, Casanova-Schmitz M. Reaction of formaldehyde in the rat nasal mucosa. In: Clary JJ, Gibson JE, Waritz RS, eds. *Formaldehyde:* toxicology, *epidemiology, and mechanisms.* New York: Marcel Dekker, 1983;211–223.
48. Casanova M, Heck Hd'A, Janszen DB. Comments on DNA-protein crosslinks, a biomarker of exposure to formaldehyde—*in vitro* and in vivo studies by Shaham et al (letter). *Carcinogenesis* 1996;17: 2097–2101.
49. Casanova M, Heck Hd'A, Everitt JI, Harrington WW Jr, Popp JA. Formaldehyde concentrations in the blood of rhesus monkeys after inhalation exposure. *Food Chem Toxicol* 1988;26:715–716.
50. Gottschling LM, Beaulieu HJ, Melvin WW. Monitoring of formic acid in urine of humans exposed to low levels of formaldehyde. *Am Ind Hyg Assoc J* 1984;45:19–23.
51. Shaham J, Bomstein Y, Meltzer A, et al. DNA-protein crosslinks, a biomarker of exposure to formaldehyde—*in vitro* and in vivo studies. *Carcinogenesis* 1996;17:121–125.
52. Fennell T. Development of methods for measuring biological markers of formaldehyde exposure. *Health Effects Institute Research Report* 1994;67:1–20.

53. Aharonson EF, Menkes H, Gatner G, Swift DL, Procter DF. Effect of respiratory airflow on the removal of soluble vapors by the nose. *J Appl Physiol* 1974;27:654–657.
54. Dallas CE, Theiss JC, Harrist RB, Fairchild EJ. Effect of subchronic formaldehyde inhalation on minute volume and nasal deposition in Sprague-Dawley rats. *J Toxicol Environ Health* 1985;16:553–564.
55. Egle L Jr. Retention of inhaled formaldehyde, propionaldehyde, and acrolein in the dog. *Arch Environ Health* 1972;25:119–124.
56. Conaway CC, Whysner J, Verna LK, Williams GM. Formaldehyde mechanistic data and risk assessment: endogenous protection from DNA adduct formation. *Pharmacol Ther* 1996;71:29–55.
57. Demkowicz-Dobrzanski K, Castonguay A. Modulation by glutathione of DNA strand breaks induced by 4-(methylnitrosamino)-1-(3-pyridyl)-1-butanone and its aldehyde metabolites in rat hepatocytes. *Carcinogenesis* 1992;13:1447–1454.
58. Casanova-Schmitz M, Heck Hd A. DNA-protein cross-linking induced by formaldehyde (FA) in the rat respiratory mucosa: dependence on FA concentration in normal rats and in rats depleted of glutathione (GSH). *Toxicologist* 1985;5:128–132.
59. Maibach H. Formaldehyde: effects on animal and human skin. In: Gibson JE, ed. *Formaldehyde toxicity.* Washington, DC: Hemisphere, 1983;166–174.
60. Bender JR, Mullin LS, Graepel GJ, Wilson WE. Eye irritation response of humans to formaldehyde. *Am Ind Hyg Assoc J* 1983;44: 463–465.
61. Kulle TJ, Sauder LR, Hebel JR, Green DJ, Chatham MD. Formaldehyde response in healthy nonsmokers. *J Air Pollution Control Assoc* 1987;37:919–924.
62. Andersen I, Molhave L. Controlled human studies with formaldehyde. In: Gibson JE, ed. *Formaldehyde toxicity.* Washington, DC: Hemisphere, 1983:154–165.
63. Horvath EP Jr, Anderson H Jr, Pierce WE, Hanrahan L, Wendlick JD. Effects of formaldehyde on the mucous membranes and lungs. A study of an industrial population. *JAMA* 1988;259:701–707.
64. Wilhelmsson B, Holmström M. Possible mechanisms of formaldehyde-induced discomfort in the upper airways. *Scand J Work Environ Health* 1992;18:403–407.
65. Broder I, Corey P, Cole P, Lipa M, Mintz S, Nethercott JR. Comparison of health of occupants and characteristics of houses among control homes and homes insulated with urea formaldehyde foam. I. Methodology. II. Initial health and house variables and exposure-response relationships. III. Health and house variables following remedial work. *Environ Res* 1988;45:141–203.
66. Berke JH. Cytologic examination of the nasal mucosa in formaldehyde-exposed workers. *J Occup Med* 1987;29:681–684.
67. Edling C, Hellquist H, Odkvist L. Occupational exposure to formaldehyde and histopathological changes in the nasal mucosa. *Br J Ind Med* 1988;45:761–765.
68. Holmström M, Wilhelmsson B, Hellquist H, Rosen G. Histological changes in the nasal mucosa in persons occupationally exposed to formaldehyde alone and in combination with wood dust. *Acta Otolaryngol* 1989;107:120–129.
69. Ballarin C, Sarto F, Giacomelli L, Battista Bartolucci G, Clonfero E. Micronucleated cells in nasal mucosa of formaldehyde-exposed workers. *Mutat Res* 1992;280:1–7.
70. Titenko-Holland N, Levine AJ, Smith MT, et al. Quantification of epithelial cell micronuclei by fluorescence in hybridization (FISH) in mortuary science students exposed to formaldehyde. *Mutat Res* 1996; 371:237–248.
71. Kerns WD, Donofrio DJ, Pavkov KL. The chronic effects of formaldehyde inhalation in rats and mice: a preliminary report. In: Gibson JE, ed. *Formaldehyde toxicity.* Washington, DC: Hemisphere, 1983:111–131.
72. Lemiere C, Desjardins A, Cloutier Y, et al. Occupational asthma due to formaldehyde resin dust with and without reaction to formaldehyde gas. *Eur Respir J* 1995;8:861–865.
73. Burge PS, Harries MG, Lam WK, O Brien IM, Patchett PA. Occupational asthma due to formaldehyde. *Thorax* 1985;40:255–260.
74. Hendrick DJ, Lane DJ. Formalin asthma in hospital staff. *Br Med J* 1975;1:607–608.
75. Hendrick DJ, Lane DJ. Occupational formalin asthma. *Br J Ind Med* 1977;34:11–18.
76. Hendrick DJ, Rando RJ, Lane DJ, Morris MJ. Formaldehyde asthma: challenge exposure levels and fate after five years. *J Occup Med* 1982; 4:893–897.
77. Schachter EN, Witek TJ Jr, Tosun T, Beck GJ. A study of respiratory effects from exposure to 2 ppm formaldehyde in healthy subjects. *Arch Environ Health* 1986;41:229–239.
78. Schachter EN, Witek TJ Jr, Brody DJ, Tosun T, Beck GJ, Leaderer BP. A study of respiratory effects from exposure to 2.0 ppm formaldehyde in occupationally exposed workers. *Environ Res* 1987;44:188–205.
79. Kilburn KH, Warshaw R, Thorton JC. Pulmonary function in histology technicians compared with women from Michigan: effects of chronic low dose formaldehyde in a national sample of women. *Br J Ind Med* 1989;46:468–472.
80. Kriebel D, Sama SR. Cocanour B. Reversible pulmonary responses to formaldhyde. A study of clinical anatomy students. *Am Rev Respir Dis* 1993;148:1509–1515.
81. Uba G, Pachorek D, Bernstein J, et al. Prospective study of respiratory effects of formaldehyde among healthy and asthmatic medical students. *Am J Ind Med* 1989;46:91–101.
82. Akbar-Khanzadeh F, Vaquerano MU, Akbar-Khanzadeh M, Bisesi MS. Formaldehyde exposure, acute pulmonary response, and exposure control options in a gross anatomy laboratory. *Am J Ind Med* 1994;26:61–75.
83. Kerfoot EJ, Mooney TF. Formaldehyde and paraformaldehyde study in funeral homes. *Am Ind Hyg Assoc J* 1975;36:533.
84. Gorski P, Krakowiak A. Formaldehyde-induced bronchial asthma—does it really exist? *Polish J Occup Med Environ Health* 1991;4: 317–320.
85. Grammer LC, Harris KE, Shaughnessy MA, et al. Clinical and immunologic evaluation of 37 workers exposed to gaseous formaldehyde. *J Allergy Clin Immunol* 1990;86:177–181.
86. Sandler SG, Sharon R, Stroup M, Sabo B. Formaldehyde-related antibodies in hemodialysis patients. *Transfusion* 1979;19:682–687.
87. Lynen R, Rothe M, Gallasch E. Characterization of formaldehyde-related antibodies in hemodialysis patients at different stages of immunization. *Vox Sang* 1983;44:81–89.
88. Maurice E, Rivory J-H, Larsson PH, Johansson SGO, Bouquest J. Anaphylactic shock caused by formaldehyde in a patient undergoing long-term hemodialysis. *J Allergy Clin Immunol* 1986;77:594–597.
89. Patterson R, Dykewicz MS, Evans R III, et al. IgG antibody against formaldehyde human serum proteins: a comparison with other IgG antibodies against inhalant proteins and reactive chemicals. *J Allergy Clin Immunol* 1989;9:359–366.
90. Dykewicz MS, Patterson R, Cugell DW, Harris KE, Wu AF. Serum IgE and IgG to formaldehyde-human serum albumin: lack of relation to gaseous formaldehyde exposure and symptoms. *J Allergy Clin Immunol* 1991;87:48–57.
91. Pross HF, Day JH, Clark RH, Lees REM. Immunologic studies of subjects with asthma exposed to formaldehyde and urea-formaldehyde foam insulation (UFFI) off products. *J Allergy Clin Immunol* 1987;79: 797–810.
92. Wantke F, Demmer CM, Tappler P, Gotz M, Jarisch R. Exposure to gaseous formaldehyde induces IgE-mediated sensitization to formaldehyde in school-children. *Clin Exp Allergy* 1996;26:276–280.
93. Potter DW, Wederbrand KS. Total IgE antibody production in BALB/c mice after dermal exposure to chemicals. *Fundam Appl Toxicol* 1995; 26:127–135.
94. Nunn AJ, Craigen AA, Venables KM, Newman-Taylor AJ. Six year follow up of lung function in men occupationally exposed to formaldehyde. *Br J Ind Med* 1990;47:747–752.
95. Schobenberg JB, Mitchell CA. Airway disease caused by phenolic (phenol formaldehyde) resin exposure. *Arch Environ Health* 1975;30: 574–577.
96. Blair A, Stewart P, O'Berg M, et al. Mortality among industrial workers exposed to formaldehyde. *J Natl Cancer Inst* 1986;76:1071–1084.
97. Walrath J, Fraumeni JF Jr. Mortality patterns among embalmers. *Int J Cancer* 1983;31:407–411.
98. Black H. Contact dermatitis from formaldehyde in newsprint. *Contact Dermatitis Newsletter* 1971;10:242.
99. Glass WI. An outbreak of formaldehyde dermatitis. *NZ Med J* 1961; 60:423–427.
100. Rycroft RJG. Occupational contact dermatitis. In: Rycroft RJG, Menne T, Frosch PJ, Benezra C, eds. *Textbook of contact dermatitis.* Berlin: Springer-Verlag, 1992;341–399.
101. Lidén S, Scheynius A, Fischer T, Johansson SG, Ruhnek-Forsbeck M, Stejskal V. Absence of specific IgE antibodies in allergic contact sensitivity to formaldehyde. *Allergy* 1993;48:525–529.

102. Cronin E. Clothing and textiles. In: Ronin E, ed. *Contact dermatitis.* Edinburgh: Churchill Livingstone, 1980;36.
103. Conolly RB, Andjelkovich DA, Casanova M, et al. *Multidisciplinary, iterative examination of the mechanism of formaldehyde carcinogenicity:* the basis for better risk assessment. *CIIT activities.* Research Triangle Park, NC: Chemical Industry Institute of Toxicology, 1995; 15(12):1–11.
104. Harrington JM, Shannon HS. Mortality study of pathologists and medical laboratory technicians. *Br Med J* 1975;1:329–332.
105. Harrington JM, Oakes D. Mortality study of British pathologists 1974–80. *Br J Ind Med* 1984;41:188–191.
106. Hall A, Harrington JM, Aw T-C. Mortality study of British pathologists. *Am J Ind Med* 1991;20:83–89.
107. Logue JN, Barrick MK, Jessup GL Jr. Mortality of radiologists and pathologists in the radiation registry of physicians. *J Occup Med* 1986;28:91–99.
108. Stroup NE, Blair A, Erikson GE.Brain cancer and other causes of death in anatomists. *J Natl Cancer Inst* 1986;77:1217–1224.
109. Walrath J, Fraumeni JF Jr. Cancer and other causes of death among embalmers. *Cancer Res* 1984;44:4638–4641.
110. Hayes RB, Blair A, Stewart PA, Herrick RF, Mahar H. Mortality of US embalmers and funeral directors. *Am J Ind Med* 1990;18:641–652.
111. Levine RJ, Andjelkovich DA, Shaw LK. The mortality of Ontario undertakers and a review of formaldehyde-related mortality studies. *J Occup Med* 1984;26:740–746.
112. Blair A, Stewart PA, Hoover RN. Mortality from lung cancer among workers employed in formaldehyde industries. *Am J Ind Med* 1990;17: 683–699.
113. Acheson ED, Gardner MJ, Pannett B, et al. Formaldehyde in the British chemical industry—an occupational cohort study. *Lancet* 1984;1:611–616.
114. Gardner MJ, Pannett B, Winter PD, Cruddas AM. A cohort study of workers exposed to formaldehyde in the British chemical industry: an update. *Br J Ind Med* 1993;50:827–834.
115. Bertazzi PA, Pesatori AC, Radice L, Zocchetti C, Vai T. Exposure to formaldehyde and cancer mortality in a cohort of workers producing resins. *Scand J Work Environ Health* 1986;12:461–468.
116. Bertazzi PA, Pesatori AC, Guercilena S, Consonni D, Zocchetti C. Cancer risk among workers producing formaldehyde-based resins: extension of follow-up. *Med Lav* 1989;80:111–122.
117. Edling C, Järvholm B, Andersson L, Axelson O. Mortality and cancer incidence among workers in an abrasive manufacturing industry. *Br J Ind Med* 1987;44:57–59.
118. Stayner LT, Elliott L, Blade L, Keenlyside R, Halperin W. A retrospective cohort mortality study of workers exposed to formaldehyde in the garment industry. *Am J Ind Med* 1988;13:667–681.
119. Andjelkovich DA, Janszen DB, Brown MH, Richardson RB, Miller FJ. Mortality of iron foundry workers: IV. Analysis of a subcohort exposed to formaldehyde. *J Occup Environ Med* 1995;37:826–837.
120. Olsen JH, Plough Jensen S, Hink M, Faurbo K, Breum NO, Møller Jensen O. Occupational formaldehyde exposure and increased nasal cancer risk in man. *Int J Cancer* 1984;34:639–644.
121. Olsen JH, Asnaes S. Formaldehyde and the risk of squamous cell carcinoma of the sinonasal cavities. *Br J Ind Med* 1986;43:769–774.
122. Hayes RB, Raatgever DW, DeBruyn A, Berin M. Cancer of the nasal cavity and paranasal sinuses and formaldehyde exposure. *Int J Cancer* 1986;37:487–492.
123. Roush GC, Walrath J, Stayner LT, Kaplan SA, Flannery JT, Blair A. Nasopharyngeal cancer, sinonasal cancer, and occupations related to formaldehyde: a case-control study. *J Natl Cancer Inst* 1987;79: 1221–1224.
124. Vaughan TL, Strader C, Davis S, Daling JR. Formaldehyde and cancers of the pharynx, sinus and nasal cavity: I. Occupational exposures. *Int J Cancer* 1986;38:677–683.
125. Vaughan TL, Strader C, Davis S, Daling JR. Formaldehyde and cancers of the pharynx, sinus and nasal cavity: II. Residential exposures. *Int J Cancer* 1986;38:685–688.
126. Blair A, Kazerouni N. Reactive chemicals and cancer. *Cancer Causes Control* 1997;8:473–490.
127. Blair A, Stewart PA, Hoover RN, et al. Cancers of the nasopharynx and oropharynx and formaldehyde exposure. *J Natl Cancer Inst* 1987; 78:191–192.
128. Walrath J, Rogot E, Murray J, Blair A. *Mortality patterns among US veterans by occupation and smoking status.* NIH Pub. No. 85-2756. Bethesda, MD: Department of Health and Human Services, 1985.
129. Conolly RB, Andersen ME. An approach to mechanism-based cancer risk assessment for formaldehyde. *Environ Health Perspect* 1993; 101(suppl 6):169–176.
130. Grafstrom RC. In vitro studies of aldehyde effects related to human respiratory carcinogenesis. *Mutat Res* 1990;238:175–184.
131. Casanova M, Deyo DF, Heck Hd'A. Covalent binding of inhaled formaldehyde to DNA in the nasal mucosa of Fischer 344 rats: analysis of formaldehyde and DNA by high-performance liquid chromatography and provisional pharmacokinetic interpretation. *Fundam Appl Toxicol* 1989;12:397–417.
132. Casanova M, Morgan KT, Steinhagen WH, Everitt JI, Popp JA, Heck Hd'A. Covalent binding of inhaled formaldehyde to DNA in the respiratory tract of rhesus monkeys: pharmacokinetics, rat-to-monkey interspecies scaling, and extrapolation to man. *Fundam Appl Toxicol* 1991;17:409–428.
133. Casanova M, Morgan KT, Gross EA, Moss OR, Heck Hd'A. DNA-protein cross-links and cell replication at specific sites in the nose of F344 rats exposed subchronically to formaldehyde. *Fundam Appl Toxicol* 1994;23:525–536.
134. Heck Hd'A, Casanova M, Steinhagen WH, Everitt JI, Morgan KT, Popp JA. Formaldehyde toxicity: DNA-protein cross-linking studies in rats and nonhuman primates. In: Feron VJ, Bosland MC, eds. *Nasal carcinogenesis in rodents:* relevance to human risk. Wageningen, The Netherlands: Pudoc, 1989:159–164.
135. Grafström RC, Fornace A, Harris CC. Repair of DNA damage caused by formaldehyde in human cells. *Cancer Res* 1984;44:4323–4327.
136. Grafström RC, Hsu IC, Harris CC. Mutagenicity of formaldehyde in Chinese hamster lung fibroblasts: synergy with ionizing radiation and N-nitroso-N-methylurea. *Chem Biol Interact* 1993;86:41–49.
137. Monticello TM, Miller FJ, Morgan KT. Regional increases in rat nasal epithelial cell proliferation following acute and subchronic inhalation of formaldehyde. *Toxicol Appl Pharmacol* 1991;111:409–421.
138. Monticello TM, Morgan KT. Cell proliferation and formaldehyde-induced respiratory carcinogenesis. *Risk Analysis* 1994;14:313–319.
139. Monticello TM, Gross EA, Morgan KT. Cell proliferation and nasal carcinogenesis. *Environ Health Perspect* 1993;101(suppl 5):121–124.
140. Zwart A, Wouterson RA, Wilmer JWGM, Spit BJ, Feron VJ. Cytotoxic and adaptive effects in rat nasal epithelium after 3-day and 13-week exposure to low concentrations of formaldehyde vapour. *Toxicology* 1988;51:87–99.
141. Reuzel PGJ, Wilmer JWGM, Woutersen RA, Zwart A, Rombout PJA, Feron VJ. Interactive effects of ozone and formaldehyde on the nasal respiratory lining epithelium in rats. *J Toxicol Environ Health* 1990; 29:279–292.
142. Morgan DP. *Recognition and management of pesticide poisonings,* 4th ed. Washington, DC: Environmental Protection Agency, 1989.
143. Hemminki K, Mutanen P, Saloniemi I, Niemi M-L, Vainio H. Spontaneous abortions in hospital staff engaged in sterilising instruments with chemical agents. *Br Med J* 1982;285:1461–1463.
144. Hemminki K, Kyyrönen P, Lindbohm M-L. Spontaneous abortions and malformations in the offspring of nurses exposed to anaesthetic gases, cytostatic drugs, and other potential hazards in hospitals, based on registered information of outcome. *J Epidemiol Community Health* 1985;39:141–147.
145. Taskinen H, Kyyrönen P, Hemminki K, Hoikkala M, Lajunen K, Lindbohm M-L. Laboratory work and pregnancy outcome. *J Occup Med* 1994;36:311–319.
146. Kilburn KH. Neurobehavioral impairment and seizures from formaldehyde. *Arch Environ Health* 1994:49:37–44.

*Environmental and Occupational Medicine,*
*Third Edition,* edited by William N. Rom.
Lippincott–Raven Publishers, Philadelphia © 1998.

# CHAPTER 81

# Styrene and Butadiene

John K. Wiencke and Piero Mustacchi

## STYRENE MONOMER

Styrene, also called cinnamene, cinnamol, ethenylbenzene, phenylethylene, styrol, styrolene, and vinylbenzene, is a colorless or yellowish oily liquid with an odor threshold of about 0.01 ppm and odor recognition near 0.1 ppm (1). Its physicochemical properties (2) are summarized in Table 1. Styrene undergoes self-polymerization and oxidation when exposed to light and air; therefore, inhibitors are added to stabilize pure styrene solutions. Styrene is widely used, ranking 21st in the top 50 chemicals produced in 1989 (3). Its annual worldwide production capacity was estimated to be over 16 million tons in 1992 (4). Styrene, when heated, polymerizes to form polystyrene (PS), a clear plastic with excellent insulating properties [2]; it is also used in the production of a variety of other resins including styrene-butadiene rubber (SBR).

### Exposure

In the United States approximately 4 million metric tons of styrene are produced annually (5); the National Institute for Occupational Safety and Health (NIOSH) estimated that 1.1 million workers are potentially exposed to it (6). The manufacture of styrene and its polymers generally occurs in closed processes in which the potential for exposure to the monomer is quite limited [time-weighted average (TWA) is generally maintained below 5 ppm or 21 $mg/m^3$] (2). The greatest source of employee exposure to styrene arises from its use in the fabrication of large items made from reinforced polyester resins (Table 2). This process, which involves the application of alternating layers of fibrous glass mats with liquid resin, is commonly called "hand layup." TWA exposures associated with manual laminating or spraying during reinforced plastics production average 20 to 300 ppm (7). The polyester resin contains approximately 40% monomeric styrene (by weight), and as much as 10% evaporates into ambient air. The application process, amount of resin consumed, and efficiency of workplace ventilation determine the workers' level of exposure. Styrene production and polymer production are associated with TWA exposures between 1 and 20 ppm with occasional short-term excursions related to line breaks, line openings, or leaks. Exposure during product fabrication, such as extruding, molding, or hot-wire cutting, is associated with TWA exposures between 0.01 and 1.0 ppm. By comparison, the mean ambient air concentrations of styrene in New Jersey, North Dakota, California, and across Canada range from 0.09 to 3.8 $\mu g/m^3$ [4.26 $\mu g/m^3$ = 1 part per billion (ppb)] (2). Finally, nonoccupational exposure to styrene can occur through the diet and tobacco smoking (2).

In addition, reinforced plastics workers may be exposed to low levels of styrene oxide (SO) (e.g., <0.5 $mg/m^3$) as a result of in situ oxidation of styrene during its polymerization (8,9). As indicated below (see Genotoxicity) recent research suggests that direct exposure to low levels of SO may be a more significant genotoxic hazard than the much larger amounts of SO arising from hepatic metabolism of styrene.

The current American Conference of Governmental Industrial Hygienists (ACGIH) threshold limit value (TLV), 50 ppm (213 $mg/m^3$), is based on the experimen-

J. K. Wiencke: Department of Epidemiology and Biostatistics, School of Medicine, University of California, San Francisco, San Francisco, California 94143-0560.
P. Mustacchi: Department of Epidemiology and Biostatistics and of Medicine, School of Medicine, University of California, San Francisco, San Francisco, California 94143-0560.

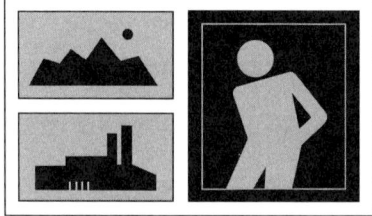

**TABLE 1.** *Physical properties of styrene*

| | |
|---|---|
| Structure | $C_6H_5$–CH=$CH_2$ |
| Freezing point | −30.6°C |
| Boiling point | 145.2°C |
| Density | 0.9060 at 20°C/4°C |
| Vapor pressure at 25°C | 6.1 mm Hg |
| Air saturated with styrene at 25°C | 8026 ppm |
| Vapor density (air=1) | 3.6 |
| Explosive limits | 1.1–6.1% |
| Solubility in $H_2O$ | 0.03% at 20°C |
| Partition coefficients | |
| Water/air | 4.38 |
| Blood/air | 32 |
| Oil/blood | 130 |
| Oil/air | 4,160 |
| Exposure standards | |
| OSHA (1989) | |
| PEL-TWO (8-hour) | 50 ppm |
| PEL-STEL (15-minute) | 100 ppm |
| NIOSH (1983) | |
| REL-TWA (8-hour) | 50 ppm |
| REL-STEL (15-minute) | 100 ppm |
| AGGIH (1986) | |
| TLV-TWA (8-hour) | 50 ppm |
| Odor threshold | Approx. 0.01 ppm |
| Odor recognition | Approx. 0.1 ppm |

Conversion factors: 1 ppm=4.26 mg/m³; 1 mg/m³=0.235 ppm.

tal induction of lymphoid and hematopoietic tumors in rodents exposed to styrene at concentrations greater than 500 ppm (2,125 mg/m³). The Swedish TLV, 26 ppm (111 mg/m³), is based on the expectation of neurologic symptoms, but a critical review of the 38 papers and related literature upon which the Swedish TLV is predicated raised questions regarding the appropriateness of the lower Swedish TLV (10).

## Environmental Monitoring

Styrene in workplace air can be determined by packed capillary column gas chromatography with a flame ionization detector. Exposure can be monitored by measuring styrene in mixed exhaled air either before or during a work shift, and by measuring the urinary concentration of mandelic or phenylglyoxylic acid or styrene in venous blood at either the end of a shift or prior to the next shift (11). An 8-hour exposure to 100 ppm styrene vapor is associated with exhalation of 2.6% of absorbed styrene, excretion of 56.9% of mandelic acid in the urine, excretion of 33.0% of phenylglyoxylic acid in urine, and a maximum of 7.5% excreted as hippurinic acid (12). For urinary mandelic acid, a level of 800 mg/g creatinine sampled at the end of a shift has been equated with a workplace exposure to the TLV-TWA of 50 ppm (13,14). An extensive study indicated a lower mandelic acid level (i.e., 584 mg/g creatinine for a 50 ppm exposure) (15). Results of an observational study of styrene in mixed exhaled air from 48 fiberglass boat builders, measured over a period of 1 year, were compared with the corresponding exposures, and indicated a linear correlation between both variables ($r^2 = 0.909$) over a range of 0 to 235 mg/m³ styrene concentrations (16,17). These results were consistent with measures of styrene in end-expired air from human volunteers exposed to short-term (100 minutes) controlled exposures of styrene (63.8–421 mg/m³). Biomarkers (such as DNA), protein adducts, and cytogenetic damage are also being evaluated as indices of styrene exposure.

**TABLE 2.** *Environmental and occupational exposure to styrene*

| | |
|---|---|
| Ambient air, New Jersey, North Dakota, California, and across Canada | 0.09–3.8 μg/m³ |
| Tobacco smoking | 18–48 μg/cigarette |
| Styrene and polymer production | <10 ppm |
| Fabricating (e.g., extruding, molding, or casting) | <10 ppm |
| Laminating | 20–300 ppm |

## Pharmacokinetics and Metabolism

Inhalation is the most significant route of exposure to styrene. Human volunteers exposed to approximately 15 and 38 ppm styrene vapor averaged 66% retention for nasal inhalation and mouth expiration, and 59% retention during exclusive mouth breathing (18). The human pulmonary styrene retention has been reported to average 61% during 8-hour exposure to 22 ppm (19); pulmonary absorption was reported to be 89% (20). The hourly styrene absorption through intact skin, initially believed to approximate 12 mg/cm²/hour (21), seems to proceed at a much slower rate (60 μg/cm²) (22), the initial value probably representing the rate of disappearance of styrene from the skin rather than its rate of absorption into the bloodstream (22). After absorption, styrene is first oxidized to styrene oxide by hepatic cytochrome P-450 isozymes (CYP2B6, CYP1A2, CYP2E1, CYP2C8) (23). SO is then converted, via epoxide hydrolases, to styrene glycol and its oxidation products, which are excreted in the urine (24,25). In humans, approximately 80% to 95% of styrene is excreted by this pathway, in contrast, in mice and rats glutathione conjugates of styrene account for about 40% of excretion products (Fig. 1). The ultimate major metabolites, mandelic acid and phenylglyoxylic acid, are used as convenient urinary and blood biomarkers of exposure (25). Styrene remains in detectable concentrations (0.1 mg/kg) in adipose tissue for up to 5 weeks after a single exposure of 2 hours to 50 ppm (26). There is no information about the persistence time of styrene in cerebral tissue (27). A number of physiologically based pharmacokinetic models have been developed for styrene in mice, rats, and humans (28–30); rodent and human models agree reasonably well

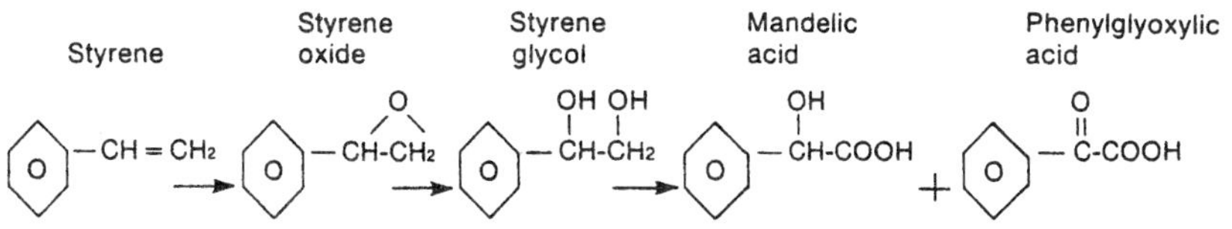


**FIG. 1.** Chemical structure and metabolism of styrene.

(reviewed in ref. 31). All of these models indicate saturation of styrene metabolism and its storage in adipose tissues at high exposure concentrations (e.g., 100 to 200 ppm for humans), whereas at low exposure concentrations the amount of styrene taken up is dependent on alveolar ventilation rates. These results have important implications for risk assessment; because SO production is saturable at high exposure levels, extrapolations based on high exposures may underestimate risks associated with SO production at low exposure levels (32).

## Acute Toxicity

### *Experimental Data*

Acute overexposure causes irritation of the eyes, mucous membranes, skin, and respiratory tract. At extreme levels, the irritant effects are severe, and depression of the central nervous system (CNS) predominates.

For single exposures, the oral median lethal dose ($LD_{50}$) in rats is approximately 500 mg/kg (slightly toxic) (33). In rats, chronic 7-hour inhalational exposures to 1,300 ppm produced eye and nose irritation (33). At 2,500 ppm, the affected animals demonstrated behavior consistent with more severe irritation with loss of consciousness after 10 to 12 hours. At levels greater than 5,000 ppm, the animals lost consciousness almost immediately and died within 8 hours. At autopsy the only significant findings among all exposed animals were limited to the lungs, where congestion, edema, exudates, and infiltrates were observed. Most deaths were attributed to styrene's effect on the CNS, but many delayed deaths were related to irritant effects on the lungs (34).

### *Human Studies*

Recognition of an otherwise unobjectionable odor follows exposure to around 60 ppm of styrene (33). Strong eye and nasal irritation but no other symptom develops at exposures of ≥600 ppm, the odor becoming objectionable at 200 to 400 ppm (33,35). However, even very low and repeated exposures (62.7 mg/m$^3$) have been associated with the occurrence of occupational asthma (36). Acute neurotoxic effects of styrene include electroencephalographic abnormalities, delayed psychomotor reaction, and impairment of color vision (37–40). Mild ocular irritation with a feeling of slight irritation and headache occur within 15 minutes of exposure at levels of approximately 376 ppm with impairment of dexterity, coordination, and Romberg test. This level of exposure for 1 to 7 hours induced no changes in hematologic or biochemical profiles (40).

## Chronic Toxicity

### *Epidemiologic Observations*

In one study, 493 workers employed at a facility that primarily manufactured and polymerized styrene were first ranked ordinally as high or low exposure and then subdivided into three groups by duration of employment <7 years, 7.1 to 20 years, and >20 years) (41). The exposure categories were validated by measurements of mandelic acid in urine and styrene in blood. Of workers in the low-exposure category, 1 of 42 (2.4%) had a blood styrene level of at least 5 ppb, while 16 of 70 (23%) of workers in the high-exposure group exceeded this level. Limited air-monitoring data were available, but they indicated that the mean TWA styrene concentrations in the purification and polymerization areas, both considered high-exposure areas, were on the order of 20 ppm. It was apparently recognized that the styrene air concentrations fluctuated widely. Mean TWA concentrations for high-exposure categories were around 5 ppm, and for low-exposure categories generally less than 1 ppm. The following outcomes were analyzed: mucous membrane irritation; ophthalmic irritation and optic neuritis; anemia, leukopenia, thrombocytopenia, and increased lymphocyte percentage; alkaline phosphatase, alanine aminotransferase [serum glutamic-pyruvic transaminase (SGPT)], serum glutamic-oxaloacetic transaminase (SGOT), and γ-glutamyl transpeptidase (GGT); pulmonary radiographs (with International Labor Office ratings and vital capacity estimates) and selected parameters from pulmonary function tests; neurologic symptoms of acute prenarcosis or sensory changes plus nerve conduction studies; carcinoembryonic antigen (CEA) level and sputum cytologic examination; mutagenicity of blood and urine *in vitro*; and karyotyping. The prevalences of these outcomes were applied to a dose-response model to look for associations with intensity of exposure, duration of employment, or both. Positive associations included (a) prenarcotic symptoms (light-headedness, dizziness, headache); (b) mucous membrane and/or eye irritation; (c) lower respiratory tract symptoms (averaging at least once a month); and (d) increased prevalence of abnormal

GGT (1.7% versus 7.2%). Duration of employment was associated with relative lymphocytosis (at least 45%), elevated GGT, and decreased peroneal nerve conduction velocity. Lymphocytosis was considered inconclusive because of the presence of benzene in the exposure inventory. The elevated GGT value was not unexpected, since one of the metabolic pathways of styrene requires this inducible enzyme. The decreased peroneal nerve conduction velocities were partially attributed to an age effect. No chronic or clinically disabling effect was noted.

The hematologic and cytogenetic variables of workers exposed to approximately 13 ppm styrene in a glass-reinforced polyester plastics product manufacturer (42) did not differ from those of referents except for a 30% excess in circulating monocytes ($p = 0.002$) (42).

The health history responses, clinical and psychological examination findings, and results of neurophysiologic tests of 96 styrene-exposed laminators were compared to those of 30 controls (43). Individual exposures were estimated by the postshift urinary mandelic acid concentration on 1 day per week for 5 weeks, then averaging the five results. The means varied from 7 to 4,715 mg/L (group median 808 mg/L). Positive findings included a higher prevalence of electroencephalographic abnormalities, defined as excessive diffuse theta activity, and local slow activity or bilateral spike-and-wave discharges among workers with urine mandelic acid concentrations greater than 0.7 g/L (30%) compared to workers with urine levels below 0.7 g/L (10%). This concentration of urine mandelic acid corresponds to 30 ppm styrene in air. A subsequent study reported changes in visuomotor accuracy when urine mandelic acid concentrations exceeded 0.8 g/L, with more pronounced visuomotor decrement plus impaired psychomotor performance when urine mandelic acid exceeded 1.2 g/L (approximately 55 ppm styrene in air) (44). The significance of the effects, in the context of toxicity or impairment, was not discussed.

The neurophysiologic effects of long-term styrene exposure were studied in workers exposed to mean concentrations of 5, 47, and 125 ppm (45). There was no statistically significant difference between groups for all motor conduction velocities, all distal motor latencies, all sensory conduction velocities, or the sensory conduction velocities, amplitudes, and durations arising from stimulation of the third finger. Statistically significant differences were noted for the sensory amplitudes arising from stimulation of the first digit only among those with exposure to approximately 47 ppm and for the sensory durations arising from stimulation of the third finger for those exposed to approximately 5 or 125 ppm. While suggesting a possible effect on peripheral sensory nerves, the lack of a dose-response relationship, the nature of the identified findings, and the inconsistency of findings across the varied nerve segments preclude definitive inference.

The motor and sensory conduction velocities of the median, ulnar, and sural nerves were studied among reinforced polyester resin workers across three exposure categories: 50 ppm or less, 51 to 100 ppm, and more than 100 ppm (46). Nineteen workers had delayed conduction of only one nerve, three had delayed conduction of two nerves, and two had delayed conduction of all three nerves. All five workers with two or more affected nerves were exposed to at least 50 ppm styrene. Also, the mean sensory conduction velocities of workers exposed to styrene at levels above 100 ppm were 8% slower than for those exposed to 50 ppm or less; however, it should be noted that the standard deviations of their test measurements were approximately 10% of the means.

A cross-sectional study of reinforced polyester resin product manufacturing workers exposed to median air concentrations of 18 ppm styrene with short-term exposures up to 600 ppm indicated that exposure up to 100 ppm caused no adverse acute or chronic effects on the CNS in terms of peripheral neuropathy, encephalopathy, or performance on neurobehavioral tests (47). Styrene has been shown to induce hearing loss in rats and is considered a probable cause of ototoxicity in humans (48); however, confounding factors do not seem to have been controlled in the human studies. A recent study on the potential ototoxicity of reinforced plastics work, which took into account numerous confounding variables, found no association between styrene and hearing loss (49).

## Carcinogenicity

### *Experimental Data*

Styrene was administered to Sprague-Dawley rats via inhalation, ingestion, intraperitoneal instillation, and subcutaneous injection (50). There were 23.3 tumors per 100 controls and 38.3 tumors per 100 exposed animals without evidence of a dose-response relationship. Female rats developed a significant treatment-related increased incidence of benign and malignant mammary tumors in all groups exposed to styrene vapor, but not among those exposed by other routes.

The administration of SO (50) (0, 50, and 250 mg/kg daily via gavage 4 to 5 days per week for 52 weeks) resulted in a dose-related increase in total and malignant tumors, the most common ones being forestomach lesions. There was no effect on mammary tumors, and other spontaneous tumors in this strain of rats. The relevance of experimentally induced forestomach tumors for humans hazards assessment of styrene monomer itself has been considered limited because (a) the route of exposure is not relevant to the human situation, where the primary route of exposure is inhalation and to a lesser extent dermal; and (b) styrene given by the oral route would not be converted to SO in the stomach because this requires a metabolic reaction that occurs primarily in the liver (51).

Rodents were administered liquid styrene via gavage during gestation (52). Their offspring were treated weekly by gavage from weaning throughout the life span at 300, 500, and 1,350 mg/kg. After 16 weeks, overt toxicity occurred in one but not in another strain of mice. The affected ones experienced premature death, multiple foci of centrilobular necrosis in the liver, splenic hypoplasia, and severe lung congestion. There was no excess of tumors among treated pregnant females, but an increased incidence of adenomas and adenocarcinomas of the lung occurred in styrene-treated weanlings.

Styrene vapor was administered to male and female rats via inhalation (53). The animals were exposed to 0, 600, or 1,200 ppm 6 hours per day, 5 days per week, males for 18.3 months and females for 20.7 months. At 600 ppm there was an increased incidence of mammary gland adenocarcinomas among female rats plus an increased incidence of leukemias and lymphocarcinomas among both males and females. These results were considered "suggestive" of an exposure-related carcinogenic effect.

Overall, the animal evidence of styrene's carcinogenicity is inconclusive. Moreover, some exposures would have saturated the normal metabolic pathways for styrene. Thus, the International Agency for Research on Cancer (IARC) has concluded that there is "limited" evidence in experimental animals that styrene is carcinogenic, whereas the evidence that styrene oxide is carcinogenic is deemed "sufficient" (54).

### *Epidemiologic Observations*

As summarized below, epidemiologic studies have suggested an increased risk of leukemia and lymphoma among workers in the SBR and plastics industries; however, concomitant exposure to other known or suspected carcinogens (e.g., benzene, 1,3-butadiene) have limited the power of these studies. For workers exposed predominantly to styrene, the data are either negative or equivocal regarding its carcinogenicity.

Among 6,678 males working at a tire-manufacturing plant in Ohio, employment for at least 5 years was associated with a relative risk of 6.2 [confidence interval (CI): 4.1–12.5] for cancer of the lymphatic and hematopoietic system (55), an observation that was not confirmed either in Germany (56) or in the United States (57). On the other hand, a study of the mortality experience of 2,904 workers involved in the development or manufacture of styrene-based products (58) identified a statistically significant excess of lymphatic leukemia cases, but none of the men with lymphatic leukemia had worked in areas where exposure to styrene was highest, and none of the leukemia cases came from SBR production plants. A follow-up study conducted a decade later identified a total of 162 cancer deaths (199 expected), of which 28 were from cancer of the lymphatic and hematopoietic system (19.5 expected). The excess of lymphatic and hematopoietic cancer had occurred mainly in workers from the polymerization, coloring, and resin extension work areas (observed 16; expected 8), but risk did not correlate with estimated intensity or duration of exposure to styrene (59).

No excess in lymphoma or leukemia (60) or in total or specific types of cancer (61) was observed, respectively, among 3,494 hand laminators or 13,920 workers in SBR manufacturing plants. On follow-up, the standardized mortality ratios (SMRs) from all causes, all cancer, and lymphatic and hematopoietic cancer were, respectively, 81, 85, and 97. Risk of lymphatic and hematopoietic cancer did not increase with duration of employment in the rubber industry or time since first employment.

A subsequent nested case-control study (62) compared the occupational exposures of 59 cases with lymphatic or hematopoietic cancer with 193 matched controls. Higher cumulative exposure was associated with an increased risk of leukemia, but this association disappeared after adjustment for concomitant exposure to butadiene (OR = 1.06; CI: 0.23–4.95). This contrasted with butadiene, which showed a significant association that persisted after styrene exposure was taken into account (OR = 7.39; CI: 1.32–41.3).

In contrast to the former studies, in which styrene exposure coexisted with other potential carcinogens, epidemiologic studies in the reinforced plastics industry predominantly involve styrene with the greatest known coexposure being acetone, which is considered noncarcinogenic in humans. Cancer mortality studies of several large cohorts of reinforced-plastics workers have been combined to assess the possible association between styrene exposure and malignant disease; 15,826 workers from 30 U.S. factories experienced significant increases in cancer mortality (all sites and several specific sites) (63), but showed no significant excess for lymphatic and hematopoietic cancers. In addition, these studies failed to show trends in cancer mortality of any type with cumulative exposure or duration of exposure. Previous smaller studies also did not find significant risks for lymphatic or hematopoietic cancers among reinforced-plastics workers (60,64).

The largest database in this industry belongs to the international historical cohort study of cancer mortality in six European countries (65); these studies involved 660 European factories employing 40,688 workers. There was no excess mortality from all neoplasms or from lymphohematopoietic cancers; however, mortality from the latter neoplasms, while increasing with time since first exposure to styrene, was not consistently associated with duration of exposure or with cumulative exposure. A borderline significant ($p = .07$) trend was reported for mortality from pancreatic cancer and cumulative styrene exposure. Results of a study among male Danish workers, some of whom were included in the larger European study, indicated a nonsignificant overall increased risk for lymphatic and hematopoietic cancer, which was concentrated in workers not included in the international cohort and among short-term workers with at least 10 years since first employment and who were employed before 1970 (66). In summary, IARC considers "inadequate" the evidence for styrene's carcinogenic potential for humans (54).

## Reproductive Toxicity

### *Animal Data*

No adverse effects on reproduction were noted in a three-generation study of rats drinking water with styrene concentrations of 0, 125, and 250 ppm (67); the latter concentration approaches the aqueous solubility limit of styrene (about 300 ppm). There was no teratogenicity in rats or rabbits exposed to 300 or 600 ppm styrene vapor 7 hours per day on days 6 through 15 of gestation for rats and days 6 through 18 for rabbits (68). Female rats were exposed to 100 ppm styrene oxide via inhalation for 3 weeks (7 hours per day, 5 days per week). After mating, they were exposed to 100 ppm daily through the 18th day of gestation (69). This experiment produced preimplantation losses of conceptuses, embryolethality, and maternal toxicity, but had no effect on malformations or ossification.

These well-conducted studies indicate that styrene oxide caused reproductive and developmental toxicities at the levels studied, but it was not established whether these were direct effects or the result of maternal toxicity.

### *Epidemiologic Observations*

A Finnish study on the occurrence of congenital malformations in children born both before and after styrene exposure provided no evidence that styrene exposure was associated with birth defects, but the small number of observations preclude definitive conclusions (70).

Another short but controversial Finnish report raised concerns about the increased frequency of spontaneous abortions among female chemical workers in general and those exposed to styrene in particular (71). For all chemical workers the abortion rate was higher than for all Finnish women at all maternal ages; but the difference was greater in younger women and greatest in the 15- to 19-year age group. The very small numbers involved (eight in the 15- to 19-years-olds) and the fact the study did not examine the many socioeconomic factors that influence abortion may have limited the value of the observation (72). In this respect, a subsequent report from the same group of investigators concluded that the odds ratio for women involved in the processing of cold and heated styrene were, respectively, 0.4 (CI: 0.1–1.2) and 0.6 (CI: 0.2–2.3). By contrast, a very significant odds ratio of 3 was observed in women employed in processing urethane. The authors concluded that neither the processing of styrene plastics nor exposure to their thermal degradation products was associated with abortion (73). However, here, too, the small size of the study population reduced to 38% the likelihood of detecting a twofold risk for exposure to thermal degradation products.

An epidemiologic study designed to have an 85% to 90% power to detect a doubling in the incidence of menstrual dysfunction showed that 174 women occupationally exposed to styrene did not differ from 449 unexposed women in the incidence of severe dysmenorrhea, intermenstrual bleeding, secondary amenorrhea, menstrual blood clots, and hypermenorrhea (74). Scandinavian data on the outcome of pregnancy in female workers in the plastic industry concluded that the odds ratio for an adverse outcome following styrene exposure was 0.8 (CI: 0.4–1.6). This result contrasts with the hazards associated with exposure to polyvinyl chloride processing (odds ratio 2.2; CI: 1.1–4.5) (75). Two cases of central nervous system defects occurred among children whose mothers had been initially exposed at work to styrene, as well as to other chemicals (76). This observation is still quoted as evidence of the developmental toxicity of styrene in humans (11), even though it is not supported by several larger and more powerful epidemiologic studies carried out by the same and other investigators (70–75,77–81).

## Genotoxicity

### *DNA and Protein Adducts*

Modification of macromolecules by styrene is thought to be mediated through its primary metabolite SO. SO reacts with a number of nucleophilic centers in DNA. It is thought this step is preceded by a ring opening of the epoxide that can generate a carbonium ion at either the 1- or 2-position of the 2-carbon sidechain of SO. Each of these substitutions may occur in two diasteriomeric forms; thus, there are four possible products of SO with each nucleophilic site (82). *In vitro* reactions of SO with either guanosine or DNA led predominantly to an N7 guanine product; other significant sites of reaction included the $N^{2-}$, $O^{6-}$ position of guanine, N1, $N^6$-position of adenine, $N^4$-, N3-, and $O^2$-positions of cytosine, and the N3-position of thymine (83). At high *in vitro* concentrations SO may produce bis-styrene-oxide DNA adducts in which two molecules of styrene react with a single nucleotide (84).

Styrene oxide also alkylates a variety of nucleophilic sites within amino acids and proteins. SO reaction products of hemoglobin and albumin have been investigated as possible biomarkers of internal dose of SO. Linear dose-responses were observed between *in vitro* SO concentration and SO-cysteine adducts in human and rat globin by the Raney nickel gas chromatography–mass spectrometry (GC-MS) method (85). The major alkylation sites for hemoglobin adduction are the β-143 and α-20 histidines (82); other sites of alkylation include the N-terminal valine. Each of these methods has been applied in animal models. In humans, early applications of DNA and protein adduct measures must be considered preliminary as they included only small numbers of subjects, with control groups not adequately matched for smoking (86–88) and other potential confounding variables. Recent studies, which have assessed multiple biomarkers and longitudinally assessed styrene and SO exposure, point to the potential usefulness of adduct measurements to document occupational styrene genotoxicity. In a study of 48 boat builders, multiple samples of air and biologic specimens were obtained from all subjects over the course of 1 year (16); SO-albumin adducts correlated positively with exposure to SO but not to styrene. SO-DNA adducts also correlated with SO-albumin adducts and sister-chromatid exchange (SCE) frequencies in peripheral blood lymphocytes, probably indicating a significant role for coexposure to SO in styrene-related genotoxicity.

### *Cytogenetic and Mutagenic Effects*

Six laboratories reported that styrene failed to manifest mutagenic activity in bacteria even with the use of metabolic activation systems, whereas two laboratories observed weak mutagenic activity in the presence of metabolic activation systems (89). Styrene did not clearly exhibit mutagenicity in tests using mammalian cells *in vitro*, even with metabolic activating systems. In human whole blood lymphocyte cultures without exogenous metabolizing systems, styrene induced an increase in SCEs and chromosome aberrations (90). The activation of styrene to SO in blood *in vitro* was thought to be mediated by oxyhemoglobin, although the relevance of this mechanism for styrene activation *in vivo* is unknown. Early *in vivo* studies of chromosome aberrations in mice, rats, or hamsters have with one exception been negative (89). In more recent animal bioassays, *in vivo* exposure to 124, 249, and 492 ppm (6 hours/day for 14 consecutive days) was reported to be a weak inducer of SCEs in both mice and rats, but produced no detectable increases in micronuclei or DNA strand breaks (91). Other studies of rats exposed to 150 to 1,000 ppm styrene (6 hours/day, 5 days/week, for 4 weeks) reported no increase in either chromosomal aberrations or SCEs in peripheral blood lymphocytes (92). *In vivo* cytogenetic studies of styrene in humans have yielded conflicting results (42,93–98); these data have been the subject of several reviews (54,101–103). The available evidence suggests that increased numbers of chromosomal aberrations are associated with relatively high styrene exposures (50–100 ppm) in reinforced plastics laminators; modest elevations in SCEs are detectable at lower concentrations (20 ppm) in workers studied longitudinally using a repeated measures design (16,17).

### Summary

Styrene is principally an irritant, and under extreme conditions, a CNS depressant. The ACGIH recommends several biologic exposure indices (13) and a TLV-TWA of 50 ppm to prevent "styrene sickness" (headache, drowsiness, fatigue, and dizziness). In 1989, the Occupational Safety and Health Administration (OSHA) revised its 8-hour personal exposure limit (PEL) to 50 ppm and its 15-minute short-term exposure limit (STEL) to 100 ppm (104).

Available studies suggest that styrene may be mutagenic after metabolic activation and that it induces enzymes involved in its metabolism. Several studies also suggest that workers exposed to styrene have increased chromosome alterations. To date, no biologic effects, such as organ-specific toxicity, carcinogenicity, or teratogenicity, that would likely be attributable to the mutagenic or clastogenic effects of styrene have been confirmed.

There are conflicting reports in the literature regarding neurologic and psychological effects of styrene at or below exposures to 50 ppm.

## 1,3-BUTADIENE

1,3-Butadiene (BD) is a colorless, noncorrosive, flammable gas. It has a mild aromatic odor and an odor threshold between 0.16 and 1.3 ppm. Its physicochemical properties are listed in Table 3. BD ranks in the top 20 synthetic organic chemicals produced in the United States, with about 3 billion pounds are produced annu-

**TABLE 3.** *Physical properties of butadiene*

| | |
|---|---|
| Structure | $CH_2$:CHCH:$CH_2$ |
| Specific gravity, liquid | 0.65 |
| Boiling point | -4.4°C |
| Vapor density | 1.9 |
| Vapor pressure at 25°C | 910 mm Hg |
| Flash point | <7°C |
| Ignition temperature | 429°C |
| Explosive limits | 2–11.5% |
| Solubility in $H_2O$ | 0.05% |
| Exposure standards | |
| OSHA | |
| PEL-TWA (8-hour) | 1,000 ppm |
| PEL-Ceiling (5 min/3 hr) | 600 ppm |
| NIOSH | |
| REL-Lowest feasible level | |
| ACGIH | |
| TLV-TWA (8-hour) | 10 ppm |
| Suspect human carcinogen | 2A(IARC) |

ally. In addition, approximately a quarter-million tons of BD monomer are imported per year (105). In the United States all BD is produced as a by-product of ethylene production, where it is used primarily in the production of styrene-butadiene rubber (SBR), and polybutadiene rubber (BR), and other polymers acrylonitrile-butadiene-styrene [(ABS) resins, SB latex, and nitrile rubber] (105). Crude BD is also available for use as feedstock.

### Exposure and Environmental Monitoring

A National Occupational Exposure Survey estimated that 52,000 workers were potentially exposed to BD in the United States in 1981 to 1983 (106); a more recent estimate indicates a much smaller number of workers potentially exposed to the compound (i.e., 9,500) (107). The current OSHA standard for BD is 1,000 ppm determined as an 8-hour TWA; in 1990, OSHA proposed a new standard that would reduce exposure to an 8-hour TWA of 2 ppm. NIOSH and the Centers for Disease Control and Prevention carried out an extent-of-exposure study of BD monomer (involving 11 plants) and polymer and end-user (involving 17 plants) industries that characterized the airborne exposures of BD for various job categories by personal sampling (107). This study utilized an improved NIOSH sampling and analytical method that is highly sensitive (e.g., detection limit of 0.005 ppm in a 25-L sample) and that minimizes interference from other $C_4$ compounds (108). Results of the study indicated that full-shift exposures in all job categories (monomer and polymer industries) were typically below 10 ppm. Of the 526 personal full-shift air samples, 2.7% contained more than 10 ppm, 10.5% more than 2 ppm but less than 10 ppm, and 86.5% less than 2 ppm. For all job categories the arithmetic mean BD concentration in air was 2.12 ppm. This study, while emphasizing that established engineering controls and work practices can be effective in minimizing BD exposure, also noted that specific activities in BD plants are associated with transient exposures exceeding 10 ppm BD (e.g., cylinder sampling, cylinder voiding, and maintenance). Consequently, further modifications of engineering controls and work practices are needed to reduce BD exposure.

Other potential sources of occupational and environmental exposure exist for BD. A limited BD exposure hazard can occur in petroleum refining and gasoline production (0.1–6.4 ppm) (109). BD is also present in motor vehicle exhaust and in urban air <0.002 ppm), and tobacco smoke (e.g., 0.3 mg/cigarette) (110).

### Pharmacokinetics and Metabolism

1,3-Butadiene metabolism involves cytochrome P-450–mediated oxidation (CYP2E1, CYP2A6) to 1,2-epoxy-3-butene (MEB) (111); the latter may be detoxified by conjugation with glutathione via glutathione S-transferase or through hydrolysis via epoxide hydrolase. MEB may also be further oxidized to diepoxybutane (DEB). MEB conversion to DEB is also mediated by CYP2E1, with minor contributions from CYP2A6 and CYP2C9 (112,113). 3,4-epoxybutane-1,2-diol can be formed by hydrolysis of MEB or through oxidation of 1,2-dihydroxy-3-butene (Fig. 2). Urinary metabolites of MEB have been detected in all mammalian species examined (rats, mice, hamsters, monkeys, and humans), indicating its importance as a metabolic intermediate of BD; however, DEB metabolites have not been detected in any species.

Several studies have investigated the pharmacokinetics of BD and related compounds in rats and mice (114,115). BD and MEB (115) in both rodent species exhibited linear pharmacokinetics at exposure concentrations below 1,000 ppm and saturation at concentrations around 2,000 ppm. Mice metabolized BD about twice as fast as rats. In rats, there was no evidence of saturation of MEB metabolism at exposure concentrations up to 5,000 ppm. In mice, saturation became apparent around 5,000 ppm. The estimated maximal metabolic rate for mice was at least seven times lower than for rats. When mice or rats were exposed to high concentrations of BD, both species exhale MEB. In mice, there was a significant depletion of nonprotein sulfhydryls in the liver that corresponded to signs of acute toxicity. Similar findings were not noted in rats.

A comparison of the uptake, metabolism, and distribution of BD in rats, mice, and monkeys showed that mice achieve higher blood concentrations of reactive metabolites than rats and that the blood concentrations of these compounds in monkeys are lower than in either rodent species (116). In one study, DEB was detected in blood and lungs of mice but not in rats (117). In contrast, researchers using a sensitive GC-MS assay detected DEB in various tissues of both rats and mice exposed to 62.5 ppm BD for 4 hours; however, levels were 40- to 160-fold lower in rats compared to mice (118). Physiologically based pharmacokinetic models have been developed for BD that accurately predict BD uptake but overestimate the blood concentrations of MEB (119–121). None of the models includes the disposition of DEB, which given its greater genotoxic potency could be an important mechanistic link to species differences in BD carcinogenesis.

The toxicokinetic interactions between BD and styrene observed in rats are reasonably well described by a model based on the assumption that BD has no effect on the metabolism of styrene, but styrene inhibits the metabolism of BD competitively. While the consulted literature does not seem to include pharmacokinetic studies of BD in humans, scaling the toxic interactions observed in rats to the human situation indicates that significant inhibition of BD metabolism would occur in people exposed to both compounds, even at low concentration (122). This would fit with the observation

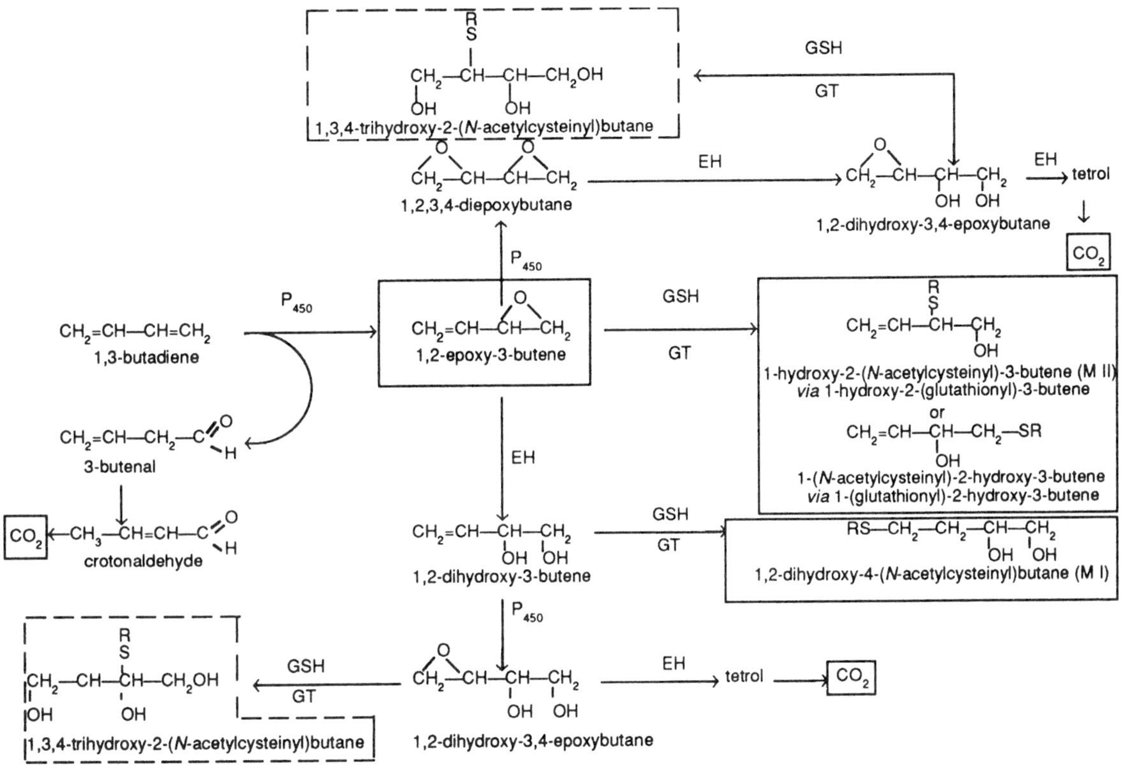


**FIG. 2.** Metabolism of 1,3-butadiene. Compounds enclosed in *boxes* have been identified *in vivo* as metabolites of 1,3-butadiene. Tentatively identified compounds are enclosed in *broken lines.* EH, epoxide hydrolase; GSH, glutathione; GT, glutathione transferase. (From ref. 174.)

that exposure to BD alone is associated with a 7.6-fold excess risk for leukemia, while this risk does not manifest in association to coexposure to mixtures of BD and styrene (123).

## Acute Toxicity

### *Experimental Data*

In the context of acute overexposure, butadiene causes CNS depression. The $LC_{50}$ for mice and rats were 122,000 and 129,000 ppm, respectively (124). Rats were exposed to BD in daily inhaled doses of 1,000, 2,000, 4,000, and 8,000 ppm for 3 months (125). Except for moderately increased salivation among those exposed to 4,000 and 8,000 ppm, no other effects were noted in the exposed animals.

### *Epidemiologic Observations*

In humans, BD is associated with irritation of the eyes, nose, and throat at concentrations of 2,000, 4,000, and 8,000 ppm for 6 to 8 hours (126). Higher levels may cause coughing, drowsiness, and fatigue. Exposure to liquid BD may cause dermatitis, but more likely frostbite because of its rapid evaporation from the skin.

## Chronic Toxicity

### *Experimental Data*

In 1985, Huff and colleagues (127) exposed mice to concentrations of 625 and 1250 ppm BD for 61 weeks (equivalent to and below the OSHA standard of 1,000 ppm) and noted reduced survival in all exposure groups in both sexes, principally because of malignant neoplasms in multiple organs. Nonneoplastic changes included ovarian and testicular atrophy. Another long-term inhalation study of BD in mice used concentrations ranging from 6.25 to 625 ppm for 6 hours per day, 5 days per week, for up to 65 weeks (128). At week 40, male mice manifested statistically significant decreases in red blood cell counts, hemoglobin, and packed red cell volume at exposure concentrations of 62.5, 200, and 625 ppm. Similar decreases were noted in female mice only in the group exposed to 625 ppm. Minimal to mild testicular atrophy was present in six of ten males exposed to 625 ppm, a finding also noted in the original study (127). Ovarian atrophy was noted at levels of 20 ppm and higher. Neoplasms were again noted in multiple organs (heart, forestomach, lung, harderian gland, mammary gland, ovary, and liver), but lymphocytic lymphoma was the principal cause of death, especially among mice exposed to 625 ppm BD. The premature mortality from this cancer at this exposure level apparently precluded expression of tumor induction at the other target organ sites.

In other studies designed to characterize exposure-response relationships, mice were exposed to BD concentrations ranging from 6.25 to 625 ppm for up variable periods (13 to 52 weeks). The study spanned 2 years. Survival was reduced in all the tested groups and the overrepresentation of lymphomas, cardiac hemangiomas, pulmonary carcinomas, and adenomas was again observed (129).

In rats exposed to 0, 1,000, or 8,000 ppm 6 hours per day, 5 days per week, for approximately 108 weeks (130,131), there were no treatment-related effects on hematopoiesis, blood chemistry, urine, gonads, or neuromuscular function. In rats, BD was a weak carcinogen that manifested a spectrum of tumors different from those seen in mice.

Species differences in the carcinogenicity of BD have been postulated to be due to the activation of an ecotropic virus in mice causing the observed excess of lymphomas (132,133); another more plausible explanation is differences in BD metabolism among species (115,116). This difference in carcinogenic potency also parallels BD's differential genotoxicity in rats and mice (see Genotoxicity, below).

### *Epidemiologic Observations*

The rubber industry is considered carcinogenic to humans (134). Its multiple potential chemical hazards include BD, but few studies have addressed the specific question of BD carcinogenicity. McMichael and co-workers (135,136) studied a cohort of rubber workers, only some of whom had potential BD exposure in the synthetics plants. They noted a 6.2-fold increase in risk for lymphatic and hematopoietic cancer (99.9% CI: 4.1–12.5) and a 3.9-fold increase for lymphatic leukemia (99.9% CI: 2.6–8.0) for workers with more than 5 years' employment in manufacturing units producing mainly SBD rubber during 1940 to 1960. A significant twofold increase was observed for gastric cancer.

Three other epidemiologic studies focused on employees in the SBR industry or in BD production (137–139). Each of these studies was updated for a 1988 symposium entitled "Symposium on the Toxicology, Carcinogenesis and Human Health Aspects of 1,3-Butadiene." The proceedings were published in 1990 (140).

Follow-up of mortality of an original study of a cohort of 2,582 male workers employed at least 6 months at a BD-manufacturing facility (137) from 1943 through 1979 was extended through 1990 (141). Down et al. (137) noted a statistically significant deficit for all causes of death and lower mortality rates than expected for most of the leading causes of death. There was, however, a statistically significant excess of mortality for lymphosarcoma among men who were employed for less than 10 years, first hired during the Second World War, and employed in jobs with potential routine exposure. The fact that SMRs decreased with increasing length of employment and were not elevated in the groups employed the longest has been used to argue against a causal relationship (141).

Meinhardt and co-workers (138) performed the initial retrospective cohort mortality study of two SBR production facilities in Port Neches, Texas with 1,662 workers employed in plant A between 1943 and 1976, and 1,094 workers employed in plant B between 1950 and 1976—all with at least 6 months employment. No historical exposure data were available, but air sampling at the time of the study (1982) revealed mean BD concentrations of 1.24 and 13.50 ppm in plants A and B, respectively. Incidentally, benzene was detected in plant A (0.10 ppm).

There were no excesses in cause-specific mortality in the overall populations in plant A or B, or in a cohort limited to those employed in plant A between 1943 and not after 1945, after which the process changed from batch to continuous feed. Lymphatic and hematopoietic cancers were responsible for nine observed deaths (versus 5.79 expected) in plant A (SMR 155) (CI: 71–295). All these deaths had occurred among men who had first been employed from 1943 through 1945. The majority of this excess was attributed to a twofold excess of leukemia (observed = 5, expected = 2.47; SMR 203, not statistically significant). The restricted group employed in plant A accounted for all nine lymphohematopoietic cancer deaths. When compared to the 4.25 expected, the SMR was 212. The majority of this excess was attributed to five leukemia deaths, compared with 1.80 expected (SMR 278).

Lemen and colleagues (142) extended the follow-up period through 1982 for plant A and 1981 for plant B. In plant A, there were two additional deaths from lymphosarcoma or reticulosarcoma, for a total of five, and one death attributed to "other neoplasms of the lymphatic and hematopoietic tissues." All three additional deaths occurred in the cohort limited to those employed between 1943 and not after 1945. In plant B, there was one additional death in the leukemia and aleukemia category, increasing the total of two deaths.

A retrospective study of 13,920 workers employed in eight U.S. and Canadian SBR facilities (139) indicated that the overall mortality rate was low compared to that of the general population, and no overrepresentation of site-specific cancers occurred. A subsequent updating of the study (143) concluded that the SMRs for all causes and all cancers were favorable when compared to those of the control population. Similarly, there was no excess of lymphopoietic cancers, including lymphosarcomas and leukemias. When employees were classified according to the job held longest, production workers (presumed to be those with highest exposure to BD) had an SMR for all deaths of 88 and a significant excess of other lymphatic cancers (SMR 656; CI: 135–1,906). When analyzed according to work area, black male production workers had a statistically significant excess of lymphopoietic cancer (SMR 532), but this finding was not observed among white male production workers or all production workers (SMRs 110 and 146, respectively, not statistically significant). When subcategories were examined, statistically significant excesses were noted for leukemia in black male production workers (SMR 656, based on three observed cases) and other lymphatic cancers in all production workers (SMR 260, based on four non-Hodgkin's lymphomas and five multiple myelomas). There was no excess of all-cause, all-cancer, or lymphopoietic cancer among maintenance workers, utility workers, or workers in the "other" category. Maintenance workers experienced fewer hematopoietic cancers, but more digestive causes that production workers. No significant increase for any other type of cancer was observed among the two other job classifications ("utility" and "other"). A nested case-control study of lymphohematopoietic cancers was carried out in the previous BD polymerization cohort (62). The study compared 59 workers with lymphopoietic cancers to 193 controls, who were matched to cases by plant, age, year of hire, duration of employment and survival to time of death of the case. Results indicated a statistically significant association of leukemia with BD exposure (odds ratio 9.4; CI: 2.1–22.9). Since the exposures to BD and to styrene were highly correlated, an attempt was made to assess their respective leukmogenic hazards (26 deaths). The RR for exposure to styrene adjusted for BD was 1.06 (CI: 0.23–4.96) where the risk for BD, adjusted for styrene, was 7.39 (CI: 1.32–41.33). The same type of analysis for the 18 deaths from "other lymphatic cancers" (including multiple myeloma and non-Hodgkin's lymphoma) yielded an RR of 0.81 (CI: 0.28–2.38 for styrene adjusted for BD and an RR of 1.68 for BD adjusted for styrene).

### Reproductive Toxicity

Morrissey and colleagues (144) reviewed and published studies and performed a series of studies of their own to evaluate the developmental and reproductive toxicity of inhaled BD. An earlier study found an increase in major skeletal defects in rat fetuses when dams were exposed to 1,000 or 8,000 ppm from days 6 through 15 of gestation. No such effects were noted at 200 ppm. This observation, however, was not confirmed in the rat study performed by Morrissey et al. Their only positive findings were a decrease in maternal weight gain between days 6 and 11 of gestation and a decrease in extragestational weight gain in dams exposed to 1,000 ppm. No toxic effects were noted at 40 or 200 ppm. In addition, there were no significant differences in the percentage of pregnant animals, number of litters with live fetuses, number of live fetuses per litter, percentage of resorptions or of malformation per litter, placental or fetal body weights, or sex ratio among exposure groups.

Small, concentration-related increases in the frequency of abnormal sperm morphology were seen 5 weeks after exposure to 1,000 or 5,000 ppm for 5 consecutive days (144).

### Genotoxicity

1,3-Butadiene and its metabolites MEB and DEB produce significant cytogenetic and mutagenic effects in a variety of *in vitro* and *in vivo* test systems. Only limited studies have been carried out in humans exposed to low levels of BD.

#### *DNA and Protein Adducts*

Inhalation and intraperitoneal injection of radiolabeled BD have been used to study total DNA binding by BD in rodents; nonradioactive BD exposures have been used to study *N*-hydroxybuteneylvaline adducts with hemoglobin (145). Levels of N-terminal valine hemoglobin adducts were increased in a dose-dependent manner in both rats and mice but were fivefold higher in mice compared with rats. In one study occupational exposure to BD at about 1 ppm was associated with the presence of hemoglobin adducts (1–3 pmol/g globin) (146).

Recent studies provide data on the structural identities of BD-related DNA modifications. BD, MEB, and DEB exposures have been shown to produce multiple covalent modifications of DNA (147,148). *In vitro* MEB forms N1- and $N^6$-adenosine and N1-inosine adducts; evidence exists that N1-adenosine adduct is the initial product of the reaction and that the N1 and $N^6$ adducts form via subsequent deamination and rearrangements, respectively (149). MEB also forms multiple adduct products with guanine; the N7-adducts formed approximately 10-fold more favorably than N1- and $N^2$- adducts (150). DEB produced a major adduct with guanine at the N7-position and three products (N3, N7, N9) with adenine (151). The N7 and N3 adducts of adenine and guanine are expected to undergo spontaneous depurination and repair and therefore their detection in urine may be useful as a biomarkers of exposure. In an *in vivo* dosimetry study in mice, skin DEB-DNA adducts exhibited a linear relationship ($r$ = 0.992) relationship between adduct level and dose (1.9–153 μmol/mouse) (152).

#### *Cytogenetic and Mutagenicity Data*

The genotoxicity of BD was reviewed and summarized in a recent working group report (145). BD is mutagenic following activation by liver microsomes in bacterial species (153). BD inhalation of 100 ppm 6 hours/day for 2 consecutive days induced micronuclei (MN) in B6C3F1 mice but not in Sprague-Dawley rats (154). SCEs were induced in bone marrow cells of B6C3F1 mice by 10-day BD inhalation at levels of 6.25,

62.5, and 625 ppm; MN in polychromatic erythrocytes were increased at 62.5 ppm, whereas bone marrow chromosomal aberrations were elevated only at 625 ppm (155,156). A subsequent study of 13-week exposures of B6C3F1 mice to 6.25 to 625 ppm also found that MNs were increased in polychromatic erythrocytes at 62.5 ppm (157). Peripheral blood and bone marrow MN increased linearly up to 200 ppm in mice exposed to BD at inhalation exposures of 1, 50, 200, 500, 1300 ppm for 6 hours/day for 5 days (158). A subsequent study confirmed the shape of the dose-response curve for MN over the same range of BD concentrations in B6C3F1 mice, but found no increases in male Wistar rats (159). The latter study is consistent with others showing that the cytogenetic response to BD is markedly different in mice and rats.

In studies by Arce and co-workers (160), BD did not induce unscheduled DNA synthesis in rat or mouse hepatocytes following exposure *in vivo*. BD also did not induce SCEs in studies *in vitro* using human whole blood lymphocyte cultures with metabolic activation (rat, mouse, and human liver homogenate). The authors noted that BD exhibited potent genotoxicity *in vivo* but weak genotoxicity *in vitro*.

The mutagenic potential and mutational spectra of BD and its metabolites has been studied in B6C3F1 mice; exposure to 625 ppm BD 6 hours/day, 5 days/week for 2 weeks resulted in a fivefold increase in the hprt mutation frequency of splenic T cells (161,162). Studies *in vitro* of human lymphoblastoid cells (TK6) showed that DEB was mutagenic at concentrations 100 times lower than BD, MEB, or MEB-diol (161,163); the predominant types of mutations induced by BD, MEB, and DEB were frameshift mutations within runs of guanine residues. The mutational spectra of BD is described as similar to that of ethylene oxide (164).

Of the four human studies of low-level BD exposure (generally <2 ppm), only one has reported a significant association of BD exposure with genotoxicity; an increased frequency of 6TG variant blood lymphocytes was observed in eight individuals in the high exposure subgroup. Urinary 1,2-dihydroxy-4-(*N*-acetylcysteinyl-S) butane was also correlated with individual 6TG-variant frequencies (reviewed in ref. 145). In another *in vivo* study, although no overall effects of BD exposures were noted for chromosomal aberrations or SCEs, a significant increase in chromosomal aberrations in blood lymphocytes was observed in workers carrying the common gene deletion polymorphism at the glutathione S-transferase theta (GSTT1) locus (165). The GSTT1 deletion polymorphism significantly affects the susceptibility of blood lymphocytes to DEB-induced chromosome damage *in vitro* and may identify a population subgroup with increased mutagen sensitivity to BD metabolites (166). Another study of low level BD exposure (<2 ppm) also failed to detect exposure-related increases in SCEs in GSTT1-positive or deleted workers (167). With reference to germ cell mutagenesis, the BD working group report concluded that the data clearly indicate that BD is a mouse germ cell mutagen that causes dominant lethal mutations in spermatozoa, structural chromosomal aberrations in spermatocytes, and sperm head abnormalities (145).

### *Comment*

Overall, the debate over the potential of BD to cause adverse human health effects has focused on the issue of lymphatic and hematopoietic cancers. The results from genotoxicity tests and long-term bioassays in mice support such an association. By contrast, the observed species differences between rodents, the inconsistency of excesses among the subcategories of lymphopoietic cancers, and the lack of coherent relationships with latency and duration of employment introduce an element of uncertainty in terms of human carcinogenesis. Nonetheless BD is currently evaluated as being probably carcinogenic to humans (group 2A) and a trans-species carcinogen for animals. For detailed discussion of these issues the reader is referred to recent reviews and commentaries (168–172), and OSHA's proposed rule for a BD standard (173).

## Summary

1,3-Butadiene is "practically nontoxic" in the context of acute inhalation overexposure. It exerts its toxic effects principally via CNS depression, with subsequent respiratory paralysis and death. Humans exposed to 2,000 to 8,000 ppm for 6 to 8 hours can expect eye, nose, and throat irritation. BD has definite carcinogenic potential in mice. Epidemiologic data are suggestive of BD carcinogenicity in humans; however, recent biomarker data also suggest that it is unlikely to produce genotoxicity in the workplace at low exposure levels in air (e.g., <2 ppm) (145). Nonetheless, overall, BD emerges as being probably carcinogenic to humans (group 2A of IARC) (54).

In 1990, OSHA proposed to reduce the PEL to 2 ppm for an 8-hour TWA and to 10 ppm for a 15-minute STEL. A 1 ppm concentration for an 8-hour TWA was proposed as an action level (173) to exempt employers from some administrative burdens such as exposure monitoring and medical surveillance. Aside from annual medical approval for use of a respirator that includes pulmonary function testing, the medical surveillance examination currently includes occupational and medical histories, a physical examination, and examination of peripheral blood cells (CBC). The purpose of these examinations is to detect persons who exhibit blood alterations characteristic of anemia or leukemia and to detect, by physical examination, non-Hodgkin's lymphoma.

## REFERENCES


1. Verschueren K. *Handbook of environmental data on organic chemicals,* 2nd ed. New York: Van Nostrand Reinhold, 1983;1055–1057.
2. Miller RR, Newhook R, Poole A. Styrene production use and human exposure. *Crit Rev Toxicol* 1994;24(S1):S1–S10.
3. Reisch MS. Top 50 chemicals production slowed markedly last year. *Chem Engineer News* 1990:68:11–15.
4. Budavari S, O'Neil MJ, Smith A, Heckelman PE. *The Merck index:* 11th ed. Rahway, NJ: Merck & Company, 1989;1397.
5. *IARC.* Some industrial chemicals. *Monographs on the evaluation of carcinogenic risk to humans,* vol 60. Lyon: IARC, 1994;233–346.
6. U.S. National Institute for Occupational Safety and Health. *National occupational exposure survey (1981–1983).* Cincinnati, OH: 1993.
7. Tossavainen A. Styrene use and occupational exposure in the plastics industry. *Scand J Work Environ Health* 1978:4(suppl 2):7–13.
8. Pfäffli P, Vainio H, Hesso A. Styrene and styrene oxide concentrations in the air during the lamination process in the reinforced plastics industry. *Scand J Work Environ Health* 1979;5:158–161.
9. Fjeldstad PE, Thurud S, Wannag A. Styrene oxide in the manufacture of reinforced polyester plastics. *Scand J Work Environ Health* 1979;5: 162–163.
10. Rebert CS, Hall TA. The neuroepidemiology of styrene: a critical review of representative literature. *Crit Rev Toxicol* 1994;24(S1): S57–S106.
11. *Documentation of threshold limit values and biological exposure indices,* 5th ed. Cincinnati, OH: ACGIH, 1986;539.
12. Guillemin MP, Bauer D. Human exposure to styrene, III. Elimination kinetics of urinary mandelic and phenylglyoxylic acids after single experimental exposure. *Int Arch Occup Environ Health* 1979;44: 249–263.
13. ACGIH. Styrene. In: *Documentation of the biological exposure indices.* Cincinnati, OH: American Conference of Government and Industrial Hygienists, 1991;159.
14. Guillemin MP, Berode M. Biological monitoring of styrene: a review. *Am Ind Hyg Assoc J* 1988;49:497–505.
15. Gallasi C, Logevinas M, Ferro G, Biocca M. Biological monitoring of styrene in the reinforced plastics industry in Emilia Romagna, Italy. *Int Arch Occup Environ Health* 1993;65:89–95.
16. Rappaport SM, Yeowell-O'Connell K, Bodell W, Yager JW, Symanski E. An investigation of multiple biomarkers among workers exposed to styrene and styrene-7,8-oxide. *Cancer Res* 1996;56:5410–5416.
17. Yager JW, Paradisin WM, Rappaport SM. Sister-chromatid exchanges in lymphocytes are increased in relation to longitudinally measured occupational exposure to low concentrations of styrene. *Mutat Res* 1993;319:155–165.
18. Fiserova-Bergerova V, Teisinger J. Pulmonary styrene vapor retention. *Ind Med Surg* 1965;34:620–622.
19. Bardodej Z, Bardodejova E. Biotransformation of ethyl benzene, styrene, and methyl styrene in man. *Am Ind Hyg Assoc J* 1970;31: 206–209.
20. Fernandez J, Caperos JR. Styrene exposure. I. Experimental study of the pulmonary absorption and excretion of human volunteers. *Int Arch Occup Environ Health* 1977;40:1–12.
21. Dutkiewicz T, Tyras H. Skin absorption of toluene, styrene and xylene by man. *Br J Ind Med* 1968;25:243.
22. Berode M, Droz PO, Guillemen MD. Human exposure to styrene. VI. Percutaneous absorption in human volunteers. *Int Arch Occup Environ Health* 1985;57:71–75.
23. Nakajima T, Elovaara E, Gonzales FJ, Gelboin FJ, Vainio H, Aoyama T. Characterization of the human cytochrome P450 isozymes responsible for styrene metabolism. In: Sorsa M, Peltonen K, Vainio H, Hemminki K, eds. *Butadiene and styrene:* assessment of health hazards. IARC Sci Publ No. 127. Lyon, France: IARC, 1993;101–108.
24. Bond JA. Review of the toxicology of styrene. *Crit Rev Toxicol* 1989; 19:227–249.
25. Summer SJ, Fennell TR. Review of the metabolic fate of the styrene. *Crit Rev Toxicol* 1994;24(S1):S11–S33.
26. Engstron J, Astwond I, Wigaeus E. Exposure to styrene in a polymerisation plant. *Scand J Work Environ Health* 1978;4:324–329.
27. Flodin U, Ekberg K, Anderson L. Neuropsychiatric effects of low exposure to styrene. *Br J Ind Med* 1989;46:805–808.
28. Ramsey JC, Andersen ME. A physiologically based description of the inhalation pharmacokinetics of styrene in rats and humans. *Toxicol Appl Pharmacol* 1984;73:159–175.
29. Filser JG, Schwegler U, Csanady GA, Greim H, Kreuzer PE, Kessler W. Species-specific kinetics of styrene in rat and mouse. *Arch Toxicol* 1993;67:517–530.
30. Csanady GA, Mendrala AL, Nolan RJ, Filser JG. A physiologic pharmacokinetic model for styrene and styrene-7,8-oxide in mouse, rat and man. *Arch Toxicol* 1994;68:143–157.
31. Sumner SF, Fennell TR. Review of the metabolic fate of styrene. *Crit Rev Toxicol* 1994;24:S11–S33.
32. Lof A, Johanson G. Dose-dependent kinetics of inhaled styrene in man. In: Sorsa M, Peltonen K, Vainio H, Hemminki K, eds. *Butadiene and styrene:* assessment of health hazards. IARC Sci Publ No 127. Lyon, France: IARC, 1993;89–99.
33. Wolf MA, Rowe VK, McCollister DD, Hollingsworth RC, Oven F. Toxicological studies of certain alkylated benzenes and benzene. *Arch Ind Health* 1956;14:387–398.
34. Spencer HC, Irish DD, Adams EM, Rowe VK. The response of laboratory animals to monomeric styrene. *J Ind Hyg Toxicol* 1942;24: 295–301.
35. Stewart RD, Dodd HC, Baretta ED, Schaffer AW. Human exposure to styrene vapor. *Arch Environ Health* 1968;16:656–662.
36. Moscato G, Biscaldi G, Cottica D, Pugliese F, Candura S, Candura F. Occupational asthma due to styrene: two case reports. *J Occup Med* 1987;29:957–960.
37. Edling C, Anundi H, Johanson G, Nilsson K. Increase in neuropsychiatric symptoms after occupational exposure to low levels of styrene. *Br J Ind Med* 1993;50:843–850.
38. Matikainen E, Forsman-Grönholm L, Pfäffli P, Juntunen J. Neurotoxicity in workers exposed to styrene. In: Sorsa M, Peltonen K, Vainio H, Hemminki K, eds. *Butadiene and styrene:* assessment of health hazards. IARC Sci Publ No. 127. Lyon, France: IARC, 1993;153–161.
39. Cherry N, Rodgers B, Venables H, Waldron HA, Wells GG. Acute behavioural effects of sytrene exposure: a further analysis. *Br J Ind Med* 1981;38:346–350.
40. Gobba F, Galassi C, Imbriani M, Ghittori S, Candela S, Cavalleri A. Acquired dyschromatopsia among styrene-exposed workers. *J Occup Med* 1991;33:761–765.
41. Lorimer WV, Lilis R, Fischbein A, et al. Health status of styrene-polystyrene polymerization workers. *Scand J Work Environ Health* 1978;4 (suppl 2):220–226.
42. Hagmar L, Högstedt B, Weilander H, Karlsson A, Rassner F. Cytogenetic and hematological effects in plastics workers exposed to styrene. *Scand J Work Environ Health* 1989;15:136–141.
43. Seppäläinen AM, Härkönen H. Neurophysiological findings among workers occupationally exposed to styrene. *Scand J Work Environ Health* 1976;3:140–146.
44. Härkönen H, Lindström K, Seppäläinen AM, Asp S, Hernberg S. Exposure-response relationship between styrene exposure and central nervous functions. *Scand J Work Environ Health* 1978;4:53–59.
45. Rosen I, Haeger-Aronsen B, Rehnostrom S, Welinder H. Neurophysiological observations after chronic styrene exposure. *Scand J Work Environ Health* 1978;4(suppl 2):184–194.
46. Cherry N, Gautrin D. Neurotoxic effects of styrene: further evidence. *Br J Ind Med* 1990;47:29–37.
47. Triebig G, Lehrl S, Weltle D, Schaller KH, Valentin H. Clinical and neurobehavioral study of the acute and chronic neurotoxicity of styrene. *Br J Ind Med* 1989;46:799–804.
48. Morata TC, Dunn DE, Sieber WK. Occupational exposure to noise and ototoxic organic solvents. *Arch Environ Health* 1994;49: 359–365.
49. Sass-Kortsak AM, Corey PN, Robertson JM. An investigation of the association between exposure to styrene and hearing loss. *Ann Epidemiol* 1995;5:15–24.
50. Conti B, Maltoni C, Perino G, Ciliberti A. Long-term carcinogenicity bioassays on styrene administered by inhalation, ingestion and injection and styrene oxide administered by ingestion in Sprague-Dawley rats, and para-methyl styrene administered by ingestion in Sprague-Dawley rats and Swiss mice. *Ann NY Acad Sci* 1988;534:203–234.
51. McConnell, Swenberg JA. Review of styrene and styrene oxide longterm animal studies. *Crit Rev Toxicol* 1994;24(S1):S49–S55.
52. Ponomarkov V, Tomatis L. Effects of long-term oral administration of styrene to mice and rats. *Scand J Work Environ Health* 1978;4(supp 2):127–135.
53. Huff JE. Styrene, styrene oxide, polystyrene, and beta-nitrostyrene/styrene carcinogenicity in rodents. *Prog Clin Biol Res* 1984;141: 227–238.

54. *IARC monographs on the evaluation of carcinogenic risks to humans,* vol 60. Lyon, France: IARC, 1994;297,339.
55. McMichael AJ, Spirtas R, Gamble JF, Tousey PM. Mortality among rubber workers: relationship to specific jobs. *J Occup Med* 1976;18: 178–185.
56. Frentzel-Beyme R, Theiss AM, Wieland R. Survey of mortality among employees engaged in the manufacture of styrene and polystyrene at the BASF Ludwigshaven works. *Scand J Work Environ Health* 1978;4(suppl 2):231–239.
57. Nicholson WJ, Selikoff J, Seidman H. Mortality experience of styrene-polystyrene polymerization workers. *Scand J Work Environ Health* 1978;4(suppl 2):247–252.
58. Ott MG, Kolesar RC, Scharnweber HC, Schneider EJ, Venable JR. A mortality survey of employees engaged in the development or manufacture of styrene-based products. *J Occup Med* 1980;22:445–460.
59. Bond GG, Bodner KM, Olsen GW, Cook RR. Mortality among workers engaged in the development or manufacture of styrene-based products—an update. *Scand J Work Environ Health* 1992;18:145–154.
60. Coggon D, Osmond C, Pannett B, Simmonds S, Winter PD, Acheson ED. Mortality of workers exposed to styrene in the manufacture of glass-reinforced plastics. *Scand J Work Environ Health* 1987;13: 94–99.
61. Matanoski GM, Santos-Burgoa C, Schwartz L. Mortality of workers in the styrene-butadiene polymer manufacturing industry, 1943–1982. *Environ Health Perspect* 1990;86:107–117.
62. Santos-Burgoa C, Matanoski GM, Zeger S, Schwartz L. Lymphohematopoietic cancer in styrene-butadiene polymerization workers. *Am J Epidemiol* 1992;136:843–854.
63. Wong O, Trent LS, Whorton MD. An updated cohort mortality study of workers exposed to styrene in the reinforced plastics and composites industry. *Occup Environ Med* 51:386–396, 1994.
64. Okun AH, Beaumont JJ, Meinhardt TJ, Crangall MS. Mortality patterns among styrene-exposed boat builders. *Am J Ind Med* 1985;8: 193–205.
65. Kogevinas M, Ferro G, Andersen A, et al. Cancer mortality in a historical cohort: study of workers exposed to styrene. *Scand J Work Environ Health* 1994;20:251–261.
66. Kolstad HA, Lynge E, Olsen J, Breum N. Incidence of lymph hematopoietic malignancies among styrene-exposed workers in the reinforced plastics industry. *Scand J Work Environ Health* 1994;20: 272–278.
67. Beliles RP, Butala JH, Stack CR, Makris S. Chronic toxicity and three-generation reproduction study of styrene monomer in the drinking water of rats. *Fundam Appl Toxicol* 1985;5:855–868.
68. Murray FJ, John JA, Balmer MF, Schwetz BA. Teratologic evaluation of styrene given rats and rabbits by inhalation or by gavage. *Toxicology* 1978;11:335–343.
69. Sikov MR, Cannon WC, Carr DB, Miller RA, Niemeier RW, Hardin BD. Reproductive toxicology of inhaled styrene oxide in rats and rabbits. *J Appl Toxicol* 1986;6:155–164.
70. Härkönen H, Tola S, Korkala ML, Hernberg S. Congenital malformations, mortality and styrene exposure. *Ann Acad Med (Singapore)* 1984;13:404–407.
71. Hemminki K, Lindbohm M-L, Hemminki T, Vainio H. Reproductive hazards and plastic industry. *Prog Clin Biol Res* 1984;141:79–87.
72. Hemminki K, Franssila E, Vainio H. Spontaneous abortion among female chemical workers in Finland. *Int Arch Occup Environ Health* 1980;45:123–126.
73. Lindbohm M-L, Hemminki K, Kyyronen P. Spontaneous abortions among women employed in the plastic industry. *Am J Ind Med* 1985; 8:579–86.
74. Lemasters GK, Hagen A, Samuels SJ. Reproductive outcomes in women exposed to solvents in 36 reinforced plastic companies. I. Menstrual dysfunction. *J Occup Med* 1985;27:490–494.
75. Albong G Jr, Bjerkedal T, Egenaes J. Delivery outcome among women employed in the plastic industry in Sweden and Norway. *Am J Ind Med* 1987;12:507–517.
76. Holmberg PC. Central nervous system defects in two children of mothers exposed to chemicals in the reinforced plastics industry. *Scand J Work Environ Health* 1977;3:212–214.
77. Holmberg PC, Nurminem M. Congenital defects to the central nervous system and occupational factors during pregnancy: a case-referent study. *Am J Ind Med* 1980;1:167–176.
78. Holmberg PC, Hernberg S, Kurppa K, Rantala K, Riala R. Oral clefts and organic solvent exposure during pregnancy. *Int Arch Occup Environ Health* 1982;50:371–337.
79. Kurppa K, Holmberg PC, Hernberg S, Rantala K, Raila R, Nurminen T. Screening for occupational exposures and congenital malformations. *Scand J Work Environ Health* 1983;9:89–93.
80. Holmberg PC, Kurppa K, Riala R, Rantala K, Knosma A. Solvent exposure and birth defects: an epidemiologic study. *Prog Clin Biol Res* 1986;220:179–185.
81. Härkönen H, Holmberg PC. Obstetric histories of women occupationally exposed to styrene. *Scand J Work Environ Health* 1982;8:74–77.
82. Phillips DH, Farmer PB. Evidence for DNA and protein binding by styrene and styrene oxide. *Crit Rev Toxicol* 1994;24(S1):S35–S46.
83. Savela K, Hesso A, Hemminki K. Characterization of reaction products between styrene oxide and deoxynucleosides and DNA. *Chem Biol Interact* 1986;60:235.
84. Kauer S, Pongracz K, Bodell WJ, Burlingame AL. Bis(hydroxyphenylethyl)deoxyguanosine adducts identified by [$^{32P}$]-postlabelling and four-sector tandem mass spectrometry: unanticipated adducts formed upon treatment of DNA with styrene 7,8-oxide. *Chem Res Toxicol* 1993;6:125–132.
85. Rappaport SM, Ting D, Jin Z, Yeowell-O'Connell K, Waidyanatha S, McDonald T. Application of Raney nickel to measure adducts of styrene oxide with hemoglobin and albumin. *Chem Res Toxicol* 1993; 6:238–244.
86. Bodell WJ, Pongracz K, Kaur S, Burlingame AL, Liu S-F, Rappaport SM. Investigation of styrene oxide-DNA adducts and their detection in workers exposed to styrene. *Prog Clin Biol Res* 1990;340C:271–282.
87. Brenner DD, Jeffrey AM, Latriano L, Wazneh L, Waraburton D, Toor M, Pero RW, Andrews LR, Walles S, Perera FP. Biomarkers in styrene-exposed boatbuilders. *Mutat Res* 1991;261:225–236.
88. Christakopoulos A, Bergmark E, Zorcec V, Norppa H, Mäki-Paakanen J, Osterman-Golkar S. Monitoring occupational exposure to styrene from hemoglobin adducts and metabolites in blood. *Scand J Work Environ Health* 1993;19:255–263.
89. Norppa H, Mäki-Paakkanen J, Jantunen K, Einisto P, Raty R. Mutagenicity studies of styrene and vinyl acetate. *Ann NY Acad Sci* 1988; 534:671–678.
90. Norppa H, Vainio H, Sorsa M. Metabolic activation of styrene by erythrocytes detected as sister chromatid exchanges in cultured human lymphocytes. *Cancer Res* 1983;43:3579–3582.
91. Kligerman AD, Allen JW, Erexson GL, Morgan DL. Cytogenetic studies of rodents exposed to styrene by inhalation. In: Sorsa M, Peltonen K, Vainio H, Hemminki K, eds. *Butadiene and styrene:* assessment of health hazards. IARC Sci Publ No 127. Lyon, France: IARC, 1993; 217–224.
92. Preston RJ, Abernethy DJ. Studies of the induction of chromosomal aberration and sister chromatid exchange in rats exposed to styrene by inhalation. In: Sorsa M, Peltonen K, Vainio H, Hemminki K, eds. *Butadiene and styrene:* assessment of health hazards. IARC Sci Publ No 127. Lyon, France: IARC, 1993;225–233.
93. Meretoja T, Vainio H, Sorsa M, Härkönen H. Occupational styrene exposure and chromosomal aberrations. *Mutat Res* 1977;56:193–197.
94. Meretoja T, Järventaus H, Sorsa M, Vainio H. Chromosome aberrations in lymphocytes of workers exposed to styrene. *Scand J Work Environ Health* 1978;4(suppl 2):259–264.
95. Fleig I, Thiess AM. Mutagenicity study of workers employed in the styrene and polystyrene processing and manufacturing industry. *Scand J Work Environ Health* 1978;4(suppl 2):254–258.
96. Theiss AM, Fleig I. Chromosome investigations on workers exposed to styrene/polyestyrene. *J Occup Med* 1978;20:747–749.
97. Mäki-Paakkanen J. Chromosome aberrations, micronuclei nd sister-chromatid exchanges in blood lymphocytes after occupational exposure to low levels of styrene. *Mutat Res* 1987;189:399–406.
98. Jablonicka A, Karelova J, Polakova H, Vargova M. Analysis of chromosomes in peripheral blood lymphocytes of styrene-exposed workers. *Mutat Res* 1988;206:167–169.
99. Deleted in proof.
100. Deleted in proof.
101. Barale R. The genetic toxicology of styrene and styrene oxide. *Mutat Res* 1991;257:107–126.
102. Norppa H, Sorsa M. Genetic toxicity of 1,3-butadiene and styrene. In: Sorsa M, Peltonen K, Vainio H, Hemminki K, eds. *Butadiene and styrene:* assessment of health hazards. IARC Sci Publ No 127. Lyon, France: IARC, 1993;185–193.

103. Scott D. Cytogenetic studies of workers exposed to styrene: a review. In: Sorsa M, Peltonen K, Vainio H, Hemminki K, eds. *Butadiene and styrene:* assessment of health hazards. IARC Sci Publ No 127. Lyon, France: IARC, 1993;275–286.
104. Air contaminants—final rule. Occupational Safety and Health. *Federal Register* 1989;54:2429–2431.
105. Morrow NL. The industrial production and use of 1,3-butadiene. *Environ Health Perspect* 1990;86:7–8.
106. U.S. National Institute for Occupational Safety and Health. *National occupational exposure survey (1981–1983).* Cincinnati, OH: 1990.
107. Fajen JM, Lunsford RA, Roberts DR. Industrial exposure to 1,3-butadiene in monomer, polymer and end-user industries. In: Sorsa M, Peltonen K, Vainio H, Hemminki K, eds. *Butadiene and styrene:* assessment of health hazards. IARC Sci Publ No 127. Lyon, France: IARC, 1993;3–13.
108. Lunsford RA, Gagnon Y, Palassis J. 1,3-butadiene (method 1024). In: *NIOSH manual of analytical methods,* 3rd ed., 2nd suppl (Publ No 84-100), Cincinnati, OH: U.S. Department of Health and Human Services, National Institute for Occupational Safety and Health, 1984.
109. CONCAWE. *A survey of exposure to gasoline vapour* (Report No. 4/87). The Hague: CONCAWE, 1987.
110. Lofroth G. Environmental tobacco smoke: overview of chemical composition and genotoxic components. *Mutat Res* 1989;22:73–80.
111. Duescher RJ, Elfarra AA. Human liver microsomes are efficient catalysts of 1,3-butadiene oxidation: evidence for major roles by cytochromes P450 2A6 and 2E1. *Arch Biochem Biophys* 1994;311: 342–349.
112. Seaton MJ, Follansbee MH, Bond JA. Oxidation of 1,2-epoxy-3-butene to 1,2:3,4-diepoxybutane by cDNA-expressed human cytochromes P450 2E1 and 3A4 and human, mouse and rat liver microsomes. *Carcinogenesis* 1995;16:2287–2293.
113. Krause RJ, Elfarra AA. Oxidation of butadiene monoxide to meso- and (+/-)-diepoxybutane by cDNA-expressed human cytochrome P450s and by mouse, rat, and human liver microsomes: evidence for preferential hydration of meso-diepoxybutane in rat and human liver microsomes. *Arch Biochem Biophys* 1997;337:176–184.
114. Bond JA, Dahl AR, Henderson RE, Birnbaum LS. Species differences in the distribution of inhaled butadiene in tissues. *Am Ind Hyg Assoc J* 1987;48:867–872.
115. Laib RJ, Filser JG, Kreiling R, et al. Inhalation pharmacokinetics of 1,3-butadiene and 1,2-expoybutane-3 in rats and mice. *Environ Health Perspect* 1990;86:57–63.
116. Dahl AR, Bechtold WE, Bond JA, et al. Species differences in the metabolism and disposition of inhaled 1,3-butadiene and isoprene. *Environ Health Perspect* 1990;86:65–69.
117. Himmelstein MW, Turner MJ, Asgharian B, Bond JA. Comparison of blood concentrations of 1,3-butadiene and butadiene epoxides in mice and rats exposed to 1,3-butadiene by inhalation. *Carcinogenesis* 1994; 15:1479–1486.
118. Thornton-Manning JR, Dahl AR, Bechtold WE, Griffith WC Jr, Henderson RF. Disposition of butadiene monoepoxide and butadiene diepoxide in various tissues of rats and mice following a low-level inhalation exposure to 1,3-butadiene. *Carcinogenesis* 1995;16: 1723–1731.
119. Kohn MC, Melnick RL. Species differences in the production and clearance of 1,3-butadiene metabolites: a mechanistic model indicates predominantly physiological, not biochemical control. *Carcinogenesis* 1993;14:619–628.
120. Johanson G, Filser JG. A physiologically based pharmacokinetic model for butadiene and its metabolite butadiene monoxide in rat and mouse and its significance for risk extrapolation. *Arch Toxicol* 1993; 93:151–163.
121. Medinsky MA, Leavens TL, Csanady GA, Gargas ML, Bond JA. In vivo metabolism of butadiene by mice and rats: a comparison of physiological model predictions and experimental data. *Carcinogenesis* 1994;15:1329–1340.
122. Filser JG, Johanson G, Kessler W, et al. A pharmacologic model to describe toxicokinetics interactions between 1,3-butadiene and styrene in rats: predictions for human exposure. *IARC Sci Publ* 1993; 127:65–68.
123. Matanoski GM, Santos-Burgoa C, Zeger SL, Schwartz L. Epidemiologic data related to health effects of 1,3-butadiene. In: Mohz V, ed. *Assessment of inhalation hazards.* Berlin: Springer-Verlag, 1989; 201–214.
124. Shugaev BB. Concentrations of hydrocarbons in tissues as a measure of toxicity. *Arch Environ Health* 1969;18:878–882.
125. Crouch CN, Pullinger DH, Gaunt IF. Inhalation toxicity studies with 1,3-butadiene. II. 3 month toxicity study in rats. *Am Ind Hyg Assoc J* 1979;40:796–802.
126. Carpenter CP, Shaffer CF, Weil CS, et al. Studies on the inhalation of 1,3-butadiene, with a comparison of its narcotic effect with benzol, toluol, and styrene, and a note on the elimination of styrene by the human. *J Ind Hyg Toxicol* 1944;26:69–78.
127. Huff JE, Melnick RL, Solleveld HA, Haseman JK, Powers M. Multiple organ carcinogenicity of 1,3-butadiene in B6C3F1 mice after 60 weeks' inhalation exposure. *Science* 1985;227:548–549.
128. Melnick RL, Huff JE, Roycroft JH, et al. Inhalation toxicology and carcinogenicity of 1,3-butadiene in B6C3F1 mice following 65 weeks of exposure. *Environ Health Perspect* 1990;86:27–36.
129. Melnick RL, Huff J, Chou BJ, Miller RA. Carcinogenicity of 1,3-butadiene in C57B2/6 x C3HF$_1$ mice at low exposure concentrations. *Cancer Res* 1990;50:6592–6599.
130. Owen PE, Glaister JR, Gaunt IF, Pullinger DH. Inhalation toxicity studies with 1,3-butadiene. 3. Two-year toxicity/carcinogenicity study in rats. *Am Ind Hyg Assoc J* 1987;48:407–413.
131. Owen PE, Glaister JR. Inhalation toxicity and carcinogenicity of 1,3-butadiene in Sprague-Dawley rats. *Environ Health Perspect* 1990;86: 19–25.
132. Irons RD, Cathro HP, Stillman WS, Steinhagen WH, Shah RS. Susceptibility to 1,3-butadiene-induced leukemogenesis correlates with endogenous ecotropic retroviral background in the mouse. *Toxicol Appl Pharmacol* 1989;101:170–176.
133. Irons RD. Studies on the mechanism of 1,3-butadiene-induced leukemogenesis. The potential role of endogenous murine leukemia virus. *Environ Health Perspect* 1990;86:49–55.
134. *IARC monograph on the evaluation of the carcinogenic risk of chemicals to humans. The rubber industry,* vol. 28. Lyon, France: IARC, 1982;230.
135. McMichael AJ, Spirtas R, Kupper LL. An epidemiologic study of mortality within a cohort of rubber workers, 1964–72. *J Occup Med* 1974;16:458–464.
136. McMichael AJ, Spirtas R, Gamble JF, Tousey PM. Mortality among rubber workers: relationship to specific jobs. *J Occup Med* 1976;18: 178–185.
137. Down TD, Crane MM, Kim KW. Mortality among workers at a butadiene facility. *Am J Ind Med* 1987;12:311–329.
138. Meinhardt TJ, Lemen RA, Crandall MS, Young RJ. Environmental epidemiologic Investigation of the styrene-butadiene rubber industry. *Scand J Work Environ Health* 1982;8:250–259.
139. Matanoski GM, Schwartz L. Mortality of workers in styrene-butadiene polymer production. *J Occup Med* 1987;29:675–680.
140. Symposium on the toxicology, carcinogenesis and human health aspects of 1,3-butadiene. *Environ Health Perspect* 1990;86:1–171.
141. Divine BJ, Wendt JK, Hartman CM. Cancer mortality among workers at a butadiene production facility. *IARC Sci Publ* 1993;127:345–362.
142. Lemen RA, Meinhardt TJ, Crandall MS, Fajen JM, Brown DP. Environmental epidemiologic investigations in the styrene-butadiene rubber production industry. *Environ Health Perspect* 1990;86:103–106.
143. Matanoski GM, Santos-Burgoa C, Schwartz L. Mortality of a cohort of workers in the styrene-butadiene polymer manufacturing industry (1943–1982). *Environ Health Perspect* 1990;86:107–117.
144. Morrissey RE, Schwetz BA, Hackett PL, et al. Overview of reproductive and developmental toxicity studies of 1,3-butadiene in rodents. *Environ Health Perspect* 1990;86:79–84.
145. Adler ID, Cochrane J, Osterman-Golkar S, Skopek TR, Sorsa M, Vogel E. 1,3-butadiene working group report. *Mutat Res* 1995;330:101–114.
146. Osterman-Golkar SM, Bond JA, Ward JB Jr, Legator MS. Use of haemoglobin adducts for biomonitoring exposure to 1,3-butadiene. *IARC Sci Publ* 1993;127:127–134.
147. Neagu I, Koivisto P, Neagu C, Kostiainen R, Stenby K, Peltonen K. Butadiene monoxide and deoxyguanosine alkylation products at the N7-position. *Carcinogenesis* 1995;16:1809–1813.
148. Koivisto P, Kostiainen R, Kilpelainen I, Steinby K, Peltonen K. Preparation, characterization and 32P-postlabeling of butadiene monoepoxide N6-adenine adducts. *Carcinogenesis* 1995;16:2999–3007.
149. Selzer RR, Elfarra AA. Characterization of N1- and N6-adenosine adducts and N1-inosine adducts formed by the reaction of butadiene monoxide with adenosine: evidence for the N1-adenosine adducts

and major initial products. *Chem Res Toxicol* 1996;9:875–881.
150. Selzer RR, Elfarra AA. Synthesis and biochemical characterization of N1-, N2-, and N7-guanosine adducts of butadiene monoxide. *Chem Res Toxicol* 1996;9:126–132.
151. Tretyakova NYU, Lin UP, Upton PB, Sangaiah R, Swenberg JA. Macromolecular adducts of butadiene. *Toxicol* 1996;113:70–76.
152. Mabon N, Moorthy B, Randerath E, Randerath K. Monophosphate 32P-postlabeling assay of DNA adducts from 1,2:3,4-diepoxybutane, the most genotoxic metabolite of 1,2-butadiene: *in vitro* methodological studies and *in vivo* dosimetry. *Mutat Res* 1996;371:87–104.
153. de Meester C, Poncelat F, Roberfroid M. The mutagenicity of BD towards Salmonella typhimurium. *Toxicol Lett* 1980;6:125–130.
154. Cunningham MJ, Choy WN, Arce GT, et al. In vivo sister chromatid exchange and micronucleus induction studies with 1,3-butadiene in B6C3F1 mice and Sprague-Dawley rats. *Mutagenesis* 1986;1:449–452.
155. Sharief Y, Brown AM, Backer LC, et al. Sister chromatid exchange and chromosome aberration analyses in mice after *in vivo* exposure to acrylonitrile, styrene, or butadiene monoxide. *Environ Mutagen* 1986; 8:439–448.
156. Tice RR, Boucher R, Luke CA, Shelby MD. Comparative cytogenetic analysis of bone marrow damage induced in male B6C3F1 mice by multiple exposures to gaseous 1,3-butadiene. *Environ Mutagen* 1987; 9:235–250.
157. Jauhar PP, Henika PR, MacGregor JT, et al. 1,3-butadiene: induction of micronucleated erythrocytes in the peripheral blood of B6C3F1 mice exposed by inhalation for 13 weeks. *Mutat Res* 1988;209:171–176.
158. Adler ID, Cao J, Filser JG, et al. Mutagenicity of 1,3-butadiene inhalation in somatic and germinal cells of mice. *Mutat Res* 1994;309: 307–314.
159. Autio K, Renzi L, Catalan J, Albrecht OE, Sorsa M. Induction of micronuclei in peripheral blood and bone marrow erythrocytes of rats and mice exposed to 1,3-butadiene by inhalation. *Mutat Res* 1994; 309:315–320.
160. Arce GT, Vincent DR, Cunningham MJ, Choy WN, Sarrif AM. *In vitro* and *in vivo* genotoxicity of 1,3-butadiene and metabolites. *Environ Health Perspect* 1990;86;75–78.
161. Cochrane JE, Skopek TR. Mutagenicity of 1,3-butadiene and its epoxide metabolites in human TK6 cells and in splenic T cells isolated from exposed B6C3F1 mice. *IARC Sci Publ* 1993;127:195–204.
162. Cochrane JE, Skopek TR. Mutagenicity of butadiene and its epoxide metabolites. II. Mutational spectra of butadiene, 1,2-epoxybutene and diepoxybutane at the hprt locus in splenic T cells from exposed B6C3F1 mice. *Carcinogenesis* 1994;15:719–723.
163. Cochrane JE, Skopek TR. Mutagenicity of butadiene and its epoxide metabolites. I. Mutagenic potential of 1,2-epoxybutene, 1,2,3,4-diepoxybutane and 3,4-epoxy-1,2-butanediol in cultured human lymphoblasts. *Carcinogenesis* 1994;15:713–717.
164. Walker VE, Skopek TR. A mouse model for the study of in-vivo mutational spectra: sequence specificity of ethylene oxide at the hprt locus. *Mutat Res* 1993;288:151–162.
165. Sorsa M, Osterman-Golkar S, Peltonen K. Saarikoski ST, Sram R. Assessment of exposure to butadiene in the process industry. *Toxicol* 1996;113:77–83.
166. Wiencke JK, Pemble S, Ketterer B, Kelsey KT. Gene deletion of glutathione S-transferase theta: correlation with induced genetic damage and potential role in endogenous mutagenesis. *Cancer Epidemiol Biomarkers Prev* 1995;4:253–259.
167. Kelsey KT, Wiencke JK, Ward J, Bechtold W, Fajen J. Sister-chromatid exchanges, glutathione S-transferase theta deletion and cytogenetic sensitivity to diepoxybutane in lymphocytes from butadiene monomer production workers. *Mutat Res* 1995;335:267–273.
168. Ott MG. Assessment of 1,3-butadiene epidemiology studies. *Environ Health Perspect* 1990;86:135–141.
169. Landrigan PJ. Critical assessment of epidemiologic studies on the human carcinogenicity of 1,3-butadiene. *Environ Health Perspect* 1990; 86:143–148.
170. Bond JA, Recio L, Andjelkovich D. Epidemiological and mechanistic data suggest that 1,3-butadiene will not be carcinogenic to human at exposures likely to be encountered in the environment or workplace. *Carcinogenesis* 1995;16:165–171.
171. Melnick RL, Kohn MC. Mechanistic data indicate that 1,3-butadiene is a human carcinogen. *Carcinogenesis* 1995;16:157–163.
172. Himmelstein MW, Acquavella JF, Recio L, Medinsky MA, Bond JA. Toxicology and epidemiology of 1,3-butadiene. *Crit Rev Toxicol* 1997; 27:1–108.
173. US Occupational Safety and Health Administration. Occupational exposure to 1,3-butadiene-proposed rule and notice of hearing. *Federal Register* 1990;55(155):32736–32826.

*Environmental and Occupational Medicine, Third Edition,* edited by William N. Rom.
Lippincott–Raven Publishers, Philadelphia © 1998.

# CHAPTER 82

# Ethylene Oxide

Anthony D. LaMontagne and Karl T. Kelsey

Ethylene oxide (EtO, ETO, EO) is the simplest chemical epoxide (molecular formula = $C_2H_4O$, molecular weight = 44.06). Its three-membered ring structure is highly strained, making it very reactive:

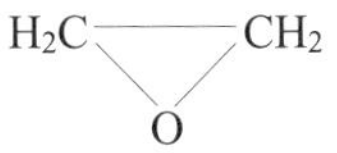


EtO, like all epoxides, reacts with a broad spectrum of nucleophiles (i.e., electron-rich centers, such as basic nitrogens) to open the ring structure and form additional compounds through a short-lived carbonium ion intermediate. This property, together with EtO's simple structure, accounts for the widespread use of EtO in industry as well as many of its hazards to humans.

Due to its high vapor pressure, EtO is a gas at room temperature and atmospheric pressure. EtO has poor warning properties: it is colorless and has an ether-like odor at concentrations above 500 to 700 ppm. Olfactory fatigue may limit a person's ability to smell EtO, but perception at concentrations below the odor threshold may occur due to mucous membrane irritation and the occurrence of a peculiar taste in the mouth. Pure EtO is highly flammable and explosive, with explosive limits ranging from 3% to 100% in air. EtO is highly soluble in water as well as lipids; thus, upon exposure, it is efficiently absorbed through the lungs and distributed through the bloodstream.

A. D. LaMontagne: Occupational Health Program, Department of Environmental Health, Harvard School of Public Health; and New England Research Institutes, Watertown, Massachusetts 02172.

K. T. Kelsey: Department of Cancer Cell Biology; and Occupational Health Program, Department of Environmental Health, Harvard School of Public Health, Boston, Massachusetts 02115-9957.

## PRODUCTION, USE, AND EXPOSURE

### Production and Use

Ethylene oxide has been produced commercially since the 1920s. It is one of the highest production volume chemicals in the United States, ranking 27th in 1991 (1). Approximately 8 to 12 U.S. chemical companies currently produce EtO through direct oxidation of ethylene in air or oxygen in the presence of a silver oxide catalyst (2,3). An alternative production process involving chlorohydrin was phased out by 1980 (3). Most EtO used in the United States is domestically produced, with the United States accounting for roughly half of world production.

Approximately 99% of the EtO produced in the United States is used as a chemical intermediate in the plants where it is produced (2). Most is used in the production of ethylene glycol (60–70%), with smaller amounts being used to produce nonionic surfactants, glycol ethers, higher glycols, ethanolamines, fuel additives, and other industrial chemicals (2). Less than 1% of the annual EtO production is used as a sterilant or fumigant in the health care manufacturing, hospital, spice, and other industries. Despite the dramatic difference in volume used, occupational exposures to EtO are higher and more widespread in its use as a sterilant than in its use as a chemical intermediate.

To protect against EtO's flammability and explosion hazards, chemical production processes are usually conducted outdoors or in enclosed or automated systems with relatively little opportunity for worker exposure, except during maintenance or under unusual circumstances. In contrast, sterilant uses in the health care industry involve pressurized and nonenclosed systems with various opportunities for direct and indirect worker exposures. EtO is favored as a sterilant because it is effective at low temperature and humidity on heat- and moisture-sensitive medical devices, and it is compatible with almost all device and packaging materials.

Ethylene oxide came into widespread use as a sterilant in hospitals in the 1950s. EtO is used in a wide variety of health care and laboratory research settings, including medical products manufacturing, hospitals (including essentially all acute care hospitals), outpatient clinics (e.g., dental, podiatry), and veterinary clinics and hospitals. As a sterilant, EtO is used in two general forms, 100% and mixtures, both of which are distributed as pressurized liquids. Small cartridges of 100% EtO containing enough for one sterilization cycle are used in negative pressure sterilizers; cartridges are placed inside the sterilizer intact and are then automatically punctured after the door is sealed. Mixtures of EtO (10–12%) and various fire and explosion-resistant diluents (e.g., carbon dioxide, various chlorofluorocarbons) are supplied in large cylinders for use in larger positive pressure sterilizers; external plumbing delivers the EtO mixture from the cylinder to the sterilizer chamber. Most new sterilizers are manufactured with built-in local exhaust ventilation and other safety features. Functionally similar machines are sometimes used in museums and libraries to fumigate books and artifacts; however, these machines tend to be older and typically have rudimentary exposure controls.

### Exposure

Various methods for the determination of EtO exposures have been developed and validated, as summarized by the National Institute for Occupational Safety and Health (NIOSH) (4,5). These methods include active pump sampling and passive dosimetry for time-weighted average (TWA) air samples, and real-time or alarm monitoring for instantaneous measurements (6,7). NIOSH has estimated that approximately 270,000 workers are potentially exposed to EtO (8). Sterilization and fumigation involve relatively high levels of exposure, with an estimated 96,000 workers potentially exposed in hospitals and 21,000 potentially exposed during the commercial sterilization of medical devices, pharmaceuticals, and spices. Health care worker exposures may occur directly due to involvement in or proximity to EtO sterilization and aeration processes, or the changing of EtO supply cartridges or cylinders. Workers outside of sterilization departments may also be exposed due to EtO residues in packaged sterile medical devices (9–11). Others who may be occupationally exposed in the health care setting include internal and external responders to EtO spills and leaks, such as in-house emergency response team members, firefighters, and hazardous materials response team members.

In the general population, patients have been widely exposed to EtO residues in EtO-sterilized medical devices (12). The public may also be exposed to EtO through consumer products and airborne releases (3,13). EtO is present in cigarette smoke, and residues remain in various pharmaceutical and cosmetic products (e.g., in polyethylene glycol additives) and foodstuffs (e.g., spices, cocoa, flour, and dried fruits) that have been treated with EtO. General population exposures to EtO have not been comprehensively characterized to date.

## TOXICOLOGY

The toxicity of EtO is unusually broad, including systemic and local, acute and chronic, and reversible and irreversible effects. EtO does not require enzymatic activation to exert toxic effects. Some effects are dependent on EtO's inherent property as an alkylator of proteins and nucleic acids (e.g., mutagenicity and sensitization), whereas others may be attributable to its anesthetic properties (e.g., acute neurotoxicity). Various detailed reviews of EtO toxicology are available to supplement the summary below (2,3,5,14–16).

### Disposition

The principal routes of exogenous EtO absorption are through the lungs and skin. Ethylene oxide occurs endogenously in small amounts as a metabolite of ethylene. EtO is hydrolyzed in the body to ethylene glycol both spontaneously and metabolically (via epoxide hydrolase). Ethylene glycol can be excreted in urine or further metabolized by alcohol and aldehyde dehydrogenases. EtO is also enzymatically deactivated via glutathione conjugation to form S-2-hydroxyethyl-glutathione, S-2-hydroxyethyl-cysteine, and S-2-hydroxyethyl-mercapturic acid. EtO does not bioaccumulate. Excretion is primarily through the urine. The half-life of absorbed EtO in humans has been estimated to be under 1 hour, assuming steady-state conditions and first-order kinetics (2).

### Effects on Mucous Membranes and Skin

In the air, EtO is an acute mucous membrane irritant. Effects can range from mild irritation from exposures around 50 to 100 ppm, to life-threatening, delayed-onset pulmonary edema from exposures in the hundreds or thousands of ppm. Skin contact with pure EtO liquid or EtO mixtures causes frostbite burns as a result of rapid vaporization. Contact with aqueous solutions can cause erythema, edema, and vesiculation, depending on dose. Resulting tissue damage can lead to residual brown pigmentation or to hypopigmentation. Repeated skin exposures to EtO can also cause allergic sensitization, as discussed in detail below.

Three cases of cataracts were reported in 1982 in workers with intermittent EtO exposures over 500 to 700 ppm (17). An epidemiologic study ($n = 55$) of cataracts among EtO-exposed Parisian hospital sterilization workers was conducted after a cluster of three cases was discovered in a separate hospital; a significant excess of cataracts was observed among EtO-exposed versus nonexposed workers (matched for age and sex), suggesting elevated cataract risks from chronic exposure to low levels as well as intermittent exposure to high levels of EtO (18). An excess incidence of cataracts was also observed in a study of EtO-exposed cynomolgus monkeys (19).

### Hematologic Effects

A 1967 Swedish study reported excesses of absolute lymphocytosis and anemia in 31 workers with high versus 26 with low EtO exposure (20). Historic case reports from the 1930s to 1950s described lymphocytosis in four EtO-exposed workers who were also acutely symptomatic with central nervous system effects [reviewed by LaMontagne et al. (21)]. Animal evidence of EtO-associated lymphocytosis is mixed, with some studies showing lymphocytosis, some showing no effect, and some showing marked lymphopenia (15,22). Animal studies of EtO-associated hemolysis are also mixed—some showing hemolysis and some showing no effect (14,15).

Recent occupational studies have also yielded inconsistent results. In 1984, Currier et al. (23) reported on 84 workers with estimated average work shift exposures below 10 ppm; no significant differences were found in leukocyte counts, percent lymphocytes, hemoglobin, hematocrit, and red blood cell count compared to controls matched on several characteristics. In 1985, Van Sittert et al. (24) examined 36 EtO production workers with estimated work shift exposures below 0.05 ppm with occasional higher excursions; they found no significant differences in leukocyte counts, percent lymphocytes, percent monocytes, and percent neutrophils compared to 35 controls. In 1990, Deschamps et al. (18) found statistically significant negative log-linear relationships between cumulative EtO exposure and blood concentrations of leukocytes, neutrophils, and lymphocytes; average concentrations of each of these cell types were not significantly different between subjects who experienced regular exposures over 5 ppm and those who did not. A 1993 study by LaMontagne et al. (21) investigated a persistent relative lymphocytosis among hospital sterilization workers exposed to work shift average EtO exposures below 1 ppm. A cross-sectional comparison with nonexposed subjects from the same hospital showed no significant differences between exposed and comparison groups in relative or absolute lymphocytosis, other white blood cell counts, red blood cell count, hemoglobin, or hematocrit. Finally, a 1995 study by Schulte et al. (25) compared hematologic parameters in 46 U.S. and 22 Mexican female hospital workers. EtO-exposure response relationships were observed between percent lymphocytes (positive) and neutrophils (negative) in the U.S. workers. In the Mexican workers, however, no relationship was found for percent lymphocytes and a positive relationship was found for neutrophils. No overall relationship was found for total leukocyte counts.

### Neurologic Effects

Ethylene oxide is structurally similar to ethyl ether and was investigated historically as an anesthetic before being abandoned because of its adverse side effects and after effects. The acute and chronic effects of EtO on the nervous system are quite uniform across species. Findings in humans are summarized below.

#### *Acute*

Very high exposures depress the central nervous system and can cause seizures or convulsions, loss of consciousness, and death. High exposures can lead to a flu-like syndrome including nausea, vomiting, and diarrhea. Other symptoms that may occur after significant acute exposure include drowsiness, confusion, lethargy, weakness, delirium, dysarthria, and ataxia.

#### *Chronic*

Chronic and acute EtO exposures have been shown to cause peripheral neuropathy (26–29). Both sensory and motor neurons can be affected, with symptoms usually including numbness in the fingers and feet and muscular weakness in the lower limbs. The syndrome is reversible with removal from exposure, apparently involving axonal degeneration with regeneration (30–32). EtO-associated chronic effects on the central nervous system have also been reported in the form of personality dysfunction or cognitive impairment (33–36), although some investigators question a causal role for EtO (37,38).

### Genotoxicity and Mutagenicity

The genotoxic and mutagenic potential of EtO has been extensively studied and reviewed (2,16,39). EtO has long been known to alkylate nucleic acids and proteins. Genotoxic and cytogenetic end points have been examined in over 100 published studies, covering a wide range of phylogenetic levels, including bacteriophages, bacteria, fungi, plants, insects, rodents, rabbits, monkeys, and humans (2). Genotoxic assays for EtO-induced chromosomal aberrations, micronuclei, unscheduled

DNA synthesis, sister-chromatid exchanges, heritable translocations, and mutations have been uniformly and strongly positive, correlating genetic damage with EtO dose (2).

In studies of workers exposed to EtO, various investigators have observed EtO-related increases in structural chromosomal changes, including chromosomal aberrations in peripheral lymphocytes (40–44). Various investigators have also shown EtO-related increases in sister-chromatid exchanges in exposed workers (40,42,43, 45–48), with some studies showing EtO-related increases in sister chromatid exchanges in workers exposed at levels below current Occupational Safety and Health Administration (OSHA) exposure limits (25,49,50). EtO exposure–related increases in mutations in the hemizygous *hprt* locus (43,51) and increases in DNA single-strand breaks (52) have also been demonstrated in exposed workers. The dose-related induction of mutations, sister-chromatid exchanges, chromosomal aberrations, and other sensitive genotoxic end points clearly suggest that EtO exposure poses a carcinogenic risk to humans.

Recent work has begun to focus on the nature of the DNA lesions induced by EtO as well as the spectrum of mutations induced in rodent cells. EtO exposure has been linked to the induction of a variety of genetic damage, including DNA base substitutions and frameshift mutations (53,54), DNA strand breaks (55), and large deletions (56), as well as DNA-protein cross-links (52,57). In systems designed to study the lesions produced by DNA alkylation, Walker et al. (53) have demonstrated that EtO produces both 7-(2-hydroxyethyl)guanine and 3-(2-hydroxyethyl)adenine adducts. While these lesions themselves are not likely to be highly promutagenic, their mutagenic potential likely derives from subsequent depurination of DNA that may cause miscoding if DNA replication occurs prior to repair of the apurinic sites (the sites where the adducts were bound). In rodents, studies of mutations at the hprt gene are consistent with this mutagenic mechanism, suggesting the involvement of both modified guanine and adenine bases in EtO-induced mutations (54).

## Carcinogenicity

Although EtO had been known to be mutagenic since the late 1940s, widespread concerns about EtO's potential human cancer risk were first spurred by a report to the Swedish government in 1959 by Ehrenberg and Gustafsson (cited in ref. 58) followed by a published study from the same group in 1967 (20). The study showed higher absolute lymphocyte counts, a higher prevalence of relative anemia, and a higher prevalence of chromosomal abnormalities (breaks and exchanges) among high versus low EtO-exposed workers. These findings led to a characterization of EtO exposure as radiomimetic (mimicking the biologic effects of ionizing radiation) as well as mutagenic.

### *Animal Studies*

Several animal studies in which EtO has been administered through various routes have shown EtO-associated increases in various solid and hematopoietic cancers (2). In the widely cited Bushy Run Study, Snellings et al. (59) reported a dose-related increase in primary brain tumors, mononuclear cell leukemia, and peritoneal mesothelioma in Fischer 344 rats exposed for 2 years at 0, 10, 33, or 100 ppm for 6 hours per day, 5 days per week. NIOSH performed a similar 2-year inhalation study in male F344 rats, confirming the Bushy Run Study findings (60). A subsequent U.S. National Toxicology Program (NTP) bioassay of EtO in mice also found clear evidence of carcinogenic activity (61). B6C3F1 mice were exposed to 0, 50, and 100 ppm EtO for 6 hours per day, 5 days per week for 2 years. EtO dose-related increases were observed in lung and harderian glands in male and female mice. In female mice, increases in malignant neoplasms were also observed in the uterus, mammary gland, and hematopoietic system. When administered to rats by gavage, EtO induced local tumors in a dose-related fashion, mainly squamous cell carcinomas of the forestomach (62).

### *Epidemiology*

In 1979, Hogstedt et al. (63) reported a cluster of three leukemias (0.2 expected) in 230 Swedish sterilization workers using 50/50 ethylene oxide/methyl formate. In a follow-up at the same worksite (64), one additional leukemia death was reported, with 0.3 expected for the 203 workers who had been employed for more than 1 year. Exposures were estimated to have been less than 30 ppm work shift TWA. In a cohort study of Swedish EtO production plant workers launched on the basis of the above-described case reports, significant excesses of stomach cancer and leukemia mortality were observed; potential confounding exposures of these workers included ethylene chlorohydrin and ethylene dichloride (65,66). The populations from the above-described Swedish studies were combined in a 1988 mortality update (total $n = 709$); statistically significant mortality excesses for leukemia [significant mortality ratio (SMR) = 921] and stomach cancer (SMR = 546) were reported (58). Consistent with the rat gavage study described above, stomach cancer excesses were speculated to be attributable to the former practice of tasting EtO reaction products (66).

A 1981 study of 767 potentially exposed U.S. EtO production workers showed an overall deficit of cancer mortality, with nonsignificant excesses of pancreatic, bladder, unspecified brain and central nervous system cancers, and Hodgkin's disease (67). A reanalysis by the U.S. Environmental Protection Agency (EPA) in 1985 (68) found statistically significant excesses of mortality from pancreatic cancer and Hodgkin's disease in EtO-exposed workers. Work shift EtO exposures were estimated to have been less than 10 ppm TWA.

In a 1989 report from Great Britain, Gardner et al. (69) assessed cancer mortality in 2,876 workers from four EtO production companies and eight hospitals where EtO was used as a sterilant. In the cohort as a whole, no significant excesses in total cancer mortality, leukemia, or stomach cancers were observed. Exposures were estimated to have been less than 5 ppm work shift TWA in almost all jobs, and less than 1 ppm in many, with occasional higher excursions.

Kiesselbach et al. (70) conducted a mortality study of 2,658 German chemical production workers exposed to EtO as well as several other hazardous substances. This cohort contained most of the smaller cohort previously studied by Thiess et al. (71). Small, nonsignificant excesses of stomach and esophageal cancer were observed. Little information was available on exposures, and many study subjects had potential exposures to other hazardous chemicals.

Mortality in a cohort of West Virginia chemical workers with exposures to EtO, chlorohydrin, and other substances was originally determined as a single group by Greenberg et al. (72) in 1990, but was subsequently split to distinguish chlorohydrin from EtO exposures to the extent feasible, and to update follow-up (73,74). Among the 278 men who worked in the chlorohydrin unit with minimal EtO exposure, substantial and significant increases in total, pancreatic, and hematopoietic cancers were observed, which increased with durations of assignment to the unit (74). The remainder of the cohort ($n = 1{,}896$) consisted of men assigned to either chlorohydrin or direct oxidation EtO production processes. Small, nonsignificant excesses of stomach, liver, and brain cancer were observed in this group (73). Trend analyses were negative, with an exception of a two- to threefold excess risk for leukemia observed among workers with more than 10 years' assignment to EtO departments. Work shift EtO exposures were estimated to have ranged from less than 1 ppm to 20 ppm TWA.

In a large mortality study of 18,254 medical product and spice sterilization workers exposed on average to less than 4 ppm work shift TWA of EtO, NIOSH investigators found no overall excesses of leukemia, brain, stomach, or pancreatic cancers (8). A small statistically significant increase in risk of non-Hodgkin's lymphoma was observed in male workers (SMR = 155), who likely had higher EtO exposures than women enrolled in the study. A positive trend was observed between hematopoietic cancer mortality and cumulative EtO exposure; this trend was strengthened by discounting EtO exposures 10 years prior to death and restricting analysis to neoplasms of lymphoid origin (75). Wong and Trent (76) conducted an independent analysis of the NIOSH cohort with extended follow-up, yielding similar results.

In a cohort study of 1,971 Italian chemical workers licensed to handle EtO, mortality excesses were observed for total cancers, hematopoietic cancers, and for lymphosarcoma and reticulosarcoma (77). When analyses were restricted to workers licensed to handle EtO only ($n = 637$), large, statistically significant excesses of hematopoietic cancers (SMR = 700) and lymphosarcoma and reticulosarcoma (SMR = 1,693) were observed. No data were available on the levels of EtO exposures or on exposures to other chemicals.

In a 1995 update of a Swedish cohort of 2,170 medical products sterilization workers, a nonsignificant increase in the incidence of hematopoietic cancers was observed (standardized incidence rate [SIR] = 1.78) (78). The risk estimate for leukemias increased, though not to statistical significance, with time since start of exposure and with higher cumulative EtO exposures. Estimated exposures were low, with a median value of 0.13 ppm-years.

Two recent studies have suggested an excess of breast cancers in women occupationally exposed to EtO (79,80). EtO-associated mammary gland tumors have also been observed in animal studies (61). In 1996, NIOSH reopened the large EtO cohort described above to test the hypothesis that EtO exposure is related to increased incidence of breast cancer.

To summarize, the epidemiologic evidence on EtO's carcinogenicity is mixed. The relatively short follow-up times and low exposure levels in many of the studies may be contributing to the difficulty of elucidating a true association, whereas confounding exposures may account for some of the associations observed to date. The compelling mechanistic, cytogenetic, and animal evidence support causal associations with a number of tumor types. A recent meta-analysis concluded that there was little evidence overall that EtO exposure elevates risks of pancreatic or brain cancers, but that there were small suggestive increases in hematopoietic and stomach cancer risks (81). In its 1994 reassessment of the mechanistic, *in vitro*, *in vivo*, and epidemiologic studies on EtO, the International Agency for Research on Cancer (IARC) reclassified EtO from its previous designation as a group 2A probable human carcinogen to a group 1 known human carcinogen (2).

### Reproductive and Developmental Toxicity

Ethylene oxide's size and solubility suggest that it readily crosses the blood-testes and fetal-placental barriers. In addition, EtO's mutagenic and genotoxic properties indicate its potential for causing heritable genetic damage, and thus both male- and female-mediated reproductive problems. Numerous mechanistic, animal, and human studies of EtO's reproductive effects have been conducted. Reviews are available to complement the summary below (39,82–84).

### *Mechanistic and Animal Studies*

Ethylene oxide causes dose- and dose-rate–related increases in dominant lethal mutations in both male and female animals exposed before mating (39,85,86). In addition to anticipated direct genetic mechanisms, novel epigenetic mechanisms have been proposed for dominant lethal mutations in exposed male animals, wherein EtO alkylates protamine in developing sperm cells, disrupting chromatin condensation, thus resulting in chromosome breakage manifesting as dominant lethal mutations (87). In studies of female mice, EtO was one of the first developmental toxicants shown to be able to cause both early pregnancy loss and later fetal death and malformation as a result of exposure soon after mating (86, 88).

A variety of effects on reproductive outcome have been observed in animal studies, depending on the timing and dose of EtO exposure, including increased embryo death near the time of implantation, increased length of pregnancy, increases in late fetal deaths, decreased litter size, decreased fetal birth weight, and structural and functional teratogenic damage (15,82,83,89). Studies of EtO-exposed male animals have shown decreases in fertility, sperm counts, and testicular weight, and increases in frequency of abnormal sperm (82–84).

### *Epidemiology*

Hemminki and colleagues (90) assessed spontaneous abortion rates among female sterilizing staff in a Finnish hospital ($n = 1{,}443$ pregnancies). A statistically significant threefold excess risk of spontaneous abortion was found among those conducting EtO sterilization duties compared to nonexposed nursing auxilliary staff. Adjustment for age, parity, decade of pregnancy, smoking, coffee and alcohol consumption, and glutaraldehye and formaldehyde exposures did not affect the results. EtO exposures were estimated to be under 0.5 ppm work shift TWA, with occasional excursions up to 250 ppm. Another study of potentially EtO exposed nurses by the same investigators was negative for excess spontaneous abortions, but EtO exposures were indirect and likely to be much lower than those in the first study (91). More recently, this group conducted a study of paternal occupational exposures and spontaneous abortions using data from Finland's nationwide Hospital Discharge Register (92). A statistically significant odds ratio of 4.7 was observed based on three spontaneous abortions among ten pregnancies involving EtO-exposed males. Exposures were described as low.

Yakubova et al. studied female workers (57 operators and 38 lab workers versus comparison group of 65 administrative staff) in an EtO production plant in the former Soviet Union (cited in ref. 15). A 33% increase in spontaneous abortion and a two- to threefold increase in pregnancy toxemia were reported. EtO exposures were reported to be well below 1 ppm work shift TWA. High levels of noise and vibration and wide variations in temperature were not addressed in the analysis.

Rowland et al. (89) investigated EtO exposure (categorical yes/no) and adverse pregnancy outcomes in a study of 1,320 pregnancies among 4,856 dental assistants registered in California. A borderline significant excess of spontaneous abortion was observed [age-adjusted relative risk (RR) = 2.5], as well as nonsignificant excesses of pre- and postterm births. A borderline significant excess (RR = 2.5) of any of the three adverse outcomes was observed after adjustment for age and exposure to nitrous oxide and mercury amalgam.

In summary, though there have been few human studies of adverse pregnancy outcomes in relation to EtO exposure, most have been positive. Further study will be required to confirm these results and estimate dose-response. Consideration of positive reproductive and developmental animal studies together with human evidence to date indicates that EtO should be treated as a potent human reproductive and developmental hazard.

## Allergic Sensitization

While most of EtO's toxic effects were established through animal and occupational studies, accumulating studies of the effects on patients from residues in EtO-sterilized medical devices established EtO as a potent sensitizing agent (12,93). Prick tests as well as radioallergosorbent (RAST) and enzyme-linked immunosorbent assays (ELISA) specific to antibodies against EtO-human serum albumin (HSA) have been developed (94). A strong relationship has been established between the presence of immunoglobulin E (IgE) and total antibodies against EtO-HSA and anaphylactic reactions to hemodialysis (95). Before 1985, approximately 5 deaths per year occurred in dialysis patients from severe anaphylactic reactions (93). EtO-HSA antibodies have also been associated with milder effects on patients, such as rash and eosinophilia, suggesting that EtO sensitization might cause other allergic diseases as well (95).

Similar methods have begun to be applied to the study of EtO-exposed workers, as for example in an assessment of EtO-HSA antibodies in seven endoscopy nurses (96). EtO's sensitizing ability also suggests a plausible mechanism for its ability to induce asthma in exposed workers. In what may prove to be sentinel cases for the industry, a number of cases of EtO-associated asthma in health care workers have been recently reported (97–99a).

## PREVENTION AND CONTROL OF EtO EXPOSURES

### Exposure Limits

Ethylene oxide was initially regulated by OSHA in 1971 for its irritant and neurotoxic properties, with a permissible exposure limit (PEL) of 50 ppm work shift TWA. On the basis of increasing evidence of EtO's potential carcinogenic and reproductive effects, a full OSHA standard on EtO was passed in 1984, with the PEL reduced to 1 ppm work shift TWA (Table 1) (100). In 1988, OSHA added a short-term excursion limit, which reduced the excess cancer risks at the 1984 work shift PEL and addressed potential dose-rate concerns (101).

Current U.S. recommended [NIOSH and American Conference of Governmental Industrial Hygienists (ACGIH)] and legally enforceable [OSHA, Food and Drug Administration (FDA), and EPA] exposure limits for EtO are listed in Table 1. The more protective NIOSH recommendation is feasibility based, and is achievable by many hospitals at the present time (82). The OSHA limits are risk-assessment based. Due to the widespread occurrence of EtO-associated adverse effects in exposed patients, the FDA has set limits for EtO as well as its two reaction products: ethylene chlorohydrin and ethylene glycol. The EPA regulates EtO as a pesticide contaminant in foodstuffs, as well as an air pollutant and hazardous waste. The EPA is drafting a National Emission Standard for EtO under the Clean Air Act; however, this regulation will affect only commercial sterilization and fumigation plants and not small users such as hospitals. Some state air pollution regulations, however, require abatement of EtO emissions even from small quantity users such as hospitals. Under Superfund and Community Right-to-Know regulations, the EPA has classified EtO as an extremely hazardous substance and requires reporting of EtO use for emergency planning, as well as reporting of any release greater than 10 lbs.

### Primary Prevention

Given the challenges of developing complete replacements for EtO as a sterilant and chemical intermediate, it appears that EtO will remain a potential occupational and environmental hazard for the foreseeable future. Substitutes for EtO as a sterilant are currently being pursued and use reduction opportunities exist; some, but not all, hospital sterilization needs can be met with alternatives, such as peracetic acid or hydrogen peroxide systems (11,102).

The OSHA 1984 EtO standard provides an integrated outline of primary and secondary control measures for EtO exposure. Personal monitoring is required, followed by specific actions on the basis of monitoring results. Employers are also required to develop means to alert employees in event of an EtO leak or spill. Detailed evaluations of the implementation and effectiveness of EtO exposure monitoring and control efforts have recently been conducted (103,104). A recent study of almost all EtO-using Massachusetts hospitals ($n = 92$) showed that most had implemented personal monitoring requirements, but that one-third of hospitals did not have EtO alarms or other means to alert employees during accidental releases (104,105). Personal EtO exposures in the health care setting have dropped steadily since NIOSH and OSHA attention became focused on EtO hazards in the late 1970s (Fig. 1), though exposures above OSHA limits continue to occur widely (103,104). Importantly, the Massachusetts hospital study also revealed that personal monitoring activities have failed to detect the widespread occurrence of accidental exposures during EtO leaks and spills. Although accidental exposures are usually short in duration, they tend to involve high exposure levels at high dose rates and are thus of concern. Quantitative assessments of routine exposures by medical surveillance providers as well as industrial hygienists should therefore be complemented by interviews with workers about accidental exposures and/or the triggering of real-time EtO alarms.

Other primary prevention measures addressed in OSHA's EtO standard include requirements for worker

**TABLE 1.** *United States exposure guidelines and legal limits for EtO*

| Agency | Setting | Title | Exposure limit (units and media) |
|---|---|---|---|
| NIOSH | Occupational | Recommended exposure limits | 0.1 ppm 8 hour TWA in air, 5 ppm 10 minute TWA in air |
| | | Immediately dangerous to life or health | 800 ppm in air |
| ACGIH | Occupational | Threshold limit value | 1 ppm 8 hour TWA in air |
| OSHA | Occupational | Permissible exposure limit | 1 ppm 8 hour TWA in air |
| | | Excursion limit | 5 ppm 15 minute TWA in air |
| FDA | Medical devices | Acceptable contaminant limits | Different limits for various devices: range from 5 ppm in intrauterine devices to 250 ppm in topical devices |
| EPA | Foodstuffs | Tolerance limit | 50 ppm (mg/kg) when used as a postharvest fumigant in raw black walnut meats, copra, and whole or ground spices |

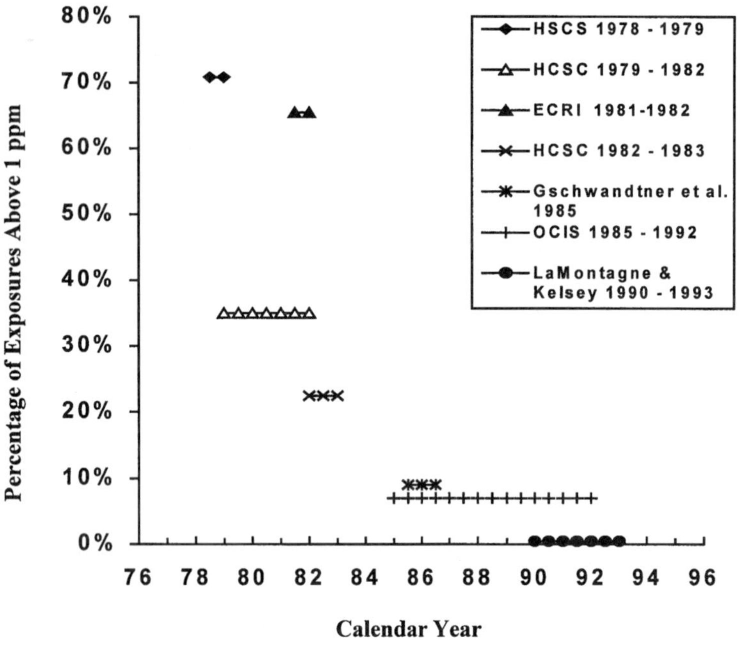


**FIG. 1.** Percentages of work shift average EtO exposures above 1.0 ppm: studies reporting data from more than 10 hospitals. Shown are percentages of exposures above 1 ppm 8-hour time-weighted average *(vertical)* versus calendar year time periods during which samples were collected *(horizontal)*. Data sources: Hospital Council of Southern California (HCSC) (103), Emergency Care Research Institute (ECRI) (103), OSHA's Computerized Information Service (OCIS) (103), Gschwandtner et al. (103a), and LaMontagne and Kelsey (104). (Adapted from ref. 103.)

health and safety training, evacuation procedures, and the use of personal protective equipment, as well as recommendations on the use of effective engineering controls. Numerous excellent practical guides to the prevention and control of EtO hazards are available (4,11,82,106). Under certain exposure and other circumstances, medical surveillance or screening for exposed workers is required.

### Medical Surveillance

Five specific circumstances or triggers in OSHA's EtO standard activate requirements for medical surveillance, and when provided, the standard states that EtO medical surveillance must include at least five components (Table 2). An evaluation of the implementation of EtO medical surveillance in Massachusetts hospitals was conducted in parallel with the exposure studies described above (107,108). Medical surveillance for EtO exposure had been provided one or more times by two-thirds of the 92 hospitals in the study. Roughly one-fourth of the providers surveyed reported observation of EtO-related symptoms or conditions, ranging from mucous membrane irritation to peripheral neuropathy (107). In an analysis of the extent to which OSHA triggers determine EtO surveillance implementation, it was found that the determinants of providing EtO medical surveillance, in order of decreasing magnitude, were accidental EtO releases, the coverage of medical surveillance issues in worker training, and the existence of voluntary, written medical surveillance policies (108). These findings highlight the interdependence of primary and secondary prevention efforts, with important roles to be played by workers, management, and medical surveillance providers. Two-thirds of providers

**TABLE 2.** *Medical surveillance requirements under OSHA's EtO standard*

| Should be provided under any of the following circumstances: | When provided, required EtO medical surveillance must include the following: |
|---|---|
| Exceeding the action level of an 8 hour TWA of 0.5 ppm for 30 or more working days per year | Medical history |
| Exposure in an accidental release | Work/exposure history |
| Observation of symptoms potentially related to EtO exposure | Physical examination with particular emphasis given to the pulmonary, hematologic, neurologic, and reproductive systems, and to the eyes and skin |
| Worker concerns over their ability to parent a healthy child | Complete blood count, with leukocyte differential |
| Before assignment to and after termination from job assignments where exposures may exceed the action level | "Any laboratory or other test which the examining physician deems necessary by sound medical practice"[a] |
| | Pregnancy testing or laboratory evaluation of fertility, "if requested by the employee"[a] |

[a]Quotations are taken from OSHA's Ethylene Oxide Standard, 29 CFR 1910.1047.

reported the performance of all five OSHA-required procedures.

## REFERENCES


1. Reisch MS. Top 50 chemicals production. *Chem Engineer News* 1991; 69:13–14.
2. IARC. Ethylene oxide. In: *IARC monographs on the evaluation of carcinogenic risks to humans, vol 60. Some industrial compounds.* Lyons, France: International Agency for Research on Cancer, World Health Organization, 1994;73–159.
3. ATSDR. *Toxicological profile for ethylene oxide.* Washington, DC: Agency for Toxic Substances and Disease Registry, U.S. Public Health Service, 1990.
4. NIOSH. *Current intelligence bulletin 52:* ethylene oxide sterilizers in health care facilities—engineering controls and work practices. Washington, DC: U.S. Department of Health and Human Services (NIOSH), 1989.
5. NIOSH. *Control technology for ethylene oxide sterilization in hospitals.* Washington, DC: U.S. Department of Health and Human Services (NIOSH), 1989.
6. Quazi AH, Ketchum NH. A new method for monitoring personal exposure to ethylene oxide in the occupational environment. *Am Ind Hyg Assoc J* 1977;38:635–643.
7. Puskar MA, Hecker LH. Field validation of passive dosimeters for the determination of employee exposures to ethylene oxide in hospital product sterilization facilities. *Am Ind Hyg Assoc J* 1989;50:30–36.
8. Steenland K, Stayner L, Greife A, et al. Mortality among workers exposed to ethylene oxide. *N Engl J Med* 1991;324:1402–1407.
9. CalOSHA. *Special studies report:* occupational exposures to ethylene oxide in hospitals, medical products industries, and spice plants. Sacramento: State of California, Department of Industrial Relations, Division of Occupational Safety and Health, 1984.
10. Gschwandtner G. Aeration of respiratory therapy items—Are you really aerating? *J Healthcare Material Manag* 1990:48–51.
11. LaMontagne AD, Kelsey KT, Christiani DC, Plantamura D. *Ethylene oxide health and safety manual:* training and reference materials on the safe use of ethylene oxide in sterilizing facilities, 2nd ed. Braintree, MA: Center for Occupational and Environmental Medicine, Massachusetts Respiratory Hospital, 1990.
12. Bommer J, Ritz E. Ethylene oxide (ETO) as a major cause of anaphylactoid reactions in dialysis (a review). *Artif Organs* 1987;11:111–117.
13. National Toxicology Program. *Ethylene oxide. Seventh annual report on carcinogens 1994:* summary. Washington, DC: National Toxicology Program, U.S. Department of Health and Human Services, Public Health Service, 1994;205–210.
14. Glaser ZR. Ethylene oxide: toxicology review and field study results of hospital use. *J Environ Pathol Toxicol* 1979;2:173–208.
15. WHO. *Environmental health criteria 55:* ethylene oxide. Geneva: World Health Organization, 1985.
16. Landrigan PJ, Meinhardt TJ, Gordon J, et al. Ethylene oxide: and overview of toxicologic and epidemiologic research. *Am J Ind Med* 1984;6:103–115.
17. Jay WM, Swift TR, Hull DS. Possible Relationship of Ethylene Oxide Exposure to Cataract Formation. *Am J Ophthalmol* 1982;93:727–732.
18. Deschamps D, Leport M, Laurent A-M, Cordier S, Festy B, Conso F. Toxicity of ethylene oxide on the lens and on leukocytes: an epidemiological study in hospital sterilisation installations. *Br J Ind Med* 1990;47:308–313.
19. Lynch DW, Lewis TR, Moorman WJ, et al. Effects on monkeys and rats of long-term inhalation exposure to ethylene oxide: major findings of the NIOSH study. In: *Inhospital ethylene oxide sterilization:* current issues in EO toxicity and occupational exposure. AAMI Technology Assessment Report No. 8-84. Arlington, VA: Association for the Advancement of Medical Instrumentation (AAMI), 1984;7–10.
20. Ehrenberg L, Hallstrom T. *Hematologic studies on persons occupationally exposed to ethylene oxide. Radiosterilization of medical products.* Report No. SM-92/96. Vienna: International Atomic Energy Agency, 1967;327–334.
21. LaMontagne AD, Christiani DC, Kelsey KT. Utility of the complete blood count in routine medical surveillance for ethylene oxide exposure. *Am J Ind Med* 1993;24:191–206.
22. Popp DM, Popp RA, Lock S, Mann RC, Hand REJ. Use of multiparamater analysis to quantitate hematological damage from exposure to a chemical (ethylene oxide). *J Toxicol Environ Health* 1986;18: 543–565.
23. Currier MF, Carlo GL, Poston PL, Ledford W. A cross-sectional study of employees with potential occupational exposure to ethylene oxide. *Br J Ind Med* 1984;41:492–498.
24. Van Sittert NJ, de Jong G, Clare MG, et al. Cytogenetic, immunological, and haematological effects in workers in an ethylene oxide manufacturing plant. *Br J Ind Med* 1985;42:19–26.
25. Schulte PA, Walker JT, Boeniger MF, Tsuchiya Y, Halperin WE. Molecular, cytogenetic, and hematologic effects of ethylene oxide on female hospital workers. *J Occup Environ Health* 1995;37:313–320.
26. Zampollo A, Zachetti O, Pisati G. On ethylene oxide neurotoxicity: report of two cases of peripheral neuropathy. *Ital J Neurol Sci* 1984;5: 59–62.
27. Fukushima T, Abe K, Nakagawa A, Osaki Y, Yoshida N, Yamane Y. Chronic ethylene oxide poisoning in a factory manufacturing medical appliances. *J Soc Occup Med* 1986;36:118–123.
28. Gross JA, Hass ML, Swift TR. Ethylene oxide neurotoxicity: report of four cases and review of the literature. *Neurology* 1979;29:978–983.
29. Finelli PF, Morgan TF, Yaar I, Granger CV. Ethylene oxide-induced polyneuropathy: a clinical and electrophysiologic study. *Arch Neurol* 1983;40:419–421.
30. Kuzuhara S, Kanazawa I, Nakanishi T, Egash T. Ethylene oxide polyneuropathy. *Neurology* 1983;33:377–380.
31. De Freitas MR, Nascimento OJ, Chimelli L. [Polyneuropathy caused by ethylene oxide. Report of a case with clinical, electrophysiological and histopathological studies]. *Arq Neuropsiquiatr* 1991;49:460–464.
32. Schroder JM, Hoheneck M, Weis J, Deist H. Ethylene oxide polyneuropathy: clinical follow-up study with morphometric and electron microscopic findings in a sural nerve biopsy. *J Neurol* 1985;232: 83–90.
33. Estrin WJ, Cavalieri SA, Wald P, Becker CE, Jones JR, Cone JE. Evidence of Neurologic Dysfunction Related to Long-Term Ethylene Oxide Exposure. *Arch Neurol* 1987;44:1283–1286.
34. Estrin WJ, Bowler RM, Lash A, Becker CE. Neurotoxicological evaluation of hospital sterilizer workers exposed to ethylene oxide. *Clin Toxicol* 1990;28:1–20.
35. Klees JE, Lash A, Bowler RM, Shore M, Becker CE. Neuropsychologic "impairment" in a cohort of hospital workers chronically exposed to ethylene oxide [see comments]. *J Toxicol Clin Toxicol* 1990;28:21–28.
36. Grober E, Crystal H, Lipton RB, Schaumberg H. EtO is associated with cognitive dysfunction. *J Occup Med* 1992;34:1114–1116.
37. Katzenstein A. Ethylene oxide and CNS dysfunction (letter). *Clin Toxicol* 1991;29:285–288.
38. Dretchen KL, Balter NJ, Schwartz SL, et al. Cognitive dysfunction in a patient with long-term exposure to ethylene oxide: role of ethylene oxide as a causal factor. *J Occup Med* 1992;34:1106–1113.
39. Dellarco VL, Generoso WM, Sega GA, et al. Review of the mutagenicity of ethylene oxide. *Environ Mol Mutagen* 1990;16:85–103.
40. Galloway SM, Berry PK, Nichols WW, et al. Chromosome aberrations in individuals occupationally exposed to ethylene oxide, and in a large control population. *Mutat Res* 1986;170:55–74.
41. Pero RW, Widegren B, Hogstedt B, Mitelman F. In vivo and *in vitro* ethylene oxide exposure of human lymphocytes assessed by chemical stimulation fo unscheduled DNA synthesis. *Mutat Res* 1981;83: 271–289.
42. Sarto F, Cominato I, Pinton AM, et al. Cytogenetic damage in workers exposed to ethylene oxide. *Mutat Res* 1984;138:185–195.
43. Tates AD, Grummt T, Toernqvist M, et al. Biological and chemical monitoring of occupational exposure to ethylene oxide. *Mutat Res* 1991;250:1–2.
44. Thiess AM, Scwegler H, Fleig I, Stocker WG. Mutagenicity study on workers exposed to alkene oxides (ethylene oxide/propylene oxide) and derivatives. *J Occup Med* 1981;23:343–347.
45. Garry VF, Hozier J, Jacobs D, Wade RL, Gray DJ. Ethylene oxide: evidence of human chromosomal effects. *Environ Mutagen* 1979;1: 375–382.
46. Lambert B, Lindblad A. Sister chromatid exchange and chromosome aberrations in lymphocytes of library personnel. *J Toxicol Environ Health* 1980;6:1237–1243.
47. Stolley PD, Soper KD, Galloway SM, et al. Sister chromatid

exchanges in association with occupational exposure to ethylene oxide. *Mutat Res* 1984;129:89–102.
48. Yager JW, Hines CJ, Spear RC. Exposure to ethylene oxide at work increases sister chromatid exchanges in human peripheral lymphocytes. *Science* 1983;219:1221–1223.
49. Schulte PA, Boeniger MF, Walker JT, et al. Biological markers in hospital workers exposed to low levels of ethylene oxide. *Mutat Res* 1992; 278:237–251.
50. Mayer J, Warburton D, Jeffrey AM, et al. Biologic markers in ethylene oxide-exposed workers and controls. *Mutat Res* 1991;248:163–176.
51. Ribeiro LR, Salvadori DF, Rios AC, et al. Biological monitoring of workers occupationally exposed to ethylene oxide. *Mutat Res* 1994; 313:81–87.
52. Popp W, Vahrenholz C, Przygoda H, et al. DNA-protein cross-links and sister chromatid exchange frequencies in lymphocytes and hydroxyethyl mercapturic acid in urine of ethylene oxide-exposed hospital workers. *Int Arch Occup Environ Health* 1994;66:325–332.
53. Walker VE, MacNeela JP, Swenberg JA, Turner MJ Jr, Fennell TR. Molecular dosimetry of ethylene oxide: formation and persistence of N-(2-Hydroxyethyl)valine in hemoglobin following repeated exposures of rats and mice. *Cancer Res* 1992;52:4320–4327.
54. Walker VE, Skopek TR. A mouse model for the study of *in vivo* mutational spectra: sequence specificity of ethylene oxide at the hprt locus. *Mutat Res* 1993;288:151–162.
55. Fuchs J, Wullenweber U, Hengstler JG, Bienfait HG, Hiltl G, Oesch F. Genotoxic risk for humans due to work place exposure to ethylene oxide: remarkable individual differences in susceptibility. *Arch Toxicol* 1994;68:343–348.
56. Lambert B, Andersson B, Bastlova T, Hou S, Hellgren D, Kolman A. Mutations induced in the hypoxanthine phosphoribosyl transferase gene by three urban air pollutants: acetaldehyde, benzo[a]pyrene diolepoxide, and ethylene oxide. *Environ Health Perspect* 1994;102 (suppl):135–138.
57. Hengstler JG, Fuchs J, Gebhard S, Oesch F. Glycolaldehyde causes DNA-protein crosslinks: a new aspect of ethylene oxide genotoxicity. *Mutat Res* 1994;304:229–234.
58. Hogstedt LC. Epidemiological studies on ethylene oxide and cancer: an updating. *IARC Sci Publ* 1988;89:265–270.
59. Snellings WM, Weil CS, Maronpot RR. A two-year inhalation study of the carcinogenic potential of ethylene oxide in Fischer 344 rats. *Toxicol Appl Pharmacol* 1984;75:105–117.
60. Lynch DW, Lewis TR, Moorman WJ, et al. Carcinogenic and toxicologic effects of inhaled ethylene oxide and propylene oxide in F344 rats. *Toxicol Appl Pharmacol* 1984;76:69–84.
61. NTP. *Toxicology and carcinogenesis studies of ethylene oxide in 6C3F1 mice, NTP TR326.* Research Triangle Park, NC, USA: National Toxicology Program, U.S. Department of Health and Human Services, Public Health Service, 1988.
62. Dunkelberg H. Carcinogenicity of ethylene oxide and 1,2-propylene oxide upon intragastric administration to rats. *Br J Cancer* 1982;46: 924–933.
63. Hogstedt C, Malmqvist N, Wadman B. Leukemia in workers exposed to ethylene oxide. *JAMA* 1979;241:1132–1133.
64. Hogstedt C, Aringer L, Gustavsson A. *Ethylene oxide and cancer—review of the literature and follow-up of two studies* (Swedish). *Arbete Halsa* 1984;49:1–32.
65. Hogstedt C, Rohlen O, Berndtsson BS, Axelson O, Ehrenberg L. A cohort study of mortality and cancer incidence in ethylene oxide production workers. *Br J Ind Med* 1979b;36:276–280.
66. Hogstedt C, Aringer L, Gustavsson A. Epidemiologic support for ethylene oxide as a cancer-causing agent. *JAMA* 1986;255:1575–1578.
67. Morgan RW, Claxton KW, Divine BJ, Kaplan SD, Harris VB. Mortality among ethylene oxide workers. *J Occup Med* 1981;23:767–770.
68. EPA. *Health assessment document for ethylene oxide.* Research Triangle Park, NC: U.S. Environ Protection Agency, Office of Research and Development, 1985.
69. Gardner MJ, Coggon D, Pannett B, Harris EC. Workers exposed to ethylene oxide: a follow up study. *Br J Ind Med* 1989;46:860–865.
70. Kiesselbach N, Ulm K, Lange HJ, Korallus U. A multicentre mortality study of workers exposed to ethylene oxide. *Br J Ind Med* 1990;47: 182–188.
71. Thiess AM, Frentzel-Beyme R, Link R, Stocker WG. *Mortality study on workers exposed to alkylene oxides (ethylene oxide/propylene oxide) and their derivatives.* Prevention of Occupational Cancer—International Symposium (Occupational Safety and Health Series No. 46. Geneva: International Labour Office, 1981:249–259.
72. Greenberg HL, Ott MG, Shore RE. Men assigned to ethylene oxide production or other ethylene oxide related chemical manufacturing: a mortality study. *Br J Ind Med* 1990;47:221–230.
73. Teta MJ, Benson LO, Vitale JN. Mortality study of ethylene oxide workers in chemical manufacturing: a 10 year update. *Br J Ind Med* 1993;50:704–709.
74. Benson L, Teta MJ. Mortality due to pancreatic and lymphopoietic cancer in chlorohydrin production workers. *Br J Ind Med* 1993;50: 710–716.
75. Stayner L, Steenland K, Greife A, et al. Exposure-response analysis of cancer mortality in a cohort of workers exposed to ethylene oxide. *Am J Epidemiol* 1993;138:787–798.
76. Wong O, Trent LS. An epidemiological study of workers potentially exposed to ethylene oxide. *Br J Ind Med* 1993;50:308–316.
77. Bisanti L, Maggini M, Raschetti R, et al. Cancer mortality in ethylene oxide workers. *Br J Ind Med* 1993;50:317–324.
78. Hagmar L, Mikoczy Z, Welinder H. Cancer incidence in Swedish sterilant workers exposed to ethylene oxide. *Occup Environ Med* 1995;52: 154–156.
79. Norman SA, Berlin JA, Soper KA, Middendorf BF, Stolley PD. Cancer incidence in a group of workers potentially exposed to ethylene oxide. *Int J Epidemiol* 1995;24:276–284.
80. Major J, Jakab MG, Tompa A. Genotoxicological investigation of hospital nurses occupationally exposed to ethylene-oxide: I. Chromosome aberrations, sister-chromatid exchanges, cell cycle kinetics, and UV-induced DNA synthesis in peripheral blood lymphocytes. *Environ Mol Mutagen* 1996;27:84–92.
81. Shore RE, Gardner MJ, Pannett B. Ethylene oxide: an assessment of the epidemiological evidence on carcinogenicity. *Br J Ind Med* 1993; 50:971–997.
82. Mortimer VD, Kercher SL. *Technical report:* control technology for ethylene oxide sterilization in hospitals. Washington, DC: DHHS (NIOSH), 1989.
83. Florack EI, Zielhuis GA. Occupational ethylene oxide exposure and reproduction. *Int Arch Occup Environ Health* 1990;62:273–277.
84. Anon. Reproductive toxicology and occupational exposure: ethylene oxide. In: Zenz C, Dickerson OB, Horvath EP, eds. *Occupational medicine,* 3rd ed. St. Louis: Mosby, 1994.
85. Generoso WM, Cain KT, Hughes LA, et al. Ethylene oxide dose and dose-rate effects in the mouse dominant-lethal test. *Environ Mutagen* 1986;8:1–7.
86. Generoso WM, Rutledge JC, Cain KT, Hughes LA, Braden PW. Exposure of female mice to ethylene oxide within hours after mating leads to fetal malformation and death. *Mutat Res* 1987;176: 269–274.
87. Sega GA, Owens JG. Binding of ethylene oxide in spermiogenic germ cell stages of the mouse after low-level inhalation exposure. *Environ Mol Mutagen* 1987;10:119–127.
88. Rutledge JC, Generoso WM. Fetal pathology produced by ethylene oxide treatment of the murine zygote. *Teratology* 1989;39:563–572.
89. Rowland AS, Baird DD, Shore DL, Darden B, Wilcox AJ. Ethylene oxide exposure may increase the risk of spontaneous abortion, preterm birth, and postterm birth. *Epidemiology* 1996;7:363–368.
90. Hemminki K, Mutanen P, Saloniemi I, Niemi ML, Vainio H. Spontaneous abortions in hospital staff engaged in sterilizing instruments with chemical agents. *Br Med J* 1982;285:1461–1463.
91. Hemminki K, Kyyronen P, Lindbohm ML. Spontaneous abortions and malformations in the offspring of nurses exposed to anaesthetic gases, cytostatic drugs, and other potential hazards in hospitals, based on registered information of outcome. *J Epidemiol Community Health* 1985;39:141–147.
92. Lindbohm ML, Hemminki K, Bonhomme MG, et al. Effects of paternal occupational exposure on spontaneous abortions. *Am J Public Health* 1991;81:1029–1033.
93. Bommer J, Barth HP, Wilhelms OH, Schindele H, Ritz E. Anaphylactoid reactions in dialysis patients: role of ethylene oxide. *Lancet* 1985: 1382–1384.
94. Grammer LC, Roberts M, Wiggins CA, et al. A comparison of cutaneous testing and ELISA testing for assessing reactivity to ethylene oxide-human serum albumin in hemodialysis patients with anaphylactic reactions. *J Allergy Clin Immunol* 1991;87:674–676.
95. Grammer LC, Patterson R. IgE against ethylene oxide-altered human

serum albumin (ETO-HSA) as an etiologic agent in allergic reactions of hemodialysis patients. *Artif Organs* 1987;11:97–99.
96. Wagner M, Kollorz W. [Occupational medicine studies of 7 ethylene oxide-exposed endoscopy nursing professionals]. *Zentralbl Bakteriol Mikrobiol Hyg [B]* 1987;185:154–163.
97. Deschamps D, Rosenberg N, Soler P, et al. Persistent asthma after accidental exposure to ethylene oxide. *Br J Ind Med* 1992;49:523–525.
98. Dugue P, Faraut C, Figueredo M, Bettendorf A, Salvadori JM. Ethylene oxide-related occupational asthma in a nurse (in French). *La Presse Med* 1991;20:1455 .
99. Jacson F, Beaudouin E, Hotton J, Moneret-Vautrin DA. Allergy to formaldehyde, latex, and ethylene oxide: triple occupational allergy in a nurse (in French). *Rev Fr Allergol* 1991;31:41–43.
99a. Verraes S, Michel O. Occupational asthma induced by ethylene oxide. *Lancet* 1995;346:1434–1435.
100. OSHA. Occupational exposure to ethylene oxide: final standard. *Federal Register* 1984;49:25734–25809.
101. OSHA. Occupational exposure to ethylene oxide;final standard. *Federal Register* 1988;53:11414–11438.
102. CHEM. Does EtO have a future in hospitals? *Healthcare Hazardous Materials Manag* 1994;7:1–6.
103. Meridian Research Inc. *Ethylene oxide:* a case study in hazard identification, *OSHA regulation, and market response. Final report.* Silver Spring, MD: Submitted to Office of Program Evaluation, OSHA, by Meridian Research, Inc., 1992.
103a. Gschwandtner GD, Kruger D, Harman P. Compliance with the EtO standard in the United States. *Healthcare Material Manag* 1986; Nov/Dec:38–41.
104. LaMontagne AD, Kelsey KT. Evaluating OSHA's ethylene oxide standard: employer exposure monitoring activities in Massachusetts hospitals from 1985–1993. *Am J Public Health* 1997;87(7):1119–1125.
105. LaMontagne AD, Needleman C. Overcoming practical challenges in intervention research in occupational health and safety. *Am J Ind Med* 1996;29:367–372.
106. IPCS. *Ethylene oxide health and safety guide:* health and safety guide, no. 16. Geneva: World Health Organization, 1985.
107. LaMontagne AD, Mangione TW, Christiani DC, Kelsey KT. Medical surveillance for ethylene oxide exposure: practices and clinical findings in Massachusetts hospitals. *J Occup Environ Med* 1996;38:144–154.
108. LaMontagne AD, Rudd RE, Mangione TW, Kelsey KT. Determinants of the provision of ethylene oxide medical surveillance in Massachusetts hospitals. *J Occup Environ Med* 1996;38:155–168.

*Environmental and Occupational Medicine,*
*Third Edition,* edited by William N. Rom.
Lippincott–Raven Publishers, Philadelphia © 1998.

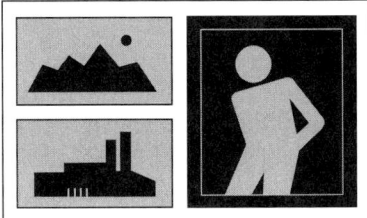

CHAPTER 83

# Pesticides

Marc B. Schenker, Samuel Louie, Louise N. Mehler, and Timothy E. Albertson

Pesticides are biocidal agents used to control a wide variety of organisms that pose a threat to health or compete for food or other materials (Table 1). Selective toxicity is the principle of pesticide use, but because organisms are similar at the cellular or subcellular level, adverse human health effects may occur.

The earliest pesticides included metals such as arsenic, mercury, and lead. Other pesticides are inorganic chemicals, such as sulfur, and organic chemicals, such as nicotine derived from plants. After the discovery of dichlorodiphenyltrichloroethane (DDT) in 1939, the world has witnessed an unprecedented increase in the search for and production of synthetic organic pesticides. Production of inorganic pesticides such as arsenicals has steadily declined since the 1940s. The prolonged ecologic half-life and lack of species selectivity of DDT and other organochlorine pesticides was recognized in the 1960s. These pesticide characteristics and concern about the effects of accumulation of organochlorines in human adipose tissue caused the banning or severe restriction of most of these agents in the United States. In their place, newer synthetic pesticides, predominantly organophosphorus compounds, have been developed and are now widely used. These agents cause less environmental damage through accumulation but are more acutely toxic to humans and other animal species.

The manufacture, distribution, and handling of pesticides in the United States is regulated under the Federal Insecticide, Fungicide, and Rodenticide Act (FIFRA). The act, administered by the Environmental Protection Agency (EPA), was passed in 1947 and has been amended several times. There are approximately 600 active pesticides ingredients, configured in more than 45,000 formulations in use today. United States production is just over 1 billion pounds of active ingredients, and worldwide approximately 4 billion pounds of pesticides are used in agriculture as well as in most household gardens today. More ominously, toxic organophosphates such as the nerve gas sarin have been used by terrorists to attack large numbers of people in cities in Japan (1).

**TABLE 1.** *Categories of pesticide agents and target organisms*

| Pesticide | Target |
|---|---|
| Acaricide | Mites |
| Algicide | Algae |
| Avicide | Birds |
| Bactericide | Bacteria |
| Defoliant | Leaves |
| Fungicide | Fungi |
| Herbicide | Weeds |
| Insecticide | Insects |
| Molluscide | Snails |
| Nematicide | Nematodes |
| Piscicide | Fish |
| Rodenticide | Rodents |

M. B. Schenker: Department of Epidemiology and Preventive Medicine, University of California, Davis, Davis, California 95616-8638.

S. Louie: Division of Pulmonary and Critical Care Medicine, Department of Internal Medicine, University of California, Davis, Davis, California 95616.

L. N. Mehler: California Pesticide Illness Surveillance Program, University of California, Davis, Davis, California 95616.

T. E. Albertson: Division of Pulmonary Critical Care Medicine, University of California, Davis, Davis, California 95616.

## EXPOSURE

### Environmental

Adverse effects of pesticides in the environment first received widespread attention in the 1960s with the publication of Rachel Carson's *Silent Spring* (2). Biomagnification of organochlorine compounds in the food chain lead to high residues, particularly in predaceous fish and birds. Elevated levels of DDT (and to a lesser degree, dieldrin) in several species of birds of prey lead to eggshell thinning and threatened species extinction. Because organochlorine compounds are not species-specific, large populations of animal species may be at risk of poisoning, which can lead to deleterious, long-term changes in the diversity of ecosystems in nature. Furthermore, pest species may develop increased tolerance or resistance to these specific pesticide compounds. Organochlorines have been largely replaced by organophosphates and carbamate compounds that rapidly hydrolyze in soil and by plants. Although organophosphates and carbamates do not accumulate significantly in the environment, they remain extremely toxic if used indiscriminately.

Environmental exposures to pesticides in humans most often result from household or garden use. The World Health Organization (WHO) has estimated that more than 3 million cases of serious acute pesticide or insecticide poisoning occur worldwide annually, the majority being caused by organophosphates used for agriculture (3). There are an estimated 220,000 deaths annually from pesticides, and 99% of these are in developing countries (3). This grim total occurs despite the fact that only 20% to 25% of the global agrochemical use is in developing countries. The easy availability of pesticides in many developing countries makes them a common means of suicides.

In 1995, there were 67,159 insecticide poisonings in the United States reported to the American Association of Poison Control Centers (4). About 90% of homes in the United States use pesticides, and exposure results from misuse or accident (5). Other environmental exposures may occur from water, air, or food. Low concentrations of pesticides have been detected in some groundwater sources, though these are not thought to pose serious health risks to the population at levels detected at this time (6).

Tolerance levels for pesticide residues in foods, the maximum residue levels allowed when pesticides are used according to the directions on the label, are set by the EPA. The levels are based on toxicologic studies that attempt to balance the risks and benefits associated with the use of pesticides on human foodstuffs (7).

Even though there is increasing public concern about pesticide residues in the food supply (e.g., Alar, a growth regulator, on apple crops), residues detected in fresh and processed foods are generally low. The Food and Drug Administration (FDA) tests a subsample of food shipments for pesticide residues; only a small percentage are found to have levels above tolerances, and most samples have no detectable residue. The FDA also conducts the Total Diet Study, testing supermarket food items considered to represent the diet of U.S. consumers. Results from these analyses indicate that in general the dietary intake of pesticide residues is within acceptable tolerance. When pesticides are used on crops for which their use is not approved or are applied in an unapproved manner, however, outbreaks of food-borne pesticide illness may occur. This was the case with the outbreak caused by aldicarb-contaminated watermelons in the western United States (8).

The EPA conducted the National Human Adipose Tissue Survey annually beginning in 1969 to monitor levels of organochlorine pesticides, polychlorinated biphenyls (PCBs), and a few other compounds in tissues collected during surgery or at autopsy. These substances tend to bioaccumulate in adipose tissue, providing an excellent medium for detecting prevalence of exposure over a long period and body burden. Detectable residues of most of these compounds are found in a large proportion of tissue samples but in very low concentrations. This program was valuable in documenting time trends in body burdens; for example, levels of DDT and its metabolites and levels of PCBs decreased from the early 1970s, reflecting decreased use in the United States (9,10).

### Occupational

Humans are exposed to pesticides in a variety of occupational settings, including agriculture, structural pest control (e.g., buildings), public health pest eradication programs, manufacture and formulation, transportation industries such as railroads and trucking, the florist industry, and hazardous waste treatment and cleanup. Many commercial products such as paints, cotton, and wood products have fungicides added to prevent degeneration. Herbicides are used heavily in maintaining roads and highways in developed countries.

Assessing exposure to pesticides in an occupational setting is a complex task. A worker may be exposed unknowingly to clothing saturated with pesticides or by direct skin contact, but these amounts do not necessarily predict the actual dose, or amount absorbed into the body. Absorption may occur through inhalation, ingestion, or direct absorption on dermal surfaces. Detailed information on rates of absorption and knowledge of the pharmacokinetics of the compound in humans is often unavailable. Relating the absorbed dose to human health effects is often difficult or impossible. Work on biologic markers of pesticides may improve assessment of exposure and dose (11).

Accurate data do not exist on the incidence of acute illnesses secondary to pesticide poisoning, and even less is known about the chronic effects of pesticide exposure. While most acute pesticide-related illnesses and deaths in the past were caused by accidental agricultural exposure or attempted suicides, toxicologists and clinicians today must be alert to the illicit use of pesticides for criminal or militant activities. Health care providers must be able to recognize the immediate health effects of pesticides to establish diagnosis quickly and to begin treatment early. The number of deaths caused by pesticide poisoning in the United States is small, but acute pesticide-related illnesses are common. For example, in California, where pesticide-related illnesses are reportable, some 2,500 to 3,000 suspected pesticide illness are reported annually, of which half occur in agriculture. Worldwide estimates for pesticide poisoning suggest the problem of acute toxicity and death is much greater in developing countries than in developed ones (3).

## IMMEDIATE HEALTH EFFECTS

### Organophosphate Insecticides

Millions of pounds of organophosphate pesticides are used worldwide in commercial farming, gardening, structural pest management, and vector control programs. The development of these agents derive from the search for new chemical warfare or nerve gas agents in the 1930s. Although the organophosphate nerve agents such as sarin, tabun, and VX have not been used as insecticides, further research has shown that related, less potent compounds can be used successfully as insecticides (Fig. 1). The worldwide use of these organophosphates compounds has increased over the last 20 years, owing to increased use in the Third World and because their use results in less severe environmental impacts than the organochlorine insecticides. Because the organophosphate insecticides are less detrimental to the environment, they have largely replaced the organochlorine insecticides.

Examples of organophosphate insecticides include parathion, chlorfenvinphos, diazinon, fenthion, diamethoate, monocrotophos, and malathion. These insecticides are commonly used in commercial farming, home gardening, pest control (e.g., flies), environmental control of vectors (e.g., mosquitoes), and the control of ectoparasites (e.g., fleas, lice). They may be combined with one or more other types of insecticides to potentiate their insecticidal action.

Organophosphate insecticides are efficiently absorbed by inhalation, ingestion, and skin penetration (12,13). Exposure by all three routes has been seen in occupational poisonings. The degree of toxicity varies considerably, depending on the route of exposure, and the exposure concentration and dose. Organophosphate insecticides vary in potency. For example, the median lethal dose ($LD_{50}$) for parathion in humans is estimated to be 3 mg/kg while that of malathion is 1,375 mg/kg.

The toxic manifestations of organophosphate insecticides result from the irreversible phosphorylation of the enzyme acetylcholinesterase (AchE) found at the nerve-nerve synapse or nerve-muscle motor end plate where anionic binding of acetylcholine normally occurs (14). The loss of function of this enzyme allows flooding of the postsynaptic receptors with acetylcholine, leading to a cholinergic crisis in severe cases (15).

#### *Acute Signs and Symptoms*

Patients acutely intoxicated with organophosphates often present with a set of signs and symptoms. Recognition of these "toxidromes" helps the astute clinician establish the chemical class of the toxicant quickly and allow vital treatment to begin early. All too often, the clinician has only a history of exposure or a toxidrome to suggest organophosphate insecticide poisoning. The dramatic accounts of the Matsumoto sarin attack in 1994 and the notorious Tokyo subway sarin attack in 1995 should serve as valuable lessons to emergency room and hospital staff and prompt simulated disaster drills to prepare health care providers (1).

The organophosphate insecticide toxidrome can develop during the chemical exposure or be delayed some 4 to 12 hours after exposure. The key aspects of this toxidrome can be divided into muscarinic, nicotinic, and central nervous system overstimulation. Muscarinic overstimulation leads to hyperactivity of the parasympathetic system, including miosis, bradycardia, and hypersecretion of salivary, lacrimal, digestive, and bronchial glands. Accumulation of acetylcholine at the nicotinic synapses leads to blockade of nerve impulses in the central nervous system, at the autonomic ganglia, and at the skeletal muscle-nerve junction. The latter effects leads to motor end plate dysfunction (16). Nicotinic effects include muscle fasciculations that can be mistaken for seizure, cramps, and generalized muscle weakness. Depression of respiratory drive, delirium, loss of consciousness, and seizures are complications of central nervous system toxicity (12,17–21) (Table 2). The mnemonic DUMBELS (diarrhea, urination, miosis, bronchospasm, emesis, lacrimation, salivation) describes the signs of cholinergic (muscarinic) excess seen with organophosphate poisoning. A garlic odor may also be noted from the exposed patient or from the container of the pesticide. Recent data have suggested visual changes, pancreatitis, and psychiatric findings are seen with acute organophosphate poisoning more commonly than previously recognized (22–25).

Establishing a diagnosis from acute or chronic low-dose exposure is particularly difficult in children. The typical muscarinic and nicotinic signs and symptoms of an acute organophosphate poisoning are often absent. Patients may present with neurobehavorial changes, hypertonicity, and even acute psychosis. To establish a preliminary diagnosis, clinicians should be aware that reliable reference laboratories are capable of detecting alkylphosphate metabolites of organophosphates in urine, but the time necessary for this assay may limit its clinical usefulness (26).

Certain organophosphate insecticides have been associated with delayed and intermediate neurotoxicity syn-

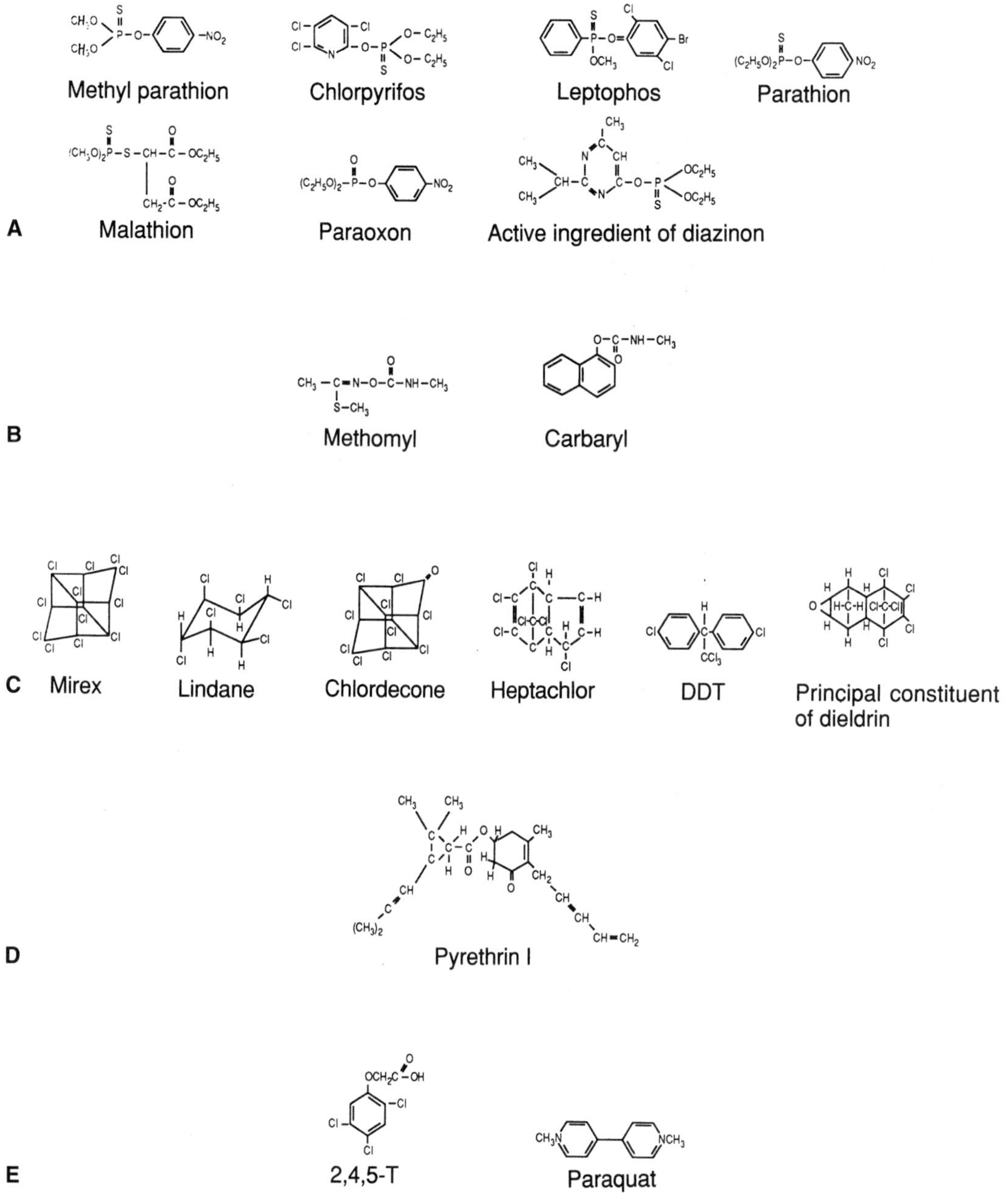


**FIG. 1.** Chemical structure of some key classes of pesticides: organophosphate insecticides **(A)**, carbamate insecticides **(B)**, organochlorine insecticides **(C)**, pyrethroid insecticides **(D)**, and herbicides **(E)**.

dromes (27–30). Characteristic manifestations include weakness, paralysis, and paresthesias in the distal lower extremities for the delayed syndrome, and weakness of proximal limb muscles and muscles of respiration, and cranial nerve paralysis in the intermediate syndrome. Development of the delayed neuropathy is not associated with inhibition of neural or neuromuscular cholinesterases, as is the acute toxicity. It has been correlated with initial phosphorylation or inhibition of the neurotoxic esterase enzyme (NTE) (31,32). Symptoms usually occur within 2 to 3 weeks, with a denervation electromyographic pattern and a progressively irreversible to slowly reversible course over 6 to 12 months. The intermediate syndrome associated with organophosphate neurotoxicity was recently described in

**TABLE 2.** *The toxidrome of acute organophosphate and carbamate insecticide poisoning*

| | |
|---|---|
| Central nervous system | |
| | Salivation[a] |
| | Incontinence[a] |
| | Convulsions[a] |
| | Headache |
| | Psychosis with delirium |
| | Nausea |
| | Dizziness |
| | Restlessness with anxiety |
| | Unconsciousness |
| Musculoskeletal system | |
| | Sweating[a] |
| | Muscle twitching with fasciculations[a] |
| | Weakness |
| | Incoordination |
| | Tremor |
| | Paralysis |
| Gastrointestinal system | |
| | Diarrhea[a] |
| | Vomiting |
| | Abdominal cramps |
| | Acute pancreatitis |
| Vision | |
| | Meiosis[a] |
| | Blurred vision |
| | Tearing |
| | Ocular pain |
| | Conjunctival injection |
| Respiratory system | |
| | Rhinorrhea[a] |
| | Pulmonary edema[a] |
| | Bronchorrhea[a] |
| | Wheezing and chest tightness[a] |
| | Respiratory muscle paralysis |
| Cardiovascular system | |
| | Bradycardia (parasympathetic stimulation)[a] |
| | Sinus arrest |
| | Early tachycardia (sympathetic ganglia stimulation) |
| | Early hypertension (sympathetic ganglia stimulation) |

[a]Key aspects of symptom complex or toxidrome.

10 patients (27). The time of onset was between 1 and 4 days after significant organophosphate insecticide poisoning, with proximal limb, neck, cranial, and respiratory muscle involvement. The electromyogram (EMG) findings were described as tetanic fade. Recovery took between 4 and 18 days; seven of ten patients had respiratory difficulty and four of ten required mechanical ventilation. Most commonly, both delayed and intermediate neurotoxicity have been seen in survivors of massive organophosphate insecticide poisonings coming from Third World countries (29). Prolonged effects of muscle blocker agents have been reported in patients poisoned by organophosphate pesticides (33,34). Persistence of organophosphates measured in blood and in tissues at autopsy in humans has been demonstrated particularly for the most lipid soluble agents such as penthion and methidathion (35). The intermediate syndrome may represent delayed organophosphate absorption or prolonged tissue half-life.

### *Laboratory Findings*

Confirmatory laboratory tests include measurements of plasma and red blood cell (RBC) cholinesterase activities, which provide a measure of the inhibition of two types of cholinesterase enzymes *in vivo*. However, these studies may be available in a limited number of diagnostic laboratories in addition to regional poison control centers. At least six different methods are available for measuring RBC and plasma cholinesterase levels. Consequently, interlaboratory variability may be great and this variability may complicate the interpretation of results (36).

Plasma cholinesterase (pseudocholinesterase) is produced by the liver. It is a phase-reactant enzyme with baseline fluctuations due to many variables. Falsely lowered activity may be due to chronic or acute liver disease, chronic alcoholism, pregnancy, malnutrition, dermatomyositis, or concomitant poisoning with carbon disulfide and organic mercury compounds. Plasma cholinesterase levels decline and return faster than RBC or "true" cholinesterase levels. The 3% of the population who are genetically deficient in this enzyme are particularly vulnerable to the neuromuscular blocker succinylcholine and may be hypersensitive to organophosphate insecticides (37). Regeneration of activity is normally related to synthesis by the liver of new enzymes and may take 7 to 60 days to return to levels found prior to organophosphate insecticide exposure. RBC cholinesterase activity regenerates even more slowly because new RBCs must be released from the bone marrow to replace those with inactivated cholinesterase enzyme (38). This slow rate of renewal (0.5% to 1% per day) can take 60 to 90 days for RBC cholinesterase levels to return to nearly baseline values.

Red blood cell cholinesterase is the preferred measurement for documenting exposure and monitoring when exposed workers can return to handling organophosphate insecticides. Generally, RBC cholinesterase levels should be greater than 75% of baseline before workers are allowed to return.

Sensitive blood and urine screens for the parent organophosphate insecticide compounds and excreted metabolites exist but they are not routinely available and often require detailed knowledge of the specific parent compound (11).

Symptoms of organophosphate insecticide toxicity are not usually seen until 50% of baseline cholinesterase activity is inhibited, although this is not a reliable threshold. The large variability in normal cholinesterase level also makes its interpretation difficult. Cases of poisoning and even deaths have been reported with depressions of less than 50%. Cholinesterase level is useful in clinical evaluation, but it must be done in association with a careful history and physical examination. Because baseline plasma cholinesterase levels are not usually available for an individual patient, serial determinations are useful in acute exposures. No clearly reliable association has been established between the magnitude of serum cholinesterase decrease and the severity of poisoning; it is simply a marker of organophosphate intoxication or poisoning. Nevertheless, most authorities consider mild exposure with minimal signs and symptoms to be associated with plasma cholinesterase levels 20% to 50% of baseline. Moderate exposure, usually resulting in muscle fasiculations and miosis, is associated with plasma cholinesterase levels of 10% to 20% of baseline. Severe poisoning with life-threatening symptoms is associated with plasma cholinesterase levels of 0% to 10% of baseline. Some authors reported that prolonged severe depression of plasma cholinesterase has been associated with poor clinical outcomes after organophosphate poisoning (35).

However, survival has been reported with extremely low plasma cholinesterase levels, leading some investigators to suggest that serum cholinesterase levels have no prognostic value in acute organophosphate poisoning. Identifying high-risk patients based on this enzyme measurement alone is not always reliable (39).

Leukocytosis with a leftward shift toward polymorphic neutrophils, hyperglycemia, ketoacidosis, glycosuria, albuminuria, and acetonuria have been reported with organophosphate poisoning, but these findings are not specific or sensitive enough for diagnostic purposes. Hyperamylasemia and other evidence of acute pancreatitis, such as computed tomographic imaging of the pancreas, have been reported following organophosphate poisoning. Recognition and appropriate therapy of acute pancreatitis when evident may lead to a better prognosis (23,25).

Large, short-term doses of organophosphates insecticides have resulted in prominent electroencephalographic (EEG) changes and convulsions in humans and other primates. Studies have shown long-term (1 to 6 years) spectral shifts in beta voltage in sarin-exposed primates or accidentally exposed workers with serial EEG determinations. The usefulness, both in terms of specificity and sensitivity, of these EEG findings in the diagnosis of organophosphate poisoning has not been established (40). Cardiac toxicity can manifest as intraventricular conduction abnormalities, atrial dysrhythmias, and repetitive ventricular tachycardia such as torsades de pointes (41).

### *Treatment*

The decision to treat a possible organophosphate poisoning is often based only on the history and physical examination findings. Initial management is directed at protecting and maintaining an open airway with respiratory support, including airway suctioning, endotracheal intubation, and mechanical ventilation with supplemental oxygen. Because organophosphates insecticides can easily cross the skin barrier, they pose a particularly insidious threat of secondary contamination to unprotected health care providers and emergency department personnel. Patients who arrive at an emergency department without having had appropriate decontamination should be decontaminated with large amounts of soap and water. Removing clothing potentially saturated with organophosphates is particularly important for both patient and health care provider. Clothing and other contaminated materials must be discarded as highly contaminated waste. Even waste water from field or hospital decontamination must be handled carefully. Gastric decontamination with lavage followed by repeated doses of activated charcoal is indicated for enteric exposure and can reduce total and continued organophosphate exposure. Hemoperfusion removes only minimal amounts of the organophosphate insecticides (35).

For acutely ill patients, atropine sulfate in doses sufficient to reverse cholinergic (muscarinic) signs and symptoms is the primary pharmacologic treatment. A specific dose limit or an arbitrary dose goal is not practical. Careful titration with atropine while monitoring reversal of excessive parasympathetic stimulation is the standard of care. Initial doses of 0.4 to 2.0 mg atropine intravenously (IV) are given every 15 minutes until evidence of "atropinization" or muscarinic blockade, such as flushing, dry mouth, dilated pupils, and tachycardia, is seen (12). Repeated doses or continuous infusion of atropine to maintain partial muscarinic blockade is needed. Evidence of cholinergic excess, including miosis, nausea, bradycardia, is used to govern atropine doses for several hours to days, depending on the severity of the organophosphate poisoning. Caution must be exercised when treating children with large doses of premixed atropine sulfate because large amounts of preservatives (e.g., alcohols) used to increase the shelf life of the drug can be toxic. Consultation with a pharmacist should allow formulation of a high-dose atropine sulfate solution that is preservative-free. Other anticholinergic agents such as glycopyrrolate have been shown to be as effective as atropine in the treatment of organophosphate poisoning (42).

Pralidoxime (Protopam, 2-PAM) is a cholinesterase reactivator available in the United States that effectively reverses the phosphorylation of the RBC and neural cholinesterase enzyme when given within 24 to 48 hours of exposure. Other oximes that act in the same manner are available in Europe. Although it is generally accepted that oximes are important in the treatment of organophosphate poisonings, some reports have rejected their usefulness (43). The sooner 2-PAM is given, the better the chances for cholinesterase reactivation. Pralidoxime is used in cases of moderate to severe organophosphate poisoning. Although 2-PAM can mitigate nicotinic and muscarinic effects of organophosphate poisoning, its actions will vary. It must usually be used concurrently with atropine sulfate. A dose of 1.0 to 2.0 g 2-PAM (20 to 50 mg/kg for children) is administered IV over 30 minutes (12). Rapid injection can cause tachycardia, laryngeal spasm, muscle rigidity, transient neuromuscular blockade, and respiratory arrest (44). Giving repeated doses of 2-PAM at intervals of 2 to 12 hours or by constant IV infusion should be considered. Keeping plasma pralidoxime concentrations above 4 mg/L, the minimum plasma concentration required for therapeutic efficacy, is recommended (45). In a recent study, loading doses of 4 mg/kg of 2-PAM followed by 3.2 mg/kg/hour kept plasma levels above 4 mg/L (45). The final decision is governed by the severity of the poisoning symptoms (46–48). Seizures may not respond to atropine and 2-PAM. These patients have been treated with IV diazepam or barbiturates. The use of IV diazepam has also been effective in the treatment of severe muscle fasciculations. Protection of the airway, aggressive control of seizures, mechanical ventilatory support if necessary, early use of 2-PAM, and titration of atropine to effect are the keys to successful treatment of severe organophosphate pesticide poisoning.

### N-Methyl Carbamates Insecticides

The carbamates, like the organophosphates, are used in commercial farming, home gardening, and control of domestic animal ectoparasites. Aldicarb, oxamyl, and methomyl are highly toxic carbamate insecticides; dioxacarb, carbaryl, and isoprocarb are less toxic. The carbamate insecticides are often used in combination with an organophosphate or pyrethroid insecticide.

Carbamate insecticides are readily absorbed by inhalation or ingestion or through the skin. The *N*-methyl carbamate esters cause reversible inhibition of acetylcholinesterase. As in the case of organophosphates, postsynaptic cholinergic receptors are flooded with acetylcholine, resulting in a characteristic toxidrome. Unlike the phosphorylated enzyme, the carbamylated acetylcholinesterase enzyme can undergo spontaneous hydrolysis *in vivo*, which reactivates the enzyme. Less severe toxidromes of shorter duration can be expected from carbamate poisoning because of this hydrolysis.

#### *Acute Signs and Symptoms*

The diagnosis of carbamate poisoning is generally made by history and clinical presentation of the patient. The clinical toxidrome of carbamate poisoning is similar to that of organophosphates (Table 2). Symptoms typically develop within 15 minutes to 2 hours after exposure and usually last less than 24 hours. Central nervous system toxicity is less predominant because the *N*-methyl carbamates do not penetrate the blood-brain barrier well. However, carbamate poisoning in children was recently found to have a greater depressant effect on the central nervous system when compared to organophosphates (49). The cause of death is often acute respiratory failure from respiratory muscle fatigue, pulmonary edema, bronchorrhea, and bronchospasm. Central nervous system depression, seizures, and ventricular arrhythmias also increase morbidity and mortality (50). Carbamate insecticide poisoning has been responsible for causing trauma-related deaths and injuries (51). When dealing with farm injuries, the clinician must consider the possibility of occult pesticide poisoning.

#### *Laboratory Findings*

Plasma and RBC cholinesterase enzyme measurements are less useful in cases of carbamate poisoning. Symptomatic patients whose blood samples are drawn within a few hours of exposure and absorption can exhibit depressed cholinesterase levels if the enzyme measurement is done rapidly. Enzyme reactivation can occur *in vitro* as well as *in vivo*, causing a rise in the enzyme activity before measurement, which makes clinical interpretation extremely difficult. Urine and blood analyses for parent compounds and metabolites have been described but are not often available (52). A radioimmunoassay has been described for carbamate insecticides that may resolve these problems if the assay becomes commercially available.

#### *Treatment*

Symptomatic treatment of the patient poisoned by carbamate insecticide includes aggressive respiratory support and atropine to reverse severe muscarinic manifestations. Because of the shorter duration of effect from *in vivo* hydrolysis, atropine treatment is usually required for less than 24 hours. The most important difference in treatment for carbamate and organophosphate poisoning involves 2-PAM. The use of 2-PAM is relatively contraindicated in carbamate poisoning because it may enhance acetylcholinesterase inactivation. After mixed or combined exposures involving both organophosphates and carbamate insecticides or in severe poisonings with an unidentified anticholinesterase agent, it is reasonable to administer 2-PAM cautiously (12).

### Organochlorine Insecticides

Most of the organochlorine pesticides have been banned in the United States, principally because of their long ecologic half-lives. Organochlorine insecticides can be classified by chemical structure (Table 3). Lindane ($\gamma$-hexachlorocyclohexane), currently the most commonly encountered organochlorine insecticide, will be used as the prototype compound for discussing acute toxicity. It is available as a garden spray, structural and environmental pest control product, and as a scabicide (Kwell). The mechanism of toxicity is related to the ability of the

**TABLE 3.** *Classification of organochlorine insecticides*

| Class | Brand names |
|---|---|
| Dichlorodiphenylethanes | Anofex, Neocid |
| DDT(1,1,1-trichloro-2,2-bis-(*p*-chlorophenyl)ethane | |
| DDD(1,1,-dichloro-2,2-bis-(*p*-chlorophenyl)ethane | Rothane |
| Dicofol | Keithane |
| Methoxychlor | Marlate |
| Hexachlorocyclohexanes | |
| Lindane (τ-hexaclorocyclohexane) | Kwell, τ-BHC, |
| Isotox | |
| Benzene hexachloride (mixed isomers) | BHC |
| Cyclodienes | |
| Endrin | Hexadrin |
| Aldrin | Aldrite, Drinox |
| Endosulfan | Thiodan |
| Dieldrin | Dieldrite |
| Toxaphene | Toxakil, Strobane-T |
| Heptachlor | Heptagram |
| Chlordane | Chlordan |
| Others | |
| Chlordecone | Kepone |
| Mirex | Dechlorane |

**TABLE 4.** *Organochlorine pesticide poisoning toxidrome*

| |
|---|
| Sensory disturbances, hyperesthesia of face and extremities, paresthesia of face and extremities |
| Headache |
| Dizziness |
| Nausea and vomiting |
| Motor disturbances, muscle, weakness, incoordination, slurred speech, tremor, myoclonic jerking, involuntary eye movements |
| Mental confusion |
| Generalized tonic-clonic convulsions |
| Coma and respiratory depression |

organochlorine to alter ion fluxes, principally in nerve tissue. Although its use is decreasing, it continues to be a source of human poisoning (53,54). Evidence suggests that lindane produces antagonism of γ-aminobutyric acid–mediated inhibition in the central nervous system.

Organochlorine insecticides are easily absorbed through the lungs, gastrointestinal tract, and skin. As much as 10% of a topical dose of lindane is systemically absorbed. Because of the relatively large surface area–to–body weight ratio of infants, lindane poisoning has been reported to result from repeated therapeutic doses of lindane scabicide shampoo. The organochlorine insecticides are metabolized slowly and are excreted principally in the feces. Lindane accumulates in organs, including fat and tissue, but to a lesser extent than many of the other organochlorine insecticide. Lindane excretion takes several days, whereas most other organochlorine insecticides have much longer elimination half-lives. Lindane is partially dechlorinated and oxidized, yielding a series of conjugated chlorophenols and other oxidation products in the urine. Many of the organochlorine insecticides, including lindane and mirex, are capable of inducing liver microsomal enzymes, e.g., cytochrome P-450–dependent monooxygenase system.

### *Immediate Signs and Symptoms*

The neural excitation caused by the organochlorine insecticides leads to their primary toxic manifestations (Table 4). The toxidrome includes disturbances of sensation, coordination, and mental status. Anorexia, malaise, headaches, myoclonic jerking, lethargy, tremor, hyperreflexia, motor hyperexcitability, oral paresthesia after ingestion, and convulsions of organochlorine pesticides have been associated with increased myocardial irritability and cardiac arrhythmias (55,56). Lindane has been rarely associated with aplastic anemia, agranulocytosis, disseminated intravascular coagulation, and proximal myopathy with myoglobinuria (57,58). A singular case of self-poisoning with 1.0 ml of intravenous thiodan resulted in refractory grand mal seizures, increased liver enzyme levels, and acute rhabdomyolysis leading to proximal myopathy and acute renal failure. Motor seizures were controlled with IV midazolam and thiopentone. Both liver and renal dysfunction resolved with supportive ICU care. Hemodialysis was not required. The patient experienced a full recovery (54).

### *Laboratory Findings*

Blood, tissue, and urine determinations of organochlorine pesticides and their metabolites are available from a limited number of laboratories. These levels are rarely useful in the clinical management of acute poisoning. The relatively rapid metabolism of lindane compared to many of the other organochlorine insecticides reduces the likelihood that the parent compound or metabolites will be detected in body fat, blood, urine, or human milk. Other organochlorine pesticides and their metabolites, such as DDT, dieldrin, mirex, and chlordecone, can remain in blood and tissue (particularly fat) for weeks or months. Persons exposed to lindane long-term at work have had fat-to-serum concentration ratios of 220:1 (59). Workers exposed to lindane had whole blood lindane levels of 0.02 to 0.45 ppm (60,61). Symptoms are unlikely in patients with whole blood lindane levels as high as 20 to 30 ppm (62). EEG abnormalities have been noted after brief or long-term organochlorine exposure (63).

### *Treatment*

Gastrointestinal decontamination with activated charcoal should be used for acute oral poisoning with organochlorine pesticides. For any exposure, skin decontamination and removal of contaminated clothing is essential. Treatment of convulsions may require ventilatory support and anticonvulsants such as diazepam, phenobarbital, or phenytoin. The organic solvents used to dispense organochlorine insecticides may result in aspiration pneumonitis and even acute respiratory failure. Because of the very long half-life of some organochlorine insecticides, e.g., chlordecone, the resin cholestyramine (3 to 8 g four times daily) has been shown to disrupt enterohepatic recirculation and significantly reduce the total body half-life of these insecticides (64). Cholestyramine has been advocated in the treatment of lindane poisoning (64). Repeated doses of activated charcoal over days to weeks may have the same effect, but this approach remains unproven, specifically with organochlorine insecticides.

## Pyrethrum and Pyrethrin Insecticides

Pyrethrum is the natural derivative or oleoresin extract of dried *Chrysanthemum cinerariaefolium* flowers, which contain six active agents or pyrethrins (Fig. 1). Although pyrethrins I through VI make up crude pyrethrum extract, pyrethrin I and II are the most active. Because of the relatively high cost, high biodegradability, and light instability of natural pyrethrum, significant efforts over the last 20 to 25 years have resulted in the production of a number of synthetic pyrethroid derivatives. The synthetic pyrethroids are divided into two classes based on function or clinical effects of toxicity. Examples of type I pyrethroid include allethrin, permethrin, and cismethrin, while representative type II pyrethroids included fenvalerate, deltamethrin, and cypermethrin. Pyrethrum and pyrethrins are usually used in combination with synergistic compounds such as piperonyl butoxide and *n*-octyl bicycloheptene dicarboximide, which retard enzymatic degradation of the pyrethroids. Commercial pesticide products with active pyrethroids often contain organophosphate or carbamate insecticides, in addition to the synergistic compounds that protect against degradation. In many of the indoor or household insecticide sprays, the pyrethrins, which cause a rapid paralytic or "knockdown" effect on insects, are often combined with longer-acting insecticides to ensure lethality. Because even the synthetic pyrethrins are expensive and have some light and heat instability, there is relatively little commercial agricultural use of these agents. Because no active crop residues result from the application of pyrethrins, new pyrethrins may be marked for agricultural use in the future. Increasingly, pyrethrins are used as human scabicides because of their better tolerance compared to organochlorine agents such as lindane.

### *Signs and Symptoms*

Pyrethroids affect nerve excitability by delaying sodium channel inactivation. This leads to type I pyrethroids causing repetitive nerve discharge. The type II pyrethroids produce an even longer delay in sodium channel closure, resulting in persistent nerve depolarization and eventual blockage of axonal conduction. The type II pyrethroids may also alter and bind γ-aminobutyric acid (GABA) receptor–mediated chloride channels.

Natural pyrethrum and its derivatives are less toxic to mammals than most other insecticides. Crude pyrethrum extracts contain dermal and respiratory allergens, which are probably other compounds than the active insecticide. These allergens produce the most common toxidrome, i.e., contact dermatitis, followed by rhinitis and asthma. An association or cross-reactivity with ragweed allergies has been noted (65). Because of the allergenic potential of pyrethrum extracts, anaphylactic or anaphylactoid reactions may occur in patients rechallenged with pyrethrum extracts or derivatives, but they have been rarely reported. The synthetic pyrethroids are less allergenic but have some irritant properties.

Systemic toxicity in mammals is reduced by rapid first-pass metabolism of pyrethrins by the liver. Pyrethrins are absorbed across the gut and by inhalation with poor bioavailability. Little dermal absorption occurs across intact skin. No modern-day pyrethrum fatalities have been reported; the estimated pyrethrum oral $LD_{50}$ is over 1 g/kg. Animals exposed to very large systemic doses of type I pyrethroids have demonstrated tremor in the limbs, which can gradually involve the entire body with increased body temperature. Clinically, the toxicity is similar to massive exposure to the organochlorine DDT. Similarly massive type II pyrethroid exposures have produced pronounced salivation, coarse whole body tremors, and choreoathetosis with terminal seizures. In humans, large absorbed doses of these pyrethroids are thought to cause incoordination, tremor, salivation, vomiting, diarrhea, and rarely death (65,66,67). The α-cyano-containing type II pyrethroids have produced a unique cutaneous paresthesia several hours after cutaneous exposure. Many workers exposed to fenvalerate described a stinging or burning paresthesia, which sometimes progressed to numbness in the exposed face, neck, forearms, and hands. In fenvalerate-exposed workers the symptoms lasted 12 to 18 hours, but rarely beyond 24 hours. They were exacerbated by sweating and exposure to water, sun, or heat. The paresthesias are thought to be caused by contact with sensory nerve endings in the skin and are not thought to be allergic (68,69).

Large exposures of people to pyrethroids are usually secondary to oral exposure to commercial products, which usually contain many other synergistic chemicals. The toxicity of these other products is often the cause of the symptoms. The synergists piperonylbutoxide and *n*-octyl bicycloheptene dicarboximide exhibit little human toxicity. Acetylcholinesterase inhibitors such as the organophosphate and carbamate insecticides combined with pyrethroids in commercial products can cause significant human toxicity and require specific treatment, which has been described elsewhere in this chapter.

### *Laboratory Findings*

No specific tests or commercially available serum or tissue assays exist for detection of pyrethrum or synthetic pyrethrin compounds or their metabolites. Confirmation of absorption or cutaneous exposure is by clinical history and examination.

### *Treatment*

Although there has been little systemic toxicity reported with pyrethroids in humans, gastrointestinal decontamination, including the use of activated charcoal, is recommended. Aggressive decontamination of the eyes with water and the skin with soap and water is suggested. Further supportive care is rarely needed. Allergic reactions or responses may require antihistamines. Pulmonary allergic reactions may require bronchodilator treatment. Preventive care should include avoidance of pyrethrum-related allergens. Pyrethrum-induced contact dermatitis may require antihistamine and topical or systemic corticosteroid administration. Type II pyrethrin-induced cutaneous paresthesias can be avoided by reducing cutaneous and volatilized exposures. Topical vitamin E oil preparations (*d*,l-a-tocopherol acetate) can modulate the cutaneous paresthesias to a greater degree than corn oil or petroleum jelly preparations (69). There is little experience treating systemic signs of pyrethroid-induced toxicity. Animal data suggest that atropine can modify pyrethroid-induced salivation and that diazepam or phenobarbital is effective against tremors and seizures. In a series of 573 cases of acute pyrethroid poisoning, one patient died after being given large doses of atropine for a condition misdiagnosed as acute organophosphate poisoning (67). In the same series, eight patients with pure pyrethroid poisoning developed atropine intoxication after receiving total atropine doses of 12 to 75 mg (67).

## Paraquat and Diquat Herbicides

Paraquat (1,1′-dimethyl-4,4′bipyridylium) is a contact herbicide considered to have low potential for environmental toxicity because it is rapidly inactivated in the soil. Commercial or technical paraquat (or diquat, a related herbicide) products range in concentration from 20% to 50%, whereas home products are usually much less concentrated (0.2% solutions to 2.5% soluble granule formulation; Table 5). Home products are often formulated in combination with other herbicides. In a recent United Kingdom 6-year study of pesticide toxicity, paraquat was the cause for 8 of the 10 reported deaths (70). Most clinical toxicity has been associated with concentrated paraquat ingestion, suicide attempts accounting for the majority of cases (71). Toxicity has resulted from inhalation, skin absorption, or even vaginal absorption (72–74). Ingestion of more than 20 mg (7.5 ml of a 20% solution) of paraquat is frequently lethal, with death caused by severe damage to the lung and other organs. The mortality rate after paraquat or diquat ingestion remains approximately 60% (75–77). Selective concentration in lungs (10 to 15 times greater than serum concentrations) accounts for this major lethal effect, although the volume of distribution for paraquat is large (2 to 8 L/kg). Paraquat has allegedly caused lung damage to marijuana smokers in the United States who obtained their marijuana from paraquat-treated Mexican plants. Diquat is not selectively concentrated in the lungs, and pulmonary injury from exposures tends to be less severe. Survivors of paraquat poisoning frequently have abnormal restrictive lung defects from pulmonary fibrosis that will rarely improve over time (78). Risk factors for paraquat toxicity from agricultural exposures in California have recently been described (79).

**TABLE 5.** *Examples of paraquat- and diquat-containing herbicide products*

| Product | Herbicide | Content (%) |
|---|---|---|
| Gramoxone | Paraquat | 29.1 |
| Paraquat Plus | Paraquat | 29.1 |
| Ortho Paraquat | Paraquat | 29.1 |
| Ortho Spot Weed and Grass Killer | Paraquat | 3.6 |
| Ortho Weed Killer Concentrate | Diquat | 35.3 |
| Ortho Diquat 2-Spray | Diquat | 35.3 |
| Ortho Diquat Water Weed | Diquat | 35.3 |
| Weedtrine D | Diquat | 8.53 |
| Dexol Weed and Grass Killer | Diquat | 0.23 |
| Frank's Weed and Grass Killer | Diquat | 0.23 |
| Scotty's Weed and Grass Killer | Diquat | 0.23 |

Adapted from ref. 92.

Damage to tissue and organs by paraquat or diquat is mediated on a molecular level by hydrogen peroxide and free radicals, including superoxide radicals ($O_2^{\pm}$) and hydroxyl radicals (·OH) in reactions that may be catalyzed by transition metal ions (80). Supplemental oxygen can increase the generation of $O_2^{\pm}$ and other free radicals in the lung, which, if not quenched by superoxide dismutase, can further free radical damage of molecular targets, e.g., proteins, lipids, and nucleic acids (81).

### *Signs and Symptoms*

Skin contact with paraquat or diquat leads to blistering, ulcerations, and discolored fingernails. Prolonged inhalation of spray droplets may cause nosebleeds, severe conjunctivitis, and severe shortness of breath. The caustic effects of paraquat result in esophageal and gastric erosions after ingestion. Extensive gastroenteritis with large amounts of mucosal sloughing can occur (Table 6). Death results from multisystem failure, including noncardiogenic

**TABLE 6.** *Paraquat toxidrome*

| Clinical finding | Prevalence (%) |
|---|---|
| Vomiting | 100% |
| Dysphagia | 100% |
| Oropharyngitis | 100% |
| Restlessness | 90% |
| Jaundice | 80% |
| Cyanosis | 45% |
| Hemoptysis | 40% |
| Diarrhea | 5% |
| Convulsions | 5% |
| Nail bed necrosis | 5% |

Adapted from ref. 86.

pulmonary edema, acute renal failure, hepatic necrosis, adrenal hemorrhage, brain damage, and myocardial necrosis (76,82–85). Paraquat poisoning in pregnancy results in high placental concentrations and fetal death (86).

### *Laboratory Findings*

Determinations of plasma paraquat levels by radioimmunoassay and various chromatographic methods is available from specialized laboratories (87). Correlation among serum levels, interval after ingestion, and clinical outcome exist (Fig. 2) (88). A qualitative colorimetric method using 1% sodium dithionite and 1N sodium hydroxide to detect paraquat in urine has been described (87). To ensure accuracy, both positive and negative controls should be tested.

In a series of 20 patients from Trinidad who were poisoned with paraquat (89), all were found to have elevated serum paraquat levels, blood urea nitrogen (BUN), and creatinine levels, as well as elevated liver function test values (bilirubin, glutamic-oxylate transaminase, and alkaline phosphatase). Hypokalemia was seen in 17 out of 20 paraquat-poisoned patients. Chest radiographs were abnormal in 45% and urine tests for paraquat were positive in 90% of these cases.

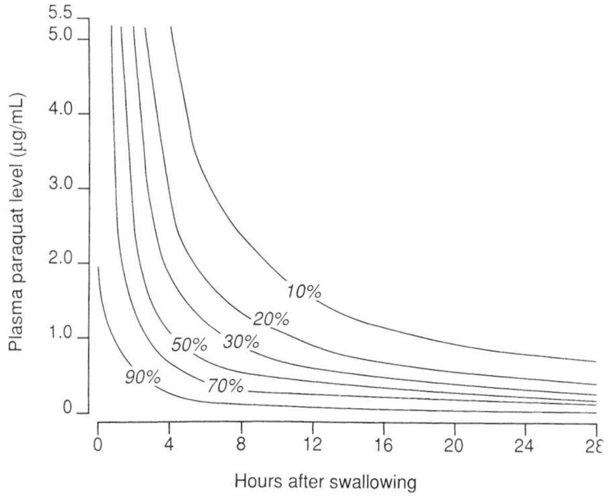


**FIG. 2.** Graph demonstrating the relationship between the plasma concentrations of paraquat in micrograms per milliliter *(ordinate)*, time after ingestion *(abscissa)*, and the probability of survival. (From ref. 88.)

Another review of 42 patients with severe paraquat poisoning found that those with serum paraquat levels above 3 µg/ml die, regardless of intervention (90). However, survival has been recently reported in a patient with a measured paraquat level of 28 µg/ml, but the patient received hemodialysis, early digestive decontamination, and antioxidant therapy (91).

### *Treatment*

Although many treatments have been studied, no proven effective antidote exists (75,89,92). Early digestive decontamination and hemodialysis followed by antioxidant therapy with low doses of deferoxamine (100 mg/kg in 24 hours) to bind transition metal catalysts (such as iron and copper) and continuous IV infusion of acetylcysteine (300 mg/kg/day for 3 weeks) may be effective in potentially fatal cases of paraquat poisoning (91). Whole lung radiation and single or bilateral lung transplants must be considered experimental (93–97). Accepted therapy includes skin and eye decontamination with copious amounts of water. Immediate administration of an absorbent after ingestion is likely to improve the outcome of a paraquat ingestion. Bentonite (75% suspension) and Fuller's earth (30% suspension) in an adult dose of 100 to 150 g each are thought to be the most effective (75,89). If these are not readily available, activated charcoal may be as effective. Because of the possible erosive changes in the esophagus, gastric intubation must be done with extreme care. Endoscopy may be required to avoid inadvertent perforation. Extracorporeal hemoperfusion (within hours of ingestion), peritoneal dialysis, and hemodialysis have been tried, with the latter two being useful in electrolyte and hemodynamic management and the former potentially useful in increasing the clearance of paraquat (75,98–103). Mechanical ventilation for acute respiratory failure (adult respiratory distress syndrome) and critical care support in an intensive care unit are often necessary in severely intoxicated patients. A poor prognosis is expected in patients with multisystem failure.

## LONG-TERM HEALTH EFFECTS

Most acute effects of pesticide toxicity are well characterized, and the mechanisms of their pathogenesis have been established in many cases. Studies on long-term effects, which develop or persist long after the exposures that may have precipitated them, typically are less consistent in their findings and often raise more questions than they answer. The ability of pesticides to cause cancer, neurotoxicity, and adverse reproductive effects has been demonstrated in laboratory animals, but unambiguous clinical or epidemiologic evidence of effects in humans exists for only a few specific agents. For most pesticides, clinical or epidemiologic data are lacking on long-term health effects or the data do not yet support clear evidence of causality.

Epidemiologic studies have focused principally on pesticide formulators and applicators as representing heavily exposed populations. Several population-based investigations have studied both cancer and reproductive outcomes, although most of these have been limited by ecologic methodology or poor estimates of pesticide exposure. In the remainder of this chapter we focus on epidemiologic studies, including pertinent laboratory and clinical results to clarify the effects of the various pesticides on health outcomes.

Issues of causation, particularly from long-term exposures, ideally require a combination of laboratory, clinical, and epidemiologic data. Laboratory studies may address the important question of biologic plausibility of associations observed in epidemiologic studies. The ability to assess exposure quantitatively through biomarkers will greatly improve the sensitivity and specificity of epidemiologic studies. Recognition of subcellular initial lesions that contribute to eventual development of degenerative diseases also will open new avenues to epidemiology. Until such studies are completed, prudent avoidance or minimization of exposure to all xenobiotics is the safest course.

## Cancer

While farmers mortality rates are lower than the general population's for all causes combined and for smoking-related cancers, numerous studies of farmers have demonstrated above average death rates from particular cancers, most not related to smoking. These studies, from several regions in the United States as well as countries in Europe, have most commonly observed increases in leukemia, non-Hodgkin's lymphoma (NHL), and multiple myeloma. Fewer studies have observed increases in Hodgkin's lymphoma and cancers of the brain, stomach, prostate, skin, and connective tissue (30,104–108). While some of these studies have linked cancer rates to pesticide use or other agricultural practices, all of the studies have serious problems of exposure misclassification. In addition, most farmers and farm workers are exposed to numerous pesticides and other potentially harmul substances, further complicating the conclusions from epidemiologic studies. The observed associations should be regarded provisionally and skeptically. Despite these difficulties, hematopoietic and lymphatic cancers consistently have been associated with farming, and in some cases have been associated with geographic areas of higher pesticide use or with specific agricultural activities, such as corn production, associated with heavy pesticide use. More recently epidemiologic studies have estimated exposure to specific pesticides (e.g., phenoxy herbicides) and evaluated their association with specific cancers (e.g., NHL).

A major epidemiologic approach to the question of pesticides and cancer has been to study occupational cohorts exposed to pesticides. Such studies have included pesticide manufacturers, structural pest control applicators, and agricultural applicators. These studies lack exact measurements of pesticide exposure in individuals, and multiple pesticide exposures often occur, especially among applicators. They do, however, target populations that experience relatively frequent, intense, and prolonged exposures (109–111). Some show small increases in mortality due to cancer at various sites, although not always increasing with increasing exposure. An increase in lung cancer mortality among arsenical manufacturers (112) is consistent with other epidemiologic data on the carcinogenicity of occupational arsenic exposure. No excess risk, however, could be detected for former users of lead arsenate (113) (long since discontinued). Small increases in lung cancer mortality have also been observed among chlordane and other organochlorine manufacturers (114–116) and among structural and agricultural applicators (117,118). Studies of these occupationally exposed cohorts generally have not shown increases in lymphatic or hematopoietic cancer mortality rates.

Recent indications that chlorinated pesticides and their contaminants may interact with hormone receptors (see Female Reproductive Effects, below) have led to speculation about a possible role in the development of cancer of the breast. This work was catalyzed by a case-control study showing increased DDE (a metabolite of DDT) in the sera of patients with breast cancer compared to controls (119). However, a larger nested case-control study conducted within a prospective cohort found no evidence of an association (120). The evidence remains contradictory and does not support a causal association (121,122).

In summary, there is consistent epidemiologic evidence for a small association of lung cancer with exposure to pesticides no longer used in developed countries. This association is established for arsenicals and is suggestive for the chlorinated hydrocarbons. Large prospective cohort studies now in progress (123) are attempting to reduce the uncertainty now prevalent.

## Neurotoxicity

In most cases of acute neurotoxicity from pesticides, recovery is complete unless convulsions or other acute injuries occur. However, there is evidence that long-term pesticide exposure may result in some chronic neurologic effects. DDT and the other organochlorines are stored in fat tissue, so cumulative exposure may occur. With DDT, symptoms of chronic and of acute toxicity are similar—anorexia, weakness, anxiety, and hyperexcitability (124). Persistent neurologic sequelae are most likely to follow acute organochlorine toxicity that is associated with convulsions (125). Polyneuropathy has been associated with chronic exposure to some organochlorine pesticides (126,127). Follow-up of adults and children years after chlordane was sprayed around the apartment complex in which they lived indicated impairment of balance, reaction time, and immediate recall, among other test results (128).

The acute neurotoxic effects of the organophosphate and carbamate insecticides, and the recently recognized intermediate syndrome, have been discussed above. A delayed neuropathy has been observed in humans days to weeks following acute organophosphate insecticide exposure. The syndrome is manifest by involvement of the longest nerve fibers, and presents with progressive weakness, ataxia, and paralysis. Pathogenesis of this irreversible syndrome appears to involve inhibition of the neurotoxic esterase enzyme (NTE) rather than of neural acetylcholinesterase (129,130), although inhibition of acetylcholinesterase has been an inevitable concomitant. One study of neurologic sequelae following organophosphate poisoning found impaired visual attention and vibrotactile sensitivity among cases compared to controls (131). While this finding is provocative, it needs to be replicated with more complete follow-up and better estimates of exposure.

The possibility that pesticide exposure may contribute to development of Parkinson's disease has been suggested following observations (132) that such exposure is more common among Parkinson's patients than among unaffected people from the same region. A similar suggestion with respect to Guillain-Barré syndrome has been reported only in the Chinese (133), in an English abstract. Both of these observed associations require further confirmation before they can be accepted as causal.

Studies of neuropsychologic effects in humans following acute organophosphate insecticide poisoning (131, 134–136) have indicated a fairly consistent constellation of subjective disturbance and subclinical deficits. Persistent symptoms following acute toxicity include headache, dizziness, nausea, visual disturbances, weakness, confusion, agitation, and insomnia. The most consistent of positive measurable results has been elevation of the threshold for vibratory sensation. These symptoms may last weeks to months following cessation of exposure, persisting long after resolution of cholinergic signs (137). Cholinesterase depression is only variably associated with these persistent symptoms.

A variety of neurobehavioral symptoms has been associated with chronic low-dose exposure to organophosphate insecticides, but careful, rigorous studies are generally lacking; some studies have failed to observe these effects. Symptoms observed among workers exposed long-term to organophosphate insecticides include fatigue, memory deficits, nervousness, malaise, vision disturbances, and loss of concentration (124). There is supportive evidence from animal studies for chronic neurologic effects of organophosphate insecticide exposure, but more carefully controlled studies are necessary in humans.

## Reproductive Toxicity

### *Male Reproduction*

Chlordecone (Kepone) was an insecticide and fungicide produced from 1958 to 1975, when production was stopped because of toxicity in production workers (138). In animal studies chlordecone causes testicular atrophy (139,140). Among the production workers in the Virginia Allied Chemical and Dye Corporation plant, chlordecone caused oligospermia and reduced sperm motility in several men, as well as neurotoxicity and several other clinical effects (138).

The study of infertility among men exposed to pesticides and other occupational agents is hindered by ignorance of the fundamental determinants and modifiers of spermatogenesis, the large individual and intraperson variability in semen parameters, and difficulty in conducting controlled epidemiologic investigations (141). Difficulties in obtaining accurate estimates of pesticide exposures further hamper studies of their potential adverse reproductive effects.

The possibility that environmental exposures including pesticides may adversely impact sexual development of the male fetus has been discussed seriously since publication of a study reporting decreasing semen quality over a 50-year period (142). Data for the earlier 30 years of the study period were sparse, and evaluation criteria may not have been comparable (143). Confirmatory and contradictory studies, including relatively strong evidence from observations of wildlife in contaminated areas, have been reviewed (144) without reaching a firm conclusion. An important source of resistance to the idea of environmental hormone disruption has been the low potency of the implicated xenobiotics. An *in vitro* study on yeast genetically altered to express a human estrogen receptor suggests synergistic effects of combined exposures (145). The area of endocrine disruptors is one of current intensive research.

### *Female Reproductive Effects*

Few human studies directly address the effect of pesticides on female reproductive outcomes. Most of the epidemiologic studies have been descriptive or ecologic and do not provide direct support for causal associations with potential pesticide exposure. Furthermore, studies that have evaluated associations between birth defects and agricultural activity or pesticide use have generally been ecologic analyses and have been inconsistent in their results. They thus have done little more than raise concern about the effects of pesticides on female reproduction (146–148).

Organochlorines, including DDT, have been implicated in a variety of adverse reproductive outcomes. The mechanism is generally thought to be interaction with estrogen receptors, either directly or indirectly by metabolism to estrogen agonists. Abnormal menses and impaired fertility have been suggested effects of the organochlorines. Epidemiologic evidence has also suggested, but not definitely implicated, DDT exposure in premature delivery and spontaneous abortion (30,149).

One study of a small but intense outbreak of congenital abnormalities provides persuasive evidence linking the event to consumption of fish treated for parasites with extraordinarily high doses of the organophosphate trichlorfon (150). Two case reports of malformations associated with prenatal exposure to organophosphates are anecdotal only, lacking any estimate of exposure magnitude (151,152).

## REFERENCES


1. Okumura T, Takasu N, Ishimatsu S, et al. Report on 540 victims of the Tokyo subway sarin attack. *Ann Emerg Med* 1996;28:129–135.
2. Carson R. *Silent spring.* Boston: Houghton Mifflin, 1962.
3. Jeyaratnam J. Acute pesticide poisoning: a major health problem. *World Health State Q* 1990;43:139–145.
4. Litovitz TL, Felberg L, White S, Klein-Schwartz W. 1995 annual report of the American Association of Poison Control Center Toxic Exposure Surveillance System. *Am J Emerg Med* 1996;14:487–537.
5. Wilkinson CF. Introduction and overview. In: Baker SR, Wilkinson CF, eds. *The effect of pesticides on human health.* Princeton: Princeton Scientific, 1990;5–33.
6. Environmental Protection Agency. *Pesticides in drinking water data base 1988 interim report.* Washington, DC: U.S. Environmental Protection Agency, 1988.
7. Nightingale SL. Pesticides and food safety. *Am Family Physician* 1989;40:289–290.
8. Goldman LR, Smith DF, Neutra RR, et al. Pesticide food poisoning from contaminated watermelons in California, 1985. *Arch Environ Health* 1990;45:229–236.
9. Robinson PE, Mack GA, Remmers J, Levy R, Mohadjer L. Trends of PCB, hexachlorobenzene, and β-benzene hexachloride levels in the adipose tissue of the U.S. population. *Environ Res* 1990;53: 175–192.
10. Strassman SC, Kutz FW. Trends of organochlorine pesticide residues in human tissue. In: Khan MAQ, Stanton RH, eds. *Toxicology of halogenated hydrocarbons. Health and ecological effects.* New York: Pergamon Press, 1981;38–49.
11. Weisskopf CP, Seiber JN, Maizlish N, Schenker M. Personnel exposure to diazinon in a supervised pest eradication program. *Arch Environ Contam Toxicol* 1988;17:201–212.
12. Zwiener RJ, Ginsburg CM. Organophosphate and carbamate poisoning in infants and children. *Pediatrics* 1988;81:121–126.
13. Peiris JB, Fernando R, De Abrew K. Respiratory failure from severe organophosphate toxicity due to absorption through the skin. *Forensic Sci Int* 1988;36:251–253
14. Besser R, Gutman L, Weilemann LS. Inactivation of endplate acetylcholinesterase during the course of organophosphate intoxications. *Arch Toxicol* 1989;63:412–415.
15. Gray AP. Design and structure-activity relationships of antidotes to organophosphorous anticholinesterase agents. *Drug Metab Rev* 1984; 15:557–589.
16. Besser R, Gutmann L, Dillmann U, Weilemann LS, Hopf, HC. Endplate dysfunction in acute organophosphate intoxication. *Neurology* 1989;39:561–567.
17. Li C, Miller WT, Jiang J. Pulmonary edema due to ingestion of organophosphate insecticide. *Am J Radiol* 1989;152:265–266.
18. Rengstorff RH. Accidental exposure to sarin: vision effects. *Arch Toxicol* 1985;56:201–203.
19. Pullicino P, Aquilina J. Opsoclonus in organophosphate poisoning. *Arch Neurol* 1989;46:704–705.
20. Morgan DP. *Recognition and management of pesticide poisonings,* 4th ed. Washington, DC: United States Environmental Protection Agency, 1989.
21. Tsao TCY, Juang YC, Lan RS, Shieh WB, Lee CH. Respiratory failure of acute organophosphate and carbamate poisoning. *Chest* 1990; 98:631–636.
22. Inoue N. Psychiatric symptoms following accidental exposure to sarin—a case report. *Fukuoka Acta Med* 1995;86:373–377.
23. Weizman Z, Sofer S. Acute pancreatitis in children with anticholinesterase insecticide intoxication. *Pediatrics* 1992;90:204–206.
24. Kato T, Hamanaka T. Ocular signs and symptoms caused by exposure to sarin gas. *Am J Ophthalmol* 1996;121:209–210.
25. Hsiao CT, Yang CC, Deng JF, Bullard MJ, Liaw SJ. Acute pancreatitis following organophosphate intoxication. *Clin Toxicol* 1996;4: 343–347.
26. Wagner SL, Orwick DL. Chronic organophosphate exposure associated with transient hypertonia in an infant. *Pediatrics* 1994;94:94–97.
27. Senanayake N N, Karalliedde L. Neurotoxic effects of organophosphate insecticides. An intermediate syndrome. *N Engl J Med* 1987; 316:761–763.
28. De Bleecker J, Neucker K, Willems J. Intermediate syndrome in organophosphate poisoning: a prospective study. *Crit Care Med* 1993;21: 1706–1711.
29. Davies JE. Changing profile of pesticide poisoning. *N Engl J Med* 1987;316:807–808.
30. Sharp DS, Eskenazi B, Harrison R, Callas P, Smith AH. Delayed health hazards of pesticide exposure. *Annu Rev Public Health* 1986;7: 441–471.
31. Johnson MK. Organophosphates and delayed neuropathy—is NTE alive and well? *Toxicol Appl Pharmacol* 1990;102:385–399.
32. Barrett DS, Oehme FW. A review of organophosphorus ester-induced delayed neurotoxicity. *Vet Hum Toxicol* 1985;27:22–37.
33. Guillermo FP, Pretel CM. Prolonged suxamethonium-induced neuromuscular blockade associated with organophosphate poisoning. *Br J Anaesth* 1988;61:233–236.
34. Weeks DB, Ford D. Prolonged suxamethonium-induced neuromuscular block associated with organophosphate poisoning. *Br J Anaesth* 1989;62:237.
35. Tsatsakis AM, Aguridakis P, Michalodimitrakis MN, et al. Experiences with acute organophosphate poisoning in Crete. *Vet Hum Toxicol* 1996;38:101–107.
36. Wilson BW, Padilla S, Henderson JD. Factors in standardizing automated cholinesterase assays. *J Toxicol Environ Health* 1996;48(2):187–195.
37. Blain PG. Aspects of pesticide toxicology. *Adverse Drug React Acute Poisoning Rev* 1990;9:37–68.
38. George ST, Varghese M, John L, Balasubramanian AS. Aryl aqlamidase activity in human erythrocyte, plasma and blood in pesticide (organophosphates and carbamates) poisoning. *Clin Chem Acta* 1985; 145:1–8.
39. Nouira S, Abroug F, Elatrous S, Boujdaria R, Bouchoucha S. Prognostic value of serum cholinesterase in organophosphate poisoning. *Chest* 1994;106:1811–1814.
40. Duffy FH, Burchfiel JL, Bartels PH, Gaon M, Sim V. Long-term effects of an organophosphate upon the human electroencephalogram. *Toxicol Appl Pharmacol* 1979;47:161–176.
41. Kiss Z, Fazekas T. Organophosphates and torsade de pointes ventricular tachycardia. *J R Soc Med* 1983;76:984–985.
42. Bardin PG, Van Eeden SF. Organophosphate poisoning: grading the severity and comparing treatment between atropine and glycopyrrolate. *Crit Care Med* 1990;18:956–960.
43. DeSilva HJ, Wijewickrema R, Senanayake N. Does pralidoxime affect outcome of management in acute organophosphorous poisoning? *Lancet* 1992;339:1136–1138.

44. Scott RJ. Repeated asystole following PAM in organophosphate self-poisoning. *Anesth Intensive Care* 1986;14:458–460.
45. Medicis JJ, Stork CM, Howland MA, Hoffman RS, Goldfrank LR. Pharmacokinetics following a loading plus a continuous infusion of pralidoxime compared with the traditional short infusion regimen in human volunteers. *Clin Toxicol* 1996;34:289–295.
46. Jovanovic D. Pharmacokinetics of pralidoxime chloride. A comparative study in healthy volunteers and in organophosphorus poisoning. *Arch Toxicol* 1989;63:416–418.
47. Farrar HC, Wells TG, Kearns GL. Use of continuous infusion of pralidoxime for treatment of organophosphate poisoning in children. *J Pediatr* 1990;116:658–661.
48. Willems J, DeBisschop HC, Colardyn F, et al. Cholinesterase reactivation in organophosphorus poisoned patients depends on the plasma concentrations of the oxime pralidoxime methylsulphate and of the organophosphate. *Arch Toxicol* 1993;67:79–84.
49. Lifshifz M, Rotenburg M, Sofer S, Tamiri T, Shahak E, Almog S. Carbamate poisoning and oxime treatment in children: a clinical and laboratory study. *Pediatrics* 1994;93:652–655.
50. Saadeh AM, Al-Ali MK, Farsakh NA, Ghani MA. Clinical and sociodemographic features of acute carbamate and organophosphate poisoning: a study of 70 adult patients in North Jordan. *Clin Toxicol* 1996;34:45–51.
51. Lee MH, Ransdell JF. A farm worker death due to pesticide toxicity: a case report. *J Toxicol Environ Health* 1984;14:239–246.
52. Miyazaki T, Yashiki M, Kojima T, Chikasue F, Ochiai A, Hidani Y. Fatal and non-fatal methomyl intoxication in an attempted double suicide. *Forensic Sci Int* 1989;42:263–270.
53. Aks SE, Krantz A, Hryhorczuk DO, Wagner S, Mock J. Acute accidental lindane ingestion in toddlers. *Ann Emerg Med* 1995;26:647–651.
54. Grimmett WG, Dzendolet I, Whyte I. Intravenous thiodan (30% endosulfan in xylene). *Clin Toxicol* 1996;34:447–452.
55. Davies JE, Dedhia HV, Morgade C, Barquet A, Maibach HI. Lindane poisoning. *Arch Dermatol* 1983;119:142–144.
56. Runhaar EA, Sangster B, Greve PA, Voortman M. A case of fatal endrin poisoning. *Hum Toxicol* 1985;4:241–247.
57. Rugman FP, Cosstick R. Aplastic anaemia associated with organochlorine pesticide: case reports and review of evidence. *J Clin Pathol* 1990;43:98–101.
58. Rao CVSR, Shreenivas R, Singh V, Perez-Atayde A, Woolf A. Disseminated intravascular coagulation in a case of fatal lindane poisoning. *Vet Hum Toxicol* 1988;30:132–134.
59. Baumann K, Angerer J, Heinrich R, Lehnert G. Occupational exposure to hexachlorocyclohexane I. Body burdens of HCH-isomers. *Int Arch Occup Environ Health* 1980;47:119–127.
60. Czegledi-Jannko G, Avar P. Occupational exposure to lindane: clinical and laboratory findings. *Br J Ind Med* 1970;27:283–286.
61. Gupta SK, Parikh JR, Shah MP. Changes in serum hexachloro-cyclohexane (HCH) residues in malaria spraymen after short-term occupational experience. *Arch Environ Health* 1982;37:41–44.
62. Samuels AJ, Milby TH. Human exposure to lindane: clinical hematological and biochemical effects. *J Occup Med* 1971;13:147–151.
63. Bernad PG. Review: EEG and pesticides. *Clin Electroencephalogr* 1989;20:ix–x.
64. Cohn WJ, Boylan JJ, Blanke RV, Fariss BS, Howell JR, Guzelian JT. Treatment of chlordecone (kepone) toxicity with cholestyramine. Results of a controlled trial. *N Engl J Med* 1978;298:243–248.
65. Feinberg S. Pyrethrum sensitization. *JAMA* 1934;102:1557–1558.
66. Paton DL, Walker JS. Pyrethrin poisoning from commercial-strength flea and tick spray. *Am J Emerg Med* 1988;6:232–235.
67. He F, Wang S, Liu L, Chen S, Zhang Z, Sun J. Clinical manifestations and diagnosis of acute pyrethroid poisoning. *Arch Toxicol* 1989;63:54–58.
68. Le Quesne PM, Maxwell IC, Butterworth STG. Transient facial sensory symptoms following exposure to synthetic pyrethroids: a clinical and electrophysiological assessment. *Neurotoxicology* 1981;2:1–11.
69. Flannigan SA, Tucker SB. Variation in cutaneous sensation between synthetic pyrethroid insecticides. *Contact Dermatitis* 1985;13:140–147.
70. Proudfoot AT, Dougall H. Poisoning treatment centre admissions following acute incidents involving pesticides. *Hum Toxicol* 1988,7:255–258.
71. Perriens J, Van Der Stuyft P, Chee H, Benimadho S. The epidemiology of paraquat intoxications in Surinam. *Trop Geogr Med* 1989;41:266–269.
72. Ong ML, Glew S. Paraquat poisoning per vagina. *Postgrad Med J* 1989;65:835–836.
73. Okonek S, Wronski R, Niedermayer W, Okonek M, Lamer A. Near fatal percutaneous paraquat poisoning. *Klin Wochenschr* 1983;61:655–659.
74. Smith JG. Paraquat poisoning by skin absorption: a review. *Hum Toxicol* 1988;7:15–19.
75. Pond SM. Manifestations and management of paraquat poisoning. *Med J Aust* 1990;152:256–259.
76. Krall J, Bagley AC, Mullenbach GT, Hallewell RA, Lynch RE. Superoxide mediates the toxicity of paraquat for cultured mammalian cells. *J Biol Chem* 1988;263:1910–1914.
77. Smith LL. Paraquat toxicity. *Philos Trans R Soc Lond* 1985;B311:647–657.
78. Bismuth C, Hall AH, Baud FJ, Barron S. Pulmonary dysfunction in survivors of acute paraquat poisoning. *Vet Hum Toxicol* 1996;38:220–222.
79. Weinbaum Z, Samuels SJ, Schenker MB. Risk factors for occupational illnesses associated with the use of paraquat (1,1′-dimethyl-4,4′-bipyridylium dichloride) in California. *Arch Environ Health* 1995;50(5):341–348.
80. Halliwell B, Gutteridge JMC. *Free radicals in biology and medicine,* 2nd ed. Oxford: Clarendon Press, 1989;306–310.
81. Shibamoto T, Taylor AE, Parker JC. $PO_2$ modulation of paraquat-induced microvascular injury in isolated dog lungs. *J Appl Physiol* 1990;68:2119–2127.
82. Barsony J, Kertesz F. Investigation of adrenal steroids and 25-hydroxy-cholecalcipherol in human gramoxone poisoning. *Arch Toxicol* 1985;8:280–283.
83. Hara H, Manabe T, Hayashi T. An immunohistochemical study of the fibrosing process in paraquat lung injury. *Virchows Arch [A]* 1989;415:357–366.
84. Hughes JT. Brain damage due to paraquat poisoning: a fatal case with neuropathological examination of the brain. *Neurotoxicology* 1988;9:243–248.
85. Vandenbogaerde J, Schelstraete J, Colardyn F, Heyndrickx A. Paraquat poisoning. *Forensic Sci Int* 1984,26:103–114.
86. Talbot AR, Fu CC. Paraquat intoxication during pregnancy: a report of 9 cases. *Vet Toxicol* 1988;30:12–17.
87. Tomita M, Suzuki K, Shimosato K, Kohama A, Ijiri I. An enzyme-linked immunosorbent assay for plasma-paraquat levels of poisoned patients. *Forensic Sci Int* 1988;37:11–18.
88. Hart TB, Nevitt A, Whitehead A. A new statistical approach to the prognostic significance of plasma paraquat concentrations. *Lancet* 1984;2:1222–1223.
89. Addo E, Ramdial S, Poon-King T. High dosage cyclophosphamide and dexamethasone treatment of paraquat poisoning with 75% survival. *W Ind Med J* 1984;33:220–226.
90. Hampson EC, Pond SM. Failure of haemoperfusion and haemodialysis to prevent death in paraquat poisoning: a retrospective review of 42 patients. *Med Toxicol Adverse Drug Exp* 1988;3:64–71.
91. Lheureux P, Ledu D, Vanbinst R, Askenasi R. Survival in a case of massive paraquat ingestion. *Chest* 1995;107:285–289.
92. Allen HM, Deck LV. Paraquat poisoning. *J Okla State Med Assoc* 1989;82:510–515.
93. Webb DB, Williams MV, Davies BH, James KW. Resolution after radiotherapy of severe pulmonary damage due to paraquat poisoning. *Br Med J* 1984;288:1259–1260.
94. Toronto Lung Transplant Group. Sequential bilateral lung transplantation for paraquat poisoning. *J Thorac Cardiovasc Surg* 1985;89:734–742.
95. Proudfoot AT, Prescott LF, Simpson D, Buckley BM, Vale JA. Radiotherapy for paraquat lung toxicity. *Br Med J* 1984;289:112.
96. Talbot AR Barnes MR. Radiotherapy for the treatment of pulmonary complications of paraquat poisoning. *Hum Toxicol* 1988;7:325–332.
97. Kamholz S, Veith FJ, Mollenkopf F, et al. Single lung transplantation in paraquat intoxication. *NY State J Med* 1984;84:82–84.
98. Williams PS, Hendy MS, Ackrill P. Early management of paraquat poisoning. *Lancet* 1984;1:627.
99. Van de Vyver FL, Giuliano RA, Paulus GJ, et al. Hemoperfusion-hemodialysis ineffective for paraquat removal in life-threatening poisoning? *Clin Toxicol* 1985;23:117–131.

100. Winchester JF, Gelfand MC, Schreiner GE. Haemoperfusion for paraquat poisoning. *Lancet* 1983;2:277.
101. Mascie-Taylor BH, Thompson J, Davison AM. Haemoperfusion ineffective for paraquat removal in life-threatening poisoning. *Lancet* 1983;1:1376–1377.
102. Talbot AR. A comparison of hemoperfusion columns for paraquat. *Vet Hum Toxicol* 1989;31:131–135.
103. Poder G, Oszvald P, Hegyi L, Mezei G, Schmidt Z. Complete recovery from paraquat poisoning causing severe unilateral pulmonary lesion. *Acta Paediatr Hung* 1985;26:53–59.
104. Schenker M, McCurdy S. Pesticides, viruses, and sunlight in the etiology of cancer among agricultural workers. In: Becker C, Coye M, eds. *Cancer prevention—strategies in the workplace.* Washington, DC: Hemisphere, 1986;29–37.
105. Blair A, Malker H, Cantor KP, Burmeister L, Wiklund K. Cancer among farmers: a review. *Scand J Work Environ Health* 1985;11: 397–407.
106. Pearce N, Reif JS. Epidemiologic studies of cancer in agricultural workers. *Am J Ind Med* 1990;18:133–148.
107. Blair A, Axelson O, Franklin C, et al. Carcinogenic effects of pesticides. In: Baker SR, Wilkinson CF, eds. *The effect of pesticides on human health.* Princeton: Princeton Scientific, 1990;201–260.
108. Council on Scientific Affairs. Cancer risk of pesticides in agricultural workers. *JAMA* 1988;260:959–966.
109. Leet T, Acquavella J, Lynch C, et al. Cancer incidence among alachlor manufacturing workers. *Am J Ind Med* 1996;30(3):300–306.
110. Ramlow JM, Spadacene NW, Hoag SR et al. Mortality in a cohort of pentachlorophenol manufacturing workers, 1940–1989. *Am J Ind Med* 1996;30(2):180–194.
111. Sathiakumar N, Delzell E, Cole P. Mortality among workers at two triazine herbicide manufacturing plants. *Am J Ind Med* 1996;29(2): 143–151.
112. Mabuchi K, Lillienfeld AM, Snell LM. Cancer and occupational exposure to arsenic: a study of pesticide workers. *Prevent Med* 1980; 9:51–77.
113. Tollestrup K, Daling JR, Allard J. Mortality in a cohort of orchard workers exposed to lead arsenate pesticide spray. *Arch Environ Health* 1995;50(3):221–229.
114. Wang HH, MacMahon B. Mortality of pesticide applicators. *J Occup Med* 1979;21:741–744.
115. Wang HH, MacMahon B. Mortality of workers employed in the manufacture of chlordane and heptachlor. *J Occup Med* 1979;21:745–748.
116. Wong O, Brocker W, Davis HV, Nagle GS. Mortality of workers potentially exposed to organic and inorganic brominated chemicals, DBCP, TRIS, PPB, and DDT. *Br J Ind Med* 1984;41:15–24.
117. Blair A, Grauman DJ, Lubin JH, Fraumeni JF Jr. Lung cancer and other causes of death among licensed pesticide applicators. *J Natl Cancer Inst* 1983;71:31–37.
118. Barthel E. Increased risk of lung cancer in pesticide-exposed male agricultural workers. *J Toxicol Environ Health* 1981;8:1027–1040.
119. Wolff MS, Toniolo PG, Lee EW, Rivera M, Dubin N. Blood levels of organochlorine residues and risk of breast cancer. *J Natl Cancer Inst* 1993;85(8):648–652.
120. Krieger N, Wolff MS, Hiatt RA, Rivera M, Vogelman J, Orentreich N. Breast cancer and serum organochlorines: a prospective study among white, black and Asian women. *J Natl Cancer Inst* 1994;86(8): 589–599.
121. Hoffman W. Organochlorine compounds: risk of non-Hodgkin's lymphoma and breast cancer? *Arch Environ Health* 1996 51(3):189–192.
122. Ahlborg UG, Lipworht L, Titus-Ernstoff L, et al. Organochlorine compounds in relation to breast cancer, endometrial cancer, and endometriosis: an assessment of the biological and epidemiological evidence. *Crit Rev Toxicol* 1995 25(6):463–531.
123. Alavanja MCR, Sandler DP, McMaster SB, et al. The Agricultural Health Study. *Environ Health Perspect* 1996 104(4):362–369.
124. Ecobichon DJ, Davies JE, Doull J, et al. Neurotoxic effects of pesticides. In: Baker SR, Wilkinson CF, eds. *The effect of pesticides on human health.* Princeton: Princeton Scientific, 1990;131–199.
125. Angle CR, McIntire MS, Meile RL. Neurologic sequelae of poisoning in children. *J Pediatr* 1968;73:531–539.
126. Onifer TM, Whisnant JP. Cerebellar ataxia and neuronitis after exposure to DDT and lindane. *Mayo Clin Proc* 1957;32:67–72.
127. Jenkins RB, Toole JF. Polyneuropathy following exposure to insecticides. *Arch Intern Med* 1964;113:691–695.
128. Kilburn KH, Thornton JC. Protracted neurotoxicity from chlordane sprayed to kill termites. *Environ Health Perspect* 1995;103: 690–694.
129. Johnson MK. The target for initiation of delayed neurotoxicity by organophosphorus esters: biochemical studies and toxicological applications. In: Hodgson E, Bend JR, Philpot RM, eds. *Reviews in biochemical toxicology.* New York: Elsevier Biomedical, 1982; 141–212.
130. Lotti M. Biological monitoring for organophosphate-induced delayed polyneuropathy. *Toxicol Lett* 1986;33:167–172.
131. Steenland K, Jenkins B, Ames RG, O'Malley M, Chrislip D, Russo J. Chronic neurological sequelae to organophosphate pesticide poisoning. *Am J Public Health* 1994;84(5):731–736.
132. Seidler A, Hellenbrand W, Robra B-P, Vieregge P, Nischan P, et al. Possible environmental, occupational, and other etiologic factors for Parkinson's disease: a case-control study in Germany. *Neurology* 1996 46(5):1275–1284
133. Zhang Z, Zhang X, Wang J, Min B, Tang X. Risk factors for Guillain-Barre syndrome in northern China: a case-control study. *Chung Kuo I Hsueh Ko Hsueh Yuan Hsueh Pao* 1995;17(4):291–295.
134. Savage EP, Keefe TJ, Mounce LM, Heaton RK, Lewis JA, Burcar PJ. Chronic neurological sequelae of acute organophosphate pesticide poisoning. *Arch Environ Health* 1988;43:38–45.
135. Levin HS, Rodnitzky RL. Behavioral effects of organophosphate pesticides in man. *Clin Toxicol* 1976;9:391–405.
136. Rosenstock L, Daniell W, Barnhart S, Schwartz D, Demers P. Chronic neuropsychological sequelae of occupational exposure to organophosphate insecticides. *Am J Ind Med* 1990;18:321–325
137. Coye MJ, Barnett PG, Midtling JE, et. al. Clinical confirmation of organophosphate poisoning by serial cholinesterase analyses. *Arch Intern Med* 1987;147:438–442.
138. Taylor JR, Selhorst JB, Houff SA, Martinez AJ. Chlordecone intoxication in man. Part I: Clinical observations. *Neurology* 1978;28: 626–630.
139. Larson PS, Engle JL Jr, Hennigar GR, Lane RW, Borzelleca JF. Acute, subchronic and chronic toxicity of chlordecone. *Toxicol Appl Pharmacol* 1979;48:29–41.
140. Epstein SS. Kepone—hazard evaluation. *Sci Total Environ* 1978;9: 1–62.
141. Schenker MB, Samuels SJ, Perkins C, Lewis EL, Katz DF, Overstreet JW. Prospective surveillance of semen quality in the workplace. *J Occup Med* 1988;30:336–344.
142. Carlsen E, Giwercman A, Keiding N, Skakkebaek NE. Evidence for decreasing quality of semen during past 50 years. *Br Med J* 1992;305: 609–613.
143. Bromwich P, Cohen J, Stewart I, Walker A. Decline in sperm counts: an artefact of changed reference range of normal? *Br Med J* 1994;309: 19–22.
144. Toppar J, Larsen JC, Christiansen P, et al. Male reproductive health and environmental xenoestrogens. *Environ Health Perspect* 1996; 104(suppl 4):741–803.
145. Arnold SF, Klotz DM, Collins BM, Vonier PM, Guillette LJ Jr, McLachlan JA. Synergistic activation of estrogen receptor with combinations of environmental chemicals. *Science* 1996;272(5267): 1489–1492.
146. Hanify JA, Metcalf P, Nebbs CL, Worsley KJ. Aerial spraying of 2,4,5-T and human birth malformations: an epidemiologic investigation. *Science* 1981;212:349–351.
147. Brogan WF, Brogan CE, Dadd JT. Herbicides and cleft lip and palate. *Lancet* 1980;2:597–598.
148. Nelson CJ, Holson JF, Green HG, Gaylor DW. Retrospective study of the relationship between agricultural use of 2,4,5-T and cleft palate occurrence in Arkansas. *Teratology* 1979;19:377–383.
149. Mattison DR, Bogumil RJ, Chapin R, et al. Reproductive effects of pesticides. In: Baker SR, Wilkinson CF, eds. *The effect of pesticides on human health.* Princeton: Princeton Scientific, 1990;297–389.
150. Czeizel AE, Elek C, Gundy S,Metneki J, et al. Environmental trichlorfon and cluster of congenital abnormalities. *Lancet* 1993;341: 539–542.
151. Romero P, Barnett PG, Midtling JE. Congenital anomalies associated with maternal exposure to oxydemeton-methyl. *Environ Res* 1989;50: 256–261.
152. Sherman JD. Chlorpyrifos (Dursban)-associated birth defects: report of four cases. *Arch Environ Health* 1996;51:5–8.

*Environmental and Occupational Medicine, Third Edition,* edited by William N. Rom.
Lippincott–Raven Publishers, Philadelphia © 1998.

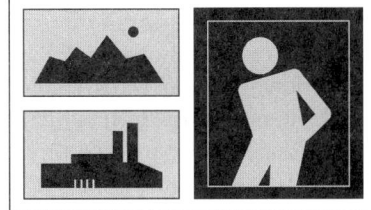

CHAPTER 84

# Health Effects of Phenoxy Herbicides and Agent Orange

Jeanne M. Stellman and Steven D. Stellman

Since the 1940s, millions of kilograms of the phenoxy herbicides 2,4-dichlorophenoxyacetic acid (2,4-D) and 2,4,5-trichlorophenoxyacetic acid (2,4,5-T) have been used throughout the world to control woody and herbaceous weeds, on broad-leafed weeds, cereal crops, pasture, and turf. These herbicides have found widespread commercial use in lawn, golf course, and roadway care, among other applications where control of broadleaf plants is desirable. Beginning in the late 1960s, the use of 2,4,5-T began to be curtailed by various governmental regulatory agencies and in 1978 the U.S. Environmental Protection Agency withdrew its registration and banned it from use (1). One particular formulation of 2,4-D and 2,4,5-T known as Agent Orange was used by U.S. military forces during the Vietnam War.

The relationship between exposure to Agent Orange and herbicides and consequent development of disease still remains a highly controversial subject with wide-ranging implications for veteran compensation, for future agricultural use of chemicals, and for potential liabilities under domestic and international law arising from past military and industrial usage (2,3). A major source of environmental anxiety is contamination of 2,4,5-T with dioxin [2,3,7,8-tetrachlorodibenzodioxin (TCDD)], an inadvertent by-product in the manufacture of many polycyclic aromatic hydrocarbons. Dioxin is a highly toxic chemical with a wide range of biologic effects (see Chapter 85). The 2,4,5-T used in the formulation of Agent Orange purchased by the military during the Vietnam War was comparatively heavily contaminated by dioxin. Estimates are that the mean concentration of TCDD in Agent Orange was 2 ppm, with the concentration ranging between 0.05 and 30 ppm (4).

## MILITARY DEFOLIATION DURING THE VIETNAM WAR

Throughout the 1960s, the United States military forces in the Republic of Vietnam undertook a massive program of defoliation. Several types and combinations of chemicals were used for the defoliation program. The mixtures were nicknamed by the color of the identification stripe that appeared on the barrel (5):

| | |
|---|---|
| Agent Orange: | Esters of 2,4-D and 2,4,5-T |
| Agent White: | Triisopropanolamine salts of 2,4-D and picloram |
| Agent Blue: | Organic arsenic (cacodylic acid) |

The ecologic consequences of the defoliation program on the Vietnamese countryside and on the Vietnamese people became a highly charged political and scientific issue almost as soon as the full-scale military policy began in 1965. As a result of social and political pressures, the United States ordered the discontinuation of the use of Agent Orange as a chemical defoliant in May 1970. The use of all other kinds of herbicides was discontinued by the end of 1971.

According to military records, more than 12 million gallons of Agent Orange were included in the 19 million gallons of total herbicides that were used in South Viet-

J. M. Stellman: Division of Health Policy and Management, Columbia University School of Public Health, New York, New York 10032.
S. D. Stellman: Division of Epidemiology, American Health Foundation, New York, New York 10017.

nam. A committee of the National Academy of Sciences that was established in 1970 to analyze the ecologic and health consequences of the spraying (6) produced a computerized record, known as the HERBS tape, of all missions flown by the U.S. Air Force's Operation Ranch Hand, the major U.S. military defoliation program (7). In the 1980s, the Department of Defense assigned to the U.S. Army and Joint Services Environmental Support Group (ESG) the task of enumerating all military use of defoliants besides those sprayed by the Air Force in Operation Ranch Hand, as recorded on the HERBS tape, primarily those used by the Army for fire and support base perimeter clearance and other road clearance and construction operations. The ESG identified and abstracted more than 1 million military records, such as Morning Reports, Operations Reports and Lessons Learned (ORLLs), inventories of the U.S. Chemical Corps, etc., and incorporated them into a second HERBS tape known as the Services HERBS tape (8). Both the NAS HERBS tape and the Services HERBS tape contain information on the type of agent used, the military purpose of the mission, its exact location (with a nominal precision of 100 m), the date of the mission, and the approximate acreage covered (9).

Over 2.3 million U.S. servicemen and -women served in Vietnam in addition to American civilians and military personnel from Australia, New Zealand, and the Republic of Korea. Despite the public health importance of possible exposure to these chemical agents, few of the studies that have been carried out on potentially exposed veteran populations meet acceptable epidemiologic standards for relating exposures to health outcomes. As will be seen, most veteran studies have relied on extremely weak surrogates for exposure, and many others are simply not informative for possible human health effects of Agent Orange. Hence, most conclusions concerning possible effects of phenoxy herbicides on veterans are based on inferences drawn from experimental studies, and from studies of occupationally exposed groups.

The most extensive set of inferences has been presented by a committee of the U.S. National Academy of Sciences Institute of Medicine (IOM). The Committee to Review the Health Effects in Vietnam Veterans of Exposure to Herbicides (referred to here simply as the IOM Committee) was created in 1992 expressly to review the available evidence in order to provide the public and policymakers with an unbiased set of conclusions concerning health effects for which sufficient evidence exists for a statistical association with Agent Orange and related herbicides. The committee has to date issued two reports, a lengthy review in 1994 plus the first of a series of anticipated biennial updates in 1996. The committee concluded that there is "sufficient evidence" that four health outcomes are associated with exposure. Three of these are rare types of cancer (soft tissue sarcoma, non-Hodgkin's lymphoma, and Hodgkin's disease), and the fourth is a skin condition, chloracne. The committee rated a large number of conditions as "inadequate/insufficient evidence" to determine whether an association exists. These included many types of cancer, including hepatobiliary, nasal and nasopharyngeal, bone, breast, female reproductive, kidney, testicular, and skin cancers, as well as a variety of reproductive outcomes.

One major potential source of data that has so far been little used is the Vietnamese population itself. Many Vietnamese civilians and former combatants lived and continue to live in areas that were heavily sprayed, and many were exposed more heavily than American forces, especially herbicide applicators who served in the Army of the Republic of Vietnam (ARVN). Schecter and colleagues (10) have recently documented significantly higher levels of TCDD in the serum of civilians living in the former South Vietnam, in comparison with serum levels in residents of the former North Vietnam, and Verger and colleagues (11) have demonstrated the feasibility of utilizing U.S. herbicide spray records for assessing exposure in Vietnamese civilians. However, few health studies have so far been carried out.

## UPTAKE, DISTRIBUTION, AND ACUTE TOXICITY

The uptake, distribution, and toxicology of 2,4,5-T and 2,4-D have been reviewed by several authorities (1,3,12,13). The extensive contamination of Agent Orange, and to a lesser extent of commercial 2,4,5-T, by dioxins greatly complicates the ability to study and define the health effects of 2,4-D and 2,4,5-T alone. The toxicology of TCDD, discussed in Chapter 85, must be considered at the same time since it is a highly toxic and pervasive contaminant of most 2,4,5-T formulations.

The physiologic distribution and molecular basis of the interactions between 2,4,5-T and 2,4,-D in humans are not fully understood. 2,4-D appears to bind covalently to liver proteins and lipids. It also accumulates in the brain. Urinary excretion is the primary route for elimination of 2,4,5-T and 2,4-D. Elimination is not first order, that is, the rate of excretion of 2,4,5-T and 2,4-D is dependent on its initial concentration (14). While the half-life of 2,4-D in humans following a single dose appears to be 18 to 20 hours (15), the half-life in humans following multiple doses is not well defined (16), all of which complicates exposure assessment in epidemiologic studies. Urinary excretion continues for several days following initial exposure. It also appears that humans store 2,4-D in the liver and kidney after high exposure, while the liver, kidney, lungs, spleen, and heart of other mammalian species have been found to have high 2,4-D levels.

The acute toxicity of 2,4-D and 2,4,5-T is species dependent. The dose lethal to 50% of an experimental group ($LD_{50}$) for 2,4-D ranges from 100 mg/kg in dogs to 540 mg/kg in chickens (12,17), while the $LD_{50}$ for 2,4,5-

T in dogs is 150 mg/kg and 500 mg/kg in rats (12). The liver appears to be a target organ for chronic toxic effects of 2,4-D. Hepatotoxicity has been observed in a number of species (15,18,19). Effects include hepatitis, local necrosis of the liver, and centrilobular atrophy and changes in liver enzymes. The central nervous system been identified as the target organ for acute response in humans (20), dogs and cats (21), and, more recently, Wistar rats (22). Both 2,4,5-T and 2,4-D have been experimentally shown to cross the blood-brain barrier (23,24).

## EXPERIMENTAL TOXICITY OF PHENOXY HERBICIDES

Chronic toxicity of phenoxy herbicides in experimental animals affects the same organ systems as the acute effects listed above, viz., liver, kidney, blood, and nervous system.

Of considerable interest are the possible mutagenicity and carcinogenicity of these chemicals in animal models. Neither 2,4-D nor 2,4,5-T is mutagenic in standard test systems. Older studies evaluating the carcinogenicity of 2,4-D are controversial because of their basic study design. Problems in design and interpretation have led to differing assessments of toxicity (25). For example, Lilienfeld and Gallo (1) have noted that the U.S. Environmental Protection Agency and the Food and Drug Administration accepted that 2,4-D is not a carcinogen, while the World Health Organization (WHO) and the International Agency for Research on Cancer (IARC) did not consider the available evidence sufficient to conclude it is so (15,26). A recent case-control study by Hayes and co-workers (27) demonstrated an increased incidence of canine malignant lymphoma related to the use of 2,4-D in lawn care by owners who kept the dogs kept as pets, while an increase in astrocytomas was observed among Fischer 344 rats receiving 2,4-D in their diets according to acceptable bioassay guidelines (28,29). These studies led the Institute of Medicine expert panel on Agent Orange effects to conclude that there is "suggestive, but not compelling evidence" that astrocytomas in rats and malignant lymphomas in dogs may be associated with 2,4-D exposure (3). Convincing experimental data demonstrating the carcinogenicity of 2,4,5-T are not available.

In a 1977 report, the IARC found 2,4-D embryotoxic to offspring of female rats treated with 2,000 ppm in the diet before and throughout pregnancy (12). Fetal anomalies were reported in offspring of several strains of mice administered 2,4-D during gestation (30). However, other studies have failed to find either reproductive or developmental effects. The IARC concluded that the herbicide 2,4,5-T was teratogenic in mice, resulting in fetal growth retardation and fetal weight reduction at doses below 20 mg/kg and in an increased incidence of cleft palate at higher doses; at doses above 45 mg/kg, cystic kidneys have been found in mice (31), a conclusion confirmed by several later studies. The chemical can also reduce the size of litters in mice (32). These experiments were carried out using 2,4,5-T not contaminated with TCDD.

### Human Studies

There are two main sources of information on clinical human health effects of phenoxy herbicides:

1. Information gleaned following industrial accidents and exposures: The populations exposed in this way have included both worker groups and community populations. Occupational groups have included workers involved in the production of chemicals, agricultural and forestry workers, and workers in the paper and pulp industry. Environmental studies of major accidental exposures involved the residents of Times Beach, Missouri, Seveso, Italy, and South Vietnamese civilians.
2. Studies of Vietnam veterans potentially exposed to Agent Orange: Several groups of veterans have formed the basis of epidemiologic studies. These include Air Force Ranch Hands who were involved in the aerial application of herbicides in Vietnam, members of the American Legion, veterans who registered for the Department of Veterans Affairs Agent Orange Registry, and participants in studies conducted by the U.S. Centers for Disease Control (CDC) in its Vietnam Experience Study (33) and Selected Cancers Study (34), among others.

## CENTRAL IMPORTANCE OF EXPOSURE ASSESSMENT AND SURROUNDING CONTROVERSIES

A difficult issue but one central to evaluation of human health effects of exposure to phenoxy herbicides is quantitative estimation of the level of exposure on an individual basis. Within the literature considered here, use of surrogate (rather than direct) measures is widespread, whether the studies be of veteran populations, industrial cohorts, or community groups. Consequently, interpretive review of the literature must emphasize the quality of exposure measures. The surrogate most frequently used in place of actual measurement of exposure is simply one's occupation or place of residence or, in the case of Agent Orange, the fact of having served in Vietnam, perhaps in a very broadly defined area in Vietnam (such as one of the four military tactical corps areas into which the then South Vietnam had been arbitrarily divided, I to IV Corps).

One frequently used surrogate for Agent Orange exposure utilizes a veteran's military occupational specialty (MOS), under the assumption that persons with combat-related specialties have an increased likelihood of exposure (35). However, this must have resulted in considerable misclassification. The relationship between Agent

Orange, Vietnam service, and combat experience is not established, although some "rule of thumb" estimates can be made. It requires approximately four support troops, who generally are not exposed to combat, for each combat soldier. Further, Stellman and colleagues (5) have found that while there is a very strong correlation between combat experience and likelihood of exposure to Agent Orange, a large number of combat veterans were not likely to have been exposed, whereas a small but distinct number of herbicide handlers and others who were not in combat situations appear to have been exposed.

A number of epidemiologic studies have relied exclusively on Vietnam service as a surrogate "exposure" measure. Such a study, by definition, can do no more than determine the relative disease rates of Vietnam veterans in comparison with non-Vietnam veterans or the nonmilitary population and cannot be considered informative on the question of Agent Orange. In addition, some published cancer studies of Vietnam veterans provided insufficient allowance for chronic disease latency to be relevant to the scientific discussion of cancer causation, for example. Such methodologic shortcomings will at worst lead to underestimates of possible health effects and false-negative studies, and, in the case of a positive study, be uninformative as to the extent of risk attributable to herbicide exposure.

### Evaluating Troop Exposure Based on Military Records

Two alternative methodologies have been used to assign potential exposure levels to Vietnam veterans. One utilizes military records to locate individual soldiers or their military units in spatial and temporal proximity to documented herbicide spraying. In addition to the herbicide dispersal data, this methodology exploits the extensive information that is also available on the physical locations of a very large number of U.S. troops during the war, and uses quantitative techniques commonly applied in environmental exposure assessment to link spray activities to troop locations. Stellman et al. (5) have developed an algorithm wherein specific troop locations in Vietnam are mathematically evaluated for proximity in time and place to known herbicidal missions, as recorded on the HERBS tapes (13). This method is similar to one later proposed by the CDC and used in its Agent Orange studies. The method does not provide an absolute measure of exposure to herbicides or TCDD, but rather is a measure of so-called exposure opportunity.

Analysis of the movements of several dozen battalions in the third combat tactical zone of Vietnam (III Corps) during the years 1966 to 1969 has shown, for example, that thousands of men appear to have been stationed within 2 km of spraying and within 1 day of the spray activity.

### Evaluating Troop Exposure Using Biomarkers

An alternative exposure assessment methodology attempts to utilize levels of TCDD in body tissues of Vietnam veterans as measures of exposure during the conflict (36). Typically, these assays are carried out on serum or adipose tissue samples collected years or decades after exposure ceased. Since the kinetics of such exposure are not understood and since such a long period of time has passed since the wartime exposure, there is a limit to the adequacy of current TCDD levels as an exposure measure. TCDD assays also provide little insight into possible levels of 2,4-D exposure. In addition to basic mechanistic issues, the most serious problem with such determinations is the length of time that has elapsed since exposure in relation to the decay rate of TCDD in the body.

The determination of TCDD half-life has been problematic. An initial estimate of 7.1 years was based on the median for 36 Air Force veterans who had two TCDD assays in serum drawn 5 years apart. A subsequent report listed a half-life of 11.3 years, which was strongly dependent on percent body fat and age (37). These calculations were based on the unwarranted assumption of a first-order reaction mechanism, despite experimental evidence to the contrary (14,15). The utility of military records and biologic measures thus remains an area of scientific controversy.

The Institute of Medicine reviewed both records-based and biomarker-based exposure methods, and concluded that neither historical exposure reconstruction nor biomarker methodology has so far been established as a completely reliable exposure assessment method; the Institute recommended that both methods be developed further (3).

## HUMAN CLINICAL EFFECTS

Although the clinical picture for both short- and long-term effects of phenoxy herbicides in humans is not well delineated, several patterns of symptoms have systematically emerged in a variety of studies. Some effects, like chloracne, an acne-like skin disease associated with exposure to a number of chlorinated hydrocarbons, have been documented for decades. Recently the first cases of industrial chloracne in women were reported among a group of Russian workers engaged in the manufacture of 2,4,5-T (38). It should be noted that while chloracne is a recognized effect of exposure, it does not uniformly result from exposure (39); absence of chloracne does not indicate absence of exposure. The causal relationship between chloracne and phenoxy herbicide exposure has been recognized by the IOM (13). A possibly causal relationship has also been recognized between exposure to herbicides and porphyria cutanea tarda (PCT). In the CDC cross-sectional health study of Vietnam veterans, the Vietnam Experience Study (VES), one Vietnam veteran (but no controls) had a pattern of urinary porphyrin levels consistent with PCT. Studies of one group of German pesticide plant workers revealed chronic hepatic porphyria, but not overt PCT (40). While the relationship to PCT is not clear, there does appear to be a consistent finding of porphyrins in the blood of some exposed people.

Clinical evaluations of exposed workers and others have found a wide range of other dermatologic, metabolic, neurologic, and behavioral effects (41). In its review of the many studies, the IOM has been unable to label these studies as more than suggestive because of the many problems in exposure assessment, assembling of control groups, and other aspects of study design that are an inherent problem in environmental and occupational exposures of this kind. Because of the large number of such studies that exist, a few are discussed here as representative of the information available on noncancer and nonreproductive health effects.

Discussion of the many potential clinical effects of phenoxy herbicides in humans, including 2,4-D and 2,4,5-T, as well as the contaminant TCDD, can be organized in four broad categories as suggested by Young et al. (4). The array of clinical manifestations associated with exposure was presented as skin manifestations, systemic effects, neurologic effects, and psychiatric effects (42). In summarizing 15 published studies, Young et al. observed that each of the following signs, symptoms, and disorders was reported in six or more individuals: headaches; sensory nerves and tracts; neuralgia or myalgia; paresis; porphyria; hyperpigmentation or hirsutism; acne; asthenia; other psychiatric problems; abdominal pain or pressure; and anorexia, nausea, vomiting, and diarrhea. Additional conditions reported in the literature and summarized by Young et al. include chloracne; mild fibrosis of the liver; elevated serum levels of transaminase, cholesterol, and triglycerides; swollen lymph glands; sexual dysfunction; depression; and bouts of anger.

A study of American Legionnaire Vietnam veterans found an array of "symptom complexes" to be dose-related to exposure. These included increased incidence of colds and upper respiratory tract problems, fatigue, neurologic symptomatology, and behavioral effects, using a military records–based Agent Orange exposure opportunity index (43,44). These findings are consistent with the studies cited by Young et al., which suggested that nonspecific symptoms or conditions, like fatigue, dizziness, and nausea might be related to chemical herbicide exposure (45).

The United States Air Force study of Air Force personnel involved in the herbicide Ranch Hand Operations has found a number of clinical differences between men who worked in Operation Ranch Hand and other Air Force personnel. In one analysis Albanese (46) reported that of 11 clinical parameters investigated in the study, six are abnormal among Ranch Handers, with five of the six abnormalities occurring in the direction predicted for an effect of dioxin exposure. These five parameters include an increased incidence of neoplasia, neurologic changes, hepatotoxicity, cardiovascular, and endocrinologic changes.

The CDC Vietnam Experience Study (VES) obtained medical histories through telephone interviews, followed by clinical examination of a sample of those interviewed. Vietnam veterans more often than non-Vietnam veterans had a history of hospitalization, hypertension, benign growths, chloracne and other skin conditions, ulcers of the stomach and duodenum, hepatitis, liver conditions other than cirrhosis, urinary tract problems, and fertility difficulties (47). The CDC study was not an Agent Orange study, but rather a study of the "Vietnam Experience," and for most analyses did not stratify the cohort of men with service in Vietnam by their exposure to combat, which is considered to be the major predictive independent variable for health and well-being outcomes (43,44).

Several clinical findings were also more prevalent in the Vietnam veterans than in the control veteran population: possible left ventricular hypertrophy, hearing loss, peripheral neuropathy, and evidence of past hepatitis B infection. Abnormal laboratory findings in the Vietnam veterans included measures of gamma-glutamyl transferase, fasting glucose, thyroid-stimulating hormone, and occult stool blood. Finally, an array of psychosocial and psychological disorders were observed, included a 15% prevalence of posttraumatic stress disorder.

## HUMAN CANCER STUDIES

Phenoxy herbicide exposures are related to at least three forms of human cancer: soft tissue sarcomas (STS), non-Hodgkin's lymphoma (NHL), and Hodgkin's disease (HD). The evidence for these associations, described below, arises chiefly from studies of occupational exposures in agricultural, forestry, and industrial workers, rather than military exposure, because it was not until recently that sufficient time had elapsed to make cancer studies of Vietnam veterans practical and valid due to latency considerations. [As a practical matter, it is not possible to determine from epidemiologic studies whether an observed association is with a specific phenoxy acid, TCDD, or both. It is noteworthy that several studies implicating phenoxy herbicides were of 2,4-D alone (48). Commercial 2,4-D is generally not as heavily contaminated with dioxin as was 2,4,5-T.] Studies have also been carried out in several populations with environmental exposure, and in some veteran groups, but with generally less reliable results.

Epidemiologic studies in occupationally exposed groups can be expected to yield the most useful data for assessing long-term health effects for a number of reasons. First, it is usually easier to characterize exposure to specific chemicals, sometimes for a subject's entire working life, because of availability of employment records, industrial hygiene measurements or other assessment of workplace exposure, and the regularity of the work process itself. Furthermore, occupational exposures to many workplace chemicals have historically been much higher than exposures to the general population. Studies differ markedly with respect to exposure information, and can be divided into those with presumptive herbicide exposure (certain agricultural and factory workers) and those where it is not possible to make any inference at all regarding exposure (some agricultural and veteran studies).

The association between cancer and phenoxy herbicide exposure has been addressed by two distinct types of studies: case-control and cohort. Positive findings have been obtained with both types. Case-control studies are usually specific for one type of cancer, and require fewer cases. Cohort studies are more readily carried out on an industrywide basis, and can yield results for many types of cancer. They are far less efficient, especially in detecting increases in rare cancers such as STS and NHL, because they require that large numbers of initially healthy subjects be followed over long time periods. One disadvantage frequently encountered in occupational epidemiology is the fragmentation of the work force, with exposures sometimes limited to small numbers of people in widely scattered workplaces. Small cohorts may lack statistical power, which increases with the size of the exposed group. For this reason, there has been an effort in several countries to assemble composite cohorts of workers in related industries with many different employers.

Three of the most important multiplant cohorts of industrial workers exposed to herbicides were assembled by the IARC in Europe, Lynge in Denmark, and Fingerhut in the United States. The IARC International Register of Workers Exposed to Phenoxy Herbicides and Their Contaminants is a cohort of 16,863 males and 1,527 females in ten countries who were employed in the production or spraying of herbicides or pesticides (49,50). A cohort of workers in facilities that produced phenoxy herbicides and other related chemicals was established by Lynge (51,52) in Denmark. This cohort contributes a large number of cases in the IARC registry. It consists of 3,390 male and 1,071 female workers involved in the manufacture of phenoxy herbicides in Denmark prior to 1982, and utilizes the Central Population Register of Denmark for ascertainment of vital status and the Danish Cancer Registry for cancer ascertainment. Another set of cohort data was contributed by the Dutch National Institute of Public Health and Environmental Protection, which has separately reported on mortality among workers from two pesticide factories producing phenoxy acid herbicides (53).

The U.S. National Institute for Occupational Safety and Health (NIOSH) developed data on a cohort of production workers from 12 chemical plants with potential exposure to TCDD, which included some phenoxy herbicide exposed workers as well (54). The American cohort consists of 5,172 male workers employed in production of TCDD-contaminated chemicals between 1942 and 1984. Several of these plants have previously been the subject of epidemiologic studies as a result of industrial accidents that released dioxin (e.g., an outbreak of chloracne in 61 workers at a Dow plant) (55).

One of the best known occupational cohorts consists of Monsanto employees exposed during an explosion of a trichlorophenol process in 1949 (56). Among 121 workers who developed verified chloracne after the accident, and who were followed-up for 30 years, there were 32 deaths [standardized mortality ratio (SMR) = 69], but for lung cancer the SMR was 175. Furthermore, there was one death from STS, one from HD, and two leukemias (SMR = 341 for hematopoietic cancers). Analysis of the mortality experience of the entire blue-collar work force of 884 men initially yielded 163 deaths (SMR = 103), but when the decedents were classified by exposure to 2,4,5-T, there were 58 deaths, of which nine were cancer: six lung, two bladder, and one STS (57). Regrettably, recent allegations of scientific misstatement in the study of Monsanto workers has raised serious questions about the utility and validity of this study (58).

Several cohorts of American industrial workers involved in manufacture of 2,4,5-T and other dioxin-contaminated products have been studied. Most groups have been too small to yield sufficient cases for analysis (59). However, in one cohort of 2,187 Dow employees, 370 deaths occurred (SMR = 93). There was 1 STS (0.4 expected) in the highest exposure group, and 5 NHL (2.6 expected). One additional worker died of STS outside the observation period. While not epidemiologically conclusive, this study adds more weight to the growing evidence (60).

**Soft Tissue Sarcoma**

Both cohort and case-control studies have provided evidence for an association between phenoxy herbicide exposure and soft tissue sarcoma (STS).

An excess of STS cases was reported among workers in the two Danish plants that manufactured phenoxy acids and other chemicals, with five cases observed [relative risk (RR) = 2.72 (0.88–6.34)]. Allowing a 10-year latency increased the risk to 3.67 (1.0–9.39) (52). In the IARC multicountry cohort, Saracci et al. (49) reported an SMR of 6.1 (1.7–15.5) among those whose deaths occurred 10 to 19 years after first exposure. Within the same cohort, Kogevinas and colleagues (50) created a nested case-control study using 11 observed cases of STS with five controls per case. A team of industrial hygienists made a detailed exposure reconstruction for cases and controls without knowledge of disease status, with special attention to cumulative exposure to phenoxy herbicides and related chemicals (61). They reported associations between STS and exposure to any phenoxy herbicide and any dioxin, as well as with cumulative exposure to TCDD and uncontaminated 2,4-D (62).

The NIOSH cohort has also reported an elevated risk for STS [SMR = 9.2, 95% confidence interval (CI) 1.9–27.0] (54). However, Collins et al. (63) have noted that all but one of the confirmed STS cases in the NIOSH study came from the Monsanto subcohort, and argued in favor of 4-aminobiphenyl rather than TCDD as the etiologic agent.

Several studies of forestry and agricultural workers carried out in different regions of Sweden have shown strong associations between exposure to phenoxy herbicides and STS. A case-control study of exposure to phenoxyacetic acids or chlorophenols among forestry workers in Northern Sweden gave an overall sixfold increase in relative risk for STS, and 5.3 for phenoxy acids only (64). A second case-control study in counties of southern Sweden, where 4-chloro-2-methylphenoxyacetic acid (MCPA) and 2,4-D have been used widely in agriculture, reported a relative risk of 8.5 for exposure to chlorophenoxy herbicides alone for more than 30 days ($n = 7$), and 5.7 for less than 30 days ($n = 7$), and 4.2 for herbicides other than 2,4,5-T (65). Yet a third registry-based study of 55 male cases in the three northernmost counties of Sweden yielded a relative risk of 3.3 ($p = .02$) for phenoxyacetic acid exposure, which rose to 4.1 if eight cases with uncertain diagnosis were removed (66). These three studies have engendered a great deal of debate and have survived more than a decade of close scrutiny from hostile reviewers, particularly in legal settings.

A population-based case-control study was conducted in northern Italy with 37 male and 31 female STS patients whose environmental exposures to phenoxy herbicides resulted mainly from rice weeding. The relative risk was 2.7 for living women, although the numbers of cases were too small to reach significance. For women under 75 years of age who had been exposed between 1950 and 1955, a highly significant risk of 15.5 was observed. Males were rarely exposed and their risk was not increased (67).

Not all epidemiologic investigations in Sweden and elsewhere have been positive (68–71). However, an excess risk of STS has been observed in a number of cohort studies, to be described below. Furthermore, the presence of negative studies does not, generally, detract from positive epidemiologic findings (12).

### Non-Hodgkin's Lymphoma and Hodgkin's Disease

Lymphatic cancers, particularly non-Hodgkin's lymphoma, have also been associated with phenoxy herbicide exposures in Sweden and the United States. In 1994 Hardell et al. (72) reported an odds ratio (OR) of 5.5 for histopathologically verified NHL (95% CI 2.7–11) in relation to exposure to phenoxyacetic acids. Among the 105 cases and 335 controls, most exposures were to a commercial mixture of 2,4-D and 2,4,5-T (similar to Agent Orange).

A National Cancer Institute research group ascertained all cases of adult NHL among Kansas residents, from 1976 to 1982 ($n = 297$). Among 200 sampled cases, the RR was 2.2 for phenoxy herbicide exposure, and 2.6 for exposure to 2,4-D alone (73).

A series of case-control studies of New Zealand farm workers initially reported elevated relative risks for certain occupational specialties (rather than specific exposures), observing, "Agricultural workers are at increased risk of developing NHL and multiply myeloma.... It is certainly plausible that exposure to phenoxy herbicides could have contributed to the excess of NHL among NZ agricultural and forestry workers" (74). In a subsequent New Zealand study in which interviews were conducted with 83 of 88 confirmed NHL cases, relative risks were calculated as 1.2 for farming, 1.5 for use of agricultural chemical sprays, 1.3 for railroad workers, 2.2 for "chemical sprayer," and 1.3 for various phenoxy herbicide exposures. As is typical in small studies, none of these risks were statistically significant, and the authors tended to discount any herbicide-cancer link (75). Their findings are nonetheless consistent with effects found in other studies. Furthermore, when other types of lymphomas were included (lymphosarcoma and reticulosarcoma), numerous RRs above 1.0 were observed, including 2.0 (0.2–21.5) for forestry sprayers and 3.2 (0.3–37.8) for railway sprayers (76).

In a study conducted in Washington State, the relative risk of NHL was significantly elevated among "men who had been farmers, 1.33 (1.03–1.7), forestry herbicide applicators, 4.80 (1.2–19.4), and for those potentially exposed to phenoxy herbicides in any occupation for 15 years or more during the period prior to 15 years before cancer diagnosis, 1.71 (1.04–2.8)" (77).

Death certificates for all HD and NHL deaths in Hancock Co., Ohio in 1958 to 1983 were analyzed via a case-control method to determine associations with specific occupations. Hancock Co. was known to have high herbicide use. Though not significant due to small numbers, the RR for NHL in farmers was 2.1 in 1958–1973, while the RR for HD was 21.2 based on three cases. The authors noted that their study "adds to the growing body of reports linking farming and malignant lymphoma, especially NHL" (78).

Hardell et al. (79) and Hardell and Bengtsson (80) reported a case-control study with 60 cases of HD. They found ORs of 2.4 (CI 0.9–6.5) for low-grade exposure to chlorophenols, and 6.5 (CI 2.7–19.0) for high-grade exposures. Persson et al. (81) studied 54 cases, with an OR of 3.8 (0.5–35.2) for exposure to phenoxy acids. In a later study that compared occupational histories of 31 HD cases with 204 controls, the OR was 7.4 (1.4–40.0) (82). The IOM Committee cites 13 additional studies in agricultural workers, but ORs were statistically significant in very few of these.

### Hepatocellular Carcinoma

Cancer of the liver, though extremely rare in Western countries, occurs at a very high rate in many Asian countries including Vietnam. The only U.S. study to address the possibility that liver cancer is related to phenoxy herbicide exposure was the CDC Selected Cancers Study, which found only eight patients who had even served in Vietnam (83) and must thus be considered uninformative. Cordier and colleagues (84) reported an elevated risk of hepatocellular carcinoma and at least 10 years military service in South Vietnam among Vietnamese veterans. However, this evidence is at best suggestive, since no actual exposure estimate was provided.

## VIETNAM VETERAN MORTALITY STUDIES

The Department of Veterans Affairs examined proportionate mortality rates (PMRs) among Army and Marine veterans, and observed that Marines had significantly high PMRs for lung cancer (PMR = 158) and non-Hodgkin's lymphoma (PMR = 210) (85).

A number of other studies of Vietnam veterans have been reported in the literature. Despite frequent references to the contrary, none, in our judgment, offers useful information about potential risks of exposure to phenoxy herbicides. For instance, while a widely cited case-control study from New York State of 281 cases of soft tissue sarcoma reported a nominal relative risk of 0.53 for Vietnam service, only 10 patients actually served in Vietnam, and no objective information about exposure was available. This study is simply not informative on Agent Orange (86). A mortality study of New York State veterans made a similar claim, but in fact had no measure of exposure other than mere presence in Vietnam (87).

The CDC's Selected Cancers study of military service in Vietnam and six types of cancer, found a significantly elevated risk (1.47) for non-Hodgkin's lymphoma, based on 99 Vietnam veterans with this malignancy, and 133 Vietnam controls. For the five other cancer sites, the numbers of patients who had served in Vietnam was so small as to be essentially meaningless: 26 cases of STS, 28 of Hodgkin's disease, eight liver cancers, three nasopharyngeal cancers, and three nasal cancers. No exposure measures for Agent Orange were utilized and hence no conclusions about a possible association can be drawn for any cancer (83).

A final group of studies is frequently cited as failing to confirm any association between cancer and herbicide exposure, but in fact careful analysis shows that none is adequate for that purpose. These include a cohort study of Finnish 2,4-D and 2,4,5-T applicators whose duration of exposure was "quite brief" (most had 2 to 7 weeks total) (88,89).

## ADVERSE HUMAN REPRODUCTIVE EXPERIENCE

The possible human reproductive health effects of exposure to phenoxyherbicides has been an area of intense interest. While not all studies on Vietnam veterans are consistent, several outcomes have consistently been observed. There appears to be a trend toward an increased incidence of miscarriages and/or birth defects among Vietnam veterans, particularly when an exposure opportunity index has been employed in the study. Increased rates of neural tube defects have led the IOM to suggest that spina bifida should be considered a positive outcome (13,47). Abnormalities in male reproductive function itself are suggested as well. These data, however, are not yet completely conclusive, and a large study, employing an acceptable exposure index, has yet to be done. Similar positive conclusions can be inferred from the reports in the Vietnamese civilian populations, despite some of their weaknesses (90).

In the early 1960s, suspicions were raised that the South Vietnamese were experiencing an increase in the congenital malformation rate as a result of the U.S. military defoliation program. These claims were first investigated by Department of Defense researchers, who carried out temporal and geographic analyses of reproductive outcomes between 1960 and 1969, using records collected from several hospitals (91). The report showed decreasing stillbirth rates for the heavily sprayed period of 1966 to 1969, compared to the 1960 to 1965 period. The negative findings of Cutting et al. (91) were strongly criticized on methodologic grounds by the National Academy of Sciences (3), which proposed a dilution effect resulting from the inclusion of Saigon to the analysis, since the Saigon area was not subjected to spraying. When Saigon was removed from the analysis, the malformation rate, molar pregnancy rate, and the stillbirth rate were all found to rise. The data, however, were considered too fraught with ascertainment and other problems to be used as the basis for a definitive study.

Several other studies of Vietnamese populations, among both South Vietnamese women and soldiers from the North, which was never sprayed with herbicides, but who served in South Vietnam, have been carried out. Some of these studies have been summarized by Constable and Hatch (90) and are derived from an international symposium on the effects of phenoxy herbicides that was held in Ho Chi Minh City (formerly Saigon) in 1983. The nine North Vietnamese studies summarized show a consistent association between presumptive paternal exposure (i.e., having served in the South prior to conception) and certain types of birth defects, particularly anencephaly and orofacial defects, although the magnitude of the risk varies. Conflicting results on paternally mediated miscarriages were found, and no association with molar pregnancies was documented, according to Constable and Hatch.

Constable and Hatch (90) also summarized the studies carried out on South Vietnamese, where both parents may have been exposed to phenoxy herbicides. These studies tended to be more consistently positive and demonstrated increased reports of miscarriage, stillbirths, molar pregnancies, and malformations. Constable and Hatch call "the evidence for an association with herbicide exposure very suggestive."

There have been several reproductive outcome studies of Vietnam veterans, both American and Australian. The CDC completed a case-control study of babies born in the metropolitan Atlanta area and concluded that Vietnam veterans in general did not have an increased risk of fathering babies with defects (all types combined) (92).

Aschengrau and Monson (93) have reported a significant increased risk of 1.7 for one or more major malformations among children born to wives of Vietnam veterans. The findings were based on a case-control study of women delivering infants at Boston Hospital for Women between 1977 and 1980. Field and Kerr (94) studied 436 Australian Vietnam veterans living in Tasmania in comparison to similar Tasmanian families fathered by nonveterans and report distinct patterns of "severe malformations and illness among veterans' children." This study is suggestive but not generalizable because of limitations in study design.

However, as with the mortality and cancer studies of Vietnam veterans discussed elsewhere, none of these reports can be considered to be Agent Orange studies, per se, since service in Vietnam is not equivalent to herbicidal exposures. Erickson et al. (92), however, did utilize an exposure opportunity index, based on military records and an expert military panel's assessment, as an exposure measure. Veterans judged to have been "exposed" to Agent Orange had significantly high risks of having children with birth defects, including spina bifida, cleft lip with or without cleft palate, and a miscellaneous constellation of neoplasms.

Two reports of a dose-related increased incidence of miscarriage among wives of Vietnam veterans also exist. Stellman et al. (43) studied a cohort of American Legionnaires who served in Southeast Asia and compared them to Vietnam era veterans with no such service. Using the exposure likelihood index described they calculated a dose-related increased risk for miscarriages among spouses of exposed veterans, with a significantly elevated rate of 1.6 among those who reported military occupations involving herbicide handling. The CDC also reported a significantly increased miscarriage rate among Vietnam veteran spouses, and using a self-reported herbicide exposure score, found that the miscarriage rate was significantly increased in the same dose-related manner as among the Legionnaires (47).

The CDC Vietnam Experience Study also found that, in comparison to non-Vietnam veterans, the Vietnam veterans experienced low sperm count, abnormal sperm morphology, and increased incidence of birth defects, which included nervous system anomalies, musculoskeletal deformities, and anomalies of the integument and hydrocephalus. Without an exposure marker, however, as stated previously, these latter data are difficult to interpret with respect to Agent Orange exposure.

The United States Air Force study of Air Force personnel involved in the herbicide Ranch Hand Operations also investigated reproductive outcomes. The 1984 report showed no significant differences compared to control groups for prematurity, miscarriages, stillbirths, or "severe" birth defects. However, the study did show an excess of "minor" defects (an unorthodox classification encompassing defects judged to be life-threatening or interfering with normal overall health or socioeconomic progress) as well as a significant excess of neonatal deaths and physical handicaps. A further analysis of the Ranch Hand data, which included all known live births and not only those births for whom maternal smoking and drinking habits were available, found a significant increase in "severe" birth defects. The birth defects odds ratio was 0.85 for Ranch Hand children born prior to Vietnam service and 1.39 for children born after (46). The 1992 and 1995 follow-up reports on this group continue to show elevated rates of birth defects, stillbirths, and spontaneous abortions. In these studies the authors attempted to relate reproductive outcomes to serum TCDD measures, which as discussed above and as noted by the IOM (13) are much fraught with difficulties. Considering the data on the outcomes themselves, however, consistently elevated rates were still observed (95).

## ACKNOWLEDGMENT

This work was supported in part by USPHS Grants CA-68384 and CA-63021 (to SDS) from the National Cancer Institute.

## REFERENCES


1. Lilienfeld D, Gallo M. 2,4-D, 2,4,5-T, and 2,3,7,8-TCDD: an overview. *Epidemiol Rev* 1989;11:28–58.
2. Committee on Government Operations (U.S. Congress), Twelfth Report. *The Agent Orange coverup*: a case of flawed science and political manipulation. House Report 101-672, August 9, 1990. Washington, DC: U.S. Government Printing Office, 1990.
3. Institute of Medicine (U.S.) Committee to Review the Health Effects in Vietnam Veterans of Exposure to Herbicides. *Veterans and Agent Orange:* health effects of herbicides use in Vietnam. Washington, DC: Institute of Medicine, 1993.
4. Young AL, Calcagani JA, Thalken CE, Trembly JW. The toxicology, environmental fate and human risk of herbicide orange and its associated dioxin. Technical Report No. TR-78-92. Brooks Air Force Base, TX: USAF Occupational and Environmental Health Laboratory, 1978.

5. Stellman SD, Stellman JM, Sommer JF Jr. Combat and herbicide exposure in Vietnam among American Legionnaires. *Environ Res* 1988;47: 112–128.
6. National Research Council. Committee on the effects of herbicides in Vietnam. *The effects of herbicides in South Vietnam:* part A. Washington, DC: National Academy of Sciences, 1974.
7. Buckingham WA. Tactical Air Command. Aerial flight operations in South East Asia 1961–1964. Washington, DC: US GPO, 1974.
8. Christian R, White JD. Battlefield records management and its relationship with the Agent Orange study. *Chemosphere* 1983;12:761–768.
9. Stellman SD, Stellman JM. Estimation of exposure to Agent Orange and other defoliants among American troops in Vietnam: a methodological approach. *Am J Ind Med* 1986;9:305–321.
10. Schecter A, Dai LC, Thuy LTB, et al. Agent Orange the Vietnamese: the persistence of elevated dioxin levels in human tissues. *Am J Public Health* 1995;85:516–522.
11. Verger P, Cordier S, Thuy LT, et al. Correlation between dioxin levels in adipose tissue and estimated exposure to Agent Orange in south Vietnamese residents. *Environ Res* 1994;65:226–242.
12. International Agency for Research on Cancer. Some fumigants, the herbicides 2,4-D and 2,4,5-T, chlorinated dibenzodioxins and miscellaneous industrial chemicals. In: *IARC monographs on the evaluation of carcinogenic risks of chemicals to man.* Lyon, France: IARC, 1977.
13. Institute of Medicine (U.S.) *Committee to Review the Health Effects in Vietnam Veterans of Exposure to Herbicides.* Veterans and Agent Orange: update 1996. Washington, DC: Institute of Medicine, 1996.
14. Gehring PJ, Betson JE. Phenoxy acids: effects and fate in mammals. *Ecol Bull* 1978;27:122–123.
15. World Health Organization. *2,4-Dichlorophenoxy (2,4-D). Environmental health criteria document 29.* Geneva: World Health Organization, 1984.
16. Ibrahim MA, Bond GG, Burke TA, et al. Weight of the evidence on the human carcinogenicity of 2,4-D. *Environ Health Perspect* 1991; 213–222.
17. Nielsen K, Kaempe B, Jensen-Holm J. Fatal poisoning in man by 2,4-dichlorophenoxyacetic acid (2,4-D): determination of the agent in forensic materials. *Acta Pharmacol Toxicol* 1965;22:224–267.
18. Palmiera CM, Morena AJ, Madeira VMC. Metabolic alterations in hepatocytes promoted by the herbicides paraquat, dinoseb and 2,4-D. *Arch Toxicol* 1994;68:24–31.
19. Palmiera CM, Morena AJ, Madeira VMC. Interactions of herbicides 2,4-D and dinoseb with liver mitochondrial bioenergetics. *Toxicol Appl Pharmacol* 1994;127:50–57.
20. Flanagan RJ, Meredith TJ, Ruprah M, Onyon LJ, Liddle A. Alkaline diuresis for acute poisoning with chlorophenoxy herbicides and ioxynil. *Lancet* 1990;335:454–458.
21. Arnold EK, Beasley VR, Parker AJ, Stedelin JR. 2,4-D toxicosis II. A pilot study of clinical pathologic and electroencephalographic effects and residues of 2,4-D in orally dosed dogs. *Vet Hum Toxicol* 1991;33: 446–449.
22. Oliveira GH, Palermo-Neto J. Effects of 2,4-dichlorophenoxyacetic acid (2,4,-D) on open-field behavior and neurochemical parameters of rats. *Pharmacol Toxicol* 1993;73:79–85.
23. Kim CS, Gargas ML, Andersen ME. Pharmacokinetic modeling of 2,4-dichlorophenoxyacetic acid (2,4-D) in rat and rabbit brain following a single dose administration. *Toxicol Lett* 1994;74:189–201.
24. Kim CS, Keizer RF, Pritchard JB. Transport of 2,4,5-trichlorophenoxyacetic acid across the blood-cerebrospinal fluid barrier of the rabbit. *J Pharmacol Exp The* 1993;267:751–757.
25. Innes JRM, Ulland BM, Valerio MG, et al. Bioassay of pesticides and industrial chemicals for mutagenicity in mice: a preliminary note. *J Natl Cancer Inst* 1969;42:1101–14.
26. International Agency for Research in Cancer. Chlorinated dibenzodioxins. In: *IARC monographs on the evaluation of the carcinogenic risk of chemicals to man,* vol 15. Lyon, France: 1977.
27. Hayes HM, New MA, Cantor KP, Jessen CR, McCurnin DM, Richardson RC. Case-control study of canine malignant lymphoma: positive association with dog owner's use of 2,4-D herbicides. *J Natl Cancer Inst* 1991;83:1226–1231.
28. Hazleton Laboratories America. *Combined toxicity and oncogenicity study in mice with 2,4-dichlorophenoxyacetic acid (2,4-D).* Final report. 1986. Prepared for the Industry Task Force on 2,4-D Research Data.
29. Hazleton Laboratories America. *Oncogenicity study in mice with 2,4,-dichlorophenoxyacetic acid (2,4-D).* Final Report. 1987. Prepared for the Industry Task Force on 2,4,-D Research Data.
30. Bionetics Research Laboratories. *Evaluation of carcinogenic, teratogenic and mutagenic activities of selected pesticides and industrial chemicals.* Vol 1, carcinogenic study. NTIS PB 223 159. Bethesda, MD: Bionetics Research Laboratories, 1968.
31. Neubert D, Dillman I. Embryotoxic effects in mice treated with 2,4,5-trichlorophenoxyacetic acid and 2,3,7,8-tetrachlorodibenzo-p-dioxin. *Naunyn Schmiedebergs Arch Exp Pathol Pharmacol* 1972;272: 243–264.
32. Umbreit TH, Hesse EJ, Gallo MA. Reproductive studies of C57B/6 male mice treated with TCDD-contaminated soil from a 2,4,5-trichlorophenoxy acetic acid manufacturing site. *Arch Environ Contam Toxicol* 1988;7:145–150.
33. Centers for Disease Control (CDC). Health status of vietnam veterans, II: physical health. *JAMA* 1988;259:2708–2714.
34. The Selected Cancers Cooperative Study Group. The association of selected cancers with service in the US military in Vietnam, I: non-Hodgkin's lymphoma. *Arch Intern Med* 1990;150:2473–2483.
35. Kang HK, Enzinger FM, Breslin P, Feil M, Lee Y, Shepherd B. Soft tissue sarcoma and military service in Vietnam: a case-control study. *J Natl Cancer Inst* 1987;79:693–699 (published erratum appears in 1987;79:1173).
36. Centers for Disease Control (CDC). *Comparison of serum levels of 2,3,7,8-tetrachloro-p-dioxin with indirect estimates of Agent Orange exposure among Vietnam veterans.* Final Report. Atlanta: CDC, 1989.
37. Wolfe WH, Michalek JE, Miner JC, et al. Determinants of TCDD half-life in Veterans of Operation Ranch Hand. *J Toxicol Environ Health* 1994;41:481–488.
38. Schecter A, Ryan JJ, Papke O, et al. Elevated dioxin levels in the blood of male and female Russian workers with and without chloracne 25 years after phenoxy herbicide exposure: the UFA "KHIMPROM" incident. *Chemosphere* 1994;27:253–258.
39. May G. TCDD: a survey of subjects ten years after exposure. *Br J Ind Med* 1982;39:128–135.
40. Jung D, Konietzko J, Reill-Konietzko G, et al. Porphyrin studies in TCDD-exposed workers. *Arch Toxicol* 1994;68:595–598.
41. Huff JE, Moore JA, Saracci R., Tomatis L. Long-term hazards of polychlorinated dibenzodioxins and polychlorinated dibenzofurans. *Environ Health Perspect* 1980;36:221–240.
42. Young AL, Reggiani G. *Agent Orange and its associated dioxin:* assessment of a controversy. Amsterdam: Elsevier, 1988.
43. Stellman SD, Stellman JM, Sommer JF Jr. Health and reproductive outcomes among American Legionnaires in relation to combat and herbicide exposure in Vietnam. *Environ Res* 1988;47:150–174.
44. Stellman JM, Stellman SD, Sommer JF Jr. Social and behavioral consequences of the Vietnam experience among American Legionnaires. *Environ Res* 1988;47:129–149.
45. Poland A, Smith D, Metter G, Possick P. A health survey of workers in a 2,4-D and 2,4,5-T plant. *Arch Environ Health* 1971;22:316–327.
46. Albanese R. *United States Air Force personnel and exposure to herbicide orange.* Brooks Air Force Base: USAF School of Aerospace Medicine, February 1988.
47. Centers for Disease Control. *Health status of Vietnam veterans,* vol 5: reproductive outcomes and child health. Atlanta: CDC, 1989.
48. Zahm SH, Weisenburger DD, Babbitt PA, et al. A case-control study of non-Hodgkin's lymphoma and the herbicide 2,4-dichlorophenoxyacetic acid (2,4-D) in eastern Nebraska. *Epidemiology* 1990;1:349–356.
49. Saracci R, Kogenvinas M, Bertazzi PA, et al. Cancer mortality in workers exposed to chlorophenoxy herbicides and chlorophenols. *Lancet* 1991;338:1027–1032.
50. Kogevinas M, Saracci R, Bertazzi PA, et al. Cancer mortality from soft-tissue sarcoma and malignant lymphomas in an international cohort of workers exposed to chlorophenoxy herbicides and chlorophenols. *Chemosphere* 1992;25:1071–1076.
51. Lynge E. A follow-up study of cancer incidence among workers in manufacture of phenoxy herbicides in Denmark. *Br J Cancer* 1985;52:259–270.
52. Lynge E. Cancer in phenoxy herbicide manufacturing workers in Denmark, 1947–87—an update. *Cancer Causes Control* 1993;4:261–272.
53. Bueno de Mesquita HB, Doornbos G, Van der Kuip DA, et al. Occupational exposure to phenoxy herbicides and chlorophenols and cancer mortality in the Netherlands. *Am J Ind Med* 1993;23:289–300.
54. Fingerhut MA, Halperin WE, Marlow DA, et al. Cancer mortality in

workers exposed to 2,3,7,8-tetrachlorodibenzo-p-dioxin. *N Engl J Med* 1991;324:212–218.
55. Bond GG. Evaluation of mortality patterns among chemical workers with chloracne. *Chemosphere* 1987;16:2117–2121.
56. Zack JA, Suskind R. The mortality experience of workers exposed to TCDD in a trichlorophenol process accident. *J Occup Med* 1980;22: 11–14.
57. Zack JA, Gaffey WR. A mortality study of workers employed at the Monsanto Company plant in Nitro, WV. In: *Human and environmental risks of chlorinated dioxins and related compounds.* New York: Plenum Press, 1983;575–591.
58. Roberts L. Monsanto studies under fire. *Science* 1991;251:626.
59. Bond GG, Ott MG, Brenner FE, Cook RR. Medical and morbidity surveillance findings among employees potentially exposed to TCDD. *Br J Ind Med* 1983;40:318–324.
60. Ott MG, Olson RA, Cook RR, Bond GG. Cohort mortality study of chemical workers with potential exposure to the higher chlorinated dioxins. *J Occup Med* 1987;29:422–429.
61. Kauppinen TP, Pannett B, Marlowe DA, et al. Retrospective assessment of exposure through modelling in a study on cancer risks among workers exposed to phenoxy herbicides, chlorophenols and dioxins. *Scand J Work Environ Health* 1994;20:262–271.
62. Kogevinas M, Kauppinen T, Winkelmann R, et al. Soft-tissue sarcoma and non-Hodgkin's lymphoma in workers exposed to phenoxy herbicides, chlorophenols and dioxins: two nested case-control studies. *Epidemiology* 1995;6:396–402.
63. Collins JJ, Strauss ME, Levinskas GJ, et al. The mortality experience of workers exposed to 2,3,7,8-tetrachloro-p-dioxin in a trichlorophenol process accident. *Epidemiology* 1993;4:7–13.
64. Hardell L, Sandstrom A. Case-control study: soft-tissue sarcomas and exposure to phenoxyacetic acids or chlorophenols. *Br J Cancer* 1979;39:711–717.
65. Eriksson M, Hardell L, Berg NO, Moller T, Axelson O. Soft-tissue sarcomas and exposure to chemical substances: a case-referent study. *Br J Ind Med* 1981;38:27–33.
66. Hardell L, Eriksson M. The association between soft tissue sarcomas and exposure to phenoxyacetic acids. A new case-referent study. *Cancer* 1988;62:652–656.
67. Vineis P, Terracini B, Ciccone G, et al. Phenoxy herbicides and soft-tissue sarcomas in female rice weeders. *Scand J Work Environ Health* 1986;13:9–17.
68. Wiklund K, Holm L-E. Soft-tissue sarcoma risk in Swedish agricultural and forestry workers. *J Natl Cancer Inst* 1987;76:229–234.
69. Hoar SK, Blair A, Holmes FF, et al. Agricultural herbicide use and risk of lymphoma and soft-tissue sarcoma. *JAMA* 1986;256:1141–1147.
70. Woods JS, Polissar L, Severson RK, Heuser LS, Kulander BG. Soft-tissue sarcoma and non-Hodgkin's lymphoma in relation to phenoxyherbicide and chlorinated phenol exposure in western Washington. *J Natl Cancer Inst* 1987;78:899–910.
71. Smith AH, Pearce NE, Fisher DO, Giles HJ, Teague CA, Howard JK. Soft tissue sarcoma and exposure to phenoxyherbicides and chlorophenols in New Zealand. *J Natl Cancer Inst* 1984;73:1111–1117.
72. Hardell L, Eriksson M, Degerman A. Exposure to phenoxyacetic acids, chlorophenols, or organic solvents in relation to histopathology, stage, and anatomical localization of non-Hodgkin's lymphoma. *Cancer Res* 1994;54:2386–2389.
73. Hoar SK, Blair A, Holmes FF, et al. Agricultural herbicide use and risk of lymphoma and soft tissue sarcoma. *JAMA* 1986;256: 1141–1147.
74. Pearce NE, Smith AH, Fisher DO. Malignant lymphoma and multiple myeloma linked with agricultural occupations in a New Zealand cancer registry-based study. *Am J Epidemiol* 1985;121:225–237.
75. Pearce NE, Smith AH, Howard JK, Sheppard RA, Giles HJ, Teague CA. Non-Hodgkin's lymphoma and exposure to phenoxyherbicides, chlorophenols, fencing work, and meat works employment: a case-control study. *Br J Ind Med* 1986;43:75–83.
76. Pearce NE, Sheppard RA, Smith AH, Teague CA. Non-Hodgkin's lymphoma and farming: an expanded case-control study. *Int J Cancer* 1987;39:155–161.
77. Woods JS, Polissar L, Severson RK, Heuser LS, Kulander BG. Soft tissue sarcoma and non-Hodgkin's lymphoma in relation to phenoxyherbicide and chlorinated phenol exposure in western Washington. *J Natl Cancer Inst* 1987;78:899–910.
78. Dubrow R, Paulson JO, Indian RW. Farming and malignant lymphoma in Hancock County, Ohio. *Br J Ind Med* 1988;45:25–28.
79. Hardell L. Relation of soft tissue sarcoma, malignant lymphoma and colon cancer to phenoxy acids, chlorophenols and other agents. Scand *J Work Environ Health* 1981;7:119–130.
80. Hardell L, Bengtsson NO. Epidemiological study of socioeconomic factors and clinical findings in Hodgkin's disease, and reanalysis of previous data regarding chemical exposure. *Br J Cancer* 1983;48: 217–225.
81. Persson B, Dahlander A-M, Fredriksson M, et al. Malignant lymphomas and occupational exposures. *Br J Ind Med* 1989;46:516–520.
82. Persson B, Fredriksson M, Ohlsen K, et al. Some occupational exposures as risk factors for malignant lymphomas. *Cancer* 1993;72: 1773–1778.
83. The Selected Cancers Cooperative Study Group. The association of selected cancers with service in the US military in Vietnam. III. Hodgkin's disease, nasal cancer, nasopharyngeal cancer, and primary liver cancer. *Arch Intern Med* 1990;150:2495–2505.
84. Cordier S, Le TB, Verger P, et al. Viral infections and chemical exposures as risk factors for hepatocellular carcinoma in Vietnam. *Int J Cancer* 1993;55:196–201.
85. Breslin P, Kang HK, Lee Y, Burt V, Shepard BM. Proportionate mortality study of Army and Marine Corps veterans of the Vietnam war. *J Occup Med* 1988;30:412–419.
86. Greenwald P, Kovasznay B, Collins DN, Therriault G. Sarcomas of soft tissues after Vietnam service. *J Natl Cancer Inst* 1984;73:1107–1109.
87. Lawrence W, Reilly AA, Quickenton P, Greenwald P, Page WF, Kuntz AJ. Mortality patterns of New York State Vietnam veterans. *Am J Public Health* 1985;75:277–279.
88. Riihimaki V, Asp S, Hernberg S. Mortality of 2,4-D and 2,4,5-T herbicide applicators in Finland. *Scand J Work Environ Health* 1982; 8:37–42.
89. Riihimaki V, Asp S, Pukkala E, Hernberg S. Mortality and cancer morbidity among chlorinated phenoxyacid applicators in Finland. *Chemosphere* 1983;12:779–784.
90. Constable JD, Hatch MC. Reproductive effects of herbicide exposure in Vietnam: recent studies by the Vietnamese and others. *Teratogen Carcinogen Mutagen* 1985;231–250.
91. Cutting RT, Phuec TH, Balb JM, et al. Congenital malformations, hydatiform moles and stillbirths in the Republic of Vietnam 1960–1969. Washington, DC: US GPO, 1970.
92. Erickson JD, Mulinare J, McClain PW, et al. Risks for fathering babies with birth defects. *JAMA* 1984;252:903–912.
93. Aschengrau A, Monson RR. Paternal military service in Vietnam and the risk of late adverse pregnancy outcomes. *Am J Public Health* 1990; 80:1218–1224.
94. Field B, Kerr C. Reproductive behaviour and consistent patterns of abnormality in offspring of Vietnam veterans. *J Med Genet* 1988;25: 819–826.
95. Wolfe WH, Michalek JE, Miner JC, et al. Paternal serum dioxin and reproductive outcomes among veterans of Operation Ranch Hand. *Epidemiology* 1995;6:17–22.

*Environmental and Occupational Medicine, Third Edition,* edited by William N. Rom. Lippincott–Raven Publishers, Philadelphia © 1998.

# CHAPTER 85

# Dioxins and Related Compounds

Ellen K. Silbergeld and Valerie M. Thomas

The dioxins and related compounds are among the most intensively studied chemicals in modern occupational and environmental health. Because of their widespread dispersal into the environment and because of their resistance to physical-chemical and biotic breakdown, most organisms tested carry measurable levels of these chemicals. The dioxins and related chemicals (Fig. 1) represent a family of structurally similar molecules, which includes polychlorinated dibenzodioxins (PCDDs), dibenzofurous (PCDFs), biphenyls (PCBs), naphthalenes (PCNs), terphenyls, azobenzenes, and azoxybenzenes. They are often grouped together for two reasons: first, they frequently arise from the same source, as discussed below, and second, they possess similar biologic properties. In this chapter the phrase "dioxins and related compounds" is used to refer to the molecules shown in Fig. 1. [The reader is also referred to the chapters on polycyclic aromatic hydrocarbons (PAHs) and PCBs for additional relevant discussion.] Typically, we discuss the tetra- through octa-chlorinated dioxins and furans, denoted PCDD/Fs. In some instances, we discuss one chlorinated dibenzodioxin, 2,3,7,8-tetrachlorodibenzodioxin (TCDD), because it is the best studied and most potent member of this chemical class. In addition, certain PCBs are also considered in this class, because of their structure and biologic properties.

For public health and clinical medicine, the dioxins are important because of their toxicity and their ubiquity. They exemplify the ongoing controversies and uncertainties about assessing risks of chemical contaminants in the workplace and general environment. Some of the most heated controversies in public policy involve the assessment of the human health risks of these compounds. Any review of this topic must note the important interplay of science and politics because of implications for legal liability by industry and for regulatory action by government. In the United States, much of the debate has been related to allegations of adverse health effects in military veterans of the Vietnam War, who were exposed to Agent Orange, a mix of herbicides that contained relatively high levels of 2,3,7,8-TCDD as a contaminant (1,2). In the early 1980s dioxins and related compounds were found in several places, such as Love Canal, New York, the Ironbound district of Newark, New Jersey, and Times Beach, Missouri, where hazardous wastes had been disposed. In the mid-1980s it was discovered that waste incineration processes could generate dioxins and related compounds, and this practically blocked development of incineration as a method for managing municipal solid waste in the United States. Soon after, the Environmental Protection Agency (EPA) reported that chlorine bleaching of wood pulp could generate dioxins and related compounds, and this increased pressure on the paper industry to change its methods of production and waste management. In every case, these disclosures lagged years after releases of dioxins from manufacture, use, and disposal. In many populations, breast milk and adipose tissue are all contaminated with these chemicals, which can be passed transplacentally from mother to offspring (3–5).

Many regulatory authorities have issued health guidance statements regarding the dioxins, as shown in Fig. 2. Most of these statements are based on assessments of the risks of these chemicals as carcinogens, calculated from studies in

E. K. Silbergeld: Departments of Epidemiology and Preventive Medicine; and Program in Human Health and the Environment, University of Maryland School of Medicine, Baltimore, Maryland 21201.

V. M. Thomas: Center for Energy and Environmental Studies, Princeton University, Princeton, New Jersey 08544-5263.

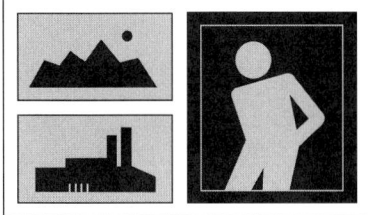

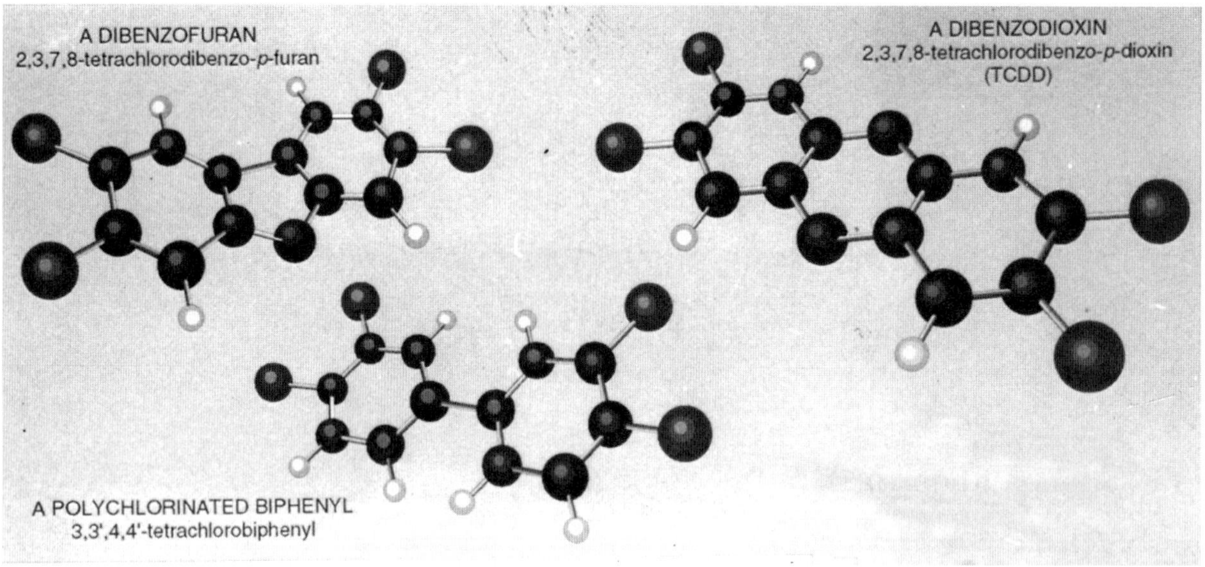


**FIG. 1.** Structures of polychlorinated dibenzo-p-dioxins, dibenzofurans, and biphenyls (6) (illustrator, James A. Perkins). (Reprinted with permission from ref. 6.)

rodents (see below). The differences among them—several orders of magnitude—arise from different assumptions as to the most appropriate way to estimate risks of chemically induced cancers at low levels of exposure, well below the range of doses used in studies of animals or experienced by occupational populations (6). There is uncertainty about the dose-response for these chemicals. In animal studies, they are among the most potent chemicals ever examined, and mechanistic research suggests that they are toxic at very low cellular concentrations (in the pico- to nanomolar range). Prudent public health policy is generally based on a recommendation to prevent all controllable sources of human exposure. However, because these chemicals are now ubiquitous in the environment, the extent to which cleanup of existing sources should be imposed remains a matter of considerable controversy.

This chapter presents a summary of current knowledge about the dioxins, and discusses health effects (epidemiology and toxicology), sources, and exposures. Decades of clinical, epidemiologic, and toxicologic research have been devoted to understanding risks of the dioxins and estimating their likelihood and magnitude in human populations. While our knowledge is not complete, we may know more about the dioxins than about almost any other toxic chemical found in the workplace and environment. Nevertheless, this knowledge has not been sufficient to end controversies over the extent to which human exposures need to be reduced.

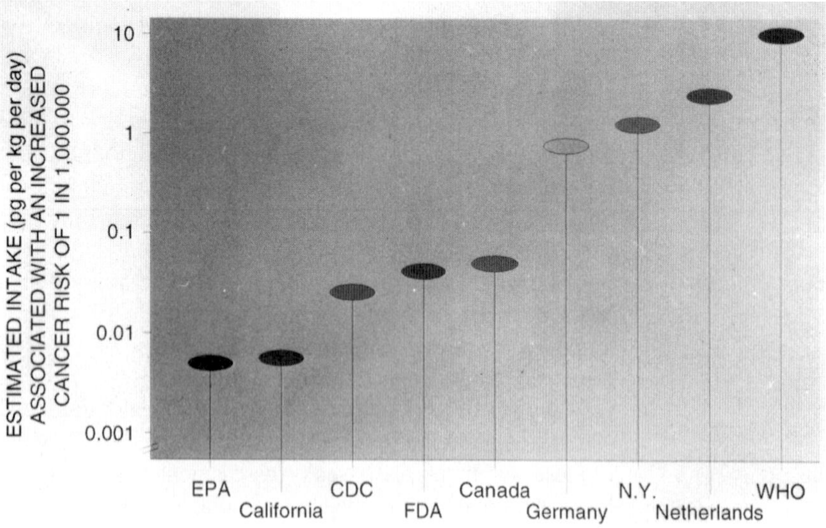


**FIG. 2.** Nine different risk estimates for the carcinogenic effects of TCDD are based on the same dose-response data in laboratory rats, and all give the daily intake believed to be associated with one additional case of cancer per million people. Yet the dioxin quantities differ by almost 2,000 times between the lowest and highest estimates, because different mathematical models were used to extend the lab data down to low doses. (Reprinted with permission from ref. 6.)

**TABLE 1.** *Effects of TCDD and related compounds in different animal species*

| Effect | Human | Monkey | Guinea pig | Rat | Mouse | Hamster | Cow | Rabbit | Chicken | Fish |
|---|---|---|---|---|---|---|---|---|---|---|
| Presence of AhR | + | + | + | + | + | + | + | + | + | + |
| Binding of TCDD: AhR Complex to the DRE | + | + | + | + | + | + | + | + | + | + |
| Enzyme induction | + | | + | + | + | + | | + | + | + |
| Acute lethality | 0 | + | + | + | + | + | + | + | + | + |
| Wasting syndrome | | + | + | + | + | + | + | + | + | |
| Teratogenesis/fetal toxicity, mortality | +/– | + | + | + | + | + | + | + | + | + |
| Endocrine effects | +/– | + | | + | + | | | | | + |
| Immunotoxicity | +/– | + | + | + | + | + | + | | + | |
| Carcinogenicity | +/– | | | + | + | + | | | | + |
| Chloracnegenic effects | + | + | | 0 | + | | | + | | |
| Porphyria | +/– | 0 | 0 | + | + | 0 | | | + | |
| Hepatotoxicity | + | + | +/– | + | + | +/– | + | + | + | |
| Edema | + | 0 | 0 | + | + | | | + | + | |
| Testicular atrophy | | + | + | + | + | | | | | |
| Bone marrow hypoplasia | | + | + | | +/– | | | | + | |

+, observed; +/–, observed to a limited extent, or +/– results; 0, not observed; blank, no data.
From ref. 3.

## HEALTH EFFECTS OF THE DIOXINS: HUMAN EPIDEMIOLOGY AND CLINICAL REPORTS

The dioxins induce a range of toxic effects, involving most of the organ systems of the body. The major health effects associated with human exposure are cancer, reproductive toxicity, immune suppression, hepatotoxicity, neurologic dysfunction, and dermatotoxicity. As shown in Table 1, these effects have been observed in many species, including humans, other mammals, birds, and fish (7). Increases in cause specific mortality (including but not limited to cancer) and a range of subclinical changes in biochemical markers are reported in humans. None of these reported associations is without controversy; however, a consensus view of the current evidence may be found in reviews of the health status of veterans exposed to Agent Orange by the Institute of Medicine, as summarized in Table 2. IOM recently concluded that there was "sufficient evidence of an association" between exposure to herbicides contaminated with TCDD and increased risk of soft tissue sarcoma, non-Hodgkin's lymphoma, Hodgkin's disease, and chloracne; limited evidence was adduced for respiratory cancers, prostate cancer, and multiple myelomas, spina bifida in children born to exposed parents, and acquired porphyria (1,2). It is interesting to note that in the Seveso, Italy cohort there was a reported decrease in incidence of breast cancer (8), consistent with animal studies (9).

Our knowledge of the human toxicity of these chemicals extends back to the earliest years of the synthetic organic chemical industry, in the late 19th century, long before the structure of dioxin was known. By the 1940s it was hypothesized that the toxicity observed in workers involved in manufacture of polychlorinated biphenyls and chlorinated naphthalenes was associated with impurities formed when the appropriate precursor molecules and conditions were present. Exposure to these contaminants was reported to cause a range of toxic effects in liver, musculoskeletal system, nervous system, and skin. Several deaths were also reported in this early literature (9).

Chloracne was one of the earliest and most frequently reported effects of exposure to these compounds. It is a

**TABLE 2.** *Association between TCDD and adverse health effects in Vietnam and other exposed populations*

| |
|---|
| Sufficient evidence of an association |
| Soft tissue sarcoma |
| Non-Hodgkin's lymphoma |
| Chloracne |
| Limited/suggestive evidence of an association |
| Respiratory cancers (lung, larynx, trachea) |
| Prostate cancer |
| Multiple myeloma |
| Spina bifida |
| Acquired porphyria |
| Inadequate or insufficient evidence for an association |
| Hepatobiliary cancers |
| Nasal/nasopharyngeal cancer |
| Bone cancer |
| Skin cancer |
| Breast cancer |
| Renal cancer |
| Testicular cancer |
| Leukemia |
| Spontaneous abortion |
| Birth defects (other than spina bifida) |
| Childhood cancer in offspring |
| Male infertility |
| Cognitive and neuropsychiatric disorders |
| Motor/coordination dysfunction |
| Immune system disorders |
| Circulatory disorders |
| Respiratory disorders |
| Skin cancer |

From ref. 2.

persistent and distinguishing acneiform dermatotoxicity, often accompanied by hyperpigmentation and hirsutism, called chloracne or perna-acne (after pernaphthalene) by Herxheimer in 1899 (9). Chloracne has persisted in highly exposed workers nearly 40 years after exposure. There was a single case of a worker who died with soft tissue sarcoma over 10 years after he was exposed to dioxins and related compounds in the (mis)management of hazardous waste in Missouri. He manifested early chloracne and toxic hepatitis with porphyrinopathic signs. During the course of his cancer, his chloracne reappeared, possibly as a consequence of cachexia, which mobilized the TCDD stored in adipose tissue (10).

Sometimes clinicians assume that there is a distinctive pathology or set of symptoms associated with a specific toxicant exposure in humans. However, this is the exception rather than the rule in cases of chemical toxicity. Few chemicals are associated uniquely with one definable outcome. Asbestos, in addition to the signature disease of mesothelioma, also induces a variety of respiratory dysfunctions in addition to tumors of the pleural cavity. Lead induces anemia, infertility, a type of toxic hepatic porphyria, renal failure, and peripheral and central neuropathy, as well as possibly increasing risks of renal cancer. The distinguishing and defining clinical characteristic of lead toxicity is an elevated level of lead in blood. For some time, it was claimed that chloracne was the signature sign of dioxin exposure, and by inference in the absence of chloracne no toxicologically significant exposure to dioxin was thought to have occurred in an individual or population (11,12). Because chloracne was considered almost diagnostic of exposure to these chemicals, many industries used surveillance of chloracne as an indicator of excessive exposure. However, not all persons similarly exposed to dioxins evince chloracne, nor was chloracne a necessary finding in all persons with other toxic sequelae of dioxin exposure (9). There are no indicative symptoms of dioxin exposure. Careful biochemical studies may provide evidence of some of the biologic responses to dioxin, such as measuring enzyme induction or direct measurement of gene products in placenta, lymphocytes, or other cells (13). Some have proposed that there may be distinctive patterns of urinary excretion of porphyrins (biologic precursors to heme) indicative of exposure to dioxin and related compounds (14), but this measurement by itself is not diagnostic of chemical exposure.

Exposure to the dioxins is generally assayed by chemical analysis of either adipose tissue (obtained by biopsy) or the lipid fraction of serum (15). Researchers at the Centers for Disease Control (CDC) determined that collection of serum after a limited fast provided something of a metabolic biopsy of the adipose tissue compartment, such that levels in serum were highly correlated with levels in adipose tissue in a large sample of the Ranch Handers (Air Force personnel involved in defoliation using Agent Orange in Vietnam). Fingerprints of specific isomers of dioxins and dibenzofurans have been used to try to identify original sources of exposure.

Over the past 60 years, many epidemiologic studies have examined the human health effects of the dioxins. These studies have generally been of three types: (1) retrospective cohort studies of workers exposed either acutely or chronically (often both) to relatively high levels of dioxins, including persons exposed in industrial accidents at chlorophenol production facilities (described in ref. 16); (2) registry and case-control studies of workers and others exposed to contaminated products, usually agricultural chemicals; and (3) prospective studies of Vietnam veterans and persons nonoccupationally exposed to these chemicals as a result of industrial releases, waste disposal, and contaminated food. Because of differences in subjects and exposures, it is difficult to compare results across studies (Table 3). The four nonoccupational cohorts that have been studied in greatest detail are the Seveso population exposed in 1976 (16); the Yusho and Yucheng cohorts exposed in 1968 and 1976 via consumption of cooking oil contaminated with a commercial PCB mixture (containing dioxins and dibenzofurans) (17); and communities living near the Great Lakes exposed to PCBs, dioxins, and related compounds through consumption of contaminated fish (18). In addition, systematic studies have been done of chemical production workers involved in the manufacture of products where dioxins and related compounds were generated (19); farmers and others employed in agriculture using herbicides contaminated with TCDD (20); and military personnel exposed to Agent Orange in Vietnam (1,2). Each of these studies has offered opportunities to investigate somewhat different aspects of human response: all of them are ongoing at present.

These studies have reported a positive association between exposures to dioxins and related compounds and a range of toxic effects related to reproductive and nervous system intoxication, as well as increases in cause-specific mortality, especially cancer and heart disease (see Table 2). The studies of community residents indicate that young children, and possibly fetuses, are at increased risk for effects on the nervous system and immune system. Some data from studies of Vietnam veterans have found associations between paternal exposure to Agent Orange and increased risks of birth defects in their children (2). Alterations in biochemical parameters of exposed human populations have also been reported, in the absence of clinical disease or defined pathophysiology, most frequently alterations in circulating levels of glucose and testosterone (21). These may be markers of early or low dose response, but at present their association with later disease is not known.

**TABLE 3.** *Epidemiologic studies of persons exposed to dioxins and related compounds*

| Exposure (sites of study) | Population studied | Chemicals involved | Type of exposure | Assessment of exposure | End points assessed |
|---|---|---|---|---|---|
| Industrial production (U.S., European Union) | Chemical workers (male) | CDD trichlorophenols, chlorinated benzenes, PCBs | High; acute and chronic | Work history; biologic monitoring | Cancer, reproduction, neurotoxicity (Japan, Taiwan), all cause mortality |
| Contaminated products (U.S., Australia) | Agricultural workers and families | TCDD 2,4,5-T and 2,4-D (also other pesticides and agricultural chemicals) | Medium to high; chronic | Residential and farming history | Cancer, reproduction |
| Contaminated products (Southeast Asia) | Vietnam veterans (male) | TCDD 2,4,5-T and 2,4-D | Low to medium; semichronic | Military records; biologic monitoring | All cause mortality, birth defects in children, other biologic effects |
| Accidental releases (Italy) | Community residents | TCDD and other dioxins, chlorinated phenols, other chemicals | Medium to high; acute | Residential location; biologic monitoring | Cancer, reproduction, immune status |
| Food contamination | Community residents (including fetal exposures) | PCBs, PCDFs, and dioxins | Low to high; chronic (low) and acute (high) | Food consumption; biologic monitoring | Reproduction, cancer, child development |

For review of all relevant studies, see refs. 1 and 2.

The available epidemiologic studies have been heatedly debated, and not all researchers are convinced of an association between these chemicals and human health risks (22). Attempts have been made to discern dose-response relationships, as shown in Table 4. These analyses are limited by lack of information on human dosimetry and toxicokinetics. With the exception of some early studies by industry on chloracne, no humans have been deliberately exposed to TCDD or related compounds. Exposure estimates are based on either evaluation of available data on occupational conditions or back calculations assuming a similar half-life across populations. In most of the studies conducted to date, exposure has been estimated by information on occupational history, food consumption, or other circumstance; in some studies, measurements of body burdens of TCDD and related compounds have been made at some point after exposure occurred (15). Toxicokinetic back calculations are then done to estimate exposure prior to measurement. The half-life of TCDD in humans is calculated to be in the range of 6 to 12 years, although the range of measured toxicokinetic parameters (half-life) in humans is great (23) and the impact of intercurrent physiologic change, such as weight loss, has not been investigated in these studies. The most that can be said is that the available data are consistent with a dose-related increase in risk (3,24). The Yusho, Yucheng, and Seveso cohorts have data on serum levels measured shortly after acute exposure episodes, as described above, and these data have been used to derive estimates of ceiling doses for specific effects (25). There is no reliable information on safe or no-effect levels of exposure for human health.

The risks of current exposures are unknown. At present, most public health officials advocate a highly prudent approach to estimating the human health risks of dioxin, and many countries have imposed occupation and environmental regulations designed to reduce exposures and ongoing releases to the maximum extent feasible. The average body burden of these chemicals in adults in the United States and Western Europe is about 10 μg/kg, while the body burdens associated with toxicity in animals are about 100 μg/kg. [These figures are expressed as toxic equivalency quantities (TEQs), a toxicity-weighted sum of the tetra- through octa-chlorinated dioxins and furans.]

## Treatment

The most important treatment for exposure to dioxin is to identify and interdict sources of exposure. Lowering body burdens of similar compounds through the use of cholestyramine (26) or fasting has been advocated, but the possibility of redistribution after mobilization from adipose tissue may have implications for toxicity (27). The toxic manifestations of dioxin must be treated as end

**TABLE 4.** *Estimated doses (and body burdens) and effects in experimental animals and humans exposed to low effect levels 2,3,7,8-TCDD*

| Effect | Species | Experimental dose | Body burden |
|---|---|---|---|
| Chloracne | Humans | | 36–3,000 ng/kg |
| Chloracne | Monkeys | 1,000 g/kg | 1000 μg/kg |
| Chloracne | Rabbits | 4 ng/kg 5 d/wk/4 wk | 220 ng/kg |
| Chloracne | Mice | 5,000 μg/kg for 3 d/wk/2 wk | 17,000 ng/kg |
| Decreased testosterone | Humans | | 13 ng/kg |
| Decreased testosterone | Rats | 12.5 μg/kg for 7 days | |
| Decreased glucose uptake by adipocytes | Guinea pigs | 30 ng/kg single dose | 30 ng/kg |
| Decreased serum glucose | Rats | 100 ng/kg/d for 30 days | 1,900 ng/kg |
| Decrease birth weight | Humans | | 1,400 ng/kg (maternal) |
| Decrease growth | Rats | 125 ng/kg/d maternal dose on gd 6–15 | 1,250 ng/kg |
| Decrease growth | Rats | 400 ng/kg maternal dose on gd 15 | 400 ng/kg |
| Altered lymphocyte subsets | Rhesus monkeys | 25 ppt in diet for 4 years | 270 ng/kg |
| Altered lymphocyte subsets | Marmosets | 0.3 ng/kg/wk for 24 weeks, 1.5 ng/kg/wk for 12 weeks | 6–8 ng/kg |
| Enhanced viral susceptibility | Mice | 10 ng/kg for 7 days | 7 ng/kg |
| Endometriosis | Monkeys | 5 ppt in diet for 4 years | 27 ng/kg |
| Decreased sperm count | Rats | 64 ng/kg maternal dose on gd 15 | 64 ng/kg |
| Cancer | Humans | | 100–7,000 ng/kg |
| Cancer | Hamsters | 100 μg/kg 6 doses (600 μg/kg total dose) | 100 ng/kg |
| Cancer | Rats | 100 ng/kg/d for 2 years | 1,400 ng/kg |
| Cancer skin tumor promotion | Mice | 7.5 ng/kg/wk for 20 weeks, dermally | 1,100 ng/kg |
| Downregulation of EGFR in placenta (maximal effect) | Humans | | 1,400 ng/kg |
| Downregulation of EGFR in liver (maximal effect) | Rats | 125 ng/kg/d for 30 weeks | 24,000 ng/kg |
| Increased placental CYP1A1 (maximal effect) | Humans | 1,400 ng/kg | |
| Increased liver CYP1A1 (maximal effect) | Rats | 125 ng/kg/d for 30 weeks | 24,000 ng/kg |
| Enzyme induction CYP1A1 (LOEL) | Rats | 1 ng/kg single dose | 1 ng/kg |
| Enzyme induction CYP1A1/1A2 (LOEL) | Mice | 1.5 ng/kg/d for 5 d/wk for 13 weeks | 23 ng/kg |

EGFR, epidermal growth factor receptor; gd, gestational day; CYP1A1, cytochrome P450 (monoxygenase) A1; LOEL, lowest observed effect level.
From ref. 3.

points in themselves, without management specifically related to etiology.

## EXPERIMENTAL TOXICOLOGY OF THE DIOXINS

The dioxins cause a range of similar effects in humans, rodents, and primates (Table 1). Thus, most of the research on health effects of the dioxins and related compounds has been conducted in experimental animals. These studies have provided important information on low-dose toxicity of the dioxins in mammals and the molecular mechanisms of toxic action. The relevance of this toxicologic literature to understanding and predicting human health effects is hotly contested. Basic research can contribute to public health and clinical medicine by providing mechanistic understanding as a context for interpreting what Bradford Hill called the biologic plausibility and context of epidemiologic findings. If toxicology is the science of great poisons, then the science of dioxin represents some of the greatest research in toxicology, which has influenced our understanding of the role of genetics in susceptibility to environmental exposures and the role of gene expression in major health end points, such as cancer.

The first such studies, in the 1930s, were undertaken by industry to determine if the toxic agent(s) was a precursor or feedstock chemical, the product itself, or some unidentified contaminant arising in production or from breakdown of the product. These studies used empirical mixtures of products and other materials collected at work sites where workers had been intoxicated. Drinker and colleagues found that exposing rats and rabbits to these mixtures produced a range of toxic effects, including death accompanied by severe wasting, jaundice, and liver necrosis. Animals were also used in a set of unpublished studies conducted by BASF in the aftermath of a process explosion in 1953. Caged rats were placed in the area where the explosion occurred; for weeks afterward, the animals rapidly died from unexplained causes (16).

In the late 1960s the chemical industry undertook studies of the PCBs and the dioxins in response to publicity about widespread environmental contamination. Toxicologic studies using purified TCDD were conducted by Kociba and colleagues (9) at Dow Chemical, starting in the 1970s. They reported that relatively low-level exposure to TCDD alone induced a range of organ toxicities, including effects on hematopoiesis, spleen, and liver. In 1978, they reported that chronic exposure to TCDD in the diet increased the rates of tumors in rats. This report, which was confirmed by an NIH bioassay, directed research on TCDD's carcinogenesis for many years (28). TCDD is a highly potent animal carcinogen in all species studied (rats, mice, monkeys, dogs, hamsters); by itself TCDD exposure increased rates of liver, lung, and thyroid cancer, and following prior exposure to a mutagenic chemical, TCDD can cause skin and liver tumors at very low doses. At about the same time Dow scientists reported that TCDD was highly teratogenic (29). Depending on species and timing of prenatal exposure, TCDD can cause structural defects in the palate, kidney, and reproductive tract (of both males and females) (18). The immune system was also found to be particularly sensitive to TCDD, with effects on B cells and T-cell subsets and cell signaling (cytokines and interleukins), which may be related to the dramatic effects of TCDD to reduce resistance to infectious disease in rats (30). TCDD at relatively low doses interferes with many end points in many organ systems in mammals, including alterations in hepatic metabolism, reproduction and development, immune system markers, a wide range of steroid and peptide hormone signaling systems, and lipid metabolism (Table 4) (3).

Mechanistic research on TCDD began with two observations, by Alan Poland and Daniel Nebert: TCDD was highly effective at inducing a set of hepatic enzymes involved in processing drugs and hormones, and this effect was highly species-specific. Moreover, slight alterations in the structure of a chlorinated dibenzodioxin (in terms of degree or position of chlorination on the molecule) greatly changed the potency of the compound. These observations led Poland to suggest, in 1982, that the toxicity of TCDD might involve an intracellular molecule, or receptor, whose expression was under genetic control and which served to recognize the presence of TCDD within cells and transduce a range of alterations in cellular function (31). Poland focused on one of the most sensitive cellular responses to dioxin, the increased transcription of messenger RNA (mRNA) for a set of enzyme proteins, the arylhydrocarbon hydroxylases (AHH). Poland's prediction was supported by inferential evidence of stereospecific binding of TCDD, with high affinity, to a cytosolic factor, which appeared to be necessary for AHH induction. This provided the nomenclature of the Ah, or dioxin, receptor (AhR or DR). In 1988 the Ah receptor was conclusively identified, and it has now been sequenced and its gene cloned (32–34). The AhR is found in all species above primitive fish, and it is present in many human tissues, including liver, skin, placenta, lung, testes, spleen, glia, and lymphocytes.

A schematic of our current understanding of the role of the Ah receptor in dioxin toxicity at the cellular level is shown in Fig. 3 (6). The receptor is similar to an intracellular steroid hormone receptor, in that it is found in cell cytosol and, after associating with dioxin (or another molecule that it recognizes) and at least one other specific protein, it is translocated to the cell nucleus where it binds to specific sites on genomic DNA with a functional effect on gene expression similar to that of steroid hor-

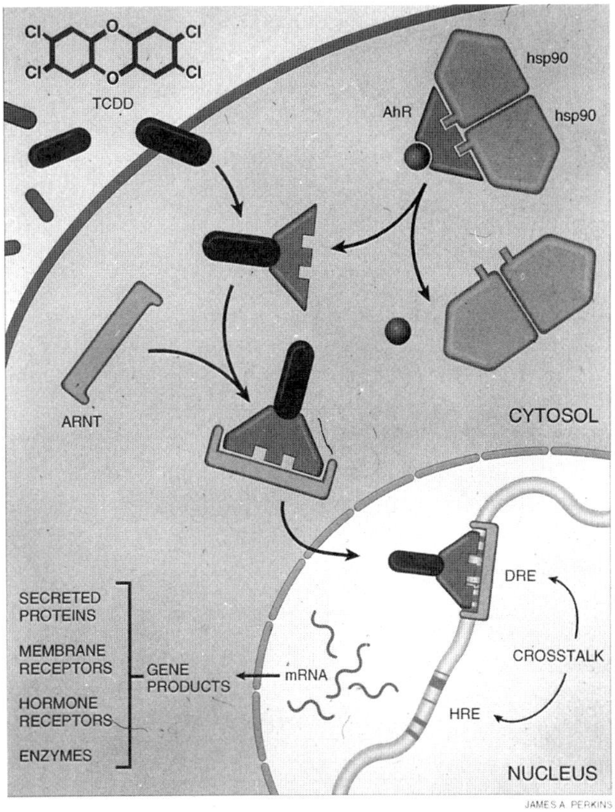


**FIG. 3.** Cellular and molecular actions of dioxins. TCDD and similar compounds diffuse across the plasma membrane and bind to a cytosolic receptor (AhR), possibly displacing an endogenous ligand. Two molecules of the chaperone protein hsp90 are displaced during the binding process. The ligand-receptor complex associates with the arylhydrocarbon receptor nuclear transporter (ARNT), and the resulting heteromeric molecule is transported to the nucleus. There it associates with dioxin response elements (DREs) in the genome to alter transcription of downstream genes. Crosstalk may occur between DRE-regulated genes and other genes regulated by endogenous hormones acting through their specific receptors on hormone response elements (HREs). Alterations in transcription change the amounts of mRNA and hence the synthesis of specific gene products. (Reprinted with permission from ref. 6.)

mones, such as the glucocorticoids, estrogen, and retinoic acid. However, the Ah receptor appears to be a wholly distinct protein; it does not recognize any endogenous hormone nor does TCDD directly displace any known hormone from its receptor (35).

The importance of understanding the molecular mechanisms of dioxin toxicity is threefold. First, it provides a rational basis for evaluating structurally similar chemicals, such as PCBs, in terms of their goodness-of-fit to the Ah receptor, relative to TCDD. This is the basis for the so-called toxicity equivalency approach of evaluating the health risks of mixtures of dioxin like chemicals, such as are found in emissions from some incinerators or in some hazardous waste streams (36,37). An integrated toxic equivalency factor (TEF) used by the EPA (1994) is shown in Table 5. While the numerical relation between total tetra- through octa-chlorinated dioxins and furans and the TEQ varies from sample to sample depending on the relative quantities of the different congeners, typically the total PCDD/F value is a factor of 60 (ranging from 50 to 100) times the TEQ value), for dioxin from combustion sources. Using such an integrated approach is important since many of these chemicals are found together in mixtures and it is reasonable to assume that risks are related to these combined exposures. Second, it assists in extrapolations across species, in that the presence of a dioxin-binding receptor in cells from different species, including humans, provides a basis for assuming similar risks of toxicity (38). In addition, the receptor mechanism may determine differences among species, based on levels of the receptor and its associated protein. Third, it has been used as a mechanistic basis for developing risk assessments to guide public policy in reducing exposures to dioxins and related compounds (13,39). By examining dose-response relationships at the level of receptor-ligand interactions, it is possible to make mathematical predictions of exposure and response at very low levels (40).

**TABLE 5.** *Proposed toxic equivalency factors for PCDDs and PCDFs by U.S. EPA*

| Congener | Factor |
|---|---|
| 2,7,8-tetraCDD | 1.0 |
| 1,2,3,7,8-pentaCDD | 0.5 |
| 1,2,3,6,7,8-hexaCDD | 0.1 |
| 1,2,3,7,8,9-hexaCDD | 0.1 |
| 1,2,3,4,7,8-hexaCDD | 0.1 |
| 1,2,3,4,6,8-heptaCDD | 0.01 |
| OctaCDD | 0.001 |
| 2,3,7,8-tetraCDF | 0.1 |
| 2,3,4,7,8-pentaCDF | 0.5 |
| 1,2,3,7,8-pentaCDF | 0.05 |
| 1,2,3,4,7,8-hexaCDF | 0.1 |
| 2,3,4,6,7,8-hexaCDF | 0.1 |
| 1,2,3,6,7,8,9-hexaCDF | 0.1 |
| 1,2,3,4,6,7,8-heptaCDF | 0.01 |
| 1,2,3,4,7,8,9-heptaCDF | 0.1 |
| OctaCDF | 0 |

From ref. 37.

Despite the depth of mechanistic knowledge of dioxin action, we still do not know how these molecular events relate to toxicity. It is widely assumed that all the toxic effects induced by dioxin require binding to the Ah receptor. Dioxin recognition elements (DREs) have been identified in the promoter region of several genes, such that the pluripotent nature of dioxin may be explained by its ability to affect a battery of genes depending on cell and developmental stage (35). How does TCDD cause cancer? At the level of the organism, it can act as a promoter, to amplify, fix, or hasten the processes of carcinogenesis; and it can also act alone, as a complete carcinogen, to increase the incidence of tumors in exposed animals (28). Complete carcinogenic chemicals are assumed to act by directly damaging DNA, either by inducing deletions or changes in base pairs or by binding to base pairs in DNA. Carcinogens that act as promoters enhance cell division, inhibit repair of genetic damage or otherwise increase the likelihood that a cell with prior genetic damage will progress to a tumor (41). These definitions are largely operational, and there is still considerable uncertainty regarding the cellular events in carcinogenesis. In human populations, it is impossible to rule out pre- or coexposure to other carcinogens in those cohorts where exposure to dioxins and related compounds has been associated with increased risks of cancer. Dioxin may induce the generation of other genotoxic agents (endogenous or exogenous) through its actions to induce hepatic microsomal metabolism reactions; or it may act in a hormone-like manner to cause cancer (similar to estrogen and diethylstilbestrol) (42).

The hormone-like actions of TCDD were first suggested in 1941 (43) and later demonstrated in studies of receptor action (42). Recently, public health concerns have focused on this mechanistic aspect of dioxin toxicity. The endocrine disruptor hypothesis links observations of altered reproduction and development in wildlife populations with compounds, such as diethylstilbestrol (DES), that are known to disrupt development and reproduction in humans exposed prenatally (44). The dioxins can disrupt endocrine function by interfering with a number of hormone mechanisms, involving estrogen, thyroid hormone, androgens, glucocorticoids, epidermal growth factor, tumor necrosis factors, and insulin (36). TCDD can alter metabolism of estrogen and testosterone, and while TCDD does not interact directly with any other known hormones or their receptors, in animals treated with TCDD and PCBs there is evidence for downregulation of steroid hormone receptors and alterations in levels of hormones in target tissues. Prenatal exposure to dioxins may alter the responsiveness of target cells to later steroid hormone programming at crucial developmental stages; this may underlie the effects of dioxin in rats on the morphologic development of the clitoris and vagina (18,57). The early finding (9) that TCDD reduced the incidence of hormone-dependent cancers in rats (mammary and pituitary) is consistent with an antiestrogenic effect, which has been demonstrated directly in terms of downregulation of the estrogen receptor (36). Based on current concepts of endocrine disruption—the property of a chemical or exposure to interfere with endogenous hormone function by affecting synthesis, release, catabolism, receptor binding, or signal transduction—the dioxins are clearly endocrine disruptors. This may mean that their most significant effects on human and nonhuman populations are on reproductive and developmental end points, and it may explain some of the most severe effects, at relatively low exposures, in Michigan children exposed before and after birth to PCBs and related compounds via the fish diets of their mothers. Alterations in early neurobehavioral development have been interpreted as suggesting endocrine disruption (44). In this way, dioxins may be prototypical endocrine disruptors, and further study of their toxic effects in human and nonhuman populations may assist us in elucidating the risks of this class of toxic agents.

## SOURCES OF DIOXINS AND FURANS

Chlorinated dioxins and furans can be present as contaminants in chlorophenols and other chlorinated organic chemicals, and can be produced both in trace quantities in the combustion of chlorinated materials and during the chlorine-bleaching of pulp and paper.

The results of two dioxin emissions inventories for the United States, based on data from the late 1980s, are shown in Fig. 4, with details of one of these inventories shown in Table 6 (45,46). There is substantial uncertainty in the determination of emission factors (emissions per kilogram of material combusted or processed); thus, emission estimates should be interpreted on an order-of-magnitude basis only. Dioxin emission measurements are expensive and not required for most dioxin sources, so

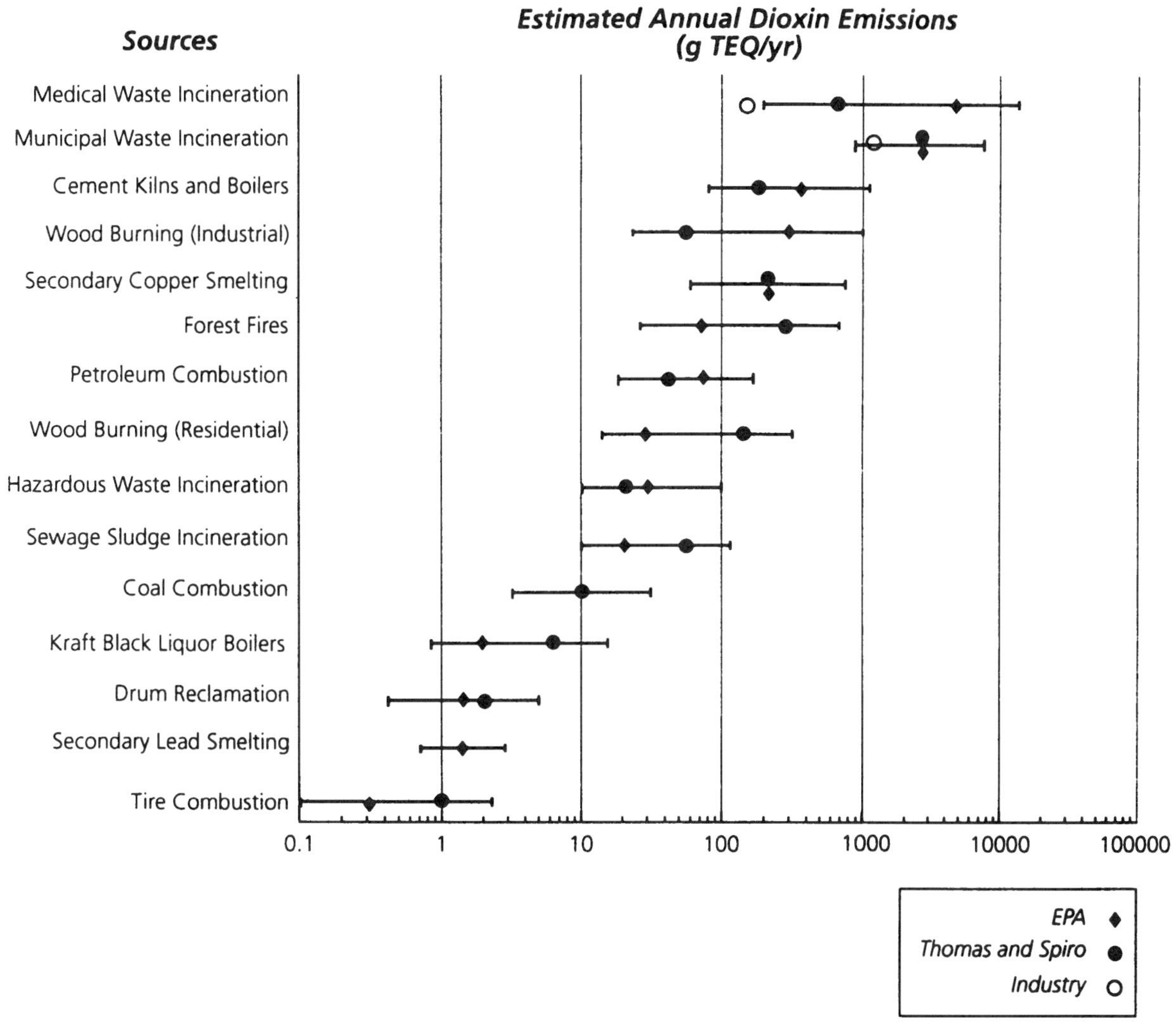


**FIG. 4.** Estimated annual U.S. toxic equivalent (TEQ) dioxin emissions from combustion. (Reprinted with permission from ref. 46.)

**TABLE 6.** *U.S. dioxin emissions inventory* (1989)

| Emission source (number of facilities tested) | Emission factor (μg/kg feed) Total | Emission factor (μg/kg feed) TEQ | Material consumed (kg/y) | PCDD/F emissions (kg/y) Total | PCDD/F emissions (kg/y) TEQ |
|---|---|---|---|---|---|
| Consumer waste | | | | | |
| MSW incinerators (14) | 10 | 0.2 | $2 \times 10^{10}$ | 200 | 3 |
| Hospital incinerators (6) | 20 | 0.35 | $2 \times 10^{9}$ | 40 | 0.7 |
| Apartment incinerators | 60 | 1 | $1 \times 10^{9}$ | 60 | 1 |
| Open garbage burning | 60 | 1 | $\sim 2 \times 10^{8}$ | 10 | 0.2 |
| Sewage sludge incinerators (3) | 1 | 0.02 | $3 \times 10^{9}$ | 4 | 0.07 |
| Industrial waste | | | | | |
| Hazardous waste incineration (35) | 3 | 0.06 | $4 \times 10^{9}$ | 10 | 0.2 |
| Copper recycling (2) | 20 | 0.4 | $7 \times 10^{8}$ | 10 | 0.2 |
| Steel recycling (9) | 0.1 | 0.004 | $3 \times 10^{10}$ | 3 | 0.1 |
| Steel drum reconditioning furnaces (3) | 30/drum | 0.5/drum | $4 \times 10^{6}$ drum/y | 0.1 | 0.002 |
| Used motor oil Burners (2) | 0.04 | 0.001 | $3 \times 10^{9}$ | 0.1 | 0.002 |
| Bleached pulp production (3) | 0.01 | 0.0002 | $3 \times 10^{10}$ | 0.4 | 0.007 |
| Tire fires (uncontrolled) | 0.09 | 0.004 | $3 \times 10^{8}$ | 0.03 | 0.001 |
| Carbon regeneration (1) | 0.06 | 0.001 | $5 \times 10^{7}$ | 0.003 | 0.00005 |
| Tire incineration (controlled) (1) | 0.009 | 0.0004 | $3 \times 10^{8}$ | 0.003 | 0.0001 |
| Biomass combustion, etc. | | | | | |
| Forest and agricultural burning | 0.4 | 0.004 | $8 \times 10^{10}$ | 30 | 0.3 |
| Residential wood burning (3) | 0.4 | 0.004 | $5 \times 10^{10}$ | 20 | 0.2 |
| Industrial wood combustion (4) | 0.05 | 0.001 | $6 \times 10^{10}$ | 3 | 0.06 |
| Structural fires | 0.4 | 0.004 | $5 \times 10^{9}$ | 2 | 0.02 |
| PCP-treated wood combustion (1) | 8 | 0.1 | $\sim 1 \times 10^{8}$ | 1 | 0.02 |
| PCB fires | 1000 | 20 | $7 \times 10^{5}$ | 0.7 | 0.01 |
| Cigarettes (1) | 0.1 | 0.002 | $5 \times 10^{87}$ | 0.05 | 0.0008 |
| Fossil fuels | | | | | |
| Oil combustion (except gasoline) | 0.003 | 0.00005 | $5 \times 10^{11}$ | 1 | 0.02 |
| Leaded gasoline (5) | 0.03 | 0.0005 | $3 \times 10^{10}$ | 1 | 0.02 |
| Unleaded gasoline (3) | 0.003 | 0.00005 | $3 \times 10^{11}$ | 0.8 | 0.01 |
| Coal combustion (1) | 0.001 | 0.00002 | $6 \times 10^{11}$ | 0.6 | 0.01 |
| Dioxin-contaminated chemicals | | | | | |
| PCP wood preservative (to air) (1) | $2 \times 10^{6}$ | | $2 \times 10^{4}$ | 10 | 0.1 |
| 2,4-D herbicide (to soil) (1) | 200 | 0.2 | $2\text{–}3 \times 10^{7}$ | 5 | 0.0005 |
| Tetrachloroethylene (to air) (4) | 10 | 0.1 | $3 \times 10^{8}$ | 3 | 0.03 |
| Total | | | $2 \times 10^{12}$ | 400 | 6.3 |

emission factors are based on a small number of measurements. Municipal waste incinerators are monitored more closely than other sources. Some sources that are likely to emit significant quantities of dioxin, such as facilities in the metals processing industries, have never been tested in the United States. And emission factors are highly variable, depending on the details of the feed material, combustion processes, and air pollution control equipment.

Figure 4 shows that the combustion of municipal solid waste and medical waste are the largest U.S. sources, as of the late 1980s. The next largest total sources include forest fires and residential wood burning, cement kilns and industrial boilers combusting hazardous wastes, and copper recycling (one of the few metals smelting industries for which U.S. dioxin emissions data are available).

Note that residential wood burning, forest fires, and agricultural fires are significant sources on a national basis only because there is so much combustion in these categories; their dioxin emission factors (emissions per kilogram of material combusted or processed) are small. The combustion of a kilogram of municipal waste is estimated to release an average of about 10 μg of PCDD/Fs (the sum of tetra- through octa-chlorinated dioxins and furans), as of 1989. This is 250 times more than from the combustion of a kilogram of firewood, which is estimated to release only about 0.4 μg of PCDD/Fs. The emissions factor, rather than the total national emissions, provides a useful indicator of local emissions potential. For example, based on the emissions factors in Table 6, the release of PCP wood preservative (used primarily on telephone poles) to air, the use of 2,4-D herbicide, and PCB fires (fires involving old PCB transformers) are highly potent local sources; the incineration of hospital waste, copper recycling, and municipal waste incineration also rank as significant local sources.

## Dioxin from Combustion

### *Municipal and Hospital Waste Incinerators*

As shown in Table 6, municipal and hospital waste incinerators have much higher dioxin emission factors than, for example, forest fires or petroleum combustion. While the formation of dioxin is not completely understood, it is increasingly clear that the high emissions from incinerators are due to several factors: the relatively high concentration of chlorine (over 1,000 ppm) due to the presence of chlorinated organic materials such as polyvinyl chloride (PVC) plastics; the presence of metals (such as copper), which can act as catalysts; and details of both the combustion and the air pollution control equipment. Dioxin formation is believed to be catalyzed, on fly ash and particulates that contain metals, in the postcombustion zone (that is, in the air pollution control equipment, in the exhaust stack, or even after the exhaust leaves the stack) (47). For both municipal and hospital waste incinerators, new EPA regulations and pollution control technology are expected to lead to much lower future emissions. Note, in addition, that the combustion of consumer waste in home fireplaces or wood stoves may be significant local sources.

### *Hazardous Waste Combustion*

Because hazardous wastes can have high chlorine concentrations, the combustion of hazardous waste has the potential for high dioxin emissions factors. However, available measurements indicate that hazardous waste incinerators, on average, have had lower dioxin emissions factors than municipal and hospital waste incinerators, presumably due to combustor design, operation, and air pollution control equipment. The emissions from any given facility depend on the details of feed material, combustion, and postcombustion conditions.

### *Metals Smelting and Recycling*

Dioxin emissions from the smelting and recycling of metals have been extensively monitored in Europe but not in the United States (48). Metals recycling smelters have the potential for significant dioxin emissions due to the presence of PVC plastic and other chlorinated compounds in the feed material. For example, secondary (recycling) copper smelters may process copper wires coated with PVC plastic, and steel drums sent for recycling may contain residues of chlorinated organic chemicals. Production of nickel and magnesium using chlorine-based processes have also produced high dioxin emissions (49).

## Dioxin from Production and Use of Chlorinated Chemicals

### *PCBs*

Polychlorinated biphenyls (PCBs) were used as heat transfer and hydraulic fluids, as dielectrics in transformers and capacitors, and as plasticizers in paints, inks, and paper. PCB production has been banned in the United States since 1976, although many PCB transformers and capacitors remain in service. In addition, household appliances such as refrigerators and air conditioners built before the early 1980s may contain PCBs. When PCBs are heated or combusted, significant concentrations of dioxins and furans can be formed. In 1981 in Binghamton, New York, a fire in an office building involving PCB transformers resulted in the contamination of the entire building (49). As a result, the EPA declared that PCB transformers must be replaced in public buildings. All PCB transformer fires must be reported to the National Response Center; about one such fire is reported each year, as of the mid-1990s.

There have been two mass poisonings stemming from the use of PCBs as a heat transfer fluid in rice oil processing. In 1968 in Japan (Yusho disease) and in 1979 in Taiwan (Yucheng disease), rice oil became contaminated with PCBs and dioxins. Thousands of people were exposed, and epidemiologic studies of these populations have contributed to the understanding of dioxin's health effects (18).

### *Chlorophenols*

Chlorophenols, which include the herbicides 2,4,5-T and 2,4-D, as well as the wood preservative pentachlorophenol (PCP), are similar in structure to dioxin, and are especially prone to dioxin contamination in the production process. In 1971 approximately 60 pounds of hexachlorophene wastes were mixed with oil and sprayed for dust control in eastern Missouri, including the residential community of Times Beach. As a result, Times Beach was permanently evacuated after a flood in 1983 (22).

### *PCP*

Pentachlorophenols, now used primarily to preserve utility poles, currently account for almost all chlorophenol production in the United States. PCP manufactured in the United States contains about 2,000 ppm of total PCDD/F. Unlike PCDD/F emissions from combustion, which typically have a fairly even distribution of dioxins and furans with different numbers of chlorine atoms, most of the dioxins in PCP are octa-chlorinated dioxins and furans, which are thought to be less toxic than the tetra-chlorinated dioxins. PCP is estimated to be among the largest sources of dioxins in the United States, amounting to nearly 3% of total PCDD/F air emissions (Table 6).

### *2,4,5-Trichlorophenol*

2,4,5-trichlorophenol was used as a herbicide in the United States from the mid-1940s until it was banned in 1984, although most uses were suspended in 1976. 2,4,5-T, in combination with another herbicide, 2,4-D (a dichlorophenol), was called Agent Orange, and was used as a defoliant during the Vietnam War (1). An estimated 1,200 kg of PCDD/F were in the Agent Orange used in Vietnam between 1965 and 1971. There have been numerous fires and accidents in 2,4,5-T plants, including the 1976 explosion in Seveso, Italy, which focused world attention on the risks of dioxin exposure.

In Love Canal, New York, approximately 200 tons of dioxin-contaminated trichlorophenols were placed in landfill over the period from the 1940s to 1970s. Later, houses and a school were built on the former landfill site. When wastes began oozing into basements and collecting in puddles on the ground in the late 1970s, the neighborhood was evacuated. The resulting national alarm was the impetus for major environmental legislation for the remediation of hazardous waste sites: the Comprehensive Environmental Response, Compensation, and Liability Act (CERCLA), commonly known as the Superfund.

### *Pulp and Paper Manufacture*

Dioxin can be formed as a by-product of chlorine bleaching of pulp and paper. Dioxin-contaminated wastes from pulp and paper bleaching, when released to streams and other water bodies, can result in highly contaminated sediments and fish, which can be a significant source of human exposure.

In addition, paper products made with chlorine-bleached pulp contain chlorinated dioxins and furans. In studies of paper products used to store or hold food, including milk cartons, coffee filters, and paper cups, on the order of 10% of the PCDD/Fs have been found to migrate from the paper into the food, based on 10- to 12-day exposure (49,50). The TCDD and TCDF levels in the paper products was in the 1 to 13 parts per trillion (ppt) range; changes in bleaching processes are expected to reduce levels in paper products to less than 2 ppt.

A number of U.S. pulp and paper manufacturers have switched from chlorine gas bleaching to chlorine dioxide bleaching, which produces less dioxin. Other manufacturers, particularly in Europe, have switched to nonchlorine bleaching processes, which do not have dioxin as a by-product.

## EXPOSURES

### Uptake and Absorption

Exposure to dioxins can occur via ingestion, inhalation, and dermal absorption. These chemicals can also be readily transferred across the placenta, and they are secreted into the breast milk of all lactating mammals. Gastrointestinal absorption of dioxins is highly efficient, especially when dioxins are in milk or fatty foods. Ingestion of soils contaminated with dioxins can result in absorption efficiencies from 30% to nearly 100% (45). Inhalation exposure occurs when dioxins are present in small particulates (such as dusts from contaminated surface soils, or emissions from imperfectly controlled incineration sources); this route of exposure is also highly efficient and dependent on particle size. Dioxins can also be absorbed dermally because of their lipophilic nature; the early occupational studies demonstrated the importance of this route of exposure in occupational settings (43).

### Retention and Excretion

These chemicals remain in the body for extended periods of time. The half-life of TCDD in humans has been calculated to be in the range of 6 to 12 years (23). They are highly stable, poorly metabolized, and preferentially stored in adipose tissue or the lipid fraction of organs. As a consequence, there is a general trend for increasing levels of dioxin with age in the general population. Excretion of TCDD is primarily in feces. TCDD is also lost from the body via breast milk, reducing body stores in the mother at the expense of exposure to the nursing infant (51).

### Pathways of Exposure

Dioxin is fat soluble and becomes concentrated in the fat of animals. For humans, the primary pathway of exposure for the general population is through the ingestion of animal foods such as fish, beef, dairy products, chicken, pork and eggs, as shown in Table 7. The average daily adult exposures are about 1 to 2 pg TEQ/kg-day. Most of the entries are based on measurements of foods from U.S. supermarkets; the fish entry is based on data from rivers and estuaries identified as free from sources of dioxin.

Table 7 shows that while there is a wide range of values, concentrations of dioxin in fish, meat, dairy prod-

**TABLE 7.** *Background adult human exposure to dioxin (USEPA, 1994)*

| Source | Concentration (TEQ) ppt ± s.d., except as noted | Media intake g/day, except as noted | Daily dioxin intake (TEQ) pg/day |
|---|---|---|---|
| Fish | 1.2 ± 1.2 | 7 | 7 |
| Beef | 0.5 ± 1 | 80 | 30 |
| Chicken | 0.2 ± 0.3 | 70 | 14 |
| Dairy | 0.4 ± 0.3 | 70 | 20 |
| Pork | 0.3 ± 0.1 | 50 | 9 |
| Egg | 0.1 ± 0.1 | 30 | 4 |
| Milk | 0.05–0.07 | 250 | 15 |
| Air | ~0.1 pg/m$^3$ | 20 m$^3$/day | 2 |
| Soil | ~8 | ~0.1 | 0.8 |
| Total | | | ~100 |

ucts, chicken, eggs, etc. are roughly comparable, and typically on the order of 0.1 to 1 ppt TEQ. By contrast, inhalation of the 0.1 pg/$m^3$ of dioxin typical of urban air constitutes only a small percentage of the average intake. These data suggest that the human exposure from individual dioxin sources, such as incinerators or paper mills, may be primarily through contamination of the food chain rather than through direct inhalation of emissions.

Food raised near dioxin sources can be expected to have higher dioxin concentrations. For example, at dairy farms located near incinerators in Vermont and in Germany, the concentration of dioxins in milk have been found to be on the order of 0.3 pg TEQ/g, several times higher than background levels (45).

Populations that may have higher dioxin exposures include breast-feeding infants and people who eat more than average quantities of fish, meat, or dairy products, especially if the food is from contaminated areas.

### Exposure from Breast Milk

Studies of U.S., German, and New Zealand women indicate that typical concentrations of dioxin in human breast milk are on the order of 8 ppt TEQ. Average exposures to infants are estimated to be about 60 pg TEQ/kg-day (45), which is significantly higher than the average adult exposure of 1 to 2 pg TEQ/kg-day. Mothers with greater than average dioxin exposure can be expected to have breast milk with higher dioxin concentrations.

### Exposure from Fish Consumption

Subsistence fishers can have fish consumption rates of 100 g/day or more, an order of magnitude more than the general population. In Sweden, fishermen and fish industry workers who consumed 700 to 1,750 g/week of salmon (30–90 pg TEQ/g) and herring (8–18 pg TEQ/g) from the Baltic Sea had blood levels of about 60 pg TEQ/g lipid, a factor of three higher than a non–fish-consuming population from the same region (52). Near a magnesium plant in Norway, which had been identified as a dioxin source, fishermen who consumed crabs from the local fjord were found to have an average dioxin consumption of about 9 pg TEQ/day from crab consumption alone, and dioxin blood concentrations seven times higher than the control group (53).

High dioxin concentrations have been found in striped bass, blue crabs, and lobsters collected from Newark Bay and the New York Bight, with levels of up to 6,200 ppt of 2,3,7,8-CDDs and -CDFs (54). The primary source of dioxin in the Newark Bay is the Diamond Shamrock superfund site, which was a major producer of the dioxin-contaminated herbicide 2,4,5-T (55). As a result of the high dioxin levels in the Newark Bay complex, New Jersey has prohibited the sale and consumption of any fish and shellfish taken from the mouth of the Passaic River and the sale or consumption of striped bass and blue crabs taken from Newark Bay and environs. Also due to dioxin contamination, New Jersey has advised that consumption of striped bass from the Hudson River be limited to no more than one meal per month; pregnant women, nursing mothers, women of child-bearing age, and young children are advised not to eat any striped bass from this area (56).

## REFERENCES


1. Institute of Medicine (IOM). *Veterans and Agent Orange.* Washington, DC: NAS Press, 1994.
2. Institute of Medicine (IOM). *Veterans and Agent Orange update 1996.* Washington, DC: NAS Press, 1996.
3. USEPA. *Health assessment document for TCDD and related compounds.* Washington, DC: EPA, 1994.
4. Schecter A. *Dioxins and human health.* New York: Plenum Press, 1994.
5. Jensen AA. PCBs, PCDDs, and PCDFs in human milk, blood and adipose tissue. *Sci Total Environ* 1987;64:259–293.
6. Silbergeld EK. Understanding risk: the case of dioxin. *Sci Amr Sci Med* 1995;2:48–47.
7. McGrath L, Cooper K, Georgopoulos P, Gallo M. Alternative models for low dose analysis of biochemical and immunological endpoints for TCDD. *Reg Toxicol Pharmacol* 1995;21:382–396.
8. Bertazzi PA, Zocchetti C, Pesatori AC, et al. Ten year mortality study of the population involved in the Seveso incident in 1976. *Am J Epidemiol* 1989;129:1187–1200.
9. Kociba RJ, Keys DG, Beyer JE, et al. Results of a two year chronic toxicity and oncogenicity study of 2,3,7,8-TCDD in rats. *Toxicol Appl Pharmacol* 1978;46:279–303.
10. Silbergeld EK. Chemicals and chloracne. In: Marzulli F, Maibach H, eds. *Dermatoxicology.* Philadelphia: Thomas and Hudson, 1996; 249–263.
11. Suskind RR. Chloracne, the hallmark of dioxin intoxication. *Scand J Work Environ Health* 1995;11:165–171.
12. Tindall JP. Chloracne and chloracnegens. *J Am Acad Dermatol* 1984; 13:539–558.
13. Clark GC, Tritscher AM, Bell DA, Lucier GW. Integrative approach for evaluating species and interindividual differences in responsiveness to dioxins and structural analogs. *Environ Health Perspect* 1992;98: 125–132.
14. Jung D, Konietzko J, Reill-Konietzko, et al. Porphyrin studies in TCDD exposed workers. *Arch Toxicol* 1994;68:595–598.
15. Ott MG, Messerer P, Zober A. Assessment of past occupational exposure to 2,3,7,8-TCDD using blood lipid analyses. *Int Arch Occup Environ Health* 1993;65:1–8.
16. Hay A. *The chemical scythe.* New York: Plenum Press, 1982.
17. Rogan WJ, Gladen BC, Hung KI, Koong SI, et al. Congenital poisoning by polychlorinated biphenyls and their contaminants in Taiwan. *Science* 1988;241:334–336.
18. Peterson RJ, Thoebald HM, Kimmel GL. Developmental and reproductive toxicity of dioxins and related compounds. *Crit Rev Toxicol* 1993; 23:283–335.
19. Flesch Janys D, Berger J, Gurn P, et al. Exposure to polychlorinated dioxins and furans and mortality in a cohort of workers from a herbicide producing plant in Hamburg, Federal Republic of Germany. *Am J Epidemiol* 1995;142:1165–1175.
20. Blair A, Mustafa D, Heineman EF. Cancer and other causes of death among male and female farmers from 23 states. *Am J Ind Med* 1993; 23:729–743.
21. Egeland GM, Sweeney MH, Fingerhut MA, Halperin WE, Wille KK, Schnoor TM. Total serum testosterone and gonadotropins in workers exposed to dioxin. *Am J Epidemiol* 1994;139:272–281.
22. Moore JA, Kimbrough RD, Gough M. The dioxin TCDD: a selective study of science and policy interaction. In: Frosch R, ed. *Keeping pace with science and engineering.* Washington, DC: NAS Press, 1993; 221–242.
23. Michalek JE, Tripathi RC, Caudill SP, Pirkle J. Investigation of TCDD

half life heterogenities in veterans of Operation Ranch Hand. *J Toxicol Environ Health* 1992;35:29–38.
24. Fingerhut MA, Halperin WE, Marlow DA, et al. Cancer mortality in workers exposed to 2,3,7,8-TCDD. *N Engl J Med* 1991;324:212–218.
25. Wilson JD. A dose-response curve for Yusho syndrome. *Regul Toxicol Pharmacol* 1987;7:364–369.
26. Cohn WJ, Boylan JJ, Blanke RV, et al. Treatment of chlordecone (kepone) toxicity with cholestyramine: results of a controlled clinical trial. *N Engl J Med* 1978;298:243–248.
27. Roberts JS, Silbergeld EK. Pregnancy, lactation and menopause: how physiology and gender affect the toxicity of chemicals. *Mt Sinai J Med* 1995;62:5;343–355.
28. Huff JE, Salmon AG, Hooper NK, Ziese L. Long-term carcinogenesis studies on 2,3,7,8-tetrachlorodibenzo-p-dioxin and hexachlorodibenzo-p-dioxins. *Cell Biol Toxicol* 1991;7:67–94.
29. Murray FJ, Smith FA, Nitschke DK, et al. Three generation study of rats given 2,3,7,8,-TCDD in the diet. *Toxicol Appl Pharmacol* 1979;50: 241–252.
30. Holsapple MP, Morris DL, Wood SC, Snyder NK. 2,3,7,8-Tetrachloro-dibenzo-p-dioxin-induced changes in immunocompetence: possible mechanisms. *Annu Rev Pharmacol Toxicol* 1991;31:73–100.
31. Poland A, Knutson JC. 2,3,7,8-TCDD and related halogenated aromatic hydrocarbons: examination of the mechanisms of toxicity. *Annu Rev Pharmacol Toxicol* 1982;22:517–554.
32. Whitlock JP. Mechanistic aspects of dioxin action. *Chem Res Toxicol* 1993;6:754–763.
33. Hankinson O. The arylhydrocarbon receptor complex. *Annu Rev Pharmacol Toxicol* 1995;35:307–340.
34. Burbach KM, Poland A, Bradfield CA. Cloning of the Ah receptor cDNA reveals a distinctive ligand-activated transcription factor. *Proc Natl Acad Sci USA* 1992;89:8185–8189.
35. Nebert DW, Puga A, Vasiliou V. Role of the Ah receptor and the dioxin inducible (Ah) gene battery in toxicity, cancer and signal transduction. *Ann NY Acad Sci* 1993;685:624–640.
36. Safe SH. Modulation of gene expression and endocrine response pathways by 2,3,7,8-TCDD and related compounds. *Pharmacol Ther* 1995;67:247–281.
37. Ahlborg UG, Becking G, Birnbaum LS, et al. Toxic equivalency factors for dioxin like PCBs, *Chemosphere* 1994;28:6–10.
38. Silbergeld EK, de Fur P. Risk assessments of dioxin-like compounds. In: Schecter A, ed. *Dioxins and human health.* New York: Plenum Press, 1994;51–78.
39. Birnbaum LS. The mechanism of dioxin toxicity: relationship to risk assessment. *Environ Health Perspect* 1994;102:157–167.
40. Kohn MC, Lucier GW, Clark GC, Tritscher AM, Portier CJ. A mechanistic model of effects of dioxin on gene expression in the rat liver. *Toxicol Appl Pharmacol* 1993;20:138–154.
41. Pitot HC, Dragan YP. Facts and theories concerning the mechanisms of carcinogenesis. *FASEB J* 1991;5:2280–2285.
42. Lucier GW. Receptor-mediated carcinogenesis. In: Vainio H, Magee PN, McGregor DB, McMichael AJ, eds. *Mechanisms of carcinogenesis in risk identification*. Lyon, France: IARC Scientific, 1992;16:87–112.
43. Thelwell Jones A. The etiology of acne with special reference to acne of occupational origin. *J Ind Hyg Toxicol* 1941;23:290–312.
44. Colborn T, vom Saal F, Soto AM. Developmental effects of endocrine disrupting chemicals in wildlife and humans. *Environ Health Perspect* 1993;101:378–384.
45. US EPA. *Estimating exposures to dioxin-like compounds.* EPA regulation 600/6-88/005Cb. Washington, DC: EPA, 1994.
46. Thomas VM, Spiro TG. An estimation of dioxin emissions in the US. *Toxicol Environ Chem* 1995;50:1–37.
47. Gullett BK, Lemieux PM. Role of combustion and sorbent parameters in prevention of polychlorinated dibenzo-p-dioxin and polychlorinated dibenzofuran formation during waste combustion. *Environ Sci Technol* 1993;28:1;107–118.
48. Lahl U. Sintering plants of steel industry: the most important thermal PCDD/F source in industrialized regions? *Organohalogen Compounds* 1993;11:311–314.
49. Fiedler H, Hutzinger O. Dioxins: sources, loads, and human exposure. *Toxicol Environ Chem* 1990;29:157–234.
50. LaFleur L. Analysis of TCDD and TCDF on the ppq-level in milk and food sources. *Chemosphere* 1990;20(10-12):1657–1662.
51. World Health Organization (WHO). Levels of PCBs, PCDDs, and PCDSs in breast milk: results of WHO-coordinated interlaboratory quality control studies and analytical field studies. In: *Environmental Health,* Series 34. Copenhagen: WHO, 1989.
52. Svensson BG, Nilsson A, Hansson M. Exposure to dioxins and dibenzofurans through the consumption of fish. *N Engl J Med* 1991;324(1): 8–12.
53. Johansen HR, Alexander J, Rossland OJ. PCDDs, PCDFs, and PCBs in human blood in relation to consumption of crabs from a contaminated fjord area in Norway. *Environ Health Perspect* 1996;104:756–764.
54. Rappe C. Levels and patterns of PCDD and PCDF contamination in fish, crabs and lobsters from Newark Bay and New York Bight. *Chemosphere* 1991;22(3-4):239–266.
55. Bopp RF. A major incident of dioxin contamination: sediments of New Jersey Estuaries. *Environ Sci Technol* 1991;25:951–956.
56. New Jersey Department of Environmental Protection. *Polychlorinated dibenzofurans, biphenyls (PCBs), chlordane, and DDT in selected fish and shellfish from New Jersey waters, 1988–1991:* results from New Jersey's Toxics in Biota Monitoring Program. Trenton, NJ: NJDEP, 1993.
57. Flaws JA, Sommer R, Silbergeld EK, et al. In utero and lactational exposure to TCDD induces genital dysmorphogenesis in the female rat. *Toxicol Appl Pharmacol* 1997;147:351–362.

*Environmental and Occupational Medicine, Third Edition,* edited by William N. Rom.
Lippincott–Raven Publishers, Philadelphia © 1998.

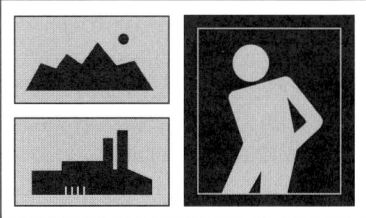

CHAPTER 86

# Pentachlorophenol and Tetrachlorophenol

Shona J. Kelly, Kay Teschke, and Clyde Hertzman

Pentachlorophenol (PCP) was first prepared by the chlorination of phenol in 1872, but was only introduced into commercial use, as a wood preservative, in the 1930s (1). Over the past 60 years, it has been adopted for multiple pesticidal uses, including as a herbicide and disinfectant. It is very toxic [mammalian oral median lethal dose ($LD_{50}$) 27–210 mg/kg] and has been responsible for numerous acute fatalities (1–3). Only in the last two decades, subsequent to its discovery as a member of the class of dioxin-contaminated substances, has pentachlorophenol's chronic toxicity come under close scrutiny.

PCP is a colorless to light brown or gray crystalline solid at room temperature with little odor (median odor threshold = 9 mg/m$^3$, pungent or phenolic scent) (2–4). These characteristics make it attractive for wood preservation compared to creosote, since PCP's presence on treated wood is indiscernible. It is nearly insoluble in water (19 mg/L at 30°C), but its commonly used sodium salt (NaPCP) is water soluble (330 g/L) (2,5). Industrial grades of PCP contain a mixture of PCP (88%), tetrachlorophenol (TCP; 4%), other chlorinated phenols (7%), and traces of diphenyl ethers, polychlorobenzenes, and other chlorinated aromatics (1,6,7). Formulations with TCP predominating were widely substituted for PCP in the 1960s and 1970s in lumber industry applications, because of sodium tetrachlorophenate's (NaTCP) greater water solubility and somewhat lesser acute toxicity (mammalian oral $LD_{50}$ 109–529 mg/kg) (2,8).

Contamination with chlorinated dibenzo-p-dioxins and dibenzofurans has generally been reported at the part-per-million level, and is highest for furans and for hexa-, hepta-, and octa-congeners (1,5,7,8). The level and composition of dioxin and furan contaminants depends on the production process; distillation purification can reduce contaminant levels by more than an order of magnitude (8,9). Combustion of PCP or PCP-contaminated substances also produces dibenzo-p-dioxins and dibenzofurans (5,9). In recent years, use of PCP and TCP has been greatly restricted in many areas of the world, including the United States, Canada, Europe, and Japan (8).

## INDUSTRIAL USES

Pentachlorophenol has been used industrially to suppress the growth of many types of undesirable microorganisms in such diverse applications as drilling fluids, adhesives, textiles, pulp and paper manufacture, soaps, laundry products, dental care products, leather tanning, mushroom culture, and cooling tower water (10). It has also been used as a house, farm, or medical disinfectant and a preharvest desiccant on seed crops (1). In Japan, its major application has been as a herbicide (1). Since 1949, it has been used in Africa and Asia as a molluscicide to control schistosomiasis (10,11). In contrast, most of the commercial use of PCP and TCP in North America and northern Europe has been as a wood preservative to protect wood from fungal growth and boring insects (10). For long-term preservation of wood from fungal decay, PCP is usually applied under pressure as a 5% solution in fuel oil, kerosene, dichloromethane, or isopropyl alcohol (10). Wood may also be treated for short-term protection against discoloring fungi during transport to markets, most commonly by spraying, dipping, or brushing with water-based formulations consisting mainly of NaTCP (8,12,13).

S. J. Kelly, K. Teschke, and C. Hertzman: Department of Health Care and Epidemiology, University of British Columbia, Vancouver, British Columbia V6T 1Z3, Canada.

## OCCUPATIONAL EXPOSURES

Occupational exposure can occur during the production and use of chlorophenols, and from contact with treated materials (6,14–20). Production workers involved in handling solidified PCP blocks, and in packing, sampling, and maintenance operations have had measurable exposures to airborne PCP and TCP (range: 0.01–16.5 mg/m$^3$) and hexa-, hepta-, and octachlorinated dioxins (range: <0.002–0.5 μg/m$^3$) (6,15). In a study comparing plasma and urinary PCP levels among pesticide formulators, house sprayers, and timber-yard operatives, the formulators had the lowest levels (mean = 1.3 mmol/L in plasma, and 40 nmol/mmol creatinine in urine), timber-yard operatives had levels two to four times higher, and sprayers had levels four to six times higher (14). Studies of employees of sawmills and other operations treating wood have found total urinary chlorophenate (TCP and PCP) levels ranging from population background levels of less than 20 μg/L to more than 1,000 μg/L (13,16,17, 19,20). The highest exposures were observed among those operating spray or dip systems or handling wet lumber downstream.

The chief routes of exposure are via skin contact and inhalation. Wild and Jones (21) compared inhalation, water intake, and dietary intake as sources of exposure among wood preservation plant workers and estimated that 79% of daily PCP absorption comes from inhalation. Although PCP and TCP have low vapor pressures ($VP_{PCP}$ = 0.00011 torr at 20°C), airborne exposures may still approach occupational standards through vaporization alone (2). Many work sites use spray application methods, which may produce aerosol mists, and manufacturing, formulating, and mixing workers may be exposed to airborne dusts (6,14,15). However, investigators who have directly measured the relative contributions of skin and inhalation sources in wood treatment workers have found skin exposures to contribute the major proportion to body burden, likely because of the greater opportunities for contact with wet treated lumber than with airborne sources (16–18). PCP and TCP are readily absorbed through the skin. Percutaneous absorption is significantly enhanced when the formulation is dissolved in organic solvents such as fuel oil (62% absorbed *in vitro*) or when it comes in contact with open cuts and scratches (22).

Because of the importance of skin absorption as a route of exposure, biologic measurements of chlorophenates in urine or blood, rather than measurements of air concentrations, are usually done to assess exposure (14, 16,17,19,20). The American Conference of Governmental Industrial Hygienists set an 8-hour time-weighted-average threshold limit value for pentachlorophenol in air of 0.5 mg/m$^3$, with a skin notation indicating the potential for significant percutaneous absorption (23). They have also established biologic exposure indices of 2 mg/g creatinine of total (free and conjugated) PCP in urine or 5 mg/L of free PCP in plasma (23).

Industrial hygiene measures for minimizing exposures include enclosing systems, automation, and other means of reducing handling of wet or dusty surfaces; mist elimination through ventilation in spray applications; employee exposure monitoring and education; and where other measures are not adequate, use of personal protective equipment, including gloves and other impervious protective clothing (8). As with all pesticides, it is also important to follow labeling information, and to wash prior to eating, drinking, or smoking. In the lumber industry, substitution with other fungicides or with kiln drying techniques has been widespread since the late 1980s (8).

## ENVIRONMENTAL EXPOSURES

PCP and TCP enter water, soil, sewage, and the food chain mainly as a result of their production and use as pesticides, though chlorination of organic matter during water treatment or bleaching processes are also potential sources (5,24). Contamination of soils around wood treatment sites is common; these sites have been shown to leach chlorophenols and contribute significantly to the levels found in surface and ground water (10,24). Disposal of sludge from PCP spray tanks and effluent treatment systems are sources of environmental exposure (25). Discharge of contaminated process water from pulp and paper mills using PCP as a slimicide led to the prohibition of this use in Sweden and elsewhere in the 1970s (5). PCP tends to distribute to soil and sediment, leading to contamination of produce and of bottom-feeding marine organisms (5,10,24). The use of treated wood chips as mulch or animal bedding has also resulted in food contamination (24).

Nonoccupational PCP and TCP exposure of humans occurs from consumption of food and water containing residues and their ubiquitous presence as an environmental contaminant. PCP has been detected in fruits, vegetables, meats, water, soils, air, and dust (5,24,26). Investigators who measured PCP residues in the air, house dust, and soil around homes estimated the median exposure of resident children via respiration and ingestion of house dust to be 0.15 and 0.04 μg/day, respectively (26). Somewhat lower inhalation intakes for adults were estimated by researchers in the United Kingdom (21). They also calculated that only 1% of the daily intake of the general population would come from inhalation, 7% from water, and 92% from the diet, largely from meat and dairy products, for a total of 4.5 mg/day (21).

Surveys have shown that 72% to 100% of urine samples from individuals not occupationally exposed contain quantifiable levels of PCP (27,28). In the U.S. National Health and Nutrition Examination Survey conducted during the period 1976 to 1980, the median urinary PCP concentration was 6.0 μg/L and the 90th percentile was 15.5 μg/L (28). In a recent Italian study and a Canadian study conducted in 1992 and 1995, median levels were lower, 3.7, 1.3, and 0.5 μg/L respectively, possibly because PCP use has been declining since the 1980s (13,27). The U.S. study found that levels in men were somewhat higher than in women, and also appeared to be higher in urban than rural residents (28). It is important to note that PCP residues in urine may also result from the metabolism of related chemicals such as hexachlorobenzene and lindane.

## METABOLISM AND TOXICITY IN HUMANS

PCP is readily and nearly completely absorbed following ingestion, dermal contact, or inhalation, though the percent absorbed depends on its form (e.g., sodium salt) and the solvent vehicle (21,29). In a human experiment on volunteers, the average half-time for absorption of an oral dose of 0.1 mg/kg was 1.3 hours (29). In blood, more than 95% of PCP is bound to plasma proteins (5,30). Little metabolism of PCP takes place in the body; some is conjugated with glucuronic acid (12–70%), and minor amounts undergo oxidative dechlorination to tetrachlorohydroquinone (29,30).

PCP is almost completely eliminated via the urine, and unchanged as the glucuronide conjugate, though some fecal elimination also occurs (~5%) (5,29,30). Human PCP kinetics have been reported to follow both one- and two-compartment elimination models (29–31). Estimates of excretion half-lives for PCP and TCP vary from several days (after acute exposures) up to 2 months (following chronic exposures) (5,29–32). Even the longest half-life estimates are short compared to those of their dioxin and furan contaminants; steady-state body burdens of chlorophenols would be reached within 6 months of chronic exposure. Finnish researchers measured tissue levels of PCP in surgical cases and fatal accident victims, and found residues in adipose tissue (median = 2 ng/g fat) and liver tissue (median = 4 ng/g fat) that reflect blood and urinary concentrations in unexposed populations (32).

PCP is toxic to humans because it uncouples oxidative phosphorylation in the mitochondria and endoplasmic reticulum, the same process that makes PCP a commercially useful pesticide (5,33). This results in increased cellular oxidative metabolism and heat production. Severe intoxications in humans are most commonly manifested by diaphoresis, tachypnea, tachycardia, and hyperpyrexia (34–37). Abdominal pain, vomiting, anorexia, weakness, metabolic acidosis, and renal and hepatic dysfunction with elevations in alkaline phosphatase, serum creatinine, and blood urea nitrogen may also be observed (35–38). Death may result from hyperpyrexia, cerebral edema, pulmonary edema, or heart failure, and is usually followed by immediate and marked rigor mortis (5,34,35). Fatalities have been reported among workers in PCP production facilities in Japan and the United States, in American, Canadian, French, and Indonesian wood preservative plants, in Australian pineapple plantations after PCP use as a herbicide, and in South African waterways after NaPCP application as a molluscicide (34). Two newborns died after their hospital diapers and bedding were washed with 23% NaPCP (38). Case reports indicate that diagnosis of PCP poisoning may easily be missed; this may especially be so where hot weather exacerbates and suggests other explanations of the symptoms.

Symptoms of intoxication may appear at urine concentrations of 2,000 μg/L (37). In fatal cases, PCP concentrations have been greater than 25,000 μg/L in urine and 28 to 640 μg/g in tissues (34,35,39). The minimum lethal dose has been estimated as 29 mg/kg (5). Poisoned individuals must be removed from further contact. Body temperature should be reduced, lost fluids replaced, and metabolic acidosis treated. Forced diuresis has been shown to reduce PCP body burden significantly (37). Blood transfusions were similarly effective in neonates who survived the hospital poisonings (38).

Case reports of nonfatal poisonings reported pancreatitis after use of wood preservative containing PCP and zinc naphthenate, and intravascular hemolysis following use of pentachlorophenol as an insecticide on furniture (36,40). Aplastic anemia developing 1 month to 2 years after industrial or home uses of PCP has also been reported (41).

With lower levels of PCP exposure, the main findings have been inflammation of the skin and mucous membranes of the eye and upper respiratory tract; these can be severe and painful if the PCP solutions contacted have concentrations greater than 1% (5,42,43). Chloracne has been observed in PCP-exposed individuals; this effect may be due to the dioxin and furan contaminants (5,14, 15,34).

A number of studies have examined effects of chronic chlorophenol exposure among occupationally exposed groups. Manufacturing workers from the United Kingdom with high PCP dust exposures were reported to have a high prevalence of chloracne (62.5%), elevated triglyceride levels, and lower levels of high-density lipoprotein (HDL) cholesterol and bilirubin, but no differences in liver enzymes (SGOT, SGPT, GGT) (15). Colosio and colleagues (13) found increased levels of serum bile acids and decreased lymphocyte response, but no clinical signs of disease in workers exposed to PCP for more than 10 years (mean urinary PCP = 127 μg/L). In a study of sawmill workers exposed to chlorophenates, the most heavily exposed group (mean urinary chlorophenates = 229 μg/L) had lower hematocrit levels and marginally lower blood leukocyte counts, but no differences in hemoglobin levels, bilirubin, glutamic-oxaloacetic transaminase (GOT), other serum markers, spirometric abnormalities, reported respiratory symptoms, or liver, kidney, or heart disease (16,44). Peripheral nerve conduction velocities were normal in chemical plant workers with urinary PCP levels ranging from 8 to 1,224 μg/L (34,45).

## EPIDEMIOLOGIC STUDIES OF CHRONIC EFFECTS

Reproductive effects have been seen in animals. In rats PCP causes decreased litter size, increased number of stillborns, and dose-related signs of embryotoxicity and fetotoxicity (46,47). In a study of paternal occupational exposure to chlorophenates and risk of congenital anomalies in offspring, Dimich-Ward et al. (48) found an increased risk of congenital anomalies of the eye, particularly congenital cataracts. Elevated risks for developing anencephaly or spina bifida and congenital anomalies of genital organs were associated with specific windows of exposure. No associations were found for low birth weight, prematurity, stillbirths, or neonatal deaths. In a related study no evidence was found for a reduction in fertility among chlorophenate-exposed males (49).

The International Agency for Research on Cancer (IARC) has determined that there is sufficient evidence of carcinogenicity in animals but insufficient evidence in humans. In their review IARC rejected all but one animal study because of "deficiencies in design, performance and/or reporting" (10). In the one study reviewed, the test animals, exposed to technical-grade PCP showed increased frequencies of benign and malignant adrenal tumors, and spleen and liver hemangiosarcomas. It was not clear whether this was due to the PCP or to its impurities.

With two exceptions there are no epidemiologic studies on the carcinogenicity of PCP in humans. Most exposed cohorts are exposed to a multiplicity of related and unrelated chemicals and PCP is rarely selected out for more detailed analysis. For example, the IARC international register of dioxin-exposed workers contains only one group exposed to PCP only. The other groups in the register had been exposed to at least seven other chemically related substances and up to 30 other chemicals.

Historically, British Columbia, Canada sawmill workers represent the world's largest identifiable occupational group exposed primarily to chlorophenols. A historical prospective cohort study of 26,000 sawmill workers exposed to industrial PCP found increased risk for non-Hodgkin's lymphoma (NHL) with increasing chlorophenate exposure ($p$ for trend = 0.04) (50). Forty percent of the cases (and all of the excess risk) occurred in workers with 20 or more years of exposure and greater than 10,000 cumulative hours of chlorophenate exposure [standardized incidence ratio (SIR) = 1.54; $p = 0.04$].

Finnish sawmill workers used a product that contained predominantly tetrachlorophenol (12) and the only increased cancer risk found by researchers was for skin cancer in males [SIR = 313; 95% confidence interval (CI) 115–680]. There were no excess cases of soft tissue sarcoma (STS), and lymphoma was nonsignificantly elevated. The population of a small town in southern Finland was exposed to chlorophenols via drinking water contaminated by a local sawmill. When residents were compared to a neighboring area, both sexes showed increased rate ratios for NHL and STS [relative risk (RR) = 2.8, 95% CI 1.4–5.6, and RR = 8.9, 95% CI 1.8–44, respectively] (51). A case-control study of residents found that people who consumed fish from the contaminated lake were at increased risk for NHL.

Several case-control studies have solicited exposure to chlorophenols from subjects with NHL or STS. In three separate studies Swedish researchers found significantly increased risk ratios varying from 2.5 to 8.8 (52–54). A New Zealand study found a nonsignificant increase in NHL for exposure to chlorophenates (55). The IARC international cohort contains 408 workers exposed to chlorophenols (56). The IARC found a nonsignificant increase for NHL and no cases of STS.

## REFERENCES


1. International Agency for Research on Cancer. Some halogenated hydrocarbons. In: *IARC monographs on the evaluation of the carcinogenic risk of chemicals to humans,* vol 20. Lyon, France: IARC. 1979.
2. U.S. National Toxicology Program, Department of Health and Human Services, Chemical Health and Safety Information. *NTP chemical repository (Radian Corporation, August 29, 1991) pentachlorophenol.* http://ntpdb.niehs.nih.gov/
3. Worthing CR, Walker SB, eds. *The pesticide manual.* Lavenham, UK: Lavenham Press, 1987.
4. Ruth JH. Odor thresholds and irritation levels of several chemical substances: a review. *Am Ind Hyg Assoc J* 1986;47:A142–151.
5. Ahlborg UG, Thunberg TM. Chlorinated phenols: occurrence, toxicity, metabolism, and environmental impact. *CRC Crit Rev Toxicol* 1980;7(1):1–35.
6. Marlow DA. Hexachlorobenzene exposure in the production of chlorophenols. In: Morris CR, Cabral JRP, ed. *Hexachlorobenzene:* proceedings of an international symposium. Lyon, France: IARC Scientific, 1986;161–169.
7. Christmann W, Koppel K, Rotard P. PCDD/PCDF and chlorinated phenols in wood preserving formulations for household use. *Chemosphere* 1989;18(1-6):861–865.
8. Teschke K, Hertzman C, Fenske R, et al. A history of process and chemical changes for fungicide application in the western Canadian lumber industry: What can we learn? *Appl Occup Environ Hyg* 1994; 9:984–993.
9. Rappe C, Marklund S, Buser H, Bosshardt H. Formation of polychlorinated dibenzo-p-dioxins (PCDDs)f and dibenzofurans (PCDFs) by burning or heating chlorophenates. *Chemosphere* 1978;3:269–281.
10. International Agency for Research on Cancer. Occupational exposures in insecticide application, and some pesticides. In: *IARC monographs on the evaluation of the carcinogenic risk of chemicals to humans,* vol 53. Lyon, France: IARC, 1991.
11. Schecter A, Jiang K, Papke O, Furst P, Furst C. Comparison of dibenzodioxin levels in blood and milk in agricultural workers and others following pentachlorophenol exposure in China. *Chemosphere* 1994; 29(9-11):2371–2380.
12. Jappinen P, Pukkala E, Tola S. Cancer incidence of workers in a Finnish sawmill. *Scand J Work Environ Health* 1989;15(1):18–23.
13. Colosio C, Maroni M, Barcellini W, et al. Toxicological and immune findings in workers exposed to pentachlorophenol (PCP). *Arch Environ Health* 1993;48(2):81–88.
14. Jones RD, Winter DP, Cooper AJ. Absorption study of pentachlorophenol in persons working with wood preservatives. *Hum Toxicol* 1986;5:189–194.

15. Baxter RA. Biochemical study of pentachlorophenol workers. *Ann Occup Hyg* 1984;28(4):429–438.
16. Enarson DA, Chan-Yeung M, Embree V, Wang R, Schulzer M. Occupational exposure to chlorophenates. *Scand J Work Environ Health* 1986;12:144–148.
17. Kauppinen T, Lindroos L. Chlorophenol exposure in sawmills. *Am Ind Hyg Assoc J* 1985;46:34–38
18. Fenske RA, Horstman SW, Bentley RK. Assessment of dermal exposure to chlorophenols in timber mills. *Appl Ind Hyg* 1987;2:143–147
19. Teschke K, Hertzman C, Dimich-Ward H, et al. A comparison of exposure estimates by worker raters and industrial hygienists. *Scand J Work Environ Health* 1989;15:424–429
20. Hertzman C, Teschke K, Dimich-Ward H, Ostry A. Validity and reliability of a method for retrospective evaluation of chlorophenate exposure in the lumber industry. *Am J Ind Med* 1988;14:703–713.
21. Wild SR, Jones KC. Pentachlorophenol in the UK environment II. Human exposure and as assessment of pathways. *Chemosphere* 1992; 24(7):847–855.
22. Horstman SW, Rossner A, Kalman DA, et al. Penetration of pentachlorophenol and tetrachlorophenol through human skin. *J Environ Sci Health* 1989;A24:229–242
23. American Conference of Governmental Industrial Hygienists. *1996 TLVs and BEIs*. Cincinnati, OH: ACGIH, 1996.
24. Agriculture Canada, Food Production and Inspection Branch. *Pentachlorophenol.* CAPCO Note 87-02. Ottawa: Agriculture Canada, 1987.
25. Lao R, Thomas R, Chiu C, Li K, Lockwood J. Analysis of PCDD-PCDF in environmental samples. In: Choudhary G, Keith L, Rappe C, eds. *Chlorinated dioxins and dibenzofurans in the total environment,* vol 2. Stoneham, MA: Butterworth, 1985;65–78.
26. Lewis RG, Fortmann RC, Camann DE. Evaluation of methods for monitoring the potential exposure of small children to pesticides in the residential environment. *Arch Environ Contam Toxicol* 1994; 26(1):37–46.
27. Thompson TS, Treble RG. Pentachlorophenol levels in human urine. *Bull Environ Contam Toxicol* 1996;56(4):520–526.
28. Kutz FW, Cook BT, Carter-Pokras OD, Brody D, Murphy RS. Selected pesticide residues and metabolites in urine from a survey of the U.S. general population. *J Toxicol Environ Health* 1992;37(2): 277–291.
29. Anonymous. Pentachlorophenol. *Rev Environ Contam Toxicol* 1988; 104:183–194.
30. Uhl S, Schmid P, Schlatter C. Pharmacokinetics of pentachlorophenol in man. *Arch Toxicol* 1986;58:182–186.
31. Kalman DA, Horstman SW. Persistence of tetrachlorophenol and pentachlorophenol in exposed woodworkers. *J Toxicol Clin Toxicol* 1983; 20:343–352.
32. Mussalo-Rauhamaa H, Pyysalo H, Antervo K. The presence of chlorophenols and their conjugates in Finnish human adipose and liver tissues. *Sci Total Environ* 1989;83:161–172.
33. Weinbach EC. Biochemical basis for the toxicity of pentachlorophenol. *Proc Natl Acad Sci USA* 1957;43(6):393–397.
34. Wood S, Rom WN, White GL, Logan DC. Pentachlorophenol poisoning. *J Occup Med* 1983;25(7):527–530.
35. Gray RE, Gilliland RD, Smith EE, Lockard VG, Hume AS. Pentachlorophenol intoxication: report of a fatal case, with comments on the clinical course and pathologic anatomy. *Arch Env Health* 1985; 40(3):161–164.
36. Hassan AB, Seligmann H, Bassan HM. Intravascular haemolysis induced by pentachlorophenol. *Br Med J* 1985;291:21–22.
37. Haley TJ. Human poisoning with pentachlorophenol and its treatment. *Ecotoxicol Environ Health* 1977;1:343–347.
38. Robson AM, Kissane JM, Elvick WH, Pundavela L. Pentachlorophenol poisoning in a nursery for newborn infants: I. Clinical features and treatment. *J Pediatr* 1969;75:309–316.
39. Bevenue A, Beckman H. Pentachlorophenol: a discussion of its properties and its occurrence as a residue in human and animal tissues. *Residue Rev* 1967;19:83–134
40. Cooper RG, Macaulay MB. Pentachlorophenol pancreatitis. *Lancet* 1982;1(8270):517.
41. Roberts HJ. Pentachlorophenol-associated aplastic anemia, red cell aplasia, leukemia and other blood disorders. *J Florida Med Assoc* 1990;77(2):86–90.
42. Sterling TD, Stoffman LD, Sterling DA, Mate G. Health effects of chlorophenol wood preservatives on sawmill workers. *Int J Health Serv* 1982;12:559–571
43. Klemmer HW, Wong L, Sato MM, et al. Clinical findings in workers exposed to pentachlorophenol. *Arch Environ Contam Toxicol* 1980;9: 715–725.
44. Embree V, Enarson DA, Chan-Yeung M, et al. Occuptional exposure to chlorophenates: toxicology and respiratory effects. *J Toxicol Clin Toxicol* 1984;22(4):317–329.
45. Triebig G, Csuzda I, Krekeler HJ, Schaller KH. Pentachlorophenol and the peripheral nervous system: a longitudinal study in exposed workers. *Br J Ind Med* 1987;44(9):638–641.
46. Exon JH, Koller LD. Effects of transplacental exposure to chlorinated phenols. *Environ Health Perspect* 1982;46:137–140.
47. Schwetz BA, Keeler PA, Gehring PJ. The effect of purified and commercial grade pentachlorophenol on rat embryonal and fetal development. *Toxicol Appl Pharmacol* 1974;28:151–161.
48. Dimich-Ward H, Hertzman C, Teschke K, et al. Reproductive effects of paternal exposure to chlorophenate wood preservatives in the sawmill industry. *Scand J Work Environ Health* 1996;22:267–273.
49. Heacock H, Hogg R, Marion SA, et al. Fertility among a cohort of male sawmill workers exposed to chlorophenate fungicides. *Epidemiology* 1998;9:56–60.
50. Hertzman C, Teschke K, Ostry A, et al. Mortality and cancer incidence among a cohort of sawmill workers exposed to chlorophenate wood preservatives. *Am J Public Health* 1997;87:71–79.
51. Lampi P, Hakulinen T, Luostarinen T, Pukkala E, Teppo L. Cancer incidence following chlorophenol exposure in a community in southern Finland. *Arch Environ Health* 1992;47(3):167–175.
52. Hardell L, Eriksson M, Degerman A. Exposure to phenoxyacetic acids, chlorophenols, or organic solvents in relation to histopathology, stage, and anatomical localization of non-Hodgkin's lymphoma. *Cancer Res* 1994;54(9):2386–2389.
53. Eriksson M, Hardell L, Berg NO, Moller T, Axelson O. Soft-tissue sarcomas and exposure to chemical substances: a case-referent study. *Br J Ind Med* 1981;38:27–33.
54. Hardell L, Eriksson M, Lennert P. A case-control study: malignant lymphoma and exposure to chemical substances, particularly organic solvents, chlorophenols and phenoxy acids (translation from Swedish). *Lakartidningen* 1980;77(4):208–210.
55. Pearce NE, Smith AH, Howard JK, et al. Non-Hodgkin's lymphoma and exposure to phenoxyherbicides, chlorophenols, fencing work, and meat works employment: a case-control study. *Br J Ind Med* 1986;43: 75–83.
56. Saracci R, Kogevinas M, Bertazzi P, et al. Cancer mortality in workers exposed to chlorophenoxy herbicides and chlorophenols. *Lancet* 1991;338(8774):1027–1032.

*Environmental and Occupational Medicine,*
*Third Edition,* edited by William N. Rom.
Lippincott–Raven Publishers, Philadelphia © 1998.

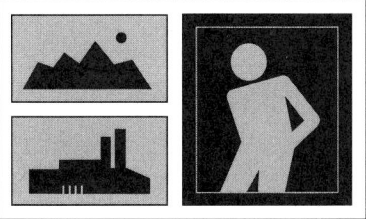

# CHAPTER 87

# Polychlorinated Biphenyls

Debie J. Hoivik and Stephen H. Safe

Polychlorinated biphenyls (PCBs) are halogenated aromatic environmental pollutants. These industrial compounds, produced by the iron-catalyzed chlorination of biphenyl, were manufactured and distributed under the trade names Aroclor, Clophen, Phenoclor, Pyralene, Kanechlor, Santotherm, and Fenclor. It is estimated that 1.5 million metric tons of PCBs were produced worldwide (1) for use in a variety of applications such as organic diluents, plasticizers, hydraulic lubricants, sealants, pesticide extenders, adhesives, heat transfer fluids, dielectric fluids for transformers and capacitors, cutting oils, dust-reducing agents and in carbonless copy paper. PCBs were marketed according to their percentage by weight chlorine content. The last two digits in their numerical designation denotes the percentage of chlorine (e.g., Aroclors 1221, 1232, and 1260 contain 21%, 32%, and 60% chlorine, respectively) (2), with the exception of Aroclor 1016, which is a redistilled version of Aroclor 1242 containing 41% chlorine (3). The chemical properties of PCBs are dependent on the degree of chlorination; the lower chlorinated mixtures are mobile, colorless oils and the higher chlorinated formulations are either immobile viscous liquids (e.g., Aroclor 1262) or an amorphous solid (e.g., Aroclor 1268). Characteristics such as physiochemical properties, chemical stability, dielectric properties, inflammability, and miscibility with other solvents (lipophilicity) make these compounds useful for diverse industrial applications.

The environmental burden of PCBs is due, in part, to direct introduction of these compounds into the environment, and contamination has resulted from either accidental release, careless disposal practices, or leakage from industrial facilities or chemical waste disposal sites. The properties that make these compounds desirable for industrial uses have also contributed to their adverse environmental impacts (stability and lipophilicity). Once released into the environment, PCBs degrade relatively slowly, undergo cycling and transport within the ecosystem and bioaccumulate and biomagnify as they move up the food chain (4–6). Commercial PCBs consist of many isomers and congeners; once in the environment biotransformation can create an even more complex undefined mixture. The environmental and human effects associated with exposure to PCBs may be due to individual components of the mixture or the additive, synergistic, or antagonistic interaction of the constituents.

## PCB ANALYSIS

Detection and analysis of PCBs became more definitive with the development of high-resolution capillary columns (7,8) and the synthesis of all 209 PCB isomers and congeners (9) for use as analytical standards. The complete congener-specific characterization of Aroclors 1016, 1242, 1254, and 1260 and Chlophen A30, A40, A50, and A60 mixtures has been achieved by high-resolution analysis (10), and this approach has been valuable for analyzing PCB extracts from biologic and environmental samples. In the commercial PCBs, 132 different PCBs have been identified, and the congener composition is dependent on the chlorine content of the mixture. The distribution of PCB congeners is also variable, since individual compounds may occur in only one formulation whereas other congeners are present in multiple mixtures. Each PCB varies in its physicochemical properties and

D. J. Hoivik and S. H. Safe: Department of Veterinary Physiology and Pharmacology, Texas A&M University, College Station, Texas 77843-4466.

this influences pharmacokinetic factors such as partitioning, uptake, and retention as well as rates of photolysis and biotransformation. Not surprisingly, the composition of PCB mixtures in biologic or environmental samples differs from the commercial products (11,12). For example, Safe and co-workers (11) compared the PCB composition in Aroclor 1260 and an extract of human. In the milk samples, 55 congeners were identified while 88 congeners were detected in the commercial preparation. Of the 55 congeners identified in the milk samples, approximately 11% were lower chlorinated congeners (e.g., 2,4,4′-trichlorobiphenyl and 2,4,4′,5-tetrachlorobiphenyl) and these compounds are only trace components of Aroclor 1260. In contrast, 2,2′,3,5′,6-pentachlorobiphenyl, 2,2′,3,4′,5′,6-hexachlorobiphenyl, 2,2′,3,4,5,5′,6-heptachlorobiphenyl, 2,2′,3,3′,4,5,6′-heptachlorobiphenyl, and 2,2′,3,3′,4,4′,5,6-octachlorobiphenyl, which compose approximately 23% of Aroclor 1260, are less than 1% of the PCBs in human breast milk samples.

In general, congeners with 2,3,6-trichloro and 2,5-dichloro substitution patterns containing two adjacent unsubstituted carbon atoms are more rapidly metabolized, and this contributes to their low levels in most environmental samples. Some of the congeners were detected at the same relative percent in the commercial mixture and the milk samples. Intersample variability in the relative levels of PCBs in breast milk samples from North America and the United Kingdom has also been observed, demonstrating how regional differences in food consumption and possibly PCB inputs can influence body burdens. For example, 2,2′,5-trichlorobiphenyl, 2,2′,4-trichlorobiphenyl, and 4,4′-dichlorobiphenyl constitute 13.7% of PCBs in milk extracts from the United Kingdom, whereas these congeners were undetected in the North American samples. These regional differences in the relative distribution of PCB congeners in breast milk (13,14) have also been reported for human adipose tissue samples (15,16).

Differences in the levels and distribution of PCBs in fish and wildlife can also be attributed to the magnitude of local and regional inputs, different rates of environmental breakdown, and the existence of short- and long-range transport processes. Analysis of most samples indicate that some compounds such as 2,2′,3,4,4′,5′-hexachlorobiphenyl, 2,2′,4,4′,5,5′-hexachlorobiphenyl, and 2,2′,3,4,4′,5,5′-heptachlorobiphenyl are routinely identified. Studies show that the PCB composition of a commercial mixture does not predict the composition in environmental and biologic samples. Thus, the challenge of risk assessment is to estimate the adverse effects of individual congeners and combinations of congeners in these mixtures, and not to rely solely on the toxicity of the commercial mixtures. Application of the toxic equivalency factor (TEF) approach (17,18) for predicting the hazards and risks associated with PCB exposure has been proposed. Two underlying assumptions for the TEF approach for risk assessment of PCBs and other halogenated aromatic hydrocarbons (HAHs) are that this family of compounds act through a common mechanism of toxicity and that the contributions of individual congeners within the mixture are additive. This relationship may or may not hold true for all congeners, and so the usefulness of the TEF approach for PCBs is currently being evaluated by various regulatory agencies.

## BIOTRANSFORMATION OF PCBs

For many chemicals, metabolism is a requirement for development of toxicity. Initial studies of PCB toxicity focused on the metabolism of these compounds (19–21) and the relative toxicity of the parent compounds and their biotransformation products. PCBs are be metabolized by cytochrome P-450 to phenols (via arene oxide intermediates), which can be conjugated or further hydroxylated to form a catechol. The arene oxide intermediate can be hydrated by epoxide hydrolase to form dihydrodiols, with subsequent dehydrogenation to yield catechols. Additionally arene oxide intermediates can be conjugated with glutathione by glutathione S-transferase and further metabolized to form methylsulfonyl metabolites. Arene oxide intermediates are electrophilic in nature and thus can covalently bind to nucleophilic cellular macromolecules (protein, DNA, RNA) and induce DNA strand breaks and DNA repair (22–24), which can contribute to the toxic response. Arene oxide intermediates are usually formed from lower chlorinated congeners or those compounds that contain two adjacent unsubstituted carbon atoms. Cytochrome P-4502 isozymes preferentially catalyze metabolism of dichlorobiphenyls with di-ortho chlorine substituents, and P-4501 isozymes primarily metabolize dichlorobiphenyls that do not contain ortho substituents (25), and both P-4501 and P-4502 isozymes catalyze metabolism of mono-ortho substituted PCBs (26). The rate and region selectivity of the initial arene oxide are dependent on the chlorine ring substitution pattern, the degree of chlorination, and the distribution and activity of the drug-metabolizing enzymes in the target organ.

Hydroxylated metabolites of PCBs are detected in the urine of laboratory animals and thus the toxicologic potential of these compounds has been evaluated. In vitro studies showed that hydroxylated metabolites of PCB congeners can inhibit or uncouple mitochondrial oxidative phosphorylation (27), compete with estradiol for the estrogen receptor and increase mouse uterine wet weight in vivo (28), inhibit cytochrome P-450 (29), and bind to prealbumin (30) and transthyretin (31), serum proteins that bind and transport thyroxine. It has been hypothesized that modulation of these cellular responses by hydroxylated PCB metabolites could contribute to their toxicity. However, in some instances the hydroxylated metabolites are relatively nontoxic. For example, after administration of 3,3′,4,4′-tetrachlorobiphenyl to rats, the major urinary metabolites formed were 3,3′,4,4′-tetrachloro-5-biphenylol and 3,3′,4′,5-tetrachloro-4-biphenylol, which displayed lower toxicity than the parent compound (32). Similar results have been reported with various other PCBs, suggesting that the toxic responses caused by PCBs are primarily associated with the parent hydrocarbons and not the hydroxylated metabolites (33,34).

Glutathione conjugates of PCBs can be biotransformed to yield methylsulfonyl metabolites, which have been identified in serum and tissue samples of humans and laboratory animals (35–38). These metabolites bind with high affinity to uteroglobin, a progesterone-binding protein (39), to a fatty acid–binding protein in chicken liver and intestinal mucosa (40) and to a lung-binding protein (41). These metabolites have been identified in relatively high concentrations in individuals accidentally exposed to PCBs (38). The binding of methylsulfonyl metabolites to these proteins may contribute to some of the toxic effects exhibited by PCBs. For example, changes in lung capacity and function have been associated with PCB exposure and methylsulfonyl PCB metabolites specifically target lung proteins (42).

## TOXICITY OF PCBs

Commercial PCBs elicit a broad range of toxic responses including acute lethality, hepatomegaly, fatty liver, porphyria, body weight loss, thymic atrophy, immunosuppressive effects, reproductive and developmental toxicity, carcinogenesis and other genotoxic responses, neurotoxicity, modulation of endocrine-derived pathways, and dermal toxicity (43). These various toxic responses are dependent on the animal species or strain used, the age and sex of the animals, the route and duration of exposure to the PCB mixture, the chlorine content and purity of the mixture, and the relative distribution of congeners within the mixture. For example, administration of Aroclor 1232, 1242, 1248, and 1254 to White Leghorn pullets decreased egg production, but Aroclors 1221 or 1268 did not (44). Administration of Clophens A60 and A30 resulted in induction of hepatocarcinogenicity with the former mixture, whereas only minimal effects were observed with the lower chlorinated Clophen A30 (45). Taken together these studies and others demonstrate that higher chlorinated mixtures of PCBs are more carcinogenic than lower chlorinated mixtures (43). This association between chlorine content and toxicity was also observed for PCB-induced immunotoxicity in mice (46).

Dermal toxicity from exposure to PCBs include alopecia, edema, distinctive hair follicles, hair loss, hyperkeratosis, and fingernail loss. The most sensitive species is the nonhuman primate, yet these effects have also been observed in some strains of mice and rabbit ears (47,48). Some PCB-induced responses are also gender-specific. For example, Aroclor 1260 induces hepatocellular adenocarcinomas and trabecular carcinomas in female but not male rats (49). In contrast, Aroclor 1254 induces gastric intestinal metaplasia and adenocarcinomas in both male and female F344 rats (50). These studies demonstrate the species and gender specific responses that occur with different PCB mixtures.

A correlation between developmental deficits such as alterations in active avoidance learning and retention of a visual discrimination task have been reported for prenatal but not postnatal exposure of rats (51) and humans (52, 53) to PCBs. These data suggest the fetus may be more susceptible to PCB-induced effects than infants and older animals.

Chronic administration of commercial PCBs to rodents results in increased incidence of hepatic neoplastic nodules and hepatocellular carcinomas (45,54). In the two-stage hepatocarcinogenesis model, PCBs also exhibit tumor-promoter activity since initiation with a carcinogen such as diethylnitrosamine, 2-acetylaminofluorene, or *N*-nitrosodiethylamine followed by repeated administration of a PCB mixture resulted in increased incidence of hepatocellular carcinoma (55), formation of neoplastic nodules (56), or lung tumors (57), respectively. In addition, PCB mixtures promote formation of enzyme altered foci (58). In the resistant hepatocyte model, Aroclor 1254 and a reconstituted PCB mixture did not initiate tumorigenesis (59) and no PCB-DNA adducts were reported in liver, lung, or kidney of exposed animals, (60) suggesting that PCB mixtures are poor initiators of carcinogenesis.

## STRUCTURE-ACTIVITY RELATIONSHIP OF PCBs

A hallmark of PCB exposure is the induction of hepatic cytochrome P-450–dependent enzyme activities (43). Commercial PCB mixtures were initially classified as mixed-type inducers since exposure to these compounds resulted in induction of both phenobarbital (CYP2A1, CYP2B1, and CYP2B2) and 3-methylcholanthrene (CYP2A1, CYP1A1, and CYP1A2) inducible P-450 isozymes (61,62). PCBs also induce P-450 isoforms, which regulate steroid metabolism (63) and those associated with lauric acid hydroxylase activity (CYP4A1) (64), and inhibit some adrenal steroid hydroxylases (65). In addition, PCB mixtures induce other enzymes associated with drug metabolism including glutathione S-transferase, epoxide hydrolase, glucuronosyl transferase, and aldehyde dehydrogenase activities. Other biochemical responses such as δ-aminolevulinic acid synthetase, hydroxymethylglutaric acid–coenzyme A (HMG-CoA) reductase, fatty acid desaturases, and lung pepsinogen isozymes are modulated after PCB exposure.

The responses elicited by PCBs are diverse and depend on a multitude of factors. Given the complex composition

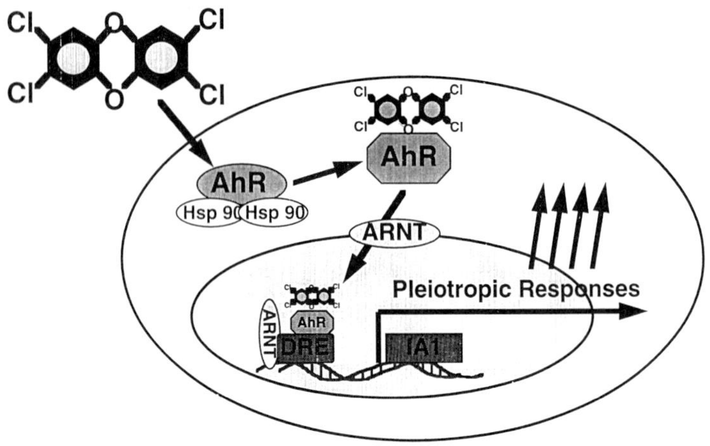


**FIG. 1.** Proposed Ah receptor–mediated mechanism of action for coplanar PCBs and other Ah receptor ligands.

of PCB mixtures, the contribution of individual components is difficult to assess. Therefore, structure-activity relationships between various structural classes of PCBs have been carried out to determine which individual components are responsible for the effects induced by PCB mixtures. The results of these studies have identified some (but not all) structural classes of compounds responsible for toxicities induced by PCB mixtures.

Induction of cytochrome P-450 (CYP1A1,CYP1A2) by 2,3,7,8-tetrachlorodibenzo-*p*-dioxin (TCDD) has been extensively investigated. In the proposed model for CYP1A1 induction, TCDD initially binds to the cytosolic aryl hydrocarbon (Ah) receptor; the resulting complex translocates to the nucleus, dimerizes with the aryl hydrocarbon receptor nuclear translocator (Arnt), and binds to specific genomic sequences (dioxin responsive elements [DRE]) prior to induction of gene transcription (Fig. 1). Coplanar PCBs have been shown to competitively bind to the Ah-receptor and induce CYP1A1 gene expression (66, 67). The compounds that exhibit this activity, such as 3,3′, 4,4′-tetrachlorobiphenyl, 3,3′,4,4′,5-pentachlorobiphenyl, 3,3′,4,4′,5,5′-hexachlorobiphenyl, and 3,4,4′,5-tetrachlorobiphenyl are all substituted in poth para and at least two meta positions (Fig. 2). The removal of any one of these substituents results in a significant loss of CYP1A1 inducible activity. Coplanar PCBs have also been reported to induce epoxide hydrolase (68) glutathione S-transferase (69) and CYP4A1-dependent activities (70). Coplanar PCBs are present in relatively low concentrations in commercial Aroclors, and their overall contribution to the Ah receptor agonist activities of commercial PCB mixtures and PCBs in environmental and human extracts is highly variable (43). Structure-toxicity relationships with TCDD and coplanar PCBs suggest that many of the toxic and carcinogenic responses elicited by PCBs, including the wasting syndrome, hepatotoxicity and porphyria, thymic atrophy, immunotoxicity, reproductive and developmental toxicity, dermal toxicity, endocrine effects, antiestrogenicity, and altered lipid metabolism, may be mediated by the Ah receptor. These responses are observed in diverse species, and the responses segregate with the Ah locus.

Introduction of a single chlorine at an ortho position of the coplanar PCBs did not eliminate CYP1A1 inducibility by these congeners (Fig. 3); however, the mono-ortho coplanar PCBs exhibited mixed-type induction of CYP isozymes (CYP1A1, CYP1A2, CYP2B1, CYP2B2, and CYP2A1). These congeners also competitively bind to the Ah receptor and thus could elicit some of the biochemical and toxic responses mediated by the Ah receptor. 2,3,3′,4,4′-pentachlorobiphenyl (pentaCB), 2,3′,4,4′,5-pentaCB and 2,3,3′,4,4′,5-hexaCB are mono-ortho coplanar PCBs that have been identified in commercial PCB mixtures and environmental extracts, and in some samples the mono-ortho substituted PCBs are major contributors to their TCDD-like activity (reviewed in ref. 43).

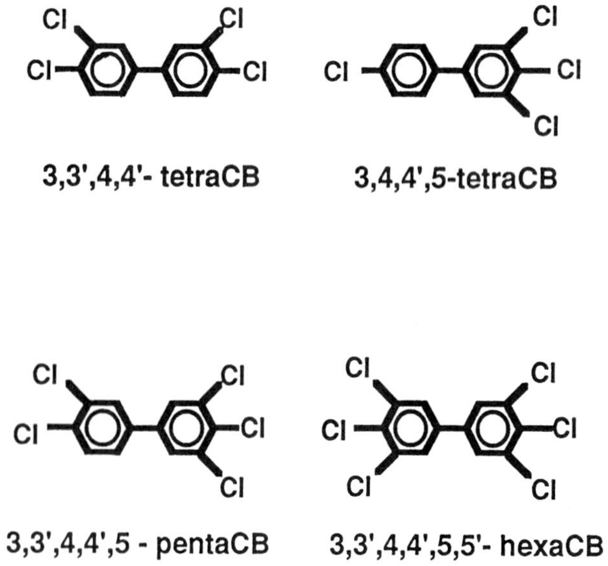


**FIG. 2.** Structures of coplanar PCBs.

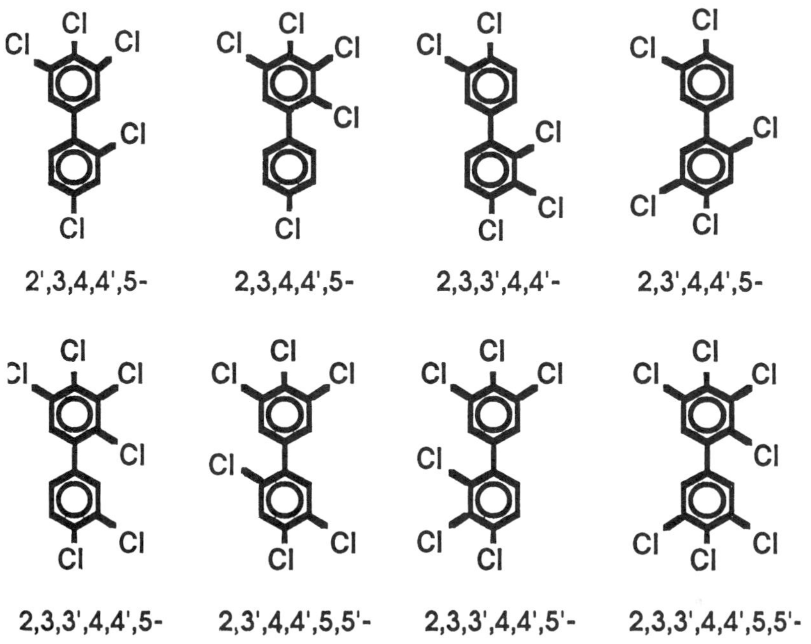


**FIG. 3.** Mono-ortho substituted PCB congeners.

Di-ortho-substituted coplanar PCBs have also been investigated for their activities as inducers of CYP1A1- and CYP1A2-dependent activity and for competitive binding to the Ah receptor. With the exception of 2,2′,4,4′,5,5′-hexachlorobiphenyl, the di-ortho substituted PCBs also exhibit Ah receptor agonist activity (67,71,72). However, these congeners are significantly weaker than the mono-ortho or coplanar PCBs, and it is unlikely that this group of compounds significantly contribute to the TCDD-like activity of most PCB mixtures (73). There is a correlation between the rank order potency for competitive displacement of [$^3$H]TCDD from the Ah receptor and induction of CYP1A1 gene expression with TCDD > coplanar PCBs (3,3′,4,4′,5-pentachlorobiphenyl, 3,3′,4,4′-tetrachlorobiphenyl, and 3,3′,4,4′,5,5-hexachlorobiphenyl) > mono-ortho substituted > diortho substituted PCBs.

2,2′,4,4′,5,5′-Hexachlorobiphenyl, a diortho substituted PCB, does not appear to induce CYP1A1 or CYP1A2 but has been shown to exhibit phenobarbital-type (CYP2A1, CYP2B1, CYP2B2) activity (74) and has been used as a prototype for investigating this type of response. Phenobarbital-like PCBs do not induce most of the responses associated with the Ah receptor, with the exception of hepatomegaly and some hepatotoxic effects (75,76). However, several of the phenobarbital-type compounds act as tumor promoters in short-term bioassays for carcinogenesis. For example, 2,2′,4,4′,5,5′-hexachlorobiphenyl increased the formation of adenosine triphosphatase (ATPase)-deficient foci in rats initiated with diethylnitrosamine (77). These congeners may mediate some of the non-Ah receptor mediated toxicities observed after exposure to PCB mixtures.

## EFFECTS OF PCBs IN HUMANS

Occupational exposure to PCBs has been associated with modulation of some biochemical activities and adverse health effects, including increased 17-hydroxycorticosteroid excretion and γ-glutamyl transpeptidase activity (78); decreased serum bilirubin and increased lymphocyte levels (79); increased skin diseases such as chloracne, folliculitis, and dermatitis; hepatomegaly (80); increased serum cholesterol; and elevated blood pressure (81). These effects vary in incidence and severity among various exposure groups, and in most studies the effects are not statistically significant and their clinical significance is questionable.

Studies of Italian capacitor workers found an increased frequency of malignancies (82) and increased mortality due to cancers of the gastrointestinal tract, hematologic neoplasms, and increased frequency of lung cancer (83). However, no clear-cut conclusion can be drawn since some of the individuals included in the study had very short exposures to PCBs or worked in areas of the plant that were not involved in PCB use or production (83). A retrospective analysis of a study of two plants manufacturing electrical capacitors in the United States also found a significant increase in the incidence of cancer, with the primary target tissues being the liver, gallbladder, and biliary tract (84). Likewise, an increased incidence of melanomas associated with PCB exposure has also been observed for capacitor manufacturing workers (85,86). In contrast, increased mortality or cancer incidence was not observed in male capacitor manufacturing workers in Sweden exposed to PCBs for an average of 6.5 years (87) or in U.S. workers (88). Thus, PCB exposure has been associated with increased incidence of some cancers; however, the variability between studies and the magnitude of these responses do not unequivocally demonstrate a linkage between cancer and occupational exposure to PCBs.

There has been some concern that the increased incidence of breast cancer in women may be due to exposure to environmental compounds such as PCBs. Initial studies comparing breast tissue levels of PCBs in cancer patients and controls indicated that higher levels were observed in the cancer patients (89,90). In contrast, comparison of blood levels of PCBs in breast cancer patients and controls in women from New York City found no significant difference in PCB levels between the patient and control groups (91). Similarly a study of white, black, and Asian women from the San Francisco Bay area found no association between exposure to PCBs and breast cancer regardless of length of follow-up, year of diagnosis, menopausal history, or estrogen-receptor status (92). In addition, meta-analysis of many studies that compared PCB levels in breast cancer patients with background levels of exposure showed there was not a significant relationship between these two variables (93). Furthermore, women occupationally exposed to relatively high levels of PCBs do not have an increased incidence of breast cancer, and therefore it is unlikely that background exposures to these compounds contribute to an increased incidence of this disease (84,94).

Two mass poisonings in Taiwan (1979) and Japan (1968) resulted in exposure of several thousand individuals including pregnant woman to PCBs by contaminated cooking oil (oil disease—"Yucheng" in Chinese and "Yusho" in Japanese). Exposed adults exhibited a broad spectrum of adverse health effects including many severe cases of chloracne. Children born to women that consumed the oil exhibited both cognitive and physical abnormalities. Physical abnormalities such as irritated or swollen gums, deformed or small nails, hyperpigmentation, acne, and conjunctivitis were detected in newborns (95). Intellectual impairment was also evident later in life, (96) and PCB-exposed Taiwanese children were shorter and weighed less than nonexposed children (95).

In these two mass poisonings relatively high levels of polychlorinated dibenzofurans (PCDFs) were also detected in the rice oil, and these compounds may be the prime etiologic agents in the poisoning incidents (97). Jacobson and co-workers (98) studied children of women who consumed Lake Michigan sports fish to determine if *in utero* or lactational exposure to PCBs influenced growth and cognitive function. In infants, higher serum and cord blood PCB levels were associated with decreased performance on Fagan's Visual Recognition Memory Test (98), and abnormalities were detected by the Brazelton Neonatal Behavioral Assessment Scale (99). Increased cord serum PCB concentrations were also associated with slower accommodation to novel stimuli in 7-month-old children (98). At age 4, umbilical cord serum PCB concentration was inversely correlated with the verbal and memory subtests of the McCarthy Memory Scales. This effect was modest but specific in that short-term and not long-term memory was affected (100). However, exposure postnatally via lactation was not related to cognitive performance in 7-month-old children (100). Prenatal PCB exposure was also associated with decreased body weight at age 4 (101).

Subsequent analysis of these same children at age 11 indicated a significant decrease in IQ scores occurred primarily in the highly exposed children. In these more highly exposed children, PCB exposure was associated with poorer verbal comprehension, freedom from distractability, focused attention, and word and reading comprehension. The serum concentration of PCBs at age 11 was unrelated to IQ or achievement measures, suggesting that in utero exposure was responsible for these neurodevelopmental effects (102). North Carolina children born to mothers with background exposure levels of PCBs were also analyzed with respect to the neurodevelopmental capabilities. Their results showed that higher PCB exposure was associated with less muscle tone and activity in infants as determined by the Brazelton Neonatal Behavioral Assessment Scale, but there was no association between PCB exposure and birth weight or head circumference in these infants (52). At 6 and 12 months of age these same North Carolina children displayed a decrease in the Bayley Psychomotor Development Index Scores with increased transplacental PCB exposure. Similarly to the Michigan children, there was no relationship between postnatal PCB exposure and these scores at the 6- or 12-month time point (103). In contrast to the findings observed in the Michigan study, there was no association between transplacental PCB exposure and McCarthy Scales of Children's Abilities at 3, 4, or 5 years of age in the North Carolina children (53).

Several recent studies have also investigated the correlation between in utero or infant exposure to PCBs and other HAHs and adverse effects in the offspring. Alaluusua and co-workers (104) correlated polychlorinated dibenzo-*p*-dioxins (PCDD)/PCDF [toxic equivalent (TEQ)] levels in breast milk with hypomineralization of teeth in children. In a study in the Netherlands it was reported that infants exposed to higher TEQ levels of PCBs/PCDDs/PCDFs in milk had decreased total thyroxine levels and lower plasma free thyroxine levels in the second week after birth (105). Correlations between umbilical cord TEQs versus altered thyroid hormone status were minimal, suggesting that in utero exposure may not contribute to this response. In a subsequent report on this group of infants there was a correlation between higher HAH (TEQ) levels in breast milk and neurodevelopmental defects in children (hypotonia) (106). In contrast, in utero levels of exposure to these compounds did not correlate with any adverse responses. An interim report on developmental neurotoxicity associated with PCB exposure in Dusseldorf, Germany indicated that there was no significant association between cord blood or milk PCB levels and neurologic optimality (107). Thus there appear to be interstudy differences on the duration of these deficits and neurodevelopmental deficits in children and correlations between the timing of exposure (peri- or postnatal) and adverse responses. Since many of the observed responses are within the range of normal and are not clinically significant, it is important that further studies be carried our in several locations to validate or invalidate the role of PCBs and other HAHs as neurodevelopmental toxins.

## RISK ASSESSMENT OF PCBs

Commercial PCBs are complex mixtures that vary in the number and relative concentration of individual congeners, making risk assessment a difficult task. Based on structure-activity relationship and mechanistic studies, it is generally accepted that many toxic responses elicited by PCBs are mediated through the Ah receptor. For Ah receptor–mediated responses, the binding between ligand and receptor is stereoselective and there is a correlation between Ah receptor–binding and –mediated toxicity. For the HAH family of chemicals TCDD is the most toxic compound and binds with the highest affinity for the Ah receptor. Based on these observations, a toxic equivalency factor (TEF) approach has been developed to estimate the toxic potency of PCB mixtures (43,108). Thus individual PCB congeners have been assigned a TEF value, which is the fractional toxicity of the congener relative to TCDD, i.e., median effective dose ($ED_{50}$) TCDD:$ED_{50}$ PCB. The toxic equivalent (TEQ) of PCBs in commercial mixtures and any extracts is defined as: $TEQ = \Sigma([PCB_i \times TEF_i]_n)$, where $PCB_i$ represent the concentration of the individual congeners, $TEF_i$ is their corresponding TEF, and $n$ is the number of congeners. The total TEQ in an environmental extract or in food also includes TEQs for the PCDD and PCDF congeners.

Toxic equivalency factor values are both response and species specific. For example, 3,3′,4,4′,5-pentachlorobiphenyl is the most active PCB congener; however, the TEF value varies depending on the end point and target organ/cell. More specifically, the inhibition of splenic plaque forming cells response to sheep red blood cells and inhibition of trinitrophenyl-lipopolysaccharide–induced antibody response in mice had TEF values for immunotoxicity that varied from 0.08 to 0.77. In contrast, the TEF value for teratogenicity in mice was between 0.07 and 0.04 (109). TEF values for the coplanar and mono-ortho coplanar PCBs were initially derived from their relative potency (using TCDD as the reference compound) as inducers of ethoxyresorufin O-deethylase (EROD) activity in rat hepatoma H4IIE cells (110). Using these values, Tanabe and co-workers (111) showed the toxic equivalency values for PCBs in most extracts from human or environmental samples exceed the TEQs for the PCDDs and PCDFs. Dewailly and co-workers (112) calculated a TEF value of 37.76 ppt for six major coplanar and mono-ortho coplanar PCBs in human milk and a value of 13.22 ppt for the 2,3,7,8-substituted PCDDs and PCDFs. Based on these calculations the TEQs for human milk samples were 74% PCBs.

A comparison of the observed and calculated $ED_{50}$ values for induction of hepatic microsomal AHH and EROD activities by Aroclors 1232, 1242, 1248, 1254, and 1260 in male Wistar rats showed there was less than a twofold difference between these values. These experimental studies confirmed that for the monitored responses there were minimal, nonadditive interactions between the PCBs in these mixtures for the induction response (113). Moreover, the in vivo log $ED_{50}$ values for AHH/EROD induction, thymic atrophy, and inhibition of body weight gain in the rat correlated with the *in vitro* log median effective concentration ($EC_{50}$) value derived from rat hepatoma cells (73), suggesting that these Ah receptor–mediated responses in the rat were essentially additive for the commercial PCB mixtures. In contrast, using a similar approach in mice, it has been shown that there were significant nonadditive (antagonistic) interactions for PCB mixtures and between PCBs and other Ah receptor agonists (114). Since both additive and antagonistic interactions for PCBs have been experimentally observed, the application of the TEF approach for PCBs should be further evaluated. For carcinogenic end points, the tumor-promoting potencies of the major congeners have not been established and thus cancer-based risk assignment of PCB mixtures also requires additional quantitative information. It has also been pointed out that humans exposed to both natural Ah receptor agonists such as indole-3-carbinol (I3C) and polynuclear aromatic hydrocarbons (PAHs) have significantly higher intakes of these compounds compared to PCBs, PCDDs, and PCDFs (115). The potential adverse human impacts of PCBs and related PAHs should be considered in parallel with the relative contributions of I3C, PAHs, and related compounds as both Ah receptor agonists and antagonists.

## ACKNOWLEDGMENTS

The financial assistance of the National Institutes of Health (P42-ESO4917, F32-ESO5734) and the Texas Agriculture Experimental Station is gratefully acknowledged. S. Safe is a Sid Kyle Professor of Toxicology.

## REFERENCES

1. DeVoogt P, Brinkman VAT. Production, properties and usage of polychlorinated biphenyls. In: Kimbrough RD, Jensen AA, eds. *Halogenated biphenyls, terphenyls, naphthalenes, dibenzodioxins and related products.* Amsterdam: Elsevier-North Holland, 1989, 3–45.
2. Hutzinger O, Safe S, Zitko V. *The chemistry of PCBs.* Boca Raton, FL: CRC Press, 1974.

3. Albro PW, Parker CE. Comparison of the composition of Aroclor 1242 and Aroclor 1016. *J Chromatogr* 1979;169:161–166.
4. Hansen L. Environmental toxicology of polychlorinated biphenyls. In: Safe S, Hutzinger O, eds. *Polychlorinated biphenyls (PCBs): mammalian and environmental toxicology, environmental toxin series.* Heidelberg: Springer-Verlag, 1987;15–34.
5. Safe S, Safe L, Mullin M. Polychlorinated biphenyls: environmental occurrence and analysis. In: Safe S, Hutzinger O, eds. *Polychlorinated biphenyls (PCBs): mammalian and environmental toxicology, environmental toxin series.* Heidelberg: Springer-Verlag, 1987;1–13.
6. McFarland VA, Clarke JU. Environmental occurrence, abundance, and potential toxicity of polychlorinated biphenyl congeners: considerations for a congener-specific analysis. *Environ Health Perspect* 1989; 81:225–239.
7. Sissons D, Welti D. Structural identification of polychlorinated biphenyls in commercial mixtures by gas liquid chromatography, nuclear magnetic resonance and mass spectometry. *J Chromatogr* 1971;60:15–21.
8. Albro PW, Corbett JT, Schroeder JL. Quantitative characterization of polychlorinated biphenyl mixtures (Aroclors 1248, 1254, and 1260) by gas chromatography using capillary columns. *J Chromatogr* 1981; 205:103–112.
9. Mullin MD, Pochini CM, McCrindle S, Romkes M, Safe S, Safe L. High-resolution PCB analysis: the synthesis and chromatographic properties of all 209 PCB congeners. *Environ Sci Technol* 1984;18: 468–476.
10. Schulz DE, Petrick G, Duinker JC. Complete characterization of polychlorinated biphenyl congeners in commercial Aroclor and Clophen mixtures by multidimensional gas chromatography-electron capture detection. *Environ Sci Technol* 1989;23:852–859.
11. Safe S, Safe L, Mullin M. Polychlorinated biphenyls (PCBs)-congener-specific analysis of a commercial mixture and a human milk extract. *J Agric Food Chem* 1985;33:24–29.
12. Duarte-Davidson RK, Burnett V, Waterhouse KS, Jones KC. A congener specific method for the analysis of polychlorinated biphenyls (PCBs) in human milk. *Chemosphere* 1991;23:119–131.
13. Dewailly E, Dodin S, Verreault R, et al. High organochlorine body burden in women with estrogen receptor-positive breast cancer. *J Natl Cancer Inst* 1994;86:232–234.
14. Hong CS, Bush B, Xiao J. Isolation and determination of mono-ortho and non-ortho substituted PCBs (coplanar PCBs) in human milk by HPLC porous graphite carbon and GC/ECD. *Chemosphere* 1992;24: 465–472.
15. Kannan N, Tanabe S, Ono M, Tatsukawa R. Critical evaluation of polychlorinated biphenyl toxicity in terrestrial and marine mammals: increasing impact of non-ortho and mono-ortho coplanar polychlorinated biphenyls from land to ocean. *Arch Environ Contam Toxicol* 1989;18:850–870.
16. Williams DT, LeBel GL. Coplanar polychlorinated biphenyl residues in human adipose tissue samples from Ontario municipalities. *Chemosphere* 1991;22:1019–2024.
17. United States Environmental Protection Agency. *Workshop report on toxicity equivalency factors for polychlorinated biphenyl congeners.* Risk assessment forum, EPA/625/3-91/020. Washington, DC: EPA, 1991.
18. Ahlborg UG, Brouwer A, Fingerhut MA, et al. Impact of polychlorinated dibenzo-p-dioxins, dibenzofurans, and biphenyls on human and environmental health with special emphasis on application of the toxic equivalency factor concept. *Eur J Pharmacol* 1992;228:179–199.
19. Sundstrom G, Hutzinger O, Safe S. The metabolism of chlorinated biphenyls—a review. *Chemosphere* 1976;5:267–298.
20. Sipes IG, Schnellmann RG. Biotransformation of PCBs: metabolic pathways and mechanisms. In: Safe S, Hutzinger O, eds. *Polychlorinated biphenyl (PCBs). Mammalian and environmental toxicology.* Environmental toxin series, vol 1. Heidelberg: Springer-Verlag, 1987; 97–110.
21. Safe S. Polyhalogenated aromatics: uptake, disposition, and metabolism. In: Kimbrough RD, Jensen AA, eds. *Halogenated biphenyls, naphthalenes, dibenzodioxins and related products,* 2nd ed. Amsterdam: Elsevier-North Holland, 1989;51–69.
22. Shimada T, Sato R. Covalent binding *in vitro* of polychlorinated biphenyls to microsomal macromolecules: involvement of metabolic activation by a cytochrome P-450 linked monooxygenase system. *Biochem Pharmacol* 1978;27:585–594.
23. Stadnicki SS, Allen JR. Toxicity of 2,2′,5,5′-tetrachlorobiphenyl and its metabolites, 2,2′,5,5′-tetrachlorobiphenyl-3,4-oxide and 2,2′,5,5′-tetrachlorobiphenyl-4-ol to cultured cells *in vitro*. *Bull Environ Contam Toxicol* 1979;23:788–796.
24. Wong A, Basrur PK, Safe S. The metabolically mediated DNA damage and subsequent repair by 4-chlorobiphenyl in Chinese hamster ovary cells. *Res Commun Chem Pathol Pharmacol* 1979;24:543–550.
25. Kaminsky LS, Kennedy MW, Adams SM, Guengerich FP. Metabolism of dichlorobiphenyls by highly purified isozymes of rat liver cytochrome P-450. *Biochemistry* 1991;20:7379–7384.
26. Preston BD, Miller JA, Miller EC. Non-arene oxide aromatic ring hydroxylation of 2,2′,5,5′-tetrachlorobiphenyl as the major metabolic pathway catalyzed by phenobarbital-induced rat liver microsomes. *J Biol Chem* 1983;258:8304–8311.
27. Ebner KV, Braselton WE. Structural and chemical requirements of hydroxylated polychlorinated biphenyl (PCBOH) for inhibition of energy dependent swelling of rat liver mitochondria. *Chem Biol Interact* 1987;63:139–155.
28. Korach KS, Sarver P, Chae K, Mclachlan JA, McKinney JD. Estrogen receptor-binding activity of polychlorinated hydroxybiphenyls: conformationally restricted structural probes. *Mol Pharmacol* 1988;33: 120–126.
29. Schmoldt A, Herzberg W, Benthe HF. On the inhibition of microsomal drug metabolism by polychlorinated biphenyl (PCBs) and related phenolic compounds. *Chem Biol Interact* 1977;16:191–200.
30. Rickenbacher U, McKinney JD, Oatley SJ, Blake CCF. Structurally specific binding of halogenated biphenyls to thyroxine transport protein. *J Med Chem* 1986;29:641–648.
31. Brouwer A, Van den Berg KJ. Binding of a metabolite of 3,4,3′,4′-tetrachlorobiphenyl to transthyretin reduces serum vitamin A transport by inhibiting the formation of the protein complex carrying both retinol and thyroxine. *Toxicol Appl Pharmacol* 1986;85:301–312.
32. Klasson-Wehler E, Brunstrom B, Rannug U, Bergman A. 3,3′,4,4′-tetrachlorobiphenyl: metabolism by the chick embryo in ovo and toxicity of hydroxylated metabolites. *Chem Biol Interact* 1990;73: 121–132.
33. Stadnicki S, Lin FSD, Allen JR. DNA single strand breaks caused by 2,2′,5,5′-tetrachlorobiphenyl and its metabolites. *Res Commun Chem Pathol Pharmacol* 1979;24:313–327.
34. Koga N, Beppu M, Yoshimura H. Metabolism in vivo of 3,4,5,3′,4′,-pentachlorobiphenyl and toxicological assessment of the metabolite in rats. *J Pharmacobiodyn* 1990;13:497–506.
35. Jensen S, Jansson B. Anthropogenic substances in seal from the Baltic: methylsulphone metabolites of PCB and DDE. *Ambio* 1976;5: 257–263.
36. Bergman A, Brandt I, Darnerud PO, Wachtmeister CA. Metabolism of 2,2′,5,5′-tetrachlorobiphenyl: formation of mono-and bis-methyl sulphone metabolites with a selective affinity for the lung and kidney tissues in mice. *Xenobiotica* 1982;12:1–7.
37. Bakke JE, Feil VJ, Bergman A. Metabolites of 2,4′,5-trichlorobiphenyl in rats. *Xenobiotica* 1983;13:555–564.
38. Haraguchi HM, Kuroki K, Masuda Y, Shigematsu N. Determination of methylio and methylsulphone polychlorinated biphenyls in tissues of patients with Yusho. *Food Chem Toxicol* 1984;22:283–288.
39. Gillner M, Lund J, Cambillau C, et al. The binding of methylsulfonyl-polychloro-biphenyls to uteroglobin. *J Steroid Biochem* 1988;31: 270–280.
40. Larsen GL, Huwe JK, Bergman A, Klasson-Wehler E, Hargis P. Methylsulfonyl metabolites of xenobiotics can serve as ligands for fatty acid binding protein in chicken liver and intestinal mucosa. *Chemosphere* 1992;25:1189–1194.
41. Lund J, Andersson O, Ripe E. Characterization of a binding protein for the PCB metabolite 4,4′-bis-(methylsulfonyl)-2,2′,5,5′-tetrachlorobiphenyl present in bronchoalveolar lavage from healthy smokers and nonsmokers. *Toxicol Appl Pharmacol* 1986;83:486–493.
42. Warshaw R, Fischbein A, Thornton J, Miller A, Selikoff IJ. Decrease in vital capacity in PCB-exposed workers in a capacitator manufacturing facility. *Ann NY Acad Sci* 1979;320:277–283.
43. Safe SH. Polychlorinated biphenyls (PCBs): environmental impact, biochemical and toxic responses, and implications for risk assessment. *Crit Rev Toxicol* 1994;24:87–149.
44. Lillie RJ, Cecil HC, Bitman J, Fries GF. Differences in response of caged white leghorn layers to various polychlorinated biphenyls (PCBs) in the diet. *Poult Sci* 1974;53:726–732.

45. Schaeffer E, Greim H, Goessner W. Pathology of chronic polychlorinated biphenyl (PCB) feeding in rats. *Toxicol Appl Pharmacol* 1984; 75:278–288.
46. Davis D, Safe S. Dose-response immunotoxicities of commercial polychlorinated biphenyls (PCBs) and their interaction with 2,3,7,8-tetrachlorodibenzo-p-dioxin. *Toxicol Lett* 1989;48:35–43.
47. Allen JR. Response of the nonhuman primate to polychlorinated biphenyl exposure. *Fed Proc* 1975;34:1675–1679.
48. Poland A, Greenlee WF, Kende AS. Studies on the mechanism of action of the chlorinated dibenzo-p-dioxins and related compounds. *Ann NY Acad Sci* 1979;320:214–230.
49. Norback DH, Weltman RH. Polychlorinated biphenyl induction of hepatocellular carcinoma in the Sprague-Dawley rat. *Environ Health Perspect* 1985;60:97–105.
50. Ward JM, Tsuda H, Tatematsu M, Hagiwara A, Ito N. Hepatotoxicity of agents that enhance formation of focal hepatocellular proliferative lesions (putative preneoplastic foci) in a rapid rat liver bioassay. *Fundam Appl Toxicol* 1989;12:163–171.
51. Lilienthal H, Neuf M, Munoz C, Winneke G. Behavioral effects of pre- and postnatal exposure to a mixture of low chlorinated PCBs in rats. *Fundam Appl Toxicol* 1990;15:457–467.
52. Rogan WJ, Gladen BC, McKinney JD, et al. Neonatal effects of transplacental exposure to PCBs and DDE. *J Pediatr* 1986;109: 335–341.
53. Gladen BC, Rogan WJ. Effects of perinatal polychlorinated biphenyls and dichlorodiphenyl dichloroethene on later development. *J Pediatr* 1991;119:58–63.
54. Kimbrough RD, Squire RA, Linder RE, Strandberg JL, Montali RJ, Burse VW. Induction of liver tumors in Sherman strain female rats by PCB Aroclor 1260. *J Natl Cancer Inst* 1975;55:1453–1459.
55. Preston BD, Van Miller JP, Moore RW, Allen JR. Promoting effects of polychlorinated biphenyls (Aroclor 1254) and polychlorinated dibenzofuran-free Aroclor 1254 on diethylnitrosamine-induced tumorigenesis in the rat. *J Natl Cancer Inst* 1981;66:509–515.
56. Tatematsu K, Nakanishi K, Murasaki G, Miyata Y, Hirose M, Ito N. Enhancing effect of inducers of liver microsomal enzymes on induction of hyperplastic liver nodules by N-2-fluorenylacetamide in rats. *J Natl Cancer Inst* 1979;63:1411–1416.
57. Anderson LM, Beebe LE, Fox SD, Issaq HJ, Kovatch RM. Promotion of mouse lung tumors by bioaccumulated polychlorinated aromatic hydrocarbons. *Exp Lung Res* 1991;17:455–471.
58. Jensen RK, Sleight SD, Aust SD, Goodman JI, Troske JE. Hepatic tumor-promoting ability of 3,3′,4,4′,5,5′-hexabromobiphenyl: the interrelationship between toxicity, induction of hepatic microsomal drug metabolizing enzymes, and tumor-promoting ability. *Toxicol Appl Pharmacol* 1983;71:163–176.
59. Hayes MA, Safe SH, Armstrong D, Cameron RG. Influence of cell proliferation on initiating activity of pure polychlorinated biphenyls and complex mixtures in resistant hepatocyte in vivo assays for carcinogenicity. *J Natl Cancer Inst* 1985;71:1037–1041.
60. Nath RG, Randerath E, Randerath K. Short-term effects of the tumor promoting polychlorinated biphenyl mixture, Aroclor 1254, on I-compounds in liver, kidney and lung DNA of male Sprague-Dawley rats. *Toxicology* 1991;68:275–289.
61. Botelho LH, Ryan DE, Levin W. Amino acid compositions and partial amino acid sequences of three highly purified forms of liver microsomal cytochrome P-450 from rats treated with polychlorinated biphenyls, phenobarbital, or 3-methylcholanthrene. *J Biol Chem* 1979;245:5635–5640.
62. Ryan DE, Thomas PE, Reik LM, Levin W. Purification characterization and regulation of five rat hepatic cytochrome P-450 isozymes. *Xenobiotica* 1982;12:727–744.
63. Goldman D, Yawetz A. Cytochrome P-450 mediated metabolism of progesterone by adrenal microsomes of PCB-treated and untreated barn owl *(Tytoalba)* and marsh turtle *(Mauremys caspica)* in comparison with the guinea-pig. *Comp Biochem Physiol* 1991;99:251–255.
64. Borlakoglu JT, Edwards-Webb JD, Dils RR, Wilkins JPG, Robertson LW. Evidence for the induction of cytochrome P452 in rat liver by Aroclor 1254, a commercial mixture of polychlorinated biphenyls. *FEBS Lett* 1989;247:327–329.
65. Goldman D, Yawetz A. The interference of Aroclor 1254 with progesterone metabolism in guinea pig adrenal and testes microsomes. *J Biochem Toxicol* 1990;5:99–107.
66. Bandiera S, Safe S, Okey AB. Binding of polychlorinated biphenyls classified as either phenobarbitone-, 3-methylcholanthrene-, of mixed-type inducers of cytosolic Ah receptor. *Chem Biol Interact* 1982;39:259–277.
67. Parkinson A, Safe S, Robertson L, Thomas PE, Ryan DE, Levin W. Immunochemical quantitation of cytochrome P-450 isozymes and epoxide hydrolase in liver microsomes from polychlorinated and polybrominated biphenyls: a study of structure activity relationships. *J Biol Chem* 1983;258:5967–5976.
68. Ahotupa M. Enhancement of epoxide-metabolizing enzyme activities by pure PCB isomers. *Biochem Pharmacol* 1981;30:1866–1869.
69. Aoki Y, Satoh K, Sato K, Suzuki KT. Induction of glutathione S-transferase P-form in primary cultured rat liver parenchymal cells by coplanar polychlorinated biphenyl congeners. *Biochem J* 1992;281: 539–543.
70. Borlakoglu JT, Clarke S, Huang SW, Kils RR, Haegle KD, Gibson GG. Lactational transfer of 3,3′,4,4′,-tetrachloro-and 2,2′,4,4′,5,5′-hexachlorobiphenyl induces cytochrome P-450IVA1 in neonates: evidence for a potential synergistic mechanism. *Biochem Pharmacol* 1992;43:153–157.
71. Stonard MD, Grieg JB. Different patterns of hepatic microsomal enzyme activity produced by administration of pure hexachlorobiphenyl isomers and hexachlorobenzene. *Chem Biol Interact* 1976; 15:365–379.
72. Parkinson A, Robertson L, Safe L, Safe S. Polychlorinated biphenyls as inducers of hepatic microsomal enzymes: structure-activity rules. *Chem Biol Interact* 1981;35:1–12.
73. Safe S. Polychlorinated biphenyls (PCBs), dibenzo-p-dioxins (PCDDs), dibenzofurans (PCDFs) and related compounds: environmental and mechanistic considerations which support the development of toxic equivalency factors (TEFs). *Crit Rev Toxicol* 1990;21: 51–88.
74. Graves PE, Elhag GA, Ciaccio PJ, Bourque DP, Halpert JR. cDNA and deduced amino acid sequences of a dog hepatic cytochrome P-450IIB responsible for the metabolism of 2,2′,4,4′,5,5′-hexachlorobiphenyl. *Arch Biochem Biophys* 1990;281:106–115.
75. Kohli KK, Gupta BN, Albro PW, Mukhtar H, McKinney JD. Biochemical effects of pure isomers of hexachlorobiphenyl: fatty livers and cell structure. *Chem Biol Interact* 1979;25:139–156.
76. Biocca M, Gupta BN, Chae K, McKinney JD, Moore JA. Toxicity of selected symmetrical hexachlorobiphenyl isomers in the mouse. *Toxicol Appl Pharmacol* 1981;58:461–474.
77. Buchmann A, Kunz W, Wolf CR, Oesch F, Robertson LW. Polychlorinated biphenyls, classified as either phenobarbital- or 3-methylcholanthrene-type inducers of cytochrome P-450, are both hepatic tumor promoters in diethylnitrosamine-initiated rats. *Cancer Lett* 1986;32:243–253.
78. Emmett EA. Polychlorinated biphenyl exposure and effects in transformer repair workers. *Environ Health Perspect* 1985;60:185–192.
79. Lawton RW, Ross MR, Feingold J, Brown JF. Effects of PCB exposure on biochemical and hematological findings in capacitor workers. *Environ Health Perspect* 1985;60:165–184.
80. Maroni M, Colombi A, Arbosti G, Cantoni S, Fao V. Occupational exposure to polychlorinated biphenyls in electrical workers. II. Health effects. *Br J Ind Med* 1981;38:55–60.
81. Kreiss K, Zack MM, Kimbrough RD, Needham LL, Smrek AL, Jones BT. Association of blood pressure and polychlorinated biphenyl levels. *JAMA* 1981;245:2505–2509.
82. Bertazzi PA, Zocchetti C, Guercilena S, Della Foglia M, Pesatori A, Ribold L. Mortality study in male and female workers exposed to PCBs. In: *Prevention of occupational cancer. International symposium.* Occupational Safety and Health Series. Geneva: ILO, 1982;46:242–262.
83. Bertazzi PA, Riboldi L, Pesatorui A, Radice L, Zocchetti C. Cancer mortality of capacitor manufacturing workers. *Am J Ind Med* 1987;11: 165–176.
84. Brown DP. Mortality in workers exposed to polychlorinated biphenyls —an update. *Arch Environ Health* 1987;42:333–339.
85. Bahn AK, Rosenwaike I, Hermann N, Grover P, Stellman J, O'Leary A. Melanoma after exposure to PCBs. *N Engl J Med* 1976;295:450.
86. Sinks T, Steele G, Smith AB, Watkins K, Shults RA. Mortality among workers exposed to polychlorinated biphenyls. *Am J Epidemiol* 1992; 136:389–398.
87. Gustavsson P, Hogstedt C, Rappe C. Short-term mortality and cancer incidence in capacitor manufacturing workers exposed to polychlorinated biphenyls (PCBs). *Am J Ind Med* 1986;10:341–344.

88. Brown DP, Jones M. Mortality and industrial hygiene study of workers exposed to polychlorinated biphenyls. *Arch Environ Health* 1981;36:120–129.
89. Falck F, Ricci A, Wolff MS, Godbold J, Deckers P. Pesticides and polychlorinated biphenyl residues in human breast lipids and their relation to breast cancer. *Arch Environ Health* 1992;47:143–146.
90. Davis DL, Bradlow HL, Wolff M, Woodruf T, Hoel DG, Anton-Culver H. Medical hypothesis: xenoestrogens as preventable causes of breast cancer. *Environ Health Perspect* 1993;101:372–377.
91. Wolff MS, Toniolo PG, Lee EW, Rivera M, Dubin N. Blood levels of organochlorine residues and risk of breast cancer. *J Natl Cancer Inst* 1993;85:648–652.
92. Krieger N, Wolff MS, Hiatt RA, Rivera M, Vogelman J, Orentreich N. Breast cancer and serum organochlorines: a prospective study among white, black, and Asian women. *J Natl Cancer Inst* 1994;86: 589–599.
93. Key T, Reeves G. Organochlorines in the environment and breast cancer. *Br Med J* 1994;308:1520–1521.
94. Safe SH. Environmental and dietary estrogens and human health: is there a problem? *Environ Health Perspect* 1995;103:346–351.
95. Rogan WJ, Gladen BC, Hung KL, et al. Congenital poisoning by polychlorinated biphenyls and their contaminants in Taiwan. *Science* 1988; 241:334–336.
96. Yu ML, Hsu CC, Gladen BC, Rogan WJ. In utero PCB/PCDF exposure: relation of developmental delay to dysmorphology and dose. *Neurotoxicol Teratol* 1991;13:195–202.
97. Kashimoto T, Miyata H, Kunita S, et al. Role of polychlorinated dibenzofuran in Yusho (PCB poisoning). *Arch Environ Health* 1981; 32:321–326.
98. Jacobson SW, Fein GG, Jacobson JL, Schwartz PM, Dowler JK. The effect of PCB exposure on visual recognition memory. *Child Dev* 1985;56:853–860.
99. Jacobson JL, Jacobson SW, Fein GG. Prenatal exposure to an environmental toxin: a test of the multiple effects model. *Dev Psychol* 1984;20:523–532.
100. Jacobson JL, Jacobson SW, Humphrey HEB. Effects of in utero exposure to polychlorinated biphenyls and related contaminants on cognitive functioning in young children. *J Pediatr* 1990;116:38–45.
101. Jacobson JL, Jacobson SW, Humphrey HEB. Effects of exposure to PCBs and related compounds on growth and activity in children. *Neurotoxicol Teratol* 1990;12:319–326.
102. Jacobson JL, Jacobson SW. Intellectual impairment in children exposed to polychlorinated biphenyls in utero. *N Engl J Med* 1996; 335:783–789.
103. Gladen BC, Rogan WJ, Hardy P, Thullen J, Tingelstad J, Tully M. Development after exposure to polychlorinated biphenyls and dichlorodiphenyl dichloroethene transplacentally and through human milk. *J Pediatr* 1988;113:991–995.
104. Alaluusua S, Lukinmaa PL, Vartiainen T, Partanen M, Torppa J, Tuomisto J. Polychlorinated dibenzo-p-dioxins and dibenzofurans via mother's milk may cause developmental defects in the child's teeth. *Environ Toxicol Pharmacol* 1996;1:193–197.
105. Koopman-Esseboom C, Morse DC, Weisglas-Kuperus N, et al. Effects of dioxins and polychlorinated biphenyls on thyroid hormone status of pregnant women and their infants. *Pediatr Res* 1994;36:468–473.
106. Huisman M, Koopman-Esseboom C, Fidler V, et al. Perinatal exposure to polychlorinated biphenyls and dioxins and its effect on neonatal neurological development. *Early Hum Dev* 1995;41:111–127.
107. Winneke G, Bucholski A, Kramer U, et al. The development neurotoxicity of PCBs: an interim report of ongoing neuroepidemiological and experimental studies. *Organohalogen Compounds* 1996;30:194–199.
108. Ahlborg UG, Becking GC, Birnbaum LS, et al. Toxic equivalency factors for dioxin-like PCBs. *Chemosphere* 1994;28:1049–1067.
109. Mayura K, Spainhour CB, Howie L, Safe S, Phillips TD. Teratogenicity and immunotoxicity of 3,3′,4,4′,5-pentachlorobiphenyl in C57BL/6 mice. *Toxicology* 1993;77:123–131.
110. Sawyer T, Safe S. PCB isomers and congeners: induction of aryl hydrocarbon hydroxylase and ethoxyreorufin O-deethylase enzyme activities in rat hepatoma cells. *Toxicol Lett* 1982;13:87–93.
111. Tanabe S, Kannan N, Wakimoto T, Tatsukawa R, Okamoto T, Masuda Y. Isomer-specific determination and toxic evaluation of potentially hazardous coplanar PCBs, dibenzofurans and dioxins in the tissues of Yusho PCB poisoning victim and in the causal oil. *Toxicol Environ Chem* 1989;24:215–231.
112. Dewailly E, Weber JP, Gingras S, Laliberte C. Coplanar PCBs in human milk in the providence of Quebec, Canada: Are they more toxic than dioxin for breast fed infants? *Bull Environ Contam Toxicol* 1991;47:491–498.
113. Harris M, Zacharewski T, Safe S. Comparative potencies of Aroclors 1232, 1242, 1248, 1254 and 1260 in male Wistar rats—risk assessment of the toxic equivalency factor (TEF) approach for polychlorinated biphenyls (PCBs). *Fundam Appl Toxicol* 1993;20:456–463.
114. Davis D, Safe S. Immunosuppressive activities of polychlorinated biphenyls in C57BL/6 mice: structure-activity relationships as Ah receptor agonists and partial antagonists. *Toxicology* 1990;63:97–111.
115. Safe S. Limitations of the toxic equivalency factor approach for risk assessment of TCDD and related compounds. *Teratogenesis Carcinog Mutagen* 1998;in press.

*Environmental and Occupational Medicine, Third Edition,* edited by William N. Rom.
Lippincott–Raven Publishers, Philadelphia © 1998.

# CHAPTER 88

# Trimellitic Anhydride

Leslie C. Grammer and Roy Patterson

The acid anhydrides are a group of reactive, low molecular weight organic chemicals that have been used for a half century as curing agents for various resins (1). In the past 15 years, the agent that has been most studied, in terms of its potential to cause immune sensitization, is trimellitic anhydride (TMA).

The acid anhydrides are named for the parent acids from which they are derived. In addition to TMA, other anhydrides used in manufacturing include hexahydrophthalic anhydride (HHPA), maleic anhydride (MA), phthalic anhydride (PA), pyromellitic dianhydride (PMDA), and tetrachlorophthalic anhydride (TCPA). All have been reported to cause occupational immune lung disease (OILD). Their structures are shown in Fig. 1.

The most common adverse health effects of the acid anhydrides are noncardiac pulmonary edema, immune sensitization, and irritation of mucous membranes and skin (2). Reports of the irritant effects and pulmonary edema have been extensive; some of the reports of pulmonary edema, pulmonary hemorrhage, and chemical pneumonitis may actually represent immune sensitization that was not evaluated (3–5). Immune sensitization, which has been studied only in the last 15 years, is probably the most important problem clinically (5). The first cases were probably reported in the 1940s, but there was no accompanying immunologic investigation (6).

L. C. Grammer: Department of Medicine, Northwestern University School of Medicine, Chicago, Illinois 60611.

R. Patterson: Department of Medicine; and Division of Allergy–Immunology, Northwestern University School of Medicine, Chicago, Illinois 60611.

## CHEMICAL USES AND REACTIVITY

The acid anhydrides, like TMA, are used principally as curing agents for alkyl and epoxy resins. Epoxy resins are essentially epichlorhydrin and bisphenol A that are cured with an acid anhydride or a reactive amine. Acid anhydrides are also used in polymers and polyesters, vinyl chloride plasticizers, surface coatings including paints, and pigments (1,5). As of the early 1990s the National Institute of Occupational Safety and Health (NIOSH) estimated that approximately 20,000 workers were exposed to TMA (5).

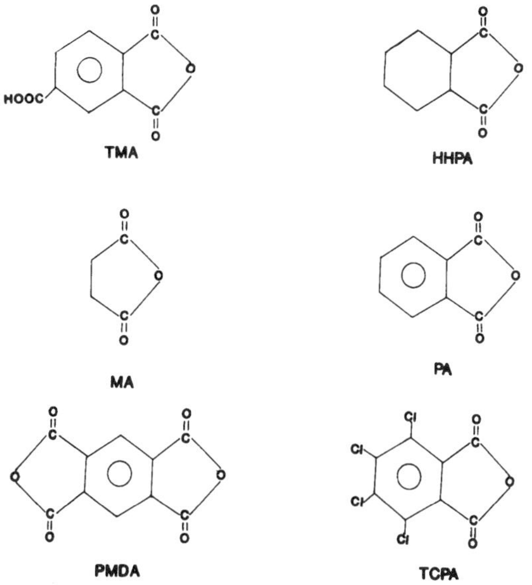


**FIG. 1.** Anhydrides that have been reported to cause occupational immune lung disease (OILD).

The current threshold limit value time-weighted average (TLV-TWA) of 0.005 ppm (0.04 $mg/m^3$) is based on studies in which rats developed intraalveolar hemorrhages at exposure levels as low as 0.01 ppm (7), approximately the vapor pressure of TMA at 25°C. Overall, the toxicity of TMA is relatively low; the median lethal dose ($LD_{50}$) for rats is 5.6 g/kg (5). Immune sensitization, the major clinical problem, occurs at much lower doses.

## CLINICAL IMMUNOLOGIC SYNDROMES

In addition to cross-linking with epichlorhydrin and bisphenol A, anhydrides can react with other chemical moieties. In particular, it is known that anhydrides react with the amino acid lysine, so proteins containing lysine may be haptenized by acid anhydrides like TMA (8). When mucosal surfaces are exposed to TMA (as by inhalation) the TMA reacts with autologous proteins in the mucus to form trimellityl (TM)-protein complexes. These TM-protein complexes are antigenic, and some workers produce antibodies against them. After reexposure to TMA and formation of TM complexes, an immune hypersensitivity reaction occurs at the site of exposure. The nature of the hypersensitivity reaction depends on the type of antibody and degree of exposure, as discussed below. Three different immune-mediated syndromes have been described in workers exposed to TMA (9). Table 1 lists their symptoms, onset, latency, and immunologic test results. Asthma-rhinitis is a syndrome of immediate-onset asthma and allergic rhinitis that is mediated by immunoglobulin E (IgE) antibody against TM-protein. Late respiratory systemic syndrome (LRSS) is a hypersensitivity pneumonitis-like syndrome followed by a flulike syndrome 4 to 12 hours after exposure. Pulmonary disease anemia (PDA) syndrome is characterized by dyspnea, hemoptysis, pulmonary infiltrates, restrictive lung function, and hemolytic anemia. It generally develops only in workers exposed to high levels of TMA fumes, such as those released when resins containing TMA are applied to hot metal. After initial description of the PDA syndrome as an immune hypersensitivity reaction, the syndrome has practically disappeared thanks to environmental control of TMA levels.

Other anhydrides have been reported to cause several immunologic syndromes. For instance, HHPA has been described to cause hemorrhagic rhinitis, which is characterized by rhinitis, nasal mucosal erosions, significant epistaxis, and high-titer IgG and IgE against HHP-HSA (10). Methylhexahydrophthalic and methyltetrahydrophthalic anhydrides (MTHPA) have been associated with contact urticaria (11). A syndrome very similar to PDA has been reported to have been induced by PMDA (12).

The most common syndromes are asthma-rhinitis and LRSS; the most lethal is PDA (13–15). The following case studies illustrate the essential features of each syndrome.

## CASE STUDY 1. ASTHMA-RHINITIS

A 50-year-old man worked in an area where TMA is flaked and bagged. After working approximately 10 months in this area he developed pruritus of the eyes and nose, lacrimation, nasal congestion, wheeze, and cough almost immediately upon entering the bagging area. This necessitated his being relocated to another area. Results of skin tests and tests *in vitro* for IgE against TM-HSA were both positive. Even now, when the wind blows TMA from the bagging area to his new work area he develops some symptoms.

## CASE STUDY 2. LATE RESPIRATORY SYSTEMIC SYNDROME

A 35-year-old woman worked in an area of a plant where epoxy resin coatings containing TMA were heated. After working approximately 6 months she noticed that she would develop cough, fever, fatigue, malaise, arthralgia,

**TABLE 1.** *Immunologic syndromes due to TMA inhalation*

| | Asthma-rhinitis | LRSS | PDA |
|---|---|---|---|
| Symptoms | Cough, dyspnea, wheeze, nasal congestion, nasal pruritus | Fever, chills, myalgia, dyspnea | Fever, dyspnea, hemoptysis, anemia |
| Onset | Immediate (minutes) | 4–12 hr | Within hours |
| Latency[a] | Weeks to months | Weeks to months | Weeks to months |
| Degree of exposure that elicits symptoms once sensitization has occurred | Minimal | Moderate | High |
| Skin test results | Positive | Negative | Negative |
| IgE-a-TM-HSA | Detectable | Absent | Absent |
| Total antibody levels against TM-HSA | Detectable | High | Very high |

[a]Work exposure period during which an immune response to TMA haptenized proteins occurs.

and dyspnea at night. By morning she felt better, took aspirin, and went to work. During a 2-week vacation she had no symptoms.

Total titer of antibody against TM-HSA was high. When she returned to work the symptoms returned, necessitating her removal from TMA exposure. She no longer has symptoms.

## CASE STUDY 3. PULMONARY DISEASE ANEMIA

A 19-year-old man worked at a plant that coated hot pipes with a material containing TMA. After 6 weeks he developed cough, dyspnea, fever, malaise, anorexia, nausea, vomiting, and hemoptysis. He had bilateral pulmonary infiltrates and hemolytic anemia. Lung biopsy showed extensive intraalveolar hemorrhage, granular pneumocyte hyperplasia, and interstitial edema. The total antibody titer against TM-HSA was very high. The patient received corticosteroids and transfusions in the hospital. Three weeks later all symptoms resolved; he has had no further exposure and no symptoms.

The immunopathogenesis of the asthma-rhinitis syndrome is the same as that of any other immediate, type I IgE-mediated process (16). TMA is inhaled and reacts with autologous proteins. The autologous protein–TM conjugate elicits a specific IgE response. This has been reported to occur with sensitization to other anhydrides such as HHPA (17) and MTHPA (18).

The IgE directed against TM protein on the surface of mast cells or basophils can be cross-linked by TM protein, causing mediator release and resultant immediate symptoms of allergic rhinitis or asthma. Workers may have both the rhinitis-asthma and the LRSS syndrome.

The immunopathogenesis of LRSS and PDA are not as clear (16,19). LRSS probably involves type III (antigen-antibody complexes) and type IV (cell-mediated) hypersensitivity, whereas PDA probably involves type II (direct cytotoxicity), type III, and type IV hypersensitivity. Using the criteria outlined in Table 1 and the immune system correlates of the probable pathogenesis of the different immunologic syndromes, several worker populations exposed to various acid anhydrides have been evaluated (19–21).

The specificity of the antibodies has been evaluated in several workers. The antibody against the anhydride-protein complex generally does not appear to be directed against the TM hapten alone; it generally behaves as if new antigenic determinants not present on hapten or carrier have been created (22).

In several reported surveillance studies of acid anhydride exposed individuals, risk factors for development of disease include level of exposure and development of antibody (23–25). TCPA, HHPA, and TMA have all been studied in that regard.

## PREVENTION

An important goal of investigations of immune sensitization to acid anhydrides is prevention of the clinical syndromes described above. Primary prevention would be desirable but probably is not possible; there are no screening tests at the present time to determine whether a given person will or will not develop an immune response when exposed to acid anhydrides. There is one report of an association of human leukocyte antigen (HLA)-DR3 with specific IgE to acid anhydrides (26). Further investigation will determine whether this is a strong enough association to make HLA screening appropriate. There is no level of acid anhydride exposure that is known to be unable to induce sensitization in any individual.

Secondary prevention—surveillance and early detection of disease—is currently the best approach to prevention. It is known that the level of immune response and the number of workers who have TMA symptoms are proportional to exposure as determined by airborne TMA concentration (27). It is also known from investigations that approximately half of workers with significant levels of antibodies have a clinical immune disease syndrome due to TMA or will develop one, and that reduction of exposure is associated with lower levels of antibody and fewer symptoms (27,28).

Consequently, a practical approach that has significantly reduced the incidence of immune disease due to TMA is periodic surveillance of exposed worker populations with serum antibody studies and questionnaires. Workers who have significant levels of antibody or report significant symptoms on questionnaires, or both, are further evaluated to determine the clinical diagnosis and whether any interventions are needed (27,28). In two studies of acid anhydride workers, it appears that early diagnosis and removal to low- or no-exposure jobs will result in a favorable outcome (29,30).

## ANIMAL MODELS OF TMA SENSITIZATION

Guinea pig models of immediate-type pulmonary responses to TMA and PA have been reported (31–33), as has passive transfer of type I airway response from humans to rhesus monkeys using serum from workers with IgE against TM-HSA (34). The latter is strong evidence for the immune mechanism of asthma-rhinitis being type I hypersensitivity. A Sprague-Dawley rat model of LRSS and PDA has also been reported, immunization occurring via TMA inhalation (35). It has been shown that antibody of various isotypes against TM proteins such as rabbit serum albumin and rabbit hemoglobin is present in serum and BAL and that both correlate with the number of hemorrhagic foci in the lung for most immunizing regimens and that antibody secreting cells develop in pulmonary lymph nodes (36,37). However, induction of tolerance is associated with prolonged TMA inhalation in the rat model (38). There is no known instance of tolerance developing in humans.

## TOXICOLOGY OF TMA OTHER THAN IMMUNOLOGIC STUDIES

Using mice in developmental toxicity tests, no effect has been reported with TMA (39). Using the Ames *Salmonella* assay, no effect was found with TMA (40).

Limited animal data are available relative to cutaneous and ocular irritation; a single application of TMA (probably 50% aqueous suspension) to rat skin produced dermatitis, and 100 mg TMA powder applied to rabbit eyes resulted in corneal corrosive lesions and chemical burns of the conjunctiva that did not reverse over 7 days (41). In extensive studies of workers with or without the immunologic diseases described above, we have not seen irritant or contact dermatitis. In the absence of allergic conjunctivitis due to TMA, irritant conjunctivitis has not been a problem with routine control of the environment.

In addition to acute toxicity studies in animals, two 90-day subacute oral toxicity studies have been performed at doses of 1,000, 5,000, and 10,000 ppm. No deaths occurred; the only effect reported was leukocytosis beginning at a dose of 5,000 ppm (41).

## OTHER ANHYDRIDES

Several other anhydrides have been reported to cause occupational asthma. There do not appear to be reports of other anhydrides causing LRSS, although systemic flu-like symptoms have been reported with PA (6). Multiple reports of occupational asthma due to PA have been published (6,15,42,43). Similarly, there are several reports of TCPA asthma (16,44,45), HHPA asthma (46), MA asthma (47), PMDA asthma (48), and MTHPA asthma (49). In some cases, specific IgE antibody has been measured *in vivo* and *in vitro*.

In summary, acid anhydrides are low molecular weight, reactive chemicals that can conjugate to human proteins, rendering the chemical-protein complex immunogenic. The major clinical problem in exposed workers appears to be immune sensitization, which can induce any of three clinical syndromes—asthma-rhinitis, LRSS, or PDA. Reduction of exposure is the industrial management of choice. Periodic surveillance appears to be useful in the early identification of workers with clinical syndromes so that they can be helped by relocation, and improved environmental control can be established to reduce the incidence of immunologic disease.

## REFERENCES


1. Venables KM. Low molecular weight chemicals, hypersensitivity, and direct toxicity: the acid anhydrides. *Br J Ind Med* 1989;46:222–232.
2. Trimellitic anhydride (TMA). *Curr Intell Bull* 1978;21:1–8.
3. Rice DL, Jenkins DE, Gray JM, Greenberg SD. Chemical pneumonitis secondary to inhalation of epoxy pipe coating. *Arch Environ Health* 1977;32:173.
4. Herbert FA, Oxford A. Pulmonary hemorrhage and edema due to inhalation of resins containing trimellitic anhydride. *Chest* 1979;76: 546–556.
5. *Trimellitic anhydride:* documentation of the threshold limit values and biologic exposure indices. Cincinnati, OH: ACGIH, 1986;606.
6. Donnat L. Syndrome d'irritation des voies aeriennes superieures et bronchiques par l'anhydride phtalique: syndrome asthmatiforme allergique. *Med Travail* 1944;16:109–114.
7. *Material safety data sheet—trimellitic anhydride.* Chicago: Amoco Chemical, 1978.
8. Butler PJG, Harris JI, Hartley BS, Leberman R. The use of maleic anhydride for the reversible blocking of amino groups in polypeptide chains. *Biochem J* 1989;112:679–689.
9. Zeiss CR, Patterson R, Pruzansky JJ, Miller MM, Rosenberg M, Levitz D. Trimellitic anhydride—induced airway syndromes: clinical and immunologic studies. *J Allergy Clin Immunol* 1977;60:96–103.
10. Grammer LC, Shaughnessy MA, Lowenthal M. Hemorrhagic rhinitis: an immunologic disease due to hexahydrophthalic anhydride. *Chest* 1993;104:1792–1794.
11. Tarvainen K, Jolanki R, Estlander T, Tupasela O, Kanerva L. Immunologic contact urticaria due to airborne methylhexahydrophthalic and methyltetrahydrophthalic anhydrides. *Contact Dermatitis* 1995;32: 204–209.
12. Czuppon AB, Kaplan V, Speich R, Baur X. Acute autoimmune response in a case of pyromellitic acid dianhydride-induced hemorrhagic alveolitis. *Allergy* 1994;49:337–341.
13. Patterson R, Addington W, Banner AS, et al. Anti hapten antibodies in workers exposed to trimellitic anhydride fumes: a potential immunopathogenetic mechanism for the trimellitic anhydride pulmonary disease—anemia syndrome. *Am Rev Respir Dis* 1979;120: 1259–1267.
14. Ahmad D, Morgan WKC, Patterson R, Williams T, Zeiss CR. Pulmonary haemorrhage and haemolytic anaemia due to trimellitic anhydride. *Lancet* 1979;1:326–328.
15. Rivera M, Nicotra MB, Byron GE, et al. Trimellitic anhydride toxicity: a cause of acute multisystem failure. *Arch Intern Med* 1981;141: 1071–1074.
16. Patterson R, Zeiss CR, Pruzansky JJ. Immunology and immunopathology of trimellitic anhydride pulmonary reactions. *J Allergy Clin Immunol* 1982;70:19–23.
17. Nielsen J, Welinder H, Ottoson H, Bensryd I, Venge P, Skerfving K. Nasal challenge shows pathogenic relevance of specific IgE serum antibodies for nasal symptoms caused by hexahydrophthalic anhydride. *Clin Exp Allergy* 1994;24:440–449.
18. Nielsen J, Welinder H, Bensryd I, Andersson P, Skerfving S. Symptoms and immunologic markers induced by exposure to methyltetrahydrophthalic anhydride. *Allergy* 1994;49:281–286.
19. Zeiss CR, Wolkonsky P, Pruzansky JJ, Patterson R. Clinical and immunologic evaluation of trimellitic anhydride workers in multiple industrial settings. *J Allergy Clin Immunol* 1982;70:15–18.
20. Grammer LC, Harris KE, Chandler MJ, Flaherty D, Patterson R. Establishing clinical and immunologic criteria for diagnosis of occupational immunologic lung disease with phthalic anhydride and tetrachlorophthalic anhydride exposures as a model. *J Occup Med* 1987;29:806–811.
21. Zeiss CR, Mitchell JH, Van Peenen PFD, Harris J, Levitz D. A twelve-year clinical and immunologic evaluation of workers involved in the manufacture of trimellitic anhydride (TMA). *Allergy Proc* 1990;11: 71–76.
22. Patterson R, Zeiss CR, Roberts M, Pruzansky JJ, Wolkonsky P, Chacon R. Human antihapten antibodies in trimellitic anhydride inhalation reactions. *J Clin Invest* 1978;62:971–978.
23. Grammer LC, Shaughnessy MA, Lowenthal M, Yarnold P. Risk factors for immunologically mediated respiratory disease from hexahydrophthalic anhydride. *J Occup Med* 1994;36:642–646.
24. Grammer LC, Shaughnessy MA, Hogan MB, Berggruen SM, Watkins DM, Yarnold PR. Value of antibody level in diagnosing anhydride induced immunologic respiratory disease. *J Lab Clin Med* 1995;125: 650–653.
25. Liss GM, Bernstein D, Genesove L, Roos JO, Lim J. Assessment of risk factors for IgE-mediated sensitization to tetrachlorophthalic anhydride. *J Allergy Clin Immunol* 1993:92:237–247.
26. Young RP, Barker RD, Pile KD, Cookson WO, Taylor AJ. The associa-

tion of HLA-DR3 with specific IgE to inhaled acid anhydrides. *Am Rev Respir Crit Care Med* 1995;151:219–221.
27. Bernstein DI, Roach DE, McGrath KG, Larsen RS, Zeiss CR, Patterson R. The relationship of airborne trimellitic anhydride—induced symptoms and immune responses. *J Allergy Clin Immunol* 1983;72: 709–713.
28. Boxer MB, Grammer LC, Harris KE, Roach DE, Patterson R. Six-year clinical and immunologic follow-up of workers exposed to trimellitic anhydride. *J Allergy Clin Immunol* 1987;80:147–152.
29. Grammer LC, Shaughnessy MA, Henderson J, et al. A clinical and immunologic study of workers with trimellitic-anhydride induced immunologic lung disease after transfer to low exposure jobs. *Am Rev Respir Dis* 1993;148:54–57.
30. Grammer LC, Shaughnessy MA, Hogan MB, et al. Study of employees with anhydride induced respiratory disease after removal from exposure. *J Occup Environ Med* 1995;37:820–825.
31. Botham PA, Rattray NJ, Woodcock DR, Walsh ST, Hext PM. The induction of respiratory allergy in guinea pigs following intradermal injection of trimellitic anhydride: a comparison with the response to 2,4-dinitrochlorobenzene. *Toxicol Lett* 1989;47:25–39.
32. Yan ZQ, Hansson GK, Skoogh BE, Lotvall JO. Induction of nitric oxide synthetase in a model of allergic occupational asthma. *Allergy* 1995;50: 760–764.
33. Sarlo K, Clark ED, Ferguson J, Zeiss CR, Hatoum N. Induction of type I hypersensitivity in guinea pigs after inhalation of phthalic anhydride. *J Allergy Clin Immunol* 1994:94:747–756.
34. Dykewicz MS, Patterson R, Harris KE. Induction of antigen-specific bronchial reactivity to trimellityl—human serum albumin by passive transfer of serum from humans to rhesus monkeys. *J Lab Clin Med* 1988;111:59–65.
35. Zeiss CR, Levitz D, Leach CL, et al. A model of immunologic lung injury induced by trimellitic anhydride inhalation: antibody response. *J Allergy Clin Immunol* 1987;79:59–63.
36. Zeiss CR, Leach CL, Levitz D, Hatoum NS, Garvin PJ, Patterson R. Lung injury induced by short-term intermittent trimellitic anhydride (TMA) inhalation. *J Allergy Clin Immunol* 1989;84:219–223.
37. Zeiss CR, Hatoum NS, Ferguson J, et al. Localization of inhaled trimellitic anhydride to lung with a respiratory lymph node antibody secreting cell response. *J Allergy Clin Immunol* 1992:90:944–952.
38. Leach CL, Hatoum NS, Zeiss CR, Garvin PJ. Immunologic tolerance in rats during 13 weeks of inhalation exposure to trimellitic anhydride. *Fundam Appl Toxicol* 1989;12:519–529.
39. Hardin BD, Schuller RL, Burg JR, et al. Evaluation of 60 chemicals in a preliminary developmental toxicity test. *Teratogenesis Carcinogen Mutagen* 1987;7:29–48.
40. NTP mutagenesis. *NTP Tech Bull* 1982;7:5–9.
41. Fielder RJ, Dale EA, Sorrie GS, et al. Trimellitic anhydride (TMA). *Toxicity Rev* 1984;8:1–20.
42. Maccia CA, Bernstein IL, Emmett EA, Brooks SM. In vitro demonstration of specific IgE in phthalic anhydride hypersensitivity. *Am Rev Respir Dis* 1976;113:701–704.
43. Bernstein DI, Gallagher JS, D'Souza L, Bernstein IL. Heterogeneity of specific IgE responses in workers sensitized to acid anhydride compounds. *J Allergy Clin Immunol* 1984;74:794–801.
44. Howe W, Venables KM, Topping MD. Tetrachlorophthalic anhydride asthma: evidence for specific IgE antibody. *J Allergy Clin Immunol* 1983;71:5–11.
45. Schlueter DP, Banaszak EF, Fink JN, Barboriak J. Occupational asthma due to tetrachlorophthalic anhydride. *J Occup Med* 1978;20: 183–188.
46. Moller DR, Gallagher JS, Bernstein DI, Wilcox TG, Burroughs HE, Bernstein IL. Detection of IgE-mediated respiratory sensitization in workers exposed to hexahydrophthalic anhydride. *J Allergy Clin Immunol* 1985;75:663–672.
47. Guerin JC, Deschamps O, Guillot YL, Chavaillon JM, Kalb JC. A propos d'un cas d'asthme a l'anhydride maleique. *Poumon Coeur* 1980;36:393–395.
48. Meadway J. Asthma and atopy in workers with an epoxy adhesive. *Br J Dis Chest* 1980;74:149–154.
49. Nielson J, Welinder H, Horstmann V, Skerfving S. Allergy to methyltetrahydrophthalic anhydride in epoxy resin workers. *Br J Ind Med* 1992; 49:769–775.

*Environmental and Occupational Medicine, Third Edition,* edited by William N. Rom.
Lippincott–Raven Publishers, Philadelphia © 1998.

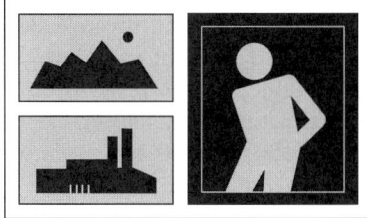

# CHAPTER 89

# Carbon Disulfide

Stephen M. Levin and Ruth Lilis

Carbon disulfide ($CS_2$) is a solvent with numerous applications in industry and agriculture. Toxic effects encompass, besides the nonspecific transitory prenarcotic and irritative effects common to most solvents, a rather unique spectrum of specific toxic effects. Toxic encephalopathy with psychotic manic-depressive manifestations, sensorimotor peripheral neuropathy, an increased incidence of atherosclerotic heart disease, and interference with normal spermatogenesis have resulted from exposure to $CS_2$ (1). Intensity of exposure is closely associated with the pattern of overt clinical effects.

## USES AND SOURCES OF EXPOSURE

Carbon disulfide is a colorless, very volatile liquid (boiling temperature 46°C). Considerable vapor is generated at room temperature; the vapor is 2.6 times heavier than air.

Approximately half is used in the production of viscose rayon and cellophane (2). Viscose production relies on the reaction of carbon disulfide with alkali cellulose (cellulose pretreated with sodium hydroxide). Cellulose xanthate and sodium trithiocarbonate ($Na_2CS_3$) are produced in this reaction. In the acid spinning bath, where filaments are formed through extrusion, coagulation and partial decomposition take place:

$$ROC^{S}{}_{SNa} + H_2CO_4 \rightarrow ROH + NaHSO_4 + CS_2$$

$$Na_2CS_3 + H_2SO_4 \rightarrow H_2S + CS_2 + Na_2SO_4$$

Carbon disulfide is generated, and exposure to $CS_2$ vapor occurs at the same time as exposure to hydrogen sulfide gas.

S.M. Levin and R. Lilis: Department of Community and Preventive Medicine, Mt. Sinai Medical Center, New York, New York 10029-6574.

The cutting of rayon filaments to staple fiber and cellophane production are known to generate higher levels of $CS_2$ exposure than other operations, such as spinning, washing, or drying of viscose.

An important application of $CS_2$ is in the manufacture of carbon tetrachloride. Other various uses are in the manufacture of neoprene cement and rubber accelerators; as a solvent for sulfur, iodine, bromine, phosphorus, selenium; and in paints, varnishes, paint-and-varnish removers, and rocket fuel.

Since the mid-1950s, an important application of carbon disulfide has been as a component in fumigants used to prevent grain infestation. A mixture of 20% carbon disulfide and 80% carbon tetrachloride (80/20 mixture) has been widely used and has resulted in cases of poisoning with severe neurologic symptoms, including extrapyramidal and cerebellar dysfunction and peripheral neuropathy (3,4). Repeated acute exposure to relatively high concentrations had occurred in the reported cases.

Elevator grain handlers and grain inspectors are among the most exposed of the 120,000 U.S. grain-processing workers, although grain farmers can also be exposed. Air concentrations of $CS_2$ have been reported to vary between 5 and 327 ppm. Exposures were found to be especially high in large export storage facilities, where some workers experienced repeated exposure to high concentrations during fumigant application. The U.S. Environmental Protection Agency (EPA) prohibited the sale or distribution of 80/20 solvent fumigants after January 1986 (5).

## ABSORPTION, DISTRIBUTION, AND BIOTRANSFORMATION

Absorption is mainly through inhalation; skin absorption has been demonstrated, but it is practically negligible. Following inhalation, about 40% of carbon disulfide is retained in the body. Recent studies using experimental exposure of humans to known concentrations of $CS_2$ have established retention values of 37% and 41% at exposures to 10 and 20 ppm, respectively. Considerable interindividual variation was observed. After four exposure periods of 50 minutes, no equilibrium was reached. The amount of adipose tissue estimated from skin-fold thickness was a significant factor in the retention of inhaled $CS_2$ (6). Most of it undergoes metabolic transformation; 10% to 30% is exhaled, and less than 1% is excreted unchanged in the urine. At the end of exposure, concentrations of carbon disulfide in exhaled air decrease rapidly; thus, for monitoring of workplace exposure the timing of sampling becomes critical (6).

Carbon disulfide disappears rapidly from the bloodstream because of its marked liposolubility, expressed in an elevated partition coefficient from blood to organs. Recently, evidence has been provided for the oxidative transformation of carbon disulfide, mediated by the mixed-function oxidase enzymes of the endoplasmic reticulum (7,8); the end product of this metabolic pathway is $CO_2$, the monooxygenated intermediate is carbonyl sulfide (COS), and atomic sulfur is generated. Atomic sulfur, thus released, is able to form covalent bonds.

## TOXIC EFFECTS: CLINICAL SYNDROMES

With high concentrations, specific toxic effects on the central nervous system are prominent and may result in severe acute or subacute encephalopathy. The clinical picture includes headache, dizziness, fatigue, excitement, depression, memory deficit, indifference, apathy, delusions, hallucinations, suicidal tendencies, delirium, acute mania, and coma. The outcome may be fatal, or in less severe cases incomplete recovery may occur with persistent psychiatric symptoms, indicating irreversible central nervous system injury.

Many such severe cases of carbon disulfide poisoning occurred, for example, in the rubber industry in France and Germany during the second half of the 19th century. As early as 1892, the first cases from the rubber industry were reported from the United States (2). Acute mania often led to admission to hospitals for the insane. With the rapid development of the viscose rayon industry, more cases of carbon disulfide poisoning occurred. Dr. Alice Hamilton (9,10) repeatedly called attention to this dangerous health hazard in the rubber and rayon viscose industries. In 1941 the first U.S. exposure standard for carbon disulfide was adopted (11). As late as 1946, persons with carbon disulfide psychosis were still admitted to state institutions for the mentally ill, often without any mention of carbon disulfide as the causative agent (10).

Chronic effects of carbon disulfide exposure were recognized later, when the massive overexposures leading to acute psychotic effects were largely eliminated.

Peripheral neuropathy of the sensorimotor type, initially involving the lower extremities but often the upper extremities as well, with distal to proximal progression, can lead to severe forms characterized by marked sensory loss, decrease in muscle strength and difficulty walking, diminished or abolished deep tendon reflexes, and muscle atrophy. Frequently, central nervous system effects can be detected in cases with toxic carbon disulfide peripheral neuropathy; fatigue, headache, irritability, somnolence, memory deficit, and changes in personality are the most common symptoms (12,13). Cerebral computed tomography has shown both focal and diffuse cerebral atrophy, cortical and central, in 15 of 16 male workers previously exposed to $CS_2$ (10 to 20 ppm, possibly with higher peaks) for at least 10 years in Norway's only rayon viscose factory (14). Cerebral blood flow examination in these workers did not reveal major abnormalities, although there was more asymmetry than in the reference group. Optic neuritis has often been reported. Constriction of visual fields has been found in less severe cases.

Electromyography and nerve conduction velocity measurements have been useful in the early detection of carbon disulfide peripheral neuropathy (15,16). Studies using electrophysiologic tests, including somatosensory evoked potentials, brain stem auditory evoked potentials, and visual evoked potentials, have revealed slowed conduction time in brain stem auditory pathways and in the visual system (17). In rats exposed to $CS_2$ inhalation (200 and 800 ppm) for 15 weeks, auditory brain stem responses were found to be delayed, suggesting a conduction dysfunction in the brain stem (18). In $CS_2$ exposed rats, visual evoked potentials (flash and pattern reversal) were shown to be decreased in amplitude, with an increase in latency. Repeated exposures had a more marked effect than acute exposure (19). Behavioral performance tests have been successfully applied for the early detection of central nervous system impairment (20).

With the recognition of toxic carbon disulfide peripheral neuropathy, efforts were made to further reduce exposure levels. While the incidence of toxic carbon disulfide peripheral neuropathy decreased, previously unsuspected cardiovascular effects of long-term carbon disulfide exposure, even at lower levels, became apparent.

Initially cerebrovascular changes, with clinical syndromes including pyramidal, extrapyramidal, and pseudobulbar manifestations, were reported with markedly increased incidence and at relatively young age in workers exposed to carbon disulfide (21).

A significant increase in mortality from coronary heart disease was well documented in workers with long-term carbon disulfide exposure at relatively low levels and led to the lowering of the threshold limit value (TLV) to 10 ppm in Finland (22–25).

Higher prevalences of hypertension and elevated cholesterol and lipoprotein levels have also been found in workers exposed to carbon disulfide and most probably contribute to the higher incidence of atherosclerotic cerebral, coronary, and renal disease (25–27).

A high prevalence of retinal microaneurysms was found in Japanese and Yugoslavian carbon disulfide–exposed workers; retinal microangiopathy was more frequent with longer carbon disulfide exposure (28,29).

A large retrospective cohort mortality study of workers exposed to $CS_2$ in the U.S. rayon industry revealed an excess of deaths from atherosclerotic heart disease among the subgroup most heavily exposed. Persons first exposed before age 30 years and who had been exposed for 15 years or more, seemed to be at highest risk (30). Reports from Finland (31) indicate that the increase in mortality from ischemic heart disease was practically eliminated by reducing $CS_2$ exposure levels to 10 ppm and by removing workers with coronary risk factors from exposure. The authors interpreted these results as indicating that the cardiotoxic effect of $CS_2$ is reversible. Follow-up of the cohort of viscose rayon workers (32) in England, the same population on which the initial report on increased coronary heart disease (CHD) deaths had been based (24), indicates a persistent high mortality rate from ischemic heart disease (IHD) in those with high $CS_2$ exposure in the spinning department. Recent exposure, during the preceding 2 years, was found to have a strong effect on IHD mortality. There was no significantly increased CHD mortality after age 65 (when exposure to $CS_2$ ceased), a fact that was interpreted as indicating that the effect of $CS_2$ is reversible and that the risk disappears after exposure ceases. The possibility that $CS_2$ might trigger clinical events in individuals at high risk of IHD was suggested, with factors related to autonomic nervous system effects on thrombus formation or on the myocardium, as possible mechanisms for $CS_2$ toxicity.

More recently, excess risk of CHD in another industry—$CS_2$ exposed rubber workers—has been reported. CHD, as defined by angina, a history of myocardial infarction, or an abnormal electrocardiogram occurred more frequently among 94 rubber workers exposed to $CS_2$ than in a nonexposed comparison group from the same plant. There was no association with duration of exposure (33).

Adverse effects of carbon disulfide exposure on reproductive function—and, more specifically, on spermatogenesis—have been reported in exposed workers, with significantly lower sperm counts and more abnormal spermatozoa than in unexposed control subjects (34). This toxic effect on spermatogenesis was confirmed in experiments on rats, where marked degenerative changes in seminiferous tubules and degenerative changes in the Leydig cells, with almost complete disappearance of spermatogonia, were found (35). Reproductive effects on women have been reported, including menstrual abnormalities, higher incidence of spontaneous abortions, and premature births (36).

## MECHANISMS OF TOXICITY

Carbon disulfide has a marked affinity for nucleophilic groups: sulfhydryl (-SH), amino ($-NH_2$), and hydroxy (-OH).

Carbon disulfide binds with amino groups of amino acids and proteins and forms thiocarbamates. These tend to undergo cyclic transformation, and the resulting thiazolidines have been shown to chelate zinc and copper (and possibly other trace metals) essential for the normal function of many important enzymes. Depletion of copper in the nervous system has been shown to occur in experimental animals. High affinity of $CS_2$ for sulfhydryl groups also may interfere with enzymatic activities.

Carbon disulfide has been shown to interfere with normal catecholamine metabolism (37). It is an inhibitor of dopamine β-hydroxylase, the enzyme responsible for the conversion of dopamine to norepinephrine. Dopamine β-hydroxylase is a copper-containing enzyme, and the copper-chelating effect of $CS_2$ may be responsible for inhibition of the enzyme. Brain norepinephrine decreases and central dopamine increases in rats after $CS_2$ administration (38).

Interference of carbon disulfide with vitamin $B_6$ and the formation of a salt of pyridoxamine dithiocarbamic acid have also been considered as a possible mechanism of toxicity.

Carbon disulfide has been found to affect liver microsomal enzymes and specifically to result in a loss of cytochrome P-450 (39–41). It is thought that oxidative desulfuration of carbon disulfide results in highly reactive sulfur, which binds covalently to the cellular macromolecules.

The carbon disulfide neurotoxic mechanism in the brain is not yet completely clear. Recently, a marked reduction in met-enkephalin immunostaining in the central amygdaloid nuclei and the globus pallidus was measured, with a parallel elevation in the lateral septal nucleus and the parietal cortex. These findings suggest that the enkephalinergic neuromodulatory system could play a role in $CS_2$ neurotoxicity (42).

Carbon disulfide is a member of the class of neuropathy-inducing xenobiotics known as neurofilament neurotoxicants. Current hypotheses propose a direct reaction of $CS_2$ with neurofilament lysine epsilon-amine moieties as a step in the mechanism of this neuropathy. A lysine-containing dipeptide and bovine serum albumin, when incubated with $^{14}CS_2$, exhibited stable incorporation of radioactivity. A specific intramolecular cross-link was also detected (43).

Covalent cross-linking of proteins by $CS_2$ has been demonstrated *in vitro* and represents a potential mechanism for the toxicity of this compound. Intraperitoneal injection of $CS_2$ in rats produced several high molecular weight proteins eluted from erythrocyte membranes, which were not present in control animals. The high molecular weight proteins were shown to be α,β-heterodimers. The production of multiple heterodimers was consistent with the existence of several preferred sites for cross-linking. Dimer formation showed a cumulative dose response in $CS_2$-treated rats (44). Covalent cross-linking of proteins has been presented as a potential molecular mechanism of $CS_2$-induced neuropathy. $CS_2$ has been shown to produce inter- and intramolecular cross-linking of the low molecular weight component of the neurofilament triplet proteins (45).

## URINARY METABOLITES AND BIOLOGIC MONITORING

Most absorbed carbon disulfide (70% to 90%) is metabolized. The biotransformation results in a number of metabolites (at least three) excreted in the urine. Two have been identified: thiocarbamide and mercaptothiazolinone (46,47).

These urinary metabolites of carbon disulfide have been found to catalyze the iodine-azide reaction (i.e., the reduction of iodine by sodium azide). The reaction is accelerated in the presence of carbon disulfide metabolites, and this is indicated by the time necessary for the disappearance of the iodine color. A biologic monitoring test was developed from these observations (48); departures from normal were found with exposures exceeding 16 ppm. It was then recommended that workers with an abnormal iodine-azide test at the end of the shift who did not recover overnight be removed (temporarily) from carbon disulfide exposure.

The first biologic monitoring method for carbon disulfide, the iodine-azide test, has low sensitivity and was shown to be unreliable at exposure levels below 15 ppm. The current TLV for $CS_2$ is 10 ppm (30 mg/m$^3$), and this made necessary biologic monitoring that is informative at relatively lower levels of exposure. A metabolite of $CS_2$, 2-thiothiazolidine-4-carboxylic acid (TTCA), was identified more recently in the urine of workers exposed to $CS_2$ (49). This metabolite is formed by conjugation with reduced glutathione after activation by P-450. The urinary concentration of TTCA was found to be quantitatively related to the uptake of $CS_2$. A high-performance liquid-chromatographic method has been developed for measurement of TTCA in urine; TTCA was easily detected even after exposure to less than 5 mg/m$^3$ (50). About 6% of the absorbed $CS_2$ is metabolized to TTCA; the correlation between urinary TTCA and air concentration of $CS_2$ was found to be as high as 0.84. A concentration of TTCA of 4 μmol/mmol creatinine in urine has been established to correspond to an exposure to 10 ppm $CS_2$ (8-hour time-weighted average). Breath monitoring of exhaled air in $CS_2$-exposed workers has benefited from the development of a transportable mass spectrometry instrument, which can measure concentrations of $CS_2$ below 1 ppm without the use of breath collection devices. A rapid first-phase elimination with a half-life of 10 minutes and a slower second elimination phase, with $CS_2$ detected in exhaled air even 16 hours after exposure, indicate the existence of at least two pharmacokinetic compartments. A monitoring strategy using preshift exhaled air samples is thought to warrant investigation (49).

## PATHOLOGY

The morphologic abnormalities underlying peripheral neuropathy produced by carbon disulfide have been studied in experiments on rats and rabbits. Axonal degeneration, characterized by multifocal paranodal and internodal fusiform axonal swelling with accumulation of neurofilaments, thinning and retraction of myelin sheets, and wallerian degeneration distal to axonal swelling, has been documented (51,52).

Axonal degeneration was also found in the central nervous system, mostly in long fiber tracts. After experimental exposure of monkeys, distal axonal swelling in retinogeniculate fibers was noted shortly after completion of exposure; changes were similar to those known to occur in corticospinal dorsal spinocerebellar fibers and peripheral nerves. Neuronal degeneration in the retina was also observed, and this persisted after termination of exposure with permanent visual acuity loss. Similar degenerative changes may explain the visual field loss and altered color vision that have been repeatedly reported and well described in humans (53). The morphologic changes and the time sequence of carbon disulfide peripheral neuropathy are of the type described as central-peripheral distal axonopathy and are very similar to that produced by *n*-hexane and methyl *n*-butyl ketone. Covalent binding of highly reactive sulfur, resulting from the oxidative desulfuration of $CS_2$ by mixed-function microsomal enzymes to thiol groups of enzymes and proteins essential for the normal function of axonal transport, is thought to be the mechanism of axonal degeneration underlying central-peripheral neuropathy induced by carbon disulfide.

The neurofilament accumulations are probably the result of a common mechanism characteristic for these toxic neuropathies, the covalent cross-linking of neurofilaments. Such features are characteristic for hexacarbon peripheral neuropathy and acrylamide peripheral neuropathy, as well as for $CS_2$ peripheral neuropathy. Covalently cross-linked masses of neurofilaments may occlude axonal transport at the nodes of Ranvier. Accumulation of neurofilaments proximal to the occlusion and degeneration of the distal axon can follow (54). In an experimental study on rats (exposure to 810 ppm), the areas most sensitive to injury were found to be the distal portions of the long fiber tracts in the spinal cord, the posterior tibial and common peroneal nerves. Large myelinated fibers were more susceptible than smaller myelinated fibers (55), a finding consistent with what has been described in other neurofilamentous axonopathies (56).

## PREVENTION

The current federal standard for a permissible level of carbon disulfide exposure is 4 ppm (12 mg/m$^3$) as an 8-hour time-weighted-average concentration, with 12 ppm as a 30-minute ceiling standard. The National Institute for Occupational Safety and Health (NIOSH) has recommended a standard of 1 ppm (3 mg/m$^3$) as a time-weighted average concentration for up to a 10-hour work shift in a 40-hour work week. NIOSH also recommended a 15-minute ceiling concentration of 10 ppm (30 mg/m$^3$).

Prevention of exposure has to rely on engineering controls and mostly on enclosed processes and exhaust ventilation. When unexpected overexposure can occur, appropriate respiratory protection has to be available and used (23). Skin contact has to be avoided and protective equipment provided; adequate shower facilities and strict personal hygiene practices are necessary. Worker education in both health hazards of carbon disulfide exposure and the importance of adequate work practices and personal hygiene has to be a part of a comprehensive preventive medicine program. Medical surveillance has to encompass assessment of neurologic function (behavioral and neurophysiologic tests are especially useful for early detection of adverse neurologic effects), cardiovascular function (electrocardiogram, including exercise electrocardiogram and ophthalmoscopic examination), renal function, and reproductive function. The urinary TTCA test is useful for biologic monitoring.

## REFERENCES


1. WHO. *Environmental health criteria 10:* carbon disulfide. Geneva: World Health Organization, 1979.
2. National Institute for Occupational Safety and Health. *Criteria for a recommended standard—occupational exposure to carbon disulfide.* DHEW publication [NIOSH] 77-156. Washington, DC: U.S. Government Printing Office, 1977.
3. Peters HA, Levine RL, Matthews CG, Sauter S, Chapman L. Synergistic neurotoxicity of carbon tetrachloride/carbon disulfide (80/20 fumigants) and other pesticides in grain storage workers. *Acta Pharmacol Toxicol* 1986;59(suppl 6):535–546.
4. Peters HA, Levine RL, Matthews CG, Chapman LJ. Extrapyramidal and other neurologic manifestations associated with carbon disulfide fumigant exposure. *Arch Neurol* 1988;45:537–540.
5. *Regulatory status of grain fumigants* (notice). 50 Federal Register. S380992.
6. Rosier J, Veulemans H, Masschelein R, Vanhoorne M, Van Peteghem C. Experimental human exposure to carbon disulfide. Respiratory uptake and elimination of carbon disulfide under rest and physical exercise. *Int Arch Occup Environ Health* 1987;59:233–242.
7. Dalvi RA, Neal RA. Metabolism in vivo of carbon disulfide to carbonyl sulfide and carbon dioxide in the rat. *Biochem Pharmacol* 1978; 27:1608–1609.
8. DeMatteis F, Seawright AA. Oxidative metabolism of carbon disulphide by the rat: effect of treatments which modify the liver toxicity of carbon disulphide. *Chem Biol Interact* 1973;7:375–388.
9. Hamilton A. *Industrial poisons used in the rubber industry.* Bulletin 179. Washington, DC: U.S. Department of Labor, Bureau of Labor Statistics; 1915;5.
10. Hamilton A. *The making of artificial silk in the United States and some of the dangers attending it.* Bulletin 10. Washington, DC: U.S. Department of Labor, Division of Labor Standards, 1937;151.
11. *Allowable concentration of carbon disulfide.* (A.S.A. Z37.3 1941). New York: American Standards Association; 1941.
12. Hamilton A, Hardy H. *Industrial toxicology.* Acton, MA: Publishing Sciences Group, 1974;262–266.
13. Lilis R. Behavioral effects of occupational carbon disulfide exposure. In: Xintaras C, Johnson BL, de Groot I, eds. *Behavioral toxicology, early detection of occupational hazards.* DHEW publication [NIOSH]. Washington, DC: U.S. Department of Health Education and Welfare, 1974;51–59.
14. Aaserud O, Gjerstad L, Nakstad P, et al. Neurological examination, computerized tomography, cerebral blood flow and neuropsychological examination in workers with long-term exposure to carbon disulfide. *Toxicology* 1988;49:277–282.
15. Manu P, Lilis R, Lancranjan I, et al. The value of electromyographic changes in the early diagnosis of carbon disulphide peripheral neuropathy. *Med Lav* 1970;61:102–108.
16. Seppalainen AM, Haltia M. Carbon disulfide. In: Schaumburg HH, Spencer PS, eds. *Experimental and clinical neurotoxicology.* Baltimore: Williams & Wilkins, 1980;356–373.
17. Rebert CS, Becker E. Effects of inhaled carbon disulfide on sensory-evoked potentials of Long-Evans rats. *Neurobehav Toxicol Teratol* 1986;8:533–541.
18. Hirata M, Ogawa Y, Okayama A, Goto S. Changes in auditory brainstem response in rats chronically exposed to carbon disulfide. *Arch Toxicol* 1992;66:334–338.
19. Herr DW, Boyes WK, Dyer RS. Alterations in rat flash and pattern reversal evoked potentials after acute or repeated administration of carbon disulfide ($CS_2$). *Fundam Appl Toxicol* 1992;18:328–342.
20. Hanninen H. Psychological picture of manifest and latent carbon disulphide poisoning. *Br J Ind Med* 1971;28:374–381.
21. Vigliani EC. Carbon disulphide poisoning in viscose rayon factories. *Br J Ind Med* 1954;11:235–244.
22. Hernberg S, Nurminen M, Tolonen M. Excess mortality from coronary heart disease in viscose rayon workers exposed to carbon disulfide. *Work Environ Health* 1973;10:93.
23. Nurminen M. Survival experience of a cohort of carbon disulphide exposed workers from an eight-year prospective follow-up period. *Int J Epidemiol* 1976;5:179–185.
24. Tiller JR, Schilling RSF, Morris JN. Occupational toxic factor in mortality from coronary disease. *Br Med J* 1968;4:407–411.
25. Tolonen M, Hernberg S, Nurminen M, et al. A follow-up study of coronary heart disease in viscose rayon workers exposed to carbon disulphide. *Br J Ind Med* 1975;32:1–10.
26. Gavrilescu N, Lilis R. Cardiovascular effects of long-extended carbon disulfide exposure. In: Brieger H, Teisinger J, eds. *Toxicology of carbon disulfide.* Amsterdam: Excerpta Medica, 1967;165.
27. Manu P, Lilis R, Nestorescu B, et al. Effects of carbon disulfide exposure on cholesterol and β-lipoprotein levels in young adults. *Med Lav* 1972;63:324.
28. Goto S, Hotta R. The medical and hygienic prevention of carbon disulphide poisoning in Japan. In: Brieger H, Teisinger J, eds. *Toxicology of carbon disulphide.* Amsterdam: Excerpta Medica, 1967;219.
29. Goto S, Sugimoto K, Hotta R, et al. Retinal microaneurysm in carbon disulphide workers in Yugoslavia. *Pravokni Lekarstvi* 1972;24:66.
30. MacMahon B, Monson RR. Mortality in the US rayon industry. *J Occup Med* 1988;30:698–705.
31. Nurminen M, Hernberg S. Effects of intervention on the cardiovascular mortality of workers exposed to carbon disulphide: a 15-year follow up. *Br J Ind Med* 1985;42:32–35.
32. Sweetnam PM, Taylor SWC, Elwood PC. Exposure to carbon disulphide and ischaemic heart disease in a viscose rayon factory. *Br J Ind Med* 1987;44:220–227.
33. Oliver LC, Weber RP. Chest pain in rubber chemical workers exposed to carbon disulphide and methaemoglobin formers. *Br J Ind Med* 1984;41:296–304.
34. Lancranjan I. Alterations of spermatic liquid in patients chronically poisoned by carbon disulphide. *Med Lav* 1972;63:29.
35. Gondzik M. Histology and histochemistry of rat testicles as affected by carbon disulfide. *Polish Med J* 1971;10:133.
36. Petrov MV. Some data on the course and termination of pregnancy in female workers of the viscose industry. *Pediatr Akusherstvo Ginekol* 1969;3:50.

37. Magos L, Jarvis JAE. The effects of carbon disulfide exposure on brain catecholamines in rats. *Br J Pharmacol* 1970;29:936–938.
38. Chester AE, Meyers FH. Central sympathoplegic and norepinephrine-depleting effects of antioxidants. *Proc Soc Exp Biol Med* 1988;187: 62–68.
39. Bond EJ, DeMatteis F. Biochemical changes in rat liver after administration of carbon disulphide, with particular reference to microsomal changes. *Biochem Pharmacol* 1969;18:2531–2549.
40. DeMatteis F. Covalent binding of sulfur to microsomes and loss of cytochrome P450 during the oxidative desulfuration of several chemicals. *Mol Pharmacol* 1974;10:849–854.
41. Wilkie IW, Seawright AA, Hrdlicka J. The hepatotoxicity of carbon disulphide in sheep. *J Appl Toxicol* 1985;5:360–367.
42. de Gandarias JM, Echevarria E, Mugica J, Serrano R, Casis, L. Changes in brain enkephalin immunostaining after acute carbon disulfide exposure in rats. *J Biochem Toxicol* 1994;9:59–62.
43. DeCaprio AP, Spink DC, Chen X, Fowke JH, Zhu M, Bank S. Characterization of isothiocyanates, thioureas, and other lysine adduction products in carbon disulfide-treated peptides and protein. *Chem Res Toxicol* 1992;5:496–504.
44. Valentine WM, Graham DG, Anthony DC. Covalent cross-linking of proteins by carbon disulfide in vivo. *Toxicol Appl Pharmacol* 1993;121:71–77.
45. Valentine WM, Amarnath V, Amarnath K, Rimmele F, Graham DG. Carbon disulfide mediated protein cross-linking by N,N-diethyldithiocarbamate. *Chem Res Toxicol* 1995;8:96–102.
46. Pergal M, Vukojevic N, Cirin-Popov N, Djuric D, Bojovic T. Carbon disulfide metabolites excreted in the urine of exposed workers: I. Isolation and identification of 2-mercapto-2-thiazolinone-5. *Arch Environ Health* 1972;25:38–41.
47. Pergal M, Vukojevic N, Djuric D. II. Isolation and identification of thiocarbamide. *Arch Environ Health* 1972;25:42–44.
48. Djuric D, Surducki N, Berkes I. Iodine-azide test on urine of persons exposed to carbon disulphide. *Br J Ind Med* 1965;22:321–323.
49. Van Doorn R, Delbressine LPC, Leijdekkers CM, Vertin PG, Henderson PTh. Identification and determination of TTCA in urine of workers exposed to carbon disulfide. *Arch Toxicol* 1981;47:51–58.
50. Campbell L, Jones AH, Wilson HK. Evaluation of occupational exposure to carbon disulphide by blood, exhaled air, and urine analysis. *Am J Ind Med* 1985;8:143–153.
51. Juntunen J, Linnoila I, Haltia M. Histochemical and electron microscope observations on the myoneural functions of rats with carbon disulfide induced polyneuropathy. *Scand J Work Environ Health* 1977; 3:36–42.
52. Seppalainen AM, Tolonen MT. Neurotoxicity of long-term exposure to carbon disulfide in the viscose rayon industry: a neurophysiological study. *Work Environ Health* 1974;11:145.
53. Eskin TA, Merigan WH, Woods RW. Carbon disulfide effects on the visual system. *Invest Ophthalmol Vis Sci* 1988;29:519–527.
54. Graham DG, Anthony DC, Szakal-Quin G, Gottfried MR, Boekelheide K. Covalent cross-linking of neurofilaments in the pathogenesis of n-hexane neuropathy. *Neuro Toxicol* 1985;6:55–64.
55. Gottfried MR, Graham DG, Morgan M, Casey HW, Bus JS. The morphology of carbon disulfide neurotoxicity. *Neuro Toxicol* 1985;6:89–96.
56. Cavanagh JB, Bennetts RJ. On the pattern of changes in the rat nervous system produced by 2,5 hexanediol. *Brain* 1981;104:297–318.

*Environmental and Occupational Medicine, Third Edition*, edited by William N. Rom.
Lippincott–Raven Publishers, Philadelphia © 1998.

CHAPTER 90

# *N*-Nitrosamines

Stephen S. Hecht

*N*-Nitrosamines, referred to as nitrosamines in this chapter, are one of the most widely studied classes of chemical carcinogens. This chapter presents representative examples of the large number of nitrosamines that have been tested for carcinogenicity in laboratory animals, and discusses the structure-activity relationships in nitrosamine carcinogenesis. Nitrosamines are likely human carcinogens. They occur widely in the human environment and are formed endogenously in humans. Nitrosamines undergo metabolic activation to intermediates that damage DNA and cause permanent mutations in critical genes involved in the cancer induction process. This chapter presents the metabolic activation and detoxification reactions of some representative nitrosamines, and discusses the role of nitrosamines in human cancer.

## CARCINOGENICITY OF NITROSAMINES

In 1954, Barnes and Magee (1) reported that *N*-nitrosodimethylamine (NDMA), the simplest dialkylnitrosamine, was a potent toxin in the rat, mouse, rabbit, and dog, causing severe hemorrhagic centrilobular necrosis of the liver. This report was followed by the seminal observation by Magee and Barnes (2) in 1956 that prolonged feeding of a diet containing 50 ppm of NDMA caused malignant hepatic neoplasia in rats. In 1937, Freund (3) had reported fatal human exposure of research chemists to NDMA. More recently, homicidal NDMA poisoning was reported in the United States and Germany (4). Acute poisoning resulted in massive hepatic necrosis. Analysis of the hepatic DNA of the American victims demonstrated the presence of adducts resulting from the metabolic activation of NDMA (5).

The initial report of NDMA carcinogenesis spurred further research into the carcinogenic properties of other nitrosamines by Druckrey, Preussmann, and Schmähl (6,7), Lijinsky (8), and others. These tests were facilitated by the ready availability of nitrosamines, which can be synthesized by simple nitrosation of the corresponding amines. The carcinogenic properties of nitrosamines have been extensively documented and reviewed (6–8). Most bioassays have been carried out in rats, hamsters, and mice. Some representative carcinogenicity data for nitrosamines in rats are summarized in Table 1. Several points are noteworthy. First, a variety of target organs are affected, and the target selectivity depends on nitrosamine structure and often on the species employed. Tumors of the liver, esophagus, lung, nasal mucosa, bladder, tongue, and forestomach are commonly induced by nitrosamines in rats. Different target organs are frequently affected in hamsters. These data are summarized in Table 2. The most notable difference between rats and hamsters is the esophagus, which is the most common target tissue in the rat but is not affected in the hamster. In contrast, the hamster pancreas is more sensitive to nitrosamine carcinogenesis than that of the rat. Nitrosamines are often the compounds of choice for the induction and study of specific types of tumors in laboratory animals (6–8). For example, *N*-nitrosomethylbenzylamine (NMBA) is widely employed to study esophageal cancer as it readily induces these tumors in rats. *N*-nitroso*bis*-2-(oxopropyl)amine is used for induction of pancreatic tumors in Syrian golden hamsters, *N*-nitrosobutyl(4-hydroxybutyl)amine reproducibly causes bladder tumors in rats, and 4-(methylnitrosamino)-1-(3-

S. S. Hecht: University of Minnesota Cancer Center, Minneapolis, Minnesota 55455.

**TABLE 1.** *Carcinogenicity of some nitrosamines in rats*

| Compound | Dose (μmol/week) | Median time to death (weeks) | Tumor types |
|---|---|---|---|
| Dialkylnitrosamines | | | |
| *N*-nitroso- | | | |
| dimethylamine (NDMA) | 45 | 31 | Liver |
| diethylamine | 44 | 26 | Esophagus, liver |
| di-n-propylamine | 35 | 31 | Esophagus, forestomach, tongue |
| di-*iso*-propylamine | 70 | 56 | Nasal |
| methylethylamine | 34 | 63 | Liver, nasal |
| methyl-n-propylamine | 14 | 28 | Esophagus, forestomach, pharynx |
| methyl-n-butylamine | 14 | 27 | Esophagus, forestomach, tongue |
| methyl-n-amylamine | 115 | 63 | Esophagus |
| methyl-n-hexylamine | 35 | 25 | Esophagus, tongue, forestomach |
| methyl-n-heptylamine | 89 | 42 | Esophagus, lung, liver |
| methyl-n-octylamine | 100 | 56 | Esophagus, lung, bladder |
| methyl-n-nonylamine | 220 | 43 | Liver, lung |
| methyl-n-decylamine | 216 | 81 | Bladder, lung |
| methyl-n-undecylamine | 215 | 48 | Liver, lung |
| methyl-n-dodecylamine | 210 | 47 | Bladder, lung |
| methyl-n-tetradecylamine | 220 | 84 | Bladder, lung |
| methylcyclohexylamine | 35 | 29 | Esophagus |
| methylphenylamine | 37 | 78 | Esophagus, forestomach |
| methylbenzylamine | 9 | 24 | Esophagus, tongue |
| diphenylamine | 4,200 | NA | Bladder |
| diethanolamine | 1870 | 58 | Liver, nasal, kidney, esophagus |
| *bis*-2-(oxopropyl)amine | 35 | 60 | Lung, thyroid, liver, kidney |
| 4-(methylamino)-1-(3-pyridyl) -1-butanone (NNK) | 1.4 | — | Lung |
| Cyclic nitrosamines | | | |
| *N*-nitroso- | | | |
| azetidine | 200 | 53 | Liver |
| pyrrolidine | 200 | 80 | Liver |
| proline | 1,000 | — | None |
| piperidine | 88 | 38 | Nasal, esophagus, liver |
| morpholine | 34 | 57 | Liver, esophagus |
| hexamethyleneimine | 87 | 27 | Esophagus, liver, nasal |
| dodecamethyleneimine | 225 | 92 | Liver |
| nornicotine | 110 | 40 | Esophagus, nasal cavity |

Adapted from ref. 8.

**TABLE 2.** *Tumors induced by nitrosamines in rats and hamsters*

| Tumor site | No. of compounds giving tumors (%) | |
|---|---|---|
| | Rats (130 nitrosamines) | Hamsters (41 nitrosamines) |
| Liver | 57 (44) | 26 (63) |
| Lung | 28 (22) | 18 (44) |
| Kidney | 8 (6) | — |
| Esophagus | 66 (51) | — |
| Nasal mucosa | 49 (38) | 25 (61) |
| Bladder | 11 (8) | 3 (7) |
| Tongue | 25 (19) | — |
| Forestomach | 25 (19) | 15 (37) |
| Pancreas | — | 11 (27) |
| Thyroid—follicular cell | 6 (5) | — |
| Trachea | 11 (8) | 11 (27) |
| Thymus | 2 (2) | — |
| Intestine | 1 (1) | — |
| Colon | 2 (2) | 1 (2) |
| Spleen | 2 (2) | — |
| No tumors | 24 (18) | — |

From ref. 8.

pyridyl)-1-butanone (NNK) is extensively used for induction of lung tumors in rats and mice.

A second important point is that nitrosamines frequently induce tumors at specific sites independent of the route of administration (6–8). Good examples are NMBA for the rat esophagus and NNK for the rat lung.

Third, some nitrosamines are extremely powerful carcinogens, inducing tumors at very low doses. For example, dose-response studies, using 4,080 rats, were carried out on NDMA and *N*-nitrosodiethylamine (NDEA) administered in the drinking water (9). At doses sufficiently high for the median time to death to be estimated, the following equation was derived: dose rate × median$^n$ = constant, where *n* was about 2.3, or 1, depending on the tumor type. At doses sufficiently low for longevity to be nearly normal (about 2.5 years), liver tumor incidence was simply proportional to dose rate. There was a linear relationship observed at doses below 1 ppm. Thus, a dose of 1 ppm caused about 25% of the rats to develop a liver neoplasm, 0.1 ppm about 2.5%, etc., with no indication of a threshold.

Approximately 200 nitrosamines have been shown to be carcinogenic (6–8). Numerous different species are responsive to nitrosamine carcinogenesis (10) (Table 3). These data, together with biochemical data indicating similar metabolic pathways in laboratory animals and humans, strongly indicate that nitrosamines are also carcinogenic in humans (7,8).

Structure-carcinogenicity relationships among nitrosamines are remarkable (6–8). This is evident from data in Table 1 for *N*-nitrosomethyl-*n*-alkylamines. Whereas NDMA and *N*-nitrosomethylethylamine give mainly liver tumors in the rat, *N*-nitrosomethyl-*n*-propylamine, *n*-butylamine, *n*-amylamine, and *n*-hexylamine (NMHA) produce mainly esophageal tumors. Higher members of this series having an even number of carbons in the alkyl chain—*N*-nitrosomethyl-*n*-decylamine, *n*-dodecylamine, and *n*-tetradecylamine—give mainly bladder tumors. *N*-nitrosomethyl-*n*-undecylamine causes tumors of the liver and lung, but not bladder. Some other relationships are illustrated in Fig. 1. NDEA produces esophageal and liver

**TABLE 3.** *Species responding to carcinogenic nitrosamines*

| Animal | Treatment | Tumors induced |
|---|---|---|
| Mammals | | |
| Mouse | NDMA, NDEA | Liver, esophagus |
| Rat | NDMA, NDEA | Liver, esophagus |
| Syrian hamster | NDMA, NDEA | Liver, nasal cavity |
| Chinese hamster | NDMA, NDEA | Lung, esophagus |
| European hamster | NDMA, NDEA | Lung, nasal cavity |
| Gerbil | NDEA | Liver, Nasal cavity |
| Guinea pig | NDMA, NDEA | Liver |
| Rabbit | NDMA, NDEA | Liver |
| Dog | NDEA | Liver |
| Pig | NDEA | Liver |
| Cat | NDEA | Liver |
| Hedgehog | NDEA | Liver, lung |
| Monkey | NDMA, NDEA | Liver |
| Fox | NDMA | Liver |
| Mink | NDMA | Liver |
| Bushbaby | NDEA | Liver |
| Shrew | NBHPA | Lung |
| Mastomys | NDMA | Liver |
| Birds | | |
| Duck | NDMA | Liver |
| Chicken | NDEA | Liver, kidney |
| Parakeet | NDEA | Liver |
| Reptiles | | |
| Python | NDEA | Liver, kidney |
| Amphibians | | |
| Frog | NDMA, NDEA | Liver, kidney |
| Newt | NDMA | Liver |
| Xenopus | NDMA | Liver, kidney |
| Fish | | |
| Guppy | NDMA | Liver |
| Zebra fish *(Brachybanio rerio)* | NDMA | Liver, esophagus |
| Medaka *(Oryzias latides)* | NDMA | Liver |
| *Rivulus ocellatus* | NDEA | Pancreas |
| *Poecilla reticulata* | NDMA, NDEA | Liver |
| Trout | NDMA, NDEA | Liver |
| Mollusk | | |
| *Unio pictorum* | NDMA, NDEA | Liver |

From ref. 8.

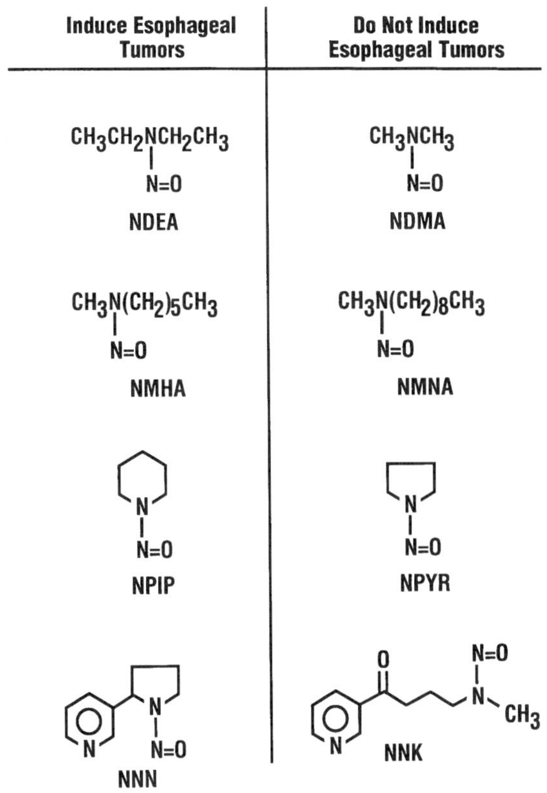


**FIG. 1.** Differing targets for carcinogenicity in rats of some structurally related nitrosamines.

tumors in rats, but in a study with over 1,000 rats per group, not a single esophageal tumor was observed in NDMA treated animals (9). As mentioned above, NMHA and three lower homologues are potent esophageal carcinogens in the rat, but *N*-nitrosomethyl-*n*-nonylamine (NMNA) gives tumors of the liver and lung. The cyclic nitrosamines *N*-nitrosopiperidine (NPIP) and *N*-nitrosopyrrolidine (NPYR) differ by only one carbon atom. NPIP produces esophageal and liver tumors in the rat, while NPYR gives liver tumors but never tumors of the esophagus. *N'*-Nitrosonornicotine (NNN) causes esophageal tumors when administered to rats in the drinking water, but the related tobacco-specific nitrosamine NNK gives no esophageal tumors in rats. Many of these relationships can be partially understood by considering tissue specific metabolic activation of these nitrosamines.

## OCCURRENCE OF NITROSAMINES

A major advance in the analysis of nitrosamines was the development of a nitrosamine selective detector (11). The N-N=O bond is thermally cleaved, and the released nitrosyl radical is oxidized by ozone to excited state $NO_2$, which returns to the ground state with emission of light in the near-infrared region of the spectrum. The emitted light is monitored by an infrared sensitive photomultiplier tube. Coupling of this detector to a gas chromatograph provides a very sensitive and reliable method for the detection and quantitation of nitrosamines, provided that they have sufficient volatility. This method has been widely applied.

There are two main sources of human exposure to nitrosamines: exogenous exposure and endogenous formation. Exogenous exposure to nitrosamines can occur in the diet, in certain occupational settings, and through the use of tobacco products, cosmetics, pharmaceutical products, and agricultural chemicals (12–14). Endogenous exposure occurs by nitrosation of amines in the body, via their acid or bacterial catalyzed reaction with nitrite, or by reaction with products of nitric oxide generated during inflammation and infection.

### Dietary Exposure

The use of nitrite as a preservative in cured or smoked meat or fish products raised concerns about nitrosamine formation, since the reaction of nitrite with amines occurs readily under a variety of conditions. Nitrite inhibits formation of a toxin by the anaerobic spore-forming bacteria *Clostridium botulinum.* Nitrite is also responsible for the pink color associated with nitrite cured meats and stabilizes the flavor of stored meats by preventing undesirable oxidation products (15). Before the introduction of process modifications and the use of ascorbate as an inhibitor, levels of nitrosamines in products such as fried bacon were up to 100 parts per billion (ppb), but this has decreased substantially. Carcinogenic nitrosamines are now generally found in concentrations of <10 ppb in cured meats; the main nitrosamines detected are NDMA and NPYR (15). Other foods and beverages that contain detectable levels of these nitrosamines, usually <10 ppb, include cheese, beer, and certain milk products. Process modifications have resulted in important reductions of the levels of nitrosamines in beer (from 5 to 20 ppb to less than 0.4 ppb). In industrialized countries, the average daily intake of NDMA and NPYR through the diet is on the order of 1 μg per person (13). The reductions in dietary nitrosamine exposure are good examples of successful cancer prevention strategies.

### Occupational Exposure

Occupational exposure to nitrosamines occurs in the rubber, leather, and metal industries (12,13,16). NDMA, NDEA, *N*-nitrosomorpholine (NMOR), and NPIP have been detected in the air of rubber factories. Accelerators and retarders employed in the vulcanization process are the sources of the nitrosamines. Workers in the rubber industry are at an increased risk for cancer, but it is uncertain whether this is due to nitrosamine exposure. Significant reductions in nitrosamine exposure have been achieved, but there is still room for improvement. In the leather tanning industry, the highest concentration of NDMA reported was 47 $\mu g/m^3$; following cleaning of the factory, NDMA concentration decreased to 0.1 to 3.4 $\mu g/m^3$. The presence of NDMA has been attributed to the use of dimethylamine sulfate in the hair removal process. Dimethylamine can be released and react with nitrogen oxides in the factory air. In the metal industry, substantial quantities of *N*-nitrosodiethanolamine (NDELA), up to 2%, have been detected in cutting fluids. NDELA is formed by the reaction of nitrite, a corrosion inhibitor, with diethanolamine or triethanolamine. NDELA levels in cutting fluids have been dramatically reduced in Germany, but may still reach high levels in other industrialized countries.

### Tobacco Products

Tobacco products are the greatest source of nonoccupational exposure to carcinogenic nitrosamines (12,13, 17–20). In commercial cigarettes, volatile nitrosamines such as NDMA and NPYR typically occur in the range of 2 to 20 ng per cigarette. Levels of these compounds in cigarette sidestream smoke, the main component of environmental tobacco smoke, are up to 100 times greater than in mainstream smoke. Tobacco-specific nitrosamines are also present in tobacco products, and their levels are much greater than those of the volatile nitrosamines. Tobacco-specific nitrosamines are formed during the curing and processing of tobacco by nitrosation of nicotine and related alkaloids of tobacco. The structures of the seven tobacco-specific nitrosamines that have been identified in tobacco products are illustrated in Fig. 2. NNK, NNN, *N'*-nitrosoanabasine (NAB), and *N'*-nitrosoanatabine (NAT) have all been identified in cigarette smoke and their levels well characterized. Typical levels per cigarette are NNK, 100 ng; NNN, 220 ng; NAB, 20 ng; and NAT, 160 ng. Among these compounds, NNK and NNN are the strongest carcinogens and are believed to play an important role in tobacco-induced cancer, as discussed below.

Levels of tobacco-specific nitrosamines are remarkably high in unburned tobacco, particularly snuff that is consumed orally in a practice called snuff-dipping. In addition to NNK, NNN, NAB, and NAT, unburned tobacco also contains NNAL, *iso*-NNAL, and *iso*-NNAC. Moreover, snuff products contain substantial amounts of nitrosamino acids. In total, 23 different nitrosamines have been identified in processed tobacco. Typical levels of tobacco-specific nitrosamines in snuff are NNK, 3.6 μg/g; NNN, 17.5 μg/g; NAT, 15.6 μg/g; and *iso*-NNAC, 1.1 μg/g.

### Cosmetics

Nitrosamines were first reported in cosmetics products in 1977 (12,21). More than 8,000 raw materials are used in formulating cosmetic products and many of these are amines and related compounds. The raw materials function as emulsifiers and thickeners. Sometimes they are contaminated with nitrosatable amines. Nitrite is sometimes present as a contaminant, and some preservatives used in cosmetics products can release nitrite. *N*-Nitrosodiethanolamine (NDELA) is the most commonly detected nitrosamine in cosmetics. It is formed by nitrosation of triethanolamine or diethanolamine. In the United States, its levels have decreased somewhat, but in 1992 there was still up to 3,000 ppb in some products. NDELA has substantial hepatocarcinogenicity in the rat. Other nitrosamines detected in cosmetics include *N*-nitrosomethyl-*n*-dodecylamine, *N*-nitrosomethyl-*n*-tetradecylamine, and *N*-nitrosomethyl-*n*-octadecylamine. Sunscreens have been found to contain 2-ethylhexyl 4-(*N*-methyl-*N*-nitrosamino)benzoate, up to 21 ppm.

### Pharmaceutical and Agricultural Products

Many drugs that are secondary or tertiary amines can potentially be nitrosated (12–14). The greatest risk for nitrosamine formation from pharmaceutical products is through endogenous nitrosation in the stomach. Administration of drugs and nitrite to laboratory animals has resulted in tumor induction, presumably by nitrosamine formation (14,22). The analgesic drug aminopyrine, which has been banned in Germany, is rapidly nitrosated to give NDMA in vivo; it also contained substantial levels of this carcinogen. Generally however, nitrosamine contamination of drugs is rare (13).

Several routes can lead to nitrosamine contamination in pesticides (12). These include the use of contaminated starting materials for synthesis, various side reactions, and the use of nitrite as a corrosion inhibitor for metal containers. Nitrosamine contamination has been limited mainly to dinitroaniline herbicides, dimethylamine salts of phenoxyalkanoic acid herbicides, diethanolamine and triethanolamine salts of acid pesticides, quarternary ammonium compounds, and morpholine derivatives. In general, the main exposure to nitrosamines in these products would be confined to workers employed in their preparation and to farmers using contaminated products (12).

### Summary of Exogenous Exposures to Nitrosamines

In nonoccupational settings, tobacco products represent by far the greatest source of carcinogenic nitrosamine

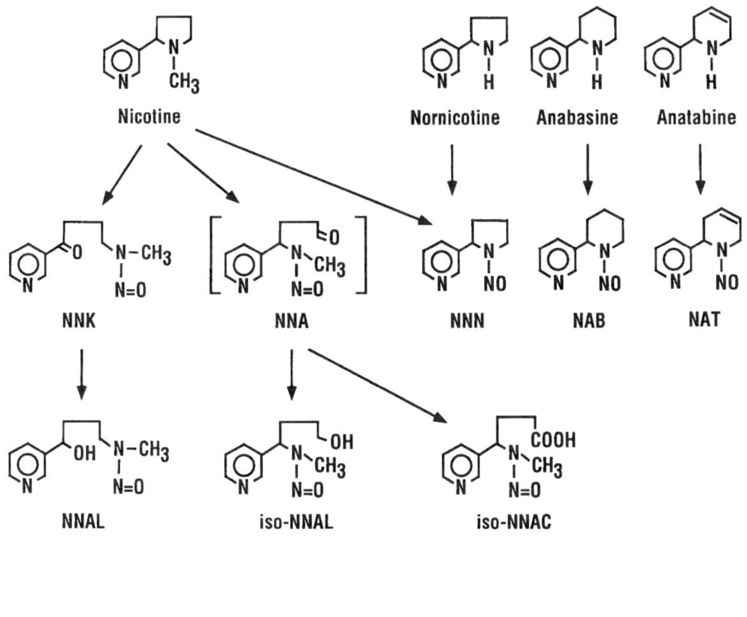


**FIG. 2.** Structures of tobacco-specific nitrosamines and their tobacco alkaloid precursors. The nitrosamines NNK, NNN, NAB, NAT, NNAL, *iso*-NNAL, and *iso*-NNAC have been detected in tobacco products.

exposure. Total exposure to volatile and tobacco-specific nitrosamines is at least 10 times greater through inhalation of cigarette smoke than by dietary exposure or by contact with other products. A person who smokes 20 cigarettes per day will inhale about 10 μg of carcinogenic nitrosamines, while dietary exposure seldom exceeds 1 μg per day. Exposure to nitrosamines through snuff-dipping is likely to be about 10 times greater than from cigarette smoking. Occupational exposures may be significant, especially in the rubber and metal-working industries.

### Endogenous Formation of Nitrosamines

Nitrosamines can readily form in the acidic environment of the stomach (14,22). Under acidic conditions, nitrite will form nitrous acid ($HNO_2$), which dimerizes with loss of water to give $N_2O_3$. This reacts with amines producing nitrosamines. Thus, animals exposed to amines and nitrite develop tumors typical of the resulting nitrosamines. However, nitrosamine formation is not limited to the acidic environment of the stomach. Activated macrophages and other cell types produce nitric oxide (NO) from arginine by the inducible NO synthase pathway (13,14,23–25). Thus, under conditions of chronic inflammation or infection, substantial amounts of NO are produced. This reacts with dissolved oxygen to give $N_2O_3$ and $N_2O_4$, which can nitrosate amines. Nitrosamine production has been confirmed in animals treated with lipopolysaccharide or infected with hepatitis virus (24,25). Bacterial strains isolated from human infections can also catalyze nitrosation of amines (13).

The endogenous formation of nitrosamines in humans has been repeatedly demonstrated by analysis of nitrosamino acids, particularly *N*-nitrosoproline (NPRO), in urine (26). Human urine contains several nitrosamino acids: NPRO; *N*-nitrososarcosine (NSAR); *N*-nitrosothiazolidine-4-carboxylic acid (NTCA); *trans*- and *cis* -isomers of *N*-nitroso-2-methylthiazolidine 4-carboxylic acid (NMTCA); 3-(*N*-nitroso-*N*-methylamino)propionic acid (NMPA); *N*-nitrosotetrahydro-4*H*-1,3-thiazine 4-carboxylic acid (NTHTCA); and *N*-nitrosoazetidine-2-carboxylic acid (NAZCA). Their structures are shown in Fig. 3. The most prevalent are NPRO, which is normally excreted in amounts of about 3 μg per day, and NTCA, NMTCA, and NSAR, total about 25 μg per day. Since NPRO is noncarcinogenic and is not metabolized, studies on its formation have been carried out in humans who ingested nitrate and proline with or without dietary nitrosation modifiers. The results of these studies demonstrated that in vivo nitrosation occurs in humans and can be inhibited by dietary constituents such as vitamins C and E. A test for endogenous nitrosation—the NPRO test—has been employed widely in studies of human populations. Using this test, elevated exposure to nitroso compounds has been demonstrated in subjects at high risk of various cancers including stomach, esophagus, oral cavity, nasopharynx, and aerodigestive tract (13,26). Endogenous nitrosation can be inhibited by ascorbic acid, which acts as a nitrite scavenger.

## METABOLIC ACTIVATION AND DETOXIFICATION OF NITROSAMINES

Nitrosamines are relatively unreactive and require enzymatic activation to intermediates which that bind to DNA, initiating the carcinogenic process (27). There are competing detoxification reactions. The metabolic activation of nitrosamines is catalyzed by members of the cytochrome P-450 enzyme family. Hydroxylation of the carbon atom next to the nitrosamino group, a reaction called α-hydroxylation, is a well-recognized metabolic activation process for many nitrosamines. This is illustrated for dialkylnitrosamines in Fig. 4. The resulting product is an α-hydroxydialkylnitrosamine, which can be generated in situ by hydrolysis of the corresponding α-acetoxynitrosamine. α-Hydroxynitrosamines have a half-life of up to 10 seconds under physiologic conditions (28). They spontaneously decompose to an aldehyde and a diazohydroxide. The latter dissociates to a diazonium hydroxide and ultimately to a carbocation, depending on the nature of the R group. The diazohydroxide and subsequent intermediates are highly electrophilic. Their major reaction is with $H_2O$, giving an alcohol, but they also react with DNA to produce a variety of alkylated

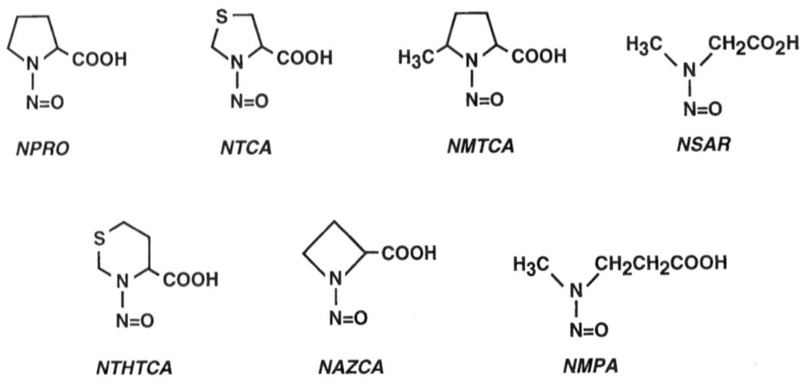


**FIG. 3.** Structures of nitrosamino acids present in human urine.

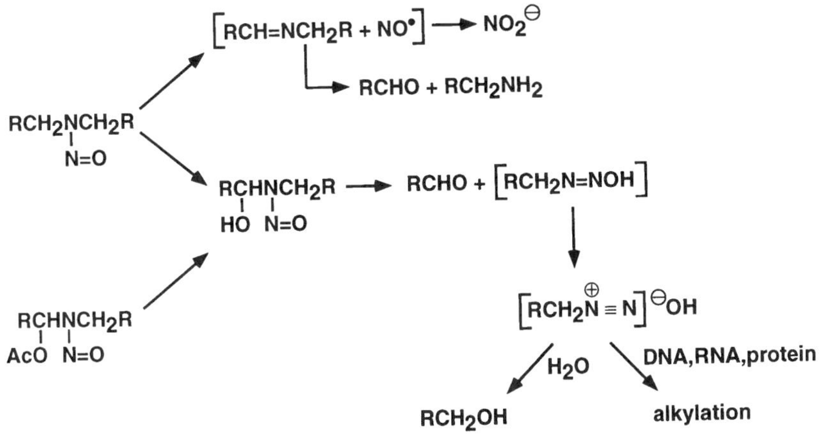


**FIG. 4.** Metabolic activation and detoxification of dialkylnitrosamines.

DNA bases. Detoxification by denitrosation competes with this metabolic activation process (29). The denitrosation is also catalyzed by cytochromes P-450 and results ultimately in the production of nitrite, an aldehyde, and a primary amine.

The reaction pathways illustrated in Fig. 4 have been most extensively studied for NDMA (R=H). Cytochrome P-450 2E1 is the major enzyme involved in the production of α-hydroxyNDMA, which fragments to yield formaldehyde and the methanediazonium ion (30). The latter is typical of alkylating agents that react with DNA and RNA at a number of different sites, including N-7, N-3, N-1, $N^2$, and $O^6$ of guanine; N-3, $O^2$, and $O^4$ of thymidine or uridine; N-3, $O^2$, or $N^4$ of cytidine; N-1, N-7, N-3, and $N^6$ of adenosine, as well as the phosphate backbone (31,32). Upon administration of NDMA to rats, 7-methylguanine is quantitatively the most significant adduct formed with DNA bases, but $O^6$-methylguanine, produced initially in one-tenth the amount as 7-methylguanine, is believed to be responsible for the carcinogenic effects of NDMA. This adduct is promutagenic, causing GC-AT transition mutations (33,34). A DNA repair protein, $O^6$-alkylguanine-DNA-alkyltransferase, can remove the methyl group from $O^6$-methylguanine, reconverting it to guanine (35). When this repair protein is depleted, $O^6$-methylguanine can accumulate, resulting in critical mutations in oncogenes and tumor suppressor genes. Such gene changes lead to derangement of normal cellular growth conrol processes, and ultimately to cancer. Thus, formation of the methanediazonium ion via α-hydroxylation is the key step in NDMA metabolic activation; in the absence of this reaction, tumors will not be formed. α-Hydroxylation is also involved in NDMA hepatotoxicity (36). Denitrosation accounts for 15% to 30% of NDMA metabolism and is thought to be a detoxification pathway (29,36).

While cytochrome P-450 2E1 is the major enzyme involved in NDMA metabolism, higher dialkylnitrosamines are not efficiently oxidized by this enzyme. Instead, a variety of other cytochrome P-450 enzymes are involved, with specificity depending on the nature of the alkyl chains (37,38). Metabolic activation of NDEA ($R=CH_3$) proceeds by α-hydroxylation, resulting in ethylation of DNA. $O^2$-Ethylthymine and $O^4$-ethylthymine are quantitatively minor adducts initially. However, they are repaired inefficiently, leading to their persistence and accumulation in hepatocyte DNA. They appear to be important in the induction of hepatocellular carcinoma by NDEA (39).

The metabolic activation of *N*-nitrosodipropylamine ($R=C_2H_5$) is more complex than that of NDMA and NDEA (27). This nitrosamine methylates DNA, in addition to the expected propylation reaction. In fact, 7-methylguanine is the major alkylation product in hepatic DNA after administration of *N*-nitrosodipropylamine to rats. The mechanism of this reaction involves initial hydroxylation of the β-carbon, followed by oxidation to give *N*-nitroso-2-oxopropylpropylamine. α-Hydroxylation on the propyl group produces 2-oxopropyldiazotate, which rearranges to give the methylating agent diazomethane. *N*-Nitrosodibutylamine ($R=CH_3CH_2CH_2$) and *N*-nitrosobutyl(4-hydroxybutyl)amine, bladder carcinogens in the rat, undergo ω, ω-1, and ω-2 oxidations. The major proximate carcinogen is believed to be *N*-nitrosobutyl-3-carboxypropylamine (40). β-Hydroxylation of this compound on the carboxypropyl chain ultimately results in loss of a 2 carbon fragment, analogous to fatty acid metabolism. Thus, Okada (40) proposed that *N*-nitrosomethylalkylamines with an even number of carbon atoms in the alkyl chain would produce *N*-nitrosomethyl-3-carboxypropylamine and would be bladder carcinogens, in contrast to those with an odd number of carbon atoms in the alkyl chain. This proposal is supported by the data in Table 1 (8).

*N*-Nitrosomethyl-*n*-amylamine is a powerful esophageal carcinogen. It undergoes hydroxylation at the 2-, 3-, and 4-positions of the amyl chain, as well as the expected α-hydroxylation reactions leading to formaldehyde and pentaldehyde (14). The latter process produces methanediazohydroxide and methylation of esophageal DNA.

NNK is a tobacco-specific nitrosamine and a potent and selective lung carcinogen in rats, mice, and hamsters

(17,18). The lung is the primary target for NNK carcinogenesis in the rat, independent of the route of administration. Thus, adenoma and adenocarcinoma of the lung are the major tumor types induced by NNK in the rat, whether it is administered by subcutaneous injection, in the drinking water, by oral swabbing, or by instillation in the bladder (8,18). The metabolism of NNK is summarized in Fig. 5 (41). The presence of the pyridine ring and carbonyl group lead to a somewhat more complex series of reactions than observed for simple dialkylnitrosamines. The major pathway of NNK metabolism in laboratory animals and humans is reduction of the carbonyl group, catalyzed by carbonyl reductase enzymes such as 11-β-hydroxysteroid dehydrogenase (42). The product, NNAL, is also a potent pulmonary carcinogen and appears to be the major transport form of NNK (43,44). Glucuronidation of NNAL produces NNAL-Gluc, which is excreted in the urine of laboratory animals and humans, and is believed to be a detoxification product of NNK (45–47). Other detoxification products are NNK-*N*-oxide and NNAL-*N*-oxide, resulting from cytochrome P-450 catalyzed oxidation of the pyridine ring. An interesting series of products is formed *in vitro*, by substitution of NNK or NNAL for nicotinamide in reduced nicotinamide adenine dinucleotide phosphate (NADPH), catalyzed by $NAD^+$ glycohydrolase (48). The α-hydroxylation pathways of NNK result in intermediates that methylate and pyridyloxobutylate DNA. The strong pulmonary tumorigenicity of NNK is associated with the formation and persistence of the resulting adducts in the Clara and type II cells of the rat lung (49,50). Studies in the A/J mouse, which is highly sensitive to lung tumor induction by NNK, have demonstrated the importance of persistent $O^6$-methylguanine in tumor formation (51). G-A mutations in codon 12 of the K-*ras* gene of these lung tumors appear to result from this persistent $O^6$-methylguanine (52).

The metabolism of cyclic nitrosamines follows pathways similar to those of acyclic nitrosamines, with one critical difference (53). α-Hydroxylation generates an intermediate in which the diazohydroxide and aldehyde functionality are in the same molecule, instead of being produced as independent moieties. These diazohydroxide aldehydes have chemical properties that are different from the simple alkylating agents. The result is a complex array of DNA modification products. This is illustrated for NPYR in Fig. 6 (54,55). Adducts *5*, *6*, *7*, *11*, and *12* to *14* have been detected *in vitro*, while adducts *5*, *6*, and *12* have been found in the liver of NPYR treated rats. These adducts as well as the major metabolites of NPYR such as 2-hydroxytetrahydrofuran (*10*) and crotonaldehyde (*9*) result from α-hydroxylation (53,56).

People who use tobacco products are exposed to substantial quantities of the cyclic nitrosamine NNN. Its metabolism is summarized in Fig. 7 (57–61). Formation of NNN-*N*-oxide by pyridine *N*-oxidation and norcotinine

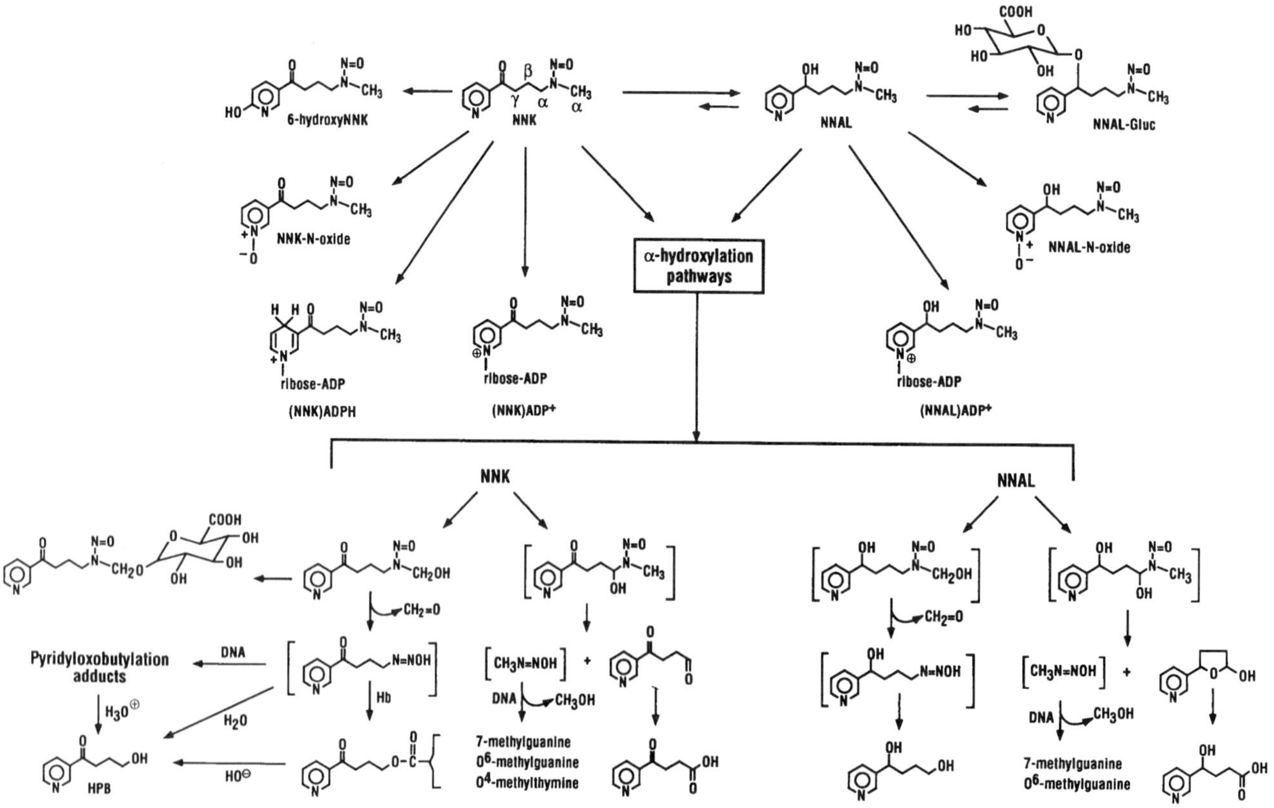


**FIG. 5.** Metabolism of NNK (see ref. 41).

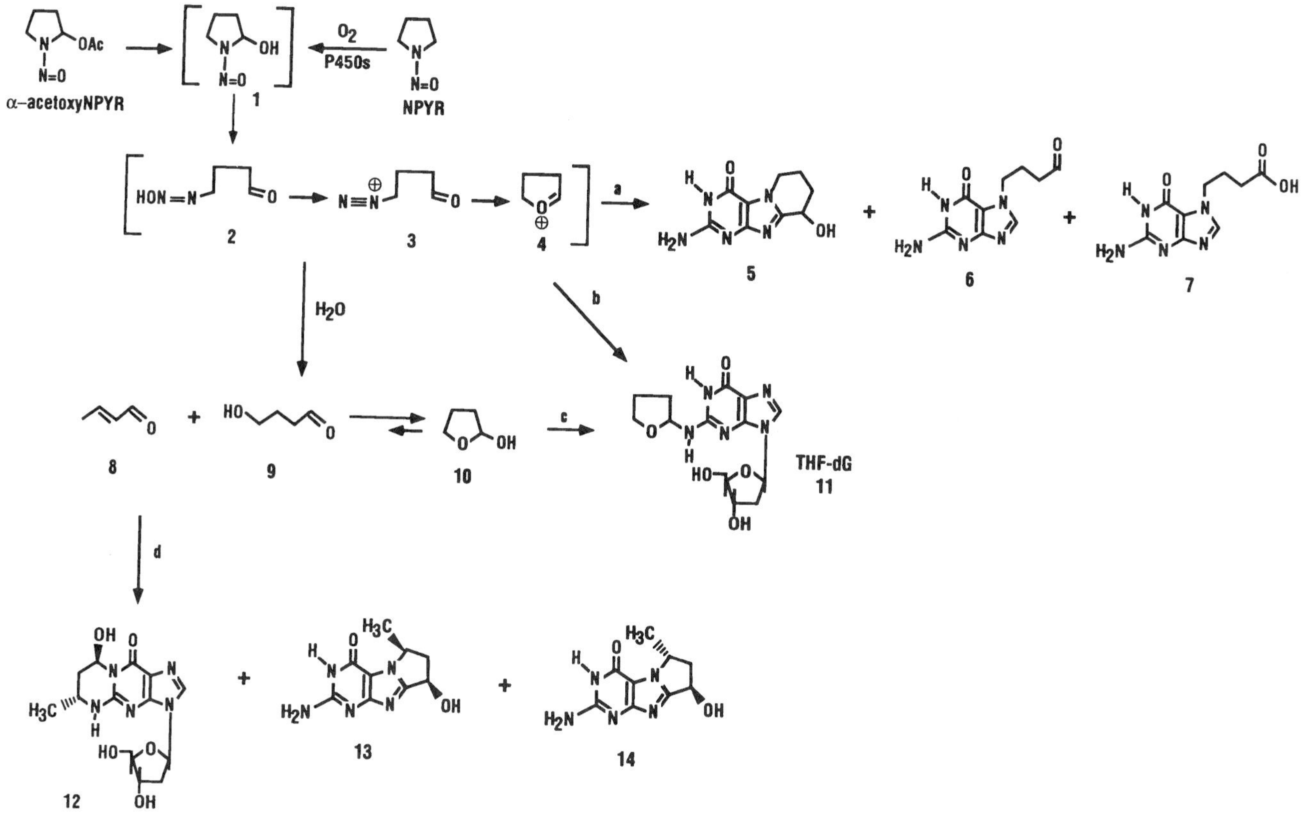


**FIG. 6.** DNA adduct formation upon α-hydroxylation of NPYR (see refs. 54, 55).

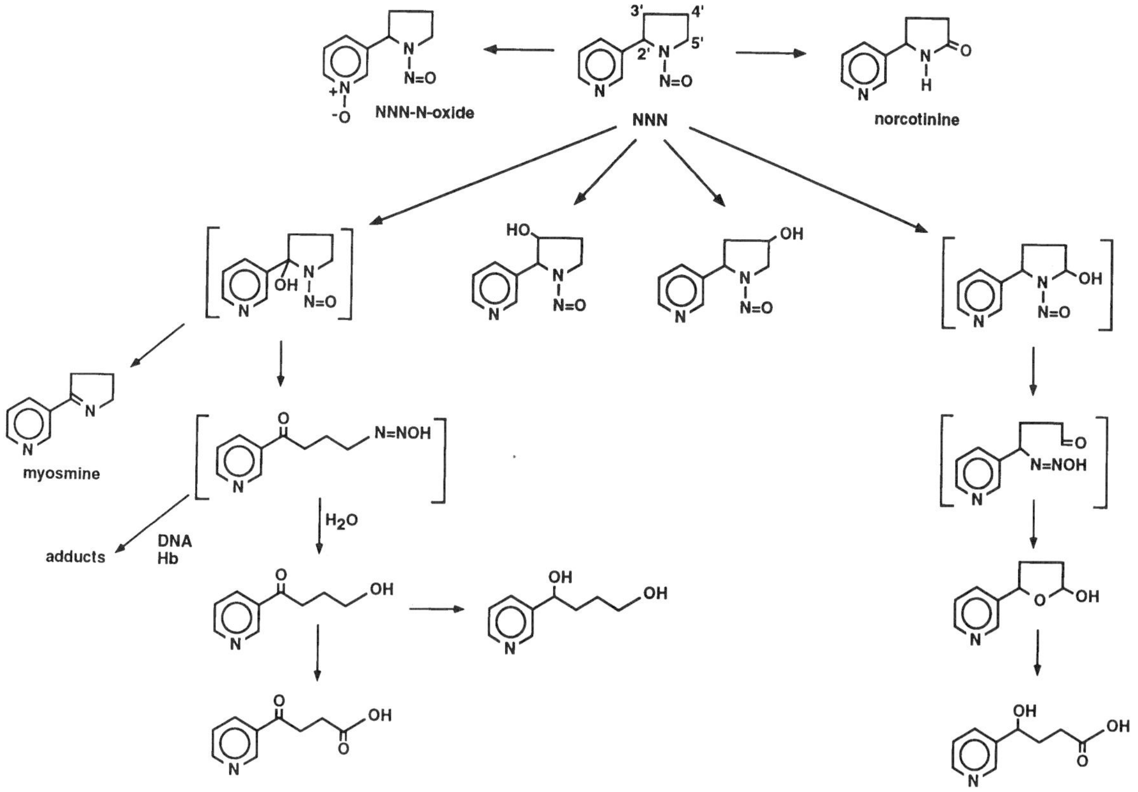


**FIG. 7.** Metabolism of NNN (see refs. 57–62).

by denitrosation and oxidation are considered to be detoxification reactions. In rodents, α-hydroxylation at the 2′ and 5′ positions of the pyrrolidine ring far exceeds β-hydroxylation at the 3′ and 4′ positions. 2′-Hydroxylation results in DNA adduct formation in the rat esophagus and is catalyzed by a high-affinity cytochrome P-450 enzyme (61,62). This reaction is probably responsible for the esophageal carcinogenicity of NNN. In rodent and human liver, 5′-hydroxylation greatly exceeds 2′-hydroxylation (60,61). The role of 5′-hydroxylation as an activation or detoxification pathway of NNN is not clear at present.

**Role of Nitrosamines in Human Cancer**

The evidence that humans would be susceptible to cancer induction by nitrosamines is overwhelming (63). As discussed above, nitrosamines are potent carcinogens that are effective in a wide variety of animal species. The same routes of metabolic activation are observed in humans and animals. Although there have been no epidemiologic studies that specifically relate nitrosamine exposure to cancer in humans, there is a large body of evidence that indicates that nitrosamines are important causative agents for several types of human cancer.

The strongest link between nitrosamine exposure and cancer induction is for cancer of the oral cavity in people who use snuff and other smokeless tobacco products (19,63–66). Snuff-dipping, the practice of placing tobacco between the cheek and gum, is an established cause of oral cancer (67). The tobacco-specific nitrosamines NNN and NNK are the most prevalent strong carcinogens in unburned tobacco (19). A mixture of NNN and NNK induces oral cavity tumors in rats (68). Exposure to NNN and NNK is so extensive through the use of snuff that the dose experienced by a snuff-dipper approaches or exceeds that employed to induce oral cavity tumors in rats (19). In the Sudan, oral consumption of *toombak*, a local tobacco product that contains extremely high levels of tobacco-specific nitrosamines, has been proposed as a cause of oral cancer in that country (69). Oral cancer is the leading cancer in India and is caused by consumption of betel quids and related preparations containing tobacco (67). These products are rich in tobacco-specific nitrosamines as well as areca-specific nitrosamines, generated by nitrosation alkaloids of the areca nut, a constituent of the betel quid (67).

The role of nitrosamines in cancer induction by tobacco smoke is more difficult to assess because tobacco smoke is a combustion product that is richer in carcinogens than is unburned tobacco. Nevertheless, there is substantial evidence that tobacco-specific nitrosamines play an important role as causative agents for cancer in smokers. Based on the concentrations of NNK in cigarette smoke, its selectivity for induction of lung tumors in rodents, and on biochemical and molecular biologic evidence, it is very likely that NNK is one of the major causes of lung cancer in smokers, particularly adenocarcinoma (17–19,70–72). Smoking is the major cause of esophageal cancer in the United States and other developed countries. Nitrosamines are powerful esophageal carcinogens and NNN is the most prevalent of these in cigarette smoke. NNN induces tumors of the esophagus in rats and is likely to play an important role in esophageal cancer induction in humans (19). Smoking is an important cause of pancreatic cancer (73,74). NNK and its metabolite NNAL are the only compounds in tobacco smoke known to induce pancreatic tumors in laboratory animals. The extensive exposure to these compounds through smoking supports their role as etiologic factors for this deadly disease.

Cancer of the esophagus occurs in very high incidences in some parts of China, South Africa, and Iran (13,14,26). Smoking and drinking, the main cause of esophageal cancer in most Western countries, is not implicated in these areas. Investigations in China have revealed correlations between esophageal cancer mortality rates and urinary nitrosamino acids, including nitrososarcosine, an esophageal carcinogen. The potential for endogenous nitrosation is also higher in high-risk areas of China (75). Nitrosamine contamination of moldy foods has been implicated as one causative factor for esophageal cancer in China and South Africa. Other studies have demonstrated the presence of $O^6$-methylguanine in esophageal DNA in high risk areas of China (76).

The incidence of cholangiocarcinoma is unusually high in Northeast Thailand, where 30% to 40% of the population is infected with the liver fluke, *Opisthorchis viverrini*. Evidence is accumulating that nitrosamines are endogenously generated in infected individuals, via nitrosating agents generated by inducible nitric oxide synthase (77). Elevated endogenous nitrosation has been observed in infected individuals and this can be blocked by ascorbic acid (13). Moreover, recent evidence indicates that cytochrome P-450 2A6, implicated in the metabolic activation of several nitrosamines, is induced in infected individuals (77).

Nasopharyngeal cancer is common in southern China (14). Its incidence was correlated with excretion of NPRO in studies carried out in China (75,78). Intake of salted fish has been strongly implicated as a causative factor (79). Nitrosamines such as NDMA have been detected in steamed salted fish, and their levels are higher in high-risk areas. Rats fed Cantonese salted dried fish developed nasal carcinoma, and nitrosamines are highly effective nasal carcinogens in rodents (8,14). Collectively, these data strongly implicate nitrosamines as causative factors for nasopharyngeal cancer (14,66).

Rates of bladder cancer are extraordinarily high in Egypt, particularly in males (64). Schistosomiasis, also known as bilharziasis, is common in the Nile valley, occurring due to work in irrigated fields. Schistomiasis infection results in elevated urinary nitrite excretion and a significant increase in urinary nitrosamines (80) This results either from bacterial nitrosation or stimulation of the NO synthase pathway due to inflammation. Certain nitrosamines are very effective bladder carcinogens, and production of bladder cancer has been noted in baboons treated with *N*-nitosobutyl(4-hydroxybutyl)amine and infected with schistosomiasis (81).

## SUMMARY

Nitrosamines are a large group of versatile carcinogens, inducing tumors at many important sites of human cancers. They are complete carcinogens that readily cause tumors without need for promoting or cocarcinogenic agents. Nitrosamines are quite selective for tumor induction at specific sites, depending on their structures. They are metabolically activated to DNA-damaging species by a simple cytochrome P-450 catalyzed hydroxylation step. There can be no question that humans exposed to sufficient amounts of nitrosamines would be susceptible to their carcinogenic effects. Human exposure does occur widely, although with the exception of tobacco products, exposures have decreased due to preventive measures. Endogenous formation of nitrosamines, however, can be extensive. Considerable evidence is available that nitrosamines are important causative agents for a number of different human cancer types including cancers of the oral cavity, lung, esophagus, pancreas, liver, nasopharynx, and bladder.

## REFERENCES

1. Barnes JM, Magee PN. Some toxic properties of dimethylnitrosamine. *Br J Ind Med* 1954;11:167–174.
2. Magee PN, Barnes JM. The production of malignant primary hepatic tumors in the rat by feeding dimethylnitrosamine. *Br J Cancer* 1956;10: 114–122.
3. Freund HA. Clinical manifestations and studies in parenchymatous hepatitis. *Ann Intern Med* 1937;10:1144–1155.
4. Cooper, SW, Kimbrough, RD, Kimbrough, LLB. Acute dimethylnitrosamine poisoning outbreak. *J Forensic Sci* 1980; 874–882.
5. Herron, DC, Shank, RC. Methylated purines in human liver DNA after probable dimethylnitrosamine poisoning. *Cancer Res* 1980;40: 3116–3117.
6. Druckrey H, Preussmann R, Ivankovic S, Schmähl D. Organotrope Carcinogen Wirkungen bei 65 verschiedenen *N*-Nitrosoverbindungen an BD-ratten. *Z Krebsforsch* 1967;69:103–201.
7. Preussmann R, Stewart BW. *N*-nitroso carcinogens. In: Searle C, ed. *Chemical Carcinogens,* 2nd ed., vol 2. ACS Monograph 182. Washington, DC: American Chemical Society, 1981;643–828.
8. Lijinsky W. *Chemistry and biology of N-nitroso compounds.* Cambridge monographs on cancer research. Cambridge, UK: Cambridge University Press, 1992;251–403.
9. Peto R, Gray R, Brantom P, Grasso P. Effects on 4080 rats of chronic administration of *N*-nitrosodiethylamine or *N*-nitrosodimethylamine: a detailed dose-response study. *Cancer Res* 1991;51:6415–6451.
10. Bogovski P, Bogovski S. Animal species in which *N*-nitroso compounds induce cancer. *Int J Cancer* 1981;27:471–474.
11. Fine DH, Rounbehler DP. Trace analysis of volatile *N*-nitroso compounds by combined gas chromatography and thermal energy analysis. *J Chromatogr* 1975;109:271–279.
12. Tricker AR, Spiegelhalder B, Preussmann R. Environmental exposure to preformed nitroso compounds. *Cancer Surv* 1989;8:251–272.
13. Bartsch H, Spiegelhalder B. Environmental exposure to *N*-nitroso compounds (NNOC) and precursors: an overview. *Eur J Cancer Prev* 1996; 5(suppl 1):11–18.
14. Mirvish SS. Role of *N*-nitroso compounds (NOC) and *N*-nitrosation in etiology of gastric, esophageal, nasopharyngeal and bladder cancer and contribution to cancer of known exposures to NOC. *Cancer Lett* 1995; 93:17–48.
15. Hotchkiss JH. Preformed *N*-nitroso compounds in foods and beverages. *Cancer Surv* 1989;8:295–321.
16. Reh BD, Fajen JM. Worker exposures to nitrosamines in a rubber vehicle sealing plant. *Am Ind Hyg Assoc J* 1996;57:918–923.
17. Hoffmann D. Hecht SS. Nicotine-derived *N*-nitrosamines and tobacco related cancer: current status and future directions. *Cancer Res* 1985; 45:935–944.
18. Hecht SS, Hoffmann D. Tobacco-specific nitrosamines, an important group of carcinogens in tobacco and tobacco smoke. *Carcinogenesis* 1988;9:875–884.
19. Hecht SS, Hoffmann D. The relevance of tobacco-specific nitrosamines to human cancer. *Cancer Surv* 1989;8:273–294.
20. Assembly of Life Sciences. *The health effects of nitrate, nitrite, and N-nitroso compounds.* Washington, DC: National Academy Press, 1981; 3–51.
21. Havery DC, Chou HJ. Nitrosamines in sunscreens and cosmetic products: occurrence, formation, and trends. In: Loeppky RN, Michejda CJ, eds. *Nitrosamines and related N-nitroso compounds:* chemistry and biochemistry. ACS Symposium Series 553. Washington, DC: American Chemical Society, 1994;20–33.
22. Mirvish SS. Formation of *N*-nitroso compounds: chemistry, kinetics, and in vivo occurrence. *Toxicol Appl Pharmacol* 1975;31:325–351.
23. Marletta MA. Mammalian synthesis of nitrite, nitrate, nitric oxidee, and *N*-nitrosating agents. *Chem Res Toxicol* 1988;1:249–257.
24. Liu RH, Baldwin B, Tennant BC, Hotchkiss JH. Elevated formation of nitrate and *N*-nitrosodimethylamine in woodchucks *(Marmota monax)* associated with chronic woodchuck hepatitis virus infection. *Cancer Res* 1991;51:3925–3929.
25. Leaf CD, Wishnok JS, Tannenbaum SR. Mechanisms of endogenous nitrosation. *Cancer Surv* 1989;8:323–834.
26. Bartsch H, Ohshima H, Pignatelli B, Calmels S. Human exposure to endogenous *N*-nitroso compounds: quantitative estimates in subjects at high risk for cancer of the oral cavity, oesophagus, stomach and urinary bladder. *Cancer Surv* 1989;8:335–362.
27. Archer MC. Mechanisms of action of *N*-nitroso compounds. *Cancer Surv* 1989;8:241–250.
28. Mochizuki M, Anjo T, Okada M. Isolation and characterization of *N*-alkyl- *N*-(hydroxymethyl)nitrosamines from *N*-alkyl-*N*-(hydroperoxymethyl) nitrosamines by deoxygenation. *Tetrahedron Lett* 1980;21: 3693–3696.
29. Streeter AJ, Nims RW, Sheffels PR, et al. Metabolic denitrosation of *N*-nitrosodimethylamine in vivo in the rat. *Cancer Res* 1990;50: 1144–1150.
30. Yang CS, Yoo JSH, Ishizaki H, Hong J. Cytochrome P-450IIE1: roles in nitrosamine metabolism and mechanisms of regulation. *Drug Metab Rev* 1990;22:147–159.
31. Margison GP, O'Connor PJ. Nucleic acid modification by *N*-nitroso compounds. In: Grover PL, ed. *Chemical carcinogens and DNA.* Boca Raton, FL: CRC Press, 1979;111–151.
32. Singer B, Grunberger D. *Molecular biology of mutagens and carcinogens.* New York: Plenum Press, 1983;68–78.
33. Loveless A. Possible relevance of 0-6 alkylation of deoxyguanosine to the mutagenicity and carcinogenicity of nitrosamines and nitrosamides. *Nature* 1969;233:206–207.
34. Loechler EL, Green CL, Essigmann JM. In vivo mutagenesis by $O^6$-methylguanine built into a unique site in a viral genome. *Proc Natl Acad Sci USA* 1984;8:6271–6275.
35. Pegg AE, Dolan ME, Moschel RC. Structure, function and inhibition of $O^6$-alkylguanine-DNA alkyltransferase. *Prog Nucleic Acid Res Mol Biol* 1995;51:167–223.
36. Lee VM, Keefer LK, Archer MC. An evaluation of the roles of metabolic denitrosation and α-hydroxylation in the hepatotoxicity of *N*-nitrosodimethylamine. *Chem Res Toxicol* 1996;9:1319–1324.
37. Lee M, Ishizaki H, Brady JF, Yang CS. Substrate specificity and alkyl group selectivity in the metabolism of *N*-nitrosodialkylamines. *Cancer Res* 1989;49:1470–1474.
38. Bellec G, Dreano Y, Lozach P, Menez JF, Berthou F. Cytochrome P-450

metabolic dealkylation of nine *N*-nitrosodialkylamines by human liver microsomes. *Carcinogenesis* 1996;17:2029–2034.

39. Swenberg JA, Hoel DG, Magee PN. Mechanistic and statistical insight into the large carcinogenesis bioassays on *N*-nitrosodiethylamine and *N*-nitrosodimethylamine. *Cancer Res* 1991;51:6409–6414.
40. Okada M. Comparative metabolism of *N*-nitrosamines in relation to their organ and species specificity. In: O'Neill JK, Von Borstel RC, Miller CT, Long J, Bartsch H, eds. *N-nitroso compounds: occurrence, biological effects and relevance to human cancer.* IARC Scientific Publications No. 57. Lyon, France: International Agency for Research on Cancer, 1984;401–409.
41. Hecht SS. Recent studies on mechanisms of bioactivation and detoxification of 4-(methylnitrosamino)-1-(3-pyridyl)-1-butanone (NNK), a tobacco-specific lung carcinogen. *CRC Crit Rev Toxicol* 1996;26: 163–181.
42. Maser G, Richter E, Friebertshauser J. The identification of 11 beta-hydroxysteroid dehydrogenase as carbonyl reductase of the tobacco-specific nitrosamine 4-(methyl)-nitrosamino-1-(3-pyridyl)-1-butanone. *Eur J Biochem* 1996;238:484–489.
43. Castonguay A, Lin D, Stoner GD, et al. Comparative carcinogenicity in A/J mice and metabolism by cultured mouse peripheral lung of N′-nitrosonornicotine, 4-(methylnitrosamino)-1-(3-pyridyl)-1-butanone and their analogues. *Cancer Res* 1983;43:1223–1229.
44. Rivenson A, Hoffmann D, Prokopczyk B, Amin S, Hecht SS. Induction of lung and exocrine pancreas tumors in F344 rats by tobacco-specific and Areca-derived *N*-nitrosamines. *Cancer Res* 1988;48:6912–6917.
45. Morse MA, Eklind KI, Toussaint M, Amin SG, Chung FL. Characterization of a glucuronide metabolite of 4-(methylnitrosamino)-1-(3-pyridyl)-1-butanone (NNK) and its dose-dependent excretion in the urine of mice and rats. *Carcinogenesis* 1990;11:1819–1823.
46. Hecht SS, Trushin N, Reid-Quinn CA, et al. Metabolism of the tobacco-specific nitrosamine 4-(methylnitrosamino)-1-(3-pyridyl)-1-butanone in the Patas monkey: pharmacokinetics and characterization of glucuronide metabolites. *Carcinogenesis* 1993;14:229–236.
47. Carmella SG, Akerkar S, Richie JP Jr, Hecht SS. Intraindividual and interindividual differences in metabolites of the tobacco-specific lung carcinogen 4-(methylnitrosamino)-1-(3-pyridyl)-1-butanone (NNK) in smokers' urine. *Cancer Epidemiol Biomarkers Prev* 1995;4:635–642.
48. Peterson LA, Ng DK, Stearns RA, Hecht SS. Formation of NADP(H) analogs of tobacco specific nitrosamines in rat liver and pancreatic microsomes. *Chem Res Toxicol* 1994;7:599–608.
49. Belinsky, SA, Foley JF, White CM, Anderson MW, Maronpot RR. Dose response relationship between $O^6$-methylguanine formation in Clara cells and induction of pulmonary neoplasia in the rat by 4-(methylnitrosamino)-1-(3-pyridyl)-1-butanone. *Cancer Res* 1990;50:3772–3780.
50. Staretz ME, Foiles PG, Miglietta LM, Hecht SS. Evidence for an important role of DNA pyridyloxobutylation in rat lung carcinogenesis by 4-(methylnitrosamino)-1-(3-pyridyl)-1-butanone: effects of dose and phenethyl isothiocyanate. *Cancer Res* 1997;57:259–266.
51. Peterson LA, Hecht SS. $O^6$-Methylguanine is a critical determinant of 4-(methylnitrosamino)-1-(3-pyridyl)-1-butanone tumorigenesis in A/J mouse lung. *Cancer Res* 1991;51:5557–5564.
52. Belinsky SA, Devereux TR, Maronpot RR, Stoner GD, Anderson MW. The relationship between the formation of promutagenic adducts and the activation of the K-*ras* proto-oncogene in lung tumors from A/J mice treated with nitrosamines. *Cancer Res* 1989;49:5305–5311.
53. Hecht SS, McCoy GD, Chen CB, Hoffmann D. The metabolism of cyclic nitrosamines. In: Scanlan RA, Tannenbaum SR, eds. *N-nitroso compounds.* Washington, DC: American Chemical Society, 1981;49–75.
54. Young-Sciame R, Wang M, Chung F-L, Hecht SS. Reactions of α-acetoxy-*N*-nitrosopyrrolidine and α-acetoxy-*N*-nitrosopiperidine with deoxyguanosine: formation of $N^2$-tetrahydrofuranyl or $N^2$-tetrahydropyranyl adducts. *Chem Res Toxicol* 1995;8:607–616.
55. Wang M, Young-Sciame R, Chung F-L, Hecht SS. Formation of $N^2$-tetrahydrofuranyl and $N^2$-tetrahydropyranyl adducts in the reactions of α-acetoxy-*N*-nitrosopyrrolidine and α-acetoxy-*N*-nitrosopiperidine with DNA. *Chem Res Toxicol* 1995;8:617–624.
56. Wang M, Chung F-L, Hecht SS. Identification of crotonaldehyde as a hepatic microsomal metabolite formed by α-hydroxylation of the carcinogen *N*-nitrosopyrrolidine. *Chem Res Toxicol* 1988;1:28–31.
57. Hecht SS, Lin D, Chen CB. Comprehensive analysis of urinary metabolites of N'- nitrosonornicotine. *Carcinogenesis* 1981;2:833–838.
58. Hecht SS, Spratt TE, Trushin N. Evidence for 4-(3-pyridyl)-4-oxobutylation of DNA in F344 rats treated with the tobacco specific nitrosamines 4-(methylnitrosamino)-1-(3-pyridyl)- 1-butanone and N′-nitrosonornicotine. *Carcinogenesis* 1988;9:161–165.
59. Carmella SG Hecht SS. Formation of hemoglobin adducts upon treatment of F344 rats with the tobacco-specific nitrosamines 4-(methylnitrosamino)-1-(3-pyridyl)-1-butanone and N′-nitrosonornicotine. *Cancer Res* 1987;47:2626–2630.
60. Hecht SS, Castonguay A, Rivenson A, Mu B, Hoffmann D. Tobacco specific nitrosamines: carcinogenicity, metabolism, and possible role in human cancer. *J Environ Sci Health* 1983;C1:1–54.
61. Murphy SE, Heiblum R, Trushin N. Comparative metabolism of N′-nitrosonornicotine and 4-(methylnitrosamino)-1-(3-pyridyl)-1-butanone by cultured rat oral tissue and esophagus. *Cancer Res* 1990;50: 4685–4691.
62. Murphy SE, Spina DA. Evidence for a high affinity enzyme in rat esophageal microsomes which alpha-hydroxylates N′-nitrosonornicotine. *Carcinogenesis* 1994;15:2709–2713.
63. Magee PN. The experimental basis for the role of nitroso compounds in human cancer. *Cancer Surv* 1989;8:207–239.
64. Preston-Martin S, Correa P. Epidemiological evidence for the role of nitroso compounds in human cancer. *Cancer Surv* 1989;8:459–473.
65. Magee PN. Nitrosamines and human cancer: introduction and overview. *Eur J Cancer Prev* 1996;5(suppl 1):7–10.
66. Reed PI. *N*-nitroso compounds, their relevance to human cancer and further prospects for prevention. *Eur J Cancer Prev* 1996;5(suppl 1): 137–147.
67. International Agency for Research on Cancer. Tobacco habits other than smoking: betel quid and areca nut chewing; and some related nitrosamines. In: *IARC monographs on the evaluation of the carcinogenic risk of chemicals to humans,* vol 37. Lyon, France: IARC, 1985;37–202.
68. Hecht SS, Rivenson A, Braley J, DiBello J, Adams JD, Hoffmann D. Induction of oral cavity tumors in F344 rats by tobacco-specific nitrosamines and snuff. *Cancer Res* 1986;46:4162–4166.
69. Idris AM, Prokopczyk B, Hoffmann D. Toombak: a major risk factor for cancer of the oral cavity in Sudan. *Prev Med* 1994;23:832–839.
70. Hoffmann D, Hecht SS. Advances in tobacco carcinogenesis. In: Cooper CS, Grover PL, eds. *Handbook of experimental pharmacology.* Heidelberg: Springer-Verlag, 1990;63–102.
71. Hoffmann D, Rivenson A, Hecht SS. The biological significance of tobacco-specific *N*-nitrosamines: smoking and adenocarcinoma of the lung. *CRC Crit Rev Toxicol* 1996;26:199–211.
72. Hecht SS, Stoner GD. Lung and esophageal carcinogenesis. In: Aisner J, Ariagada R, Green MR, Martini N, Perry MC, eds. *Textbook on thoracic oncology.* Baltimore, MD: Williams and Wilkins, 1996;25–50.
73 International Agency for Research on Cancer. *Tobacco smoking IARC monographs on the evaluation of the carcinogenic risk of chemicals to humans,* vol 38. Lyon, France: International Agency for Research on Cancer, 1986.
74. Fuchs CS, Colditz GA, Stampfer MJ, et al. A prospective study of cigarette smoking and the risk of pancreatic cancer. *Arch Intern Med* 1996;156:2255–2260.
75. Wu Y, Chen J, Ohshima H, et al. Geographic associations between urinary excretion of *N*-nitroso compounds and oesophageal cancer mortality in China. *Int J Cancer* 1993;54:713–719.
76. Umbenhauer D, Wild CP, Montesano R, et al. $O^6$-Methyldeoxyguanosine in oesophageal DNA among individuals at high risk of oesophageal cancer. *Int J Cancer* 1985;36:661–665.
77. Satarug S, Lang, MA, Yongvanit P, et al. Induction of cytochrome P-450 2A6 expression in humans by the carcinogenic parasite infection, *opisthorchiasis viverrini. Cancer Epidemiol Biomarkers Prev* 1996;5: 795–800.
78. Zeng, Y, Ohshima H, Bouvier G, et al. Urinary excretion of nitrosamino acids and nitrate by inhabitants of high- and low-risk areas for nasopharyngeal carcinoma in southern China. *Cancer Epidemiol Biomarkers Prev* 1993;2:195–200.
79. Yu MC, Mo CC, Chong W-X, Yeh F-S, Henderson BE. Preserved foods and nasopharyngeal carcinoma: a case-control study in Guangxi, China. *Cancer Res* 1988;48:1954–1959.
80. Tricker AR. Excretion of *N*-nitrosamines in patients with bacterial bladder infections or diversions of the urinary tract. *Eur J Cancer Prev* 1996;5(suppl 1):95–99.
81. Hicks RM. Nitrosamines as possible etiologic agents in Bilharzial bladder cancer. In: Magee PN, ed. *Nitrosamines and human cancer.* Banbury Report 12. Cold Spring Harbor, NY: Cold Spring Harbor Laboratory, 1982;455–469.

*Environmental and Occupational Medicine, Third Edition,* edited by William N. Rom.
Published by Lippincott–Raven Publishers,
Philadelphia, 1998.

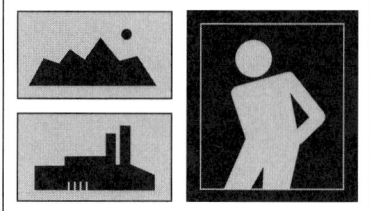

CHAPTER 91

# The Bhopal Disaster

James M. Melius

In 1984, one of the world's worst industrial disasters occurred in India (1). On December 3 of that year, a Union Carbide of India, Ltd. chemical plant located in Bhopal, India released over 30 tons of methyl isocyanate and other chemicals into the air over the city. Initial reports indicated that thousands of people had died and that many more were suffering severe medical effects from this exposure. As medical and disaster relief teams from throughout India rushed to Bhopal to help these victims, the world slowly learned more about the scope and cause of this disaster. Over 12 years later, we now have some results from the medical follow-up of these victims and can begin to recognize the longer term consequences from this disaster. We can also appreciate some of the impact of this tragedy on preventing similar disasters.

The Union Carbide of India plant had been built in Bhopal, India several years before the disaster. It manufactured a number of pesticides for nearby agricultural areas of central India. As part of the pesticide manufacturing process, the plant produced methyl isocyanate in a batch process. The methyl isocyanate was stored in stainless steel tanks and later reacted with other chemicals to produce carbamate pesticides. At the time of the incident, one of the storage tanks contained over 40 tons of methyl isocyanate. The most likely cause of the accident was that a quantity of water entered this storage tank some time on December 2, 1984 (2). The water reacted with the methyl isocyanate in an exothermic reaction leading to the buildup of heat and pressure in the storage tank. Workers on the evening shift at the plant reportedly noticed this pressure buildup, but the pressure did not reach catastrophic levels until around midnight. At around 12:30 the pressure was so great that a pressure release valve on the tank gave way, venting approximately 30 tons of methyl isocyanate and reaction by-products.

The plant was designed so that a release of methyl isocyanate would be prevented or mitigated by a number of safety mechanisms. The storage tanks were refrigerated to slow down any reaction. The release valves directed the vented methyl isocyanate to a caustic scrubber, which would cause a caustic solution to react with the methyl isocyanate to neutralize it. The vented methyl isocyanate was directed through a flare tower, which would burn it. There was also a water cascade system that would hose water over the storage tank area. Unfortunately, the refrigeration system, caustic scrubber, and flare tower were not operational at the time of the incident. The water cascade system would not reach the top of the tower, where the methyl isocyanate and reaction products were being released.

Gradually, over the next few hours in the early morning of December 3, the plant released approximately 30 tons of methyl isocyanate and reaction products into the air around the plant. Weather conditions in the early morning hours further contributed to the disaster. Winds were very light and blowing in the direction of the more heavily populated areas of Bhopal. The air was dry, and there was a temperature inversion, which kept the released methyl isocyanate close to the ground as it spread over the city, which was located on a flat plain near a lake.

The location of the plant near populated areas also enhanced the consequences from the release. It was located only a mile or so from the major population center of the city called Old Bhopal. The railway station was less than a mile from the plant. Directly across the street

J. M. Melius: New York State Laborer's Health and Safety Trust Fund, Albany, New York 12211.

from the plant, and approximately 100 yards from where the methyl isocyanate was released, there was a settlement of several thousand people living in poorly constructed housing, mainly shacks. As this cloud of methyl isocyanate and reaction products spread over the area around the plant, the health consequences were immediate. Thousands of people living in the area near the plant were affected. Some died in their sleep. Others suffering from the acute irritative properties of the methyl isocyanate (e.g., eye irritation, respiratory distress) struggled to escape. There was no organized evacuation; people just struggled to get away from the irritating gas without knowing in what direction to run. As the methyl isocyanate cloud spread over the city, more and more people were affected, and escape became increasingly difficult. Although methyl isocyanate concentrations decreased with distance from the plant, concentrations were sufficient to cause acute irritative symptoms in people living several miles from the plant. Gradually, over the night, the methyl isocyanate cloud dispersed.

The scale of the disaster, and the lack of information about what chemical had been released, made provision of medical care very difficult. The identity of the chemical released was not confirmed for medical care providers until a few days after the disaster. During the night, thousands of people made their way to nearby hospitals. The major hospital in the area treated an estimated 15,000 people during the night of the incident, and many thousands more were treated in other health care facilities in the city (1). Given the difficult circumstances, physicians in these hospitals did an excellent job of providing care (3). A standard protocol was established for those with ocular symptoms. Respiratory problems were treated symptomatically, but many people coming to the hospital were so severely affected that they died almost immediately.

In the days after the incident, it was estimated that nearly 100,000 people sought medical care for health problems caused by the exposure. Medical and disaster relief groups came from throughout India to assist. Temporary tent hospitals were set up throughout the city. In addition, medical teams went door to door in the severely affected areas to help provide medical care.

How many people died from the incident is difficult to estimate. Entire families died, leaving no survivors, and the high death toll and dislocation in the residential areas near the plant made accurate counts very difficult to obtain. Many deaths were not recorded at the time. The usual estimate of immediate deaths is on the order of 2,000 to 2,500, but some information supports a higher toll.

## METHYL ISOCYANATE TOXICITY

Methyl isocyanate is a clear, colorless liquid. It has a boiling point of 39°C and a vapor pressure of 348 mm Hg. It is used primarily as an intermediate in the production of carbamate pesticides and is not a common industrial chemical. Due to this limited use and the more complete information available on other, more widely used isocyanate compounds, relatively few studies had been conducted on the toxicity of methyl isocyanate prior to the Bhopal incident. However, after the disaster, the National Institute of Environmental Health Sciences, Union Carbide, and some university groups began further toxicologic studies of this chemical (4). These studies have provided considerable toxicologic information to help understand the health consequences of this disaster.

Methyl isocyanate is a very reactive chemical. Upon contact with exposed tissue, the methyl isocyanate may react to carbamylate hydroxyl groups, sulfhydryls, and imidazoles. This reaction in turn can interfere with enzyme activities. In addition, in aqueous solutions, methyl isocyanate may hydrolyze. This hydrolysis is a very exothermic reaction and directly could destroy tissue. These would appear to be the two major mechanisms for the acute toxicity of methyl isocyanate (4).

The immediate reactivity of methyl isocyanate limits its capacity for reacting with nonrespiratory tissues. Thus, while some studies have shown effects from direct exposures of tissue to methyl isocyanate (5,6) and others have shown evidence of some tissue uptake of methyl isocyanate in exposed animals (7,8), the clinical significance of these findings is not clear. More recent research has focused on mechanisms (e.g., carbamoylation, glutathione conjugation, or hydrolysis) that might account for toxic effects in distant tissues (9–11). The production of antibodies to methyl isocyanate in guinea pigs injected with the compound and the finding of low levels of these antibodies in the blood of people exposed in Bhopal does not appear to be clinically significant (12). Thus, most toxic effects from exposure to methyl isocyanate appear to be due to contact with the eye and respiratory tissues. Further work is needed to assess whether other mechanisms are a significant source for the clinical effects seen in exposed persons.

### Eye Effects

Since the Bhopal disaster, several animal studies have been conducted that attempt to re-create the type of exposure that occurred in Bhopal by exposing animals to high levels of methyl isocyanate over short periods of time (i.e., 15 minutes to 16 hours) (4,13). These studies have shown that such acute exposures cause severe eye irritation with erosion of the corneal epithelium (14). However, no evidence of permanent eye damage was found at the doses used in these studies (15).

### Pulmonary Effects

Methyl isocyanate is a sensory and pulmonary irritant. Inhalation exposure at levels of 30 to 200 ppm leads to respiratory distress with delayed breathing accompanied by a reduction in arterial pH and arterial oxygen levels (16). These effects appear to be due to small airway obstruction. Acute exposure is also followed by the development of other pulmonary changes that persist for months after initial exposure: intraluminal fibrosis, mild bronchitis and bronchiolitis, and mucous plugs that lead to obstructive changes in pulmonary function studies (17). Chronic alveolitis also developed in mice acutely exposed to methyl isocyanate, possibly related to damaged pulmonary clearance mechanisms (18,19). A 2-year follow-up of acutely exposed rats has shown persistent pulmonary fibrosis in animals exposed to 10 ppm or less for a single 2-hour period (20). This finding has been confirmed in other studies that have also demonstrated evidence of persistent activation of macrophages even after exposure has ceased (21,22).

### Other Health Effects

Other organ systems may be affected by methyl isocyanate, although some of these effects may be secondary to the pulmonary damage. Exposure of rats to 9 to 15 ppm methyl isocyanate for 3 hours on the 8th day of gestation led to resorption of over 75% of the implants (23). Preliminary findings from a 2-year follow-up of acutely exposed rats has shown an increase in the occurrence of pheochromocytomas of the adrenal medulla and, in only the male rats, adenomas of the pancreas. The significance of these findings is unclear (20).

## CLINICAL EFFECTS

The medical consequences of the Bhopal disaster are only partially documented in the medical literature. Several factors play a role in this delay and in some of the shortcomings in the published reports. The scope of the disaster made complete documentation of the immediate medical findings in this enormous group of people nearly impossible. Many of the dead never made it to a hospital and were buried or cremated without documentation. The need to provide emergency medical care to thousands of victims limited attempts to systematically collect information. People went to many different medical providers, often traveling great distances. Some were only seen at temporary medical facilities set up in the city.

Other events also disrupted the follow-up. Thousands of people left the city approximately 2 weeks after the incident when the government announced that it was going to restart the manufacturing process at the plant to get rid of the remaining methyl isocyanate (1). Many of these people never returned to Bhopal. This evacuation combined with the social disruption of a disaster of this scale severely limited the capability to comprehensively follow the population. Frustration with the limited therapy available to victims with persistent health problems after the incident and the confusion caused by the attempts to obtain legal compensation for the victims also contributed to the limited follow-up reported in some of the studies. Thus, despite the exceptional attempts of the Indian government scientists and other medical groups to collect scientific information on the victims from Bhopal, these limitations must be acknowledged in reviewing the available medical literature on the medical consequences of this exposure.

Studies of those acutely affected by the incident documented eye irritation and respiratory symptoms such as dyspnea and chest pain as being the most common health problems (24,25). Fear of permanent eye damage in the many thousands of people with acute eye irritation was a major concern immediately after the disaster. Respiratory tract problems obviously accounted for most of the immediate deaths as well as the most serious ill residents after the incident. Many less seriously ill persons also had respiratory symptoms. Thus, most of the initial follow-up focused on the eyes and respiratory systems. As time went by, other concerns emerged including the possibility of other long-term health consequences such as cancer. These concerns led the Indian government scientists and other physicians to conduct a series of health studies to attempt to comprehensively address the health effects of this exposure.

### Ophthalmologic Effects

A high prevalence of immediate eye complaints was documented among Bhopal residents living in communities near the plant and in those hospitalized after the incident (24,25). These complaints were characterized by photophobia, eye watering, edema of the lids, and corneal ulcerations. A study of children hospitalized after the incident also showed a high rate of eye symptoms similar to those seen in the adults although most did not have corneal involvement (26). Follow-up studies of the affected patients has shown some persistent eye problems such as chronic conjunctivitis and refractive changes, and possibly an increased risk of eye infections (27,28). Other forms of serious permanent eye damage were not found to be more prevalent than expected.

### Pulmonary Effects

The major clinical manifestations from methyl isocyanate exposure were pulmonary. Most of the dead appeared to die from pulmonary causes. Among hospitalized persons, respiratory tract problems also accounted for most of the morbidity and delayed fatalities. Of 978 patients hospitalized at one facility immediately after the disaster, 70 died, most in the first few days after the incident and most from respiratory failure or complications from this condition (24). Examination of records on 544 of these hospitalized patients showed that over 80% had physical findings of respiratory disease (mostly rhonchi and crepitations). More than 80% of the 500 patients who received chest x-rays at this hospital had evidence of pulmonary edema (29).

A community survey of 446 residents of the area near the plant conducted approximately 3 to 4 months after the incident reported persistent respiratory symptoms in over 70% of those with such symptoms immediately after the incident, accompanied by persistent or worsening pulmonary function test results in many (30). A community survey of 164 children living near the plant conducted 100 days after the incident found that over 80% complained of cough and more than 45% of breathlessness (31).

Clinical follow-up of the exposed residents confirmed the respiratory effects from the exposure. Follow-up of 82 patients with persistent symptoms approximately 1 to 2 months after the incident demonstrated a high prevalence of restrictive pulmonary function defects (78%); evidence of an obstructive defect in some (29%); and an inability to maintain normal minute ventilation and oxygen uptake at rest (55%) in this group (32). Flow rate and flow volume abnormalities were also found in many of these people. Follow-up of some of this population 3 to 6 months after the incident found improvement for some but persistent restrictive defects and symptoms for many others (33). Karol and colleagues (12) demonstrated antibodies to methyl isocyanate in some people exposed at Bhopal, but these antibodies were at low levels and were not persistent.

One early study reported on examination of bronchoalveolar lavage (BAL) in 36 patients from Bhopal conducted 18 to 24 months after the incident (34). This study demonstrated alveolitis characterized by accumulation of macrophages and neutrophils (smokers only) in the severely exposed group. Follow-up studies by this same research group have included additional BAL studies 2 to 7 years after the Bhopal exposure for 44 patients, including 20 who were originally examined as part of the first study (35). Twelve of these patients were found to have elevated fibronectin levels. Elevated levels were more likely to occur in patients with more severe exposures and were associated with radiographic abnormalities and abnormal decline in pulmonary function. In these patients, the initial macrophage alveolitis had progressed to a macrophage/neutrophilic alveolitis.

A later report from this research group reported on pulmonary function and BAL results in 60 patients evaluated 1 to 7 years after exposure (36). The study found a correlation between lung inflammation (total inflammatory cells, etc.) and impaired pulmonary function with severity of exposure as estimated by acute symptoms and death in family members at the time of the incident. In nonsmokers, BAL neutrophils and other measures of persistent lung inflammation were negatively correlated with pulmonary function. Although the number of patients followed is small, these results suggest that irreversible and progressive lung damage has occurred in severely exposed Bhopal victims.

These pulmonary findings largely parallel the findings from the recent toxicologic studies. The pattern of chronic or persistent health effects is similar to fibrosing bronchiolitis obliterans, which has been documented in other incidents of acute exposure to high concentrations of an irritating gas (37). While the follow-up clinical information supports the occurrence of this condition in some people after the incident, the prevalence and extent of this disorder cannot be ascertained from the available data.

### Other Health Effects

Immediate and follow-up medical studies have focused on a number of other health outcomes. One difficult issue concerned the possibility that cyanide could somehow be responsible for some of the medical consequences from the exposure. It was thought that cyanide could result from the metabolism or biologic transformation of the methyl isocyanate or from a chemical reaction occurring when the methyl isocyanate was released from the plant. While several studies have supported some role for cyanide, others have not confirmed this, and no firm conclusion can be made (3). However, it should be noted that nearly all of the clinical manifestations seen in the Bhopal victims can be explained by exposure to methyl isocyanate alone or from complications resulting from the effects of methyl isocyanate exposure or from the stress of this incident. As noted above, some studies have suggested ways for methyl isocyanate exposure to affect distant tissues, but the actual contribution of these pathways is uncertain.

Neurologic problems—muscle weakness, tremors, depression, and somnolence—were commonly noted in patients right after the incidence (24,38). Many of these findings were transitory and could be explained as secondary to respiratory distress or to the psychological and physical stress from the incident. Further follow-up of the exposed population demonstrated a high prevalence of psychological symptoms (22% of those with medical problems), and the mental health needs of the population were a significant focus of the follow-up effort (39,40).

Reproductive effects were also a concern. One follow-up study showed a high incidence of spontaneous abortions (24.2%) among pregnant women exposed to the methyl isocyanate compared to women living in another area (5.6%) (41). Another study involving some of the same population confirmed this high incidence of spontaneous abortion and an increased incidence of neonatal mortality (42,43). Cytogenetic studies of exposed populations have shown some differences in comparing the exposed residents to other groups (44–46). The implications of these findings are uncertain and await further follow-up study.

## PREVENTION

The available medical studies of the Bhopal victims have significant limitations. Study populations are not well defined in terms of exposure, and follow-up is uneven. These limitations arise largely from the difficulties arising from the disaster as described above and the difficulty of organizing large follow-up studies under those circumstances.

Compensation issues contribute to this difficulty. There was considerable confusion and delay in obtaining compensation for the victims of the disaster. This effort involved court proceedings and appeals in both the United States and India. As might be expected with a disaster of this scope, even after funds were available for compensating the victims, there were difficulties in setting up a mechanism for distributing the funding. By 1990, the Indian commission handling the claims had medical claims for over 350,000 reported victims of the disaster (47).

While the currently available medical studies do not provide a full assessment of the health effects resulting from the methyl isocyanate release in Bhopal, the data do indicate the occurrence of significant medical problems for a large number of people residing in that city at the time of the incident. More than 2,000 people died and tens of thousands suffered immediate health problems. Chronic respiratory problems have been documented in some of the survivors. While the epidemiologic follow-up of the victims has not been as comprehensive as one would hope, the circumstances of the tragedy made any comprehensive follow-up very difficult. The extent and severity of these respiratory problems need to be further documented (especially in children) as well as the occurrence of other health problems related to this exposure. We can hope that further follow-up medical studies will provide this information and will add to the limited information on the long-term medical consequences of this type of exposure.

The Bhopal incident also has some clear lessons for the prevention of similar industrial accidents (1,48). There are many steps that could have been taken to prevent or ameliorate the damage from this incident. Better design of facilities handling or manufacturing toxic materials is needed. Even if all of the safety devices at the Bhopal plant (such as the flare tower) had been properly operating, it is not clear whether a release of that magnitude would have been significantly reduced. There was an alternative manufacturing process for the pesticides manufactured at the plant that did not involve the production of methyl isocyanate. This production process was used at some other plants producing these pesticides.

Proper work procedures as well as training and education for the staff managing and operating the plant also are very important. People must understand the chemical properties and toxicity of the materials that they are working with and the appropriate procedures for handling and preventing mishaps.

Locating the plant near a populated area also contributed to the high morbidity and mortality from this incident. While certain types of industrial facilities typically are located away from population centers (e.g., munitions plants), most are not. Even when plants are built in isolated areas, people often move to these areas to be closer to their jobs or as part of the expansion from urban centers. The Union Carbide of India plant was originally located close to the urban areas of Bhopal, and more people moved to the area near the plant, drawn by the economic activity there. Land-use planning and control need to account for the potential hazards of this type of land use.

Emergency planning is very important for preventing significant morbidity and mortality should this type of accident occur. In the Bhopal incident, very little emergency planning was evident. The evacuation of the effected areas was unplanned and chaotic. While the medical personnel did an admirable job of responding to the many patients overwhelming their facilities, the health care providers did not have adequate information about the chemicals involved in the incident. Preparation for this type of incident must include adequate information about the substances that could be released and the quantities and potential spread of these materials. Evacuation must be planned, and adequate means available to accomplish it. Residents must be aware of the plan and know what to do. Emergency response personnel must also be trained and properly equipped. Medical facilities must also be prepared with information about the medical effects from exposure, appropriate training for personnel, and adequate equipment and medical supplies.

Preventing and responding to this type of industrial accident requires the cooperation of industry, unions, and many levels of government. In response the Bhopal incident, recent United States legislation has mandated the development of community emergency plans for this type of incident. This law requires facilities handling or storing hazardous materials to provide information about these materials to the community to help develop these plans. These provisions were strengthened with the recent changes in the Clean Air Act, which included requirements for preventive assessment of potential hazards for facilities handling certain types of chemicals. Overall, industry in the United States and throughout the world has implemented efforts to better prevent this type of incident.

The Bhopal disaster provides many lessons about the potential hazards from the storage and handling of hazardous materials. The thousands of victims of that disaster provide a compelling argument for better efforts to prevent this type of accident and for efforts to better understand the health impacts from acute exposure to high concentrations of irritating gases.

## REFERENCES

1. Parrish RG, Falk H, Melius JM. Industrial disasters: classification, investigation and prevention. In: Harrington JM, ed. *Recent advances in occupational health,* vol 3. London: Churchill Livingstone, 1987;155–168.

2. Mehta PS, Mehta AS, Mehta SJ, Makhijani AB. Bhopal tragedy's health effects: a review of methyl isocyanate toxicity. *JAMA* 1990;264: 2781–2787.
3. Tachakra SS. The Bhopal disaster. *J R Soc Health* 1987;107:1–2.
4. Bucher JR. Methyl isocyanate: a review of health effects research since Bhopal. *Fundam Appl Toxicol* 1987;9:367–379.
5. Segal A, Solomon JJ, Li FJ. Isolation of methylcarbamoyl-adducts of adenine and cytosine following *in vitro* reaction of methyl isocyanate with calf thymus DNA. *Chem Biol Interact* 1989;69:359–372.
6. Anderson D, Goyle S, Phillips BJ, Tee A, Beech L, Butler WH. Effects of methyl isocyanate on rat muscle cells in culture. *Br J Ind Med* 1988; 45:269–274.
7. Bhattaccharya BK, Sharma SK, Jaiswal DK. In vivo binding of C 14 labeled methyl isocyanate to various tissue proteins. *Biochem Pharmacol* 1988;37:2489–2493.
8. Ferguson JS, Kennedy AL, Stock MF, Brown WE, Alarie Y. Uptake and distribution of C 14 during and following exposure to C 14 methyl isocyanate. *Toxicol Appl Pharmacol* 1988;94:104–117.
9. Pearson PG, Slatter JG, Rashed MS, Han DH, Baillie TA. Carbamoylation of peptides and proteins *in vitro* by S-(N-methylcarbamoyl) glutathione and S- (N-methylcarbamoyl) cysteine, two electrophilic S-linked conjugates of methyl isocyanate. *Chem Res Toxicol* 1991;4:436–444.
10. Jaeevaratnam K, Sugendran K, Vaidyanathan CS. Do the hydrolysis products, methylamine and N,N-dimethylurea, play a role in the methyl isocyanate-induced haematological and biochemical changes in rabbits? *Hum Exp Toxicol* 1993;12:135–139.
11. Slatterer JG, Rashed MS, Pearson PG, Han DH, Baillie TA. Biotransformation of methyl isocyanate in the rat, evidence for glutathione conjugation as a major pathway of metabolism and implications for isocyanate mediated toxicities. *Chem Res Toxicol* 1991;4:157–161.
12. Karol MH, Taskar S, Gangal S, Rubanoff BF, Kamat SR. The antibody response to methyl isocyanate: experimental and clinical findings. *Environ Health Perspect* 1987;72:169–175.
13. Dodd DE, Frank FR, Fowler EH, Troup CM, Milton RM. Biological effects of short-term, high-concentration exposure to methyl isocyanate. I. Study objectives and inhalation exposure design. *Environ Health Perspect* 1987;72:13–19.
14. Salmon AG, Kerr-Muir M, Andersson N. Acute toxicity of methyl isocyanate: a preliminary study of the dose response for eye and other effects. *Br J Ind Med* 1985;42:795–798.
15. Gupta BN, Stefanski SA, Bucher JR, Hall LB. Effect of methyl isocyanate (MIC) gas on the eyes of Fischer 344 rats. *Environ Health Perspect* 1987;72:105–108.
16. Fedde MR, Dodd DE, Troup CM, Fowler EH. Biological effects of short-term, high concentration exposures to methyl isocyanate. III. Influence on gas exchange in the guinea pig lung. *Environ Health Perspect* 1987;72:13–19.
17. Bucher JR, Boorman GA, Gupta BN, Uraih LC, Hall LB, Stefanski SA. Two-hour methyl isocyanate inhalation exposure and 91-day recovery: a preliminary description of pathologic changes in F344 rats. *Environ Health Perspect* 1987;72:71–75.
18. Boorman GA, Uraih LC, Gupta BN, Bucher JR. Two-hour methyl isocyanate inhalation and 90-day recovery study in B6C3F1 mice. *Environ Health Perspect* 1987;72:63–69.
19. Boorman GA, Brown R, Gupta BN, Uraih LC, Bucher JR. Pathologic changes following acute methyl isocyanate inhalation and recovery in B6C3F1 mice. *Toxicol Appl Pharmacol* 1987;87:446–456.
20. Bucher JR, Uraih LC, Hildebrandt PK, Sauer RM, Seely JC. Carcinogenicity and pulmonary pathology associated with a single 2-hour inhalation exposure of laboratory rodents to methyl isocyanate. *J Natl Cancer Inst* 1989;81:1586–1587.
21. Jeevaratnam K, Sriramachari S. Comparative toxicity of methyl isocyanate and its hydrolytic derivatives in rats. I. Pulmonary histopathology in the acute phase. *Arch Toxicol* 1994;69:39–44.
22. Sriramachari S, Jeevaratnam K. Comparative toxicity of methyl isocyanate and its hydrolytic derivatives in rats II. Pulmonary histopathology in the subacute an chronic phases. *Arch Toxicol* 1994;69:45–51.
23. Varma DR, Ferguson JS, Alarie Y. Reproductive toxicity of methyl isocyanate in mice. *J Toxicol Environ Health* 1987;21:265–275.
24. Misra NP, Pathak R, Gaur KJ, et al. Clinical profile of gas leak victims in acute phase after Bhopal episode. *Ind J Med Res* 1987;86(suppl): 11–19.
25. Andersson N, Kerr-Muir M, Mehra V, Salmon AG. Exposure and response to methyl isocyanate: results of a community based survey in Bhopal. *Br J Ind Med* 1988;45:469–475.
26. Dwivedi PC, Raizada JK, Saini VK, Mittal PC. Ocular lesions following methyl isocyanate contamination: the Bhopal experience (letter). *Arch Ophthalmol* 1985;103:1627.
27. Andersson N, Ajwani MK, Mahashabde S, et al. Delayed eye and other consequences from exposure to methyl isocyanate: 93% follow up of exposed and unexposed cohorts in Bhopal. *Br J Ind Med* 1990;47: 553–558.
28. Khurrum MA, Ahmad SH. Long term follow up of ocular lesion of methyl-isocyanate gas disaster in Bhopal. *Ind J Ophthalmol* 1987;35: 136–137.
29. Sharma PN, Gaur KJ. Radiological spectrum of lung changes in gas exposed victims. *Ind J Med Res* 1987;86(suppl):39–44.
30. Naik SR, Acharya VN, Bhalerao RA, et al. Medical survey of methyl isocyanate gas affected population of Bhopal. Part II. Pulmonary effects in Bhopal victims as seen 15 weeks after M.I.C. exposure. *J Postgrad Med* 1986;32:185–191.
31. Irani SF, Mahashur AA. A survey of Bhopal children affected by methyl isocyanate gas. *J Postgrad Med* 1986;32:195–198.
32. Kamat SR, Mahashur AA, Tiwari AK, et al. Early observations on pulmonary changes and clinical morbidity due to the isocyanate gas leak at Bhopal. *J Postgrad Med* 1985;31:63–72.
33. Kamat SR, Patel MH, Kolhatkar VP, Dave AA, Mahashur AA. Sequential respiratory changes in those exposed to the gas leak at Bhopal. *Ind J Med Res* 1987;86(suppl):20–38.
34. Vijayan VK, Pandey VP, Sankaran K, Mehrotra Y, Darbari BS, Misra NP. Bronchoalveolar lavage study in victims of toxic gas leak at Bhopal. *Ind J Med Res* 1989;90:407–414.
35. Vijayan VK, Sankaran K, Sharma SK, Misra NP. Chronic lung inflammation in victims of toxic gas leak at bhopal. *Resp Med* 1995;89: 105–111.
36. Vijayan VK, Sankaran K. Relationship between lung inflammation, changes in lung function and severity of exposure in victims of the Bhopal tragedy. *Eur Respir J* 1996;9:1977–1982.
37. Weill H. Disaster at Bhopal: the accident, early findings and respiratory health outlook in those injured. *Bull Eur Physiopathol Respir* 1987; 23:587–590.
38. Bharucha EP, Bharucha NE. Neurological manifestations among those exposed to toxic gas at Bhopal. *Ind J Med Res* 1987;86(suppl):59–62.
39. Sethi BB, Sharma M, Trivedi JK, Singh H. Psychiatric morbidity in patients attending clinics in gas affected areas in Bhopal. *Ind J Med Res* 1987;86(suppl):45–50.
40. Murthy RS, Isaac MK. Mental health needs of Bhopal disaster victims & training of medical officers in mental health aspects. *Ind J Med Res* 1987;86(suppl):51–58.
41. Bhandari NR, Syal AK, Kambo I, et al. Pregnancy outcome in women exposed to toxic gas at Bhopal. *Ind J Med Res* 1990;92:28–33.
42. Varma DR. Epidemiological and experimental studies on the effects of methyl isocyanate on the course of pregnancy. *Environ Health Perspect* 1987;72:153–157.
43. Varma DR. Pregnancy Complications in Bhopal Women Exposed to Methyl Isocyanate Vapor. *J Environ Sci Health* 1991;A26:1437–1447.
44. Goswami HK. Cytogenetic effects of methyl isocyanate exposure in Bhopal. *Hum Genet* 1986;74:81–84.
45. Ghosh BB, Sengupta S, Roy A, Maity S, Ghosh S, Talukder G, Sharma A. Cytogenetic studies in human populations exposed to gas leak at Bhopal, India. *Environ Health Perspect* 1990;86:323–326.
46. Goswami HK, Chandorkar M, Bhattacharya K, et al. Search for chromosomal variations among gas-exposed persons in Bhopal. *Hum Genet* 1990;84:172–176.
47. Dhara R, Dhara R. Bhopal - A Case Study of International Disaster. *Int J Occup Environ Med* 1995;1:58–69.
48. Jasanoff S. The Bhopal disaster and the right to know. *Soc Sci Med* 1988;27:1113–1123.

*Environmental and Occupational Medicine, Third Edition*, edited by William N. Rom.
Lippincott–Raven Publishers, Philadelphia © 1998.

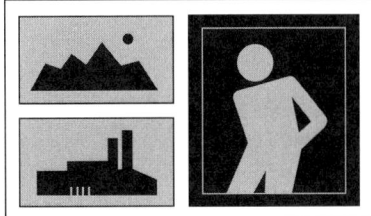

CHAPTER 92

# Health Effects of Dibromochloropropane

M. Donald Whorton

Dibromochloropropane (DBCP), a brominated, organochlorine nematocide, was widely used until 1977 on citrus, grapes, peaches, pineapples, soybeans, and tomatoes. In Central America and Israel, banana trees were treated with DBCP. DBCP was usually applied by adding the liquid to irrigation water or by metering the materials into the ground by injection. Once in the ground, it volatilized and fumigated the soil. DBCP was less acutely toxic than earlier soil fumigants and did not damage plants. By 1975, 25 million pounds were being produced in the United States every year. The bulk of the U.S. production was applied in the coastal states, particularly California's San Joaquin Valley, and in the Southern Atlantic Coast states.

In 1977, DBCP was found to cause infertility and sterility in exposed workers. The affected men were otherwise completely healthy (1). In the United States, the Occupational Safety and Health Administration (OSHA) rapidly set an exposure standard for DBCP, while the Environmental Protection Agency (EPA) severely restricted its use. Application of DBCP to anything but pineapples in Hawaii was banned by the EPA in 1979. In 1982, the EPA exempted the peach crop in the southern Atlantic Coast states (2). However, in 1985, it extended the ban to all U.S. crops.

Since 1977 DBCP's targeting of the male reproductive tract has been much studied. This chapter summarizes the animal and human investigations of the reproductive effects of DBCP.

## ANIMAL STUDIES

The immediate and delayed effects of DBCP toxicity have been investigated in a variety of animal species. Most studies have used rats, mice, rabbits, guinea pigs, or monkeys (3–25).

DBCP targets spermatogenesis in male animals, causing a decrease in sperm count and motility and alterations in morphology. The level of follicle-stimulating hormone (FSH) is increased, in response to the disruption in spermatogenesis. The luteinizing hormone (LH) level also increases, although testosterone remains stable. DBCP is directly toxic to posttesticular sperm, possibly via a disruption in the energy-generating ability of posttesticular sperm. Fertility of exposed animals is decreased, and a dominant lethal effect may occur. Changes in spermatogenesis may be reversible, depending on the extent and duration of DBCP exposure.

Results of animal studies have been consistent in showing marked interspecies differences in the extent of reproductive effects at a given does (milligram per kilogram body weight) of DBCP. Mice are relatively resistant to DBCP's toxic reproductive effects, rats are more susceptible, and rabbits are the most sensitive of these species.

Similar effects have been seen when rats, the most extensively studied species, have been administered equivalent doses of DBCP via gavage, subcutaneous injection, or intraperitoneal injection. Mild and reversible damage to the seminiferous tubules of rats has been noted after a cumulative injected does as small as 60 mg/kg (10).

Three investigators have exposed animals to DBCP via inhalation. Moderate and reversible testicular effects were noted in rabbits that inhaled 1.0 ppm for 14 weeks, producing a cumulative dose of 490 mg/kg (23). Saegusa and colleagues (9) noted slight testicular atrophy after rats were exposed to 3 ppm for 24 hours per day for 14 consecutive days (cumulative dose 670 mg/kg). In this

M.D. Whorton: Environmental Services Health Sciences, Alameda, California 94501.

study, testicular toxicity was not observed in rats that received less than 1 ppm for a cumulative inhalation dose of 225 mg/kg. Torkelson and colleagues (3) found adverse testicular effects at the lowest test dose of 5 ppm (cumulative dose 820 mg/kg).

Research by Kluwe and associates (6,7,11,13) suggests that toxicity of DBCP is cumulative. A dose that may not immediately result in toxicity may produce adverse reproductive effects when given repeatedly over time. However, a "no observable effect" level may exist for reproductive toxicity.

## HUMAN STUDIES

The discovery of the adverse testicular effects in humans is interesting. The problem was observed in 1977 by the wives of workers of the California pesticide formulation plant, not by physicians or scientists. The number of workers in the particular area of the factory in which DBCP was processed was small, but they were young enough to want children and noted that very few children were conceived after they had started to work in that area of the factory. The catalyst for action by the workers was a free-lance film crew that was making a film at the factory. After considerable discussion, one of the workers convinced five co-worker volunteers to submit semen samples for analyses. All the sperm samples were grossly abnormal—azoospermic or severely oligospermic (fewer than 20 million sperm cells per milliliter of seminal fluid). The worker's results were sent to a physician who had been a consultant to the local union. The physician, who had not seen the men previously, examined them and repeated the semen analysis. The results were the same as the original ones. That information led the company and the union to agree jointly to allow the same physician to examine the remainder of the workers in that area of the factory.

A common factor in all the workers tested was exposure to DBCP. Since 1962, the company had regularly formulated DBCP in a special agricultural chemical division (ACD). Air levels of DBCP in early 1977 had been measured at 0.4 ppm for an 8-hour time-weighted average (TWA8) in this division, lower than the 1 ppm recommended by Torkelson's group (3).

The initial study of the 25 nonvasectomized workers in the ACD revealed that 14 of them were azoospermic or oligospermic. There was a striking relationship between the duration of DBCP exposure and sperm count: all 11 men with sperm counts below 1 million had worked in the ACD at least 3 years; none with sperm counts above 40 million had worked there more than 3 months. The mean levels of FSH and LH were significantly higher in those with sperm counts no greater than 1 million, as compared with those sperm counts of more than 40 million. However, testosterone levels were similar in the two groups, and no other significant abnormalities were found by medical examinations and laboratory analyses.

Of the 100 chemicals used in the plant, four had been shown to be toxic to the male reproductive system. Because of the relative quantities of production, the agent most suspected in this facility was DBCP (26). On the basis of the reported findings, the two producers of DBCP conducted medical evaluations of their workers and found similar results. The association between expo-

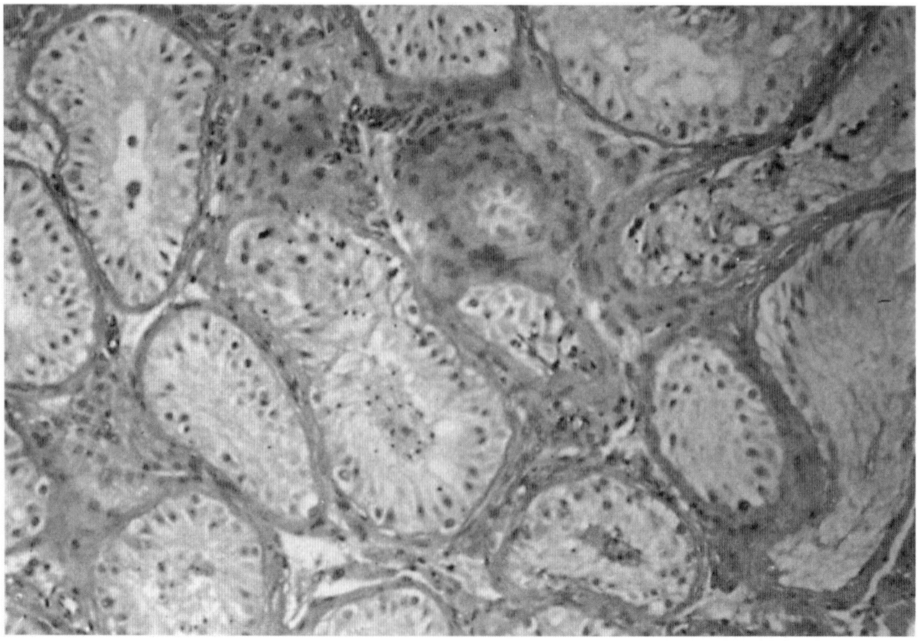

**FIG. 1.** Photomicrograph of a testicular biopsy specimen from a DBCP-exposed worker with a sperm count of 1 million cells per milliliter, which was zero 3 months later (×100).

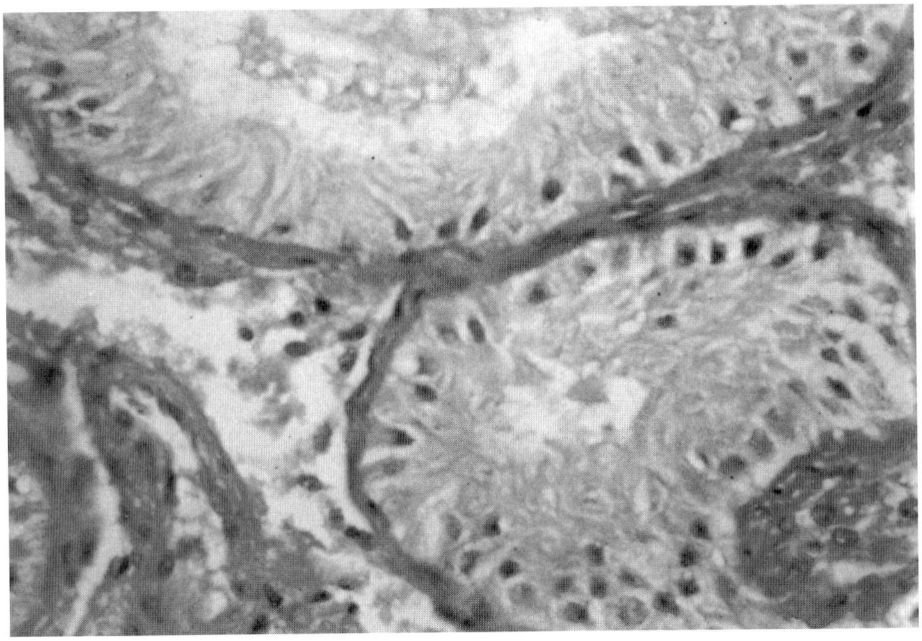

**FIG. 2.** Same specimen as in Fig. 1 (400×). Note the lack of sperm development. The worker had a recovery of 30 million cells per milliliter of semen a year later.

sure to DBCP and testicular dysfunction was strengthened when it was found that the only toxicant exposure common to the workers at the three plants was DBCP.

In 1978 Biava and colleagues (27) published the results of testicular biopsies performed in 10 of the affected Lathrop chemical plant workers. The testicular biopsies revealed the seminiferous tubules to be the site of damage. In severely affected men, the seminiferous tubules were devoid of spermatogenic cells. In the less severely affected, moderate to marked diminution of sperm formation was observed. Sertoli cells were well preserved in both groups. There was no evidence of inflammation, and only minimal evidence of fibrosis and interstitial changes (Figs. 1 and 2).

Other studies of male workers conducted during the period 1977 to 1978 are summarized in Table 1. While methods, exposure assessment, and group ascertainment differed among the studies, profound effects on spermatogenesis were evident in all studied groups (26,28–31).

Adverse reproductive effects were directly related to the duration of exposure to DBCP. It is difficult to determine the actual dose level of DBCP that cause adverse reproductive effects in occupational settings. Workers may have been exposed to DBCP via inhalation or dermal absorption. However, there are few historic air measurement data; in addition, skin exposure to DBCP cannot be quantitated. For many of the worker studies, dermal exposures may be the more important route of entry.

In addition to DBCP production plant workers, reproductive toxicity has been reported in DBCP applicators, formulators, farmers, and pineapple workers in the United States and from Central America (30,32,33). These data contrast with two National Institute for Occupational Safety and Health (NIOSH) Health Hazard Assessments in 1981 (34,35). Both of these studies failed to show any effects among pineapple workers. A cross-sectional study of Hawaiian pineapple workers was performed in 1981 (34). Workers had not been exposed to DBCP for at least 5 or 6 months. No significant difference were found in sperm count or morphology between the 27 exposed and 23 unexposed workers, but semen samples were provided by only 44% of men exposed to DBCP and 22% of unexposed ones. Because of the low participation rate, it is not known whether results were truly representative.

In a separate 1981 study, Hawaiian pineapple workers were followed longitudinally (35,36). Semen analyses

**TABLE 1.** *Summary of studies of male workers conducted during the period of 1977 to 1978*

| Subjects (*n*) | "Spermia" status: Azoospermia (%) | Oligospermia (%) |
|---|---|---|
| Factory workers (114) | 13.2 | 17.5 |
| Factory workers (64) | 6.1 | 11.0 |
| Factory workers (71) | 1.4 | 15.5 |
| Factory workers (86) | 34.9 | 23.3 |
| Applicators (74) | 8.1 | 20.3 |
| Factory workers (23) | 52.2 | 26.1 |
| Applicators (53) | 3.8 | 37.7 |
| Factory workers (23) | 39.1 | 47.8 |
| Totals (508) | 15.7 | 22.1 |

Data from refs. 26–31,38a,39a.

were performed before, at the midpoint, and shortly after the end of the season. The results were correlated with work history logs and industrial hygiene data. While exposure to DBCP ranged from none detected to 0.62 ppm, most were below 1 ppb. Sixty-two exposed workers and 29 unexposed workers provided serial semen samples. Age, alcohol drinking, smoking, marijuana use, and years of work in pineapples fields were not found to be significant confounding variables. Longitudinal sperm counts were not significantly different between exposure groups (mean difference for field, maintenance, and unexposed workers were 1.0, 1.2, and 1.2 million cells per milliliter, respectively).

Thrupp (33) reported that 1,500 male workers from the Atlantic banana-growing region of Costa Rica were found to be either sterile or infertile due to DBCP exposures. This number represents from 20% to 25% of the banana workers in Costa Rica. There are also other reported cases of sterility and infertility among banana workers from other Central American countries. The magnitude of the problem in Central American workers remains unknown due to the lack of any systematic reporting.

Investigators have published the results of 2-, 4-, 5-, and 8-year follow-up of DBCP-affected men (37–42). In most men initially diagnosed as oligospermic, function was recovered within 12 to 16 months after the last exposure. For men made azoospermic by DBCP, particularly in the presence of an elevated FSH level, spermatogenesis was not recovered. DBCP has resulted in a permanent destruction of their germinal epithelium.

Researchers in Israel followed pregnancy outcomes of wives of DBCP-exposed workers. Kharrazi et al. (43) reported an increase in spontaneous abortion rate among pregnancies that occurred while the male partner was exposed to DBCP, as compared to pregnancies that occurred before exposure. Goldsmith, Potashnik, and coworkers (44,45) did not find an increase in the spontaneous abortion rate among wives of DBCP exposed men, but they did note a decrease in the male-female ratio of offspring. They suggested that DBCP may be particularly toxic to Y chromosome–bearing sperm cells.

In 1987, Wong and co-workers (46) reported the results of the investigation of the relationship between DBCP contamination in drinking water and birth rates in Fresno County. They developed methods to estimate DBCP contamination of drinking water (47) and used birth rates as practical means of assessing fertility. Results were analyzed by two methods: the indirect method of adjustment [the standardized birth ratio (SBR)] and a direct method of comparison. Evaluating reproductive performance via the SBR has been described by Wong and colleagues (48). In the Fresno study, the expected births by census tract were adjusted for five age groups, two racial groups, two ethnic groups (Hispanic and non-Hispanic), and five parity groups. During the years 1978 through 1982, 45,914 women in Fresno County bore 46,328 live babies. The SBRs by DBCP exposure categories, after adjustment, showed no clear trend by exposure level. The lowest SBR was found in the lowest DBCP exposure category. The birth ratios of the seven DBCP exposure categories were compared directly using the Mantel-Haenszel chi-square test. Again, there was no trend in relative birth ratios by exposure category.

In addition to birth rates, Whorton et al. (49) also evaluated birth weights, birth defects (as reported on the birth certificate), and gender by census tracts as categorized by DBCP levels in the drinking water. They did not find any correlation between birth outcomes and DBCP contamination. In addition, they did not find any difference in gender ratios in relation to DBCP contamination.

The negative findings in these epidemiologic studies were felt by the authors to be consistent with the dose-response relationship to occupational studies. Based on estimated DBCP levels in drinking water, the total dose from water was far below the doses associated with infertility in workplace settings. The authors concluded that the amount of DBCP in the drinking water of Fresno County has had no major adverse impact on birth rates there.

Whereas adverse testicular effects have been the only pathologic findings in humans associated with DBCP, the chemical does cause other effects in animals. For public health considerations the most important of these other findings is carcinogenesis. Olson and co-workers (50) reported gastric squamous carcinoma in both rats and mice that were subjected to repeated gavage with DBCP. In addition, the female rats also developed mammary adenocarcinoma. Weisburger (51) showed the same results in long-term feeding studies of rats and mice. Van Duuren's group (52) showed an increase in skin papillomas as well as lung and stomach tumors with dermally applied DBCP. Finally, Reznik and co-workers (53) reported increased prevalence of nasal cavity tumors in rats long exposed to DBCP by inhalation. The animal data show DBCP to be carcinogenic in the four animal studies.

There have been three formal epidemiologic studies of workers exposed to DBCP: Hearn et al. (54) with an update by Olsen et al. (55), Wong et al. (56), and Delzell et al. (57). All were small cohorts of workers exposed to DBCP. These studies did not report any elevation of overall cancer or consistent cancer sites. Only Olsen et al. reported a statistical elevation of lung cancer (3 observed with 0.9 expected) among 81 workers with at least 1 year of exposure to DBCP. Both Wong and Delzell reported less than the expected numbers for lung cancer. To date, the worker studies do not show an increase in overall cancer or specific cancer types.

Surveys conducted in 1979 detected DBCP in groundwater in the San Joaquin Valley in California. DBCP had been used heavily in this region until 1978, and it was thought likely that groundwater contamination was due to percolation of DBCP from agricultural areas. An unpublished study by Jackson and colleagues (58) compared patterns of DBCP water contamination with cancer mortality in San Joaquin Valley County. The human cancers selected were those of stomach, esophageal, liver, kidney, and female breast, as well as lymphoid leukemia; 1,257 county residents had such terminal cancers between 1970 and 1979. Sources of drinking water were identified and DBCP levels measured. The authors assumed that current DBCP levels were representative of past concentrations. Census tracts were then aggregated into three categories: low (0 to 0.05 ppb), medium (>0.05 to 1.0 ppb), and high (>1.0 ppb) DBCP exposure levels. Census data were used to compute age- and sex-specific mortality rates for each cancer. Statistically significant trends of increasing risk with increasing DBCP exposure were noted for male stomach cancer, all stomach cancers, and all lymphoid leukemias. The authors noted that the "high DBCP" census tracts also were more rural, more Hispanic, and of a lower socioeconomic status than the "low DBCP" tracts. Owing to the possible role of confounding factors, the lack of information on past DBCP water levels, and the long latency of cancers, the authors stated that DBCP exposure may not be the sole explanation for these findings. The authors recommended further research into the extent and effects of environmental DBCP contamination.

Wong and co-workers (59) studied Fresno County residents for gastric cancer and leukemia, using both ecologic and case-control methods. The ecologic analyses found no correlation between gastric cancer and leukemia (including the lymphatic varieties), mortality rates, and DBCP concentrations in drinking water by census tract in Fresno County for the period 1960 to 1983. The gastric cancer case-control study found no relation between gastric cancer and DBCP in drinking water, but found that Hispanics in the county experienced a relative risk of gastric cancer of 2.77 when compared with non-Hispanics. A similar case-control study found no relation between all leukemia and lymphatic leukemia and DBCP in drinking water. Farm workers, however, did appear to have an increased risk of leukemia.

## SUMMARY

Studies of men exposed occupationally to DBCP have shown that in humans DBCP targets the male reproductive system. Mild to moderate effects may be reversible over time, but in exposed men with both azoospermia and elevated FSH level, follow-up evaluations have generally revealed permanent destruction of germinal epithelium.

Dose levels in human studies are difficult to determine, owing in part to few air measurements plus the inability to quantitate skin exposure. In many of the worker studies the more important route of entry may be transdermal (60).

Pregnancy outcomes among wives of DBCP-exposed workers have shown no change in birth weight, incidence of congenital malformation, or growth and development of offspring. Chromosome analysis of ten children conceived during or after paternal exposure to DBCP has been normal; however, the ratio of male to female offspring was lower. This suggest that DBCP may be particularly toxic to Y chromosome–bearing sperm cells. The single human study that showed an increase in spontaneous abortion is consistent with the animal-dominant lethal studies.

One community study investigated the live birth rate among residents exposed to small quantities of DBCP in drinking water. The negative results of this study are consistent with animal research: small quantities of DBCP in drinking water do not produce a peak or constant does that is detrimental to the reproductive system.

In contrast to the positive animal studies, the limited number of available human studies on the carcinogenicity of DBCP have not shown it to be carcinogenic. This is especially true for the standardized mortality ratio studies and case-control studies. There are also differences in potential doses for each of the studies. Like the reproductive studies, workers' exposure levels are generally much higher than those of the community.

## REFERENCES


1. Whorton D, Krauss RM, Marshall S, Milby TH. Infertility in male pesticide workers. *Lancet* 1977;2:1259–1261.
2. Whorton D, Foliart DE. Mutagenicity, carcinogenicity and reproductive effects of dibromochloropropane (DBCP). *Mutat Res* 1983;123: 12–20.
3. Torkelson TR, Sadek SE, Rowe VK. Toxicologic investigations of 1,2-dibromo-3-chloropropane. *Toxicol Appl Pharmacol* 1961;3:545–559.
4. Ruddick JA, Newsome WH. A teratogenicity and tissue distribution study on dibromochloropropane in the rat. *Bull Environ Contam Toxicol* 1979;21:483–487.
5. Teramoto S, Saiato R, Aoyama H, Shirasu Y. Dominant lethal mutation induced in male rats by 1,2-dibromo-3-chloropropane (DBCP). *Mutat Res* 1980;77:71–78.
6. Kluwe WM. Acute toxicity of 1,2-dibromo-3-chloropropane in the F344 male rat. II. Development and repair of the renal, epididymal, testicular, and hepatic lesions. *Toxicol Appl Pharmacol* 1981;59-84–95.
7. Kluwe WM. Acute toxicity of 1,2-dibromo-3-chloropropane in the F344 male rat. I. Dose-response relationships and differences in routes of exposure. *Toxicol Appl Pharmacol* 1981;59:71–83.
8. Rao KS, Burek FJ, John JA, Schwetz BA, Bell TJ. Toxicologic and reproductive effects of inhaled 1,2-dibromo-3-chloropropane in rats. *Fundam Appl Toxicol* 1983;3:104–110.
9. Saegusa J, Hasegawa H, Kawai K. Toxicity of 1,2-dibromo-3-chloropropane (DBCP). I. Histopathological examination of male rats exposed to DBCP vapour. *Ind Health* 1982;20:315–323.
10. Shemi D, Sod-Moriah UA, Kaplanski J, Potashnik G, Yanai-Inbar. I. Suppression and recovery of spermatogenesis in dibromochloropropane-treated rats. *Andrologia* 1982;14:191–199.
11. Kluwe WM, Lamb JC, Greenwell A, Harrington FA. 1,2-dibromo-3-chloropropane (DBCP)-induced infertility in male rats mediated by a posttesticular effect. *Toxicol Appl Pharmacol* 1983;71:294–298.
12. Warren DW, Wisner JR, Nazir A. Effects of 1,2-dibromo-3-chloropropane on male reproductive function in the rat. *Biol Reprod* 1984; 31:454–463.
13. Kluwe WM, Weber H, Greenwall A, Harrington F. Initial and residual toxicity following acute exposure of developing male rats to dibromochloropropane. *Toxicol Appl Pharmacol* 1985;79:54–68.
14. Amann RP. Detection of alterations in testicular and epididymal function in laboratory animals. *Environ Health Perspect* 1986;70:149–158.
15. Johnston RV, Mensik DC, Taylor HW, Jersey GC, Dietz FK. Single-generation drinking water reproduction study of 1,2-dibromo-3-chloro-

propane in Sprague-Dawley rats. *Bull Environ Contam Toxicol* 1986; 37:531–537.
16. Saegusa J. Age-related susceptibility to dibromochloropropane. *Toxicol Lett* 1986;36:45–50.
17. Oakberg EF, Cummings CC. Lack of effect of dibromochloropropane on the mouse testis. *Environ Mutagen* 1984;6:621–625.
18. Osterloh J, Letz G, Pond S, Becker C. An assessment of the potential testicular toxicity of 10 pesticides using the mouse sperm morphology assay. *Mutat Res* 1983;116:407–415.
19. Lee IP, Suzuki K. Induction of unscheduled DNA synthesis in mouse germ cells following 1,2-dibromo-3-chloropropane (DBCP). *Mutat Res* 1979;68:169–173.
20. Generoso WM, Cain KT, Hughes LA. Tests for dominant-lethal effects of 1,2-dibromo-3-chloropropane (DBCP) in male and female mice. *Mutat Res* 1985;156:103–108.
21. Sasaki YF, Imanishi H, Watanabe M., et al. Mutagenicity of 1,2-dibromo-3-chloropropane (DBCP) in the mouse spot test. *Mutat Res* 1986;174:145–147.
22. Russel LB, Hunsicker PR, Cacheiro NL. Mouse specific-locus test for the induction of heritable gene mutations by dibromochloropropane (DBCP). *Mutat Res* 1986;170:161–166.
23. Rao KS, Burek FJ, John JA, et al. Toxicologic and reproductive effects of inhaled 1,2-dibromo-3-chloropropane in male rabbits. *Fundam Appl Toxicol* 1982;2:241–251.
24. Foote RH, Schermerhorn EC, Simkin ME. Measurement of semen quality, fertility, and reproductive hormones to assess dibromochloropropane (DBCP) effects in live rabbits. *Fundam Appl Toxicol* 1986;6: 628–637.
25. Foote RH, Berndtson WE, Rounsaville TR. Use of quantitative testicular histology to asses the effect of dibromochloropropane (DBCP) on reproduction in rabbits. *Fundam Appl Toxicol* 1986:6:638–647.
26. Whorton D, Milby TH, Krauss RM, Stubbs HA. Testicular function in DBCP-exposed pesticide workers. *J Occup Med* 1979;21:161–166.
27. Biava CG, Smuckler EA, Whorton D. The testicular morphology of individuals exposed to dibromochloropropane. *Exp Mol Pathol* 1978; 29:448–458.
28. Milby TH, Whorton, D. Epidemiological assessment of occupationally related, chemically induced sperm count suppression. *J Occup Med* 1980:22(2):77–82.
29. Lipschultz LI, Ross CE, Whorton D, et al. Dibromochloropropane and its effects on testicular function in man. *J Urol* 1980:124:464–468.
30. Glass RI, Lyness RN, Mengle DC, Powell KE, Kahn E. Sperm count depression in pesticide applicators exposed to dibromochloropropane. *Am J Epidemiol* 1979;109:346–351.
31. Potashnik G, Yanai-Inbar I, Sacks MI, Israeli R. Effect of dibromochloropropane on human testicular function. *Isr J Med Soc* 1979;15: 438–442.
32. Takahashi W, Wong L, Rogers BJ, Hale RW. Depression of sperm counts among agricultural workers exposed to dibromochloropropane and ethylene dibromide. *Bull Environ Contam Toxicol* 1981;27: 551–558.
33. Thrupp LA. Sterilization of workers from pesticide exposure: the causes and consequences of DBCP-induced damage in Costa Rica and Beyond. *Int J Health Serv* 1991;21:731–757.
34. Coye MJ, Albrecht WB, Whorton DM. *NIOSH health hazard evaluation,* report 80-162. HETA 81-040-1315. Lanai, HI: Dole Pineapple Corp., 1983.
35. Coye MJ, Albrecht WB, Sinks T. *NIOSH health hazard evaluation,* report 81-162. HETA 81-162-1935. Maui Kahuli, HI: Maui Pineapple Company, 1990.
36. Landrigan PJ, Melius JM, Rosenberg MJ, Coye MJ, Binkin NJ. Reproductive hazards in the workplace. *Scand J Work Environ Health* 1983;9:83–88.
37. Whorton D, Milby TH. Recovery of testicular function among DBCP workers. *J Occup Med* 1980;22(3):177–179.
38. Lantz GD, Cunningham GR, Huckins C, Lipschultz LI. Recovery from severe oligospermia after exposure to dibromochloropropane. *Fertil Steril* 1981;35:46–53.
38a. Sandifer SH, Wilkins RT, Loadholt CB, Lane LG, Eldridge JC. Spermatogenesis in agricultural workers exposed to dibromochloropropane (DBCP). *Bull Environ Contam Toxicol* 1979;23:703–710.
39. Potashnik G. A four-year reassessment of workers with dibromochloropropane-induced testicular dysfunction. *Andrologia* 1983;15:164–170.
39a. Marquez EM. 1,2-dibromo-3-chloro-propano (DBCP) nematicida con accion, esterilizante en el hombre. *Salud Publica Mex* 1978;2:551–558.
40. Eaton M, Schenker M, Whorton MD, et al. Seven-year follow-up of workers exposed to 1,2-dibromo-3-chloropropane. *J Occup Med* 1986; 28:1145–1150.
41. Potashnik G, Yanai-Inbar I. Dibromochloropropane (DBCP): an 8-year reevaluation of testicular function and reproductive performance. *Fertil Steril* 1987;47:317–323.
42. Olsen GW, Lanham JM, Bodner KM, Hylton DB, Bond GG. Determinants of spermatogenesis recovery among workers exposed to 1,2-dibromo-3-chloropropane. *J Occup Med* 1990;32:979–984.
43. Kharrazi M, Potashnik G, Goldsmith JR. Reproductive effects of dibromochloropropane. *Isr J Med Sci* 1980;16:403–406.
44. Goldsmith JR, Potashnik G, Israeli R. Reproductive outcomes in families of DBCP-exposed men. *Arch Environ Health* 1984;39:85–89.
45. Potashnik G, Goldsmith J, Insler V. Dibromochloropropane-induced reduction of the sex ratio in man. *Andrologia* 1984;16:213–218.
46. Wong O, Whorton D, Gordon N, Morgan RW. An epidemiological investigation of the relationship between DBCP contamination in drinking water and birth rates in Fresno County, California. *Am J Public Health* 1988;78:1–4.
47. Whorton MD, Morgan RW, Wong O, Larson S. Problems associated with collecting drinking water quality data for community studies: a case example, Fresno County, California. *Am J Public Health* 1987;77 (11):1–5.
48. Wong O, Morgan RW, Whorton MD. An epidemiologic surveillance program for evaluating occupational reproductive hazards. *Am J Ind Med* 1985;7:295–306.
49. Whorton MD, Wong O, Morgan RW, Gordon N. An epidemiologic investigation of birth outcomes in relation to dibromochloropropane contamination in drinking water in Fresno County, California, USA. *Int Arch Occup Environ Health* 1989;61:403–407.
50. Olson WA, Habermann RT, Weisburger EK, Ward JM, Weisburger JH. Induction of stomach cancer in rats and mice by halogenated aliphatic fumigants. *J Natl Cancer Inst* 1973;51:1993–1995.
51. Weisburger EK. Carcinogenicity studies on halogenated hydrocarbons. *Environ Health Perspect* 1977;21:7–16.
52. Van Duuren BL, Goldschmidt BM, Loewengart G, et al. Carcinogenicity of halogenated olefinic and aliphatic hydrocarbons in mice. *J Natl Cancer Inst* 1979;63:1433–1439.
53. Reznik G, Reznik-Schuller H, Ward JM, Stinson SF. Morphology of nasal cavity tumours in rats after chronic inhalation of 1,2-dibromo-3-chloropropane. *Br J Cancer* 1980;42:772–781.
54. Hearn S, Ott MG, Kolesar RC, Cook RR. Mortality experience of employees with occupational exposure to DBCP. *Arch Environ Health* 1984;39(1):49–55.
55. Olsen GW, Bodner KM, Stafford BA, Cartmill JB, Gondek MR. Update of the mortality experience of employees with occupational exposures to 1,2-dibromo-3-chloropropane (DBCP). *Am J Ind Med* 1995;28: 399–410.
56. Wong O, Brocker W, Davis HV, Nagle GS. Mortality of workers potentially exposed to organic and inorganic brominated chemicals, DBCP, TRIS, PBB, and DDT. *Br J Ind Med* 1984;41(1):15–24.
57. Delzell E, Cole P, Satiakumar N, Adjepong Y. *A follow-up study of mortality among workers at the shell denver chemical plant.* Birmingham: University of Alabama, 1993.
58. Jackson RJ, Greene CJ, Thomas JT, Murphy EL, Kaldor J. *Literature review on the toxicological aspects of DBCP and epidemiological comparison of patterns of DBCP drinking water contamination with mortality rates from selected cancers in Fresno County, California 1970–1979.* Sacramento, CA: Epidemiology Studies of the California Department of Health Services, 1982.
59. Wong O, Morgan RW, Whorton MD, Gordon N, Khiefets L. Ecological analyses and case-control studies of gastric cancer and leukemia in relation to DBCP in drinking water in Fresno County, California. *Br J Ind Med* 1989;46:521–528.
60. Whorton D, Wong O. Reproductive Effects of Dibromochloropropane (DBCP) on Humans. A case study in occupational medicine. *Chinese J Occup Med* 1996;3:191–206.

*Environmental and Occupational Medicine, Third Edition,* edited by William N. Rom.
Published by Lippincott–Raven Publishers,
Philadelphia, 1998.

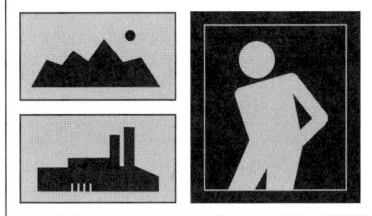

CHAPTER 93

# Vinyl Chloride and Polyvinyl Chloride

Henry Falk and N. Kyle Steenland

The announcement by the B. F. Goodrich Company in early 1974 of several cases of hepatic angiosarcoma (HAS) among its polyvinyl chloride (PVC) polymerization workers set off a rapid chain of events that had a dramatic impact on the field of occupational health. First, vinyl chloride monomer (VCM: $H_2c$ = CHCL), the starting material in the production of PVC resins, to which tens of thousands of workers had been exposed in recent decades, was transformed from a relatively innocuous industrial substance to a carcinogen that produces a fatal malignancy. Second, human epidemiologic data and animal experimental evidence for the carcinogenicity of VCM appeared almost simultaneously, providing definitive results that quickly brought about sharply lower occupational standards and changed industrial and environmental practices in many countries. Third, because of the many consumer uses of VCM and vinyl plastics, concern spread beyond the traditional confines of occupational health to the general public.

Several excellent review articles and conference proceedings highlight the multifaceted research stimulated by the first report of HAS induced by VCM (1–6). More recent reviews have focused on the toxicologic and occupational mortality data (7,8). In recent years there has been rapidly expanding knowledge on the mechanisms of carcinogenicity of VCM. This chapter focuses principally on the medical and epidemiologic findings.

H. Falk: Division of Environmental Hazards and Health Effects, National Center for Environmental Health, Centers for Disease Control and Prevention, Atlanta, Georgia 30341-3724.

N. K. Steenland: National Institute for Occupational Safety and Health, Cincinnati, Ohio 45226.

## PVC POLYMERIZATION

Worldwide demand and production capacity for PVC continues to grow; 1996 global demand was estimated at about 44 billion pounds per year, and production capacity is increasing at a rate of close to 4% per year. Growth is most rapid in Asia, particularly China (9). PVC has been used principally in building and construction (particularly PVC pipe, electrical wire and cable, and flooring), home furnishings, recreational products (e.g., records and toys), packaging (e.g., film sheet, bottles), apparel, and transportation materials (e.g., automobile tops, upholstery, mats), besides a variety of other products, including medical tubing (3,7).

The PVC industry, begun in the United States in the early 1940s, consists of three separate processes. The first step is vinyl chloride monomer production, usually by direct chlorination or oxychlorination of ethylene. This is done in a closed system, although leaks or breaks in the process may lead to high levels for brief periods. In the United States, ten companies (15 plants) were engaged in this process in 1976 (slightly fewer in 1988); several thousand U.S. workers have been employed in this phase of the industry (3,7). The second step is polyvinyl chloride polymerization, in which gaseous VCM (boiling point −13.5°C) is liquefied under pressure in large polymerization reactors or vessels and chemically reacts to form PVC polymer (2). The polymerization reaction can be carried out in several different ways—suspension, emulsion, bulk, or solution polymerization—to produce polymer or copolymer particles of different size and quality (3). In 1976 there were 22 companies (39 plants) that polymerized PVC in the United States; tens of thousands of U.S. workers have been employed in this phase of the industry. The highest exposures to VCM occurred in these plants, particularly because of the need to open and clean reactor vessels between reactions, a process that allows residual unreacted monomer to escape from the vessel. At one time workers were lowered into reaction vessels to clean them manually, and undoubtedly they were exposed to peak VCM exposure levels of several thousand parts per million (ppm). That practice was phased out in the late 1960s and 1970s, after the identification of acroosteolysis (AOL) in these VCM-exposed workers. The third step, PVC compounding and fabricating, involves compounding PVC resins with a variety of substances, such as pigments, plasticizers, fillers, antistatic agents, and stabilizers, and then making them into the various products. Many more fabricating workers are employed than polymerization workers, but VCM exposures have been considerably lower, arising principally from retained unreacted monomer (levels of which have been considerably reduced in recent years). Emissions and effluents from VCM and PVC production plants are the main sources of VCM released into the environment, although multiple smaller sources exist (7).

## HEALTH EFFECTS

Two very uncommon diseases, AOL and hepatic angiosarcoma (HAS), are clearly linked to work in PVC polymerization plants. HAS actually represents the end stage of a hepatic fibrotic precursor lesion (described in detail below). The earliest references in the literature to liver disease or findings suggestive of AOL in VCM-exposed workers date from 1949 and have been summarized (4,5,10). The liver findings in these early reports were described as hepatitis-like changes, hepatomegaly, and abnormalities on liver function tests. Detailed descriptions of AOL appeared in 1966 and 1967, and during the early 1970s the characteristic liver disease and its pathogenesis were described by Lange and co-workers and by Marsteller and associates in Germany, as well as by Creech and co-workers and Popper and Thomas in the United States (22,27–31).

### Acroosteolysis

In 1967 Harris and Adams (11) described two cases of AOL in Britain. The main findings included symptoms of Raynaud's phenomenon, osteolysis in the terminal phalanges of some of the fingers, and thickening of the skin or raised nodules on the hands and forearms. One case that included puffiness of the face was initially interpreted as scleroderma. The lytic lesions of the terminal phalanges of the fingers gave the appearance of clubbing (pseudoclubbing); additional findings suggestive of a systemic effect included lytic lesions of the feet, cortical erosion in the patella, and widening and marginal sclerosis of the sacroiliac joint.

In 1967 Wilson and colleagues (12) described 31 cases of AOL (fewer than 3% of the polymerization workers) in a U.S. company. They observed the same primary triad of Raynaud's phenomenon, sclerodermatoid lesions on hands and forearms, and lytic lesions of the terminal phalanges of the fingers; systemic manifestations, such as radiographic abnormalities in the feet, were not seen. AOL was subdivided into a mild stage (loss of cortex of one or more tufts of the distal phalanges), an advanced stage (more severe lytic destruction with complete loss of the tuft and a portion of the shaft of the distal phalanx), and a healing stage (fragmentation of the tuft or shaft and subsequent bony or fibrous union; Fig. 1). AOL was observed to occur primarily in workers who cleaned reactors, leading to restriction of manual activity of some workers, although in others the process improved spontaneously.

An epidemiologic study of 5,011 U.S. employees reported in 1971 identified 25 definite and 16 possible cases of AOL (13). Of the 25 patients, 24 had Raynaud's phenomenon and all 25 patients had cleaned reactors at some point, leading to the conclusion that manual cleaning of reactors was important in causation (14).

Other reports also pointed to some systemic changes in skin, bones, and sacroiliac joints (2,15–19). Rats dosed orally with VCM for 2 years were shown to develop thickening of the skin, with evidence of increased collagen synthesis (20); this provides some further support for the systemic nature of the skin findings. Vascular changes in the digital arteries of the hand associated with AOL, including narrowing of the lumen and partial or total occlusion, have been demonstrated by arteriography (21,22). In immunologic studies of workers with vinyl chloride disease, some of whom had evidence of Raynaud's phenomenon or AOL, Ward and colleagues (23) identified a number of abnormalities, including evidence of circulating immune complexes and their deposition in vessels. The hypothesis that these immune changes may be related to the pathogenesis of AOL and to other aspects of VCM-induced disease needs further study. The relationship of AOL to other environmentally induced sclerodermatoid disorders has been reviewed (24).

A puzzling aspect is that AOL was not described in detail until the 1960s. Unlike HAS, which has a latency period of approximately 20 years, AOL can have a very short latency period of 1 to 2 years and thus should have occurred in the 1940s and 1950s. Either the disease was missed during those years or it did not occur because of unidentified factors that are yet to be explained. One author suggested that AOL first occurred after the introduction of vinyl chloride–vinyl acetate copolymers (3). Unfortunately, such exposure information is lacking in virtually all published reports of AOL.

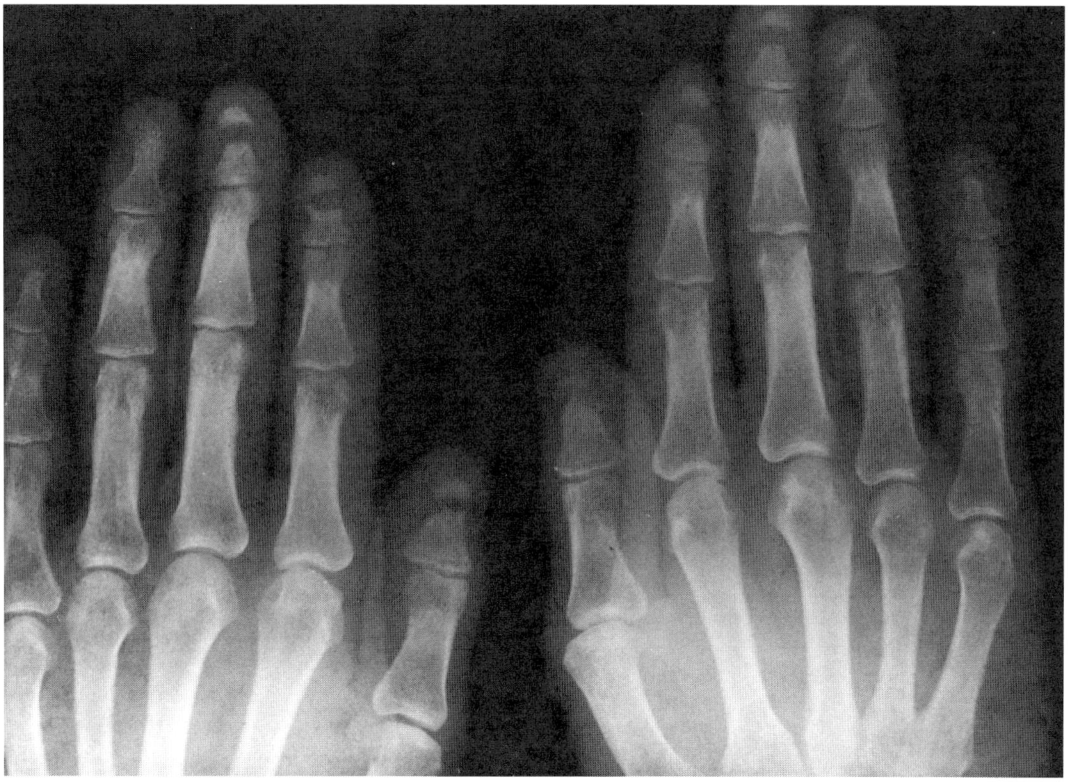

**FIG. 1.** Radiograph of long-term polyvinyl chloride polymerization worker's hand shows marked acroosteolysis, November 1964. (Courtesy of Dr. John Creech, B. F. Goodrich Company, Louisville, Kentucky.)

With the reduction of exposures that have occurred in this industry over the last two decades, case reports of AOL are now rare.

### Liver Disease

Studies carried out during the 1960s in Romania reported hepatomegaly in vinyl chloride workers (reversible in some after cessation of VCM exposure), which was often associated with abnormalities of liver function tests (25). The spectrum of VCM-induced liver disease began to emerge from studies of PVC polymerization workers in Germany, starting in 1972. Lange and co-workers (22) described workers with hepatic fibrosis, splenomegaly, and thrombocytopenia—all findings suggestive of portal hypertension—in the absence of significant hepatic parenchymal damage. In a subsequent report, 81% of 70 workers studied were noted to have thrombocytopenia, 67% had increased Bromsulphalein (BSP) sodium retention, and 57% had splenomegaly; 14% had increased serum enzyme levels, indicating hepatic damage (25). Histologic studies demonstrated activation of hepatic sinusoidal cells and hepatic (particularly perisinusoidal) fibrosis, with less extreme changes in hepatocytes (26); fibrosis of the liver capsule was clearly visualized at laparoscopy (27).

In 1974 Creech and Johnson (28) first reported hepatic angiosarcoma following VCM exposure when they described three cases among PVC polymerization workers at the B. F. Goodrich plant in Louisville, Kentucky. Subsequent detailed studies at that plant identified additional cases of HAS and cases of nonmalignant hepatic disease, consisting principally of hepatic fibrosis, portal hypertension, and splenomegaly (29). Study of pathology specimens from VCM-exposed workers at various stages of liver disease and of serial biopsies in a number of workers who ultimately developed HAS enabled Popper and colleagues (30–32) to establish the morphologic progression and pathogenesis of HAS, which are similar to those seen in HAS from other causes known and unknown.

The earliest findings in the precursor stage are areas of combined hyperplasia of hepatocytes and sinusoidal cells associated with an excess of reticulin and with sinusoidal dilatation. These changes can progress to hepatic fibrosis, portal hypertension (33), and occasionally peliosis hepatitis or hepatocellular carcinoma (34,35); the hyperplastic sinusoidal cells become increasingly atypical and eventually undergo malignant transformation in the development of HAS (Fig. 2). Hepatocellular injury is not a feature of the early stages of this sequence, although it does appear in the later ones. Therefore, the hepatic dis-

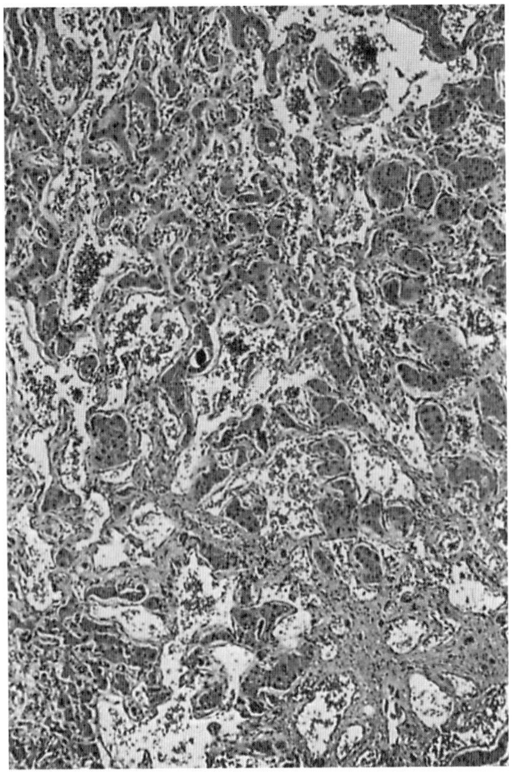

**FIG. 2.** Trabecular angiosarcoma in a VCM worker. Note cords of hyperplastic hepatocytes, sometimes surrounding bile plugs. These cords are surrounded by layers of angiosarcoma cells. The sinusoidal spaces are dilated (hematoxylin eosin stain, ×60). (Courtesy of Dr. Hans Popper, Mt. Sinai School of Medicine, New York.)

ease caused by VCM is quite distinct from that caused by most previously identified hepatotoxins (36).

An increased frequency of abnormalities of standard liver function tests, particularly in VCM-exposed workers whose clinical findings are compatible with VCM-related hepatic disease, has been reported in a number of studies (25,37). Liver function abnormalities, however, are a relatively late finding (38), and a number of cross-sectional studies of actively employed PVC polymerization workers have not detected gradual decrements in function (39–41). Nevertheless, when incorporated into ongoing medical surveillance, standard liver function tests have been valuable in identifying VCM-induced hepatic disease, particularly when multiple abnormalities or prolonged abnormalities on repeated examination have been observed (42,43). As a result, periodic screening with standard liver function tests was included in the National Institute for Occupational Safety and Health (NIOSH) recommendations and U.S. regulations (44).

There is a generally perceived need for the development of reliable screening tests for the early stages of VCM-induced hepatic disease. Proposed measures have included sensitive clearance tests to detect very early loss of hepatic function (45–48) or of increased liver endothelial cell activity (49), scintigraphy and other means of detecting altered hepatic architecture (50–53), and capillary microscopy in vivo (54). The degree of reversibility of the hepatic fibrotic precursor lesion has not been determined (55), but withdrawal from exposure is prudent, in the hope of preventing progression. Survival of patients with untreated HAS continues to be very poor and has been estimated to average 6 months or less. Dannaher and co-workers (56) reported on the use of chemotherapy in cases of VCM-associated HAS to improve the duration and quality of survival.

### Pulmonary Effects

Lilis and colleagues (10) reported a decrease in pulmonary function in PVC polymerization workers exposed to VCM and PVC dust. Gamble and associates (57) found no evidence of such a decrease, but they did demonstrate a temporary loss of pulmonary function during the course of a single work shift. A report from England described some deterioration of lung function, slight abnormalities of the chest radiograph, and complaints of slight dyspnea associated with exposure to PVC dust (58). Baser and co-workers (59) reported pulmonary function abnormalities and increased respiratory tract symptoms in PVC fabrication workers (59). Reports of respiratory function decreases in PVC fabrication workers continue to occur, most recently from Asia and Africa (60–62).

Cases of pneumoconiosis induced by PVC resin also have been reported, and a report from Italy described 20 cases of PVC pneumoconiosis in workers exposed to PVC dust (63–65). Ultrastructural evaluation of lung biopsy material demonstrated apparent PVC particles in pulmonary macrophages and giant cells (63,65). The respective roles of retained VCM, PVC dust, and PVC additives such as plasticizers in the development of these pulmonary changes need to be clarified.

## CYTOGENETIC STUDIES

Particularly during the late 1970s there were a number of reports of increased frequencies of chromosome aberrations in cytogenetic studies of peripheral lymphocytes from VCM-exposed workers. Subsequent studies reported apparently conflicting results and difficulties in reconciling these findings, although the various methods, particularly of measuring VCM exposure and of choosing of control groups, were not always comparable. Giri (66) has recently reviewed the genetic toxicology literature, and concluded that VCM, particularly following metabolic activation or directly from its active metabolites, has significant mutagenic activity and can directly interact with DNA, leading to chromosomal aberrations and sister-chromatid exchanges. The bulk of the literature supports this conclusion, and Giri interprets the smaller number of negative studies as being limited by small sample size, inadequate exposure, or presence of confounding factors. The positive studies have been in workers with relatively long periods of exposure to VCM, and often to the high levels seen before 1975. Several reports have demonstrated the disappearance of cytogenetic abnormalities in groups of workers followed periodically after cessation of exposure (67). Fucic and co-workers (68,69) have explored the localization of chromosome breaks in human lymphocytes and the potential relation to oncogenic activation. In any event, it is uncertain how to interpret these cytogenetic findings in terms of health risk to individual workers. Also, potential confounding factors in the industrial setting demand consideration in greater detail.

## REPRODUCTIVE EFFECTS

As part of a cross-sectional medical screening of PVC polymerization workers, Infante and colleagues (70) noted increased reporting of fetal loss by wives of VCM-exposed workers. A number of methodologic issues have been raised concerning that report, and, clearly, data on spontaneous abortions obtained directly from the workers' wives would have been preferable (71). High rates of congenital anomalies of the central nervous system have been reported in communities with PVC polymerization plants (72,73); subsequent case-control studies have not been able to confirm that the excess of defects is related to VCM exposure (73,74). Nevertheless, the ever-expanding literature on the mutagenic effects of VCM in microbial and mammalian test systems raises concern about possible genetic or reproductive effects, although teratogenicity (production of major congenital anomalies) has not been identified in animal systems (5).

## OTHER EFFECTS

A number of other findings, including hypertensive changes and symptoms such as headaches and fatigue (possibly related to the anesthetic effect of large doses), have been reported (22,25,37,39,40). Peripheral neuropathy was reported in a group of workers in Italy (75); a variety of neurologic findings were reported from a plant in Poland (76).

## CANCER

### Hepatic Angiosarcoma Registry

Two initial reports from NIOSH, in 1975 and 1978, summarized the worldwide distribution of, as it was then known as, VCM-related cases of HAS (77,78). The great majority of those cases occurred in PVC polymerization workers; 64 had been identified to NIOSH as of October 1977. At that time, 23 cases had been identified in the United States, 10 in Canada, nine in the Federal Republic of Germany, eight in France, and most of the remainder from nine European countries. For those 64 cases, the latency period (interval from first exposure to diagnosis) ranged from 9 to 38 years (median 21); the length of exposure ranged from 4 to 31 years (median 18); and the age at diagnosis ranged from 37 to 71 years (median 49). The majority of cases were diagnosed after 1973.

A world register of HAS due to VCM has been maintained since 1974 on behalf of the Association of Plastic Manufacturers in Europe (79). In 1985, Forman and co-workers (80) published an interim analysis of data in the registry. Through 1984, 118 cases had been reported. The number of deaths appeared to have peaked in the 1975 to 1979 period (9.2 per year). Mean age at diagnosis was 52 years. Twelve countries had reported at least one case. Most came from the United States, 35 cases; West Germany, 26; France, 18; Canada, 10; and the United Kingdom, 9.

The most recent tabulation from the register shows 173 deaths through October 1993 (81). The period of peak occurrence is still 1975 to 1979, and has been diminishing since then (approximately 5 cases/year from 1990 to 1993). Western Europe has reported 106 cases; North America, 57; and the remainder of the world, 10.

Cases of HAS have been reported in persons exposed to lesser concentrations of VCM than PVC polymerization workers, for example, PVC fabricating workers and residents near PVC plants (77,82,83), but, because of the relatively large numbers of persons potentially exposed to lower levels, additional epidemiologic studies are needed to evaluate the associations. In a study of Thorotrast-induced HAS, the initially reported cases involved exposure to large doses and relatively short latency periods, while a larger number of cases that appeared later were associated with smaller doses and longer latency periods (84). Thus, it is important to follow trends of VCM-related cases of HAS in the future, to observe shifts in epidemiologic patterns. In nationwide reviews of HAS in the United States (1964 to 1974) and the United Kingdom (1963 to 1977), some 6% to 7% of pathologically confirmed cases occurred among PVC polymerization workers (12 of 168 in the United States; two of 35 in the United Kingdom) (81,85).

### Occupational Cohort Studies

Studies on animals exposed to VCM have identified a multiplicity of tumors, in addition to HAS, (see below). As a result, a series of cohort mortality studies, principally of PVC polymerization workers, have evaluated the risk for all malignant neoplasms in these groups. Some of the primary difficulties in conducting and interpreting these studies (particularly the early cohort studies reported in the 1970s) included the relative youth of the

PVC industry (most of the workers in the various cohort studies had not passed through the age of peak cancer incidence), the relatively few deaths among workers who had been long exposed and quite some time earlier in some of the studies, and the difficulty of precisely quantifying past exposure to VCM, PVC, and other chemicals used in the polymerization processes such as other monomers used to produce copolymers (8). Doll (8) provided a comprehensive overview of the cohort mortality studies in 1988. His analysis combined data from the largest and most recent studies in four countries (United States, United Kingdom, Canada, Italy), each of which fulfilled the criteria of providing substantial numbers of observations more than 25 years after first exposure and covering a period long enough for more than 10% of the workers to have been expected to die. Doll's conclusion was that only HAS can be definitively related to VCM exposure in these cohorts. The increases previously noted for three other sites (brain, lung, and lymphatic and hematopoietic tissue) are in his analysis either insignificant or only weakly suggestive of a small effect.

Most epidemiologic data published since the 1988 Doll (8) review have tended to confirm the view that the only cancer outcome caused by exposure to vinyl chloride is liver cancer, particularly angiosarcoma. Two large studies were done, one in the United States and one in Europe. Wu et al. (86) studied 4,835 workers at a single VC/PVC manufacturing plant, 3,635 (75%) of whom had been exposed to VC, and 1,181 (24%) of whom had died (86). This study was an update of an earlier study of Waxweiler et al. (87). Among those exposed to VC, the lung, brain, liver, and hematopoietic cancer standardized mortality ratios (SMRs) were 1.15 (0.95–1.39), 1.45 (0.79–2.48), 3.33 (2.02–5.21), and 0.78 (0.48–1.21) based on 80, 10, 14, and 15 deaths, respectively. Nested case-control studies of lung, brain, and liver cancer within the entire cohort, using estimated rankings of cumulative exposure, showed that only liver cancer was associated with increased exposure to VC. Furthermore, when liver cancers were categorized by angiosarcomas and other liver cancers, based on the death certificate and medical records, only angiosarcoma showed a positive dose-response. The nested case-control studies showed no risk for exposure to PVC dust.

Simonato et al. (88) conducted a mortality study 14,351 subjects (1,438 dead) in 19 plants manufacturing VC or PVC in England, Sweden, Norway, and Italy. These plants included some that had been studied previously but that were updated. Lung cancer, brain cancer, liver cancer, and hematopoietic cancer had SMRs of 0.97 (0.82–1.14), 1.07 (0.59–1.80), 2.86 (1.83–4.25), and 0.89 (0.60–1.29), respectively, based on 144, 14, 24, and 29 deaths. A nested case-control study for liver cancer showed a significant positive dose-response with estimated cumulative VC exposure. A second nested case-control study of angiosarcomas showed an even steeper does-response.

Three other smaller studies have been published since the 1988 Doll (8) review. Laplanche et al. (89) updated earlier work in a 7-year follow-up for 1,100 VC-exposed subjects and 1,100 nonexposed subjects for morbidity and mortality. These workers were aged 40 to 55 and exposed at time of baseline in 1980. There were only 82 deaths in this group; three angiosarcomas occurred in the exposed and none in the nonexposed. Morbidity data indicated an excess of Raynaud's disease in the exposed versus nonexposed (14 versus 1 case), and an excess of cardiovascular disease, which was primarily due to more hypertension in the exposed (55 versus 34 cases). The excess hypertension, while apparently associated with higher exposures, did not lead to a significant excess of myocardial infarction in exposed versus the nonexposed (21 versus 16 cases). Smulevich et al. (90) studied 3,232 workers producing VC and PVC between 1939 and 1977. They found 288 deaths, with a significant four- to five-fold excess of both leukemia and other hematopoietic cancers, each based on five deaths. However, there were no deaths from liver cancer, which might have been expected. Furthermore, considering the literature as a whole, there appears little support for excesses of hematopoietic cancers or lymphomas among VC-exposed workers. Finally, Hagmar et al. (91) studied 2,031 workers in a PVC processing plant with low exposures to VC (1–10 ppm). Among the 149 deaths, no angiosarcomas were observed. Using morbidity data, lung cancer (rate ratio 1.86, 0.99–3.18) and brain cancer (rate ratio 2.29, 0.84–4.98) were elevated.

Although one cannot completely exclude a causal role for VC exposure and other cancers, the epidemiologic data suggest the risk is limited to angiosarcoma. These data suggest that the risk of angiosarcoma is concentrated among workers with higher exposures, e.g., at least 1 year above 50 ppm, although one cannot exclude some increase in risk for workers with lower exposures. As current exposures for workers are generally below 1 ppm, one can anticipate minimal risk for currently exposed workers.

Several reports suggest the occurrence of cases of primary liver cancer or hepatocellular carcinoma (92,93), which might be expected based on animal studies, but the number of cases is very small. It should be noted that for individual plants actual historical exposures to VCM, PVC, and other copolymers and additives are not certain, and that unique or unusual exposures may have occurred at some of the plants. Such information could be lost in a large meta-analysis.

### Experimental Studies

In 1971 Viola and co-workers (94) first demonstrated the carcinogenicity of VCM in rats exposed to 30,000 ppm for 12 months. Hepatocarcinogenicity, particularly HAS, was reported later in a series of experiments by

Maltoni (95,96) and reproduced in other laboratories (5,7). VCM has been reported to produce HAS at doses as low as 25 ppm in rats, and a variety of tumors, including Zymbal gland carcinomas, nephroblastomas, nonhepatic angiosarcomas, and skin, brain, lung, and mammary tumors, have been produced in multiple species (including rats, mice, and hamsters) (7,95). Hepatocellular carcinomas also have been observed after exposure of newborns to VCM. The carcinogenicity data for animals has been reviewed in the Agency for Toxic Substances and Disease Registry (ATSDR) toxicologic profile for vinyl chloride (7).

A metabolite of vinyl chloride, rather than VCM itself, is the ultimate carcinogenic substance (97). In bacterial and other test systems, the mutagenicity of VCM is much increased by the addition of a metabolizing system (e.g., rat liver microsome), and an evaluation of animal carcinogenicity data suggested a closer link between HAS formation and the amount of VCM metabolized than the VCM exposure concentration (98). Although a number of mutagenic metabolites are formed, the reactive epoxide (chloroethylene oxide) formed during oxidative metabolism of the VCM double bond appears of greatest concern. Recent studies have demonstrated the formation of DNA adducts by the reactive metabolites of VCM (99–107), and such data have been used in the development of models to predict cancer risk (108,109). The short-lived active metabolites are formed in the hepatocytes but are carcinogenic in the adjacent sinusoidal cells, which, unlike the hepatocytes, appear to have limited ability for detoxification (110).

The most exciting developments in recent years are those that begin to explain how DNA damage may initiate the carcinogenic process. Several possibilities have been suggested, including (a) mutations in *ras* oncogenes and expression of their encoded p21 proteins, (b) mutation of the p53 tumor suppressor gene, and (c) detection of Kaposi's sarcoma-associated herpesvirus-like DNA sequences in angiosarcoma (111–115). There is also the possibility that mutant p21 or p53 in serum could serve as a biomarker for detection of disease.

The evidence for the carcinogenicity of vinyl chloride raised considerable concern about the safety of a number of structurally related halogenated hydrocarbons (116,117). Studies on animals indicate some evidence for carcinogenicity of vinylidene chloride (118), vinyl bromide (116), and trichloroethylene and tetrachloroethylene. Green (119) has summarized the differences between VCM and these structurally related chemicals: in short, he states that VCM produces more tumors, in more species, more consistently, and at lower doses, and by a direct genotoxic mechanism, and therefore has more marked carcinogenic properties. For some of these related compounds, however, only limited data are available on potential human carcinogenicity (119).

## OCCUPATIONAL STANDARDS

In the United States, the Occupational Safety and Health Administration (OSHA) requires that a worker's exposure to VCM not exceed 1 ppm (8-hour time-weighted average) [permissible exposure limit (PEL) TWA]. The ceiling concentration limit for 15 minutes or less is 5 ppm [short-term exposure limit (STEL) 15 minutes] (44). In general, except in the Scandinavian countries, European VCM exposure standards are somewhat higher than in the United States (5).

## REFERENCES


1. Berk PD, Martin JF, Young RS, et al. Vinyl chloride—associated liver disease. *Ann Intern Med* 1976;84:717–731.
2. Gauvain S, Barnes AW, Williamson KS, et al. Vinyl chloride. *Proc R Soc Med* 1976;69:275.
3. Milby TH, ed. *Vinyl chloride:* an information resource. DHEW publication (NIOSH) 78-1599. Washington, DC: U.S. Government Printing Office; 1978.
4. Selikoff IJ, Hammond EC, eds. Toxicity of vinyl chloride—polyvinyl chloride. *Ann NY Acad Sci* 1975;246:1–337.
5. Vinyl chloride, polyvinyl chloride, and vinyl chloride-vinyl acetate copolymers. *IARC Monogr Eval Carcinog Risk Chem Hum* 1979;19: 377.
6. Waxweiler RJ, Landrigan PJ, Infante P, et al., eds. Conference to reevaluate the toxicity of vinyl chloride, poly (vinyl chloride) and structural analogs. *Environ Health Perspect* 1981;41:1–231.
7. *Toxicological profile for vinyl chloride.* Atlanta, GA: Agency for Toxic Substances and Disease Registry; 1997.
8. Doll R. Effects of exposure to vinyl chloride—an assessment of the evidence. *Scand J Work Environ Health* 1988;14:61–78.
9. Layman PL. PVC global outlook brightens as substitution by competitors levels off. *Chem Eng News* 1996(May 6);22–25.
10. Lilis R, Anderson H, Miller A, et al. Pulmonary changes among vinyl chloride polymerization workers. *Chest* 1976;69:299–303.
11. Harris DK, Adams WGF. Acroosteolysis occurring in men engaged in the polymerization of vinyl chloride. *Br Med J* 1967;2:712–714.
12. Wilson RH, McCormick WE, Tatum CF, et al. Occupational acroosteolysis. *JAMA* 1967;201:577–581.
13. Dinman BD, Cook WA, Whitehouse WM, et al. Occupational acroosteolysis: I. An epidemiological study. *Arch Environ Health* 1971;22: 61–73.
14. Cook WA, Giever PM, Dinman DD, et al. Occupational acroosteolysis: II. An industrial hygiene study. *Arch Environ Health* 1971;22: 74–82.
15. Dodson VN, Dinman BD, Whitehouse WM, et al. Occupational acroosteolysis: III. A clinical study. *Arch Environ Health* 1971;22: 83–91.
16. Hahn E, Aderka D, Suprun H, et al. Occupational acroosteolysis in vinyl chloride workers in Israel. *Isr J Med* Sci 1979;15:218–222.
17. Johnston ENM. Vinyl chloride disease. *Br J Dermatol* 1978;99: 45–48.
18. Markowitz SS, McDonald CJ, Fethiere W, et al. Occupational acroosteolysis. *Arch Dermatol* 1972;106:219.
19. Ostlere LS, Harris D, Buckley C, Black C, Rustin MHA. Atypical systemic sclerosis following exposure to vinyl chloride monomer. A case report and review of the cutaneous aspects of vinyl chloride disease. *Clin Exp Dermatol* 1992;17:208–210.
20. Knight KR, Gibbons R. Increased collagen synthesis and cross-link formation in the skin of rats exposed to vinyl chloride monomer. *Clin Sci* 1987;72:673–678.
21. Falappa P, Magnavita N, Bergamaschi A, Colavita N. Angiographic study of digital arteries in workers exposed to vinyl chloride. *Br J Ind Med* 1982;39:169–172.
22. Lange CE, Jühe S, Stein G, et al. So-called vinyl chloride disease: Is it an occupational systemic sclerosis? *Int Arch Arbeitsmed* 1974;32: 1–32.
23. Ward AM, Udnoon S, Watkins J, et al. Immunological mechanisms in the pathogenesis of vinyl chloride disease. *Br Med J* 1976;1:936–938.

24. Haustein UF, Ziegler V. Environmentally induced systemic sclerosis-like disorders. *Int J Dermatol* 1985;24:147–151.
25. Veltman G, Lange GE, Jühe S, et al. Clinical manifestations and course of vinyl chloride disease. *Ann NY Acad Sci* 1975;246:6–17.
26. Gedigk P, Muller R, Bechtelsheimer H. Morphology of liver damage among polyvinyl chloride production workers: a report on 51 cases. *Ann NY Acad Sci* 1975;246:278–285.
27. Marsteller HJ, Lelbach W, Muller R, et al. Unusual splenomegalic liver disease as evidenced by peritoneoscopy and guided liver biopsy among polyvinyl chloride production workers. *Ann NY Acad Sci* 1975;246:95–134.
28. Creech JL Jr, Johnson MN. Angiosarcoma of liver in the manufacture of polyvinyl chloride. *J Occup Med* 1974;16:150–151.
29. Falk H, Creech JL Jr, Heath CW Jr, et al. Hepatic disease among workers at a vinyl chloride polymerization plant. *JAMA* 1973;230: 59–63.
30. Popper H, Thomas LB. Alterations of liver and spleen among workers exposed to vinyl chloride. *Ann NY Acad Sci* 1975;246:172–194.
31. Popper H, Thomas LB, Telles NC, et al. Development of hepatic angiosarcoma in man induced by vinyl chloride, Thorotrast, and arsenic: comparison with cases of unknown etiology. *Am J Pathol* 1978;92:349–376.
32. Thomas LB, Popper H, Berk PD, et al. Vinyl chloride—induced liver disease from idiopathic portal hypertension (Banti's syndrome) to angiosarcomas. *N Engl J* Med 1975;292:17–22.
33. Blendis LM, Smith PM, Lawrie BW, et al. Portal hypertension in vinyl chloride monomer workers: a hemodynamic study. *Gastroenterology* 1978;75:206–211.
34. Dietz A, Langbein G, Permanetter W. (Vinyl chloride—induced hepatocellular carcinoma.) *Klin Wochenschr* 1985;63:325–331.
35. Evans DMD, Jones Williams W, Kung ITM. Angiosarcoma and hepatocellular carcinoma in vinyl chloride workers. *Histopathology* 1983; 7:377–388.
36. Popper H, Gerber MA, Schaffner F, et al. Environmental hepatic injury in man. *Prog Liver Dis* 1979;6:605–638.
37. Lilis R, Anderson H, Nicholson WJ, et al. Prevalence of disease among vinyl chloride and polyvinyl chloride workers. *Ann NY Acad Sci* 1975;246:22–41.
38. Tamburro CH. Relationship of vinyl monomers and liver cancers: angiosarcoma and hepatocellular carcinoma. *Semin Liver Dis* 1984;4: 158–169.
39. Waxweiler RJ, Falk H, McMichael A, et al. *A cross-sectional epidemiologic survey of vinyl chloride workers.* DHEW publication (NIOSH) 77-177. Washington, DC: U.S. Government Printing Office, 1977.
40. Kotseva K. Five year follow up study of the incidence of arterial hypertension and coronary heart disease in vinyl chloride monomer and polyvinyl chloride production workers. *Int Arch Occup Environ Health* 1996;68:377–379.
41. Wyatt RH, Kotchen JM, Hochstrasser DL, et al. An epidemiologic study of blood screening tests and illness histories among chemical workers involved in the manufacture of poly-vinyl chloride. *Ann NY Acad Sci* 1975;246:80–87.
42. Makk L, Creech JL, Whelan JG Jr, et al. Liver damage and angiosarcoma in vinyl chloride workers: a systematic detection program. *JAMA* 1974;230:64–68.
43. Ho SF, Phoon WH, Gan SL, Chan YK. Persistent liver dysfunction among workers at a vinyl chloride monomer polymerization plant. *J Soc Occup Med* 1991;41:10–16.
44. United States Occupational Safety and Health Administration. 39 *Federal Register* 35, 890, 1974.
45. Liss GM, Greenberg RA, Tamburro CH. Use of serum bile acids in the identification of vinyl chloride hepatotoxicity. *Am J Med* 1985;78: 68–76.
46. Studniarek M, Durski K, Liniecki J, Brykalski D, Poznanska A, Gluszcz M. Effects of vinyl chloride on liver function of exposed workers, evaluated by measurements of plasma clearance of the 99mTc-N-2, 4-dimethylacetanilido—iminodiacetate complex. *J Appl Toxicol* 1989;9:213–218.
47. Tamburro CH. Health effects of vinyl chloride. *Tex Rep Biol Med* 1978;37:126–144;146–151.
48. Li GY, Wang T, Huggins EM Jr, et al. Cholylglycine measured in serum by RIA and interleukin-1 beta determined by ELISA in differentiating viral hepatitis from chemical liver injury. *J Occup Med* 1992;34:930–933.
49. Froment O, Marion MJ, Lepot D, Contassot JC, Trepo C. Immunoquantitation of Von Willebrand factor (factor VIII-related antigen) in vinyl chloride exposed workers. *Cancer Lett* 1991;201–206.
50. Fitzgerald EJ, Griffiths TM. Computerized tomography of vinyl chloride—induced angiosarcoma of liver. *Br J Radiol* 1987;60:593–595.
51. Tamburro CH, Makk L, Popper H. Early hepatic histologic alterations among chemical (vinyl monomer) workers. *Hepatology* 1984;4: 413–418.
52. Whelan JG Jr, Creech JL, Tamburro CH. Angiographic and radionuclide characteristics of hepatic angiosarcoma found in vinyl chloride workers. *Radiology* 1976;118:549–557.
53. Williams DMJ, Smith PM, Taylor KJW, et al. Monitoring liver disorders in vinyl chloride monomer workers using gray-scale ultrasonography. *Br J Ind Med* 1976;33:152–157.
54. Maricq HR, Darke CS, Archibald RM, et al. In vivo observations of skin capillaries in workers exposed to vinyl chloride: an English-American comparison. *Br J Ind Med* 1978;35:1–7.
55. Berk PD, Martin JF, Waggoner JG. Persistence of vinyl chloride—induced liver injury after cessation of exposure. *Ann NY Acad Sci* 1975;246:70–77.
56. Dannaher CL, Tamburro CH, Yam LT. Chemotherapy of vinyl chloride-associated hepatic angiosarcoma. *Cancer* 1981;47:466–469.
57. Gamble J, Liu S, McMichael AJ, et al. Effect of occupational and nonoccupational factors on the respiratory system of vinyl chloride and other workers. *J Occup Med* 1976;18:659–670.
58. Soutar CA, Copland LH, Thornley PE, et al. Epidemiological study of respiratory disease in workers exposed to polyvinyl chloride dust. *Thorax* 1980;35:644–652.
59. Baser ME, Tockman MS, Kennedy TP. Pulmonary function and respiratory symptoms in polyvinylchloride fabrication workers. *Am Rev Respir Dis* 1985;131:203–208.
60. El-Gamal M, Kordy MN, Ibrahim MA. Study of respiratory symptoms and lung function in polyvinyl chloride fabrication workers. *Saudi Med J* 1995;16:36–41.
61. Ng TP, Lee HS, Low YM, Phoon WH, Ng YL. Pulmonary effects of polyvinyl chloride dust exposure on compounding workers. *Scand J Work Environ Health* 1991;17:53–59.
62. Oleru UG, Onyekwere C. Exposures to polyvinyl chloride, methyl ketone and other chemicals—the pulmonary and non-pulmonary effect. *Int Arch Occup Environ Health* 1992;63:503–507.
63. Arnaud A, Pommier DeSanti P, Garbe L, et al. Polyvinyl chloride pneumoconiosis. *Thorax* 1978;33:19–25.
64. Mastrangelo G, Manno M, Marcer G, et al. Polyvinyl chloride pneumoconiosis: epidemiological study of exposed workers. *J Occup Med* 1979;21:540–542.
65. Studnicka MJ, Menzinger G, Drlicek M, Maruna H, Neumann MG. Pneumoconiosis and systemic sclerosis following 10 years of exposure to polyvinyl chloride dust. *Thorax* 1995; 50:583–585.
66. Giri AK. Genetic toxicology of vinyl chloride-A review. *Mutat Res* 1995;339:1–14.
67. Fucic A, Barkovic D, Garaj-Vrhovac V, et al. A nine-year follow up study of a population occupationally exposed to vinyl chloride monomer. *Mutat Res* 1996;361:49–53.
68. Fucic A, Hitrec V, Garaj-Vrhovac V, Barkovic D, Kubelka D. Relationship between locations of chromosome breaks induced by vinyl chloride monomer and lymphocytosis. *Am J Ind Med* 1995;27: 565–571.
69. Fucic A, Horvat D, Dimitrovic B. Localization of breaks induced by vinyl chloride in the human chromosomes of lymphocytes. *Mutat Res* 1990;243:95–99.
70. Infante PF, Wagoner JK, McMichael AJ, et al. Genetic risks of vinyl chloride. *Lancet* 1976;1:734–735.
71. Clemmesen J. Mutagenicity and teratogenicity of vinyl chloride monomer (VCM)—epidemiological evidence. *Mutat Res* 1982;98: 97–100.
72. Infante P. Oncogenic and mutagenic risks in communities with polyvinyl chloride production facilities. *Ann NY Acad Sci* 1976;271: 49–57.
73. Theriault G, Iturra H, Gingras S. Evaluation of the association between birth defects and exposure to ambient vinyl chloride. *Teratology* 1983;27:359–370.
74. Edmonds LD, Anderson CE, Flynt JW Jr, et al. Congenital central nervous system malformations and vinyl chloride monomer exposure: a community study. *Teratology* 1978;17:137–142.
75. Perticoni GF, Abbritti G, Cantisani TA, Bondi L, Mauro L. Polyneu-

ropathy in workers with long exposure to vinyl chloride—electrophysiological study. *Electromyogr Clin Neurophysiol* 1986;26:41–47.
76. Langauer-Lewowicka H, Kurzbauer H, Byczkowska Z, Wocka-Marek T. Vinyl chloride disease—neurological disturbances. *Int Arch Occup Environ Health* 1983;52:151–157.
77. Lloyd JW. Angiosarcoma of the liver in vinyl chloride/polyvinyl chloride workers. *J Occup Med* 1975;17:333–334.
78. Spirtas R, Kaminski R. Angiosarcoma of the liver in vinyl chloride/polyvinyl chloride workers: 1977 update of the NIOSH register. *J Occup Med* 1978;20:427–429.
79. Purchase IFH, Stafford J, Paddle GM. Vinyl chloride: an assessment of the risk of occupational exposure. *Food Chem Toxicol* 1987;25: 187–202.
80. Forman D, Bennett B, Stafford J, Doll R. Exposure to vinyl chloride and angiosarcoma of the liver: a report of the register of cases. *Br J Ind Med* 1985;42:750–753.
81. Lee FI, Smith PM, Bennett B, Williams DMJ. Occupationally related angiosarcoma of the liver in the United Kingdom 1972-1994. *Gut* 1996;39:312–318.
82. Baxter PJ, Anthony PP, MacSween RNM, et al. Angiosarcoma of the liver: annual occurrence and aetiology in Great Britain. *Br J Ind Med* 1980;37:213–221.
83. Brady J, Liberatore F, Harper P, et al. Angiosarcoma of the liver: an epidemiologic survey. *J Natl Cancer Inst* 1977;59:1383–1385.
84. Falk H, Telles NC, Ishak KG, et al. Epidemiology of Thorotrast-induced hepatic angiosarcoma in the United States. *Environ Res* 1979;18:65–73.
85. Falk H, Herbert J, Crowley S, et al. Epidemiology of hepatic angiosarcoma in the United States, 1964–1974. *Environ Health Perspect* 1981;41:107–113.
86. Wu W, Steenland K, Brown D, et al. Cohort and case-control analyses of workers exposed to vinyl chloride: an update. *J Occup Med* 1989;31: 518–523.
87. Waxweiler R, Smith A, Falk H, et al. Excess lung cancer risk in a synthetic chemical plant. *Environ Health Perspect* 1981;41:159–165.
88. Simonato L, L'Abbe K, Andersen A, et al. A collaborative study of cancer incidence and mortality among vinyl chloride workers. *Scand J Work Environ Health* 1991;17:159–169.
89. Laplanche A, Clavel-Chapelon F, Contassot J, Lanouziere C, French VCM group. Exposure to vinyl chloride monomer: results of a cohort study after a seven year follow up. *Br J Ind Med* 1992;49:134–137.
90. Smulevich V, Fedotova I, Filatova V. Increasing evidence of the rise of cancer in workers exposed to vinyl chloride. *Br J Ind Med* 1988;45: 93–97.
91. Hagmar L, Akesson B, Nielsen J, et al. Mortality and cancer morbidity in workers exposed to low levels of vinyl chloride monomer at a polyvinyl chloride processing plant. *Am J Ind Med* 1990;17: 553–565.
92. Lelbach WK. A 25-year follow-up study of heavily exposed vinyl chloride workers in Germany. *Am J Ind Med* 1996; 29:446–458.
93. Pirastu R, Comba P, Reggiani A, Foa V, Masina A, Maltoni C. Mortality from liver disease among Italian vinyl chloride monomer/polyvinyl chloride manufacturers. *Am J Ind Med* 1990;17:155–161.
94. Viola PL, Bigotti A, Caputo A. Oncogenic response of rat skin, lungs, and bones to vinyl chloride. *Cancer Res* 1971;31:516–519.
95. Maltoni C. Vinyl chloride carcinogenicity: an experimental model for carcinogenesis studies. In: Hiatt HH, Watson JD, Winsten JA, eds. *Origins of human cancer:* incidence of cancer in humans. Cold Spring Harbor Conference on Cell Proliferation, vol 4. Cold Spring Harbor, NY: Cold Spring Harbor Laboratory, 1977;A119–146.
96. Maltoni C, Cotti G. Carcinogenicity of vinyl chloride in Sprague-Dawley rats after prenatal and postnatal exposure. *Ann NY Acad Sci* 1988;534:145–159.
97. Gwinner LM, Laib RJ, Filser JG, Bolt HM. Evidence of chloroethylene oxide being the reactive metabolite of vinyl chloride towards DNA: comparative studies with 2, 2′-dichloro-diethylether. *Carcinogenesis* 1983;4:1483–1486.
98. Gehring PJ, Watanabe PG, Park CN. Resolution of dose-response toxicity data for chemicals requiring metabolic activation: example-vinyl chloride. *Toxicol Appl Pharmacol* 1978;44:581–591.
99. Bolt HM, Laib RJ, Peter H, Ottenwalder H. DNA adducts of halogenated hydrocarbons. *J Cancer Res Clin Oncol* 1986;112:92–96.
100. Eberle G, Barbin A, Laib RJ, Ciroussel F, Thomale J, Bartsch H, Rajewsky F. 1, N6-Etheno-21-deoxyadenosine and 3, N4-etheno-21-deoxycytidine detected by monoclonal antibodies in lung and liver DNA of rats exposed to vinyl chloride. *Carcinogenesis* 1989;10: 209–212.
101. Fedtke N, Boucheron JA, Turner MJ Jr, Swenberg JA. Vinyl chloride—induced DNA adducts. I: Quantitative determination of N2, 3-ethenoguanine based on electrophore labeling. *Carcinogenesis* 1990; 11:1279–1285.
102. Fedtke N, Boucheron JA, Walker VE, Swenberg JA. Vinyl chloride-induced DNA adducts. II: Formation and persistence of 7-(21-oxoethyl) guanine and N2, 3-ethenoguanine in rat tissue DNA. *Carcinogenesis* 1990;11:1287–1292.
103. Swenberg JA, Fedtke N, Ciroussel F, Barbin A, Bartsh H. Etheno adducts formed in DNA of vinyl chloride-exposed rats are highly persistent in liver. *Carcinogenesis* 1992; 13:727–729.
104. La DK, Swenberg JA. DNA Adducts: biological markers of exposure and potential applications to risk assessment. *Mutat Res* 1996;365: 129–146.
105. Ballering LAP, Nivard MJM, Vogel EW. Characterization by two-endpoint comparisons of the genetic toxicity profiles of vinyl chloride and related etheno-adduct forming carcinogens in Drosophila. Carcinogenesis 1996;17:1083–1092.
106. Dosanjh MK, Chenna A, Kim E, Fraenkel-Conrat H, Samson L, Singer B. All four known cyclic adducts formed in DNA by the vinyl chloride metabolite chloroacetaldehyde are released by a human DNA glycosylase. *Proc Natl Acad Sci USA* 1994;91:1024–1028.
107. Singer B. DNA damage: chemistry, repair, and mutagenic potential. *Regul Toxicol Pharmacol* 1996;23:2–13.
108. Reitz RH, Gargas ML, Andersen ME, Provan WM, Green TL. Predicting cancer risk from vinyl chloride exposure with a physiologically based pharmacokinetic model. *Toxicol Appl Pharmacol* 1996; 137:253–267.
109. Clewell HJ, Gentry PR, Gearhart JM, Allen BC, Andersen ME. Considering pharmacokinetic and mechanistic information in cancer risk assessments for environmental contaminants: examples with vinyl chloride and trichloroethylene. *Chemosphere* 1995;31:2561–2578.
110. Ottenwalder H, Bolt HM. Metabolic activation of vinyl chloride and vinyl bromide by isolated hepatocytes and hepatic sinusoidal cells. *J Environ Pathol Toxicol* 1980;4:411–417.
111. DeVivo I, Marion MJ, Smith SJ, Carney WP, Brandt-Rauf PW. Mutant c-ki-ras p21 protein in chemical carcinogenesis in humans exposed to vinyl chloride. *Cancer Causes Control* 1994;5:273–278.
112. Soini Y, Welsh JA, Ishak KG, Bennett WP. p53 mutations in primary hepatic angiosarcomas not associated with vinyl chloride exposure. *Carcinogenesis* 1995;16:2879–2881.
113. Trivers GE, Cawley HL, DeBenedetti VMG, et al. Anti-p53 antibodies in sera of workers occupationally exposed to vinyl chloride. *J Natl Cancer Inst* 1995;87:1400–1407.
114. Kemp CJ. Hepatocarcinogenesis in p53-deficient mice. *Mol Carcinogenesis* 1995;12:132–136.
115. McDonagh D, Liu J, Gaffey MJ, Layfield LJ, Azumi N, Traweek ST. Detection of Kaposi's sarcoma-associated herpesvirus-like DNA sequences in angiosarcoma. *Am J Pathol* 1996;149:1363–1368.
116. Bolt HM, Laib RJ, Stockle G. Formation of preneoplastic hepatocellular foci by vinyl bromide in newborn rats. *Arch Toxicol* 1979;43:83–84.
117. Bogdanffy MS, Makovec GT, Frame SR. Inhalation oncogenicity bioassey in rats and mice with vinyl fluoride. *Fundam Appl Toxicol* 1995;26:223–238.
118. Cotti G, Maltoni C, Lefemine G. Long-term carcinogenicity bioassay on vinylidene chloride administered by inhalation to Sprague-Dawley rats—new results. *Ann NY Acad Sci* 1988;534:160–168.
119. Green T. Chloroethylenes: a mechanistic approach to human risk evaluation. *Annu Rev Pharmacol Toxicol* 1990;30:73–89.

*Environmental and Occupational Medicine, Third Edition,* edited by William N. Rom.
Lippincott–Raven Publishers, Philadelphia © 1998.

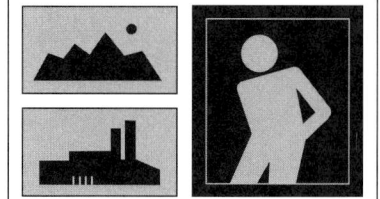

# CHAPTER 94

# Polycyclic Aromatic Hydrocarbons

Jan Schwarz-Miller, Michael D. Goldstein, and Paul W. Brandt-Rauf

Polycyclic aromatic hydrocarbons (PAHs) are widely dispersed in nature and are formed during combustion of organic material and high-temperature processing of crude oil, coal, coke, or other industrial carbon compounds. PAHs contain multiple benzene rings (i.e., three or more aromatic rings that share a pair of carbon atoms). Typical PAH chemical structures are illustrated in Fig. 1. They are important to occupational health because many of the substituted compounds are potent carcinogens, and many processes in a variety of workplaces are contaminated with PAHs.

Benzo[*a*]pyrene (BaP) is one of the most important carcinogens of the group. Often, it is measured to indicate the presence or absence of PAHs, though the correlation between BaP content and the actual carcinogenicity of the compound may be weak. Anthracene and phenanthrene are not carcinogenic, but methyl additions may render the compounds carcinogenic (1). Figure 2 illustrates the sites of methylation that produce carcinogenic activity in benzanthracene (1). The 7,12-dimethylbenzanthracene is a very potent carcinogen.

Technically, naphthalene is not considered a PAH because it has only two fused benzene rings. It is the single most abundant constituent of coal tar and is used as a moth repellent, an insecticide, and in various chemicals. It is a skin irritant, and vapors may cause headache, nausea, diaphoresis, and vomiting. It can cause hemolytic anemia as well.

Exposure to coal tars, pitches, asphalt fumes, and carbon black all lead to exposure to PAHs. Tars and pitches are black or brown, liquid or semisolid products derived from coal, petroleum, wood, shale oil, or other organic materials. Generally, pitches are solid residues from heated and distilled tars. Coal tar is condensed from the effluent of coke oven plants. Asphalt is the residuum remaining after the fractional distillation of crude oil. Asphalt fumes are defined as the cloud of small particles created by condensation from the gaseous state after the

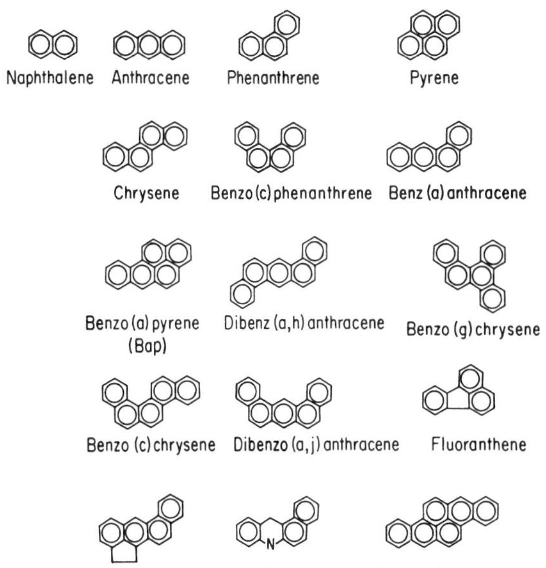


**FIG. 1.** Polycyclic aromatic hydrocarbons.

J. Schwarz-Miller: Division of Environmental Health Sciences, Occupational Medicine Atlantic Health System, Columbia University School of Public Health, Morristown, New Jersey 07962.

M. D. Goldstein: Columbia University School of Public Health, New York, New York 10032.

P. W. Brandt-Rauf: Division of Environmental Health Sciences, Columbia University School of Public Health, New York, New York 10032.

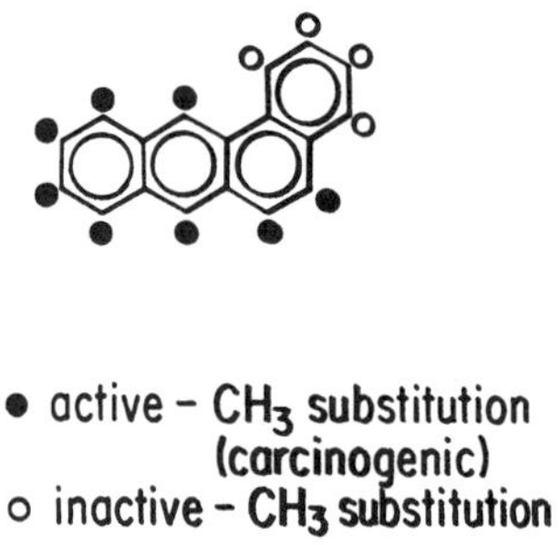


**FIG. 2.** Benzanthracene.

volatilization of asphalt (2). Creosote is distilled from coal tar and used in wood preservation, naphtha, oils, and other chemicals.

## POPULATIONS AT RISK

### Historical Perspective

The era of scientific inquiry into environmental carcinogenesis began in 1775, when Sir Percival Pott (3) described cancer of the scrotum in English chimney sweeps. The soot in the chimneys contaminated the workers' pants and, consequently, the skin in contact with the pants. Pott wrote that the disease "seems to derive its origin from a lodgement of soot in the rugae of the scrotum" (3).

In 1910, Wilson described 35 cases of cancer of the scrotum in Manchester, England. Twenty-five were among mulespinners from cotton textile factories, and five had once been mulespinners (4). Southam and Wilson (5) reviewed all 141 cases of cancer of the scrotum seen at the Royal Infirmary of Manchester from 1902 to 1922. The patients were predominantly mulespinners; only one was a chimney sweep. The work environment of mulespinners was very hot and humid; they wore a single layer of clothing. Their job was to lean over a carriage bar containing spinning cotton spindles that were lubricated twice daily with oil refined from shale (shale oil). Balancing on the left leg, they leaned over the bar, exposing their pants to the splashing mineral oil. Ninety percent of the scrotal cancers appeared on the anterior aspect of the left side of the scrotum. In 1908, cancer of the scrotum receive statutory recognition in England: "Scrotal epithelioma occurring in chimney sweeps and epitheliomatous cancer or ulceration of the skin occurring in the handling or use of pitch, tar, and tarry compounds was added to the third schedule of the Workman's Compensation Act" (6).

From 1900 to 1921 Scott (7) reported 65 workers with epithelioma among Scottish shale oil workers. The epitheliomas occurred predominantly on the scrotum or upper extremities, and the risk increased with duration of exposure. Substitution of refined petroleum lubricant oil for shale oil was required in Great Britain in 1953, and use of the spinning mule has been virtually eliminated.

Leitch (8) was among the first to show oil shale's carcinogenicity with skin-painting experiments on animals, and in 1933 Cook and co-workers (9) identified BaP as a carcinogenic constituent of coal tar.

Waldron and co-workers (10) reported 344 cases of scrotal cancer in the West Midlands between 1936 and 1976. About 70% of the men affected had been exposed to mineral oil; 89 worked as tool setters and tool fitters, and some 7% to 8% were exposed to tar and pitch.

### Occupational and Environmental

Epidemiologic studies have implicated PAHs in a variety of other cancers including lung and other respiratory, bladder, skin, lymphatic and hematopoietic, buccal cavity, esophagus, stomach, colon, pancreatic, kidney, laryngeal, and brain cancers. PAH exposure occurs in a variety of occupations and settings. These include, but are not limited to, coke ovens, gas-generation facilities, crude petroleum refineries, aluminum-reduction work, roofing, asphalt work, carbon black production, coal-conversion and oil-shale-retorting processes, and the myriad jobs in which cutting oils are used.

Coke oven workers are exposed to myriad PAHs during the coking of coal, and they have an elevated rate of cancer mortality. A number of studies have shown an increased rate of lung cancer in these workers (11–15). Lloyd (11) reported that men employed as coke oven workers had a lung cancer mortality rate more than twice that predicted by the experience of all steel workers and that the risk increased with both the duration of employment and level of exposure. He also reported an excess mortality of cancer of the kidney. The lung cancer risk was greater for workers employed on top of the coke ovens, compared to those working at the sides, reflecting more exposure to PAHs formed during high-temperature carbonization. The National Institute for Occupational Safety and Health (NIOSH) found that the BaP level on the top of the coke oven was 18 $\mu g/m^3$ for an 8-hour time-weighted average (TWA) versus 7 $\mu g/m^3$ at the side (12). Redmond and colleagues (13) evaluated the mortality of 1,852 coke plant workers with more than 5 years' employment and found significant elevations in standardized mortality ratios (SMRs) from cancer of the respiratory and genitourinary systems. Among the topside workers with at least 15 years' experience, eight of the 29 died of a respiratory cancer. This represents almost 16 times greater relative risk (14). They also found that coke plant workers who were not oven workers had excess mortality from cancer of the colon, pancreas, buccal cavity, and pharynx (13). Bertrand and colleagues (15) reported that mortality due to lung cancer was 2.51 times higher than expected in two coke oven plants. In 1976 the Occupational Safety and Health Administration (OSHA) set a permissible exposure limit to coke oven emissions of 150 μg/$m^3$ benzene-soluble fraction of total particulate matter (BSFTPM). The standard went into effect in 1977.

Workers in gas generation facilities have been found to have increased rates of cancers. Kawai and co-workers (16) reported a 33-fold increase in lung cancer risk among male workers exposed to tar fumes while employed at the gas-generation facility of a Japanese steel mill. The risk was even greater among workers employed longer than 20 years. Sir Richard Doll and colleagues (17–19) extended those observations with their studies of a London gas company. The number of deaths from lung cancer was approximately double that for male inhabitants of London of the same age. In following those with more than 5 years' employment, Doll's group found that the most heavily exposed carbonizers had 69% more lung cancers and four times as many bladder cancers as minimally exposed or unexposed workers. The absolute increase in mortality from lung cancer was 160; for bladder cancer, 23; and for scrotum and skin cancer, 12 per 100,000 per year. Both Kawai and Doll's groups concluded that smoking could not account for the observed increases. Lawther and colleagues (20) reported the BaP level to be 3 μg/$m^3$ as the 8-hour TWA exposure in an English gasworks.

PAHs are thought to be responsible for excessive cancer risk among aluminum reduction workers. Coal tar pitch is employed as a binder in the pots during the electrolytic production of aluminum by the Söderberg process. Vertical electrodes in this process may release pitch volatiles, exposing aluminum potroom workers to PAHs. Milham (21) found elevated SMRs for lung, lymphatic and hematopoietic, and pancreatic cancers in a cohort study of a Washington plant, and Gibbs and Horowitz (22) found a dose-response relationship between lung cancer mortality and tar-years and years of exposure in Quebec.

Ronnenberg and Langmark (23) evaluated eight separate investigations of aluminum plant workers (47,000 men) and three investigations of carbon plant workers (4,700 men). They concluded that there was an increased risk of bladder cancer in men who work in Söderberg potrooms. This association increased with increasing duration of exposure to coal tar pitch volatiles. The results were not as convincing for lung cancer. Two of the studies showed statistically significant excess of lung cancers, but the authors caution that these results and the bladder cancer results, may be biased secondary to both inadequate smoking histories and inadequate assessments of exposures to other occupational carcinogens. Details of some of the studies that they reviewed are described below.

Thériault's group (24,25) conducted a case-control study on all cases of bladder cancer in men in areas with aluminum plants in Quebec between 1970 and 1979. They identified individuals who had worked in aluminum plants and found that there was a statistically significant association between bladder cancer risk and cumulative exposure. Armstrong et al. (24) analyzed these data with improved smoking histories and estimates of exposure and concluded that, among individuals employed in the Söderberg potrooms, there was an increased relative risk of bladder cancer that was tied to each year of exposure to BaP and to benzene soluble material. Gibbs and Horowitz (22) conducted a mortality study in workers at three aluminum plants in Quebec. Cumulative exposure to tar exposure was calculated and a statistically significant association was seen between exposure and lung and bladder cancer. When comparing the lung cancer deaths to local rather than regional mortality rates, the association was not found for lung cancer. In the tar exposed population there were also statistically significant increases in deaths reported from pneumonia, bronchitis, and gastric and esophageal cancer, but not from leukemias or cancers of the pancreas, larynx, and brain. There also was increased mortality due to Hodgkin's disease as well as excess deaths from a category defined as "other malignancies."

Rockette and Arena (26) investigated the mortality data of 21,829 men who worked for at least 5 years between 1946 and 1977 in U.S. aluminum plants. These men worked in both prebake and Söderberg plants. The data were broken down by the work area and length of employment. They found statistically significant excesses of death due to pancreatic cancer, leukemia, and lung cancer. These findings were specific to certain areas of the plants and required prolonged exposures. Interestingly, mortality from lung cancer was only found after 25 years of exposure in workers employed for at least 25 years in the carbon area of one prebake plant. Armstrong et al. (24) were interested in analyzing the contribution of smoking to lung cancer mortality in the Gibbs and Horowitz (22) cohort. They obtained more detailed smoking histories, controlled for smoking, and still found a clear excess in lung cancer risk among the workers with higher exposures to coal tar pitch volatiles. Tremblay et al. (25) conducted a nested case-control study on aluminum plant workers and were able to add 69 new cases of bladder. They concluded that there is excess risk of developing bladder cancer among men employed in Söderberg potrooms. They stated that this conclusion was not confounded by smoking, but they could not ensure that there were not other contributing exposures. Both the Armstrong and Tremblay groups thought that the combination of smoking and occupational exposure to coal tar pitch volatiles could act additively or multiplicatively in the development of bladder and lung cancer.

Roofers and asphalt workers may be exposed to coal tar and/or bitumen fumes. Bitumens are obtained as residuals from nondestructive distillate of crude petroleum oil. Bitumens are dark solid or semisolid materials predominantly composed of asphaltenes, straight and branched aliphatic hydrocarbons, naphthene aromatics, and resins. The amount of PAHs in bitumens varies, but the amount is substantially lower than is found in coal tars and coal-tar pitches.

Roofers have been found to have elevated cancer rates. Menck and Henderson (27) found that roofers' rate of lung cancer mortality was five times that of the general population. Hammond and co-workers (28) performed a mortality study of roofers exposed to hot fumes from roofing materials, including coal tar, pitch, and asphalt. They reported excess mortality for cancer of the lung, stomach, bladder, and skin (except malignant melanoma) and for leukemia in roofers with at least 20 years' exposure. Smoking habits were not evaluated. Partanen and Boffetta (29) conducted a review and meta-analysis of epidemiologic studies of asphalt workers and roofers. In the aggregate analysis of the roofers there were significant excesses of lung cancer [relative risk (RR) of 1.8], stomach cancer (RR of 1.7), nonmelanoma skin cancer (RR of 4.0), and leukemia (RR of 1.7).

Highway maintenance workers and road pavers as well as many other types of workers are exposed to asphalt fumes. Asphalt fumes are primarily an irritant of mucous membranes, especially of the conjunctiva and upper respiratory tract. The amounts of BaP found in asphalt fumes from two different hot-mix asphalt plants ranged from 3 to 22 ng/m$^3$; this is approximately 0.03% of the amount of coke oven emissions (2). Hansen (30) performed a historical cohort study of unskilled asphalt workers. They were found to have an increased number of deaths due to respiratory and urinary bladder cancer. An increased risk of digestive cancer was also seen in the last 5 years of the data. In addition, three cases of brain cancer were found (SMR = 500). It has been suspected that the increased cancer mortality may be due to exposure to bitumen fumes, to which roofers are also exposed. Both Knecht and Woitowitz (31) and Hansen (32) report increased incidence of cancer mortality due to bitumen fumes, and both state that the amount of PAH released from bitumen is minimal and is not likely to be the cause of the increased cancer. Jongeneelen and associates (33) measured ambient PAH level exposure of road workers applying bitumen and reported moderate levels in air. Partanen and Boffetta (29) conducted a review and meta-analysis of epidemiologic studies of asphalt workers and roofers. They found that the aggregate relative risk in road pavers and highway maintenance workers for cancers of the lung (RR of 9), stomach (RR of 1.1), bladder (RR or 1.2), skin (RR of 2.2), and leukemias (RR of 1.3) were lower than for roofers. One of the studies identified a significantly higher risk of skin cancer.

Carbon black is more than 85% elemental carbon in nearly spherical colloid form obtained by the thermal combustion of hydrocarbons in an oxygen-deficient atmosphere (34). About 93% of carbon black is used in pigmenting and reinforcing rubber, principally in tire manufacturing. PAHs constitute 0.1% to 1.5% of carbon black, and NIOSH estimated 88 ppm of suspect PAH carcinogens in one sample (34). Also PAHs are absorbed onto carbon black particles and may be eluted by human plasma. Robertson and Ingalls (35) reviewed the mortality experience of four carbon black producers between 1935 and 1974, covering 34,739 person-years at risk. No excess of cancer or heart disease was noted among 190 deaths. Robertson and Inman (36) updated this study and included 20 years of additional mortality experience. The preliminary results of the update confirmed the findings of the initial study, which had not been considered definitive because 68% of the person-years were among persons younger than 45 years of age. In the follow-up study 20% of the additional person-years were in retirees at least 65 years of age. NIOSH recommends that occupational exposure levels of carbon black be less than 3.5 mg/m$^3$ and of PAHs no more than 0.1 mg/m$^3$, measured as the cyclohexane-extractable fraction over an 8-hour work shift in a 40-hour workweek. Hodgson and Jones (37) conducted a retrospective mortality study of 1,422 carbon black workers employed between 1947 and 1980 with a minimum of 12 months' exposure. A statistically insignificant increase in lung cancer mortality was found, which was not associated with the length of exposure or environmental levels. There continues to be no good evidence that carbon black is a carcinogen, but owing to shortcomings with the current epidemiologic studies, a definitive conclusion is premature.

PAHs may be a hazard in the coal conversion and oil shale—retorting processes in the synthetic fuels program. The Department of Energy estimates that by the year 2000 coal gasification will provide $8.6 \times 10^{15}$ BTU per year in the United States, employing 140,000 workers (38).

Cutting oils may cause a variety of skin conditions, including oil acne and folliculitis, primary skin irritation, and allergic contact dermatitis. Long-term exposure may lead to skin cancer, mainly scrotal cancer. The poorly refined oils have a high content of polycyclic aromatic compounds (39). The higher the PAH content, the more carcinogenic is the oil. Roy et al. (40) demonstrated that all the lubricating oils that caused skin cancer in mice contained more than 1% PAH. There are conflicting results regarding increased rates of cancers other than of the scrotum in those exposed to cutting oils. Waldron (41) found an excess of tumors of the bronchus, larynx, stomach, skin, and lip. Jarvholm and co-workers' (42) study of 792 men exposed to cutting oils did not reveal excessive numbers of these cancers. Eisen et al. (43) reported that exposure to metal working fluid in automotive workers was associated with an almost twofold excess in laryngeal cancer risk. The authors question whether this association is due to the PAH content of the oils or the sulfuric additive (43).

Certain genetic predispositions make people more sensitive or resistant to exogenous exposures and endogenous processes. Several cytochrome P-450 enzymes, responsible for metabolically activating carcinogens and medications, express wide interindividual variation whose genetic coding has been identified as polymorphic and linked to cancer risk. For example, a restriction fragment length polymorphism for cytochrome P-4501A1(CYP1A1), which metabolizes polycyclic aromatic hydrocarbons, has been associated with an increased lung cancer risk (44,45). Detoxifying enzymes such as the glutathione transferases may also affect the metabolic fates of PAHs. The GSTM1 null genotype is a common form of glutathione transferase deficiency (46) and may result in raised cancer risks among affected individuals (who lack sufficient levels of these enzymes).

A number of recent studies have focused on the metabolism of PAHs in relation to the risk for breast cancer (47,48). One investigation (49) revealed no increased risk with the null GSTM1 genotype but did find an elevated breast cancer risk among women with the CYP1A1 polymorphism (odds ratio of 1.61). Others have theorized that PAHs may have estrogen-mimicking qualities and thereby increase the risk of breast cancer (50).

Adduct formation, the covalent binding of metabolically activated diol epoxides to deoxyribonucleic acid (DNA), is thought to be a critical event in the process of carcinogenesis. Techniques have been developed to measure benzo[*a*]pyrene diol epoxide—DNA adducts and antibodies to these adducts. A number of researchers have utilized this technique in high risk populations. Harris and co-workers (51,52) determined the levels of benzo[*a*]pyrene diol epoxide—DNA adducts in peripheral blood lymphocytes and antibodies to the adducts in serum from coke oven workers. Harris's group studied 41 workers who had been employed for a minimum of 5 years (51); 76% (31/41) of the workers had adduct formation. Antibodies to the adducts were found in 11 employees. Haugen and colleagues (52) investigated 38 topside coke oven workers and demonstrated adduct formation in 34% (13/38). Antibodies were detected in 12 of the workers. In a study by Kriek et al. (53) 47% of coke oven workers had detectable levels of PAH-DNA adducts in their white blood cells compared with 27% of controls. Perera and colleagues (54) classified 35 foundry workers into low-, medium-, and high-exposure groups and included an additional 10 unexposed persons as controls (54); 20% of the controls, 72% of the low-exposure group, and 100% of the medium- and high-exposure groups were found to exhibit adduct formation on the enzyme-linked immunosorbent assay (ELISA) technique. The three exposed groups all had statistically significant average adduct levels that were higher than those in the control group. Hemminki and colleagues (55) compared adduct formation in three different groups. They included coke oven workers, persons living near the coke ovens, and residents of rural Poland. The levels of DNA adducts from the white blood cells of the coke oven workers and the local population were both elevated, and essentially the same, whereas the rural population had significantly lower levels. This study indicates that environmental pollution due to PAHs must be considered a source of increased risk of cancer.

PAHs are mutagenic. Three were tested in vivo with three cytologic tests utilizing bone marrow from Chinese hamsters (56). Two carcinogens—7,12-dimethylbenz[*a*]anthracene (7,12-DMBA) and 3,4-benzo[*a*]-pyrene—and a noncarcinogen (phenanthrene) induced an elevated rate of sister-chromatid exchanges, but only the carcinogens induced chromosome aberrations and only 7,12-DMBA induced micronuclei.

Animal studies have focused on the role that oncogenes may play in PAH-related cancers. Several of these investigations have implicated the *ras* oncogene in PAH-related tumor induction (57,58). In one investigation (59), papillomas were induced in mouse skin by several different PAHs. Specific PAHs were found to induce specific base mutations in the c-H-*ras* oncogene. The authors conclude that these mutations in the oncogene are responsible for the resultant papilloma formation. The use of oncogenes to study human populations with exposures to PAHs has been limited to date. It should be noted, however, that in the aforementioned foundry worker cohort adduct study, selected persons in the high levels of exposure to PAHs have also been found to have elevated expression of oncogene protein in their serum compared to unexposed controls (60). It is possible, therefore, that increased PAH-DNA adducts contribute to an increased risk of cancer via pathways that include oncogene activation.

**Monitoring/Regulatory Issues**

The medical surveillance of employees exposed to PAHs on a regular basis is no simple task. The primary difficulty lies in the fact that most exposed individuals have come in contact with substances containing mixtures of various PAHs. Therefore, surveillance programs have to date relied on the evaluation of urinary metabolites of the various PAH compounds. More recently, researchers have begun to focus on the use of PAH DNA adducts as a measure of exposure.

1-Hydroxypyrene (a metabolite of pyrene) has been found in the urine of workers exposed to PAHs and may be a useful indicator of exposure (61). Elevated levels were found in the urine of a worker employed in a wood-preserving plant and in a number of workers who were employed as asphalt road resurfacers. In another study, the concentration of PAHs in the personal air samples of 24 Danish foundry workers was measured and correlated to levels of urinary 1-hydroxypyrene and β-naphthylamine (62). The authors determined that 1-hydroxypyrene is a useful and direct biomarker of low-dose occupational exposure to PAH compounds. They suggest that β-naphthylamine may also be used to estimate PAH exposures.

Research into the use of adducts as a surveillance tool in PAH exposed populations has received a good deal of attention recently (63,64). The formation of PAH DNA adducts was studied in peripheral blood lymphocytes from Polish men with occupational and environmental exposures. Results revealed high adduct level cells in 13.6%, 11.5%, and 3.7% of coke oven workers, environmentally exposed individuals, and rural controls, respectively. The authors conclude that their immunohistochemical adduct analysis technique is a promising addition to biomonitoring studies (65).

PAH industrial hygiene measurements are often determined using one of two methods. The first, total benzene soluble material, includes all particulate coal tar pitch volatiles. The second method involves specific testing for benzo[*a*]pyrene, used as an indicator for PAHs in general. The current American Conference of Government Industrial Hygienists (ACGIH) threshold limit value for benzene soluble material is 0.2 $mg/m^3$. Notably, however, a recent study of aluminum workers in Canada indicates that after 40 years of exposure at the current hygiene standard, the risk model predicts a lifelong excess risk for lung cancer of 3.8% (24).

## REFERENCES


1. Hueper WC, Conway WD. *Chemical carcinogenesis and cancers.* Springfield, IL: Charles C Thomas, 1964.
2. National Institute for Occupational Safety and Health. *Asphalt fumes:* criteria for a recommended standard. DHEW publication (NIOSH) 78-106. Washington, DC: U.S. Government Printing Office, 1977.
3. Pott P. Cancer scroti. In: *The chirurgical works of Percival Pott.* London: Hawes, Clarke, and Collins, 1775;734–736.
4. Lee WR, McCann JK. Mulespinners cancer and the wool industry. *Br J Ind Med* 1967;24:148–151.
5. Southam AH, Wilson SR. Cancer of the scrotum: the etiology, clinical features, and treatment of the disease. *Br Med J* 1922;2:971–973.
6. Henry SA. *Cancer of the scrotum in relation to occupation.* London: Oxford University Press, 1946.
7. Scott A. On the occupation cancer of the paraffin and oil workers of the Scottish shale oil industry. *Br Med J* 1922;2:1108–1109.
8. Leitch A. Paraffin cancer and its experimental production. *Br Med J* 1922;2:1104–1106.
9. Cook JW, Hewett CL, Heiger I. The isolation of cancer-producing hydrocarbons from coal tar. *J Chem Soc* 1933;1:396–398.
10. Waldron HA, Waterhouse JAH, Tesseman N. Scrotal cancer in the West Midlands. *Br J Ind Med* 1984;41:437–444.
11. Lloyd JW. Long-term mortality study of steelworkers: V. Respiratory cancer in coke plant workers. *J Occup Med* 1971;13:53–68.
12. Bridbord K, French JC. Carcinogenic and mutagenic risks associated with fossil fuels. In: Jones PW, Freudenthal RI, eds. *Carcinogenesis:* polynuclear aromatic hydrocarbons. New York: Raven, 1978;3: 451–463.
13. Redmond CK, Strobino BR, Cypess RH. Cancer experience among coke by-product workers. *Ann NY Acad Sci* 1976;271:102–115.
14. Redmond CK. Cancer mortality among coke oven workers. *Environ Health Perspect* 1983;52:67–73.
15. Bertrand JP, Chau N, Patris A, et al. Mortality due to respiratory cancers in the coke oven plants of the Lorraine coal mining industry (Houilleres du Bassin de Lorraine). *Br J Ind Med* 1987;44:559–565.
16. Kawai M, Amamoto H, Harada K. Epidemiologic study of occupational lung cancer. *Arch Environ Health* 1967;14:859–864.
17. Doll R. The causes of death among gas workers with special reference to cancer of the lung. *Br J Ind Med* 1952;9:180–185.
18. Doll R, Fisher REW, Gammon EJ, et al. Mortality of gas workers with special reference to cancers of the lung and bladder, chronic bronchitis, and pneumoconiosis. *Br J Ind Med* 1965;22:1–12.
19. Doll R, Vessey MP, Beasley RWR, et al. Mortality of gas workers: final report of a prospective study. *Br J Ind Med* 1972;29:394–406.
20. Lawther PJ, Commins BT, Waller RE. A study of the concentrations of polycyclic aromatic hydrocarbons in gas works retort houses. *Br J Ind Med* 1965;22:13–20.
21. Milham S. Mortality in aluminum reduction plant workers. *J Occup Med* 1979;21:475–480.
22. Gibbs GW, Horowitz I. Lung cancer mortality in aluminum reduction plant workers. *J Occup Med* 1979;21:347–353.
23. Ronneberg A, Langmark F. Epidemiologic evidence of cancer in aluminum reduction plant workers. *Am J Ind Med* 1992;22:573–590.
24. Armstrong B, Tremblay C, Baris D, Thériault G. Lung cancer mortality and polynuclear aromatic hydrocarbons: a case control study of aluminum production workers in Arvida, Quebec, Canada. *Am J Epidemiol* 1994;139:250–262.
25. Tremblay C, Armstrong B, Thériault G, Brodeur J. Estimation of risk of developing bladder cancer among workers exposed to coal tar pitch volatiles in the primary aluminum industry. *Am J Ind Med* 1995;27: 335–348.
26. Rockette HE, Arena VC. Mortality studies of aluminum reduction plat workers: potroom and carbon department. *J Occup Med* 1983;25: 549–557.
27. Menck HR, Henderson BE. Occupational differences in rates of lung cancer. *J Occup Med* 1976;18:797–801.
28. Hammond EC, Selikoff IJ, Lawther PL, Seidman H. Inhalation of benzopyrene and cancer in man. *Ann NY Acad Sci* 1976;271:116–124.
29. Partanen T, Boffetta P. Cancer risk in asphalt workers and roofers: review and meta-analysis of epidemiologic studies. *Am J Ind Med* 1994;26:721–740.
30. Hansen ES. Cancer mortality in the asphalt industry: a ten-year follow-up of an occupational cohort. *Br J Ind Med* 1989;46:582–585.
31. Knecht U, Woitowitz HJ. Risk of cancer from the use of tar bitumen in road works. *Br J Ind Med* 1989;46:24–30.
32. Hansen ES. Cancer incidence in an occupational cohort exposed to bitumen fumes. *Scand J Work Environ Health* 1989;15:101–105.
33. Jongeneelen FJ, Scheepers PTJ, Groenendijk A, et al. Airborne concentrations, skin contamination, and urinary metabolite excretion of polycyclic aromatic hydrocarbons among paving workers exposed to coal tar–derived road tars. *Am Ind Hyg Assoc* J 1988;49:600–607.
34. National Institute for Occupational Safety and Health. *Carbon black:* Criteria for a recommended standard. DHEW publication (NIOSH) 78-204. Washington, DC: U.S. Government Printing Office, 1978.
35. Robertson JM, Ingalls TH. A mortality study of carbon black workers in the United States from 1935–1974. *Arch Environ Health* 1980;35: 181–186.
36. Robertson JM, Inman KJ. Mortality in carbon black workers. *J Occup Environ Med* 1996;35:569–570.
37. Hodgson JT, Jones RD. A mortality study of carbon black workers employed at five United Kingdom factories between 1947 and 1980. *Arch Environ Health* 1985;40:261–268.
38. National Institute for Occupational Safety and Health. *Recommended health and safety guidelines for coal gasification pilot plants.* DHEW publication (NIOSH) 78-120. Washington, DC: U.S. Government Printing Office, 1978.
39. Mackerer CR. Health effects of oil mists: a brief review. *Toxicol Ind Health* 1989;5:429–440.
40. Roy TA, Johnson SW, Blackburn GR, Mackerer CR. Correlation of mutagenic and dermal carcinogen activities of mineral oils with polycyclic aromatic compound content. *Fundam Appl Toxicol* 1988;10:466–476.
41. Waldron HA. The carcinogenicity of oil mist. *Br J Cancer* 1975;32: 256–257.
42. Jarvholm B, Lavenius B. Mortality and cancer morbidity in workers exposed to cutting fluids. *Arch Environ Health* 1987;42:361–366.
43. Eisen EA, Tolbert PE, Hallock MF, Monson RR, Smith TJ, Woskie SR. Mortality studies of machining fluid exposure in the automobile industry III: a case-control study of larynx cancer. *Am J Ind Med* 1994;26: 185–202.

44. Quan T, Reiners JJ Jr, Bell AO, Hang N, States JC. Cytotoxicity and genotoxicity of benzopyrene-trans-7,8- dihydrodiol in Cyp1A1-expressing human fibroblasts quantitatively correlate with Cyp1A1 expression level. *Carcinogenesis* 1994;15 (9):1827–1832.
45. Shields PG, Caporaso NE, Falk RT, et al. Lung cancer, race and a Cyp1A1 genetic polymorphism. *Cancer Epidemiol Biomarkers Prev* 1993;2(5):481–485.
46. Lin JM, Han CY, Hardy S. Effects of isothioacyanates on tumorigenesis by benzo-a-pyrene in Murine tumor bottles. *Cancer Lett* 1993; 74(3):151–159.
47. Hecht SS, el-Bayoumy K, Rivenson A, Amin S. Potent mammary carcinogenicity in female Cd rats of a fjord region diol-epoxide of benzo-c-phenanthrene compared to a bay region diol-epoxide of benzo-a-pyrene. *Cancer Res* 1994;54(1):21–24.
48. Calaf G, Russo J. Transformation of human breast epithelial cells by chemical carcinogens. *Carcinogenesis* 1993;14(3):483–492.
49. Ambrosone CB, Freudenheim JL, Graham S, et al. Cytochrome P4501A1 and glutathione S-transferase (MI) genetic polymorphisms and post menopausal breast cancer risk. *Cancer Res* 1995;55(16):3483–3485.
50. Davis DL, Bradlow HL, Wolff M, Woodruff T, Hoel DG. Medical xenoestrogens as preventable causes of breast cancer. *Environ Health Perspect* 1993;101(5):372–377.
51. Harris CC, Vahakangas K, Newman MJ, et al. Detection of benzo(a)pyrene diol epoxide–DNA adducts in peripheral blood lymphocytes and antibodies to the adducts in serum from coke oven workers. *Proc Natl Acad Sci USA* 1985;82:6672–6676.
52. Haugen A, Becher G, Benestad C, et al. Determination of polycyclic aromatic hydrocarbons in the urine, benzopyrene diol epoxide–DNA adduct in lymphocyte DNA, and antibodies to the adducts in sera from coke oven workers exposed to measured amounts of polycyclic aromatic hydrocarbons in the work atmosphere. *Cancer Res* 1986;46: 4178–4183.
53. Kriek E, Van Schooten FJ, Hillebrand MJ, et al. DNA adducts as a measure of lung cancer risk in humans exposed to polycyclic aromatic hydrocarbons. *Environ Health Perspect* 1993;99:71–75.
54. Perera FP, Hemminki K, Young TL, Brenner D, Kelly G, Santella RM. Detection of polycyclic aromatic hydrocarbon—DNA adducts in white blood cells of foundry workers. *Cancer Res* 1988;48:2288–2291.
55. Hemminki K, Grzybowska E, Chorazy M, et al. DNA adducts in humans environmentally exposed to aromatic compounds in an industrial area of Poland. *Carcinogenesis* 1990;11:1229–1231.
56. Bayer U. In vivo induction of sister chromatid exchanges by three polyaromatic hydrocarbons. In: Jones DW, Freudenthal RI, eds. *Carcinogenesis:* Polynuclear aromatic hydrocarbons. New York: Raven, 1978; 3:423–428.
57. Ronai ZA, Gradia S, el-Bayoumy K, Amin S, Hecht SS. Contrasting incidence of ras mutations in rat mammary and mouse skin tumors. *Carcinogenesis* 1994;15(10):2113–2116.
58. DiGiovanni J, Bletran L, Rupp A, Harvey RG, Gill RD. Further analysis of c-Ha-ras mutations in papillomas initiated by several polycyclic aromatic hydrocarbons and papillomas from uninitiated, promoter-treated skin in SENCAR mice. *Mol Carcinog* 1993;8(4):272–279.
59. Chakravarti V, Pelling JC, Cavalieri EL, Rogan EG. Relating aromatic hydrocarbon-induced DNA adducts and c-H-Ras mutations in mouse skin papillomas. *Proc Natl Acad Sci USA* 1995;92 (22):10422–10426.
60. Brandt-Rauf PW, Smith S, Perera FP, et al. Serum oncogene proteins in foundry workers. *J Soc Occup Med* 1990;40:11–14.
61. Jongeneelen FJ, Anzion RBM, Scheepers PTJ, et al. 1-Hydroxypyrene in urine as a biological indicator of exposure to polycyclic aromatic hydrocarbons in several work environments. *Ann Occup Hyg* 1988;32: 35–43.
62. Hansen AM, Omland O, Paulsen OM, et al. Correlation between work process-related exposure to polycyclic aromatic hydrocarbons and urinary levels of alpha-naphthol, beta naphthylamine and 1-hydroxypyrene in iron foundry workers. *Int Arch Occup Environ Health* 1994;65(6):385–394.
63. Rojas M, Alexandrov K, van Schooten FJ, Hillebrand M, Krick E, Bartsch H. Validation of a new fluorometric assay for benzo-a-pyrene DNA adducts in human white blood cells. *Carcinogenesis* 1994;15(3): 557–560.
64. DiGiovanni J, Beltran L, Rupp A, Harvey RG, Gill RD. Further analysis of c-Ha-ras mutations in papillomas initiated by several polycyclic aromatic hydrocarbons. *Mol Carcinog* 1993;8(4):272–279.
65. Motykiewicz G, Malusecka E, Grzybowska E, et al. Immuno histochemical quantitation of polycyclic aromatic hydrocarbon-DNA, adducts in human lymphocytes. *Cancer Res* 1995;55:1417–1422.

*Environmental and Occupational Medicine, Third Edition,* edited by William N. Rom.
Lippincott–Raven Publishers, Philadelphia © 1998.

CHAPTER 95

# Petroleum Refining Industry

Myron A. Mehlman and William N. Rom

Crude oil, known as petroleum, is a combination of two words, the Greek word *petra,* which means "rock," and the Latin word *oleum,* meaning "oil." Petroleum products are derivatives of crude oil and thousands of chemical compounds ranging from volatile gases, such as methane, to liquids and solids at room temperatures. The principal elements of petroleum are carbon and hydrogen; in addition crude oils also contain sulfur, oxygen, metals (vanadium, nickel, iron, and arsenic), and hydrogen sulfide ($H_2S$), present as dissolved gas. During heating, $H_2S$, which is extremely toxic, is released. The principal hydrocarbons in crude oil are paraffins, olefins, naphthenes, and aromatics. For a detailed description and composition of crude oils, see Domask (1).

The refining processes that extend, yield, and modify the character of gasoline are catalytic cracking, coking, alkylation, and catalytic reforming. Gasoline is one of the better-known complex mixtures of petroleum chemicals to which humans are exposed (2). It consists of more than 150 hydrocarbons with a boiling range of approximately 40° to 180°C. The gasoline hydrocarbons are composed of about 50% to 70% alkanes (paraffins), which consist of straight-chain hydrocarbons of the $C_4$ to $C_{12}$ range; isoparaffins, which are branched-chain hydrocarbons of about the same size; alkenes (olefins), approximately 5% of which are unsaturated linear and branched-chain hydrocarbons; and naphthenics, which are saturated cyclics. Aromatics, which are the most dangerous carcinogenic chemicals in gasoline, are present at 30% to 40% and consist mainly of benzene, toluene, ethylbenzene, and xylene. Other blending agents and additives are also present in gasoline (2). Both tetraethyl and tetramethyl lead, which are strong neurotoxins from gasoline, have been phased out in recent years; however, alcohols, such as ethanol, methanol, *tert*-butyl alcohol, and methyl tertiary butyl ether (MTBE), are being added at 5% to 20% to the gasoline.

## TOXICITY OF GASOLINE

Humans come in contact with both liquid and vapors of gasoline. There is a substantial amount of vapor released from gasoline, which results in human exposure to gasoline vapors at retail service stations and adjacent populated areas, as well as to workers in refineries. Exposure to gasoline vapors in high concentration has occurred from the intentional sniffing of vapors for hallucinatory effects (3). Symptoms from exposure include eye irritation, dizziness, excitement, intoxication, nausea, anesthesia, and muscular weakness, and liver and kidney damage may occur. Death has resulted following exposure to vapors for 5 minutes at 5,000 ppm (3).

Information related to the carcinogenicity of petroleum products has been obtained from animal skin painting studies (4). The studies show that the carcinogenic activity of petroleum products, among others, resides in polynuclear aromatic hydrocarbons of the 3 to 7 ring-size range. Studies on carcinogenicity of various gasoline components are summarized in Table 1.

Mice were exposed for 2 years to gasoline vapors at concentrations of 67 (low), 292 (medium), and 2,056

M. A. Mehlman: Department of Environmental and Community Medicine, University of Medicine and Dentistry of New Jersey–Robert Wood Johnson Medical School, Piscataway, New Jersey 08855.

W. N. Rom: Division of Pulmonary and Critical Care Medicine, Departments of Medicine and Environmental Medicine; and Chest Service, Bellevue Hospital Center, New York University Medical Center, New York, New York 10016.

**TABLE 1.** *Unit cancer risk from gasoline*

| Pollutant | Unit risk[a] | Health effects summary | Comments |
|---|---|---|---|
| Gasoline vapor | | Kidney tumors in rats, liver tumors in mice | Gasoline test samples in the animal studies were completely volatilized and therefore may not be completely representative |
| Plausible upper limit[b] | | | |
| Rat studies | $3.5 \times 10^3$ | | |
| Mice studies | $2.1 \times 10^3$ | | |
| Maximum likelihood estimates | | | |
| Rat studies | $2.0 \times 10^3$ | | |
| Mice studies | $1.4 \times 10^3$ | | |
| Benzene[c] | $1.4 \times 10^3$ | Human evidence of leukemogenicity, zymbal gland tumor in rats; lymphoid and other cancers in mice | EPA: listed as a hazardous air pollutant, emission standards proposed to support causal association between exposure and cancer |
| Ethylene dibromide | $4.2 \times 10^1$ | Evidence of carcinogenicity in animals by inhalation and gavage; rats: nasal tumors; mice: liver tumors | EPA: suspect human carcinogen; recent restrictions on pesticidal uses |
| Ethylene dichloride | $2.8 \times 10^1$ | Evidence of carcinogenicity in animals. Rats: circulatory system, forestomach, and glands; mice: liver, lung, glands, and uterus | EPA: suspect human carcinogen; draft health assessment document released for review, March 1984 |

[a]Unit cancer risk factor is in terms of the probability of cancer incidence (occurrence) in a single individual for a 70-year lifetime of exposure to 1 ppm of pollutant.
[b]Confidence interval of 95%.
[c]Derived from human epidemiologic data, U.S. EPA.

(high dose) ppm (Table 2) (4,5). The results showed a significant increase in malignant tumors in the female mice at a high dose of exposure (Table 2).

## OXYFUELS AND METHYL TERT-BUTYL ETHER (MTBE) HEALTH EFFECTS

The 1990 amendments to the Clean Air Act mandated that gasoline be reformulated to reduce ambient carbon monoxide and ozone levels in nonattainment areas. Oxygenated gasoline (oxyfuel) is conventional gasoline to which a minimum of 2.7% oxygen by weight is added to reduce carbon dioxide. Reformulated gasoline also must contain 2% oxygen by weight but has different components to reduce hydrocarbon emissions in order to diminish ozone production. The amendments stated that oxyfuel was to be used year-round in areas with the most severe ozone problems. Chemicals that can be used to oxygenate fuels are methyl *tert*-butyl ether (MTBE), ethyl *tert*-butyl ether (ETBE), *tert*-amyl methyl ether (TAME), and *tert*-butyl alcohol (TBA). MTBE is the predominant chemical additive constituting 15% by volume. Approximately 17 billion pounds of MTBE were produced in the United States. in 1995 (12th among industrial chemicals based on volume). Ethanol is second to MTBE in use as an oxygenate (6).

Exposures to MTBE may occur in the manufacture and transport of the chemical, and service station workers, mechanics, and drivers who pump their own gas or are exposed from unburned gasoline vapors. There is also the potential for exposure through contamination of drinking water from leaking underground gasoline storage tanks.

The oxidative metabolism of MTBE is by cytochrome P-450 enzymes to *tert*-butyl alcohol and formaldehyde

**TABLE 2.** *Incidence of liver tumors in male and female mice exposed to whole vaporized gasoline*

| Test group | Animals examined | Total tumors | Adenomas | Carcinomas | % Carcinomas |
|---|---|---|---|---|---|
| Control | 108 | 31 | 13 | 18 | 16.6 |
| Low dose | 94 | 28 | 8 | 20 | 21.2 |
| Medium dose | 101 | 34 | 9 | 25 | 24.7 |
| High dose | 110 | 53 | 13 | 40 | 36.4 |

(7). MTBE is cleared rapidly (minutes) in the blood of humans, whereas TBA is more persistent (several hours) (8). Acute inhalation exposures to humans for up to 1 hour over dose ranges from 1.4 to 50 ppm have not been associated with any health effects (8).

Methyl tertiary butyl ether has been documented to be carcinogenic in rodents. A 2-year cancer bioassay demonstrated that inhalation of high concentrations of MTBE vapors increased the incidence of kidney cancer in male F-344 rats and liver cancer in female CD-1 mice (9,10). Rats that were chronically exposed to oral doses of MTBE were found to have an increase in the incidence of interstitial cell tumors of the testes as well as an increase in lymphohematopoietic tumors in female rats (11). TBA fed to male F-344 rats in their drinking water also caused kidney tumors (12). Neither MTBE nor TBA is mutagenic, raising the possibility that their carcinogenicity is through nongenotoxic mechanisms. Both chemicals cause damage to renal proximal tubular cells and bind to a unique rat renal protein, α2u-globulin, that can be identified as protein droplets and in lysosomes (13). Chemical binding to this protein retards hydrolysis and the excess protein is lethal to the cells, resulting in cytotoxicity, restorative cell proliferation, and cancer. Since this protein is not found in humans, these data are not considered relevant by the U.S. Environmental Protection Agency (EPA) to mandate quantitative risk assessment (6). α2u-Globulin is a low molecular weight protein synthesized in the liver of male rats but not by hepatocytes of female rats or by mice of either sex. The finding that the severity of chronic nephropathy was also increased in female rats exposed to MTBE does not support the hypothesis that α2u-globulin alone accounted for the kidney lesions observed in these studies.

Studies conducted in Alaska by Moolenar et al. (14) during and after the period MTBE was used in motor fuels showed that humans experienced numerous symptoms when exposed to gasoline containing MTBE. MTBE was introduced into gasoline in Alaska in mid-October 1992 and was discontinued on December 11, 1992, by order of the governor of Alaska. Most complaints emanated from Fairbanks, where cars were left to idle for long periods of time in the frigid winter. Those exposed in the fall were compared to those exposed in February and March 1993 and various symptoms were compared; there was no unexposed group. The ambient air concentrations in the workplace for 8-hour, time-weighted averages were a mean of 0.37 mg/m$^3$ (0.02–2.92 mg/m$^3$) during the fall and a mean of 0.13 mg/m$^3$ (0–0.51 mg/m$^3$) during the late winter. Reported health complaints are listed in Table 3. Headache, eye irritation, burning sensation of the nose or throat, dizziness, and spaciness or disorientation were the most frequent health complaints that were observed in those exposed to gasoline containing MTBE (15).

Lioy et al. (16) conducted a study on the methods for measuring concentrations of MTBE associated with automobile use. They measured exposure patterns in the interior of a car during stop-and-go commuter travel and also during gasoline refueling at attendant-assisted and self-service gas stations. The average concentration of MTBE reported in the cabin of cars after 1 hour of driving was 6 parts per billion (ppb) (1–160 ppb); when personally refueling a vehicle, exposures to MTBE were 10 ppb to 14,000 ppb over 5-minute intervals.

**TABLE 3.** *Health complaints of occupationally exposed workers in December 1992 compared to February 1993*

| Complaint | Fall 1992 (%) (*n* = 18) | Winter 1993 (%) (*n* = 28) |
|---|---|---|
| Headache | 72 | 4 |
| Eye irritation | 67 | 7 |
| Burning sensation of nose or throat | 50 | 0 |
| Dizziness | 44 | 0 |
| Spaciness or disorientation | 33 | 0 |

The Health Effects Institute (HEI) conducted a review of the scientific literature of oxygenated gasoline (17). According to the HEI review, symptoms reported in a number of communities where the oxygenated reformulated gasoline was used included eye irritation, burning sensations in the nose and throat, headaches, nausea, vomiting, cough, spaciness, disorientation, and dizziness, among others. In conclusion, the review stated that although more thorough research was needed, some individuals exposed to emissions from automotive gasoline containing MTBE may experience acute symptoms such as headache or eye and nose irritation.

## EPIDEMIOLOGIC STUDIES OF WORKERS IN THE PETROLEUM INDUSTRY

Crude petroleum, its fractions, and the PAHs produced in the refining process are all capable of causing cancer in laboratory animals, especially liver, lung, and kidney. Early human reports have demonstrated in case series that cancers of the skin, scrotum, lung, bladder, and gastrointestinal tract occurred after exposure to petroleum oils. Hanis and colleagues (18) reported a larger Canadian refinery cohort with 10 years' follow-up focusing on cancer mortality. They found a three times excess of esophageal and stomach cancer and two times excess for lung cancer among exposed compared to unexposed workers; in addition, increasing risks of both cancers occurred with increasing duration of employment. Thériault and Goulet (19) suggested brain cancer might be associated with refinery work, and confirmed suspicions about digestive system cancer, but neither of these findings was statistically significant.

Thomas et al. (20) examined records of workers from the Oil, Chemical, and Atomic Workers International Union (OCAW). A total of 3,105 males whose deaths were reported by OCAW local unions in Texas between 1947 and 1977 were analyzed. Approximately 40% of the deceased were under 50 years of age at the time of death, and 40% of the deceased were union members for less than 10 years. Proportional mortality ratios (PMRs), adjusted for age and calendar time using the U.S. general population, were analyzed, and there were significant increases in cancer rates for digestive and respiratory systems, brain, and skin. In 1982, Thomas et al. (21) extended their previous studies of union members in Texas refineries, and demonstrated a significant increase in cancer of the stomach, pancreas, prostate, brain, and hematopoietic and lymphatic systems (including leukemia).

A retrospective cohort study over an 8-year period of 8,666 refinery employees in Louisiana revealed elevated standardized mortality ratios (SMRs) for cancer of the kidney, testis, brain, pancreas, and lymphopoietic sites, but none of these was statistically significant (22). Because of the possibility of brain cancer in workers in the petrochemical industry, Austin and Schattner (23) performed a retrospective cohort mortality study of 6,588 white male employees who had been employed for more than 1 day between 1941 and 1977. They found no excess cancer mortality nor increases in cancer of the lung or liver. However, they confirmed 16 cases of brain cancer with an elevated but nonsignificant SMR. Upon further inspection, one was metastatic, and nine were of the glioblastoma multiforme histologic type. Although these tumors occurred with long latency, no specific exposure or job title appeared to be associated with this cluster.

Blot and colleagues (24) correlated age-adjusted white-male cancer mortality over a 20-year period in U.S. counties with petroleum industries. They compared 39 petroleum industry counties where at least 100 persons were employed in refineries to 117 counties without refineries and matched by geographic region and various demographic indicators. Cancer mortality in the petroleum industry counties was significantly increased overall and of the following sites: nasal cavity and sinuses, lung, skin, testes, stomach, and rectum. Low mortality was observed for brain cancer. In contrast, Hearey et al. (25) used Kaiser Foundation data to survey their members living near the petrochemical plants in the San Francisco Bay Area and found no association between mortality at any cancer site and proximity to the industry. This study was based on incident cases, and used a large prepaid health plan, which would minimize bias in case ascertainment. In 1989, the International Agency for Research on Cancer (IARC) reported that gasoline is "a possible human carcinogen" (26).

## CARCINOGENICITY OF CRUDE OIL

Crude oil is known to be carcinogenic. Distillate fractions of crude oil boiling between 120° and 1,070°F contain chemicals that are potentially carcinogenic. A highly carcinogenic fraction that boils between 700° and 1,070°F contains polynuclear aromatic compounds (PNAs). Table 4 shows the chemical analysis of distillate fractions with boiling temperatures of 120° to 350°F from crude oils with low and high sulfur contents. Benzene levels, but not those of toluene and other alkylbenzenes, were similar in crude oils with both low and high sulfur contents. Concentrations of PNAs, such as benz[*a*]anthracene and benzo[*a*]pyrene, were higher in the distillates from crude oils with high sulfur contents. The percentage of animals that developed cancers from the various fractions ranged between 22% and 98% (4).

3-Methylcholanthrene, a polycyclic hydrocarbon and a component of crude oil, increase dermal benzo[*a*]pyrene-3-hydroxylase and diphenoloxizole hydroxylase (27). Crude oil from Kuwait applied to the skin of rats caused an increase in the activities of both these enzymes, equivalent to the activity of 3-methylcholanthrene alone.

Benzene, a significant component of gasoline, has been shown to be a carcinogen in both animals and humans (28). Benzene has been used as a solvent and in inks, rubber, lacquers, paint remover, and many other products. Total benzene usage today is approximately 11 billion gallons per year, and an estimated 238,000 people are occupationally exposed to benzene in petrochemical plants, petroleum refineries, and other operations. Benzene is currently classified by the EPA and IARC as a human carcinogen. In numerous studies, Maltoni et al. (29–34) demonstrated that benzene caused tumors in rats and mice, including lymphomas, and leukemias, and cancers of the zymbal gland, oral cavity, lung, skin, nasal cavity, forestomach, mammary gland, ovary and uterus. Huff et al. (35) expanded these studies using a broader dose range; they reported numerous cancers, occurring at a lower dosage of various organs and tissues.

Infante and White (36) calculated the relative risk and excess risk of death from leukemia for workers exposed to benzene for an occupational lifetime. The relative risk of death from leukemia for exposures at 10 ppm range from 9 to 170 per 1,000 workers exposed and at exposures of 1 ppm the range was from 1 to 17 per 1000 workers exposed.

Crude oil contains a high concentration of sulfur, depending on the sources of the crude. $H_2S$ is a colorless, highly toxic gas with a characteristic obnoxious odor like that of rotten eggs, even at very low concentrations. It is flammable in air, can explode, and can be ignited by static discharge. $H_2S$ is produced by decomposition of

**TABLE 4.** *Analysis of distillate fractions with boiling range of 120°F to 350°F*

| | Crude C (0.21%) | Crude D (2.54%) |
|---|---|---|
| Average molecular weight | 125 | 111 |
| | Hydrocarbon composition (%) | |
| Butanes | 0.0 | 0.3 |
| Pentanes | 0.2 | 2.2 |
| 6- to 12-carbon paraffins | 16.9 | 69.2 |
| Total paraffins | 17.1 | 71.7 |
| Monocycloparaffins | 51.7 | 18.7 |
| Dicycloparaffins | 23.8 | 0.6 |
| Total cycloparaffins | 75.5 | 19.3 |
| Benzene | 0.5 | 0.5 |
| Toluene | 0.5 | 1.8 |
| Ethylbenzene, xylenes | 1.3 | 1.8 |
| 9- to 11-carbon alkylbenzenes | 4.8 | 3.4 |
| Indans/tetralins | 0.3 | 0.1 |
| Naphthalenes | 0.0 | 0.0 |
| Total aromatics | 7.4 | 9.0 |
| | Polynuclear aromatics (ppb) | |
| Pyrene | 0.42 | 6.11 |
| Benzo[*a*]anthracene | 0.07 | 0.45 |
| Benzo[*a*]pyrene | 0.10 | 0.20 |
| Benzo[*e*]pyrene | 0.06 | 0.39 |
| Benzo[*g,h,i*]perylene | 0.16 | 0.21 |
| | Nonhydrocarbon elements (ppm) | |
| Nitrogen | 1 | 1 |
| Oxygen | <100 | <100 |
| Sulfur | 140 | 260 |
| Chloride | 3.3 | 4.3 |

organic material by bacteria, and is also a significant constituent of petroleum crude. In the workplace (namely, oil refineries), it is one of the leading causes of sudden death.

## ACUTE REFINERY INDUSTRY HAZARDS

1. Marathon Oil, Texas City Refinery, October 30, 1981. A release of hydrogen fluoride gas resulted in the evacuation of 3,000 people, and 800 people were treated for acute health effects.
2. Shell Oil Refinery, Norco, Louisiana, May 5, 1988. The emission of a toxic vapor cloud that ignited and exploded killing seven people and injuring up to 5,000 others.
3. Phillips Petroleum, Pasadena, Texas, October 23, 1989. Twenty-three workers killed and 232 people injured after a valve on a polyethylene reactor was left open, venting gases that caught fire and exploded.
4. Exxon Refinery, Baton Rouge, Louisiana, December 24, 1989. Two workers were killed and seven injured as a result of an explosion from escaped ethane and propane gases.
5. Atlantic Richfield, Channel View, Texas, July 5, 1980. An explosion in a compressor killed 17 workers.

## OIL SPILLS AND THEIR AFTERMATH

Until 1983, approximately 6 million metric tons of crude oil entered marine environments annually. Since that time, the amount of crude oil entering marine environments has increased significantly as a result of major spills such as that of the *Exxon Valdez,* that in Kuwait, and many others. Crude oil in marine environments causes major damage to fish, wildlife, and the entire marine ecosystem. Birds and other species ingest oil from man-caused spills, resulting in the increase of enzymatic activities in various tissue and organs. The presence of carcinogens, such as benzo[*a*]pyrene and many others, in crude oil poses a danger of increased risk for cancer similar to that of individual chemical compounds or greater due to interactions and enzyme inductions.

Numerous spills of varying magnitudes have occurred at facilities and by ships owned by Shell, Texaco, Mobil, Union Oil, Hess, and other oil industry corporations. On March 24, 1989, the *Exxon Valdez* oil tanker carrying approximately 45 million gallons of crude oil ran aground in the Prince William Sound off the pristine coast of Alaska, releasing some 11 million gallons of crude oil into the waters of the Sound. The investigation of the *Exxon Valdez* disaster revealed many shortcuts in the race to develop Alaska's North Slope. First, the wilderness of the Brooks Range of northern Alaska had to be breached to allow for the pipeline and haul road. Environmentalists were bitterly opposed, but lost to overwhelming economic and strategic interests of developing the rich North Slope oil fields. Second, the Yukon River had to be bridged. Third, designs were necessary to prevent earthquake damage to the pipeline, and to allow migratory animals to pass. The oil industry favored the shipping lanes from Alaska to the U.S. West Coast rather than an overland route via Canada to the U.S. Northwest. Prince William Sound was particularly hazardous for navigation due to many islands and rocky reefs. These islands, in the face of a major spill, would slow the natural cleansing process that takes place on beaches exposed to heavy surf. The gravel beaches of the Sound along the rocky shoreline absorbed the oil, and then leaked it back into the Sound over years. The frigid Alaskan waters slows the breakdown of crude oil that otherwise dissipates in warmer seas. The oil industry was ill-prepared with necessary containment booms and suction pumps to scoop up spilled oil, allowing heavy seas to spread the slick over 300 miles to Kodiak Island and beyond.

Prince William Sound was home to whales, porpoises, seals, sea lions, and an estimated 10,000 sea otters before the spill. Some 400,000 resident birds are joined in the spring by a million migrating sea birds, and 10 million water fowl and shore birds. Five species of salmon spawn in the Sound's rivers, and area fisherman harvest 120 million dollars per annum in salmon, herring, shrimp, and halibut. The oil industry and government agencies had no emergency response plan; ill-conceived plans became unkept promises. A civil lawsuit collectively representing Native Americans, fishermen, and the Prince William Sound communities successfully sued Exxon, resulting in an award assessing punitive damages of $5 billion (37). Exxon has appealed.

Oil drenched or spattered 1,200 miles of the shoreline, killing at least 100,000 birds including 150 bald eagles. At least 1,000 sea otters perished. Exxon hired 11,000 workers spending approximately $2.1 billion on the inefficacious cleanup. High-pressure hoses and hot water hoses were used to clean beaches and direct oil to skimmers. Special nitrogen-phosphorus fertilizers were spayed on select oil-laden shores to stimulate oil-eating bacteria to hasten bioremediation. The most volatile components of the crude evaporated in the first 20 hours, leaving a thicker mousse-like crude behind. When dispersants were mobilized, high winds spread the slicks, making this strategy unworkable as well as the attempted containment with large booms. Approximately 10% of the oil spilled was accounted for in the cleanup efforts.

As a result of public outrage against such spills, the oil companies, under the auspices of the American Petroleum Institute, established a high-level committee, consisting of top oil-industry executives, to develop strategies to control oil spills similar to the *Valdez* disaster. According to the EPA, since the Alaska spill in March 1989, more than 11,000 oil spills have occurred in the United States alone. This includes the discovery of a major spill by Mobil in which more than 17 million gallons of oil were spilled over a period of many years in Brooklyn, New York. The aftermath of oil spills, especially the cleanup process, results in high human exposure to various carcinogenic elements of oil. In 1990, Congress passed the Oil Pollution Control Act, which mandated U.S. oil companies to convert to double-hull tankers by the year 2015.

## REFERENCES


1. Domask WG. Introduction to petroleum hydrocarbons, chemistry and composition in relation to petroleum-derived fuels and solvents. In: Mehlman MA, ed. *Advances in modern environmental toxicology,* vol 7. Princeton, NJ: Princeton Scientific, 1984;1–26.
2. Page NP, Mehlman MA. Health effects of gasoline refueling vapors and measured exposures at service stations. *Toxicol Ind Health* 1989;5: 869–890.
3. Poklis A, Burkett C. Gasoline sniffing: a review. *Clin Toxicol* 1977;11: 35–41.
4. Lewis SC, King RW, Cragg ST, Hillman DW. Skin carcinogenic potential of petroleum hydrocarbons II. Crude oil, distillate fractions and chemical class subfractions. In: Mehlman MA, ed. *Advances in modern environmental toxicology,* vol 6. Princeton, NJ: Princeton Scientific, 1984;139–50.
5. Mehlman MA, Hemstreet CP III, Thorpe JJ, Weaver NK. Renal effects of petroleum hydrocarbons. In: Mehlman MA, ed. *Advances in modern environmental toxicology,* vol 7. Princeton, NJ: Princeton Scientific, 1984;1–281.
6. Borghoff SJ, Prescott-Mathews JS, Poet TS. The mechanism of male rat kidney tumors induced by methyl tert-butyl ether and its relevance in assessing human risk. *CIIT Activities, Chemical Industry Institute of Toxicology* 1996;16:1–10.
7. Brady JF, Xiano F, Ning SM, Yang CS. Metabolism of methyl-tertiary-butyl ether by rat hepatic microsomes. *Arch Toxicol* 1990;64:157–160.
8. Cain WS, Leaderer BP, Ginsberg GL, et al. Acute exposure to low-level methyl-tertiary-butyl ether (MTBE): human reactions and pharmacokinetic response. *Inhal Toxicol* 1996;8:21–48.
9. Chun JS, Burleigh-Flayer HD, Kintigh WJ. *Methyl-tertiary-butyl ether:* vapor inhalation oncogenicity study in Fischer 344 rats. BRRC report no. 91N0013B. Export, PA: Bushy Run Research Center, 1992.
10. Burleigh-Flayer HD, Chun JS, Kintigh WJ. *Methyl-tertiary-butyl ether:* vapor inhalation oncogenicity study in CD-1 mice. Report no. 91N0013A. Export, PA: Bushy Run Research Center, 1992.
11. Belpoggi F, Soffritti M, Maltoni C. Methyl-tertiary-butyl ether (MTBE) —a gasoline additive—causes testicular and lymphohaematopoietic cancers in rats. *Toxicol Ind Health* 1995;11:119–149.
12. National Toxicology Program (NTP). *Technical report on the toxicology and carcinogenesis studies of t-butyl alcohol in F344/N rats and B6C3F1 mice.* NTP technical report no. 436. Research Triangle Park, NC: National Toxicology Program, 1995.
13. U.S. Environmental Protection Agency (U.S. EPA). *Alpha$_{2u}$-globulin:* association with chemically induced renal toxicity and neoplasia in the male rat. Washington, DC: EPA, 1991.
14. Moolenar RL, Hefflin BJ, Ashley DL. Methyl tertiary butyl ether in human blood after exposure to oxygenated fuel in Fairbanks, Alaska. *Arch Environ Health* 1994;49:402–409.
15. U.S. EPA. *Assessment of potential health risks of gasoline oxygenated with methyl tertiary butyl ether* (MTBE). EPA 600/R-93/206. Washington, DC: Office of Research and Development, 1993.
16. Lioy PJ, Weisel CP, Jo W-K, Pellizzari E, Raymer JR. Microenvironmental and personal measurements of methyl-tertiary butyl ether (MTBE) associated with automobile use activities. *J Expos Anal* 1994; 4:427–441.

17. Health Effects Institute (HEI). *Review of the potential health effects of oxygenates added to gasoline.* Cambridge, MA: The Health Effects Institute, 1995.
18. Hanis N, Stavraky KM, Fowler JL. Cancer mortality in oil refinery workers. *J Occup Med* 1979;21:167–174.
19. Theriault G, Goulet L. A mortality study of oil refinery workers. *J Occup Med* 1979;21:367–370.
20. Thomas TL, Decoufle P, Mouré-Eraso R. Mortality among workers employed in petroleum refining and petrochemical plants. *J Occup Med* 1980;22:97–103.
21. Thomas TL, Waxweiler RJ, Moure RE, Itaya S, Fraumeni JF. Mortality patterns among workers in three Texas oil refineries. *J Occup Med* 1982;24:135–141.
22. Hanis NM, Holmes TM, Shallenberger LG, Jones KE. Epidemiologic study of refinery and chemical plant workers. *J Occup Med* 1982;24: 203–212.
23. Austin SG, Schnatter R. A cohort mortality study of petrochemical workers. *J Occup Med* 1983;24:305–312.
24. Blot WJ, Brinton LA, Fraumeni JF Jr, Stone BJ. Cancer mortality in U.S. counties with petroleum industries. *Science* 1977;198:51–53.
25. Hearey CD, Ury H, Siegelaub A, Ho MKP, Salomon H, Cella RL. Lack of association between cancer incidence and residence near petrochemical industry in the San Francisco Bay Area. *J Natl Cancer Inst* 1980; 64:1295–1299.
26. International (IARC) Report. *Occupational exposures in petroleum refining:* crude oil and major petroleum fuels, vol 45. Lyon, France: IARC, 1989.
27. Rahimtula AD, O'Brien PJ, Payne JE. Induction of xenobiotic metabolism in rats on exposure to hydrocarbon-based oils. In: Mehlman MA, ed. *Advances in modern environmental toxicology,* vol 6. Princeton, NJ: Princeton Scientific, 1984;71–79.
28. Maltoni C. Myths and facts in the history of benzene carcinogenicity. In: Mehlman MA, ed. *Advances in modern environmental toxicology,* vol 4. Princeton, NJ: Princeton Scientific, 1983;1–21.
29. Maltoni C, Scarnato C. First experimental demonstration of the carcinogenic effects of benzene. Long-term bioassays on Sprague-Dawley rats by oral administration. *Med Lav* 1979;70:352–357.
30. Maltoni C. Benzene: a multipotential carcinogen. *Acta Oncol* 1982;3: 1–4.
31. Maltoni C,Conti B, Scarnato C. Squamous cell carcinoma of the oral cavity in Sprague-Dawley rats, following exposure to benzene by ingestion. *Med Lav* 1982;73:441–445.
32. Maltoni C, Cotti G, Valgimigli L, Mandrioli A. Zymbal gland carcinomas in rats following exposure to benzene by inhalation. *Am J Ind Med* 1982;3:11–17.
33. Maltoni C, Conti B, Cotti G. Benzene: a multipotential carcinogen. Results of long-term bioassays performed at the Bologna Institute of Oncology. *Am J Ind Med* 1983;4:589–630.
34. Maltoni C, Conti B, Perino G, Dimai V. Further evidence of benzene carcinogenicity: results on Wistar rats and Swiss mice, treated by ingestion. *Ann NY Acad Sci* 1987;534:412–426.
35. Huff JE, Melnick RL, Solleveld HA, Haseman JK, Powers M, Miller RA. Multiple organ carcinogenicity of 1,3-butadiene in $B_7C_3F_1$ mice after 60 weeks of inhalation exposure. *Science* 1985;227: 548–549.
36. Infante P, White M. Projections of leukemia risk associated with occupational exposure to benzene. *Am J Ind Med* 1985;7:403–413.
37. Labedoff D. *Cleaning up.* New York: The Free Press, 1997;1–321.

*Environmental and Occupational Medicine, Third Edition*, edited by William N. Rom.
Lippincott–Raven Publishers, Philadelphia © 1998.

CHAPTER 96

# Occupational Hazards in the Microelectronics Industry

Joseph LaDou and Timothy J. Rohm

The fundamental discoveries that initiated the microelectronics industry first occurred about 50 years ago. The principal discovery was that of the transistor, a small, low-power amplifier that was to replace the cumbersome, inefficient vacuum tube. This development revolutionized the electronics industry and led to the introduction of many hundreds of solid state electronics products now commonly used throughout the world.

Microelectronics is a major international industry. Its explosive growth has resulted in a world market for semiconductor devices alone that is valued at more than $140 billion. The microelectronics industry work force may exceed a million workers. Until a few years ago, we thought of semiconductor manufacturing as the activity of only a few regions such as Silicon Valley (in Northern California), Route 128 outside Boston, Kyushu Island in Japan, and a few areas of Western Europe. There are now many active Asian and European producers of microelectronics devices creating a global competition for product development and distribution (Fig. 1) (1).

The microelectronics industry is difficult to characterize. There are many products and there are many more manufacturing processes (2). Thousands of different chemicals and other materials have been used in the

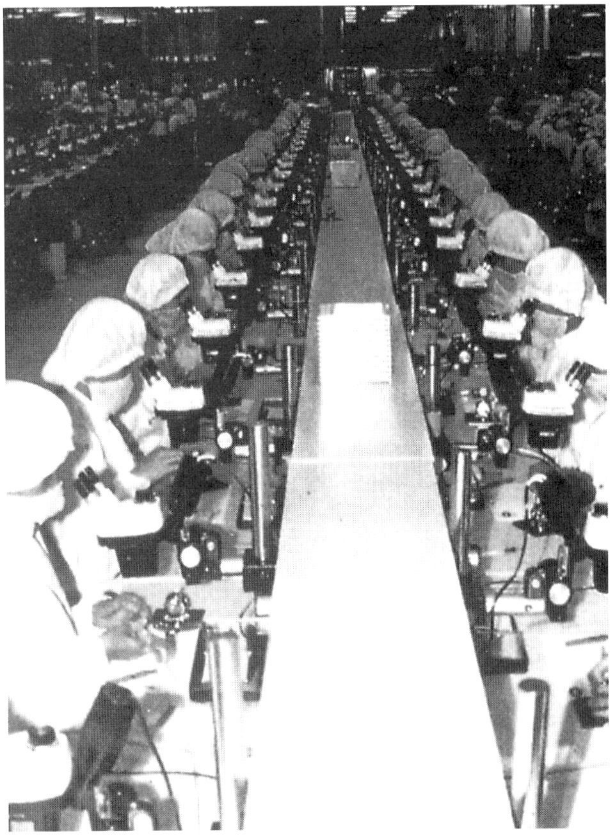

**FIG. 1.** The incredible obedience of Asian workers brings many companies to Malaysia, Thailand, Indonesia, and other countries, to manufacture their semiconductor products.

J. LaDou: Division of Occupational and Environmental Medicine, University of California School of Medicine, San Francisco, California 94143-0924.
T. J. Rohm: University of California, Santa Cruz, Santa Cruz, California 95192-0100.

**TABLE 1.** *Agents used in cluster analyses of semiconductor exposures*

| |
|---|
| Chemical agents |
| Ethylene-based glycol ethers (EGE) (including 2-methoxyethanol, 2-methoxyethyl acetate, and 2-ethoxyethyl acetate) |
| Xylene |
| *n*-butyl acetate (nBA) |
| Propylene glycol monomethyl ether acetate |
| Acetone |
| Isopropanol |
| Methanol |
| Antimony compounds |
| Arsenic compounds |
| Boron compounds |
| Phosphorus compounds |
| Fluoride compounds |
| Physical agents |
| Extremely low-frequency magnetic fields |
| Radiofrequency radiation |

From ref. 18.

microelectronics industry. The manufacturing settings share many characteristics, but no two are the same. And many of the older technologies are sent to newly industrialized countries as newer technologies are installed in the more highly developed industries of Japan, the United States, and European countries. Thus, worldwide, older problems with occupational health and safety and environmental contamination problems are still present. And new problems are introduced by technologies that are finding their first applications in many countries.

What was once thought to be the first "clean industry," is actually one of the most chemical-intensive industries ever conceived. Common worker exposure hazards are listed in Table 1. And because of its rapid development and its penchant for industrial secrecy, it is one of the least understood. Because an industry is characterized as "high technology" does not mean that occupational health and safety problems are any less common than in older industries. In our experience to date, occupational health and safety problems and difficulties with environmental contamination and public health are as common and as serious as in any other manufacturing industry.

## SEMICONDUCTOR MANUFACTURING

A microelectronics circuit consists of an assembly of electrical components such as transistors, capacitors, and resistors on or near the surface of a semiconducting substrate such as silicon or gallium arsenide (GaAs). The first transistor was developed by Walter Brattain, John Bardeen, and William Shockley in 1947. Since the development of the transistor, methods have been devised for incorporating thousands of the devices on semiconducting substrates to produce circuits that act as amplifiers, microprocessors, and other electrical devices whose dimensions are measured in millimeters (3).

The operation of an integrated circuit depends on the ability to control the movement of charged carriers through an electrical pathway (circuit) constructed on or just below the surface of a semiconducting material such as silicon. The circuit is fabricated by introducing impurities (dopants) in stringently controlled concentrations in precisely defined areas of the semiconducting material (substrate). By any measure, the substrate of choice is silicon, although other materials such as gallium arsenide, germanium, and certain organic compounds are used to construct special devices such as light-emitting diodes. The dimensions of the areas in which dopants are introduced are measured in microns and the concentrations of dopants are measured in units of atoms per cubic centimeter.

Improvements in the design and production of semiconductors have resulted in devices that combine more components in a single device. Many state-of-the-art semiconductor companies are preparing for the use of 300-cm (11.8-inch) wafers. Use of 300 cm-wafers in place of the 8-inch wafers now in use represents a doubling of the surface area. Hence, twice as many devices may be obtained from a 300 cm-wafer than an 8-inch wafer. Automation of many of the production processes and the use of larger silicon wafers allow the production of many more devices using the same number of process steps. Automation decreases the number of workers required to produce semiconductors. However, hazards associated with the automated process equipment still need to be considered.

### Circuit Design

The design of integrated circuits requires a thorough knowledge of electrical circuitry as well as special knowledge of the properties of semiconductor-based devices. Normally, the designer or design team develops a circuit to serve a particular function. The desired circuit may function as an amplifier, memory device, microprocessor, or any one of a large number of other devices. Computer-aided design of microelectronics devices is now the method of choice for producing circuits. The design is three dimensional, as the function of semiconductor devices requires that regions of materials with different electrical properties be placed above and below one another as well as side by side.

The product of a computer-aided design circuit is a computer tape that contains the circuit elements for each plane of the device. It is installed in a pattern generator, which takes each plane in turn, breaks down the pattern into rectangular blocks, and photographically reproduces the blocks at 10× magnification on a chromium-coated plate called a reticule. The reticule is then transferred to a step-and-repeat system, where it is projected onto a mask plate at actual size and exposed. The system then moves to a new position and repeats the process of exposure until the mask is covered with identical images of the original pattern.

The circuit diagrams of each level of the circuit are treated in the same manner. The result is a collection of glass plates, each bearing multiple images of one level of the circuit.

## Silicon Production

Silicon is the material of choice for construction of integrated circuits, but only extremely pure silicon can be used in the process. To obtain silicon of the required purity, "chemically pure" silicon is converted to a silicon halide or trichlorosilane ($SiCl_3H$). This material is then purified by fractional distillation in quartz vessels. Next, the silicon halide or trichlorosilane is reconverted to elemental silicon by reduction with hydrogen:

$$SiX_4 + 2H_2 = Si + 4HX \qquad [1]$$

or

$$SiHCl_3 + H_2 = Si + 3HCl \qquad [2]$$

The pure silicon is then further purified (impurities $<10^{-9}$ atom percent) by zone refining. Germanium is prepared in a similar manner.

The superpure silicon is then remelted in a vessel in an inert atmosphere. For particular applications, doping materials may be added to the melt to produce a substrate with different electrical properties. A silicon ingot is slowly drawn from the melt by using a seed crystal of silicon with a particular crystal structure attached to the end of a rod. The drawing rod or the vessel containing the melt, or both, may be rotated. If both the rod and the melt vessel are rotated, the directions of rotation are opposite. The result of this process is a cylindrical silicon ingot, 2 to 8 inches in diameter, that may be several feet in length (depending on the amount of material in the melt and on luck).

The ingot is then ground to a uniform diameter and a longitudinal section of the cylinder is removed to produce a flat. After the crystal structure of the ingot is verified by x-ray diffraction, the ingot is sliced into individual wafers with multiple inner-diameter diamond saw blades. The thickness of the wafers after slicing ranges from 15 to 40 mil (1 mil = $10^{-3}$ inch = 25.4 μm) depending on their diameter. The larger-diameter wafers need to be thicker to provide mechanical stability during processing.

The wafers are then ground (lapped) on special machines that rotate them while applying considerable pressure. A grinding slurry containing fine silica, water, and surfactants is used to remove the damaged surface that results from sawing. After lapping, wafers are etched with a mixture of nitric acid ($HNO_3$), hydrofluoric acid (HF), and acetic acid ($CH_3COOH$) to remove debris resulting from the lapping procedure and to reduce the thickness of the wafer. Finally, one side of the wafer is polished in another dedicated grinding machine using an aqueous mixture of colloidal silica and sodium hydroxide as the polishing medium. The result of this procedure is a wafer with a mirror-like surface that, after a final cleaning with an aqueous solution of hydrofluoric acid and surfactants, is ready for processing into integrated circuits. Most semiconductor manufacturers purchase wafers from firms that specialize in their production (Fig. 2).

The preparation of gallium arsenide as a substrate material begins with chemically pure gallium and arsenic. The elements, along with dopants such as silicon, tellurium, or chromium, are combined at high tem-

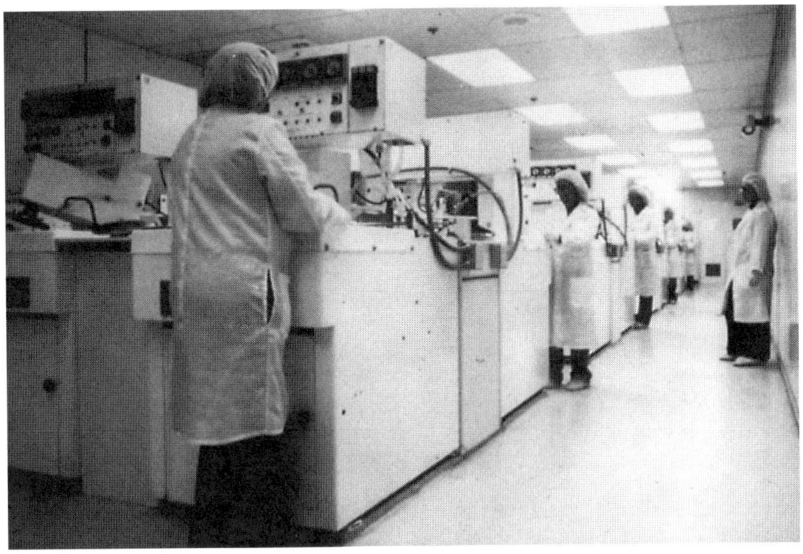

**FIG. 2.** Wafer manufacture does not require clean room conditions of semiconductor fabrication. Exposure to heat, dusts, chemicals, and radiation are common in these work settings.

peratures to form bulk polycrystalline gallium arsenide or single-crystal ingots. Preparation of single-crystal gallium arsenide is more difficult than preparation of single-crystal silicon, owing to the physical properties of the starting materials and the product. Arsenic is a solid at standard temperature and pressure, having a melting point of 814°C at 36 atmospheres. Gallium has a melting point of 29°C and a boiling point of 1,983°C. Gallium arsenide has a melting point of 1,238°C. Therefore, combining elemental arsenic and gallium requires the use of resistance furnaces that provide the temperature zones appropriate for each of the starting materials to vaporize and the product to condense. It is further necessary that all air be excluded from the system, a step that is accomplished by placing the materials in a quartz tube, evacuating the tube, and sealing it with a hydrogen-oxygen torch.

There are two popular methods of producing single-crystal gallium arsenide, which differ by the temperatures used in the resistance furnaces. The horizontal Bridgeman system consists of a two-zone furnace, one end heated to 615°C and the other to 1,240°C. The basic principle in horizontal Bridgeman involves traversing two heated zones (one above the melting point of gallium arsenide and one below) over a boat of gallium arsenide, which allows the material to assume the same structure as the seed crystal; the seed crystal is never melted in the process. In the gradient freeze method of gallium arsenide production the starting materials are heated to approximately 1,260°C. After they have combined, the ampoule is allowed to cool in a precise manner that produces single-crystal gallium arsenide.

Besides these methods, the liquid-encapsulated Czochralski technique is becoming increasingly popular. In the Czochralski process, bulk gallium arsenide is melted in a quartz vessel within a graphite receptor. The surface of the melt is covered with molten boron oxide ($B_2O_3$) and the melt chamber is pressurized with argon to prevent dissociation of the gallium arsenide. In a manner similar to that of the formation of silicon ingots, an ingot of single-crystal gallium arsenide is pulled from the melt using a seed crystal attached to the end of a puller.

The ingots of gallium arsenide produced in the methods just outlined are then sandblasted to remove exterior contaminants and oxides. The operation is carried out in a glove box using silicon carbide or calcined alumina as the abrasive medium. After the crystal structure of the ingot has been determined by x-ray diffraction, the ends of the ingot are cropped off. Gallium arsenide wafers are sliced from the ingots using automated saws with inner-diameter diamond saw blades. The wafers are then polished and cleaned in much the same way as are silicon wafers. Other methods of gallium arsenide wafer production are under investigation. Notable among these is an epitaxial layer technique, in which thin layers of material are deposited one on top of the other to yield a material with the proper electrical characteristics.

The recent development of gallium arsenide on silicon substrates for production of electronic and optical devices warrants consideration. Techniques for the deposition of gallium arsenide on silicon have made it possible to combine the unique electronic properties of gallium arsenide with the low cost, strength, size, and weight of silicon. The increased use of gallium arsenide may result in more worker exposure to the raw materials used in its manufacture than to the gallium arsenide itself. The hazards of gallium arsenide arise mainly from the use of elemental arsenic as a raw material. Gallium arsenide itself was originally considered physiologically inert; however, gallium arsenide administered to rats orally and by intratracheal instillation resulted in increased blood arsenic levels.

## Photolithography

Photolithographic processes are used to transfer the circuit patterns on the photomasks (masks) to the surface of the substrate. This is done by coating the substrate, which is normally covered with a thin coating of silicon dioxide (oxide), with a light-sensitive material known as photoresist. There are two types of photoresists, positive and negative, based on the behavior of the material when it is exposed to energy. When exposed to energy, positive photoresists weaken and negative photoresists are strengthened. The energy required to effect these changes may be ultraviolet light, electron beam, or x-radiation. The photoresists are formulated to react with the particular wavelength of energy to be used in the photolithographic process.

By far the majority of semiconductor devices are produced in processes in which ultraviolet light is used in the photolithographic process. The most common negative photoresists contain two components: a nonphotosensitive material and a photosensitive material that cross-links when exposed to ultraviolet light.

The nonphotosensitive material is a polymer formed by the condensation of isoprene (2-methyl-1,3-butadiene) to form the cyclized poly(*cis*-isoprene) material. The photosensitive material used in negative photoresists is a bisarylazide. The most common solvent for negative photoresists is a mixture of ethylbenzene and xylenes. Typical photoresist preparations contain about 20% of the polymer-photosensitive material in the solvent.

Positive photoresists generally contain three components: resin, photosensitive component, and a tertiary solvent mixture. The resin used in positive photoresists is a low molecular weight Novolak resin formed by the condensation of phenol and formaldehyde. The sensitizers used in the commercial positive photoresists are *o*-naphthoquinone diazines or benzoquinone diazides.

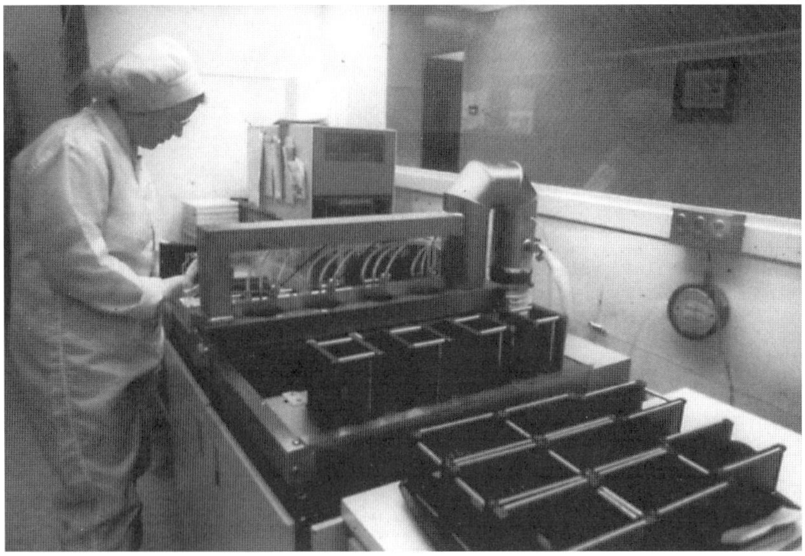

**FIG. 3.** Photoresist is applied to the surface of wafers by a device that provides only limited protection for this woman of childbearing age from the carrier solvent in the chemical preparation. This is one of many possible contacts for women with glycol ethers.

There is a 1:1 ratio of resin to the photosensitive compound. Like the negative photoresists, the resin-photosensitive material is suspended in the solvent at a concentration of about 20%. The most common solvent system for positive photoresists is a mixture of xylene, Celloslove acetate, and *n*-butyl acetate.

A popular resist for electron beam processing is poly(methyl methacrylate). This material reacts positively (i.e., is weakened) when exposed to the energy of the electron beam. Other positive electron beam resists contain poly(butene-1-sulfone), cross-linked poly(methacrylamide), or poly(methylmethacrylate-co-acrylonitrile) as the polymer. Negative electron beam resists contain polymeric materials such as poly(glycidylmetharcylate-co-ethylacrylate) or epoxidized poly(butadiene).

The photoresists are most often applied to the wafer by delivering 1 to 2 ml of the preparation to the center of the wafer, then spinning the wafer at high speed to spread the material over the surface and produce a thin, uniform coating. This spinner process is carried out automatically under local ventilation, which protects the wafer surface from redeposition of droplets of excess material (Figs. 3 and 4). After the photoresist coating has been applied, the wafer goes through a "soft-bake" process, during which the solvents evaporate from the photoresist. The soft bake is generally carried out in a continuous process oven, which is ventilated to an air-scrubbing system that collects the solvent vapors.

Following the soft bake, the wafer is exposed. The exposure process most often used involves placing the

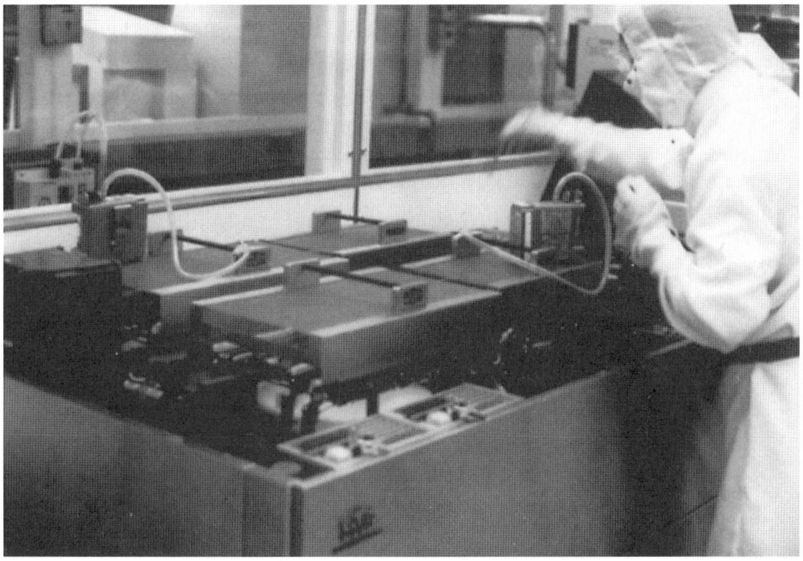

**FIG. 4.** Photoresist is applied by a safer, more closed system. Area samplers are placed on the equipment, while the worker's breathing zone is being sampled for glycol ether (the carrier solvent of the photoresist material) by a personal monitor not shown in the photograph.

photoresist-coated wafer in proximity to the appropriate photomask and directing energy through the mask onto the surface of the wafer. During the exposures, the chemical process of either bond making or bond breaking takes place, depending on the composition of the photoresist. It is crucial that the photomask be properly aligned and that the intensity and duration of the incident energy be precisely controlled.

After exposure, the wafers are developed by immersion in a solution that dissolves the photoresist material, which in the case of negative photoresists was not exposed or in the case of positive photoresists has been exposed (Fig. 5). Those for developing negative-reacting photoresists are mixtures of aliphatic hydrocarbons (deodorized kerosene, Stoddard solvent), and xylene. For positive-reacting photoresists, the developer is usually an aqueous solution of sodium hydroxide. Following development, the wafers go through a "hard-bake" process, during which the photoresist that remained on the wafer is set, much like the finish on an automobile.

Next, the wafers are immersed in an etchant solution, which removes the material that is not protected by photoresist. In most cases, the material that is removed is silicon dioxide, and hydrofluoric acid is the etchant.

After the etch step, the photoresist material is removed either by wet (liquid) chemical processes or by plasma ashing. Two types of chemical solutions are used to remove hardened photoresists. Positive resists may be removed with aqueous solution of sodium or potassium hydroxide. Negative photoresists are removed with mixtures of one or more of the sulfonic acids, an organic solvent such as tetrachloroethylene, Stoddard solvent, or a mixture of naphthalene, *o*-dichlorobenzene, and phenol. Following resist removal and rinsing with deionized water, the surface of the wafer has etched on it the pattern for one layer of the pattern of conducting zones that will make up the devices and connecting pathways of the integrated circuits.

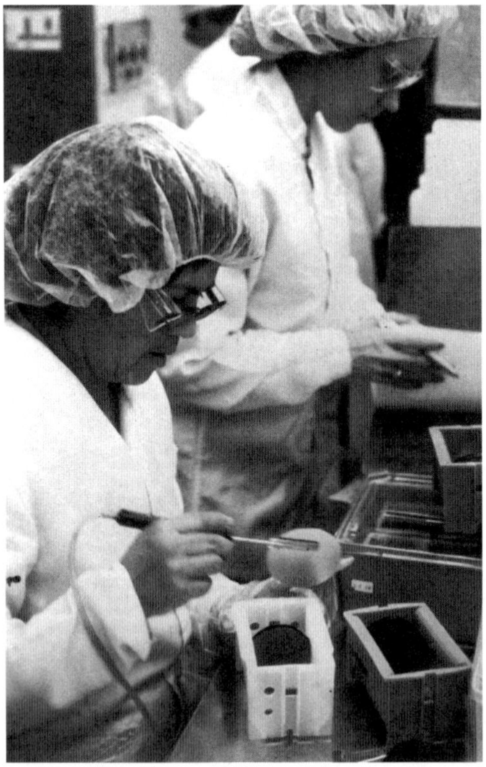

**FIG. 5.** Wafers are transferred from quartz boats to Teflon containers for chemical treatment phases. Note the use of a suction wand for holding the wafer. This device has prevented many ergonomic complaints.

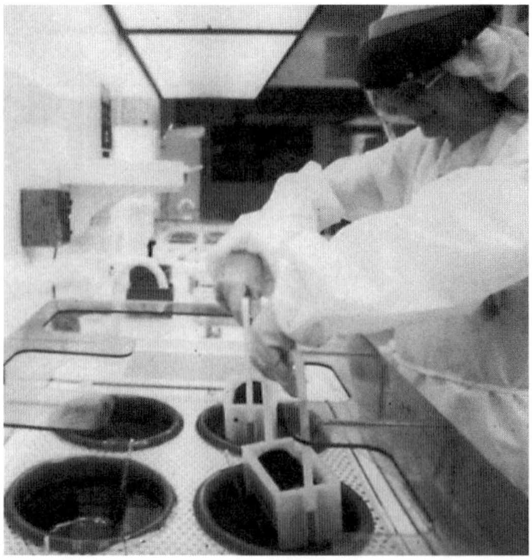

**FIG. 6.** Wet etching with hydrofluoric acid is the principal cause of chemical burns in the microelectronics industry. Wet etching is still common in smaller companies and in older technologies. This worker is properly gowned, gloved, and protected from splash by splash guards, face shield, and safety glasses.

The dopants are next added to the areas of the substrate that are not protected by the protective layer of silicon dioxide or other materials. The methods used to introduce the impurities (dopants) are described in the following sections. After the addition of dopants, the protective coating of silicon dioxide is removed with aqueous solutions of hydrofluoric acid (Figs. 6–8). The process of masking, doping, and silicon growth is repeated as many as ten times, until the entire circuit has been constructed on the substrate.

## Dopants

Dopants are impurities added to the semiconductor crystal to form electrical junctions or boundaries between *n* and *p* regions in the semiconductor crystal. An *n*-type region in a semiconductor crystal is an area containing an excess of electrons for conduction of electricity. A *p*-type region in the crystal contains an excess of electron holes

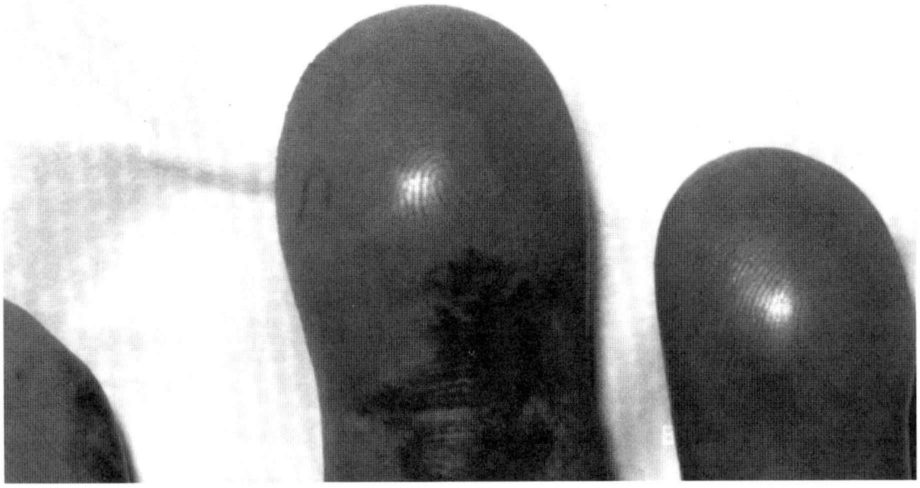

**FIG. 7.** Hydrofluoric acid burns of fingers from a porous leak in acid-resistant work gloves. Subungual burns result in painful swelling of the distal phalanges.

or acceptors. The difference in the electric potentials in the two regions allows the flow of electrons in the circuit. Junctions are necessary in all semiconductor circuits and provide the basis of function. The dopants are deposited selectively (in both quantity and location) in the semiconductor device, forming the junctions.

The most common methods of doping semiconductor devices are through diffusion and ion implantation (Fig. 9). The materials commonly used as *n*-type dopants are the oxides of antimony, arsenic and phosphorus, arsine, phosphine, phosphorus oxychloride, and phosphorus pentafluoride. The most commonly used materials for *p*-type dopants are the halides of boron, boron trioxide, boron nitride, diborane, and silicon tetrabromide.

## Plasma Processes

Plasma processes involve subjecting the surface of a silicon, or other substrate, wafer to a plasma of highly reactive chemical species in order to remove or deposit materials on the surface of the substrate. The plasma is produced in a reaction chamber in which a gas or vapor is irradiated by radiofrequency energy, typically 13.56 MHz. The plasma contains highly reactive chemical species that react with materials on the surface of the substrate. In some applications, the plasma process is used to remove photoresists or other materials from the surface of the substrate by converting the materials to the gaseous form. These applications are referred to as plasma cleaning or plasma stripping processes or, more commonly, as cleaning or stripping processes. In other applications, materials are deposited on the surface of the substrate. These applications are referred to as chemical vapor deposition (CVD) processes.

The chemical reactions that take place in a plasma involve highly energetic and reactive chemical species that are observed only in the plasma. The plasma has been referred to as the fourth state of matter as plasma chem-

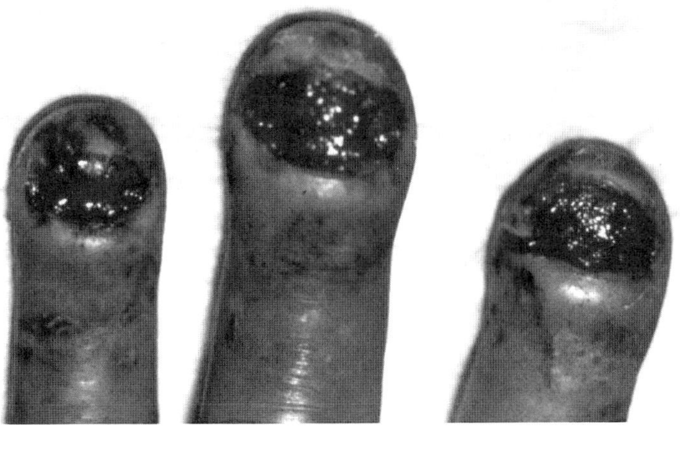

**FIG. 8.** Burn ulcers must be exposed by nail removal to allow healing of the subungual HF burns.

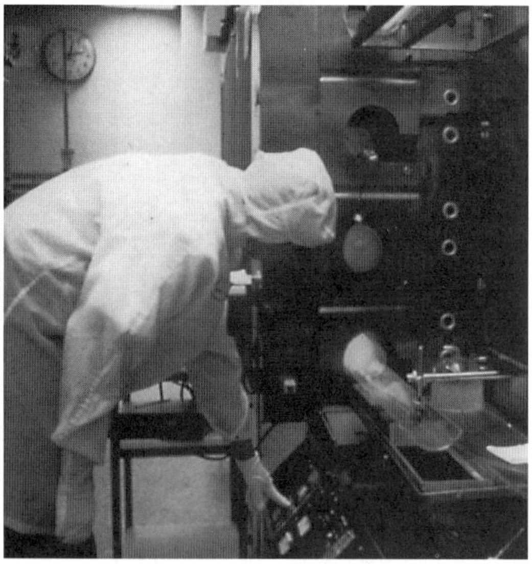

**FIG. 9.** Diffusion furnaces may serve as a source of exposure to toxic dopant gases. Poor ergonomic placement of the control buttons on this furnace requires the worker to bend over, bringing the breathing zone near the openings of the furnace.

istry is, in many ways, unique. Chemical species and reactions observed in a plasma are distinct from those that are observed in reactions in the gas, liquid, or solid states (4).

When irradiated in a plasma chamber, materials such as nitrogen trifluoride produce highly energetic fluorine species that combine with silicon dioxide to form volatile silicon tetrafluoride. When a mixture of silane and ammonia are irradiated, silicon nitride is deposited on the wafer surface. Many different chemical reactions occur within the plasma environment, where gases are ionized and therefore act differently than in their normal state. Every gas forms several different new molecules and radicals, which react with the desired layer in order to generate a volatile product (e.g., $SiF_4$). As a result of these chemical gas components, many other by-products are also formed. Hydrogen fluoride (HF) is released during the silicon nitride etch process. Hydrogen cyanide is also a dangerous exposure possibility with nitride etch. The most common volatile product of plasma etching is silicon tetrafluoride. If the equipment is used properly, manufacturing workers should not be exposed to hazardous gases. This implies that the flow rate of the scrubber exhaust and the duration of the pump-down at the end of the process are efficient in cleaning the etch chamber from the gases before it is opened (Fig. 10). The waste products from the reaction chamber may present a chemical hazard. The waste products are normally pumped from the chamber after the process has reached the desired end point. The waste materials may dissolve in the pump fluids or pass through the pumps. The exhaust from the pumps used to evacuate plasma chambers is commonly scrubbed with water prior to release to the atmosphere.

### Chemical Vapor Deposition

Chemical vapor deposition is a process whereby thin layers of crystalline silicon, silicon dioxide, and silicon nitride are deposited on the surface of the semiconductor wafer. The formation of these compounds is based on chemical reactions between the heated substrate (wafer) and the decomposition of various process gases fed into the system. The purpose of chemical vapor deposition is the formation of a stable compound on the wafer substrate to act as a mask (silicon nitride, silicon dioxide), or as a new layer for further junction forma-

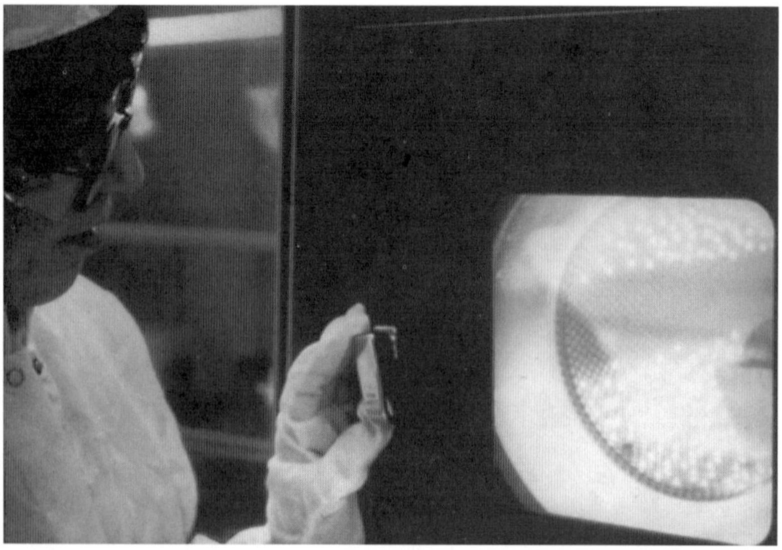

**FIG. 10.** Replacing wet etching with dry plasma etching removes the hazard of chemical burns. Newer hazards are introduced in the form of decomposition products created in the plasma field, and the microwave emitted by the radiofrequency (RF) power source of the dry plasma device.

tion (polycrystalline silicon, silicon dioxide), or as an insulating layer between two or more conductive layers.

A special type of chemical vapor deposition is called passivation. Here a protective layer of silicon dioxide or silicon nitride is deposited over the surface of the wafer as a last fabrication step prior to nonfabrication processing. This protective layer will help insulate the circuit from the chemical and electrical conditions in the environment.

There are several ways in which thin layers are deposited on the wafer in chemical vapor deposition, and each has many applications: low-pressure chemical vapor deposition, medium-temperature chemical vapor deposition, low-temperature chemical vapor deposition, and low-temperature plasma-enhanced chemical vapor deposition.

The basic components found in almost all chemical vapor deposition systems are the reaction chamber, the gas control section, time and sequence control, a heat source for substrates, and effluent handling.

The types of materials used in the chemical vapor deposition process depend on the compound deposited on the surface of the wafer. A combination of gases or vapors may be used. Popular sources of silicon to form silicon dioxide, silicon nitride, or silicon include silane ($SiH_4$) and tetraethylorthosilicate ($Si(OC_2H_5)_4$), which is commonly referred to as TEOS. Silane is a pyrophoric gas that has been the cause of hundreds of fires in semiconductor plants. Tetraethylorthosilicate is a combustible liquid with a flash point of 116°F. No threshold limit value (TLV) has been established for TEOS.

The most common source for nitrogen to form silicon nitride is ammonia ($NH_3$). Ammonia is an irritating gas with a TLV of 25 parts per million (ppm). Other gases in use in chemical vapor deposition processes include arsine ($AsH_3$), which is a toxic gas with a TLV of 50 parts per billion (ppb), phosphine ($PH_3$), which is a pyrophoric, toxic gas with a TLV of 300 ppb, and diborane ($B_2H_6$), which is a toxic gas with a TLV of 100 ppb.

### *Reaction Chamber*

The reaction chamber provides a controlled envelope in which the reaction occurs. There are several types of reaction chamber systems. Among the most common ones are horizontal, vertical, cylindrical or barrel, and gas-blanketed downflow systems. The names for these systems are derived from the orientation of the reaction chamber and the process gas flow within each.

### *Gas Control Section*

The gas flow-control section carefully limits and mixes the process gases into the reaction chamber. The sophistication of the mass flow controller increases with the degree of precision needed for the reaction.

### *Time and Sequence Control*

A time and sequence control device is necessary to operate a chemical vapor deposition unit. Its complexity can vary much, from an operator pushing buttons to a fully automated programmable sequencer or computer control.

### *Heat Source for Substrates*

The heating sources for chemical vapor deposition units are of two types: cold-wall and hot-wall systems. Cold-wall systems are those in which deposition reactions occur slowly on the walls of the reaction chamber but much faster on the susceptor and wafers. In cold-wall systems heat is usually produced by radiofrequency radiation or ultraviolet energy. Hot-wall systems use thermal resistance heating, as in a diffusion furnace, so the walls are as hot as the susceptors and wafers. The advantages of cold-wall systems are that less deposition occurs on the walls of the chamber and, since the mass energy transfer is much smaller, the wafers can be heated and cooled more rapidly than in a hot-wall system.

### *Effluent Handling*

In this process effluents are the unreacted gases and carrier gases not used in the chemical vapor–deposition process. Effluents exit the system through a series of vacuum pumps and undergo a variety of treatments before being released into the atmosphere.

## Metallization

Subsequent to device fabrication in the silicon substrate, connections must be made to link the circuits together, a process called metallization. Metallization puts conductive electrical interconnects on silicon between resistive and capacitive areas in one layer, as well as a number of other layers in the circuit, providing paths for electric current.

Conductive films are put on circuits as a substitute for conventional solder and wire connections, and also to provide external connections to the circuit. The methods of metallization are diverse, but the general requirements of conductive films are low sheet resistance, low contact resistance, ability to adhere to the wafer substrate, and resistance to atmospheric attack. The most common metals used for metallization are aluminum (most used), nickel, chromium, nichrome, gold, germanium, copper, silver, titanium, tungsten, platinum, and tantalum.

Metallization is often accomplished by a vacuum deposition technique. Such systems have the following characteristics: a chamber that can be evacuated sufficiently for the deposition, vacuum pumps, instrumentation for monitoring the vacuum levels and other system variables, and a method for depositing the metal layers. The five most common methods for depositing metal layers are filament evaporation, electron beam evaporation (e-beam), flash evaporation, induction evaporation, and sputtering.

#### *Filament Evaporation*

Filament evaporation is the simplest method. The process is generally carried out in a bell jar, in which evaporation takes place from a filament or boat heated by thermal resistance. As the temperature rises, the metal to be deposited is melted and wets the filament. As the current through the filament is increased further, the metal vaporizes. The metal vapor condenses on the surface of the wafers, which are arranged near the filament or boat. Because materials thus deposited are highly contaminated, this method is often used for coating only backsides of wafers (5).

#### *Electron-Beam Evaporation*

e-Beam uses a focused beam of electrons to heat the material to be deposited. The material is evaporated from a water-cooled crucible and deposited on the wafer substrate. Since the e-beam is focused only on the deposition material, the process is associated with little contamination.

#### *Flash Evaporation*

In the process of flash evaporation, wire from a spool is fed to a heated ceramic bar, where it evaporates. This method is similar to a filament evaporation because the material is heated by thermal resistance.

#### *Induction Evaporation*

Induction evaporation uses radiofrequency radiation to evaporate metal in a crucible for deposition.

#### *Sputtering*

Sputtering is the final vacuum deposition method discussed here. In sputtering, ions of an inert gas are introduced into a low-vacuum atmosphere. An electric field is utilized to ionize the atoms in the chamber and draw them to one plate, called the target. The target is made of the material to be deposited on the wafer substrate. When the ions strike the target, atoms from it are dislodged and strike the wafer substrate facing it. The target atoms are thus deposited, or sputtered, on the surface of the wafer. Sputtering can be done with either direct current or radio frequency, to produce the electric field, and can be used to deposit almost any material (Fig. 11).

### Encapsulation

Epoxy Novolak resin formulations are used to encapsulate approximately 90% of all integrated circuits that are produced. The epoxy Novolak resins are nearly physically inert, as are practically all fully polymerized materials. There are, however, potential hazards associated with their use, owing to the presence of unreacted starting materials (monomers), solvents, curing agents, and additives. A brief review of the preparation of typical epoxy or epoxy Novolak formulations will serve to illustrate the source of the contaminants (6).

The basic epoxy resin system consists of epichlorohydrin (chloro-2,3-epoxypropane) combined with bisphenol A (4,4′-isopropylidenediphenol) to form the diglycidylether of bisphenol A. Bisphenol A is produced by the reaction of acetone and phenol. Epoxidized Novolak resins may be prepared by reacting a Novolak, such as bisphenol F, with epichlorohydrin. Bisphenol F is formed by the reaction of phenol and formaldehyde.

Normally, prior to curing, diluents and flame retardants are added to the resin. Materials commonly added

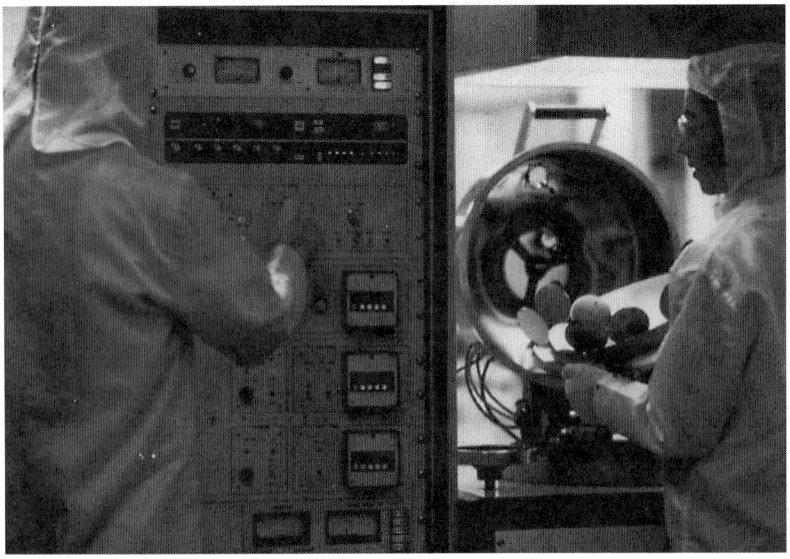

**FIG. 11.** Sputtering chamber with wafers in a planetary for metal deposition. Equipment such as this requires high voltage and has been the source of fatal accidents in the semiconductor industry.

as fillers are fused silica, alumina, or quartz. Common flame retardants are the halogenated derivatives of bisphenol A–tetrachlorobisphenol A and tetrabromobisphenol A, antimony trioxide, and alumina trihydrate. Acid anhydrides and Novolaks are the most common curing agents for epoxy resin systems, although modified amines and amides may be used. The toxic properties of common starting materials, monomers, and selected curing agents and additives are not present in the completely polymerized product.

Beryllium oxide (beryllia) is often used for ceramic encapsulation of semiconductor devices. As with the epoxy formulation described above, there is little if any health hazard associated with the finished product under normal conditions. However, the process of device encapsulation (packaging) and operations involving crushing or grinding the finished product could possibly expose workers to the toxicant by inhalation.

### Solder and Fluxes

Although they are not often considered part of the semiconductor manufacturing process, solder and fluxes are used extensively in the final stages of the manufacture of semiconductor devices. The solders used most often are alloys containing approximately 60% tin and 40% lead. The soldering is carried out in automated devices known as wave solder units. In these units, the parts requiring solder are drawn through a vessel (solder pot) containing molten solder. The solder wets the metal of the lead frame, bonding it to any electrical connections to the semiconductor device. Wave solder units are routinely used to solder integrated circuits (ICs) to circuit boards.

The solder in wave solder units is heated to just above its melting point, approximately 328°F, well below the boiling point of lead, 1,740°F. Formation of lead fume is therefore highly unlikely. The soldering pens used throughout the electronics industry are designed to produce temperatures between 600°F and 800°F. Formation of measurable lead fume from these devices is also unlikely.

The organic soldering fluxes in common use in the semiconductor industry contain ethanol, propanol, or isopropanol as the major ingredient. The organic fluxes also contain one or more of the following ingredients at the approximate concentrations indicated: resin (37%), organic acids (10%), organic phosphates (2%), surfactants (5%), and formic acid (5%).

Inorganic fluxes are sometimes used. Most often they are dilute aqueous solutions of hydrochloric or phosphoric acid with an organic acid such as glutamic acid.

### Recent Advances

As mentioned earlier, the semiconductor industry is in the process of converting manufacturing equipment to accommodate larger silicon wafers. However, there are many facilities in which fabrication is carried out using smaller wafers—4, 6, and 8 inches in diameter. No matter the size of the wafer, the processes used to construct the microelectronics circuitry on the surface of the wafer is the same for a given device.

Automation of fabrication processes has advanced markedly during the past few years. This has resulted in fewer workers at risk for exposure to process chemicals in the fabrication area. However, the introduction of automated process equipment has introduced new hazards associated with the equipment and the process chemicals used in the equipment.

There have been significant advances in the equipment used for the detection of airborne contaminants in semiconductor fabrication facilities. Currently, electrochemical sensors as well as detectors that use chemically impregnated paper to detect the presence of fugitive process gases are in use in many facilities. Such detectors are available for ammonia, hydrides (arsine, diborane, germane, phosphine, and silane), mineral acids (hydrogen, bromide, hydrogen chloride, and hydrogen fluoride), and chlorine. Other types of detectors are available for carbon monoxide, nitrogen trifluoride, and ozone. Although these detectors are used primarily to detect leaks of process gases in storage areas or process equipment, they also serve to warn employees of the presence of the gases in the work area. The sensors can detect their target gases at concentration levels at or below their TLVs.

## OCCUPATIONAL HEALTH

Microelectronics is a light manufacturing industry, and as such, causes fewer injuries than heavier manufacturing industries (Fig. 12). Occupational illnesses occur, how-

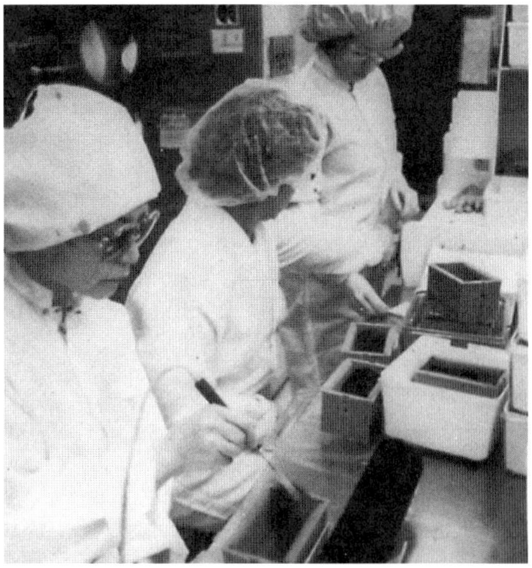

**FIG. 12.** Most microelectronics workers are women. Production workers in the United States are usually of childbearing age, and for many English is not their first language, which may affect ability to understand and implement health and safety instructions.

**TABLE 2.** *Workloss occupational illnesses as percent of all reported injuries and illnesses*

| | 1992 (%) | 1993 (%) | 1994 (%) | 1995 (%) |
|---|---|---|---|---|
| All manufacturing industries | 5.4 | 5.7 | 6.2 | 6.2 |
| Electronic components and accessories | 8.2 | 8.0 | 9.9 | 9.7 |
| Semiconductor and related devices | 8.9 | 9.4 | 10.9 | 12.8 |

Source: Bureau of Labor Statistics, U.S. Department of Labor, April 1997.

ever, at a higher rate in electronics workers, and particularly the semiconductor industry, whose workers represent about a quarter of all electronics workers. This disturbing fact first became apparent in California where Silicon Valley companies produced the major source of reliable data during the early years of the industry. Now that semiconductor manufacture is found in many regions of the United States, national figures are available. They tell the same story that California data presented in years prior. Table 2 shows recent experience with occupational illnesses severe enough to result in time lost from work. In 1995 the average in all manufacturing industries for work loss due to occupational illness was 6.2% of workers. The electronics industry produced a much higher prevalence of occupational illness cases, 9.7% of workers. The semiconductor component of electronics workers had the highest rate of occupational illness in 1995, 12.8%. A study of reporting of occupational illnesses in California found that semiconductor companies properly reported less than half their cases according to Occupational Safety and Health Administration (OSHA) reporting criteria (7).

A similar prevalence of occupational illness is found in national data presented in Table 3. Occupational illnesses in 1995 as a percent of all work-loss injuries and illnesses for the average of manufacturing industries was 13.7%; for the electronics industry, 22.3%; and for the semiconductor industry, 30.0%. This increase in occupational illness is consistent from year to year, and does not appear to be altered by changes in the environmental engineering of the plants, or the health and safety systems developed to protect workers from occupational illnesses.

Occupational illnesses as a percent of all reported illnesses and injuries include the larger numbers of non–work-loss cases. Here, again, the manufacturing industry average in 1995 is 14.3%, electronics industry 20.5%, and semiconductor industry 30.2%.

When employers in California report that an occupational illness is related to exposure to toxic materials, the condition is coded as a systemic poisoning. In California, exposure to toxic materials is twice as likely to be a cause of occupational illness in electronics workers as it is in other manufacturing industries. National figures parallel this distressing fact. Table 4 shows the percent of work-loss injuries and illnesses involving exposure to caustic, noxious, or allergenic substances in recent years. The manufacturing industry average in 1995 is a prevalence of 2.6%. Compare that with the electronics industry experience in the same year at 7.2%, and the semiconductor industry experience of 9.3%.

Occupational illness data may be the result of the widespread use of toxic materials in the semiconductor industry. The manufacture of integrated circuits requires the use of many metals, chemicals, and toxic gases in a wide variety of combinations and plant settings. The majority of semiconductor fabrication facilities do photolithography, wet and dry etching, thin film technologies including metal deposition, and ion implantation (Table 5).

Table 6 shows that virtually all fabrication facilities use photoresist chemicals, chemical strippers, etchants, and diffusion furnaces. Most fabrication facilities use ion implantation, chemical vapor deposition, and thin-film sputter technologies. Moreover, the technology underlying this industry is continually changing. This fast-paced change, as well as the stringent security precautions of the industry, have added to the difficulty of instituting proper health and safety measures in the microelectronics industry.

The Semiconductor Industry Association (SIA)-sponsored study conducted by the University of California, Davis, gives a picture of semiconductor worker exposure that was not available until recently. For example, despite repeated industry assertions that glycol ether exposure was phased out of the clean rooms, 63% of semiconductor fabrication facilities used ethylene-based glycol ethers in recent years, 75% used aromatic solvents, 67% used arsine gas, 93% used phosphine gas, and 64% used diborane gas; 68% of photomask workers are exposed to ethylene-based glycol ethers, 72% to xylene, and 83% to electromagnetic fields (>2 milligauss time-weighted

**TABLE 3.** *Occupational illnesses as percent of all workloss injuries and illnesses*

| | 1992 (%) | 1993 (%) | 1994 (%) | 1995 (%) |
|---|---|---|---|---|
| All manufacturing industries | 12.6 | 13.1 | 13.8 | 13.7 |
| Electronic components and accessories | 18.2 | 18.1 | 22.1 | 22.3 |
| Semiconductor and related devices | 19.6 | 20.9 | 22.9 | 30.0 |

Source: Bureau of Labor Statistics, U.S. Department of Labor, April 1997.

**TABLE 4.** *Percent of work-loss injuries and illnesses involving exposure to caustic, noxious, or allergenic substances*

| | 1992 | 1993 | 1994 | 1995 |
|---|---|---|---|---|
| All manufacturing industries | 2.7 | 2.8 | 2.7 | 2.6 |
| Electronic components and accessories | 8.3 | 8.4 | 8.8 | 7.2 |
| Semiconductor and related devices | 8.7 | 12.6 | 6.0 | 9.3 |

Source: Bureau of Labor Statistics, U.S. Department of Labor, June 1997.

**TABLE 5.** *Process groups in 44 semiconductor fabrication rooms (Fabs), identified during site visits by study industrial hygienists*

| Process group | Fabs with process group (*n*) |
|---|---|
| Photolithography | 28 |
| Wet and dry etching | 34 |
| Masking | 13 |
| Diffusion | 38 |
| Thin film or metals | 32 |
| Ion implantation | 15 |
| Epitaxy | 4 |
| Chemical vapor deposition | 4 |

From ref. 19.

**TABLE 6.** *Percentages of subjects exposed to agents at any level, by work group in semiconductor health study*

| | | Fabrication room work groups[a] | | | | |
|---|---|---|---|---|---|---|
| | | Masking | | Dopants and thin film | | |
| Exposure | Outside fabrication rooms ($n = 444$) % | Photolithography ($n = 227$) % | Etching ($n = 130$) % | Furnace ($n = 123$) % | TFII[b] ($n = 92$) % | Fabrication room supervisors and engineers ($n = 54$) % |
| Photoresist and developer solvent | | | | | | |
| Ethylene glycolethers | 0 | 68 | 42 | 16 | 21 | 18 |
| Propylene-based glycolethers | 0 | 31 | 13 | 8 | 8 | 6 |
| Xylene | 0 | 72 | 45 | 19 | 21 | 24 |
| *n*-butyl acetate | 0 | 69 | 44 | 16 | 18 | 22 |
| Fluoride | 1 | 31 | 75 | 82 | 52 | 37 |
| Cleaning solvents | | | | | | |
| Acetone | 18 | 39 | 29 | 21 | 19 | 16 |
| Isopropyl alcohol | 25 | 75 | 76 | 76 | 82 | 49 |
| Methanol | 3 | 17 | 21 | 15 | 27 | 14 |
| Dopants | | | | | | |
| Antimony | 0 | 4 | 7 | 20 | 16 | 2 |
| Arsenic | 0 | 8 | 13 | 36 | 29 | 6 |
| Boron | 0 | 11 | 19 | 64 | 39 | 16 |
| Phosphorous | 0 | 9 | 18 | 76 | 39 | 18 |
| Radiation | | | | | | |
| ELF-MF (>2mG TWA)[c] | 22 | 83 | 80 | 86 | 84 | 51 |
| Radiofrequency | 0 | 28 | 55 | 31 | 51 | 59 |

[a]Some subjects worked in more than one group.
[b]TFII, thin film and ion implantation.
[c]ELF-MF, extremely–low-frequency magnetic fields; mG, milligauss; TWA, time-weighted average.
From ref. 21.

average). Workers etching silicon wafers sustained similar exposures to chemical and physical hazards.

The high rates of occupational illness in electronics workers, and the association of these illnesses with toxic materials, provide ample reason for implementing occupational health and safety programs for these companies, particularly for semiconductor manufacturers. To date, few model programs of occupational health have been developed. In most companies the safety component is much better developed than the health component. Most semiconductor companies lack medical departments other than nurse stations. Only a few physicians are employed by semiconductor companies, and most of them on a part-time, consulting basis.

**Epidemiologic Studies**

As a result of the environmental contamination of public water supplies in San Jose, California by microelectronics companies, the state Department of Health Services conducted an investigation. Widespread use of underground chemical storage tanks had resulted in leakage of solvents and other chemicals into groundwater. An initial epidemiologic study of reproductive outcome measures in the population that drank contaminated water showed increases in the rates of spontaneous abortion and congenital malformations of infants exposed during pregnancy (8). A follow-up study of greater power covering more years of exposure failed to confirm the initial findings (9).

However, workers in the microelectronics industry were exposed to much greater concentrations of chemicals than persons exposed through drinking water. Since the large majority of microelectronics workers are women of childbearing age, the risk of adverse reproductive outcomes was examined among semiconductor workers in Massachusetts. Personal interviews were conducted with manufacturing workers, spouses of male workers, and an internal comparison group of nonmanufacturing workers (10). Elevated rates of spontaneous abortion were observed for women working in clean rooms (31.3 for photolithographic workers, 38.9 for diffusion workers, and 17.8 for unexposed women). No other significant differences in reproductive outcome were identified. The authors stressed the tentative nature of their findings and called for more definitive studies.

IBM, then the largest U.S. manufacturer of integrated circuits, engaged the School of Hygiene and Public Health at Johns Hopkins University to conduct a reproductive study with IBM employees (11). The retrospective portion of the IBM study, conducted at facilities in New York and Vermont, was reported in 1992 as showing an increased spontaneous abortion rate for women workers in two specific clean-room areas. Although other workers exposed to glycol ethers (diethylene glycol dimethyl ether and ethylene glycol monoethyl ether acetate) were not found to have similar increases in abortion rate, the association of glycol ether exposure and spontaneous abortion in the retrospective portion of the study caused IBM to notify its employees worldwide of the findings and to announce to the media that the study would lead to more restrictive handling of glycol ethers at IBM facilities. The prospective study of IBM employees analyzed work functions assuming significant ethylene glycol ether exposures with some jobs. The study lacked personal sampling data on the exposed workers. Analyses of groups of processes and the chemicals required for each process within the clean room revealed significant associations between spontaneous abortion and several compounds (11). It was difficult, however, to identify specific agents because several processes were conducted together as a group, and many chemicals were used in a process. Nevertheless, the analysis strongly suggested that the ethylene-based glycol ether (EGE) photoresist chemicals used in the Clean Mix and Photo/Apply processes were associated with an increased risk of miscarriage. Stratified analyses indicated that no single chemical demonstrated a significant additional effect after adjustment for use of photoresist.

In a small prospective study, Schenker et al. (12) could not demonstrate an association of reproductive outcomes with exposure to a group of chemicals, with so few pregnancies among exposed workers. There were only six pregnancies among women who worked with processes that required any use of EGE-based Photoresists and solvents. Even though four of these six pregnancies resulted in spontaneous abortion (66.7%), when compared to the rate of pregnancy loss among women in non–clean room areas (43.8%), the relative risk of spontaneous abortion of 1.5 (associated with work requiring EGE) was not statistically significant.

Correra and colleagues (13) point out that "lack of specific measurements of exposure to EGE for study subjects was one limitation of the study." They also caution that "the nature of semiconductor manufacturing made it difficult for us to address the question of whether the associations noted were specific to EGE; in particular, work with the photoresist mixture entailed use of hexamethyldisilazane, *n*-butyl acetate, *n*-methyl-2-pyrrolidine, and xylene at the same time."

As an example of the complexities posed by semiconductor chemicals, observe the formulation of a DQN Photoresist. Novolak resin is a phenol-formaldehyde resin. Small amounts of formaldehyde and substituted phenols contaminate the finished resin and therefore are also present in the final photoresist formulation. It is possible that these monomers are partially vaporized in the soft-bake process, though the more likely exposure would occur through skin contact with the liquid photoresist. Besides formaldehyde released by the photoresist soft-bake process (12), other contact sensitizers have been recognized in resins based on phenol and formaldehyde. Para-tertiarybutyl phenol (PTBP) has been the most widely documented (14).

Despite differences in location, demographics, period of recall, inclusion of multiple pregnancies per woman, and exposure assessment methods, the IBM historical cohort results were remarkably similar to those of the SIA study (12,13).

The prospective reproductive study demonstrated an increased risk of spontaneous abortion with a relative risk of 1.34 (13). Here, a group of women workers submitted daily urine specimens to be analyzed for human chorionic gonadotropin (hCG) levels that would detect abortions that might otherwise be missed even by the women workers. The study was conducted for only 6 months, so pregnancy outcomes such as birth weight and birth defects were not observed. The sample size was too small to implicate any of the chemicals associated with abortion in the retrospective portion of the study. There were only 20 pregnancies in the fabrication worker group during the study period. Unfortunately, no attempt was made to analyze the urine specimens for glycol ether metabolites to document exposure in these workers.

The reproductive findings in semiconductor industry studies indicate that other health problems should be evaluated, including cancer and a variety of chronic illnesses. The SIA and IBM studies show how important it is to open this industry to further health research both in the United States and in Japan, Germany, Malaysia, and the many other countries where this high-risk manufacturing process is now being conducted (15–17).

## REFERENCES


1. LaDou J, ed. The microelectronics industry. State-of-the-art reviews. *Occup Med* 1986;1(1).
2. Harrison M. Semiconductor manufacturing hazards. In: Sullivan JB, Krieger GR, eds. *Clinical principles of environmental health.* Baltimore: Williams & Wilkins, 1992.
3. Van Zant P. *Microchip fabrication:* a practical guide to semiconductor processing, 3rd ed. New York: McGraw-Hill, 1997.
4. Chen FF. Semiconductors open a new niche for plasma researchers. *Science* 1995;270:1292.
5. Bauer S, Wolff I, Werner N, Schmidt R, Blume R, Pelzing M. Toxicological investigations in the semiconductor industry: IV. Studies on the subchronic oral toxicity and genotoxicity of vacuum pump oils contaminated by waste products from aluminum plasma etching processes. *Toxicol Ind Health* 1995;11(5):523–541.
6. Goosey MT. Introduction to plastics and their important properties for electronic applications. In: Goosey MT, ed. *Plastics for electronics.* New York: Elsevier Applied Sciences, 1985.
7. McCurdy SA, Schenker MB, Samuels SJ. Reporting of occupational injury and illness in the semiconductor manufacturing industry. *Am J Public Health* 1991;81(1):85.
8. Rudolph L, Swan SH. Reproductive hazards in the microelectronics industry. State-of-the-art reviews. *Occup Med* 1986;1:135–143.
9. Wrensch M, Swan SH, Lipscomb J, et al. Pregnancy outcomes in women potentially exposed to solvent-contaminated drinking water in San Jose, California. *Am J Epidemiol* 1990;131:283–300.
10. Pastides H, Calabrese EJ, Hosmer DW, Harris DR. Spontaneous abortion and general illness symptoms among semiconductor manufacturers. *J Occup Med* 1988;30:543–551.
11. Gray R. *Final report retrospective and prospective studies of reproductive health among IBM employees in semiconductor manufacturing.* Baltimore: Johns Hopkins University School of Hygiene and Public Health, 1993.
12. Schenker MB, Gold EB, Beaumont JJ, et al. Association of spontaneous abortion and other reproductive effects with work in the semiconductor industry. *Am J Ind Med* 1995;28:639–659.
13. Correra A, Gray RH, Cohen R, et al. Ethylene Glycol Ethers and Risks of Spontaneous Abortion and Subfertility. *Am J Epidemiol* 1996; 143(7):707–717.
14. Bruze M. Contact dermatitis from phenol-formaldehyde resins. In: Maibach HI, ed. *Occupational and industrial dermatology,* 2nd ed. Chicago: Year Book Medical Publishers, 1987.
15. LaDou J. Health issues in the global semiconductor industry. *Ann Acad Med Singapore* 1994;23(5):765–769.
16. Schenker M. Occupational lung diseases in the industrializing and industrialized world due to modern industries and modern pollutants. *Tubercle Lung Dis* 1992;73:27–32.
17. LaDou J. In many areas of the world, the migration of reproductive hazards precedes the development and implementation of reproductive policy. *Int J Occup Environ Health* 1996;2(1):73–75.
18. Hines CJ, Selvin S, Samuels SJ, et al. Hierarchical cluster analysis for exposure assessment of workers in the semiconductor health study. *Am J Ind* Med 1995;28:715.
19. Hammond SK, Hines CJ, Hallock MF, et al. Tiered exposure-assessment strategy in the semiconductor health study. *Am J Ind Med* 1995; 28:670.
20. Hallock MF, Hammond SK, Hines CJ, et al. Patterns of chemical use and exposure control in the semiconductor health study. *Am J Ind Med* 1995;28:687.
21. Swan SH, Beaumont JJ, Hammond KS, et al. Historical cohort study of spontaneous abortion among fabrication workers in the semiconductor health study: agent level analysis. *Am J Ind Med* 1995;28:751–769.

*Environmental and Occupational Medicine,*
*Third Edition,* edited by William N. Rom.
Lippincott–Raven Publishers, Philadelphia © 1998.

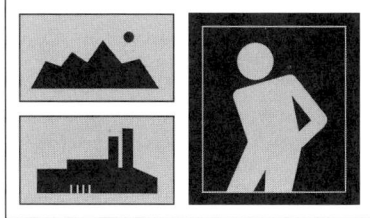

CHAPTER 97

# Ionizing Radiation

Arthur C. Upton

Within weeks after Roentgen's discovery of the x-ray in 1895, radiation injuries began to be encountered in those working with the early radiation equipment (1). During the century since then, the study of such injuries has received continuing impetus from the expanding uses of radiation in medicine, science, industry, and nuclear energy.

In historical perspective, the effects of ionizing radiation have received more study than those of any other hazardous environmental agent. As a result, our experience with radiation has been strategically important in addressing other environmental and occupational causes of disease.

## NATURE AND PROPERTIES OF IONIZING RADIATION

Ionizing radiations are of two broad types: electromagnetic and particulate. The electromagnetic radiations include roentgen rays (or x-rays) and gamma rays, which possess no mass or charge and which are characterized by extremely short wave length and high frequency (Fig. 1). The particulate radiations consist of electrons, protons, neutrons, alpha particles, negative pi-mesons, heavy charged ions, and other atomic particles varying in mass and charge. Both types of ionizing radiation differ from other forms of radiant energy in being able to disrupt the atoms and molecules on which they impinge, thereby producing ions, free radicals, and, in turn, biochemical lesions.

As ionizing radiation penetrates matter, it gives up its energy by colliding with atoms and molecules in its path. Such collisions are clustered so closely together along the path of an alpha particle that the particle typically has only enough energy to traverse a few cells, whereas the collisions are separated so far apart along the path of an x-ray that the radiation can traverse the entire body (Fig. 2). The average rate at which energy is deposited per unit length of path, i.e., the linear energy transfer (LET) of the radiation, is customarily expressed in kiloelectron volts per micrometer (keV/μm) (4).

In general, the higher the LET of the radiation, the more likely it is to deposit enough energy in a critical site within the cell, e.g., a deoxyribonucleic acid (DNA) molecule or a chromosome, to cause an irreparable molecular lesion. Alpha particles and other high-LET radiations are typically more potent, therefore, than low-LET radiations such as x-rays (4).

Within the body, the distribution and retention of each internally deposited radionuclide is governed by its physical and chemical properties, i.e., the amount of radioactivity remaining in situ decreases with time through both physical decay and biologic removal. The physical half-lives of radionuclides vary from less than a second in the case of some radionuclides to billions of years in the case of others. Biologic half-lives also vary, tending to be longer for bone-seeking radionuclides (such as radium, strontium, or plutonium) than for radionuclides that are deposited predominantly in soft tissue (such as iodine, cesium, or tritium) (5).

## QUANTITIES AND UNITS OF MEASURE

Following the recommendation of the International Commission on Radiological Units and Measurements (6), the International System (SI) of units has come into increasingly wide use in place of the centimeter-gram-

A. C. Upton: Department of Environmental and Community Medicine, University of Medicine and Dentistry of New Jersey–Robert Wood Johnson Medical School, Piscataway, New Jersey 08855-1179.

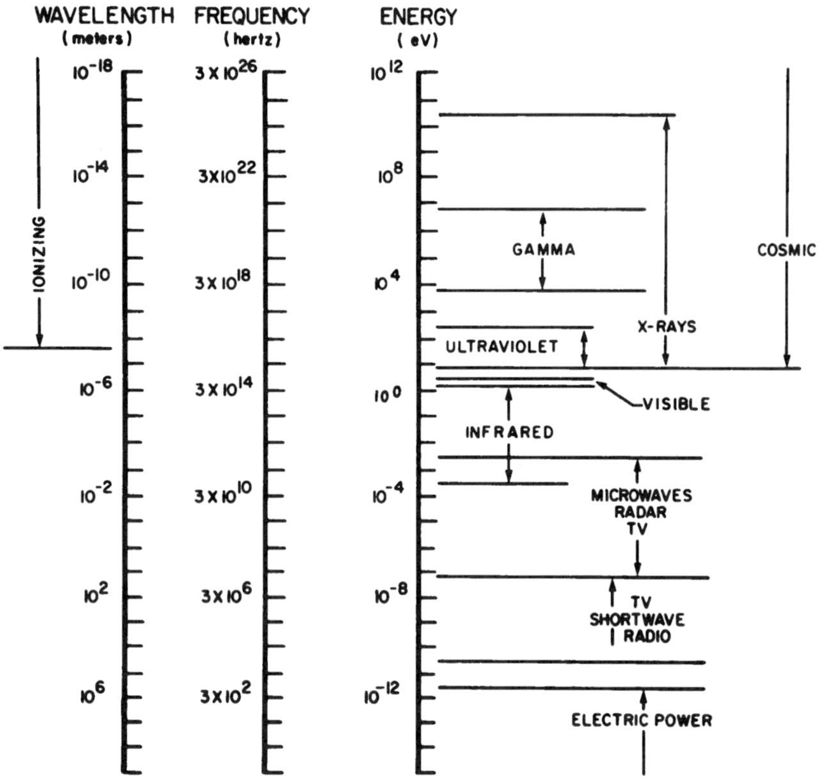


**FIG. 1.** The electromagnetic spectrum. (From ref. 2.)

second (cgs) system (7). The SI unit for expressing the dose of radiation that is absorbed in tissue is the gray (Gy): 1 Gy = 1 joule per kilogram of tissue (Table 1). The corresponding cgs unit is the radiation absorbed dose (rad): 1 rad = 100 erg per gram of tissue = 0.01 Gy.

To enable doses of radiations of differing potencies to be normalized in terms of risk, another unit, i.e., the equivalent dose, also is used in radiologic protection (Table 1). This unit is the sievert (Sv): 1 sievert is equivalent to the dose in gray multiplied by an appropriate relative biological effectiveness (RBE)-dependent quality factor (Q), so that, in principle, 1 Sv of any given type of radiation represents the dose that is equivalent in biologic effectiveness to 1 Gy of gamma rays. The corresponding cgs unit is the rem: 1 rem = 0.01 Sv.

The unit for expressing the collective effective dose to a population is the person-Sv; 1 sievert to each of 100 people = 100 person-Sv = 10,000 person-rem (Table 1).

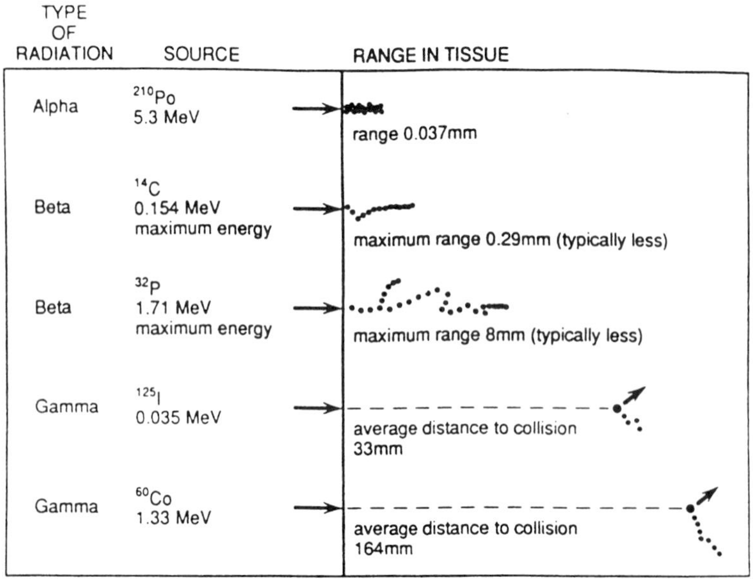


**FIG. 2.** Differences among various types of ionizing radiation in penetrating power in tissue. (Reprinted by permission from ref. 3.)

**TABLE 1.** *Quantities and dose units of ionizing radiation*

| Quantity being measured | Definition | Dose unit[a] |
|---|---|---|
| Absorbed dose | Energy deposited in tissue (1 joule/kg) | Gray (Gy) |
| Equivalent dose | Absorbed dose weighted for the relative biologic effectiveness of the radiation | Sievert (Sv) |
| Effective dose | Equivalent dose weighted for the sensitivity of the exposed organ(s) | Sievert (Sv) |
| Collective effective dose | Effective dose applied to a population | Person (Sv) |
| Committed effective dose | Cumulative effective dose to be received from a given intake of radioactivity | Sievert (Sv) |
| Radioactivity | One disintegration per second | Becquerel (Bq) |

[a]The units of measure listed are those of the International System, introduced in the 1970s to standardize usage throughout the world (ICRP, 1990). They have largely supplanted the earlier units, namely, the rad (1 rad = 100 erg per g = 0.01 Gy), the rem (1 rem = 0.01 Sv), and the curie (1 Ci = $3.7 \times 10^{10}$ disintegrations per second = $3.7 \times 10^{10}$ Bq).

The unit for expressing the amount of radioactivity in a given sample of matter is the becquerel (Bq); 1 Bq corresponds to that quantity of radioactivity in which there is one atomic disintegration per second. The cgs unit used for the same purpose is the curie (Ci); one Ci represents that quantity of radioactivity in which there are $3.7 \times 10^{10}$ atomic disintegrations per second (1 Ci = $3.7 \times 10^{10}$ Bq).

Historically, the unit used for measuring exposure to x-rays is the roentgen. One roentgen (R), defined loosely, is the amount of x-radiation that produces one electrostatic unit of charge in 1 cubic centimeter of air under standard conditions of temperature and pressure. Exposure of the surface of the skin to 1 R of x-rays typically deposits a dose of slightly less than 10 mGy (1 rad) in the underlying epidermis.

## SOURCES AND LEVELS OF IONIZING RADIATION IN THE ENVIRONMENT

Ionizing radiation from natural, as well as artificial, sources is ubiquitous in the human environment (Table 2). Natural background radiation comes from three main sources: (a) cosmic rays, which originate in outer space; (b) terrestrial radiation, which emanates from radium and other radioactive elements in the earth's crust; and (c) internal radiation, which is emitted by potassium-40 and other naturally occurring radionuclides normally present in the body (Table 2). The dose received from all three sources by a person living at sea level in the United States averages about 0.94 mSv per year to all soft tissues other than the lung (Table 2). The intensity of cosmic radiation varies with altitude by a factor of two or more, however, so that a person residing at a high elevation (e.g., Denver) may receive twice as large a dose from this source as one who resides at sea level. The radiation from the earth's crust also varies markedly from one geographic region to another, depending on local variations in the content of radioactive material in soil and subterranean rock. The doses from these sources are far smaller in any event than the average dose to the bronchial epithelium from radon in indoor air (Table 2); in heavy smokers, moreover, portions of the respiratory tract may also receive as much as 200 mSv additional radiation per year from the polonium that is normally present in tobacco smoke (8,9).

Of various artificial sources of ionizing radiation to which members of the U.S. population are exposed, the most important is the use of x-rays in medical diagnosis (Table 2). Far less important, barring accidents, are "technologically enhanced" sources (such as the use of radionuclide-containing minerals in phosphate fertilizers

**TABLE 2.** *Average amounts of ionizing radiation received annually from different sources by a member of the U.S. population*

| Source | Dose[a] (mSv) | (mrem) | (%) |
|---|---|---|---|
| Natural | | | |
| Radon[b] | 2.0 | 200 | 55 |
| Cosmic | 0.27 | 27 | 8 |
| Terrestrial | 0.28 | 28 | 8 |
| Internal | 0.39 | 39 | 11 |
| Total natural | 2.94 | 294 | 82 |
| Artificial | | | |
| X-ray diagnosis | 0.39 | 39 | 11 |
| Nuclear medicine | 0.14 | 14 | 4 |
| Consumer products | 0.10 | 10 | 3 |
| Occupational | <0.01 | <1.0 | <0.3 |
| Nuclear fuel cycle | <0.01 | <1.0 | <0.03 |
| Nuclear fallout | <0.01 | <1.0 | <0.03 |
| Miscellaneous[c] | <0.01 | <1.0 | <0.03 |
| Total artificial | 0.63 | 63 | 18 |
| Total natural and artificial | 3.57 | 357 | 100 |

[a]Average effective dose to soft tissues, excluding bronchial epithelium.
[b]Average effective dose to bronchial epithelium alone.
[c]Department of Energy facilities, smelters, transportation, etc.
Adapted from refs. 8 and 9.

**TABLE 3.** *Workers who may be exposed occupationally to ionizing radiation*

| |
|---|
| Aircraft pilots and crews |
| Atomic energy plant workers |
| Cathode ray tube makers |
| Dental assistants |
| Electron microscope makers |
| Electron microscopists |
| Electrostatic eliminator operators |
| Fire alarm makers |
| Gas mantle makers |
| High-voltage TV repairmen |
| Industrial fluoroscope operators |
| Industrial radiographers |
| Klystron tube operators |
| Liquid level gauge operators |
| Luminous dial painters |
| Nuclear submarine workers |
| Oil well loggers |
| Ore assayers |
| Petroleum refinery workers |
| Physicians |
| Pipeline weld radiographers |
| Plasma torch operators |
| Radar tube makers |
| Radiologists |
| Radium handlers |
| Reactor workers |
| Thorium alloy workers |
| Thorium ore producers |
| Underground metal miners |
| Uranium miners and mill workers |
| Workers near gamma ray sources |
| X-ray diffraction apparatus operators |
| X-ray technicians and aides |
| X-ray tube makers |

Modified from ref. 10.

and building materials), atomic weapons fallout, nuclear power production, and consumer products (color television sets, smoke detectors, luminescent clock and instrument dials, etc.; see Table 2).

Workers in various occupations (Table 3) are exposed to additional ionizing radiation, doses of which vary with the nature of the occupation, particular work assignment, and working conditions (Table 4). The annual dose equivalent received occupationally in the United States averages less than 20 mSv (200 mrem), and less than 0.1% of radiation workers exceed the maximum permissible dose limit (50 mSv) in any given year (12).

**TABLE 4.** *Estimated numbers of U.S. workers exposed occupationally to ionizing radiation*

| Types of work | No. of workers exposed annually | Average dose per year |
|---|---|---|
| Nuclear energy[a] | 62,000 | 8.4 |
| Naval reactor | 36,000 | 2.2 |
| Healing arts | 500,000 | 1.2 |
| Research | 100,000 | 1.2 |
| Manufacturing and industrial | 7,000,000 | 0.07 |

[a]Including entire nuclear fuel cycle.
From ref. 11.

## NATURE AND TYPES OF RADIATION INJURIES

For purposes of radiologic protection, it is customary to distinguish between radiation injuries that have dose thresholds and those that are assumed to lack dose thresholds. The former (so-called nonstochastic or deterministic effects) include various acute and chronic tissue reactions (e.g., erythema of the skin, depression of the blood count, oligospermia, cataract of the lens) that result from the killing of large numbers of cells in affected organs (13). Injuries of the latter type, on the other hand, include mutagenic and carcinogenic effects, which are viewed as stochastic, or probabilistic, effects that can result from radiation-induced changes in single cells within affected organs.

### Effects of Radiation at the Cellular Level

#### *Gene Mutation*

Of the various molecules that radiation may damage within the cell, DNA is the most critical, since damage to a single gene may irreparably alter or kill the cell. A dose of radiation large enough to kill the average dividing cell (1 or 2 Sv) suffices to cause dozens of lesions in its DNA, most of which are reparable, depending on the effectiveness of the cell's DNA repair processes (14). In fact, thousands of such lesions are thought to be produced each day in the DNA of every cell by natural background radiation, oxidative metabolic reactions, and other causes (15).

Mutagenic effects of radiation have not yet been documented in human germ cells, but they have been investigated extensively in human somatic cells and in the germ cells of many other species, in which their frequency approximates $10^{-5}$ to $10^{-6}$ per locus per Sv, depending on the locus in question and the conditions of irradiation (9,16). The magnitude of the increase per unit dose is so small that the absence of detectable mutagenic effects on the children of the atomic bomb survivors is not surprising in view of the limited numbers of such children and the comparatively small average gonadal dose received by their parents (9,16). On the basis of present knowledge, the dose of ionizing radiation that would be required to double the frequency of heritable mutations in the human population is estimated to exceed 1 Sv (9), from which it is inferred that less than 1% of the total burden of genetically related human diseases is attributable to natural background irradiation.

#### *Chromosome Aberrations*

By breaking chromosomes and/or interfering with their normal segregation to daughter cells at the time of cell division, irradiation can alter the number and structure of chromosomes in the cell. If two or more chromosome breaks occur close enough together in space and time, the broken ends from one break point may be joined incorrectly with those from another, giving rise to translocations, inversions, rings, dicentrics, and other types of chromosome rearrangements. With high-LET irradiation, the frequency of such "two-event" aberrations increases steeply as a linear function of the dose and is virtually independent of the dose rate (Fig. 3), whereas with low-LET irradiation it increases less abruptly, as a linear-quadratic function of the dose, and is highly dependent on the dose rate, i.e., the linear dose term predominates at low doses and low dose rates, whereas the quadratic term predominates at high doses and high dose rates (Fig. 3).

In human lymphocytes irradiated in culture, the frequency of two-event chromosome aberrations approximates 0.1 aberration per cell per seivert in the low-to-intermediate dose range (Fig. 3). It is not astonishing, therefore, that the frequency of such aberrations has been observed to be increased in radiation workers and persons residing in areas of high natural background radiation, as well as in persons exposed accidentally or therapeutically to large doses of radiation, for whom it can serve as a crude biologic dosimeter (18).

### *Cytotoxic Effects*

In general, the radiosensitivity of cells varies in proportion to their rate of proliferation and inversely in relation to their degree of differentiation, as noted early in this century by Bergonie and Tribondeau. Relatively few types of cells (e.g., lymphocytes and oocytes) are radiosensitive in a nonproliferative state. Although any cell can be killed by a large-enough dose of radiation (hundreds or thousands of gray), a dose of only 1 to 2 Gy suffices to render most human clonogenic cells incapable of proliferating (19,20).

The survival of cells, as measured by their ability to proliferate, tends to decrease exponentially with increasing dose (Fig. 4). With high-LET radiation, the dose-survival curve is characteristically steeper than with low-LET radiation and is relatively independent of the dose rate (Fig. 4), whereas with low-LET radiation the curve usually has an initial shoulder in the low-dose region, which reappears between successive exposures as a result of repair of radiation damage during the interim (Fig. 4).

### *Effects on Tissues and Organs*

Tissues in which cells proliferate rapidly are generally the first to manifest injury (2,19,20). Mitotic inhibition is typically detectable within minutes after intensive irradi-

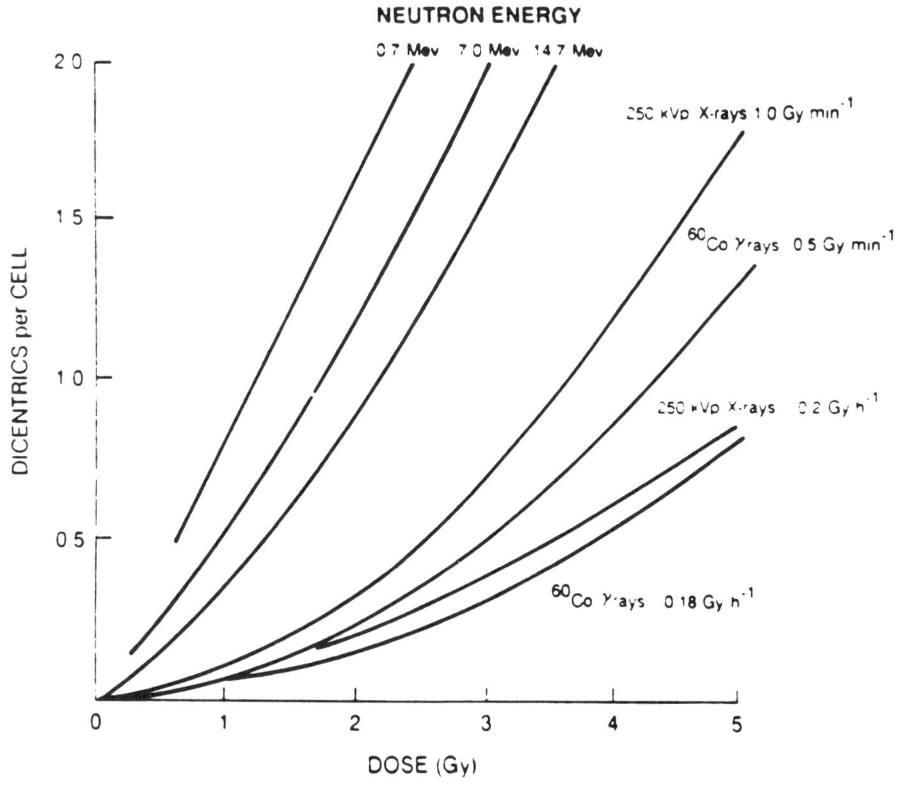


**FIG. 3.** Frequency of dicentric chromosome aberrations in human lymphocytes in relation to dose, dose rate, and quality of irradiation *in vitro*. (From ref. 17.)

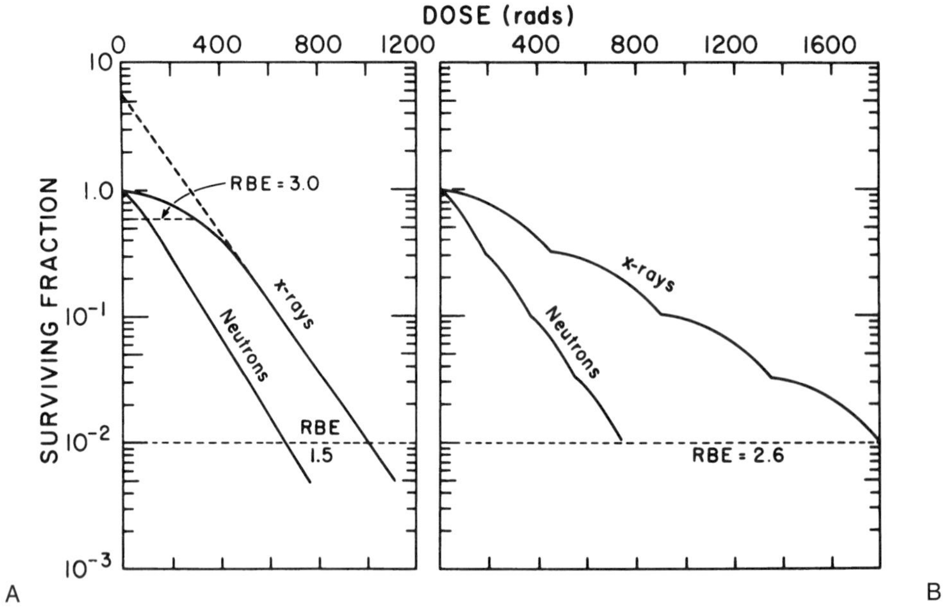


**FIG. 4.** Typical dose-survival curves, single **(A)** and fractionated **(B)**, for mammalian cells exposed to x-rays and fast neutrons. (From ref. 20.)

ation, in contrast to scarring, tissue breakdown, and other degenerative changes, which may not appear until months or years later. If a dose of radiation is absorbed gradually enough, its damaging effects may be offset to varying degrees by the compensatory proliferation of stem cells that escape injury, so that a larger dose of radiation can be tolerated if it is spread out in time than if it is absorbed in a single brief exposure (2,13).

Because of the great multiplicity and diversity of ways in which irradiation can affect different organs (2,20), only those effects that are of particular relevance to occupational and accidental irradiation are described in the following sections.

*Skin*

The earliest outward reaction of the skin is erythema, which results from dilatation of blood capillaries by substances released from injured cells in the overlying epidermis. The severity of the erythema increases with the area as well as the depth of skin that is irradiated. The threshold dose for erythema in an area greater than 10 $cm^2$ varies from about 6 to 8 Gy delivered in a single, brief exposure to more than 30 Gy delivered in multiple exposures over a period of several weeks. After rapid exposure to a dose of 6 Gy, the erythema may become evident within hours, typically lasts only a few hours, and is followed 2 to 4 weeks later by one or more waves of deeper and more persistent erythema (2,13, 19).

For epilation, the threshold is lower: a dose of 3 to 5 Gy delivered in a single, brief exposure suffices to cause temporary shedding of hair from the scalp (2,13).

*Blood-Forming Tissues*

Hematopoietic cells are highly radiosensitive, undergoing degenerative changes within minutes after a dose of 1 Sv, while mature leukocytes, erythrocytes, and platelets are radioresistant. A dose of 3 to 5 Sv acute whole-body irradiation suffices to kill enough hematopoietic cells to cause profound depression of the white blood cell and platelet counts within 3 to 5 weeks (Table 5), whereas a dose of 0.5 to 1.0 Sv is not large enough to depress the count severely. A dose of 10 Sv of whole-body irradiation, which is lethal when received within minutes or days, can be tolerated when accumulated gradually over a period of weeks or months or when delivered to only a small fraction of the hematopoietic marrow (2,13,16).

Lymphocytes, like hematopoietic cells, are highly radiosensitive. A dose of 3 to 5 Sv of intensive whole-body irradiation suffices to cause prompt lymphopenia, with profound depression of the immune response (2,13,16).

*Gastrointestinal Tract*

Germinative cells in the epithelium of the small intestine can be killed in sufficient numbers by intensive irradiation to cause denudation and ulceration of the overlying mucosa. When a large part of the small intestine is exposed acutely to a dose in excess of 10 Gy, a fulminating dysentery-like reaction is produced, which may terminate fatally within several days (Table 5).

*Reproductive Organs*

Immature spermatogonia are among the most radiosensitive cells in the body. As a result, rapid expo-

**TABLE 5.** *Major forms and features of the acute radiation syndrome*

| Time after irradiation | Cerebral form (>50 Sv) | Gastrointestinal form (10-205v) | Hematopoietic form (2–10 Sv) | Pulmonary form (>6 Sv to lungs) |
|---|---|---|---|---|
| First day | Nausea<br>Vomiting<br>Diarrhea<br>Headache<br>Disorientation<br>Ataxia<br>Coma<br>Convulsions<br>Death | Nausea<br>Vomiting<br>Diarrhea | Nausea<br>Vomiting<br>Diarrhea | Nausea<br>Vomiting |
| Second week | | Nausea<br>Vomiting<br>Diarrhea<br>Fever<br>Erythema<br>Prostration<br>Death | | |
| Third to sixth week | | | Weakness<br>Fatigue<br>Anorexia<br>Fever<br>Hemorrhage<br>Epilation<br>Recovery (?)<br>Death (?) | |
| Second to eighth month | | | | Cough<br>Dyspnea<br>Fever<br>Chest pain<br>Respiratory failure (?) |

Modified from ref. 16.

sure of both testes to a dose of only 0.15 Sv suffices to depress the sperm count temporarily, and permanent sterility may result from a dose in excess of 4 Sv (2, 13).

Oocytes also are radiosensitive. A dose of 1.5 to 2.0 Sv to both ovaries may cause temporary sterility, and a dose of 2.0 to 3.0 Sv permanent sterility, depending on age at the time of irradiation (2,13).

### *Lens of the Eye*

Irradiation of the lens can cause the formation of lens opacities within a matter of months, depending on the dose (2,13). Although a posterior subcapsular opacity may become detectable microscopically after a dose of 0.6 to 1 Sv received in a single, brief exposure, the threshold for a vision-impairing cataract is estimated to vary from about 2 to 3 Sv if received in a few minutes to as much as 5.5 to 14 Sv if received over a period of months. The occurrence of radiation cataracts in pioneer cyclotron physicists provided the first evidence of the relatively high cataractogenic effectiveness of neutrons (13).

## THE ACUTE RADIATION SYNDROME

Intensive irradiation of a major part of the hematopoietic system, the gastrointestinal tract, the lung, or the brain can cause the acute radiation syndrome. The prodromal symptoms—anorexia, nausea, and vomiting—typically begin within a few hours after irradiation. Except at the highest doses, these symptoms usually subside by the end of the first day and are followed by a symptom-free interval until the onset of the main phase of the illness (Table 5).

In the intestinal form of the syndrome, the main phase of the illness characteristically begins 2 to 3 days after irradiation, with abdominal pain, fever, and increasingly severe diarrhea, dehydration, prostration, and toxemia. The reaction progresses rapidly, culminating within several days in a fatal, shocklike state (Table 5).

In the hematopoietic form of the syndrome, the main phase of the illness is related to leukopenia and thrombocytopenia, which typically do not give rise to symptoms until the second to third week after irradiation. When injury of the marrow is sufficiently extensive, death from infection or hemorrhage may result during the fourth to sixth week after irradiation (Table 5).

In the pulmonary form, an acute pneumonitis develops in the irradiated area within 1 to 3 months after a dose of 6 to 10 Sv to the lung (Table 5). If extensive, the process may terminate in respiratory failure, or it may lead to pulmonary fibrosis and cor pulmonale months or years later (2,13).

A fourth form of radiation sickness, the cerebral form, can result from acute exposure of the brain to a dose in excess of 50 Sv. In this reaction, anorexia, nausea, and vomiting begin almost immediately after irradiation, to be followed within minutes or hours by increasing drowsiness, confusion, ataxia, convulsions, loss of consciousness, and death (Table 5).

### Carcinogenic Effects

Irradiation has been observed to increase the incidence of cancers of various types in radiotherapy patients, early radiologists, radium dial painters, underground hardrock miners, and atomic bomb survivors, depending on the conditions of exposure (2,9,16,22). Such cancers have not appeared until years or decades after irradiation, however, and none has shown features identifying it as having resulted from radiation specifically, as opposed to some other cause. These findings, are complemented by extensive experimental data on radiation carcinogenesis in laboratory animals (9).

Excesses of many types of malignancy are evident in atomic bomb survivors (Fig. 5), in whom the overall incidence of cancer appears to have increased in proportion to the radiation dose (Fig. 6). However, the data do not suffice to define precisely the shape of the dose-incidence curve in the low-dose domain. Hence the carcinogenic risks of low-level irradiation can be estimated only by extrapolation, based on assumptions about the relationship between incidence and dose. Of the available dose-incidence data for the various cancers, the most extensive pertain to leukemia, cancer of the female breast, and cancer of the thyroid gland.

#### *Leukemia*

All major forms of leukemia, except the chronic lymphocytic form, have been observed to be increased in frequency after irradiation of the whole body or a large part of the hematopoietic system. The increase has typically appeared within 2 to 5 years after irradiation, has been dose dependent, and has persisted 15 years or longer, depending on the hematologic type of leukemia and age at irradiation (9,21,23,25). In atomic bomb survivors, patients treated with spinal irradiation for ankylosing spondylitis, and women treated with pelvic irradiation for menorrhagia, the overall excess of all forms of leukemia (other than the chronic lymphocytic form) averaged over the first 25 years after irradiation has approximated 1 to 3 cases per 10,000 persons per year per sievert to the bone marrow (2,9,16). A comparable excess has been observed in occupationally exposed workers, based on combined analyses of the data from several different cohorts (26). The data do not suffice to define the shape of the dose-incidence curve unambiguously, but they appear to be most consistent with a linear-quadratic dose-incidence relationship (2,9,23).

Leukemia has also been observed to be increased in frequency in British and American children who were exposed prenatally during radiographic examination of

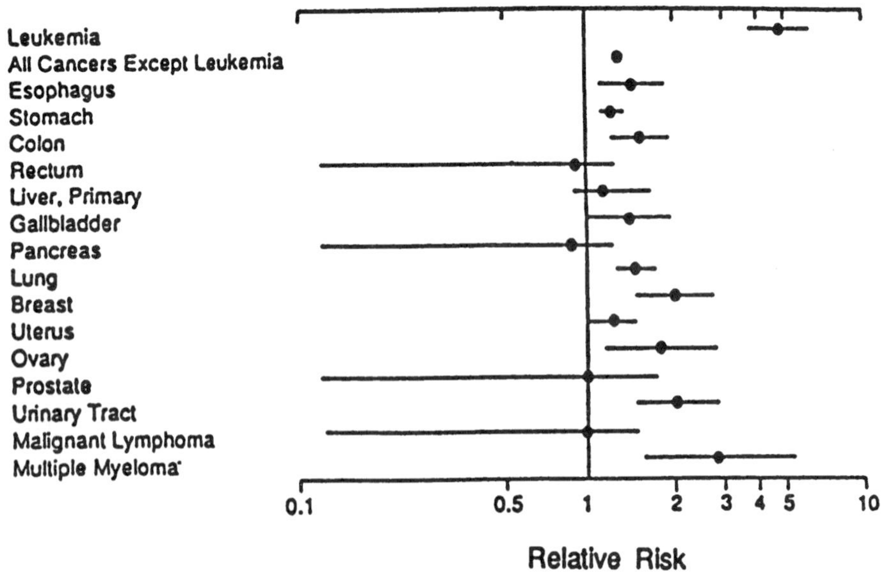


FIG. 5. Relative risk of different cancers in atomic bomb survivors at 1 Gy exposure (shielded kerma), 1950–1985, with 90% confident intervals. (Modified from ref. 21.)

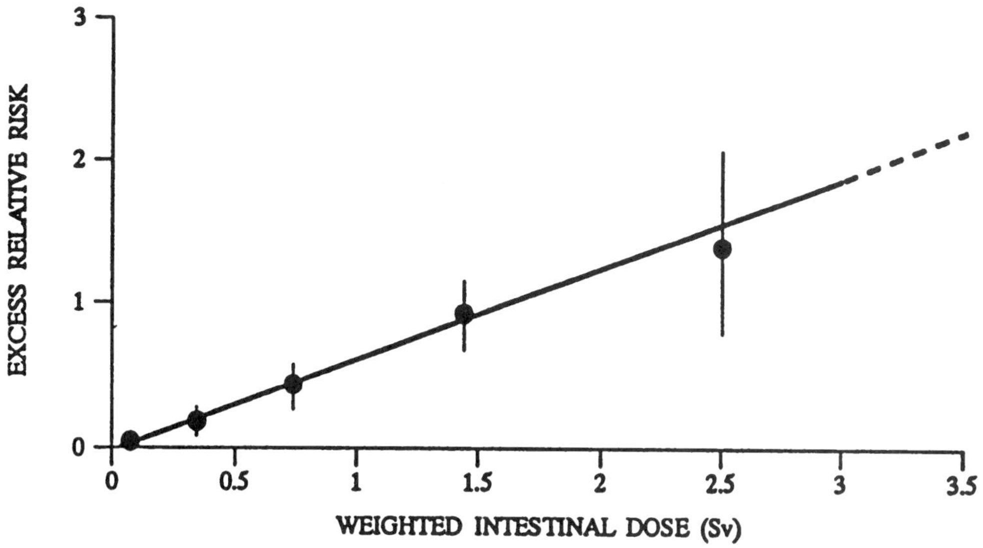


**FIG. 6.** Dose-response relationship for total incidence of cancer, all types excluding leukemia, in atomic bomb survivors, 1958–1987. (From ref. 25, based on data from ref. 24.)

their mothers, the excess corresponding roughly to a 5% increase in the relative risk of childhood leukemia per millisievert, or to approximately 25 cases per 10,000 children at risk per sievert per year during the first 10 years of life (2,9). Although no such increase was evident in Japanese children exposed prenatally to atomic bomb radiation, the lack of an excess in this population is not incompatible with the increase noted above, in view of the limited numbers of children in question (9,16,25).

The possibility that the excesses of leukemias and lymphomas in children residing in the vicinity of some of the nuclear plants in the United Kingdom may have been caused by heritable oncogenic effects resulting from the occupational irradiation of their fathers has been suggested by a case-control study (27), but arguing against this hypothesis are (a) the lack of any comparable excess in larger numbers of children born outside of Seascale, England, to fathers who had received similar or even larger doses of occupational radiation at the same facility; (b) the lack of similar excesses in French, Canadian, or Scottish children born to fathers with comparable occupational exposures; (c) the lack of an excess in the children of atomic bomb survivors; and (d) the lack of excesses in U.S. counties containing nuclear plants (28).

### *Cancer of the Breast*

A dose-dependent increase in the incidence of cancer of the breast has been observed in women who survived atomic bomb irradiation, women who were given radiation therapy to the breast for acute postpartum mastitis or other benign diseases, women who were examined repeatedly by fluoroscopy of the chest during treatment for pulmonary tuberculosis with artificial pneumothorax, and women who worked as radium dial painters (2,9,16). In all four groups of women, the incidence of carcinoma of the breast was observed to become elevated within 5 to 10 years after irradiation, depending on age at exposure, and to remain elevated for the duration of follow-up. Averaged over all ages, the magnitude of the dose-dependent excess is similar in each group, in spite of marked differences among the groups in the rapidity with which the total doses were received (9). The observation of comparably large carcinogenic effects in the women who accumulated their doses in many small and widely separated increments implies that successive exposures are additive in their cancer-causing effects on the breast and that there may be little or no threshold for such effects (2,9,29).

Susceptibility appears to be highest in childhood and to decrease markedly with age at the time of irradiation, little if any cancer excess being detectable in women exposed after age 40 (30). Furthermore, in atomic bomb survivors of any given cohort whose tumors appeared relatively early, the excess was larger than in those whose tumors appeared later, suggesting that the former may have constituted a genetically susceptible subgroup (31). In women irradiated during infancy or childhood, the excess did not become evident until 30 to 40 years later, implying that expression of the carcinogenic effects of radiation on the breast depended on their being promoted by age-related hormonal stimulation (30).

### *Thyroid Gland*

Tumors of the thyroid gland have been observed to be increased in frequency in atomic bomb survivors, patients given radiation therapy to the neck in infancy for thymic enlargement and other nonneoplastic conditions, patients given x-ray therapy to the scalp in childhood for treatment of tinea capitis, Marshall islanders exposed to radioactive fallout from a weapons test in 1954, children exposed to fallout from nuclear weapons detonated at the Nevada test site, children exposed to radioactivity released in the Chernobyl accident, and other populations exposed to external irradiation of the thyroid (2,9,25,32). The induced neoplasms have consisted chiefly of papillary adenomas and carcinomas, have caused a relatively low rate of mortality, and have been preceded by latent periods of 10 to 25 years or longer. Susceptibility to the induction of such tumors appears to be appreciably higher in females than in males, and to be markedly higher in childhood than in adult life (2,9,25).

In persons who received x-ray therapy to the neck in infancy, the incidence of thyroid cancer has been observed to be increased after a dose as low as 65 mSv, and the observed dose-incidence relationship appears to be consistent with a linear, nonthreshold function, corresponding to an excess of approximately 4 cancers per 10,000 person-yr-Sv (2,9,25). No excess has been evident, however, in patients who have received as much as 0.5 Gy to the thyroid from iodine-131 administered for diagnostic purposes, implying that such radiation is substantially less carcinogenic to the thyroid than external x- or gamma-radiation, possibly because of spatial and temporal differences in the distribution of the radiation within the gland (2,25).

### Effects of Prenatal Irradiation on Growth and Development

During critical stages of organogenesis, as little as 0.25 Sv has been observed to cause malformations of many types in experimental animals, and such effects have been reported after intensive prenatal irradiation in human infants, as well (2,33). In atomic bomb survivors who were irradiated in utero, for example, a dose-dependent increase in the prevalence of severe mental retardation (Fig. 7) and dose-dependent decreases in IQ scores and scholastic performance (2 9,33) were experienced by those who were exposed between the 8th and 15th week (and to a lesser extent between the 16th and 25th week) after conception.

#### *Risks from Low-Level Irradiation*

Although the existing evidence does not suffice to define precisely the dose-incidence relationship for the carcinogenic effects of low-level radiation or to exclude the possible existence of a threshold for such effects at low doses, the aggregate epidemiologic and experimental

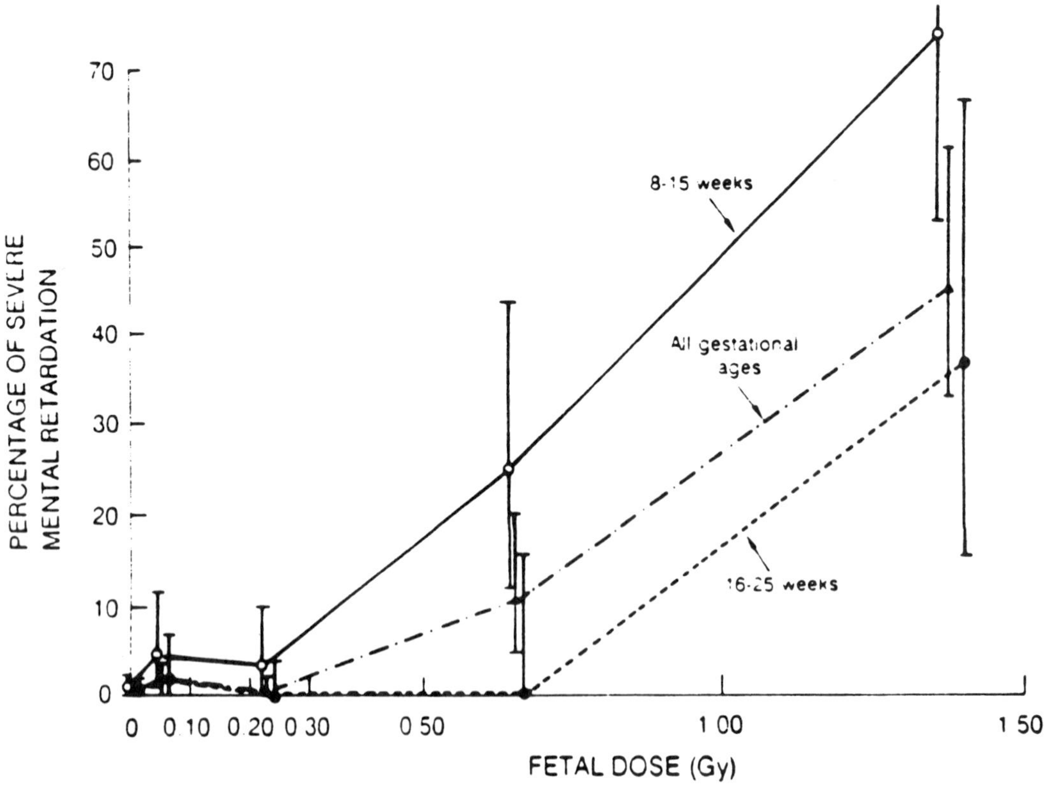


**FIG. 7.** The frequency of severe mental retardation in relation to radiation dose in prenatally irradiated atomic bomb survivors. (Reprinted with permission from ref. 42.)

data argue against the likelihood of a threshold for every type of cancer. Attempts to estimate the risks of radiation-induced cancers from low doses have, therefore, generally been based on the conservative assumption that the overall incidence of cancer varies as a linear, nonthreshold function of the dose (2,7,9,16,25).

Extrapolations based on this assumption have yielded a range of risk estimates for cancers of different organs (Table 6), from which it has been inferred that less than 3% of all cancers in the general population are attributable to natural background radiation, although a larger percentage—perhaps up to 10%—of lung cancers may be attributable to inhalation of naturally occurring radon (9,25). In radiation workers, moreover, the risk of leukemia appears to increase with the cumulative dose in a manner consistent with the estimate tabulated (26), as noted above, even though the lifetime risk of cancer attributable to occupational irradiation is estimated to average less than 1% of the natural baseline risk (9).

The probability that a given cancer arising in a previously irradiated person was caused by the radiation in question cannot be determined with certainty; however, the probability may be assumed to increase with the radiation dose that was received, all other things being equal. Hence, given sufficient knowledge of the dose, when it was received, and the extent to which other risk factors may also have contributed, it is possible to arrive at a crude estimate of the probability that the cancer resulted from the exposure in question. The rationale and methodology for making this type of estimate was set forth in a report mandated by the U.S. Congress for the purpose of aiding in the adjudication of compensation cases arising out of the exposure of U.S. citizens to nuclear weapons fallout from the Nevada test site (35).

**TABLE 6.** *Estimated lifetime risks of cancer attributable to 0.1 Sv (10 rem) rapid irradiation*

| Type or site of cancer | Excess cancer deaths per 100,000 (No.) | (%)[a] |
|---|---|---|
| Stomach | 110 | 18 |
| Lung | 85 | 3 |
| Colon | 85 | 5 |
| Leukemia (excl. CLL) | 50 | 10 |
| Urinary bladder | 30 | 5 |
| Esophagus | 30 | 10 |
| Breast | 20 | 1 |
| Liver | 15 | 8 |
| Gonads | 10 | 2 |
| Thyroid | 8 | 8 |
| Osteosarcoma | 5 | 5 |
| Skin | 2 | 2 |
| Remainder | 50 | 1 |
| Total | 500 | 2 |

[a]Percentage of the spontaneous, baseline rate in the general population.
CLL, chronic lymphocytic leukemia.
Modified from refs. 7 and 34.

## MANAGEMENT AND PREVENTION OF RADIATION INJURY

### Radiation Protection

Inasmuch as the primary goal of occupational and environmental medicine is the prevention of avoidable injury, radiation protection programs strive to minimize unnecessary exposure to ionizing radiation. Pursuit of this goal is guided by two major principles, the principle of justification and the principle of optimization. The principle of justification holds that any amount of radiation, no matter how small, carries some risk of harm, and hence that no exposure can be justified unless it is accompanied by a commensurate benefit, either to the person(s) directly exposed or to society as a whole. The principle of optimization holds that the dose to any exposed person(s) should be kept as low as reasonably achievable (ALARA), all social and economic costs considered (7).

To protect against excessive radiation exposure, operating limits have been placed on the doses that may be delivered to radiation workers and members of the public. Such exposure limits, or maximum permissible doses, have been reduced repeatedly over the past 60 years, apace with evolution of knowledge of the risks of low-level irradiation. The dose limits now recommended (Table 7) are considered sufficiently restrictive to protect completely against radiation-induced impairment of organ function (e.g., depression of hematopoiesis, impairment of fertility, radiation cataract), even in the most sensitive members of the population (7,13,36). The limits are not assumed, however, to prevent all mutagenic and carcinogenic effects of radiation (since thresholds for these effects may not exist), but they are intended to restrict the risks of such effects to levels that are acceptably low (7,36).

Achievement of the goal of minimizing unnecessary radiation exposure of workers and other persons requires careful design of the workplace, equipment, and work procedures; thorough training and supervision of workers; and implementation of an appropriate radiation protection program, including systematic health physics oversight and monitoring.

Increasing attention is now being given to limitation of the doses involved in medicine and dentistry, because the average dose to the population from the medical and dental uses of radiation is now an appreciable fraction of that which is received from natural sources (see Table 2). Methods for reducing such doses include reducing the number of radiographs per patient; limiting the size of the field exposed; reducing the duration and intensity of exposure per radiograph; using radiography in preference

**TABLE 7.** *Recommended limits for exposure to ionizing radiation*[a]

| Type of exposure[b] | Maximum permissible dose (mSv) |
|---|---|
| A. Occupational exposures | |
| 1. For protection against stochastic effects | |
| a. Annual (effective dose) | 50 |
| b. Cumulative (effective dose) | Age × 10 |
| 2. For protection against nonstochastic effects in individual organs | |
| a. Lens of the eye (annual effective dose) | 150 |
| b. All other organs (annual effective dose) | 500 |
| 3. Planned special exposure (effective dose) | 100 |
| 4. Emergency exposure | [c] |
| B. Public exposures | |
| 1. Continuous or frequent exposure (effective dose/year) | 1 |
| 2. Infrequent exposure (effective dose/year) | 5 |
| 3. Remedial action recommended when: | |
| a. Effective dose | >5 |
| b. Exposure to radon and its decay products | >0.007 $Jhm^{-1}$ |
| C. Education and training exposures[b] | |
| 1. Effective dose (annual) | 1 |
| 2. Equivalent dose (lens of eye, skin, extremities) (annual) | 50 |
| D. Exposure of the embryo-fetus | |
| 1. Total equivalent dose | 5 |
| 2. Equivalent dose in any one month | 0.5 |

[a]Including natural background radiation exclusive of that from internally deposited radionuclides.
[b]Sum of internal and external exposures, excluding medical irradiation.
[c]Effective dose in any one planned event, or cumulative effective dose in planned special exposures over a working lifetime should not exceed 100 mSv (10 rem). Short-term exposure to more than 100 mSv (10 rem) is justified only in life-saving, emergency situations.
(From ref. 36.)

to fluoroscopy whenever practicable; shielding tissues outside the field, especially the gonads or the fetus; proper selection, installation, calibration, and operation of apparatus; and proper training of physicians and dentists in requesting radiologic examinations, and of staff engaged in performing them. In the use of radiographic techniques for mass screening of populations, assessment of the risk-benefit relationship is particularly important, since only diseased persons benefit directly while the risks are distributed over all screenees (37).

### Radiation Accidents

In spite of elaborate precautions, some 285 nuclear reactor accidents (excluding the Chernobyl accident) were reported between 1945 and 1987 in various countries, causing more than 1,350 persons to be irradiated, 33 of whom were injured fatally (38). The Chernobyl accident itself, owing to inadequate containment of the reactor and other design and operating flaws, released enough radioactivity to necessitate the evacuation of thousands of people and farm animals from the surrounding area, and it caused radiation sickness and burns in more than 200 emergency personnel and firefighters, injuring 31 fatally (16). Accidents involving medical and industrial gamma ray sources, which have been more numerous than reactor accidents, also have also resulted in injuries and loss of life. In 1987, for example, the improper disposal of a cesium-137 radiotherapy source in Goiania, Brazil, led to the irradiation of dozens of unsuspecting victims, four of whom were injured fatally as a result (39).

From the foregoing, it follows that in any situation where people may be irradiated accidentally, plans for coping with such an accident should be in place. The plans should include delineation of lines of authority for managing an accident, knowledge of the local medical facilities capable of evaluating and treating radiation accident victims, plans for handling and transporting radioactive victims, and some instruction on the hazards of radiation for those employed at the site (40,41).

In managing the radiation accident victim, sound medical judgment should come first. Thus, even victims who are heavily irradiated or contaminated should be evaluated for other forms of injury, such as burns, mechanical trauma, or smoke inhalation. In addition, persons who handle or examine a potentially contaminated victim should wear gloves, mask, and other protective clothing, to guard against self-contamination with radioactivity. Detailed records should be kept of all examinations, measurements, procedures, findings, personnel, and times involved.

If radioactive contamination is detected, the victim should be isolated and the contaminated area sealed off as soon as possible. Contaminated clothing should be removed promptly, isolated in a plastic bag, and labeled to denote radioactivity. Contaminated parts of the body should be isolated with paper or plastic, monitored for radioactivity, rinsed thoroughly, and monitored again. During the rinsing, care should be taken to avoid abrading contaminated skin, and the rinse water should be isolated as radioactive waste. If radioactive material may have been inhaled, the victim should rinse the oral and nasal cavities with water, taking care not to inhale or swallow more radioactivity in the process, and the rinse water and any other secretions should be collected in plastic bags, labeled, and isolated for subsequent examination.

The management of radiation injuries themselves depends on the severity of the injuries and the organs that are affected (see Table 5). Because the signs and symptoms of radiation injury are nonspecific, pertinent information from the victim's exposure record, medical history, physical examination, and laboratory data must be synthesized and integrated. Inasmuch as the nature and severity of injury depend inevitably on the size and anatomic distribution of the radiation dose, evaluation of the latter is paramount. In the absence of physical dosimetry, cytogenetic analysis of circulating lymphocytes can serve as a useful biologic dosimeter (18).

## REFERENCES


1. Upton AC. Historical perspective on radiation carcinogenesis. In: Upton AC, Albert RE, Burns FJ, Shore RE, eds. *Radiation carcinogenesis.* New York: Elsevier Science, 1986;1–10.
2. Mettler FA Jr, Upton AC. *Medical effects of ionizing radiation.* New York: WB Saunders, 1995.
3. Shapiro J. *Radiation protection:* a guide for scientists and physicians, 3rd ed. Cambridge, MA: Harvard University Press, 1990.
4. International Commission on Radiation Units and Measurements (ICRU). *The quality factor in radiation protection.* Report of a Joint Task Group of the ICRP and the ICRU. ICRU report 40. Bethesda, MD: International Commission on Radiation Units and Measurements, 1986.
5. International Commission on Radiological Protection (ICRP). *Limits for intakes of radionuclides by workers.* Publication 30. Oxford: Pergamon Press, 1979.
6. International Commission on Radiation Units and Measurements (ICRU). *Radiation quantities and units.* Report 33. Bethesda, MD: ICRU, 1980.
7. International Commission on Radiological Protection. *1990 recommendations of the International Commission on Radiological Protection.* ICRP publication 60. Ann. ICRP 21., No. 1–3. Oxford: Pergamon Press, 1991.
8. National Council on Radiation Protection and Measurement (NCRP). *Ionizing radiation exposure of the population of the United States.* Report 93. Bethesda, MD: NCRP, 1987.
9. National Academy of Sciences Advisory Committee on the Biological Effects of Ionizing Radiation. *The effects on populations of exposure to low levels of ionizing radiation* (BEIR V). Washington, DC: National Academy of Sciences, 1990.
10. Kahn K, Ryan K, Sabo A, Boyce P. Ionizing radiation. In: Levy BS, Wegman DH, eds. *Occupational health.* Boston: Little, Brown, 1983; 189–206.
11. Interagency Task Force on the Health Effects of Ionizing Radiation. *Report of the work group on science.* Washington, DC: U.S. Department of Health, Education, and Welfare, 1979.
12. National Council on Radiation Protection and Measurement (NCRP). *Exposure of the U.S. population from occupational radiation.* Report 101. Bethesda. MD: NCRP, 1989.
13. International Commission on Radiological Protection (ICRP). *Nonstochastic effects of ionizing radiation.* Publication 41. Annals of the ICRP, vol 14(3). Oxford: Pergamon Press, 1984.
14. Ward JF. Radiation Mutagenesis: the initial DNA lesions responsible. *Radiat Res* 1995;142:362–368.
15. Ward JF. DNA damage produced by ionizing radiation in mammalian cells: identities, mechanisms of formation and reparability. *Prog Nucleic Acids Res Mol Biol* 1988;35:96–128.
16. United Nations Scientific Committee on the Effects of Atomic Radiation (UNSCEAR). *Sources, effects and risks of ionizing radiation.* Report to the General Assembly, with annexes. New York: United Nations, 1988.
17. Lloyd DC, Purrott RJ. Chromosome aberration analysis in radiological protection dosimetry. *Radiat Protect Dosim* 1981;1:19–28.
18. International Atomic Energy Agency (IAEA). *Biological dosimetry:* chromosomal aberration analysis for dose assessment. Technical report no. 260. Vienna, IAEA, 1986.
19. United Nations Scientific Committee on the Effects of Atomic Radiation (UNSCEAR). *Ionizing radiation:* sources and biological effects. Report to the General Assembly, with annexes. New York: United Nations, 1982.
20. Hall EJ. *Radiobiology for the radiologist,* 4th ed. Philadelphia: JB Lippincott, 1994.
21. Shimizu Y, Kato H, Schull WJ. Studies of the mortality of A-bomb survivors. 9. Mortality 1950–1985: Part 2. Cancer mortality based on the recently revised doses (DS 86). *Radiat Res* 1990;121:120–141.
22. Trott K, Streffer C. Occupational radiation carcinogenesis. In: Schrerer E, Streffer C, Trott K, eds. *Occupational risks.* New York: Springer-Verlag, 1990;61–74.
23. Pierce DA, Shimizu Y, Preston DL, Vaeth M, Mabuchi K. Studies of the mortality of atomic bomb survivors. Report 12, part 1. Cancer: 1950–1990. *Radiat Res* 1996;146:1–27.
24. Thompson DE, Mabuchi K, Ron E, et al. Cancer incidence in atomic bomb survivors. Part II: solid tumors 1958–87. *Radiat Res* 1994;137: S17–S67.
25. United Nations Scientific Committee on the Effects of Atomic Radiation (UNSCEAR). *Sources and effects of ionizing radiation.* UNSCEAR 1994 Report to the General Assembly, with annexes. New York: United Nations, 1994.
26. Cardis E, Gilbert ES, Carpenter L, et al. Effects of low doses and low dose rates of external ionizing radiation: cancer mortality among nuclear industry workers in three countries. *Radiat Res* 1995;142:117–132.
27. Gardner MJ, Hall A, Snee MP, Downes S, Powell CA, Terell JD. Results of case-control study of leukemia and lymphoma among young people near Sellafield nuclear plant in West Cumbria. *Br Med J* 1990;300: 423–429.
28. Wakeford R. The risk of childhood cancer from intrauterine and preconceptional exposure to ionizing radiation. *Environ Health Perspect* 1995;103:1018–1025.
29. Howe GR, McLaughlin J. Breast cancer mortality between 1950 and 1987 after exposure to fractionated moderate-dose-rate ionizing radiation in the Canadian fluoroscopy cohort study and a comparison with breast cancer mortality in the atomic bomb survivors study. *Radiat Res* 1996;145:694–707.
30. Tokunaga M, Land C, Tukapa S, Nishimori I, Soda M, Akiba S. Incidence of female breast cancer in atomic bomb survivors. 1950–1985. *Radiat Res* 1994;138:209–223.
31. Tokunaga M, Land C, Aoki Y, et al. Proliferative and non-proliferative breast disease in atomic bomb survivors. *Cancer* 1993;72:1657–1665.
32. Kreisel W. International program on the health effects of the Chernobyl accident. *Stem Cells* 1995;suppl 1:33–39.
33. United Nations Scientific Committee on the Effects of Atomic Radiation (UNSCEAR). *Genetic and somatic effects of ionizing radiation.* Report to the General Assembly, with Annexes. New York: United Nations, 1986.
34. Puskin JS, Nelson CB. Estimates of radiogenic cancer risks. *Health Phys* 1995;69:3–101.
35. Rall JE, Beebe GW, Hoel DG, et al. *Report of the National Institutes of Health Working Group to Develop Radioepidemiological Tables.* NIH publication 85–2478. Washington, DC: U.S. Government Printing Office, 1985.

36. National Council on Radiation Protection and Measurements (NCRP). *Limitation of exposure to ionizing radiation.* Report No. 116. Bethesda, MD: NCRP, 1993.
37. National Council on Radiation Protection and Measurement (NCRP). *Mammography—a user's guide.* Report No. 85. Washington, DC: NCRP, 1986.
38. Lushbaugh CC, Fry SA, Ricks RC. Nuclear reactor accidents: preparedness and consequences. *Br J Radiol* 1987;60:1159–1183.
39. United Nations Scientific Committee on the Effects of Atomic Radiation (UNSCEAR). *Sources and effects of ionizing radiation.* Report to the General Assembly, with annexes. New York: United Nations, 1993.
40. Huber CF, Fry S. *The medical basis for radiation accident preparedness.* New York: Elsevier/North Holland, 1980.
41. *What the general practitioner (MD) should know about medical handling of overexposed individuals.* IAEA-TECDOC-366. Vienna: International Atomic Energy Agency, 1986.
42. National Academy of Sciences. *Health effects of exposure to low levels of ionizing radiation.* Washington, DC: National Academy Press, 1990.

*Environmental and Occupational Medicine, Third Edition,* edited by William N. Rom.
Lippincott–Raven Publishers, Philadelphia © 1998.

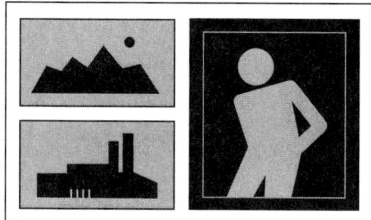

CHAPTER 98

# Diseases of Uranium Miners and Other Underground Miners Exposed to Radon

Jonathan M. Samet and Douglas W. Mapel

Malignant respiratory disease in underground miners was first described in metal ore miners in the Central European region of Schneeberg (1). For centuries, the incidence of fatal pulmonary disease among miners in the Erz mountains was high; this problem was chronicled as early as the 1500s by Agricola. In the late 19th century, Harting and Hesse (1) showed that these miners developed respiratory tract malignancy, and in 1913 Arnstein (2) reported that the malignancy was primary cancer of the lung. In 1929, underground miners at Joachimsthal, Czechoslovakia—the current Czechoslovakian side of the Erz mountains—were found to have similar lung cancer problems (3). High concentrations of radon were measured in both locations and radon was considered even then by some researchers to be a cause of lung cancer in the miners, although it was not accepted universally (4).

During the late 1940s and early 1950s, uranium mining burgeoned throughout the world as ore was mined for the production of nuclear weapons, and later for the growing nuclear power industry. In the late 1940s, the United States Public Health Service implemented a study of uranium miners in the Colorado Plateau region, the principal site of uranium mining in the country. By the late 1950s, that study had demonstrated excess rates of lung cancer in those miners (5). An excessive rate of lung cancer was subsequently demonstrated in many other groups of underground miners exposed to radon, including uranium miners and miners of other materials in radon-contaminated mines (5).

As the biologic basis of respiratory carcinogenesis was understood and the lung dosimetry of radon and its short-lived progeny was described, it was recognized that alpha-particle emissions from inhaled radon progeny, not from radon itself, caused lung cancer in radon-exposed miners. Radon decays with a half-life of 3.82 days into a series of solid, short-lived radioisotopes that collectively are referred to as radon daughters, radon progeny, or radon decay products (Fig. 1). Two of those decay products, polonium-218 and polonium-214, emit alpha particles, which are high-energy and high-mass particles consisting of two protons and two neutrons that are very damaging to tissue. When the alpha emissions take place within the lung as inhaled radon progeny decay, the DNA of cells lining the airways may be damaged and lung cancer may ultimately result. Animal studies demonstrated that radon alone through its progeny could induce cancer in the respiratory tract (5). Thus, as evidence emerged supporting the biologic plausibility of radon as a respiratory tract carcinogen and the scope of the epidemiologic data expanded, radon was confirmed as an occupational carcinogen and regulations to limit exposure were implemented in many countries.

In the United States, most underground uranium mines had shut down by the late 1980s, but occupational exposure to radon progeny remains a concern for many other types of underground miners and other underground workers. Worldwide, uranium mining continues with documented production in Canada, Australia, South

J. M. Samet: Department of Epidemiology, The Johns Hopkins University School of Hygiene and Public Health, Baltimore, Maryland 21205.
D. W. Mapel: Department of Epidemiology and Cancer Control, University of New Mexico, Albuquerque, New Mexico 87131-5306.

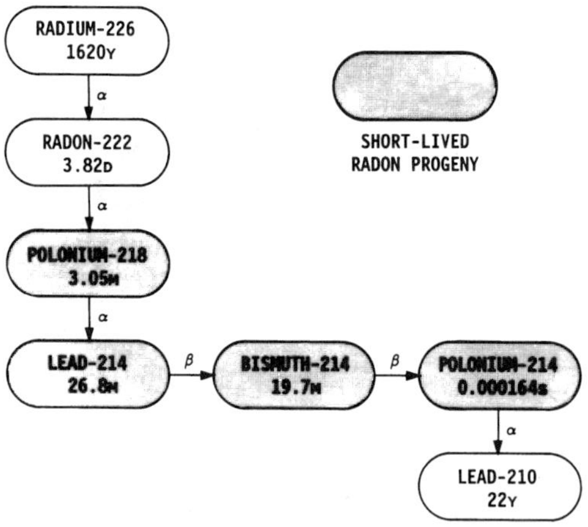


**FIG. 1.** Radon daughter decay chart.

Africa, and other African countries (6). Thus, at the close of the 20th century, radon in underground mines remains a significant occupational hazard.

We are also becoming aware of the large numbers of persons who mined uranium both in Western countries and in the former Soviet bloc, during an era when exposures were extremely high (7). These former miners have now reached the age range when lung cancer rates are extremely high, and for a substantial proportion it will be their cause of death. In the United States, former miners who worked during the years that uranium was mined for the Atomic Energy Commission are compensated by the Radiation Exposure Compensation Act, passed in 1990, which offers an apology to these former miners. The Presidential Commission on Radiation Experiments found the exposures received by the miners to have been unethically high and questioned conducting an epidemiologic study when risks could be lowered by ventilation (8).

Radon progeny have also emerged as a significant cause of lung cancer for the general population. An inert gas, radon occurs naturally as a decay product of radium-226, the fifth daughter of uranium-238. Because both radium-226 and uranium-238 are present in most soils and rocks, radon is continually generated in the earth, with some atoms entering the surrounding air or water. Thus, radon is ubiquitous in outdoor and indoor air. As information on air quality in indoor environments accumulated during the 1970s and 1980s, it became clear that radon and its decay products are invariably present in indoor environments and in some dwellings may reach unacceptably high concentrations, equivalent to those in mines. In fact, radon is the greatest source of radiation exposure in the United States from natural background radiation (9). An extensive body of literature now addresses the risks of indoor radon, a topic covered elsewhere in this volume. The epidemiologic studies of uranium and other miners have been the principal basis for estimating the risks of indoor radon, and the epidemiologic data have been extensively analyzed to develop risk models.

## EXPOSURE TO RADON AND THE RESPIRATORY DOSIMETRY OF RADON PROGENY

For historic reasons, the concentration of radon progeny in underground mines is generally expressed in working levels (WLs): 1 WL is any combination of radon progeny in 1 L of air that ultimately releases $1.3 \times 10^5$ MeV of alpha energy during decay (10). Concentrations of radon are also frequently expressed as picocuries per liter (pCi/L), a unit for the rate of decay, and 200 pCi/L is equivalent to 1 WL at 50% equilibrium between radon and its progeny. Exposure to 1 WL for 170 hours equals 1 working level month (WLM) of exposure, a unit developed to describe exposure sustained by miners during the average number of hours spent underground.

The relationship between exposure to radon progeny, measured as WLM, and dose to target cells, measured as rem or sieverts, in the respiratory tract is extremely complex and depends on both biologic and nonbiologic factors (11,12). Factors that influence the dosimetry of radon progeny include the physical characteristics of the inhaled air, the amount of air inhaled, breathing patterns, and the biologic characteristics of the lung (13) (Table 1).

Radon is an inert gas, but its progeny are solid, charged particles. While most of the progeny attach to larger aerosols immediately after forming, a variable proportion of the activity remains in a smaller size mode, historically referred to as the "unattached fraction." The unattached decay products, while not attached to larger particles, appear to form aggregates; water molecules and other chemical species may be part of the clusters (14). The fraction of unattached radon progeny in inhaled air is an important determinant of the dose received by target cells at a particular concentration in inhaled air; as the unattached fraction increases, the dose also increases because of the efficient deposition of the unattached progeny in the larger airways. The size distribution of particles in the inhaled air also affects the dose to the airways because particles of different sizes deposit preferentially in different generations of airways.

The amount of inhaled radon decay products varies directly with the minute ventilation (i.e., the total volume of air inhaled each minute). However, the deposition of radon progeny within the lung does not depend simply on the minute ventilation; it varies with the flow rate in each airway generation, which depends on both tidal volume and breathing frequency. The proportions of mouth and of nose breathing also influence the relationship between exposure and dose. With nasal breathing, a large proportion of the unattached radon progeny is deposited in the nose, whereas oral deposition of unattached progeny is less efficient.

**TABLE 1.** *Physical and biologic factors influencing dose to target cells in respiratory tract from radon exposure*

| Physical factors | Biologic factors |
|---|---|
| Fraction of radon daughters unattached to particles | Tidal volume and respiratory frequency |
| Aerosol size distribution | Partitioning of breathing between the oral and nasal routes |
| Equilibrium of radon with its progeny | Bronchial morphometry |
| | Mucociliary clearance rate |
| | Thickness of mucus |
| | Location of target cells |

From ref. 13.

Computer models have been developed to (1) describe the relation between exposure to radon progeny and the dose of alpha radiation to target tissues, and (2) assess the consequences on that relation of the physical and biologic factors listed in Table 1. Those complex models generally incorporate biologic factors, including geometry of airways, deposition, ventilation pattern, mucociliary clearance, and location of the target cells, as well as physical factors, including the unattached fraction and the aerosol size distribution (11,12). With the use of such models, factors for converting WLM to an absorbed radiation dose can be calculated, but the range of published dose-conversion factors is wide (12). These models have proved useful for comparing exposure-dose relations for exposures in homes and in mines as risk relations observed in miners are extended to the population generally.

## EPIDEMIOLOGIC STUDIES OF RADON AND LUNG CANCER IN MINERS

The causal association between exposure to radon progeny and lung cancer has been firmly established through epidemiologic investigations of underground miners. Studies of mining populations from around the world have found that the risk of developing lung cancer increases in direct proportion to the cumulative exposure to radon progeny. These studies have also provided data on factors that modify the exposure-response relationship, which include smoking, the intensity of radon exposure, and the time since last exposure. The full impact of the exposure to radon progeny on these mining cohorts is yet to be seen, since not all miners have been followed for their full life span.

The risk of lung cancer among miners exposed to radon progeny should be considered in the context of the extensive literature on lung cancer in the general population. Lung cancer, once considered a rare disease, has become the leading cause of cancer death in the United States and in many other developed countries (15). Most lung cancers are caused by cigarette smoking, and only 5% to 10% of the total occur in lifelong nonsmokers (16). For cigarette smokers, the risk of developing lung cancer increases with the number of cigarettes smoked daily and with the number of years of smoking. When cigarette smoking is combined with exposure to other pulmonary carcinogens such as radon progeny, the two agents may interact to produce synergistically a risk for developing lung cancer that is much greater than the sum of the risks from the exposures individually. Because cigarette smoking is the major cause of lung cancer, investigations of the relationship between exposure to radon progeny and lung cancer have addressed the possible confounding and modifying effects of smoking to the extent possible with the limited data available on smoking.

The World Health Organization classification system divides lung cancer into four basic histologic types: adenocarcinoma, squamous cell carcinoma, small-cell carcinoma, and large-cell carcinoma (17). Among nonsmokers, adenocarcinoma accounts for up to 75% of the total, while small-cell carcinoma is very rare (18). Among smokers, the risk for developing any of the four histologic types is increased, although squamous cell carcinoma and small-cell carcinoma have the strongest association with tobacco use.

### Studies of Miners

The relationship between radon progeny and lung cancer has been investigated in about 20 mining populations, including not only uranium miners but miners of other types of ores who were exposed to radon either from the ore itself or from radon dissolved in mine water. These studies have shown that the risk for lung cancer increases proportionally with the cumulative exposure to radon progeny. Most of these have been cohort studies involving follow-up of miners from a particular mine or mining region, although some case-control studies have also been reported. Of the cohort studies, 11 have had sufficient data on individual radon exposure and sufficient incidences of lung cancer deaths to allow more detailed analysis of the dose-response relationship (Table 2). These studies were included in a pooled analysis reported recently by Lubin et al. (19,20). Although the studies differ somewhat in the nature of the mining populations and in their methods, and not all include detailed smoking histories from all miners, the crude estimates of excess relative risk (ERR) per WLM of radon progeny exposure have been remarkably consistent.

**TABLE 2.** *Selected studies of exposure to radon progeny and lung cancer in underground miners*

| Location and type of mining | Number of miners | Lung cancer deaths | SMR (95% CI) | ERR/WLM (95% CI) |
|---|---|---|---|---|
| Colorado Plateau, USA uranium (23,46) | 4,146 | 155 | 4.8 (4.1–5.7) in non-Hispanic whites, 4.2 (2.1–7.1) in Native Americans | 0.42% (0.3–0.7) |
| New Mexico, USA uranium (43) | 3,469 | 68 | 4.0 (3.1–5.1) | 1.72% (0.6–6.7) |
| Ontario, Canada uranium (59) | 21,346 | 152 | 2.3 (1.9–2.6) | 0.89% (0.5–1.5) |
| Port Radium, Canada uranium (60) | 2,103 | 57 | 2.3 (1.7–2.9) | 0.19% (0.1–0.6) |
| Beaverlodge, Canada uranium (60) | 8,487 | 65 | 1.9 (1.5–2.4) | 2.21% (0.9–5.6) |
| Czechoslovakia[a] uranium (35,61) | 4,042 | 574 | 4.7 (4.3–5.1) | 0.34% (0.2–0.6) |
| France uranium (62) | 1,785 | 45 | 2.1 (1.6–2.8) | 0.36% (0.1–1.3) |
| Australia[b] uranium (63) | 931 | 32 | 2.2 (1.5–3.0) | 5.1% (1.0–12.2) |
| Malmberget, Sweden iron (37) | 1,294 | 50 | 3.9 (2.9–5.1) | 0.95% (0.1–4.1) |
| Newfoundland, Canada fluorspar (44) | 1,772 | 113 | 5.3 (4.3–6.3) | 0.76% (0.4–1.3) |
| Yunnan Province,China tin (45) | 17,143 | 981 | Not available | 0.16% (0.1–0.2) |
| Total | 66,518 | 2,292 | 3.6 (3.4–3.8) | 0.49% (0.2–1.0) |

SMR, standardized mortality ratio, or the observed number of lung cancer deaths in the study cohort divided by the expected number of lung cancer deaths determined from state, provincial, or national registries; ERR, excess relative risk per WLM exposure.

[a]Miners who began mining before 1957.

[b]Underground miners with follow-up only.

(From ref. 19.)

Analysis of data from the miner cohorts has also shown that in addition to the cumulative WLM radon exposure, the rate at which the exposure is accrued is a determinant of lung cancer risk. This has been described as the inverse dose-rate effect or protraction enhancement, wherein miners who have incurred their exposure at low concentrations over long periods of time have a higher risk than miners who incurred the same total exposure over shorter periods (20). The inverse dose-rate effect was found in all cohorts listed in Table 2 except for the French uranium miners cohort. It has been suggested that the inverse dose-rate effect may depend on the total cumulative dose, and the available data suggest that this effect may not be significant for those with exposure of less than 50 WLM; however, this observation is limited by the small number of miners with low cumulative radon exposure. The inverse dose-rate effect hypothesis is supported by biologic models of α-particle radiation injury (21), and animal studies have also shown that longer durations of radon exposure at lower concentrations induced more lung cancers than shorter durations at higher concentrations (22).

Together, tobacco smoking and exposure to radon progeny appear to carry a joint risk that is greater than the sum but less than the product of the relative risks of the two independent factors (19,20). Analysis of the smoking-radon interaction has been limited by a lack of information about tobacco use in the epidemiologic studies of miners; only six of the cohorts listed in Table 2 have data on smoking, and a seventh has derived smoking data from a related case-control study. The Colorado Plateau cohort has the most extensive smoking information; data in this cohort are consistent with an intermediate or fully multiplicative smoking-radon interaction, although the data are best fit by a submultiplicative model (23). A nested case-control analysis of the Colorado Plateau data has also found that the relative timing of the two exposures affects risk, with persons who began using cigarettes after starting work in the mines having a significantly higher lung cancer risk than those who were already regular smokers before becoming miners (24). This suggests that smoking may be a promoter of radon-initiated cells, an effect that has been observed in animal studies (25). Data from each of the other cohorts with smoking information fit either additive or multiplicative interactive models (19).

An elevated risk for lung cancer has also been shown in miners who have never smoked cigarettes. A follow-up study of 516 white nonsmoking miners from the Colorado Plateau cohort showed 14 lung cancer deaths with only 1.1 expected, based on the never smokers in the study of U.S. veterans (26). Native-American miners in the Colorado Plateau cohort, mostly Navajos, were almost all nonsmokers or very light smokers; a follow-up study of 757 members of this group identified 34 deaths from lung cancer when only 10.2 were expected [standardized mortality ratio (SMR) 3.3, 95% confidence interval (CI) 2.3–4.6] (27), confirming an earlier case-control study of lung cancer in Navajo men (28). A pooled analysis of the 2,798 never-smoking miners in the 11 miner groups (Table 2) found that the estimated ERR/WLM for nonsmokers (0.0103, 95% CI 0.002–0.057) was almost three times that of smokers (0.0034, 95% CI 0.001–0.015), which is consistent with the submultiplicative interaction between smoking and radon in the full data set (19).

The majority of the studies in Table 2 have shown that the risk for developing lung cancer after exposure to radon decreases as time since exposure increases (19). In the pooled analysis, risks from exposure 25 years or more previously were only about 30% of those received in the last 5 to 14 years. Attained age also modifies the cancer risk, with older miners having a relatively lower risk than younger miners (23). The age at which a miner is first exposed to radon does not appear to have a consistent effect on risk overall, but the data are limited at younger ages. In the Chinese cohort of tin miners, which had some miners who started working during childhood, the ERR/WLM for those who started mining before age 20 was almost three times the ERR/WLM for those who started after age 20.

The histopathology of lung cancer has been described in some of the mining cohorts to determine if radon exposure is associated with a particular histologic type of lung cancer. Although most of these studies have found that miners exposed to radon progeny have an unusually high prevalence of small-cell carcinomas, radon cannot be linked to any particular histologic type because the risk for all types appears to be elevated (5,29). Small-cell and squamous cell carcinomas were found to account for the largest proportion of tumors in the Colorado Plateau and Chinese mining cohorts, although both of these cohorts also showed increased risk for adenocarcinoma. Miners in the Czech cohort had more small-cell, squamous cell, and lung cancers other than adenocarcinomas than expected, while the risk for adenocarcinoma was not increased. Because these studies were in mining populations with high prevalence rates of tobacco use, the effects of radon and of smoking on the distribution of histologic types cannot be readily separated. Two studies of nonsmoking miners have found a higher prevalence of small-cell cancers than would be expected, although the distribution of histologic types overall was not different from that of the general population (27,30). Longitudinal observations of Colorado Plateau miners by Saccomanno and associates (31,32) found that the proportion of small-cell cancer declined from 76% in 1964 to 22% in the late 1970s, while squamous cell carcinomas increased concurrently (31). The majority of the small-cell cancers during the early decades of the Colorado Plateau study were in miners with cumulative exposures above 1,200 WLM. Recent analysis compared the location of lung cancers within the lung in the miners with locations in an age-matched nonmining control group. Squamous cell and small-cell cancers were significantly more likely to be located in the central lung zones in miners, while there was no difference in the distribution of adenocarcinomas in the miners and the controls (32).

The search for signatures of radon-related lung cancer has now moved to the molecular level. Mutational spectra in the tumor suppressor gene p53 and in the oncogene *ras* have been examined using lung cancer tissue from New Mexico uranium miners. Vahakangas et al. (33) reported a pattern of *ras* mutations distinct from that typically seen in smokers. Taylor et al. (34) did not confirm this finding in Colorado Plateau uranium miners but did find an apparent mutational hot spot in the p53 gene.

In addition to radon, underground miners may also be exposed to other agents that are known or suspect causes of lung cancer, including arsenic, diesel exhaust, and silica. Limited data are now available on the effects of arsenic exposure and silica.

Arsenic is an established pulmonary carcinogen that is present in the Czech uranium (35) and the Chinese tin mines (36). The Chinese tin miners were exposed to arsenic in the ore, estimated at 1.34% by weight. Independent effects of radon progeny and arsenic exposure were found and the lung cancer risk from radon progeny was reduced with control for arsenic. The two principal mines where the Czech miners worked, Jachymov and Hormé Slavkov, had differing arsenic content, 0.5% and 0.01%, respectively. The lung cancer risks were approximately twofold higher in miners who had worked in Jachymov, and a cumulative arsenic exposure index, lagged by 5 years, was associated with lung cancer risk (35).

Silica exposure, ubiquitous for underground miners, is a suspected cause of lung cancer, either by acting as a specific carcinogen or through nonspecific effects on the lung, including inflammation and fibrosis. Two studies have found no association between the radiographic presence of silicosis and increased lung cancer risk (37,38). Finkelstein (39) conducted a case-control study nested within a cohort of Ontario uranium miners. Silicosis was associated with increased risk, but only 31 lung cancer cases were included in the analysis.

### Risk Modeling

Risk modeling techniques have been applied to the data from the studies of miners to estimate the excess lifetime risk of lung cancer associated with radon progeny exposure. Those risk models have been used as a basis for projecting the consequences of occupational standards and for estimating the risks of indoor radon. This chapter reviews three of the most recent risk models applicable to the occupational setting: those of the National Council on Radiation Protection (NCRP) and Measurements (12), the Biological Effects of Ionizing Radiation (BEIR) IV, Committee of the National Research Council (5), and the National Institute for Occupational Safety and Health (NIOSH) (40). Other risk models are reviewed in the report of the BEIR IV Committee (5).

The BEIR IV model is now supplanted by a model based on a pooled analysis of data from 11 cohorts of radon-exposed underground miners (Table 2). With the publication of additional studies and the opportunity to work with the team investigating the Czechoslovakian uranium miners, the U.S. National Cancer Institute analyzed data from 11 studies of underground miners (41).

The cohorts included uranium, tin, iron, and fluorspar miners. Various methods were used to estimate exposure to radon progeny; six studies had some data on cigarette smoking, and only a few studies had information on exposures other than radon progeny. The pooled data set included over 2,700 lung cancer deaths among 68,000 miners followed for nearly 1.2 million person-years of observation. A full description of the analysis has been published as a National Cancer Institute Monograph (41).

The data were analyzed with Poisson regression methods comparable to those used by the BEIR IV Committee. Most analyses were based on a linear excess relative risk (ERR) model:

$$RR = 1 + \beta w \quad [1]$$

where RR is relative risk, β is a parameter measuring the unit increase in ERR per unit increase in $w$, and $w$ is cumulative exposure to radon progeny in WLM. As in the BEIR IV analysis, cumulative exposure was also divided into the amounts received during windows defined by time since exposure.

As in the BEIR IV analysis, ERR was linearly related to cumulative exposure to radon progeny. The ERR/WLM varied significantly with other factors; it decreased with attained age, time since exposure, and time after cessation of exposure, but was not affected significantly by age at first exposure. Over a wide range of total cumulative exposures to radon progeny, lung cancer risk increased as exposure rate declined. This finding of an exposure rate effect in the pooled analysis confirms the pattern reported from the Colorado Plateau study (23), and supports the prior hypothesis of an inverse dose-rate effect (42). The inverse exposure rate has potentially significant implications for risk estimation at typical indoor levels using the miner studies.

Information on tobacco use was available from six cohorts. The combined data were consistent with a relationship between additive and multiplicative for the joint effect of smoking and exposure to radon progeny. Over 50,000 person-years, including 64 lung cancer deaths, were accrued by miners who were identified as never smokers. In this group, there was a linear exposure-response trend that was about threefold greater than observed in the smokers.

Two sets of models were preferred by the report's authors; the sets differ in being either categorical or contiguous in the parameterization of the variables. Each includes one model (TSE/age/WL–cat model) incorporating radon progeny exposure during three time since exposure (TSE) windows and variables for effect modification by attained age and exposure rate, and one model (TSE/age/DUR–cat model) similarly incorporating exposure in the same windows and variables for attained age and duration (DUR) of exposure. The selected exposure-windows were 5 to 14 years, 15 to 24 years, and 25 or more years before the attained age; exposures during these windows are $w_{5-14}$, $w_{15-24}$, and $w_{25+}$, respectively. The two categorical models are given below.

TSE/age/WL–cat model:

$$RR = 1 + \beta(w_{5-14} + \theta_2 w_{15-24} + \theta_3 w_{25+}) \times \phi_{age} \times \gamma_{WL} \quad [2]$$

where $\beta = 0.0611$, $\theta_2 = 0.81$, $\theta_3 = 0.40$,

$\phi_{age}$ = 1.00 for age < 55 years
0.65 for 55 ≤ age < 65 years
0.38 for 65 ≤ age < 75 years
0.22 for 75 ≤ age years,

$\gamma_{WL}$ = 1.00 for WL < 0.5
0.51 for 0.5 ≤ WL < 1.0
0.32 for 1.0 ≤ WL < 3.0
0.27 for 3.0 ≤ WL < 5.0
0.13 for 5.0 ≤ WL < 15.0
0.10 for 15.0 ≤ WL.

TSE/age/DUR–cat model:

$$RR = 1 + \beta(w_{5-14} + \theta_2 w_{15-24} + \theta_3 w_{25+}) \times \phi_{age} \times \gamma_{DUR} \quad [3]$$

where $\beta = 0.0039$, $\theta_2 = 0.76$, $\theta_3 = 0.31$,

$\phi_{age}$ = 1.00 for age < 55 years
0.57 for 55 ≤ age < 65 years
0.34 for 65 ≤ age < 75 years
0.28 for 75 ≤ age years,

$\gamma_{DUR}$ = 1.00 for DUR < 5 years
3.17 for 5 ≤ DUR < 15 years
5.27 for 15 ≤ DUR < 25 years
9.08 for 25 ≤ DUR < 35 years
13.6 for 35 ≤ DUR.

The models are similar to the BEIR IV model with an additional term for either rate of exposure or duration of exposure. In applying this model, uncertainty arises as to the most biologically appropriate extrapolation of the exposure rate effect to typical levels of indoor exposure.

## DISEASES OTHER THAN LUNG CANCER

Underground mines may contain a variety of respiratory toxins such as silica dust and diesel fumes; exposure to these toxins may cause pulmonary fibrosis, silicosis, and other nonmalignant respiratory diseases in underground miners. Radon is also thought to be a cause of nonmalignant respiratory disease, based on animal studies showing evidence of pulmonary fibrosis and emphysema in animals exposed to high concentrations of radon (5). A lack of individual exposure data for silica dust in any of the mining cohorts limits the analysis of the relative contributions of silica dust, radon, and other toxins to the nonmalignant respiratory disease. Miners in the Colorado Plateau, New Mexico, Newfoundland, and Czech cohorts have been found to have an increased risk of death from nonmalignant respiratory diseases when compared to the general population (43–45). Miners in the Chinese cohort were also found to have an increased risk of death from nonmalignant respiratory disease with prolonged mining exposure. These studies have not addressed the contribution of smoking to mortality from nonmalignant respiratory disease; however, two studies of Native-American miners from New Mexico and the Colorado Plateau have found an increased incidence of obstructive lung disease and death from nonmalignant respiratory disease in this population, which traditionally uses very little tobacco (27,46). Miners in the Colorado Plateau, New Mexico, and Czech cohorts have also had an increased risk of death from tuberculosis, probably reflecting the increased virulence of *Mycobacterium tuberculosis* in persons with silica-related lung disease.

Early studies of Colorado Plateau uranium miners indicated pulmonary function abnormalities related to exposure (47,48). Those studies were carried out with methods that would no longer be considered acceptable.

A survey of nonmalignant respiratory diseases was conducted in the early 1980s on 192 long-term New Mexico uranium miners (49). After controlling for cigarette smoking, the duration of underground uranium mining activity was associated with reduction of air flow. Review of radiographs showed abnormalities compatible with silicosis in 9% of the miners surveyed.

Mapel and colleagues (50) analyzed cross-sectional data from 1,359 New Mexico uranium miners. Quantitative estimates of radon progeny exposure were not available. Years of underground uranium mining was associated with lower lung function in the Native-American miners, and risk of radiographic pneumoconiosis was predicted by duration of working underground for Hispanic and Native-American miners.

A case series reported by Archer and colleagues (46) provides evidence that uranium miners may develop a fibrotic lung disorder distinct from silicosis. Archer and colleagues identified 22 miners from 400 referred for evaluation as possibly having radiation-related interstitial fibrosis of the lung. All had evidence of diffuse radiographic abnormalities in the lower lung fields and five had interstitial fibrosis and honeycombing on lung biopsy. Archer et al. concluded that there is a radiation-caused diffuse interstitial fibrosis in uranium miners.

Concern has been expressed over the possibility of cancers other than lung cancer resulting from underground mining exposure. Slight increases in risk of death from lymphomas (45), cancers of the buccal cavity, pharynx, and salivary glands (44), and stomach cancer (37) have been found in individual studies. However, no increased risk of death from cancers other than lung cancer has been found in the Colorado Plateau, New Mexico, French, Beaverlodge, Eldorado, or Czech cohorts (51).

Darby and colleagues (52) pooled data from 10 of the 11 cohorts included in the pooled analysis conducted by Lubin et al (19,20) and added data from the study of Cornish tin miners. For all nonlung cancers combined, the overall SMR was close to unity. Twenty-eight individual cancer groupings were examined without clear evidence for a link of any site to exposure to radon progeny.

Mortality studies of the cohorts in Table 2 have consistently found an increased risk of death from trauma, including motor vehicle accidents and other external causes of death, in underground miners. Miners in the Czech cohort had an increased risk of death from cirrhosis and cardiovascular diseases (35), although in the Colorado Plateau and New Mexico cohorts these same risks were decreased. It is suggested that these risks reflect the inherent risk of trauma in underground mining and lifestyle factors, and are not due to any particular exposure in the mines.

An excessive mortality rate from nonmalignant renal disease was reported in one analysis of data from the Colorado Plateau study (53). Mortality from chronic and unspecified nephritis was elevated more than threefold. That finding has not been replicated, and it cannot be readily interpreted as a direct consequence of exposure to radon decay products (5).

In a series of papers in the 1960s, Muller and colleagues (54–56) described reproductive outcomes in children of Czechoslovakian uranium miners. The secondary sex ratio (male to female births) was found to decline following underground employment. In the 1980s, descriptive data from New Mexico were considered to show adverse reproductive effects of the uranium-mining industry related to effects on the miners or to effects on those living near mines and mills (57). Descriptive studies showed changes in the secondary sex ratio for counties in New Mexico where uranium was mined; high rates of congenital malformations and spontaneous abortion were reported for Shiprock Indian Health Services Hospital, which cares for Navajos in an area of uranium mining and milling (57). A follow-up survey of reproductive outcome in the children of uranium miners did not show evidence of adverse effects (58).

## SUMMARY

Underground uranium miners and other miners exposed to radon progeny have sustained a high burden of radiation-caused excess lung cancer. The risks have been well documented and an extensive epidemiologic database has served as the basis for developing risk models. These data have also highlighted the risks of cancer in the miners and motivated compensation programs. Fortunately, radon-exposed miners do not experience excess risk for other cancers, but they have developed pneumoconiosis from silica exposure and possibly nonspecific fibrosis as well. There is a need for continued monitoring for lung cancer risk in past and current uranium miners.

## REFERENCES


1. Harting FH, Hesse W. Der Lungenkrebs, die bergkrankheit in den schneeberger gruben. *Viertel Gerichtl Med Oeff Sanitaetswes* 1879;31: 102–132,313–337.
2. Arnstein A. On the so-called "Schneeberg Lung Cancer." *Verhandl Deutsch pathol Gesellsch* 1913;16:332–342.
3. Pirchan A, Sikl H. Cancer of the lung in the miners of Jachymov. *Am J Cancer* 1932;16:681–722.
4. Lorenz E. Radioactivity and lung cancer: a critical review of lung cancer in the miners of Schneeberg and Joachimsthal. *J Natl Cancer Inst* 1944;5:1–15.
5. National Research Council (NRC), Committee on the Biological Effects of Ionizing Radiation. *Health risks of radon and other internally deposited alpha-emitters: BEIR IV. Washington, DC: National Academy Press, 1988.*
6. *United Nations Scientific Committee on the Effects of Atomic Radiation (UNSCEAR).* Sources, *effects and risks of ionizing radiation.* Annex F—radiation carcinogenesis in man. New York: United Nations Press, 1988.
7. Kahn P. A grisly archive of key cancer data: meticulous medical records of former East German uranium workers tell a horror story, but they could help settle some long-standing arguments about risks from low-level radiation. *Science* 1993;259:448–451.
8. Advisory Committee on Human Radiation Experiments. *Final report.* Washington, DC: U.S. Government Printing Office, 1995.
9. National Council on Radiation Protection and Measurements (NCRP). *Exposure of the population in the United States and Canada from natural background radiation.* Bethesda, MD; National Council on Radiation Protection and Measurements, 1987.
10. Holaday DA, Rushing DE, Coleman RD, Woolrich PF, Kusnetz HL, Bale WF. *Control of radon and daughters in uranium mines and calculations on biologic effects.* Washington, DC: U.S. Government Printing Office, 1957.
11. James AC. Lung dosimetry. In: Nazaroff WW, Nero AV Jr, eds. *Radon and its decay products in indoor air.* New York: John Wiley, 1988; 259–309.
12. National Council on Radiation Protection and Measurements (NCRP). *Evaluation of occupational and environmental exposures to radon and radon daughters in the United States.* Bethesda, MD; NCRP, 1984.
13. Samet JM. Radon and lung cancer. *J Natl Cancer Inst* 1989;81: 745–757.
14. Phillips CR, Khan A, Leung HMY. The nature and determination of the unattached fraction of radon and thoron progeny. In: Nazaroff WW, Nero AV Jr, eds. *Radon and its decay products in indoor air.* New York: John Wiley, 1988.
15. Mason TJ. The descriptive epidemiology of lung cancer. In: Samet JM, ed. *Epidemiology of lung cancer.* New York: Marcel Dekker, 1994; 51–70.
16. Wu-Williams AH, Samet JM. Lung cancer and cigarette smoking. In: Samet JM, ed. *Epidemiology of lung cancer.* New York: Marcel Dekker, 1994;71–108.
17. World Health Organization. WHO histological typing of lung tumors. *Am J Clin Pathol* 1982;77:123–136.
18. Churg A. Lung cancer cell type and occupational exposure. In: Samet JM, ed. *Epidemiology of lung cancer.* New York: Marcel Dekker, 1994; 413–436.
19. Lubin JH, Boice JD Jr, Edling C, et al. Lung cancer in radon-exposed miners and estimation of risk from indoor exposure. *J Natl Cancer Inst* 1995;87:817–827.
20. Lubin JH, Boice JD Jr, Edling C, et al. Radon-exposed underground miners and inverse dose-rate (protraction enhancement) effects. *Health Phys* 1995;69:494–500.
21. National Research Council (NRC), Committee on Health Effects of Exposure to Radon (BEIR VI), Commission on Life Sciences. *Health effects of exposure to radon:* time for reassessment? Washington, DC: National Academy Press, 1994.
22. Cross FT. Evidence of lung cancer from animal studies. In: Nazaroff WW, ed. *Radon and its decay products in indoor air.* New York: John Wiley, 1988.
23. Hornung RW, Meinhardt TJ. Quantitative risk assessment of lung cancer in U.S. uranium miners. *Health Phys* 1987;52:417–430.
24. Thomas D, Pogoda J, Langholz B, Mack W. Temporal modifiers of the radon-smoking interaction. *Health Phys* 1994;66:257–262.
25. Gray RG, Lafuma J, Parish SE, Peto R. Lung tumors and radon inhalation in over 2000 rats: approximate linearity across a wide range of doses and potentiation by tobacco smoke. In: Thompson RC, Mahaffey JA, eds. *Lifespan radiation effects studies in animals:* What can they tell us? Proceedings of the 22nd Hanford Life Sciences Symposium, September 27–29, 1983, Richland, WA. Springfield, VA: National Technical Information Service, 1986;592–607.
26. Roscoe MS, Steenland K, Halperin WE, Beaumont JJ, Waxweiler RJ. Lung cancer mortality among nonsmoking uranium miners exposed to radon daughters. *JAMA* 1989;262:629–633.
27. Roscoe RJ, Mason TJ. Uranium miners—low dose investigation. A joint NIOSH-NCI project, 1983.
28. Samet JM, Kutvirt DM, Waxweiler RJ, Key CR. Uranium mining and lung cancer in Navajo men. *N Engl J Med* 1984;310:1481–1484.
29. National Research Council (NRC), Panel on Dosimetric Assumptions Affecting the Application of Radon Risk Estimates. *Comparative dosimetry of radon in mines and homes.* Companion to BEIR IV Report. Washington, DC: National Academy Press, 1991.
30. Saccomanno GS, Huth GC, Auerbach O, Kuschner M. Relationship of radioactive radon daughters and cigarette smoking in the genesis of lung cancer in uranium miners. *Cancer* 1988;62:1402–1408.
31. Saccomanno GS. The contribution of uranium miners to lung cancer histogenesis. *Recent Results Cancer Res* 1982;82:43–52.
32. Saccomanno GS, Auerbach O, Kuschner M, et al. A comparison between the localization of lung tumors in uranium miners and in nonminers from 1947 to 1991. *Cancer* 1996;77:1278–1283.
33. Vahakangas KH, Samet JM, Metcalf RA, et al. Mutations of p53 and ras genes in radon-associated lung cancer from uranium miners. *Lancet* 1992;339:576–580.
34. Taylor JA, Watson MA, Devereox RT, Michaels R, Saccomanno GS, Anderson M. Mutational hotspot in p53 gene in lung tumors from uranium miners. *Lancet* 1994;343:86–87.
35. Tomasek L, Swerdlow AJ, Darby SC, Placek V, Kunz E. Mortality in uranium miners in West Bohemia: a long-term cohort study. *Occup Environ Med* 1994;51:308–315.
36. Xuan X, Lubin JH, Li JY, Blot WJ. A cohort study in southern China of workers exposed to radon and radon decay products. *Health Phys* 1993; 64:120–131.
37. Radford EP, Renard St Clair KG. Lung cancer in Swedish iron ore miners exposed to low doses of radon daughters. *N Engl J Med* 1984;310: 1485–1494.
38. Samet JM, Pathak DR, Morgan MV, Coultas DB, Hunt WC. Silicosis and lung cancer risk in underground uranium miners. *Health Phys* 1994; 66:450–453.
39. Finkelstein MM. Silicosis, radon, and lung cancer risk in Ontario miners. *Health Phys* 1995;69:396–399.
40. U.S.Department of Health and Human Services (USDHHS), National Institute for Occupational Safety and Health (NIOSH). *A recommended standard for occupational exposure to radon progeny in underground mines.* Washington, DC: U.S. Government Printing Office, 1988.
41. Lubin JH, Boice JD Jr, Edling C, et al. *Radon and lung cancer risk:* a joint analysis of 11 underground miners studies. Bethesda, MD: U.S. Department of Health and Human Services, Public Health Service, National Institutes of Health, 1994.
42. Darby SC, Doll R. Radon in houses: How large is the risk? *Radiat Prot Aust* 1990;8:83–88.
43. Samet JM, Pathak DR, Morgan MV, Key CR, Valdivia AA. Lung cancer mortality and exposure to radon decay products in a cohort of New Mexico underground uranium miners. *Health Phys* 1991;61:745–752.
44. Morrison HI, Semenciw RM, Mao Y, Wigle DT. Cancer mortality among a group of fluorspar miners exposed to radon progeny. *Am J Epidemiol* 1988;128:1266–1275.
45. Xiang-Zhen X, Lubin JH, Jun-Yao L, et al. A cohort study in southern china of tin miners exposed to radon and radon decay products. *Health Phys* 1993;64:120–131.
46. Archer VE, Gillam JD, Wagoner JL. Respiratory disease mortality among uranium miners. *Ann NY Acad Sci* 1976;271:280–293.
47. Archer VE, Brinton HP, Wagoner JK. Pulmonary function of uranium miners. *Health Phys* 1964;10:1183–1194.
48. Archer VE, Wagoner JK, Lundin FE. Lung cancer among uranium miners in the United States. *Health Phys* 1973;23:351–371.
49. Samet JM, Young RA, Morgan MV, Humble CG, Epler GR, McLoud T. Prevalence survey of respiratory abnormalities in New Mexico uranium miners. *Health Phys* 1984;46:361–370.

50. Mapel DW, Coultas DB, James DS, Hunt WC, Stidley CA, Gilliland FD. Ethnic differences in non-malignant respiratory disease prevalence among uranium miners. *Am J Public Health* 1997;87:833–838.
51. Tomasek L, Darby SC, Swerdlow AJ, Placek V, Kunz E. Radon exposure and cancers other than lung cancer among uranium miners in West Bohemia. *Lancet* 1993;341:919–923.
52. Darby SC, Whitley E, Howe GR, et al. Radon and cancers other than lung cancer in underground miners: a collaborative analysis of 11 studies. *J Natl Cancer Inst* 1995;87:378–384.
53. Waxweiler RJ, Roscoe RJ, Archer VE, Thun MJ, Wagoner JK, Lundin FE. Mortality follow-up through 1977 of the white underground uranium miners cohort examined by the United States Public Health Service. In: Gomez M, ed. *Radiation hazards in mining:* control, *measurement and medical aspects.* New York: American Institute of Mining, Metallurgical, and Petroleum Engineers, 1981.
54. Muller C, Kubat M, Marsalek J. Study on the fertility of the miners in Joachimsthal. *Zentralbl Gynakol* 1962;2:63–68.
55. Muller C, Reiicha V, Kubat M. On the question of the genetic effects of the ionizing rays on the miners of Joachimsthal. *Zentralbl Gynakol* 1962;15:558–560.
56. Muller C, Ruzicka L, Bakstein J. The sex ratio in the offsprings of uranium miners. *Acta Univ Carol [Med]* 1967;13:599–603.
57. Wiese WH. Birth effects in the four corners area. Albuquerque, NM: University of New Mexico School of Medicine, 1981.
58. Survey of reproductive outcomes in uranium and potash mine workers: results of first analysis. In: *International conference on the health of miners,* vol 14. Cincinnati: American Conference of Government Industrial Hygienists, 1986;187–192.
59. Kusiak RA, Ritchie AC, Muller J, Springer J. Mortality from lung cancer in Ontario uranium miners. *Br J Ind Med* 1993;50:920–928.
60. Howe GR, Naire RC, Newcombe HG, Miller AB, Burch JD. Lung cancer mortality (1950–1980) in relation to radon daughter exposure in a cohort of workers at the Eldorado Port Radium uranium mine: possible modification of risk by exposure rate. *J Natl Cancer Inst* 1987;79: 1255–1260.
61. Sevc J, Tomasek L, Kunz E, et al. A survey of the Czechoslovak follow-up of lung cancer mortality in uranium miners. *Health Phys* 1993;64:355–369.
62. Tirmarche M, Raphalen A, Allin F, Chameaud J, Bredon P. Mortality of a cohort of French uranium miners exposed to relatively low radon concentrations. *Br J Cancer* 1993;67:1090–1097.
63. Woodward A, Roder D, McMichael AJ, Crouch P, Mylvaganam A. Radon daughter exposures at the Radium Hill uranium mine and lung cancer rates among former workers, 1952–87. *Cancer Cause Cont* 1991;2:213–220.

*Environmental and Occupational Medicine, Third Edition,* edited by William N. Rom.
Lippincott–Raven Publishers, Philadelphia © 1998.

# CHAPTER 99

# Nonionizing Radiation

Roy E. Shore

The term *nonionizing radiation* designates a wide spectrum of electromagnetic radiation frequencies (from 0 Hz to over $10^{15}$ Hz; Fig. 1) and, therefore, potentially a variety of health effects. Several types of nonionizing radiation have been the subject of considerable public attention and controversy in recent years. This chapter reviews the research literature concerning various types of nonionizing radiation to provide a perspective on the perceived risks. Some of the main experimental findings are briefly summarized (although this literature is too extensive to describe comprehensively), after which the principal epidemiologic studies are reviewed, since these often drive public perception and risk estimates. Because this review provides little coverage of industrial hygiene, dosimetry, engineering, and basic biologic aspects of these radiations, references are given to other sources that provide such coverage. A number of types of nonionizing radiation are reviewed, including extremely low frequency and static electromagnetic fields, lasers, ultraviolet radiation, radiofrequency and microwave radiation, and ultrasound. Studies of video display terminals are the subject of another chapter, so they will not be covered here.

## EXTREMELY LOW FREQUENCY ELECTROMAGNETIC FIELDS

Extremely low frequency electromagnetic fields (EMFs) are usually defined to include 1 to 3,000 Hz, but the ones of most interest are the 50- to 60-Hz fields associated with alternating currents in electric power distribution systems. In the United States there are more than 300,000 miles of overhead electric transmission lines, of which about 67,000 miles carry at least 345 kV. The magnetic field under a maximally loaded 765-kV line may reach a few tenths of a gauss (G) (2) [10,000 G = 1 tesla (T)]. Ranges of measured EMF exposures for a variety of home and occupational settings are shown in Fig. 2. Measurements in offices have ranged from 1 mG to about 100 mG. At the other extreme, near spot welding machines and electrosteel furnaces, fields range up to 17 G and 80 G, respectively (3). The average EMF in homes is about 1 mG (ranging up to several milligauss), while the magnetic field for a person lying under an electric blanket may be 10 to 20 mG, or up to 50 mG close to certain household appliances such as microwave ovens, vacuum cleaners, hair dryers, food mixers, and shavers (3–5). Even moderate use of electric blankets can double one's residential EMF exposure (6). The magnitude and range of EMF from power lines and household appliances are very different; for appliances the magnetic fields are confined mainly to a distance of a meter or two, whereas fields from high-voltage power lines have a range on the order of 50 to 150 m (7).

Reviews of dosimetric, physical interaction, and biologic aspects of EMF are found elsewhere (3,9–12).

### Biologic Effects

*In vitro* experiments suggest that EMF exposures have the potential to affect cell function in a variety of ways (12):

- Modulation of ion and protein flow across the cell membrane (e.g., calcium homeostasis)
- Chromosome damage and interference with DNA synthesis and RNA transcription

R. E. Shore: Department of Environmental Medicine, New York University Medical Center, New York, New York 10016.

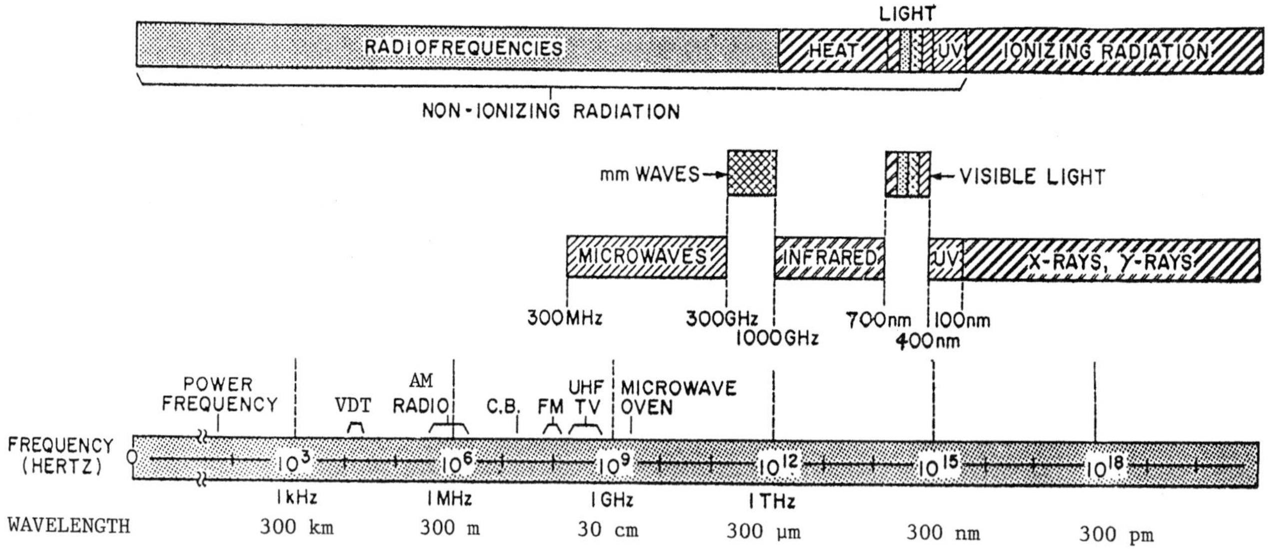


**FIG. 1.** Electromagnetic spectrum in terms of frequency, wavelength and uses. (Adapted from ref. 1, with permission.)

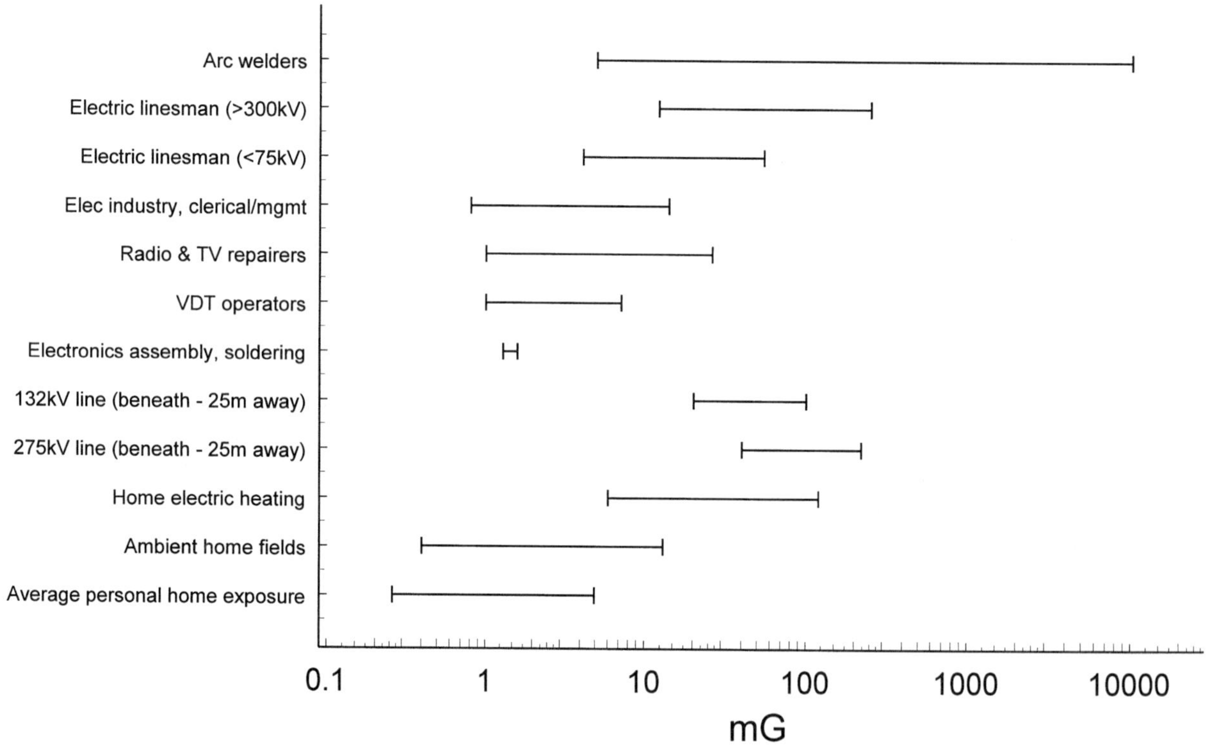


**FIG. 2.** Ranges of EMF exposures in milligauss for various domestic and occupational settings or powerline proximity. (Values taken from ref. 8.)

- Interaction with the cell response to different hormones and enzymes, including those involved in cell growth processes and stress responses
- Interaction with the cell response to chemical neurotransmitters
- Interaction with the immune response of cells
- Interaction with cancerous cells.

However, some of these effects have been found in only one laboratory and have not been replicable by other investigators (12). Extremely low frequency EMF does not appear to act directly on the deoxyribonucleic acid (DNA) structure, but may perhaps interfere with ribonucleic acid (RNA) transcription (12). Because the cell membrane is a primary site of action of magnetic fields, processes governed by the cell membrane, such as immune function and cell-cell communication, may be sensitive to EMF effects (13).

### Reproductive and Teratogenic Effects

There have been a few positive reports of reproductive and teratogenic effects of EMF in experimental animals, but the findings have been inconsistent in different species and have tended not to be replicable (2,12,14,15).

Nordstrom and co-workers (16) found an apparent association between EMF exposure due to paternal work at an electrical substation and congenital malformation frequency in offspring. There were several methodologic flaws in the study, however (2, 9), and another study failed to replicate the findings (17). Wertheimer and Leeper (18,19) have also reported that fetal losses are related to the use of ceiling heating cables, heated water beds, and electric blankets, but the studies contain methodologic weaknesses and interpretive problems. In contrast, Dlugosz et al. (20) found an inverse association between congenital defects and electric bed heating. Other studies have evaluated fetal growth, perinatal mortality, sperm morphology, sex ratio, or fertility, with generally negative results (14). A good-quality study by Bracken et al. (21) found no association between maternal electrical bed heating and birth weight or fetal growth retardation.

### Hematopoietic, Immune System, and Endocrine Effects

A number of experimental studies have been conducted on the effects of electrical fields on the hematopoietic system (9). Some have shown changes in average values of hematologic parameters, but all within the normal range, and most studies used field strengths much greater than those to which humans are likely to be exposed. Similarly, many studies have been performed on the relation of electrical fields to blood chemistry and endocrine parameters. Of the many parameters studied, possible effects have been seen for corticosterone, testosterone, and melatonin (9). Nordstrom and co-workers (16) reported a high frequency of chromosome breaks in the lymphocytes of workers at an electrical substation, but this was not confirmed in another study (17). Melatonin has become a subject of scrutiny by a number of investigators because of its possible role in oncogenesis, immune function, and neuromodulation (13,22,23). Alterations in various immune system cells by EMF exposure have been reported in experiments, but whether the changes are of clinical significance is unclear (9,13).

### Neurologic and Behavioral Effects

Frey (13) summarized recent biologic and mechanistic studies of EMF and neural function. Adey (24) reported that EMF affects the binding affinity *in vivo* of brain tissue for calcium ions. Thomas and colleagues (25) studied neurobehavioral function and found that EMF exposure did not cause learning impairment, nor did it potentiate the impairing effects of a psychoactive drug. Most other studies of learning or cognition in EMF-exposed workers have, similarly, shown no effects (26–28). A recent study suggested that occupational EMF exposure may be a risk factor for Alzheimer's disease (29), although this finding has not yet been replicated.

A psychiatric outcome has been studied by Perry and colleagues (30), who compared measured EMF at the doors of the homes of 598 suicide cases and matched controls and found the fields were higher, on average, for the suicide cases. Several methodologic weaknesses of this study have been pointed out by Michaelson (31). Another study did not show an excess of suicide among workers in various electrical and electronics occupations (32). Poole et al (33) reported an association between proximity to a high-voltage electric line and depressive symptoms and headaches, but the study suffered from possible selection bias and biased reporting because of polarized community attitudes toward the line. A natural experiment in a study of workers near a 400 kV line on a day when the power was on and another day when it was off, unbeknown to them, showed no differences in self-reported psychological states (34).

### Carcinogenic Effects

#### *Residential EMF Exposure*

In 1979 Wertheimer and Leeper (35) reported that childhood cancers, especially leukemia, were associated with residential high-current configurations (HCC), which were defined by the size of the wires in the electric line and proximity of the house to wires, transformers, and power stations. This generated considerable interest even though the study was of limited method-

**TABLE 1.** *Leukemia and nervous-system cancer in relation to home EMF exposures*

| First author (reference) | Type of cancer and study[a,b] (Ages) | No. of high-exposure cases/ total cases | Relative risk (95% conf. interval) | Definition of high magnetic field exposure[b] |
|---|---|---|---|---|
| Childhood leukemia | | | | |
| Myers (182) | Leukemia/lymphoma, C-C (child) | 11/180 | 1.1 (0.5–2.5) | <50m from powerline |
| Tomenius (36) | Leukemia, C-C (0–18) | 4/243 | 0.3 (0.1–1.0) | ≥3 mG[c] |
| Savitz (37) | Leukemia, C-C (0–14) | Leuk: 65/231 | A) 1.6 (1.0–2.5); B) 1.0 (0.6–2.0); C) ALL: 1.3 (0.7–2.3) | A) HCC[d]; B) ≥2 mG[c]; C) HCC |
| Coleman (183) | Leukemia, C-C (0–17) | 14/84 | 1.5 (0.7–3.4) | <50m from power substation |
| London (38) | Leukemia, C-C (0–10) | 42/211, 16/164 | A) 2.2 (1.1–4.3); B) 1.5 (0.7–3.3) | A) HCC; B) ≥2.68 mG[c] |
| Olsen (184) | Leukemia, cohort (0–14) | 4/833 | 1.0 (0.3–3.3) | ≥1 mG[c] |
| Feychting (39) | Leukemia, cohort | A) 7/38; B) 4/24 | A) 2.7 (1.0–6.3); B) 0.6 (0.2–1.8) | Mag. field ≥2 mG; A) Estimated; B) Measured |
| Verkasalo (185) | Leukemia, cohort (0–19) | 3/35 | 1.2 (0.3–3.6) | ≥4 mGy-years[e] |
| Tynes (186) | Leukemia, nested C-C (0–14) | 9/148 | 1.1 (0.5–2.3) | Estimated time wtd. mag. field ≥0.5 mG[e] |
| Adult leukemia | | | | |
| Coleman (183) | Leukemia, C-C | 15/190 | 0.9 (0.5–1.7) | <50 m from power substation |
| Severson (41) | ANLL, C-C | A) 29/97; B) 23/133 | 1.5 (0.8–2.7); 1.0 (0.5–2.0) | Two different definitions of HCC |
| Wertheimer (187) | Leukemia, C-C | 23:23[f] | 1.0 (0.6–1.8) | HCC |
| Youngson (188) | Myeloid leukemia, C-C | A) 76/801; B) 9/801 | A) 1.3 (0.9–1.9); B) 3.0 (0.8–11) | A) Power-line distance <100 m; B) ≥1 mG[c] |
| Feychting (189) | A&C) AML; B&D) CML; cohort | A) 5/77; B) 6/63 | A) 1.9 (0.6–4.7); B) 2.7 (1.0–6.4); C) 1.1 (0.4–2.4); D) 1.5 (0.7–3.2) | A&B) ≥30 mG-y[e]; C&D) ≥2 mG[c] |
| Li (73) | A) Leukemia; B) AML; C) ALL. C-C | A) 97/870; B) 41/415; C) 17/126 | A) 1.4 (1.0–1.9); B) 1.1 (0.7–1.7); C) 1.7 (1.0–3.1) | >2 mG[e]; A) Trend $p = 0.04$ |
| Brain cancer | | | | |
| Wertheimer (35) | Nerv. syst., C-C (0–19) | 30/66 | 2.4 (1.1–5.4) | HCC |
| Savitz (37) | Brain, C-C (0–14) | 20/59 | 2.0 (1.1–3.8) | HCC |
| Tomenius (36) | Nerv. syst., C-C (0–18) | 13/294 | 3.9 (1.2–12.7) | >3 mG |
| Feychting (39) | CNS, cohort (0–15) | A) 7/38; B) 5/23 | A) 2.7 (1.0–6.3); B) 1.5 (0.4–4.9) | Mag. field ≥2 mG; A) Estimated; B) Measured |
| Olsen (184) | CNS, cohort (0–14) | 3/624 | 1.0 (0.3–3.7) | ≥1 mG[c] |
| Verkasalo (185) | Nerv. syst., cohort (0–19) | 7/39 | 2.3 (0.9–4.8) | ≥4 mG-y |
| Gurney (190) | Brain, C-C (0–19) | | 0.9 (0.5–1.5) | HCC; no association with electric blankets, water beds or electric heating |
| Preston-Martin (191) | Brain, C–C (0–19) | A) 31/281; B) 16/281 | A) 1.2 (0.6–2.2); B) 1.2 (0.5–2.8) | A) HCC; B) >2 mG[c]; trend $p = 0.98$ |
| Preston-Martin (192) | Brain, C-C (0–19) | 53/485 | 0.9 (0.6–1.2) | In utero exposure to electric blanket or heated water bed |
| Wertheimer (187) | Nerv. syst., C-C (adult) | 25:11[c] | 2.3 (1.1–4.8) | HCC |
| Feychting (189) | CNS, cohort (adult) | A) 6/228; B) 22/132 | A) 0.7 (0.3–1.5); B) 0.8 (0.5–1.3) | A) ≥30 mG-y[e]; B) ≥2 mG[c] |
| Tynes (186) | Brain, nested C-C (0–14) | 12/156 | 1.2 (0.6–2.4) | Estimated time wtd. mag. field ≥0.5 mG[e] |
| Li (73) | Brain, C-C (adult) | 71/577 | 1.1 (0.8–1.6) | >2 mG[d] |

[a]"Leukemia" means all types of leukemia; ALL, acute lymphocytic leukemia; ANLL, acute nonlymphocytic leukemia; AML, acute myeloid leukemia; CML, chronic myeloid leukemia; Nerv. syst., brain/nervous system tumor; CNS, central nervous system tumor.

[b]C-C, case-control study; cohort, cohort study.

[c]Measured magnetic fields.

[d]HCC, high current configuration based on types of wires and the distance from wires, transformers, and substations to a house.

[e]Estimated cumulative magnetic-field exposure based on distance to high-voltage line, line load records, etc.

[f]Matched study; values given are numbers of pairs in which case or control (case:control) had higher wiring code "exposure."

ologic quality. A number of additional studies have since examined childhood leukemia and residential EMF, of which a sampling of the largest or best is shown in Table 1. None has found a relationship as strong as that originally reported by Wertheimer and Leeper. It is of interest to obtain a summary index of the association between childhood leukemia and either measurements of residential EMFs or estimates based on HCC or other power-line metrics. An overall analysis of the childhood leukemia data in Table 1 showed that for the HCC/power-line estimates there was a weak positive association [overall relative risk (RR) = 1.6, 95% confidence interval (CI) = 1.1–2.1], but there was no association for measured EMFs (overall RR = 0.9, 95% CI = 0.5–1.4). Although these analyses are not definitive (e.g., the tables do not comprehensively cover the available studies), they nevertheless suggest that any association is either weak or nonexistent.

The studies of residential exposure to EMF and adult leukemia (Table 1) do not provide convincing evidence of a relationship; only a single RR out of several in one study was significantly elevated. Similarly, the studies of residential EMF and nervous system cancers, shown in Table 1, do not show consistently elevated RRs; an overall analysis of these data yielded an RR = 1.3 for HCC/power-line assessments and an RR = 1.1 for measured EMF levels.

One problem encountered in this literature is selectivity in interpretation. For example, various reviews of these studies have cited the Tomenius study (36) as showing a significant elevation in cancer among EMF-exposed children and have ignored the facts that (a) for childhood leukemia, the main hypothesized cancer-EMF association, the relative risk was 0.3; and (b) the mean measured EMFs outside the residences of cancer patients and controls were virtually identical (0.68 and 0.67 mG, respectively). It was only when Tomenius divided the distribution of exposures at 3 mG that a statistically significant difference was seen for "all cancers." Similarly, the Savitz et al. (37) study is sometimes cited as showing positive results (based on the HCC results shown in Table 1), even though the RR was 1.0 based on measured levels in the living areas of the homes with the usual appliances turned on. Likewise, London et al. (38) found a statistically significant ($p = 0.02$) exposure-response trend for leukemia with wire codes but no trend for home EMF measurements, and Feychting and Ahlbom (39) similarly found a positive trend ($p = 0.02$) for leukemia with a transmission-line estimate of EMF exposure but a trend in the negative direction for home EMF measurements.

There are probably several reasons for the discrepancy in results between measured fields and wiring codes. Electromagnetic fields in homes are affected by variations in the appliances used, in home wiring, and in EMFs from water-pipe grounds (40), so that wiring codes represent only some fraction of home EMF exposures. In support of this view, two studies have compared the two indices of exposure and found that the HCC codes account for only 15% to 20% of the variation in measured field levels (37,41), suggesting that wiring codes are a poor surrogate for actual measurements. Feychting and Ahlbom (39) found that a more sophisticated estimate of transmission-line EMFs predicted 49% of the variation in measured home EMF levels. Another line of evidence suggesting that wire codes may capture only a fraction of the variation in residential EMFs is the finding by Feychting et al. (42) that 91% of those with transmission-line estimates ≥2 mG also had spot measurements ≥2 mG, but over 40% of those with spot measurements ≥2 mG had transmission-line estimates of <1 mG. In other words, while high EMF from outside wiring does produce high EMF levels in the home, one cannot infer that low-EMF outside wiring means low EMF levels in the home, apparently because of other sources of EMFs. They also found that for spot measurements, but not for transmission-line based estimates of EMFs, the fields were higher in apartments than in one-family homes, again showing the lack of predictiveness of wire-code metrics.

On the other hand, some have asserted that wiring codes are better estimates of EMF exposure than short-term EMF measurements because the wiring codes provide a stable, long-term index of exposure, whereas short-term (e.g., 5-minute or even 24-hour) measurements are subject to considerable measurement error due to short-term fluctuations in EMF levels. Available data, however, indicate that short-term measurements are reasonably stable and predictive. For instance, Savitz's group (43,44) found that spot measurements made in a series of homes and then repeated after 5 years correlated 0.74. They reported that contemporary spot measurements were better predictors of the spot measurements 5 years previously than were contemporary wire codes. They also found unreliability or instability in about 10% of the wire codes when recoded after 5 years because of changes in wire configurations, errors in coding, etc. Friedman et al. (45) reported that measured EMFs in children's bedrooms correlated well ($r = 0.76$) with personal EMF dosimeter measurements while the child was at home. However, they noted that at-home personal EMF dosimetry did not correlate as well ($r = 0.59$) with total personal EMF dosimetry for older children, a fact that would limit the predictiveness of any type of residential dosimetry.

### *Occupational EMF Exposure*

A number of the main studies of occupational EMF exposure and leukemia are shown in Table 2. Most of the studies did not show statistically significant elevations in risk. To generate a summary figure, the EMF-exposed leukemia cases were summed across all the studies. The observed and expected cases numbered 1,540 and 1,337

**TABLE 2.** *Leukemia in relation to occupational EMF exposure*

| Population studied (reference) | Study type[a] | Relative risk (95% confidence interval) (no. of cancers observed)[b] | Exposure groups and comments[c] |
|---|---|---|---|
| Wisconsin death cert. (193) | PMR | 1.0 (0.8–1.3) (81) | Elec occup; deaths 1963–78 |
| Thames cancer registry (194) | PIR | 1.2 (1.0–1.4) (113) | Elec occup; registry, 1961–79 |
| Brit. Columbia death cert. (195) | PMR | 1.1 (0.9–1.4) (65) | Elec occup; deaths, 1950–84 |
| U.S. Navy (48) | SIR | 1.5 (0.9–2.2) (19) | Electricians; electronics tech; radio & sonar operators |
| Coal miners (196) | Case-cont | 2.5 (1.8–3.5) (32) | Exposed = coal mining 25+ yr; possible sampling biases |
| Finnish cancer registry (49) | SIR | 1.2 (0.7–1.9) (17) | Elec occup |
| U.S. death cert (197) | Case-cont | 1.0 (0.8–1.2) (76) | Elec occup; deaths in 16 states |
| Telephone workers (46) | SIR | A) 7.0 (1.4–20) (3); B) 1.1 (0.2–3.5) (2) | A) Cable splicers, & B) central office techs (two highest exposure groups) |
| England-Wales tumor registry (198) | PMR (total leuk.) & case-cont (AML) | A) 1.0 (0.8–1.2) (85); B) 2.3 (1.4–3.7) (36) | A) All leukemia; B) AML; 1970–73 registry |
| England tumor registry (199) | PIR | 1.2 (1.1–1.4) (217) | 1981–87 registry; jobs in elec/ electronic industry |
| Washington State elec occup (200) | PMR | 1.4 (1.1–1.6) (146) | Elec occup |
| New Zealand elec workers (201) | Case-cont | 1.6 (1.0–2.5) (21) | Elec occup |
| Electricians, Naval shipyard (202) | Case-cont | 3.0 (1.3–7.0) (11) | |
| Swedish elec utility workers (50) | SMR | 1.1 (0.7–1.5) (26) | Power linesmen and power station operators |
| Swedish telephone operators (53) | SIR | 1.0 (0.5–1.8) (12) | |
| Los Angeles tumor registry (203) | PIR | 1.3 (0.9–1.8) (35) | Elec occup |
| Danish elec occup (69) | SIR | 1.6 (1.2–2.2) (39) | Based on census industry/ occup. codes |
| Los Angeles elec workers (204) | Case-control | 1.2 (1.0–1.5) (121) | RR per 10 mG increase in estimated mean magnetic field |
| Swedish train drivers/conductors (54) | SIR | 1.2 (0.7–1.9) (20) | Excess claimed for lymphatic leukemia; exposure levels of ~100 mG of 16 Hz EMF |
| Quebec/France pulsed EMF elec utility workers (55) | Nested case-cont | 0.7 (0.4–1.2) (95) | Expos. to pulsed EMFS; RR <1 for myeloid leukemia also |
| Canadian/French elec utility workers (56) | Nested case-cont | A) 1.5 (0.7–3.1) (140); B) 1.5 (0.3–7.6) (47) | A) All leukemia; B) AML; based on cumulative exposure-response |
| U.S. elec utility workers (57) | Poisson regression—mortality | 1.01 (0.9–1.1) (164) | RR per μT-year; no association for AML either |

[a]SMR (SIR), standardized mortality (or incidence) ratio; PMR (PIR), proportional mortality (or incidence) ratio; Case-cont, case-control study.
[b]Statistics for total leukemia are given unless noted otherwise.
[c]Elec, electric(al); Occup, occupation; AML, acute myeloid leukemia.

respectively, which gives an RR of 1.15. This suggests that if there is any association between occupational exposure to EMF and leukemia in adults it must be small. It is notable that, of 12 cohort studies of workers in electrical and electronics occupations, only one has shown a significant elevation in overall leukemia risk (46–57).

The studies of brain cancer and occupational EMF exposure provide little support for an association. Kheifets et al. (58) recently reviewed this literature and conducted a meta-analysis of the 29 relevant studies they could identify. Overall they found a pooled RR of 1.2 (95% CI = 1.1–1.3), but when they restricted the analysis to the 12 cohort studies, the strongest type of study design, RR = 1.04 (95% CI = 1.0–1.1). When they grouped occupations according to estimated EMF exposure levels, based on reported EMF measurements, they did not find a positive exposure-response relationship for brain tumors.

Several studies have investigated childhood brain tumors and paternal occupational EMF exposure with mixed results. These were recently reviewed by Heath (59). The nominal elevation in RR shown in several of the case-control studies is probably an artifact, because a genuine effect would require a germline mutation in the father, and the evidence suggests that EMFs do not cause mutations.

Interest has been generated in the hypothesis that EMF exposure may cause breast cancer because it reduces melatonin secretion by the pineal gland (60). There have been a few reports of excess male breast cancer in various electrical occupations (61–63) but also several negative studies (56,64,65) and six additional electrical-worker studies that found no cases of breast cancer (66). Of more concern than male breast cancer, in terms of its public health implications, is whether female breast cancer may be associated with EMF exposure. One large study of female death certificate data reported a modest association between breast cancer mortality and history of electrical occupation (RR = 1.4, 95% CI = 1.0–1.8) (67). However, an independent, more detailed analysis of much the same database found no consistent exposure-response relationship (68), and several other studies of female breast cancer, including cohort studies of electrical workers, have been negative (51,52,69,70). In addition, several studies of female breast cancer and residential EMF exposure have been mostly negative (71–74).

There are several problems in getting accurate and unbiased estimates of the association between EMFs and cancer. Other exposures or risk factors could bias the results, particularly in occupational studies, where exposure to carcinogenic chemicals is a possibility. There may also be a problem in selectivity of reporting, in which negative findings are less likely to be published either because of editors' lack of enthusiasm for such studies or because these studies are not submitted by investigators who may view negative results as unpublishable. Either of these problems could lead to overestimates of EMF effects based on the published literature. On the other hand, it is also possible that the relationships observed may be underestimates. When studies are based on crude exposure surrogates such as broad occupational categories, there is the potential for dilution of effects because many of the putatively exposed persons may have had little or no exposure. Similarly, random error in imputing exposure levels in the residential studies would probably lead to underestimates of the association.

In summary, at face value there appears to be a weak association of EMF with childhood leukemia risk. However, there is also the possibility of positive or negative bias in the epidemiologic data, effects of which cannot be disentangled. Thus, while there is a suggestion of an association, the evidence is not strongly convincing. The collective results for residential EMFs and brain cancer or adult leukemia do not provide substantial evidence for associations, nor do the data on occupational EMF exposure and various cancers.

## MAGNETIC RESONANCE IMAGING AND OTHER STATIC MAGNETIC FIELDS

The static magnetic field of the earth, to which humans are constantly exposed, is about 0.5 G. A few industrial processes (e.g., electric welding machines, induction furnaces) can subject workers to much larger static fields of up to 100 G, while magnetic resonance imaging (MRI) may briefly expose patients as much as 20,000 G. Reviews of MRI and static magnetic fields may be found elsewhere (75–78).

There has been less research on the health effects of static magnetic fields than on low-frequency EMF. There have been numerous negative experimental studies of MRI examining various outcomes: neurobehavioral or psychological outcomes, cardiac effects, reproductive and teratogenic effects, mutagenesis or cytogenetic abnormalities, and immune system effects (75). On the other hand, there have been isolated reports of associations between MRI and chromosome aberrations, malformations of chick embryos, altered insulin release, changes in serum glutamyl transpeptidase, increased nerve excitability, altered rat behavior, and altered blood-brain barrier permeability (76,77). Kanal and colleagues (79) conclude that, while there is no definitive evidence of deleterious biologic effects of MRI, the issue is not settled and further research is needed. A nationwide survey of the reproductive experience of women who worked at MRI facilities as compared to employees at other jobs showed no evidence among the MRI workers of excess spontaneous abortions, infertility, premature delivery, or low birth weight (80).

Several studies have been conducted of workers exposed to static magnetic fields. Workers exposed to strong static magnetic fields in an electrolysis cell room of a chloralkali plant, where the fields ranged from 40 to 290 G, were studied (81). For employees who had worked in the room at least 5 years, the observed-expected cancer mortality ratio was 5/6.3, which equals 0.8 (95% CI 0.3–1.9). Marsh and colleagues (82) studied the health of 320 persons working near electrolysis cells and found no major health effects.

Milham (83) reported an excess of leukemia mortality among workers in the aluminum industry, but four other reports have not shown significant excesses (81,84–86). One study also reported a negative finding for brain cancer mortality among electrolysis process workers (84).

## RADIOFREQUENCY AND MICROWAVE RADIATION

The radiofrequency (RF) range encompasses about 3 kHz to 300 GHz, which includes the microwave frequencies of approximately 300 MHz to 300 GHz. Microwave and RF equipment are found in many industries with such diverse uses as drying; gluing; plastic processing; sterilization; radio, television, and microwave transmitters; radar; and diathermy. The largest consumer use by far is microwave ovens. Ambient exposure levels from radio and TV transmission are very low. A survey conducted in 15 U.S. cities found that 95% of persons receive RF exposures of less than 0.1 $\mu W/cm^2$ from radio and TV sources, which is at least two orders of magnitude below the population limit (87). Summaries of RF dosimetry, and physical and biologic interactions are given elsewhere (88–93).

To address issues of the biologic effects of radiation over the RF range, one needs an exposure metric of specific absorption rates (SARs), the rate at which electromagnetic energy is absorbed by a volume of tissue. SARs turn out to be complex functions of carrier frequency, modulation, electric-field and magnetic-field strengths, and zone of irradiation (near or far field). In addition, the energy absorption may be highly nonuniform, owing to layers of tissue having different water content and dielectric properties, to reflective tissue surfaces and to body cavities. This complexity has meant that the exposure levels in many historical biologic studies have been inadequately defined, and the studies are therefore difficult to interpret or compare.

For a number of years the upper limit of whole-body averaged SAR has been set at 0.4 W/kg over 0.1 hour for occupational exposure, and 0.08 W/kg averaged over ½ hour for general population exposure (94). For a 2.45-GHz source, such as a microwave oven or diathermy machine, a power density of 5 mW/cm$^2$ to a human body surface would translate into approximately 0.4 W/kg (94).

The literature on the biologic effects of RF, and especially microwave, radiation is voluminous. Unfortunately, inadequate attention to defining exposure levels, to possible thermal effects, to developing dose-response data, and, in human studies, to adequate control groups has meant that the types of effects and exposure levels at which they occur are still rather poorly defined.

A number of macromolecular and cellular effects of RF irradiation have been studied, including effects on enzymes, mitochondria, calcium transport, cell growth, cell replication rates, cell survival time, chromosome aberrations, cell mutations, cell transformation (to a premalignant state), and growth rates of tumors. An extensive review of these end points is given elsewhere (89), with the conclusion that most or all of the effects seen are due to thermal changes and are therefore unlikely to occur at the lower human exposure levels of primary concern.

### Reproductive or Teratogenic Effects

Most of the experimental studies of adverse reproductive outcomes or teratogenesis have used power densities sufficient to produce significant thermal effects, so the validity of extrapolating such findings to human experience is uncertain (89). Several more recent studies have been performed using lower power densities in which the thermal effects would be minimal. Two studies of long-term maternal microwave irradiation of rats by Jensh (95,96) found no effects on maternal gestational weight gain, birth weight, litter size, fetal resorption rate, or fetal abnormality rate. However, offspring of irradiated animals did show subtle long-term neurobehavioral and developmental deficits (97). Another maternal study found no differences except a small increase in one type of birth defect (98). A recent study of long-term microwave irradiation of male mice showed no increase in chromosome aberrations in spermatogonia and no decline in their mates' pregnancy rate or in preimplantation or postimplantation survival (99).

Several human studies have examined possible reproductive detriment following microwave irradiation. Rubin and Erdman (cited in ref. 100) reported that women who had been treated by diathermy for pelvic inflammatory disease showed no observed interference with ovulation or conception. Barron and Baraff (101) found no changes in fertility among male radar workers. Among female physical therapists, the relations between miscarriages and reported microwave or shortwave diathermy equipment use during the first trimester of pregnancy or in the 6 months preceding pregnancy were examined (102). They reported an exposure-response gradient for use of microwave diathermy equipment but not for shortwave diathermy. Critics have pointed out, however, that the results are not very plausible because shortwave diathermy would be more likely than microwave diathermy to penetrate to the embryo or early fetus (103). Kallen et al. (104) studied 2,018 Swedish physiotherapists and found that the incidences of perinatal death, serious malformations, short gestational duration, and low birth weight were below expectation in this group. In a nested case-control study they found a suggestive association between adverse pregnancy outcomes (dead or malformed infant) and work with shortwave equipment during pregnancy. However, a later study based on an overlapping cohort found no exposure-related gradients in reproductive risks (105). Another study found no association between shortwave irradiation among female physiotherapists and birth weight or gender ratio of offspring (106).

A preliminary report of a study received much publicity when it purported to show an association between Down syndrome and paternal occupational exposure to radar (107). However, when the study was subsequently enlarged and more detailed exposure information was obtained, the suggested excess was not confirmed (108).

Two studies have been conducted of congenital defects among offspring of physical therapists exposed in varying degrees to diathermy machines. A study of male physiotherapists found no association between diathermy exposure and congenital defects in offspring (109). On the other hand, a study of female physiotherapists found a statistically significant association between reported frequency of work with or near diathermy machines during pregnancy and a grouping of congenital malformations and perinatal deaths (104). Closer inspection of the results, however, revealed that there was little commonality among the eight malformations, and one of the three perinatal deaths was clearly unrelated to exposure (due to Rh factor incompatibility). There was also an indication of recall bias; two of the three "unrelated" exposure items they included as a methodologic check showed trends suggestive of recall bias.

### Hematopoietic, Immune Systems, and Neuroendocrine Effects

The National Council on Radiation Protection and Measurements has reviewed the experimental literature on adverse effects of radiofrequency and microwave radiation on the hematopoietic and immune systems and concluded there was no clear evidence of nonthermogenic effects (89; see also ref. 110). Neuroendocrine effects appear to be related to nonspecific stress and to metabolic changes (111), and there are thresholds at or above SARs of 4 W/kg (10 times the maximum allowable occupational exposure level) for these effects.

There have been few evaluations of these systems in human studies, although there are a number of reports from Eastern Europe that are difficult to interpret because of methodologic deficiencies (110,112), and they will not be reviewed here. The study of the U.S. embassy in Moscow, conducted because of microwaves the Soviets had beamed at the embassy, found no excess of morbidity due to blood diseases in comparison with that in employees at other Eastern European U.S. embassies (113). Although high lymphocyte counts were found among the Moscow embassy employees, they proved not to correlate with microwave exposure.

A Polish study conducted medical examinations of about 500 workers exposed to high levels (average power density over 0.2 $mW/cm^2$) and 330 exposed to low levels (114). No differences between the two groups were found for a class of conditions that included endocrine and hematopoietic disorders. Barron and Baraff (101) conducted medical examinations of 335 radar workers and 100 controls and found no meaningful difference between the two groups in red cell, white cell, or differential count, nor did they find any abnormal level of globulins among the exposed workers. A study of 20,700 U.S. Navy personnel with potentially high exposure to radar showed no excess of endocrine, metabolic or allergic diseases or hematopoietic diseases as compared with 20,100 personnel exposed to low levels (115).

### Neurologic, Behavioral, and Psychological–Psychiatric Effects

Experimental disruption of the blood-brain barrier has been reported in rats from high-power microwave exposures (SAR over 200 W/kg) (116), but lower-level exposures do not appear to affect the blood-brain barrier (117). Efflux in vivo of calcium ions from cat brains produced by amplitude-modulated RF energy at certain "frequency windows" has been reported, but the significance of this finding is unknown (118).

A number of animal studies have documented behavioral impairment following short-term exposure to microwaves at levels that produce thermal and metabolic stress effects (89). Thresholds of behavioral impairment appear to be in the range of whole-body averaged SARs of 4 to 8 W/kg, which are 10 to 20 times the permitted occupational level (94). At lower exposure levels investigators generally have not found impairment on tests that index nervous system development (119). A recent study at lower microwave exposure levels showed that exposure did not affect learning but it did disrupt performance of a previously acquired task (i.e., memory). The animals performance levels returned to baseline after exposure ceased (119). A major gap in the experimental database on behavioral effects is that most microwave studies have used short-term exposure; little is known of the effects of long-term low-level exposure (89).

Prior to the establishment of worker safety limits for RF and microwave radiation, there were reports of uncontrolled studies from a number of Eastern European and other countries of autonomic and central nervous system disturbances and "radio wave sickness," which was a complex of symptoms including headache, dizziness, loss of memory and concentration, irritability, sleep disturbance, weakness, decrease in libido, chest pains, tremor of hands, hypochondria, depression, and anxiety (1,88). Since these symptoms are also typical of stress situations, the question can be raised of whether they resulted from microwave radiation or from other stressors in the work environment. Silverman (120) has provided an excellent review of these and other studies of neurologic and psychiatric effects.

Human studies with adequate control groups have generally failed to demonstrate neurologic and psychiatric effects of microwave exposure (101,113–115). Whether the discrepancy between these findings and those of the older clinical studies is due to lower exposure levels in recent decades or to inadequacies of the older studies is not known. A limitation of some of the more recent studies (113,115) is that they consist of only records and reports of neuropsychiatric morbidity, which may underdetermine these end points in comparison with a standardized neuropsychiatric examination. Nevertheless, the controlled studies have more credence than the earlier inadequately controlled clinical ones.

### Cataractogenic Effects

A review of the experimental literature concluded that no well-documented studies show lens changes or cataracts to result from exposure levels less than about 10 $mW/cm^2$. The threshold for irreversible changes is about 150 $mW/cm^2$ for a single 100-minute exposure (1). Most mechanistic studies have concluded that thermal effects are central to cataractogenesis, although there may be photochemical effects as well (121). A recent review of the subject indicated the heat-labile antioxidant enzymes, such as glutathione peroxidase, are inactivated so that protein sulfhydryl groups are oxidized and high molecular weight aggregates are formed. These changes alter the orderly structure of the lens's cells, which is crucial for its translucency (122). A comparison of continuous and pulsed microwave exposure indicates that the average power level rather than peak power level is the determinant of ocular injury (123).

The first case of microwave cataractogenesis was reported in 1952 in a 20-year-old radar worker, and, in all, more than 50 reported cases presumably have been induced by microwaves (89). Most studies conducted more recently have failed to find any microwave-associated ocular disease. Findings of three medical record-based studies have been negative: the aforementioned study of 20,000 Naval radar workers (115), a case-control study of 2,900 Army and Air Force veterans with cataracts and 2,100 without cataracts (124), and the Moscow U.S. embassy study (113). Of the studies that included ocular examinations, two showed suggestive effects. An Australian study (125) showed an increased prevalence of posterior subcapsular opacities among a group of 53 radio linemen, but the power densities around their work areas were sometimes very high (up to 3900 mW/cm$^2$). In a larger study in the United States in the early 1960s, Cleary et al. (124) found an apparent association between (subclinical) lenticular opacities and estimated microwave exposure, but measured power densities were not available. On the other hand, ocular examination studies by a number of other investigators have shown no increase in lenticular opacities or other ocular damage related to microwave exposure (101,114, 126–129). In these studies the workers generally were exposed to power densities less than 10 mW/cm$^2$, so the data suggest that maintaining exposure below this level affords protection against cataractogenic effects.

### Cancer Induction

Only a few human studies have evaluated cancer as an end point. Neither the Moscow U.S. embassy study (113) nor a Polish evaluation of radar workers (114) showed any evidence of excess cancer induction among exposed persons, but these studies were too small, and the embassy exposure levels too low, to have much statistical power to detect carcinogenic effects. In a case-control study of 424 adult brain tumor deaths and 381 control deaths, next of kin were interviewed about occupational exposure to microwave or RF sources. Once they removed persons who had received EMF exposures through electronics or electrical jobs, there was no association with microwave or RF exposure (25). A recent study of occupational factors for breast cancer did not find support for an association with RF fields (68). A U.S. Air Force study showed a borderline risk for brain tumors in relation to RF/microwave exposure (RR = 1.4, 95% CI = 1.0–1.9) (130). The best cancer study to date is a U.S. Naval study in which about 20,000 persons who potentially had high microwave exposures were compared to 20,000 with little exposure (115). No increase in total cancer rate was found in the exposed group, although there was a suggestion of more leukemias. An updated follow-up of this population would be valuable to provide further evidence on this question. Another study found what appeared to be a gradient of risk for several cancers in relation to proximity to a TV and FM-radio transmitter, but an attempt to replicate it near other transmitters did not support the initial findings (131,132).

### Cellular Telephones and Brain Tumors

Most portable cellular telephones currently employ signals in the 804- to 894-MHz range, although those in the near future will use higher frequencies (1,800–2,200 MHz) and lower average power levels. Cellular telephones automatically adjust their power levels to maintain a connection; thus, calls from telephones farther from the cell site or those with obstructions between the telephone and the cell cite will result in increased power output. The magnetic field specific absorption rate (SAR) attenuates rapidly in tissue, with a half-value layer of about 1.5 cm, so the tissues with the largest exposure are the glial/meningeal tissue at the outermost surface of the lower anterior portion of the parietal lobe and the bone marrow overlaying it, the acoustic nerve and the parotid gland, and only on the side of the head where the telephone is placed (133). At this point, substantial epidemiologic studies of cellular telephones and brain tumors have not yet been reported, although several studies will be completed in the next year or two.

## ULTRAVIOLET RADIATION

Although as early as 1894 Unna hypothesized that sunlight causes skin cancer, it was not until 1928 that Findlay confirmed it by producing skin cancer on an animal using ultraviolet radiation (UVR) (134). UV-B has both initiating and promoting actions in skin carcinogenesis (135). The carcinogenic action of UV-B is thought to be associated with the formation of pyrimidine dimers, which, when misrepaired, result in point mutations. Defects in the repair of these dimers is a primary reason for the great susceptibility of xeroderma pigmentosum patients to skin cancer (136). A good summary of experimental studies of the biologic effects of UVR is found elsewhere (137).

UV-B damage to the skin also causes photoaging—wrinkling, mottled pigmentation, coarseness, telangiectasia, laxity, and atrophy of the skin. Although this is usually of limited medical significance, it is of economic import; in the United States more than $12 billion is spent annually on cosmetics to camouflage aging skin.

About 3% of the sun's electromagnetic output is emitted as UVR, but only a fraction reaches the surface of the earth. UV-C (240 to 290 nm) is virtually eliminated by ozone in the stratosphere and troposphere, while only a fraction of UV-B (290- to 320-nm wavelengths) reaches the earth's surface. The reliability of temporal data on stratospheric ozone concentrations is limited, but it has been estimated that concentrations have declined about 2% over the past 20 years, at least in part because of increases in environmental chlorofluorocarbons (138). This 2% decrease is thought to increase the biologically effective solar radiation by approximately 4%, which in turn will likely increase nonmelanotic skin cancer by 6% to 12% and cutaneous melanoma by about 3% to 4% (139). Chlorofluorocarbons (CFCs) are a primary concern because of their capacity to destroy stratospheric ozone. CFCs have been banned as spray-can propellants in the United States, and they are being phased out in other applications, such as air conditioning and refrigeration. CFC production had been growing worldwide at a rate of 5% per year (140) until an international agreement was reached to limit their production. Even so, they will continue to accumulate in the upper atmosphere for many years because of the slow rate at which existing CFCs will be released into the environment and their slow degradation (138).

The projected effects of ozone depletion on skin cancer risk, however, pale in comparison to the changes in rates that are already occurring, apparently owing to lifestyle changes in patterns of sun exposure. The incidence of both nonmelanotic skin cancer and cutaneous melanoma has been rising at an annual rate of 3% to 8% in Caucasian populations in the United States, Europe, and Australia since the 1960s (139,141). Stated differently, rates of cutaneous malignant melanoma have risen by a factor of 3.5 and of squamous cell carcinoma by a factor of 3 over the past 25 years (142). Interestingly, this rise in rates is not just a generational effect (i.e., where a new generation has higher rates); rather, the increase is being seen in adults of all ages.

## Cutaneous Malignant Melanoma

Because there is no good animal model for cutaneous malignant melanoma, most of our knowledge about its causation has come from epidemiologic studies. These studies generally have not found that melanoma risk is related to cumulative long-term sun exposure. Several of the epidemiologic studies have found that the frequency of severe sunburns, especially in childhood and adolescence, is predictive of malignant melanoma risk (143). Similarly, studies of migrants to Australia, where the level of insolation is high, have shown that migration at early ages confers much more melanoma risk than migration in adulthood (143).

Genetic factors appear to play a significant role in the causation of cutaneous malignant melanoma. There is appreciable evidence that the dysplastic nevus syndrome, or at least a tendency toward developing nevi, is a major risk factor for melanoma. In one large study, persons with five or more raised nevi on their arms, who also had a history of severe sunburn episodes in childhood, had 24 times the melanoma risk of those who had neither risk factor (144).

There has been concern about exposure to artificial sources of UVR. Appreciable UVR is given off by welding equipment. Gas arc lamps, including fluorescent bulbs, are another source. Early suntan lamps of the low-pressure mercury type emitted approximately 65% of their energy as UV-B. The newer tanning lamps emit 95% to 99% of their energy as UV-A, which is less carcinogenic. There is little information on whether suntan lamps pose a risk of skin cancer. One study found an elevated melanoma risk among suntan lamp users and showed a dose-response relationship with amount of use (145); however, the study did not control for amount of exposure to natural sunlight, which one might suspect would be correlated with suntan lamp use and would confound the results. Common fluorescent lights, which emit fairly low levels of UV-B and UV-C, became a matter of concern after a couple of early studies suggested they conferred risk for malignant melanoma. However, a number of other studies have now shown essentially negative results for this source of exposure (144,146).

## Nonmelanotic Skin Cancer

Nonmelanotic skin cancer appears to be more related to cumulative long-term sun exposure than melanoma is. For example, one study found that persons with evidence of severe actinic skin damage had ten times as much risk of basal cell carcinomas as those with no actinic damage (135). There is evidence from migrant studies and case-control studies that repeated exposure in childhood may be important in the causation of nonmelanotic skin cancers (147,148). Several studies have shown that persons who receive a psoralen plus UV-A (PUVA) for the treatment of psoriasis have great risk of cutaneous squamous cell carcinomas, particularly of the scrotum (149–151). However, several European studies have not demonstrated induction of squamous cell cancer by PUVA (152,153). The discrepancy among the studies may have occurred because of differences in the intensity and duration of treatment or in other factors.

Prevention of skin cancer is a topic of importance, given the high and rising rates of skin cancers. Since over 60% of the total solar UV-B that reaches the earth does so between 10 A.M. and 3 P.M., added sun protection during these hours is clearly important (154). It has been estimated that about three-fourths of nonmelanotic skin cancers (and probably an appreciable fraction of melanomas) could be prevented if adequate sunscreen protection were routinely applied to children (148). Older sunscreen formulations were effective mainly against UV-B. The long periods of sunbathing that are possible without burning when a person uses a sunscreen may allow the skin to receive unnaturally large doses of UV-A, so it was recognized that formulations that protect against both UV-B and UV-A were needed, and they have now become available. It is thought that regular use of a sunscreen with a sun protection factor (SPF) of 15 or higher for the first two decades of life could decrease lifetime risk of nonmelanotic skin cancer by 70% to 80% (139).

Ultraviolet radiation also damages the eye. UV-A causes corneal damage and cortical opacities, while UV-B leads to both cortical and anterior pole opacities (155,156). Both acute and chronic UVR can have cataractogenic effects (157). A wavelength of 300 nm is most effective in producing cataracts. UV-A in the range 325 to 440 nm and blue light are especially damaging to the retina (158,159).

## EXPOSURE TO ULTRASOUND

Ultrasound is commonly classified as nonionizing radiation, even though it is mechanical and not electromagnetic. The first ultrasound device was invented in 1917. The earliest use of ultrasound was in detecting submarines, but today it has many industrial and laboratory uses, such as cleaning and degreasing, plastic welding, liquid extraction, atomization, and homogenization (160). Ultrasound has been used in medical diagnostics and therapy for more than 50 years. Therapeutic uses include treatment of Meniere's disease, cataract surgery, renal lithotripsy, and physical therapy for joint and soft tissue ailments (161). Diagnostic ultrasonography is valuable for detecting brain lesions, thyroid abnormalities, intraocular pathology, functional and morphologic abnormalities of the heart, and hepatic, pancreatic, renal, and obstetric disease. Detailed reviews of the physical, biologic, and safety aspects of ultrasound can be found elsewhere (160–165).

Experimental studies have presented a variety of findings concerning hazardous effects on different organs and physiologic processes. Ultrasound exposure of the uterus of mice led to a reduction in fetal weight (166,167), although the levels were such that this may have been attributable to temperature elevation (168). Above a rather high threshold level, central nervous system lesions can also be produced in mice by ultrasound. The threshold is age dependent, being about a fourth as high for neonatal mice as for adults (164). There have been both negative and positive reports of ultrasound's effects on spermatogenesis, fertility, and dominant lethal mutations (169).

Ultrasonography is widely used by obstetricians to monitor fetal growth and development. More than half of all pregnant women in the United States undergo at least one ultrasound examination. Because the developing organism is thought to be especially susceptible to adverse effects, most human studies of possible hazards from ultrasound have been directed toward exposure *in utero*.

Several studies have examined birth weight and other indicators of status at birth in relation to fetal ultrasound exposure. Most findings have been negative (170,171). In the one study that was apparently positive (172), the association between sonography and low-birth weight likely occurred because pregnancies examined with multiple sonograms had more maternal and fetal risk factors to begin with. Of six randomized controlled trials of the effects of ultrasound, only one suggested that it was associated with lower birth weight, while two of them found that ultrasound was instrumental in detecting fetuses that were small for gestational age, so that mothers received more active interventions and had fewer low birth weight children (173–178). Other studies have examined height and weight at later ages (up to 12 years) and have found no differences between ultrasound-exposed and -unexposed children (170,171,179). Several studies of chromosome abnormalities following ultrasound exposure have also been negative (161).

A few studies have looked at a variety of developmental, neurologic, behavioral, and psychometric outcomes at various ages in relation to fetal ultrasound exposure. Scheidt (180) found no differences between ultrasound-exposed and unexposed groups for history of infections, hearing loss, history of convulsions or paralysis, developmental delay, or behavioral indicators of central nervous system damage. Another study reported no evidence of speech disorders, hearing disorders, or developmental problems [cited in reference (161)].

The most extensive study, by Stark and colleagues (171), evaluated Apgar scores, gestational age, head circumference, birth weight and length, congenital anomalies, and infections among newborns in relation to fetal ultrasound exposure. The children were followed up, and at age 7 to 12 years were evaluated for auditory discrimination ability, nerve deafness, visual acuity, color perception, history of childhood diseases and hospitalizations, intelligence test scores, verbal and arithmetic achievement scores, reading disability, and behavioral deficits. Among this battery of measures the only adverse effect possibly seen was a greater frequency of dyslexia, as assessed by the reading test, among ultrasound-exposed children. This finding may represent a false-positive result associated with the many statistical tests performed.

One of the randomized controlled trials of ultrasound has now followed the children until 8 to 9 years of age (181). The authors obtained information on intelligence and on reading, spelling, and arithmetic performance in school for 2,000 study children and found no differences between the ultrasound-screened group and the controls. A subsample of 600 was administered specific tests for dyslexia; the relative risk for dyslexia among the screened children was only 0.8.

In summary, the human findings on the possible risks from ultrasound exposure are virtually all negative, although the modest samples sizes, patient selection factors, and other study limitations temper the conclusions that can be drawn. It is to be hoped that the randomized trials of fetal ultrasound screening (173–175) will provide follow-up for their populations with a broad range of evaluations that can provide answers about possible ultrasound risks that would not be confounded by patient selection factors. Another need is to more thoroughly evaluate the effects of ultrasound exposure during the first trimester of pregnancy, to determine whether teratogenesis or other effects might be caused by exposure during this critical period of organogenesis. Studies until now have had very few subjects with first-trimester exposure. In conclusion, the data now available give little cause for concern about adverse ultrasound effects at presently used power levels. However, continued comprehensive follow-up of the children born in the randomized trials will be valuable.

## REFERENCES


1. Petersen RC. Bioeffects of microwaves: a review of current knowledge. *J Occup Med* 1983;25:103–111.
2. Kavet RI, Banks R. Emerging issues in extremely-low-frequency electric and magnetic field health research. *Environ Res* 1986;39:386–404.
3. Electric Power Research Institute. *Electric and magnetic field fundamentals.* Palo Alto, CA: EPRI, 1989.
4. Savitz DA, John E, Kleckner R. Magnetic field exposure from electric appliances and childhood cancer. *Am J Epidemiol* 1990;131:763–773.
5. Theriault G. Cancer risks due to exposure to electromagnetic fields. *Recent Results Cancer Res* 1990;120:166–180.
6. Meyer RE, Aldrich T, Easterly C. Effects of noise and electromagnetic fields on reproductive outcomes. *Environ Health Perspect* 1989;81: 193–200.
7. Florig HK, Nair I, Morgan M. *Briefing paper 1:* sources and dosimetry of power-frequency fields. Technical Report, DER Contract SP117. Tallahassee, Florida: Dept. of Environmental Regulation, 1987.
8. Doll R, Beral V, Cox R, et al. *Electromagnetic fields and the risk of cancer.* Report of an advisory group on non-ionising radiation. Documents of the NRPB, vol 3(1). Chilton, Didcot, England: National Radiological Protection Board, 1992.
9. WHO. *Extremely low frequency (ELF) fields.* Environmental health criteria no. 35. Geneva: World Health Organization, 1984.
10. Kaune WT. Physical interaction of 1-Hz to 100-kHz electric and magnetic fields with living organisms. In: *Nonionizing electromagnetic radiations and ultrasound.* Proceedings No. 8. Bethesda, MD: National Council on Radiation Protection and Measurements, 1988; 129–160.
11. Tenforde TS. Biological interactions and potential health effects of extremely-low-frequency magnetic fields from power lines and other common sources. *Annu Rev Public Health* 1992;13:173–196.
12. U.S. Congress. *Biological effects of power frequency electric & magnetic fields—background paper.* OTA-BP-E-53. Washington, DC: U.S. Gov't Printing Office, 1989.
13. Frey AH. Electromagnetic field interactions with biological systems. *FASEB J* 1993;7:272–281.
14. Brent R, Gordon W, Bennett W, Beckman D. Reproductive and teratologic effects of electromagnetic fields. *Reprod Toxicol* 1993;7:535–580.
15. Graves HB. Biological effects of power frequency electric fields: an overview. In: *Nonionizing electromagnetic radiations and ultrasound.* Proceedings no. 8. Bethesda, MD: National Council on Radiation Protection and Measurements, 1988:162–178.
16. Nordstrom S, Birke E, Gustavsson L. Reproductive hazards among workers at high voltage substations. *Bioelectromagnetics* 1983;4: 91–101.
17. Bauchinger MR, Hauf R, Schmid E, Drisp J. Analysis of structural chromosome changes and SCE after occupational long-term exposure to electric and magnetic fields from 380 kV systems. *Radiat Environ Biophys* 1981;19:235–238.
18. Wertheimer N, Leeper E. Possible effects of electric blankets and heated waterbeds on fetal development. *Bioelectromagnetics* 1986;7: 13–22.
19. Wertheimer N, Leeper E. Fetal loss associated with two seasonal sources of electromagnetic field exposure. *Am J Epidemiol* 1989;129: 220–224.
20. Dlugosz L, Vena J, Byers T, Sever L, Bracken M, Marshall E. Congenital defects and electric bed heating in New York State: a register-based case-control study. *Am J Epidemiol* 1992;135:1000–1011.
21. Bracken MB, Belanger K, Hellenbrand K, et al. Exposure to electromagnetic fields during pregnancy with emphasis on electrically heated beds: association with birthweight and intrauterine growth retardation. *Epidemiology* 1995;6:263–270.
22. Wilson BW, Anderson L. ELF electromagnetic-field effects on the pineal gland. In: Wilson B, Stevens R, Anderson L, eds. *Extremely low frequency electromagnetic fields:* the question of cancer. Columbus, OH: Battelle Press, 1989;159–186.
23. Stevens RG, Wilson B, Anderson L. The question of cancer. In: Wilson B, Stevens R, Anderson L, eds. *Extremely low frequency electromagnetic fields:* the question of cancer. Columbus, OH: Battelle Press, 1989;361–370.
24. Adey WR. Frequency and power windowing in tissue interactions with weak electromagnetic fields. *Proc IEEE* 1980;68:119–125.
25. Thomas TL, Stolley P, Stemhagen A, et al. Brain tumor mortality risk among men with electrical and electronics jobs: a case-control study. *J Natl Cancer Inst* 1987;79:233–238.
26. Broadbent D, Broadbent M, Male J, Jones M. Health of workers exposed to electric fields. *Br J Ind Med* 1985;42:75–84.
27. Baroncelli P, Battisti S, Checcucci A, et al. A health examination of railway high-voltage substation workers exposed to ELF electromagnetic fields. *Am J Ind* Med 1986;10:45–55.
28. Knave B, Gamberale F, Bergstrom S, et al. Long-term exposure to electric fields: a cross-sectional epidemiologic investigation of occupationally exposed workers in high-voltage substations. *Scand J Work Environ Health* 1979;5:115–125.
29. Sobel E, Davanipour Z, Sulkava R, et al. Occupations with exposure to electromagnetic fields: a possible risk factor for Alzheimer's disease. *Am J Epidemiol* 1995;142:515–524.
30. Perry FS, Reichmanis M, Marino A, Becker R. Environmental power-frequency magnetic fields and suicide. *Health Phys* 1981;41: 267–277.
31. Michaelson SM. Influence of power frequency electric and magnetic fields on human health. *Ann NY Acad Sci* 1987;502:55–75.
32. Baris D, Armstrong B. Suicide among electric utility workers in England and Wales. *Br J Ind Med* 1990;47:788–792.
33. Poole C, Kavet R, Funch D, Donelan K, Charry J, Dreyer N. Depressive symptoms and headaches in relation to proximity of residence to an alternating-current transmission line right-of-way. *Am J Epidemiol* 1993;137:318–330.
34. Gamberale F, Olson B, Eneroth P, Lindh T, Wennberg A. Acute effects of ELF electromagnetic fields: a field study of linesmen working with 400 kV power lines. *Br J Ind Med* 1989;46:729–737.
35. Wertheimer N, Leeper E. Electrical wiring configurations and childhood cancer. *Am J Epidemiol* 1979;109:273–284.
36. Tomenius L. 50 Hz electromagnetic environment and the incidence of childhood tumors in Stockholm County. *Bioelectromagnetics* 1986;7: 191–208.
37. Savitz DA, Wachtel H, Barnes F, John E, Tvrdik J. Case-control study of childhood cancer and exposure to 60-Hz magnetic fields. *Am J Epidemiol* 1988;128:21–38.
38. London SJ, Thomas D, Bowman J, Sobel E, Cheng T, Peters J. Exposure to residential electric and magnetic fields and risk of childhood leukemia. *Am J Epidemiol* 1991;134:924–937.
39. Feychting M, Ahlbom A. Magnetic fields and cancer in children residing near Swedish high-voltage power lines. *Am J Epidemiol* 1993;138: 467–481.
40. Bracken TD, Kheifets L, Sussman S. Exposure assessment for power frequency electric and magnetic fields (EMF) and its application to epidemiologic studies. *J Expos Anal Environ Epidemiol* 1993;3:1–22.
41. Severson RK, Stevens R, Kaune W, et al. Acute nonlymphocytic

leukemia and residential exposure to power frequency magnetic fields. *Am J Epidemiol* 1988;128:10–20.
42. Feychting M, Kaune W, Savitz D, Ahlbom A. Estimating exposure in studies of residential magnetic fields and cancer: importance of short-term variability, time interval between diagnosis and measurement, and distance to power line. *Epidemiol* 1996;7:220–224.
43. Dovan T, Kaune W, Savitz D. Repeatability of measurements of residential magnetic fields and wire codes. *Bioelectromagnetics* 1993;14: 145–159.
44. Savitz D, Pearce N, Poole C. Update on methodological issues in the epidemiology of electromagnetic fields and cancer. *Environ Res* 1993; 15:558–566.
45. Friedman D, Hatch E, Tarone R, et al. Childhood exposure to magnetic fields: residential area measurements compared to personal dosimetry. *Epidemiology* 1996;7:151–155.
46. Matanoski G, Elliot E. Cancer incidence among New York Telephone Company workers, 1976–1980. Presented at DOE/EPRI Contractors Review, November 14, 1989, Portland, OR.
47. Olin R, Vagero D, Ahlbom A. Mortality experience of electrical engineers. *Br J Ind Med* 1985;42:211–212.
48. Garland FC, Shaw E, Gorham E, Garland C, White M, Sinsheimer P. Incidence of leukemia in occupations with potential electromagnetic field exposure in United States Navy personnel. *Am J Epidemiol* 1990;132:293–303.
49. Juutilainen J, Pukkala E, Laara E. Results of epidemiological cancer study among electrical workers in Finland. *J Bioelectric* 1988;7: 119–121.
50. Tornqvist S, Norell S, Ahlbom A, Knave B. Cancer in the electric power industry. *Br J Ind Med* 1986;43:212–213.
51. Vagero D, Olin R. Incidence of cancer in the electronics industry: using the new Swedish cancer environment registry as a screening instrument. *Br J Ind Med* 1983;40:188–192.
52. Vagero D, Ahlbom A, Olin R, Sahlsten S. Cancer morbidity among workers in the telecommunications industry. *Br J Ind Med* 1985;42: 191–195.
53. Wiklund K, Einhorn J, Eklund G. An application of the Swedish Cancer-Environment Registry. Leukemia among telephone operators at the Telecommunications Administration in Sweden. *Int J Epidemiol* 1981;10:373–376.
54. Alfredsson L, Hammar N, Karlehagen S. Cancer incidence among male railway engine-drivers and conductors in Sweden, 1976–90. *Cancer Caus Cont* 1996;7:377–381.
55. Armstrong B, Theriault G, Guenel P, Deadman J, Goldberg M, Heroux P. Association between exposure to pulsed electromagnetic fields and cancer in electric utility workers in Quebec, Canada, and France. *Am J Epidemiol* 1994;140:805–820.
56. Theriault G, Goldberg M, Miller A, et al. Cancer risks associated with occupational exposure to magnetic fields among electric utility workers in Ontario and Quebec, Canada, and France: 1970–1989. *Am J Epidemiol* 1994;139:550–572.
57. Savitz DA, Loomis D. Magnetic field exposure in relation to leukemia and brain cancer mortality among electric utility workers. *Am J Epidemiol* 1995;141:123–134.
58. Kheifets L, Afifi A, Buffler P, Zhang Z. Occupational electric and magnetic field exposure and brain cancer: a meta-analysis. *J Occup Environ Med* 1995;37:1327–1341.
59. Heath C. Electromagnetic field exposure and cancer: a review of epidemiologic evidence. *CA* 1996;65:29–44.
60. Stevens R. Electric power use and breast cancer: a hypothesis. *Am J Epidemiol* 1987;125:556–561.
61. Tynes T, Andersen A. Electromagnetic fields and male breast cancer (letter). *Lancet* 1990;336:1596.
62. Matanoski GM, Breysse P, Elliott E. Electromagnetic field exposure and male breast cancer. *Lancet* 1991;337:737.
63. Demers PA, Thomas D, Rosenblatt K, et al. Occupational exposure to electromagnetic fields and breast cancer in men. *Am J Epidemiol* 1991;134:340–347.
64. Loomis DP. Cancer of breast among men in electrical occupations. *Lancet* 1992;339:1482–1483.
65. Rosenbaum P, Vena J, Zielezny M, Michalek A. Occupational exposures associated with male breast cancer. *Am J Epidemiol* 1994;139:30–36.
66. Trichopoulos D. Are electric or magnetic fields affecting mortality from breast cancer in women? *J Natl Cancer Inst* 1994;86:885–886.
67. Loomis DP, Savitz D, Ananth C. Breast cancer mortality among female electrical workers in the United States. *J Natl Cancer Inst* 1994;86:921–925.
68. Cantor KP, Dosemeci M, Brinton L, Stewart P. Re: Breast cancer mortality among female electrical workers in the United States. *J Natl Cancer Inst* 1995;87:227–228.
69. Guenel P, Raskmark P, Andersen J, Lynge E. Incidence of cancer in persons with occupational exposure to electromagnetic fields in Denmark. *Br J Ind Med* 1993;50:758–764.
70. Coogan P, Clapp R, Newcomb P, et al. Occupational exposure to 60-hertz magnetic fields and risk of breast cancer in women. *Epidemiology* 1996;7:459–464.
71. McDowall ME. Mortality of persons resident in the vicinity of electricity transmission facilities. *Br J Cancer* 1986;53:271–279.
72. Schreiber GH, Swaen G, Meijers J, Slangen J, Sturmans F. Cancer mortality and residence near electricity transmission equipment: a retrospective cohort study. *Int J Epidemiol* 1993;22:9–15.
73. Li C-Y, Theriault G, Lin R. Residential exposure to 60-Hertz magnetic fields and adult cancers in Taiwan. *Epidemiology* 1997;8:25–30.
74. Vena JE, Graham S, Hellmann R, Swanson M, Brasure J. Use of electric blankets and risk of postmenopausal breast cancer. *Am J Epidemiol* 1991;134:180–185.
75. Shellock FG. Biological effects and safety aspects of magnetic resonance imaging. *Magn Reson Q* 1989;5:243–261.
76. Beers GJ. Biological effects of weak electromagnetic fields from 0 Hz to 200 Hz: a survey of the literature with special emphasis on possible magnetic resonance effects. *Magn Reson Imaging* 1989;7: 309–331.
77. Budinger TF. Safety of NMR in vivo imaging and spectroscopy. In: *Nonionizing electromagnetic radiations and ultrasound.* Proceedings no. 8. Bethesda, MD: National Council on Radiation Protection and Measurements, 1988;265–283.
78. WHO. *Magnetic fields.* Environmental Health Criteria 69. Geneva: World Health Organization, 1987.
79. Kanal E, Shellock F, Talagala L. Safety considerations in MR imaging. *Radiology* 1990;176:593–606.
80. Kanal E, Gillen J, Evans J, Savitz D, Shellock F. Survey of reproductive health among female MR workers. *Radiology* 1993;187:395–399.
81. Barregard L, Jarvholm B, Ungethum E. Cancer among workers exposed to strong static magnetic fields. *Lancet* 1985;2:892.
82. Marsh JL, Amstrong T, Jacobson A, Smith R. Health effects of occupational exposure to steady magnetic fields. *Am Ind Hyg Assoc J* 1982;43:387–394.
83. Milham S. Mortality in aluminum reduction plant workers. *J Occup* Med 1979;21:475–480.
84. Mur JM, Moulin J, Meyer-Bisch C, Massin N, Coulon J, Loulergue J. Mortality of aluminum reduction plant workers in France. *Int J Epidemiol* 1987;16:257–264.
85. Rockette HE, Arena V. Mortality studies of aluminum reduction plant workers: potroom and carbon department. *J Occup Med* 1983;25: 549–557.
86. Budinger TF, Bristol K, Yen C, Wong P. Biological effects of static magnetic fields. Presented at 3rd Annual Meeting of Society for Magnetic Resonance in Medicine, New York, 1984:
87. Janes DE, Jr. Radiation surveys—measurement of leakage emissions and potential exposure fields. *Bull NY Acad Med* 1979;55: 1021–1041.
88. WHO. *Radiofrequency and microwaves.* Environmental health criteria 16. Geneva: World Health Organization, 1981.
89. NCRP. *Biological effects and exposure criteria for radiofrequency electromagnetic fields.* NCRP report no. 86. Bethesda, MD: National Council on Radiation Protection and Measurements, 1986.
90. NCRP. *Radiofrequency electromagnetic fields. Properties, quantities and units, biophysical interaction, and measurements.* Report no. 67. Bethesda, MD: National Council on Radiation Protection and Measurements, 1981.
91. Stuchly MS. Interaction of radiofrequency and microwave radiation with living systems: a review of mechanisms. *Radiat Environ Biophys* 1979;16:1–14.
92. Wilkening GM. Protection against nonionizing electromagnetic radiation, an evolutionary process. In: *Radiation protection today—the NCRP at sixty years.* Proceedings No. 11 (1989).Bethesda, MD: National Council on Radiation Protection and Measurements, 1990;235–249.
93. Tell RA. The state of the art in measuring electromagnetic fields for hazard assessment. In: *Radiation protection today—the NCRP at sixty years.* Proceedings No. 11 (1989).Bethesda, MD: National Council on Radiation Protection and Measurements, 1990;251–261.
94. Wilkening GM. Biomedical effects of microwave radiation. *Bull NY Acad Med* 1979;55:1047.

95. Jensh RP. Studies of the teratogenic potential exposure of rats to 6000-MHz microwave radiation. I. Morphologic analysis at term. *Radiat Res* 1984;97:272–281.
96. Jensh RP, Weinberg I, Brent R. An evaluation of the teratogenic potential of protracted exposure of pregnant rats to 2450-Mz microwave radiation: I. Morphologic analysis at term. *J Toxicol Environ Health* 1983;11:23–35.
97. Jensh RP. Studies of the teratogenic potential of exposure of rats to 6000-MHz microwave radiation. II. Postnatal psychophysiologic evaluations. *Radiat Res* 1984;97:282–301.
98. Berman E, Kinn J, Carter H. Observations of mouse fetuses after irradiation with 2.45-GHz microwaves. *Health Phys* 1978;35:791–801.
99. Saunders RD, Kowalczuk C, Beechey C, Dunford R. Studies of the induction of dominant lethals and translocations in male mice after chronic exposure to microwave radiation. *Int J Radiat Biol* 1988;53: 983–992.
100. Leonard A, Berteaud A, Bruyere A. An evaluation of the mutagenic, carcinogenic and teratogenic potential of microwaves. *Mutat Res* 1983;123:31–46.
101. Barron C, Baraff A. Medical considerations of exposure to micro waves (radar). *JAMA* 1958;168:1194–1199.
102. Ouellet-Hellstrom R, Stewart W. Miscarriages among female physical therapists who report using radio- and microwave-frequency electromagnetic radiation. *Am J Epidemiol* 1993;138:775–786.
103. Hocking B, Joyner K. Re: "Miscarriages among female physical therapists who report using radio- and microwave-frequency electromagnetic radiation" (Letter). *Am J Epidemiol* 1995;141:273–274.
104. Kallen B, Malmquist G, Moritz U. Delivery outcome among physiotherapists in Sweden: Is non-ionizing radiation a fetal hazard? *Arch Environ Health* 1982;37:81–85.
105. Taskinen H, Kyyronen P, Hemminki K. Effects of ultrasound, shortwaves, and physical exertion on pregnancy outcome in physiotherapists. *J Epidemiol Commun Health* 1990;44:196–201.
106. Guberan E, Campana A, Faval P, et al. Gender ratio of offspring and exposure to shortwave radiation among female physiotherapists. *Scand J Work Environ Health* 1994;20:345–348.
107. Sigler A, Lilienfeld A, Cohen B, et al. Radiation exposure in parents of children with mongolism (Down's syndrome). *Bull Johns Hopkins Hosp* 1965;117:374–399.
108. Cohen BH, Lilienfeld A, Kramer S, et al. Parental factors in Down's syndrome—results of the second Baltimore case-control study. In: Hook E, Porter I, eds. *Population cytogenetics, studies in humans.* New York: Academic Press, 1977;301–352.
109. Logue JN, Hamburger S, Silverman P, Chiacchierini R. Congenital anomalies and paternal occupational exposure to shortwave, microwave, infrared, and acoustic radiation. *J Occup Med* 1985;27: 451–452.
110. Smialowicz RJ. Hematologic and immunologic effects of nonionizing electromagnetic radiation. *Bull NY Acad Med* 1979;55:1094–1118.
111. Lu S, Lotz W, Michaelson M. Advances in microwave-induced neuroendocrine effects: the concept of stress. *Proc IEEE* 1977;68:73–77.
112. Cleary SF. Recapitulation: biomedical effects. *Bull NY Acad Med* 1979;55:1119–1125.
113. Pollack H. Epidemiologic data on American personnel in the Moscow embassy. *Bull NY Acad Med* 1979;55:1182–1186.
114. Czerski P, Siekierzynski M, Gidynski A. Health surveillance of personnel occupationally exposed to microwaves. I. Theoretical considerations and practical aspects. *Aerospace Med* 1974;45:1137–1142.
115. Robinette CD, Silverman C, Jablon S. Effects upon health of occupational exposure to microwave radiation (radar). *Am J Epidemiol* 1980; 112:39–53.
116. Lin JC, Lin M. Microwave hyperthermia-induced blood-brain barrier alterations. *Radiat Res* 1982;89:77–87.
117. Justesen DR. Microwave irradiation and the blood-brain barrier. *Proc IEEE* 1967;68:60–67.
118. Wilkening GM, Sutton C. Health effects of nonionizing radiation. *Med Clin North Am* 1990;74:489–507.
119. O'Connor ME. Behavioral effects regarding exposure to nonionizing electromagnetic radiation. In: *Nonionizing electromagnetic radiations and ultrasound.* NCRP proceedings no. 8. Bethesda, MD: National Council on Radiation Protection and Measurements, 1988;65–78.
120. Silverman C. Nervous and behavioral effects of microwave radiation in humans. *Am J Epidemiol* 1973;97:219–224.
121. Carpenter RL, Hagan G, Donovan G. Are microwave cataracts thermally caused? In: Hazzard DG, ed. *Symposium on biological effects and measurements of radio frequency/microwaves.* U.S. DHEW publication (FDA)77-8026. Rockville, MD: Food and Drug Administration, 1977;352–372.
122. Lipman RM, Tripathi B, Tripathi R. Cataracts induced by microwave and ionizing radiation. *Surv Ophthalmol* 1988;33:200–210.
123. Birenbaum L, Grosof G, Rosenthal S, Zaret M. Effect of microwaves on the eye. *IEEE Trans Biomed Eng* 1969;16(1):7–14.
124. Cleary SF, Pasternack B, Beebe G. Cataract incidence in radar workers. *Arch Environ Health* 1965;11:179–182.
125. Hollows FC, Douglas J. Microwave cataract in radiolinemen and controls. *Lancet* 1984;2:406–407.
126. Appleton B. Microwave cataracts. *JAMA* 1974;229:407–408.
127. Siekierzynski M, Czerski P, Gidynski A, et al. Health surveillance of personnel occupationally exposed to microwaves. III. Lens translucency. *Aerospace Med* 1974;45:1146–1148.
128. Shacklett DE, Tredici T, Epstein D. Evaluation of possible microwave-induced lens changes in the United States Air Force. *Aviat Space Environ Med* 1975;46:1403–1406.
129. Hathaway JA, Stern N, Soles O, Leighton E. Ocular medical surveillance on microwave and laser workers. *J Occup Med* 1977;19:683–688.
130. Grayson J. Radiation exposure, socioeconomic status, and brain tumor risk in the US Air Force: a nested case-control study. *Am J Epidemiol* 1996;143:480–486.
131. Dolk H, Shaddick G, Walls P, et al. Cancer incidence near radio and television transmitters in Great Britain. I. Sutton Coldfield transmitter. *Am J Epidemiol* 1997;145:1–9.
132. Dolk H, Elliott P, Shaddick G, Walls P, Thakrar B. Cancer incidence near radio and television transmitters in Great Britain. II. All high power transmitters. *Am J Epidemiol* 1997;145:10–17.
133. Rothman K, Chou C, Morgan R, et al. Assessment of cellular telephone and other radio frequency exposure for epidemiologic research. *Epidemiology* 1996;7:291–298.
134. Gordon D, Silverstone H. Worldwide epidemiology of premalignant and malignant cutaneous lesions. In: Andrade R, Gumport S, Popkin G, Rees T, eds. *Cancer of the skin, biology-diagnosis-management,* vol 1. Philadelphia: Saunders, 1976;405–434.
135. Rogers GS, Gilchrest B. The senile epidermis: environmental influences on skin ageing and cutaneous carcinogenesis. *Br J Dermatol* 1990;122 (Suppl):55–60.
136. Editorial. Sunlight, DNA repair, and skin cancer. *Lancet* 1989;1: 1362–1363.
137. WHO. *Ultraviolet radiation.* Environmental health criteria no. 14. Geneva: World Health Organization, 1979.
138. Kripke ML. Impact of ozone depletion on skin cancers. *J Dermatol Surg Oncol* 1988;14:853–857.
139. Gloster H, Brodland D. The epidemiology of skin cancer. *Dermatol Surg* 1996;22:217–226.
140. Jones RR. Ozone depletion and cancer risk. *Lancet* 1987;2:443–446.
141. Armstrong B, Kricker A. Skin cancer. *Dermatol Clin* 1995;13:583–594.
142. Glass AG, Hoover R. The emerging epidemic of melanoma and squamous cell skin cancer. *JAMA* 1989;262:2097–2100.
143. Elwood JM. Melanoma and ultraviolet radiation. *Clin Dermatol* 1992;10:41–50.
144. Osterlind A, Tucker M, Stone B, Jensen O. The Danish case-control study of cutaneous malignant melanoma. II. Importance of UV-light exposure. *Int J Cancer* 1988;42:319–324.
145. Walter SD, Marrett L, From L, Hertzman C, Shannon H, Roy P. The association of cutaneous malignant melanoma with the use of sunbeds and sunlamps. *Am J Epidemiol* 1990;131:232–243.
146. International Radiation Protection Association. Fluorescent lighting and malignant melanoma. *Health Phys* 1990;58:111–112.
147. Marks R. Skin cancer—childhood protection affords lifetime protection. *Med J Aust* 1987;147:475–476.
148. Stern RS, Weinstein M, Baker S. Risk reduction for non-melanoma skin cancer with childhood sunscreen use. *Arch Dermatol* 1986;122: 537–545.
149. Stern RS, Lange R, Members of Photochemotherapy Follow-up Study. Nonmelanoma skin cancer occurring in patients treated with PUVA five to ten years after first treatment. *J Invest Dermatol* 1988;91:120–124.
150. Stern RS, Members of Photochemotherapy Follow-up Study. Genital tumors among men with psoriasis exposed to psoralens and ultraviolet A radiation (PUVA) and ultraviolet B radiation. *N Engl J Med* 1990;322:1093–1097.
151. Henseler T, Christophers E, Honigsmann H, Wolff K, al. e. Skin tumors in the European PUVA study. Eight-year follow-up of 1,643 patients treated with PUVA for psoriasis. *J Am Acad Dermatol* 1987; 16:108–116.

152. Eskelinen A, Halme K, Lassus A, Idanpaan-Heikkila J. Risk of cutaneous carcinoma in psoriatic patients treated with PUVA. *Photodermatol* 1985;2:10–14.
153. MacKie RM, Fitzsimons C. Risk of carcinogenicity in patients with psoriasis treated with methotrexate or PUVA singly or in combination. *J Am Acad Dermatol* 1983;9:467–469.
154. Urbach F, Bailar J, Gori G, Demopoulos H, Garfinkel L. Ultraviolet radiation and skin cancer in man. *Prev Med* 1980;9:227–230.
155. Zuclich JA. Cumulative effects of near-ultraviolet induced corneal damage. *Health Phys* 1980;38(5):833–838.
156. Schmitt C, Schmidt J, Wegener A, Hockwin O. Ultraviolet radiation as a risk factor in cataractogenesis. In: Hockwin O, Sasaki K, Leske M, eds. *Risk factors for cataract development.* New York: Karger, 1989; 169–172.
157. Lerman S. Human ultraviolet radiation cataracts. *Ophthalmic Res* 1980;12:303–314.
158. West SK, Rosenthal F, Bressler N, et al. Exposure to sunlight and other risk factors for age-related macular degeneration. *Arch Ophthalmol* 1989;107:875–879.
159. AMA Council On Scientific Affairs. Harmful effects of ultraviolet radiation. *JAMA* 1989;262:380–384.
160. WHO. *Ultrasound.* Environmental health criteria #22. Geneva: World Health Organization, 1982.
161. Ziskin MC. Ultrasound: medical applications and medical exposures. In: Sinclair WK, ed. *Nonionizing electromagnetic radiations and ultrasound.* Proceedings No. 8. Bethesda, MD: National Council on Radiation Protection and Measurements, 1986;308–328.
162. Carson PL. Medical ultrasound fields and exposure measurements. In: *Nonionizing electromagnetic radiations and ultrasound.* Proceedings No. 8. Bethesda, MD: National Council on Radiation Protection and Measurements, 1988;287–307.
163. NCRP. *Biological effects of ultrasound:* mechanisms and clinical implications. NCRP report no. 74. Bethesda, MD: National Council on Radiation Protection and Measurements, 1983.
164. Dunn F. Biological effects of ultrasound. In: Sinclair WK, ed. *Nonionizing electromagnetic radiations and ultrasound.* Proceedings no. 8. Bethesda, MD: National Council on Radiation Protection and Measurements, 1986;329–346.
165. NCRP. *Protection in nuclear medicine and ultrasound diagnostic procedures in children.* Report no. 73. Bethesda, MD: National Council on Radiation Protection and Measurements, 1983.
166. Stolzenberg SJ, Torbit C, Edmonds P, Taenzer J. Effects of ultrasound on the mouse exposed at different stages of gestation: acute studies. *Radiat Environ Biophys* 1980;17:245.
167. Hande MP, Devi P. Teratogenic effects of repeated exposures to x-rays and/or ultrasound in mice. *Neurotoxicol Teratol* 1995;17:179–188.
168. O'Brien WD. Dose-dependent effect of ultrasound on fetal weight in mice. *J Ultrasound Med* 1983;2:1–8.
169. Brent RL, Jensh R, Beckman D. Medical sonography: reproductive effects and risks. *Teratology* 1991;44:123–146.
170. Lyons EA, Dyke C, Toms M, Cheang M. In utero exposure to diagnostic ultrasound: a 6-year follow-up. *Radiology* 1988;166(3):686–693.
171. Stark CR, Orleans M, Haverkamp A, Murphy J. Short- and long-term risks after exposure to diagnostic ultrasound in utero. *Obstet Gynecol* 1984;63:194–200.
172. Moore RM, Diamond E, Cavalieri R. The relationship of birth weight and intrauterine diagnostic ultrasound exposure. *Obstet Gynecol* 1988;71:513–517.
173. Saari-Kemppainen A, Karjalainen O, Ylostalo P, Heinonen O. Ultrasound screening and perinatal mortality: controlled trial of systematic one-stage screening in pregnancy. *Lancet* 1990;336:387–391.
174. Bakketeig LS, Eik-Nes S, Jacobsen G, et al. Randomised controlled trial of ultrasonographic screening in pregnancy. *Lancet* 1984;2: 207–210.
175. Wladimiroff JW, Laar J. Ultrasonic measurement of fetal body size. *Acta Obstet Gynecol Scand* 1980;59:177–179.
176. Waldenstrom U, Axelsson O, Nilsson S, Fall GEO, Lindeberg S, Sjodin Y. Effects of routine one-stage ultrasound screening in pregnancy: a randomised controlled trial. *Lancet* 1988;2:585–588.
177. Ewigman B, LeFevre M, Hesser J. A randomized trial of routine prenatal ultrasound. *Obstet Gynecol* 1990;76:189–194.
178. Newnham JP, Evans S, Michael C, Stanley F, Landau L. Effects of frequent ultrasound during pregnancy: a randomised controlled trial. *Lancet* 1993;342:887–891.
179. Macdonald W, Newnham J, Gurrin L, Evans S, Western Australian Pregnancy Cohort Working Group. Effect of frequent prenatal ultrasound on birthweight: follow up at 1 year of age. *Lancet* 1996; 348:482.
180. Scheidt PC, Stanley F, Bryla D. One-year follow-up of infants exposed to ultrasound in utero. *Am J Obstet Gynecol* 1978;131:743–748.
181. Salvesen KA, Bakketeig L, Eik-Nes S, Undheim J, Okland O. Routine ultrasonography in utero and school performance at age 8-9 years. *Lancet* 1992;339:85–89.
182. Myers A, Clayden A, Cartwright R, Cartwright S. Childhood cancer and overhead powerlines: a case-control study. *Br J Cancer* 1990;62: 1008–1014.
183. Coleman MP, Bell C, Taylor H, Primic-Zakelj M. Leukemia and residence near electricity transmission equipment: a case-control study. *Br J Cancer* 1989;60:793–798.
184. Olsen JH, Nielsen A, Schulgen G. Residence near high voltage facilities and risk of cancer in children. *Br Med J* 1993;307:801–805.
185. Verkasalo P, Pukkala E, Hongisto M, et al. Risk of cancer in Finnish children living close to power lines. *Br Med J* 1993;307:895–899.
186. Tynes T, Haldorsen T. Electromagnetic fields and cancer in children residing near Norwegian high-voltage power lines. *Am J Epidemiol* 1997;145:219–226.
187. Wertheimer N, Leeper E. Magnetic field exposure related to cancer subtypes. *Ann NY Acad Sci* 1987;502:43–54.
188. Youngson J, Clayden A, Myers A, Cartwright R. A case/control study of adult haematological malignancies in relation to overhead powerlines. *Br J Cancer* 1991;63:977–985.
189. Feychting M, Ahlbom A. Magnetic fields, leukemia, and central nervous system tumors in Swedish adults residing near high-voltage power lines. *Epidemiology* 1994;5:501–509.
190. Gurney J, Mueller B, Davis S, Schwartz S, Stevens R, Kopecky K. Childhood brain tumor occurrence in relation to residential power line configurations, electric heating sources, and electric appliance use. *Am J Epidemiol* 1996;143:120–128.
191. Preston-Martin S, Navidi W, Thomas D, Lee P, Bowman J, Pogoda J. Los Angeles study of residential magnetic fields and childhood brain tumors. *Am J Epidemiol* 1996;143:105–119.
192. Preston-Martin S, Gurney J, Pogoda J, Holly E, Mueller B. Brain tumor risk in children in relation to use of electric blankets and water bed heaters. *Am J Epidemiol* 1996;143:1116–1122.
193. Calle EE, Savitz D. Leukemia in occupational groups with presumed exposure to electrical and magnetic fields (letter). *N Engl J Med* 1985; 313:1476–1477.
194. Coleman M, Bell J, Skeet R. Leukaemia incidence in electrical workers (letter). *Lancet* 1983;1:982–983.
195. Gallagher RP. Occupational electromagnetic field exposure, solvent exposure, and leukemia (letter). *J Occup Med* 1990;32:64–65.
196. Gilman PA, Ames R, McCawley M. Leukemia risk among U.S. white male coal miners. *J Occup Med* 1985;27:669–671.
197. Loomis DP, Savitz D. Mortality from brain cancer and leukemia among electrical workers. *Br J Ind Med* 1990;47:633–638.
198. McDowall ME. Leukaemia mortality in electrical workers in England and Wales. *Lancet* 1983;1:246.
199. Fear N, Roman E, Carpenter L, Newton R, Bull D. Cancer in electrical workers: an analysis of cancer registrations in England, 1981–87. *Br J Cancer* 1996;73:935–939.
200. Milham S. Mortality in workers exposed to electromagnetic fields. *Environ Health Perspect* 1985;62:297–300.
201. Pearce N, Reif J, Fraser J. Case-control studies of cancer in New Zealand electrical workers. *Int J Epidemiol* 1989;18:55–59.
202. Stern F, Waxweiler R, Beaumont J, et al. A case-control study of leukemia at a naval nuclear shipyard. *Am J Epidemiol* 1986;123: 980–992.
203. Wright WE, Peters J, Mack T. Leukaemia in workers exposed to electrical and magnetic fields (letter). *Lancet* 1982;2:1160–1161.
204. London SJ, Bowman J, Sobel E, et al. Exposure to magnetic fields among electrical workers in relation to leukemia risk in Los Angeles County. *Am J Ind Med* 1994;26:47–60.

*Environmental and Occupational Medicine, Third Edition*, edited by William N. Rom.
Published by Lippincott–Raven Publishers, Philadelphia, 1998.

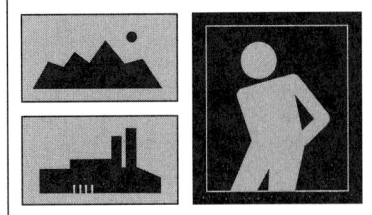

CHAPTER 100

# Occupational Health Aspects of Work with Video Display Terminals

Soo-Yee Lim, Steven L. Sauter, and Teresa M. Schnorr[1]

In 1973, Hultgren and Knave first recognized the potential health risks of video display terminal (VDT) use. Since that time, VDTs have become almost ubiquitous in the workplace, and an enormous amount of research has examined their effects on both the design of jobs and the health of workers. The National Institute for Occupational Safety and Health (NIOSH), alone, has conducted several dozen health hazard evaluations and published more than 50 scientific reports on the subject (1). It is not possible to address all of the research findings to date in this chapter; rather, the chapter focuses on key studies to summarize current views on the risks of VDT use. Ergonomic and organizational countermeasures are also discussed. While closure is emerging on some issues (e.g., effects on vision), uncertainty in other areas seems to be increasing. For example, it is becoming increasingly apparent that musculoskeletal disorders among VDT users are not a simple function of biomechanics alone. Data strongly suggest that psychosocial factors play an important etiologic role, although their relative importance and mechanisms of effect are not well understood.

This chapter addresses four health end points: visual system dysfunction, musculoskeletal disorders, stress, and adverse pregnancy outcomes. For each end point we summarize findings on the nature, prevalence, and causes of health or functional disturbances in VDT work; a description of recommendations, as available, for control of these effects is also provided.

## VISUAL SYSTEM DYSFUNCTION

Until recent years, visual system disturbances such as sore, aching, irritated, or tired eyes, and blurred or double vision were at the focus of health concerns in VDT work. Headache is often included in this cluster. Together, these types of disturbances are often referred to loosely as asthenopia, visual fatigue, or simply eyestrain, the expression used in this chapter.

Reviews of field studies of VDT operators suggest that prevalence rates of 50% or more for at least occasional experience of certain eyestrain symptoms are typical (2–4). By far, ocular discomfort symptoms, as opposed to visual imperception, are the most common problems. In one of the first NIOSH studies of VDT users, for example, 75% of VDT users reported occasional aching or burning eyes at work, whereas 39% reported blurred vision (5). (The rates were 27% and 5%, respectively, for frequent or constant problems.) In perhaps the largest epidemiologic study of VDT users ever conducted (over 20,000 Italian workers), burning eyes was the most common symptom (reported by more than 30% of participants). Only half this number reported blurred vision (6).

Eyestrain problems are by no means unique to VDT work. They were described in antiquity (7) and have proliferated in modern times with the increasing near vision job demands associated with the expanding information sector of the economy. Carmichael and Dearborn (8) recognized this growing problem in 1947: "There is probably no single way in which the demands made by modern

S.-Y. Lim and S. L. Sauter: Applied Psychology and Ergonomics Branch, National Institute for Occupational Safety and Health, Cincinnati, Ohio 45226-1998.
T. M. Schnorr: Industrywide Studies Branch, National Institute for Occupational Safety and Health, Cincinnati, Ohio 45220-1998.

[1]Dr. Schnorr prepared the section of this chapter on reproductive effects.

industrial civilization upon the human organism differ more from those of earlier times than in the requirements made upon the eyes" (p. 1). In this regard, many studies of VDT users have shown that prevalence rates for eyestrain are often comparable to the rates among clerical workers who do not use VDTs (5,9,10).

### Health Implications

While eyestrain from VDT use can be a painful and debilitating problem, there is little evidence of pathophysiologic or enduring functional changes in the visual system that can be connected with VDT use. In a comprehensive review of studies seeking objective correlates (e.g., changes in accommodation, vergence, heterophoria, acuity, flicker sensitivity) of reported eyestrain among VDT users, the World Health Organization (WHO) found little consistent evidence of dysfunction (4). In contrast, other studies found shifts in tonic accommodation and vergence following near work and VDT work [see Tyrell and Leibowitz (11) for a review]. Also, the potential for color perception abnormalities following video display viewing is generally acknowledged, but such effects are not known to persist.

With regard to organic disease of the eyes, cataract development in VDT work was once a major concern. This possibility has been discounted, however, by the National Research Council (3), and findings of several subsequent epidemiologic studies have been generally supportive of this position (12–15). In the above-mentioned Italian epidemiologic study of 20,000 VDT users (16), researchers found no connection between the use of video terminals and the early appearance of cataracts, nor with any of nine other pathologic ophthalmic conditions (ocular hypertension, hypertensive retinopathy, etc.). Electromagnetic radiation is the only known VDT-dependent risk factor for cataractogenesis. WHO (4), however, claimed that radiation emissions from VDTs cannot be considered as a credible cause of cataract formation in VDT operators.

In a 1990 reappraisal of risks to the eyes, the WHO concluded, "There is no evidence of damage or permanent impairment to the visual system of persons working with VDTs" (30). This WHO conclusion was based almost entirely on cross-sectional or acute exposure studies. There are, however, some prospective findings that provide supportive evidence. A 2-year study of Dutch telephone operators, for example, showed no deterioration in optometric measures of visual function (17). A more recent, 6-year longitudinal study of visual health comparing VDT users to controls in Australia concluded that there is no convincing evidence to support the hypothesis that VDT use could be harmful to the eyes (18). In comparing year 1 and year 4 data, the study showed no significant differences in the two groups in visual acuity, or in abnormalities of the lens (opacities), cornea, aqueous humor, iris, or pupil. Age, however, seemed to be related to some of the eye abnormalities.

### Etiology and Control

As suggested above, eyestrain is a rather imprecise concept. Symptoms are nonspecific and objective signs are lacking. Duke-Elder and Abrams (19) define eyestrain in terms of the symptoms resulting from the "conscious striving" to see. According to this definition, any aspect of the visual environment or of the individual that impairs the legibility or visibility of a visual display is liable to lead to eyestrain.

As summarized below, knowledge exists on ways to maximize the visual quality of displays and on appropriate vision correction to minimize eyestrain among VDT users. Application of this technology alone, however, may be only partially effective in controlling eyestrain from VDT use. The reason is that psychological or motivational factors can intervene to influence the conscious efforts of seeing. This is probably one explanation why eyestrain is unlikely when reading a newspaper or interesting novel, even though the print may be small or of poor quality. In this regard, the very nature of VDT jobs must be considered in assessing potential for eyestrain in VDT work. A recent survey of Swedish public employees found, for example, that eye discomfort among VDT users was related to work organization factors such as lack of work control, high work pace, and time pressure (20).

There are three classes of variables that could influence the legibility and visibility of VDT displays: (1) visual capabilities of VDT users, (2) physical characteristics of the video display, and (3) workplace lighting (which interacts with display characteristics). Only a synopsis of key measures to optimize these variables for VDT work is possible here. Numerous texts provide a more extensive treatment of this subject, as well as quantitative design specifications for high-quality displays (2,21–25).

#### *Vision Correction*

Miscorrected or uncorrected problems may be an important cause of eyestrain among VDT users (26–28). Hypermetropes and presbyopes may be at special risk (27,28). In correcting the vision of VDT users it is of primary importance to remember that the viewing distance for VDT images is usually greater, in the neighborhood of 48 to 65 cm (29), than the distance for reading hard copy. This poses a special problem for presbyopes who use reading glasses or bifocals because the video display is usually at an intermediate distance between the far point of near vision and the near point of far vision. Such persons often require special lenses to see clearly without extraordinary effort. Similarly, the customary (lower lens) placement of the near-vision bifocal is often problematic, necessitating an uncomfortable backward tilt and forward flexion of the head for display viewing.

WHO recommends an eye examination for all VDT operators before they begin work, and subsequent examinations beyond age 40 years, especially for persons who report musculoskeletal or eyestrain symptoms (30). WHO recommends that the examiner be trained in visual ergonomics and that examinations include both refraction and visual acuity. WHO cautions against the tinting of eyeglasses for control of glare in the VDT environment. This action could result in unsatisfactory foreground-background contrast on the video display.

## DESIGN FEATURES

Video display and workplace design features are believed to influence visibility, legibility, and comfort video display viewing. The American National Standard for Human Factors Engineering of Visual Display Terminal (21) provides perhaps one of the most comprehensive and authoritative guidelines to maximize these parameters. This standard, prepared by the American National Standards Institute (ANSI) and the Human Factors and Ergonomics Society is presently undergoing revision, and an update is anticipated in 1997 or 1998.

### Display Characteristics

#### *Character Contrast*

A strong character-to-background contrast ratio is one of the most important conditions for comfortable viewing of a video display. In this regard it is critical that screen reflections, both sharp and diffuse, be minimized. The best solution is to reduce excess or stray room lighting (see Workplace Lighting, below); alternatively, filters that can be placed over the display may attenuate reflections. However, these filters (examples include "micromesh" filters, "neutral density" filters, "polarizing" filters) should not be employed without prior testing, since character brightness or sharpness also may be excessively reduced.

#### *Character Sharpness*

Character blur can lead to excessive and futile efforts of the eye to bring characters into focus. The culprit may be an aging VDT, a maladjusted focus control, or excessive character brightness (character brightness is often increased intentionally to overcome contrast problems), resulting in radiation of light ("bloom") around the edge of characters, which creates blur.

#### *Character Design*

Small or tightly spaced characters and unusual fonts are difficult to discern and create problems in distinguishing among characters, impairing legibility and comfort.

#### *Image Stability*

Image instability may result in blur or annoying flicker of the display. VDT images that are created using cathode ray tube technology are inherently unstable, owing to the screen "refresh" process necessary to create the image. However, this type of problem is becoming increasingly rare as VDT technology improves. Excessive character brightness, resulting, possibly, from efforts to improve contrast, increases the ability to detect the instability in video displays.

#### *Color*

Characters formed by colors at the ends of the spectrum (blues and reds), are less visible than green, yellow, and white characters. Excessive numbers of colors on the display may also add to confusion, and when the colors are widely separated on the spectrum (e.g., simultaneous use of both reds and blues), some blurring may be perceived.

#### *Image Contrast Polarity*

At present, there seems to be little consensus that displays with dark characters on a light background are more or less stressful to the eyes than displays with light characters on a dark background.

#### *Workplace Lighting*

The lighting requirements for reading from hardcopy and from video displays are different. Within limits, increases in ambient illumination increase the legibility of paper documents, and in this regard a bright visual environment is desirable in the conventional office setting. A bright office environment, however, creates a risk in VDT work, since it increases the opportunity for screen reflections (diffuse or sharp glare), which are at best annoying and at worst obscure the display. A number of measures, including reorienting VDTs, selective removal of light fixtures, or use of partitions or blinds, may be helpful in controlling room lighting in offices where VDTs are used. The ANSI (21) guidelines suggests the use of a mixture of general and task lighting in the VDT workplace. Task or local lighting can improve the visibility of printed matter, while not impairing the visibility of the video display.

With regard to lighting systems for VDT use, "lensed-indirect up-lighting systems" that distribute the light over a broad area of the ceiling to provide diffuse office lighting was rated more favorably, produced fewer glare problems, and resulted in improved eye comfort in comparison to a parabolic down-lighting system, which uses ceiling recessed fixtures and louvers that direct the light downward (31).

## MUSCULOSKELETAL DISORDERS

Musculoskeletal discomfort is as prevalent as, or more prevalent than, eyestrain in VDT work, and has become the primary focus of VDT-related health concerns in recent years. Early NIOSH studies showed a prevalence rate exceeding 75% for the "occasional" experience of back, neck, and shoulder discomfort among VDT users (5,32). In a later NIOSH survey of nearly 1,000 VDT users in two state agencies (33), prevalence rates of 20% to 25% for "almost daily" discomfort in the upper torso were observed. A 1989 NIOSH Health Hazard Evaluation of newspaper employees found that 40% of the 834 participants reported symptoms that met the study case definition for any cumulative trauma disorder during the past year (34). In two more recent NIOSH studies of VDT users, one in the newspaper industry and one in the telecommunications industry, prevalence rates for upper extremity disorders defined by symptoms alone were of a similar magnitude (35,36). (Prevalence rates based on objective signs were reduced to approximately one-half the rates for symptom measures.)

The neck, back, and brachial plexus seem to be a primary site of musculoskeletal discomfort among VDT users. A 1982 Bell System study (10) found neck discomfort to be exceeded only by headache in VDT operators. Neck discomfort was also the only symptom that distinguished VDT operators from controls. Neck pain, followed by shoulder pain, was the most prevalent musculoskeletal symptom in a study of more than 1,500 VDT users in Massachusetts (37). Analyzing VDT users' responses to questionnaires published in a safety and health trade journal, Evans (38) found "painful/stiff neck or shoulders" to be the most common complaint (53% of 4,000 respondents). In the Italian study of more than 20,000 VDT users, back pain and, second, neck pain, were the most prevalent musculoskeletal symptoms (6). Neck-shoulder problems were also most prevalent in studies conducted by Bergquist et al. (39). Recent NIOSH studies indicate, however, that pain at the hand and wrist is also prevalent (36,40). With regard to upper extremity problems in VDT work, much of the current scientific attention seems to focus on carpal tunnel syndrome. Yet NIOSH research suggests that the risk of carpal tunnel syndrome per se in VDT work may be relatively low (35).

As with eyestrain, numerous studies fail to show a significant increase in musculoskeletal symptoms among VDT users in comparison to controls performing related tasks (5,41–43). A recent Scandinavian study found increased risk only for hand and wrist problems (39). (However, most of the studies showed that the prevalence of musculoskeletal discomfort were high in absolute terms for both VDT and non-VDT operators.)

### Health Implications

Regarding the long-term health risks associated with musculoskeletal discomfort in VDT use, WHO (4) has concluded that injury from repeated stress to the musculoskeletal system is possible. Dramatizing this possibility, an epidemic of repetition strain injury (RSI) affecting VDT operators swept Australia in the last decade. Five-year prevalence rates approaching 35% were recorded in some Australian organizations (44). Japan experienced a similar phenomenon during the 1970s (45). Some earlier studies suggested that disabling musculoskeletal disorders are becoming a problem among VDT users in the United States (46,47). A recent report by the Office Ergonomic Research Committee (48) indicated that repeated traumas are still growing but their growth rate started to slow down in 1993 and 1994. However, current recording systems make it difficult to determine whether musculoskeletal injuries to VDT users are increasing or decreasing, and the relative contribution of these types of injuries to the rather dramatic increase in cumulative trauma disorders in the United States during the 1980s and 1990s.

Hadler (49) and others (50–54) have argued that musculoskeletal discomfort reported by VDT users represents merely use-associated fatigue or pain, and not underlying pathology. These sources argue that cultural or social conditioning fosters illness beliefs and behaviors among persons who suffer musculoskeletal discomfort (a process referred to as "social iatrogenesis") and that disability then ensues. According to Cleland (52) and The Royal Australian College of Physicians (54), these conditioning forces involve, in part, widely held but false assumptions in the medical and legal community about the seriousness of musculoskeletal discomfort and its relationship to biomechanical demands of VDT work.

Beliefs that musculoskeletal discomfort among VDT users is a benign condition, or that the epidemic spread of disabling musculoskeletal disorders among VDT users is not related to physical job demands, have been challenged by a number of investigators (55–57). Contrary to this viewpoint, several studies have suggested a link between biomechanical stresses and musculoskeletal problems in VDT and keyboard work. Duncan and Ferguson (58) found awkward postures of the upper extremities to be significantly more common among telegraphers with diagnosed myalgia or cramp than among their asymptomatic peers. Hunting and associates (59) reported that deviant postures and lack of arm-hand support were associated with increased discomfort and clinical signs (e.g., pain with palpation and isometric contraction) in both VDT operators and typists. Maeda and colleagues (60) found relatively strong correlations of upper extremity and head tilt angles with arm-hand and shoulder discomfort among accounting machine operators.

Subsequent NIOSH research adds to this evidence. In one study, up to 38% of the variance in musculoskeletal discomfort among VDT data entry operators could be explained by objective measures of posture and workstation ergonomics (33). In a NIOSH study of newspaper employees (34), typing time and speed were significant predictors of upper extremity symptoms. A second NIOSH study among newspaper workers also found a relationship between typing time and hand/wrist disorders (36). Other factors such as static work postures, hand positions, use of lower arm support, repeated work movements, and keyboard or VDT vertical positioning were found to be associated with various upper-body muscular problems (61).

## Etiology and Control

Some VDT operators commonly remain seated in fixed, sometimes awkward postures for long periods of time, possibly resulting in increased biomechanical stresses on the back, neck, shoulders, and upper extremities. Additionally, repetition is a concern. Keystroke rates as high as 20,000 per hour are not uncommon for some VDT operators. Some of the biomechanical stresses imposed on VDT operators are subject to control through the careful design and configuration of workstations (chair, table, VDT, etc.). This section begins by discussing measures for reducing biomechanical stresses at the VDT workstation. More detailed, technical specifications are available from several authoritative sources (21,24,62,63). Below is a selective set of chair and workstation characteristics that should be considered in the design of VDT workstations.

### *Chair Characteristics*

#### *Back Rest*

A slightly reclining posture is not uncommon for VDT operators and can help to minimize the muscular effort of continuous sitting in an upright posture (64). A slight recline may also reduce lumbar disk forces during sitting (65). To accommodate a reclining posture in VDT work, it is important that the chair have a tall back rest, and that the back rest tilt backward independently of the seat pan. A slightly protruding lumbar support is important in either the upright or reclining seated posture. Vertical adjustability of the back rest will help ensure proper positioning of the lumbar support.

#### *Arm Rests*

Adjustable arm rests may help to reduce loads in the back, neck, and shoulders that are created when the arms and hands are suspended over the keyboard (66).

#### *Chair Base*

Chairs with five spokes or castors in the base will help to ensure stability.

#### *Seat Pan*

Height adjustability of the seat pan will help to achieve a comfortable working level vis-à-vis the keyboard (about elbow level).

#### *Footrest*

It is believed that seat pan heights above popliteal height may create uncomfortable thigh pressure or possibly circulatory impairment in the lower extremities. In this regard, many chairs do not adjust low enough for women of small stature, and a footrest may therefore be necessary.

#### *Padding*

Padding can be helpful to minimize pressure points at the chair pan, back rest, and arm rests. A rounded ("waterfall") forward edge of the seat pan may also be desirable in this regard.

### *Workstation Characteristics*

#### *Keyboard Height*

It is generally believed that loads on the shoulders and elbow flexors can be minimized by positioning the keyboard (home row) at elbow height or perhaps slightly lower (33,67). Some evidence indicates, however, that slight elevation of the table or keyboard may be inconsequential, or even preferred by some workers (68,69).

#### *Knee Envelope*

With a thick keyboard or tabletop (e.g., a desk with a pencil drawer), it may be impossible to lower the keyboard to a comfortable height without sacrificing leg room. Restriction of leg and knee room by the table top, table legs, or "modesty panels" beneath the table may lead to highly constrained or awkward working postures. (Constrained postures may also result when the work surface area is too small or designed in such a way as to prevent flexibility in positioning of the keyboard, video display, or other work materials.)

#### *Display Height*

Height adjustability of the VDT above the work surface can help minimize biomechanical stresses from awkward head postures in viewing the display. There is general agreement that the primary viewing area of the display should not be positioned above the horizontal line of sight. Views differ on the permissible declination of line of sight; but extreme, downward head tilt should probably be avoided.

*Arm/Hand Rests*

Cushioned and broad support surfaces (e.g., chair arm rest or wrist rest) for the upper extremities can help to minimize compression or irritation at the wrist, forearm, or elbow.

### *Adjustability*

Implicit in the foregoing discussion is that adjustability of chair and worktable components is important for achieving a comfortable working posture. Not uncommonly, important components of workstations are not adjustable or the mechanisms are difficult to operate. This becomes a special concern when the same furniture is used by several workers. For example, it is unlikely that the workers will bother readjusting the heights of chairs to fit their individual needs unless the chairs have an automatic mechanism that can be operated from the sitting position.

In addition to workstation design, the importance of work organization cannot be overstated as a control measure for biomechanical stresses in VDT work. Work organization (i.e., the way tasks are performed and managed) represents a form of administrative influence over the exposure of VDT operators to biomechanical stressors, including repetition. Examples of promising organizational interventions for VDT jobs include increased rest pauses (70), job rotation, or expansion of jobs to include nonkeyboard work. Work organization is closely intertwined with factors that influence the psychosocial environment and stress at work. Thus, in addition to an influence on exposure to biomechanical stressors, work organization may influence musculoskeletal comfort via other mechanisms.

### *Work Organization*

One of the most significant developments in the study of work-related musculoskeletal disorders has been the implication of psychosocial factors as causal agents. In the most general use of the term, psychosocial factors refer to aspects of the job or individual, or of broader socioeconomic conditions, that result in psychological demands on the individual (and hence can lead to psychological stress). Among the conditions in the workplace that lead to psychological demand and stress are aspects of work organization such as the scheduling of work, aspects of job design (e.g., the complexity of tasks), co-worker and supervisory relationships, management practices, and organization climate/culture. To date, over a dozen major studies have established significant associations between these types of organizational factors and musculoskeletal problems in VDT work (5,36,40,61,71–74). For example, in a NIOSH study of upper-extremity disorders among telephone directory assistance operators, factors such as heavy information processing demands, lack of supervisory support, and time pressure were predictive of objective signs of tendinitis and other neuromuscular and skeletal conditions (35). More recently, Lim (75) found that work pressure and lack of control over work pace were predictive of discomfort, especially in the neck and shoulder regions.

Although extant data strongly suggest an influence of workplace psychosocial stressors on musculoskeletal problems in VDT workers, the mechanisms underlying these effects are still uncertain. In recent years, theoretical frameworks to explain these linkages have been developed by several investigators (75–78). Mechanisms that are common to most of these models are discussed in the following sections. Although knowledge regarding these mechanisms is incomplete, all of these suspected effects stem originally from work organization problems in the VDT workplace.

*Physical Mechanisms*

As discussed above, it is probable that work organization directly influences biomechanical demands. For example, the complexity of a VDT task is directly related to the degree of repetition in the task (e.g., data entry work is less complex and more repetitive than general secretarial work), thereby influencing biomechanical stresses to the upper extremities. Psychological demand and job stress also vary as a function of task complexity, but their association with biomechanical stress is merely coincidental in this case.

*Psychophysiologic Mechanisms*

It is well established that VDT or keyboard work can give rise to muscle tension in excess of the demands of keying (79–81). This effect is part of the generalized autonomic adjustment of the body to stress, which also includes increased catecholamine secretion, reduced peripheral circulation, and a variety of other psychophysiologic responses (82). The possible contribution of these effects, especially stress-related muscle tension, to musculoskeletal function and comfort among VDT users is a subject of study by several investigators (81,83,84).

*Perceptual and Cognitive Mechanisms*

A broad body of research in health psychology suggests that cognitive factors, including psychological stress, are influential in the detection symptoms and in the attribution of symptoms as job-related disease

(85,86). It is plausible that these processes are instrumental in the development of musculoskeletal problems in VDT work; e.g., stress-related arousal may sharpen sensitivity to normally subthreshold musculoskeletal sensations. [Note: This mechanism would incorporate the iatrogenic hypothesis posed by Hadler (49) and others.] However, to date no studies have directly investigated this mechanism in the context of VDT work and health.

## JOB STRESS

Until the advent of the industrial revolution, goods were produced by craft workers. Craft workers participate in all aspects of the production process and exercised considerable control over the pace of the job and the way it was performed. With the advent of mass production technology, the organization of work changed dramatically. Mechanization created more standardized, narrow, and repetitive job tasks. Individual control over the work process was replaced by machine pacing and piece work, and workers' identification with the final product was reduced. Occupational stress researchers have come to recognize these conditions as the building blocks for ill health (87).

The nature of office work has been changing in a similar manner. Prior to the advent of the typewriter, office work could still be classified largely as "craft" work. Clerical workers or secretaries were fully and independently responsible for all of the transactions and support functions in the office, the work was varied, and multiple skills were required. Although this form of office work can still be found today, the information age and the mechanization of office work—abetted by the typewriter—resulted in major changes in the nature of office jobs. [See Giuliano (88) for an excellent review of the evolution of office work.] The industrial office functions much like a manufacturing assembly line. Documents are delivered and processed in a serial fashion by successive groups of clerks or information specialists, each performing a very narrow or specialized operation in a standardized fashion. Few workers understand, or could perform, all steps of the job. Piecework, creating heavy workload demand, is common.

Computerization holds the potential for a positive transformation of industrial office work. VDTs make it easier for a single person to create, modify, store, retrieve, deliver, or otherwise process information (i.e., accomplish a skilled and varied task that may otherwise have required numerous separate transactions involving several persons). For example Johansson and Aronsson (89) reported that VDTs enabled agents to obtain a more complete picture of an insurance case and to independently process a claim.

In many cases, however, the introduction of computerization to the office has served only to intensify negative attributes of industrial-age office work. Computerization, for example, has subjected office workers to electronic monitoring of their performance, creating implicit or explicit expectations for heightened productivity and perceptions of increased supervisory control.

Early NIOSH investigations (5,32) were among the first to examine systematically the change in the content and organization of office work associated with the introduction of VDT technology. These studies showed that, in contrast to peers who did not use VDTs, VDT users reported increased work pressure, reduced autonomy, and increased management control over work processes. Furthermore, both studies showed increased disruptions in working relationships between VDT users and their peers and supervisors.

Subsequent studies and reviews of the literature (see refs. 4 and 90 for a comprehensive review) tend to confirm the general pattern of results observed in the earlier NIOSH investigations (although these are effects evident mainly for clerical work). More recent studies highlight additional VDT work-related stress factors, including concerns with computer breakdown and response delays, physical immobility (13), excessive repetition (91), and electronic performance monitoring. For example, electronic performance monitoring of telecommunications workers was associated with increased problems with supervisors and higher levels of reported stress. The combination of electronic performance monitoring was especially problematic when performance standards were enforced, and monitored employees who were barely able to meet the performance standard were the most affected.

### Health Effects

There is growing evidence that long-term exposure to the types of unfavorable working conditions that have been observed among some VDT users might have serious health consequences. Accumulating epidemiologic data, for example, suggest that the combination of heavy work-load demands and reduced worker autonomy or control may create a risk for affective disorders and cardiovascular disease.

Although an unusual prevalence of chronic, stress-related psychological or somatic disorders has yet to be documented among VDT users, acute disturbances have been reported in many investigations. A high prevalence of irritability, anxiety, and depressive states among VDT operators was reported in several early studies (32). VDT work is associated with complaints of daily psychological stress. Cardiovascular and neurohormonal responses indicative of increased autonomic arousal have also been reported in persons who perform various types of VDT work. Schleifer and Okogbaa (92) found suppression of sinus arrhythmia and significant elevations in both diastolic and systolic blood pressure when VDT operators worked under incentive pay compensation schedules. Elevations in both blood pressure and catecholamine excretion among VDT operators were reported in relation to faulty computer function (89). Additionally, Tanaka and colleagues (93) reported age-related elevations in catecholamine excretion under conditions of demanding VDT work (e.g., poor display quality).

Recent prospective studies have improved upon the quality of studies of stress and health in VDT work (39,94). In a longitudinal study of office workers, Carayon et al. (94) were able to show that task clarity and ambiguity of job future were associated with worker strain over the 3-year periods. Furthermore, the study also showed that there were different job factors in addition to the above two factors associated with worker strain at each time period (i.e., each year) of the study.

In some sense it may be inappropriate to identify many of these later investigations as studies of VDT work, i.e., implying that the outcomes noted are VDT-related or VDT-specific. Unlike conditions in the 1980s where VDT users worked side by side with office workers who did not use VDTs (thereby enabling studies to reliably attribute outcomes to VDT use), computerization and VDT work is an integral aspect of modern office work and a growing feature of many other jobs. Thus, it is becoming progressively more difficult to disentangle, both methodologically and conceptually, the influence of VDTs from the conditions of modern work.

### Controlling Stress in VDT Work

The National Research Council (3) concluded that stress and dissatisfaction in VDT work have resulted from failure to apply to jobs "well-established principles of good design and practice" (p. 2). These principles have been summarized in generic form by NIOSH (97), and described in more specific terms for application in VDT use by Galitz (96), the WHO Regional Office for Europe (90), and Sauter (95).

There is strong convergence among the prescriptions offered by these sources for the design of VDT work. Most sources emphasize, for example, that VDT jobs should be challenging, within the limits of workers' capabilities, and have inherent meaning and value to workers. In this regard, tasks should be sufficiently varied or complex to sustain interest and to utilize acquired skills. Additionally, tasks should have closure, so that each work cycle can be associated with a distinct and meaningful work product. By way of example, most VDT data entry jobs represent the antithesis of most of these conditions.

Most sources emphasize also that the job should provide some opportunities for worker discretion about the way work is organized and performed (e.g., prioritizing, scheduling, and pacing tasks or subtasks). In VDT work it is important that this discretion extend to the physical configuration or design of the workstation.

A third key concern is the social environment at work. VDT jobs and facilities should be designed to enable interpersonal interaction for purposes of both emotional support and concrete assistance in performing tasks. Teamwork or task sharing may help serve this end and help sustain interest in work. Modern offices are often configured in open layouts in which individual office cubicles are created by movable partitions. Depending on the types and positioning of the partitions, this type of open layout can be conducive to workplace interaction. However, this design needs to be balanced against the need for privacy.

Equal in importance to the design of the job is the manner in which VDT technology is introduced to the workplace. Most recommendations emphasize the need for (a) early communications to workers to avoid stressful misunderstandings or uncertainty, (b) early participation of workers to impart a sense of control and to utilize their subject matter expertise, (c) gradual change emphasizing steps with the greatest potential for success and confidence building, (d) training and social or technical support to minimize error and frustration, and (e) avenues of redress to deal with problems while they are still benign (96).

Based on events at the Federal Express Corporation, Westin (98) provides an excellent case example of the design of VDT jobs that conform to these general guidelines. Key to the success of the project was (a) the early formulation of a corporate "people-technology" policy, which espoused, "It is the policy of Federal Express Corporation to systematically incorporate human factors, ergonomics, and job/task design criteria with the development or modification of electronic technology applications"; and (b) development of a standing, labor-management task force to carry out this mandate. Examples of job design specifications under the people-technology policy include teamwork, rotating and combining tasks, and increased deregulation and individual control of work. Importantly, the task force whose responsibility it was to ensure that all design criteria were met was composed of management representatives from all relevant departments (e.g., facilities management, management information systems, safety and health, human resources, risk management), as well as worker participants from the affected production areas.

## REPRODUCTIVE EFFECTS

Video display terminals were first associated with adverse reproductive outcomes in 1980, when a cluster of birth defects was observed among women using VDTs at the Toronto Star newspaper (99). The appearance of several clusters led several investigators to conduct epidemiologic studies of the reproductive risk of VDT work (100–115).

Three characteristics of VDT use have been proposed as possible explanations for the observed association between VDT use and adverse pregnancy outcomes:

physical stress, psychological stress, and exposure to electromagnetic fields. Electromagnetic field exposure has been regarded as the most plausible mechanism for possible reproductive effects of VDTs. Two types of electromagnetic fields are produced by the VDT: extremely low frequency (ELF) and very low frequency (VLF) fields. Some review articles offer a detailed review of the literature on VDT use (116) or electromagnetic field exposure (117,118) and reproductive health. This chapter summarizes the VDT literature (100–115). As discussed below, these studies have largely shown no relationship between VDT use and adverse pregnancy outcomes.

### Health Effects

Most of the large epidemiologic studies of pregnancy outcomes among office workers have not shown a relationship between VDT use and spontaneous abortion. Of the ten studies of spontaneous abortion, eight have shown no relationship to VDT use (100–107). Most of these studies examined potential risk in relation to weekly hours of VDT use and did not attempt to distinguish between specific risk factors (physical stress, psychological stress, and electromagnetic fields) that might be associated with the VDT. One study that did collect data on job stress and ergonomic work load found that neither factor was correlated significantly with spontaneous abortion (103). A greater risk of spontaneous abortion for women in clerical jobs who reported using a VDT for 20 hours or more during pregnancy was found in one study (108). However, two other studies that examined risk by occupational title did not observe an increased risk for clerical workers (104,106).

Two studies have been conducted that made measurements of electromagnetic fields produced by the VDT (105,109). In one study that measured the electromagnetic fields in the workplace of both VDT users and nonusers, no increased risk of spontaneous abortion was found (105). Measurements of the electromagnetic fields indicated that women seated at VDTs had higher VLF magnetic field exposures than the nonusers or the general population. ELF magnetic field exposures were similar for women seated at VDTs and women who did not use VDTs and also fell within the range of residential exposures. A second study conducted laboratory measurements of electromagnetic fields of the VDTs and found an increased risk of spontaneous abortion among women who used VDT models with ELF magnetic fields measurements over 3 mG at a distance of 50 cm (109). These high emitting VDTs had ELF fields that were about three times higher than the average levels found in other studies in the United States, Canada, Australia, and Sweden (105,116,119,120), suggesting that the exposures VDT operators in this study may not be typical of most VDT users.

Birth defects were also associated with VDT use in some cluster reports, but this association with VDT use was not observed consistently in the five epidemiologic studies that examined birth defects (111). Two studies found no increased risk of major malformations among moderate or heavy VDT users (108,111). A third study found no increased risk for major malformations as a group but found a significantly higher risk for hydrocephalus (110). A fourth study observed an increasing risk of major malformations with increasing weekly hours of VDT use but no greater risk for specific defects (101). A fifth study found an overall excess risk of malformations as well as an increased risk of renal defects (106). Most of these studies had relatively low statistical power to detect increased risks for specific defects, and none measured the electromagnetic fields.

Some investigators have also examined the relationship of VDT use with low birth weight, preterm delivery, or fecundity (15,106,112–115). Most found no increased risk associated with VDT use (106,112–114). One study found a slight, elevation in risk for intrauterine growth retardation in association with more VDT use (104). Another found a slightly increased risk associated with prolonged waiting time to pregnancy among women with greater VDT use (115).

In summary, the weight of the evidence thus far indicates that VDTs in themselves do not increase the risk for adverse pregnancy outcomes. To examine further whether high electromagnetic field exposure constitutes a risk factor for adverse pregnancy outcomes, future studies should focus on populations with higher electromagnetic field exposures than VDT users. In these studies, electromagnetic field exposures should be measured and fully characterized in the workplace to account for all sources of exposure.

## REFERENCES


1. National Institute for Occupational Safety and Health. *NIOSH publications on video display terminals.* Cincinnati: National Institute for Occupational Safety and Health, 1987.
2. Dainoff MJ. Occupational stress factors in visual display terminal (VDT) operation: a review of empirical research. *Behav Inform Technol* 1982;1:141–176.
3. National Research Council. *Video displays, work, and vision.* Washington, DC: National Academy Press, 1983.
4. World Health Organization. *Visual display terminals and workers' health.* WHO Offset Publication No. 99. Geneva: World Health Organization, 1987.
5. Sauter SL, Gottlieb MS, Jones KC, Dodson VN, Rohrer KM. Job and health implications of VDT use: initial results of the Wisconsin-NIOSH study. *Communications of the Association of Computing Machinery* 1982;26:284–294.
6. Rubino GF, di Bari A, Turbati M. Epidemiological analysis of discomfort signs. *Boll Oculist* 1989;68:113–123.
7. Ramazzini B. *De Morbis Artificum,* Wright WC, trans. Chicago: University of Chicago Press, 1940.
8. Carmichael L, Dearborn WF. *Reading and visual fatigue.* Cambridge, MA: Houghton, Mifflin, 1947.
9. Gould JD, Grischkowsky N. Doing the same work with hard copy and with cathode-ray tube (CRT) computer terminals. *Hum Factors* 1984;26:323–327.
10. Starr SJ, Thompson CR, Shute SJ. Effects of video display terminals on telephone operators. *Hum Factors* 1982;24:699–711.
11. Tyrell RA, Leibowitz HW. The relation of vergence effort to reports of

visual fatigue following prolonged near work. *Hum Factors* 1990;32: 341–357.
12. Boos SR, Calissendorff BM, Knave BG, Nyman KG, Voss M. Work at video display terminals. An epidemiological health investigation of office employees. III. Ophthalmological examination. *Scand J Work Environ Health* 1985;11:475–481.
13. Canadian Labor Congress. *Toward a more humanized technology:* Exploring the impact of VDTs on the health and working conditions of Canadian office workers. Ottawa: CLC Labour Education Studies, 1982.
14. Frank AL. *Effects on health following occupational exposure to video display terminals.* Report No. 40536-0084. Lexington: University of Kentucky, Department of Preventive Medicine and Environmental Health, 1984.
15. Smith AB, Tanaka S, Halperin W. Correlates of ocular and somatic symptoms among video display terminal users. *Hum Factors* 1984; 26:143–156.
16. Bonomi L, Bellucci R. Considerations on the ocular pathology in 30,000 personnel of the Italian telephone company (SIP) using VDTs. *Boll Oculist* 1989;68:96–97.
17. Degroot JP, Kamphuis A. Eyestrain in VDU users: physical correlates and long-term effects. *Hum Factors* 1983;25:409–413.
18. Cole BL, Maddocks JD, Sharpe K. *The prevalence of ocular disease in VDU users.* The SEC-VDU study. Bulletin number 4. Melbourne, Australia: Victorial College of Optometry, University of Melbourne, Australia, 1994.
19. Duke-Elder S, Abrams D. Ophthalmic optics and refraction. In: Duke-Elder S, ed. *System of ophthalmology.* St. Louis: CV Mosby, 1970.
20. Aronsson G, Stromberg A. Work content and eye discomfort in VDT work. *Int J Occup Safety Ergonom* 1995;1(1):1–13.
21. American National Standards Institute. *American National Standard for human factors engineering of visual display terminal workstations.* ANSI/HFS Standard No. 100-1988. Santa Monica, CA: Human Factors Society, 1988.
22. Boyce PR. *Human factors in lighting.* New York: Macmillan, 1981.
23. IBM. *Human factors of workstations with visual displays,* 3rd ed. San Jose, CA: International Business Machines, 1984.
24. Sauter SL, Chapman LJ, Knutson SJ. *Improving VDT work:* causes and control of health concerns in VDT use. Madison: University of Wisconsin, Department of Preventive Medicine, 1986.
25. Shurtleff DA. *How to make displays legible.* La Mirada, CA: Human Interface Design, 1980.
26. Schleifer LM, Sauter SL, Smith RJ. Ergonomic predictors of visual system complaints in VDT data entry work. *Behav Inform Technol* 1990;9:273–282.
27. Scullica L, Rechichi C. The influence of refractive defects on the appearance of asthenopia in subjects employed at video terminals (epidemiological survey on 30,000 subjects). *Boll Oculist* 1989; 68:25–48.
28. Sheedy JE, Parsons S. Vision and the video display terminal: clinical findings. In: Sauter SL, Dainoff MJ, Smith MJ, eds. *Promoting health and productivity in the computerized office:* models of successful ergonomic intervention. London: Taylor and Francis, 1990; 197–206.
29. Piccoli B, Braga M, Zambelli PL, Bergamasch, A. Viewing distance variation and related ophthalmological changes in office activities with and without VDUs. *Ergonomics* 1996;39(5):719–728.
30. World Health Organization. *Update on visual display terminals and workers' health.* Geneva: World Health Organization, 1990.
31. Hedge A, Sims WR Jr, Becker FD. Effects of lensed-indirect and parabolic lighting on the satisfaction, visual health, and productivity of office workers. *Ergonomics* 1995;38(2):260–280.
32. Smith MJ, Cohen BGF, Stammerjohn LW. An investigation of health complaints and job stress in video display operations. *Hum Factors* 1981;23:387–400.
33. Sauter SL, Schleifer LM, Knutson SJ. Work posture, workstation design and musculoskeletal discomfort in a VDT data-entry task. *Hum Factors* 1991;22(2):151–167.
34. National Institute for Occupational Safety and Health (NIOSH). *HETA Report 89-250-2046.* Melville, NY: Newsday. Cincinnati: National Institute for Occupational Safety and Health, 1990.
35. NIOSH. *HETA Report 89-299-2230, US West communications:* Phoenix, Arizona, Minneapolis, Minnesota, Denver, and Colorado, 1992. Cincinnati, OH: National Institute for Occupational Safety and Health, 1992.
36. NIOSH. *Health hazard evaluation report on Los Angeles Times, Los Angeles, CA, 1993.* HETA 90-013-2277. Cincinnati, OH: National Institute for Occupational Safety and Health, 1993.
37. Rossignol AM, Morse EP, Summers VM, Pagnotto LD. Video display terminal use and reported health symptoms among Massachusetts clerical workers. *J Occup Med* 1987;29:112–118.
38. Evans J. Women, men, VDU work and health: a questionnaire survey of British VDU operators. *Work Stress* 1987;1:271–283.
39. Bergquist U, Kanve B, Voss M, Wibom R. A longitudinal study of VDT work and health. *Int J Hum Comput Interact* 1992;4(2): 197–219.
40. Hales TR, Sauter SL, Peterson MR, et al. Musculoskeletal disorders among visual display terminal users in a telecommunications company. *Ergonomics* 1994;37(10):1603–1621.
41. Bolinder G. *Dataterminalarbete vid Karolinska Sjukhuset.* (VDT work at the Karolinska Hospital.) (In Swedish). Solna: National Board of Occupational Safety and Health, 1983.
42. Knave BG, Wibom RI, Voss M, Hedstrom LD, Bergquist UOV. Work at video display terminals. An epidemiological health investigation of office employees. I. Subjective symptoms and discomforts. *Scand J Work Environ Health* 1985;11:457–466.
43. Grieco E, Occhipinti, Colombini D. Work postures and musculoskeletal disorders in VDT operators. *Boll Oculist* 1989;68:99–112.
44. Hocking B. Epidemiological aspects of "repetition strain injury" in Telecom Australia. *Med J Aust* 1987;147:218–222.
45. Nakaseko M, Tokunaga R, Hosokawa M. History of occupational cervicobrachial disorder in Japan. *J Hum Ergol (Tokyo)* 1982;11:7–16.
46. Eisen DJ, LeGrande D. Repetitive strain injury in 3 U.S. communications-industry offices. Paper presented at the Second International Scientific Conference—Work with Display Units, Montreal, Canada, 1989 (September).
47. Pasternak J. Computeritis. *Los Angeles Times Magazine* 1989 (March 12);19–22,42–44.
48. Office Ergonomics Research Committee. Betterndorf RF (executive secretary). *Musculoskeletal disorders in the U.S. office workforce.* Manchester Center, VT: Office Ergonomics Research Committee, 1996 (Jan. 4).
49. Hadler NM. The Australian and New Zealand experience with arm pain and backache in the workplace. *Med J Aust* 1986;144:191–195.
50. Bell DS. "Repetition strain injury": an iatrogenic epidemic of simulated injury. *Med J Aust* 1989;151:280–284.
51. Brooks PM. Occupational pain syndromes. *Med J Aust* 1986;144: 170–171.
52. Cleland L. "RSI:" a model of social iatrogenesis. *Med J Aust* 1987; 147:236–239.
53. Kiesler S, Finholt T. The mystery of RSI. *Am Psychol* 1988;43: 1004–1015.
54. Royal Australian College of Physicians. Repetitive strain injury/occupational overuse syndrome: a statement by the Royal Australian College of Physicians. *RCAP Fellowship Affairs* 1988;1:6–7.
55. Bammer G, Martin B. The arguments about RSI: an examination. *Community Health Stud* 1988;12:348–358.
56. Quinter JL. The pain of RSI. The central issue. *Aust Fam Physician* 1989;18:1542–1545.
57. Dennett X, Fry HJH. Overuse syndrome: a muscle biopsy study. *Lancet* 1988;1:905–908.
58. Duncan J, Ferguson D. Keyboard operating posture and symptoms in operating. *Ergonomics* 1974;17:651–662.
59. Hunting W, Laubli T, Grandjean E. Postural and visual loads at VDT workplaces I. Constrained postures. *Ergonomics* 1981;24:917–931.
60. Maeda K, Hunting W, Grandjean E. Factor analysis of localized fatigue complaints of accounting-machine operators. *J Hum Ergol (Tokyo)* 1982;37–43.
61. Bergqvist B, Wolgast E, Nilsson B, Voss M. Musculoskeletal disorders among visual display terminal workers: individual, ergonomic, and work organizational factors. *Ergonomics* 1995;38(4):763–776.
62. Donkin SW. *Sitting on the job. How to survive the stresses of sitting down to work—a practical handbook.* Boston: Houghton Mifflin, 1986.
63. Kroemer KHE. VDT workstation design. In: Helander M, ed. *Handbook of human-computer interaction.* Amsterdam: Elsevier Science (North Holland), 1988.

64. Grandjean E, Hunting W, Piderman M. VDT workstation design: Preferred settings and their effects. *Hum Factors* 1983;25: 161–176.
65. Andersson GBJ, Ortengren R. Lumbar disc pressure and myoelectric back muscle activity II. Studies on an office chair. *Scand J Rehabil Med* 1974;6:115–121.
66. Sihvonen T, Baskin K, Hanninen O. Neck-shoulder loading in word-processor use. Effect of learning, gymnastics and arm supports. *Int Arch Occup Environ Health* 1989;61:229–233.
67. Bendix T, Jessen F. Wrist support during typing—a controlled electromyographic study. *Appl Ergonom* 1986;17:162–168.
68. Arndt R. Working posture and musculoskeletal problems of video display terminal operators—review and reappraisal. *Am Ind Hyg Assoc J* 1983;44:437–446.
69. Cushman WH. Data entry performances and operator preferences for various keyboard heights. In: Grandjean E, ed. *Ergonomics and health in modern offices.* London: Taylor and Francis, 1983.
70. Swanson NG, Sauter SL, Chapman LJ. The design of rest breaks for video display terminal work: a review of the relevant literature. In: Mital A, ed. *Advances in industrial ergonomics and safety,* vol 1. New York: Taylor and Francis, 1989;895–898.
71. Faucett J, Rempel D. VDT-related musculoskeletal symptoms: interactions between work posture and psychosocial work factors. *Am J Ind Med* 1994;26(5):597–612.
72. Lim SY, Carayon P. An integrated approach to cumulative trauma disorders in computerized offices: the role of psychosocial work factors, psychological stress, and ergonomic risk factors. In: Smith MJ, Salvendy G, eds. *Advances in human factors/ergonomics, vol 19A:* Human computer interaction: *applications and case Studies.* Proceedings of the Fifth International Conference on Human-Computer Interaction, (HCI International 93), vol 1. Amsterdam, The Netherlands: Elsevier Science, 1993;880–885.
73. Lim SY, Carayon P. Psychosocial work factors and upper extremity musculoskeletal discomfort among office workers. In: Grieco A, Molteni G, Piccoli B, Occhipinti E, eds. *Work with display units.* Amsterdam, The Netherlands: Elsevier Science, 1994;57–62.
74. Westgaard RH, Jensen JL, Hansen K. Individual and work-related risk factors associated with symptoms of musculoskeletal complaints. *Int Arch Occup Environ Health* 1993;64:405–413.
75. Lim SY. An integrated Approach to cumulative trauma disorders in the office environment: the role of psychosocial work factors, psychological stress, and ergonomic risk factors. Ph.D. dissertation 1994, University of Wisconsin–Madison, Madison, WI.
76. Bongers PM, Winter CR de, Kompier MAJ, Hildebrandt VH. Psychosocial factors at work and musculoskeletal disease: a review of the literature. *Scand J Work Environ Health* 1993;(19)5:297–312.
77. Sauter SL, Swanson NG. An ecological model of musculoskeletal disorders in office work. In: Moon SD, Sauter SL, eds. *Beyond biomechanics:* psychosocial aspects of musculoskeletal disorders in office work. London: Taylor & Francis, 1996;3–21.
78. Smith MJ, Carayon P. Work organization, stress, and cumulative trauma disorders. In: Moon SD, Sauter SL, eds. *Beyond biomechanics:* psychosocial aspects of musculoskeletal disorders in office work. London: Taylor & Francis, 1996;23–42.
79. Lundervold A. Electromyographic investigations during typewriting. *Acta Physiol Scans* 1951;24(84):226–232.
80. Westgaard RH, Bjorklund R. Generation of muscle tension additional to postural muscle load. *Ergonomics* 1987;30(6):911–923.
81. Waersted M, Bjorklund RA, Westgaard, RH. Shoulder muscle tension induced by two VDU-based tasks of different complexity. *Ergonomics* 1991;34(2):137–150.
82. Frankenhaeuser M, Gardell B. Underload and overload in working life: outline of a multidisciplinary approach. *J Hum Stress* 1976;2:35–46.
83. Theorell T. Possible mechanisms behind the relationship between the demand-control-support model and disorders of the locomotor system. In: Moon SD, Sauter SL, eds. *Beyond biomechanics:* psychosocial aspects of musculoskeletal disorders in office work. London: Taylor & Francis, 1996;65–73.
84. Waersted M, Bjorklund RA, Westgaard RH. The effect of motivation on shoulder- muslce tension in attention-demanding tasks. *Ergonomics* 1994;37(2):363–376.
85. Pennebaker JW, Hall G. *The psychology of physical symptoms.* New York: Springer-Verlag, 1982.
86. Cioffi D. Beyond attentional strategies: a cognitive-perceptual model of somatic interpretation. *Psychol Bull* 1991;109(1):25–41.
87. Levi L. *Preventing work stress.* Reading, MA: Addison-Wesley, 1981.
88. Giuliano VE. The mechanization of office work. *Sci Am* 1982;247: 149–164.
89. Johansson G, Aronsson G. Stress reactions in computerized administrative work. *J Occup Behav* 1984;5:159–181.
90. World Health Organization. Work with visual display terminals: psychosocial aspects and health. Report on a World Health Organization meeting. *J Occup Behav* 1989;31:957–968.
91. Stellman JM, Klitzman S, Gordon GC, Snow BR. Work environment and the well-being of clerical and VDT workers. *J Occup Behav* 1987; 8:95–114.
92. Schleifer LM, Okogbaa GO. System response time and method of pay: cardiovascular stress effects in computer-based tasks. *Ergonomics* 1990;33:1495–1509.
93. Tanaka T, Fukumoto T, Yamamoto S, Noro K. The effects of VDT work on urinary excretion of catecholamines. *Ergonomics* 1988;31: 1753–1763.
94. Carayon P, Yang CL, Lim SY. Examining the relationship between job design and worker strain over time in a sample of office workers. *Ergonomics* 1995;38(6):1199–1211.
95. Sauter SL, Murphy LR, Hurrell JJ. Prevention of work-related psychological disorders. A national strategy proposed by the National Institute for Occupational Safety and Health (NIOSH). *Am Psychol* 1990;45:1146–1158.
96. Galitz WO. *Human factors in office automation.* Atlanta: Life Office Management Association, 1980.
97. National Institute for Occupational Safety and Health. Stress: some principles, definitions and problems. In: *Health issues—video display terminals.* National Institute for Occupational Safety and Health manual. Cincinnati: National Institute for Occupational Safety and Health, 1984;41–53.
98. Westin A. Organizational culture and VDT policies: a case study of the Federal Express Corporation. In: Sauter SL, Dainoff MJ, Smith MJ, eds. *Promoting health and productivity in the computerized office:* models of successful ergonomic intervention. London: Taylor & Francis, 1990;147–168.
99. Bergquist UO. Video display terminals and health. *Scand J Work Environ Health* 1984;10(suppl 2):62–67.
100. Ericson A, Kallen B. An epidemiological study of work with video screens and pregnancy outcome: I. A registry study. *Am J Ind Med* 1986;9:447–457.
101. Ericson A, Kallen B. An epidemiological study of work with video screens and pregnancy outcome: II. A case-control study. *Am J Ind Med* 1986;9:459–475.
102. Bryant HE, Love EJ. Video display terminal use and spontaneous abortion risk. *Int J Epidemiol* 1989;18(1):132–138.
103. Nielsen CV, Brandt LP. Spontaneous abortion among women using video display terminals. *Scand J Work Environ Health* 1990;16: 323–328.
104. Windham GC, Fenster L, Swan SH, Neutra RR. Use of video display terminals during pregnancy and the risk of spontaneous abortion, low birthweight, or intrauterine growth retardation. *Am J Ind Med* 1990; 18:675–688.
105. Schnorr TM, Grajewski BA, Hornung RW, et al. Video display terminals and the risk of spontaneous abortion. *N Engl J Med* 1991; 324:727–733.
106. McDonald AD, McDonald JC, Armstrong B, Cherry N, Nolin AD, Robert D. Work with visual display units in pregnancy. *Br J Ind Med* 1988;45:509–515.
107. Roman E, Beral V, Pelerin M, Hermon C. Spontaneous abortion and work with visual display units. *Br J Ind Med* 1992;49:507–512.
108. Goldhaber M, Polen M, Hiatt R. The risk of miscarriage and birth defects among women who use visual display terminals during pregnancy. *Am J Ind Med* 1988;13:695–706.
109. Lindbohm M-L, Hietanen M, Kyyronen P, et al. Magnetic fields of video display terminals and spontaneous abortion. *Am J Epidemiol* 1992;188:1041–1051.
110. Brandt LPA, Nielsen CV. Congenital malformations among children of women working with video display terminals. *Scand J Work Environ Health* 1990;16:329–333.
111. Kurppa K, Holmberg PC, Rantala K, Nurminen T, Saxen L. Birth

defects and exposure to video display terminals during pregnancy. *Scand J Work Environ Health* 1985;11:353–356.
112. Nurminen T, Kurppa K. Office employment, work with video display terminals, and course of pregnancy. *Scand J Work Environ Health* 1988;14:293–298.
113. Bracken MB, Belanger K, Hellenbrand K, et al. Exposure to electromagnetic fields during pregnancy with emphasis on electrically heated beds: association with birthweight and intrauterine growth retardation. *Epidemiology* 1995;6:263–270.
114. Nielsen CV, Brandt LP. Fetal growth, pre-term birth and infant mortality in relation to work with video display terminals during pregnancy. *Scand J Work Environ Health* 1992;18:346–350.
115. Brandt LP, Nielsen CV. Fecundity and the use of video display terminals. *Scand J Work Environ Health* 1992;18:298–301.
116. Delpizzo V. Epidemiological studies of work with video display terminals and adverse pregnancy outcomes (1984–1992). *Am J Ind Med* 1994;26:465–480.
117. Shaw GM, Croen LA. Human adverse reproductive outcomes and electromagnetic field exposures: review of epidemiologic studies. *Environ Health Perspect* 1993;101(suppl 4):107–119.
118. Savitz DA. Exposure assessment strategies in epidemiological studies of health effects of electric and magnetic fields. *Sci Total Environ* 1995;168:143–153.
119. Haes DL, Fitzgerald MR. Video display terminal very low frequency measurements: the need for protocols in assessing VDT user dose. *Health Phys* 1995;68:572–578.
120. Kavet R, Tell R. VDTs: field levels, epidemiology and laboratory studies. *Health Phys* 1991;61:47–57.

*Environmental and Occupational Medicine, Third Edition,* edited by William N. Rom.
Lippincott–Raven Publishers, Philadelphia © 1998.

# CHAPTER 101

# Occupational Exposure to Noise

Robert J. McCunney and John D. Meyer

Damage to human hearing from exposure to noise can take two forms: acute, which is secondary to a loud noise such as a blast, and chronic, which is due to long-term exposure to hazardous noise levels. Noises hazardous to human hearing are present in a variety of environments, including military service, civilian occupations, especially manufacturing, and leisure-time pursuits. Noise-induced hearing loss (NIHL) was recognized as early as the publication of Bernardo Ramazini's text on diseases of workers in the 18th century.

Recent estimates indicate that 30 million people in the United States work where noise exposure levels of 85 dB or greater may present a hazard to hearing (1). A review of data from the 1977 National Health Interview Survey and the National Occupational Hazard Survey indicated that approximately 3.2% of people had some degree of hearing loss. The proportion of those with hearing loss increased with age; within age groups, rates were consistently greater for those who worked in industries defined as noisy (2). The Occupational Safety and Health Administration (OSHA) has estimated that 17% of production workers have at least some mild hearing impairment (3).

Hearing loss, however, is not limited to persons exposed to noise at work. As many as 25% to 40% of people older than 65 years have some degree of hearing loss (2). The National Institute for Occupational Safety and Health (NIOSH) has suggested that nearly one of every four workers older than 55 years who have been exposed to high noise levels (beyond 90 dB) have some degree of material impairment (4).

Clearly, noise is a major occupational health risk. In fact, NIOSH has identified NIHL as one of the 10 leading work-related disorders (5). NIOSH recommended the following measures to prevent hearing loss:

1. Develop new technology that leads to quieter processes.
2. Develop noise control strategies at the source of existing operations.
3. Develop hearing conservation programs and effective hearing protection devices.

The importance of a proper assessment of the need for a hearing conservation program to aid in the prevention of NIHL cannot be overemphasized. Although the cost of worker's compensation claims for NIHL varies among states, one survey suggests that the average cost per claim is approximately $15,000 (6). NIHL has other potential impacts on the operation of a business, for example in the form of fines levied against the business for violation or noncompliance with the standards of the OSHA hearing conservation amendment.

## INDUSTRIES THAT EXPOSE WORKERS TO NOISE-INDUCED HEARING LOSS

Although certain work duties in virtually any industry can present a risk to hearing, some industries have a greater proportion of workers at risk of NIHL. In the petroleum, lumber, and food-processing industries, as many as 25% of the work force may be exposed to levels beyond the OSHA permissible exposure level of 90 dB [8-hour time-weighted average ($TWA_8$)]. Manufacture of furniture, metals, rubber, and plastics also presents risks

R. J. McCunney: Environmental Medical Services, Massachusetts Institute of Technology, Cambridge, Massachusetts 02139.
J. D. Meyer: Institute of Occupational and Environmental Health, West Virginia University School of Medicine, Morgantown, West Virginia 26506-9190.

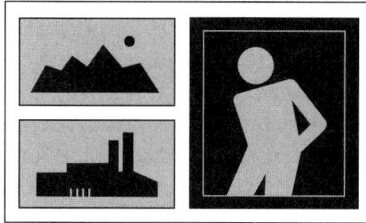

to human hearing if workers are not properly protected from hazardous levels of noise.

The effects of environmental noise on human health has also aroused concern. However, ambient noise from road traffic, aircraft, and construction activities has not yet attracted well-controlled epidemiologic studies (7). Such evaluations present substantial scientific challenges in study design, implementation, and analysis, especially in controlling for confounding factors. Nonetheless, attempts have been made to determine the effect of traffic noise on sleep (8), cardiovascular disease risk (7), and hypertension (9). In the latter study, inhabitants of areas near aircraft and automobile traffic had higher rates of hypertension when compared to subjects living in another, less noisy, area.

## THE ROLE OF THE OCCUPATIONAL PHYSICIAN

Physicians who provide occupational health services are faced with a number of challenges in the evaluation of NIHL (10). They must conduct clinical evaluations of workers who report symptoms of hearing loss. Interpreting the results of audiometric testing, evaluating the effectiveness of a hearing conservation program, and providing assistance in the selection of hearing protection devices are all functions mandated by the OSHA hearing conservation standard with which the occupational health physician must be comfortable and conversant. Finally, the physician must aid in facilitating referrals to appropriate specialists such as otolaryngologists and audiologists when such consultation is indicated.

## OSHA REGULATIONS

A standard to help prevent NIHL in American industries was issued by OSHA in 1983 (3). This regulation requires employers to assess the level of noise in a facility, to reduce noise when it exceeds certain levels, and to provide employees with appropriate medical testing, education, training, and hearing protection devices. Physicians can participate in any or all of these activities and provide a medical perspective in efforts designed to prevent hearing damage from noise. The OSHA standard requires employers to implement noise control measures when levels exceed 90 dB ($TWA_8$) and to support a hearing conservation program when levels are beyond 85 dB (Table 1). An approach to assessing the need for a hearing conservation program is outlined later in this chapter.

**TABLE 1.** *Decibel levels of noises in different environments*

| | Community | |
|---|---|---|
| Industrial and military | Outdoor | Indoor |
| Uncomfortably loud (over 100 dB) | | |
| Diesel engine room (125 dB) | 50 hp siren at 100 ft (125 dB) | Live rock-and-roll band (114 dB) |
| Armored personnel carrier (13 dB) | Thunderclap overhead (120 dB) | |
| Oxygen torch (121 dB) | Jet plane at ramp (117 dB) | |
| Scraper-loader (117 dB) | Chain saw (110 dB) | |
| Compactor (116 dB) | Jet flyover at 1,000 ft (103 dB) | |
| Riveting machine (110 dB) | | |
| Textile loom (106 dB) | | |
| Electric furnace area (100 dB) | | |
| Loud (80 to 99 dB) | | |
| Farm tractor (98 dB) | Power mower (96 dB) | Inside subway car, 35 mph (95 dB) |
| Newspaper press (97 dB) | Compressor at 20 ft (94 dB) | Shouted conversation (90 dB) |
| Cockpit of propeller aircraft (88 dB) | Rock drill at 100 ft (92 dB) | Food blender (88 dB) |
| Milling machine (85 dB) | Motorcycles at 25 ft (90 dB) | Garbage disposer (80 dB) |
| Cotton spinning (83 dB) | Propeller aircraft flyover at 1,000 ft (88 dB) | |
| Lathe (81 dB) | | |
| Tabulating (80 dB) | Diesel truck, 40 mph at 50 ft (84 dB) | Diesel train, 40 to 50 mph at 100 ft (83 dB) |
| Moderately loud (60 to 79 dB) | | |
| | Passenger car, 65 mph at 25 ft (77 dB) | Clothes washer (78 dB) |
| | | Living room music (76 dB) |
| | Auto traffic near freeway (64 dB) | Dishwasher (75 dB) |
| | Air conditioning unit at 20 ft (60 dB) | Television (70 dB) |
| | | Vacuum cleaner (70 dB) |
| Quiet (40 to 59 dB) | | |
| | Large transformer at 200 ft (58 dB) | Normal conversation (50 dB) |
| | Light traffic at 100 ft (50 dB) | |
| Very quiet (20 to 39 dB) | | |
| | Rustling leaves (20 dB) | |

## NOISE AND HEALTH

In occupational medical practice, noise presents three fundamental risks to health:

1. Acutely, through blasts, explosions, or other high-impulse noises that lead to hearing deficits.
2. Chronically, through continued exposure to unsafe levels of noise that lead to sensorineural hearing impairment.
3. Through extraauditory effects, including alterations in blood pressure and adverse influences on existing illnesses such as hyperlipoproteinemia and diabetes.

### Acute Acoustic Trauma

Exposure to intense levels of noise can cause permanent damage to the middle and inner ear. In one review of 52 cases of acute acoustic trauma (AAT) (11), the most common symptoms were hearing loss (95%) and tinnitus (70%). Most of the cases were thought to have been exposed to noise levels in the range of 140 to 160 dB. Military service accounted for the majority (45%); about one in four had bilateral damage.

Results of audiometric evaluation in AAT may reflect conductive hearing loss secondary to traumatic rupture of the tympanic membrane, disruption of the ossicular chain, and mechanical damage to the oval window, as well as sensorineural loss from cochlear hair cell disruption. Higher-frequency pure tone hearing loss is more common in AAT, with frequencies between 4,000 and 8,000 Hz most affected, (12,13). A period of weeks to months may be required for hearing to stabilize; the pathologic process resulting in progression of hearing loss from AAT appears not to extend beyond a year unless other factors are present (14). Even if the audiometric results return to normal, however, permanent damage may have occurred to the sensory cells of the inner ear, and continued exposure to noise may result in further deterioration of hearing (14). An interesting finding of evaluations of AAT is that most people do not seek medical attention immediately following the blast explosion or traumatic event. It appears that tinnitus, rather than pain or decreased hearing acuity, was the symptom most likely to prompt people to seek a medical evaluation (11,15).

Military operations present the greatest risks for suffering an acute injury to the ear. A survey of World War II casualties (16) indicated that aural injuries accounted for 5.8% of the patients treated at a U.S. military hospital in Paris. Relatively little information is available on the extent of occupationally related acute hearing damage that progresses to the sensorineural pattern typical of NIHL.

Unusual explosions have also occurred in certain settings, especially in concert with terrorist activities. One such event in Belfast, Northern Ireland was described (17). Nearly a year after an explosive blast in a restaurant, 30% of those present suffered from high-frequency sensorineural hearing loss. (Hearing loss was defined as >30 dB at 4,000 and 8,000 Hz in one or both ears.)

In the Falkland Islands war (18), military personnel who operated heavier weapons suffered greater hearing loss than those not so exposed. Soldiers operating the heavier artillery, on average, had at least 5 dB loss in each ear at certain frequencies. Blast injuries are particularly difficult to prevent in military operations because of the reluctance of personnel to wear hearing protection devices for fear that they will interfere with communications and place their lives at risk.

On physical examination the ear is usually normal unless the tympanic membrane is ruptured, which occurs in approximately a third of cases of AAT. Damage to the cochlea, vestibular system, and ossicles of the inner ear can also occur. The diagnostic use of the auditory brain stem response has been found to be effective in the clinical evaluation of a blast injury to the ear (19). Note that it is not necessarily the ear exposed to the blast that sustains the injury, since blast waves may bounce off walls and surrounding objects to cause an injury in the ear not directly exposed to the source.

Complications following such injuries include persistent perforation of the tympanic membrane, permanent hearing loss, and cholesteatoma. About 10% to 20% of tympanic membrane ruptures require surgical correction (20), with the remainder generally healing without intervention. The patient with a persistent perforation should be advised to keep water, foreign bodies, and other potential contaminants out of the external auditory meatus. Large perforations and those that appear not to be healing mandate referral to an otolaryngologist.

Although prevention of AAT should be emphasized, these injuries can rarely be predicted. Where prevention fails, proper treatment depends on access to medical care. A number of treatment measures have been attempted that are based on the premise that the blast has caused metabolic disturbances in the sensory cells of the inner ear. Evaluation of the effectiveness of medications, however, is impeded by the lack of preexposure audiometric values (21).

In a review of medicinal therapy for AAT, no convincing evidence was noted to support the use of vitamin A, B, or E, nicotinic acid, papaverine hydrochloride, or a number of other substances (22). Dextran has been widely used by the German military with variable results, which may have been in part due to better pretreatment thresholds in the treated subjects. Reports suggest that following the injury, treatment must be given promptly if the intervention is to be effective. More recent reports indicate a lack of efficacy of dextran (23,24,25). The strength of these claims is difficult to evaluate in light of the absence of clinically controlled double-blind evaluations.

A thorough understanding of the mechanisms of AAT would enhance both prevention and treatment. Animal studies have suggested that certain pathologic features are consistent within species, especially the acute mechanical failure associated with AAT. Consistent findings include separation of the organ of Corti from the basilar membrane and disturbances in function of the tympanic membrane and ossicles (26). In an attempt to understand the effect of various military operations on the hearing of troops, the U. S. Army sponsored an evaluation of 67 sheep and pigs that were exposed to military operations while they were positioned in an armored vehicle (27). Tympanic membrane rupture was a consistent finding in the animals; the authors concluded, "The prevalence and severity of ear drum injury is greater for large anti-armor artillery and that the injury correlated with increasing peak pressure" and therefore blast intensity (27).

### Chronic Hearing Loss

Prolonged exposure to noise primarily damages the inner ear, especially the hair cells of the organ of Corti (28) (Fig. 1). Cochlear blood vessels, the stria vascularis, and nerve endings associated with the hair cells can also be damaged. Initially, the hair cells of the basal turn of the cochlea are affected; this area is responsible for perception of higher-frequency sound. Eventually, disruption of the medial and apical areas occurs as well.

Although the risk of suffering NIHL tends to increase with advancing age as well as with length of employment, most noise-related effects occur within the early phases of exposure to noise (29). In fact, most of the damage that occurs to the hearing mechanism tends to occur within the first 10 years. Presbycusis, the impairment of hearing due to advancing age, results in diminished hearing ability usually beginning in the mid-40s and continuing thereafter. People who suffer from sensorineural hearing loss, however, do not usually recognize early changes in their ability to hear. Nonetheless, early changes can usually be documented by audiometric monitoring. A study of army helicopter pilots indicated that only one of four who exhibit decrements on audiometric monitoring was aware of any hearing deficit (30). Early symptoms of NIHL reflect a person's ability to distinguish higher-pitched consonant sounds. For example, the word *fist* may sound like *fish.* Speech is recognized as less intelligible as opposed to lower in volume. This latter point accounts for the lack of efficacy of hearing amplification devices in the treatment of people whose hearing is impaired due to noise.

### *Risk Factors*

The major risk factor for suffering noise-induced hearing loss is prolonged unprotected exposure to levels of noise beyond 85 dB. A number of other risk factors, however, have been proposed, including hyperlipoproteinemia (31,32), diabetes (33), solvents (34), cigarette smoking (35), eye color (36), and thyroid abnormalities (37).

The contribution to hearing loss from lipid abnormalities remains uncertain. A review of 100 patients with bilateral sensorineural deficit found the prevalence of hyperlipoproteinemia to be lower than in the general population (31). These results, however, differ from other, later results indicating a significant correlation of elevated low-density-lipoprotein cholesterol with noise-induced hearing loss (32).

A significant issue in occupational medicine is whether workers with diabetes are at greater risk of NIHL. Non–insulin-dependent diabetes may increase the risk of severe hearing loss in those with occupational exposure to noise (38). Imprecise data, especially regarding the duration and severity of disease, and small sample sizes of workers with insulin-dependent diabetes mellitus (IDDM), have hampered attempts to draw a link between IDDM and NIHL (33). The cause of diabetes-induced hearing loss, however, is yet to be fully determined, but it

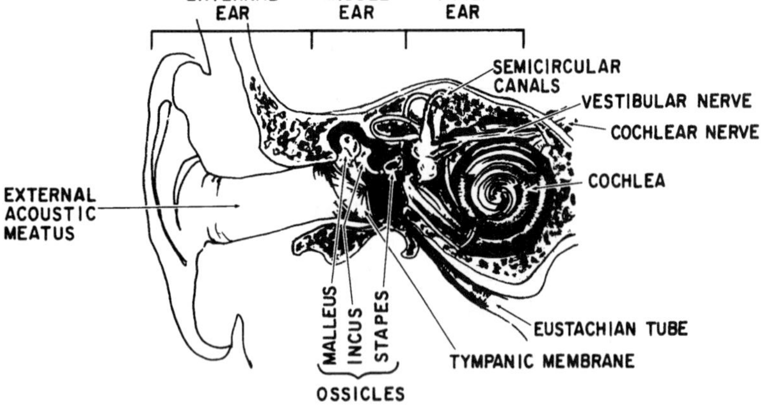


**FIG. 1.** Illustration of a cross section of the human auditory system. High noise levels can damage the tympanic membrane, middle ear conducting system, and sensor cells in the inner ear (cochlea).

appears to be due to metabolic disturbances that affect nerve function. Despite the possibility of increased risk of NIHL among diabetic patients, most occupational physicians do not feel that scientific evidence warrants restricting people with this disorder from noisy work if appropriate measures for reducing noise exposure are followed (32).

An investigation of more than 2,000 noise-exposed white males in an aerospace company indicated that cigarette smokers have an approximately 40% greater risk of NIHL (35). In fact, the major risk factors for this cohort were smoking, a noisy hobby such as guns, and number of years worked at a noisy plant. These results give credence to the theory that susceptibility to NIHL may be due to relative ischemia of the vasculature of the inner ear. The contribution of ischemia, however, to the development of NIHL is difficult to discern in light of conflicting scientific evidence, especially regarding people with diabetes. For example, patients with diabetic retinopathy had no greater prevalence of sensorineural hearing impairment than controls (39,40). Other studies assessing the contribution of cigarette smoking to the development of NIHL have shown mixed results. Some evaluations (41,42) have shown a strong association between smoking and NIHL, others a dose-response relationship significant only at heavy smoking levels (43), and still others demonstrate no association (44,45).

After noise, the exposure of most concern in the workplace setting is industrial solvent exposure. Selective midfrequency hearing deficits have been demonstrated in rats exposed to toluene, styrene, xylenes, and trichloroethylene (46). Solvent abusers, with exposure primarily to toluene, have also demonstrated balance disorders and hearing impairment (47). Epidemiologic studies of hearing loss in solvent-exposed workers have been more variable, possibly because of the role of other factors, such as workplace noise, aging, and smoking, on the results. High-frequency hearing loss has been described in workers exposed to mixed solvents and noise (34,48). Several cohorts of workers exposed to solvents in the absence of noise have also shown abnormalities on pure-tone audiometry or on evoked cortical response audiometry, indicating an effect on more central pathways of the auditory response (49).

### Mechanisms of Noise-Induced Hearing Loss

How noise actually damages hearing has been the subject of a variety of research efforts. Most investigations have been conducted on animals and have attempted to determine the cellular and vascular damage secondary to noise. The first detailed description of abnormalities in the inner ear associated with sensorineural hearing loss was published in 1934 (50). Since then, research has indicated that the effects of noise tend to occur in the organ of Corti, within the cochlea of the inner ear (51). This structure has three outer rows and one inner row of hair cells, with the tectorial membrane suspended above them. The hair cells contain cilia that project toward the tectorial membrane. The energy transmitted from the tympanic membrane via the ossicles to the cochlea vibrates the cilia and is then coded into nerve impulses in the acoustic nerve. The hair cells are quite susceptible to the trauma of loud noise. The cell bodies swell with repeated exposure to loud noise and ultimately the hair cells are destroyed (51). Studies have indicated that the vascular supply of the basilar membrane is disrupted when high noise levels are applied (52). Capillary vasoconstriction in response to loud noise may result in diminished oxygen tension and local hypoxia within the cochlea.

A variety of animal investigations have been performed that confirm the mechanisms described above. In a transmission electron microscopic study, edema and swelling of the afferent nerve endings below the inner hair cells were noted (53). Following an acute reaction, in which the hair cell was distended, a cytoplasmic protrusion occurred that indicated cell damage. These changes to the afferent nerve fibers were also noted in an investigation of guinea pigs. In general, most investigators agree that a combination of mechanical, metabolic, and vascular factors are involved in the destructive changes that lead to NIHL. Eventually, the organ of Corti breaks down with separation of segments of sensory cells from the basilar membrane, leading to elimination of sensory structures and replacement by a single flat cell layer (54).

In a study of rats, mean cochlear blood flow was much lower in noise-exposed groups than in those not exposed to noise (55). In fact, an interesting finding of potential clinical application was noted: rats that were spontaneously hypertensive tended to have a greater decrease in blood supply than those that were not hypertensive. This finding may have some relevance in evaluating the extraauditory health risks associated with noise, such as hypertension. This observed reduction in cochlear blood flow could lead to hypoxia, and ultimately disruption in inner ear metabolism. This finding that hypertensive rats were at greater risk for NIHL was confirmed by another study (56). It remains unclear, however, whether the decrease in blood supply associated with impaired hearing is either a primary or secondary pathologic response. Another animal investigation noted vasoconstriction of the cochlear blood vessels in response to exposure to high noise levels (57). These authors also proposed impaired blood flow in the inner ear capillary as the major mechanism leading to NIHL.

According to some authors, the pathologic abnormalities associated with NIHL can be differentiated from those due to presbycusis (58). Certain morphologic abnormalities, for example, appear to be different. Noise disrupts the outer and inner hair cells of the organ of Corti; ultimately degeneration of nerve fibers and ganglion cells occurs. Presbycusis, by contrast, causes abnormalities over the entire auditory system.

### Extraauditory Effects of Noise

The extraauditory effects of noise, most notably hypertension, remain an area of active interest regarding health implications of noise. Investigative results, however, have varied regarding the relationship to hypertension of long-term noise exposure. The basis of the proposed relationship between noise and hypertension is grounded in the stress response, that is, as a result of noise, release of adrenocortical hormones and sympathomimetic mediators leads to increased heart rate and eventually higher blood pressure. Investigations have been hampered because the prevalence of hypertension and presbycusis, as well as NIHL, tends to increase with age.

A number of investigations have been conducted into the relationship between noise and hypertension. One approach involves correlating noise levels with blood pressure measurements, which has been attempted in some cross-sectional evaluations. For example, the blood pressure of certain noise-exposed groups can be compared to a similarly matched group of workers not exposed to loud noise. Another approach is to evaluate the blood pressure of people with sensorineural hearing loss and compare their measurements to those of matched controls without NIHL. An investigation of nearly 200 workers in a quiet plant (less than 81 dB) in comparison to others in a noisy plant (greater than 90 dB) observed no difference in mean systolic or diastolic blood pressure (58). A strong relationship, however, was noted between severe NIHL (defined as a hearing threshold of 65 dB or more at 3,000, 4,000, 6,000, and 8,000 Hz) and high blood pressure (defined as diastolic pressure more than 90 mm Hg or a physician's prescribing hypertensive medication). The rate of hypertension among older workers with severe NIHL was twice as great as for those without hearing loss. The authors noted the clinical difficulties in distinguishing presbycusis from sensorineural hearing loss. They found that subjects with NIHL were impaired in both ear- and bone-conducted sound and exhibited the traditional 4,000-Hz dip on audiometric evaluation. This study, however, was the first effort in which NIHL proved to be a biologic marker for hypertension, even when traditional risk factors were controlled. These results are consistent with other evaluations that suggest that the duration of noise exposure required to cause hypertension is greater than that needed to cause NIHL.

A study of 245 retired metal assembly workers showed a significant relationship between hypertension and NIHL (defined as more than 65 dB loss at 3,000, 4,000, or 6,000 Hz) (59). Note that these definitions of severe NIHL are not identical to standard threshold shifts that may be detected in audiometric evaluations. The authors also suggested that a threshold of occupational noise exposure may be necessary to increase the risk of hypertension. High-frequency hearing loss has also been associated with elevations in serum cholesterol (60), which may lead to impaired blood supply to the inner ear. In fact, a model for an apparent interaction between hypercholesterolemia and NIHL has been proposed (61).

An investigation of automotive workers, however, found no relationship between mean blood pressure and hearing loss at 4,000 Hz among white workers (62). Among the 119 blacks in the study a higher prevalence of hypertension (32%) was noted than in the 150 whites (22%). (These percentages are similar to age- and race-adjusted rates for hypertension in the United States.) The authors noted other interesting findings. In particular, they found no correlation between years of exposure and hearing loss; as a result of this finding, they suggested that the exposure years may not accurately reflect cumulative noise exposure. Moreover, because of blacks' higher risk of hypertension, the authors suggested they may also be more susceptible to sensorineural hearing loss. This study was the first to address the relationship between occupational noise exposure and hypertension among black workers in the United States. A study of nearly 500 people who worked in a textile plant and were exposed to levels of noise beyond 100 dB revealed that approximately a third had hypertension. The authors noted, however, that the relation of arterial hypertension to noise exposure was not strong (63). Studies of human volunteers have tended to support a relationship between noise and diastolic blood pressure elevations in both normotensive and hypertensive volunteers (64).

Fifteen healthy normotensive medical students exposed to 95 dB noise for 20 minutes exhibited significant elevations in diastolic blood pressure (65). This elevation in diastolic blood pressure secondary to noise is confirmed by other investigations (66). The authors proposed that noise activates the sympathetic nervous system and elevates blood pressure by increasing total peripheral resistance. Animal studies support the concept that vasoconstriction of the cochlear vessels plays an important role in causing NIHL. An interesting aspect of this mechanism is that different strains of rats have marked differences in susceptibility for contracting hypertension due to noise (65). In a review of the animal literature, Pillsbury (67) claimed a significant relationship between hypertension, noise, hyperlipoproteinemia, and hearing loss.

Various hormonal responses have also been described secondary to noise; effects range from increased levels of urinary catecholamines to increased concentration of 17-hydroxycorticoids (68,69). Increased postshift urinary cortisol excretion has been noted in workers exposed to high ambient noise levels compared with those wearing hearing protection equipment (69). These findings bolster the hypothesis that noise acts as a general stressor in the setting of normal work demands.

### Pregnancy and Noise

Exposure to noise has resulted in teratogenic effects on laboratory rats, including reduced fertility and enlargement of the ovaries (70,71). In a case-control study in Finland, approximately 1,200 women were evaluated (72). Results showed no relationship between occupational noise exposure (greater than 80 dB) and risk of either premature birth or low birth weight. Only approximately 3% of the study group, however, reported any exposure to noise at work during their pregnancy. Moreover, approximately two-thirds of the noise-exposed women were on sick leave during their pregnancy.

It is unclear what effect exposure to noise during pregnancy may have on the unborn child, in terms of increased rate of miscarriage, low birth weight, or prematurity. Most evaluations have been conducted on women living in the vicinity of airports (73). Exposure to noise in utero may affect hearing later in life (74). In a study of 131 offspring of Quebec women, there was a threefold increase in the risk of high-frequency hearing loss in the children whose mothers were exposed in utero to noise in the range of 85 to 95 dB, and a significant increase in the risk of hearing loss at 4,000 Hz when there was a strong component of low-frequency noise exposure (74).

## CLINICAL EVALUATION OF HEARING IMPAIRMENT

Physicians who practice occupational medicine are likely to find themselves asked to assess hearing impairment, prevent further deterioration of hearing, and recommend patients for further evaluation and treatment. Human hearing has a remarkable capability for differentiating sounds ranging from a rustling leaf to the blast of armaments. In fact, the ear can hear frequencies as low as 20 Hz and as high as approximately 20,000 Hz (10). The early symptoms of NIHL tend to be subtle and may not be readily recognized by the patient. As NIHL progresses, the person's ability to distinguish softer sounds is usually disrupted first. For example, the sounds of birds and other high-frequency sounds such as voices may be difficult to discern. People with high-pitched voices, such as children and some women, may speak in a way that presents difficulties for a person with NIHL. In general, the amplitude of the sound is not affected as much as its clarity. As noted earlier, people with NIHL initially have difficulty with higher-pitched sibilant consonant sounds, such as distinguishing the word *fish* from *fist.*

Since the primary effect of NIHL is on the inner ear, the astute physician must be aware of other symptoms of inner ear disease, especially vertigo. Vertigo is often the first symptom of inner ear disorders. Both vertigo and high-pitched tinnitus can be early signs of acoustic neuroma. Its presence may also suggest Meniere's disease. Vertigo, however, is seldom associated with NIHL or presbycusis. Nevertheless, NIHL rarely, if ever, produces profound deafness (75), but the condition tends to be progressive. Hearing handicaps are usually noticed when the threshold hearing level of important (speech frequencies such as 500, 1,000, 2,000, and 3,000 Hz) averages more than 25 dB.

The diagnosis of NIHL is straightforward when the physician incorporates a clear occupational history of noise exposure with the results of an audiometric evaluation. The audiometric results may indicate the need for further evaluation with more detailed diagnostic studies. The major pathologic entities in the differential diagnosis of NIHL are presbycusis and ototoxicity (76), although more than 40 genetic and metabolic syndromes can cause deafness (77). Physicians evaluating the contribution of workplace noise to hearing loss should also consider nonoccupational causes such as target shooting, motorcycle riding, hunting, loud music, and portable radios. It has been shown, for example, that personal stereos with headphones can generate noise levels well beyond OSHA standards (78). The major drugs associated with deafness include furosemide and aminoglycoside antibiotics (gentamicin, for example). Analgesics, such as salicylates and antihistamines, as well as tricyclic antidepressants have been associated with ototoxicity. Salicylates, in particular, are well known to cause reversible tinnitus.

In evaluating a hearing-impaired person, the physician is advised to review the results of pure-tone audiometric testing, which assesses the ability to hear various standardized frequencies. During the test, tone levels are increased in volume until the person recognizes the sound. The decibel reading at which the person first recognizes the sound at each frequency is recorded; this value is termed the hearing threshold for that frequency. Threshold levels above 25 dB are abnormal, and are especially important when the speech frequency ranges (500 to 4,000 Hz) are affected.

Early impairment due to NIHL tends to occur at 4,000 Hz, with preservation of hearing at higher frequencies (8,000 Hz). These findings are typical of NIHL, with this 4,000-Hz notch persisting and deepening with increased hearing loss secondary to noise (Fig. 2). With presbycusis, the audiometric pattern has a similar decrement in the 4,000-Hz range; however, the loss tends to be greater still in the 8,000-Hz range, and no notch is noted. The audiometric findings of hearing loss due to ototoxicity are similar to those of presbycusis.

Despite the differences described for audiometric results, differentiating NIHL from presbycusis can be a difficult exercise. Moreover, presbycusis and NIHL can act concurrently to affect hearing. People with NIHL, however, tend to show high-frequency hearing deficits for both ear and bone conduction of sound, reflecting the sensorineural character of the hearing loss.

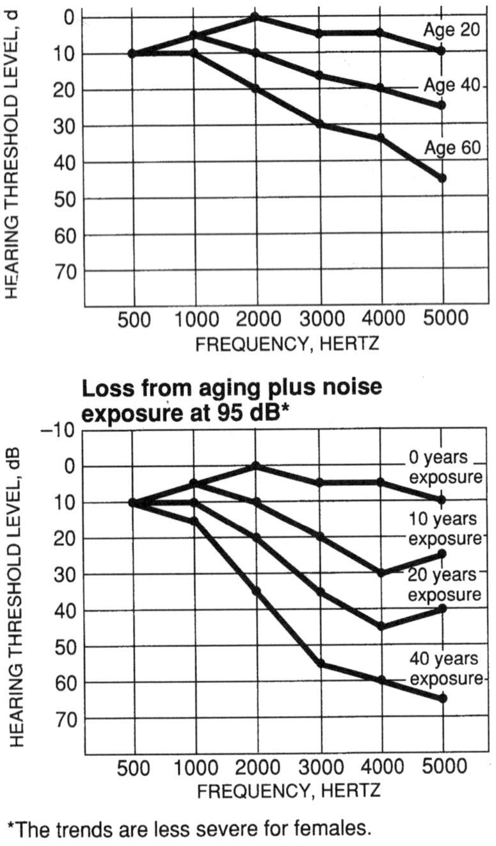


**FIG. 2.** Audiogram results depicting hearing loss from aging and noise.

Other diagnostic and screening tools used to identify hearing impairment and distinguish between differing etiologies have been described (79). To assess the degree of hearing impairment among people over 65 years of age, a handheld audioscope was combined with the Hearing Handicap Inventory for the Elderly (HHIE), a self-administered ten-item questionnaire designed to assess emotional and social problems associated with impaired hearing. The audioscope can be inserted into the ear and delivers a 40-dB tone at frequencies of 500, 1,000, 2,000, and 4,000 Hz. In this evaluation of 178 patients, the audioscope proved to be a sensitive and reliable test for the detection of hearing impairment in persons older than 65 years. The same study, when coupled with the HHIE, was 83% accurate in diagnosing NIHL.

Another screening test that has been used in the occupational setting is the W-22MAX, which assesses speech discrimination of words that are presented with a competing sound (59). This procedure attempts to determine a person's ability to communicate in everyday life by assessing both psychosocial impairment and biologic damage to the hearing mechanism. Words are presented on an audiotape in the presence of background noise. The percentage of the words correctly identified in the better ear is the W-22MAX score for speech discrimination. In the study described above (59) the authors claimed that the W-22MAX may be a more sensitive index of both the psychosocial and biologic components of NIHL through its capacity to measure both noise-related damage to the cochlea as well as to determine the degree of communication handicap. Further work with speech discrimination testing in occupational groups exposed to noise would be valuable.

Another diagnostic study used to evaluate hearing loss is the auditory brain stem response, which tracks the brain stem response to auditory stimuli (80). This test may be especially valuable in assessing persons who report hearing loss but whose audiometric test results are equivocal.

### Disposition and Follow-Up

After reviewing diagnostic studies, especially the audiometric evaluation, the physician can formulate an opinion as to the cause of hearing loss and whether therapy may be effective. Unfortunately, treatment measures for NIHL tend to be ineffective, since the primary problem is not the amplification of sound but the distinguishing of various types of sounds. Thus, amplification devices that correct other types of hearing impairment by increasing transmission of sound in the middle ear are largely ineffective. Nonetheless, the physician should be aware of the need for otologic referral in evaluating hearing loss (81). Consultation with an otolaryngologist may be necessary when reviewing audiometric monitoring tests of a hearing conservation program or for clinical evaluation of individual patients (81) (see Table 1). Some points to remember in the evaluation of suspected NIHL include the following (75):

1. Chronic NIHL is usually symmetric; other otologic disorders, especially the more serious, as well as treatable, types, are often asymmetric.
2. NIHL usually develops gradually; other otologic disorders may progress rapidly.
3. NIHL usually causes high-frequency threshold shifts.
4. Regardless of the cause, a pure-tone threshold average in excess of 25 dB in either ear is likely to cause hearing difficulties.

### Determination of Impairment

Occupational physicians may also be asked to evaluate hearing impairment, an area for which several sets of guidelines have been proposed (82,83). One approach considers a person hearing impaired if either of two factors is present:

1. A 40-dB loss in *both* ears at *either* the 1,000- *or* 2,000-Hz frequency.

2. A 40-dB loss in *one* ear at the 1,000- *and* 2,000-Hz frequency.

Along similar lines, the American Academy of Otolaryngology has published a formula for calculating hearing impairment based on pure-tone hearing loss at various frequencies (83). These criteria have been adopted by the AMA in the *Guides to the Evaluation of Permanent Impairment,* to aid physicians in the process of disability determination (84). The guidelines assign a 1.5% impairment of monaural hearing for every decibel that the average hearing level (the mean thresholds measured at frequencies of 500, 1,000, 2,000, and 3,000 Hz) exceeds a 25-dB threshold. Impairment does not begin until an average hearing loss of 25 dB has been reached, and is considered complete at a threshold average of 92 dB. Calculation of binaural hearing impairment, as well as whole-person impairment resulting from hearing loss, is made from tables provided in the guides. Another approach has been recommended for military personnel that uses a mathematical model to evaluate a soldier's ability to hear when performing certain military tasks (85).

## HEARING CONSERVATION PROGRAMS

OSHA promulgated a standard that requires employers to determine the noise levels in certain operations, to institute noise control measures where appropriate, and to provide audiometric monitoring, education, and training for the exposed employees (3). According to the standard, the permissible daily exposure limit for noise is 90 dB(A). (All noise levels described in the OSHA standard refer to $TWA_8$; dB(A) refers to decibels weighted according to the A scale, which reduces the weight given to low-frequency sound and reflects sound discrimination by the ear.) An exchange rate of 5 dB for every doubling or halving of the exposure time is used to modify the TWA for louder noise exposures. For example, workers would be permitted only a 4-hour exposure to noise at 95 dB, and a 2-hour exposure at 100 dB. A ceiling or short-term (15 minute) exposure limit of 115 dB is the maximum value beyond which noise exposure is not permitted regardless of duration. Some European countries use an exchange rate of 3 dB for every halving of the exposure time. Acoustically, this approach is considered to have a firmer mathematical foundation, since, as a logarithmic measurement, an increase of 3 dB represents a doubling of sound wave pressures. Exposure to noise beyond the 90 dB $TWA_8$ must be reduced, principally by engineering controls such as equipment modification, enclosure, sound-absorbent surroundings, and improved maintenance. Administrative procedures such as rotating workers and mandatory use of hearing-protection devices may also be necessary.

Hearing conservation programs (HCP) are required when workers are exposed to levels above 85 dB. The fundamentals of an HCP include the following measures (3,86): noise level assessment, noise control measures, audiometric monitoring, education and training, and hearing-protection devices.

### Noise-Level Assessment

The first step in assessing the need for an HCP is to measure the ambient noise level. Assessments are customarily performed by an industrial hygienist or a similar professional. Measurements performed in the occupational setting usually consist of overall levels that are obtained either through a sound-level meter or a noise dosimeter (87). According to OSHA, monitoring of certain areas of a facility that generate noise is required to identify employees who need to be enrolled in the HCP or who require hearing protection. These measurements can also be effective in determining the amount of attenuation required of the hearing-protection devices may be used. Moreover, noise assessments help to acquaint employees and employers with the level of noise in the facility. Generally, OSHA allows area surveys to assess individual exposure if the work force is located in the same general area and the noise levels are relatively stable throughout the work shift. Settings in which impulse or impact noises are present require different approaches.

When area surveys are not appropriate, individual measurements must be made with a personal dosimeter. This particular approach, although capable of yielding more accurate results, tends to be more time-consuming and complicated. Generally, an employee wears the noise dosimeter on the shirt collar throughout a work shift. Accurate measurements depend on reliable calibration of the monitoring device. In certain circumstances it is worthwhile to assess noise at the ear (10). An approach to monitoring noise exposure in workers who wear communication headsets has also recently been introduced (88). This first step, assessing the noise levels encountered in work, is one of the more critical determinants in evaluating the need for an HCP. Once noise levels are determined, they need to be reevaluated at intervals, especially if new processes or plant equipment are introduced into an operation. It is essential that these noise measurements be accurately recorded and available for review, especially by regulatory agencies such as OSHA. The occupational physician who is asked to participate in an audiometric monitoring program should obtain results of noise level assessments, the date of the measurements, and an assessment of whether they reflect normal operations.

In work settings where noise levels exceed 90 dB, engineering controls should be employed (89). Machinery design, enclosures, and noise-control products can be effective in reducing noise at its source. The importance of noise-control measures cannot be overemphasized. One author, for example, has claimed that "prevention of occupational deafness, if it is to be taken seriously, requires a decisive shift to engineering noise control" (29).

**Audiometric Monitoring**

Audiometric monitoring, evaluation of the ability to hear pure-tone frequencies, is essential to preventing NIHL. Periodic audiometric monitoring is a notable example of an effective screening tool that can reduce the risk of occupational illness, because workers with early decrements on audiometric tests usually do not describe hearing difficulties. As an example, one study of army helicopter pilots noted that nearly three out of four soldiers with abnormal audiometric test results (as reflected by a significant threshold shift) were unaware of any hearing loss (30).

Occupational physicians who participate in HCPs are often responsible for interpreting audiometric test results. General principles of medical surveillance apply to HCPs, and the occupational physician is charged with (a) determining the acceptability of the results, (b) assessing alterations in hearing reflected by those results, (c) recommending follow-up actions to evaluate hearing abnormalities, and (d) communicating aggregate results to management and to others with a need to know. Physicians should ensure that the audiometric equipment is properly calibrated according to criteria of the Council for Accreditation in Occupational Hearing Conservation. These guidelines also stipulate training requirements for the person performing the audiometric test, the proper calibration of the audiometer, and the efficacy of the sound control booth. Occupational hearing tests are conducted in many settings, including in the plant, at clinical facilities, and in mobile vans. It is essential that the results be reliable and based on proper testing procedures with functioning equipment.

For employees covered under the OSHA standard, baseline audiometric monitoring is required within 6 months of their hiring. Periodic audiometric test results will eventually be compared to the baseline values; thus, if any abnormalities are noted in this evaluation, the worker should be retested after a 14-hour period without exposure to noise. The OSHA standard mandates yearly audiometric examinations for employees exposed at or above the action level of 85 dB. Records of audiometric testing must be maintained by the employer for the duration of the affected worker's employment.

The physician interpreting audiometric results looks for deviations from the baseline values. A standard threshold shift (STS) refers to a significant hearing decrement as documented by audiometry. As defined by OSHA, an STS refers to an average of 10 dB or greater change from baseline for the average of hearing thresholds at 2,000, 3,000, and 4,000 Hz in either ear. An employee with this change should be retested within 30 days to see if the shift persists. If the increased hearing thresholds persist, the new audiogram, reflecting the STS, is used as a new baseline to measure any further hearing decrements. The employee with a confirmed STS needs to be informed and evaluated to ensure that hearing protection devices fit properly and are being used as directed. Management also needs to be apprised of an STS. Confirmed STSs with an average decrement of 25 Hz or greater in either ear must be recorded as an occupational illness on the OSHA 200 Log form (90). In some cases the physician must address the contribution of presbycusis to hearing impairment. The OSHA standard (3) includes recommended calculations to determine the contribution of age to hearing impairment. More recently, the validity of applying population-derived statistics to individual audiometric results has been challenged, and NIOSH, in a revised criteria document, has recom-

**TABLE 2.** *Example of audiometric thresholds obtained on worker who exhibited progressive noise-induced hearing*

| | Frequency (Hz)[a] | | | | | | | | | | | |
|---|---|---|---|---|---|---|---|---|---|---|---|---|
| | Left ear | | | | | | Right ear | | | | | |
| Thresholds[b] on: | 500 | 1,000 | 2,000 | 3,000 | 4,000 | 6,000 | 500 | 1,000 | 2,000 | 3,000 | 4,000 | 6,000 |
| Reference | 5 | 0 | 0 | 10 | 10 | 5 | 0 | 5 | 5 | 10 | 10 | 10 |
| 1st annual | 0 | 0 | 0 | 10 | 10 | 10 | 5 | 5 | 5 | 10 | 15 | 10 |
| 2nd annual | 5 | 5 | 0 | 10 | 15 | 10 | 0 | 5 | 5 | 15 | 20 | 15 |
| 3rd annual | 0 | 5 | 5 | 15 | 15 | 15 | 5 | 5 | 5 | 15 | 25 | 10 |
| 4th annual | 5 | 5 | 10 | 15 | 20 | 20 | 0 | 5 | 5 | 20 | 25 | 15 |
| 5th annual | 0 | 5 | 15 | 25 | 30 | 25 | 10 | 10 | 10 | 15 | 25 | 20 |
| 6th annual | 5 | 10 | 20 | 35 | 40 | 30 | 10 | 10 | 15 | 20 | 35 | 25 |
| 7th annual | 0 | 10 | 30 | 45 | 50 | 40 | 15 | 15 | 20 | 30 | 40 | 35 |
| 8th annual | 5 | 15 | 35 | 50 | 55 | 40 | 15 | 20 | 30 | 45 | 55 | 40 |
| 9th annual | 10 | 25 | 40 | 60 | 70 | 50 | 15 | 35 | 45 | 55 | 65 | 50 |
| 10th annual | 10 | 35 | 55 | 70 | 85 | 60 | 20 | 40 | 50 | 65 | 80 | 55 |
| 11th annual | 15 | 40 | 65 | 80 | 95 | 80 | 10 | 45 | 60 | 75 | 90 | 70 |

[a]*Frequency* is a measure of the pitch of a sound and is expressed in Hertz (Hz). Higher frequencies (4,000, 6,000 Hz) are usually first affected in noise-induced hearing impairments.

[b]*Thresholds* are recorded in decibels (dB), and the quantities shown under frequency indicate the softest intensity level at which the person could hear the different test tones. (Note: 0 dB is audiometric "zero," and deviations from optimum normal are recorded in dB hearing levels greater than 0.)

mended that audiograms no longer be adjusted to account for the effects of presbycusis (1).

The importance of periodic audiometric monitoring in preventing NIHL cannot be overemphasized. Audiometry serves as an effective tool for surveillance if used regularly and properly (91). Especially in the early years of noise exposure, decrements in hearing can occur without being noticed by the worker (30). Table 2 illustrates a case of progressive, albeit subtle, changes that occurred over a 10-year period, ultimately leading to serious hearing impairment in both ears. The audiometric test value that is most reflective of hearing acuity is in the frequency range below 3,000 Hz. Although there is no requirement for outside referral in the OSHA regulations, the reviewing or examining physician may find it appropriate to help workers obtain more detailed audiometric evaluations. Although audiometric screening has been effective among occupationally exposed groups, this testing has not been valuable as a screening tool in the general population because of the low prevalence of hearing loss in younger cohorts (92).

### Hearing Protection Devices

The fundamental approach to reducing the risk of NIHL is to control noise at its source. In some cases, however, this approach is not feasible, so it is essential to provide hearing-protection devices. These are of three basis types: insert, which are devices inserted directly into the ear canal; semiinsert, which are devices that cover entry into the ear canal; and muffs, which completely encapsulate the ear itself. Hearing-protection devices provide various levels of attenuation (noise reduction). No single type of hearing protection can be considered the single best choice for all users; different workers will choose different devices because of such factors as personal comfort and variations in the anatomic structure of their ears. Thus it is essential to offer employees a variety of hearing-protection devices, to ensure that all can comfortably wear them. During the audiometric evaluation it is worthwhile to acquaint or reeducate the employee in the proper use of the hearing-protection device. When such a device is fitted at the time of the audiometric evaluation, the external canal can be evaluated more thoroughly.

Most hearing-protection devices provide 15- to 30-dB attenuation. When insert plugs are combined with muffs, an additional 10- to 15-dB protection can be obtained, a result noted clinically in a study of army helicopter pilots (30). A noise reduction rating (NRR), which reflects attenuation of environmental noise, must be assigned by the manufacturer of the hearing protection device. Efficacy of these devices in the workplace, however, is dependent on many variables, and attenuation of noise under actual working conditions may be 25% to 75% of the labeled NRR. For a comprehensive review of hearing-protection devices, including selection, fitting, and care, the best source remains Berger (93).

### Education and Training

Physicians may also participate in various educational and training programs designed to acquaint managers and employees with the health implications of long-term exposure to high noise levels. Such educational sessions can be of great benefit in motivating employers and supervisors, and impressing on them the importance of noise control measures and proper use of hearing-protection devices. Employees also need to be apprised of the nature and consequences of NIHL, and of the importance of wearing hearing-protection devices and participating in annual audiometric monitoring programs. A thorough discussion of the importance of education, training, and motivation can be found in Gasaway (94).

## REFERENCES

1. National Institute for Occupational Safety and Health. *Criteria for a recommended standard. Occupational noise exposure.* Revised criteria 1996. Washington: USDHHS, 1996.
2. Moss AJ, Parsons VL. Current estimates from the National Health Interview Survey—United States, 1985. *Vital Health Stat* 1986;160:1–182.
3. 29 CFR 1910.95. *Occupational noise exposure.* Washington, DC: U.S. Government Printing Office, 1996.
4. Leading work-related diseases and injuries—United States. *JAMA* 1986;255:2133.
5. Centers for Disease Control. Leading work-related diseases and injuries—United States. *MMWR* 1983;32:24–26;32.
6. Alleyne BC, Dufresne RM, Nasim K, Reesal MR. Costs of workers' compensation claims for hearing loss. *J Occup Med* 1989;31:134–138.
7. Babisch W, Ising H, Gallacher JEJ, Elwood PC. Traffic noise and cardiovascular risk. The Caerphilly study, first phase. Outdoor noise levels and risk factors. *Arch Environ Health* 1988;43:407–414.
8. Stevenson DC, McKellar NR. The effect of traffic noise on sleep of young adults in their homes. *Acoustical Soc Am* 1989;85(2):768–771.
9. Von Eiff AW, Friedrich G, Neus H. Traffic noise. A factor in the pathogenesis of essential hypertension. *Contrib Nephrol* 1982;30:82–86.
10. Gasaway DC. Noise-induced hearing loss. In: McCunney RJ, ed. *A practical approach to occupational and environmental medicine.* Boston: Little,Brown, 1994;230–247.
11. Axelsson A, Hamernik RP. Acute acoustic trauma. *Acta Otolaryngol (Stockh)* 1987;104:225–233.
12. Hanner P, Axelsson A. Acute acoustic trauma. An emergency condition. *Scand Audiol* 1988;17:57–63.
13. Ylikoski J. Acute acoustic trauma in Finnish conscripts. Etiological factors and characteristics of hearing impairment. *Scand Audiol* 1989;-18:161–165.
14. Segal S, Harell M, Shahar A, Englender M. Acute acoustic trauma: dynamics of hearing loss following cessation of exposure. *Am J Otol* 1988;9:293–298.
15. Melinek M, Naggan, L, Altman M. Acute acoustic trauma — A clinical evaluation and prognosis in 433 symptomatic soldiers. *Isr J Med Sci* 1976;12:560–569.
16. Hepskind MM. Auditory impairment due to battle incurred acoustic trauma. In: DeBakey M, ed. *Surgery in WWII. Ophthalmology and otolaryngology.* Washington, DC: Office of the Surgeon General, 1967; 489–511.
17. Kerr AG. Trauma and the temporal bone. *J Laryngol Otol* 1980; 94:107–110.
18. Brown JR. Noise-induced hearing loss sustained during land operations in the Falkland Islands campaign, 1985. *J Soc Occup Med* 1985; 35:44–54.
19. Pratt H, Goldsher M, Netzer A, Shenhav R. Auditory brainstem evoked potentials in blast injury. *Audiology* 1985;24:297–304.
20. Phillips Y, Zajtchuk J. Blast injuries of the ear in military operations. *Ann Otol Rhinol Laryngol* 1989;98:3–8.
21. Chait RJ. Blast injury of the ear: historical perspective. *Ann Otol Rhinol Laryngol* 1989;98:9–11.

22. Melnick W. Medicinal therapy for hearing loss resulting from noise exposure. *Am J Otolaryngol* 1984;5:426–431.
23. Ward WD. Endogenous factors related to susceptibility to damage from noise. *Occup Med State Art Rev* 1995;10:561–575.
24. Tschopp K, Probst R. Acute acoustic trauma: a retrospective study of influencing factors and different therapies in 268 patients. *Acta Otolaryngol (Stockh)* 1989;108:378–384.
25. Martin G, Jakobs P. Clinical comparison of dextran 40 and xantinol-nicotine in the therapy of acoustic traumas. *Laryngol Rhinol Otol* 1977; 56:860–863.
26. Roberto M, Hamernik R, Turrentine G. Damage of the auditory system associated with acute blast trauma. *Ann Otol Rhinol Laryngol* 1989;98: 23–34.
27. Phillips Y, Hoyt R, Mundie T, Dodd K. Middle ear injury in animals exposed to complex blast waves inside an armored vehicle. *Ann Otol Rhinol Laryngol* 1989;98:17–22.
28. Berger EH, Ward WD, Morril JC, Roiyster LH, eds. *Noise and hearing conservation manual.* Akron, OH: American Industrial Hygiene Association, 1986.
29. Atherly GA. Prevention of occupational deafness. A coming crisis? *J Occup Med* 1989;31:139–140.
30. Fitzpatrick D. An analysis of noise-induced hearing loss in army helicopter pilots. *Aviat Space Environ Med* 1988;59:937–941.
31. Lowry L, Isaacson S. Study of 100 patients with bilateral sensorineural hearing loss for lipid abnormalities. *Ann Otol* 1978;87:404–408.
32. Pyykko I, Koskimies K, Starck J, Pekkarinen J, Inaba R. Evaluation of factors affecting sensory neural hearing loss. *Acta Otolaryngol (Suppl)* 1988;449:155-158
33. Hodgson MJ, Talbot E, Helmkamp JC, et al. Diabetes, noise exposure, and hearing loss. *J Occup Med* 1987;29:576–579.
34. Barregard L, Axelsson A. Is there an ototraumatic interaction between noise and solvents? *Scand Audiol* 1984;13:151–155.
35. Barone J, Peters J, Garabrant D, Bernstein L, Krebsbach R. Smoking as a risk factor in noise-induced hearing loss. *J Occup Med* 1987;29: 741–745.
36. Carter NL. Eye colour and susceptibility to noise-induced permanent threshold shift. *Audiology* 1980;19:86–93.
37. Meyerhoff WL. The thyroid and audition. *Laryngoscope* 1976;86: 483–489.
38. Ishil EK, Talbott EO, Findlay RC, D Antonio JA, Kuller LH. Is NIDDM a risk factor for noise-induced hearing loss in an occupationally noise exposed cohort? *Sci Total Environ* 1992;127:155–165.
39. Gibbin KP, Davis CB. A hearing survey in diabetes mellitus. *Clin Otolaryngol* 1981;6:345–350.
40. Miller JJ, Beck L, Davis A, et al. Hearing loss in patients with diabetic retinopathy. *Am J Otolaryngol* 1983;4:342–346.
41. Thomas GB, Williams CE, Hoger NG. Some nonauditory correlates of the hearing threshold levels of an aviation noise-exposed population. *Aviat Space Environ Med* 1981;9:531–536.
42. Chung DY, Willson GN, Gannon RP, et al. Individual susceptibility to noise. In: Hamernik RP, Henderson D, Salvi R, eds. *New perspectives on noise-induced hearing loss.* New York: Raven, 1982;511–519.
43. Virokannas H, Anttonen H. Dose-response relationship between smoking and impairment of hearing acuity in workers exposed to noise. *Scand Audiol* 1995;24:211–216.
44. Drettner B, Hedstrand H, Klockhoff I, et al. Cardiovascular risk factors and hearing loss. *Acta Otolaryngol* 1975;79:366–371.
45. Siegelaub AB, Friedman GD, Adour K, et al. Hearing loss in adults. *Arch Environ Health* 1984;29:107–109.
46. Crofton KM, Lassiter TL, Robert CS. Solvent-induced ototoxicity in rats: an atypical selective mid-frequency hearing deficit. *Hearing Res* 1994;80:25–30.
47. Morata TC, Nylen P, Johnson A-C, Dunn DE. Auditory and vestibular functions after single or combined exposure to toluene. A review. *Arch Toxicol* 1995;69:431–443.
48. Morata TC, Dunn DE, Kretschmer LW, Lemasters GK, Keith RW. Effects of occupational exposure to organic solvents and noise on hearing. *Scand J Work Environ Health* 1993;19:245–254.
49. Johnson A-C, Nylen P. Effects of industrial solvents on hearing. *Occup Med State Art Rev* 1995;10:623–640.
50. Crowe SJ, Guild SR, Polvogt LM. Observations on the pathology of high-tone deafness. *Bull Johns Hopkins Hosp* 1934;54:315–379.
51. Alexiou NG, Gladfelter T, Saraceno C. Noise-induced hearing loss: a preventable occupational disease. *J Fam Practice* 1986;22:407–414.
52. Hawkins JE. The role of vasoconstriction in noise-induced hearing loss. *Otol Rhinol Laryngol* 1971;80:903–914.
53. Fredelius L. Time sequence of degeneration pattern of the organ of Corti. *Acta Otolaryngol* 1988;106:373–385.
54. Bohne AB. Mechanisms of noise damage in the inner ear. In: Henderson D, Hamernik RP, Dosanjh DS, Mills JH, eds. *Effects of noise on hearing.* New York: Raven Press, 1976:41–68.
55. Hillerdal M, Jansson B, Engstron B, Hultcrantz E, Borg E. Cochlear blood flow in noise-damaged ears. *Acta Otolaryngol (Stockh)* 1987; 104:270–278.
56. Borg E. Noise-induced hearing loss in normotensive and spontaneously hypertensive rats. *Hearing Res* 1982;8:117–130.
57. Nakai Y, Masutani H. Noise-induced vasoconstriction in the cochlea. *Acta Otolaryngol (Stockh)* 1988;447:23–27.
58. Talbott E, Helmkamp J, Matthews K, Kuller L, Cottington E, Redmond G. Occupational noise exposure, noise-induced hearing loss, and the epidemiology of high blood pressure. *Am J Epidemiol* 1985;121: 501–514.
59. Talbott E, Findlay R, Kuller L, et al. Noise-induced hearing loss: a possible marker for high blood pressure in older noise-exposed populations. *J Occup Med* 1990;32(8):690–697.
60. Morizono T, Paparella M. Hypercholesterolemia and auditory dysfunction. Experimental studies. *Ann Otol Rhinol Laryngol* 1978;87:804–814.
61. Axelsson A, Lindgren F. Is there a relationship between hypercholesterolemia and noise-induced hearing loss? *Acta Otolaryngol (Stockh)* 1985;100:379–386.
62. Tarter S, Robins R. Chronic noise exposure, high-frequency hearing loss, and hypertension among automotive assembly workers. *J Occup Med* 1990;32(8):685–689.
63. Belli S, Sani L, Scarficcia G, Sorrentino R. Arterial hypertension and noise: a cross-sectional study. *Am J Ind Med* 1984;6:59–65.
64. Schulte W, Heusch G, Eiff AW. The influence of experimental traffic noise on autonomous function of normotensives and hypertensives after stress. *Basic Res Cardiol* 1977;72:575–580.
65. Andren L, Lindstedt G, Bjorkman M, Borg KO, Hansson L. Effect of noise on blood pressure and "stress" hormones. *Clin Sci* 1982;62:137–141.
66. Mosskov Jl, Ettema JH. Extraauditory effects in short-term exposure to aircraft and traffic noise. *Int Arch Occup Environ Health* 1977; 40:165–173.
67. Pillsbury HC. Hypertension, hyperlipoproteinemia, chronic noise exposure: Is there synergism in cochlear pathology? *Laryngoscope* 1986;96:1112–1135.
68. Arguelles AK, Martinez MA, Pucciarelli E, Disisto MV. Endocrine and metabolic effects of noise in normal, hypertensive and psychotic subjects. In: Welch BL, Welch AS, eds. *Physiological effects of noise.* New York: Plenum, 1970;43–55.
69. Melamed S, Bruhis S. The effects of chronic industrial noise exposure on urinary cortisol, fatigue, and irritability. *J Occup Environ Med* 1996;38:252–256.
70. Geber WF. Developmental effects of chronic maternal audiovisual stress on the rat fetus. *J Embryol Exp Morphol* 1966;16:1–16.
71. Geber WF. Cardiovascular and teratogenic effects of chronic intermittent noise stress. In: Welch BL, Welch AS, eds. *Physiological effects of noise.* New York: Plenum, 1970;85–90.
72. Hartikainen-Sorri AL, Sorri M, Anttonen H, Tuimala R, Laara E. Occupational noise exposure during pregnancy: a case-control study. *Int Arch Occup Environ Health* 1988;60:279–283.
73. Edmonds LD, Layde PM, Erickson JD. Airport noise and teratogenesis. *Arch Environ Health* 1979;34:243–247.
74. Lalande NM, Hetu R, Lambert J. Is occupational noise exposure during pregnancy a risk factor of damage to the auditory system of the fetus? *Am J Ind Med* 1986;10:427–435.
75. Dobie RA. Noise-induced hearing loss: the family physician's role. *Am Fam Physician* 1987;36:141–148.
76. Keeve JP. Ototoxic drugs and the workplace. *Am Fam Physician* 1988;38:177–181.
77. Konigsmark BW, Gorlin RJ. *Genetic and metabolic deafness.* Philadelphia: Saunders, 1976.
78. Catalano PJ, Levin SM. Noise-induced hearing loss and portable radios with headphones. *Int J Pediatr Otorhinolaryngol* 1985;9:59–67.
79. Lichtenstein MJ. Validation of screening tools for identifying hearing-impaired elderly in primary care. *JAMA* 1988;259:2875–2878.
80. DeWeese DD, Saunders WH. Evaluation of hearing. In: *Textbook of otolaryngology,* 6th ed. St Louis: CV Mosby, 1982;279–295.

81. *Otologic referral criteria for occupational hearing conservation programs.* Rochester, MN: American Academy of Otolaryngology—Head and Neck Surgery; 1983.
82. Ventry IM, Weinstein B. Identification of elderly people with hearing problems. *ASHA* 1983;25:37–42.
83. Ward WD. The American Medical Association/American Academy of Otolaryngology formula for determination of hearing handicap. *Audiology* 1983;22:313–324.
84. American Medical Association. *Guides to the evaluation of permanent impairment,* 4th ed. Chicago: American Medical Association 1993.
85. Price G, Kalb J, Garinther G. Toward a measure of auditory handicap in the army. *Ann Otol Rhinol Laryogol* 1989;98:42–51.
86. Guidelines for the conduct of an occupational hearing conservation program. *J Occup Med* 1987;29(12):981–982.
87. Berger EH, Ward WD, Morill JC, Royster LH. *Noise and hearing conservation manual,* 4th ed. Akron, OH: American Industrial Hygiene Association, 1986.
88. Van Moorhem WK, Woo KS, Liu S, Golias E. Development and operation of a system to monitor occupational noise exposure due to wearing a headset. *Appl Occup Environ Hyg* 1996;11:261–265
89. Nabelek IV. Noise measurement and engineering controls. In: Feldman AS, Grimes CT, eds. *Hearing conservation in industry.* Baltimore: Williams & Wilkins, 1985;27–76.
90. Driscoll D, Morrill J. A position paper on a recommended criterion for recording occupational hearing loss on the OSHA Form 200. *Am Ind Hyg Assoc J* 1987;48:714–716.
91. Franks JR. Management of hearing conservation data with microcomputers. In: Lipscomb DM, ed. *Hearing conservation in industry, schools, and the military.* Boston: Little, Brown, 1988.
92. Berwick DM. Screening in health fairs. *JAMA* 1985;254:1492–1498.
93. Berger EH. Hearing protection devices. In: Berger EH, Ward WD, Morrill JC, Royster LH, eds. *Noise and hearing conservation manual.* Akron, OH: American Industrial Hygiene Association, 1986.
94. Gasaway DC. *Hearing conservation:* a practical manual and guide. Englewood Cliffs, NJ: Prentice-Hall, 1985.

*Environmental and Occupational Medicine, Third Edition,* edited by William N. Rom.
Lippincott–Raven Publishers, Philadelphia © 1998.

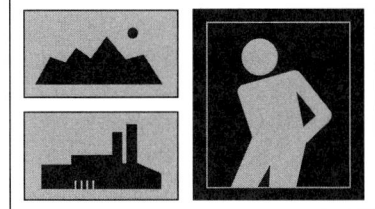

# CHAPTER 102

# Dysbarism

Rafael E. de la Hoz and Bruce P. Krieger

*Dysbarism* is the collective term used to describe the pathologic changes that occur when the human body is exposed to environmental pressure changes (alternobaric exposure). Those altered pressures are translated into unphysiologic behavior of gases in organs and tissues. Failure to adequately or timely adapt to those changes, can generate (depending on a number of exposure and individual factors) the different clinical syndromes of dysbarism. Alternobaric exposure is a concern in a number of occupational and recreational activities, such as diving, compressed air work (as in tunnel construction and caisson work), as well as in aviation, mountain climbing, and high-altitude flying.

## HISTORICAL PERSPECTIVE

Diving has been an important human activity since antiquity and, as such, the quest for increased depths and durations has been ongoing since then. Although reports of dysbaric disorders began earlier, their experimental study was not possible until the 17th century, when diving bells were introduced for salvage operations. In 1650, von Guericke developed the air pump, which permitted simulation of high-altitude environments in special gas chambers. Sir Robert Boyle (1627–1691) experimented with live animals exposed to this gas chambers and noted bubbles floating in the vitreous humor of their eyes. In 1667, Redi, an Italian naturalist, reported on the death of animals when air was injected into neck veins. In the 19th century, Augustus Siebe manufactured the first diving suit with a surface air supply, and Ammussat observed that the speed of death of air-injected animals was related to the size of the injured vein and the relationship of this vein to the heart when air was injected. In 1818, Bauchene reported the first case of fatal air embolism in a human (1). In the 1840s, decompression sickness (DCS) was first recognized in France in men who were working in the compressed air environments of tunnels and caissons. A French scientist, Paul Bert (1833–1886), was the first to hypothesize that "caisson disease" resulted from the development of air bubbles in body tissues and fluids after decompression from a hyperbaric exposure (2). Bert also determined that the gas in those bubbles was nitrogen (3). In 1930, a Dutch physician named Jongbloed recognized that the joint symptoms that he experienced after self-experimenting with hyperbaric exposure were the same as those observed in men after rapid decompression from diving or caisson work. During World War II, Jacques Cousteau and Emile Gagnon developed a demand regulator that automatically delivered breaths at any depth, the self-contained underwater breathing apparatus ("scuba"). Hyperbaric chamber treatment techniques were also refined during World War II because of the demands of submarine technology and higher flying aviation. At the same time, Behnke (2) recognized that the symptoms felt at high altitude were analogous to those associated with caisson work, thus identifying a link between aviation and diving hazards. By 1960, a classification scheme for decompression sickness based on symptoms experienced by tunnel workers had been formulated (4).

## ALTERNOBARIC EXPOSURES

Exposure to altered environmental pressures followed by a return to atmospheric pressure occurs in a number of

R. E. de la Hoz: Chest Service and Occupational Medicine Clinic, Bellevue Hospital Center, New York University Medical Center, New York, New York 10016.
B. P. Krieger: Division of Pulmonary Medicine, University of Miami School of Medicine, Mt. Sinai Medical Center, Miami Beach, Florida 33140.

settings. When the rapidity of the pressure changes exceeds that of the compensatory and adaptive mechanisms of the human body, dysbaric disorders can result, depending in part on interindividual differences in responses and susceptibility. This chapter focuses on compressed air work and diving.

Compressed air work is carried out during tunnel construction and caisson work. A caisson is a watertight chamber used in construction work to construct bridge and tunnel foundations under water. The chamber is placed over the site of the proposed underwater foundation, and air is pumped in at a pressure sufficient to displace the water and allow work to be performed under dry conditions (Fig. 1). In the United States, working pressures for compressed air have varied from 3.1 to as high as 6.1 atmosphere absolute (ATA) (5,6). Part of this work can now be done with mechanical devices.

There are three main diving methods, which have been sequentially developed during man's quest for deeper and more prolonged dives: breath-hold diving, scuba diving, and saturation diving. Breath-hold diving is the simplest and oldest of all. Once the diver holds his breath and descends, the increased pressure that he is exposed to is applied to his entire body. The duration of the dive is limited by that of the breath-hold, and specifically the rate of $PaCO_2$ rise. This diving modality is currently limited to specific groups of divers in some parts of the world, like Asian fishers and some competitive divers (7).

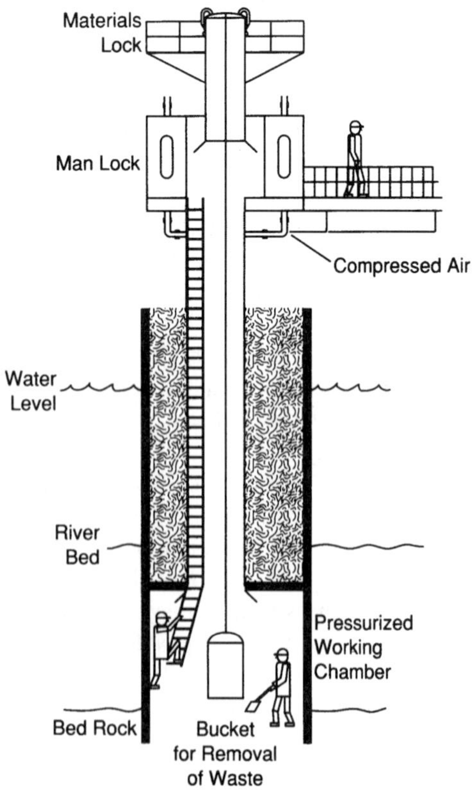


**FIG. 1.** Schema of a caisson. (Courtesy of I. H. Thomas.)

Scuba diving allows descent deeper into the water and for a considerable longer duration than breath-hold diving. Scubas provide a breathing mixture (air, oxygen, helium-oxygen, helium-nitrogen-oxygen, hydrogen-nitrogen-oxygen) upon demand at the ambient pressure to which the diver is exposed. This allows the maintenance of ambient pressure within the respiratory tract. Dive computers calculate saturation and desaturation of tissues. Their purpose is to maximize the time underwater by pushing dives to the limit of a decompression model different from the more conservative one used to derive decompression tables. They therefore decrease safety margins and may increase the probability of dysbarism (8). Recreational scuba diving has gained immense popularity in many industrialized countries, where it is by far more widespread than commercial and military diving. Recreational diving is currently restricted to depths of 39 m (3).

Saturation diving was developed to permit commercial divers, especially in the oil industry, to perform complex and economically profitable tasks during prolonged periods and at increased depths. Saturation diving allows for an increase in the ratio of time spent underwater to the total diving time, which is the sum of underwater plus decompression time. In this modality, divers descend in a diving bell where they are gradually compressed to the pressure level encountered at the depths where they are released (which usually exceed 200 to 300 m). Breathing mixtures have high partial pressures of inspired oxygen ($PIO_2$), and an inert gas other than nitrogen (usually helium) is added. The compression and descent phase of this diving modality is long enough for the diver's tissues to become fully saturated with the inert gas that is being breathed. Once saturated, the diver can remain underwater for an indefinitely long period, without further increasing his obligated decompression time. Stays of 10 to 14 days are usual, with decompressions of approximately the same duration.

The technical refinements of scuba and saturation diving have allowed increased human activity underwater under hyperbaric conditions. With these modalities, divers are exposed to breathing mixtures that are usually hyperbaric, hyperoxic, and have an increased gas density. Furthermore, the surrounding environment can be hypothermic, physical activity can be strenuous, and the specific tasks performed underwater may also expose commercial or technical divers to potentially injurious toxins and physical agents. The compromises that are made are felt to be "acceptable," although long-term, close follow-up is necessary to exclude unforeseen deleterious consequences.

## PATHOPHYSIOLOGY OF DYSBARISM

Whereas body tissues are nearly incompressible, the physical behavior of gases is affected by three factors:

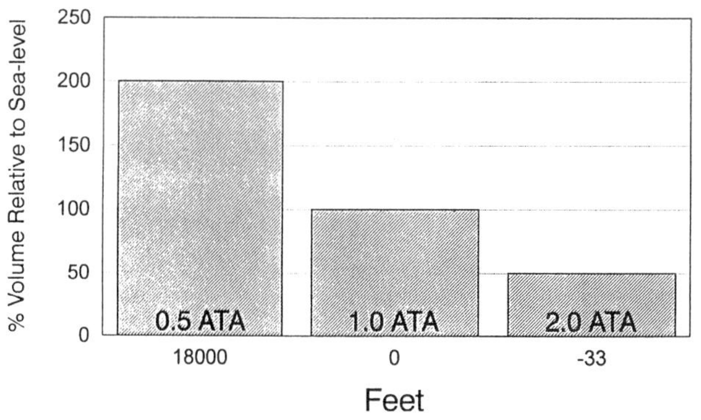


**FIG. 2.** Changes in gas volumes in relation to ambient pressure.

pressure, volume, and temperature (9). The interrelationship between these factors is determined by Boyle's, Dalton's, and Henry's laws, three fundamental gas laws. Comprehension of these concepts is essential to the understanding of dysbaric disorders, which in this chapter are classified according to their pathophysiology.

### Barometric Pressure and Gas Laws

Pressure is defined as force applied per unit area. Commonly used units and equivalent pressures are 1 atmosphere (atm), 760 mm Hg, 33 feet (or 10 m) of sea water (fsw), 34 feet of fresh water, and 14.7 pounds per square inch (psi). The sea of air under which we normally reside is defined (at sea level) as 1 atmosphere (atm) of barometric pressure. Hyperbaric exposures add to the ambient pressure and hypobaric exposures subtract from it. Absolute pressure is the sum of ambient pressure plus any additionally applied pressure. It is measured in atmosphere absolute (ATA) units. For instance, under 33 feet (or 10 m) of sea water, 1 atm is added to the ambient pressure and the absolute pressure is 2 ATA.

Boyle's law states that the volume *(V)* of a given mass of gas is inversely proportional to its pressure *(P)*: $PV =$ K (a constant). In the human body, hyperbaric exposures (compression, diving descent) cause a contraction in gas volume, and hypobaric exposures (decompression, ascent after diving) cause an expansion. A doubling of pressure to 2 ATA results in the volume being halved; similarly, a decrease of pressure to 0.5 ATA is associated with a doubling of volume (Fig. 2). The diameter of a sphere or bubble is also affected by the pressure change but to a lesser extent than volume (Table 1). Whereas the volume change is more important in predicting barotrauma, the bubble diameter change is the important factor for restoring circulation to embolized areas during recompression therapy.

Dalton's law states that the total pressure ($P_T$) exerted by a mixture of n gases is the absolute sum of each individual gas: $P_T = P_1 + P_2 + P_3 + \cdots + P_n$. This law forms the physical principle of hyperbaric (recompression) therapy and the hypoxemia that occurs under hypobaric conditions (Table 2).

Henry's law provides the physiologic basis for understanding decompression sickness, nitrogen narcosis, and the formation of bubbles when a bottle of champagne is uncorked. This law states that the amount of gas that dissolves in a liquid at a given temperature is directly proportional to the partial pressure of that gas. Boyle's, Dalton's, and Henry's law together describe the ideal gas law: $PV = nRT$ ($P$ = pressure; $V$ = volume; $n$ = number of moles of gas; R = universal gas constant, at $T$ = absolute temperature). This law allows the prediction of the behavior of gases in response to changes in environmental pressures.

### Behavior of Gases During Compression and Decompression

As predicted by the gas laws, the volume of gases within the body change during hyperbaric and hypobaric exposures. If the gas volume changes provoked exceed compensatory mechanisms of the body, the major dysbaric disorders—decompression sickness (DCS) and barotrauma—may result. In both conditions pathologic changes result from the formation of gas bubbles. In barotrauma, changes in gas volumes within air-filled anatomic structures are involved, and gas may be directly injected into arteries. In DCS gas bubbles form within tissues and their vasculature, where they cause most of the damage. Explaining the behavior of

**TABLE 1.** *Effects of gas laws on hypo- and hyperbaric exposures*

| | Ambient pressure | | | | |
|---|---|---|---|---|---|
| Distance from sea level (ft) | (ATA) | (PSI) | (mm Hg) | Bubble volume | Diameter |
| +18,000 | 0.5 | 7.35 | 380 | 200% | 126% |
| +6,000 | 0.8 | 11.76 | 608 | 125% | 107% |
| 0 | 1 | 14.70 | 760 | 100% | 100% |
| −33 | 2 | 29.40 | 1,520 | 50% | 79% |
| −66 | 3 | 44.1 | 2,280 | 33% | 69% |
| −99 | 4 | 58.8 | 3,040 | 25% | 63% |
| −132 | 5 | 73.5 | 3,800 | 20% | 59% |
| −165 | 6 | 88.2 | 4,560 | 17% | 55% |

ATA, atmosphere absolute; PSI, pounds per square inch.

**TABLE 2.** *Gas pressures under hypo- and hyperbaric conditions*

| Distance from sea level (ft) | Pressure (ATA) | $PO_2$ (mm Hg) | $P_N$ (mm Hg) | $P_T$ (mm Hg) |
|---|---|---|---|---|
| +24,000 | 0.388 | 62 | 233 | 295 |
| +8,000 | 0.743 | 119 | 446 | 565 |
| 0 | 1.0 | 160 | 600 | 760 |
| -33 | 2.0 | 320 | 1,200 | 1,520 |
| -66 | 3.0 | 480 | 1,800 | 2,280 |
| -99 | 4.0 | 640 | 2,400 | 3,040 |
| -132 | 5.0 | 800 | 3,000 | 3,800 |
| -165 | 6.0 | 960 | 3,600 | 4,560 |

ATA, atmosphere absolute; $PO_2$, oxygen tension; $P_N$, nitrogen tension; $P_T$, total gas tension.

gases in the body under these circumstances takes into account the phenomena of compression versus decompression, and gas behavior at the level of tissues and of air-filled organs.

Compression in a hyperbaric environment causes tissue uptake and saturation with gases. When ambient pressure rises, the partial pressure of a given gas (e.g., nitrogen) in a tissue and the total pressure of gas in an air-filled organ rise proportionally. Compression of gas in the latter is the direct cause of barotrauma of descent. Compression also results in the development of a gradient that causes a net flow of nitrogen from pulmonary alveoli to the blood and subsequently into body tissues. The rate of gas uptake is most rapid immediately following a pressure increase and reaches a plateau as tissue saturation is approached. The time that it takes to achieve equilibrium in gas uptake is a function of (a) the solubility of the gas in the tissue and (b) the rate at which the gas is delivered to that tissue by blood. Tissue perfusion varies. Well-perfused tissues such as the brain can achieve equilibrium with a gas within minutes; they are relatively "fast" tissues. On the other hand, poorly perfused tissues such as adipose tissue, joints, and tendons, which also have a high solubility for gases, require more time to reach equilibrium and are called "slow" tissues. Tissues acquire gases exponentially, and a range of half-times (from 5 to 75 minutes) has been estimated to describe that process in different body tissues. Much longer half-times, however, are believed to occur for some tissues under specific circumstances (8). The latter is important, because decompression tables are based on those half-time estimates. Increased tissue perfusion, and thus gas uptake, as observed during exercise, active heating, immersion, and supine position, may all increase the risk for dysbarism (in particular DCS) (8).

When ambient pressure is lowered during decompression, the rate of escape of gas from tissue is believed to be similar to the rate of uptake, but in reverse, as long as bubbles do not form. If the reduction of ambient pressure to a level lower than the total gas pressure in tissues is too rapid, formation of microbubbles within tissues is favored. These bubbles immediately appear because the pressure of the dissolved gas cannot decrease fast enough by diffusion alone. Reversal of tissue supersaturation with gas must therefore be controlled during ascent (decompression) in order to minimize bubble formation and growth, the development of DCS, gas expansion within air-filled organs, and barotrauma of ascent.

In the case of barotrauma of ascent, gas bubbles are formed from the injection of rapidly expanding gas into the arteries. In the case of DCS, the exact site of initial bubble formation and the microcirculatory events related to intravascular bubbles following rapid decompression remain unclear. Formation of bubbles primarily in the venous circulation, tissues themselves, and/or arteries, have been hypothesized. Bubbles are thought to originate on preformed bubble nuclei. The latter may exist in microscopic hydrophobic spaces (e.g., between endothelial cells), or be generated by shear forces exerted on moving tissues. Once bubbles develop on those nuclei, their size can increase as a function of several factors, including exchange of gas with adjacent blood, presence of surfactant, and coalescence or disintegration of bubbles resulting from collision (10). The high fat content of the nervous tissue, combined with the high liposolubility of nitrogen, may account for its vulnerability (8,11). Histologic studies on rapidly decompressed animals demonstrated relative abundance of intravascular gas bubbles in fat-rich tissues and organs. In the spinal cord, the white matter, rather than the gray matter, is usually affected. A number of observations have established the presence of bubbles in almost all tissues, intra- and extravascularly, and even intracellularly. Progressive stages of bubble formation in fat tissue range from the enlargement of fat cells by inclusions of microbubbles to the rupture of gas-filled cells generating extracellular and extravascular pockets of gas in the tissue.

Regardless of the origin of the gas bubbles three main interrelated mechanisms have been invoked to explain their pathologic effects in tissues: (a) mechanical obstruction with reduced blood flow, (b) surface activity at the gas-liquid interface of the bubbles, and (c) injury of vascular endothelia. These three mechanisms can then trigger local and systemic inflammatory effects. Bubbles have been shown to have surface activity due to the abnormal gas-liquid interface. Denaturation and reorientation of globular plasma proteins are believed to occur upon contact with that interface and be associated with loss of function, aggregation of proteins, and coating of blood cells that favor their aggregation (12). Those phenomena may explain several of the observed changes in the blood during decompression, which include sludging and rouleaux formation of red cells in small vessels, neutrophil aggregation, platelet clumping, and a decrease in the number of circulating red and white cells and platelets (13–15). In addition, and possibly through activation of kinin and complement pathways, several inflammatory phenomena may result, such as increased capillary permeability and fluid extravasation. All these alterations contribute to producing microcirculatory compromise, endothelial damage, and local inflammatory tissue damage (8,13).

Some of the manifestations of DCS are similar to those of systemic inflammatory conditions characterized by complement activation. This led some to hypothesize that complement activation may mediate DCS, perhaps underlie interindividual differences in susceptibility to it, and possibly even explain its occasional recurrence after initially successful resolution with hyperbaric treatment (8). Complement activation may also mediate some of the observed changes in blood elements and vascular endothelial injury. In animal studies, air bubbles have been observed to activate complement by the alternative pathway (16). In humans, activation of complement by the alternative pathway has also been demonstrated in plasma samples incubated with air (17) and nitrogen bubbles (18), and in individuals subjected to decompression (17,19). Furthermore, subjecting some of those individuals to a series of pressure profiles severe enough to cause bubble formation in blood vessels revealed that complement-activation seemed to correlate with susceptibility to DCS (17). The functional and clinical relevance of decompression-associated complement activation, however, remains to be determined (8,19).

### Cardiovascular and Pulmonary Effects of Gas Embolization

The physiologic consequences of gas embolization to the heart and lungs is due to mechanical factors as well as secondary effects of released mediators (as described above). Cardiovascular collapse may ensue due to a combination of acute right heart failure and hypoxemia-related myocardial infarction. If even a small amount (< 0.1 ml) of air enters a coronary artery, ventricular fibrillation and infarct can result (20). Ultimately, poor oxygen delivery results in multisystem organ failure and death.

Mechanical obstruction of the pulmonary arterial system and the right heart may result from simple lodging of bubbles causing an "air-lock" phenomenon. Vortex flow around a partially obstructing embolus is postulated to cause a "whipping" type action that results in a blood-froth mixture. The latter enhances platelet aggregation, fibrin formation, and coalescence of intravascular fat (21). Proximal deposition of these fibrin strands interspersed with conglomerations of red cells may play a major role in the obstruction of the pulmonary vasculature (1). Transient pulmonary vasoconstriction has also been detected in a canine model of venous gas emboli (1). These mechanisms resulted in a brisk rise in pulmonary vascular resistance (PVR) prior to a fall in cardiac output when bubbles were injected into the venous system of sheep (22). This sequence of events lends further support to the hypothesis that vasoactive mediators may be involved in the subsequent changes following gas emboli.

In the lungs, airways resistance ($R_{aw}$) increases when gas emboli are composed of air, oxygen, or nitrogen but not when they contain only carbon dioxide ($CO_2$) or the inert gases helium, neon, argon, or xenon (1). As a result of the significant increases in $R_{aw}$, lung water, and PVR, there is maldistribution of ventilation relative to perfusion. The ventilation/perfusion ($\dot{V}/\dot{Q}$) ratio imbalances result in hypoxemia due to low $\dot{V}/\dot{Q}$ areas as well as areas of physiologic shunting ($\dot{V}/\dot{Q} = 0$). The $\dot{V}/\dot{Q}$ maldistribution that occurs during venous gas embolism also causes increased areas of dead space (elevated $\dot{V}/\dot{Q}$ ratios). This explains the finding of a drop in end-tidal $CO_2$ concentration ($ETCO_2$) following venous gas embolization as areas of high $\dot{V}/\dot{Q}$ experience a "washout" of $CO_2$ from the poorly or nonperfused alveoli. The decrease in $ETCO_2$ is exaggerated when the cardiac output is also decreased (1).

### Cardiopulmonary Effects of Diving

The physiologic effects of submersion have been studied in a head-out immersion model during which the subject is submersed up to the neck (23,24). This induces an asymmetric pressure on the subject's body that is proportional to the vertical distance that is immersed. Venous return is augmented due to compression of the extremities by the relative high density of water and an increase in abdominal pressure relative to intrathoracic pressure. Right atrial pressure rises, which stimulates release of atrial natriuretic factor (ANF), which contributes to the diuresis and natriuresis that usually accompanies head-out immersion. However, this shift can acutely reduce circulating blood volume, which is further compromised by sweating, the cold pressor response, and any associated alcohol intake.

The increase in intrathoracic pressure during head-out immersion experiments induces several pulmonary changes, including (a) a 70% decrease in expiratory reserve volume (ERV); (b) smaller reductions in vital capacity, since there is an increase in inspiratory capacity that partially compensates for the large decrease in ERV;

(c) a small, but statistically significant, decrease in residual volume caused by an increase in intrathoracic blood volume; (d) a 60% increase in the work of breathing partly due to an increase in nonelastic airways resistance; and (e) a form of "negative-pressure ventilation," since the thorax and lungs experience greater than 1 ATA while the oropharynx and nose are surrounded by only 1 ATA (at sea level) (9,23).

During breath-hold diving, the entire body is exposed to the increased ambient pressure. Breath-hold diving is associated with decreased intrathoracic pressure (relative to ambient pressure) and chest elastic recoil, and increased work of breathing (25). Increased venous return to the heart also results, which causes an increase in cardiac output that probably contributes to counteracting the pressure exerted on the thoracic cage (7). Distribution of pulmonary perfusion may also improve (24). At the end of a prolonged dive, marked hypoxemia and hypercapnia occur (25), the latter being the usual stimulus for resumption of ventilation. Ventilatory responses to hypercapnia and hypoxia have been shown to be altered in elite breath-hold divers, Japanese pearl divers, and submarine escape training instructors (26,27). Most studies have described a blunted response to hypercapnia with variable tolerance to hypoxia. Whether these traits are genetic or adaptive has not been determined, but they do contribute to the breath-hold diver's longer underwater performance. Hyperventilation before a dive produces a larger depletion of the body $CO_2$ reserves than increases in those of $O_2$. By retarding the hypercapnic stimulus, predive hyperventilation prolongs the apnea time and favors the development of a more severe hypoxemia than would result otherwise, thus increasing the risk of syncope and death (25).

By contrast, scubas maintain atmospheric pressure within the respiratory tract. They expose the lungs, however, to breathing mixtures that are more dense, hyperbaric, and hyperoxic in comparison to atmospheric air. The increased work of breathing, with decreased expiratory flow rates in direct proportion to the ambient pressure, has been well documented by several investigators in the past (28). Furthermore, mouthpieces, masks, and helmets all add dead space (i.e., increased pulmonary ventilation/perfusion ratio) to the total ventilation required for adequate respiratory gas exchange (8).

Different studies have documented pulmonary functional changes in scuba divers and, more recently, in saturation divers. The results generally suggest definite but mild degrees of overinflation and obstructive impairment. Cross-sectional ventilatory functional studies in divers with prolonged exposure to hyperbaric environments demonstrated significant increases in forced vital capacity (FVC) and forced expiratory volume in 1 second ($FEV_1$). Other studies detected decreases in air flow rates at low lung volumes suggestive of obstructive impairment (29–31), and decreased diffusion capacity uncorrected (32,33) or corrected for alveolar volume (DL/VA) (30). Hyperoxia, hyperbaria, and venous gas microembolism appear to be independent contributors to the described pulmonary functional changes (32,34). Although these changes may result (at least in part) from occupational self-selection or from respiratory muscle training (30,35,36), they have also been suggested to indicate small airways dysfunction (37,38).

## NITROGEN NARCOSIS AND HIGH-PRESSURE NERVOUS SYNDROME (HPNS)

Nitrogen narcosis has been most commonly described in deep diving while breathing compressed air. It has also been described in compressed air workers. The resulting increased partial pressure of nitrogen in compressed air generates a large additional nitrogen load, which (due to its lipid solubility) easily saturates the brain tissue. This allows nitrogen to exert narcotic effects, which have also been described for other "inert" gases (e.g., hydrogen) in close correlation with their lipid solubility. The term *inert gas narcosis* is sometimes used when referring to this condition, which sets clear limits on compressed air diving—to depths of about 50 m (13).

The clinical syndrome of nitrogen narcosis is quite similar to alcohol intoxication, and Cousteau coined the term *"l'ivresse des grandes profondeurs"* (or "rapture of the depths") to describe it. It is characterized by the development of abnormal behavior, euphoria, as well as impaired judgment, intellectual functions, neuromuscular coordination, and performance. The symptoms may begin at depths of 20 to 30 m. At depths greater than 90 m (10 ATA), loss of consciousness can occur. The risk for drowning accidents and death is very high, particularly because of the euphoria and impaired judgment. Individual susceptibility to this condition varies, and there is also some evidence for adaptation from frequent exposures (25). The narcotic effect is believed to be exacerbated by cold water, hypercarbia, fatigue, strenuous activity, and alcohol consumption. Upon decompression (ascent), rapid and complete recovery occurs.

High-pressure neurologic syndrome (HPNS) was described when breathing mixes of helium-oxygen began to be used to allow deep dives (exceeding depths of 100 m) while avoiding the development of nitrogen narcosis. Increased environmental pressure by itself causes HPNS, although there are interindividual differences in susceptibility. HPNS is characterized by hyperexcitability of the central nervous system. Clinically, symptoms include opsoclonus, headache, vertigo, fatigue, euphoria, nausea, and vomiting. Signs include decreased manual dexterity, tremors of hands and arms, myoclonus, dysmetria, and hyperreflexia.

The pathogenesis of HPNS is still unclear, but it involves a number of disturbances in neural transmission, in particular enhanced subcortical release of glutamate (with excitation of *N*-methyl-D-aspartate receptors) and decreased serotoninergic activity. Electroencephalography reveals increased theta activity. At compressions of more than 30 ATA sleep disturbances are observed consisting of awake periods, increased sleep stages I and II, and decreased REM periods (39). Brain stem auditory evoked potential studies during saturation dives have demonstrated increased neural transmission times, suggestive of enhanced synaptic excitability (40). A puzzling observation has been that the effects of high environmental pressure (which explains HPNS) and anesthesia (which nitrogen narcosis resembles) are mutually antagonistic (8).

Prevention of HPNS may be achieved by reducing the speed of compression, and by adding nitrogen (5–10%) or hydrogen to the heliox breathing mixture (8). Although anticonvulsants (especially barbiturates) have anti-HPNS activity, they are of no practical use in diving. Serotonin receptor antagonists may provide an additional approach to the prevention of HPNS (39). Resolution without long-term sequelae seems to be the rule.

## DECOMPRESSION SICKNESS

Decompression sickness (DCS) is probably the most frequent dysbaric disorder. DCS occurs upon return from a hyperbaric (e.g., during a diver's ascent) or from a hypobaric exposure [hypobaric or altitude DCS, e.g., in aviators (41)]. DCS is a probabilistic phenomenon with clear interindividual differences in susceptibility (8).

Decompression sickness symptoms are frequently concurrent, and sometimes difficult to differentiate clinically from those of barotrauma of ascent. This is not surprising, given that both conditions result from the formation and the pathologic effects of gas bubbles. Furthermore, treatment for the two conditions is essentially the same. The terms *decompression illness* and *decompression disorders* are being increasingly used to include both DCS and barotrauma (42). A descriptive clinical classification has been recently proposed that does not attempt to differentiate between these two entities or ascribe the observed clinical features to a given disease mechanism (8,43). This chapter, however, follows the traditional approach of discussing these two entities separately.

## CLINICAL PRESENTATION

Decompression sickness encompasses a broad spectrum of clinical disorders, involving several organ systems with different degrees of severity. The diagnosis of DCS is a clinical one. Multiple organ involvement is more frequent in DCS than in barotrauma of ascent, but the signs and symptoms of both conditions can be quite similar and often occur concurrently. Although symptoms of DCS usually occur within 6 hours from ascent, they are frequently not present immediately upon surfacing, and delayed presentations (24 hours) have been described. In contrast, symptoms of barotrauma and arterial gas embolism have a sudden and rapid onset upon surfacing. In practice, any neurologic or cardiovascular symptom or sign that occurs within 15 minutes of reaching the surface should be assumed to be due to barotrauma and arterial gas embolism until proven otherwise (44). Both conditions can relapse after initial successful hyperbaric treatment, but this occurs slightly more frequently with DCS than with barotrauma.

On the basis of severity of clinical presentation and the presence or absence of neurologic involvement, decompression sickness has been traditionally classified into two types (4): type I (mild; peripheral limb and joint pain, cutaneous involvement, no neurologic symptoms), and type II (serious; primarily neurologic including vestibular, cerebral, and spinal involvement, as well as other systemic symptoms). The symptoms of type I disease may mask or antedate the more serious type II manifestations. Although studies differ widely on the relative frequency of the two types of disease (41,45–47), type II disease probably occurs in as many as 80% of DCS patients.

### *Spinal Cord and Brain*

Central nervous system (CNS) manifestations of decompression sickness reflect potentially very ominous complications resulting in permanent neurologic damage. The spinal cord, particularly the lower thoracic and upper lumbar (T12-L1) segments and its dorsal and lateral columns, is by far the most frequently affected CNS structure. There is some evidence, however, that cerebral damage may be more prevalent in DCS than was once thought (48,49). The predilection for spinal cord in DCS remains unexplained, and it sharply contrasts with the predilection of barotrauma with arterial gas embolism for the brain.

Morphologic studies in humans with DCS have been limited. Four stages of damage to the spinal cord have been described in humans: hyperacute, acute, subacute, and chronic (13). In the hyperacute phase, abrupt decreases in external pressure and formation of bubbles within tissues leads to an explosive effect. If the pressure changes are less severe, gradual accumulation of bubbles in the white matter may be seen instead. The acute stage generally occurs 10 to 48 hours following rapid decompression. Infarcts are found in the lateral, ventral, and dorsal columns of the white matter. Early myelin degeneration, and changes in the structure of neurons in the gray matter are also observed at this stage, with associated vascular injury and microthrombi. The subacute stage is characterized by lipid phagocytosis, replacement of cells by astrocytes, and progressive nerve fiber (wallerian) degeneration.

The chronic stage is marked by the progressive organization of white matter infarcts.

The typical presentation of DCS in the CNS begins with transient back pain radiated to the anterior chest or abdomen soon after rapid decompression. Multifocal lesions probably explain the frequently observed combinations of sensory and motor deficits at multiple sites (11). Subsequently, paresthesias and hypesthesias develop in the legs. Without medical intervention this situation progresses to urinary retention, lower extremity paresis, and eventually paralysis. Detection of subclinical neurophysiologic abnormalities may be possible by using somatosensory evoked potentials (SSEPs) (50).

Although neurologic DCS has been regarded as predominantly a spinal cord disease, on rare occasions it involves the brain. Clinically detectable manifestations of brain damage include visual disturbances, hemiplegia, and unconsciousness (51). Patients with classic spinal cord manifestations have been reported to have concomitant cerebral perfusion defects (48). A recent study using single photon emission tomography (SPET) reported statistically significant abnormal brain textures in divers who had experienced DCS in the past, compared to divers who had not. Overlapping results between the two groups, however, were evident (49), and the significance of these findings remains unclear.

### *Pulmonary System*

Under normal conditions the lungs work well in filtering out most gas microbubbles (52). In most cases of DCS, no pulmonary symptoms occur, even though bubbles may be detected in the venous circulation. However, the relationship between degree of pulmonary embolization and pulmonary symptoms remains unknown. Morphologic studies of the lungs' response to decompression showed no alteration in the bronchoscopic and histologic appearance of the airway mucosa. Pulmonary edema has been noted on histologic examination of the lung parenchyma. In addition, small autopsy series of patients who succumbed to acute decompression sickness frequently demonstrated fat emboli to the lungs and peripheral organs.

The pulmonary syndrome, called "the chokes" by divers, develops in 2% to 8% of DCS patients and is characterized by paroxysmal cough, substernal chest pain, and dyspnea. Early physical signs include respiratory distress, tachypnea, cyanosis, and in severe cases, hypotension and shock.

Without appropriate therapeutic intervention (i.e., recompression) patients suffering from this syndrome may progress to noncardiogenic pulmonary edema, circulatory collapse, and death. Recompression results in essentially complete reversal of symptoms, usually within minutes. In a case report, complete radiographic resolution of pulmonary edema was documented to occur within a few hours of recompression treatment (53).

### *Osteoarticular System*

It has been said that bone is the organ that limits human exposures to compressed air (2). Indeed, involvement of bones in DCS occurs very frequently, and includes an acute pain condition (known as the "bends"), and the late, chronic complication of dysbaric osteonecrosis or aseptic bone necrosis.

The bends are one of the most frequent and typical manifestation of decompression sickness. They consist of pain felt in the joints, or in both muscles and bones. The pain has been described as dull, throbbing, gradual in onset, variable in progression and severity, and occasionally preceded by paresthesias (2). The affected extremity is usually held in a semiflexed position, and less intense pains are referred to by divers as the "niggles." It is believed that the bends are caused by air embolism most likely affecting the bone marrow, and to be related to later development of chronic dysbaric osteonecrosis. The diagnosis of this condition is based on its clinical features. Evaluation includes a search for involvement of other organ systems, and treatment is the same as for all DCS (as discussed below).

Dysbaric osteonecrosis (caisson disease) is a late and chronic complication of exposure to hyperbaric environments. Caisson disease was first recognized at the beginning of the century in men who had worked in caissons. It was later described in divers and, rarely, in aviators exposed to hypobaric environments. Adherence to recognized decompression procedures does not completely prevent bone necrosis. The lack of early symptoms (and few late ones) and its long latency (months or even years after the initial exposure) also contribute to the persistence of this occupational hazard (54,55).

Incidence and prevalence of dysbaric osteonecrosis among occupationally exposed workers have varied over time. In divers, prevalence seems to correlate with exposure dose (e.g., in terms of amount of pressure, and number and duration of dives). Statistically significant correlations have also been suggested between the presence of definite osteonecrotic lesions and number of episodes of decompression sickness, as well as body weight (55). In the United Kingdom, the Medical Research Council Decompression Sickness Registry, based on 10-year longitudinal data on 4,980 commercial divers, estimated the prevalence of dysbaric osteonecrosis at 4.2%, and the highest incidence at 6/1,000/year of diving experience. When the comparison has been possible, dysbaric osteonecrosis has been found more frequently in compressed air workers than in divers (54–56). Among compressed air workers the incidence of bone lesions also appears to be related to exposure dose (intensity of hyperbaric exposure and number of hyperbaric experiences). No lesions have been reported in workers exposed to less than 2.4 ATA, and osteonecrosis is most common when the pressure exceeds 3.6 ATA. At least 50% of experienced compressed air workers who have been exposed for many years have bone lesions (54,55). Yet, there is evidence that even a single hyperbaric exposure can result in osteonecrosis. Men without previous exposure to compressed air who suffered at least one attack of the bends were more likely to have a bone lesion than those who had not suffered such attacks. Conversely, not all men with radiographic evidence of osteonecrosis were thought to have experienced acute decompression sickness (55,56). Furthermore, in the absence of any additional hyperbaric exposure, new lesions may develop in previously normal areas, and existing lesions may progress (57).

Dysbaric osteonecrosis usually develops only in portions of long bones and in sites where fatty bone marrow is found in mature adults. The most common sites are the distal end of the femur and the proximal end of the humerus, tibia, and femur (54,55) (Fig. 3). At each of these sites two types of lesions can occur. Juxtaarticular (JA) lesions are situated adjacent to the joint surface, more frequently in the femoral and humeral heads and seldom near the articular surfaces of the knee or elbow joints. Head, neck, or shaft (HNS) lesions, are situated in the remaining parts of the bone that lie at a distance from the joint surface. HNS lesions most frequently affect the medullary cavity of the lower femoral and upper tibial shaft, but may involve the neck and head of the femur and humerus (55,58) and are often bilateral and symmetric. While HNS lesions usually remain symptom free, JA lesions may cause pain and limitation of movement due to damage to the adjacent joint surface (54,58,59). Structural failure of the joint may result, and osteoarthritis may develop, causing marked disability. In divers, joint damage was estimated to occur in 14.5% of previously identified JA lesions (55).

While the characteristics of the osteonecrotic lesions that occur in divers and compressed air workers are essentially indistinguishable, their emphasis and distribution varies in the two groups. JA lesions have been described to occur more commonly in compressed air workers than in divers and have a predilection for the femoral head. In contrast, JA lesions in divers occur more frequently in the humeral head. When HNS lesions occur, their location is more often in the humerus in compressed air workers and in the lower femur in divers.

The precise cause of dysbaric osteonecrosis is not known. It is believed to result from occlusion of multiple end arteries in the bones by intravascular gas bubbles that develop during decompression (54); experimental evidence, however, is insufficient (58). Alternatively, it has been hypothesized that rapidly expanding nitrogen gas would cause bone marrow adipose tissue damage with disruption of lipids and lipoproteins. The latter would then lead to local release of intravascular procoagulant factors (60) and the blood changes discussed before.

No satisfactory experimental animal model exists for dysbaric osteonecrosis. Within just a few hours of arterial occlusion, the absence of osteocytes from the bone lacunae can be recognized. As repair of a necrotic area takes place, granulation tissue grows from the living

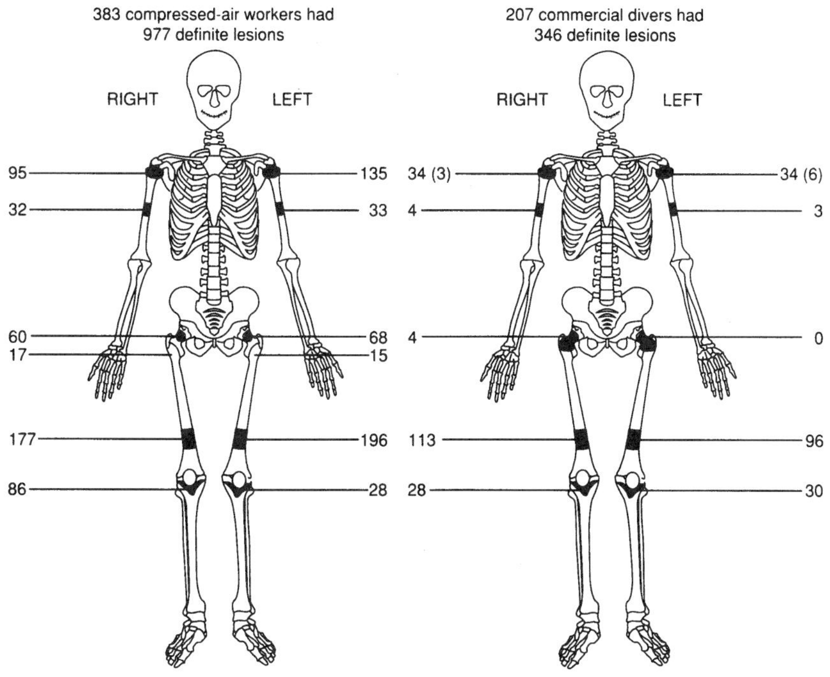


**FIG. 3.** Distribution of bone lesions in compressed air workers and commercial divers. Figures in parentheses indicate the number of affected joints that had structural failure or secondary osteoarthritis, or required surgical treatment. (From ref. 55.)

bone into the necrotic area and new bone is laid over the dead trabeculae without prior resorption of latter. This formation of new bone and failure of resorption creates an area of thickened trabeculae that is separate from the dead bone and marrow. If the area of bone necrosis is not too extensive, it may be completely repaired. This buildup of the trabeculae takes at least 5 months after the ischemic episode to appear and is the first point at which radiographic changes appear. As time passes the changes become more pronounced, the dense areas growing larger. Structural failure of the articular surface, easily detectable by radiography, may eventually occur and can lead to secondary osteoarthritis. The time from the first radiographic indication to the point of structural failure can range from several months to a few years; the patient remains symptom free until the articular surface is no longer intact. If bone death is not extensive and complete repair occurs, the radiographs return to normal (13,54,56).

Mesenchymal malignancies have very rarely been reported in association with preexisting osteonecrosis, regardless of the etiology. In the majority of reported cases (including all of those associated with dysbaric disorders), malignant fibrous hystiocytomas have been the histologic type. Tumors have developed in the distal femur, femoral head, and distal tibia, and all reported cases have been associated with HNS lesions, with long (about 20-year) latencies between last exposure and diagnosis (61,62).

Because the first changes leading to osteonecrosis are only slightly different from the normal variation in the trabeculae, early radiographic diagnosis requires high-quality radiographs and skilled interpretation. Routine bone surveys should include the proximal ends of the humerus and femur and the shafts of the femur and tibia. The most common radiographic abnormalities (in order of descending frequency) are calcified areas in the shaft of the bone, juxtaarticular dense areas and spherical segmental opacities, and linear opacities. A generally accepted classification developed by the British Medical Research Council Decompression Sickness Registry is used for clinical and surveillance purposes. It first classifies the lesions according to their location (JA or HNS), and then describes the patterns of altered bone density and structural failure (54,58).

On radiographs, some difficulty may be experienced in distinguishing dense areas of aseptic bone necrosis from the bone islands that are commonly found in the normal skeleton (47). However, bone islands are usually composed of uniformly dense compact bone and are ovoid or oblong. Lesions of aseptic osteonecrosis are usually irregular and have thickened trabeculae running through them. Also, as mentioned previously, they are often multiple and bilateral (56) (Fig. 4). Radiographic changes due to dysbaric osteonecrosis must also be differentiated from those of other conditions such as Gaucher's disease, sickle cell anemia, the arthropathy of steroid therapy, alcoholism, radiotherapy, some hemoglobinopathies, and osteoblastic metastases. Most of these causes of bone necrosis are rare in relatively young and healthy persons; therefore, when osteonecrosis occurs in a person exposed to a hyperbaric environment, as long as the other causes are ruled out, it can be attributed to work (54,56).

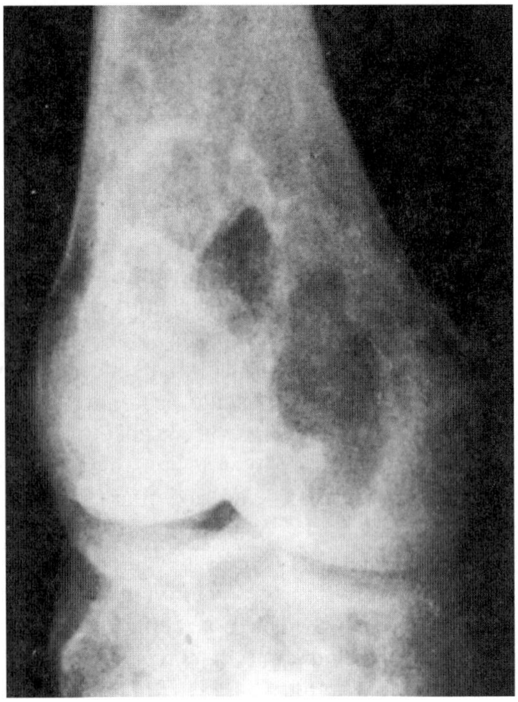

**FIG. 4.** Aseptic bone necrosis seen after many years of caisson work. (From ref. 90.)

Additional imaging techniques may be useful in the diagnosis of dysbaric osteonecrosis. These include computed tomography (CT), bone scintigraphy, and magnetic resonance imaging (MRI) (54). CT gives much better definition than conventional radiography. In the early stages of osteonecrosis, CT allows clearer identification of the thickened trabeculae. Structural failure is also more easily identified with CT (57). Bone scintigraphy with $^{99m}$technetium-labeled diphosphonate seems more sensitive than traditional radiographic methods (63). With bone scintigraphy the necrotic area of bone produces a "cold" lesion resulting from decreased or absent uptake of radioisotope from the hypometabolic area. During revascularization, radioisotope uptake increases, producing a "hot" lesion. While bone scintigraphy is a powerful tool in that it can identify areas of osteonecrosis within several weeks of ischemia, it is not without limitations. What bone scintigraphy possesses in sensitivity, it lacks in predictive value. Many bone diseases show the characteristic hot spots that occur in osteonecrosis. Moreover, fewer than half the lesions shown by bone scintigraphy progress to positive radiographic evidence of osteonecrosis (54). MRI has enhanced the detection of osteonecrosis thanks to its ability to image in multiple planes and to more clearly identify soft tissue and bone marrow. On MRI necrotic areas appear as homogeneous areas of decreased signal intensity in the JA area within just a few days. As revascularization occurs, so does an increase in the signal intensity. MRI can be helpful in the detection of early lesions. However, like bone scintigraphy, MRI lacks positive predictive value (54). Therefore, traditional radiography, in conjunction with CT, still remains the easiest, most readily available method of diagnosing dysbaric osteonecrosis. Bone scintigraphy may prove to be useful in early detection and thus have a role in periodic surveillance. MRI may be useful in clarifying equivocal radiographic appearances. Further work will determine the role of bone scintigraphy and MRI in early detection (54).

### *Other Involved Systems*

The skin is very frequently affected in DCS. Cutaneous pruritus, erythema, nonspecific macular eruptions, and cutis marmorata are common presentations of cutaneous DCS. Inner ear decompression sickness (64) is more common when helium-oxygen breathing mixtures are used for diving. Symptoms usually begin during decompression (ascent) or shortly after after surfacing from a dive. Those symptoms include sensorineural hearing loss, tinnitus, and/or vertigo during or shortly after decompression, which are similar to those of inner ear barotrauma (discussed below). The latter, however, usually occurs during compression or after a shallow dive, and may be associated with middle ear barotrauma. Treatment is the opposite for both conditions (recompression for inner ear DCS but not for barotrauma). Explosion of teeth, especially if they have been previously repaired, has been described after rapid decompression and it is more frequently consider a form of barotrauma of ascent. Ocular signs and symptoms occur in about 7% of all DCS cases (45,65), and may include nystagmus, diplopia, visual field defects, cortical blindness, convergence insufficiency, central retinal artery occlusion, and optic neuropathy. Fluorescein angiography findings similar in appearance to those of choroidal ischemia have been documented in divers, but their significance remains to be established (65). The hematopoietic system is affected even beyond the intravascular changes in blood components and plasma volume that have been discussed above. Bone marrow infarction has been recognized as a complication of decompression sickness. This is a consequence of bubble-induced swelling of fat cells in the marrow rather than direct toxicity to the hematopoietic series (13). Nephrotic syndrome due to minimal-change glomerulonephritis was described in association with DCS in one case report (66).

## Treatment and Prognosis

Ideally, DCS should be prevented by decompression schedules (e.g., the one developed by the U.S. Navy) that estimate the degree and duration of safe decompression to be allowed for gas equilibration during return to a normobaric environment. Those schedules are developed and revised according to both empiric data and mathematical models of gas elimination in the body. Not surprisingly, current schedules, even when strictly followed, do not completely prevent DCS (6,11,67,68). Furthermore, it may be impossible to eliminate the risk (3). Surveillance with periodic radiographic examinations is necessary for persons at risk for dysbaric osteonecrosis.

Decompression sickness is a true medical emergency, especially when neurologic manifestations occur. The primary treatment for decompression sickness (as well as barotrauma) is to administer hyperbaric therapy accompanied by 100% oxygen (51,69). The recompression pressure causes bubbles to become smaller, and breathing pure oxygen produces a gradient by which inert gas in bubbles and tissues can diffuse out of the body. Treatment protocols (decompression tables) usually consist of series of timed exposures to increased atmospheric pressure with alternating 100% oxygen and air breathing (to avoid oxygen toxicity). The use of helium-oxygen mixes during recompression seems promising and m ay be used more frequently in the future (8,11,70). Rapid transport of the victim to a recompression facility is the single most important measure, and the probability of recovery greatly decreases with delays (71,72). If transportation is by air, either pressurized or low-flying unpressurized aircraft are preferred (44). Portable one-person recompression chambers have been devised to initiate treatment immediately while transporting the patients, but are not widely available. If transportation delays cannot be avoided, intermittent administration of 100% oxygen and air is recommended. Additional supportive measures include the use of corticosteroids to reduce nerve tissue edema (71) and volume expansion (intravenous fluids). Their beneficial effects, however, have not yet been substantiated (8).

Treatment can be extremely effective if begun early, when symptoms are just developing, and tissue damage is only mild. Hyperbaric oxygen therapy has achieved successful results in as many as 98% of cases of neurologic DCS (41). If treatment is delayed, tissue damage increases; even if all bubbles disappear with hyperbaric therapy, healing requires days to weeks and may not be complete. By a still unknown mechanism, however, some patients [30–50% (44)] relapse after having responded favorably to recompression treatment, long after bubbles may have persisted (3). Repeated recompression treatment is indicated in case of relapses, or until no further clinical improvement is observed. Somatosensory evoked potential testing may provide a tool to monitor neurophysiologic improvement during recompression treatment (50).

In most cases the aftereffects of decompression sickness resolve within weeks of initial treatment, yet little is known of subsequent health complications of this disorder. Permanent neurologic defects can result (67,73), even with prompt and adequate recompression (11). In a study of U.S. Navy divers that compared postdecompression sickness hospitalization rates with those for a matched sample of divers who had no recorded diving accidents, divers who had suffered from decompression sickness had significantly higher rates than matched controls for total hospitalizations, symptoms (vertigo, abnormal involuntary movement, limb or joint pain, chest pain, abdominal pain, syncope, and headache), and disorders of the arteries and veins (arterial embolism and thrombosis, phlebitis and thrombophlebitis, occlusion of precerebral arteries, and aneurysm) (74). Other manifestations may not appear for many years. There is controversy, however, about the nature, frequency, and extent of neurologic sequelae of neurologic DCS and arterial gas embolism, which may be difficult to document objectively (75,76).

At the present time, there is still no consensus about recommendations for divers who have had DCS. It is probably advisable that diving not be resumed until 4 weeks after an episode of DCS and that it be discontinued if long-term sequelae remain after treatment.

Treatment of dysbaric osteonecrosis is mainly symptomatic. Attempts at repairing and revascularizing necrotic areas of bone in the femoral and humeral heads have been largely unsuccessful. Patients with severe structural failure frequently require prosthetic articular replacement (54). Workers with definite JA osteonecrotic lesions should be advised to stop their exposures, and should be followed even if they do. On the other hand, data does not support a similar recommendation for workers with definite HNS lesions. The probability (albeit small) of neoplastic transformation in the site of bone infarction needs to be kept in mind during long-term follow-up.

## BAROTRAUMA

Barotrauma is the second leading cause of death in scuba divers (drowning is the first). Barotrauma may occur during descent or ascent whenever a gas-filled space, such as pulmonary alveoli, middle ear, paranasal sinuses, stomach, or dental fillings, fails to equalize its internal pressure relative to changes in ambient pressure. As noted in Table 1, the most dramatic changes in pressure and volume occur under hyperbaric conditions, but the hypobaric environment of aviation and space flight can also predispose the aviator to complications of barotrauma. Manifestations of barotrauma of descent are usually referred to as "the squeeze," and those of barotrauma of ascent as "reverse squeeze." Recreational divers refer to the pulmonary complications of barotrauma as "bubble trouble." The main forms of barotrauma are summarized in Table 3.

**TABLE 3.** *Clinical forms of barotrauma*

| |
|---|
| Barotrauma of descent |
| Middle-ear squeeze |
| Paranasal and sinus squeeze |
| Inner ear squeeze |
| Dental filling squeeze |
| Face squeeze |
| Barotrauma of ascent |
| Gastric rupture |
| Pneumothorax |
| Pneumomediastinum |
| Subcutaneous emphysema |
| Pneumopericardium |
| Arterial gas embolism |

### Barotrauma of Descent

The middle ear is commonly affected in divers and air travelers. As the ambient pressure is altered by high altitude or diving, the tympanic membrane (TM) is displaced outward or forced inward because of the compressibility of middle ear air. If the pressure across the TM is equalized by normally patent eustachian tubes, or by forcing air into the tubes by a controlled Valsalva maneuver, there will be no net displacement of the TM and no barotrauma. If the eustachian tube or sinus osmium is blocked, it is not possible to restore gas pressure equilibrium across the TM and intense pain and hemorrhage can result. Blockage is most frequently due to mucosal edema from infections or allergies. Middle ear barotrauma can be associated with usually transient peripheral facial nerve paralysis due to compression of vasa nervorum and neurapraxia. If the inner ear is affected, perforation of the oval window may result in symptoms of tinnitus, vertigo, hearing loss, and nystagmus. Temporal relation with and the characteristics of the dive help differentiate this inner ear barotrauma from inner ear DCS (see above), which is important in view of their different treatments.

Together with the middle ear, the paranasal sinuses are the most common targets of barotrauma in divers, and the frontal sinuses are more frequently affected. Symptoms of sinus barotrauma include severe pain overlying the sinus or adjacent teeth, sometimes associated with bloody nasal discharge. Submucosal hemorrhage in the ear or paranasal sinuses may be severe enough that surgical drainage is required. Prevention of these conditions can be accomplished by the judicious use of systemic or nasal decongestant and antiinflammatory steroid sprays. Unsatisfactory symptom control and/or failure to equalize middle ear pressure by a Valsalva maneuver contraindicate a hyperbaric exposure.

During descent, facial barotrauma (face squeeze) can occur if the diver does not exhale through his nose into the mask. The latter allows equalization of the gas pressure in the space between the mask and the face, and the ambient pressure. The manifestations include facial mucocutaneous edema and/or ecchymosis, which does not require treatment. Dental barotrauma, characterized by implosion of teeth (especially poorly filled ones), can also occur during descent.

### Barotrauma of Ascent

The ears are rarely affected on ascent because the eustachian tubes normally function as one-way valves, allowing air to escape from the middle ear but not to enter it. Although less frequent than barotrauma of descent, barotrauma of ascent is associated with the most serious and potentially lethal complications: pulmonary barotrauma and arterial gas embolism (AGE).

When transpulmonary (intratracheal minus alveolar) pressure exceeds 100 cm $H_20$, gas can escape along perivascular sheaths and rupture into the pulmonary interstitial tissue (interstitial emphysema), mediastinum (pneumomediastinum), pleural spaces (pneumothorax), subcutaneous tissues (subcutaneous emphysema), or the pulmonary veins or the left atrium (paradoxically through a patent foramen ovale) causing arterial gas embolism. Excessive transpulmonary pressure gradients are most common under hyperbaric conditions, such as scuba diving, during which the scuba apparatus allows the diver to maintain near-normal lung volumes despite being exposed to hyperbaric intraalveolar pressures. According to Boyle's law, if a scuba diver ascends from a salt water dive of only 33 feet too rapidly or without exhaling, alveolar volume will double (Table 1, Fig. 2). This differs from breath-hold diving during which the volume cannot exceed total lung capacity at sea level. Less significant volume expansion occurs at altitude (Fig. 2). However, even small volume changes may cause barotrauma if individual lung units have prolonged time constants (resistance × compliance) due to obstruction or bronchospasm or if the diver fails to exhale during ascent.

Short of rupturing, overdistention of the lung with resulting local injury results in the relatively mild pulmonary overinflation syndrome. Patients may complain of hemoptysis, with or without chest pain. Chest radiographs may reveal a small pleural effusion. Injury is localized to the overdistended area and requires only symptomatic treatment.

Symptoms of mediastinal emphysema include dysphagia, cough, dyspnea, and pleuritic chest pain that may radiate to the shoulders. Mediastinal emphysema can only be detected radiographically, unless it extends to the subcutaneous tissues of the neck (subcutaneous emphysema). A pneumothorax, especially if under tension, is clinically detectable by a characteristic physical examination: diminished ipsilateral breath sounds, hyperresonance to percussion, and deviation of the trachea to the contralateral side. Concomitant signs include tachypnea, tachycardia, hypertension, and cyanosis. If a pneumopericardium is also present, a harsh pericardial rub (Hamman's "crunch") may be auscultated. Treatment of a pneumothorax involves administering high-flow oxygen and placement of a chest tube. Concomitant injuries may require hyperbaric oxygen therapy.

Arterial gas embolism (AGE) is the most life-threatening syndrome of barotrauma. AGE and decompression sickness share similar pathophysiology (formation of arterial gas bubbles) and treatment (decompression). However, they differ in the source of the gas bubbles, and in that DCS requires a transition to an environment with lower ambient pressure, whereas AGE occurs isobarically. Although it is much less frequent than DCS, AGE accounts for a disproportionately higher number of deaths from diving.

Clinically, there are two main presentations of AGE: (a) isolated central nervous system (CNS) symptoms and (b) cardiovascular collapse. In divers, the CNS manifestations predominate (95% of reported cases of AGE). Cardiovascular collapse is thought to be due to either acute myocardial ischemia after coronary artery embolization or neurogenic-mediated hypertension and cardiac dysrhythmias if the embolus lodges within the cerebral arterial circulation.

The neurologic manifestations of AGE are diverse. In contrast to DCS, the brain is the most frequent target of AGE, and symptoms and signs are noticed immediately upon surfacing, almost without exception. Simultaneous embolization of multiple brain arteries occurs, and this explains the diversity of the neurologic clinical findings. Symptoms include vertigo, a feeling of apprehension, confusion, and faintness. Signs progress rapidly and range from sensory disturbances and aphasia to hemiplegia, cortical blindness, hemianopias, confusion, coma, and seizures. Rare, but classic, signs include marbling of the skin of the upper torso, gas in the retinal arteries, and sharply demarcated areas of pallor on the tongue (Leibermeister's sign) (20).

Five percent of individuals with AGE die almost immediately and 35% stabilize or deteriorate. The majority (60%) improve within minutes because of redistribution of emboli to the venous circulation (44). Interestingly, within 1 hour of initial embolization, approximately 15% of AGE cases recover completely, but frequently relapse. Relapse may be due to the interactions between air and blood elements, and triggering of the inflammatory mediator cascades discussed above (see Pathophysiology).

Treatment is very similar to that of DCS. Despite the severity of AGE manifestations, recompression in a hyperbaric chamber frequently reverses them. Delays in transporting patients to a treatment facility is directly proportional to mortality and frequency of long-term sequelae. A few issues are relevant to the treatment of AGE. Patients are transported in a head-down and left lateral decubitus position and that position is also maintained during hyperbaric treatment. The recommended starting compression is usually higher in AGE than in DCS, to ensure immediate bubble size reduction (8). Relapse after an initial complete recompression treatment is frequent (about 30%), although usually less so in AGE patients than in those with DCS. Hyperbaric treatment is indicated for relapses, and is continued daily until there is no evidence of further improvement. Although administration of large doses of corticosteroids has been recommended in the treatment of AGE, its therapeutic value is unclear (8). Cardiac antiarrhythmic medication infusions are being increasingly used. Chest radiograph to exclude tension pneumothorax and continuous ECG monitoring during hyperbaric treatment are also indicated.

As with DCS, there is no agreement on the nature, extent, and frequency of long-term neurologic sequelae from episodes of AGE. Long-term follow-up should include careful neuropsychological assessments. All individuals who have suffered AGE should permanently refrain from diving.

## OTHER DYSBARIC DISORDERS

Oxygen-diving–induced middle ear underaeration is a condition of unknown pathogenic mechanism, believed to be different from middle ear barotrauma. It occurs in divers in the morning hours after diving the previous day with a pure oxygen breathing mixture. The pathogenesis is still unclear. Middle ear negative pressure has been demonstrated by tympanography. Transient pain and hearing deficit are the usual complaints, and effusions can be observed by otoscopic examination. The process is self-limited (77).

## MEDICAL EVALUATION OF PROSPECTIVE DIVERS

Diving requires strenuous activity in an alien, hyperbaric, environment. The medical evaluation of individuals wishing to dive needs to focus on conditions that either limit the ability to exercise, are exacerbated by exercise, or can be provoked or worsened by alterations of ambient pressure, volume, or temperature. Any contraindication for hyperbaric treatment also contraindicates diving. Table 4 lists those conditions that are believed to be disqualifying for diving. The major diseases that require exclusion are obstructive lung disease and cardiac conditions. The type of diving (recreational versus commercial) influences the rigidity of the standards used to evaluate candidates. Specific standards have been developed by the U.S. Navy, the Occupational Safety and Health Administration, and scuba certifying organizations depending on the activities planned (51).

**TABLE 4.** *Medical conditions that may disqualify individuals from diving*

| |
|---|
| Pulmonary disease |
| Obstructive lung disease |
| Asthma (see text) |
| Bullous or cystic lung disease |
| Bronchiectasis |
| Cystic fibrosis |
| Chronic obstructive pulmonary disease |
| Predisposition to pulmonary barotrauma |
| Previous pneumothorax |
| Previous thoracic surgery |
| Eosinophilic granuloma |
| Pulmonary lymphangioleiomyomatosis |
| Pulmonary hemorrhage |
| Cardiac diseases |
| Intracardiac shunts, unrepaired |
| Coronary artery disease |
| Exercise-induced tachyarrhythmias |
| Dysrhythmias, not controlled |
| Neurologic diseases |
| History of seizure disorder (except febrile seizures in infancy) |
| Recurrent episodes of syncope |
| Ophthalmologic and otolaryngologic conditions |
| Meniere's disease |
| Middle ear prosthesis |
| Visual disturbance, severe |
| External ear canal obstruction |
| Unilateral vestibular organ damage |
| Failure to voluntarily equalize middle ear pressures (e.g., by Valsalva maneuver) |
| Recent eye surgery (for guidelines, see ref. 65) |
| Presence of hollow orbital implant |
| Obstructed nasal and paranasal passages (e.g., upper respiratory infections) |
| Miscellaneous |
| Previous episode AGE or sequelae from DCS |
| Poor physical conditioning |
| Psychological instability |
| Drug dependency |
| Insulin-dependent diabetes mellitus |
| Sickle-cell disease or trait |
| Caries (including poorly filled ones) |

The elderly should undergo appropriate cardiopulmonary exercise testing prior to diving. The older diver should also be warned about an increased risk of hypothermia.

Obstructive lung disease or previous pulmonary barotrauma place the diver at risk because of hyperinflation, which may occur during ascent, and because of limited exercise tolerance. Similarly, exercise-induced cardiac dysrhythmias are a potential danger for divers. Intracardiac shunts predispose to paradoxical venous emboli followed by arterial gas embolization. Unfortunately, patent foramen ovale (demonstrated by echocardiography during a Valsalva maneuver) is a very common condition in the general population. One study noted a prevalence of 24% in a group of divers who had no symptoms of decompression sickness, compared to two-thirds of divers who had (78). Another study documented patent foramen ovale in 18 of 30 divers who had experienced arterial gas embolism (79).

Asthma poses a vexing problem when an afflicted individual wants to dive. Exercise or hyperventilation of cold, dry air may provoke airway constriction that can cause nonuniform ventilation distribution and localized pulmonary hyperinflation. Even when asymptomatic and well controlled, asthmatics show evidence of abnormal ventilation distribution as assessed by frequency dependence of compliance testing (80). Hyperinflation and air trapping theoretically predispose the diver to barotrauma during ascent. Whether the hypothetical concerns of increased risk of barotrauma in asthmatics translates into an increased number of diving accidents in asthmatic divers has not been conclusively documented, and remains a controversial issue. Until recently, most experts disqualified diving candidates who had an asthma attack after the age of 12 (81,82). Recently, various arguments have questioned this dictum based on epidemiologic data (82–84). Of 100 scuba diving fatalities in New Zealand and Australia, 7% occurred in asthmatics, whereas the incidence of asthma in those countries is 12% to 20% (82). However, there was a strong bias during the decade studied (1980–1990) to exclude asthmatics from the dying population, which may explain the underrepresentation of asthmatics in mortality figures. In a questionnaire study of 10,400 certified divers, 8.3% had a history of asthma and 3.3% currently had asthma at the time of the study (82). In studies of active asthmatic divers, Farrell and Glanville (85) reported no statistically increased incidence of barotrauma compared to nonasthmatic divers. Using data collected by the Divers Alert Network (DAN), Moon (81) reported that 5.3% of 696 randomly selected members had asthma and 1.9% had experienced wheezing or had used bronchodilators in the previous 12 months ("current" asthma). The estimated risk ratio for arterial gas embolism was 1.25 (95% confidence interval 0.8–2.1) for asthmatic divers, and 1.65 (0.8–3.6) for current asthmatics (81). However, a small sample size may have limited the ability to detect statistically significant risk ratios. In any case, data from the United States led to an estimation of less than one episode of arterial gas embolization per 250,000 dives. Asthmatics would therefore face a less than twofold increase in risk of a very infrequent event (84).

Realizing that a significant number of recreational and commercial divers have active or past history of asthma, the Undersea and Hyperbaric Medical Society recently sponsored a conference on asthmatic divers (86). Given the fact that many asthmatics dive without experiencing the theoretically increased risk of dysbarism, the experts focused on identifying which asthmatics should be excluded from diving. The panel concluded that (a) previous policies that excluded all asthmatics from diving may paradoxically increase the risk of dysbarism in asthmatic divers by discouraging them from obtaining an appropriate assessment of their fitness to dive; (b) pulmonary function testing (PFT) is the best method of evaluating an asthmatic's fitness to dive; (c) asthma that is controlled (no symptoms, normal PFT), even if inhaled (not systemic) steroids are required, does not preclude safe diving; and (d) acute asthma, as evidenced by symptoms (dyspnea, chest tightness, cough, nocturnal awakenings), signs (wheezing, coughing), or PFT abnormalities, would preclude diving until the symptoms have normalized and returned to the individual's baseline for a minimum of 3 weeks (9). Airway hyperreactivity, a physiologic hallmark of asthma, may be best assessed in divers by bronchoprovocation testing (87) with exercise (which simulates the activity of diving); inhalation of cold dry air, methacholine, or histamine are other available methods (86).

Most experts discourage diving during pregnancy (88). Pregnant women may incur difficulties when diving due to the physiologic changes that they undergo. Congested mucous membranes may prevent equilibration of the middle ear and sinuses. Abnormal temperature regulation may predispose to hypothermia. In addition, the increase in body fat may predispose to decompression sickness. Of more concern is the fate of the fetus, which can be adversely affected by a decrease in oxygen delivery. Surveys of women who scuba dived during their pregnancies showed a fetal complication rate similar to the general population but statistically increased when compared to women divers who refrained from diving when pregnant (89).

A previous history of dysbaric disorder is also a consideration. Divers who have suffered DCS should refrain from any diving until 4 weeks after complete recovery. Divers who have sequelae from DCS or who have experienced AGE (with or without sequelae) should not dive at all (44,65).

## SUMMARY

Dysbaric disorders result from exposure to altered environmental pressure, their rapid changes, and/or from the resulting abnormal behavior of gases in the body. The inverse relationship between the pressure and the volume of a gas explains the translation of changed environmental pressures into changes in gas volumes within the human body. Although most dysbaric disorders result from abnormal gas behavior in the body, exposure to an increased environmental pressure per se (during compression or descent) causes high-pressure neurologic syndrome (HPNS). If the hyperbaric exposure is combined with compressed air breathing, nitrogen narcosis may occur. The immediate compression of gas volumes in air-filled organs due to hyperbaric exposure explains barotrauma of descent. On the other hand, a rapid sequence of pressure changes, exceeding the capacity or the rapidity of the compensatory and adaptive mechanisms of the human body, can cause the formation of gas bubbles and the most frequent dysbaric disorders. If the source of the bubbles is in the tissues (and/or their vasculature), decompression sickness (DCS) can occur. If the bubbles form in overpressurized lungs and escape directly into the pulmonary interstitium or the arteries, barotrauma of ascent and arterial gas embolism result.

The altered pressure to which an individual may be exposed must be gradually returned to normal according to recommended schedules, so that the risk of dysbaric disorders can be reduced. The complete elimination of that risk remains elusive, due in good part to the poor understanding of the basis for differences in interindividual susceptibility (3).

Dysbarism continues to be significant today as hyperbaric environments are being increasingly used in commercial, recreational, and military spheres. Despite the development of mechanical devices, human exposure to compressed air environments is still necessary in tunnel construction or caisson work. In the past several decades, especially after the oil crisis of 1973, commercial diving has reached a new level of importance in the search for and extraction of petroleum oil from the ocean floor. Commercial dives are being made regularly to increasing depths in many parts of the world. Simulated experimental dives to 400 to 650 m and for extended periods of time in hyperbaric chambers are providing information that will increase the current limits of commercial and professional diving. Moreover, recreational and sports diving (snorkel diving, underwater hockey, breath-hold diving, and scuba diving) have gained immense popularity in several countries during the last decade. Around the world, most scuba diving is recreational. Although specific depth limits are established for recreational diving, dysbarism still occurs in that setting. Furthermore, the military operational or training use of hyperbaric environments, in aerospace and submarine conditions, continues to make dysbarism an ongoing problem.

## REFERENCES


1. Wilson MM, Curley FJ. Gas embolism: Part I. Venous gas emboli. *J Intensive Care Med* 1996;11:182–204.
2. Behnke AR. Decompression sickness incident to deep sea diving and high altitude ascent. *Medicine* 1945;24:381–402.
3. Moon RE, Vann RD, Bennet PB. The physiology of decompression illness. *Sci Am* 1995;273:70–77.
4. Golding FC, Griffiths P, Hempleman HV, Paton WDM, Walder DN. Decompression sickness during construction of the Dartford tunnel. *Br J Ind Med* 1960;17:167–180.
5. Nellen JR, Kindwall EP. Aseptic necrosis of bone secondary to occupational exposure to compressed air: roentgenologic findings in 59 cases. *Am J Roentgenol 1972;*115:512–524.
6. Downs GJ, Kindwall EP. Aseptic necrosis in caisson workers: a new set of decompression tables. *Aviat Space Environ Med* 1986;57:569–574.
7. Wang YT. Diving (underwater) for pulmonary pearls. *Singapore Med J* 1993;34:14–15.
8. Madsen J, Hink J, Hyldegaard O. Diving physiology and pathophysiology. *Clin Physiol* 1994;14:597–626.
9. Krieger PB. Diving complications. *Pulmon Crit Care Update* 1993;9:1–6.
10. Hills BA. Air embolism: fission of microbubbles upon collision in plasma. *Clin Sci Mol Med* 1974;45:629–634.
11. Aharon-Peretz J, Adir Y, Gordon CR, Kol S, Gal N, Melamed Y. Spinal cord decompression sickness in sport diving. *Arch Neurol* 1993;50: 753–756.
12. Lee WH, Hairston P. Structural effects on blood proteins at the gas-blood interface. *Fed Proc* 1971;30:1615–1620.
13. Calder IM. Dysbarism—a review. *Forensic Sci Int* 1986;30:237–266.
14. Philp RB. A review of blood changes associated with compression-decompression: relationship to decompression sickness. *Undersea Biomed Res* 1974;1:117–150.
15. Barnard EEP, Wethersby PK. Blood cell changes in asymptomatic divers. *Undersea Biomed Res* 1981;8:187–198.
16. Ward CA, Koheil A, McCullough D, Johnson WR, Fraser WD. Activation of complement at plasma-air or serum-air interface of rabbits. *J Appl Physiol* 1986;60:1651–1658.
17. Ward CA, McCullough D, Fraser WD. Relation between complement activation and susceptibility to decompression sickness. *J Appl Physiol* 1987;62:1160–1166.
18. Shastri KA, Logue GL, Lundgren CE. In vitro activation of human complement by nitrogen bubbles. *Undersea Biomed Res* 1991;18: 157–165.
19. Pekna M, Ersson A. Complement system response to decompression. *Undersea Hyperbaric Med* 1996;23:31–34.
20. Wilson MM, Curley FJ. Gas embolism: Part II. Arterial gas embolism and decompression sickness. *J Intensive Care Med* 1996;11:261–283.
21. O'Quin RJ, Lakshminarayan S. Venous air embolism. *Arch Intern Med* 1982;142:2173–2176.
22. Neuman TS, Spragg RG, Wagner PD, Moser KM. Cardiopulmonary consequences of decompression stress. *Respir Physiol* 1980;41: 143–153.
23. Craig AB, William DE. Effect of immersion in water on vital capacity and residual volume of the lungs. *J Appl Physiol* 1965;23:423–425.
24. Linér MH. Cardiovascular and pulmonary responses to breath-hold diving in humans. *Acta Physiol Scand* 1994;151(suppl 620):1–32.
25. Héritier F, Feihl F. La plongéee: bases physiques et physiologiques. *Rev Med Suisse Romande* 1994;114:505–516.
26. Grassi B, Ferretti G, Costa M, et al. Ventilatory responses to hypercapnia and hypoxia in elite breath-hold divers. *Respir Physiol* 1994; 97:323–332.
27. Linér MH, Linnarsson D. Tissue oxygen and carbon dioxide stores and breath-hold diving in humans. *J Appl Physiol* 1994;77:542–547.
28. Wood LDH, Bryan AC. Effect of increased ambient pressure on flow-volume curve of the lung. *J Appl Physiol* 1969;27:4–8.
29. Davey IS, Cotes JE, Reed JW. Relationship of ventilatory capacity to hyperbaric exposure in divers. *J Appl Physiol* 1984;56:1655–1658.
30. Crosbie WA, Reed JW, Clarke MC. Functional characteristics of the large lungs found in commercial divers. *J Appl Physiol* 1979;46:639–645.
31. Thorsen E, Segadal K, Kambestad BK, Gulsvik A. Pulmonary function one and four years after a deep saturation dive. *Scand J Work Environ Health* 1993;19:115–120.
32. Zeljko D, Eterovic D, Denoble P, Krstacic G, Tocilj J, Gosovic S. Effect of a single air dive on pulmonary diffusing capacity in professional divers. *J Appl Physiol* 1993;74:55–61.
33. Cotes JE, Davey IS, Reed JW, Rooks M. Respiratory effects of a single saturation dive to 300 m. *Br J Ind Med* 1987;44:76–82.
34. Thorsen E, Segadal K, Kambestad BK. Mechanisms of reduced pulmonary function after a saturation dive. *Eur Respir J* 1994;7:4–10.
35. Crosbie WA, Clarke MB, Cox RAF, et al. Physical characteristics and ventilatory function of 404 commercial divers working in the North Sea. *Br J Ind Med* 1977;34:19–25.
36. Cotes JE. Respiratory effects of diving [editorial]. *Eur Respir J* 1994; 7:2–3.
37. Thorsen E, Segadal K, Kambestad BK, Gulsvik A. Divers' lung function: small airways disease? *Br J Ind Med* 1990;47:519–523.
38. Thorsen E, Kambestad BK. Persistent small-airways dysfunction after exposure to hyperoxia. *J Appl Physiol* 1995;78:1421–1424.
39. Jain KK. High-pressure neurological syndrome (HPNS). *Acta Neurol Scand* 1994;90:45–50.
40. Lorenz J, Brooke ST, Petersen R, Török Z, Wenzel J. Brainstem auditory evoked potentials during a helium-oxygen saturation dive to 450 meters of seawater. *Undersea Hyperbaric Med* 1995;22:229–240.

41. Wirjosemito SA, Touhey JE, Workman WT. Type II altitude decompression sickness (DCS): U.S. Air Force experience with 133 cases. *Aviat Space Environ Med* 1989;60:256–262.
42. Elliott DH, Moon RE. Manifestations of the decompression disorders. In: Bennett PB, Elliott DH, eds. *The physiology and medicine of diving,* 4th ed. London: WB Saunders, 1993:481–505.
43. Smith DJ, Francis TJR, Pethybridge RJ, Wright JM, Sykes JJW. An evaluation of the classification of decompression disorders. *Undersea Biomed Res* 1993;20:17–18.
44. Gorman DF. Decompression sickness and arterial gas embolism in sports scuba divers. *Sports Med* 1989;8:32–42.
45. Rivera JC. Decompression sickness among divers: an analysis of 935 cases. *Milit Med* 1964;129:314–335.
46. Lam TH, Yau KP. Manifestations and treatment of 793 cases of decompression sickness in a compressed air tunneling project in Hong Kong. *Undersea Biomed Res* 1988;15:377–388.
47. Erde A, Edmonds C. Decompression sickness: a clinical series. *J Occup Med* 1975;17:324–328.
48. Adkisson GH, Hodgson M, Smith F, et al. Cerebral perfusion deficits in dysbaric illness. *Lancet* 1989;2:119–122.
49. Staff RT, Gemmell HG, Duff PM, et al. Texture analysis of divers' brains using 99Tcm-HMPAO SPET. *Nucl Med Commun* 1995;16:438–442.
50. Murrison A, Glasspool E, Francis J, Sedgwick M. Somatosensory evoked potentials in acute neurological decompression illness. *J Neurol* 1995;242:669–676.
51. Strauss RH. Diving medicine. *Am Rev Respir Dis* 1979;119:1001–1023.
52. Butler BD, Hills BA. The lung as a filter for microbubbles. *J Appl Physiol* 1979;47:537–543.
53. Zwirevich CV, Müller NL, Abboud RT, Lepawsky M. Noncardiogenic pulmonary edema caused by decompression sickness: rapid resolution following hyperbaric therapy. *Radiology* 1987;163:81–82.
54. Davidson JK. Dysbaric disorders: aseptic bone necrosis in tunnel workers and divers. *Baillieres Clin Rheumatol* 1989;3:1–23.
55. Decompression Sickness Panel-Medical Research Council (UK). Aseptic bone necrosis in commercial divers. *Lancet* 1981;2:384–388.
56. McCallum RI, Walder DN. Bone lesions in compressed air workers—with special reference to men who worked on the Clyde Tunnels 1958 to 1963. *J Bone Joint Surg* 1966;48B:207–235.
57. Van Blarcom ST, Czarnecki DJ, Fueredi GA, Wenzel MS. Does dysbaric osteonecrosis progress in the absence of further hyperbaric exposure? A 10-year radiologic follow-up of 15 patients. *Am J Roentgenol* 1990;155:95–97.
58. Gregg PJ, Walder DN. Caisson disease of bone. *Clin Orthop* 1986;210:43–54.
59. Decompression Sickness Panel-Medical Research Council (UK). Decompression sickness and aseptic necrosis of bone: investigations carried out during and after the construction of the Tyne Road Tunnel (1962–66). *Br J Ind Med* 1971;28:1–21.
60. Jones JP, Ramírez S, Doty SB. The pathophysiologic role of fat in dysbaric osteonecrosis. *Clin Orthop* 1993;296:256–264.
61. Kitano M, Iwasaki H, Yoh SS, Kuroda K, Hayashi K. Malignant fibrous histiocytoma at site of bone infarction in association with DCS. *Undersea Biomed Res* 1984;11:305–314.
62. Torres FX, Kyriakos M. Bone infarct-associated osteosarcoma. *Cancer* 1992;70:2418–2430.
63. Williams ES, Khreisat S, Ell PJ, King JD. Bone imaging and skeletal radiology in dysbaric osteonecrosis. *Clin Radiol* 1987;38:589–592.
64. Neblett LM. Otolaryngology and sport scuba diving: update and guidelines. *Ann Otol Rhinol Laryngol* 1985;115:1–12.
65. Butler FK. Diving and hyperbaric ophthalmology. *Surv Ophthalmol* 1995;39:347–366.
66. Yin PD, Chan KW, Chan MK. Minimal change nephrotic syndrome presenting after acute decompression. *Br Med J* 1986;292:445–446.
67. Hughes JS, Eckenhoff RG. Spinal cord decompression sickness after standard U. S. Navy air decompression. *Milit Med* 1986;151:166–168.
68. Bennett PB, Elliott DH. *The physiology and medicine of diving,* 4th ed. London: WB Saunders, 1993.
69. Robin ED, Gabb G. Hyberbaric oxygen: a therapy in search of diseases. *Chest* 1987;92:1074–1082.
70. Melamed Y, Shupak A, Bitterman H. Medical problems associated with underwater diving. *N Engl J Med* 1992;326:30–35.
71. Leitch DR, Green RD. Pulmonary barotrauma in divers and the treatment of cerebral arterial gas embolism. *Aviat Space Environ Med* 1986;57:931–938.
72. Lim EBH, How J. A review of cases of pulmonary barotrauma from diving. *Singapore Med J* 1993;34:16–19.
73. DiLibero RJ, Pilmanis A. Spinal cord injury resulting from scuba diving. *Am J Sports Med* 1983;11:29–33.
74. Hoiberg A. Consequences of U.S. Navy diving mishaps: decompression sickness. *Undersea Biomed Res* 1986;13:383–394.
75. Murrison AW, Glasspool E, Pethybridge RJ, Francis TJR, Sedgwick EM. Electroencephalographic study of divers with histories of neurological decompression illness. *Occup Environ Med* 1995;52:451–453.
76. Murrison AW, Glasspool E, Pethybridge RJ, Francis TJR, Sedgwick EM. Neurophysiological assessment of divers with medical histories of neurological decompression illness. *Occup Environ Med* 1994;51:730–734.
77. Shupak A, Attias J, Aviv J, Melamed Y. Oxygen diving-induced middle ear under-aeration. *Acta Otolaryngol* 1995;115:422–426.
78. Wilmshurst PT, Byrne JC, Webb-Peploe MM. Relation between interatrial shunts and decompression sickness in divers. *Lancet* 1989;2:1302–1306.
79. Moon RE, Camporesi EM, Kisslo JA. Patent foramen ovale and decompression sickness in divers. *Lancet* 1989;1:513–514.
80. Woolcock AJ, Vincent NJ, Macklem PT. Frequency dependence of compliance as a test for obstruction in the small airways. *J Clin Invest* 1969;48:1097–1106.
81. Moon RE. The case that asthmatics should not dive. In: Elliott DH, ed. *Are asthmatics fit to dive?* Kensington, MD: Undersea and Hyperbaric Medical Society, 1997;45–50.
82. Neuman TS. The case for asthmatics to dive. In: Elliott DH, ed. *Are asthmatics fit to dive?* Kensington, MD: Undersea and Hyperbaric Medical Society, 1997;39–43.
83. Harries M. Why asthmatics should be allowed to dive. In: Elliott DH, ed. *Are asthmatics fit to dive?* Kensington, MD: Undersea and Hyperbaric Medical Society, 1997;7–12.
84. Neuman TS, Bove AA, O'Connor RD, Kelsen SG. Asthma and diving. *Ann Allergy* 1994;73:344–350.
85. Farrell PJ, Glanville P. Diving practices of scuba divers with asthma. *Br Med J* 1990;300:166
86. Elliott DH, ed. *Are asthmatics fit to dive?* Kensington, MD: Undersea and Hyperbaric Medical Society, 1997.
87. Palmeiro EM, Hopp RJ, Biven RE, Bewtra AK, Nair NN, Townley RG. Probability of asthma based on methacholine challenge. *Chest* 1992;101:630–633.
88. Creswell JE, St. Leger-Dowse M. Women and scuba-diving. *Br Med J* 1991;302:1590–1591.
89. Bolton ME. Scuba diving and fetal well-being: a survey of 208 women. *Undersea Biomed Res* 1980;7:183–189.
90. Jacobson HG. *The radiology of skeletal disorders.* Baltimore: Williams & Wilkins, 1971.

*Environmental and Occupational Medicine, Third Edition*, edited by William N. Rom.
Lippincott–Raven Publishers, Philadelphia © 1998.

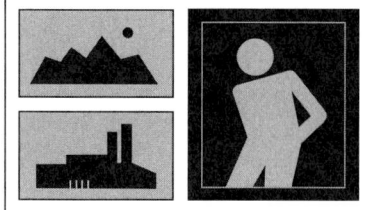

# CHAPTER 103

# High-Altitude Illnesses

William N. Rom

High-altitude environments (above 3,000 m) have fascinated both physicians and physiologists because of high-altitude acclimatization and illnesses, and especially the physical grandeur of the high peaks. Human voyages into these environments were first motivated by adventure to explore and climb, subsequently by employment in metal mines in Colorado and Bolivia, and more recently through aerospace travel. Father José de Acosta (1) in 1590 visited the Bolivian Andes and noted "strange intemperature" among his companions. It was not noted in everyone and was greater among those who "mount[ed] from the sea" than among those who ascended from plateaus. Partial acclimatization on plateaus probably accounted from this difference. Even Mt. Everest has been climbed solo without oxygen, pushing to the ultimate man's physical endurance and acclimatization (2).

Thousands of workers, resident at sea level, will work in newly developed Chilean mines over the next few years, spending 1 week working at around 4,500 m and 1 week resting at low altitude.

## ACCLIMATIZATION

Human beings are at a disadvantage at high altitude because of the diminished ambient pressure of oxygen. Decreased pressure reduces the gradient along which oxygen traverses from alveolus to cell, despite the fact that oxygen remains at 20.93% of air. The partial pressure of oxygen at 5,500 m (18,000 ft) is half that at sea level (3). Adaptive mechanisms intervene in the acclimatization process at all stages of the oxygen transport system: alveolar ventilation, pulmonary diffusion, circulation, and tissue diffusion (4).

Hyperventilation is usually noted first on ascent and is proportional to the altitude or degree of hypoxic stimulus. The increase in ventilation occurs in hours and reaches a maximum in 3 to 4 days. The increase is primarily in tidal volume, and minute ventilation exceeds that of a sea level resident acutely exposed to altitude at all elevations (4). The effect of the ventilatory response is to elevate the alveolar and arterial $pO_2$ and increase the diffusion gradient between the blood and tissues. A respiratory alkalosis is invariably present. The response is mediated by the carotid and aortic chemoreceptors, which respond to hypoxemia. After acclimatization, when the sojourner is given oxygen, ventilation does not return to sea-level values.

Theoretically, the resulting alkalemia and cerebrospinal fluid alkalosis would limit further increase in ventilation, since central chemoreceptors would inhibit ventilation. However, central chemoreceptors are subsequently "reset" by the transport of hydrogen ions into and bicarbonate ions out of the cerebrospinal fluid, thus restoring pH to normal and allowing further ventilatory response to hypoxia (3,5). The role of the cerebrospinal fluid in regulating the ventilatory response to altitude is not universally accepted. After several years at high altitude, ventilation slowly declines, yet it continues to exceed that of high-altitude natives. Thus, for any altitude sojourners appear to have a decreased sensitivity of their peripheral chemoreceptors to hypoxia.

Pulmonary diffusion also may be increased at altitude (at least in natives) by several mechanisms: (a) increased lung volumes, which increase alveolar surface area for gas exchange; (b) pulmonary hypertension, which results

W. N. Rom: Division of Pulmonary and Critical Care Medicine, Departments of Medicine and Environmental Medicine: and Chest Service, Bellevue Hospital Center, New York University Medical Center, New York, New York 10016.

in capillary recruitment; and (c) erythrocytosis, which increases the absolute number of red blood cells in the capillary bed available for gas exchange. However, the diffusion capacity usually has not been found to be increased (3).

The cardiac output increases transiently owing to a tachycardia, since stroke volume does not change (4). With acclimatization, cardiac output both at rest and with exercise does not differ significant from sea-level values at the same work level. There is a reduction in the maximal cardiac output that can be attained with exercise, and this is more pronounced in sojourners than in natives. There also is a drop in arterial saturation with exercise at altitude that is proportional to the altitude. Studies of newcomers to high altitudes have shown a reduction in aerobic capacity from 20% to 60% of that at sea level, depending on the altitude (3). Mean pulmonary artery pressure rises progressively during the first 24 hours at altitude to approximately double the baseline value (6).

Major adaptive responses occur within the blood. Hypoxia is an important stimulus of red blood cell production, and erythropoiesis is increased within hours after ascent. Erythropoietin rapidly increases, but declines to an intermediate value between the sea level and peak value at altitude after a few days (7). Although erythrocytosis of altitude increases oxygen-carrying capability, the increased RBC mass decreases viscosity. Erythropoietin is transcriptionally activated in human hepatoblastoma cells when exposed to hypoxia in vitro (8). Hypoxia-inducible factor 1 (HIF-1), a nuclear protein whose DNA binding activity is induced by hypoxia, binds to a 3′ enhancer sequence as well as to promoter elements on the erythropoietin gene. HIF-1 is induced by hypoxia in many other cells and is involved in transcriptional regulation of genes encoding glycolytic enzymes in hypoxic cells (9). HIF-1 may therefore play a general role in activating homeostatic responses to hypoxia. Endothelial cells upregulate messenger RNA (mRNA) for the vascular permeability factor, vascular endothelial growth factor (VEGF), within 12 hours after exposure to hypoxia, and the VEGF protein accumulates within 24 hours (10). There is a HIF-1 binding motif in the vascular endothelial growth factor promoter (10). Hypoxia also prolongs the half-life of the mRNA for vascular endothelial growth factor, and increases receptors for VEGF, which may enhance its activity on the endothelium (11,12). VEGF may be a mediator of hypoxia increasing pulmonary vascular leakage in altitude illness.

Several adaptive mechanisms also may occur at the tissue level: (a) there may be more capillaries opened up to deliver oxygen, (b) myoglobin in muscle increases with greater diffusion of oxygen, (c) mitochondrial density may increase, and (d) increased cytochrome concentration at altitude acts to keep oxygen uptake constant (4,13).

The American Medical Research Expedition to Mt. Everest in 1981 gathered measurements at extreme altitudes on climber-scientists (13–15). The barometric pressure on the summit (8,848 m, 29,028 ft) was 253 torr and an alveolar gas sample obtained by Dr. Chris Pizzo revealed the $Paco_2$ to be 7.5 mm torr (13,16). Hyperventilation was maximal: a respiratory rate of 85/minute defended a $Pao_2$ of 35 mm torr, resulting in a calculated pH of 7.7 to 7.8, an extreme respiratory alkalosis that was not compensated by kidney excretion of bicarbonate (17). It is this extreme lowering of $Paco_2$ that is able to compensate against extreme hypoxia and thus maintain arterial, and therefore tissue $Pao_2$, enabling humans to reach the summit of Mt. Everest without supplemental oxygen. The respiratory alkalosis at extreme altitude is acute, and after several days kidney bicarbonate excretion decreases the ability to maintain this acute adjustment, explaining, at least in part, why climbers can remain at extreme altitudes for only a few days. Furthermore, at the summit there was a large calculated $Po_2$ difference between alveolar gas and end-capillary blood of about 7 torr, indicating diffusion limitation of oxygen transfer (13,17).

All of the lowlanders experienced periodic breathing at sleep (Cheyne-Stokes breathing) and the apneas could be abolished with supplemental oxygen (18). Interestingly, the Sherpas did not experience sleep apneas at altitude, in keeping with their blunted ventilatory response. Episodes of apnea at altitude are primarily central nonobstructive, and occur more often during sleep than while awake. With acclimatization individuals sleep better probably due to the higher arterial oxygen percent saturation. The most severe hypoxia at altitude occurs during sleep. Acetazolamide improves oxygen saturation during sleep while reducing arousals and episodes of periodic breathing. Periodic breathing at 6,300 m during sleep averaged 72% of the time in study subjects, with average minimal arterial oxygen saturation of 63% and values of $Pao_2$ during apneic episodes in our study on the order of 33 torr (18).

The magnitude of the hypoxic ventilatory response at sea level was evaluated in the Mt. Everest Research Expedition climbers and roughly correlated as a predictor with the maximum altitude attained or with the highest camp at which the climbers slept (19). Nine climbers were evaluated for hypoxic ventilatory response (HVR) at sea level, 5,400 m, and 6,300 m. Their sea level HVR correlated with that obtained at 5,400 m after acclimatization. The three climbers with highest HVR reached the summit in rank order while all of those with lower HVR did not reach the summit and had a lower maximal altitude attained, thus affirming the predictive value of HVR for relative climbing success. At 6,300 m maximal exercise studies were performed with reduced $O_2$ mixtures (16% and 14%) to stimulate the summit of Mt. Everest (20). Maximal $O_2$ uptake fell dramatically as the inspired $O_2$ was reduced, but two subjects were able to reach an uptake of 1 l/min at the lowest inspired $PO_2$ (20). Theoretical analysis predicted an uptake only half this amount, suggesting Mt. Everest would only be adequate for basal metabolism at rest. Above 7,400 m, work levels became very restricted, and ventilation and heart rate actually declined despite an increase in respiratory frequency to very high levels. Clearly, humans are at their limit of physical endurance at the summit of Mt. Everest without supplemental oxygen.

Erythrocytosis is seen at an altitude with the mean hemoglobin concentration at 6,300 m being 18.8 g/dl with a mean hematocrit of 53.4% (21). The concentration of 2,3-diphosphoglycerate (2,3-DPG) showed a mean increase of about 0.2 mol per mole of hemoglobin, and this increase caused a rightward shift of the oxygen dissociation curve, the partial pressure of oxygen at which hemoglobin is half-saturated ($P_{50}$) increasing by 1 or 2 torr (13,21). However, above 6,300 m there is a progressively increased respiratory alkalosis, with the pH above 7.4, causing a leftward shift of the oxyhemoglobin dissociation curve actually enhancing the loading of oxygen by the pulmonary capillaries (21).

Mountaineers have frequently noted mental lapses at altitude such as increased difficulty in performing serial-7 subtractions and mild deterioration in the ability to learn, remember, and express information verbally. An objective evaluation of 35 mountaineers before and 1 to 30 days after ascent to extreme altitude revealed significant declines in visual long-term memory, and twice as many verbal expression errors after than before ascent (22). Both measures correlated with a more vigorous response to hypoxia, possibly due to decreased cerebral blood flow caused by hypocapnia that more than offsets the increase in arterial oxygen saturation. These impairments were transient and not detectable a year later; the exception was a finger-tapping test that measured motor coordination that is under control of the cerebellum, a region of the brain more sensitive to the effects of hypoxia.

There is a progressive decrease in platelets of up to 25% at 6,000 m, with sequestration and destruction of platelets in the pulmonary vasculature (13,23). There are alterations in the pituitary-thyroid axis with increases in serum thyroxine ($T_4$) concentrations, persistent elevations of serum triiodothyronine, and paradoxical increased levels of thyroid-stimulating hormone (TSH) (24). The electrocardiogram at extreme altitude was consistent with raised pulmonary artery pressure showing right bundle branch conduction disturbances and right ventricular hypertrophy (25).

Hematologic parameters have been compared in Andean natives and Himalayan Sherpas living at 3,700 m, matched for age and acclimatized Western sojourners. No significant differences were observed in regard to erythropoietin levels, $P_{50}$, position of the oxyhemoglobin curve, or 2,3-DPG, but the hematocrit and hemoglobin were slightly higher in the Andean natives (26,27). Chronic mountain sickness has only been observed in the latter population. The observation of sleep apnea with hypoxemia in Andean natives but not in Himalayan highlanders may explain the difference in erythrocytosis (28). Winslow and colleagues (26) evaluated the oxyhemoglobin dissociation curve *in situ* among 45 Andean natives at 4,540 m, finding that increased $P_{50}$ resulting from increased red cell 2,3-DPG concentration was offset by compensated respiratory alkalosis, with the net result that the position of the curve closely approached that of persons who live at sea level. Their mean hemoglobin was 20.2 g/dl, hematocrit 61%, and $Pa{O_2}$ 51 torr.

## ACUTE MOUNTAIN SICKNESS

Acute mountain illnesses are a spectrum from acute mountain sickness (AMS) to high-altitude pulmonary edema (HAPE) to cerebral edema (CE). In 1913, Ravenhill accurately described AMS (normal puna), HAPE (cardiac puna), and cerebral edema (nervous puna) (29,30). Referred to as *"soroche"* or *"puno"* in the Andes, AMS is characterized by cardinal symptoms, including headache, insomnia, dyspnea, anorexia, and fatigue that develop during the first 24 hours at altitude (31–33). Headache is the most prominent symptom, producing at times severe, incapacitating pain. Rather than the diuresis commonly seen on ascent to high altitude, an antidiuresis may be a prominent feature. The vital capacity is reduced and pulmonary rales are detected in 20% to 30% of affected persons (34). Neurologic symptoms (memory deficits, vertigo, tinnitus, and auditory and visual disturbances) may impair work proficiency, and anorexia, nausea, or even vomiting may occur (35). Abrupt exposure to moderate altitude (3,000 m) causes AMS in approximately 30% of individuals, and to high altitude (4,500 m) in 75% (34). The reduced partial pressure of oxygen is considered the primary stimulus for the development of AMS, and those who are more susceptible have lower hypoxic ventilatory drives than others (34). Relative hypoventilation at altitude would increase cerebral blood flow, both by lowering $Pa{O_2}$ and raising $Pa{CO_2}$. In most cases, AMS is self-limiting; symptoms diminish after 3 to 7 days.

In Nepal, Hackett and Rennie (32) found an incidence of AMS of 53% in 278 unacclimatized hikers at 4,243 m over a 4-week period. Twelve developed HAPE or CE; 11 of them had flown without taking acetazolamide. Acetazolamide reduced the incidence and severity of AMS in a double-blind study among persons who flew to 2,800 m and subsequently hiked, but had no effect on those who hiked up to that altitude. Hackett and Rennie also emphasized that slow ascent was protective.

Prevention or amelioration of AMS can be achieved by climbing slowly (350 m ascent per/day), by acclimatizing to an intermediate altitude (e.g., 2,000 to 3,000 m), or by using acetazolamide (Diamox). Administration of acetazolamide prior to and during ascent ameliorates the symptoms of AMS but does not prevent HAPE (36).

Acetazolamide reduces cerebrospinal fluid production and pressure, raises cerebrospinal fluid hydrogen ion concentration, and inhibits carbonic anhydrase in the kidneys resulting in excretion of bicarbonate ions. The resultant metabolic acidosis is a stimulus to increase the rate and depth of breathing, resulting in a higher oxygen tension in subjects taking the drug. Furthermore, it decreases sleep hypoxemia by stimulating increased ventilation, thus reducing arousals and episodes of periodic breathing (37). In a double-blind placebo-controlled trial in 64 climbers on Mount Rainier (4,392 m), acetazolamide (10 mg/kg/24 hours) reduced the frequency of AMS from 67% to 16% (36). On the summit, AMS was less common in climbers receiving acetazolamide, and they experienced less headache, nausea, drowsiness, dyspnea, and dizziness, and a greater sense of well-being. Minute ventilation was 50% greater and vital capacity 16% greater than in the placebo group, and more climbers in the treatment group made the summit (36). Side effects of acetazolamide that are common include distal paresthesias, especially of the fingers, which may be bothersome, interfering with sleep; gastrointestinal distress; and increased frequency of urination. Treatment of AMS with acetazolamide (500 mg) at 4,200 m on Mt. McKinley improved the symptom score, reduced the alveolar-arterial gradient, and improved $Pa_{O_2}$ over 24 hours compared to placebo (38). These improvements were most likely secondary to an increase in minute ventilation. Additional hypobaric chamber studies have found dexamethasone an effective prophylactic agent in reducing the symptoms of AMS and in treating the disorder, but have noted hyperglycemia to occur (39,40). A placebo-controlled trial conducted at 4,559 m found that dexamethasone significantly reduced symptoms in climbers with moderate to severe AMS (41). Dexamethasone was also effective in reducing AMS symptom score in new arrivals to an altitude of 2,700 m but was not effective at 2,050 m (42). Acetazolamide would be preferable to corticosteroids for the treatment of AMS since it has fewer side effects. Voluntary hyperventilation every 10 to 15 minutes may reduce symptoms, especially headache. Proper fluid intake to maintain a copious urine output also is essential at high altitudes. Treatment includes oxygen and descent, with recovery being more rapid with the latter (32).

## HIGH-ALTITUDE PULMONARY EDEMA

High-altitude pulmonary edema occurs in climbers and skiers following rapid ascent (6–48 hours) to altitudes above 2,500 to 4,000 m (incidence approximately 0.5–1.5%) (43–45). It was first reported in the English-language literature by Aspen internist Dr. Charles Houston (46) in 1960. Heavy exertion and lack of acclimatization are predisposing factors. Slow ascent for lowlanders averaging 300 m per day is recommended to prevent HAPE. Symptoms include dry cough, dyspnea disproportionate to the effort exerted, fatigue, and confusion or other mental changes. Symptoms are often more prominent and may be initially manifest at night, when sleep aggravates arterial unsaturation. Previous episodes of AMS, HAPE, or difficulty at altitude may be present in about 12% of subjects (47). Frequent clinical signs include tachypnea, tachycardia, pink-frothy sputum, obtundation or frank unconsciousness, oliguria, cyanosis, hypotension, hemoptysis, mild fever, and bilateral pulmonary rales. Signs of infection are absent. HAPE is more common in adolescents and following reascent to high altitude by denizens who travel briefly to lower elevations (48,49). HAPE affects both sexes, and there is no background of preexisting cardiac or pulmonary disease. Hultgren and Marticorena (43) found that in Peru, 20% of patients with HAPE had experienced at least one previous episode, suggesting that some people are more susceptible to HAPE. However, some climbers with a history of HAPE have no difficulty on subsequent climbs. Radiographic features begin with a patchy, peripheral distribution rapidly becoming homogeneous and central as well as peripheral (50). The lower quadrants, especially the right one, are more severe. Over 90% of cases are characterized by homogeneous air space disease. Electrocardiograms may show acute right heart strain. The pulmonary arteries may be prominent. Singh et al. (33) noted a definite time lag, ranging from 6 to 96 hours between arrival at altitude and onset of symptoms. During this time lag, affected persons were oliguric compared with unaffected persons.

The pathophysiologic mechanisms of HAPE center around the concepts of high perfusion and flow to affected lung segments, and/or stress failure of pulmonary capillaries leading to interstitial and alveolar edema. Capillary congestion and thrombi consisting of platelets, leukocytes, and fibrin are seen (51). Heath et al. (52) described the formation and protrusion of multiple endothelial vesicles into the pulmonary capillaries in rats exposed to a simulation of altitude of the summit of Mt. Everest. These edema vesicles could form and disappear rapidly, could obstruct pulmonary blood flow, and were also observed in alveolar epithelial cells.

Physiological studies have shown a normal left ventricular filling pressure, low cardiac output, arterial unsaturation, elevated pulmonary artery pressure, and normal to low pulmonary capillary wedge pressure. There is a raised alveolar/arterial oxygen gradient that cannot be corrected by 100% oxygen (53). There is a high correlation of HAPE with pulmonary hypertension caused by hypoxic pulmonary vasoconstriction. HAPE is characterized physiologically by uneven pulmonary vasoconstriction leading to overperfusion in some areas, with increased hydrostatic vascular pressure followed by capillary stress failure and interstitial and alveolar edema. The hypoxia also activates endothelial cells, and mediators may be released that increase endothelial cell permeability (54). Hultgren (47) developed the overperfusion hypothesis of HAPE in the 1970s, suggesting nonhomogeneous obstruction of the pulmonary vascular bed was caused by hypoxic vasoconstriction and possibly intravascular thromboses. Thus, during periods of exercise and increased pulmonary blood flow, unobstructed areas of the pulmonary circulation (particularly capillaries) would be subjected to high pressure and flow, resulting in interstitial and alveolar edema. Hultgren et al. (55) have shown that when subjects with a history of HAPE are brought to higher altitudes, excessive pulmonary hypertension developed before the onset of symptoms or findings of edema. Children with a past history of HAPE in Leadville, Colorado had a threefold greater mean pulmonary artery pressure when breathing 16% $O_2$ compared to unaffected controls (56). West et al. (57) suggested that interstitial edema causes increased pulmonary vascular resistance with precapillary vessel closure. Further evidence of the importance of high flow is anatomical variation, e.g. the association between unilateral high-altitude pulmonary edema and absence of pulmonary artery on the opposite side (58), and anomalous pulmonary venous drainage or even pulmonary thromboembolism (59,60). Against this are the facts that pulmonary artery pressures in those who previously had HAPE are not increased when breathing hypoxic mixtures at sea level; very high pulmonary artery pressures occur in exercising subjects at high altitude without HAPE; and the patchy inhomogeneous pattern on chest radiographs rapidly becomes homogeneous (54).

West and his colleagues (61–65) have linked the concept of hypoxic pulmonary vasoconstriction and severe pulmonary hypertension with stress failure of pulmonary capillaries, leading to HAPE. The blood air membrane in the lung is extremely thin with a harmonic mean of ~0.6 μm, but half the area is 0.2 to 0.4 μm (61). The membrane is made up of the capillary endothelial cell, basement membrane (predominantly type IV collagen), and the type I alveolar epithelial cell. Under extreme exercise, the transmural pressure at the base of the lungs in arterial capillaries nearly reaches that which causes stress failure (40 mm Hg). In situ perfused rabbit lungs with increased transmural pressures produces breaks in the capillary endothelium and epithelium, with the basement membrane remaining intact in about half the breaks attesting to the great strength of type IV collagen. Most of these breaks are elongated and diamond- or rectangular-shaped, with most oriented perpendicular to the capillary axis (Fig. 1). The dimensions are approximately 4 μm in length by 1 μm in width. The orientation of the breaks suggested that surface tension of the alveolar lining layer played an important role in protecting the blood-gas barrier against stress (63). Almost no breaks occurred at intercellular junctions, although many were seen within 1 mm of the junctions. This finding suggested that the junctions have considerable mechanical strength. The breaks were highly variable, consistent with the weak-link theory that a structure fails when its weakest link gives way. Lowering the transmural pressure reversed these ultrastructural changes, suggesting that cells can move along their underlying matrix by rapid disengagement and reattachment of cell adhesion molecules, causing breaks to open or close within minutes (64). Stress failure of pulmonary capillaries results in a high-permeability form of edema, or even frank pulmonary hemorrhage (65). The pulmonary hypoxic vasoconstriction is uneven, exposing capillaries not protected by the vasoconstriction to very high pressure. This may explain the patchy distribution of HAPE. Furthermore, the exposed basement membranes caused by vascular endothelial cell disruption may cause the vascular thrombi and fibrin clots in the lung noted at postmortem in HAPE. Lastly, exercise at high altitude is a provocative factor in HAPE, presumably by raising pulmonary vascular pressure (65).

Because HAPE is associated with fluid accumulation in the alveoli, mechanisms of increased vascular permeability have been evaluated. Atrial natriuretic peptide may increase vascular permeability and cause dilation of preterminal arterioles with right-to-left shunting, characteristic of ventilation/perfusion mismatch seen in HAPE (66). Five skiers with HAPE had elevated levels of arterial natriuretic factor that normalized after descent to Denver and recovery (66). In addition, four of six mountaineers, who had previous HAPE, when brought to 4,559 m developed fluid retention and significant increase in atrial natriuretic peptide that correlated with right atrial cross section (67).

Bronchoalveolar lavage (BAL) studies at 4,400 m on Mt. McKinley have shed light on the mechanisms of HAPE (68). Six individuals with HAPE had striking increases in total cells per milliliter compared to four controls ($346 \times 10^3$ vs. $73 \times 10^3$ cells/ml) that were 67% alveolar macrophages, 25% neutrophils, and 7% lymphocytes (68). The lavage total protein was strikingly increased (616 mg/dl vs. 12 mg/dl), which included large molecules such as immunoglobulins G and M. The protein concentrations were in the range of acute respiratory distress syndrome, consistent with the concept that HAPE is a high-protein, high-permeability type of pulmonary edema. Thromboxane, a potent mediator of pulmonary vasoconstriction, was also increased in lavage fluid; such a mediator of vasoconstriction could promote hypoxic ventilation/perfusion mismatches (69). Lastly, leukotriene $B_4$, a potent neutrophil chemoattractant, was increased in lavage fluid. Although neutrophils and high molecular weight proteins are observed in BAL from HAPE, recovery with rest, oxygen, and descent is rapid without sequalae, differentiating the disorder from acute respiratory distress syndrome. Four individuals with AMS were also lavaged, and cell differentials and protein concentrations did not differ from controls, suggesting not only different mechanisms for the two disorders but also that AMS may not develop into HAPE (69).

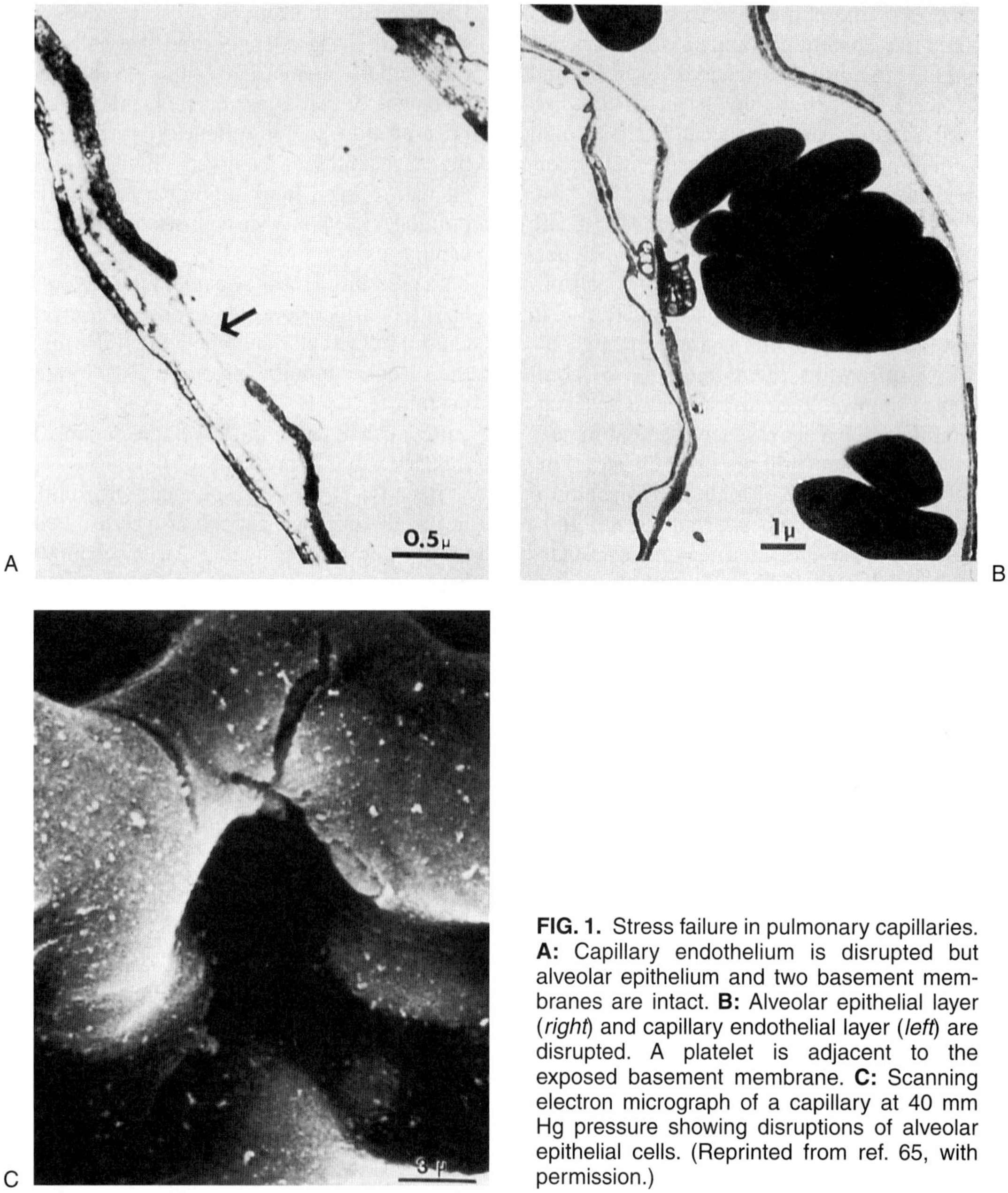


**FIG. 1.** Stress failure in pulmonary capillaries. **A:** Capillary endothelium is disrupted but alveolar epithelium and two basement membranes are intact. **B:** Alveolar epithelial layer (*right*) and capillary endothelial layer (*left*) are disrupted. A platelet is adjacent to the exposed basement membrane. **C:** Scanning electron micrograph of a capillary at 40 mm Hg pressure showing disruptions of alveolar epithelial cells. (Reprinted from ref. 65, with permission.)

Physiological studies on climbers with a history of HAPE have found a diminished hypoxic ventilatory response; three climbers with HAPE on Mt. McKinley had severe hypoxia a high-frequency, low-tidal volume pattern of breathing, and a low hypoxic ventilatory response (70,71). In a review of published studies, 77% of those susceptible to altitude illness had low acute ventilatory responses to hypoxia, whereas 23% had normal hypoxic ventilatory responses (72). Among those studied who were nonsusceptible to altitude illness, only 25% had low hypoxic ventilatory responses.

Anholm et al. (73) showed that there was a small but statistically significant decrement in forced vital capacity (FVC) and pulmonary flow rates at 2,835 m within the first 12 hours of ascent. They studied 126 individuals daily for 3 days, finding the greatest differences for FVC between the first and third days, which correlated with symptoms (cough, headache, dyspnea, insomnia). The pulmonary function findings also include decrements in flow rates that suggested a subclinical amount of interstitial edema; thus, the edema response to high altitude may be more widespread than originally thought, but clinically apparent in only a few.

Lack of recognition of the syndrome or failure of insisting on early descent or in provision of oxygen has resulted in numerous deaths. When symptoms of cough, difficulty in breathing, and mental confusion arise, descent and oxygen administration, the cornerstones of therapy, may be lifesaving. Modern helicopters may assist in high-altitude rescues, even as high as 6,000 m. If HAPE is in the early stages, oxygen will increase arterial oxygen saturation, lower pulmonary artery pressure, and reduce heart and respiratory rate. A field trial of positive expiratory airway pressure was helpful in increasing arterial oxygen saturation, raising $Pa_{CO_2}$, and decreasing the respiratory rate in four climbers with HAPE at 4,400 m, but its long-term effects need to be evaluated since there is a risk of barotrauma or worsening cerebral edema (74,75). In a retrospective analysis of 166 cases of HAPE, the overall mortality rate was 11%, and when descent was impossible and oxygen unavailable, it was 44% (76). Thus a simple drug regimen would be desirable. Digitalis compounds have no effect, and morphine may be counterproductive, since it depresses ventilation when respiration is needed. Nifedepine was effective in six climbers with HAPE at 4,559 m, reducing AMS symptom score, improving oxygenation, reducing the A-a gradient and pulmonary artery pressure, and progressively clearing alveolar edema (76). Given prophylactically, nifedipine prevents HAPE in susceptible persons going to high altitudes (77). Bärtsch and colleagues (77) reported that 7 of 11 subjects with a history of HAPE who received placebo but only 1 of 10 subjects who received nifedipine every 8 hours had pulmonary edema at 4,559 m. Subjects on nifedipine had significantly lower mean systolic pulmonary artery pressure, alveolar-arterial pressure gradient, and acute mountain sickness symptom score. Nifedipine does not prevent acute mountain sickness, however (78). Dexamethasone or intravenous corticosteroids have not proven to be beneficial once HAPE has developed. Diuretics, particularly furosemide, have been advocated as both efficacious and preventive. However, their use in oliguric, severely hypovolemic individuals with a possible pulmonary capillary leak syndrome, often in an unconscious state, may exacerbate the pathophysiology rather than be therapeutic (33,44,45,47). Inhaled nitric oxide (NO) is a novel approach to treating HAPE because it attenuates the pulmonary vasoconstriction produced by short-term hypoxia (79). Ten mountaineers susceptible to HAPE inhaled NO at 40 ppm for 15 minutes and had improved arterial oxygen saturation from 67% to 73% with a shift of pulmonary perfusion from edematous to nonedematous regions of the lung (79). There was also a threefold decrease in pulmonary artery pressure compared to mountaineers not susceptible to HAPE at 4,559 m.

## CEREBRAL EDEMA

In humans at high altitude, cerebral blood flow and cerebrospinal fluid pressure increase (80). Edematous brain tissue was noted by Singh et al. (33) upon histologic examination. Swelling of the brain may be responsible for most of the symptoms of AMS. Cerebral blood flow is increased by the stimulus of reduced oxygen saturation, but this response is diminished by concomitant hypocapnia; periodic sleep apnea may cause $Pa_{CO_2}$ to rise and result in a further increase of cerebral blood flow (80). Neurologic problems associated with cerebral edema (CE) are headache, irritability, insomnia, nausea and vomiting, cranial nerve palsies, paralysis, hallucinations, seizures, stupor, and coma. The cerebellum is particularly sensitive to hypoxia, which may give rise to truncal ataxia. Papilledema is present in about half of the patients.

## RETINAL HEMORRHAGE

Schumacher and Petajan (81) reported retinal hemorrhage in 36% of 39 subjects exposed to altitudes at or above 3,700 m, being more common in subjects with altitude headache. They postulated that the hemorrhages were not an accompaniment of increased intracranial pressure per se, but were probably related to increased retinal blood flow and dilation of retinal capillaries, arteries, and veins at high altitudes due to reduced arterial oxygen saturation. Frayser et al. (82) reported 9 of 25 subjects with retinal hemorrhage with only one symptomatic (scotoma owing to a macular hemorrhage); acetazolamide or furosemide did not prevent retinal hemorrhage. No evidence of major alterations in intraocular pressure occurs at high altitudes (83). About 60% of patients with altitude cerebral edema have retinal hemorrhages.

## CHRONIC MOUNTAIN SICKNESS

Chronic mountain sickness (CMS, Monge's disease) refers to loss of pulmonary acclimatization observed in long-term Andean residents above 4,000 m and the development of chronic cor pulmonale with neurologic symptoms (84). Monge's disease is due to alveolar hypoventilation and is characterized by cyanosis, extreme erythrocytosis, very low values of arterial oxygen saturation, pulmonary hypertension with muscularization of pulmonary arteries, and right enlargement (84). Central depression of ventilation by chronic cerebral hypoxia and increased respiratory rate with reduced tidal volume (raising $V_D/V_T$) contribute to alveolar hypoventilation in CMS. Marked arterial desaturation occurred at sleep, providing a strong stimulus to the erythrocytosis seen in this disorder. Descent to sea level results in amelioration and disappearance of many of the abnormal findings. In addition, phlebotomy improves the condition. Treatment with the respiratory stimulant medroxyprogesterone increased tidal volume and minute ventilation, resulting in lowered $Pa_{CO_2}$ and raised $Pa_{O_2}$ during waking and sleeping hours, and the hematocrit declined to normal values (85). CMS

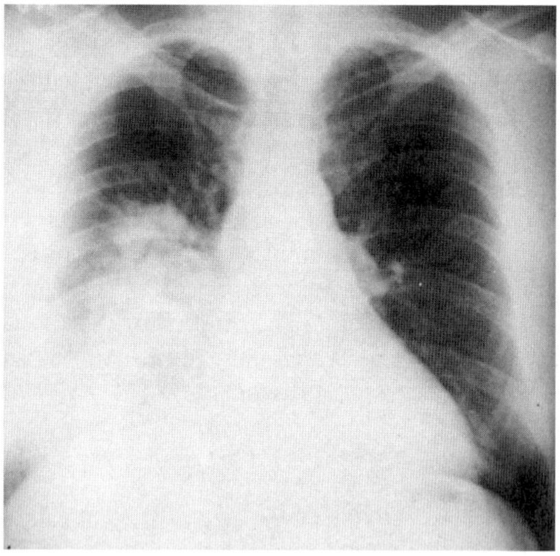

**FIG. 2.** PA chest x-ray of unilateral right lower lobe and right middle lobe HAPE.

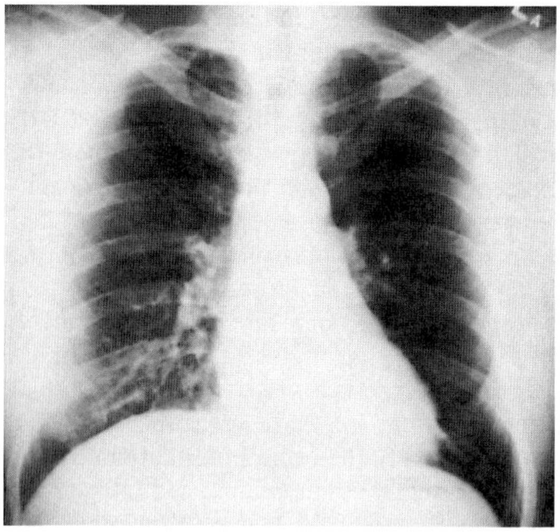

**FIG. 3.** Clearing of HAPE on chest x-ray after descent.

has also been reported in Han Chinese who have emigrated to Lhasa, Tibet; a recent study evaluating the hypothesis that depression of the hypoxic ventilatory response in CMS results from increased release of endogenous opioids found no improvement in ventilation following intravenous naloxone, an opioid inhibitor (86).

Sherpas and Tibetans seem uniquely adapted to their high-altitude environment, probably reflecting genetic selection. For example, chronic mountain sickness does not occur among them. Tibetan newborns have higher oxygen saturation values than Han Chinese (87). In contrast to the Quechua Indians of Peru, Tibetans and Sherpas lack smooth muscle in the small pulmonary arteries, and have a normal resting pulmonary artery pressure (88). Interestingly, their cardiac muscle utilizes glucose and aerobic metabolism generating 36 adenosine triphosphate (ATP) molecules per glucose molecule rather than anaerobic glycolysis seen in lowlanders, who only generate two ATP molecules per glucose molecule metabolized (89). The yield per $O_2$ molecule is up to 60% higher with glucose than free fatty acids, suggesting a unique biochemical adaptation to hypobaria in Sherpas.

## CASE REPORT: HIGH-ALTITUDE PULMONARY EDEMA (HAPE)

A 48-year-old man from Seattle, Washington, flew to Salt Lake City, Utah, and went skiing at Alta, Utah (base elevation 2,750 m, summit 3,750 m). He complained of dyspnea on the night of arrival and felt light-headed. He

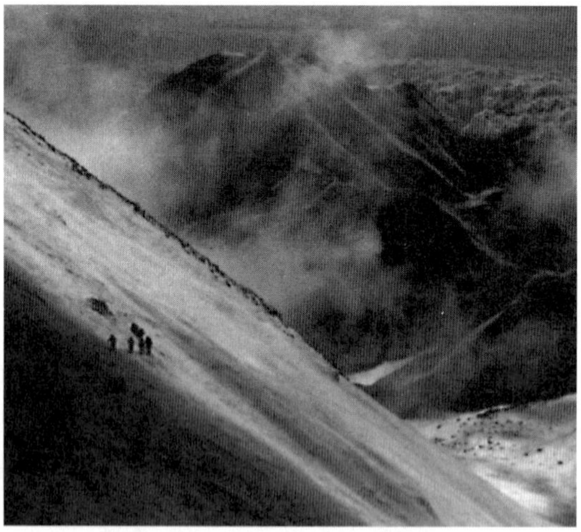

**FIG. 4.** Denali Pass (6,000 m), Mt. McKinley, Alaska. Mountaineering on high peaks such as Mt. McKinley has resulted in an incidence of 0.5 to 1.5% of high altitude pulmonary edema. *See color plate between pages 1384 and 1385.*

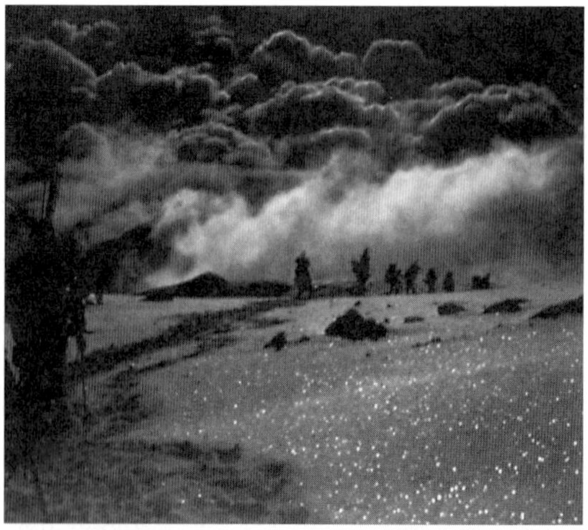

**FIG. 5.** High-altitude mountaineering on Mt. McKinley, Alaska. *See color plate between pages 1384 and 1385.*

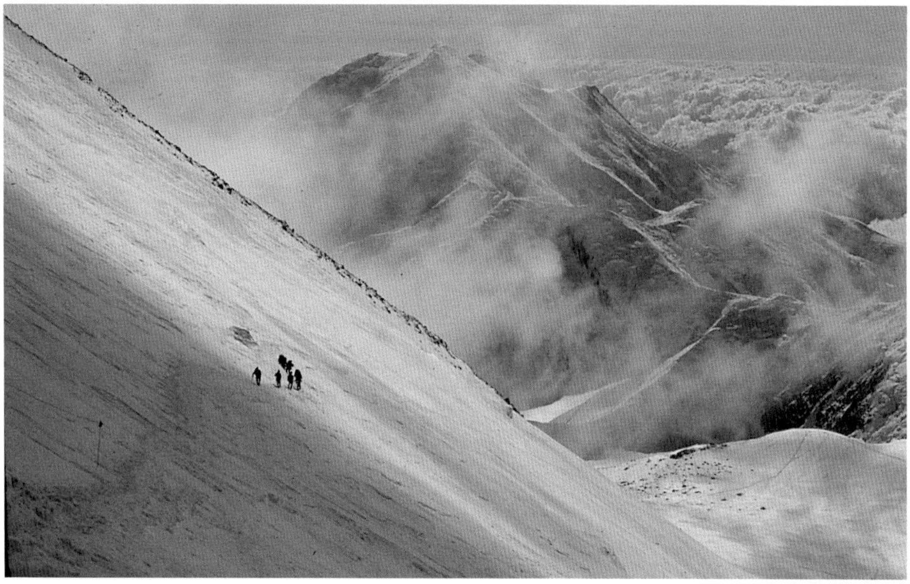

**COLOR PLATE 103–4.** Denali Pass (6,000 m), Mt. McKinley, Alaska. Mountaineering on high peaks such as Mt. McKinley has resulted in an incidence of 0.5 to 1.5% of high altitude pulmonary edema.

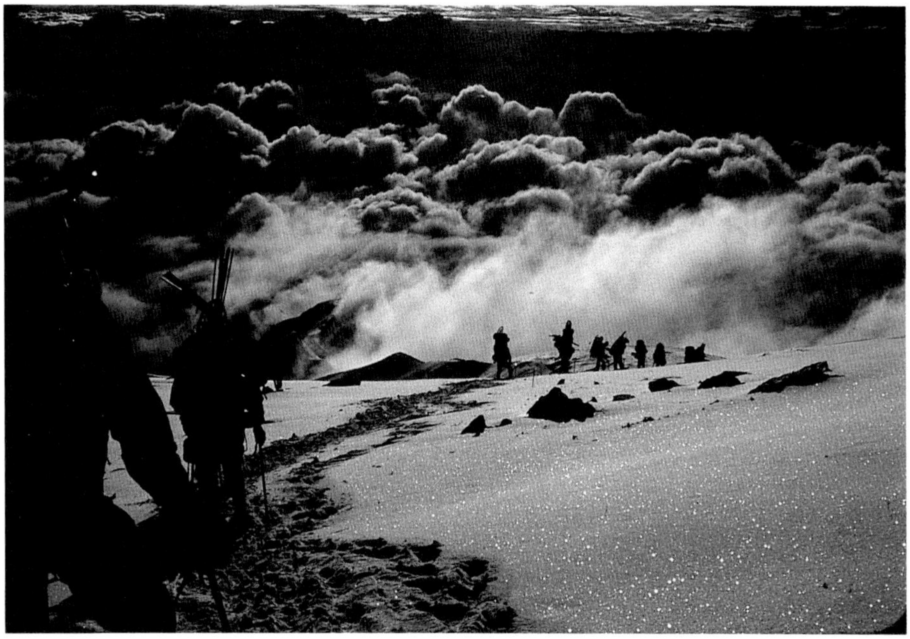

**COLOR PLATE 103–5.** High-altitude mountaineering on Mt. McKinley, Alaska.

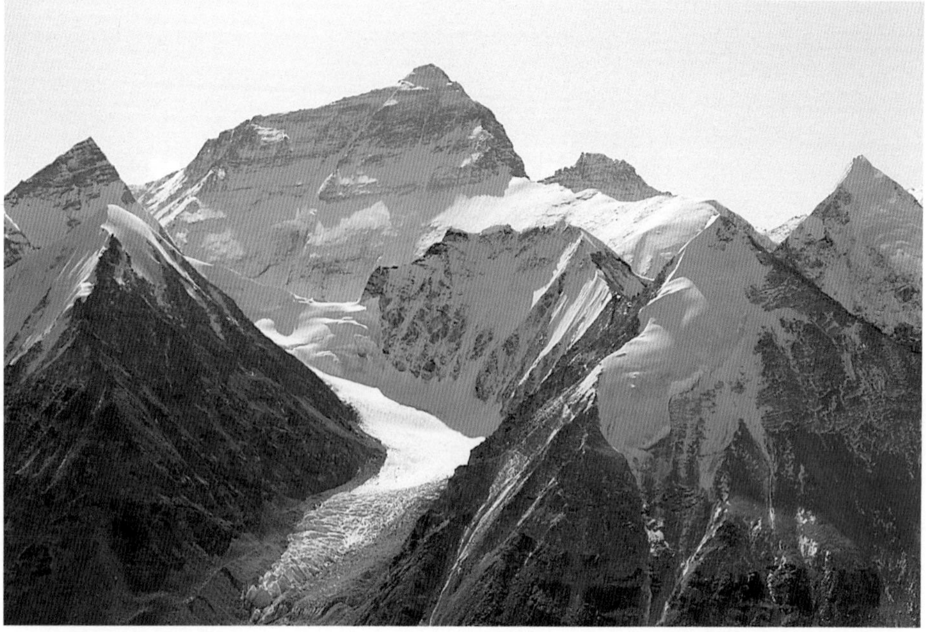

**COLOR PLATE 103–6.** Extreme altitude at 6,600 m in the West Rongbuk Valley in Tibet looking at the North Face of Mt. Everest.

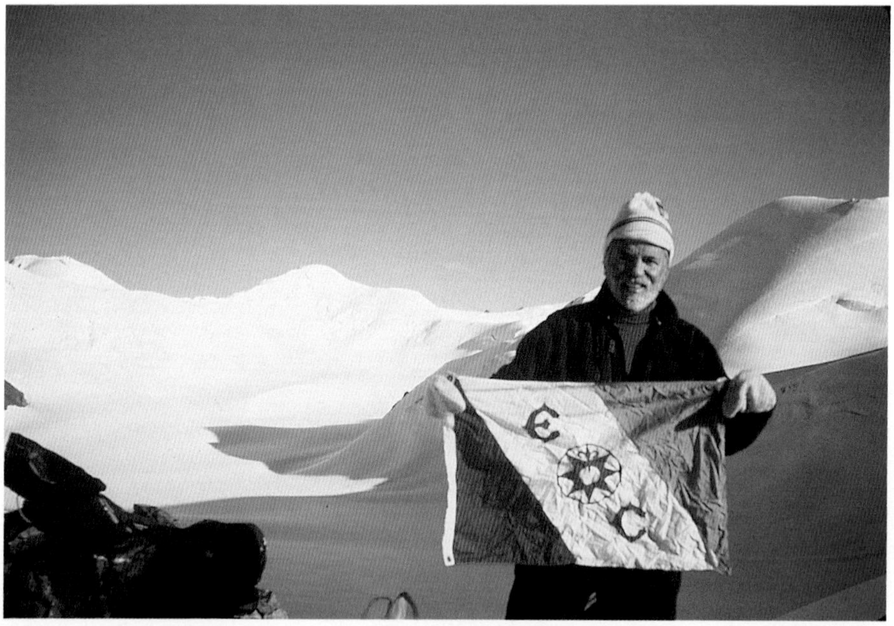

**COLOR PLATE 103–7.** First American ascent of Mount Geladaintong (6,621 m) at the source of the Yangtze River in Tibet. Author is holding Explorer's Club flag.

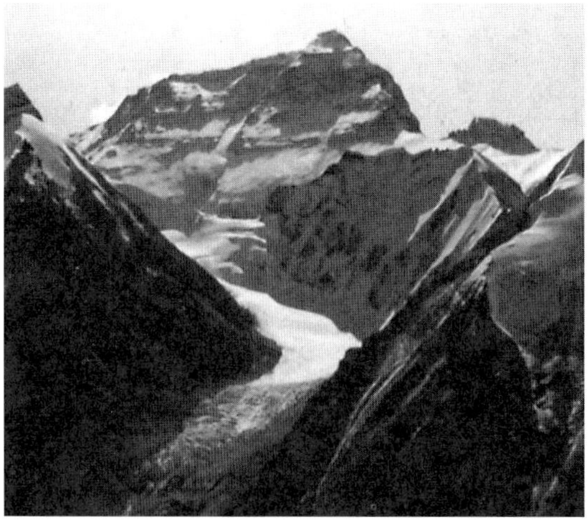

**FIG. 6.** Extreme altitude at 6,600 m in the West Rongbuk Valley in Tibet looking at the North Face of Mt. Everest. *See color plate between pages 1384 and 1385.*

skied hard the next day and was more dyspneic the following evening. He spent a restless night unable to sleep because of dyspnea. The following morning he was hospitalized, and he complained of fatigue and visual disturbances. He had no hemoptysis or leg pain. He had been in excellent health with no prior history of heart disease. On examination, bilateral rales were heard, with the right lung greater than the left. His white blood cell count was 11,400, the electrocardiogram was normal, and his arterial blood gases were pH 7.44, $Pa_{O_2}$ 59 mm torr, and $Pa_{CO_2}$ 31 mm torr.

The patient had noted previously that he experienced more fatigue and dyspnea while skiing or hiking at high altitudes than did his peers. He had no previous hospitalizations or episodes of HAPE and was an active jogger. He also was an ex-smoker, having stopped 12 years prior to admission. His chest radiograph (Fig. 2) showed unilateral right lower lobe and right middle lobe pulmonary edema that progressively cleared over 3 days (Fig. 3) as his clinical symptoms disappeared. HAPE is known to occur predominantly in the right middle lobe area (Figs. 4–7). High-altitude mountaineering is increasing in popularity.

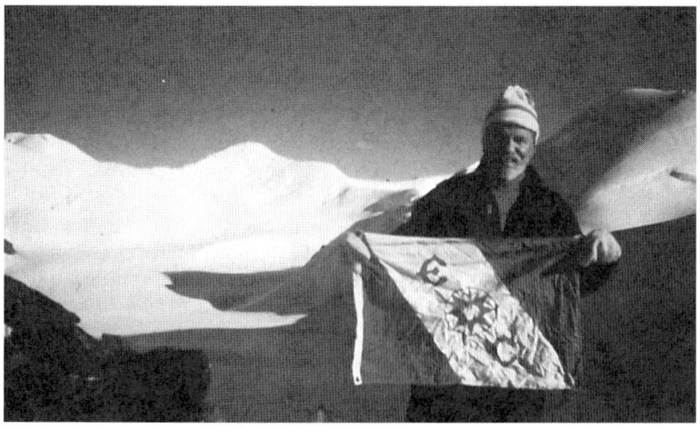

**FIG 7.** First American ascent of Mount Geladaintong (6,621 m) at the source of the Yangtze River in Tibet. Author is holding Explorer's Club flag. *See color plate between pages 1384 and 1385.*

## REFERENCES


1. de Acosta J. *Historia natural y moral de las Indias, en qu se tratan las cosas notables de cielo, y elementos, metales, plantas, y animales dellas:* y los ritos, *y ceremonias, leyes, y gobierno, y guerras de los Indios.* Seville, Spain: Juan de Leon, 1590;759–770.
2. Sutton JR, Pugh LGCE. Climbing Everest without oxygen. *Semin Respir Med* 1983;5:213–216.
3. Friasancho AR. Functional adaption to high altitude hypoxia. Changes occurring during growth and development are of major importance in man's adapting to high altitudes. *Science* 1975;187: 313–319.
4. Lenfant C, Sullivan K. Adaption to high altitude. *N Engl J Med* 1971; 284:1298–1309.
5. Severinghaus JW, Mitchell RA, Richardson BW, et al. Respiratory control at high altitude suggesting active transport regulation of cerebrospinal fluid pH. *J Appl Physiol* 1963;18:1155–1166.
6. Kronenberg RS, Safar P, Lee J, et al. Pulmonary artery pressure and alveolar gas exchange in man during acclimatization to 12,470 ft. *J Clin Invest* 1971;50:827–837.
7. Mairbäurl H, Schobersberger W, Oelz O, Bärtsch P, Eckardt U, Bauer C. Unchanged in vivo $P_{50}$ at high altitude despite decreased erythrocyte age and elevated 2,3-diphosphoglycerate. *J Appl Physiol* 1990;68: 1186–1194.
8. Wang GL, Semenza GL. Purification and characterization of hypoxia-inducible factor 1. *J Biol Chem* 1995;270:1230–1237.
9. Semenza GL, Roth PH, Fang H-M, Wang GL. Transcriptional regulation of genes encoding glycolytic enzymes by hypoxia-inducible factor 1. *J Biol Chem* 1994;269:23757–23763.
10. Namiki A, Brogi E, Kearney M, et al. Hypoxia induces vascular endothelial growth factor in cultured human endothelial cells. *J Biol Chem* 1995;270:31189–31195.
11. Levy AP, Levy NS, Goldberg MA. Post-transcriptional regulation of vascular endothelial growth factory by hypoxia. *J Biol Chem* 1996; 271:2746–2753.
12. Brogi E, Schatteman G, Wu T, et al. Hypoxia-induced paracrine regulation of vascular endothelial growth factor receptor expression. *J Clin Invest* 1996;97:469–476.
13. West JB. Human physiology at extreme altitudes on Mount Everest. *Science* 1984;223:784–788.
14. West JB. *Everest. The testing place.* New York: McGraw-Hill, 1985.
15. West JB. High living: lessons from extreme altitude. *Am Rev Respir Dis* 1984;130:917–923.
16. West JB, Lahiri S, Maret KH, Peters RM, Pizzo CJ. Barometric pressures at extreme altitudes on Mt. Everest: physiological significance. *J Appl Physiol* 1983;54:1188–1194.
17. West JB, Hackett PH, Maret KH, et al. Pulmonary gas exchange on the summit of Mount Everest. *J Appl Physiol* 1986;61:280–287.
18. West JB, Peters RM Jr, Aksnes G, Maret KH, Milledge S, Schoene RB. Nocturnal periodic breathing at altitudes of 6,300 and 8,050 m. *J Appl Physiol* 1986;61:280–287.
19. Schoene RB, Lahiri S, Hackett PH, et al. Relationship of hypoxic ventilatory response to exercise performance on Mount Everest. *J Appl Physiol* 1983;55:678–687.
20. West JB, Boyer SJ, Graber DJ, et al. Maximal exercise at extreme altitudes on Mount Everest. *J Appl Physiol* 1983;55:688–698.
21. Winslow RM, Samaja M, West JB. Red cell function at extreme altitude on Mount Everest. *J Appl Physiol* 1984;56:109–116.
22. Hornbein TF, Townes BD, Schoene RB, Sutton JR, Houston CS. The cost to the central nervous system of climbing to extremely high altitude. *N Engl J Med* 1989;32:1714–1719.
23. Gray GW, Bryan AC, Freedman MH, et al. Effect of altitude exposure on platelets. *J Appl Physiol* 1975;39:648–651.
24. Mordes JP, Blume D, Boyer S, Zheng M-R, Braverman LE. High-altitude pituitary-thyroid dysfunction on Mount Everest. *N Engl J Med* 1983;308:1135–1138.
25. Karliner JS, Sarnquist FF, Graber DJ, Peters RM Jr, West JB. The elec-

trocardiogram at extreme altitude: experience on Mt. Everest. *Am Heart J* 1985;109:505–513.
26. Winslow RM, Mone CC, Statham NJ, et al. Variability of oxygen affinity of blood: human subjects native to high altitude. *J Appl Physiol* 1981;51:1411–1416.
27. Winslow RM, Chapman KW, Gibson CC, et al. Different hematologic responses to hypoxia in Sherpas and Quecha Indians. *J Appl Physiol* 1989;66:1561–1569.
28. Beall CM, Strohl KP, Brittenham GM. Reappraisal of Andean high altitude erythrocytosis from a Himalayan perspective. *Semin Respir Med* 1983;5:195–201.
29. Houston CS. A brief history of research in altitude illness. *Semin Respir Med* 1983;5:103–108.
30. Ravenhill TH. Some experiences of mountain sickness in the Andes. *J Trop Med* 1913;20:313–320.
31. Johnson TS, Rock PB. Acute mountain sickness. *N Engl J Med* 1988; 319:841–845.
32. Hackett PH, Rennie D. The incidence, importance, and prophylaxis of acute mountain sickness. *Lancet* 1976;2:1149–1154.
33. Singh I, Khanna PK, Srivastava MC, Lal M, Roy SB, Subramanyam CSV. Acute mountain sickness. *N Engl J* Med 1969;280:175–183.
34. Hackett PH, Rennie D. Acute mountain sickness. *Semin Respir Med* 1983;5:132–140.
35. Wilson R. Acute high-altitude illness in mountaineers and problems of rescue. *Ann Intern Med* 1973;78:421–428.
36. Larson EB, Roach RC, Schoene RB, Hornbein TF. Acute mountain sickness and acetazolamide. Clinical efficacy and effect on ventilation. *JAMA* 1982;248:328–332.
37. Sutton JR, Houston CS, Mansell AL, et al. Effect of acetazolamide on hypoxemia during sleep at high altitude. *N Engl J Med* 1979;301: 1329–1331.
38. Grissom CK, Roach RC, Sarnquist FH, Hackett PH. Acetazolamide in the treatment of acute mountain sickness: clinical efficacy and effect on gas exchange. *Ann Intern Med* 1992;116:461–465.
39. Rock PB, Johnson TS, Larsen RF, Fulco CS, Trad LA, Cymerman A. Dexamethasone as prophylaxis for acute mountain sickness. Effect of dose level. *Chest* 1989;95:568–573.
40. Johnson TS, Rock PB, Fulco CS, Trad LA, Spark RF, Maher JT. Prevention of acute mountain sickness by dexamethasone. *N Engl J Med* 1984;310:683–686.
41. Levine BD, Yoshimura K, Kobayashi T, Fukushima M, Shibamoto T, Ueda G. Dexamethasone in the treatment of acute mountain sickness. *N Engl J Med* 1989;321:1707–1713.
42. Montgomery AB, Luce JM, Michael P, Mills J. Effects of dexamethasone on the incidence of acute mountain sickness at two intermediate altitudes. *JAMA* 1989;261:734–736.
43. Hultgren HN, Marticorena EA. High altitude pulmonary edema. Epidemiologic observations in Peru. *Chest* 1978;74:372–376.
44. Gray GM. High altitude pulmonary edema. *Semin Respir Med* 1983;5: 141–150.
45. Kleiner JP, Nelson WP. High altitude pulmonary edema. A rare disease? *JAMA* 1975;234:491–495.
46. Houston CS. Acute pulmonary edema of high altitude. *N Engl J Med* 1960;263:478–480.
47. Hultgren HN. High altitude medical problems. *West J Med* 1979;131: 8–23.
48. Scoggin CH, Hyers TM, Reeves JT, Grover RF. High-altitude pulmonary edema in the children and young adults of Leadville, Colorado. *N Engl J Med* 1977;297:1269–1272.
49. Rennie D. Give me air!—But not much. *N Engl J Med* 1977;297: 1285–1287.
50. Vock P, Brutsche MH, Nanzer, Bärtsch P. Variable radiomorphologic data of high altitude pulmonary edema. *Chest* 1991;100:1306–1311.
51. Bärtsch P, Waber U, Haeberill A, et al. Enhanced fibrin formation in high-altitude pulmonary edema. *J Appl Physiol* 1987;63:752–757.
52. Heath D, Moosavi H, Smith P. Ultrastructure of high altitude pulmonary oedema. *Thorax* 1973;28:694–700.
53. Coates G. High-altitude pulmonary edema. *Semin Respir Med* 1981;3: 108–111.
54. Richalet J-P. High altitude pulmonary oedema: still a place for controversy? *Thorax* 1995;50:923–998.
55. Hultgren HN, Grover RF, Hartley LH. Abnormal circulatory response to high altitude in subjects with a previous history of high-altitude edema. *Circulation* 1971;44:759–770.
56. Fasules JW, Wiggins JW, Wolfe RR. Increased lung vasoreactivity in children from Leadville, Colorado, after recovery from high altitude pulmonary edema. *Circulation* 1985;72:957–962.
57. West JB, Dollery CI, Heard BE. Increased pulmonary vascular resistance in the dependent zone of the isolated dog lung caused by perivascular edema. *Circ Res* 1965;17:191–206.
58. Hackett PH, Creagh CE, Grover RF, et al. High-altitude pulmonary edema in persons without the right pulmonary artery. *N Engl J Med* 1980;302:1070–1073.
59. Derks A, Bosch FH. High-altitude pulmonary edema in partial anomalous pulmonary venous connection of drainage with intact atrial septum. *Chest* 1993;103:973–974.
60. Nakagawa S, Kubo K, Koizumi T, Kobayashi T, Sekiguchi M. High-altitude pulmonary edema with pulmonary thromboembolism. *Chest* 1993;103:948–950.
61. West JB, Tsukimoto K, Mathieu-Costello O, Prediletto R. Stress failure in pulmonary capillaries. *J Appl Physiol* 1991;70:1731–1742.
62. Tsukimoto K, Mathieu-Costello O, Prediletto R, Elliott AR, West JB. Ultrastructural appearances of pulmonary capillaries at high transmural pressures. *J Appl Physiol* 1991;71:573–582.
63. Costello ML, Mathieu-Costello O, West JB. Stress failure of alveolar epithelial cells studied by scanning electron microscopy. *Am Rev Respir Dis* 1992;145:1446–1455.
64. Elliott AR, Fu Z, Tsukimoto K, Prediletto R, Mathieu-Costello O, West JB. Short-term reversibility of ultrastructural changes in pulmonary capillaries caused by stress failure. *J Appl Physiol* 1992;73: 1150–1158.
65. West JB, Mathieu-Costello O. Stress failure of pulmonary capillaries: role in lung and heart disease. *Lancet* 1992;340:762–767.
66. Cosby RL, Sophocles AM, Durr JA, Perrinjaquet CL, Yee B, Schrier RW. Elevated plasma atrial natriuretic factor and vasopressin in high-altitude pulmonary edema. *Ann Intern Med* 1988;109:796–799.
67. Bärtsch P, Pfluger N, Audetat M, et al. Effects of slow ascent to 4559 m on fluid homeostasis. *Aviat Space Environ Med* 1991;62:105–110.
68. Schoene RB, Hackett PH, Henderson WR, et al. High altitude pulmonary edema. *JAMA* 1986;256:63–69.
69. Schoene RB, Swenson ER, Pizzo CJ, et al. The lung at high altitude: bronchoalveolar lavage in acute mountain sickness and pulmonary edema. *J Appl Physiol* 1988;64:2605–2613.
70. Hackett PH, Roach RC, Schoene RB, Harrison GL, Mills WJ Jr. Abnormal control of ventilation in high-altitude pulmonary edema. *J Appl Physiol* 1988;64:1268–1272.
71. Viswanathan R, Sabramanian S, Lodi STK, et al. Further studies on pulmonary edema of high altitude: abnormal responses to hypoxia of men who had developed edema of high altitude. *Respiration* 1978;36: 216–222.
72. Selland MA, Stelzner TJ, Stevens T, Mazzeo RS, McCullough RE, Reeves JT. Pulmonary function and hypoxic ventilatory response in subjects susceptible to high-altitude pulmonary edema. *Chest* 1993; 103:111–116.
73. Anholm JD, Houston CS, Hyers TM. The relationship between acute mountain sickness and pulmonary ventilation at 2,835 meters (9,300 ft). *Chest* 1979;75:33–36.
74. Schoene RB, Roach RC, Hackett PH, Harrison G, Mills WJ Jr. High altitude pulmonary edema and exercise at 4,400 meters on Mount McKinley. Effect of expiratory positive airway pressure. *Chest* 1985; 87:330–333.
75. Larson EB. Positive airway pressure for high-altitude pulmonary oedema. *Lancet* 1985;1:371–373.
76. Oelz O, Maggirorini M, Ritter M, et al. Nifedipine for high altitude pulmonary oedema. *Lancet* 1989;2:1241–1244.
77. Bärtsch P, Maggiorini M, Ritter M, Noti C, Vock P, Oelz O. Prevention of high-altitude pulmonary edema by nifedipine. *N Engl J Med* 1991; 325:1284–1289.
78. Hohenhaus E, Niroomand F, Goerre S, Vock P, Oelz O, Bärtsch P. Nifedipine does not prevent acute mountain sickness. *Am J Respir Crit Care Med* 1994;150:857–860.
79. Scherrer U, Vollenweider L, Delabays A, et al. Inhaled nitric oxide for high-altitude pulmonary edema. *N Engl J Med* 1996;334:624–629.
80. Dickinson JG. High altitude cerebral edema: cerebral acute mountain sickness. *Semin Respir Med* 1983;5:151–158.
81. Schumacher GA, Petajan JH. High altitude stress and retinal hemorrhage. Relation to vascular headache mechanisms. *Arch Environ Health* 1975;30:217–221.
82. Frayser R, Houston CS, Bryan AC, Rennie ID, Gray G. Retinal hemorrhage at high altitude. *N Engl J Med* 1970;282:1183–1184.

83. Sutton JR. High altitude retinal hemorrhage. *Semin Respir Med* 1983; 5:159–163.
84. Kryger MH, Grover RF. Chronic mountain sickness. *Semin Respir Med* 1983;5:164–168.
85. Hryger M, McCullough RE, Collins D, Scoggin CH, Weil JV, Grover RF. Treatment of excessive polycythemia of high altitude with respiratory stimulant drugs. *Am Rev Respir Dis* 1978;1217:455–464.
86. Sun SF, Huang SY, Zhang JG, et al. Decreased ventilation and hypoxic ventilatory responsiveness are not reversed by naloxone in Lhasa residents with chronic mountain sickness. *Am Rev Respir Dis* 1990;142: 1294–1300.
87. Niermeyer S, Yang P, Shanmina, Krolkar, Zhuang J, Moore LG. Arterial oxygen saturation in Tibetan and Han infants born in Lhasa, Tibet. *N Engl J Med* 1995;333:1248–1252.
88. Gupta ML, Rao KS, Anand IS, Banerjee AK, Boparai MS. Lack of smooth muscle in the small pulmonary arteries of the native Ladakhi. Is the Himalayan highlander adapted? *Am Rev Respir Dis* 1992;145: 1201–1204.
89. Hochachka PW, Clark CM, Holden JE, Stanley C, Ugurbil K, Menon RS. $^{31}P$ magnetic resonance spectroscopy of the Sherpa heart: a phosphocreatine/adenosine triphosphate signature of metabolic defense against hypobaric hypoxia. *Proc Natl Acad Sci USA* 1996;93:1215–1220.

*Environmental and Occupational Medicine, Third Edition,* edited by William N. Rom.
Lippincott–Raven Publishers, Philadelphia © 1998.

# CHAPTER 104

# Hot and Cold Work Environments

Kathleen A. Delaney and Lewis R. Goldfrank

Workers who labor under adverse environmental conditions may suffer serious physical injury from the effects of extreme elevation or depression of body temperature. Hyperthermia in particular has been associated with many occupational deaths (1–3). Environmental temperature extremes may be constant and predictable, like those that prevail in an underground mine, foundry, or ice-making plant, or can vary with the seasons in outdoor occupations such as surface mining, roofing, farming, or construction. Sporadic unintentional exposures such as cold water immersion in the fishing industry or exposure to intense heat during firefighting also occur.

## THE PHYSIOLOGY OF THERMOREGULATION

Heat transfer between the body and the environment is affected by many variables. The net gain or loss of heat by the body *(S)* is represented by the heat equation $S = M - W - E \pm R \pm C_1 \pm C_2$, where $S$ is the change in heat storage, $M$ is metabolic heat, $W$ is work done in the environment, $E$ is evaporative heat loss, $R$ is heat gained or lost by radiation, $C_1$ is heat gained or lost by convection, and $C_2$ is heat gained or lost by conduction. Radiant heat is transferred from a hot body (the sun, a smelter, a burning oil well) to another body (the skin, for example) without heating the air between them. During convection, body heat is transferred to air molecules, and during evaporation, to water molecules. Both convection and evaporation are increased by air movement. Conductive heat gain (or loss) involves the transfer of heat directly from one body to another. Conduction is the major mechanism of heat loss during water immersion (4). Despite exposure to a wide range of environmental temperatures, the human body maintains a core temperature of 37°C (98.6°F) with a very narrow range of normal variation. That is, under most conditions, the net heat change *(S)* is zero (5,6). The advantage conferred by such tight thermoregulation is undoubtedly related to the temperature dependence of critical metabolic processes such as the maintenance of membrane integrity, enzyme function, and electrolyte gradients (7). The pathophysiologic effects of extremes of body temperature clearly demonstrate the importance of normothermia. The body tolerates hyperthermia less well than hypothermia: organ injury becomes evident as tissue temperatures approach 41.7°C (107°F) (8,9) whereas under controlled circumstances patients have survived temperatures as low as 9°C (48.2°F) (10). The most consequential effects of hypothermia are caused by reversible depression of important physiologic processes, although cell injury also occurs, particularly in prolonged ischemic states (11). Extreme body temperature disturbances result when (a) exposure to extreme environmental temperatures overloads maximally functioning thermoregulatory processes, (b) endogenous heat production is greater than the body's capacity to dissipate heat or is inadequate to maintain body temperature, or (c) medical illness, drugs, or toxins interfere with normal thermoregulation (4,8,12).

The core temperature is most accurately defined as the temperature of the blood perfusing the hypothalamus. Although it may be higher than the rectal temperature, the rectal temperature is the closest approximation of the core temperature readily available to the clinician. Body temperature regulation is governed by central autonomic

K. A. Delaney: Division of Emergency Medicine, University of Texas Southwestern Medical Center, Dallas, Texas 75235-8579.
L. R. Goldfrank: Department of Emergency Medicine, Bellevue Hospital Center, New York University Medical Center; and New York City Poison Center, New York, New York 10016.

responses to core temperature changes and by central and peripheral responses to changes in the temperature of the skin, which facilitate the loss or preservation of body heat (5,13). Skin cooling generates afferent impulses to the spinal cord and hypothalamus from cold-sensitive neurons in the skin. Cutaneous vasoconstriction occurs, followed by shivering, piloerection, and mobilization of fat and glucose stores. The intensity of these responses is augmented by the cooling of core blood. They result in decreased loss of heat to the environment and increased metabolic heat production (5).

Heat-sensitive hypothalamic neurons increase their firing rate in response to an increase in the temperature of core blood, leading to dilatation of cutaneous vessels and the initiation of sweating (5). The intensity of both these responses is moderated by skin temperature (4,14). Sweating is mediated by parasympathetic (cholinergic) fibers. The effectors responsible for cutaneous vasodilatation remain poorly characterized, but it appears to be closely linked to the onset of sweating (15). Cutaneous vasodilatation facilitates the conductive transfer of heat from blood to skin, where it is cooled by the mechanisms of convection and evaporation discussed above.

## WORK IN A HOT ENVIRONMENT

### Physiologic Responses to Exercise in the Heat

The capacity to significantly increase blood flow to a dilated cutaneous vascular bed is a requirement for the effective loss of metabolic heat produced during exercise. In a healthy worker the increased circulatory demand is met by a rate-related increase in cardiac output and sympathetically mediated renal and splanchnic vasoconstriction (13). The ability to dissipate heat through increases in cutaneous blood flow is ultimately limited by the maximum achievable cardiac output, which is a function of the maximal heart rate, the intravascular volume, and the amount of renal and splanchnic vasoconstriction that can be achieved and maintained (8,13). Preexisting volume depletion has serious deleterious effects and limits the potential cardiovascular response to the increased circulatory demands of heat stress (9,16,17,18). Volume depletion has been commonly associated with the development of both heat exhaustion and heat stroke (18).

Competing needs to maintain perfusion of exercising muscle, perfusion of skin in the service of heat loss, and adequate blood pressure represent a major cardiovascular challenge in exercising heat-stressed workers. Failure to meet these demands may result in collapse due to heat exhaustion, or heat stroke, the most severe manifestation of heat illness associated with life-threatening body temperature elevation.

Some of the physiologic processes associated with collapse during work in the heat, with or without a dangerous elevation of body temperature, have been elucidated in human and animal studies, and some remain speculative. When an individual achieves a maximal heart rate during exercise yet heat storage continues to rise, further increases in cardiac output cannot occur and the body's hemodynamic response may be inadequate to maintain blood pressure and muscle perfusion in the context of the increased circulatory demands of thermoregulation. Volume depletion, which occurs during exercise as a result of sweat losses and fluid shifts into muscle, further exacerbates this progressive hemodynamic compromise (9,16–18). Volume depletion also impairs the ability to sweat (19). There appears to be considerable individual variation in the distribution of blood flow that occurs in response to these hemodynamic stresses during exercise in the heat. Frequently, the physiologic response of blood pressure maintenance is preserved while the capacity to dissipate heat is lost (8,9,13,20). Failure to maintain cutaneous vasodilatation despite elevated body temperatures was demonstrated in a sheep model of exertional heat stroke. Collapse was preceded by redistribution of blood flow from skin to muscle, resulting in increased blood pressure, increased peripheral vascular resistance, and rapid elevation of the body temperature (8). A sudden loss of splanchnic vasoconstriction has been demonstrated to precede cutaneous vasoconstriction and rapid temperature rise in a rat model of heat stroke (9). A dramatic decrease in cardiac output associated with rapidly rising rectal temperature was noted at the point of collapse of one subject in a hazardous military study that exposed healthy men to a dry environment at 160°F. Whether this person's collapse was a result of vascular redistribution of blood flow or of primary cardiac failure was not determined (21). Some individuals appear capable of maintaining a significant degree of cutaneous vasodilatation and collapse without dangerous elevation of the core temperature (9,22).

Whether or not thermoregulatory failure is an obligatory antecedent of heat stroke in humans is not clear. A wide pulse pressure, suggesting vasodilatation and decreased peripheral vascular resistance, and copious sweating are frequently noted in victims of exertional heat stroke (21–24). On the basis of such clinical observation it is generally accepted that some cases of heat stroke may occur when the amount of heat produced during strenuous exercise exceeds the dissipation capacity of a normally functioning thermoregulatory system (9,25, 26). Other individuals exhibit clear evidence of thermoregulatory failure, as manifested by the cessation of sweating in 25% to 50% of healthy patients with exertional heat stroke (26,27).

### Effects of the Environment

The efficiency of these thermoregulatory mechanisms in promoting heat loss is significantly affected by environmental conditions. Transfer of heat by convection from the skin surface to the air requires a temperature gradient between air and the body surface, which is lost as the environmental temperature approaches the temperature of the skin. Evaporative heat loss is impaired by high ambient humidity. An obligatory rise in body temperature occurs in persons exposed to conditions of 100% humidity and an ambient temperature that exceeds the skin temperature. The rate of body temperature increase under these circumstances is a function of the intensity of activity (18). These extremes of temperature and humidity approximate environmental conditions in protective garments when the air temperature equals or exceeds the body temperature and convection and evaporation do not occur. Dramatic rises in body temperature can occur during intense physical labor, overwhelming thermoregulatory mechanisms and producing life-threatening elevations of body temperature (18,28,29). Very intense ambient heat may cause heat stroke in the absence of exercise (21).

The magnitude of the risk to workers of an overly warm environment can be predicted by examination of air temperature, wind velocity, amount of radiant heat, and humidity. Historically, much creative effort has been expended to develop a quantitative predictor of the probable physiologic response and risk of these environmental factors for workers and athletes (30–34). As might be expected, complex variables are involved and attempts to account for all of them produce a cumbersome tool. Simplification increases the applicability of such an index but limits its predictive accuracy (30). The most widely used heat index today is the wet bulb globe temperature (WBGT), which is calculated from information obtained with three different devices. The dry bulb temperature (DBT) is the air temperature taken from a thermometer placed in shade. The wet bulb temperature (WBT) is taken by a thermometer whose bulb is in contact with a wet wick. When ambient humidity is low, the WBT is substantially lower than the DBT, reflecting the effects of evaporation. As humidity increases, the WBT approaches the DBT. In the early 1900s the WBT was used by Haldane to predict heat stress in the humid tin mines or Cornwall, England (30). The WBT's reliability decreases when radiant heat is substantial. The black globe temperature (BGT) is given by a thermometer whose bulb is in an airtight black globe exposed to the sun. Because the black globe absorbs radiant heat and may gain or lose heat to the surrounding air by convection and radiation, the BGT may be higher than the DBT, or lower, as when clouds block the sun or wind velocity increases convective heat loss. The WBGT is calculated by the following formulas, which weighs the importance of the contributions of the three measurements to heat risk:

$$WBGT = WBT \times 0.7 + DBT \times 0.1 + BGT \times 0.2 \text{ (outdoors)} \quad [1]$$

$$WBGT = WBT \times 0.7 + BGT \times 0.3 \text{ (indoors)} \quad [2]$$

The WBGT predicts the rate of rise of the rectal temperature in healthy acclimatized persons during exercise. As might be expected, it does not correlate with the rate of rise of rectal temperature in persons who exercise in heavy protective clothing (34). The WBGT has been adopted as a guide to the modification of exertional activity during heat stress in the military, by athletic organizations, and in industry (31,35–37). Guidelines for heat exposure based on the WBGT as recommended by the American Conference of Governmental Industrial Hygienists are presented in Table 1. The goal of exercise modification guidelines is that a well-acclimatized worker whose salt and fluid intake is adequate and while wearing the usual work uniform can perform the normal job and maintain a rectal temperature below 38°C (100.4°F). Many variables affect the applicability of these guidelines in any individual work setting that are independent of the individual worker. Implementation requires analysis of work loads, type of clothing necessary for the job, and assessment of exposure to other sources of heat such as infrared or microwave radiation (30). In addition, there are many variables that are dependent on the individual worker, such as body habitus and the effects of medications and acute or chronic illness on heat tolerance.

**TABLE 1.** *Permissible heat exposure threshold (WBGT) limit values in °C*

| Work-rest regimen | Work load | | |
|---|---|---|---|
| | Light | Moderate | Heavy |
| Continuous work | 30.0 | 26.7 | 25.0 |
| 75% work, 25% rest each hour | 30.6 | 28.0 | 25.9 |
| 50% work, 50% rest each hour | 31.4 | 29.4 | 27.9 |
| 25% work, 75% rest each hour | 32.2 | 31.1 | 30.0 |

Note: Higher heat exposures than shown in this table are permissible if the workers have been undergoing medical surveillance and it has been established that they are more tolerant to work in heat than the average worker. Workers should not be permitted to continue their work when their core body temperature exceeds 38.0°C.

### Risk Factors for Heat Stroke in Healthy Persons

Heat stroke is the most serious manifestation of heat illness. An extreme historical example of its effects is represented by Wilcox's 1920 account of 462 heat stroke deaths in a single month among British troops training in the Persian Gulf (38). The largest modern experiences of heat injury come from studies of miners (39–42), military recruits (22,23,26,27,43), athletes (28,29,44), and Mecca pilgrims (45–49). Analyses of case series of heat stroke reveals identifiable factors that may predict who is most likely to be intolerant of heat. Risk factors for heat stroke include sleep deprivation, obesity, poor physical conditioning, lack of acclimatization, dehydration, febrile illness, and skin disorders that affect sweating. Heavy protective gear also confers a significant risk (3,33,34). Abuse of ethanol leads to dehydration, alters vascular reactivity, and impairs perception, increasing the risk of heat stroke. Cases of exertional heat stroke in otherwise healthy persons have also been related to the use of medications that impair the normal thermoregulatory response. Specific effects of drugs on thermoregulation are discussed in the following section. Although a history of heat stroke has been regarded as a risk factor for repeated heat stroke, suggesting the possibility of resultant or predisposing thermoregulatory dysfunction (50), a recent study of ten persons with a history of heat stroke demonstrated that 90% of them were able to acclimatize normally following subsequent exposure to heat (51). This study was limited by the number of patients evaluated. Although it suggests that persistent heat intolerance is not an obligatory consequence of heat stroke, it is likely that persons with persistent antecedent risk factors for heat stroke remain at increased risk.

### Effects of Drugs and Toxins on Heat Tolerance

Many commonly used drugs and toxins impair normal thermoregulatory processes and have been associated with the development of heat stroke. Drugs with anticholinergic effects such as antihistamines, phenothiazines, and cyclic antidepressants impair sweating. β-adrenergic receptor antagonists and calcium-channel antagonists decrease cardiac contractility and limit the maximal cardiac output. They may also alter the normal vascular distribution of blood flow in response to heat exposure. The volume depletion associated with the use of diuretics also limits the ability to increase the cardiac output and has significant effects on heat tolerance (16) and on sweating (19). Widely used over-the-counter agents with α-adrenergic effects such as phenylephrine or phenylpropanolamine limit cutaneous vasodilatation as do sympathomimetic agents such as amphetamines and cocaine, resulting in heat stroke during exertion (52–55). Sporadic cases of exertional heat stroke in otherwise healthy individuals have been related to the therapeutic use of medications that blunt the normal thermoregulatory response (28,53,56–61). Therapeutic doses of lithium and fluoxetine have also been associated with exertional heat stroke, possibly due to interference with hypothalamic thermoregulatory mechanisms (57).

### Medical Illnesses that Predispose to Heat Stroke

It should be evident from the preceding discussion of the physiologic mechanisms of heat loss that a number of common medical conditions can interfere with heat dissipation. Cardiac disease of any cause limits the maximal cardiac output and impairs the capacity to increase cutaneous circulation (62). Diabetic or atherosclerotic vascular disease impairs vasodilatation. Patients with diseases of the central nervous system, spinal cord, or peripheral nervous system also exhibit inadequate thermoregulatory responses. Lastly, extensive cutaneous disorders, such as psoriasis, extensive scarring or burns, or even sunburn and heat rash, decrease the ability to sweat adequately and may alter vasodilatation (63).

### Clinical Manifestations of Heat Stroke

The single clinical finding that distinguishes heat stroke from other forms of heat-related illness is altered mental status caused by heat injury to the brain. Other clinical criteria frequently used to define heat stroke include a temperature greater than 41.1°C (106°F) and the absence of sweating (24,32,43). The absence of sweating when noted at the onset of heat stroke suggests thermoregulatory failure and occurs in 25% to 50% of healthy patients who suffer exertional heat stroke (25–27), but absence of sweating is not required to make the diagnosis of heat stroke. Heat stroke victims frequently sweat profusely, suggesting that thermoregulatory mechanisms are at least partly functional (22,23,26, 63). It has been difficult to define the lowest core temperature necessary for the development of tissue injury, as many patients have, appropriately, had cooling initiated prior to determination of the temperature (25). In addition, the rectal temperature does not reflect the temperature of vulnerable tissues such as the liver and brain, which may be much higher (18). In studies of heat stroke in a rat model, a median lethal core temperature of 41.5°C has been reported (9). A patient with an initial recorded rectal temperature of 46.5°C (115.7°F) recovered completely (64). At best, it can be stated that at some temperature very near 42°C the onset of protein coagulation and lipid liquefaction occur. How long the temperature is elevated may be as critical as the absolute degree of elevation. Autopsy studies of patients who died of heat stroke demonstrate that all body tissues are susceptible to heat injury, which is histologically manifest as cellular swelling, coagulation necrosis, and hemorrhage (26,27,65).

Clinical evidence of neurologic injury is present by definition in patients with heat stroke. Its manifestations range from mild confusion to psychosis, seizures, and coma (22,23,26,27,43,66). Mortality is correlated with the height of the temperature, the duration of temperature elevation, and duration of coma longer than 3 hours (25, 26). Extensive cerebral edema with gross and microscopic hemorrhage is reported in patients who die soon after the onset of heat stroke (26,27,65). Although complete neurologic recovery is the rule in survivors of heat stroke, deficits may persist (32,67).

Most patients with exertional heat stroke have tachycardia, and approximately 50% have systolic blood pressure below 100 mm Hg (22–24,26). In Malamud et al.'s (27) detailed report of 125 military basic training fatalities, 60% were hypotensive at first evaluation. Two types of hemodynamic patterns are evident. A hyperdynamic state is most common, with vasodilation and a wide pulse pressure suggesting a low peripheral resistance and a high cardiac output (22–24,68). These patients are usually not substantially volume depleted and their hypotension responds to cooling and moderate fluid administration (24,68,69). Studies utilizing right heart catheterization demonstrate low systematic vascular resistance (SVR), normal pulmonary capillary wedge pressure (PCWP), pulmonary vascular resistance (PVR), and elevated cardiac output, suggesting that the hyperdynamic state is not associated with significant cardiac or pulmonary dysfunction (68,70). Less commonly, patients with heat stroke manifest a hypodynamic state with clinical evidence of low cardiac output, hypotension, and increased peripheral resistance. Significant volume depletion, myocardial dysfunction, or peripheral vascular failure may be the cause (24,70–72). Recent studies suggest a role for elevated endotoxins and tissue cytokines (interleukins, tumor necrosis factor, interferon) in the development of hemodynamic collapse, metabolic acidosis, and multiorgan failure in heat stroke (48,73).

Respiratory alkalosis and lactic acidosis are commonly noted in patients with heat stroke (22,24,74). Lactic acidosis resolves rapidly with cooling and hydration (43). Serum sodium varies as a function of the patient's hydration status (22). Another consistent and predictable laboratory abnormality noted in patients with heat stroke is an elevation of lactic dehydrogenase (LDH), which reflects diffuse tissue injury. Elevation of creatine phosphokinase (CPK), a measure of muscle injury, and the aspartate aminotransferase (AST) and alanine aminotransferase (ALT), markers of liver injury, are also anticipated. The diagnosis of heat stroke is suspect and unlikely in the absence of demonstrable elevation of these enzymes (25, 26,41). Hypophosphatemia has been attributed to renal phosphate losses induced by thermal effects on the renal tubules (75) and hyperventilation on cellular phosphate gradients (76). Serum potassium is initially low or normal in most cases and decreases in the first 24 hours, reflecting the aldosterone-induced total body potassium deficit that occurs early in heat exposure (22,26,77). Apparent normalization of a previously low serum potassium value may occur in the setting of rhabdomyolysis. When significant rhabdomyolysis is present, hyperkalemia, hypocalcemia, and hyperphosphatemia may be noted. The hypocalcemia has been attributed to extensive calcium binding to injured muscle tissue (18,78,79).

Coagulation disturbances are very common in heat stroke and are multifactorial (80). Thrombocytopenia appears early and has been attributed to the presence of disseminated intravascular coagulation (DIC) (65,81), to increased clearance of heat-injured platelets in the absence of other evidence of DIC (80), and to megakaryocyte injury (27). Early elevation of the prothrombin time has been attributed to direct heat injury to clotting factors (82). DIC is the most severe form of coagulation disturbance, seen in the setting of extensive vascular intimal injury (64,83). Primary fibrinolysis has been described (84) and attributed to the effects of heat-induced platelet activation (85). Coagulation disturbances related to liver injury are evident 2 to 3 days into the clinical course, concurrent with the delayed presentation of other clinical evidence of liver injury (42,80).

Renal failure occurs in as many as 10% of patients with exertional heat stroke and is strongly correlated with the presence of rhabdomyolysis and hypotension (26,78). The major pathologic process is precipitation of myoglobin in the renal tubules, although in severe cases there is also direct heat injury to the renal parenchyma (27,39,65). It is important to note that myoglobinuric renal failure also occurs as a consequence of muscle injury related to intense exertion in persons who do not have severe hyperthermia (86). Compartment syndromes associated with rhabdomyolysis have also been reported in this setting (87).

Noncardiogenic pulmonary edema (NCPE) was reported in 23% of 52 consecutive cases of heat stroke observed during the Mecca pilgrimages in 1985. In those patients NCPE appeared to be closely linked with the presence of DIC and was associated with a high mortality (88). In a series of 125 military fatalities, 58% of autopsy specimens showed evidence of hemorrhagic NCPE (27). The incidence of NCPE in exertional heat stroke is not often reported in clinical studies that include many survivors; it may be uncommon in survivors, or underdiagnosed. Acute pulmonary edema has been attributed to excessive fluid administration during resuscitation (69,89). Most patients with heat stroke do not show elevation of the PCWP when studied with right heart catheterization (68,71).

Direct thermal injury to the gastrointestinal mucosa commonly leads to diarrhea. Vomiting is also common (26,27). Major gastrointestinal hemorrhage occurs, particularly when there is an associated coagulopathy. The liver is frequently injured, as reflected by elevation of hepatic enzymes, which is noted within hours of the injury. In patients who survive, clinical evidence of liver injury such as jaundice and coagulation disturbances are manifest 2 to 3 days following the thermal insult (42,80, 90). Patients discharged prematurely from medical care following rapid clinical recovery from heat stroke have presented with hepatic failure several days later (90).

Heat stroke causes diffuse myocardial injury with nonspecific electrocardiographic ST and T wave changes and occasionally demonstrable elevations of myocardial specific CPK. Acute myocardial infarction is rarely reported in young healthy patients (22,40,91). Ischemic changes related to the territory of a single coronary artery were reported in 21% of older heat stroke victims, possibly related to underlying coronary artery disease in the setting of significant cardiovascular stress (47). Reversible prolongation of the QT interval has been reported in 50% to 60% of cases (22,47). In fatal cases petechiae and subendocardial hemorrhages and necrosis are evident on pathologic examination of the heart (27, 40). Clinical evidence of right-sided heart failure has been observed with elevated central venous pressures (18,24) and abnormal radionucleotide ventriculograms (72). Right ventricular dilatation is frequently reported at autopsy (27,40).

## Other Heat-Related Illnesses

### *Heat Syncope*

Heat syncope is a potential problem for workers who must stand for long periods in a hot environment. It is a consequence of venous pooling in persons unacclimatized to heat, and is usually observed in the absence of any substantial exertion. Prior to loss of consciousness, the pulse rate is significantly elevated but the core temperature is not. Orthostatic pulse and blood pressure changes are evident, which improve with acclimatization (92,93). Its occurrence may endanger workers operating at heights where balance and station are critical or those who operate machinery. When loss of consciousness occurs during more substantial exercise in the heat, a diagnosis of heat stroke should be assumed.

### *Heat Exhaustion*

Heat exhaustion occurs during exercise in the heat, resulting in collapse or inability to continue work. It is differentiated from heat stroke by the presence of a normal mental status and by somewhat lower body temperatures, usually not exceeding 105°F. Salt and water depletion are common, and either hyponatremia or hypernatremia may be noted. Heat stroke has been observed in persons returned to their work environment after (presumably inadequate) treatment of heat exhaustion. Heat exhaustion is treated by rest, cooling, and oral or intravenous administration of sodium-containing fluids (18,22).

### *Heat Cramps*

Heat cramps are extremely painful muscle contractions that occur in well-acclimatized, physically fit persons as a consequence of sodium depletion following intense use of the involved muscle (18,94). Severe heat cramps are adequately treated by rest and oral administration of salt-containing fluids.

## Management of Patients with Heat Stroke

The most critical steps in the management of heat stroke are the recognition of the possibility of temperature elevation and immediate, on-site initiation of rapid cooling. Because the duration of temperature elevation is a critical factor in the development of cellular injury, cooling must be initiated concurrently with major resuscitative procedures such as management of respiratory failure or cardiac arrest. Cooling must take precedence over all other resuscitative or diagnostic procedures.

In addition to preventative measures employing the use of heat indexes, gradual conditioning, and increased emphasis on hydration, early detection of heat stroke and rapid cooling of soldiers at the training site have led to a significant decrease in military basic training heat stroke casualties (22,23,25,31). Early detection in the military setting has been facilitated by education of soldiers to recognize subtle behavioral signs possibly attributable to heat injury. Any person who becomes irrational or confused or collapses during exercise should be considered to have heat stroke. Problems of detection in the work environment occur when early behavioral aberrations are not recognized, when collapse due to heat stroke occurs unexpectedly in a person laboring in a cool environment, when temperature measurement is delayed or inaccurate axillary or oral temperatures are not confirmed by a core temperature measurement, and when thermometers are used that do not register temperatures higher than 105°F. Rapid recovery may lead to failure to hospitalize and detect delayed complications such as renal failure, coagulopathy, or liver injury.

Following the initiation of cooling at the work site or athletic field, the patient should be transported to a medical facility. The cooling process must be continued en route. When advanced medical support is available, protective intubation of the comatose patient is desirable, as aspiration of gastric contents is a common problem.

Theoretical considerations predict that evaporative cooling techniques using tepid water and fans will be more efficacious than ice water immersion because they minimize the vasoconstriction and shivering that occur when skin contacts ice water. Cooling devices using this technique are favored by the physicians who handle mass heat casualties during the Mecca pilgrimages (45,46). Others have demonstrated that despite these theoretical drawbacks, ice water immersion is very effective. Military use of ice water immersion has significantly decreased the mortality and morbidity of heat stroke in basic training (95). Regardless of the technique used, it must be readily available and rapidly instituted. Shivering and agitation, which do increase heat production, may be effectively controlled by small doses of an intravenous benzodiazepine titrated to effect. Hypotension should be treated with volume resuscitation and careful monitoring of urine output.

Rapid onset of heat stroke with exertion is not uncommon. In these cases, the extent of volume depletion is limited. The average amount of fluid required for resuscitation has been reported to be between 1,000 and 1,400 ml in several studies (24,68,69,89). Patients who have reported symptoms consistent with heat exhaustion prior to collapse may be significantly dehydrated (26). Vasopressors with $\alpha$-adrenergic effects are contraindicated in the management of hypotension owing to their potential to impair cooling (32,71). Insertion of a Swan-Ganz catheter may provide very useful information when hypotension persists in the heat stroke patient (70,71). The establishment of adequate urine output is especially important in preventing myoglobinuric renal failure. The use of sodium bicarbonate and mannitol infusions to decrease the precipitation of myoglobin has been widely recommended, although their efficacy in preventing myoglobinuric renal failure independent of volume administration has not been established (96,97). Blood glucose levels below 65 mg/dl have been reported in 5 of 12 heat stroke patients (22). Because of this high incidence of hypoglycemia in patients with heat stroke, it would be prudent to administer 0.5 to 1.0 g/kg dextrose empirically after blood sampling for glucose when a rapid and reliable determination of blood glucose is not available. All patients who suffer heat stroke should be closely observed for the development of renal, hepatic, and coagulation abnormalities.

Dantrolene, which specifically blocks the release of calcium from the sarcoplasmic reticulum, has been used to treat severe muscle rigidity in patients with a congenital disturbance of muscle calcium regulation who develop the rare disorder malignant hyperthermia during the induction of general anesthesia (98,99). Dantrolene has also been anecdotally reported to offer benefit for patients with severe rigidity and hyperthermia associated with the neuroleptic malignant syndrome (100). Although there is no pharmacologic rationale for the use of dantrolene in the treatment of exertional heat stroke, where neuromuscular rigidity is uncommon, it has been frequently recommended as a first-line therapeutic measure (101,102). Although one small clinical study suggested that an increased cooling rate occurred in patients given dantrolene in addition to external cooling measures (45), two subsequent studies have not demonstrated any difference (49,52). Pending more extensive and convincing clinical investigations, dantrolene should not be routinely administered in cases of exertional heat stroke. It should never be used as a primary intervention, as cooling should be effectively achieved long before dantrolene would be expected to exert its pharmacologic effects. Dantrolene may be useful as a second-line agent when persistent neuromuscular rigidity is present in patients who do not respond rapidly to aggressive external cooling and sedation with a benzodiazepine.

### Prevention of Heat Stroke

Public education resulting in behavioral changes has had dramatic public health impact in the prevention of heat injury in athletes, military recruits, and the workplace. Preventive measures, including use of the WBGT to guide training schedules, close observation of the behavior of military recruits, education about and restriction of the use of ethanol, enforced rests and fluids protocols, and special guidelines for detection and acclimatization of potentially heat-sensitive recruits, have dramatically decreased the incidence of heat stroke in military personnel (22,23,25,31,95). The establishment of acclimatization regimens has similarly decreased the incidence of heat stroke fatalities among Bantu miners in South Africa (39). Adherence to similar guidelines of the American College of Sports Medicine has decreased the incidence of heat illness among athletes (33,103,104). Thirst is well known to be an inadequate measure of fluid needs. To avoid dehydration, workers must drink beyond their thirst (105). Education of workers with regard to the need to (a) drink adequately, (b) rest periodically in a cool environment, (c) take off or work at a slower pace when ill, and (d) avoid ethanol prior to and during work is important. Workers and supervisors should also be aware of the meaning of early signs of neurologic impairment, such as irritability, confusion, or clumsiness. A ready means of cooling should be available at every work site where heat injury might occur.

## HYPOTHERMIA IN THE WORKPLACE

Environmental factors play a predominant role in the development of hypothermia in healthy persons working in the cold. Heat is lost from the body primarily by the processes of evaporation, conduction, and convection. Wind velocity and ambient air temperature are major determinants of convective heat loss. Significant hypothermia can occur with air temperatures as high as 65°F, particularly when clothing is wet. Water immersion may precipitate a very significant loss of body heat.

### Risk Factors for Hypothermia

In addition to environmental exposure, risk factors for hypothermia include exhaustion, immobilization by injury or entrapment, use of ethanol or drugs or toxins that impair judgment, and inadequate protective clothing.

Certain drugs may also inhibit an adequate thermoregulatory response to severe cold stress. Hypothermia commonly occurs in association with ethanol abuse. In addition to its effects on judgment, ethanol increases heat loss through vasodilatation, and may also impair shivering. Other agents with central sedative effects such as barbiturates and opiates also impair shivering. α-Adrenergic receptor-antagonist agents, such as chlorpromazine or direct-acting vasodilators such as hydralazine prevent vasoconstriction and are associated with hypothermia in animal models (54,106). Centrally acting α-adrenergic agonist drugs such as clonidine and guanabenz appear to interfere with central mechanisms of thermoregulation and have been associated with the development of hypothermia in the overdose setting (107). β-antagonist drugs impair mobilization of glucose and increase hypothermia in animal models (54).

Medical illnesses are exacerbated by exposure to cold. Angina occurs during exercise in cold as a result of increased afterload and sympathetic response. Ischemic effects secondary to peripheral vascular disease in patients with diabetes, atherosclerosis, or Raynaud's disease may be exacerbated by exposure to cold.

### Effects of Cold Exposure

Prolonged exposure or acute immersion injuries may cause life-threatening hypothermia. Shivering is violent at the onset of acute cold exposure then ceases as body temperature approaches 27°C (80.6°F). Vasoconstriction shunts blood from the periphery to the core and results in diuresis and volume depletion. This central shunting of blood leads to significant differences between the temperature of the core blood and that of the periphery. These temperature gradients account for the development of cold injury to the extremities in the absence of core hypothermia. Such temperature gradients have also been postulated to account for decreases in core temperature observed when the extremities are aggressively rewarmed, an effect that has been attributed to the central return of cold blood following dilatation of peripheral vessels by local rewarming.

The metabolic rate declines at approximately 6% for every degree centigrade decrease in body temperature, resulting in a decreased oxygen requirement. The observed protective effect of hypothermia on vital organs is historically attributed to this metabolic sparing effect (108–110). Recently it has also been shown that in addition to decreasing metabolic oxygen requirements, hypothermia inhibits the release of glutamate in ischemic brain tissue (111). Hypothermia has also been shown to slow the decline in adenosine triphosphate (ATP) availability noted during myocardial ischemia and to increase the time to ischemic contracture of the underperfused myocardium (112,113).

### Effects of Hypothermia on the Heart

Following an initial sympathetically mediated tachycardia, the heart rate declines in proportion to the decrease in temperature. Hypothermia does not depress the contractile force of the myocardium so that the stroke volume remains normal. Any decreased myocardial oxygen demand is mediated by this hypothermia induced bradycardia (114–118). The cause of increased myocardial contractility in the hypothermic heart has been suggested by the demonstration in vitro of elevated myocardial intracellular calcium concentrations (118–121). Fatalities due to hypothermia in humans are primarily a result of depression of the myocardial conduction system. However, the protective effects of hypothermia on the heart are limited, and myocardial necrosis is a well-documented complication of hypothermia both in patients undergoing cardiac surgery (122,123) and in fatal cases of unintentional hypothermia (124). Even mild hypothermia has been associated with cardiac injury (125). Conduction disturbances in the atrioventricular (AV) node are manifest as progressive bradycardia leading to asystole. Myocardial conduction disturbances are evident on the ECG as QT and QRS prolongation, and the "J" or Osborne wave, a characteristic sharp upward deflection of the ST segment rising steeply from the downsloping QRS segment that is pathognomonic of hypothermia (126–130). Electrophysiologic studies of the cold myocardium demonstrate that hypothermia decreases the diastolic resting membrane potential, decreases the magnitude of the phase one inward sodium current, and increases the duration of the action potential (121,131–133). These effects are likely related to dysfunction of components of the myocardial conductive apparatus such as the functional proteins of the membrane ion channels, electrolyte gradients, lipid structures, and the ATP-dependent sodium/potassium pump (131,132).

As body temperature declines below 28°C (82.4°F) potentially fatal dysrhythmias increase in frequency. Ventricular fibrillation is most often an iatrogenic event, related to stimulation of the cold ventricle by movement of the patient, or perhaps by shifts of colder blood from the periphery to the warmer endocardium (134–136). An important early study showed that the risk of fibrillation increased as the temperature difference between the right and left ventricles increased (137). More recently, cardiac physiologists have proposed that regions of intramyocardial temperature variability create areas of different refractoriness and conductivity, leading to reentry dysrhythmias (131).

### Neurologic Effects of Hypothermia

Neurologic depression is predictable and a direct function of body temperature. Clumsiness, ataxia, slowed responses to stimuli, and dysarthria are noted at temperatures ranging from 35°C (95°F) to 32.2°C (90°F) (138). These neurologic effects of mild hypothermia place the exposed worker at risk of injury from machinery or falls. Significant mental status depression in patients with temperatures above 89°F should suggest head injury, a drug or toxin, or another complicating cause. An incoherent verbal response may be elicited at temperatures as low as 27°C (80.6°F) and purposeful motor responses occur as low as 20°C (68°F) (138). A patient whose body temperature is lower than 20°C (68°F) is unresponsive to stimuli. The pupils may be fixed and the still-living patient may appear dead (139).

### Other Effects of Cold Exposure

Complications of cold exposure not necessarily associated with core hypothermia include impairment of manual dexterity, frost nip, and frostbite. Frostnip is a painful area where vasoconstriction is evident but ice crystal formation has not occurred. Signs and symptoms of frostnip resolve with rewarming and permanent tissue damage does not occur. Frostbite is associated with varying degrees of irreversible tissue damage in exposed areas of the hands, feet, or face that occurs as a consequence of ischemia caused by vasoconstriction and structural injury to cells caused by ice crystal formation. Freeze-thaw cycles are particularly injurious. Frostbite is graded as superficial when partial- (first degree) or full-thickness (second degree) dermal injury is present, and deep when subcutaneous (third degree) or bone, muscle, and tendon involvement (fourth degree) are present. Permanent functional impairment of the hands or feet may result (140).

### Management of Cold Disorders

Most patients with hypothermia respond to simple passive measures that decrease heat loss and facilitate heat retention, such as removal of wet clothing and insulation with blankets. Active external rewarming is accomplished by the application of warm blankets to the trunk (10,141). In cases when cardiac arrest has occurred, CPR with rapid core rewarming may be lifesaving. Cardiopulmonary bypass or partial (fem-fem) bypass is effective for rapid core rewarming (142–145); however, when cardiopulmonary bypass is not available, hemodialysis (146, 147), peritoneal dialysis (148,149), or thoracic lavage (150,151) have been associated with survival.

Several caveats apply in the management of the profoundly hypothermic patient. The first is that prolonged cardiopulmonary resuscitation associated with rapid rewarming of patients with ventricular fibrillation or asystole has resulted in neurologically intact survival despite circulatory arrest lasting as long as 4 hours (124, 139,152,153). The longest reported ice water submersion that resulted in intact survival was 66 minutes (154). Patients with unintentional hypothermia have survived temperatures as low as 14.2°C (57.6°F) (144). Defibrillation is frequently unsuccessful until the patient's temperature reaches 30°C (86°F), so repeated attempts at defibrillation at lower temperatures are unwarranted if one or two attempts are not successful (124,155). Bretylium has been anecdotally reported to be useful in the treatment of ventricular fibrillation associated with hypothermia (156,157). Repeated administration of cardiac drugs should be avoided during cardiopulmonary resuscitation, as drug metabolism is altered during hypothermia, with the possibility of toxic drug effects being manifest after the patient is rewarmed (155). A final caveat in managing the significantly hypothermic patient is that physical stimulation may convert an effective sinus bradycardia to ventricular fibrillation (134–136). This risk begins to increase as the body temperature declines below 28°C (82.4°F) (110,134,136). Unnecessary movement and stimulation of hypothermic patients should be avoided. Although in rare cases intubation has resulted in the precipitation of ventricular fibrillation, the benefit of the maintenance of oxygenation and ventilation is significant and intubation should be preformed when indicated (11,158,159). The adequacy of ventilation is best determined using the uncorrected arterial blood gases (109,113,134).

Experimental studies demonstrate that arterial pressure increases with cooling to temperatures near 27°C (80.6°F) (115,160). Many patients with accidental hypothermia who present with temperatures above 25°C (77°F) have a normal blood pressure. These patients require fluid support during rewarming. Hypotension does occur in profound exposure-related hypothermia as a consequence of bradycardia and cold-induced diuresis. Due to decreased metabolic demands tissue perfusion may be adequate in the hypothermic patient in spite of very low blood pressures (113,134). Lactic acidosis is not reliable as a measure of the adequacy of blood pressure. Although it does occur when perfusion is inadequate, it is also a consequence of shivering, and of "washout" of the peripheral microcirculation as perfusion improves during resuscitation. Attempts to raise the blood pressure by fluid administration are worthwhile and should be guided by measurement of urine output and continuous assessment of oxygenation and pulmonary function (155). Pharmacologic or electrical attempts to increase heart rate theoretically increase myocardial oxygen demand. A recent abstract suggests that increasing the heart rate may increase the rewarming rate of hypothermic subjects (161). The utility of vasopressor agents has not been clearly demonstrated. Theoretical contraindications to pressors in the profoundly hypothermic patient include the accumulation of unmetabolized pharmacologically active agents, and an increased risk of frostbite injury due to vasoconstriction. Chest compressions should not be initiated in the field if there is any detectable movement, pulse, or cardiac rhythm, any one of which suggests a degree of cardiac function likely to sustain life in a profoundly hypothermic patient. The institution of chest compressions in these patients increases the likelihood of precipitating ventricular fibrillation and inducing myocardial injury (124,136). In the hypothermic patient who has suffered cardiac arrest, chest compressions are effective in establishing blood flow and should be initiated at the same rate as in the normothermic patient (160).

Lactic acidosis is common and multifactorial (139,142, 159,162,163). It does not require specific treatment beyond standard resuscitative measures. Hypokalemia is frequently attributed to renal potassium losses and to sympathetically medicated intracellular shifts. Rats given potassium supplements to correct hypokalemia during resuscitation became hyperkalemic following rewarming (164). Significant hyperkalemia is not routinely described in survivors of hypothermia.

An association of severe hyperkalemia with failed resuscitation in severe unintentional hypothermia has been reported. Six avalanche victims who died despite rewarming with cardiopulmonary bypass had serum potassiums levels of 6.8, 9.4, and greater than 12 mEq/L (165). In the description of the resuscitation of ten young mountaineers trapped for 72 hours in a snow cave on Mt. Hood, potassium levels of 5.3 mEq/L and 6.7 mEq/L were measured in the two survivors and ">8" (20–33 mEq/L where precisely measured) were recorded in all nonsurvivors (139). Potassium levels of this magnitude are likely related to generalized membrane failure in patients with irreversible death rather than a potentially treatable manifestation of hypothermia. This seems clearest in the Mt. Hood cases, where the nonsurvivors sustained no trauma, were in asystole, and had temperatures ranging from 3°C to 12°C (generally regarded as nonsurvivable) with one outlier at 19.7°C. These data suggest that serum potassium measurements greater than 10 mEq/L indicate a very poor prognosis for the success of prolonged resuscitation in profoundly hypothermic patients.

Excessive bleeding due to cold-induced coagulopathy may be a problem in managing the hypothermic patient. Trauma surgeons have long recognized the significance of this coagulation disturbance. Since blood specimens used for coagulation studies in the hospital laboratory are routinely warmed to 37°C prior to determinations of the protime (PT) and partial thromboplastin time (PTT), the coagulopathy may frequently go unrecognized (166,167). Patients resuscitated from prolonged severe hypothermia rarely manifest DIC (139). A recent study of dogs cooled below 10°C showed that bleeding was a major complication and cause of death at this temperature (168).

Frostbite should be treated with rapid local rewarming of frostbitten extremities by immersion in warm water (104° to 110°F) to minimize tissue loss. It is important not to attempt to rewarm areas of frostbite in the field if there is any danger of refreezing. Frostbitten areas should never be rubbed, as the frozen tissue is particularly susceptible to trauma. Surgical debridement of injured tissue prior to ischemic delineation of dead tissue may result in unnecessary tissue loss (169,170).

### Prevention of Hypothermia

The occurrence of hypothermia and other cold-related injuries during day-to-day activities in a cold environment is readily prevented by adherence to a few simple recommendations:

1. Educate employees with regard to the risks and prevention of hypothermia.
2. Provide heated shelters and regular rest periods so that workers can rewarm periodically.
3. Maintain a work rate slow enough to preclude heavy sweating.
4. Use appropriate protective equipment, including the use of nonconducting surfaces, to prevent frostbite of hands, feet, and face.
5. Provide an on-site means of warming hands, face, and feet to prevent frostbite and the loss of dexterity.
6. Wear enough protective clothing. A good method is to use three layers: an outer layer that breaks the wind and allows some ventilation (usually Goretex or nylon); a middle layer of wool, down, or synthetic pile that absorbs sweat and retains its insulating capacity when wet; and an inner layer of cotton or synthetic weave that allows ventilation and escape of moisture. Assure the availability of replacement clothing.
7. Avoid using ethanol to keep warm and other mind-altering drugs that impair judgment and coordination. Smoking leads to vasoconstriction and theoretically increases the risk of dermal injury due to cold exposure. Encourage adequate nutrition.
8. Prevent dermal injury secondary to drying of the skin by frequent application of protective emollients and use of windbreaking clothing.
9. Closely observe employees for evidence of impairment or alteration of consciousness.

## SUMMARY

Exposure to extremes of cold or heat in the occupational environment may have serious health consequences. Prevention of heat- and cold-related injury is best achieved by (a) analysis of the risks posed by constant or changing environmental conditions and appropriate adjustment of work rates and exposure times; (b) education and monitoring of workers' fluid intake, drug, toxin and alcohol use, and rest periods; (c) provision of protective facilities and equipment, such as rewarming or cooling areas, hand warmers, and a readily available water supply; and (d) identification of workers at risk of heat- or cold-related injury because of acute or chronic medical illness, drug or toxin use, body habitus, or lack of adequate acclimatization. The special needs of workers whose jobs require wearing protective clothing in a hot environment must be recognized. Early recognition and treatment, particularly of heat stroke, significantly decreases morbidity and mortality and mandates the availability of treatment facilities at the work site.

## REFERENCES


1. Fatalities from occupational heat exposure. *MMWR* 1984;33:410–412.
2. Sherman R, Copes R, Stewart RK, et al. Occupational death due to heat stroke: report of two cases. *Can Med Assoc* J 1989;140:105–107.
3. Cole RD. Heat stroke during training with nuclear, biological and chemical protective clothing: case report. *Milit Med* 1983;148: 624–625.
4. Stolwijk JAJ. Responses to the thermal environment. *Fed Proc* 1977; 36:1655–1658.
5. Hensel H. Neural processes in thermoregulation. *Physiol Rev* 1973; 53:948–1007.
6. Mackowiak PA, Wasserman SS, Levine MM. A critical appraisal of 98.6°F, the upper limit of the normal body temperature, and other legacies of Carl Reinhold August Wunderlich. *JAMA* 1992;268: 1578–1580.
7. Hochachka PW. Defense strategies against hypoxia and hypothermia. *Science* 1986;231:234–241.
8. Hales JRS, Khogali M, Fawcett AA, Mustafa MKY. Circulatory changes associated with heatstroke: observations in an experimental animal model. *Clin Exp Pharmacol Physiol* 1987;14:761–777.
9. Hubbard RW. An introduction: the role of exercise in the etiology of exertional heatstroke. *Med Sci Sports Exerc* 1990;22:2–5.
10. Harnett RM, Pruitt JR, Sias FR. A review of the literature concerning resuscitation from hypothermia: Part I, The problem and general approaches. *Aviat Space Environ Med* 1983;5:425–434.
11. Delaney KA. Hypothermic Sudden Death. In: Paradis NA, Halperin HR, Nowak RM, eds. *Cardiac arrest:* the science and practice of resuscitation medicine. Baltimore: Williams and Wilkins, 1996; 745–760.
12. Vassallo SU, Delaney KA. Pharmacologic effects on thermoregulation: mechanisms of drug-related heatstroke. *J Toxicol Clin Toxicol* 1989;27:199–224.
13. Rowell LB. Cardiovascular aspects of human thermoregulation. *Circ Res* 1983;52:367–379.
14. Nadel ER, Bullard RW, Stolwijk AJ. Importance of skin temperature in the regulation of sweating. *J Appl Physiol* 1971;31:80–87.
15. Johnson JM, Brengelmann GL, Hales JRS, et al. Regulation of the cutaneous circulation. *Fed Proc* 1986;45:2841–2850.
16. De Garavilla L, Durkot MJ, Ihley TM, et al. Adverse effects of dietary and furosemide-induced sodium depletion on thermoregulation. *Aviat Space Environ Med* 1990;61:1012–1017.
17. Gisolfi CV, Wenger CB. Temperature regulation during exercise: old concepts, new ideas. *Exerc Sport Sci Rev* 1984;12:339–373.
18. Knochel JP. Environmental heat illness: an eclectic review. *Arch Intern Med* 1974;133:841–863.
19. Nielsen B, Hansen G, Jorgenesen O, Nielsen E. Thermoregulation in exercising man during dehydration, and hyperhydration with water and saline. *Int J Biometeorol* 1971;15:195–200.
20. Johnson JM, Rowell LB, Brengelman GL. Modification of the skin blood flow-body temperature relationship by upright exercise. *J Appl Physiol* 1974;37:880–886.
21. Gold J. Development of heat pyrexia. *JAMA* 1960;173:1175–1182.
22. Costrini AM, Pitt MA, Gustafson AB. Cardiovascular and metabolic manifestations of heatstroke and severe heat exhaustion. *Am J Med* 1979;66:296–302.
23. Beller GA, Boyd AE. Heatstroke: a report of 13 consecutive cases without mortality despite severe hyperexia and neurologic dysfunction. *Milit Med* 1975;140:464–467.
24. O'Donnell TF, Clowes GHA. The circulatory abnormalities of heatstroke. *N Engl J Med* 1972;287:734–737.
25. Shapiro Y, Seidman DS. Field and clinical observations of exertional heat stroke patients. *Med Sci Sports Exerc* 1990;22:6–14.
26. Shibolet S, Coll R, Gilat T, Sohar E. Heatstroke: its clinical picture and mechanism in 36 cases. *Q J Med* 1967;36:525–548.
27. Malamud N, Haymaker W, Custer RP. Heatstroke: a clinicopathologic study of 125 fatal cases. *Milit Med* 1946;99:397–444.
28. Wyndham CH. Heat stroke and hyperthermia in marathon runners. *Ann NY Acad Sci* 1977;301:129–139.
29. Robinson S. Temperature regulation in exercise. *Pediatrics* 1963: 691–702.
30. Lee DHK. Seventy-five years of searching for a heat index. *Environ Res* 1980;22:331–356.
31. Minard D. Prevention of Heat Casualties in Marine Corps Recruits: period of 1955–60, with comparative incidence rates and climatic heat stresses in other training categories. *Milit Med* 1961;136:261–272.
32. Clowes GHA, O'Donnell TF. Current concepts: heatstroke. *N Engl J Med* 1974;291:564–566.
33. Squire DL. Heat illness: fluid and electrolyte issues for pediatric and adolescent athletes. *Pediatr Clin North Am* 1990;37:1085–1109.
34. Tilley RI, Standerwick JM, Long GJ. Ability of the wet bulb globe temperature index to predict heat stress in men wearing NBC protective clothing. *Milit Med* 1987;152:554–556.
35. *Documentation of the threshold limit values,* 4th ed. Cincinatti, OH: American Conference of Governmental Industrial Hygienists, 1980; 451–455.
36. *Criteria for a recommended standard:* occupational exposure to hot environments. USDHEW Publication (NIOSH) HSM 72-10269. Washington, DC: U.S. Government Printing Office, 1972.
37. American College of Sports Medicine. Prevention of thermal injuries during distance running (position statement). *Physician Sports Med* 1984;12:43–51.
38. Wilcox WH. The nature, prevention and treatment of heat hyperpyrexia. *Br Med J* 1920;1:392–397.
39. Kew MC, Abrahams C, Levin NW, et al. The effects of heat stroke on the function and structure of the kidney. *Q J Med* 1967;36:277–300.
40. Kew MC, Tucker RBK, Bersohn I, Seftel HC. The heart in heat stroke. *Am Heart J* 1972;77:324–335.
41. Kew M, Bersohn I, Seftel M. The diagnostic and prognostic significance of serum enzyme changes in heat stroke. *Trans R Soc Trop Med Hyg* 1971;65:325–330.
42. Kew M, Bersohn I, Seftel H, Dent G. Liver damage in heatstroke. *Am J Med* 1970;49:192–202.
43. O'Donnell TF. Acute heat stroke. *JAMA* 1975;234:824–828.
44. O'Donnell TF. The hemodynamic and metabolic alterations associated with acute heat stress injury in marathon runners. *Ann NY Acad Sci* 1977;301:262–29.
45. Channa AB, Seraj MA, Saddique AA, et al. Is dantrolene effective in heatstroke patients? *Crit Care Med* 1990;18:290–292.
46. Weiner JS, Khogali M. A physiological body-cooling unit for treatment of heat stroke. *Lancet* 1980;1:507–509.
47. Akhtar MJ, al-Nozha M, al-Harthi S, Nou MS. Electrocardiographic abnormalities in patients with heat stroke. *Chest* 1993;104:411–414.
48. Bouchama A, Parhar RS, el-Yazigi A, Sheth K, al-Sediary S. Endotoxemia and release of tumor necrosis factor and interleukin 1a in acute heatstroke. *J Appl Physiol* 1991;70:2640–2644.
49. Bouchama A, al-Sediary S, Siddiqui S et al. Elevated pyrogenic cytokines in heatstroke. *Chest* 1993;104:1498–1502.
50. Shapiro Y, Magazinik A, Udassin R, et al. Heat intolerance in former heat stroke patients. *Ann Intern Med* 1979;90:913–916.
51. Armstrong LE, De Luca JP, Hubbard RW. Time course of recovery and heat acclimation ability of prior exertional heat stroke patients. *Med Sci Sports Exerc* 1990;22:36–48.
52. Watson JD, Ferguson C, Hinds CJ, et al. Exertional heat stroke induced by amphetamine analogues. *Anaesthesia* 1993;48:1057–1060.
53. Kew MC, Hopp M, Rothberg A. Fatal heatstroke in a child taking appetite suppressant drugs. *South Afr Med J* 1982;62:905–906.
54. Maickel RP. Interaction of drugs with autonomic nervous function and thermoregulation. *Fed Proc* 1970;29:1973–1979.
55. Coper H, Lison H, Rommelspacher H, et al. The influence of adrener-

gic receptor blocking agents, amphetamine and 6-aminonicotinamide on thermoregulation. *Arch Exp Pathol Pharmacol* 1971;270:378–392.
56. Squires LA, Neumeyer AM, Bloomberg J, Krishnamoorthy KS. Hyperpyrexia in an adolescent desipramine treatment. *Clin Pediatr* 1992;31:635–636.
57. Albukrek D, Moran DS, Epstein Y. A depressed workman with heatstroke. *Lancet* 1996;347:1016.
58. Weaving EA, Berro VE, Kew MC. Heat stroke during a "run for fun." *S Afr Med J* 1980;57:753–754.
59. Zellman S, Guillan R. Heatstoke in phenothiazine-treated patients: a report of three fatalities. *Am J Psychiatr* 1970;126:1787–1790.
60. Sarnquist F, Larson CP. Drug-induced heatstroke. *Anesthesiology* 1973;39:348–350.
61. Whitworth JAG, Wolfman MJ. Fatal heat stroke in a long distance runner. *Br Med J* 1983;287:948.
62. El Sherif N, Shahwan L, Sorour AH. The effect of acute thermal stress on general and pulmonary hemodynamics in the cardiac patient. *Am Heart J* 1970;79:305.
63. Epstein Y. Heat intolerance: predisposing factor or residual injury? *Med Sci Sports Exerc* 1990;22:29–35.
64. Slovis CM, Anderson GF, Casolaro A. Survival in a heat stroke victim with a core temperature in excess of 46.5°C. *Ann Emerg Med* 1982; 11:269–271.
65. Chao TC, Sinniah R, Pakiam JE. Acute heatstroke deaths. *Pathology* 1981;13:145–156.
66. Carter BJ, Cammermeyer M. A phenomenology of heat injury: the predominance of confusion. *Milit Med* 1988;153:118–126.
67. Mehta AC, Baker RN. Persistent neurological deficits in heatstroke. *Neurology* 1970;20:336–340.
68. Damash NS, Al Harthi SS, Akhtar J. Invasive evaluation of patients with heat stroke. *Chest* 1993;103:1210–1214.
69. Seraj MA, Channa AB, Al-Harthi SS, et al. Are heatstroke victims fluid depleted? Importance of monitoring central venous pressure as a simple guideline for fluid therapy. *Resuscitation* 1991;21:33–39.
70. Vera ZA, Cross CE. Cardiovascular alterations in heat stroke. *Chest* 1993;103:987–988.
71. Sprung CL. Hemodynamic alterations of heatstroke in the elderly. *Chest* 1979;75:362–366.
72. Zahger D, Moses A, Weiss AT. Evidence of prolonged myocardial dysfunction in heat stroke. *Chest* 1989;95:1089–1091.
73. Gathiran P, Wells M, Raidoo D, et al. Portal and systemic arterial plasma lipopolysaccharide concentration in heat-stressed primates. *Circ Shock* 1988;25:223–230.
74. Stoneham MD, Price DJA. Acid-base disturbances and heat-stress in the armed forces. *Lancet* 1992;339:870–871.
75. Guntupalli KI, Sladen A, Selker RG, et al. Effects of induced total-body hyperthermia on phosphorous metabolism in humans. *Am J Med* 1984;77:250–254.
76. Knochel JP, Caskey JH. The mechanism of hypophosphatemia in acute heatstroke. *JAMA* 1977;238:425–426.
77. Knochel JP, Dotin LN, Hamburger RJ. Pathophysiology of intense physical conditioning in a hot climate. *J Clin Invest* 1972;51:242–255.
78. Vertel RM, Knochel JP. Acute renal failure due to heat injury. *Am J Med* 1967;43:435–451.
79. Gabow PA, Kaehny WD, Kelleher SP. The spectrum of rhabdomyolysis. *Medicine* 1982;61:141–152.
80. Mustafa KY, Omer O, Khogali M, et al. Blood coagulation and fibrinolysis in heatstroke. *Br J Haematol* 1985;61:517–523.
81. Weber MB, Blackely JA. The haemorrhagic diathesis of heatstroke. *Lancet* 1969;2:1190–1192.
82. Beard ME, Hickton CM. Haemostasis in heatstroke. *Br J Haematol* 1982;52:269–274.
83. Sohal RS, Sun SC, Colcolough HL, Burch GE. Heatstroke: an electron microscopic study of endothelial cell damage and disseminated intravascular coagulation. *Arch Intern Med* 1968;122:43–47.
84. Meikle AW, Graybill JR. Fibrinolysis and hemorrhage in a fatal case of heatstroke. *N Engl J Med* 1967;276:911–913.
85. Gader AMA, Al-Mashhadani SA, Al-Harthy SS. Direct activation of platelets by heat is the possible trigger of the coagulopathy of heat stroke. *Br J Haematol* 1990;74:86–92.
86. Schrier RW, Hano J, Deller HI, et al. Renal, metabolic, and circulatory responses to heat and exercise. *Ann Intern Med* 1970;73:213–223.
87. Amundson DE. The spectrum of heat-related injury with compartment syndrome. *Milit Med* 1989;154:450.
88. El-Kassimi FA, Al-Mashhadani S, Abdullah AK, Akhtar J. Adult respiratory distress syndrome and disseminated intravascular coagulation complicating heat stroke. *Chest* 1986;90:571–574.
89. Al-Harthi SS, Akhtar J, Nouh MS, Al-Nozha MM. Evaluation of fluid deficit in pilgrims with heat stroke by hemodynamic monitoring. *Emirates Med J* 1989;7:153–157.
90. Chobanian SJ. Jaundice occurring after resolution of heat stroke. *Ann Emerg Med* 1983;12:102–103.
91. Knochel JP, Beisel WR, Herndon EG, et al. The renal, cardiovascular, hematologic and serum electrolyte abnormalities of heat stroke. *Am J Med* 1961;30:299–309.
92. Wyndham CH, Benade AJA, Williams CG, et al. Changes in central circulation and body fluid spaces during acclimatization to heat. *J Appl Physiol* 1968;25:586–593.
93. Ahvartz E, Styrdom NB, Kotze H. Orthostatism and heat acclimation. *J Appl Physiol* 1975;39:590–595.
94. Talbott JH. Heat cramps. *Medicine* 1965;14:323–376.
95. Costrini, AM. Emergency treatment of exertional heatstroke and comparison of whole body cooling techniques. *Med Sci Sports Exerc* 1990;22:15–18.
96. Eneas JF, Schoenfeld PY, Humphreys MH. The effect of infusion of mannitol-sodium bicarbonate on the clinical course of myoglobinuria. *Arch Intern Med* 1979;139:801–805.
97. Ron D, Taitelman U, Michaelson M, et al. Prevention of acute renal failure in traumatic rhabdomyolysis. *Arch Intern Med* 1984;144:277–280.
98. Ward A, Chaffman MO, Sorkin EM. Dantrolene: a review of its pharmacodynamic and pharmacokinetic properties and therapeutic use in malignant hyperthermia, the neuroleptic malignant syndrome and an an update of its use in muscle spasticity. *Drugs* 1986;32:130–167.
99. Britt BA. Etiology and pathophysiology of malignant hyperthermia. *Fed Proc* 1979;38:44–48.
100. Guze BH, Baxter LR. Current concepts: neuroleptic malignant syndrome. *N Engl J Med* 1985;313:163–166.
101. Lydiatt JS, Hill GE. Treatment of heat stroke with dantrolene. *JAMA* 1981;246:41–42.
102. Larner AJ. Dantrolene for exertional heatstroke. *Lancet* 1992;339:182.
103. Murphy RJ. Heat illness in the athlete. *Am J Sports Med* 1984;12: 258–261.
104. Elias SR, Roberts WO, Thorson DC. Team sports in hot weather: guidelines for modifying youth soccer. *Physician Sports Med* 1991; 19:67–78.
105. Moroff SV, Bass DE. Effects of overhydration on man's physiological responses to work in the heat. *J Appl Physiol* 1965;20:267–270.
106. Kollias J, Bullard RW. The influence of chlorpromazine on physical and chemical mechanisms of temperature regulation in the rat. *J Pharmacol Exp Ther* 1964;145:373–381.
107. Perrone J, Hoffman RS, Jones B, Hollander JE. Guanabenz induced hypothermia in a poisoned elderly female. *J Toxicol Clin Toxicol* 1994; 32:445–449.
108. Hynson JM, Sessler DI, Moayeri A, McGuire J. Absence of nonshivering thermogenesis in anesthetized adult humans. *Anesthesiology* 1994;79:695–703.
109. Hering JP, Schröder T, Singer D, Hellige G. Influence of pH management on hemodynamics and metabolism in moderate hypothermia. *J Thor Cardiovasc Surg* 1992;104:1388–1395.
110. Wong KC. Physiology and pharmacology of hypothermia. *West J Med* 1983;138:227–232.
111. Busto R, Globus MYT, Dietrich WD, et al. Effect of mild hypothermia on ischemia-induced release of neurotransmitters and free fatty acids in rat brain. *Stroke* 1989;20:904–910.
112. Wittnich C, Maitland A, Vincente W, Salerno T. Not all neonatal hearts are equally protected from ischemic damage during hypothermia. *Ann Thorac Surg* 1991;52:1000–1004.
113. Swain JA, McDonald TJ, Balaban RS, Robbins RC. Metabolism of the heart and brain during hypothermic cardiopulmonary bypass. *Ann Thorac Surg* 1991;51:105–109.
114. Buckberg GD, Brazier JR, Nelson RL et al. Studies of the effect of hypothermia on regional myocardial blood flow and metabolism during cardiopulmonary bypass: I. The adequately perfused beating, fibrillating and arrested heart. *J Thorac Cardiovasc Surg* 1977;73: 87–95.
115. Orts A, Alcaraz C, Delaney KA, et al. Bretylium tosylate and electrically induced cardiac arrhythmias in dogs. *Am J Emerg Med* 1992;10: 311–316.

116. Covino BG, Beavers W. Changes in cardiac contractility during immersion hypothermia. *Am J Physiol* 1958;195:433–436.
117. Badeer H, Khachadurian A. Role of bradycardia and cold per se in increasing mechanical efficiency of hypothermic heart. *Am J Physiol* 1958;192:331.
118. Rebeyka IM, Diaz J, Augustine JM, et al. Effect of rapid cooling contracture on ischemic tolerance in immature myocardium. *Circulation* 1991;84(suppl 3):389–393.
119. Svensson OLO, Wohlfart B, Johansson BW. Hypothermic effects on action potential and force production of hedgehog and guinea pig papillary muscles. *Cryobiology* 1988;25:445–450.
120. Mattiazzi AR, Nilsson E. The influence of temperature on the time course of the mechanical activity in rabbit papillary muscle. *Acta Physiol Scand* 1976;97:310–318.
121. Shattock MJ, Bers DM. Inotropic response to hypothermia and the temperature dependence of ryanodine action in isolated rabbit and rat ventricular muscle: implication of excitation-contraction coupling. *Circ Res* 1987;61:761–767.
122. Hottenrott CE, Towers B, Kurkji HJ, et al. The hazard of ventricular fibrillation in hypertrophied ventricles during cardiopulmonary bypass. *J Thorac Cardiovasc Surg* 1973;66:742–753.
123. Brazier JR, Cooper N, McConnell DH, Buckberg GD. Studies of the effects of hypothermia on regional myocardial blood flow and metabolism during cardiopulmonary bypass. III. Effects of temperature, time and perfusion pressure in fibrillating hearts. *J Thorac Cardiovasc Surg* 1977;73:102–108.
124. Splittgerber FH, Talbert JG, Sweezer WP, Wilson RF. Partial cardiopulmonary bypass for core rewarming in profound accidental hypothermia. *Am Surg* 1986;52:407–411.
125. Frank SM, Beattie C, Christopherson R, et al. Unintentional hypothermia is associated with postoperative myocardial ischemia. *Anesthesiology* 1993;78:468–476.
126. Patel A, Getsos J. Osborne waves of hypothermia. *N Engl J Med* 1994; 330:680.
127. Osborne L, Lamal El-Din AS, Smith JE. Survival after prolonged cardiac arrest and accidental hypothermia. *Br Med J* 1984;289:881–882.
128. Okada M, Nishimura F, Yoshino H, et al. The J wave in accidental hypothermia. *J Electrocardiol* 1983;16:23–28.
129. Okada M. The cardiac rhythm in accidental hypothermia. *J Electrocardiol* 1984;17:123–128.
130. Trevino A, Razi B, Beller BM. The characteristic electrocardiogram of accidental hypothermia. *Arch Intern Med* 1971;127:470–472.
131. Bjornstad H, Pal M. Cardiac electrophysiology during hypothermia: implications for medical treatment. *Arch Med Res* 1991;50:Suppl 6: 71–75.
132. Bjornstad H, Tande PM, Refsum H. Class III antiarrhythmic action of d-sotalol during hypothermia. *Am Heart J* 1991;191:1429–1436.
133. Jacobs HK, South FE. Effects of temperature on cardiac transmembrane potentials in hibernation. *Am J Physiol* 1976;230:403–409.
134. Delaney KA, Howland MA, Vassallo S, Goldfrank LR. The assessment of acid-base disturbances in hypothermia and their physiological consequences. *Ann Emerg Med* 1989;18:72–82.
135. Lloyd EL, Mitchell B. Factors affecting the onset of ventricular fibrillation in hypothermia. *Lancet* 1974;2:1294–1296.
136. Zell SC, Kurtz KJ. Severe exposure hypothermia: a resuscitation protocol. *Ann Emerg Med* 1985;14:339–345.
137. Mouritzen CV, Anderson MN. Myocardial temperature gradients and ventricular fibrillation during hypothermia. *J Thorac Cardiovasc Surg* 1965;49:937–944.
138. Fishbeck KH, Simon RP. Neurological manifestations of accidental hypothermia. *Ann Neurol* 1981;10:384–387.
139. Hauty MG, Esrig BC, Hill JG, Long WB. Prognostic factors in severe accidental hypothermia: experiences from the Mt. Hood tragedy. *J Trauma* 1987;27:1107–1112.
140. Rabold M. Frostbite and other localized cold-related injuries. In: Tintinalli JE, Ruiz E, Krome RL, eds. *Emergency medicine:* a comprehensive study guide. New York: McGraw-Hill; 1996; pp 843–846.
141. Danzl DF, Pozos RS. Accidental hypothermia. *N Engl J Med* 1994; 331:1756–1760.
142. Letsou GV, Kopf GS, Elefteriades JA, Carter JE, Baldwin JC, Hammond GL. Is cardiopulmonary bypass effective for treatment of hypothermic arrest due to drowning or exposure? *Arch Surg* 1992; 127:525–528.
143. Waters DJ, Belz M, Lawse D, Ulstad D. Portable cardiopulmonary bypass: resuscitation from prolonged ice-water submersion and asystole. *Ann Thorac Surg* 1994;57:1018–1019.
144. Dobson JAR, Burgess JJ. Resuscitation of severe hypothermia by extracorporeal rewarming in a child. *J Trauma* 1996;40:483–485.
145. Antretter H, Bonatti J, Dapunt OE. Accidental hypothermia (letter). *N Engl J Med* 1995;332;1033–1034.
146. Murray PT, Fellner SK. Accidental hypothermia (letter). *N Engl J Med* 1995;332:1034.
147. Hernandez E, Praga M, Alcazar JM. Accidental hypothermia (letter). *N Engl J Med* 1995;332;1034.
148. Davis FM, Judson JA. Warm peritoneal dialysis in the management of accidental hypothermia: report of five cases. *NZ Med J* 1981;94: 207–209.
149. Jessen K, Hagelsten JO. Peritoneal dialysis in the treatment of profound accidental hypothermia. *Aviat Space Environ Med* 1978;49: 426–429.
150. Iversen RJ, Atkin SH, Jaker MA et al. Successful CPR in a severely hypothermic patient using continuous thoracostomy lavage. *Ann Emerg Med* 1990;19:1335–1337.
151. Hall KN, Syverud SA. Closed thoracic cavity lavage in the treatment of severe hypothermia in human beings. *Ann Emerg Med* 1990;19: 204–205.
152. Southwick FS, Preston DH. Recovery after prolonged asystolic cardiac arrest in profound hypothermia. *JAMA* 1980;243:1250–1253.
153. Althaus U, Aeberhard P, Schupback P, et al. Management of profound accidental hypothermia with cardiorespiratory arrest. *Ann Surg* 1982; 195:492–495.
154. Bolte RG, Black PG, Bowers RS, et al. The use of extracorporeal rewarming in a child submerged for 66 minutes. *JAMA* 1988;260: 377–379.
155. Reuler JB. Hypothermia: pathophysiology, clinical settings and management. *Ann Intern Med* 1978;89:519–527.
156. Buckley JJ, Bosch OK, Bacaner MB. Prevention of ventricular fibrillation during hypothermia with bretylium tosylate. *Anesth Analg* 1971;50:587–593.
157. Danzl DF, Sowers MB, Vicario SJ, et al. Chemical ventricular defibrillation during hypothermia with bretylium tosylate. *Ann Emerg Med* 1982;11:698–699.
158. Gillen JP, Vogel MFX, Holterman RK, Skeindzielewski JJ. Ventricular fibrillation during orotracheal intubation of hypothermic dogs. *Ann Emerg Med* 1986;15:412–416.
159. Danzl DF, Pozos RS. Multicenter hypothermia survey. *Ann Emerg Med* 1987;16:1042–1045.
160. Maningas PA, DeGuzman LR, Hollenbach SJ, et al. Regional blood flow during hypothermic arrest. *Ann Emerg Med* 1986;15:390–396.
161. Lombino D, Dixon R, Rusnaic R, Dougherty J. Transcutaneous pacing in a hypothermic dog model (Abstract). *Ann Emerg Med* 1991;20: 459.
162. Siebke H, Breivik H, Rod T. Survival after 40 minute submersion without cerebral sequelae. *Lancet* 1975;1:1275–1277.
163. Miller JW, Danzl DF, Thomas DM. Urban accidental hypothermia: 135 cases. *Ann Emerg Med* 1980;9:456–461.
164. Sprung JJ, Cheng EY, Gamulin S, et al. Effects of acute hypothermia and B-adrenergic receptor blockade on serum potassium concentration in rats. *Crit Care Med* 1991;19:1545–1551.
165. Schaller MD, Fischer AP, Perret CH. Hyperkalemia. A prognostic factor during acute severe hypothermia. *JAMA* 1990;264:1842–1845.
166. Rohrer MJ, Natale AM. Effect of hypothermia on the coagulation cascade. *Crit Care Med* 1992;20:1402–1405.
167. Johnston TD, Chen Y, Reed R, II. Functional equivalence of hypothermia to specific clotting factor deficiencies. *J Trauma* 1994;37:413–417.
168. Haneda K, Sands M, Thomas R, et al. Prolongation of the safe interval of hypothermic circulatory arrest: 90 minutes. *J Cardiovasc Surg* 1983;24:15–21.
169. Lapp NL, Juergens JL. Frostbite. *Mayo Clin Proc* 1965;40:932–938.
170. Washburn B. Frostbite. *N Engl J Med* 1962;266:974–989.

*Environmental and Occupational Medicine, Third Edition,* edited by William N. Rom.
Lippincott–Raven Publishers, Philadelphia © 1998.

# CHAPTER 105

# Occupational Exposure to Vibration

Donald E. Wasserman

Probably since earliest time, when humans first took to the sea, the debilitating and incapacitating effects of vibrating motion have been known. With the beginning of the Industrial Revolution came vibrating hand tools and automated machinery. Raynaud's phenomenon first appeared in 1911 to 1918 in some workers who used vibrating hand tools. Post–World War II, with the introduction of modern aircraft, ships, vehicles, etc., emerged a myriad of studies to determine how vibration affects the ability of human beings to function and perform work. It is now apparent that occupational vibration affects the worker's health and the ability to work safely (1).

Approximately 8 million workers in the United States are exposed to occupational vibration (2). Of these, 6.8 million are principally associated with vehicular operation (e.g., truck and bus driving, farming, construction) where vibration impinges on the entire body. The remaining 1.2 million workers are users of gasoline powered tools (e.g., chain saws, brush cutters, etc.), and users of pneumatic and electrical hand tools. Vibration impinges locally and principally on the upper limbs when using the aforementioned tools. The former vibration is referred to as whole-body vibration (WBV), and is usually transmitted to the entire human body through some supporting structure, such as a vehicle seat or a building floor; the latter vibration is referred to as segmental or hand-arm vibration (HAV) and usually is applied locally to specific body parts, for example the hands, by a vibrating tool. The generic term *vibration* refers to back-and-forth, up-and-down, side-to-side linear motion that emanates from and returns to some defined reference position. Rotational motion (pitch, yaw, and roll) also occurs, but is rarely measured in occupational situations. Although WBV and HAV are usually distinct, some workers may be exposed to both types of vibration, depending on the job. For example, a worker using a pneumatic jackhammer or road ripper tool with outstretched arms receives principally HAV, whereas if the worker operates the tool so that it is placed in contact with the abdomen, the vibration reverts to WBV (3,4).

A person who works at the same job with vibration exposure for 20 hours per week, 50 weeks per year, for 30 years, that person can receive up to 30,000 hours of cumulative vibration exposure. Thus it is imperative to monitor and minimize both the acute and chronic effects of the vibration exposure on workers.

## TERMINOLOGY

To understand vibration's effects on humans it is important to be familiar with some terms. Vibration frequency, expressed in Hertz (Hz), describes the cyclic nature of vibration. One Hertz means that one complete cycle of measurable vibrating source motion occurs in 1 second, two Hertz means that two cycles of source motion occur in 1 second, etc. For WBV, the 1-Hz to 80-Hz band (range) is of interest; for HAV the band is from 5 to 5,000 Hz. In the occupational setting, usually more than one vibration frequency is simultaneously present, thus constituting a "vibration spectrum" that must be analyzed. Vibration motion per se is characterized as a "vector quantity," which consists of both a direction and a magnitude. Three mutually perpendicular (linear) vectors at each vibrating point are usually measured. Each vector magnitude can be expressed either as (a) vibration displacement, which refers to the distance traversed between the normal resting position of an object and its position at

D. E. Wasserman: Human Vibration and Biomedical Engineering Consultant, Biodynamics, Cincinnati, Ohio 45242-6437.

a given time in its vibratory cycle (in units of inches, feet, centimeters, millimeters, etc.); (b) velocity (speed) of a moving object, which refers to the time rate of change of displacement (in units of feet per second, meters per second, etc.); or (c) a moving object's speed, which usually changes over time; this time rate of change of speed or velocity is acceleration and is expressed in gravitational units *(g)*, or in meters per second per second ($1g = 9.81$ m/sec/sec). Acceleration has been the most frequently used measure of vibration intensity or magnitude, owing in part to its ease of measurement, and from this one parameter both vibration velocity and displacement can be mathematically derived. Resonance refers to the optimum condition of maximum transfer (or coupling) of vibration energy from the vibrating source to the receiver (e.g., the human body) accompanied by an actual amplification of the incoming vibration by the human body per se; thus in a resonant situation the body uncontrollably acts in concert with the incoming vibration, exacerbating the effects (5).

## WHOLE-BODY VIBRATION

Epidemiology and laboratory studies have shown that WBV is a form of cumulative trauma; it can be regarded as a generalized stressor and may affect multiple body parts and organs, depending on the vibration stimuli characteristics. Thus vibration exposure time, direction, and intensity are important, and the human resonance is especially important since resonance represents the Achilles' heel of human response to vibration. When the vibration impinges vertically on the body, the principal WBV resonance occurs in the 4- to 8-Hz band (nominally 5 Hz). When the vibration impinges horizontally or laterally, WBV resonance occurs in the 1- to 2-Hz band. These resonances are due principally to the response of the upper trunk and torso. The head-shoulder system can resonate in the frequency range of 20 to 30 Hz, and the eyeballs can resonate in the 60- to 90-Hz range. The hand-arm system appears to resonate in the 150- to 200-Hz range. Other body parts can resonate at other frequencies.

The significance of resonance can best be described by a simple example. If a 5-Hz vibration magnitude of 1*g* were applied to a human subject's buttocks, one could expect to measure as much as a 1.5*g* vibratory magnitude at the cranial level. Thus the body has intensified the actual acceleration applied by a factor of 1.5. The concern is that many vehicles, for example, contain 5-Hz vibration components that reach the body, as do higher-frequency tool components that reach the resonance of the hand-arm system and can stimulate this response (5).

With regard to WBV medical effects, studies of human subjects have shown that during WBV exposure oxygen consumption and pulmonary ventilation increase (6–8). One study of 78 Russian concrete workers exposed to WBV showed marked changes in bone structure involving spine deformations, intervertebral osteochondrosis, and calcification of the intervertebral disks and Schmorl's nodes (9). Hypoglycemia, hypocholesterolemia, and low blood ascorbic acid levels in concrete workers exposed to WBV have also been reported (10,11). In an early study of agricultural and forestry workers, a rare clinical description of so-called WBV sickness is found (12):

"The first stage is marked by epigastralgia, distention, nausea, loss of weight, drop in visual acuity, insomnia, disorders of the labyrinth, colonic cramps, etc. The second stage is marked by more intense pain concentrated in the muscular and osteoarticular systems. Objective examinations of the workers disclosed muscular atrophy and tropic skin lesions. it is apparent that it is difficult to determine the critical moment at which pathologic changes set in, especially due to differences in individual sensitivity to vibration."

In the early 1970s the National Institute for Occupational Safety and Health (NIOSH) conducted several morbidity records studies in the following groups of U.S. workers: bus drivers, truck drivers, and heavy equipment operators. The study of bus drivers revealed a statistically significant excess of venous, bowel, respiratory, muscular, and back disorders in a population of 1,448 interstate bus drivers exposed to WBV who were compared to office workers and general population control groups (13). The study concluded that the combined effects of WBV, body posture, postural fatigue, and poor dietary habits contributed to the occurrence of these disorders. The study of truck drivers examined 3,205 drivers and a control group of unexposed air traffic controllers (14). The study conclusions indicated that WBV, forced body posture, cargo handling, and poor eating habits contributed to significant excesses of back pain, spine deformities, strains, sprains, and hemorrhoids among the truck drivers. The first study of heavy equipment operators (15) found that WBV-exposed workers had an excess of certain musculoskeletal diseases, including slipped disks, limb fractures, male genital diseases (prostate), ischemic heart disease, and obesity of nonendocrine origin. A study of farm tractor drivers revealed that, in many cases, the effects of WBV were exacerbated by poor seats, poor seating posture, and long working hours (16). A recent critical review of WBV epidemiology studies with regard to the back concluded, "The most frequently reported adverse effects (of WBV) are: low back pain, early degeneration of the lumbar spinal system, and herniated lumbar disks....It must be concluded that long-term exposure to WBV is harmful to the spinal system" (17). Particularly disturbing are recent reports suggesting that WBV-exposed female workers experience a high risk of menstrual disorders, abortion, varicosities, and hyperemesis gravidarum (18).

Most whole-body vibration researchers would agree that hard-tissue (mostly lumbar) spinal disorders are the most frequently reported disorders associated with occupational WBV exposures. But these lumbar spine disorders must be tempered with the patient's work history of lifting heavy objects and related activities that can confound the diagnosis.

Finally, it is important to note that kinetosis can appear in the very low WBV frequency vibration range of 0.1 to 1 Hz (19) and rarely are there carryover effects on workers after the exposure ceases.

Through the years there have been many human performance studies of WBV. Most have used young, physically fit military personnel, such as jet aircraft pilots, for short time periods (up tp 30 minutes) in simulated military situations (20). Studies of vibration have shown that the lowest subjective discomfort-tolerance level occurs around the 5-Hz resonance frequency. Manual tracking capability is also most seriously affected at 5 Hz. Visual acuity is severely impaired in the 1- to 25-Hz range (21,22). Performance of tasks such as pattern recognition, reaction time, and monitoring appear not to be affected by WBV exposure (22). Laboratory studies using simulated heavy equipment driving tasks that compared the effects of a mixture of multiple vibratory frequencies (i.e., a limited spectrum) showed that human subjects performed worse under the mixed-vibration conditions containing a 5-Hz resonant frequency gradually improving as the mixture was replaced by nonresonant single sinusoidal vibration (23).

### Whole-Body Vibration Control

Currently there are three WBV standards in use in the United States, International Standards Organization (ISO) 2631 (24), American National Standards Institute (ANSI) S3.18, and American Conference of Government Industrial Hygienists-Threshold Limit Values (ACGIH-TLV) for WBV. Both of the latter standards were derived from, and are similar to, the ISO 2631 standard. All of these standards (a) attempt to codify what is known about WBV, (b) define uniform methods of gathering and analyzing three axes vibration data, and (c) compare the analysis results to health and safety guidelines prescribed by these standards. In addition to using these standards, the following measures to minimize WBV worker exposure effects should be considered:

1. Do not remain on a vibrating surface any longer than absolutely necessary.
2. If possible, locate machine controls remotely, a short distance from the vibrating surface.
3. In the case of vehicles, use vibration-isolated suspended or air-ride seats. Mechanically isolate other vibrating sources from workers.
4. Carefully maintain vibration sources to prevent excessive vibration from developing.
5. Do not lift objects immediately after emerging from a vehicle after a lengthy ride; rather, first walk around for a few minutes.

## HAND–ARM VIBRATION

Hand–arm vibration (HAV), or segmental vibration, unlike WBV, appears as locally applied cumulative trauma to the fingers and hands of exposed workers using gasoline powered, pneumatic, or electrical hand tools such as chain saws, chipping hammers, grinders, jackhammers, jack-leg type drills, etc. Extensive use of such tools (especially in cold environments) has been causally linked to Raynaud's phenomenon of occupational origin, also variously called "dead hand" or "vibration white fingers" (VWF) and most recently termed hand–arm vibration syndrome (HAVS). This condition is characterized by tingling, numbness, and blanching of the fingers with probable loss of muscle control and reduction of sensitivity to heat and cold with accompanying pain on return of the circulation (25).

Historically, the condition of blanching, numbness, and tingling in the fingers of clinical patients was first reported in 1862 by the French physician Maurice Raynaud in his M.D. thesis, "Local Asphyxia and Symmetrical Gangrene of the Extremities" (26), which describes "a condition, a local syncope, where persons, who are ordinary females, see under the least stimulus one or more fingers becoming white and cold all at once. The determining cause is often the impression of cold. The cutaneous sensibility also becomes blunted and then annihilated." This is primary Raynaud's disease. Raynaud's phenomenon affects up to 10% of the general population and 5% or 6% of the working male population. These blanching attacks usually affect the fingers symmetrically and are relatively trivial in the early stages of the disease. In later stages the attacks become severe and painful, leading to blue, cold fingers wherein the skin becomes atrophic, later ulcerated, and finally gangrenous. Raynaud also noted that the number and severity of blanching attacks increased during times of emotional stress.

In 1911 Loriga in Italy first described the initial association of vibrating hand tools and Raynaud's symptoms in the hands of miners who used pneumatic hand tools (27). In 1918, the famous study of Dr. Alice Hamilton was reported (28). She studied stone cutters using pneumatic hammers in the Oolitic limestone quarries of Bedford, Indiana. She reported:

> Among men who use the air hammer for cutting stone there appears very commonly a disturbance in the circulation of the hands which consists in spasmodic contraction of the blood vessels of certain fingers, making them blanched, shrunken, and numb. These attacks come on under the influence of cold, and are most marked, not while the man is at work with the hammer, but usually in the morning or after work. …The fingers affected are numb and clumsy when the vascular spasm persists. As it passes over there may be decided discomfort and even pain, but the hands soon become normal in appearance and as a usual thing the men do not complain of discomfort between the attacks. …The condition is undoubtedly caused by the use of the air hammer; it is most marked in those branches of stonework where

> the hammer is most continuously used and it is absent only where the air hammer is used little or not at all. Stonecutters who do not use the air hammer do not have this condition of the fingers. ...Men who have given up the use of the air hammer for many years may still have their fingers turn white and numb in cold weather. ...The trouble seems to be caused by three factors: long-continued muscular contraction of the fingers in holding the tool, the vibration of the tool, and cold. It is increased by too continuous use of the air hammer, by grasping the tool too tightly, by using a worn, loose air hammer, and by cold in the working place. If these factors can be eliminated the trouble can probably be decidedly lessened.

In the 1930s, reports by Seyring (29), who studied fettlers in iron foundries, by Telford and co-workers (30), who described men working with electrically driven rotating tools in a warm environment, and by Hunt (31), who studied riveters using pneumatic tools, all showed that VWF was on the increase. In 1939, Leys (32) reported diffuse scleroderma and Raynaud's phenomenon in a pneumatic hammer operator. In 1947, Agate and Druett (33) examined 230 men who were grinding excess metal from small castings; of this total, 163 (71%) had a history of white fingers, later to be called VWF. With further research into VWF in the 1950s, signs and symptoms associated with vibrating tools were reported in other systems, such as the peripheral nerves, bones, joints, and muscles. The association of VWF with these disabilities became known later as hand-arm vibration syndrome.

In 1962 and 1964, Ashe and colleagues (34,35) at Ohio State University investigated a small group of hard-rock drillers from Saskatchewan, seven of whom were examined in the hospital. As part of these investigations, arteriography and biopsy of the digital arteries were performed. Results showed that, in the worst cases, extensive damage to the digital artery intima with narrowing of the lumen had occurred as a result of the vibration exposure.

From 1964 on, a significant number of vibration syndrome cases appeared in the United Kingdom, up to 90% in the logging and forestry industries, where gasoline-powered chain saws had been in widespread use for some 12 to 14 years. The clinical state of the hands of workers using these chain saws was deteriorating to such an extent that the British Forestry Commission, in 1971, issued workers newly designed antivibration (A/V) saws, which were based on the best available vibration criteria of the time for 6 to 7 hours per day, 5 days per week exposure (25).

In the United States there were no studies after the 1918 Hamilton study until 1946, when Dart (36) described the effects of vibrating hand tools on 112 workers in the aircraft industry. He noticed that these workers complained of pain, swelling, and increased vascular tone in the hands, as well as tenosynovitis. The lack of U.S. studies then resumed until the aforementioned Ashe studies.

In the early 1970s, NIOSH estimated that some 1.2 million U.S. workers were exposed to occupational hand-arm vibration (1). In 1975 NIOSH sponsored an international hand-arm conference, where the epidemiologic, medical, clinical, physiologic, and engineering aspects of vibration syndrome and vibration measurements were discussed in depth (37). This conference became the catalyst for NIOSH's work through the mid-1980s. In particular, NIOSH conducted a series of comprehensive studies of pneumatic tool users, chippers, and grinders in foundries and shipyards, and repeated the 1918 Hamilton study, 60 years later in Bedford, Indiana. The results of the foundry and shipyard studies (38–41), showed that high prevalences of vibration syndrome ranged from (1) approximately 50% in exposed foundry workers, with a latent interval (i.e., between first vibration exposure and appearance of the first white fingertip) of some 1 to 2.4 years to (2) 20% with a latent interval of some 20 years in a shipyard. The differences in prevalences and corresponding latent intervals between the former and latter were attributed, to a large extent, to the fact that the foundries studied used the incentive system (i.e., piecework) but the shipyard did not. The repeat of the Bedford study (42) showed a similar prevalence of vibration syndrome to that found by Dr. Hamilton (83%). Sadly, virtually nothing had changed in 60 years except the victims! In response to these findings, NIOSH in 1983 issued a warning to the medical community about the consequences of HAV exposure (43).

### Medical Assessment (53)

It is important that primary Raynaud's disease, as originally described by Raynaud, be distinguished from secondary Raynaud's phenomenon. Secondary Raynaud's (Table 1) may arise from (a) exposure to vibration; (b) trauma, such as lacerations and fractures of the fingers and hands; (c) frostbite; (d) occlusive vascular disease, such as arteriosclerosis; (e) intoxication, as from ergot or nicotine; and (f) neurogenic causes such as poliomyelitis. It is also necessary to exclude causes of reduced blood flow to the fingers from compression of the main blood vessels at the outlet of the thorax (e.g., cervical rib or "thoracic outlet" syndrome). In addition, connective tissue disorders, such as scleroderma, polyarteritis nodosa, and rheumatoid arthritis, may cause secondary Raynaud's phenomenon (Table 1). It is recognized that it may not be possible to eliminate confounding conditions during the diagnostic process, since on occasion scleroderma and sclerodactyly with vibration-induced Raynaud's have occurred simultaneously in patients (32,44) as have carpal tunnel syndrome (CTS) and primary Raynaud's (45,46).

Some years ago Taylor (25) and Pelmear developed a white finger grading system, which bears their names and became widely used in many countries (Table 2). Their system tended to emphasize the vascular component of HAVS. In 1986 a meeting was held in Stock-

**TABLE 1.** *Exclusion criteria and differential diagnosis for hand–arm vibration syndrome*

| | |
|---|---|
| Primary | |
| Raynaud's disease | Constitutional white finger |
| Secondary | |
| Raynaud's phenomenon connective-tissue disease | Scleroderma, systematic lupus erythematous, dermatomyositis, polyarteritis nodosa, mixed connective-tissue disease |
| Trauma | |
| Direct to the extremities | Following injury, fracture, or operation; occupational origin, vibration; frostbite and immersion syndrome |
| To proximal vessels by compression | Thoracic outlet syndrome (cervical rib, scalenus anterior muscle), costoclavicular and hyperabduction syndromes |
| Occlusive vascular disease | Thromboangiitis obliterans, arteriosclerosis, embolism, thrombosis |
| Dysglobulinemia | Cold hemagglutination syndrome; cryoglobulinemia, macroglobulinemia |
| Intoxication | Acro-osteolysis, ergot, nicotine |
| Neurogenic | Poliomyelitis, hemiplegia, syringomyelia |
| Other | Carpal tunnel syndrome |

holm, Sweden, at which a modified Taylor-Pelmear system was adopted with the concurrence of Drs. Taylor and Pelmear. The modified system, called the Stockholm system (47), came about in recognition that although the majority of HAVS subjects have a combination of neurologic and vascular signs and symptoms, it became necessary to separate these two components and stage or classify each independently, since it is possible that the neurologic component of the syndrome can progress independently of the peripheral space vascular component in some patients.

Given that the Taylor-Pelmear system has been used for many years and that the literature is replete with studies that use it, and given the relative newness of the Stockholm system (Table 3), both systems will be addressed here.

The Taylor-Pelmear system was developed for grading HAVS patients and uses the results of the physical examination, occupational health history, history of social impairment (as a direct consequence of induced white finger), and the degree of interference with hobbies; the HAVS patient is placed into one of the following categories (see Table 2): The initial symptoms of HAVS are tingling or numbness after vibration exposure. In stage 1, as vibration exposure time increases, finger blanching attacks begin and increase in number, duration, and severity. They occur at first mainly in cold temperatures, and especially during the early morning, either at home, with chores, or en route to work as a result of exposure to the elements (e.g., grasping a cold steering wheel, driving a motorcycle), or during morning rest breaks. Workers who work outside in all weather conditions (e.g., forestry workers) are most prone to early morning attacks. Workers may report interference both at work and during hobby and leisure activities (e.g., gardening, fishing, woodworking, auto maintenance, etc.). All such activities have one common factor: a reduced environmental temperature, which triggers an HAVS attack. The latent period to finger blanching is defined as the time interval from when the worker began using the vibrating tool(s) to the appearance of the first white fingertip; also note that thumbs generally do not blanch during an HAVS attack.

In stage 2 there is a limitation of hobby activities. In stage 3, there is a definite cessation of hobby activities as well as interference with work, particularly in outdoor jobs such as forestry, and especially in the winter; difficulty with fine manual dexterity; difficulty in feeling and

**TABLE 2.** *Stage assessment for HAVS[a] (Taylor–Pelmear classification system)*

| Stage | Condition of fingers | Work and social interference |
|---|---|---|
| OO | No tingling, numbness, or blanching of fingers | No complaints |
| OT | Intermittent tingling | No interference with activities |
| ON | Intermittent numbness | No interference with activities |
| OTN | Intermittent tingling and numbness | No interference with activities |
| 1 | Blanching of a fingertip with or without tingling and/or numbness | No interference with activities |
| 2 | Blanching of one or more fingers beyond tips, usually during winter | Possible interference with activities outside work; no interference at work |
| 3 | Extensive blanching of fingers; frequent episodes in both summer and winter | Definite interference at work, at home, and with social activities; restriction of hobbies |
| 4 | Extensive blanching of most fingers; frequent episodes in both summer and winter | Occupation usually changed because of severity of signs and symptoms |

[a]Complications are not used in this grading system.

**TABLE 3.** *Stockholm-revised vibration syndrome classification system*

| Stage | Grade | Description |
|---|---|---|
| Vascular component[a] | | |
| 1 | Mild | Occasional blanching attacks affecting tips of one or more fingers |
| 2 | Moderate | Occasional attacks distal and middle phalanges of one or more fingers |
| 3 | Severe | Frequent attacks affecting all phalanges of most fingers |
| 4 | Very severe | As in stage 3 with trophic skin changes (tips) |
| Sensorineural component[a] | | |
| | OSN | Vibration exposed—no symptoms |
| | 1SN | Intermittent or persistent numbness with or without tingling |
| | 2SN | As in 1SN with reduced sensory perception |
| | 3SN | As in 2SN with reduced tactile discrimination and manipulative dexterity |

[a]The staging is made for each hand. The final grade of the disorder is indicated by the stage and the number of affected fingers in each hand (e.g., stage/hand/no. of digits).

Note: This Stockholm Classification System is based on:
(a) Removal of the unquantifiable areas—difficulty at work, home, and hobby activities.
(b) Discarding the seasonal component.
(c) The syndrome to be separated into two major areas—vascular and sensorineural.
(d) Separate staging of each hand.

picking up small coins; difficulty in buttoning/unbuttoning clothing; finger clumsiness with increasing joint stiffness. In stage 4, the severity of the HAVS and interference with work, social activities, and hobbies are so intense that the patient changes occupation; tissue necrosis of the fingers can appear in rare instances with increased vibration and cold exposure in this stage.

It is to be noted that the preceding sequence of increasing stages of HAVS severity arises from the cumulative trauma effects of the impinging vibration on the hands, usually from prolonged and regular use of vibrating tools found in industry. The aforementioned latent interval is related to the vibration (acceleration) intensity; the shorter the latent interval, the more severe will be the HAVS if vibration exposure continues.

The Stockholm system (47) is shown in Table 3 and requires the examining physician to do extensive work/hobby histories in order to estimate the patient's vibration dose. Vascular, neurologic, and musculoskeletal objective tests must be performed in order to separately stage each hand for neurologic and for vascular damage. The following tests for HAVS are recommended (48,49):

- Vascular component tests: cold provocation tests; Doppler artery delineation; Allen and Louis-Prusik tests.
- Neurologic component tests: two-point discrimination and depth sense (aesthesiometry); vibrotactile threshold tests; light-touch, pain, and temperature appreciation and dexterity tests; Moberg and pinch tests.
- Musculoskeletal tests: dynamometer grip force and pinch tests.
- Differential diagnosis (neuropathy and polyneuropathy): Tinel's and Phalen's tests; nerve conduction velocity for median, ulnar, motor, and sensory nerves of the Tinel and Phalen tests (which indicate the degree of CTS symptoms).

### Hand–Arm Vibration Control

It is beyond the scope of this presentation to describe in detail the various methods for controlling HAVS in the workplace except to briefly mention them. Totally controlling HAVS usually is multifaceted and involves several measures (5,49,50).

The first line of control is better tool design (or tool redesign) that incorporates the engineering principles of vibration damping and isolation together with good ergonomic design. Currently there are many reduced vibration [or so-called antivibration (A/V)] gasoline-powered chain saws and related forestry and professional landscaping tools available; unfortunately, this is not the case for most pneumatic tools, except for a single major Swedish company with virtually a complete line of effective A/V tools. Although new A/V tools employing ergonomic principles are beginning to appear on the market, most tool companies have a few A/V tools at most in their complete lines.

The second line of control is A/V gloves, which use special viscoelasic materials to damp a broad spectrum of vibration. These gloves are also intended to keep the hands warm and dry and prevent cuts and lacerations. The main design challenge is allowing sufficient sensory feedback and dexterity with a minimum grip strength (in order to reduce vibration coupling into the hand).

The third line of control is hand–arm vibration standards, of which there are three in use in the United States (ACGIH-TLV, ANSI S3.34, NIOSH HAVS criteria document 89-106). Although all of these standards try to protect workers from the harmful effects of hand–arm vibration, these standards emphasize (weight) the lower vibration frequencies more than the high-frequency spectral components (51–53). As a result, some of these standards are in the process of being revised accordingly.

The fourth and final line of control is work practices and medical surveillance (5,43,49,50):

1. Any worker whose hands may be exposed to vibratory hand tools should, prior to employment, be physically examined and questioned about:
   a. Signs and symptoms of primary Raynaud's disease or Raynaud's phenomenon.
   b. Detailed history of vibration exposure (which should be recorded); on the basis of present medical evidence, it is not advisable to allow workers with primary Raynaud's disease to use vibratory hand tools.
2. A/V tools should be used when and where possible; all tools should be carefully maintained according to manufacturer's recommendations. Worn-out tools should be discarded and replaced with new ones, preferably A/V tools.
3. Workers are advised as follows:
   a. Use only full-finger A/V gloves at all times when using vibrating hand-tools. A/V gloves with fingertip material removed expose the fingertips to vibration and thus do not adequately protect the finger-hand system despite the fact that finger dexterity is improved.
   b. Wear adequate clothing to keep the body core temperature at a stable, acceptable level.
   c. Keep the hands warm before and during work.
   d. Do not allow the hands to become wet and chilled. Should this happen, dry and warm the hands and put on a pair of dry, warm A/V gloves. This may require carrying an extra pair of gloves.
   e. Do not smoke while using vibrating hand tools. Nicotine acts as a vasoconstrictor, reducing the blood supply to the fingers and hands.
   f. Let the tool do the work, grasping it as lightly as it is safe to do so, allowing the tool to rest on the workpiece where and when possible.
   g. Use only ergonomically designed A/V tools where and when possible.
   h. Use the tool only when absolutely necessary, operating at reduced speed when possible.
   i. Should signs of tingling, numbness, or white or blue fingers occur, see a physician promptly.
4. The hazard of HAVS can be reduced if continuous vibration exposure over long time periods is avoided. Therefore, a 10-minute vibration-free rest break for every hour of continuous vibration exposure is recommended.

## ACKNOWLEDGMENT

This chapter is dedicated to the late and venerable HAVS pioneer and colleague, William Taylor, M.D., whose inspiration, clinical, and epidemiology studies led the HAVS area for many years.

## REFERENCES

1. Wasserman DE, Badger DW. *Vibration and the worker's health and safety.* DHEW/NIOSH publication no. 77. Washington, DC: U.S. Government Printing Office, 1973.
2. Wasserman DE, Badger DW, Doyle TE, Margolies L. Industrial vibration: an overview. *J Am Soc Safety Engr* 1974;19:38–40.
3. Shields PG, Chase KH. Primary torsion of the omentum in a jackhammer operator: another vibration related injury. *J Occup Med* 1988;30: 892–894.
4. Wasserman DE. Jackhammer usage and the omentum. *J Occup Med* 1989;31:563.
5. Wasserman DE. *Human aspects of occupational vibration.* Amsterdam: Elsevier, 1987.
6. Duffner LR, Hamilton LH, Schmitz MA. Effects of whole-body vertical vibration on respiration in human subjects. *J Appl Physiol* 1962;17: 913–917.
7. Ernsting J. *Respiratory effects of whole-body vibration.* Publication no. 179. Farnborough, England: Royal Airforce Institute of Aviation Medicine, 1961.
8. Hood WB, Murray RH, Urschel CW. Cardiopulmonary effects of whole-body vibration in man. *J Appl Physiol* 1966;21:1725–1731.
9. Rumjancey GI. Bone structure changes in the spinal column of prefabricated concrete workers exposed to whole-body (50 Hz) vibration. *Gig Tr Prof Zabol* 1966;10:6–9.
10. Puskina NM. Biochemical blood values in workers exposed to vibration. *Gig Tr Prof Zabol* 1961;2:29–30.
11. Andreeva-Galanina ED. Towards a solution to the problem of degeneration and regeneration of peripheral nerves following experimental exposure to vibration. *Gig Tr Prof Zabol* 1969;4–9.
12. Jakubouski R. General characteristics of vibration of various workplaces in agriculture and forestry. *Med Wiej* 1969;4:47–50.
13. Gruber G, Zipperman HH. *Relationship between whole-body vibration and morbidity patterns among motor coach operators.* DHEW/NIOSH publication no. 75-104. Washington, DC: U.S. Government Printing Office, 1974.
14. Gruber G. *Relationship between whole-body vibration and morbidity patterns among interstate truck drivers.* DHEW/NIOSH publication no. 77-167. Washington, DC: U.S. Government Printing Office, 1976.
15. Milby TH, Spear RC. *Relationship between whole-body vibration and morbidity patters among heavy equipment operators.* DHEW/NIOSH publication no. 74-131. Washington, DC: U.S. Government Printing Office, 1974.
16. Berry CM. Agricultural hazards. In: Clayton GD, Clayton FE, eds. *Patty's industrial hygiene.* New York: Wiley, 1978.
17. Hulshof C. Whole-body vibration and low-back pain. A review of epidemiologic studies. *Int Arch Occup Environ Health* 1987;59:205–220.
18. Seidel H, Heide R. Long term effects of whole-body vibration: a critical survey of the literature. *Int Arch Occup Environ Health* 1986;58:1–12.
19. Guignard JC, McCauley M. Motion sickness incidence induced by complex periodic waveforms. Proceedings of the 21st Meeting of the Human Factors Society, 1977.
20. Goto D, Kanda H. *Motion sickness in the actual environment.* Document ISO TC 108/SC4/WG 2-63. Geneva: International Standards Organization, 1977.
21. Grether WF. Vibration and human performance. *Hum Factors* 1971;13: 203–205.
22. Shoenberger RW. Human response to whole-body vibration. *Percept Motor Skills* 1972;34(monograph suppl 1):127–153.
23. Cohen HH, Wasserman DE, Hornung R. Human performance and transmissibility under sinusoidal and mixed vertical vibration. *Ergonomics* 1977;20:207–216.
24. International Standards Organization. *Guide for the measurement and evaluation of human exposure to whole-body vibration* (ISO 2631). Geneva: ISO, 1978.
25. Taylor W. *The vibration syndrome.* London: Academic, 1974.
26. Raynaud M. Local asphyxia and symmetric gangrene of the extremities. (M.D. Thesis, Paris). In: *Selected monographs.* London: New Sydenham Society, 1888.
27. Loriga G. Pneumatic tools: occupation and health. In: *Encyclopedia of hygiene, pathology, and social welfare,* vol 2. Geneva: International Labor Office, 1934.
28. Hamilton A. *A study of spastic anemia in the hands of stonecutters.* Industrial Accident and Hygiene Series, Bureau of Labor Statistics/

Department of Labor report no. 19, bulletin 236. Washington, DC: U.S. Government Printing Office, 1918.
29. Seyring M. Disease resulting from work with compressed air tools. *Arch Gewerbepathol Gewerbehyg* 1930;1:359–361.
30. Telford ED, McCann MB, MacCormack DH. Dead hands in the users of vibrating tools. *Lancet* 1945;5:359–362.
31. Hunt JJ. Raynaud's phenomenon in workmen using vibrating instruments. *Proc R Soc Med* 1936;30:171–172.
32. Leys D. Diffuse scleroderma and Raynaud's phenomenon from the use of a pneumatic hammer. *Lancet* 1939;2:692.
33. Agate JN, Druett NA. A study of portable vibrating tools in relation to the clinical effects they produce. *Br J Ind Med* 1947;4:141–163.
34. Ashe WF, Cook WT, Old JW. A study of portable vibrating tools in relation to the clinical effects they produce. *Arch Environ Health* 1962;5:333–343.
35. Ashe WF, Williams N. Occupational Raynaud's. *Arch Environ Health* 1964;9:425–429.
36. Dart EE. Effects of high speed vibrating tools on operators engaged in the airplane industry. *Occup Med* 1946;1:515–550.
37. Wasserman DE, Taylor W, eds. *Proceedings of the International Occupational Hand-Arm Vibration Conference.* DHEW/NIOSH publication no. 77-170. Washington, DC: U.S. Government Printing Office, 1977.
38. Wasserman DE, Taylor W, Behrens V, Samueloff S, Reynolds D. *Vibration white finger disease in U.S. workers using chipping and grinding hand tools, vol 1, epidemiology.* DHEW/NIOSH publication no. 82-118. Washington, DC: U.S. Government Printing Office, 1982.
39. Wasserman DE, Reynolds D, Behrens V, Taylor W, Samueloff S, Basel R. *Vibration white finger disease in U.S. workers using chipping and grinding hand tools, vol 2, engineering.* DHEW/NIOSH publication no. 82-101. Washington, DC: U.S. Government Printing Office, 1982.
40. Behrens V, Wasserman DE, Taylor W, Samueloff S, Reynolds D. Vibration syndrome in chipping and grinding workers. *J Occup Med* 1984;26:765–788.
41. Taylor W, Wilcox T, Wasserman DE. *Health hazard evaluation report—Neenah Foundry Co.* DHEW/NIOSH report no. HHE-80-189-870. Washington, DC: U.S. Government Printing Office, 1981.
42. Taylor W, Wasserman DE, Behrens V, Samueloff S, Reynolds D. Effects of the airhammer on the hands of stonecutters; the limestone quarries of Bedford, Indiana revisited. *Br J Ind Med* 1984;41:289–295.
43. Fishman S, Wasserman DE, Behrens V. *Vibration syndrome, Current intelligence.* Bulletin no. 38. DHEW/NIOSH publication no. 83-110. Washington, DC: U.S. Government Printing Office, 1983.
44. Blair HM, Headington JT, Lynch PJ. Occupational trauma, Raynaud's phenomenon and sclerodactylia. *Arch Environ Health* 1974;28:80–82.
45. Conner DE, Kolisek FR. Vibration induced carpal tunnel syndrome. *Orthop Rev* 1986;15:49–50.
46. Wieslander G, Norback D, Gothe CJ, Juhlin L. Carpal tunnel syndrome and exposure to vibration, repetitive wrist movements, and heavy manual work. *Br J Ind Med* 1989;46:43–47.
47. Gemne G, Pyykko I, Taylor W, Pelmear PL. The Stockholm Workshop Scale for the Classification of Cold-Induced Raynaud's Phenomenon in the Hand-Arm Vibration Syndrome (revision of the Taylor-Pelmear Scale). *Scand J Work Environ Health* 1987;13:275–283.
48. Taylor W, Pelmear PL. Objective tests and dose/response relationships for the assessment of hand-arm vibration syndrome. *J Low Frequency Noise Vibration* 1989;8:69–74.
49. Pelmear PL, Taylor W, Wasserman D. *Hand-arm vibration:* a comprehensive guide for occupational health professionals. New York: Van Nostrand-Reinhold, 1992.
50. Wasserman DE. The control aspects of occupational hand-arm vibration. *Appl Ind Hyg* 1989;4:F22–26.
51. Pelmear PL, Leong D, Taylor W, Nagalingam M, Fung D. Measurement of vibration of hand-held tools: Weighted or unweighted? *J Occup Med* 1989;31:902–908.
52. Wasserman DE. To weight or not to weight... that is the question. *J Occup Med* 1989;31:909.
53. Starck J, Pekkarinen J, Pyykko I. Physical characteristics of vibration in relation to vibration-induced white finger. *J Am Ind Hyg Assoc* 1990;4:179–184.

*Environmental and Occupational Medicine, Third Edition,* edited by William N. Rom.
Published by Lippincott–Raven Publishers, Philadelphia, 1998.

CHAPTER 106

# Shift Work: Health and Performance Effects

Roger R. Rosa and Michael J. Colligan

Broadly defined, shift work involves work at times other than normal daylight hours of approximately 7:00 A.M. to 6:00 P.M. Because 24-hour operations are an inevitable component of numerous industries, night work or shift work is a necessary condition of employment for a significant segment of the American work force. Critical 24-hours operations include police and fire protection, medical care, transportation, communications, and energy and water utilities. Other industries require continuous processing or operate around the clock to optimize capital investment in machinery and other production materials. Estimates of the number of persons doing shift work range from 10% to 25% of all those employed (i.e., at least 11 million workers) (1,2).

Almost all occupations or industries have employees engaged in shift work. The U.S. Bureau of Labor Statistics (2) has reported that 2% to 10% of employees in all occupations work evening, night, or rotating shifts. These kinds of schedules happen quite often among, for example, police and firefighters. More than half of them work evenings and nights, and about one-fourth rotate shifts. Many transportation and public utility workers, about one-fifth, also work shifts. Long-haul truckers often make their best time in the evening or at night. Lately, many materials must be delivered "just in time," or just before they are used in manufacturing, which has forced truckers to take trips at any hour of the day or night.

Because of the necessity of 24-hour operations, shift workers often live at variance with the conventional pattern of human activity, which is highest in the day and evening hours. These deviations from the daytime (or diurnal) activity pattern place the shift worker in opposition to many human functions that oscillate within a 24-hour period. Physiologic processes (e.g., metabolic rate), psychological processes (e.g., short-term memory), and social processes (e.g., family interaction) all have demonstrated rhythmic increases and decreases in daily activity. These patterns are called circadian rhythms because they cycle about once a day (3).

Deviation from the normal daytime pattern (i.e., peak activity during the night) does not readily result in changes in circadian rhythms. The relative persistence of circadian rhythms has important implications for work scheduling, because working at night requires coping with physiologic, psychological, and social processes that are not in synchrony with a nighttime schedule (4). Consequently, shift work potentially can affect diverse aspects of worker health, efficiency, and well-being.

Previous research has examined the relationship between shift scheduling and physical and psychological health, safety, productivity, efficiency, job satisfaction, marital harmony, domestic stability, and social adjustment. The resulting literature has not been consistent, in some cases indicating positive effects associated with shift work, in other cases negative effects, and in still others no effect at all. Some of these inconsistencies may be attributed to limitations inherent in field research designs, but others reflect the subtleties and complexities of shift work's impact on worker adjustment (5–7). Extraneous conditions involving ergonomic and organizational factors, job demands, workers' personalities, sociodemographic characteristics, geographic location, recreational resources, housing arrangements, sociometric patterns, and social support may act to influence or modulate the

R. R. Rosa: Division of Biomedical and Behavioral Science, National Institute for Occupational Safety and Health, Cincinnati, Ohio 45226.

M. J. Colligan: Education and Information Division, National Institute for Occupational Safety and Health, Cincinnati, Ohio 45226.

effects of shift work. Nonetheless, perusal of the literature suggests that some generalizations about the risks potentially associated with shift work can be made.

Night and shift work have been associated with both immediate risk to worker or public safety and long-term risk to worker health and well-being. The immediate risks are related to reduced alertness as a result of both night work and poor sleep. The long-term risks may be a result of increasing intolerance to the stress and strain of constantly switching from a daytime to a nighttime orientation.

## IMMEDIATE EFFECTS

### Sleep

The most direct and consistent effect of shift work is the periodic reduction in the quantity, and impairment of the quality, of sleep. Both retrospective cross-sectional surveys and prospective sleep-diary types of studies have indicated that night-shift workers (i.e., day sleepers) consistently obtain less sleep than day- or evening-shift workers. Furthermore, night-shift workers often report their daytime sleep to be lighter, more fragmented, and less restful than sleep at night (8). Electroencephalographic (EEG) studies of shift workers' sleep have confirmed the self-reports (9). The general pattern of decreased total sleep time during the day (when working nights) is apparent whether the worker has a permanent night schedule or rotates shifts. Rotators, however, obtain less sleep, overall, than their counterparts on permanent schedules. Increasing experience with shift work apparently does not result in adaptation of sleep patterns, since older shift workers still show decreased daytime sleep (10).

Whether routine reductions in the length and quality of sleep result in long-term compromises to health is unclear. Poor sleep is a persistent complaint among shift workers and likely contributes to a general malaise or reduction in well-being sometimes experienced by these persons. Some researchers suggest that this malaise may be a factor in the development of other chronic conditions observed in association with shift work (11).

#### *Sleep Loss, Performance, and Safety*

The immediate deleterious effects of sleep loss have been demonstrated more consistently than long-term effects. Sleep loss makes people sleepier while awake, which may affect the shift worker's ability to perform activities safely and efficiently, both on and off the job. Increased sleepiness (or decreased alertness) in shift workers on the job has been demonstrated with subjective reports (12), objective performance testing (13), and EEG recordings showing brief, on-the-job sleep episodes (14). As would be expected, sleepiness is most apparent during night shift, and poor daytime sleep appears to be a contributing factor (15).

### Circadian Rhythms, Performance, and Safety

In addition to sleep loss, the nighttime downturn in other endogenous circadian processes also can contribute to reduced alertness and performance loss in shift workers. In the normal diurnal situation, these circadian processes are in synchrony with the sleep-wake cycle. Consequently, alertness and arousal are highest and performance is most efficient during the day. During the night, on the other hand, alertness is lowest, which allows for optimal sleep (3,16). In shift workers, these processes may be asynchronous with the sleep-wake cycle, and often they do not adapt to night work at the same rate as the sleep-wake cycle (4). Therefore, there are some night shifts when the worker experiences decreased alertness and performance efficiency both from sleep deprivation and from the asynchrony of other circadian rhythms. There will be other night shifts when a normal amount of sleep is obtained but loss of alertness and compromised performance will be experienced because other circadian rhythms have not adapted to the nighttime orientation. Consequently, a night worker experiencing a combination of sleep deprivation and unadapted (i.e., diurnally oriented) circadian rhythms is likely to be at higher risk for operational errors or accidents than a day worker. In support of this proposition, separate studies have indicated that meter reading errors at a gas works, and single-vehicle accidents believed to be fatigue-related, were most common between midnight and 7:00 A.M. (17).

### Social and Familial Disruptions

In his chapter on social problems of shift work, Walker (18) quotes Bunnage's conclusion, "Shift work interferes with the social and family life of shift workers more than it facilitates them." Because shift workers often work in the evening or sleep during the day, they frequently must sacrifice participation in social and family activities that commonly occur at those times. Furthermore, because most shift workers work in continuously operating organizations, they regularly are required to work weekends and holidays, when much social and family interaction occurs (18,19). Consequently, too little time with family and friends is the most frequent and most negatively rated complaint among shift workers. The extent to which such disruptions occur depends both on the worker's schedule and the degree of flexibility in the worker's social contacts and leisure pursuits (18,19). Solitary or time-flexible pursuits such as gardening, golf, or woodworking would be less disrupted by night work or rotating shift work than participatory or time-inflexible activities such as social clubs or team sports. Shift work often conflicts with child care and school activities and may place an extra burden on the spouse who must support these activities in the shift worker's absence. Thus, the work schedule affects not only the worker's social adjustment but also the family's adjustment. The children, for example, are forced to be quiet at inconvenient times so that the shift worker can sleep.

## LONG-TERM EFFECTS

### Health

Research into the health effects of shift work has involved a variety of strategies. Absenteeism (20), self-report health inventories, physical examination and physiologic monitoring (21), and mortality (22) all have been used in shift work investigations. For the most part, these studies have involved comparisons of day workers to shift workers on select health indices using cross-sectional samples, retrospective record searches, or short-term prospective designs (23). The findings have been contradictory, making it difficult to assert categorically that shift work causes certain illnesses (24).

Many researchers have focused on gastrointestinal and digestive disorders, on the assumption that shift work interferes with normal eating patterns (25) and because there is a circadian rhythm to gastric secretion (26). It has been proposed, however, that sociocultural differences in eating habits make generalizations difficult (27). Approximately 20 to 30% of the working population may be unable to adapt to shift work because of nervous diseases and digestive complaints. Weed (28) emphasized the need to control for crossover effects and selective attrition (the "survivor" or "healthy worker" effect) in shift-worker studies. Studies of workers who have left shift work indicate persistent health complaints attributed to the former work schedule (29).

The role of shift work in the causation of other illnesses is not clear. The incidence of cardiovascular disease and of nervous disorders appears to be no greater among shift workers than among the general population. Later studies have emphasized increased complaints of job stress and more frequent use of alcohol, sleeping pills, and tranquilizers (1). It is possible that the stresses associated with shift work have an indirect impact on health by, for example, exaggerating preexisting health problems, altering the dose-response characteristics of prescribed medication as a result of circadian variability (30), or increasing worker susceptibility to physical and chemical exposures in the workplace (30).

Recent intensive studies of the incidence of ischemic heart disease and cardiovascular risk factors in shift workers have produced stronger associations than previous studies. In a Swedish study of paper mill workers followed for 15 years, increasing risk of ischemic heart disease was associated with increasing exposure to shift work (31). This association was independent of age and smoking history. In a cross-sectional study by the same group, coronary atherosclerosis risk factors such as smoking and serum triglycerides were observed to be higher in shift workers than in day workers (32). It is not clear, however, which specific work schedule or other occupational factors related to shift work are precursors of higher cardiovascular risk. Disruptions of sleep-wake cycles and other circadian and social rhythms, as well as higher overall levels of perceived stress, need more focused consideration in regard to their cardiovascular risk potential.

## COUNTERMEASURES

Efforts to promote adaptation to, or ease the difficulties of coping with, shift work are relatively new. A sampling of interventions reviewed by Rosa and colleagues (33) include designing new work schedules, devising sleep strategies, altering circadian rhythms with bright light, optimally timing physical activity, improving physical conditioning, introducing pharmacologic aids, planning dietary regimens, applying stress reduction techniques, organizing social support groups, and providing family counseling. Empirical evaluations and applications of some techniques have begun, but the efficacy of most remains hypothetical.

With respect to work schedule design, for example, there are ongoing debates about the relative advantages of fixed versus rotating shifts (34), rapid (i.e., every few days) versus slow (several days or weeks) shift rotation (35), shift timing (36,37), and the use of compressed workweeks (38,39). In the compressed workweek schedule, longer (i.e., 10- to 12-hour) shifts are used so that fewer consecutive shifts are needed to complete a week's work. These schedules are popular because of the extra off-duty days, but there are persistent concerns about excessive fatigue from the longer shifts (especially 12-hour night shifts) (38–40). Sleep strategies involve napping either before or during the night shift (41). Opportunities for napping during the night shift have been permitted in other countries but not in the United States. Laboratory studies using appropriately timed exposure to bright light have indicated that circadian rhythms can be "phase-shifted" (i.e., the time of peak activity can be shifted) more rapidly than usual (42). However, only a few workplace applications have been attempted and results have been equivocal (42–44). Intense physical activity also can phase-shift circadian rhythms (45), but it is not clear whether the required level of exercise is agreeable to the average worker. Improved physical conditioning has beneficial effects on worker well-being, but it probably does not directly influence adaptation to shift work (46,47). Various pharmacologic compounds reliably induce sleep or alertness at desired times (48), or shift circadian rhythms (49), but the potential for adverse side effects in some compounds makes long-term use questionable. Dietary routines to promote alertness or relaxation have been proposed, but recommendations from different researchers have directly contradicted each other

(27). Stress reduction, social support, and family counseling generally have beneficial effects on well-being, but organized treatment plans and outcome studies for shift workers have yet to be devised (50).

## REFERENCES


1. Gordon NP, Cleary PD, Parker CE, Czeisler CA. The prevalence and health impact of shift work. *Am J Public Health* 1986;76:1225–1228.
2. Mellor EF. Shift work and flextime: How prevalent are they? *Monthly Labor Rev* 1986;109:14–21.
3. Minors DS, Waterhouse JM. Introduction to circadian rhythms. In: Folkard S, Monk TH, eds. *Hours of work:* temporal factors in work scheduling. Chichester: John Wiley, 1985;1–14.
4. Åkerstedt T. Adjustment of physiological and circadian rhythms and the sleep-wake cycle to shift work. In: Folkard S, Monk TH, eds. *Hours of work:* temporal Factors in work scheduling. Chichester: John Wiley, 1985;185–198.
5. Colligan MJ. Methodological and practical issues related to shift work research. *J Occup Med* 1980;22:163–166.
6. Colligan MJ, Smith MJ, Hurrel JJ, Tasto D. Shift work: a record study approach. *Behav Res Meth Inst* 1979;11:5–8.
7. Johnson LC, Tepas DI, Colquhoun WP, Colligan MJ, eds. *Biological rhythms, sleep, and shift work.* New York: Spectrum, 1981.
8. Lavie P, Chillag N, Epstein R, et al. Sleep disturbances in shift workers: a marker for maladaptation syndrome. *Work Stress* 1989;3:33–40.
9. Walsh JK, Tepas DI, Moss PD. The EEG sleep of night and rotating shift workers. In: Johnson LC, Tepas DI, Colquhoun WP, Colligan MJ, eds. *Biological rhythms, sleep, and shift work.* New York: Spectrum, 1981;371–381.
10. Tepas DI, Duchon JC, Gersten AH. Shift work and the older worker. *Exp Aging Res* 1993;19:295–320.
11. Naitoh P, Kelly TL, Englund C. Health effects of sleep deprivation. *Occup Med* 1990;5:209–238.
12. Folkard S, Monk TH, Lobban MC. Short and long-term adjustment of circadian rhythms in "permanent" night nurses. *Ergonomics* 1978;21: 785–799.
13. Wilkinson R, Allison S, Feeney M, Kaninska Z. Alertness of night nurses: two shift systems compared. *Ergonomics* 1989;32:281–292.
14. Torsvall L, Åkerstedt T, Gillander K, Knutsson A. Sleep on the night shift: 24-hour EEG monitoring of spontaneous sleep-wake behavior. *Psychophysiology* 1989;26:352–358.
15. Åkerstedt T. Sleepiness as a consequence of shift work. *Sleep* 1988;11: 17–34.
16. Monk T, Folkard S. Circadian rhythms and shiftwork. In: Hockey R, ed. *Stress and fatigue in human performance.* Chichester: John Wiley, 1983;97–121.
17. Mitler MM, Carskadon MA, Czeisler CA, Dement WC, Dinges DF, Graeber RC. Catastrophes, sleep, and public policy: consensus report. *Sleep* 1988;11:100–109.
18. Walker J. Social problems of shiftwork. In: Folkard S, Monk TH, eds. *Hours of work:* temporal factors in work scheduling. Chichester: John Wiley, 1985;211–226.
19. Colligan MJ, Rosa RR. Shift work effects on social and family life. *Occup Med* 1990;5:315–322.
20. De La Mare G, Walker J. Shift working: the arrangement of hours on night work. *Nature* 1969;208:1127–1128.
21. Wojtczak-Jaroszowa J. *Physiological and psychological aspects of night and shift work.* DHEW publication (NIOSH) 78-113. Washington, DC: U.S. Government Printing Office, 1977.
22. Taylor PJ, Pocock SJ. Mortality of shift and day workers 1956–68. *Br J Ind Med* 1972;29:201–207.
23. Ottmann W, Karvonen Ml Schmidt KH, Knauth P, Rutenfranz J. Subjective health status of day- and shift-working policemen. *Ergonomics* 1989;32:847–854.
24. Scott AJ, LaDou J. Shift work: effects on sleep and health with recommendations for medical surveillance and screening. *Occup Med* 1990; 5:273–299.
25. Stewart AJ, Wahlquist ML. Effect of shift work on canteen food purchase. *J Occup Med* 1985;27:552–554.
26. Moore JC, Englert E. Circadian rhythms of gastric acid secretion in man. *Nature* 1970;226:1261–1262.
27. Tepas DI. Do eating and drinking habits interact with work schedule variables? *Work Stress* 1990;4:203–211.
28. Weed DL. Historical roots of the healthy worker effect. *J Occup Med* 1986;28:343–347.
29. Koller M, Kundi M, Cervinka R. Field studies at an Austrian oil refinery. I: Health and psychosocial well-being of workers who drop out of shift work. *Ergonomics* 1978;21:835–847.
30. Smolensky MH, Reinberg A. Clinical chronobiology: relevance and applications to the practice of occupational medicine. *Occup Med* 1990;5:239–272.
31. Knutsson A, Åkerstedt T, Jonsson BG, Orth-Gomer K. Increased risk of ischaemic heart disease in shift workers. *Lancet* 1986;2:89–92.
32. Knuttson A, Åkerstedt T, Jonsson BG. Prevalence of risk factors for coronary artery disease among day and shift workers. *Scand J Work Environ Health* 1988;14:317–321.
33. Rosa RR, Bonnet MH, Bootzin RR, et al. Intervention factors for promoting adjustment to nightwork and shiftwork. *Occup Med* 1990;5: 391–415.
34. Knauth P, Rutenfranz J. Experimental shiftwork studies of permanent night, and rapidly rotating, shift systems. *Int Arch Occup Environ Health* 1976;37:125–137.
35. Knauth P. Speed and direction of shift rotation. *J Sleep Res* 1995; 4(suppl 2):41–46.
36. Kecklund G, Åkerstedt T. Effects of timing of shifts on sleepiness and sleep duration. *J Sleep Res* 1995;4(suppl 2):47–50.
37. Rosa RR, Härmä M, Pulli K, Mulder M, Näsman, O. Rescheduling a three-shift system at a steel rolling mill: effects of a 1-hour delay of shift starting times on sleep and alertness in younger and older workers. *Occup Environ Med* 1996;53:677–685.
38. Colligan MJ Tepas DI. The stress of hours of work. *Am Ind Hyg Assoc J* 1986;47:686–695.
39. Rosa RR. Extended workshifts and excessive fatigue. *J Sleep Res* 1995; 4(suppl 2):51–56.
40. Rosa RR, Colligan MJ, Lewis P. Extended work days: effects of 8-hour and 12-hour rotating shift schedules on performance, subjective alertness, sleep patterns, and psychosocial variables. *Work Stress* 1989;3: 21–32.
41. Rosa RR. Napping at home and alertness on the job in rotating shiftworkers. *Sleep* 1993;16:727–735.
42. Eastman CI, Boulos A, Terman M, Campbell SS, Dijk D-J, Lewy AJ. Light treatment for sleep disorders: consensus report. *J Biol Rhythms* 1995;10:157–164.
43. Budnick LD, Lerman SE, Nicolich MJ. An evaluation of scheduled bright light and darkness on rotating shiftworkers: trial and limitations. *Am J Ind Med* 1995;27:771–782.
44. Costa G, Ghirlanda G, Minors DS, Waterhouse JM. Effect of bright light on tolerance to night work. *Scand J Work Environ Health* 1993;19: 414–420.
45. Eastman CI, Hoese EK, Youngstedt SD, Liu L. Phase-shifting human circadian rhythms with exercise during the night shift. *Phys Behav* 1995;58:1287–1291.
46. Härmä MI, Ilmarinen J, Knauth P, Rutenfranz J, Hanninen 0. Physical training intervention in female shift workers: I. The effects of intervention on fitness, fatigue, sleep, and psychosomatic symptoms. *Ergonomics* 1988;31:39–50.
47. Härmä MI, Ilmarinen J, Knauth P, Rutenfranz J, Hanninen O. Physical training intervention in female shift workers: II. The effects of intervention on the circadian rhythms of alertness, short-term memory, and body temperature. *Ergonomics* 1988;31:51–63.
48. Walsh JK, Muehlbach MH, Schweitzer PK. Hypnotics and caffeine as countermeasures for shiftwork-related sleepiness and sleep disturbance. *J Sleep Res* 1995;4(suppl 2):80–83.
49. Arendt J, Deacon S, English J, Hampton S, Morgan L. Melatonin and adjustment to phase shift. *J Sleep Res* 1995;4(suppl 2):74–79.
50. Penn PE, Bootzin RR. Behavioral techniques for enhancing alertness and performance in shift work. *Work Stress* 1990;4:213–226.

*Environmental and Occupational Medicine, Third Edition,* edited by William N. Rom.
Lippincott–Raven Publishers, Philadelphia © 1998.

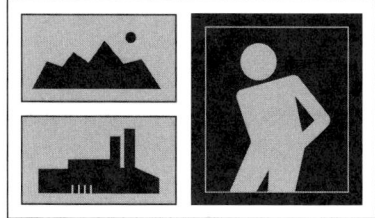

# CHAPTER 107

# Sleep Disorders and Work

Joyce A. Walsleben, Edward B. O'Malley, and David M. Rapoport

The world of sleep revolves around the light/dark cycles of day and night. The interaction of numerous physiologic processes governed by endogenous circadian pacemakers produce rhythmic changes in one's alertness, mood, and performance across the 24-hour day (1). For most of us, adequate sleep during the nighttime hours and alert functioning during the day is expected. Yet many of us are aware of the postlunch dip in functioning, and many have experienced the fatigued aftermath of a poor or short night's sleep. These normal occurrences highlight the two drives that interact to regulate the sleep/wake system: (a) circadian rhythm and (b) the need for adequate sleep. Unfortunately, little concern is given these "normal" experiences until something major goes wrong. Even then society is generally uninformed regarding the need for sleep, the consequences of poor sleep, and the potential for improvement. Society rewards irregular hours and heroic work schedules with promotions and perquisites, reinforcing the notion that increased hours of wakefulness at the expense of lost sleep is not only acceptable but, in many cases, necessary for success. We mistakenly believe that we can sacrifice our need for sleep without consequences.

As an example, a poll based on telephone interviews of 1,027 adults conducted by the Gallup Organization in October 1995 (2) and sponsored by the National Sleep Foundation found that over 50% of persons with symptoms of chronic sleep disorders (insomnia or sleep apnea) do not consider their sleeplessness enough of a problem to warrant consultation with a physician. One in four persons contacted believed that sleep and success are mutually exclusive. In fact, 20% of the persons polled believe that less sleep allows more productivity. Little concern is given to the impact of sleepiness on the quality of performance.

J. A. Walsleben: Division of Pulmonary and Critical Care Medicine; and New York University Sleep Disorders Center, New York University Medical Center, New York, New York 10016.

E. B. O'Malley: Division of Pulmonary and Critical Care Medicine, New York University Medical Center, New York, New York 10016; and Norwalk Hospital Sleep Disorders Center, Norwalk, Connecticut 06856.

D. M. Rapoport: Division of Pulmonary and Critical Care Medicine, New York University Sleep Disorders Center, New York University Medical Center, New York, New York 10016.

## SLEEP AND PERFORMANCE

The connection between sleep and performance has a long history. In 1896, Patrick and Gilbert (3) were the first to study performance as a critical probe of CNS function. They observed that sustained behavioral wakefulness (90 hours) resulted in decreased sensory acuity, reaction time, motor speed, and memory. They also noted the occurrence of uncontrollable napping and semiwake dreams in their sleep-deprived subjects. To be sure, these consequences remain true today and have been the subject of much research.

We now know that sleepiness is not a linear function of our time awake. Rather sleepiness is modulated by a circadian rhythm that acts as a pacemaker to promote sleep at night and wakefulness during the day. Within the 24-hour cycle there are two major nadirs for alertness, during which many people may feel slowed or sleepy. The stronger nadir occurs at night, between 10 P.M. and 8 A.M., peaking around 4 A.M.; the second occurs between 2 P.M. and 4 P.M. The subjective and objective signs of sleepiness are also modulated by a homeostatic drive influenced by the number of hours of preceding wakefulness. The longer we have been awake (the fewer hours we have slept), the more our drive for sleep increases. The homeostatic drive for sleep interacts with the circadian pacer so that we feel sleepier at times of the circadian nadir. Sleep need is also individually determined. The average amount required is 7 to 8 hours per 24-hour period. If sleep is curtailed, as frequently occurs with today's societal demands, sleep loss accumulates (4). This accumulation can be likened to a debt. For instance, a person who requires 7 hours of nightly sleep for optimal alertness but only captures 6 hours per night will incur a 5-hour sleep debt by week's end. Eventually, when the debt is large enough, or unmasked by boring or passive tasks, one can no longer maintain wakefulness and involuntary episodes of sleep will occur. These episodes, called microsleeps, may be as brief as 5 to 10 seconds in duration and often go unnoticed.

In terms of performance, however, the microsleeps are critical. A driver of an automobile who experiences a 5-second microsleep at 60 mph travels 440 feet! Vigilance and memory formation suffer during these episodes as well. Lapses in performance occur at a rate 3 to 10 times greater in persons who have been awake longer than 14 hours (5,6). Combined with an increasing sleep debt, performance is at its worst during the circadian nadirs. This is important information for supervisors who develop work schedules. Time on task, repetitiveness, and task attention also influence performance. The need for sleep may be unmasked and hard to combat when tasks are long, tedious, or boring. Repetitive tasks increase habituation in a sleepy brain and consequently unmask or augment underlying sleepiness (7). Motivation also plays a role; it can improve performance during short tasks, but is no guarantee if the sleep debt is large.

The fundamental effects of sleep loss permeate all levels of performance and negatively impact the workplace. Performance deficits can be subtle and first emerge as lapses, omissions, and cognitive deficits (8). These may be expressed as slowed or inappropriate decision making, perseveration, and poor overall job performance. Lapses in thought, memory, and speed occur that affect immediate and recall memory, perhaps due to faulty encoding (9) and decreased discriminability (10).

### The Cost of Sleepiness to Society

The impact on society from sleep deprivation is just beginning to be recognized (11). As has been noted, poor sleep quality or lack of adequate sleep results in impaired daytime function. For a worker involved with technology, precision machinery, transportation, or critical decision making, the effects of accumulated sleep loss can be sadly tragic. There are numerous examples of major accidents linked to sleepiness that have affected society over the last several years.

Upon investigation of the tanker *Exxon Valdez* crash in 1989, the National Transportation Safety Board (NTSB) found that a probable cause of the grounding of the *Exxon Valdez* was the failure of the third mate to properly maneuver the vessel because of fatigue and excessive workload (12). Total monetary cost of this crash was over $8 billion for cleanup, losses, and legal suits.

On August 18, 1993, an American International Airways flight to Guantanamo Bay, Cuba crashed/mile short of the runway. Three crew members sustained serious injury and the plane was lost. During the subsequent investigation the NTSB, it was noted that the crew had been on duty for 18 hours, having flown for 9 hours (13). Although this was well within the allowed maximum workday of 24 hours with 12 hours of flight time, investigators noted that the crash reflected the crew's poor judgment due to effects of fatigue and lack of vigilance.

The presidential commission investigating the disastrous launch of the spaceship *Challenger* in 1986 noted that time pressure, particularly that caused by launch scrubs and turnarounds, increased the potential for sleep loss and judgment errors, and that working excessive hours, while admirable, raises serious questions when it jeopardizes job performance, particularly when critical management decisions are at stake (14).

Local newspapers count driver deaths from single vehicle accidents occurring in the early morning hours, in the absence of other causes, on a weekly basis. Investigators note that the likely cause is that the driver fell asleep. The pervasiveness of this issue was highlighted by a recent telephone survey sponsored by the New York State (NYS) Governor's Task Force on Drowsy Driving. One thousand randomly selected licensed drivers in NYS were interviewed. Results showed that 24.7% of respondents reported falling asleep while driving; 4.7% reported actual crashes due to drowsiness or sleeping while driving. The likelihood of driving while sleepy increased with longer work hours. Thirty-nine percent of respondents who worked between 41 and 50 hours per week and 44.1% of those working over 50 hours reported falling asleep at the wheel compared to 23.6% of those working 36 to 40 hours (15).

While many of today's workers are reducing sleep times, others cannot enjoy the pleasure of a full night's sleep even though they try. It is well recognized that upwards of 30% to 49% of adult Americans will suffer from a sleep disorder during their work career. Presently there are over 80 known sleep disorders categorized by the International Classification of Sleep Disorders (16). This chapter discusses the major sleep disorders likely to produce sleepiness among working adults.

## INSOMNIA

Insomnia is generally defined as the subjective sense that sleep is difficult to initiate or maintain, or that sleep itself is nonrefreshing. Prevalence studies have shown that about one-third of the adult population experiences insomnia (nearly 10% as a chronic problem) (17). Many sufferers report daytime consequences similar to those associated with chronic sleep deprivation: fatigue, performance decrements, and mood disturbances (18). The daytime impairments result in decreased worker productivity, higher accident rate, and increased morbidity, with augmented use of medical facilities (19). These findings present an obvious cause for concern in the workplace.

### Pathophysiology

Insomnia often results from a combination of factors. The underlying causes are generally listed as the 5 P's: physical, psychological, psychiatric, pharmacologic, and physiologic. Physical factors like pain, illness, hormonal changes, and environmental disturbances can play a causative role in insomnia by acting to heighten the arousal system. Psychological stressors and active psychiatric disease can directly affect the body's ability to initiate or maintain sleep. Pharmacologic factors may cause insomnia in several ways: as a side effect of medications prescribed for other illnesses, through the arousing properties of caffeine and other central nervous system (CNS) stimulants, as a direct effect of ethanol ingestion, or indirectly as a rebound effect following withdrawal of CNS depressants initially prescribed as sleep aids. Finally, physiologic, or circadian changes such as those involving jet travel or rotating shift work can severely disrupt the sleep/wake cycle.

### Diagnosis

It is important to note that the complaint of insomnia is a symptom, not a disorder itself. Thus, careful evaluation of potential causes is indicated. Duration, accompanying symptoms, and the premorbid state are all critical factors important for accurate diagnosis. The principal diagnostic tools are subjective assessment of sleep quantity and quality. Diaries of sleep/wake activity are crucial to the investigation of symptoms and causes. Frequently, just the act of completing a diary encourages the individual to look more closely at behavioral influences or acknowledge that the symptoms are not as severe as previously thought. Objective polysomnography (the electrophysiologic recording of multiple parameters used to record sleep) may be used to exclude other physical causes of sleep disruption or document the individual's complaints.

### Treatment

Where possible, treatment should be addressed toward correction of the underlying cause, particularly when there are associated medical/psychiatric issues. Simple changes in routine, living situation, and food intake may be effective. In all cases, education regarding the mechanics of sleep, i.e., sleep promoting and interfering behaviors, is important (Table 1).

**TABLE 1.** *Techniques of good sleep hygiene*

| |
|---|
| Secure a calm, safe, and quiet environment |
| Settle disagreements with bed partner before bedtime |
| Plan a worry time during the day to reduce worries at night |
| Maintain regular wake time |
| Exercise regularly during late afternoon |
| If lying in bed awake and upset, get up but remain in quiet, darkened area |
| Limit use of alcohol, caffeine, and tobacco, especially late in day |
| Avoid naps unless they are regularly scheduled |

Specific treatment regimens are generally implemented in accordance with the time course of symptoms. Transient insomnia, lasting a few days to a couple of weeks, is usually associated with transmeridian travel, a brief illness, or a stressful event (next day examination or presentation), and hypnotics can be used as the main therapy (20,21). The most effective are the benzodiazepines and drugs with a similar chemical structure or agonist-like compounds. Short-term insomnia, lasting several weeks to a month, is usually associated with more traumatic life events that can be either negative (death of a loved one, divorce, or sudden hospitalization) or positive (marriage, job promotion, or birth of a child). Although hypnotic therapy is indicated over the short term, behavioral therapies and education are important to prevent the development of chronic insomnia. The longer insomnia persists, the more complex are its causes and treatment.

Long-term or chronic insomnia may last months to years (22). There are well-recognized effective behavioral treatments available to address the symptoms of chronic insomnia: sleep restriction, cognitive therapy, relaxation therapies, stimulus control, and biofeedback (22). These therapies have common modes of action and relieve insomnia by either reducing emotional/somatic arousal (cognitive and relaxation therapy, biofeedback) or improving sleep efficiency (sleep restriction, stimulus control). Behavioral therapies typically require a 6- to 8-week program to be effective. Hypnotics should not be viewed as the sole source of treatment particularly in the case of chronic insomnia. Rather, medication should be utilized as reinforcement for the educational and behavioral techniques.

There are also a number of safety concerns regarding the use of hypnotics. Each hypnotic has the potential to produce side effects, which include extended sedation, performance decrements, and amnesia (23), particularly in the elderly. These can usually be controlled through adequate dosage and selection of specific drug. Additionally, hypnotic agents have the potential to worsen other illnesses, especially respiratory-related disorders and depression. Risk of overdose leading to serious outcomes exist especially if the drug is combined with alcohol. Hence, tolerance and abuse potential should be closely monitored. Care should be given to match the symptom to the pharmacologic action of the drug; short half-life drugs can be used successfully for symptoms of poor sleep initiation, while longer acting drugs can be used for sleep maintenance problems or for associated daytime anxiety. Finally, there are classes of individuals for whom hypnotic therapy is counterindicated. These include the fragile elderly, pregnant women, and those needing to respond to emergencies in the night, such as firefighters or physicians.

Unfortunately, over 40% of people with complaints of insomnia have been reported to self-medicate with over-the-counter (OTC) products and/or alcohol (2). The use of these products is not without risk. Most OTCs produce anticholinergic side effects, e.g., dry mouth or oversedation, that may prove annoying or outright dangerous when taken with other medications. The sedating nature of alcohol, for instance, is contraindicated in patients with breathing disorders. Furthermore, while alcohol may hasten sleep onset, the body's metabolizing of alcohol through the night leads to fragmented sleep and profound REM sleep rebound and nightmares (24,25). Since rapid tolerance develops to the hypnotic properties of alcohol, there is also danger of escalating doses and potential dependence.

Finally, natural products such as L-tryptophan, an amino acid precursor to serotonin, and melatonin, a neurohormone secreted by the pineal gland in the dark, along with herbs such as valerian root, have captured public attention and are being freely used as sleep aids. While their known physiologic actions suggest a use in sleep/wake control, scientific evidence is mixed on these substances as regards both efficacy and risk (26–28). Not all natural products are safe in synthetic form, when taken in larger than physiologic doses, or at incorrect circadian times (29). Furthermore, there is a risk of contamination by impurities when production is not regulated by the Food and Drug Administration (FDA) (30).

## NARCOLEPSY

Narcolepsy is a debilitating lifelong central nervous system disorder of excessive daytime sleepiness affecting 0.03% to 0.05% of the worldwide population, effectively 1:2,500 Americans, with higher estimates among the Japanese (31). Symptoms are rare in prepubertal children, with onset peaking in the second decade, but continuing into the fifth decade of life. Frequently, the onset appears to be invoked by stressful life occurrences, e.g., death of a loved one, divorce. There is a pentad of primary symptoms that have been noted, although not all must be present for diagnosis. These symptoms include severe sleepiness, characterized by frequent sleep attacks during which the person cannot fight sleep; cataplexy, which is reversible motor inhibition, triggered by internal or external emotionally ladened stimuli, resulting in partial or complete sudden loss of muscle tone; hypnagogic hallucinations, which are sleep onset–related auditory, visual, or tactile sensations that may be pleasant or frightening, lasting seconds to minutes; sleep paralysis, characterized by areflexia of skeletal muscles, which may be partial or complete, noted at sleep onset or offset; and severely fragmented nocturnal sleep. All persons with narcolepsy are pathologically sleepy; 65% to 90% develop cataplexy, 30% to 60% develop hallucinations and sleep paralysis, and 50% develop fragmented nocturnal sleep. It is important to note that although persons with narcolepsy appear sleepier than others, they do not show higher total amounts of sleep on objective testing. Rather, they slide from sleep to wake and back in unconsolidated episodes across the 24-hour day. Although many persons with narcolepsy were misdiagnosed as having psychiatric illnesses in the past, there is no evidence to show that there is any more psychopathology in this group compared to any other (32).

### Pathophysiology

Research using the dog model of narcolepsy indicates that brain neurotransmitter dysfunction is involved in the pathophysiology of this disorder (33). Both the cholinergic and noradrenergic systems are involved. It has been noted that there is an upregulation of brain stem M2-cholinergic receptors and a decrease in the release of monoamines in narcoleptic dogs. Additionally, there is a strong association with the class II antigen of the major histocompatibility complex human leukocyte antigen (HLA) DR2 subtypes DR15 (DRB1*1501) and DQ6 (DQB1*0602), which suggests strong genetic involvement. While not conclusive or necessary for the diagnosis of narcolepsy, the best marker across ethnic groups is the DQB1-0602 (34). Currently, the pathophysiology of narcolepsy is felt to be multifactorial, involving other suspected pathogenic environmental factors such as viral infections, head trauma, and use of recreational dopaminergic drugs.

### Diagnosis

Accurate diagnosis of narcolepsy requires objective polysomnographic testing including a nocturnal polysomnogram (NPSG) followed by Multiple Sleep Latency Testing (MSLT) (35). The MSLT performed during the day provides four or five 20-minute opportunities for the patient to try to sleep. Latency to sleep onset is scored as well as the presence of REM sleep should it occur. Positive MSLT, following a night in which other sleep disorders are excluded, requires a mean latency to sleep of under 8 minutes with two REM onset naps. There is question as to whether the presence of cataplexy as a diagnostic marker could circumvent the need for full polysomnography. Although cataplexy may be a pathog-

**TABLE 2.** *Treatment rationale for narcolepsy*

| |
|---|
| Sleepiness |
|   Dopaminergic agonists |
|     CNS stimulants (amphetamine, methylphenidate, pemoline) |
|     Noradrenergic agonists (amphetamine) |
|   Adenosine receptor antagonist: methylxanthines |
|     Caffeine, theophylline |
|   Other wake-promoting agents (modafinil) |
| Cataplexy |
|   Catecholamine reuptake blockers |
|   Serotonin reuptake blockers |
|   Centrally acting cholinergic antagonists |

nomonic feature, which in the presence of sleepiness suggests the diagnosis, cataplexy is rarely witnessed in the clinical setting. Therefore, the clinician must rely on the patient's report. Since the diagnosis of narcolepsy usually requires lifelong treatment with stimulants, most states require objective testing rather than accepting patient reports as a prerequisite for treatment.

### Treatment

Thorough treatment of this disorder is very individualized and involves the understanding of both the clinician's expectations for outcome as well as the patient's and family's goals. Therapy typically involves the combination of pharmacologic and behavioral techniques. CNS stimulants, when tolerated, improve the symptoms of daytime sleepiness (36,37). Drug choice depends on expected outcome and the patient's reaction and side effects. Full daytime wakefulness may not be desired or, conversely, may be required by the patient's needs. Controversy regarding the prevalence and severity of stimulant therapy side effects exists. The presence of side effects may be associated with dosage and other factors such as general health. Side effects may include tolerance, changes in heart rate and blood pressure, possibility of abuse, and, in very rare cases, psychosis.

Antidepressant drugs improve the REM sleep–related symptoms of cataplexy, hallucinations, and sleep paralysis (Table 2). These drugs have norepinephrine (NE) reuptake blocking properties as well as anticholinergic effects. Although useful for cataplexy, they may be poorly tolerated due to their anticholinergic effects.

Behavioral techniques help to improve the symptom of sleepiness with and without pharmacologic therapy. Short (20-minute) daytime naps are refreshing. Regular sleep hours and daytime schedules help to reinforce nocturnal sleep.

## OBSTRUCTIVE SLEEP APNEA

The most common disorder resulting in daytime sleepiness among adult workers is obstructive sleep apnea syndrome (OSAS). OSAS is characterized by repetitive episodes of cessation of airflow during sleep, which result in brief arousals. Daytime consequences include excessive sleepiness, cardiovascular changes, and cognitive deficits (Fig. 1). Estimated prevalence suggests that 9% of females and 24% of males have more than five apneic episodes per hour, while 2% to 4% of the working adult public suffers from at least mild to moderate symptoms of this disease (38). The disorder is found more frequently in overweight males. However, it has been noted in obese females, particularly children and postmenopausal women. OSAS may also occur, especially in the mild form, in the absence of obesity. It has become

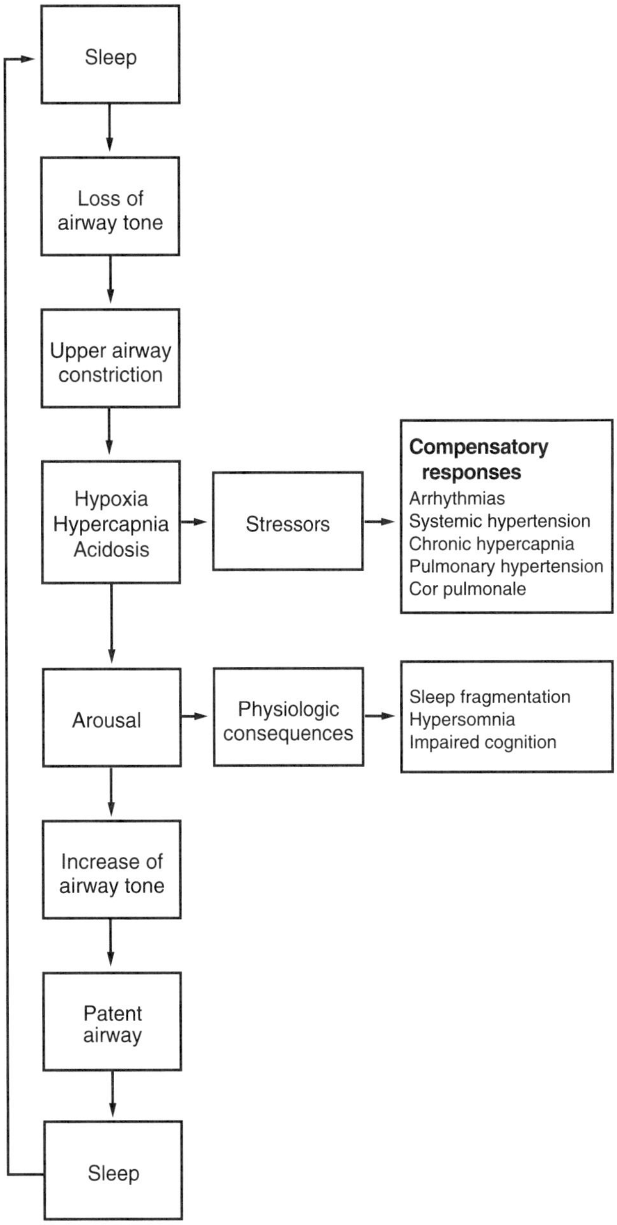


**FIG. 1.** Consequences of obstructive sleep apnea syndrome.

clear over the last two decades that OSAS is a frequent cause of morbidity (39).

### Pathophysiology

Obstructive apnea involves the actual cessation (apnea) or the reduction of airflow (hypopnea) for brief periods (10–60 seconds). It occurs repetitively during sleep, most frequently in response to complete or partial blockage of the upper airway. The blockage may be the result of changes in muscle tone that occur with sleep and the following factors: reclining position, blockage of the airway in the presence of redundant tissue or enlarged tonsils and adenoids, anatomically small airway passage, and changes in the arousal threshold occurring with the ingestion of alcohol or sedating drugs. Each apneic event may alter blood oxygenation and cerebral blood flow (CBF) (40). Depending on the oxyhemoglobin saturation curve, brief events of apnea can result in significant oxygen desaturations. Of note, each apneic event is ended by a brief, often undetected, electroencephalographic (EEG) arousal (41). Although the arousals are believed to result in the symptom of excessive daytime sleepiness, it is still not clear how the oxygen desaturations interact to impact daytime symptoms of cognitive impairment and sleepiness.

More recently, a broader spectrum of sleep-disordered breathing has been recognized. Sensitive testing paradigms have allowed sleep researchers to note subtle changes in airflow that, although not constituting complete apnea, appear to share the same pathophysiology and consequences as that of OSAS. This subtle form has been labeled upper airway resistance syndrome (UARS) (42).

### Symptoms

Typical symptoms of untreated OSAS and UARS include loud, sporadic snoring, excessive sleepiness, and restless sleep. The onset of either disorder is insidious. Persons seldom can mark the beginning of the syndrome. However, bed partners are usually sensitive to a marked worsening of nocturnal symptoms following illness, alcohol/sedative use, or weight gain. Patients typically present to the physician at the urging of either bed partners who observe the symptoms or co-workers/supervisors who deal with the prominent daytime consequences such as excessive sleepiness. Cardiovascular symptoms, such as hypertension and strokes, are thought to be correlated with sleep apnea. Other consequences of OSAS include loss of memory, irritability, depression, and impotence.

### Treatment

Treatment options now include mechanical support to the airway, such as the continuous positive airways pressure (CPAP) device; surgical repairs of the upper airway—uvulopalatopharyngoplasty (UPPP) or laser-assisted UPPP (LAUP); dental devices designed to increase airway space by extending the mandible; and behavioral techniques such as weight loss or position changes during sleep (43). Of these, nasal CPAP appears to be the most successful in obliterating the respiratory events. The essential components of the CPAP device include (a) a source of pressurized air that is individually titrated to affect change in the patient's airway; (b) a tight-fitting nasal or full-face interface (mask, nasal prongs) held in place by fitted headgear; and (c) a connecting hose and intentional leak port positioned near the face. The air pressure acts as a pneumatic splint to hold the airway open. The patient breathes and sleeps well once individually titrated therapeutic CPAP pressures are reached. While CPAP has been shown to be highly effective, compliance is an issue. Overall there appears to be about an 50% to 85% compliance rate, with most patients utilizing the device at least 4 hours per night. Research shows immediate return of symptoms once the device is discontinued (44).

In the past, tracheostomy was the preferred surgical technique to bypass the site of airway closure. It is still used today in cases of life-threatening disease that are not amenable to other therapies. However, other surgeries have advanced and are now state of the art for appropriate patients. The UPPP consists of surgical removal of the uvula, a portion of the soft palate, tonsils and adenoids if present, and portions of the lateral pharyngeal wall, in an effort to enlarge the anteroposterior dimension of the upper airway (45). The LAUP is gaining recognition as an alternative to UPPP in some patients. This procedure is carried out in stages and may offer reduced surgical morbidity; however, no data exist yet to document this claim. Alternative, highly invasive surgeries have also shown good results in certain patients. These surgeries include mandibular advancement often in conjunction with UPPP and hyoid myotomy-suspension (46). If surgical repair is undergone, it is important to note the need for follow-up review of the disease status. Surgery removes the person's ability to snore, but may not impact on the quality/quantity of apnea.

## IMPACT OF SLEEPINESS ON THE WORKPLACE

The impact of sleepiness on the workplace may be insidious or profound, depending on the amount of sleep loss and the job duties. Multiple factors contribute to fatigue. Not the least of these is the economic loss suffered by workers and industry who can't or are not willing to meet the demands of modern society. We have become a 24-hour culture that demands 24-hour service in mail, fresh produce, repair parts, transportation, and entertainment. Competition to capture key contracts is keen and we believe that one cannot be "caught sleeping."

While there are no job restrictions for people with untreated insomnia, complaints should be taken seriously to ensure peak performance at positions that require heightened vigilance for long periods of time. Additionally, the employer of an insomniac must also be concerned about the impact of hypnotic therapy and any sedating hangover effects among workers, especially if they are involved in areas that require a rapid response time or, conversely, in areas where activity is monotonous (47).

The global impact of narcolepsy on the workplace will depend, in part, on the person's age at symptom onset and diagnosis. Sadly, these two variables may be separated in time by many years. Research indicates that it is not uncommon for patients to visit several physicians and have upward of 15 years between symptom onset and accurate diagnosis. In cases such as this, one can assume that education has been negatively affected leading to poor job marketability and performance. Additionally, patients are often confronted at work with conflicts regarding the use of stimulants and the need for periodic naps. The American Disability Act of 1990 addresses some of this concerns and offers protection to people with this disorder. Despite this, there will be certain jobs for which a person with narcolepsy would be unfit, such as occupations requiring long periods of driving or monotonous attention to critical dials and gauges. If cataplexy is uncontrolled, occupations that entail episodes of intense emotional excitement should be avoided. Early diagnosis, adequate treatment, and supportive vocational counseling are critical in improving the quality of life in persons with this disease.

The impact of untreated OSAS on the workplace can be serious because of the effects of unrecognized nightly sleep loss as one awakens hundreds of times to breathe. Job performance may be sporadic and declining. Unfortunately, the effects of sleep apnea are the most insidious and may be accepted as general consequences of aging or job boredom.

Wake-time gaps in attention and deficits in performance are most critical in the transportation industry because of its far-reaching range of activities. Of note, it is becoming clear that the commercial driver who is male, middle-aged, and overweight/obese fits the apneic profile, and employers should be aware of the potential that these workers may be sleep deprived. While the data on vehicular crashes and sleep disorders are mixed, several small retrospective studies have indicated an increased risk of vehicular crashes in persons with untreated sleep apnea and narcolepsy (48,49). The commercial driver incurs a greater risk.

Many municipalities are now engaged in assessment of driving risk for the sleep disordered and the challenge of how to limit it, particularly among commercial drivers (50). The federal government is reevaluating hours of service contracts to assess the impact on sleepiness. Currently drivers may drive continuously for 10 hours and remain at work for 16 hours. It has been argued that this schedule does not provide adequate rest time since drivers may spend time off on personal issues or socializing and not sleep. The U.S. Federal Aviation Administration (FAA) in collaboration with the NASA Ames Research Center developed the NASA Ames Fatigue Countermeasure Program, which provides educational tools/workshops designed to teach pilots and others how to recognize fatigue and correct it. Furthermore, addressing sleep apnea, the agency notes that symptoms may present a risk to safe flying, and it demands a complete polysomnographic evaluation including daytime tests of alertness [Maintenance of Wakefulness Test (MWT)] before return to work. Additionally, the American Automobile Association (AAA) has established an educational program called the AAA Foundation for Traffic Safety. The American Trucking Association has also designed a teaching module designed to educate drivers about the symptoms, danger, and prevention of sleepiness.

Professional societies are also involved in the discussion of driving rights and responsibilities as they pertain to sleep disordered patients. An ad hoc committee of the American Thoracic Society was formed to study the issue of behavioral morbidity among those with sleep apnea. The committee noted that under present circumstances and inability to offer objective assessment of risk, categorical reporting of all patients with sleep apnea is undesirable. Patients would be discouraged from seeking needed help. The committee suggested that physicians should be encouraged to review risk, educate the patient regarding risk, and follow up on treatment effects. Furthermore, the committee suggests (a) the physician should report the patient to the motor vehicle department if the diagnosis is severe apnea, and there has been a history of motor vehicle accidents, and either the condition is untreatable or the patient refuses treatment; (b) the physician must consider a patient's increased occupational exposure to driving and, in cases of commercial drivers, may consider reporting more freely (51).

## CONCLUSION

Sleep deprivation and sleep disorders are prevalent in society today. Survival in this economic environment forces many workers to endure extended hours, extra shifts, and second jobs, all of which serve to decrease available time to sleep. Detrimental effects on performance are noted within the workplace and at home. Lack of performance or errors of judgment have already cost our society billions of dollars. Industry would be wise to heed these facts and endeavor to establish workplaces that encourage regular hours, foster stress reduction, and provide adequate nutritional and rest breaks. These will benefit both worker and industry. Additionally, the improved recognition and treatment of sleep disorders should aid in reducing these costs, as well-treated patients have the potential to return to normal function.

## REFERENCES


1. Borbely AA. Sleep homeostasis and models of sleep regulation. In: Kryger MH, Roth T, Dement WC, eds. *Principles and practice of sleep medicine.* Philadelphia: Saunders, 1994;309–320.
2. *Sleep 1995.* Gallup Survey. Washington, DC: National Sleep Foundation, 1995.
3. Patrick GT, Gilbert JA. On the effects of loss of sleep. *Psychol Rev* 1896;3;469–483.
4. Carskadon MA, Dement WC. Cumulative effects of sleep restriction on daytime sleepiness. *Psychophysiology* 1981;18:107–113.
5. Dinges DF. Probing the limits of functional capability: The effects of sleep loss on short-duration tasks. In: Broughton RJ, Ogilvie R, eds. *Sleep arousal and performance.* Boston: Birkhauser, 1992;176–188.
6. Dinges DF, Broughton RJ, eds. *Sleep and alertness:* chronological, *Behavioral and medical aspects of napping.* New York: Raven Press, 1989;322.
7. Naitoh P. Signal detection theory as applied to vigilance performance. *Sleep* 1983;6:359–361.
8. Williams HL, Lubin A, Goodnow JJ. Impaired performance with acute sleep loss. *Psychol Monogr Gen Appl* 1959;73:1–26.
9. Polzella DJ. Effects of sleep deprivation on short term recognition and memory. *J Exp Psychol* 1975;104:194–200.
10. Babkoff H, Genser SG, Sing HC, et al. The effects of progressive sleep loss on a lexical decision task. Response lapses and response accuracy. *Behav Res Meth Instr Comput* 1985;17:614–622.
11. Mitler MM, Carskadon MA, Czeisler CA, et al. Catastrophes, sleep and public policy. *Sleep* 1988;11:100–109.
12. National Transportation Safety Board. *Marine accident report—grounding of the U.S. tank ship Exxon Valdez on Bligh reef, Prince William Sound, near Valdez, Alaska, March 24, 1989.* NTSB/MAR-90/04. Washington, DC: NTSB, 1990;1–256.
13. National Transportation Safety Board. *Aircraft accident report:* uncontrolled collision with terrain. American International Airways flight number 808, Douglas DC-8-61, N814 CK-US Naval Air Station, Guantanamo Bay, Cuba August 18, 1993. NTSB/AAR-94/04. Washington, DC: NTSB, 1994.
14. *Report of the presidential commission on the space shuttle Challenger accident,* vol 2, appendix G. Washington, DC: U.S. Government Printing Office, 1986.
15. McCartt AT, Ribner SA, Pack AI, Hammer MC. The scope and nature of the drowsy driving problem in New York State. Presented at the 39th Annual Meeting of the Association for the Advancement of Automotive Medicine, Chicago, Illinois, 1994.
16. Diagnostic Classification Steering Committee. Thorpy MJ, Chairman. *International classification of sleep disorders:* diagnostic and coding manual. Rochester, MN: American Sleep Disorders Association, 1990.
17. National Commission on Sleep Disorders Research. *Wake up America:* a national sleep alert. Executive report of the National Commission on Sleep Disorders Research. Washington, DC: U.S. Government Printing Office, 1993.
18. Mendelson WB, Garnett D, Linnoila M. Do insomniacs have impaired daytime functioning? *Biol Psychiatr* 1984;19:1261–1263.
19. Addison RG, Thorpy MJ, Roehrs TA, et al. Sleep/wake complaints in the general population. *Sleep Res* 1991;20:112.
20. Consensus Development Panel, Freedman D, Chair. Drugs and insomnia: the use of medications to promote sleep. *JAMA* 1984;251:2410–2414.
21. Woods J, Katz J, Winger G. Abuse liability of benzodiazepines. *Pharmacol Rev* 1987;39:251–419.
22. Lacks P, Morin CM. Recent advances in the assessment of insomnia. *J Consult Clin Psychol* 1993;60:586–594.
23. Mamelak M, Csima A, Price V. A comparative 25-night sleep laboratory study on the effects of quazepam and triazolam on chronic insomniacs. *J Clin Pharmacol* 1984;24:65–75.
24. Peeke SC, Callaway E, Jones RT, et al. Combined effects of alcohol and sleep deprivation in normal young adults. *Psychopharmacology* 1980; 67:179–187.
25. Zwyghwizen-Doorenbos A, Roehrs T, Lamphere J, et al. Increased daytime sleepiness enhances ethanol's sedative effects. *Neuropsychopharmacology* 1988;1:279–286.
26. Dollins AB, Zhdanova IV, Wurtman RJ, et al. Effect of inducing nocturnal serum melatonin concentrations in daytime on sleep, mood, body temperature and performance. *Proc Natl Acad Sci USA* 1994;91: 1824–1828.
27. Tzischinsky O, Dagan Y, Lavie P. The effects of melatonin on the timing of sleep in patients with delayed sleep phase syndrome. In: Toitou Y, Arendt J, Pevet P, eds. *Melatonin and the pineal gland.* Amsterdam: Elsevier Science, 1993.
28. Mendelson WB. *Human sleep research and clinical care.* New York: Plenum Press, 1987.
29. Carmen JS, Post RM, Buswell R, Goodwin FK. Negative effects of melatonin ion depression. *Am J Psychiatry* 1987;133:1181–1186.
30. Kilbourne EM. Eosinophilia myalgia syndrome: coming to grips with a new illness. *Epidemiol Rev* 1992;14:16–36.
31. Hublin C, Partinen M, Kaprio J, et al. Epidemiology of narcolepsy. *Sleep* 1994;17:S7–12.
32. Aldrich MS. Narcolepsy. *Neurology* 1992;42(suppl 6):34–43.
33. Nishimo S, Reid MS, Dement WC, Mignot E. Neuropharmacology and neurochemistry of canine narcolepsy. *Sleep* 1994;17:S84–92.
34. Mignot E, Lin X, Arrigoni J, et al. DQB1*0602 and DQA1*0102 (DQ1) are better markers than DR2 for narcolepsy in Caucasian and black Americans. *Sleep* 1994;17:S60–67.
35. Association of Professional Sleep Societies, APSS Guidelines Committee, MA Carskadon, chairperson. Guidelines for the Multiple Sleep Latency Test (MSLT): a standard measure of sleepiness. *Sleep* 1986;9: 519–524.
36. Mitler MM, Aldrich MS, Koob GF, et al. ASDA Standards of Practice: narcolepsy and its treatment with stimulants. *Sleep* 1994;17(4): 352–371.
37. Standards of Practice Committee of the American Sleep Disorders Association. ASDA Standards of Practice: practice parameters for the use of stimulants in the treatment of narcolepsy. *Sleep* 1994;17(4): 348–351.
38. Young T, Palta M, Dempsey J, et al. The occurrence of sleep disordered breathing among middle-aged adults. *N Engl J Med* 1993;328: 1230–1235.
39. He J, Kryger MH, Zorick FJ, Roth T. Mortality and apnea index: experience in 385 male patients. *Chest* 1988;94:9–14.
40. Balfors EM, Franklin KA. Impairment of cerebral perfusion during obstructive sleep apnea. *Am J Respir Crit Care Med* 1994;150: 1587–1591.
41. O'Malley EB, Norman RG, Walsleben JA, Rapoport DM. Upper airway obstructive events and location of EEG arousal activity. *Sleep Res* 1996:321.
42. Guilleminault C, Stroohs R, Clerk A, et al. From obstructive sleep apnea syndrome to upper airways resistance syndrome: consistency of daytime sleepiness. *Sleep* 1992;15:S13–16.
43. Rapoport DM. Treatment of sleep apnea syndrome. *Mt Sinai J Med* 1994;61(2):123–130.
44. Kribbs NB, Getsy J, Dinges DF. Investigation and management of daytime sleepiness in sleep apnea In: Saunders NA, Sullivan CE, eds. *Sleep and breathing.* New York: Marcel Dekker, 1992;2.
45. Fujita S, Conway W, Zorick F, Roth T. Surgical correction of anatomic abnormalities in obstructive sleep apnea syndrome: uvulopalatopharyngoplasty. *Otolaryngol Head Neck Surg* 1981;89:923–934.
46. Riley RW, Powell NB, Guilleminault C. Obstructive sleep apnea syndrome: a surgical protocol for dynamic upper airway reconstruction, *J Oral Maxillofacial Surg* 1993;51:742–747.
47. Nicholson AN. Hypnotics and occupational medicine. *J Occup Med* 1990;32(4):335–341.
48. Findley LJ, Levinson MP, Bonnie RJ. Driving performance and automobile accidents in patients with sleep apnea. *Clin Chest Med* 1992;13; 427–435.
49. George C, Nickerson P, Hanly P, et al. Sleep apnoea patients have more automobile accidents. *Lancet* 1987;8556:447.
50. Pakola SJ, Dinges DF, Pack AI. Review of regulations and guidelines for commercial and noncommercial drivers with sleep apnea and narcolepsy. *Sleep* 1995;18:787–796.
51. American Thoracic Society Ad Hoc Committee. Sleep apnea, sleepiness and driving risk. *Am J Respir Crit Care Med* 1994;150:1463–1473.

*Environmental and Occupational Medicine, Third Edition,* edited by William N. Rom.
Lippincott–Raven Publishers, Philadelphia © 1998.

CHAPTER 108

# Ergonomics

Manny Halpern

Introduced over 125 years ago, the term *ergonomics* is derived from Greek and literally means the study of work. The formal study of human work began at the turn of the century with time and motion measurements developed by Frank and Lillian Gilbreth and Frederick Taylor. However, it was not until World War II that the need to optimize human performance and safety was fully realized. In its broadest sense, ergonomics is a multidisciplinary study of the laws that govern the interaction between people, machines, and their environment.

As a multidisciplinary science, the study of ergonomics evolved in four main areas:

1. *Human factors engineering* is concerned with the information processing requirements of the interaction between people, machines, and the environment. By studying the design of displays and controls, human factors engineers focus on enhancing performance and reducing errors.
2. *Anthropometry* is the science of measurement and the art of application that establish the physical geometry, mass properties, and strength capabilities of the human body. Thus, important information is available to design furniture, machines, tools, and clothes.
3. *Occupational biomechanics* is the application of the laws of physics and engineering concepts to study the physical interaction of workers with their tools, machines, and materials. By assessing the forces acting on the body, important information is available about the tolerance of the musculoskeletal system and the risk of overexertion injuries.
4. *Work physiology* is concerned with the responses of the body to the metabolic demands of work. By measuring the activity of the cardiovascular, respiratory, and muscular systems at work, information is available to prevent whole-body and localized fatigue.

M. Halpern: Occupational and Industrial Orthopaedic Center, New York University Medical Center, New York, New York 10016.

As an applied science, the goal of the occupational ergonomics endeavor is to fit the job to the worker. Thus, the National Institute for Occupational Safety and Health (NIOSH) defines ergonomics as "the discipline that strives to develop and assemble information on people's capacities and capabilities for use in designing jobs, products, workplaces, and equipment." This definition states further that through job design, a "best fit" between the human and imposed job conditions would "ensure and enhance worker health, safety, comfort, and productivity."

The capabilities and limitations of the worker concern both the worker and the industry. The Occupational Safety and Health Act of 1970, the Americans with Disabilities Act of 1990, and the workers' compensation laws provide the legal framework of these concerns. Beyond that, market forces play a considerable role in introducing ergonomic interventions. An estimated $34.3 billion were spent in 1989 on workers' compensation in the United States. Many of these expenses are the results of musculoskeletal injuries and illnesses. The financial consequences of these disorders were estimated at $61 billion for direct medical costs and $65 billion for indirect costs, including lost work days and lowered productivity (1).

## WORK-RELATED MUSCULOSKELETAL DISORDERS

Musculoskeletal disorders can be characterized as work-related diseases. The World Health Organization (WHO) defines these diseases as multifactorial. Work contributes significantly, though not exclusively, to the causation of the disease. When some of the outcomes are of uncertain pathogenesis and may consist of symptoms without obvious clinical signs, the word *disorder* is more appropriate (2). As loss in productivity and absence from work may occur even at a preclinical stage, the term *work-related musculoskeletal disorders* (WRMDs) is used here. WRMDs can be partially caused by adverse work conditions and exacerbated by workplace exposures, and they can impair work capacity (3). In view of the multifactorial nature of WRMDs and the trend toward multidisciplinary treatment of these disorders, it is reasonable to suggest that ergonomics, as the study of human work, may play a role in identifying the etiology of the disorders, the rehabilitation of injured employees, and their return to work.

Most of what we know about the etiology of WRMDs comes from epidemiologic studies. These studies show that the musculoskeletal disorders are not unique to any occupational group. Reported occupations range from furniture movers and meat processors, to apparel workers or assemblers in the manufacturing industries, to data entry operators in offices. The common trait of these groups is intense occupational exposure to specific work attributes. The attributes that are associated with increased probability of WRMD are considered risk factors.

The Occupational Safety and Health Administration (OSHA) logs of illnesses and injuries at work offer an overview of the distribution of WRMD in the United States. Table 1 summarizes the latest data from private industry, although a similar picture emerges from the records of the previous 3 years. The data collected by the Bureau of Labor Statistics (4) show that the back is the body part affected most often. These back injuries are probably caused mainly by overexertion, of which lifting is the major event attributed to the injury. It is also probable that many of the back injuries are sprains and strains. Disorders of the upper extremities such as the wrist constitute a small number of the cases reported in the private industry. However, they are of concern because they imply a relatively long absence from work. Though rare, nerve impingement disorders such as carpal tunnel syndrome (CTS) require an absence of 30 days in half of the cases. Repetitive motions are the main event associated with these cases.

**TABLE 1.** *The distribution of WRMD in the private industry in the U.S. in 1994*

| | % of cases in private industry (2,236,600) | Days away from work (median) |
|---|---|---|
| Nature of injury | | |
| Sprains and strains | 43.1% | 6 |
| Carpal tunnel syndrome | 1.7% | 30 |
| Body part | | |
| Back | 27.1% | 6 |
| Wrist | 4.9% | 13 |
| Event | | |
| Overexertion | 27.4% | 6 |
| Repetitive motions | 4.1% | 18 |

From ref. 5.

The studies that investigated exposure to physical workload assumed a biomechanical etiology of WRMDs. This approach was adopted by NIOSH in the proposed national strategy for the prevention of musculoskeletal injuries (6). It is also the approach of the current injury surveillance systems. Broad categories of physical workload, such as static posture, manual handling, repetitive work, and excessive force, frequently appear in reviews of epidemiologic studies (6–8). Several environmental factors such as exposure to vibrating vehicles or powered handtools have been associated with WRMDs. Also, exposure to cold temperature may exacerbate WRMDs. Biologically plausible responses to exposure to physical risk factors have been suggested (3,9), but are not well substantiated. Based on a review of 22 studies that provide evidence of dose-response relationship (expressed as odds ratios), Armstrong et al. (3) hypothesized several exposure-dose variables relevant to muscle, tendon, and nerve disorders. These variable are work load, work location, work frequency, work duration, muscle force, muscle contraction velocity, frequency and duration, muscle length, joint position, and compartment pressure.

Increasingly, investigators try to incorporate variables from other domains. The biopsychosocial model of disease hypothesizes that biologic, psychological, and social factors operate and interact at all stages of health and illness (10). The WHO definition of WRMD implicitly acknowledges that psychosocial factors play a role in the development, progress, and treatment of the disease. Exposure to stressful events, therefore, should be considered in planning intervention strategies.

Several models have been developed to explain the health effects of physical and psychosocial stressors, and numerous measures have been suggested based on these models. The variable methodologies make it difficult to draw any overall conclusions about the epidemiologic evidence and its association with musculoskeletal disorders. The primary limitation of the available studies relates to causality of WRMD. Nonetheless, work-load exposure and perceived work stress should be measured simultaneously. Their analysis should take into account the interaction between physical and psychosocial factors, and the multicollinearity between some of the psychosocial factors. Recent regulatory efforts, for example those undertaken by ANSI (11), acknowledge that certain attributes of work organization are linked to WRMD. They advise that prevention programs view stressful time-related and job-related events as risk factors that need to be measured and modified.

## ERGONOMIC INTERVENTION

In practice, ergonomics is a process of problem solving. The process requires answers to several questions:

Where is the problem?—the jobs or positions targeted for intervention;
What is the problem?—the specific risk factors for WRMD present on the job, their magnitude, and the body parts at risk;
Why is there a problem?—the possible ergonomic root causes of the risk factors, i.e., hazards that may exacerbate WRMD;
What to do?—prioritizing hazard control measures.

The following sections provide an overview of the methods used to obtain answers to these questions. Based on a literature review, Wilson (12) lists general approaches that have been commonly used in ergonomics and other disciplines. The analyses of tasks and work activity demands are of particular relevance to the prevention of musculoskeletal disorders. The methods that follow these approaches, the techniques, and their measures or outcomes, are summarized in Table 2. These methods serve throughout the process of solving ergonomic problems.

### Where Is the Problem: Selecting the Target of Intervention

Several criteria may be used to choose a target for an ergonomic intervention. The problems that need to be addressed vary from high injury rates or employee turnover, to errors or low-quality output. Injury prevention programs require that a surveillance system be set up to allow a timely identification of jobs or positions with high WRMD rates, though there are no established incidence rates that would trigger an intervention. Relative risk and attributable risk statistics establish how much occupational factors increase the risk of injury and how many cases might be prevented by a control program. However, in many workplaces the number of employees at risk is too small and unstable, and the work situation too variable to allow rigorous statistical analyses. Often continued surveillance is warranted, and a comparison population is needed or data have to be pooled to overcome some of the statistical problems.

Health surveillance may be characterized as passive or active. Passive systems include OSHA-mandated recording of injuries in the line of duty or classical public health methods such as a review of clinical visits or insurance

**TABLE 2.** *A classification of methods, techniques, and outcome measures used in ergonomics to analyze tasks and work activity demands relevant to the development of musculoskeletal disorders*

| Method | Technique | Outcome measure |
|---|---|---|
| Task analysis | • Ability requirements | • Requirements for hiring and training |
| | • Knowledge description | |
| | • Flowchart, link and time diagrams | • Task sequences, times, error rates, critical phases |
| Expert analysis | • Checklist walkthrough Delphi | |
| | • Method study techniques, expert systems | |
| Archives, database | • Medical records, accident/injury reports | • Incidence, severity, risk factors |
| Physical workload | • Indirect observation, e.g., Borg scale, psychophysical techniques | • "Subjective" ratings (rates of perceived exertion) |
| | • Biomechanical models | • Moments and force estimates to compare with criteria |
| | • Performance records, secondary or alternative tasks of psychomotor performance, physical changes | • Performance decrement |
| Posture analysis | • Biochemical models | • Angular configuration to compare with norms or criteria |
| | • Optical methods (motion analysis) | • Motion patterns in space |
| | • Direct angle measurement (goniometry) | • Opinions of discomfort |
| | • Observation (live, video) | |
| | • Self-rated questionnaires | • "Objective" data to be interpreted against norms or criteria |
| Physiologic analysis | • HR, HR variability, $O_2$ uptake, air analysis, GSR, ECG, EMG, EEG, ERP | |
| Mental workload | • Primary/secondary/alternative task, subjective assessment, physiologic response | • Performance decrement, load (subjective or objective) |
| Stress assessment | • Physiologic responses (GSR, etc.) | |
| | • Indirect observation techniques | |
| Job and work attitude measurements | • Indirect observation, especially rating scales informal group or individual interviews | • Satisfaction, needs, important job characteristics |

HR, heart rate; ECG, electrocardiography; EEG, electroencephalography; EMG, electromyography; ERP, event related potentials; GSR, galvanic skin response.
Adapted from ref. 12.

claims. Active systems include the administration of health interviews, symptom surveys, or physical examinations. Several studies indicate that OSHA logs underreport the prevalence of musculoskeletal disorders, particularly subacute problems of the upper extremities. These studies suggest further that symptom surveys provide a fairly accurate description of the magnitude of the problems, i.e., high sensitivity and moderate specificity, depending on the definition of false-positive cases (13, 14).

An active surveillance system is useful for proactive interventions. When passive systems do not provide sufficient data, as in new work situations, surveys of risk factors may help identify potential problem areas on the job even before musculoskeletal disorders develop. The surveys consist of walkthrough evaluations, informal interviews, and checklists. These job surveys serve, therefore, as screening tools for typical risk factors of WRMD. Hazard surveillance can be conducted by ergonomics experts during job inspections and interviews with workers, or by a team of workers, supervisors, or safety and health personnel trained to identify ergonomic hazards. The main purpose of this activity is to prioritize jobs or positions for a detailed analysis (11).

### What Is the Problem: Describing the Exposure to Risk Factors

Unfavorable working conditions have a potentially harmful effect on the body, thus acting as a stressor. The mere presence of a stressor on the job may not be sufficient for measuring the risk or for designing an ergonomic intervention. The next step is to document and evaluate the exposure to specific risk factors. The documentation includes information on the objectives of the job, production standards, staffing, materials, tools, and the work environment. Traditional industrial engineering methods such as motion time measurements serve to describe the tasks and their basic elements (15, 16).

The choice of method is a tradeoff between the state of the knowledge, the available time and resources, and the level of detail desired. The most cursory task analysis involves a description of process flow, using functional terms such as *transportation, operation, inspection,* and *storage.* This analysis may be sufficient for addressing layout of a facility. To document the actions performed, a more detailed analysis is used, usually plotting activities against time. The activities are described as lifting, turning, carrying, walking, standing, or sitting. This level of analysis is sufficient when the whole body is engaged and the metabolic demands of the job are of concern (Table 3). The activities of the upper extremities require a more detailed analysis. In many cases it is sufficient to describe the task operationally as "grasp part" or "hold part." In micromotion studies fundamental operations are recorded for each hand (Table 4). This level of analysis may be needed for identifying specific assembly operations that we seek to improve.

The methods used in ergonomic interventions that aim to prevent WRMD are primarily risk factor assessments. The assessment characterizes the stresses that act on the worker. The assessment established the circumstances under which people are affected and how severe the problems are. What are the stresses associated with WRMD? The generic risk factors are the following (2, 17):

Excessive force
Awkward postures
Contact between the body and vibrating surfaces
Contact pressure with soft tissue, e.g., sharp edges or hard surfaces
Metabolic cost involved in oxygen consumption and cardiovascular activity
Ambient temperature

The dimensions of the exposure—magnitude, duration, repetitiveness (frequency)—are necessary to assess the risk.

The biomechanical and physiologic stresses are interrelated. Joint moments or force caused by external loads must be resisted internally by the muscles and ligaments surrounding the joint. Posture as the configuration of the body in space is related to force exertions in several ways, as summarized in Table 5.

**TABLE 3.** *Example of energy expenditure in a sequence of tasks*

| Order | Task | Description | Metabolic cost (kcal/min) |
|---|---|---|---|
| 1 | Lifting | 25 lb, 4 times, floor to 30-in height | 1.52 |
| 2 | Turning 180 degrees | 25 lb, 4 times | 0.28 |
| 3 | Carrying | 25 lb, against thigh, 4 times, 10 ft 15 2.5 mph | 1.15 |
| 4 | Setting object on conveyor | 25 lb, 4 times | 0.35 |
| 5 | Turning 180 degrees | 4 times, 0 lb | 0.20 |
| 6 | Walking back | 4 times, 10 ft at 3 mph | 0.40 |
| 7 | Maintaining posture | Standing | 1.53 |
| Total | | | 5.43 |

Source: Energy Expenditure Program, University of Michigan, 1988.

**TABLE 4.** *Gilbreth table of work elements*

| Element | Description |
|---|---|
| Search | Looking for something with the eyes or hand |
| Select | Locating an object mixed with others |
| Grasp | Touching or gripping an object with the hand |
| Reach | Moving the hand to some object or location |
| Move | Moving an object from one location to another |
| Hold | Exerting force to hold an object at a fixed location |
| Position | Moving an object in a desired orientation |
| Inspect | Examining an object by sight, touch, sound |
| Assemble | Joining together two or more objects |
| Disassemble | Separating two or more objects |
| Use | Manipulating a tool or device with the hand |
| Unavoidable delay | Interrupting work activity because of factors beyond the worker's control |
| Avoidable delay | Interrupting work activity because of some factor under the worker's control |
| Plan | Performing a mental process that precedes movement |
| Rest | Interrupting work activity to overcome fatigue |

Adapted from ref. 15.

A more detailed analysis of the dimensions of these stressors may warrant using task-specific methods. A large body of literature evolved in two categories of tasks: manual materials handling and tasks involving the upper extremities. Handling activities such as lifting, pushing, or pulling of loads are involved in most of the overexertion injury claims. Several methods have been developed to assess exertions that exceed the worker's capabilities using biomechanical, physiologic, and psychophysical criteria.

Biomechanical criteria deal with forces and moments acting on the body joints and soft tissues. To estimate the forces and moments we need information on the posture adopted during the handling activities, the speed of movement, the weight of the load, as well as anatomical and physiologic data (e.g., moment arm of the muscles involved, pattern of muscle recruitment). Several biomechanical models have been developed to simulate physical requirements and resulting forces. Unlike static models, the dynamic models take into account the effect of moments of inertia and acceleration, thus predicting higher stress on the spine. As the incidence rates for low back pain are related to the compressive forces on the L5/S1 vertebral disk, the biomechanical criterion of maximal back compression appears to be a good predictor of the risk of back incidents and overexertion injuries in general (18). Figure 1 provides an example of the application of a static biomechanical model (3D Static Strength Prediction Program SSPP version 2.0, University of Michigan, Center for Ergonomics, 1991) to calculate the compression load and moment of force on the lower back while handling a 20-lb weight. Holding the object close to the body, the compression force on the disks at L5/S1 is well below the biomechanical safety criterion. The moment of force and the compression force increased when the posture changed due to a larger horizontal distance of the load away from the body. Since the weight of the object has not changed, the increased stress is due to the additional effect of the weight of the trunk.

Psychophysical criteria are derived from workers perception of acceptable loads. The acceptable level of stress has been measured under controlled conditions and rates of perceived exertions have been developed. The Borg

**TABLE 5.** *The effects of posture as a mechanical stressor*

| Postural aspect | Physiologic effect |
|---|---|
| Body segment inclined with respect to the line of gravity | A moment of force acts on a joint and is countered by muscles and ligaments |
| Joint angle close to the extreme range of motion | Compression of blood vessels and nerves against bony structures (mainly in the extremities)<br>Passive stabilization through ligaments (mainly in the spine) |
| Joint posture outside the optimal working range | Muscles act at a mechanical disadvantages<br>Reduced blood supply |
| Change of posture | Lack of change requires static muscle contraction resulting in reduced blood supply<br>Fast and frequent motions reduce recovery time |

Adapted from ref. 2.

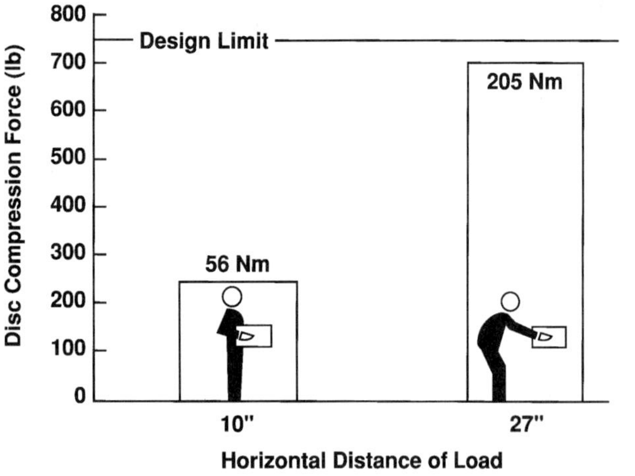


**FIG. 1.** Application of a static biomechanical model to assess the stress on the lower back. Disk compression force [in pounds (lbs)] and moment of force at L5S1 [in newton-meters (Nm)] while handling a 20-lb weight in two situations (load at 10 inches and 27 inches away from the body). The design limit corresponds to the action limit in the 1981 NIOSH Work Practice Guide.

scales in Table 6 are one of the most commonly used instruments to measure perceived exertion (19). Applying the paradigm of threshold measurements in experimental psychology to handling activities, researchers also study the willingness to engage in physical effort and determine maximum acceptable weights and forces. This paradigm is used in strength testing for worker selection but it has also been used extensively to develop criteria for acceptable loads in manual materials handling (18).

The physiologic criteria for manual materials handling have been derived from measurements of energy consumption and fatigue. They assume that the intensity of effort and endurance time are related to the aerobic capacity for dynamic work performed by large muscle groups. The Energy Expenditure Model (20) further assumes that the energy expended on the job is the sum of the demands of the tasks comprising it. Table 3 shows an example of energy expenditure in a job. Only a few workers can be expected to expend 5.43 kcal/min for an 8-hour shift. To reduce the metabolic cost, the intervention should target the carrying and walking tasks.

Based on the biomechanical, psychophysical, and physiologic criteria, ergonomic design recommendations have been developed to assess the risk of the occupational factors associated with WRMD. The criteria, the acceptable limits, and the methods used to evaluate them are summarized in Table 7. These criteria apply to manual materials handling tasks that affect mainly the lower back. It is possible to quantify the exposure of the upper extremities to occupational risk factors. However, similar criteria still need to be developed for tasks involving the upper extremities (11). As smaller muscle groups are needed in tasks involving the upper extremities, the main thrust of the research is directed toward biomechanical and psychophysical criteria.

There is evidence of a relationship between repetitive force exertions and pain or WRMD of the upper extremities. Frequency of motion, velocity, and acceleration are all related; as force equals mass times acceleration, an increase in each may increase the load on the tissues of the extremity (21). Considerable effort has been directed toward establishing criteria for force exertions. In controlled studies, localized muscle fatigue was induced by increasing the duration of the exertion. A special case involves isometric contractions typical to static work. It has been suggested that exertions below 15% of maximum voluntary contraction (MVC) might be maintained indefinitely without fatigue, though current studies show that fatigue can occur during contractions as low as 5% of MVC. Frequently repeated isometric exertions showed that 10% of MVC was unacceptable for repeated 5-sec-

**TABLE 6.** *Borg scales for subjective rating of perceived exertion (RPE)*

| Borg's RPE scale | | Borg's CR-10 scale | |
|---|---|---|---|
| 6 | No exertion at all | 0 | Nothing at all |
| 7 | | 0.5 | Extremely weak (just noticeable) |
| 8 | Extremely light | | |
| 9 | Very light | 1 | Very weak |
| 10 | | 2 | Weak (light) |
| 11 | Light | 3 | Moderate |
| 12 | | 4 | |
| 13 | Somewhat hard | 5 | Strong (heavy) |
| 14 | | 6 | |
| 15 | Hard | 7 | Very strong |
| 16 | | 8 | |
| 17 | Very hard | 9 | |
| 18 | | 10 | Extremely strong (almost maximal) |
| 19 | Extremely hard | | |
| 20 | Maximal | | Maximal |

From ref. 19.

**TABLE 7.** *Criteria for assessing the risk of WRMD, their acceptable limits, and the methods used to assess the exposure*

| Criteria | Acceptable limit | Method |
|---|---|---|
| Compressive force on L5/S1 vertebral disk | ≤770 lbs | Biomechanical models, e.g., static strength prediction programs |
| Strength | >75% of population capable | Psychophysical tables of maximum acceptable weights and forces |
| Energy expenditure | ≤3.1 kcal/min (whole body, materials handling near floor level)<br>≤2.2 kcal/min (arm work, materials handling at bench height) | Energy expenditure models, e.g., energy expenditure program |
| Heart rate | 100–105 bpm (whole body)<br>90–95 bpm (arm work) | |
| Postural stress | Avoid activities beyond the neutral position of a body joint | Posture analysis; see Table 2 |
| Force exertion | Acceptable level depends on maximal voluntary contraction, exertion time, and recovery time | Physical work load or physiologic analysis; see Table 2 |
| Perceived stress | Light | Borg scale |

Adapted from ref. 18.

ond exertions. Where nerve impingement is of concern, another possible biomechanical criteria may be used: intrajoint pressure. Several studies suggest a dose-response relationship between intrajoint pressure, repetitive wrist motions, or awkward postures of the wrist, and impairment. This criterion would be equivalent to vertebral disk compression limits, and threshold levels have been suggested for carpal tunnel syndrome (21).

Contact stress is another mechanical factor specific to tasks involving the upper extremities. These stresses are the result of pressure exerted on a body part as it comes in contact with various surfaces. Duration of exertion and pressure intensity are related to pain thresholds for different parts of the hand. Similarly, some studies showed that intrajoint pressure is related to contact stress on the wrist. Further studies are needed to determine the acceptable pressure-time combinations for other tissues in the elbow and shoulders (21).

Several environmental factors have been associated with WRMD. Exposure to vibration entails sustaining mechanical stimuli with a variety of effects on the body, ranging from degradation of motor functions, to the development of disorders affecting the musculoskeletal, vascular, and nervous systems. Vibration is a vector quantity with properties of amplitude and frequency. According to the points of entry, vibration is defined as whole-body when the exposure is through the feet or buttocks, and segmental when the exposure occurs at the hands. Various body tissues have characteristic responses to vibration, where the spine responds at 4 to 8 Hz by increasing vertebral disk pressure, while the muscles respond to higher frequencies through different neural pathways, such as the tonic vibration reflex. An increase in oxygen consumption was also measured in response to exposure to whole-body vibration (21,22).

In addition to vibration, skin exposure to cold temperature under 20°C is known to result in loss of tactile sensitivity, which can lead to excessive force exertions and loss of manual dexterity. The vasoconstrictive effects of cold have also been associated with vascular disorders such as secondary Raynaud syndrome or vibration white finger (21).

### Why Is There a Problem? Describing Ergonomic Root Causes

Once exposure to occupational risk factors has been characterized, we can identify possible ergonomic hazards that may have caused the exposure. The risk factors, e.g., excessive force exertion or awkward posture, may be attributed to several types of ergonomic hazards. The possible root causes and the relevant design parameters are summarized in Table 8. The table demonstrates multifactorial nature of the risk factors: an ergonomic hazard may induce several types of stress, and a certain stress may have its roots in several causes, as discussed in the following subsections.

#### *Workstation Design*

Awkward posture during work activities can be caused by inappropriate layout of objects in the workstation or by inappropriate dimensions of the workstation. The biomechanical and psychophysical design criteria for manual materials handling tasks rely mainly on workstation dimensions as direct means to control posture and consequently the compressive forces acting on the spine. For example, the neutral position of the trunk is standing upright without twisting or bending sideways. Deviations from the neutral position occur when objects are not read-

**TABLE 8.** *A summary of the various risk factors for WRMD (stressors), their possible ergonomic root causes, and their specific design parameters*

| Root cause | Design parameter | Stressor |
|---|---|---|
| Workstation design | Layout of objects | Posture |
| | Dimensions of work benches | |
| | Placement of controls | |
| | Material and shape of work surface | Contact stress |
| | Terrain | Oxygen consumption, vibration |
| Tool design | | |
| Manual and powered handtools | Weight | Force |
| | Size | Posture |
| | Shape | Contact stress |
| | Engine/handle | Vibration |
| Chairs | Seat height | Posture |
| | Seat size | Contact stress |
| | Back, arm, and foot supports | Force, oxygen consumption |
| | Upholstery materials | Vibration |
| Controls | Size and shape | Contact stress |
| | Displacement | Posture |
| | Actuation force | Force |
| Visual displays | Image quality | Posture |
| Product design | Object weight | Force |
| | Size and shape | Posture |
| | Material properties (e.g., liquid, hardness) | |
| | Coupling (e.g., handles) | Contact stress |
| Work Technique | Skill and experience | Force and posture |
| | Individual strength and endurance | Oxygen consumption |
| Work organization | Piece rate wages and quotas | Force (repetitiveness, duration) |
| | Rest breaks and overtime | Oxygen consumption |
| | Pace and control | |

ily accessible. Trunk flexion can be caused by reaching objects placed below the level of the hands when standing with the arms hanging down, or by reaching for objects placed too far in front of the body. The trunk may be bent sideways or twisted when reaching objects placed to the side or behind the worker's body.

The placement of hand and foot controls or visual displays directly affect the posture of the extremities and head. Similarly, work benches that are designed too high or too low may result in awkward hand, arm, and shoulder positions. Hard workstation surfaces with sharp edges may also cause contact stresses. In precision tasks such as sewing or dentistry, viewing conditions may force the head, neck, arms, and trunk into awkward positions depending on the placement of the work object (23).

In tasks performed outdoors such as construction, mining, firefighting, or law enforcement, the environment and terrain constitute the workstation and affect the posture, the forces that need to be exerted, oxygen consumption, and the vibration of vehicles used.

### *Tool Design*

Since most tools are operated by the hand, their weight, size, and shape directly determine the magnitude of the force exerted and contact stresses. They may also indirectly affect the posture of the hand, arm, and shoulders. These effects are magnified in powered hand tools, where the vibration of the engine and the damping properties of the handles confound the force exertion and contact stresses, while exhaust outlets may directly expose the skin to cold temperatures.

Grip strength is greatest when the wrist is straight. Since the design of the workstation also influences wrist posture, the design of the grip of a tool has to be considered in the context of the task and workstation. For example, a pistol handle is appropriate to vertical surfaces at elbow height. At this height, a pistol handle is inappropriate for horizontal surfaces because the wrist cannot be aligned with the forearm. However, a pistol handle is appropriate for horizontal surfaces below elbow height.

Chairs can be viewed as work tools and their height with respect to the workstation directly affects the posture of the trunk. Their shape, size, and material determine contact stresses and skin temperature at the thighs, buttocks, and back. When seats are used on vibrating platforms, the damping properties of the materials would also influence muscle contraction, trunk posture oxygen consumption, and contact stress (24).

Controls of machines can also be classified as work tools. The shape, size, displacement, and actuation force directly determine force exertion, posture, and the contact stresses of the extremities. The quality of the images on visual displays such as computer screens also affects posture, independently of the placement of the display in the workstation. For example, small text characters may be illegible on low-resolution screens with low contrasts between character and background, thus inducing the user to bend closer to the screen.

### *Product Design*

In many situations the work object or the product that is being handled directly affects posture and force exertion. In manual materials handling, the weight of the load, its size, shape, and the interface with the hand determine the risk factors of WRMD, namely the awkwardness of the posture, the forces acting on the spine and other joints, as well as contact stresses on the hand.

The NIOSH lifting equation (25) attempts to combine these features with workstation design parameters in order to determine the acceptability of a task. The acceptability is expressed as a recommended weight limit (RWL). This limit is based on a multiplicative model that weighs each of the six task variables. The weights are expressed as multipliers that serve to decrease the maximum load to be lifted under ideal conditions (51 lbs). The task variables are horizontal and vertical lifting distance, asymmetry angle, frequency of lifting, and a hand-load coupling assessment.

In assembly tasks, the design of the product affects the sequence of operations, the repetitiveness, and force exertion in addition to the posture and contact stresses. For example, the type of screw fastener head and screw tip needed can affect screwdriver feed force. A Phillips-head screwdriver requires more than six times the force needed for a slotted screw with an equivalent diameter head. Material hardness is also important for self-tapping screws (26).

In addition to increased process cost, the quality of assembly parts such as screws may also affect injury rates. It should be pointed out that health outcomes might not be manifested among the workers at the manufacturing stage but later in the maintenance stage. The relationship between products that are hard to assemble or difficult to maintain and the impact on health outcomes needs further research.

### *Work Technique*

Practitioners of ergonomics have often observed individual variability in work techniques. Even in structured tasks such as assembly operations, workers adopt individual techniques to carry out the task. The variability within and between individuals performing various tasks is usually considered in motion time measurements and cycle time data. However, the variability in terms of posture and force has rarely been studied formally.

In manual materials handling, individuals have considerable freedom to vary the way they perform the task. The assisted one-hand lift is practiced in manufacturing and warehousing where large containers are used to handle loads that are frequently under 30 lbs, which can be grasped with one hand. By resting one hand on top of the container while bending over and handling parts with the other hand, the worker reduces the stress to the lower back by involving the shoulders, arm, and hip. The two-hand squat is another technique that can be used to lift compact loads that can be brought in between the knees and close to the body.

Some studies estimated that 20% to 40% of the lifting motions are due to individual worker handling technique (27,28,29). It is possible that mainly twisting motions can be avoided using a different handling technique such as turning the entire body (29). Good muscle coordination is one of the hallmarks of experienced workers. A jerky motion can characterize a poorly coordinated activity. Jerk is defined as changes in acceleration. A highly skilled movement is therefore defined as one with low variability in acceleration. Recent findings regarding the increased risk of back injury in high-acceleration lifting (30) suggest that worker technique may be important in the high-risk operations.

### *Work Organization*

Certain organizational parameters determine the exposure to risk factors at work. The duration of a task, the work/rest schedule, and the length of a work shift define the dose and the permissible exposure. For example, an NIOSH-sponsored committee developing work practice guidelines for manual materials handling reviewed the literature on work capacity and duration. The group concluded that a person could work only 4 minutes at intensity equal to maximal physical capacity. As the duration of work increases, the intensity of work must decrease. For a typical 8-hour work shift the average rate should not exceed a third of the individual work capacity (31).

It is less clear how other organizational parameters constitute a hazard. It is conceivable that piece rate payments may motivate workers to work faster and for longer hours. Production quotas may have the same effect. The relationship between these parameters and the occurrence of WRMD requires further studies.

## What to Do: Ergonomics Controls

Having established the possible ergonomic causes of the stressors, the ergonomist is in a position to determine possible controls. The multifactorial nature of WRMD implies that several categories of ergonomic hazards induce a variety of stressors. It follows therefore that several solutions are often possible. The preferable solution would effectively control all the risk factors identified on the job by modifying the workstation design and the tools, redesigning the work objects, and/or reorganizing the work.

**TABLE 9.** *Example of ergonomic design principles and guidelines to reduce exposure to risk factors for musculoskeletal disorders*

| Principle | Guideline |
|---|---|
| 1. Design the workstation and tools to accommodate a variety of user sizes | Provide easily adjustable features |
| 2. Place objects within easy reach and view | Frequently used objects should be placed close to the center between hip and chest height |
| 3. Design tools and work objects to operate at optimal force exertions | Reduce forces at the source by changing the weight, size and shape of the objects |
| | Provide grips appropriate to the task |
| | Use mechanical aids such as hoists and balancers to hold the weight |
| | Use gravity chutes to eliminate the need to lower work objects |
| | Use carts or conveyor belts to eliminate the need to carry objects |
| 4. Train material handlers in safe practices | Plan the lift by: |
| | prearranging objects within easy reach |
| | reorienting objects so the largest dimension is vertical |
| | getting help if the weight is not within one's capabilities |
| | preparing the destination |
| | selecting an unobstructed course of action |
| | stepping close to the object before lifting or pulling it close before lifting |
| | Face the object |
| | Balance the load in both hands |
| | Pivot instead of twist |
| | Avoid very fast and jerky motions |
| 5. Tasks should have a variety of stresses distributed among different body segments | Consider job rotation and enrichment techniques |

To deal with multiple risk factors, numerous root causes, and a variety of solutions, professional and administrative strategies need to be developed. To maintain sufficient room for maneuvering, ergonomists prefer to establish principles of design rather than set up standard solutions. The previous section provided examples showing it is meaningless to claim that a workstation, tool, or product is ergonomically designed. We must always examine the tasks that need to be performed with the equipment, the physical and organizational environment in which the equipment is put to use, and the characteristics of the people who are going to use it. Broad principles of design such as those listed in Table 9 give us guidelines to create new devices and evaluate existing conditions. The technical specifications need to be developed with the task and user in mind.

The choice of the controls also implies that we need to devise strategies of prioritization. Solutions usually take one of two forms. The quick fixes are implemented when a preliminary job survey identifies an obvious risk factor. Where several solutions are possible, prioritization can be based on several factors. To maximize safety, a typical scheme might be as follows (22):

1. Fix immediately (imminent danger of injury).
2. Fix soon (no immediate danger).
3. Fix when equipment is shut down.
4. Redesign and fix if cost-benefit ratio is acceptable.
5. Redesign the next time equipment is built or purchased.

One of the divisions of Boeing Company applies the following considerations (32):

*Benefit*: Since risk is viewed as the severity of the stressor, improvement is the reduction in exposure to the stressor. A matrix of risk and improvement can be constructed, where low risk and little improvement yield low benefits and high risk and large improvements yield high benefits.
*Impact*: The number of people affected by the intervention.
*Feasibility*: The development required for implementing a control. Some solutions are available off the shelf; others require a time range.
*Cost*: Dollar values can be estimated or classified on a range from low to high.

Weights can be assigned to the scores of these factors and summed up for each solution. The solutions are then prioritized according to the rank order of the scores.

The last phase of the process is ascertaining that the problem has been resolved. Any good intervention should include a follow-up evaluation. The criteria for evaluation must be compatible with the considerations that led to selecting the solution. If the benefits are given high weights, the reduction in exposure to the stressor should be measured. Similarly, we need to measure whether the target audience was reached, whether solutions were implemented within the planned time frame, or whether the budget allocated was sufficient. It is also critical that we use valid measures to evaluate the effectiveness of the intervention. For example, a training program that aimed at reaching a large audience and adopted a lecture format should be evaluated first by the increase in knowledge; if practice were included in the training, a valid measure would be the change in performance. The time frame for follow-up is important. Employee or user satisfaction should be measured at the right time interval, to avoid the confounding effect of introducing a change in the job. Many manufacturing operations also change rapidly in response to market conditions and this change confounds the measurements. Changing WRMD rates or reducing health care costs requires additional considerations. As WRMDs take a while to develop, we need to allow some time to resolve the condition. An ergonomic program also increases employee awareness of the work-relatedness of musculoskeletal disorders, leading to increases in clinical visits or complaints. Similarly, early intervention is also likely to increase the number of clinical visits. New measures may have to be implemented in these cases, such as monitoring the severity, chronicity, or recurrence rates.

From an investment viewpoint, some health and safety costs are unavoidable but others are preventable. For example, in a retrospective cross-sectional study of 469 Danish steel workers, Suadicani et al. (33) used a self-administered questionnaire and a standard job classification system to calculate the odds ratio for 1-year prevalence of low back pain. The risk of a recent pain attributable to physical work conditions was about 30%, and 35% for domestic recreational activities; the lifetime risk attributable to lifting was 47%. Others have also estimated that up to 25% of low back injuries in industry could be prevented if workplaces were properly designed (22). Justifying ergonomics within a firm is a difficult process as health and safety costs are not defined precisely and accounting systems are rarely designed for specific investments. New techniques are developed that allow us to estimate the health and safety cost associated with cost objects such as a workstation, a production line, a department, or a product, rather than specific employees. Benefits resulting from an ergonomics investment may result in costs avoided as well as real cost savings (34).

Changing the conditions at work may introduce new risk factors. Some of these are inadvertently introduced when ergonomic interventions shift the stress from one body part to another. Others are introduced by new technologies. The ergonomic process of problem solving becomes one of continuous improvement.

## PREVENTION

### Primary Prevention

Adopting the established practices in controlling exposure to hazardous materials, NIOSH lists four areas of strategies to control and prevent musculoskeletal injuries (5):

- Engineering controls to redesign tools, tasks, and workstation design.
- Administrative controls:
  - Work practices (job rotation or enrichment, limited overtime, work/rest cycles)
  - Safe work practice training, including body mechanics
  - Worker placement evaluation (employee selection).
- Personal protective equipment (PPE), such as gloves, padding, and wrist rests.
- Medical management to minimize the impact of the health problems.

The ergonomic principles listed in Table 9 can also be classified into these categories; the first three are engineering controls and the last two are administrative.

The goal of NIOSH's intervention strategy is to eliminate, reduce, or control the presence of ergonomic hazards. To achieve this goal, NIOSH recommends a tiered hierarchy of controls, where engineering changes are viewed as the first preference, administrative changes are a second preference, and personal protective equipment is the last choice. These strategies fall under the category of primary prevention, i.e., measures taken to prevent the clinical manifestation of a disease before it occurs (22). While the exposure to the ergonomic hazards can be demonstrably reduced, we still need evidence demonstrating the effectiveness of primary prevention strategies in controlling WRMD.

The increase in reported cases of WRMD and the increase in workers' compensation costs in the United States prompted some regulatory efforts. Until 1991, attempts to standardize or control exposure to WRMD risk factors were limited to specific tasks or situations. American and international standards on exposure to vibration have been available. In 1981 NIOSH issued a work practice guide for manual lifting. The approach to hazard control was coupled to the *action limit,* a resultant term that denoted the recommended weight limit derived from the lifting equation. In 1988, The Human Factors Society, together with ANSI, issued ergonomic guidelines for computer workstations [video display terminals (VDTs)]. These were not specifically aimed at addressing WRMDs, though they contained technical standards for workstation design, chairs, keyboards, and monitors (ANSI/HFS 100-1988). The International Standards Organization has also established a technical committee for ergonomics (ISO TC 159), with a subcommittee for standardizing the terminology, methodology, and data on anthropometry and biomechanics. Another subcommittee standardizes the dimensions of control stations that affect postures. The subcommittee for human systems interaction issued standards for VDT workplaces (ISO 9241), which will supersede existing directives and guidelines in place in the European Community regarding furniture, hardware, software, and environments for VDT stations (35).

In an attempt to broaden the approach to prevention of WRMD, NIOSH sponsored a conference to develop a national strategy for occupational musculoskeletal injury prevention (5). Consequently, the lifting guide was revised in 1991 (25). The revised equation reflected new findings and provided methods for addressing issues not covered by the previous guide: lifts of objects with less than optimal couplings between the object and the worker's hands. It also added to the biomechanical criteria equations for asymmetrical lifting tasks, and guidelines for multiple task exposure.

Following high-profile citations under the general duty clause, as well as improper reporting of injuries, OSHA issued in 1993 guidelines for managing ergonomics programs (36). These were limited to the meatpacking industry. This industry was targeted because of high incidence and severity of WRMDs of the upper extremities, or cumulative trauma disorders (CTD). OSHA further emphasized that this was not a standard or regulation. OSHA's approach focused on ergonomics as a process. The guidelines consisted of a discussion on the importance of management commitment and employee involvement, recommended program elements, and detailed guidance and examples for the program elements.

OSHA later attempted to expand the scope of the guide to the general industry. The program may include guidelines for the following elements:

1. Management commitment and employee involvement
    - 1.1. Commitment by top management
    - 1.2. Employee involvement
    - 1.3. Written program
    - 1.4. Regular program review and evaluation.
2. Program elements
    - 2.1. Work site analysis
    - 2.2. Hazard prevention and control
        - 2.2.1. Engineering controls
        - 2.2.2. Work practice controls
        - 2.2.3. Personal protective equipment (PPE)
        - 2.2.4. Administrative controls
    - 2.3. Medical management
        - 2.3.1. Periodic workplace walkthrough
        - 2.3.2. Symptom survey
        - 2.3.3. Identification of restricted duty jobs
        - 2.3.4. Health surveillance
        - 2.3.5. Employee training and education
        - 2.3.6. Early reporting of symptoms
        - 2.3.7. Appropriate medical care
        - 2.3.8. Accurate record keeping
        - 2.3.9. Periodic program evaluation
    - 2.4. Training and education
        - 2.4.1. General training
        - 2.4.2. Job specific training
        - 2.4.3. Training for supervisors
        - 2.4.4. Training for managers
        - 2.4.5. Training for engineers and maintenance personnel

A similar approach was adopted by the ANSI-accredited committee for controlling CTD (11). The working draft is limited to CTD of the upper extremities, although many of the concepts are applicable to other parts of the body. Specific recommendations for other body parts may be added as separate sections. If approved, ANSI's voluntary standards will outline management responsibilities, a written program, training, and employee involvement as essential requirements. The process is driven by surveillance of hazards and health outcome. The standards will state when a detailed job analysis should be initiated, and how to prioritize interventions. In setting priorities, the following information should be considered:

- Jobs where work-related CTD have been identified as individual cases
- Jobs where the incidence and severity of CTD are higher compared with other departments, facilities, or other groupings
- Jobs where proactive job surveys suggested further job analysis and possible intervention.

The job design aims to reduce the exposure to risk factors. The process is seen to continue until health and hazard surveillance data indicate that the problem is under control.

**Secondary Prevention**

The measures taken to arrest the development of a disease while it is still in the early symptomatic stage are called secondary prevention (22). Ergonomic accommodations for employees who developed WRMDs fall under this category. There are three principal ways to accommodate impaired or disabled employees:

1. *Client matching* is the simplest and most effective way to return a person with a disability to work. It involves ensuring that the job requirements are consistent with the present abilities of the employee. If employees cannot return to their previous jobs, an alternative job is found that they can perform without risk of reinjury. This strategy does not attempt to fit the job to the worker, as it hardly requires any modifications in the job. The ergonomic methods for analyzing job demands can be used in the matching process (37,38).
2. *Job restructuring* is an administrative control to reduce exposure to a risk factor. In secondary prevention it entails assigning restricted duties to the employee. For example, restructuring the job by assigning heavy-lifting tasks to another person would enable a worker with low back pain to work while

recovering from the injury. Here too the ergonomic methods for analyzing job demands can be used to reassign the tasks.

3. *Job modifications and redesign* usually involve providing assistive technology to enable individuals to perform the required tasks. Occasionally, some tasks can be eliminated in the process of introducing new technology. Other employees may also benefit from similar devices. All the ergonomic methods described above can be used in this process. However, more detailed knowledge is required about the residual abilities and limitations of the individual.

Many health and safety problems can be attributed to failure to anticipate the capacity and behavior of the worker population. Accidents, musculoskeletal disorders, and localized and whole-body fatigue are common examples of these problems. Ergonomics is the application of epidemiology, anthropometry, biomechanics, physiology, psychology, and engineering to the evaluation and design of work. This discipline can contribute to the prevention of injuries while maximizing productivity. As part of occupational injury prevention efforts, ergonomics is a problem-solving process of continuous improvement.

## REFERENCES


1. Frymoyer JD. Cost and control of industrial musculoskeletal injuries. In: Nordin M, Andersson GBJ, Pope MH, eds. *Musculoskeletal disorders in the workplace.* Philadelphia: Mosby, 1997;62–71.
2. Wells R. Task analysis. In: Ranney D, ed. *Chronic musculoskeletal injuries in the workplace.* Philadelphia: WB Saunders, 1997;41–63.
3. Armstrong TJ, Buckle P, Fine LJ, Hagberg M, Jonsson B. A conceptual model for work-related neck and upper-limb disorders. *Scand J Work Environ Health* 1993;19:73–84.
4. Bureau of Labor Statistics. *Characteristics of injuries and illnesses resulting from absences from work, 1994.* BLS News. USDL-96-163. Washington, DC: BLS, 1996.
5. NIOSH. *A national strategy for occupational musculoskeletal injuries:* implementation issues and research needs—1991 conference summary. NIOSH publication no. 93-101. Washington, DC: DHHS, 1992.
6. Kilbom Å. Repetitive work of the upper extremity: part II—the scientific basis (knowledge base) for the guide. *Int J Ind Ergon* 1994;14:59–86.
7. Riihimaki H. Low back pain, its origin and risk indicators. *Scand J Work Environ Health* 1991;17:81–90.
8. Winkel J, Westgaard R. Occupational and individual risk factors for shoulder-neck complaints: Part II—The scientific basis (literature review) for the guide. *Int J Ind Ergon* 1992;10:85–104.
9. Sjøgaard G, Jensen BR. Muscle pathology with overuse. In: Ranney D, ed. *Chronic musculoskeletal injuries in the workplace.* Philadelphia: WB Saunders, 1997;17–40.
10. Weiser S. Psychosocial aspects of occupational musculoskeletal disorders. In: Nordin M, Andersson GBJ, Pope MH, eds. *Musculoskeletal disorders in the workplace.* Philadelphia: Mosby, 1997;51–61.
11. American National Standards Institute. Accredited Standards Committee. *Control of cumulative trauma disorders,* working draft. Z-365. Itasca. IL: National Safety Council, 1997.
12. Wilson JR. A framework and a context for ergonomics methodology. In: Wilson JR, Corlett EN, eds. *Evaluation of human work,* 2nd ed. New York: Taylor & Francis, 1995;1–39.
13. Fine LJ, Silverstein BA, Armstrong TJH, Anderson CA, Sugano DS. The detection of cumulative trauma disorders of the upper extremities in the workplace. *J Occup Med* 1986;28:675–678.
14. Maizlish N, Rudolph I, Dervin K, Sankaranarayan M. Surveillance and prevention of work-related carpal tunnel syndrome: an application of the Sentinel Events Notification system for Occupational Risks. *Am J Ind Med* 1995;27(5):715–729.
15. Putz-Anderson V. *Cumulative trauma disorders.* New York: Taylor & Francis, 1988.
16. Niebel B. *Motion and time study.* Homewood, IL: Richard D. Irwin, 1986.
17. Magnusson M. Posture. In: Nordin M, Andersson GBJ, Pope MH, eds. *Musculoskeletal disorders in the workplace.* Philadelphia: Mosby, 1997; 74–84.
18. Garg A. Manual materials handling: the science. In: Nordin M, Andersson GBJ, Pope MH, eds. *Musculoskeletal disorders in the workplace.* Philadelphia: Mosby, 1997;85–119.
19. Borg G. Borg scales for subjective rating of perceived exertion. *Scand J Work Environ Health* 1990;16:55–58.
20. Garg A, Chaffin DB, Herrin GD. Prediction of metabolic rates for manual materials handling jobs. *Am Ind Hyg Assoc J* 1978;38:661–674.
21. Armstrong TJ and Martin BJ. Adverse effects of repetitive loading and segmental vibration. In: Nordin M, Andersson GBJ, Pope MH, eds. *Musculoskeletal disorders in the workplace.* Philadelphia: Mosby, 1997;134–151.
22. Pope MH, Andersson GBJ. Prevention. In: Nordin M, Andersson GBJ, Pope MH, eds. *Musculoskeletal disorders in the workplace.* Philadelphia: Mosby, 1997;244–249.
23. Hazelgrave C. What do we mean by a "working posture"? *Ergonomics* 1994;37(4):781–799.
24. Pope MH. Whole-body vibration. In: Nordin M, Andersson GBJ, Pope MH, eds. *Musculoskeletal disorders in the workplace.* Philadelphia: Mosby, 1997;127–133.
25. NIOSH. *Revised NIOSH lifting equation.* Publication no. 94-110. Cincinnati, OH: NIOSH, 1994.
26. Radwin RG, Oh S, and Carlson-Dakes C. Biomechanical aspects of hand tools. In: Nordin M, Andersson GBJ, Pope MH, eds. *Musculoskeletal disorders in the workplace.* Philadelphia: Mosby, 1997; 466–479.
27. Hale A and Mason I. L'evaluation du role d'une formation kinetique dans la prevention des accidents de manutention. *Le Travail Humain* 1986;49(3):195–208.
28. Drury CG. Influence of restricted space on manual materials handling. *Ergonomics* 1985;28:167–175.
29. Chaffin DB, Gallay LS, Wooley CB, Kuciemba SR. An evaluation of the effect of a training program in worker lifting postures. *Int J Ind Ergon* 1986;1:127–136.
30. Marras WS, Lavender SA, Leurgans SE, et al. The role of dynamic three dimensional trunk motion in occupationally related low back disorders: the effects of workplace factors, trunk position and trunk motion characteristics on the risk of risk of injury. *Spine* 1993;18:616–641.
31. NIOSH. *Work practices guide for manual lifting.* Publication no. 81-122. Cincinnati, OH: NIOSH, 1981.
32. Faville B. One approach for an ergonomics program in a large manufacturing environment. *Int J Ind Ergon* 1996;18:373–380.
33. Suadicani P, Hansen K, Fenger AM, Gyntelberg F. Low back pain in steelplant workers. *J Occup Med.* 1994;44(4):217–221.
34. Riel PE, Imbeau D. Justifying investments in industrial ergonomics. *Int J Ind Ergon* 1966;18:349–361.
35. Smith WJ. *ISO and ANSI:* ergonomic standards for computer products. Upper Saddle River, NJ: Prentice Hall, 1996.
36. OSHA. *Ergonomics program management guidelines for meatpacking plants.* DOL/OSHA 3123. Washington, DC: OSHA, 1993.
37. Halpern N. Prevention of low back pain in the workplace: Basic ergonomics in the workplace and the clinic. *Baillieres Clin Rheumatol* 1992;6(3):705–730.
38. Halpern M. A computerized medical standards system to help place impaired employees. *Methods of Information in Medicine,* 1996;35: 317–323.

*Environmental and Occupational Medicine, Third Edition,* edited by William N. Rom.
Lippincott–Raven Publishers, Philadelphia © 1998.

# CHAPTER 109

# Biomechanics

Nihat Özkaya

Bioengineering is a unique interdisciplinary field in which principles and methods from engineering, basic sciences, and technology are applied to design, test, and manufacture equipment for use in medicine and to understand, define, and solve problems in physiology and biology. Biomechanics is an important part of bioengineering that considers the applications of classical mechanics to the analysis of biologic systems. Different aspects of biomechanics utilize different parts of applied mechanics. For example, the principles of statics have been applied to analyze the magnitude and nature of forces involved in various joints and muscles of the musculoskeletal system. The principles of dynamics have been utilized for motion description, gait analysis, and segmental motion analysis, and have many applications in sports mechanics. The principles of solid mechanics provide the necessary tools for developing the field of constitutive equations for biologic systems that are used to evaluate their functional behavior under different load conditions. The principles of fluid mechanics have been used to investigate blood flow in the circulatory system, air flow in the lung, and joint lubrication.

Research in biomechanics is aimed to improve our knowledge of a very complex structure, the human body. Ongoing research activities in biomechanics can be divided into three areas: experimental studies, model analysis, and applied research. Experimental studies in biomechanics are used to determine the mechanical properties of biologic materials, including the bone, cartilage, muscle, tendon, ligament, skin, and blood as a whole or parts constituting them. The theoretical studies in the form of mathematical model analysis have also been an important component of research in biomechanics. In general, a model that is based on experimental findings can be used to predict the effect of environmental and operational factors without resorting to laboratory experiments.

The ultimate goal of research in biomechanics must be to apply the knowledge gained for the benefit of the human being. For example, musculoskeletal injury and illness is acknowledged by health and safety experts as one of the primary occupational hazards in industrialized countries. Such injuries may be combatted by learning how the musculoskeletal system adjusts to common work conditions and by developing guidelines to assure that manual work conforms more closely to the physical limitations of the human body and to natural body movements. The need to enhance the worker's performance while minimizing the risk of musculoskeletal injuries has led to an applied discipline, occupational biomechanics, which may be defined as a field concerned with the mechanical behavior and response of the human musculoskeletal system to physical work. This field has developed because of an awareness that occupational musculoskeletal injuries are usually the result of a physical mismatch between workers' physical abilities and the tasks required of them. In this sense, occupational biomechanics provides a foundation for the field of ergonomics. Ergonomics is concerned with adapting jobs and workplaces to the worker by designing tasks, workstations, tools, and equipment so as to improve worker's health, safety, productivity, and efficiency.

Occupational biomechanics deals with work-related factors that can lead to injury or illness. These include psychosocial factors such as work satisfaction and men-

N. Özkaya: Department of Environmental Medicine, New York University Medical Center; Occupational and Industrial Orthopedic Center, Hospital for Joint Diseases, New York, New York 10014.

tal demands that may contribute to fatigue, carelessness, and compensatory injuries, and environmental factors such as excessive and/or repetitive force, constrained posture, vibration, and extreme temperature variations. For example, low back pain is a costly occupational problem that can have many contributing factors—from work stress to vibration to constrained postures—that also influence prevention and treatment options. These and other occupational hazards are covered in detail in other chapters of this volume.

## BASIC CONCEPTS

### Scalars, Vectors, and Tensors

Most of the concepts in mechanics are either scalar or vector. A scalar quantity has a magnitude only. Concepts such as mass, energy, power, mechanical work, and temperature are scalar quantities. For example, it is sufficient to say that an object has 80 kg of mass. A vector quantity, on the other hand, has both a magnitude and a direction associated with it. Force, moment, velocity, and acceleration are examples of vector quantities. To describe a force fully, one must state how much force is applied and in which direction it is applied. The magnitude of a vector is also a scalar quantity. The magnitude of any quantity (scalar or vector) is always a positive number corresponding to the numerical measure of that quantity.

There are various notations used to refer to vectors. In this chapter, letters with an underbar will be used to indicate vector quantities. For example, $\underline{F}$ is be used to refer to a force vector. On the other hand, $F$ without the underbar indicates the magnitude of a force vector or a scalar quantity. Graphically, a vector is represented by an arrow such that the orientation of the arrow indicates the line of action, the arrowhead denotes the direction and sense, and the base of the arrow corresponds to the point of application of the vector. If there is a need for showing more than one vector in a single drawing, then the length of each arrow must be proportional to the magnitude of the vector it represents.

Both scalars and vectors are special forms of a more general category of all quantities in mechanics, called tensors. Scalars are also known as "zero-order tensors," whereas vectors are "first-order tensors." Concepts such as stress and strain, on the other hand, are "second-order tensors." In this definition, the order corresponds to the power $n$ in $3^n$. For scalars, $n$ is 0, and therefore, $3^{\circ} = 1$, or only one quantity (magnitude) is necessary to define a scalar quantity. For vectors, $n$ is 1, and therefore, $3^1 = 3$. That is, three quantities (components in three directions) are necessary to define a vector quantity in three-dimensional space. On the other hand, $n$ is 2 for second-order tensors, and since $3^2 = 9$, nine quantities (three components in three planes) are needed to define concepts like stress and strain.

### Force Vector

Force can be defined as mechanical disturbance or load. When an object is pushed or pulled, a force is applied on it. A force is also applied when a ball is thrown or kicked. In all of these cases, the force is associated with the result of muscular activity. A force acting on an object may deform the object, change its state of motion, or both. Although forces may cause movement, it does not necessarily follow that force is always associated with motion. For example, a person sitting on a chair applies his or her weight on the chair, and yet the chair remains stationary. Forces may be classified in various ways according to their effect on the objects they are applied or according to their orientation as compared to one another. For example, a force may be internal or external, normal (perpendicular) or tangential, tensile, compressive, or shear, gravitational (weight), or frictional. Any two or more forces acting on a single body may be coplanar (acting on a two-dimensional plane surface), collinear (have a common line of action), concurrent (lines of action intersecting at a single point), or parallel. Note that weight is a special form of force. The weight of an object on Earth is the gravitational force exerted by Earth on the mass of that object. The magnitude of the weight of an object on Earth is equal to the mass of the object times the magnitude of the gravitational acceleration which is about 9.8 meters per second squared ($m/s^2$). For example, a 10-kg object weighs about 98 newtons (N) on Earth. The direction of weight is always vertically downward.

### Torque and Moment Vectors

The effect of a force on the object it is applied upon depends on how the force is applied and how the object is supported. For example, when pushed, an open door will swing about the edge along which it is hinged to the wall. What causes the door to swing is the torque generated by the applied force about an axis that passes through the hinges of the door. If one stands on the free end of a diving board, the board will bend. What bends the board is the moment of the body weight about the fixed end of the board. In general, torque is associated with the rotational and twisting action of applied forces, while moment is related to the bending action. However, the mathematical definition of moment and torque is the same.

Torque and moment are vector quantities. The magnitude of the torque or moment of a force about an axis is equal to the magnitude of the force times the length of the shortest distance between the axis and the line of action of the force, which is known as the lever or moment arm. Consider a person on an exercise apparatus who is holding a handle that is attached to a cable (Fig. 1). The cable is wrapped around a pulley and attached to a weight pan. The weight in the weight pan stretches the cable such that the magnitude $F$ of the tensile force in the cable is equal to the weight of the

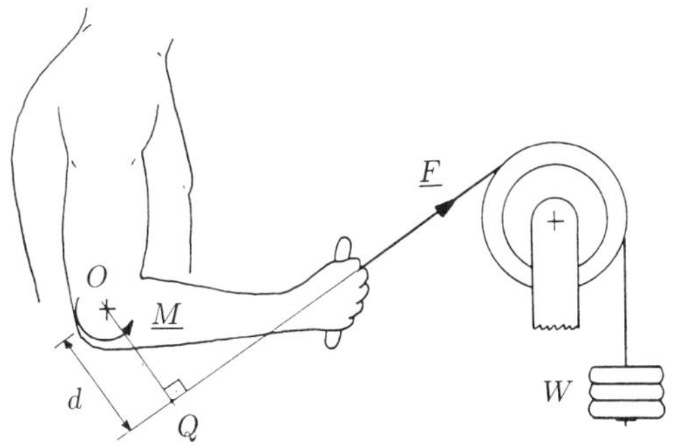


**FIG. 1.** Definition of torque.

weight pan. This force is transmitted to the person's hand through the handle. At this instant, if the cable attached to the handle makes an angle θ with the horizontal, then the force $\underline{F}$ exerted by the cable on the person's hand also makes an angle θ with the horizontal. Let $O$ be a point on the axis of rotation of the elbow joint. To determine the magnitude of the moment due to force $\underline{F}$ about $O$, extend the line of action of force $\underline{F}$ and drop a line from $O$ that cuts the line of action of $\underline{F}$ at right angles. If the point of intersection of the two lines is $Q$, then the distance $d$ between $O$ and $Q$ is the lever arm, and the magnitude of the moment $\underline{M}$ of force $\underline{F}$ about the elbow joint is $M = dF$. The direction of the moment vector is perpendicular to the plane defined by the line of action of $\underline{F}$ and line $OQ$, or for this two-dimensional case, it is counterclockwise.

### Newton's Laws

There are relatively few basic laws that govern the relationship between applied forces and corresponding motions. Among these, the laws of mechanics introduced by Sir Isaac Newton (1642–1727) are the most important. Newton's first law states that an object that is originally at rest will remain at rest or an object in motion will move in a straight line with constant velocity if the net force acting on the object is zero. Newton's second law states that an object with a nonzero net force acting on it will accelerate in the direction of the net force and that the magnitude of the acceleration will be proportional to the magnitude of the net force. Newton's second law can be formulated as $\underline{F} = m\underline{a}$. Here, $\underline{F}$ is the applied force, $m$ is the mass of the object, and $\underline{a}$ is the linear (translational) acceleration of the object upon which the force is applied. If there is more than one force acting on the object, then $\underline{F}$ represents the net or the resultant force (the vector sum of all forces).

An alternative formulation of Newton's second law of motion is $\underline{M} = I\underline{\alpha}$, where $\underline{M}$ is the net or resultant moment of all forces acting on the object, $I$ is the mass moment of inertia of the object, and $\underline{\alpha}$ is the angular (rotational) acceleration of the object. The mass $m$ and mass moment of inertia $I$ in these equations of motion are measures of resistance to changes in motion. The larger the inertia of an object, the more difficult it is to set it in motion or to stop it if it is already in motion.

Newton's third law states that to every action there is a reaction and that the forces of action and reaction between interacting objects are equal in magnitude, opposite in direction, and have the same line of action. This law has important applications in constructing free-body diagrams.

### Free-Body Diagrams

Free-body diagrams are constructed to help identify the forces and moments acting on individual parts of a system and to ensure the correct use of the equations of mechanics to analyze the system. For this purpose, the parts constituting a system are isolated from their surroundings and the effects of surroundings are replaced by proper forces and moments.

The human musculoskeletal system consists of many parts that are connected to one another through a complex tendon, ligament, muscle, and joint structure. In some analyses, the objective may be to investigate the forces involved at and around various joints of the human body for different postural and load conditions. Such analyses can be carried out by separating the body into two parts at the joint of interest and drawing the free-body diagram of one of the parts. For example, consider the arm illustrated in Fig. 1. Assume that the forces involved at the elbow joint are to be analyzed. As illustrated in Fig. 2, the entire body is separated into two at the elbow joint and

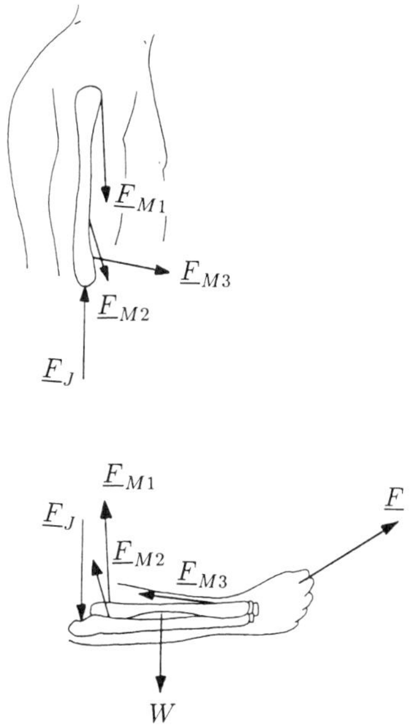


**FIG. 2.** Forces involved at and around the elbow joint and the free-body diagram of the lower arm.

the free-body diagram of the forearm is drawn (Fig. 2). Here, $\underline{F}$ is the force applied to the hand by the handle of the cable attached to the weight in the weight pan, $\underline{W}$ is the total weight of the lower arm acting at the center of gravity of the lower arm, $\underline{F}_{M1}$ is the force exerted by the biceps on the radius, $\underline{F}_{M2}$ is the force exerted by the brachioradialis muscles on the radius, $\underline{F}_{M3}$ is the force exerted by the brachialis muscles on the ulna, and $\underline{F}_J$ is the resultant reaction force at the humeroulnar and humeroradial joints of the elbow. Note that the muscle and joint reaction forces represent the mechanical effects of the upper arm on the lower arm. Also note that as illustrated in Fig. 2 (which is not a complete free-body diagram), equal magnitude but opposite muscle and joint reaction forces act on the upper arm as well.

### Conditions for Equilibrium

Statics is an area within applied mechanics that is concerned with the analysis of forces on rigid bodies in equilibrium. A rigid body is one that is assumed to undergo no deformations. In reality, every object or material may undergo deformation to an extent when acted upon by forces. In some cases the amount of deformation may be so small that it may not affect the desired analysis. In such cases, the object may assumed to be rigid. In mechanics, the term *equilibrium* implies that the body of concern is either at rest or moving with constant velocity. For a body to be in a state of equilibrium, it has to be both in translational and rotational equilibrium. A body is in translational equilibrium if the net force (vector sum of all forces) acting on it is zero. If the net force is zero, then the linear acceleration (time rate of change of linear velocity) of the body is zero, or the linear velocity of the body is either constant or zero. A body is in rotational equilibrium if the net moment (vector sum of the moments of all forces) acting on it is zero. If the net moment is zero, then the angular acceleration (time rate of change of angular velocity) of the body is zero, or the angular velocity of the body is either constant or zero. Therefore, for a body in a state of equilibrium, the equations of motion (Newton's second law) take the following special forms: $\underline{F} = 0$ and $\underline{M} = 0$.

It is important to remember that force and moment are vector quantities. For example, with respect to a rectangular (Cartesian) coordinate system, force and moment vectors may have components in the *x, y,* and *z* directions. Therefore, if the net force acting on an object is zero, then the sum of forces acting in each direction must be equal to zero ($\Sigma F_x = 0$, $\Sigma F_y = 0$, $\Sigma F_z = 0$). Similarly, if the net moment on an object is zero, then the sum of moments in each direction must also be equal to zero ($\Sigma M_x = 0$, $\Sigma M_y = 0$, $\Sigma M_z = 0$). Therefore, for three-dimension force systems, there are six conditions of equilibrium. For two-dimensional force systems in the *xy* plane, only three of these conditions ($\Sigma F_x = 0$, $\Sigma FM_y = 0$, $\Sigma M_x = 0$) need to be checked. The other three would be satisfied automatically. Note that one has to pay extra attention to the directions of forces and moments while applying these conditions. For example, while using the translational equilibrium condition in the *x* direction ($\Sigma F_x = 0$), the forces acting in the positive *x* direction must be added together and the forces acting in the negative *x* direction must be subtracted. The use of the equations of equilibrium will be demonstrated in the next section.

## BIOMECHANICS OF SKELETAL JOINTS

The human body is rigid in the sense that it can maintain a posture, and flexible in the sense that it can change its posture and move. The flexibility of the human body is due primarily to the joints or articulations of the skeletal system. The primary function of joints is to provide mobility to the musculoskeletal system. In addition to providing mobility, a joint must also possess a degree of stability. Since different joints have different functions, they possess varying degrees of mobility and stability. Some joints are constructed so as to provide a high degree of mobility. For example, the construction of the shoulder joint (a ball-and-socket type joint) enables the arm to move in all three planes. However, this high level of mobility is achieved at the expense of reduced stability, increasing the vulnerability of the joint to injuries, such as dislocations. On the other hand, the elbow joint (a hinge joint) provides movement only in one plane, but is more stable and less prone to injuries than the shoulder joint. The nature of motion about a joint and the stability of the joint are dependent on factors such as the manner in which the articulating surfaces fit together, the structure and length of the ligaments around the joint, and the degree to which the muscles that cross the joint can be stretched.

Movement of human body segments is achieved as a result of forces generated by skeletal muscles that convert chemical energy into mechanical work. A skeletal muscle is attached, via tendons, to at least two different bones controlling the relative motion of one segment with respect to the other. When its fibers contract under the stimulation of a nerve, the muscle exerts a pulling effect on the bones to which it is attached. The result of a muscle contraction is always tension. Muscles can only exert a pull. Muscles cannot exert a push. A muscle can cause movement only while its length is shortening. If the length of a muscle increases during a particular movement, then the tension generated by the muscle contraction is aimed at controlling the movement of the body segments associated with that muscle. If a muscle contracts but there is no segmental motion, then the tension in the muscle balances the effects of externally applied forces such as those due to gravity.

The principles of statics (equations of equilibrium) can be applied to investigate the muscle and joint forces involved at and around the joints for various postural positions of the human body and its segments. The immediate purpose of such analysis is to provide answers to questions such as: What tension must the neck extensor muscles exert on the head to support the head in a specified position? When a person bends, what would be the force exerted by the erector spinae on the fifth lumbar vertebra? How does the compression at the elbow, knee, and ankle joints vary with externally applied forces and with different segmental arrangements? How does the force on the femoral head vary with loads carried in the hand? What are the forces involved in various muscle groups and joints during different exercise conditions?

To help understand possible uses of the equations of equilibrium, consider the arm illustrated in Fig. 3. The elbow is flexed at a right angle and an object is held stationary in the hand. The free-body diagram of the lower arm is shown in Fig. 3. For practical reasons, it is assumed that the biceps is the primary flexor muscle and that the line of action of the tension in the biceps is vertical. In Fig. 3, $W_1$ is the weight of the lower arm, $W_2$ is the weight of the object held in the hand, $F_M$ is the magnitude of the muscle tension in the biceps, $F_J$ is the elbow joint reaction force, $O$ represents the center of the elbow joint, $A$ is where the biceps is attached to the radius, $B$ is the center of gravity of the lower arm, and $C$ is the center of gravity of the weight held in the hand. The distances between $O$ and $A$, $B$, and $C$ are measured as $a$, $b$, and $c$. Note that weights are always directed vertically downward. Since the direction of the muscle tension is also vertical, the direction of the joint reaction force has to be in the vertical (a parallel force system) so that the lower arm remains in equilibrium.

Consider the rotational equilibrium of the lower arm about the elbow joint center at $O$. Relative to $O$, there are three moment-producing forces: $\underline{F}_M$, $\underline{W}_1$, and $\underline{W}_2$. The lever or moment arms of these forces relative to $O$ are $a$, $b$, and $c$, respectively. The moments produced by these forces are either clockwise or counterclockwise. For the rotational equilibrium of the lower arm, the net moment about an axis that passes through $O$ must be equal to zero. Assuming that counterclockwise moments are positive, then $aF_M - bW_1 - cW_2 = 0$. Dividing all terms by $a$ and rearranging the order of terms will yield $F_M = (bW_1 + cW_2)/a$. Therefore, if the weight of the object held in the hand, total weight of the lower arm, and positions of $A$, $B$, and $C$ relative to $O$ are known, then the magnitude of the muscle tension in the biceps can be calculated. Once $F_M$ is known, then the translational equilibrium condition in the vertical direction can be utilized to determine the magnitude of the elbow joint reaction force $F_J = F_M - W_1 - W_2$.

For example, if $a = 4$ cm, $b = 15$ cm, $c = 35$ cm, $W_1 = 20$ N, and $W_2 = 80$ N, then $F_M = 775$ N and $F_J = 675$ N. The magnitude of the muscle force is quite significant in that to maintain the flexed position of the arm, the biceps is required to exert a force about ten times larger than the weight of the object held in the hand. This is due to the fact that relative to the elbow joint, the length of the lever arm of the muscle force is much smaller than the length of the lever arm of the load held in the hand. The smaller the lever arm, the greater the muscle force required to balance the rotational effect of the load held in the hand about the elbow joint.

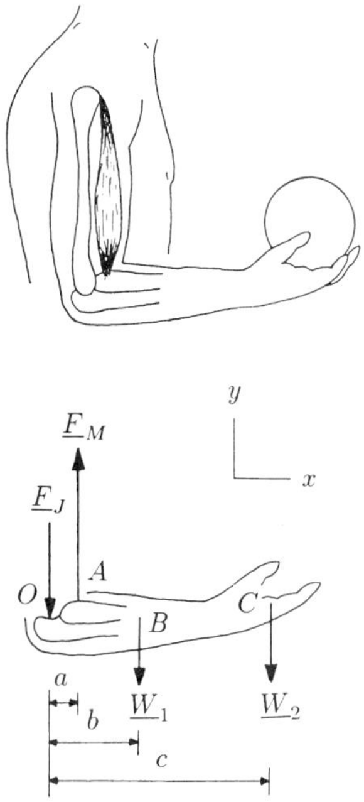


**FIG. 3.** A simple mechanical model of the lower arm.

The elbow is a diarthrodial joint. A ligamentous capsule encloses the articular cavity, which is filled with synovial fluid, a thick, viscous material. The primary function of this fluid is to lubricate the articulating surfaces, thereby reducing the frictional forces that may develop while one articulating surface moves over the other. The synovial fluid also nourishes the articulating cartilages. Another function of the synovial fluid is to distribute the forces involved at the joint over a relatively large surface area (Fig. 4). A common property of fluids is that they exert pressures (force per unit area) that are distributed over the surfaces they contact. The fluid pressure always acts in a direction toward and perpendicular to the surface it touches, having a compressive effect on the surface. The small arrows in Fig. 4 represent the synovial fluid pressure. In a two-dimensional sense, the fluid pressure has components in the horizontal and vertical directions. The fact that the joint reaction force at the elbow acts vertically downward on the ulna implies that the horizontal components of these vectors cancel out, but their vertical components add up to form the resultant force $\underline{F}_J$. Therefore, the joint reaction force $\underline{F}_J$ corresponds to the resultant of the distributed force system (pressure) applied through the synovial fluid.

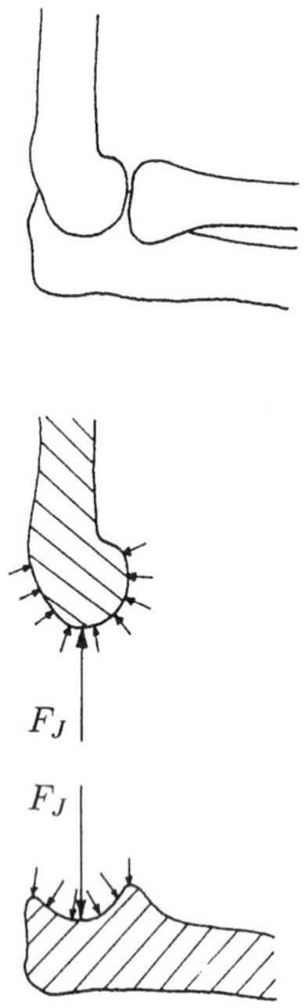


**FIG. 4.** Explaining the joint reaction force.

In general, the unknowns in static problems involving the musculoskeletal system are the magnitudes of joint reaction forces and muscle tensions. The mechanical analysis of a skeletal joint requires that we know the vector characteristics of tensions in the muscles, the proper locations of muscle attachments, the weights of body segments, and the locations of the centers of gravity of the body segments. The mechanical model of the lower arm presented above is obviously a simple one. The most critical weakness of this model is the assumption that the biceps is the only muscle group that maintains the flexed position of the arm. The reason for making such an assumption is to reduce the system under consideration to a statically determinate one. This model can be improved by considering the contributions of other elbow flexors such as the brachioradialis and the brachialis (Fig. 2). However, that will increase the number of unknowns (two additional muscle tensions) and make the model a statically indeterminate one. To analyze the improved model, one would need additional information related to the muscle forces. This information can be gathered through electromyography measurements of muscle signals or by applying certain optimization techniques. A similar analysis can be made to investigate forces involved at and around other major joints of the musculoskeletal system.

## MECHANICAL PROPERTIES OF MATERIALS

There are many reasons why it is important to know the deformation characteristics and mechanical properties of materials. One of the tasks of an engineer (mechanical, civil, electrical, or biomedical) is to determine the safest and most efficient operating condition for a machine, a structure, a piece of equipment, or a prosthetic device. This task can be accomplished by assessing the proper operational environment through force analyses, making the correct structural design, and choosing the material to sustain the forces involved in that environment. The primary concern of a design engineer is to make sure that when loaded, a machine part, a structure, a piece of equipment, or a device will not break or deform excessively. Knowing the mechanical properties of materials can also enable us to construct material functions and constitutive equations. These equations can be used along with physical laws in the form of governing equations to predict the behavior of the material under different load and environmental conditions without resorting to tedious and expensive laboratory experiments.

### Modes of Deformation

When acted upon by externally applied forces, objects may translate in the direction of the net force and rotate in the direction of the net torque acting on them. If an object is subjected to externally applied forces but is in static equilibrium, then it is most likely that there is some local shape change within the object. Local shape change under the effect of applied forces is known as deformation. The extent of deformation an object may undergo is dependent on many factors including the material properties; size and shape of the object; environmental factors such as heat and humidity; and the magnitude, direction, and duration of applied forces.

One way of distinguishing forces is by observing their tendency to deform the object they are applied upon. For example, the object is said to be in tension if the body tends to elongate, and in compression if it tends to shrink in the direction of the applied forces. Shear loading differs from tension and compression in that it is caused by forces acting in directions tangent to the area resisting the forces causing shear, whereas both tension and compression are caused by collinear forces applied perpendicular to the areas on which they act. It is common to call tensile and compressive forces normal or axial forces, whereas shearing forces are tangential forces. Objects also deform when they are subjected to forces that cause bending and torsion, which are related to the moment and torque actions of applied forces.

A material may respond differently to different loading configurations. For a given material, there may be different physical properties that must be considered while analyzing the response of that material to tensile loading as compared to compressive or shear loading. The mechanical properties of materials are established through stress analysis by subjecting them to various experiments such as uniaxial tension and compression, torsion, and bending tests.

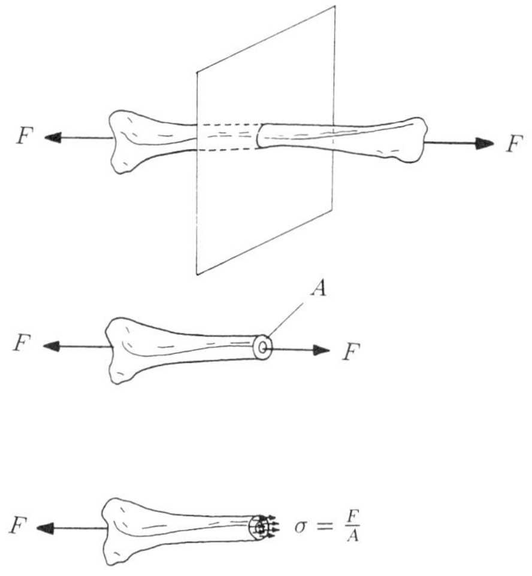


**FIG. 5.** Definition of normal stress.

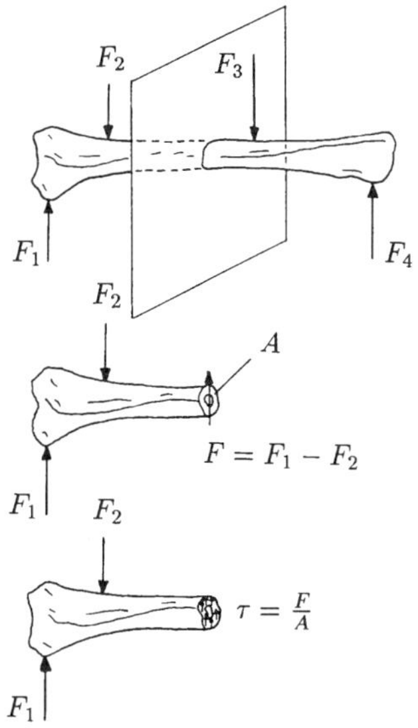


**FIG. 6.** Definition of shear stress.

## Normal and Shear Stresses

Consider the whole bone in Fig. 5, which is subjected to a pair of tensile forces of magnitude *F.* The bone is in static equilibrium. To analyze the forces induced within the bone, the method of sections can be applied by hypothetically cutting the bone into two pieces through a plane perpendicular to the long axis of the bone. Since the bone as a whole is in equilibrium, the two pieces must individually be in equilibrium as well. This requires that at the cut section of each piece there is an internal force that is equal in magnitude but opposite in direction to the externally applied force (Fig. 5). The internal force is distributed over the entire cross-sectional area of the cut section, and $F$ represents the resultant of the distributed force (Fig. 5). The intensity of this distributed force (force per unit area) is known as stress. For the case shown in Fig. 5, since the force resultant at the cut section is perpendicular to the plane of the cut, the corresponding stress is called a normal or axial stress. It is customary to use the symbol σ (sigma) to refer to normal stresses. Assuming that the intensity of the distributed force at the cut section is uniform over the cross-sectional area $A$ of the bone, then $\sigma = F/A$. Normal stresses that are due to forces that tend to stretch (elongate) materials are more specifically known as tensile stresses, whereas those that tend to shrink them are known as compressive stresses. According to the Standard International (SI) unit system, stresses are measured in newtons per square meter ($N/m_2$), which is also known as Pascal (Pa).

There is another form of stress, called shear stress, which is a measure of the intensity of internal forces acting tangent (parallel) to a plane of cut. For example, consider the whole bone in Fig. 6. The bone is subject to a number of parallel forces that act in planes perpendicular to the long axis of the bone. Assume that the bone is fictitiously cut into two parts through a plane perpendicular to the long axis of the bone (Fig. 6). If the bone as a whole is in equilibrium, then its individual parts must be in equilibrium as well. This requires that there has to be an internal force at the cut section that acts in a direction tangent to the cut surface. If the magnitudes of the external forces are known, then the magnitude $F$ of the internal force can be calculated by considering the translational and rotational equilibrium of one of the parts constituting the bone. The intensity of the internal force tangent to the cut section is known as the shear stress. It is customary to use the symbol τ (tau) to refer to shear stresses (Fig. 6). Assuming that the intensity of the force tangent to the cut section is uniform over the cross-sectional area $A$ of the bone, then $\tau = F/A$.

## Normal and Shear Strains

Strain is a measure of the degree of deformation. As in the case of stress, two types of strains can be distinguished. A normal strain is defined as the ratio of the change (increase or decrease) in length to the original (undeformed) length, and is commonly denoted with the symbol ε (epsilon). Consider the whole bone in Fig. 7.

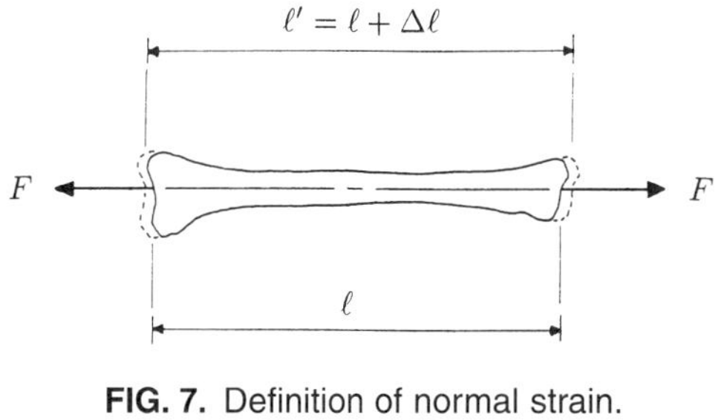


**FIG. 7.** Definition of normal strain.

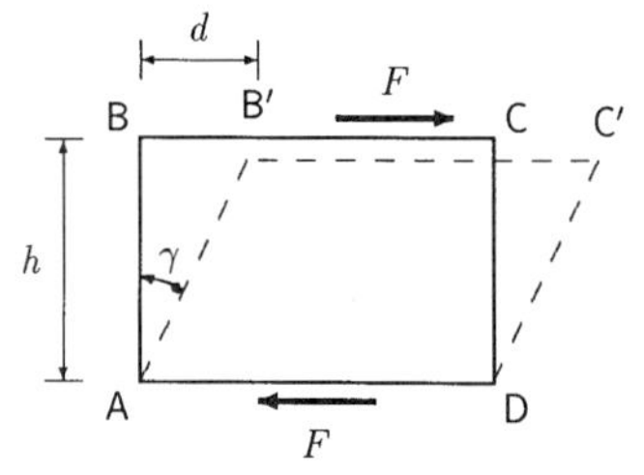


**FIG. 8.** Definition of shear strain.

The total length of the bone is $l$. If the bone is subjected to a pair of tensile forces, the length of the bone may increase to $l'$, or by an amount $\Delta l = l' - l$. The normal strain is the ratio of amount of elongation to the original length, or $\varepsilon = \Delta l/l$. If the length of the bone increases in the direction in which the strain is calculated, then the strain is tensile and positive. If the length of the bone decreases in the direction in which the strain is calculated, then the strain is compressive and negative.

Shear strains are related to distortions caused by shear stresses and are commonly denoted with the symbol $\gamma$ (gamma). Consider the rectangle *(ABCD)* shown in Fig. 8, which is acted upon by a pair of tangential forces that deform the rectangle into a parallelogram *(AB′C′D)*. If the relative horizontal displacement of the top and the bottom of the rectangle is $d$ and the height of the rectangle is $h$, then the average shear strain is the ratio of $d$ and $h$, which is equal to the tangent of angle $\gamma$. The angle $\gamma$ is usually very small. For small angles, the tangent of the angle is approximately equal to the angle itself measured in radians. Therefore, the average shear strain is $\gamma = d/h$.

Strains are calculated by dividing two quantities measured in units of length. For most applications, the deformations and consequently the strains involved may be very small (e.g., 0.001). Strains can also be given in percentages (e.g., 0.1%).

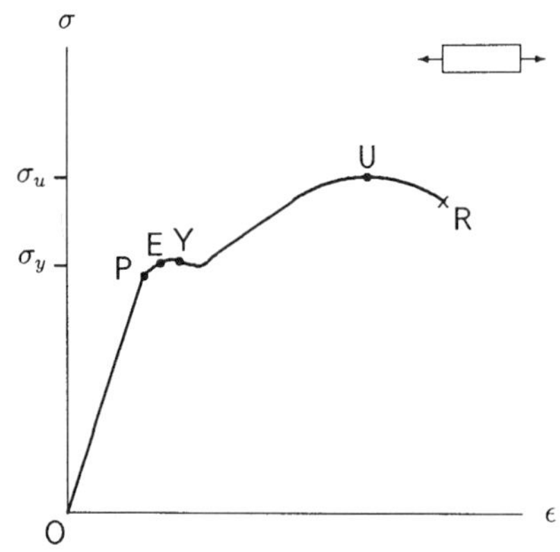


**FIG. 9.** Stress–strain diagrams.

## Stress-Strain Diagrams

Different materials may demonstrate different stress-strain relationships. Consider the stress-strain diagram shown in Fig. 9. There are six distinct points on the curve, which are labeled as *O, P, E, Y, U,* and *R*. Point *O* is the origin of the stress-strain diagram, which corresponds to the initial (no load, no deformation) state. Point *P* represents the proportionality limit. Between *O* and *P,* stress and strain are linearly proportional and the stress-strain diagram is a straight line. Point *E* represents the elastic limit. Point *Y* is the yield point and the stress $\sigma_y$ corresponding to the yield point is called the yield strength of the material. At this stress level, considerable elongation (yielding) can occur without a corresponding increase of load. *U* is the highest stress point on the stress-strain diagram. The stress $\sigma_u$ is the ultimate strength of the material. The last point on the stress-strain diagram is *R,* which represents the rupture or failure point. The stress at which the failure occurs is called the rupture strength of the material. For some materials, it may not be easy to distinguish the elastic limit and the yield point. The yield strength of such materials is determined by the offset method, which is applied by drawing a line parallel to the linear section of the stress-strain diagram that passes through a strain level of about 0.2%. The intersection of this line with the stress-strain curve is taken to be the yield point, and the stress corresponding to this point is called the apparent yield strength of the material.

Note that a given material may behave differently under different load and environmental conditions. If the curve shown in Fig. 9 represents the stress-strain relationship for a material under tensile loading, there may be a similar but different curve representing the stress-strain relationship for the same material under compressive or shear loading. Also, temperature is known to alter the relationship between stress and strain. For some materials, the stress-strain relationship may also depend on the rate at which the load is applied on the material.

## Elastic and Plastic Deformations

Elasticity is defined as the ability of a material to resume its original (stress-free) size and shape upon removal of applied loads. In other words, if a load is applied on a material such that the stress generated in the material is equal to or less than the elastic limit, then the deformations that took place in the material will be completely recovered once the applied loads are removed. An elastic material whose stress-strain diagram is a straight line is called a linearly elastic material. For such a material, the stress is linearly proportional to strain. The slope of the stress-strain diagram in the elastic region is called the elastic or Young's modulus of the material, which is commonly denoted by *E*. Therefore, the relationship between stress and strain for linearly elastic materials is

$\sigma = E\varepsilon$. This equation that relates normal stress and strain is called a material function. For a given material, different material functions may exist for different modes of deformation. For example, some materials may exhibit linearly elastic behavior under shear loading. For such materials, the shear stress $\tau$ is linearly proportional to the shear strain $\gamma$ and the constant of proportionality is called the shear modulus or the modulus of rigidity. If $G$ represents the modulus of rigidity, then $\tau = G\gamma$. Combinations of all possible material functions for a given material form the constitutive equations for that material.

Plasticity implies permanent deformations. Materials may undergo plastic deformations following elastic deformations when they are loaded beyond their elastic limits. Consider the stress-strain diagram of a material under tensile loading (Fig. 9). Assume that the stresses in the specimen are brought to a level greater than the yield strength of the material. Upon removal of the applied load, the material will recover the elastic deformation that had taken place by following an unloading path parallel to the initial linearly elastic region. The point where this path cuts the strain axis is called the plastic strain, which signifies the extent of permanent (unrecoverable) shape change that has taken place in the material.

### Material Properties Based on Stress-Strain Diagrams

The stress-strain diagrams of two or more materials can be compared to determine which material is relatively stiffer, harder, tougher, more ductile, or more brittle. For example, the slope of the stress-strain diagram in the elastic region represents the elastic modulus that is a measure of the relative stiffness of materials. The higher the elastic modulus, the stiffer the material and the higher its resistance to deformation. A ductile material is one that exhibits a large plastic deformation prior to failure. A brittle material, such as glass, shows a sudden failure (rupture) without undergoing a considerable plastic deformation. Toughness is a measure of the capacity of a material to sustain permanent deformation. The toughness of a material is measured by considering the total area under its stress-strain diagram. The larger this area, the tougher the material. The ability of a material to store or absorb energy without permanent deformation is called the resilience of the material. The resilience of a material is measured by its modulus of resilience, which is equal to the area under the stress-strain curve in the elastic region.

Although they are not directly related to the stress-strain diagrams, there are other important concepts used to describe material properties. For example, a material is called homogeneous if its properties do not vary from location to location within the material. A material is called isotropic if its properties are independent of direction. A material is called incompressible if it has a constant density.

### Multiaxial Deformations

When an object is subjected to a pair of tensile forces, the length of the object in the axial direction (direction in which the force is applied) will increase, and there will be positive stress and strain in the axial direction. For most materials, especially for incompressible materials, the gain in length in one direction is compensated by a decrease in the dimensions in the lateral directions (directions perpendicular to the axial direction), indicating the presence of negative strains in the lateral directions. In a more general sense, when an object is subjected to externally applied forces and moments in three mutually perpendicular directions, stresses and strains may be induced within the material in all three directions. For example, consider the rectangular bar in Fig. 10, which is subjected to forces and moments in the $x$, $y$, and $z$ directions. Let $P$ be a point within the bar. Stresses acting at point $P$ can be analyzed by constructing a cubical material element around point $P$. In Fig. 10, there are three normal stresses ($\sigma_{xx}$, $\sigma_{yy}$, $\sigma_{zz}$) and three corresponding normal strains ($\varepsilon_{xx}$, $\varepsilon_{yy}$, $\varepsilon_{zz}$). There are also six shear stresses ($\tau_{xy}$, $\tau_{yx}$, $\tau_{yz}$, $\tau_{zy}$, $\tau_{zx}$, $\tau_{xz}$), and the stress tensor has a total of nine components. However, the condition of static equilibrium requires that $\tau_{xy} = \tau_{yx}$, $\tau_{yz} = \tau_{zy}$, and $\tau_{zx} = \tau_{xz}$. Therefore, there are only three independent shear stresses ($\tau_{xy}$, $\tau_{yz}$, $\tau_{zx}$) and three corresponding shear strains ($\gamma_{xy}$, $\gamma_{yz}$, $\gamma_{zx}$). Note that the subscripts of these stress and strain components are such that the first index represents the direction normal (perpendicular) to the plane on which the stress or strain is measured, and the second index corresponds to

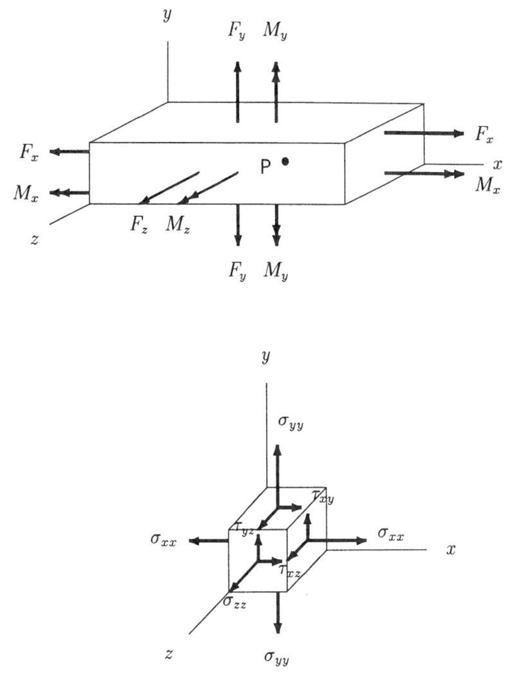


**FIG. 10.** Stress as a second-order tensor.

the direction along which the stress or strain is measured. Also note that these stress and strain tensor components are related.

It is important to note that components of the stress and strain tensors at a material point may vary with respect to the coordinate system adapted and with respect to the orientation of the material element constructed around the point. However, if the state of stress (or strain) with respect to one coordinate frame is known, then the state of stress with respect to another coordinate frame can be determined through appropriate coordinate transformations.

### Principal Stresses

There are infinitely many possibilities of constructing elements around a given point within a structure. Among these possibilities, there may be one element for which the normal stresses are maximum and minimum. These maximum and minimum normal stresses are called the principal stresses, and the planes whose normals are in the directions of the maximum and minimum stresses are called the principal planes. On a principal plane, the normal stress is either maximum or minimum, and the shear stress is zero. It is known that fracture or material failure occurs along the planes of maximum stresses, and structures must be designed by taking into consideration the maximum stresses involved. Failure by yielding (excessive deformation) may occur whenever the largest principal stress is equal to the yield strength of the material or failure by rupture occurs whenever the largest principal stress is equal to the ultimate strength of the material. For a given structure and loading condition, the principal stresses may be within the limits of operational safety. However, the structure must also be checked for critical shearing stress, called the maximum shear stress. The maximum shear stress occurs on a material element for which the normal stresses are equal.

Consider the solid circular shaft in Fig. 11, which is under pure torsion. Torsion is one of the fundamental modes of loading resulting from the twisting action of applied forces. Due to the externally applied torque $\underline{M}$ (represented with a double-headed arrow), the shaft deforms in such a way that the straight line *AB* on the outer surface of the shaft that is parallel to the center line of the shaft is twisted into a helix *AB′*. Also consider a plane perpendicular to the center line of the shaft (transverse plane *abcd* in Fig. 11), which cuts the shaft into two circular cylinders. Since the shaft as a whole is in equilibrium, its individual parts have to be in equilibrium as well. This condition requires the presence of internal shearing forces distributed over the cross-sectional area of the shaft (Fig. 11). The intensity of these internal forces is the shear stress τ. The magnitude of this shear stress is related to the magnitude of the applied torque, the cross-sectional area of the shaft, and the radial distance between the center line and the point at which the shear stress is to be determined. For a given shaft and applied torque, the torsional shear stress τ is a linear function of the radial distance *r* measured from the center of the shaft. At the center of the shaft, $r = 0$ and $\tau = 0$. The stress-free center line of the solid circular shaft is called the neutral axis. The magnitude of the shear stress is maximum on the circumference of the shaft where $r = r_0$ and $\tau = 2M/\pi r_0^3$.

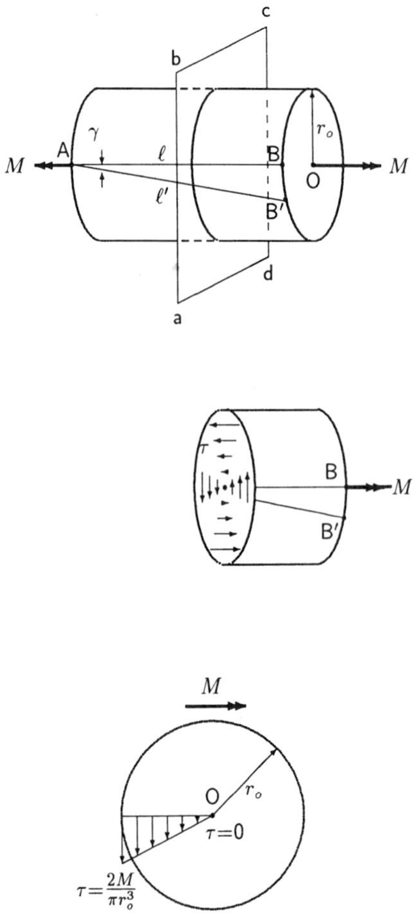


**FIG. 11.** Shear stress distribution for a solid cylindrical shaft under pure torsion.

The shear stress discussed herein is that induced in the transverse planes. For a shaft subjected to torsional loading, shear stresses are also developed along the longitudinal planes (planes that cut the shaft into two semicylinders). This is illustrated in Fig. 12*A* on a material element that is obtained by cutting the shaft with two transverse and two longitudinal planes. The transverse and longitudinal stresses are denoted with $\tau_t$ and $\tau_l$, respectively, and the equilibrium of the material element requires that $\tau_t$ and $\tau_l$ must be numerically equal. A shaft subjected to torsion not only deforms in shear but is also subjected to normal stresses. This can be explained by the fact that the straight line *AB* deforms into a helix *AB′* (Fig. 11), which indi-

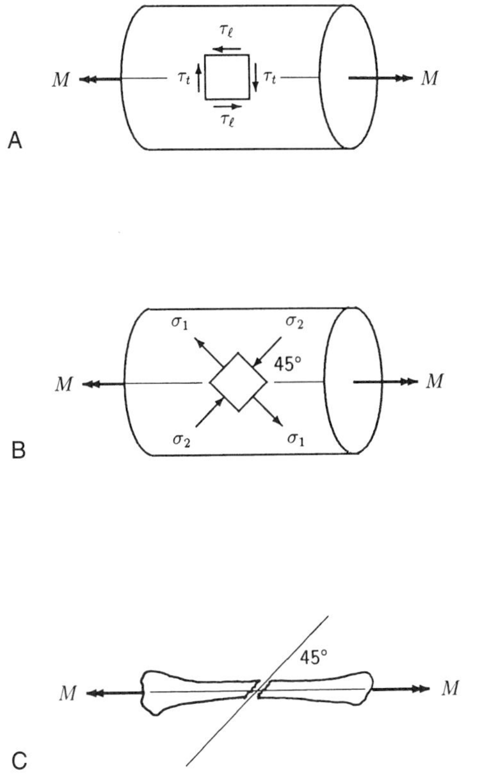


**FIG. 12.** Transverse ($\tau_t$) and longitudinal ($\tau_l$) stresses on a cylindrical shaft under pure torsion **(A)**, principal stresses ($\sigma_1$ and $\sigma_2$) on a cylindrical shaft under pure torsion **(B)**, and spiral fracture pattern for a bone subjected to pure torsion **(C)**.

cates an increase in length and the presence of tensile stresses. Consider the material element in Fig. 12*B*. The normals of the sides of this material element make an angle 45 degrees with the center line of the shaft. It can be proven that the only stresses induced on the sides of such an element are normal stresses (tensile stress $\sigma_1$ and compressive stress $\sigma_2$). The absence of shear stresses on this material element indicates that the normal stresses present are the principal (maximum and minimum) stresses, and that the planes on which these stresses act are the principal planes. For structures subjected to pure torsion, material failure occurs along one of the principal planes. This can be demonstrated by twisting a piece of chalk until it breaks into two pieces. A careful examination of the chalk will reveal the occurrence of the fracture along a spiral line normal to the direction of maximum tension. For circular shafts, the spiral lines make an angle of 45 degrees with the neutral axis (center line). The same fracture pattern has been observed for long bones subjected to pure torsion (Fig. 12*C*). Torsional fractures are usually initiated at regions of the bones where the cross sections are the smallest. Some particularly weak sections of human bones are the upper and lower thirds of the humerus, femur, and fibula, the upper third of the radius, and the lower fourth of the ulna and tibia.

## Fatigue and Endurance

Principal and maximum shear stresses are useful in predicting the response of materials to static loading configurations. Loads that may not cause the failure of a structure in a single application may cause fracture when applied repeatedly. Failure may occur after a few or many cycles of loading and unloading, depending on factors such as the amplitude of the applied load, mechanical properties of the material, size of the structure, and operational conditions. Fracture due to repeated loading is called fatigue.

There are several experimental techniques developed to understand the fatigue behavior of materials. Consider the bar shown in Fig. 13. Assume that the bar is made of a material whose ultimate strength is $\sigma_u$. This bar is first stressed to a mean stress level $\sigma_m$ and then subjected to a stress fluctuating over time, sometimes tensile and other times compressive (Fig. 13). The amplitude $\sigma_a$ of the stress is such that the bar is subjected to a maximum tensile stress less than the ultimate strength of the material. This reversible and periodic stress is applied until the bar fractures and the number of cycles $N$ to fracture is recorded. This experiment is repeated on specimens having the same material properties by applying stresses of varying amplitude. A typical result of a fatigue test is

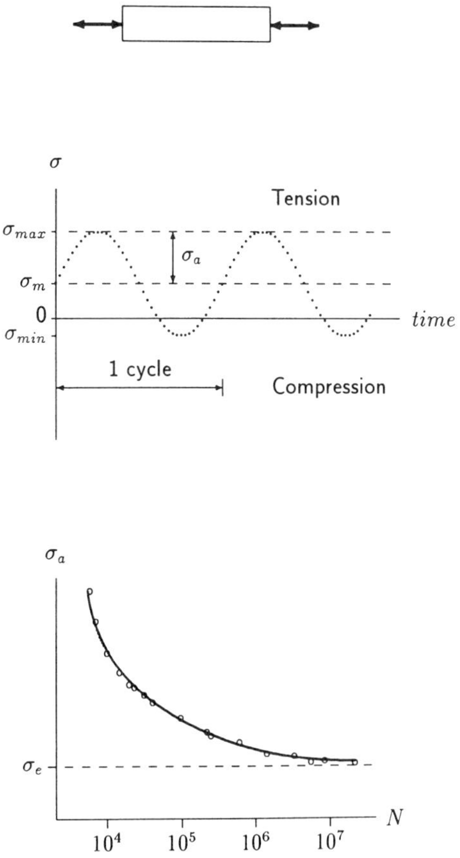


**FIG. 13.** Fatigue and endurance.

plotted in Fig. 13 on a stress amplitude versus number of cycles to failure diagram. For a given $N$, the corresponding stress value is called the fatigue strength of the material at that number of cycles. For a given stress level, $N$ represents the fatigue life of the material. For some materials, the stress amplitude versus number of cycles curve levels off. The stress $\sigma_e$ at which the fatigue curve levels off is called the endurance limit of the material. Below the endurance limit, the material has a high probability of not failing in fatigue no matter how many cycles of stress are imposed upon the material.

The fatigue behavior of a material depends on several factors. The higher the temperature in which the material is used, the lower the fatigue strength. The fatigue behavior is very sensitive to surface imperfections and presence of discontinuities within the material that can cause stress concentrations. The fatigue failure starts with the creation of a small crack on the surface of the material, which can propagate under the effect of repeated loads, resulting in the rupture of the material.

Orthopedic devices undergo repeated loading and unloading due to the activities of the patients and the actions of their muscles. Over a period of years, a weight-bearing prosthetic device or a fixation device can be subjected to a considerable number of cycles of stress reversals due to normal daily activity. This cyclic loading and unloading can cause fatigue failure of the device.

### Viscoelasticity

When they are subjected to relatively low stress levels, many materials such as metals exhibit elastic material behavior. They undergo plastic deformations at high stress levels. Elastic materials deform instantaneously when they are subjected to externally applied loads and resume their original shapes almost instantly when the applied loads are removed. For an elastic material, stress is a function of strain only, and the stress-strain relationship is unique (Fig. 14). Elastic materials do not exhibit time-dependent behavior. There is a different group of materials, such as polymer plastics, metals at high temperatures, and almost all biologic materials, that exhibits

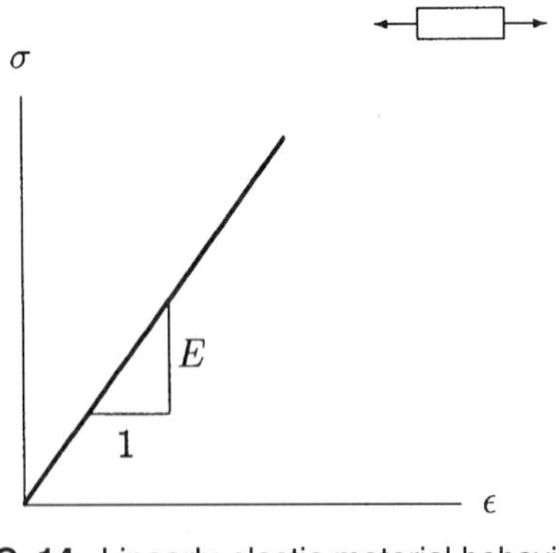

**FIG. 14.** Linearly elastic material behavior.

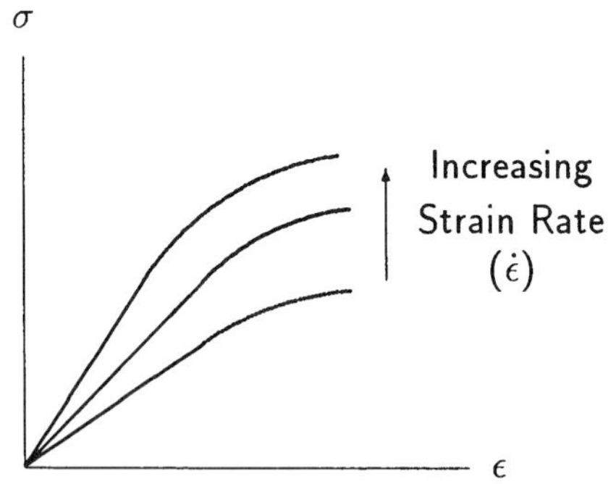

**FIG. 15.** Strain rate-dependent viscoelastic material behavior.

gradual deformation and recovery when they are subjected to loading and unloading. Such materials are called viscoelastic. The response of viscoelastic materials is dependent on how quickly the load is applied or removed. The extent of deformation that viscoelastic materials undergo is dependent on the rate at which the deformation-causing loads are applied. The stress-strain relationship for a viscoelastic material is not unique, but is a function of time or the rate at which the stresses and strains are developed in the material (Fig. 15). The word *viscoelastic* is made of two words. Viscosity is a fluid property and is a measure of resistance to flow. Elasticity is a solid material property. Therefore, viscoelastic materials possess both fluid- and solid-like properties.

For an elastic material, the energy supplied to deform the material (strain energy) is stored in the material as potential energy. This energy is available to return the material to its original (unstressed) size and shape once the applied load is removed. The loading and unloading paths for an elastic material coincide, indicating no loss of energy. Most elastic materials exhibit plastic behavior at high stress levels. For elasto-plastic materials, some of the strain energy is dissipated as heat during plastic deformations. For viscoelastic materials, some of the strain energy is stored in the material as potential energy and some of it is dissipated as heat regardless of whether the stress levels are small or large. Since viscoelastic materials exhibit time-dependent material behavior, the differences between elastic and viscoelastic material responses are most evident under time-dependent loading conditions.

There are several experimental techniques designed to analyze the time-dependent aspects of material behavior. As illustrated in Fig. 16, a creep and recovery test is conducted by applying a load on the material, maintaining the load at a constant level for a while, suddenly removing the load, and observing the material response. Under a creep and recovery test, an elastic material will respond by an instantaneous strain that would remain at a constant level until the load is removed (Fig. 16). At the instant when the load is removed, the deformation will instantly and completely recovered. To the same constant loading

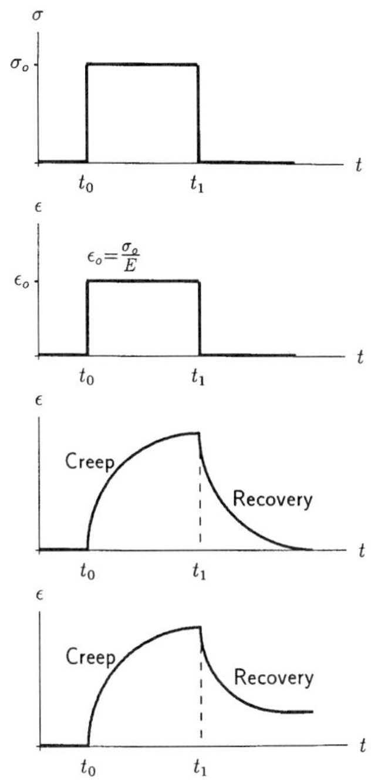


**FIG. 16.** Creep and recovery test.

condition, a viscoelastic material will respond with a strain increasing and decreasing gradually. If the material is viscoelastic solid, the recovery will eventually be complete (Fig. 16). If the material is viscoelastic fluid, complete recovery will never be achieved and there will be a residue of deformation left in the material (Fig. 16). As illustrated in Fig. 17, a stress relaxation experiment is

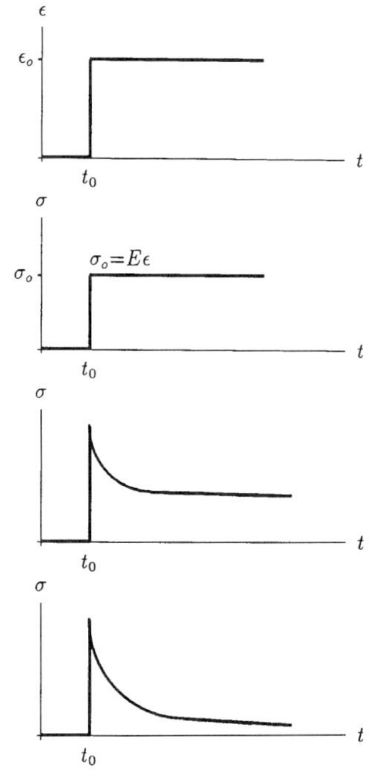


**FIG. 17.** Stress relaxation experiment.

conducted by straining the material to a level and maintaining the constant strain while observing the stress response of the material. Under a stress relaxation test, an elastic material will respond by a stress developed instantly and maintained at a constant level (Fig. 17). That is, an elastic material will not exhibit a stress relaxation behavior. A viscoelastic material, on the other hand, will respond with an initial high stress level that will decrease over time. If the material is a viscoelastic solid, the stress level will never reduce to zero (Fig. 17). As illustrated in Fig. 17, the stress will eventually reduce to zero for a viscoelastic fluid.

## BIOMECHANICS OF BIOLOGIC TISSUES

### Biomechanics of Bone

Bone is the primary structural element of the human body. Bones form the building blocks of the skeletal system, which protects the internal organs, provides kinematic links, provides muscle attachment sites, and facilitates muscle actions and body movements. As compared to other structural materials, bone is unique in that it is self-repairing. Bone can also alter its shape, mechanical behavior, and mechanical properties to adapt to the changes in mechanical demand. The major factors that influence the mechanical behavior of bone are the composition of bone, the mechanical properties of the tissues composing the bone, the size and geometry of the bone, and the direction, magnitude, and the rate of applied loads.

In biologic terms, bone is a connective tissue that binds together various structures of the body. In mechanical terms, bone is a composite material with various solid and fluid phases. Bone consists of cells and an organic mineral matrix of fibers and a ground substance. Bone also contains inorganic substances in the form of mineral salts. The inorganic component of bone makes it hard and relatively rigid, and its organic component provides flexibility and resilience. At the macroscopic level, all bones consist of two types of tissues. The cortical or compact bone tissue is a dense material forming the outer shell (cortex) of bones and the diaphysial region of long bones. The cancellous or trabecular bone tissue consists of thin plates (trabeculae) in a loose mesh structure that is enclosed by the cortical bone. Bones are surrounded by a dense fibrous membrane called the periosteum. The periosteum covers the entire bone except for the joint surfaces that are covered with articular cartilage.

Bone is a nonhomogeneous material because it consists of various cells, organic and inorganic substances with different material properties. Bone is an anisotropic material because its mechanical properties in different directions are different. Bone possesses viscoelastic material properties. The mechanical response of bone is dependent on the rate at which the loads are applied.

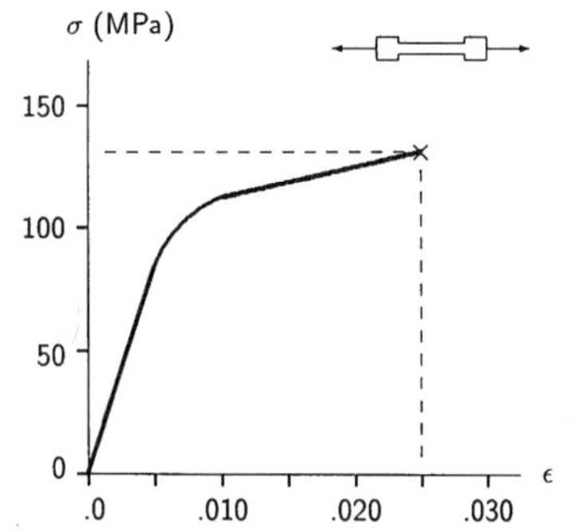


**FIG. 18.** Stress–strain diagram for the human cortical bone loaded in the longitudinal direction at a strain rate of $\dot{\varepsilon} = 0.05\ s^{-1}$.

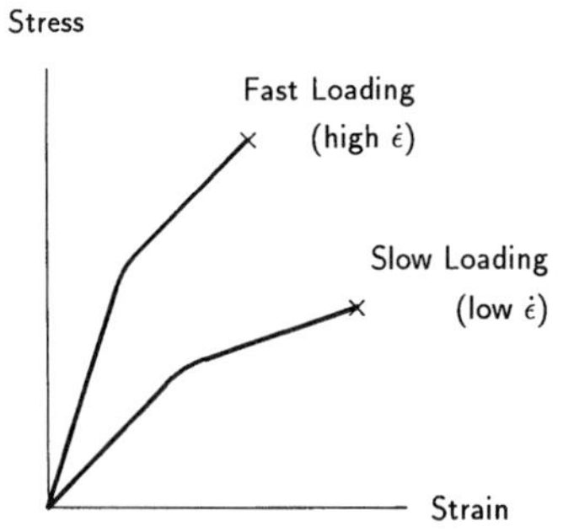


**FIG. 19.** The strain rate-dependent material behavior of the cortical bone.

Bone can resist rapidly applied loads much better than slowly applied loads. Bone is stiffer and stronger at higher strain rates. The mechanical response of bone can be observed by subjecting it to tension, compression, bending, and torsion. If the purpose is to investigate the mechanical response of a specific bone tissue (cortical or cancellous), then the tests are performed using bone specimens. Testing an entire bone, on the other hand, attempts to determine the "bulk" properties of that bone. The tensile stress-strain diagram for the cortical bone is shown in Fig. 18, which has three distinct regions. In the initial linearly elastic region, the stress-strain curve is nearly a straight line and the slope of this line is equal to the elastic modulus of the bone, which is about 17 GPa ($17 \times 10^9$ Pa). In the intermediate region, the bone exhibits nonlinear elasto-plastic material behavior. Material yielding also occurs in this region. The yield strength of the cortical bone is about about 110 MPa ($110 \times 10^6$ Pa). In the final region, the bone exhibits a linearly plastic material behavior and the stress-strain diagram is another straight line. The slope of this line is the strain hardening modulus of the bone tissue, which is about 0.9 GPa. The bone fractures when the tensile stress is about 128 MPa, for which the tensile strain is about 0.026. The tensile ultimate strength of the human cortical bone is about 128 MPa.

The mechanical responses of bone tissues depend on the rate at which the loads are applied. This viscoelastic nature of bone tissues is demonstrated in Fig. 19 for the cortical bone. The cortical bone that is subjected to rapid loading (high $\dot{\varepsilon}$) has a greater elastic modulus and ultimate strength than a bone tissue that is loaded slowly (low $\dot{\varepsilon}$). Furthermore, the energy absorbed by the bone tissue increases with an increasing strain rate. The stress-strain behavior of the bone tissue is also dependent on the orientation of the bone with respect to the direction of loading. This anisotropic material behavior of bone is demonstrated in Fig. 20. Notice that the cortical bone has a larger ultimate strength (stronger) and a larger elastic modulus (stiffer) in the longitudinal direction than in the transverse direction. Furthermore, bone specimens loaded in the transverse direction fail in a more brittle manner as compared to bone specimens loaded in the longitudinal direction. The bone strength is highest under compressive loading in the longitudinal direction (direction of osteon orientation) and lowest under tensile loading in the transverse direction (direction perpendicular to the longitudinal direction). The elastic modulus of cortical bone in the longitudinal direction is higher than its elastic modulus in the transverse direction. Therefore, cortical bone is stiffer in the longitudinal direction than in the transverse direction.

There are several factors that may affect the structural integrity of bones. For example, the size and geometry of a bone determine the distribution of the internal forces throughout the bone, thereby influencing its response to externally applied loads. The larger the bone, the larger the area upon which the internal forces are distributed and the smaller the intensity (stress) of these forces. Consequently, the larger the bone, the more resistant the bone to applied loads. A common characteristic of long bones is their tubular structure in the diaphysial region. Tubular structures are more resistant to torsional and bending loads as compared to solid cylindrical structures. Furthermore, a tubular structure can distribute the internal forces more evenly over its cross section as compared to a solid cylindrical structure of the same cross-sectional area. Certain skeletal conditions such as osteoporosis can reduce the structural integrity of bone by reducing its apparent density. Small decreases in bone density can

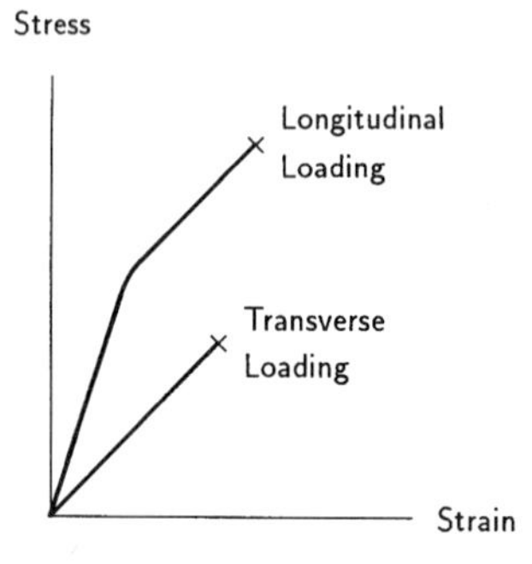


**FIG. 20.** The direction-dependent stress–strain material behavior of the bone tissue.

generate large reductions in bone strength and stiffness. As compared to a normal bone with the same geometry, an osteoporotic bone may deform easier and fracture at lower loads. The density of bone can also change with aging, after periods of disuse, or after chronic exercise, thereby changing its overall strength. Certain surgical procedures that alter the normal bone geometry may also reduce the strength of bone. Bone defects such as screw holes reduce the load-bearing ability of bone by causing stress concentrations around the defects.

When bones are subjected to moderate loading conditions, small deformations may occur that are only present while the loads are applied. When the loads are removed, bones exhibit elastic material behavior by resuming their unstressed shapes and positions. Large deformations occur when the applied loads are high. Bone fractures when the stresses generated in any region of bone are larger than the ultimate strength of bone. Fractures caused by tensile forces are observed in bones with a large proportion of cancellous bone tissue. Fractures due to compressive loads are commonly encountered in the vertebrae of the elderly whose bones are weakened as a result of aging. Bone fractures caused by compression occur in the diaphysial regions of long bones. Compressive fractures are identified by their oblique fracture pattern. Long bone fractures are usually caused by torsion and bending. Torsional fractures are identified by their spiral oblique pattern, whereas bending fractures are usually identified by the formation of "butterfly" fragments. Fatigue fracture of bone occurs when the damage caused by repeated mechanical stress outpaces the bone's ability to repair itself to prevent failure. Bone fractures caused by fatigue are common among professional athletes and dedicated joggers. Clinically, most bone fractures occur as a result of complex, combined loading situations rather than simple loading mechanisms.

### Biomechanics of Soft Tissues

Examples of soft tissues include muscles, tendons, ligaments, skin, articular cartilage, and cardiovascular tissues. From a mechanical point of view, all soft tissues are composite materials. Among the common components of soft tissues, collagen and elastin fibers have the most important mechanical properties affecting the overall mechanical behavior of the tissues in which they appear. Collagen is a protein made of crimped fibrils that aggregate into fibers. The mechanical properties of collagen fibrils are such that each fibril can be considered a mechanical spring and each fiber an assemblage of springs. The primary mechanical function of collagen fibers is to withstand axial tension. Because of their high length-to-diameter ratios (aspect ratio), collagen fibers are not effective under compressive loads. Whenever a fiber is pulled, its crimp straightens, and its length increases. Like a mechanical spring, the energy supplied to stretch the fiber is stored in the fiber, and it is the release of this energy that returns the fiber to its unstretched configuration when the applied load is removed. The individual fibrils of the collagen fibers are surrounded by a gel-like ground substance, which consists largely of water. The collagen fibers possess a two-phase, solid-fluid, or viscoelastic material behavior. The geometric configuration of collagen fibers and their interaction with the noncollagenous tissue components form the basis of the mechanical properties of soft tissues. Among the noncollagenous tissue components, elastin is another fibrous protein with material properties that resemble the properties of rubbers. Elastin and microfibrils form the elastic fibers that are highly extensible, and their extension is reversible even at high strains. Elastin fibers possess a low-modulus elastic material property, while collagen fibers show a higher-modulus viscoelastic material behavior.

### Biomechanics of Skeletal Muscles

Skeletal muscles are attached via tendons to at least two bones causing and/or controlling the relative movement of one bone with respect to the other. When its fibers contract under the stimulation of a nerve, the muscle exerts a pulling effect on the bones to which it is attached. Contraction is a unique ability of the muscle tissue, which is defined as the development of tension in the muscle. Muscle contraction can occur as a result of muscle shortening (concentric contraction), muscle lengthening (eccentric contraction), or without any change in the muscle length (static or isometric contraction).

The skeletal muscle is composed of muscle fibers and myofibrils. Myofibrils are made of contractile elements, actin and myosin proteins. Actin and myosin appear in bands or filaments. Several relatively thick myosin filaments interact across cross-bridges with relatively thin actin filaments to form the basic structure of the contractile element of the muscle, called the sarcomere. Many sarcomere elements connected in a series arrangement form the contractile element (motor unit) of the muscle. It is within the sarcomere that the muscle force (tension) is generated, and where muscle shortening and lengthening takes place. The active contractile elements of the muscle are contained within a fibrous passive connective tissue, called fascia. Fascia encloses the muscles, separates them into layers, and connects them to tendons.

The force developed by a muscle is dependent on many factors, including the number of motor units within the muscle, the number of motor units recruited, the manner in which the muscle changes its length, and the velocity of muscle contraction. For muscles, two different forces can be distinguished. Active tension is the force produced by the contractile elements of the muscle and is a result of voluntary muscle contraction. Passive tension is the force developed within the connective muscle tissue

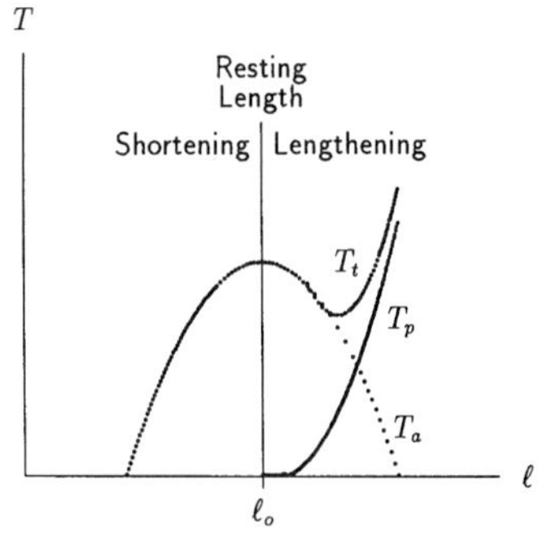


FIG. 21. Muscle force $T$ versus muscle length $l$.

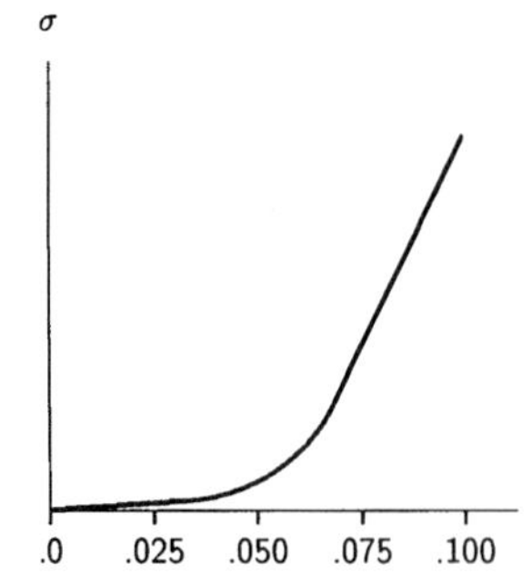


FIG. 22. Tensile stress–strain relationship for tendon.

when the muscle length surpasses its resting length. The net tensile force in a muscle is dependent on the force-length characteristics of both the active and passive components of the muscle. A typical tension versus muscle length diagram is shown in Fig. 21. The number of cross-bridges between the filaments is maximum, and therefore, the active tension ($T_a$) is maximum at the resting length of the muscle. As the muscle lengthens, the filaments are pulled apart, the number of cross-bridges is reduced, and the active tension is decreased. At full length, there are no cross-bridges and the active tension reduces to zero. As the muscle shortens, the cross-bridges overlap and the active tension is again reduced. When the muscle is at its resting length or less, the passive (connective) component of the muscle is in a loose state with no tension. As the muscle lengthens, a passive tensile force ($T_p$) starts building up in the connective tissues. The force-length characteristic of this passive component resembles that of a nonlinear spring. Passive tensile force increases at an increasing rate as the length of the muscle increases. The overall, total, or net muscle force ($T_t$) that is transmitted via tendons is the sum of the forces in the active and passive elements of the muscle. Note here that for a given muscle, the tension-length diagram is not unique but is dependent on the number of motor units recruited. The magnitude of the active component of the muscle force can vary depending on how the muscle is excited, and is usually expressed as a percentage of the maximum voluntary contraction.

### Biomechanics of Tendons and Ligaments

Tendons and ligaments are fibrous connective tissues. Tendons help execute joint motion by transmitting mechanical forces (tensions) from muscles to bones. Ligaments join bones and provide stability to the joints. Unlike muscles that are active tissues and can produce mechanical forces, tendons and ligaments are passive tissues and cannot actively contract to generate forces.

Around many joints of the human body, there is insufficient space to attach more than one or a few muscles. Therefore, to accomplish a certain task, one or a few muscles must share the burden of generating and withstanding large loads. The stress due to these loads is largest at regions closer to the bone attachments where the cross-sectional areas of the muscles are small. As compared to muscles, tendons are stiffer, have higher tensile strengths, and can endure larger stresses. Therefore, around the joints where the space is limited, muscle attachments to bones are made by tendons that are capable of supporting very large loads with very small deformations. This property of tendons enables the muscles to transmit forces to bones without wasting energy to stretch tendons.

The mechanical properties of tendons and ligaments depend on their composition that can vary considerably. Figure 22 shows a typical tensile stress-strain diagram for tendons. The shape of this curve is the result of the interaction between elastic elastin fibers and the viscoelastic collagen fibers. At low strains (up to about 0.05), less stiff elastic fibers dominate and the crimp of the collagen fibers straightens, requiring very little force to stretch the tendon. The tendon becomes stiffer when the crimp is straightened. At the same time, the fluid-like ground substance in the collagen fibers tends to flow. At higher strains, the stiff and viscoelastic nature of the collagen fibers begins to take an increasing portion of the applied load. Tendons are believed to function in the body at strains of up to about 0.04, which is believed to be their yield strain. Tendons rupture at strains of about 0.1 (ultimate strain) or stresses of about 60 MPa (ultimate stress). The time-dependent, viscoelastic nature of the tendon is illustrated in Fig. 23. When the tendon is stretched

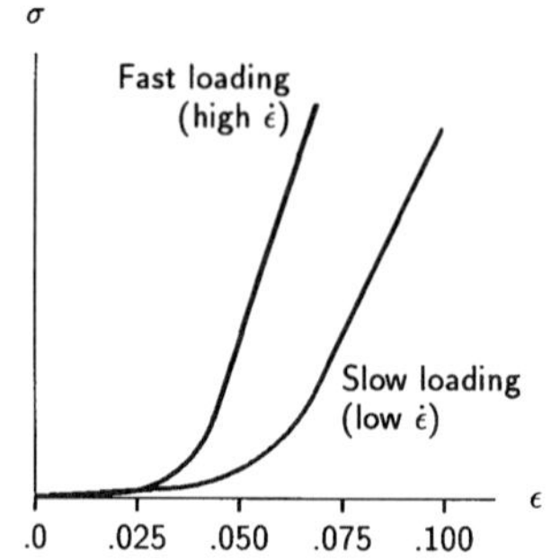


FIG. 23. The strain rate-dependent material behavior of tendon.

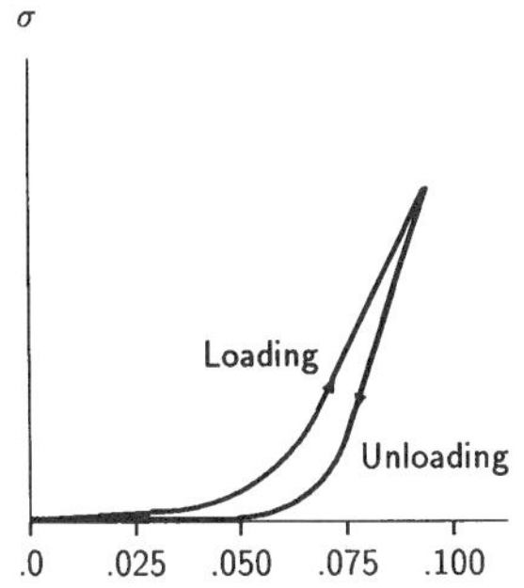


**FIG. 24.** The hysteresis loop of stretching and relaxation modes of tendon.

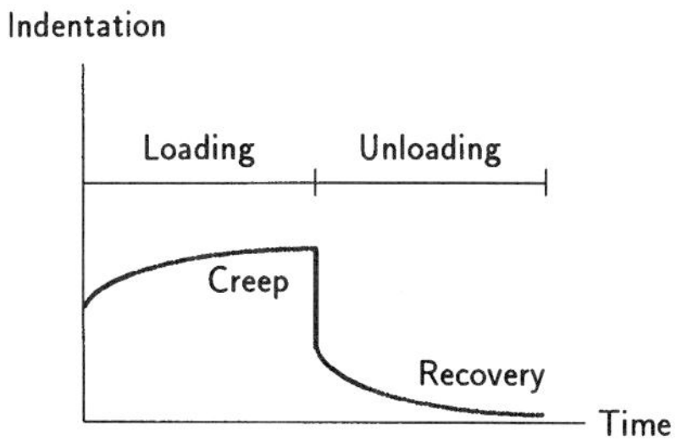


**FIG. 25.** The indentation test.

rapidly, there is less chance for the ground substance to flow, and consequently, the tendon becomes stiffer. The hysteresis loop shown in Fig. 24 demonstrates the time-dependent loading and unloading behavior of the tendon. Note that more work is done in stretching the tendon than is recovered when the tendon is allowed to relax, and therefore, some of the energy (the area enclosed by the hysteresis loop) is dissipated in the process.

The mechanical role of ligaments is to transmit forces from one bone to another. Ligaments also have a stabilizing role for the skeletal joints. The composition and structure of ligaments depend on their function and position within the body. Like tendons, they are composite materials containing crimped collagen fibers surrounded by ground substance. As compared to tendons, they often contain a greater proportion of elastic fibers, which accounts for their higher extensibility but lower strength and stiffness. The mechanical properties of ligaments are qualitatively similar to those of tendons. Like tendons, they are viscoelastic and exhibit hysteresis, but deform elastically up to strains of about 0.25 and stresses of about 5 MPa. They rupture at a stress level of about 20 MPa.

### Biomechanics of Articular Cartilage

Cartilage covers the articulating surfaces of bones at the diarthrodial (synovial) joints. The primary function of cartilage is to facilitate the relative movement of articulating bones. Cartilage reduces stresses applied to bones by increasing the area of contact between the articulating surfaces and reduces bone wear by reducing the effects of friction. Cartilage is a two-phase material consisting of about 75% water and 25% organic solid. A large portion of the solid phase of the cartilage material is made up of collagen fibers. The remaining ground substance is mainly proteoglycan (hydrophilic molecules). Collagen fibers are relatively strong and stiff in tension, while proteoglycans are strong in compression. The solid-fluid composition of cartilage makes it a viscoelastic material.

The mechanical properties of cartilage under various loading conditions have been investigated using experimental techniques such as indentation and confined compression tests. In an indentation test, a small cylindrical indentor is pressed into the articulating surface, and the resulting deformation is recorded. A typical result of an indentation test is shown in Fig. 25. When a constant magnitude load is applied, the material initially responds with a relatively large elastic deformation. The applied load causes pressure gradients to occur in the interstitial fluid, and the variations in pressure cause the fluid to flow through and out of the cartilage matrix. As the load is maintained, the amount of deformation increases at a decreasing rate. The deformation tends toward an equilibrium state as the pressure variations within the fluid are dissipated. When the applied load is removed (unloading phase), there is an instantaneous elastic recovery that is followed by a more gradual recovery leading to complete recovery.

During daily activities, the articular cartilage is subjected to tensile and shear stresses as well as compressive stresses. Under tension, cartilage responds by realigning the collagen fibers that carry the tensile loads applied to the tissue. The tensile stiffness and strength of cartilage depend on the collagen content of the tissue. The higher the collagen content, the higher the tensile strength. Shear stresses on the articular cartilage are due to the frictional forces between the relative movement of articulating surfaces. However, the coefficient of friction for synovial joints is so low (of the order 0.001–0.06) that friction has an insignificant effect on the stress resultants acting on the cartilage.

Both structural (such as intraarticular fracture) and anatomical abnormalities (such as rheumatoid arthritis and acetabular dysplasia) can cause cartilage damage, degeneration, wear, and failure. These abnormalities can change the load-bearing ability of the joint by altering its mechanical properties. The importance of the load-bearing ability of the cartilage and of maintaining its mechanical integrity may become clear if we consider that the magnitude of the forces involved at the human hip joint is about five times body weight during ordinary walking. The hip contact area over which these forces are applied is about 15 $cm^2$ (0.0015 $m^2$). Therefore, the compressive stresses involved are of the order 3 MPa for an 85-kg person.

## SUMMARY

Bioengineering is a young and dynamic field of study that has developed worldwide from the recognition that the theories and methods developed in conventional engineering can be useful for understanding and solving problems in physiology and medicine. Biomechanics is an important part of bioengineering that considers the applications of classical mechanics to biologic problems. In the theoretical and practical advances made in the field of biomechanics, there has usually been cooperation between life scientists, physicians, engineers, and basic scientists. Such a cooperation requires a certain amount of common vocabulary. For example, the engineer must learn some anatomy and physiology, and the medical personnel need to understand the basic concepts of the physical science and mathematics involved.

## FURTHER READINGS

Black J. *Orthopaedic biomaterials in research and practice.* New York: Churchill Livingstone, 1988.

Burstein AH, Wright TM. *Fundamentals of orthopaedic biomechanics.* New York: Williams & Wilkins, 1995.

Chaffin DB, Andersson GBJ. *Occupational biomechanics,* 2nd ed. New York: Wiley, 1991.

Fung YC. *Biomechanics: motion, flow, stress, and growth.* New York: Springer-Verlag, 1990.

Hay JG, Reid JG. *Anatomy, mechanics and human motion,* 2nd ed. Englewood Cliffs, NJ: Prentice-Hall, 1988.

Mow VC, Hayes WC. *Basic orthopaedic biomechanics.* New York: Raven Press, 1991.

Mow VC, Ratcliff A, Woo SL-Y, eds. *Biomechanics of diarthrodial joints.* New York: Springer-Verlag, 1990.

Nahum AM, Melvin J, eds. *The biomechanics of trauma.* Norwalk, CT: Appleton-Century-Crofts, 1985.

Nordin M, Frankel VH, eds. *Basic biomechanics of the musculoskeletal system,* 2nd ed. Philadelphia: Lea & Febiger, 1989.

Özkaya N, Nordin M. *Fundamentals of biomechanics:* equilibrium, *motion, and deformation.* New York: Van Nostrand Reinhold, 1991.

Schmid-Schönbein GW, Woo SL-Y, Zweifach BW, eds. *Frontiers in biomechanics.* New York: Springer-Verlag, 1985.

Skalak R, Chien S, eds. *Handbook of bioengineering.* New York: McGraw-Hill, 1987.

Williams M, Lissner HR. *Biomechanics of human motion,* 3rd ed. (B. LeVeau, ed.) Philadelphia: Saunders, 1992.

Winter DA. *Biomechanics and motor control of human behavior,* 2nd ed. New York: Wiley, 1990.

Winters JM, Woo SL-Y, eds. *Multiple muscle systems.* New York: Springer-Verlag, 1990.

*Environmental and Occupational Medicine, Third Edition,* edited by William N. Rom.
Lippincott–Raven Publishers, Philadelphia © 1998.

CHAPTER 110

# Firefighters' Health and Safety

Scott Barnhart and George P. Pappas

Firefighters are exposed to extremely hazardous environments. Potentially lethal products of combustion combine with uncontrolled thermal stresses, psychological pressures, biologic agents, and ergonomic strains to make firefighting physically demanding and dangerous. In the U.S. approximately 270,000 career firefighters and 840,000 volunteer firefighters provide fire suppression, education, and emergency services to their communities (1). Despite recognition of the risks of fighting fires, firefighters continue to experience elevated rates of injuries, illnesses, and chronic diseases. The National Fire Protection Association reported 566 firefighter deaths and approximately 600,000 injuries in the line of duty between 1990 and 1995 (1). This chapter discusses the hazards faced by firefighters, reviews the epidemiology of firefighter illness and injury, examines the pulmonary effects of fighting fires, and identifies areas of focus for future research that may improve firefighter health and safety.

## HAZARDS OF FIREFIGHTING

### Products of Combustion and Chemical Exposures

Products of combustion include particulates and gases, and are the major source of firefighters exposures to toxic chemicals. They are determined by the type of material burned, the temperature of the fire, and the presence or absence of oxygen in the combustion environment (2). Modern dwellings contain a bewildering array of natural and synthetic materials. The burning of a typical urban structure containing woods, paints, glues, plastics, and synthetic materials in furniture, carpeting, and insulation liberates hundreds of chemicals. The combustion products of several common materials are presented in Table 1 (3). Firefighting is often considered to have two stages: a knockdown stage, when the fire is brought under control; and an overhaul stage, when smoldering fires are extinguished. Potentially harmful materials have been detected during all phases of fire suppression (4). Studies of controlled fires under laboratory conditions, structural fires, and forest fires offer insight into combustion products commonly encountered by firefighters (2–10).

Particulates generated during fires are a complex mixture of partial and complete combustion products of the original substance with additional compounds adsorbed on the surface (10). Measurement and analysis of particulates found in firefighting environments are limited. Personal breathing-zone sampling of Boston firefighters revealed median total particulate concentrations of 21.5 $mg/m^3$, with 15% of samples exceeding 100 $mg/m^3$ (8). In residential fires, total particulate concentrations ranged from undetectable to 560 $mg/m^3$ during knockdown, and up to 45 $mg/m^3$ during overhaul (4). A furnished tenement fire with dense smoke generated particles with mass median diameter of 1 $\mu m$ during knockdown and 10 $\mu m$ during overhaul (4). Diesel exhaust from vehicles in fire stations has also been identified as a significant source of particulate exposure (11).

Among the most toxic products of combustion is carbon monoxide, which displaces oxygen from hemoglobin and is a significant contributor to many fire associated fatalities. Carbon monoxide is present in nearly all fire environments as a result of incomplete combustion. Personal sampling devices worn by firefighters at structural fires have demonstrated CO levels ranging from 0 to

S. Barnhart and G. P. Pappas: Department of Medicine, University of Washington/Harborview Medical Center, Seattle, Washington 98104.

**TABLE 1.** *Products of combustion*

| Source | Major combustion products |
|---|---|
| Wood | Carbon monoxide, carbon dioxide, hydrogen, methane, acetic acid, alcohols, tars, aldehydes, ketones |
| Cotton | Carbon monoxide, hydrogen cyanide, nitrogen oxides, aldehydes, ketones |
| Wool | Carbon monoxide, carbon dioxide, hydrogen cyanide, hydrogen sulfide, benzene, toluene, carbon disulfide, carbonyl sulfide |
| Polyester | Carbon monoxide, carbon dioxide, methane, benzene, saturated and unsaturated hydrocarbons |
| Nylon | Carbon monoxide, carbon dioxide, hydrogen cyanide, ammonia, nitrogen oxides, low molecular weight alkanes and alkenes, assorted lactams and nitriles |
| Polyurethane foams | Carbon monoxide, hydrogen cyanide, carbon dioxide, acetonitrile, acrylonitrile, pyridine, benzonitrile, low molecular weight hydrocarbons |
| Polyvinyl chloride | Carbon monoxide, carbon dioxide, hydrogen chloride, benzene, saturated aromatic hydrocarbons, phosgene |
| Urea-formaldehyde | Carbon monoxide, carbon dioxide, hydrogen cyanide, ammonia |

Adapted from ref. 3.

27,000 ppm (4,6–10,12). In a study of 22 fires, CO was the most common contaminant measured during knockdown (4). Approximately 10% of CO samples exceeded 1,500 ppm, a concentration immediately hazardous to life. During overhaul CO levels were lower, ranging from background to 82 ppm. After an active shift, nonsmoking firefighters were found to have mean blood carboxyhemoglobin levels 2% greater than unexposed nonsmoking controls (13). Carbon monoxide levels found in forest fires are lower than those in structural fires, largely due to superior ventilation and lack of confinement (14).

Hydrogen cyanide is formed during the combustion of wool, paper, silk, and nitrogen-containing synthetic polymers and is another important cause of smoke inhalation fatalities (15). Hydrogen cyanide interferes with cellular respiration and has been detected in up to 50% of residential fires, especially fires involving vehicles, mattresses, or upholstered furniture (4,8,9). Small elevations in serum thiocyanate have been demonstrated in firefighters wearing respiratory protection after active duty (16).

Carbon dioxide is produced during the combustion of all organic materials, and can act as an asphyxiant by displacing oxygen from the environment. Personal sampling measurements at residential fires revealed $CO_2$ concentrations from 350 to 5,410 ppm during knockdown and 130 to 1,420 ppm during overhaul, although concentrations of up to 70,000 ppm have been described (4,17). Irritant gases such as hydrogen chloride can be generated by the decomposition of chlorine containing plastics such as polyvinyl chloride, acrylics and flame retardants (2–10). Acrolein, a highly toxic aldehyde and respiratory irritant, has repeatedly been measured at hazardous levels in over half of residential fires (4,9). Other potentially toxic agents measured in firefighting environments include nitrogen oxides; sulfur dioxide and sulfuric acid; hydrogen fluoride; formaldehyde; metals such as lead, chromium, and arsenic; and a broad spectrum of volatile organic chemicals (3–10,18). Increasingly, firefighters are participating in responses to hazardous materials spills, providing potential exposure to thousands of chemicals used in industry.

Firefighters are also exposed to a wide variety of potential carcinogens. Benzene, a recognized leukemia causing agent, is detectable at nearly all fires (4,6,9). Polycyclic aromatic hydrocarbons (PAHs) in soots, tars, and diesel exhaust; arsenic in wood preservatives; formaldehyde in wood smoke; and asbestos in building insulation are other carcinogens commonly found in the fire atmosphere (9,10). Specific incidents can result in exposures to uncommon but potent carcinogens, including pesticides, polychlorinated biphenyls, and dioxins. Detailed assessment of firefighters' exposures to carcinogens is difficult to perform given the episodic, unpredictable, and complex nature of firefighter exposures.

As protection against a potentially lethal environment, the Occupational Safety and Health Administration (OSHA) requires firefighters to use self-contained breathing apparatus (SCBA) respirators designed to provide protection factors of 10,000 when fighting structural fires (contaminants inside the face piece are reduced to 1/10,000 of ambient concentrations) (19). Actual protection factors provided by these respirators are not well characterized. Although decreased face-piece fit, possible respirator overbreathing from extreme physical exertion, and patterns of respirator use may result in lower levels of protection, the use of SCBA respirators has served to dramatically reduce firefighter exposures (20). Most firefighters wear their respirators during knockdown of structural fires, but some may not wear the respirator during overhaul or for nonstructural fires, when potentially harmful exposures may still be present (4). The use of SCBA respirators has dramatically altered firefighter exposures over the past 20 years. For this reason, studies from periods when SCBA use was limited may not be generalizable to situations where SCBA use is more common.

## Biologic Hazards

Firefighters are increasingly involved in rescue operations and the provision of emergency medical services. In this capacity, firefighters are at risk for communicable diseases transmitted by blood, respiratory secretions, or other infectious materials. A study of infectious disease exposures in 650 dual-trained firefighter/emergency medical technicians found an overall incidence rate of 4.4 infectious exposures per 1,000 emergency medical services calls (21). Many populations served by emergency medical service personnel have elevated rates of blood-borne communicable diseases such as hepatitis B, hepatitis C, and human immunodeficiency virus (HIV) (22,23). Although no studies have documented increased rates of transmission of these diseases to firefighters, the prevalence of hepatitis B among emergency service personnel in several major metropolitan areas is elevated, and significant correlations have been observed between hepatitis B infection and years of work in emergency medical service (24,25). Firefighters are included in the OSHA blood-borne pathogens standard, and should be educated about risks of blood-borne infection and means of prevention (26). Vaccination with hepatitis B is required by OSHA for firefighters who have a potential exposure to blood or other infectious materials. In addition, firefighters are at risk for diseases spread by airborne droplets such as tuberculosis. Firefighters should be knowledgeable about tuberculosis prevention and enrolled in purified protein derivative (PPD) screening programs, in accordance with Centers for Disease Control and Prevention (CDC) guidelines for health care workers (27).

### Physical Hazards

Firefighters are exposed to extremes of heat. Between 1990 and 1995, over 25,000 firefighters sustained physical or chemical burns, resulting in significant morbidity and mortality. In addition, over 20,000 firefighters experienced heat exhaustion or frostbite (1). Heavy turnout gear, SCBAs, and barrier clothing used for hazardous materials incidents can increase the work of firefighting and impede body temperature control mechanisms, further contributing to thermal stress.

Firefighters are also subject to loud noise exposures from sirens, engines, air horns, and pumps. Exposures during emergency response operations can approach 115 dB for brief periods of time, although firefighters' 8-hour time-weighted average noise exposures are frequently beneath the OSHA permissible exposure level of 90 dB (28). Audiometric testing of firefighters has consistently demonstrated excess hearing loss compared to controls, with greater deficits among senior personnel (29,30). Firefighters should be educated about hearing protection and enrolled in hearing conservation programs to minimize noise-induced hearing loss.

### Stress and Shift Work

In the course of their work, firefighters are routinely placed in demanding situations and high-risk environments. As such, firefighting is recognized as one of the most stressful occupations. Although the stresses inherent to firefighting are clear, the physical and emotional consequences of those stresses are less obvious. Stress has been suggested as a cause of cardiovascular disease among firefighters. However, the mechanisms for stress-induced cardiovascular effects remain poorly defined, and there is still debate as to whether firefighters have elevated rates of cardiovascular mortality.

Recent interest has focused on the psychological sequelae of involvement in traumatic fire and rescue events. Following a severe polyvinyl chloride (PVC) chemical fire, firefighters combating the blaze demonstrated higher measures of postincident psychological distress than unexposed firefighter controls (31). Increased rates of self-reported psychological distress and alcohol use have also been reported in firefighter populations (32). However, the relationship of traumatic events to firefighters' long-term psychological and emotional well-being has yet to be determined (33).

Firefighters typically work long shifts and are subject to fatigue, alterations in mood, and sleepiness as a consequence of shift work (34). With the flexibility of their work schedule, firefighters may seek additional employment opportunities for their off hours, placing them at risk for further occupational exposures, injuries, and illnesses.

### Injuries

Firefighting has one of the highest rates of injuries of all occupations, with 41% of firefighters reporting work-related injuries in 1993 (35). Statistics from 1995 describe 94,500 firefighter injuries that required medical attention or resulted in at least 1 day of restricted activity (36). The most common injuries were musculoskeletal, including sprains, strains, and muscle pains, including back pain. Firefighter tasks, such as carrying hoses and victims, and climbing ladders, frequently require heavy lifting, twisting, stretching, and exerting efforts, activities that have been identified in ergonomic studies as risk factors for injury (37). Physical fitness programs for firefighters may be effective in reducing injury rates (38). Lacerations and burns (physical and chemical) are also frequently reported. These injuries result in lost work hours, significant medical expenses, and even premature disability (35).

### Reproductive Hazards

Firefighters are regularly exposed to chemical and physical hazards that could influence reproductive health. Products of combustion such as acrolein, benzene, carbon monoxide, and formaldehyde are associated with reproductive toxicity in animal models, although human data are lacking (39). Heat is a reproductive toxin, affecting spermatogenesis and fertility in heat-exposed cohorts; however, the effects of heat on the reproductive health of firefighters has not been studied (40). Lifting also poses a risk for pregnant women, especially in the later stages of pregnancy (41). Offspring of firefighters were found to have increased risk of ventricular septal defects and atrial septal defects in one case-control study, but additional data on the reproductive health of firefighters are needed (42).

## EPIDEMIOLOGY

Firefighters are exposed to many agents that could potentially cause cardiovascular, respiratory, and malignant disease. Attempts to establish associations between firefighters and occupational diseases have yielded conflicting results, reflecting the challenges encountered in studying this population. Firefighters are selected for their abilities to perform strenuous tasks. This healthy worker population of firefighters may demonstrate lower rates of disease than a normal comparison population, masking exposure-response associations (43). To control for this, some studies rely on comparisons of firefighters to policemen, a group presumed to be similar in physical abilities and socioeconomic status. The occupational exposures experienced by firefighters may vary greatly, influenced by the types of fires encountered, job responsibilities, and use of personal protective equipment. Data on nonoccupational risk factors such as cigarette smoking are rarely available. Firefighters who experience health problems related to their work may choose to leave their position, creating a survivor effect of individuals more resistant to the effects of firefighter exposures. Despite these difficulties, many important observations about the health of firefighters have been made. Overall, firefighters have repeatedly been shown to have all-cause mortality rates less than or equal to reference populations (44–54). However, several specific causes of morbidity and mortality warrant further discussion.

### Cardiovascular Disease

Early U.S. Vital Statistics data suggested an increased cardiovascular mortality among firefighters (55). Recognition that firefighters were exposed to carbon monoxide, smoke, physical and psychological stress, and the subsequent demonstration of ECG abnormalities in a small number of firefighters led to additional investigations of this association (56). The epidemiologic data are summarized in Table 2 (44–53,57–59). The majority of studies show risks of cardiovascular disease less than or equal to comparison populations. Although this may be due to the healthy worker effect, studies using police officers for comparison populations similarly show no excess risk. Several studies found increasing risk of cardiovascular disease with increasing duration of employment. In one positive study, Bates (59) reported excess circulatory disease mortality in a cohort of 646 Toronto firefighters between the ages of 45 and 54; however, a subsequent study of 5,995 Toronto firefighters including Bates's cohort found no significant elevations in circulatory system standardized mortality ratios (SMRs) and no trend by duration of employment (49). Although firefighters may sustain acute myocardial injuries as a result of carbon monoxide poisoning, the weight of the epidemiologic evidence does not support an excess of cardiovascular mortality.

### Malignant Diseases

#### *Brain Cancer*

Epidemiologic data provide substantial support for an association between firefighting and brain cancer, which

**TABLE 2.** *Cardiovascular risk estimates among firefighters*

| Author | Population | Year | Risk ratio | 95% confidence interval (CI) |
|---|---|---|---|---|
| Musk et al. | 5,655 Boston firefighters | 1978 | 0.86 | NA |
| Dibbs et al. | 171 Boston firefighters | 1982 | 0.5 | 0.2–1.4 |
| Feuer et al. | New Jersey (PMR) | 1986 | 1.01 vs. police | |
| | | | 1.02 vs. New Jersey pop. | |
| | | | 1.09 vs. U.S. pop. | |
| Vena et al. | 1,867 Buffalo firefighters | 1987 | 0.92 | 0.81–1.04 |
| **Demers et al.** | **4,546 northwest firefighters** | **1992** | **0.79 vs. U.S. pop.** | **0.72–0.87** |
| | | | 0.86 vs. police | 0.74–1.00 |
| Heyer et al. | 2,289 Seattle firefighters | 1990 | 0.78 | 0.68–0.92 |
| Sardinas et al. | 306 Connecticut firefighters | 1986 | 1.07 | 0.91–1.23 |
| **Bates** | **596 Toronto firefighters** | **1987** | **1.73** | **1.12–2.66** |
| Guidotti | 3,328 Alberta firefighters | 1993 | 1.03 | 0.88–1.21 |
| Burnett et al. | 27 U.S. states (PMR) | 1994 | 1.01 | 0.97–1.05 |
| Tornling et al. | 1,116 Stockholm firefighters | 1994 | 0.84 | 0.71–0.98 |
| **Beaumont et al.** | **3,066 San Francisco firefighters** | **1991** | **0.89** | **0.81–0.97** |
| Aronson et al. | 5,995 Toronto firefighters | 1994 | 0.99 | 0.89–1.10 |

Risk ratio is expressed by authors as standardized mortality ration (SMR), proportionate mortality ratio (PMR), standardized incidence ratio (SIR), mortality odds ratio (MOR), or RR, with no excess risk equal to 1.

Note: **Bold** type in Tables 2–7 indicates statistically significant result.

**TABLE 3.** *Brain cancer risk estimates for firefighters*

| Author | Population | Year | Cases | Risk ratio | 95% CI |
|---|---|---|---|---|---|
| **Aronson et al.** | **5,955 Toronto firefighters** | **1994** | **14** | **2.01** | **1.10–3.37** |
| Burnett et al. | 27 U.S states (PMR) | 1994 | 38 | 1.03 | 0.73–1.41 |
| Tornling et al. | 1,116 Stockholm firefighters | 1994 | 5 | 2.79 | 0.91–6.51 |
| Guidotti | 3,328 Alberta firefighters | 1993 | 3 | 1.46 | 0.30–4.28 |
| Demers et al. | 4,546 northwest firefighters | 1992 | 18 | 1.63 vs. police | 0.70–3.79 |
| | | | **18** | **2.07 vs. population** | **1.23–3.28** |
| Beaumont et al. | 3,066 San Francisco firefighters | 1991 | 5 | 0.81 | 0.26–1.90 |
| **Grimes et al.** | **Honolulu firefighters (PMR)** | **1991** | **3** | **3.78** | **1.22–11.71** |
| Heyer et al. | 2,289 Seattle firefighters | 1990 | 3 | 0.95 | 0.20–2.79 |
| Sama et al. | 315 Massachusetts firefighters | 1990 | 5 | 1.52 vs. police | 0.39–5.92 |
| | Case control study | | | 0.86 vs. population | 0.34–2.15 |
| Vena et al. | 1867 Buffalo firefighters | 1987 | 6 | 2.36 | 0.86–5.13 |
| Musk et al. | 5655 Boston firefighters | 1978 | 8 | 1.03 | |

are summarized in Table 3 (44,46–53,60,61). The latency period for the development of brain cancer can be short, with increased risks demonstrated after 5 to 9 years of employment in Toronto firefighters (49). Among northwestern U.S. firefighters, risks were greatest in firefighters with 10 to 19 years of employment (SMR = 3.53), although no consistent association between duration of employment and risk was found (48). In a cohort of Buffalo firefighters, a statistically significant fourfold excess of brain cancer was seen among firefighters with latencies of less than 29 years (46). A study of Stockholm firefighters found increased risk of brain cancer that was most pronounced among firefighters with advanced age, long employment, and a high exposure index (53). A review of epidemiologic studies assessing firefighters' cancer risks concluded that there is adequate support for a causal relationship between firefighting and brain cancer, with cumulative relative risk of 1.44 (62). Occupational exposures to PAHs, benzene, pesticides, vinyl chloride, and polychlorinated biphenyls (PCBs) have been associated with increased risks of brain cancer, and many of these chemicals may be present in the fire environment (2–10). However, current firefighter exposure assessments are not adequate to determine which agent(s) may be responsible for the increased mortality from brain cancer.

### *Cancers of the Hematopoietic and Lymphatic Systems*

Increased risks of leukemia and lymphoma have been described in several epidemiologic studies of firefighters (Table 4) (45,47–49,51,52,61). Risks of leukemia are often two to three times that of comparison populations, and greatest in older age groups (45,58). Leukemia risk is also associated with long duration of employment and long latency (47,48). Twofold risks of non-Hodgkin's lymphoma have also been reported by investigators in the United States and Canada (49,61). However, the wide variety of tumors included under the rubric of leukemia and lymphoma in mortality studies precludes the assessment of causal associations for these conditions (62). Benzene is detected in most fire environments, and has been associated with leukemia and multiple myeloma in occupational cohort studies (6,8,9). Given established exposures to benzene, there is biologic plausibility for firefighters to be at increased risk of these malignancies.

Increased risks for multiple myeloma have also been reported. Heyer and co-workers (47) found an overall

**TABLE 4.** *Leukemia risk estimates for firefighters*

| Author | Year | Cases | Risk ratio | 95% CI |
|---|---|---|---|---|
| Aronson et al. | 1994 | 4 myeloid | 1.20 | 0.33–3.09 |
| | | 4 lymphatic | 1.90 | 0.52–4.88 |
| Burnett et al. | 1994 | 61 | 1.19 | 0.91–1.53 |
| Demers et al. | 1992 | 15 | 0.80 vs. police | 0.38–1.70 |
| | | 15 | 1.27 vs. population | 0.71–2.09 |
| Beaumont et al. | 1991 | 7 | 0.61 | 0.22–1.33 |
| Heyer et al. | 1990 | 7 | 1.73 | 0.70–3.58 |
| Sama et al. | 1990 | 6 | 2.67 vs. police | 0.62–11.54 |
| | | | 1.12 vs. population | 0.48–2.59 |
| **Feuer et al.** | **1986** | **4** | **2.76 vs. police** | |
| | | | 1.86 vs. U.S. population | |
| | | | 1.77 vs. New Jersey population | |

**TABLE 5.** *Bladder cancer risk estimates for firefighters*

| Author | Year | Cases | Risk ratio | 95% CI |
|---|---|---|---|---|
| Aronson et al. | 1994 | 7 | 1.28 | 0.51–2.63 |
| Burnett et al. | 1994 | 37 | 0.99 | 0.70–1.37 |
| Guidotti | 1993 | 4 | 3.16 | 0.86–8.08 |
| Demers et al. | 1992 | 2 | 0.16 vs. police | 0.02–1.24 |
| | | 2 | 0.23 vs. population | 0.03–0.83 |
| Beaumont et al. | 1991 | 5 | 0.57 | 0.19–1.35 |
| **Sama et al.** | **1990** | **26** | **2.11 vs. police** | **1.07–4.14** |
| | | | **1.59 vs. population** | **1.02–2.50** |
| **Vena and Fielder** | **1987** | **9** | **2.86** | **1.30–5.40** |

SMR of 225 [95% confidence interval (CI) 47–660] for multiple myeloma among Seattle firefighters, with higher risks in firefighters with long duration of employment. A 27-state mortality study found a proportionate mortality ratio (PMR) of 148 (95% CI 102–207) (51). A review of firefighter epidemiology found support for a causal association between firefighting and multiple myeloma (pooled SMR = 1.51, 95% CI 91–235) (62).

### *Cancers of the Genitourinary System*

The epidemiologic data suggest firefighters are at increased risk for cancer of the bladder (Table 5) (46, 48–52,61). Buffalo firefighters were found to have nearly a threefold risk of bladder cancer, with an association between increasing latency and increased risk (46). Alberta firefighters had a threefold risk of bladder cancer, with significant association seen among firefighters over 60 years of age and latency greater than 40 years (50). Firefighters are exposed to PAHs as products of combustion, and these chemicals have been associated with bladder cancer in occupational cohort studies (4). Increased risk of kidney, prostate, and testicular cancer have also been noted in epidemiologic investigations; however, additional studies are needed to clarify the risk of these malignancies (50,51,53).

### *Skin Cancer*

Several investigators have found increased risk of firefighter mortality from skin cancer (Table 6) (45,48,49,51, 52,61). Skin cancer mortality is usually from malignant melanoma, as other types of skin cancer are rarely fatal. A 1990 review of firefighter epidemiology calculated a statistically significant pooled risk estimate of 1.73 for melanoma (62). However, the authors cautioned that additional data on confounding variables (such as sun exposure), dose-response relationships, and occupational risks for melanoma are necessary before a causative association can be established.

### *Cancers of the Digestive System*

Several epidemiologic studies have shown an excess of colon and rectal carcinomas among firefighters (Table 7) (46–49,51–53,61,63). Increased risk of colon cancer has been associated with long duration of employment and long latency (46). Increased rates of colon cancer have been found in asbestos workers, and this is one postulated mechanism for the excess of colorectal cancers described in firefighters. Firefighters have also been noted to have an excess of cancers of the esophagus, liver, pancreas, and stomach; however, the lack of consistency argues for viewing the results cautiously.

### *Lung Cancer*

Inhalational exposure to asbestos, PAHs, and formaldehyde have made lung cancer a primary focus in epidemiologic evaluations of firefighters. Despite clear evidence of carcinogenic exposures, there has been no consistent demonstration of lung cancer excess among

**TABLE 6.** *Skin cancer risk estimates for firefighters*

| Author | Year | Cases | Risk ratio | 95% CI |
|---|---|---|---|---|
| Aronson et al. | 1994 | 2 | 0.73 | 0.09–2.63 |
| **Burnett et al.** | **1994** | **38** | **1.63** | **1.15–2.23** |
| Demers et al. | 1992 | 6 | 1.12 vs. police | 0.27–4.76 |
| | | 6 | 0.98 vs. population | 0.36–2.13 |
| Beaumont et al. | 1991 | 7 | 1.69 | 0.68–3.49 |
| Sama et al. | 1990 | 18 | 1.38 vs. police | 0.60–3.19 |
| | | | **2.92 vs. population** | **1.70–5.03** |
| Feuer et al. | 1986 | 4 | 1.35 vs. police | |
| | | | **2.70 vs. U.S. population** | |
| | | | 1.90 vs. New Jersey population | |

**TABLE 7.** *Rectal cancer risk estimates for firefighters*

| Author | Year | Cases | Risk ratio | 95% CI |
|---|---|---|---|---|
| Aronson et al. | 1994 | 13 | 1.71 | 0.91–2.93 |
| **Burnett et al.** | **1994** | **37** | **1.48** | **1.05–2.05** |
| Tornling et al. | 1994 | 8 | 2.07 | 0.89–4.08 |
| Demers et al. | 1992 | 8 | 0.89 vs. police | 0.30–2.66 |
| | | 8 | 0.95 vs. population | 0.41–1.87 |
| **Orris** | **1992** | **34** | **1.64** | **1.14–2.30** |
| Beaumont et al. | 1991 | 13 | 1.45 | 0.77–2.49 |
| Heyer et al. | 1990 | 2 | 0.65 | 0.08–2.37 |
| Sama et al. | 1990 | 22 | 0.97 vs. police | 0.50–1.88 |
| | | 22 | 1.35 vs. population | 0.84–2.19 |
| Vena and Fielder | 1987 | 7 | 2.08 | 0.83–4.28 |

firefighters. The majority of studies have failed to demonstrate any statistically significant associations between firefighters and lung cancer, although lung cancer rates elevated relative to the general population have been noted (50,64,65). Guidotti (50) found an SMR of 142 in a cohort study of Alberta firefighters, with significant excess in a subcohort of Edmonton firefighters with over 35 years of experience. Heyer et al. (47) found no overall increase in respiratory cancer risk, but did note an elevated SMR of 177 for firefighters over 65 years of age. No excess of lung cancer was found by Demers et al. (48) in a subsequent mortality study of 4,546 northwest U.S. firefighters (SMR 0.92, 95% CI 0.69–1.19). At present, there are limited data to support an association between firefighter exposures and lung cancer. However, given the limited data on firefighters occupational exposures and smoking habits, additional work is needed.

## Respiratory Disease

Toxic combustion products can have profound effects on the respiratory system, causing acute symptoms, physiologic changes, and chronic diseases. Respiratory irritants such as hydrochloric acid, phosgene, ammonia, oxides of nitrogen, aldehydes, and sulfur dioxide can cause direct damage to the proximal airways, distal airways, and alveolar-capillary membrane. The combustion products of synthetic materials in modern furniture and building materials may produce smoke that is more toxic than that produced in the past. Clinical manifestations of smoke inhalation can range from mild irritant symptoms of the upper and lower airways to life-threatening adult respiratory distress syndrome; irritant-induced asthma, bronchiolitis obliterans, bronchiectasis, chronic bronchitis, airway injuries, and pulmonary fibrosis have also been described (65). The frequency, severity, and duration of smoke exposures appear to be important determinants of clinical outcomes, as well as individual susceptibility factors (65–68). Chemical composition, water solubility, particle size, and temperature characteristics of the combustion products also influence the pulmonary effects (65,68). Although the complexities of exposure assessment and unpredictable nature of fires have permitted only limited evaluations of acute dose-response relationships and even less refined assessments of the long-term effects of smoke inhalation, many important observations have been made about the acute and chronic effects of smoke inhalation in firefighters.

### *Acute Effects*

Following exposures to smoke, firefighters have demonstrated acute changes in pulmonary function including decreased oxygenation, reductions in spirometry, and increased airway reactivity. The finding of mild hypoxemia in two firefighters who responded to a building fire containing dense smoke from polyvinyl chloride combustion prompted Genovesi and co-workers (69) to evaluate an additional 19 firefighters involved in the same incident. Mild to moderate hypoxemia ($pO_2$ 54–102, mean $pO_2$ 71) was documented in 19 of 21 mostly asymptomatic firemen, and resolved within 24 hours. Detailed pulmonary function tests performed on the same individuals 1 month later showed no significant abnormalities or differences from matched nonfirefighter controls, suggesting a single episode of smoke inhalation does not necessarily result in permanent impairment (70). Musk et al. (68) followed 39 firefighters over a 6-week period with pulmonary function tests and exhaled carbon monoxide levels, in conjunction with sampling of smoke at fire scenes. Following smoke exposure the forced expiratory volume in 1 second ($FEV_1$) declined by an average of 0.05 L, with 30% of declines in excess of 0.1 L. The decline in $FEV_1$ was related to particulate exposures, firefighters' report of exposure severity, and symptoms of cough, eye irritation, or phlegm. Of interest, the use of a SCBA was associated with large decreases in $FEV_1$ (0.21 L), suggesting the equipment was put on too late, removed too early, leaking, or associated with heavier exposure. The importance of appropriate SCBA use was again demonstrated by Brandt-Rauf and co-workers (71), who studied a cohort of 77 firefighters with pre- and postfire spirometry and industrial hygiene sampling of the fire environment. Statistically significant reductions in $FEV_1$ and forced vital capacity (FVC) were demonstrated only for firefighters who did not wear respiratory protective equipment. Personal monitoring data from unprotected firefighters documented exposures to sulfur dioxide and other combustion products at concentrations sufficient to cause decrements in pulmonary function.

Several studies have examined changes in firefighters lung function in conjunction with measures of airway reactivity. Sheppard and co-workers (72) measured baseline airway reactivity to methacholine in 29 firefighters, and then followed preshift, postshift, and postfire spirometry over an 8-week period. Significant declines in $FEV_1$ and/or FVC were more frequent following work shifts with fires, and occurred regardless of firefighters' baseline airway reactivity. Sherman and co-workers (73) performed spirometry and methacholine challenge testing before and after firefighting activities in 18 Seattle firefighters. Firefighting was associated with acute reductions in $FEV_1$ ($3.4\% \pm 1.1\%$) and forced expiratory flow after 25% to 75% of vital capacity had been expelled ($FEF_{25-75}$), and an acute increase in airway responsiveness. Increased airway responsiveness has been identified as a risk factor for the development of chronic obstructive pulmonary disease. The finding of increased airway responsiveness in firefighters suggests that they may be at risk for accelerated loss of ventilatory function. Chia and co-workers (74) exposed 10 new firefighter recruits and 10 experienced firefighters with normal airway reactivity to smoke in a chamber without respiratory protection. Following exposure, the new recruits maintained normal airway reactivity. However, 80% of the experienced firefighters developed increased airway reactivity. The authors suggested smoke-induced chronic injury or inflammation of the pulmonary epithelium in experienced firefighters may lead to increased risk of airway reactivity. Evaluating 13 victims of smoke inhalation 3 days after the fire, Kinsella and co-workers (75) found 12/13 (92%) to have airway reactivity, which was strongly correlated with carboxyhemoglobin levels. Repeat assessment 3 months later showed most to have improvement in airway reactivity, but not $FEV_1$ or specific conductance. The authors speculated that airway obstruction following smoke inhalation may be more common and persistent than generally recognized.

Recent studies of fire victims using bronchoalveolar lavage have provided insights into the cellular and biochemical effects of smoke inhalation. Following smoke inhalation, significant numbers of neutrophils are recruited to the airways (76). Neutrophils are capable of releasing proteolytic enzymes and inflammatory cytokines, which may contribute to injury of the airway epithelium and the development of bronchospasm and airway hyperreactivity (65). In patients with inhalation injury and cutaneous burns, increased numbers of both alveolar macrophages and neutrophils have been demonstrated in the airways; the alveolar macrophage may further contribute to the inflammatory response by elaborating additional cytokines such as tumor necrosis factor and interleukin-1, interleukin-6, and leukotriene $B_4$ (65,77). Although preliminary, these findings suggest potential mechanisms for the decrements in lung function and increases in airway reactivity demonstrated in epidemiologic investigations.

### *Chronic Effects*

Longitudinal studies of lung function in firefighters have provided conflicting results. Peters and co-workers (77) reported accelerated loss of $FEV_1$ and FVC over a 1-year follow-up of Boston firefighters. Rates of decline were more than twice the expected rate (77 ml/year vs. 30 ml/year for FVC), and were significantly related to the frequency of fire exposure. However, in subsequent follow-up studies at 3-, 5-, and 6-year intervals, investigators found rates of decline comparable to the general population, which were unrelated to indices of occupational smoke exposure (78–80). There was evidence of survival bias in the cohort, as firefighters with respiratory difficulties were selectively moved to lesser exposed jobs. The authors concluded that selection factors within the fire department and increased use of personal respiratory protective equipment were important in reducing the effects of smoke inhalation; significant attrition in follow-up cohorts may also have influenced the results. A 5-year study of firefighters participating in the Normative Aging Study found firefighters to have greater rates of decline in $FEV_1$ and FVC than nonfirefighters (18 ml/year and 12 ml/year, respectively) (81). It is important to note that the participants in these studies were evaluated before routine use of respiratory protective equipment, and may have sustained very significant smoke exposures (81). Two more recent studies of firefighters from the United Kingdom have not shown evidence for longitudinal decline in lung function (82,83). Overall, the evidence suggests that firefighters using appropriate respiratory protective equipment do not have accelerated loss of ventilatory function, although additional research is needed in this area. It is important to note that wildland firefighters, who do not typically wear protective respiratory equipment, have been shown to have decrements in lung function and increased airway responsiveness after a season of fighting fires (84).

The effects of frequent smoke exposure on mortality from nonmalignant chronic respiratory conditions have also been investigated. Studies comparing firefighters to U.S. population controls have demonstrated reduced chronic respiratory disease mortality rates in firefighters, despite evidence of acute and chronic pulmonary effects of smoke inhalation (42,46–48,51–56). However, these studies are susceptible to the healthy worker effect, where selection of healthy workers results in mortality rates lower than a general reference population. In a PMR study of New Jersey firefighters, Feuer and Rosenman (45) found an excess of nonmalignant respiratory disease compared to police controls (PMR = 1.98, $p$ <.05). Rosenstock and co-workers (54) compared a cohort of firefighters from the northwestern U.S. to police, and found an increased SMR of 141 for nonmalignant respiratory disease, as opposed to a deficit when compared to U.S. rates. However, a subsequent study of the same cohort with a longer period of follow-up found risks of nonmalignant respiratory disease to be of lower magnitude (incidence density ratio 1.11, 95% CI 0.71–1.73) (48). There is need for additional research on the chronic effects of smoke inhalation using appropriate control groups, especially in the context of changing firefighter exposures.

## CONCLUSION

Despite the long-standing recognition of the dangers of fighting fires, firefighters continue to sustain elevated rates of injury and illness. Although substantial progress has been made in protecting respiratory health through the use of personal protective equipment, firefighters continue to demonstrate increased rates of fatal and nonfatal injuries, hearing loss, and certain malignancies. Newly appreciated risks of communicable disease and reproductive toxicity warrant further investigation. In addition, the healthy worker effect may result in underestimation of firefighters health risks. Given their important role in protecting society, the health of firefighters should receive additional attention. Respiratory and malignant disease may be reduced by conscientious use of respiratory protective equipment through all stages of firefighting activities. Future efforts should be targeted toward preventing injury and illness, and protecting firefighters health and well-being.

## REFERENCES


1. National Fire Protection Association. Quincy, MA: NFPA, 1996.
2. Terrill JB, Montgomery RR, Reinhardt CF. Toxic gases from fires. *Science* 1978;200:1343–1347.
3. Orzel RA. Toxicological aspects of fire smoke: polymer pyrolysis and combustion. *Occup Med* 1993;8:415–429.
4. Jankovic J, Jones W, Burkhart J, Noonan G. Environmental study of firefighters. *Ann Occup Hyg* 1991;35:581–602.
5. Anonymous. Plastic trees create new hazards for both firemen and public. *JAMA* 1975;234:1211–1213.
6. Brandt-Rauf PW, Fallon Jr LF, Tarantini T, et al. Health hazards of fire fighters: exposure assessment. *Br J Ind Med* 1988;45:606–612.
7. Lowry WT, Juarez BS, Petty CS, Roberts B. Studies of toxic gas production during actual structural fires in the Dallas area. *J Forensic Sci* 1985;30:59–72.
8. Gold A, Burgess WA, Clougherty EV. Exposure of firefighters to toxic air contaminants. *Am Ind Hyg Assoc J* 1978;39:534–539.
9. Treitman RD, Burgess WA, Gold A. Air contaminants encountered by firefighters. *Am Ind Hyg Assoc J* 1980;41:796–802.
10. Lees PSL. Combustion products and other firefighter exposures. *Occup Med* 1995;10:691–706.
11. Froines JR, Hinds WC, Duffy RM, et al. Exposure of firefighters to diesel emissions in fire stations. *Am Ind Hyg Assoc J* 1987;48: 202–207.
12. Burgess WA, Reinhard S, Lynch JJ, Buchanan P. Minimum protection factors for respiratory protective devices for firefighters. *Am Ind Hyg Assoc J* 1977;38:18–23.
13. Radford EP, Levine MS. Occupational exposures to carbon monoxide in Baltimore firefighters. *J Occup Med* 1976;18:628–632.
14. Materna BL, Jones JR, Sutton PM, et al. Occupational exposures in California wildland fire fighting. *Am Ind Hyg Assoc J* 1992;53:69–76.
15. Shusterman DJ. Clinical smoke inhalation injury: systemic effects. *Occup Med* 1993;8:469–503.
16. Levine MS, Radford EP. Occupational exposures to cyanide in Baltimore fire fighters. *J Occup Med* 1978;20:53–56.
17. Burgess WA, Treitman RD, Gold A. *Air contaminants in structural fire fighting.* NFPCA grant 7X008. Boston: Harvard School of Public Health, 1979.
18. Atlas EL, Donnelly KC, Giam CS, McFarland AR. Chemical and biological characteristics of emissions from a fireperson training facility. *Am Ind Hyg Assoc J* 1985;46:532–540.
19. *Code of Federal Regulations,* 2. 29 CFR 1910.156. Washington, DC: U.S. Government Printing Office, Office of the Federal Register, 1992.
20. Burgess JL, Crutchfield CD. Quantitative respirator fit tests of Tucson fire fighters and measurement of negative pressure excursions during exertion. *Appl Occup Environ Hyg* 1995;10:29–36.
21. Reed E, Daya MR, Jui J, Grellman K, Gerber L. Occupational infectious disease exposures in EMS personnel. *J Emerg Med* 1993;11:9–16.
22. Jui J, Modesitt S, Fleming D, et al. Multicenter HIV and hepatitis B seroprevalence study. *J Emerg Med* 1990;8:243–251.
23. Kelen GD, Green GB, Purcell RH, et al. Hepatitis B and hepatitis C in emergency department patients. *N Engl J Med* 1992;327:1032.
24. Valenzuela TD, Hook 3d EW, Copass MK, Corey L. Occupational exposure to hepatitis B in paramedics. *Arch Intern Med* 1985;145: 1976–1977.
25. Pepe PE, Hollinger FB, Troisi CL, Heiberg D. Viral hepatitis risk in urban emergency medical services personnel. *Ann Emerg Med* 1986; 15:454–457.
26. Occupational Safety and Health Administration. Occupational exposure to bloodborne pathogens: final rule, 29 CRF Part 1910.1030. FR 56:64052, 1991.
27. Centers for Disease Control and Prevention. Guidelines for preventing the transmission of *Mycobacterium tuberculosis* in health care facilities. *MMWR* 1994;43(RR-13):1–133.
28. Reischl U, Bair HS, Reischl P. Fire fighter noise exposure. *Am Ind Hyg Assoc J* 1979;40:482–489.
29. Tubbs RL. Occupational noise exposure and hearing loss in fire fighters assigned to airport fire stations. *Am Ind Hyg Assoc J* 1991;52:372–378.
30. Tubbs RL. *Health hazard evaluation:* Pittsburgh Bureau of Fire. HHE report 8-0290-2460. Cincinnati: National Institute of Occupational Safety and Health, 1994.
31. Markowitz JS, Gutterman EM, Link B, Rivera M. Psychological response of firefighters to a chemical fire. *J Hum Stress* 1987;40:84–93.
32. Boxer PA, Wild D. Psychological distress and alcohol use among fire fighters. *Scand J Work Environ Health* 1993;19:121–125.
33. Gist R, Woodall SJ. Occupational stress in contemporary fire service. *Occup Med* 1995;10:763–787.
34. Paley MJ, Tepas DI. Fatigue and the shiftworker: firefighters working on a rotating shift schedule. *Hum Factors* 1994;36:269–284.
35. International Association of Fire Fighters. *Death and injury survey, 1993.* Washington, DC: International Association of Fire Fighters, 1994.
36. Karter MJ Jr, LeBlanc PR. 1995 US firefighter injuries. *NFPA J* 1996; Nov/Dec:103–112.
37. Department of Health and Human Services. *Proposed national strategy for the prevention of musculoskeletal injuries.* DHHS publication 89–129. Washington, DC: National Institute for Occupational Safety and Health, 1986.
38. Hilyer JC, Brown KC, Sirles AT, Peoples L. A flexibility intervention to reduce the incidence and severity of joint injuries among municipal firefighters. *J Occup Med* 1990;32:631–637.
39. McDiarmid MA, Lees PS, Agnew J, et al. Reproductive hazards of fire fighting. II. Chemical hazards. *Am J Ind Med* 1991;19:447–472.
40. Agnew J, McDiarmid MA, Lees PS, Duffy R. Reproductive hazard of fire fighting. I. Non-chemical hazards. *Am J Ind Med* 1991;19: 443–445.
41. Evanoff BA, Rosenstock L. Reproductive hazards in the workplace: a case study of women firefighters. *Am J Ind Med* 1986;9:503–515.
42. Olshan AF, Teschke K, Baird PA. Birth defects among offspring of firemen. *Am J Epidemiol* 1992;135:1318–1320.

43. Gilbert ES. Some confounding factors in the study of mortality and occupational exposures. *Am J Epidemiol* 1982;116:177–188.
44. Musk AW, Monson RR, Peters JM, Peters RK. Mortality among Boston firefighters, 1915–1975. *Br J Ind Med* 1978;35:104–108.
45. Feuer E, Rosenman K. Mortality in police and firefighters in New Jersey. *Am J Ind Med* 1986;9:517–527.
46. Vena JE, Fiedler RC. Mortality of a municipal-worker cohort: fire fighters. *Am J Ind Med* 1987;11:671–684.
47. Heyer N, Weiss NS, Demers P, Rosenstock L. Cohort mortality study of Seattle fire fighters: 1945–1983. *Am J Ind Med* 1990;17:493–504.
48. Demers PA, Heyer NJ, Rosenstock L. Mortality among firefighters from three northwestern United States cities. *Br J Ind Med* 1992;49: 664–670.
49. Aronson KJ, Tomlinson GA, Smith L. Mortality among fire fighters in metropolitan Toronto. *Am J Ind Med* 1994;26:89–101.
50. Guidotti TL. Mortality of Urban firefighters in Alberta. *Am J Ind Med* 1993;23:921–940.
51. Burnett CA, Halperin WE, Lalich NR, Sestito JP. Mortality among fire fighters: a 27 state survey. *Am J Ind Med* 1994;26:831–833.
52. Beaumont JL, Chu GST, Jones JR, et al. An epidemiologic study of cancer and other causes of mortality in San Francisco firefighters. *Am J Ind Med* 1991;19:357–372.
53. Tornling G, Gustavsson P, Hogstedt C. Mortality and cancer incidence in Stockholm fire fighters. *Am J Ind Med* 1994;25:219–228.
54. Rosenstock L, Demers P, Barnhart S. Respiratory mortality among firefighters. *Br J Ind Med* 1990;47:462–465.
55. Guralnick L. *Mortality by occupation and cause of death among men 20–64 years of age.* United States 1950 Vital Statistics, Special Reports 53. Washington, DC: U.S. Department of Health, Education and Welfare, Public Health Service, National Vital Statistics Division, 1950;279.
56. Barnard RJ, Gardner GW, Diaco NV, Kattus AA. Near-maximal ECG stress testing and coronary artery disease risk factor analysis in Los Angeles city fire fighters. *J Occup Med* 1975;17:693–695.
57. Dibbs E, Thomas HE, Wess ST, Sparrow D. Fire fighting and coronary heart disease. *Circulation* 1982;5:943–946.
58. Sardinas A, Miller JW, Hansen H. Ischemic heart disease mortality of firemen and policemen. *Am J Public Health* 1986;76:1140–1141.
59. Bates JT. Coronary artery disease deaths in the Toronto Fire Department. *J Occup Med* 1987;29:132–135.
60. Grimes G, Hirsch D, Borgeson D. Risk of death among Honolulu fire fighters. *Hawaii Med J* 1991;50:82–85.
61. Sama SR, Martin TR, Davis LK, Kriebel D. Cancer incidence among Massachusetts firefighters, 1982–1986. *Am J Ind Med* 1990;18:47–54.
62. Howe GR, Burch JD. Fire fighters and risk of cancer: an assessment and overview of the epidemiologic evidence. *Am J Epidemiol* 1990; 132:1039–1050.
63. Orris P, Kahn G, Melius J. Mortality study of Chicago firefighters. *Revue Epidemiol Sante Publique* 1992;40(suppl 1):S90–91.
64. Golden AL, Markowitz SB, Landrigan PJ. The risk of cancer in firefighters. *Occup Med* 1995;10:803–820.
65. Haponik EF. Clinical smoke inhalation injury: pulmonary effects. *Occup Med* 1993;8:431–468.
66. Loke J, Farmer W, Matthay RA, Putman CE, Smith GJW. Acute and chronic effects of fire fighting on pulmonary function. *Chest* 1980;77: 369–373.
67. Large AA, Owens GR, Hoffman LA. The short-term effects of smoke exposure on the pulmonary function of firefighters. *Chest* 1990;97: 806–809.
68. Musk AW, Smith J, Peters JM, McLaughlin E. Pulmonary function in firefighters: acute changes in ventilatory capacity and their correlates. *Br J Ind Med* 1979;36:29–34.
69. Genovesi MC, Tashkin DP, Chopra S, Morgan M, McElroy C. Transient hypoxemia in firemen following inhalation of smoke. *Chest* 1977;71: 441–444.
70. Tashkin DP, Genovesi MG, Chopra S, Coulson A, Simmons M. Respiratory status of Los Angeles firemen. *Chest* 1977;71:445–449.
71. Brandt-Rauf PW, Cosman B, Fleming Fallon L, Tarantini T, Idema C. Health hazards of firefighters: acute pulmonary effects after toxic exposures. *Br J Ind Med* 1989;46:209–211.
72. Sheppard D, Distefano S, Morse L, Becker C. Acute effects of routine firefighting on lung function. *Am J Ind Med* 1986;9:333–340.
73. Sherman CB, Barnhart S, Miller MF, et al. Firefighting acutely increases airway responsiveness. *Am Rev Respir Dis* 1989;140: 185–190.
74. Chia KS, Jeyaratman J, Chan TB, Lim TK. Airway responsiveness of firefighters after smoke exposure. *Br J Ind Med* 1990;47:524–527.
75. Kinsella J, Carter R, Reid WH, Campbell D, Clark CJ. Increased airway reactivity after smoke inhalation. *Lancet* 1991;337:595–596.
76. Clark CJ, Pollock AJ, Reid WH, Campbell D, Gemmel C. Role of pulmonary alveolar macrophage activation in acute lung injury after burns and smoke inhalation. *Lancet* 1988;2:872–874.
77. Peters JM, Theriault GP, Fine LJ, Wegman DH. Chronic effect of fire fighting on pulmonary function. *N Engl J Med* 1974;291:1320–1322.
78. Musk AW, Peters JM, Wegman DW. Lung function in firefighters, a three year follow up of active subjects. *Am J Public Health* 1977;67: 626–629.
79. Musk AW, Peters JM, Berstein et al. Lung function in firefighters: a six year follow up in the Boston fire department. *Am J Ind Med* 1982;3:3–9.
80. Musk AW, Peters JM, Wegman DW. Lung function in firefighters, a five year follow-up of retirees. *Am J Public Health* 1977;67:630–635.
81. Sparrow D, Bosse R, Rosner B, Weiss ST. The effect of occupational exposure on pulmonary function. *Am Rev Respir Dis* 1982;125: 319–322.
82. Douglas DB, Douglas RB, Oakes D, Scott G. Pulmonary function of London firemen. *Br J Ind Med* 1985;42:55–58.
83. Horsfield K, Guyatt AR, Cooper FM, Buckman M, Cumming M. Lung function in west Sussex firemen: a four year study. *Br J Ind Med* 1988;45:116–121.
84. Liu D, Tager IB, Balmes JR, Harrison RJ. The effect of smoke inhalation on lung function and airway responsiveness in wildland fire fighters. *Am Rev Respir Dis* 1992;146:1469–1473.

*Environmental and Occupational Medicine,*
*Third Edition,* edited by William N. Rom.
Lippincott–Raven Publishers, Philadelphia © 1998.

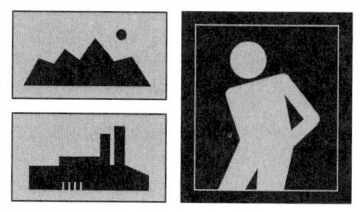

# CHAPTER 111

# Occupational Hazards in the Visual and Performing Arts

Michael McCann

In recent years, concern about occupational hazards has extended beyond industry. Office workers, teachers, and public employees all have their own occupational hazards, and so do visual and performing artists.

## VISUAL ARTS

Professional artists and crafters, art teachers, hobbyists, and children are exposed to a wide variety of hazardous chemicals (1,2) (Table 1). Unfortunately, artists often use them without taking adequate precautions, and often without even knowing that they are hazardous. Since about half of artists work at home, they also can expose spouses and children (3).

Examples of diseases of artists due to exposure to art materials include lead poisoning in a stained-glass artist (4), chromium sensitization in a fiber artist (5), neuropathy in a silk-screen artist (6), heart attacks from methylene chloride in a furniture refinisher (7), respiratory problems in photographers (8), and mesothelioma in jewelers (9). Other hazards in the visual arts include eye damage by ultraviolet or infrared radiation (from welding, foundries, kilns, and carbon arcs); hearing loss from noisy machinery; hazards from inadequately guarded machines; damage to the fingers and hands (Raynaud's phenomenon) from vibrating pneumatic tools; and ergonomic problems (damage to muscles, tendons, joints, and nerves) from poorly designed tools and repetitive motions (1,2,10).

M. McCann: Center for Safety in the Arts, New York, New York 10011.

### Epidemiologic Studies

Few epidemiologic studies have specifically examined artists. A proportionate mortality ratio (PMR) study of 1,746 white professional artists conducted by the National Cancer Institute found that deaths from arteriosclerotic heart disease and from cancers of all sites combined were significantly elevated for painters, and to a lesser degree for other artists (11). For male painters, rates of leukemias and cancers of the bladder, kidney, and colorectum were significantly elevated. Proportionate cancer mortality ratios had a similar pattern, but risk estimates were reduced. A case-control study of bladder cancer patients found an overall relative risk estimate of 2.5 for artistic painters (11), confirming a twofold excess of bladder cancer deaths in the PMR study. The case-control study also found the risk to increase with length of employment as an artistic painter.

In other male artists, PMRs for bladder cancer and leukemia were not significantly elevated, though they were for colorectal and kidney cancer. A preliminary report found that the risk of colon or prostate cancer was significantly elevated for sculptors (12). Some of these results are supported by death certificate surveys in which all art specialties are grouped together (13–16).

### Nature of the Problem

From a public health point of view there are four main aspects to the occupational hazards in the visual arts: (a) chemicals that are too toxic, (b) inadequate labeling, (c) lack of training in schools, and (d) misdiagnosis of occupational illnesses.

**TABLE 1.** *Occupational hazards in the visual arts*

| Technique | Material/process | Hazard |
|---|---|---|
| Airbrush | Pigments | Lead, cadmium, manganese, cobalt, mercury, etc. |
| | Solvents | Mineral spirits, turpentine |
| Batik | Wax | Fire, wax, decomposition fumes |
| | Dyes | See Dyeing |
| Ceramics | Clay dust | Silica |
| | Glazes | Silica, lead, cadmium, and other toxic metals |
| | Slip casting | Talc, asbestiform materials |
| | Kiln firing | Sulfur dioxide, carbon monoxide, fluorides, infrared radiation, burns |
| Commercial art | Rubber cement | *n*-hexane, heptane, fire |
| | Permanent markers | Xylene, propyl alcohol |
| | Spray adhesives | *n*-hexane, heptane, 1,1,1-trichloroethane, fire |
| | Airbrushing | See Airbrush |
| | Typography | See Photography |
| | Photostats, proofs | Alkali, propyl alcohol |
| Computer art | Ergonomics | Carpal tunnel syndrome, tendinitis, poorly designed workstations |
| | Video display | Glare, ELF radiation |
| Drawing | Spray fixatives | *n*-hexane, other solvents |
| Dyeing | Dyes | Fiber-reactive dyes, benzidine dyes, naphthol dyes, basic dyes, disperse dyes |
| | Mordants | Vat dyes, ammonium dichromate, copper sulfate, ferrous sulfate, oxalic acid, etc. |
| | Dyeing assistants | Acids, alkalis, sodium hydrosulfite |
| Electroplating | Gold, silver | Cyanide salts, hydrogen cyanide |
| | Other metals | Cyanide salts, acids |
| Enameling | Enamels | Lead, cadmium, arsenic, cobalt, etc. |
| | Kiln firing | Infrared radiation, burns |
| Fiber arts | Animal fibers | Anthrax and other infectious agents |
| (see also Batik | Synthetic fibers | Formaldehyde |
| and Weaving) | Vegetable fibers | Molds, allergens, dust |
| Forging | Hammering | Noise |
| | Hot forge | Carbon monoxide, polycyclic aromatic hydrocarbons, infrared radiation, burns |
| Glassblowing | Batch process | Lead, silica, arsenic, etc. |
| | Furnaces | Heat, infrared radiation, burns |
| | Coloring | Metal fumes |
| | Etching | Hydrofluoric acid, ammonium hydrogen fluoride |
| | Sandblasting | Silica |
| Holography | Lasers | Nonionizing radiation, electrical hazards |
| (see also | Developing | Bromine, pyrogallol |
| Photography) | | |
| Intaglio | Acid etching | Hydrochloric and nitric acids, nitrogen dioxide, chlorine gas, potassium chlorate |
| | Solvents | Alcohol, mineral spirits, kerosene |
| | Aquatint | Rosin dust, dust explosion |
| | Photoetching | Glycol ethers, xylene |
| Jewelry | Silver soldering | Cadmium fumes, fluoride fluxes |
| | Pickling baths | Acids, sulfur oxides |
| | Gold reclaiming | Mercury, lead, cyanide |
| Lapidary | Quartz gemstones | Silica |
| | Cutting, grinding | Noise, silica |
| Lithography | Solvents | Mineral spirits, isophorone, cyclohexanone, kerosene, gasoline, methylene chloride, etc. |
| | Acids | Nitric, phosphoric, hydrofluoric, hydrochloric, etc. |
| | Talc | Asbestiform materials |
| | Photolithography | Dichromates, solvents |
| Lost wax casting | Investment | Cristobalite |
| | Wax burnout | Wax decomposition fumes, carbon monoxide |
| | Crucible furnace | Carbon monoxide, metal fumes |
| | Metal pouring | Metal fumes, infrared radiation, molten metal, burns |
| | Sandblasting | Silica |
| Painting | Pigments | Lead, cadmium, mercury, cobalt, manganese compounds, etc. |
| | Oil, alkyd | Mineral spirits, turpentine |
| | Acrylic | Trace amounts ammonia, formaldehyde |
| Paper making | Fiber separation | Boiling alkali |
| | Beaters | Noise, injuries, electrical hazards |
| | Bleaching | Chlorine bleach |
| | Additives | Pigments, dyes, etc. |
| Pastels | Pigment dusts | See Painting pigments |

ELF, extremely low frequency.

**TABLE 1.** Continued.

| Technique | Material/process | Hazard |
|---|---|---|
| Photography | Developing bath | Hydroquinone, monomethyl-p-aminophenol sulfate, alkalis |
| | Stop bath | Acetic acid |
| | Fixing bath | Sulfur dioxide, ammonia |
| | Intensifier | Dichromates, hydrochloric acid |
| | Toning | Selenium compounds, hydrogen sulfide, uranium nitrate, sulfur dioxide, gold salts |
| | Color processes | Formaldehyde, solvents, color developers, sulfur dioxide |
| | Platinum printing | Platinum salts, lead, acids, oxalates |
| Relief printing | Solvents | Mineral spirits |
| | Pigments | See Painting pigments |
| Screen printing | Pigments | Lead, cadmium, manganese, and other pigments |
| | Solvents | Mineral spirits, toluene, xylene |
| | Photoemulsions | Ammonium dichromate |
| Sculpture, clay | | See Ceramics |
| Sculpture, lasers | Lasers | Nonionizing radiation, electrical hazards |
| Sculpture, neon | Neon tubes | Mercury, cadmium phosphors, electrical hazards, ultraviolet radiation |
| Sculpture, plastics | Epoxy resin | Amines, diglycidyl ethers |
| | Polyester resin | Styrene, methyl methacrylate, methyl ethyl ketone peroxide |
| | Polyurethane resins | Isocyanates, organotin compounds, amines, mineral spirits |
| | Acrylic resins | Methyl methacrylate, benzoyl peroxide |
| | Plastic fabrication | Heat decomposition products (e.g., carbon monoxide, hydrogen chloride, hydrogen cyanide, etc.) |
| Sculpture, stone | Marble | Nuisance dust |
| | Soapstone | Silica, talc, asbestiform materials |
| | Granite, sandstone | Silica |
| | Pneumatic tools | Vibration, noise |
| Stained glass | Lead came | Lead |
| | Colorants | Lead-based compounds |
| | Soldering | Lead, zinc chloride fumes |
| | Etching | Hydrofluoric acid, ammonium hydrogen fluoride |
| Weaving | Looms | Ergonomic problems |
| | Dyes | See Dyeing |
| Welding | General | Metal fumes, burns, sparks |
| | Oxyacetylene | Carbon monoxide, compressed gases |
| | Arc | Ozone, nitrogen dioxide, fluoride and other flux fumes, ultraviolet and infrared radiation, electrical hazards |
| | Metal fumes | Oxides of copper, zinc, lead, nickel, etc. |
| Woodworking | Machining | Injuries, wood dust, noise, fire |
| | Glues | Formaldehyde, resorcinol, epoxy |
| | Paint strippers | Methylene chloride, toluene, methyl alcohol, etc. |
| | Paints and finishes | Mineral spirits, toluene, turpentine, ethyl alcohol, etc. |
| | Preservatives | Chromated copper arsenate, pentachlorophenol, creosote |

### *"Do Not Use" Chemicals*

Many chemicals are used in arts and crafts that are too toxic for common use. Examples include known carcinogens (asbestos, cadmium in silver solders, lead and zinc chromate pigments), leaded ceramics glazes and copper enamels, *n*-hexane in rubber cement and spray adhesives, and cyanide compounds in electroplating baths. For most of these, adequate substitutes are available or could be made available with minimal effort.

### *Inadequate Labeling*

Until 1988 only acute-hazard labeling was required on art materials under the Federal Hazardous Substances Act (FHSA). Attempts to get a federal law mandating chronic hazard labeling of art materials began in the late 1970s and congressional hearings were held in 1980. As a result of this movement, the art materials industry adopted a voluntary labeling standard; however, it was largely limited to fine-art paints and some ceramics materials.

During the early to mid-1980s, California, Oregon, Tennessee, Illinois, Florida, Virginia, and Connecticut passed laws for chronic hazard labeling and banned the use of toxic art materials in elementary schools. Because labeling requirement varied from state to state, and because art material manufacturers who conformed to the voluntary standard were often at a competitive disadvantage to nonconforming manufacturers, many manufacturers and their trade associations supported a federal labeling law. In 1988 Congress passed the Labeling of Hazardous Art Materials Act (17). This law amended the FHSA to require chronic hazard labeling on all art materials and to allow the Consumer Product Safety Commission (CPSC) to get a court injunction against any school that purchased chronically toxic art materials for use in elementary schools. A major innovation in this law, as opposed to the Occupational Safety and Health Administration (OSHA) Hazard Communication Standard, for example, was that it required the CPSC to develop criteria for chronic hazards, rather than leaving it up to individual manufacturers. Unfortunately, the regulations promulgated by the CPSC did not require manufacturers to follow the CPSC chronic hazards guidelines.

### *Lack of Training*

Art students should learn the hazards of art materials and processes when they first learn techniques, and schools should have a safe working environment. Unfortunately, a major problem is that teachers and administrators themselves often are ignorant of the hazards. In addition, most secondary schools and colleges have not had a health and safety program and have not established adequate ventilation, storage, and handling procedures. Only in the last few years has this begun to change, with schools bringing consultants in to lecture on art hazards or to make recommendations for improvements in ventilation and other safety measures.

### *Misdiagnosis*

A final problem area is improper diagnosis of illnesses caused by exposure to hazardous art materials. Most artists go to physicians who are not trained in the toxic effects of chemicals, and many such physicians are reluctant to believe that art materials can cause occupational illnesses. Misdiagnosing lead poisoning as a psychosomatic disorder is just one example of what can happen (4).

The growth, over recent years, of occupational health clinics has provided a referral for artists with illnesses suspected to be caused by exposure to art materials.

## Children and Other High-Risk Groups

Art materials are commonly used by children in daycare centers, elementary school, and the home; by hospital patients in art and occupational therapy programs; by disabled persons in schools and institutions; and by the elderly in community centers and nursing homes. Age or certain medical problems can render such persons more susceptible to toxic chemicals, and special care should be taken to ensure that they use safe appropriate art materials (18,19). It is still all too common to find lead glazes, solvents, and other toxic materials in elementary school art classrooms.

In many instances art materials have caused illnesses in persons at special risk. During 1991, the American Association of Poison Control Centers received reports of 318 incidents of ceramic glaze ingestion, including one fatal case, in the United States (20,21). This included more than ten cases of lead poisoning from ingestion of ceramic glazes in nursing homes when the glazes were handed out in medication cups to elderly nursing home residents (22). Another example involved seizures from turpentine in a kindergarten student (23). Children in particular may be at risk from art materials used by parents or siblings. In one instance an 18-month-old child was reported to have contracted lead poisoning by playing near the parents while they were making stained glass. Awareness of many of these cases come through calls to poison control centers or to the Center for Safety in the Arts. Unfortunately, few end up in the medical literature.

## PERFORMING ARTS

A wide variety of performers—actors, dancers, musicians, and singers—are subject to occupational illnesses and injuries: skin irritation and allergies from theatrical makeup, respiratory irritation from fogs and smoke used on stage and motion picture sets, performance anxiety (stage fright), electrical hazards from lighting, accidents involving rigging, fire hazards from special effects pyrotechnics, and injuries from falls, stunts, and other risky situations (24–27). Many such injuries are peculiar to particular groups of performers. Even minor physical problems can often affect a performer's peak performance capability, and result in lost time, or even lost jobs. In recent years the diagnosis and treatment of injuries to performers has led to the new field of arts medicine, originally an offshoot of sports medicine (28).

The technical crew—stage carpenters, scenic artists, electricians, special effects experts, and camera crew—face, in addition to many of these same hazards, a wide variety of chemical hazards from materials used in scene, prop, and costume shops. Materials commonly used include paints, dyes, solvents, polyurethane, and polyester resins. Many of the same materials are used in the visual arts.

### Dance

The main occupational hazards facing dancers are acute trauma from a single injury (e.g., collisions, sprained ankles, pulled muscles) and overuse injuries resulting from repetitive motions (e.g., chronic back and knee problems) (29,30). The most common injuries to dancers are those of the musculoskeletal system—muscles, tendons, ligaments, joints, and bones—especially inflammation. Certain types of bone injuries are also common in dancers. Improper techniques and training methods may contribute to injuries. Other dance hazards include poor dance floors, stress, performance anxiety, and poor nutrition. Many studies have found high rates of injury among dancers (31).

Precautions include dancing on the proper type of suspended floor, proper warm-up exercises and other types of training techniques, and good nutrition. Allowing adequate time for healing and gradually getting back into shape is a crucial part of ensuring that a minor injury does not become more serious. In some instances, medication or surgery may be necessary.

### Music

Instrumentalists face a variety of occupational hazards. Several studies have shown that many musicians, including orchestra players, have noise-induced hearing loss (32,33). Sound level measurements in the orchestra pits of nine Broadway shows in New York City showed excessive sound levels (34). Again, overuse is a major problem for instrumentalists. The problems can include inflammation of the muscles, tendons, ligaments, and joints (tendinitis, arthritis); disorders of muscle control; and nerve entrapment due to inflammation of surrounding tissues (e.g., carpal tunnel syndrome) (35,36). Such injuries can be permanently disabling. Many result from repetitive motions of particular parts of the body. Examples include tendinitis of the arms in string players, and right-hand problems, especially of the fourth and fifth fingers, in pianists. In some instances, injuries occur because a musician is working beyond his or her physical capabilities.

Solutions to the noise problems have included special ear plugs and plastic shields placed behind the most exposed orchestra members. Solutions to the other types of musicians' occupational hazards include good posture, holding the instrument properly, and good practice technique. In particular, length of practice time is important if an injury occurs; treatment can include rest, proper exercises, and other physical therapy, medication, and sometimes surgery.

Singers can develop a variety of voice problems such as vocal cord damage from overuse and misuse, artificial fogs or smoke on stage, stage dust, and infections. Minor and temporary respiratory tract irritation, which for most people is not normally considered a problem, can drastically affect voice quality and pose a major problem for singers (37,38).

### Theater

The most common complaints of actors have revolved around the use of fogs and smoke on stage, stage temperature, problems with makeup (especially shared makeup), and injuries from stage fights, falls, trapdoors, and falling sets or lights (22).

One PMR study of screen and stage actors was published in 1985 (39). PMRs for cancer of the lung, esophagus, and bladder were significantly elevated for women, and the lung cancer rate for stage actresses was 3.8 times that for screen actresses. These observations are probably related to higher rates of smoking in actresses (similar to that found in women artists). Males had significant increases in PMRs for pancreas and colon cancer, although the increases were not significant when proportionate cancer mortality ratios (PCMRs) were calculated. Mortality from testicular cancer was twice the expected rate, by both methods. PMRs for suicide and non–motor vehicle accidents were significantly elevated in both men and women, and cirrhosis of the liver in men. These are probably reflections of the stress of the acting profession.

A 1993 survey of injuries among 313 performers in 23 Broadway shows in New York City found that 55.6% reported at least one injury, with a mean of 1.08 injuries per performer (40). For Broadway dancers, the most frequent sites of injury were the lower extremities (52%), back (22%), and neck (12%), with raked or slanted stages being a significant contributing factor. For actors, the most frequent sites of injuries were the lower extremities (38%), the lower back (15%), and vocal cords (17%). The use of fogs and smoke on stage was listed as a major cause.

In 1991, the National Institute for Occupational Safety and Health (NIOSH) investigated the health effects of the use of smoke and fogs in four Broadway shows. All the shows used glycol-type fogs, although one also used mineral oil. A questionnaire survey of 134 actors in these shows with a control group of 90 actors in five shows not using fogs found significantly higher levels of symptoms in actors exposed to fogs, including upper respiratory symptoms such as nasal symptoms, irritation of mucous membranes, and lower respiratory symptoms such as coughing, wheezing, breathlessness, and chest tightness. A follow-up study could not demonstrate a correlation between fog exposure and asthma, possibly due to the low number of responses.

There have been no similar studies of stagehands or scenic artists.

### Motion Picture and Film Production

Motion picture production has many of the same risks for actors and technical crews as the theater, but the safety risks are much greater, largely owing to the more dangerous stunts performed in motion pictures and to the often inadequate emergency medical care.

The Center for Safety in the Arts compiled a list of 40 fatalities that occurred from 1980 to 1989 in American motion picture and television film production (25), both in the United States and abroad. Sources include NIOSH, the National Traumatic Occupational Fatality Database, the California Division of Labor Statistics and Research, and news clippings from the "Cinema: Accidents" file of the New York Public Library for the Performing Arts located at Lincoln Center. Of these 40 fatalities, 30 were related to stunts, though only 10 involved stunt performers. The other casualties were actors, camera operators, pilots, and others on the set.

Accurate statistics on the number of accidents and Illnesses in motion picture and television film production are difficult to obtain. It is also difficult to correlate information from various sources, since they use different definitions of the industry. National statistics reported for the motion picture production and services industry for 1986 included 4,240 recordable occupational illnesses and injuries in full-time workers, with 1,600 involving lost workdays. The data for 1985 was about the same in total injuries but 10% higher for lost workday injuries.

California statistics for disabling, nonfatal injuries in motion picture production resulting in more than one lost workday for the years 1980 through 1988 indicate an increase in injuries and illnesses, from 2,588 in 1980–1982, to 2,962 in 1983–1985, to 2,968 in 1986–1988, a 15% increase overall. During this same period, California also had 13 fatalities directly related to film production, an incidence 1.5 fatalities per 1,000 injuries. This is three times higher than the 1988 California average of 0.5 fatalities per 1,000 injuries, and higher than the rates for manufacturing and construction.

The Screen Actors Guild (SAG) has also done studies, based on accident reports submitted by member companies of the Alliance of Motion Picture and Television Producers (AMPTP). A study of injuries and illnesses in SAG members from 1982 through 1984 reported 600 were injured, 53% of them stunt performers. About 80% of the injuries occurred while filming, and 80% on location rather than in the studio. More recent data are not available.

The demand for realism and increasingly more dangerous stunts is one cause of this high rate of injuries and deaths. For example, 18 of the 30 stunt-related fatalities since 1980 were caused by helicopter accidents. A second cause is inadequate or no advance planning for emergencies. This includes lack of adequate on-site emergency medical care, no provision for emergency transportation, and failure to locate beforehand hospitals with properly staffed and equipped emergency rooms. Solutions include requiring that motion picture producers have independent review of proposed stunts, adequate safety procedures, proper qualifications for stunt helicopter pilots, and adequate emergency medical care on location.

## REFERENCES


1. McCann M. *Artist beware,* 2nd ed. New York: Lyons and Burford, 1992.
2. McCann M. *Health hazards manual for artists,* 4th ed. New York: Lyons and Burford, 1993.
3. McCann M, Hall N, Klarnet R, et al. Reproductive hazards in the arts and crafts. Presented at 1986 Annual Conference of the Society for Occupational and Environmental Health Conference on Reproductive Hazards in the Environment and Workplace, Bethesda, MD, 1986.
4. Feldman R, Sedman T. Hobbyists working with lead. *N Engl J Med* 1975;292:929.
5. Chromium sensitization in an artist's workshop. *MMWR* 1982;31:111.
6. Prockup L. Neuropathy in an artist. *Hosp Pract* 1978 November;89.
7. Stewart R, Hake C. Paint remover hazard. *JAMA* 1976;235:398–401.
8. Kipen HM, Lerman Y. Respiratory abnormalities among photographic developers: a report of 3 cases. *Am J Ind Med* 1986;9:341–347.
9. Driscoll RJ, Mulligan WJ, Schultz D, et al. Malignant mesothelioma: a cluster in a native American population. *N Engl J Med* 1988;318: 1437–1438.
10. Norris RN. Physical disorders of visual artists. *Art Hazards News* 1990;13:1.
11. Miller AB, Silverman DT, Hoover RN, et al. Cancer risk among artistic painters. *Am J Ind Med* 1986;9:281–287.
12. Miller AB, Blair A, McCann M. Mortality patterns among professional artists: a preliminary report. *J Environ Pathol Toxicol Oncol* 1985;6: 303–313.
13. Guralnick L. Mortality by occupation and cause of death among men 20–64 years of age, U.S 1950. *Vital Statistics* 1963;53(3).
14. Petersen GR, Milham S Jr. Occupational mortality in the state of California 1959–61. DHHS(NIOSH) publication 80-104. Washington, DC: U.S. Government Printing Office, 1980.
15. Miller AB. The etiology of bladder cancer from an epidemiology viewpoint. *Cancer Res* 1977;37:2939–2942.
16. Englund A. Cancer incidence among painters and some allied trades. *J Toxicol Environ Health* 1980;6:1267–1273.
17. McCann M. Congress passes labeling act. *Art Hazards News* 1988; 11(9):1.
18. Babin A, Peltz PA, Rossol M. *Children's art supplies can be toxic.* New York: Center for Safety in the Arts, 1989.
19. McCann M. *Teaching art safely to the disabled.* New York: Center for Safety in the Arts, 1987.
20. Litovitz TL, Holm KC, Baily KM, et al. 1991 Annual report of the American Association of Poison Control Centers National Data Collection System. *Am J Emerg Med* 1992;10:452–491.
21. Lead ingestion and ceramic glazes. *MMWR* 1992;41:1.
22. Vance MV, Curry SC, Bradley JM, et al. Acute lead poisoning in nursing home and psychiatric patients from the ingestion of lead-based ceramic glazes. *Arch Intern Med* 1990;150:2085–2092.
23. Nerby D. Turpentine and young children. *Art Hazards News* 1983; 6(10):3.
24. Rossol M. *Stage fright:* health and safety in the theater, 2nd ed. New York, Allworth Press, 1991.
25. Rossol M. Ill effects of theatrical special effects. *Med Probl Perf Art* 1986;1:49–56.
26. Psychological issues in performing arts medicine. *Med Probl Perf Art* 1990;5(1).
27. McCann M. *Lights! Camera! Safety! A health and safety manual for motion picture and television production.* New York: Center for Safety in the Arts, 1991.
28. Lederman RJ. Performing arts medicine. *N Engl Med J* 1989;320:246.
29. Daum MC. *Musculoskeletal problems in dancers.* New York: Center for Safety in the Arts, 1988.
30. Ryan AJ, Stephens RE. *Dance medicine. A comprehensive guide.* Chicago: Pluribus, 1987.
31. Bowling A. Injuries to dancers: prevalence, treatment and perceptions of causes. *Br Med J* 1989;298:731–734.
32. Axelsson A, Lindgren F. Hearing in classical musicians. *Acta Otolaryngol* 1981;377(suppl):3–74.
33. Daum MC. *Hearing loss in musicians.* New York: Center for Safety in the Arts, 1988.
34. Babin A. Orchestra pit sound level measurements in Broadway shows. Presented at 124th Annual Meeting of the American Public Health Association, New York, 1996.
35. Daum MC. *Musculoskeletal problems in musicians.* New York: Center for Safety in the Arts, 1988.
36. Harman SE. Bibliography of occupational disorders in instrumental musicians. *Med Probl Perf Art* 1987;2:155–162; 1988;3:163–165.
37. Sataloff R. Common diagnoses and treatments in professional voice users. *Med Probl Perf Art* 1987;2:15–20.
38. Daum MC. *Occupational hazards in music.* New York: Center for Safety in the Arts, 1988.
39. Depue RH, Kagey BT. A proportionate mortality study of the acting profession. *Am J Ind Med* 1985;8(1):57–66.
40. Evans RW, Evans RI, Carvajal S, et al. A survey of injuries among Broadway performers. *Am J Public Health* 1996;86:77–80.

*Environmental and Occupational Medicine, Third Edition,* edited by William N. Rom.
Published by Lippincott–Raven Publishers, Philadelphia, 1998.

CHAPTER 112

# Sick Building Syndrome and Building-Related Illness

Kathleen Kreiss

Since the late 1970s, consultants and public health agencies at the local, state, and federal levels have been barraged with requests for investigative assistance to determine the origins of and solutions to complaints of office workers regarding their indoor building environments. The most frequent constellation of building-associated complaints is called *sick building syndrome.* It consists of mucous membrane irritation of eyes, nose, and throat; headache; unusual tiredness or fatigue; and, less frequently, dry or itchy skin. The hallmark of these complaints is their tight temporal association with building occupancy, and their rapid resolution, within minutes to hours, when affected office workers leave implicated buildings. Sick building syndrome is distinguished from more medically serious building-related illness by its subjective nature, reversibility, and high prevalence within implicated buildings and across the nonindustrial building stock in North America and Europe. Building-related illnesses include asthma, hypersensitivity pneumonitis, inhalation fever, and infection. In contrast to sick building syndrome, these building-related illnesses are uncommon and may result in substantial medical morbidity. Building-related asthma and hypersensitivity pneumonitis are usually accompanied by sick building syndrome complaints among co-workers. Whether similar etiologies contribute to sick building syndrome and these building-related illnesses is still speculative.

K. Kreiss: Epidemiology Investigations Branch, Division of Respiratory Disease Studies, National Institute for Occupational Safety and Health, Morgantown, West Virginia 26505.

## EPIDEMIOLOGY OF BUILDING-RELATED RISK FACTORS

Despite more than two decades of public health investigation of sick building syndrome, scientific research regarding cause and effective intervention or prevention has been meager. The historical origins of this inattention from the scientific community are of interest for other occupational and environmental problems of uncertain etiology.

The initial approach to building complaints was dominated by an industrial hygiene conceptual framework with applicability to the industrial environment. Since the late 1970s and even currently, building investigators typically measured air concentrations of pollutants of building material origin, such as formaldehyde or volatile organic compounds. Finding individual chemicals in low concentrations, in comparison to permissible exposure limits, frequently led to allegations that building occupants had no verifiable basis for complaint and therefore had mass psychogenic illness. Mass psychogenic illness, however, is not a diagnosis of exclusion and has criteria for diagnosis (1). The endemic nature of sick building syndrome within implicated buildings, its high prevalence in "nonproblem" buildings, and its symptom constellation are not explicable by hysteria resulting from hyperventilation and a visible person-to-person chain of transmission. However, building occupants whose complaints about indoor environmental quality have been ignored or for whom investigation has not resulted in effective remediation are often anxious and turn to nonscientific explanations of their symptoms.

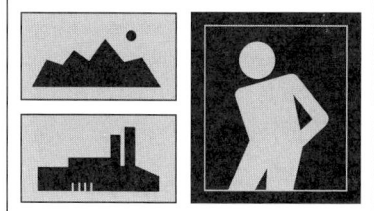

The industrial hygiene conceptual approach to problem building investigation resulted in measurement of carbon dioxide concentration and the guidance that levels should be kept below 1,000 ppm. Of course, $CO_2$ could not cause the symptoms composing sick building syndrome even at the highest levels found in office buildings. However, $CO_2$, a product of human metabolism, served as a marker of ventilation rate in relation to occupancy, with increases above the 350 ppm found in outdoor air being typical of indoor environments. The underlying assumption of this ventilation hypothesis for sick building syndrome was that human occupants were the source of the deterioration of indoor environmental quality. Indeed, this assumption was the basis of the earliest ventilation standards, which sought to ameliorate body odor from assembled groups indoors in the decades before current hygiene practices, indoor plumbing, and personal deodorants. The popularity of this approach to problem building investigation derived from the observation that building-related complaints surfaced after the energy crisis in the early 1970s. The American Society of Heating, Refrigeration, and Air-Conditioning Engineers had lowered its consensus standard for ventilation rate in occupied spaces from 20 cubic feet of outdoor air per minute (cfm) per person to 5 cfm per person in 1975. The $CO_2$ concentration is often still used as an indication of ventilation adequacy for removing nonoccupant produced air pollutants, although scientific data do not support such use, and relationships between $CO_2$ and actual ventilation rates are complex (2).

Advances in scientific understanding of indoor environmental quality complaints were made by European investigators beginning in the 1980s (3–5). Taking an epidemiologic approach, they showed that building-associated symptoms were common in buildings not recognized as having indoor environmental problems. Complaint rates varied substantially from building to building and were associated with building types and characteristics. Most interesting from the point of view of etiology and prevention was the finding that ventilation system type was important in determining risk of occupant complaints, with mechanical ventilation and/or air-conditioning conferring a severalfold risk in comparison to buildings with natural ventilation (6,7). This finding shifted the research emphasis from affected persons to ventilation engineering and building design concerns. The association of air-conditioning with risk of symptom prevalence also dovetailed nicely with the findings of human panel studies that evaluated subjective air quality, odor, and stuffiness of buildings in relation to ventilation system activity and occupancy (8,9). In some buildings, operation of the ventilation system resulted in deterioration of subjective air quality, suggesting that ventilation systems could be sources of complaints rather than the solution to them.

These findings called into question the simple guidance, now obsolete, that carbon dioxide levels be maintained below 1,000 ppm. Today we know that building materials, furnishings, equipment, and ventilation systems produce irritant pollutants that can interact to produce even more irritating chemicals (10). Controlling nonhuman pollutant levels requires ventilation without regard to control of human bioeffluents, as indicated by $CO_2$ levels. Experimental studies evaluating symptom prevalence rates in relation to ventilation rate have mixed results with regard to level of ventilation. At ventilation rates substantially above the current standard of 20 cfm per person set by the American Society of Heating, Refrigeration, and Air-Conditioning Engineers, a doubling of ventilation rate had no effect on the symptoms composing sick building syndrome (11). However, starting with low ventilation rates of about 20 cfm per person or less, several experimental studies have documented statistically significant improvement in symptom prevalence with increases in ventilation rate (12,13). In summary, minimum ventilation levels are likely important for dilution of the suspected indoor pollutants resulting in sick building syndrome, as long as the ventilation system is not itself the source of the pollutants (14). In cross-sectional studies, ventilation rates above 30 cfm per person are associated with further reduction of occupant symptoms (15), suggesting that the current ventilation and $CO_2$ guidelines may not be health protective.

The association of air cooling and or humidification with occupant complaints spawned the hypothesis that moisture in the ventilation system could support microbial amplification and dissemination in the indoor environment. Air cooling may chill the air stream below the dew point within duct work. Humidification obviously increases the moisture available for saprophytic fungi.

Modern duct work is commonly lined with sound-dampening materials, such as fibrous glass, which can support microbial growth when damp and which collect dirt, providing additional carbon sources for microbial proliferation. Despite many attempts to demonstrate associations between microbial burden in indoor air and sick building syndrome symptom prevalences, the evidence is still inconclusive.

Available methods of measuring microbial pollution in buildings are limited. No correlations have been consistently found for total viable bacteria or fungi and complaint rates (12), but sampling times of minutes, used in quantitative sampling methods, may be unrepresentative. A Dutch study reported that gram-negative rods had several times higher concentration in supply air in buildings characterized by higher complaint rates when compared to mechanically ventilated buildings in which occupants had complaint rates typical of naturally ventilated buildings (16). Similarly, gram-negative bacteria in carpet dust have been shown in one study to be related to symptom prevalence (17).

Viability of microbes may not be important for biologic effect of an allergic, toxic, or inflammatory nature.

Endotoxin, a constituent of the cell walls of gram-negative bacteria, has potent biologic effects. Contradictory data exist for the association of endotoxin with complaint prevalence (18); two reports document an association (16,19). Analytical methods for the low levels of endotoxin in the air of nonindustrial environments are problematic, and endotoxin activity was not shown to be correlated with symptoms in one study that showed strong correlations with viable gram-negative organisms in carpet dust (17). Fungal spore counts are independent of viability but may not be representative because of short duration samples. Analytic methods for mycotoxins generally require prior knowledge of the type of mycotoxin sought and relatively large amounts of material, but mycotoxins have been demonstrated in wipe samples of building surfaces with obvious fungal growth. Newer approaches for assessing fungal biomass with ergosterol and β-1,3-glucans, constituents of fungal membranes and cell walls respectively, may be promising as a means of assessing fungal microbial contamination in relation to symptom prevalence (19,20).

In addition to the associations between occupant complaint rates and both air-conditioning and low ventilation rates, epidemiologic approaches have identified a few workspace risk factors for sick building syndrome. Carpets, textile wall materials, and increased numbers of workers in an office space are supported as risk factors in most studies (12,18,21–26). Inconsistent or sparse reports make the associations of sick building syndrome with the following building and workspace factors open to further investigation: humidification, mechanical ventilation without air-conditioning, newer construction, poor ventilation system maintenance, negative ionization, improved office cleaning, proximity of photocopiers, and environmental tobacco smoke (12). In systematic investigations by the National Institute for Occupational Safety and Health (NIOSH) of 2,435 respondents in 80 buildings with perceived problems, the relative risk of having multiple symptoms of sneezing, eye irritation, and other nasal symptoms was increased in the presence of maintenance deficiencies of heating, ventilation, and air-conditioning (HVAC) systems, the presence of suspended ceiling panels, daily surface dusting, and interior pesticide application (27).

Apart from measuring ventilation rates, no measurements of indoor environmental quality have been consistently shown to be associated with some symptom of the sick building syndrome. Measurements consistently shown not to be associated with complaint rates include carbon monoxide, carbon dioxide, formaldehyde, total particles, viable fungi, air velocity, and noise. Measurements remaining open to further investigation because of sparse evidence or inconsistent findings among studies include total volatile organic hydrocarbons, respirable particulates, floor dust, endotoxins, β-1,3-glucan, low negative ions, high temperature, low humidity, and light intensity and glare (12).

Although specific measurements are not available to determine the likelihood that building occupants will avoid the sick building syndrome, the epidemiologic findings to date do lay a foundation for intervention studies (28). The risk factors of air-conditioning, carpet, respirable particulates, carpet or floor dust, and office and HVAC maintenance may all be related as affecting sources or reservoirs of biologically active agents from microorganisms or building fabric. Intervention studies to lower respirable particulates, maintain HVAC systems, and clean office environments are beginning to be conducted with blind and crossover designs (29).

## EPIDEMIOLOGY OF PERSONAL AND JOB RISK FACTORS

The study of sick building syndrome is challenging because of the psychosocial milieu in which building complaints arise. Although the body of epidemiologic research clearly documents environmental risk factors for the syndrome, investigators of problem buildings have a common experience of polarization, suspicion, and controversy surrounding their efforts. Job stress or dissatisfaction has been consistently demonstrated to be related to sick building syndrome in investigations of occupants in buildings not known to have indoor air complaints (12). It remains uncertain whether this association is a cause or an effect of sick building syndrome.

Researchers have documented an invariable female gender predisposition to report building-associated symptoms (3,5,11–13,23,25). Whether this female predominance reflects overexposure to unknown etiologic agents in building microenvironments, higher susceptibility, job dissatisfaction, or lower threshold for observation or reporting remains in dispute. Smokers have inconsistently shown increased risk of sick building syndrome (12).

Respondent reports of asthma or allergies are consistently associated with sick building syndrome (11–13,23,25), but no prospective studies exist to establish whether this personal factor is an outcome, a confounder, or a predisposing factor for reports of mucous membrane symptoms in relation to building occupancy. Among occupants of problem buildings, physician diagnosis of asthma since building occupancy was statistically associated with outdoor air intake within 25 feet of vehicular traffic, dirty HVAC filters, debris inside the air intake, the presence of cloth partitions, and renovation (especially the installation of new drywall in the preceding 3 months) (27). These environmental associations with the development of asthma during building occupancy suggest that asthma may be a result of exposures predictive of sick building syndrome.

The job-related risk factor consistently demonstrated to be associated with sick building syndrome has been video display terminal use. Inconsistent associations have been found with clerical jobs, use of carbonless copy paper, and photocopier use (12).

The study of sick building syndrome has been complicated by the subjective nature of the complaints. In the face of associations with job stress and dissatisfaction, investigators have feared that classification of cases was unreliable. For eye irritation complaints, however, breakup time of the tear film, eye epithelial damage, and interblink interval have been shown to correlate with subjective complaints and with experimental manipulations of the environment (29,30). Other research methods, such as nasal resistance studies, are being evaluated for their utility in corroborating sick building syndrome complaints. The consistency of building-related complaints across nations and their similar environmental associations make the effort to find objective measures of less concern than formerly, when a substantial portion of the indoor air scientific community wondered whether the complaints were of purely psychosocial origin. Research is proceeding regarding likely mechanisms, such as mediator release associated with inflammatory and toxic effects of microbial constituents expected to be associated with sick building syndrome (31).

## MAGNITUDE OF SICK BUILDING SYNDROME

European investigators surveying buildings not known to have indoor environmental complaints found a substantial subset with symptom complaint rates similar to those demonstrable in buildings being investigated for complaints (3–5,7,16). Comparable information for the United States population is meager, with only preliminary information available from studies of nonproblem office buildings (32,33). A random sample telephone survey of the U.S. population documented that about one-fourth of office workers perceived indoor air quality problems to exist in their office environments and 20% of all respondents reported their work performance to be hampered by the air quality (34).

Although sick building syndrome is not considered medically serious by most physicians, the comfort of a substantial sector of nonindustrial workers is compromised by the office building stock. Cost estimates of productivity loss related to discomfort and illness are substantial, in comparison to the energy cost savings of decreasing ventilation or savings on ventilation system capacity and maintenance and housekeeping (35). Solution of this common problem likely depends on many disciplines, including architects, general contractors, ventilation engineers, building operations personnel, physicians, industrial hygienists, epidemiologists, and microbiologists. Although specific etiologies have defied scientific documentation, the epidemiologic findings to date suggest interventions that should be evaluated in experimental studies, such as lowering respirable particulates, maintaining an immaculate ventilation system and duct work, and appropriate housekeeping.

## BUILDING-RELATED ILLNESSES

Building-related illnesses, such as hypersensitivity pneumonitis and asthma, often occur against a backdrop of sick building syndrome complaints among other building occupants. Their recognition is important because they are often medically serious, require cessation of exposure to improve prognosis, and serve as sentinel events for others at risk. When building occupants report building-related chest symptoms such as shortness of breath with exertion, cough, and wheezing or chest tightness, asthma or hypersensitivity pneumonitis should be suspected. These chest symptoms are not typical of sick building syndrome, although cough can be of either sinus or chest origin. Profound malaise and sick fatigue are characteristic of granulomatous lung disease, such as hypersensitivity pneumonitis, and are not characteristic of asthma or sick building syndrome. Physician recognition of building-associated asthma and hypersensitivity pneumonitis may be poor, and the building investigator may need to suggest referral of building occupants with building-related chest symptoms to specialists with an interest in early diagnosis of disease from building-associated etiologies. Persons with building-related asthma or hypersensitivity pneumonitis may have symptom exacerbation with reentry into an implicated environment even after environmental remediation (36–39), presumably because of the immunologic potentiation of response to even low levels of antigen exposure.

Outbreaks of building-associated hypersensitivity pneumonitis have been reported in association with contaminated spray water humidification systems and contaminated air-conditioning systems (37,40–43), including duct work (44). Hypersensitivity pneumonitis also can occur endemically in water-damaged buildings (45) in which wet furnishings support microbial growth or in buildings with moisture incursion from below-grade walls (36). In contrast to the frequency of water damage to buildings from roof leaks, plumbing mishaps, and basement flooding, reports of hypersensitivity pneumonitis are infrequent. This may indicate low-risk, reversible disease, or poor recognition of building-related granulomatous or interstitial lung disease by clinicians who seldom inquire about building risk factors for these lung diseases in sporadic cases. In industrial settings, outbreaks of interstitial lung disease are more likely to be recognized in relation to water spray processes, humidification systems, or air-conditioning systems. These have been reported from the stationery industry (46), printing works (47), photographic film industry (48), swimming pools with water spray features (49), and textile industry (50).

Building-related asthma is recognized even less frequently than hypersensitivity pneumonitis. Outbreak investigations and case reports document water incursion (36), cool mist vaporizers (51), and humidifiers (52,53) as factors in etiology. As with hypersensitivity pneumonitis, recognition of possible cause by clinicians may be lacking. There are population-based studies of asthma that implicate residential dampness as a risk factor for asthma (54–57).

Building-related illness includes inhalation fevers. Pontiac fever is a self-limited illness with high attack rate associated with serologic immunity to *Legionella* antigen (58). Humidifier fever has been attributed to endotoxins (59), *Bacillus subtilis* (60), and amoebae (61–64).

## INFECTION

From a public health viewpoint, the most important condition influenced by buildings is communicable respiratory infection, such as influenza and tuberculosis. Compelling evidence exists that infection transmission for respiratory disease is affected by ventilation characteristics. A landmark study in this regard was the observation that military recruits housed in energy-efficient barracks had a 51% increase in incidence of febrile respiratory disease when compared to recruits housed in old barracks, presumably with greater air infiltration (65). Higher increases to 250% were documented in epidemic years when trainees were not immunized against adenovirus. Military troops housed in air-conditioned buildings in Saudi Arabia had excess symptoms of sore throat and cough compared to troops housed in outdoor environments, and this was attributed to increased infection transmission indoors (66). Similarly, epidemic pneumococcal disease has been documented in an overcrowded jail, in which median ventilation was only 6.1 cfm per inmate (67). In office worker populations, a Swiss investigator found that absenteeism due to respiratory illness was greater in a fully air-conditioned building than in a naturally ventilated building with a similar population (68). Tuberculosis transmission has long been known to be affected by ventilation patterns and rates (69). Despite the considerable burden of preventable infection associated with building environments, insufficient research exists in this area to support educational efforts for architects and ventilation engineers. Our understanding of microbial etiology in the case of infection has put this set of diseases in the purview of infectious disease specialists, with scant consideration by the many disciplines required to pursue preventive strategies of an environmental nature.

Apart from building ventilation characteristics enhancing transmission of communicable disease, building structures have been implicated as sources of noncommunicable infections. The classic example of building-related infection is *Legionella* pneumonia, and there is increasing evidence that potable water supplies in buildings, rather than aerosols, may be the ultimate reservoir and means of transmission of the organism (70–72). Infection of immunocompromised patients with *Mycobacterium avium* complex has also been shown to be associated with this organism in potable water supplies (73) and indoor swimming pools (74). Systemic fungal infections in immunocompromised hosts have occurred in hospital settings with saprophytic fungi colonizing ventilation duct work or disseminated in renovation dusts (75–79). Laboratory techniques and molecular epidemiology are allowing us to understand the implications of building environments as risk factors for both common and new agents of infection (67,73).

## SUMMARY

Occupational and environmental health professionals have a unique contribution to make in the assessment of indoor environmental problems. We do not yet know enough to recommend specific measurements of office building air concentrations to assure occupant health prospectively or in response to intervention in a problem building. Nevertheless, we have promising leads from the epidemiology of building-related symptoms to pursue research using new methods of assessment of environment and microbial burden. We also have promising leads for intervention studies without knowing specific etiologies. The science of indoor environmental quality does not support the uncritical application of either recommended ventilation rates or carbon dioxide measurements as assessment of whether the building is acceptable to occupants.

Careful assessment of the nature of health complaints can result in the recognition of building-related asthma or hypersensitivity pneumonitis. These diseases require a different clinical management and public health investigation than does sick building syndrome alone. Finally, the study of indoor environmental quality points toward potential opportunities to lower morbidity from infections that are impacted by ventilation rates and building operation practices.

## REFERENCES

1. Guidotti TL, Alexander RW, Fedoruk MJ. Epidemiologic features that may distinguish between building-associated illness outbreaks due to chemical exposure or psychogenic origin. *J Occup Med* 1987;29:148–150.
2. Persily A, Dolls WS. *The relation of $CO_2$ concentration to office building ventilation.* Standard technical publication 1067. Philadelphia: American Society of Testing and Materials, 1990.
3. Finnegan MJ, Pickering CAC, Burge PS. The sick building syndrome: prevalence studies. *Br Med J* 1984;289:1573–1575.
4. Skov P, Valbj rn O, Danish Indoor Climate Study Group. The "sick" building syndrome in the office environment: the Danish town hall study. *Environ Int* 1987;13:339–349.
5. Burge S, Hedge A, Wilson S, Bass JH, Robertson A. Sick building syndrome: a study of 4373 office workers. *Ann Occup Hyg* 1987;31(4A):493–504.
6. Mendell MJ, Smith AH. Consistent pattern of elevated symptoms in air-conditioned office buildings: a reanalysis of epidemiologic studies. *Am J Public Health* 1990;80:1193–1199.

7. Jaakkola JJK, Miettinen P. Type of ventilation system in office buildings and sick building syndrome. *Am J Epidemiol* 1995;141:755–765.
8. Fanger PO. Introduction of the olf and decipol units to quantify air pollution perceived by humans indoors and outdoors. *Energy Build* 1988; 12:1–6.
9. Fanger PO, Lauridsen J, Bluyssen P, Clausen G. Air pollution sources in offices and assembly halls, quantified by the olf unit. *Energy Build* 1988;12:7–19.
10. Weschler CJ, Hodgson AT, Wooley JD. Indoor chemistry: ozone, volatile organic compounds, and carpets. *Environ Sci Technol* 1992;26: 2371–7.
11. Menzies R, Tamblyn R, Farant J-P, Hanley J, Nunes F, Tamblyn R. The effect of varying levels of outdoor-air supply on the symptoms of sick building syndrome. *N Engl J Med* 1993;328:821–827.
12. Mendell MJ. Non-specific symptoms in office workers: a review and summary of the epidemiologic literature. *Indoor Air* 1993;3:227–236.
13. Jaakkola JJK, Heinonen OP, Seppanen O. Mechanical ventilation in office buildings and the sick building syndrome: an experimental and epidemiological study. *Indoor Air* 1991;2:111–121.
14. Jaakkola JJK, Miettinen P. Ventilation rate in office buildings and sick building syndrome. *Occup Environ Med* 1995;52:709–714.
15. Stenberg B, Eriksson N, Höög J, Sundell J, Wall S. The sick building syndrome (SBS) in office workers. A case-referent study of personal, psychosocial and building-related risk indicators. *Int J Epidemiol* 1994; 23:1190–1197.
16. Teeuw KB, Vandenbroucke-Grauls CMJE, Verhoef J. Airborne gram-negative bacteria and endotoxin in sick building syndrome. *Arch Intern Med* 1994;154:2339–2345.
17. Gyntelberg F, Suadicani P, Nielsen JW, et al. Dust and the sick building syndrome. *Indoor Air* 1994;4:223–238.
18. Hodgson MJ, Frohliger J, Permar E, et al. Symptoms and microenvironmental measures in nonproblem buildings. *J Occup Med* 1991;33: 527–533.
19. Rylander R, Persson K, Goto H, Yuasa K, Tanaka S. Airborne beta-1,3-glucan may be related to symptoms in sick buildings. *Indoor Environ* 1992;1:263–267.
20. Miller JD, Young JC. The use of ergosterol to measure exposure to fungal propagules in indoor air. *Am Ind Hyg Assoc J* 1997;58:39–43.
21. Norback D, Torgen M. A longitudinal study relating carpeting to sick building syndrome. *Environ Int* 1989;15:129–135.
22. Norback D, Torgen M, Edling C. Volatile organic compounds, respirable dust, and personal factors related to the prevalence and incidence of sick building syndrome in primary schools. *Br J Med* 1990; 47:733–741.
23. Skov P, Valbjørn O, Pedersen BV, Danish Indoor Climate Study Group. Influence of personal characteristics, job-related factors and psychosocial factors on the sick building syndrome. *Scand J Work Environ Health* 1989;15:286–295.
24. Skov P, Valbjørn O, Pedersen BV, Danish Indoor Climate Study Group. Influence of indoor climate on the sick building syndrome in an office environment. *Scand J Work Environ Health* 1990;16:1–9.
25. Zweers T, Preller L, Brunekreef B, Boleij JSM. Health and indoor climate complaints of 7043 office workers in 61 buildings in the Netherlands. *Indoor Air* 1992;2:127–136.
26. Jaakkola JJK, Tuomaala P, Seppänen O. Textile wall materials and sick building syndrome. *Arch Environ Health* 1994;49:175–191.
27. Seiber WK, Stayner LT, Malkin R, et al. The National Institute for Occupational Safety and Health indoor environmental evaluation experience: Part three: Associations between environmental factors and self-reported health conditions. *Appl Occup Environ Hyg* 1996;11(12): 1387–1392.
28. Bourbeau J, Brisson C, Allaires. Prevalence of the sick building syndrome symptoms in office workers before and after being exposed to a building with an improved ventilation system. *Occup Environ* Med 1996;53:204–210.
29. Wyon D. Sick buildings and the experimental approach. *Environ Technol* 1992;13:313–322.
30. Franck C, Bach E, Skov P. Prevalence of objective eye manifestations in people working in office buildings with different prevalences of the sick building syndrome compared with the general population. *Int Arch Occup Environ Health* 1993;65:65–69.
31. Norn S, Clementsen P, Kristensen KS, Stahl Skov P, Bisgaard H, Gravesen S. Examination of mechanisms responsible for organic dust-related diseases: mediator release induced by microorganisms. A review. *Indoor Air* 1994;4:217–222.
32. Nelson NA, Kaufman JD, Burt J, Karr C. Health symptoms and the work environment in four nonproblem United States office buildings. *Scand J Work Environ Health* 1995;21:51–59.
33. Mendell MJ, Fisk WJ, Deddens JA, et al. Elevated symptom prevalence associated with ventilation type in office buildings. *Epidemiology* 1996;7:383–389.
34. Woods JE. Cost avoidance and productivity in owning and operating buildings. In: Cone JE, Hodgson MJ, eds. Problem buildings: Building-associated illness and the sick building syndrome. *Occup Med State Art Rev* 1989;4:575–592.
35. Fisk WJ, Rosenfeld AH. Estimates of improved productivity and health from better indoor environments. *Indoor Air* 1997;7:158–172.
36. Hoffman RE, Wood RC, Kreiss K. Building-related asthma in Denver office workers. *Am J Public Health* 1993;83:89–93.
37. Bernstein RS, Sorenson WG, Garabrant D, Reaux C, Treitman RD. Exposures to respirable, airborne Penicillium from a contaminated ventilation system: clinical, environmental and epidemiologic aspects. *Am Ind Hyg Assoc J* 1983;44:161–169.
38. Marinkovich VA, Hill A. Hypersensitivity alveolitis. *JAMA* 1975;231: 944–947.
39. Solley GO, Hyatt RE. Hypersensitivity pneumonitis induced by Penicillium species. *J Allergy Clin Immunol* 1980;65:65–70.
40. Hodgson MJ, Morey PR, Simon JS, Waters TD, Fink JN. An outbreak of recurrent acute and chronic hypersensitivity pneumonitis in office workers. *Am J Epidemiol* 1987;125:631–638.
41. Banaszak EF, Thiede WH, Fink JN. Hypersensitivity pneumonitis due to contamination of an air conditioner. *N Engl J Med* 1970;283: 271–276.
42. Arnow PM, Fink JN, Schlueter DP, et al. Early detection of hypersensitivity pneumonitis in office workers. *Am J Med* 1978;64:236–242.
43. Ganier M, Lieberman P, Fink J, Lockwood DG. Humidifier lung an outbreak in office workers. *Chest* 1980;77:183–187.
44. Hales CA, Rubin RH. Case records of the Massachusetts General Hospital, Case 47-1979. *N Engl J Med* 1979;301:1168–1174.
45. Hodgson MJ, Morey PR, Attfield M, et al. Pulmonary disease associated with cafeteria flooding. *Arch Environ Health* 1985;40:96–101.
46. Friend JAR, Gaddie J, Palmer KNV, Pickering CAC, Pepys J. Extrinsic allergic alveolitis and contaminated cooling-water in a factory machine. *Lancet* 1977;1:297–300.
47. Pickering CAC, Moore WKS, Lacy J, Holfor-Strevens VC, Pepys J. Investigation of a respiratory disease associated with an air-conditioning system. *Clin Allergy* 1076;6:109–118.
48. Woodard ED, Friedlander B, Lasher RJ, Font W, Kinney R, Hearn T. Outbreak of hypersensitivity pneumonitis in an industrial setting. *JAMA* 1988;259:1965–1969.
49. Lynch DA, Rose CS, Way D, King TE, Jr. Hypersensitivity pneumonitis: sensitivity of high-resolution CT in a population-based study. *AJR* 1992;159:469–472.
50. Reed CE, Swanson MC, Lope M, et al. Measurement of IgG antibody and airborne antigen to control an industrial outbreak of hypersensitivity pneumonitis. *J Occup Med* 1983;25:207–210.
51. Solomon WR. Fungus aerosols arising from cool-mist vaporizers. *J Allergy Clin Immunol* 1974;54:222–228.
52. Finnegan MJ, Pickering CAC. Building related illness. *Clin Allergy* 1986;16:389–405.
53. Burge PS, Finnegan M, Horsfield N, Emory D. Occupational asthma in a factory with a contaminated humidifier. *Thorax* 1985;40:248–254.
54. Brunekreef B. Damp housing and adult respiratory symptoms. *Allergy* 1992;47:498–502.
55. Dales RE, Burnett R, Zwanenburg H. Adverse health effects among adults exposed to home dampness and molds. *Am Rev Respir Dis* 1991;143:505–509.
56. Spengler J, Neas L, Nakai S, et al. Respiratory symptoms and housing characteristics. *Indoor Air* 1994;4:72–82.
57. Dekker GC, Dales R, Bartlett S, Brunekreef B, Zwanenburg H. Childhood asthma and the indoor environment. *Chest* 1991;100:922–926.
58. Kaufmann AF, McDade JE, Patton CM, et al. Pontiac fever: isolation of the etiologic agent *(Legionella pneumophila)* and demonstration of its mode of transmission. *Am J Epidemiol* 1981;114:337–347.
59. Rylander R, Haglind P, Lundholm M, Mattsby I, Stenqvist K. Humidifier fever and endotoxin exposure. *Clin Allergy* 1978;8:511–516.

60. Parrott WF, Blyth W. Another causal factor in the production of humidifier fever. *J Soc Occup Med* 1980;30:63–68.
61. Edwards JH. Microbial and immunological investigations and remedial action after an outbreak of humidifier fever. *Br J Ind Med* 1980;37:55–62.
62. Edwards JH, Griffiths AJ, Mullins J. Protozoa as sources of antigen in "humidifier fever." *Nature (Lond)* 1976;264:438–439.
63. Ashton I, Axford AT, Bevan C, Cotes JE. Lung function of office workers exposed to humidifier fever antigen. *Br J Ind Med* 1981;38:34–37.
64. Cockroft A, Edwards J, Bevan C, et al. An investigation of operating theatre staff exposed to humidifier fever antigens. *Br J Ind Med* 1981;138:144–151.
65. Brundage JF, Scott RMcN, Lednar WM, Smith DW, Miller RN. Building-associated risk of febrile acute respiratory diseases in army trainees. *JAMA* 1988;259:2108–2112.
66. Richards AL, Hyams KC, Watts DM, Rozmajzl PJ, Woody JN, Merrell BR. Respiratory disease among military personnel in Saudi Arabia during Operation Desert Shield. *Am J Public Health* 1993;83:1326–1329.
67. Hoge CW, Reichler MR, Dominguez EA, et al. An epidemic of pneumococcal disease in an overcrowded, inadequately ventilated jail. *N Engl J Med* 1994;331:643–648.
68. Guberan E. Letter to the editor. *Br Med J* 1985;290:321.
69. Nardell EA, Keegan J, Cheney SA, Etkind SC. Airborne Infection. Theoretical limits of protection achievable by building ventilation. *Am Rev Respir Dis* 1991;144:302–306.
70. Yu VL. Could aspiration be the major mode of transmission for *Legionella? Am J Med* 1993;95:13–15.
71. Blatt SP, Parkinson MD, Pace E, et al. Nosocomial legionnaires' disease: aspiration as a primary mode of disease acquisition. *Am J Med* 1993;95:16–22.
72. Stout JE, Yu VL, Muraca P, Joly J, Troup N, Tompkins LS. Potable water as a cause of sporadic cases of community-acquired legionnaires' disease. *N Engl J Med* 1992;326:151–155.
73. von Reyn CF, Maslow JN, Barber TW, Falkinham JO, Arbeit RD. Persistent colonization of potable water as a source of Mycobacterium avium infection in patients with AIDS. *Lancet* 1994;343:1137–1141.
74. von Reyn CF, Arbeit RD, Tosteson ANA, et al., and the International MAC Study Group. The international epidemiology of disseminated Mycobacterium avium complex infection in AIDS. *AIDS* 1996;10:1025–1032.
75. Arnow PM, Sadigh M, Costas C, Weil D, Chudy R. Endemic and epidemic aspergillosis associated with in-hospital replication of Aspergillus organisms. *J Infect Dis* 1991;164:998–1002.
76. Fox BC, Chamberlin L, Kulich P, Rae EJ, Webster LR. Heavy contamination of operating room air by Penicillium species: identification of the source and attempts at decontamination. *Am J Infect Control* 1990;18:300–306.
77. Arnow PM, Andersen RL, Mainous PD, Smith EJ. Pulmonary aspergillosis during hospital renovation. *Am Rev Respir Dis* 1978;118:49–53.
78. Krasinski K, Holzman RS, Hanna B, Greco MA, Graff M, Bhogal M. Nosocomial fungal infection during hospital renovation. *Infect Control* 1985;6:278–282.
79. Opal SM, Asp AA, Cannady PB, Jr, Morse PL, Burton LJ, Hammer PG 2d. Efficacy of infection control measures during a nosocomial outbreak of disseminated aspergillosis associated with hospital construction. *J Infect Dis* 1986;153:634–637.

*Environmental and Occupational Medicine, Third Edition,* edited by William N. Rom.
Lippincott–Raven Publishers, Philadelphia © 1998.

CHAPTER 113

# Cigarette Smoking and Cancer

Stephen S. Hecht

Cigarette smoking is the leading cause of avoidable cancer death in the United States and worldwide. Nearly 170,000 cancer deaths were attributed to cigarette smoking in the United States in 1995 (1). The epidemiologic evidence linking smoking and cancer is beyond dispute. This chapter describes the established relationship of smoking to cancers of the lung and other organs. The chemistry of cigarette smoke has been thoroughly investigated and many carcinogenic agents have been characterized. The role of these carcinogens in causing cancers associated with smoking is also discussed, and many of the relevant mechanisms of tumor induction, which are now well understood, are described. Our understanding of mechanisms of tumor induction by cigarette smoke carcinogens forms the basis for new strategies to prevent cancer in addicted smokers.

## EPIDEMIOLOGY OF SMOKING AND CANCER

In 1950, Wynder and Graham (2) in the United States and Doll and Hill (3) in England published the first large-scale studies linking smoking and lung cancer. In 1964, the U.S. Surgeon General (4) concluded that cigarette smoking was causally related to lung cancer; this was reaffirmed in 1989 (5). In 1986, the International Agency for Research on Cancer (6) evaluated the relationship between smoking and cancer and concluded that cigarette smoking was the predominant cause of lung cancer worldwide. All three main types of lung cancer—squamous cell, small cell, and adenocarcinoma—are caused mainly by tobacco smoking. Major prospective studies have consistently demonstrated a dose-response between increasing numbers of cigarettes consumed daily and relative risk for lung cancer (1,5,6). These data, based on over 20 million person years of observation, are summarized in Table 1 (1).

The incidence of lung cancer also depends on the duration of smoking (1,5,6). The greatest risk is among those who start smoking in adolescence and continue throughout their lives. Cessation of smoking gradually decreases the risk of lung cancer. Data on the relative risk of developing lung cancer by time since stopping and total duration of smoking are summarized in Table 2 (1).

Patterns of lung cancer incidence in the United States follow patterns of cigarette consumption (1,5,6). In the early part of the 20th century, lung cancer was a rare disease. The first modern blended cigarette was introduced in the United States in 1913. Until then, most tobacco was consumed as chewing tobacco or smoked as cigars or pipes. The advent of machine-made cigarettes together with mass marketing led to a sharp increase in cigarette consumption during and after World War I. This increase continued until 1950. The increase in lung cancer in men and women can be seen to follow trends in their uptake of cigarette smoking, with an approximate 20-year delay. Lung cancer is now the leading cause of cancer death in both men and women in the United States. Recently, due to decreased smoking in the past three decades, there has been a downturn in lung cancer death rates among U.S. men (7).

While cigarette smoking has been definitively established as the major cause of lung cancer, a number of perplexing and challenging scientific issues remain to be solved (8). Since 1975, the incidence of adenocarcinoma has greatly increased in the United States. The ratio of adenocarcinoma to squamous cell carcinoma was 1:2.3

S. S. Hecht: University of Minnesota Cancer Center, Minneapolis, Minnesota 55455.

**TABLE 1.** *Lung cancer mortality ratios in men and women, by number of cigarettes smoked daily, major prospective mortality studies*

| | Men | | Women | |
|---|---|---|---|---|
| Study, population | Cigarettes/day | Ratio | Cigarettes/day | Ratio |
| ACS 25-state study, 1 million | Nonsmokers | 1.00 | Nonsmokers | 1.00 |
| | All smokers | 8.53 | All smokers | 3.58 |
| | 1–9 | 4.62 | 1–9 | 1.30 |
| | 10–19 | 8.62 | 10–19 | 2.40 |
| | 20–39 | 14.69 | 20–39 | 4.90 |
| | 40+ | 18.71 | 40+ | 7.50 |
| British doctors' study, 40,000 | Nonsmokers | 1.00 | Nonsmokers | 1.00 |
| | All smokers | 14.90 | All smokers | 5.00 |
| | 1–14 | 7.50 | 1–14 | 1.28 |
| | 15–24 | 14.90 | 15–24 | 6.41 |
| | 25+ | 25.40 | 25+ | 29.71 |
| U.S. veterans' study, 290,000 | Nonsmokers | 1.00 | | |
| | All smokers | 11.28 | | |
| | 1–9 | 3.89 | | |
| | 10–19 | 9.63 | | |
| | 21–39 | 16.70 | | |
| | 40+ | 23.70 | | |
| Japanese study, 270,000 | Nonsmokers | 1.00 | Nonsmokers | 1.00 |
| | All smokers | 3.76 | All smokers | 2.03 |
| | 1–9 | 2.06 | 1–9 | 2.25 |
| | 10–19 | 4.00 | 10–19 | 2.56 |
| | 20+ | 6.24 | 20+ | 4.47 |
| ACS 50-state study, 1.2 million | Nonsmokers | 1.00 | Nonsmokers | 1.00 |
| | All smokers | 22.36 | All smokers | 11.94 |
| | 1–20 | 18.80 | 1–10 | 5.50 |
| | 20+ | 26.90 | 11–19 | 11.20 |
| | | | 20 | 14.20 |
| | | | 21–30 | 20.40 |
| | | | 31+ | 22.00 |

From ref. 1.

**TABLE 2.** *Relative risk of developing lung cancer, by time, since stopping smoking and total duration of smoking behavior*

| | Duration of smoking habit | | | |
|---|---|---|---|---|
| Time since stopping smoking | 1–19 years | 20–39 years | 40–49 years | >50 years |
| Men | | | | |
| 0 | 1.0[a] | 2.2 | 2.8 | 3.0 |
| 1–4 | 1.1 | 2.1 | 3.3 | 3.8 |
| 5–9 | 0.4 | 1.5 | 2.2 | 2.8 |
| 10+ | 0.3 | 1.0 | 1.6 | 2.7 |
| Women | | | | |
| 0 | 1.0[b] | 2.1 | 2.7 | 5.2 |
| 1–4 | 1.0 | 2.3 | 2.1 | 7.1 |
| 5–9 | 0.4 | 2.0 | 1.1 | 1.7 |
| 10+ | 0.4 | 0.8 | 2.3 | |

[a]Baseline category; risk for people who had never smoked relative to that for current smokers who had smoked for 1 to 19 years was 0.3.

[b]Baseline category; risk for people who had never smoked relative to that for current smokers who had smoked for 1 to 19 years was 0.6.

From ref. 1.

among white males in 1969 to 1971, whereas it was 1:1.4 in 1984 to 1986. This changing histology of cigarette smoke–induced lung cancer is not well understood. Adenocarcinoma is particularly prominent in women and in nonsmokers exposed to environmental tobacco smoke. There are important geographic and ethnic differences in lung cancer that require investigation. Lung cancer incidence in Japan is considerably lower than would be expected by comparison to U.S. rates in spite of a dramatic increase in smoking. Diet may be one factor that enhances risk in the United States; laboratory studies have shown that a high-fat diet similar to that consumed in the United States can enhance lung cancer induction by constituents of tobacco smoke. In the United States, lung cancer rates among African-Americans are substantially higher than among Caucasians in spite of the fact that African-Americans smoke less. Some evidence suggests that ethnic differences in the metabolism of tobacco smoke carcinogens may be involved in these differences. Recent studies have also indicated that there are gender differences in susceptibility to cigarette smoke, with women apparently being at greater risk than men, for a given level of cigarette consumption. It has been proposed that hormonal effects may mediate these differences.

In addition to its firmly established and widely recognized role as a major cause of lung cancer, cigarette smoking is also an important cause of bladder cancer, cancer of the renal pelvis, oral cancer, oropharyngeal cancer, hypopharyngeal cancer, laryngeal cancer, esophageal cancer, and pancreatic cancer (6). Other cancers that may be caused by smoking include renal adenocarcinoma, cancer of the cervix, myeloid leukemia, and stomach cancer. Relative risks for major smoking-related cancers are summarized in Table 3 (1,6).

**TABLE 3.** *Relative risks for major smoking-related cancer sites among male and female smokers: ACS 50-state study, 4-year follow-up*

| Cancer site | Current smokers | Former smokers |
|---|---|---|
| Males | | |
| Lung | 22.36 | 9.36 |
| Oral | 27.48 | 8.80 |
| Esophagus | 7.60 | 5.83 |
| Larynx | 10.48 | 5.24 |
| Bladder | 2.86 | 1.90 |
| Pancreas | 2.14 | 1.12 |
| Kidney | 2.95 | 1.95 |
| Females | | |
| Lung | 11.94 | 4.69 |
| Oral | 5.59 | 2.88 |
| Esophagus | 10.25 | 3.16 |
| Larynx | 17.78 | 11.88 |
| Bladder | 2.58 | 1.85 |
| Pancreas | 2.33 | 1.78 |
| Kidney | 1.41 | 1.16 |
| Cervix | 2.14 | 1.94 |

From ref. 1.

According to a major evaluation of causes of cancer death in the United States in 1981, smoking was responsible for 30% of all cancer death (9). A similar evaluation carried out in 1995 came to essentially the same conclusion (1). The 1995 data are summarized in Table 4. These data demonstrate the enormous impact of smoking on death rates from cancers of various sites.

Establishing whether there exists cause and effect between environmental tobacco smoke and lung cancer has been more difficult, given the limitations of conventional epidemiologic studies (10,11). Environmental tobacco smoke is mainly a composite of the smoke generated between puffs, called sidestream smoke, and a minor portion of mainstream smoke constituents that are exhaled by a smoker. Although, as discussed below, the levels of certain carcinogens in environmental tobacco smoke are greater than in mainstream smoke per gram of tobacco burned, environmental tobacco smoke is diluted by air. Therefore, the carcinogen dose received by a nonsmoker exposed to environmental tobacco smoke may be only 1%

**TABLE 4.** *1995 U.S. cancer deaths caused by cigarette smoking*

| Site and ICD disease category | 1995 cancer deaths expected | Smoking attributable risk, % | Estimated deaths due to smoking |
|---|---|---|---|
| Males | | | |
| Oral, 140–149 | 5,480 | 90.6 | 4,965 |
| Esophagus, 150 | 8,200 | 76.6 | 6,282 |
| Pancreas, 157 | 13,200 | 25.9 | 3,419 |
| Larynx, 161 | 3,200 | 79.6 | 2,547 |
| Lung, 162 | 95,400 | 89.4 | 85,288 |
| Bladder, 188 | 7,500 | 43.8 | 3,285 |
| Kidney, 189 | 7,100 | 45.1 | 3,202 |
| Total cancer deaths expected | 289,000 | | 108,988 |
| Females | | | |
| Oral, 140–149 | 2,890 | 58.5 | 1,691 |
| Esophagus, 150 | 2,700 | 71.5 | 1,931 |
| Pancreas, 157 | 13,800 | 31.0 | 4,278 |
| Larynx, 161 | 890 | 85.5 | 761 |
| Lung, 162 | 62,000 | 76.1 | 47,182 |
| Cervix, 180 | 4,800 | 30.6 | 1,469 |
| Bladder, 188 | 3,700 | 34.2 | 1,265 |
| Kidney, 189 | 4,600 | 10.7 | 492 |
| Total cancer deaths expected | 258,000 | | 59,069 |
| Total male and female cancer deaths expected in 1995 | | | 547,000 |
| Total excess deaths due to cigarette smoking | | | 168,057 |
| Percent of cancer deaths due to cigarette smoking in 1995 | | | 30.7 |

From ref. 1.

of machine-made cigarettes of that received by an active smoker. Thus, the risk for cancer will be less. Conventional epidemiologic studies of environmental tobacco smoke and lung cancer have typically found relative risks between 1 and 2. The National Research Council, the U.S. Surgeon General, and the Environmental Protection Agency, among others, have concluded that environmental tobacco smoke is a cause of lung cancer, and a recent study has provided further evidence supporting this conclusion (10–13). However, further epidemiologic studies using appropriate biomarkers of environmental smoke uptake need to be performed to confirm its role in lung cancer induction (14).

In spite of the well-known adverse effects of cigarette smoking, 25% (46 million people) of the U.S. adult population were smokers in 1993 (15). The prevalence of cigarette smoking among adults in the United States decreased 40% from 1965 to 1990 (from 42.4% to 25.5%) (15). Smoking prevalence among different birth cohorts of men and women in the United States has been analyzed in detail and can be seen to result from uptake of the habit in early adulthood, mainly in response to targeted marketing (1). Smoking is more prevalent in lower socioeconomic strata and is generally inversely proportional to level of education (15). There are hundreds of millions of smokers worldwide, and smoking is increasing in many countries. Many smokers are addicted to nicotine and do not stop, even after attending smoking-cessation programs. Thus, cigarette smoking remains a major international health hazard, not only with respect to lung cancer but for several other cancer types and causes of mortality. Based on studies in Great Britain, it has been estimated that about half of all regular cigarette smokers will eventually be killed by their habit (16).

## CHEMISTRY OF TOBACCO SMOKE

When cigarette tobacco is burned, mainstream smoke and sidestream smoke are generated. Mainstream smoke is the material drawn from the mouth end of a cigarette during puffing. Sidestream smoke is the material released into the air from the burning tip of the cigarette plus the material that diffuses through the paper. The material emitted from the mouth end of the cigarette between puffs is sometimes also considered as sidestream smoke (17).

The mainstream smoke emerging from the cigarette is an aerosol containing about $1 \times 10^{10}$ particles per milliliter, ranging in diameter from 0.1 to 1.0 μm (mean diameter 0.2 μm) (6,18). For chemical analysis, the smoke is arbitrarily separated into a vapor phase and a particulate phase, based on passage through a glass-fiber filter pad called a Cambridge filter. This retains 99.7% of all particles with diameters of 0.1 mm and above. Individual smoke components of which more than 50% appear in the vapor phase of fresh mainstream smoke are considered volatile smoke components, while all others are considered particulate phase components. Standardized machine smoking conditions have been used for measurement of cigarette smoke constituents. These conditions are also arbitrary, and it is recognized that each smoker may puff in ways that are widely different from the standardized conditions, thereby changing the yield of individual smoke constituents. Tables 5 and 6 list major types of components identified in the vapor phase and particulate phase of cigarette smoke (17,18). These tables summarize representative data but are not complete, as cigarette smoke is known to contain approximately 4,000 identified compounds. Many of the components are present in higher concentration in sidestream smoke than in mainstream smoke; this is especially true of nitrogen-containing compounds. However, a person's exposure to sidestream smoke is generally far less than to mainstream smoke because of dilution with room air.

Carcinogens in tobacco and tobacco smoke are listed in Table 7, along with the evaluations of the International Agency for Research on Cancer (IARC) of their carcinogenicity in laboratory animals and humans (18). This list focuses on those compounds that have been evaluated by the IARC as carcinogenic in animals. However, it should be noted that there are many related compounds that either have not been evaluated or may have some carcinogenic activity. These include various other polycyclic aromatic hydrocarbon (PAH) isomers and alkylated PAH as well as other nitrosamines, aza-arenes, and aromatic amines. Nevertheless, the 60 compounds listed in Table 7 represent the important carcinogens in tobacco and cigarette smoke. Structures of some of these carcinogens are illustrated in Fig. 1.

## TUMOR INDUCTION BY CIGARETTE SMOKE AND ITS CONDENSATE IN LABORATORY ANIMALS

Experimental studies evaluating the ability of cigarette smoke and its condensate to cause cancer in laboratory animals have been summarized by the IARC and in an earlier publication (6,19). These studies have collectively demonstrated "that there is sufficient evidence that inhalation of tobacco smoke as well as topical application of tobacco smoke condensate cause cancer in experimental animals" (6).

The Syrian golden hamster has been the model of choice for inhalation studies of cigarette smoke because it has a low background incidence of spontaneous pulmonary tumors and little interfering respiratory infection (6). Inhalation of cigarette smoke has repeatedly caused carcinomas in the larynx of hamsters and this model system has been widely applied. It is the most reliable model for induction of tumors by inhalation of cigarette smoke. Studies in mice, rats, and dogs have been less frequent.

There are a number of operational problems inherent in inhalation studies of cigarette smoke (6). The smoke must be delivered in a standardized fashion and this has been

**TABLE 5.** *Major constituents of the vapor phase of nonfilter cigarettes*

| Compound[a] | Mainstream smoke (MS) concentration/cigarette (% of total effluent) | SS/MS[b] ratio |
|---|---|---|
| Nitrogen | 280–320 mg (56–64%) | |
| Oxygen | 50–70 mg (11–14%) | |
| Carbon dioxide | 45–65 mg (9–13%) | 8–11 |
| Carbon monoxide | 14–23 mg (2.8–4.6%) | 2.5–4.7 |
| Water | 7–12 mg (1.4–2.4%) | |
| Argon | 5 mg (1.0) | |
| Hydrogen | 0.5–1.0 mg | |
| Ammonia | 10–130 μg | 40–170 |
| Nitrogen oxides [$NO_x$] | 100–600 μg | 4–10 |
| Hydrogen cyanide | 400–500 μg | 0.1–0.25 |
| Hydrogen sulfide | 20–90 μg | |
| Methane | 1.0–2.0 mg | |
| Other volatile alkanes (20) | 1.0–1.6mg[c] | |
| Volatile alkenes (16) | 0.4–0.5 mg | |
| Isoprene | 0.2–0.4 mg | |
| Butadiene | 25–40 μg | |
| Acetylene | 20–35 μg | |
| Benzene | 12–50 μg | 5–10 |
| Toluene | 20–60 μg | 5.6–8.3 |
| Styrene | 10 μg | |
| Other volatile aromatic hydrocarbons (29) | 15–30 μg | |
| Formic acid | 200–600 μg | 1.4–1.6 |
| Acetic acid | 300–1,700 μg | 1.9–3.6 |
| Propionic acid | 100–300μg | |
| Methyl formate | 20–30 μg | |
| Other volatile acids (6) | 5–10 μg[c] | |
| Formaldehyde | 20–100 μg | 0.1–50 |
| Acetaldehyde | 400–1,400 μg | |
| Acrolein | 60–140 μg | 8–15 |
| Other volatile aldehydes (6) | 80–140 μg | |
| Acetone | 100–650 μg | 2–5 |
| Other volatile ketones (3) | 50–100 μg | |
| Methanol | 80–180 μg | |
| Other volatile alcohols (7) | 10–30 μg[c] | |
| Acetonitrile | 100–150μg | |
| Other volatile nitriles (10) | 50–80μg[c] | |
| Furan | 20–40 μg | |
| Other volatile furans (4) | 45–125 μg[c] | |
| Pyridine | 20–200 μg | 6.5–20 |
| Picolines (3) | 15–80 μg | 3–13 |
| 3-Vinylpyridine | 10–30 μg | 20–40 |
| Other volatile pyridines (25) | 20–50 μg[c] | |
| Pyrrole | 0.1–10 μg | |
| Pyrrolidine | 10–18 μg | |
| *N*-Methylpyrrolidine | 2.0–3.0 μg | |
| Volatile pyrazines (18) | 3.0–8.0 μg | |
| Methylamine | 4–10 μg | 4.2–6.4 |
| Other aliphatic amines (32) | 3–10 μg | |

[a]Numbers in parentheses represent the individual compounds identified in a given group.
[b]Sidestream smoke/mainstream smoke ratio.
[c]Estimate.
Adapted from refs. 17,18.

**TABLE 6.** *Major constituents of the particulate matter of nonfilter cigarettes*

| Compound[a] | Mainstream smoke (MS) μg/cigarette | SS/MS[b] ratio |
|---|---|---|
| Nicotine | 1,000–3,000 | 2.6–3.3 |
| Nornicotine | 50–150 | |
| Anatabine | 5–15 | <0.1–0.5 |
| Anabasine | 5–12 | |
| Other tobacco alkaloids (17) | n.a. | |
| Bipyridyls (4) | 10–30 | |
| *n*-Hentriacontaine [$n$-$C_{31}H_{64}$] | 100 | |
| Total nonvolatile hydrocarbons (45)[b] | 300–400[c] | |
| Naphthalene | 2–4 | |
| Naphthalenes (23) | 3–6[c] | |
| Phenanthrenes (7) | 0.2–0.4[c] | |
| Anthracenes (5) | 0.05–0.1[c] | |
| Fluorenes (7) | 0.6–1.0[c] | |
| Pyrenes (6) | 0.3–0.5[c] | |
| Fluoranthenes (5) | 0.3–0.45[c] | |
| Carcinogenic polynuclear aromatic hydrocarbons (11)[a] | 0.1–0.25 | 2–4 |
| Phenol | 80–160 | 1.6–3.0 |
| Other phenols (45)[c] | 60–180[c] | |
| Catechol | 200–400 | 0.6–0.9 |
| Other catechols (4) | 100–200[c] | |
| Other dihydroxybenzenes (10) | 200–400[c] | |
| Scopoletin | 15–30 | |
| Other polyphenols (8)[c] | n.a. | |
| Cyclotenes (10)[c] | 40–70[c] | |
| Quinones (7) | 0.5 | |
| Solanesol | 600–1,000 | |
| Neophytadienes (4) | 200–350 | |
| Limonene | 30–601 | |
| Other terpenes (200–250)[c] | | |
| Palmitic acid | 100–150 | |
| Stearic acid | 50–75 | |
| Oleic acid | 40–110 | |
| Linoleic acid | 60–150 | |
| Linolenic acid | 150–250 | |
| Lactic acid | 60–80 | |
| Indole | 10–15 | |
| Skatole | 12–16 | |
| Other indoles (13) | n.a. | |
| Quinolines (7) | 2–4 | 8–11 |
| Other aza-arenes (55) | n.a. | |
| Benzofurans (4) | 200–300 | |
| Other *O*-heterocyclic compounds (42) | n.a. | |
| Stigmasterol | 40–70 | |
| Sitosterol | 30–40 | |
| Campesterol | 20–30 | |
| Cholesterol | 10–20 | |
| Aniline | 0.36 | 30 |
| Toluidines | 0.23 | 19 |
| Other aromatic amines (12) | 0.25 | 30 |
| Tobacco-specific nitrosamines (4) | 0.34–2.7 | 0.5–4 |
| Glycerol | 120 | |

[a]Numbers in parentheses represent individual compounds identified in a given group.
[b]Sidestream smoke/mainstream smoke ratio.
[c]Estimate.
Adapted from refs. 17,18.

**TABLE 7.** *Carcinogens in tobacco and cigarette smoke*

| Compound | In processed tobacco (per gram) | In mainstream smoke (per cigarette) | IARC evaluation: evidence of carcinogenicity | |
|---|---|---|---|---|
| | | | In laboratory animals | In humans |
| PAH | | | | |
| Benz[*a*]anthracene | | 20–70 ng | Sufficient | |
| Benzo[*b*]fluoranthene | | 4–22 ng | Sufficient | |
| Benzo[*j*]fluoranthene | | 6–21 ng | Sufficient | |
| Benzo[*k*]fluoranthene | | 6–12 ng | Sufficient | |
| Benzo[*a*]pyrene | 0.1–90 ng | 20–40 ng | Sufficient | Probable |
| Dibenz[*a,h*]anthracene | | 4 ng | Sufficient | |
| Dibenzo[*a,i*]pyrene | | 1.7–3.2 ng | Sufficient | |
| Dibenzo[*a,l*]pyrene | | Present | Sufficient | |
| Indeno[1,2,3-*cd*]pyrene | | 4–20 ng | Sufficient | |
| 5-Methylchrysene | | 0.6 ng | Sufficient | |
| Aza-arenes | | | | |
| Quinoline | | 1–2 μg | | |
| Dibenz[*a,h*]acridine | | 0.1 ng | Sufficient | |
| Dibenz[*a,j*]acridine | | 3–10 ng | Sufficient | |
| 7H-dibenzo[*c,g*]carbazole | | 0.7 ng | Sufficient | |
| Nitrosamines | | | | |
| *N*-Nitrosodimethylamine | ND–215 ng | 0.1–180 ng | Sufficient | |
| *N*-Nitrosoethylmethylamine | | 3–13 ng | Sufficient | |
| *N*-Nitrosodiethylamine | | ND–25 ng | Sufficient | |
| *N*-Nitrosopyrrolidine | 5–50 ng | 3–60 ng | Sufficient | |
| *N*-Nitrosodiethanolamine | 50–3,000 ng | ND–68 ng | Sufficient | |
| *N*-Nitrososarcosine | 20–120 ng | | Sufficient | |
| *N′*-Nitrosonornicotine (NNN) | 0.3–89 μg | 0.12–3.7 μg | Sufficient | |
| 4-(Methylnitrosamino)-1-(3-pyridyl)-1-butanone (NNK) | 0.2–7 μg | 0.08–0.77 μg | Sufficient | |
| *N′*-Nitrosoanabasine | 0.01–1.9 μg | 0.14–4.6 μg | Limited | |
| *N*-Nitrosomorpholine | ND–690 ng | | Sufficient | |
| Aromatic amines | | | | |
| 2-Toluidine | | 30–200 ng | Sufficient | Inadequate |
| 2-Naphthylamine | | 1–22 ng | Sufficient | Sufficient |
| 4-Aminobiphenyl | | 2–5 ng | Sufficient | Sufficient |
| Heterocyclic aromatic amines[a] | | | | |
| AαC | | 25–260 ng | Sufficient | |
| MeAαC | | 2–37 ng | Sufficient | |
| IQ | | 0.26 ng | Sufficient | Probable |
| Trp-P-1 | | 0.29–0.48 ng | Sufficient | |
| Trp-P-2 | | 0.82–1.1 ng | Sufficient | |
| Glu-P-1 | | 0.37–0.89 ng | Sufficient | |
| Glu-P-2 | | 0.25–0.88 ng | Sufficient | |
| PhIP | | 11–23 ng | Sufficient | Possible |
| Aldehydes | | | | |
| Formaldehyde | 1.6–7.4 μg | 70–100 μg | Sufficient | Limited |
| Acetaldehyde | 1.4–7.4 μg | 18–1,400 μg | Sufficient | Inadequate |
| Miscellaneous organic compounds | | | | |
| 1,3-Butadiene | | 20–75 μg | Sufficient | Probable |
| Isoprene | | 450–1,000 μg | Sufficient | Possible |
| Benzene | | 12–70 μg | Sufficient | Sufficient |
| Styrene | | 10 μg | Limited | Possible |
| Vinyl chloride | | 1–16 ng | Sufficient | Sufficient |
| DDT[b] | 20–13,400 ng | 800–1,200 ng | Sufficient | |
| DDT[b] | 7–960 ng | 200–370 ng | Sufficient | |
| Acrylonitrile | | 3.2–15 μg | Sufficient | Limited |
| Acrylamide | | Present | Sufficient | Probable |
| 1,1-Dimethylhydrazine | 60–147 μg | | Sufficient | |
| 2-Nitropropane | | 0.73–1.21 μg | Sufficient | |
| Ethyl carbamate | 310–375 ng | 20–38 ng | Sufficient | |
| Ethylene oxide | | 7 μg | Sufficient | Limited |
| Di(2–ethylhexyl) phthalate | Present | 20 μg | Sufficient | |
| Furan | | 18–30 μg | Sufficient | Inadequate |

*Continued on next page*

**TABLE 7.** *Continued*

| Compound | In processed tobacco (per gram) | In mainstream smoke (per cigarette) | IARC evaluation: evidence of carcinogenicity: In laboratory animals | IARC evaluation: evidence of carcinogenicity: In humans |
|---|---|---|---|---|
| Miscellaneous organic compounds | | | | |
| Benzo[*b*]furan | | Present | Sufficient | Inadequate |
| Inorganic compounds | | | | |
| Hydrazine | 14–51 ng | 24–43 ng | Sufficient | Inadequate |
| Arsenic | 500–900 ng | 40–120 ng | Inadequate | Sufficient |
| Nickel | 2,000–6,000 ng | 0–600 ng | Sufficient | Limited |
| Chromium | 1,000–2,000 ng | 4–70 ng | Sufficient | Sufficient |
| Cadmium | 1,300–1,600 ng | 41–62 ng | Sufficient | Limited |
| Lead | 8–10 μg | 35–85 ng | Sufficient | Inadequate |
| Polonium–210 | 0.2–1.2 pCi | 0.03–1.0 pCi | Sufficient | Sufficient |

[a]Abbreviations for heterocyclic amines: AαC, 2-amino-9H-pyrido(2,3-*b*)indole; MeAαC, 2-amino-3-methyl-9H-pyrido(2,3-*b*)indole; IQ, 2-amino-3-methylimidazo(4,5-*b*)quinoline; Trp-P-1, 3-amino-1,4-dimethyl-5H-pyrido(4,3-*b*)indole; Trp-P-2, 3-amino-1-methyl-5H-pyrido-(4,3-*b*)indole; Glu-P-1, 2-amino-6-methyl(1,2-*a:3′,2′-d*)imidazole; Glu-P-2, 2-aminodipyrido-(1,2- *a:3′,2′-d*)imidazole; PhIP, 2-amino-1-methyl-6-phenylimidazo(4,5-*b*)pyridine.

[b]During the last decade, DDT and DDE have been drastically reduced in U.S. cigarette tobacco (<60 ng and <13 ng).

ND, not detected; PAH, polycyclic aromatic hydrocarbons.

Updated by D. Hoffmann from ref. 18.

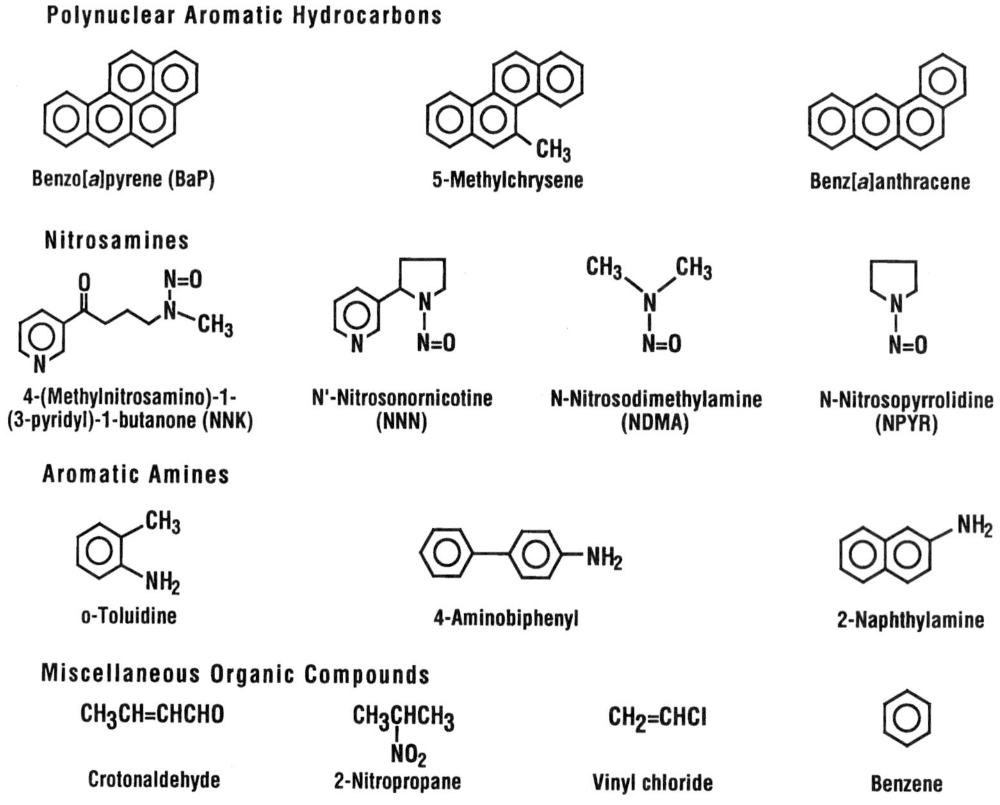


**FIG. 1.** Structures of representative carcinogens in tobacco smoke.

accomplished in different ways. Both whole-body exposure and nose-only exposure designs have been used. Generally, a 2-second puff from a burning cigarette is diluted with air and forced into the chamber. Animals undergo avoidance reactions and do not inhale the smoke the way humans do. Thus, the dose to the lung is less than in humans, and this partially explains the occurrence of larynx tumors rather than lung tumors in hamsters. Unlike humans, rodents are obligatory nose breathers. Their nasal passages are more complex than those of humans, thereby affecting particle deposition in the respiratory tract. Tobacco smoke is irritating and toxic, creating further problems in inhalation studies with rodents.

Inhalation studies have been summarized (6). As stated above, various experiments reproducibly demonstrated that cigarette smoke, especially its particulate phase, caused laryngeal carcinomas in hamsters. Some experiments with mice resulted in low incidences of lung tumors. Respiratory tract tumors were produced in one long-term exposure of rats to cigarette smoke. Studies in rabbits and dogs were equivocal. Treatment-related tumors other than those of the respiratory tract have not been consistently observed. The gaseous phase of cigarette smoke has shown no consistent respiratory carcinogenicity.

Experiments in which cigarette smoke condensate (CSC) has been tested for tumor induction have been summarized (6,19). CSC is produced by passing smoke through cold traps and recovering the material in the traps by washing with a volatile solvent that is then evaporated. Some volatile and semivolatile constituents may be lost during this process. CSC is roughly equivalent to cigarette total particulate matter (TPM), the material collected on a Cambridge filter that has had smoke drawn through it. The word *tar,* which is often used in official reports on cigarette brands, is equivalent to TPM but without nicotine and water.

Cigarette smoke condensate generation and collection techniques have been standardized (6). The most widely used test system for carcinogenicity of CSC is mouse skin. Consistently, CSC induces benign and malignant skin tumors in mice. This test system has been widely used to evaluate the carcinogenic activities of cigarettes of different designs and to investigate mechanisms of carcinogenesis by cigarette smoke. For example, mouse skin studies led to the identification of carcinogenic PAH in cigarette smoke as well as the demonstration that CSC has cocarcinogenic and tumor-promoting activity (20). The overall carcinogenic effect of CSC on mouse skin appears to depend on the composite interaction of the tumor initiators such as PAH, tumor promoters, and cocarcinogens. Tumors are not induced by the PAH alone, using doses equivalent to their concentrations in CSC (20).

There are drawbacks to the mouse skin assay. Since CSC lacks volatile and semivolatile components, contributions of these compounds to total activity is lost. Furthermore, mouse skin is insensitive to certain carcinogens in tobacco smoke, such as nitrosamines, which show high organoselectivities for tissues such as lung. Mouse skin, on the other hand, is a relatively sensitive tumor induction site for PAH. Mouse skin studies also ignore the complexity of the respiratory system, where different cell types are known to respond differently to various carcinogens in tobacco smoke.

Cigarette smoke condensate has also been tested by direct injection into the rodent lung, generally in a lipid vehicle. This caused squamous cell carcinomas of the lung in rats. Tumors were not observed in rats treated with the vehicle (6).

## ASSOCIATION OF CIGARETTE SMOKE CARCINOGENS WITH LUNG CANCER IN SMOKERS

The role of specific carcinogens of tobacco smoke in human cancers can be assessed by considering the amounts of the carcinogens in tobacco products, their target tissues and carcinogenic potency in laboratory animals, and biochemical evidence that humans respond in similar ways to laboratory animals. Likely causative agents for lung cancer in smokers are summarized in Table 8.

**TABLE 8.** *Smoking and lung cancer: causative agents*

| Carcinogens | Modifying agents |
|---|---|
| Strong evidence[a] | |
| NNK | Cocarcinogens (catechols) |
| PAH (benzo[*a*]pyrene, benzo[*b,j,* and *k*]fluoranthenes, 5-methylchrysene, dibenz[*a,h*]anthracene, indeno[1,2,3-*cd*]pyrene) | Tumor promoters (phenols and others)<br>Toxic aldehydes (acrolein)<br>Diet |
| Weak evidence | |
| Oxidative damage and free radicals | |
| $^{210}$Po, Cr, Cd, Ni | |
| Aldehydes | |

[a]Criteria: Animal carcinogenicity, presence in tobacco smoke, biochemical studies in animal and human lung.
Modified from ref. 18.

PAHs such as benzo[*a*]pyrene (BaP), which are formed by the incomplete combustion of tobacco during smoking, are well recognized carcinogens that have been shown to induce tumors of the lung in laboratory animals exposed by inhalation, instillation in the trachea, or implantation in the lung (21–23). Squamous cell carcinomas of the lung are frequently induced by a carcinogenic PAH such as BaP. Considering the amounts of these compounds in cigarette smoke and their carcinogenic potency, one can plausibly argue that they are important in lung cancer induction (18). This argument is bolstered by biochemical studies that have demonstrated that human lung tissue can metabolize PAH by pathways that lead to covalent modification of DNA (adduct formation) and by the detection of the relevant DNA adducts in lung tissue of smokers, as discussed below. Moreover, a recent study indicated that an ultimate carcinogen of BaP can cause mutational changes in the *p53* gene similar to those observed in lung tumors from smokers (24).

4-(Methylnitrosamino)-1-(3-pyridyl) -1-butanone (NNK), a nitrosamine formed from the major tobacco constituent nicotine during the processing of tobacco and during smoking, is a powerful and organ-selective lung carcinogen in laboratory animals (25). NNK is one of a family of nicotine-derived nitrosamines that are collectively called tobacco-specific nitrosamines. Adenocarcinoma of the lung is the main type of lung cancer induced by NNK. The total amount of NNK required to produce lung cancer in rats is similar to the total amount of this compound to which a smoker would be exposed in a lifetime of smoking (26,27). These data support the role of NNK in the induction of human lung cancer, particularly adenocarcinoma. Moreover, human lung tissue metabolically activates NNK in the same way as rodent tissue, although there are quantitative differences (28). DNA adducts specific to NNK and the related nitrosamine, *N′*-nitrosonornicotine (NNN), have been detected in smokers' lungs, and metabolites of NNK are present in smokers' urine (27,29). As stated earlier, the ratio of adenocarcinoma to squamous cell carcinoma in smokers has been increasing in the past three decades. Changes in the cigarette have been such that the levels of NNK have been increasing over this time period while levels of BaP have been decreasing (8,30). The increase in human exposure to NNK, which induces adenocarcinoma, and the decrease in exposure to BaP, which induces squamous cell carcinoma, may account in part for the increase in adenocarcinoma of the lung being observed in smokers.

Table 8 lists some other tobacco smoke constituents that could be involved in lung cancer induction; the evidence suggesting a role for these compounds is weaker than that discussed above for PAH and NNK.

Polonium-210 is present in cigarette mainstream smoke and is a strong pulmonary carcinogen, which induces tumors of the lung upon inhalation in rats or upon intratracheal instillation in Syrian golden hamsters (18). The significance of polonium-210 in tobacco-induced lung cancer has been questioned based on comparisons of doses experienced by smokers versus those in miners. It has been estimated that about 1% of the lung cancer risk associated with cigarette smoking could be ascribed to polonium-210.

Chromium, cadmium, and nickel are all present in cigarette smoke (18). Calcium chromate is carcinogenic in rats, inducing lung tumors after instillation. Cadmium chloride aerosols produce adenocarcinoma and squamous cell carcinoma in rats. Nickel subsulfide yields lung cancer in rats upon inhalation. Since levels of exposure to chromium, cadmium, and nickel compounds in cigarette smoke may be comparable to those of some PAH, these metals may play some role in lung cancer induction.

Inhalation studies of formaldehyde and acetaldehyde have demonstrated that they are respiratory carcinogens in the rat, inducing mainly nasal cavity tumors (18). There may be a direct effect of these compounds on the lung upon inhalation in tobacco smoke. Although they are weak respiratory carcinogens, levels of formaldehyde and acetaldehyde in cigarette smoke are at least 1,000 times greater than those of PAH and nitrosamines.

Cigarette smoke contains some stable free radicals and is known to induce oxidative damage (18,31). Products resulting from oxidative damage to both lipids and DNA have been detected in smokers, and their levels are higher than in nonsmokers (32,33). Although the direct role of such products in carcinogenesis is unclear, it is worth noting that 8-oxoguanine, a DNA adduct detected at elevated levels in smokers, has miscoding properties associated with the cancer-induction process as discussed below.

## ASSOCIATION OF CIGARETTE SMOKE CARCINOGENS WITH OTHER CANCERS IN SMOKERS

PAHs and the tobacco-specific nitrosamines NNK and NNN are the most likely causative agents for oral cavity cancer in smokers, although the evidence is not as strong as for the role of PAH and NNK in lung cancer induction (18). Certain PAHs such as 7,12-dimethylbenz[*a*]-anthracene (DMBA) can reproducibly induce oral tumors in Syrian golden hamsters (34). DMBA is not a constituent of tobacco smoke but other PAHs may have similar activity, although BaP is not a potent oral carcinogen. A mixture of NNN and NNK induced oral tumors in rats, and other nitrosamines may also have similar activity (35). DNA adducts have been detected in exfoliated oral mucosal cells of smokers and these may result partially from PAH (36). There is a strong synergy between cigarette smoking and alcohol consumption for causation of oral cavity and esophageal cancer (37). While the mechanism of this synergistic effect has not been thoroughly delineated, available evidence indicates that one major factor is competitive inhibition by ethanol of hepatic carcinogen clearance, resulting in greater delivery of carcinogen to extrahepatic tissues. A second factor that may be important is induction of carcinogen activating enzymes by ethanol.

Nitrosamines are the only well-characterized esophageal carcinogens in cigarette smoke (18). The rat esophagus is a common major target tissue for cancer induction by several nitrosamines, notably NNN and *N*-nitrosodiethylamine among those present in smoke. Considering the quantities of these carcinogens present in tobacco smoke as well as their carcinogenic potencies, they are the most likely causative agents for esophageal cancer in smokers. The enhancement of nitrosamine-induced esophageal carcinogenesis by ethanol has been demonstrated in rats, and esophageal DNA adducts are also increased by ethanol administration in the monkey (38–41).

The aromatic amines 4-aminobiphenyl and 2-naphthylamine are human bladder carcinogens (42). These compounds can also induce bladder cancer in laboratory animals, and they are the only tobacco smoke constituents known to do so (18). Hemoglobin adducts of aromatic amines have been detected in smokers' blood, and adduct levels may be predictive of cancer risk (43). The presence of aromatic amine DNA adducts in exfoliated urinary bladder cells and biopsy tissues of smokers has been demonstrated (44). Epidemiologic studies have noted a relationship between carcinogen exposure, inefficient detoxification, and higher risk for bladder cancer (45). Collectively, these data provide strong evidence for the role of aromatic amines in bladder cancer induction in smokers.

NNK and its major metabolite NNAL are the only known pancreatic carcinogens to which smokers are exposed (46). Therefore, they may play some role in the induction of pancreatic cancer in humans. Benzene causes leukemia in humans; its relatively high concentrations in cigarette smoke indicate that it may be a principal causative agent for leukemia in smokers (42).

## CIGARETTE SMOKE TUMOR PROMOTERS AND COCARCINOGENS

Tumor promoters are substances that enhance tumorigenicity when applied after a carcinogen. Cocarcinogens enhance tumorigenicity when applied simultaneously with a carcinogen. In general, tumor promoters and cocarcinogens do not possess tumorigenic activity themselves. The tumor-promoting activity of cigarette smoke and CSC has been clearly demonstrated (6,19,20). Inhalation studies have shown that animals treated with a single dose of a PAH such as BaP or DMBA by intratracheal administration, followed by inhalation of cigarette smoke, have higher incidences of respiratory tumors than animals treated with the PAH alone or cigarette smoke alone (6). Experiments with CSC have shown that it is a tumor promoter on mouse skin, in animals treated with an initiating dose of a PAH (19,20). Fractionation studies demonstrated that the majority of the tumor-promoting activity resides in the weakly acidic fraction (20). Further studies localized this activity to subfractions of the weakly acidic fraction containing phenolic compounds, but the structure of the tumor promoter(s) has not been determined (47).

Cigarette smoke condensate also has considerable cocarcinogenic activity, particularly in its weakly acidic fraction (48). The major cocarcinogen in cigarette smoke is catechol (1,2-dihydroxybenzene), which is strongly cocarcinogenic with BaP (48,49). Other cocarcinogens present in tobacco smoke include methylcatechols, pyrogallol, decane, undecane, pyrene, benzo[*e*]pyrene, and fluoranthene (19,20,49).

## MECHANISMS OF TUMOR INDUCTION BY CIGARETTE SMOKE CARCINOGENS

The carcinogens of cigarette smoke form the link between nicotine addiction and cancer. This is illustrated for lung cancer in Fig. 2. Nicotine addiction is the reason people continue to smoke (50). Each cigarette contains the carcinogens discussed above; for lung cancer, PAH and NNK are the most important. These compounds require metabolic activation to exert their carcinogenic effects. Detoxification pathways are protective. The balance between metabolic activation and detoxification in part determines risk for cancer. DNA adducts are formed as a result of the metabolic activation process. If these persist unrepaired in critical regions of genes, they can cause permanent deleterious changes in oncogenes, tumor suppressor genes, and other important cellular growth control systems such as Ki-*ras*, *p53*, *Rb*, *p16*$^{INK4a}$, and DNA methyltransferase (51–55). The result is derangement of normal cellular growth control processes

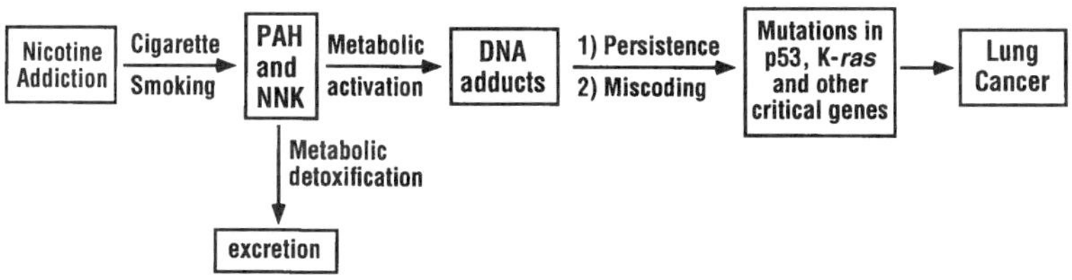


**FIG. 2.** Scheme linking nicotine addiction and lung cancer via cigarette smoke carcinogens.

and cancer. Mechanisms of DNA modification by representative cigarette smoke carcinogens are discussed below.

### Metabolism of Some Cigarette Smoke Carcinogens to DNA Reactive Products

Metabolism is the key to understanding the mechanisms by which carcinogens interact with DNA. Figure 3 summarizes some known metabolic reactions of BaP, a representative PAH. Metabolic reactions of PAH are complex (56). The initial reactions involve formation of a series of arene oxides, catalyzed by cytochrome P-450 enzymes, principally P-450 1A1 and 1A2, although others including members of the 2C and 3A families are also involved (57,58). There is a great deal of selectivity in the formation of these arene oxides; depending on the PAH, only certain ones will be formed and generally with a high degree of stereoselectivity (i.e., one optical isomer of each arene oxide frequently predominates). The arene oxide may rearrange spontaneously to phenols. Some phenols, such as 6-hydroxyBaP, are formed by direct hydroxylation. Competing with the rearrangement of arene oxides to phenols is their hydration to *trans*-dihydrodiols, catalyzed by epoxide hydrolase, as well as conjugation with glutathione catalyzed by different forms of glutathione-S-transferases (GST). Arene oxides are electrophiles and they react with DNA in vitro. Thus it was widely believed that they were ultimate carcinogens of PAH, but DNA-binding studies carried out in vivo did not support this hypothesis (56).

The *trans*-dihydrodiols formed by hydration of arene oxides can be conjugated as glucuronides or, in some cases, undergo further oxidation to diol epoxides. The epoxide ring can be added to the molecule on the same side as the benzylic hydroxyl group, giving a *syn*-diol epoxide, or on the opposite side, producing an *anti*-diol epoxide. Each *syn* or *anti* diol epoxide can exist in two optically isomeric (enantiomeric) forms. Thus, a racemic *trans*-dihydrodiol can be oxidized to four diol epoxides.

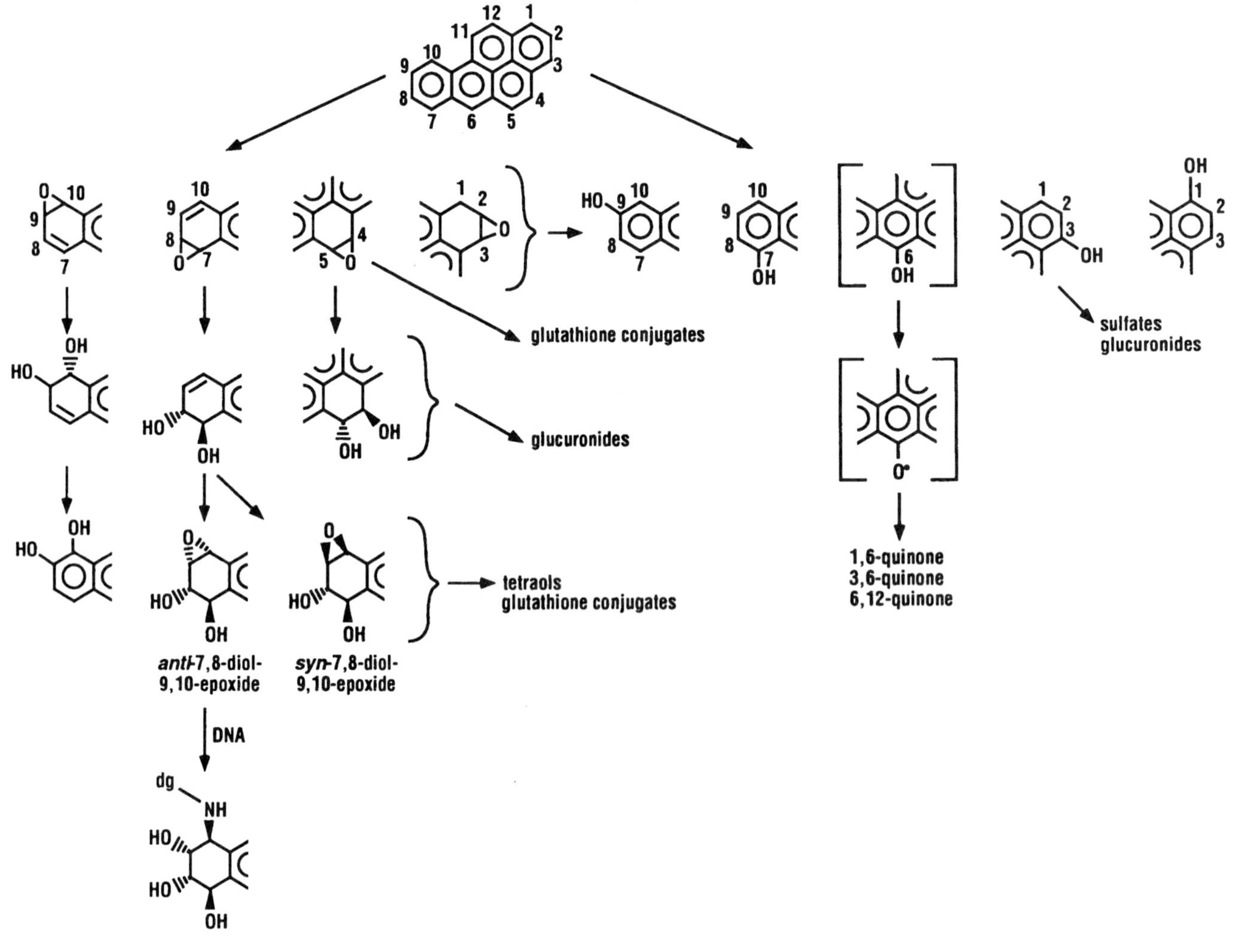


**FIG. 3.** Metabolism of benzo[*a*]pyrene (BaP).

Diol epoxides in which the epoxide ring is in the bay region of a PAH are major ultimate carcinogens of a number of PAH (59,60). Steric factors play a major role in the reactivity of diol epoxides with DNA, influencing the extent of the reaction, the types of adducts that are formed, and their mutagenicity and carcinogenicity. In general, the *anti* diol epoxides are more effective carcinogens and, among these, the *R,S,S,R* diol epoxide enantiomers are the most effective. DNA adducts formed from the *R,S,S,R* diol epoxides result predominantly from *trans*-addition of the exocyclic amino groups of deoxyguanosine or deoxyadenosine to the benzylic position of the epoxide ring (60).

Among the many reactions illustrated in Fig. 3, only formation of the *R,S,S,R* enantiomer of the *anti*-7,8-diol-9,10-epoxide (illustrated in the figure), has been conclusively shown to be a metabolic activation pathway. All other reactions represent probable detoxification pathways. Quantitatively, the metabolic activation pathway resulting in the formation of a diol epoxide ultimate carcinogen is a minor one, but the diol epoxide is highly carcinogenic and mutagenic and the DNA adducts that are formed cause somatic mutations and are plausibly responsible for many of the carcinogenic effects of BaP.

Pathways of NNK metabolism are summarized in Fig. 4 (61,62). Reduction of the carbonyl group, catalyzed by carbonyl reductase enzymes such as 11β-hydroxysteroid dehydrogenase (63), is a major metabolic pathway. This produces NNAL, which is also a potent pulmonary carcinogen (46,64). NNAL can be conjugated as its O-glucuronide, NNAL-Gluc, which is believed to be a detoxification product of NNK. NNAL-Gluc has been detected in smokers' urine after exposure to NNK (27,65). Oxidation of the pyridine ring at the nitrogen produces NNK-*N*-oxide, which is generally regarded as a detoxified metabolite of NNK. Likewise, NNAL is converted to NNAL-*N*-oxide. Other reactions involving the pyridine ring include 6-hydroxylation of NNK and formation of metabolites in which the pyridine ring of NNK or NNAL displaces nicotinamide from nicotinamide adenine dinucleotide phosphate (NADP) or reduced NADP (NADPH) (62). The major metabolic activation pathways result from cytochrome P-450 catalyzed oxidation adjacent to the *N*-nitroso group, a process called α-hydroxylation. Human cytochromes P-450 1A2, 2A6, and 3A4 are involved in this reaction (62,66). This leads to intermediates that are unstable and spontaneously decompose to produce aldehydes and diazohydroxides

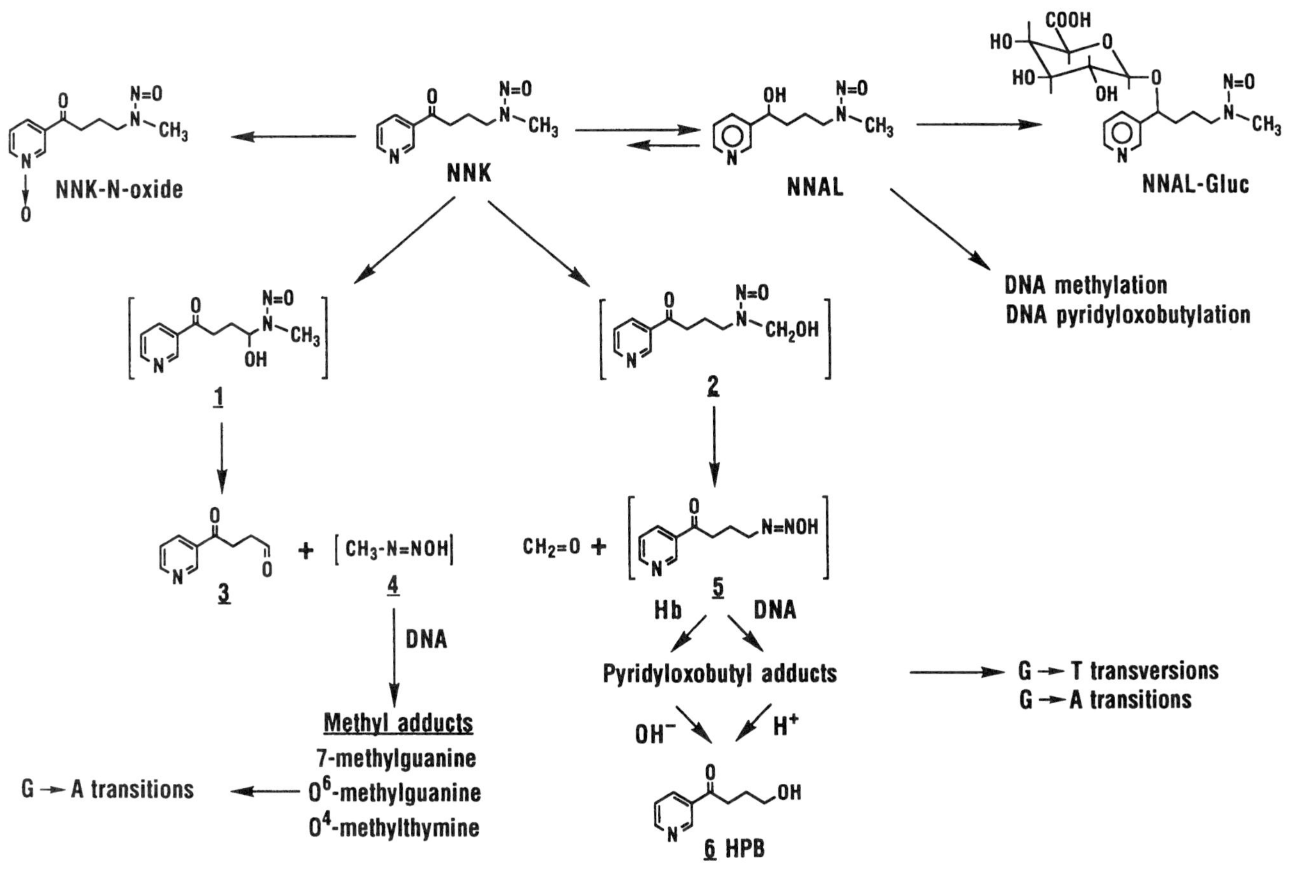


FIG. 4. Metabolism of 4-(methylnitrosamino)-1-(3-pyridyl)-1-butanone (NNK).

(R–N=N–OH). The diazohydroxides are electrophiles with very high reactivity toward DNA.

Methanediazohydroxide methylates DNA forming at least 13 different adducts among which 7-methylguanine, $O^6$-methylguanine, and $O^4$-methylthymidine have been detected in the DNA isolated from tissues of animals treated with NNK (67). $O^6$-methylguanine is known to cause miscoding, leading to a G to A transition (purine to purine) mutation (68). The other diazohydroxide produced from NNK also reacts with cellular macromolecules such as DNA and globin, giving adducts that can be hydrolyzed to 4-hydroxy-1-(3-pyridyl)-1-butanone (HPB). These adducts are structurally uncharacterized but are present in the DNA of animals treated with NNK. They have been shown to cause both G to A transition mutations and G to T transversion (purine to pyrimidine) mutations in DNA (69). Both pathways are regarded as metabolic activation modes for NNK and both are important in the induction of tumors by this compound. NNAL has similar metabolic activation pathways. The $\alpha$-hydroxylation pathways and conversion to NNAL are generally the major metabolism routes seen for NNK in rodents.

In comparing the metabolic activation pathways of PAH and nitrosamines, one interesting difference is that metabolic activation of the latter involves only one enzymatic step—$\alpha$-hydroxylation. The diol epoxide metabolites of PAH are generally more stable than the $\alpha$-hydroxy and diazohydroxide metabolites of nitrosamines. The latter react mainly at their site of formation, although evidence exists for their transport, e.g., by glucuronidation (70). Diol epoxides of PAH can be transported to sites other than those at which they are formed (71). Although $\alpha$-hydroxylation of nitrosamines generally exceeds diol epoxide formation from PAH, both types of compounds modify DNA to similar extents in laboratory animals.

Cr[VI] is one of the more extensively studied metals known to induce lung cancer (72,73). Cr[VI] is taken up by cells via passive anion transport channels and reduced intracellularly, resulting ultimately in Cr[III]. Various forms of DNA damage result from this process including the formation of Cr-DNA adducts, DNA-protein crosslinks, and DNA strand breaks. The mechanisms by which these effects occur are a subject of some controversy, but it seems clear that reductive metabolism of Cr[VI] is necessary. Some studies in vitro have demonstrated the formation of 8-oxodeoxyguanosine in DNA, upon exposure to Cr[VI] and reducing agents. This presumably results from the generation of reactive oxygen species such as hydroxyl radical associated with Cr[VI] metabolism, but the relevance of this process in vivo in the lung is not clear.

Hydroxylation of the amino nitrogen to form a hydroxylamine, catalyzed by hepatic cytochrome P-450 1A2, is considered to be the major metabolic activation pathway of aromatic amine bladder carcinogens, as well as the heterocyclic aromatic amines of tobacco smoke (43). The hydroxylamine can reach the bladder, where it forms a nitrenium ion that reacts with epithelial DNA. The major adducts result from the binding of the nitrenium ion to C-8 of deoxyguanosine. *N*-acetylation of the parent amine and hydroxylation of the ring carbons are generally considered to be detoxification pathways for aromatic amine bladder carcinogens (74).

### Cigarette Smoke Carcinogens: DNA Adduct Formation and Repair

Representative structures of some of the deoxyguanosine adducts that could form in lung DNA upon exposure to cigarette smoke are illustrated in Fig. 5. In DNA, deoxyguanosine is generally the most reactive with metabolically activated carcinogens, although reactions at this site are never exclusive. As discussed above, 7-methyldeoxyguanosine (structure 1*)* and $O^6$-methyldeoxyguanosine (structure 2) would typically be formed, among other methylated adducts, by nitrosamines such as NNK. 8-Oxodeoxyguanosine (structure 3) is formed as a result of reaction with active oxygen species associated with cigarette smoke. A large number of DNA adducts will be formed from the PAH of cigarette smoke. Only two

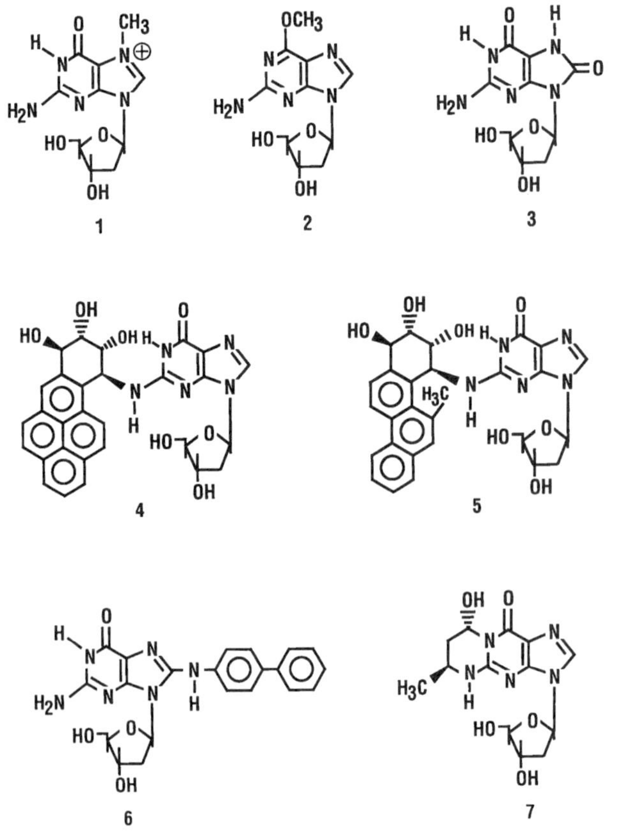

**FIG. 5.** Same DNA adducts that can form in tissues exposed to cigarette smoke.

of these (structures 4 and 5), derived from BaP and 5-methylchrysene, are illustrated. The aminobiphenyl adduct 6 is typical of those formed by aromatic amines whereas the exocyclic propanodeoxyguanosine adducts such as 7 are produced from α,β-unsaturated aldehydes such as crotonaldehyde and acrolein.

Techniques have been developed to assess individually the miscoding consequences of specific DNA adducts such as those illustrated in Fig. 5 (75). Results from studies on $O^6$-methyldeoxyguanosine (structure 2) are illustrative. During DNA replication, this adduct is recognized by DNA polymerases as deoxyadenosine, resulting in the incorporation of thymidine in the newly synthesized strand. In the next round of replication, this thymidine is paired with deoxyadenosine resulting in the permanent conversion of what was originally a G-C base pair to an A-T base pair. In contrast to $O^6$-methyldeoxyguanosine, the most common point mutation associated with adducts such as structures 3 to 7 of Fig. 5 is a G-C to T-A transversion. G to T transversions are also associated with some types of DNA damage that is structurally uncharacterized, for example the pyridyloxobutylation of DNA by NNK.

Since cigarette smoke is a complex mixture that contains carcinogens likely to produce a mixture of adducts that may, in simplified form, resemble those illustrated in Fig. 5, and since most of the adducts in Fig. 5 produce G to T transversions, it might be assumed that G to T transversions would be perhaps the most common mutations found in genes of tumors taken from smokers. This is in fact observed as discussed below. This simplified view of tobacco carcinogenesis assumes that all adducts would be formed and would persist in DNA to equal extents. This is not the case. The formation of different adducts depends on the metabolic activation and detoxification processes for the carcinogens of cigarette smoke, whereas the persistence of the adducts depends on their repair and the extent of cell replication, which can in turn be influenced by toxic constituents of cigarette smoke.

Two relevant DNA repair processes involved in lung carcinogenesis are the alkyltransferase pathway that removes alkyl groups from the $O^6$ position of deoxyguanosine and the excision repair pathway that removes sterically bulky adducts and alkyl adducts formed at the 7 position of guanine or 3 position of adenine from DNA (76–78). Repair of mutagenic $O^6$-alkylguanines is carried out by the repair protein $O^6$-alkylguanine-DNA-alkyltransferase. This protein removes the alkyl group from the $O^6$ position of guanine and transfers it to a cysteine acceptor site in the protein, regenerating the original DNA structure in a single step. The cysteine site of the protein is not regenerated. Therefore, new protein must be synthesized to continue repair. In this stoichiometric process, the cellular levels of protein and $O^6$-alkylguanine adduct are critical.

Excision repair can be broadly classified into nucleotide excision repair and base excision repair (76). In nucleotide excision repair, sterically bulky adducts such as those formed from PAH are removed from DNA. A section of the damaged DNA strand is excised, probably in reactions involving several proteins, and a new strand is synthesized by DNA polymerase using the undamaged strand as a template. Adducts such as 7-methylguanine are frequently removed by base excision repair. The damaged base is removed by a glycosylase, leaving an abasic site in DNA. The abasic site is a substrate for an endonuclease. Then, resynthesis of the DNA and ligation occur.

Many studies have indicated that certain types of adducts are preferentially removed from the transcribed strand of DNA. This leads to a bias in favor of mutations resulting from unrepaired adducts in the nontranscribed strand (76).

### Consequences of DNA Adduct Formation and Persistence

Oncogene activation and tumor suppressor gene inactivation are two events that are thought to be involved in the multistep carcinogenic process. In some cases, these genes are activated or inactivated by mutations resulting from DNA adducts. One of the most consistently detected activated oncogenes associated with smoking is the Ki-*ras* gene, isolated from adenocarcinoma of the lung (51). Point mutations in codon 12 of this oncogene, which are sufficient for its activation, have been most commonly detected. The normal codon 12 of the Ki-*ras* oncogene is GGT. In the activated Ki-*ras* genes detected in adenocarcinoma, the observed mutations are GGT→TGT (58%), GGT→ GTT (16%) and GGT→ GAT (19%). It has been reasonably hypothesized that these mutations arise from direct interaction of metabolically activated carcinogens of tobacco smoke with the Ki-*ras* gene, by mechanisms such as those discussed above. The prevalence of G-T transversions is consistent with the prevalence of G-T transversion-producing compounds in tobacco smoke. It has been proposed that the types of mutations seen in codon 12 of the activated Ki-*ras* gene could be a signature of a particular carcinogen. Thus, in mouse lung tumors, NNK induces mainly G to A transition mutations in codon 12 of the Ki-*ras* gene while BaP induces mainly G to T transversions (69,79,80). Accordingly, one could propose that the mutations in the activated Ki-*ras* gene from human lung adenocarcinomas arise mainly from BaP. Although this reasoning is attractive, it is probably naive because of the large variety of G to T transversion-producing compounds present in tobacco smoke.

The most commonly mutated gene found in human cancers is the *p53* tumor suppressor gene (52). Among the tobacco related cancers, the most extensive database exists for lung cancer, in which mutations in the *p53* gene have been detected in approximately 50% of tumors. In contrast to the Ki-*ras* gene, the mutations are scattered over several exons of this large gene. A wide variety of mutations has been seen in lung cancer from smokers including the ubiquitous G-T transversions in approximately 31% and G-A transitions in about 24%; in adenocarcinoma these percentages are approximately 23% and 32%. Since *p53* mutations have not been commonly observed in tumors from laboratory animals treated with tobacco smoke carcinogens, it is difficult to attempt to associate specific mutations with specific carcinogens. However, the large variety of mutations that is seen could well result from direct interaction of metabolically activated carcinogens with this gene. Importantly, mutations in the *p53* gene from lung tumors have a bias toward the nontranscribed strand, consistent with its slower repair. In addition, there appears to be a direct relationship between pack-years of smoking and G-T transversions in the *p53* gene. As mentioned above, the ultimate carcinogen of BaP gives a similar spectrum of *p53* mutations as observed in lung tumors from smokers (24).

## BIOMARKERS OF CIGARETTE SMOKE CARCINOGENS

The metabolic activation and detoxification of lung carcinogens vary among people. Both higher extents of metabolic activation and lower extents of detoxification will presumably be associated with higher risk for lung cancer (Fig. 2). Biomarkers that are quantitative measures of parameters reflecting carcinogen metabolic activation or detoxification are now becoming available (81–87).

Biomarkers related to the uptake and metabolic activation of PAH and nitrosamines, the major lung carcinogens to which humans are exposed, have been developed. These include urinary metabolites, DNA adducts, and hemoglobin adducts. Urinary metabolites can provide a profile of metabolic activation and detoxification of a carcinogen. Adducts are a measure of the internal dose of the carcinogen. Although DNA is considered the important target in carcinogenesis, proteins such as hemoglobin have been employed as surrogates for adduct measurement because of their availability.

PAH-DNA adducts in human tissues have been determined by a variety of methods, including immunoassay, $^{32}$P-postlabeling, synchronous fluorescence spectroscopy and other fluorescence techniques, and gas chromatography–mass spectrometry (GC-MS) (86,87). Among these, immunoassay and $^{32}$P-postlabeling have been applied most widely; however, they lack specificity to individual PAH carcinogens, which makes results difficult to evaluate. The more specific methods have been employed less extensively. Presently available data on PAH-DNA adducts indicate that there are a variety of exposure sources including certain occupations, diet, and tobacco smoke (84–87). Biomarkers of NNK uptake and metabolism have the advantage of being specific to tobacco smoke, since NNK is formed from nicotine while PAHs are present in any mixture resulting from incomplete combustion of organic matter (25). Presently available biomarkers for NNK include hemoglobin adducts, DNA adducts, and urinary metabolites (27,29,81,82). The hemoglobin adducts and DNA adducts are formed by metabolic activation of NNK and are not entirely specific to this carcinogen, since they are also produced by activation of NNN. The hemoglobin and DNA adducts are determined by GC-MS of HPB released upon hydrolysis (81,82). DNA adduct levels are higher in the lungs of smokers than nonsmokers (29). Hemoglobin adducts are higher in some smokers than in nonsmokers (81,82). Since the hemoglobin adducts of NNK and NNN result from metabolic activation, they could be biomarkers of risk.

Urinary metabolites of NNK are readily quantifiable and provide important information on both dose and metabolic activation of this lung carcinogen (27,65). In rodents and primates, NNK is extensively metabolized and virtually all the metabolites are excreted in the urine within 24 hours (25,61,62). The major metabolite of NNK in almost all animal and human tissues is its carbonyl reduction product NNAL (25,28,61,62,64). In humans, NNAL and NNAL-Gluc are excreted in urine, with the latter predominating as determined by GC with a nitrosamine selective detector (27,65). The total levels of NNAL and NNAL-Gluc provide an estimate of NNK exposure in a person. An interesting and potentially useful parameter is the ratio of NNAL-Gluc to NNAL, which has been shown to vary at least tenfold in smokers (65). NNAL-Gluc is presumed to be a detoxification product of NNAL; consequently, this ratio might provide a measure of detoxification potential upon exposure to NNK.

NNAL and NNAL-Gluc in urine can provide information on the exposure of nonsmokers to environmental tobacco smoke. Subjects exposed to sidestream tobacco smoke had increased levels of NNAL and NNAL-Gluc in their urine, providing evidence that nonsmokers exposed to sidestream smoke take up and metabolize a lung carcinogen (88). It is interesting to note that NNK and NNAL induce primarily pulmonary adenocarcinoma in rodents, which is the prevalent tumor type observed in nonsmokers exposed to environmental tobacco smoke.

Although biomarkers of carcinogen uptake, metabolic activation, and detoxification have not yet been applied in large epidemiologic studies of lung cancer, the presently available results from pilot and transitional studies indicate that this will be an important approach toward understanding mechanisms of cancer induction (14,84,85). These biomarkers are based on metabolic transformations of established lung carcinogens and therefore can potentially provide essential specific information relevant to lung cancer etiology.

## CARCINOGEN METABOLIZING ENZYMES AS BIOMARKERS

Another approach to assessing risk upon exposure to lung carcinogens is consideration of the enzymes that metabolically activate and detoxify them (56,83–85,89). Cytochrome P-450 enzymes are most commonly involved in the metabolic activation of carcinogens (56). Cytochromes P-450 1A1 and 1A2 are involved in the activation of BaP and perhaps other PAHs, while cytochrome P-450 1A2 is involved in the activation of aromatic amines and NNK.

Cytochrome P-450 2E1 is important in the metabolic activation of *N*-nitrosodimethylamine (NDMA) but not NNK. Cytochrome P-450 1A1 is inducible by exposure to tobacco smoke, and correlations have been observed between the activity of this enzyme and PAH-DNA adducts in smokers lungs (87). Polymorphisms in the cytochrome P-450 1A1 and 2E1 genes have been associated with lung cancer in certain populations, which may reflect increased carcinogen metabolic activation by some genotypes (85). Another cytochrome P-450 enzyme that has been studied in connection with lung cancer risk is cytochrome P-450 2D6, which metabolizes the drug debrisoquine. Extensive metabolizers of debrisoquine are at higher risk for lung cancer according to some epidemiologic studies, but others have found no relationship (85). The relationship of these findings to metabolism of lung carcinogens is presently obscure. GSTs are involved in the detoxification of metabolites of BaP and other PAH. Human GSTs can be classified into at least three genetically distinct groups called mu, alpha, and pi. The null phenotype of GST mu has been associated with increased risk for bladder cancer and for lung cancer in some studies (85). Collectively, biomarkers may have great promise for assessing individual risk for cancer development upon exposure to carcinogens.

## CHEMOPREVENTION OF TOBACCO-RELATED CANCER

Avoidance of tobacco products is clearly the best way to prevent tobacco-related cancers. Smoking-cessation programs have enjoyed some success in this regard, particularly with the advent of the nicotine patch (90,91). Political pressure, especially related to the potentially harmful effects of environmental tobacco smoke, has also had an impact on decreasing smoking. However, approximately 25% of the adult population in the United States continues to smoke, and many of these people are addicted to nicotine. For the addicted smoker who has failed smoking cessation, chemoprevention may be a way to reduce the risk for cancer. Chemoprevention involves administration of a nontoxic agent capable of blocking or reversing any of the steps illustrated in Fig. 2.

Chemoprevention of lung cancer and other tobacco-related cancers in humans is attractive because epidemiologic studies have consistently demonstrated a protective effect of vegetables and fruits against these cancers (92). This indicates that there are compounds in vegetables and fruits that can inhibit carcinogenesis by NNK, PAH, and other carcinogens. There are already a substantial number of compounds that have been shown to inhibit lung carcinogenesis induced by NNK and BaP in rats and mice, and many of these are naturally occurring (93–96). Phenethyl isothiocyanate (PEITC) is a relatively nontoxic compound that occurs in watercress as a thioglucoside conjugate. It is released upon chewing of the watercress. PEITC is an effective inhibitor of lung cancer induced by NNK in both rats and mice (97,98). Its major mode of action is inhibition of metabolic activation of NNK by selectively inhibiting cytochrome P-450 enzymes of the lung. PEITC does not inhibit carcinogenesis by BaP, but a related naturally occurring isothiocyanate, benzyl isothiocyanate (BITC), is a good inhibitor of BaP induced lung tumorigenesis in mice (99). Other isothiocyanates are known inhibitors of tumor development at other sites (100). Notable among these is sulforaphane, a constituent of broccoli (101).

Some of the other compounds that have been shown to inhibit lung carcinogenesis by NNK include butylated hydroxyanisole, an antioxidant used in food preservation; d-limonene, a constituent of orange juice and other citrus products; and diallyl sulfide, a constituent of garlic.

Inhibition of NNK carcinogenesis has also been observed in animals treated with green and black tea, as well as its major polyphenolic constituents. Inhibitors of lung tumorigenesis induced by BaP include β-naphthoflavone, butylated hydroxyanisole, ethoxyquin, diallyl sulfide, and *myo*-inositol. It seems likely that properly designed combinations of some of these inhibitors will be effective chemopreventive agents against lung cancer in humans.

A number of human trials are already in progress, and several of these have centered on β-carotene as a potential chemopreventive agent for lung cancer. The results have not been encouraging, as β-carotene had an enhancing effect on lung cancer, while vitamin E as well as a combination of β-carotene and vitamin E had no inhibitory effect (102,103). However, it should be noted that animal studies have not demonstrated efficacy against lung cancer for these two agents (96,104,105). On the other hand, 13-*cis*-retinoic acid was effective in preventing second cancers in individuals with cancer of the head and neck, induced primarily by smoking (106). In future trials, it will be important to carefully select chemopreventive agents based on their effectiveness in animal studies and on known mechanisms of action that would be applicable to smokers. In addition, smokers may need to be selected based on their biomarker profiles and smoking history.

## CARDIOVASCULAR DISEASE

Hypertension, cigarette smoking, and hypercholesterolemia are the three major independent risk factors for coronary artery disease. When these risk factors are present in combination, the risks are multiplicative. As an isolated risk factor in males, cigarette smoking increases the likelihood of developing coronary artery disease by 70%. Smoking appears to play a particularly important role in the genesis of the most feared manifestation of coronary artery disease—sudden death. The risk of developing coronary artery disease rises with increasing exposure to cigarette smoke. Autopsy studies show a dose-dependent increase in coronary atherosclerosis and myocardial arteriolar wall thickening in smokers compared with nonsmokers. Acute effects from smoking may promote a lethal or nonfatal coronary event by creating an imbalance between oxygen supply and demand, precipitating a dysrhythmia or stimulating increased platelet adhesiveness. Cessation of smoking reduces the risk of developing coronary artery disease, an effect that is measurable within 1 year.

Cigarette smoking, hypertension, and hypercholesterolemia are also major risk factors for arteriosclerotic peripheral vascular disease. Cessation of smoking improves the prognosis of this disorder and has a salutary impact on its surgical treatment. The mortality from abdominal aortic aneurysm is two to five times higher in current smokers. Nonsyphilitic aortic aneurysm, Buerger's disease, and subarachnoid hemorrhage in women all occur more frequently in smokers than in nonsmokers. Each year, an estimated 18% of the 150,000 stroke deaths in the United States are due to cigarette smoking. Women who use oral contraceptives and smoke have an increased risk for both myocardial infarction and stroke, especially in older age groups.

## CHRONIC OBSTRUCTIVE PULMONARY DISEASE (COPD)

Cigarette smoking has been identified as the most important cause of chronic bronchitis and emphysema. The mortality ratio for COPD, i.e., emphysema and chronic bronchitis, comparing smokers with nonsmokers, ranges from 2.3 to 24.7. COPD is also much more prevalent in smokers than in nonsmokers. Both the increased mortality ratio and the increased prevalence of COPD among smokers are dose related. Smokers have an increased frequency of cough, sputum production, and pulmonary function abnormalities. Even in teenage smokers, subtle pulmonary function abnormalities are demonstrable. In older individuals, pathologic evidence of chronic bronchitis and emphysema occurs much more commonly in smokers than in nonsmokers. Smoking hastens the onset of clinically significant COPD in patients with $\alpha_1$-antitrypsin deficiency. Current studies suggest that cigarette smoking contributes to the development of COPD by promoting an imbalance of pulmonary protease-antiprotease activity. Cessation of smoking is associated with improved pulmonary function, decreased cough and sputum production, and a reduced risk of dying from COPD.

## PREGNANCY

Smoking even less than 10 cigarettes per day doubles the risk of low birth weight. Infants whose mothers smoke during pregnancy weigh, on average, 170 g less and are more likely to be born preterm than infants whose mothers are nonsmokers. Maternal smoking during pregnancy increases the likelihood of spontaneous abortion, placenta previa, abruptio placentae, preterm rupture of membranes, and sudden infant death syndrome. Maternal smoking during pregnancy also may adversely affect an infant's long-term growth, intellectual development, and behavioral characteristics. Smoking-related fetal hypoxia is thought to mediate some of these effects.

## PEPTIC ULCER DISEASE

The mortality rate and prevalence of peptic ulcer disease are greater in cigarette smokers than in nonsmokers. Smoking also impairs peptic ulcer healing and increases recurrence rate. Impaired pancreatic bicarbonate secretion and pyloric reflux have been demonstrated in smokers, effects that may contribute to the pathogenesis of peptic ulcer disease.

## SUMMARY

Cigarette smoking is the major avoidable cause of cancer in the United States and worldwide. Studies in laboratory animals have conclusively shown that the particulate phase of cigarette smoke is carcinogenic to the respiratory tract and other organs. Many of the carcinogens in cigarette smoke have been characterized. Among them, PAH and the tobacco-specific nitrosamine NNK are the most important causes of lung cancer. Aromatic amines, nitrosamines, and PAH are involved in other cancers associated with smoking. Tumor promoters and cocarcinogens also contribute to the carcinogenicity of cigarette smoke. The pathways by which cigarette smoke carcinogens are detoxified or metabolically activated to reactive electrophiles are well understood. The electrophiles react with DNA and the resultant damage, if unrepaired, leads to permanent mutations. The consequences of such mutations include activated oncogenes or inactivated tumor suppressor genes. These processes are crucial in lung tumor induction by cigarette smoke. Biomarkers are being developed that can specifically monitor such processes in people and perhaps predict susceptibility for cancer. For those who are addicted to nicotine and have failed in smoking cessation programs, chemoprevention may be a feasible approach to prevent or delay the onset of tobacco-induced lung cancer. However, avoiding tobacco products is the best way to prevent tobacco-related cancers.

## REFERENCES


1. Shopland DR. Tobacco use and its contribution to early cancer mortality with a special emphasis on cigarette smoking. *Environ Health Perspect* 1995;103(suppl 8):131–142.
2. Wynder EL, Graham EA. Tobacco smoking as a possible etiologic factor in bronchiogenic carcinoma. A study of six hundred and eighty-four proved cases. *JAMA* 1950;143:329–336.
3. Doll R, Hill AB. Smoking and carcinoma of the lung. Preliminary report. *Br Med J* 1950;2:739–748.
4. United States Surgeon General. *Smoking and health.* USPHS publication no. 1103. Washington, DC: Department of Health, Education and Welfare, 1964.
5. United States Surgeon General. *Reducing the health consequences of smoking. Twenty-five years of progress.* USPHS publication no. (CDC) 89-8411. Rockville, MD: Department of Health and Human Services, 1989.
6. International Agency for Research on Cancer. *Tobacco smoking. In: IARC monographs on the evaluation of the carcinogenic risk of chemicals to humans,* vol 38. Lyon, France: International Agency for Research on Cancer, 1986.
7. Cole P, Rodu B. Declining cancer mortality in the United States. *Cancer* 1996;78:2045–2048.
8. Wynder EL, Hoffmann D. Smoking and lung cancer: scientific challenges and opportunities. *Cancer Res* 1994;54:5284–5295.
9. Doll R, Peto R. *The causes of cancer:* quantitative estimates of avoidable risks of cancer in the United States today. *J Natl Cancer Inst* 1981;66:1191–1308.
10. U.S. Environmental Protection Agency. *Respiratory health effects of passive smoking:* lung cancer and other disorders. Washington, DC: Office of Health and Environmental Assessment and Office of Research and Development, U.S. EPA, 1992.
11. National Research Council, National Academy of Sciences. *Environmental tobacco smoke:* measuring exposures and assessing health effects. Washington, DC: National Academy Press, 1986.
12. United States Surgeon General. *The health consequences of involuntary smoking.* DHHS publication no. (PHS) 87-8398. Washington, DC: DHHS, 1986.
13. Fontham ET, Correa P, Reynolds P, et al. Environmental tobacco smoke and lung cancer in nonsmoking women. A multicenter study. *JAMA* 1994;271:1752–1759.
14. Hecht SS. Environmental tobacco smoke and lung cancer: the emerging role of carcinogen biomarkers and molecular epidemiology (editorial). *J Natl Cancer Inst* 1994;86:1369–1370.
15. Anonymous. Cigarette smoking among adults—United States, 1993. *MMWR* 1994;43:925–930.
16. Doll R, Peto R, Wheatley K, Gray R, Sutherland I. Mortality in relation to smoking: 40 years' observations on male British doctors. *Br Med J* 1994;309:901–911.
17. Guerin MR, Jenkins RA, Tomkins BA. *The chemistry of environmental tobacco smoke:* composition and measurement. Boca Raton, FL: Lewis, 1992;43–62.
18. Hoffmann D, Hecht SS. Advances in tobacco carcinogenesis. In: Cooper CS, Grover PL, eds. *Handbook of experimental pharmacology.* Heidelberg: Springer-Verlag, 1990;94:63–102.
19. Wynder EL, Hoffmann D. Tobacco and tobacco smoke. *Studies in experimental carcinogenesis.* New York: Academic Press, 1967.
20. Hoffmann D, Wynder EL. A study of tobacco carcinogenesis. XI. Tumor initiators, tumor accelerators, and tumor promoting activity of condensate fractions. *Cancer* 1971;27:848–864.
21. Wolterbeek APM, Schoevers EJ, Rutten AAJJL, Feron VJ. A critical appraisal of intratracheal instillation of benzo[a]pyrene to Syrian golden hamsters as a model in respiratory track carcinogenesis. *Cancer Lett* 1995;89:107–116.
22. Stanton MF, Miller E, Wrench C, Blackwell R. Experimental induction of epidermoid carcinoma in the lungs of rats by cigarette smoke condensate. *J Natl Cancer Inst* 1972;49:867–877.
23. Thyssen J, Althoff J, Kimmerle G, Mohr U. Inhalation studies with benzo[a]pyrene in Syrian golden Hamsters. *J Natl Cancer Inst* 1981; 66:575–577.
24. Denissenko MF, Pao A, Tang M, Pfeifer GP. Preferential formation of benzo[a]pyrene adducts at lung cancer mutational hotspots in p53. *Science* 1996;274:430–432.
25. Hecht SS, Hoffmann D. Tobacco-specific nitrosamines, an important group of carcinogens in tobacco and tobacco smoke. *Carcinogenesis* 1988;9:875–884.
26. Hecht SS, Hoffmann D. 4-(Methylnitrosamino)-1-(3-pyridyl)-1-butanone, a nicotine-derived tobacco-specific nitrosamine, and cancer of the lung and pancreas in humans. In: Brugge, J, Curran T, Harlow E and McCormick F, eds. *Origins of human cancer:* a comprehensive review. Cold Spring Harbor, NY: Cold Spring Harbor Laboratory Press, 1991;745–755.
27. Carmella SG, Akerkar S, Hecht SS. Metabolites of the tobacco-specific nitrosamine 4- (methylnitrosamino)-1-(3-pyridyl)-1-butanone in smokers' urine. *Cancer Res* 1993;53:721–724.
28. Castonguay A, Stoner GD, Schut HAJ, Hecht SS. Metabolism of tobacco-specific N- nitrosamines by cultured human tissues. *Proc Natl Acad Sci USA* 1983;80:6694–6697.
29. Foiles PG, Akerkar SA, Carmella SG, et al. Mass spectrometric analysis of tobacco-specific nitrosamine-DNA adducts in smokers and non-smokers. *Chem Res Toxicol* 1991;4:364–368.
30. Hoffmann D, Rivenson A, Murphy SE, Chung F-L, Amin S, Hecht SS. Cigarette smoking and adenocarcinoma of the lung: the relevance of nicotine-derived N-nitrosamines. *J Smoking Relat Disord* 1993;4: 165–189.
31. Church DF, Pryor WA. Free radical chemistry of cigarette smoke and its toxicological implications. *Environ Health Perspect* 1985;64: 111–126.
32. Morrow JD, Frei B, Longmire AW, et al. Increase in circulating products of lipid peroxidation (F2-isoprostanes) in smokers. *N Engl J Med* 1995;332:1198–11203.
33. Loft S, Vistisen K, Ewertz M, Tjonneland A, Overvad K, Poulsen HE. Oxidative DNA damage estimated by 8-hydroxydeoxyguanosine excretion in humans: influence of smoking, gender and body mass index. *Carcinogenesis* 1992;13:2241–2247.
34. Solt DB, Polverini PJ, Claderon L. Carcinogenic response of hamster buccal pouch epithelium to 4 polycyclic aromatic hydrocarbons. *J Oral Pathol* 1987;16:294–302.
35. Hecht SS, Rivenson A, Braley J, DiBello J, Adams JD, Hoffmann D. Induction of oral cavity tumors in F344 rats by tobacco-specific nitrosamines and snuff. *Cancer Res* 1986;46:4162–4166.
36. Foiles PG, Miglietta LM, Quart AM, Quart E, Kabat GC, Hecht SS. Evaluation of $^{32}$P-postlabeling analysis of DNA from exfoliated oral mucosa cells as a means of monitoring exposure of the oral cavity to genotoxic agents. *Carcinogenesis* 1989;10:1429–1434.
37. McCoy GD, Wynder EL. Etiological and preventive implications in alcohol carcinogenesis. *Cancer Res* 1979;39:2844–2850.
38. von Gibel W. Experimentelle Untersuchung zur Synkarzinogenese beim Osophagus-Karzinom. *Arch Geschwulstforsch* 1967;30:181–189.
39. Aze Y, Toyoda K, Furukawa F, Mitsumori K, Takahashi M. Enhancing effect of ethanol on esophageal tumor development in rats by initiation of diethylnitrosamine. *Carcinogenesis* 1993;14:37–40.
40. Anderson LM, Carter JP, Logsdon DL, Driver CL, Kovatch RM. Characterization of ethanol's enhancement of tumorigenesis by N-nitrosodimethylamine in mice. *Carcinogenesis* 1992;13:2107–2111.
41. Anderson LM, Souliotis VL, Chhabra SK, Moskal TJ, Harbaugh SD, Kyrtopoulos SA. N-nitrosodimethylamine-derived $O^6$-methylguanine in DNA of monkey gastrointestinal and urogenital organs and enhancement by ethanol. *Int J Cancer* 1996:66;130–134.
42. International Agency for Research on Cancer. *Overall evaluations of carcinogenicity:* an updating of IARC monographs volumes 1 to 42, supplement 7. Lyon, France: International Agency to Research on Cancer, 1987;91–92,120–122,261–263.
43. Landi MT, Zocchetti C, Bernucci I, et al. Cytochrome P-4501A2: enzyme induction and genetic control in determining 4-aminobiphenyl-hemoglobin adduct levels. *Cancer Epidemiol Biomarkers Prev* 1996:5;693–698.
44. Talaska G, Schamer M, Skipper P, et al. Detection of carcinogen-DNA adducts in exfoliated urothelial cells of cigarette smokers: association with smoking, hemoglobin adducts, and urinary mutagenicity. *Cancer Epidemiol Biomarkers Prev* 1991;1:61–66.
45. Bell DA, Taylor JA, Paulson DF, Robertson CN, Mohler JL, Lucier GW. Genetic risk and carcinogen exposure: a common inherited

defect of the carcinogen-metabolism gene glutathione-S-transferase M1 (GSTM1) that increases susceptibility to bladder cancer. *J Natl Cancer Inst* 1993:85;1159–1164.
46. Rivenson A, Hoffmann D, Prokopczyk B, Amin S, Hecht SS. Induction of lung and exocrine pancreas tumors in F344 rats by tobacco-specific and Areca-derived N-nitrosamines. *Cancer Res* 1988;48: 6912–6917.
47. Hecht, SS, Thorne RL, Maronpot RR, Hoffmann D. Tumor-promoting subfractions of the weakly acidic fraction. A study of tobacco carcinogenesis, XIII. *J Natl Cancer Inst* 1975;55:1329–1336.
48. Hecht SS, Carmella S, Mori H, Hoffmann D. Role of catechol as a major cocarcinogen in the weakly acidic fraction of smoke condensate. A study of tobacco carcinogenesis. XX. *J Natl Cancer Inst* 1981; 66:163–169.
49. Van Duuren BL, Goldschmidt BM. Cocarcinogenic and tumor-promoting agents tobacco carcinogenesis. *J Natl Cancer Inst* 1976;56: 1237–1242.
50. United States Surgeon General. *The health consequences of smoking:* nicotine addiction. DHHS publication no. (CDC) 88-8406. Rockville, MD: Department of Health and Human Services, 1988.
51. Rodenhuis S, Slebos RJC. Clinical significance of ras oncogene activation in human lung cancer. *Cancer Res* [Suppl] 1992;52: 2665s–2669s.
52. Greenblatt MS, Bennett WP, Hollstein M, Harris CC. Mutations in the p53 tumor suppressor gene: clues to cancer etiology and molecular pathogenesis. *Cancer Res* 1994;54:4855–4878.
53. Kratzke RA, Greatens TM, Rubins JB, et al. Rb and p16INK4a expression in resected non-small cell lung tumors. *Cancer Res* 1996: 56;3415–3420.
54. Belinsky SA, Nikula KJ, Baylin SB, Issa JJ. Increased cytosine DNA-methyltransferase activity is target-cell-specific and an early event in lung cancer. *Proc Natl Acad Sci USA* 1996:93;4045–4050
55. Minna JD. The molecular biology of lung cancer pathogenesis. *Chest* 1993;103:449s–456s.
56. Thakker DR, Yagi H, Levin W, Wood AW, Conney AH, Jerina DM. Polycyclic aromatic hydrocarbons: metabolic activation to ultimate carcinogens. In: Anders MW, ed. *Bioactivation of foreign compounds.* New York: Academic Press, 1985;177–242.
57. Guengerich FP, Shimada T. Oxidation of toxic and carcinogenic chemical by human cytochrome P-450 enzymes. *Chem Res Toxicol* 1991;4: 391–407.
58. Yun C-H, Shimada T, Guengerich FP. Roles of human liver cytochrome P-4502C and 3A enzymes in the 3-hydroxylation of benzo(a)pyrene. *Cancer Res* 1992;52:1868–1874.
59. Conney AH. Induction of microsomal enzymes by foreign chemicals and carcinogenesis by polycyclic aromatic hydrocarbons: G.H.A. Clowes Memorial Lecture. *Cancer Res* 1982;42:4875–4917.
60. Dipple A. Reactions of polycyclic aromatic hydrocarbons with DNA. In: Hemminki K, Dipple A, Shuker DEG, Kadlubar FF, Segerbäck D, Bartsch H, eds. *DNA adducts:* identification and biological significance. Lyon, France: International Agency for Research on Cancer, 1994;107–129.
61. Hecht SS. Metabolic activation and detoxification of tobacco-specific nitrosamines-a model for cancer prevention strategies. *Drug Metab Rev* 1994;26:373–390.
62. Hecht SS. Recent studies on mechanisms of bioactivation and detoxification of 4-(methylnitrosamino)-1-(3-pyridyl)-1-butanone (NNK), a tobacco-specific lung carcinogen. *CRC Crit Rev Toxicol* 1996;26: 163–181.
63. Maser G, Richter E, Friebertshauser J. The identification of 11 beta-hydroxysteroid dehydrogenase as carbonyl reductase of the tobacco-specific nitrosamine 4-(methylnitrosamino)-1-(3-pyridyl)-1-butanone. *Eur J Biochem* 1996:238:484–489.
64. Castonguay A, Lin D, Stoner GD, et al. Comparative carcinogenicity in A/J mice and metabolism by cultured mouse peripheral lung of N'-nitrosonornicotine, 4-(methylnitrosamino)-1-(3-pyridyl)-1-butanone and their analogues. *Cancer Res* 1983;43:1223–1229.
65. Carmella SG, Akerkar S, Richie JP Jr, Hecht SS. Intraindividual and interindividual differences in metabolites of the tobacco-specific lung carcinogen 4-(methylnitrosamino)-1-(3-pyridyl)-1-butanone (NNK) in smokers' urine. *Cancer Epidemiol Biomarkers Prev* 1995;4: 635–642.
66. Patten CJ, Smith TJ, Murphy SE, et al. Kinetic analysis of the activation of 4-(methylnitrosamino)-1-(3-pyridyl)-1-butanone by heterologously expressed human P-450 enzymes and the effect of P-450-specific chemical inhibitors on this activation in human liver microsomes. *Arch Biochem Biophys* 1996;332:127–138.
67. Hecht SS, Peterson LA, Spratt TE. Tobacco-specific nitrosamines. In: Hemminki K, Dipple A, Shuker DEG, Kadlubar FF, Segerbäck D, Bartsch H, eds. *DNA adducts:* identification and biological significance. Lyon, France: International Agency for Research on Cancer, 1994;91–106.
68. Loechler, EL, Green CL, Essigmann JM. In vivo mutagenesis by $O^6$-methylguanine built into a unique site in a viral genome. *Proc Natl Acad Sci USA* 1984;81:6271–6275.
69. Ronai Z, Gradia S, Peterson LA, Hecht SS. G to A transitions and G to T transversions in codon 12 of the Ki-ras oncogene isolated from mouse lung tumors induced by 4-(methylnitrosamino)-1-(3-pyridyl)-1-butanone (NNK) and related DNA methylating and pyridyloxobutylating agents. *Carcinogenesis* 1993;14:2419–2422.
70. Murphy SE, Spina DA, Nunes MG, Pullo DA. Glucuronidation of 4-(hydroxymethyl)- nitrosamino-1-(3-pyridyl)-1-butanone, a metabolically activated form of 4-(methylnitrosamino)-1-(3-pyridyl)-1-butanone, by phenobarbital treated rats. *Chem Res Toxicol* 1995;8: 772–779.
71. Ginsberg GL, Atherholt TB. DNA adduct formation in mouse tissues in relation to serum levels of benzo(a)pyrene-diol-epoxides after injection of benzo(a)pyrene or the diol-epoxide. *Cancer Res* 1990;50: 1189–1194.
72. Klein, CB, Frenkel K, Costa M. The role of oxidative processes in metal carcinogenesis. *Chem Res Toxicol* 1991;4:592–604.
73. Standeven AM, Wetterhahn KE, Is there a role for reactive oxygen species in the mechanism of chromium (VI) carcinogenesis? *Chem Res Toxicol* 1991;4:616–625.
74. Badawi AF, Hirvonen A, Bell DA, Lang NP, Kadlubar FF. Role of aromatic amino acetyltransferases, NAT 1 and NAT 2, in carcinogen-DNA adduct formation in the human urinary bladder. *Cancer Res* 1995;55:5230–5237.
75. Basu AK, Essigmann JM. Site-specifically modified oligodeoxynucleotides as probes for the structural and biological effects of DNA-damaging agents. *Chem Res Toxicol* 1988;1:1–18.
76. Scicchitano DA, Hanawalt PC. Intragenomic repair heterogenicity of DNA damage. *Environ Health Perspect* 1992;98:45–51.
77. Belinsky SA, Dolan ME, White CM, Maronpot RR, Pegg AE, Anderson MW. Cell specific differences in $O^6$-methylguanine-DNA methyltransferase activity and removal of $O^6$-methylguanine in rat pulmonary cells. *Carcinogenesis* 1988;9:2053–2058.
78. Peterson LA, Liu X-K, Hecht SS. Pyridyloxobutyl DNA adducts inhibit the repair of $O^6$-methylguanine. *Cancer Res* 1993;53: 2780–2785.
79. Belinsky SA, Devereux TR, Maronpot RR, Stoner GD, Anderson MW. The relationship between the formation of promutagenic adducts and the activation of the K-*ras* proto-oncogene in lung tumors from A/J mice treated with nitrosamines. *Cancer Res* 1989;49:5305–5311.
80. You M, Candrian U, Maronpot RR, Stoner GD, Anderson MW. Activation of the Ki-*ras* protooncogene in spontaneously occurring and chemically induced lung tumors of the strain A mouse. *Proc Natl Acad Sci USA* 1989;86:3070–3074.
81. Hecht SS, Carmella SG, Murphy SE, Foiles PG, Chung FL. Carcinogen biomarkers related to smoking and upper aerodigestive tract cancer. *J Cell Biochem* [Suppl] 1993;17F:27–35.
82. Hecht SS, Carmella SG, Foiles PG, Murphy SE. Biomarkers for human uptake and metabolic activation of tobacco-specific nitrosamines. *Cancer Res* [Suppl] 1994;54:1912s–1917s.
83. U.S. Department of Health and Human Services, Biomarkers in human cancer, Part I. *Environ Health Perspect* 1992;98:5–278.
84. U.S. Department of Health and Human Services, Biomarkers in human cancer, Part II. *Environ Health Perspect* 1993;99:5–390.
85. Perera FP. Molecular epidemiology: insights into cancer susceptibility, risk assessment, and prevention. *J Natl Cancer Inst* 1996;88:496–509.
86. Kaderlik KR, Kadlubar FF. Metabolic polymorphisms and carcinogen-DNA adduct formation in human populations. *Pharmacogenetics* 1995;5:S108–S17.
87. Bartsch H. DNA adducts in human carcinogenesis: etiological relevance and structure-activity relationship. *Mutat Res* 1996;340:67–79.
88. Hecht SS, Carmella SG, Murphy SE, Akerkar S, Brunnemann KD, Hoffmann D. A tobacco-specific lung carcinogen in the urine of men exposed to cigarette smoke. *N Engl J Med* 1993;329:1543–1546.

89. Kato S, Bowman E, Harrington AM, Blomeke B, Shields PG. Human lung carcinogen-DNA adduct levels mediated by genetic polymorphisms in vivo. *J Natl Cancer Inst* 1995;87:902–907.
90. Hennrikus DJ, Jeffery RW, Lando HA. The smoking cessation process: longitudinal observations in a working population. *Prev Med* 1995;24:235–244.
91. Kenford SL, Fiore MC, Jorenby DE, Smith SS, Wetter D, Baker TB. Predicting smoking cessation—who will quit with and without the nicotine patch. *JAMA* 1994;271:589–594.
92. Potter JD, Steinmetz K. Vegetables, fruit and phytoestrogens as preventive agents. In: Stewart BW, McGregor D, Kleihues P, eds. *Principles of chemoprevention.* Lyon, France: International Agency for Research on Cancer, 1996;61–90.
93. Wattenberg L, Lipkin M, Boone CW, Kelloff GJ, eds. *Cancer chemoprevention.* Boca Raton, FL: CRC Press, 1992.
94. Wattenberg LW. Chemoprevention of cancer by naturally occurring and synthetic compounds. In: Wattenberg L, Lipkin M, Boone CW, Kelloff GJ, eds. *Cancer chemoprevention.* Boca Raton, FL: CRC Press, 1992:19–39.
95. Morse MA, Stoner GD. Cancer chemoprevention: principles and prospects. *Carcinogenesis* 1993;14:1737–1746.
96. Hecht SS. Approaches to chemoprevention of lung cancer based on carcinogens in tobacco smoke. *Environ Health Perspect* 1997;105 (Suppl 4):955–963.
97. Hecht SS, Trushin N, Rigotty J, Carmella SG, Borukhova A, Akerkar SA, Rivenson A. Complete inhibition of 4-(methylnitrosamino)-1-(3-pyridyl)-1-butanone induced rat lung tumorigenesis and favorable modification of biomarkers by phenethyl isothiocyanate. *Cancer Epidemiol Biomarkers Prev* 1996;5:645–652.
98. Morse MA, Amin SG, Hecht SS, Chung F-L. Effects of aromatic isothiocyanates on tumorigenicity, $O^6$-methylguanine formation, and metabolism of the tobacco-specific nitrosamine 4-(methylnitrosamino)-1-(3-pyridyl)-1-butanone in A/J mouse lung. *Cancer Res* 1989;49:2894–2897.
99. Lin J-M, Amin S, Trushin N, Hecht SS. Effects of isothiocyanates on tumorigenesis by benzo[a]pyrene in murine tumor models. *Cancer* Lett 1993;74:151–159.
100. Hecht, SS. Chemoprevention by isothiocyanates. *J Cell Biochem* [Suppl] 1995;22:195–209.
101. Zhang Y, Talalay P, Cho CG, Posner GH. A major inducer of anticarcinogenic protective enzymes from broccoli: isolation and elucidation of structure. *Proc Natl Acad Sci USA* 1992;89:2399–2403.
102. Anonymous. The effect of vitamin E and beta carotene on the incidence of lung cancer and other cancers in male smokers. The Alpha-Tocopherol, Beta-Carotene Cancer Prevention Study Group. *N Engl J Med* 1994;330:1029–1035.
103. Huttunen JK. Evaluation of human trial findings. In: Stewart BW, McGregor D, Kleihues P, eds. *Principles of chemoprevention.* Lyon, France: International Agency for Research on Cancer, 1996; 271–276.
104. Castonguay A, Pepin P, Stoner GD. Lung tumorigenicity of NNK given orally to A/J mice: its application to chemopreventive efficacy studies. *Exp Lung Res* 1991;17:485–499.
105. Beems RB. The effect of β-carotene on BP-induced respiratory tract tumors in hamsters. *Nutr Cancer* 1987;10:197–204.
106. Hong WK, Lippman SM, Itri LM, et al. Prevention of second primary tumors with isotretinoin in squamous-cell carcinoma of the head and neck. *N Engl J Med* 1990;323:795–801.

*Environmental and Occupational Medicine, Third Edition,* edited by William N. Rom.
Lippincott–Raven Publishers, Philadelphia © 1998.

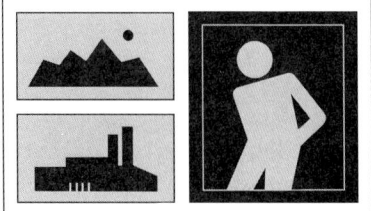

CHAPTER 114

# Community Air Pollution

William E. Lambert, Jonathan M. Samet, and Douglas W. Dockery

## THE SCOPE OF THE PROBLEM

Particles and gases are continuously emitted into the atmosphere by human activities. People are exposed outdoors, in their homes, at work, in public places, and while in transit. Despite increasing restrictions on emissions, and increased awareness of the large contribution of indoor sources to total exposure, exposures to outdoor (ambient) air pollution continue to be a public health concern. Exposure to airborne pollutants is causally associated with a number of respiratory and cardiovascular health effects, ranging from acute irritation and inflammation of the respiratory tract to serious chronic diseases such as emphysema, chronic bronchitis, and childhood asthma. In addition, there are effects for which evidence is suggestive of an association but further research is needed for confirmation, including premature death from respiratory and cardiac diseases. Because many persons living in urban areas of the United States are exposed to outdoor air pollution, the number of people adversely affected may be large.

In the more developed countries, little time is spent outdoors, with an average of less than 1 hour per day for adults (1). Because of the high proportion of time spent indoors, the presence of indoor sources, and reduced air exchange in enclosed spaces, indoor environments are important settings for exposure. Nevertheless, certain groups may spend large proportions of time outdoors, such as children, and adults who work in outdoor occupations. Further, outdoor locations may be the sole or predominant source of exposure to some pollutants, such as ozone, and the movement of polluted outdoor air into buildings and vehicles provides opportunities for exposure in enclosed settings. Thus, protection of outdoor air quality is relevant to exposures received by many segments of the population in varied settings.

During the second half of the 20th century increasing public health and regulatory concern has been directed at outdoor air pollution. This concern followed recognition of the substantial morbidity and mortality that may result from outdoor air pollution. From the 1930s through the 1950s, episodes of excess mortality at times of extremely high levels provided dramatic evidence that air pollution can cause excess deaths (2) (Table 1). For example, the London Fog of 1952 resulted in several thousand excess deaths (3). In subsequent years, epidemiologic and toxicologic research on health effects, in addition to expanded air quality monitoring, have provided the scientific basis for air quality regulation, and comprehensive programs for air quality management are now in place in the United States and other countries.

Outdoor air is community property; maintenance of acceptable air quality has required complex governmental initiatives affecting industry, transportation, and even personal lifestyles. The broad goals of such initiatives include the protection of human health and the prevention of environmental degradation. Beginning in the 1950s, in the United States and some other countries, deterioration of visibility and the evidence of adverse effects on health led to research and regulatory programs that had their

W. E. Lambert: Epidemiology and Cancer Control Program/New Mexico Tumor Registry, University of New Mexico Health Sciences Center, Albuquerque, New Mexico 87131-5306.

J. M. Samet: Department of Epidemiology, The Johns Hopkins University School of Hygiene and Public Health, Baltimore, Maryland 21205.

D. W. Dockery: Department of Environmental Health, Harvard University School of Public Health, Boston, Massachusetts 02115.

**TABLE 1.** *Acute air pollution episodes and attributed mortality*

| Place | Date | Excess deaths (no.) |
|---|---|---|
| Meuse Valley, Belgium | December 1930 | 63 |
| Donora, PA | October 1948 | 20 |
| London, England | December 1952 | 3,500 |
| New York, NY | November 1953 | 200 |
| London, England | December 1962 | 700 |
| Osaka, Japan | December 1962 | 60 |

Modified from ref. 10.

foundation in the research findings. The United States Congress enacted the first national legislation, the Air Pollution Control Act, in 1955. In passing the Clean Air Act of 1963, the federal government established its right over the states to legislate air pollution on the constitutional basis of interstate commerce. The Motor Vehicle Air Pollution Control Act of 1965 established a process for implementing national emissions standards for new motor vehicles.

The Clean Air Act Amendments of 1970 and the establishment of the U.S. Environmental Protection Agency (EPA) changed the course of pollution control in the United States. Congress charged the EPA with establishing National Ambient Air Quality Standards (Table 2) and gave the agency enforcement authority. Congress imposed federal mobile source emission standards on manufacturers, and states had to establish air pollution implementation plans to reach compliance with federal criteria. After reviewing the scientific evidence for health and welfare effects, the EPA promulgated regulations on criteria pollutants, which currently are carbon monoxide, nitrogen dioxide, lead, particulate matter, sulfur dioxide, and ozone. The EPA is required periodically to review the relevant evidence and prepare large compendia of information (the so-called criteria documents), and to set standards for each of these pollutants. The act was amended in 1977 and again in 1990. The 1990 amendments are far-reaching and address hazardous air pollutants, acid rain, and stratospheric ozone depletion. Many other important regulatory issues are addressed in the latest amendments, including nonattainment of federal standards and sanctions that permit enforcement and compliance. An initial list of hazardous pollutants includes 189 compounds, principally carcinogens, for which the EPA must set emissions standards.

The literature on the health effects of air pollution is voluminous, and thus this chapter is selective, of necessity, in its citations. Comprehensive reference lists are included in the criteria documents of the EPA. A review of the health effects of air pollution by the American Thoracic Society includes the more recent and significant references through 1995 (4,5). A 1996 monograph addresses particulate air pollution (6).

## TRENDS IN AIR QUALITY

In the United States, Canada, and other Western countries, standardized outdoor monitoring for several pollutants has been conducted since the 1950s. The ambient concentrations of some pollutants have decreased, and many cities that were once badly polluted by local fossil fuel–burning industries now have much cleaner air because control technologies have been put into place or factories have closed. In the United States there have been decreases in the ambient concentrations of total suspended particulates (TSP), sulfur dioxide, lead, and carbon monoxide (7). Ambient levels of organic carbon compounds, such as benzo[*a*]pyrene, have also been reduced. These decreases probably reflect many factors, including controls on emissions from power plants, fac-

**TABLE 2.** *National ambient air quality standards, 1987 outdoor concentration ranges, and principal health effects attributable to increased pollutant levels*

| Pollutant | Primary standards[a] | Averaging time | Concentration range |
|---|---|---|---|
| Ozone[b] | 0.12 ppm (235 μg/m$^3$) | 1 hr | 0.80–0.20 ppm |
| Particulate matter[b] ($PM_{10}$) | 50 μg/m$^3$ | Annual (arithmetic mean) | 30–80 μg/m$^3$ |
| | 150 μg/m$^3$ | 24 hr | — |
| Sulfur oxides ($SO_2$) | 0.03 ppm (80 μg/m$^3$) | Annual (arithmetic mean) | 0.002–0.019 ppm |
| | 0.14 ppm (365 μg/m$^3$) | 24 hr | — |
| Nitrogen dioxide | 0.053 ppm (200 μg/m$^3$) | Annual (arithmetic mean) | 0.01–.04 ppm |
| Carbon monoxide | 9 ppm (10 mg/m$^3$) | 8 hr | 3–13 ppm |
| | 35 ppm (40 mg/m$^3$) | 1 hr | — |
| Lead | 1.5 μg/m$^3$ | Quarterly average | 0.1–0.5 μg/m$^3$ |

[a]Primary standard: standard to protect against adverse health effects. 5th–95th percentiles: data represent range of 2nd highest concentration.

[b]Standards are pending revision.

$PM_{10}$, particulate matter equal or less than 10 μm in diameter. Reported as total suspended particulate matter, data not available for $PM_{10}$.

tories, and vehicles, the construction of new power plants and factories in locations away from urban centers, the burning of cleaner fuels, and a decline in manufacturing-related industries.

Levels of some other pollutants either have shown no change or have increased. For example, in 1991, the EPA estimated 69 million people live in counties that exceeded the National Ambient Air Quality Standard for ozone (0.12 ppm, 1-hour average) (8). Ozone pollution now affects many regions of the United States other than Southern California, where it was first identified. In spring and summer most of the population east of the Mississippi experiences ozone concentrations above 0.10 ppm for at least 1 hour per day. The pervasive problem of ozone pollution reflects population growth and urban sprawl. Although newer cars emit smaller amounts of hydrocarbons and nitrogen oxides, the precursors of photochemical pollution or smog, increasing numbers of motor vehicles and miles driven offset the lower emissions per car (8).

Although levels of sulfur dioxide have declined, the problem of acid pollution by sulfate and nitrate species has become increasingly prominent in the United States and Canada (9). Through complex chemical reactions, nitrogen oxides and sulfur oxides can be converted to acidic gases and particles. Common acidic species include sulfuric acid, ammonia bisulfate, acidic particles, and nitrous and nitric acid gases. Concentrations of sulfate are highest in the central portion of the eastern United States, where sulfur-containing fuels, principally coal, are burned in power plants and industry (10).

With population growth and increasing urbanization in developing countries, outdoor air pollution has become an increasingly important public health concern in many large cities and particularly in the so-called mega-cities, such as Mexico City (11). Uncontrolled emissions from industry, motor vehicles, and polluting cooking and heating fuels cause the outdoor air of many of the cities of Eastern Europe, Asia, Africa, and South America to resemble that of London, Pittsburgh, and New York City 40 years ago. Unfortunately, such extremely polluted conditions can cause excess deaths, and air pollution–related morbidity seems likely to occur in developing countries.

## TOTAL PERSONAL EXPOSURE

Perhaps because of the different sources of outdoor and indoor air pollution, and the separate regulatory approaches and control strategies for outdoor air and for the workplace, the home, and other indoor environments, exposures and health effects have been addressed separately for outdoor and indoor air. However, the concept of total personal exposure to air pollution is more relevant for the protection of public health. Total personal exposure represents the time-weighted average of pollutant concentrations in microenvironments—physical settings that have relatively uniform concentrations of air pollutants during the time people spend there (12). The contribution of outdoor pollutants to total personal exposure varies from pollutant to pollutant. For ozone and aerosols, for example, exposure experienced in outdoor locations probably makes the predominant contribution in most urban areas. For other pollutants, such as nitrogen dioxide, both indoor and in-transit exposures may make substantial contributions to total personal exposure. A 1991 National Research Council report (12) advocates reduction of personal exposure by directing controls and other interventions at the major contributing microenvironments rather than simply implementing universal controls or focusing control efforts principally on outdoor sources.

## RESEARCH METHODS

### Exposure Assessment

For regulatory purposes, monitoring networks for the principal pollutants are maintained throughout the United States. Through the early 1970s, pollutant measurements at such monitoring sites were generally considered adequate to represent the exposure of persons living nearby in conducting observational investigations. Thus, many epidemiologic studies used outdoor monitoring data to classify subjects' exposure. The pitfall of exposure misclassification introduced by such simplistic approaches became apparent as the spatial and temporal variations of pollution levels in urban areas were characterized and the bias and loss of statistical power arising from measurement error went unrecognized (2,13).

Strategies for assessing exposure to outdoor pollution have become increasingly sophisticated since the 1970s. In a series of studies in western Pennsylvania, data from an extensive monitoring network within a relatively small geographic region were used in a computer model to estimate exposure at homes and schools (14,15). In the study of the health effects of air pollution in six U.S. cities conducted by Harvard University, exposure to pollutants in outdoor air was estimated from data obtained with monitors in the areas where subjects lived (16). Indoor and personal monitoring have also been used in this study to improve the characterization of personal exposures of these populations and to validate the strategy applied to the full population (17,18).

Increasingly, research designs incorporate approaches for estimating personal exposures, whether for the purpose of epidemiologic investigation or for characterizing population patterns of exposure. Approaches to personal exposure assessment can be categorized as direct and indirect (12). In the direct method a personal monitor placed on the subject provides either a continuous or an integrated assessment of exposure. Passive monitors have been developed for several outdoor pollutants, including ozone, nitrogen dioxide, carbon monoxide, and volatile organic compounds. Active samplers, using small pumps, are available for particles. Biomarkers represent another direct approach. For carbon monoxide, carboxyhemoglobin level and concentration of the gas in end-tidal air can be measured. Similarly, levels of volatile organic compounds can be measured in blood or breath. Indirect approaches combine area monitoring with a record of the locations where a subject spends time and the time spent in each site. Personal exposure is estimated by summing the respective products of concentrations of pollutant in various microenvironments and the time spent in each.

### Research Approaches

Achieving full and confident understanding of the health effects of outdoor air pollution has proved difficult. The relevant data may include information on exposures and complementary findings on health from toxicologic investigations, controlled human exposures, and epidemiologic studies. Each of these research approaches has specific strengths and weaknesses in evaluating the effects of outdoor air pollution on human health. Animal studies provide the opportunity to evaluate pathogenic mechanisms of injury by pollutants and to use methods that would not be ethical or practical to apply to human subjects (19). Closely controlled exposure-response data can be collected using a wide array of biologic outcome measures in multiple species, but regardless of the scope and quality of animal data, uncertainty is introduced by extrapolating findings from animal models to humans. Differences in respiratory tract morphology, regional deposition of pollutants in the lung, and interspecies differences in biologic and physiologic sensitivity to given concentrations of pollutants contribute to the uncertainty of such extrapolation.

Human exposure experiments permit strict control of the exposure and of the characteristics of exposed persons. These studies typically involve small and homogeneous groups of subjects who inhale pollutants through a mouthpiece, mask, or chamber air (20). In addition to ensuring control of exposure, the outcome measures can be carefully characterized, even by using relatively invasive tests such as fiberoptic bronchoscopy. As previously noted, ethical and practical considerations limit the use of laboratory exposure studies of humans. Exposures must be at concentrations below the levels that are likely to produce unacceptable short-term or long-term effects. Feasibility usually limits exposure to a few hours, and chronic effects cannot be readily addressed. The participants are volunteers; those individuals most likely to be affected by inhaled pollutants, i.e., having severe lung disease, cannot be readily and ethically studied. Despite these constraints, controlled clinical testing has been used extensively, for example, in investigation of the acute effects of exposure to nitrogen dioxide, sulfur dioxide, and ozone in persons with asthma (21).

Epidemiologic studies examine the relation between exposure and health effects in the community setting, typically in large populations. Descriptive approaches of varying designs may be used. Ecologic studies have been performed that involved the correlation of disease indicators for geographic units. Death or hospitalization rates in comparison communities, with estimates of pollution exposure for these areas have been used (22–24). Time series designs have also been used to compare variation of disease outcome measures with pollution concentrations; for example, Samet and co-workers (25) assessed the effects of 24-hour concentrations of outdoor pollutants on the numbers of daily emergency room visits in Steubenville, Ohio, and time series analyses of daily mortality have raised concern that current levels of particulate pollution are causing excess deaths. New methods for analysis of the time series data have strengthened this approach (26).

In the community setting, cross-sectional and longitudinal designs are most often used. Questionnaire and tests of pulmonary function that can readily be implemented in the field setting (e.g., portable spirometers and peak flow meters) usually assess symptom and illness histories. These epidemiologic approaches have limitations. Accurate estimation of exposure to a pollutant is typically difficult and limited by feasibility and cost, and many outdoor pollutants occur as components of complex mixtures. Potential confounding factors include environmental agents other than the pollutant of concern (e.g., cigarette smoking) and factors that influence the susceptibility of subjects (e.g., health status, medication). Data on confounding and modifying factors may not be readily available.

### Risk Assessment

Health risk assessment is increasingly used as a method for developing a summary estimate of the impact of air pollutants and other environmental agents on the health of the nation. The concepts of health risk assessment, a four-step process, were described in a 1983 report by a committee of the National Research Council (27). The first step is hazard identification: agents that pose a risk are identified through controlled human studies, animal bioassay, or epidemiologic observations. Second, the dose-response relationship is established to quantify the risk per unit exposure. Third, the magnitude and frequency of human exposure is determined. Fourth, by combining the dose-response relationship with the data on exposure, the magnitude of the health problem is estimated. The Clean Air Act amendments of 1990 mandated two additional activities on risk assessment: the National Research Council's Committee on Risk Assessment Methodology (28), and the Presidential Commission on

Risk Assessment. The report of the latter emphasized the need to consider variability and uncertainty in risk assessment, while the former called for greater public engagement of the risk assessment process.

The task of assembling and synthesizing data and constructing a risk model is useful for identifying uncertainties in the scientific evidence that may require resolution. When risk assessments are performed on various pollutants, the relative hazards can be compared and used as a basis for establishing priorities (29).

## EXPOSURES AND HEALTH EFFECTS OF SPECIFIC OUTDOOR AIR POLLUTANTS

### Carbon Monoxide

#### *Sources and Exposure*

Because of its many sources, carbon monoxide (CO) is a ubiquitous air pollutant in the urban environment. It is produced during the combustion of carbonaceous material, including gasoline, natural gas, oil, coal, wood, and tobacco. The principal source of carbon monoxide in outdoor air is motor vehicle emissions. In some areas of the country, wood burned for heating may be an important contributor to ambient levels. The concentrations of carbon monoxide in ambient air vary much, owing to the great spatial and temporal variability associated with its sources (30).

Substantial data on the personal exposures of urban dwellers are available from the U.S. EPA monitoring surveys of residents of Denver, Colorado, and Washington, D.C. (31), and from other studies. Low ambient levels (less than 1 ppm) are typically observed in outdoor settings away from active roadways, such as some parks and recreation areas. Outdoor concentrations tend to increase with motor vehicle density (e.g., downtown areas) and tend to be elevated in the air of the passenger compartments of motor vehicles (32). Exposure to carbon monoxide is greatest during commuting and in proximity to operating motor vehicles (31). The concentration in the passenger compartment of an automobile typically averages 5 ppm. Outdoor levels near roadways and parking areas average 3 to 4 ppm. Relatively higher levels may be encountered traveling in heavy traffic: peak levels to 50 ppm may occur in a background of approximately 10 ppm (32). Because of the reliance on motor vehicles for transportation in urban areas, automobile exhaust represents the single greatest contributing source to total personal exposure (31).

In comparison to exposure during travel in automobiles, indoor levels in residences and public buildings are generally low. In the absence of unvented combustion appliances, indoor levels are usually equal to local outdoor concentrations. During the winter of 1982–1983, residential exposure in Washington, D.C., and Denver averaged less than 2 ppm (31). The most commonly used unvented natural gas appliance, the cooking range, is not a strong source, even if the residence is poorly ventilated (31). Neither has tobacco smoke been found to be an important source of carbon monoxide exposure in homes (31). Carbon monoxide can accumulate because of the presence of stronger sources, including improperly vented or malfunctioning furnaces, kerosene space heaters (33), and charcoal fires for heating (34). In public buildings concentrations of 2 to 4 ppm have been found to be typical (31). The fact that this level is slightly higher than those in private residences is probably attributable to the activity of motor vehicles in the areas immediately surrounding public buildings. Levels exceeding the 9-ppm 8-hour federal standard for ambient air have been observed in a Honolulu shopping mall with an attached garage (35). Elevated indoor levels were also observed in a Washington, D.C. office building with an underground parking garage (36).

Personal exposure to high levels of carbon monoxide in outdoor settings may occur during the use of equipment and appliances powered by small gasoline engines (37). Important sources include lawn mowers, edgers and trimmers, chain saws, and snow blowers. These tools may be used for prolonged sessions of work, and because they are handheld, the user is close to the exhaust plume. Further, high concentrations of carbon monoxide may accumulate when such equipment is used in sheltered or partially enclosed areas. High levels have also been measured in the air of ice hockey rinks, which is contaminated by emissions from resurfacing machines (37).

#### *Health Effects*

When inhaled, carbon monoxide diffuses across the lung epithelium into the blood and reversibly binds to hemoglobin, taking over binding sites for oxygen. Hemoglobin's affinity for carbon monoxide is approximately 200 times greater than that for oxygen (38). Additionally, in the presence of carbon monoxide, allosteric changes take place on the hemoglobin molecule (39), causing leftward shift of the oxyhemoglobin dissociation curve (40) (Fig. 1). Thus, inhalation of carbon monoxide decreases the oxygen-carrying capacity of the blood and also the ability of tissues to extract oxygen from the hemoglobin at low partial pressures. Tissues that are most sensitive to low oxygen stress—the brain (41) and the heart (42)—are regarded as particularly vulnerable to hypoxia induced by the presence of carbon monoxide. Carbon monoxide may also interfere with intracellular oxygen transport in muscle; it has been shown to bind to myoglobin and cytochrome P-450 (43).

Sustained exposure to high concentrations of carbon monoxide, particularly indoors, may lead to poisoning, and ultimately death. A carboxyhemoglobin saturation level of 50% is generally regarded as sufficient to cause coma and death (43). Analysis of death certificate data

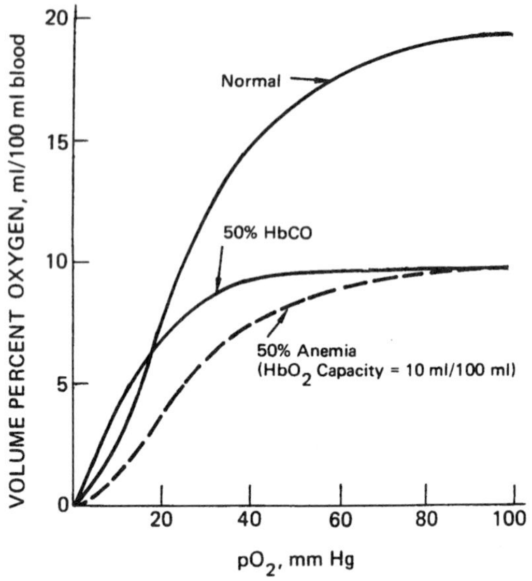


**FIG. 1.** Oxyhemoglobin dissociation curve for blood containing nominal levels of carbon monoxide, and blood 50% saturated with carbon monoxide. The effect of 50% anemia is presented for comparison. (From ref. 40.)

for 1977 through 1988 indicate that 11,547 deaths occurred nationally from carbon monoxide exposures that could not be attributed to suicide, homicide, or house fire (44). Most of these deaths were associated with asphyxiation by indoor exposures to exhaust from running autos, but 1,199 deaths were attributed to the use of coal, kerosene, or wood in a heating appliance (e.g., wood-burning stoves, kerosene space heaters), and another 1,047 deaths were attributed to carbon monoxide exposure from improperly vented furnaces and heaters using natural gas fuels. Fortunately, there appears to be a decreasing trend in the annual incidence rates of unintentional carbon monoxide poisoning associated with nonvehicular sources. The clinical manifestations of subacute poisoning (less than 50% saturation) reflect the underlying hypoxic processes associated with high carboxyhemoglobin levels. They range from headache, fatigue, and flu-like symptoms to chest pain, cardiac arrhythmia, and myocardial infarction. The sequelae and diagnosis of subacute carbon monoxide poisoning are well described elsewhere (45–48).

Most outdoor levels are too low to produce clinical symptoms but outdoor carbon monoxide does penetrate indoors and can contribute to elevating carboxyhemoglobin saturation levels. In the 1976 to 1980 National Health and Nutrition Examination Survey, the wintertime mean carboxyhemoglobin level in nonsmokers was 1.2%, and levels in excess of 2% were observed in 3% to 4% of the general population (49). This finding indicates that a substantial proportion of the population was exposed at the time to carbon monoxide levels that exceed the 9-ppm 8-hour and 35-ppm 1-hour federal standards for ambient air. These time-averaged standards were chosen to keep carboxyhemoglobin levels from rising above 2%.

Low-level exposures have been the focus of most recent health effects studies. In particular, these studies have tended to focus on subpopulations whose cardiovascular or respiratory health is compromised. Susceptible groups include people with ischemic heart disease (IHD), peripheral vascular disease, and chronic obstructive pulmonary disease (COPD). For each of these groups, exercise testing has been used to evaluate exercise capacity after exposures to carbon monoxide sufficient to elevate carboxyhemoglobin levels into the 2% to 6% range. Most of the studies employed double-blind crossover experimental designs, comparing exercise performance after exposure to carbon monoxide to performance after exposure to clean air. The responses evaluated in heart patients include the interval to onset of angina pectoris and ST-segment depression on the electrocardiogram (ECG), and in patients with intermittent claudication, reduction in interval to leg pain. In the testing of COPD patients, the maximum distance walked during progressive treadmill exercise has been used. In most studies, the subject selection criteria have involved testing to demonstrate the reproducibility of the specific response during exercise testing and have excluded current smokers.

In patients with exertional angina, earlier onset of angina pectoris and ST-segment depression have been consistently observed at carboxyhemoglobin levels of 2% to 4% by several investigative teams (50–52). In the largest of these studies, the Health Effects Institute multicenter carbon monoxide study (52), 5% and 12% decreases in the time to onset of ST-segment depression were observed at carboxyhemoglobin levels of 2% and 4%, respectively. Significant decreases in time to onset of angina, 4% and 7%, were also demonstrated at these respective carboxyhemoglobin levels. Findings for the objective ECG end point and subjective end point of chest pain yielded consistent results and are compatible with the hypothesis that an elevated carboxyhemoglobin level impairs the response of the myocardium to increased metabolic demands.

Another manifestation of myocardial ischemia is ventricular arrhythmia (53,54). Myocardial hypoxia caused by carbon monoxide has been postulated to be a mechanism of sudden death (55). Animal models (56–58) have provided limited and mixed information on the arrhythmogenic potential of carbon monoxide. The experimental design in these studies included induction of myocardial infarction followed by exposure to produce carboxyhemoglobin levels as high as 20%. Current evidence suggests no effect at carboxyhemoglobin levels up to 5% to 6% in patients with coronary artery disease and no baseline ectopy at rest (59), but is inconclusive for patients with baseline ectopy (60,61). Clinical studies have used carboxyhemoglobin levels more typical of the urban exposure range. Sheps and colleagues (60) investigated the arrhythmogenic potential of carbon monoxide in a group of 41 men and women with clinically established ischemic heart disease and a mixed history of ventricular ectopy. A 32% increase in the rates of ventricular arrhythmia during cycle exercise was observed after chamber exposure to 200 ppm carbon monoxide for 1 hour (mean carboxyhemoglobin 5.3%) relative to filtered room air but not after exposure to 100 ppm for 1 hour. At neither level of exposure was there a significant difference in the rate of ventricular ectopy as measured by ambulatory ECG during the 6 hours after exposure and exercise.

Epidemiologic studies provide limited support for the hypothesis that ambient carbon monoxide aggravates myocardial ischemia. Several studies have reported associations between ambient carbon monoxide levels and hospital admissions for cardiorespiratory disease (62–65); however, causal inferences cannot confidently be made. Most of the investigations have relied on estimates of personal exposure derived from measurements made at outdoor monitoring stations. Because correlations between central site measurements and personal exposures are poor for carbon monoxide (31), substantial exposure misclassification probably occurred in these designs. Furthermore, the study designs may have been confounded by unknown or uncontrolled factors, including cigarette smoking and medications.

In an occupational study (66) of tunnel and bridge workers in New York City, employment records and historical monitoring records were used to retrospectively classify exposure during the period 1952 to 1981. Exposure classification was validated by personal monitoring of contemporary workers. A standardized mortality ratio of 1.35 for cardiovascular causes of death was observed for the high exposure group (tunnel workers) when compared to the low exposure group (bridge workers). This statistical association was supported by the observed decrease in mortality among workers transferred from tunnels to bridges. The results of this study imply that short-term repeated carbon monoxide exposure may be associated with excess mortality from heart disease.

Controlled clinical studies have also been conducted on patients with COPD. Subjects with severe COPD are believed to be at risk for development of elevated carboxyhemoglobin levels because of reduced ability to eliminate carbon monoxide owing to decreased ventilatory capacity. However, the evidence for effects of carbon monoxide on exercise performance in this potentially susceptible subgroup is limited. Calverley and co-workers (67) observed a 7% reduction in the distance walked in 12 minutes after exposure to 200 ppm carbon monoxide for 20 to 30 minutes; however, because the order of exposure and testing was not randomized, the effect could be attributed to fatigue.

Because of the sensitivity of the central nervous system to hypoxia, several clinical studies have evaluated the impairment of vigilance, perception, and the performance of complex tasks after exposure to low concentrations of carbon monoxide. The results of these investigations have been inconsistent (68) and are potentially attributable to methodologic differences in the neurobehavioral end-point measurements and differences in carbon monoxide exposure protocols and measurement of carboxyhemoglobin levels. Varying effects on visual perception (69), auditory perception (70), manual dexterity (71), and vigilance (68) have been reported, but in normal subjects clinically important neurobehavioral deficits have not been observed below 10% carboxyhemoglobin.

Finally, limited animal toxicology data have implicated carbon monoxide as an agent that causes lower birth weight and increased fetal and neonatal mortality (72). A case-control study of birth weight and maternal exposure to ambient carbon monoxide during the last trimester of pregnancy demonstrated an odds ratio of 1.5 at a mean neighborhood outdoor level of at least 3 ppm, compared to lower levels (73). The accuracy of this finding is limited by failure to control for maternal smoking and potential misclassification of personal exposure because outdoor monitoring data were used.

The findings of controlled exposure studies, when viewed with the evidence for widespread exposures to carbon monoxide in urban populations, suggest that several groups may be at risk for adverse health effects. Although concentrations of carbon monoxide in the outdoor environment are generally low, the prolonged exposure may nevertheless lead to development of carboxyhemoglobin levels at which health effects have been clinically demonstrated for susceptible persons. Because of the prevalence of cardiovascular disease, chronic respiratory disease, and pregnancy in the population, these adverse health effects assume public health importance.

## Nitrogen Dioxide

### *Sources and Exposure*

High-temperature combustion processes generate nitric oxide (NO) and, to a lesser extent, nitrogen dioxide ($NO_2$). In turn, nitric oxide is converted to nitrogen dioxide through oxidation reactions involving oxygen, ozone, and organic compounds (74). Nitrogen dioxide is highly reactive and in the presence of sunlight combines with hydrocarbons to form ozone and other photochemical species. Additionally, nitrogen dioxide may react with aerosols to form nitrous and nitric acids and contribute to secondary acidic particles (75).

The principal source of nitric oxide and nitrogen dioxide in outdoor air is motor vehicle emissions, but power plants and fossil fuel-burning industries may also contribute. In most U.S. cities, ambient levels of nitrogen dioxide vary with traffic density. For example, in the Los Angeles area, Spengler and colleagues (76) used passive diffusion samplers to obtain 48-hour integrated mean measurements of outdoor air at the homes of a population-based sample of Los Angeles residents. In coastal, mountain, and desert areas, where traffic density is lowest, nitrogen dioxide concentrations ranged from 0.007 to 0.040 ppm. In highly urbanized areas of the Los Angeles basin nitrogen dioxide concentrations averaged 0.011 to 0.065 ppm. Lower ambient levels than those in Los Angeles have been measured in Boston, Massachusetts (77), Portage, Wisconsin (78), and Albuquerque, New Mexico (79). During the winter, mean outdoor levels range from 0.007 to 0.015 ppm. These lower levels are probably attributable to lower traffic density and weather differences. In 1997, all areas in the United States reporting $NO_2$ monitoring data were in attainment of the National Ambient Air Quality Standard for $NO_2$.

Indoor levels of nitrogen dioxide are determined by air exchange, the infiltration of outdoor air, and the presence and strength of indoor sources. The contribution of outdoor exposures to indoor residential concentrations has been estimated at approximately 50% by regression models (76,78,79). Unvented combustion sources, including cooking ranges (80) and kerosene space heaters (81), emit nitric oxide and nitrogen dioxide, adding to the background from outdoor air. Because over half of the residences in the United States have gas cooking stoves and Americans spend a large proportion of time in their homes (81), the residential environment is generally regarded as the most important source of the population's total exposure to nitrogen dioxide (76,77,82).

### *Health Effects*

Inhaled nitrogen dioxide is postulated to combine with water in the lung to form nitric and nitrous acids, which are believed to damage the lung epithelium via oxidation mechanisms (83). Dosimetric modeling suggests that nitrogen dioxide is absorbed principally in the large and small airways and that little is deposited in the alveoli (84,85). At extremely high concentrations, greater than 200 ppm, nitrogen dioxide causes extensive lung injury, including fatal pulmonary edema and bronchopneumonia (86).

Oxidant injury also occurs at lower concentrations, affecting the defense mechanisms of the lung, including mucociliary clearance, particle transport and detoxification by alveolar macrophages, and local immunity (87,88). In animal experiments involving challenge with bacteria and viruses, exposure to nitrogen dioxide reduces clearance of infecting pathogens and increases mortality. In these infectivity studies, the adverse effects have been demonstrated at concentrations that are an order of magnitude greater than those generally found in the urban setting. Further, it is difficult to extrapolate the results of these animal studies to humans.

Few infectivity studies have been done on human subjects. In one example, Goings and colleagues (89) investigated the effects of acute nitrogen dioxide exposures of 1 to 3 ppm on 152 young, nonsmoking adults. A randomized crossover design was used, which included a placebo exposure. Following 2-hour exposures on 3 successive days, subjects were inoculated intranasally with live attenuated influenza A virus. Respiratory tract symptoms were tracked, and nasal washings and blood sera were collected before inoculation and daily for 4 days thereafter. Few subjects developed respiratory symptoms as a result of this exposure. During the first 2 years of the investigation there were no statistically significant differences in antibody titers in either the serum or nasal wash specimens. However, in year 3, 90% of subjects developed an antibody response to exposure, compared to 70% of those exposed to placebo. While these results are suggestive of an effect, they are limited by the small sample size and the possibility that susceptibility to infection may have varied across the 3 years because of immunity acquired from natural influenza infections.

From a public health perspective the relatively high concentrations and lengthy exposures used in animal and clinical studies are not representative of exposure in the community. Daily average personal exposure levels as high as 0.065 ppm may occur (76). Few data exist on the frequency and level of transient elevated exposures during daily activities. Brief exposure to concentrations as high as 0.500 ppm may be experienced while cooking with a gas stove or driving in traffic (90); elevated levels are also expected when an unvented gas space heater is operated, but such elevated levels generally are not sustained.

Several epidemiologic studies have attempted to examine the relation between respiratory tract illness and symptoms and ambient levels. In an early study, Shy and colleagues (91,92) tracked the respiratory tract symptoms of 871 families (4,043 individuals) selected from five schools situated near a munitions factory in Chattanooga, Tennessee. The mean 24-hour ambient nitrogen dioxide level in the high-exposure area was 0.083 ppm, 0.063 ppm in the intermediate area, and 0.043 ppm in the low area. Total suspended particulate and sulfate concentrations were similar across the three areas. Responses to biweekly questionnaires indicated that the rates of acute respiratory tract illness were higher among the families living in the relatively high-exposure area, although the rates were not consistently correlated with the exposure gradient among the three schools in the high-exposure area. Differences in family size, income, or education could not explain the observed associations. Parental smoking habits did not appear to influence the illness rates among children. The effects on the parents of smoking status were not reported.

In a subsequent study in the same Chattanooga community, Pearlman, Shy, and colleagues (93) focused on lower respiratory tract infections in 3,217 schoolchildren and infants. Physician office records were used to validate parents' reports of illness. A history of one or more episodes of bronchitis was reported significantly more often for schoolchildren who lived for 2 or 3 years in the areas of high and intermediate levels of ambient nitrogen dioxide. This pattern was not observed in the infants, and no significant difference in incidence rates was observed in the areas of high and intermediate levels of nitrogen dioxide. The incidence of croup and pneumonia did not differ significantly among the three exposure areas. Controls for socioeconomic status and parental smoking were not mentioned.

More recently, in a large study of air pollution in Switzerland, respiratory symptoms of 625 children were monitored on a daily basis (94). Symptom incidence rates were not associated with indoor and outdoor $NO_2$ concentrations but duration of symptom episodes was associated with outdoor $NO_2$ concentration.

The relation between respiratory illness and symptoms and nitrogen dioxide exposure has been studied more frequently in the indoor setting. Reports of serious respiratory illness (95,96) and hospitalization before age 2 years for respiratory tract illness (97) have been reported to be more common among children from homes with gas stoves; however, in other cross-sectional studies no association has been observed between type of cooking stove and current respiratory tract symptoms or illness history (98). The results of prospective study designs are similarly inconsistent (99–101). Difficult methodologic problems have limited the informativeness of these studies (101). Small sample size, inadequate control of potential confounding factors (e.g., presence of other children in the household, day-care attendance, breast-feeding, exposure to tobacco smoke, socioeconomic status), and potential misclassification of exposure and outcome call into question the validity and limit the interpretation of these investigations.

These methodologic concerns were addressed in a large prospective cohort study of infants in Albuquerque, New Mexico (102). Exposures to nitrogen dioxide and respiratory illnesses were monitored from birth to 18 months of age in over 1,000 infants. In multivariate analyses that controlled for potential confounding factors, no consistent trends in incidence or duration of illness were observed by level of nitrogen dioxide exposure.

A meta-analysis of studies conducted to 1990, however, showed a significant effect of nitrogen dioxide on the respiratory health of children (103). This meta-analysis can be questioned because it grouped infants, preschoolers, and schoolchildren, and used diverse health end points (104).

Decreases in lung function as the result of low-level nitrogen dioxide exposure have not been consistently demonstrated in epidemiologic studies of indoor exposure in the general population (15,105–109). Clinical studies suggest that short-term exposure may affect pulmonary function and the degree of nonspecific airways responsiveness in asthma patients and in normal subjects (82). For example, Frampton and co-workers (110) reported that 3-hour exposure during exercise of subjects without airway hyperactivity to 1.5 ppm nitrogen dioxide increases airway reactivity to carbachol. In this study, intermittent peak exposures were simulated by repeated 15-minute exposures to 2.0 ppm nitrogen dioxide; this schedule did not alter airway reactivity. However, there has been little consistency across studies reported to date (5). Of ten studies of asthmatics considered in the review by the American Thoracic Society, nine showed no effect of nitrogen dioxide exposure. Varying approaches to subject selection and small sample sizes constrain interpretation of these studies. Older persons and persons with COPD have also been investigated with little indication of heightened susceptibility (111).

The results of the epidemiologic and clinical studies of the effects of outdoor and indoor exposures must be cautiously interpreted (82). In outdoor air, nitrogen dioxide does not occur in isolation but as part of a complex mixture of pollutants, so failure to control for the effects of other toxicants may confuse interpretation of the effect. Studies have been mostly limited to nitrogen dioxide and other gaseous products associated with it, such as nitrous acid (10,74), may be directly responsible for the health effects. The contribution of nitrogen dioxide to secondary particles and its role in the formation of ozone may be more relevant to public health than any direct effect of the gas.

## Ozone

### *Sources and Exposure*

Ozone ($O_3$) is an oxidant gas generated in the atmosphere by chemical reactions of volatile organic compounds (VOCs) and nitrogen oxides ($NO_x$) in the presence of sunlight (74). Ambient levels of ozone vary from area to area and by time of day, depending on the mix of precursor compounds and meteorologic conditions (112).

In most urban areas, the major source of $NO_x$ emissions is motor vehicles and utility and industry boilers. VOCs are emitted in auto exhaust and through the evaporation of solvents and gasoline. In some regions, such as the southeastern United States, natural vegetation may produce substantial quantities of VOCs (113). Efforts to reduce ozone levels by implementing controls on manmade sources have had limited success because they require humans to make basic changes in a wide variety of activities, including transportation, electrical power generation, fossil fuel use, industrial processes, and manufacturing (8). In approximately 100 urban areas the concentrations of ozone exceed the National Ambient Air Quality Standard currently set at a peak 1-hour average concentration of 0.12 ppm (8). The National Research Council (113a) has argued that further reductions in ozone concentrations will only be possible with targeted, site-specific $NO_x$ controls.

Elevated concentrations of ozone are most often observed in summer, when sunlight is most intense and temperatures highest, conditions that increase the rate of photochemical smog formation (112). Substantial diurnal variations are commonly observed with ozone levels generally being lowest in the morning hours, accumulating through midday, and decreasing rapidly after sunset (114). This diurnal pattern in many urban areas reflects the production of ozone at the ground level by sunlight. Similar diurnal patterns are observed in rural areas as transported ozone is mixed down to the ground by convection in the middle of the day.

While ozone concentrations may be elevated in outdoor air, they are substantially lower indoors where ozone reacts rapidly with surfaces (114,115). As outdoor air moves into buildings ozone is removed by reactions with water on walls, fabric, and other surfaces. The lower indoor concentrations are attributed to the reaction of ozone with surfaces. Mechanical ventilation systems also remove ozone during conditioning processes. For these reasons, staying indoors or closing automobile windows and using air conditioning are generally recognized to protect against exposure to ambient ozone (116).

For many people outdoor exposure is limited because the majority of time is spent indoors. However, the occupations and activities of some groups are expected to place them at risk for high exposure because they spend a lot of time outdoors. These groups include construction and landscape workers, public works employees, and children playing outdoors. Furthermore, the increased breathing rates associated with many of these outdoor activities increase the delivery of large doses of ozone to the lung. During periods of high ozone concentration, health agencies issue warnings to avoid exertion when outdoors, and the outdoor activities of schoolchildren are canceled (116).

There is considerable variability in ozone levels across the United States. High levels are most common in Southern California. One population exposure model (117), which combined data on subjects' activity patterns and locations with outdoor monitoring data, estimated that virtually every person in Los Angeles is exposed to concentrations exceeding the 120 parts per billion (ppb) standard for at least 1 hour each year. Because health effects vary with exercise level, estimates of exposure were made by level of exertion. At low exercise levels, it was estimated that 97% of the population of the Los Angeles area was exposed to ozone levels in excess of 120 ppb for 22 hours per person per year; 30% of the population of Los Angeles was estimated to spend 14 hours exercising vigorously at exposure levels in excess of the annual standard. These estimates indicate that prolonged exposures to high ozone concentrations are probable for a large proportion of the population living in Los Angeles.

### *Health Effects*

Short-term exposures to ozone, at concentrations frequently observed in the ambient air, have been shown to produce immediate but transient decreases in lung function and increases in respiratory symptoms in both healthy adults and susceptible subgroups of the population (118). Long-term exposure is suspected to contribute to the development of chronic lung diseases, including asthma and chronic bronchitis, and to accelerate aging of the lung. In the remainder of this section the evidence on the health effects of ozone is reviewed. More complete reviews are available elsewhere (119–121).

The effects of ozone on lung function have been evaluated in numerous experimental studies in which exercising human subjects have been exposed in chambers. Decrements in measures of lung function and physical performance, and aggravation of respiratory tract symptoms, have been clearly demonstrated at exposure levels as low as 120 ppb. In healthy young adult subjects, intense and sustained exercise is required to provoke changes in forced expiratory volume in 1 second ($FEV_1$) and in forced vital capacity (FVC) (122–124). Significant losses in lung function, and symptoms of cough and pain with deep breathing, have been observed after prolonged exposure to concentrations of 120 and 80 ppb. In extended exposures (6.6 hours), healthy young adults performing moderate exercise had an average 7% decline in $FEV_1$ after exposure to ozone concentrations of 80 ppb (125). The individual changes in $FEV_1$ relative to exercise in clean air ranged from -26% to +8%, indicative of the great between-person variability in response observed in most studies. These results suggest that athletes, outdoor workers, and others who engage in prolonged exercise outdoors may be at risk for adverse health effects at ozone concentrations near the ambient standard and typical of summertime levels in some cities.

Similar acute, reversible changes in $FEV_1$ and FVC have been observed in exercising children exposed to concentrations as low as 0.12 ppm (126,127). The results of clinical studies on other subgroups posited to be susceptible have been mixed. The lung function and symptom responses of asthmatics and patients with COPD do not appear to differ from those of healthy subjects (128–130).

Transient respiratory symptoms, including cough, throat irritation, and pain on respiration are reported after these controlled exposures to $O_3$. The time course of the increased symptoms is similar to that for lung function changes. Moreover, there is considerable between-subject variability in respiratory symptoms, as in the lung function response.

Ozone exposure produces increased airway responsiveness as measured by reduction in lung function following challenge with bronchoconstricting drugs such as methacholine or histamine. Ozone concentrations as low as 200 ppb for 1 hour or 80 ppb for 6.6 hours have been reported to cause small but statistically significant increases in bronchial responsiveness in healthy young adults (125,131).

There is evidence from human studies that alveolar macrophage antimicrobial defense functions are impaired after exposure to $O_3$. Moderately exercising adults exposed to 80 ppb ozone for 6.6 hours have reduced pulmonary macrophage function (131).

The acute respiratory tract effects of short-term variations in ambient ozone have been evaluated in several epidemiologic studies. In so-called summer camp studies on children who were spending large amounts of time outdoors, short-term decrements in $FEV_1$ and peak expiratory flow have been associated with exposure to ozone. A reanalysis of six of these studies found a combined estimate of a 0.50 ml decrease in $FEV_1$/ppb $O_3$ (132). These effects are similar in magnitude to those seen under controlled exposure conditions. A recent study analyzed air pollution effects among moderate to severe asthmatic children attending summer asthma camps in Connecticut (133). Ozone exposures (maximum 1 hour 160 ppb) were associated with decreased peak flow, increased respiratory symptoms, and increased medication use.

Numerous studies in the eastern United States and Canada have reported that ambient $O_3$ exposures are associated with increased hospital admissions (134–137) and emergency room visits (138,139).

Schwartz (140–144) has analyzed the association between daily respiratory hospital admissions among the elderly based on Medicare data and ozone exposures in several U.S. cities. Positive, generally statistically significant associations were found with ozone exposures for pneumonia, for COPD, and for all respiratory admissions.

Epidemiologic associations have also been reported between ozone episodes and increased acute mortality. These analyses have been controversial since in many cases apparent associations with ozone were apparently due to failure to consider concurrent particle exposures (145,146). Recently, Samet et al. (147) have analyzed daily mortality in Philadelphia for the years 1973 to 1980 to assess the effects of multiple air pollutants (TSP, ozone, sulfur dioxide, nitrogen dioxide, and carbon monoxide). They report statistically significant associations between ozone and daily mortality that are independent of the effects of the other pollutants. A 20-ppb increase in daily mean ozone was associated with a 1.9% increase in total daily mortality, 1.1% increase in cardiovascular mortality (not statistically significant), 2.5% increase in respiratory mortality (not significant), and 2.5% in other causes. Verhoeff et al. (148) reported positive, statistically significant associations between daily mortality in Amsterdam and ozone exposures 2 days prior. These positive ozone associations were also seen after adjusting for particulate matter smaller than 10 μg aerodynamic diameter ($PM_{10}$), although they were no longer statistically significant. Thus there is new suggestive evidence that the daily mortality may be associated with ozone exposures, independently of the effects of particulate air pollution.

The evidence for widespread exposure of the population to ozone concentrations linked with acute changes by clinical studies has raised concern for possible long-term effects. The results of animal studies show that chronic low-level exposure to ozone can produce both air space enlargement and subtle fibrosis of the small airways (121). These findings indicate the importance of and support for the need for additional longitudinal and cross-sectional populations studies to look for evidence of excessive obstructive airways impairment, not only among residents of perennially $O_3$-polluted areas such as the Los Angeles basin, but also in the majority of U.S. metropolitan areas where elevated ozone exposures are still observed.

## Lead

### *Sources and Exposure*

Of the several metals present in motor vehicle exhaust, lead has received the greatest attention. The use of akyl-lead fuel additives in gasoline has resulted in widespread dispersion of this metal throughout the biosphere (149). Humans may develop a significant body burden from inhaling airborne lead (150). Inhaled lead aerosols, like other particles, are deposited in the lung by diffusion, sedimentation, and impaction. About 20% to 60% of inhaled lead particles are deposited in the adult human respiratory tract (151). The amount of deposition varies with rate and depth of respiration, and the age and sex of the person, which determines the size of the airways. Most of the deposited lead is cleared by phagocytosis by alveolar macrophages and absorption into the systemic circulation (152). Lead particles ingested by macrophages are also cleared by the mucociliary blanket and swallowed. Approximately 10% are absorbed in the gastrointestinal tract by adults, and more by children (151). Airborne lead can also contribute to exposure through household dust and garden soil contamination from the fallout of airborne lead particles. Exposure to nonairborne lead may occur via contaminated drinking water or food or, in older housing, lead-based paints (when children eat paint chips or flakes) (150).

The removal of lead from gasoline has resulted in a significant reduction in both outdoor airborne lead con-

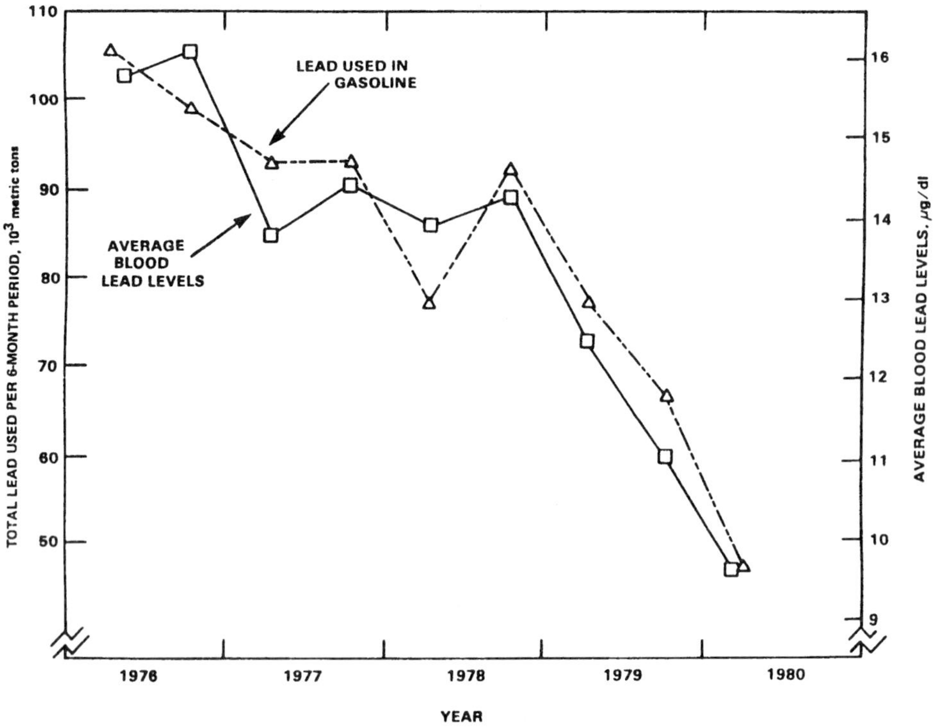


**FIG. 2.** Parallel decreases in blood lead and lead used in gasoline during 1976–1980. (From ref. 150.)

centrations and blood lead levels as measured in random samples of the population. Comparison of the mean blood levels observed in the second National Health and Nutrition Examination Survey conducted between 1976 and 1980 demonstrated a 37% decline in average blood lead levels as the total amount of lead used in gasoline was reduced by approximately half (150) (Fig. 2). Decreases in blood lead levels have also been observed near stationary sources that have reduced their emissions (153). Blood leads for the U.S. population have continued to decline with geometric means of 2.9 µg/dl reported for phase I of the National Health and Nutrition Examination Surveys (NHANES III) (conducted from October 1988 to September 1991) compared to 12.8 µg/dl for NHANES II (1976–1980) (154). The prevalence of blood lead levels greater than or equal to 10µg/dl decreased from 77.8% to 4.4% between these surveys. The Centers for Disease Control and Prevention (CDC) has recently reported that blood lead levels were further declined in phase 2 of NHANES III (1991–1994) to a geometric mean of 2.3 µg/dl with 2.2% of the sample above 10 µg/dl (CDC. Update: Blood lead levels—United States, 1991–1994. *MMWR* 1997;46:141–146). The decrease of lead in blood suggests that a substantial portion of personal exposure is associated with the inhalation and ingestion of airborne lead. The contribution of airborne lead to total blood levels has been estimated in the range of 7% to 40%, and 25% to 40% of inhaled lead is retained in bone tissue (151).

### *Health Effects*

Children are considered particularly susceptible to the adverse effects of lead because of smaller body size, higher rates of absorption through ingestion, and continuing growth. Animal and epidemiologic studies have demonstrated that low-level exposure has adverse effects on the development and function of the central nervous system. Low levels of lead in the blood have been associated with various behavioral disorders, including distractibility, inability to follow simple directions, and lower scores on IQ tests (155–159).

These associations are found even among asymptomatic children and after controlling for potential confounding factors (150). The literature on the neurobehavioral effects of long-term exposure of children to low levels of lead have been reviewed by several authors (160,161) and agencies (150,162). These meta-analyses have found a two-point decline in mean IQ associated with each 10- to 20-µg/dl increase in blood lead.

Lippmann (163) has suggested that the sensitivity of the brain to lead during the period of maximal brain growth and differentiation, in the first 2 years of life, may enhance the long-term consequences. Bellinger and colleagues (156) followed a cohort of healthy infants born to relatively affluent families after unremarkable pregnancies. Children were assigned to one of three exposure groups by the lead level in umbilical cord blood. The mental development test scores of the group with the highest cord blood levels were lower than those of the other two groups. In continued follow-up of these children, intellectual and academic performance at 10 years was inversely associated with blood leads measured at 24 months (164). Needleman and colleagues (155) reported on a cohort of 132 young adults whose levels of dentine lead were measured in primary school. Young people whose childhood dentine levels were greater than 20 ppm were found to be at a markedly higher risk of dropping out of high school (adjusted odds ratio 7.4) and having reading disabilities (adjusted odds ratio 5.8) than the low lead exposure group, whose dentine lead levels had been less than 10 ppm. Other measures of performance affected included vocabulary and grammatical reasoning, absenteeism, hand-eye coordination (poorer), and reaction time (slowed). Needleman and colleagues (165) have recently reported that school-aged boys with self-reported antisocial and delinquent behaviors had higher body burdens of lead measured by x-ray fluorescence of tibia bone at age 12 years. These studies suggest that lead has effects on neurobehavioral function that persist or are observed long after exposure.

Experimental studies have shown that exposures to moderate levels of lead increase blood pressure in vivo in animals (166). In various population studies blood lead concentrations in adults have been associated with increased blood pressure. This association was evaluated in the NHANES II random stratified sample of the U.S. population (167,168). From this survey, carefully standardized measurements of blood pressure measurements were available to compare to blood lead levels. The analysis was restricted to white males between age 20 and 74 years, and statistical adjustments were made for age, body mass index, nutritional factors, and blood chemistry. Significant increases in systolic and diastolic blood pressure were associated with increasing blood lead levels. A recent meta-analysis examined the results from 15 general population studies of the association of blood lead and blood pressure (169). Consistent, positive associations were found in all these studies. The combined effect estimate across all these studies indicated that a reduction in blood lead from 10 μg/dl to 5 μg/dl would be associated with a 1.25 mm Hg decrease in systolic blood pressure. Because blood lead levels were observed to decrease by 37% across the period of 1976 to 1980 covered by NHANES II, Pirkle and colleagues (167) estimated that this reduction in lead exposure would lead to a 17.5% reduction in the prevalence of hypertension (diastolic pressure at least 90 mm Hg) in white males aged 40 to 59 years.

The reduction of lead in air has greatly reduced exposure not only through respiration but also through swallowed dust, food, water, and beverages contaminated with lead deposited from air. However, some lead exposure will continue to occur from natural sources of lead and from past deposition of lead onto soil and into other media. Lead will continue to be an important public health concern despite reduced air exposures in the U.S. The body burden of lead will continue to have long-term sequelae. Moreover, leaded gasoline continues to be an important source of lead exposure in many parts of the world.

### Sulfur Oxides, Particulates, and Acid Aerosols

The sources, exposures, and health effects of sulfur oxides, particulate matter, and acid aerosols are presented together because, though these pollutants are physically distinct, they often have common sources, principally combustion processes (170). Primary particles come directly from combustion sources while secondary particles form from condensation and chemical reactions of gases released by combustion (6). The acid aerosols are generated by chemical reactions involving the combustion emissions, and sulfur and nitrogen oxides (75). Primary particles come directly from combustion sources, while secondary particles are formed in the atmosphere by physical and chemical processes. Further, particulate matter, sulfur oxides, and acid aerosols (e.g., sulfuric acid) may be surrogates for the actual cause of the observed health effects, possibly hydrogen ion ($H^+$), metals, or volatile organics (163,171). Thus, while sulfur dioxide is directly regulated under the Clean Air Act, many of the health effects of concern for this pollutant are likely to reflect the combined action of the diverse components of the pollutant mixture created by fossil fuel combustion.

#### *Sources and Exposure*

Sulfur is a natural contaminant of fossil fuels. Sulfur dioxide is produced by industrial processes involving fossil fuel combustion and by coal- and oil-fired power plants. Emissions increased steadily over the past century, to a peak of 32 million tons in 1970, and declined following enactment that year of the Clean Air Act. Although stable at 23 million tons per year, sulfur dioxide emissions are expected to increase during the next several decades (172).

Sulfur and nitrogen oxides released into the atmosphere from anthropogenic sources are oxidized during airborne transport to sulfuric and nitric acid (173). Reactions can occur when the pollutants exist as gases, are dissolved in liquids, or adhere to the surfaces of particles and water droplets. The specific physicochemical pathways followed depend on the concentration and mix of pollutants, and various physical factors such as wind speed and mixing, sunlight intensity, temperature, and liquid water content of the air mass.

Until the recent use of tall stacks, sulfur oxides were released from smokestacks relatively close to the ground, and deposition and reactions with the landscape occurred close to the stack (10). Under these release conditions, reactions with surfaces tended to remove the sulfur oxides within short distances of the source. Following the passage of the 1970 Clean Air Act in the United States, many sources of sulfur dioxide emissions, particularly large power plants located in rural areas, installed tall stacks that release the pollutants above the inversion layer to reduce mixing to the ground. Consequently, the effect of local removal processes has been reduced and the production of acid aerosols through homogeneous gas- and aqueous-phase reactions in plumes has been facilitated. Thus, the scope of concern for adverse effects of sulfur oxides has moved from local to regional exposure. Further, the seasonal cycle of elevated concentrations has changed from winter to summer, when substantial acid aerosol and sulfate concentrations are associated with increased electrical power generation and more intense sunlight.

Particulate matter, released into the ambient air from a variety of sources, is composed of dust and pollen, and of soot and aerosols from combustion activities such as agricultural burning, transportation, manufacturing, and power generation. Typically, suspended particles in the atmosphere are bimodally distributed with respect to size. The larger fraction, 3 to 30 μg in aerodynamic diameter, usually consists of geologic (crustal) materials, generally of natural origin and alkaline in total pH. Biologic particles, including pollens and spores, are found among these large particles. The smaller particles, less than 3 μg aerodynamic diameter, are mainly anthropogenic and generally are composed of acid condensates of combustion processes. Sulfate and nitrate aerosols are found in this size range and generally make up the largest fraction of these particles by mass. Particles less than 2 to 3 μm in aerodynamic diameter tend to deposit in the airways and alveoli of the lung, while larger particles deposit in the upper airway.

The regulation of particulate pollution has evolved over the past several decades from considering total suspended particulates (TSP), which included all suspended particles with only an ill-defined upper size limit, to a size-restricted inhaled particle standard (174). Larger particles are removed in the upper airways but small particles may be deposited deep in the lungs, in the terminal bronchioles and alveolar air spaces. In 1987, the EPA restricted the National Ambient Air Quality Standard to $PM_{10}$. This cutoff point focused monitoring and regulatory effort on a more biologically relevant size fraction of particles than TSP. Refinements in the classification of inhalable particulate matter continue and there are now substantial data on specific acidic sulfate aerosols, including sulfuric acid ($H_2SO_4$), ammonium bisulfate ($NH_4HSO_4$), and letovicite $(NH_4)_3H(SO_4)_2$. From the perspective of public health, acidic species, metals, and other constituents of particles are thought to be the cause of adverse effects of air pollution, rather than the particles generally.

In 1997, the EPA proposed two new standards, annual and 24-hour standards for particulate matter less than 2.5 μm in aerodynamic diameter. The proposal for these standards reflected new evidence on health effects and the understanding that particles in this size range penetrate into the airways and alveoli of the lung. These standards would be added to the existing standards for $PM_{10}$.

## *Health Effects*

The exposure of humans and animals to sulfur dioxide, particles, and acid aerosols has been associated with respiratory morbidity and mortality. These pollutants may be directly responsible for the health effects or may be surrogate measures of the toxic components of particulate matter (163,171). This section emphasizes the newer epidemiologic evidence, particularly in relation to particles and acid aerosols. Extensive reviews of the earlier literature, which tended to use less refined measures of exposure, have been published (2,170); newer studies are covered in a recent book (6).

### *Ambient Exposure and Mortality*

Historically, high concentrations of particles and sulfur dioxide have been associated with substantial short-term increases in morbidity and mortality in the air pollution episodes (see Table 1). The sudden increases in morbidity and mortality that accompanied these episodes, and the frequency and severity of respiratory tract complaints, left little doubt that pollution exposure caused the adverse effects.

For example, during the December 1952 air pollution episode in London, England, there were an estimated 4,000 excess deaths in the metropolitan area, including 2,000 in London County (3,175). British Smoke measurements of particles had a maximum 24-hour average of about 4,000 μg/m$^3$; sulfur dioxide reached a maximum value of 1.5 ppm and an average of 0.95 ppm. These levels are at least tenfold greater than peaks found in most cities in the United States at present. Exactly 10 years later, in December 1962, a similar air pollution episode occurred (176). Sulfur dioxide concentrations peaked at about 1.5 ppm and averaged about 0.80 ppm during the episode. Particle concentrations were about 20% of those during the 1952 episode, but total excess deaths in this episode were only estimated to be 350 in London County. Thus, while sulfur dioxide concentrations were similar to the 1952 episode, particle concentrations and the number of excess deaths in the 1962 episode were much lower than in the earlier episode. This contrast suggests that excess deaths may have been more closely associated with particulate than with sulfur dioxide air pollution. The putative agent, sulfuric acid, would be expected to be present in the particulate fraction of the pollutant mixture (171).

These historic episodes were characterized by sulfur oxide and particulate pollution in the presence of fog, conditions known to favor catalytic oxidation and subsequent formation of acid aerosols. Commins and Waller (177) observed sulfuric acid concentrations as high as 199 $\mu g/m^3$ for 24 hours in February 1959, and 347 $\mu/m^3$ in December 1962. Regular daily measurements began during the winter of 1963–64 and continued through the winter of 1971–72. The highest concentrations occurred during the winter months, maximum daily means ranging from 20 to 30 $\mu/m^3$. In a recent reanalysis of the London mortality data for 1963 to 1972, stronger statistical associations of daily mortality with pollution were observed for sulfuric acid than for British Smoke or sulfur dioxide (24).

The acid component of the particulate fraction has been further implicated in another analysis of daily mortality in London during 1952 to 1972 (178). A significant positive association with both particulate and sulfur dioxide pollution was observed. When both pollutants were considered jointly, the association of particle levels was independent of sulfur dioxide concentration, while the sulfur dioxide effect was substantially diminished after controlling for particulate pollution.

Fortunately, air pollution episodes of this magnitude are no longer seen in the United States or Western Europe. However, particulate and sulfur oxide concentrations can be extremely high in many developing East European countries, and transport of this pollution to Western Europe during unusual meteorologic conditions in January 1985 was associated with increased respiratory tract morbidity in the United Kingdom (179) and in West Germany (180).

While days of extremely high air pollution with particles and sulfur oxides are now rare in developed countries, many studies reported during the 1990s have shown associations between daily mortality counts and measures of particulate air pollution (181,182). These time series studies have consistently demonstrated these associations at current levels of particulate pollution, after controlling for weather, season, and other factors. The consistency among these studies in showing association of mortality with particulate air pollution, across a range of levels of other pollutants, has led to the hypothesis that fine particles are causing this effect (182,183). The association does not appear to reflect methodologic limitations or uncontrolled confounding (147,184).

The extent to which this pattern of daily association reflects life shortening by particulate pollution has been controversial. Two studies indicate increased mortality for persons living in more polluted cities, even after taking account of potential confounding factors (185,186). In follow-up studies of 8,111 adults in the Harvard Six Cities Study, Dockery et al. (185) found about a 25% increased risk of dying over the 14 to 16 years of follow-up in residents of the most polluted city (Steubenville, OH) compared with the least polluted city (Portage, WI). Among 500,000 participants in the American Cancer Society's Cancer Prevention Study II (CPS-II), mortality was similarly associated with particulate pollution (186). In both studies, cardiopulmonary mortality was more strongly associated with particulate pollution than was total mortality, as would be expected on a clinical basis. These two studies have been interpreted as evidence that air pollution is not just advancing the time of death by days but having a longer-term effect on mortality. The studies of mortality figured centrally in the proposal for a new particulate matter standard by the EPA.

Mechanisms that could underlie the acute and chronic effects of particulate air pollution are presently unclear (187). Emphasis has been placed on the fine particles because of their deposition in the airways and alveoli. Seaton and colleagues (188) have hypothesized that alveolar deposition of ultrafine particles causes inflammation and release of systemically active cytokines. Airways inflammation and effects on lung defenses have also been postulated.

### *Ambient Exposure and Morbidity*

The findings on mortality are complemented by evidence on morbidity measures, including use of medical care facilities and individual-level effect indicators such as symptom rates and lung function levels. Particle exposure has been associated with increased hospitalization for respiratory tract illness and with other evidence of respiratory morbidity. Morbidity effects have been observed in association with previously described episodes of severe pollution. In London during the 1952 fog, hospitalization rates rose dramatically. During the 1985 European episode, increased hospitalization and ambulance calls were reported in Germany (180), and reduced pulmonary function was reported in children living in the Netherlands examined 16 days after an episode (189). This latter finding is consistent with the pattern of change in pulmonary function among children in Steubenville, Ohio, before, during, and following particulate and sulfur dioxide pollution episodes (190).

Many studies of morbidity from combustion-related air pollution, including particles, sulfur oxides, and acidic aerosols, have been reported (5). These studies have addressed acute and chronic effects and have been conducted at the population and individual levels. The principal study designs include time series and cross-sectional analyses of medical care usage in populations and cohort and cross-sectional studies of the respiratory health of individual participants, selected in some studies on the basis of heightened susceptibility to air pollution, e.g., asthmatics.

Several studies have been particularly informative. A series of studies was conducted in the Utah Valley, a region with winter episodes of high particulate pollution arising from operation of a steel mill and low sulfur dioxide, nitric oxide, and ozone concentrations. Hospital admissions of children for respiratory illnesses doubled in this community in winters when violations of $PM_{10}$ standards were recorded and dropped when the mill was temporarily closed (191,192). Schwartz and co-authors (189) reported an association between $PM_{10}$ concentrations and daily rates of lower respiratory tract symptoms in a diary study of school children in the Harvard Six Cities Study; during the time of the study, $PM_{10}$ concentrations were well below the ambient standard at all times. Dockery and colleagues (193) have also reported an association between chronic cough, bronchitis, and chest illness rates in schoolchildren in the Harvard study with various measures of particulate pollution, including TSP, $PM_{15}$, $PM_{2.5}$, and sulfate. The associations with sulfur dioxide were also positive, though weaker.

Suggestive epidemiologic evidence for an association between morbidity and elevated acid concentrations comes from the Harvard Six Cities Study. Questionnaire reports of bronchitis, chronic cough, and a composite measure of lower respiratory tract illness were reported to be associated with various indicators of particulate pollution (193); however, the strength of the statistical associations appears to be substantially improved when direct measures of aerosol acidity are substituted in the analyses for the measures of particle pollution (194).

Methods to measure acid aerosols in outdoor air were developed only recently; however, the preliminary data suggest that measurements of strong acid species and hydrogen ion may correlate more closely with respiratory symptoms than measurements of particulate matter. The ongoing epidemiologic studies, which directly measure acid aerosol exposure and response, will provide important information needed to evaluate the extent of the impact on respiratory tract health.

### Controlled Human Exposure Studies

Although these epidemiologic studies suggest that particulate matter may be a more relevant indicator of the toxicologic agent in the mixture of sulfur dioxide and particles, there is clear evidence from controlled-exposure studies that sulfur dioxide alone can have important health effects. Accidental exposure to high concentrations can cause severe airways obstruction and pulmonary dysfunction for up to a year (195). Exposure studies using bronchoalveolar lavage have demonstrated an increase in macrophages and mast cells, both indicators of inflammatory processes (196).

Clinical studies of asthmatics have consistently demonstrated bronchoconstriction in response to inhaled sulfur dioxide (197). At exposures as low as 0.5 ppm study subjects experienced moderate to severe wheezing, sometimes requiring ending the exercise protocol. Following exposure to 1.0 ppm sulfur dioxide during moderate exercise, adolescents with asthma demonstrate a 23% decrease in $FEV_1$, a 67% increase in total respiratory resistance, and a 50% decrease in maximal flow rate (198). The clinical symptoms typically associated with sulfur dioxide exposure are shortness of breath, wheezing, and cough (199). Symptoms usually resolve within 30 minutes of the exposure and can be reversed immediately with $\beta_2$-agonist by inhaler. Subjects without clinical asthma who have allergies and exercise-induced bronchospasm are also sensitive to sulfur dioxide. Koenig and co-workers (200) exposed adolescents with allergic rhinitis to 1 ppm sulfur dioxide during exercise. This 10-minute exposure induced a 35% increase in the work of nasal breathing.

Although the concentrations used in these studies are higher than those that generally occur in urban areas, the results have raised concern. Stagnant weather conditions can produce brief, ground-level sulfur dioxide concentrations of 1.0 ppm. Although these high concentrations usually last less than an hour and therefore would not necessarily violate the 24-hour averaged standard for sulfur dioxide, sensitive persons who may be exposed could be expected to suffer severe effects.

Acidic aerosols have also been studied. Controlled exposure to sulfuric acid alone, or in combination with sulfur dioxide, has been shown to cause increased airways resistance and decreases in pulmonary flow parameters. While no changes in pulmonary function have been observed among normal subjects after brief exposures to as much as 1,000 $\mu g/m^3$ sulfuric acid (201), adolescent asthma patients with exercise-induced bronchospasm showed reductions in $FEV_1$, maximal flow at 50% of expired vital capacity, and total airways resistance after exposure to 100 $\mu g/m^3$ during exercise (202). Adult asthmatics exposed to 450 and 1,000 $\mu g/m^3$ sulfuric acid also show reduced specific airway conductance ($SG_{aw}$) and $FEV_1$ (203). In these studies the degree of bronchoconstriction increased with acidity (e.g., lower concentrations of sulfuric acid than of ammonium sulfate are required to induce a response. Individual change in $SG_{aw}$ in response to 1,000 $\mu g/m^3$ sulfuric acid correlated closely with responsiveness as assessed with nonspecific challenge by carbachol. By contrast, exposure to an $H_2SO_4$ aerosol at a concentration of 90 $\mu g/m^3$ did not adversely affect ventilatory function of older persons with COPD.

There have been only limited clinical studies of soluble and insoluble particles (187). Exposures of healthy volunteers to $H_2SO_3$ aerosols at concentrations below 1,000 $\mu g/m^3$ do not affect lung function (203). Acidic aerosols do adversely affect persons with asthma as does $SO_2$. Little information is available from clinical studies on older persons with chronic heart and lung disease, the group presumed at risk for mortality from exposure to particulate pollution. Toxicologic research involving animal models of chronic heart and lung disease is now in progress and should provide further understanding of the toxicity of these pollutants.

The information provided by controlled human exposure studies has helped to clarify the role of hydrogen ion as a cause of respiratory health effects in sensitive persons, but there is little evidence on particles. Further research is needed, and innovative approaches must be developed and used that characterize the responsiveness of subjects in the laboratory and follow their exposure and response to acid aerosols in the community setting.

## CLINICAL ISSUES

### Susceptible Populations

The likelihood of an adverse response to an inhaled pollutant depends on the degree of exposure to the pollutant and the individual characteristics of the exposed person that determine susceptibility. The concept of susceptibility is highly relevant to public health protection and to the care of individual patients. Factors that determine susceptibility (Table 3) include sex, age, pregnancy, and the presence of cardiovascular or lung disease, airways responsiveness, and $\alpha_1$-antitrypsin deficiency. Exposure to other agents, such as cigarette smoke, may also influence susceptibility for certain air pollutants.

**TABLE 3.** *Risk factors for susceptibility to air pollution*

| Factor | Potential mechanism | Consequences |
|---|---|---|
| Infancy | Immature lung defense mechanisms | Increased risk for respiratory infection |
| Advanced age elder | Impaired respiratory defenses, reduced functional reserve | Increased risk for infection; increased risk for clinically significant effects on function |
| Asthma | Increased airways responsiveness | Increased risk for exacerbation and respiratory symptoms |
| COPD | Reduced lung function | Increased risk for clinically significant effects on function |
| IHD | Impaired myocardial oxygenation | Increased risk for myocardial ischemia |
| Cigarette smoking | Impaired defense and clearance; lung injury | Increased damage through synergism |

COPD, chronic obstructive pulmonary disease; IHD, ischemic heart disease.

### *Control Approaches*

Control of outdoor pollution requires complex societal strategies as exemplified in such legislation as the Clean Air Act and its amendments; however, adverse effects of outdoor pollution may also be reduced through individual actions. Modifying time use to limit time spent outdoors during episodes of high pollution represents an effective strategy for some pollutants. For example, ozone levels in buildings are lower than outdoor levels. Acidic aerosols can penetrate indoors but neutralization by ammonia produced by occupants, pets, and household products may reduce concentrations. Vigorous exercise outdoors, which increases the amount of inhaled air and so the dose of pollution delivered to the respiratory tract, should also be avoided at times of high outdoor pollution and near active roadways.

For persons with underlying lung disease that increases susceptibility to inhaled pollution, alteration of therapy may be appropriate if symptoms have increased at a time of high pollution. In the laboratory, cromolyn sodium and bronchodilating agents may block acute responses to some pollutants. Respiratory protective equipment could potentially reduce exposure to particles and gases, but such devices add to the work of breathing and are not tolerated well by persons with respiratory diseases. The use of air cleaners indoors has not been shown to reduce exposure to outdoor air pollution that enters indoor spaces.

## REFERENCES

1. Ott WR. Exposure estimates based on computer generated activity patterns. *J Toxicol Clin Toxicol 1989;*21:7–128.
2. Shy CM, Goldsmith JR, Hackney JD, Lebowitz MD, Menzel DB. Health effects of air pollution. *ATS News* 1978;6:1–63.
3. Brimblecombe P. *The big smoke. A history of air pollution in London since medieval times.* New York: Methuen, 1987.
4. Bascom R, Kesavanathan J, Swift DL. Human susceptibility to indoor contaminants. [Review]. *Occup Med* 1995;10:119–132.
5. American Thoracic Society, Committee of the Environmental and Occupational Health Assembly, Bascom R, Bromberg PA, Costa DA, et al. Health effects of outdoor air pollution. Part 1. *Am J Respir Crit Care Med* 1996;153:3–50, 477–498.
6. Wilson R, Spengler JD, eds. *Particles in our air. Concentrations and health effects.* Cambridge, MA: Harvard University Press, 1996.
7. U.S. Environmental Protection Agency (EPA). *National air quality and emissions trends report, 1992.* EPA-454/R-93-031. Research Triangle Park, NC: Office of Air and Radiation/Office of Air Quality Planning and Standards, 1993.
8. Office of Technology Assessment. *Catching our breath:* next steps to reducing urban ozone. Washington, DC: U.S. Government Printing Office, 1989.
9. U.S. Environmental Protection Agency (EPA), Office of Health and Environmental Assessment. *An acid aerosols issue paper. Health effects and aerometrics.* EPA-600/8-88-005F. Washington, D.C. U.S. Government Printing Office, 1989.
10. Wilson R, Colome SD, Spengler JD, Wilson DG. *Health effects of fossil fuel burning:* assessment and mitigation. Cambridge, MA: Ballinger, 1980.

11. Smith KR. *Biofuels, air pollution, and health. A global review.* New York: Plenum Press, 1987.
12. National Research Council (NRC), Committee on Advances in Assessing Human Exposure to Airborne Pollutants. *Human exposure assessment for airborne pollutants:* advances and opportunities. Washington, DC: National Academy Press 1991.
13. Shy CM, Kleinbaum DG, Morgenstern H. The effect of misclassification of exposure status in epidemiological studies of air pollution health effects. *Bull NY Acad Med* 1978;54:1155–1165.
14. Schenker MB, Samet JM, Batterman S, Gruhl J, Speizer FE. Health effects of air pollution due to coal combustion in the Chestnut Ridge region of Pennsylvania: Results of cross-sectional analysis in adults. *Arch Environ Health* 1983;38:325–330.
15. Vedal S, Schenker MB, Samet JM, Speizer FE. Risk factors for childhood respiratory disease. *Am Rev Respir Dis* 1984;130: 187–192.
16. Ferris BG Jr, Speizer FE. Effects of sulfur oxides and respirable particles on human health: Methodology and demography of populations in study. *Am Rev Respir Dis* 1979;120:767–779.
17. Spengler JD, Ferris BG Jr, Dockery DW, Speizer FE. Sulfur dioxide levels and nitrogen dioxide levels inside and outside homes and the implications on health effects research. *Environ Sci Technol* 1979;13: 1276–1280.
18. Spengler JD, Dockery DW, Turner WA, Wolfson JM, Ferris BG Jr. Long-term measurements of respirable sulfates and particles inside and outside homes. *Atmos Environ* 1981;15:23–30.
19. Mauderly JL, Samet JM. General environment. In: Crystal RG, West JB, eds. *The lung:* scientific foundations. New York: Raven Press, 1991;1947–1960.
20. Frank R, O'Neil JJ, Utell MJ, Hackney JD, Van Ryzin J, Brubaker PE. *Inhalation toxicology of air pollution:* clinical research considerations. Philadelphia: American Society for Testing and Materials, 1985.
21. Bromberg PA. Asthma and automotive emissions. In: Watson AY, Bates RR, Kennedy D, eds. *Air pollution, the automobile and public health.* Washington, DC: National Academy Press, 1988;465–498.
22. National Research Council (NRC), Commission on Life Sciences, Board on Toxicology and Environmental Health Hazards, Committee on the Epidemiology of Air Pollutants. *Epidemiology and air pollution.* Washington, DC: National Academy Press, 1985.
23. Bates DV, Sizto R. Air pollution and hospital admissions in southern Ontario: The acid summer haze effect. *Environ Res* 1987;43:317–331.
24. Thurston GD, Ito K, Lippmann M, Hayes C. Reexamination of London, England, mortality in relation to exposures to acidic aerosols during 1963–1972 winters. *Environ Health Perspect* 1989;79:73–82.
25. Samet JM, Speizer FE, Bishop Y, Spengler JD, Ferris BG Jr. The relationship between air pollution and the emergency room visits in an industrial community. *J Air Pollut Control Assoc* 1981;31:236–240.
26. Zeger SL, Diggle PJ. Semiparametric models for longitudinal data with application to CD4 cell numbers in HIV seroconverters. *Biometrics* 1994;50:689–699.
27. National Research Council (NRC), Committee on the Institutional Means for Assessment of Risks to Public Health. *Risk assessment in the federal government:* managing the process. Washington, DC: National Academy Press, 1983.
28. National Research Council (NRC), Committee on Risk Assessment of Hazardous Air Pollutants. *Science and judgment in risk assessment.* Washington, DC: National Academy Press, 1994.
29. U.S. Environmental Protection Agency (EPA), Scientific Advisory Board, Relative Risk Reduction Strategies Committee. *Reducing risk:* setting priorities and strategies for environmental protection. Washington, DC: U.S. Government Printing Agency, 1990.
30. Ott WR, Flachsbart PG. Measurement of carbon monoxide concentrations in indoor and outdoor locations using personal exposure monitors. *Environ Int* 1982;8:295–304.
31. Akland GG, Hartwell TD, Johnson TR, Whitmore RW. Measuring human exposure to carbon monoxide in Washington, D.C., and Denver, Colorado, during the winter of 1982–1983. *Environ Sci Technol* 1985;19:911–918.
32. Flachsbart PG, Howes JE, Mack GA, Rodes CE. Carbon monoxide exposures of Washington commuters. *J Air Pollut Control Assoc* 1987;37:135–142.
33. Cooper KR, Alberti RR. Effect of kerosene space heater emissions on indoor air quality and pulmonary function. *Am Rev Respir Dis* 1984; 129:629–631.
34. Kim YS. Seasonal variation in carbon monoxide poisoning in urban Korea. *J Epidemiol Commun Health* 1985;39:79–81.
35. Flachsbart PG, Brown DE. *Surveys of personal exposure to vehicle exhaust in Honolulu microenvironments.* University of Hawaii at Manoa, Honolulu, HI: Department of Urban and Regional Planning, 1985.
36. Wallace LR. Carbon monoxide in air and breath of employees in an underground office. *J Air Pollut Control Assoc* 1983;33:678–682.
37. Lambert WE, Colome SD, Kleinman MT. Carbon monoxide exposure patterns in Los Angeles among a high-risk population. Paper No. 91-138.4. Presented at the 84th Annual Meeting of the Air and Waste Management Association, 1991.
38. Douglas CG, Haldane JS, Haldane JBS. The laws of combustion of hemoglobin with carbon monoxide and oxygen. *J Physiol* 1912;44: 275–304.
39. Stryer L. *Biochemistry.* San Francisco: WH Freeman, 1975.
40. National Research Council (NRC), Committee on Medical and Biological Effects of Environmental Pollutants. *Carbon monoxide.* Washington, DC: National Academy Press, 1977.
41. Beard RR, Grandstaff NW. Carbon monoxide and human functions. In: Weiss B, Laties VG, eds. *Behavioral toxicology.* New York: Plenum Press, 1975.
42. Ayres SM, Gianelli S, Mueller H. Myocardial and systemic responses to carboxyhemoglobin. *Ann NY Acad Sci* 1970;174:268–293.
43. Coburn RF. Mechanisms of carbon monoxide toxicity. *Prev Med* 1979;8:310–322.
44. Cobb N, Etzel RA. Unintentional carbon monoxide-related deaths in the United States, 1979 through 1988. *JAMA* 1991;266:659–663.
45. Kelley JS, Sophocleus GJ. Retinal hemorrhages in subacute carbon monoxide poisoning. Exposure in homes with blocked furnace flues. *JAMA* 1978;239:1515–1517.
46. Dolan MC, Haltom TL, Barrows GH, Short CS, Ferriell KM. Carboxyhemoglobin levels in patients with flulike symptoms. *JAMA* 1987;16:782–786.
47. Kirkpatrick JN. Occult carbon monoxide poisoning. *West J Med* 1987; 146:52–56.
48. Heckerling PS, Leikin JB, Maturen A, Perkins JT. Predictors of occult carbon monoxide poisoning in patients with headache and dizziness. *Ann Intern Med* 1987;107:174–176.
49. Radford EP, Drizd TA. *Blood carbon monoxide levels in persons 3–74 years by age, United States, 1976–80.* National Center for Health Statistics: Advance Data from Vital and Health Statistics No. 76. Hyattsville, MD: U.S. Government Printing Office, 1982.
50. Anderson EW, Andelman RJ, Strauch JM, Fortuin NJ, Knelson JH. Effect of low-level carbon monoxide exposure on onset and duration of angina pectoris. A study in ten patients with ischemic heart disease. *Ann Intern Med* 1973;79:46–50.
51. Kleinman MT, Davidson DM, Vandagriff RB, Caiozz VJ, Whittenberger JL. Effects of short-term exposure to carbon monoxide in subjects with coronary artery disease. *Arch Environ Health* 1989;44:361–369.
52. Allred EN, Bleecker ER, Chaitman BR, et al. Short-term effects of carbon monoxide exposure on the exercise performance of subjects with coronary artery disease. *N Engl J Med* 1989;321:1426–1432.
53. Carboni GP, Lahiri A, Cashman PMM, Raftery EB. Mechanisms of arrhythmias accompanying ST-segment depression on ambulatory monitoring in stable angina pectoris. *Am J Cardiol* 1987;60: 1246–1253.
54. Hausmann D, Nikutta P, Trappe JH, Daniel W, Wenzlaff P, Lichtlen PR. Incidence of ventricular arrhythmias during transient myocardial ischemia in patients with stable coronary artery disease. *J Am Cardiol* 1990;16:49–54.
55. Goldsmith JR, Landaw SA. Carbon monoxide and human health. *Science* 1968;162:1352–1359.
56. DeBias DA, Banarjee CM, Birkhead NC, Greene CH, Scott SD, Harrer WV. Effects of carbon monoxide inhalation on ventricular fibrillation. *Arch Environ Health* 1976;31:42–46.
57. Foster JR. Arrhythmogenic effects of carbon monoxide in experimental acute myocardial ischemia: Lack of slowed conduction and ventricular tachycardia. *Am Heart J* 1981;102:876–882.
58. Verrier RL, Mills AK, Skornik WA. *Acute effects of carbon monoxide on cardiac electrical stability.* Research report 35. Cambridge, MA: Health Effects Institute, 1990.
59. Hinderliter AL, Adams KF Jr, Price CJ, Herbst MC, Koch G, Sheps

DS. Effects of low-level carbon monoxide exposure on resting and exercise induced ventricular arrhythmias in patients with coronary artery disease and no baseline ectopy. *Arch Environ Health* 1989;44:89–93.
60. Sheps DS, Herbst MC, Hinderliter AL, et al. Production of arrhythmias by elevated carboxyhemoglobin in patients with coronary artery disease. *Ann Intern Med* 1990;113:343–351.
61. Dahms TE, Younis LT, Wiens RD, Zarnegar S, Byers SL, Chaitman BR. Effects of carbon monoxide exposure in patients with documented cardiac arrhythmias. *J Am Coll Cardiol* 1993;21:442–450.
62. Cohen SI, Deane M, Goldsmith JR. Carbon monoxide and survival from myocardial infarction. *Arch Environ Health* 1969;19:510–517.
63. Hexter CA, Goldsmith JR. Carbon monoxide: association of community air pollution with mortality. *Science* 1971;172:265–267.
64. Kurt TL, Mogielnicki RP, Chandler JE, Hirst K. Ambient carbon monoxide levels and acute cardiorespiratory complaints: an exploratory study. *Am J Public Health* 1979;69:360–363.
65. Morris RD, Naumova EN, Munasinghe RL. Ambient air pollution and hospitalization for congestive heart failure among elderly people in seven large U.S. cities. *Am J Public Health* 1995;85:1361–1365.
66. Stern FB, Haplerin WE, Hornung RW, Ringenburg VL, McCammon CS. Heart disease mortality among bridge and tunnel officers exposed to carbon monoxide. *Am J Epidemiol* 1988;128:1276–1288.
67. Calverley PMA, Leggett RJE, Flenley DC. Carbon monoxide and exercise tolerance in chronic bronchitis and emphysema. *Br Med J* 1981;283:878–880.
68. Benignus VA, Otto DA, Prah JD, Benignus G. Lack of effects of carbon monoxide on human vigilance. *Percept Mot Skill* 1977;45: 1007–1014.
69. Horvath SM, Dahms TE, O'Hanlon JF. Carbon monoxide and human vigilance. *Arch Environ Health* 1971;23:343–347.
70. Beard RR, Wertheim GA. Behavioral impairment associated with small doses of carbon monoxide. *Am J Public Health* 1967;57: 2012–2022.
71. McFarland RA. Low level exposure to carbon monoxide and driving performance. *Arch Environ Health* 1973;27:355–359.
72. Longo LD. The biological effects of carbon monoxide on the pregnant woman, fetus, and newborn infant. *Am J Obstet Gynecol* 1977;129: 69–103.
73. Alderman BW, Baron AE, Savitz DA. Maternal exposure to neighborhood carbon monoxide and risk of low infant birth weight. *Public Health Rep* 1987;102:410–414.
74. Atkinson R. Atmospheric Transformations of Automobile Emissions. In: Watson AY, Bates RR, Kennedy D, eds. *Air pollution, the automobile and public health.* Washington, DC: National Academy Press, 1988;99–132.
75. Spengler JD, Brauer M, Koutrakis P. Acid air and health. *Environ Sci Technol* 1990;24:946–956.
76. Spengler J, Ryan PB, Schwab M, et al. An overview of the Los Angeles personal monitoring study. In: *Total exposure assessment methodology:* a new horizon. Proceedings of the EPA/Air and Wase Management Association Specialty conference, November 1989, Las Vegas, NV. Pittsburgh, PA: AWMA, 1990:66–85.
77. Ryan PB, Spengler JD, Schwab M, Billick IH. Nitrogen dioxide exposure studies: I. The Boston personal monitoring study: In: *Total exposure assessment methodology:* a new horizon. Proceedings of the EPA/Air and Waste Management Association Specialty conference, November 1989, Las Vegas, NV. Pittsburgh, PA: AWMA, 1990:38–65.
78. Quackenboss JJ, Spengler JD, Kanarek MS, Letz R, Duffy CP. Personal exposure to nitrogen dioxide: Relationship to indoor/outdoor air quality and activity patterns. *Environ Sci Technol* 1986;20:775–783.
79. Marbury MC, Harlos DP, Samet JM, Spengler JD. Indoor residential NO2 concentrations in Albuquerque, New Mexico. *J Air Pollut Control Assoc* 1988;38:392–398.
80. National Research Council (NRC), Committee on Indoor Pollutants. *Indoor pollutants.* Washington, DC: National Academy Press, 1981.
81. Traynor GW, Apte MG, Carruthers AR, Dillworth JF, Grimsrud DT, Thompson WT. Indoor air pollution and interroom pollutant transport due to unvented kerosene-fired space heaters. *Environ Int* 1987; 159–166.
82. Samet JM, Utell MJ. The risk of nitrogen dioxide: What have we learned from epidemiological and clinical studies? *Toxicol Indust Health* 1990;6:247–262.
83. Mustafa MG, Tierney DF. Biochemical and metabolic changes in the lung with oxygen, ozone, and nitrogen dioxide toxicity. *Am Rev Respir Dis* 1978;118:1061–1090.
84. Goldstein E, Goldstein F, Peek NF, Parks NJ. Absorption and transport of nitrogen oxides. In: Lee SD, editor. *Nitrogen oxides and their effects on health.* Ann Arbor, MI: Ann Arbor Science, 1980;143–160.
85. Miller FJ, Overton JH, Myers ET, Graham JA. Pulmonary dosimetry of nitrogen dioxide in animals and man. In: Schneider T, ed. *Air pollution by nitrogen oxides.* New York: Elsevier Scientific, 1982:
86. Lowry T, Schuman LM. "Silo-filler's disease"—a syndrome caused by nitrogen dioxide. *JAMA* 1956;162:153–160.
87. Gardner DE. Oxidant-induced enhanced sensitivity to infection in animal models and their extrapolations to man. *J Toxicol Environ Health* 1984;13:423–439.
88. Morrow PE. Toxicological data on $NO_2$: An overview. *J Toxicol Environ Health* 1984;13:205–227.
89. Goings SAJ, Kulle TJ, Barscom R. Effect of nitrogen dioxide exposure on susceptibility to influenza A virus infection in healthy adults. *Am Rev Respir Dis* 1989;139:1075–1081.
90. Harlos DP. *Acute exposure to nitrogen dioxide during cooking or commuting.* Dissertation. Boston, MA: Harvard School of Public Health, 1988.
91. Shy CM, Creason JP, Pearlman ME, McClain KE, Benson FB, Young BB. The Chattanooga school children study. Part I: Effects of community exposure to nitrogen dioxide. *J Air Pollut Control Assoc* 1970; 20:539–581.
92. Shy CM, Creason JP, Pearlman ME, McClain KE, Benson FB, Young BB. The Chattanooga school children study. Part II: Effects of community exposure to nitrogen dioxide. *J Air Pollut Control Assoc* 1970; 20:582–588.
93. Pearlman ME, Finklea JF, Creason JP, Shy CM, Young MM, Horton RJM. Nitrogen dioxide and lower respiratory illness. *Pediatrics* 1971; 47:391–398.
94. Braun-Fahrlander C, Ackermann-Liebrich U, Schwartz J, Gnehm HP, Rutishauser M, Wanner. Air pollution and respiratory symptoms in preschool children. *Am Rev Respir Dis* 1992;145:42–47.
95. Speizer FE, Ferris BG Jr, Bishop YM, Spengler JD. Respiratory disease rates and pulmonary function in children associated with $NO_2$ exposure. *Am Rev Respir Dis* 1980;121:3–10.
96. Melia RJ, Florey CV, Altman DG, Swan AV. Association between gas cooking and respiratory disease in children. *Br Med J* 1977;2: 149–152.
97. Ekwo EE, Weinberger MW, Lachenbruch PA, Huntley WH. Relationship of parental smoking and gas cooking to respiratory disease in children. *Chest* 1983;84:662–668.
98. Schenker MB, Samet JM, Speizer FE. Risk factors for childhood respiratory disease: The effect of host factors and home environmental exposures. *Am Rev Respir Dis* 1983;128:1038–1043.
99. Keller MD, Lanese RR, Mitchell RI, Cote RW. Respiratory illness in households using gas and electricity for cooking. I. Survey of incidence. *Environ Res* 1979;19:495–503.
100. Keller MD, Lanese RR, Mitchell RI, Cote RW. Respiratory illness in households using gas and electricity for cooking. II. Symptoms and objective findings. *Environ Res* 1979;19:504–515.
101. Berwick M, Zagraniski RT, Leaderer BP, Stolwijk JA. Respiratory illness in children exposed to unvented combustion sources. In: Berglund B, Lindvall T, Sundell J, eds. *Indoor air, vol 2:* radon, *passive smoking, particulates and housing epidemiology.* Stockholm: Swedish Council of Building Research, 1984;255–260.
102. Samet JM, Lambert WE, Skipper BJ, et al. Nitrogen dioxide and respiratory illness in children. Part I: Health outcomes. *Res Rep Health Eff Inst* 1993;1–32;discussion 51–80.
103. Hasselblad V, Kotchmar DJ, Eddy DM. Synthesis of environmental evidence: Nitrogen dioxide epidemiology studies. *J Air Waste Manage Assoc* 1992;42:662–671.
104. Li Y, Powers TE, Roth HD. Random-effects linear regression meta-analysis models with application to the nitrogen dioxide health effects studies. *J Air Waste Manage Assoc* 1994;44:261–70.
105. Samet JM, Marbury MC, Spengler JD. Health effects and sources of indoor air pollution. Part I. *Am Rev Respir Dis* 1987;136: 1486–1508.
106. Ware JH, Dockery DW, Spiro A, III. Passive smoking, gas cooking, and respiratory health of children living in six cities. *Am Rev Respir Dis* 1984;129:366–374.
107. Berkey CS, Ware JH, Dockery DW. Indoor air pollution and pul-

monary function growth in preadolescent children. *Am J Epidemiol* 1986;123:250–260.
108. Brunekreef B, Houthuijs D, Dijkstra L, Boleij JJM. Indoor nitrogen dioxide exposure and children's pulmonary function. *J Air Waste Manage Assoc* 1990;40:1252–1256.
109. Jarvis D, Chinn S, Luczynska CM, Burney P. Association of respiratory symptoms and lung function in young adults with use of domestic gas appliances. *Lancet* 1996;347:426–432.
110. Frampton MW, Morrow PE, Cox C, Gibb FR, Speers DM, Utell MJ. Effects of nitrogen dioxide exposure on pulmonary function and airway reactivity in normal humans. *Am Rev Respir Dis* 1991;143:522–527.
111. Morrow PE, Utell MJ, Bauer MA, Speers DM, Gibb FR. Effects of near ambient levels of sulfuric acid aerosol on lung function in exercising subjects with asthma and COPD. *Ann Occup Hyg* 1994; 38(suppl):933–938.
112. Logan JA. Tropospheric ozone: seasonal behavior, trends, and anthropogenic influence. *J Geophys Res* 1985;90:10463–10482.
113. Chameides WL, Lindsay RW, Richardson J, Kiang CS. The role of biogenic hydrocarbons in urban photochemical smog. *Science* 1988; 241:1473–1475.
113a. National Research Council, Committe on Tropospheric Ozone Formation and Measurement. *Rethinking the ozone problem in urban and regional air pollution.* Washington, DC: National Academy Press, 1991.
114. Yocum JE. Indoor-outdoor air quality relationships: a critical review. *J Air Pollut Control Assoc* 1982;32:500–520.
115. Gold DR, Allen G, Damokosh A, Serrano P, Hayes C, Castillejos M. Comparison of outdoor and classroom ozone exposures for school children in Mexico City. *J Air Waste Manage Assoc* 1996;46(4): 335–342.
116. South Coast Air Quality Management District. *Playing it safe on smoggy days.* El Monte, CA: SCAQMD, 1990.
117. McGurdy TR. *National estimates of exposure to ozone under alternative national standards.* Research Triangle Park, NC: U.S. EPA Office of Air Quality Planning and Standards, 1986.
118. *Catching our breath:* next steps to reducing urban ozone. Washington, DC: U.S. Government Printing Office, 1989.
119. U.S. Environmental Protection Agency (EPA). *Air quality criteria for ozone and other photochemical oxidants.* Washington, DC: U.S. EPA Environmental Criteria and Assessment Office, 1986.
120. U.S. Environmental Protection Agency (EPA). *Review of the national ambient air quality standards for ozone:* preliminary assessment of scientific and technical information, draft staff paper. Washington, DC: U.S. EPA Office of Air Quality Planning and Standards, 1988.
121. Lippmann M. Health effects of ozone. A critical review. *J Air Pollut Control Assoc* 1989;39:672–695.
122. McDonnell WF, Horstman DH, Hazucha MJ, Seal E, Sallam SA, House DE. Pulmonary effects of ozone exposure during exercise: dose response characteristics. *J Appl Physiol* 1983;5:1345–1352.
123. Avol EL, Linn WS, Venet TG, Shamoo DA, Hackney JD. Comparative respiratory effects of ozone and ambient oxidant pollution exposure during heavy exercise. *J Air Pollut Control Assoc* 1984;31:666–668.
124. Folinsbee LJ, McDonnell WF, Horstman DH. Pulmonary function and symptom responses after 6.6 hour exposure to 0.12 ppm ozone with moderate exercise. *J Air Pollut Control Assoc* 1988;38:28–35.
125. Horstman DH, Folinsbee LJ, Ives PJ, Abdul-Salaam S, McDonnell WF. Ozone concentration and pulmonary response relationships for 6.6 hour exposures with five hours of moderate exercise to 0.08, 0.10, and 0.12 ppm. *Am Rev Respir Dis* 1990;142:1158–1163.
126. McDonnell WF, Chapman RS, Leigh MW, Strope GL, Collier AM. Respiratory responses of vigorously exercising children to 0.12 ppm ozone exposure. *Am Rev Respir Dis* 1985;132:875–879.
127. Avol EL, Linn WS, Shamoo DA, et al. Short-term respiratory effects of photochemical oxidant in exercising children. *J Air Pollut Control Assoc* 1987;37:158–162.
128. Linn WS, Shamoo DA, Venet TG, et al. Response to ozone in volunteers with chronic obstructive pulmonary disease. *Arch Environ Health* 1983;38:278–283.
129. Koenig JQ, Covert DS, Marshall SG, Belle GV, Pierson WE. The effects of ozone and nitrogen dioxide on pulmonary function in asthmatic adolescents. *Am Rev Respir Dis* 1987;136:1152–1157.
130. Kehrl HR, Hazucha MJ, Solic JJ, Bromberg PA. Responses of subjects with chronic obstructive pulmonary disease after exposures to 0.30 ppm ozone. *Am Rev Respir Dis* 1985;131:719–724.
131. Devlin RB, McDonnell WF, Mann R, et al. Exposure of humans to ambient levels of ozone for 6.6 hours causes cellular and biochemical changes in the lung. *Am J Respir Cell Mol Biol* 1991;4:72–81.
132. Kinney PL, Thurston GD, Raizenne M. The effects of ambient ozone on lung function in children: a reanalysis of six summer camp studies. *Environ Health Perspect* 1996;104:170–174.
133. Thurston GD, Lippmann M, Scott MB, Fine JM. Summer haze air pollution and children with asthma. *Am J Respir Crit Care Med* 1997; 155:654–660.
134. Bates D, Sizto R. Air pollution and hospital admissions for southern Ontario: the summer haze effect. *Environ Res* 1987;43:317–331.
135. Thurston GD, Ito K, Kinney PL, Lippmann M. A multiyear study of air pollution and respiratory hospital admissions in three New York State metropolitan areas: Results for 1988 and 1989 summers. *J Exp Anal Environ Epidemiol* 1992;2:429–450.
136. Thurston GD, Ito K, Hayes CG, Bates DV, Lippmann M. Respiratory hospital admissions and summertime haze air pollution in Toronto, Ontario: Consideration of the role of acid aerosols. *Environ Res* 1994; 65:271–290.
137. Burnett RT, Dales RE, Raizenne ME, Krewski D, Summers PW, Roberts GR. Effects of low ambient levels of ozone and sulfates on the frequency of respiratory admissions to Ontario hospitals. *Environ Res* 1994;65:172–194.
138. Cody RP, Weisel CP, Birnbaum G, Lioy PJ. The effect of ozone associated with summertime photochemical smog on the frequency of asthma visits to hospital emergency departments. *Environ Res* 1992; 58:184–194.
139. White MC, Etzel RA, Wilcox WD, Lloyd C. Exacerbations of childhood asthma and ozone pollution in Atlanta. *Environ Res* 1994;65: 56–68.
140. Schwartz J. Air pollution and hospital admissions for the elderly in Birmingham, Alabama. *Am J Epidemiol* 1994;139:589–590.
141. Schwartz J. Air pollution and hospital admissions for the elderly in Minneapolis/St. Paul, Minnesota. *Arch Environ Health* 1994;49: 366–374.
142. Schwartz J. Short-term fluctuations in air pollution and hospital admissions of the elderly for respiratory disease. *Thorax* 1995;50: 531–538.
143. Schwartz J. Particulate air pollution and daily mortality in Detroit. *Environ Res* 1991;56:204–213.
144. Schwartz J, Morris R. Air pollution and hospital admissions for cardiovascular disease in Detroit, Michigan. *Am J Epidemiol* 1995;142: 23–35.
145. Kinney PL, Ito K, Thurston GD. A sensitivity analysis of mortality: PM10 associations in Los Angeles. *Inhal Toxicol* 1995;7:59–69.
146. Burja-Aburto VH, Loomis DP, Bangdiwala SI, Shy CM, Rascon-Pacheco RA. Ozone, suspended particulates, and daily mortality in Mexico City. *Am J Epidemiol* 1997;145:258–268.
147. Samet JM, Zeger SL, Kelsall JE, Xu J, Kalkstein LS. Air pollution, weather, and mortality in Philadelphia 1973–1988. In: Health Effects Institute Report, ed. *Particulate air pollution and daily mortality:* analyses of the effects of weather and multiple pollutants. The Phase I.B Report of the Particle Epidemiology Evaluation Project. Cambridge, MA: Health Effects Institute, 1997.
148. Verhoeff AP, Hoek G, Schwartz J, Van Wijnen JH. Air pollution and daily mortality in Amsterdam. *Epidemiology* 1996;7:225–230.
149. Settle DM, Patterson CC. Magnitude and sources of precipitation and dry deposition fluxes of industrial and natural leads to the North Pacific at Eniwetok. *J Geophys Res* 1982;87:8857–8869.
150. U.S. Environmental Protection Agency (EPA). *Air quality criteria for lead.* EPA-600/8-83-028. Research Triangle Park, NC: Environmental Criteria and Assessment Office, 1986.
151. Schlesinger RB. Biological deposition for airborne particles: Principles and application to vehicular emissions. In: Watson AY, Bates RR, Kennedy D, eds. *Air pollution, the automobile, and public health.* Washington, DC: National Academy of Sciences, 1988; 239–298.
152. Morrow PE, Beiter H, Amato F, Gibb FR. Pulmonary retention of lead: An experimental study in man. *Environ Res* 1980;21:373–384.
153. Gottlieb K, Kohler JR. Blood lead levels in children from lower socioeconomic communities in Denver, Colorado. *Arch Environ Health* 1994;49:260–266.
154. Pirkle JL, Brody DJ, Gunter EW, et al. The decline of blood lead lev-

els in the United States: the National Health and Nutrition Examination Surveys (NHANES). *JAMA* 1994;272:284–291.
155. Needleman HL, Schell A, Bellinger D, Leviton A, Allred EN. The long-term effects of exposure to low doses of lead in childhood: an 11-year follow-up report. *N Engl J Med* 1990;322:83–88.
156. Bellinger D, Needleman MC, Bromfield R, Nimtz M. A follow-up study of the academic attainment and classroom behavior of children with elevated dentine lead levels. *Biol Trace Elem Res* 1984;6: 207–223.
157. Silva PA, Hughes P, Williams S, Faed JM. Blood lead, intelligence, reading, attainment, and behaviour in eleven-year-old children in Dunedin, New Zealand. *J Child Psychol Psychiatry* 1986;29:43–52.
158. Schwartz J, Otto D. Blood lead, hearing thresholds, and neurobehavioral development in children and youth. *Arch Environ Health* 1987; 42:152–160.
159. Winneke G, Kramer U, Brockhus A, et al. Neurophysical studies in children with elevated tooth lead concentrations. *Int Arch Occup Environ Health* 1983;51:231–252.
160. Needleman HL, Gatsaris CA. Low-level lead exposure and the IQ of children. A meta-analysis of modern studies. *JAMA* 1990;263: 673–678.
161. Schwartz J. Low-level lead exposure and children's IQ: a meta-analysis and search for a threshold. *Environ Res* 1994;65:42–55.
162. World Health Organization. *Environmental health criteria on inorganic lead.* Geneva: WHO, 1995.
163. Lippmann M. Background on health effects of acid aerosols. *Environ Health Perspect* 1989;79:3–6.
164. Bellinger D, Stiles KM, Needleman HL. Low-level lead exposure, intelligence and academic achievement: a long-term follow-up study. *Pediatrics* 1992;90:855–861.
165. Needleman HL, Reiss JA, Tobin MJ, Biesecker GE, Greenhouse JB. Bone lead levels and delinquent behavior. *JAMA* 1994;272:284–291.
166. Bellinger D, Schwartz J. Effects of lead in children and adults. In: Steenland K, Savitz DA, eds. eds. *Topics in environmental epidemiology.* New York: Oxford University Press, 1997;314–349.
167. Pirkle JL, Schwartz J, Landis JR, Harlan WR. The relationship between blood lead levels and blood pressure and its cardiovascular risk implications. *Am J Epidemiol* 1985;121:246–258.
168. Schwartz J. The relationship between blood lead and blood pressure in the NHANES II survey. *Environ Health Perspect* 1989;79:3–6.
169. Schwartz J. Lead, blood pressure, and cardiovascular disease in men. *Arch Environ Health* 1995;50:31–37.
170. U.S. Environmental Protection Agency (EPA). *Air quality criteria for particulate matter and sulfur oxides.* Research Triangle Park, NC: Office of Health and Environmental Assessment, U.S. EPA, 1982.
171. Amdur MO. Sulfuric acid: what the animals tried to tell us. *Appl Ind Hyg* 1989;4:189–197.
172. Office of Technology Assessment. *Acid rain and transported air pollutants.* New York: UNIPUB, 1985.
173. Calvert JG, Lazrus A, Kok GL, et al. Chemical mechanisms of acid generation in the troposphere. *Nature* 1985;317:27–35.
174. U.S. Environmental Protection Agency (EPA). Proposed revisions to the nation's ambient air quality standards for particulate matter. *Federal Register* 1987;10408-35:49.
175. Logan WPD. Mortality in the London fog incident, 1952. *Lancet* 1953;1:336–338.
176. Scott JA. The London fog of December, 1962. *Med Officer* 1963;109: 250–252.
177. Commins BT, Waller RE. Observations from a 10-year study of pollution at a site in the city of London. *Atmos Environ* 1967;1:49–68.
178. Schwartz J, Marcus A. Mortality and air pollution in London: A time series analysis. *Am J Epidemiol* 1990;131:185–194.
179. Ayres J, Fleming D, Williams M, McInnes G. Measurement of respiratory morbidity in general practice in the United Kingdom during the acid transport event of January 1985. *Environ Health Perspect* 1988; 79:83–88.
180. Wichmann HE, Mueller W, Allhoff P, et al. Health effects during a smog episode in West Germany in 1985. *Environ Health Perspect* 1989;79:89–99.
181. Dockery DW, Pope CA. Acute respiratory effects of particulate air pollution [Review]. *Annu Rev Public Health* 1994;15:107–132.
182. Pope CA III, Kalkstein LS. Synoptic weather modeling and estimates of the exposure-response relationship between daily mortality and particulate air pollution. *Environ Health Perspect* 1996;104: 414–420.
183. Dockery DW, Pope CA III. Acute respiratory effects of particulate air pollution. *Annu Rev Public Health* 1994;15:107–132.
184. Samet JM, Zeger SL, Berhane K. *The association of mortality and particulate air pollution. Particulate air pollution and daily mortality:* replication and validation of selected studies. Cambridge, MA: Health Effects Institute, 1995.
185. Dockery DW, Pope CA III, Xu X, et al. An association between air pollution and mortality in six U.S. cities. *N Engl J Med* 1993;329: 1753–1759.
186. Pope CA III, Thun MJ, Namboodiri MM, et al. Particulate air pollution as a predictor of mortality in a prospective study of U.S. adults. *Am J Respir Crit Care Med* 1995;151:669–674.
187. Utell MJ, Samet JM. Airborne particles and respiratory disease: clinical and pathogenic considerations. In: Wilson R, Spengler JD, eds. *Particles in our air:* concentrations and health effects. Cambridge MA: Harvard University Press, 1996;169–188.
188. Seaton A, MacNee W, Donaldson K, Godden D. Particulate air pollution and acute health effects. *Lancet* 1995;345:176–178.
189. Schwartz J, Dockery DW, Ware JH, et al. Acute effects of acid aerosols on respiratory symptoms reporting in children. Paper no. 89-92.1. Presented at the 82nd Annual Meeting of the Air Pollution Control Association, 1989.
190. Dockery DW, Ware JH, Ferris BG Jr, Speizer FE, Cook NR, Herman SM. Change in pulmonary function associated with air pollution episodes. *J Air Pollut Control Assoc* 1982;32:937–942.
191. Pope CA III. Respiratory disease associated with community air pollution and a steel mill, Utah Valley. *Am J Public Health* 1989;79: 623–628.
192. Pope CA III. Respiratory hospital admissions associated with PM10 Pollution in Utah, Salt Lake, and Cache Valleys. *Arch Environ Health* 1991;46:90–97.
193. Dockery DW, Speizer FE, Stram DO, Ware JH, Spengler JD, Ferris BG Jr. Effects of inhalable particles in respiratory health of children. *Am Rev Respir Dis* 1989;139:587–594.
194. Speizer FE. Studies of acid aerosols in six cities and in a new multicity investigation: design issues. *Environ Health Perspect* 1989;79: 61–67.
195. Rabinovitch S, Greyson ND, Weiser W, Hoffstein V. Clinical and laboratory features of acute sulfur dioxide inhalation poisoning: two-year follow-up. *Am Rev Respir Dis* 1989;139:556–558.
196. Sanstrom T, Stjernberg N, Andersson M, et al. Cell response to bronchoalveolar lavage fluid after exposure to sulfur dioxide. *Am Rev Respir Dis* 1989;140:1828–1831.
197. Horstman D, Folinsbee LJ. Sulfur dioxide-induced bronchoconstriction in asthmatics exposed for short durations under controlled conditions: a selected review. In: Utell MJ, Frank R, eds. *Susceptibility to inhaled pollutants.* Philadelphia: American Society for Testing and Materials, 1989.
198. Koenig JQ, Pierson WE. Pulmonary effects of inhaled sulfur dioxide in atopic adolescents: a review. In: Frank R, O'Neil JJ, Utell MJ, eds. *Inhalation toxicology of air pollution:* clinical research considerations. Philadelphia: American Society for Testing and Materials, 1985.
199. Koenig JQ, Covert DS, Pierson WE. Acid aerosols and asthma: a review. In: Utell MJ, Frank R, eds. *Susceptibility to inhaled pollutants.* Philadelphia: American Society for Testing and Materials, 1989.
200. Koenig JQ, McManus MS, Bierman CW. Chlorpheniramine—sulfur dioxide interactions of lung and nasal function in allergic adolescents. *Pediatr Asthma Allerg Immunol* 1988;2:199–205.
201. Utell MJ. Effects of inhaled acid aerosols on lung mechanics: An analysis of human exposure studies. *Environ Health Perspect* 1985; 63:39–44.
202. Koenig JQ, Pierson WE, Horike M. The effect of inhaled sulfuric acid on pulmonary function in adolescent asthmatics. *Am Review Respir Dis* 1983;128:221–225.
203. Utell MJ, Morrow PE. Latent development of airway hyperactivity in human subjects after sulfuric acid aerosol exposure. *J Aerosol Sci* 1983;14:202–205.

*Environmental and Occupational Medicine,*
*Third Edition,* edited by William N. Rom.
Lippincott–Raven Publishers, Philadelphia © 1998.

CHAPTER 115

# Indoor Air Pollution

Jonathan M. Samet, John D. Spengler, and Clifford S. Mitchell

Throughout the 20th century pollution of outdoor air has been a focus of public health concern. Dramatic episodes of outdoor air pollution showed that high levels of pollutants in industrialized areas increased the death rate; epidemiologic studies demonstrated that lower levels were associated with morbidity, primarily reflecting effects on the respiratory tract (1). In many developed countries regulations have been implemented to reduce emissions of pollutants that have proven adverse health effects, and improvements in air quality have been made. Unfortunately, in many less developed countries outdoor air pollution is an increasing problem, as polluting industries have moved from developed to developing nations.

As the 20th century ends, indoor air pollution has been recognized as a significant public health problem for both more developed and less developed societies. In developed countries, where most time is spent indoors, personal exposure to potentially hazardous air pollutants largely reflects indoor sources. Modern building techniques that incorporate many synthetic materials and mechanical heating, ventilating, and air conditioning systems tend to broaden the range of exposures and to increase pollutant concentrations indoors. In undeveloped and developing countries, reliance on biomass fuels for heating and cooking exposes a large proportion of the world's population to smoke indoors (2). Biologic pollutants, including infectious organisms and allergens, are of concern throughout the world.

This chapter provides an overview of indoor air pollution, with emphasis on developed countries. The principal indoor air pollutants are reviewed, and sources, concentrations, and health effects are covered. The scope of the review of health effects is limited; other chapters in this volume address some of these pollutants in more detail. In addition, several books provide more comprehensive reviews of indoor air pollution (3–5). Indoor air pollution in developing countries was also reviewed recently (2,6).

This chapter emphasizes adverse health effects of individual indoor air pollutants. However, the most common response to inadequate indoor air quality is probably perceived discomfort, which may have diverse concomitant manifestations. Ensuring human comfort has always been the principal focus of the design and operation of residential and nonresidential buildings. Some of the physical elements of comfort include temperature, temperature gradient, draftiness, humidity, noise, odors, and lighting. More subjective factors also influence an occupant's perception of the indoor environment; for example, perception of an indoor space might be influenced by furnishings, ability to control temperature and lighting, the presence of windows, cleanliness, and perception of hazards. We have inadequate understanding of the roles of these diverse physical and psychological factors as they determine responses to indoor environments—and even less information on the interaction of indoor air pollution with other characteristics of the indoor environment. Indoor air pollution and comfort are reviewed elsewhere (7,8).

J. M. Samet: Department of Epidemiology, The Johns Hopkins University School of Hygiene and Public Health, Baltimore, Maryland 21205.

J. D. Spengler: Department of Environmental Health; and Environmental Science and Engineering Program, Harvard School of Public Health, Boston, Massachusetts 02115-6021.

C. S. Mitchell: Department of Environmental Health Sciences, The Johns Hopkins University School of Hygiene and Public Health, Baltimore, Maryland 21205.

## PERSONAL EXPOSURE

In developed countries, patterns of time use and activity place children and adults in diverse indoor and outdoor environments throughout the day, each of which may have its peculiar set of air contaminants. Perhaps because of the distinct sources that contaminate outdoor and indoor air and the separate regulatory mechanisms for outdoor air, the workplace, and the home, the health effects of outdoor and indoor air pollution have often been addressed separately.

However, the concept of total personal exposure is more relevant for health; personal exposure to air pollution represents the time-weighted average of pollutant concentrations in microenvironments (environments that have relatively homogeneous air quality) where time is spent (9,10). Thus, for an office worker relevant microenvironments might include home, office, car, outdoors at home, outdoors at work, and during commuting. For some pollutants (e.g., ozone, acid aerosols) outdoor environments may make the predominant contribution to total personal exposure; for others (e.g., radon, formaldehyde) indoor locations are most important. Studies of time-activity patterns demonstrate that residents of more developed countries spent most time indoors; thus, personal exposure to many pollutants occurs predominantly indoors (11,12).

## SOURCES AND CONCENTRATIONS

Indoor pollutants can be categorized by type of source, such as combustion, and by pollutant group, such as volatile organic compounds (VOCs) and fibers (Table 1). Sources can be further characterized by pollutants emitted, by locations, and by rate and pattern of emissions. For some pollutants, the presence of a potential source does not necessarily indicate exposure. For example, the presence of fibrous asbestos-containing material in a building may not be an exposure hazard unless the material is disturbed or inadequately maintained. Pollutant species are typically described under the broad

**TABLE 1.** *Sources of common indoor contaminants*

| Contaminant | Source |
|---|---|
| Asbestos: chrysotile, crocidolite, amosite, tremolite | Some wall and ceiling insulation installed between 1930 and 1950; old insulation on heating pipes and equipment; old wood stove door gaskets; some vinyl floor tiles; drywall joint-finishing material and textured paint purchased before 1977; cement asbestos millboard and exterior wall shingles; some sprayed and troweled ceiling finish plaster installed between 1945 and 1973; fire retardant sprayed onto some structural steel beams |
| Combustion by-products: carbon monoxide, nitrogen- and sulfur dioxide, particulate soot, nitrogenated compounds | Gas ranges; wood and coal stoves; fireplaces; backdraft of exhaust flues; candles and incense |
| Tobacco smoke: carbon monoxide, nitrogen- and carbon dioxide, hydrogen cyanide, nitrosamines, aromatic hydrocarbons, benzo[*a*]pyrene, particles, benzene, formaldehyde, nicotine | Cigarettes, pipes, cigars |
| Formaldehyde | Some particleboard, plywood, pressboard, paneling; some carpeting and carpet backing; some furniture and dyed materials; UFFI, some household cleaners and deodorizers; combustion gas, tobacco, wood; some glues and resins; tobacco smoke; cosmetics; permanent-press textiles |
| Microbiologic organisms: fungal spores, bacteria, virus, pollens, arthropods, protozoa | Mold, mildew and other fungi; humidifiers with stagnant water; water-damaged surfaces and materials; condensing coils and drip pans in HVAC systems; refrigerator drainage pans; some thermophilics on dirty heating coils; animals, rodents, insects, humans |
| Radon: radon gas, $^{210}$Bi, $^{218}$Po, $^{210}$Po, $^{210}$Pb | Soil, rocks, water (gas diffuses through cracks and holes in the foundation and floor), well water; natural gas used near the source wells; some building materials such as granite |
| Volatile organic compounds: alkanes, aromatic hydrocarbons, esters, alcohols, aldehydes, ketones | Solvents and cleaning compounds, paints, glues and resins, spray propellants, fabric softeners and deodorizers, combustion, dry-cleaning fluids, some fabrics and furnishings, stored gasoline, out-gassing from water, some building materials, waxes and polishing compounds, pens and markers, binders and plasticizers |

source headings of combustion, evaporation, abrasion, biologic, and radon. Table 1 lists the major indoor sources and contaminants.

## Combustion

The principal combustion sources indoors include tobacco smoking, which generates environmental tobacco smoke (ETS), unvented combustion appliances, and wood stoves and fireplaces. Combustion sources emit inorganic gases ($H_2O$, NO, $NO_2$, CO, $CO_2$) and particles. In addition, depending on fuel type and pyrolysis conditions, combustion sources can also emit hydrocarbon gases, vapors, and organic particles. Most liquid and solid fuels contain impurities or additives that may result in emissions of metals, mercaptans, sulfur oxides, or particles as the fuels burn. The particles, containing partially burned carbon soot or minerals, are readily visible when released from oil-, wood-, or kerosene-fueled appliances. Gas appliances may emit very small particles, in the submicron range, as may burning tobacco products. Because some combustion sources burn at temperatures high enough (over 900°C) to produce atomic nitrogen, they can produce nitrogenated species in the effluent.

Unvented gas combustion is a ubiquitous source of nitrogen dioxide and carbon monoxide in residences; almost half the homes in the United States have gas stoves. Many studies indicate that gas ranges can raise indoor nitrogen dioxide concentrations above ambient levels (13). The levels are nearly always higher in homes with gas ranges than in homes with electric ranges in the same community (14–16). Typically, kitchens have the highest levels; short-term peaks associated with cooking are superimposed on the more stable background from pilot lights. Levels drop off in rooms remote from the kitchen. Higher levels may be found in small city apartments and where the oven is used for space heating.

Gas stoves emit carbon monoxide at about 10 times the rate of nitrogen dioxide, but under typical conditions concentrations do not exceed 10 ppm over the cooking period. Nevertheless, the extreme conditions that result in elevated nitrogen dioxide concentrations also cause higher carbon monoxide levels. Concentrations of 25 to 50 ppm have been measured in kitchens in New York City (17).

About 11% of the U.S. population is potentially exposed to gas or kerosene space heater emissions, which include particles, carbon monoxide, and nitrogen dioxide—and sulfur dioxide if sulfur-containing fuel is burned. Leaderer and colleagues (18) conducted a survey of indoor air quality in a small number of homes in Connecticut. The sulfur dioxide levels were less than 2 $\mu g/m^3$ inside homes without kerosene space heaters but 60 to 150 $\mu g/m^3$ in homes where such heaters were operated. In Connecticut at the time, commercial kerosene apparently contained a measurable amount of sulfur. Kerosene space heaters and gas ranges emit particulate matter (19,20). Bioassays have shown that kerosene heaters produce a carbonaceous particle—principally from nitrated polycyclic aromatic hydrocarbons—that is very mutagenic (21).

In some regions of the United States wood stoves are a prevalent source of primary heat in homes; but overall, about 6% of homes have wood stoves and 19% fireplaces. Emissions from wood stoves and fireplaces are vented to the outdoors, but during start-up and stoking, and if the system is not airtight, emissions can contaminate the indoor air. Under such instances, transient elevations of particle levels may occur, but on average an increase in particulate matter of only a few micrograms per milliliter can be attributed to the presence of a home wood- or coal-burning stove (22).

Significant exposure to combustion products may occur in many other settings. Internal combustion gasoline or propane engines are sometimes used indoors. For example, exhaust emissions from ice-resurfacing machines may contaminate skating rinks with carbon monoxide and nitrogen dioxide. Offices, hotels, hospitals, schools, shopping centers, and department stores often have adjacent or lower-level garages. Buildings with attached garages and offices connected to warehouses that use gasoline or propane forklifts can have elevated concentrations of combustion-related emissions. Negative pressures on lower floors of sealed high-rise buildings may result in entrainment of garage or roadside emissions. In more developed countries, nearly everyone spends time in automobiles or buses and is exposed to vehicle exhaust.

The burning of tobacco products is a ubiquitous source of a large number of indoor contaminants (23). Tobacco burning produces a complex mixture of gases, vapors, and particulate matter. More than 4,500 compounds have been identified from burning tobacco, 50 of which are known or suspected carcinogens (23). Tobacco smoke can be classified as mainstream (MS), sidestream (SS), or environmental (ETS). MS smoke is the emissions inhaled by the smoker during active smoking, when the temperature of the burning cone of the tobacco may reach 900°C. Myriad compounds are generated by combustion at these high temperatures. SS smoke refers to the emissions from the smoldering cigarette; as the cigarette smolders the cone temperature may drop as low as 400°C. Approximately half the tobacco in a cigarette is consumed by smoldering and the remainder by active puffing. Because pyrolysis conditions differ during puffing and smoldering, the components of MS and SS smoke differ to some extent, both qualitatively and quantitatively; many toxic compounds are present at higher concentrations in SS (23).

Environmental tobacco smoke, the combination of exhaled MS and SS (23), consists principally of SS, which undergoes modification with dilution and aging after formation. Components with high vapor pressures may volatilize from particles and enter the vapor phase. For example, nicotine is emitted in the SS particle phase, but then evaporates to the vapor phase. Particles may change size and number as they age, gain water, and form aggregates. The concentration of ETS cannot be measured directly. Concentrations of individual ETS components can be measured and used as surrogates for this complex mixture; nicotine and respirable particles are the most widely used indices of ETS (23,24). The concentrations of ETS constituents vary among indoor locations and over time. The number of smokers and the pattern of smoking determine the source strength for generation of ETS. The concentrations of ETS components to which nonsmokers are exposed depend further on the degree of dilution of the smoke. In smoky bars, waiting areas, restaurants, automobiles, airplanes, or even in the home, short-term concentrations of ETS can be quite high. Concentrations of particles of respirable size in rooms contaminated by ETS can range from 100 to more than 1,000 μg/ml. In closed environments the nicotine level can range from a few $\mu g/m^3$ to more than 100 (23).

### Volatile Organic Compounds

Modern furnishings, construction materials, and consumer products contaminate indoor air with numerous vapor-phase organic compounds (VOCs). In a recent Environmental Protection Agency (EPA) study of air quality in ten public-access buildings, more than 500 VOCs were identified (25,26). To some extent the characteristics of volatile and semivolatile organic compounds overlap. Volatile organic compounds exist as vapors over the normal range of air temperatures and pressures, whereas semivolatile ones exist as liquids or solids but also evaporate. Termiticides, such as chlordane and heptachlor, are injected into the ground as liquids but are effective against termites because of emanating vapors. Many semivolatile insecticides and pesticides have similar physical properties. Some higher molecular weight organic molecules occur as particulate matter in air.

Formaldehyde, used in hundreds of products, is one of the most ubiquitous indoor organic vapors. Formaldehyde is added to medicines, cosmetics, and toiletries, and to some food containers as a preservative. The largest single use of formaldehyde is in producing urea and phenol-formaldehyde resins, which are used to bond laminated wood products and to bind wood chips in particle board. These wood products are widely used in homes and offices, as shelving, counters, bookcases, cabinets, floors, and wall covers. Formaldehyde has been used as a carrier solvent in the dying of textiles and paper products and is particularly effective on synthetic fibers. In the mid-1970s, urea formaldehyde foam insulation (UFFI) became a popular insulation material. UFFI emits formaldehyde in an initial burst and then continuously at a lower level (27). Improper installation or formulation results in sustained release of formaldehyde UFFI and higher indoor concentrations (28,29).

### Asbestos

Asbestos consists of several fibrous inorganic materials characterized by chemical formulation and crystalline structure. Because of its high tensile strength and thermal properties, asbestos has been used extensively in building materials since the beginning of this century. The broad-use categories in buildings are thermal and acoustic insulation, fire protection, and the reinforcement of building products. Asbestos has been used in acoustic ceiling tiles and vinyl floor tiles, paints, and wall and ceiling plaster. Until it was restricted in the late 1970s asbestos materials were used to coat pipes, boilers, and steel structural beams.

The use of asbestos in the United States has decreased since 1973, coincident with the banning of certain applications by the EPA. However, asbestos-containing materials are still present in many homes, offices, and schools. Based on surveys, the EPA has estimated that 20% of the nation's buildings, about 733,000 not including schools and residential buildings of fewer than ten units, contain some asbestos materials (30); 16% have thermal insulation containing asbestos. Separate surveys in New York City suggest that 67% (158,000) of the buildings contain asbestos (30,31).

Occupant risk is determined by exposures to airborne fibers rather than the presence of asbestos materials in the building. At present, information is lacking on the relationship between the presence of asbestos materials and indoor concentrations of airborne asbestos fibers. This relationship cannot be readily evaluated because of the episodic fashion in which much of the asbestos is released into indoor air. Water damage or mechanical damage, in addition to normal aging of binders, is thought to release fibers indoors. The episodic nature of fiber release and gravitational settling reduce the likelihood that elevated concentrations will be detected by area-integrated monitoring. The available database on airborne asbestos concentrations in buildings demonstrates extremely low average values under normal building use conditions (32).

Results of monitoring buildings for asbestos cannot be readily compared across studies because different sampling, analysis, and counting criteria have been used. Phase-contrast microscopy (PCM), the most widely used method in the occupational setting, identifies fibers with a length-to-aspect ratio of 3:1. Because it is typically used at 400×, this method underestimates fibers thinner than 0.25μm, and the method is not specific for asbestos fibers. It may overestimate concentrations of larger fibers. On the other hand, transmission electron microscopy (TEM) is used at a magnification of 20,000× and can positively differentiate asbestos fibers from other fibers and classify asbestos fibers by type. Typically, TEM counts five times the number of fibers detected by PCM. Some investigators use an indirect method of TEM that transfers fibers to a counting stage. This method tends to further fracture fiber bundles and, so, yields higher counts. Furthermore, interlab comparison studies indicate that not only do results vary among laboratories but even the technicians handling, preparing, and counting TEM-analyzed fibers may introduce important variations.

Surveys conducted by the EPA of fibers in commercial buildings demonstrate very low fiber concentrations under normal conditions. The 1991 Literature Review Panel Report of the Health Effects Institute—Asbestos Research compiled all published data as well as previously unpublished information on buildings sampled for litigation and other reasons. The report included 1,377 measurements made by TEM in 198 buildings. For the fibers greater than 5 μm in length, considered most relevant to disease causation, the mean and median concentrations were about 0.001 fibers (f)/ml, three or more orders of magnitude lower than concentrations in the occupational settings where diseases were found to be caused by asbestos in workers.

In a survey of 73 schools, fiber concentrations averaged 0.0002 f/cc (31). These observations, and the growing awareness of removal costs, led the EPA to publish new recommendations that encourage management in place and worker protection (33).

## Radon

Radon-222, a noble gas, is produced in the decay of naturally occurring uranium-238. Its half-life is 3.8 days, and it decays into a series of short-lived progeny—polonium-218, lead-214, bismuth-214, and polonium-214—all of which have a half-life shorter than 30 minutes (34). The principal source of radon in buildings is natural radon gas in soil (35). The soil gas penetrates through sump pump wells, drains, cracks, utility access holes, and foundations into the air in homes. The driving pressure for entry of soil gas comes from the pressure gradient established across the soil by a house; the gradient varies with atmospheric pressure, wind flow over a structure, and buoyancy of air within the structure. Generally, building materials and potable water do not harbor significant amounts of radon; however, potable water drawn from wells in areas where soil and rocks are rich in radium may be an important source of radon (36).

There are now extensive data on radon concentrations in homes in the United States and other countries. In the United States, the EPA has completed the National Residential Radon Survey, which involved 6,000 randomly selected homes (U.S. EPA 1992). The average value was about 1.25 picocuries per liter (pCi/L), but the distribution of concentrations was approximately log normal and about 4% of homes were estimated to exceed the EPA's action guideline of 4 pCi/L as the annual average concentration. The average concentration is about two orders of magnitude lower than the mines where miners historically had high rates of radon-caused lung cancer. Levels in some homes, however, range as high as those in uranium and other mines. The data collected by the screening protocol of the EPA, which uses a short-term test methods and conditions intended to screen for high concentrations, provide an upwardly biased picture of radon concentrations. The National Residential Radon Survey has now provided data from a nationally representative sample that have been collected with a long-term protocol.

## Microbiologic Contaminants

Microbiologic contaminants take a wide variety of forms (37) (Table 2). Pollens from trees, grasses, and other plants are familiar to the general public through their association with allergens and clinical syndromes of allergy. Microbiologic contaminants of indoor air also include microbial cells such as viruses and bacteria in addition to fungal spores, protozoans, algae, animal dander and excreta, and insect excreta and fragments. Volatile metabolites of living and decaying organisms should also be considered. The contaminants may be viable organisms that multiply in an infected host, or the organisms may live in dust, soil, water, oil, organic films, food, vegetative debris, or wherever the microclimate provides conditions that support growth. Bathroom walls and window casements as well as damp basements are sites where water condenses.

Microbiologic contamination has also been found in many other locations. For example, the use of cool mist humidifiers in the home can result in microbiologic contamination. Ultrasonic humidifiers can also disseminate bacteria if tap water is used and becomes contaminated. Humidification by steam in a central air-handling system usually does not present a problem, since biocides are added to most steam supplies; however, the addition of

**TABLE 2.** *Common bioaerosols, related diseases, and typical sources*

| Bioaerosol | Examples of diseases | Common sources |
|---|---|---|
| Pollens<br>Spores<br>Plant parts | Hay fever<br>Allergic rhinoconjunctivitis<br>Asthma<br>Upper airway irritation | Plants, trees, grasses, ferns harvesting, cutting<br>Shiploading |
| Fungi | Asthma, allergic diseases<br>Infection<br>Toxicosis<br>Tumors | Plant material, skin, leather, oils, bird, bat, and animal droppings; feathers, soil nutrients, glues, wool |
| Bacteria | Endotoxicosis<br>Tuberculosis<br>Pneumonia, respiratory and wound infections, legionellosis, Q and Pontiac fever | Humans, birds and animals (e.g., saliva, blood, dental secretions, skin, vomit, urine, feces)<br>Water sprays and surf, humidifiers, hot tubs, pools, drinking water, cooling towers |
| Other allergens<br>Insects<br>Anthropods<br>Algae | Asthma<br>Dermatitis<br>Hypersensitivity<br>Pneumonitic | Mite excreta, insect parts (cockroach, spider, moth, midge)<br>Dander and saliva from cats, dogs, rabbits, mice, and rats<br>Bird serum<br>Farm animal dander |
| Viruses | Respiratory infections, colds, measles, mumps, hepatitis A, influenza, chicken pox,<br>Hanta virus | Infected humans<br>Animal excreta<br>Insect vectors<br>Protozoa[a] |

[a]Protozoa in the form of free-living amoebae can be direct-acting pathogens or allergens; they also can interact with bacteria (e.g., *Legionella* growth within amoebae).
Adapted from ref. 97.

moisture to dust-contaminated ducts has led to biologic contamination.

## HEALTH EFFECTS

### Environmental Tobacco Smoke

Nonsmokers are exposed to ETS, the mixture of SS smoke from the smoldering cigarette and exhaled MS smoke. This complex mixture contains many of the injurious agents inhaled by active smokers, though the concentrations are diluted. Nonsmokers exposed involuntarily to ETS often have detectable levels of nicotine and of cotinine, a metabolite of nicotine, in body fluids (13,23), demonstrating that nonsmokers absorb and metabolize ETS components. Studies of smoking parents and their children provided the first evidence that passive smoking has adverse effects. Maternal smoking was found to place infants at increased risk for lower respiratory tract infections, and smoking by household members, particularly the mother, was shown to increase the incidence of chronic respiratory symptoms and reduce the level of lung function in children (23,38). Other studies showed that environmental tobacco smoke irritates the upper respiratory tract and eyes (23,39).

A new adverse effect of ETS, increased risk of lung cancer for exposed nonsmokers (passive smokers), was first reported in 1981 (40,41). Since then, many studies have addressed this association; pooling of the data indicates that nonsmokers married to smokers have about a 25% greater risk of lung cancer than those married to "never smokers" (38,42,43).

In 1986, reports published by the U.S. Surgeon General and the National Research Council comprehensively reviewed the available evidence on the health effects of ETS. Both concluded that the children of parents who smoke are at greater risk of respiratory infection than children of nonsmokers and have higher rates of respiratory symptoms and slower lung growth. Although the underlying basis for the judgment differed somewhat between the two reports, both agreed that ETS causes lung cancer in nonsmokers. The Surgeon General's report based this finding largely on the qualitative similarities between the exposure for active and involuntary smokers, the extensive evidence on active smoking and lung cancer, and the supporting epidemiologic data on involuntary smoking. The Committee of the National Research Council based its conclusion principally on careful review of the epidemiologic evidence and the biologic plausibility of the association. The Surgeon General's report also concluded that simply separating smokers and nonsmokers in the same air space does not protect nonsmokers from ETS. This conclusion implies that, to eliminate exposure of nonsmokers to ETS, it is necessary to prohibit smoking indoors or to supply separate, ventilated areas.

In a 1992 report, the EPA conducted a risk assessment on ETS as a carcinogen and also evaluated the effects on children (U.S. EPA 1992). Based on a review of the epidemiologic evidence, including a quantitative synthesis using meta-analysis, as well as of the supporting toxicologic data, the EPA classified ETS as a class A carcinogen, a designation applied to agents causally linked to cancer in humans. The risk assessment estimated the annual number of lung cancer deaths attributable to ETS as 2,000 in never smokers.

Some questions concerning the health effects of ETS remain unanswered. Several studies have suggested that ETS exposure reduces lung function in adult nonsmokers (44,45) and increases risk for ischemic heart disease (46). The American Heart Association (AHA) has concluded that ETS exposure is a major preventable cause of cardiovascular disease and death (47). The AHA's Council on Cardiopulmonary and Critical Care has estimated that 35,000 to 40,000 cardiovascular disease deaths occur annually consequent to ETS exposure. The evidence supporting this conclusion comes from epidemiologic evidence, supporting animal experiments, and mounting understanding of potential mechanisms (48). Other proposed associations of involuntary smoking with disease include increased risk for cancers at sites other than the lung, younger age at menopause, increased risk for sudden infant death syndrome, and reduced birth weight. While additional research will be conducted on these and other putative associations of ETS with disease, the available evidence, and the firm conclusions of the reports of the Surgeon General and the National Research Council, have provided a strong impetus for reduction of involuntary smoking.

### Nitrogen Dioxide

Nitrogen dioxide is an oxidant gas that at high concentrations causes lung injury. Toxicologic studies have shown that it reduces the efficacy of lung defense mechanisms against infection (49). Some studies suggest that short-term exposure may exacerbate asthma (50). Thus, the potential health effects of exposure to nitrogen dioxide indoors include increased respiratory tract infection from effects of defense mechanisms, increased respiratory tract symptoms and reduced lung function from direct inflammation, and deterioration of the health status of persons with chronic respiratory diseases, particularly asthma.

In 1977, Melia and coworkers (51) in the United Kingdom reported that children living in homes with gas stoves had a higher prevalence of respiratory tract symptoms than children from homes with electric stoves. These investigators speculated that this effect might result from elevated concentrations of nitrogen oxides released by combustion of natural gas. Since that publication, numerous studies have assessed respiratory effects of nitrogen dioxide from gas stoves, but the evidence on respiratory illnesses, respiratory symptoms, and lung function level in children and adults remains inconclusive, in spite of the number of such studies (13,50). A meta-analysis using data from 11 studies found that a long-term increase in $NO_2$ exposure of approximately 15 parts per billion (ppb), consistent with the presence of a gas stove in the home, is associated with a 20% increase in the risk of respiratory illness in children (52). A cross-sectional study of women in England also indicated adverse respiratory effects (53). On the other hand, a large study of children under the age of 2 years found no association between indoor $NO_2$ exposure and respiratory illness (54).

Inflammation from exposure to an oxidant gas, such as $NO_2$, would be expected to worsen the status of persons with asthma. The evidence for such effects has been conflicting (50), and the exposures typically found in indoor and outdoor environments are not like to cause clinically relevant effects for most asthmatics. However, several recent studies indicate that $NO_2$ exposure in combination with allergens may adversely affect asthmatics, possibly by increasing the permeability of the respiratory epithelium to allergens. Two studies showed that exposure to $NO_2$ increases the response to challenge with specific allergen, such as ragweed, at levels as low as 0.40 ppm (55,56). These studies support a hypothesis that indoor exposure to $NO_2$ could increase the adverse effects of common indoor allergens.

### Wood Smoke

Since the 1970s there has been a resurgence of residential wood burning in the United States. In many communities where wood burning is prevalent, wood smoke has become a visible pollutant in outdoor air. The use of fireplaces and wood stoves can potentially increase indoor concentrations of smoke pollutants, by reentrainment of outdoor air or by direct leakage into indoor air. Limited data suggest that properly maintained and operated wood stoves and fireplaces have little effect on indoor air quality.

Only a few studies have addressed the health effects of wood burning in more developed countries. Data from less developed countries, where exposure is substantially more intense, suggest that wood smoke can cause chronic lung disease (2,6). A study in Michigan showed a markedly increased prevalence of respiratory symptoms in children from homes with wood stoves, in comparison with control children (57). This finding has not yet received adequate confirmation. Further investigation is needed to describe the impact of wood burning on indoor air quality and to assess potential health effects.

### Biologic Agents

Biologic agents represent an extremely diverse group that cause disease primarily through infection and immune mechanisms (58), but they may also release irritants and toxins. The potential for transmission of many infectious diseases through inhalation of indoor air has been recognized for many years (59). Case reports of individual patients, and of problem buildings, continue to indicate the potential of biologic agents in indoor air to cause disease. Hypersensitivity pneumonitis and humidifier fever have been linked to central and room humidifiers, contaminated heating and cooling systems, moisture-damaged building materials, cool mist vaporizers, and automobile air conditioning systems (60). Legionnaires' disease, an acute bacterial infection caused by *Legionella pneumophila,* was first described following the 1976 epidemic in Philadelphia. Airborne transmission of this organism from contaminated water in cooling towers is well documented.

Asthma may be exacerbated by allergens in outdoor and indoor air. New immunochemical methods and sampling techniques have facilitated the study of allergens in indoor air. For example, the major allergen house dust mite has been characterized, and its concentration measured in homes (61). Preventive trials have been undertaken to assess the benefits of control of indoor allergens for persons with asthma.

### Formaldehyde and Other Volatile Organic Compounds

While widespread exposure to formaldehyde and other volatile organic compounds has been well documented, controversy remains concerning the health effects of these indoor pollutants, which include carcinogens and mutagens (e.g., benzene), irritants (e.g., formaldehyde and terpenes), and neurotoxins (e.g., aromatic compounds). Formaldehyde is known to be toxic at high concentrations and to be irritating to the respiratory tract (62). Associations with respiratory morbidity and neurobehavioral impairment, demonstrated in some studies, have not yet been conclusively established (63). Formaldehyde causes nasal cancer in rats exposed to high concentrations and is a suspected occupational carcinogen (64). While formaldehyde exposure in the indoor environment must also be considered as potentially carcinogenic, little relevant evidence is available (13,63). The other volatile organic compounds may also have short- and long-term health effects, but definitive human data are largely lacking (65). The volatile organic compounds are considered as contributing to sick-building syndrome.

### Building-Related Illnesses

Since the early 1970s numerous outbreaks of work-related health problems have been described among employees in offices that are not directly contaminated by industrial processes (66). In some of these outbreaks a specific causal factor and illness can be identified, such as hypersensitivity pneumonitis associated with a contaminated ventilation system. In many outbreaks, however, the symptom pattern is nonspecific and a cause cannot be identified. Because many such outbreaks have occurred in newer sealed office buildings, the outbreaks are often referred to as "tight building" or "sick building syndrome."

The problem of sick building syndrome emerged largely during the 1980s. Investigations of outbreaks have shown that the symptoms are nonspecific but are often related to the respiratory tract, that a high proportion of the work force may be affected, and that no apparent cause other than inadequate ventilation can be found (67,68). Volatile organic compounds have been considered one possible cause of sick building syndrome, but additional investigation is needed.

### Radon

Exposure to radon progeny, the short-lived decay products of radon, has been causally linked to increased risk of lung cancer in uranium and other underground miners (69). Measurements made in the 1970s showed that radon was present in most homes and could reach concentrations as high as those in underground mines where excess rates of lung cancer were documented in miners. The problem of radon in the domestic environment received little attention in the United States until the finding in the mid-1980s that many homes in a geologic region known as the Reading Prong had radon concentrations much higher than are permitted in uranium mines. Subsequently, many homes throughout the United States have been found to have high levels of radon, and exposure to radon has been considered as a potentially important cause of lung cancer in smokers and nonsmokers in the general population.

The hazard posed by exposure to radon progeny in indoor air has been addressed principally through risk estimation procedures (70,71), although ecologic and case-control studies have been published recently. The risks for the general population are projected by extrapolating risks observed in the studies of miners. A number of risk assessment models have been developed; they differ in their underlying assumptions and in the quantitative conclusions, and their results are subject to diverse uncertainties (69,72). Nevertheless, use of each of the models leads to the conclusion that radon contributes significantly to the burden of lung cancer in the population, annually causing an estimated 10,000 to 20,000 cases, or possibly more, in the United States (70). The burden of radon-related lung cancer in the general population reflects in part the synergism between radon and cigarette smoking, assumed in several of the models on the basis of the data from underground miners (70).

## CONTROL

### Policy

It is now clear that protecting public health requires satisfactory outdoor and indoor air quality (73). Moreover, the public also expects a degree of indoor air quality that ensures comfort. The elements of comfort include, among other factors, temperature, temperature gradients, draftiness, humidity, noise, odors, and lighting. We do not yet have comprehensive data on the bounds for these factors that constitute acceptable indoor environmental quality; we lack comprehensive criteria for acceptable indoor air quality.

The Clean Air Act provides a regulatory framework for the United States that is designed to achieve and maintain lower pollutant levels in outdoor air, meeting standards established to prevent adverse health effects. We lack a comparable comprehensive legal, regulatory, administrative, and technical framework for approaching the problem of indoor air pollution. Indoor air pollution has diverse sources: indoor air quality problems may result from natural sources, poor building design, inadequate building maintenance, structural components and furnishings, consumer products, and occupant activities. Neither standards nor guidelines developed for outdoor air or for the workplace should be applied directly to indoor environments.

The U.S. government has not yet established a framework for policy on indoor air, as it has for outdoor air. Sexton (74) addressed the sequence of steps needed to develop responsible and effective control strategies (Table 3). The government has several options for controlling an indoor air pollution problem, ranging from taking no action to implementing specific rules and regulations. The federal government has so far pursued voluntary industry codes and standards for kerosene space heaters and has offered an "action guideline" for radon; it has also provided guidance on handling asbestos in schools and in public and commercial buildings, and has now moved to begin eliminating further use of asbestos. Indoor air pollution by environmental tobacco smoke has been handled by some states and municipalities, and public education to alter behavior has been undertaken by other government agencies.

Existing statutory authorities in the United States do not provide a single federal agency with jurisdiction over indoor air (74) (Table 4). The EPA is responsible for ambient air (outdoor air) through the Clean Air Act. Under the provisions of Title IV of the Superfund Amendments and Reauthorization Act of 1986, Radon and Indoor Air Quality Research, Congress directed the EPA to establish a research program to address radon and other indoor pollutants. The research program was mandated to address data gathering, to coordinate research activities, and to assess federal actions on mitigation of environmental and health risks associated with indoor air.

In its 1987 report to Congress on indoor air quality, as mandated by Title IV of the Superfund Amendments and Reauthorization Act, the EPA outlined policy objectives and strategy, which have remained as a blueprint over the next ten years. Research was proposed to refine understanding of health effects; emphasis was placed on obtaining data for risk assessment. The agency also planned to identify and assess methods for mitigating high-priority problems. The proposed strategy for control was multifaceted and included regulating under existing authorities, augmenting government and private capabilities to manage indoor air quality problems, referring problems to other federal agencies that have regulatory authority, and requesting regulatory authority from Congress. The agency stated a clear preference for avoiding regulation and achieving its goals through research and development, dissemination of information, and technical assistance and training.

In addition to the EPA, other federal agencies are also involved in ensuring indoor air quality. The National Institute for Occupational Safety and Health (NIOSH) conducts health hazard evaluations of workplaces consid-

**TABLE 3.** *Summary of the major steps in addressing indoor air quality problems*

| |
|---|
| Problem definition |
| Emission sources |
| Dilution |
| Indoor concentrations |
| Activity patterns |
| Exposures |
| Health consequences |
| Health risk assessment |
| Number of people exposed |
| Severity of exposure |
| Dose-response relationship |
| Applicability of mitigating measures |
| Ventilation |
| Source removal |
| Source modification |
| Air cleaning |
| Behavior adjustment |
| Resolution of policy issues |
| Building "publicness" |
| Conservation benefits |
| Voluntary versus involuntary risks |
| Importance of short- and long-term health effects |
| Public versus private responsibility |
| Local, state, or federal intervention |
| Appropriate government responses |
| Alternative government responses |
| No action |
| More research |
| Public information |
| Economic incentives |
| Moral suasion |
| Legal liability |
| Guidelines |
| Rules and regulations |

**TABLE 4.** *Federal laws potentially applicable to indoor air*

| |
|---|
| National Environmental Policy Act: A broad act that establishes as a national goal "to assure for all Americans safe, healthful, productive, and aesthetically and culturally pleasing surroundings." |
| Clean Air Act: Gives EPA regulatory authority over outdoor air. |
| Toxic Substances Control Act: Provides EPA with authority to collect and develop data on the risks of chemicals and to restrict manufacturing, distribution, and use of toxic chemicals, including indoor air contaminants. |
| Federal Insecticide, Fungicide, and Rodenticide Act: Provides EPA with authority to collect data, to monitor, and to regulate use of pesticides, including those used indoors. |
| Asbestos Hazard Emergency Response Act and the Asbestos School Hazard Detection and Control Act: Requires EPA to develop regulations detailing methods for handling asbestos in schools. The Detection and Control Act creates a task force for the problem. |
| Superfund Amendments and Reauthorization Act, Title IV: Radon Gas and Indoor Air Quality Research Act: Requires EPA to establish a research program. |
| Safe Drinking Water Act: Authorizes EPA to perform research on contaminants of drinking water. The regulatory authority extends to contaminants in public water supplies that have adverse effects through indoor air pollution. |
| Consumer Product Safety Act: Provides Consumer Product Safety Commission to require labeling for hazardous household products. |
| Occupational Safety and Health Act: As a national policy, "to assure as far as possible every working man and woman in the nation safe and healthy working conditions." |
| National Manufactured Housing Construction and Safety Standards Act of 1974: The state directs the Department of Housing and Urban Development to establish standards for construction and safety of manufactured housing (e.g., mobile homes). Features related to indoor air pollution have been regulated. |
| Department of Energy Organization Act of 1977: Requires integration of national environmental protection goals in developing energy programs. Mandates research on energy technologies and programs. |
| Energy Reorganization Act of 1974: Charged the Energy Research and Development Association (ERDA) with research on environmental, biomedical, physical, and safety research related to energy. |
| Atomic Energy Act: Authorizes research relevant to radon and nonionizing radiation. |
| Energy Conservation and Production Act: Has the goal of reducing energy demand, but the Department of Energy must consider potential health consequences. |

ered to be unhealthy; many evaluations have been conducted in nonindustrial settings to evaluate problems related to indoor air quality. In 1994, the Occupational Safety and Health Administration (OSHA) proposed broad regulations on indoor air quality that would establish plans for management of indoor air quality and complaints related to indoor air quality in the work environment (Federal Register 1994). The proposed regulations would require the banning of smoking in the workplace or the provision of separately ventilated smoking areas. The Department of Energy oversees energy conservation activities and it is charged with considering the health consequences of energy conservation programs. It also has its own program of research in several areas. Under the Consumer Product Safety Act, the Consumer Product Safety Commission has authority to regulate injurious products. The commission has addressed asbestos, urea formaldehyde foam insulation, biologic dissemination from humidifiers, unvented combustion appliances, and the efficacy of CO detectors for the home. The Department of Housing and Urban Development sets building standards for agency-funded projects and standards for materials for mobile homes. Federal activities on indoor air are coordinated through the congressionally mandated Interagency Committee on Indoor Air Quality (IAQ). Operating outside of the Interagency Committee on IAQ are the activities of the Federal Aviation Administration (FAA) and the Federal Trade Commission (FTC). The FAA has the authority to set airplane cabin air quality standards under their broadly defined responsibilities for safety and health. To date, only an ozone limit has been set, but there is no requirement to monitor and there is no enforcement provision. The FTC has investigated the legitimacy of advertising claims made by the manufacturers of filters and home air cleaners.

### Control Techniques

The broad approaches to limiting the health effects of indoor air pollution include removal and control of sources, increased rate of exchange of indoor with outdoor air, and air cleaning (Table 5) (68). Sources may be removed, relocated, or mitigated; for many pollutants source removal and control represents the most effective and economical approach. For example, tobacco smoking can be restricted or eliminated in indoor spaces, and household products that release volatile organic compounds can be stored outside the occupied area and their use minimized. Building materials and furnishings can be selected for low emission rates. Ventilation may be increased throughout a structure or in a specific area that has inadequate ventilation or particularly strong sources. The American Society for Heating, Refrigeration, and Air Conditioning Engineers (ASHRAE) publishes consensus guidelines for ventilation requirements in its Standard 62 (75). The specified level of ventilation is intended to be sufficient to achieve healthy indoor air quality. However, as the complexity of the relationship of indoor air quality with health has been appreciated, it has become evident that provision of ventilation alone cannot assure air quality that is safe for all persons in the population (76). A wide variety of air-cleaning devices are available, which operate by filtration, adsorption, absorption, electrostatic precipitation, or other principles. These devices have not yet been shown to be effective for specific health conditions such as asthma and allergic rhinitis.

**TABLE 5.** *Pollutant control measures*

| Pollutant | Measures and materials | Ventilation and design |
|---|---|---|
| Respirable particles | High-efficiency filters, tight-sealing doors and grates, properly drafting chimney, electrostatic precipitators | Zone and ventilate for smoking; supply outside combustion air to heater and fireplace; relocate air intakes; maintain filter system |
| Nitric oxide, nitrogen dioxide | Remove gasoline engines; pilotless ignition | Place effective hood vent over source; isolate garage from indoor space |
| Carbon dioxide | Check static pressure in return air ducts to make sure return is not overriding fresh-air intake | Isolate garage from indoor space |
| Agents from biologic sources | Insulate to prevent condensation; damp-proof foundation, ducts; proper drainage of drip pans under condenser coils; add bactericides to steam and water for humidifiers and cooling towers; proper maintenance of filters and ducts; routine cleaning; discard water-damaged floor covering; do not use cool-mist humidifiers and vaporizers | Maintain inside relative humidity of 35% to 50%; exhaust bath and kitchen; vent crawl spaces |
| Formaldehyde | Substitute products such as phenolic resin plywood; seal sources; remove materials | Increase air exchange to house or office |
| Radon and radon daughters | Vapor barrier around foundation; damp-proof basement and crawl space; seal cracks and holes in floor traps and drains; install charcoal water-scrubber for well water; seal foundation completely | Vent crawl space; vent sump hole to exterior; depressurize subslab; vent bathroom and laundry to exterior |
| Volatile organic compounds | Substitute products; isolate storage area; apply only according to specifications; do not locate transformers indoors | Use only with adequate ventilation; ventilate laundry, shop; provide separate ventilation to storage area |
| Asbestos | Remove; use injection sealant; wrap pipes with plastic duct tape | Ventilation does not provide adequate protection |

Modified from ref. 96.

Radon, a ubiquitous indoor pollutant, warrants special consideration; the level of radon in a home can be measured inexpensively, and effective mitigation techniques are available. Thus, as recommended by the EPA, homeowners should be encouraged to test the radon level in their homes, particularly in regions where some homes are known to have high concentrations. Should it be demonstrated that elevated concentrations exist, there are a variety of mitigation strategies to follow. An effective and cost-efficient approach is to seal all cracks in the foundation and then depressurize the subslab area. Depressurization is a deliberate attempt to create controlled entrance of radon. Directed through inexpensive plastic piping, the subslab air is vented away from the house.

## Building-Related Illnesses and Sick Building Syndrome

The entities of building-related illness (BRI) and sick building syndrome (SBS) need to be conceptually separated. The former is a term applied to a host of conditions in which specific exposures in the indoor environment, often to the biologic and physical agents discussed above, lead to specific illnesses, many of which are readily diagnosed, treated, and prevented. The latter term applies to a syndrome of symptoms (Table 6), often occurring in groups of building occupants in newer sealed office buildings. Despite considerable research and a great deal of interest in the popular press, SBS continues to challenge and frustrate health care providers, indoor air quality professionals, and affected persons. Satisfying etiologic explanations, effective therapies, and prevention modalities for SBS remain few, and several authors have argued that the term as such should be discontinued, since in many cases other clinical diagnoses can be applied (77).

**TABLE 6.** *Clinical characteristics of the sick building syndrome*

| | |
|---|---|
| Mucous membrane irritation | Eye, nose, and throat irritation |
| Central nervous system symptoms | Headaches |
| | Fatigue and lethargy |
| | Irritation |
| Chest tightness | |
| Skin complaints | Dryness |
| | Itching |
| | Erythema |
| Odor sensitivity | |

Modified from ref. 77.

The entity of SBS has been diagnosed since the early 1970s, when outbreaks of work-related health problems were described among employees in offices that are not directly contaminated by industrial processes (66). The syndrome received increasing recognition during the 1980s. Outbreak investigations and epidemiologic surveys have shown that symptoms are nonspecific but are often related to the respiratory tract, that a high proportion of the work force in mechanically ventilated office buildings can be affected by one or more symptoms, and that often no apparent cause other than inadequate ventilation can be found. Risk factors associated with the development of symptoms consistent with sick-building syndrome include female gender, a history of asthma or rhinitis, occupation (clerical workers are at increased risk compared with managers), high psychosocial work load, and jobs involving use of carbonless copy paper and visual display terminals (67,77,78). Building-related factors that may contribute to occupant comfort and the development of symptoms include inadequate outside air supply or distribution of air inside the building; inadequate filtration of outdoor contaminants; contamination of insulation; poor maintenance; or physical environmental factors including temperature, lighting, noise, or vibration (77,79–81).

The clinical presentation of individuals diagnosed with SBS is highly variable. Patients may complain only of irritation, or they may have a wide range of symptoms (82). By definition, symptoms are present when the patient is in the building, and resolve when exposure ceases. Persistence of symptoms during time outside of the building should increase suspicion that another underlying problem is involved. In some individuals, symptoms will initially be present only in the building, but over time the symptoms become more generalized, triggered by a variety of chemical exposures. Eventually, some of these patients may become indistinguishable from patients with multiple chemical sensitivity (83,84).

Individuals diagnosed with SBS usually do not have evidence of any abnormality of respiratory function. The upper respiratory tract has been the focus of considerable attention as a likely target organ. The presence of lower respiratory tract symptoms, particularly cough, wheeze, or dyspnea, should prompt examination for the presence of airways hyperresponsiveness (85).

Thus far, a common etiology for individuals diagnosed with SBS remains elusive, although volatile organic compounds, bioaerosols such as bacterial endotoxins or β-1,3-glucan, work organization and other psychosocial factors, and unpleasant odors have all been suggested as possible causal or contributing factors (77,86–88). There is also disagreement as to whether and under what circumstances the amount of building ventilation affects the development of SBS. Experiments in which building ventilation (specifically, percentage of fresh versus recirculated air) is altered without the knowledge of the occupants have not shown any change in symptom reporting, although perception of air quality does correlate with symptoms (89,90). However, in other cases improvements in building ventilation systems (including relative humidity and fresh air intake) have been associated with decreases in symptom reporting (77,91,92). Recent efforts to examine baseline indoor air quality in large numbers of office buildings, combined with population-based assessments of symptoms, may help to clarify the differences between sick buildings (buildings where occupants develop SBS) and nonsick buildings (93,94).

In conclusion, the condition known as sick building syndrome remains poorly defined, without any proven etiology, diagnostic test, or treatment. It is likely that many individuals who have been diagnosed with SBS have some other underlying and treatable medical condition. The term *sick building syndrome* should probably be reserved for epidemiologic, rather than clinical, purposes.

### Clinical Approach to the Patient with Indoor Air Problems

The clinical evaluation of patients with health problems related to indoor environments offers distinct challenges. A patient presenting with nonspecific respiratory complaints may not suspect a link to a particular environment. Another patient may be concerned about a potential indoor exposure even in the absence of specific symptoms. In yet another case, the patient may have a specific condition—asthma, hypersensitivity pneumonitis, Legionnaires' disease—that suggests a potential contribution from the indoor environment. In each case, the physician must consider the possible role of the indoor environment.

Diagnosis of an indoor air-related health problem typically involves the following elements: (a) a history suggestive of an indoor air problem, based on symptoms that are temporally or geographically related to the indoor environment; (b) a diagnosis of a specific condition that is often associated with indoor environments, such as Legionnaires' disease; and (c) evaluation of the indoor environment by an industrial hygienist, to document the nature and extent of sources and exposures. In some cases, diagnosis may involve use of a questionnaire to determine whether others in the building are experiencing similar symptoms. When questionnaires are used, it is important to consider the use of previously validated questionnaires and appropriate control populations (4).

Although patients may in some cases be convinced of not only the diagnosis but also its relationship to a specific indoor exposure or environment, the physician should remain a diagnostic skeptic. It is especially important to identify specific treatable and preventable conditions, not only for the patient but for others who may be potentially exposed to the same conditions.

Laboratory testing should focus on the diagnosis of specific conditions, based on the presenting symptoms.

Spirometry can be very useful in separating obstructive or restrictive pathology from symptoms that involve only the upper respiratory tract. The presence of an elevated white count may suggest infection or hypersensitivity pneumonitis. Total serum immunoglobulin E (IgE) may be elevated in allergic disorders such as asthma and rhinitis. For allergic conditions where an exposure is well documented or a particular agent is suspected, the use of specific antibody testing through radioallergosorbent tests (RASTs) or epicutaneous tests is appropriate. However, the use of broad antigen panels, while identifying individuals with a broad range of allergies, may not help determine the specific agent to which the person is reacting in the indoor environment.

Characterizing the responsible exposure will often require consultation with an industrial hygiene professional, an indoor air quality expert, and a heating, ventilation, and air conditioning (HVAC) engineer. The evaluation of the indoor environment in most cases involves interviews with the occupants, a walkthrough evaluation, and sampling for common indoor pollutants including organics, bioaerosols, and, in some cases, particular substances such as pesticides or combustion products. Measurements of temperature and humidity should be compared with ASHRAE standards. Ventilation rates, including air velocity and air changes per hour, should be measured. The HVAC system should be inspected carefully, including the air supply ducts, air handling units, cooling towers, and air intakes (which can sometimes inadvertently be located near external sources of pollutants). The building should be examined for water leaks and other defects, which often contribute to the development of bioaerosols and other indoor air pollutants. Other potential sources of indoor pollutants include photocopy machines (ozone, toner, VOCs), building construction material such as resin-containing particle boards (formaldehyde), and carpeting. Measurements of indoor air quality are rarely informative by themselves. If the setting is a workplace, and exposure to a particular chemical agent is at issue, the material safety data sheets should be reviewed. Other factors may also be involved, including lighting of work areas, noise and/or vibration, ergonomics, and, importantly, work organization (95).

Once the diagnosis is established, management involves three aspects: (a) medical management of the patient, (b) administrative management of the patient, and (c) administrative management of the building-related problem. Medical management of the patient involves appropriate treatment for the particular condition (e.g., asthma or rhinitis). Administrative management of the patient is often complex, involving decisions related to return to work and workers compensation. In cases involving building-related illnesses, identification and removal of the exposure is paramount. In cases involving SBS, a search for a unique cause is often frustrating, and while correctable building-related problems such as inadequate ventilation may improve the situation, they may not completely resolve it.

## CONCLUSIONS

The sources of indoor air pollution are diverse. Natural and man-made sources pollute indoor environments that can then produce disease through diverse mechanisms: inflammatory, immune, infectious, and carcinogenic (96). The spectrum of effects ranges from acute dysfunction to subtle effects on function. Control of indoor air pollution requires broad-based government policy; strategies for individual pollutants may rely on source modification and control, increased ventilation, and air cleaning.

## REFERENCES


1. Wilson R, Spengler JD, eds. *Particles in our air:* concentrations and health effects. Cambridge, MA: Harvard University Press, 1996.
2. Smith KR. *Biofuels, air pollution, and health. A global review.* New York: Plenum Press, 1987.
3. Samet JM, Spengler JD. *Indoor air pollution. A health perspective.* Baltimore: Johns Hopkins University Press, 1991.
4. Maroni M, Seifert B, Lindvall T, eds. *Indoor air quality. A comprehensive reference book.* Amsterdam: Elsevier, 1995.
5. Gammage RB, Berven BA. *Indoor air and human health,* 2nd ed. Boca Raton, FL: Lewis-CRC Press, 1997.
6. Chen BH, Hong CJ, Pandey MR, Smith KR. Indoor air pollution in developing countries. *World Health Stat Q* 1990;43:127–138.
7. Spengler JD, Samet JM. A perspective on indoor and outdoor air pollution. In: Samet JM, Spengler JD, eds. *Indoor air pollution. A health perspective.* Baltimore: Johns Hopkins University Press, 1991.
8. Godish T. *Sick buildings:* definition, diagnosis and mitigation. Boca Raton, FL: Lewis (CRC Press), 1995.
9. National Research Council (NRC), Commission on Life Sciences, Board on Toxicology and Environmental Health Hazards, Committee on the Epidemiology of Air Pollutants. *Epidemiology and air pollution.* Washington, DC: National Academy Press, 1985.
10. Sexton K, Ryan PB. Assessment of human exposure to air pollution: methods, measurements, and models. In: Watson AY, Bates RR, Kennedy D, eds. *Air pollution, the automobile, and public health.* Washington, DC: National Academy Press, 1988, 207–238.
11. Szalai A. *The use of time:* daily activities of urban and suburban populations in twelve countries. The Hague: Mouton, 1972.
12. Chapin FS Jr. *Human activity patterns in the city.* New York: Wiley-Interscience, 1974.
13. Samet JM, Marbury MC, Spengler JD. Health effects and sources of indoor air pollution. Part I. *Am Rev Respir Dis* 1987;136:1486–1508.
14. Spengler JD, Schwab M, Ryan PB, et al. Personal exposure to nitrogen dioxide in the Los Angeles Basin. *Air Waste* 1994;44:39.
15. Spengler JD, Duffy CP, Letz R, Tibbits TW, Ferris BG, Jr. Nitrogen dioxide inside and outside 137 homes and implications for ambient air quality standards and health effects research. *Environ Sci Technol* 1983;17:164–168.
16. Marbury MC, Harlos DP, Samet JM, Spengler JD. Indoor residential $NO_2$ concentrations in Albuquerque, New Mexico. *J Air Pollut Control Assoc* 1988;38:392–398.
17. Sterling TD, Kobayashi D. Use of the gas ranges for cooking and heating in urban dwellings. *J Air Pollut Control Assoc* 1981;29:238–241.
18. Leaderer BP, Zangraniski RT, Berwick M, Stolwijk JAJ, Qing-Shan M. Residential exposure to $NO_2$, $SO_2$, and HCHO associated with unvented kerosene space heaters, gas appliances, and sidestream tobacco smoke. In: Berglund B, Lindvall T, eds. *Indoor air.* Stockholm: Swedish Council for Building Research, 1984, 151–156.
19. Girman JR, Apte MG, Traynor GW, Allen JR, Hollowell CD. Pollutant emission rates from indoor appliances and sidestream cigarette smoke. *Environ Int* 1982;8:213–221.

20. Traynor GW, Allen JB, Apte MG, Girman JR, Hollowel CD. Pollutant emissions from portable kerosene-fired space heaters. *Environ Sci Technol* 1983;17:369–371.
21. Traynor GW, Apte MG, Sokol HA, Chuang JC, and Mumford JL. Selected organic pollutant emissions from unvented kerosene heaters. Presented at the 79th Annual Meeting of the Air Pollution Control Association, Minneapolis, MN, 1986; Air Pollution Control Association; Pittsburgh, PA.
22. Sexton K, Spengler JD, Treitman RD. Effects of residential wood combustion on indoor air quality: a case study in Waterbury, Vermont. *Atmos Environ* 1984;18:1371–1383.
23. U.S. Surgeon General. *The health consequences of involuntary smoking.* [CDC] 87-8398. Rockville, MD: U.S. Government Printing Office, 1986.
24. Guerin MR, Jenkins RA, Tomkins BA, Center for Indoor Air Research, eds. *The chemistry of environmental tobacco smoke:* composition and measurement. Chelsea, MI: Lewis, 1992.
25. Sheldon LS, Handy RW, Hartwell TD, Whitmore RW, Zelon HS, Pellizzari EE. *Indoor air quality in public buildings,* vol 1. Washington, DC: U.S. Environmental Protection Agency, 1988.
26. Sheldon LS, Zelon HS, Sickles J, Eaton C, Hartwell TD. *Indoor air quality in public buildings,* vol 2. Washington, DC: U.S. Environmental Protection Agency, 1988.
27. Allan GG, Dutkiewicz J, Gilmartin EJ. Long-term stability of urea-formaldehyde foam insulation. *Environ Sci Technol* 1980;14:1237.
28. Wolkoff P. Volatile organic compounds—sources, measurements, emissions, and the impact on indoor air quality. *Indoor Air* 1995;3:9–73.
29. Brown SK, Sim MR, Abramson MJ, Gray CN. Concentrations of volatile organic compounds in indoor air—a review. *Indoor Air* 1994;4: 123–134.
30. U.S. Environmental Protection Agency (EPA). *Study of asbestos-containing materials in public buildings:* a report to Congress. Washington, DC: U.S. Government Printing Office, 1988.
31. Price B. Assessing asbestos exposure potential in buildings. Paper presented at the Symposium on Health Effects of Exposure to Asbestos in Buildings, December 14–16, 1988, Harvard University.
32. Health Effects Institute, Asbestos Research Committee, Literature Review Panel. *Asbestos in public and commercial buildings:* A literature review and a synthesis of current knowledge. Cambridge, MA: Health Effects Institute, 1991.
33. U.S. Environmental Protection Agency (EPA). *Managing asbestos in place:* a building owner's guide to operations and maintenance programs for asbestos-containing materials. Washington, DC: U.S. EPA, Office of Pesticides and Toxic Substances, 1990.
34. Evans RD. Engineers' guide to the elementary behavior of radon daughters. *Health Phys* 1969;17:229–252.
35. Nazaroff WW, Nero AV Jr. *Radon and its decay products in indoor air.* New York: Wiley, 1988.
36. Nazaroff WW, Doyle SM, Nero AV Jr, Sextro RG. Radon entry via potable water. In: Nazaroff WW, Nero AV Jr, eds. *Radon and its decay products in indoor air.* New York: Wiley, 1988, 131–157.
37. Burge H. Bioaerosols: prevalence and health effects in the indoor environment. *J Allergy Clin Immunol* 1990;86:687–701.
38. National Research Council (NRC), Committee on Passive Smoking. *Environmental tobacco smoke:* measuring exposures and assessing health effects. Washington, DC: National Academy Press, 1986.
39. Samet JM, Cain WS, Leaderer BP. Environmental tobacco smoke. In: Samet JM, Spengler JD, eds. *Indoor air. A health perspective.* Baltimore: Johns Hopkins University Press, 1991, 131–169.
40. Hirayama T. Nonsmoking wives of heavy smokers have a higher risk of lung cancer: a study from Japan. *Br Med J* 1981;282:183–185.
41. Trichopoulos D, Kalandidi A, Sparros L, MacMahon B. Lung cancer and passive smoking. *Int J Cancer* 1981;27:1–4.
42. U.S. Environmental Protection Agency (EPA). *Environmental equity:* reducing risk for all communities. Report to the Administrator from the EPA Environmental Equity Workgroup. Draft, publication no. 230-DR-92-002. Washington, DC: EPA, 1992;
43. Wald NJ, Nanchakal K, Thompson SG, Cuckle HS. Does breathing other people's tobacco smoke cause lung cancer? *Br Med J* 1986;293: 1217–1222.
44. White JR, Froeb HF. Small airways dysfunction in nonsmokers chronically exposed to tobacco smoke. *N Engl J Med* 1980;302: 720–723.
45. Kauffmann F, Tessier JS, Oriol P. Adult passive smoking in the home environment: a risk factor for chronic airflow limitation. *Am J Epidemiol* 1983;117:269–280.
46. Glantz SA, Parmley WW. Passive smoking and heart disease: epidemiology, physiology, and biochemistry. *Circulation* 1991;83:1–12.
47. Taylor AE, Johnson DC, Kazemi H. Environmental tobacco smoke and cardiovascular disease: a position paper from the council on cardiopulmonary and critical care, American Heart Association. *Circulation* 1992;86:1–4.
48. Glantz SA, Parmley WW. Passive smoking and heart disease. Mechanisms and risk. *JAMA* 1995;273:1047–1053.
49. Morrow PE. Toxicological data on $NO_2$: an overview. *J Toxicol Environ Health* 1984;13:205–227.
50. Samet JM, Utell MJ. The risk of nitrogen dioxide: What have we learned from epidemiological and clinical studies? *Toxicol Ind Health* 1990;6:247–262.
51. Melia RJ, Florey CV, Altman DG, Swan AV. Association between gas cooking and respiratory disease in children. *Br Med J* 1977;2: 149–152.
52. Hasselblad V, Kotchmar DJ, Eddy DM. Synthesis of environmental evidence: nitrogen dioxide epidemiology studies. *J Air Waste Manage Assoc* 1992;42:662–671.
53. Jarvis D, Chinn S, Luczynska C, Burney P. Association of respiratory symptoms and lung function in young adults with use of domestic gas appliances. *Lancet* 1996;347:426–432.
54. Samet JM, Lewitt EM, Warner KE. Involuntary smoking and children's health. *Crit Health Issues Child Youth* 1994;4:94–114.
55. Devalia JL, Rusznak C, Herdman MJ, Trigg CJ, Tarraf H, Davies RJ. Effect of nitrogen dioxide and sulfur dioxide on airway responses of mild asthmatic patents to allergen inhalation. *Lancet* 1994;344: 1668–1671.
56. Tunnicliffe WS, Burge PS, Ayres JG. Effect of domestic concentrations of nitrogen dioxide on airway responses to inhaled allergen in asthmatic patients. *Lancet* 1994;344:1733–1736.
57. Honicky RE, Osborne JS, Akpom CA. Symptoms of respiratory illness in young children and the use of wood-burning stoves for indoor heating. *Pediatrics* 1985;75:587–593.
58. Lebowitz MD. Indoor bioaerosol contaminants. In: Lippmann M, ed. *Critical reviews of environmental toxicants—human exposures and their health effects.* New York: Van Nostrand Reinhold, 1992, 331–359.
59. Burge HA, Feeley JC. Indoor air pollution and infectious diseases. In: Samet JM, Spengler JD, eds. *Indoor air pollution. A health perspective.* Baltimore: Johns Hopkins University Press, 1991, 273–284.
60. Weissman DN, Schuyler MR. Biological agents and allergic diseases. In: Samet JM, Spengler JD, eds. *Indoor air pollution. A health perspective.* Baltimore: Johns Hopkins University Press, 1991, 285–305.
61. Platts-Mills TAE, Chapman MD. Dust mites: immunology, allergic disease, and environmental control. *J Allergy Clin Immunol* 1987;80: 755–775.
62. National Research Council (NRC), Committee on Aldehydes. *Formaldehyde and other aldehydes.* Washington, DC: National Academy Press, 1981.
63. Leikauf GD. Formaldehydes and other aldehydes. In: Lippmann M, ed. *Critical reviews of environmental toxicants—human exposures and their health effects.* New York: Van Nostrand Reinhold, 1992, 299–300.
64. Kerns WD, Donofrio DJ, Pavkov KL. The chronic effects of formaldehyde inhalation in rats and mice: a preliminary report. In: Gibson JE, ed. *Formaldehyde toxicity.* New York: Hemisphere, 1983, 111–131.
65. Wallace LA. Volatile organic compounds. In: Samet JM, Spengler JD, eds. *Indoor air pollution. A health perspective.* Baltimore: Johns Hopkins University Press, 1991, 252–272.
66. Kreiss K. The epidemiology of building-related complaints and illness. In: Cone JE, Hodgson MJ, eds. *Problem buildings:* building-associated illness and the sick building syndrome. Philadelphia: Hanley and Belfus, 1989, 575–592.
67. Hodgson MJ. Clinical diagnosis and management of building-related illness and the sick building syndrome. In: Cone JE, Hodgson MJ, eds. *Problem buildings:* building-associated illness and the sick building syndrome. Philadelphia: Hanley and Belfus, 1989, 593–606.
68. American Thoracic Society. Environmental controls and lung disease. *Am Rev Respir Dis* 1990;142:915–939.
69. National Research Council (NRC), Committee on the Biological Effects of Ionizing Radiation. *Health risks of radon and other internally deposited alpha-emitters: BEIR IV.* Washington, DC: National Academy Press, 1988.

70. Samet JM. Radon and lung cancer. *J Natl Cancer Inst* 1989;81: 745–757.
71. Puskin JS, Nelson DB. EPA's perspective on risks from residential radon exposure. *J Air Pollut Control Assoc* 1989;39:915–920.
72. National Research Council (NRC) and Committee on Risk Assessment of Hazardous Air Pollutants.National Research Council (NRC), Committee on Risk Assessment of Hazardous Air Pollutants, eds. *Science and judgment in risk assessment.* Washington, DC: National Academy Press, 1994.
73. Samet JM. Indoor air pollution: a public health perspective. *Indoor Air* 1993;219–226.
74. Sexton K. Indoor air quality: an overview of policy and regulatory issues. *Sci Technol Human Values* 1986;2:53–67.
75. American Society of Heating Refrigerating and Air Conditioning Engineers (ASHRAE). *Ventilation for acceptable indoor air quality.* ASHRAE standard 62-1989. Atlanta: American Society of Heating, Refrigerating, and Air Conditioning Engineers (ASHRAE), 1989.
76. Cain WS, Samet JM, Hodgson MH. The quest for negligible health risk from indoor air. *ASHRAE J* 1995;37:38–44.
77. Hodgson M. The sick-building syndrome. *Occup Med* 1995;10: 167–175.
78. Apter A, Bracker A, Hodgson M, Sidman J, Leung WY. Epidemiology of the sick building syndrome. *J Allergy Clin Immunol* 1994;94:277–288.
79. Woods JE. Cost avoidance and productivity in owning and operating buildings. *Occup Med* 1989;4(4):753–770.
80. Spaul WA. Building–related factors to consider in indoor air quality evaluations [review]. *J Allergy Clin Immunol* 1994;94:385–389.
81. Nordstrom K, Norback D, Akselsson R. Influence of indoor air quality and personal factors on the sick building syndrome (SBS) in Swedish geriatric hospitals. *Occup Environ Med* 1995;52:170–176.
82. Hodgson M. The medical evaluation. *Occup Med* 1995;10:177–194.
83. Welch LS, Sokas R. Development of multiple chemical sensitivity after an outbreak of sick-building syndrome. *Toxicol Ind Health* 1992;8: 47–50.
84. Salvaggio JE. Psychological aspects of "environmental illness," "multiple chemical sensitivity," and building-related illness. *J Allergy Clin Immunol* 1994;94:366–370.
85. Hodgson M, Storey E. Patients and the sick building syndrome. *J Allergy Clin Immunol* 1994;94:335–343.
86. Skov P, Valbjorn O, Pedersen BV. Danish Indoor Climate Study Group: influence of personal characteristics, job-related factors and psychosocial factors on the sick building syndrome. *Scand J Work Environ Health* 1989;15:286–295.
87. Bauer RM, Greve KW, Besch EL, et al. The role of psychosocial factors in the report of building-related symptoms in sick building syndrome. *J Consult Clin Psychol* 1992;60(2):213–219.
88. Ryan CM, Morrow LA. Dysfunctional buildings or dysfunctional people: an examination of the sick building syndrome and allied disorders. *J Consult Clin Psychol* 1992;60(2):220–224.
89. Jaakkola JJ, Tuomaala P, Seppanen O. Textile wall materials and sick building syndrome. *Arch Environ Health* 1994;49:175–181.
90. Menzies R, Tamblyn R, Farant JP, Hanley J, Nunes F. The effect of varying levels of outdoor-air supply on the symptoms of sick building syndrome. *N Engl J Med* 1993;328:821–827.
91. Bourbeau J, Brisson C, Allaire S. Prevalence of the sick building syndrome symptoms in office workers before and after being exposed to a building with an improved ventilation system. *Occup Environ Med* 1995;30:285–295.
92. Reinikainen LM, Jaakkola JJ, Seppanen O. The effect of air humidification on symptoms and perception of indoor air quality in office workers: a six-period cross-over trial. *Arch Environ Health* 1992;47: 8–15.
93. Crandall MS, Sieber WK, Malkin R. Teichman KY, eds. *HVAC and building environmental findings and health symptom associations in 80 office buildings.* IAQ 96: paths to better building environments. Atlanta: American Society of Heating, Refrigerating, and Air-Conditioning Engineers, 1996;103.
94. Womble SE, Ronca EL, Girman JR, Brightman HS, Teichman KY, eds. *Developing baseline information on buildings and indoor air quality* (BASE '95). IAQ 96: paths to better building environments. Atlanta: American Society of Heating, Refrigerating, and Air-Conditioning Engineers, 1996;109.
95. U.S. Environmental Protection Agency (EPA). *Building air quality:* a guide for building owners and facility managers. EPA/400/91/033. Washington, DC: EPA, 1991.
96. Samet JM, Marbury MC, Spengler JD. Health effects and sources of indoor air pollution. Part II. *Am Rev Respir Dis* 1988;137:221–242.
97. Burge HA. *Bioaerosols.* Boca Raton, FL: Lewis Press, 1995.

*Environmental and Occupational Medicine, Third Edition,* edited by William N. Rom.
Published by Lippincott–Raven Publishers, Philadelphia, 1998.

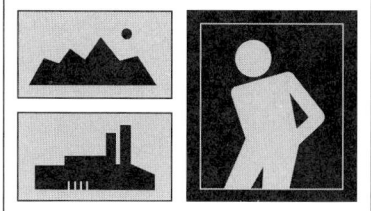

# CHAPTER 116

# Air Pollution: Human Health Studies

Robert B. Devlin

Community air pollution is an age-old problem that has been with us for as long as civilization, dating back to black linings on the caves inhabited by our ancestors. Although the 1930s, 1940s, and 1950s saw several major air pollution inversions in which increased mortality was associated with air pollution (1–3), these episodes did not generate sufficient political or public interest to attract real interest in defining the effects of air pollution on humans. The passage of the Clean Air Act in 1963 and its subsequent amendments in 1970, along with the formation of the Environmental Protection Agency (EPA), led to the implementation of National Ambient Air Quality Standards (NAAQS) for several major air pollutants, including $O_3$, sulfur and nitrogen oxides, carbon monoxide, particulate matter, and lead. These events focused substantial research interest on assessing the health effects of air pollution, which has continued to the present day.

The effects of air pollution on human health are a complex issue and the database for assessing the risk posed by air pollutants has been obtained using a multidisciplinary approach: epidemiology, animal toxicology, and human inhalation studies. Each of these approaches has advantages and limitations. Epidemiologic investigations examine exposure of people to complex mixtures of pollutants as they exist in the real world. They can study large numbers of people, including subgroups that may be susceptible to the effects of air pollutants such as elderly people with underlying cardiopulmonary disease. They can also study the effects of chronic exposure to air pollution. Outcome measures are usually assessed by questionnaires, examination of death certificates, hospital records, doctor visits, etc., and many outcomes associated with air pollution are considered adverse (e.g., mortality, increased emergency room visits, increased use of medication). However, epidemiology studies frequently have difficulty attributing effects to a specific component of air pollution, and they struggle with potential confounders such as cigarette smoking or occupational factors. In addition, sophisticated measurements of physiologic, cellular, and biochemical response cannot be routinely made in these studies.

In contrast, inhalation studies with animals can be used to study pathogenic mechanisms of pollutant injury, and can use invasive methods or study toxic pollutants that would not be practical or ethical to apply to humans. Specifically bred or treated animals can approximate various human diseases such as emphysema or pulmonary hypertension, although there is some question as to how well these models replicate the human disease state. Animal studies are also well suited to study the chronic effects of pollutants since animals can be exposed for months or even years to pollutants. Interpretation of animal studies is complicated by difficulty in extrapolating findings from animals to humans, especially at high exposure levels frequently used in animal studies.

Human exposure studies allow exposure to precise levels of individual pollutants and can examine interactions among groups of pollutants or interactions with variables such as exercise, temperature, and humidity. They also permit detailed characterization of exposure-response relationships using environmentally relevant pollutant concentrations. In addition to subjective measurements of effects (symptoms), traditional physiologic effects can be assessed as well as airway reactivity, small airway func-

R. B. Devlin: Clinical Research Branch, National Health and Environmental Effects Research Laboratory, U. S. Environmental Protection Agency, Research Triangle Park, North Carolina 27711.

tion, or mucociliary clearance. Biologic end points can also be measured using a variety of sophisticated immunologic, biochemical, and molecular end points on samples of respiratory tract cells and fluid removed by bronchoalveolar lavage. For practical and ethical reasons, controlled human exposure studies usually focus on effects in small homogeneous groups of healthy individuals or people with mild disease (e.g., mild asthmatics), and are limited to studying pollutants that do not cause dangerous or irreversible effects. Usually only acute effects are assessed in controlled human exposure studies, with a typical exposure being 1 to 8 hours for 1 to 5 days.

The focus of this chapter is on the use of controlled human exposure studies to assess the health effects of criteria air pollutants, especially $O_3$, nitrogen dioxide, and respirable urban air particulate matter ($PM_{10}$). A comprehensive review of the biologic response to all six criteria pollutants, as assessed by epidemiology, animal toxicology, and human exposure studies, can be found elsewhere (4,5).

## OZONE

Ozone is a major component of photochemical smog present in the troposphere. It is distinct from the $O_3$ layer in the stratosphere, which is 10 km above the earth's surface, and it is formed by a series of sunlight-driven reactions involving nitrogen oxides and hydrocarbons. The EPA has classified $O_3$ as a criteria pollutant and established a NAAQS of 0.12 ppm averaged over 1 hour (not to be exceeded more than three times in a 3-year period). However, tens of millions of U.S. residents reside in areas that are not in compliance with the current standard.

### Changes in Lung Function

Early controlled exposure studies showed that relatively high levels of $O_3$ could cause alterations in lung function in subjects at rest (6,7). However, in a seminal study, Bates et al. (8) showed that subjects exposed to relatively low concentrations of $O_3$ (similar to what is present in many urban areas) while undergoing intermittent exercise also exhibited lung function changes. The addition of intermittent exercise, designed to mimic moderate outdoor activity, emphasized the idea that individuals are often active when exposed to air pollution, and exercise may be an important factor in delivering air pollutants to target tissues deep in the lung. An exercise regimen of some sort has been incorporated into virtually all subsequent controlled exposure studies of humans to air pollutants. In fact, humans exposed to relatively high levels of $O_3$ (0.4 ppm) while at rest do not show measurable lung inflammation or changes in lung function (9).

Over the past 20 years, more than 100 controlled human exposure studies have clearly documented three types of physiologic lung responses to acute $O_3$ exposure: (a) irritant cough and substernal pain upon inspiration; (b) decrements in forced vital capacity (FVC) and forced expiratory volume in 1 second ($FEV_1$), due primary to decreased inspiratory capacity rather than airway obstruction; and (c) increased bronchial reactivity to nonspecific bronchoconstrictors such as histamine or methacholine. These changes are usually transient and resolve within 24 hours following a single acute exposure to $O_3$.

Dose-response studies of humans exposed to varying concentrations of $O_3$ (0.12–0.40 ppm) for 2 hours while undergoing intermittent exercise suggest a sigmoidal relationship with a few or no effects observed below 0.12 ppm and a plateau of response at higher concentrations (10–12). Most of these studies used exposure durations of 1 to 2 hours, presumably to replicate conditions in the Southern California basin at that time, in which $O_3$ levels rise sharply at midday and then begin to subside. However, in some urban areas $O_3$ levels may not exceed the NAAQS standard of 0.12 ppm, but may nevertheless remain elevated at slightly lower concentrations (0.08–0.10 ppm) for several hours. Studies designed to mimic these conditions have shown that humans exposed to levels of $O_3$ as low as 0.08 ppm for 6.6 hours while performing light exercise experience significant alterations in lung function and airway reactivity (13). These data, together with data from panel studies that demonstrate an association between decrements in lung function and outdoor $O_3$ concentration in children attending summer camps (14), have led the EPA to propose changing the current NAAQS 1-hour standard to one that would use a longer averaging time and lower $O_3$ concentration. These concentration-response studies at different exercise levels and for different durations have also been instrumental in shifting emphasis from a simplistic concentration-response evaluation of exposure data to a more complex risk analysis that takes into account activity patterns, duration of exposure, pollutant concentration, respiratory tract uptake, and other factors.

### Lower Respiratory Tract Injury and Inflammation

The recent use of bronchoalveolar lavage (BAL) as a research tool in humans has afforded the opportunity to sample cells and fluid lining the respiratory tract following exposure of humans to air pollutants. In 1986, Seltzer et al. (15) used BAL to demonstrate that humans exposed to 0.40 and 0.60 ppm $O_3$ for 2 hours had significant increases in neutrophils polymorphic nuclear leukocytes (PMNs) and several prostaglandins 3 hours following exposure. This initial study was extended by Koren et al. (16), who demonstrated that humans exposed to 0.4 ppm $O_3$ for 2 hours followed by BAL 18 hours later had increased BAL levels of PMNs, influx of plasma components into the airways, mild edema, epithelial cell injury, decreased phagocytic capacity of alveolar macrophages, and increases in a number of soluble mediators involved in lung injury and repair including interleukin-6 (IL-6), prostaglandin $E_2$ ($PGE_2$), thromboxane, clotting and coagulation factors, fibronectin, complement, elastase, and α-antitrypsin. Other studies have demonstrated $O_3$-induced changes in IL-8 (17), substance P (18), and antioxidants (19). Lung cell damage, inflammation, and decreased macrophage function have been reported in humans exposed to as little as 0.08 ppm $O_3$ for 6.6 hours (20). Ozone-induced lung injury and inflammation occurs within an hour of exposure (17) and is not resolved by 24 hours (16). Some inflammatory mediators are preferentially expressed immediately after exposure (IL-6, $PGE_2$) and others not until 24 hours (fibronectin, plasminogen activator). Recent studies have incorporated methods to sample cells and fluid specifically from the large airways (21,22), airway epithelial cells obtained by brush scraping (23), and endobronchial biopsy specimens (22,24).

### Mechanisms of Lung Function and Inflammatory Changes

Ozone-induced reductions in FVC and $FEV_1$ are primarily due to a neurally mediated decrease in inspiratory capacity (25), mediated via C-fibers (26), rather than a bronchoconstrictive process. Pretreatment of humans with antiinflammatory agents (e.g., ibuprofen) prior to $O_3$ exposure diminishes acute spirometric responses as well as $PGE_2$ (27), suggesting that the $O_3$ effect on inspiratory capacity may be mediated through prostaglandins released by airway epithelial cells (28,29), which in turn stimulate intraepithelial sensory nerve endings (30). Human alveolar macrophages exposed to $O_3$ *in vitro* produce some of the compounds found in the BAL of humans following *in vivo* $O_3$ exposure (31,32), but high concentrations of $O_3$ (1.0 ppm) are required to elicit a response, suggesting that secondary interactions between macrophages and other cells/products may be required for complete elaboration of macrophage-derived products. However, human airway epithelial cells exposed to low concentrations of $O_3$ (0.1 ppm) secrete increased amounts of many mediators found in the BAL fluid of $O_3$-exposed human including inflammatory cytokines [tumor necrosis factor (TNF), IL-6, IL-8], eicosanoids (prostaglandins, leukotrienes), platelet activating factor, lactate dehydrogenase (LDH), and fibronectin (28,29,33). These data suggest that epithelial cells are the primary target of $O_3$ and that products released by these cells initiate a cascade of events leading to lung function changes and inflammation.

### Effects of Repeated Ozone Exposure

In 1956 Stokinger et al. (34) demonstrated that rats preexposed to low concentrations of $O_3$ developed "tolerance" and were protected from a subsequent lethal $O_3$ dose. Difference in the magnitude of lung function decrements in controlled exposure studies done in Los Angeles and Chapel Hill, North Carolina, suggested that people exposed to $O_3$ on a regular basis may be less responsive than those living in an unpolluted environment (35). This notion led to studies that demonstrated that exposure of humans to $O_3$ for 5 consecutive days results in attenuation of the lung function response by the fifth day (36,37). The attenuation lasted for 7 to 10 days (38). Some indicators of inflammation (PMNs, IL-6, $PGE_2$) are also attenuated after 5 days of $O_3$ exposure, but indicators of cell injury (LDH, sloughing of epithelial cells) continue to progress, indicating that attenuation of lung function and inflammation is not necessarily a beneficial compensatory response and may well mask underlying tissue damage (39). In addition, attenuation of some inflammatory mediators is not reversed even after 3 weeks, suggesting that processes involved in reversal of lung function changes may differ from those involved in reversal of inflammatory mediators. Although controlled exposure studies are not well suited to study longer durations of exposure, Linn et al. (40) demonstrated that residents of Los Angeles who showed $O_3$-induced decrements of lung function in the spring were less responsive in the late summer or early fall at the end of the $O_3$ season; they regained their sensitivity by the following spring. This study suggests that long-term exposure to $O_3$ causes an alteration in the sensitivity to $O_3$ (at least as measured by lung function decrements), which may take some time to reverse. Rats and monkeys exposed to $O_3$ for up to 2 years have thickened airway epithelium and persistent inflammatory lesions (41–43); similar responses in humans may play a role in the seasonal response to $O_3$.

### Susceptible Subpopulations

Federal law requires that ambient air-quality standards protect the most sensitive subgroups within the population. Consequently, much research has focused on identifying and characterizing individuals who display increased sensitivity to $O_3$. Ozone-induced decrements do not vary with gender (44,45) or race (46). Children appear to have reductions in lung function similar to those in young adults (47,48), while elderly people (>50 years) have somewhat smaller $O_3$-induced responses (49,50). Cigarette smokers appear to be less responsive to $O_3$ as assessed by spirometry (51,52), but they have inflammatory responses similar to nonsmokers (53).

Several recent epidemiology studies have reported associations between variations in cardiopulmonary mortality and air pollutants, including $O_3$. Death certificates suggest that elderly people with preexisting lung disease, e.g., chronic obstructive pulmonary disease (COPD), may be susceptible to even small increases in ambient air pollution. However, controlled exposure studies have not found that individuals with COPD are particularly susceptible to $O_3$ (54–56). The subjects were generally middle-aged or older and some were current cigarette smokers; both factors are associated with a reduced response to $O_3$. In addition, most of these individuals had limited capacity for exercise, and consequently these studies were done at relatively low, minute ventilations. Only individuals with mild COPD were tested in these clinical studies and they may not be reflective of the COPD population identified in the epidemiology studies. It is also possible that a single pollutant (e.g., $O_3$) may not be sufficient to induce enhanced effects in individuals with COPD, but that a mixture more representative of outdoor air pollution (e.g., $O_3$ plus particles) might be required.

Epidemiology studies have associated increased probability of asthma attacks (57,58) and hospital visits or emergency room visits by asthmatics (59–62) with high levels of summer haze pollutants, including $O_3$. However, controlled exposure studies have not generally shown asthmatics to have enhanced $O_3$ responsiveness compared with nonasthmatic individuals (63–65). These studies usually involved mild asthmatics performing mild exercise, and only spirometric changes were studied. Recent data demonstrate that if more intense exercise is used (66) or more severe asthmatics are studied (67), asthmatics show increased airway (66) and decreased lung function (67). Even if $O_3$-induced decrements in lung function of mild asthmatics are similar to those of healthy individuals, they nevertheless represent a further decline in lung volumes and flows that are already diminished. If an asthmatic begins with a lower baseline level of lung function than a healthy individual, then the clinical consequences of an $O_3$ exposure may be greater for an asthmatic even if absolute decrements are similar.

Another way in which $O_3$ could exacerbate attacks in asthmatics is to increase their response to allergens. In 1991 Molfino et al. (68) reported that allergic asthmatics exposed to 0.1 ppm $O_3$ for 1 hour while at rest required twofold less allergen to induce bronchoconstriction than after exposure to air. Although this initial study had design flaws and was not able to be replicated (69), it nevertheless has stimulated further interest in this area. Two recent studies have shown that asthmatics exposed to higher concentrations of $O_3$ (0.2 ppm for 3 hours or 0.16 ppm for 7 hours) while undergoing mild exercise require less allergen to induce bronchoconstriction (70,71). Recent studies have also reported that $O_3$ induces a more pronounced inflammatory response in asthmatics (72) as well as increased numbers of eosinophils (73).

Animal studies have suggested that genetic factors can play a major role in responsiveness to $O_3$. There are numerous examples of large interstrain differences in response to $O_3$ and recently a single autosomal recessive genetic locus has been identified in mice that confers susceptibility to the $O_3$-induced influx of PMNs into the lung (74). A wide variability also exists in human responses to $O_3$. Controlled exposure studies have shown that $O_3$-induced decrements in lung function can vary by more than an order of magnitude (11,36) and that the response of each individual is reproducible over time (75). Reproducibility over time suggests that a genetic component may contribute to the degree of $O_3$ responsiveness. Large variations are also seen in accumulation of inflammatory markers such as PMNs, IL-6, and $PGE_2$ in the BAL fluid of humans exposed to $O_3$ (20), but it is not known if individual differences are reproducible over time. Interestingly, those individuals with the largest decrements in lung function do not necessarily have the largest increases in inflammatory mediators and there is no correlation between changes in lung function and inflammatory mediators (76), suggesting that separate mechanisms (or genes) may underlie these two responses to $O_3$. Studies with identical and fraternal twins are currently under way to determine the contribution of genetic and environmental factors to $O_3$ responsiveness.

## NITROGEN DIOXIDE

Nitrogen dioxide is a highly reactive gas that, together with sunlight and hydrocarbons, participates in the formation of $O_3$. It is relatively insoluble in water and when inhaled it penetrates to the periphery of the lung, where its toxicity is thought to be due to its oxidative capabilities. Since $NO_2$ is an essential precursor of $O_3$, reduction of outdoor $NO_2$ levels plays a part in efforts to reduce $O_3$. Outdoor levels in the United States typically range from 0.015 to 0.056 ppm and are usually below the current NAAQS standard of 0.053 ppm (annual arithmetic mean). In contrast to other criteria pollutants, levels of $NO_2$ are also generated in indoor air that may exceed outdoor concentrations. Major indoor sources include gas cooking ranges (77) and kerosine heaters (78). Since more than half of U.S. residents have a gas cooking stove, and people spend more time indoors than outdoors, the indoor environment is considered the major source of $NO_2$ exposure (79). Levels as high as 0.5 ppm have been reported in the vicinity of an operating gas stove (80) and peak levels may exceed 2.0 ppm (81).

### Changes in Lung Function and Airway Responsiveness

Concern over possible health effects associated with $NO_2$ exposure arises from epidemiology studies that link the incidence of acute respiratory illness in children with indoor $NO_2$ levels (82). Controlled exposure studies examining responses of healthy volunteers to $NO_2$ levels ranging from 0.3 to 4.0 ppm have generally failed to show alterations in lung function or airway resistance (83–86). Some studies have reported that acute exposure to 1.5 to 2.0 ppm $NO_2$ causes small but significant increases in nonspecific airway reactivity to methacholine (86) or carbachol (87).

## Lower Respiratory Tract Injury and Inflammation

Unlike $O_3$, exposure of humans to $NO_2$ concentrations even an order of magnitude greater than that found in outdoors ambient air (2.0 ppm) does not cause a significant inflammatory response as measured by increased PMNs in BAL fluid (88–90). However, exposure of humans to 2.0 ppm (91) or 3.5 ppm (92) $NO_2$ results in increased PMNs in cells recovered from the first wash ("bronchial fraction") of the BAL. Low levels of $NO_2$ (0.30 ppm) fail to induce an inflammatory response in asthmatics or people with COPD, as assessed by induced sputum (93). In addition, asthmatics exposed to 0.4 ppm $NO_2$ did not have increased nasal resistance or levels of eosinophilic cation protein (ECP), myeloperoxidase (MPO), or IL-8 in nasal lavage fluid; however, allergen challenge after $NO_2$ exposure, but not air exposure, increased levels of ECP in nasal lavage fluid (94). Taken as a whole, these studies indicate that $NO_2$ is a much less potent inducer of inflammation than $O_3$.

There is some evidence that $NO_2$ exposure may alter the balance of immune cells in the lung, particularly lymphocytes and natural killer cells. These cells play a key role in host defense against respiratory viruses by eliminating infected host cells. Significant increases in both lymphocytes and mast cells were reported in humans exposed to 2.25 to 5.0 ppm $NO_2$ for 20 minutes (95). In contrast, humans exposed to 1.5 ppm (96) or 4.0 ppm (97) $NO_2$ for several consecutive days were reported to have decreased BAL levels of natural killer cells, B lymphocytes, alveolar macrophages, and T cytotoxic suppressor lymphocytes. However, repeated exposure of humans to lower, more relevant levels of $NO_2$ (0.6 ppm) failed to find any changes in T or B lymphocytes or alveolar macrophages, and found a slight increase in natural killer cells (89). These studies indicate that single exposures to $NO_2$ may increase lymphocytes in the lung, while repeated exposures may decrease these immune cells. However, the clinical significance of small changes in lymphocyte subsets after exposure of humans to high $NO_2$ concentrations is unclear.

## Changes in Host Defense/Infectivity

Epidemiology studies associating $NO_2$ exposure with respiratory illness are supported by acute and chronic animal exposure studies that demonstrated enhanced mortality in animals challenged with bacteria (reviewed in ref. 98) or virus (99). Impairment of macrophage function appears to play a role in this effect (100,101), as does decreased mucociliary clearance (102). Only a limited number of controlled human exposure studies have addressed the effects of $NO_2$ on respiratory infections. Over a 3-year period, 152 healthy volunteers were exposed to 1.0, 2.0, or 3.0 ppm $NO_2$ for 3 consecutive days and an attenuated cold-adapted influenza virus was administered intranasally after the second exposure (103). Viral infection was measured by virus recovery or an increase in serum/nasal wash influenza antibody titers. There were no significant differences in infection between air and $NO_2$-exposed individuals, although there was a trend toward more infection in $NO_2$-exposed subjects in the third year of the study.

Another approach has been to obtain alveolar macrophages from volunteers exposed to $NO_2$ and examine them *in vitro* for changes in function related to host defense capability. Alveolar macrophages removed from humans exposed to 2.0 ppm $NO_2$ for 4 hours had impaired phagocytic activity as well as decreased superoxide anion production (91). Macrophages removed from individuals exposed to 0.60 ppm $NO_2$ for 3 hours tended to inactivate influenza virus less effectively than macrophages from individuals exposed to air (90). This effect was observed in cells from four of the nine subjects studied; macrophages from the same four subjects also released elevated amounts of IL-1. These limited data point out the utility of using controlled exposures followed by *in vitro* challenge with microorganisms as a way to assess the effects of air pollutants on host defense capability in the lung.

## Susceptible Subpopulations

A report in 1976 (104) directed attention to the possibility that a brief exposure of mild asthmatics to relatively low levels of $NO_2$ (0.1 ppm) might enhance in a subset of the cohort (13 of 20 subjects) their subsequent responsiveness to bronchial challenge with a bronchoconstricting drug such as histamine or methacholine. However, these results were not confirmed in subsequent studies with adults or adolescent asthmatics exposed to low concentrations of $NO_2$ (64,105,106) or adult asthmatics exposed to levels as high as 4.0 ppm (107). Two laboratories reported decrements in lung function and airway reactivity in subsets of asthmatics exposed to 0.30 ppm $NO_2$ (108,109), but were unable to confirm these observations in subsequent studies (110,111). The inconsistent results of these studies is not well understood. Although factors such as exposure concentration, duration, level of exercise, severity of asthma, and use of medication may account for some of the discrepancies, it is clear that asthmatics have a wide range of response to $NO_2$. Results may differ simply because of the number of "responders" present in different studies. In this regard, Bauer et al. (108) reported that 7 of 15 subjects had a significant reduction in $FEV_1$ and airway reactivity after exposure to 0.30 ppm $NO_2$. The same seven subjects were included in a follow-up to this "positive" study, and although the follow-up study was conducted 1 year later (and included a total of 20 asthmatics) and was "negative," the same seven individuals were equally responsive to $NO_2$ in this second study (112). The consistency of responses of asthmatics to $NO_2$ across a 1-year interval suggests that some asthmatics are inherently responsive to $NO_2$ and suggests the need for additional studies designed to identify which asthmatics may be susceptible to $NO_2$.

Few studies have examined the response of people with COPD to $NO_2$. Linn et al. (113) found no lung function changes in subjects exposed to 0.5 to 2.0 ppm $NO_2$ for 1 hour, nor did Vagaggini et al. (93) in COPD subjects exposed to 0.30 ppm $NO_2$ for 1 hour. However, Morrow et al. (114) reported progressive decrements in lung function in a group of COPD patients exposed to 0.30 ppm $NO_2$ for 4 hours, which may reflect a difference in the severity of disease between the two cohorts or the difference in the duration of exposure. It is worth noting the changes in lung function observed in COPD patients were of the "restrictive" pattern seen with $O_3$ rather than the "obstructive" changes observed in asthmatics exposed to $NO_2$.

There is no evidence to suggest that elderly people are particularly sensitive to $NO_2$ (114), but two studies suggest that smokers may be. Smokers exposed to 0.3 ppm $NO_2$ experienced a significant drop in $FEV_1$ that was greater than that experienced by nonsmokers (114), and smokers exposed to 3.5 ppm $NO_2$ are reported to have increased BAL levels of both PMNs and alveolar macrophages (92).

## PARTICLES AND ACIDIC AEROSOLS

Early epidemiology studies of severe air pollution episodes in the U.S. and Europe demonstrated that exposure to very high levels of urban air particles can result in increased mortality and morbidity (1–3) During the past decade, several epidemiologic studies using improved statistical techniques and more precise and extended particle monitoring data have reported statistically significant positive correlations between daily (or a several-day average) concentrations of $PM_{10}$ and increased mortality and morbidity. More than two dozen analyses and reanalyses of these studies report a 2% to 8% increase in relative risk of mortality for every 50 $\mu g/m^3$ increase in the 24-hour average $PM_{10}$ concentration (115). The observed increases in mortality and morbidity, while statistically significant, are still small compared to risks found in epidemiologic studies of occupational or other risk factors. However, because of the large fraction of the population potentially exposed to elevated $PM_{10}$ levels, it has been estimated that 60,000 excess mortalities in the United States each year may be attributable to $PM_{10}$. In general, these studies report higher mortality rates attributable to respiratory and cardiovascular causes than for total nonaccidental mortality, as well as increased mortality in those older than 65.

Several potential mechanisms have been proposed to provide biologic plausibility to the notion that acute exposure to relatively low levels of fine particles can result in a rapid increase in mortality and morbidity. $PM_{10}$ has been reported to cause a variety of effects in humans or animals, including respiratory symptoms, inflammation, changes in mucociliary clearance of particles, decrements in lung function, and morphologic changes in lung tissue. Many of these effects could contribute to pulmonary or cardiopulmonary events that could result in $PM_{10}$-associated mortality. Events that cause hypoxemia such as bronchoconstriction, impaired diffusion, edema, and inflammation can lead to cardiac arrhythmia. $PM_{10}$-induced acute inflammation can lead to production of numerous cytokines and other proinflammatory compounds, edema, and epithelial cell injury that may not be perceptible to normal healthy individuals, but could lead to cardiopulmonary stress in some elderly individuals or those with underlying pulmonary disease. Repeated induction of inflammation and lung injury could also lead to chronic lung injury such as the initiation or progression of COPD.

Despite the impressive epidemiologic evidence linking $PM_{10}$ levels with increased mortality and morbidity, animal toxicologic and controlled human exposure studies have not yet provided compelling evidence pointing to a specific component or components of $PM_{10}$ that may be responsible for the health effects reported in the epidemiology literature. $PM_{10}$ pollution is a complex mixture of organic and inorganic constituents whose composition can vary widely depending on the time of year and geographical location. Particulate matter exists over a wide range of sizes and geometries. In general, however, it can be depicted as discrete solid particles, as agglomerated chains of such particles, or as dispersed liquid droplets. Nevertheless, there are several properties or components of $PM_{10}$ that may be responsible for increased mortality/morbidity. These include particle size, particle acidity, transition metals present on particles, bioaerosols, and organic compounds found on particles.

### Acidic Aerosols

Of these components, controlled human exposure studies have focused primarily on particle acidity. Here is a brief summary of some of the more important findings from these studies. More than 20 controlled exposure studies of healthy human and asthmatic volunteers to acidic aerosols have been performed. They are in general agreement that healthy subjects experience no decrements in lung function at levels up to 1,000 $\mu g/m^3$ (an order of magnitude higher than ambient levels), although exposures at the highest concentrations were associated with mild increases in symptoms (reviewed in ref. 4). It is possible that a large portion of the inhaled acid is neutralized by ammonia present in the mouth and respiratory tract. In human studies the size of the acidic aerosol was not a critical factor in response (116–118). Several studies have suggested that asthmatics are more sensitive than healthy subjects to acid aerosols (4), and that adolescent asthmatics may experience small decrements in lung function even at exposure levels lower than 100 μg/m$^3$ (119,120).

Healthy subjects exposed to relatively modest concentrations of acidic aerosols experience accelerated clearance in large bronchi, but slower clearance in small airways (121–123). Interestingly, while macrophages from humans exposed to acidic aerosols have altered phagocytic function, acid exposures do not appear to induce an acute neutrophilic inflammation (124,125). Altered mucociliary clearance and phagocytic capability may render some individuals more susceptible to infections, and contribute to the observed increase in morbidity associated with $PM_{10}$.

Despite the extensive epidemiologic database indicting acid as an air pollutant of potential concern, the clinical data have not been widely acknowledged as sufficient evidence to account for the mortality/morbidity effects ascribed to $PM_{10}$. Perhaps acid alone is too simple a metric for assessment. Guinea pigs exposed to acid-coated zinc oxide particles had significant reductions in total lung volume and vital capacity (126), airway responsiveness (127), and increased inflammatory mediators (128) compared with animals exposed to zinc oxide or acid alone. However, it remains to be seen whether humans respond in an analogous fashion and whether such exposures are realistic in the general ambient environment.

### Other Particle Components

Considerably less is known about the response of humans to other potentially active agents present in particulate pollution. Animal exposure studies and *in vitro* toxicology have provided considerable evidence that transition metals present on particles may lead to lung damage and inflammation (reviewed in ref. 129), likely via formation of reactive oxygen species, but there is little data available from human studies. Instillation of iron oxide into the lungs of humans results in a significant inflammatory response at 24 hours that has largely subsided by 48 hours (130). In nonsmokers an association has been reported between exposure to fuel oil ash, which contains high concentrations of transition metals, and upper airway inflammation manifested by increased numbers of PMNs (131), as well as decrements in $FEV_1$ (132).

Diesel exhaust particles have been reported to stimulate increased immunoglobulin E (IgE) production following instillation into nasal passages of volunteers (133), and it was suggested that polyaromatic hydrocarbons (PAHs) present on the particles were responsible for the response. Exposure of volunteers to 300 μg/m$^3$ diesel exhaust resulted in a pronounced inflammatory response and inflammation in the airway mucosa (134), and it was postulated that particulate components within the diesel exhaust were responsible for the effects. In contrast, eye and nose irritation and airway resistance increased after exposure of humans to diesel exhaust but were primarily associated with gas phase products (135). Studies in which humans are directly exposed to concentrated urban air particles are currently under way and should yield important information about clinical effects induced by these particles.

## REFERENCES


1. Firket J. The causes of accidents which occurred in the Meuse Valley during the fogs of December 1930. *Bull Acad R Med Belg* 1931;11: 683–741.
2. Schrenk HH, Heimann H, Clayton GD, Gafafer WM, Wexler H. *Air pollution in Donora, PA. Epidemiology of the unusual smog episode of October 1948:* preliminary report. Public Health Service bulletin no. 306. Washington, DC: Public Health Service, 1949.
3. Martin AE. Mortality and morbidity statistics and air pollution. *Proc R Soc Med* 1964;57:969–975.
4. Bascom R, Bromberg PA, Costa DL, et al. Health effects of outdoor air pollution. Part 1. *Am J Respir Crit Care Med* 1996;153:3–50.
5. Bascom R, Bromberg PA, Costa DL, et al. Health effects of outdoor air pollution. Part 2. *Am J Respir Crit Care Med* 1996;153:477–498.
6. Young WA, Shaw DB, Bates DV. Pulmonary function in welders exposed to ozone. *Arch Environ Health* 1963;7:337–340.
7. Young WA, Shaw DB, Bates DV. Effects of low concentrations of ozone on pulmonary function in man. *J Appl Physiol* 1964; 19:765–768.
8. Bates DV, Bell G, Burnham C, et al. Short term effects of ozone on the lung. *J Appl Physiol* 1972;32:176–181.
9. Hatch GE, Slade R, Harris LP, et al. Ozone dose and effect in humans and rats: a comparison using oxygen-18 labeling and bronchoalveolar lavage. *Am J Respir Crit Care Med* 1994;150:676–686.
10. Kulle TJ, Sauder LR, Hebel JR, Chatham MD. Ozone response relationships in healthy nonsmokers. *Am Rev Respir Dis* 1985;132:36–41.
11. McDonnell WF, Horstman DH, Hazucha MJ, et al. Pulmonary effects of ozone exposure during exercise: dose response characteristics. *J Appl Physiol* 1983;5:1345–1352.
12. Linn WS, Avol EL, Shamoo DA, et al. A dose response study of healthy, heavily exercising men exposed to ozone at concentrations near the ambient air quality standard. *Toxicol Ind Health* 1986;2: 99–112.
13. Horstman DH, Folinsbee LJ, Ives PJ, Abdul-Salaam S, McDonnell WF. Ozone concentration and pulmonary response relationships for 6.6 hr exposures with 5 hr of moderate exercise to 0.08, 0.10, and 0.12 ppm. *Am Rev Respir Dis* 1990;142:1158–1163.
14. Spektor DM, Lippmann M, Lioy PJ, et al. Effects of ambient ozone on respiratory function in active, normal children. *Am Rev Respir Dis* 1988;137:313–320.
15. Seltzer J, Bigby BG, Stulbarg M, et al. $O_3$-induced change in bronchial reactivity to methacholine and airway inflammation in humans. *J Appl Physiol* 1986;60:1321–1326.
16. Koren HS, Devlin RB, Graham DE, et al. Ozone-induced inflammation in the lower airways of human subjects. *Am Rev Respir Dis* 1988; 139;407–415.
17. Devlin, RB, McDonnell WF, Becker S, et al. Time-dependent changes of inflammatory mediators in the lungs of humans exposed to 0.4 ppm ozone for 2 hr: a comparison of mediators found in bronchoalveolar lavage fluid 1 and 18 hr after exposure. *Toxicol Appl Pharmacol* 1996; 138:176–185.
18. Hazbun ME, Hamilton R, Holian A, Eschenbacher WL. Ozone-induced increases in substance P and 8-epi-prostaglandin F2 alpha in the airways of human subjects. *Am J Respir Cell Mol Biol* 1993;9: 568–72.
19. Slade R, Crissman K, Norwood J, Hatch G. Comparison of antioxidant substances in bronchoalveolar lavage cells and fluid from humans, guinea pigs, and rats. *Exp Lung Res* 1993;19:469–84.
20. Devlin RB, McDonnell WF, Mann R, et al. Exposure of humans to ambient levels of ozone for 6.6 hours causes cellular and biochemical changes in the lung. *Am J Respir Cell Mol Biol* 1991;4:72–81.
21. Schelegle ES, Siefkin AD, McDonald RJ. Time course of ozone-

induced neutrophilia in normal humans. *Am Rev Respir Dis* 1991;143: 1353–1358.
22. Aris RM, Christian D, Hearne PQ, Kerr K, Finkbeiner WE, Balmes JR. Ozone-induced airway inflammation in human subjects as determined by airway lavage and biopsy. *Am Rev Respir Dis* 1993;148: 1363–1372.
23. Quay J, Becker S, Koren HS, Clapp WA, Schwartz DA. Comparison of cytokine (IL-1β, SIL-1RA, IL-6 and TNFα) expression in human bronchial epithelium and in alveolar macrophages exposed to endotoxin-contaminated grain dust. *Am Rev Respir Dis* 1993;147:A19.
24. Krishna MT, Springall DR, Meng Q-H, et al. Effects of 0.2 ppm ozone on the sensory nerves in the bronchial mucosa of healthy humans (abstract). *Am J Respir Crit Care Med* 1996;153:A700.
25. Hazucha MJ, Bates DV, Bromberg PA. Mechanism of action of ozone on the human lung. *J Appl Physiol* 1989;67:1535–1541.
26. Coleridge JCG, Coleridge HM, Schelegle ES, Green JF. Acute inhalation of ozone stimulates bronchial C-fibers and rapidly adapting receptors in dogs. *J Appl Physiol* 1993;74:2345–2352.
27. Hazucha MJ, Madden M, Pape G, et al. Effects of cyclooxygenase inhibition on ozone-induced respiratory inflammation and lung function changes. *Eur J Appl Physiol* 1996;73:17–27.
28. Devlin RB, McKinnon KP, Noah T, Becker S, Koren HS. Ozone-induced release of cytokines and fibronectin by alveolar macrophages and airway epithelial cells. *Am J Physiol* 1994;266: L612–L619.
29. Leikauf GD, Driscoll KE, Wey HE. Ozone-induced augmentation of eicosanoid metabolism in epithelial cells from bovine trachea. *Am Rev Respir Dis* 1988;137:435–442.
30. Coleridge HM, Coleridge JC, Baker DG, Ginzel KH, Morrison MA. Comparison of the effects of histamine and prostaglandin on afferent C-fiber endings and irritant receptors in the intrapulmonary airways. *Adv Exp Med Biol* 1978;99:291–305.
31. Madden MC, Eling TE, Dailey LA, Friedman M. The effect of ozone exposure on rat alveolar macrophage arachidonic acid metabolism. *Exp Lung Res* 1991;17:47–63.
32. Becker S, Madden MC, Newman SL, Devlin RB, Koren HS. Modulation of human alveolar macrophage properties by ozone exposure *in vitro*. *Toxicol Appl Pharmacol* 1991;110:403–415.
33. Samet JM, Noal TL, Yankaskas JR, McKinnon K, Dailey LA, Friedman M. Effect of ozone on platelet-acting-factor production in phorbol-differentiated HL60 cells, a human bronchial epithelial cell line (BEAS S6), and primary human bronchial epithelial cells. *Am J Respir Cell Mol Biol* 1992;7:514–522.
34. Stokinger HE, Wagner WD, Wright PG. Studies on ozone toxicity. I Potentiating effects of exercise and tolerance development. *Arch Ind Health* 1956;14:158–162.
35. Hackney JD, Linn WS, Buckley RD, Hislop HJ. Studies on adaptation to ambient oxidant air pollution: effects of ozone exposures in Los Angeles residents vs. new arrivals. *Environ Health Perspect* 1976;18: 141–146.
36. Horvath SM, Gliner JA, Folinsbee LJ. Adaptation to ozone: duration of effect. *Am Rev Respir Dis* 1981;123 496–499.
37. Hackney JD, Linn WS, Mohler JG, Collier CR. Adaptation to short-term respiratory effects of ozone in men exposed repeatedly. *J Appl Physiol* 1977;43:82–85.
38. Kulle TJ, Sauder LR, Kerr DH, Farrell BP, Bermel MS, Smith DM. Duration of pulmonary function adaptation to ozone in humans. *Am Ind Hyg Assoc* 1982;43:832–837.
39. Devlin RB, Folinsbee, LJ, Biscardi F, et al. Inflammation and cell damage induced by repeated exposure of humans to ozone. *Inhal Toxicol* 1997;9:211–235.
40. Linn WS, Avol EL, Shamoo DA, et al. Repeated laboratory ozone exposures of volunteer Los Angeles residents; an apparent seasonal variation in response. *Toxicol Ind Health* 1988;4:505–520.
41. Tyler WS, Tyler NK, Last JA, Gillespie MJ, Barstow TJ. Comparison on daily and seasonal exposures of young monkeys to ozone. *Toxicology* 1988;50:131–144.
42. Barr BC, Hyde DM, Plopper CG, Dungworth DL. Distal airway remodelling in rats chronically exposed to ozone. *Am Rev Respir Dis* 1988;137:924–938.
43. Barry BE, Miller FJ, Crapo JD. Effects of inhalation of 0.12 and 0.25 parts per million ozone on the proximal alveolar region of juvenile and adult rats. *Lab Invest* 1985;53:692–704.
44. Gibbons SI, Adams WC. Combined effects of ozone exposure and ambient heat on exercising females. *J Appl Physiol Respir Environ Exerc Physiol* 1984;57:450–456.
45. Lauritzen SK, Adams WC. Ozone inhalation effects consequent to continuous exercise in females: comparison to males. *J Appl Physiol* 1985;59:1601–1606.
46. Seal E Jr, McDonnell WF, House DE, et al. The pulmonary response of white and black men and women to six concentrations of ozone. *Am Rev Respir Dis* 1993;147:804–810.
47. McDonnell WF, Chapman RS, Leigh MW, Strope GL, Collier AM. Respiratory responses of vigorously exercising children to 0.12 ppm ozone exposure. *Am Rev Respir Dis* 1985;132:875–879.
48. Avol EL, Linn WS, Shamoo DA, et al. Short-term respiratory effects of photochemical oxidant in exercising children. *J Air Pollut Control Assoc* 1987;37:158–162.
49. Drechsler-Parks DM, Bedi JF, Horvath SM. Pulmonary function response of older men and women to ozone exposure. *Exp Gerontol* 1987;22:91–101.
50. Seal E Jr, McDonnell WF, Chapman RS, House DE. The effect of menstrual cycle and age on the pulmonary response to ozone (abstract). *Am Rev Respir Dis* 1993;147:A637.
51. Kerr HD, Kulle TJ, McIlhany ML, Swiderski P. Effects of ozone on pulmonary function in normal subjects: an environmental chamber study. *Am Rev Respir Dis* 1975;111:763–773.
52. Frampton MW, Morow PE, Torres A, Cox C, Voter KZ, Utell MJ. Ozone responsiveness in smokers and nonsmokers. *Am J Respir Crit Care Med* 1997;155:116–121.
53. Torres A, Utell MJ, Morow PE, Frampton MW. Airway inflammation in smokers and nonsmokers with varying responsiveness to ozone. *Am J Respir Crit Care Med* 1997;156:728–736.
54. Solic JJ, Hazucha MT, Bromberg PA. The acute effects of 0.2 ppm ozone in patients with chronic obstructive pulmonary disease. *Am Rev Respir Dis* 1982;125:664–669.
55. Hackney JD, Linn WS, Fischer A, et al. Effects of ozone in people with chronic obstructive lung disease (COLD). *Adv Modern Environ Toxicol* 1983;5:205–211.
56. Kehrl HR, Hazucha MJ, Solic JJ, Bromberg PA. Responses of subjects with chronic obstructive pulmonary disease after exposures to 0.30 ppm ozone. *Am Rev Respir Dis* 1985;131:719–724.
57. Contant CF Jr, Stock TH, Buffler PA, Holguin AH, Gehan BM, Kotchmar DJ. The estimation of personal exposures to air pollutants for a community-based study of health effects in asthmatics—exposure model. *J Air Pollut Control Assoc* 1987;37:587–594.
58. Whittemore AS, Korn EL. Asthma and air pollution in the Los Angeles area. *Am J Public Health* 1980;70:687–696.
59. Cody RP, Weisel CP, Birnbarm G, Lioy PJ. The effect of ozone associated with summertime photochemical smog on the frequency of asthma visits to hospital emergency departments. *Environ Res* 1992;58: 184–194.
60. Thurston GD, Ito K, Kinney PL, Lippman M. A multi-year study of air pollution and respiratory hospital admissions in three New York state metropolitan areas: results for 1988 and 1989 summers. *J Expo Anal Environ Epidemiol* 1992;2:429–450.
61. Thurston GD, Ito K, Hayes CG, Bates DV, Lippmann M. Respiratory hospital admissions and summertime haze air pollution in Toronto, Ontario: consideration of the role of acid aerosols. *Environ Res* 1994; 65:271–290.
62. White MC, Etzel RA, Wilcox WD, Lloyd C. Exacerbations of childhood asthma and ozone pollution in Atlanta. *Environ Res* 1994;65: 56–68.
63. Linn WS, Buckley RD, Spier CE, et al. Health effects of ozone exposure in asthmatics. *Am Rev Respir Dis* 1978;117:835–843.
64. Koenig JQ, Covert DS, Morgan MS, et al. Acute effects of 0.12 ppm ozone or 0.12 ppm nitrogen dioxide on pulmonary function in healthy and asthmatic adolescents. *Am Rev Respir Dis* 1985;132:648–651.
65. Koenig JQ, Covert DS, Marshall SG, Van Belle G, Pierson WE. The effects of ozone and nitrogen dioxide on pulmonary function in healthy and asthmatic adolescents. *Am Rev Respir Dis* 1987;136: 1152–1157.
66. Kreit JW, Gross KB, Moore TB, Lorenzen TJ, D'Arcy J, Eschenbacher WL. Ozone-induced changes in pulmonary function and bronchial hyperresponsiveness in asthmatics. *J Appl Physiol* 1989; 66:217–222.
67. Horstman DH, Ball BA, Brown J, Gerrity TR, Folinsbee LJ. Comparison of pulmonary response of asthmatic and non-asthmatic subjects

performing light exercise while exposed to a low level of ozone. *Toxicol Ind Health* 1995;11369–85.

68. Molfino NA, Wright SC, Katz I, et al. Effect of low concentrations of ozone on inhaled allergen responses in asthmatic subjects. *Lancet* 1991;338:199–203.
69. Ball BA, Folinsbee LJ, Peden DB, Kehrl HR. Allergen bronchoprovocation of patients with mild allergic asthma after ozone exposure. *J Allergy Clin Immunol* 1996;93:563–572.
70. Jorres RD, Nowak D, Magnussen H. The effect of ozone exposure on allergen responsiveness in subjects with asthma or rhinitis. *Am J Respir Crit Care Med* 1996;153:56–64.
71. Kehrl HR, Ball B, Folinsbee L, Peden D, Horstman D. Increased specific airway reactivity of mild allergic asthmatics following 7.6 hr exposures to 0.16 ppm ozone. *Am Rev Respir Dis* 1993;147(4):A731.
72. Scannell C, Chen L, Aris RM, et al. Greater ozone-induced inflammatory responses in subjects with asthma. *Am J Respir Crit Care Med* 1996;154:24–29.
73. Peden DB, Boehlecke B, Horstman D, Devlin R. The effect of prolonged ozone exposure on inflammatory mediators in asthmatics. *Am Rev Respir Dis* 1993;147(4):A731.
74. Kleeberger SR, Bassett DJP, Jakab GJ, Levitt RC. A genetic model for evaluation of susceptibility to ozone-induced inflammation. *Am J Physiol (Lung Cell Mol Physiol)* 1990;258:L313–L320.
75. McDonnell WF, Horstman DH, Abdul-Salaam S, House DE. Reproducibility of individual responses to ozone exposure. *Am Rev Respir Dis* 1985;131:36–40.
76. Balmes JR, Chen LL, Scannell C, et al. Ozone-induced decrements in FEV1 and FVC do not correlate with measures of inflammation. *Am J Respir Crit Care Med* 1996;153:904–909.
77. National Academy of Sciences Commission on Life Sciences. *Indoor pollutants.* Washington, DC: National Academy Press, 1981.
78. Traynor GW, Apte MG, Carruthers AR, et al. The effects of infiltration and insulation on the source strengths and indoor air pollution from combustion space heating appliances. *J Air Pollut Control Assoc* 1988;38:1011–1015.
79. U.S. Environmental Protection Agency. *National air quality and emissions trends report.* Report 450-R-92-001. Research Triangle Park, NC: Office of Air Quality and Planning Standards, 1991.
80. Goldstein IF, Lieber K, Andrews LR, et al. Acute respiratory effects of short-term exposures to nitrogen dioxide. *Arch Environ Health* 1988; 43:138–142.
81. Leaderer BP, Stolwijk JAJ, Zagraniski RT, Quing-Shang MA. Field study of indoor air contaminant levels associated with unvented combustion sources (abstract). 77th Annual Meeting of the Air Pollution Control Association 1984;33.3.
82. Samet JM, Marbury MC, Spengler JD. Health effects and sources of indoor air pollution. Part I. *Am Rev Respir Dis* 1987;136;1486–1508.
83. Linn WS, Solomon JC, Trim SC, et al. Effects of exposure to 4 ppm nitrogen dioxide in healthy and asthmatic volunteers. *Arch Environ Health* 1985;40:234–238.
84. Hackney JD, Theide FC, Linn WS, et al, Experimental studies on human health effects of air pollutants. Part IV. Short-term physiological and clinical effects of nitrogen dioxide exposures. *Arch Environ Health* 1978;33:176–180.
85. Kerr HD, Kulle TJ, McIlhany ML, Swiderzsky P. Effects of nitrogen dioxide on pulmonary function in human subjects: an environmental chamber study. *Environ Res* 1979;19:392–404.
86. Mohsenin V. Airway responses to 2.0 ppm nitrogen dioxide in normal subjects. *Arch Environ Health* 1988;43:242–246.
87. Frampton MW, Morrow PE, Cox C, Gibb FR, Speers DM, Utell-MJ. Effects of nitrogen dioxide exposure on pulmonary function and airway reactivity in normal humans. *Am Rev Respir Dis* 1991;143:522–527.
88. Frampton MW, Finkelstein JN, Roberts NJ Jr, Smeglin AM, Morrow PE, Utell MJ. Effects of nitrogen dioxide exposure on bronchoalveolar lavage proteins in humans. *Am J Respir Cell Mol Biol* 1989;1: 499–505.
89. Rubinstein I, Reiss TF, Bigby BG, Stites DP, Boushey HA Jr. Effects of 0.60 ppm nitrogen dioxide on circulating and bronchoalveolar lavage lymphocyte phenotypes in healthy subjects *Environ Res* 1991; 55:18–30.
90. Frampton MW, Smeglin AM, Roberts NJ Jr, Finkelstein JN, Morrow PE, Utell MJ. Nitrogen dioxide exposure *in vivo* and human alveolar macrophage inactivation of influenza virus in vitro. *Environ Res* 1989; 48:179–192.
91. Devlin R, Horstman D, Becker S, Gerrity T, Madden M, Koren H. Inflammatory response in humans exposed to 2.0 ppm $NO_2$ (abstract). *Am Rev Respir Dis* 1992;145:A455.
92. Helleday R, Sandstrom T, Stjernberg N. Differences in bronchoalveolar cell response to nitrogen dioxide exposure between smokers and nonsmokers. *Eur Respir J* 1994;7:1213–1220.
93. Vagaggini B, Paggiaro PL, Giannini D, et al. Effect of short-term $NO_2$ exposure on induced sputum in normal, asthmatic and COPD subjects. *Eur Respir J* 1996;9:1852–1857.
94. Wang JH, Devalia JL, Duddle JM, Hamilton SA, Davies RJ. Effect of six-hour exposure to nitrogen dioxide on early-phase nasal response to allergen challenge in patients with a history of seasonal allergic rhinitis. *J Allergy Clin Immunol* 1995;96:669–676.
95. Sandstrom T, Stjernberg N, Eklund A, et al. Inflammatory cell response in bronchoalveolar lavage fluid after nitrogen dioxide exposure of healthy subjects: a dose-response study. *Eur Respir J* 1991;4: 332–339.
96. Sandstrom T, Ledin MC, Thomasson L, Helleday R, Stjernberg N. Reductions in lymphocyte subpopulations after repeated exposure to 1.5 ppm nitrogen dioxide. *Br J Ind Med* 1992;49:850–854.
97. Sandstrom T, Helleday R, Bjermer L, Stjernberg N. Effects of repeated exposure to 4 ppm nitrogen dioxide on bronchoalveolar lymphocyte subsets and macrophages in healthy men. *Eur Respir J* 1992; 5:1092–1096.
98. Gardner DE. Oxidant-induced enhanced sensitivity to infection in animal models and their extrapolations to man. *J Toxicol Environ Health* 1984;13:423–439.
99. Rose RM, Fuglestad JM, Skornik WA, et al. The pathophysiology of enhanced susceptibility of murine cytomegalovirus respiratory infection during short-term exposure to 5 ppm nitrogen dioxide. *Am Rev Respir Dis* 1988;137:912–917.
100. Goldstein E, Eagle MC, Hoeprich PD. Effect of nitrogen dioxide on pulmonary bacterial defense mechanisms. *Arch Environ Health* 1973; 26:202–204.
101. Jakab GJ. Modulation of pulmonary defense mechanisms by acute exposures to nitrogen dioxide. *Environ Res* 1987;42:215–228.
102. Helleday R, Huberman D, Blomberg A, Stjernberg N, Sandstrom T. Nitrogen dioxide exposure impairs the frequency of the mucociliary activity in healthy subjects. *Eur Respir J* 1995;8:1664–1668.
103. Goings SAJ, Kulle TJ, Bascom R, et al. Effect of nitrogen dioxide exposure on susceptibility to influenza A virus infection in healthy adults. *Am Rev Respir Dis* 1989;139:1075–1081.
104. Orehek J, Massari JP, Gayrard P, Grimaud C, Charpin J. Effect of short-term, low-level nitrogen exposure on bronchial sensitivity of asthmatic patients. *J Clin Invest* 1976;57:301–307.
105. Hazucha MJ, Ginsberg JF, McDonnell WF, et al. Effect of 0.1 ppm nitrogen dioxide on airways of normal and asthmatic subjects. *J Appl Physiol Respir Environ Exerc Physiol* 1983;54:730–739.
106. Koenig JQ, Pierson WE, Marshall SG, Covert DS, Morgan MS, Van Belle G. The effects of ozone and nitrogen dioxide on lung function in healthy and adolescent asthmatics. *Res Rep Health Effect Inst* 1988; 14:5–24.
107. Linn WS, Shamoo DA, Avol EL, et al. Dose-response study of asthmatic volunteers exposed to nitrogen dioxide during intermittent exercise. *Arch Environ Health* 1986;41:292–296.
108. Bauer MA, Utell MJ, Morrow PE, Speers DM, Gibb FR. Route of inhalation influences airway responses to 0.30 ppm nitrogen dioxide in asthmatic subjects (abstract). *Am Rev Respir Dis* 1985;133: A171.
109. Roger LJ, Horstman DH, McDonnell WF, et al. Pulmonary effects in asthmatics exposed to 0.3 ppm $NO_2$ during repeated exercise. *Toxicologist* 1985;5:70.
110. Mohsenin V, Gee BL. Acute effect of nitrogen dioxide exposure on the functional activity of alpha-1-protease inhibitor in bronchoalveolar lavage fluid of normal subjects. *Am Rev Respir Dis* 1987;136: 646–650.
111. Roger LJ, Horstman DH, McDonnell WF, et al. Pulmonary function, airway responsiveness, and respiratory symptoms in asthmatics following exercise in $NO_2$. *Toxicol Ind Health* 1990;6:155–171.
112. Morrow PE, Utell MJ. Responses of susceptible subpopulations to nitrogen dioxide. *Res Rep Health Effect Inst* 1989;23:1–44.
113. Linn WS, Shamoo DA, Spier CE, et al. Controlled exposures of volunteers with chronic obstructive pulmonary disease to nitrogen dioxide. *Arch Environ Health* 1985;40:313–317.

114. Morrow PE, Utell MJ, Bauer MA, et al. Pulmonary performance of elderly normal subjects and subjects with chronic obstructive pulmonary disease exposed to 0.3 ppm nitrogen dioxide. *Am Rev Respir Dis* 1992;145:291–300.
115. U.S. Environmental Protection Agency. *Air quality criteria for particulate matter,* vol 1. Report 600/P-95/001cF. Washington, DC: EPA Office of Research and Development, 1996.
116. Avol EL, Linn WS, Whynot JD, et al. Respiratory dose-response study of normal and asthmatic volunteers exposed to sulfuric acid aerosol in the sub-micrometer size range. *Toxicol Ind Health* 1988;4:173–118.
117. Avol EL, Linn WS, Wightman LH, Whynot JD, Anderson KR, Hackney JD. Short-term respiratory effects of sulfuric acid in fog: a laboratory study of healthy and asthmatic volunteers. *JAPCA* 1988; 38:258–263.
118. Linn WS, Avol EL, Anderson KR, Shamoo DA, Peng RC, Hackney JD. Effect of droplet size on respiratory responses to inhaled sulfuric acid in normal and asthmatic volunteers. *Am Rev Respir Dis* 1989;140:161–166.
119. Koenig JQ, Pierson WE, Horike M. The effects of inhaled sulfuric acid on pulmonary function in adolescent asthmatics. *Am Rev Respir Dis* 1983;128:221–225.
120. Koenig JQ, Covert DS, Pierson WE. Effects of inhalation of acidic components on pulmonary function in allergic adolescent subjects. *Environ Health Perspect* 1989;79:173–178.
121. Leikauf GD, Yeates DB, Wales KA, Spektor D, Albert RE, Lippmann M. Effects of sulfuric acid aerosol on respiratory mechanics and mucociliary particle clearance in healthy nonsmoking adults. *Am Ind Hyg Assoc J* 1981;42:273–282.
122. Leikauf GD, Spektor DM, Albert RE, Lippman M. Dose-dependent effects of submicrometer sulfuric acid aerosol on particle clearance from ciliated human lung airways. *Am Ind Hyg Assoc J* 1984;45:285–292.
123. Spektor DM, Yen BM, Lippmann M. Effect of concentration and cumulative exposure of inhaled sulfuric acid on tracheobronchial particle clearance in healthy humans. *Environ Health Perspect* 1989;79: 167–72.
124. Frampton MW, Morrow PE, Cox C, et al. Sulfuric acid aerosol followed by ozone exposure in healthy and asthmatic subjects. *Environ Res* 1992;69:-1–14.
125. Becker S, Devlin RB, Koren HS, Roger LB. Exposure of humans to $HNO_3$ causes alveolar macrophage activation. *Inhal Toxicol* 1996; 8:185–200.
126. Amdur MO, Chen LC. Furnace-generated acid aerosols: speciation and pulmonary effects. *Environ Health Perspect* 1989;79:147–150.
127. Chen LC, Miller PD, Amdur MO, Gordon T. Airway hyperresponsiveness in guinea pigs exposed to acid-coated ultrafine particles. *J Toxicol Environ Health* 1992;35:165–174.
128. Chen LC, Miller PD, Amdur MO. Effects of sulfur oxides on eicosanoids. *J Toxicol Environ Health* 1989;28:99–109.
129. Devlin RB, Ghio A, Costa DL. Particle Lung Interactions. In: Gehr P, Heyder J, eds. *Lung biology in health and disease.* New York: Marcel Dekker, 1997;in press.
130. Lay J, Bennet WD, Gerrity TR, Devlin RB. Particle-cell interaction in the human lung. *J Aerosol Med* 1993;6:30.
131. Hauser R, Elreedy S, Hoppin JA, Christiani DC. Airway obstruction in boilermakers exposed to fuel oil ash. A prospective investigation. *Am J Respir Crit Care Med* 1995;152:1478–84.
132. Hauser R, Elreedy S, Hoppin JA, Christiani DC. Upper airway response in workers exposed to fuel oil ash: nasal lavage analysis. *Occup Environ Med* 1995;52:353–358.
133. Diaz-sanchez D, Dotson AR, Takenaka H, Saxon A. Diesel exhaust particles induce local IgE production *in vivo* and alter the pattern of IgE messenger RNA isoforms. *J Clin Invest* 1994;94:1417–1425.
134. Salvi SS, Blomberg A, Rudell B, et al. Acute inflammatory changed in the airways of healthy human subjects following short-term exposure to diesel exhaust. *Am Rev Respir Dis* 1997;155:A425.
135. Rudell B, Ledin MC, Hammarstrom U, Stjernberg N, Lundback B, Sandstrom T. Effects on symptoms and lung function in humans experimentally exposed to diesel exhaust. *Occup Environ Med* 1996; 53:658–662.

*Environmental and Occupational Medicine, Third Edition,* edited by William N. Rom.
Lippincott–Raven Publishers, Philadelphia © 1998.

# CHAPTER 117

# Acid Rain

Kathleen C. Weathers and Gene E. Likens

Through the ever-increasing dependence on energy-intensive activities, from the burning of fossil fuels for electricity, to the use of energy to produce goods and services, humans have had large and measurable impacts on the world's ecosystems. Human use of fossil fuels ultimately is the source of many air pollution–related problems. This chapter focuses on one air pollution problem—acid rain—and specifically the altered cycles of sulfur (S) and nitrogen (N) that lead to it. It is important to note, however, that there are many other air pollutants that are also of ecological and environmental concern, and that several of these air pollutants can enhance the effects of acid rain. Tropospheric ozone ($O_3$), for example, is both intimately connected to the emission of nitrogen oxides ($NO_X$) (1,2) and is an air pollutant that can cause considerable environmental damage. Furthermore, heavy metals, such as lead, cadmium, and mercury, are also emitted into the atmosphere by human activity, deposited to diverse ecosystems, and can have deleterious effects.

Acid rain—the result of emissions of sulfur and nitrogen oxides—is one of the few ecological issues that has captured the interest of scientists, politicians, lawmakers, industry, and the general public alike. The term *acid rain* appeared in the literature over 100 years ago. It was used by an English chemist in an 1872 publication entitled "Air and Rain: The Beginnings of Chemical Climatology," in reference to the acidic nature of rainwater collected and analyzed from England (3–5). However, it was in the late 1960s and early 1970s that the term was brought to the attention of scientists and the public (6–8). The next two decades saw an exponential rise in interest about—and research on—acid rain. During this era of acid rain research, our understanding of the atmospheric chemistry, patterns of deposition, and ecological and environmental effects of acidic deposition grew dramatically (9).

Acid rain crosses geographic and political boundaries (e.g., state, national, and international); thus, its environmental, economic, political, and legal ramifications are extraordinarily complex and often vexing. This chapter provides a general overview, basic background, and sources of information on the topic of acid rain: its sources, delivery to ecosystems, ecological effects, and the relationship between sources and sinks of acid deposition. The chapter is not intended to be an exhaustive review, as thousands of scientific papers, reports, and general articles have been written on acid rain, nor will it address many of the nonscientific complexities of the topic. Furthermore, although acid rain now affects most of the world, the focus of this chapter will be primarily on North America.

## ACID RAIN VERSUS ACID DEPOSITION

*Acid rain* is the popular term (6) for rain, snow, sleet, and hail that is abnormally acidic due to human activities, primarily the burning of fossil fuels. However, this term is underrepresentative: there is more to acid rain than acid and rain! First, a large variety of nutrients, acids, and other pollutants are delivered to the Earth via rain and snow (wet deposition). In addition, though wet deposition is often the primary way in which these chemicals are deposited to ecosystems, there are other mechanisms. Acids are also delivered to ecosystems via the deposition of dry particles and gases (dry deposition) and, in many high elevation and coastal areas, through cloud or fog

K. C. Weathers and G. E. Likens: Institute of Ecosystem Studies, Millbrook, New York 12545.

water, or rime ice deposition (occult or cloud deposition). Thus the term acid deposition is used frequently to refer to all forms of deposition. Throughout this chapter we will use the terms *acid rain* and *acid* (or *acidic*) *deposition* interchangeably; however, we use both terms in the more inclusive sense.

## SOURCES AND CHEMICAL REACTIONS

Acid rain is caused by the emissions of gaseous sulfur oxides [primarily sulfur dioxide ($SO_2$)], and nitrogen oxides ($NO_x$) [primarily nitric oxide (NO) and nitrogen dioxide ($NO_2$)], which originate from the combustion of coal, oil, and other organic matter, and from smelting processes. These primary pollutants (i.e., those emitted directly from smokestacks, or tail pipes of combustion engines) are further oxidized and then hydrolyzed in the atmosphere to form secondary pollutants, such as the strong, mineral acids sulfuric ($H_2SO_4$) and nitric ($HNO_3$) (1,7,10–12). Though hydrochloric acid (HCl) is a strong mineral acid found in the atmosphere in both gaseous and aqueous forms, it usually constitutes a relatively small portion of the acidity in acid rain falling on industrialized parts of the world and will not be considered further here (13–15).

### Sulfur

Sulfur oxides ($SO_x$) are emitted from smokestacks and chimneys along with other gases and particulate matter

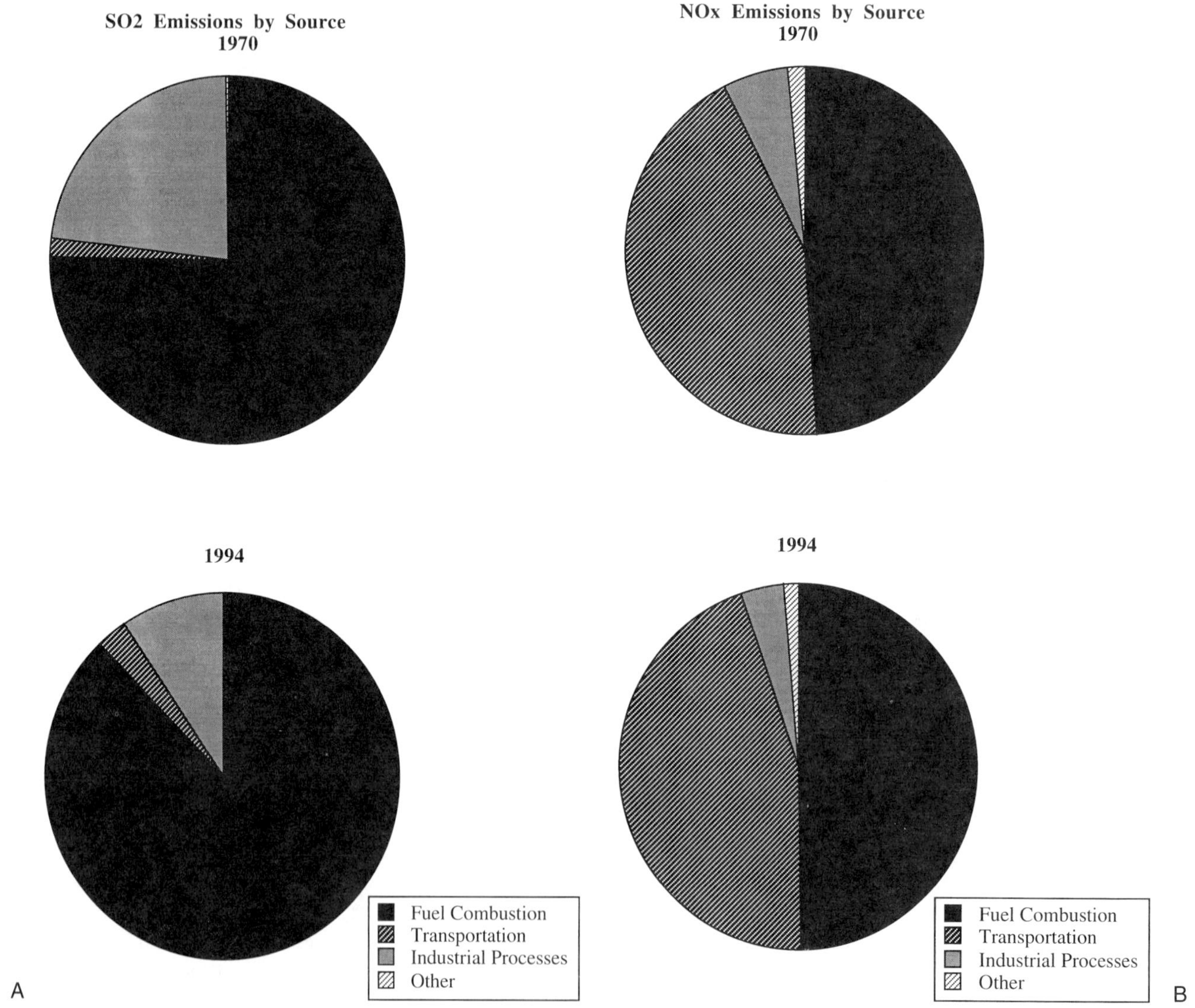


**FIG. 1. A,B:** Sulfur dioxide and nitrogen oxide emissions in the United States by source for 1970 and 1994. Sources include fuel combustion (electric utilities, industrial, other), transportation (on-and off-highway), miscellaneous (wildfires and other combustion), and industrial processes (chemical, petroleum, and other industries, metals processing, solvent utilization, storage and transport, and waste disposal and recycling) (18).

when sulfur contained in coal and oil is oxidized by combustion. In North America, approximately 97% of $SO_x$ emissions are sulfur dioxide ($SO_2$) while ~3% are sulfate ($SO_4^{2-}$) (16). Though there are some natural sources of sulfur oxides, including volcanic activity and sea spray (15), in many parts of the world, the burning of fossil fuels is the primary source of $SO_2$ in the atmosphere. In fact, in the eastern United States it is estimated that over 90% of sulfur emitted to the atmosphere is the result of human activity (3,17).

In the United States, electric utilities and nonutility point sources are the main contributors to $SO_2$ emissions. For example, in 1970, over three-fourths of anthropogenically produced sulfur dioxides were from fuel combustion, including electric utilities (56%) concentrated primarily in the midwestern United States, especially the Ohio and Tennessee River Valleys. Approximately one-fourth were from industrial processes, such as chemical and petroleum industries, and a small fraction of $SO_2$ emissions came from transportation sources (Fig. 1*A*). In 1994, the major source of $SO_2$ was fuel combustion (88%), while industrial processes declined to 10% (18). Temporal trends show that total sulfur dioxide emissions rose from 20 million tons in 1940, to a high of 31 million tons in 1970 and decreased to 21 million tons in 1994 (Fig. 2). Under mandated reductions through the U.S. Clean Air Act Amendments (CAAA) of 1990, sulfur dioxide emissions are projected to decrease to about 10 million tons below the 1980 values by the year 2000 (~10 million tons), with contributions from electric utilities declining and non–point utility sources and miscellaneous categories increasing (19).

After emission, gaseous $SO_2$ either can be deposited directly to the surface of the Earth through such processes as direct deposition to vegetation or other materials, or absorption through stomata in vegetation (16), or it can react in the atmosphere where it is oxidized in the plume or in the ambient atmosphere to sulfuric acid aerosols or sulfates. Chemical reactions occur either (a) in the gas phase with hydroxyl (OH) radicals, (b) in the liquid phase with hydrogen peroxide ($H_2O_2$) or ozone ($O_3$), (c) on the surfaces of solids with oxygen and/or air with or without metal catalysis, or combinations of all three (10). The general reactions for sulfuric acid formation are:

$$SO_2 + H_2O \rightarrow H_2SO_4 \leftrightarrow H^+ + HSO_4^- \leftrightarrow 2H^+ + SO_4^{2-} \quad [1]$$

## Nitrogen

Documenting the importance of nitrogen in the mineral nutrition of plants as well as its delivery from the atmosphere to ecosystems occurred as early as the mid-1800s (20). Though 78% of the atmosphere is nitrogen (1,21), it is in the form of dinitrogen ($N_2$), which is tightly bonded and unavailable to plants or for atmospheric chemical reactions in the absence of a source of energy to break the chemical bonds. It is the oxidized (e.g., $N_2O$, $NO$, $NO_2$, $HNO_3$, $NO_3^-$) and reduced ($NH_3$, $NH_4^+$) forms of N that are most reactive in the atmosphere and biosphere, and these nitrogenous compounds are made increasingly more available through anthropogenic activities (1,2,10,22). In recent decades, much ecological research has been focused on the cycling of nitrogen, primarily because nitrogen is thought to limit plant growth in many regions of the world (2,23), but also because increasingly high rates of nitrogen deposition are now considered to be a pollution problem in Europe and parts of the United States (24,25).

Nitrogen oxides (generally referred to as $NO_x$) are the other important precursors to acid rain. Nitrogen oxide emissions are the result of either (a) thermal reactions when combustion temperatures are raised high enough to

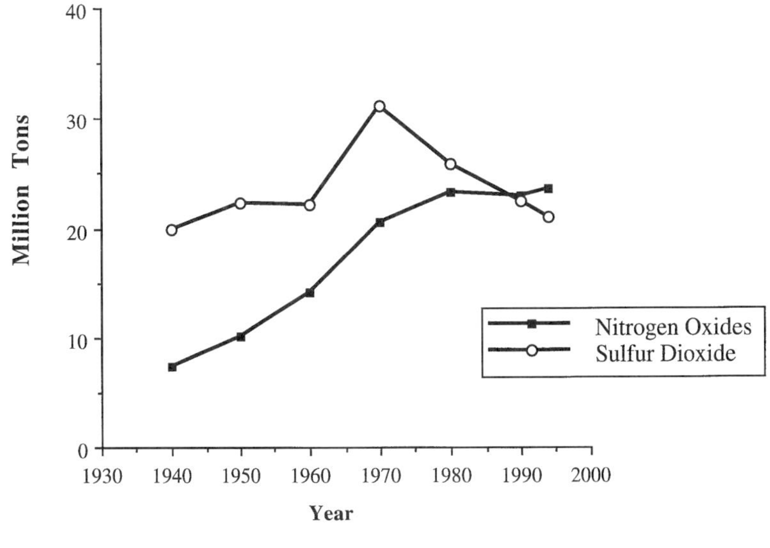


**FIG. 2.** Sulfur dioxide and nitrogen oxide emission trends from 1940–1994 (18).

oxidize atmospheric $N_2$ (thermal $NO_x$) or (b) the oxidation of nitrogenous compounds in fuel (fuel $NO_x$) (1), though fossil fuels (e.g., coal or oil) normally contain much lower concentrations of nitrogen than of sulfur. Thus an important source of the nitrogen for NO emissions is often atmospheric nitrogen ($N_2$). The resultant $NO_x$ can be deposited to surfaces as $NO_2$, or further oxidized, often through reacting with hydroxyl radicals, and hydrolyzed to nitrate ($NO_3^-$) and nitric acid ($HNO_3$) (26). The generalized reaction for nitric acid formation, a strong mineral acid in acidic deposition, is:

$$NO_x + H_2O \rightarrow HNO_3 \leftrightarrow H^+ + NO_3^- \quad [2]$$

In 1970, the primary anthropogenic sources of nitrogen oxides were fuel combustion (49%) and transportation (44%) (Fig. 1*B*) and total emissions were 20.6 million tons. By 1994, $NO_x$ emissions had increased to 23.6 million tons (Fig. 2), exceeding emissions of $SO_2$, and fuel combustion contributed 50% of the total, while transportation contributed 45% (Fig. 1b). Although the CAAA included a provision for reductions in $NO_x$ emissions, nitrogen was not the main focus of regulation in this amendment, primarily because nitrogen was not perceived to be a critical environmental problem. In fact, U.S. $NO_x$ emissions are still rising (Fig. 2) and nitrogen emissions are also expected to increase worldwide over the next decade (2,27,28).

### Reduced Nitrogen and Other Cations

The acid-base status of a solution is the result of its complete chemistry, not simply its hydrogen ion, sulfate, nitrate, and chloride content. The pH of precipitation, then, is a result of its total ionic composition, which is in turn a result of the sulfur and nitrogen content, as well as other substances that are emitted to the atmosphere, react, and subsequently are delivered to the Earth in precipitation. In fact, some of these compounds are important in neutralizing the acidity in rain. For example, reduced nitrogenous compounds such as ammonia and ammonium ($NH_3$ and $NH_4^+$), which are the result of both combustion and agricultural activities (15,21), often combine with $NO_3^-$ as $NH_4NO_3$ or sulfate as $(NH_4)_2SO_4$ and are transported long distances. Atmospheric calcium, sodium, potassium, and magnesium, often referred to as base cations, are a result of sea spray, the suspension of dirt and dust particles (from roads, for example), anthropogenic emissions, and a variety of other sources (13,15,29), and neutralize the acidity of precipitation as well.

### Transport

As noted above, sulfur and nitrogen oxides may be transported very long distances in the atmosphere either as primary pollutants or as secondary pollutants. Indeed, an early solution to local air pollution problems in urban and industrialized areas was to increase the height of chimneys and smokestacks in order to reduce local, ground-level concentrations of particulate air pollutants (3–5,7,9). One of the results of this control measure was that air pollutants, particularly gases, were introduced into the atmosphere at a greater height and thereby were transported greater distances downwind. The average height of chimneys and smokestacks increased dramatically within the United States after about 1950: over 400 smokestacks taller than 60 m were built in the 1970s and many were extended to greater than 300 m in height (3,7). The operating philosophy was "dilution is the solution to pollution." Local pollution issues were therefore made into regional air pollution problems. This fact led to one of the most contentious and politically vexing aspects of the acid deposition issue (3,9,30). That is, pollutants generated in one area could be deposited in a far distant area with little recourse for the recipient. Moreover, it was difficult to trace quantitatively the individual sources of the pollutants.

## ACID DEPOSITION

Deposition is the amount of a substance that is deposited to a surface. Its units are usually an amount (e.g., kg, Eq, mol) per unit area (e.g., ha, $m^2$) per unit time (e.g., year, day). The actual delivery of acidic droplets, particles, and gases to the Earth–atmospheric deposition–is the result of a three-stage process: (a) emission of primary pollutants; (b) chemical reactions (e.g., formation of secondary pollutants) and transport in the atmosphere; and (c) deposition to the Earth's surface (1). It is the third stage, the delivery of these pollutants to–and their interaction with–ecosystems, materials, and humans, that results in measurable and important effects.

Research over the past two decades at locations such as the Hubbard Brook Experimental Forest (HBEF), New Hampshire, which has the longest continuous record of precipitation chemistry in North America, has shown that although rain and snow may account for much of the total deposition to a variety of ecosystems, in some regions dry deposition and/or cloud, fog, or rime ice deposition can contribute approximately one-third to two-thirds of the total depositional load (9,28,31–41). For example, dry deposition averages about 30% of total deposition at the HBEF (33). For several sites in other parts of North America, dry deposition can contribute, on average, 50% of the total deposition of sulfur (S) and nitrogen (N) (16,22). For many high-elevation or coastal areas in the northeastern United States, cloud or fog water accounts for 50% to 80% of the total S and N deposited (35,42–44) (Fig. 3). The relative contribution of each of these processes (wet, dry, and cloud) depends on many factors, such as frequency and amount of rain and snow, presence of cloud cover, the condition and architecture of impaction surfaces, elevation, and wind speeds (28,35,40,41,45).

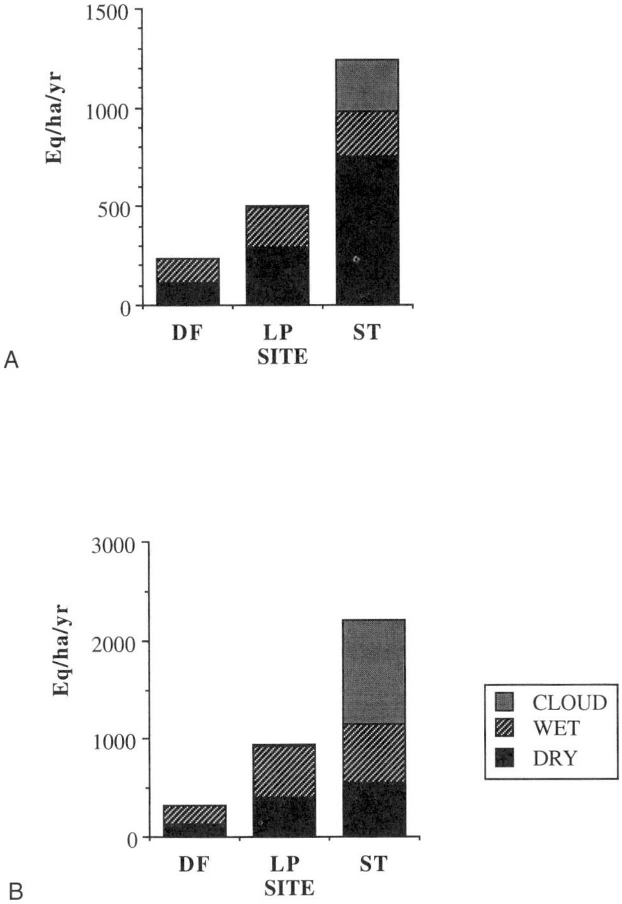


**FIG. 3. A:** Cloud, wet, and dry deposition of nitrogen from three sites in North America. **B:** Cloud, wet, and dry deposition of sulfur from three sites in North America. DF, Douglas fir site, Thompson Forest, Washington; LP, loblolly pine site, Oak Ridge, Tennessee; ST, red spruce site, Smoky Tower, Great Smoky Mountains National Park, Tennessee (88).

Although many advances have been made over the last decade, the techniques for measuring and quantifying dry and cloud deposition are still being refined. In future years more accurate total deposition measurements are likely to be available and geographic variation in their relative contributions will be better documented (see below). The data gathered to date, however, have made clear that there is in fact more to acid rain than rain: dry and cloud water deposition usually are very important contributors to total acid deposition.

## WHAT'S THE "NORMAL" pH OF RAIN?

This question has been at the core of heated debates (usually more political than scientific) that have focused on what the background pH of rain should have been in the absence of human-caused emissions. We have seen from the previous sections that currently, throughout much of the world, acid deposition is a result of sulfuric and nitric acids—strong mineral acids—that tend to release hydrogen ion ($H^+$), which is a measure of acidity. Acidity is usually expressed as pH, and that pH is based on a logarithmic scale (pH = -log (concentration of $H^+$). Early in the acid rain debate, in the absence of much actual data, the "background" pH of precipitation was considered to be approximately 5.6, the lowest pH possible as a result of carbonic acid formation in pure water under normal atmospheric conditions (7,46):

$$CO_2 + H_2O \rightarrow H_2CO_3 \leftrightarrow H^+ + HCO_3^- \leftrightarrow 2H^+ + CO_3^2 \quad [3]$$

It was not until the early 1980s that a group of scientists decided to measure the chemistry of rainwater collected from some of the most remote locations on Earth to test this assumption (46–48). They surmised that, in the absence of appropriate historical data, rainwater from these locations was likely to be as representative of "preindustrial" rain as possible. Indeed, their data showed that the chemical concentrations from these sites were the lowest in the world, and suggested that the background pH of rain is more likely 5.1 to 5.3 than 5.6, or about ten times less acidic, and less concentrated in sulfate and nitrate, than rain collected from the northeastern United States (Fig. 4). The additional acidity (between pH 5.6 and 5.1–5.3) was thought to be the result of natural emissions of S and N from, for example, volcanoes, lightning, wildfires, and stratospheric transport, in combination with other cations and anions in solution (46–48). Further, they found that precipitation in remote sites was far more likely to be dominated by naturally occurring organic acids, such as formic and acetic acids, than that collected from eastern North America (6,43,46–49). Thus preindustrial rain has been shown to be quite different from postindustrial rain; human activities have led to acid deposition.

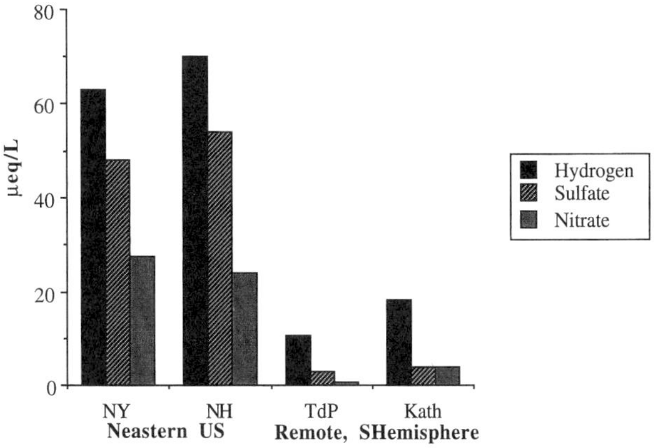


**FIG. 4.** Volume-weighted average hydrogen, sulfate, and nitrate ion concentrations in precipitation from two sites in the northeastern United States (NY, Millbrook, New York; NH, HBEF, New Hampshire) and the southern hemisphere (TdP, Torres del Paine, Chile; Kath, Katherine, Australia) (49,89).

## TRENDS AND PATTERNS OF ACID DEPOSITION

### Rates of Increase

It has been difficult to examine changes in precipitation acidity over time in North America and elsewhere because no continuous records of rain pH are available that extend from before industrialization to the present. The data that do exist provide a somewhat sketchy picture for trends in precipitation acidity in the United States, a fact that has contributed to considerable debate over whether, or how long, rain has been acidic. We now know that by the mid-1950s much of the eastern United States, and particularly the northeastern United States, was being subjected to acid precipitation (3,7,30,50,51). It appears that the southeastern and much of the midwestern United States were not receiving acid precipitation during this time period. However, 10 years later, in the mid-1960s, the acidity had spread to the southeast and midwestern United States (3,7,50,52). Thus, over the last two to three decades, there has been a significant spread of acid precipitation, with the northeastern United States receiving most of the acidity (7,30,38,53,54).

Currently, the average pH of rain throughout North America, in Europe, and other parts of the world is between 4 and 5 (100 μEq/L and 10 μEq $H^+$/L) (7,55–57), though precipitation events have been reported with pHs much lower than this (e.g., pH 2.85 at HBEF). At our research site in the mid–Hudson River Valley, New York, the 11-year volume-weighted average pH of rain water is approximately 4.2, though pHs vary seasonally (Fig. 5).

### Sulfuric versus Nitric Acid

In the United States, the relative contribution of sulfur and nitrogen to acidity in precipitation is a function of several factors, such as distance from sources (e.g., proximity to Midwestern coal-burning facilities), wind direction, and presence of neutralizing particles or gases in the air. Recent data from the HBEF suggest that sulfuric acid, measured as sulfate in precipitation samples, contributes approximately half of the acidity in rainwater, while nitric acid, measured as nitrate in precipitation samples, contributes slightly less than half (14). In contrast, precipitation data from a monitoring site in Oregon, which is relatively much less polluted by $SO_2$ and $NO_x$ and much more influenced by sea salt, show that nitrate often contributes 10% and sulfate only 18%, while chloride (from sea salt) contributes ~70% of the acidity (55).

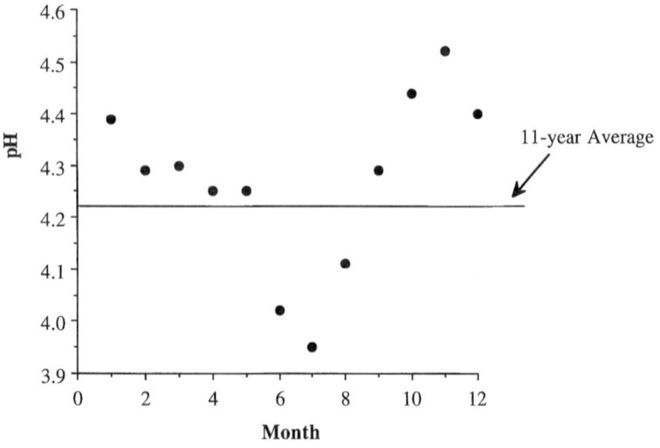


FIG. 5. Monthly volume-weighted average pH of precipitation from Millbrook, New York. *Line* shows the 11-year, volume-weighted average pH. Data from IES Environmental Monitoring Program.

### Geographic Distribution of Acid Deposition

Of the three forms of atmospheric deposition (wet, cloud, and dry), quantifying wet inputs is the most straightforward. Rain and snow can be collected in chemically inert, clean polyethylene buckets, chemically analyzed and multiplied by rain amount rather simply to measure rates of wet deposition. Wet deposition collections began as early as the 1800s in England and France (Rothamsted, England 1880–1920, France 1876–1907) (cf. ref. 5); however, routine monitoring of wet deposition was a much later occurrence.

Monitoring programs now exist that are designed to measure and quantify atmospheric deposition in its various forms. Most of these programs were begun in the late 1970s in North America, and until recently, included only rain monitoring. One of the goals of these networks has been to gather sufficient data to quantify the deposition of pollutants and nutrients over large geographic regions. As a result, data now exist that show the geographic distribution of deposition of various ions in precipitation (Fig. 6). It is clear from these data that for the United States, wet deposition of various pollutants and nutrients varies across the country. For example, there are much higher rates of sulfate and nitrate deposition in most of the eastern vs western United States (Fig. 6). This pattern is, in part, a result of proximity to sources, predominant wind direction, and amount of precipitation deposited.

As noted above, cloud water is another form of wet deposition. Although there are virtually no continuous records available for cloud-water deposition, we do know that cloud-water samples collected from remote locations in North America show similar geographic patterns in rainwater (Fig. 7), and are often several times more acidic (lower in pH) and more concentrated in other ions than rain water collected at the same time from those same locations (36). In addition, average cloud water from the northeastern United States is about 40 times more acidic than rainwater from remote areas of the world (28). Extremely acid (<pH 3.0), regional cloud events have been measured (38), and cloud water pHs often occur in the 3 range (Fig. 6) (36). At times these acidic cloud-

water events have occurred in combination with high concentrations of other air pollutants, such as ozone (38).

Within the last several years, there has been a concerted effort to colocate dry with wet deposition monitoring sites to provide information on wet plus dry deposition over a wide geographic region. Although the data are somewhat limited, they have been used to model wet and dry deposition over the northeastern United States, showing an increase in total deposition from northeast to southwest (53).

## EFFECTS

The effects of acid deposition are highly variable: some are direct and demonstrable, while others are indirect and less clear. Here we give a brief overview of some of the better understood and well-documented effects of acidic deposition (Table 1).

### Aquatic Ecosystems

Some of the first and most obvious effects of acid deposition were observed in freshwater ecosystems. Tens of thousands of lakes and streams in North America and Europe are more acid than they were a few decades ago as a result of acid deposition (58–61). These freshwaters are in sensitive regions, such as areas with hard bedrock, thin acid soils, and little neutralizing capacity, and their acidification has resulted in losses of fish and other aquatic organisms (19,58,62,63). The evidence showing that strong mineral acidity has caused ecological changes has come from many sources, including (a) historical changes in chemistry and biology of freshwaters (58,64), (b) experimental manipulations (64), and (c) measurements made in aquatic ecosystems receiving acid deposition (61). For example, analyses of historical changes in alkalinity of lakes in the Adirondack Mountain region of New York State showed highly significant acidification of a large number of those lakes during recent decades (19,60). Some 80% of 274 lakes studied became acidified during the last 50 to 60 years (60). These changes were attributed to acid deposition and were not explainable by other factors such as changes in land use.

Surface water acidification as a result of acid rain has had demonstrable effects on organisms at several trophic levels, including fish, zooplankton, and benthic organisms (58,62,63,65–69). The chemical constituents that consistently appear to have an effect on freshwater organisms, and that are a result of acid deposition, are monomeric aluminum ($Al^{3+}$), calcium, and hydrogen (as indicated by pH) (62). Fish as well as invertebrates are affected by acidification, primarily through physiologic disturbances. In waters where mobile, monomeric aluminum species are present, direct effects on gills (e.g., lesions and disturbance of respiratory function) and ion regulation disturbances have been observed (62,69).

### Terrestrial Ecosystems

Although terrestrial effects can be quite obvious and dramatic when examined near the source, for example, in close proximity to an active smelter (70,71), the response of terrestrial ecosystems to regional acid deposition has been debated widely. The effect of acid deposition on long-lived species, such as trees, and highly heterogeneous systems, such as soils, and within the context of other simultaneous stresses, such as disease, ozone, and drought, can be difficult to quantify in general, but particularly difficult when effects exhibit significant time lags. Demonstrating cause and effect of acid deposition has been more difficult in the case of terrestrial ecosystems than for acidic deposition's effects on aquatic ecosystems.

#### *Soils*

Soils require hundreds to thousands of years to develop (72). Exchange sites on negatively charged clay particles in soils often are dominated by such ions as aluminum, calcium, magnesium, potassium, and sodium. Excess hydrogen ion from acidic deposition has been shown to displace these cations, which are subsequently removed from the soil through leaching. This displacement represents a change in the nutrient and acid/base status of the soils, since calcium, for example is an essential plant nutrient that is usually taken up by plant roots from the soil (13,73,74). It is now known from long-term studies in Europe (75) and studies in the northeastern United States, such as at the HBEF, that rain at pH 4.6 can affect soils in ways that rain at pH 5.6 cannot. For example, common alumina minerals are essentially insoluble at pH 5.6, but are quite soluble at 4.6, in fact, 1000 times more soluble. Increased leaching of aluminum from soil occurs at these lower pHs, and dissolved aluminum is toxic to organisms (see above). In addition, a buildup of aluminum in the soil can affect a plant's biogeochemical function as well as result in toxicity (76–78). We now know that some soils in regions of high acid deposition are significantly affected by acid deposition (73,78,79).

#### *Forests*

Forest decline can be defined as a measurable reduction in the health of a forest ecosystem, which is characterized by unexpected changes in growth, reproduction, and death of trees, and has been noted in many parts of the industrialized world. In the decline areas, forest trees are either dying, generally unhealthy, or growing slowly. This condition has become widespread in Europe and

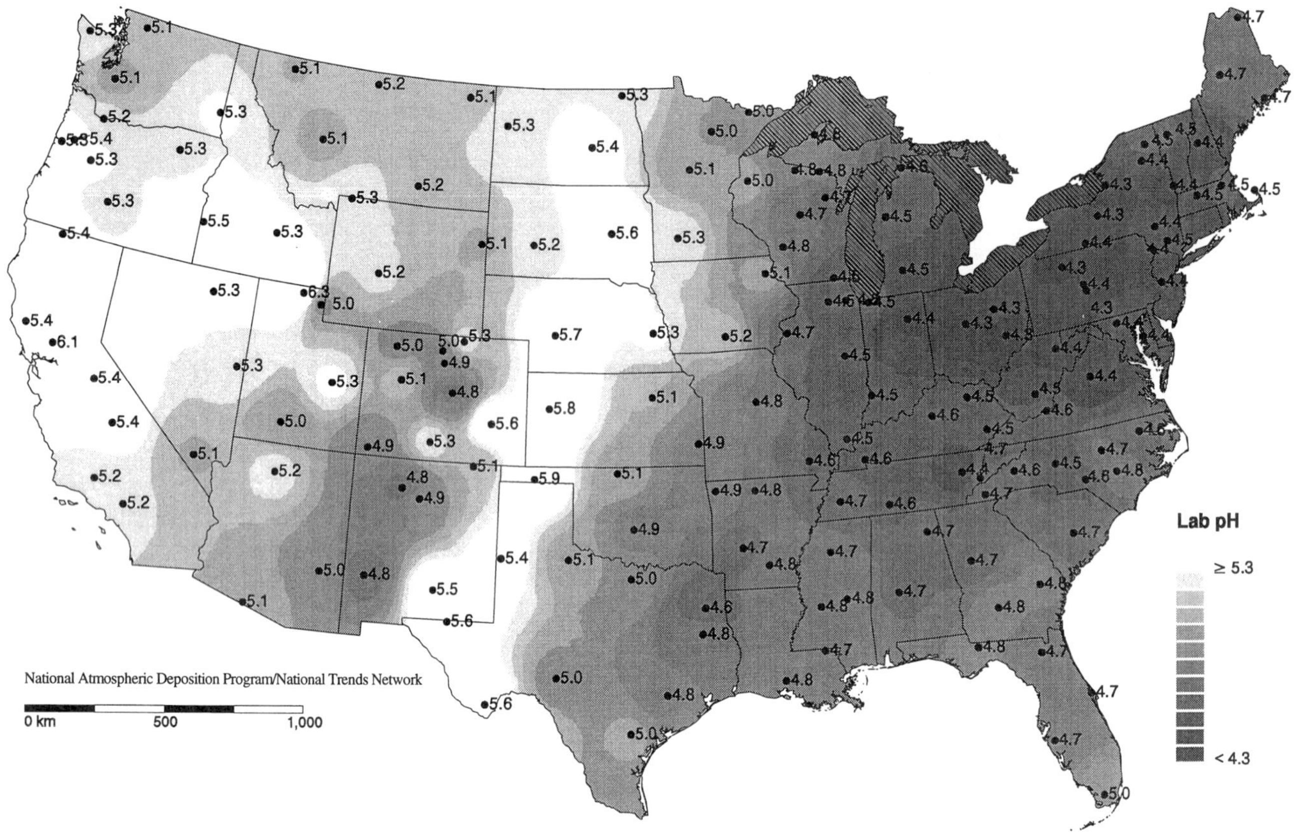
National Atmospheric Deposition Program/National Trends Network
0 km
500
1,000
Lab pH
≥ 5.3
< 4.3

A

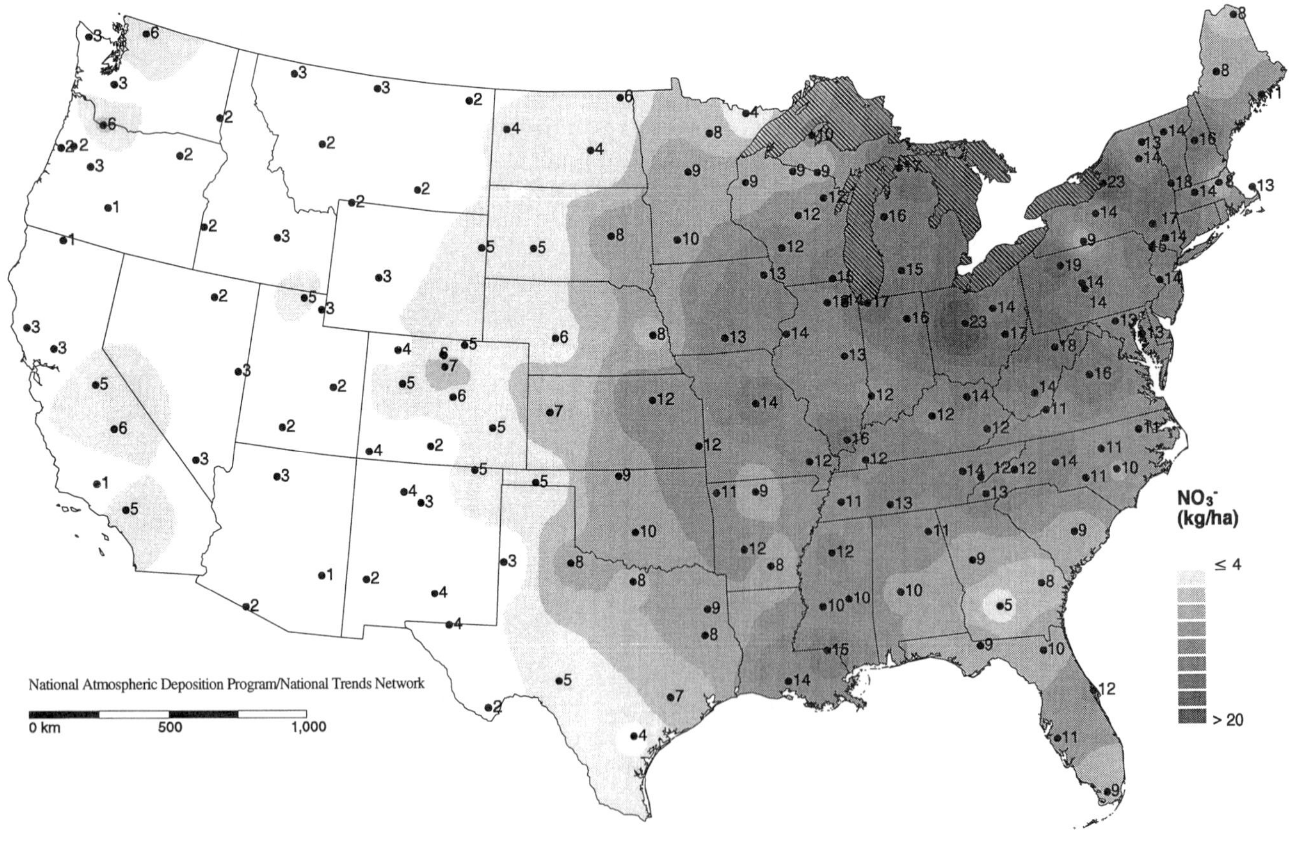
National Atmospheric Deposition Program/National Trends Network
0 km
500
1,000
$NO_3^-$ (kg/ha)
≤ 4
> 20

B

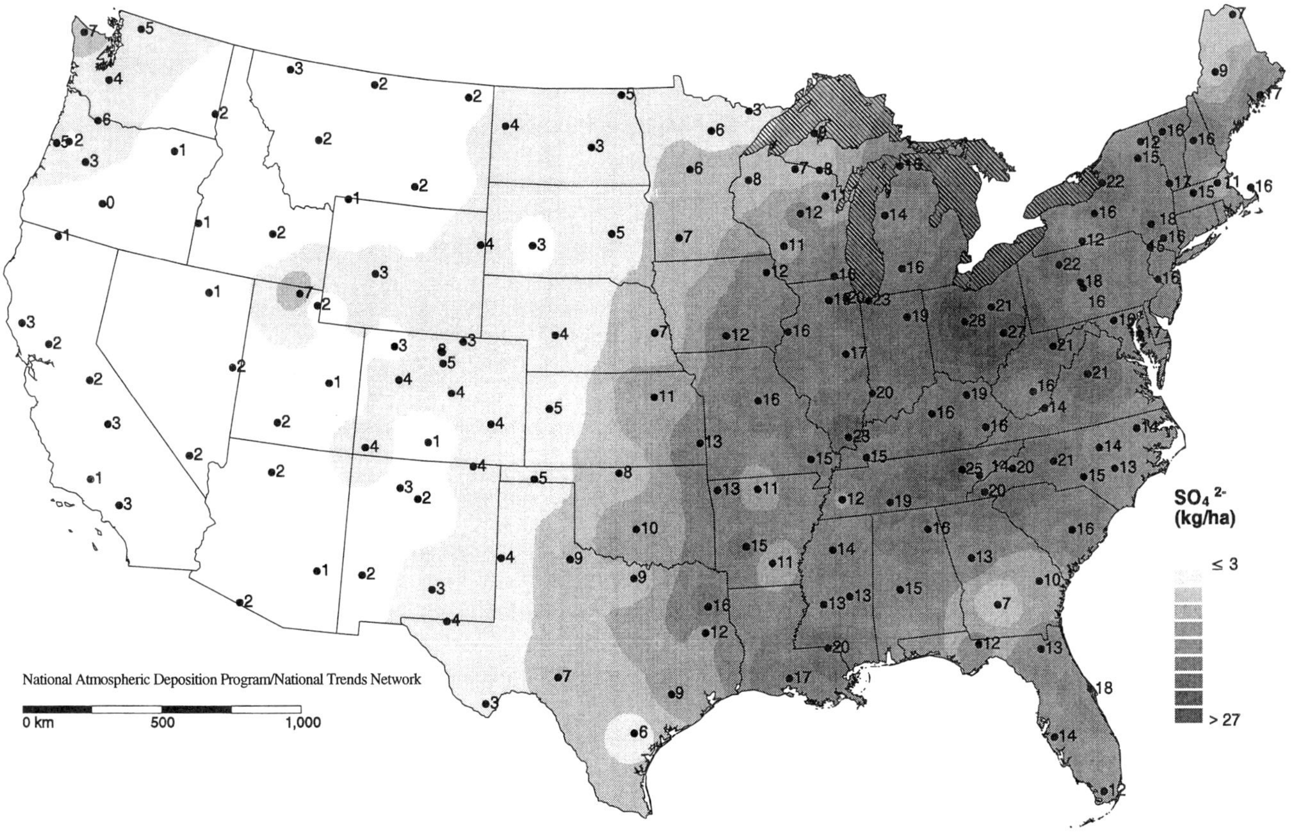


C

**FIG. 6.** Geographic distribution of pH **(A)**; and nitrate **(B)** and sulfate **(C)** deposition (kg/ha). Data from National Atmospheric Deposition Program (NRSP-3)/National Trends Network, 1996. NADP/NTN Coordination Office, Natural Resource Ecology Laboratory, Colorado State University, Fort Collins, Colorado.

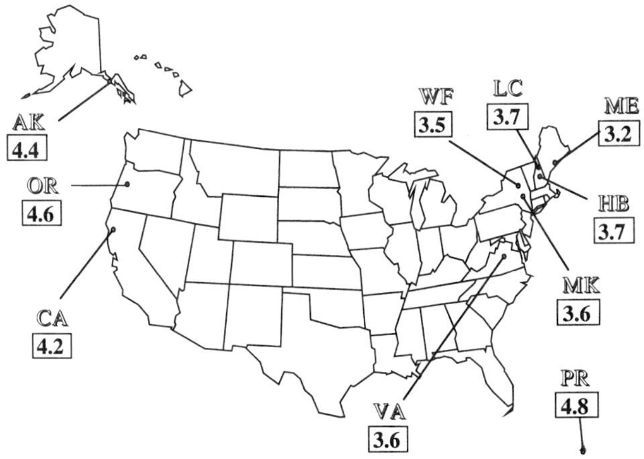


**FIG. 7.** Average pH for cloud water collected during 1984–1985 as part of the Cloud Water Project of the Institute of Ecosystem Studies (37). AK, Juneau, Alaska; OR, Mary's Peak, Oregon; CA, Arcata, California; VA, Blue Ridge Mountains, Virginia; PR, Pico del Este, Puerto Rico; MK, Mohonk Mountain, New York; HB, Hubbard Brook, New Hampshire; ME, Acadia National Park, Maine; LC, Lakes-of-the-Clouds, New Hampshire; WF, Whiteface Mountain, New York.

parts of North America (80–82), but the causes are complex and controversial (83). Many, if not most, terrestrial ecosystems are likely to be stressed simultaneously by acid rain, acid cloud or fog water, ozone, toxic metals, the global climate, hydrocarbons, disease, exotic pests, as well as land-use changes (30,81–84). Interactive effects of various pollutants as well as the interaction between pollutants and other stresses have been proposed as causes of forest decline. Another complicating factor is that many years may be required before symptoms of stress become obvious as damage to trees or forest. Although these interactions are admittedly complex and it is difficult, if not impossible, to assign absolute cause and effect, it is clear that air pollution can stress forest ecosystems.

### Health Effects

Extreme air pollution events within cities have been of concern for centuries (4), and increasingly polluted conditions have been the norm in many cities worldwide. In fact, urban pollution episodes have not only resulted in increased morbidity and mortality (63), but ultimately they influenced the passage of the Clean Air Act in the United States and similar legislation elsewhere in the world (4).

**TABLE 1.** *Examples of effects of acid precipitation*

| System | Biogeochemical effects | Biotic effects | Affected regions (examples) |
|---|---|---|---|
| Freshwater | Loss of alkalinity<br>Increases in aluminum | Species losses (e.g., some species of fish, invertebrates, phytoplankton), physiologic disturbances | Eastern United States, Canada, parts of Germany, western Scotland, Wales, Norway, Sweden, Finland |
| Soils | Increased leaching of base cations, aluminum<br>Changes in soil solution chemistry | | Parts of eastern United States, Europe |
| Forests | Unlikely single cause for forest decline<br>Acid deposition may contribute to nutrient deficiencies, dead and dying trees, Al toxicity, general stress | | Parts of Europe, Northeastern United States, Canada |
| Humans | Acidic aerosols may contribute to increased mortality, morbidity, pulmonary changes, mucociliary alterations, bronchitis | | Metropolitan areas worldwide |

After centuries of experience, it is now well known that persons who have respiratory ailments are particularly sensitive to acidic aerosols, such as sulfates ($SO_4^=$) and sulfuric acid ($H_2SO_4$) (63). Acidic aerosols, "can alter mucociliary clearance of lungs in normal and asthmatic humans," and "chronic exposure may contribute to the development of chronic bronchitis" (63). In addition, pulmonary function in some humans has been shown to be negatively affected. Although additional experimentation and observation is ongoing (63), there is little doubt that acidic aerosols can also have deleterious effects on humans.

## RELATIONSHIP BETWEEN SOURCES AND SINKS

### Emission and Deposition

It should now be evident that in many parts of the world human activities are the major source of emissions of nitrogen and sulfur oxides. Thus reducing human-caused emissions is one obvious way to control acidic deposition. In the United States, the 1990 CAAA specifically addressed acid rain and proposed to reduce sulfur dioxide emissions by 50% by the year 2000, based on 1980 levels. However, pollutants often travel long distances and are chemically transformed in the process between emission and deposition. A logical question and one that has been asked is, "What is the relationship between reduction in emission of primary pollutants that lead to acid deposition and the chemical concentrations and deposition of those components in rain?" Two examples illustrate the relationship.

Data from the long-term precipitation chemistry record at HBEF suggest that reductions in $SO_2$ emission in the United States are reflected in both sulfate concentration and deposition in rainwater, indicating that reduction in emissions is closely related to the amount of sulfur deposited to ecosystems (56). Similarly, after leaded gasoline was banned in the eastern United States, there was a steep and significant decrease in lead concentration in precipitation from the HBEF (56). These are persuasive examples of how a reduction in source results in decreasing deposition, despite the complicated chemical and transport processes involved between emission and deposition.

### *Is the Clean Air Act Adequate?*

Although the CAAA addressed emissions, it is not clear that this regulation will be enough to protect ecosystems (13). Emissions may need to be reduced even more if the goal is to reduce acid rain and its effects. The 1990 CAAA focused primarily on reducing sulfur emissions and less on nitrogen emissions. Currently at HBEF, the nitric acid inputs in atmospheric deposition are almost as large as the sulfuric acid additions. This has changed since the mid-1960s when about 75% of the acidity in rain and snow was from sulfuric acid and some 10% to 20% was from nitric acid. If these trends continue, we expect $NO_3^-$ to exceed $SO_4^=$ in 2015!

Current measurements in Millbrook, New York, and at 25 monitoring sites throughout New York State operated by the Department of Environmental Conservation show no significant improvement in acid rain since 1987, in spite of the 1990 CAAA (85). There are several possible reasons for this: (a) Emissions of $SO_2$ have only decreased by about 2 million tons per year (or the total 10 million tons required by the CAAA) and $NO_x$ emissions have not decreased at all (Fig. 2). (b) Some states are claiming credit for reductions in emissions from motor vehicles against state inventories. These credits avoid placing controls on emissions leading to long-range transport, which result in acid rain falling in New York State. (c) Because the CAAA allows emission sources to buy and sell pollution credits from other sources, significant reduction credits have been purchased from sources that do not contribute acid rain to the northeastern United States, and thus avoid controls on sources that do (85). Thus from an ecological perspective, the jury is still out on the answer to the question, Is the Clean Air Act adequate?

## CONCLUSIONS

From the initial awareness of acid rain, there have been major controversies, often spawned by vested interests, rather than by science, although the scientific components are indeed complex. Acid deposition is one of the most complex and difficult environmental problems ever faced by humans because of its ecological as well as political and economic ramifications, and its global dimensions.

Ecological research initiated in the 1960s and 1970s led to the discovery of acid rain in North America, suggesting that acid rain was indeed a regional issue (6–8,30,50). Since the early 1970s, tens-of-thousands of scientific papers and reports have been published, and hundreds of meetings to discuss the topic have been held. As a result, a great deal is known about the science of acid deposition (9,17,64). For example, acid rain is common over large regions of the industrialized world: all of eastern North America, parts of western North America, most of Europe and Asia, and in parts of the Southern Hemisphere as well (7,28,47,48,86). Air pollution worldwide, as characterized by increasing emissions of nitrogen or sulfur oxides, is on the rise (2,18,27).

Acid deposition has been shown to have biologic as well as biogeochemical effects. For example, some freshwater ecosystems in sensitive areas have become acidified and lost biotic diversity (58). Some soils have become acidified and base cations as well as aluminum have leached from them. Finally, the respiratory systems of many humans have been compromised by acidic aerosols.

The variability and complexity of ecological results regarding acid deposition have led to controversy, albeit some of this controversy has been fueled by vested interests, about how widespread or uniform the effects of acid rain are. However, the biologic variability and complexity are both understandable and expected when dealing with natural ecological systems just as no two humans respond in exactly the same way to the common cold.

Some 20 years ago, scientists thought that the acid rain issue consisted only of the effects of anthropogenic sulfuric acid in rain on lakes and streams. Now it is known that the problem is much more complicated and serious. Considerations must be given as well to nitrogen pollution, and air pollution's effects on forests, soils, structures, and human health, and to the multiplying, interactive effects with other pollutants such as tropospheric ozone and toxic metals (86–88).

The common root cause of three of the most urgent environmental problems (acid deposition, atmospheric ozone, and global warming) is increasing consumption of fossil fuels. Solving these problems in the immediate future will challenge our best minds and talents.

## ACKNOWLEDGMENT

This is a contribution to the program of the Institute of Ecosystem Studies.

## REFERENCES

1. Seinfeld JH. *Atmospheric chemistry and physics of air pollution.* New York: Wiley, 1986.
2. Vitousek PM, Aber JD, Howarth RW, et al. Human alteration of the global nitrogen cycle: causes and consequences. *Issues Ecol* 1997;1:1–15.
3. Likens GE. Acid rain: The smokestack is the "smoking gun." *Garden Magazine* 1984(July/August), 12–18.
4. Brimblecombe P. *The big smoke:* a history of air pollution in London since medieval times. London and New York: Metheun, 1987.
5. Erisman JW, Draaijers GPJ. *Atmospheric deposition in relation to acidification and eutrophication.* Amsterdam: Elsevier, 1995.
6. Likens GE, Bormann FH, Johnson NM. Acid rain. *Environment* 1972;14:33–40.
7. Likens GE, Wright RW, Galloway JN, Butler TJ. Acid Rain. *Sci Am* 1979;241:39–47.
8. Likens GE, Bormann FH. Acid rain: A serious regional environmental problem. *Science* 1974;184:1176–1179.
9. Weathers KC, Lovett GM. Acid deposition research and ecosystem science: Synergistic successes. In: Pace ML, Groffman PM, eds. *Successes, limitations, and frontiers in ecosystem science,* the VII Cary Conference. New York: Springer-Verlag, in press.
10. Finlayson-Pitts BJ, Pitts JN Jr. *Atmospheric chemistry:* fundamentals and experimental techniques. New York: Wiley, 1986.
11. Mohnen V. The challenge of acid rain. *Sci Am* 1988;259:30–38.
12. Aber JD, Melillo JM. *Terrestrial ecosystems.* Philadelphia: WB Saunders, 1991.
13. Likens GE, Driscoll CT, Buso DC. Long-term effects of acid rain: Response and recovery of a forest ecosystem. *Science* 1996;272:244–246.
14. Likens GE, Bormann FH. *Biogeochemistry of a forested ecosystem,* 2nd ed. New York: Springer-Verlag, 1995.
15. Schlesinger WS. *Biogeochemistry:* an analysis of global change. San Diego: Academic Press, 1991.
16. Lindberg SE. Atmospheric deposition and canopy interactions of sulfur. In: Johnson SW, Lindberg SE, eds. *Atmospheric deposition and forest nutrient cycling:* a synthesis of the integrated forest study. New York: Springer-Verlag, 1992;74–90.
17. Driscoll CT, Galloway JN, Hornig JF, et al. *Is there scientific consensus on acid rain?* Excerpts from six governmental reports. Ad Hoc Committee on Acid Rain: Science and Policy. Millbrook, NY: Institute of Ecosystem Studies, 1985.
18. Council on Environmental Quality (CEQ). *Environmental quality:* 25th anniversary report. Washington, DC: Council on Environmental Quality, 1997.
19. National Acid Precipitation Assessment Program (NAPAP). *1992 report to Congress.* Washington, DC: NAPAP, 1993.
20. Boussingault JB. Recherches sur la quantité de l acide nitrique contenue dans la pluie, le brouillard, la rosée. *Compt Rend* 1858;46: 1123–1130,1175–1183.
21. Warneck P. *Chemistry of the natural atmosphere.* San Diego: Academic Press, 1988.
22. Lovett GM. Atmospheric deposition and canopy interactions of nitrogen. In: Johnson DW, Lindberg SE, eds. *Atmospheric deposition and forest nutrient cycling.* New York: Springer-Verlag, 1992;152–166.
23. Vitousek PM, Howarth RW. Nitrogen limitation on land and in the sea: How can it occur? *Biogeochemistry* 1991;13:87–115.
24. Durka W, Schulze E-D, Gebauer G, Voerkelius S. Effects of forest decline on uptake and leaching of deposited nitrate determined from $^{15}N$ and $^{18}O$ measurements. *Nature* 1995;372:765–767.
25. Aber JD, Nadlehoffer KJ, Stuedler P, Melillo JM. Nitrogen saturation in northern forest ecosystems. *Bioscience* 1989;39:378–386.
26. Tanner RL. Sources of acids, bases, and their precursors in the atmosphere. In: Lindberg SE, Page AL, Norton SA, eds. *Acidic precipitation,*

*vol 3:* sources, *deposition, and canopy interactions.* New York: Springer-Verlag, 1990;1–19.
27. Galloway JN. Acid deposition: Perspectives in time and space. *Water Air Soil Pollut* 1995;85:15–24.
28. Weathers KC, Likens GE. Clouds in southern Chile: An important source of nitrogen-limited ecosystems? *Environ Sci Tech* 1997;31: 210–213.
29. Hedin LO, Likens, GE. Atmospheric dust and acid rain. *Sci Am* 1996;275:88–92.
30. Likens GE. Some aspects of air pollution effects on terrestrial ecosystems and prospectus for the future. *Ambio* 1989;18:172–178.
31. Eaton JS, Likens GE, Bormann FH. Throughfall and stemflow chemistry in a northern hardwood forest. *J Ecol* 1973;61:495–508.
32. Lindberg SE, Lovett GM, Richter DD, Johnson DW. 1986. Atmospheric deposition and canopy interactions of major ions in a forest. *Science* 1986;231:141–145.
33. Likens GE, Bormann FH, Hedin LO, Driscoll CT, Eaton JS. Dry deposition of sulfur: A 23-yr record for the Hubbard Brook Forest ecosystem. *Tellus* 1990;42B: 319–329.
34. Lovett GM, Likens GE, Nolan SS. Dry deposition of sulfur to the Hubbard Brook Experimental Forest: A preliminary comparison of methods. In: Schwartz SE, Slinn WGN, eds. *Proceedings of the Fifth International Conference on Precipitation Scavenging and Resuspension.* Victoria, Canada: Hemisphere, 1992;1391–1401.
35. Lovett GM. Atmospheric deposition of nutrients and pollutants in North America: An ecological perspective. *Ecol Appl* 1994;4:629–650.
36. Weathers, KC, Likens, GE, Bormann, FH, et al. Cloud water chemistry from ten sites in North America. *Environ Sci Tech* 1988;22:1018–1026.
37. Weathers, KC, Likens, GE, Bormann, FH, et al. Chemical concentrations in cloud water from four sites in the eastern United States. In: Unsworth MH, Fowler D, eds. *Acid deposition at high elevation sites.* Kluwer Academic, 1988;345–357.
38. Weathers KC, Likens GE, Bormann FH, et al. A regional acidic cloud/fog water event in the eastern United States. *Nature* 1986;319: 657–658.
39. Hultberg H, Likens GE. Sulphur deposition to forested catchments in northern Europe and North America Large-scale variations and long-term dynamics. In: Schwartz SE, Slinn WGN, eds. *Fifth International Conference on Precipitation Scavenging and Atmosphere-surface Exchange, vol 3:* the Summers volume: *applications and appraisals.* Washington, DC: Hemisphere, 1992;1343–1365.
40. Weathers KC, Lovett GM, Likens GE. Cloud deposition to a spruce forest edge. *Atmos Environ* 1995;29:665–672.
41. Lovett GM, Weathers KC. Controls on atmospheric deposition at the landscape and regional scales. In: Mohrer GMJ, Cerny M, eds. *Atmospheric deposition and forest management.* NATO-ASI series. Kluwer Academic, in press.
42. Miller EK, Friedland AJ, Arons EA, et al. Atmospheric deposition along an elevated gradient at Whiteface Mt., NY, USA. *Atmos Environ* 1993;27A:2121–2136.
43. Vong RJ, Sigmon JT, Mueller SF. Cloud water deposition to Appalachian forests. *Environ Sci Tech* 1991;25:1014–1021.
44. Lovett GM, Kinsman JD. Atmospheric pollutant deposition to high elevation ecosystems. *Atmos Environ* 1990;244:2767–2786.
45. Weathers KC, Lovett GM, Likens GE. The influence of a forest edge on cloud deposition. In: Schwartz SE, Slinn WGN, eds. *Proceedings of the Fifth International Conference on Precipitation Scavenging and Resuspension.* Washington, DC: Hemisphere, 1992;1415–1423.
46. Galloway JN, Likens GE, Hawley ME. Acid precipitation: Natural vs. anthropogenic components. *Science* 1984;226:829–831.
47. Galloway JN, Keene WC, Likens GE. Processes controlling the composition of precipitation at a remote southern hemisphere location: Torres del Paine National Park, Chile. *J Geophys Res* 1996;101: 6883–6897.
48. Likens GE, Keene WC, Miller JM, Galloway JN. Chemistry of precipitation from a remote, terrestrial site in Australia. *J Geophys Res* 1987;92(D11):13299–13314.
49. Likens GE. Some consequences of long-term human impacts on ecosystems. *Rev Chil Historia Natural* 1991;64:597–614.
50. Cogbill CV, Likens GE. Acid precipitation in the northeastern United States. *Water Resources Res* 1974;(10):1133–1139.
51. Cogbill CV, Likens GE, Butler TJ. Uncertainties in historical aspects of acid precipitation: Getting it straight. *Atmos Environ* 1984;18(10): 2261–2270.
52. Likens GE, Butler TJ. Recent acidification of precipitation in North America. *Atmos Environ* 1981;15(7):1103–1109.
53. Ollinger SV, Aber JD, Lovett GM, Millham SE, Lathrop RG, Ellis JM. A spatial model of atmospheric deposition for the northeastern U.S. *Ecol Appl* 1993;3:459–472.
54. Husar RB, Sullivan TJ, Charles DF. Historical trends in atmospheric sulfur deposition and methods for assessing long-term trends in surface water chemistry. In: Charles DF, Christie S, eds. *Acidic deposition and aquatic ecosystems:* regional case studies. New York: Springer-Verlag, 1990;65–82.
55. National Atmospheric Deposition Program (NADP). *NADP/NTN annual data summary:* precipitation chemistry in the United States 1994. Fort Collins CO: National Resource Ecology Laboratory, Colorado State University, 1996.
56. Likens GE. *The ecosystem approach:* its use and abuse. Oldendorf/Luhe, Germany: Ecology Institute, 1992.
57. Galloway JN, Likens GE, Edgerton ES. Acid precipitation in the northeastern United States: pH and acidity. *Science* 1976;194:722–724.
58. Schindler DW. Effects of acid rain on freshwater ecosystems. *Science* 1988;239:149–157.
59. Last FT. Critique. In: Last FT, Watling R, eds. Acidic deposition: its nature and impacts. *Proc R Soc Edinburgh* 1991;97B:273–324.
60. Asbury CE, Vertucci FA, Mattson MD, Likens GE. Acidification of Adirondack lakes. *Environ Sci Tech* 1989;23:362–365.
61. Schindler DW, Frost TM, Mills KH, et al. Comparisons between experimentally- and atmospherically- acidified lakes during stress and recovery. In: Last FT, Watling R, eds. *Proc R Soc Edinburgh* 1991;97B: 193–226.
62. Havas M, Rosseland BO. Response of zooplankton, benthos, and fish to acidification: An overview. *Water Air Soil Pollut* 1995;85:51–62.
63. Irving PM, ed. *Acid deposition:* state of science and technology. Summary report of the U.S. National Acid Precipitation Assessment Program. Washington: NAPAP, 1991.
64. Charles DF, ed. *Acidic deposition and aquatic ecosystems.* New York: Springer-Verlag, 1991.
65. Hall RJ, Driscoll CT, Likens GE. Importance of hydrogen ions and aluminum in regulating the structure and function of stream ecosystems: An experimental test. *Freshwater Biol* 1987;18:17–43.
66. Hall RJ, Driscoll, CT, Likens GE, Pratt JM. Physical, chemical and biological consequences of episodic aluminum additions to a stream. *Limnol Oceanogr* 1985;30(1):212–220.
67. Havas M, Likens GE. Toxicity of aluminum and hydrogen ions to *Daphnia catawba*, *Holopedium gibberum*, *Chaoborus punctipennis*, and *Chironomus anthrocinus* from Mirror Lake, New Hampshire. *Can J Zool* 1985;63:1114–1119.
68. Drabløs D, Tollan A, eds. SNSF project. Ecological impact of acid precipitation. Proceedings of an International Conference, March 11–14, 1980, Sandefjord, Norway.
69. Baker JL, Schofield CL. Aluminum toxicity to fish in acidic waters. *Water Air Soil Pollut* 1982;18:289–309.
70. Perrin N. A landscape made by hand. *Invention Technol* 1988;Winter:66–70.
71. Hutchinson TC, Havas M, eds. *Effects of acid precipitation on terrestrial ecosystems.* New York: Plenum Press, 1980.
72. Brady NC. *The nature and property of soils,* 8th ed. New York: Macmillan, 1974.
73. Reuss JO, Johnson DW. *Acidification of soils and waters.* New York: Springer-Verlag, 1986.
74. Johnson DW, Cresser MS, Nilsson SI, et al. Soil changes in forest ecosystems: Evidence for and probable causes. *Proc R Soc Edinburgh* 1991;97B:81–116.
75. Tamm CO, Hallbäcken L. Changes in soil acidity in two forest areas with different acid deposition: 1920s–1980s. *Ambio* 1986;17:56–61.
76. Cronan CS, Grigal DF. Use of calcium/aluminum ratios as indicators of stress in forest ecosystems. *J Environ Qual* 1995;24:209–226.
77. Ulrich B. Effects of acidic precipitation on forest ecosystems in Europe. In: Adriano DC, Havas M, eds. *Acidic precipitation, vol 2:* biological and ecological effects. New York: Springer-Verlag, 1989;189–272.
78. Ulrich B, Mayer R, Khenna PK. Soil acidity and its relations to acid deposition. In: Ulrich B, Pankrath J, eds. *Effects of accumulation of air pollutants in forest ecosystems.* Boston: D. Reidel, 1983;127–146.
79. Fernandez IJ. Effects of acid precipitation on soil productivity. In: Adriano DC, Havas M, eds. *Acidic precipitation, vol 2:* biological and ecological effects. New York: Springer-Verlag, 1989;61–83.

80. Schulze E-D, Lange OL, Oren R, eds. *Forest decline and air pollution:* a study of spruce (Picea abies) on acid soils. Berlin: Springer-Verlag, 1989.
81. Eager C, Adams MB, eds. *Ecology and decline of red spruce in the eastern United States.* New York: Springer-Verlag, 1992.
82. Smith WH. *Air pollution and forests:* interaction between air contaminants and forest ecosystems, 2nd ed. New York: Springer-Verlag, 1990.
83. Skelly JM, Innes JL. Waldsterben in the forests of central Europe and eastern North America: fantasy or reality? *Plant Dis* 1994;78: 1021–1032.
84. Johnson AH, McLaughlin SB, Adams MB, et al. Synthesis and conclusions for epidemiological and mechanistic studies of red spruce decline. In: Eager C, Adams MB, eds. *Ecology and decline of red spruce in the eastern United States.* Ecological studies 96. New York: Springer-Verlag, 1992;384–411.
85. New York State Department of Environmental Conservation. New York State atmospheric deposition monitoring network wet deposition 1993 executive summary, July 1996;1–4.
86. Rodhe H, Grennfelt P, Wisniewski J, et al. Acid reign '95 Conference summary statement. *Water Air Soil Pollut* 1995;85:1–14.
87. Likens GE. Limitations to intellectual progress in ecosystem science. In: Pace ML, Groffman PM, eds. *Successes, limitations, and frontiers in ecosystem science,* the VII Cary Conference. New York: Springer-Verlag, in press.
88. Johnson DW, Lindberg SE. *Atmospheric deposition and forest nutrient cycling:* a synthesis of the Integrated Forest Study. New York: Springer-Verlag, 1992.
89. Kelly VK. Environmental monitoring program, 1984–1993 summary report. *Occas Pub Institute Ecosystem Studies* 1995;9:1–20.

*Environmental and Occupational Medicine,*
*Third Edition,* edited by William N. Rom.
Lippincott–Raven Publishers, Philadelphia © 1998.

CHAPTER 118

# Organismic Responses to Contaminated Aquatic Systems: Four Case Histories from the Hudson River

Isaac I. Wirgin and John R. Waldman

## BIOAVAILABILITY AND BIOACTIVITY OF POLLUTANTS IN AQUATIC SYSTEMS

Aquatic ecosystems, such as that of the Hudson River, can be extremely sensitive to the effects of environmental contaminants. Water soluble, and particularly water insoluble, xenobiotics have the opportunity to accumulate to unusually high concentrations in aquatic environments. Unlike compartments in terrestrial systems, which often serve as transient depositories of pollutants and for which concentrations of xenobiotics are relatively low, aquatic systems are final sinks for contaminants, which often accumulate to extraordinarily high concentrations. This occurs despite the dynamic nature of aquatic systems; tidal action, wave action, and currents serve to transport pollutants from their sources and to dilute ambient concentrations of pollutants. Yet, despite high concentrations of xenobiotics in some aquatic systems, episodes of acute lethality directly attributable to chemical exposures are rarely observed. Most frequently, sublethal effects are discovered, which may impact the organism's ability to reproduce, develop normally, or to withstand disease. Xenobiotics that damage DNA or alter gene expression in natural populations, while not overtly toxic, can be particularly pernicious because of the potential transmission of the response to subsequent generations. In some instances, selection for resistant genotypes in highly exposed populations may have occurred to ameliorate the effects of xenobiotics.

Many pollutants are persistent in the aquatic environment. This is particularly true for lipophilic contaminants, which tend to concentrate in dissolved or particulate organic and inorganic matter in the water column, settle to the bottom, and aggregate in the organic carbon-rich sediments where they often are resistant to physical, chemical, or biologic degradation, and can be extremely long-lived. The toxicity of many aquatic pollutants is regulated by the extent to which the chemicals bind to the sediments. Physical, chemical, and biologic factors that characterize the sediments and overlying waters can modulate xenobiotic bioavailability. For example, organic carbon concentration, acid volatile sulfide concentration, and particle size of the sediment, interactions of xenobiotics, and characteristics of the overlying water such as salinity and temperature can impact the bioavailability of xenobiotics. The species composition of the macrobenthos and resulting degree of bioturbation of the sediments can also significantly influence the bioavailability of sediment-borne contaminants. Thus, despite the presence of high concentrations of contaminants in sediments, availability of xenobiotics to the lower rungs of the food chain can be limited. Furthermore, bioavailability of contaminants is not necessarily always predictive of tissue loads. Rates of uptake and rates of elimination of contaminants can differ among taxa within an ecosystem and even

I. I. Wirgin: Department of Environmental Medicine, New York University Medical Center, Tuxedo, New York 10987.
J. R. Waldman: Hudson River Foundation, New York, New York 10011.

among populations of a single species at different geographic sites. At the same time, elevated tissue loads of contaminants do not necessarily translate into elevated levels of overt or chronic toxicity. Genetic differences among species or individuals may result in differing sensitivities to xenobiotics.

The actions of toxicants in the aquatic environment can be viewed from two perspectives: that of ecosystem or wildlife health, and that of human health. For evaluation of ecosystem health, biologic end points are identified in sentinel species or tester organisms that can be measured and compared between suspected impacted systems and clean reference waterways. Endemic species are preferred for testing because of their environmental relevance, but on occasion, well-characterized, sensitive alternative models are used. This latter approach allows for comparisons among heterogeneous aquatic systems from disjunct geographic locales.

Attention can be focused on organisms ranging from the bottom of the phylogenetic scale through fishes and marine mammals. Often bioeffects are evaluated in bottom-dwelling invertebrates because of their high levels of exposure, inability to migrate from contaminated sites, ease with which they can be handled under laboratory conditions, opportunity for large samples size to provide statistical power in data analyses, and their importance at the base of food webs. Analysis of responses in higher-level vertebrate organisms may be more technically demanding and expensive, yet it provides the ability to interpret results in mechanistic frameworks derived from mammalian models and allows for extrapolations to human responses. Unfortunately, mechanisms of response to xenobiotics often differ between invertebrate and vertebrate taxa. For example, in vertebrates (including fishes and marine mammals), the aromatic hydrocarbon receptor (AhR) pathway is believed to mediate most, if not all, toxic responses to aromatic hydrocarbon compounds such as 2,3,7,8-tetrachlorodibenzo-*p*-dioxin (TCDD). However, to date, studies have failed to confirm the presence of an AhR homologue in invertebrate taxa (1), although binding of a TCDD analogue to lower molecular weight cytosolic proteins has been described in several aquatic invertebrate species, but not in others (2).

Responses that can be measured run the gamut of biologic organization from the biochemical to the community levels. Biochemical and molecular responses offer the advantage of potentially revealing a direct cause-and-effect relationship between chemical exposure and biologic effect. The chemical identity of xenobiotic inducers can often be inferred from molecular responses, and responses to xenobiotics and model chemicals are frequently dose responsive in representative feral populations. Unfortunately, while biochemical responses can be rapidly and relatively inexpensively assessed, they offer the disadvantages of not being immediately predictive of adverse biologic impacts on the organismic or population levels. On the other hand, measurements of impacts on the population or community levels are readily interpretable as to their adverse consequences, but are very difficult to ascribe to exposure to single chemicals or contaminated environments. Processes that regulate population abundance or community diversity are complex, making it difficult to relate reduced performance to xenobiotic exposure. Perhaps the only workable strategy to relate xenobiotic exposure and molecular responses to higher level biologic effects is to establish mechanistic links across levels of biological organization. If a sufficient number of these are established, then perturbation at the molecular level with a degree of certainty can be predictive of adverse impacts on the organismic or population levels.

## CHARACTERISTICS OF THE HUDSON RIVER ESTUARY

The Hudson River and New York Harbor are almost legendary for the degree and diversity of toxic pollution they have received. Boyle (3), in a treatise on the river, comments, "To those who know it, the Hudson River is the most beautiful, messed up, productive, ignored, and surprising piece of water on the face of the earth." Writing in 1951, Mitchell (4) commenced his classic article on New York Harbor thusly, "The bulk of the water...is oily, dirty, and germy. Men on the mud suckers, the big harbor dredges, like to say that you could bottle it and sell it for poison. The bottom of the harbor is dirtier than the water. In most places it is covered with a blanket of sludge that is composed of silt, sewage, industrial wastes, and clotted oil." However, this legacy, unfortunate though it may be, makes the Hudson estuary a natural laboratory for examination of the effects of contaminants on aquatic biota.

New York City and portions of the Hudson River Valley have extremely high population densities that have inflicted profound damage in the form of contamination of the Hudson River estuary. Passage of the Clean Water Act in 1972 and strong environmental activism helped alleviate pollution in the region such that obviously degraded conditions as noted by Boyle and Mitchell, on the whole, no longer exist, but their residues do, together with reduced, less tractable, but still important non–point-contaminant sources.

The Hudson River originates in the Adirondack Mountains in northern New York. Because much of its valley is near sea level, the river is tidal far inland (248 km from the tip of Manhattan), to the Federal Dam at Troy, New York, just north of the capital city of Albany (Fig. 1). The river drains a total of 34,680 square kilometers and has an annual freshwater flow of about 550 cubic meters per second; however, tidal flow can be 10 to 100 times greater than freshwater flow (5). Salinity ranges from polyhaline [18 to 30 parts per trillion (ppt)] at the mouth of the estu-

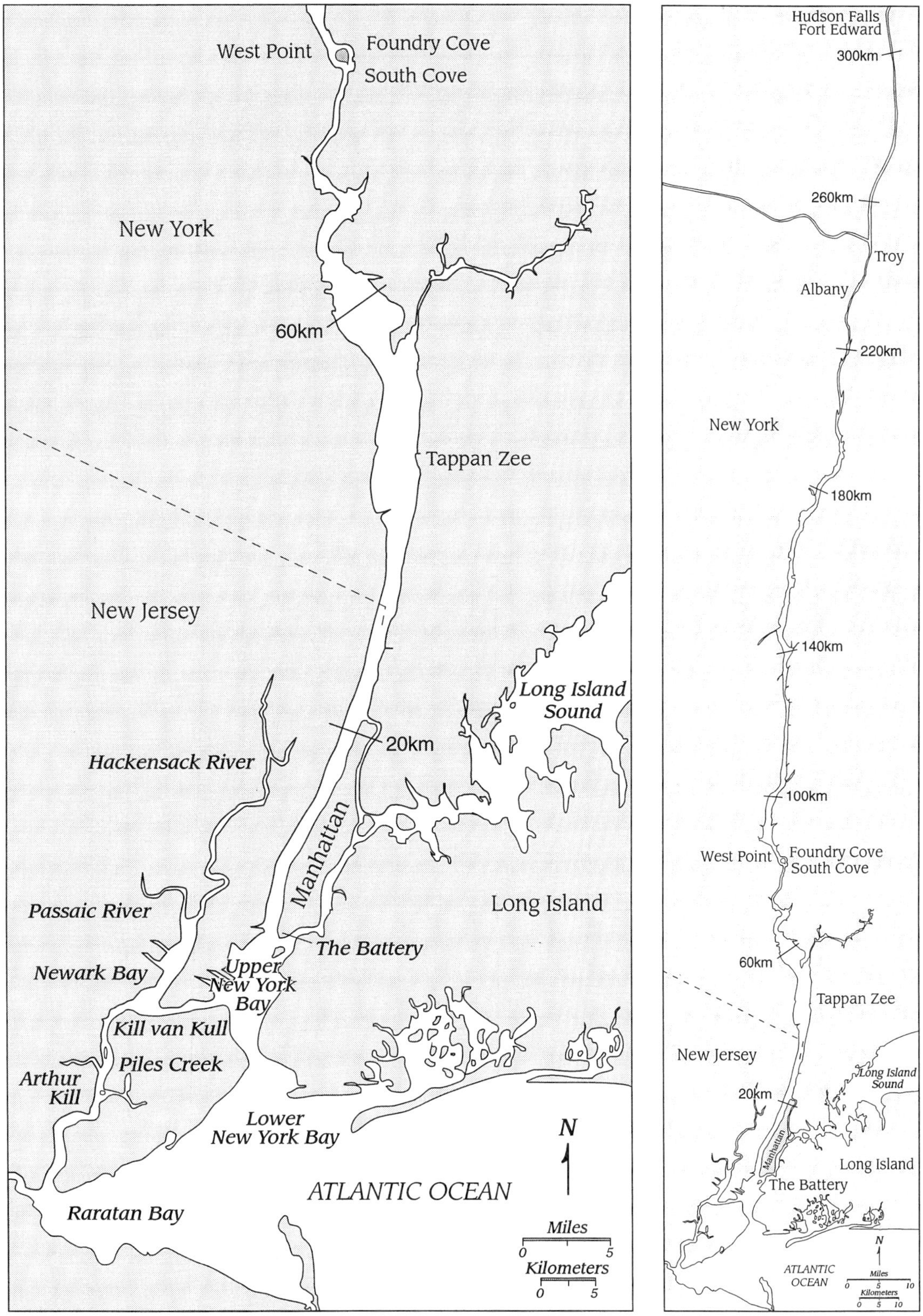


**FIG. 1.** A map of the Hudson River estuary from Lower New York Bay to Hudson Falls, New York, depicting all the locales described in the text.

ary, to fresh above the salinity intrusion (0.5 ppt), which may reach 95 km inland during drought conditions. The river north of the Battery at lower Manhattan is home to more than 200 fish species (6); until contamination became prevalent, many of these fishes, and several invertebrates, supported important fisheries within the estuary (7). The human population along the Hudson estuary is concentrated near its mouth, in the New York City metropolitan region, which had approximately 15 million people in 1980 (8). Population densities are much lower north of the New York City region, with a mixture of towns, small cities, and farmland until the Albany region at the head of tide, which has a population of about half a million.

Tarr and Ayres (8) chronicled the historical flow of pollution into the Hudson system. Raw sewage was the primary insult to the estuary in the late nineteenth century as municipalities sought to cope with sanitary and stormwater wastes. But as industry developed, the Hudson system was used as a convenient receptacle for increasing quantities and varieties of discharges. In the early part of the twentieth century, much of the industrial contamination in the metropolitan area was in the form of oil, soap, soda, bleach, acids and bases, and copper and lead. A survey in the 1950s found that of total industrial wastes, 65% came from the petroleum industry, 14% from utilities, and 10% from the chemical industry. Polychlorinated biphenyls (PCBs) entered the estuary primarily at two nearby General Electric plants above the head of tidewater north of Troy, New York.

Today, the chief toxics of concern in the Hudson estuary are PCBs, polycyclic aromatic hydrocarbons (PAHs), heavy metals, and dioxins (9). There is abundant evidence that concentrations of these contaminants in the water column generally are low and that the water quality of the Hudson estuary is improving (9,10). But decades of contamination have left substantial residues in the sediments. Sediments from five sites in New York Harbor were ranked among the ten most toxic sites in the United States (11); unusually high concentrations of dioxins, furans, PCBs and selected heavy metals are found in sediments from Newark Bay and its tributaries. Highly contaminated deposits of PCBs remain in "hot spots" in the river north of Albany.

The high degree of contamination of the Hudson River Estuary has made it an excellent natural laboratory for observing contaminant effects on feral populations of aquatic organisms. In this chapter, we provide case histories of four disparate interactions between single or classes of contaminants and particular organisms that are unique to or have been especially well documented in the Hudson system. These include (a) cadmium and an oligochaete worm (*Limnodrilus hoffmeisteri*), (b) methylmercury and mummichog (*Fundulus heteroclitus*), (c) aromatic hydrocarbons and Atlantic tomcod (*Microgadus tomcod*), and (d) PCBs and striped bass (*Morone saxatilis*).

## EVOLUTIONARY RESISTANCE TO CADMIUM BY AN OLIGOCHAETE WORM

Heavy metals are released into the environment in three ways: (a) by production processes, (b) by fossil-fuel combustion, and (c) by dissipation of intermediate or final products, i.e., via "consumptive" uses, such as in gasoline additives (8). The Hudson Highlands, approximately 70 to 90 km north of the river's mouth, never became urbanized or industrialized. However, Foundry Cove, a tidal freshwater bay, 87 km upriver from the river's mouth and immediately opposite the U.S. Military Academy at West Point, witnessed one of the most dramatic episodes of metal contamination ever reported in a natural ecosystem. Beginning in 1953 and continuing until 1971, a nickel-cadmium battery plant in Cold Spring, New York, directly discharged cadmium (Cd), nickel (Ni), and sometimes cobalt (Co) precipitates into a tidal creek from which it spread into the broader expanse of Foundry Cove and periodically into the main stem of the Hudson River (12). In total, it is estimated that 179 metric tons (MT) of Cd were discharged from the factory, of which 51 MT of particulates and 1.6 MT of solubles went into Foundry Cove and the remainder was discharged directly into the Hudson River.

Cadmium concentrations in superficial sediments from the tidal creek immediately adjacent to the discharge site exceeded 100,000 ppm Cd and also contained equimolar concentrations of Ni and about 10% of that concentration of Co. Within the larger expanse of the cove, a gradient in levels of sediment Cd concentrations was observed ranging between 500 and 10,000 ppm and it was estimated that approximately 30% of the cove in 1975 had surface sediment Cd concentrations that exceeded 1,000 ppm (Fig. 2) (13). Although export of water-borne Cd occurred from Foundry Cove to the main stem of the Hudson River through a narrow channel, the magnitude of loss (0.8% of Cd lost annually) was believed insufficient to contaminate the main river channel or to significantly decrease Cd concentrations within Foundry Cove within the near future. Instead, it was believed that burial of Cd was occurring in the cove and accounted for any major reductions observed in superficial Cd concentrations (12). In 1972 and 1973, the top 30 cm of sediments in the cove were dredged, but it is believed that only 10% of the Cd load within the cove was removed in this process. By the 1980s, Foundry Cove was designated a federal Superfund Site and remediation costing $91 million and including dredging, draining, and treating of contaminated sediments was completed in the winter of 1994.

When evaluated in the 1970s, concentrations of Cd were significantly elevated both in filtrates of Foundry Cove water and in water-borne particulates, but not to remarkably high levels, perhaps due to chemical characteristics of the sediments, such as the acid volatile sulfide phase, which modulates the bioavailability of metals such

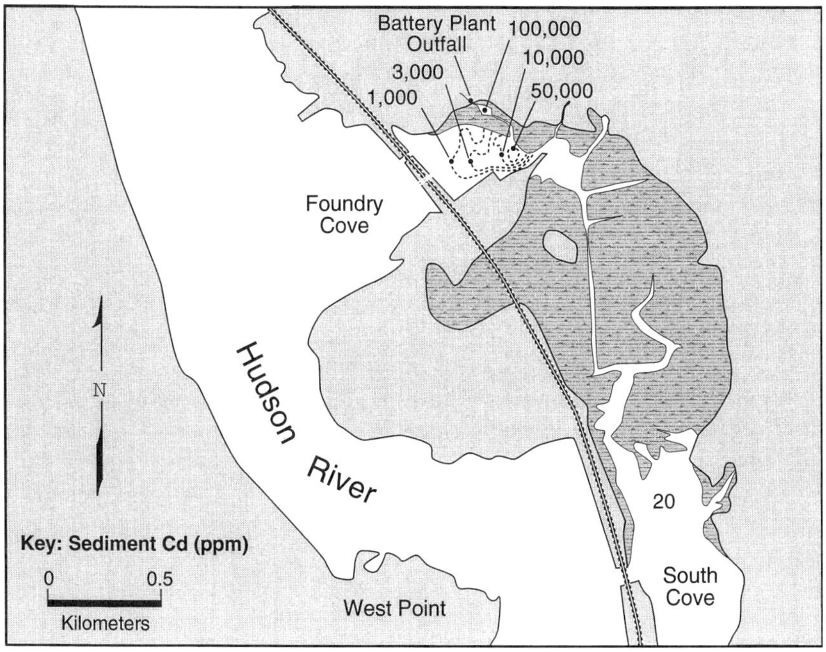


**FIG. 2.** A map of Foundry Cove and South Cove depicting cadmium concentrations (ppm) in surficial sediments in 1983 as described (13).

as Cd to benthic invertebrates (14). With few exceptions, Cd concentrations in water filtrates from Foundry Cove did not exceed the 10 μg/L Cd allowed in drinking water (15,16). Initial studies confirmed the bioavailability of Cd to plant and animal species that are endemic to Foundry Cove. Elevated tissue concentrations of Cd were detected in cattails (*Typha angustifolia*), blue crabs (*Callinectes sapidus*), and banded killifish (*Fundulus diaphanus)* from Foundry Cove and concentrations in cattails were inversely related to their distance from the source of effluent discharge (15,17). In fishes, the organs that bioaccumulated the highest concentrations of Cd included intestines, liver, and kidney. The failure of Cd to bioaccumulate in muscle suggested that Cd wasn't available to human consumers of fish from the Hudson River. However, concentrations in the hepatopancreas of blue crabs from nearby Hudson River sites was sometimes remarkably high and potentially posed a threat to humans who consumed this popular resource species. For example, levels of Cd in the hepatopancreas of crabs from Stony Point, New York (19 Km south of Foundry Cove), averaged 8.7 to 18.2 μg Cd/g tissue compared to 0.39 μg Cd/g tissue in crabs from a relatively clean bay in southern New Jersey (18).

Based on controlled laboratory exposures, ingestion of contaminated foods or sediments was probably the dominant route of exposure to Cd in crabs and fish from Foundry Cove. However, biomagnification of Cd levels did not occur in organisms representative of the top of the food chain, and laboratory experiments demonstrated the depuration of Cd from these tissues to control levels (15). Finally, acute toxicity was not observed in goldfish (*Carassius auratus*) or banded killifish exposed to environmentally relevant levels of Cd through either the water or food routes (15), and equilibrium tissue concentrations were an order of magnitude less than those that elicited Cd-induced toxicity in other fish species or mammals. This indicated the inability of bioavailable Cd, by itself, to elicit overt toxicity in feral populations of killifish within Foundry Cove.

Ecological surveys showed no decrease in the overall abundance of macrobenthos at three sites in Foundry Cove (500 ppm and 7,000 ppm Cd in surface sediments), including the highly polluted tidal creek (50,000 ppm Cd), compared to a much cleaner control site 2 km to the south, South Cove (20 ppm Cd) (Fig. 2) (13). However, the diversity of macrobenthic taxa was decreased at the highly polluted tidal creek compared to less polluted sites in Foundry Cove and South Cove. Further analysis revealed the density of two benthic species, the oligochaete worm *Limnodrilus hoffmeisteri* and an insect *Tanypus neopunctipennis*, were significantly elevated and could explain the overall abundance of macrobenthos within the tidal creek in the face of reduced species diversity (13). Bioavailability of both Cd and Ni to *L. hoffmeisteri* was demonstrated when gut content analysis revealed elevated body burdens of both metals (19). It was postulated that both species had acquired resistance to metal-induced toxicity.

Controlled laboratory exposures of *L. hoffmeisteri* collected from a site in Foundry Cove (7,000 ppm Cd) and a site in South Cove (20 ppm) to contaminated Foundry Cove sediments (7,000 or 50,000 ppm) or metal spiked water (Cd, Ni, Co) confirmed the resistance of the Foundry Cove population (20). Additionally, it was found that the degree of resistance varied directly with the sediment cadmium concentration at the collection site. The heritability of the resistance phenotype was next addressed. Worms collected from Foundry Cove and South Cove were mated and their offspring were reared for two generations in metal-free sediments and then tested for survival for 28 days in contaminated Foundry Cove sediments. Little difference was observed in tolerance between Foundry Cove collected worms and their laboratory-reared offspring; however, their survival was significantly elevated over that of the offspring of South Cove worms. These results demonstrated that resistance to metal-induced toxicity in *L. hoffmeisteri* was a genetic adaptation and not the result of single-generational physiologic acclimation.

Selection experiments were conducted with South Cove worms exposed to water-borne metals to determine if resistance to these agents could develop under controlled laboratory conditions and if so, the number of generations needed. After only three generations of Cd selection, the difference in resistance between the selected and control lines was 66% of the difference in resistance between field collected worms from Foundry Cove and South Cove (20). Thus, development of resistance under controlled laboratory conditions was remarkably rapid and could explain most of the resistance to metal toxicity observed in natural populations in Foundry Cove. Interestingly, the extent of resistance of the *L. hoffmeisteri* population in Foundry Cove was revisited 2 years after the completion of remediation in 1994. Measurable resistance in the population decreased within four to six generations of the completion of remediation, suggesting either the import of worms from elsewhere or that selective pressure for resistant genotypes was strong and costs associated with tolerance were high (21).

The fact that resistance developed so rapidly and almost certainly resulted from exposure to this suite of metals provided a model to explore the mechanisms whereby resistance was operative. Initial studies investigated the possibility of reduced bioaccumulation of metals either through reduced uptake or more efficient elimination. Studies with arsenite-resistant bacterial strains (22) and a zinc resistant annelid population (23) suggested that elevated rates of efflux of metals, perhaps mediated by the multidrug resistance gene (24), could provide heritable resistance to exposure to toxicants such as Cd. Unexpectedly, when exposed to water- or sediment-borne Cd, *L. hoffmeisteri* collected from Foundry Cove and their laboratory-reared naive offspring exhibited significantly increased accumulation of Cd compared to worms that were collected from the South Cove reference site (13,25). Thus, reduced bioaccumulation of toxicants did not occur in worms from Foundry Cove and was not responsible for their resistance.

It was demonstrated that concentrations of Cd were significantly higher in the cytosol than in other subcellular fractions that were isolated from Cd-treated worms from either Foundry Cove or South Cove (25). Was bioaccumulated Cd in the cytosol of *L. hoffmeisteri* uniformly distributed, protein-bound, or compartmentalized? When exposed to water or sediment-borne Cd, worms from both Foundry Cove and South Cove exhibited increased expression of very low molecular weight proteins and somewhat larger proteins (16 kd) whose molecular size fell within the upper range of that of vertebrate metallothioneins (25). Metallothioneins have been characterized in a variety of aquatic taxa, including several invertebrate species (26), and are probably ubiquitous in the animal kingdom. Metallothioneins can be induced by a variety of metals, including Cd, and are believed to function in the binding and intracellular transport of essential metals, and perhaps in the detoxification of environmentally damaging metals such as Cd. Associations between reduced metal-induced toxicity and (a) preexposure of aquatic invertebrates to nontoxic concentrations of metallothionein inducers (26), (b) increased expression of metallothionein in recombinant yeast cells (27), (c) levels of metallothionein expression in larval turbot (*Scopthalmus maximus*) (28), and (d) metallothionein gene amplification in Cu-resistant natural populations of *Drosophila melanogaster* (29) all suggest a protective role for metallothionein against metal-induced toxicity. The fact that Cd, in Cd-exposed worms was complexed with induced proteins also supports, but does not prove, a protective role for these metallothionein-like proteins in *L. hoffmeisteri*. Increased protein binding of Cd in the resistant worms is suggestive of lowered Cd availability and perhaps toxicity to cellular organelles. However, attempts to confirm the identity of the Cd-binding protein as metallothionein have failed because of an inability to purify sufficient quantities for characterization and the hypervariability of metallothionein gene structure among even closely related invertebrate taxa.

After exposure to water-borne Cd, Foundry Cove worms, their offspring, and South Cove worms all had high levels of cytosolic Cd associated with a particulate subcellular pool (25). Electron microprobe studies demonstrated that the amount of Cd sequestered in these subcellular granules was greater in worms from Foundry Cove and their offspring than in worms from South Cove, thus suggesting this as a mechanism protecting against Cd-induced cellular toxicity. Sequestration of Cd was apparently by two distinct mechanisms, both of which involved compartmentalization of Cd in cytosolic granules. Very dense granules containing high concentrations of Cd and S in a 1:1 ratio were observed in the gut wall and the body wall. Compartmentalization of Cd with Ca-P in less dense granules was observed in the chloragog tissues surrounding the gut, suggesting that this interaction may provide a mechanism to sequester toxic metals and excrete them via the gut.

The high levels of protein bound and sequestered Cd in the cytosol of *L. hoffmeisteri* and perhaps other organisms from Foundry Cove may have adverse consequences for higher trophic levels in the Hudson River food chain. Compartmentalization suggests that Cd is persistent and in high concentrations in prey organisms from contaminated sites and may be readily bioavailable to predators. This hypothesis was tested by preparing food pellets from the cytosol and other subcellular fractions of Cd-treated *L. hoffmeisteri* and then feeding the pellets to a natural predator, the grass shrimp *Palaemonetes pugio* (30). Not surprisingly, the cytosolic fraction provided the highest concentration of bioavailable Cd to shrimp and the transfer of cytosolic-bound Cd was highly efficient (65–80%). This indicates that while sequestration of Cd in the cytosol may serve to reduce toxicity to the prey organism, in this case *L. hoffmeisteri*, it also serves to efficiently transfer high levels of Cd to a predator and thus increase potential risk to organisms at higher trophic levels.

It should be remembered that of all taxa initially investigated in Foundry Cove, only *L. hoffmeisteri* provided evidence of resistance to metal toxicity; in fact several taxa were absent from the most polluted site. No evidence of genetic resistance to metal exposure was observed in the insect species, *T. neopunctipennis*, perhaps due to high levels of gene flow with adjacent populations from less polluted sites. Thus, evolution of resistance to toxicity should not be considered a justification for release of environmental pollutants. Furthermore, elevated levels of sequestered Cd in resistant worms provided an efficient mechanism to transfer Cd to higher levels of the food chain and serve as a possible route to export Cd from the Foundry Cove environment.

## METHYLMERCURY TOXICITY IN MUMMICHOG FROM NEWARK BAY

The lower Hudson River estuary, particularly its western arm extending into Newark Bay, New Jersey, and branching into the lower Hackensack and Passaic rivers, is urbanized and industrialized. As a result, sediments in this area contain some of the highest concentrations of xenobiotics within the entire Hudson River estuary (31) and within any U.S. coastal water (32). For example, the lower Passaic River, Hackensack River, and Newark Bay sediments contain concentrations of dioxins and furans that exceed those of any U.S. estuary. Similarly, the Kill van Kull and Arthur Kill waterways connecting upper New York Bay and Raritan Bay with Newark Bay have experienced a series of major oil spills within the past decade; these waterways also are ringed by power generating stations, chemical factories, and sewage plants. Bioavailability of both halogenated and nonhalogenated aromatic hydrocarbon compounds to resident shellfish and finfish populations within this area has been documented (31,33). Yet despite elevated concentrations of these toxicants in the Newark Bay region, fauna is abundant, and richness does not appear significantly diminished compared with other estuarine systems in the Virginian province. However, it should also be noted that concentrations of toxicants such as TCDD are sometimes elevated in migratory resource species such as bluefish (*Pomatomus saltatrix*), striped bass, and weakfish (*Cynoscion regalis*), which use the Newark Bay area seasonally as feeding and nursery areas (31,33). Thus, the impacts of Newark Bay contaminated sediments may on occasion extend out into coastal ecosystems and to human consumers of these valuable resource species.

In addition to elevated levels of organic contaminants, the lower Hudson River estuary contains concentrations of 12 metals that are among the highest in any U.S. estuary, that exceed predicted biologic effect levels, and that warrant concern for aquatic life and human health (31). Of these metals, only concentrations of mercury exceeded predicted effects levels in all three media: water, sediment, and biota. Mercury levels in the sediments of Newark Bay and its tributaries are as high as 1,750 ppm in Berry's Creek, but generally range from 1 to 20 ppm (31). Populations of mummichogs (*Fundulus heteroclitus*) thrive in this region and have provoked a series of studies on Hg toxicity, and possible resistance of a mummichog population in Piles Creek, a backwater of the Arthur Kill (34). Mummichog have a restricted home range and thus their exposure histories are believed reflective of their site of capture. Mummichog in the Hudson River estuary do not exhibit tumors, but mummichog from the Elizabeth River, Virginia, do have a high prevalence of hepatocellular carcinomas, probably due to extremely high sediment concentrations of creosote-derived PAHs (35). Throughout their extensive Atlantic coast distribution, mummichog exhibit unusually high levels of genetic variation, perhaps conferring increased potential to respond to environmental heterogeneity and pollutant exposure (36).

Studies have shown that concentrations of organic methylmercury biomagnify in aquatic food chains, can be extremely high in top predatory fish, and that consumption of some species can pose a threat to human populations. Many studies have demonstrated that inorganic mercury entering aquatic ecosystems is methylated by microorganisms in aquatic sediments, that methylmercury compounds are very efficiently absorbed yet poorly eliminated, and that they bioaccumulate to high levels in fish tissues. As expected, mummichog from Piles Creek exhibited 7.5-fold higher levels of Hg than fish from cleaner eastern Long Island, New York; however, bioconcentration factors for Hg and (other metals) were lower in Piles Creek fish (37), suggesting exclusion or more rapid elimination of Hg in fish from the contaminated Piles Creek site. Exposure of naive mummichogs embryos (prehatched) under controlled laboratory conditions to methylmercury resulted in teratogenic craniofacial, cardiovascular, and skeletal malformations (38), and, following hatch in their larvae, reduced prey capture ability (39), reduced swimming performance, and reduced predator avoidance (40). Similarly, exposure of mummichog sperm to methylmercury resulted in reduced motility and fertilization success (41). Thus, as expected, young life stages and adult mummichog exhibited neurologic and other impairments consistent with methylmercury exposures. Additionally, cytogenetic alterations induced by methylmercury treatment of mummichog embryos were observed, probably due to a decreased mitotic rate (42).

However, embryos of offspring of mummichogs collected from the Long Island clean environment exhibited varied sensitivities to methylmercury exposures; both tolerant and sensitive families were observed when evaluated at these teratogenic, behavioral, and cytogenetic end points. Furthermore, when mummichog embryos derived from Piles Creek parents were experimentally exposed to methylmercury, they demonstrated uniformly more tolerant responses at these end points (34). Additional experiments demonstrated that methylmercury-treated sperm from Piles Creek mummichogs were more motile and viable than similarly treated sperm obtained from males from a clean site. Moreover, the effects of methylmercury exposure on the prey-capture ability of Piles Creek mummichog was less than in Long Island fish (43). These results suggested that resistance to methylmercury (and perhaps other toxicants) had developed in the Piles Creek population.

Studies were initiated to determine the mechanistic basis of tolerance in embryos from Piles Creek. It was demonstrated that resistance was transmitted through eggs; however, multigenerational studies to confirm that tolerance was a heritable genetic adaptation were not performed. No association was observed between levels of metallothionein expression during sensitive embryonic stages and susceptibility to methylmercury induced toxicity (44). At the time of hatching, levels of metallothionein were higher in tolerant than in sensitive larvae, but the onset of increased gene expression was too late to account for the variation in embryonic tolerance to methylmercury. However, it was observed that the bioaccumulation of methylmercury was lower in experimentally treated resistant embryos than in sensitive embryos, perhaps due to differences in chorionic permeability. This observation was consistent with the maternal transfer of resistance because the chorion of the developing embryo is derived from the female gamete. Additionally, the rate of development of Piles Creek embryos was more rapid during the most sensitive early life stages than in sensitive populations, perhaps providing a narrower temporal window to incur damage.

Increased tolerance to methylmercury exposure in the Piles Creek population was not without its costs. Resistance to methylmercury toxicity in Piles Creek fish did not extend to later life stages; if anything, Piles Creek larvae and adults were more sensitive to methylmercury toxicity than fish from a cleaner site. Increased sensitivity to Hg toxicity, reduced life expectancy, reduced larval growth (45), reduced ability to capture prey in the absence of methylmercury (43), and reduced brain concentrations of serotonin and its metabolites were also observed in adult mummichog from the resistant population (46).

## NEOPLASIA IN NORTH AMERICAN FISH POPULATIONS AND IN DOMESTICATED SPECIES

To the general public, one of the most obvious and alarming manifestations of environmental degradation is an elevated prevalence of cancer in feral organisms in their region. Some species of both feral and domesticated fish have proved exquisitely sensitive to chemically induced neoplasia. The most common target tissue for tumor development in feral fish populations has been the epithelium and affected sites have included the liver, pancreas, and gastrointestinal and epidermal tissues. Of 19 epizootic neoplasias of likely chemical etiology in North American fish populations, 6 were in epidermis and the remaining 13 were in liver (47). In contrast, the development of spontaneous tumors in feral and domestic fish is relatively rare compared to that observed in rodent models. Thus, development of tumors in domestic and feral fish can with some certainty be assigned a chemical etiology.

Much of the metabolic machinery that processes environmental procarcinogens is the same in fishes and mammals. Many phase I enzymes, including cytochrome P-450s (which oxidize PAHs to more hydrophilic and reactive forms), are conserved in fishes. As in mammals, ultimately these electrophilic metabolites can covalently bond to cellular macromolecules such as DNA and cause mutations, or alternatively, be eliminated from the body by phase II enzyme-catalyzed conjugation with carrier molecules such as glutathione, glucuronic acid, and amino acids. The most intensively studied of the cytochrome P-450 subfamilies in fishes, cytochrome P-4501A (CYP1A), has been demonstrated to convert PAHs such as benzo[*a*]pyrene (B[*a*]P) (48) and dimethylbenz[*a*]anthracene (DMBA) (49) to reactive metabolites that are similar to those observed in mammals. The formation of DNA adducts is believed prerequisite to the initiation of chemical carcinogenesis in fish, and elevated levels of bulky PAH hepatic DNA adducts, detected by $^{32}P$ postlabeling analysis, have been observed in many species of feral fish from impacted sites (50,51). Additionally, elevated levels of hydroxyl radical–induced mutagenic base modifications have been reported in hepatic neoplasms (52), nonneoplastic hepatic lesions (53), and neoplasm-free hepatic tissues (54) in English sole (*Parophrys vetulus*) from contaminated sites in Puget Sound, Washington. Studies with the domesticated rainbow trout (*Oncorhyncus mykiss*) model also have established a direct relationship between levels of hepatic

DNA adducts, frequencies of K-*ras* oncogene activation, and incidence of liver neoplasms (55). Compared to mammalian models, however, the capacity for DNA repair is probably diminished in fish. After an initial period of rapid DNA repair, hepatic DNA adducts are far more persistent in both environmentally exposed (56) and chemically treated (57) fish than in rodents.

One of the first observations of liver tumors in a domesticated species was in the Shasta hatchery strain of rainbow trout, which exhibited sensitivity to dietary aflatoxin $B_1$ induced carcinogenicity (58). Yet, despite their proclivity to chemically induced liver and kidney neoplasms, spontaneous tumors are rare in rainbow trout fed control diets. The absence of background tumors allows for statistical precision when evaluating the carcinogenic potential of low doses of experimental chemicals. Exposure of domesticated small aquarium species, such as medaka (*Oryzias latipes*) and guppy (*Poecilia reticulata*), to PAHs, nitroso compounds, and aromatic amines under controlled laboratory conditions has elicited elevated levels of hepatic tumors (48). Furthermore, the progression of histologic pathologies in livers from treated fish follows the multistage process predicted from carcinogenesis studies in rodents. The spectrum of hepatocellular proliferative lesions progresses from foci of cellular alteration with altered enzyme activities to adenomas and finally to invasive, poorly differentiated, hepatocellular carcinomas.

However, attempts to elicit overt hepatic neoplasms in cancer-prone feral species with PAHs under controlled laboratory conditions have not been successful. This may result from the inability to expose and rear sensitive young life stages to maturity, the inability of hatchery-reared feral fish to experience the rates of growth and sexual maturation experienced by natural populations, or the failure to expose fish to the mixtures of tumor initiators and promoters found in many contaminated environments. However, aromatic hydrocarbon-rich extracts prepared from contaminated sediments from locales in Puget Sound, Washington, did induce presumptive preneoplastic foci of cellular alteration in naive 2-year-old English sole that were collected from a reference site (59). Furthermore, organic extracts prepared from contaminated sediments from tributaries of the Great Lakes caused skin tumors when painted on mice (60) and preneoplastic lesions and liver tumors when injected in rainbow trout sac fry (61,62). Additionally, PAH and aromatic compound–enriched nonpolar fractions prepared from contaminated Great Lakes sediments were highly mutagenic in Ames tester strains after activation by liver enzymes (62). In summary, these studies demonstrate that some PAHs can act as complete carcinogens in sensitive domesticated fish, that sediments from contaminated sites often have mutagenic activity and carcinogenic activity in sensitive models, and that induction of tumors in cancer-prone feral species probably requires exposure to environmental mixtures that contain both tumor initiators and promoters.

The initial report of an epizootic of liver neoplasms in North American fish populations occurred in bottom-dwelling white suckers (*Catostomus commersoni*) and brown bullhead (*Ictalurus nebulosus*) from Deep Creek Lake, Maryland (63), and followed by approximately two decades the onset of the exponential growth of industries in North America that synthesized organic chemicals. Since then, epizootics of neoplasia have been reported in feral populations from freshwater, marine, and estuarine waters throughout North America. The highest prevalences of neoplasia were observed in bottom-dwelling species from Puget Sound, Washington, tributaries of the Great Lakes, the Elizabeth River, Virginia, Boston Harbor, Massachusetts, and the Hudson River, New York (47) (Table 1). Conspecific populations from more pristine reference sites exhibited either sig-

**TABLE 1.** *Characterization of selected epizootic neoplasias in North American fish populations*

| Species | Location | Neoplasm(s) | Prevalence of tumors (%) | When sampled | Reference |
|---|---|---|---|---|---|
| Atlantic tomcod (*Microgadus tomcod*) | Hudson River, New York | HHC | 52 | 1985–1989 | 72 |
| Winter flounder (*Pseudopleuronectes americanus*) | Boston Harbor, MA | HHC<br>CCC | 8 | 1984 | 105 |
| | New Bedford Harbor, MA | HHC<br>CCC | 32 | 1985–1989<br>1989 | 106 |
| English sole (*Pleuronectes vetulus*) | Eagle Harbor, WA | HHC<br>CCC | 18 | 1979–1985 | 107 |
| | Duwamish Waterway, WA | Mixed | 17 | 1979–1985 | |
| Mummichog (*Fundulus heteroclitus*) | Elizabeth River, VA | HHC | 35 | 1989 | 35 |
| Brown bullhead (*Ictalurus nebulosus*) | Black River, OH | CCC | 39 | 1982 | 66 |
| | | HHC | 10 | 1987 | |
| | | Epidermal papillomas<br>Papillary carcinomas | 30 | 1980 | 108 |
| | | Squamous carcinomas | 20 | 1980 | |
| White sucker (*Catostomus commersoni*) | Lake Ontario, ONT (tributaries) | Epidermal papillomas | 60 | No data | 109 |

HCC, hepatocellular carcinomas; CCC, cholangiocellular carcinomas; mixed, hepatocellular/cholangiocellular carcinomas.

nificantly lower prevalences or an absence of neoplasms. A direct relationship between the prevalence of hepatic lesions, including preneoplastic lesions and neoplasms, and PAHs in sediments, stomach contents, and bile was observed in winter flounder from the Atlantic coast and in three species of marine fish—English sole (*Pleuronectes vetulus*), starry flounder (*Platichthys stellatus*), and white croaker (*Genyonemus lineatus*) from the Pacific coast (64,65). Additionally, populations of fish from all of these sites exhibited high levels of bulky hepatic DNA adducts further implicating PAHs as a causative agent of these epizootics (50). PCB exposure was not a risk factor for liver disease in winter flounder from the Atlantic coast, but it was a risk factor for hepatic lesions in sole and flatfish from the Pacific coast. Confirmation of the significance of PAHs in eliciting hepatic tumors in natural populations of brown bullhead was documented when a significant decline in liver neoplasms was observed following the closing of a coking plant on the Black River, a tributary of Lake Erie, Ohio. After the closing of the plant, sediment concentrations of PAHs declined 99%, whole-body burdens of PAHs in bullheads declined 75% to 97%, and the prevalence of hepatic neoplasms decreased from 39% to 10% (66). These data strongly supported a cause-and-effect relationship between PAH exposure and liver cancer in this population of fish.

## ATLANTIC TOMCOD, LIVER CANCER, AND AROMATIC HYDROCARBONS

Atlantic tomcod is a very common bottom-dwelling species in the Hudson River, whose overall distribution extends from Labrador to New Jersey (67). The Hudson River supports their southernmost spawning population, and as a result they may be thermally stressed during summer. Tomcod are not a commercially important species; however, recreational fishermen frequently target them within the Hudson River estuary. They are a dominant finfish within the Hudson River, and as such have been used as an indicator species of environmental quality (68). Atlantic tomcod are anadromous, yet spend their entire life cycles within the confines of their natal estuaries (69). Within the Hudson River estuary, adult tomcod undergo upriver winter spawning migrations to approximately 40 to 90 km north of the river's mouth in New York City, and juveniles and postspawning adults then drop back to more saline reaches of the estuary for summer feeding in upper New York Bay and Newark Bay. Tomcod are opportunistic feeders; their diet consists of many available bottom-dwelling and potentially contaminated food species. Tomcod also have unusually high liver lipid concentrations that serve to bioaccumulate many xenobiotics of concern, due to their lipophilic nature (70). As a result of their life history and physiology, the exposure history of tomcod potentially integrates contaminant levels from throughout the lower Hudson River estuary and make tomcod an excellent sentinel species.

Atlantic tomcod collected in the early 1980s from the Hudson River exhibited one of the highest prevalences of neoplasia in any feral population of aquatic or terrestrial species. For example, more than 50% of 1-year-old Hudson River tomcod exhibited hepatocellular carcinomas and more than 90% of 2-year-olds displayed these lesions (71). In contrast, less than 5% of tomcod from the Pawcatuck River, Rhode Island (71), or the Saco River, Maine, exhibited liver lesions (72). To date, liver tumors have not been detected in tomcod from more pristine rivers in the Canadian Maritime provinces, although other diseases have been observed (73). The frequency and severity of liver tumors in Hudson River tomcod increased directly with the age and length of the fish such that within an age class the frequency of tumors was significantly higher in larger fish (71). All of these factors suggest an environmental etiology to the elevated level of neoplasia in the Hudson River population.

Over the same period, the tomcod population in the Hudson River exhibited a truncated age-class structure compared with tomcod from other rivers. When investigated in the early 1980s, more than 95% of the Hudson River spawning population was composed of 1-year-old fish and almost all of the remaining fish were 2-year-olds (71). In comparison, the spawning aggregations of tomcod in other rivers were primarily composed of 2- to 4-year-old fish and tomcod up to 7 years of age have been reported from more northerly populations. Thus, it has been suggested that the elevated prevalence of hepatic tumors in the Hudson River population may have contributed to its truncated age structure; however, this hypothesis was not tested in controlled laboratory experiments.

Studies were conducted to determine the etiology of hepatic neoplasia in the Hudson River tomcod population. Clearly, tomcod from the Hudson River are exposed to among the highest concentrations of sediment bound aromatic hydrocarbon contaminants, including PAHs, PCBs, and dioxins, of any estuary in the United States (32). Bioavailability of these compounds to tomcod was confirmed by high hepatic concentrations of PCBs, including the more toxic coplanar congeners (71,74) and elevated levels of PAH metabolites in bile (75). Dioxin concentrations have yet to be measured in tomcod tissues; however, their levels are highly elevated in sympatric finfishes in the lower Hudson River estuary (76). Surprisingly, neoplasms have rarely been reported in sympatric species of Hudson River fish, although bioaccumulation and bioactivity of cancer-initiating agents in causing hepatic DNA damage are as high as in tomcod (77).

Did exposure and bioaccumulation of these compounds in Hudson River tomcod result in molecular alterations associated with early stages of chemical carcinogenesis? Cytochrome P-4501A1 (CYP1A1)–encoded enzyme activities are necessary to oxidize environmental procarcinogens to reactive electrophiles, which can then adduct to cellular DNA and initiate genetic lesions. Furthermore, in fishes, CYP1A1 transcription is induced by exposure to a variety of aromatic hydrocarbon compounds, including dioxins, furans, coplanar PCB congeners, and PAHs. When hepatic CYP1A1 messenger RNA (mRNA) expression was compared between tomcod from the Hudson River and four other less impacted populations in New England and Atlantic Canada, levels of gene expression were approximately 28-fold higher in Hudson River tomcod than in fish from the most pristine river, the Margaree, Nova Scotia. Furthermore, overall levels of CYP1A1 mRNA expression generally corresponded to known sediment contaminant levels in the five rivers (75). These results confirmed both the exposure of Hudson River tomcod to high levels of environmental procarcinogens and tumor promoters and their ability to elicit a carcinogenically relevant response. Subsequently, $^{32}P$ postlabeling analysis was used to determine if this exposure to environmental aromatic hydrocarbons resulted in elevated levels of overall hepatic DNA damage in tomcod from the Hudson River (Fig. 3). Tomcod from the Hudson River exhibited 40-fold higher levels of hepatic DNA adducts than tomcod from the most pristine river, demonstrating that tomcod from the Hudson River are exposed to extraordinarily high levels of environmental PAHs and that these compounds are active in initiating DNA damage (75).

During Northern blot screening of tomcod CYP1A1 mRNA, a polymorphism in the size of the CYP1A1 transcript was detected in a moderate percentage (10%) of Hudson River tomcod and was absent in tomcod from the four other rivers (78). DNA analysis, using Southern blot hybridizations, revealed that this polymorphism was genetically encoded, only observed in a heterozygous state, and only present in tomcod from the Hudson River. Further characterization of the CYP1A1 variant and common alleles revealed that the polymorphism resulted from a 606-bp deletion in the 3 untranslated region (3-UTR) of the cDNA (79). Studies using in vitro mammalian models have demonstrated that the nucleotide sequence of 3-UTRs probably impacts mRNA stability, and therefore translational efficiencies of mRNAs, and ultimately levels of gene expression. Thus, the CYP1A1 polymorphism in the Hudson River tomcod population may serve a selective advantage in reducing levels of gene expression, and therefore CYP1A1-mediated DNA damage or promotion of initiated cells.

Activation of *ras* oncogenes in tumor DNAs by point mutations at selected hot spots is a signature of exposure of rodents to model PAHs and is also common in certain human cancers. The sensitivity of domesticated rainbow trout to mutations at codons 12 and 13 and 61 and 62 of K-*ras* has been observed in hepatic tumors resulting from treatment with the cancer-causing food contaminant, aflatoxin B1, and PAHs, some of which are of environmental concern (58). Additionally, levels of hepatic DNA adducts and frequencies of K-*ras* activation were often dose responsive in chemically treated trout (55). This suggests that many of the molecular mechanisms of carcinogenesis are conserved between fish and mammals.

The NIH3T3 transfection assay was used to evaluate the ability of tomcod liver tumor DNAs to transform

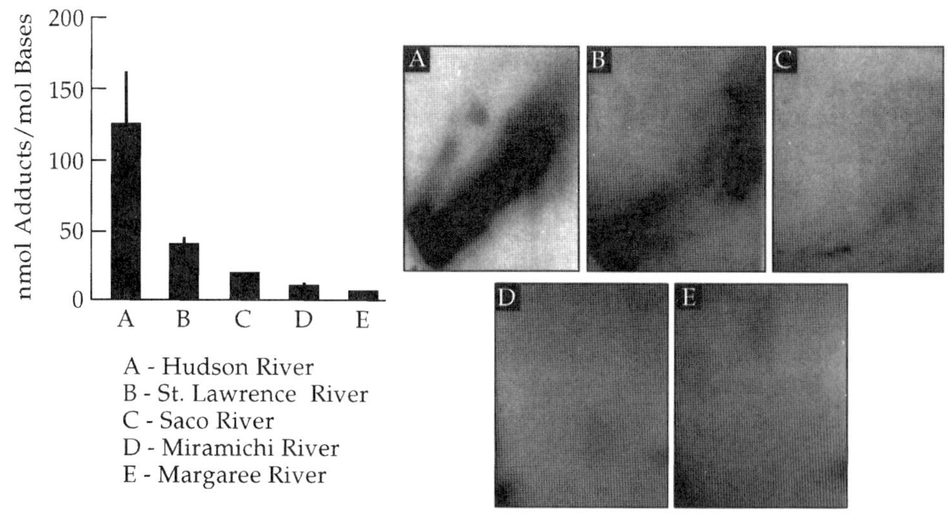


**FIG. 3.** Levels of hepatic DNA adducts in Atlantic tomcod from five rivers (Hudson, St. Lawrence, Saco, Miramichi, and Margaree) along the Atlantic coast of North America. Levels of DNA adducts were detected by the nuclease P1 version of the 32P-postlabeling assay.

mouse fibroblasts in vitro (80). Six of nine tumor DNAs proved positive, whereas DNAs from normal liver tissues failed to elicit foci. The anchorage independence of these transformed cells was confirmed and their tumorigenicity was demonstrated in nude mouse tumor assays. Furthermore, in Southern blot analysis, DNAs isolated from these nude mouse tumor DNAs exhibited an exogenous tomcod K-*ras* oncogene. An activated K-*ras* oncogene was also reported in winter flounder from a site in Boston Harbor highly polluted with PAHs (81). Polymerase chain reaction (PCR) analysis of a panel of DNAs from the winter flounder hepatic lesions revealed mutations at the 12th codon of K-*ras*, a site consistently mutated in tumor DNAs from rodents treated with chemical carcinogens and in human tumor DNAs. In contrast, PCR analysis of Hudson River tomcod liver and tumor DNAs revealed a high frequency of mutations in the 16th codon of K-*ras*; these mutations resulted in the substitutions of glycine and glutamic acids for the normal lysine residue (82). These results in two species of feral fish demonstrate that environmental exposures to xenobiotics can elicit mutations at the same carcinogenically relevant loci, and sometimes, although not always, at the same mutational hot spots, as observed in mammals.

Controlled laboratory experiments were conducted with tomcod from the Hudson River and the cleaner Miramichi River, New Brunswick, to determine threshold values for induction of CYP1A1 mRNA and to evaluate the dose-responsiveness of gene expression to treatment with 3,3′,4,4′-tetrachlorobiphenyl (TCB), TCDD, and two nonhalogenated aromatic hydrocarbons: B[*a*]P and β-naphthoflavone (β-NF) (83). Not surprisingly, CYP1A1 mRNA was induced at low, environmentally relevant, exposure concentrations of all four chemicals in tomcod from the Miramichi River, and levels of gene expression were dose-responsive. In contrast, only the two nonhalogenated compounds (B[*a*]P and β-NF) induced CYP1A1 mRNA expression in tomcod from the Hudson River (74,83). These results suggested that prior exposure history of Hudson River tomcod may inhibit further gene induction and that separate molecular pathways mediate CYP1A1 transcription in tomcod for nonhalogenated PAH compounds versus halogenated aromatic compounds such as TCB or TCDD.

In mammals, CYP1A1 transcription is mediated by activation of the aromatic hydrocarbon receptor (AhR) pathway. A battery of additional genes, several of which are important in the processing of xenobiotics, have been identified, whose transcription is also mediated by the AhR pathway (84). In fact, it is believed that most, if not all, toxic consequences resulting from exposure to aromatic hydrocarbon compounds are mediated by the AhR pathway. Briefly, xenobiotics such as TCDD enter the cell and bind to AhR in the cytoplasm, are translocated to the nucleus where heterodimerization with a second protein (aromatic receptor nuclear translocator, ARNT) and perhaps other proteins occurs, and the AhR complex then binds to enhancer elements within the regulatory region of CYP1A1 and a host of other genes in the AhR battery and thereby activate their transcription. Studies have identified AhR in liver tissue in several taxa of bony and elamobranch fish, but not in more primitive jawless fish (85). It is possible that inhibition of CYP1A1 transcription in tomcod from the Hudson River maps exclusively to the CYP1A1 locus; however, it is more likely that inhibition results from downregulation of the AhR pathway through either genetic or epigenetic mechanisms.

Enhancer elements [dioxin responsive elements (DREs)] whose core sequence was identical to those in mammals were characterized in the 5′ regulatory region of CYP1A1 in tomcod (86). Levels of inducible protein binding (presumably AhR complex) to the DREs were compared between tomcod from resistant (Hudson) and nonresistant (Miramichi) populations to determine if noninducibility of CYP1A1 was due to variation in expression or structure of AhR (87). Differences in levels of protein binding to DREs were observed between tomcod from the Hudson and the Miramichi rivers. Levels of AhR complex binding were significantly lower in tomcod from the Hudson River treated with TCB, compared with similarly treated tomcod from the Miramichi River. However, levels of protein binding to DREs were very similar in B[*a*]P-treated tomcod from the two rivers. In total, these results suggest that inhibition of CYP1A1 transcription probably represents downregulation of AhR, implications of which extend to a cascade of biological responses mediated by this pathway. Additionally, DNA analysis of AhR structure in tomcod from the Hudson and other rivers (87) has indicated high levels of variability in the 3 end of AhR cDNA, polymorphisms that can possibly influence levels of gene expression. It can be envisioned that AhR downregulation can serve to attenuate the DNA damaging effects of CYP1A1 activities, cancer-promoting activities of slowly metabolized dioxins and PCBs, or perhaps other toxicologic consequences of exposure.

Initial evidence suggests that downregulation of AhR may be a common occurrence in Atlantic coast estuarine fish from contaminated locales. Recently, inhibition of CYP1A1 transcription was also observed in a second species of fish, mummichog, from several highly contaminated Atlantic coast sites, including New Bedford Harbor, Massachusetts (PCBs) (88); Newark Bay, New Jersey (PCBs, dioxins, and furans) (89); and the Elizabeth River, Virginia (PAHs) (90). Interestingly, resistance to TCDD and creosote-induced lethality also was found in the Newark Bay and the Elizabeth River mummichog populations. Resistance to neoplasia and associated early mortality may also be occurring in the Hudson River tomcod population. Recent observations (1995–1996) suggest that the prevalence of hepatic tumors has significantly decreased and the age structure of the Hudson

River population has expanded (91). Heritability of inhibition of CYP1A1 induction and resistance to overt lethality has been demonstrated in the offspring of controlled laboratory crosses of mummichog from the resistant populations in Newark Bay (92) and the Elizabeth River (93), suggesting that resistance in these populations probably results from genetic adaptations.

However, there may be a cost associated with AhR downregulation–mediated resistance. Although an endogenous ligand for AhR has yet to be identified, untreated AhR-defective murine hepatoma cells exhibited altered morphology, decreased albumin synthesis, and a prolonged doubling time compared with wild-type mouse hepatoma cells (94). Similarly, an AhR-deficient mouse line showed decreased accumulation of lymphocytes in the spleen and lymph nodes and impaired liver development. Livers were reduced in size by 50% and exhibited bile duct fibrosis (95). Thus, it can be envisioned that downregulation of AhR function in natural populations may be associated with costs resulting in adverse impacts on higher level biologic processes in the absence of xenobiotics.

## PCBs AND STRIPED BASS

The Hudson River contains the greatest quantity of PCBs in the United States. The major source of this contamination was two General Electric capacitator production facilities located along the nontidal Hudson River north of the Federal Dam at Troy. It has been estimated that about 75,000 tons of PCBs were used at these plants, of which at least 500 tons accumulated in the proximal river (8). Roughly 50% to 60% of this was immobilized at dump sites from dredging that occurred between 1978 and 1980. However, due to removal of a flood-damaged dam directly below the discharge sites and periodic spring flooding events, some of the most highly contaminated sediments were washed downstream as far as New York City. It has been estimated that up to 75% of the PCBs in the lower river originate from sites upriver of Troy.

The Hudson River supports one of the two large, migratory striped bass populations of the Atlantic coast (the other occurring in the Chesapeake Bay). Striped bass was a primary commercial species within the Hudson River until commercial harvests were banned in 1976 because of PCB contamination of their flesh (96); this fishery remains closed. The Long Island, New York, commercial fishery for striped bass was terminated in 1985 for the same reasons; however, later it was reopened along the eastern portion of Long Island where PCB testing showed lower average concentrations in striped bass flesh. PCB levels of Hudson River striped bass have received intense interest because of the discomfiture experienced by the commercial fishermen who lost significant income as a result of the harvest bans, because of concerns about recreational fishermen who may ignore health advisories concerning consumption of striped bass, and because PCB body burdens of these fish provide a data-rich currency with which to model the movement of PCBs within the system and its biota.

Due to harvest restrictions to help protect the depleted Chesapeake Bay stock of striped bass and because of reduced commercial harvest, the abundance of the Hudson River stock increased dramatically since 1976. In response to this increase, the recreational fishery for striped bass within the Hudson River also intensified, although it remains primarily a catch-and-release effort. Health advisories have been in place in both New York and New Jersey waters of the Hudson River since 1976. Presently, the public is advised to eat no more than half a pound per week of any fish from the Hudson estuary, and none from the area of the PCB hot spots, between Hudson Falls and the Federal Dam at Troy, New York.

The movements of striped bass between the heavily PCB-contaminated Hudson River and the much less contaminated coastal waters is of major importance in understanding patterns and rates of PCB uptake and depuration and of human health risks. Striped bass of the Hudson River are facultatively anadromous, meaning that many, but not all, individual fish migrate to ocean waters before returning to the Hudson to spawn (97). Striped bass that leave the Hudson River may range as far north as the Bay of Fundy and south to Cape Hatteras, North Carolina (98). Young-of-the-year striped bass are largely restricted to the estuary, but usage of coastal waters increases with age and size (97,98). However, a small portion of the population appears to remain residential within the river (97). Thus, the variable life history modes within the Hudson River's striped bass population provides the opportunity for PCB uptake versus depuration scenarios.

Thomann et al. (99) have modeled the fate and accumulation of PCBs in striped bass of the Hudson River estuary. The model includes a large number of striped bass age classes, food web interactions, and movements in and out of the Hudson estuary. PCB homologues were used in the model because the authors believed that use of total PCBs could obscure fundamental mechanisms, whereas a congener-based model (209 possible congeners) would be overly complex. Thomann et al. predicted future striped bass PCB concentrations under two scenarios: (a) no action, where trends in upstream and downstream loading were assumed to continue; and (b) an instantaneous elimination of the upstream load applied in 1987 to simulate the effect of possible upstream dredging of hot spots. Under the no-action alternative, 50% of the striped bass would be expected to be below 2 μg/g (net weight) (the federal level for human consumption) in about 5 years (1992), and another 12 years (2004) would be required for 95% of the fish to be below 2 μg/g. However, the times until these benchmarks were achieved under the alternative scenario were not significantly different from the no action-alternative. This result points to the importance of controlling downstream PCB sources, such as nonpoint runoff and atmospheric inputs.

By 1994, PCB levels in striped bass (100) were showing a continuum from unsafe levels near Albany (mean = 6.41 ppm), to just below 2 ppm in the Tappan Zee region (~1.9 ppm), to lower levels along the south shore of Long Island (~1.2 ppm). The lower PCB levels found in striped bass outside of the Hudson River is partly due to inclusion of individuals from more southerly stocks, which have a lower probability of PCB concentrations above 2 ppm than do Hudson River specimens (96). Although dredging of the PCB hot spots still has not occurred, a final decision by the U.S. Environmental Protection Agency (EPA) is expected by 1998. The analysis by Thomann et al. (99) notwithstanding, interest in the dredging alternative has increased because of new PCB inputs upriver. In 1991, sudden increases to extremely high levels of PCBs concentrations in the water column (>4,000 ng/L) were found in the vicinity of the former General Electric site at Ft. Edward; high concentrations (~500 ng/L) in the water column continued through 1992 (100).

Despite concerns about the effects on human health of consuming PCB-contaminated Hudson River striped bass, there is no convincing evidence to date of a detrimental effect of PCBs on striped bass at the population level. The Hudson River striped bass population is estimated to have grown at about 8% per year since the mid-1970s (98). Monosson et al. (101) did use a close relative of striped bass, the white perch (*Morone americana*), as a surrogate for the species in laboratory testing of the effects of a highly toxic coplanar PCB congener, 3,3′,4,4-tetrachlorobiphenyl (TCB). TCB was injected intraperitoneally at one of three doses (0.2, 1.0, and 5.0 mg/kg of body weight). TCB delayed or suppressed ovarian growth and oocyte growth, resulted in fewer mature fish in the group receiving the highest TCB dose, and decreased larval survival. These results suggest that high PCB body burdens have the potential to cause reproductive impairment in moronids (white perch and striped bass).

PCB research on the Hudson River has focused on the fate, transport, and contamination of its fishes. Most studies of the effects of PCBs on human health have been conducted on the Great Lakes basin. Evidence suggests that consumption of contaminated finfish species has resulted in elevated serum levels of PCBs in families that consume particularly large amounts of sport fish from the Great Lakes. Furthermore, correlations were observed between maternal serum and umbilical cord serum concentrations of PCBs, suggesting the transplacental transfer of maternal PCBs. Evidence suggests that in utero or postpartum exposure via maternal milk is responsible in infants for lower birth weight, reduced gestational age, smaller head circumference, and adverse effects on cognitive, motor, and development behavior (102).

Human health risks from eating contaminated striped bass remain a major concern despite the health advisories. Recreational fishing, particularly among minority groups, often occurs partly for subsistence; also, fish may be distributed to nonfishermen who have less knowledge of the health risks posed. Many of these anglers either are not aware of health advisories or choose to ignore them (103). For example, in a survey conducted in the New Jersey portion of New York Harbor, Belton et al. (104) found that approximately 25% of anglers interviewed knew of official health warnings but ate their catch anyway, and another 25% knew of the warnings, ate their catch, and claimed it was safe to do so.

## CONCLUSIONS

Hudson River sediments have some of the highest concentrations of metal and aromatic hydrocarbon contaminants within any aquatic system in the world. Bioaccumulation of these xenobiotics is evident in a variety of taxa. Biologic responses, including pathologic manifestations of exposure at the molecular, cellular, and organismic levels, have been observed in populations from highly contaminated sites. Yet, there is little evidence of diminishment of population abundances or species diversity due to exposure to these chemicals. In fact, for many of its valuable resource finfish species, the Hudson River supports the largest and most viable populations along the North American Atlantic coast. Resistance to xenobiotic exposure apparently is occurring in some populations from highly impacted Hudson River sites. DNA damage is extensive in Hudson River populations resulting in somatic cell mutations, and population-specific germ line polymorphisms suggest the intergenerational transmission of variant, and perhaps resistant, genotypes. Whereas this strategy assists the survival of individuals and populations, it is associated with costs that probably diminish population performance and may eventually have adverse consequences on the community level. Additionally, bioassays using resistant organisms from the Hudson River or other contaminated sites may provide misleading false-negative results because of increased tolerance to xenobiotics in these impacted populations.

The major effects of the contamination of the Hudson River on its surrounding human population are twofold. First is the elimination or diminution of many of its resource species as commercially available food sources. Of its many fishes, only American shad *Alosa sapidissima* can legally be harvested for sale; the only other remaining commercial fishery is for blue claw crab. Recreational fisherman still are permitted under present regulations to keep a portion of their catch, but the incentive to do so and to enjoy the river is tempered by devitalizing health advisories on their consumption.

Nonetheless, selected human groups do eat fish and shellfish from the Hudson River. The second major consequence of contamination of the Hudson River on humans is its detrimental effect on health. There has been little study of the consequences of the Hudson system's toxic legacy on residents of the region. However, based on research from other contaminated systems, it is reasonable to assume that high concentrations of cadmium, mercury and other heavy metals, dioxins, PAHs, PCBs, and other xenobiotics have diminished human health in the Hudson River region.

## REFERENCES


1. Hahn ME, Poland A, Glover E, Stegeman JJ. Photoaffinity labeling of the Ah receptor: phylogenetic survey of diverse vertebrate and invertebrate species. *Arch Biochem Biophys* 1994;310:218–228.
2. Brown DJ, Clarke GC, Van Beneden RJ. Halogenated aromatic hydrocarbon-binding proteins identified in several invertebrate marine species. *Aquat Toxicol* 1997;37:71–78.
3. Boyle RH. *The Hudson River:* a natural and unnatural history. New York: Norton, 1969.
4. Mitchell, J. *The bottom of the harbor.* Boston: Little, Brown, 1959.
5. Moran MA, Limburg KE. The Hudson River ecosystem. In: Limburg KE, Moran MA, McDowell WH, eds. *The Hudson River Ecosystem.* New York: Springer-Verlag, 1986;6–39.
6. Smith CL, Lake TR. Documentation of the Hudson River fish fauna. *American Museum Novitates* 1990;2981:1–17.
7. McKenzie Jr CL, History of the fisheries of Raritan Bay, New York and New Jersey. *Mar Fish Rev* 1990;52:1–45.
8. Tarr JA, Ayres RU. The Hudson-Raritan basin. In: Turner BL II, Clark WC, Kates RW, Richards JF, Mathews JT, Meyer WB, eds. *The earth as transformed by human action.* Cambridge: Cambridge University Press, 1990;623–639.
9. Suszkowski DJ. Conditions in New York/New Jersey Harbor Estuary. In: *Proceedings of cleaning up our coastal waters:* an unfinished agenda. Riverdale, NY: Manhattan College, 1990;105–131.
10. Brosnan TM, O'Shea ML. Long-term improvements in water quality due to sewage abatement in the lower Hudson River. *Estuaries* 1996; 19:890–900.
11. Long ER, Morgan LG. *The potential for biological effects of sediment-sorbed contaminants tested in the National Status and Trends Program.* National Oceanic and Atmospheric Administration Technical Memorandum NOS OMA 52. Seattle, WA: National Oceanic and Atmospheric Administration, 1990.
12. Knutson AB, Klerks PL, Levinton JS. The fate of metal contaminated sediments in Foundry Cove, New York. *Environ Pollut* 1987;45: 291–304.
13. Klerks PL, Levinton JS. Effects of heavy metals in a polluted aquatic ecosystem. In: Levin SA, Harwell MA, Kelly JR, Kimball KD, eds. *Ecotoxicology:* problems and approaches. New York: Springer-Verlag, 1989;41–67.
14. Ankley GT, Phipps GL, Leonard EN, et al. Acid-volatile sulfide as a factor mediating cadmium and nickel bioavailability in contaminated sediments. *Environ Toxicol Chem* 1991;10:1299–1307.
15. Hazen RE. *Cadmium in an aquatic ecosystem.* Ph.D. thesis. New York: New York University, 1981.
16. Hazen RE, Kneip TJ. Biogeochemical cycling of cadmium in a marsh ecosystem. In: Nriagu JO, ed. *Cadmium in the environment.* New York: Wiley, 1980;399–424.
17. Kneip TJ, Hazen RE. Deposit and mobility of cadmium in a marsh-cove ecosystem and the relation to cadmium concentration in biota. *Environ Health Perspect* 1979;28:67–73.
18. Wiedow MA. *Distribution and binding of cadmium in the blue crab (Callinectes sapidus): implications on human health.* Ph.D. thesis. New York: New York University, 1981.
19. Klerks P. *Adaptation to metals in benthic macrofauna.* Ph.D. thesis. Stony Brook, NY: State University of New York, 1987.
20. Klerks PL, Levinton JS. Rapid evolution of metal resistance in a benthic oligochaete inhabiting a metal-polluted site. *Biol Bull* 1989;176: 135–141.
21. Suatoni L, Levinton J. Personal communication, 1997.
22. Beppu M, Arima K. Decreased permeability as the mechanism of arsenite resistance in *Pseudomonas pseudomallei. J Bacteriol* 1964; 88:151–157.
23. Bryan GW, Hummerstone LG. Adaptation of the polychaete *Nereis diversicolor* to estuarine sediments containing high concentrations of zinc and cadmium. *J Mar Biol Assoc UK* 1973;53:839–857.
24. Kurelec B. The multixenobiotic resistance mechanism in aquatic organisms. *Crit Rev Toxicol* 1992;22:23–43.
25. Klerks PL, Bartholomew PR. Cadmium accumulation and detoxification in a Cd-resistant population of the oligochaete *Limnodrilus hoffmeisteri. Aquat Toxicol* 1991; 19:97–112.
26. Roesijadi G, Fellingham GW. Influence of Cu, Cd, and Zn preexposure on Hg toxicity in the mussel *Mytilus edulis. Can J Fish Aquat Sci* 1987;44:680–684.
27. Thiele DJ, Walling JJ, Hamer DH. Mammalian metallothionein is functional in yeast. *Science* 1986;231:854–856.
28. George SG, Hodgson PA, Tyler P, Todd K. Inducibility of metallothionein mRNA expression and cadmium tolerance in larvae of a marine teleost, the turbot (*Scopthalmus maximus*). *Fundam Appl Toxicol* 1996;33:91–99.
29. Maroni G, Wise J, Young JE, Otto E. Metallothionein gene duplications and metal tolerance in natural populations of *Drosophila melanogaster. Genetics* 1987;117:739–744.
30. Wallace WG, Lopez GR. Relationship between subcellular cadmium distribution in prey and cadmum trophic transfer to a predator. *Estuaries* 1996;19:923–930.
31. Squibb KS, O'Connor JM, Kneip TJ. New *York/New Jersey Harbor estuary program module 3.1:* Toxics characterization report. New York: Institute of Environmental Medicine, NYU Medical Center, 1991:188.
32. Progress report: *A summary of selected data on chemical contaminants in sediments collected during 1984, 1985, 1986, and 1987.* National Status and Trends Program for Marine Environmental Quality. NOAA Technical Memorandum NOS OMA 44. Rockville, MD: National Oceanic and Atmospheric Administration 1980.
33. O'Keefe P, Hilker D, Meyer C, et al. Tetrachlorodibenzo-*p*-dioxins and tetrachlorodibenzofurans in Atlantic coast striped bass and in selected Hudson River fish, waterfowl and sediments. *Chemosphere* 1984;13: 849–860.
34. Weis JS, Weis P. Tolerance and stress in a polluted environment. *Bioscience* 1989;39:89–95.
35. Vogelbein WK, Fournie JW, Van Veld PA, Huggett RJ. Hepatic neoplasms in the mummichog *Fundulus heteroclitus* from a creosote-contaminated site. *Cancer Res* 1990;50:5978–5986.
36. Gonzalez-Villasenor LI, Powers DA. Mitochondrial-DNA restriction-site polymorphisms in the teleost *Fundulus heteroclitus* support secondary intergradation. *Evolution* 1990;44:27–37.
37. Khan AT, Weis JS. Bioaccumulation of heavy metals in two populations of mummichog (*Fundulus heteroclitus*). *Bull Environ Contam Toxicol* 1993;51:1–5.
38. Weis P, Weis JS. Methylmercury teratogenesis in the killifish, *Fundulus heteroclitus. Teratology* 1977;16:317–326.
39. Weis JS, Weis P. Effects of embryonic exposure to methylmercury on larval prey-capture ability in the mummichog, *Fundulus heteroclitus. Environ Toxicol Chem* 1995;14:153–156.
40. Weis JS, Weis P. Swimming performance and predator avoidance by mummichog (*Fundulus heteroclitus*) larvae after embryonic or larval exposure to methylmercury. *Can J Fish Aquat Sci* 1995;52: 2168–2173.
41. Khan AT, Weis JS. Effects of methylmercury on sperm and egg viability of two populations of killifish (*Fundulus heteroclitus*). *Arch Environ Contam Toxicol* 1987;16:499–505.
42. Perry DM, Weis JS, Weis P. Cytogenetic effects of methylmercury in embryos of the killifish, *Fundulus heteroclitus. Arch Environ Contam Toxicol* 1988;17:569–574.
43. Weis JS, Khan AA. Reduction in prey capture ability and condition of mummichogs from a polluted habitat. *Trans Am Fish Soc* 1991;120: 127–129.
44. Weis P. Metallothionein and mercury tolerance in the killifish, *Fundulus heteroclitus. Mar Environ Res* 1984;14:153–166.
45. Toppin SV, Heber M, Weis JS, Weis P. Changes in reproductive biology and life history of *Fundulus heteroclitus* in a polluted environment. In: Vernberg WB, Calabrese A, Thurberg FP, Vernberg FJ, eds. *Pollution physiology of estuarine organisms.* Columbia, SC: University of South Carolina Press, 1987;171–184.

46. Smith GM, Khan AT, Weis JS, Weis P. Behavior and brain chemistry correlates in mummichogs (*Fundulus heteroclitus*) from polluted and unpolluted environments. *Mar Environ Res* 1995;39:329–333.
47. Harshbarger JC, Clark JB. Epizootiology of neoplasms in bony fish of North America. *Sci Total Environ* 1990;94:1–32.
48. Hawkins WE, Walker WW, Overstreet RM. Carcinogenicity tests using aquarium fish. In: Rand GM, ed. *Fundamentals of aquatic toxicology:* effects, environmental fate, and risk assessment. Washington, DC: Taylor and Francis, 1995;421–446.
49. Miranda CL, Henderson MC, Williams DE, Buhler DR. In vitro metabolism of 7,12- dimethylbenz[a]anthracene by rainbow trout liver microsomes and trout P-450 isoforms. *Toxicol Appl Pharmacol* 1997; 142:123–132.
50. Stein J, Reichert W, Varanasi U. Molecular epizootiology: assessment of exposure to genotoxic compounds in teleosts. *Environ Health Perspect* 1994;102:19–23.
51. Maccubbin AE, Black JJ, Dunn BP. $^{32}$P-postlabeling detection of DNA adducts in fish from chemically contaminated waterways. *Sci Total Environ* 1990;94:89–104.
52. Malins DC, Ostrander GK, Haimanot R, Williams P. A novel DNA lesion in neoplastic livers of feral fish: 2,6-diamino-4-hydroxy-5-formamidopyrmidine. *Carcinogenesis* 1990;11:1045–1047.
53. Malins DC, Polissar NL, Garner MM, Gunselman SJ. Mutagenic DNA base modifications are correlated with lesions in nonneoplastic hepatic tissue of the English sole carcinogenesis model. *Cancer Res* 1996;56:5563–5565.
54. Malins DC, Gunselman SJ. Fourier-transform infrared spectroscopy and gas chromatography–mass spectrophometry reveal a remarkable degrees of structural damage in the DNA of wild fish exposed to toxic chemicals. *Proc Natl Acad Sci USA* 1994;91:13038–13401.
55. Fong AT, Dashwood RH, Cheng R, et al. Carcinogenicity, metabolism and Ki-ras proto-oncogene activation by 7,12-dimethylbenz[a]anthracene in rainbow trout embryos. *Carcinogenesis* 1993;14:629–635.
56. French BL, Reichert WL, Hom T, Nishimoto M, Sanborn HR, Stein JE. Accumulation and dose-response of hepatic DNA adducts in English sole (*Pleuronectes vetulus*) exposed to a gradient of contaminated sediments. *Aquat Toxicol* 1996;36:1–16.
57. Stein JE, Reichert WL, French B, Varanasi U. $^{32}$P-postlabeling analysis of DNA adduct formation and persistence in English sole (*Pleuronectes vetulus*) exposed to benzo[a]pyrene and 7H- dibenzo[c,g]carbazole. *Chem Biol Interact* 1993;88:55–69.
58. Bailey GS, Williams DE, Hendricks JD. Fish models for environmental carcinogenesis: the rainbow trout. *Environ Health Perspect* 1996; 104(suppl 1):5–21.
59. Schiewe MH, Weber DD, Myers MS, et al. Induction of foci of cellular alteration and other hepatic lesions in English sole (*Parophrys vetulus*) exposed to an extract of an urban marine sediment. *Can J Fish Aquat Sci* 1991;48:1750–1760.
60. Black JJ, Fox H, Black P, Bock F. Carcinogenic effects of river sediment extracts in fish and mice. In: Jolley RL, Bull RJ, Davis WP, Katz S, Roberts MH, Jacobs VA, eds. *Water chlorination:* chemistry, environmental impact, and health effects. New York: Plenum Press, 1985; 415–427.
61. Metcalfe CD, Cairns VW, Fitzsimons JD. Experimental induction of liver tumors in rainbow trout (*Salmo gairdneri*) by contaminated sediment from Hamilton Harbor, Ontario. *Can J Fish Aquat Sci* 1988;45: 2161–2167.
62. Balch GC, Metcalfe CD, Huestis SY. Identification of potential fish carcinogens in sediment from Hamilton Harbor, Ontario, Canada. *Environ Toxicol Chem* 1995;14:79–91.
63. Dawe CJ, Stanton MF, Schwartz FJ. Hepatic neoplasms in native bottom-feeding fish of Deep Creek Lake, Maryland. *Cancer Res* 1964; 24:1194–1201.
64. Johnson LL, Stehr CM, Olson OP, et al. Chemical contaminants and hepatic lesions in winter flounder (*Pleuronectes americanus*) from the northeast coast of the United States. *Environ Sci Technol* 1993;27: 2759–2771.
65. Myers MS, Stehr CM, Olson OP, et al. Relationships between toxicopathic hepatic lesions and exposure to chemical contaminants in English sole (*Pleuronectes vetulus*), starry flounder (*Platichthys stellatus*), and white croaker (*Genyonemus lineatus*) from selected marine sites on the Pacific coast, USA. *Environ Health Perspect* 1994;102: 200–215.
66. Baumann PC, Harshbarger JC. Decline in liver neoplasms in wild brown bullhead catfish after coking plant closes and environmental PAHs plummet. *Environ Health Perspect* 1995;103:168– 170.
67. Bigelow H, Schroeder W. Fishes of the Gulf of Maine. *US Fish Wildl Serv Fish Bull* 1953; 74:1– 577.
68. McLaren JB, Peck TH, Dey WP, Gardinier M. Biology of Atlantic tomcod in the Hudson River estuary. In: Barnthouse LW, Klauda RJ, Vaughan DS, Kendall RL, eds. Science, law, and Hudson River power plants. *Am Fish Soc Monogr* 1988;4:102–112.
69. Klauda RJ, Moos RE, Schmidt RE. Life history of Atlantic tomcod, *Microgadus tomcod*, in the Hudson River estuary, with emphasis on spatio-temporal distribution and movements. In: Smith CL, ed. *Fisheries research in the Hudson River.* Albany, NY: State University of New York Press, 1988;219–251.
70. Cormier SM, Racine RN, Smith CE, Dey WP, Peck TH. Hepatocelluar carcinoma and fatty infiltration in the Atlantic tomcod, *Microgadus tomcod* (Walbaum). *J Fish Dis* 1989;12:105–116.
71. Dey WP, Peck TH, Smith CE, Kreamer G-L. Epizoology of hepatic neoplasia in Atlantic tomcod (*Microgadus tomcod*) from the Hudson River estuary. *Can J Fish Aquat Sci* 1993;50:1897–1907.
72. Cormier SM, Racine RN. Histopathology of Atlantic tomcod: a possible monitor of xenobiotics in northeast tidal rivers and estuaries. In: McCarthy JF, Shugart LR, eds. *Biomarkers of environmental contamination.* Boca Raton, FL: 1990;59–71.
73. Courtenay S. Personal communication, 1996.
74. Wirgin II, Kreamer G-L, Grunwald C, Squibb K, Garte SJ. Effects of prior exposure history on cytochrome P-4501A mRNA induction by PCB congener 77 in Atlantic tomcod. *Mar Environ Res* 1992;34: 103–108.
75. Wirgin II, Grunwald C, Courtenay S, Kreamer G-L, Reichert WL, Stein JE. A biomarker approach to assessing xenobiotic exposure in Atlantic tomcod from the North American Atlantic coast. *Environ Health Perspect* 1994;102:764–770.
76. Rappe C, Bergqvist P-A, Kjeller L-O, et al. Levels and patterns of PCDD and PCDF contamination in fish, crabs, and lobsters from Newark Bay and the New York Bight. *Chemosphere* 1991;22:239–266.
77. Stein J, Wirgin I. Unpublished data.
78. Wirgin I, Kreamer G-L, Garte SJ. Genetic polymorphism of cytochrome P-4501A in cancer-prone Hudson River tomcod. *Aquat Toxicol* 1991;19:205–214.
79. Roy NK, Kreamer G-L, Konkle B, Grunwald C, Wirgin I. Characterization and prevalence of a polymorphism in the 3 untranslated region of cytochrome P-4501A1 in cancer-prone Atlantic tomcod. *Arch Biochem Biophys* 1995;322:204–213.
80. Wirgin I, Currie D, Garte SJ. Activation of the K-*ras* oncogene in liver tumors of Hudson River tomcod. *Carcinogenesis* 1989;10:2311–2315.
81. McMahon G, Huber LJ, Moore MJ, Stegeman JJ. Mutation in c-Ki-ras oncogenes in diseased livers of winter flounder from Boston Harbor. *Proc Natl Acad Sci USA* 1990;87:841.
82. Roy NK, Wirgin I. Unpublished data.
83. Courtenay SC, Grunwald CM, Kreamer G-L, Fairchild WL, Arsenault J, Wirgin I. A comparison of the dose and time response of cytochrome P-4501A1 mRNA induction in chemically treated Atlantic tomcod from two populations. *Aquat Toxicol* submitted.
84. Sutter TR, Greenlee WF. Classification of members of the Ah gene battery. *Chemosphere* 1992;25:223–226.
85. Hahn ME, Stegeman JJ. Phylogenetic distribution of the Ah receptor in non-mammalian species: implications for dioxin toxicity and Ah receptor evolution. *Chemosphere* 1992;25:931–937.
86. Roy NK, Konkle B, Wirgin I. Characterization of *CYP1A1* gene regulatory elements in cancer- prone Atlantic tomcod. *Pharmacogenetics* 1996;6:273–277.
87. Roy NK, Wirgin I. Characterization and expression of the aromatic hydrocarbon receptor gene and its expression in Atlantic tomcod. *Arch Biochem Biophys* 1997;344:373–386.
88. Nacci D, Coiro, L, Kuhn-Hines A, Munns Jr WR. Resistance to chemical stressors in embryo- larval fish from a marine Superfund site. *SETAC* 1996;262.
89. Prince R, Cooper KR. Comparisons of the effects of 2,3,7,8-tetrachlorodibenzo-p-dioxin on chemically impacted and non-impacted subpopulations of *Fundulus heteroclitus*. II. Metabolic considerations. *Environ Toxicol Chem* 1995;14:589–596.
90. Van Veld PA, Westbrook DJ. Evidence for depression of cytochrome P-4501A in a population of chemically resistant mummichog (*Fundulus heteroclitus*). *Environ Sci* 1995;3:221–234.

91. Young J. Personal Communication, 1997.
92. Cooper KR. Chemical impacts on *Fundulus heteroclitus* from Newark Bay compared to fish from Tuckerton, New Jersey. *SETAC* 1996;63.
93. Vogelbein WK, Williams CA, Van Veld PA, Unger MA. Acute toxicity resistance in a fish population with a high prevalence of cancer. *SETAC* 1996;64.
94. Ma Q, Whitlock JP. The aromatic hydrocarbon receptor modulates the Hepa 1c1c7 cell cycle and differentiated state independently of dioxin. *Mol Cell Biol* 1996;16:2144–2150.
95. Fernandez-Salguero P, Pineau T, Hilbert DM, et al. Immune system impairment and hepatic fibrosis in mice lacking the dioxin-binding Ah receptor. *Science* 1995;268:722–726.
96. Fabrizio MC, Sloan RJ, O'Brien JF. Striped bass stocks and concentrations of polychlorinated biphenyls. *Trans Am Fish Soc* 1991;120: 541–551.
97. Secor DH, Piccoli PM. Age- and sex-dependent migrations of striped bass in the Hudson River as determined by chemical microanalysis of otoliths. *Estuaries* 1996;19:778–793.
98. Waldman JR, Dunning DJ, Ross QE, Mattson MT, Range dynamics of Hudson River striped bass along the Atlantic Coast. *Trans Am Fish Soc* 1990;119:910–919.
99. Thomann RV, Mueller JA, Winfield RP, Huang C-R. Model of fate and accumulation of PCB homologues in the Hudson estuary. *J Environ Engineer* 1991;117:161–178.
100. Sloan RB, Young B, Hattala K. PCB paradigms for striped bass in New York State. *New York State Department of Environmental Conservation Technical Report* 1995;95-1.
101. Monosson E, Fleming WJ, Sullivan CV. Effects of the planar PCB 3,3′,4,4′-tetrachlorobiphenyl (TCB) on ovarian development, plasma levels of sex steroid hormones and vitellogenin, and progeny survival in the white perch (*Morone americana*). *Aquat Toxicol* 1994;29:1–19.
102. Jacobson JL, Jacobson SW. Intellectual impairment in children exposed to polychlorinated biphenyls in utero. *N Engl J Med* 1996;335:783–789.
103. Barclay B. *Hudson River angler survey.* Poughkeepsie, NY: Hudson River Sloop Clearwater, 1993.
104. Belton T, Roundy R, Weinstein N. Urban fishermen: managing the risks of toxic exposure. *Environment* 1986;28:18–20,30–37.
105. Murchelano RA, Wolke RE. Epizootic carcinoma in the winter flounder, *Pseudopleuronectes americanus*. *Science* 1985;228:587–589.
106. Gardner GR, Pruell RJ, Folmar LC. A comparison of both neoplastic and non-neoplastic disorders in winter flounder (*Pseudopleuronectes americanus*) from eight areas in New England. *Mar Environ Res* 1989:28:393–397.
107. Malins DC, McCain BB, Landahl JT, et al. Neoplastic and other diseases in fish in relation to toxic chemicals: an overview. *Aquat Toxicol* 1988;11:43–67.
108. Baumann PC, Smith WS, Parland WK. Tumor frequencies and contaminant concentrations in brown bullheads from an industrialized river and a recreational lake. *Trans Am Fish Soc* 1987;116:79–86.
109. Hayes MA, Smith IR, Rushmore TH, et al. Pathogenesis of skin and liver neoplasms in white suckers from industrially polluted areas in Lake Ontario. *Sci Total Environ* 1990;94:105–123.

*Environmental and Occupational Medicine, Third Edition,* edited by William N. Rom.
Lippincott–Raven Publishers, Philadelphia © 1998.

CHAPTER 119

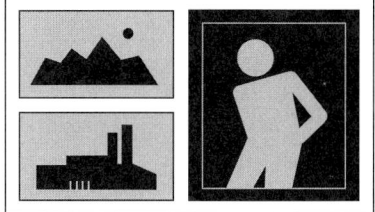

# Fate and Bioaccumulation of PCBs in Aquatic Environments

Kevin J. Farley and Robert V. Thomann

Polychlorinated biphenyls (PCBs) represent a family of compounds produced commercially by the direct chlorination of biphenyl (1). In this process, chlorines can be placed at any or all of the ten available sites on the biphenyl structure (e.g., as shown in Fig. 1), and a total of 209 PCB congeners are theoretically possible. Until its production ban in 1977, PCBs were manufactured in the United States by the Monsanto Chemical Company and marketed under the trade name Aroclor. Aroclors typically contained only about half of the 209 possible PCB congeners (due to steric hinderances in their commercial synthesis) and were defined by their degree of chlorination. For example, Aroclors 1221, 1232, 1242, 1248, 1254, and 1260 contained 21%, 32%, 42%, 48%, 54%, and 60% chlorine by weight. Aroclor 1016 was a redistilled version of Aroclor 1242, with a chlorine content of 41% (2). Aroclors were used widely as heat transformer fluids, dielectric fluids for transformers and capacitors, hydraulics lubricants, solvent extenders, plasticizers, flame retardants, and in carbonless copy paper (2).

Through their manufacture and use, PCBs have been released into aquatic environments and are a concern at a number of sites including the Hudson River in New York (3–11), New Bedford Harbor in Massachusetts (12,13), the Fox River and Green Bay in Wisconsin (14,15), and Lake Hartwell in South Carolina (16), as well as in the Great Lakes (17–20). Because of their hydrophobic nature and moderate to low vapor pressures, PCBs tend to accumulate in sediments, and, to a lesser extent, in water and air phases. Low concentrations of PCBs present in the water and air phases typically do not present a significant human health risk through water ingestion or inhalation. However, the hydrophobic nature of PCBs causes them to bioaccumulate in aquatic food chains where they may pose a serious risk to human health through the consumption of contaminated seafood.

In PCB site evaluations, mathematical models have been used as an integral part of the overall analysis to examine present pathways of exposure, to project future exposure levels, and to determine the effectiveness of various management alternatives (such as source reduction, dredging, and capping). The general modeling approach used in determining the temporal and spatial

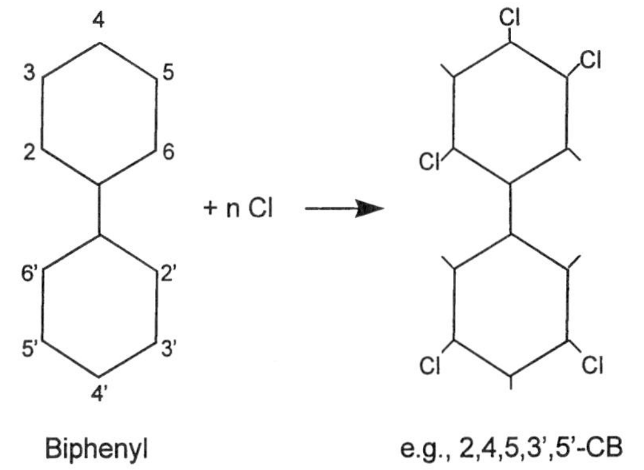


**FIG. 1.** Synthesis of PCBs (e.g., 2,4,5,3′,5′-pentachlorobiphenyl) by the direct chlorination of biphenyl.

K. J. Farley and R. V. Thomann: Department of Environmental Engineering, Manhattan College, Riverdale, New York 10471.

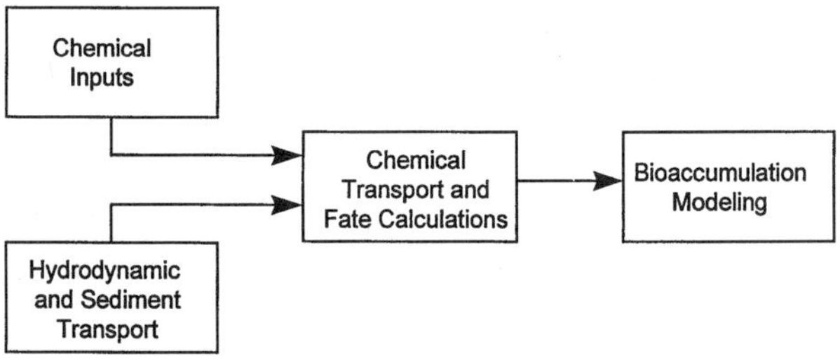


**FIG. 2.** General modeling framework.

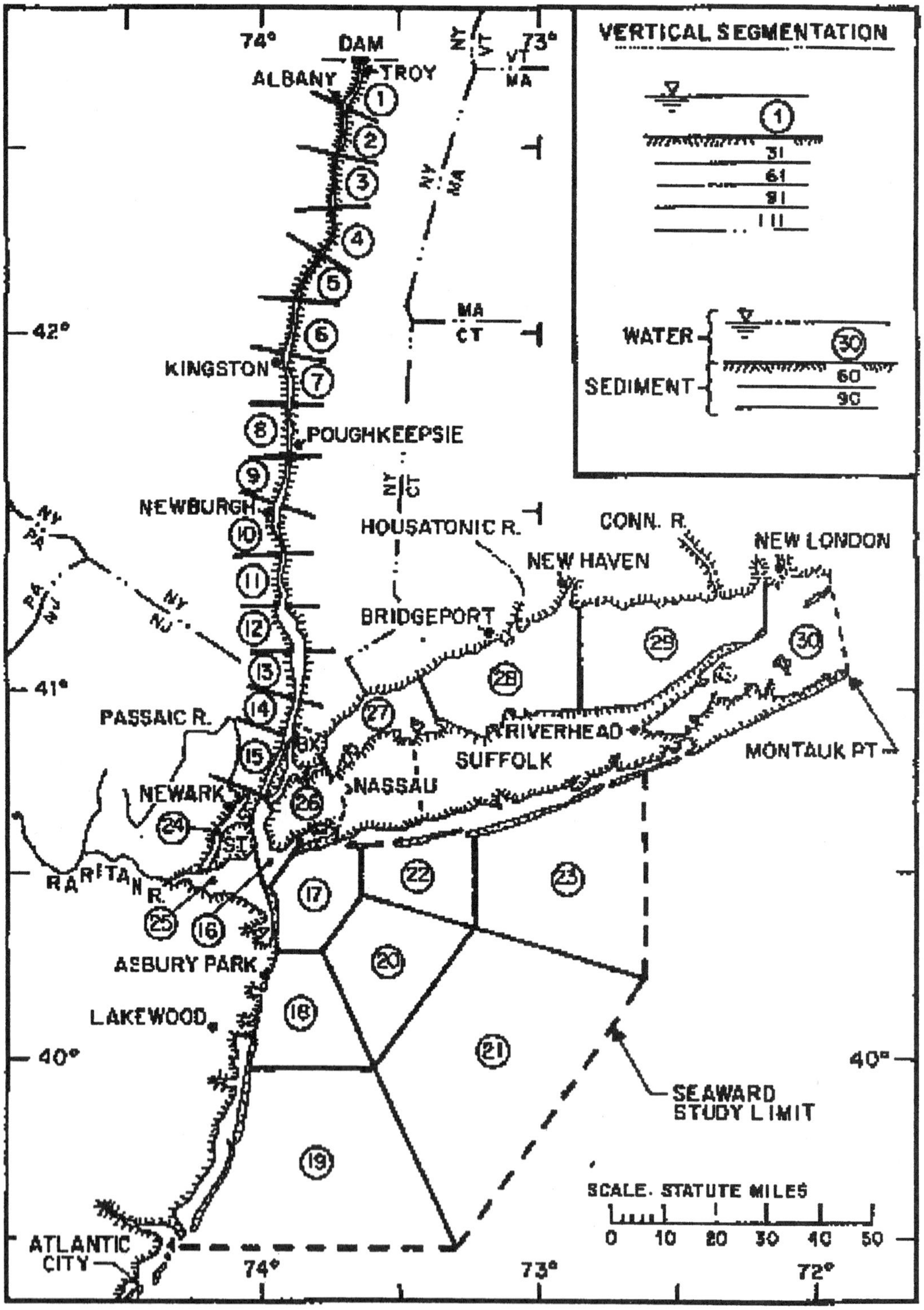


**FIG. 3.** Hudson River Estuary (with finite difference segmentation for the PCB model shown).

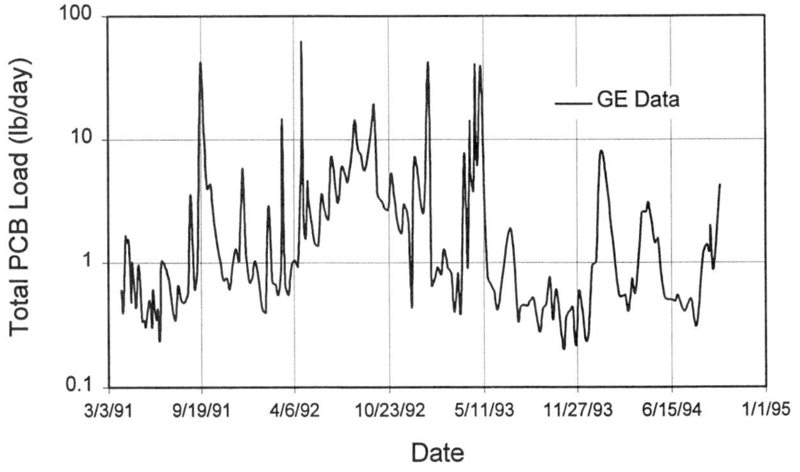


**FIG. 4.** Total PCB load from the Upper Hudson at Fort Edwards (river mile 194.4). (Data from General Electric.)

distributions of PCBs in water, sediments, and fish is based on mass conservation principles (21). As shown in Fig. 2, the modeling framework consists of four distinct parts: specification of chemical inputs, hydrodynamic and sediment transport, chemical transport and fate calculations, and bioaccumulation modeling. After a brief background on PCB contamination in the Hudson River Estuary, these modeling aspects are discussed with specific application to PCBs in the Hudson River Estuary.

## BACKGROUND

The Hudson River Estuary (and the associated tidal portion of the Hudson River) is located in the eastern portion of New York State and extends from Federal Dam at Troy (river mile 157) to the Battery in New York City (river mile 0) (Fig. 3). At Federal Dam, the estuary is fed by waters from the Upper Hudson and Mohawk Rivers. From approximately 1947 to 1977, General Electric (GE) facilities along the Upper Hudson at Hudson Falls (river mile 197) and nearby Fort Edwards (river mile 195) used PCBs in the manufacturing of electrical capacitors. According to the U.S. Environmental Protection Agency (EPA) (9), 0.2 to 1.3 million pounds of PCBs were discharged from the GE facilities into the Upper Hudson River between 1957 and 1975. Downstream migration of PCBs over the 40-mile stretch between Hudson Falls and Federal Dam was greatly enhanced in 1973 with the removal of the Fort Edwards Dam (river mile 195) and subsequent high water discharges in April 1974 and April 1976 (8). In 1976, the New York State Department of Environmental Conservation (NYDEC) imposed a ban on fishing in the Upper Hudson River and on commercial fishing for striped bass in the estuary due to the potential risk posed by consumption of PCB-contaminated fish.

Although PCB use at the GE facilities was curtailed in 1977, recent data on PCB loads (Fig. 4) show that inputs of approximately one pound per day of PCBs continue to enter the Upper Hudson. The current upstream loads are primarily attributed to PCB oil seeps

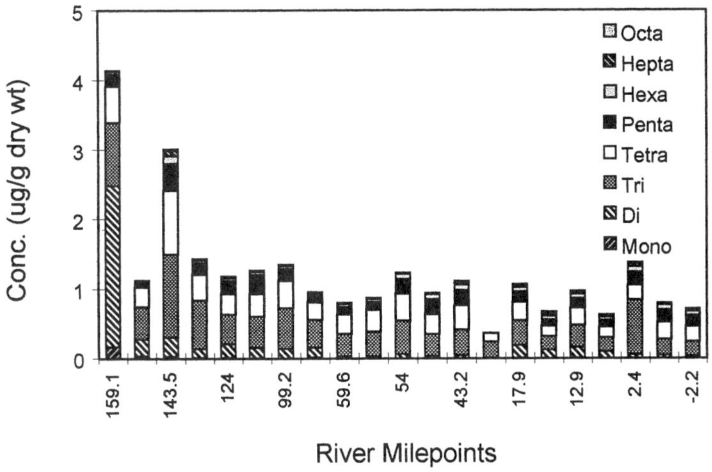


**FIG. 5.** PCB concentrations and homologue distributions for surface sediments in the Hudson River Estuary (8/92–11/92). [Data from TAMS/Gradient (10).]

through the fractured bedrock underlying the Hudson Falls facility. In addition to the Upper Hudson source, PCB sources from wastewater treatment plant discharges, rainfall runoff, and direct atmospheric sources may also be important. For example, PCB loadings from New York City wastewater treatment plant effluents and combined sewer overflows were estimated to be on the order of 0.55 pounds per day from 1994–1995 monitoring data (22).

Concentrations of PCBs in surface sediments (0–2 cm) in the Hudson River Estuary are given in Fig. 5. In this plot, total PCB concentrations are subdivided into homologues (i.e., groups with similar number of chlorines substituted on the biphenyl structure) and are presented for mono- through octa-chlorobiphenyl (CB). The data show a gradient in PCB concentrations from the upper portions of the estuary down into New York Harbor, particularly for the lower chlorinated homologues. This decrease in PCB sediment concentrations suggests dilution of PCB-contaminated sediments by cleaner, downstream sediment sources and/or PCB loss from the estuary by volatilization and/or degradation. An increase in total PCB sediment concentrations is also evident around river mile 0 and reflects PCB source loading from the New York City area. Dissolved water column concentrations in the upper and mid-estuary region are in the range of 10 to 20 ng/L (10,23).

PCB homologue concentrations in white and yellow perch from an August 1993 survey of the estuary are presented in Fig. 6. Although the gradient in PCB perch concentrations does not seem to be as dramatic as the PCB sediment gradient (Fig. 5), PCB perch concentrations varied from a high of 11 μg/g wet weight in the upper portion of the estuary to a low of 2 μg/g wet weight further downstream. In comparison to the surface sediment data (Fig. 5), the perch data show a clear shift to higher chlorinated compounds. Based on NYDEC data (10), PCB concentrations for 2- to 5-year-old striped bass in the 1993 mid-estuary fish collections had a median concentration of 1.8 μg/g wet weight with a 5 and 95 percentile range of 0.59 and 5.54 μg/g/ wet weight.

## MODEL DEVELOPMENT

Based on the available information for PCB contamination in the Hudson River, the purpose of our studies is to construct a model for evaluating the transport, fate, and subsequent food-chain bioaccumulation of PCBs in the estuary. Toward this end, PCB concentration in striped bass was chosen as the final end point, with particular emphasis in model development given to management questions related to (a) the relative impacts of PCBs sources from the Upper Hudson and from wastewater discharges from the New York City area, (b) the impact of PCB-contaminated sediments on dredged material disposal, and (c) a time projection for the reopening of the Hudson River striped bass fishery.

Long-term time scales (seasons and decades) were chosen for model application based on the decades-long extent of PCB inputs, the long-term memory of the sediment, the life span of striped bass, and the long-term projection period. The geographic extent of the model was specified from the Federal Dam at Troy out into the New York Bight and Long Island Sound with large spatial segmentation of the water column (see Fig. 3) based on estuarine mixing behavior and the migration patterns of striped bass. Underlying each water column segment was placed 2 to 14 sediment segments with thicknesses ranging from 0.5 cm (in low deposition zones) to 2.5 cm (in high deposition zones) for a total of 30 water column segments and 120 sediment segments. The geometry of each segment is given in Thomann et al. (6).

Although total PCB concentration was used as a state variable in many previous model studies, e.g., New Bedford Harbor (12), this approach was not considered adequate for this study based on the large differences in

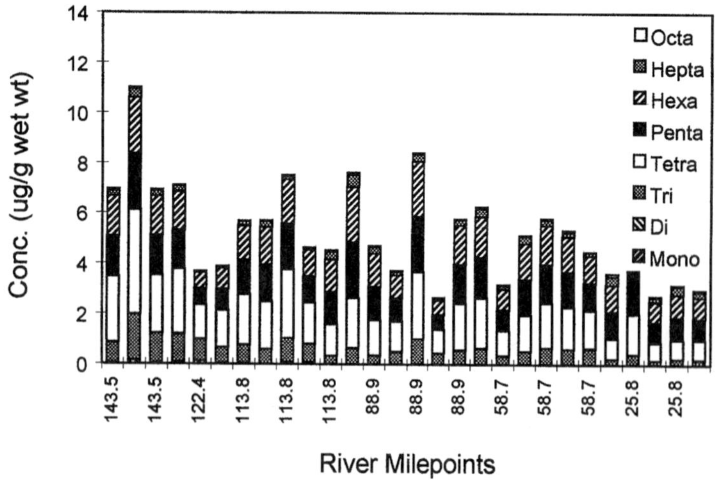


**FIG. 6.** PCB concentrations and homologue distributions for white and yellow perch in the Hudson River Estuary (8/93). [Data from TAMS/Gradient (10)].

physical-chemical and biochemical behavior of PCB congeners. However, modeling the transport, fate, and bioaccumulation of a large number of congeners over decadal time periods in a 150-segment model was not considered tractable. As a compromise solution, model calculations presented below were performed for the five PCB homologue groups (di-CB through hexa-CB) that contain the largest mass of PCBs. With this as a basis for modeling PCBs in the Hudson River Estuary, descriptions of PCB inputs, hydrodynamic and sediment transport, transport and fate calculations, and bioaccumulation modeling are given below.

## PCB INPUTS

In most contamination studies, direct information on chemical inputs is not available and various estimates are employed in calculating loads. For PCB contamination in the Hudson River Estuary, estimates of PCB loadings over Federal Dam at Troy for 1947 to 1975 were determined from PCB concentrations in sediment cores upstream of the dam (6). For 1976 to the present, PCB loads over the dam were determined from measured water column concentrations and flows (e.g., see Fig. 4 for recent loads from the Upper Hudson). Downstream PCB loads were determined from few measurements of PCBs in wastewater treatment plant effluents, wastewater treatment plant influents (to estimate loads from combined sewer overflows), tributaries, and rainfall (to estimate direct atmospheric inputs). Of the downstream loads, discharges from New York City and New Jersey wastewater treatment plants and combined sewer overflows, which accounted for PCB loading of 0.77 pounds per day in 1994–95 (11), appear to be most significant.

## HYDRODYNAMIC AND SEDIMENT TRANSPORT

Hydrodynamic transport in estuaries can be determined from simple hydrodynamic calculations, e.g., for the James River Estuary (24), complex hydrodynamic models, e.g., for Chesapeake Bay (25), or from observations and simple flow balance calculations. For the Hudson River Estuary PCB model, we used the latter approach and defined flow in the estuary for average annual and seasonal flow conditions using U.S. Geological Survey (USGS) river and tributary inflow records, surface runoff estimates, wastewater treatment plant discharge, and in the case of net circulation in the New York Bight, using observation of McLoughlin et al., as contained in O'Connor et al. (26). Dispersion coefficients, which describe horizontal mixing between adjacent water column segments, were calibrated using measured salinity concentrations. A summary of flows and dispersion coefficients for average-annual hydrologic conditions are given in Thomann et al. (6).

Sediment transport models describing particle settling, coagulation, resuspension, and burial have been applied to rivers and estuaries with some success (27), but these models typically require large data collection efforts for model parameterization and calibration. Solids balances have also been used in a number of studies such as our application for the Hudson River Estuary. In this approach, solids transport in a given segment is defined by the following mass balance equations:

$$V_i \frac{dm_i}{dt} = \Sigma Q_{ij} m_j - \Sigma Q_{ij} m_i + \Sigma E_{ij}(m_j - m_i) + W_m - w_s A_{s_i} m_i + w_u A_{s_i} m_{sed_i} \quad [1]$$

$$V_{sed_i} \frac{dm_{sed_i}}{dt} = w_s A_{s_i} m_i - w_{u_i} A_{s_i} m_{sed_i} - w_{b_i} A_{s_i} m_{sed_i} \quad [2]$$

where Equation 1 represents the change in the mass of solids in water column segment $i$ with time and is equal to the mass rate of solids flowing into and out of segment $i$, plus the mass rate of solids dispersing into and out of segment $i$, plus the input of solids from external sources (e.g., tributary inflow), minus the loss of solids from the water column by settling, plus the gain of solids to the water column by resuspension. Equation 2 is a similar expression for the change in the mass of solids in a surface sediment segment with time, which is equal to the addition of solids by settling from the overlying water, minus losses of solids by resuspension and burial. (A complete listing of terms used in the equations is given in the appendix to this chapter.) For the Hudson River application, the settling velocity for solids was specified as 10 ft/day. This value was used along with estimates of solids loadings from rivers, surface runoff, treatment plant discharges, and barge disposal (6), sediment deposition rates [based on studies by Bopp (28)], and harbor dredging [taken from Olsen et al. (29)] to calibrate solids transport in the model study area.

## CHEMICAL TRANSPORT AND FATE

Following evaluations for hydrodynamic and sediment transport, the transport and fate of toxic organic chemicals (such as PCBs) in estuaries can be expressed by a set of mass conservation equations—one for each water column and sediment segment. For a vertically well-mixed water column, the mass conservation equation for total (i.e., dissolved plus particulate) concentration of a specific chemical constituent (e.g., a PCB homologue) can be written for each water column segment as

$$V_i \frac{dC_i}{dt} = \Sigma Q_{ij} C_j - \Sigma Q_{ij} C_i + \Sigma E_{ij}(C_j - C_i) + W_{c_i} - w_{s_i} A_{s_i} m_i \Gamma_i + w_{u_i} A_{s_i} m_{sed_i} \Gamma_{sed_i} - k'_f A_{s_i} (C_{dissed_i} - C_{dis_i}) + k'_v A_{s_i} \left(\frac{P_c(MW)}{K_H} - C_{dis_i}\right) - k_i V_i C_{dis_i} \quad [3]$$

where the first term represents the time rate of change of the dissolved plus particulate chemical concentration in the water column; the second and third terms represent the mass rate of chemical flowing into and out of segment $i$, respectively; the fourth term represents chemical entering or leaving segment $i$ by dispersion; the fifth term represents chemical input into segment $i$ from an external source (e.g., tributary input or wastewater discharge); the sixth term represents chemical loss from the water column by settling; the seventh term represents chemical gain from resuspension; the eighth term represents diffusive exchange between dissolved concentrations in the water column and pore waters; the ninth term represents the transfer of chemical across the air-water interface (i.e., volatilization); and the last term represents transformation losses from the water column (e.g., by aerobic degradation).

Similar equations can be written for chemical concentrations in the sediments. For example, total (dissolved plus particulate) concentration for a chemical constituent in a stationary surface sediment layer can be written as

$$V_{\mathrm{sed_i}} \frac{dC_{\mathrm{sed_i}}}{dt} = w_{\mathrm{si}} A_{\mathrm{s_i}} m_{\mathrm{i}} \Gamma_{\mathrm{i}} - w_{\mathrm{u_i}} A_{\mathrm{s_i}} m_{\mathrm{sed_i}} \Gamma_{\mathrm{sed_i}} - w_{\mathrm{b_i}} A_{\mathrm{s_i}} m_{\mathrm{sed_i}} \Gamma_{\mathrm{sed_i}} - k'_{\mathrm{f}} A_{\mathrm{si}} (C_{\mathrm{dis_{sed_i}}} - C_{\mathrm{dis_i}}) + k'_{\mathrm{f}} A_{\mathrm{s_i}} (C_{\mathrm{dis_{deep\ sed_i}}} - C_{\mathrm{dis_{sedi}}}) - k_{\mathrm{sed_i}} V_{\mathrm{sed_i}} C_{\mathrm{dis_{sed_i}}} \qquad [4]$$

where the first term represents the change in the total (dissolved plus particulate) chemical mass with time; the second term represents the gain of chemical by settling from the overlying water; the third and fourth terms represent the loss of chemical by resuspension and burial into deeper sediments, respectively; the fifth and sixth terms represent diffusive exchange of dissolved chemical with the overlying water and deeper sediment pore water, respectively; and the last term represents transformation losses from the sediments (e.g., by anaerobic dechlorination). Chemical gain, for example, by dechlorination of higher chlorinated congeners, is also possible.

Since sorption plays an important role in determining the partitioning of chemical between the dissolved and particulate phases, its definition is essential in describing the various flux terms in Equations 3 and 4. In modeling studies, sorption reactions are usually assumed to be fast compared to other environmental processes and are typically modeled as instantaneous (or equilibrium) reactions (30–32). Dissolved and particulate phase concentrations of a chemical constituent can then be expressed in terms of the total chemical concentrations using the equilibrium partitioning relationship ($K_{\mathrm{d}} = \Gamma/C_{\mathrm{dis}}$) and the total mass concentration equation ($C = \phi C_{\mathrm{dis}} + \Gamma m$) as

$$C_{\mathrm{dis}} = \frac{C}{\phi + K_{\mathrm{d}} m} \qquad [5]$$

$$C_{\mathrm{part}} = \Gamma m = \frac{K_{\mathrm{d}} m C}{\phi + K_{\mathrm{d}} m} \qquad [6]$$

where $\phi$ is the porosity (and is approximately equal to 1 in the water column). Similar expressions can be written for dissolved and particulate phase chemical concentrations for the sediment layers.

For contaminant transport studies, chemical partitioning of hydrophobic organic contaminants in the water column is considered to be a function of the fraction organic carbon on the suspended solids and the octanol-water partitioning coefficient (33) ($K_{\mathrm{d}} = f_{\mathrm{oc}} K_{\mathrm{ow}}$). For the Hudson River Estuary, the fraction organic carbon for Hudson River suspended solids was taken as 0.072, based on data from Olsen et al. (29), and log $K_{\mathrm{ow}}$ values for the PCB homologues are given in Table 1. Following the findings of Brownawell and Farrington (34), PCB partitioning in sediments is considered to be controlled by chemical binding to fraction organic carbon of the sediments and the dissolved organic carbon (DOC) in the porewater. For the Hudson Estuary, the fraction organic carbon of the sediments is taken as 0.024, based on data from Olsen et al. (29), and DOC in the porewater is taken as 10 mg/L.

Volatilization rate coefficients are typically calculated using the two-layer model of the air-water interface (32). For rivers and estuaries, mass transfer coefficients for the water side of the interface can be calculated using the O'Connor-Dobbins (35) formula. Mass transfer coefficients for the air side of the interface are often estimated from water evaporation rates (with a correction for differences in the molecular dif-

**TABLE 1.** *Homologue-specific octanol-water partition coefficients, bioconcentration factors, and chemical assimilation efficiencies for the Hudson River Estuary striped bass food chain bioaccumulation model*

| | | | | BCF [L/kg(wet)] | | |
|---|---|---|---|---|---|---|
| Homologue | Log $K_{ow}$ [L/kg] | Log BCF [L/kg (lipid)] | Chemical assimilation efficiency | Zooplankton and small fish $f_{lipid}$ = 6% | White perch $f_{lipid}$ = 4% | Striped bass $f_{lipid}$ = 7% |
| di-CB | 4.9 | 4.9 | 0.71 | 4.8 | 3.2 | 5.6 |
| tri-CB | 5.4 | 5.4 | 0.80 | 15.1 | 10.0 | 17.6 |
| tetra-CB | 5.8 | 5.8 | 0.80 | 37.9 | 25.2 | 44.2 |
| penta-CB | 6.2 | 6.2 | 0.63 | 95.1 | 63.4 | 110.9 |
| hexa-CB | 6.7 | 6.7 | 0.35 | 300.7 | 200.5 | 350.4 |

fusivity of the organic chemical and water vapor in air). For PCBs in the Hudson River Estuary, transfer through the water side of the interface was assumed to control the overall transfer rate. In our initial studies (6,7), oxygen transfer rates were used in calculating transfer rates through the water side of the interface. In subsequent work, we have used the results of a sulfur hexafluoride and helium-3 tracer study by Clark et al. (36) in calculating the transfer rates. In both cases, molecular diffusivity corrections were made based on the dependency given in the O'Connor-Dobbins formula.

Dissolved chemical exchange between porewater and the overlying water column is dependent on the detailed hydrodynamic structure at the water-sediment interface and can be greatly enhanced by bioturbation. For most applications, the porewater exchange rate coefficient ($k'_f$) is specified by some multiple (e.g., 10 to 100 times) of molecular diffusivity divided by the thickness of the sediment segment. For our applications, we found that settling and resuspension of particle-bound PCB dominated the chemical transfer rates across the water-sediment interface and that the transport and fate of the PCB homologues were not sensitive to the selection of the porewater exchange rate coefficient.

Transformations of toxic organic chemicals can occur in the aquatic systems by hydrolysis, photolysis, biodegradation, and reductive dechlorination reactions. Although PCBs were originally thought to be refractory organic compounds, a number of studies have shown that certain PCB congeners may be degraded under aerobic conditions or microbially dechlorinated under anaerobic conditions in aquatic environments (1). The major conclusion from the aerobic degradation studies (37–39) is that biodegradation of PCBs can occur by the attack of a dioxygenase enzyme at an unchlorinated 2,3 (or 5,6) site or at an unchlorinated 3,4 (or 4,5) site. These attacks result in cleavage of the biphenyl ring and can be carried out by a variety of naturally occurring bacteria. Congeners with chlorines at both ortho (2,6) positions on either ring are generally not degraded as well as congeners lacking this characteristic.

Under anaerobic conditions, organisms leave the biphenyl ring intact while removing chlorines from the ring, thereby producing less chlorinated congeners. Although details of the dechlorination process are not fully understood, reductive dechlorination has been shown to proceed primarily through the selective removal of meta (3,5) and para (4) chlorines (1,40–44). In the Hudson, aerobic degradation and anaerobic dechlorination have been observed in the upper river (above the Federal Dam at Troy). However, in the estuary, aerobic degradation and anaerobic dechlorination are not thought to be important—for aerobic degradation, due to low oxygen concentrations in sediments, and for anaerobic dechlorination, possibly due to PCB concentrations being below a threshold value.

## BIOACCUMULATION MODELING

The accumulation of toxic organic chemicals in aquatic organisms has been modeled at several levels of detail. In the simplest formulation, a partition coefficient [i.e., the bioconcentration factor (BCF)] is used to define the chemical concentration in the organism relative to its dissolved concentration in water. A more complex formulation is the food chain model (45). In this approach, the chemical accumulation within a given organism in the food chain is viewed as a dynamic process that depends on direct uptake from the water, ingestion of contaminated prey, depuration (from urine excretion and egestion of fecal matter), and metabolic transformation of the chemical within the organism.

Model equations for the uptake and release of toxic organic chemicals into a given organism are typically written in terms of microgram of chemical per gram weight of organism ($v_k$) (45). The general form of this equation is given as

$$\frac{dv_k}{dt} = k_{u_k} C_{dis} - k_{b_{kl}} v_k + \Sigma \alpha_{kl} I_{kl} v_l - [k_e + k_m + k_g] v_k \qquad [7]$$

where the first term represents the change in chemical concentration in organism $k$ with time on a microgram of contaminant per gram weight of organism basis; the second term represents the direct uptake of chemical from the water phase by diffusion across an external cell or gill membrane; the third term represents back-diffusion of the chemical across the membrane; the fourth term represents chemical uptake through the ingestion of contaminated food or prey and is dependent on the chemical assimilation efficiency ($\alpha_{kl}$) and the consumption rate ($I_{kl}$) for organism $k$ feeding on organism $l$; and the last term represents decreases in chemical concentrations in organism $k$ due to excretion ($k_e$), metabolic transformation ($k_m$), and growth dilution ($k_g$). In this equation, growth dilution is included as a loss term to account for the reduction in $v_k$ due to the increase in the size of the organism.

In applying this model to striped bass in the Hudson River Estuary, Thomann et al. (6,7) developed a time-variable, age-dependent striped bass food chain model. The model included a five-component, pelagic food chain that consisted of phytoplankton, zooplankton, small fish, seven age classes of white perch, and 17 age classes of striped bass (Fig. 7). Based on feeding studies where stomach contents of striped bass were examined (46–48), the 0- to 2-year-old striped bass are assumed to feed on zooplankton; 2- to 6-year-old striped bass are assumed to feed on a mixture of small fish and 0- to 2-year-old perch; and 7- to 17-year-old striped bass are assumed to feed on 2- to 5-year-old white perch.

For the lower levels of the food chain, PCB homologue concentrations in phytoplankton are considered to be in equilibrium with dissolved water concentrations and are described using a constant BCF value of 30

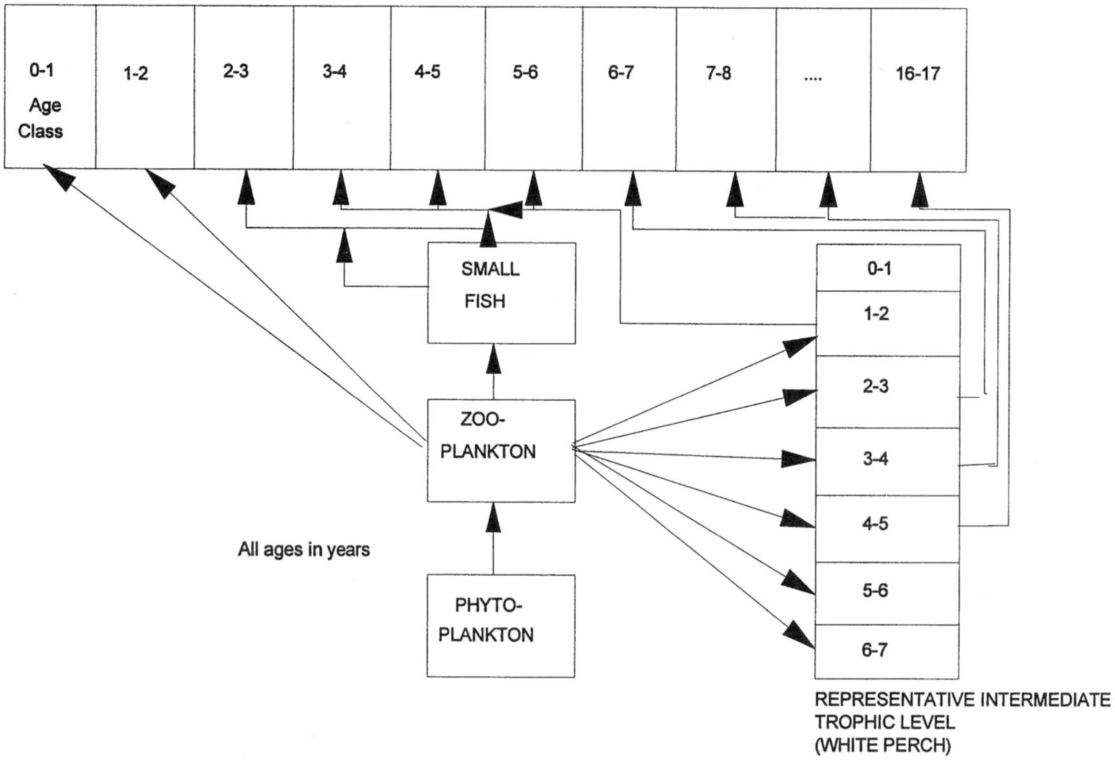


**FIG. 7.** Five component, pelagic food chain for the Hudson River Estuary PCB bioaccumulation model.

L/g(wet) for all PCB homologues. The phytoplankton are then preyed upon by a zooplankton compartment, the characteristics of which are considered to be represented by zooplankter *Gammarus*. The small fish compartment is meant to reflect a mixed diet of fish of about 10 g in weight and includes 0 to 1 year old tomcod and herring. The white perch is considered as a representative size-dependent prey of the striped bass and is assumed to feed exclusively on zooplankton.

Growth rates and respiration rates for striped bass and other food chain compartments were estimated using formulations given in Thomann and Connolly (17) and Connolly and Tonelli (49). Details are given in Thomann et al. (6). BCF values and assimilation efficiencies for zooplankton, small fish, white perch, and striped bass are given in Table 1 as a function of PCB homologue. Uptake rate coefficients ($k_u$) were determined as a function of the respiration rate and weight of the organism, as well as the $K_{ow}$ of the PCB homologue (6). The excretion rate was calculated as the ratio of the uptake rate coefficients ($k_u$) and the BCF values.

In bioaccumulation model calculations for the Hudson, migration of striped bass adds a further complication in specifying time-dependent exposure concentrations. Migration patterns used in the initial calculations were assigned using Waldman (50) and are described in Thomann et al. (6,7). In summary, striped bass are born on May 15 of each year and the yearlings are assumed to remain in the mid-estuary (as defined by river mile points 18.5 to 78.5); 2- to 5-year-old striped bass are considered to migrate from the mid-estuary into New York Harbor in June and spend the summer months (July through September) in Long Island Sound and the New York Bight. Lastly, 6- to 17-year-old striped bass are assumed to spend most of their year in the open ocean, but migrate into Long Island Sound and the New York Bight around March 15 and return to the mid-estuary in around April 15. They remain in the mid-estuary until the middle of July.

## HUDSON RIVER ESTUARY PCB MODEL RESULTS

### Model Calibration and Previous Modeling Results

The PCB homologue model for the Hudson River Estuary was initially run using a long-term average annual hydrology and coefficients discussed previously. Model calibration was performed for the period of 1946 (before PCB contamination) through 1987 using total PCB and Aroclor data for the water column, sediments, and striped bass. Details of the calibration are given in Thomann et al. (6,7). Model projections were then made assuming exponentially decreasing loads from the Upper Hudson and the downstream sources. Results of this work indicated that, under a no-action alternative, 50% of the

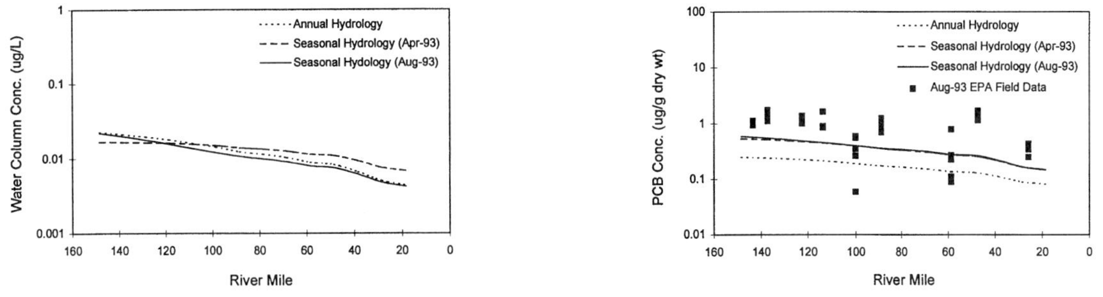


A B

**FIG. 8.** Average-annual hydrology and seasonal hydrology model results for dissolved PCB water column concentrations **(A)** and PCB surface sediment concentrations **(B)** for 1993. [Data from TAMS/Gradient (10).]

striped bass would be below the Food and Drug Administration (FDA) limit of 2 μg of total PCB/g of fish (wet weight) by 1992 and 95% of the striped bass would be below the FDA limit by 2004.

## PCB Transport and Fate Calculations

As an extension of the initial modeling studies, a post-audit evaluation of PCB homologue model calculations was performed using water column, sediment, striped bass, and loading data that have been collected since the 1987 model calibration. In this evaluation, we found that the model provided a good description of PCB water column and striped bass data. The model calculations, however, tended to underestimate PCB accumulations in surface sediments (see dotted line in Fig. 8*B*).

As a follow-up, preliminary model calculations were performed using the SEDAN model (51) to examine the effects of seasonal hydrology on PCB transport and fate in the estuary. For the seasonal study, 50% of the flow, 85% of the solids, and 68% of the PCBs transported over Federal Dam at Troy and into the estuary were attributed to a 2-month spring high-flow period based on information given in Limno-Tech et al. (9). Solids loading to the estuary, sediment deposition rates, and volatilization rates were also decreased by a factor of two based on more recent estimates.

Model results are given in Fig. 8 for the seasonal hydrology simulation (as shown by the solid and dashed lines) and the average annual hydrology simulation (as shown by the dotted line). As shown in Fig. 8*A*, dissolved PCB concentrations in the water column are not dramatically different in the upper and mid-estuary for the two flow descriptions. PCB surface sediment concentrations, however, are two to three times higher for the seasonal hydrology simulation and correspond more closely to the observed concentrations.

Using the seasonal hydrology results as a guide, it appears that a disproportionate amount of toxic organic contaminants (such as PCBs) enter estuaries during periods of high flow. Because hydraulic residence times in estuaries are shorter during high-flow periods, contaminant loss by volatilization and/or degradation are minimized and most of the incoming contaminant load is accumulated in sediments. During low-flow periods (and longer residence times in estuaries), toxic organic contaminants may be lost from the water column by volatilization and/or degradation. As the contaminant is lost from the water column, it is replenished by desorption from contaminated sediments that are continually being resuspended by tidal motion. For PCBs in the Hudson, the net result of seasonal hydrology is a decrease in volatilization losses and an increase in transport of PCBs from the Upper Hudson to the lower estuary.

## Striped Bass Bioaccumulation Results

Post-audit model calculations for 2- to 5-year-old striped bass are shown by the solid line in Fig. 9. These results are based on expected striped bass migrations patterns where 2- to 5-year-olds remain in the mid-estuary from November to May and migrate to the New York Bight and Long Island Sound in the summer. Although the model predictions provide a good indication of the median PCB concentrations, the wide range in the 5 and 95 percentile values for observed PCB concentrations in striped bass is somewhat disturbing. The wide range of measured PCB concentrations may in part be explained by variations in striped bass migration patterns as discussed below.

In a recent study, Secor and Piccoli (52) have shown that strontium/calcium ratios in striped bass otoliths can be used to estimate the life history (in terms of salinity environment) for individual striped bass. Representative results of their work (Fig. 10) show a wide range in

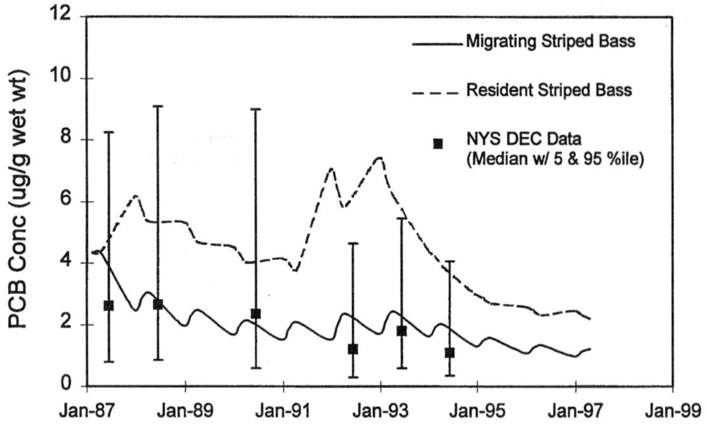


**FIG. 9.** Model results for PCB concentrations in 2- to 5-year-old striped bass in the mid-estuary. Results are shown for the migrating striped bass population and a resident (nonmigrating) striped bass subpopulation. [Data are from NYS DEC, as reported in TAMS/Gradient (10).]

migration behavior for two male striped bass. One striped bass (Fig. 10*A*) is shown to have followed a somewhat expected migration pattern, spending his first few years in the mid-estuary and migrating out to ocean waters later in life. The other striped bass (Fig. 10*B*) is shown to have never left the tidal freshwater region of the estuary. One possibility is that this latter migration behavior is representative of a subpopulation of male striped bass.

Since the male subpopulation would have continuous exposures to high PCB concentrations, they are expected to have higher PCB accumulations. Our breakdown of PCB concentrations in female and male striped bass (Fig. 11) shows a higher PCB average concentration and a more noticeable presence of outliers for males (as indicated by the open circles on Fig. 11). These results are consistent with the notion of a portion of the male population stays in the estuary year round while the remainder of the males and all or most of the females follow a seasonal migration pattern.

To examine the effect of limited migration behavior on PCB accumulation in striped bass, model calculations were performed for a subpopulation of striped bass migrating between the tidal freshwater Hudson (river mile 78.5 to 153.5) and the mid-estuary. Results of this calculation are shown by the dashed line in Fig. 9 and as expected show much higher PCB accumulations. These results correspond reasonably well to the 95 percentile concentrations for PCBs in striped bass and may help to explain the high end of the measured PCB distribution. These calculations underscore the importance of properly identifying the migratory behavior of species such as striped bass, bluefish, and shad in PCB and other exposure assessment studies.

## CONCLUSIONS

In the Hudson River and other PCB-contaminated waterways, human exposure to PCBs is primarily through the consumption of contaminated seafood. Mathematical models for the transport, fate, and bioaccumulation of PCBs have been used at a number of sites as a complement to monitoring data to project future concentrations in fish and to determine the effectiveness of various management alternatives for site restoration. For the Hudson River Estuary, elevated concentrations of PCBs in striped

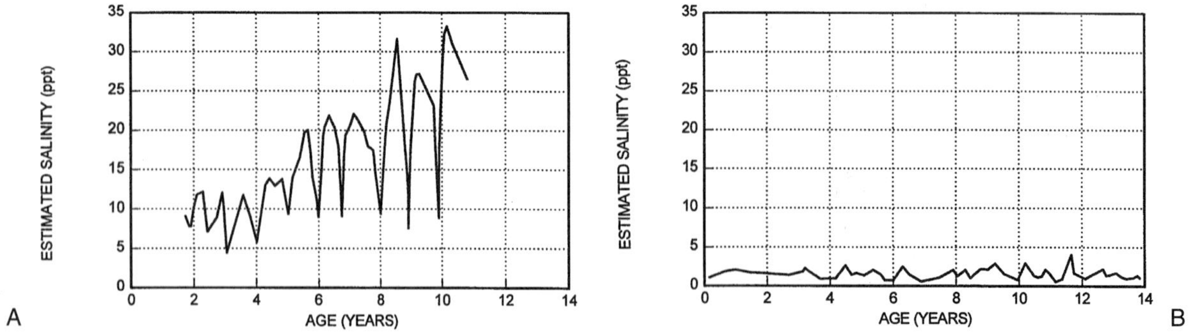


**FIG. 10. A,B:** Migration time histories (as a function of salinity regions) for male striped bass. Salinity regions are estimated from strontium:calcium ratios in striped bass otoliths. [Data from Secor and Piccoli (52).]

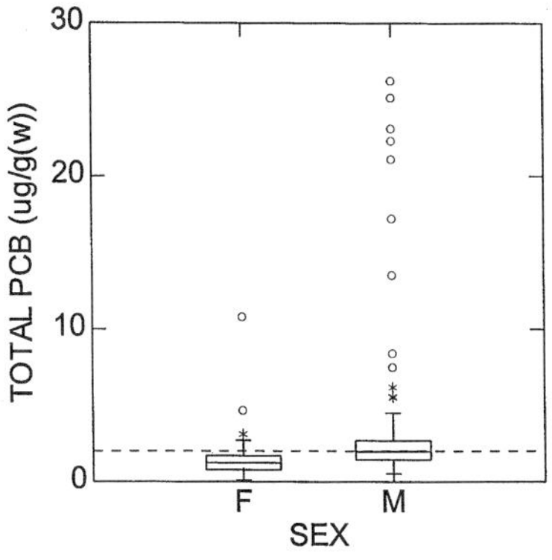


**FIG. 11.** Total PCB concentration distributions in female and male striped bass from the mid-estuary in 1993. Data from NYS DEC, as reported in TAMS/Gradient (10), are presented in "box and whisker" plot, with "o" representing outliers of the distribution. *Dashed line* represents the present FDA limit.

bass are due to continuing inputs to the estuary and the long-term retention of PCBs in sediments. The loads appear to be dominated by PCB inputs from the Upper Hudson, with wastewater treatment plants in the New York City area making significant contributions to concentrations in New York Harbor and the lower estuary.

Using the Hudson as an example, the transport, fate, and bioaccumulation of PCBs and other hydrophobic organic chemicals in estuaries is expected to be controlled by seasonal hydrology and migration patterns. In our scenario for the Hudson, a large portion of the PCB load is transported into the estuary and deposited in sediments during high flows in the spring. For low to moderate flows that usually occur during the remainder of the year, the sediments serve as a source of PCBs to the overlying water via desorption from contaminated sediments during tidal resuspensions. Because of the longer-term retention of PCBs in sediments, surface sediment PCB concentrations and dissolved PCB concentrations in the overlying water do not show large seasonal variations in our model calculations. Since food chain accumulations are ultimately driven by dissolved PCB concentrations and accumulation in lower trophic species, seasonal variations in PCB exposure concentrations are not expected to be significant for resident fish populations. Seasonal migration patterns, however, will affect their bioaccumulation of PCBs, e.g., in striped bass. New information on migrating patterns, which suggests migrating and resident subpopulations of striped bass, is important and may help explain the large variations in observed PCB concentrations in striped bass.

## ACKNOWLEDGMENTS

Support for this work was provided by the Hudson River Foundation, the Port Authority of New York and New Jersey, and the U.S. Environmental Protection Agency, Region II. The work of our research assistants, David Interdonato and Michael Carroll, is gratefully acknowledged. Views expressed in this chapter do not necessarily reflect the beliefs or opinions of our sponsoring agencies.

## REFERENCES

1. Abramowicz DA. Aerobic and anaerobic biodegradation of PCBs: a review. *Crit Rev Biotechnol* 1990;10:241–251.
2. Safe SH. Polychlorinated Biphenyls (PCBs): environmental impact, biochemical and toxic responses, and implications for risk assessment. *Crit Rev Toxicol* 1994;24:87–149.
3. Bopp RF, Simpson HJ, Olsen CR, Kostyk N. Polychlorinated biphenyls in sediments of the Tidal Hudson River. *Environ Sci Technol* 1981;15: 210–216.
4. Bopp RF, Simpson HJ, Olsen CR, Trier RM, Kostyk N. Chlorinated hydrocarbons and radionuclide chronologies in sediments of the Hudson River and Estuary, New York. *Environ Sci Technol* 1982;16:666–676.
5. Bopp RF, Simpson HJ, Deck BL, Kostyk N. The persistence of PCB components in sediments of the lower Hudson. *Northeast Environ Sci* 1984;3:179–183.
6. Thomann RV, Mueller JA, Winfield RP, Huang C-R. *Mathematical model of the long-term behavior of PCBs in the Hudson River estuary.* Riverdale, NY: Manhattan College, 1989.
7. Thomann RV, Mueller JA, Winfield RP, Huang C-R. Model of fate and accumulation of PCB homologues in Hudson Estuary. *J Environ Engr* 1991;117:161–178.
8. Chillrud SN. *Transport and fate of particle associated contaminants in the Hudson River basin.* New York: Columbia University, 1996;277.
9. Limno-Tech/Menzie Cura and Associates/The CADMUS Group. *Further site characterization and analysis, vol 2B—preliminary model calibration report Hudson River PCBs reassessment RI/FS.* Phase 2 report, review copy. New York: U.S. Environmental Protection Agency, Region II, 1996.
10. TAMS/Gradient. *Further site characterization and analysis database report.* Phase 2 report, review copy. New York: U.S. Environmental Protection Agency, Region II, 1995.
11. TAMS/The Cadmus Group/Gradient. *Further site characterization and analysis, vol 2C—data evaluation and interpretation report, Hudson River PCBs reassessment RI/FS.* Phase 2 report, review copy. Kansas City: U.S. Environmental Protection Agency, Region II and U.S. Army Corps of Engineers, Kansas City District, 1997.
12. Connolly JP. Application of a food chain model to polychlorinated biphenyl contamination of the lobster and winter flounder food chains in New Bedford Harbor. *Environ Sci Technol* 1991;25:760–770.
13. Garton LS, Bonner JS, Ernest AN, Autenrieth RL. Fate and transport at the New Bedford Harbor Superfund Site. *Environ Toxicol Chem* 1996; 15:736–745.
14. Velleux M, Endicott D. Development of a mass balance model for estimating PCB export from the lower Fox River to Green Bay. *J Great Lakes Res* 1994;20:416–434.
15. Velleux M, Endicott D, Steuer J, Jaeger S, Patterson D. Long-term simulation of PCB export from the Fox River to Green Bay. *J Great Lakes Res* 1995;21:359–372.
16. Farley KJ, Germann GG, Elzerman AW. Differential weathering of PCB congeners in Lake Hartwell, South Carolina. In: Baker L, ed. *Chemistry of lake watersheds.* Washington, DC: American Chemical Society, 1994.
17. Thomann RV, Connolly JP. Model of PCB in the Lake Michigan trout food chain. *Environ Sci Technol* 1984;18:65–71.
18. Oliver BG, Niimi AJ. Trophodynamic Analysis of polychlorinated biphenyl congeners and other chlorinated hydrocarbons in the Lake Ontario ecosystem. *Environ Sci Technol* 1988;22:388–397.
19. Gobas FAPC. A model for predicting the bioaccumulation of hydrophobic organic chemicals in aquatic food webs: application to Lake Ontario. *Ecol Model* 1993;69:1–17.
20. Gobas FAPC, Z'graggen MN, Zhang X. Time response of the Lake Ontario ecosystem to virtual elimination of PCBs. *Environ Sci Technol* 1995;29:2038–2046.
21. O'Connor DJ, Connolly JP, Garland EJ. Mathematical models—fate, transport, and food chain. In: Levin SA, Harwell JR, Kelly JR, Kimball KD, eds. *Ecotoxicology:* problems and approaches. New York: Springer-Verlag, 1989;222–243.

22. Chen I. *New York/New Jersey Harbor PCBs loading, a review of the PCB report submitted by New York City Department of Environmental Protection.* New York: U.S. Environmental Protection Agency, Region 2, Water Management Division, 1995.
23. Brownawell BJ. Personal communication, 1997.
24. O'Connor DJ, Mueller JA, Farley KJ. Distribution of Kepone in the James River Estuary. *J Environ Engr* 1983;109:397–413.
25. Johnson B, Kim K, Heath R, Hsieh B, Butler L. Validation of a three-dimensional hydrodynamic model of Chesapeake Bay. *J Hydraul Engr* 1993;119:2–20.
26. O'Connor DJ, Thomann RV, Salas HJ. *Water quality:* MESA New York Bight atlas monograph 27. Albany, NY: Hydroscience for New York Sea Grant Institute, 1977.
27. Gailani J, Ziegler CK, Lick W. Transport of suspended solids in the Lower Fox River. *J Great Lakes Res* 1991;17:479–494.
28. Bopp RF. *The geochemistry of polychlorinated biphenyls in the Hudson River.* Univ. Micro. Intern. New York: Columbia University, 1979;191.
29. Olsen CR, Larsen IL, Brewster RH, Cutshall NH, Bopp RF, Simpson HJ. *A geochemical assessment of sediment and contaminant distributions in the Hudson-Raritan Estuary.* Rockville, MD: NOAA, 1984.
30. Ambrose RB, Wool TA, Connolly JP, Schnaz RW. *WASP4:* a hydrodynamic and water quality model—model theory, *user's manual and programmer's guide.* Athens, GA: U.S. EPA Environmental Research Laboratory, 1988.
31. Mossman DJ, Schnoor JL, Stumm W. Predicting the effects of a pesticide release to the Rhine River. *J Water Pollut Control Fed* 1988;60: 1806–1812.
32. O'Connor DJ. Models of toxic sorptive substances in freshwater systems. I: basic equations. *J Environ Engr* 1988;114:507–531.
33. Karickhoff SW. Semi-empirical estimation of sorption of hydrophobic pollutants on natural sediments and soils. *Chemosphere* 1981;10: 833–846.
34. Brownawell BJ, Farrington JW. Biogeochemistry of PCBs in interstitial waters of a coastal marine sediment. *Geochem Cosmochem Acta* 1986; 50:157–169.
35. O'Connor DJ, Dobbins WE. Mechanisms of reaeration in natural streams. *Trans ASCE* 1958;641:123.
36. Clark JF, Schlosser P, Stute M, Simpson HJ. SF6-3He tracer release experiment: a new method of determining longitudinal dispersion coefficients in large rivers. *Environ Sci Technol* 1996;30:1527–1532.
37. Bedard DL, Unterman R, Bopp LH, Brennan MJ, Haberl ML, Johnson C. Rapid assay for screening and characterizing microorganisms for the ability to degrade polychlorinated biphenyls. *Appl Environ Microbiol* 1986;51:761–768.
38. Bedard DL, Haberl ML, May RJ, Brennan MJ. Evidence for novel mechanisms of polychlorinated biphenyl metabolism in Alcaligenes eutrophus H850. *Appl Environ Microbiol* 1987;53:1103–1112.
39. Bedard DL, Wagner RE, Brennan MJ, Haberl ML, Brown JF. Extensive degradation of Aroclors and environmentally transformed polychlorinated biphenyls by Alcaligenes eutrophus H850. *Appl Environ Microbiol* 1987;53:1094–1102.
40. Quensen JF, Tiedje JM, Boyd SA. Reductive dechlorination of polychlorinated byphenyls by anaerobic microorganisms from sediments. *Science* 1988;242:752–754.
41. Abramowicz DA, Brennan MJ, Dort HMV, Gallagher EL. Factors influencing the rate of polychlorinated biphenyl dechlorination in Hudson River sediments. *Environ Sci Technol* 1993;27:1125–1131.
42. Rhee G-Y, Sokol RC, Bush B, Bethoney CM. Long-term study of the anaerobic dechlorination of Aroclor 1254 and without biphenyl enrichment. *Environ Sci Technol* 1993;27:714–719.
43. Rhee G-Y, Bush B, Bethoney CM, DeNucci A, Oh H-M, Sokol RC. Reductive dechlorination of Aroclor 1242 in anaerobic sediments: pattern, rate and concentration dependence. *Environ Toxicol Chem* 1993; 12:1025–1032.
44. Rhee G-Y, Bush B, Bethoney CM, DeNucci A, Oh H-M, Sokol RC. Anaerobic dechlorination of Aroclor 1242 as affected by some environmental conditions. *Environ Toxicol Chem* 1993;12:1033–1039.
45. Thomann RV, Connolly JP, Parkerton TF. An equilibrium model of organic chemical accumulation in aquatic food webs with sediment interaction. *Environ Toxicol Chem* 1992;11:615–629.
46. O'Connor JM. PCBs: dietary dose and burdens in striped bass from the Hudson River. *Northeast Environ Sci* 1984;3:152–158.
47. Gardinier MN, Hoff TB. Diet of striped bass in Hudson River Estuary. *New York Fish Game J* 1982;29:152–165.
48. Setzler EM, Boynton WR, Wood KV, et al. *Synopsis of biological data on striped bass, Morone saxatilis (Waldbaum).* Rockville, MD: U.S. Department of Commerce, 1980.
49. Connolly JP, Tonelli R. Modelling Kepone in the striped bass food chain of the James River Estuary. *Estuary Coast Shelf Sci* 1985;20: 349–366.
50. Waldman JR. *1986 Hudson River striped bass tag recovery program.* New York: Hudson River Foundation, 1988.
51. Marshall MJ, Farley KJ. *Sediment contamination in streams and rivers.* Clemson, SC: South Carolina Water Resources Research Institute, 1997.
52. Secor DH, Piccoli PM. Age-and sex dependent migrations of the Hudson River Striped Bass population determined from otolith chemical microanalysis. *Estuaries* 1996;19:778–793.

## APPENDIX A: NOTATIONS

The following symbols and abbreviations are used in this chapter:

$A_s$ = surface area ($m^2$)
BCF = bioconcentration factor (L/kg)
$C$ = total (dissolved plus particulate) concentration (μg/L)
$C_{dis}$ = dissolved chemical concentration (μg/L)
$C_{part}$ = particulate chemical concentration (μg/L)
$E_{ij}$ = bulk dispersion coefficient for mixing between segments $i$ and $j$ ($m^3$/sec)
$f_{lipid}$ = fraction of organism mass that is comprised of lipids (g lipid/g wet weight)
$f_{oc}$ = fraction organic carbon for suspended solids and sediments (g organic carbon/g dry weight)
$K_d$ = equilibrium partition coefficient (L/kg)
$K_H$ = Henry's constant (atm-$m^3$/mol)
$K_{ow}$ = octanol-water partition coefficient (L/kg)
$k$ = chemical transformation rate coefficient (1/day)
$k_b$ = back-diffusion rate coefficient across organism membrane or gill (1/day)
$k_e$ = chemical excretion rate coefficient (1/day)
$k_{f'}$ = porewater-water column exchange rate coefficient (m/day)
$k_g$ = growth dilution rate coefficient (1/day)
$k_m$ = chemical metabolic rate coefficient (1/day)
$k_u$ = chemical uptake rate coefficient across organism membrane or gill [L/g(wet)/day]
$k_{v'}$ = volatilization rate coefficient (m/day)
$I_{kl}$ = consumption rate of organism $k$ feeding on organism $l$ [g(wet) prey/g(wet) predator/day]
MW = molecular weight (g/mol)
$m$ = solids concentration (mg/L)
$Q_{ij}$ = flow rate from segment $i$ to segment $j$ ($m^3$/sec)
$t$ = time (days)
$V$ = volume ($m^3$)
$W_C$ = chemical input rate from external sources, e.g., tributaries, effluent discharges (kg/day)
$W_m$ = solids input rate from external sources, e.g., tributaries (kg/day)
$w_b$ = burial rate for solids (cm/yr)

$w_s$ = solids settling velocity (m/day)
$w_u$ = solids resuspension velocity (m/day)
$\alpha_{kl}$ = chemical assimilation efficiency for organism $k$ feeding on organism $l$ (dimensionless)
$\Gamma$ = solid phase chemical concentration (μg/g)
$v$ = biota chemical concentration [ug/g(wet)]
$\phi$ = porosity (dimensionless)

The following subscripts are used in this chapter:

$i,j$ = segment descriptors for spatial segments
$k,l$ = descriptors for trophic levels in the food chain
*sed* = surface (active) sediment layer
*deep sed* = deep sediment layer underlying the surface sediment

*Environmental and Occupational Medicine, Third Edition,* edited by William N. Rom.
Published by Lippincott–Raven Publishers, Philadelphia, 1998.

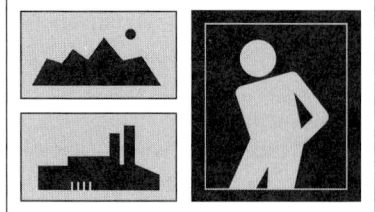

CHAPTER 120

# Persian Gulf War Health Issues

Stephen C. Joseph, Kenneth C. Hyams, Gary D. Gackstetter, Edward C. Mathews, and Relford E. Patterson

The many scientific and public controversies that have arisen out of what have come to be called Persian Gulf illnesses (PGIs) illustrate perhaps more sharply than other recent controversial issues in science and public policy a number of long-standing dilemmas. In addition to those that are concerned principally with military operational and intelligence issues, three more generic sets of dilemmas are especially noteworthy.

The first concerns the existing limits to both accuracy and precision in medical nosology and diagnosis. What are the defining boundaries of fatigue? How may "headache, otherwise undefined" be differentiated from patient to patient? Which collections of symptoms are coherent enough to form a case definition in a circumstance of unclear etiology, absent objective physical and laboratory findings? With PGI, as with chronic fatigue syndrome, fibromyalgia, multiple chemical sensitivity, and other unclear and perhaps nonexistent syndromes, clinicians and epidemiologist alike gain new humility for the current limits of their arts and sciences.

Second, more relevant to epidemiologic puzzle-breaking, is the reality that most new dilemmas of this sort in both military and occupational settings permit only retrospective analysis during the time of hottest debate, and perhaps forever. It is not possible to construct a military campaign on a prospective double-blind basis. Much time and effort is spent, after the fact, in attempting to prove the elusive negative. This becomes especially difficult when partisans of one hypothesis or another allege increasing strings of multifactorial causation.

Third, rational approaches to science and public policy in circumstances of high emotion and high decibels are tenuous to sustain. We have the responsibility to ensure that political agendas and media sensationalism do not crowd out well-considered analyses. As a society, what is our answer to the question: "How should the public interest, the patient's right to assert and advocate, and the responsibilities of government, industry, the press, and science be fairly balanced?" This may, indeed, be the salient public health question of our time.

To any but the most casual observer or most true-believing advocate, the Persian Gulf illnesses saga offers a rich mix of all the issues above. The final chapter will not be written for some considerable time to come.

## BACKGROUND

More than 7 years following the Persian Gulf War, there are persistent questions about the health consequences of the Persian Gulf War experience for veterans and their families. The Departments of Defense (DoD) and Veteran Affairs (VA), the scientific community, the general public, and government officials have become increasingly concerned about occupational and environmental health issues related to the Gulf War. Questions have arisen about possible hazardous exposures and related health effects, including the possible existence of a unique war-related clinical syndrome. However, shortcomings in several areas have

S. C. Joseph, G. D. Gackstetter: Office of the Assistant Secretary of Defense for Health Affairs, Department of Defense, The Pentagon, Washington, D.C. 20301-1200.
K. C. Hyams: Epidemiology Division, Naval Medical Research Institute, Bethesda, Maryland 20889-5607.
E. C. Mathews: Department of Internal Medicine, Wilford Hall Medical Center, Lackland Air Force Base, Texas 78236-5300.
R. E. Patterson: Department of Preventive Medicine and Biometrics, Uniformed Services University of the Health Sciences, Bethesda, Maryland 20814.

complicated efforts to precisely determine relationships between hazardous exposures, which may have occurred during the Gulf War, and subsequent health outcomes. Some of the health concerns of Persian Gulf War veterans may never be completely resolved because of a scarcity of data involving lost medical records, limited baseline health data, imprecise records of troop locations, limited exposure measurements, and incomplete data concerning the health effects of some potential health risks. Any discussion of Gulf War veterans' health issues could cover a wide variety of complex topics regarding health care–seeking behavior, the public's perception of risks, issues of chronic health effects following difficult to quantify exposures, disease causation, and work-relatedness of disease. Detailed discussions of each of these topics are beyond the scope of this chapter. Nonetheless, there are important areas within these topics that warrant consideration. This chapter provides an overview of Gulf War health issues by briefly summarizing information regarding military occupational exposures, epidemiology of veterans' illnesses including the results of systematic clinical evaluations, and a historical review of postwar syndromes. It is hoped that the information presented herein will prove useful to health professionals involved in the care of Gulf War veterans.

Between August 1990 and March 1991, in addition to other coalition forces, the United States deployed 697,000 troops to the Persian Gulf region, the British 51,000 troops, and the Canadians 4,500 troops (1). To deal with a broad range of health threats to such a large combat force, coalition forces established an extensive health care network (2,3), and preventive medicine effort, which included monitoring of water and food supplies, field sanitation, infectious disease control programs, and medical surveillance (4,5).

Medical preparedness was a high priority before and during this military campaign. The incidence of disease and nonbattle injuries (DNBI) was substantially less than in any previous major conflict involving U.S. military personnel (1,4,6). In addition, the rates of both combat and noncombat deaths were lower than in other modern wars. There were 147 U.S. combat deaths during the 39-day air war and 4 days of ground fighting; more deaths (225) were due to nonbattle causes, primarily motor vehicle and training accidents, during 12 months of deployment (7).

Following the end of hostilities on February 28, 1991, the health of Gulf War troops remained a priority for the DoD, VA, and the Department of Health and Human Services (HHS) (8). The U.S. government implemented a concerted program that included readjustment counseling for families, health registries, specialized health care centers, and research studies of war-related health problems (9–11). Health care has been made available for all Gulf War veterans experiencing health problems possibly related to the war, either through the DoD or the VA.

After returning home, some U.S., British, and Canadian Gulf War veterans began reporting combinations of nonspecific symptoms, which did not fit readily into a common diagnosis (12–14). The most common physical symptoms involve multiple organ systems and various combinations of the following: fatigue, headache, joint pain, sleep disturbances, memory problems, shortness of breath, impaired concentration, and other symptoms. These symptoms have not been associated with a characteristic set of clinical signs (15). Without a defined symptom complex or specific case definition, it is difficult to accurately determine the number of veterans who report illnesses possibly resulting from Gulf War service. However, estimates range from a few thousand within 1 to 2 years after the war, increasing to 49,000 by 1995, to more than 100,000 in 1997 (11). There also have been concerns about possible occurrences of sudden deaths, various illnesses, and offsprings' birth defects in the veteran population (9).

The physical symptoms reported by Gulf War veterans share similarities with the diversity of health problems associated with prior war syndromes (16). Also analogous to prior war syndromes, there has been uncertainty as to whether or not the symptoms reported by Gulf War veterans represent organic diseases or manifestations of psychological illnesses (16). In previous conflicts, unexplained somatic symptoms among war veterans usually have been attributed to psychological factors, rather than to hazardous environmental exposures (16).

## OCCUPATIONAL EXPOSURES OF MILITARY SERVICE

Military service is associated with a variety of potential occupational hazards. An overview of these hazards and the preventive medicine programs in place to mitigate them provides an important perspective for considering the health aspects of service in the Gulf War. Military personnel are required to perform multiple combat and noncombat duties that may place them at risk for occupational and environmental illnesses and/or injuries (17). Service personnel routinely perform occupational duties that may involve potentially hazardous exposures that are similar to those in civilian industrial settings. However, unlike the civilian workplace, there are inherent, sometimes unpredictable hazards associated with combat and combat-support operations resulting from the threats of the enemy's weaponry, operation of sophisticated weapons systems, and the natural battlefield environment. Additionally, military personnel, especially when they are deployed, are exposed to a large number of drugs, biologicals, and chemicals to which their civilian counterparts in the United States are not exposed (18).

### The Combat Environment

Military units regularly participate in realistic training exercises, including deployments to locations within their geographic areas of responsibility, to enhance their combat readiness skills. Both the military training environment and the natural battlefield environment commonly involve extremes in temperature, humidity, other harsh weather conditions, inadequate water supplies, and other environmental stressors (19). The operation of military equipment and weapons systems can be associated with potentially hazardous exposures to noise, vibration, nonionizing radiation from communications and radar tracking equipment, and laser target designators (19,20). Combustion products from vehicles, propellants from ammunition, solvents, and chemical warfare agents are just some of the chemical toxicants that may be present under battlefield conditions (19,20). Biologic hazards include venomous bites from insects and reptiles, arthropod-borne diseases and pathogenic microorganisms and their toxins and enzymes, as well as potential biologic warfare agents. Psychological stressors related to fear and isolation are frequently characteristic of combat situations. Situations may arise involving simultaneous exposures to multiple categories of potential hazards. For example, tank, aircraft, and submarine crews may be exposed to a variety of simultaneous hazards including blast injury, acoustical energy, toxicants in the air, extremes in barometric pressure, oxygen deficiency, and whole-body vibration (20). In the combat environment all resources are directed toward winning the battle as quickly and decisively as possible, which minimizes the number of casualties. Occupational exposures cannot be closely monitored unless there is reason to believe these may adversely effect the military mission or cause serious harm to our troops.

### Preventive Medicine Support of Military Operations

The DoD promotes the health and safety of its military members and civilian employees under provisions of the Occupational Safety and Health Act of 1970 and various DoD directives and instructions (20). DoD occupational safety and health programs for both military and DoD civilian employees are directed toward maintaining health and fitness, enhancing combat effectiveness, minimizing illness and injury, and eliminating loss of life. These occupational health programs identify work-related hazards, assess human health risks, conduct medical screening, provide diagnostic evaluations, provide consultation to line commanders, and communicate health risk information to the entire chain of command. Depending on their occupational specialty, some civilians and service members participate in occupational health surveillance programs (e.g., hearing conservation, respiratory protection, protection against blood-borne pathogens, pesticide application) as a result of identified occupational health hazards in the workplace. Also, all military members receive periodic medical examinations to ensure fitness for duty.

It is impractical to conduct extensive workplace monitoring on the battlefield or in combat simulated training; instead, the services conduct detailed health hazards assessments as part of their materiel acquisition processes (20). These programs assess the hazards associated with the operation and maintenance of military equipment to ensure that military personnel are not exposed to unnecessary health risks. In the field, during training exercises and in combat, military preventive medicine personnel are often present to identify health hazards and threats, and to place them in proper perspective relative to the military operational task at hand. Preventive medicine teams usually include physicians trained in preventive, occupational, or aerospace medicine; veterinarians; entomologists; sanitary engineers; industrial hygienists; and other military public health specialists. In general, protection is provided through instruction to avoid or reduce health threats, personal protective equipment and clothing, repellents, prophylactic medications and vaccines, sanitation and hygiene programs, and pest management operations (19,20). Prior to military operations, anticipated biologic, chemical, physical, and psychological hazards are identified and appropriate interventions designed to eliminate or reduce health threats.

## POTENTIAL GULF WAR HEALTH HAZARDS

A variety of physical, chemical, biologic, and psychosocial hazards commonly associated with military operations were present in the Persian Gulf environment, in addition to hazards unique to the Persian Gulf War (Table 1) (21). Any assessment of Gulf War veterans' health hazards is limited because comprehensive exposure data were not collected during the conflict. In addition, civilian occupational exposures are potential confounders in the evaluation of health problems among Gulf War veterans since a large proportion of this population served in the reserves/National Guard and also had non-

**TABLE 1.** *Potential health hazards associated with deployment to the Persian Gulf*

| |
|---|
| Accidents and injuries |
| Infectious diseases |
| Leishmaniasis |
| Biologic warfare |
| Immunizations |
| Pyridostigmine bromide prophylaxis |
| The desert environment |
| Heat stress |
| Sand |
| Oil-well fire smoke |
| Depleted uranium |
| Chemical warfare agents |
| Psychological factors |

military jobs. The following exposures constitute the major recognized potential health hazards resulting from this wartime deployment.

### Accidents and Injuries

Deployed military personnel were at high risk of injury while hurriedly preparing and transporting equipment and supplies, training, and eventually fighting a war. Accidents were a leading cause of mortality during this deployment (7). Training and sports-related activities were common causes of morbidity (5,22,23). Musculoskeletal problems are frequent in military populations and may be related to requirements for constant physical conditioning and the military's emphasis on physical fitness (24,25).

### Infectious Diseases

Along with accidents and injuries, travelers'-type diarrhea and acute upper respiratory infections were common problems (4,5). These infectious diseases are routinely encountered when troops are crowded together during deployments. Also, arthropod-borne infections were anticipated, particularly sandfly fever and cutaneous leishmaniasis, because these diseases had caused high morbidity among allied troops stationed in the Persian Gulf during World War II. In fact, a total of just 32 cases of cutaneous and viscerotropic leishmaniasis, seven cases of malaria, and one case of West Nile fever were diagnosed among U.S. troops (4). Also, there were three cases of Q fever, but no case of sandfly fever or brucellosis was identified (4). The very low number of serious infectious diseases has been attributed to cold weather conditions during the height of the buildup in December and January, the appropriate use of pesticides, and deployment to barren desert locations (4,6).

The only chronic infectious disease associated with this war was viscerotropic leishmaniasis caused by *Leishmania tropica*, a parasite species that typically causes cutaneous and not systemic disease (26). Because just 12 cases have been diagnosed and 11 of these cases had readily detectable signs of pathology, viscerotropic leishmaniasis has not been considered to be a major cause of undiagnosed symptoms (11). Nevertheless, specific diagnostic tests, which are under development by DoD, are needed to determine the prevalence of latent infection among Gulf War veterans.

A previously unidentified or emerging infectious disease has been considered as a possible cause of chronic symptoms in Gulf War veterans (27). However, no clinical sign or laboratory abnormality indicative of a systemic infectious process has been demonstrated among veterans (9,14). Although Iraq maintained an active biologic warfare research program, agents of biologic warfare, like anthrax and botulinum toxin, are designed to be highly lethal in very small quantities and would not be expected to cause chronic illness without acute symptoms proximal to the time of exposure or characteristic pathology (11).

### Immunizations

A possible side effect from immunizations is another hypothesized cause of long-term morbidity among Gulf War veterans (9). Deployed troops were provided with routine booster immunizations, and immune globulin was administered for hepatitis A prophylaxis. Primary vaccination series were administered during basic training or boot camp, when troops are initially inducted into the military. Two additional, nonlive vaccines were administered: approximately 8,000 U.S. troops received an botulinum toxoid used under investigational new drug (IND) provisions of the Food and Drug Administration (FDA), and about 150,000 individuals received one or two doses of an FDA-licensed anthrax vaccine (1). The vaccinations given to U.S. troops have a long record of safety when administered alone or in combination, and are not known to cause chronic symptomatology (28).

### Desert Environment

The first 2 months of the deployment were especially dangerous for ground troops because of the hot desert environment, with daily high temperatures up to 108°F (1,5,21). Initial preventive medicine efforts therefore concentrated on providing potable water and ensuring adequate hydration. These efforts resulted in very few heat casualties (5). By the time the war began in January, troops had to endure cold weather conditions with mean daily high temperatures of 65°F and mean low temperatures of 45°F (21).

Blowing sand also was considered a potential health threat in the desert. Air sampling after the war indicated that respirable and nonrespirable particulate matter concentrations exceeded U.S. standards (29,30). Nevertheless, most respiratory complaints among troops were not associated with exposure to the outdoor environment, and an increased rate of pulmonary disease has not been reported among guest workers living in the Persian Gulf (31,32).

### Oil-Well Fire Smoke

The Iraqi military ignited over 600 oil well fires during their retreat from Kuwait in February 1991 (1). These fires had the potential of producing a major ecological disaster and a serious health threat over wide areas of Kuwait and Saudi Arabia. Consequently, extensive atmospheric monitoring was conducted shortly after the war by the U.S. Army, U.S. Environmental Protection Agency (EPA), and other international agencies.

Ground-level pollutant concentrations from air sampling were found to be much lower than anticipated (11,30). Measured levels of pollutant gases and polycyclic aromatic hydrocarbons (PAHs) were comparable to concentrations measured in large U.S. cities, possibly due to the rapid rise of smoke into a consolidated superplume, which prevented contaminants from reaching high concentrations in the breathing zone at ground level. The results of a health risk assessment conducted by the Army concluded that the potential for long-term health effects was minimal (30). The major risk was considered to be from the inhalation of volatile organic compounds (VOCs), particulate heavy metals, and PAHs. However, the predicted carcinogenic risk levels were estimated not to exceed three cases per million exposed population. This level was within the EPA range of acceptable excess risk. Also, the predicated noncarcinogenic risk was low, ranging from 0.6 to 2.0 hazard indices (HI) in Saudi Arabia and from 2.0 to 5.0 HI in Kuwait (a HI of greater than 1 indicates increased risk for a general population that includes young children and elderly persons) (11,30). Analysis of biologic samples from deployed troops, local inhabitants, and autopsy cases, to date, do not indicate a risk from atmospheric pollution (9,11,30,33). One study found an increase in sister-chromatid exchanges in soldiers deployed from Germany to the Persian Gulf, but the cause for the genic stress was not determined (34).

### Depleted Uranium

In the war with Iraq, the U.S. military used some munitions containing depleted uranium (DU) as the penetrator in artillery and antitank shells because of DU's enhanced armor-piercing capability (1). Also, DU's high density and strength make it an ideal component of the armor on tanks and other combat vehicles. DU is a by-product of the uranium enrichment process and is composed of three isotopes, $^{238}U$ (99.75%), $^{235}U$ (0.25%), and $^{234}U$ (0.0005%). Although the chemical and physical properties of natural uranium and DU are essentially identical, their radiologic properties differ since DU is roughly 60% as radioactive as natural uranium. A health risk is presented when this heavy metal enters the body as shrapnel or is inhaled following aerosolization from combustion or impact with armor (11). Soldiers potentially exposed included those who worked on battle damaged vehicles that may have been contaminated with DU dust. Some service members were struck by friendly fire and retain DU shell fragments. The VA is following 32 wounded soldiers who retain DU shell fragments. To date, these soldiers have not developed the types of immunologic, neurologic, or renal disease that could result from radiation exposure or heavy metal intoxication.

### Pesticides

As is routine in overseas military deployments, pesticides and insect repellents were utilized by U.S. forces to prevent the transmission of rodent- and insect-borne diseases. The vast majority of pesticides were applied by trained, certified applicators, using EPA-registered products, including organophosphates, carbamates, chlorinated hydrocarbons, anticoagulants, and boric acid (9,11). Although most of the deployment took place during the cool winter months (when insect vector numbers are at their seasonal low), the U.S. military did have insect repellents *n,n*-diethyl-m-toluamide (DEET) and permethrin available for use. In addition to the official products, troops frequently used commercial insect repellents purchased in the U.S. The epidemiology of pesticide use by the military has not been characterized in published reports; however, no cases of acute pesticide poisoning were known to have occurred among U.S. troops in the Gulf (1,11).

### Pyridostigmine Bromide

U.S. troops were supplied with one or two blister packs of 30-mg tablets (21 to a pack) of pyridostigmine bromide (PB) as pretreatment for chemical warfare (CW) nerve agent exposure. One tablet of PB was to be self-administered every 8 hours when the risk of a CW attack was deemed to be high during the air and ground war. It is estimated that approximately 250,000 U.S. troops took at least one 30-mg tablet of PB (11). Although licensed since the 1950s for the treatment of myasthenia gravis, PB required clearance by the FDA to be used in an IND status for CW prophylaxis (9).

Pyridostigmine bromide, a carbamate, reversibly binds to the enzyme acetylcholinesterase (AChE), preventing the organophosphate nerve agent from irreversibly binding to and inactivating AChE. By protecting a portion of the enzyme from nerve agent inactivation, the ability to survive a potentially lethal exposure to chemical nerve agent (e.g., soman) is increased when PB has been used prior to postexposure treatment with atropine and praxlidoxime chloride (2-PAM). Minor acute gastrointestinal and urinary discomfort was commonly reported with the use of PB, but serious side effects requiring discontinuation of the drug occurred in less than 0.1% of troops (35). PB has not been considered a likely cause of chronic illness after the war because of the low doses involved, short half-life of PB, and long record of safety using this drug in much higher doses (1,11,15).

A basic toxicology study of the acute interactions of PB, DEET, and permethrin when administered orally to rats was conducted by the U.S. Army (11). Because lethality was the end point, very high doses were administered orally. The investigators noted a potential synergism of effect when PB was combined with DEET and permethrin. More recently, a study by Abou-Donia et al. (36) indicated that at high, nonlethal doses, of the same three compounds, acute synergistic neurotoxic effects occur in a chicken model. The relevance of high-dose acute toxicity studies in hens to the potential for chronic effects in humans from subclinical exposures is unknown. The DoD and VA are supporting several studies to address these scientific questions (10).

### Chemical Warfare Agents

Iraq had an extensive arsenal of CW nerve and blister agents (e.g., mustard agent) that had been employed during the Iran-Iraq war. During the war there were several reports by coalition forces of nerve and mustard agent detections at very low levels for brief periods of time (1,11). A source of CW agents has not been verified that can account for these detections. Several days after the end of hostilities up to 100,000 troops may have been exposed to subclinical levels of CW agents from the destruction of unmarked CW weapons at a munitions storage facility in Iraq.

Data regarding the long-term health effects related to nerve agent exposure are limited (1). Minor electroencephalographic changes have been noted more than a year after symptomatic exposure (37); however, the clinical significance of such findings are unclear. A study examining the long-term or delayed health effects of anticholinesterases tested on 1,400 military volunteers in the 1960s and 1970s was unable to rule out the possibility that some agents produced long-term adverse health effects in some individuals (38). However, current scientific evidence indicates that acute subclinical exposure to organophosphate nerve agents does not cause long-term neurophysiologic health effects (1,11,21). On the other hand, blister agents like mustard agent cause acute inflammation of the skin and mucosal surfaces and can pose a long-term risk of pulmonary disease and cancer.

Current findings suggest that CW agents are not a primary cause of chronic symptoms of Gulf War veterans. First, there were no reports of acute toxicity compatible with exposure to either CW agents or pesticides during the deployment. Second, the types of chronic neurologic and pulmonary pathology expected from exposure to pesticides or CW agents have not been observed in clinical evaluations of over 100,000 veterans by the DoD and VA (9,14). However, additional research is needed to thoroughly understand any potential long-term health effects of very low level exposure to CW agents, pesticides, and/or repellents (1,11). In particular, further investigation of the possible combined effects among these chemical agents and PB is needed.

### Psychological Stressors

The psychological stressors associated with deployment to a war zone were an important health risk for military personnel deployed to the Gulf. Troops often had the added burden of having to leave behind family and civilian jobs because a larger proportion of this combat force was composed of slightly older reservists/National Guard personnel (17%) and women (7%) than in previous wars (11,39).

Troops were rushed into a harsh desert environment where they were crowded into warehouses and tents, with little privacy, a limited diet, and primitive sanitary facilities (1,5). Typically, military personnel were isolated from local populations and had few opportunities for recreation. Contributing to the tensions of the deployment, coalition forces initially were outnumbered by the Iraqi army, and throughout the 5-month buildup period there was mounting uncertainty about Iraq's willingness to use chemical and biologic weapons (9).

After hostilities began, the lives of coalition troops were directly threatened in combat and from Scud missile attacks. Following an unexpectedly short war, the rapid return home of troops and subsequent readjustment provided another period of stress (39). Finally, widespread reports of unexpected deaths, mystery illnesses, and birth defects have contributed to the health concerns of Gulf War veterans (11).

### Other Exposures

Additional health hazards included potential exposure to microwaves; isocyanate containing, chemical-agent–resistant coating (CARC) paint; petroleum products (principally diesel, leaded gasoline, and jet fuels, which sometimes were used in tent heaters or sprayed on the ground to dampen dust and blowing sand); and chemical agent decontamination solution containing propylene and ethylene glycol. Most of these exposures involved small numbers of troops and are not known to cause chronic symptoms without acute or measurable pathology (9,11).

## EPIDEMIOLOGIC INVESTIGATIONS, CLINICAL CARE, AND RESEARCH

Early reports of illnesses among troops from an Army and a Navy reserve unit led to initial clinical and epidemiologic investigations. These epidemiologic investigations were conducted before widespread publicity addressed this issue (1,11,40). Both of the initial field investigations were conducted to verify cases, identify exposures of interest, and establish a case definition. Patient interviews, written surveys, physical examinations, and medical record reviews were conducted. In both of these initial investigations, patients reported a broad range of symptoms and exposures. Also, onset of symptoms usually varied from weeks to months following the war. Patients did not present with consistent symptoms, and diagnoses were diverse, spanning multiple organ systems. A case definition(s) could not be constructed for a unique war-related illness. Additionally, neither investigation resulted in confirmation that linked the symptoms and illnesses reported by Gulf veterans to any exposures. Although difficult to document as an exposure, stress was recognized a potential contributing factor. The investigators reasoned that the emotional impact of the deployment itself was a plausible explanation for some of the medical problems noted.

Several large-scale research investigations have found that Gulf War veterans are subject to stress-related conditions, which have been associated with physical symptoms (11,41–45). Prior studies have demonstrated that diverse somatic symptoms—physical complaints, cognitive difficulties, and sleep disturbances—are common manifestations of stress associated with war and other traumatic experiences (46–49). These nonspecific symptoms also are reported frequently in the general population and among clinic outpatients (50,51).

Subsequent studies involving larger populations and comparison groups have found that Gulf War veterans self-report higher rates of diverse symptoms but did not identify a unique disease or demonstrate a consistent demographic, exposure, or geographic risk factor (45,52,53). Large epidemiologic studies also have found no overall increase among veterans in mortality or hospitalization rates for medical causes and no overall increase in birth defects (54–57). Consistent with mortality studies involving Vietnam War veterans, Gulf War veterans have had increased mortality from external causes, principally motor vehicle accidents (54).

### Clinical Examinations

In June 1994, the DoD implemented the Comprehensive Clinical Evaluation Program (CCEP) to provide examinations to veterans concerned about their health. This large clinical program was designed primarily to provide medical care rather than as a research study. Nevertheless, because the CCEP included systematic clinical evaluations, extensive clinical data were obtained that provide considerable insight into the nature of illnesses being experienced by Gulf War veterans (58).

The DoD has provided medical examinations to Gulf War veterans using a two-phased clinical approach comparable to one used by the VA Registry Program. Phase I of the CCEP contains a self-administered exposure checklist, a standardized provider-administered symptoms questionnaire, and a physical examination similar in scope to an inpatient medical admission workup. The phase I laboratory panel includes a complete blood count, urinalysis, and blood chemistries. Patients who do not have a clearly defined diagnosis that explains their symptoms are referred to medical specialists in one of 14 DoD medical centers for a more definitive diagnostic workup and evaluation. Components of the phase II evaluation include administration of the Structured Clinical Interview for the *Diagnostic and Statistical Manual* (DSM-III-R), the Clinician Administered Posttraumatic Stress Disorder (PTSD) Scale, and additional laboratory tests. An independent panel of experts from the Institute of Medicine has reviewed the CCEP clinical protocol and concluded that it is a thorough, systematic approach to the diagnosis of a wide spectrum of diseases (58).

In April 1996 DoD reported data derived from the examination of 18,598 participants, which included information on self-reported exposures, symptoms, and diagnostic outcomes. CCEP participants were asked to responded to a checklist of 25 possible exposures. The most frequently self-reported environmental exposures included passive cigarette smoke (88%), diesel and other fuels (88%), pyridostigmine bromide tablets (74%), oil fire smoke (71%), tent heater fumes (70%), and personal pesticide use (66%). Possible exposures that were self-reported least often include nerve gas/nerve agent (6%), mustard/blistering agents (2%), and wounded in combat (2%). Nearly one-third of the CCEP participants indicated they were current smokers, smoking an average of 15 cigarettes per day. CCEP participants report a wide variety of symptoms spanning multiple organ systems in no consistent, clinically apparent pattern. The most frequently reported chief complaints were joint pain (11%), fatigue (10%), headache (7%), dermatitis (7%), and memory loss (4%). CCEP participants were asked to record up to eight symptoms. The proportion of CCEP participants listing the following symptoms included joint pain (49%), fatigue (47%), headache (39%), memory loss (34%), sleep disturbance (32%), rash/dermatitis (31%), difficulty concentrating (27%), depression (23%), muscle pain (21%), diarrhea (18%), dyspnea (18%), abdominal pain (17%), and/or hair loss (12%). When participants were asked to recall a date of onset, over one-half of all patients could not recall or did not list when their symptoms began. Among those who did list a date of onset, the 9-month interval after the Gulf War was the average time period listed.

Among the first 20,000 self-referred veterans enrolled in this clinical case series, the types of primary and secondary diagnoses varied widely (Table 2), with a total of 1,263 separate ICD-9-CM codes required to categorize primary diagnoses (14). The most common diagnoses involved the following three broad International Classification of Diseases–Clinical Modification (ICD-9-CM) categories: (a) musculoskeletal diseases; (b) mental disorders; and (c) symptoms, signs, and ill-defined conditions.

No distinctive pulmonary, renal, or immunologic disease was diagnosed that would indicate exposure to a common environmental health hazard. Also, a characteristic neurologic disease was not identified among over 800 veterans who had extensive neurophysiologic and neuropsychological testing, which included nerve con-

**TABLE 2.** *Frequency of primary and secondary diagnoses by broad ICD-9-CM categories among the first 20,000 self-referred Gulf War veterans evaluated by DoD in the Comprehensive Clinical Evaluation Program (CCEP)*

| | Percent with diagnosis | |
|---|---|---|
| Category (ICD-9-CM code) | Primary | Secondary |
| Diseases of the musculoskeletal system and connective tissue (710–739) | 18.6 | 29.5 |
| Mental disorders (290–319) | 18.3 | 17.9 |
| Symptoms, signs, ill-defined conditions (780–799) | 17.8 | 32.6 |
| Diseases of the respiratory system (460–519) | 6.8 | 10.8 |
| Diseases of skin and subcutaneous tissue (680–709) | 6.3 | 13.7 |
| Diseases of the digestive system (520–579) | 6.2 | 14.1 |
| Diseases of nervous system and sense organs (320–389) | 5.8 | 12.3 |
| Infectious and parasitic diseases (001–139) | 2.6 | 6.4 |
| Diseases of the circulatory system (390–459) | 2.2 | 5.9 |
| Endocrine, nutritional, and metabolic diseases, and immunity disorders (240–279) | 2.1 | 6.1 |
| Diseases of the genitourinary system (580–629) | 1.3 | 4.2 |
| Injury and poisoning (800–999) | 0.8 | 2.4 |
| Neoplasms (140–239) | 0.8 | 2.1 |
| Diseases of the blood and blood-forming organs (280–289) | 0.6 | 2.6 |
| Congenital anomalies; certain conditions originating in the perinatal period (740–779) | 0.2 | 0.9 |

duction studies and electromyography on 300 veterans; and EEGs, electromyography, and muscle biopsies on a smaller population (14,59,60). Lastly, no indication was found of a systemic infectious disease (except for previously identified viscerotropic leishmaniasis) or of transmission of an infectious disease among 831 family members evaluated in the CCEP.

The CCEP participants with either a primary or secondary diagnosis within the symptoms, signs, and ill-defined conditions category varied substantially in clinical presentation, and no characteristic laboratory abnormality or physical sign was identified, including a skin rash or fever (14,61). Additionally, as a group, veterans within this category were not severely disabled compared to CCEP participants in other diagnostic categories.

Although the DoD and VA have clinically examined more than 10% of all U.S. veterans, registry findings have to be carefully qualified since a rare or mild illness could have been missed even in a very large clinical case series where an appropriate comparison or control population was not available to characterize illness rates. Nevertheless, the massive size of the CCEP cohort and the systematic approach of the CCEP examination provide substantial insight toward characterizing the nature of these veterans' symptoms, illnesses, and health concerns. The data for the CCEP cannot be used to test for possible associations between exposures and health effects; however, it can be combined with other information to identify promising directions for more definitive research (58).

### Gulf War Health Research

The DoD, VA, and HHS have initiated an extensive and coordinated research program to study Gulf War health problems (8–10). A document entitled "A Working Plan for Research on Persian Gulf Veterans' Illnesses" was published in 1995 and revised in 1996 (10). The Working Plan details relevant research questions, catalogues research projects that address these questions, and lists some initial findings.

Researchers have had to contend with the inherent limitations of conducting studies after an extraordinary wartime experience. In general, only retrospective analyses of wartime health risks and outcomes are possible. Recall and selection bias remain a problem in studies that rely on self-reports, especially if the study population(s) have been the focus of widespread publicity about possible adverse exposures and illnesses (62). In addition to self selection and recall bias, confounding and chance findings from multiple comparisons are major considerations when conducting research studies that involve a large number of potential hazardous exposures and health outcomes that lack objective measures. While recognizing these limitations, the U.S. government has continued to pursue an extensive basic science, clinical, and epidemiologic research program to evaluate Gulf War health issues (8,10,11).

Several studies have demonstrated that while objective measures remained consistent between study and comparison groups, in certain groups of Persian Gulf veterans there is a greater prevalence of self-reported symptoms when compared to nondeployed veterans (52,63). Investigators have demonstrated in 1,498 Seabees (Construction Battalion personnel) an increase of self-reported symptoms among deployed versus nondeployed Seabees, with no physical correlates (63). Of interest, objective measures, such as clinical laboratory results, pulmonary function tests, or hand-grip strength test results were not significantly different between study and comparison groups (52,63). Investigators with the Centers for Disease

Control and Prevention (CDC) and the State of Pennsylvania have also demonstrated an increase of symptoms, but no differences in serology or other lab data, between groups of deployed versus nondeployed Air National Guardsmen in Pennsylvania (52). Investigators suspect that symptom patterns in the latter study bear a similarity to chronic fatigue syndrome; however, the severity of symptoms appear less debilitating than in chronic fatigue syndrome. Although clinical examinations were not conducted, in a study where a large number of both Persian Gulf veterans and nondeployed Service members were surveyed, Persian Gulf veterans self-reported significantly higher rates of symptoms than nondeployed individuals (45). Gulf War veterans also report that symptoms have adversely impacted their lives (45). Because each of these studies were restricted to very specific military units or a specific state of residence, generalizing the findings to all veterans is difficult. These findings, in selected groups of veterans, are consistent with the findings of DoD's CCEP and VA's Persian Gulf Registry program.

### Persian Gulf Veteran Morbidity and Mortality

Gray et al. (55) have shown that hospitalization rates and discharge diagnoses among active duty service members who served in the Persian Gulf were similar to those who were not deployed to the Persian Gulf. Although this study did not include those veterans who had separated from the military, the study does suggests that as a group Persian Gulf veterans are not experiencing a greater incidence of major illnesses. From death certificates, investigators Kang and Bullman (54) studied the mortality experience of Persian gulf veterans since the war. The study included all deaths from May 1, 1991 to September 30, 1993, recording cause-specific mortality for the 695,516 U.S. troops deployed for the Persian Gulf War compared to 746,291 nondeployed U.S. service members. The adjusted mortality rate ratio for deaths from all causes was 1.09 [95% confidence interval (CI) 1.01–1.16], implying a small increase in all-cause mortality among Persian Gulf War veterans. The excess deaths were attributed to external causes, including all accidents and motor vehicle accidents. It is important to note that despite the small increase in overall mortality for deployed veterans when compared to nondeployed military, the mortality risk from all causes for deployed veterans was half of that expected from the U.S. civilian population.

Focusing on specific categories of illness, research to determine the prevalence of organic neuropsychological and/or neurologic deficits in Persian Gulf veterans is a priority. Early studies of neuropsychological and neurologic outcomes suggest that self-selected Persian Gulf veterans demonstrate subtle differences from controls. Goldstein et al. (64) found that Persian Gulf Registry participants may have small, clinically insignificant neuropsychological deficits that could be related to the presence of psychological comorbidity. Another study of 14 British Gulf War veterans with unexplained illness also found possible indications of neurologic injury compared to 13 healthy controls (65). This study, by Jamal et al., found that Persian Gulf veterans with self-report symptoms showed evidence of small alterations in peripheral nervous system function. However, interpretation of these findings is difficult because of the small sample size and the possibility that the findings are confounded by several biases, including that of selection, recall, and misclassification.

The findings of a clinical and epidemiologic study of another reserve Seabee battalion also suggested that some veterans may have neurologic impairment (66–68). From a Battalion of 606 veterans, 249 (41%) elected to participate in the study. Neurologic testing was done on only 23 (4%) of the most ill study subjects (67). Test results were usually within normal limits and a panel of six neurologists could not identify a unique syndrome. However, the investigators did report that test findings were "significantly more in the abnormal direction" compared to a control population. Also, an accompanying cross-sectional survey found a possible association between self-reported chemical exposures in the Gulf and three postulated neurologic illnesses that were identified by factor analysis of self-reported symptoms (66,68). The Haley et al. (66–68) studies suggest that some members of their study population have symptoms associated with neuropsychological impairment representing chronic neurotoxicity caused by low-dose exposure to chemical agents. These studies raise important questions but have limitations that substantially weaken the authors' conclusions (62).

Conversely, these findings of possible neurologic impairment among Gulf War veterans have not been confirmed by four other clinical studies that involved a larger total number of veterans but no comparison study subjects (11,59,60,69,70). Additionally, a pilot clinical program at the Birmingham, Alabama, VA Medical Center conducted neuropsychological tests on veterans from the VA Persian Gulf Registry who self-report exposure to environmental hazards including chemical weapons. Preliminary evidence does not show any pattern to indicate a common, identifiable neuropathologic process (70).

### Adverse Birth Outcomes

In addition to the CDC-State of Mississippi study (56), computerized DoD hospital medical records of 33,998 children born to men and women who served in the Persian Gulf War were compared to those of 41,463 children born to military service members who were not deployed (57). The study noted that children born to Persian Gulf War veterans were not at increased risk of birth defects in general, or of specific serious congenital malformations as defined by the CDC (57). Because the study was based on records of live births, other reproductive outcomes, such as spontaneous abortions or miscarriages, could not be evaluated. However, the study did note that the proportion of veterans identified as having children since the war was not associated with Gulf War service, implying no reduction in fertility, and that the ratio of male babies to female babies did not vary between deployed and nondeployed study groups (57).

### Novel Hypotheses

Media and other reports of symptoms and illnesses of Gulf War veterans began shortly after and have continued sporadically since the end of the Gulf War. These reports, quoting scientists, advocacy groups, and various other individuals, have offered numerous explanations as to the cause or causes and the severity of illnesses. Speculation has ranged from a septicemia resulting from an invasive mycoplasma or bacterial cocci that can only be detected by special staining techniques of urine sediments to endogenous retrovirus infections and to brain stem pathology. To date, none of these hypotheses has met the generally accepted principles of peer-reviewed scientific investigation, such as randomized design, double-blinded methodologies, appropriate control groups, statistical rigor, known sensitivities and specificities of laboratory tests, and independent confirmation. However, until appropriate scientific methods have been applied and these hypotheses tested in a systematic way, the possibility remains that some of these hypotheses may eventually explain a portion of the conditions within subpopulations of Gulf War veterans.

## POSTWAR SYNDROMES

A review of prior war-related illnesses offers an important perspective on Gulf War health questions (16). The possible medical and psychological responses individuals have after being exposed to the stress of a war environment were noted after all major wars since the Civil War, including World Wars I and II (71–76). Systematic medical studies of war syndromes began during the U.S. Civil War when J. M. DaCosta evaluated soldiers for a poorly understood condition characterized by shortness of breath, palpitations, chest pain, fatigue, headache, diarrhea, and disturbed sleep. Another illness associated with the Civil War, "nostalgia," was characterized by obsessive thoughts of home and a variety of physical symptoms. A condition very similar to the one described by DaCosta became a major problem during World War I when British and U.S. soldiers presented with an unexplained illness characterized by shortness of breath, palpitations, chest pain, fatigue, headache, difficulty concentrating, forgetfulness, and nightmares (16). To care for these troops, specialized health care centers were established, a concerted research program was instituted, and pensions were provided for disabled veterans. By the end of WW I there was considerable controversy as to whether DaCosta's syndrome was primarily a medical or psychiatric illness. Another illness associated with WWI was acute combat stress reaction, which was popularly known as "shell shock." At the beginning of WWII, the controversy over the nature and causes of effort syndrome in World War I had not been resolved, but clinical studies eventually indicated a psychological etiology among WWII troops (16). A better understanding also was developed during WWII of acute combat stress reaction (now called battle or operational fatigue), which frequently was associated with fatigue, palpitations, diarrhea, headache, difficulty concentrating and remembering, and disturbed sleep.

Acute combat stress reaction continued to be an important problem during the Korean Conflict and Vietnam War. A high prevalence of PTSD, depression, and substance abuse was found among veterans of the Vietnam War (77,78), in addition to other personal and social difficulties (79,80). In a comparison with contemporaries who did not serve in Vietnam, Vietnam veterans also reported more physical symptoms and illnesses (81), and a lower general state of health (82), although physical abnormalities usually were not associated with these reports. Other studies have also found a correlation between levels of PTSD symptoms and reported physical health problems (83,84); however, part of this is expected due to the relation of combat injury to PTSD.

After the Vietnam War, the most controversial health issues were PTSD and the potential toxic effects of exposure to Agent Orange, namely, 2,4,5,-trichlorophenoxyacetic acid (2,4,5-T), which contained the contaminant 2,3,7,8-tetrachlorodibenzo-p-dioxin (2,3,7,8-TCDD). Analogous to prior war-related illnesses, Vietnam veterans who had PTSD or who may have been exposed to Agent Orange had higher self-reported rates of somatic complaints (Table 3).

This brief historical review illustrates that since the Civil War there have been two general categories of poorly understood and controversial war-related illnesses: one postulated to be caused by organic disease and another due to wartime stress. The diagnosis of these syndromes has been problematic because they were identified by similar nonspecific symptoms (Table 3). Over time, unexplained symptoms among war veterans have been attributed primarily to psychological factors, rather than to hazardous environmental exposures, because a disease process was not identified and stress and psychological illness frequently cause chronic physical symptoms (16). The symptoms reported by Gulf War veterans are similar to the diversity of physical complaints associated with prior war syndromes (16). Also analogous to prior war syndromes, there remains uncertainty whether

**TABLE 3.** *Somatic symptoms commonly associated with war-related medical and psychological illnesses*

| Symptoms | War and illness | | | | | |
|---|---|---|---|---|---|---|
| | Civil War, DaCosta's syndrome | WW I, effort syndrome | WW II, combat stress reaction | Vietnam, Agent Orange exposure | Vietnam/ other conflicts, PTSD | Persian Gulf, unexplained illnesses |
| Fatigue or exhaustion | + | + | + | + | + | + |
| Shortness of breath | + | + | + | | + | + |
| Palpitations and tachycardia | + | + | + | | + | |
| Precordial pain | + | + | | | + | + |
| Headache | + | + | + | + | + | + |
| Muscle or joint pain | | | | + | + | + |
| Diarrhea | + | | + | + | + | + |
| Excessive sweating | + | + | + | | | |
| Dizziness | + | + | + | + | + | |
| Fainting | + | + | | | | |
| Disturbed sleep | + | + | + | + | + | + |
| Forgetfulness | | + | + | + | + | + |
| Difficulty concentrating | | + | + | + | + | + |

+, a commonly reported symptom.
Reprinted with permission from ref. 16; the American College of Physicians is not responsible for the accuracy of the translation.

these symptoms represent an organic disease or are due to psychological factors.

## HEALTH CONSEQUENCES OF THE GULF WAR

### Persian Gulf Illnesses

Many of the concerns regarding the health consequences of the Gulf War have focused around three fundamental issues: (a) whether or not veterans are experiencing illnesses at a higher frequency than would be expected; (b) whether or not Gulf War veterans are experiencing a unique illness or syndrome; and (c) whether or not the illnesses being experienced by veterans are the result of some aspect of their Gulf War experiences.

As mentioned earlier in the chapter, epidemiologic studies and clinical case series confirm that groups of Gulf War veterans report experiencing various combinations of physical symptoms; and that there is evidence to suggest that the rates of these symptoms are higher when compared with groups of non–Gulf War veterans. However, these observations have occurred without detection of clinically significant abnormal physical findings, laboratory tests, or diagnostic procedures. Gulf War veterans presenting with varying combinations of physical symptoms (ranging from discrete to nonspecific) for evaluation in the clinical programs provided by the federal government usually have been diagnosed with the types of illnesses commonly seen in primary care practice (50,85). Medical practitioners have made these diagnoses in the absence of definitional criteria for a unique syndrome, using standard professional practice methods and diagnostic criteria. Finally, as a group, initial studies have indicated that the overall hospitalization and mortality experience of Gulf War veterans has been favorable compared to that of the general population.

Although limited, studies of outpatient practice have identified symptom patterns similar to those observed among Gulf War veterans (86). However, diagnostic coding of patients' presenting problems in primary care settings is a complex process. Evidence indicating that about half of all diagnoses in primary care visits do not resolve into codable diagnostic entries (87) may provide an important context for interpreting the diagnostic information related to the evaluation of Gulf War veterans. The degree to which veterans' symptoms, illnesses, and conditions differ from what might be expected in a comparable military or civilian populations will require further study.

### Causes of Gulf War Veterans' Illnesses

Gulf War veterans do not appear to be experiencing a single disease or syndrome, but rather multiple illnesses with overlapping symptoms and causes (15). Inability to find a comprehensive answer to the causes of fatigue, headache, memory problems, and other generalized, nonspecific symptoms experienced by Gulf veterans who do not have conditions that fit defined diagnostic criteria reflect limitations that currently exist in primary care practice as observed in other adult populations. The fundamental causes of nonspecific symptoms are not well understood in the general population (51,88). The physical symptoms reported by some Gulf War veterans who do not have clearly defined diagnoses have been compared to other symptom-based conditions, including chronic fatigue syndrome, fibromyalgia, and allergy/sensitivity disorders (21,52,89). Because objective and specific diagnostic criteria have not been defined for these postulated conditions, it currently has not been possible to establish a relationship with veterans' illnesses (90).

Six expert panels have reviewed Gulf War risk factors that may have contributed to the development of Persian Gulf illnesses (1,11,15,21,91) (Table 4). None of the panels has identified a unique syndrome or a single environmental exposure as a likely cause of illnesses among widespread groups of veterans. However, these deliberations were conducted with limited data to quantitatively characterize possible dose-response relationships for some potential health hazards. In one of the most extensive scientific reviews conducted to date, the Presidential Advisory Committee considered the short-term and long-term health consequences of various exposure scenarios, including high-level to low-level exposure, single to multiple exposures, and chronic or continuing exposure. Their assessment included an extensive review of the scientific literature and consideration of possible health effects independent of whether exposures were undocumented, lack precision, were known. The panel did not identify a physical or chemical risk factor as a likely cause of Gulf War veterans' illnesses. It did endorse continued investigation into areas of uncertainty about Gulf War risk factors including the long-term effects of low-level exposures to chemical warfare agents and the synergistic effects of exposures to pyridostigmine bromide and other risk factors.

The interpretation and application of the conclusions of the various expert panels regarding Persian Gulf risk factors must be done with caution. Patients' health problems result from a combination of many different factors, only some of which may be work-related. Any assessment as to whether an individual's illness might be related to their Persian Gulf experience should carefully weigh all of the causal factors that have occurred over the period of time of interest. As in most occupational health settings, the following fundamental principles are worthy of consideration: clinically, most occupational or environmental illnesses are indistinguishable from those of nonenvironmental origin; many illnesses of occupational or environmental cause are multifactorial, with nonenvironmental factors also contributing to the disease process; and, finally, individuals differ in their clinical susceptibility to hazardous exposures. Given these principles and the complexity of the Gulf War environment, it is plausible that the Gulf War experience was a contributing or aggravating factor in the development of some illnesses among veterans.

**TABLE 4.** *United States expert review panels that have evaluated Gulf War health issues*

| |
|---|
| Defense Science Board Task Force on Persian Gulf War Health Effects (1) |
| Department of Veterans' Affairs Persian Gulf Expert Scientific Committee (113) |
| National Institutes of Health Technology Assessment Workshop Panel: The Persian Gulf Experience and Health (15) |
| Institute of Medicine, Committee to Review the Health Consequences of Service During the Persian Gulf War (21,91) |
| Institute of Medicine, Committee on the DoD Persian Gulf Syndrome Comprehensive Clinical Evaluation Program (58) |
| Presidential Advisory Committee on Gulf War Veterans' Illnesses (11) |

In December 1996, the Presidential Advisory Committee on Gulf War Veterans' Illnesses concluded that stress is likely to be an important contributing factor in the development of the broad range of illnesses currently being reported by Gulf War veterans (11). The conclusion was based on the recognition that veterans experienced extraordinarily stressful circumstances during and since the Gulf War, on diagnoses of psychiatric disorders and forms of mental illnesses that have a stress component, and on the realization that stress is known to affect the brain, immune system, cardiovascular system, and various hormonal responses.

Relatively few individuals were exposed to actual combat during the Persian Gulf conflict, the circumstance found to be most clearly associated with development of PTSD and other psychiatric problems after involvement in a war (92,93). Although this was generally true, there were several extraordinarily stressful circumstances in the Gulf War setting, including theater-wide threats of Scud missile attacks. Significantly higher levels of mental health symptoms were noted among deployed as compared to nondeployed personnel in a study involving Army, Navy, and Marine reservists, and these symptoms seemed to be correlated with higher levels of stress exposure (94,95). Observing or handling human remains is also very stressful and was a part of Persian Gulf experience for some service members. Previous studies have indicated increased psychological distress in people exposed to dead bodies following a disaster (96,97). A comparison of Gulf War participants who handled remains and those who did not found significantly higher levels of intrusive and avoidant symptoms in the former (98). Eight months following the Gulf War, considerable psychopathology was found among a group of Army reservists who served in a war zone and performed grave-registration duty (99). Higher levels of psychopathology were found among reservists who did grave-registration work in the Persian Gulf, as compared to in the United States (100). During the Persian Gulf War, Reserve and National Guard units experienced some stressors to a higher degree than active duty members: minimal preparation time for deployment, family and vocational disruption, and financial distress resulting from loss of civilian employment (39). Findings of Israeli researchers provide further data to indicate that the stress of the Gulf War extended beyond direct combat experiences. Moderate levels of psychological distress were found in many soldiers who were not in direct combat (101). These difficulties were attributed to a combination of factors, including fear of impending missile attacks, the impression created by the news media that the population of Israel was experiencing acute distress, and a low level of trust in Army authorities.

### Individual and Community Responses to Traumatic Events

The trauma of armed conflict is not unique in causing or contributing to the development of health problems. The symptoms and conditions reported previously by groups of individuals who have experienced high levels of trauma and disaster stress (102) are similar in many respects to those reported by Gulf War veterans (14,24). Physical symptoms and psychiatric morbidity have been found in nonmilitary groups following natural catastrophes, with higher rates of somatic symptoms reported in both man-made and natural disaster populations (103,104). The correlation of PTSD with somatic complaints has been seen in these situations as well (105). Additionally, neuropsychiatric symptoms, including weakness, fatigue, malaise, anxiety, depressed or irritable mood, difficulty concentrating, distractibility, and memory impairment are commonly experienced by members of groups following acute or chronic exposure to a wide range of noxious substances in occupational and environmental settings (106). These symptoms may result from the direct toxic effect of exposure on the central nervous system, from psychological or emotional reactions to exposure, or from a combination of both (106). Finally, the media, community forums, and governmental actions can markedly influence a community's reactions to plausible environmental threats (107). Since the end of the Gulf War, the media, advocacy groups, and other community forums have placed considerable attention and emphasis on health problems of Persian Gulf veterans, sometimes implicating one or more exposures as a possible cause. In many instances these information sources appeared credible and authoritative and helped influence how veterans attribute their illnesses to their wartime experiences even before thorough assessment and evaluations could be performed.

### Clinical Care

Because Gulf War veterans have been found to be subject to a wide diversity of illnesses that affect other adult populations, specific guidelines for diagnosis and treatment cannot be recommended. Each veteran has to be cared for as an individual, as in other outpatient settings (108,109). As in any clinical evaluation, a thorough environmental and occupational history, general health history, review of symptoms, and complete physical examination are essential. A history of workplace and wartime occupational risks is useful, but documentation generally is not available to quantify hazardous exposures among individual veterans. Clinicians should inquire about the specific scope of duties related to the veteran's military occupational specialty, lifetime deployment history, and the availability of military medical and immunization records. Diagnostic tests and specialty consultation have proven helpful when there is clinical evidence of a distinctive illness (58). No specific therapy has been found effective for veterans with nonspecific symptoms, but supportive care and a structured physical rehabilitation program has proven beneficial among some patients (24,58). Depressive and anxiety disorders may represent comorbid conditions and as such require appropriate diagnoses and treatment. Some Gulf War veterans evaluated through the CCEP have clinical presentations that appear to overlap with the symptom presentations described in fibromyalgia and chronic fatigue syndrome. Referrals to consultants with expertise in managing patients with chronic fatigue, chronic pain, and related disorders may be of benefit in severely impaired veterans (58).

## PREVENTION

The health issues raised by the Persian Gulf War have focused attention on the unique health threats of military deployments and the necessity for improved health surveillance of service personnel. The inability to resolve uncertainties regarding long-term, chronic health sequelae of Gulf War veterans is due in part to a deficiency of objective measures of health status and exposure information needed to evaluate potential health risks. The DoD has acted upon the recommendations of various scientific review panels, advisory groups, other federal agencies, and its own internal reviews of Gulf War health issues to develop a comprehensive medical surveillance policy for deployments. The policy incorporates lessons learned derived from the department's deployment experience not only in the Persian Gulf, but in Somalia and Haiti, as well. Components of the surveillance policy specify development of enhanced capabilities to identify populations at risk, conduct standardized health screening before and after deployments, assess and document hazardous exposures, and monitor health outcomes subsequent to deployments. The policy reflects the importance of targeting occupational and/or traumatic stressors within the war zone and the ensuing health problems of deployed personnel (110). Elements of the surveillance policy have been implemented in Bosnia including monitoring of air, soil, and water in geographic areas where U.S. forces are concentrated, health screening to identify medical and psychiatric conditions prior to departure from the theater (111), and deployment of combat stress management teams. The surveillance plan and other related programs will be used to develop intervention programs to help prevent or minimize the development of health problems after future deployments.

## CONCLUSIONS

During the Gulf War, U.S. military forces were very successful in maintaining the health of deployed troops and preventing combat deaths. Because troops experienced unprecedented low rates of morbidity and mortality, controversy over veterans' health was unforeseen just after the war. Among Gulf War veterans, there are clearly individuals who are experiencing symptoms and illnesses with real consequences. Various expert panels have concluded that Gulf War veterans do not appear to be experiencing a single disease or syndrome, but rather illnesses with overlapping symptoms and causes. To date, the results of epidemiologic studies, clinical care programs, and focused research efforts have provided some reassurance that veterans have diagnosable and treatable conditions; and initial studies suggest that the overall mortality and hospitalization of Gulf War veterans appears favorable compared to the general population.

However, as in previous conflicts, epidemiologic research has been hampered by inherent problems in research design and difficulties of measuring wartime exposures and long-term health outcomes (112). Scientific panels have been unable to identify a direct causal link between the symptoms and illnesses reported by Gulf War veterans and certain occupational and environmental exposures. Given the complexity of the Persian Gulf environment and the multiple variables that affect susceptibility to illness or injury, it is likely that Gulf War experiences have been a contributing or aggravating factor in the development of some veterans' illnesses. Although stress has been cited as an important contributing factor to a broad range of illnesses, a clearer understanding of the relationship between stress and the development of organic disease is needed (11,62). The health experiences of Gulf War veterans share similarities with the experiences of veterans of prior military conflicts and groups that have experienced traumatic events or hazardous exposures. The development of comprehensive surveillance programs by DoD and sponsorship of prioritized research to better understand the health consequences of stress and the possible interactions of drugs, biologicals, and chemicals in U.S. military forces represent major efforts to prevent adverse health consequences resulting from military operations.

## ACKNOWLEDGMENT

The views expressed in this manuscript are those of the authors and are not to be taken as the official opinion of the Department of Defense.

## REFERENCES

1. Department of Defense. *Report of the Defense Science Board Task Force on Persian Gulf War Health Effects, June 1994.* Washington, DC: Office of the Under Secretary of Defense for Acquisition and Technology, 1994.
2. Blanck RR, Bell WH. Special reports: medical aspects of the Persian Gulf war. Medical support for American troops in the Persian Gulf. *N Engl J Med* 1991;324:857–859.
3. Medicine in the Gulf War. *US Med* 1991;27:1–113.
4. Hyams KC, Hanson K, Wignall FS, et al. The impact of infectious diseases on the health of U.S. troops deployed to the Persian Gulf during Operations Desert Shield and Desert Storm. *Clin Infect Dis* 1995; 20:1497–1504.
5. Wasserman GM, Martin BL, Hyams KC, Merrill BR, Oaks HG, McAdoo HA. A survey of outpatient visits in a United States Army forward unit during Operation Desert Shield. *Milit Med* 1997;162: 374–379.
6. Lindsay GC, Dasey C. Operations Desert Shield/Storm infectious disease rates: a fortuitous anomaly. *United States Army Medical Research and Development Command News* 1992(February):5–6.
7. Writer JV, Defraites RF, Brundage JF. Comparative mortality among U.S. military personnel in the Persian Gulf region and worldwide during Operations Desert Shield and Desert Storm. *JAMA* 1996;275: 118–121.
8. Beach P, Blanck RR, Gerrity T, et al. Coordinating Federal efforts on Persian Gulf war veterans. *Fed Pract* 1995;12:9–11,15.
9. Persian Gulf Veterans Coordinating Board. Unexplained illnesses among Desert Storm veterans: a search for causes, treatment, and cooperation. *Arch Intern Med* 1995;155:262–268.
10. Persian Gulf Veterans Coordinating Board. *A working plan for research on Persian Gulf veterans' illnesses, first revision.* Washington, DC: Department of Veterans Affairs, 1996.
11. *Presidential Advisory Committee on Gulf War Veterans' Illnesses. Final report.* ISBN 0-16-048942-3. Washington, DC: U.S. Government Printing Office, 1996.
12. Revell T. The Gulf war syndrome (letter). *Br Med J* 1995;310:1073.
13. Robinson A. Veterans worry that unexplained medical problems a legacy of service during Gulf War. *Can Med Assoc J* 1995;152: 944–947.
14. Joseph SC, and the Comprehensive Clinical Evaluation Program Evaluation Team. A comprehensive clinical evaluation of 20,000 Persian Gulf war veterans. *Milit Med* 1997;162:149–155.
15. National Institutes of Health Technology Assessment Workshop Panel. The Persian Gulf experience and health. *JAMA* 1994;272:391–395.
16. Hyams KC, Wignall FS, Roswell R. War syndromes and their evaluation: from the U.S. Civil War to the Persian Gulf War. *Ann Intern Med* 1996;125:398–405.
17. Gaydos JC, Thomas RJ, Sack DM, Patterson RE. Armed forces, Emergency and security services. In: Stellman JM, ed. *ILO encyclopedia of occupational safety and health,* 4th ed. Geneva: International Labor Office, 1998;in press.
18. Institute of Medicine. *Interactions of drugs, biologics, and chemicals in U.S. military forces.* Washington, DC: National Academy Press, 1996.
19. Legters LJ, Llewellyn CH, Military Medicine. In: Maxey, Rosenau, Last, eds. *Public health and preventive medicine.* East Norwalk, CT: Appleton and Lange, 1992;1141–1157.
20. Deeter DP, Gaydos JC, eds. *Occupational health, the soldier and the industrial base, textbook of military medicine series.* Washington, DC: Walter Reed Army Medical Center, 1993.
21. Institute of Medicine. *Health consequences of service during the Persian Gulf war:* initial findings and recommendations for immediate action. Washington, DC: National Academy Press, 1995.
22. Stong GC, Hope JW, Kalenian MH. Medical evacuation experience of two 7th Corps medical companies supporting Desert Shield/Desert Storm. *Milit Med* 1993;158:108–113.
23. Hines JF. A comparison of clinical diagnoses among male and female soldiers deployed during the Persian Gulf war. *Milit Med* 1993;158: 99–101.
24. Department of Defense. *Comprehensive clinical evaluation program for Gulf War veterans:* CCEP report on 18,598 participants. Washington, DC: Office of the Assistant Secretary of Defense for Health Affairs—Clinical Services, 1996.

25. Armed Forces Epidemiological Board. *Injuries in the military, a hidden epidemic.* Aberdeen, MD: U.S. Army Center for Health Promotion and Preventive Medicine, 1995.
26. Magill AJ, Grogl M, Gasser RA, Sun W, Oster CN. Visceral infection caused by Leishmania tropica in veterans of Operation Desert Storm. *N Engl J Med* 1993;328:1383–1387.
27. Nicolson GL, Rosenberg-Nicolson NL. Doxycycline treatment and Desert Storm. *JAMA* 1995;273:618–619.
28. White CS, Adler WH, McGann VG. Repeated immunization: possible adverse effects. Reevaluation of human subjects at 25 years. *Ann Intern Med* 1974;81:594–600.
29. *Interim report:* Kuwait oil fire health risk assessment, no. 39.26-L192-91, 5 May–15 September 1991. Aberdeen Proving Ground, MD: Department of the Army, U.S. Army Environmental Hygiene Agency, 1991.
30. *Final report:* Kuwait oil fire health risk assessment, no. 39.26-L192-91, 5 May–3 Dec 1991. Aberdeen Proving Ground, MD: Department of the Army, U.S. Army Environmental Hygiene Agency, 1991.
31. Korenyi-Both AL, Molnar AC, Korenyi-Both AL, et al. Al Eskan disease: Desert Storm pneumonitis. *Milit Med* 1992;157:452–462.
32. Richards AL, Hyams KC, Watts DM, Rozmajzl PJ, Woody JN, Merrell BR. Respiratory disease among military personnel in Saudi Arabia during Operation Desert Shield. *Am J Public Health* 1993;83:1326–1329.
33. Coombe MD, Drysdate SF. Assessment of the effects of atmospheric oil pollution in post war Kuwait. *J R Army Med Corps* 1993;139: 95–97.
34. McDiarmid MA, Jacobson-Krane D, Loloder K, Deeter DP. Short communication: increased frequencies of sister chromatid exchange in soldiers deployed to Kuwait. *Mutagenesis* 1995;10(3):263–265.
35. Keeler JR, Hurst CG, Dunn MA. Pyridostigmine used as a nerve agent pretreatment under wartime conditions. *JAMA* 1991;266:693–695.
36. Abou-Donia MB, Wilmarth KR, Jensen KF, et al. Neurotoxicity resulting from coexposure to pyridostigmine bromide, DEET, and permethrin: implications of Gulf War chemical exposures. *J Toxicol Environ Health* 1996;48:35–56.
37. Duffy FH, Burchfiel JL, Bartels PH, Gaon M, Sim VM. Long-term effects of an organophosphate upon the human electroencephalogram. *Toxicol Appl Pharmacol* 1979;47:161–176.
38. Institute of Medicine, Division of Health Promotion and Disease Prevention. *Committee on the Evaluation of the Comprehensive Clinical Evaluation Program—Nerve Agents.* Washington, DC: National Academy Press, 1997.
39. Malone JD, Paige-Dobson B, Ohl C, DiGiovanni C, Cunnion S, Roy MJ. Possibilities for unexplained chronic illnesses among reserve units deployed in Operation Desert Shield/Desert Storm. *South Med J* 1996;89:1147–1155.
40. DeFraites RF, Wanat ER, Norwood AE, et al. *Report, investigation of a suspected outbreak of an unknown disease among veterans of Operation Desert Shield/Storm,* 123d Army Reserve Command, Fort Benjamin Harrison, Indiana, April, 1992. Washington, DC: Epidemiology Consultant Service (EPICON), Division of Preventive Medicine, Walter Reed Army Institute of Research, June 15, 1992.
41. Sutker PB, Uddo M, Brailey K, et al. War-zone trauma and stress-related symptoms in Operation Desert Shield/Storm (ODS) returnees. *J Soc Issues* 1993;49:33–49.
42. Stretch RH, Bliese PD, Marlowe DH, et al. Post-traumatic stress disorder symptoms among Gulf War veterans. *Milit Med* 1996;161: 407–410.
43. Labbate LA, Snow MP. Posttraumatic stress symptoms among soldiers exposed to combat in the Persian Gulf. *Hosp Community Psychiatry* 1992;43:831–833.
44. Ross MC, Wonders J. An exploration of the characteristics of post-traumatic stress disorder in reserve forces deployed during Desert Storm. *Arch Psychiatr Nurs* 1993;7:265–269.
45. The Iowa Persian Gulf Study Group. Self-reported illness and health status among Gulf war veterans. *JAMA* 1996;277:238–245.
46. Grinker RR, Spiegel JP. The syndrome of "Operational Fatigue" (War Neuroses) in returnees. In: *Men under stress.* York, PA: Maple Press, 1945.
47. The Centers for Disease Control Vietnam Experience Study: health status of Vietnam veterans. II. Physical health. *JAMA* 1988;259: 2708–2714.
48. Bremner JD, Scott TM, Delaney RC, et al. Deficits in short-term memory in posttraumatic stress disorder. *Am J Psychiatry* 1993;150: 1015–1019.
49. Yehuda R, Keefe RSE, Harvey PD, et al. Learning and memory in combat veterans with posttraumatic stress disorder. *Am J Psychiatry* 1995;152:137–139.
50. Kroenke K, Price RK. Symptoms in the community: prevalence, classification, and psychiatric comorbidity. *Arch Intern Med* 1993;153: 2474–2480.
51. Kroenke K, Wood DR, Mangelsdorff AD, Meier NJ, Powell JB. Chronic fatigue in primary care: prevalence, patient characteristics, and outcome. *JAMA* 1988;260:929–934.
52. Centers for Disease Control and Prevention. Unexplained illness among Persian Gulf War veterans in an Air National Guard unit: preliminary report—August 1990–March 1995. *MMWR* 1995;44: 443–447.
53. Stretch RH, Wright KM, Bliese PD, et al. Physical health symptomatology of Gulf War-era service personnel from the states of Pennsylvania and Hawaii. *Milit Med* 1995;160:131–136.
54. Kang HK, Bullman TA. Mortality among U.S. veterans of the Persian Gulf War. *N Engl J Med* 1996;335:1498–1504.
55. Gray GC, Coate BD, Anderson CM, Kang HK, Berg SW, Wignall FS, Knoke JD, Barrett-Connor E. The postwar hospitalization experience of U.S. veterans of the Persian Gulf War. *N Engl J Med* 1996;335: 1505–1513.
56. Penman AD, Currier MM, Tarver RS. No evidence of increase in birth defects and health problems among children born to Persian Gulf War veterans in Mississippi. *Milit Med* 1996;161:1–6.
57. Cowan DN, DeFraites RF, Gray GC, Goldenbaum MB, Wishik SM. A records-based evaluation of the risk of birth defects among children of Gulf War veterans. *N Engl J Med* 1997;336:1650–1656.
58. Institute of Medicine, Division of Health Promotion and Disease Prevention, Committee on the DoD Persian Gulf Syndrome Comprehensive Clinical Evaluation Program. *Evaluation of the U.S. Department of Defense Persian Gulf Comprehensive Clinical Evaluation Program.* Washington, DC: National Academy Press, 1996.
59. Newmark J, Clayton WL. Persian Gulf illnesses: preliminary neurological impressions. *Milit Med* 1995;160:505–507.
60. Amato AA, McVey A, Cha C, et al. Evaluation of neuromuscular symptoms in veterans of the Persian Gulf War. *Neurology* 1997;45: 4–12.
61. Krivda SJ, Roy MJ, Chung RCY, James WD. Cutaneous findings in Gulf War veterans. *Arch Dermatol* 1996;132:846–847.
62. Landrigan PJ. Illness in Gulf war veterans: causes and consequences. *JAMA* 1997;277:259–261.
63. Kaiser KS, Hawksworth AW, Gray GC. A comparison of self-reported symptoms among active duty Seabees: Gulf War veterans versus era controls (Abstract). 123rd Meeting and Exhibition of the American Public Health Association, Session 2198, 1995.
64. Goldstein G, Beers SR, Morrow LA, Shemansky WJ, Steinhauer SR. A preliminary neuropsychological study of Persian Gulf veterans. *J Int Neuropsych Soc* 1996;2:368–371.
65. Jamal GA, Hansen S, Apartopoulos F, et al. The "Gulf War syndrome". Is there evidence of dysfunction in the nervous system? *J Neurol Neurosurg Psychiatry* 1996;60:449–451.
66. Haley RW, Kurt TL, Horn J. Is there a Gulf war syndrome? Searching for syndromes by factor analysis of symptoms. *JAMA* 1996;277:215–222.
67. Haley RW, Horn J, Roland PS, et al. Evaluation of neurologic function in Gulf War veterans: a blinded case-control study. *JAMA* 1996;277: 223–230.
68. Haley RW, Kurt TL. Self-reported exposure to neurotoxic chemical combinations in the Gulf war: a cross-sectional epidemiologic study. *JAMA* 1996;277:231–237.
69. Axelrod BN, Milner IB. Neuropsychological findings in a sample of Operation Desert Storm veterans. *J Neuropsychiatry Clin Neurosci* 1997;9:23–28.
70. Kotler-Cope S, Milby JB, Roswell R, et al. *Neuropsychological deficits in Persian Gulf war veterans:* a preliminary report. Chicago: International Neuropsychological Society, 1996.
71. Glass AJ. Army Psychiatry before World War II. In: Anderson RS, Glass AJ, Bernucci RJ, eds. *Neuropsychiatry in World War II; vol 1:* Zone of interior. Washington, DC: Office of the Surgeon General, Department of the Army, 1966.
72. Dobson M. Post-traumatic stress disorder in Australian World War II

veterans attending a psychiatric outpatient clinic [letter]. *Med J Aust* 1993;159(3):212.
73. Hovens JE, Falger PR, Op den Velde W, Schouten EG, De Groen JH, Van Duijn H. Occurrence of current posttraumatic stress disorder among Dutch World War II resistance veterans according to the SCID. *J Anxiety Dis* 1992;6(2):147–157.
74. Macleod AD. Post-traumatic stress disorder in World War Two veterans. *N Z Med J* 1991;104(915):285–288.
75. Hovens JE, Op den Velde W, Falger PR, Schouten EG, De Groen JH, Van Duijn H. Anxiety, depression and anger in Dutch Resistance veterans from World War II. *Psychother Psychosom* 1992;57(4):172–179.
76. Molgaard CA, Poikolainen K, Elder JP, et al. Depression late after combat: a follow-up of Finnish World War Two veterans from the seven countries east-west cohort. *Milit Med* 1991;156(5):219–222.
77. Breslau N, Davis GC. Post-traumatic stress disorder: the etiologic specificity of wartime stressors. *Am J Psychiatry* 1987;144:578–583.
78. Faustman W, White P. Diagnostic and psychopharmacological treatment characteristics of 536 inpatients with post-traumatic stress disorder. *J Nerv Ment Dis* 1989;177:154–159.
79. Figley CR. Psychosocial adjustment among Vietnam veterans: an overview of the research. In: CR Figley, ed. *Stress disorders among Vietnam veterans:* theory, *research, and treatment.* New York: Brunner/Mazel, 1978;57–70.
80. Stretch RH. Psychosocial readjustment of Canadian Vietnam veterans. *J Consult Clin Psychol* 1991;59(1):188–189.
81. Kulka RA, Schlenger WE, Fairbank JA, Hough RL, et al. *National Vietnam veterans readjustment study (NVVRS): description, current status, and initial PTSD prevalence estimates.* Washington, DC, Veterans Administration, 1988.
82. The Centers for Disease Control Vietnam Experience Study: health status of Vietnam Veterans II. Physical Health. *JAMA* 1988;259: 2708–2714.
83. Stretch RH. Post-traumatic stress disorder among Vietnam and Vietnam era veterans. In: Figley C, ed. *Trauma and its wake, vol 2:* traumatic stress theory, *research and intervention.* New York: Brunner/Mazel, 1986;156–192.
84. Litz BT, Keane TM, Fisher L, Marx B, Monaco V. Physical health complaints in combat-related Post-Traumatic Stress Disorder: a preliminary report. *J Traumatic Stress* 1992;5:131–141.
85. Kroenke K, Arrington ME, Mangelsdorff AD. The prevalence of symptoms in medical outpatients and the adequacy of therapy. *Arch Intern Med* 1990;160:1685–1689.
86. Kroenke K, Mangelsdorff D. Common symptoms in ambulatory care: incidence, evaluation, therapy, and outcome. *Am J Med* 1989;86: 262–266.
87. Starfield B. *Primary care—concept, evaluation, and policy.* New York: Oxford University Press, 1992.
88. Marpie R, Lucey C, Kroenke K, et al. A prospective study of the concerns and expectations in patients presenting with common symptoms; and The 2-week outcome in patients presenting with common physical complaints. [Abstract] *Clin Res* 1993;41:579A.
89. Hollander DH. Beef allergy and the Persian Gulf syndrome. *Med Hypotheses* 1995;45:221–222.
90. Reyes M, Gary HE, Dobbins JG, et al. Surveillance for chronic fatigue syndrome—Four U.S. cities, September 1989 through August 1993. *MMWR Surveillance Summaries* 1997;46:1–13.
91. Institute of Medicine. *Health consequences of service during the Persian Gulf war:* recommendations for research and information systems. Washington, DC: National Academy Press, 1996.
92. Fontana A, Rosenheck R. A casual model of the etiology of PTSD. Paper presented at the annual meeting of the International Society for Traumatic Stress Studies, Washington, DC, 1991.
93. Green BL, Lindy JD, Grace MC, Gleser GC. Multiple diagnosis in post-traumatic stress disorder: the role of war stressors. *J Nerv Ment Dis* 1989;177:329–335.
94. Perconte ST, Dietrick A, Wilson AT, Spiro KJ, Pontius EB. Psychological and war stress symptoms among deployed and nondeployed reservists following the Persian Gulf war. *Milit Med* 1993;158: 516–521.
95. Wynd CA, Dziedzicki RE. Heightened anxiety in Army Reserve nurses anticipating mobilization during Operation Desert Storm. *Milit Med* 1992;157(12):630–634.
96. Miles MS, Demi AS, Mostyn-Aker P. Rescue workers' reactions following the Hyatt Hotel disaster. *Death Education* 1984;8:315–331.
97. Ursano RJ, McCarroll JE. The nature of a traumatic stressor: handling dead bodies. *J Nerv Ment Dis* 1990;178:396–398.
98. McCarroll JE, Ursano RJ, Fullerton CS. Symptoms of post-traumatic stress disorder following recovery of war dead. *Am J Psychiatry* 1993; 150(12):1875–1877.
99. Sutker PB, Uddo M, Brailey K, Allain AN, Errera P. Psychological symptoms and psychiatric diagnoses in Operation Desert Storm troops serving graves registration duty. *J Traumatic Stress* 1994;7: 159–171.
100. Sutker PB, Uddo M, Brailey K, Vasterling JJ, Errera P. Psychopathology in war-zone deployed and nondeployed Operation Desert Storm troops assigned graves registration duties. *J Abnorm Psychol* 1994; 103:383–390.
101. Solomon Z, Margalit C, Waysman M, Bleich A. In the shadow of the Gulf War: psychological distress, social support and coping among Israeli soldiers in a high risk area. *Isr J Med Sci* 1991;11–12:687–695.
102. Ursano RY, McCaughey BG, Fullerton CS. Trauma and Disaster. In: Ursano RY, McCaughey BG, Fullerton CS, eds. *Individual and community response to trauma and disaster.* New York: Cambridge University Press, 1994;3–27.
103. Fleming R, Baum A, Girsiel MM, Gatchel RJ. Mediating influences of social support on stress at Three Mile Island. *J Hum Stress* 1982;8: 14–22.
104. Pennebaker JW, Newtson D. Observation of a unique event: the psychological impact of the Mount Saint Helens volcano. *New Directions for Methodology of Social and Behavioral Science* 1983;15:93–109.
105. McFarlane AC. The phenomenology of post-traumatic stress disorder following a natural disaster. *J Nerv Ment Dis* 1988;176:22–29.
106. Schottenfeld RS, Psychologic sequelae of chemical and hazardous materials exposures. In: Sullivan JB, Krieger GR, eds. *Hazardous materials toxicology, clinical principles of environmental health.* Baltimore, MD: Williams and Wilkins, 1992;463–468.
107. Schwartz SP, White PE, Hughes RG. Environmental threats, communities, and hysteria. *J Public Health Policy* 1985;6:58–77.
108. Campion EW. Disease and suspicion after the Persian Gulf War. *N Engl J Med* 1996;335:1525–1527.
109. David A, Ferry S, Wessely S. Gulf war illness: New American research provides leads but no firm conclusions. *Br Med J* 1997;314: 239–240.
110. Dobson M, Marshall, RP. Surviving the war zone experience:preventing psychiatric casualties. *Milit Med* 1997;162:283–287.
111. United States General Accounting Office. *Report to congressional requesters, defense health care, medical surveillance improved since Gulf War, but mixed results in Bosnia.* GAO/NSIAD-97-136. Washington, DC: GAO, 1997.
112. Goldberg J, Eisen SA, True WR, Henderson WG. Health effects of military service—lessons learned from the Vietnam experience. *Ann Epidemiol* 1992;2:841–853.
113. Department of Veterans Affairs. *VA Persian Gulf Expert Scientific Committee report (February 19, 1996).* Department of Veterans Affairs Secretary's Responses and Action Plan. Washington, DC: Department of Veterans Affairs, 1996.

*Environmental and Occupational Medicine, Third Edition,* edited by William N. Rom.
Lippincott–Raven Publishers, Philadelphia © 1998.

# CHAPTER 121

# Hazardous Waste

Frank L. Mitchell

Hazardous waste is an inevitable result of modern life. Large numbers of new chemicals, and chemically related processes are introduced each year. After use, they and their by-products have often been discarded in ways that give insufficient consideration to the effects they may ultimately have on the environment or to people. Although past major events such as those at Love Canal, Times Beach, Missouri, and Bhopal, India, have brought wide publicity and attention, few communities have not had to deal, in one way or another, with hazardous waste issues.

The public, worried about the risks from these materials, is confronting health professionals and public officials with questions about the human effects those substances may cause. They want to know whether the land they live on might have been contaminated by chemical wastes, and if so, whether the contaminants can reach them through their water supplies, their food, or the air. They also want information about the potential consequences of such exposure to themselves and future generations.

Today's health professional needs to have an understanding of the scientific issues of hazardous wastes in the environment and their political and social implications.

## LEGISLATIVE ACTIONS

Concern about uncontrolled hazardous materials in the environment has been reflected in federal legislation. While a number of laws have addressed specific aspects of waste material disposal, relatively few have attempted to deal with the overall problem.

F. L. Mitchell: Department of Environmental and Occupational Health, Emory University School of Public Health, Atlanta, Georgia 30327.

The Resource Conservation and Recovery Act (RCRA) was passed in 1976 (1). An outgrowth of the Solid Waste Disposal Act of 1965, RCRA's purpose was to create guidelines for the prudent management and disposal of hazardous waste. It was an attempt to make sure that hazardous materials would be disposed of in a controlled and regulated manner by closely tracking hazardous wastes from cradle to grave. There are specific and stringent control procedures established by RCRA, including manifest systems for tracking hazardous wastes and a permit system that contains standards for waste handling and disposal. If all its provisions were carried out, RCRA could eliminate uncontrolled hazardous waste in the future by ensuring that all these wastes would be properly handled in carefully regulated disposal sites (1). An addition to RCRA, the Hazardous and Solid Waste Amendments (HSWA), was passed in 1984. HSWA established rigid requirements for landfills and other hazardous waste management facilities and severely restricted the land disposal of hazardous wastes. HSWA also gave the U.S. Environmental Protection Agency (EPA) the authority to require nonhazardous waste sites to conform to the same standards as required for hazardous wastes. The EPA has also significantly increased its enforcement activities under RCRA (2). Ironically, although many sites were managed according to the requirements of RCRA, about 4,000 of these facilities are now leaking and in need of cleanup (3).

In December 1980, Congress passed the Comprehensive Environmental Response, Compensation, and Liability Act of 1980 (CERCLA), commonly known as the Superfund (4). CERCLA was called the Superfund because it established the $1.6 billion Hazardous Waste Trust Fund, derived from taxes on crude oil and 42 commercial chemicals. The law had several purposes:

- To identify and characterize where hazardous materials had been or might in the future be released into the environment.
- To establish priorities for cleaning up the worst existing hazardous waste sites.
- To remediate those sites not cleaned up by the responsible parties.
- To advance the United States' scientific capability to deal with hazardous waste management, treatment, and disposal.

The law placed the majority of the regulatory and remedial responsibility with the EPA, but also created the Agency for Toxic Substances and Disease Registry (ATSDR) as a part of the U.S. Public Health Service. Its responsibilities include conducting health assessments at each of the hazardous waste sites listed on the National Priorities List (NPL); developing priority lists of the most commonly found hazardous substances at Superfund sites and to prepare toxicologic profiles on each; carrying out health studies and registries where indicated; and preparing educational materials for physicians and other health providers (4,5).

CERCLA was renewed and extensively modified in 1986 by the Superfund Amendments and Reauthorization Act (SARA), which contained a number of provisions: an increase of the amount of the trust fund to $8.5 billion; a review every 5 years after any remedial action to determine if the action was successful in protecting human health; mandatory schedules for cleanup activities; and guarantees of greater citizen input and involvement in most activities in the law (4).

Other legislation playing a role in hazardous waste include the Clean Air Act; the Clean Water Act; the Safe Drinking Water Act; the Federal Insecticide, Fungicide, and Rodenticide Act; the Toxic Substances Control Act; the National Environmental Policy Act; and others (2).

## INTERNATIONAL

Many countries have increased the attention given to hazardous waste. The problem has grown in importance for a number of reasons; two examples are (a) the attention focused on the environmental problems in Eastern Europe after the breakup of the Soviet Union, and (b) the worldwide interest in the actions taken at the United Nations Conference on Environment and Development (UNCED), held in 1992 in Rio de Janeiro, Brazil (6–8). Other activities include cooperation between the United States and Canada on hazardous waste issues around the Great Lakes (5), and the Organization for Economic Cooperation and Development (OECD) providing the basis for European Community legislation that recommends controls for the transportation and disposal of hazardous wastes. OECD also established the International Wastes Identification Code (IWIC) that will help to more adequately identify and track the movement of hazardous waste materials throughout the world (6). A number of other nations are also increasing their activities related to hazardous waste (7,8).

## THE NATURE AND EXTENT OF HAZARDOUS WASTE

Although hazardous waste has been defined in a number of ways, it is, in essence, any uncontrolled chemical or other material that is capable of producing adverse health effects. These effects can be caused directly, through contact, ingestion, or inhalation of the toxicant, or indirectly, from fire, explosion, or other secondary effects. In this chapter, hazardous wastes are defined as those materials that have been discarded or abandoned in such a way that they can reach or affect humans.

About 6 billion tons of waste are produced in the United States each year, and about 250 million tons are classed as hazardous. Of that 250 tons, over 6% is industrial waste and over 93% is agricultural and mining waste. A very small amount is accounted for by municipal and utility waste. These figures exclude high-level radioactive waste (1).

The EPA maintains two listings that help to define the size of the uncontrolled hazardous waste problem in the United States. The CERCLA Information System (CERCLIS) lists those sites where releases of hazardous substances have been or need to be investigated. The listing includes all known sites, whether active or inactive, and whether they have had remediation or may need further remediation (4). At the end of 1995, the EPA inventory listed about 15,000 sites. Although the list at one time contained nearly 33,000 sites, 24,000 sites were removed by the EPA in 1995 because they presented little or no threat to health or the environment (9).

The second list, the National Priorities List (NPL), was established by the Clean Water Act of 1972, and incorporated into Superfund. This list, which is updated at least annually, identifies those abandoned or uncontrolled hazardous waste sites requiring long-term remediation. They are grouped according to such categories as the type and toxicity of materials, the numbers of people potentially exposed, the pathways through which they might be exposed, and the location of nearby, possibly vulnerable, groundwater. There are about 1,300 sites on the NPL, including more than 150 federal facilities (4,10). The federal listings require special mention because these 150 facilities represent a much higher number of sites. For example, a study by the National Research Council in 1994 lists 17,482 contaminated sites at 1,855 Department of Defense installations (10). Another agency, the Department of Energy, has some facilities that consist of very large expanses of land. These facilities may include many individual sites containing mixed wastes that are toxicologically very complex and that will be very difficult to remediate.

Neither the NPL nor the CERCLIS itemizes those sites that are certified and operated under the mandate of RCRA, but, as previously noted, a large number of those sites will also require cleanup.

## CLEANUP COSTS

Although they cannot be estimated with accuracy, the resources needed to clean up hazardous waste sites in the United States will be large by any standard. In 1988, the EPA estimated the costs of a cleanup for the average site on the NPL to be $21–30 million, with a number of the larger sites requiring upward of $300 million (4). In 1991, the EPA estimated the cost of cleaning up nonfederal NPL sites could exceed $30 billion (3).

Other publications have estimated cleanup costs from $500 billion to $1 trillion (11,12).

## SITE CHARACTERIZATION

Hazardous waste sites take many forms. They can include both abandoned and active facilities. Of the 1,300 sites listed on the NPL, one source estimates that 42% are landfills or treatment, storage, and disposal facilities (TSDF), 31% are abandoned manufacturing facilities, 8% are waste recycling services, 5% are mining sites, 4% government installations, and the remainder are in miscellaneous categories (13).

Hazardous waste sites are found in rural settings, in cities, in residential areas, and in parks. They can cover very extensive surface areas, or be invisible. The only indication of contamination may be the discovery of contaminated groundwater. Although the source of the contamination can usually be identified, there have been occasions when no cause of contamination was found.

The contaminants at Superfund sites are often industrial chemicals. They may have arrived from numerous sources over many years, or could have been the result of one illegal dumping incident. In the past, some businesses and governmental agencies did not always make sure that their waste materials were disposed of in an environmentally safe manner, even by earlier standards. Little or no attention may have been given to the long-term consequences of disposal. In some cases, although arrangements may have been made with a contractor to remove waste from the facility, the company had no idea where it went or what happened to it. Some contractors would move the waste to an isolated site and merely dump it onto the ground. On other occasions, the waste would be buried in drums or poured into a pit dug into the ground. There are instances where waste was dumped into abandoned mine sites or down old wells.

However, not all industrial sites have occurred because of intentional mishandling or carelessness. The regulations and laws governing the treatment and disposal of hazardous wastes have become increasingly strict. Companies that disposed of hazardous waste in ways that conformed to all laws and regulations in force at an earlier time, as is the case with many RCRA sites, have been involved in extensive cleanup operations at the same site years later because of leakage or other contamination.

Waste materials from mining operations (tailings) have also been left to accumulate in large mounds in the open that have, in a number of cases, grown so large as to become geographical landmarks. Mine tailings can blow freely and be carried miles away, or even stay where they were placed and present a threat through skin contact.

Old and worn out trailers have been filled with waste and then abandoned in isolated spots or buried in huge pits. In all too many cases, buried drums and other containers have deteriorated, allowing their contents to move through the soil to reach the surface or groundwater supplies and aquifers. Contamination can travel miles from the point of the original pollution to reach rivers, streams, and lakes where the living organisms (biota) can serve as a route of exposure to humans through the food chain.

Rural areas have their own problems with hazardous materials. The agricultural industry uses a great number of materials that, if not carefully handled, can become hazardous wastes (14).

Of the more than 2,000 substances found at hazardous waste sites, about 700 have been detected in media (air, water, soil) (15). If the contaminated media have been found to have reached human populations, that pathway is said to be completed. In 1994, the ATSDR published a list of those substances found most frequently in com-

**TABLE 1.** *Substances found most often (1% of 1,356) in completed exposure pathways (15)*

| | |
|---|---|
| Trichloroethylene | 45% |
| Lead | 42% |
| Tetrachloroethylene | 34% |
| Arsenic | 29% |
| Benzene | 27% |
| 1,1,1-Trichloroethane | 24% |
| Cadmium | 23% |
| Chromium | 23% |
| Chloroform | 19% |
| Manganese | 18% |

**TABLE 2.** *Most frequent binary combinations of contaminants in soil (16)*

| Number of sites | Contaminant 1 | Contaminant 2 |
|---|---|---|
| 243 | Chromium | Lead |
| 212 | Arsenic | Lead |
| 209 | Cadmium | Lead |
| 158 | Arsenic | Chromium |
| 138 | Arsenic | Cadmium |
| 130 | Tetrachloroethylene | Trichloroethylene |
| 129 | Lead | Zinc |
| 124 | Ethyl benzene | Toluene |
| 124 | Lead | Nickel |

**TABLE 3.** *Most frequent binary combinations of contaminants in air (16)*

| Number of sites | Contaminant 1 | Contaminant 2 |
|---|---|---|
| 42 | Benzene | Toluene |
| 32 | Benzene | Trichloroethylene |
| 31 | Benzene | Tetrachloroethylene |
| 27 | Tetrachloroethylene | Toluene |
| 25 | Ethyl benzene | Toluene |
| 25 | Toluene | Trichloroethylene |
| 23 | 1,1,1-Trichloroethane | Trichloroethylene |
| 23 | Toluene | Total xylenes |
| 22 | 1,1,1-Trichloroethane | Tetrachloroethylene |

pleted exposure pathways at Superfund sites. They are shown in Table 1 (15).

Knowing what chemicals are most common in hazardous waste sites is only a small part of the problem, because many sites contain multiple contaminants, both in the sense of separate compounds and in the sense of mixtures. These mixtures can vary widely in their potential effects. In some sites, more than 100 chemicals have been identified in the air, the water, and the soil. Johnson and DeRosa (16) developed Tables 2, 3, and 4 showing the most frequently found binary combinations:

These tables show that the contaminants most commonly found by ATSDR at hazardous waste sites are volatile organic compounds (VOCs), which were found in 74% of site assessments. Other classes of materials frequently found are inorganics (found at 71% of sites), halogenated pesticides (found at 37% of sites), and polychlorinated aromatic hydrocarbons (PAHs), found at 25% of the sites having public health assessments (16). Knowing the types of compounds most frequently found has allowed the development of methodologies to more rapidly characterize sites, which, in turn, has allowed more efficient remediation plans to be put in place.

As part of its congressional mandate, the ATSDR carries out public health assessments (PHAs) on hazardous waste sites. Health assessments are defined by the agency to be "An evaluation of data and information on the release of hazardous substances into the environment in order to assess any current or future impact on public health..." (17). The PHA program thus provides an opportunity to evaluate the degree of potential human exposure from hazardous waste sites, and therefore some idea of the health effects they may produce.

The ATSDR PHA process classifies hazardous waste sites into the following categories (17):

Urgent public health hazard: Sites that present a public health hazard as a result of short-term exposures to hazardous substances.

Public health hazard: Sites that present a public health hazard as a result of long-term exposures to hazardous substances.

Indeterminate public health hazard: Sites with incomplete information.

No apparent public health hazard: Sites where human exposure to contaminated media is occurring or has occurred in the past but exposure is below a level of a health hazard.

No public health hazard: Sites that do not present a public health hazard.

Unclassified: Sites with data that are inadequate for site characterization.

Assignment to a category is not based on risk-based derivations but rather on the professional judgment of the ATSDR staff, based on the site findings. This scheme differs from, but is complementary to, the EPA's Hazard Ranking System (HRS). The PHA does not take into account ecological or environmental effects; it is based solely on human health impact (13). However, of 1,719

**TABLE 4.** *Most frequent binary combinations of contaminants in water (16)*

| Number of sites | Contaminant 1 | Contaminant 2 |
|---|---|---|
| 279 | Tetrachloroethylene | Trichloroethylene |
| 225 | Chromium | Lead |
| 213 | 1,1,1-Trichloroethane | Trichloroethylene |
| 206 | Lead | Trichloroethylene |
| 204 | Cadmium | Lead |
| 202 | Benzene | Trichloroethylene |
| 194 | Arsenic | Lead |
| 172 | 1,2-Dichloroethane, *trans* | Trichloroethylene |
| 161 | Benzene | Trichloroethylene |

**TABLE 5.** *Most commonly detected contaminants (18)*

| Substance | Sites (number) | Percent of sites evaluated |
|---|---|---|
| Metals (inorganics) | 564 | 59 |
| Volatile organic (VOC) | 518 | 54 |
| Polycyclic aromatics (PAH) | 187 | 20 |
| Polychlorinated biphenyls (PCB) | 162 | 17 |
| Phthalate | 106 | 11 |
| Pesticides | 82 | 9 |
| Dioxins | 47 | 5 |

public health assessments on more than 1,300 Superfund sites, 23% represented a health hazard, according to ATSDR's public health assessment criteria. Of the 136 sites for which public health assessments were conducted and advisories issued for fiscal years 1993 and 1994, ATSDR classified 54% as health hazards (13).

An older analysis of the first 951 Superfund site health assessments showed that the majority of the sites were related to either industrial facilities (31%) or landfills (30%) (18). As in a previously cited study (15), the most commonly detected contaminants (Table 5) were inorganics and VOCs.

The survey estimated that 4.1 million people live within a 1-mile radius of the 785 sites for which population data were available (18). Of that population, 18% live near sites that were concluded to be a "public health concern" or a "probable health concern"; 80% lived around sites designated as a "potential health concern," a category used when data were deemed by the ATSDR to be insufficient to completely characterize the exposures and/or health threat.

More than 600 substances were identified in various media on the 951 sites studied, but the actual number may be much larger due to deficiencies in the data (18). An "occurrence" was defined as (a) the presence of the substance at "elevated" levels, or (b) the suspicion of off-site migration, or (c) the presence of substances where direct human contact could occur.

## HUMAN HEALTH EFFECTS

Excepting acute releases of hazardous materials, the concentration of chemicals in the environment around hazardous waste sites is typically very low; however, the dose of a chemical (which considers the route, concentration of the materials and the time over which it is received) that a person may actually receive is very site specific. The target organ and the ultimate effects, can differ depending on whether the exposure is through groundwater, surface water, air, or direct contact. Other variables affecting the dose are the specific substances involved and whether they are mixed with other chemicals that can alter their usual characteristics. The persistence and stability of the chemical are also important.

The two most common sources of toxicologic information used to evaluate sites are animal experiments and studies of worker populations. Although both are useful, few were designed to address the type of exposure found at most hazardous waste sites. When these sources of information are being used, the limitations and inherent problems of extrapolations become apparent. As a result of these difficulties, epidemiologic techniques have been investigated that may help to better define health effects potentially associated with hazardous waste sites.

A number of epidemiologic studies have been carried out. These have been summarized by Johnson (13), who noted that while many of these studies are negative in the sense that statistically significant increases in adverse health effects were not found, he noted that both positive and negative results of such studies can be due to many factors, including the misclassification of study participants, inadequate exposure data, inappropriate choice of comparison data or groups, and errors in statistical analysis.

In his review, Johnson (13) cited two opposing views of the potential for health effects from hazardous waste sites:

> The National Research Council (NRC), in 1991, after reviewing much of the literature on the public health implications of hazardous waste, noted that "in spite of the complex limitations of epidemiologic studies of hazardous waste sites, several investigations at specific sites have documented a variety of symptoms of ill health in exposed persons, including low birth weight, cardiac anomalies, headache, fatigue, and a constellation of neurobehavioral problems." The NRC concluded that the overall impact of hazardous wastes in the United States is unknown because of limitations in identifying, assessing, or ranking hazardous waste sites (HWS) exposures and their potential effects on public health (19).
>
> In contrast, Grisham (20) concluded that little evidence existed to support the proposition that chemical wastes were adversely affecting the health of communities.

The ATSDR's National Exposure Registry (NER) (21,22) is composed of groups of persons having documented exposure to substances of priority to ATSDR and for which there are gaps in information. Each group is designated a subregistry. The NER, and its component subregistries, is one attempt to evaluate the public health effects of chemicals found on hazardous waste sites and has reported findings on noncancer chronic disease morbidity relevant to the impact of hazardous waste sites on human health. For example, the subregistry of persons exposed to trichloroethylene (TCE) consists of 4,280 persons living near 13 sites in Indiana, Illinois, and Michigan (23). The levels of TCE, although varying in concentration from site to site, and accompanied by differing levels and numbers of co-contaminants, was considered by the ATSDR as the primary contaminant. The duration of registrants' exposure to TCE varied from months to several years, but ceased when they were provided with an alternative water supply, in most cases, a municipal water system.

The TCE registrants are surveyed periodically on an ongoing basis to obtain their self-reported health status, and these data are compared to the results of the National Health Interview Survey (NHIS), an annual, population-based survey of the United States, and the National Household Survey on Drug Abuse (23). Although the ATSDR reported the TCE subregistry cohort as having a higher rate of some reported adverse health outcomes (stroke, liver disease, diabetes, blood disorders, urinary tract disorders, and skin rashes), it is important to remember that the results are based on self-reported data, and do not imply a causal relationship between TCE exposure and those health effects. As noted by the ATSDR (23), that conclusion could be reached only following detailed examinations, objective data gathering efforts, and more definitive epidemiologic investigations. However, efforts such as the ATSDR health registries may be able to contribute new information, as will other long-term investigations.

As noted by one author (13), a problem of some studies at hazardous waste sites is the application of inappropriate toxicologic analysis. Often this is the result of gaps in information concerning the effects of chemicals at low dosage levels. This issue can be very difficult to deal with and can be a primary cause of difficulty in interpreting whether health effects are a result of exposure. The issue can also be fundamental in litigation situations.

It is true that science does not know as much as we would like about the effect of chemicals at very low levels. Not as much may be known, for example, about the potential effects of a substance at very low environmental levels as may be known about its effects at higher, more occupationally relevant levels. Therefore, while extrapolating the information known about higher levels can be useful in the evaluation of health effects at a given site, it can also be very misleading. The question of what effects are produced by low-level chemical exposure is an area of significant research and one that will not be soon resolved. It is therefore essential that the information available for a site be carefully evaluated in relation to the conditions found at that site, and that any conclusions reached are clearly identified as site-specific.

One method used to evaluate the effects of low-level chemical exposure is quantitative risk assessment (QRA). There are a number of variations of the quantitative risk assessment process, but in general, it uses elements such as the evaluation of the hazard, the dose-response relationships of the hazard, exposure assessment, and risk characterization combined in a mathematical way to produce an estimation of risk from the substance in question (24). Since it is based on a number of carefully drawn assumptions, QRA is complex and can be difficult to understand. Due to the nature of the process, it is usually inappropriate to apply a risk assessment calculation to a site unless it was developed for that site. QRA is sometimes confused with the PHA process used by ATSDR and a number of states. Although based on much of the same site information, the two processes are complementary and look at the data in different ways. This allows a broader-based review and characterization of a site and having both available on a given site will assist decision-makers in developing appropriate remediation (25).

## PHYSICIAN RESPONSE AND EDUCATION

Due to the limitations on the uses of traditional sources of information, it can be difficult to evaluate the potential health risk of a given environmental exposure, even for those dealing with these situations on a daily basis. For others, evaluating the potential risks to health from a site can be quite frustrating. Since it is often physicians to whom people turn when they have questions about a possible exposure, it is important that the physician be prepared to supply appropriate answers.

In 1988, the Institute of Medicine (IOM), part of the National Academy of Sciences, published a report on the role of the primary care physician in occupational and environmental health (26). The report concludes, in part, that private physicians are often not knowledgeable of the effects of many chemicals found in hazardous waste sites. Further, these physicians have no idea of where to get this information. As a result, when questioned on issues of chemicals in the environment, the answers that are given are often unintentionally wrong or misleading.

Compared to only a few years ago, much more information from both federal agencies and other sources is available to assist the physician. Two series of publications are the ATSDR-produced *Case Studies in Environmental Medicine,* and the ATSDR's *Toxicologic Profiles,* which supply in-depth information on a large number of substances found at hazardous waste sites (27,28). The IOM also published, in 1995, the book *Environmental Medicine:* Integrating a Missing Element into Medical Education (29). It describes efforts to include environmental information into the medical curriculum and contains all of the ATSDR's *Case Studies,* along with a number of other papers that will help orient a physician to environmentally related health effects.

The occupationally trained physician often has an advantage in environmental situations, but the diagnosis of adverse effects due to environmental exposures cannot always be equated to the diagnosis of work-related effects. Exposure standards or guidelines for workplace exposure are set at levels that should not cause symptoms in the normal, healthy individual working a normal workweek and supplied with protective equipment or administrative controls where appropriate. While these exposure guidelines may not be protective in all cases, they have been very effective for many years. However, while the levels for many chemicals found in the workplace are typically in the parts per million range, the levels for many of the same chemicals at hazardous waste sites are often magnitudes lower, e.g., in the parts per billion or even parts per trillion range, which the conventional guidelines were not intended to consider.

Current knowledge suggests that the earliest recognizable effects of low-level chemical exposures tend to be common to many conditions. Signs and symptoms such as headache, malaise, minor skin irritations, and respiratory complaints are also frequent, and may fall within the range of complaints that are often a part of any medical office. Some illnesses, and many cancers, may have latency periods of 20 to 40 years before the first signs or symptoms appear. The physician must therefore be very detailed in his clinical evaluation to understand and clarify these vague complaints. He must be able to relate clinical symptoms and signs to the dose of chemical received, which, as previously noted, must include (a) the concentration of the material, (b) the time over which the concentration was received, and (c) the route by which the material was absorbed. While these cannot always be determined with accuracy, their importance cannot be overstated, and the physician must realize that the strength of any conclusions will be diminished in direct proportion to missing or unknown data. Finally, the physician must also understand that merely establishing an association in time or place between a putative toxic material and human health effects is not enough to establish causation.

## BIOMARKERS

The relative inability to detect early signs of environmentally related adverse effects has led to an increased interest in chemical testing. Without overt disease or specific symptoms, the only way to identify subtle pathophysiologic changes in a particular organ system is to look for alterations in the cells and metabolic products of tissues that make up that system (30). These biologic indicators of chemical exposure have been termed biomarkers, and they are the subject of extensive investigation (31–33).

The National Research Council of the National Academy of Sciences has defined three types of biomarkers (34):

A *biomarker of exposure* is one that measures an exogenous substance, its metabolite, or the product of a reaction between that substance and the organism.

A *biomarker of effect* is an alteration within an organism that can be recognized as an established or potential impairment or disease.

A *biomarker of susceptibility* is a measure of the organism's ability to respond to an exposure to an exogenous substance.

Perhaps the major importance of biomarkers is their potential ability to detect or measure points along a continuum from a causal exposure to overt disease (35). They can be a measure of an individual's ability to respond to a chemical challenge or to determine whether the individual has been exposed to a substance in a sufficient amount to have caused some change to occur. Therefore, as opposed to the traditional view of disease being either present or absent, the health status can be viewed as a progression of events from exposure to clinically apparent abnormalities.

To use the example of lead, an exposure to the metal can lead to an internal dose (blood lead levels), a biologically effective dose (lead level in bone marrow cells), an early biologic effect (inhibition of δ-aminolevulinic acid dehydrogenase), altered structure/function (accumulation of zinc protoporphyrin), and finally, clinical disease (anemia, developmental abnormalities) (35).

The ability to detect and measure these intermediate steps could possibly be very useful in evaluating environmental disease, but a subcommittee of two federal health agencies, looking at these issues, made the point that using laboratory tests in environmental studies requires "special emphasis upon developing reference ranges and validating their sensitivity and specificity for biologic health endpoints" (30). The subcommittee report quoted Thomas (36), who listed the following desirable characteristics of a biomarker:

1. Relative specificity to a narrow range of toxicants;
2. Relative absence in unexposed persons;
3. Measurable by minimally invasive means;
4. Inexpensive to collect and analyze;
5. High analytic sensitivity, specificity, and reproducibility.

The federal subcommittee report further noted that data for the predictive value of most biomarkers are not available, underlining that the study of biomarkers is still an area of rapid growth and change (30).

Many investigators feel that biomarkers may prove to be of prime importance in the detection and tracking the results of exposure to toxicants in the environment. They have obvious potential to detect changes caused by environmental exposures while they are still subclinical, which will allow intervention to lessen or avoid harmful effects.

## EMERGENCY CHEMICAL RELEASES

Even when properly handled, hazardous wastes can become a threat because of incidents during transportation, storage, or other handling. To use one measure, the quantities of hazardous materials that are transported in the United States are immense. Each year, over 1.5 billion tons are conveyed throughout the United States by land, sea and air. In only one year, 1982, 467,000 trucks transported 927 million tons of hazardous materials. In that same year, 115,600 rail tank cars moved 73 million tons, and 4,909 tanker barges transported 549 million tons.

There are over 500,000 shipments per day (37). It is inevitable that a certain number of these shipments will have unplanned incidents, which can have a significant impact on the environment.

Emergency situations can also occur in well-managed stationary facilities or in abandoned, poorly controlled sites, or from deteriorated containers.

In 1990, the ATSDR, in cooperation with five state health departments, initiated the Hazardous Substances Emergency Events Surveillance System (HSEES) as an active surveillance program (38,39). The HSEES system, now including 14 states, actively seeks emergency event information from agencies and local departments within the state.

As defined by ATSDR, a hazardous substance emergency event is the uncontrolled or illegal release, or threatened release, of a hazardous substance or of its by-products. Only events are included that would require cleanup, neutralization, or removal. Events are also included when a threat of a release could affect the health of employees, responders, or the general public. Not included are events involving only petroleum products. Victims are defined as persons who suffered at least one injury, or died, as a result of the event (40).

The 12 states participating in the HSEES system in 1994 reported 4,244 events; 79% of the events occurred at fixed facilities and 21% were transportation-related (40). Seventeen percent of the events occurred on a weekend. In 90% of the events, a single substance was released. The most commonly released substances were volatile organic compounds (19% of events), other inorganic substances (16%), and acids (10%). Of the 4,244 events, 4,145 resulted in a total of 2,178 victims and 20 deaths; 574 events led to evacuation of people. Of the 20 deaths, 8 persons died in fixed-facility events, and 12 died in transportation events. The population groups showing the greatest frequency of injury were employees (45% of injuries), the general public (44%), and responders (11%) (40).

Exposures from unplanned or emergency chemical events tend to be acute. Although serious effects can be caused from some materials, there is, in the usual case, a brief time of exposure, and the actual dose received is typically small. Health effects are therefore frequently those of irritation and are usually without long-term consequences. However, careful follow-up should be considered to ensure that is the case, and exposed persons should be cautioned to return to their health provider if delayed symptoms occur during the next several days.

## HAZARDOUS WASTE WORKERS

In general, hazardous waste workers are involved in site remediation or response to hazardous material incidents.

Estimates of the numbers of workers involved in such activities have varied widely. In 1989, OSHA (41) estimated that up to 1.758 million employees could be involved, while Warhit (42) in 1995 gave a considerably lower estimate of about 200,000 workers divided among federal and nonfederal sites. The estimates are uncertain because of the often temporary nature of the work, the use of employees in remediation activities who may have been hired for other duties, and how the work is classified, i.e., whether the work is reported as related to hazardous waste.

First responders to emergency chemical events may also have intermittent, but intense, exposure to hazardous materials. These personnel may normally work in a variety of occupations such as emergency medical technicians (EMTs), firemen, police, hospital emergency room personnel, and others. Although difficult to estimate with accuracy, Johnson (43), reporting on ATSDR attempts to identify these workers, has suggested that over 400,000 may be involved, but also noted that there are in excess of one million firefighters and the amount of their involvement cannot be known. There are also a very large number of law enforcement officers and transportation workers who may become involved in emergency response situations.

Regardless of their actual number, these employees work in unpredictable situations, often outside, in terrain that is frequently unfavorable. The equipment they wear to protect them from contact with hazardous materials is cumbersome and can produce its own hazards. In the past, this equipment has not always been appropriate to these employees' specific exposures, nor have they always had training available to teach them how to properly utilize it (44).

## HAZARDOUS WASTE WORKER REGULATIONS (HAZWOPER)

The Federal standards developed for general industry and construction also apply to hazardous waste operations, but both the Occupational Safety and Health Administration (OSHA) and the EPA have issued regulations applying specifically to hazardous waste workers (41,45). The EPA regulation, which is identical to the OSHA requirements, applies to state and local government employers in states that do not have delegated OSHA programs (45). These two regulations (29 CFR 1910.120 and 40 CFR 311) are together known as the worker protection standards for *haz*ardous *w*aste *op*erations and *e*mergency *r*esponse (HAZWOPER). In situations where a conflict appears to exist between general industry standards and HAZWOPER during covered operations, the latter takes precedence (41).

In addition to HAZWOPER, there are other regulations that may have application in particular circumstances. For example, the OSHA standard for occupational exposure to blood-borne pathogens may be pertinent to workers at an emergency situation involving injuries (46).

HAZWOPER became effective on March 6, 1990. The regulation applies to work carried out on federal sites, sites that are a part of a federal mandate (e.g., Superfund or RCRA sites), areas that are designated as uncontrolled hazardous waste sites, and during emergency response operations at releases of hazardous substances.

HAZWOPER includes a wide range of requirements aimed at protecting the health and safety of hazardous waste workers. It requires a site-specific safety and health plan, which must discuss all phases of the anticipated work, the specific hazards expected to be encountered, their pathways, and emergency procedures. Generic plans are not adequate. Worker training is also required, with the number of hours varying depending on the exact work anticipated and the number of days per year worked (41).

Other subjects covered by HAZWOPER include engineering controls, work practices, personal protective equipment, and decontamination procedures.

The regulation requires a medical surveillance program to be offered to all employees who are potentially exposed to hazardous substances for more than 30 days per year, who must use a respirator for more than 30 days per year, who are injured from exposure to hazardous substances during an emergency incident, or who are members of a hazardous materials (HazMat) team (41).

HAZWOPER requires that medical examinations be provided prior to assignment and at least once every 12 months, unless the physician believes a longer interval is appropriate; however, the interval may not exceed 2 years. Examinations must also be provided upon termination of employment, transfer to a noncovered assignment, as soon as possible following overexposure or the appearance of signs or symptoms compatible with possible overexposure, or when deemed medically necessary by the examining physician (41).

Detailed records must be kept of all examinations, and maintained in the same way as other OSHA-mandated medical records (41).

The only specified requirements for the examinations are:

- A medical and work history, with special emphasis on symptoms relating to the handling of hazardous materials.
- The evaluation of fitness for wearing any required respirator under any conditions (e.g., extreme temperatures) that may be expected at the work site (41).

Beyond these two requirements, the regulation states only that the content of the examination is to be determined by the attending physician. A good general reference for further information is the *Occupational Safety and Health Guidance Manual for Hazardous Waste Site Activities,* a document produced jointly by OSHA, the National Institute for Occupational Safety and Health (NIOSH), EPA, and the U.S. Coast Guard (47). Because it was published in 1985, it does not cover HAZWOPER, but it does cover a wide number of related topics.

## HAZARDOUS WASTE WORKER MEDICAL SURVEILLANCE

When developing a medical surveillance program for hazardous waste workers, the physician must keep in mind their unique employment conditions.

The history should detail any past adverse effects of chemical exposures and the circumstances of any previous heat stress episodes. Any previous history of problems while wearing personal protective equipment should be investigated, as should any continuing exposures to chemicals such as secondary employment or hobbies. The physician should also be aware of any condition that might contraindicate the wearing of respirators, such as asthma, other pulmonary conditions, or severe claustrophobia, which can cause problems in fully enclosed suits and respirators. Any allergies or history of atopy should also be detailed (44).

The physical examination should evaluate the worker's general capacity for hard work. Overall fitness is of prime importance. Obesity, lack of physical exercise, and any history or evidence of back or other musculoskeletal problems should be thoroughly documented (44).

A complete pulmonary function evaluation should be carried out at the initial examination to help determine the worker's ability to wear any respirator, up to those that are full-face, supplied. Other factors that might affect the ability to properly wear respirators should be noted. These include facial hair and scars, or perforated eardrums and contact lenses. Vision tests should also be carried out and, if necessary, lenses prescribed to wear inside full-face respirators. Contact lenses should not be worn inside respirators. Auditory acuity should also be evaluated in the range of 500 to 8,000 Hz.

Some physicians perform extensive baseline laboratory testing for a number of chemicals. Others believe that since these workers are often on a large number of sites with little consistency of exposure, such testing would only rarely be of use in an exposure situation. A compromise often used is a general laboratory screen including hepatic and renal function tests, along with the usual pulmonary function, vision, and auditory tests (44, 47).

The protective clothing worn by hazardous waste workers may include full-coverage suits, full-face masks, and self-contained breathing apparatus (SCBA). The equipment can severely compromise vision and movement, meaning that accidents and trauma can be more of a danger than chemical exposure. Table 6 presents the four levels of clothing worn while doing hazardous waste remediation work.

PPE becomes more difficult and stressful to use as its ability to protect from chemical contamination increases.

**TABLE 6.** *Personal protective equipment (PPE) used by hazardous waste workers*

| Level | Clothing | Respirator |
|---|---|---|
| A | Fully encapsulating, chemical-resistant suit and outer gloves; hard hat and safety shoes/boots | Pressure-demand full-face SCBA or supplied-air respirator with escape SCBA |
| B | Chemical-resistant clothing and boots; inner and outer gloves; hard hat and safety shoes/boots | Pressure-demand full-face SCBA or supplied-air respirator with escape SCBA |
| C | Chemical-resistant clothing and boots; inner and outer gloves; hard hat and safety shoes/boots | Full-face piece, air-purifying canister-equipped respirator |
| D | Coveralls; hard hat and safety shoes/boots; safety goggles or splash goggles | None |

The equipment, particularly in levels B and A, essentially eliminates both radiation and evaporation as physiologic heat control, which leads to heat stress, perhaps the most important and constant threat to the workers.

Even in cool weather, workers in protective equipment must be closely monitored for the effects of heat stress, and appropriate measures must be in place to administer treatment, if necessary. One study demonstrated that the use of protective clothing caused increases in heart rates of from 40% to 60%, with some increasing as much as 80% (the mean being an increase in the mean from 84 at work arrival, to 137 after approximately 3 hours of work). Oral temperatures did not increase, but how the core temperatures may have been affected is not known (48). The workers in this study were not wearing the most protective totally encapsulating suits and were not using supplied-air respirators. Both add considerable weight, thus significantly increasing the work effort and the potential for heat stress.

Adaptation to work performed in PPE should be planned for and carried out through initially shortening the periods of work, and more frequent rest periods. Health care should be immediately available by trained personnel such as emergency medical technicians and nurses, and as a part of the site safety plan arrangements should be made with a local hospital for any needed further care (49).

In summary, the most important step to assure the health and safety of hazardous waste workers is preparation. To help ensure that employees are protected to the extent possible, many companies go far beyond the requirements of the HAZWOPER regulations. A well thought out program of training, surveillance, and preparation can be very effective in preventing injury to these workers.

## BIOREMEDIATION

The method most frequently used to remediate hazardous waste sites has been excavation of the contaminated soil followed by transportation to an appropriate landfill for final disposal. However, these actions are very costly and even higher expenses are incurred to develop and provide long-term maintenance of the landfills that themselves can begin to leak. In addition, finding areas where new landfills can be established is a major problem.

Incineration has been used at a number of sites, but the contaminated material must be excavated and transported to the incinerator, or an incinerator must be erected at the site. Both are expensive, and there have been many concerns about air pollution resulting from incinerators that are not optimally maintained.

Beyond these problems, there is also concern about the complex contamination at some sites, particularly federal facilities, and the great difficulties of moving the contaminated materials to other areas for disposal.

For all these reasons, considerable attention has been given to alternative methods of remediating waste sites, particularly *in situ*, and one of the most promising is the process of bioremediation.

Bioremediation involves the use of organisms to convert bioavailable hazardous substances to less toxic or more easily handled by-products. The organisms can either be "natural" or genetically modified. While bioremediation has the advantage of not having to move the contaminated material to a different site for treatment, it requires new and different skills.

The Superfund Act (CERCLA) gave to the U.S. Geological Survey (USGS) the mandate to conduct a program to investigate the many issues involved in bioremediation. Other agencies, such as the EPA and the Department of Energy are also involved (50,51).

One of the more important findings of the USGS program has been the confirmation that microorganisms in shallow aquifers affect the fate and transport of virtually all kinds of toxic substances. Those studies also showed that microorganisms naturally present in the soils were actively consuming fuel-derived toxic compounds and transforming them into carbon dioxide. Further, the rate of that transformation could be greatly increased by the addition of nutrients. Therefore, the USGS began a program of treating contaminated soils with nutrients to see if treatment would increase the rate of degradation. These experiments were highly successful, with contamination being decreased at some sites by 75%. The nearer to the source of nutrients, the higher was the rate of degradation (51).

For some sites, an experimental approach has been used to excavate the contaminated soil, form mounds on top of plastic liners, and trickle surfactants and detergents through the soil, which causes the toxicants to be gathered at the bottom. Aerobic or anaerobic treatment can then be used to degrade the detergents and contaminants (52). This two-stage treatment offers the possibility of greater control throughout the process and would allow faster treatment of deeper contamination. However, it would also seem to add considerable expense.

While still considered by most to be somewhat experimental, bioremediation has been successfully used in some applications:

The Argonne National Laboratory has used bioremediation techniques in a pilot program to clean up 13,000 pounds of soil containing 2,4,6-trinitrotoluene (TNT) (53).

The City of San Francisco has successfully bioremediated soils contaminated with various hydrocarbon fuels at a cost of $16 to $22 per cubic yard, which was said to have been 10 times cheaper than incineration techniques (54).

However, as with every other innovation, there are a number of concerns that must be considered before widespread use can proceed. For example, since the U.S. Supreme Court has ruled that new forms of life can be patented, there may not be full information publicly available about the biologic activity of genetically altered or created microorganisms. Thus, the potential effects may not be predictable by scientists who are not part of the company owning the organism (54).

The effects of adding a very large number of microorganisms to an area of soil that could be quite extensive is not yet well understood. Although the idea that the microorganisms would become so adapted to the toxicant that they would die out when the contaminant is gone is attractive, but that theory needs further confirmation (54).

The fact that no federal regulations currently exist covering the use of genetically engineered organisms causes some to be concerned about the introduction of bioremediation practices that are not completely understood.

However, there is little doubt that interest in bioremediation will increase in the future. One investment group has estimated that demand for bioremediation will grow at a rate of 16% per year based on cost advantages over other hazardous waste treatments and support by government agencies (55). Such an estimate seems credible, based on the near impossibility of establishing enough landfills to dispose of the soil known to be contaminated, and the difficulty of assuring that those landfills will not leak in the future.

On a federal level, the Department of Energy (DOE) has established a Natural and Accelerated Bioremediation Research program (NABIR). This will be a 10-year effort to find microorganisms and plants that could detoxify metals, radionuclides, and radioactive mixtures at the sites owned by DOE. Interestingly, the NABIR will also include a project to examine the societal aspects of bioremediation (56).

## COMMUNITY INVOLVEMENT

In 1988, Congress passed a free-standing addition to the Superfund Amendment and Reauthorization Act (SARA) known as Title III, or the Emergency Planning and Community Right to Know Act (4). While primarily concerned with planning for chemical emergencies, the act also had the effect of forcing community involvement in many related issues through requirements for state-level planning commissions, notification to these commissions of chemical releases, and the establishment of specific ways that facilities having hazardous substances must report to the commissions the presence, amounts, location, and emergency response characteristics of those substances. These requirements have helped to more accurately identify the type, amount, and location of hazardous materials and the degree of impact on specific communities.

## THE FUTURE OF HAZARDOUS WASTE MANAGEMENT

In coming years, the hazardous waste problem will be addressed in three major ways:

- The continuation of efforts to remediate existing sites, utilizing new technologies to help ensure that cleanups will be permanent.
- The continuation of research to define the human effects of hazardous waste.
- The attempt to avoid such problems in the future.

In addition, there will be more legislative action at all levels of government and within the community of nations. Many of the sites are of such size and complexity that governments will have to be involved in their remediation. Indeed, some of the largest and most complex sites in the United States are current or former federal facilities.

The EPA is currently reevaluating the ways in which responsible parties are defined and the extent to which they will be included in liability for the hazardous waste sites. However, because of the enormous cleanup costs, there will be much effort expended to further clarify many issues of liability, which will probably lead to increased litigation. This may affect the speed and type of remediation responses, and therefore the amount of potential exposure to the affected populations.

Research is needed to further define the human effects resulting from exposure to hazardous waste. A number of avenues will be explored. Among the most important will be the investigation of biomarkers as early indicators of exposure; the effects of exposure on reproduction and development; and increased numbers of pilot medical studies, epidemiologic investigations, and population registries at hazardous waste sites to further define the human effects.

Perhaps one of the most difficult issues for the future will be the question of how to avoid or prevent hazardous waste situations. Whatever steps will be taken cannot be those of governments or scientists alone. They will be determined by society as a whole. Until we can agree to both limit the production of hazardous waste and on ways to dispose of it in environmentally acceptable terms, the problem will remain and grow larger. Although everyone agrees that these wastes must be properly handled, there is great resistance to almost every effort to establish new waste sites or treatment facilities. No matter what scientific tests are performed, there will be considerable resistance to the establishment of additional sites regardless of how remote they may be. Therefore, although science and engineering must continue to look for new ways to treat and dispose of hazardous waste, until societal understanding and agreement is reached, the issue will not go away.

## REFERENCES


1. U.S. Environmental Protection Agency. The birth of a program. *EPA J* 1987(January-February);14–35.
2. Morgan, Lewis, Bockius. *Environmental deskbook.* Philadelphia: Morgan, Lewis, & Bockius, 1996.
3. Habicht H. Plans, problems and promises for the years ahead. *Hazard Mat Control* 1991;60:3.
4. Lucero E, Moertl K, Holmes R, Arnstein C. *Superfund handbook,* 3rd ed. Chicago: ENSR, 1989.
5. Agency for Toxic Substances and Disease Registry. FY 1993 *Agency profile and annual report: Oct. 1, 1992 to Sept. 30, 1993.* Atlanta: ATSDR, 1994.
6. Cortina de Nava C. Worldwide overview of hazardous waste. In: Hazardous waste and public health: *International Congress on the Health Effects of Hazardous Waste.* Princeton: Princeton Scientific, 1994.
7. Rummel-Bulska I. The Basel Convention: a global approach for the management of hazardous waste. In: *Hazardous waste and public health:* International Congress on the Health Effects of Hazardous Waste. Princeton: Princeton Scientific, 1994.
8. Maltezou SP. Hazardous waste problems in selected countries in eastern Europe. In: *Hazardous waste and public health:* International Congress on the Health Effects of Hazardous Waste. Princeton: Princeton Scientific, 1994.
9. Browner C. Testimony to the Subcommittee on Commerce, Trade, and Hazardous Materials, Committee on Commerce, U.S. House of Representatives, Washington, D.C., October 1995.
10. U.S. Environmental Protection Agency. National Priority List for uncontrolled hazardous waste sites. *Federal Register* 1994;59:43314.
11. Russell M, Colglazier EM, English MR. *Hazardous waste remediation:* the task ahead. Knoxville: University of Tennessee, 1991;A-3,10.
12. U.S. Congressional Budget Office. *The total costs of cleaning up nonfederal Superfund sites.* Washington, DC: GPO, 1994.
13. Johnson BL. Hazardous waste: human health effects. In: *Hazardous waste and public health:* International Congress on the Health Effects of Hazardous Waste. Princeton: Princeton Scientific, 1994.
14. Clean Sites. *Hazardous waste sites and the rural poor.* Alexandria, VA: Clean Sites, 1990.
15. Agency for Toxic Substances and Disease Registry. Priority list of hazardous substances that will be the subject of toxicological profiles. *Federal Register* 1994;59:9486–9487.
16. Johnson BL, DeRosa CT. Chemical mixtures released from hazardous waste sites: implications for health risk assessment. *Toxicology* 1995; 105:145–156.
17. Agency for Toxic Substances and Disease Registry. *Public health assessment guidance manual.* Boca Raton, FL: Lewis, 1992.
18. Susten AS. Findings from ATSDR's health assessments. J *Environ Health* 1992;55:17–21.
19. National Research Council. *Environmental epidemiology:* public health and hazardous wastes, vol 1. Washington, DC: National Academy Press, 1991;114:20–21.
20. Grisham J, ed. *Health aspects of the disposal of waste chemicals.* New York: Pergamon Press, 1986.
21. Gist GL, Burg JR, Radtke TM. The site selection process for the National Exposure Registry. *J Environ Health* 1994;56:7.
22. Gist GL, Burg JR. Methodology for selecting substances for the National Exposure Registry. *J Exposure Anal Environ Epi* 1995;5: 197.
23. Burg JR, Gist GL, Allred SL, Radtke TM, Pallos LL, Cusack CD. The National Exposure Registry—morbidity analysis of noncancer outcomes from the trichloroethylene subregistry baseline data. *Int J Occup Med Toxicol* 1995;4:237.
24. Committee on the Institutional Means of Risks to Public Health, National Research Council. *Risk assessment in the federal government:* managing the process. Washington, DC: National Academy Press, 1983.
25. Mitchell FL, McKinnon H. Risk assessment and public health assessment. Presented at the First International Congress on the Health Effects of Hazardous Waste, Atlanta, May, 1993.
26. Institute of Medicine. *Role of the primary care physician in occupational and environmental medicine.* Publication no. IOM-88-05. Washington, DC: National Academy Press, 1988.
27. Agency for Toxic Substances and Disease Registry. *ATSDR case studies in environmental medicine,* numbers I–XX. Atlanta: ATSDR.
28. Agency for Toxic Substances and Disease Registry. *Toxicological profiles.* Atlanta: ATSDR.
29. Pope AM, Rall DP, Eds. *Environmental medicine:* integrating a missing element into medical education. Washington, DC: Institute of Medicine, National Research Council Press, 1995.
30. CDC/ATSDR Subcommittee on Biomarkers of Organ Damage and Dysfunction. *Biomarkers of organ damage or dysfunction for the renal, hepatobiliary, and immune systems.* Atlanta, GA: CDC/ATSDR, 1990.
31. Needleman H. Introduction: biomarkers in neurodevelopmental toxicology. *Environ Health Perspect* 1987;74:149–152.
32. Kimbrough RD. Early biological indicators of chemical exposure and their significance for disease. In: Fowler BA, ed. *Mechanisms of cell injury:* implications for human health. New York: Wiley, 1987; 291–301.
33. Cullen MR. The role of clinical investigations in biological markers research. *Environ Res* 1989;50:1–10.
34. National Academy of Sciences. *Biologic markers in reproductive toxicology.* Washington, DC: National Academy Press, 1989.
35. Schulte PA. A conceptual framework for the validation and use of biologic markers. *Environ Res* 1989;48:129–144.
36. Thomas R. New study: biologic markers of disease. *CLS Lifelines* 1986;12(1–2):12–13.
37. U.S. Department of Transportation, Research and Special Programs Administration, personal communication, 1990.
38. Hall HI, Dhara VR, Kaye WE, Price-Green P. Surveillance of hazardous substance releases and related health effects. *Arch Environ Health* 1994;49:45.
39. Hall HI, Price-Green P, Dhara VR, Kaye WE. Health effects related to releases of hazardous substances on the Superfund priority list. *Chemosphere* 1995;31:2455.
40. Agency for Toxic Substances and Disease Registry. *Hazardous substances emergency event surveillance:* annual report. Atlanta: ATSDR Division of Health Studies, 1995.
41. U.S. Department of Labor, Occupational Safety and Health Administration. *Hazardous waste operations and emergency response:* final rule. *Federal Register,* March 6, 1989. Washington, DC: U.S. Government Printing Office, 1989;54:9294–9336.
42. Warhit EB. *Labor demand projections for the waste remediation market.* Indiana, PA: National Environmental Education and Training Center, 1995.
43. Johnson BL. Worker safety and health. In: *Hazardous waste and public health.* Chelsea, MI: Ann Arbor Press, in press.

44. Mitchell FL. Hazardous waste workers. In: Zenz C, Dickerson OB, Horvath EP, eds. *Occupational medicine,* 3rd ed. St. Louis: Mosby, 1994;937–942.
45. EPA. *Hazardous waste operations and emergency response.* EPA OSWER publication no. 9285.2-09FS. Washington, DC: EPA, 1991.
46. OSHA. *Occupational exposure to bloodborne pathogens:* precautions for emergency responders. OSHA publication no. 3130. Washington, DC: Occupational Safety and Health Administration, 1992.
47. National Institute for Occupational Safety and Health, Occupational Safety and Health Administration, U.S. Coast Guard, U.S. Environmental Protection Agency. *Occupational safety and health guidance manual for hazardous waste site activities.* Publication no. DHHS (NIOSH) 85-115. Atlanta: U.S. Department of Health and Human Services, 1985.
48. Paull JM, Rosenthal FS. Heat strain and stress for workers wearing protective suits at a hazardous waste site. *Am Ind Hyg Assoc J* 1987;48: 458–463.
49. Favata EA, Buckler G, Gochfeld M. Heat stress in hazardous waste workers: evaluation and prevention. In: Gochfeld M, Favata EA, eds. *Occup Med State Art Rev* 1990;5:79–91.
50. U.S. Environmental Protection Agency. *Bioremediation resource matrix.* Publication EPA/542-B-93-004a. Washington, DC: United States Environmental Protection Agency, Office of Solid Waste and Emergency Response, 1993.
51. U.S. Geological Survey. *Bioremediation:* nature's way to a cleaner environment. Fact sheet FS-054-95. Reston, VA: United States Department of the Interior, U.S. Geological Survey, 1995.
52. Gray GGH. *Bioremediation of contaminated soils.* Ontario: University of Waterloo, Technology Transfer and Licensing Office, Office of Research, September 1996.
53. U.S. Department of Energy. *Bacteria's sweet-tooth for molasses provides cleanup solution to TNT-contaminated soil.* News release, October 9. Argonne, IL: U.S. Department of Energy, Argonne National Laboratory, 1996.
54. Rachel's Hazardous Waste News. *New alternatives to incineration.* Annapolis: Rachel's Hazardous Waste News #306, October 1992.
55. Freedonia Group. *Bioremediation.* News release, May 5. Cleveland: The Fredonia Group-Environmental, 1995.
56. Kaiser J. DOE serves up remediation funds. *Nature* 1996;274:1074.

*Environmental and Occupational Medicine, Third Edition,* edited by William N. Rom.
Lippincott–Raven Publishers, Philadelphia © 1998.

CHAPTER 122

# Biologic and Medical Implications of Global Warming

Paul R. Epstein and Alexander Leaf

For several years the evidence has been quite overwhelming that human activities are causing global warming. The production and release of some 5 to 6 billion metric tons of carbon dioxide into the atmosphere each year, largely from the burning of fossil fuels, together with other gases capable of absorbing infrared radiations are causing a global warming. Carbon dioxide is normally present in the atmosphere. If there were no gases in the atmosphere capable of absorbing infrared radiation, the surface of the earth would be about 40°C colder, the oceans would be frozen over, and life as we know it would not be possible (1). But today the concentration of carbon dioxide in the atmosphere, about 360 ppm, is some 25% to 30% higher than it has been at any time within the past 160,000 years (2).

In 1995 environmental ministers from over 150 nations issued a "Berlin Mandate," acknowledging the need to strengthen the Framework Convention on Climate Change (FCCC). They launched a new round of negotiations aimed at reaching agreement in late 1997 on binding commitments by the industrialized countries to reduce emission of heat-trapping gases by the year 2005. [The First Assessment of the Intergovernmental Panel on Climate Change (IPCC) calls for a 60% reduction in greenhouse gas (GHG) emissions to stabilize atmospheric concentrations (3).] The Alliance of Small Island States, concerned about the threat to their very existence from climate change–induced rising sea levels and more intense storms, has called upon industrialized countries to cut their greenhouse-gas emissions by 20% below 1990 levels by the year 2005. (The most recent proposals call for a 15% reduction by 2010.) The reason for urgency is the recognition of the threatening consequences to the health of humans and other biologic systems to which the man-made climate changes must lead. This chapter focuses on the consequences of the global warming to the health of human and other biologic systems. Our emphasis is on human health effects, but the biosphere is a highly integrated system and there is much interdependence between the human and nonhuman bioses.

Before discussing the specifics of the changes imposed by global warming on living things, it is important to summarize the socioeconomic factors that will compound with the global warming to cause the potential health problems. It is generally understood that the rapid growth in human population underlies many of the problems we will consider (4). Figure 1 shows the dramatic rate of increase in the world's human population. Despite the reduced rate of increase, in the developed, industrialized countries, we are still adding some 90,000,000 persons annually to the world's population (5). Predictions from the United Nations suggest that if serious efforts are made to control the rate of increase, by 2050 the total population will level off at some 8 billion; if that effort is not maximal, the population may reach 10 to 12 billion; and if nothing is done to reduce present rates, 20 billion may be reached (4). And the birth rates do not tell the whole story. As the absolute numbers of women of reproductive age increases, a decrease in birth rate can be masked since the final number of humans added is the product of rate times numbers of potential producers.

P. R. Epstein: Center for Health and the Global Environment, Harvard Medical School, Boston, Massachusetts 02115.
A. Leaf: Department of Medicine, Massachusetts General Hospital, Harvard Medical School, Charlestown, Massachusetts 02129.

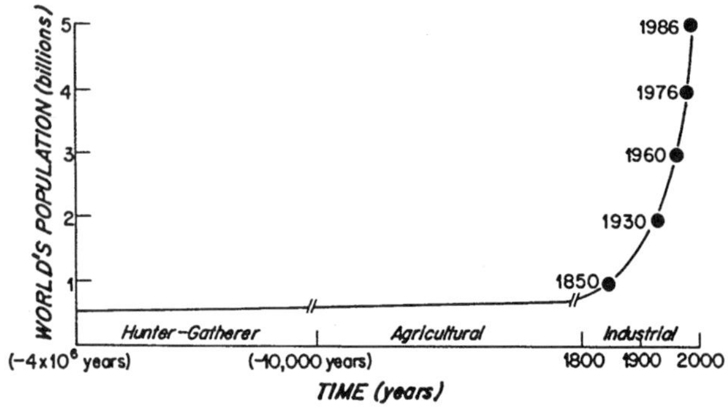


**FIG. 1.** The world's population growth.

When China's population increased to more than 1 billion despite the low birth rate achieved by dint of strict communal measures (which the West has criticized), the annual absolute number of newborns was still enormous. Whereas in 1960 one-third of the world's population lived in the industrialized, developed countries, by 1995 these countries made up only one-sixth of the population; 83% were in the developing countries. The gulf between the affluent and the impoverished has increased both relatively in total numbers and in actual wealth. Further, the proportion of the population living in urban areas has greatly increased (6), with all the associated problems of poverty, crowding, pollution, and stress.

Examination of World Bank figures indicate that equity (land distribution, income) within a society is directly correlated with a nation's ability to control its population growth.

It is the combination of the huge growth in population and efforts to attain higher standards of living that have created the need for more energy sources, supplied largely from burning of fossil fuels, that today adds some 6 billion metric tons of carbon dioxide, the major greenhouse gas, to the atmosphere annually. Chlorofluorocarbons (especially efficient absorbers of infrared radiation) in aerosols and refrigerants, and methane (from decaying organic matter and cattle flatus) plus water vapor also accumulate in the atmosphere and contribute to the greenhouse effect. Together these gases trap reradiated heat from the earth: increases lead to global warming. The annual average global temperature has risen gradually from about 14.5°C in 1886, when reliable records began, to 15.4°C in 1995, and the rise correlates closely with the increase in atmospheric heat-trapping greenhouse gases (2). Both trends are now accelerating, resulting in predictions of a 1° to 3.5°C increase in the next century (2). The mean global increase may not seem impressive, but the warming equals the increase that has occurred since the last ice age and is occurring at a greatly increased rate. Warming toward the poles may exceed the average; thus warming can affect the heavily populated and large agriculture producing areas of the middle and higher latitudes disproportionately to the tropics and will cause more extremes of hot weather to occur.

The effects of global warming on human health are both direct and indirect and include the following:

1. Heat stress
2. Weather disasters, rising sea levels, environmental refugees and crowding
3. Land and water scarcity
4. Food sufficiency and nutritional health
5. Noninfectious respiratory diseases and air pollution
6. Infectious diseases
   a. vector borne
   b. nonvector borne

## HEAT STRESS

Heat stress is the most direct health effect of global warming. An increase in average temperature will probably increase the number and severity of extreme heat waves in some areas. Climate change would exacerbate an already large urban heat island effect. Mid-latitude cities that experience irregular heat waves appear to be most susceptible—cities such as Washington, D.C., St Louis, Chicago, and New York. A mean rise of 2° to 5°C in the next 50 to 100 years will increase the number of days with temperatures over 38°C (100.4°F). Washington, D.C., which now averages 1 to 2 days a year with temperatures over 38°C, may be expected to average some 12 such days by the middle of the next century (7). This would cause an increase in illness and death, particularly among the very young, the elderly, the frail, and the chronically ill. The deaths of 726 people that were attributed to the heat wave in Chicago in the summer of 1995 may be an extreme recent example (8), but it serves as a possible indicator of what might occur if climate changes occur, as predicted.

A crucial element in the 1995 heat wave was the lack of letup at night. Minimum temperatures (TMINs, nighttime and winter) are projected to increase more rapidly than average temperatures with global warming (9). And there is evidence that TMINs are already rising disproportionately (9). A warmed atmosphere holds more water vapor (6% more for each 1°C), thus we are observing increased cloudiness (and night time and winter warming), increased humidity in heat waves, and more extreme precipitation events.

Tropical and subtropical cities seem less susceptible. Populations have acclimatized to hot weather and lifestyles have adapted. The magnitude of the increases in mortality is not yet clear. People in mid-latitude cities may also acclimatize. Air conditioning could reduce the number of sufferers, but air conditioning expends much energy and increases the consumption of fossil fuels that create the greenhouse warming. The increase in mortality may also be offset to some extent by a decrease in winter deaths from hypothermia and cold. (The majority of winter mortality is due to infectious diseases transmitted person-to-person, e.g., influenza, where there is no direct correlation with ambient temperatures.) Despite these uncertainties, the 1995 National Academy of Sciences Conference on Human Health and Global Climate Change (10) states there is a clear need to develop an adequate warning system to alert the public and government agencies when oppressive air masses are expected—extended periods of extreme high temperature, light winds, high humidity, and intense solar radiation. This is recommended, in addition to the urgent need to increase the efficiency of our use of available energy and to reduce dependence for energy supplies on fossil fuels.

## WEATHER DISASTERS, RISING SEA LEVELS, ENVIRONMENTAL REFUGEES, AND CROWDING

Global warming is expected to be associated with more frequent and more severe storms with heavy precipitation and flooding. The increased temperature of the air and of the oceans will result in more evaporation, creating more clouds and more rain and snow. But this effect will not be general. It will occur mainly in coastal areas, while the interior of continents are expected to become drier and hotter, leading to increased droughts.

In the past 100 years, sea levels have risen 10 to 25 cm. Even the expected rise of sea level by one-half to 1 m due to thermal expansion of oceans and the melting of glaciers and icecaps (1) will inundate large population centers and much fertile land. Over half the world now lives in coastal regions and, as population increases further, so will this percentage. Already over 70% of the people of Southeast Asia live near the coast (11), while the increases in upland populations are less (11). The expected rise may create 50 million environmental refugees worldwide, double or triple the numbers of refugees and nationally displaced persons created by wars, droughts, and famine today (12). Mainland coastal regions as well as low islands will be in danger. Cities built on barrier islands and the fertile plains that typically surround river deltas are in jeopardy. Low-lying countries, such as Bangladesh, will be most severely affected. Coastal storms today already cause flooding and havoc in that densely populated country with its impoverished millions. Similarly, storms surges and storms are affecting Caribbean and Pacific Island nations: Losses of barrier reefs, and submergence of coral reefs and wetlands further increase the vulnerability to subsequent storms, tidal surges, and to gradual sea level rise (SLR). A substantial part (some 18% to 34%) could disappear, displacing 15% to 35% of its population. In Egypt, where only 4% of its land is arable, and that mainly along the banks of the lower Nile and its delta, these areas are at risk of inundation. Food production would drop severely and 8.5 million people could be displaced from their homes (11). In these crowded countries there is no place for displaced persons to move and no new land on which to grow crops. In addition, land will be rendered unfit for agriculture by the rising salinity of water tables.

Large areas of the wetlands, which filter nutrients and pollutants and nourish the world's fisheries, will be destroyed. The United States, with more than 19,000 km of coastline, will not be spared. For example, much of Florida sits on porous limestone. Pumping down the aquifer to water the citrus and other crops, facilitates ocean water to seep under the land. Miami has such a porous aquifer that a protective dike against rising sea levels would have to start more than 45 m (150 ft) beneath the surface to prevent salt water from welling up behind it (7). Displaced people and less arable land will compound the task of feeding the world's population.

## LAND AND WATER

Other factors are moving at an even faster pace to reduce the world's croplands. The rapid urbanization of the world's population causes cities to expand into the countryside. The urban share of global population is expected to rise from 43% in 1990 to 61% in 2025 (6). Cities must house, transport, employ, and provide recreation for their citizens, and these all require land. Industrialization, which often occurs in or around cities, is growing rapidly in developing countries and requires considerable area for factories and supporting infrastructure (6). In the developing world, Latin America and Africa can still absorb urban expansion without a net loss of agricultural land, but Asia cannot.

China's rapid industrialization during the decade 1986 to 1996 created 200 new cities, and more that 100 million peasants migrated from rural areas to cities in search of a better life, a worldwide phenomenon. In 1988 and 1989, just prior to China's double-digit economic growth, the country lost more than 1 million hectares of cultivated land, 16% of which was converted to urban and industrial use, The rest was lost to natural disasters, restoration of forests and grasslands, or to orchards or fish ponds. China has already paved over 435,000 hectares of cropland in this decade, as a conservative estimate, enough to feed 10 million Chinese (5). A 1990 World Bank study of Indonesia reported some 10,000 hectares of agricultural land are needed each year just for house lots. A U.S. Department of Agriculture report states that the island of Java loses nearly 20,000 hectares annually to urban growth—enough to grow rice for some 378,000 Indonesians each year. In crowded Bangladesh, cropland around Dhaka continues to disappear as farmers earn more selling their land for development than they could by farming. Metropolitan Bangkok is projected to expand by 51,000 hectares between 1984 and 2000, an increase of 40%. If 80% of this expansion engulfs farmland in Thailand, the loss will represent rice enough to feed 344,000 people (6).

These are just a few examples of what is and will be happening in the crowded lands of Asia. But the situation is further worsened by the fact that urban expansion often claims the best croplands. Cities historically are founded near rich agricultural lands and as they grow some of a country's most fertile land is taken out of production. In the United States just over 18% of all rural land is classified as prime farmland, but within 50 miles of the largest urban areas 27% of farmland is prime. Of the 2.4 million hectares of prime U.S. farmland lost on a net basis between 1982 and 1992, two-thirds were converted to rural and urban development (6). In developed countries a further sizable loss occurs due to construction of roads. It was estimated already a decade ago that in the United States an area the size of the state of Oklahoma had already been covered by concrete. If developing countries become as dependent on automobiles as we are, similar losses of actual or potential agricultural lands will occur.

Agricultural lands can cease production if watered by overdrawn aquifers. India, Saudi Arabia, and the United States overpump water from aquifers faster than the water is replenished by rainfall to irrigate extensive tracts of agricultural land. As aquifers are depleted, continued pumping becomes economically impractical. Saudi Arabia cut its wheat and barley area by more than a fifth from 1994 to 1996, partly from concern for water depletion (5). During the decade ending in 1992, farmers drawing water from the huge Ogallala aquifer in the United States lost three times more irrigated hectares than they gained. In five High Plains states and three in the western United States irrigated area fell by nearly 10% over this decade as aquifer levels dropped (6).

As already mentioned, the rise in sea levels will inundate coastal lands, reducing farmland. Global warming is expected to raise sea levels by 10 to 120 cm (4–47 inches) by 2100. A World Bank study projects a loss of 9.2 million hectares covering 48 cities, which would be flooded in China, if sea levels rise 50 to 100 cm. This would displace 67 million people. In India 570,000 hectares and 7 million people are at risk of inundation (6).

Forests, one of the "sinks" for carbon in the global carbon cycle, are being demolished at an unprecedented rate to provide fuel. In Nepal, for example, this leaves denuded areas, which are then eroded by the monsoons, while the rains and soils cause flooding and mudslides below in India. In Brazil forests are cut down for timber or for pasture and farmland. In the tropics the lush rain forests grow on a shallow surface of good soils. The rapid decay of vegetation there provides nutrients that are promptly absorbed and reassimilated into the forest coverage. When forests are cut to provide timber for export, pasture lands for cattle, and farmlands for the impoverished populace, large tracts of the denuded land are quickly depleted of their limited nutrients and left to be eroded by rains and winds and converted by the hot sun to desert. The populace moves on to destroy more forests. Each year 6 million hectares (27.2 million acres) of productive land turn into desert, creating in three decades an area roughly the size of Saudi Arabia (3). More than 11 million hectares (29 million acres) of forest are destroyed each year—in three decades an area roughly the size of India (4). In 1990 a U.N. report on global land degradation, known as the GLASOD study (6), found that more than 15% of agricultural land degraded between 1945 and 1990 was made essentially irretrievably unproductive. At modest grain production rates this land could have fed more than 1.5 billion peoples, more than one-quarter of the world's population today. GLASOD reported that nearly one-sixth of the world's vegetated area has suffered some degree of soil degradation since World War II. More than three-quarters of this abuse has been caused by agriculture and livestock production or by converting forests to cropland. Abuse of farmland ranges from salting and waterlogging, found on poorly managed irrigated lands, to compaction caused by the use of heavy machinery and to pollution from the excessive application of pesticides or manure. But erosion is by far the most common type of land degradation, accounting for 84% of affected areas according to the U.N. study.

Climate modeling, though greatly improved in the last decade, does not yet allow sufficient spatial resolution to permit prediction over areas less than several hundred kilometers square. Nevertheless, gross predictions have been made indicating that in contrast to coastal areas, interiors of continents will suffer less precipitation with resulting hotter, drier, arid conditions unfavorable to growth of much of present-day agriculture. In the United States, the southwestern desert will shift north to cover the Midwestern grain belt, which will move into Canada. Temperatures favorable for growing grains will move from mid-Europe and the middle United States to Canada and Siberia, but whether the fertile soils, adequate rainfall, and the other essentials of optimal growth will exist in the higher latitudes, is uncertain. California will be hard hit by drought. Southern California is expected to have a drier winter, the season when most of the precipitation falls. Even if total precipitation levels remain unchanged, the warmer temperatures will cause more of the winter's precipitation to fall as rain, which will mean quick runoffs, winter flooding, and less melting snow to support water needs in the summer. As summer supplies of fresh water shrink in the San Francisco Bay area, sea water will further infiltrate the aquifer beneath the Sacramento delta, and this will be amplified by the rising sea level (7).

## FOOD SUFFICIENCY AND NUTRITIONAL HEALTH

The discussion so far has been a necessary prelude to understanding the issues of food sufficiency and health.

Food, water, and health—three basic needs—are intimately related. It is the combined effects of climate change, population increase, and expectations of a higher standard of living that lead to water and land scarcity for crop production, posing serious questions about food sufficiency and possible diets. Of these three factors it may well be the last two that are most important and would alone have eventually resulted in the same threatening situation. But global warming will most probably accelerate the urgency of the problem.

There are those who have argued that the increased ambient temperature and atmospheric carbon dioxide will improve crop yield and compensate thereby for the deleterious effects of the factors just discussed. Since carbon dioxide is a reactant in photosynthesis, plant growth from this factor alone would be expected to accelerate plant and crop growth. The effect of warming within the limits of temperature tolerance would also be expected to enhance plant growth. However, other conditions must be present along with the green house warming effect and the increased $CO_2$ concentrations for the latter to improve crop yields. Water is one such required ingredient and its availability will likely be lacking. There have now been several field experiments testing the effects on plant growth of simply increasing ambient $CO_2$ concentrations and these so far show variable effects, are preliminary, and leave much uncertainty on this issue. A climate modeling simulation for a scenario in which $CO_2$ concentrations doubled, a condition predicted to exist after a period of 60 to 70 years, was made by the IPCC (3). Here are the conclusions from an analysis of this study (13):

> Under the scenarios of climate change derived from the experiments doubling $CO_2$ levels, it is estimated that global food production will decrease, and without farm-level adaptation the adverse effect could be severe. With adaptation the negative global impact would be reduced but it would not disappear, even on an assumption that the beneficial direct physiologic $CO_2$ effects on crop growth will be fully realized. Perhaps, more importantly, climate change may increase potential production in the developed world but reduce it in developing nations, and agricultural adaptation does little to lessen that disparity. Cereal prices, and the population at risk of hunger in developing countries, would thus increase.

Though such a study lacks predictive credibility, it suggests that positive effects of $CO_2$ on plant growth do not necessarily extrapolate to increased crop yields.

Furthermore, the warming will accelerate insect growth, more frequent breeding, and earlier migration. Plant growth can be limited by many factors and attack by insects is a major one. In the northern boreal forests warm years are often associated with pest outbreaks. An example has been cited from the effect of warming on the spruce budworm (2). This is an insect that attacks new growth on conifers and has been gradually moving westward across Canada destroying more forest than any other insect pest. It is estimated that a single outbreak can produce 7,200 trillion individual budworms. With standard insect mutation rates this should create some billions of genetic variants among which adaptation to any environmental change should be likely. With global warming some regions of the Canadian forests may become both warm and dry, but for any possible climate scenario there will likely be a strain of budworms preadapted to those conditions. In the case of insects and parasites that destroy crops, global warming may allow some that require warm environments to move northward, and infect crops in areas that previously had been too cold for them and their high mutation rates make them genetically adaptable to changing conditions.

Another aspect of climate change—climate instability and extreme weather events—will also affect agriculture. Prolonged droughts (as in the U.S. southwest during the summer of 1996) or killing frosts (Florida, late 1996) may markedly alter linear projections based only on shifting agricultural zones.

There have also been arguments that new, or more plentiful fertilizers and pesticides will increase crop yields. It was the combination of high-yield grains, increased irrigation, and more and more pesticides that accounted for the unprecedented "green revolution," which occurred between 1950 and 1990. In that interval the world's grain harvest increased from 631 million tons to 1,780 million tons, almost tripling (5). Since 1990, however, there has been a considerable reduction in the rate of increase, which has not kept up with the population increase so that the actual grain production per person has fallen (5). With smaller returns from increases in fertilizer use, global fertilizer use today has plateaued. Increasing use apparently is no longer able to compensate for or replace the depletion of nutrients from soil degradation. Fertilizers cannot provide other essential factors for optimal plant growth, such as organic materials, insects, microorganisms, water, and trace elements (5). Also strains of insects and parasites resistant to the pesticides have evolved, frustrating even the use of increased amounts of pesticides. By 1994, 520 insects and mites, 150 plant diseases, and 113 weeds had developed resistance to one of more pesticides meant to prevent them (4). In addition, at least 17 insects were resistant to all major classes of insecticides, and several plant diseases were immune to most fungicides used against them (14). Development of new classes of pesticides is a slow process, generally requiring a decade or more. Reducing the use of pesticides and adopting integrated pest management has been shown to increase crop production.

Meanwhile both the fertilizers and pesticides have become major environmental polluters. The increase in nitrogen and phosphorus from fertilizers has thrown the nitrogen cycle and phosphorus balance out of kilter. Phosphorous and nitrogen leached from farm fields wind up in rivers, lakes, and the ocean, where they cause algal growth and kill fish. Such erosion has become the largest source of water pollution in the United States (6).

Pollution of rivers, lakes, and ocean with leached pesticides have poisoned potable water supplies and killed fish, shell fish, and other aqueous food sources, often contaminating the survivors, making them unfit for human consumption.

Other pollutants have been accumulating in the troposphere that are injurious to plants. These are largely the result of industrial processes and consumption of fossil fuels, such as sulfur dioxide and nitrogen oxides (the chief contributors to acid rain). Ammonia, hydrogen sulfide, and dimethyl sulfide are also toxic to vegetation, killing forests, and poisoning fresh water in lakes and streams. The acidification of the environment threatens large areas of Europe and North America. Central Europe receives more than 1 g of sulfur on every square kilometer of ground each year (4). A 7-year U.S. study reported that air pollution is reducing U.S. crop output by at least 5% (15). Western Europe with similar dependence on automobiles and fossil fuels will suffer similar crop losses. Eastern Europe and China with their heavy dependence on coal may have even larger crop losses (13). Industrial nitrogen oxides and both natural and industrial hydrocarbons are thought to be responsible for toxic levels of tropospheric ozone. The enlarging ozone hole in the stratosphere allows more ultraviolet-B to enter the troposphere where it reacts with nitrogen oxides and hydrocarbons, creating tropospheric ozone. Ozone is a major contributor to smog and is highly toxic to plants. High levels of ozone are observed over the eastern United States during summer at concentrations high enough to damage crops (16), Thus the chlorofluorocarbons that are responsible for depleting the thin ozone shield in the stratosphere result paradoxically also in an increase in ozone at ground level.

Many seem to expect a quick technological fix to save us from serious food deficiency. Genetic engineering as a means to facilitate adaptation of crops to the changes in the environment is a favorite hope and indeed may afford some welcome surprises, as might a return to farming native, indigenous crops rather than concentrating agriculture production on one or a few common grains or crops for marketing. But whether these will be adequate and thrive on degraded soils on reduced, available arable lands with diminished water is not known. Will currently successful native crops adapt to climate changes? These are uncertainties which leave considerable potential risk for the welfare of the predicted future huge populations.

What is the present status of food sufficiency in the world today and what may that augur for the future? Grains provide more than 50% of the world's human foods and, therefore, the availability of grains, especially when expressed on a per person basis, is our best index of food sufficiency (6). We have already referred to the unprecedented tripling of grain production between 1950 and 1990. Since then the rate of growth has slowed considerably and the yield per person has fallen from an all-time high level of 346 kg per person in 1984 to 313 kg in 1996, a decline of 7%. With this decline world grain reserves had fallen to their lowest ever. An excellent harvest in 1990 swelled the grain reserves to 342 million tons, which fell by 1996 to 240 million tons, sufficient to sustain consumption for only 50 days (5).

As usual, the declines have especially affected the developing world, where impoverished multitudes already live on the verge of starvation. With 86 million fewer tons of grain in 1993 than in 1992 and with 90 million more people to share the harvest, per capita grain output dropped nearly 7%. At 303 kg per person, it was down 12% from the historic high of 346 kg per person in 1984 (15). The short-fall is experienced predominantly in the developing world. In 1990, there were 530 million people or about 10% of the population with an income insufficient either to procure or produce its food requirement (13) and the numbers are predicted to rise. Between the peak of production in 1984 and 1988 world grain production per person fell 14%, while in Africa since 1967 the decline has been 27% (17).

But some figures showing current and near future population and grain production estimates (5) indicate that the problem is not going away: The Middle East with a population of 243 million in 1995 is projected to increase to 544 million by 2030, forcing this water-short region to import most of its grain (5). North Africa—Morocco through Egypt—already facing a water shortage, will grow from its 136 million in 1995 to 239 million by 2030. These countries already import half or more of their grain (5). Over the same 35-year period sub-Saharan Africa is projected to grow from 585 million to 1.45 billion. With its poor prospects for increasing grain production, it will have to become dependent largely on grain imports, if such are available and affordable (5). India, already close to 1 billion, is projected to increase its population to 1.45 billion. Already facing groundwater depletion, it will likely need to import heavily. Neighboring Pakistan, now at the limits of its water resources, will grow from 132 million in 1995 to 312 million in 2030 (5). As Mexico with its 1995 population of 94 million, already having a grain deficit, increases to 150 million in 2030, its deficit can only increase. Brazil, which is already the largest grain importer in the Western Hemisphere, will increase from 161 million in 1995 to 210 million in 2030. With its poor endowment of agriculture resources, adequate expansion of its own production of crops is unlikely (5). China, which is increasingly importing grains, is projected to import some 200 million tons by 2030, an amount equal to total current world grain exports (5).

There is a wide range in levels of food consumption in different countries. In the United States, average annual grain consumption per person is some 800 kg, most of which is consumed indirectly as beef, pork, poultry, eggs, and dairy products. In India the average annual grain consumption is only 200 kg, but this is almost entirely consumed directly. Neither the fat-rich diet of Americans or the Indian diet dominated by starchy grains, mainly rice, provide the healthiest diets. Judged on longevity of the populace, the Mediterranean diet with some 400 kg of grains, vegetables, fruits, and vegetable oils or the rice, fish, and vegetables of the traditional Japanese diet would seem to be the healthiest. As Brown (5) points out, if the 1996 grain harvest of 1.82 billion tons can be increased to 2 billion tons, that would be enough grain to support 2.5 billion Americans or 10 billion Indians.

With affluence, populations change from traditional to American diets. The high livestock consumption of grains is expensive, as in the United States it takes 6.9 kg of grain to produce a kg of pork, 4.8 kg for a kg of beef, 2.8 kg for a kg of chicken, 3.0 kg for a kg of cheese, and 2.6 kg for a kg of eggs (18). Even fish farming consumes grains. Since it requires some 2 to 3 kg of fish entrails to produce 1 kg of fish, grains are a more available feed for fish, and are gradually replacing marine foods in the aquaculture industry.

The high fat intake that results from large meat consumption in the United States and Western industrialized countries contributes to heart disease, obesity, hypertension, diabetes, and certain cancers. The associated high protein intake may contribute to osteoporosis because of the acid load to be excreted from the catabolism of the excess protein. Thus, the high meat consumption by affluent populations are deleterious to the health as well as to the availability of food for the poor in the developing countries.

With its recent and very rapid industrialization China is becoming affluent even as its own crop production is becoming limited. The Chinese are eating more meats, which increase disproportionately their need to import grains. With affluence they are able to buy a larger portion of the world's grain exports to satisfy their expanded food preferences. This has the potential to reduce the affordability of grain imports by impoverished developing countries, increasing the malnutrition and starvation in these countries (19).

In many nations (e.g., Japan) fish accounts for well over half of the protein consumed. Fisheries are under multiple stresses—from overharvesting, coastal pollution, and changes in ocean temperatures (see below). With the oceanic fish catch no longer expanding and the rise in land productivity at 1% per year the important question, Is how can the world's food production system support a population that continues to grow at a projected rate of 1.5%? Without taking into account the overarching problem of population growth, one cannot talk rationally about food sufficiency. Food insufficiency with famine and starvation have always led to instability of governments and social institutions with wars and flagrant human rights abuses, not healthy conditions for humans. Malnutrition is a recognized cause of diminished immune competence, which will amplify the other major health impediment created by environmental change and global warming, namely infectious diseases.

## NONINFECTIOUS RESPIRATORY DISEASES

It has long been appreciated that some occupations were associated with high incidences of noninfectious respiratory diseases: silicosis with coal mining, asbestosis with ship building during World War II, berylliosis with early fluorescent lights, and so forth. Recently it has become increasingly evident that particulate matter of $<1.5$ μm can cause respiratory irritation and inflammation if present chronically in the inspired air. The same industrial processes that produce greenhouse gases will produce increased urban air pollutants, which can pose major health risks. Levels of fine particulates (from fossil fuel and wood smoke) and ground-level ozone, a powerful respiratory irritant (from photochemical reactions), are known to be associated with hospitalizations for respiratory diseases and also for heart disease and general mortality increases. With hot weather, which will increase in frequency during summers in populated urban areas in the industrialized mid-latitudes, the industrial pollutants combined with automobile exhausts produce inflammatory pulmonary diseases, exacerbating asthma and eventually chronic obstructive pulmonary disease. In the United States, where air pollution is relatively low compared to Mexico City and several Asian cities, it nevertheless contributes to 70,000 excess deaths and a million additional hospitalizations annually. In the future, as global increases in energy production lead to higher levels of particulates, and increases in temperature and ultraviolet radiation accelerate the reactions that produce ozone and other secondary pollutants, the health effects of air pollution on a global scale are predicted to worsen (8).

## CLIMATE CHANGE AND INFECTIOUS DISEASES

### Background

According to *The World Health Report 1996: Fighting Disease, Fostering Development* (World Health Organization), (20) 30 diseases new to medicine have emerged in the past two decades. In addition there is the resurgence of old diseases: multidrug-resistant tuberculosis—exacerbated by HIV/AIDS—causes 3 million deaths annually, while diphtheria, whooping cough, and measles are increasing, particularly where social systems have deteriorated. Malaria, dengue ("breakbone") fever, yellow fever, rodent-borne viruses, and cholera are also appearing with increased frequency; and these diseases, requiring animals or water as vectors for transmission, will reflect changes in the environment and in social systems.

### Climate Change and Vector-Borne Disease

Outbreaks of vector-borne diseases are clearly multifactorial—involving compounding social, biologic, and environmental factors. Periurban sprawl, poor sanitation, and proliferating nonbiodegradable (and other) water containers—and social inequities in general—provide the setting for the resurgence of dengue fever in Latin America, for example.

But meteorological factors play a role. In general terms, climate circumscribes the range at which vector-borne diseases (VBDs) can occur, while weather influences the timing of outbreaks (21).

In the tropics, rain is the limiting factor; in the extratropics and at high altitudes, temperature and precipitation are key parameters. (Cloud cover also plays a role.)

Two characteristics of climate change are germane: (a) the gradual rise in average global temperatures over the past 100 years (about 0.6°C), and (b) the disproportionate rise in minimum temperatures (TMINs)—i.e., nighttime and winter—in relation to the gradual rise in average global temperatures (4). As above, the lack of relief at night evidently played a significant role in the 1995 Chicago heat-wave deaths. Both aspects of global warming can impact mosquito activity, biting rates, breeding sites, and ability to overwinter.

#### *Montane Regions*

Mountain regions—where winter temperature isotherms may first noticeably shift in response to global warming, and where physical and biologic responses may be most easily detected—can be sentinel areas to examine for climate change (22,23).

Consistent with model projections of new areas that could sustain vector-borne disease transmission with global warming (24,25), insect-borne diseases (e.g., malaria and dengue fever) are being reported at high altitudes in Africa, Asia, and Latin America (26–29). Highland malaria is becoming a problem for rural areas in Papua New Guinea and for urban centers in Central Africa (30). Malaria, for example, has appeared in Nairobi. In 1995, dengue fever blanketed the Americas, crossing mountain ranges that previously presented barriers to spread, and moving from the Pacific to the Atlantic coast.

A relevant finding comes from the work of Parmesan (31), who reported a population shift in Edith's Checkerspot butterflies in 1996. The level of population extinctions at the far southern end of its range (in Mexico) is four times as great than at the far northern end of its range (in Canada); and about two-and-a-half times as great at lower elevations as compared to populations above 8,000 feet.

Additionally, upward migration of plants has been documented on 26 Alpine peaks (32) and has been observed in Alaska, the U.S. Sierra Nevada, and New Zealand (33). These biologic findings are occurring in tandem with widespread physical changes: montane glaciers are in retreat in Argentina, Peru, Alaska, Iceland, Norway, the Swiss Alps, Kenya, the Himalayas, Indonesia, and New Zealand (34,35).

The clearest signal comes from the report by Diaz and Graham (36) that the freezing level (0°C isotherm) in the mountains (30°N to 30°S latitudes) has shifted upward approximately 500 feet (i.e., almost 2°F adiabatically) since 1970.

Paleoclimatic fossil data (37) demonstrate shifts in isotherms—especially TMINs—were key to large geographic shifts of beetles at the end of the last ice age (10,000 years ago). These records indicate that insects change distribution in response to climatic changes much more rapidly than do grasses, shrubs, forests, and large mammals. "Beetles are better climatic indicators than bears" (37a). A disproportionate rise in TMINs can allow insects to overwinter and to be more active at night.

Anophelines transmitting *Plasmodium falciparum,* and *Aedes aegypti* carrying dengue and yellow fevers have known thresholds for survival (e.g., approximately the 16°C and 10°C winter isotherms, respectively) (38). Thus models, incorporating vectorial capacity, of the geographic areas conducive to maintaining VBDs (e.g., involving insects and snails) uniformly indicate spread to higher altitudes and higher latitudes under global warming (2× $CO_2$) scenarios (23–25,39–42). Mosquitoes, in particular, are highly sensitive to climatic factors (43–47). Seasonality of transmission may also increase in areas now on the margins of areas with bioclimatic (temperature and moisture) conditions conducive for vector survival.

These considerations hold as well for agricultural pests that are stenotherms, requiring specific temperature thresholds for survival (48,49). Assessment of food availability with climate change must include projections for the potential redistribution of crop pests, as well as the impacts of extreme weather events (e.g., floods, prolonged drought; see below).

In this decade autochthonous (locally transmitted) malaria has occurred at high latitudes. Malaria has occurred in New Jersey (1991) and Queens, New York (1993) during hot, wet summers (50), in Texas (1995), Michigan (1996), and Florida (1996) (50a). Elsewhere, dengue fever has appeared in Australia (Torres Strait) and malaria has reinvaded the Kwazulu-Natal province of South Africa. These findings are consistent with the model projections. But the consistency of highland changes with other physical and biologic data provides the most convincing evidence that climate change appears to have begun.

### Climate Variability and Epidemics

A third characteristic of climate change—climatic variability and the observed increase in extreme weather events (51)—also contributes to disease outbreaks and epidemic clusters. Changes in climate variability can affect the timing, intensity, and spatial patterns of weather. Since the mid-1800s a global warming trend has been documented, and periods of warming may be associated with increased variability. The IPCC projects that more intense heat waves and extreme precipitation events may accompany the warming trend.

Data from the National Climatic Data Center—this nation's main repository for meteorological data—indicate that, since the 1970s, extreme weather events have increased in the continental United States. Droughts have become longer and bursts of precipitation more intense (>2 inches over 24 hours) (52). Such events were greater in the 1980s than the 1970s, and more so in the 1990s than in the 1980s.

Extreme events—floods, storms, droughts, and uncontained fires—can be devastating for agriculture, for human settlements, and for health. Heat waves and winter storms both usher in cardiac deaths. Floods spread bacteria, viruses, and chemical contaminants, foster the growth of fungi, and favor insect breeding. Prolonged droughts interrupted by heavy rains favor population explosions of insects and rodents. Extreme weather events (most often associated with El Niño/La Niña changes in Pacific surface ocean temperatures) have been accompanied by malaria outbreaks in Asia, harmful algal blooms (HABs) in the United States and Asia, and waterborne diseases (like typhoid, hepatitis A, bacillary dysentery, and cholera) in Latin America and in Asia.

In August 1995, for example, the eastern Pacific Ocean turned cold, initiating a La Niña event that would last until late 1996. Along the Caribbean coast of Colombia in South America a June 1995 heat wave was followed by the heaviest August rainfall in 50 years (after years of drought that accompanied the previous prolonged El Niño, 1990–1995). The heat and flooding precipitated a cluster of diseases involving mosquitoes (Venezuelan equine encephalitis and dengue fever), rodents (leptospirosis), and toxic algae (killing 350 tons of fish) (53).

### Underlying Mechanism: Understanding Biologic Controls

Insect, rodents, weeds, and microorganisms are opportunistic species (*r*-strategists); they reproduce rapidly, they have huge broods, small body sizes, and wide-ranging appetites, and they are good at dispersal and colonization of new—and especially disturbed—environments. *K*-strategists represent the carrying capacity of the environment, i.e., they level off asymptotically in response to resource depletion and generation of wastes. *K*-strategists (like large predators) also fare well in stable environments. The relative balance among functional groups (e.g., predators and prey, scavengers and decomposers) helps keep opportunistic organisms from overgrowing environments (51,54). In degraded environments, opportunists can become dominant, just as opportunistic infections (OIs) take advantage in patients with weakened immune systems.

Owls, coyotes, and snakes, for example, eat rodents; and rodents can devour grains (55) and carry Lyme disease ticks, hantaviruses, arenaviruses (hemorrhagic fevers), human plague, and leptospirosis bacteria. Control of mosquito populations is naturally performed by reptiles, birds, spiders, ladybugs, and bats—and fish that consume their larvae in ponds. Mosquitoes provide nourishment for these animals—but some carry malaria, yellow fever, dengue fever, and several types of encephalitis.

Several aspects of global change tend to reduce predators disproportionately, releasing prey from their biologic controls. Among the most widespread are the following: (a) habitat loss and fragmentation, (b) monocultures in agriculture and aquaculture, (c) excessive use of toxic chemicals, (d) excess ultraviolet radiation, and (e) climate change and weather instability.

Fragmentation of wilderness into smaller patches, compounded by "edge effects," (56) reduces the habitat for large predators, favoring pests (57). Monocultures, with reduced genetic and species diversity, show increased vulnerability to infections and invasions of exotic species. Excessive use of pesticides harms birds and "helpful" insects. *Silent Spring* (58) referred to the absence of bird calls in spring, and the resulting resurgence of herbivores—that had themselves evolved resistance to the pesticides. (An evolutionary change compounded by a deficiency in the coevolved, regulatory, biologic control system.)

At all scales a diversity of responses to stress is essential for resilience and resistance. Animal groups sometimes viewed as "redundant" may also be seen as "insurance" species, ensuring resilience and vigor in the face of disease, starvation, and environmental change.

### Rodents: "Nasty" Synergies

Rodents are a growing problem in the United States, Latin America, Africa, Europe, Asia, and Australia, and altered climate variability is contributing. Rodents—preeminent opportunists—are believed to be the fastest-reproducing mammal; they eat everything humans do, thrive on contaminated water and food, and are even great swimmers. Rodents consume 20% of world's growing and stored grain—13% in the United States, and up to 75% in some African nations. Rodents also can carry diseases.

For the hantavirus in the United States, prolonged drought in the U. S. Southwest reduced predator populations of rodents, while the heavy rains of 1993 (the Mississippi River floods) precipitated a tenfold increase in rodent populations (54). A relatively "new" disease (hantavirus pulmonary syndrome)—the virus perhaps present, but at low levels—emerged, apparently transmitted through rodent excreta. The case fatality rate has been close to 50%. Krebs et al. (59) and Stenseth (60) describe a similar synergy in Canadian snowshoe hares. Added food supplies double populations; caging out predators triples them; together, these interventions lead to an 11-fold increase.

In southern Africa in 1994, rodent populations exploded in the aftermath of 1993 and 1994 rains (54), and plague followed in Malawi and Mozambique (61), and in Zambia in 1997. In 1994 plague resurged in India following a blistering summer (124°F), leaving animals prostate across the north and creating furnaces for fleas in houses with stored grains. The unusually heavy monsoons following the heat wave led to population crowding in Surat, and an apparent outbreak of pneumonic (person-to-person) plague. Malaria and dengue fever upsurges also followed in the wake of flooding (62).

Rodent-borne hantaviruses have resurged in several European nations, particularly in former Yugoslavia, and rodent-borne diseases like leptospirosis are increasingly reported in United States urban centers, where sanitation has declined. In late 1996, hantavirus infection emerged in western Argentina. (At least ten deaths occurred, frightening off tourists and threatening the livelihood of the region.) A combination of stresses contributed to the sudden appearance of several viral hemorrhagic fevers in rural Latin America: Junin, Argentina (1953); Machupo, Bolivia (1962 and 1996); Guaranito, Venezuela; and Sabiá, Brazil (63). In Bolivia, land clearing shifted Calomys mice populations from forest to field where they became dominant. Heavy applications of DDT—meant to eradicate malaria—helped reduce predators. When cats were reintroduced to the area in 1962, the epidemic of Bolivian hemorrhagic fever—which had killed 10% to 20% of the small local population—was abated (64).

### Ocean Warming and Marine Coastal Ecosystems

The oceans are the main memory and repository for the climate system. The oceans absorb and circulate heat, and thus may be modulating long-term warming of the atmosphere. But deep ocean warming can contribute to sea level rise (through thermal expansion), increase the hydrological cycle (thus alter precipitation patterns), and can affect marine life (65).

Deep ocean warming has been reported from the Atlantic, Pacific, and Indian Oceans (66–68), and near the poles (67,69,70). Ocean warming increases the hydrological cycle (35) and has encouraged marine fauna to shift northward—since the 1930s—along the California coast (71).

Warming—in the presence of sufficient nutrients—may also be contributing to the proliferation of coastal algal blooms. Harmful algal blooms of increasing extent, duration, and intensity—and involving new species—are being reported from nations throughout the globe. Indeed, "the worldwide increase in coastal algal blooms may be one of the first biologic signs of global change" (T. Smayda, personal communication, 1995).

Coasts throughout the world are subject to increasing pressures, and the rate of human population growth near shores is double over all population growth globally. These pressures include (a) excessive nutrients (eutrophication)—from sewage, fertilizers, and aerosolized acid (nitrogen) precipitation; (b) reduced acreage of wetlands—"nature's kidneys" that filter nitrogen and other wastes; (c) overfishing, which can reduce predation; (e) chemical pollutants and excess UV-B penetration, which may increase mutation levels; and (e) warming, which, with stratification in the water column, increases algal growth and photosynthesis, and can help shift the species composition of algae to more toxic species (cyanobacteria and dinoflagellates) (72).

All these factors favor the growth of coastal algae. Warming may also reduce the immune systems of sea mammals and coral and encourage the growth of opportunistic infections (such as distemper viruses in sea mammals). The warming related to coral bleaching may do so through stimulation of the *Vibrio* bacterial growth and by reducing the defenses of the coral polyps (73).

Cholera is more widespread today than ever before, and there is evidence that it can be harbored in marine plankton. In 1991, cholera reached the Americas. During the first 18 months over 500,000 cases occurred in Latin America, with 5,000 deaths.

### Costs of Climate Variability and Disease Outbreaks

The impacts of disease on humans, agriculture, and livestock can also be costly. The 1991 cholera epidemic cost Peru over $1 billion ($750 million in seafood exports, $250 million in lost tourist revenues) (74). After the plague outbreak in India in 1994, the airline and hotel industries lost from $2 to $5 billion (D. Gubler, personal communication, 1994). Cruise boats are turning away from islands racked by dengue fever, threatening that region's $12 billion tourist industry (employing over 500,000 people). The global resurgence of malaria, dengue fever, and cholera—and emergence of relatively new diseases like Ebola, *Escherichia coli* 0157:H7, and "Mad Cow" disease—can affect eating habits, trade, tourism, and politics.

### Health Hazards of Fossil Fuel Dependency

From an ecosystem/human health perspective, assessing the consequences of fossil fuel use can be treated with a "life-cycle analysis." The related activities include extraction, mining, refining, transport, and combustion.

The impacts of oil extraction in Ecuadorian forests at the headwaters of the Amazon (over 330 wells), for example, may be felt throughout the pathway of that great basin (and the cultures inhabiting it). Extraction, refining, and transport (leaks far outstripping spills) have untold consequences for water quality and marine biodiversity. Combustion causes acid precipitation, harming forests and statues and contributing nitrogen fertilizing coastal algae—depreciating coastal fisheries. Combustion also causes local air pollution and the growing urban dilemma of respiratory disease.

Then there are the global impacts, for burning fossilized and living resources (timber) is altering atmosphere chemistry, enhancing the normal greenhouse effect, and may be destabilizing the climate system itself.

### Applications of Climate Forecasting

There are several implications of the connections of disease to climate change and climate variability:

1. Surveillance and response capability can be enhanced with health early warning systems of climate conditions (whether or not climate is changing) conducive to outbreaks—to facilitate early, environmentally sound public health interventions (e.g., vaccinations, clean-ups, *Bacillus thuringiensis israeliensis (Bti)* applications, etc.). The El Niño signal can provide early warning of conducive weather conditions for specific regions of the globe (71,75).
2. Broader awareness among scientists and policy makers as to the growing environmental and social vulnerabilities to the spread of emerging infections diseases (EIDS), and the role of human activities (e.g., land-use change and others), altering social and biological controls over opportunistic pests and pathogens.
3. Increased awareness among policy makers concerning the health and long-term costs of current energy policies—the respiratory and cardiovascular impacts of air pollution being well documented. Now the aggregate of emissions appears to be heating up the climate system; and this could play an increasing role in the future in stimulating disease vectors and infectious organisms.

## CONCLUSIONS

We are using Earth's resources and generating wastes at rates beyond the capacity of global biogeochemical systems to recycle them. Human activities affecting forestry and fisheries, utilizing fossil fuels and petrochemicals, must all be examined in light of their impacts on biodiversity and on global life-support systems.

Since the glaciers receded from North America and Europe 10,000 years ago, the earth's climate has been relatively stable and hospitable. The end of the last ice age ushered in the agricultural revolution and the recolonization of the northern plains in the U.S. Average temperature has been 15°C during the past 10,000 years (the Holocene), whereas it was about 5° to 10°C cooler during the last ice age in the mid-latitudes. Ice caps have also been relatively stable. The Earth's average temperature is now approaching 16°C, thus raising the potential for a nonlinear change in ice cap size, and thus in sea level and the climate regime itself. Are the changes in the distribution of disease one indicator that the global system is unstable?

Epidemics in the past (Justinian, medieval, and in the mid-1800s) grew out of deteriorating social conditions, and contributed to major changes in the organization of society (76). Sanitary and environmental reform grew out of the triple epidemics (TB, smallpox, and cholera) besetting the Dickensian cities of the 19th century. And the health professions and earliest epidemiologists played a significant role in calling attention to the environmental deterioration underlying the epidemics.

We have entered a period of social, ecological, and climatic transition. Will we heed the symptoms of environmental dysfunction, and take corrective measures before the resilience of those systems is exceeded? Today, health professionals can play a central role in examining and exposing these connections (77).

Solutions, however, do not lie with individual actions. Changes in national priorities and international agreements will be necessary. The Montreal Protocol for eliminating chlorofluorocarbons (CFCs) is one example of such an accord; the United Nations Convention on the Laws of the Seas (UNCLOS) is another aspect of governance over "the commons." A strong Framework Convention on Climate Change (FCCC, or the Climate Treaty) will be essential, for the carbon and global heat budget are central to all living systems. Significant positive incentives (financial instruments) may be needed in the FCCC to drive development of renewable energy sources and energy-efficient technologies. But it will take an aroused public to reject the fallacious "scientific" arguments raised by self-interest groups to preserve the status quo.

Development and distribution of renewables, and the process of environmental restoration may provide the economic and technological stimuli needed to address the underlying inequities, well into the next century.

The global resurgence of infectious disease across a wide taxonomic range during the last quarter of the 20th century is one consequence of compounding global-scale changes in physical, chemical, biologic, and social systems. Indeed, we may be vastly underestimating the true costs of "business as usual," as well as underestimating the benefits to society as a whole of efficiently using the resources we have inherited.

## ACKNOWLEDGMENT

The highly informative publications of the Worldwatch Institute are excellent resources on all aspects of global environmental and socioeconomic influences on the state of our planet. Many citations and references to specific Worldwatch publications are included in this chapter. We are grateful for their permission to make these citations.

## REFERENCES


1. McElroy MB. The challenge of global change. *Bull Am Acad Arts Sci* 1989;42:24–38.
2. Bright C. Tracking the ecology of climate change. In: Brown LR, et al., eds. *State of the world 1997.* World Watch Institute. New York: W.W. Norton, 1997;78–94.
3. Houghton JT, Callender BA, Varney SK, eds. *Climate change:* the supplementary report to the IPCC scientific assessment. Cambridge: Cambridge University Press, 1992.
4. World Commission on Environment and Development. *Our common future.* Oxford: Oxford University Press, 1987.
5. Brown LR. Facing the prospect of food scarcity. In: Brown LR, et al., eds. *State of the world 1997.* World Watch Institute. New York: W.W. Norton, 1997;23–41.
6. Gardner G. Preserving agricultural resources. In: Brown LR, et al., eds. *State of the world 1996.* World Watch Institute. New York: W.W. Norton, 1996;78–94.
7. Revkin AC. Endless summer: living with the greenhouse effect. *Discover* 1988;October:50–61.
8. Phelps PB. Direct effects on human health. In: Setlow V, Pope E, eds. *Conference on human health and global climate change:* summary of the proceedings. National Science and Technology Council. Institute of Medicine/National Academy of Sciences. Washington, DC: National Academy Press, 1996:9:13–14.
9. Karl TR, Jones PD, Knight RW, et al. A new perspective on recent global warming: asymmetric trends of daily maximum and minimum temperature. *Bull Am Meteorol Soc* 1993;74:1007–1023.
10. Kalkstein LS, Greene JS. An evaluation of climate/mortality relationships in large U.S.cities and the possible impacts of climate change. *Environ Health Perspect* 1997;105:84–93.
11. Weber P. Coral reefs in decline. In: Brown LR, Kane H, Roodman DM, eds. *Vital signs 1994:* the trends that are shaping our world. World Watch Institute. New York: W.W. Norton, 1994;122–123.
12. Jacobson JL. Abandoning homelands: the threat of inundation. In: Brown LR, et al., eds. *State of the world 1989.* World Watch Institute. New York: W.W. Norton, 1989;71–76.
13. Parry ML, Rosenzweig C. Food supply and risk of hunger. In: Epstein PR, Sharp D, eds. *Health and climate change.* London: Lancet 1994; 23–25.
14. Weber P. Resistance to pesticides growing. In: Brown LR, Kane H, Roodman DM, eds. *Vital signs 1994:* the trends that are shaping our world. World Watch Institute. New York: W.W. Norton, 1994;92–93.
15. Brown LR. Reexamining the world food prospect. In: Brown LR, et al., eds. *State of the world 1989.* World Watch Institute. New York: W.W. Norton, 1989;41–58.
16. Seinfeld JH. Urban air pollution: state of the science. *Science* 1989; 243:745–752.
17. USDA, Economic Research Service. *Production, supply, and demand view.* Washington, DC: USDA;1995.
18. Durning AT, Brough HB. Reforming the livestock economy. In: Brown LR, et al., eds. *State of the world 1992.* World Watch Institute. New York: W.W. Norton, 1992;70.
19. Brown LR. Nature's limits: the China factor. In: Brown LR, et al., eds. *State of the world 1995.* World Watch Institute. New York: W.W. Norton, 1995;16–20.
20. World Health Organization. *The world health report 1996:* fighting disease, *fostering development.* Geneva: WHO, 1996.
21. Dobson A, Carper R. Biodiversity. *Lancet* 1993;342:1096–1099.
22. MacArthur RH. *Geographical ecology.* New York: Harper & Row, 1972.
23. Maskell K, Mintzer IM, Callander BA. Basic science of climate change. *Lancet* 1993;342:1027–1031.
24. Martens WJM, Rotmans J, Niessen LW. *Climate change and malaria risk:* an integrated modelling approach. GLOBE report series no. 3 RIVM report No. 461502003. Bilthoven, The Netherlands: Global Dynamics and Sustainable Development Programme, 1994.
25. Matsuoka Y, Kai K. An estimation of climatic change effects on malaria. *J Global Environ Engineer* 1994;1:1–15.
26. Loevinsohn M. Climatic warming and increased malaria incidence in Rwanda. *Lancet* 1994;343:714–718.
27. Rozendaal J. *Assignment report:* Malaria. World Health Organization. Pt. Moresby. Papua New Guinea. Geneva: WHO, 1996.
28. Koopman JS, Prevots DR, Marin MAU, et al. Determinants and predictors of dengue infection in Mexico. *Am J Epidemiol* 1991;133: 1168–1178.
29. Suarez MF, Nelson MJ. Registro de altitud del Aedes Aegypti en Colombia. *Biomedica* 1981;1:225.
30. Epstein PR. Look to weather for clues to malaria comeback. *New York Times* 1997(13 January):A16.
31. Parmesan C. Climate and species' range. *Nature* 1996;382:765–766.
32. Grabherr G, Gottfried N, Pauli H. Climate effects on mountain plain. *Nature* 1994;369:447.
33. Yoon CK. Warming moves plants up peaks, threatening extinction. *New York Times* 1994(21 June):C4.
34. Thompson LG, Mosley-Thompson E, Davis ME, et al. Late glacial stage and Holocene tropical ice core records from Huascaran, Peru. *Science* 1995;269:46–50.
35. Intergovernmental Panel on Climate Change (IPCC). In: Houghton JT, Meiro Filho LG, Callandar BA, Harris N, Kattenberg A, Maskell K, eds. *Climate change '95:* the science of climate change. Contribution of Working Group I to the Second Assessment Report of the IPCC. Cambridge, UK: Cambridge University Press, 1996.
36. Diaz HF, Graham NE. Recent changes in tropical freezing heights and the role of sea surface temperature. *Nature* 1996;383:152–155.
37. Elias SA. *Quaternary insects and their environments.* Washington, DC: Smithsonian Institution Press, 1994 (based on work of R. Coope and others).

37a. Moore PD. Bears versus beetles. *Nature* 1986;320:385–386.

38. Patz JA, Epstein PR, Burke TA, Balbus JM. Global climate change and emerging infectious diseases. *JAMA* 1996;275:217–223.
39. Reisen WK, Meyer RP, Preser SB, Hardy JL. Effect of temperature on the transmission of western equine encephalomyelitis and St. Louis encephalitis viruses by *Culex tarsalis* (*Diptera:* Culicadae). *J Med Entomol* 1993;30:151–160.
40. Reeves WC, Hardy JL, Reisen WK, Milby MM. Potential effect of global warming on mosquito-borne arboviruses. *J Med Entomol* 1994; 31:323–332.
41. Martin PH, Lefebvre MG. Malaria and climate: sensitivity of malaria potential transmission to climate. *Ambio* 1995;24:200–209.
42. Focks DA, Daniels E, Haile DG, Keesling LE. A simulation model of the epidemiology of urban dengue fever: literature analysis, model development, preliminary validation, and samples of simulation results. *Am J Trop Med Hyg* 1995:53:489–506.
43. Gill CA. The role of meteorology and malaria. *Ind J Med Res* 1920;8: 633–693.
44. Gill CA. The relationship between malaria and rainfall. *Ind J Med Res* 1920;37:618–632.
45. Billett JD. Direct and indirect influences of temperature on the transmission of parasites from insects to man. In: Taylor AER, Muller R, eds. *The effects of meteorological factors upon parasite.* Oxford: Blackwell Scientific, 1974;79–95.
46. Burgos JJ. Analogias agroclimatologicas utiles para la adaptacion al posible cambio climatico global de America del Sur. *Rev Geofisica* 1990;32:79–95.
47. Burgos JJ, Curto de Casas SI, Carcavallo RU, Galindez GI. Global Climate change in the distribution of some pathogenic complexes. *Entomol Vectores* 1994;1:69–82.
48. Dahlstein DL, Garcia R, eds. *Eradication of exotic pests:* analysis with case histories. New Haven, CT: Yale University Press, 1989.
49. Sutherst RW. Impact of climate change on pests and diseases in Australasia. *Search* 1990;21:230–232.
50. Zucker JR. Changing patterns of autochthonous malaria transmission in the United States: a review of recent outbreaks. *Emerg Infect Dis* 1996;2:37–43.

50a. ProMED, reported by Roger Spitzer. Malaria, autochthonous. Florida: ProMED Archives, 1996.

51. Epstein PR, Dobson A, Vandermeer J. Biodiversity and emerging infectious diseases: integrating health and ecosystem monitoring. In: Grifo F, Rosenthal J, eds. *Biodiversity and human health.* New York: Island Press, 1997;60–86.

52. Karl TR, Knight RW, Plummer N. Trends in high-frequency climate variability in the twentieth century. *Nature* 1995;377:217– 220.
53. Epstein PR, Pena OC, Racedo JB. Climate and disease in Colombia. *Lancet* 1995;346:1243–1244.
54. Epstein PR. 1995. Emerging diseases and ecosystem instabilities: new threats to public health. *Am J Public Health* 85:168–72.
55. Epstein PR, Chikwenhere GP. Biodiversity questions. *Science* 1994; 265:1510–1511.
56. Skole D, Tucker C. Tropical deforestation and habitat fragmentation in the Amazon: satellite data from 1978 to 1988. *Science* 1993;260: 1905–1910.
57. Molineaux L. The epidemiology of human malaria as an explanation of its distribution, including some implications for its control. In: Wernsdorfer WH, McGregor I, eds. *Malaria, principles and practice of malariology,* vol 2. New York: Churchill-Livingstone, 1988;913–998.
58. Carson R. *Silent spring.* Boston: Houghton Miflin, 1962.
59. Krebs CJ, Boutin S, Boonstra R, et al. Impact of food and predation on the snowshoe hare cycle. *Science* 1995;269:1112–1115.
60. Stenseth NH. Snowshoe hare populations squeezed from below and above. *Science* 1995;269:1061–1062.
61. Barreto A, Aragon M, Epstein PR. Bubonic plague in Mozambique, 1994. *Lancet* 1995;345:983–984.
62. Epstein PR. Climate change played a role in India's plague. *New York Times* 1994(13 November).
63. Coimbra TLM, Nassar ES, Burattini MN, et al. New arenavirus isolated in Brazil. *Lancet* 1994;343:391–392.
64. Garrett L. *The coming plague:* newly emerging diseases in a world out of balance. New York: Farrar, Straus, and Giroux, 1994.
65. Epstein PR, Ford TE, Puccia, Da Possas C. Marine ecosystem health: implications for public health. In: Wilson ME, Levins R, Spielman A, eds. *Disease in evolution.* New York: Academy of Sciences, 1993.
66. Parrilla G, Lavin A, Bryden H, Garcia M, Millard R. Rising temperatures in the sub-tropical North Atlantic Ocean over the past 35 years. *Nature* 1994;369:48–51.
67. Thwaites T. Are the antipodes in hot water? *New Scientist* 1994(12 November):21.
68. Bindoff NL, Church JA. Warming of the water column in the southwest Pacific. *Nature* 1992;357:59–62.
69. Travis J. Taking a bottom-to sky "slice" of the Arctic Ocean. *Science* 1994;266:1947–1948.
70. Regaldo A. Listen up! The world's oceans may be starting to warm. *Science* 1995;268:1436–1437.
71. Hales S, Weinstein P, Woodward A. Dengue fever in the South Pacific: driven by El Nino Southern Oscillation? *Lancet* 1996;348:1664–1665.
72. Barry JP, Baxter CH, Sagarin RD, Gilman SE. Climate-related, long-term faunal changes in a California rocky intertidal community. *Science* 1995;267:672–675.
73. Kushmaro A, Loya Y, Fine M, Rosenberg E. Bacterial infection and coral bleaching. *Nature* 1996;380;396.
74. Epstein PR, Nutter F. *Assessing the costs of climate change.* World Wide Web Newsletter: Center for Health and the Global Environment. Boston: Harvard Medical School, 1997.
75. Bouma MJ, Sondorp HE, van der Kaay HJ. Climate change and periodic epidemic malaria. *Lancet* 1994;343:1440.
76. Epstein PR. Pestilence and poverty—historical transitions and the great pandemics (Commentary). *Am J Prev Med* 1992;8:263–265.
77. Leaf A. Potential health effects of a global climate and environmental changes. *N Engl J Med* 1989;321:1577–1583.

## FURTHER READING

Levins R, Auerbuch T, Brinkmann V, et al. New and resurgent diseases: the failure of attempted eradication. *The Ecologist* 1995;25:21–26.

*Environmental and Occupational Medicine,*
*Third Edition,* edited by William N. Rom.
Lippincott–Raven Publishers, Philadelphia © 1998.

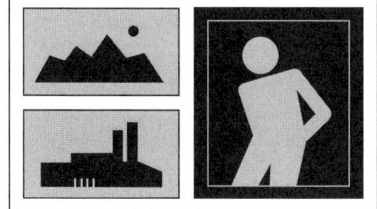

CHAPTER 123

# Chlorofluorocarbons and Destruction of the Ozone Layer

Mario J. Molina and Luisa T. Molina

It was first proposed in 1974 that stratospheric ozone could be depleted as a consequence of the release of chlorofluorocarbons (CFCs) to the environment (1,2). The CFCs are industrial chemicals that have been used in the past as coolants for refrigerators and air conditioners, propellants for aerosol spray cans, foaming agents for plastics, and cleaning solvents for electronic components, among other uses. These chemicals are also known under trademarks such as Freon (DuPont) and Genetron (Allied Signal). The CFCs are fully halogenated hydrocarbons; the three most common ones are listed in Table 1.

One of the two important properties that makes the CFCs commercially valuable is their volatility, which can be assessed from their boiling points (Table 1); they can be readily converted from a liquid to a vapor, and vice versa. The other important property is their chemical inertness: they are nontoxic, nonflammable, noncorrosive, and unreactive with most other substances. Thus, they do not decompose inside a spray can or a refrigerator. In fact, it is their chemical inertness that creates a global scale problem by enabling them to reach the stratosphere, where they decompose, releasing chlorine atoms that affect the ozone layer.

## ATMOSPHERIC OZONE

Ozone ($O_3$) molecules are made from three oxygen atoms, instead of the two of normal oxygen molecule ($O_2$), which makes up 21% of the air we breathe. The average concentration of ozone in the atmosphere is about 300 parts per billion by volume (ppbv), although most of it (~90%) is contained in the stratosphere, where it is present at levels of several parts per million by volume (ppmv) (Fig. 1). Even though it occurs in such small quantities, ozone plays a vital role in supporting life on Earth. It is continuously being made by the action of solar radiation on molecular oxygen, predominantly in the upper stratosphere and at low latitudes; it is also continuously being destroyed throughout the atmosphere by a variety of chemical processes. The basic ozone formation-destruction mechanism consists of the following reactions, which were first suggested by Chapman (3) in the 1930s:

$$O_2 + h\nu \rightarrow O + O \qquad [1]$$

$$O + O_2 \rightarrow O_3 \qquad [2]$$

$$O_3 + h\nu \rightarrow O + O_2 \qquad [3]$$

$$O + O_3 \rightarrow O_2 + O_2 \qquad [4]$$

Molecular oxygen absorbs solar radiation at wavelengths ~200 nm and releases oxygen atoms (reaction 1), which rapidly combine with oxygen molecules to form ozone (reaction 2). In reactions 1 and 3, $h\nu$ denotes a solar photon. Ozone absorbs solar radiation very efficiently at wavelengths ~200 to 300 nm; it is destroyed by this absorption process (reaction 3), but the oxygen atoms produced by this reaction readily regenerate the ozone molecule by reaction 2. Thus, the net effect of reactions 2 and 3 is the conversion of solar energy to heat, without the destruction of ozone. This process leads to an increase of temperature with altitude, which is the feature that gives rise to the stratosphere; the inverted temperature

M. J. Molina and L. T. Molina: Department of Earth, Atmospheric and Planetary Sciences, Massachusetts Institute of Technology, Cambridge, Massachusetts 02139.

**TABLE 1.** *Physical properties of some common CFCs*

| Compound | Formula | Vapor pressure −13°C | (atm) 27°C | Boiling point |
|---|---|---|---|---|
| CFC-11 | $CFCl_3$ | 0.22 | 1.12 | 23.8°C |
| CFC-12 | $CF_2Cl_2$ | 1.93 | 6.75 | −29.8°C |
| CFC-113 | $CFCl_2CClF_2$ | 0.08 | 0.47 | 47.4°C |

profile in this layer is responsible for its large stability toward vertical movements (Fig. 2). In contrast, in the lowest layer—the troposphere—temperature decreases with altitude, and winds disperse atmospheric trace components very efficiently on a global scale in this lower layer, on a time scale of months within each hemisphere and about a year or two between the two hemispheres.

Most of the time oxygen atoms make ozone (as in reaction 2), but occasionally they destroy ozone (as in reaction 4). However, the calculated ozone concentration based on Chapman's mechanism was considerably higher than the observed amount; thus, there must be other reactions that contribute to the reduction of the ozone concentration. In the early 1970s Crutzen (4) and Johnston (5) independently suggested that trace amounts of nitrogen oxides ($NO_x$)—formed in the stratosphere through the decay of chemically stable nitrous oxide ($N_2O$), which originates from soil-borne microorganisms—control the ozone abundance through a catalytic cycle consisting of the following reactions:

$$NO + O_3 \rightarrow NO_2 + O_2 \quad [5]$$

$$NO_2 + O \rightarrow NO + O_2 \quad [6]$$

$$O_3 + h\nu \rightarrow O + O_2 \quad [3]$$

$$\text{Net: } 2\ O_3 \rightarrow 3\ O_2$$

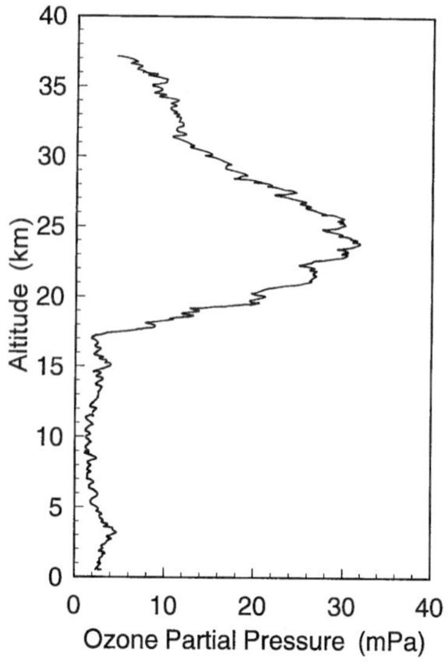


**FIG. 1.** Typical atmospheric temperatures and pressures as a function of altitude.

The species NO and $NO_2$ are still present after these three reactions have occurred, but two molecules of ozone have been destroyed. These species have an odd number of electrons; they are free radicals and are chemically very reactive. Although the concentration of NO and $NO_2$ is small (several ppbv), each radical pair can destroy thousands of ozone molecules before being temporarily removed, mainly by reaction with hydroxyl (OH) radical to form nitric acid:

$$OH + NO_2 \rightarrow HNO_3 \quad [7]$$

Ozone is also present in the troposphere (Fig. 1); some of it is generated there by photochemical reactions, and some is transported from the stratosphere. The ingredients for its photochemical formation are $NO_x$, hydrocarbon fragments, and solar radiation; thus, $NO_x$ plays a dual role, destroying or generating $O_3$ depending on the altitude. Ozone is a key component of urban smog, where it is present in amounts that are relatively small on a global scale, but very significant on a local scale because of the human health effects resulting from breathing air containing ozone at levels above a few tenths of 1 ppmv (6).

Other free radicals that destroy stratospheric ozone are OH and $HO_2$, derived from the water molecule, and that participate in cycles such as the following:

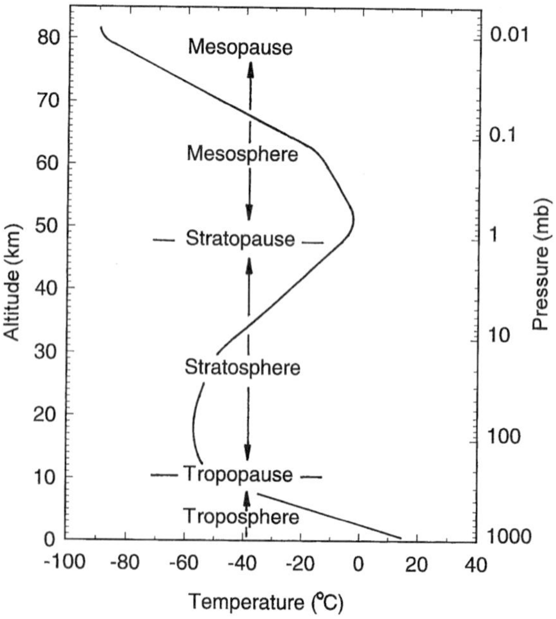


**FIG. 2.** Typical atmospheric ozone profile: millipascals of ozone vs. altitude.

$$OH + O_3 \rightarrow HO_2 + O_2 \quad [8]$$

$$HO_2 + O_3 \rightarrow OH + 2O_2 \quad [9]$$

$$\text{Net: } 2\,O_3 \rightarrow 3\,O_2$$

Chlorine atoms are also very efficient catalysts for ozone destruction and may participate in a very similar catalytic cycle (1,2,7):

$$Cl + O_3 \rightarrow ClO + O_2 \quad [10]$$

$$ClO + O \rightarrow Cl + O_2 \quad [11]$$

$$O_3 + h\nu \rightarrow O + O_2 \quad [3]$$

$$\text{Net: } 2\,O_3 \rightarrow 3\,O_2$$

However, only small amounts of chlorine compounds of natural origin exist in the stratosphere: the only important source is methyl chloride ($CH_3Cl$), which is present at a level of less than 1 ppbv. This species is produced at the Earth's surface by biological activity and also to some extent by biomass burning; most of the $CH_3Cl$ is destroyed in the troposphere, but a few percent reaches the stratosphere. There are large natural sources of inorganic chlorine compounds at the Earth's surface, e.g., NaCl and HCl from the oceans; however, these compounds are water soluble and are removed very efficiently from the atmosphere by clouds and rainfall long before they reach the stratosphere.

## THE CHLOROFLUOROCARBONS

In the 1930s, Thomas Midgley (8) invented the CFCs during a search for nontoxic substances that could be used as coolants in home refrigerators. The CFCs soon replaced the toxic ammonia and sulfur dioxide as the standard cooling fluids. Subsequently, the CFCs found uses as propellants for aerosol sprays, blowing agents for plastic foam, and cleansers for electronic components. All this activity doubled the worldwide use of CFCs every 6 to 7 years and the annual industrial usage eventually reached about 700,000 metric tons by early 1970s.

In 1973, using the newly developed electron capture detector, Lovelock and co-workers (9) were able to detect measurable levels of CFCs in the atmosphere over the South and North Atlantic. Rowland and Molina (1,2) decided to investigate the ultimate atmospheric fate of these wonder compounds. After carrying out a systematic search of chemical and physical processes that might destroy the CFCs in the lower atmosphere, they concluded that the only significant sink was solar ultraviolet (UV) photolysis in the middle stratosphere (~25–30 km).

The CFCs are practically insoluble in water, and thus are not removed by rainfall. Furthermore, they are inert toward the OH radical; reaction with this radical to form water is the process that initiates the oxidation of hydrocarbons in the lower atmosphere, which eventually leads to $CO_2$ and water. Thus, the CFCs are not removed by the common atmospheric cleansing mechanisms that operate in the lower atmosphere. Because CFC molecules are transparent from 230 nm through the visible wavelengths, they are effectively protected below 25 km by the stratospheric ozone layer that shields the Earth's surface from UV light. Instead, they rise into the stratosphere, where they are eventually destroyed by the short wavelength (~200 nm) solar UV radiation. Because transport into the stratosphere is very slow, the residence time for the CFCs in the environment is of the order of 50 to 100 years.

The destruction of CFCs by solar radiation leads to the release of chlorine atoms, which participate in ozone destruction cycles: these atoms attack ozone within a few seconds (as in reaction 10) and are regenerated on a time scale of minutes (as in reaction 11). These cycles may be temporarily interrupted, e.g., by reaction of chlorine monoxide (ClO) with $HO_2$ or $NO_2$ to produce hypochlorous acid (HOCl) or chlorine nitrate ($ClONO_2$), respectively; or by reaction of the Cl atom with methane ($CH_4$) to produce the relatively stable hydrogen chloride (HCl):

$$ClO + HO_2 \rightarrow HOCl + O_2 \quad [12]$$

$$ClO + NO_2 \rightarrow ClONO_2 \quad [13]$$

$$Cl + CH_4 \rightarrow HCl + CH_3 \quad [14]$$

The chlorine-containing product species HCl, $ClONO_2$, and HOCl function as temporary inert reservoirs: they are not directly involved in ozone depletion, but they are eventually broken down by reaction with other free radicals or by absorption of solar radiation, thus returning chlorine to its catalytically active free radical form. At low latitudes and in the upper stratosphere, where the formation of ozone is fastest, a few percent of the chlorine is in this active form; most of the chlorine is in the inert reservoir form, with HCl being the most abundant species. The temporary chlorine reservoirs remain in the stratosphere for several years before returning to the troposphere, where they are rapidly removed by rain or clouds. There are two reasons for this long stratospheric residence time: (a) transport is very slow in the vertical direction, because of the inverted temperature profile; and (b) there is no rain in the stratosphere, and clouds do not normally form there, thus preventing the rapid removal of water-soluble compounds such as the chlorine reservoir species. This is due to the fact that a large fraction of the water vapor present at lower altitudes condenses on its way up into the stratosphere, making it very dry. A schematic representation of these processes is presented in Fig. 3.

Besides chlorine, bromine also plays an important role in stratospheric chemistry. There are industrial sources of brominated hydrocarbons as well as natural ones. The halons are fully halogenated hydrocarbons, produced industrially as fire extinguishers; examples are $CF_3Br$

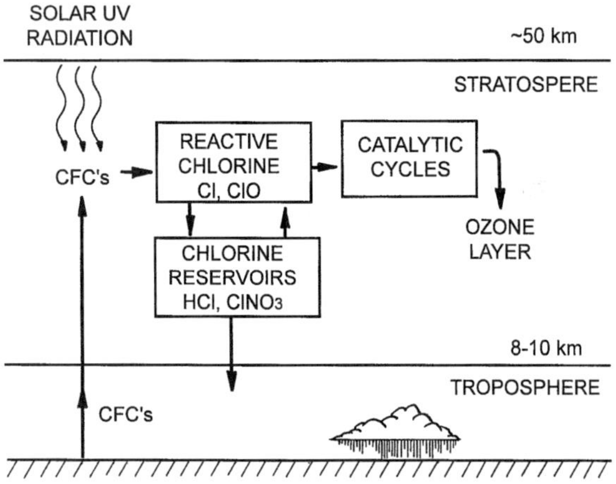


**FIG. 3.** Schematic representation of the CFC-ozone depletion hypothesis.

and $CF_2ClBr$. Methyl bromide ($CH_3Br$) is both natural and man-made; it is used as an agricultural fumigant. These sources release bromine to the stratosphere at pptv levels, compared with ppbv for chlorine. On the other hand, bromine atoms are about 50 times more efficient than chlorine atoms for ozone destruction on an atom-per-atom basis (10); a large fraction of the bromine compounds is present as free radicals, because the temporary reservoirs are less stable and are formed at considerably slower rates than the corresponding chlorine reservoirs. In contrast, fluorine atoms abstract hydrogen atoms very rapidly from methane and from water vapor, forming the very stable hydrogen fluoride (HF) molecule, which serves as a permanent inert fluorine reservoir. Hence, fluorine free radicals are extremely scarce and the effect of fluorine on stratospheric ozone is negligible.

Our understanding of the effects of chlorine and bromine on stratospheric ozone can be examined by comparing predictions of computer models of the atmosphere with actual observations. The models typically incorporate information on the rates of over a hundred chemical and photochemical reactions, as well as information on atmospheric motions and on natural levels of a variety of compounds. Because of the complexity of the system, calculations were carried out initially with one-dimensional models, averaging the motions and concentrations of species over latitude and longitude and leaving only their dependency on altitude and time. Two-dimensional models, in which the averaging is over longitude only, are now being used extensively; more recently, three-dimensional models have been developed. The models can be further tested with measurements of atmospheric trace species conducted as a function of time of day, season, and latitude.

Various fundamental aspects of the CFC-ozone depletion hypothesis were verified in the late 1970s and early 1980s, following the initial publication of the Molina-Rowland article (1). Measurements of the atmospheric concentrations of the CFCs indicated that they accumulate in the lower atmosphere and that they reach the stratosphere in the amounts predicted. Chlorine atoms and ClO radicals were found in the stratosphere, together with other species such as HCl, $ClONO_2$, HOCl, O, NO, $NO_2$, OH, $HO_2$, etc., with observed concentrations in reasonable agreement with the model predictions. On the other hand, a decrease in stratospheric ozone levels was not observable at that time because of the large natural variability of this species. However, the ozone levels in the Antarctic stratosphere dropped dramatically in the spring months starting in the early 1980s, as first reported by Farman and co-workers (11) in 1985; their data is presented in Fig. 4. Subsequently it became evident that ozone was being depleted in the Northern Hemisphere as well, particularly at high latitudes and in the winter and spring months. More recently, it has been possible to show by examination of the ozone records that significant changes have also taken place in the lower stratosphere at mid-latitudes (10), as shown in Fig. 5. Furthermore, satellite measurements have directly confirmed conclusions that the bulk of the chlorine present in the stratosphere is of human origin (12).

The depletion of ozone over Antarctica—the ozone hole—was not predicted by the atmospheric sciences community. However, the cause of this depletion has become very clear in recent years: laboratory experiments, field measurements over Antarctica, and model calculations have shown unambiguously that the ozone hole can indeed be traced to the man-made CFCs.

## POLAR OZONE CHEMISTRY

The polar stratosphere is unique in several ways. First of all, ozone is not generated there, because the short

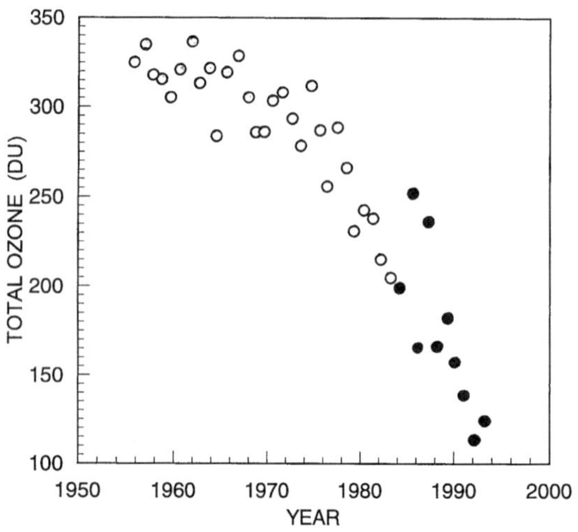


**FIG. 4.** Average total amount of ozone measured in October over Halley Bay, Antarctica, by Farman et al. (11) *(open circles)*, and by Jones and Shanklin (27) *(solid circles)*. A Dobson unit (DU) is equivalent to a milli-atmosphere centimeter; the global average total ozone column is about 300 DU.

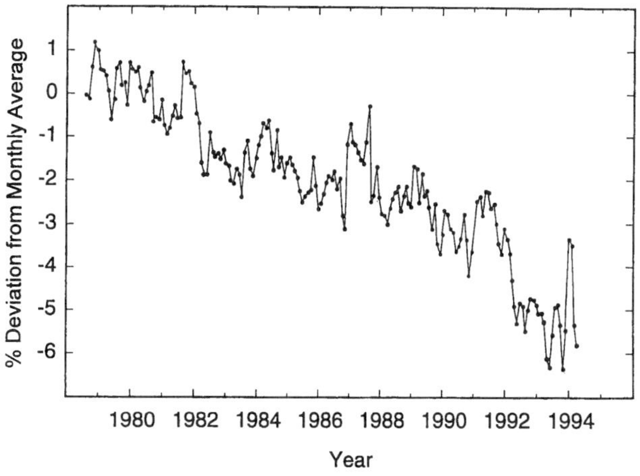


**FIG. 5.** Trend in global ozone values averaged between 60° north and 60° south. (Adapted from ref. 10.)

wavelength solar radiation that is absorbed by molecular oxygen is scarce, as a consequence of the solar inclination (large solar zenith angles). In addition, the total ozone column abundance at high latitudes is large because ozone is transported toward the poles from higher altitudes and lower latitudes. Furthermore, the prevailing temperatures over the stratosphere above the poles in the winter and spring months are the lowest throughout the atmosphere, particularly over Antarctica. Thus, ozone is expected to be rather stable over the poles if one considers only gas phase chemical and photochemical processes, because regeneration of ozone-destroying free radicals from the reservoir species would occur only very slowly at those temperatures.

Another important feature of the polar stratosphere is the seasonal presence of polar stratospheric clouds (PSCs). As mentioned above, the stratosphere is very dry—water is present only at a level of a few ppmv, a level comparable to that of ozone itself. Over the poles, a somewhat larger amount of water is present, resulting from the oxidation of methane. Furthermore, the temperature can drop to below −85°C over Antarctica in the winter and spring months, leading to the formation of ice clouds, which are known as type II PSCs. The presence of trace amounts of nitric and sulfuric acids enables the formation of polar stratospheric clouds a few degrees above the frost point (which is the temperature at which ice can condense from the gas phase); these acids can form cloud particles consisting of crystalline hydrates, known as type I PSCs.

Solomon et al. (13) first suggested that PSCs could play a major role in the depletion of ozone over Antarctica by promoting the release of photolytically active chlorine from its reservoir species. This occurs mainly by the following reaction:

$$HCl + ClONO_2 \rightarrow Cl_2 + HNO_3 \quad [15]$$

Laboratory studies have shown that this reaction occurs very slowly, if at all, in the gas phase (14,15); however, in the presence of ice surfaces, it proceeds with remarkable efficiency (16). The product $Cl_2$ is immediately released to the gas phase and decomposes readily even with the faint amount of sunlight present over Antarctica in the early spring:

$$Cl_2 + h\nu \rightarrow Cl + Cl \quad [16]$$

The following are also chlorine activation reactions promoted by PSCs:

$$ClONO_2 + H_2O \rightarrow HOCl + HNO_3 \quad [17]$$

$$HOCl + HCl \rightarrow Cl_2 + H_2O \quad [18]$$

The net effect of these two reactions is reaction 15. The catalytic effect of ice to promote reactions 15 and 18 was surprising at first, because there was little precedent for ice-induced chemistry. The reaction mechanism could be explained by assuming that the HCl molecule is incorporated very efficiently into the ice surface at low temperatures, even when its gas phase concentration is below the ppb level. HCl is taken up very efficiently by liquid water, forming hydrochloric acid as it dissolves. However, HCl is only barely soluble in the ice matrix; when dilute hydrochloric acid solutions freeze, almost pure water ice forms, as the ice crystals reject impurities. On the other hand, experimental observations (16,17), as well as recent theoretical calculations (18), indicate that HCl solvates readily on the ice surface and forms hydrochloric acid. Compared to the crystal, the ice surface is disordered—it behaves more like a liquid than a solid—thus explaining the high affinity of ice for HCl. As a consequence, chlorine activation reactions on the surfaces of ice crystals proceed through ionic mechanisms analogous to those in aqueous solutions.

The presence of PSCs also leads to the removal of nitrogen oxides ($NO_x$) from the gas phase; the source for these free radicals in the polar stratosphere is nitric acid, which condenses in the cloud particles. Furthermore, some of the particles consist of large enough ice crystals to fall out of the stratosphere, permanently removing the nitric acid, a process referred to as denitrification. This process turns out to have important consequences: the nitrogen oxides normally interfere with the catalytic ozone loss reactions involving chlorine oxides, mainly by scavenging chlorine monoxide to form chlorine nitrate, as in reaction 13. In the absence of nitrogen oxides, chlorine radicals destroy ozone much more rapidly.

The catalytic cycles such as those involving reactions 10 and 11 are efficient only in regions where ozone is being produced, because they require the presence of free oxygen atoms, which are scarce at high latitudes. Several different cycles have been suggested as being at work over Antarctica, such as the following one involving chlorine peroxide (ClOOCl) (19):

$$ClO + ClO \rightarrow ClOOCl \quad [19]$$

$$2\,[Cl + O_3 \rightarrow ClO + O_2] \quad [10]$$

$$ClOOCl + h\nu \rightarrow 2Cl + O_2 \quad [20]$$

$$\text{Net: } 2\,O_3 \rightarrow 3\,O_2$$

No free oxygen atoms are involved in this cycle. The key is the combination of two ClO radicals to form ClOOCl, which then photolyses to release molecular oxygen and free chlorine atoms. The species ClOOCl had not been characterized previously; its geometry is now well established from submillimeter wave spectroscopy (20). It is thermally unstable at room temperature, but it is stable below about −60°C. Laboratory studies (21,22) have shown that the photolysis products are indeed chlorine atoms rather than ClO radicals, which are the products of the thermal decomposition reaction.

Another important cycle operating in the polar stratosphere involves bromine free radicals in synergism with chlorine free radicals (23):

$$ClO + BrO \rightarrow Cl + Br + O_2 \quad [21]$$

$$Cl + O_3 \rightarrow ClO + O_2 \quad [10]$$

$$Br + O_3 \rightarrow BrO + O_2 \quad [22]$$

$$\text{Net: } 2\,O_3 \rightarrow 3\,O_2$$

As is the case with the chlorine peroxide cycle, this cycle does not require the presence of free oxygen atoms; furthermore, it can in principle operate in the dark, as there is no photolytic step. However, reaction 21 has other channels that prevent the continuous production of the free halogen atoms in the absence of light (15):

$$ClO + BrO \rightarrow BrCl + O_2 \quad [23]$$

$$\rightarrow Br + OClO \quad [24]$$

On the other hand, both products BrCl and OClO decompose readily in sunlight. In fact, the presence of OClO at night has been used as an indication of the occurrence of the ClO + BrO reaction, as this is likely to be the main source for OClO (24).

## FIELD MEASUREMENTS OF ATMOSPHERIC TRACE SPECIES

Farman et al. (11) conducted their measurements of rapid ozone loss in the stratosphere over Antarctica from the ground, using a relatively simple instrument developed in the 1920s by Dobson and co-workers (25). This instrument—the Dobson spectrophotometer—measures the intensity of solar radiation at two different wavelengths, one strongly absorbed by ozone and the other one not absorbed. Farman et al.'s findings were subsequently confirmed by satellite data from the total ozone mapping spectrometer (TOMS) (26), which measures ozone by a similar principle, namely by monitoring at two such wavelengths the attenuation of solar radiation that has been back-scattered from the atmosphere below the ozone layer. More recent measurements from ground-based Dobson instruments (27), shown in Fig. 4, as well as from satellites, indicate that the extent of ozone depletion over Antarctica in the spring months continued to increase after 1985. On the other hand, this trend is not expected to continue, since more than 99% of the ozone is destroyed in the lower stratosphere (28), where the chlorine and bromine free radical chemistry takes place, and hence the ozone hole cannot get any deeper (Fig. 6).

Several expeditions were launched in the years following the initial discovery of the ozone hole to measure trace species in the stratosphere over Antarctica (e.g., ref. 29). The results provided strong evidence for the occurrence of the chemical reactions described above, and hence for the crucial role played by industrial chlorine in the depletion of ozone. At the time that ozone is strongly depleted in the polar stratosphere (during the spring), a large fraction of the chlorine is present as a free radical (Fig. 7). Anderson et al. (30) measured ppbv levels of chlorine monoxide, which were strongly inversely corre-

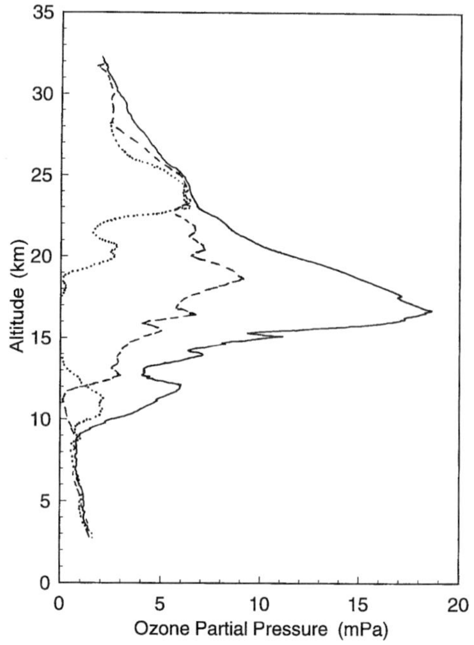


**FIG. 6.** Balloon measurements of ozone profiles over Amundsen-Scott Station at the South Pole in 1993. *Solid line*, August 23; *dashed line*, September 13; *dotted line*, October 16. (Adapted from ref. 28.)

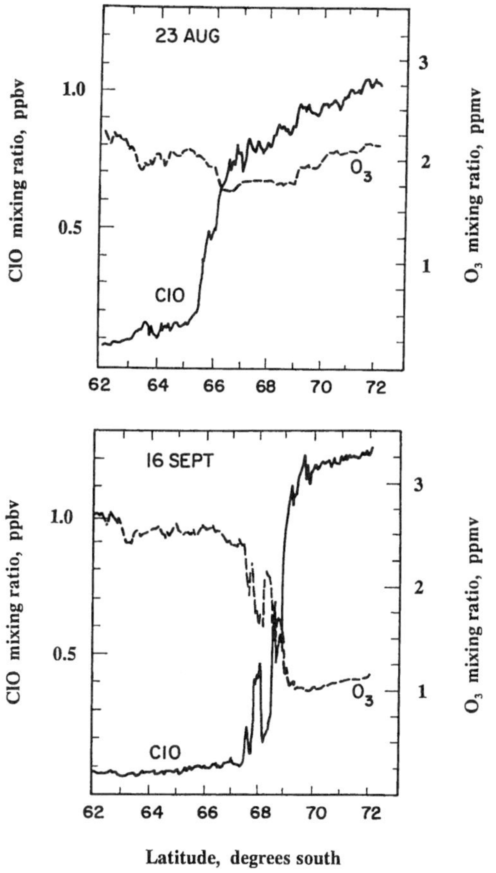


**FIG. 7.** Aircraft measurements conducted on August 23 and September 16, 1987, of chlorine monoxide by Anderson et al. (30), and of ozone by Proffitt et al. (31).

lated with ozone loss monitored by Proffitt et at. (31). An analysis of these measurements indicates that the chlorine peroxide cycle (reactions 8, 19, 20) accounts for about three-fourths of the observed ozone loss, with the bromine cycle (reactions 8, 21, 22) accounting for the rest (30). Furthermore, $NO_x$ levels were found to be very low and nitric acid was shown to be present in the cloud particles (29).

Atmospheric field measurements have also been conducted in the Arctic stratosphere (32), indicating that a large fraction of the chlorine is also activated there. Nevertheless, ozone depletion is less severe over the Arctic and is not as localized, because the temperatures are not as low as over Antarctica; the active chlorine does not remain in contact with ozone long enough and at low enough temperatures to destroy it before the stratospheric air over the Arctic mixes with warmer air from lower latitudes. This warmer air also contains $NO_2$, which passivates the chlorine. On the other hand, as expected, cold winters lead to significant ozone depletion—30% or more—over large areas, as was the case over northern Europe in 1995–1996. Furthermore, as mentioned earlier, ozone is also being depleted to some extent at mid-latitudes (Fig. 5).

Much has been learned about the chemistry of the polar stratosphere through laboratory studies, field measurements, and modeling calculations; however, questions remain such as the chemical identity and the formation mechanism of the various cloud particles that are present in the polar stratosphere. Also, the observed mid-latitude ozone loss is larger than predicted from the models. Hence, additional research needs to be carried out to improve the reliability of the predictions of ozone depletion in the next few decades.

## OZONE DEPLETION AND UV-B RADIATION

Depletion of stratospheric ozone leads to increases in the level of solar UV radiation reaching the Earth's surface predominantly at wavelengths ~290 to 315 nm, the so-called UV-B radiation. At shorter wavelengths atmospheric ozone absorbs essentially all the solar photons (UV-C), and at longer wavelengths (UV-A, 315–400 nm) the absorption is negligible. UV-B radiation is also partially shielded by clouds, by dust, and by air pollution. With a clear sky, each 1% reduction in the total ozone column results in an increase of about 1.3% in the intensity of UV-B at ground level. This increase is well documented by direct measurements under the Antarctic ozone hole, where the UV-B levels can exceed the maximum summer values measured at San Diego, California (33) (Fig. 8). At other latitudes, where ozone depletion is less severe, the UV radiation increases are correspondingly smaller and more difficult to establish because of the lack of direct long-term measurements; however, UV radiation increases were evident, for example, during the winter of 1992–1993, when low ozone values prevailed over Europe (34).

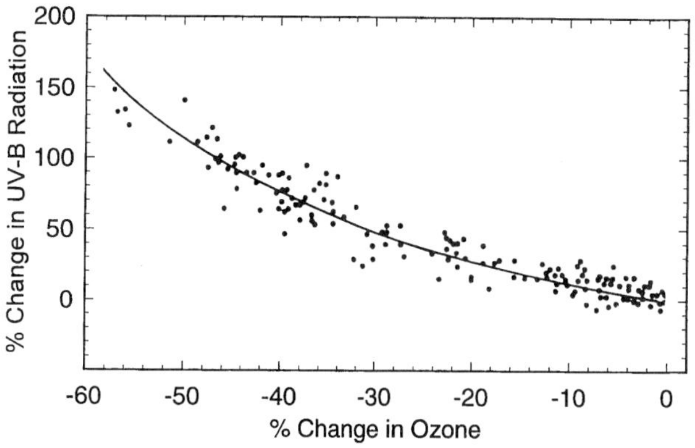


**FIG. 8.** Spring vs. autumn increase in UV-B radiation over South Pole, Antarctica, vs. change in total ozone column, both measured at the same solar zenith angle in 1991–1992. (Adapted from ref. 10.)

## BIOLOGIC EFFECTS OF ULTRAVIOLET RADIATION

The environmental and health effects of stratospheric ozone depletion have been summarized in several assessment reports that form part of the information on which the parties to the Montreal Protocol based their decisions regarding the protection of the ozone layer (35,36). UV-B radiation can induce acute skin damage in humans, such as sunburn. Other potential risks of increased UV-B radiation on human health include increases in the morbidity and incidence of skin cancer, eye diseases, and infectious diseases (37). Investigations of human epidemiology as well as animal experiments have established that UV-B radiation is a key risk factor for development of nonmelanoma skin cancer in light-skinned populations. The two main types of this cancer are basal cell carcinoma and squamous cell carcinoma; it is estimated that a sustained 1% decrease in stratospheric ozone would result in an increase of about 2% in the incidence of these types of cancer. For cutaneous melanoma the situation is less clear; there are indications that the risk increases with sunlight exposure, but there is uncertainty about the relative importance of UV-B radiation. The mechanism responsible for the UV damage is reasonably well understood at the molecular level; there is a peak in the absorption spectrum of the DNA molecule around 260 nm, but the spectrum extends beyond 320 nm. Absorption of a photon damages the DNA molecule; some efficient repair mechanisms exist, but the damage may lead eventually to faulty replication and mutation (e.g., ref. 38).

Numerous experiments have shown that the cornea and lens of the eye can also be damaged by UV-B radiation, and that chronic exposure to this radiation is associated with the risk of cataract of the cortical and posterior subcapsular forms (37). In addition, studies in human subjects show that exposure to UV-B radiation can suppress the induction of some immune responses, and experiments in animals indicate that such exposure decreases the immune response to skin cancers and some infectious agents. The reason is that the immune system has some components that are present in the skin, which makes it susceptible to the effects of UV-B radiation (39,40). Unfortunately, there are very limited data about the actual importance of these immune effects on infectious diseases in humans.

Terrestrial plants can also be affected by UV-B radiation, although the response varies to a large extent among different species. In addition to plant growth, the changes induced by UV radiation can be indirect, affecting, for example, the timing of developmental phases or the allocation of biomass to the different parts of the plant (41). Aquatic ecosystems can also be damaged by UV-B radiation; for example, there is evidence for impaired larval development and decreased reproductive capacity in some amphibians, shrimp, and fish (42). Furthermore, there is direct evidence of UV-B effects under the ozone hole on the productivity of natural phytoplankton communities in Antarctic waters (43). On the other hand, there is not enough information to reliably assess the potential damage on other terrestrial or aquatic ecosystems resulting from ozone depletion.

## INTERNATIONAL REGULATIONS

Following the publication of the Molina-Rowland hypothesis, the National Academy of Sciences issued two reports in 1976, which stated that the atmospheric sequence outlined by Molina and Rowland was essentially correct (44,45). The United States and some other countries responded in late 1970s by banning the sale of aerosol spray cans containing CFCs; this caused a temporary pause in the growing demands for CFCs. But worldwide use of the chemicals continued and the production rate began to rise again. In September 1987, an international agreement limiting the production of CFCs was approved under the auspices of the United Nations Environment Programme (UNEP). At that time the expeditions to the Antarctic stratosphere were just beginning to gather the data that would eventually firmly link the CFCs to the depletion of polar ozone. This agreement, the Montreal Protocol on Substances that Deplete the Ozone Layer, initially called for a reduction of only 50% in the manufacture of CFCs by the end of the century. In view of the strength of the scientific evidence that emerged in the following years, the initial provisions were strengthened through the London and the Copenhagen amendments to the protocol in 1990 and 1992, respectively. The production of CFCs in industrialized countries was phased out at the end of 1995, and other compounds such as the halons, methyl bromide, carbon tetrachloride, and methyl chloroform ($CH_3CCl_3$) were also regulated.

Developing countries are allowed to continue CFC production temporarily, to facilitate their transition to the newer CFC-free technologies. An important feature of the Montreal Protocol was the establishment of a funding mechanism to help these countries meet the costs of complying with the protocol and with its subsequent amendments. It involves the creation of the Multilateral Fund, financed by the industrialized countries; the implementing agencies include UNEP, the United Nations Industrial Organization (UNIDO), the United Nations Development Programme (UNDP), and the World Bank.

So far, the provisions of the Montreal Protocol have been successfully enforced. Chlorine levels are expected to peak before the end of the century; in fact, atmospheric measurements indicate that the abundance of chlorine contained in the CFCs and other chlorocarbons is beginning to decline in response to the Montreal Protocol regulations (46). On the other hand, because of the long residence times of the CFCs in the atmosphere, relatively high chlorine levels in the stratosphere—with the conse-

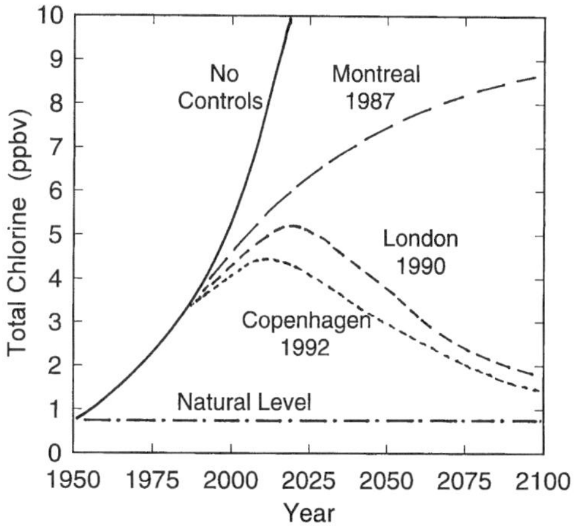


**FIG. 9.** Measured and projected chlorine concentrations in the stratosphere according to the provisions of the Montreal Protocol and subsequent amendments.

quent ozone depletion—are expected to continue well into the next century, as indicated in Fig. 9.

A significant fraction of the former CFC usage is being dealt with by conservation and recycling. Furthermore, roughly a fourth of the former use of CFCs is being temporarily replaced by hydrochlorofluorocarbons (HCFCs)—compounds that have similar physical properties to the CFCs, but their molecules contain hydrogen atoms and are less stable in the atmosphere. A large fraction of the HCFCs released industrially reacts in the lower atmosphere with the OH radical before reaching the stratosphere, forming water and an organic free radical that rapidly photo-oxidizes to yield water-soluble products, which are then removed from the atmosphere mainly by rainfall. Some hydrofluorocarbons (HFCs), which do not contain chlorine atoms, are also being used as CFC replacements, e.g., HFC-134a ($CF_3$–$CH_2F$), for automobile air conditioning. About half of the CFC usage is being replaced by not-in-kind compounds; for example, CFC-113—used extensively as a solvent to clean electronic components—is being phased out by CFC-free cleaning technologies such as soap and water or terpene-based solvents; there are also new technologies to manufacture clean electronic boards to begin with.

It is now clear that human activities can lead to serious environmental problems not just on a local, but also on a global scale. One of the key steps in any rational approach to addressing global environmental issues is to promote internationalism—a widespread understanding that all of our human problems are interconnected. Regional and international cooperation will be essential to the solution of environmental problems. The formulation of the Montreal Protocol sets a very important precedent for addressing global environmental problems. It demonstrates how the different sectors of society—scientists, industry people, policy makers, and environmentalists—can work together and can be very productive by functioning in a collaborative mode rather than in an adversary mode.

## REFERENCES


1. Molina MJ, Rowland FS. Stratospheric sink for chlorofluoromethanes: chlorine-atom catalyzed destruction of ozone. *Nature* 1974;249: 810–812.
2. Rowland FS, Molina MJ. Chlorofluoromethanes in the environment. *Rev Geophys Space Phys* 1975;13:1–35.
3. Chapman S. A theory of upper atmospheric ozone. *Mem R Meteorol Soc* 1930;3:103.
4. Crutzen PJ. The influence of nitrogen oxides on atmosphere ozone content. *Q J R Meteorol Soc* 1970;96:320–325.
5. Johnston HS. Reduction of stratospheric ozone by nitrogen oxide catalysts from supersonic transport exhaust. *Science* 1971;173:517–522.
6. Rom WN, ed. *Environmental and occupational medicine,* 2nd ed. Boston: Little, Brown, 1992.
7. Stolarski RS, Cicerone R. Stratospheric chlorine: a possible sink for ozone. *Can J Chem* 1974;52:1610–1650.
8. Midgley T. From the Periodic Table to production. *Ind Engr Chem* 1937;29:241–244.
9. Lovelock JE, Maggs RJ, Wade RJ. Halogenated hydrocarbons in and over the Atlantic. *Nature* 1973;241:194–196.
10. World Meteorological Organization. *Scientific assessment of ozone depletion:* 1994. WMO Global Ozone Research and Monitoring Project, report no. 37, Geneva: WMO, 1995.
11. Farman JC, Gardiner BG, Shanklin JD. Large losses of total ozone in Antarctica reveal seasonal $ClO_x/NO_x$ interactions. *Nature* 1985;315: 207–210.
12. Russell JM III, Luo M, Cicerone RJ, Deaver LE. Satellite confirmation of the dominance of chlorofluorocarbons in the global stratospheric chlorine budget. *Nature* 1996;379:526–529.
13. Solomon S, Garcia RR, Rowland FS, Wuebbles DJ. On the depletion of Antarctic ozone. *Nature* 1986;321:755–758.
14. Molina LT, Molina MJ, Stachnick RA, Tom RD. An upper limit to the rate of the HCl + $ClONO_2$ reaction. *J Phys Chem* 1985;89:3779–3781.
15. DeMore WB, Sander SD, Golden DM, et al. *Chemical kinetics and photochemical data for use in the stratospheric modeling.* Evaluation no. 11, JPL publication no. 94-26. Pasadena, CA: NASA Jet Propulsion Laboratory, 1994.
16. Abbatt JPD, Beyer KD, Fucaloro AF, et al. Interaction of HCl vapor with water-ice: implications for the stratosphere. *J Geophys Res* 1992; 97:15819–15826.
17. Molina MJ. The probable role of stratospheric 'ice' clouds: heterogeneous chemistry of the ozone hole. In: Calvert JG, ed. *Chemistry of the atmosphere:* the impact of global change. Oxford, UK: Blackwell Scientific, 1994.
18. Gertner BJ, Hynes JT. Molecular dynamics simulation of hydrochloric acid ionization at the surface of stratospheric ice. *Science* 1996;271: 1563–1566.
19. Molina LT, Molina MJ. Production of $Cl_2O_2$ from the self-reaction of the ClO radical. *J Phys Chem* 1987;91:433–436.
20. Birk M, Friedl RR, Cohen EA, Pickett HM, Sander SP. The rotational spectrum and structure of chlorine peroxide. *J Chem Phys* 1989;91: 6588–6597.
21. Cox RA, Hayman GD. The stability and photochemistry of dimers of the ClO radical and implications for Antarctic ozone depletion. *Nature* 1988;332:796–800.
22. Molina MJ, Colussi AJ, Molina LT, Schindler RN, Tso T-L. Quantum yield of chlorine-atom formation in the photodissociation of chlorine peroxide (ClOOCl) at 308 nm. *Chem Phys Lett* 1990;173:310–315.
23. McElroy MB, Salawitch RJ, Wofsy SC, Logan JA. Reduction of Antarctic ozone due to synergistic interactions of chlorine and bromine. *Nature* 1986;321:759–762.
24. Solomon S, Mount GH, Saunders RW, Schmeltekopf AL. Visible spectroscopy at McMurdo Station, Antarctica. *J Geophys Res* 1987;92: 8329–8338.
25. Dobson GMB, Harrison DN. Measurement of the amount of ozone in the Earth's atmosphere and its relation to other geophysical conditions. *Proc R Soc Lond* 1926;110:660–693.

26. Stolarski RS, Bloomfield P, McPeters RD, Herman JR. Total ozone trends deduced from Nimbus 7 TOMS data. *Geophys Res Lett* 1991;18: 1015–1018.
27. Jones AE, Shanklin JD. Continued decline of total ozone over Halley, Antarctica, since 1985. *Nature* 1995;376:409–411.
28. Hofmann DJ, Oltmans SJ, Lathrop JA, Harris JM, Vomel H. Record low ozone at the South Pole in the spring of 1993. *Geophys Res Lett* 1994; 21:421–424.
29. Tuck AF, Watson RT, Condon EP, Margitan JJ, Toon OB. The planning and execution of ER-2 and DC-8 aircraft flights over Antarctica, August and September 1987. *J Geophys Res* 1989;94:11,181–222.
30. Anderson JG, Toohey DW, Brune WH. Free radicals within the Antarctic Vortex: the role of CFCs in Antarctic ozone loss. *Science* 1991;251: 39–46.
31. Proffitt MH, Steinkamp MJ, Powell JA, et al. In situ ozone measurements within the 1987 Antarctic ozone hole from a high-altitude ER-2 aircraft. *J Geophys Res* 1989;94:16,547–555.
32. Turco R, Plumb A, Condon E. The Airborne Arctic Stratospheric Expedition: prologue. *Geophys Res Lett* 1990;17:313–316.
33. Madronich S, McKenzie RL, Caldwell MM, Björn LO. Changes in ultraviolet radiation reaching the Earth's surface. *Ambio* 1995;24:143–152.
34. Seckmeyer G, Mayer B, Erb R, Bernhard G. UVB in Germany higher in 1993 than in 1992. *Geophys Res Lett* 1994;21:577–580.
35. van der Leun J, Tang X, Tevini M. Environmental effects of ozone depletion: 1994 assessment. *Ambio* 1995;24:138.
36. Biggs RH, Joyner MEB, eds. *Stratospheric ozone depletion/UV-B radiation in the biosphere.* New York: Springer-Verlag, 1994.
37. Longstreth JD, de Grujil FR, Kripke ML, Takizawa Y, van der Leun JC. Effects of solar radiation on human health. *Ambio* 1995;24:153–165.
38. Brash DE, Rudolph JA, Simon JA, et al. A role for sunlight in skin cancer: UV-induced p53 mutations in squamous cell carcinoma. *Proc Natl Acad Sci USA* 1991;88:10,124–128.
39. De Fabo EC, Noonan FP. Mechanism of immune suppression by ultraviolet irradiation in vivo. I. Evidence for the existence of a unique photoreceptor in skin and its role in photoimmunology. *J Exp Med* 1983; 157:84–98.
40. Cooper KD, Oberhelman L, Hamilton TA, et al. UV exposure reduces immunization rates and promotes tolerance to epicutaneous antigens in humans—relationship to dose, CD1a-DR$^+$ epidermal macrophage induction and Langerhans cell depletion. *Proc Natl Acad Sci USA* 1992;89:8497–8501.
41. Caldwell MM, Teramura AH, Tevini M, Bomman JF, Björn LO, Kulandaivelu G. Effects of increased solar ultraviolet radiation on terrestrial plants. *Ambio* 1995;24:166–173.
42. Häder DP, Worrest RC, Kumar HD, Smith RC. Effects of increased solar ultraviolet radiation on aquatic ecosystems. *Ambio* 1995;24: 174–180.
43. Smith RC, Prézelin BB, Baker KS, et al. Ozone depletion: ultraviolet radiation and phytoplankton biology in Antarctic waters. *Science* 1992; 255:952–959.
44. National Research Council. *Halocarbon:* environmental effects of chlorofluoromethane release. Washington, DC: National Academy of Sciences, 1976.
45. National Research Council. *Halocarbons:* effects on stratospheric ozone. Washington, DC: National Academy of Sciences, 1976.
46. Montzka SA, Butler JH, Myers RC, et al. Decline in the tropospheric abundance of halogen from halocarbons: implications for stratospheric ozone depletion. *Science* 1996;272:1318–1322.

# SECTION III

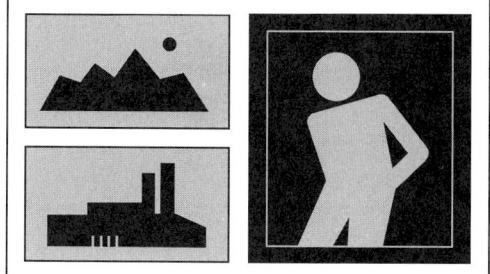

## Control of Environmental and Occupational Diseases and Exposures

*Environmental and Occupational Medicine, Third Edition,* edited by William N. Rom.
Lippincott–Raven Publishers, Philadelphia © 1998.

# CHAPTER 124

# Environmental Law and the Science of Ecology

Jeffrey G. Miller

Intuitively, the purpose of environmental law is to protect and promote stable and healthy ecosystems. Yet few environmental statutes have that as their goal, and if they occasionally serve that end, they often do so serendipitously. This is not altogether surprising, however, because the science of ecology is in its infancy and the knowledge so far developed simply cannot support the massive and complex body of law protecting the environment.

This situation highlights a central tension of environmental policy: the demand and perceived need for meaningful action in the face of the frequent lack of knowledge and data to support such action. On the one hand, it seems foolish to take action requiring an expenditure of billions of dollars to avoid a danger, when there is inadequate knowledge and data to clearly establish either the existence of the danger or whether the expenditures will avert the danger. Lack of hard information often provides a respectable and quasi-scientific cloak for those who oppose environmental action on other grounds (usually because it will cost them, their clients, or their constituents money). On the other hand, it seems foolish not to act, even in the face of scientific uncertainty, when the cost of acting is small compared to the damage that would occur if the danger does come to pass. But with insufficient knowledge, how can the risk or its cost be measured? Indeed, how can it be known that the action will avert the danger? The question of how much knowledge is needed to warrant action is central to many important contemporary environmental issues. It dominated the policy debate on acid rain for over a decade, until Congress finally acted in 1990 to require acid rain controls on coal fired power plants. It dominates the policy debate today on whether to increase the stringency of air standards for small particulates and ozone. It promises to dominate the debate for the next few years on the need to control greenhouse gases to avert global warming.

This tension reflects one of the concepts developed by the infant science of ecology: the law of unintended consequences. Simply stated, when an ecologic system is not fully known or understood, changing a variable or introducing a new factor is likely to produce unforeseen and unintended consequences. This is a corollary of the central law of ecology: all factors in an ecologic system are interrelated (1). Change one of those factors enough, and changes in other factors will occur as a consequence. If the system is well enough understood, the consequential changes may be predicted. If it is not, the consequential changes are likely to be unpredictable.

Our knowledge of ecosystems is limited to a few of the more simple ones, such as the relationship between wolves, owls, lemmings, and lemming forage on the tundra. In some areas lemmings are the chief food of wolves and owls, and the relative abundance of lemmings as a food supply is the chief variable in the population of those predators. At the same time, the presence and number of predators and the abundance of lemming forage limit the lemming population. As these variables change, predictable results occur. For instance, as the lemming population grows, the predator population will grow with it and the abundance of lemming forage will decrease proportionately. At some point lemming forage will be depleted enough that it will not support the lemming population, which then contracts rapidly, causing predator populations to decrease and forage abundance to increase. Consumption of forage by lemmings destroys their cover, making them easier prey for predators. Moreover, as the cover is destroyed, the shade it provides the permafrost disappears,

J. G. Miller: Pace University School of Law, Center for Environmental Legal Studies, White Plains, New York 10603.

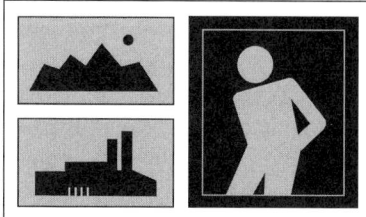

melting the permafrost. Plant nutrients that had been trapped on the surface of the permafrost then leach beyond the reach of forage vegetation, increasing the disappearance of the lemmings' food (James Utter, Pace University School of Law, White Plains, New York, personal communication, 1990). Of course, the system is more complicated than this (1), but it is nevertheless a simple system and is understood enough to predict the consequence of changing one variable and even of introducing some new ones. But as the systems become more complex, our ability to predict the consequences of changing a variable diminishes greatly and even disappears. Hence the law of unintended consequences.

Environmental law and regulation pose a policy dilemma. The development of civilization has upset most of the Earth's ecosystems in known and unknown ways by changing variables and introducing new ones. As a result, many of those ecosystems are stressed, some to the point of collapse. Yet we do not fully understand either the ecosystems or the changes in them we have wrought. We want to alleviate the stress and avoid the collapse, but if we do not understand the ecosystems or the consequences of our actions in the first place, how can we know what actions will alleviate the stress and avoid the collapse? To do nothing invites complete ecologic collapse, which is unthinkable. Action is necessary. But because of our incomplete knowledge, out best intended corrective actions may be ineffectual and sometimes even counterproductive. It is hoped we can learn from our experiences and mistakes and improve both our diagnoses and cures.

The concerns that lead to the demand for environmental protection often are reactions to symptoms that ecologic systems are under stress and may be collapsing, for instance, the extinction of species, destructive forest fires, and rampant algae blooms. Where the ecosystems involved are relatively simple, we may understand them and be able to arrest or reverse a perceived imbalance. Whooping cranes were becoming extinct because of their loss of habitat. Protecting the relatively small areas of their breeding and wintering habitats enabled this endangered population to grow and stabilize. Bald eagles and peregrine falcons were on the brink of extinction through reproductive failure because DDT made their egg shells so brittle they broke when parent birds incubated them. Banning DDT enabled the species to rebound. Unusually destructive fires swept through the lodgepole pine forests of Yellowstone National Park. The severity of the fires resulted from the accumulation of downed timber in the forests, an accumulation assured by the success of previous efforts to contain and extinguish forest fires. This ignored the natural role of fire in promoting healthy lodgepole pine forests. Fires are necessary not only to clear downed timber and undergrowth to promote lodgepole growth, but also to release lodgepole seeds, enabling new growth. Controlled burning may be the answer, both for the promotion of healthy forests and the avoidance of massive fires. Algae blooms in Lake Erie grew to massive proportions, threatening to choke the lake, because of unlimited discharges to the Great Lakes system of their chief nutrients: phosphorus and nitrogen. Algae was brought under control in the lake by limiting introduction of the two nutrients by a combination of the treatment of municipal wastewater and changes in agricultural practices, and by changes in the composition of household detergents.

Where ecosystems are more complex, our knowledge is often too limited to deal with what we perceive as problems. For instance, despite reducing industrial and municipal pollutants formerly discharged to the Great Lakes' system by 85% to 95% in an effort to restore the lakes' water quality, the biota of the lakes is still plagued by heavy concentrations of some toxic pollutants. In part, this result was predictable, because the discharge of pollutants to surface waters from other sources (e.g., many agricultural activities) was unregulated. But these other discharges could not wholly explain the range and concentrations of pollutants in the system. Eventually they were discovered to originate in air pollutants from power plants and industries both within the system and well beyond it. The Environmental Protection Administration (EPA) reports, for instance, that 55% of nitrogen and 22% of sulfate loadings in Lake Superior are from atmospheric deposition (2). Even this is simple, compared to understanding the causes and antidotes to global warming. While there appears to be a consensus that gradual global warming is a real phenomenon, there does not appear to be a consensus on the role that human activity plays in it. While emissions of carbon dioxide from the burning of fossil fuel clearly can cause atmospheric warming through the "greenhouse" effect, emissions of particulate matter clearly can cause atmospheric cooling through deflecting light from the atmosphere. Which is dominant? Indeed, is the warming observed a product of human forces acting on the atmosphere or of cyclical changes in ocean currents?

Both these anecdotal examples and the underlying principles of ecology suggest that environmental problems are interrelated and are best addressed in a comprehensive, integrated manner, based on adequate knowledge. Our response to environmental problems, however, has not been an integrated one, nor has it always been based on adequate knowledge. The results of our efforts, predictably, are less than might be desired and often have unintended and unforeseen consequences.

## ENVIRONMENTAL STATUTES: CATEGORIES AND THEMES

Environmental law is statutory and regulatory law. In the absence of a statute addressing a particular aspect of environmental degradation, individual instances of environmental damage might support common law tort actions such as negligence, trespass, or nuisance. For instance, in the absence of the Clean Air Act (CAA), emissions from factories that damage the productivity of nearby farms might be successfully attacked using tort law (3,4). But these actions are usually for damages to individual interests, not to the environment. They address single instances of damages, not systematic damage. They are in reaction to damage that has already occurred, not to the threat of future harm. They seek money damages, not prevention of future harm. Hence the need for addressing broader problems with comprehensive legislation and regulation. The common law causes of action, however, have not been extinguished by environmental legislation, but continue to operate alongside it. The legislation seeks to regulate present and future action to prevent future environmental damage, while the common law provided a remedy for individuals nonetheless damaged by environmental insults.

### Natural Resource Management

Environmental law began in the late 19th century with legislation managing natural resources of either particular economic value (forests, minerals, grasslands) or particular aesthetic, historic, or ecologic value (parks, monuments, wildlife sanctuaries). This branch of environmental law dominated the field until the 1970s. Emblematic of its dominance were the names of government and professional organizations important in the field. Federal environmental laws were enforced within the Lands and Natural Resources Division of the Department of Justice, only recently renamed the Environment and Natural Resources Division. The section of the American Bar Association devoted to environmental law, the Section on Natural Resources, Energy, and Environment, only recently added the word *environment* to its name.

Early natural resource legislation had a conservation focus, but usually conservation was practiced to ensure a continued supply of an economic resource rather than a healthy ecosystem. Rather than protect ecosystems, these statutes managed their exploitation. Legislation establishing national parks or protecting migratory bird species was a significant exception, but even its purpose was to provide exploitation of ecosystems for educational, recreational, or hunting use rather than to protect them for their intrinsic value. Modern natural resource management legislation has moved somewhat from serving narrow commercial interests, such as managing national forests exclusively for timber production, to providing for broader interests, such as managing national forests for multiple purposes, including recreation.[a] Some more recent natural resource management legislation actually provides ecosystem protection, albeit for rather special kinds of ecosystems such as wilderness areas, endangered species habitats, and coral reefs.[b]

[a]Compare 16 U.S.C. §475 (1994), enacted in 1897, authorizing the establishment of national forests to improve and protect forests for watershed protection and for a continuous supply of timber with 16 U.S.C. §528 (1994), enacted in 1976, authorizing national forests for outdoor recreation, range use, timbering, watershed protection, and fish and wildlife management.

### Pollution Control and Waste Management

With the advent of the 1970s, pollution control and waste management began to dominate the field of environmental law. The new field built on the conservation ethic that underlay and was developed by the earlier natural resource management law. Indeed, the new branch of environmental law reflects the older law's ambivalence about the purpose of conserving the environment, namely whether conservation is intended primarily to benefit human economy and society or the environment itself. Here are the most notable of the pollution and waste control statutes:

National Environmental Policy Act of 1969 (NEPA) required that decisions to undertake major federal activities significantly affecting the environment be made only after a study of the alternatives and their environmental affects (5).

Clean Air Act of 1970 (CAA) replaced earlier, ineffective legislation requiring controls on sources of air pollution (6).

Clean Water Act of 1972 (CWA) replaced earlier, ineffective legislation requiring controls on point sources of water pollution (7).

Federal Insecticide, Fungicide, and Rodenticide Act of 1972 (FIFRA) amended earlier regulation of pesticide manufacture to make protection of the environment and human health as important as ensuring farmers of the efficacy of the products they purchased (8).

Safe Drinking Waste Act of 1974 (SDWA) provided for federal standards to be met by public water suppliers (9).

Resource Conservation and Recovery Act of 1976 (RCRA) regulated transport, treatment, storage, and disposal of solid and hazardous waste (10).

Toxic Substances Control Act of 1976 (TSCA) required premanufacturing review of new chemicals, and authorized regulation of existing chemicals to protect public health and the environment (11).

Comprehensive Environmental Response and Liability Act of 1980 (CERCLA or Superfund) authorized and funded federal cleanup of hazardous waste contamination and recovery of costs from those responsible (12).

Emergency Planning and Community Right to Know Act of 1986 (EPCRKA), enacted as part of amendments to CERCLA, provided public information on the location of hazardous chemicals and encouraged the development of local response capability for releases of hazardous chemicals (13).

[b]See the Wilderness Act of 1964, 16 U.S.C. §§1131–1136 (1994); the Endangered Species Act, 16 U.S.C. §§1531–1544 (1994); and the Marine Protection, Research and Sanctuaries Act, 33 U.S.C. §§1401–1445 (1994).

Oil Pollution Act of 1990 (OPA) augmented earlier legislation authorizing and funding federal cleanup of oil spills and recovery of costs from those responsible (14).

There are a number of other, more limited statutes of this nature, such as those regulating ocean dumping[c] or asbestos-related activities,[d] which either stand alone or amend the principal statutes. There are also significant related statutes that are not discussed here, such as the Occupational Health and Safety Act (15) and the Federal Food, Drug, and Cosmetic Act (16).

While these statutes have much in common, it is their lack of commonality that is most remarkable and that ultimately inhibits rational and comprehensive environmental protection. Each statute has a single focus: one sort of environmental insult, one category of product, or one set of actors. Nothing provides for integration of the different statutes, except similar vague purposes to protect the public health and the environment and administration by the EPA or different parts of it, and its state counterparts. The EPA has 17 separate offices, headed by the highest level civil servants, serving under four presidentially appointed assistant administrators, implementing the statutes considered here. The statutes lack a common focus, a common regulatory strategy, and a common understanding about how much protection should be afforded by environmental legislation. Indeed, the statutes are at times senselessly inconsistent. Worse, in the aggregate they do not address all environmental problems. For instance, they provide no comprehensive protection of groundwater quality[e] and virtually no regulation to prevent global warming.[f] The statutes establish no priorities, either individually or in the aggregate, a particularly troublesome problem since the expenditures that could be made to protect the public health and environment are virtually limitless, while the public's view of what should be spent for the public good is limited. The statutes often fail to make hard choices, but defer them to the EPA. They establish impossible tasks, both for the EPA and the regulated public, and require the tasks to be accomplished within equally impossible deadlines. They entrust their implementation to the EPA and counterpart state agencies, establishing bureaucratic redundancy and rivalry that often impedes their administration. When, predictability, their mandates are not met, Congress amends them again and again, providing ever more detailed requirements. As a consequence, the requirements they impose do not stand still, but are ever changing. Despite these severe handicaps, the EPA has done a remarkable job of making progress on many environmental fronts. Trends in environmental improvement and degradation are summarized in *Environmental Quality,* a publication of the Council on Environmental Quality. The publication began as an annual summary, but has become less frequent as the importance of that organization has waned.

### *Single-Focus Legislation*

The single focus of the statutes ignores the basic principle of ecology: the interrelatedness of all ecologic factors. Predictably, the single focus of the statutes severely inhibits their ability to provide comprehensive environmental protection in an efficient manner. Most human activity, even day-to-day living, produces waste. Once waste is produced, it must be disposed of somewhere in or on land, air, or water. Wise legislation would seek both to reduce the amount of waste produced and to direct wastes nevertheless produced to the place where they can be recycled or disposed of in a manner that causes the least harm to the environment. It would do so with an eye to costs, so that society's resources are spent first to alleviate the worst harms and risks, not squandered to address small problems or problems whose cure costs more than the problems being cured. Single-focus legislation cannot accomplish these goals, but has the tendency to push problems from one part of the environment to another. Air stripping of volatile organic pollutants from industrial wastewater, for instance, solves a water pollution problem, but only by pushing the pollutants from the water into the air. Air pollution control strategies that fail to take into account the water pollution resulting from fallout of airborne pollutants on large bodies of water may make it impossible to achieve water quality objectives for them.

Wise environmental policy would devote always limited resources to achieving the maximum environmental good for the resources expended. Single-focus legislation makes that impossible. The demands of each piece of legislation must be met, no matter how insignificant the problem it addresses in comparison with problems addressed by other legislation (17). Recent legislation on medical wastes is a good example (18). Worse, single-focus legislation institutionalizes the single-focus view, making integration and priority setting ever more difficult. Single-focus statutes become the focus of single congressional subcommittees, single implementing divisions in the EPA and its state counterparts, single organi-

[c]This was a major purpose of the MPRSA.

[d]This authority was added to TSCA in 1986, 15 U.S.C. §§2641–2655 (1994).

[e]There are bits and pieces of groundwater protection in several of the statutes. Both RCRA and CERCLA protect groundwater from contamination by hazardous waste disposal, and SDWA protects it from contamination by wastes disposed in wells. But these are only small part of the causes of groundwater contamination. Pesticides and nitrates from normal agricultural use, for instance, are a widespread source of groundwater contamination, the EPA, *Water Quality Inventory,* supra, pp. 119–129.

[f]Congress has addressed several gases that deplete the upper atmosphere ozone layer, especially chlorofluorocarbons (CFCs), in 1990 amendments to the CAA, 42 U.S.C. §§7671–7671q (1994), replacing earlier, more general authority on the subject enacted in 1977. The EPA's authority to address more common global warming gases, such as carbon dioxide, however, are more tenuous.

zations of state agencies, single professional groups, and single parts of law and other professional firms. Thus the Clean Air Act is the focus of single subcommittees in the Senate and in the House, and it is administered by a single assistant administrator in the EPA and her counterparts in state agencies. The state air pollution administrators have their own organization, and there is a national association of air pollution professionals. The American Bar Association has an air pollution subcommittee. Professionals who work in air pollution tend not to work on other pollution problems. The CAA is sufficiently voluminous and complex that few pretend to deal with it as a whole, much less with other pollution programs. But the single focus misses many opportunities for efficiency and effectiveness that integration offers.

The CAA is a good example of many of the concerns discussed thus far. It was enacted in its modern form in 1970, at a time when our knowledge of the mechanics of air pollution was much more elementary than it is today. We then assumed that the effects of air pollution were local. This led to the assumption that plans sufficient to prevent adverse effects of air pollution in the area of its origin would address all its adverse effects. This led to the assumption that air pollution control plans should be developed at the state and local level, which conveniently dovetailed with a political desire not to erect a large federal superstructure to administer the statute. One consequence of this was the development of local air pollution control strategies that utilized tall smokestacks on power plants to shoot pollutants high enough to avoid polluting their surrounding areas. Today we know, of course, that this whole structure was built on a false assumption. Air pollution effects are not only local, but regional and even national. Sulfur oxides shot high in the sky by copper smelters in the Southwest and coal burning power plants in the Midwest cause acid rain problems in the Northeast and parts of Canada. The tall stacks that solved local problems, exacerbated a regional problem, a good example of the law of unintended consequences when acting in the absence of knowledge of an ecosystem.

At the same time, much progress was made in controlling air pollution as a result of the 1970 legislation. Incomplete knowledge of the mechanics of air pollution would not have been a good excuse for taking no action at all. Indeed, complete knowledge may not be always necessary to frame responsive action. Sufficient knowledge was available in 1970 that common air pollutants had significant adverse health effects and that they could be largely controlled at affordable costs. To do nothing until the mechanics of air pollution were completely understood would have prolonged needlessly many of the health threats posed by it. Indeed, sufficient knowledge was available by the late 1970s to recognize that acid rain was a significant problem and that its control would require significant curtailment of sulfur oxide emissions by Midwestern coal-burning power plants. Action to reduce those emissions could have been taken at any time, but Congress did not act on that knowledge until 1990. While regulation was fought under the guise that multibillion dollar expenditures could not be justified in the absence of complete knowledge of the mechanics of acid rain, the real issues were political and economic. When Congress finally acted in 1990, its knowledge of the underlying science was not significantly different than it had been in 1980 and the costs of controls were far less than had been anticipated.[g]

When action is taken on the basis of incomplete knowledge, it is important to revisit the action as knowledge is developed. Better knowledge may require adjustments in control strategies. Early air pollution control efforts, for instance, focused on particulate matter regardless of its size or nature. Those control efforts resulted in air that was healthier and visibly cleaner. As knowledge of the health effects of particulate matter grew, however, it became apparent that smaller particulates posed greater heath threats than larger particulates. The EPA modified its particulate standard in the late 1970s to target "particles with an aerodynamic diameter less than or equal to a nominal 10 micrometers" (the $PM_{10}$ standard) (19). The EPA is once again examining more recent health studies to determine whether it should target even smaller particulates. The data underlying the studies that are the most suggestive of such a strategic shift, however, have not been subject to peer review. Moreover, newer monitoring techniques may be able to distinguish between different small particulates by type and origin, enabling control strategies not to focus on small particulates in general, but rather on those small particulates that in fact pose health problems. This would assure that expenditures for control achieve the maximum health benefits. This situation suggests that further regulation be deferred while further knowledge is developed.

The single focus aspect of the CAA has inhibited the EPA's ability to deal with all sources that contribute to air pollution and has led it to ignore secondary impacts of air pollution. Most other means of waste disposal have air pollution impacts, but the EPA's air pollution office has largely ignored them because they are under the purview of other offices. A graphic example is the use of a process called air stripping to remove volatile organics from con-

[g]For a survey of knowledge on the subject a decade before legislative action, see *Acid Precipitation,* hearings before the Subcommittee on Health and the Environment, Committee on Energy and Commerce, House of Representatives Nos. 97–99 and 100 (1980). With regard to costs, the costs of treatment were made more palatable by allowing the regulated power plants to trade tons of reduction in sulfur oxide emissions. Thus one plant, for which reduction costs were unusually high, could buy from a second plant, for which reduction costs were unusually low, reduction over and above the reduction otherwise required of the second plant. The second plant's additional reduction would then be credited against the first plant's reduction requirements. When these "credits" were first traded on the Chicago commodities exchange, it was anticipated that they would cost $1,000 a ton, reflecting the expected cost of reduction. Today they are traded at less than $100 a ton, reflecting much lower than anticipated costs of reduction.

taminated water. The process essentially accelerates the evaporation of volatile chemicals into the atmosphere. Because it is an effective way to remove contaminants from industrial wastewater, it is the basis for regulations promulgated by the EPA's water pollution program requiring water pollution control by some industries. It is also used in the EPA's Superfund cleanup program to remove contaminants from groundwater at some hazardous waste sites. The EPA's air office long ignored these developments because its primary focus was not surface water pollution or groundwater pollution. It could have influenced the other EPA offices to choose different treatment technology or to require air pollution controls on air stripping at the outset. It eventually did so, but only after years of chasing volatile organic pollution from water to air.

Another aspect of the CAA's single focus is the curious fact that it concerns only outdoor air pollution, ignoring the contamination of indoor air. Indoor air pollution has a greater probability of affecting human health than outdoor air because so many people spend the majority of their lives indoors. Moreover, the confinement of buildings inhibits the dispersion of pollutants that takes place naturally outdoors. Tobacco smoke, radon, cooking gases, formaldehyde glues, and other such air pollutants pose few health problems when they occur in the open air, but when confined in buildings they have very real health effects. Unable to deal with these problems under the CAA, the EPA may be causing massive expenditures on air pollution controls that have far less health benefits than similar expenditures on improvements in indoor air.

On the other hand, the focus of the air office on controls to protect the public from the health effects of inhaling air pollution has led it to ignore the effects of air pollutants on other aspects of the environment. It could have regulated sulfur oxide emissions to prevent secondary effects, such as acid rain and acid deposition. But it did not do so until legislation required it. It continues to ignore the secondary effects of emissions of toxic air pollutants on major water bodies into which they fall, such as the Great Lakes or Chesapeake Bay, despite conclusive evidence that such emissions bear large responsibility for degraded water quality.

The EPA's stewardship of the CAA has been cautious, to the point of being viewed as ineffectual by some. This results from many factors. The single focus of the legislation and the EPA's implementation of it is a factor. The split of responsibility between the EPA and the states and the EPA's frequent deferral to the states is another factor. The many requirements laid on the EPA by the legislation controlling it, with no way for it to establish effective priorities is another. The unrealistic deadlines established by environmental legislation is another.

The EPA's slow implementation of the CAA has resulted in repeated congressional intervention to make the requirements of the statute ever more explicit and detailed. Congress has amended the statute no fewer than ten times since the seminal 1970 enactment. The 1990 amendments alone fill more than 300 small-print pages. The detail of their prescriptions is exemplified by their ban on chlorofluorocarbon-propelled plastic party streamers and noise horns (20). In its length and complexity the statute rivals the Internal Revenue Code. It is inaccessible and incomprehensible to all but a few professionals specializing in it, which compounds its single-focus shortcomings.

The single focus of environmental legislation is under fire from both the academic and business communities. Two major studies, headed by two former EPA administrators, William Ruckelshaus and William Reilly, are currently investigating how to reform environmental legislation to provide more efficient and effective programs. Integration of the statutes and their administration is a common thrust of both studies. Although there may be considerable support for integration, the one institution that can achieve it has a vested interest in the perpetuation of single-focus legislation. Under the current committee structure of Congress, jurisdiction over the environmental statutes is spread among several committees and subcommittees in each chamber. To integrate the legislation, many of those committees and subcommittees in each chamber would have to lose jurisdiction. Loss of jurisdiction is loss of power, anathema to congressmen. The 104th Congress trumpeted its intention to reform the congressional committee structure, although not with the intent of promoting the integration of environmental legislation. Its efforts did not result in sufficient change to suggest that Congress could accomplish the internal restructuring necessary to integrate environmental legislation.

### *Public Health Focus*

Although pollution control and waste management are intuitively aimed at ecologic protection and enhancement, their legislative purposes are often to protect public health. Thus, the first stated purpose of the CAA is to "promote the public health and welfare"; nowhere in its purpose clauses is there a reference to the broader environment (21). Almost all other major pollution and waste control statutes that have purpose or policy clauses state their intent to protect and promote health and the environment.[h] The sole exception is the Clean Water Act, whose only stated purpose is to "restore and maintain the chemical, physical and biological integrity of the Nation's waters"(22).

While purpose clauses may be only hortatory, the emphasis on protecting health is clear and explicit in the driving forces of many of the statutes, i.e., the provisions that establish the criteria the EPA is to use in promulgating environmental standards. For instance, the basic standards in the CAA are the National Ambient Air Quality

[h]See, for instance, the policy statements set forth in TSCA, 15 U.S.C. §§2601 (b).

Standards (NAAQS). The criterion the CAA establishes for the EPA to use in promulgating primary NAAQS is nothing more or less than the protection of public health, with an adequate margin of safety (23). In establishing these standards, the EPA looks to observed effects of pollution on the most sensitive portion of the population, unusually the very young and the very old and those who suffer from pulmonary problems (24). The EPA does have authority to promulgate secondary standards to protect public welfare (25), but it has promulgated the same standards as primary and secondary NAAQS for all but one pollutant (26).

This emphasis on the protection of human health in standard setting pervades environmental law. It is sometimes tempered by other considerations. Pesticides, for instance, are to be registered for the uses requested by their manufacturers unless they pose "an unreasonable risk to man or the environment, taking into account the economic, social, and environmental benefits of the use of the pesticide" (27). And the TSCA authorizes regulation of chemicals that pose an "unreasonable risk" of injury to health or the environment (28).

In addition to establishing environmental standards at levels that protect health, most of the statutes follow the lead of the CAA in authorizing the EPA to seek injunctive relief from the courts when pollution presents an imminent and substantial endangerment to health, whether or not the statute is being violated (29,30). As interpreted by both the EPA and the courts, dangers need be neither close at hand nor life threatening to justify judicial relief (31). The objective of addressing endangerment to health from the release of hazardous substances into the environment from wastes disposed of long ago is the cornerstone of the Superfund environmental cleanup program.

Establishing environmental standards to protect health requires predicting what health effects will result from exposure to different levels of a pollutant. We are not able to do this for many pollutants because experimentation with humans is not feasible and because epidemiologic data are scarce and often inconclusive. Consequently, the EPA and its sister agencies have developed a risk assessment process to predict the increased incidence of cancers that would result from exposure to different levels of a pollutant in the environment (32). Risk assessment is a two-step process. The first step is to determine the possible size of the population exposed to the pollutant, the possible routes or methods of exposure, and the possible level of exposure. The second step is to determine how many excess cancers may be caused by the hypothesized exposure. Few of these factors are known with any certainty, and assumptions must be made throughout the process. Each assumption is made conservatively, assuming the worst. For instance, in the case of contaminated soil, it might be assumed that children would swallow it at a rate of six tablespoons a day, each day, for 70 years. The cumulative multiplication of such conservative assumptions results in overpredicting risk.

The method used in the risk assessment process to determine carcinogenicity has drawn the most fire, probably because it is employed in contexts far beyond setting environmental standards, such as regulating food additives under the Federal Food, Drug, and Cosmetic Act and establishing safe worker exposure levels under the OHSA act. This method exposes experimental animals to several different concentrations of the pollutant of concern under controlled conditions to determine at which concentration, if any, the toxicant will produce cancer. A control group, which is not exposed to the pollutant, is maintained to ensure that cancers in the exposed animals can be attributed to the pollutant. Assuming the exposure at one or more concentrations is found to induce cancer, the results are extrapolated to humans using one of several mathematical models.

While the method is far from satisfactory, it is the best that has been available. It is time-consuming and expensive, often taking 2 or 3 years and costing in excess of a million dollars to test one pollutant. Small irregularities in handling the experimental animals can invalidate the results. Indeed, irregularities at a leading testing laboratory cast doubt on regulatory clearances for hundreds of products that were based on studies it had conducted.[i] Perhaps the greatest controversy surrounding the method in the regulatory context arises because exposing experimental animals to pollutants in the very low range to which humans are exposed to them (parts per million or billion, or even less) usually does not produce observable cancers during the animals' short lives. Consequently the animals are exposed to very high concentrations of the pollutants, often to as much as they can tolerate without experiencing mortality from causes other than cancer. While the results may demonstrate animal carcinogenicity at extremely high dose levels, extrapolating that to predict human carcinogenicity at extremely low dose levels is open to doubt. Indeed, some investigators doubt that the results have any predictive value. The impossibility of determining cancer rates in experimental animals at the extremely low dose levels to which humans are normally exposed makes it impossible to determine whether there are threshold exposures below which cancer is not induced. The EPA bridges this gap by a policy assumption that there are not threshold exposures for carcinogens: any exposure may result in a cancer. Moreover, the method does not utilize recent advances in the understanding of carcinogenesis, such as the role of chemicals as inducers or promoters. While

[i]The registrations of 200 pesticides were thrown into doubt because they were supported by tests done by Industrial Biotest (IBT), after IBT was found to have routinely conducted spurious tests and to have produced falsified data. Four company executives ultimately were jailed. See Bosso CJ, ed. *Pesticides and Politics*. Pittsburgh: University of Pittsburgh Press, 1987; 199–200.

this method appears to be overpredictive, it assesses risk for only one carcinogen at a time and fails to take into account the cumulative or possibly synergistic effects of the multitude of carcinogens to which most of us are exposed on a continual basis.

### *The Road from Protecting Ecosystems to Protecting Public Health*

If ecosystem protection is the natural province of environmental law, how was it diverted to the protection of public health? The journey was directed in part by historical developments and in part by political imperative. Prior to the creation of the EPA, most of the environmental statutes were products of traditional natural resource management concerns. Water pollution abatement, for instance, was entrusted to the Department of Interior and its counterpart state agencies, and it focused on protection of fish and other aquatic life. Pesticide regulation was entrusted to the Department of Agriculture and its state counterparts, and it focused on the promotion of agricultural production. Both programs were yanked out of torpor by environmental crises. The Cuyahoga River in Cleveland, Ohio, became so polluted that it reportedly caught fire and eventually burned a fireboat sent to extinguish the flames. Of greater ecologic significance was the choking of Lake Erie at the same time by alga blooms 40 miles long, nourished by organic pollutants, nitrogen and phosphorus from surrounding farms and municipal wastewater. Expert predictions of the death of the lake and media pictures of the burning river prompted passage of the modern version of the CWA and the transfer of its administration to the new EPA. Rachel Carson's *Silent Spring* and the tailspin in the bald eagle population, whose eggs were made so brittle by DDT that they broke when the parent eagles roosted on them, prompted the overhaul and updating of the pesticide laws to protect the environment as well as farmers and transferring their administration to the EPA. Of course, DDT had accumulated in human fatty tissue as well and was often found in human milk, raising initial concerns over the effects of pesticides on human health.

The focus of earlier environmental law on the well-being of the nonhuman population was a logical outgrowth of the natural resource conservation roots and composition of the environmental advocacy groups. The largest membership groups, the Sierra Club, the Natural Wildlife Federation, and the Audubon Society, were composed largely of those whose interests centered on preservation of natural areas for recreational use: as breeding grounds for birds, fish, and other game; for camping and wilderness travel; or just to be there. Some of these concerns were aesthetic and had an element of elitism about them, particularly when it came to preservation of resources for economically unproductive purposes. The Wilderness Act, for instance, was opposed as being antidemocratic, setting aside significant parts of the nation's land mass and resources for the few with the economic means and leisure time to get to them.[j] Since most of the areas accorded wilderness protection were located far from urban areas, they were indeed remote from the concerns of most voters. The recession and Arab oil embargo of the 1970s put environmentalists on the defensive. To be politically salable, environmental initiatives needed a more compelling focus.

Air pollution control was the major exception to this pattern. Concern with air pollution as a matter for government regulation grew out of an incident in Donora, Pennsylvania, in which 20 people died in 1948 from severe air pollution from steel mills during a protracted temperature inversion. This concern was increased by recognition of the adverse health impact of soot-laden London fog, which during the famous "killer smog" episode of 1952 was thought to be responsible for some 1,600 additional deaths from pulmonary causes. Prior to the creation of the EPA, the federal air pollution program was vested in the Public Health Service, a part of the then Department of Health, Education, and Welfare. At the state level it was typically a part of a department of public health. From the beginning of regulation, air pollution standards have been established to protect public health.

Most environmental legislation since the mid-1970s has been driven by concern over human exposure to toxic chemicals in the environment and has focused on that exposure. This coincided with two scientific developments that made it possible. The first was recognition of the importance of cancer as a cause of human deaths and a growing, though still far from complete, understanding of the mechanics of cancer. This included an appreciation of the role that toxic chemicals could play in the causing and promoting cancer. The second was a rapid development in chemical analytic instrumentation. As late as the 1960s chemicals in the environment could often be detected and measured only in parts per million at best. The 1970s saw the development and widespread dissemination of instrumentation that made possible the detection of most chemical substances present in the environment in concentrations of parts per billion or even smaller concentrations. This suddenly enabled the detection and measurement of a legion of carcinogens or suspected carcinogens in water, food, and other matter to which we are commonly exposed (33).

This set the stage for exploiting fear of cancer from exposure to chemicals in the environment as a stalking-horse to seek the enactment of a wide range of environmental legislation. Thus TSCA was enacted in reaction to discovery that polychlorinated biphenyls (PCBs) were ubiquitous in the environment, leading to the closure of the Hudson River fisheries, among other consequences. The Safe Drinking Water Act (SDWA) was enacted after the new analytical technology made possible a study demon-

[j]Senator Barry Goldwater was a vehement foe of the legislation on this ground.

strating the presence of hundreds of toxic chemicals in low concentrations in public water supply intakes on the Ohio, Mississippi, and other large rivers. The RCRA was enacted specifically to protect the public from exposure to toxic chemicals in the environment. The Superfund was enacted in reaction to Love Canal and similar incidents in which public exposure to chemicals disposed of earlier was thought to pose a pervasive public health problem.

This directed the development, growth, and emphasis of environmental law toward environmental problems that could also be characterized as public health problems, particularly as carcinogenic health problems. Emblematic of this trend was the decision of the EPA in the late 1970s to cease seeking funding from Congress to implement the Noise Control Act (34) because noise was perceived to be more of a nuisance than a real public health problem. While studies demonstrated mental health impacts from noise, they were not carcinogenic and therefore somehow less important.

Of course, more typical environmental conservation concerns continued to surface and to be reflected in legislative action. Concern with the preservation of scenic vistas by the Sierra Club, for instance, prompted litigation, and later legislation, to prevent air in relatively pristine areas from significant degradation and to protect vistas in and from national parks and monuments from being befouled by air pollution (35). Recent legislation aimed at acid rain control is rooted in concerns for the effect of acid deposition on the aquatic biota and forests. Of course, the air pollution giving rise to both of these concerns may also have public health consequences.

The next probable focus of significant legislation, global warming, has both environmental and public health aspects (36). There seems little doubt that the effects of increased emissions of carbon dioxide from fossil fuel combustion (mostly from energy generation and transportation) will culminate in the so-called greenhouse effect, which in turn could result in gradual warming of the Earth's atmosphere, with all the consequences that will entail. While increased carbon dioxide emissions have no apparent direct health effects, increased emissions of other greenhouse gases may. Moreover, the secondary effects of desertification, flooding, and decreases in arable land could have significant, even catastrophic, health effects. Global warming is a classical ecological problem. Change one variable (carbon dioxide) in a complex and not well understood ecosystem and unforeseen consequences are likely to follow. Some of those consequences, such as increased cloud cover, could even prevent or delay a temperature increase.

### *Costs, Priorities, and Regulatory Reform*

Pollution control is not cheap. The United States spends about 2% of its gross national product on environmental protection. It could easily spend more, but there are, and always will be, limits on how much people are willing to spend on this or any other public benefit. Some environmentalists assume that as long as government itself does not foot the bill, the opportunities for requiring industry to do so are virtually limitless. After all, shouldn't the polluter pay? This overlooks two factors. First, we all are polluters, not just industry. Having industry bear the cost of controlling industrial pollution may do little or nothing to clean up the municipal landfill or sewage treatment plant. Second, even for industrial pollution, the public ultimately pays the bill for both the consequences of pollution and for its control. For instance, if hospitals dispose of their wastes in an uncontrolled manner, the public exposed to the wastes absorbs the cost in adverse health and other impacts. When the hospitals are required to dispose of their wastes in a controlled manner at a higher cost, the public absorbs the higher cost in higher bills for medical services and insurance.

If the amount we are willing to spend on environmental control is limited, which it always is, then it would be prudent public policy to spend those limited funds to secure the greatest environmental benefits. This suggests two primary foci in determining where and how to spend limited resources. The first focus is on priorities. If we can't do everything, or do everything at once, then what should we do, or do first? All other things being equal (which they seldom are) our priority should be to address the problems that cause the greatest adverse impacts. The second focus is on efficiency. If we can't do everything or do everything at once, what remedial alternatives should we choose for the problems we address? All other things being equal, our choices should be the most efficient ones available, because they leave the most funds available to address other environmental concerns.

We don't either prioritize or make efficient choices very well. Most of the blame for this can be attributed to the single-focus, crisis-driven nature of environmental legislation. Congress tells the EPA and the states to abate air pollution, control water pollution, provide safe drinking water, review all new chemicals, assure the efficacy and safety of all pesticides, stop disposal of most hazardous waste on land, cleanup contamination from uncontrolled waste disposal from the past, etc., all without establishing priorities between these various tasks. While prioritization among them occurs of necessity during annual budget allocations, those allocations are not accomplished by any measured comparison of the benefits to be achieved from expenditures for the different programs. Indeed, the allocation that does take place often is driven by court orders secured by environmental groups suing the EPA for not accomplishing a congressionally mandated aspect of one of the programs. Even within a single program, choices between subprogram elements are seldom made by a measured comparison of the benefits to be achieved by each subprogram.

This difficulty in prioritization is driven directly by Congress. Congress mandates EPA action under dozens of statutes but does not authorize it to prioritize among those actions. And Congress mandates what the EPA addresses within each environmental sector, often with no weighing of the importance of adverse consequence of different environmental problems within each sector. The CAA, for instance, does not authorize the EPA to regulate the air pollution most responsible for lung cancer—indoor pollution from tobacco smoke, radon, and other pollutants (37). The CAA authorizes the EPA to regulate only pollution of the outdoor air. This keeps it focused on emissions from industrial and other large pollution sources and away from the emissions from everyday living, a politically easy focus for both Congress and the EPA. To be sure, the sulfur oxide, particulate, and ozone-causing pollutants to which the CAA and EPA devote most of their attention are ubiquitous in the outdoor environment and do cause adverse health effects. Moreover, public exposure to them is involuntary and largely unavoidable. But neither Congress nor the EPA have calculated the comparative health benefits from spending all or part of the billions of dollars a year we now spend on outdoor air pollution control on indoor air pollution control instead.

Even with the outdoor air pollutants the CAA does address, the CAA does not establish priorities. It places the same emphasis on controlling emissions of a handful of so-called criteria pollutants, e.g., sulfur dioxide, particulates, and ozone-causing pollutants, as it does on controlling emissions of 189 so-called toxic pollutants, e.g., ethylene dibromide and quinoline. This ignores the fact that the entire population is exposed to the criteria pollutants, often in concentrations that pose adverse health effects, while there may be only a handful of people exposed to a toxic pollutant. Indeed, the greatest health effects of toxic pollutants are in the workplaces in which they are used or emitted, but the CAA authorizes control only to protect people beyond the fence line.

The difficulty of making efficient choices between pollution control alternatives can also be attributed to Congress. It typically directed the EPA to promulgate standards for pollution control that protect public health or require the best control technology, with little or no regard to cost. The CAA, for instance, directs that air pollution standards are to be established at levels that are protective of public health, with an adequate margin of safety, and makes no mention of costs as a consideration (38). While the CWA directed the EPA to establish initial standards for industrial treatment of waste that considered the costs of the treatment in relation to the pollution reduction benefits achieved, it required the EPA to establish subsequent standards considering costs in an unspecified manner as one of many factors (39).

The call for regulatory reform had developed in reaction to the high costs of environmental protection. Regulatory reform is nothing new, but has been with environmental protection since it began to impose meaningful resource demands and management constraints. Until recently regulatory reform measures have resulted primarily from initiatives by the Office of Management and Budget focusing on the cost/benefit and cost/efficiency of alternatives for particular regulatory measures. More recently Congress has entered the fray, undertaking modest measures at establishing priorities and imposing more ambitious procedures on administrative agencies to promote more cost-effective regulatory choices. The latter is an especially attractive political path for Congress, for it forces the EPA, not Congress, to make all the hard choices.

The first steps by Congress toward establishing priorities focused solely on the timing of regulatory standards rather than on a choice between alternative regulatory standards. But at least Congress began to recognize that everything could not be done at once. Examples of this are in the CAA amendments of 1990, in which Congress established a schedule for the EPA to promulgate toxic air pollution standards for 189 pollutants, allowing the EPA to promulgate them in several groups over 10 years and to determine which air pollutants to consider at each stage in the schedule (40). This was modeled after a similar provision in the RCRA amendments of 1984.[k] Recently, Congress has given the EPA more discretion in determining the pollutants for which it will promulgate standards. For instance, in 1996 Congress amended the SDWA to require the EPA every 5 years to review five contaminants found in public water supplies to determine whether maximum contaminant levels (MCLs) should be established for them (41). This replaced a scheme under which the EPA was to establish MCLs for 25 new pollutants every 3 years, essentially setting in motion an almost endless progression of standards, with little or no regard to how much any standard was needed, by a comparative or any other measure.

Since the beginning of serious environmental regulation in the early 1970s, the White House Office of Management and Budget (OMB) has been leery of the impact of environmental protection on both the federal budget and the economy as a whole. Indeed, President Nixon vetoed the CWA in 1972 because of his belief that federal payments for the construction of local sewage treatment plants was a "budget buster." His veto was handily overridden by Congress. Ironically, he will be remembered in history in part because he presided over the birth of modern environmental protection. Not long after, the Nixon/Ford OMB began a focused review of costs and constraints of environmental and social welfare regulations proposed by the EPA and its sister

[k]There Congress enacted a phased schedule for the EPA to determine how and whether hazardous wastes could be disposed in on land based treatment and disposal facilities, 42 §U.S.C. 6924 (d) to (g) (1994).

agencies. This was formalized in a series of executive orders,[l] requiring federal agencies proposing and promulgating regulations to develop regulatory impact analyses. Those analyses were to determine the costs and benefits of proposed regulations and to consider alternative approaches to the regulations and differences in the costs and benefits of the various approaches. The executive orders also required the agencies to consult with the OMB and secure its approval of the proposal and promulgation of major regulations not otherwise exempted from such review.

Congress did not use a consistent approach to the role that cost or cost/benefit analysis played in establishing environmental standards. It usually avoided consideration of the issue for standards determining how clean the environment should be, but often considered it to varying degrees in determining how much pollution control would be required of individual sources of pollution.[m] Recently, it has become more willing to assign a greater role for cost in determining the levels at which environmental standards should be established. For example, in the 1996 SDWA amendments discussed above, Congress required the EPA to determine if the benefits of a proposed MCL justify its costs and, if not, to establish the MCL at a level for which its benefits do justify its costs.

As Congress became interested in regulatory reform, however, it began to explore generic approaches much like those already imposed by the executive orders discussed above. When the Republicans recaptured Congress in 1994, regulatory reform was one of their major rallying cries. Indeed, regulatory reform was one of the ten major reforms in the Contract with America that the House Republicans attempted to enact. The proposed legislation started with the models of the executive orders, but pushed further, requiring that the costs of regulations bear a reasonable relation to their benefits. While the executive orders did not require regulations to be cost-effective if the existing legislation authorizing the regulations required protection without regard to cost, the proposed legislation would have amended the existing legislation to require that cost be taken into account. While the executive orders did not allow the courts to overturn regulations because they did not comport with the orders, the proposed legislation would have required them to overturn regulations not in compliance with it. Most importantly, the proposed legislation would have required the establishment of a risk assessment procedure that is less prone to overprediction. Finally, the proposed legislation would have increased the opportunity for the subjects of federal enforcement actions to recover their attorneys' fees when the governmental actions were ill-founded.

The focus on risk analysis in the proposed regulatory reform legislation is also reflected in a greater willingness by Congress to deal with the issue in existing legislation. For example, in 1996 it amended the Food, Drug, and Cosmetic Act (42) to replace a prohibition against the presence of any carcinogenic pesticide residue in processed food with a prohibition against more than a negligible amount of such pesticide residue, the same measure it had applied and continues to apply for pesticide residue in raw food (43). This amendment followed the recommendations of a study by the National Academy of Sciences (33). The study concluded that there was no justification for banning carcinogenic pesticide residues in minute quantities in canned tomato paste but not on raw tomatoes, and that the risk posed by such residues might be small in comparison to their public health benefits.

The regulatory reform legislation of the 104th Congress was not enacted, in large part because of public reaction to the negative effects of the proposed legislation on environmental protection. Other aspects of the Contract with America affecting environmental regulation were enacted. An example was the so-called unfunded-mandate legislation creating a point of order barring consideration on the floor of either chamber of Congress a bill that would mandate state or local action without the federal funds to finance it (44).

Despite the failure of regulatory reform legislation in the 104th Congress, pressure for regulatory reform will continue and will be felt in many ways. The OMB will continue to promote cost-effective regulation within the executive branch. And there will continue to be legislative proposals for more extensive cost-effectiveness requirements and overhaul of the risk assessment process. Moreover, Congress will continue to address the most imbalanced emphasis of public health over costs as it revisits each of the environmental statutes on a periodic basis, as it has just done with the SDWA.

## INDIVIDUAL STATUTES

Having seen something of the origins of environmental law and the interplay between that law and health policy in a general way, we turn to a discussion of the major environmental statutes. The discussion is necessarily a very rudimentary one. The leading treatise on the subject surveys the statutes in two volumes, and barely scratches the surface.[n] In this review, priority is given to environmental programs that have a health impact and that may provide information relevant to health professionals.

[l]President Regan's Executive Order 12,291, 46 Fed. Reg. 13,193 (1981), 3 CFR 123 (1982), is probably the most expansive of these orders. President Clinton's version, Executive Order 12,866, 58 Fed. Reg. 51,735, 3 CFR 638 (1994), retreats from OMB's tight lock on the regulation issuing agencies.

[m]Thus the CWA does not require any economic consideration in establishing water quality standards to be achieved in surface water, 33 U.S.C. §1313 and 1314 (a), but does in establishing standards for treating contaminated water by pollution sources, 33 U.S.C. §1314 (b).

[n]Novak R. *Law of Environmental Protection.* New York: Clark Boardman, 1987. See also Cooke SM, *The Land of Hazardous Waste,* New York: Matthew Bender, 1997; Grad F. *Treatise on Environmental Law,* New York: Matthew Bender, 1997; Rogers W. *Environmental Law,* St. Paul, MN: West Publishing Co., 1997; and Stever D. *Law of Chemical Regulation and Hazardous Waste.* New York; Clark Boardman, 1996 (updated annually).

## National Environmental Policy Act

The National Environmental Policy Act (NEPA) was enacted in 1969, on the heels of the first Earth Day, which sent millions to the streets to demonstrate for a better environment. In a way NEPA was a cheap response, for it required no action beyond considering environmental consequences when the government undertook new actions. But in another way, NEPA was a profound response, in that it focused the government's attention on environmental consequences and in some respects altered the way the government does business. The concepts pioneered by the act have been adopted widely, by many states and throughout the world.

NEPA's requirement is simple: no new major federal action significantly affecting the environmental may proceed without assessing the environmental consequences and the comparative environmental consequences of alternatives to the proposed action (45). Environmental consequences include effects on human health and safety. The act establishes a process by which the assessment takes place: the development of an environmental impact statement. The process involves participation and review at all levels of government and allows participation by interested public groups. The assessment is to be part of the decision-making process by the government entity that decides on the proposed action.

NEPA does not require federal agencies to make environmentally sound decisions or to avoid environmentally detrimental actions. As long as the agency complies with the process requirements and produces a viable impact assessment, it may proceed with the proposed action as it likes (46). The process, however, allows all interested parties to have their say and affords them time to effectively mobilize their political forces. Anyone who attempts to avoid or short-circuit the process may be stopped by a lawsuit commenced by concerned citizens, giving them additional time, and ammunition, to kill a project politically.

NEPA offers health professionals the opportunity to make sure the health consequences of proposed actions are recognized before the actions are taken, and to participate in the assessment of those consequences. It is not likely to produce any original research on health issues. An environmental impact statement may be a good starting point for understanding a completed project that is thought to be having adverse health effects. On the other hand, NEPA can stall projects advocated by health professionals while the assessment process is completed, educating opponents and offering them time and opportunities to mobilize whatever political forces they can muster.

## Clean Air Act

In its modern incarnation the CAA dates from 1970, when it supplanted an ineffectual and unsophisticated first-generation attempt to deal with air pollution. As presently constituted, after all of its amendments, the act consists of five basic programs: (a) the underlying program designed to achieve health-based ambient air quality standards; (b) programs dealing with new sources of pollution; (c) a program dealing with toxic emissions that begins with technology-based requirements and supplements them, where necessary, with health-based requirements; (d) an acid rain program aimed primarily at Midwestern coal-burning power plants; and (e) programs for controlling emissions from motor vehicles. In a sense, all of the programs are related, and in many ways the last four programs are subsidiary to the first.

### *NAAQSs and State Implementation Plans*

The basic program requires the EPA to establish national ambient air quality standards (NAAQSs) for pollutants widely present in the air, at levels sufficient to protect public health, with an adequate margin of safety (47). The EPA interprets "adequate margin of safety" to require that NAAQSs be set at levels that provide absolute health protection to the most sensitive part of the population. If an NAAQS were being established for a carcinogen, this interpretation, coupled with the EPA's no-threshold assumption for carcinogenesis, would mean the NAAQSs would have to be set at zero.

After NAAQSs are promulgated, the states are to develop state implementation plans (SIPs) to achieve the NAAQSs (48). SIPs are state statutes, regulations, and even permits designed to reduce emissions from sources in the state sufficient to achieve and maintain the NAAQSs. The SIPs are forwarded to the EPA for approval as sufficient to achieve the NAAQSs. The EPA is supposed to promulgate a SIP for an area where a state does not itself develop an approvable SIP. The EPA has been reluctant to do so, however. The local focus of the SIPs and EPA's deference to the states developing them has allowed deterioration in regional air quality from long-range transport of pollutants, even while they have brought about improvements in air quality from locally generated pollutants.[o] The EPA has promulgated NAAQSs for six common pollutants: particulate matter, sulfur oxides, carbon monoxide, ozone, nitrogen dioxide, and lead (49). Its Office of Air Planning and Standards, in Research Triangle Park, North Carolina, keeps an up-to-date inventory of studies on health effects from these air pollutants and others.

### *New Source Requirements*

The EPA is required to promulgate standards for new stationary sources of air pollution (as opposed to mobile sources such as vehicles), establishing for each category

[o]See generally Conservation Foundation. *State of the Environment,* supra, pp. 54–88.

of sources the best technologic system of continuous emissions reduction, considering cost, non-air health and environmental impact, and energy requirements (50). It has done so for more than 60 categories of sources, such as coal-fired power plants, cement plants, and municipal incinerators. When this requirement was added in 1970 it was thought that the new source requirements would be the driving force for clean air, as replacement of the industrial infrastructure resulted in the construction of cleaner facilities. This has not occurred, in part because the EPA has not always been aggressive in establishing stringent new source requirements, and because where the EPA has established more stringent standards for new sources than for existing ones, modernization has been discouraged.

Larger new air pollution sources may be subject to a variety of other requirements, depending on whether they are located in areas that have attained the NAAQS or in ones that have yet to attain it (51). They include theoretically more stringent technology-based requirements, and in the case of new sources in areas that have not yet attained the NAAQS, requirements to reduce emissions from other sources in the area by more than the amount of the emissions that will result from the new source. These offsets allow new development (and new air pollution) to proceed no matter how polluted an area is, but ensure that air quality will improve even thought new sources of pollution are constructed. The reviews that take place when permits are issued for these new sources are also intended to enhance attainment of the NAAQS elsewhere as a result of emissions from the new sources. These measures to prevent adverse effects from long-range transport have been singularly unsuccessful in the past, largely because the EPA has lacked the political will to implement them strictly. They were strengthened by the 1990 amendments, one hopes to the point where they will prove effective.

### *Air Toxics*

The 1970 CAA also included a provision for the EPA to promulgate standards for emissions of hazardous air pollutants from different categories of sources, to protect public health. Both these standards and NAAQSs were calculated to protect public health with an ample margin of safety. But NAAQSs are ambient standards, to be achieved in the air we breathe by emission requirements imposed on air pollution sources in SIPs. The hazardous standards, by contrast, are applicable directly to air pollution sources, without implementation through SIPs. NAAQS are to be developed for ubiquitous pollutants, hazardous standards for local pollutants. Every time a NAAQS is promulgated for a new pollutant, all states must promulgate SIPs to either attain or maintain the NAAQS. To do this in all states for a hazardous pollutant emitted in only a few would be a wasteful exercise, hence the different implemented mechanisms.

In the 20 years following the enactment of this provision, the EPA promulgated emission standards for only seven hazardous pollutants: mercury, beryllium, asbestos, vinyl chloride, benzene, arsenic, and radionuclides (52). Three factors stymied the EPA from proceeding further: (a) the requirement that the standard protect health with an ample margin of safety, (b) the application of the standards at the smokestack, and (c) the EPA's cancer policy. The EPA had already interpreted protection of health with an ample margin of safety to require absolute protection for the most sensitive population, when applying the same concept in the context of NAAQS. For carcinogens, absolute safety would require zero discharge, as a consequence of the EPA's assumption that there is no safe threshold for carcinogens. Because pollution control rarely eliminates all of a target pollutant, a zero emissions requirement would likely cause any industry subject to it to close and move to a country with less stringent standards. The EPA's reaction was paralysis.[p]

Judicial review of the standard the EPA set for vinyl chloride reversed the EPA's absolutist reading of the "margin of safety" requirement in 1987, giving some hope that the EPA could escape from its paralysis (53). But before this possibility was tested, reacting both to demands by environmentalists that the EPA was doing nothing in the face of the "air toxics" crisis and to the EPA's lament that the 1970 standard-setting criteria were impractical, Congress changed the program. To appease the environmentalists, it mandated that the EPA set standards on 189 specified chemicals over a 10-year schedule (54). To enable the EPA to do so without shutting down American industry, the standards are to require the maximum degree of emission reduction achievable, taking cost and other factors into account. Resort to a technology-based standard rather than a health-based one rescues the EPA from its earlier dilemma. But 8 years after each standard is promulgated, the EPA is to determine whether a health risk remains from the pollutants still being emitted. If so, it is to promulgate a second standard to protect public health, with an ample margin of safety, taking cost and other factors into account. Unless the EPA changes its cancer policy, it will be forced into this second round of standard setting for carcinogens, but costs and other factors may allow it to retreat from a zero emissions standard. In the meantime, the EPA is to report to Congress on methods of determining the risk remaining, to assess the significance of the risk, and to recommend legislative adjustments. The EPA is to develop this report in a public process, inviting participation from interested parties.

The new measure continues the trend of environmental legislation, to require possibly huge expenditures in the name of public health protection with no regard to the seriousness of the perceived health problem and with no

[p]Rogers W. *Environmental Law;* supra, §3 20

regard to the value of the health benefits that derive from the measures required. It exacerbates this trend by imposing these standards for a large number of pollutants over a set period and then potentially requiring a second, more protective standard thereafter. It softens the measure somewhat by allowing costs and other factors to be taken into account. Perhaps more significantly, it invites the EPA to reexamine the viability of this whole approach and the significance of the health impact at issue and to suggest corrective measures.

Of significance to health professionals is the health effects information, which the EPA has collected on the seven pollutants for which it promulgated hazardous emission standards under the old scheme and which it will collect on 189 pollutants under the new scheme (though not in a systematic way until the end of the 1990s). The responsible office, again, is the Office of Air Planning and Standards, in Research Triangle Park, North Carolina.

### *Acid Rain*

For reasons already discussed, the former NAAQS and SIP processes did not control long-range transport of pollutants, and in some ways encouraged it. As a result, uncontrolled or partially uncontrolled coal-burning power plants in the Midwest emitted millions of tons of sulfur oxides a year, many of which landed in the Northeast and Canada in the form of acid rain or dry deposits that ultimately have the same effect. To address this problem Congress required that national sulfur oxide emissions be reduced by 10 million tons over a 10-year period, from their high of 20 million tons a year in 1980 (55). It did so by specifying exactly how many tons each of 120 Midwestern power plants is allowed to emit. The EPA is supposed to issue "allowances" to each plant for its requisite number of tons. Plants are allowed to buy and sell these allowances, the net effect being that the 10 million ton reduction theoretically will be achieved by the plants for which it is cheapest to control emissions. In essence, other plants may purchase "overcontrol" from plants that can control cheaply. Nitrogen dioxide emissions are to be reduced by 2 million tons a year in a similar scheme.

### *Motor Vehicle Emissions*

Motor vehicles emit significant or even preponderant percentages of several of the pollutants—ozone, carbon monoxide, nitrogen dioxide, and lead—for which NAAQSs have been promulgated. These NAAQSs cannot be achieved in urban areas without significant controls on motor vehicle emissions. Yet few states have the capacity to regulate them, and the automobile manufacturers understandably prefer one regulator to 50. As a result, emission standards for motor vehicles are established either by Congress itself in the CAA, or by the EPA for vehicles Congress has not regulated (56). Because California regulated automobile emissions before the federal government did and because it has the worst smog problem in the country, it has always been allowed to establish emission standards that are more stringent than the federal ones. Other states that do not meet the ozone NAAQSs have been allowed to adopt the California standards, but none has.

Automobile manufacturers chose to meet early emission standards by using catalytic converters, which were inactivated by lead. Hence Congress authorized the EPA to regulate fuel additives, and the EPA initiated phasing out of lead in gasoline, which was supported and strengthened by the promulgation (as a result of a lawsuit by an environmental group) of the lead NAAQS (57).

The federal emission standards focused on motor vehicles at the manufacturing stage, but the fact that an automobile comes off the line with adequate emission controls is no guarantee that the control device will perform well in use. That may require good maintenance, avoidance of leaded fuel, or other measures; hence the importance of emissions inspections, which are required in SIPs of states that do not meet the NAAQS for ozone. Even with all these programs in place there are at least 40 urban areas in the country that do not meet the ozone NAAQS. The SIPs for these areas must contain a variety of measures to further reduce ozone-producing emissions, from providing enhanced emissions inspection programs to requiring fleets to operate non–gasoline-powered vehicles (58).

### *Other*

The CAA has been difficult to enforce in many instances because of difficulties both in determining what requirements apply to a particular source and whether the source is in compliance with the requirements. The difficulty in determining what requirements apply to a given source stems from the facts that states are constantly amending SIPs and providing variances to individual sources, and that none of these actions is effective at the federal level unless and until approved by the EPA. The SIPs are constantly in flux. In addition, a source may be subject to requirements from SIPs developed for different pollutants and to requirements from other parts of the CAA, such as new source requirements. The difficulty in determining compliance stems from the fact that, for many sources, until recently the chief method for determining compliance was a stack test. These are cumbersome, rather expensive measurements that cannot be done on a surprise basis or continuously. Surrogate compliance tests were often only approximations.

The 1990 amendments and scientific advance have dealt with these problems. In the future, all air pollution requirements applicable to a source must be set forth in a single permit, and the permit must require the source to periodically test its compliance and report the results to the government. In the meantime, in-stack monitoring devices have been developed to measure many stack gases, and a laser-based remote sensor has been developed that enables inspectors to determine compliance from off the premises. Violations of the CAA are subject to a full range of civil and criminal sanctions and are subject to enforcement by citizens.

### *Clean Water Act*

The CWA was grafted onto an older, ineffective program in 1972. It regulates pollutants discharged to surface waters through "point sources"—pipes, ditches, fissures, and other discrete conveyances (59). Pollution sources are required to treat their wastes to meet the most stringent of two sets of requirements, based on either technologic feasibility or attainment of desired levels of water quality.

About half the pollution load from these sources comes from municipally operated sewage treatment plants. They are subject to a set of technology-based standards that, roughly, require at least 85% removal of organic and solid matter as well as chlorination and other controls. Industries that discharge wastes to the public treatment plants are required to install the best available treatment for removal of toxic pollutants and are prohibited from discharging wastes that will interfere with or pass through the public treatment works and cause them to violate their permits.

Industries that discharge directly into surface waters are subject to several levels of technology-based requirements, the most stringent of which is the best available treatment for toxic pollutants. Toxic pollutants under the CWA are pollutants that are toxic to parts of the biota, although they may very well be harmful to humans as well. Best available treatment normally requires removal in excess of 85%, often in excess of 99% of regulated pollutants, and may even require cessation of the discharge. Technology-based standards are established by the EPA in regulations for whole industries, broken down into subcategories of industries that produce similar wastes from similar processes. For instance, the pulp and paper industry is regulated as 25 different subcategories (e.g., the tissue from wastepaper subcategory) (60). The translation of these industrial subcategory standards to discharge limitations for an individual factory is accomplished fairly easily in a permit.

The process of deriving treatment requirements to attain given water quality is a more complicated four-step process (61). First, the state establishes the desired highest use for a surface water (e.g., drinking water without treatment or warm-water fish propagation). Uses that devote water to waste disposal are no longer allowed. Second, the state adopts scientific criteria for water quality to support the designated use (e.g., at least 5.0 ppm dissolved oxygen or no more than 0.05 ppm chromium). Criteria have been developed by the EPA based on the scientific literature and some experimentation of its own. Although the EPA's criteria have not been adopted in formal rules, the EPA has been successful in persuading states to adopt them. Third, the state must determine how much of a pollutant may be discharged into a body of water without violating the criteria (e.g., 5 pounds of chromium a day may be discharged without exceeding the 0.05 ppm criterion). This is known as a maximum daily loading and is developed from field data. Its size clearly depends on the volume of the receiving waters, which normally varies substantially over the course of a year. The convention is to calculate the load based on the flow during the lowest flow for 7 consecutive days during a 10-year period. The last step is to determine how much of the pollutant may be discharged by a given point source. That is easy if the criterion is not being exceeded: all sources may continue at their present levels. But if the criterion is being exceeded, the difference between the total daily discharges and the maximum daily loading must be eliminated. This is easy if only one source is discharging the pollutant. But if there are several sources, how should the required reduction be allocated among them? What if the required loading could not be achieved even if all industrial discharge was eliminated? Neither the CWA, the EPA regulations, nor the EPA policy indicate how the difference should be divided between sources that discharge the pollutant. That is left to the state and could easily be a political decision.

Individual discharge limitations are developed for each source in a permit. Permits require sources to test their effluents, often continuously, to determine compliance, and to report the results to the government. These reports are public information and self-reporting of violations can be used by the government and private citizens as proof of violations in enforcement actions.

Most point sources have installed the technology necessary to meet their requirements, and current violations tend to result from faulty operation or maintenance. The EPA's emphasis for new treatment requirements is to achieve water quality criteria in those areas where they have not been met and to ensure that individual discharges do not cause toxicity to target organisms in 96-hour bioassays.

This program has been successful in restoring water quality in areas where industrial and municipal wastes were the chief causes of water pollution. For instance, Atlantic salmon have returned to many of the rivers in the Northeast, where in the early 1970s they spawned only in one small river in Maine. Where other pollution sources such as agriculture or air pollution are significant contributors to water pollution, advances are less discernible.[q]

[q]Conservation Foundation. *State of the Environment,* supra, pp. 82–106.

The CWA has a free-standing program that prohibits spills of oil and hazardous substances into surface waters (62). If such spills occur, the EPA and the Coast Guard may perform cleanup operations and recover their costs from the source of the spill. This program was the model for the Superfund. In addition, tank farms and other facilities that store material that can be spilled into surface waters must develop and implement programs to prevent spills and contain and remove them if they occur. The inadequacy of the response plan during the recent *Exxon Valdez* spill indicates this program has not been enforced vigorously. Remedial oil spill legislation was recently enacted, expanding this program considerably and containing new requirements, such as double hulls for ships that carry oil products.[r]

Information on the pollutants discharged from individual sources is readily available in permit applications in state water pollution offices and in the Water Division in the EPA's 10 regional offices. Information on the effects of pollutants on the biota is available from its Office of Water Regulations and Standards in Washington.

### *Federal Insecticide, Fungicide, and Rodenticide Act*

The Federal Insecticide, Fungicide, and Rodenticide Act (FIFRA) dates back to 1947 legislation designed to ensure the efficacy of products for agricultural customers, predominantly, but not entirely, farmers and other growers. Doctors and hospitals that use germicides were among the beneficiaries of the program. In 1972 Congress substantially amended the earlier effort to focus on health and environment, as well as on efficacy.

The main regulatory tool of FIFRA is the registration of pesticides (63). Registration is both product- and use-specific. To be registered for a particular use the pesticide must (a) be efficacious for that use, (b) carry a label with directions for the use, (c) perform the use without unreasonably adverse effects on health and the environment, and (d) not result in such effects when used in common practice. Because the registration decision turns on whether adverse health and environmental effects from a pesticide are reasonable, FIFRA is a balancing statute. It weighs the usefulness of pesticides against their detrimental effects. Almost by definition they have some adverse effects, but their benefits in providing an abundant food supply, preserving food from decay, or ridding premises of pests may outweigh those effects. Adverse effects may be avoided or minimized by requiring pesticide labels to give directions on how registered uses can be accomplished safely. Pesticides may be registered for general or restricted use. Restricted-use pesticides may be applied only by applicators who are trained and licensed by the state. Recent amendments to FIFRA require previously registered pesticides to be reregistered so that they are reviewed using contemporary data and criteria. Registration may be canceled if data developed subsequent to the registration would justify a decision not to register. Distributing an unregistered pesticide or failing to comply with the directions on the label is a violation of FIFRA.

Pesticides have both active and inert ingredients. These terms must be understood in their pesticide context. A so-called inert ingredient is not really inert; it just is not pesticidal and is used for another purpose, for instance as a carrier. Inert ingredients in pesticides may be as harmful as active ingredients to health and the environment.

The focus of the EPA's registration activities is currently generic reregistration of each active ingredient. Under this approach, the EPA reviews the available data on each chemical used as an active ingredient, identifies data gaps that must be filled, and publishes a generic standard that sets forth the uses for which the ingredient will be authorized. These standards are interim standards, however, to be used until the data gaps are filled. The process will not be completed until after the year 2000. In the meantime, new products are registered on a conditional basis and will be revised after a standard is established for the active ingredient and any data gaps are filled.

The data that the EPA requires for registration include residue chemistry; environmental fate; degradation, metabolism, mobility, dissipation, and accumulation studies; acute, chronic, and subchronic effects on humans and other nontarget species; teratogenicity and mutagenicity studies; and pesticide spray-drift evaluation. Moreover, pesticide registrants have a continuing obligation to provide postregistration data to the EPA whenever the registrant becomes aware of data that suggest adverse effects. This includes incomplete toxicologic studies and individual incident reports.

The EPA has a tremendous bank of information on health effects of registered pesticides. Although much of this is available to the public, the security maintained for business confidential information submitted to the EPA under FIFRA is extraordinarily tight. Indeed, a longer prison term may be imposed for disclosing business confidential FIFRA information than for violating the substantive requirements of FIFRA. This has an inhibiting effect on the EPA personnel who deal with requests for FIFRA information. Nevertheless, most of the health data are publicly available and even confidential information may be released to doctors and others to the extent necessary to treat or prevent illness. The office to contact for such information is the Health Effects Division in the Office of Pesticide Programs in Washington, D.C.

### *Safe Drinking Water Act*

The Safe Drinking Water Act (SDWA) contains two primary related regulatory programs. The first establishes

[r]The Oil Pollution Act, Pub. L 101–380. Aug 18, 1990, 104 Stat 484. Although parts of the new act are freestanding, it also amends the CWA's oil pollution program.

standards to be met by public drinking water sources. The second regulates injection of contaminants into wells. The connecting link is that uncontrolled underground injection may contaminate aquifers that serve as drinking water supplies.

The drinking water regulatory program is designed to ensure that public water supplies meet drinking water standards. Water suppliers that serve as few as 25 people, e.g., a small trailer park, are regulated. Regulated suppliers must treat water to meet drinking water standards at the tap, must test their water for compliance with the standards, must report the test results to the regulatory agencies, and must inform their customers of violations of the standards. Variances and exemptions are available for some sources (64).

Drinking water standards are to be established for contaminants that the EPA believes may have an adverse impact on human health and that are likely to be present in public water supplies. For each such contaminant, the EPA is to establish a maximum contaminant level goal (MCLG) at a level at which no known or anticipated adverse health effects occur. For carcinogens, using the EPA's no-threshold assumption, this is zero. Then the EPA is to establish a maximum contaminant level (MCL) as close to the MCLG as can be justified by weighing the benefits against the costs. The MCLG and the MCL are known as the primary drinking water standards, but public water suppliers need only comply with the MCLs. The EPA is also authorized to promulgate secondary drinking water standards to protect public welfare. The EPA has promulgated standards for turbidity, several radioactive elements, microbial contaminants, and almost 70 organic and inorganic chemicals (65). It is required to review another five contaminants every 5 years to determine whether it should establish standards for them. The EPA also issues health advisories on contaminants not present in enough public water supplies to warrant establishing a standard, but present in enough of them to warrant advising the public on safe levels of the contaminant. These advisories include "suggested no-adverse-response levels" (SNARLs) (66).

The public water supply program has a number of provisions that deal with specific contamination problems. For example, SDWA prohibits using lead in pipes, solder, or flux (67). It also requires states to establish well-head protection programs to protect the aquifers feeding drinking-water well fields from being contaminated by activity on the surface above the wells.

Although SDWA requires the EPA to establish the primary drinking water standards, SDWA contemplates that states assure drinking water suppliers comply with the standards. All but a handful of states do administer the program, making the EPA's role one of an overseer and an enforcer of last resort.

The underground injection program requires owners and operators of wells that will pump material underground to obtain authorization by permit or regulation. The most common types of underground injection are for waste disposal, enhanced recovery of oil and gas, and mining of dissolvable minerals. Permits are issued only if the applicant demonstrates that injection will not result in contamination of underground drinking water sources and that the wells meet technical standards designed to assure they do not leak. The permits require periodic testing of the wells to ensure that they are not leaking. A few wells subject to the program inject hazardous wastes. They are also subject to additional regulatory requirements under RCRA. These programs may be administered by states that meet the requirements established for state administration in SWDA.

### *Toxic Substances Control Act*

The Toxic Substances Control Act (TSCA) was enacted in 1976 on a clean slate. It required the EPA to establish an inventory of chemicals manufactured or processed in the United States (68). Chemicals not on the inventory could not thereafter be manufactured, imported, or processed without premanufacture notification (PMN) of the EPA. Chemicals covered do not include those regulated under FIFRA, the Federal Food, Drug, and Cosmetic Act, or the Atomic Energy Act. Information required in a PMN includes chemical descriptions of the material and its by-products; volume and types of uses expected; manufacturing process and locations; worker and environmental exposure; and health, safety, and environmental fate and effects test data known to the submitter or reported in the literature. The PMN is not required to demonstrate either efficacy or lack of adverse health or environmental effect. The EPA publishes a notice of its receipt of PMNs in the *Federal Register.* If the EPA takes no action for 90 days after the submission (or after an additional 90-day extension that the EPA may grant itself), the chemical is added to the inventory and the submitter is free to manufacture, import, or process it. On the other hand, the EPA can prevent this by order, rule, or court action if it determines that unconditioned manufacture, processing, distribution, use, or disposal of the chemical may present an unreasonable risk of injury to health or the environment or that available data are insufficient for the EPA to determine that the chemical will not pose an unreasonable risk.

For any chemical on the inventory the EPA is authorized to promulgate a regulation requiring manufacturers, importers, or processors of the chemical to perform testing to determine whether it presents an unreasonable risk of injury to health or the environment. If it does, the EPA may also promulgate regulations to prevent the manufacture, processing, distribution, use, or disposal of a chemical from causing such an unreasonable risk. The EPA has used these authorities sparingly. Manufacturers, importers, and processors of a chemical have a continuing obligation to report to the EPA any information that comes to their attention supporting the conclusion that it presents a substantial risk of injury to health or the environment.

In addition to its general regulatory authority, the EPA is charged specifically with responsibility for regulating PCBs, asbestos, and radon (69). The EPA's Health and Environmental Review Division in the Office of Toxic Substances is the repository of information on health effects of chemicals in the inventory and of chemicals under PMN review.

### *Resource Conservation and Recovery Act*

The Resource Conservation and Recovery Act (RCRA) was enacted in 1976, grafted on earlier legislation under which the EPA gave technical assistance to states on solid waste disposal and established guidelines for federal solid waste minimization and disposal programs. RCRA deals both with hazardous and nonhazardous solid wastes. Its main emphasis, however, is on hazardous waste.

RCRA creates a cradle-to-grave regulatory scheme to manage storage, transport, and disposal of hazardous waste, administered by the EPA or by states that have approved programs. Generators of hazardous waste must dispose of it at facilities designated for that particular waste (70). If the permitted disposal site is not located on the generator's facility, the generator must transport the waste to the disposal site, accompanied by a RCRA manifest to document proper disposition (71). If the waste is stored for any appreciable time prior to disposal, the storage facility must have a permit and must meet standards designed to prevent release of waste into the environment. Exacting standards are established in regulations for the common types of storage and disposal facilities: incinerators, landfills, and surface impoundments, among others. These requirements include prohibitions on disposal of particular wastes in particular types of facilities (e.g., no liquid wastes may be disposed in landfills). Closure and postclosure requirements are also established, to avoid release of the waste into the environment after the disposal facilities are closed. Permitted facilities must identify onsite pre-RCRA disposal areas and take remedial measures, if necessary, to ensure they do not release hazardous wastes into the environment. Hazardous waste generators are to certify they have taken measures to minimize the generation of hazardous waste. The high cost of disposal, however, creates an incentive for waste minimization quite apart from the requirement. It is generally thought that, as a result, hazardous waste generation has declined by some 25% since the system became effective.

Wastes covered by this system include those that are (a) corrosive; (b) ignitable; (c) reactive; (d) capable of releasing in excess of specified amounts of heavy metals, pesticides, or organic contaminants; (e) contained on a list of over 100 specific industrial wastes; or (f) contained on a list of several hundred specific discarded commercial chemical products. These categories are broad and sweeping and contain some wastes that are not truly hazardous. The EPA's regulations contain a procedure for "delisting" such wastes, to remove them from the RCRA system. Delisting, however, is an expensive and time-consuming procedure with an uncertain rate of success.

While RCRA establishes a comprehensive program for regulating hazardous waste disposal, it deals with nonhazardous waste disposal only by requiring states to bring their municipal landfills into conformity with standards established by the EPA (72). The EPA cannot enforce the standard against violating landfills, unless it finds the state does not have a solid waste regulatory program meeting RCRA standards. As a practical matter, municipal landfills subject to these standards may be used by generators of hazardous waste who dispose of it in quantities small enough to escape hazardous waste regulation. In addition, the landfills contain the residues of household products that would be classified as hazardous wastes if they were discarded by industries in larger quantities. Moreover, when municipal waste decomposes, it releases chemicals that are also produced by decomposition of hazardous wastes. It is not surprising that the composition of leachates from industrial and municipal landfills is similar. Increasing attention to control of municipal waste disposal can be expected because of the similarity of environmental effects. This is reinforced by the crisis in much of the Northeast over the rapid exhaustion of existing landfill capacity, coupled with the inability to locate new landfills in the face of local opposition, especially to disposal of waste generated out of state. These two factors are likely to combine in the near future to force federal legislation dealing more explicitly with municipal waste disposal.[s]

The RCRA program has not generated a significant amount of health effects data. Permit files in the EPA regional offices or state offices, however, contain considerable information on the specific chemicals present at particular storage or disposal sites and on how, if at all, those chemical are released into the environment.

### *Comprehensive Environmental Response, Compensation, and Liability Act (Superfund)*

The RCRA is designed to prevent current hazardous waste disposal from causing future health and environmental problems. The Superfund is designed to remediate environmental releases from pre-RCRA hazardous waste disposal. The Superfund authorizes the EPA to pursue one of two avenues for remediation. The first is to sue responsible parties to require them to perform the remediation work (73). Responsible parties include generators of the hazardous substances found at the offending site,

[s]For a discussion of probable future congressional focus on municipal landfills, see a RCRA roundtable *Environ Forum* 1991:30–31.

transporters who took the substances to the site, current owners or operators of the site, and owners and operators of the site at the time the hazardous substances were disposed there. The second avenue is for the EPA to remediate the site itself and to sue the responsible parties to recover its costs (74). Whichever route the EPA chooses, the resulting process and remedial action are approximately the same and the responsible parties ultimately bear the cost of cleanup. There may be hundreds of responsible parties at a site. The EPA never pursues all of them, often only a handful. But the parties the EPA pursues have the right to pursue the remaining responsible parties to recover their contribution to remedial costs (86).

There are over 30,000 sites on the EPA's Comprehensive Environmental Response Compensation and Liability Information System (CERCLIS) list for Superfund evaluation; currently some 1,300 have been placed on the National Priority List (NPL) for Superfund action (75). When a site is placed on the first list, it is evaluated to determine whether any immediate action (removal of leaking drums, fencing) is necessary to prevent serious adverse effects, and a hazard evaluation is completed to determine whether the site should be placed on the NPL. Once a site is on the NPL a remedial investigation is conducted to determine the nature and extent of contamination and the routes of exposure to people and the environment. Then a remedial feasibility study is done to determine alternative remedial actions and their cost. The EPA then chooses a remedial option in a public notice and comment procedure, after which remedial action is taken.

The Agency for Toxic Substances and Disease Registry (ATSDR) of the Public Health Service is to perform a health assessment for all sites on the NPL and for sites for which physicians so petition. The assessments are to determine potential human health risk at the sites, to help decide what remedial action should be taken and whether additional health information, including epidemiologic studies and registries of exposed persons, should be developed. In addition, ATSDR is to develop toxicologic profiles of the 100 or more most common hazardous substance found at Superfund sites.[t]

### *Emergency Planning and Community Right to Know Act*

The Emergency Planning and Community Right to Know Act (EPCRKA) was enacted a part of the 1986 amendments to the Superfund. It has two essential elements. The first is a program to establish response teams at the local level to deal with emergency situations involving hazardous substances. The second is a sort of national mass balance of hazardous substances to be performed by the EPA. Both produce information useful in determining to which chemicals humans may have been exposed.

Facilities where hazardous substances are stored or used must notify the local emergency planning organization and fire department of the existence, location, and volume of the materials (76). They must report releases of substances both to the local authorities and to the EPA's National Response Center. They must also furnish local authorities with Materials Safety Data Sheets required under the Occupational Safety and Health Administration (OSHA) Act for chemicals kept or used at the facility. They must report annually to the EPA the quantities of some 300 chemicals used by them and their disposition into the environment. The EPA maintains a computerized codification of the latter information, which is publicly available (a specific statutory requirement). These several reporting requirements apply to different sets of chemicals with different reporting thresholds. The reason for the differences is not apparent.

Most of this information is available from local emergency authorities or fire departments or from the EPA's Toxic Chemical Release Inventory in Washington, D.C. Although some of the information may be submitted as business confidential information, health professionals are entitled to most of it where necessary for health care. More information can be had from the EPA's Emergency Planning and Community Right to Know Hotline at 800-535-0202.

[t]See Siegel MR. Integrating public health into superfund: What has been the impact of the agency for toxic substances and disease registry? *Environ Law Reporter* 1990;20:10013–10020; and Johnson BC. Implementation of Superfund's health-related provisions by ATSDR. *Environ Law Reporter* 1990;20:10277–10282.

## REFERENCES


1. Odum E. *Fundamentals of ecology.* Sunderland, MA: Sinauer Associates, 1989.
2. *National water quality inventory,* 1988 Report to Congress, 440-4-90-003, 1988;39.
3. *Martin v. Reynolds Metals Co.*, 221 Or. 86, 342 F. 2d 7909 (1959).
4. *Boomer v. Atlantic Cement Co.*, 26 N.Y. 2d 219, 257 N.E. 2d 870, 309 N.Y.S. 2d 312 (1970).
5. 42 U.S.C. §§4321–4370a (1994).
6. 42 U.S.C. §§7401–7671q (1994).
7. 33 U.S.C. §§1251–1387 (1994).
8. 7 U.S.C. §§136–136y (1994).
9. 42 U.S.C. §§300f–300j-26 (1994).
10. 42 U.S.C. §§6901–6992k (1994).
11. 15 U.S.C. §§2601–2671 (1994).
12. 42 U.S.C. §§9601–9675 (1994).
13. 42 U.S.C. §§11001–11050 (1994).
14. 33 U.S.C. §§2701–2761 (1994).
15. 29 U.S.C. §§651–667 (1994).
16. 21 U.S.C. §§301–394 (1994).
17. Science Advisory Board. *Reducing risk:* setting priorities and strategies for environmental protection. EPA publication SAB-EC-90-021. Washington, DC: EPA, 1990.
18. 42 U.S.C. §§6992–6992k (1994).
19. 40 CFR §50.6 (c) (1996).
20. 42 U.S.C. §7671i (b) (1).
21. 42 U.S.C. §7401 (b) (1).
22. 33 U.S.C. §1251 (a).
23. 42 U.S.C. §7409 (b) (1).
24. *Lead Industries Assn. v. EPA,* 647 F.2d 1130 (D.C.Cir. 1980).

25. 42 U.S.C. §7409 (b) (2).
26. 40 CFR Part 50 (1996).
27. 7 U.S.C. §§136a (c) (5) and 136 (bb).
28. 15 U.S.C. §2605 (a).
29. 42 U.S.C. §7603.
30. CWA, 33 U.S.C. §1364.
31. Cook S. *The law of hazardous waste.* New York: Matthew Bender, §15.01 (2) (e).
32. *Principles of risk assessment:* a nontechnical review. Washington, DC: EPA, 1985.
33. National Research Council. *Regulating pesticides in food.* Washington, DC: National Academy Press, 1987.
34. 42 U.S.C. §§4901–4918 (1994).
35. Rogers W. *Environmental law.* St. Paul, MN: West Publishing Co., 1987.
36. *Intergovernmental panel on climate change: the IPCC scientific assessment.* Cambridge, England, Cambridge University Press, 1990.
37. Courch WR. Risk assessments and comparisons: An introduction. *Science* 1987;236:267–270.
38. 42 U.S.C. §7409 (b) (1994).
39. 33 U.S.C. §1314 (b) (1994).
40. 42 U.S.C. §7412 (e).
41. Pub. L. No. 104–182, 110 Stat. 1613.
42. 21 U.S.C. §§301–394.
43. Pub. L. 104–170, §402 (b), 110 Stat. 1489, 1513.
44. Pub. L. 104–4, 109 Stat. 48.
45. 42 USC §4332 (C).
46. *Strycker's Bay Neighborhood Council, Inc. v. Karlen,* 444 US 223 (1980).
47. 42 USC §7409, 40 CFR part 50.
48. 42 USC §7410, 40 CFR parts 51–52.
49. 40 CFR part 50.
50. 42 USC §7411, 40 CFR part 60.
51. 42 USC §7501-08 (for new major sources in areas not yet attaining NAAQS—nonattainment areas) and 42 USC §7470–7491 (for new major sources in areas attaining NAAQS—prevention of significant deterioration areas).
52. 40 CFR part 61.
53. *Natural Resources Defense Council v. EPA,* 824 F2d 1146 (DC cir. 1987).
54. 42 USC §7412.
55. 42 USC §7651–7651o.
56. 42 USC §7521.
57. 42 USC §7545.
58. 42 USC §7511–7511f.
59. 33 USC §1311 (a), 1362 (14).
60. 40 CFR part 430.
61. 33 USC §1313.
62. 33 USC §1321, 40 CFR parts 112-114.
63. 7 USC §136a.
64. 42 USC §§300g-300g-5.
65. 40 CFR §§141.13, .15–.16, and .61–.63 (1996).
66. Stever D. *Chemical regulation*, supra note n; pp. 7–33, 34.
67. 42 USC §300g-6.
68. 15 USC §2607 (b).
69. 15 USC §2605 (e) (PCBs), 2641–55 (asbestos, 2661–71 (radon).
70. 42 USC §6922, 6925; 40 CFR part 262.
71. 42 USC §6922 (a) (5), 6923; 40 CFR §262.20 to 23.
72. 42 USC §6941–6949a, 40 CFR parts 256, 257.
73. 42 USC §9606.
74. 42 USC §9604, 9607.
75. 40 CFR part 300, Appendix B, as amended from time to time in the *Federal Register.*
76. 42 USC §11002; 40 CFR Part 355.

*Environmental and Occupational Medicine, Third Edition,* edited by William N. Rom.
Published by Lippincott–Raven Publishers, Philadelphia, 1998.

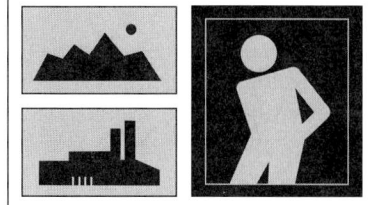

CHAPTER 125

# OSHA and the Regulatory Agencies

John Howard

Federal governmental regulation of occupational safety and health is a relatively recent phenomenon. Prior to the passage of the Occupational Safety and Health (OSH) Act in 1970, no nationwide law existed that protected the safety and health of American workers. Although some states had effective workplace safety laws, the degree of worker protection varied widely from state to state. By the late 1960s, both the business and labor communities believed that a comprehensive occupational health and safety statute was needed at the federal level. In 1968, Congress began active consideration of national occupational safety and health legislation, and on December 29, 1970, President Nixon signed the Williams-Steiger Occupational Safety and Health Act (OSH Act) into federal law.

In passing the OSH Act, Congress wanted "to assure, as far as possible, every working man and woman in the country safe and healthful working conditions." Unlike previous federal workplace health and safety legislation that regulated working conditions for specific types of occupations or industries, the OSH Act did not focus on specific industries or occupations. Instead, the OSH Act delegated responsibility for the development of specific workplace health and safety standards to the Secretary of Labor. Shortly after passage of the OSH Act, the Secretary established the Occupational Safety and Health Administration (OSHA) as a separate agency within the U.S. Department of Labor to administer all aspects of the OSH Act, including standards development and standards enforcement. Even though OSHA was not specifically mentioned in the Act, the Act did mandate the creation of a National Institute for Occupational Safety and Health (NIOSH) within the U.S. Department of Health and Human Services (DHHS) to support the new regulatory scheme with scientific research.

Nearly 30 years have elapsed since the passage of the act and the creation of OSHA. The regulation of workplace safety and health has become a pervasive aspect of doing business in the United States, Employers, workers, labor unions, lawyers, and physicians all face the daunting task of understanding a myriad of federal and state regulatory requirements for workplace safety, often in the absence of adequate knowledge of the overall framework of workplace health and safety law. This chapter presents an overview of the OSH Act as the centerpiece of the federal government's efforts to protect the health and safety of American workers and also reviews the laws enforced by other federal regulatory agencies that impact the field of occupational safety and health.

## EMPLOYER DUTIES UNDER THE OSH ACT

The duty of employers to provide a safe and healthful workplace is defined in two ways under the OSH Act. First, employers have a "general duty" to keep their workplaces free from recognized hazards likely to cause death or serious physical harm. Second, employers have a duty to comply with specific occupational safety and health standards promulgated by OSHA (1).

### General Duty Clause

To prove that an employer violated the general duty clause of the OSH Act, OSHA must show that (a) the employer failed to render the workplace free of a hazard, (b) the hazard was recognized by the employer or the employer's industry, (c) the hazard caused or was likely to

J. Howard: Division of Occupational Safety and Health, California Department of Industrial Relations, San Francisco, California 94105.

cause death or serious physical harm, and (d) there existed a feasible means to eliminate or materially reduce the hazard.

The requirement that the cited condition be recognized as a hazard is judged from the perspective of what is generally known in the particular industry where the hazard exists. In other words, knowledge of a hazard will be imputed to the cited employer on the basis that others in the employer's industry knew of the hazard, even if the particular employer is personally unaware of such information. This type of knowledge is called "constructive knowledge," and is based on the legal concept that a reasonable person in the employer's position would have known, or should have known, about a particular hazard.

Since the general duty clause is not available when a specific standards exists to address the hazard, OSHA utilizes the general duty clause primarily to cite employers for hazards that are not yet covered by a specific standard. Yet in the case of ergonomic hazards, OSHA has not been successful in using the general duty clause. In *Pepperidge Farms*, a case involving 173 instances of general duty clause violations, OSHA was unable to prove that there were specific and feasible steps the employer could have taken to correct the hazards in a cookie manufacturing plant associated with the development of cumulative trauma disorders (2).

### Occupational Safety and Health Standards

Employers also have the duty to comply with specific standards promulgated by OSHA. Even though OSHA adopted many of its earliest standards from private sector standard-setting organizations ("consensus" standards), OSHA now adopts standards through a lengthy rule-making process (3). Rule making requires that OSHA give the public notice of the proposed standard through publication in the *Federal Register,* provide the public an "opportunity to comment" on the proposed standard, and furnish written responses to the public's comments. After the standard development process is completed, the new standards are published in volume 29 of the Code of Federal Regulations (CFR) and become legally binding on all employers under federal jurisdiction. States with their own programs are required to adopt standards that are "at least as effective" as those adopted by OSHA within 6 months of federal promulgation (4).

OSHA also has the authority to adopt temporary standards on an emergency basis, but has done so infrequently. To issue a emergency temporary standard, OSHA must make two determinations: that "employees are exposed to grave danger from exposure to substances or agents determined to be toxic or physically harmful or from new hazards," and that "such an emergency standard is necessary to protect employees from such danger."

OSHA's notice and comment rule making has been consistently criticized for being a slow and cumbersome process. For example, critics point out that OSHA has promulgated only about two dozen standards for carcinogenic substances despite there being several hundred such chemicals in use today. One solution is to streamline new health standards by adopting generic standards on the topics that reoccur in each health standard, e.g., exposure assessment methodology, medical surveillance, and employee training.

Several different, and often confusing, terms are commonly used to describe OSHA's workplace standards. Standards are sometimes classified as safety standards or health standards to indicate what expertise is required to address the hazard, e.g., safety engineering or industrial hygiene. Another way of classifying OSHA standards is to refer to them as vertical or horizontal standards. Vertical standards apply exclusively to a specific industry, while horizontal ones apply to a particular hazard across all industries. Standards can also be described as specification or performance standards. Specification standards set forth specific instructions about how an employer must comply, whereas performance-oriented standards set forth a performance goal, but leave it to the employer how to achieve that goal. Even though the overwhelming preference of employers when a standard is being developed is that a performance-oriented approach should be used, it is not uncommon to hear complaints after a performance-oriented standard is adopted that OSHA has provided no specific guidance on how to comply!

### Variances

Employers can be exempted from complying with a standard by seeking and obtaining a variance from OSHA. After completing a variance application, OSHA gives the employer an opportunity to request a hearing on the issues contained in the employer's variance. Variances can be granted on a temporary basis (up to 6 months) or permanently. Temporary variances are granted to employers who have a legitimate need for more time in order to comply with a standard. Permanent variances are granted to employers who can demonstrate to OSHA's satisfaction that the employer has an equally effective way to ensure employee protection as that required by the relevant standard.

Variances seem to be an unavoidable fact of life with standards that are specification-oriented, but are largely unnecessary when performance-oriented approaches to standard development are used. The flexibility written into a performance standard takes the initial decision about how to ensure safety out of the hands of OSHA and places it in the hands of the employer. Therefore, there is no need for an employer to ask OSHA's approval to "vary" from the performance set forth in the standard.

**Judicial Review of OSHA Standards**

Within 60 days of its promulgation, an OSHA standard can be challenged by "any person who may be adversely affected by a standard." Most of OSHA's health standards, and some its safety standards, have been subject to judicial review. When a challenge is lodged, implementation of the standard is usually "stayed," in whole or in part, pending review by the court. Many court decisions have been favorable to OSHA, but some standards have been vacated altogether. For example, in a significant setback to OSHA's effort to streamline the standards development process, the entire 1989 Air Contaminants Standard was struck down by the Eleventh Circuit Court of Appeals (5).

Over the past 30 years, two legal challenges to OSHA's health standards have reached the U.S. Supreme Court—the benzene (6) and the cotton dust (7) cases. The decisions in these two cases have greatly influenced how OSHA goes about developing its occupational health standards.

In 1980, the U.S. Supreme Court rejected OSHA's first benzene standard because OSHA had failed to demonstrate scientifically that the 1 ppm permissible exposure limit (PEL) in the new standard would eliminate a "significant risk" of harm in the workplace. Since the Supreme Court's benzene decision, OSHA has spent considerable effort to establish that a significant risk exists with respect to the hazard to be prevented for each new health standard. Since the benzene decision, OSHA provides extensive epidemiologic evidence of risk (and how the risk will be reduced by the provisions of the new standard) every time it regulates a new workplace health risk.

Section 6(b)(5) of the OSH Act requires that OSHA adopt standards for exposure to toxic substances that will protect employees "to the extent feasible." Section 29 U.S.C. §655(b)(5) states in part that "The Secretary, in promulgating standards dealing with toxic materials or harmful physical agents under this subsection, shall set the standard which most adequately assures, *to the extent feasible,* on the basis of the best available evidence, that no employee will suffer material impairment of health or functional capacity even if such employee has regular exposure to the hazard dealt with by such standard for the period of his working life." In setting its first standard for asbestos in the early 1970s, OSHA's view was that feasibility issues (either economic or technological) may legitimately be considered when setting a PEL. Thus, in the asbestos standard, OSHA mandated phased-in compliance over a 4-year period. OSHA's phased-in compliance view, based on feasibility considerations, was challenged, but a court of appeals agreed with OSHA's position. Then, in 1981, the feasibility issue reached the U.S. Supreme Court.

In the cotton dust case, the Supreme Court agreed that to meet the Act's requirements of feasibility, OSHA was indeed required to determine that the affected industry "will maintain long-term profitability and competitiveness" even after complying with the provisions of an OSHA standard. In an important limitation on how far OSHA had to go in providing evidence that compliance with a standard was feasible, the Supreme Court in the cotton dust case ruled that the OSH Act does not require OSHA to perform formal cost-benefit analysis in developing health and safety standards.

**Information Management Duties**

Employers have several obligations under the OSH Act to manage workplace safety and health information. Employers with 11 or more employees are required to gather and maintain information regarding work-related injuries and illnesses, i.e., record-keeping duties. Employers must maintain a log and summary of all recordable occupational injuries and illnesses in their establishment. Each recordable injury and illness must be entered in the log and summary no later than 6 days after receiving information that such an injury or illness has occurred. The term *recordable occupational injury or illness* includes (a) a fatality (regardless of the time between injury and death, or the length of the illness); (b) a lost workday case, other than a fatality, that results in lost workdays; and (c) a nonfatal case, without lost workdays, that results in the loss of consciousness, restriction of work or motion, transfer to another job or termination of employment, or medical treatment (other than first aid), and any diagnosed occupational illness that is reported to the employer but that is not classified as a fatality or a lost workday case.

In addition to record-keeping responsibilities, employers also have an obligation to report fatalities or multiple hospitalization incidents. Within 8 hours after the death of any employee from any work-related incident, or the inpatient hospitalization of three or more employees as a result of a work-related incident, employers must report the fatality, or multiple hospitalization, by telephone or in person to the OSHA area office nearest the site of the incident or by using the OSHA toll-free central telephone number. The employer has the obligation to report even if the work-related fatality or hospitalization occurs up to 30 days after the incident. Lastly, employers have specific reporting and recording responsibilities that are set forth in many occupational health standards, e.g., occupational noise, ionizing radiation, asbestos, inorganic arsenic, lead, blood-borne pathogens, and cotton dust.

## ENFORCEMENT OF THE OSH ACT

**Types of Inspections**

The first step in the enforcement of the OSH Act is an inspection of the workplace. Workplace inspections are most often initiated by an employee complaint, by a report of a fatality or serious injury, or as part of an OSHA program designed to eliminate a hazard in a particular industry. OSHA usually does not give the employer advanced notice of an inspection. However, if an employer refuses to consent to an inspection, the U.S. Supreme Court has ruled that the Fourth Amendment of the U.S. Constitution requires OSHA to obtain a warrant, based on "probable cause," before conducting an inspection (8). The warrant must be supported either by probable cause that a specific violation exists or by administrative probable cause. Administrative probable cause is a special legal concept applicable to OSHA inspections and requires that an establishment be selected for general schedule, or programmed, inspection by means of specific neutral criteria.

During an inspection, OSHA compliance officers review any records an employer is required to maintain, including their safety and health management program, and then conduct a "walkaround" to physically identify workplace hazards that are a violation of OSHA safety and health standards. Following the physical inspection of the workplace, the compliance officer conducts an exit conference at which time potential violations and civil penalties are discussed with the employer.

### Violations and Civil Penalties

OSHA's uses a "first instance" citation method. After a standard goes into legal effect, employers can be cited for a violation of the standard even if it is the employer's first instance of noncompliance. An employer's noncompliance with safety and health standards can result in one of nine types of violations. Violations are classified as *de minimis,* regulatory, nonserious, serious, repeat, and failure to abate. In addition, the classification of "willful" can be added to a violation that is regulatory, nonserious, or serious.

A *de minimis* violation is one that has no direct or immediate relationship to safety and health. No penalties are assessed for a *de minimis* violation. A nonserious violation has no statutory definition, but has been judicially defined to be one that has "a direct and immediate relationship to safety and health, but it not of such a relationship that the result injury or illness is death or serious physical harm." Also included in the category of nonserious violations are regulatory violations. Examples of these include an employer's failure to post a notice that informs employees of their rights under the OSH Act. A serious violation is one that poses "a substantial probability that death or serious physical harm could result...unless the employer did not, and could not with the exercise of reasonable diligence, know of the presence of the violation." Both nonserious and serious violations carry a statutory maximum penalty of $7,000 for each violation.

The most severe civil penalties can be levied for willful and repeated violations. At issue in a willful violation is whether the employer acted with "an intentional disregard of, or plain indifference to," the OSH Act. For an employer to be cited for a repeated violation, OSHA must show when citing the employer for a repeated violation that there was a final order of the Occupational Safety and Health Review Commission for the previous violation and that there exists "substantial similarity" between the two violations. The statutory maximum penalty for a willful or a repeated violation is $70,000 per violation.

Each citation OSHA issues must "fix a reasonable time for abatement of the violation." OSHA can issue a failure-to-abate violation when the employer fails to correct a citation whose abatement period has expired. If an employer appeals the citation, the Act provides that the abatement period for that citation does not begin to run until a final order of the review commission is entered. Staying abatement until the adjudication of a contested citation is completed is a controversial feature of the OSH Act. Labor advocates have argued that permitting the abatement of serious hazards to be stayed increases the chances that employees will be injured while legal proceedings are pending. Furthermore, in the case of short-term construction projects, the cited employer is able to "fight the citation" until the project is completed, thereby escaping abatement altogether. On the other hand, employers argue that OSHA is frequently unable to prove the existence of a cited violation. In those cases, they assert that it would be a waste of their resources to abate a condition that was not a violation. When a final order of the review commission is entered, though, and the employer has not yet corrected the violation, OSHA can impose on the employer a penalty of up to $7,000 for each day that the violation remains uncorrected.

### Citation Contestation Proceedings

The act grants employers who have received an OSHA citation the right to contest, before a neutral party, (a) the existence of the violation, (b) the classification of the violation, or (c) the reasonableness of the proposed civil penalty. The employer has 15 days from receipt of the citation to file an appeal with the review commission. Once filed, the review commission assigns the case for a adjudicative hearing presided over by an administrative law judge (ALJ) employed by the review commission to hear contested cases. At the hearing, OSHA carries the burden of proving the existence of the violation, its classification, and the reasonableness of the civil penalty.

Even if OSHA carries its burden of proving the violation, the employer still has the opportunity to present affirmative defenses to the violation. The most common affirmative defense presented by employers is called the "independent employee act" defense. The employer must show that the violation occurred because of unpreventable employee misconduct despite the employer's best efforts to maintain an effective safety program that was effectively communicated and enforced.

At the administrative hearing, the ALJ can affirm or vacate the violation, the proposed penalty, or both. If either party loses at the administrative hearing stage, an appeal can be filed requesting that the review commission itself hear the case. Since such appeals are discretionary, the review commission is under no obligation to accept the employer's invitation to review the case. If the review commission does hear the case, the losing party can then appeal to the United States Court of Appeals in the circuit where the violation took place, where the employer has its principal place of business, or in the Court of Appeals for the District of Columbia. Ultimately, an aggrieved party can request that the Supreme Court review its case, but such requests are rarely granted.

### Criminal Prosecution

Even though the major emphasis in the OSH Act is on civil enforcement through monetary penalties, the OSH Act does provide for criminal prosecution of an employer under certain conditions. Criminal liability occurs if the employer "willfully violates any standard, rule or order promulgated pursuant to section 6" and the violation "caused death to any employee." Since the violation must be of a section 6 standard, criminal liability cannot be imposed for violations of the general duty clause. Usually, a direct causal connection must be demonstrated between the violation and the death of the employee for criminal liability to be triggered.

Criminal penalties under section 17(e) include 6 months' imprisonment or a $10,000 fine, or both, for the first conviction and 1 year's imprisonment or a $20,000 fine, or both, for any second or subsequent convictions. Over the last 30 years, criminal prosecutions under the act have been uncommon. During the 1980s, OSHA was criticized for a lack of interest in referring willful fatality cases to the U.S. Department of Justice for criminal prosecution. In the 1990s, though, OSHA began to refer more cases to the Department of Justice for criminal prosecution than it had in the past (9).

Some states that operate their own state OSHA plans have criminal provisions that are somewhat broader that found in the federal OSH Act. For instance, Minnesota permits fines up to $10,000 and imprisonment of up to 6 months for any willful or repeated violation, and California provides for a fine not exceeding $5,000 or up to 6 months' imprisonment for employers who knowingly or negligently commit serious violation or a repeated or failure-to-abate violation that creates a real and apparent hazard to employees.

Aside from the OSH Act, several states, such as California, Illinois, Michigan, Texas, and Washington, have utilized their state's general criminal laws to file murder and manslaughter charges against employers allegedly responsible for workplace fatalities (10). Even in states under federal OSHA jurisdiction, most courts have ruled that the OSH Act does not preempt such state criminal law prosecutions.

In an expansion of state criminal liability, California in 1989 enacted the Corporate Criminal Liability Act, which applies to any corporation or limited liability company, and to any person who is a manager and has authority for the safety of a product or a business practice. If such a person has "actual knowledge of a serious concealed danger," he or she is required by law to report the information to the California OSHA program and to warn "affected employees in writing" of the concealed danger. The act provides for strict criminal penalties, including imprisonment for up to 3 years and/or a fine of up to $25,000 for individual managers and $1,000,000 for corporations.

## EMPLOYEE RIGHTS UNDER THE OSH ACT

### Participation Rights

Employees, or their representatives, can request that OSHA initiate a workplace inspection by filing a complaint. During an inspection, the act allows an employee representative to accompany OSHA during the physical inspection of the workplace. When no authorized employee representative exists (such as at a nonunion workplace), OSHA is required to consult with "a reasonable number of employees concerning matters of health and safety in the workplace." Also, employee representatives have the right to be present in the opening and closing conferences of an OSHA inspection either separately or jointly with the employer at the discretion of the employer. Affected employees must also be given notice of variance applications and afforded an opportunity to participate in the variance hearing.

Employees also have rights to participate in citation contestation proceedings. For instance, employees have the right to object to the time fixed in the citation for abatement. If an employee files a notice of contest alleging that the abatement time is unreasonable, the review commission must hold a hearing on the matter. Also, when an employer files a notice of contest, affected employees or their representatives have the right to participate in the contestation proceedings as legal parties to the action. However, if OSHA reaches a settlement with the employer and withdraws the citation, employee parties are legally powerless to challenge OSHA's decision.

### Job Protection Rights

Employees are protected by the OSH Act from discharge or discrimination for filing a complaint with OSHA, instituting any proceeding or testifying in any proceeding related to the act, or exercising any of the employee's rights under the act. Job protection rights afforded by Section 11(c)(1) are broadly stated in that the discrimination prohibition is directed at "persons" not just employers, e.g., labor unions, employment agencies, or other employers. The type of employee activities that are protected by the Act have also been broadly interpreted. Employees are protected when they participate in an OSHA inspection, when they file a notice of contest challenging the time fixed in a citation for abatement, and when they participate in a variance hearing or in a judicial challenge to a standard.

However, employees have only 30 days from the date that the discharge or discrimination occurs to file a complaint with the secretary of the Department of Labor. The Secretary has 90 days to conduct an investigation and to notify the complainant of the results. The Secretary can decide to bring legal action in federal district court against the person allegedly responsible for the job-related retaliation, and the courts can order all appropriate relief including restoration of the employee to the employee's former position with back pay.

Even though an employee's right to refuse hazardous work is not expressly provided for in the OSH Act, OSHA promulgated in 1973 a regulation containing a limited right to refuse hazardous work. The OSHA regulation requires that, to be protected, the employee's refusal must satisfy the following four conditions: (a) employee's refusal must be made in good faith, (b) a reasonable person in the employee's place would conclude that a real danger of death or serious physical harm exists, (c) insufficient time exists to eliminate the hazard through the act's usual enforcement mechanisms, and (d) the employee (where possible) must have sought from the employer (and failed to achieve) abatement of the hazardous condition. In *Whirlpool Corp. v. Marshall*, the U.S. Supreme Court unanimously rejected an employer's challenge of the validity of the OSHA refusal of hazardous work regulation in the case of two employees who refused to work on an elevated wire mesh screen 2 weeks after another employee had fallen to his death through the screen after filing an OSHA complaint (11).

### Information Rights

The OSH Act requires that employers "keep their employees informed of their protections and obligations" through "posting of notices or other appropriate means." OSHA has developed a notice that informs employees of their protections and obligations and lists the various OSHA offices throughout the country and furnishes it free of charge to employers. Once the notice is furnished by OSHA, employers are then required to "post and keep posted" the OSHA notice (or more commonly, OSHA poster). Employers must also provide to employees access to the log and summary of recordable occupational injuries and illnesses for each establishment in which the employee works, or worked in the past.

Employees also have a right of access (for examination and copying) to their exposure and medical records. Two limitations exist on the employee's right of access to exposure and medical records. First, the employer can request that the employee designate in writing a representative to receive the requested information if a physician representing the employer believes that direct employee access to the information regarding a specific diagnosis of a terminal illness or psychiatric condition could be detrimental to the employee's health. Second, employers can protect "trade secret" information by deleting information about the manufacturing process or the percentage of a chemical substance in a mixture, but must inform the employee of the deletion. Lastly, OSHA's Hazard Communication Standard provides employees with the right to know about any hazardous substances used in the workplace.

## CONSULTATION

Aside from its standards development and enforcement goals, the OSH Act also aims to reduce workplace injuries and illnesses "by encouraging employers and employees in their efforts to reduce the number of occupational safety and health hazards at their places of employment, and to stimulate employers and employees to institute new and to perfect existing programs for providing safety and healthful working conditions." To carry out this responsibility under the act, OSHA is able to enter into cooperative agreements with states to provide consultative assistance to the employers in that state. OSHA has consultation agreements with all states and these agreements are governed by specific federal regulations.

Consultative assistance is provided free of charge upon employer request and is based on cooperative interaction between the employer and the consultant. Consultation activities are conducted independently from enforcement activities and consultation programs must have managerial staff separate from enforcement. Even though the focus of a consultation is on making the employer's management program for preventing workplace injury and illness as effective as possible, consultants may also identify hazards that are in violation of an OSHA standard during the performance of an on-site consultation visit.

Lastly, the Voluntary Protection Program (VPP) has been an important adjunct to OSHA's consultation mission. VPP recognizes the achievements of employers who have exemplary safety and health programs and whose rates of workplace injury and illness are far below others in their industry. Increasingly popular among employers, successful entry into VPP also exempts employers from programmed inspections.

## STATE PROGRAMS

When Congress passed the OSH Act in 1970, it was in the belief that federal protection needed to be provided to

America's workers since in many states standards development and standards enforcement was weak or absent altogether. At the same time, though, Congress realized that some states had administered effective occupational safety and health programs for many years and such efforts should be encouraged. Thus, even though the Act sets forth a comprehensive, nationwide approach to worker protection, states are encouraged "to assume the fullest responsibility for the administration and enforcement of their occupational safety and health laws." In addition to encouragement, the OSH Act provides financial "grants to the states to assist them in administering and enforcing [occupational safety and health] programs" (12).

The OSH Act allows states to assume responsibility for administering their own workplace safety and health programs, but only if states submit, and obtain approval of, a state plan that meets rigorous federal criteria. Many of the problems that have arisen between OSHA and the states over the past 30 years have had their origin in some of these criteria. For instance, states must assure OSHA that they will "devote adequate funds to the administration and enforcement of standards" and that they will have enough qualified personnel for enforcement. Much discussion—and even a court of appeals case (13)—has arisen over how many compliance personnel states must have to receive final approval of their plan. In 1992, OSHA threatened to decertify the North Carolina OSHA program for what OSHA perceived as the state's failure to provide enough compliance personnel for their program.

Another criterion that has proven to be a contentious issue between OSHA and the states is the requirement for states to provide standards that are "at least as effective" in providing safe and healthful employment as those adopted by OSHA. After federal OSHA has adopted a standard, states have 6 months to adopt a standard as effective as the federal one. Most states simply adopt the identical standard that OSHA has developed. But some states, such as California, Michigan, Oregon, Hawaii, Minnesota, and Washington, often adopt standards that are more protective than their federal counterparts. Review and approval of the state's version of the new OSHA standard is a time-consuming and tedious task for both the state and OSHA. Also, some states will often develop and adopt occupational safety and health standards that OSHA has not yet adopted.

Out a total of 56 jurisdictions eligible to establish their own occupational safety and health programs, 25 states operate their own programs (14). In states without approved plans, responsibility for workplace safety and health remains with OSHA. Even in states under the jurisdiction of the federal OSH Act, OSHA has no jurisdiction over those states' public sector employees (state, county, and city employees) since the OSH Act makes clear that the word *employer* does not include "any state or political subdivision of a state." Labor unions that represent public sector employees have sought to amend the public sector employee exclusion found in the OSH Act. Their belief is that the coverage of the Act needs to be extended to public sector employees specifically excluded from federal coverage because state workplace safety protections are inadequate in many of those states covered by OSHA.

States are required to submit any new standards or enforcement regulations that they develop to OSHA for approval as well as respond to any federally initiated changes. In addition, the performance of states with respect to standards adoption and standards enforcement activities is closely monitored by OSHA. Despite the many requirements imposed on states by the federal government, states with their own programs benefit from a higher level of local participation in workplace safety and health activities by employers, employees, labor unions, and others within the state.

## NIOSH

The OSH Act also established the National Institute for Occupational Safety and Health (NIOSH) in the Department of Health and Human Services. The act gave NIOSH a set of broad responsibilities pertaining to occupational safety and health, including conducting research, experiments, and demonstrations relating to occupational safety and health. NIOSH is authorized to develop and establish recommended occupational safety and health standards to OSHA, but since NIOSH does not have the authority to adopt a standard, OSHA determines which of the NIOSH recommended standards it will adopted. Since 1970, NIOSH has issued far more proposals for a recommended standard than OSHA has acted upon.

NIOSH is also responsible for developing criteria for safe exposure to toxic substances and harmful physical agents and for publishing an annual list of all known toxic substances and the concentrations at which toxicity is known to occur. Like OSHA, NIOSH also has the authority to enter workplaces to conduct investigations of occupational safety and health problems and to question employers and employees about those problems. If an employer refuses entry, NIOSH must obtain an inspection warrant to gain entry to the workplace in order to collect information and medically examine workers. Generally, though, NIOSH conducts its worksite investigations (called health hazard evaluations) with the full cooperation of employers and employees.

NIOSH must also conduct educational programs to provide an adequate supply of safety and health professionals to carry out the purposes of the act. NIOSH has established 12 regional education resource centers (ERCs) in universities throughout the United States to provide residency training for physicians in occupational medicine, graduate training in industrial hygiene and safety, and nondegree programs in various occupational safety and health topics such as pulmonary function testing (15). Lastly, NIOSH produces a considerable literature on occupational health and safety. To obtain a catalog, contact the NIOSH Publications Office, 4676 Columbia Parkway, MS C-13, Cincinnati, Ohio 45226.

## OTHER FEDERAL AGENCIES AND STATUTES

### Mine Safety and Health Administration

All mines are subject to the jurisdiction of the Mine Safety and Health Administration (MSHA) of the Department of Labor under the statutory authority of the Federal Mine Safety and Health Act (Mine Act) (16). Like the OSH Act, the Mine Act provides for adopting standards by MSHA to protect the safety and health of employees engaged in mining operations by conducting inspections, issuing citations, and imposing civil and criminal penalties on mine operators. A number of important differences exist between the OSH and Mine Acts.

Unlike the OSH Act's provision that allows the abatement time to be stayed pending the outcome of a contested case, the Mine Act requires mine operators to begin immediately correcting the violative condition even if the mine operator contests the citation. Another difference is that OSHA must seek injunction relief in an appropriate federal district court before ordering employees to be removed from exposure to an imminent danger. Under the Mine Act, an MSHA inspector can order that all miners be withdrawn from the area of a mine affected by an imminent danger. The Mine Act also provides for pay for miners who participate in an MSHA inspection or who are out of work as a result of closure order issued by MSHA. OSHA has no comparable provisions even though there was an unsuccessful effort by OSHA in 1977 to provide equivalent benefits.

### Environmental Protection Agency

The Environmental Protection Agency (EPA) administers several federal statutes that grant it the authority to regulate occupational safety and health. Among these statutes are the Toxic Substances Control Act (TSCA) (17) and the Federal Insecticide, Fungicide, and Rodenticide Act (FIFRA) (18).

Under TSCA, EPA has the authority to regulate the manufacturing, processing, distribution, use, and disposal of chemical substances and mixtures. TSCA also requires EPA to publish a chemical substances inventory. Under its TSCA authority, EPA has promulgated regulations pertaining to employee health and safety in the manufacture and use of toxic substances. In 1986, Congress enacted the Asbestos Hazard Emergency Response Act (AHERA) as Title II of TSCA to address the problem of asbestos in schools, public buildings, and commercial buildings.

Under FIFRA, the EPA regulates the registration and labeling of hazardous pesticides and conducts inspections of industries manufacturing or using hazardous pesticides. Also under FIFRA, the EPA issues regulations governing the use of agricultural pesticides in the workplace. Under the OSH Act, this exercise of EPA jurisdiction over worker safety effectively precludes OSHA from issuing standards for farm workers exposed to pesticides. In 1985, the EPA first issued regulations to protect farm workers from the harmful effects of pesticides and updated these regulations in 1992 (19). The EPA's new pesticide standard protects not only farm workers who perform hand labor operations in fields treated with pesticides, but also workers who handle pesticides in forests, nurseries, and greenhouses. The new regulation prohibits application of pesticides in such a manner so as to expose workers to unsafe conditions, adds new sections for decontamination and emergency medical duties, and prescribes specific time intervals for employee reentry into pesticide-applied areas.

## FUTURE CHALLENGES

As the 21st century nears, the OSH Act faces a number of challenges. The most fundamental challenge to the Act's future survival is determining how effective the Act has been in "assuring safe and healthful working conditions." Despite nearly 30 years of standard development and enforcement activities, the quantity and quality of empirical evidence about how effective these activities have been in eliminating occupational injuries and illnesses is scant. If the OSH Act is to survive its current critics, it is imperative that OSHA develop ways to measure injury and illness outcomes, rather than continuing to rely on activity measurements as an index of the act's effectiveness and relevance to the American workplace.

Hazards that were important when the OSH Act was new—and the manufacturing sector of the American economy was still robust—are now being overtaken by newer hazards that have arisen from the dramatic changes in the American workplace. For instance, the typical American office has been transformed "from a paper-handling to a electronic-processing operation" (20). Associated with the appearance of computer workstations has been a sharp rise in the number of musculoskeletal injuries (MSIs) involving the upper extremity. These and other MSIs involving the low back now account for majority of claims in the workers' compensation insurance system. As America moves from the industrial to the information age, OSHA will need to develop regulatory strategies to address MSIs if it is to have any positive impact on injury reduction in the 21st century. In addition to the challenge of MSI injury reduction, OSHA also faces the challenge of addressing other emerging hazards such as workplace stress and workplace violence.

Even the way people are employed today and in the next century will provide a challenge to OSHA. Instead of working for just one employer, an increasing number of Americans are now contract employees. As such, they are sent by a primary employer—temporary agency or employee leasing firm—to work at a site controlled by a secondary employer. In these "dual employer" situations, the primary employer often assumes that the secondary employer is ensuring that worker protections are implemented when, in fact, neither is doing so. Even what constitutes a "workplace" will change in the 21st century. By the year 2000, it is estimated that 20% of American workers will work from their home, as opposed the traditional workplace envisioned by the Act in 1970.

As America moves from the Industrial Age to a new Information Age, the flexibility of the OSH Act drafted in 1970 "to assure, as far as possible, every working man and woman in the country safe and healthful working conditions" will be tested in numerous ways. But, as this chapter has shown, the fundamental structure of the Act is sound, and the commitment of employers, employees, labor unions, and occupational safety and health professionals will ensure that the protections guaranteed by the Act will survive.

## REFERENCES

1. OSHA's workplace safety and health regulations and standards are mainly codified at Parts 1900–1910, 1926 and 1953 of the Code of Federal Regulations (CFR).
2. OSHRC Doc. No. 89-0265 (Rev Comm'n J., March 25, 1993, review directed, Sept. 13, 1993).
3. OSHA rule making conforms to the provisions of the United States Administrative Procedures Act which is codified at 5 U.S.C. §706.
4. 29 C.F.R. §1953.23(a)(2).
5. *AFL-CIO v. OSHA,* 965 F.2d 962 (11th Cir. 1992).
6. *Industrial Union Department, AFL-CIO v. American Petroleum Institute,* 448 U.S. 601, 100 S. Ct. 2844 (1980).
7. *American Textile Manufacturers' Institute, Inc. v. Donovan,* 452 U.S. 490 (1981).
8. *Marshall v. Barlow's Inc.,* 436 U.S. 307 (1978).
9. Bor VL, Feitshans IL, eds. *Occupational safety and health law: 1995 supplement.* Washington, DC: The Bureau of National Affairs, 1995; 101.
10. Bokat SA, Thompson HA, eds. *Occupational safety and health law.* Washington, DC: The Bureau of National Affairs, 1988;327–328.
11. 445 U.S. 1 (1980).
12. 29 U.S.C. §672(g) limits the federal contribution to no more than "50 percent of the total cost to the State of the program."
13. *AFL-CIO v. Marshall,* 570 F.2d 1030 (D.C.Cir. 1978). In this case, a unanimous panel held that the secretary's regulations and program directives establishing numerical staffing requirements, or "benchmarks," for each state plan failed to meet the criteria set forth in the OSH Act for enforcement staffing. On remand, the district court issued an order to the Secretary on December 5, 1978, specifying a number of factors to be taken into account in developing "benchmark" staffing for each state—which states would have to meet before receiving final approval under Section 18(c) of the act.
14. 29 U.S.C. §653(7) defines the term *State* as "a State of the United States, the District of Columbia, Puerto Rico, the Virgin Islands, American Samoa, Guam, and the Trust Territory of the Pacific Islands." Under this statutory definition, the states that administer their own occupational safety and health programs are Alaska, Arizona, California, Hawaii, Indiana, Iowa, Kentucky, Maryland, Michigan, Minnesota, Nevada, New Mexico, North Carolina, Puerto Rico, South Carolina, Oregon, Tennessee, Utah, Vermont, Virgin Islands, Virginia, Washington and Wyoming.
15. Rom WN. Medicine re-enters the workplace. A new era in occupational medicine? *N Engl J Med* 1979;300:672–673.
16. Pub. Law No. 95-164, 91 Stat. 1290 (1977), 30 U.S.C. §801 et seq.
17. 15 U.S.C. §§2601 et seq.
18. 7 U.S.C. §§136 et seq.
19. 40 C.F.R. §§170 et seq.
20. Rifkin J. *The end of work.* New York: Putnam, 1995;146.

*Environmental and Occupational Medicine, Third Edition*, edited by William N. Rom.
Lippincott–Raven Publishers, Philadelphia © 1998.

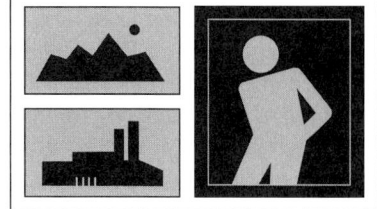

CHAPTER 126

# Economic Issues in Occupational Safety and Health

Nicholas A. Ashford and Robert F. Stone

An understanding of economic aspects of occupational safety and health is important for several reasons: (a) economic forces explain, in part, the behavior of employers and workers regarding workplace hazards; (b) imperfections in the job market help explain the need for government intervention; and (c) economic mechanisms and policies can be introduced by government to improve worker safety and health.

Following a description of the market for safety and health, this chapter investigates the following three issues: (a) imperfections in the job market that induce suboptimal levels of occupational safety and health; (b) the need for government intervention, and the various forms that such government involvement can take; and (c) the logic and limitations of using cost-benefit analysis to fashion government policy concerning occupational safety and health.

## THE MARKET FOR SAFETY AND HEALTH

In our society, the preferred mechanism for conducting economic and social activities is the private market—and usually with good reason. A well-functioning market system possesses two important properties. First, under suitable conditions, a market system is economically efficient in the following sense: resources are allocated where they are most highly valued; the appropriate mix of goods and services, embodying the desired bundle of characteristics (for example, size, color, and style for clothing), is produced; and all possible mutually beneficial exchanges will take place, so that further improvements in the welfare of any member of society cannot be attained without making at least one other member worse off. Second, consistent with libertarian values, marketplace transactions are entirely voluntary; only if the interested parties are able to negotiate to mutual advantage will a market exchange occur.

For some economic activities, of course, no marketplace exists. For instance, in the case of environmental hazards, the party releasing a pollutant and those parties at risk are generally economic strangers. There is no market mechanism through which polluters and citizens can effectively negotiate to reduce the environmental risk, at least not prior to an environmental release. Occupational hazards, however, take place within the context of a labor market that permits, and sometimes requires, the employer and the employee to bargain over workplace health and safety conditions to their mutual advantage. Our natural starting point then is to consider whether the unfettered market—which includes the courts, to enforce the agreed-upon terms of real or implied market transactions—promotes the socially desired degree of occupational health and safety, and if not, why not.

### The Idealized Job Market

Filling a specific job vacancy in a market system represents the intersection of employer demand and worker supply, where each job embodies a particular combination of workplace characteristics, such as salary and other

N. A. Ashford: School of Engineering, Massachusetts Institute of Technology, Cambridge, Massachusetts 02139.
R. F. Stone: Center for Technology, Policy and Industrial Development, Massachusetts Institute of Technology, Cambridge, Massachusetts 02139.

worker benefits, job content (affecting worker job satisfaction), and job-related risks to worker health and safety. According to economic theory, a job market operating under ideal conditions will reduce workplace hazards to their socially optimal level.

Employers compete among themselves in the job market to attract workers, who will obviously choose the most desirable job in terms of the bundle of workplace characteristics provided. Therefore, in order to hire workers to perform relatively unpleasant tasks, employers must offer some offsetting benefit, such as a higher wage rate. Similarly, to induce workers to accept hazardous jobs, employers must offer to compensate the risk. Risk compensation is typically evaluated in terms of a wage premium for risk, but it may equally well take the form of insurance benefits, employer assumption of liability for worker injuries and illness, or some combination of the above. The magnitude of the compensation required to attract applicants for hazardous jobs depends on the amount of extra risk involved and the extent of worker preferences for risk avoidance. If workers are relatively risk-averse, they will demand more compensation to accept any specified level of job hazard. However, since workers compete with each other for jobs, the risk premium and other risk benefits an individual worker can command are limited to the extent that other workers require less risk compensation to accept hazardous work.

So far in the discussion, job hazards have been treated as fixed. In reality, job hazards and other working conditions are variables under the control of the employer. Safety equipment, engineering controls, and related employer investments can reduce the level of workplace risk and allow an employer to lower, by a commensurate amount, the risk compensation he must offer his workers. An employer will find it profitable to increase the level of workplace safety so long as the associated savings in worker risk compensation exceed the cost of the hazard reduction, evaluated at the margin.

Thus, according to economic theory, the operation of the private market provides an allocatively efficient level of occupational risk and is capable of providing the socially optimal level of occupational risk as well. However, as we will examine later in more detail, four conditions must be satisfied for the marketplace to function as postulated by economic theory. First, workers must be fully informed about their job opportunities, including the degree of risk present in alternative work environments. Second, those parties engaging in marketplace transactions concerning the level of job risk must bear all of the costs and derive all of the benefits of their actions—that is, the job market must not create externalities. Third, the job market must be competitive so that individual employers or workers—or small groups of employers, or workers, acting in concert—are not able to influence the wage level or the wage premium for risk. Fourth, since market outcomes vary depending on the preexisting distribution of wealth and other social parameters concerned with justice and equity, for the market-derived level of occupational risk to be socially optimal (not just allocatively efficient), the moral and distributional setting in which the market functions must be socially acceptable. Unfortunately, these idealized conditions are seldom met.

### Performance of the Job Market: The U.S. Experience

Until the beginning of the 20th century, the magnitude of occupational risk in the United States was determined almost entirely by the unconstrained workings of the private job market. Unfortunately, its performance fell far short of the accomplishments ascribed to economic theory's ideally functioning market.

Rapid industrialization in this country was accompanied by a noticeable increase in workplace injuries. Despite extremely hazardous working conditions in many industries, employers, with rare exception, failed to introduce even the most rudimentary health and safety measures. Nor were workers compensated for the job risks they encountered. Wages for hazardous work were largely undifferentiated from wages for less hazardous but otherwise equivalent work, and employers generally offered no wage-loss, medical, or impairment benefits to workers sustaining job-related injuries (1).

Other than workers' compensation, itself a quasi-market insurance system, the job market operated with limited government intervention from 1910 to 1970, when the Occupational Safety and Health Act was passed. How did the private job market perform?

After a downward trend for some decades, the occupational injury rate began rising in the mid-1950s. By 1970, annual deaths from workplace injuries were estimated to exceed 14,000, with another 2.2 million workers suffering disabling injuries (2). Data on occupational diseases were far less reliable, but even more disturbing. The most commonly cited figures were 390,000 cases of occupational illness annually, resulting in 100,000 fatalities each year, but the actually number of cases and deaths from occupational disease might reasonably have been half or twice those amounts (3). Regardless, the magnitude of occupational risks resulting from marketplace decisions were unnecessarily high and, by almost any standard, far exceeded the social optimum.Furthermore, despite workers' compensation and tentative evidence that workers received a (modest) wage premium for the risks they assumed, worker benefits were not nearly commensurate with workplace hazards, particularly risks of occupational disease (4).

## IMPERFECTIONS IN THE JOB MARKET

What accounts for the job market's disappointing performance? Recall that the efficient and socially optimal functioning of the private market relies, according to economic theory, on four conditions: full information, lack of externalities, perfect competition, and a just and equitable social setting. The failure of the job market to produce socially desirable outcomes reflects the violation of those conditions.

### Imperfect Information

The economist's model of an idealized market system assumes that the participants are fully informed of their options, or able to acquire needed information costlessly. Applied to the job market, this means that workers and employers must know the consequences of any decisions they might make, including the associated workplace risks, in order to negotiate to best advantage. Workers unaware of job hazards would not seek compensation for the risks they bear, and as a result, employers would have insufficient incentives to invest in safer working conditions. Similarly, if employers overestimate the cost of eliminating workplace hazards, then the level of occupational risk to which workers are exposed would exceed the social optimum.

Both experimental and market-related evidence suggests that individuals have considerable difficulty in processing information about low-probability, high-consequence events—such as occupational risks—in a rational manner. For example, individuals systematically underestimate less-publicized risks and risks over which they exercise some control (e.g., some 80% of drivers believe they drive more safely than the average driver), and for life-threatening risks they are inexperienced in valuing, a priori, undesirable outcomes (5). In addition to these problems of risk perception, most individuals are unable to comprehend or rationally act on risk information when presented in the technical language preferred by most risk analysts—such as a 1/100,000 versus a 1/10,000 annual risk of worker death.

Despite these defects in the information process, the private job market may function tolerably in response to many occupational safety hazards. Some working conditions are inherently unsafe and commonly recognized as such. For example, workers can reason that activities involving explosive materials are dangerous. Furthermore, workers develop some, albeit limited, knowledge of the workplace safety hazards confronting them from their own and their co-workers' on-the-job injury experience.

It is in the area of occupational disease that informational deficiencies most seriously compromise the performance of the private job market. Whereas the relationship between an occupational accident and the resultant injury is both obvious and immediate, the connection between the work environment and job-related disease generally is not. Most diseases have multiple potential causes and may be the result of synergistic effects, making it virtually impossible to determine whether an individual's disease is job related rather than an "ordinary disease of life" resulting from lifestyle, genetic, physiologic, or other (nonoccupational) environmental factors. This problem is compounded by the fact that there is frequently a long latency period—sometimes 20 years or more—between exposure to the occupational health hazard and the manifestation of the consequent disease. As a result, a worker usually cannot rely on his knowledge or "intuition" to draw a connection between workplace conditions and a chronic disease, as he could in the case of an acute injury. For example, would a worker attribute his heart attack to cigarette smoking, excess weight, hypertension, or genetic predisposition, or to occupational factors such as exposure to carbon disulfide, on-the-job noise, or other job-related stress?

An additional area of imperfect information in the job market concerns the productivity losses associated with occupational disease. For example, most employers do not realize the extent to which respiratory disorders of occupational origin increase the rate of worker absenteeism or that occupational noise stress adversely affects the quality of workmanship and magnifies the risk of workplace accidents (3). As a result, employers usually underinvest in technologies to reduce such occupational hazards.

### Externalities

Externalities arise when the actions of economic agents impose costs or bestow benefits on other parties that are direct (not those caused indirectly by price adjustments) and that are not recognized in market transactions. The presence of externalities undermines the efficiency of the market because, given the resulting divergence between social and private costs, the market imparts inaccurate signals to economic agents. Workplace health and safety hazards involve significant externalities since many of the costs of occupational injury and illness are borne not by those whose market decisions determine the level of occupational risk, but by the rest of society.

The way in which workers' compensation is financed is one source of externalities. Most employers do not self-insure, but are either class-rated, based on industry-wide safety and health performance, or experienced-rated, which is a class rating adjusted by the individual employer's safety and health performance. These employers' payments to workers' compensation do not fully reflect the costs of their employees' work-related injuries and illnesses. Such risk-spreading features of workers' compensation dampen employers' incentives to improve workplace health and safety (6).

An even larger source of externalities arises from the injury and illness costs not covered by workers' compensation. The dominant problem is that a worker suffering from an occupational disease is rarely awarded any workers' compensation at all because the worker's disease is usually not recognized as job related. To qualify for workers' compensation, a worker must demonstrate by a "preponderance of evidence" (that it is more likely than not) that he was exposed to a workplace hazard and that such exposure caused (or significantly contributed to) the disease (i.e., "arose out of and in the course of employment"). Because of the informational deficiencies, identified earlier, concerning the relationship between occupational hazards and disease, it is often impossible to meet this test, especially for diseases with multiple etiologies.Even if a causal relationship between a hazardous exposure and a disease is known, the worker's history of exposure may be unknown, since exposure frequently occurs a decade or more before disease symptoms appear. The net effect is that fewer than 5% of severely disabled workers who believe their disease is job-related receive workers' compensation benefits—and many workers are themselves unaware their disease is or may be due to exposure to occupational hazards (7,8).

### Imperfect Competition

The economist's idealized market system is predicated on a model of perfect competition. That is, the market for each commodity is assumed to contain such a large number of buyers and such a large number of sellers that no individual economic agent is able, through his actions, to influence the price of the commodity. Each buyer and seller therefore treats prices as given and makes maximizing decisions by comparing marginal gains or losses against the corresponding market price. As a result, the market transmits accurate information about tastes and technology in the form of prices, and prices act as signals in guiding the market decisions of economic agents. The allocative efficiency of the decentralized market system relies on these conditions.

Because of the large number of buyers and sellers of labor services, the job market is frequently considered representative of the economist's conception of a perfectly competitive market. In reality, the job market is not one market, but many markets differentiated by occupation, geography, and other factors. To a greater or lesser degree, many of these job markets violate the conditions necessary for perfect competition, and wages in these markets generally do not adequately reflect the market value of labor services to employers.

A more pervasive source of imperfect competition in job markets is related to the fact that workers are not indifferent between continuing to perform at their present job and being fired, since contrary to the model of perfect competition, they cannot costlessly secure a similar job at the same wage with another employer. Intrafirm promotion and training opportunities, health insurance coverage, pension rights, and wages often depend on job tenure, making the opportunity cost of voluntary job changes prohibitively high. Employers derive market power from the fact that a portion of the compensation they provide to their employees is not transferable to other jobs (since the employees cannot effectively signal their dissatisfaction about workplace risks by threatening to quit). As a consequence, job hazards will be socially excessive.

### Market-Transmitted Injustices or Inequities

Market transactions do not take place in a vacuum. They occur in a social setting with a preexisting distribution of wealth and a specified set of individual rights and obligations that affect market outcomes.

The economist's idealized market system allocates resources efficiently; in an efficient market, it is impossible to reallocate resources in a way that makes someone better off without making someone else worse off. Economists refer to such an allocation of resources as "Pareto optimal" (or, more accurately, "Pareto efficient"). However, as indicated above, the Pareto-optimal allocation of resources generated by the market depends on the preexisting distribution of wealth.

If the initial endowment of wealth were distributed in a socially undesirable manner, then the resulting market outcome would, in all likelihood, not be socially optimal. The poor would sustain too many injuries and illnesses. A socially preferred outcome could, as a rule, be achieved by some more equitable, nonmarket reallocation of resources, even though there would be associated efficiency losses.

In addition, some individual actions are circumscribed by rights and duties that take precedence over market opportunities. Market transactions in such circumstances may be socially unacceptable on ethical grounds, regardless of their voluntary nature. For example, we do not permit individuals to sell themselves into slavery or to bring their children into factories to assist them in earning wages for the family. Similarly, the right to vote and criminal penalties are privileges and sanctions, respectively, which cannot be transferred to others, through the market or otherwise.

The preceding considerations about social justice and equity, applied to the job market, potentially challenge the legitimacy, much less the optimality, of the market-determined level of workplace risk. For example, a socially unacceptable distribution of wealth could (and sometimes does) create a large class of impoverished individuals whose financial desperation makes them willing to perform highly dangerous work. In that case, reducing workplace risk toward the level that would obtain under a more equitable distribution of wealth would be socially preferable to the market-derived level of risk. Furthermore, permitting financially desperate individuals, under such circumstances, to exchange their health and safety for money would be morally unacceptable—even if they consented to and benefited from the transactions—if the source of the financial desperation were itself deemed unjust (in the same sense that "voluntary" blackmail transactions are, nonetheless, morally unacceptable).

## GOVERNMENT INTERVENTION TO REMEDY MARKET IMPERFECTIONS

The preceding discussion demonstrates that the conditions necessary for the private market to produce socially optimal outcomes are violated in the job market. The various defects in the unfettered job market—imperfect information, externalities, imperfect competition, and potential inequities—result in a socially excessive level of workplace risk and create a need for government intervention to correct the market failure.

Government intervention to promote social health and safety objectives is often perceived as taking only one form: the imposition, by the applicable regulatory authority, of mandatory health and safety standards. In reality, the range of policy instruments through which government intervention can be effected is considerably more extensive than simply mandatory standards. Other possible policy instruments include research, education and training, economic charges, financial and tax incentives, insurance (including workers' compensation), and liability rules. These various policy instruments are not necessarily mutually exclusive or independent of one another; they may interact in complex ways to promote workplace health and safety.

One way to categorize policy instruments is according to the market defects they attempt to remedy. Consider, for instance, imperfect information in the job market. Government-conducted or government-sponsored research in the fields of toxicology, epidemiology, and occupational medicine is only one of several policy tools whose purpose is to address imperfect information. Another is government research to improve the knowledge base concerning the prevention of work-related injury and disease. Several other policy instruments attempt to rectify information-dissemination deficiencies in the job market through right-to-know legislation and regulation. Other examples of information-enhancing interventions include government-supported training and education of occupational physicians and nurses, industrial hygienists, safety engineers, business managers, and other professionals concerned with occupational health and safety; direct worker training and education in hazard recognition and control; and government-conducted or government-funded demonstration projects to inform firms of available hazard-reducing technologies.

A diverse set of policy instruments might be deployed to remove job-market externalities created by workplace hazards. One practical approach would be to levy an economic charge on the employer based on the amount of hazardous material present in the workplace, or better yet, on the level of worker exposure to hazardous substances. Other ways of removing externalities caused by workplace hazards include modifying the workers' compensation system and the tort system so that employers and suppliers responsible for workplace injuries and disease pay a larger share of the associated costs. For example, the workers' compensation system might increase the degree of experience-rating and institute employer deductibles or copayments, and both the workers' compensation system and the tort system might relax evidentiary requirements to establish the worker-relatedness of the individual's illness. Finally, rather than removing externalities, the government may provide employers with positive tax incentives or financial assistance to stimulate investment in occupational health and safety—thereby neutralizing employer disincentives occasioned by the externalities. These policy instruments include investment tax credits, accelerated depreciation, government loan programs, and direct subsidies or grants to firms making investments to reduce occupational hazards.

Government policies to address imperfect competition in the job market tend to be the identical policies that remedy social inequities transmitted through the job market. For example, government programs to train the unemployed or to retrain workers have the dual effect of improving job mobility—that is, increasing competition among employers in the job market—and enhancing the equity of (primarily) disadvantaged citizens. Similarly, programs to redistribute wealth to the poorest members of society also provide them the economic resources to acquire job skills or to move to areas where job opportunities are more favorable—that is, these programs expand their occupational and geographic mobility.

In contrast to mandatory health and safety standards, the aforementioned policy instruments attempt to correct, to the extent possible, the functioning of the job market rather than to supplant the market process. Maintaining market-like private incentives may offer significant efficiency gains in a decision-making arena as potentially complex and dynamic as the workplace. Whereas a well-functioning job market can provide the socially preferred level of workplace health and safety at lowest cost, mandatory standards (e.g., specification standards for safety equipment) may lock in uniform technological choices that, for many employers, are neither statically nor dynamically efficient.

Nevertheless, workplace health and safety standards may, in some cases, preserve much of the flexibility of the market. For example, the imposition of a hazard communication standard, which requires that dangerous substances in the workplace be clearly labeled (and that workers receive training concerning them), attempts to ensure that workers have access to job-risk information (and can understand it), but entrusts the determination of occupational health and safety outcomes to the workings of the market. Similarly, performance standards specifying the maximum allowable level of worker exposure to designated hazardous substances allow the firm to select the low-cost means of compliance.

Even so-called design or engineering standards, which specify the precise characteristics that the workplace or workplace equipment must meet, may contain flexible elements. The regulatory authority may make fine distinctions in applying design standards, for instance on the basis of firm size, new versus existing plants, or the nature of the production process. Similarly, the regulatory authority can target inspection rates and the size of penalties for regulatory violations according to policy-relevant attributes (e.g., the expected magnitude of health consequences associated with a specific violation). In addition, the firm may be permitted compliance exemptions on the basis of desirable market performance. An obvious example is the innovation waiver, which encourages firms to develop new technologies that are either more effective than the design standard, less costly, or both (9).

## COST-BENEFIT ANALYSIS

The various types of government intervention identified above are, separately and in combination, capable of reducing the socially excessive level of workplace risk produced by the defective functioning of the private job market, but they will normally impose social costs as well. Government decision makers have the responsibility of identifying which, if any, public policies concerning workplace health and safety will, on balance, make society "better off" in some meaningful sense, and of selecting from among them the policy or mix of policies that will provide the largest social improvement. The key underlying issue is what analytic technique is appropriate for evaluating social states before and after the enactment of (alternative) government policies.

During the past two decades, cost-benefit analysis has become the dominant method used by policy makers to evaluate government intervention in the areas of health and safety. As conceived in theory, cost-benefit analysis (a) enumerates all possible consequences, both positive and negative, that might arise in response to the implementation of a candidate government policy; (b) estimates the probability of each consequence occurring; (c) estimates the benefit or loss to society should each occur, expressed in monetary terms; (d) computes the expected social benefit or loss from each possible consequence by multiplying the amount of the associated benefit or loss by its probability of occurrence; and (e) computes the net expected social benefit or loss associated with the government policy by summing over the various possible consequences. The reference point for these calculations is the social state in the absence of the government policy, termed the "baseline."

All of the consequences of a candidate policy are described fully in terms of the times during which they occur. What cost-benefit analysis does is translate all of these consequences into "equivalent" monetary units (since a dollar in an earlier time period could be invested to earn interest over time) by discounting each to present value and aggregating them into a single dollar value intended to express the net social effect of the government policy.

The cost-benefit calculation can be expressed in simple mathematical terms by the following equation:

$$V = \sum_{i=1}^{n} \sum_{j=1}^{m} \frac{(B_{ij} - C_{ij})}{(1+r)^i} \quad [1]$$

where $B_{ij}$ and $C_{ij}$ are the $j$th type of policy benefit and cost, respectively, in the $i$th year after the policy is introduced and $B$ and $C$ are expressed in monetary units; $r$ is the appropriate discount rate; and $V$ is the (discounted) present value of the policy.

When there is only one policy option, cost-benefit analysis dictates that option should be implemented only if its anticipated net social effect is positive. In general, however, numerous policies or sets of policies are possible, where each policy can be differentiated according to the various features—type of policy instrument, policy level or stringency, firms covered, etc.—that compose it. In this situation, according to the cost-benefit criterion, the policy with the largest expected net social benefit, when compared to the baseline, should be implemented.

As a decision-making tool, cost-benefit analysis offers several compelling advantages. First, cost-benefit analysis clarifies choices among alternatives by evaluating consequences in a systematic and rational manner. Second, it professes to foster an open and fair policy-making process by making explicit the estimates of costs and benefits and the assumptions on which those estimates are based. Third, by expressing all of the gains and losses in monetary terms, discounted to their present value, cost-benefit analysis permits the total impact of a policy to be summarized using a common metric and represented by a single dollar amount.

As a practical matter, however, cost-benefit analysis possesses several serious limitations. The remainder of this chapter explores these limitations. We note, however, the ensuing dissection of cost-benefit analysis is not intended to suggest a wholesale rejection of the technique, but to caution against the uncritical application of an imperfect methodology and the unqualified acceptance of its results.

### Problems in Estimating Public Policy Benefits

The benefits of a specific government policy concerning occupational health and safety are generally the reduced social costs associated with a decrease in the number (or severity) of job-related injuries and illnesses, where the decrease is brought about by the policy in question. Prominent examples of policy benefits include reductions in medical expenses, productivity losses, physical disability, pain and suffering, and loss of life. Estimation of the policy benefits in cost-benefit analysis is a formidable task because it is difficult to predict the reduced risk of injury and disease and to monetize the associated benefits.

There are many problems in trying to determine the effects of a government policy on the incidence of job-related injuries and disease. The baseline occupational risks may not be scientifically established. In most cases, the precise relationship between exposure and disease is simply not known. Estimating the effects of the policy on worker exposure levels may also be rather uncertain, depending as it does on assumptions about firm and worker behavior as well as on technical production relationships.

Additionally, many of the benefits of government policy, such as reductions in physical disability, pain and suffering, and loss of life, have no clearly defined economic value (as compared to the market prices established for labor and medical services). The traditional methods of monetizing these benefits—surveys and market studies—have been, to a large extent, unsuccessful. Interviews and questionnaires asking individuals what they would be willing to pay for a stated reduction in risk have inherent limitations since answers to hypothetical questions have been shown to be poor indicators of a person's behavior. Imputing the value of risk reduction from an individual's market behavior is also a seriously flawed approach (10). Individual actions are normally undertaken for a variety of reasons, and it is difficult to isolate what portion is motivated by a desire to reduce the risk of bodily impairment, pain and suffering, or a premature death. Furthermore, consumers are rarely well-informed about the risks confronting them and have a well-documented history of being unable to process the risk information at their disposal in an expected manner (11–13). As a result, the assumption of economic efficiency underlying attempts to value risks from consumer market decisions is untenable in practice.

Where policy analysts have most frequently turned to derive the value of a reduction in risk is the job market itself. Recall that, according to economic theory, the risk-compensating wage premium represents the workers' valuation of job risk. But the same job market imperfections that produce a socially excessive level of workplace risk and create a need for government intervention also undermine the usefulness of the risk premium as a measure of the worker's risk valuation. For example, job-related diseases that the worker does not know about will not be reflected in the wage premium for risk. Moreover, workers may have difficulty in understanding risk information. In theory, they are just as likely to overreact as underreact to hazard information, but in practice, worker risk perception appears to be dominated by an "it-can't-happen-to-me" attitude (3). This results in known risks being understated and therefore undervalued. Another job market defect, externalities, causes the observed wage premium for risk to measure only the worker's valuation of an incremental risk, but not the value family members, friends, and other interested parties attach to the risk. Furthermore, models of the risk-compensating wage differential assume a perfectly competitive job market; violation of this assumption means that the resulting estimates will "misinterpret" the true wage premium for risk. This is a particularly serious problem, since there may be no way to adjust the estimates to correct for the misspecification.

### Problems in Estimating Public Policy Costs

Although the costs imposed by a government policy seem rather easy to identify and to express in economic terms, they are usually no more certain or reliable than the benefits. One reason is that policy analysts rarely have access to detailed, independent information about actual and potential production relationships and associated costs in an industry. Instead, they must depend to a large extent on industry-provided data to develop estimates of the costs to industry of complying with the public policy. Since higher compliance costs make a policy less attractive, industries adversely affected by the policy may choose to inflate their reported compliance costs.

In addition, compliance cost estimates often fail to take three significant factors into account: (a) economies of scale, which reflect the fact that an increase in the level of production of compliance technology often reduces unit costs; (b) the ability of industry to learn over time to comply more cost-effectively—what the management scientists refer to as the learning curve; and (c) compliance costs based on present technological capabilities ignore the role played by technological innovation in reducing those costs (9). The last factor is particularly crucial: a recent retrospective analysis of eight Occupational Safety and Health Administration (OSHA) regulations issued between 1974 and 1989 concluded that the agency's estimates of economic impacts systematically and significantly overestimated compliance costs by ignoring the innovative response of industry to the enacted standards (14).

### Problems of Equity and Ethics

Policy decisions regarding the level of workplace risk rely fundamentally on considerations of equity and concern for individual justice. Yet, traditional cost-benefit analysis is unable to address these issues or, relatedly, to assess whether implementation of a government policy truly constitutes an improvement in social welfare.

The economist's normative standard is Pareto optimality—achieving a situation in which it is impossible to make someone better off without making someone else worse off (because all mutually beneficial exchanges will already have occurred). The cost-benefit criterion closely resembles the test of Pareto optimality. If the net effects of a government policy are positive, then those who gain as a result of the policy *could* pay off those who lose and still have some benefits left over for themselves. Potentially, no one loses and at least some gain. But a *potential* Pareto is not the same as an *actual* Pareto improvement unless the redistribution of benefits to the losers actually takes place. Hence, cost-benefit analysis carries no normative weight as a measure of a policy's effects on social welfare.

For some types of government policy, of course, the distributional consequences are negligible; in such instances, the cost-benefit criterion may serve as a reasonable indicator of real Pareto improvements. However, many workers risk their health and safety, and frequently their lives, to perform tasks for which, because of market imperfections, they are inadequately compensated. Furthermore, the workers at risk are not a random cross section of the general population; they represent a disproportionate share of the poor and unskilled, that sector of society with the smallest preexisting endowment of wealth. Thus, for government policies involving workplace hazards, the distributional effects are likely to be substantial, in which case cost-benefit analysis will be an unsatisfactory measure of Pareto improvements.

In addition, certain policy effects are not intrinsically economic, but concern more fundamental social attributes, such as individual rights and justice. The procedure of quantifying and monetizing these attributes, as part of a cost-benefit analysis, is more likely to obfuscate and misconstrue their essential qualities than to clarify their values. (For example, what monetary value should society place on protecting all workers equally, although it may be less costly and more cost-effective to protect workers in new plants more than workers in old plants?)

Whether, and to what extent, policies concerning workplace health and safety involve individual rights is assuredly a controversial matter. The central issue seems to revolve around whether workers voluntarily accept job risks (for which they are compensated). Clearly, "voluntary" and "involuntary" are not absolutes; these terms must be evaluated within a specific social context and relative to some operational standard. Nevertheless, voluntary transactions would seem to require some acceptable degree of information and the absence of coercion or desperation. Therefore, to the extent that workers have no desirable job opportunities because of their social background and education, are denied pertinent information about job hazards or are unable to assess risks rationally, and are unable to respond to acquired and understood risk information because of geographic or occupational immobility or other employment impediments, these workers cannot be said to have voluntary choices (15).

### Other Misuses and Abuses

In addition to the inherent limitations of cost-benefit analysis already discussed, the use of cost-benefit analysis, in practice, has raised a host of other interrelated problems, among them suboptimization, quantification bias, "bottom-line" myopia, and the politicization of cost-benefit analysis as a decision-making tool.

*Suboptimization* has been defined as discovering the best way to do things that might better be left undone (16). Cost-benefit analysis could fall prey to suboptimization for either of two reasons. First, the cost-benefit analysis might unwittingly neglect superior policy options. For instance, policies concerned with the design of personal protective equipment to reduce worker exposure to hazardous materials may ignore the possibility of redesigning the production process so as to remove the workplace hazard entirely. Second, cost-benefit analysis is an "instrumental technique," concerned not with selecting ultimate societal ends, but merely with helping to choose the best means to achieve those ends (17). A policy satisfying the cost-benefit criterion might still be socially undesirable because the policy objective itself is suboptimal. For example, a policy to limit worker risks in disposing of radioactive wastes from nuclear power plants overlooks the larger question of whether nuclear power production is a socially desirable activity. If not, then the best policy to limit worker exposure to radioactive wastes is not to create them in the first place.

*Quantification bias* refers to the tendency of many policy analysts to identify policy effects that are difficult to quantify or to express in monetary terms—such as distributional impacts or violations of individual rights—but to omit these effects entirely in the ensuing cost-benefit calculations. What this does, in essence, is to impose a value of zero on those policy effects for which no objective economic value is available, even though those effects may be of larger social significance than all of the monetized consequences combined. An illustration of quantification bias is the practice, popularized in recent years by some economists, of evaluating a regulation based solely on its cost per life saved. The problem with this approach is that it ignores all other benefits of a regulation, such as environmental amenities as well as reductions in the number of injuries. For instance, according to this approach, the most inefficient regulation, by far, is OSHA's 1987 formaldehyde standard (18). Yet when the benefits of injury reduction are included, the formaldehyde standard—which prevents approximately 30,000 illnesses for every life saved—has been demonstrated to be enormously cost-effective and socially beneficial (19).

*"Bottom-line" myopia* concerns the double-edged property of cost-benefit analysis to be able to express the total (expected) effect of a policy in a single dollar amount. The summary cost-benefit value makes alternative government policies commensurate and facilitates comparisons among them, but it does so at a price. Collapsing the various consequences of a policy into a single, bottom-line value does not reveal the myriad assumptions and data on which that value is based; it compresses them and removes them from view. As a practical matter, policy makers and the public are apt to accept the summary value of cost-benefit analysis as gospel without considering the plausibility of the underlying assumptions and the accuracy of the supporting data, particularly when such information is not readily available. Similarly, the uncertainty surrounding the estimates of the costs and the benefits, the sensitivity of the expected policy impacts to specific assumptions and data, and the "confidence interval" that represents the range within which the true effect of the policy will probably fall are all matters to be considered in making policy decisions, but they are suppressed by the reduction of the cost-benefit details to a single bottom-line value. For example, even minute changes in the (often controversial) choice of discount rate reflecting the time value of money may have a profound effect on the estimated impact of a policy. But unless this information accompanies the bottom-line value, the results of the cost-benefit analysis, for policy-making purposes, are liable to be misleading and misunderstood. In that case, rather than promoting rational, candid policy making, cost-benefit analysis exposes the policy-making process to potential abuse.

*The politicization of cost-benefit analysis* is one of the ways in which the policy-making process can be abused. Political groups, in the hope of furthering ideological or special interests, may endeavor to influence both the cost-benefit estimates of policy impacts and how those estimates are used in policy making. In the former case, policy analysts with a vested interest in the outcome might attempt to "construct" the cost-benefit analysis so as to arrive at a predetermined outcome. Note that unless the underlying assumptions and data are revealed and subject to public scrutiny, the manipulation of the estimation procedure is liable to go unnoticed. In the latter case, the abuse of the policy-making process is normally accomplished by imposing a cost-benefit decision rule on the policy maker that, in effect, circumvents government checks and balances. Using the cost-benefit criterion as a decision rule for policies whose estimated impacts have been influenced by politically motivated "guidance" subverts rather than promotes the democratic process. Democratic policy making is threatened with replacement by political tactics whose purpose is to reorient legislative mandates to serve narrow interests. The policy maker's ability to make decisions is compromised, and his accountability eroded. In short, as a decision rule, cost-benefit analysis no longer clarifies and facilitates the democratic process, but becomes a substitute for it.

## CONCLUSIONS

We have described above the various theoretical and practical shortcomings of cost-benefit analysis, although its basic objective and approach—to help evaluate government policy by enumerating all of its consequences—are arguably desirable. Unfortunately, many of the admitted limitations of cost-benefit analysis are, in fact, unavoidable by-products of any such systematic approach to decision making. For example, the imprecision of the cost-benefit estimates of policy impacts involving workplace hazards simply mirrors the technical uncertainties and the social complexities surrounding the problem. Obviously, more accurate estimates of impacts could be achieved by improved scientific methods and knowledge, but the same could be said for any policy evaluation technique, not just cost-benefit analysis.

The fact that an objective, unambiguously correct assessment of policy impacts cannot be guaranteed reinforces the importance of the process by which a particular assessment is performed. It is in this area—the evaluative process—that cost-benefit analysis is most vulnerable. The process of conducting a cost-benefit analysis forces the policy analyst to make explicit assumptions and data choices. However, in practice, collapsing the policy impacts ultimately into a single, bottom-line value has tended to conceal the underlying assumptions and supportive data from public examination.

One way to remedy this problem is for policy analysts to acknowledge the limitations of their craft and to provide policy makers and the public not merely the bottom-line expected value, but in addition, a meaningful critique of the policy evaluation exercise, including uncertainties, confidence intervals, and the sensitivity of the results to specific assumptions and data choices. Even if this were to be done, however, the specter of political misuse and abuse of cost-benefit analysis remains a viable threat.

A possible method for defusing the threat is to have the policy analyst calculate the various policy consequences without translating the various economic, health, and other effects into a single dollar metric; without discounting them to present value; and without summing the benefits and costs accruing to actors in order to come up with a net benefit or a benefit-to-cost ratio. The consequences, when presented in disaggregated form, permit decision makers to examine the real policy trade-offs, guided by the social expression of preferences provided in the law. Such a "trade-off" analysis avoids unnecessarily obscuring the differences between noncommensurables such as economic commodities, risks to life, and individual rights, or between those who benefit and those who suffer from the public policy (20). This type of analysis not only exposes to public scrutiny the policy analyst's disaggregated estimates, and the assumptions and data on which they are based; it also forces the policy maker to comply with legislative mandates and to make explicit his value judgments and trade-offs, thereby preventing him from abdicating responsibility for his decisions. In this way, instead of compromising congressional intent, economic analysis can contribute to furthering legislative goals in occupational health and safety, environmental preservation, economic growth, and technological advance.

## ACKNOWLEDGMENT

This chapter draws heavily from Chapter 5 of reference 20.

## REFERENCES

1. *Preventing illness and injury in the workplace.* (OTA-H-256). Washington, DC: U.S. Congress, Office of Technology Assessment, 1985.
2. *Accident facts.* Washington, DC: United States National Safety Council, 1972.
3. Ashford NA. *Crisis in the workplace:* occupational disease and injury. Cambridge, MA: MIT Press, 1976.
4. Ashford NA, Stone RF. *Cost-benefit analysis in environmental decision-making:* theoretical considerations and applications to protection of stratospheric ozone. Washington: DC: U.S. Environmental Protection Agency, 1988.
5. Slovic P, Fischhoff B, Lichtenstein S. Informing the public about the risks from ionizing radiation. *Health Phys* 1981;41:589–598.
6. Ashford NA. Workers' compensation. In: Rom WN, ed. *Environmental and occupational medicine,* 3rd ed. Philadelphia: Lippincott–Raven, 1998.
7. *An interim report to the Congress on occupational diseases.* Washington, DC: United States Department of Labor, 1980.
8. Viscusi WK. Liability for occupational accidents and illnesses. In: Litan RE, Winston C, eds. *Liability:* perspectives and policy. Washington, DC: Brookings Institution, 1988.
9. Ashford NA, Ayers C, Stone RF. Using regulation to change the market for innovation. *Harvard Environ Law Rev* 1985;9:419–465.
10. Fischer GW, Willingness to pay for probabilistic improvements in functional health status: a psychological perspective. In: Mushkin SJ, Dunlop DW, eds. *Health:* What is it worth? Measures of health benefits. New York: Pergamon Press, 1979.
11. Tversky A, Kahneman D. Judgment under uncertainty: heuristics and biases. *Science* 1974;185:458–468.
12. Fischhoff B. Cost benefit analysis and the art of motorcycle maintenance. *Policy Sci* 1977;8:177–202.
13. Machina MJ. Choice under uncertainty: problems solved and unsolved. *J Econ Perspect* 1987;1:121–154.
14. *Gauging control technology and regulatory impacts in occupational safety and health—an appraisal of OSHA's analytic approach.* (OTA-ENV-635). Washington, DC: U.S. Congress, Office of Technology Assessment, 1995.
15. Caldart CC. Promises and pitfalls of workplace right-to-know. *Semin Occup Med* 1986;1:81–90.
16. Boulding KE. Fun and games with the gross national product: the role of misleading indicators in social policy. In: Roelofs RT, Crowley JN, Hardesty DL, eds. *Environment and society.* Englewood Cliffs, NJ: Prentice-Hall, 1974.
17. Tribe LH. Technology assessment and the fourth discontinuity. *Southern Cal Law Rev* 1973;46:3.
18. Viscusi WK. Economic foundations of the current regulatory reform efforts. *J Econ Perspect* 1996;10:119–134.
19. Stone RF. Correspondence: benefit-cost analysis. *J Econ Perspect* 1997;11:187–188.
20. Ashford NA, Caldard CC. *Technology, law, and the working environment.* Washington, DC: Island Press, 1996.

*Environmental and Occupational Medicine, Third Edition,* edited by William N. Rom.
Lippincott–Raven Publishers, Philadelphia © 1998.

# CHAPTER 127

# Risk Assessment

Roger O. McClellan

Risk assessment is the process of characterizing and quantifying potential adverse effects on humans of exposure to chemicals, physical agents, or situations that pose a health hazard. The concept of risk assessment is not new—we have always had to make decisions about risks in the course of our daily lives. Relatively new, however, is the shift from concern for immediate hazards with readily discernible linkages between a specific hazardous situation and an adverse outcome to situations where there are only probabilistic linkages between exposure to an agent and the occurrence of an adverse effect over a long period of time. The legendary coal miners' canary illustrates a readily discernible linkage between poor air quality and acute asphyxiation. The need to set standards for toxic materials for protection against lung cancer risks of 1 in $10^6$ over a lifetime represents the other extreme. The heavy cigarette smoker who knows that the odds of developing lung cancer late in life are 1 in 10 and yet continues to smoke represents an intermediate paradox.

Risk assessment as it is now practiced has multiple roots. One of these roots was the early concern for the safety of workers and the use of human experience to establish workplace practices that minimized the potential for adverse effects on health. Examples are the earliest threshold limit values established by the American Conference of Governmental Industrial Hygienists (ACGIH). A second root relates to the field of food safety in which the results of controlled animal studies were extrapolated to humans using safety factors. The third root relates to the radiation field, where major use was made of quantitative analyses to estimate potential adverse consequences of radiation exposure.

R. O. McClellan: Chemical Industry Institute of Toxicology, Research Triangle Park, North Carolina 27709.

The earliest safety models, including those for radiation exposure, were based on the assumption of a threshold relationship between exposure or dose and the health response of concern. Over time there was a subtle but important change in terminology with the word *risk* being used instead of *safety.* With this model, no response is expected below a specified exposure or dose, while responses are expected above the threshold. Two new discoveries emerged in the mid–20th century that challenged the threshold dose-response model. The first was the discovery that radiation is an effective genetic toxicant. The second was the discovery that DNA is the genetic material that transfers encoded information for cell structure and function from generation to generation of both cells and organisms.

For radiation it was soon recognized that genetic damage was produced in the form of mutations in both germ and somatic cells. Mutations in germ cells could be transmitted to subsequent generations, while mutations in somatic cells could be transmitted to cell progeny and ultimately result in cancer. Observations relating dose to response were soon made, and various empirical and biologically based models were developed to describe dose-response relationships over the range of observations. Most significantly, linear extrapolations to lower doses were made on the theoretical assumption that the smallest quantity of radiation dose had an associated level of calculable risk for induction of mutations, cancer, and genetic defects. Moreover, the risk for a population could be calculated by summing the risk for the individuals in the population no matter how small the individual's risks might be. The calculated levels of risk were frequently for readily measurable exposures that nonetheless had associated levels of risk well below those that could actually be observed and differentiated from the background level of cancer. Because of statistical limitations imposed on the development of experimental or epidemiologic observations, the possibility could not be excluded that the actual risk was zero at some low level of dose.

Quantitation of exposure-dose-response relationships in the field of chemical toxicology and carcinogenesis generally lagged behind those in the radiation field. However, the concept soon emerged that certain chemicals had electrophilic characteristics and associated interactions with DNA that mimicked those of radiation and were therefore capable of causing genetic mutations and cancer in a manner analogous to that of radiation. For risk assessment purposes, as will be noted later, a major default assumption emerged: chemicals, like radiation, could also produce calculable levels of risk at the lowest levels of exposure.

With the above as background, let us now examine the risk paradigm and how it is used to assess occupational and environmental risks.

## RISK PARADIGM

The risk paradigm, as now widely used in the United States and increasingly in other countries, is depicted schematically in Fig. 1 (1,2). It consists of four interrelated activities: risk research, risk assessment, risk management, and risk communication. This formalized structure was heavily influenced by recommendations of a 1983 National Research Council (NRC) report, *Risk Assessment in the Federal Government:* Managing the Process (1). The report delineated the four-step risk assessment process: (a) hazard identification—Does the agent cause an adverse effect?; (b) dose-response assessment—What is the relationship between dose and incidence in humans?; (c) exposure assessment—What exposures are currently experienced or anticipated under different conditions?; and (d) risk characterization—What is the estimated incidence of the adverse effect in a given population?

In Fig. 1, the dose-response component has been expanded to include exposure-dose-response linkages based on recognition that exposure and dose are not always equivalent. In dealing with airborne materials, physical and chemical characteristics such as particle size and valence state can markedly influence the dose (the quantity of the material or its metabolites) reaching a critical organ or tissue.

The risk paradigm has also been expanded to explicitly include a feedback loop from risk assessment to risk research. The feedback loop serves as a reminder that the major uncertainties identified when risk is characterized represent research needs that, if addressed, can reduce the uncertainty in future risk assessments. And finally, the paradigm has been expanded to explicitly include risk communication, an essential but often overlooked portion of the risk paradigm.

Another committee of the NRC reviewed the U.S. Environmental Protection Agency (EPA) approach to assessing the risks of a large number of hazardous air pollutants and produced a report, *Science and Judgment in Risk Assessment* (2) that endorsed the risk paradigm laid out in 1983. The report also emphasized the importance of characterizing both uncertainty (the limits of what we know and do not know) and variability (the range of measurements of what we do know). It also emphasized the value of the feedback loop in helping to

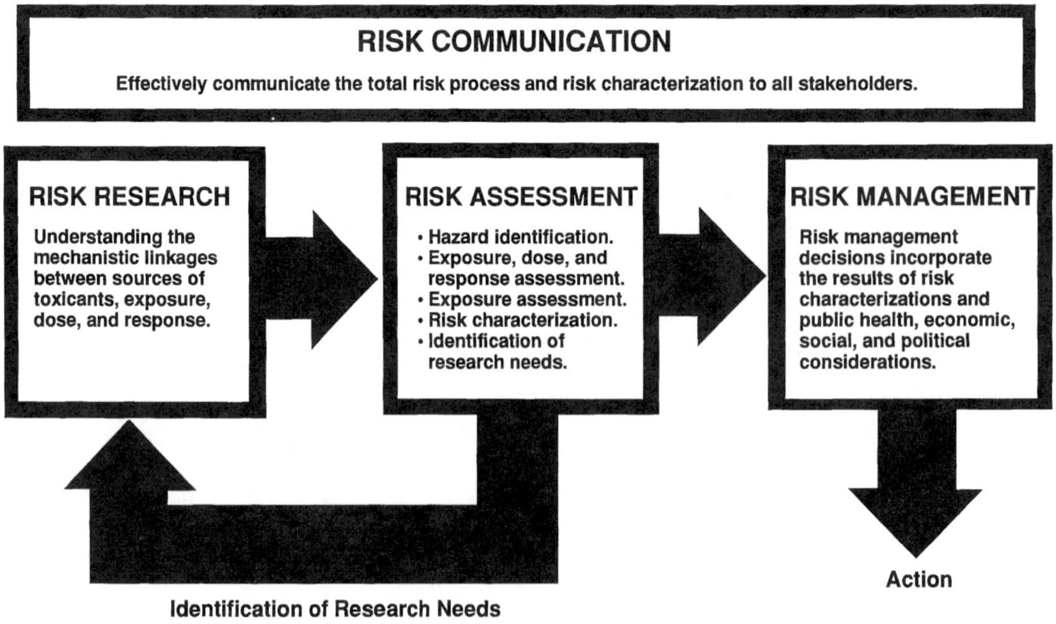


**FIG. 1.** The risk paradigm expanded from versions published by the National Research Council (1,2).

improve the scientific information available for assessing human risks of chemical exposures.

Approaches to assessing the health risks of exposure can be divided into those for which the primary concern is cancer and those for which the concerns are for adverse functional changes and diseases other than cancer. The EPA has developed guidelines for assessing the risk of cancer (3) and recently proposed revised cancer risk guidelines (4). Guidelines are available for other effects such as neurotoxicity (5), immunotoxicity (6), reproductive toxicity (7), developmental toxicity (8), and inhalation toxicity (9).

## SOURCES OF INFORMATION

There are various sources of information for conducting human risk assessments (Fig. 2). Since the goal is to develop risk assessments for humans, maximum use should be made of any human data that are available, including results from epidemiologic studies. Such data frequently have two limitations: first, exposures have usually been poorly characterized; second, statistical limitations preclude positive observations at low exposure levels and minimize the interpretation of negative findings. If there is strong evidence that exposure to the material will not cause irreversible effects, conducting controlled exposure studies in humans may be ethically feasible.

The findings of adverse effects in the past from exposure to specific agents or work processes has served as a warning, and increasingly a proactive approach is being used to assess the human health risks of new products and technologies at an early stage before the material or process is widely used and there is potential for the occurrence of adverse human experience. This proactive approach places an emphasis on obtaining toxicologic information from in vitro studies of cells and tissues from humans and laboratory animals and from in vivo studies conducted with various species of laboratory animals.

Ultimately, the success of the proactive approach will be judged by the outcome of future epidemiologic studies done for surveillance purposes. Studies with a negative outcome, while not precluding some level of effect below statistical limits of detection, will still be reassuring. Positive studies that detect a statistically significant association between human exposure and adverse health outcome will represent a failure of our proactive approach to adequately control human exposure. Should such untoward circumstances be detected, the circumstances can be critically evaluated to provide input for revisions in our approach to proactive toxicologic evaluation, risk assessment, and exposure control. For example, the unfortunate experience with the pharmaceutical agent thalidomide stimulated a change in our approach to assessing developmental toxicity.

Figure 2 has purposefully been drawn to emphasize the integrative nature of the process of hazard or risk characterization. One of the major challenges that is increasingly being encountered is how to utilize data from in vitro assays in the risk assessment process. This can be illustrated with two different kinds of assays, one for mutagenicity and the other for endocrine modulating activity. Recognition of the key role of mutagenicity in the complex process of carcinogenicity stimulated the development of mutagenicity assays. Perhaps the best known of these is the Ames assay developed by Bruce

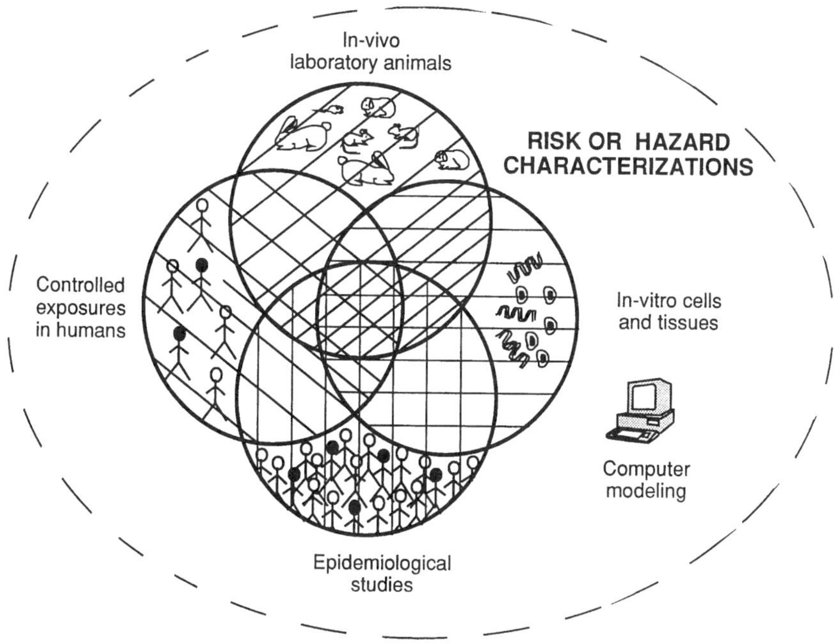


**FIG. 2.** Schematic representation of sources of information for a proactive approach to risk or hazard characterization.

Ames and associates (10). This assay system uses strains of *Salmonella* bacteria that have induced mutations to assay for a test agent's potential to reverse-mutate the cells. The results of the assay are typically reported in qualitative fashion as positive or negative for mutagenicity. Many individuals view the mutagenicity findings as indicative of the cancer-causing potential of the chemical. More recently, concern has developed for chemicals having the potential to mimic naturally occurring hormones. This has led to legislation calling for development of screening tests. One approach that has been reported uses yeast strains with DNA introduced from humans or laboratory animals to encode for hormone receptors such as those for estrogen, androgen, and progesterone (11). These systems, such as the estrogen receptor assay, are exquisitely sensitive for detection of binding of both naturally occurring and synthetic chemicals to the hormone receptor at potencies equal to that of estradiol down to five or six orders of magnitude less than that of estradiol. Ultimately, in vitro findings such as those from the *Salmonella* and yeast assays must be interpreted for their relevance in assessing human risks in vivo at plausible levels of human exposure.

A somewhat similar situation arises in the interpretation of the results of in vivo laboratory animal studies. Such studies frequently use as the highest dose level the maximum tolerated dose (MTD) of the chemical, a quantity that produces some evidence of toxicity but minimal mortality in short-term studies of up to 90 days. The MTD is selected without concern for the relevance of the animal exposure level to human exposures, which are frequently many orders of magnitude lower than plausible human exposures. The objective of the earliest studies conducted by the National Toxicology Program (NTP) was to detect carcinogens without concern for exposure-response relationship issues. The experimental design using the MTD was intended to maximize statistical power when only 50 animals per sex and species (typically mice and rats) could be used at each exposure level. The legacies of this program are many cancer bioassay results that are qualitatively evaluated as indicating no, equivocal, some, or clear evidence of carcinogenicity, as will be discussed later. The significance of the carcinogenic responses in rodents exposed at the MTD for human risk assessment has been a topic of much debate (12).

## CANCER CLASSIFICATION SCHEMES

Cancer caused by chemicals and radiation has been a dominant concern in the fields of occupational and environmental health during the past 30 years. Early cancer risk assessments focused on whether or not a chemical or an industrial occupation posed a carcinogenic hazard based on epidemiologic evidence. Later, the assessments were broadened to include evidence for carcinogenic hazard based on laboratory animal studies. As multiple sources of evidence were considered, the process became more complex, and the need for a more formalized structure arose.

On the international front, the International Agency for Research on Cancer (IARC) initiated a program in 1969 to evaluate the carcinogenic hazards of agents and occupations. The results of the evaluations are published in a series of monographs (13,14). The IARC program has had major international impact because of the prominence of the organization as an arm of the World Health Organization and the authoritative nature of the reviews. Although IARC is not a regulatory agency per se, the IARC classifications are widely used as basis for action by government agencies around the world.

The IARC approach to evaluation of carcinogenic hazards is briefly described in the preamble to each monograph. The actual evaluations are carried out by international working groups of experts with assistance from the IARC staff. In the monographs, the term *carcinogenic* is used to denote an agent or a process that is capable of increasing the incidence of malignant neoplasms under some exposure condition.

The IARC evaluation considers four types of data: (a) exposure data, (b) human carcinogenicity data, (c) experimental animal carcinogenicity data, and (d) other data relevant to an evaluation of carcinogenicity and its mechanisms. The monographs summarize all the information used in the evaluations and do not necessarily summarize all the published studies.

The epidemiologic evidence is classified into four categories:

1. *Sufficient evidence of carcinogenicity*—a causal relationship has been established between exposure to the agent and human cancer.
2. *Limited evidence of carcinogenicity*—a positive association between exposure to an agent and human cancer is considered to be credible, but chance, bias, or confounding could not be ruled out with reasonable confidence.
3. *Inadequate evidence of carcinogenicity*—the available studies are of insufficient quality, consistency, or statistical power to permit a conclusion regarding the presence or absence of a causal association.
4. *Evidence suggesting lack of carcinogenicity*—there are several adequate studies covering the full range of doses to which human beings are known to be exposed; these studies must be mutually consistent in not showing a positive association between exposure and any studied cancer at any observed level of exposure.

The IARC evaluation process also gives substantial weight to carcinogenicity data from laboratory animals. The preamble to the IARC report notes that all known human carcinogens that have been studied adequately in experimental animals have produced positive results in one or more animal species (15,16). The preamble also notes that for some 24 agents or exposure situations (including cyclophosphamide, estrogens, and vinyl chloride), the evidence of carcinogenicity was first established or became highly suspect from studies in laboratory animals and was then confirmed in human studies (17). The preamble to the IARC report (18) goes on to state:

> Although this association cannot establish that all agents and mixtures that cause cancer in experimental animals also cause cancer in humans, nevertheless, in the absence of adequate data on humans, it is biologically plausible and prudent to regard agents and mixtures for which there is sufficient evidence of carcinogenicity in experimental animals as if they presented a carcinogenic risk to humans. The possibility that a given agent may cause cancer through a species-specific mechanism which does not operate in humans should also be taken into consideration. [p. 21]

The IARC classifies the strength of the animal evidence of carcinogenicity in experimental animals in a manner analogous to that used for human data. Particular attention is to be given to mechanistic data that may strengthen the plausibility of the conclusion that the agent being evaluated is carcinogenic to humans. Experimental animal evidence is placed in one of four categories much as is done for human evidence. Category 1, sufficient evidence of carcinogenicity, is used when the working group considers that a causal relationship has been established between an agent and an increased incidence of malignant neoplasms or an appropriate combination of benign and malignant neoplasms in (a) two or more species of animals or (b) two or more independent studies in one species carried out at different times, in different laboratories, or under different protocols. A single study in one species might be considered under exceptional circumstances to provide sufficient evidence when malignant neoplasms occur to an unusual degree with regard to incidence, site, type of tumor, or age at onset.

Supporting evidence includes a range of information such as structure-activity correlations, toxicologic information, and data on kinetics, metabolism, and genotoxicity from laboratory animals, humans, and lower levels of biologic organization such as tissues and cells.

In 1991, the IARC convened a special panel to consider how mechanistic data should be used in the classification process. The panel recommended that mechanistic data should be used (19), and subsequent IARC reports have included this statement: "Special attention is given to measurements of biologic markers of carcinogen exposure or action, such as DNA or protein adducts, as well as markers of early steps in the carcinogenic process, such as protooncogene mutation, when these are incorporated into epidemiologic studies focused on cancer incidence or mortality" (14). Such measurements are viewed as allowing inferences to be made about putative mechanisms of action (19–21).

Finally, all the relevant data are integrated, and the agent is categorized on the strength of the evidence derived from studies in humans and experimental animals and other studies, as shown in Table 1 (14).

The EPA uses a cancer classification scheme similar to that of the IARC as described in the agency's 1986 guide-

**TABLE 1.** *International Agency for Research on Cancer carcinogen evaluation scheme*

| Category | Human evidence | Experimental animal evidence |
|---|---|---|
| Group 1: The agent (mixture) is carcinogenic to humans; the exposure circumstance entails exposures that are carcinogenic to humans | (a) Sufficient<br>(b) Less than sufficient | No animal evidence required<br>Sufficient evidence and strong evidence in exposed humans that the agent (mixture) acts through a relevant mechanism of carcinogenicity |
| Group 2a: The agent (mixture) is probably carcinogenic to humans; the exposure circumstance entails exposures that are probably carcinogenic to humans | (a) Limited<br>(b) Limited<br>(c) Inadequate | None<br>Sufficient<br>Sufficient and strong evidence that the carcinogenesis is mediated by a mechanism that also operates in humans |
| Group 2b: The agent (mixture) is possibly carcinogenic to humans; the exposure circumstance entails exposures that are possibly carcinogenic to humans | (a) Limited<br>(b) Inadequate<br>(c) Inadequate | Less than sufficient<br>Sufficient<br>Limited together with supporting evidence from other relevant data |
| Group 3: The agent (mixture or exposure circumstance) is not classifiable as to its carcinogenicity | (a) Inadequate<br>(b) Inadequate | Inadequate or limited<br>Sufficient and strong evidence that the mechanism of carcinogenicity in experimental animals does not operate in humans |
| Group 4: The agent (mixture) is probably not carcinogenic to humans | (a) Lack of carcinogenicity<br>(b) Inadequate | Lack of carcinogenicity<br>Lack of carcinogenicity consistently and strongly supported by a broad range of other relevant data |

Abstracted from ref. 14.

**TABLE 2.** *U.S. Environmental Protection Agency (EPA) cancer categorization scheme*

| | Animal evidence | | | | |
|---|---|---|---|---|---|
| Human evidence | Sufficient | Limited | Inadequate | No data | No evidence |
| Sufficient | A[a] | A | A | A | A |
| Limited | B1[b] | B1 | B1 | B1 | B1 |
| Inadequate | B2 | C[c] | D[d] | D | D |
| No data | B2 | C | D | D | E[e] |
| No evidence | B2 | C | D | D | E |

[a]Group A: Human carcinogen.
[b]Group B: Probable human carcinogen.
B1. Limited evidence of carcinogenicity from epidemiology studies.
B2. Inadequate human evidence but positive animal evidence.
[c]Group C: Possible human carcinogen.
[d]Group D: Not classifiable as to human carcinogenicity.
[e]Group E: Evidence of noncarcinogenicity for humans.
From ref. 3.

lines for cancer risk assessment (Table 2) (3). A key difference between the IARC and EPA guidelines is in how data from both positive and negative studies are interpreted and used. The IARC process uses a strength-of-evidence approach in which one or two positive studies are taken as limited or sufficient evidence of carcinogenicity irrespective of how many well-conducted negative studies exist. The EPA approach uses a weight-of-evidence approach that weighs all the evidence and takes into account the strengths and weaknesses of all studies. The EPA process reports results as an alphanumeric categorization rather than using the numeric categorization of the IARC.

Partly as a response to recommendations of an NRC committee (2), the EPA proposed revised cancer risk assessment guidelines in 1996 (4). One proposed change from the 1986 guidelines is the addition of a narrative statement to complement the alphanumeric characterization. A narrative statement would be expected to more adequately describe the evidence for carcinogenic risk, including conditions under which the laboratory animal studies were done and the relevance to human exposure conditions. For example, any nonphysiologic method of administering the agent such as intraperitoneal or intratracheal instillation would be noted. Likewise, the relationship between the dosage or exposure level studied and plausible human exposures would be noted. The proposed revisions of the guidelines were still under consideration in early 1997. Examples of possible narrative statements for two important occupational exposure agents, fiber glass and carbon black, have been published (22,23).

The NTP also uses a classification scheme somewhat similar to that of the IARC. In its reports on the results of animal bioassays, it classifies the results as clear evidence, some evidence, equivocal evidence, or inadequate study of carcinogenic activity. Beyond interpreting the results of animal bioassays, the NTP plays a prominent role through its publication of the *Biennial Report on Carcinogens.* In this report, agents are listed either as human carcinogens or as reasonably anticipated to be human carcinogens, or are not listed (24). In 1996, the NTP announced that it was going to use mechanistic data in classifying agents, much as the IARC has done since 1991 (25). Although the NTP is not a regulatory agency, the *Biennial Report on Carcinogens* is widely used by other agencies as a basis for regulatory decisions on listed chemicals.

The various carcinogen classification schemes only provide input into the first component of risk assessment, i.e., hazard identification. Because the classification schemes do not provide information on carcinogenic potency, they are not adequate for fully characterizing risk even when exposure is known. This is readily apparent from considering two compounds, benzene and bis(chloromethyl)ether, classified as human carcinogens by both the IARC (category 1) and EPA (group A). The EPA has estimated the inhalation unit risk, the upper 95% confidence of the lifetime cancer risk per $\mu g/m^3$, as $8.3 \times 10^{-6}$ for benzene and $6.8 \times 10^{-2}$ for bis(chloromethyl)ether. Thus, despite their similar carcinogen classification at similar levels of exposure measured in $\mu g/m^3$, they would pose markedly different risks.

The characterization of risk and, ultimately, the provision of guidance for setting occupational or environmental exposure limits require information on the exposure-dose-response relationship for the compound. Two fundamentally different relationships have been used: a threshold model and a linear, no-threshold model. Both these approaches will be discussed.

## THRESHOLD DOSE-RESPONSE APPROACHES

### Threshold Limit Values

The earliest risk assessments for occupational exposure to airborne materials were much less formal than those conducted today and focused on alterations in function and structure. A threshold was assumed to exist for the exposure-response relationship so that level of exposure could be defined below which no effects would be observed—hence the term *threshold limit value* (TLV). The TLVs are usually expressed as a time-weighted average (TWA) for a normal 8-hour workday and a 40-hour workweek.

The TLV values are set by the ACGIH for a number of compounds. The TLV values are regularly reevaluated and the current values published in a regularly updated document (26). The ACGIH also makes available detailed supporting information in a separate document (27). As defined in the introduction to the ACGIH documents, TLVs refer to airborne concentrations of substances and represent conditions under which it is believed that nearly all workers may be repeatedly exposed day after day without adverse health effects. The document goes on to note that individuals vary in their susceptibility and that a small portion of individuals may be affected at levels below the TLV. The document also emphasizes the harmful effects of smoking. Since TLVs are specifically intended to provide guidance for occupational exposures, the document contains appropriate admonishments about not using TLVs for purposes such as the setting of community air pollution indices or estimating toxic potential. The document also notes that there is not a fine line between safe and dangerous concentrations of an agent. The TLVs are developed within a structure that implies a threshold relationship between exposure and health effect; therefore, values are established that accord relative safety in contrast to higher exposures, which have a higher degree of hazard.

The ACGIH also establishes biologic exposure indices (BEIs) to complement the TLVs. The BEIs are reference values used in assessing the concentration of appropriate determinants in biologic specimens collected from workers at specified times relative to chemical exposures. The measured value (such as methyl chloroform concentration in exhaled air or trichloroethanol in blood or urine) relative to the BEI gives an indication of the extent to which compliance with the TLV for the compound has been established.

The earliest TLVs, such as the TLV for crystalline silica (quartz), were developed using human data since substantial human data were available on the materials of interest. As additional compounds were considered by the ACGIH, it soon became apparent that the human data alone were not sufficient for establishing TLVs; accordingly, the incorporation of experimental animal data into the process was necessary. Since the animal data were of uncertain relevance to humans, safety factors were introduced into the extrapolation procedure. The use of these factors will be discussed in greater detail later when the establishment of reference dose concentrations and uncertainty factors is considered.

Examples of TLV listings for some widely encountered materials are shown in Table 3 (26).

**TABLE 3.** *Adopted threshold limit values from 1995–1996 handbook*

| | | | Adopted values | | | |
|---|---|---|---|---|---|---|
| | | | TWA | | STEL/Ceiling (C) | |
| Substance | CAS no. | Year adopted | ppm | mg/m | ppm | mg/m$^3$ |
| Ammonia | 7664-41-7 | 1976 | 25 | 17 | 35 | 24 |
| bis(chloromethyl)ether[a] | 542-88-1 | 1981 | 0.001, A1 | 0.0047, A1 | — | — |
| Caprolactam | 105-60-2 | | | | | |
| Dust | | 1974 | — | 1 | — | 3 |
| Vapor | | 1992 | 5 | 23 | 10 | 46 |
| Carbon dioxide | 124-38-9 | 1986 | 5,000 | 9,000 | 30,000 | 54,000 |
| Carbon monoxide[b] | 630-08-0 | 1992 | 25 | 29 | — | — |
| Chlorine | 7782-50-5 | 1989 | 0.5 | 1.5 | 1 | 2.9 |
| Chloroform[a,c] | 67-66-3 | 1986 | 10, A2 | 49, A2 | | |
| Cyclohexane | 110-82-7 | 1987 | 300 | 1,030 | — | — |
| Ethylene glycol aerosol[d] | 107-21-1 | 1995 | — | — | C39.4, A4 | C100, A4 |
| Formaldehyde[a] | 50-00-C | 1992 | — | — | C0.3, A2 | C0.37, A2 |
| Paraquat | 4685-14-7 | | | | | |
| Total dust | | 1978 | — | 0.5 | — | — |
| Respirable fraction | | 1978 | — | 0.1 | — | — |
| Perchloroethylene[a,b,c] | | | | | | |
| (tetrachloroethylene) | 127-18-4 | 1993 | 25, A3 | 170, A3 | 100, A3 | 685, A3 |
| Trichloroethylene[a,b,c] | 79-01-6 | 1993 | 50, A5 | 269, A5 | 100, A5 | 537, A5 |

CAS, chemical abstract service; STEL, short-term exposure limit; TWA, time-weighted average.
[a]Substances identified by other sources as a suspected or confirmed human carcinogen (see text of ACGIH document for code).
[b]Identifies substances for which there are also biologic exposure indices.
[c]Substances for which the TLV is higher than the OSHA Permissible Exposure Limit, the National Institute for Occupational Safety and Health (NIOSH) recommended exposure limit, or both.
[d]1995–1996 adoption.
Modified from ref. 26.

**TABLE 4.** *Comparison of risk assessment and risk management estimates*

| Estimate | NAS paradigm | Exposure scenario | Effect level | Population | Database | Dosimetry | SF or UF |
|---|---|---|---|---|---|---|---|
| ACGIH TLV-TWA | Management | 8 h/day, 40 h/wk, 40 yr | Impairment of health or freedom from irritation; narcosis; nuisance; stress | Healthy worker | Industrial experience; experimental human and animal | No | SF |
| NIOSH REL | Characterization | 10 h/day, 40 h/wk, "working lifetime" | Impairment of health or functional capacity and technical feasibility | Healthy worker | Medical; biologic; chemical; trade | No | SF |
| OSHA PEL | Management | 8 h/day, 40 h/wk, 45 yr | Impairment of health or functional capacity and technical feasibility | Healthy worker | Medical; biologic; chemical; trade | No | SF |
| EPA RfC | Dose-response | 24 h/day, 70 yr | NOAEL | General population, including susceptible | Occupational; experimental human and animal | Yes | UF |
| ATSDR MRL | Dose-response | 24 h/day, 70 yr | NOAEL | General population, including susceptible | Occupational; experimental human and animal | No | UF |

MRL, minimal risk level; NAS, National Academy of Sciences; NOAEL, no-observed-adverse-effect level; PEL, permissible exposure limit; REL, recommended exposure limit; SF, safety factor; UF, uncertainty factor for explicit extrapolations applied to data.
From ref. 30.

### Inhalation Reference Concentration Methodology

To provide guidance for evaluating noncancer health effects of airborne materials, the EPA has developed an inhalation reference concentration (RfC) methodology (28–30). Jarabek (30) has reviewed the methodology in detail and defined an RfC as "an estimate (with uncertainty spanning perhaps an order of magnitude) of a continuous inhalation exposure to the human population (including sensitive subgroups) that is likely to be without appreciable risk of deleterious noncancer health effects during a lifetime." In Table 4, the EPA RfC methodology is compared with several other approaches, including the TLV approach just discussed, for assessing and managing noncancer risks of airborne materials. All five approaches have in common the use of safety factors or uncertainty factors for making extrapolations to humans from data developed in laboratory animals when sufficient human data are not available. The EPA RfC approach is unique among the five in having provision for using dosimetry data to make extrapolations. Provision for a dosimetry adjustment is an especially significant advance in view of the extent to which there are marked species differences for exposure-dose relationships for many airborne materials that may be hazardous.

The RfC methodology is intended to provide guidance for noncancer toxicity, that is, adverse health effects or toxic end points other than cancer and gene mutations due to effects of environmental agents on the structure and function of various organ systems. This includes both respiratory and extrarespiratory effects that occurred when the respiratory tract is the portal of entry. An assumption inherent in the methodology is that a threshold exists in the relationship between exposure (or dose) and noncancer responses. This assumption contrasts sharply with the nonthreshold relationship between exposure and response that is a key default assumption in the 1986 EPA cancer risk assessment guidelines. The noncancer responses are defined by both continuous incidence and severity scales above the threshold, which contrasts with the quantal or dichotomous nature of the cancer response. The RfC is intended to estimate a benchmark level for continuous exposure; thus when data for less than continuous exposure are used, it is normalized to exposure for 24 hours/day for a lifetime of 70 years.

The RfC methodology focuses on the establishment of either a no-observed-adverse-effect level (NOAEL) or a lowest-observed-adverse-effect level (LOAEL) as the starting point for deriving exposure limits (Fig. 3).

All the exposure-toxicity data for a chemical are initially arrayed and examined to select the prominent toxic effect. The toxicity profile of concern is defined as the

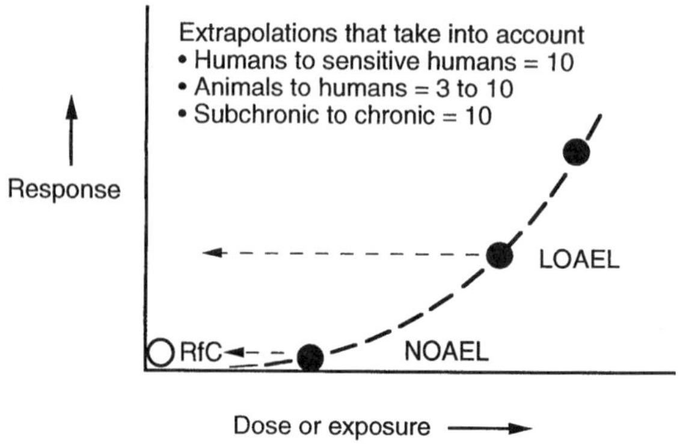


**FIG. 3.** Schematic representation of exposure-response relationships used for establishing guidance or standards for reagents and effects with threshold exposure-response relationships.

critical effect pertinent to the mechanisms of action of the chemical that is at or just below the threshold level for more serious effects. The chosen critical effect is generally characterized by the lowest NOAEL, adjusted to the human equivalent concentration (HEC), that is representative of the threshold region for the entire data array. The RfC is then derived from $NOAEL_{(HEC)}$ for the critical effect by application of appropriate uncertainty factors (Table 5).

One criticism of this approach is that it does not utilize all the data on a chemical. Crump (31) has described an approach that utilizes all the data to define the lower 95% confidence limit on the dose associated with a given level of response, say 10%, to establish a benchmark dose. This approach may be used for either cancer or noncancer data.

## NATIONAL AMBIENT AIR QUALITY STANDARDS

The establishment of National Ambient Air Quality Standards (NAAQSs) for criteria air pollutants represents an important example of the use of a threshold exposure-response relationship. Under the Clean Air Act (CAA), the EPA is required to develop primary NAAQSs for the

**TABLE 5.** *Guidelines for the use of uncertainty factors in deriving inhalation reference concentration (RfC)*

| Standard uncertainty factors (UF) | Processes considered in UF purview |
|---|---|
| H = Human to sensitive human: Use a tenfold factor when extrapolating from valid experimental results from studies using prolonged exposure to average healthy humans. This factor is intended to account for the variation in sensitivity among the members of the human population. | Pharmacokinetics-pharmacodynamics<br>Sensitivity<br>Differences in mass (children, obese)<br>Concomitant exposures<br>Activity pattern<br>Does not account for idiosyncrasies |
| A = Animal to human: Use a threefold factor when extrapolating from valid results of long-term studies on experimental animals when results of studies of human exposure are not available or are inadequate. This factor is intended to account for the uncertainty in extrapolating animal data to the case of average healthy humans. Use of a threefold factor is recommended with default dosimetric adjustments. More rigorous adjustments may allow additional reduction. Conversely, judgment that the default may not be appropriate could result in an application of a tenfold factor. | Pharmacokinetics-pharmacodynamics<br>Relevance of laboratory animals model<br>Species sensitivity |
| S = Subchronic to chronic: Use a tenfold factor when extrapolating from less than chronic results on experimental animals or humans when there are no useful long-term human data. This factor is intended to account for the uncertainty in extrapolating from less than chronic NOAEL to chronic NOAEL. | Accumulation-cumulative damage<br>Pharmacokinetics-pharmacodynamics<br>Severity of effect<br>Recovery<br>Duration of study<br>Consistency of effect with duration |
| L = $LOAEL_{[HEC]}$ to $NOAEL_{[HEC]}$: Use a tenfold factor when deriving an RfC from a $LOAEL_{[HEC]}$, instead of a $NOAEL_{[HEC]}$. This factor is intended to account for the uncertainty in extrapolating from $LOAEL_{[HEC]}$ to $NOAEL_{[HEC]}$. | Severity<br>Pharmacokinetics-pharmacodynamics<br>Slope of dose-response curve<br>Trend, consistency of effect<br>Relationship of end points<br>Functional vs. histopathologic evidence<br>Exposure uncertainties |
| D = Incomplete to complete database: Use up to a tenfold factor when extrapolating from valid results in experimental animals when the data are "incomplete." This factor is intended to account for the inability of any single animal study to adequately address all possible adverse outcomes in humans. | Quality of critical study<br>Data gaps<br>Power of critical study and supporting studies<br>Exposure uncertainties |
| Modifying factor (MF): Use professional judgment to determine whether another uncertainty factor (MF) that is ≤10 is needed. The magnitude of the MF depends on the professional assessment of scientific uncertainties of the study and database not explicitly treated above (e.g., the number of animals tested or quality of exposure characterization). The default value of the MF is 1. | |

*Note:* Assuming that the range of the UF is distributed log-normally, reduction of a standard tenfold UF by half (i.e., $10^{-5}$) results in a UF of 3. Composite UF for derivation involving four areas of uncertainty is 3,000 in recognition of the lack of independence of these factors. Inhalation reference concentrations are not derived if all five areas of uncertainty are invoked.

From ref. 30.

criteria air pollutants that shall be ambient air quality standards, the attainment and maintenance of which in the judgment of the administrator, based on such criteria and allowing an adequate margin of safety, are required to protect public health [Section 109(b)1, Clean Air Act Amendments of 1970] (32). The intent is to have nationwide standards for major air pollutants that are widely distributed and arise from multiple sources. The current criteria pollutants are listed in Table 6. The agency is also required to promulgate secondary or welfare standards for each criteria pollutant to protect against the effects of these pollutants on vegetation, buildings, visibility, and other aspects of general welfare. Implementation of the NAAQSs is primarily the responsibility of state and regional authorities.

The Clean Air Act and the associated legislative history clearly leave the impression that the exposure-response relationship for the criteria air pollutants has a threshold, or hockey-stick–shaped, exposure-response relationship, i.e., the reference to setting the standard with an adequate margin of safety below the level with effects. Moreover, it has been noted that an adequate margin of safety is intended to protect against effects that have not yet been uncovered by research and effects whose medical significance is a matter of disagreement.

The primary NAAQSs are intended to protect against adverse effects and not necessarily against all identifiable effects of air pollutants. The question of what constitutes an adverse effect has been the subject of extensive debate. Although the Congress did not rigorously define adverse effects, the debate on the legislation did provide some general guidance by referring to cancer, metabolic and respiratory disease, impairment of mental processes, headache, dizziness, and nausea. An American Thoracic Society (ATS) committee (33) has developed guidelines for defining adverse respiratory health effects identified in epidemiologic studies. The ATS guidelines, which have been used by the EPA, emphasize the importance of distinguishing between reversible and irreversible changes. The guidelines also give weight to determining when there are departures from normal trends associated with growth and aging as revealed by serial measurements.

The CAA (32) also requires consideration of sensitive population groups, noting that the NAAQS should protect "particularly sensitive citizens as bronchial asthmatics and emphysematics who in the normal course of daily activity are exposed to the ambient environment." The Congress gave further guidance in noting that a standard is statutorially sufficient whenever there is an absence of adverse effects on the health of a statistically related sample of persons in sensitive groups from exposure to the ambient air. The reference to a subpopulation with an absence of adverse effect again implies the existence of a threshold in the exposure-response relationship. A statistically related sample is defined as the number of persons necessary to test in order to detect a deviation in the health of any persons within such sensitive group which is attributable to the condition of the ambient air.

As may be noted from consideration of Table 6, the NAAQSs are set to protect against a broad range of health effects. All the effects are attributable to pollutants entering the body via respiration, i.e., the respiratory tract is the portal of entry. In some cases, such as with ozone and particulate matter (PM), the principal effects are also found in the respiratory tract. In other cases, the effects are observed

**TABLE 6.** *National Ambient Air Quality Standards as of December 31, 1997*

| Pollutant | Sensitive population | Health effects | Averaging time | Primary standard[a] |
|---|---|---|---|---|
| Particles ($PM_{10}$)[b] | Individuals with preexisting respiratory disease | Changes in mortality in sensitive populations, increase in respiratory symptoms, reduced pulmonary function | 24-hour | $PM_{10}$-150 μg/m$^3$<br>$PM_{2.5}$-65 μg/m$^3$ |
| | | | Annual | $PM_{10}$-50 μg/m$^3$<br>$PM_{2.5}$-15 μg/m$^3$ |
| Sulfur dioxide | Asthmatics | Increased respiratory symptoms, reduced pulmonary function | 24-hour | 0.140 ppm |
| | | | Annual | 0.003 ppm |
| Carbon monoxide | Individuals with heart disease | Aggravation of angina pectoris | 8-hour | 9.000 ppm |
| | | | 1-hour | 35.000 ppm |
| Nitrogen dioxide | Young children and asthmatics; individuals with preexisting respiratory disease | Increased pulmonary symptoms, reduced pulmonary function | Annual | 0.053 ppm |
| Ozone | None identified | Increased respiratory symptoms, reduced pulmonary function | 8-hour | 0.008 ppm |
| Lead | Fetuses and young children | Neurobehavioral development, impaired heme synthesis | Quarterly | 1.5 μg/m$^3$ |

[a]μg/m$^3$, micrograms per cubic meter; ppm, parts per million.
[b]Under review for potential revision, EPA has proposed adding $PM_{2.5}$ standards; 24-hour, 50 μg/m$^3$; and annual, 15 μg/m$^3$.

in other systems, e.g., the effects of carbon monoxide on the cardiovascular and nervous systems and the effects of lead on the hematopoietic and central nervous system.

Under the CAA, the EPA is charged with reviewing and updated the criteria every 5 years, a schedule the EPA has rarely met. The process of setting the NAAQS has been reviewed in detail elsewhere (34). Suffice it to note that the EPA Office of Research and Development, with broad input from the scientific community, prepares an updated criteria document such as those recently completed on ozone and PM (35,36). These documents are encyclopedic compilations of everything known about the pollutant under consideration and are excellent reference sources. The criteria documents are reviewed for their completeness and accuracy by the EPA Clean Air Scientific Advisory Committee (CASAC).

The CASAC, whose existence is mandated under the CAA, consists of experts on health and air quality matters. Using information in the criteria document, the EPA Office of Air Quality, Planning, and Standards (OAQPS) then prepares a staff position paper on the pollutant. These documents are much briefer than the criteria documents. They focus on synthesizing and integrating the data relevant to establishing the appropriate exposure metric and offer ranges of exposure levels and options for the form of the potential NAAQS. The staff papers are excellent references for the most critical data available on exposure-response relations for the criteria pollutants. Examples are the recent staff position papers on ozone and PM (37,38). The staff position papers are also reviewed by CASAC. The CASAC consideration of the documents concludes with a closure letter to the EPA administrator that comments on the scientific adequacy for regulatory purposes of the material contained in the documents. Brief synopses of the CASAC review of the ozone and PM documents and the advice to the administrator have been published (39,40).

In 1997 the EPA revised the NAAQS for both ozone (41) and PM (42). In proposing NAAQS, the EPA administrator is expected to rely solely on the scientific information contained in the criteria documents and staff position papers. Under the CAA, the administrator is not allowed to consider any costs that may arise as a result of the NAAQS being proposed. Costs can only be considered with regard to the implementation schedule for a given NAAQS. The primary ozone NAAQS up until 1997 was set at 120 parts per billion (ppb) averaged over a 1-hour period, with a region considered to be in attainment if the standard is not exceeded more than once in a 3-year period. In 1997 a new primary NAAQS for ozone was changed to 80 ppb averaged over 8 hours, with attainment considered to be achieved when the 3-year average of the annual fourth highest daily maximum 8-hour average $O_3$ concentration is less than or equal to 80 ppb (41). The proposed standard is viewed as being more health-relevant since ozone exposures at concentrations below 120 ppb do produce alterations in pulmonary function when protracted over a number of hours.

The data now available on ozone strongly suggest that there is no absolute threshold above 40 ppb, taken as the background ozone level absent human activity, where a bright line can be drawn that separates levels of exposure producing effects from those where effects are not observed. This is apparent from consideration of data from the New York City area on estimated hospital admissions for asthmatics, one of the critical health end points for ozone (39). Out of approximately 15,000 hospital admissions of asthmatics, an estimated 1,065 cases are due to ozone, and about 677 are due to ozone exposures below the background concentration of 40 ppb. These values are obviously highly uncertain and are developed based on the assumption of a linear relationship between ozone exposure and response extending down to a hypothetical zero level of ozone.

The EPA revised the PM standard in 1997 (42). The original PM standard set in 1971 under the CAA used a total suspended particulate (TSP) metric (24 hours, 260 $\mu g/m^3$; annual, 75 $\mu g/m^3$). As shown schematically in Fig. 4 (5,43), this included substantial mass related to larger particles that had a low probability of being inhaled and deposited in the respiratory tract. Recognition of the importance of particle size as a determinant of particle-induced disease led to a revision of the PM NAAQS in 1987 with use of a $PM_{10}$ metric; the 10-μm size point represents the size of particles collected with a 50% collection efficiency at 10 μm. The primary NAAQS for PM was set at 24 hours, 150 $\mu g/m^3$ and annual average 50 $\mu g/m^3$. An emerging body of data reviewed in the PM criteria document and staff paper indicate that the smaller particles in the $PM_{10}$ range may be more toxic than the larger particles. The smallest particles arise primarily from combustion processes or secondary chemical reactions in the atmosphere, while the larger particles are formed primarily by mechanical processes such as construction, unpaved roads, and erosion of soil. This has led the EPA to propose the use of a $PM_{2.5}$ metric in addition to retention of the $PM_{10}$ metric (42). The $PM_{2.5}$ cut point represents the size of particles collected with 50% collection efficiency at 2.5 μm. The new rule establishes two new $PM_{2.5}$ standards: (1) an annual standard set at 15 $\mu g/m^3$ based on the 3-year average of annual arithmetic mean $PM_{2.5}$ concentrations from single or multiple community-oriented monitors; and (2) a 24-hour standard of 65 $\mu g/m^3$ based on the 3-year average of the 98th percentile of 24-hour concentrations at each population-oriented monitor within an area. The rule revises two $PM_{10}$ standards: (1) a 24-hour $PM_{10}$ standard set at 150 $\mu g/m^3$ for the 3-year average of the 99th percentile of the 24-hour concentrations at each monitor within an area; and (2) an annual $PM_{10}$ standard set at 50 $\mu g/m^3$ for the 3-year average of the annual arithmetic mean $PM_{10}$ concentration at each monitor within an area.

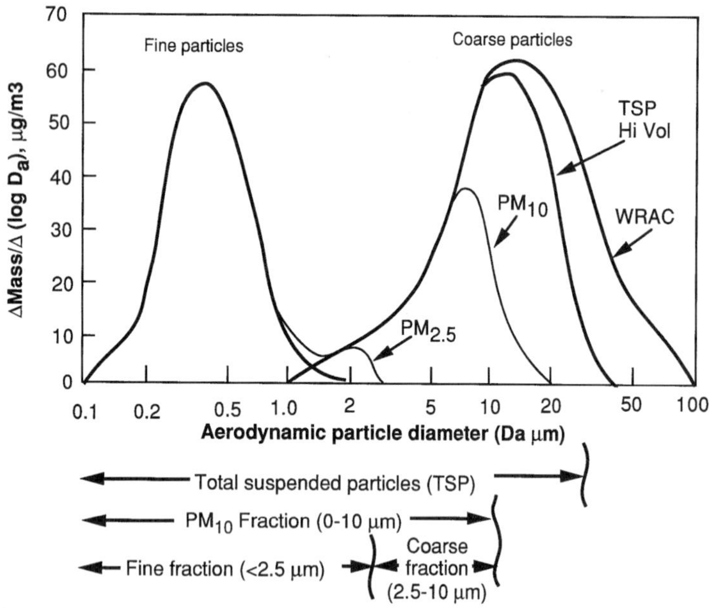


**FIG. 4.** Sampling fractions for an idealized ambient particulate mass distribution. (Adapted from ref. 43.)

There is much controversy surrounding the introduction of a new $PM_{2.5}$ metric. One point of controversy is the size cut. Some have concluded that a $PM_{1.0}$ metric would be more appropriate if the goal is to reduce the number of smallest particles arising from combustion. Resolution of this controversy has been stymied by the relatively modest amount of $PM_{2.5}$ and $PM_{1.0}$ data available since most of the data have been collected for regulatory compliance purposes (i.e., TSP or $PM_{10}$ measurements when these metrics were the standard). Another point of controversy relates to interpretation of the health effects at low concentrations of PM. The EPA has interpreted the available data as indicating a 4% increase in daily mortality for a 50 µg/m$^3$ increase in PM concentration with no evidence for a threshold concentration.

## HAZARDOUS AIR POLLUTANTS

In addition to providing for regulation of criteria pollutants, the CAA also requires regulation of pollutants arising from location sources that have hazardous properties, hence the term *hazardous air pollutants* (HAP). The 1970 version of the CAA specified that regulations for HAP should be established to protect public health with an ample margin of safety. If, as will be discussed later, one assumes that even the smallest intake of a carcinogenic chemical has calculable risk of causing cancer, then there is no level of exposure that is without some level of risk. This raises the critical issue of what is an acceptable exposure level. Because of controversy over how to set HAP standards, only seven HAP standards (arsenic, asbestos, benzene, beryllium, mercury, vinyl chloride, and radionuclides) were developed from 1970 to 1990. The history of how these standards were developed has been reviewed by Albert (44).

Largely due to the slow pace of regulation, Congress radically changed the approach to regulating the HAP in the CAA amendments of 1990 (45). The new approach uses two phases. The first phase is technology-based and requires the use of maximum achievable control technology (MACT) for the regulation of various categories of sources of 189 HAP listed in this act. This phase depends on installation of control equipment, process changes, operator training, and substitution of materials to reduce emissions of the HAPs. The second phase is based on health risk and requires an assessment of the residual risk after use of MACT. If the residual risks over a lifetime exceed more than $10^{-6}$ for individuals in a population, then further action will be required.

In Table 7, 10 of 189 chemicals (or mixtures) identified in the CAA amendments of 1990 are listed. A complete list may be found as an appendix in *Science and Judgment in Risk Assessment* (2). Table 7 shows some of the kinds of data available on the HAP. The toxic release inventory data shown are calculated releases and should not automatically be assumed to equate to actual exposures. Many factors such as the stability of the chemical in air, atmospheric chemistry, meteorologic conditions, and location of people relative to plant sources influence the actual exposure of individuals.

In Table 7, only summary information is given. A comprehensive compilation of information on most of these chemicals can be found in the EPA's Integrated Risk Information System (IRIS), an on-line database originally developed for internal EPA use (46,47). It contains the rationale for the risk status of each chemical, including reference concentration values and cancer classification, if available, and bibliographic documentation for over 500 chemicals. The IRIS database is one of the databases available through the Toxicology Data

**TABLE 7.** *Data on selected hazardous air pollutants (from a total of 189 listed in the Clean Air Act Amendments of 1990)*

| | | | | | | | Genetic toxicity data[g] | | | | | | |
|---|---|---|---|---|---|---|---|---|---|---|---|---|---|
| | | | | | | | Mammalian | | | Bacterial | | | |
| | | | | | | | *In vivo* | | *In vitro* | | | | |
| Chemical name | 1991 TRI emissions[a] (tons, yr) | IUR[b] per μg/m³ | OUR[c] per μg/L | EPA[d] WOE | RfC[e] (mg/m³) | IARC[f] WOE | S | G | M | C | S | E | R-D data[h] |
| Acetaldehyde | 3,540.5 | 2.2E-6 | | B2 | 9.0E-3 | 2B | + | | | + | + | + | X |
| Acrylonitrile | 1,094.4 | 6.8E-5 | 1.5E-5 | B1 | 2.0E-3 | 2A | − | − | + | +− | + | + | X |
| Asbestos | 6.3 | 2.3E-1 | Fib/ML | A | | 1 | − | | −+ | +− | − | − | |
| 1,3-Butadiene | 1,975.2 | 2.8E-4 | | B2 | | 2B | + | | | | + | | X |
| Benzene | 8,737.2 | 8.3E-6 | 8.3E-7 | A | UR | 1 | | +− | −+ | − | − | − | X* |
| Cadmium compounds | 34.7 | 1.8E-3 | | B1 | UR | 2A | − | − | + | +− | | + | |
| Caprolactam | | | | | | 4 | | | − | −+ | | | X |
| Carbon tetrachloride | 773.4 | 1.5E-5 | 3.7E-6 | B2 | | 2B | | − | | | − | + | X |
| Carbon disulfide | 44,669.6 | | | | UR | | + | + | | | − | | X* |
| Chlorine | 38,804.7 | | | D | | | | | | | | | |
| Chloroform | 9,541.4 | 2.3E-5 | 1.7E-7 | B2 | UR | 2B | − | | − | − | − | − | X |
| Chromium compounds | 278.2 | 1.2E-2 | | A | UR | 1 | + | + | + | + | + | + | |
| Formaldehyde | 5,109.2 | 1.3E-5 | | B1 | | 2A | +− | − | + | + | + | + | X* |
| Glycol ethers | 21,957.1 | | | | | | | | | | | | |
| Hydrazine | 14.2 | 4.9E-3 | 8.5E-5 | B2 | | 2B | − | | − | | + | + | |
| Hydrochloric acid | 41,460.7 | | | | 7.0E-3 | | | | | | | | X |
| Methanol | 99,841.5 | | | UR | | | | | | | | | X |
| Methyl chloroform (1,1,1-trichloroethane) | 68,753.1 | | | D | UR | 3 | | | | | | | X |
| Methyl ethyl ketone (2-butanone) | 51,710.9 | | | D | 1.0E+0 | | | | | | | | X |
| Methyl isobutyl ketone (hexone) | 13,599.3 | | | | UR | | | | | | | | X |
| Methyl tert butyl ether | 1,519.1 | | | | 5.0E-1 | 3 | | | | | | | X |
| Methylene chloride (dichloromethane) | 39,669.2 | 4.7E-7 | 2.1E-7 | B2 | UR | 2B | − | | − | + | + | | X |
| Nickel | 121.6 | 4.8E-4 | | A | UR | 1 | + | − | +− | + | + | − | |
| Propylene oxide | 533.3 | 3.7E-6 | 6.8E-6 | B2 | 3.0E-2 | 2A | + | − | + | + | + | + | |
| Styrene | 14,238.2 | | | UR | 1.0E+0 | 2B | +− | | | + | + | | X* |
| Tetrachloroethylene (perchloroethylene) | 8,343.7 | | | | | 2B | | − | + | | − | − | X |
| Toluene | 99,260.1 | | | D | 4.0E-1 | | + | | − | | | − | X* |
| Trichloroethylene | 17,529.2 | | | UR | UR | 3 | + | − | +− | +− | + | + | X |
| Vinyl acetate | 2,743.2 | | | UR | 2.0E-1 | 3 | | | | + | − | | X |
| Vinyl chloride | 523.7 | 8.4E-5 | 5.4E-5 | A | | 1 | + | − | + | | + | + | X |
| Xylenes (isomers and mixture) | 57,776.5 | | | D | NV | | − | | | − | − | − | X |

[a]TRI, 1991 Toxic Release Inventory data in tons/year.
[b]IUR, Inhalation unit risk estimate per μg/m³. Source is the EPA Integrated Risk Information System (IRIS) database.
[c]OUR, Oral unit risk per μg/L. Source is the EPA IRIS database.
[d]EPA/WOE, EPA Weight-of-Evidence Cancer Classification. Source is the EPA IRIS.
[e]RfC Workgroup; V, verified on IRIS, concentration given in mg/m³; NV, not verified; UR, under review.
[f]IARC/WOE, International Agency for Research on Cancer Classification.
[g]Genetic toxicity data; mammalian *in vivo:* S, somatic, G, germ cell; mammalian *in vitro:* M, mutation, C, chromosome aberration; bacterial: S, *Salmonella typhi,* E, *Escherichia coli* (EPA Genetic Activity Profile database provided by Dr. Michael Waters, EPA, current as of 1992).
[h]Reproductive-developmental toxicity data provided by Dr. John Vandenburg, EPA; X, data available, X*, some human data available.
Adapted from ref. 2.

Network (TOXNET) of the National Library of Medicine, which can be accessed via the Internet (telnet://toxnet.nim.nih.gov).

## QUANTITATIVE ESTIMATES OF CANCER RISK

A number of the HAPs are regulated based on concern for their cancer-causing potential. The methodology used by the EPA for assessing cancer risk will first be reviewed and then illustrated using the HAP formaldehyde.

The basic approach used by the EPA in assessing cancer risk is outlined in guidelines released in 1986 (3) and proposed for revision in 1996 (4). Albert (44) has reviewed how these practices developed within the EPA. As noted early in this chapter, the NRC report *Risk Assessment in the Federal Government:* Managing the Process (1) had a profound influence on how EPA risk assessment practices developed, especially those for cancer-causing agents. More recently, the NRC produced the report *Science and Judgment in Risk Assessment* (2) in response to a congressional request made in the CAA amendments of 1990. An annotated review of the report is available (48). The 1994 NRC report generally endorsed continued EPA use of the risk assessment paradigm laid out in the 1983 NRC report. However, the report did offer a number of recommendations for improvements, many of which the EPA has included in its proposed revisions to its cancer risk assessment guidelines. In particular, the 1994 NRC report advocated that increased attention be given to characterizing uncertainty and variability in the risk assessment process. The report also gave substantial attention to the topic of default options.

Default options or inferences were defined in the 1983 NRC report as "the option chosen on the basis of risk assessment policy that appears to be the best choice in the absence of data to the contrary" (1, p. 63). Three key default options are as follows (the number in parentheses refers to the EPA 1986 cancer risk assessment guidelines) (3):

1. Laboratory animals are a surrogate for humans in assessing cancer risks; positive cancer bioassay results in laboratory animals are taken as evidence of a chemical's cancer-causing potential in humans (IV).
2. Humans are as sensitive as the most sensitive animal species, strain, or sex evaluated in a bioassay with appropriate study design characteristics (III.A.1).
3. Chemicals act like radiation at low exposures (doses) in inducing cancer; that is, intake of even one molecule of a chemical has an associated probability for cancer induction that can be calculated, so the appropriate model for relating exposure-response relationships is the linearized multistage model (III.A.2).

The first two default options are an essential part of any carcinogen classification scheme that utilizes data from animal species such as those reviewed earlier in this chapter. The third option is concerned with extrapolation from observations made at high exposure concentrations to lower exposure concentrations whether the data are from positive epidemiologic investigations or laboratory animal studies. Positive epidemiologic studies with quantitative exposure data are available for only a very few agents. Thus the use of this default option in practice most typically involves two extrapolations: from laboratory animals to humans and from high to low levels of exposure.

To avoid underestimating risk, the EPA has selected default options that are scientifically plausible and conservative. This is not an unreasonable position to take in the absence of data to the contrary. The critical issue becomes one of determining the kind and weight of the scientific evidence required to depart from a default.

In one of the two appendixes to *Science and Judgment in Risk Assessment,* Finkel (49) advocates the use of "plausible conservatism" in choosing and altering defaults. He argues that the EPA should assemble all the available data and models that are deemed plausible by knowledgeable scientists and then "from this 'plausible set,' EPA should adopt (or should reaffirm) as a generic default that model or assumption which tends to yield risk estimates more conservative than the other plausible choices" (p. 613). In contrast, McClellan and North (50) argued that "plausible conservatism" has a role in the initial selection of default options but is not an appropriate criterion to use for determining when to depart from a default option and use specific scientific information. They argue that such a test places an excessively high hurdle on the introduction of new science and tends to freeze risk characterizations at the level determined by conservative default options.

In conducting science-based risk assessments, McClellan and North (50) go on to advocate building on the general principles outlined in the 1983 NRC report. They argue for full use of scientific information, including a closer linkage between the components of research and risk assessment, in the science-based risk paradigm (Fig. 1). As discussed earlier in this chapter, the risk assessment process is envisioned as yielding both risk characterizations and identification of research needs. The latter are derived from considering the major uncertainties in the science undergirding the risk characterization. If these uncertainties can be reduced through further research, they serve as a basis for creating the agenda and priorities for subsequent research. As conservative default options are replaced over time with specific scientific information, there should be a general reduction in the estimated risk levels and a tightening of the bounds of uncertainty. This is illustrated below with the formaldehyde example of cancer risk assessment.

Formaldehyde, a naturally occurring constituent of the mammalian body and a major commodity chemical, is one of the 189 listed hazardous air pollutants (Table 7). For details on the toxicity and carcinogenicity of formaldehyde, the reader is referred to reviews by Heck et al. (51) and the IARC (52).

The irritancy of formaldehyde is well known to all who have worked with it. Its irritancy was the basis for establishing the early TLV for formaldehyde (Table 3). In the early 1970s, concern developed for the potential carcinogenicity of formaldehyde. This led to a life span study with mice and rats conducted by the Chemical Industry Institute of Toxicology (CIIT). In the CIIT study, both species were exposed to 14.3, 5.6, 2.0, or 0 ppm of formaldehyde for 6 hours per day and 5 days per week for 2 years. At the highest exposure concentration, 14.3 ppm, over 50% of the rats developed nasal tumors (53). This was clearly a significant finding since spontaneous nasal tumors are quite rare in rats. At the next lower level, 5.6 ppm, only two tumors were observed in 153 rats. No tumors were observed at the lowest exposure concentration or in control rats. In the mice, a marginally significant increase in nasal tumor incidence was observed only at the highest exposure concentration. The data on exposure and cancer response for the rats are striking in their nonlinearity. If the response was proportional to the exposure concentration based on the results of 14.3 ppm, 40 rats out of 153 would have been expected to have tumors at 5.6 ppm compared to the two observed. At 2.0 ppm, 15 cases would be expected based on a linear response compared to none observed. Thus the data suggested a threshold for response, an observation that has major implications for extrapolating the rat findings to humans. To understand the basis for the findings, a major experimental program was initiated at CIIT. It focused on two areas: establishing an appropriate biologic marker of effective dose and exploring the role of cell proliferation in the carcinogenic response. In parallel, a series of interrelated epidemiologic studies was conducted on a population of foundry workers who had been exposed to high levels of formaldehyde. A key finding was the absence of an increase in nasal tumors (54).

Both the animal and epidemiologic data have been used to classify formaldehyde as to its carcinogenicity. Both the EPA (55) and the IARC (52) have classified formaldehyde as a probable human carcinogen, group B1 by the EPA and group 2A by the IARC. The classification is based on (a) sufficient animal evidence, (b) limited human evidence, and (c) supporting information such as structure-activity relationships that associate formaldehyde with genotoxic activity and carcinogenicity, including formation of DNA adducts and cytotoxicity.

To fully characterize risk, it is necessary to look beyond the cancer classification and consider quantitative estimates of the carcinogenic potency of formaldehyde. The first estimates by the EPA (55) used the air concentration of formaldehyde as the exposure metric. The observed rat tumor data (53) were fit with a linearized multistage model and extrapolated to lower levels of exposure (GLOBAL 83 or 86, ICF Clement Associates, Rushton, LA), as advocated by the EPA cancer risk assessment guidelines (3). This yielded a cancer unit risk of $1.6 \times 10^{-2}$ per ppm.

Noting the nonlinearity in the exposure-response relationship discussed earlier, Casanova et al. (56,57) conducted research that led to the development of sensitive techniques for measuring the delivered dose of formaldehyde for comparison with the air concentration. The metric they used was the DNA-protein cross-link. Rats were studied because the most significant excess of nasal tumors was observed in that species. With the EPA default options, data from the most sensitive species evaluated are used for the human risk assessment. Monkeys were studied as a primate species intermediate in size between rats and humans. The results are summarized in Fig. 5. Two key points can be made concerning the data. First, for both rats and monkeys, the relationship between air concentrations of formaldehyde and DNA-protein cross-links is clearly nonlinear, with fewer cross-links per unit of exposure at low compared to high concentrations of formaldehyde. Second, the rate of DNA-protein cross-link formation at a given level of formaldehyde exposure, say at 2.0 ppm, is less in monkeys than in rats. Casanova et al. (57) used rat data as input to a pharmacokinetic model with physiologic parameters for rats and monkeys. The model yielded DNA-protein cross-link predictions for the monkeys that were in excellent agreement with the measured values. This gives confidence to the use of similar models for extrapolating the monkey and rat data to humans. Using the rat DNA-protein cross-link data as the exposure (or, more correctly, dose) metric yielded a cancer unit risk estimate of $2.8 \times 10^{-3}$ per ppm. When the monkey data were used, the estimate was further reduced to $3.3 \times 10^{-4}$ per ppm. The EPA cancer unit risks represent the upper 95% confidence limit.

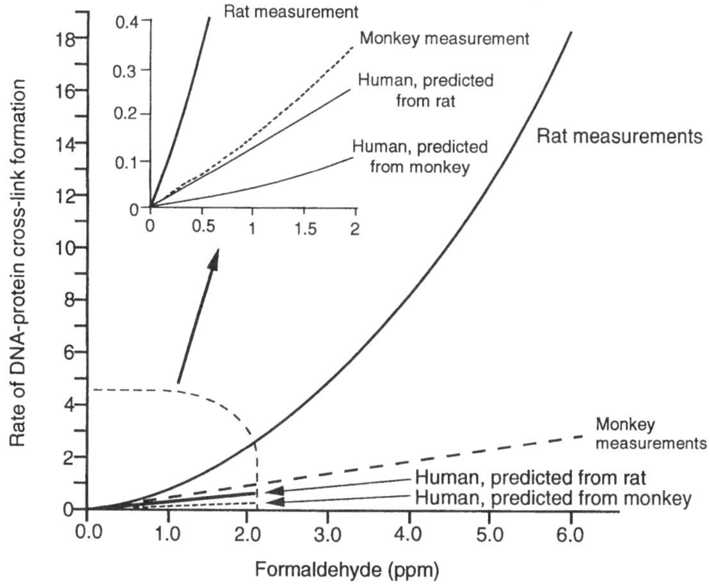


**FIG. 5.** Delivered dose of formaldehyde, as measured by DNA-protein cross-links in rats and monkeys and predicted for humans.

This is an excellent example of how specific science can be introduced into the risk assessment process to reduce uncertainty, the kind of iterative approach advocated in the 1994 NRC report. Because the original estimates of risk were based on conservative assumptions, the later estimates using more data to replace the assumptions produce lower estimates of risk.

More refined estimates of risk can be expected as additional scientific information is developed on the mechanism by which formaldehyde causes cancer in rats. Conolly et al. (58) proposed a strategy for incorporating data on DNA-protein cross-links, cell proliferation, and putative preneoplastic changes into a biologically based model for assessing human cancer risks. The strategy builds on the approach advocated by Moolgavkar (59). He proposed a model that incorporates cell proliferation arising secondary to cytotoxicity or mitogenic stimulation and mutations as they arise from DNA damage from interaction of the chemical with DNA or spontaneous DNA damage. Such biologically based models are likely to have an important role in the future, at least for assessing risks of a few chemicals for which substantial mechanistic data become available. For example, the results of the studies on cell proliferation in rats and monkeys chronically exposed to formaldehyde have been reported (60–62). Not unexpectedly, a marked increase in cell proliferation was observed in the nasal tissue of both species. The data indicate a threshold in response with no major differences in cell proliferation in the animals exposed at the lowest concentrations as compared to controls.

Butterworth et al. (63) pointed out that biologically based approaches to risk assessment are not dependent on having detailed mechanistic data. They note that significant progress can be made by considering the mode of action of the chemical in inducing cancer. The mode of action considers the potential of the chemical for (a) interacting with and damaging DNA, thereby causing mutations; (b) causing cytotoxicity, thereby producing compensatory cell proliferation; or (c) direct mitogenic stimulation via receptor-mediated events.

## RISK COMMUNICATION

As noted early in this chapter, risk communication is often overlooked as a part of the risk paradigm. For practitioners of environmental and occupational medicine, however, risk communication is a critical aspect of their professional practice. Risk communication is the process of communicating to workers, local citizens, plant managers, regulatory authorities, and others the nature and extent of risks associated with particular operations.

Effective risk communication poses several challenges. One of the major challenges is the need to communicate to a diverse audience, many members of which may not be particularly knowledgeable about the technical details of the topics under discussion. However, they do have a clear stake in the matter under consideration: their health, their livelihood, and their sense of well-being may all be at stake. A second challenge that is frequently encountered relates the quest for certainty. This is illustrated with the question, Is my workplace environment safe? The question can rarely be answered with a yes or no response. Safety is a relative term. This leads to a third challenge, the need to use quantitative concepts when communicating risk. What is the level of exposure? What is the potency of the toxic agent for causing adverse effects? What is the likelihood of a toxicant-induced effect occurring? What are the severity and duration of the toxicant-induced effect? How do the likelihood and severity of the toxicant-induced effect compare to the overall prevalence and severity of the health effect influenced by other factors. These other factors include the individual's or population's genetic makeup, age, social habits (e.g., smoking, diet), occupation, and environment.

## ACKNOWLEDGMENTS

Grateful acknowledgment is made of the assistance of the following individuals in preparing this chapter: for scientific review, Drs. William Bunn, Rory Conolly, and Paul Schlosser; for scientific editing, Dr. Barbara Kuyper; for word processing, Linda Smith; and for graphics, Stan Piestrak.

## REFERENCES

1. National Research Council (NRC). *Risk assessment in the federal government:* Managing the process. Washington: National Academy Press, 1983.
2. National Research Council (NRC), Committee on Risk Assessment of Hazardous Air Pollutants. *Science and judgment in risk assessment.* Washington: National Academy Press, 1994.
3. U.S. Environmental Protection Agency (EPA). Guidelines for carcinogen risk assessment. *Fed Reg* 1986;51:33992–34003.
4. U.S. Environmental Protection Agency (EPA). Proposed guidelines for carcinogenic risk assessment. *Fed Reg* 1996;61:17959–18011.
5. U.S. Environmental Protection Agency (EPA). Proposed guidelines for neurotoxicity risk assessment. *Fed Reg* 1995;60:52032–52056.
6. U.S. Environmental Protection Agency (EPA), Office of Prevention, Pesticides and Toxic Substances. *Biochemical test guidelines:* immunotoxicity. Report no. EPA/712-C-96 280. Washington, DC: EPA, 1996.
7. U.S. Environmental Protection Agency (EPA). Guidelines for reproductive toxicity risk assessment. *Fed Reg* 1996;61(212):56274–56322.
8. U.S. Environmental Protection Agency (EPA). Guidelines for developmental toxicity risk assessment. *Fed Reg* 1991;56(234): 63798–63826.
9. U.S. Environmental Protection Agency (EPA), Office of Prevention, Pesticides and Toxic Substances. Health effects test guidelines: acute inhalation toxicity. Report no. EPA/712-C-96 193. Washington, DC: EPA, 1996.
10. Ames BN, McCann J, Yamasek E. Methods for detecting carcinogens as mutagens with the *Salmonella*/mammalian microsome mutagenicity test. *Mutat Res* 1975;31:347–364.
11. Gaido KW, Leonard LS, Lovell S, et al. Evaluation of chemicals with endocrine modulating activity in a yeast-based steroid hormone receptor gene transcription assay. *Toxicol Appl Pharmacol* 1997;143: 205–212.
12. McConnell EE. Maximum tolerated dose in particulate inhalation studies. A pathologist's point of view. *Inhal Toxicol* 1996;8(suppl):111–124.

13. International Agency for Research on Cancer (IARC). *Overall evaluations of carcinogenicity:* an updating of IARC monographs [IARC monographs on the evaluation of carcinogenic risks to humans, supplement 70, vols 1 to 42]. Lyon, France: IARC, 1987.
14. International Agency for Research on Cancer (IARC). *Printing processes and printing inks, carbon black and some nitro compounds* [IARC monographs on the evaluation of carcinogenic risks to humans, vol 65]. Lyon, France: IARC, 1996.
15. Wilbourn J, Haroun L, Heseltine E, Kaldor J, Partensky C, Vainio H. Response of experimental animals to human carcinogens: an analysis based upon the IARC monographs programme. *Carcinogenesis* 1986;7: 1853–1863.
16. Tomatis L, Aitio A, Wilbourn J, Shuker L. Human carcinogens so far identified. *Jpn J Cancer Res* 1989;80:795–807.
17. Vainio H, Wilbourn J, Tomatis L. Identification of environmental carcinogens: the first step in risk assessment. In: Mehlman MA, Upton A, eds. *The identification and control of environmental and occupational diseases:* hazards and risks of chemicals in the oil refining industry. Princeton: Princeton Scientific, 1994;1–19.
18. International Agency for Research on Cancer (IARC). *Some industrial chemicals* [IARC monographs on the evaluation of carcinogenic risks to humans, vol 60]. Lyon, France: IARC, 1994.
19. International Agency for Research on Cancer (IARC). *A consensus report of an IARC monographs working group on the use of mechanisms of carcinogenesis in risk identification.* IARC intern. tech. rep. no. 91/002). Lyon, France: IARC, 1991.
20. Vainio H, Heseltine E, McGregor D, Tomatis L, Wilbourn J. Working group on mechanisms of carcinogenesis and the evaluation of carcinogenic risks. *Cancer Res* 1992;52:2357–2361.
21. Vainio H, Magee P, McGregor D, McMichael A, ed. *Mechanisms of carcinogenesis in risk identification.* IARC scientific publications no. 116]. Lyon, France: IARC, 1992.
22. McClellan RO. Evaluation of the potential health risks of man-made fibers using fibrous glass as an example. *J Occup Health Safety—Aust NZ* 1996;12:247–257.
23. McClellan RO. Lung cancer in rats from prolonged exposure to high concentrations of particles: implications for human risk assessment. *Inhal Toxicol* 1996;8(suppl):193–226.
24. National Toxicology Program (NTP). *Seventh annual report on carcinogens,* 2 vols. Washington, DC: U.S. Department of Health and Human Services, Public Health Services, 1994.
25. National Toxicology Program (NTP). Revised criteria and process for listing substances in the biennial report on carcinogens. *Fed Reg* 1996; 61(188):50499–50500.
26. American Conference of Governmental Industrial Hygienists (ACGIH). *Threshold limit values and biological exposure indices for 1995–1996.* Cincinnati, OH: ACGIH, 1995.
27. American Conference of Governmental Industrial Hygienists (ACGIH). *Documentation for the threshold limit values and biological exposure indices for 1991.* Cincinnati, OH: ACGIH, 1991.
28. Barnes DG, Dourson M. Reference dose (RfD): description and use in health risk assessments. *Regul Toxicol Pharmacol* 1988;8: 471–486.
29. U. S. Environmental Protection Agency (EPA). *Methods for derivation of inhalation reference concentration and application of inhalation dosimetry.* Report no. EPA/600/8 90/066F. Washington, DC: EPA, 1994.
30. Jarabek AM. Inhalation RfC methodology: dosimetric adjustments and dose-response estimation of noncancer toxicity in the upper respiratory tract. In: Miller F, ed. *Nasal toxicity and dosimetry of inhaled xenobiotics:* implications for human health. Washington: Taylor & Francis, 1995;301–325.
31. Crump KS. An improved procedure for low-dose carcinogenic risk assessment from animal data. *J Environ Pathol Toxicol Oncol* 1984;5: 339–348.
32. Clean Air Act Amendments of 1970, Public Law no. 91 604;84 STAT.1676 1713, 1970.
33. Andrews C, Buist S, Ferris BG, et al. Guidelines as to what constitutes an adverse respiratory health effect, with special reference to epidemiologic studies of air pollution. *Am Rev Respir Dis* 1985;131: 666–668.
34. Lippmann M. Criteria and standards for occupational exposures to airborne chemicals. *Clin Podiatr Med Surg* 1987;4:619–628.
35. U.S. Environmental Protection Agency (EPA). *Air quality criteria for ozone and other photochemical oxidants.* Research Triangle Park, NC: EPA, 1995.
36. U.S. Environmental Protection Agency (EPA). *Air quality criteria for particulate matter,* 3 vols. Washington, DC: EPA, 1996.
37. U.S. Environmental Protection Agency (EPA). *Review of the national ambient air quality standards for ozone:* assessment of scientific and technical information. OAQPS staff paper, Office of Air Quality Planning and Standards. Washington, DC: EPA, 1995.
38. U.S. Environmental Protection Agency (EPA). *Review of the national ambient air quality standards for particulate matter:* policy assessment of scientific and technical information. OAPQS staff paper. Washington, DC: EPA, 1996.
39. Wolff GT. The scientific basis for a new ozone standard. *Environ Manag* 1996(September);27–32.
40. Wolff GT. The scientific basis for a particulate matter standard. *Environ Manag* 1996(October);26–31.
41. U.S. Environmental Protection Agency (EPA). National Ambient Air Quality Standards (NAAQS) for ozone. Final rule. *Fed Reg* 1997; 62(138):38856–38896.
42. U.S. Environmental Protection Agency (EPA). National Ambient Air Quality Standards for particulate matter. Final rule. *Fed Reg* 1997; 62(138):38652–38760.
43. Wilson WE, Suh HH. Fine and coarse particles: concentration relationships relevant to epidemiological studies. *J Air Waste Manag Assoc* 1997;47:1238–1249.
44. Albert RE. Carcinogen risk assessment in the U.S. Environmental Protection Agency. *Crit Rev Toxicol* 1994;24:75–85.
45. Clean Air Act Amendments of 1990, Public Law no. 101 549; 104 STAT.2399, 1990.
46. U.S. Environmental Protection Agency (EPA). *IRIS background paper:* integrated risk information system. Washington, DC: EPA Office of Health and Environmental Assessment, Office of Research and Development, 1993.
47. Griffin WA. Toward an improved information resource for risk assessment: EPA's integrated risk information system (IRIS). *CIIT Activities* 1994;14:1–7.
48. McClellan RO. A commentary on the NRC report Science and Judgment in Risk Assessment. *Regul Toxicol Pharmacol* 1994;20: S142–S168.
49. Finkel AM. The case for plausible conservatism in choosing and altering defaults. Appendix N-1. In: *Science and judgment in risk assessment,* National Research Council, Committee on Risk Assessment of Hazardous Air Pollutants. Washington: National Academy Press, 1994; 601–627.
50. McClellan RO, North DW. Making full use of scientific information in risk assessment. Appendix N-2. In: *Science and judgment in risk assessment,* National Research Council, Committee on Risk Assessment of Hazardous Air Pollutants. Washington: National Academy Press, 1994;629–640.
51. Heck Hd'A, Casanova M, Starr T. Formaldehyde toxicity new understanding. *Crit Rev Toxicol* 1990;20:397–426.
52. International Agency for Research on Cancer (IARC). *Occupational exposures to wood dusts and formaldehyde* [IARC monographs on the evaluation of carcinogenic risks to humans, vol 62]. Lyon, France: IARC, 1995.
53. Kerns WD, Pavkov KL, Donofrio DJ, Gralla EJ, Swenberg JA. Carcinogenicity of formaldehyde in rats and mice after long-term inhalation exposure. *Cancer Res* 1983;43:4382–4392.
54. Andjelkovich DA, Janszen DB, Brown MH, Richardson RB, Miller FJ. Mortality of iron foundry workers. IV. Analysis of a subcohort exposed to formaldehyde. *J Occup Environ Med* 1995;37:826–837.
55. U.S. Environmental Protection Agency (EPA), Office of Pesticides and Toxic Substances. *Formaldehyde risk assessment update.* Washington, DC: EPA, 1991.
56. Casanova M, Deyo DF, Heck Hd'A. Covalent binding of inhaled formaldehyde to DNA in the nasal mucosa of Fischer-344 rats: analysis of formaldehyde and DNA by high-performance liquid chromatography and provisional pharmacokinetic interpretation. *Fundam Appl Toxicol* 1989;12:397–417.
57. Casanova M, Morgan KT, Steinhagen WH, Everitt JI, Popp JA, Heck Hd'A. Covalent binding of inhaled formaldehyde to DNA in the respiratory tract of rhesus monkeys: pharmacokinetics, rat-to-monkey interspecies scaling, and extrapolation to man. *Fundam Appl Toxicol* 1991; 17:409–428.

58. Conolly RB, Morgan KT, Andersen ME, Monticello TM, Clewell HJ. A biologically-based risk assessment strategy for inhaled formaldehyde. *Comments Toxicol* 1992;4(4):269–293.
59. Moolgavkar SH. Carcinogenesis modeling: from molecular biology to epidemiology. *Annu Rev Public Health* 1986;7:151–169.
60. Monticello TM, Morgan KT, Everitt JI, Popp JA. Effects of formaldehyde gas on the respiratory tract of rhesus monkeys. Pathology and cell proliferation. *Am J Pathol* 1989;134:515–527.
61. Monticello TM, Miller FJ, Morgan KT. Regional increases in rat nasal epithelial cell proliferation following acute and subchronic inhalation of formaldehyde. *Toxicol Appl Pharmacol* 1991;111:409–421.
62. Monticello TM, Morgan KT. Cell proliferation and formaldehyde-induced respiratory carcinogenesis. *Risk Anal* 1994;14:313–319.
63. Butterworth BE, Conolly RB, Morgan KT. A strategy for establishing mode of action of chemical carcinogens as a guide for approaches to risk assessments. *Cancer Lett* 1995;93:129–146.

*Environmental and Occupational Medicine, Third Edition,* edited by William N. Rom.
Lippincott–Raven Publishers, Philadelphia © 1998.

# CHAPTER 128

# Workers' Compensation

Nicholas A. Ashford

At the turn of the century, pressure began to mount to shift the impact of occupational injury from the worker to the employer and society in general. This pressure came both from increased numbers of successful lawsuits brought by workers against employers for injuries suffered on the job and from increased public awareness that an unfair burden was being placed on workers as the country began a new period of industrialization. The first workers' compensation laws were passed by nine states in 1911, and most of the remaining states quickly followed. At the time these laws were enacted, occupational disease was considered a far less pressing problem than injury. It was not until 1917 that Massachusetts and California became the first states to compensate occupational disease. Unfortunately, it took until 1976 for all 50 states to have some form of occupational disease coverage (1), although that coverage fell far short of addressing most of the serious job-related health problems (2–6).

The primary purpose of a workers' compensation system is to cover the costs of medical care and rehabilitation and to provide compensation for lost wages resulting from workplace illness and injury. The agreement embodied in the state programs is that the employee relinquishes the right to sue an employer for damages in return for fair and timely compensation for occupational injury. To receive compensation, the worker need not prove employer negligence but only that the injury or illness was caused by the job. Most states limit compensation to two-thirds of previous wages and cover all medical costs (2).

Within each state program, three fundamental provisions characterize the operation of the compensation programs: first, all worker claims are handled by the state compensation boards; second, the insurer is entitled to contest permanent disability claims; and third, in any contested case the burden of persuasion is on the worker (7). These provisions establish a one-sided, no-fault system that sometimes operates to the detriment of workers (5,8).

In addition to rapid and fair compensation, workers' compensation programs have two other objectives. One is to internalize the cost of workplace disease and injury so that employers will bear the burden of maintaining hazardous workplaces and have an incentive to improve job safety and health conditions. The other objective is to mitigate the costs to a single employer of a catastrophic financial loss by spreading the risk through an insurance pool. These three goals of the workers' compensation system work somewhat at cross-purposes.

Employers avoid major catastrophic costs through risk spreading, which is accomplished in three ways. The largest firms, which constitute about 1% of employers and 10% to 15% of employees, are self-insured. Risk spreading is accomplished in these firms because of the large number of employees. The smallest firms, constituting 85% of employers and 15% of employees, are class rated. Class rating sets a payroll tax deduction based on industry illness and injury history. The third mechanism used by the remainder of firms, which constitute 14% of employers and about 70% of employees, is experience rating, which is class rating further adjusted to individual experience (9). While these mechanisms promote the goal of risk spreading, they impair attainment of the goal of internalization of injury and illness costs. Since, in most cases, the full cost of disease and injury does not fall on an individual employer, risk spreading, in fact, removes a considerable portion of the incentive to improve job health and safety (2).

N. A. Ashford: School of Engineering, Massachusetts Institute of Technology, Cambridge, Massachusetts 02139.

Even if the risk spreading effects of the insurance system did not weaken the employer's impetus to improve job health and safety conditions, little actual incentive exists for an employer to internalize the costs of harm of chronic occupational disease. The employer faces a choice: reduce health hazards today or pay compensation costs 20 to 30 years from now. The cost of capital—the interest-earning capacity of money—makes it economically attractive to avoid compliance costs today, even if higher workers' compensation benefits, measured in nominal terms, might have to be paid decades later. If the costs of workers' compensation were the only incentive an employer faced, the employer would probably profit by postponing preventive measures to improve health and safety.

This chapter reviews some of the inequities arising from variations among state systems and discusses efforts to ameliorate them. General trends and costs of workers' compensation programs, the problems of occupational disease coverage, and alternative mechanisms for compensating occupationally diseased victims are also examined.

## INEQUITIES AND STATE VARIATIONS

Prompted by the 1972 study of the National Commission on State Workmen's Compensation Laws, the 1976 Democratic platform promised nationwide minimum standards for workers' compensation programs. The national commission, composed of representatives from labor, industry, and state and federal governments, investigated the status of compensation programs in all 50 states and issued a unanimous report calling for 84 revisions in state systems (10).

Among the problems the commission found were that many employees had no coverage at all; occupational diseases were not covered adequately; there were arbitrary limits on medical and physical rehabilitation services, as well as on the duration or total amount of benefits; there were inadequate cash benefits for temporary, permanent, total, and partial disabilities and for death dependents; coverage of work-related diseases with latency periods was limited by filing restrictions; and in some cases, filing jurisdictions were unclear and provided very different compensation schedules. The commission specified 19 changes that they considered essential. Their report concluded that the states should be given some time to straighten out their programs but that Congress should act by 1975 if all states had not then resolved the most severe problems of workers' compensation.

In the years since the national commission's report, many states have updated, expanded, and improved their programs. These improvements have included expanded coverage to all employees, longer periods for filing claims, full medical benefits for occupational disease, and broader representation of labor's concerns as reflected in the composition of the state compensation boards. While the states' record of compliance with the commission's 19 essential recommendations has clearly shown improvement (an average compliance score of 12.7 out of 19.0 in 1992 compared with 6.8 in 1972), most gains (12.0) had already been achieved by 1980 (11). As of 1988, only some 30 states were in full compliance, and the commission's chairman expressed his continued disappointment, concluding "the quest for adequate workers' compensation benefits is far from over" (12).

In recent years, many states have further increased workers' compensation benefits. Nevertheless, workers' compensation benefits still vary significantly among the states. For instance, in 1995, the maximum state benefits for both temporary total disability and permanent total disability ranged from $817 in Iowa to $253 in Mississippi (13). In 29 jurisdictions, permanent total disability payments were at least 100% of the state's average wage, although in 10 states the payments were no more than 75% of the average wage (13). Although the differences among states in workers' compensation benefits paid to workers have narrowed significantly in recent years (as measured by benefits paid per 100,000 workers), it appears that the primary cause is a substantial reduction in benefits paid by the more generous states rather than an increase in benefits paid by the less generous states (14).

Since 1976, members of Congress have sought to renew the promise of fair and adequate coverage for occupational injury and disease through the imposition of nationwide standards. Characteristically, labor and employers have found themselves on opposite sides of this issue. Labor has vigorously supported nationwide standards as a way to remove the inequities and injustices of the current program, and employers have tended to believe that states can resolve the problems without national interference (9). In the past few years, after escalating costs and inadequate benefits, labor, management, and insurers have all been calling for major reforms (15).

In the past, consensus for a federal solution was reached only after a work-related disease became a pressing problem for industry, and then the solution typically involved the federal government's absorbing most of the compensation costs. The black lung program is a prominent example.

## TRENDS AND COSTS IN COVERAGE

Although workers' compensation programs are supposed to provide coverage for all workers, the national commission found that 15% of the 1972 work force was not covered. By 1980 the percentage of uncovered workers declined to around 10% (16). Workers who are not covered include casual workers, some small business workers, domestic workers, farm workers, self-employed workers, and state and local government workers.

It is estimated that in 1978 there were 7.8 million workers' compensation awards in the following categories:

| | |
|---|---|
| Medical payments | 6 million |
| Temporary disability benefits | 1.3 million |
| Partial disability benefits | 0.42 million |
| Permanent total disability benefits | 2,600 |
| Death benefits | 7,800 |

Although the incidence of occupational injuries and illnesses originally declined after the passage of the Occupational Safety and Health (OSH) Act, from 10.9 cases per 100 workers in 1972 to 7.6 cases per 100 workers in 1983, it has edged up in recent years, to 8.9 cases per 100 workers in 1992 (17). Even more troubling is the fact that, per 100 workers, the rate of injuries involving time lost from work—injuries that are presumptively more severe—has increased by approximately 20% between 1972 and 1992, and the average time lost as a result of these injuries has steadily increased over the period, by approximately 65% in total (6,17).

The fastest growing category of occupational disease, by far, has been musculoskeletal problems resulting from cumulative or repetitive trauma, such as carpal tunnel syndrome (6). Of the 368,000 new cases of occupational disease reported by employers in 1991, some 61% were cumulative or repetitive trauma cases, up from 18% in 1981 (18). In that year, musculoskeletal disorders accounted for 43% of all occupational injuries and illnesses reported by the Bureau of Labor Statistics (18).

Ignoring musculoskeletal disorders, only 5% of occupational diseases are covered by workers' compensation programs (16), and occupational disease accounts for only about 1% of all workers' compensation claims (15).

The costs of workers' compensation have been escalating since the national commission's report and the subsequent state efforts to improve programs. In 1970, total costs were about $4.9 billion; by 1978, costs had escalated to $15.8 billion. This increase was due to inflation in medical costs as well as to improvements in coverage. At the same time that payments were increasing by more than threefold, workers' compensation costs as a percentage of payroll increased by 62%, from 1.11% to 1.80%; 60% of premiums were paid out in compensation, and 40% were used to pay overhead, legal fees, and to provide a cash surplus for insurance carriers (16).

After the mid-1980s workers' compensation insurance costs were driven by rising medical expenses rather than by rising cash benefits for workers (15). From 1990 to 1993 alone, the medical component of workers' compensation benefits increased from 40.9% of total workers' compensation benefits to 50% (6). By 1993, workers' compensation programs cost $57.3 billion, up from $25.1 billion in 1984, and the share of costs paid out in compensation had increased to 73% (19,20). Meanwhile, workers' compensation costs as a percentage of payroll rose to a peak of 2.40% in 1991 and then dipped back slightly to 2.30% in 1993 (20).

Theoretically, workers' compensation payments are intended to provide for two-thirds wage replacement in individual cases. In reality, however, they do not operate this way. Total lost income for occupational disease was estimated to be around $11.4 billion for 1978, and since at most 3% of the $15.8 billion awarded in 1978 was for work-related disease, nearly $11 billion of lost wages was not compensated by workers' compensation programs. If one considers all sources of compensation, only 40% of the earnings lost because of disease is compensated in individual cases, and only 5% of the compensation is provided by workers' compensation programs. The remainder comes from Social Security, welfare, pensions, veterans' benefits, and private insurance.

Work-related *injuries* are covered at a rate of about 60%, the majority of this compensation coming from workers' compensation programs (16). The total compensation from all sources for wages lost from work-related injuries averages around 60%. In 1980, for workers totally disabled by *disease,* the average lifetime compensation in individual cases was $9,700, which is 12.6% of the $77,000 they would normally have expected in adjusted lifetime earnings (16). In very few individual cases does the compensation meet the two-thirds wages goal, and the aggregate figures show an even more dismal picture.

Among the reasons for failure of state programs to cover occupational disease and injury adequately are these:

Payments are subject to low ceilings.
No cost-of-living increases are provided.
Payments for severe permanent disability are lower than those for temporary disability.
There are restrictions on medical care services and total amounts compensated.
Nonpecuniary losses, such as pain and suffering, are never compensated.
Many occupational diseases are not covered at all.
Ten percent of all workers are excluded from coverage.

An additional complicating factor is that compensation is based on the extent of disability as judged by physicians. This arrangement sets up a contest between the worker and employer to find physicians who will provide the most desired judgments.

## PROBLEMS IN OCCUPATIONAL DISEASE COVERAGE

The problems are most severe for occupational disease coverage. Workers' compensation programs did not originally cover work-related diseases, and in 1972 only 41 states provided a reasonable range of coverage. Even today, 21 states limit occupational disease coverage to diseases that are peculiar to or characteristic of a worker's occupation, subject to review by the state workers' compensation boards.

Injuries resulting from accidents were the focus of the original workers' compensation systems. The "risk of the accident had to be peculiar to employment or not common to the general public" (21). When the states expanded their coverage to include occupational disease, they often changed the language so that the disease itself and not the risk of the disease was covered. As a result, in many cases, coverage is limited to diseases peculiar to the occupation and ordinary diseases of life are excluded, whatever their cause. This restriction effectively eliminates coverage for much occupationally related disease.

The burden of persuasion for establishing the connection between workplace conditions and disability is also more difficult to meet with occupational disease (8). Illness, particularly cancer and other chronic diseases, often develops many years after exposure and is not usually traceable to exposure in the workplace.

The distinctions between disease and accident compensation are striking. Sixty percent of all disease claims are initially denied, while only 10% of accident claims receive the same treatment (5,8). In addition, there is more than a 1-year average delay in any compensation for disease victims when it is awarded. Furthermore, work-related disease claims are typically burdened by significant litigation costs; legal assistance is required for 77% of all disease claims but only 24% of all injury claims. Compensation also varies; in 1980 survivor death benefits averaged $3,500 for disease victims and $57,500 for injury victims. Finally, workers' compensation claims are contested at an average rate of 60% for respiratory disease, 55% for heart ailments, and only 10% for accidents (5,11). The majority of uncontested compensated disease claims are for minor ailments or problems readily apparent as workplace induced (16).

As stated earlier, ordinary diseases of life are usually excluded from coverage. These include infectious diseases, many heart ailments, and many diseases with a work-related element. Work-related diseases are not generally covered by workers' compensation for several reasons. One reason is that very often occupational diseases have multiple causes, and it is therefore difficult to trace the cause to the workplace. A second reason is that many diseases have a long latency period, which tends to obscure the precise cause of the disease and the exact place of employment where critical exposure occurred. Problems of multiple causation and latency are compounded by statutes of limitations that apply to claims in most states (5). There are, in addition, jurisdictional problems with disease victims who have changed jobs during the period when the disease was developing. Moreover, many states have set minimum exposure requirements; a worker must be exposed for a specific time period before a disease can be attributed to an occupational cause (21). Finally, a major reason that work-related diseases are not covered by workers' compensation is that workers and medical personnel often do not recognize that a disease results from workplace exposure. They therefore neglect to investigate a particular workplace or occupation as a potential source of disease.

Cancer and respiratory tract disease compensation deficiencies continue to be a critical problem today. To obtain compensation for occupationally induced cancer, workers must prove that the disease is work related, and the standard of proof for this demonstration is difficult to meet (8). The courts have accepted some cancers as occupationally induced—mesothelioma caused by asbestos, leukemia caused by benzene, and angiosarcoma of the liver caused by vinyl chloride are three that are increasingly recognized—but other job-related cancers, such as asbestos-induced lung cancer, are less readily accepted, especially if the worker also happens to have been a smoker. In meeting the standard of proof for causation, animal models are not sufficient demonstration that a cancer is occupationally related. Only one of every 79 persons who dies of occupational cancer in the United States receives workers' compensation (8).

Even a nonneoplastic respiratory tract disease such as byssinosis (brown lung) is, for compensation purposes, barely recognized as occupationally related, even though studies of textile workers leave little doubt about the contribution of cotton-dust exposure to byssinosis.

Self-insured employers are subject to the largest losses from successful claims, and they contest at a higher rate than other employers. From the viewpoint of employers the stakes are high: permanent disability from occupational disease accounts for only 5% of the claims but 50% of the costs. To the extent that insurance carriers respond to pressure from employers to keep payouts and, hence, premiums at a minimum, occupational disease will continue to be excluded as much as possible. It is also true that insurance carriers (especially noncompetitive carriers) who operate more or less on a percentage-of-cash-flow basis do face a counterincentive to include occupational disease in order to increase profits. Why, then, is there so much resistance? The answer probably lies in the fact that the occupational disease problem is already large and threatens to become larger (given the history of exposure to harmful substances) and in the great uncertainty involved in setting premium payments for disease. The prospect of large, uncertain payouts in the future would discourage any substantial increase in scheduled payouts for diseases.

In sum, significant scientific, legal, and economic barriers exist to the incorporation of occupational disease into the workers' compensation system. Other avenues to make the victim whole must be pursued, at least as supplements to the currently inadequate state programs.

## ALTERNATIVE COVERAGE FOR OCCUPATIONAL DISEASE

There are two additional means by which workers can obtain payments for general occupational disease. In 1980 the Social Security Disability Income Insurance Program provided 53% of the compensation to occupational respiratory disease victims, and it was their major provider of relief (16). Occupational disease costs this program about $2.2 billion annually, and 47% of all disease-afflicted workers received some form of compensation. Although Social Security compensation is low, it is substantially easier to obtain than workers' compensation: 83.6% of all claims are allowed on initial application (16). Nevertheless, workers often do encounter difficulties under the Social Security program, including 5-month delays in payment, restrictions on recency of employment, and 2-year delays in Medicare coverage.

The second means is third-party liability suits brought in the state and federal courts. These are suits brought against manufacturers of harmful substances that an employee uses in the workplace. Workers are generally prevented from suing their employers directly, unless the employer is also the manufacturer. Through this system, workers are able to bring suits against manufacturers or suppliers one step back in the process. Conversely, employers who purchased the harmful substances for use in the workplace may be able to sue manufacturers for the costs of employee compensation.

Although third-party suits are costly for employees, they are appealing because they provide compensation for lost wages, disfigurement, medical and legal expenses, and pain and suffering. On average, the possible awards are much higher than standard workers' compensation claims.

Product liability suits can be brought for three major causes: manufacturing defects, design defects, and inadequate warnings. To receive recovery, a worker must show an injury, a manufacturing or design defect, and a causal link between the two.

A manufacturer can use the following defenses in the negligence suit: contributory negligence, assumption of risk, and misuse of the product. For a suit brought under a breach of warranty, a manufacturer may use the assumption of risk and misuse of the product. However, in such cases, "defendants usually escape liability only when the plaintiff assumes the risk by voluntarily and unreasonably proceeding to encounter a known danger" (21).

At one time, product liability suits were the greatest concern to machine tool manufacturers and were confined to injury claims. Because of the reduction in third-party liability problems that would accompany national standards, machine tool manufacturers are now one of the few industrial groups that support national workers' compensation standards. The use of third-party liability suits in disease claims is well established in the asbestos exposure area and is now being tested in other areas of chemical exposure. The courts have been considering several issues with respect to worker suits: the producer's awareness of effects, the severity of effects, the user's assumption of risk, and the technological feasibility of instructions and warnings. Unfortunately, a number of factors also limit recovery under this system, including statutes of limitation and the expense and time involved in obtaining recovery through private legal action. These suits are most successful where the link between exposure to a harmful substance and occupational disease is acknowledged as a matter of science or medical knowledge. In cases where the link is weak or allegedly complicated by other possible causes, such as smoking or drinking, recovery in the courts meets the same obstacle it does in the workers' compensation system—the problem of causality. Advances in epidemiology, biologic markers (22), and improved diagnoses by physicians are essential to the recognition of occupational disease in both systems.

In addition to the aforementioned programs to provide payment to victims of occupational disease in general, systems may be designed for a specific disease. An example is the black lung compensation system enacted by Congress in 1977. This system operates as a no-fault mechanism to award those suffering from black lung with compensation and medical care in lieu of state workers' compensation benefits. This substance-by-substance approach arises after a problem has reached crisis magnitude, and it relies on a public bailout of the associated industries. While satisfying the social goal of compensating workers, it provides little incentive for prevention of future harm from new hazards.

## PROSPECTS FOR THE FUTURE

Compensation for occupational disease will, unfortunately, continue to be a problem that is addressed inadequately by state workers' compensation systems. The Social Security system will probably continue to provide assistance to occupationally diseased workers. In terms of specific diseases, workers' compensation systems will never cover the myriad adverse health effects caused by exposure to chemicals in general. Minimum federal compensation standards would improve the situation for many workers, and private lawsuits may benefit others. However, by and large, since causality remains a difficult problem, most occupational diseases will, sadly, not be paid for by the employer, by the consumer of that employer's products, or by manufacturers of harmful substances (5). Instead, the public and the worker will continue to bear the burden. These considerations are one more reason why a strong federal regulatory effort to limit worker exposure to toxic substances is needed.

## REFERENCES


1. Solomons ME. Workers' compensation for occupational disease victims: federal standards and threshold problems. *Albany Law Rev* 1977;41:Sections I, IV, V (part A) and VI.
2. Ashford NA. *Crisis in the workplace:* occupational disease and injury. Cambridge, MA: MIT Press, 1976.
3. Ashford NA, Caldart CC. *Technology, law, and the working environment.* Washington, DC: Island Press, 1996.
4. Barth PS, Hunt HA. *Workers' compensation and work-related illnesses and disease.* Cambridge, MA: MIT Press, 1980.
5. Boden LI. Workers' compensation. In: Levy BS, Wegman DH, eds. *Occupational health:* recognizing and preventing work-related disease. Boston: Little, Brown, 1995;201–220.
6. Spieler EA. Perpetuating risk? Workers' compensation and the persistence of occupational injuries. *Houston Law Rev* 1994;39:119–264.
7. Reuter M. The shame of workmen's compensation. *Nation* 1980;230: 298.
8. Caldart CC. Are workers adequately compensated for injury resulting from exposure to toxic substances? In: Homburger F, Marquis JK, eds. *Chemical safety regulation and compliance.* Basel: Karger, 1985; 92–98.
9. Odlin WS. The workers' compensation controversy: a status report. *Job Safety Health* 1977;5:16.
10. Burton JF Jr. Workers' compensation reform. *Labor Law J* 1976;27: 399.
11. Burton JF Jr. The twentieth anniversary of the National Commission on State Workmen's Compensation Laws: a symposium. *John Burton's Workers' Compensation Monitor* 1992(Nov./Dec.);5:1–5.
12. Burton J. *New perspectives in workers' compensation.* Ithaca, NY: Industrial Relations Press, 1988.
13. *State workers' compensation laws.* Washington, DC: United States Department of Labor, 1995.
14. Burton JF Jr, Blum F. Workers' compensation benefits paid to workers: the 1996 update. *John Burton's Workers' Compensation Monitor* 1996 (Nov./Dec.);9:13–27.
15. Thompson R. Reforming workers compensation. Editorial Research Reports, Washington D.C. *Congressional Q* 1990;1:206–219.
16. *An interim report to Congress on occupational diseases.* Washington, DC: United States Department of Labor, 1980.
17. Rhinehart, L. State initiatives on injury and illness prevention: comprehensive OSHA reform needed. *John Burton's Workers' Compensation Monitor* 1994(Oct./Nov.);7:3–9.
18. *Injuries and illnesses in the United States by industry 1991.* Washington, DC: Bureau of Labor Statistics, United States Department of Labor, 1993.
19. Burton JF Jr. Workers' compensation, twenty-four-hour coverage, and managed care. *John Burton's Workers' Compensation Monitor* 1996 (Jan./Feb.);9:11–22.
20. Burton JF Jr. Workers' compensation benefits and costs: significant developments in the early 1990s. *John Burton's Workers' Compensation Monitor* 1995(May/June);8:1–11.
21. Compensating victims of occupational disease. *Harvard Law Rev* 1980; 93:916–937.
22. Ashford NA, Spadafor CJ, Hattis DB, Caldart CC. *Monitoring the worker for exposure and disease:* scientific, legal and ethical considerations in the use of biomonitors. Baltimore: Johns Hopkins University Press, 1990.

*Environmental and Occupational Medicine, Third Edition*, edited by William N. Rom.
Lippincott–Raven Publishers, Philadelphia © 1998.

CHAPTER 129

# International Occupational and Environmental Health

Joseph LaDou

The Industrial Revolution is occurring all over again and in many different regions of the world. It affects many more workers than ever before, yet the statistical record of its impact is no more precise than it was a century ago. In the absence of an international record-keeping system, there is no way of knowing the extent of human suffering resulting from global industrialization. The International Labour Office (ILO) estimates that 220,000 worker fatalities and 125 million workplace injuries occur each year. There is general agreement that if the developing countries continue their current rate of industrial growth, these figures will double by the year 2025.

The World Health Organization (WHO) estimates that 10 million cases of occupational disease occur each year worldwide. The global epidemic of occupational diseases is occurring almost exclusively in the developing countries. Far too little effort is being made in the developing countries to prevent occupational disease. The failure of the developed countries to protect the health of Third World workers is likely to be a scandal of epic proportion.

The positive economic and social results of industrial activity in developing countries are accompanied by serious environmental degradation. The major cities of developing countries are now reeling from the impact of air pollution, the absence of sewage treatment and water purification, and the growing quantities of hazardous waste buried in or left on the soil or dumped into rivers or the oceans. In many countries, there are no environmental regulations, or if they exist at all, there is little or no enforcement. Except in the most developed countries, there is no serious effort to measure the environmental health impact of industrialization.

The experience of developed countries with the costs of occupational health and safety and environmental programs is that a very substantial financial burden is being shifted to newly industrialized countries. Many developing countries ignore or deny occupational disease and workers' rights to compensation. The cost of future accidents such as Bhopal, mitigation of environmental damage, and effects on the public health are not often discussed with candor in the Third World. Thus the greatest challenge of contemporary occupational and environmental medicine is in the international arena.

## THE GLOBAL INDUSTRIAL COMMUNITY

Foreign companies and investors from developed countries today account for almost two-thirds of industrial investment and development in the Third World. For many countries, such investment is the primary source of new jobs. About one-sixth of the world's foreign direct investment (FDI) is directed to companies in the developing world, up from 5% just 10 years ago. The countries of Asia (excepting Japan), Latin America, and Eastern Europe are referred to as the emerging market, a term coined by a World Bank official in 1981 to enhance the attractiveness of investment in the Third World (1). Multinational corporations have tripled their annual investment in the developing world in the past 7 years, while sharply cutting back on new investments in industrialized nations (2). The shift indicates that business growth prospects are

J. LaDou: Division of Occupational and Environmental Medicine, Department of Medicine, University of California School of Medicine, San Francisco, California 94143-0924.

brighter in Asia and Latin America than in the United States, Japan, and Western Europe.

Most investment in developing countries goes to Asia. Both Japan and the United States have significantly realigned their investment strategies toward Asia in recent years. United States corporations are prominent in China, Hong Kong, Indonesia, the Philippines, Taiwan, and Thailand. From 1980 to 1994, the movement of American money into stocks of foreign corporations increased 16-fold, to $1.5 trillion. The internationalization of portfolio investing has fed a swell in the world's pool of exchange-listed securities. By the end of 1995 the total value of the world's equities was $18 trillion (1).

Among industrialized nations, Japan is a prime source of foreign direct investment. Japanese companies and investments are found in almost every country in the world. With limited land and great population density, Japan has a pressing need to export many of its industries.

European nations invest heavily in the global industrial community. They also have exported hazardous and environmentally outmoded industries to Africa and the Middle East, Latin America, and Central Europe. In Asia, Western European corporations are the largest investors in Bangladesh, India, Pakistan, Singapore, and Sri Lanka (3).

China and India, with the world's largest populations, have had dramatic policy reversals in recent years, and as a result have welcomed industries from many countries. Thousands of foreign corporations now operate in China, and many more are moving into India. Within a generation, China will overtake the United States as the world's largest economy. The combination of growing economic power and shared culture led Hong Kong, Taiwan, and Singapore Chinese to invest heavily in their homeland. Chinese citizens of other countries have supplied much of the capital responsible for the growth of the mainland in the 1990s. China's economy has grown annually by double-digit percentages, and may continue to do so.

The optimistic prospects for Asia's new industrial powers are real in the long term, but can also be exaggerated. China's economy, for instance, has been growing annually by double-digit percentages, but it starts from a very weak base—per capita income of $490 compared with the $24,750 in the United States (4). Measured in hard currency, China's gross national product is roughly equal to New York State's, considerably smaller than California's.

"Greater China" is a rapidly growing cultural and economic reality and has begun to become a political one. The economy of East Asia is increasingly China-centered and Chinese-dominated. Chinese in Southeast Asia dominate the economies of their adopted countries. Chinese make up 1% of the population of the Philippines but are responsible for 35% of the sales of domestically owned firms. In Indonesia, Chinese are 2% to 3% of the population, but own roughly 70% of the private domestic capital. Chinese are 10% of the population of Thailand but own nine of the ten largest business groups, and are responsible for about one-third of the population of Malaysia but almost totally dominate the economy. Outside Japan and Korea, the East Asian economy is basically a Chinese economy (5).

Despite the Asian success stories of China, Taiwan, Korea, and Singapore, global industry continues to primarily benefit the economies of the developed countries. As global trade expanded vigorously in recent years, the developed countries actually increased their commanding share of total exports, from 63% to 72%, while most regions other than Asia suffered shrinkage in exports.

## INCENTIVES FOR GLOBALIZATION OF INDUSTRY

The usual explanation for the migration of industry from developed to developing countries is the lower cost of labor. Few question that the low cost of labor is the principal reason for the rapid growth of industry in the developing world. Labor costs are a small fraction in developing countries of what they are in the developed countries. For instance, the *Financial Times* on March 7, 1994, reported the following comparisons of manufacturing labor costs per hour:

| | |
|---|---|
| West Germany | $24.90 |
| Former East Germany | $17.30 |
| Japan | $16.90 |
| United States | $16.40 |
| France | $16.30 |
| United Kingdom | $12.40 |
| Singapore | $5.10 |
| South Korea | $4.90 |
| Hong Kong | $4.20 |
| Hungary | $1.80 |
| Czech Republic | $1.10 |
| China | $0.50 |

Japanese manufacturers now make more color televisions overseas than in Japan. Matsushita's decision to manufacture televisions in Malaysia, where wages are just 6% to 7% of those offered in Japan, was said to be the result of competition with Korea's Goldstar. In fact, its Japanese competitors, Toshiba, Sony, and Panasonic, already manufacture abroad in less expensive sites, from Wales to Baja California.

This conventional wisdom of labor costs is increasingly questioned by a number of economists. A World Bank study suggests that labor intensity is not so important a factor in explaining the migration of industry as is commonly accepted. Only 15% of the products of environmentally outmoded industries are manufactured by labor intensive production processes (6). Environmentally outmoded industries are defined as those incurring the highest level of pollution abatement and control expenditures in the United States.

Low-cost labor is not the only incentive for migration of industry to developing countries. The more a multinational locates itself in many countries, the more opportunity it has to avoid taxation. The major opportunity for tax evasion occurs through intrafirm trade in which the company, as both buyer and seller, decides for itself the price of goods moving between its subsidiaries and assigns the costs of overhead and debt deductions to suit its own advantage. Tax collectors from competing countries struggle to unwind the complexities of "transfer pricing," but without much success.

The average multinational firm with subsidiaries in more than five regions uses income shifting to reduce its taxes to about half of what they would otherwise be. American companies with subsidiaries in low-tax countries paid relatively low U.S. taxes per sales or assets, lower than the multinationals with branches in high-tax countries. Thus, tax arbitrage provides another incentive, along with cheaper labor, to relocate in such low-tax havens as Singapore, Hong Kong, South Korea, and Taiwan (6).

Global industry does not have to look far for new markets for products, and for workers to assemble them. Virtually all of the world's population growth is occurring in the Third World. At present, the labor force in developing countries totals around 1.76 billion, but it will rise to more than 3.1 billion in 2025—implying a need for 38 to 40 million new jobs every year (7).

The spectacular rates of economic growth in East Asia are being matched by equally spectacular rates of population growth in the Islamic countries. Population expansion in the Balkans, North Africa, and Central Asia has been significantly greater than that in the neighboring countries and in the world generally. In major Arab countries (Algeria, Egypt, Morocco, Syria, Tunisia) the number of people in their early twenties seeking jobs will expand until about 2010. In just 20 years, entrants into the job market will increase by 30% in Tunisia; by about 50% in Algeria, Egypt, and Morocco; and by over 100% in Syria (5).

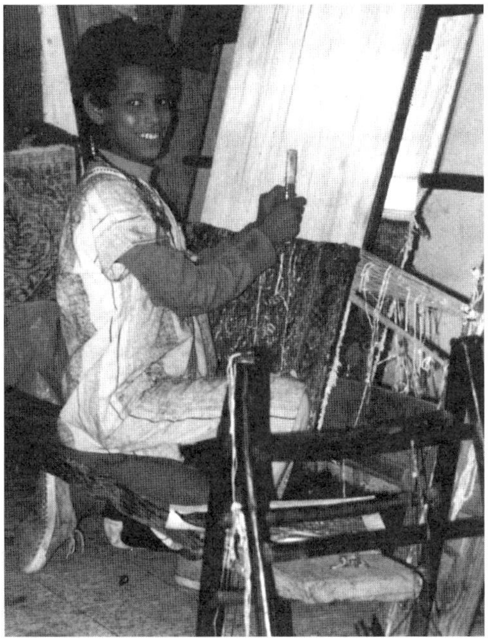

**FIG. 1.** Egyptian boys are often sold to carpet manufacturers for whom they will tie knots for their entire youth. The child is often grown up before the carpet is completed.

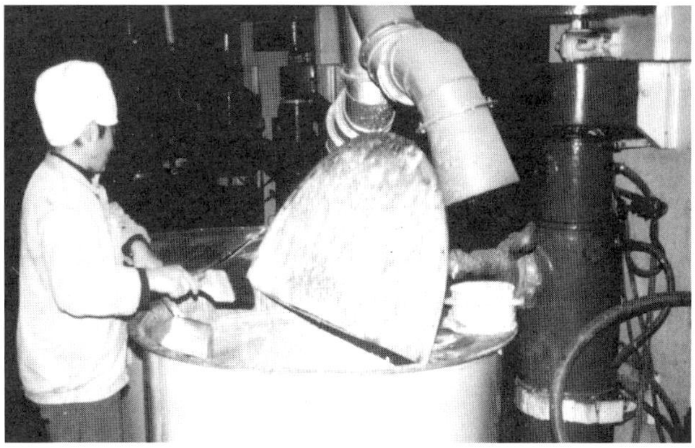

**FIG. 2.** Chinese paint manufacturer still employs benzene as a solvent and a cleaning agent. This worker will need to scour the inside of the paint drum with benzene.

Moreover, children account for up to 11% of the work force in some countries in Asia, up to 17% in Africa, and up to a quarter in Latin America. Children are the most easily exploited of all workers, and in the developing world their numbers are ever increasing. The worldwide population of children under 14 who work full-time exceeds 250 million. Children are often exposed to heat stress, noise, poor lighting, explosives, flying glass, radioactive substances, industrial machinery, pesticides, herbicides, benzene, asbestos, carbon monoxide, and all the other risks associated with work in developing countries (8). Many work settings, such as the thousands of carpet factories of Asia and the Middle East, subject children to slavery (Figs. 1 and 2).

Unfortunately, the Third World's lack of health and safety standards and of pollution control regulations provide another powerful incentive for industry to migrate to developing countries.

## WORKING CONDITIONS IN DEVELOPING COUNTRIES

The work force of developing nations is accustomed to working in small industry settings. Generally, the smaller the industry, the higher the rate of workplace injury and illness. These workplaces are characterized by unsafe buildings and other structures, old machinery, poor ventilation, and noise; workers have limited education, skill, and training. Protective clothing, respirators, gloves,

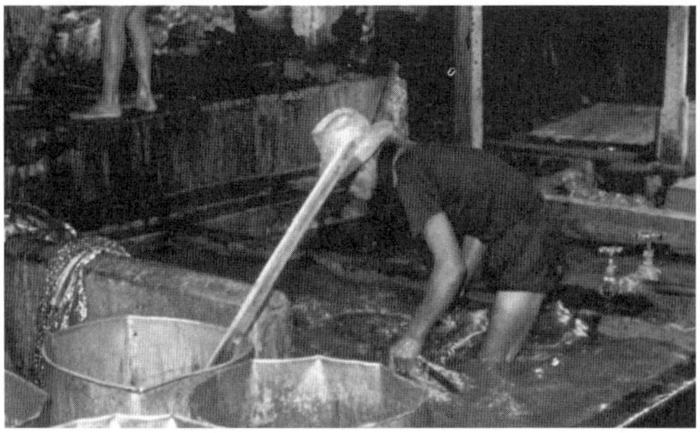

**FIG. 3.** Indonesian dye workers wade in pools of hazardous chemicals for the length of workdays.

hearing protectors, and safety glasses are seldom available. The companies are often inaccessible to inspections by government health and safety enforcement agencies. In many instances, they operate as an "underground industry" of companies not even registered with the government for tax purposes (Figs. 3 and 4).

Multinational corporations may well be the dominant institution of the late 20th century. There are about 35,000 multinational corporations, with 147,000 foreign affiliates. The total annual sales of the 350 biggest multinational corporations are equal to one-third of the combined gross domestic products of the industrial world, and exceed by far that of the developing world. They can be a powerful force in the provision of occupational health and safety in developing countries. In that capacity, they may be more influential than governments and even the local cultures. All too often, the multinational corporations influence the governments of countries where they operate, taking advantage of free-trade privileges, wages as low as 11cents an hour, and a near-total absence of unions. They may even have sanctioned forced labor in some areas of the world (1).

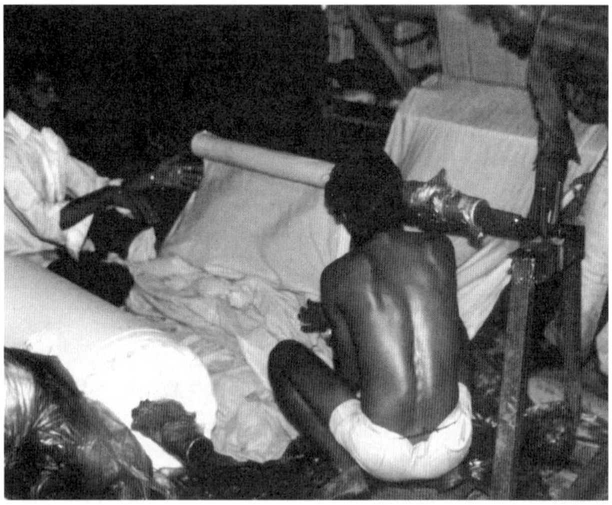

**FIG. 4.** Indian workers exposed to toxic dyes receive no governmental protection and no benefits in the event of occupational illness.

The major multinationals grew in sales from $721 billion in 1971 to $5.2 trillion in 1991, claiming a steadily growing share of commerce (one-third of all manufacturing exports, three-fourths of commodity trade, four-fifths of the trade in technology and management services). Yet the human labor required for each unit of their output has diminished dramatically (4). During the last generation the world's 500 largest multinational corporations grew sevenfold in sales. Yet the worldwide employment by these global firms remained virtually unchanged. This being the case, worker demands for better working conditions are not likely to occur (9).

The asbestos industry serves as a good example of the influence of multinational corporations on governments. Canada and other asbestos-exporting countries are looking to the developing countries as a major market for asbestos. Increased use of asbestos in developing countries offsets market losses in the developed countries. Quarterly publications of the Asbestos Institute of Canada describe aggressive sales efforts in Asia, Africa, and Latin America. Unfortunately, conditions of current asbestos use in Asia, Africa, Latin America, and Eastern Europe resemble those that existed in the industrialized nations before the consequences of breathing asbestos dust was recognized. This exploitation of ignorance and poverty has the strong backing of the government of Canada and a number of other governments.

The European multinational corporations Eternit (of Belgium) and Saint Gobain (France) present a deplorable history of exploitation in Brazil. They opened huge and profitable markets, not only in Brazil but elsewhere in Latin America and the countries where Brazilian asbestos is exported. Brazil is now the fifth largest producer and consumer of asbestos in the world, after Russia, Canada, Kazakhstan, and China. More than half of Brazil's asbestos is mined by the European consortium created by Eternit and Saint Gobain. Brazil exports about 70,000 tons of asbestos per year, principally to India, Thailand, Nigeria, Angola, Mexico, Uruguay, and Argentina.

While asbestos use in the United States is about 100 g per citizen per year, asbestos use in Brazil averages 1,400 g per citizen per year. As in other third-world countries, the consumption is increasing at an annual rate of about 7%, while the industrialized countries are phasing out their use of asbestos. In Brazil, there are some 3,000 manufactured products containing asbestos. It is mainly used in asbestos-cement, friction materials, the textile industry, and in plastic, chemical, and furniture products (10).

The world's experience with the industrial use of asbestos leads to the conclusion that the only way to assure an end to asbestos-related disease is to ban asbestos. This approach, which has been taken in many developed countries, is even more necessary in develop-

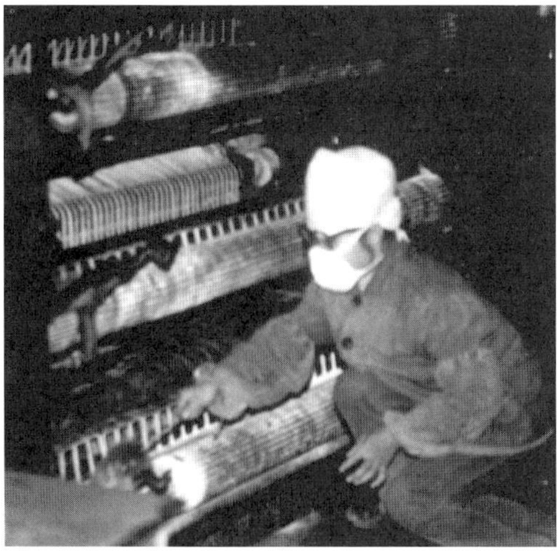

**FIG. 5.** Chinese asbestos workers may create a silent epidemic of asbestos-related diseases since they are seldom evaluated and their illnesses are not reported.

ing countries, where stringent regulation and enforcement is not a viable alternative to a ban (Fig. 5).

An international meeting was held in 1994 in Sao Paulo. The meeting called for a global asbestos ban. The conference was held in a very tense atmosphere. The Canadian government, the French Asbestos Committee, and Brazilian asbestos manufacturers were outspoken in their opposition to the meeting (10).

A medical expert from the ILO spoke against the proposed asbestos ban. He was later identified as an official of the Quebec Asbestos Mining Association and the Asbestos Institute of Canada. A labor expert representing the French Ministry of Labor and the International Commission on Occupational Health (ICOH) was actually an employee of Saint Gobain Corporation. These dual credentials demonstrate the common problem of multinational corporations penetrating governmental institutions and professional organizations with their separate agendas (10).

At the end of the Sao Paulo meeting, the Sao Paulo Declaration called on all governments to place an immediate ban on the use of asbestos in any form, to promote the use of substitute products that have been proven harmless, while maintaining and creating jobs, and to dismantle safely all structures containing asbestos and to provide health care and compensation benefits for asbestos victims. It created a Worldwide Ban Asbestos Network, composed of associations in Europe, America, and Asia, with the common objective of an asbestos-free world. Nothing has come of these calls for help (10).

## THE ENVIRONMENTAL IMPACT OF INDUSTRIALIZATION

Developing countries seldom have enforceable occupational and environmental regulations. They are concerned with overwhelming problems of unemployment, malnutrition, and infectious diseases, often to the exclusion of environmental hazards (Fig. 6). About 450 million people live in extreme poverty and malnutrition, while another 880 million live in what can only be described as absolute poverty (11). Newly industrialized countries are eager for the financial benefits that foreign companies and foreign investors bring them. However, these benefits bring profound social and ecological problems.

In the developed countries, industry provides jobs, pays taxes that support community services, and is subject to environmental and occupational health laws. As industrialized nations enact laws to limit the environmental hazards associated with many industrial operations, production costs rise and undermine competitive advantages. To offset this problem, manufacturers move many of their hazardous operations to the newly industrialized countries. They are welcomed because the creation of an infrastructure in many developing nations relies on industrial expansion by foreigners. When industry migrates to developing nations, companies not only take advantage of lower wages, but also benefit from the low tax rates in communities that are not spending much on such things as sewage systems, water treatment plants, schools, and public transportation. When companies establish plants in developing countries, their tax burden is a small fraction of what it would be in most developed countries. Some migrating companies try to introduce their own corporate or home country's environmental and occupational health and safety standards in the host country. Unfortunately, less conscientious companies simply conform to the standards of the host country. Consequently, worker injury and fatality rates are much higher in newly industrialized countries than in the developed nations.

The positive economic and social results of industrial activity in Third World countries are accompanied by seri-

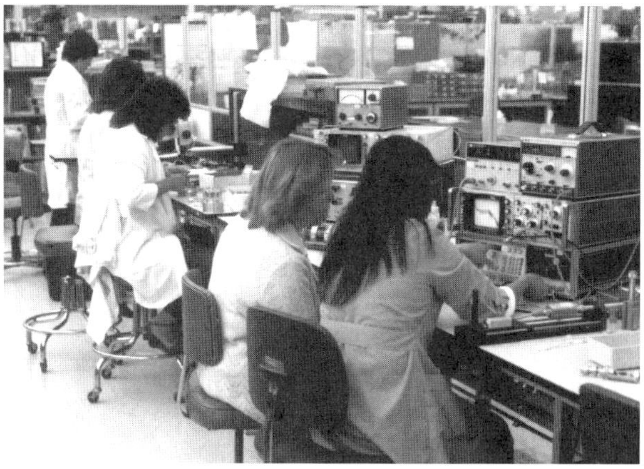

**FIG. 6.** Mexican electronics workers in border plants are mostly women of childbearing age. They are not informed about the reproductive hazards of electronics manufacturing, although employers go to considerable means to discourage pregnancy.

ous environmental degradation. The World Bank reports that the amount of sulfur dioxide, nitrogen dioxide, and total suspended particulates in the air—three of the most significant industrial pollutants—increased by a factor of ten in Thailand, eight in the Philippines, and five in Indonesia in the past decade. Five of the seven cities in the world with the worst air pollution are in Asia. With energy demand doubling in Asia every 12 years, Asian countries will produce in the next 10 years more sulfur dioxide than Europe and America combined (12).

The worldwide use of pesticides is inexcusably inefficient. Nearly 3 million tons of synthetic pesticides are used each year. Most all of this use occurs without the approval of environmental health experts, or in spite of their efforts to control the misuse of pesticides. Moreover, despite the profligate use of pesticides, pests and spoilage still destroy 25% to 50% of crops before and after harvest. Incomprehensibly, that proportion is higher than average crop losses before synthetic pesticides were introduced to global farming (Fig. 7).

Pests can be effectively controlled without heavy application of pesticides by using integrated pest management (IPM). This approach involves various strategies such as developing and planting pest-resistant strains of crops, encouraging natural enemies of pests, following mixed cropping, destroying crop wastes where pests shelter, as well as the discrete and tightly controlled use of synthetic pesticides. IPM is generally a vast improvement over the heavy use of pesticides from both economic and environmental perspectives (13).

Because of the widespread misuse of many pesticides in the developing countries, they especially will benefit from the application of IPM. Indonesia, for example, has had remarkable success with IPM. In 1986, responding to a presidential decree, Indonesia banned 57 of 66 pesticides used on rice. Pesticide subsidies, which were as high as 80%, were phased out over 2 years, and some of the resources saved were diverted into IPM. Since then, more than 350,000 farmers have been trained in IPM techniques, insecticide use has decreased by 60%, the rice harvest has risen more than 15%, and farmers and the Indonesian government have saved more than $1 billion. Pesticide use no doubt could be greatly reduced everywhere by wider adoption of integrated pest management (14).

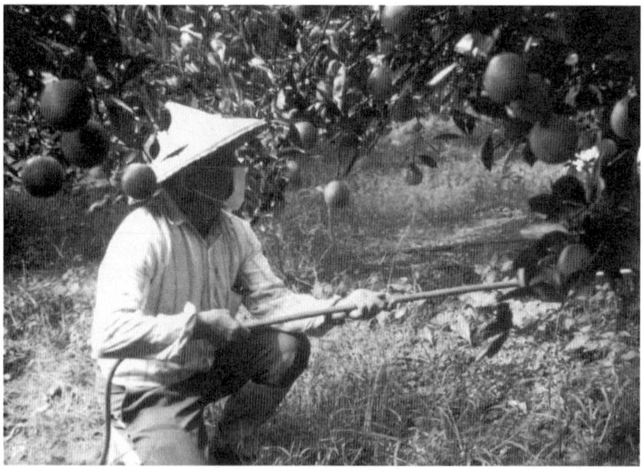

**FIG. 7.** Taiwanese orchard sprayers apply pesticides banned in developed countries that go unregulated in developing countries.

## INTERNATIONAL STANDARDS

The proposition that human dignity is indivisible does not suppose that everyone will become equal or alike or perfectly content in his or her circumstances. It does insist that certain well-understood social principles exist internationally, and that they are enforceable and ought to be the price of admission to the global system. The idea is very simple: every man, woman, and child, regardless of where he or she lives or of his or her place or on the chain of economic development, is entitled to respect as an individual being.

Developing countries often collude with industries to thwart regulation. In many developing countries, opponents of regulation argue that it is a matter of national sovereignty that allows each nation to develop its own standards. In other cases, there is resentment of any foreign influence, especially from the nations that have already increased their standards of living from the industrial activities that are now being regulated. Developing nations often take the position that after they have the standard of living of the developed nations, they will then adopt stricter regulatory policies. When developed nations are asked to provide developing nations with industries whose technology is environmentally benign, interest in industrial migration lessens dramatically.

Developed countries adopt similar standards for recommended exposure levels for workers that cannot be exceeded without regulatory or legal action. In developing countries, exposure standards are often nonexistent, not enforced, or too lax to be of use. International standards can and should be developed. Developing countries, and particularly the foreign companies that manufacture in them, can be given a reasonable period of time to comply with the standards that are enforced throughout most of the developed world. If this is not done, workers in these countries will pay an inordinate portion of the cost of industrialization.

The most logical international standard of occupational health and safety is the development of an international workers' compensation insurance system. Workers in all countries are entitled to the basic benefits of workers' compensation law. Workers' compensation insurance provides economic incentives for employers to provide a safe and healthful work environment. Workers in all countries, regardless of the ownership of the company, should receive this benefit. At present, only 16% of workers in Africa, 43% in Latin America, and 23% in Asia enjoy protection under social security systems (15).

Developing countries do not have large, well-funded environmental groups or agencies of government responsible for the environment such as exist in developed countries. Enforcement requires the training of personnel and the consistent support of governments that, until recently, placed so much emphasis on industrial expansion that the issue of environmental protection was not even a consideration. This is changing, but there are few examples of active enforcement of laws in the developing countries.

## VOLUNTARY GUIDELINES

There have been many efforts to control the behavior of industry. The Organization for Economic Cooperation and Development (OECD) Guidelines for Multinational Enterprises, the U.N. Code of Conduct on Transnational Corporations, and the ILO Tripartite Declaration of Principles Concerning Multinational Enterprises and Social Policy attempt to provide a framework of ethical behavior (16).

Multinational corporations agree to operate plants according to more strict home-based regulatory standards and thereby set the best example possible in the developing countries. When these corporations bring their home health and safety practices to the developing world, they are a powerful force for improvement in working conditions in newly industrialized countries. They are also a particularly powerful force for raising the living standards and working conditions of women and child workers (17).

Concern about transboundary air and water pollution has led to several different international agreements to regulate such environmental degradation and its possible adverse health effects. These agreements are the result of efforts by the United Nations' WHO and ILO; the OECD; and by the trade provisions of the North American Free Trade Agreement (NAFTA) and the General Agreement on Tariffs and Trade (GATT).

The movement of hazardous waste across national boundaries has attracted special international attention. In 1989, the Basel Convention on the Control of Transboundary Movement of Hazardous Wastes and Their Disposal was adopted at a conference of more than 115 countries and went into effect in 1992. The Basel Convention prohibits the movement and disposal of hazardous waste only if all involved countries—including any transit countries—give their written consent.

Efforts are under way to harmonize the multitude of different occupational and environmental health and safety regulations that exist among the world's economies. However, harmonization may prove elusive. The GATT views stringent health and safety regulations as nontariff barriers, while others—concerned about exploited workers—view lax regulations as a subsidy to production. Another hurdle is that enforcement of environmental regulations is nonexistent in some countries and differs markedly even among industrialized countries. For instance, while American regulatory systems carry the threat of fines and jail, European regulatory systems are in large part only advisory.

Nevertheless, international trade may improve rather than compromise occupational and environmental health. If a superior technology, designed in an industrialized country, was deployed and perfected first in a developing country, then such a technology could eventually compete with the older, less-desirable technologies in both the donor and the recipient countries. The receiving country could then be given an equity share in subsequent sales both back to the exporting country and to other developing countries. But as some point out, such an approach requires a deliberate industrial policy for the environment, not the current collection of laissez-faire trade practices.

The World Bank, the major lender to developing countries, has often been criticized for pressing money on poor countries regardless of need or benefit. The bank is the biggest single lender to the Third World. It holds more than 11% of the Third World's long-term foreign debt, public and private. But the bank does much more than lend money; to a great degree it also decides how its loans will be spent. It proposes, designs, and oversees the implementation of the projects it funds. It requires its borrowers to adopt the economic and other domestic policies it considers conducive to successful development.

The World Bank, through its massive projects and its profound influence on government policies, has a great impact on poor people (18). In 1972, the bank pointed out that 800 million people lived in absolute poverty. Despite massive World Bank lending, that number has since increased by 60% to 1.3 billion, out of a world population of 5.5 billion. Moreover, 80% of the world's population live in developing countries, and they are growing ever poorer in relation to the developed countries. One reason for this is the large debt already accumulated in developing countries. In 1994, for example, the developing world received $167.8 billion in foreign loans and paid out $169.5 billion in debt service—a net transfer from the poor to the rich nations of $1.7 billion.

Dam building is the world's most popular form of development. Since independence, India—with considerable help from the World Bank—has built more than 1,500 large dams. India is now one of the most dammed nations on earth—and many more dams and irrigation projects are planned or under way. So far most have been failures. Seventy percent of the large irrigation projects started since independence are still incomplete. Bank-funded development projects across the world have displaced millions of people, pushing many into destitution (18).

In some industrialized countries, governments have promoted the use of environmental auditing as a systematic way for manufacturers to evaluate the effectiveness of their environmental management systems, to verify compliance with environmental requirements, and to assess risks from regulated and unregulated materials and practices. Environmental auditing, however, remains a little used environmental risk management tool, even in the developed countries. This is largely because manufacturers are concerned that they cannot protect the confidentiality of the company's internal efforts at compliance when disclosure of those audit results is demanded in legal proceedings.

Throughout the world, efforts are under way to internationalize product quality standards through the International Standards Organization (ISO). ISO 9000 and 14000 standards are beginning to be used as benchmarks for product sales in the international marketplace. Structurally, the ISO 14000 series of Environmental Management Standards (EMSs) are a set of voluntary standards and guidance reference documents that include environmental management systems, environmental audits, ecolabeling, environmental performance evaluations, life cycle assessment, and environmental aspects in product standards. The EMSs do not directly establish requirements for environmental compliance or specific levels of environmental performance. Rather, the emphasis is on management standards, much like the ISO 9000 Quality Management Standards (QMSs) series. However, the EMS specification document addresses compliance indirectly through a commitment to both compliance with environmental laws and prevention of pollution.

The increasing emphasis on international environmental standards occurs because (a) foreign facilities become subject to foreign environmental laws with potential sanctions for noncompliance, particularly in the United States and Europe; and (b) the adoption of GATT by most of the trading countries in the world has raised the specter of potential trade sanctions against those countries or regions that have adopted stringent environmental laws that might be construed as trade barriers to importing countries with less rigorous environmental laws. Many companies based in the United States and Europe perceive that the development of international environmental management standards might be the only mechanism for avoiding or minimizing arbitration before the World Trade Organization.

## INTERNATIONAL LABOR

A fledgling labor movement is struggling to be born across the developing countries, though it is still much too weak to threaten the powerful interests that control global industry. The development of these labor institutions may be understood, in time, as a pivotal social question for those societies—their best available mechanism for developing civil society and mature social relations as well as more equitable economic terms (19).

Many developed countries say that they support the concept of free labor, but, in practice, they do not. Major governments like the United States take their cues from the multinationals and are unwilling to press the labor issue against even the most abusive cases (20). International organized labor often expresses its solidarity with exploited foreign workers, but offers little in the way of direct support to the international labor movement.

The global industrial system pays little attention to organized labor. Industries in developing countries thrive on low-cost and disposable labor, more often than not with the collaboration of governments and their politicians. Firms extract the cost advantage until such time as upward wage pressures develop. Then they move on to other, poorer countries, and repeat the process (3).

Imposing rules for minimal wage and working conditions may be the only way to rescue workers in the poorest economies from the their hopeless condition. In reality, global labor rights are far too threatening to the present industrial growth strategies of most developing countries to stand much chance of acceptance.

## RESOURCES

### International Agencies

The *International Labor Office* (ILO) brings governments, employers, and trade unions together for united action in the cause of social justice and better working and living conditions. The ILO establishes international labor standards, technical guides, and codes of practice. During the past 10 years the ILO has assisted many countries to define and implement a coherent occupational safety and health policy, establish or strengthen specialized institutions and services, organize appropriate training, and encourage tripartite participation. Cooperation with international organizations is an essential feature of ILO activities. For information, contact Chief, Occupational Safety and Health Branch, ILO, 4, Route des Morillons, CH-1211 Geneva 22, Switzerland; telephone 41 22 799 67 16, fax 41 22 799 68 78; E-mail: takala@hq1.illo.ch.

The *International Occupational Safety and Health Information Center* (CIS) of the International Labor Office offers access to literature published worldwide in the field of occupational safety and health through a bibliographic database available on a subscription basis. CIS operates in collaboration with more than a hundred national OSH institutions around the world. These organizations can be accessed on their Internet home pages through hyperlinks. For information, contact: ILO/BIT-CIS, CH 1211 Geneva 22, Switzerland; telephone 41 22 799 67 40, fax 41 22 798 62 53, E-mail: 100043.2440@compuserve.com. Home page: http://turva.me.tut.fi/cis/home.html.

The *United Nations Development Program* (UNDP) is the world's largest source of grant funding for development cooperation. Its funds, which totaled $1.9 billion in 1995, come from yearly voluntary contributions from member states of the U.N. or its related agencies. Through a network of 136 offices worldwide, UNDP works with 175 governments to build developing countries capacities for sustainable human development. UNEP activities focus on four priority areas: poverty elimination, creation of jobs and sustainable livelihoods, advancement of women, and protection and regeneration of the environment. Environmental objectives are included in almost all of the country programs approved for UNDP funding. For information, contact UNDP, 1 United Nations Plaza, New York, NY 10017.

The *United Nations Environment Program* (UNEP) was established in 1972 and given by the United Nations a broad and challenging mandate to stimulate, coordinate, and provide policy guidance for sound environmental actions throughout the world. From the global headquarters in Nairobi, Kenya, and seven regional and liaison office worldwide, UNEP carries out a program laid down and revised every 2 years by a governing council of representatives from its 58 member states. UNEPs programs stimulate action on major environmental problems and promote environmentally sound management at both the national and international levels. Activities are grouped under five program areas: sustainable management and use of natural resources, sustainable production and consumption, a better environment for human health and well-being, globalization and the environment, and global and regional servicing and support. For information, contact the UNEP Regional Office for North America, Room DC2-0803, 2 United Nations Plaza, New York, NY 10017.

The *World Health Organization Office of Occupational Health* assists countries in protecting and promoting the health of the working population by developing appropriate national programs based on the principles and objectives of the WHO Global Strategy for Occupational Health for All. WHO Collaborating Centers exchange experience in occupational health between industrialized and developing countries with regional and country projects. The Office of Occupational Health reviews standards and criteria, particularly industrial hygiene guides, and coordinates research and epidemiologic studies on occupational health. It assists in the development of information systems. For information, contact Chief Medical Officer, Office of Occupational Health, WHO, CH-1211 Geneva 27, Switzerland; telephone 41 22 791 4806, fax 41 22 791-4806; E-mail: mikheevm@who.ch.

**U.S. Government Agencies**

The missions and bureaus of the *Agency for International Development* (AID) receive technical assistance from the Environment Health Project (EHP) when it addresses the growing health problems created by environmental pollution and degradation in developing countries. EHP provides technical assistance with water and sanitation, wastewater, solid waste, toxic and hazardous waste, air pollution, food hygiene, occupational health, injury, and tropical diseases in 80 projects in 22 countries.

The project is organized as a consortium of specialized organizations headed by Camp Dresser & McKee International Inc., all with staff and consultants experienced in developing countries and fluent in foreign languages. The consortium gives EHP access to expertise in disciplines vital to sustainable development: public participation, financial management, health and information system development, institution-building, and policy making. For information, contact EHP, 1611 North Kent Street, Suite 300, Arlington, VA 22209-2111; telephone (703) 247-8730, fax (703) 243-9004; E-mail: ehp@access.digex.com. Home page: http://www.access.digex.net/~ehp.

The *Bureau of International Labor Affairs* (U.S. Department of Labor) assists in formulating international economic, trade, and immigration policies affecting American workers. The bureau represents the United States on delegations to multilateral and bilateral trade negotiations, and on such international bodies as the International Labor Organization (ILO), the Organization for Economic Cooperation and Development (OECD), the World Trade Organization (WTO), and other United Nations Organizations.

The bureau's Office of Foreign Relations provides technical assistance to developing countries and to countries in transition from communism through the organization and delivery of U.S. skills, resources, technology, and personnel to address labor-related problems. For information, contact BILA, 200 Constitution Avenue, N.E.,Washington, D.C. 20210.

The *Fogarty International Center* (FIC) of the National Institutes of Health (NIH) collaborates with the National Institute of Environmental Health Sciences (NIEHS), the National Institute for Occupational Safety and Health (NIOSH), and the Centers for Disease Control and Prevention (CDC) to develop international training and research programs related to environmental health for foreign health scientists, clinicians, epidemiologists, toxicologists, engineers, industrial hygienists, chemists, and allied health workers from developing countries and emerging democracies. Awards to U.S. and foreign universities support programs in more than 20 developing countries. For information, contact Division of International Training and Research, Fogarty International Center, NIH Bldg. 31, room B2C32, 9000 Rockville Pike, Bethesda, MD 20892-2220; telephone (301) 496-1653, fax (301) 402-2056; E-mail: jbreman@nih.gov.

The *National Center for Environmental Health* (NCEH) is part of the CDC. Created in 1980, NCEH provides national leadership through science and service to promote health and quality of life by preventing and controlling disease, birth defects, disability, and death resulting from interactions between people and their environment. NCEH collaborates with international groups and foreign governments, and provides technical support to CDC activities related to populations affected by complex humanitarian emergencies in foreign countries. Functions include preliminary assessment, epidemiologic assistance, development of public health prevention and emergency preparedness programs and contingency plans, and design and implementation of operational and formative research projects to develop more effective public health and nutritional interventions among emergency-affected populations. For information, contact NCEH Office of Communication, 4700 Buford Hwy NE, Atlanta, GA 30341-3724; telephone (770) 488-7030; E-mail: http;//www.cdc.gov.

The *International Health Programs* (IHP) is a division of the U.S. Department of Energy (DOE) Office of Health Studies. It supports research that advances the knowledge of the health effects of ionizing radiation from workplace exposure and environmental contamination in the United States and abroad. Results of this research serve as the basis for radiation health protection standards worldwide. The major programs of IHP are in the former Soviet Union, in Japan, and in the Marshall Islands. IHP administers the DOE Health Effects Fellowship Program of postdoctoral fellowships in radiobiology, epidemiology, environmental sciences, genetics, medical and health physics, and public health policy. During the second year of the fellowship, research is conducted at various international and related national programs supported by the DOE. During a 5-year period, approximately 30 fellows are trained under this program. For information, contact Office of International Health Programs, EH-63/270CC, U.S. Department of Energy, 19901 Germantown Road, Germantown, MD 20874-1290; telephone (301) 903-1846, fax (301) 903-1413; E-mail: joseph.weiss@hq.doe.gov. Home page: http://tis-nt.eh.doe.gov.ihp.

## REFERENCES


1. Fishman TC. The joys of global investment. *Harper's Magazine* 1997;294(1761):35.
2. United Nations. *1995 world investment report.* New York: United Nations Conference on Trade and Development, 1995.
3. United Nations Centre on Transnational Corporations. *Transnational corporations in world development:* trends and prospects. New York: United Nations, 1988.
4. Greider W. *One world, ready or* not. New York: Simon & Schuster, 1997.
5. Huntington SP. *The clash of civilizations and the remaking of world order.* New York: Simon & Schuster, 1996.
6. Low P, Yeats A. Do "dirty" industries migrate? In: Low P, ed. *International trade and the environment.* Washington, DC: World Bank, 1992, Chapter 6.
7. Kennedy P. *Preparing for the twenty-first century.* New York: Random House, 1993.
8. International Labour Conference, Child Labour. *Targeting the intolerable.* Geneva: ILO, 1996.
9. LaDou J. The role of multinational corporations in providing occupational health and safety in developing countries. *Int Arch Occup Environ Health* 1996;68(6):363.
10. Giannasi F, Thebaud-Mony A. Asbestos in Brazil. In: Peters GA, Peters BJ, eds. *Sourcebook on Asbestos Diseases, vol 10: current asbestos: legal, medical and technical research.* Salem, NH: Butterworth, 1994, Chapter 10.
11. Rantanen J. Development of an occupational health and safety program in Third World countries. In: Reich RR, Okubo T, eds. *Protecting workers' health in the Third World.* New York: Auburn House, 1992, Chapter 2.
12. Goldemberg J. Energy needs in developing countries and sustainability. *Science* 1995;269:1058.
13. Wargo J. *Our children's toxic legacy:* how science and law fail to protect us from pesticides. New Haven, CT: Yale University Press, 1996.
14. Ehrlich PR, Ehrlich AH. *Betrayal of science and reason.* Washington, DC: Island Press, 1996.
15. Kjellstrom T. Issues in the developing world. In: Rosenstock L, Cullen MR, eds. *Textbook of clinical occupational and environmental medicine.* Philadelphia: WB Saunders, 1994, Chapter 3.
16. Fleming LE, Herzstein JH, Bunn B, eds. *Issues in international occupational and environmental medicine.* Beverly, MA: OEM Press, 1996.
17. LaDou J. Women workers: international issues. *Occup Med: State of the Art Reviews* 1993;8:673–683.
18. Caulfield C. *Masters of illusion:* the World Bank and the poverty of nations. New York: Henry Holt, 1996,
19. Shahi G, Levy BS, Lawrence R, Binger A, Kjellstrom T, eds. *International perspectives in environment, development, and health:* toward a sustainable world. New York: Springer, 1997.
20. Frumkin H. Workers in the Global Economy. In: Wallace RB, ed. *Maxcy-Rosenau-Last public health and preventive medicine,* 14th ed. Stamford, CT: Appleton & Lange, 1997, Chapter 34B.

*Environmental and Occupational Medicine, Third Edition,* edited by William N. Rom.
Lippincott–Raven Publishers, Philadelphia © 1998.

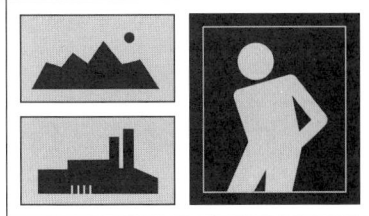

# CHAPTER 130

# Child Labor

Philip J. Landrigan, Susan H. Pollack, and Renate Belville

Child labor is defined as paid employment of children younger than 18 years. It is a common phenomenon in American society (1). According to data from the U.S. Department of Labor, more than 4 million children in the United States were legally employed in 1993, a substantial increase over a decade earlier (2). Illegal child labor is also widespread. Despite the popular belief that this problem was remedied long ago, it has persisted in the United States and appears to be on the rise (3) (Fig. 1).

Internationally, child labor is an enormous social and public health problem (4–7). According to the International Labour Office (ILO), at least 200 million children are employed worldwide. ILO estimates that in developing countries alone there are at least 120 million children between the ages of 5 and 14 years who are fully employed (5). Of these, 61% are found in Asia, 32% in Africa, and 7% in Latin America. Although Asia has the largest number of child workers, Africa has the highest prevalence with approximately 40% of young children employed. The ILO (5) observes:

> Rural children, in particular girls, tend to begin their economic activity at an early stage, at 5, 6, or 7 years of age. In some countries, children under 10 years of age are estimated to account for 20% of child labour in the rural areas and around 5% in urban centres. Their number can be much higher in certain occupations and industries, for example, in domestic service and home-based industries. Children are also conspicuously present in scavenging and rag-picking or in marginal economic activities in the streets and are exposed to drugs, violence, criminal activities, and physical and sexual abuse.

In some countries, children constitute 15% to 25% of the total work force. Children are employed as rug weavers in the Middle East, as underground tin miners in South America, and as metal workers, fireworks makers, textile weavers, and glass blowers. In nations around the world at least one million children are employed in forced prostitution (7).

## HISTORICAL BACKGROUND

Modern-day child labor began in Europe and America during the 1700s as a consequence of the need created by the Industrial Revolution for large numbers of workers. In that era, "Most mill owners preferred to hire children rather than adults. Above all, they were cheaper ... but also more tractable, and as labor unions developed, less likely to strike" (8). Children as young as 11, especially girls, were sent by their families to work in the mills because wages they could earn far exceeded the income of their parents at home on farms (9).

The hazards and horrors of child labor in the 18th and 19th centuries were chronicled by Charles Dickens in *Hard Times* (10) and by Frances Trollope in *The Life and Adventures of Michael Armstrong, the Factory Boy* (11). "Six-year old girls in the mines [of Scotland] did work that later, in times of relative enlightenment, was turned over to ponies" (12). In the mines of Pennsylvania and the mills of Massachusetts and South Carolina conditions were no different (13):

> In the spring of 1903, [in] Kensington, Pennsylvania,...75,000 textile workers were on strike. Of this number

P. J. Landrigan and R. Belville: Department of Community and Preventive Medicine, Mt. Sinai Medical Center, New York, New York 10029-6574.
S. H. Pollack: Department of Pediatrics, University of Kentucky College of Medicine, Lexington, Kentucky 40536.

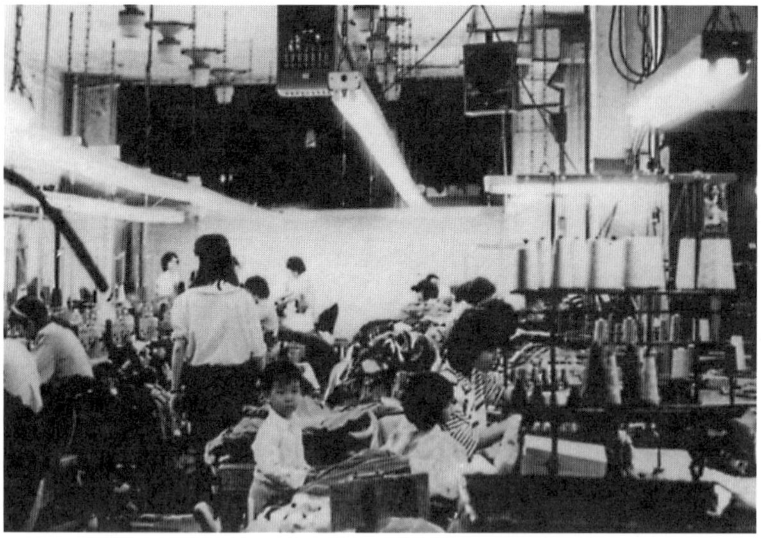

**FIG. 1.** Child workers in a garment industry sweatshop in New York City, 1989. (Courtesy of Dani Steele, photographer.)

> at least 10,000 were little children. The workers were striking for more pay and shorter hours. Every day little children came into Union Headquarters, some with their hands off, some with the thumb missing, some with their fingers off at the knuckle. They were stooped little things, round shouldered and skinny.

Drawings of children being beaten in the cotton mills, lowered on ropes into the coal mines, and carrying 50-pound rocks on their backs up mine ladders sparked great popular revulsion against the worst abuses of child labor (14).

In the United States, despite federal and state legislation, child labor continued to be a major problem during the first third of the 20th century. Inadequate enforcement of existing statutes contributed to the problem. The need for enforcement was tragically demonstrated by the Triangle Shirtwaist Fire in New York City in 1911. Late in the afternoon, one Saturday in March, a fire broke out on the eighth floor of a building that housed the Triangle Shirtwaist Company. Having recently lost their strike for a 40-hour workweek, 500 women and children on the seventh, eighth, and ninth floors of the building were still laboring at the end of their 59-hour week. Since "the factory doors were locked each day to keep the workers in and the union organizers out" and since the interior doors opened inward, fire escapes seemed the only recourse, but they broke under the weight of the desperate workers. The fire-engine ladders reached only to the sixth floor. Ultimately, 146 young women, many not yet aged 18, lost their lives that day, only 8 years after the passage of landmark child labor legislation and fire protection laws in New York. Many of those killed were the sole providers for widowed mothers and siblings (15).

In 1938, after several unsuccessful attempts to pass legislation regulating child labor, the Fair Labor Standards Act was enacted. It remains the major federal legislation governing child labor in the United States today. This legislation established uniform federal standards for minimum wage, overtime pay, and maintenance of records on wages and hours for employees of all ages. Additionally, it established child labor standards, including lists of permitted work hours and prohibited occupations, and it raised the age limit for full-time work to 16 years.

Under the Fair Labor Standards Act no child under age 16 years may work during school hours, and a ceiling is set on the number of hours of employment permissible for each school day and each school week. Employment in any hazardous nonagricultural occupation is prohibited for anyone younger than 18 years. No child under age 18 may work in mining, logging, brick and tile manufacture, roofing, or excavating, as a helper on a vehicle, or on power-driven machinery. Meat-processing machinery, delicatessen slicers, and supermarket box crushers are specifically prohibited.

In agriculture, where the restrictions are much less stringent, hazardous work is prohibited only until age 16, and all work on family farms is totally exempted. According to the law, however, no child under age 16 working on a nonfamily farm is allowed to drive a tractor with an engine over 20 horsepower or to handle or apply category I or II pesticides or herbicides (16).

To combat child labor internationally, the ILO has established the International Programme on the Elimination of Child Labour (IPEC) (5). IPEC serves as an international clearinghouse and assists countries worldwide to reduce child labor. A particular need is for reliable benchmark statistics in each member nation on the extent and severity of child labor; IPEC has developed survey methodologies to collect such data. In parallel, the United Nations Children's Fund (UNICEF) oversees implementation of the International Convention on the Rights of the Child, an international bill of rights for children (6). Additionally, international codes of conduct have been developed for various industries, beginning with the apparel industry; these international compacts are intended to prevent the import into the United States of goods produced overseas by children under sweatshop conditions (4).

With currently pending proposals for the international harmonization of trade regulations, opportunity exists to control child labor, particularly in export markets. But also there exists the countervailing danger that harmonization could occur at the level of least restrictive regulation.

## CURRENT EXTENT OF CHILD LABOR IN THE UNITED STATES

Paid employment is common among children and adolescents in the United States, and is especially common in the later teen years. The U.S. Department of Labor estimates that 2.1 million 16- and 17-year-olds, nearly 1 million 15-year-olds, and another million younger children are legally employed (2). An additional number are employed illegally (3). Some relevant statistics are the following (17):

- Children under age 15 work as news carriers, on farms, in retail stores, and in family businesses.
- 42% of 16- and 17-year-olds reported in 1993 that they had been employed at some time during the past year.
- 16- and 17-year-olds report working on average of 24 hours per week for 25 weeks of the year.
- By graduation from high school, 80% of adolescents in the United States have worked. The most common jobs are in fast-food restaurants, grocery stores, farms, nursing homes, and factories.
- Low-income teens are more likely to be employed in high-risk jobs such as agriculture, manufacturing, and construction.

A reconvergence of economic and social factors similar to those that produced the major increases in child labor at the beginning of the Industrial Revolution has produced the current increase in prevalence of child labor (1):

- *Increased child poverty.* More American children live below the poverty line today than 20 years ago. For those American children who live in conditions of poverty, financial need constitutes a compelling reason to seek employment.
- *Massive immigration.* More immigration into the United States has occurred in the past ten years than in any 10-year period in this century except the decade between 1900 and 1910. Illegal immigrants, particularly children without parents, are highly vulnerable to exploitation in the workplace (4). The recent surge of immigration has lead to the reemergence of illegal immigrant sweatshops in large cities such as New York, Chicago, and Los Angeles (1,18,19).
- *Growing frequency of student-workers (20).* Student-workers are a phenomenon unique to North America. These student-workers, employed after school, on weekends, and during vacation are employed in all industrial sections, but especially frequently in the fast-food and service industries.
- *Relaxation of child labor law enforcement.* Relaxation has occurred since 1980 in enforcement of federal child labor laws, including relaxation of the provisions limiting the maximum permissible hours of work and the prohibitions against use of dangerous machinery. Repeal of the ban on industrial homework, which was created 40 years ago to protect working women and children from industrial exploitation in piecework industries, has further undermined the historic intent of child labor laws. There are fewer than 1000 federal labor inspectors for 113 million workers.

Illegal employment of children occurs today in all industrial sectors in the United States. Sweatshop conditions are increasingly common (18,19). A sweatshop is defined as any establishment that routinely and repeatedly violates wage, hour, and child labor laws as well as the laws protecting occupational safety and health (18). Traditionally, these shops have been considered fringe establishments, such as those in the garment and meatpacking industries. Increasingly, however, restaurants and grocery stores, not typically considered sweatshops, are also fulfilling the definition (19).

Health and safety conditions in sweatshops are often very poor. Fire hazards may be created by blocked exit doors, accumulations of combustible materials, and inadequate ventilation; electrocution hazards result from overloaded electrical connections, workstations located close to exposed wire, and bare fuse boxes. The large number of fire code violations being discovered by the inspectors of the Garment Industry Task Force of the New York State Department of Labor suggests that sweatshop workers, including children, are at very high risk of dying in a fire if these conditions are not corrected (21). The Triangle Shirtwaist tragedy could be repeated.

## RISKS

The hazards of child labor fall into two categories: (1) threats to education and development; and (2) risks of injury, illness, and toxic exposure.

### Developmental Risks

One of the principal hazards of child labor is interference with school performance. Employed children risk having too little time for homework and being overtired on school days; teachers of children in areas where preholiday employment is common or industrial homework is escalating have reported declines in the academic performance of previously adequate students. These children are described as falling asleep at their desks, and they are unable to learn (21). Even if they maintain their academic standing, working children are able to participate less than their peers in after-school activities and sports. Child labor also interferes with play, which is very important for normal development throughout childhood, and relaxation and freedom from fatigue are necessary for children to grow and learn (22). And work can increase the exposure of adolescents to drugs and alcohol (23).

### Health Risks

Injuries, the leading cause of death in children older than 1 year, account for 45% of all deaths of 5- to 14-year-old children in the United States. Approximately 10,000 children die from injuries each year (24). Injuries are the leading cause of potential years of life lost (YPLL) in the United States (25).

Injuries associated with child labor appear to pose a significant public health problem (26). Data reported by the Centers for Disease Control and Prevention (CDC) indicate that in 1993 child and adolescent workers in the United States sustained an estimated 21,620 injuries involving lost workdays (26). The Bureau of Labor Statistics of the U.S. Department of Labor reports that each year between 1992 and 1995 an average of 180 work-related traumatic deaths occurred among working children and adolescents (27). Young farm workers had the largest number of deaths. Workers in jobs that interact with the public such as retail sales clerks also had high numbers of worked-related fatalities; homicide accounted for over 70% of deaths in these occupations (27). Data collected by the National Electronic Injury Surveillance System (NEISS) in the United States indicate that injury rates in 16- and 17-year-old workers are exceeded in the entire work force only by those in 18- and 19-year-olds (28).

Illustrating the importance of the workplace as a source of injury for children and adolescents, a recent review of adolescent visits to emergency rooms in Massachusetts found that work accounted for 7% to 13% of all emergency visits for 14- to 17-year-olds, and for 14% to 26% of visits among 17-year-olds; (29) the fraction of injuries due to work exceeded the fraction due to sports. Comparable data have been reported for Texas (30), Connecticut (31), Saskatchewan (32), and North Carolina (3). Illegal employment has been shown to be especially dangerous, accounting for over 70% of all injuries to working children (33).

The fast food industry is among the most rapidly growing and largest employers of youth in the United States today. Lacerations and burns are common hazards in fast food establishments. There is also a risk of electrocution, although this may have been reduced by changes mandated subsequent to the death by electrocution in 1987 of a teenaged worker in a hamburger restaurant; the source was a power outlet on a wet floor in an improperly grounded building (34).

The delivery of pizzas and other hot food items has proven to be extremely hazardous to working children. The rash promise made by a Midwestern pizza company that all pizzas would be delivered within 30 minutes of the time of placing an order has been shown to encourage reckless driving by young, often inexperienced motor vehicle operators. A total of 20 fatalities, among children working in pizza delivery and the persons with whom they collided, were documented within a single year to be

**TABLE 1.** *Proportion of permanent disability by type of injury among workers' compensation awards to children under 18 in New York State: 1980–1987*

| Type of injury | Degree of disability[a] (%) | Total injury awards |
|---|---|---|
| Amputation | 100 | 121 |
| Fracture | 68 | 1,935 |
| Dislocation | 66 | 148 |
| Multiple trauma | 53 | 564 |
| Laceration | 52 | 3,340 |
| Gunshot wound | 50 | 16 |
| Freezing | 50 | 6 |
| Other | 22 | 3,917 |
| Total | | 10,047 |

[a]Includes 35 deaths from fracture (6), multiple trauma (6), gunshot (3), laceration (2), poisoning (2), electric shock (1) and unclassified injury (15).

**TABLE 2.** *Distribution of work-related injuries in children by age and SIC in New York State: 1980–1987*

| | | Age | | |
|---|---|---|---|---|
| Major economic sector | Total (%) | ≤13 (%) | 14–15 (%) | 16–17 (%) |
| Retail | 53 | 4 | 17 | 62 |
| Services | 18 | 3 | 21 | 18 |
| Manufacturing | 14 | 91 | 41 | 7 |
| Agriculture | 5 | 1 | 11 | 4 |
| Wholesale | 3 | 1 | 2 | 3 |
| Public administration | 2 | — | 5 | 2 |
| Construction | 2 | — | 1 | 2 |
| Transp./comm./electr. | 1 | [a] | 1 | 1 |
| Finance/insurance/real estate | 1 | — | 1 | 1 |
| Other | 1 | [a] | — | [a] |
| Total | 100 (10,047) | 100 (391) | 100 (972) | 100 (8,684) |

[a]Data not available.

associated with the ill-conceived delivery policies of this firm (35).

In the years 1980 to 1987, workers' compensation awards were made to 10,047 children under age 18 years in New York State for work-related injury; 44% of these resulted in some degree of permanent disability. There were 35 deaths (36) (Table 1). These injuries and deaths occurred in a wide range of industries (Table 2).

### Chronic Illness

Little information is available on the incidence or severity of work-related illness caused in children by toxic occupational exposures. However, children are known to experience a variety of toxic exposures at work. These exposures include formaldehyde and dyes in the garment industry, solvents in paint shops, organophosphate and other pesticides in agricultural work and lawn care, asbestos in building abatement, and benzene in pumping unleaded gasoline. Given the wide occurrence of these exposures, it is not inconceivable that some still undefined fraction of adolescent asthma might be related to occupational exposures to dusts or formaldehyde or that some cases of leukemia in children and adolescence may be the consequence of occupational exposure to benzene in unleaded gasoline; previous studies have shown unequivocally that workers exposed early in life to asbestos can later develop malignancies such as mesothelioma. Noise exposure in adolescence may begin the sequence of destructive events in the auditory system that lead to noise-induced hearing loss in adult life (37).

### Health Risks of Agricultural Child Labor

Rural children are employed extensively in agriculture, both on family farms and commercially. The hazards to health associated with agricultural work include lacerations, amputations, and crush injuries from farm machinery; blunt trauma from large animals; motor vehicle accidents involving farm vehicles on public roads; risk of suffocation in grain elevators and silos; and exposure to pesticides. Small physical size and inexperience may, however, superimpose additional risk for young workers. Although the numbers of children working in agriculture are not so large as in other sectors, the potential hazards (especially those involving machinery and large animals), coupled with the historical lack of regulation of agriculture, combine to create an important problem, particularly in rural states. Agriculture has come to surpass mining as the most dangerous occupation (38). Perhaps for this reason, much of the scanty literature available on work-related injury and illness in children focuses on agriculture (39,40).

Data on injury in adolescent workers are provided by a 1985 paper by Rivara (41):

> Nearly 300 children and adolescents die each year from farm injuries, and 23,500 suffer nonfatal trauma. The fatality rate increases with age of the child; the rate for 15- to 19-year-old boys is double that of young children and 26-fold higher than for girls. More than half (52.5%) [of those injured] die without ever reaching a physician; an additional 19.1% die in transit to a hospital, and only 7.4% live long enough to receive inpatient care. The most common cause of fatal and nonfatal injury is farm machinery. Tractors accounted for one half of these machinery-related deaths, followed by farm wagons, combines, and forklifts.

## PREVENTION

Child labor has reemerged in the United States and has become a serious health hazard (40). Prevention of injury and illness in working children requires the following actions:

1. Development of better data to define the extent and severity of the problem of child labor and its associated injuries and illnesses. Absence of these data is a major impediment to prevention. Their collection will permit identification of particularly dangerous industries and occupations and help target prevention.
2. Education of children, parents, teachers, physicians, and the business community about the hazards of child labor. Physicians and other health providers must learn to inquire routinely about work as a possible source of trauma in any injured child or adolescent.
3. Review of existing regulations to determine whether there are areas that require strengthening or modification to be more appropriate to current conditions.
4. Discontinuation of the poorly considered federal initiative to relax certain labor regulations that protect children at work, particularly the regulations limiting industrial homework. This relaxation will lead inevitably to increased child labor.
5. Stricter enforcement of existing law and regulations by state and federal agencies.

## REFERENCES


1. Pollack SH, Landrigan PJ, Mallino DL. Child labor in 1990: prevalence and health hazards. *Annu Rev Public Health* 1990;11:359–375.
2. U.S. Department of Labor, Bureau of Labor Statistics. *Employment and earnings,* vol 41, no 1. Washington, DC: U.S. Department of Labor, 1994.
3. Dunn KA, Runyan CW. Deaths at work among children and adolescents. *Am J Dis Child* 1993;147:1044–1047
4. CQ Researcher: child labor and sweatshops. *Congressional Q* 1996;6: 721–744.
5. International Labour Office. *Child labour:* targeting the intolerable. Geneva: ILO, 1996.
6. United Nations Children's Fund (UNICEF). *The state of the world's Children—1997.* Oxford, UK: Oxford University Press, 1997.
7. U.S. Department of Labor, Bureau of International Labor Affairs. *Forced labor:* the prostitution of children. Washington, DC: U.S. Department of Labor, 1996.

8. Trattner WI. *Crusade for the children:* a history of the National Child Labor Committee and child labor reform in America. Chicago: Quadrangle, 1970.
9. Rossner J. *Emmeline.* New York: Pocket Books, 1980.
10. Dickens C. *Hard times.* New York: Norton, 1854.
11. Trollope F. *The life and adventures of Michael Armstrong, the factory boy.* London: Colburn, 1840.
12. McPhee J. *The crofter and the laird.* New York: Farrar, Straus, Giroux, 1970.
13. Zinn H. *A people's history of the United States.* New York: Harper, 1980;43–44.
14. Hunter D. *The diseases of occupations,* 5th ed. London: English University Press, 1974.
15. Wertheimer BM. *"We were there"—the story of working women in America.* New York: Pantheon, 1977.
16. National Child Labor Committee. *Child labor and related law compendium.* New York: NCLC, 1986.
17. Children's Safety Network. *Protecting working teens—a public health resource guide.* Newton, MA: Education Development Center, 1995.
18. *Sweatshops and child labor violations:* a growing problem in the United States. Washington, DC: U.S. General Accounting Office, 1989.
19. *Sweatshops in the U.S.—opinions on their extent and possible enforcement actions.* GAO/HRD 88-130BR. Washington, DC: U.S. General Accounting Office, 1988.
20. Postol T. Public health and working children in twentieth century America: an historical overview. *J Public Health Policy* 1993;14:348–354.
21. New York State Department of Labor. Hearings on child labor law (Albany, Buffalo, Manhattan, Hauppauge, and Syracuse), 1988.
22. Cohen S. *Social and personality development in childhood.* New York: Macmillan, 1976;163–186.
23. Greenberger E, Steinberg L. *When teenagers work:* the psychological and social costs of adolescent employment. New York: Basic Books, 1986.
24. Waller AE, Baker SP, Szocka A. Childhood injury deaths: national analysis and geographical variations. *Am J Public Health* 1989;79:310–315.
25. Centers for Disease Control and Prevention. Years of potential life lost before age 65—United States, 1987. *MMWR* 1989;38:27–29.
26. Centers for Disease Control and Prevention. Work-related injuries associated with child labor—United States, 1993. *MMWR* 1996;45:464–468.
27. Derstine B. Job-related fatalities involving youths, 1992–95. *Compensation and Working Conditions* 1996(December);40–42.
28. Suruda AJ. Injuries to working children. *West J Med* 1994;161:62–63.
29. Brooks DR, Davis LK, Gallagher SS. Work-related injuries among Massachusetts children: a study based on emergency department data. *Am J Ind Med* 1993;24:313–324.
30. Cooper SP, Rothstein MA. Health hazards among working children in Texas. *South Med J* 1995;88:550–554.
31. Banco L, Lapidus G, Braddock M. Work-related injury among Connecticut minors. *Pediatrics* 1992;89:957–960.
32. Glor ED. Survey of comprehensive accident and injury experience of high school students in Saskatchewan. *Can J Public Health* 1989;80:435–440.
33. Landrigan PJ, Belville R. The dangers of illegal child labor. *Am J Dis Child* 1993;147:1029–1030.
34. National Institute for Occupational Safety and Health, Division of Safety Research, FACE Program, Jan. 22, 1988.
35. Kelly M. A deadly delivery program. *Boston Globe* 1989 (July 19);21.
36. Belville R, Pollack SH, Godbold JH, Landrigan PJ. Occupational injuries among working adolescents in New York State. *JAMA* 1993;269:2754–2759.
37. Broste SK, Hansen DA, Strand RL, Steuland DT. Hearing loss among high school farm students. *Am J Public Health* 1989;79:619–622.
38. Swanson JA, Sachs MI, Dahlgren KA, Tinguely SJ. Accidental farm injuries in children. *Am J Dis Child* 1987;141:1276–1279.
39. Cogbill TH, Busch HM, Stiers GR. Farm accidents in children. *Pediatrics* 1988;76:562–566.
40. Fatalities associated with improper hitching to farm tractors—New York, 1991-1995. *MMWR* 1996;45:307–311.
41. Rivara FP. Fatal and nonfatal farm injuries to children and adolescents in the United States. *Pediatrics* 1985;76:567–573.

*Environmental and Occupational Medicine, Third Edition,* edited by William N. Rom.
Lippincott–Raven Publishers, Philadelphia © 1998.

# CHAPTER 131

# Environmental Justice

George Friedman-Jiménez and Luz Claudio

One of the great challenges of the 21st century will be development of more efficient and sustainable means of industrial production to better meet the needs of human society, while at the same time minimizing the negative environmental impact of that production on individuals and populations, and on the planet. In the process of creating social and economic benefits to society, industrial production also generates environmental contaminants, some of which are hazardous to human health and/or impact negatively on quality of life. The nature and magnitude of environmental contamination, and who is exposed to it, depend not only on scientific and technological factors, but also reflect economic, political, social, and many other influences. A limited body of evidence suggests that the burden of exposure to environmental and occupational hazards is not randomly distributed in the population, but tends to be disproportionately concentrated among low-income and minority communities (1,2).

Perceptions of substantial and disproportionate impact of environmental and occupational hazards on these communities have given rise to a movement to bring about environmental justice as part of the larger goal of achieving social and economic justice. One observation that has generated some of the concern about environmental injustice is that, in many cases, those who tend to suffer the greatest negative impact on health and quality of life caused by environmental contamination from industrial production are not the same people who derive the greatest amount of the economic and social benefits created by that production. A principal objective of environmental justice is provision of adequate protection from environmental hazards for all people, regardless of age, ethnicity, gender, health status, social class, or race.

Over the past decade, the environmental justice issue has become a high priority at the national level. Some of the responses of the federal government to this issue have included presidential executive order 12898, "Federal Actions to Address Environmental Justice in Minority Populations" (3); a large public symposium sponsored by the Department of Health and Human Services, the Environmental Protection Agency (EPA), and the Department of Energy (4,5); a federally funded study currently under way by the Institute of Medicine (6); and a variety of requests for proposals from federal environmental health science funding agencies for development of research and interventions related to environmental justice. This chapter briefly reviews several examples of environmental justice issues, major knowledge gaps and challenges to environmental and occupational medicine, and some of the approaches that have been proposed to address these challenges in the future.

## EXAMPLES THAT ILLUSTRATE ENVIRONMENTAL JUSTICE ISSUES IN COMMUNITY AND WORKPLACE

Environmental and occupational hazards and the diseases they cause can affect members of all communities and all racial, ethnic, and socioeconomic groups. Some evidence suggests that low-income and minority communities and workers may be more exposed and/or more affected than the general population. Since 1987, the environmental justice discussion has expanded beyond its

G. Friedman-Jiménez: Bellevue Hospital Center, New York University Medical Center, New York, New York 10016.
L. Claudio: Department of Environmental and Occupational Medicine, Mt. Sinai Medical Center, New York, New York 10029.

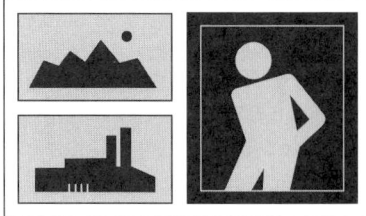

initial focus on siting of hazardous waste facilities to include a range of environmental hazards, in both community and occupational settings (7,8). Available information and data sets are not adequate to systematically review the question of racial and socioeconomic influences on environmental exposure and disease. Most of the evidence consists of studies of specific diseases or environmental and occupational hazards, sometimes limited to a particular community or workplace situation. A few selected examples presented below illustrate some of the medical, scientific, and public health issues of the environmental justice discussion.

**Siting of Toxic Waste Facilities**

One specific example of environmental justice concern about dumping of hazardous waste in a minority community is the uranium ore discarded on Navajo lands in New Mexico during the 1950s (9). Investigation by the Agency for Toxic Substance and Disease Registry (ATSDR) found high enough radiation levels in private residences to cause health concern, and the discarded ore was removed by the EPA and the Navajo Superfund office. This and other cases led to a more general concern about siting practices for hazardous waste facilities.

The Commission for Racial Justice of the United Church of Christ published in 1987, and updated in 1994, a report, "Toxic Wastes and Race in the United States" (8,10,11). The major finding of these studies was that communities that had one or more commercial hazardous waste facilities had significantly higher proportions of racial minority populations than communities with no commercial hazardous waste facilities. In the United States in 1993, for example, people of color (defined as everyone except non-Hispanic whites) constituted 14.4% of residents in zip code areas with no commercial hazardous waste facilities, 29.5% of residents in areas with one facility, and 45.6% of residents in areas with three or more facilities, or an incinerator, or a large landfill. In 1980, a similar trend had been evident. Lower per capita income was associated with having commercial hazardous waste sites as well. The original study was one of the important factors in motivating a substantial response to the environmental justice issue from the federal government.

**Urban Asthma**

Elevated and rising asthma prevalence, hospitalization, and mortality are reported to occur in urban low-income and minority communities (12,13). For example, in New York City, African-American, Latino, and low-income populations were found to have three to five times higher hospitalization and mortality rates from asthma compared with the general New York City population (14). Excesses are reported among adults as well as children, and have increased rapidly in the past 15 years. The time trends strongly suggest that changes in nongenetic factors are important in increasing expression of asthma in these populations.

There is some evidence that exposure to environmental factors associated with asthma may be more common or more intense for urban African-American, Latino, and low-income communities than for the general population (15). For example, racial/ethnic disparities in community exposure to air pollution have been reported, with Latinos and African-Americans more likely than whites to live in areas that exceed National Ambient Air Quality Standards for particulates, sulfur dioxide, and ozone. Wernette and Nieves (16) reported that 15% of whites, 17% of African-Americans, and 34% of Latinos live in geographic areas out of compliance with these standards for particulate matter. The respective percentages of whites, African-Americans, and Latinos living in nonattainment areas were 7%, 12%, and 6% for sulfur dioxide and 52%, 62%, and 71% for ozone. These differences among the races in exposure to ambient air pollution may contribute to some degree to the reported differences in asthma hospitalization and mortality rates.

Most people spend most of their time indoors, and indoor air contaminants may differ systematically by population group (17,18). Goldstein et al. (19) reported that indoor air levels of nitrogen dioxide and carbon monoxide in homes of a predominantly African-American and Latino study group were higher than levels reported in other indoor air studies. The elevated levels were largely due to use of gas stoves for heating the apartment. Aeroallergen exposures related to housing conditions and other socioeconomic factors may differ systematically by racial group as well (20).

Sexton et al. (21) reviewed the relation of race and social class to air pollution and its health effects. They listed relevant associations that have been reported between asthma and specific explanatory variables including race, gender, poverty, maternal smoking, low birth weight, neonatal intensive care, maternal age at birth, maternal education, living in a large family and/or small space, not residing with biologic parent, and nutritional status. These factors are in addition to, or overlap with, specific environmental, infectious, and medication-related factors. They concluded that, despite the absence of systematically collected data, the available evidence suggests that many disadvantaged and minority groups may be exposed to poor outdoor air quality, as well as high levels of indoor air contaminants at home and work. They recommended that areas (such as inner cities) and populations (such as occupational groups) that seem to be at high risk should be identified, and special emphasis placed on understanding and reducing exposures.

### Lead Exposure and Toxicity

There is some evidence indicating that African-American children are more likely to be exposed to environmental lead, to have elevated blood lead levels, and, as a result, to suffer toxic effects of lead, than white children (22,23). Since regulation and removal of lead from gasoline, persisting disparities in exposure and blood lead levels may be predominantly due to lead-based paint in poor condition in low-income housing that is not owner occupied (24). Additional sources include lead persisting in soil, lead dust released during repainting of steel structures, and dust brought home on clothing of family members who work in jobs with poorly controlled lead exposures. It has been reported that higher percentages of people of color live in areas with high levels of airborne lead, with 6% of the white, 9% of the African-American, and 18% of the Latino population living in areas that failed to attain EPA air quality standards for lead (16). Nutritional and dietary factors associated with poverty may also contribute to disparities in the blood lead levels of minority children. African-American children are reported to have lower calcium intakes than white children. Thus, it is possible that they absorb ingested lead more efficiently, since dietary calcium blocks absorption of lead from the gastrointestinal tract (24). The extent to which this effect actually contributes to elevated blood lead levels is unclear.

### Gauley Bridge Disaster

Some of the most evident examples of environmental injustice have occurred in occupational settings. One of the most extreme of these was the Gauley Bridge disaster (also known as the Hawk's Nest incident), reported to be the worst industrial disaster ever to have occurred in the United States (25). In 1931 to 1932, a tunnel was drilled through a mountain in Gauley Bridge, West Virginia. Although dust respirators and wet drilling were both available technologies at that time, for reasons of cost and expediency neither was used in the project. In a 7-year period, over 700 deaths occurred, largely from acute silicosis attributable to work in the tunnel. An estimated 76% of the deaths occurred among African-Americans, mostly migrant workers. These estimates did not include deaths due to chronic silicosis, which would have occurred after the study period.

African-Americans made up 20% of the local population, 66% of the total tunnel project work force, and 80% of the workers who actually worked inside the tunnel, where silica dust exposures were the highest. Over 60% of the African-American workers had worked inside the tunnel, compared with 30% of the white workers. This is a well-documented example of disproportionate hiring of African-American workers into the most hazardous subset of jobs in a hazardous industry. Most of these hundreds of deaths from environmental lung disease could have been prevented by utilizing protective technology that existed at the time.

### Outbreak of Toxic Liver Disease in Manufacturing Workers

A more recent example of disproportionate excess risk of environmentally induced disease in the workplace is an outbreak of toxic liver disease among predominantly Latino urban manufacturing workers (26,27). This example illustrates a variety of issues, including the increasing inclusion of occupational health in the environmental justice discussion. A Latino man was seen in an emergency room with nausea, abdominal pain, headache, and abnormal liver function tests. A well-trained physician assistant who spoke Spanish took a brief occupational history and referred him to the affiliated occupational and environmental medicine clinic. The patient reported that he worked as a production worker in a factory that produced urethane-coated waterproof fabric, and that other workers in the plant had similar symptoms. The production process utilized large machines that coated the fabric with a solution containing urethane and a solvent.

After making a presumptive clinical diagnosis of possible toxic liver disease in the individual patient, the occupational and environmental medicine clinic negotiated with the plant management to conduct a medical survey of the workers in the factory. They found that 35 (76%) of the production workers and 1 (8%) of the nonproduction workers had abnormal liver function tests. Although the aminotransferase liver function tests indicated liver inflammation, they could not identify the specific environmental etiology of the liver disease. Using simple field epidemiology methods, unprotected skin contact with the solvent dimethylformamide (DMF) was identified as the cause of the outbreak.

Of the 46 production workers, 93% were Latino (mostly monolingual Spanish-speaking from Puerto Rico), whereas of the 12 nonproduction workers, only 33% were Latino. Being Latino was strongly and significantly associated with toxic liver disease due to DMF exposure in this study. It was well known to the workers that something in the production jobs was making them sick. However, few other jobs were available in other parts of the plant, or in other businesses in the area that would hire monolingual Spanish speaking workers, or that would provide nearly unlimited overtime work. The production process had not changed for over 10 years, and the turnover of workers was extremely high, due to symptoms consistent with the toxic liver disease. It is likely that the outbreak had been ongoing for most of these years, although it had not been identified previously by any occupational disease or hazard surveillance, nor by the community primary care physicians who cared for individual workers one at a time. Although hepatotoxicity of DMF was suspected from prior animal studies, efficient skin absorption leading to hepatotoxicity in humans had not been previously described.

In response to recommendations made by the clinic, and in compliance with detailed health and safety language in the contract negotiated by the union, the DMF was substituted with a different solvent, the production process was modified to eliminate skin contact with the solvent, and ongoing medical monitoring of the workers was initiated. With these changes, the outbreak of toxic liver disease ended completely and has not recurred. The combination of the initial field epidemiology and the preventive intervention trial (eliminating the DMF exposure and clinically monitoring changes in health outcome) provided definitive evidence of the hepatotoxicity of DMF in humans. Interventions to change the production process eliminated the causal exposure and successfully prevented further liver disease among the workers. The turnover of workers was greatly reduced, morale improved, and productivity and profitability of the plant remained high, even after accounting for the substantial up-front investment required to change the production process.

This case of environmentally induced, work-related disease illustrates a variety of important points:

- disproportionate employment of a specific ethnic group (Puerto Rican) in a high-risk workplace;
- exemplary recognition and clinical and preventive public health follow-up of a sentinel case;
- failure of existing occupational and environmental disease and hazard surveillance systems, and local primary care physicians, to identify a severe and longstanding outbreak of clinically diagnosable liver disease;
- the appropriate role of clinical environmental and occupational medicine, at the specialist and primary care levels, in identifying environmental diseases not identified by existing surveillance systems;
- objective medical diagnosis and ongoing medical monitoring using well-validated biologic markers of effect;
- ability of an epidemiologic study, followed by a carefully monitored preventive intervention trial, to support strong causal inference regarding the etiologic agent;
- empowerment of an affected population of workers through effective organizing;
- primary prevention of disease by appropriate modification of the manufacturing process;
- decreased time lost from work and preservation of productivity and profitability through control of the epidemic;
- a win-win solution resulting from collaboration of an open-minded management, a public health– and prevention-oriented environmental and occupational medicine clinic and organized representatives of the affected population.

## KNOWLEDGE GAPS AND CHALLENGES

Some of the issues and problems that have been recurrent themes in the environmental justice discussion challenge the limits of current knowledge and methods in environmental and occupational medicine. Among the most salient challenges is the difficulty in establishing the existence of a causal relationship between environmental exposures and adverse health outcomes. Areas of difficulty in establishing causal relationships include (27a):

1. incomplete understanding of etiology of many diseases;
2. complex interrelationships among multiple nonenvironmental and environmental causes;
3. distinction between exacerbation and cause of disease;
4. exposure and dose assessment;
5. mixed and/or repeated exposures to a diversity of chemical, biologic, and physical agents;
6. lack of effective surveillance and reporting systems for environmental diseases and exposures;
7. long latency periods;
8. multiple target organs or systems;
9. lack of sufficiently predictive clinical diagnostic and screening tests, especially for early or subclinical biologic effects of environmental agents;
10. inherent variability in biologic susceptibilities to environmentally induced illness.

Understanding mechanisms of human environmental exposure and disease causation sufficiently to intervene effectively at the appropriate levels and prevent exposure and disease is the central scientific challenge posed by the environmental justice discussion. Mechanisms are fundamental processes or factors that determine exposure, dose, or effects. They may be understood at different levels, from the biologic to the chemical and physical, to the sociological (21). Although molecular pathogenetic mechanisms are currently receiving the greatest research attention, preventive interventions can be effective at a variety of levels, from small to large, from simple to complex.

One example of this is the control of lead toxicity over the past several decades. Although the precise mechanisms are incompletely understood, existence of significant disparities in lead exposure and toxicity has been well documented. Understanding that lead from gasoline was the principal environmental source led to effective regulation and control of this source, which produced substantial and widespread decreases in lead exposure and toxicity. Understanding of mechanisms of indoor exposure, as well as absorption, transport, storage, and excretion of lead in the human body has and will continue to lead to improvements in treatment and prevention of lead toxicity. Much of our understanding of mechanisms, as well as causes of disparities in exposure and toxicity, has come as a result of appropriate utilization of the blood lead level, a well-validated biomarker of recent absorbed dose. Use of this biomarker has strengthened the scientific foundation of regulatory, public health, and clinical approaches to reducing the burden of lead toxicity. Similarly, biomarkers of exposure to other toxicants could potentially make important contributions to effective and equitable control of other environmental and occupational hazards.

Other potentially important levels of mechanisms are incompletely understood as well. Often, racial, cultural, and socioeconomic factors are simply treated as "noise," and either ignored or controlled in epidemiologic and exposure assessment studies. There are no animal or tissue culture toxicologic models for their impact on human health. In some cases, however, information about these factors may help facilitate understanding the mechanisms of disease causation and exposure, and may turn out to be important in designing preventive strategies. Race has often been used in health studies as a surrogate for a constellation of socioeconomic factors, preventing the studies from distinguishing effects of those factors from effects of race and ethnicity (28). Influence of socioeconomic status, race, ethnicity, and racism on health and environmental health is the subject of an ongoing debate among researchers (21,29–31). It is clear, however, that environmental and occupational medicine research to address issues related to environmental justice will need to incorporate improved measures of these factors into sound research designs in human populations.

Many of the research challenges posed by environmental justice issues are illustrated by the example of urban asthma. First, the clinical diagnosis of asthma is not entirely clear-cut, and diagnostic methods and accuracy may vary among different population groups (32). The complex, interacting web of causation of asthma may include the environmental exposures of primary research interest, plus other toxic, allergenic, dietary, and infectious exposures, genetic and acquired susceptibility factors, and racial and socioeconomic factors. Environmental agents may induce new-onset asthma or aggravate preexisting asthma, and may come from outdoor or indoor sources at home, work, school, or other locations. Time-activity patterns may be complicated and existing technology is not adequate to characterize the levels and variability over time and location of many of these environmental agents.

Inborn and acquired variations in susceptibility to effects of environmental exposures in minority populations have been reviewed by Rios et al. (33). Susceptibility can be affected by genetic factors (e.g., sickle cell trait may increase susceptibility to toxic effects of carbon monoxide), dietary factors (e.g., lower calcium intake among African-American children may act to increase gastrointestinal absorption of ingested lead), other lifestyle factors (e.g., smoking increases lung cancer susceptibility in asbestos-exposed workers), or other environmental exposures (e.g., concurrent solvent exposure may increase likelihood of hearing loss due to high-level noise). Additional factors may include compromised health status (e.g., people with diabetes may be less able to detoxify organic solvents), as well as social inequality of access to health care (e.g., poor primary care control of asthma may increase susceptibility to particulate air pollution), and education and communication skills (e.g., non–English-speaking workers may not be able to read health and safety warnings at work). It is expected that greater understanding of the determinants of variation of susceptibility in human populations will facilitate more equitable prevention of environmentally and occupationally induced diseases.

There is a great paucity of environmental and occupational medicine research that specifically includes low-income and minority communities and workers (2). For example, in one systematic review of 116 occupational cancer epidemiology studies in four journals, only 14 studies (12%) provided data on a nonwhite group. The authors concluded that the published literature contributes little to understanding the complex relationships between occupation, cancer, and race (34). There are inadequate data on the relationships among environmental, racial, ethnic, and other socioeconomic determinants of adverse health outcomes. One reason is exclusion of numerical minority subgroups from studies, with rationale given that the smaller numbers of subjects would have provided unacceptably low statistical power to test the primary study hypotheses in these groups, and since they may differ systematically from the majority group, a combined analysis would not have been appropriate. Other reasons include difficulties in long-term follow-up (e.g., migrant farm workers); inadequate measurement, classification, and reporting of data on race, ethnicity, and relevant socioeconomic variables (35,36); and difficulty in research access to high-risk workplaces that employ low-wage workers (e.g., apparel sweatshops or other small businesses).

Some of the mechanisms acting to increase risk of environmental and occupational diseases among minority workers and communities were reviewed by Frumkin and Walker (2). In addition to disparities in exposures and susceptibility to environmental agents in the community and workplace, the authors point out that the racial/ethnic and socioeconomic disparities that exist in access to health care in general may extend to occupational and environmental illnesses, although further research is needed to clarify this.

## PROPOSED APPROACHES TO ACHIEVING ENVIRONMENTAL JUSTICE

A variety of approaches have been proposed to address the knowledge gaps and challenges outlined in the previous section. Recommendations made at the 1994 symposium are summarized, followed by discussion of a public health framework for integrating the various approaches.

### Recommendations from 1994 Environmental Justice Symposium

A 1994 symposium on Health Research and Needs to Ensure Environmental Justice, sponsored by several federal agencies, was attended by over 1,000 people including representatives from community and labor organizations, academia, business, and government. One product of this conference was a set of recommendations for achieving environmental justice (37). These recommendations reflect general agreement, although not complete consensus, of the participants.

From the perspective of environmental and occupational medicine, most of the important recommendations could be summarized in an overarching recommendation to develop more effective and timely public health interventions that will prevent environmental and occupational diseases, and that directly, equitably, and sustainably benefit low-income and minority communities and workers. Where the scientific basis for these interventions is inadequate, more and better environmental and occupational health science research should be done that includes these populations, and that is specifically designed to support public health decision making and preventive interventions.

With regard to research, a focus on human health effects was strongly emphasized. Essential components of the recommended research approach included epidemiology, toxicology, molecular biology, exposure assessment, public health surveillance, and clinical research in occupational and environmental medicine. A need was stressed for improvement and further development of methodologies to address the scientific challenges of studying human health effects of low-dose and mixed exposures, racial and socioeconomic factors, interactions of susceptibility and exposure factors, and exposures among small groups of people. Development of new molecular technologies and tools was encouraged, with the specific objective of addressing the public health needs of at-risk workers and communities.

Participatory approaches to research and educational programs were advocated. To this end, it was recommended that partnerships be developed between community members, basic science researchers, and health care providers that involve the high-risk communities and workers as active participants in environmental health science research and educational activities. It was felt that utilization of the local knowledge of community members and workers about their diseases and exposures could improve the quality of the science, and that active community involvement could help ensure that communities benefit from the research and its applications, and facilitate better communication and more trusting relationships between communities and researchers.

Increased support was also recommended for other occupational and environmental medicine activities, including (a) increased training of health care providers; (b) development of more effective surveillance methods; (c) better inclusion of people of color and/or low income as subjects in epidemiologic and clinical studies; (d) improved access of these populations to medical monitoring and treatment of occupational and environmental diseases; (e) increased recruitment, retention, and promotion of people of color and members of affected communities as junior and tenured faculty in institutions conducting research and education in environmental health science, (f) increased environmental health science research and education activities at historically black colleges and universities (HBCUs) and other minority institutions. Recognizing the merits of a multidisciplinary approach, recommendations were made to promote interagency coordination among different federal agencies, as well as state, local, and tribal government agencies involved in environmental and occupational health issues. Pollution prevention and abatement of known hazards were advocated. Finally, legal and legislative recommendations included enacting, strengthening, and/or enforcing legislation such that it provides equal protection of the law to all people against environmental problems.

### A Public Health Approach

A public health approach to addressing the major environmental justice issues would include a broad range of disciplines, including risk communication and management, education, surveillance, clinical environmental and occupational medicine, and research.

Clear communication about environmental hazards and risks is key to meaningful involvement of community residents and workers in risk management decisions (38). The complexity of the issues, diversity in perceptions of risk, and the great uncertainties that exist can easily lead to misunderstandings between concerned communities and professionals attempting to address the relevant issues. Risk communication is a field that has been well developed and general principles have been reviewed (39,40). These risk communication methods need to be more widely utilized, in a culturally sensitive manner, in low-income and minority communities, and greater inclusion of involved communities and workers in risk assessment and management processes, including risk communication, has been advocated (38,41). Environmental risk management, with integral involvement of stakeholders (including representatives of communities and workers), has been proposed as an approach to improving these links (38). In the proper ethical and political context, this approach has great potential to contribute to economically sustainable and equitable improvement of public health.

In order for broad stakeholder involvement to be successful, there is a need for education of the various parties involved. Some of the educational approaches that have been proposed include parent education, school-based education of children, community outreach by specially trained social workers and nurses, community-based patient-physician alliances, and indigenous outreach workers who are members of the target community trained to educate their peers (15,42). Bidirectional education has been proposed, including education of environmental health researchers and public health practitioners in the value of community residents and workers understanding of exposure pathways, health and disease beliefs, and perceptions of risk. Another educational approach is to increase opportunities in the environmental health sciences for young minority students early in their careers, thus increasing the roster of minority environmental scientists (43).

Continuing medical education of primary health care providers is important, as well, in order to implement the recommendation of the Institute of Medicine that "at a minimum, all primary care physicians should be able to identify possible occupationally or environmentally induced conditions and make the appropriate referrals for follow-up" (44). This education will need to explicitly include those primary care providers who serve low-income and minority communities and workers. In addition, adequate numbers of physicians with specialty training in environmental and occupational medicine and who are accessible to these communities and the primary care physicians who serve them will be important to provide ongoing clinical backup and medical education. Successful application of this approach was demonstrated by the clinic and medical center that recognized and eliminated the outbreak of toxic liver disease.

Following the lead of public health surveillance for infectious diseases, effective methods of surveillance are being developed for occupational diseases. Recently, public health surveillance has been proposed for environmental diseases and hazards as well (45,46). The particular need for improved methods and implementation of surveillance for environmental and occupational diseases in low-income populations is illustrated by the example of the outbreak of toxic liver disease. The majority of people in the exposed group had symptomatic and objectively documentable environmentally-caused adverse health outcomes. Improved occupational disease and hazard surveillance mechanisms need to be developed that would, at the very least, be capable of more rapidly recognizing such an obvious outbreak of occupational disease in low income and minority workers.

The focus on human health research challenges the discipline of epidemiology to address some of its limitations, particularly its imprecision in determining risk when studying small groups or low-level exposures. Increased use of emerging molecular, exposure assessment, and information management tools in epidemiology may be able to substantially increase the ability of epidemiology to accurately quantify excess risk in human populations. Specifically, the promise of biomarkers of exposure, susceptibility, and biologic effect to increase the resolving power of epidemiology for limited sample sizes, and, importantly, to increase the degree of confidence in reassuring society if a study finds no effect, is beginning to be realized (47,48). While recognizing the importance of incorporating these new tools, however, some scientists have cautioned that epidemiology must also retain its population perspective. They have pointed out that social, cultural, and economic differences between populations are frequently treated as extraneous factors in epidemiologic studies of risk factors. These population differences may, in fact, be primary and critical determinants of exposure, susceptibility, and disease, and understanding them may be key to prevention of those diseases (49,50). This warning is particularly appropriate for epidemiologic research related to environmental justice issues.

At present the environmental risk management process tends to rely heavily on animal toxicology data, and some scientists have called for an expanded role of epidemiology in this process (51,52). They point out that epidemiology is the discipline most directly relevant to human health; it can investigate the effects of environmental exposures as actually experienced by the population, and it can characterize effects across the full range of human susceptibility. Research in human subjects, both epidemiologic and clinical, complements animal and in vitro toxicology and risk assessment. Each of these approaches plays a critical role in protection of human health.

Demonstration trials of preventive interventions can potentially address several of the difficulties enumerated in the environmental justice discussion. These include difficulties of evaluating possible causal relationships between suspected environmental agents and adverse health outcomes in humans, questions about interspecies and dose-level extrapolations, technical difficulties of complex mixtures of toxicants, communities' and workers' frequent distrust of research, and their concern that research results often seem far removed from the bottom line objective of reducing environmental risk. Well-designed, hypothesis driven, clinically monitored trials of preventive interventions can sometimes provide stronger evidence supporting or refuting hypothesized causal relationships between environmental agents and adverse health outcomes in humans than traditional epidemiologic, toxicologic, or clinical studies. Intervention trials have the advantage of combining a relatively strong, quasi-experimental research methodology with a public test of a concrete intervention that the community members or workers can observe and understand, and in which they can often actively participate. An illustration of a successful demonstration trial of a preventive intervention is the well-designed before-and-after medical monitoring of the coated fabric factory workers when dimethylformamide was substituted for by a less toxic solvent, discussed earlier. Intervention effectiveness research is one of the 21 priority areas of the National

Institute for Occupational Safety and Health (NIOSH) National Occupational Research Agenda (53). The National Institute of Environmental Health Sciences (NIEHS) supports community-based prevention/intervention research as well, and this approach is being explored by other national research agencies.

It is important to ensure that low-income and minority communities and workers are appropriately included in environmental and occupational health science research. The National Institutes of Health (NIH) Revitalization Act of 1993 (54) and the subsequent NIH guidelines on inclusion of women and minorities as subjects in clinical research (55) directed NIH to monitor inclusion of minorities and women in NIH-funded clinical research, broadly defined as encompassing all research involving human subjects. It is considered that a clinical study without appropriate numbers of women or minority subjects may be scientifically flawed, as would one without an appropriate control group or one with serious methodological weaknesses (56). In addition, interpopulation differences may be of substantial clinical and public health importance, and failing to investigate them may severely limit the generalizability of the study and its usefulness to those different groups. Thus, broad inclusion of minority groups and women in clinical research is considered an issue both of scientific merit and of equity. For human studies of environmental hazards, methods of ensuring appropriate inclusion might include multicenter collaboration, oversampling of numerical minority subgroups, targeting of high-risk populations or occupational groups, and developing clinical research based in health care facilities known to and trusted by the community. Initial assessment of NIH experience with the inclusion policy suggests that it is working. Level of compliance with the 1994 guidelines in applications for extramural funding is high, and procedures are in place to monitor and measure actual inclusion in funded studies (57).

The complexity of determinants of exposure and disease in humans provides a compelling reason to develop more collaborative multidisciplinary and multilevel approaches to research. Sexton et al. (27a) have proposed a central role for research to better inform decision making related to environmental justice, and have framed the environmental justice discussion in terms of risk and understanding of mechanisms of exposure and disease. They suggest that research to investigate whether environmental justice is being achieved should also investigate whether certain segments of the population are disproportionately more exposed and/or more susceptible to environmental agents. Public policy decision making, especially that related to environmental justice, would benefit from better understanding of mechanisms of exposure and of disease causation at many levels. Different levels could be, for example, a nation with certain industries and regulatory laws; a community concerned about effects of a variety of pollutants; an individual resident with a certain time-activity pattern of exposures to airborne agents from multiple sources; the individual's medical history of respiratory disorders; the individual's lung, environmental, and genetic factors in up- and down-regulation of a cytokine mechanism involved in pulmonary inflammatory response; or a specific genetic mutation. Preventive interventions could target levels from the molecular level (e.g., chemoprevention or gene therapy), to the exposure pathway level (e.g., preventing children from ingesting lead-containing dust at home), to the lifestyle level (e.g., asbestos-exposed worker quitting smoking), to the societal level (e.g., equitable enforcement of regulation of known occupational and environmental toxins).

With multilevel understanding of exposure pathways and disease causation, preventive strategies that intervene at the levels thought most promising (given current science and technology) can be designed and tested for effectiveness. Careful investigation of influences of race, ethnicity, and socioeconomic status, and their complex interrelationships with health outcomes, environmental and occupational exposures, biomarkers, and other important factors will be important. Susser and Susser (58) have proposed a multilevel approach to epidemiology, termed eco-epidemiology, which could provide an integrating framework for public health–oriented research conducted to address some of the complex scientific, social, and public health challenges posed by environmental justice issues. Regardless of the details of the particular approach taken, it is clear that a public health response to these complex environmental justice issues will need to be based on scientifically sound, multidisciplinary, collaborative research.

## CONCLUSION

In spite of the inadequacy of information to date, it is clear that inequities and injustices related to environmental and occupational hazards continue to exist, and need to be addressed. Successfully linking mechanistic research on environmental exposures and diseases with the prevention and public health needs of society, specifically the high-risk communities and workers of concern, will be a great challenge. In the process of addressing issues of social and economic justice, the environmental justice discussion has raised a number of fundamental issues in environmental and occupational medicine that highlight major data and knowledge gaps. It is likely that efforts to address these difficult environmental justice issues will lead to advancement in methods of diagnosis, prevention, and treatment of environmental and occupational diseases, as well as in understanding of mechanisms of environmental exposure and disease causation.

Different approaches have been proposed, variously emphasizing risk management, education and communication, medical care, regulatory enforcement, preventive interventions, and multidisciplinary collaborative research. These approaches all have merit and are not mutually exclusive. A public health framework for research and informed prioritizing and decision making could integrate all the necessary elements of these approaches. Placing the emphasis on public health may be the most direct and sustainable means to achieve reasonable and measurable improvements in environmental and occupational health, which will benefit the diverse members of our society in a just and equitable manner.

## REFERENCES


1. Walker B, Goodwin N, Warren R. Environmental Health of African-Americans. *J Natl Med Assoc* 1995;87:123–129.
2. Frumkin H, Walker D. Minority workers and communities. In: *Maxcy-Rosenau textbook of public health and preventive medicine,* 14th ed. 1997;in press.
3. Clinton W. Presidential Executive Order 12898 "Federal Actions to Address Environmental Justice in Minority Populations and Low Income Populations". February 11, 1994. *W Comp Pres Docs* 1994;30: 276-9 F14.
4. *Symposium on health research and needs to ensure environmental justice:* part 1; *executive summary and proceedings.* Sponsored by National Institutes of Health, Centers for Disease Control and Prevention, Environmental Protection Agency, Agency for Toxic Substance and Disease Registry, Department of Energy. February, 1994.
5. *Symposium on health research and needs to ensure environmental justice:* part 2; *recommendations.* Sponsored by National Institutes of Health, Centers for Disease Control and Prevention Environmental Protection Agency, Agency for Toxic Substance and Disease Registry, Department of Energy, February, 1994.
6. Institute of Medicine. *Report of commissioned study on environmental justice:* research, *health policy and educational needs.* Manuscript in preparation, forthcoming, 1998.
7. Bullard RD, Wright BH. Environmental Justice for all: community perspectives on health and research needs. *Toxicol Ind Health* 1993;9(5): 821–841.
8. Commission for Racial Justice, United Church of Christ. *Toxic wastes and race in the United States.* New York: United Church of Christ, 1987.
9. Johnson B, Coulberson S. Environmental epidemiologic issues and minority health. *Ann Epidemiol* 1993;3:175–180.
10. Deleted in proof.
11. Goldman BA, Fitton L. *Toxic wastes and race revisited.* New York: Center for Policy Alternatives, 1994.
12. Weitzman M, Gortmaker S, Sobol A. Racial, social, and environmental risks for childhood asthma. *Am J Dis Child* 1990;144:1189–1194.
13. Weiss KB, Wagener DK. Changing patterns of asthma mortality: identifying target populations at high risk. *JAMA* 1990;264:1683–1687.
14. Carr W, Zeitel T, Weiss K. Variations in asthma hospitalizations and deaths in New York City. *Am J Public Health* 1992;82:54–65.
15. Claudio L, Torres T, Sanjurjo E, Sherman LR, Landrigan PJ. Environmental health sciences education—a tool for achieving environmental equity and protecting children. *Environ Health Perspect* 1998;106.
16. Wernette DR, Nieves LA. Minorities and air pollution: a preliminary geodemographic analysis, 1991. Presented at the Socioeconomic Research Analysis Conference, Baltimore MD, June 27–28, 1991.
17. Samet JM, Marbury MC, Spengler JD. Health effects and sources of indoor air pollution, part I. *Am Rev Respir Dis* 1987;136:1486–1508.
18. Samet JM, Marbury MC, Spengler JD. Health effects and sources of indoor air pollution, part II. *Am Rev Respir Dis* 1988;137:221–242.
19. Goldstein IF, Andrews LR, Hartel D. Assessment of human exposure to nitrogen dioxide, carbon monoxide and respirable particulates in New York inner-city residences. *Atm Envir* 1988;22:2127–2139.
20. Chapman MD, Pollart SM, Luczynska CM, Platts-Mills TAE. Hidden allergic factors in the etiology of asthma. *Chest* 1988;94:185–190.
21. Sexton K, Gong H, Bailar JC, Ford JG, Gold DR, Lampert WE, Utell MJ. Air pollution health risks: do race and class matter? *Toxicol Ind Health* 1993;9:843–878.
22. Mahaffey KR, Annest JL, Roberts J, Murphy RS. National estimates of blood lead levels, United States, 1976–1980: association with selected demographic and socioeconomic factors. *N Engl J Med* 1982;307: 573–579.
23. Lanphear BP, Weitzman M, Eberly S. Racial differences in urban children's environmental exposure to lead. *Am J Public Health* 1996;86: 1460–1463.
24. Sargent JD, Brown MJ, Freeman JL, Bailey A, Goodman D, Freeman DH. Childhood lead poisoning in Massachusetts communities: its association with sociodemographic and housing characteristics. *Am J Public Health* 1995;85:528–534.
25. Cherniak M. *The Hawk's Nest incident:* America's worst industrial disaster. New Haven, CT: Yale University Press, 1986.
26. Redlich CA, Beckett WS, Sparer J, et al. Liver disease associated with occupational exposure to the solvent dimethylformamide. *Ann Intern Med* 1988;108:680–686.
27. Friedman-Jiménez G, Ortiz J. Occupational health. In: Molina CW, Aguirre-Molina M, eds. *Latino health in the U.S.: a growing challenge.* Washington DC: American Public Health Association, 1994;341–389.

27a. Sexton K, Olden K, Johnson B. Environmental Justice: the central role of research in establishing a credible scientific foundation for informed decision making. *Toxicol Ind Health* 1993;9:685–727.

28. Montgomery LE, Carter-Pokras O. Health status by social class and/or minority status: implications for environmental equity research. *Toxicol Ind Health* 1993;9:729–773.
29. Freeman HP. Poverty, race, racism and survival. *Ann Epidemiol* 1993;3: 145–149.
30. Krieger N, Rowley DL, Herman AA, Avery B, Phillips MT. Racism, sexism and social class: implications for studies of health, disease, and well-being. *Am J Prev Med* 1993;9(6 suppl):82–122.
31. Warren RC. The morbidity/mortality gap: What is the problem? *Ann Epidemiol* 1993;3:127–129.
32. Gergen P. Editorial: Social class and asthma-distinguishing between the disease and the diagnosis. *Am J Public Health* 1996;86:1361–1362.
33. Rios R, Poje GV, Detels R. Susceptibility to environmental pollutants among minorities. *Toxicol Ind Health* 1993;9:797–820.
34. Kipen H, Wartenberg D, Scully PF, et al. Are non-whites at greater risk for occupational cancer? *Am J Ind Med* 1991;19(1):67–74.
35. Feinleib M. Data needed for improving the health of minorities. *Ann Epidemiol* 1993;3:199–202.
36. Montgomery LE, Carter-Pokras O. Health status by social class and/or minority status: implications for environmental equity research. *Toxicol Ind Health* 1993;9:729–773.
37. *Symposium on health research and needs to ensure environmental justice:* recommendations. Sponsored by National Institutes of Health, Centers for Disease Control and Prevention, Environmental Protection Agency, Agency for Toxic Substance and Disease Registry, Department of Energy, February, 1994.
38. Presidential/Congressional Commission on Risk Assessment and Risk Management. *Framework for environmental health risk management, Final Report,* vol 1. Washington DC: Riskworld, 1997.
39. National Research Council. *Improving risk communication. Report of the committee on risk perception and communication.* Washington, DC: National Academy Press, 1989.
40. Goldstein, BD, Gotsch AR. Risk communication. In: Rosenstock L, Cullen MR, eds. *Textbook of clinical occupational and environmental medicine.* Philadelphia: WB Saunders, 1994;68–76.
41. Shulte P. Risk communication and minority groups. In: Johnson BL, Williams RC, Harris CM, eds. *Proceedings of the National Minority Health Conference:* focus on environmental contamination. Princeton, NJ: Princeton Scientific, 1990.
42. Claudio L. From the laboratory to the community: commitment to outreach. *Environ Health Perspect* 1997;105:278–281.
43. Claudio L. Increasing minority participation in environmental health sciences. *Environ Health Perspect* 1997;105:174–176.
44. Institute of Medicine, National Academy of Sciences. *Role of the primary care physician in occupational and environmental medicine.* Washington DC: National Academy Press, 1988.
45. Thacker SB, Stroup DF, Parrish RG, Anderson HA. Surveillance in environmental public health: issues, systems, and sources. *Am J Public Health* 1995;85:633–637.
46. Levy B. Editorial: Toward a holistic approach to public health surveillance. *Am J Public Health* 1995;85:624–625.
47. Hulka BS, Wilcosky TC, Griffith JD. *Biological markers in epidemiology.* New York: Oxford Press, 1990.
48. Shulte P, Perera F. *Molecular epidemiology.* San Diego: Academic Press, 1993.
49. McMichael AJ. The health of persons, populations and planets: epidemiology comes full circle. *Epidemiology* 1995;6:633–636.
50. Pearce N. Traditional epidemiology, modern epidemiology, and public health. *Am J Public Health* 1996;86:678–683.

51. Hertz-Picciotto I. Epidemiology and quantitative risk assessment: a bridge from science to policy. *Am J Public Health* 1995;85:48–50.
52. Samet JM, Burke TA. Epidemiology and risk assessment. In: Brownson RC, Pettiti D, eds. *Applied epidemiology:* theory to practice. New York: Oxford University Press, 1998.
53. *National occupational research agenda.* DHHS (NIOSH) Publication No., 96–115. Washington, DC: National Institute for Occupational Safety and Health, Public Health Service, Centers for Disease Control and Prevention, US Department of Health and Human Services, 1996.
54. National Institutes of Health Revitalization Act of 1993 (Public Law 103–143), United States Code, Title 42, Section 289, Subsection (a)(1), 10 June 1993.
55. US Department of Health and Human Services, National Institutes of Health. NIH Guidelines on the inclusion of women and minorities as subjects in clinical research. *Federal Register* 59, 14508–14513 (28 March 1994).
56. Hayunga EG, Costello MD, Pinn VW. Women and minorities in clinical research, part 4: Demographics of study populations. *Appl Clin Trials* 1997;6:41–45.
57. Hayunga EG, Pinn VW. Women and minorities in clinical research, part 2: Implementing the 1994 NIH Guidelines. *Appl Clin Trials* 1996;5: 34–40.
58. Susser M, Susser E. Choosing a future for epidemiology: from black box to Chinese boxes and eco-epidemiology. *Am J Public Health* 1996; 86:674–677.

*Environmental and Occupational Medicine,*
*Third Edition,* edited by William N. Rom.
Lippincott–Raven Publishers, Philadelphia © 1998.

CHAPTER 132

# Industrial Hygiene Measurement and Control

Beverly S. Cohen

The tremendous advances in understanding the causes of occupational disease that occurred in the 20th century have resulted in increased urgency to identify and control occupational exposure to toxicants. The industrial hygienist is dedicated to the anticipation, recognition, evaluation, and control of workplace hazards. Workplace hazards include "all environmental factors or stresses which may cause sickness, impaired health and well-being, or significant discomfort and inefficiency among workers or among citizens of the community" (1).

The profession of industrial hygienist began with the formation of the American Conference of Governmental Industrial Hygienists (ACGIH) and the American Industrial Hygiene Association (AIHA) in 1938 and 1939 (2). The ACGIH was initially a conference held by governmental industrial hygienists to provide a medium for exchange of ideas and information by those who worked in the field. The efforts of these hygienists, together with many physicians, chemists, engineers, nurses, and others who studied both the causes and prevention of occupational disease, culminated in passage of the Occupational Safety and Health (OSH) Act of 1970, which stimulated both industrial hygiene research and increased efforts to train professionals who could apply their knowledge and skills to effect a noticeable reduction in the tragic toll of occupational disease. The application of the knowledge gained from efforts to improve the industrial environment has been increasingly applied in offices and other workplaces, homes, and outdoors, for the protection of all.

The industrial hygienist seeks to control exposure to chemical and physical hazards such as ionizing and non-ionizing radiation, noise, and mechanical stress. As the nature of the work force changes and diversifies, with the growth of service industries relative to heavy industry, attention has also focused on work-induced psychological stress. In areas such as health care, concern has grown over exposure of medical personnel to biologic agents, including viable aerosols (e.g., fungi and viruses), drugs, and anaesthetic or sterilant gases.

Traumatic injuries associated with the construction and transportation industries, as well as from contact with machines and tools have come under new scrutiny, as have musculoskeletal disorders associated with lifting and repetitive forceful motion.

B. S. Cohen: Department of Environmental Medicine, New York University Medical Center, New York, New York 10987.

## IDENTIFICATION OF WORKER EXPOSURE

### Routes of Exposure

The first step in an industrial hygiene evaluation of a workplace is to identify the potential for exposure to harmful agents. Toxic materials may enter the body via ingestion, skin absorption, or inhalation, in order of increasing importance.

Ingestion is not generally an important route in the occupational environment. An exception may be in cases of extreme carelessness, including the contamination of cigarettes with material previously deposited on the hands. The inhalation of cigarette smoke itself is usually a greater hazard.

Skin absorption can be a significant route of exposure in the industrial environment, where large quantities of chemicals are processed. Significant potential for skin contact exists also for laboratory, medical, and maintenance personnel. Dermal contamination may occur by direct contact with liquid or powder reservoirs, but also by deposition of airborne contaminants. Intact skin is a good barrier for many materials but is permeable to many others such as organic solvents, and cuts and abrasions provide pathways for absorption. In addition, occupational skin diseases, which are about 15% to 20% of all reported occupational diseases, are largely contact (allergic and irritant) dermatitis (3).

Inhalation is the principal route by which toxicants gain entry to the body. For this reason, plus the potential for deposition onto skin, an industrial hygiene evaluation will pay particular attention to contaminants that are, or may become, airborne. Substantial effort has always been directed toward developing and improving air-sampling methods and programs.

### Air-Sampling Programs

An air-sampling program must be designed to answer specific questions, otherwise it may not fulfill the need for which it was initiated. A prospective epidemiologic program, for example, requires random sampling in order for statistical predictions to be valid. Sampling for worker protection, on the other hand, will require selection of persons at maximum risk. Reasons for sampling are varied and may include the following:

- health risk evaluation, to measure worker exposure in order to estimate the risk of undesirable health effects and the need for control measures;
- environmental protection, to determine the amount of any toxic or hazardous materials released to the environment;
- compliance, to ensure that exposure levels for workers or environmental releases are within regulatory limits and to satisfy legislative monitoring requirements;
- process control, to evaluate the performance of engineering or other process controls and to ensure that contaminant control remains adequate;
- source identification, to find and control contaminant sources;
- documentation of exposure, to maintain records of exposure for prospective studies or for institutional protection against future legal action.

Five of these represent efforts to improve air quality and working conditions.

**TABLE 1.** *Industrial hygiene sampling protocols*

| Purpose | Types of samples |
|---|---|
| Health risk evaluation | Personal |
| Environmental protection | Area, environmental |
| Compliance | Personal, environmental, stack |
| Process control | Area, personal, stack |
| Source identification | Area, stack |
| Documentation of exposure | Personal |

The sampling strategy for each of the stated purposes requires different protocols and sampling systems (Table 1). The types of samples noted in Table 1 refer to whether a personal exposure sample should be collected in the breathing zone of a worker or whether an area, stack, or other environmental sample is preferable. Sampling from exhaust stacks is commonly done for process and emission control. Health protection requires personal exposure monitoring.

### Preliminary Survey

An industrial hygiene evaluation starts with a preliminary survey, which will reveal process points at which there is potential for dermal or inhalation exposure. It will be the basis for determining whether sampling is needed and for the design of a sampling program, providing the information needed to decide what, when, and where to sample. The following discussion refers primarily to identification of chemical hazards (Table 2) but is applicable with some modification to other stresses. These include ionizing and nonionizing radiation, noise, thermal, ergonomic, and visual stresses.

The first step is to become familiar with the process, the chemicals that are used, and any intermediate products. A thorough understanding of the process flow provides orientation to points at which exposure is possible. It is particularly important to know the physical state of the material at each point in the process, in order to assess the potential for release to the environment as well as to decide how sources may be sampled. Texts are available that describe process flows for many types of facilities (4–6). Details of site-specific plant operations are obtained from the plant personnel. A list of chemicals and radioactive materials that come into the facility is also obtained. As a result of the Occupational Safety and Health Administration (OSHA) Hazard Communications Standard (29 CFR 1910.1200), a set of material safety data sheets should be available for any site. These note all chemicals used at the facility and provide basic toxicity data for each.

A walk-through survey of the premises permits observation of all plant operations. Possible sources and potential contaminants from specific types of processes can be identified (Table 3). The walk-through provides an important opportunity to meet plant personnel and to identify and talk with engineers, foremen, and other workers. They know the process problems that may be encountered and they are aware of complaints or symptoms among the workers. During the walk-through survey job activities are reviewed with plant personnel to learn where workers are deployed and exactly how they carry out their job assignments. Control measures, too, are reviewed. Not all control measures are actually used; whether local exhaust ventilation is in working condition and in use should be determined, as well as whether personal protective devices such as clothing, respirators, and

**TABLE 2.** *Target organ effects of chemical hazards*[a]

| | Signs and symptoms | Chemicals |
|---|---|---|
| Hepatoxins (produce liver damage) | Jaundice, hepatomegaly | Carbon tetrachloride, nitrosamines |
| Nephrotoxins (produce kidney damage) | Edema, proteinuria | Halogenated hydrocarbons, uranium |
| Neurotoxins (produce their primary toxic effects on the nervous system) | Narcosis, behavioral changes, decrease in motor functions | Mercury, carbon disulfide |
| Agents that act on the blood of hematopoietic system (decrease hemoglobin function, deprive body tissues of oxygen) | Cyanosis, loss of consciousness | Carbon monoxide, cyanides |
| Agents that damage the lung (irritate or damage the pulmonary tissue) | Cough, tightness in chest, shortness of breath | Silica, asbestos |
| Reproductive toxins (affect the reproductive capabilities, including chromosome damage and tetratogenesis) | Birth defects, sterility | Lead, DBCP |
| Cutaneous hazards (affect the dermal layer of the body) | Defatting of the skin, rashes, irritation | Ketones, chlorinated compounds |
| Ocular hazards (affect the eye or visual capacity) | Conjunctivitis, corneal damage | Organic solvents, acid |

[a]A chemical health hazard, as defined by the Federal Hazard Communication Standard (CFR 1910.1200), "means a chemical for which there is statistically significant evidence, based on at least one study conducted in accordance with established scientific principles, that acute or chronic health effects may occur in exposed employees. The term 'health hazard' includes chemicals which are carcinogens, toxic or highly toxic agents, reproductive toxins, irritants, corrosives, sensitizers, hepatoxins, nephrotoxins, neurotoxins, agents which act on hematopoietic system, and agents which damage the lungs, skin, eyes, or mucous membranes" (OSHA 1985). (Modified from 29 CFR 1910-1200, Appendix A.)

shielding are actually used. It is also instructive to note the general state of housekeeping. Consideration must be given to whether situations are set up for continuous or intermittent exposure, and the potential for exposure to uncommon episodes, which may or may not be predictable (7).

When a preliminary survey has been completed a report should be written that covers all employees or work situations. All pertinent information should be included—names, social security numbers, jobs, location at the work site, potential exposure, applicable exposure limits, complaints, controls, and notes about whether any action is required. The report of the preliminary survey forms the basis for decisions about both monitoring and sampling. Monitoring refers to the observation of exposure distribution; sampling refers to obtaining specific measurements.

## Decision-Making Criteria

Criteria must be established upon which the decisions will be based when sampling results are evaluated. Criteria for worker exposure measurements are most frequently selected by reference to established standards. These may be OSHA permissible exposure limits (PELs) or National Institute of Occupational Safety and Health (NIOSH) recommended exposure limits (RELs), but preferably the most recent ACGIH threshold limit values (TLVs) should be used. TLVs for chemical substances refer to airborne concentrations of substances and "represent conditions under which it is believed that nearly all workers may be repeatedly exposed day after day without adverse health effects" (8) (Table 4). The TLVs for chemical substances and physical agents are revised annually to take into account the most recent knowledge from human and animal studies together with industrial experience. Standards are based on varying factors such as health impairment, narcosis, irritation, and other forms of stress as appropriate. OSHA amended its air contaminants standard in 1989 (9). The PEL was made more protective for 212 substances, and PELs were set for 164 new substances not previously regulated by OSHA. Many of the PELs were based on then current TLVs. OSHA also incorporated short-term exposure limits (STELs), established a designation for skin, and added ceilings where appropriate (Table 4). However, the new standards were set aside by the courts and revisions are now planned for small groups of individual agents. The OSHA limits for air contaminants are given in Title 29 of the Code of Federal Regulations part 1910.1000, subpart Z (see also refs. 9,10).

Threshold limit values may be designated in units of parts per million (ppm) or mass per unit volume, usually milligrams per cubic meter ($mg/m^3$). Parts per million is a volume fraction such that concentration, $C$, in ppm:

$$C_{\text{ppm}} = \frac{10^6 v}{V}, \qquad [1]$$

where $v$ is the volume of contaminant present in a total volume and $V$ the volume of air plus the contaminant C.

**TABLE 3.** *Potentially hazardous operations and associated air contaminants*

| Process types | Contaminant type | Contaminant examples |
|---|---|---|
| Hot operations | | |
| Welding | Gases (g) | Chromates (p) |
| Chemical reactions | Particulates (p) (dust, fumes, mists) | Zinc and compounds (p) |
| Soldering | | |
| Melting | | Manganese and compounds (p) |
| Molding | | |
| Burning | | Metal oxides (p) |
| | | Carbon monoxide (g) |
| | | Ozone (g) |
| | | Cadmium oxide (p) |
| | | Fluorides (p) |
| | | Lead (p) |
| | | Vinyl chloride (g) |
| Liquid operations | | |
| Painting | Vapors (v) | Benzene (v) |
| Degreasing | Gases (g) | Trichloroethylene (v) |
| Dipping | Mists (m) | Methylene chloride (v) |
| Spraying | | |
| Brushing | | 1,1,1-Trichloroethylene (v) |
| Coating | | |
| Etching | | Hydrochloric acid (m) |
| Cleaning | | Sulfuric acid (m) |
| Dry cleaning | | Hydrogen chloride (g) |
| Pickling | | Cyanide salts (m) |
| Plating | | Chromic acid (m) |
| Mixing | | Hydrogen cyanide (g) |
| Galvanizing | | TDI, MDI (v) |
| Chemical reactions | | Hydrogen sulfide (g) |
| | | Sulfur dioxide (g) |
| | | Carbon tetrachloride (v) |
| Solid operations | | |
| Pouring | Dusts | Cement |
| Mixing | | Quartz (free silica) |
| Separations | | Fibrous glass |
| Extraction | | |
| Crushing | | |
| Conveying | | |
| Loading | | |
| Bagging | | |
| Pressurized spraying | | |
| Cleaning parts | Vapors (v) | Organic solvents (v) |
| Applying pesticides | Dusts (d) | Chlordane (m) |
| | Mists (m) | Parathion (m) |
| Degreasing | | Trichloroethylene (v) |
| Sand blasting | | 1,1,1-Trichloroethane (v) |
| Painting | | |
| | | Methylene chloride (v) |
| | | Quartz (free silica, d) |
| Shaping operations | | |
| Cutting | Dusts | Asbestos |
| Grinding | | Beryllium |
| Filing | | Uranium |
| Milling | | Zinc |
| Molding | | Lead |
| Sawing | | |
| Drilling | | |

From ref. 7.

**TABLE 4.** *Terms as defined in the regulatory text (29 CFR 1910.1000) for limiting employee exposure to air contaminants*

*Time-weighted average* ($TWA_8$): The employee's average airborne exposure in any 8-hour work shift of a 40-hour workweek, which shall not be exceeded.

*Short-term exposure limit* (STEL): The employee's 15-minute TWA exposure, which shall not be exceeded at any time during a workday unless another time limit is specified in a parenthetical notation below the limit. If another time period is specified, the TWA exposure over that time limit shall not be exceeded at any time during the working day.

*Ceiling:* The employee's exposure, which shall not be exceeded during any part of the workday. If instantaneous monitoring is not feasible, the ceiling shall be assessed as a 15-minute TWA exposure, which shall not be exceeded at any time over a workday.

*Skin Designation:* To prevent or reduce skin absorption, an employee's skin exposure to substances listed in Table Z-1-A (29 CFR 1910.1000) with the designation "skin" following the substance name, shall be prevented or reduced to the extent necessary in the circumstances through the use of gloves, coveralls, goggles, or other appropriate personal protective equipment, engineering controls, or work practices.

Adapted from ref. 9.

When $v$ is less than 0.005 $V$ the contaminant volume may be neglected in the denominator (11). To convert $C_{\text{ppm}}$ to $C$ (mg/m$^3$) at 760 torr barometric pressure and 25°C, a conversion factor may be applied as follows:

$$C(mg/m^3) = \frac{C_{ppm}M}{24.45}, \qquad [2]$$

where $M$ is the gram molecular weight of the contaminant.

To determine whether control measures are required, the measured exposure is compared with an appropriate limit. In the case of a mixture of contaminants that act on the same organ system the equivalent exposure is computed as follows:

$$E_{\text{m}} = \frac{C_1}{L_1} + \frac{C_2}{L_2} + \ldots + \frac{C_n}{L_n}, \qquad [3]$$

where $E_{\text{m}}$ is the equivalent exposure for the mixture, $C$ is the concentration of a particular contaminant, and L is the exposure limit for that substance. The value of $E_{\text{m}}$ should not exceed unity (9).

Biologic monitoring of workers is sometimes used to supplement air monitoring. Results of biologic monitoring are evaluated by comparing with biologic exposure indices (BEIs), reference values that "represent the levels of determinants which are most likely to be observed in specimens collected from a healthy worker who has been exposed to chemicals to the same extent as a worker with inhalation exposure to the TLV" (8). Determinant(s) measured in biologic specimens obtained from a worker at a specified time may be the chemical itself, a metabolite, or a "characteristic reversible biochemical change induced by the chemical" (8).

The discussion about monitoring that follows applies to either air sampling or biologic monitoring. As of this writing BEIs have been adopted by ACGIH for 36 chemicals and proposed for two more.

Standards for exposure to radioactive contaminants must be in accord with the most recent federal guidelines. These or other appropriate standards may be used to establish decision-making criteria at various points in the sampling strategy. In radiation protection the goal is to reduce exposure to levels as low as reasonably achievable (ALARA) below specified limits. It is based on the concept that exposure to any amount of ionizing radiation confers some degree of risk, however small, of carcinogenesis. The ALARA is not generally applied in industrial hygiene, but it is a worthwhile ultimate goal for any workplace.

When results of air sampling measurements are compared with decision criteria, it is important to recognize that sufficient information for health protection will not be available until after the true exposure distribution can be estimated with some confidence. For this reason action levels, levels at which certain control or added monitoring requirements take effect, are set at half the exposure limit.

Preliminary source sampling may be advisable for evaluating the potential for exposure of personnel. A determination that no hazardous emissions could cause overexposure may lead to a strategy of source monitoring for unusual releases rather than personal exposure monitoring.

## EVALUATION AND MONITORING

### Exposure Monitoring

Leidel and Busch (12) suggest that the exposure monitoring strategy be divided into initial monitoring and exposure distribution monitoring. The following discussion is based on the chapter "Statistical Design and Data Analysis Requirements," by N. A. Leidel and K. A. Busch (12). Further details on decision points in such monitoring programs may be found in this reference. It is highly recommended for step-by-step guidance on the statistical aspects of establishing and executing a monitoring program.

#### *Initial Monitoring*

The initial monitoring should be carried out as an exposure screening program to obtain exposure estimates for workers at maximum risk, those expected to be most exposed. Thus, the workers to be sampled are selected in a nonrandom manner and it is assumed that no other worker can be exposed to more than the amount measured. Professional judgment must be used to identify these persons for each process.

**TABLE 5.** *Sample size for a maximum-risk subgroup*

Sample size for top 10% ($\tau$ = 0.1) and confidence 0.90 ($\alpha$ = 0.1) (use $n = N$ if $N \leq 7$)

| | | | | | | | | | | | | | |
|---|---|---|---|---|---|---|---|---|---|---|---|---|---|
| Size of group ($N$) | 8 | 9 | 10 | 11–12 | 13–14 | 15–17 | 18–20 | 21–24 | 25–29 | 30–37 | 38–49 | 50 | ∞ |
| Required no. of measured employees ($n$) | 7 | 8 | 9 | 10 | 11 | 12 | 13 | 14 | 15 | 16 | 17 | 18 | 22 |

Sample size for top 10% ($\tau$ = 0.1) and confidence 0.95 ($\alpha$ = 0.05) (use $n = N$ if $N \leq 11$)

| | | | | | | | | | | | | |
|---|---|---|---|---|---|---|---|---|---|---|---|---|
| Size of group ($N$) | 12 | 13–14 | 15–16 | 17–18 | 19–21 | 22–24 | 25–27 | 28–31 | 32–35 | 36–41 | 42–50 | ∞ |
| Required no. of measured employees ($n$) | 11 | 12 | 13 | 14 | 15 | 16 | 17 | 18 | 19 | 20 | 21 | 29 |

Sample size for top 20% ($\tau$ = 0.2) and confidence 0.90 ($\alpha$ = 0.1) (use n = N if N ≤ 5)

| | | | | | | |
|---|---|---|---|---|---|---|
| Size of group ($N$) | 6 | 7–9 | 10–14 | 15–26 | 27–50 | 51–∞ |
| Required no. of measured employees ($n$) | 5 | 6 | 7 | 8 | 9 | 11 |

Sample size for top 20% ($\tau$ = 0.2) and confidence 0.95 ($\alpha$ = 0.05) (use $n = N$ if $N \leq 6$)

| | | | | | | | | |
|---|---|---|---|---|---|---|---|---|
| Size of group ($N$) | 7–8 | 9–11 | 12–14 | 15–18 | 19–26 | 27–43 | 44–50 | 51–∞ |
| Required no. of measured employees ($n$) | 6 | 7 | 8 | 9 | 10 | 11 | 12 | 14 |

From ref. 7.

If it is not possible to identify the maximum risk workers, random sampling must be carried out. Enough workers selected at random from a group should be sampled so that at least one is from the highest 10% or 20% of the exposure distribution (7). Table 5 may be used to find the required number of employees to be selected at random for groups of various sizes, in order to obtain the confidence shown that at least one employee will be from the highest 10% or 20% exposure group.

### *Monitoring for Exposure Distribution*

More extensive monitoring is needed to determine the actual exposure distribution of a population of workers. The results of an exposure distribution-monitoring program are used to judge whether we can be confident that almost all the exposures are below the desired control limit. One approach is the lognormal probability plot used to approximate the distribution. It is a first approach, which may be adequate for certain estimates. To use this method a sample of about six to ten exposure estimates should be taken. The cumulative distribution is then plotted on lognormal probability paper. If the distribution is lognormal, the data points approximate a straight line. If the line is clearly curved or kinked, additional information is needed and the cited texts (7,12) should be consulted. An idea of the variability will be obtained from the set of samples, since a geometric standard deviation can be derived, and the fraction of samples that can be expected to exceed a given level can be determined from the probability plot (Fig. 1).

### *Individual Worker Exposure*

Air sampling to evaluate the exposure of an individual worker in an industrial environment should provide an accurate assessment of the concentration of the contaminant in the air the worker inhales. It is not yet clear, however, how to measure the true exposure of a worker, but research and new technical developments are improving the prospects for obtaining good exposure measurements. The importance of measuring the fraction of airborne

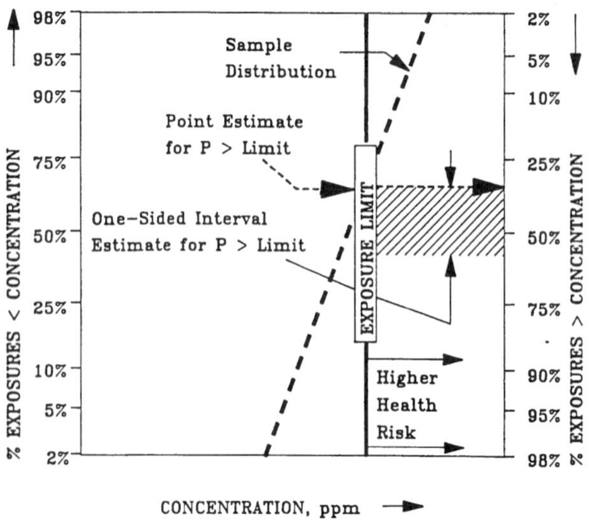


**FIG. 1.** Interval estimate for true proportion (P) of TWA exposures exceeding an exposure limit. (From ref. 37.)

particles that can enter the respiratory tract (13) has stimulated the investigation of new aerosol samplers that closely mimic inhalation patterns.

The term *exposure* here refers to the average air concentration of a contaminant to which a worker is exposed in the course of the workday or some other given work period. The estimates of airborne concentration, or exposure, must ultimately be translated into an inhalation dose. This conversion adds its own uncertainties as a result of the model used to estimate lung deposition and the variability of biologic parameters such as breathing pattern, lung morphometry, dissolution, and clearance rates. Workplace air may be sampled by continuous air monitors for general area surveillance and to monitor for unexpected contaminant release, but general air samples collected to monitor the work environment are not useful for determining the inhalation exposure of personnel. When measurements are made to determine worker exposure, the air near the worker's nose must be sampled.

The concentration of airborne contaminants in the workplace varies both in space and time. Some of the variability results from production processes, ventilation patterns, work practices, and production schedules. The concentration of a contaminant to which a worker is exposed further varies as the worker moves through a normal daily routine of work, rest breaks, and meals.

In most workplaces processes differ from location to location, and the ultimate variations in toxicant concentration resulting from the mix of production processes will be complex. Mechanical resuspension of settled dusts will be superimposed on process contaminant sources. Mixing and dilution will result from the opening and closing of windows and doors. Overhead doors for vehicles are commonly in active use during the workday, as are doors for personnel. Ventilation systems and local exhausts, which may be used as needed, also contribute to variability. Clearly, substantial variability in airborne contaminant concentration is to be expected over time at a given work position and at different locations at any given time. As a result of the spatial and temporal concentration variations in the workplace, individual exposures will differ with job assignment.

An alternative framework has been recommended by the AIHA Exposure Assessment Strategies Committee (14). The group prepared a complete step-by-step program for workplace exposure assessment. A basic construct of the program is the assignment of every worker to a homogeneous exposure group (HEG) such that the probability distribution of exposures is the same for all members of the group. The manual also contains a useful set of appendices that include a working example for a hypothetical plant, and useful statistical information and tables.

Another useful source for guidance on occupational sampling strategy is the ACGIH Air Sampling Instruments text (15).

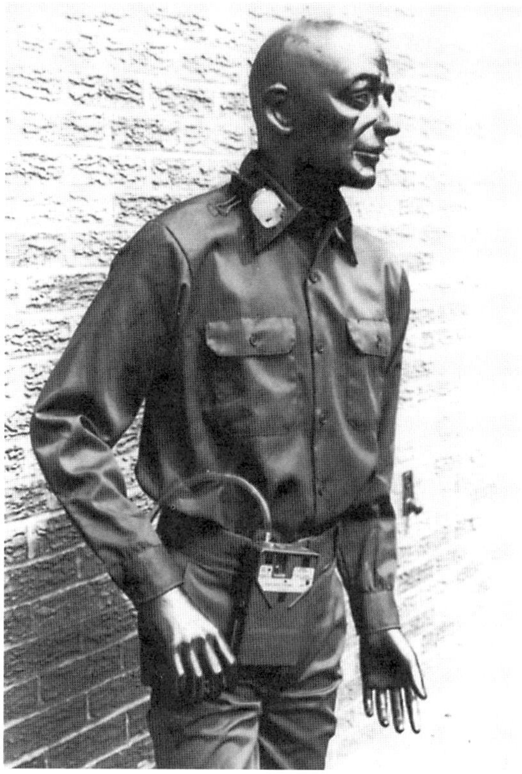

**FIG. 2.** A filter cassette clipped to the lapel and connected to a small pump worn at the belt is demonstrated on a mannequin. (From ref. 38.)

## Air Sampling Methods and Instruments

Two methods are in common use to measure exposure. A personal sampler may be placed near the worker's nose, usually on the lapel of the work clothing, to sample for a full shift (Fig. 2). This method ensures that the monitor travels with the worker, and it is assumed that the sample collected is representative of the inhaled air. This method complies with the requirements of NIOSH that a monitor be placed in the breathing zone of a worker, defined as a 2-foot-diameter sphere around the head. The concentration in such a sphere is not normally uniform, and a question remains as to the best location for a personal monitor (16). A second method is to collect samples of all the different atmospheres to which a worker is exposed during the shift and simultaneously to do a time and motion study of the worker. When the worker is near a source of contaminant the sample is collected as close to the nose as possible. Concentrations measured by these samples are then appropriately combined, based on the time and motion study to give a time-weighted average (TWA) exposure estimate. The computation method for an 8-hour exposure period is as follows:

$$E = (C_aT_a + C_bT_b + \ldots + C_nT_n)/8, \qquad [4]$$

where $E$ is the equivalent exposure for the work shift, $C$ is the concentration during any period of time $T$, where the concentration remains constant, and $T$ is the duration in hours of the exposure at concentration $C$.

This method is also useful when concentrations are too low to be sampled satisfactorily with low-flow personal monitors. The two methods are expected to produce equivalent results, but comparative measurements of the exposure of workers determined by each of the two methods may not agree. The principal cause of the discrepancy between inhalation exposure as estimated by TWAs and as measured by lapel-mounted monitors has been shown, in a beryllium production facility, to be dust resuspended from work clothing into the lapel monitors (17,18). In that industry, a significant contribution to measurement error was also introduced by fluctuations in the flow rate of some of the samplers caused by variations in line voltage.

The results of air-sampling measurements will form the basis for decisions about whether further action is needed. Such decisions determine how well people are protected from hazardous exposure, and if mitigating action is required there may be substantial expense involved. It is therefore essential that reliable and representative samples be obtained. A reliable sample can be obtained only with equipment that is known to be properly calibrated and in good working order. In addition, the precision and accuracy of all the observed data should be evaluated and a cumulative measurement error determined. The detection limits of the system can be evaluated from the measurement error.

Air-sampling instruments are designed either for detection of airborne particles or for gases and vapors and are classified in various ways. Some samplers measure concentration directly; in others samples are collected and returned to the laboratory for analysis; some are "grab" samplers that collect an instantaneous sample, measuring the concentration at one point in space and time, and others provide time-integrated values. Further classification of air-sampling instruments may depend on whether sampling is active or passive (i.e., whether a pump is required), whether large or small volumes of air are required, or on detection method (optical, electrochemical).

Air-sampling equipment may vary in complexity from a small, completely passive monitor that adsorbs any contaminant molecules that diffuse onto a collection substrate (Fig. 3), through a simple sampling train consisting of a collector and an air mover, to self-contained, completely automated sampling instruments with real-time sensors and data-recording and storage capabilities. Many have built-in alarms to warn of conditions such as low oxygen content in a confined space. The first two types of samplers represent systems in which the quantity of contaminant and air volume sampled are determined separately and the concentration calculated from the measurements. A few instruments and methods used for personal sampling of worker exposure will be discussed below, but the reader is referred to the ACGIH publication Air Sampling Instruments for Evaluation of Atmospheric Contaminants (19) for detailed information on selection of sampling equipment and calibration methods.

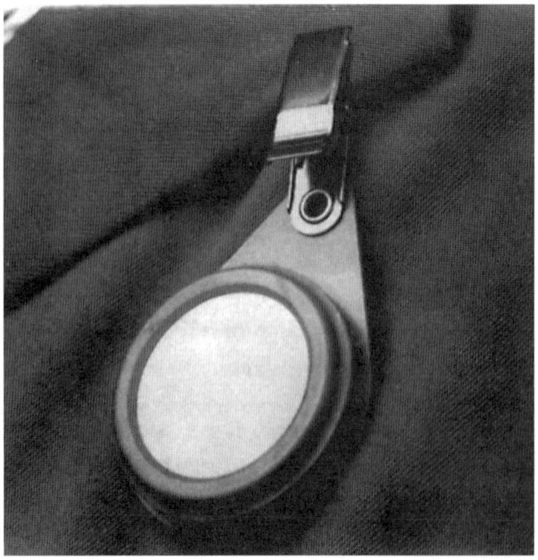

**FIG. 3.** Passive diffusion monitor (3M Corporation) vapors diffuse through the 32-mm diameter membrane to a charcoal substrate.

### *Sampling Train*

A simple sampling train should begin with the collector, followed by a flow monitor and an air mover (Fig. 4). It is preferable to have the collector first in the sampling train, to avoid losses, although certain systems may require a probe prior to the collector. The air mover should be last, so that air leaks will not perturb the measurement. If a probe is used, it is essential to ensure that it does not bias the sample. Flow calibration is required for any sampler with an air mover. The calibration may be done with a primary standard or with a secondary standard calibrated against a primary standard. Primary standards provide direct measures of volume (e.g., spirometers). When combined with time, these provide measures of flow. Bubble meters or frictionless piston meters are primary standards now available as relatively rugged field instruments. A bubble meter consists of a

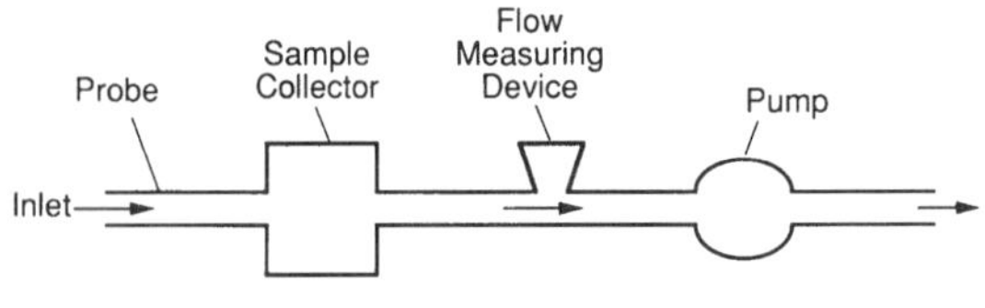


**FIG. 4.** Components of a simple air-sampling train.

transparent tube that has accurate volume markings. A soap film bubble is placed across the tube and the volume displacement of the bubble per unit time measures the flow. Secondary standards include wet-test and dry gas meters and a variety of devices that measure flow directly. They are usually simpler to use. Mass flow meters, which measure the amount of heat transferred between two sensors, are reliable and simple and are used with feedback loops to control flow in many contemporary instruments. The precision of most field flow instruments is about 5%.

The problem of drawing a representative sample into the inlet of a sampler has received substantial attention in recent years. Inlet efficiency is not generally a problem for gases and vapors, although line losses must always be considered, collection efficiency must be established, and sample stability ensured. Collection efficiency must be established with standard atmospheres. Reference methods are available for generating standard atmospheres (11,19). For aerosols the situation is more complex. Whether airborne particles can penetrate the inlet of a given monitor depends on particle size, inlet size, sampling velocity, sampler shape and orientation, and ambient air velocity. Theoretical criteria and models for accurate sampling have been summarized by several authors (20,21). Quantitation of the collected contaminant may be simple (e.g., weighing a filter) or complex, requiring chemical recovery from the collection substrate, followed by an appropriate analytical measurement (e.g., gas chromatography with mass spectrometry). Additional considerations for quantitation of collected sample include sample stability, especially if samples will be transported or stored, interferences of either cocontaminants or material introduced by the substrates, and efficiency of recovery. Stringent quality control measures are required to obtain valid measurements of trace quantities of either gaseous or particulate matter. Calibration standards should be traceable to the National Institute of Standards Technology (NIST).

### *Particle Size Separation*

When sampling airborne particles it is frequently necessary or useful to determine the particle size distribution or to fractionate the particles into specific size ranges. One of the primary reasons for measuring the size distribution of aerosol particles is to assess potential health effects. The size of a particle determines the probability that it may be inhaled and also where in the respiratory tract it is likely to be deposited. Other reasons for obtaining particle size information include the evaluation of the efficacy of pollution control technology and the assessment of environmental impact. Atmospheric transport, deposition to surfaces, and resuspension of deposited particles are size-dependent processes. Measurement of particle size may also be used to assist in the identification of sources of worker exposure.

### *Aerosol Particles*

Airborne particles may range in size from 0.001 to over 100 μm in diameter. When evaluating the behavior of a particle in air it is customary to refer to the aerodynamic size, which is a mathematical combination of factors that determine the aerodynamic behavior of a particle. These include the particle's shape and density as well as its geometric diameter. The hazard that may result from inhalation of airborne particles is critically determined by the particle size. It is obvious that the size of a particle determines how much toxic material it contains, but in addition the aerodynamic behavior of a particle determines the probability that it will be inhaled in the first place and where in the respiratory tract it may be deposited. Inhaled particles are deposited in the respiratory tract by impaction, diffusion, sedimentation, or interception; the latter is important at branch points along the airways and for elongated particles such as asbestos fibers. The aerodynamic diameter ($d_{ae}$) determines which deposition mechanism is dominant. The efficiency with which particles are deposited in the total respiratory tract is minimal at $d_{ae}$, about 0.5 μm. It increases for smaller particles because deposition by diffusion becomes more important, and for larger particles because deposition by impaction and sedimentation then become more important. There is about a 50% probability that a particle larger than about 30 μm will be inhaled in the first place.

Knowledge gained during the past 30 years or so has largely determined where in the respiratory system particles are deposited based on their aerodynamic properties, the morphometry of the respiratory tract, and breathing parameters. These are important considerations because of the tendency of many occupational diseases to be associated with material deposited in particular regions of the respiratory tract. The fact that only particles small enough to pass beyond the tracheobronchial tree and reach the gas-exchange region of the lung were important in the production of pneumoconiosis in hard rock miners was recognized in the middle of the 20th century. Since that time criteria for exposure of certain groups of workers, such as miners and asbestos workers, have included requirements that limit exposure to particles of certain sizes.

The ACGIH has concluded, "Because the biological effects of inhaled aerosols depend on particle size, it will frequently be necessary to take into account the particle sizes present in the environment and the size-selective characteristics of samplers in industrial hygiene evaluations of workplace atmospheres" (22). The three aerosol mass fractions recommended for sampling shown in Fig.

**TABLE 6.** *Respiratory tract regions*

| Region | Anatomic structures |
|---|---|
| Head airways | Nose, mouth, nasopharynx, oropharynx, laryngopharynx |
| Tracheobronchial tree | Larynx, trachea, bronchi, bronchioles (to terminal bronchioles) |
| Gas-exchange region | Respiratory bronchioles, alveolar ducts, alveolar sacs, alveoli |

From ref. 40.

5 are the fractions that reach specific subdivisions of the respiratory tract as defined in Table 6.

A large variety of samplers are available that segregate particles by size or provide a measurement related to particle size. These may utilize the optical, inertial, diffusive, or electrical properties of the particles. One popular device for size-fractionating particles is known as a cascade impactor. It segregates particles onto individual collection plates according to their aerodynamic properties. The separated size fractions can then be analyzed by chemical, physical, or radiometric means. This permits determination of the size fraction with which a specific material is associated, information that is needed to properly assess respiratory hazard from airborne particles (23). Single particle optical counters are among the most commonly used instruments for measuring particle size distributions. They operate by sensing the quantity of light scattered from a single particle, which is related to the size and composition of the particle. Because of the dependence on composition, the particle size measured may differ from the aerodynamic size. Particles smaller than about 0.3 μm cannot be detected optically, and electrical mobility classification or diffusion batteries (24) must be used.

### *Aerosol Sampling*

Personal monitoring for airborne particles is normally carried out by active sampling onto a filter. The collecting filter and precollector, if there is one, are placed in a small lapel holder, and air is drawn through by a belt-mounted pump (see Fig. 2). Total mass collected on the filter may be determined, or collected material may be analyzed for a specific chemical or radioactive component. Diameters of collected particles may be determined by microscopic observation.

Many types of filter media are commercially available, including fiber filters made from a variety of materials such as cellulose, glass, and plastic. Membrane filters of cellulose nitrate or cellulose acetate are popular for air sampling. Polycarbonate sheets with uniform pores and plastic foam filters are also useful for special purposes. Information on filter properties and criteria for selection of an appropriate filter are given elsewhere (25). Ideally, measurement of personal exposure to airborne particles

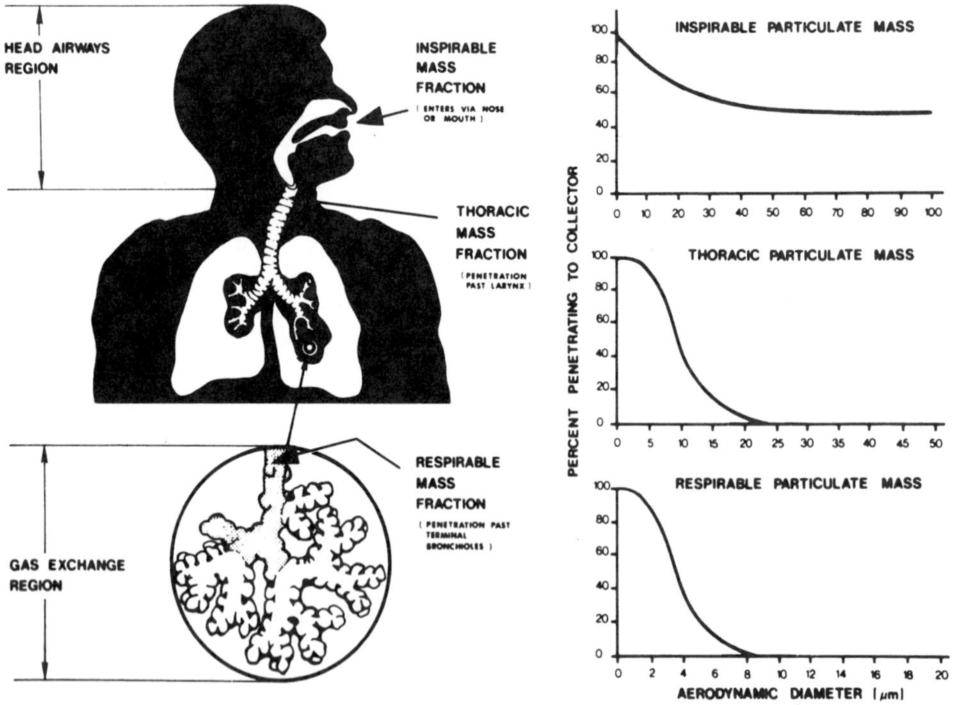


**FIG. 5.** The three aerosol mass fractions recommended for use in particle size-selective aerosol sampling by the ACGIH Air Sampling Procedures Committee. (From ref. 39.)

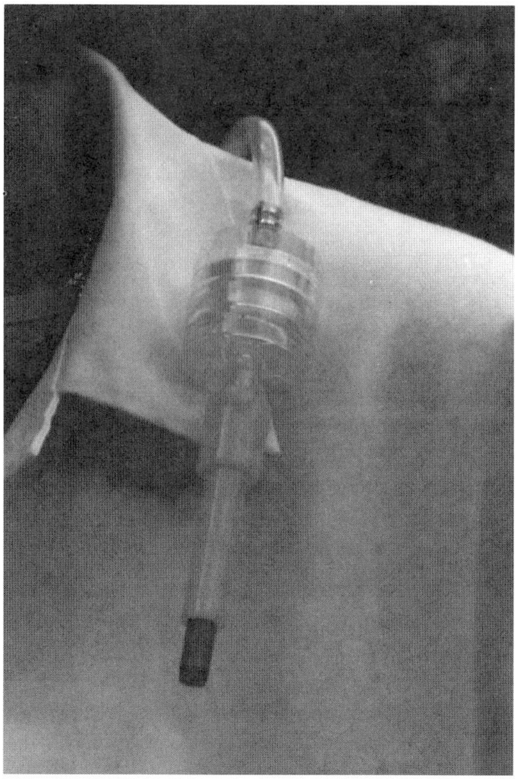

**FIG. 6.** A 10-mm nylon cyclone precedes a filter collector for monitoring respirable particle mass.

should incorporate the recommendations of the ACGIH (8). Adequate personal samplers for all three mass fractions are just becoming available. A reasonably small sampler has recently been developed that separates particle mass by virtual impaction into three fractions, as shown in Fig. 5 (25a). To sample the respirable or thoracic fraction, the filter is preceded by a device that removes a specific fraction of the large particles (13). The preselector most commonly used in the United States to measure respirable particulate mass is a miniature cyclone 10 mm in diameter (Fig. 6), which directs the air along a spiral path and forces large particles out of the air stream onto the walls. Other precollectors include a multiorifice personal impactor (26). A complete discussion may be found elsewhere (13). A personal sampler for the inhalable fraction (Fig. 7) has been developed (27). The inlet is 15 mm in diameter and the design flow rate is 2 L per minute. A few personal samplers are also available that fractionate the airborne particles according to size (28). Small, passive, personal dust monitors that optically sense and automatically record concentrations over an 8-hour shift are also available but less common.

### *Sampling for Gases and Vapors*

Personal sampling for exposure to gases and vapors has been simplified in recent years by the invention of passive personal monitors. The first of these was described by Palmes and Gunnison (29). Typically they are very small (a few $cm^3$), lightweight (about 50 g) samplers that require no power source and have no mechanical parts (see Fig. 3). Contaminant gases diffuse along a tube or through a semipermeable membrane to be collected by adsorption onto a substrate at the back of the sampler. Samples of organic vapors are generally collected onto charcoal. The sampler may be returned to a laboratory for desorption and analysis of the collected material. The amount of material collected during a known exposure period *(T)* is related to the airborne concentration by Fick's law of dif-

A 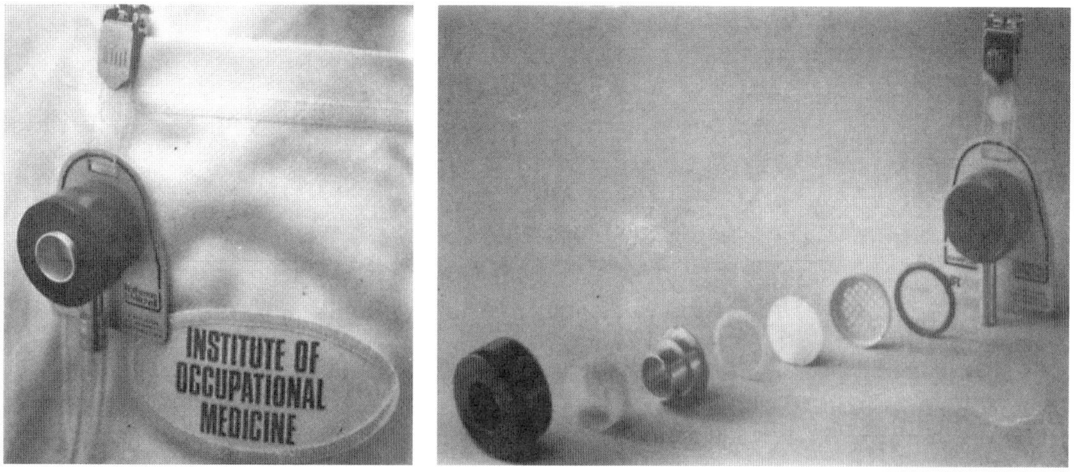 B


**FIG. 7.** Institute of Occupational Medicine personal monitor **(A)** for inhalable particle mass; exploded view **(B)**. (From ref. 21.)

fusion. Concentration *(C)* is determined from the net mass *(M)* recovered from the sorbent as follows:

$$C = \frac{ML}{\varepsilon DAT}, \qquad [5]$$

where $L$ is the length of the diffusion path, $\varepsilon$ the efficiency with which the mass is recovered from the substrate, $D$ the diffusivity of the contaminant molecules, and $A$ the cross-sectional area of the diffusion path.

A factor $k$ is usually supplied by the manufacturer for each compound where

$$k = \frac{L}{DA} \qquad [6]$$

and

$$C = \frac{kM}{ET}. \qquad [7]$$

These passive diffusion samplers have revolutionized personal monitoring for exposure to gases and vapors by providing inexpensive, convenient, and accurate measurements.

Small, active samplers that require a pump to draw air over or through a collection medium are also used for monitoring personal exposure to gases and vapors. The sample collector is clipped to the lapel and a small pump worn on the belt may be used to draw air through tubes containing solid sorbents (Fig. 8*A*). In practice, a plastic cylindrical holder is used to shield the glass collector tube (Fig. 8*A*) from breakage. Various sorbents are used, depending on the gas or vapor to be collected—activated charcoal, silica gel, porous polymers, ambersorbs, coated sorbents, and molecular sieves (30). For certain soluble gases air may be bubbled through an appropriate liquid sorbent contained in a midget impinger or midget bubbler (Fig. 8*B*).

Detector tubes are not personal samplers but are very useful for screening and quick estimation of airborne concentrations of gases and vapors. Such stain tubes have been in use for many years and are available for more than 100 compounds. A small quantity of air is pulled by a handheld pump through a small tube containing an adsorption medium that reacts with the contaminant to produce a color change or stain. The intensity of color change or length of stain is proportional to the concentration of the contaminant. A major drawback with detector tubes is that other substances often interfere with the chemical reaction; thus care should be exercised when using detector tubes where multiple contaminants are present. NIOSH requires an accuracy of ±35% at half the exposure standard and ±25% at one to five times the standard. Pumps and tubes from different manufacturers should not be interchanged, since this may affect accuracy.

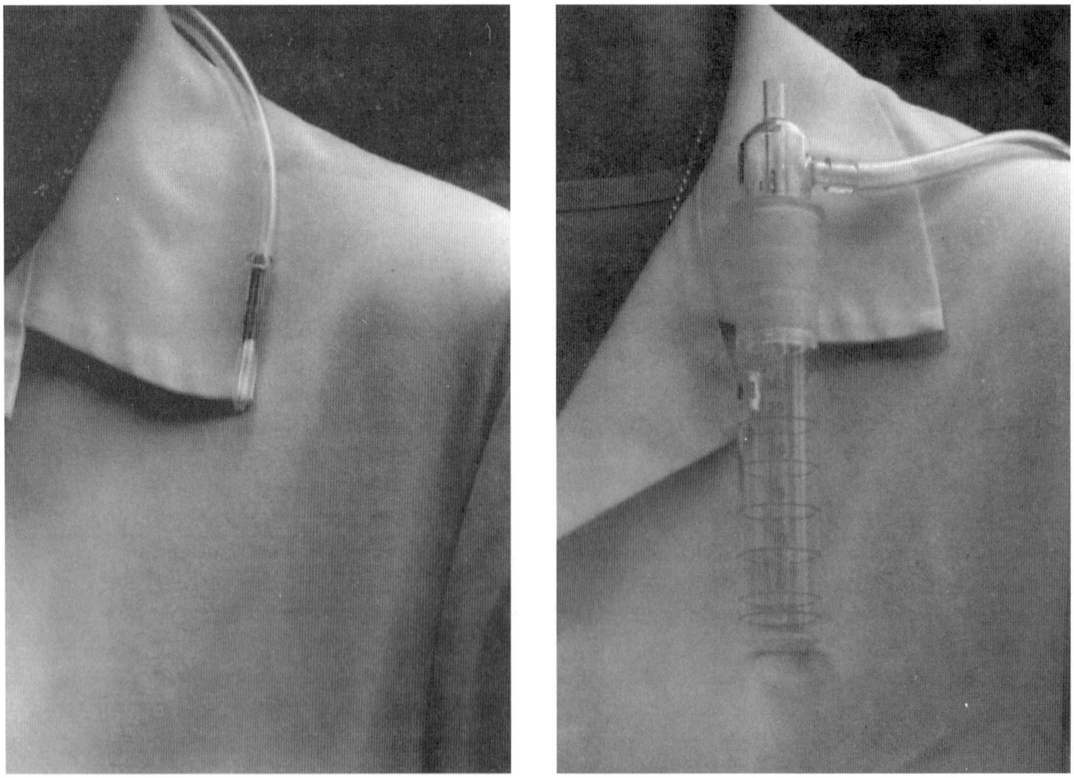

A B

**FIG. 8.** Sample collectors for gases and vapors. **A:** Charcoal sorbent tube. **B:** Midget impinger. Air is drawn through the collector by a small pump.

#### *Viable Aerosols*

Sampling methods for bioaerosols follow the same principles as those for sampling any aerosol but have additional requirements that depend on the processing that will be required. If, for example, microbiologic assays are needed, sampling trains must be sterile and appropriate substrates must be provided. Collectors containing liquid substrates, such as those described previously, may be used with isotonic solutions. Other samplers currently available include cascade impactors, which utilize collection dishes prefilled with agar for collecting size-segregated samples of microorganisms. Sampling protocols for bioaerosols have not been studied as thoroughly as those for nonviable particles. Some guidance is available from a manual developed by the ACGIH Committee on Bioaerosols (31). The guidance provided is designed for investigation of building-related complaints that might be caused by airborne living organisms. Further information is provided elsewhere (32).

## CONTROLLING WORKERS' EXPOSURE

Reduction of exposures to toxicants in the workplace may be accomplished by engineering or administrative controls, adjustment of work practices, personal protective equipment, or a combination of these.

### Engineering Controls

Engineering controls are the most desirable and most reliable means for reducing workplace exposure, and often the most cost-effective choice. Controls are relatively permanent improvements. They do not require worker cooperation, and once they are implemented only routine maintenance is needed. Engineering controls include (a) the substitution of less toxic or less hazardous process materials, (b) the isolation of potential sources of exposure, and (c) ventilation.

The substitution of less toxic material for any potentially hazardous compound used in production should always be considered. For example, substitution of a relatively nonvolatile solvent for one that is volatile may greatly reduce solvent air concentrations. It is, of course, essential to consider the relative toxicity of the substituted solvent. Substitution may also include altering chemical reactions that are part of the process in order to avoid toxic intermediates. If substitution is feasible, this simple step can result in the complete elimination of a serious hazard.

Enclosure, or isolation, of potential sources is another engineering control that can provide cost-effective exposure reduction. If it has been observed that skin contamination may occur by direct chemical contact, efforts must be made to enclose or otherwise contain the process. The most satisfactory industrial hygiene resolution is to physically remove the possibility of dermal contact. Source isolation may also be very effective for reducing excessive noise. For radioactive sources, isolation with appropriate shielding is the method of choice.

Ventilation is an extremely flexible and effective engineering control method for reducing air concentrations of toxic contaminants. Ventilation can reduce the concentration of airborne vapors and particles available for inhalation and also for deposit onto exposed skin or onto work clothing with subsequent penetration to the dermal surface. Ventilation may be defined as "a method for providing control of an environment by strategic use of air flow" (33). The air flow that is provided for climate control in any enclosed space reduces contaminant concentrations by diluting them with clean incoming air. In an industrial environment the general ventilation can be designed to provide enough air changes per unit time to dilute contaminant concentration to any desired level. If it is necessary to heat, cool, humidify, or otherwise condition the incoming air, it may be desirable to limit the air exchange rate, and a combination of dilution, ventilation, and other controls may be preferred.

Local exhaust ventilation can be provided directly at the source of a contaminant by installing a hood at the point of emission. Hoods vary from small, open evacuating ducts to enclosure hoods that completely surround a contaminant source. The hood may be independent or part of a large network of exhaust ducts.

The Committee on Industrial Ventilation of the ACGIH publishes the *Industrial Ventilation: A Manual of Recommended Practice* (34). The manual contains basic information on general principles of ventilation, hood design, design procedures for ventilation systems, air-cleaning devices, fans, and system-testing procedures, among other topics. It also contains design criteria, tables, and illustrative diagrams that are invaluable aids for the design of a ventilation system.

Once a ventilation system is installed for contaminant control, routine maintenance is essential to assure ongoing proper operation of the control system.

### Administrative Controls

Administrative controls include limiting the number of hours a worker spends at a particular job or location, and rotating workers. While it is not desirable to use administrative controls in lieu of engineered reduction of airborne contaminant concentration, they can be effective and may be needed (e.g., while engineering controls are being installed). Administrative controls are useful for controlling exposure to heat or cold. Rest breaks in a cool environment are a recommended control strategy for workers subject to heat stress, and heated warming shelters are recommended when work is performed continuously in the cold (8).

### Work Practices

Controlling exposure through work practices refers to the use of prescribed operating procedures for specific jobs. Proper procedures for routine process operation, for startup and shutdown of a process, and for emergency shutdown are important for safe operation of an industrial process. Unnecessary exposure to hazardous materials can be controlled by developing proper standard operating procedures and training of workers to comply with the protocols. However, hazard control by job protocol is less dependable than engineering control, since fatigue or time pressure may result in less attention to detail. This can lead to serious consequences, such as entering a confined space with dangerous levels of asphyxiants or no oxygen. Process control is also now regulated by OSHA rules: Process Safety Management of Highly Hazardous Chemicals (29 CFR Part 1926.64).

### Personal Protective Equipment

Personal protection equipment, particularly respiratory protection, is considered by most industrial hygienists to be a last resort for controlling worker exposure. Equipment ranges from gloves, to heavy work clothing and safety shoes, to completely impermeable suits with self-contained breathing apparatus.

Protective clothing and gloves provide barriers between skin and potentially hazardous airborne materials, but no clothing is truly impervious (34), and few materials are available that provide relatively impermeable barriers for extended periods. Requirements for protective clothing depend on the chemical, potential exposure time, environmental conditions (e.g., permeation rate depends on temperature), and other factors. If chemical contact may result from only occasional accidental splashes and clothing may be changed quickly, less stringent requirements may apply. Extensive guidance on selecting and evaluating clothing protective against chemicals will be found in Roder (35). Recommendations for appropriate clothing are available (36), but these guidelines should not be used without testing representative samples from specific garments because of manufacturing differences in materials and garments (35). Roder also recommends that testing be done under anticipated work conditions, because of differences in generic materials and because observations from tests of individual chemicals cannot predict the behavior of mixtures.

The least desirable industrial hygiene control is the use of respiratory protective devices, though they may be useful for occasional brief tasks that can result in heavy inhalation exposure such as changing hood filters and similar maintenance operations. They are often essential for emergency releases. Many types of respiratory protective devices are available, varying in size from those that cover about a quarter of the face through full face pieces. Some rely on filtering or purifying of ambient air; some use supplied air. Many use replaceable air-purifying cartridges that protect against airborne particles or specific gases or vapors. To operate properly, a respirator must cover both nose and mouth and fit properly; otherwise contaminated air can leak into the inspired air volume. Proper selection and leak testing of respirators are critical if the wearer is to be protected from inhaling contaminated air, and the amount of protection provided by any specific respirator must be evaluated by trained personnel.

### Employee Education

Worker training and education is an essential component of programs to control worker exposure. OSHA's Hazard Communication Standard (29 CFR 1919.1200; 1983, revised 1987) addresses worker training on the hazards of exposure to chemical contaminants. It requires employers to have a written hazard communication program and to disseminate information on any chemicals present in a workplace. Material safety data sheets (MSDS) must be available for each hazardous chemical an employee may be exposed to. The MSDS must contain information on the chemical hazard and ways to protect against it. Informed employees can protect themselves from hazards and ensure that proper work practices reduce potential exposure as much as possible.

If sampling or monitoring programs have been undertaken, employees should be informed of the results. Video recording of concentrations measured by air sampling instruments during specific work practices are beginning to gain favor for worker training. These systems, which display the concentration readings overlaid on videotapes of work in progress, can provide effective visual evidence of the impact of specific work practices on exposure.

## SUMMARY

The design of an industrial hygiene sampling program must be based on professional judgment and scientific method. When the reason for undertaking a program is clear, a preliminary survey provides the input needed for specific sampling decisions. Decision criteria must be established to evaluate sampling results. A statistical approach is necessary if inferences are to be drawn from sampling data. Personal monitoring should be used to assess worker exposure. To relate sampling data to health effects, it is important to obtain a reliable and representative sample and to sample the relevant fraction of an airborne contaminant. Interpretation of sampling results requires professional judgment and awareness of the limitations of current equipment. Engineering controls are the preferred method for reducing the potential of hazardous exposure. Other options include administrative control and personal protective equipment. Employee education and training are essential for maintaining a safe and healthy work environment.

## REFERENCES


1. AIHA. *Who's who in industrial hygiene.* Fairfax, VA: American Industrial Hygiene Association, 1996.
2. Corn JK. Historical review of industrial hygiene. *Ann Am Conf Ind Hyg* 1983;5:13–17.
3. NIOSH. *National occupational research agenda.* DHHS (NIOSH) Publication No. 96-115. Washington, DC: National Institute for Occupational Safety and Health, CDC, PHS, USDHHS, 1996.
4. Cralley LV, Cralley LJ, eds. *Industrial hygiene aspects of plant operations, process flows.* New York: Macmillan, 1982;1.
5. Cralley LV, Cralley LJ, eds. *Industrial hygiene aspects of plant operations, unit operations and product fabrication.* New York: Macmillan, 1984;2.
6. Cralley LV, Cralley LJ, eds. *Industrial hygiene aspects of plant operations, engineering considerations in equipment selection layout and building design.* New York: Macmillan, 1985;3.
7. Leidel NA, Busch KA, Lynch JR. *Occupational exposure sampling strategy manual.* NIOSH publication 77-173. Cincinnati, OH: U.S. Department of Health, Education and Welfare, 1977.
8. ACGIH. *1996 threshold limit values for chemical substances and physical agents and biological exposure indices.* Cincinnati, OH: American Conference of Governmental Industrial Hygienists, 1996.
9. OSHA. *Air contaminants—permissible exposure limits.* OSHA 3112. Document (OSHA) 929 022 000009. Washington, DC: U.S. Government Printing Office, 1989.
10. ACGIH. *Guide to occupational exposure values.* Cincinnati, OH: American Conference of Governmental Industrial Hygienists, 1996.
11. Nelson GO. *Gas mixtures:* preparation and control. Chelsea, MI: Lewis Publishers, 1992.
12. Leidel NA, Busch KA. Statistical design and data analysis requirements. In: Cralley LJ, Cralley LV, eds. *Patty's industrial hygiene and toxicology,* 2nd ed. New York: Wiley, 1985;3A:395–507.
13. Lippmann M. Size-selective health hazard sampling. In: Cohen BS, Hering SV, eds. *Air sampling instruments for evaluation of atmospheric contaminants,* 8th ed. Cincinnati, OH: American Conference of Governmental Industrial Hygienists, 1995;81–119.
14. Hawkins NC, Norwood SK, Rock JC, eds. A strategy for occupational exposure assessment. Akron, OH: American Industrial Hygiene Association, 1991.
15. Rock JC. Occupational air sampling strategies. In: Cohen BS, Hering SV, eds. *Air sampling instruments.* Cincinnati, OH: American Conference of Governmental Industrial Hygienists, 1995;19–44.
16. Malek RM, Daisey JM, Cohen BS. Investigation of breathing zone concentration variations for organic vapors. Presented at the American Industrial Hygiene Conference, May 22–27, 1983, Philadelphia, PA.
17. Cohen BS, Harley NH, Lippmann M. Bias in air-sampling techniques used to measure inhalation exposure. *Am Ind Hyg Assoc J* 1984;45: 187–192.
18. Bohne JE Jr, Cohen BS. Aerosol resuspension from fabric: implications for personal monitoring in the beryllium industry. *Am Ind Hyg Assoc J* 1985;46:73–79.
19. Cohen BS, Hering SV, eds. *Air sampling instruments for evaluation of atmospheric contaminants,* 8th ed. Cincinnati, OH: American Conference of Governmental Industrial Hygienists, 1995.
20. Hinds WC. Sampler efficiencies: inspirable mass fraction. In: *Particle size—selective sampling in the workplace, report of the ACGIH Technical Committee on Air Sampling Procedures.* Cincinnati, OH: American Conference of Industrial Hygienists, 1985.
21. Vincent JH. *Aerosol sampling, science and practice.* New York: Wiley, 1989.
22. ACGIH. *Particle size—selective sampling in the workplace.* Cincinnati, OH: American Conference of Governmental Industrial Hygienists, 1985.
23. Cohen BS. The first forty years. In: Lodge JP, Chan TL, eds. *Cascade impactor—sampling and data analysis.* Akron, OH: American Industrial Hygiene Association, 1986;1–21.
24. Cheng YS. Diffusion batteries and denuders. In: Cohen BS, Hering SV, eds. *Air sampling instruments for evaluation of atmospheric contaminants,* 8th ed. Cincinnati, OH: American Conference of Governmental Industrial Hygienists, 1995;511–526.
25. Lippmann M. Sampling aerosols by filtration. In: Cohen BS, Hering SV, eds. *Air sampling instruments,* 8th ed. Cincinnati, OH: American Conference of Governmental Industrial Hygienists, 1995;247–278.

25a.Keady PB. *A new size-selective personal practice sampler:* description and performance. 1998 Applied Workshop Occupational & Environmental Exposure Assessment. Chapel Hill, NC: ACGIH, 1998.

26. Marple VA, Rubow KL. Theory and design guidelines. In: Lodge JP, Chan TL, eds. *Cascade impactor:* sampling and data analysis. Akron, OH: American Industrial Hygiene Association, 1986.
27. Mark D, Vincent JH. A new personal sampler for airborne total dust in workplaces. *Ann Occup Hyg* 1986;30:89–102.
28. Marple VA, Rubow KL. Impactors for respirable dust sampling. In: Marple VK, Liu BY, eds. *Aerosols in the mining and industrial environment.* Ann Arbor, MI: Ann Arbor Science, 1983;3:847–860.
29. Palmes ED, Gunnison AF. Personal monitoring device for gaseous contaminants. *Am Ind Hyg Assoc J* 1973;34:78–81.
30. Eller PM, ed. *NIOSH manual of analytical methods.* 4th ed. Cincinnati, OH: U.S. Department of Health and Human Services, 1994.
31. ACGIH. *Guidelines for the assessment of bioaerosols in the indoor environment.* Cincinnati, OH: American Conference of Governmental Industrial Hygienists, 1989.
32. Macher JM, Chatigny MA, Burge HA. Sampling airborne microorganisms and aeroallergens. In: Cohen BS, Hering SV, eds. *Air sampling instruments.* Cincinnati, OH: American Conference of Governmental Industrial Hygienists, 1995;586–617.
33. Soule RD. Industrial hygiene engineering controls. In: Clayton GD, Clayton FE, eds. *Patty's industrial hygiene and toxicology,* 3rd ed. New York: Wiley, 1978;1:771–823.
34. ACGIH. *Industrial ventilation:* a manual of recommended practice, 22nd ed. Cincinnati, OH: American Conference of Governmental Industrial Hygienists, 1995.
35. Roder MM. *A guide for evaluating the performance of chemical protective clothing (CPC).* Publication (NIOSH) 26505-2888. Morgantown, WV: U.S. Department of Health and Human Services, 1990.
36. Schwope AD, Costas PP, Jackson JO, Stull JO, Weitzman DJ. *1987 guidelines for the selection of chemical protective clothing,* vols 1 and 2, 3rd ed. Publications AD A179 516, AD A179 164. Arlington, VA: National Technical Information Service (NTIS), 1987.
37. Leidel NA, Busch KA. Evolution of sampling strategies over the last decade, 1975 to 1985. Presented at Workshop on Exposure Assessment. Washington, DC, December 1986.
38. Cohen BS, Chang AE, Harley NH, Lippmann M. Exposure estimates from personal lapel monitors. *Am Ind Hyg Assoc J* 1982;43:239–243.
39. *AIHA respiratory protection manual.* Akron, OH: American Industrial Hygiene Association, 1991.
40. Phalen RF. Introduction and recommendations, airway anatomy and physiology. In: *Particle size-selective sampling in the workplace.* Report of the ACGIH Technical Committee on Air-Sampling Procedures. Cincinnati, OH: ACGIH, 1985.

*Environmental and Occupational Medicine,*
*Third Edition,* edited by William N. Rom.
Lippincott–Raven Publishers, Philadelphia © 1998.

# CHAPTER 133

# Respirators

Philip Harber

Properly employed, respiratory personal protective devices (respirators) can be a very effective component of a worker protection program. Respirators are devices worn to improve the healthfulness of inhaled air. In most cases, they do so by decreasing the level of hazardous agents in the inspired air. In other situations, they add oxygen to the air stream or modify the inspired air conditions (e.g., by heating frigid air).

Use of respirators must be considered only one component in a respiratory protection program, and their use must be coordinated with the other aspects. Respirators generally are employed in occupational settings; however, they may be used in home settings by hobbyists with potential toxic exposures or in military operations for protection against chemical, biologic, and radiologic (CBR) warfare agents. They have also been used by civilian populations threatened by CBR attack (e.g., by Israeli civilians during the Persian Gulf War); there have been few formal studies of their use under such circumstances. This chapter focuses on use in the occupational setting.

## USE OF RESPIRATORS

Use of respirators is not the method of choice for controlling exposures. Respirators do not provide foolproof protection. Respirator-based protection is completely dependent on voluntary compliance by the worker. Furthermore, protection by respirator use requires an ongoing multifaceted program to assure proper maintenance and utilization. The cost of the respirator itself is only a small part of the total cost of an effective program.

P. Harber: Occupational and Environmental Medicine Program, Department of Medicine, University of California, Los Angeles, Los Angeles, California 90095.

Respirators may be used for protection against a large variety of inhaled agents. The respiratory system may serve as route of entry even if the target organ for toxicity is not the lungs themselves (for example, lead). In other instances, the respiratory system is the target organ; both the upper respiratory tract (nose) and lower respiratory systems may be targeted.

In the traditional "hierarchy of controls" for prevention, other methods are preferable. Elimination of the toxic agent or substitution of a less toxic agent can be more efficacious. Engineering controls, such as enclosure of the process producing airborne toxic materials or local exhaust ventilation, do not rely on worker compliance. Administrative controls, which directly reduce the potential for worker exposure, are also often preferable.

There are, however, situations in which respirator use is needed. Respirators are often required when the work is of a varied nature, preventing the construction of adequate engineering controls (for example, in construction). Respirators are also commonly needed during maintenance and repair operations when ventilation controls are disengaged or nonoperative. Respirators also are frequently needed when relatively infrequent operations are conducted (e.g., transfers of liquid raw materials). Personal respiratory protection may be needed for emergency and unplanned events (e.g., as part of the emergency response to a spill). Finally, there are some routine operations for which product substitutions or engineering controls are not financially feasible.

## TYPES OF RESPIRATORS

There are many types of respirators. The appropriate device must be used to achieve adequate protection and be sufficiently comfortable for use by the worker (1,2).

There are several ways to characterize respirators, as summarized in Table 1. There are two fundamental methods by which the respirator can supply air with reduced contaminants: *air purifying* respirators use ambient air and filter or adsorb the contaminants; *atmosphere supplying* respirators use an independent air supply rather than relying on removal of contaminants from the air in the environment. Most respirators in use are air purifying respirators. Generally, atmosphere supplying respirators provide a higher level of protection.

Air purifying respirators decrease contaminant levels by one of several mechanisms: Filtration may remove particles by passing air through small pores. The filtration process is often assisted by electrostatic characteristics, in which particles with surface charges interact with charges within the respirator filter matrix. Sorbent respirators adsorb the chemical agent to the material with which the respirator matrix is impregnated.

The physical design varies. The mask itself may be the filtration or sorbent matrix. In other designs, cartridges or canisters containing the media are attached to the mask; these must be selected to provide the proper filter/absorbent combination for the particular environmental exposure. In a gas mask design, a canister is attached by a hose to the mask, whereas cartridges attach directly to the mask.

**TABLE 1.** *Respirator characterization*

| |
|---|
| Contaminant reduction |
| Air purifying: use ambient air by partially reducing contaminant concentration |
| Atmosphere supplying: provide clean air from an independent source |
| Physical design |
| Air purifying |
| Mask only |
| Cartridge |
| Canister |
| Atmosphere supplying |
| Self-contained breathing apparatus (SCBA) |
| Air line: air via a hose |
| Combined air line with backup tank |
| Pressure dynamics |
| Air purifying |
| Negative pressure |
| Powered air purifying respirator (PAPR) |
| Air hood |
| Atmosphere supplying |
| Continuous flow |
| Demand: air flow only during inspiration |
| Pressure demand: attempts to maintain mask pressure positive throughout respirator cycle |
| Fit type |
| Tight fitting |
| Loose fitting |
| Mask type |
| Quarter mask |
| Half mask |
| Full-face mask |
| Other (e.g., air hat) |

Air purifying respirators generally require that the user generate negative pressure to "suck air through" the filtration/absorbent unit. However, some air purifying devices are fitted with a fan that blows air through the device, relieving the user of the necessity to do this. These are known as powered air purifying respirators (PAPRs).

The service life of the devices must be considered. As loading of filtration devices increases by extended use, particularly in a very dusty environment, the air flow resistance increases. Similarly, devices depending on chemical sorbents may exhaust the sorbent capacity, and "breakthrough" of toxic contaminants into the inspired air will occur (3).

Atmosphere supplying respirators use an independent air source. In a self-contained breathing apparatus (SCBA), the worker carries an air tank, generally on the back. An air-line respirator supplies air via a long hose from a source at a distance from the contaminated air. In selected instances (typically for short-term use during escape), a chemical oxygen generator is employed, usually from a source such as potassium permanganate. Because atmosphere supplying respirators are typically used in the more hazardous settings, a small backup air tank may be employed when an air-line respirator is used; the air tank is activated if the supplied air hose becomes nonoperable or the external compressor ceases to function properly.

Supplied air respirators require two particular concerns. For an air-line respirator, one must assure that the air source is itself not contaminated. The compressor should not entrain outside air if there is contamination. A tank-based system has a limited service life, and the length of work that can be accommodated using an air tank decreases as work level and hence ventilation rate increases.

Pressure dynamics is another characterization of respirators. As the worker inhales, pressure within the mask may be negative relative to the atmospheric pressure, allowing inward movement of contaminated air if there are any gaps between the mask and the facial surface. To decrease this possibility, respirators may be utilized in the positive pressure mode in very toxic atmospheres. When used in this manner, sufficiently high air flow is provided to maintain the pressure in the mask positive to ambient pressure. However, with high exertion rates, negative mask pressure can still occur if the user's inspiratory flow rate exceeds the supply rate (4).

The fit type of the respirator represents another categorization. Most require a tight fit against the sealing surface of the face. Some, however, are loose fitting. For example, welders' and sandblasters' hoods do not require tight fits; instead, sufficient air flow is provided to keep contaminated air from entering the breathing zone to an unacceptable degree. Air hats also do not require a tight facial seal.

Tight fitting respirators, which are the most common, require that the facial seal remain excellent. If there is a break in the seal between the mask and the face, contaminated air can enter. In many situations, leakage around the mask is a more important source of contamination than transmission through the mask and the sorbent/filter media.

Face masks may be characterized as quarter mask (covering nose to mid-chin), half mask (nose to under chin), or full-face mask (forehead to under chin). The larger masks are more protective. This is particularly true for a full-face mask respirator, which obviates the possibility of a leakage at the facial seal surface above the nose. Occasionally, mouthpiece-only devices are used for limited-time emergency escape (e.g., in mining situations); such small devices are carried by the miner or worker and therefore cannot contain a large mask.

## RESPIRATOR FIT

Most respirators require a tight seal between the mask and the user's face. The overall efficacy of the respirator in decreasing the concentration of inhaled toxins is described by its protection factor (PF). The protection factor is the ratio of the contaminant concentration outside the mask to the concentration inside the mask. Higher protection factors imply a greater degree of protection. There are several protection factor types:

Assigned protection factor (APF): The APF is assigned to the particular type of respirator device without direct measurement in the subject. Assignments are made based on published studies and/or professional judgment (5).

Measured protection factor (MPF): The protection factor for the individual worker is measured in a clinical laboratory test setting with the worker wearing the actual respirator under optimal conditions.

Workplace protection factor (WPF): The WPF reflects the actual protection afforded in "real-life use." It is determined using measurements made in actual workplace conditions.

Examples of assigned protection factors for different types of masks are shown in Table 2. There can be significant differences among the APF, MPF, and WPF (6–8). For example, a worker often has an MPF that is greater than the APF. However, the WPF, which most accurately reflects the actual protection afforded, may be significantly lower than the APF or MPF because of factors such as inadequate beard shaving.

### Fit Testing and Checking

Every time a user dons a respirator, he or she should perform a fit check to qualitatively estimate if the tight-fitting mask leaks. For example, if there are inspiratory valves, the worker occludes them and sucks in. If air still enters, there is a significant leak.

**TABLE 2.** *Assigned protection factors*

| Type | Factor |
|---|---|
| Air purifying | |
| Half mask | 10 |
| Full facepiece | 100 |
| Powered air purifying | |
| Half mask | 50 |
| Full facepiece | 100–1000 |
| Atmosphere supplying | |
| SCBA (demand mode) full facepiece | 100 |
| Air-line (demand mode) full facepiece | 100 |
| Air-line (pressure demand) full facepiece | 1,000 |
| SCBA (pressure demand) full facepiece | Up to 10,000 |

From ref. 11.

Fit testing is a procedure for measuring the adequacy of fit; it is typically performed when a worker first starts to use one type of respirator. There are two types of fit tests—qualitative and quantitative. A qualitative fit test depends on detection of a tracer material by the subject. For example, saccharine, bittrex, or irritant smoke is placed outside the mask. If the user indicates by cough or verbal statement that the material is detected, the mask is considered to fit inadequately.

In a quantitative fit test, the concentration of a marker substance inside and outside the mask is measured under laboratory conditions for the specific user. The ratio represents the MPF for that individual. In the past, material such as dioctyl phthalate (DOP) was used, but now natural aerosols are used most commonly. Individual Occupational Safety and Health Administration (OSHA) standards prescribe which fit testing method should be utilized. Quantitative fit testing is mandated under certain circumstances.

There can be significant differences between the assigned protection factor and the actual workplace protection factor. For example, differences in individual facial configurations, growth of a beard or stubble, or failure to optimally seat the respirator on the face can all lead to significant differences.

## RESPIRATORY PROTECTION PROGRAM

Respirator use requires a complete program (9–11). Several major components are listed in Table 3. It is nearly always inappropriate to recommend use of a respirator unless all the components are in place, including written procedures. Therefore, clinicians who are asked to perform "medical certification for respirator use" should ascertain that the employer has established the other program components. A single individual should be responsible for the overall respiratory protection program; often this is an industrial hygienist or occupational medicine physician.

**TABLE 3.** *Components of respiratory protection programs*

| |
|---|
| Assessment of whether respirators are needed |
| Exposure assessment |
| Respirator selection |
| Medical assessment of users |
| Training |
| Cleaning and maintenance |
| Program audit |
| Written procedures; designated program director |

Respirator selection, discussed in detail in the next section, must be based on knowledge of the specific exposures in the workplace. Medical certification involves determining whether specific workers can safely and effectively employ respirators. A training program is needed for both users and for their supervisors; respirator use is highly contingent on proper worker cooperation. A formal respirator maintenance program is necessary to assure that respirators are maintained in proper working order and that cartridges are replaced periodically as necessary. A regular audit of program efficacy is also required.

The respiratory protection program should be operated in conjunction with an overall occupational health surveillance program. Although the medical aspects of respirator use can be handled independently, much of the information collected is also useful for other aspects of occupational respiratory surveillance.

Numerous regulations apply. In the United States, OSHA has promulgated regulations for respirator use; most are included in 29 CFR 1910 and 1926. In addition, the respirator aspects of OSHA standards for specific agents (e.g., asbestos) have been consolidated in section 1910. For specific requirements for respirator programs, the program director should consult the appropriate standards carefully. In the United States, actual certification of respirator types is the responsibility of the National Institute for Occupational Safety and Health (NIOSH). Historically, other agencies in the United States such as the Mine Safety and Health Administration (MSHA), the Department of Agriculture (DOA), and the Nuclear Regulatory Commission (NRC) have also been involved in respirator certification. States may also promulgate specific relevant regulations.

In the United States, it is generally held that an employer must have a full respiratory protection program in place even if the respirator is used solely at the discretion and choice of the individual worker. Thus, if a patient follows physician advice and uses a respirator at work, this generally obligates the employer to establish a complete respiratory protection program.

## RESPIRATOR SELECTION

Respirator selection is a complex process. Generally, selection of the appropriate respirator type should be done by a certified industrial hygienist or an occupational-environmental medicine specialist. NIOSH periodically publishes updated "respirator decision logic" manuals (1), which provide specific algorithms for guiding respirator selection. Two groups of considerations affect respirator selection—the first relates to the exposure situation per se, and the second to individual worker characteristics and preferences.

The first step is determination of whether respirators should be used at all. One must first ask if use of personal respiratory protection is the optimal technique or if engineering controls, process elimination, or product substitution would be more effective.

The second step is evaluating the level of contaminant reduction that is necessary. This defines the respirator class that is needed to provide adequate protection factors to sufficiently reduce exposure.

The nature of work-site exposures should be determined, including those that occur regularly, during temporary shutdown for maintenance, and during unexpected potential emergencies (e.g., spills, leaks, fires). The air concentrations should be determined. The workplace air concentration is then compared to the level that is permitted. Under OSHA regulations, this is described by the permissible exposure level (PEL). The ratio of the actual workplace exposure level to the permissible exposure defines the degree of reduction that the respirator must afford. Hence, if the workplace level reaches 100 ppm and the PEL is 10 ppm, a respirator that can reliably produce a tenfold (100:10) reduction is necessary. The nature of the agent and its time course of inducing toxic effects must be considered. For agents that produce a toxic effect on a cumulative basis, the 8-hour time-weighted average (TWA) is the appropriate metric; for other agents, short-term peaks of exposure are particularly hazardous, and therefore the short-term exposure limits (STEL) define necessary protection. Generally, a safety factor of tenfold is added rather than directly relying on the measured workplace to PEL ratio.

Because single-use disposable respirators have a maximum assigned protection factor of 10 ppm, they cannot be used in many exposure situations if a safety factor of 10 is added. Further, when fit testing is performed, one assumes that the fit test may misestimate the actual workplace protection by a factor of ten. Hence, fit testing for single-use respirators is not feasible since their protection factor is only ten at most.

The third step is consideration of two special circumstances—"immediately dangerous to life and health" (IDLH) and poor warning properties—related to the exposure. IDLH circumstances occur when there is a reasonable likelihood that the exposure would produce irreversible health effects, such as with radioactive exposures, highly toxic materials, and oxygen-deficient atmospheres. Under such circumstances, an atmosphere supplying rather than air purifying respirator is generally required. In particularly hazardous situations, dual protection is necessary to assure safety; for example, if an air-line respirator is used, a small supplementary air tank is necessary to allow escape if the air supply should fail. For nearly all IDLH circumstances (except oxygen deficiency), full-face mask with positive pressure mode operation is employed to avoid inward movement of contaminants during inspiration.

The second concern is related to the warning properties of the contaminant agent (12). As discussed earlier, respirator filtration/sorbent media eventually become exhausted and may allow breakthrough of the contaminant. For some materials (e.g., chlorine, ammonia), this will be obvious to the user. On the other hand, some materials (e.g., carbon monoxide) are poorly detectable, and the respirator user will not be driven to change the exhausted media before toxic exposure occurs. In particular, end of service life indicators (if available) are necessary if air purifying respirators are employed with agents with poor warning properties.

The fourth step is to consider the work situation as a guide to respirator type selection. For example, air-line respirators cannot be used where considerable mobility is necessary. Workers may tolerate certain respirator types for a brief period, but would not be able to use uncomfortable or bulky devices for a longer period. Powered air purifying devices require considerable maintenance to assure the batteries are always charged.

The fifth group of considerations relates to the individual user. These include both medical impairment–related considerations and personal preference. Medical considerations are discussed in a subsequent section. User preference cannot be ignored, since ultimately worker protection depends completely on proper voluntary utilization by the worker.

The sixth step is programmatic consideration. Respirator selection must be made in view of the overall program goals and resources. Particularly expensive types (purchase, maintenance, and/or training) may not be justified in some circumstances. In addition, since respirators are only a part of the worker's protection program, their integration with other protective measures must be considered (e.g., protective suits). From a programmatic standpoint, the utilization of too diverse an array of respirator types in any workplace may create significant supervision and training problems.

The seventh step is to look at past experience. Respirator programs must be periodically evaluated.

### Additional Considerations

The paradigm described above is consistent with most regulatory approaches. However, there are several factors other than the ratio of acceptable concentration to workplace air concentration that determine the degree of protection necessary. Such considerations are rarely directly included in regulatory requirements.

The physical state, rather than the mass concentration per se, may affect the biologic effect of an inhaled agent. Particle size very significantly affects the penetration of the agent, and a greater degree of respiratory protection is necessary if small size particles (e.g., fumes) are generated (13). For fibers, the dimensions and charge affect uptake and clearance; they also affect the air concentration to human toxicity relationship in a manner not always reflected by regulation. Greater degrees of respiratory protection are advisable when there is likely to be longer duration of exposure for a particular worker (either on a short-term basis or over a working lifetime). The level of exertion is also a major determinant of dose. Heavier exertion is associated with greater ventilation and therefore a greater dose delivered to the body. In addition, heavy exertion may increase the negative in-mask pressure and lead to a greater degree of leakage.

Personal susceptibility must also be considered. Types of respiratory protection that are suitable for most individuals may be inadequate for highly sensitive persons. Persons with preexisting lung disease may be more sensitive to additional inhaled material. Similarly, for agents having target organs elsewhere in the body, preexisting disease or personal susceptibility factors are important considerations.

Therefore, in most circumstances, the regulatory requirements should be considered as the minimum degree of protection to be afforded, and greater respiratory protection may be needed in particular work situations or for specific individuals.

## MEDICAL CONSIDERATIONS

The determination of whether an individual should use a respirator and, if so, which is the optimal type, is based on an understanding of how respirators affect users (14–16). While in the past much emphasis was placed on the effects on the pulmonary and cardiac systems, more recent work has suggested that a broader perspective is needed. Research has also suggested that respirators are generally well tolerated (17,18). This section briefly reviews the major effects of respirator use, which are listed in Table 4.

Respirators often impede work performance, and this may be a major factor with noncompliance (19–21). At the very least, respirator use imposes significant financial cost for the various aspects of the program, including purchase, training, maintenance, and audit. The device may also decrease work performance by impeding mobility. Interference with communication is a burden for supervisors and for use in health care settings. Although rarely admitted, the presence of a worker in a respirator is often interpreted to imply that a hazardous material is present, and therefore their use may tend to be eschewed in publicly visible situations.

**TABLE 4.** *Potential adverse effects of respirator use*

| |
|---|
| Interference with work performance |
| Psychological effects |
| Cardiovascular effects |
| Pulmonary effects |
| Ventilatory loads |
| Psychophysical effects |
| Musculoskeletal |
| Vision |
| Communication |
| Skin |
| Thermal effects |
| Nasal effects |
| Infection |

Three psychological considerations are relevant—fear of exposure, psychological stress, and health orientation. First, respirator use may imply to some workers that a significant chemical or other hazard exists. Such fear can be best handled through assuring (if valid) that inappropriate exposures will not occur and communicating this with an adequate worker training program.

Second, psychological stress induced by the mask itself may be due to a sense of claustrophobia or other reactions, which Morgan (22) has estimated are experienced by 10% of users. In some but not all circumstances, stress may be managed by psychological interventions. In other settings, use of alternative respirator types not depending on tight fit may be helpful.

The third psychological factor is worker health orientation. Workers must pursue safe and healthful behaviors. There has been only limited research addressing psychological and social determinants of adequate respirator use (23–25). Worker training programs that focus only on imparting knowledge and not affecting attitudes may inadequately motivate workers to protect themselves with such devices.

Some respirators (heavy SCBAs) impose increased cardiac loading by virtue of weight; carrying a 35-pound respirator is no different than carrying any other 35-pound weight. Studies have shown that during submaximal exercise, cardiac effects of most types are limited (26,27). Although there has been concern that pleural pressure swings induced by breathing through the resistance of a respirator may produce effects on cardiac output and blood pressure homeostasis, this has not been convincingly demonstrated to be a significant factor. Thermal stress induced by respirator use in conjunction with impermeable clothing can affect the cardiovascular system (28–31).

Pulmonary effects have been well demonstrated (14,15,27,32). Although early studies emphasized the impact of effects on respiratory physiology, more recent studies have emphasized the ability to compensate for these physiologic loads (16–18). Inspiratory resistance is common, and expiratory resistance also occurs if exhalation valves are not provided. Dead space loading occurs because much of the air exhaled into the mask is rebreathed during the next breath; this imposes a carbon dioxide load (33–35). Furthermore, some atmosphere supplying respirators, particularly those that generate oxygen operating in a closed circuit mode, do not fully scrub the carbon dioxide and allow significant inhaled levels. Threshold loading, representing a pressure that must be generated to open a valve, is usually small but can become more significant if the valve system partially malfunctions in an SCBA or air purifying respirator.

Studies have demonstrated that respirator type loading decreases maximal exercise capability but has less physiologic impact at lower exercise levels. The respiratory pattern adapts to the loads imposed. Inspiratory resistance loading leads to prolongation of the inspiratory phase and a change in the duty cycle (inspiratory to total respiratory cycle time ratio). This decreases the peak pressure and peak ventilatory work rate, increasing tolerance (36).

Respiratory psychophysiology is affected. Some individuals have higher degrees of psychophysiologic sensitivity to resistance loading (36). Further, there is evidence of short-term adaptation of sensitivity, decreasing the awareness of such effects as respirator loading persists (37).

Overall, the direct ventilatory loading imposed by most modern respirators is tolerated by workers. In very marginal situations, the small additional load imposed by the respirator may interfere with ventilation. On the other hand, there is considerable evidence that the psychophysiologic aspects of respirator use, affecting the sensation of breathing, may be an important determinant of the effect of respirators and the ability to use them effectively.

For these reasons, reliance on tests of ventilatory function and mechanics may be misleading. The measurement of forced expiratory volume in 1 second ($FEV_1$) and similar spirometry parameters need not correlate very well with sensation-based pulmonary limitation. Spirometry, however, is an effective means of detecting individuals with moderate to severe respiratory disease that might interfere with respirator use or place the individual at greater risk of inhaled toxins. The maximal voluntary ventilation (MVV) has also historically been considered important (32,38,39). This test is predicated on the belief that ventilatory limitation is the critical limiting factor for respirator use, a finding that is not uniformly borne out in research studies.

There are other pulmonary considerations; although individuals with asthma may be particularly dependent on use of respirators when exposed to unexpected irritant atmospheres, it is not known whether such individuals are particularly prone to adverse effects either physiologically or psychophysiologically. Chronic productive coughs may also create problems for respirator users, as it is difficult to eliminate sputum when wearing a mask.

Some respirators impose significant musculoskeletal burdens. Certain SCBA types may weigh as much as 35 pounds and present problems to the individuals with back or knee problems. In addition, considerable agility is necessary to don certain respirator types that require over-the-shoulder straps. Therefore, persons with upper extremity impairments may not be able to don protective equipment sufficiently quickly in emergency situations. Furthermore, the decreased mobility induced by use of air-line respirators (necessitating a hose attachment) requires compensatory agility on the part of the user in many circumstances.

Respirators may affect vision. The face piece of full face mask respirators may fog. This may be partially averted by use of an inserted nose-mouth cup that diverts exhaled moist air from the face piece (40). In the past, contact lenses were considered to be contraindicated for respirator users. There were concerns that toxic materials might become concentrated beneath impermeable lenses. Since such hard lenses are rarely used now, this is less of a concern. However, individuals who are subject to dislodging of contact lenses may still be unable to use a respirator safely since they cannot safely remove the mask to readjust the lens. In such circumstances, special insert spectacles may be made available. OSHA technically does not allow contact lens use, so regulation and enforcement policies should be consulted.

Respirators can impede communication and may interfere with the ability to give verbal instructions, creating significant hazards in transportation and other applications. Special diaphragms or electronic communication devices may overcome this. Respirators also may impede receptive auditory function because some devices (e.g., sandblasters' hoods) create significant noise within the hood. Indeed, many workers may turn down air supply to limit the noise.

The skin at the sealing surface of the tight-fitting mask may be affected. Theoretically, individuals may be allergic to a component of the mask material. Sweating occurs at the sealing surface, and this may be irritating to certain individuals. It is held that pseudobarbae follicularis may prevent proper use in some individuals. The necessity to shave regularly is also viewed by some as burdensome. It is not necessary to remove all facial hair, only the hair that contacts the sealing surface of the respirator.

Respirators can have significant thermal effects on users. These include both physiologic and comfort effects (28–30,41,42). Heat loading is particularly important when the respirator is used in combination with impermeable clothing (such as in nuclear industry and hazardous waste work). The combined thermal stress can be significant (31). The respirator may also affect comfort significantly. The temperature and humidity of air striking the face has been shown to affect respiratory comfort. Particularly when there are concomitant thermal loads to the body and to the face, users may be adversely affected (28). Heat loading occurs because of rebreathing of exhaled heated air in many respirators; with oxygen-generating escape respirators, which depend on exothermic reactions, heat loading may be almost intolerable.

Nasal effects may be mediated by the thermal changes. In addition, pressure loading and resistance loading affect the normal switch from oral-nasal to oral breathing routes (43). Normal individuals switch from nasal to oral breathing at high exercise levels (44,45), and respirator users may be forced to do this at lower levels. This may bypass the "air conditioning" effect of nasal breathing and lead to subjective or perhaps physiologic impact in some individuals. Odors associated with the respirator may also be of subjective concern, although this has not been well studied.

There are concerns about cross-infection if the same device is used by different workers. Although optimally, each worker should be assigned a personal respirator when possible, this is not always feasible. Appropriate decontamination after each use can prevent cross-infection. Furthermore, respirators may be a potential source of biologic contamination if they are soiled from contagious sources (e.g., patients). Therefore, respirators that are soiled by body fluids should be decontaminated or disposed of as appropriate.

## MEDICAL EVALUATION FOR RESPIRATOR USE

Much has been written about medical evaluation (certification) for respirator use, but there is not an adequate consensus. Medical assessment occurs at three different settings:

(1) prior to respirator use,
(2) periodically during use, and
(3) for special causes in selected workers.

In the past, most emphasis has been given to routine testing of most or all users before use. This practice is predicated on the assumption that there are sufficiently predictive tests to determine who is likely to be unable to use the devices safely and effectively. In actuality, such test procedures have not yet been delineated. Indeed, respirator use is unique in occupational health because the actual outcome is difficult to measure in research settings (16). Furthermore, because the respirators may impose a wide variety of loads and the effect will differ significantly among different persons, it is not surprising that no simple test or test combination has been demonstrated to be adequately predictive.

A committee of experts (10) has recently reviewed the medical certification concerns and concluded that there should be decreased emphasis on preuse testing. In many settings, a questionnaire asking about respiratory and other health conditions, and in particular about prior use of respirators and tolerance thereof, may be the central component of preuse medical evaluation. In selected situations, such as IDLH use, hands-on medical examination by a physician or nurse practitioner may be helpful. Such clinical evaluation is needed when there are other major stressors or risks (the aging worker, concomitant cardiopulmonary or psychiatric disease, heat stress, or very high exertion levels). In these situations, many consider a limited exercise test to be warranted. However, if such a test is performed, its purpose should be carefully defined—Is it to be a sensitive test for cardiac disease or is it designed to determine ability to do the actual job?

In marginal cases, observation of the worker using the respirator in the workplace or during work simulation may be needed. This is the most job relevant test and is most likely to be consistent with the implications of the Americans with Disability Act.

Physicians performing medical certification—whether based on questionnaire or hands-on—must be personally responsible for each evaluation and should be available to answer questions about specific settings. Computer algorithms, generic rules, and simple algorithms cannot replace good clinical judgment. To adequately perform such evaluation, the physician must know the nature of the hazards, the type of respirator to be used, use frequency and duration, the presence of any concomitant stressor (e.g., heat), and the potential consequences of failure to adequately use respirator-based protection. Furthermore, the physician should be assured that a complete respiratory protection program is in place at the work site. In many circumstances, as discussed above, the overall program direction is not the physician's responsibility. Physicians should avoid accepting responsibility and liability by performing medical examinations if this inappropriately implies endorsement of the health and safety of the workplace.

Periodic evaluation of users is also advisable. On a regular basis, users should be assessed for both subjective and physiologic effect. Because of the limited predictive validity of preuse assessment, many feel that new users should be reassessed several months after use begins. Indeed, this may provide more information in many circumstances than the preplacement assessment. For regular users with prior experience, the periodicity should be determined based on the nature of the hazard, the risk of the patient, personal susceptibility, and resource availability. Periodic assessment may in many instances be limited to administration of a questionnaire.

Special examinations of selected users focus on individuals who have expressed difficulty with respirator use. Under such circumstances, more intensive assessment of the user is warranted. For example, observation of use at the work site or in a simulated work-site setting, and exercise testing using the respirator may be advisable. Careful assessment of psychological factors and workplace social influences affecting respirator use is also important. As is the case for all fitness for duty evaluations, such detailed evaluations should be done with a full understanding of the individual's medical condition as well as the work condition. The author has found it useful to explicitly ask for the patient's opinion.

Often, respirator medical evaluations are not performed in an isolated fashion, but may be integrated with other surveillance programs. When this is the case, data acquisition for the respirator program should be done in a manner compatible with data management for the remainder of the surveillance program.

The respirator medical certification and surveillance program should not substitute for careful assessment of the overall efficacy of workplace protection programs. Thus, simply meeting requirements for a respirator medical evaluation should not imply that additional agent specific medical assessments are unnecessary. For example, while chest radiography has no role in respirator evaluation per se, it may be the cornerstone of asbestos exposed worker assessment.

## RESPIRATORS FOR BIOAEROSOL PROTECTION—SPECIAL CONSIDERATIONS

Bioaerosols include living organisms or their products. The paradigm for respirator selection described earlier, which depends on the ratio of air concentration to acceptable concentration in the worker's in-mask breathing zone is often difficult to apply. For antigenic substances, such as those that induce occupational rhinitis and asthma due to animal antigens, extremely low doses may affect a sensitized worker. Furthermore, measurement of air concentrations is more difficult than for most radiologic and chemical agents. The effective dose for living organisms is also difficult to assess. Theoretically, a very small number of organisms may enter a worker and reproduce, leading to disease. The "minimal effective dose" therefore cannot be assessed in a manner comparable to determining acceptable workplace chemical exposure levels. However, limited laboratory studies (46) and theoretical models (47) provide insights. The risk of tuberculosis infection is related to the duration and magnitude of exposure, and therefore greater respiratory protection is needed when there are frequent exposures in a high-prevalence medical center or prison. Respiratory protection of health care workers is complicated by the frequency of unsuspected sources. Hence, administrative and training programs for the early suspicion and isolation of suspect cases must be central, and respiratory protection per se should play a vital, but secondary, role (48). Where there is a reasonable anticipated risk and engineering controls are infeasible as the sole method, personal respiratory protection should be used. The newer U.S. particulate respirator classification (84 CFR 1986) has made such devices financially feasible for health care and similar settings by decreasing the need for expensive high-efficiency particulate air (HEPA) devices.

## SUMMARY

Respirators may be an effective component of workplace protection (1,2,9–11,49). However, respirator use must be part of a complete respiratory protection program including program audit and exposure assessment. Inappropriate use of respirators can lead to a false sense of security and potential exposures.

## REFERENCES


1. *NIOSH respirator decision logic.* Publication 87-108. Washington, DC: U.S. Department of Health and Human Services, Public Health Service, Centers for Disease Control, National Institute for Occupational Safety and Health, Division of Standards Development and Technology Transfer, 1987.
2. Colton CE, Birkner LR, Brosseau LM. *Respiratory protection:* a manual and guideline, 2nd ed. Akron: American Industrial Hygiene Association, 1991.
3. Tanaka S, Tanaka M, Kimura K, Nozaki K, Seki Y. Breakthrough time of a respirator cartridge for carbon tetrachloride vapor flow of workers respiratory patterns. *Ind Health* 1996;34:227–236.
4. Dahlback GO, Novak L. Do pressure-demand breathing systems safeguard against inward leakage? *Am Ind Hyg Assoc J* 1983;44:336–340.
5. Nelson TJ. The assigned protection factor according to ANSI. *Am Ind Hyg Assoc J* 1996;57:735–740.
6. Johnston AR, Myers WR, Colton CE, Birkner JS, Campbell CE. Review of respiratory performance testing in the workplace: issues and Concerns. *Am Ind Hyg Assoc J* 1992;53:705–712.
7. Campbell DL, Noonan GP, Merinar TR, Stobbe JA. Estimated workplace protection factors for positive-pressure self-contained breathing apparatus. *Am Ind Hyg Assoc J* 1994;55:322–329.
8. Nelson TJ. The assigned protection factor of 10 for half-mask respirators. *Am Ind Hyg Assoc J* 1995;56:717–724.
9. Bollinger NJ, Shultz RH. *NIOSH guide to industrial respiratory protection.* Publication 87-116. Morgantown, WV: U.S. Department of Health, Education, and Welfare, Public Health Service, Centers for Disease Control, National Institute for Occupational Safety and Health, Division of Safety Research, U.S.G.P.O., 1987;1–112.
10. Harber P, Barnhart S, Boehlecke BA, et al. American thoracic society: respiratory protection guidelines. *Am J Respir Crit Care Med* 1996;154: 1153–1165.
11. American National Standard Institute. *American National Standard for respiratory protection.* ANSI, Z88.2 1992. New York: ANSI, 1992.
12. American Industrial Hygiene Association. *Odor thresholds for chemicals with established occupational health standards.* Akron: American Industrial Hygiene Association, 1989.
13. Hinds WC. *Aerosol technology. Properties, behavior, and measurements for airborne particles.* New York: Wiley, 1982.
14. Harber P. Medical evaluation for respiratory use. *J Occup Med* 1984;26:496–502.
15. Hodous TK. Screening prospective workers for the ability to use respirators. *J Occup Med* 1986;28:1074–1080.
16. Harber P, Brown C, Beck J. Respirator physiology research: answers in search of the question. *J Occup Med* 1991;33:38–44.
17. Hodous TK, Petesonk L, Boyles C, Hankinson J, Amandus H. Effects of added resistance to breathing during exercise in obstructive lung disease. *Am Rev Respir Dis* 1983;128:943–948.
18. Hodous TK, Boyles C, Hankinson JL. Effects of industrial respirator wear during exercise in subject with restrictive lung disease. *Am Ind Hyg Assoc J* 1986;47:176–180.
19. Raven PB, Davis TO, Shafer CL, Linnebur AC. Maximal Stress test performance while wearing a self-contained breathing apparatus. *J Occup Med* 1977;19:802–806.
20. Craig FN, Blevings WV, Cummings G. Exhausting work limited by external resistance and inhalation of carbon dioxide. *J Appl Physiol* 1970;29:847–851.
21. Stemler FW, Craig FN. Effects of respiratory equipment on endurance in hard work. *J Appl Physiol* 1977;42:28–32.
22. Morgan WP. Psychological problems associated with the wearing of industrial respirators: a review. *Am Ind Hyg Assoc J* 1983;44:671–677.
23. White MC, Baker EL, Larson MB, Wolford R. The role of personal beliefs and social influences as determinants of respirator use among construction painters. *Scand J Work Environ Health* 1988;14:239–245.
24. Nuutinen J, Terho EO, Husman K, Kotimaa M, Harkonen R, Nousiainen H. Protective value of powered dust respirator helmet for farmers with farmer's lung. *Eur J Respir Dis* 1987;152:212–220.
25. Aiba Y, Kobayashi K, Suzuki J, et al. A questionnaire survey on the use of dust respirators among lead workers in small scale companies. *Ind Health* 1995; 33:35–41.
26. Arborelius M. Dahlback GO, Data PG. Cardiac output and gas exchange during heavy exercise with a positive pressure respiratory protective apparatus. *Scand J Work Environ Health* 1983;9:471–477.
27. Louhevaara VA. Physiological effects associated with the use of respiratory protective devices: a review. *Scand J Work Environ Health* 1984; 10:275–281.
28. Nielsen R, Gwosdow AR, Berglund LG, DuBois AB. The effect of temperature and humidity levels in a protective mask on user acceptability during exercise. *Am Ind Hyg Assoc J* 1987;48:639–645.
29. DuBois AB, Harb ZF, Fox SH. Thermal discomfort of respiratory protective devices. *Am Ind Hyg Assoc J* 1990;51:550–554.
30. Babb T. Turner N, Saupe K, Pawelczyk J. Physical performance during combinations of hypercapnic resistive, and hot air breathing. *Am Ind Hyg Assoc J* 1989;50:105–111.
31. White MK, Vercruyssen M, Hodous TK. Work tolerance and subjective responses to wearing protective clothing and respirators during physical work. *Ergonomics* 1989;32:1111–1123.
32. Raven PB, Dodson AT, Davis TO. The physiological consequences of wearing industrial respirators: a review. *Am Ind Hyg Assoc J* 1979;40: 517–534.
33. Harber P, Shimozaki S, Barrett T, Loisides, Fine G. Effects of respirator dead space, inspiratory resistance and expiratory resistance ventilatory loads. *Am J Ind Med* 1989;16:189–198.
34. Bentley RA, Griffin OG, Love RG, Muir DC, Sweetland KF. Acceptable levels of the breathing resistance of respiratory apparatus. *Arch Environ Health* 1973;27:273–280.
35. Hermansen L, Vokac Z, Lereim P. Respiratory and circulatory response to added air flow resistance during exercise. *Ergonomics* 1972;15:15–24.
36. Shimozaki S, Harber P, Barrett T, Loisides P. Subjective tolerance of respirator loads and its relationship to physiological effects. *Am Ind Hyg Assoc J* 1988;49:108–116.
37. Epstein Y, Keren G, Lerman Y, Shefer A. Physiological and psychological adaptation to respiratory protective devices. *Aviat Space Environ Med* 1982;53:663–665.
38. Morgan WP, Raven PB. Prediction of distress for individuals wearing industrial respirators. *Am Ind Hyg Assoc J* 1985; 46:363–368.
39. Wilson JR, Raven PB. Clinical pulmonary function tests as predictors of work performance during respirator wear. *Am Ind Hyg Assoc J* 1989; 50:51–57.
40. Zelnick SD, McKay RT, Lockey JE. Visual field loss while wearing full-face respiratory protection. *Am Ind Hyg Assoc J* 1994;55:315–321.
41. Lind AR. The influence of inspired air temperature or tolerance to work in the heat. *Br J Ind Med* 1955;12:126–130.
42. James R, Rukes-Dobos F, Smith R. Effects of respirators under heat/work conditions. *Am Ind Hyg Assoc J* 1984;45:399–404.
43. Harber P, Beck J, Hsu P, Luo J. Nasal-oral flow partition with respirator use. *Am Rev Respir Dis* 1991;143:A104
44. Niinimaa V, Cole P, Mintz S, Shephard RJ. The switching point from nasal to oronasal breathing. *Resp Physiol* 1980;42:61–71.
45. Niinimaa V, Cole P, Mintz S, Shephard RJ. Oronasal distribution of respiratory airflow. *Resp Physiol* 1981;43:69–75.
46. Chen SK, Vesley D, Brosseau LM, Vincent JH. Evaluation of single-use masks and respirators for protection of health care workers against mycobacterial aerosols. *Am J Infect Control* 1994;22:65–74.
47. Nicas M. Refining a risk model for occupational tuberculosis transmission. *Am Ind Hyg Assoc J* 1996;57:16–22.
48. Blumberg HM, Watkins DL, Berschling JD, Antle A, Moore P, White N, Hunter M, Green B, Ray SM, McGowan JE Jr. Preventing the nosocomial transmission of tuberculosis. *Ann Intern Med* 1995;122: 658–663.
49. Boehlecke BA. Respirators. In: Harber P, Schenker MB, Balmes JR, eds. *Occupational and environmental respiratory disease.* St. Louis: Mosby-Year Book, 1996;963–971.

*Environmental and Occupational Medicine,*
*Third Edition,* edited by William N. Rom.
Lippincott–Raven Publishers, Philadelphia © 1998.

CHAPTER 134

# The Occupational Health Service

Jean Spencer Felton

## HISTORICAL BACKGROUND

Although certain discrete activities by physicians serving commerce and industry have been noted prior to the beginning of the 20th century, the formalization of a medical department in the industrial setting had its initiation in the early 1900s. Preventive medicine concerns for the worker had no enforcing mandates, and the few efforts at the provision of on-site health services could be traced to humanitarian employers. The passage of workers' compensation legislation in some of the states gave impetus to the development of medical programs at the work site.

The employment of persons with disabilities, women, and older workers during the industrial buildup before and during World War II, and the need for maximum utilization of the work force, swelled the number of health professionals in industry. Many practitioners of medicine, nursing, and industrial hygiene remained after the war in the growing medical departments to aid in their development of programs capable of preventing illness among workers exposed to, or in contact with, hazardous materials. As industry proclaimed its newfound social conscience in the late 1960s, it became apparent that there was a greater need for a progressive program support from the medical department, requiring more effort in employee counseling and in the understanding of worker behavior.

With the passage of the Occupational Safety and Health (OSH) Act in 1970, new legislation mandated full attention to the medical surveillance of employees potentially exposed to hazardous substances. The act required that any standard established under the law "shall prescribe the type and frequency of medical examinations or other tests which shall be made available ... to employees exposed to ... hazards in order to most effectively determine whether the health of such employees is adversely affected by such exposure" (1). With the passage of the Rehabilitation Act of 1973, which made the hiring of "handicapped" workers obligatory for the federal government and its contractors, medical departments in industry found they had new functional charges and different, considerably more pro-worker responsibilities. More recently, in-plant health services have had to meet new challenges brought on by a fluctuating economy, a changing international balance, mergers of large corporations, the downsizing of long-established companies, telecommuting of workers, and a continuing transfer abroad of goods manufacture and assembly. The enactment of the Family and Medical Leave Act of 1993 added responsibilities to the Occupational Health Service (OHS) in the form of medical certification of illness and the determination of the severity of health conditions.

Long after a medical activity in a company became relatively commonplace came the realization that there were other sites of productive human activity besides the industrial plant, and that there were groups of employees seeking medical oversight who were not located in the prototypical large installation, turning out marketable goods and services for consumption throughout the world. New to the concept of occupational medicine were workers in agriculture, education, the armed services, research, business, and even homemaking and the health professions. In keeping with this increased horizontal coverage, industrial medicine rightfully became occupa-

J. S. Felton: Department of Medicine, University of California, Irvine; and Department of Preventive Medicine, University of Southern California, Los Angeles, Mendocino, California 95460.

tional medicine, and the older medical department in industry became the Occupational Health Service, implying a move from care for employment-generated injury to the preservation of the worker's health. Because of the difficulty of separating the area of one's work environment from that of one's home or community, concerned professional societies and monograph authors have viewed this particular medical arena as Occupational and Environmental Medicine, the title aptly given this present work.

An OHS is an organizational unit of a commercial, industrial, or hospital enterprise whose activities are targeted toward the appraisal, maintenance, restoration, or improvement of the health of the worker, his or her productivity, and his or her fulfilling interaction with work and living communities, seen as a positive psychic reward from the labor and an enhanced quality of life. Whereas representatives of the various disciplines who compose the department's staff may function toward one particular facet of the overall goal, the total effort of all members should be seen in an increase in the health, well-being, and sense of self-worth of every employee who has contact with the professional OH team.

## OBJECTIVES

The objectives of an OHS are the following:

1. To protect the health and well-being of workers against the stressors and potential health hazards of the work environment.
2. To place job applicants or current employees in work commensurate with their physical and emotional capacities, work that can be performed without endangering the worker or fellow employees and without damaging property.
3. To provide emergency medical care for injured or ill workers and definitive care and rehabilitation for those with work-generated injuries or illnesses, in keeping with the medical, surgical, or psychotherapeutic expertise of the staff, medical department policy, managerial policy, and the availability of community resources.
4. To maintain or improve the health of the worker through promotional, educational, counseling, or informational activities, preventive health measures including fitness or wellness programs, and periodic clinical reviews of health status.

## POSITION IN ORGANIZATION

In many industrial plants the OHS may be placed in an organizational position that limits its usefulness, as within the department of safety or risk management, or employee relations (human resources). Whenever the OHS is organizationally distant from the manager's office, it is not likely to be consulted on the possible hazards of new products or new work processes. Its needs may be attenuated, misinterpreted, or even countered by intervening officials who may poorly understand the functions of an OHS.

Ideally, the department should be placed organizationally as close to the head of the installation as possible, whether president, plant manager, or division chief. Such proximity avoids the multiplication of layers between the medical arm and the person who establishes policy, either alone or with the approval of the board of directors.

Of second choice is the placement of the OHS so that the director reports to the chief executive officer (CEO). The advantage in this position is that the CEO is usually more accessible than the president.

The third choice is industrial relations, which is probably the situation in the majority of companies in the United States. A wise and discerning head will take pride in the OHS and will do everything within his or her authority to support and advance the programs proffered by the medical unit. One unfortunate factor is at play here. Most heads of industrial relations or human resources hold Master of Business Administration (MBA) degrees, having completed a curriculum lacking in any inclusion of OH principles. The graduate, on assumption of departmental duties, has responsibility for a function—the OHS—for which there has been no preparation and, absent any understanding of industry's health needs, may negate much of what an active OHS is likely to offer.[1]

## STAFF RESOURCES

Many disciplines are represented on the OH team (Table 1). It is this group that works collectively to bring substance to the objectives listed previously. The National Institute for Occupational Safety and Health (NIOSH) Educational Resource Centers train as a team the specialists in occupational medicine, industrial hygiene, occupational health nursing, and safety.

A medical facility has its own pyramidal hierarchy, in that at the top there is a corporate medical director (CMD) who must assume responsibility for what is done by subordinates. Reporting to the CMD are directors of nursing and industrial hygiene, and in a few instances, the director of safety.

[1]There has been some curricular change. The Management Institute for Environment and Business (MEB) has been working with business schools across the United States and more recently in Latin America to develop materials and programs for integrating environmental issues into business school education. Some 25 such schools have committed resources and class time to addressing environmental factors in business through MEB's leadership program. The efforts have resulted in the integration of the environment into exciting classes, the creation of new classes and the establishment of internships dedicated to environmental management issues (125).

**TABLE 1.** *Personnel of occupational health service*

| |
|---|
| Physicians[a] |
| Corporate medical director |
| Plant or regional medical director |
| Occupational medical specialist |
| Staff physician |
| Nurses[b] |
| Occupational health nurse |
| Nurse practitioner |
| Professional nurse |
| Licensed vocational nurse |
| Industrial hygienists[c] |
| Certified industrial hygienist |
| Industrial hygienist |
| Industrial hygiene engineer |
| Industrial hygiene chemist |
| Industrial hygiene technologist |
| Clerical and other support staff |
| Ambulance driver |
| Maintenance personnel |
| Receptionist |
| Records clerks and computer operators |
| Secretaries |
| Workers' compensation clerks |
| Other professionals |
| Administrator |
| Biostatistician |
| Clinical psychologist |
| Environmentalist |
| Epidemiologist |
| Health educator |
| Medical records administrator |
| Optician |
| Optometrist |
| Pharmacist |
| Physical therapist |
| Sanitarian |
| Toxicologist |
| Technical staff members |
| Clinical laboratory technologist |
| Emergency medical technician |
| Physical therapy technologist |
| Radiology technologist |

[a]A physician at any level may be certified by the American Board of Preventive Medicine in the subspecialty of occupational medicine.

[b]All but the licensed vocational nurse may be certified by the American Board for Occupational Health Nurses.

[c]All but the industrial hygiene technologist may be certified by the American Board of Industrial Hygiene.

The OH team concept is threaded through every undertaking in the delivery of services. The physician and the nurse plan programs together; the industrial hygienist may obtain work histories; and the medical director and the health educator outline employee orientation efforts for the year ahead. With the possible exception of rehabilitation, OH is the one arena of professional exercise where combined energies are needed for solidarity in programming.

Particularly necessary is parallelism in the efforts of the clinician and the industrial hygienist because of the interaction between the worker and the work environment. The health appraisal and the environmental evaluation must mesh for an understanding of the effects, good or bad, of occupational exposure to toxicants on the employee. A change in physiologic response or an anatomic alteration indicates something awry in the workplace, and for accurate formulation of the diagnosis of a possible occupational illness, measurements are needed for workroom air or energy levels. Similarly, if excessive quantities of toxic materials are encountered in the air of the work site, effects should be sought in the exposed employee by means of clinical and laboratory investigation. To neglect one or the other, or to have a failure of communication between the two disciplines, does a great disservice to the workers at risk.[2]

## PROGRAM ELEMENTS

Services can be divided into the following categories: evaluative/preventive, therapeutic, rehabilitative, administrative, research, and others as determined by extent of facilities and locale. In another scheme, program elements or services can be divided into those offered employment applicants, well employees, and ill or injured employees. A combination of the two systems appears in Tables 2 and 3.

Complete documentation of the work history, particularly as it relates to possible past toxicant exposure, an accurate estimate of the current body burden of any hazardous substance(s), and a good evaluation of present health status should all be accomplished to establish a reliable baseline for future comparison.

A word of caution: any injury attendant upon the preplacement examination or incurred subsequent to initial immunization is considered identical to an occupational injury with employer liability, even though the applicant's employment contract may still be incomplete, pending results from the medical examination, all in keeping with the boundaries established by the Americans with Disabilities Act of 1990 (ADA).

The essence of Table 2 is the true preventive medical segment of an OH program. The periodic examination may bring to light long-standing congenital or anomalous changes that during the employment procedure were accepted without a question of relationship to job performance skills. Referral for surgical reconstruction or rehabilitation can be accomplished at this time, an action appreciated by most employees.

[2]An excellent example of cross-disciplinary cooperation has been related in a joint study of a dozen workers complaining of job-related dermatitis. Described is an excellent combined effort by industrial hygienists and extramural physicians to define the etiology of the dermatomes (126).

**TABLE 2.** *Occupational health service program for well employees*

| |
|---|
| Evaluative and preventive services |
| Initial and interval health and work histories |
| Initial and periodic medical examination |
| Determination of health status classification |
| Health education activities, including wellness or fitness programs |
| Environmental surveillance |
| Plant sanitation |
| First-aid training |
| Immunization procedures |
| Diagnostic laboratory procedures, including measure of use of controlled substances |
| Fitting, issue, and testing of personal protective devices |
| Treatment services |
| Emergency treatment of untoward reaction to venipuncture or other examination procedure |
| Emergency treatment of untoward reaction to immunizing injection |
| Rehabilitative services |
| Referral for correction of impairment that precludes or limits work performance |
| Reasonable accommodation of applicant or employee with a disability |
| Administrative services |
| Recommendations to human resources department regarding placement |
| Initiation and maintenance of health record, either by manual or computer method, to include previous medical records, if available |
| Entry into statistical record of examinations and procedures completed, resultant findings, and changes in health classification status |
| Entry into statistical record of health education activities (single or group), wellness-program efforts, environmental surveillance procedures, and pertinent sanitation reviews |
| Entry into statistical record of number and kind of employees completing first-aid, cardiopulmonary resuscitation or Heimlich maneuver training |
| Maintenance, review, and recording of results of bioassays conducted on employees at hazard contact risk |
| Maintenance of supplies for examinations, surveillance, training, health education, administration, and first-aid and antidote cabinets |
| Research services |
| Conduct of research projects involving study of current employees either in conjunction with university personnel or as individual departmental activity |
| Other services |
| Provision of educational field experience for graduate students involving work with current employees |
| Provision of orientation program for new employees descriptive of services offered by the OHS |
| Conduct of "right-to-know" sessions and such other specific informative conferences as mandated by federal, state, or local law |

Although OM is primarily preventive and its practitioners interventionists, it must be recognized that heavy industry offers a critical environment where harm may ensue through mechanical failure or workers' inattention to accepted protocol. Accidents do occur, and they produce injuries. Each medical service must be prepared to provide emergency treatment, and the extent of care given will be in keeping with the factors indicated earlier. It may be that all injured workers will be prepared for transport to community specialists, and only those workers with minor burns, contusions, or lacerations will be seen intramurally. The skills needed by the staff will be dictated by the kind of illnesses or injuries seen most frequently.

## HEALTH EXAMINATIONS

An extensive study conducted in Canada concluded that the annual health examination had insufficient rationale to warrant its continued exercise (2). It was recommended that a periodic review be substituted and that certain toxicant exposures be listed,[3] in a sense, recommending periodic examinations in some work situations. A comparable but more recent Australian review of the screening of asymptomatic persons indicated no specific examinations based on job-related exposure. However, it was stated that in persons presenting with a history of

[3]Examples of the conditions reviewed by the task force as leaving sufficient scientific evidence to warrant periodic examination are smoking—workers in asbestos, silica, uranium, coal, and grain industries; cancer of the bladder—workers exposed to bladder carcinogens and smokers; cancer of the skin—outdoor workers and those in contact with polycyclic aromatic hydrocarbons; and tuberculosis—persons exposed to the disease through their work (2). In the most recent updating of the study (127) occupational exposure is either down-played or omitted as an indication for inclusion of a procedure in the periodic health examination. Screening for bladder cancer, as an example, is indicated in a footnote: "High-risk groups are males >60 years of age who smoke or have smoked, and were employed in a trade that may have exposed them to aromatic amines" (p. 836). In the discussion of intervention against lung cancer, no mention is made of fibrogenic pulmonary or pleural disease, or its human and financial costs when found in a worker.

**TABLE 3.** *Occupational health service program for ill or injured employees*

- Evaluative and preventive services
  - Determination and recording of altered baseline data, such as vision screening in eye-injured employees or pulmonary function evaluation in employees subjected to inhalation of toxic vapors, fumes, mists, etc.
  - Evaluation of extent of illness or injury for the determination of disposition
  - Determination of preventive measures to be taken to preclude repetition of injury-producing accident
- Treatment services
  - Emergency or definitive medical care for occupational illness
  - Emergency or definitive medical care for occupational injury
  - Emergency medical care for nonoccupational illness
  - Emergency medical care for nonoccupational injury
  - Ambulance transportation
  - Referral to local sources of specialty care or consultation
  - Counseling for acute emotional disorder
  - Counseling for substance abuse
  - Short-term counseling and referral for treatment of chronic illness states or impairment caused by illness or injury residue
  - Interviews with illness- or injury-absence recidivists
  - Physical therapy for injured employees
- Rehabilitative services
  - Referral for surgical correction of disabling congenital anomaly
  - Referral to community sources of care for substance abuse, in conjunction with supportive in-plant counseling
  - Referral to local sources of care or consultation in anaplastology, low vision devices, orthotics, reconstructive surgery, prosthetics, self-help devices, or sensory aids
  - Communication with or referral to, ostomy groups, lost-chord groups, voluntary health agencies, rehabilitation nurses, other self-help groups, or sources of home health care
  - Referral for training in independent living
  - Referral for social casework therapy
  - Referral for speech therapy
  - Debriefing of employees returning form foreign service
- Administrative services
  - Maintenance of health records by manual or computer method
  - Preparation and forwarding of first reports of injury or other workers' compensation or accident reports, and subsequent reports of progress or closure
  - Entry into statistical record of illnesses or injuries treated, with associated diagnoses and identifying variables
  - Entry into statistical record of illnesses or injuries resulting in absence from work, with duration of absences, diagnoses, and identifying variables
  - Maintenance of mandated OSHA or state report forms of occupationally incurred injuries or illnesses
  - Maintenance of statistical record of deaths of employees by diagnosis and identifying variables, for later epidemiologic review
  - Clinical photography of injury lesions, when indicated, at first visit, at intervals, and at time of discharge as "well"
  - Maintenance of supplies for patient treatment
  - Notification of local health authority of animal bites sustained by employees or of a diagnosis of a reportable disease
  - Notification of plant executive, local authorities, and next of kin in the event of death of an employee at the work site or en route for care
- Research services
  - Research projects involving special studies of employees with occupational illnesses or injuries
- Other services
  - Consultation with managerial personnel regarding problems in group morale, lowered productivity, disaffection, anger, increased turnover, harassment, etc.
  - Consultation with supervisors regarding absence control efforts for individual workers
  - Educational field experience for graduate students involving work with ill or injured employees

**TABLE 4.** *Variety of periodic medical examinations performed in the occupational health service*

| |
|---|
| Mandatory examinations, complete |
| Preplacement medical examination |
| Periodic medical examination, general |
| Periodic medical examination, specific |
| Hazardous exposure, asbestos |
| Hazardous exposure, ionizing radiation |
| Hazardous exposure, lead |
| Hazardous exposure, mercury |
| Hazardous exposure, other |
| Promotion medical examination |
| Foreign travel or assignment, examination prior to |
| Return-to-work examination, postinjury |
| Return-to-work examination, postillness |
| Motor vehicle operator examination |
| Locomotive engineer examination |
| Physical fitness examination, determination of |
| Disability retirement examination |
| Flight personnel examination |
| Job transfer examination |
| Mandatory examinations, partial |
| Placement, subsequent to |
| Crane operation vision test |
| Hazardous exposure, noise—audiometry |
| Microwave exposure—slit-lamp examination |
| Courtesy examinations |
| Camp counseling, prior to |
| Teaching, extramural, prior to |
| Disability insurance, report for |

chemical exposure, the investigation was best covered by OH and safety services (3). British writers concerned with the fitness for work indicate that periodic review of individual health may be undertaken in some circumstances and will relate to specific requirements, for example, regular assessment of visual acuity in some jobs (4).

The kinds of medical examinations carried out in an OHS may vary, but Table 4 shows the spectrum of periodic evaluations that is possible, and in some settings obligatory. Certain of the examinations are performed as a courtesy; the service is offered to reduce time off work.

## PREPLACEMENT MEDICAL EXAMINATION

The content of the preplacement examination varies, but the history obtained as part of the process should offer a complete chronology of past work performed. The health history can be the traditional type, but if ill health can be correlated with certain work activities, the issue should be pursued in detail.

Formerly, certain radiographic examinations—of the chest, old fracture sites, and the lumbosacral spine—were performed on nearly every applicant for physically demanding jobs and on many other applicants for lighter work, but the custom diminished remarkably because of the exposure to ionizing radiation that such studies entail (5). Although some employers still believe that spine radiographs serve as predictors of serious back injuries, current opinion leans toward the belief that the defects discovered are not etiologically related to the soft tissue injuries of the back presented by workers (6). A cautionary note is in order regarding chest radiography. Although tuberculosis until recent years has been considered a conquered disease, there has been a recrudescence of much pulmonary infection with the influx of refugees in the United States, particularly from Southeast Asia (7,8). It is wise to obtain chest radiographs on all such persons seeking employment, a group readily classified as a "selected population shown to have a significant yield of previously undiagnosed disease" (9).

The clinical laboratory test procedures that are included will be determined by their cost, the desire for as complete a health status baseline as possible, and the need for the evidence such tests would offer of the health of target organs that possibly were challenged or assaulted in previous employment. A bioassay to determine body burdens of retained hazardous substances is a valuable measurement for note at the time of contact with a worker's first known toxicant whose effect is cumulative.

Many job aspirants have noted the preplacement protocol to be the most complete examination they have ever experienced, and they deserve a full translation in understandable language of the findings of both the physical investigation and the various laboratory studies. Health counseling should be carried out where deficits have been identified and, if the applicant agrees, a report of the results should be forwarded to the individual's family physician. Certain positions, particularly assignments in law enforcement and firefighting, may require testing maximal physical strength and endurance and cardiovascular stress testing as part of the preplacement examination (10). The objective is to discover asymptomatic coronary artery disease or dysrhythmias that might place the incumbent in severe physical jeopardy at the time of great physical or functional demand.

Applicants displaying borderline findings—minimal hypertension, moderate hyperlipidemia, overweight, or evidence of a high cardiac risk profile—should be counseled in precautionary corrective measures.

With the increased acceptance of persons with disabilities, more work applicants are seen who have compensated deficits, postillness or postinjury residua, or static impairments that require "reasonable accommodation" according to law.[4] Such candidates should be

[4]*Reasonable accommodation*, in general, is the effort made by the employer who is a recipient of federal funds in any form to accommodate the person with a disability through the provision of accessible facilities, job restructuring, modified work schedules, special devices, provision of readers, etc. See *Federal Register* 42822680, Section 84.12, 1977, Reasonable Accommodation (regulations to section 504 of the Rehabilitation Act of 1973 and the Americans with Disabilities Act of 1990 (ADA).

interviewed at some length to determine their need for special parking, ingress to the work site, rapid egress in case of emergency, and particular requirements that may be dictated by blindness, hearing deficit, wheelchair use, and the like. Baseline clinical photographs in color are desirable in cases of amputation, arthritic joint changes, burn scars or keloids, and areas of pigmentation or depigmentation, for example, so that in the event of injury, comparisons can be made. If the referral of such an employee has come from a rehabilitation agency, contact should be maintained with the counselor concerned, so that the success attained on the job will become known.

An applicant will be classified on completion of the examination in accordance with a commonly employed scheme:

Health status 1 implies that the person presents no detectable defect that would limit performance in any position and that there are no anatomic or physiologic variations of any consequence.

Health status 2 indicates that, on examination, changes were detected that warranted notation but did not limit current, and probably not future, performance of the assigned tasks. Such findings might include a deviated nasal septum, a functional heart murmur, hypertrophied tonsils, a single varix, or an old healed burn scar.

Health status 3 informs the individual, the OHS, and the human resources department that the candidate can perform the job being sought but cannot be asked to undertake certain tasks such as climbing high ladders, operating motorized equipment, working a rotating shift, working where acute vision is required, and the like.

Health status 4 designates the applicant as medically unfit for any position because of a severe disorder (e.g., generalized, acute, untreated rheumatoid arthritis, a terminal malignant growth, or diabetic gangrene of a lower extremity).

Health status 5 is the classification given a person who is acutely ill or has an upper respiratory infection with fever, acute specific urethritis, or some clinical disorder that, with treatment, will clear and allow reexamination and placement within a few days.

A candidate's acceptance may be deferred for a period while hypertension is brought under clinical control, a hernia is repaired, or an acute ingrown toenail is treated. Such action does not imply disability but means that a readily remediable condition has been found that should be regulated, treated, or corrected before the applicant begins work.

The same classification can be used for periodic examinations, and if, because of aging or other intervening circumstances, there should be a change from one health status class to another, such action should be taken. The OHS should assist management, so that a change of this type will not jeopardize the individual's job.

## PERIODIC GENERAL MEDICAL EXAMINATIONS

Such examinations are conducted on persons who are not necessarily at risk, apart from contact with stressors that accompany performance in any job. Executives may be examined annually or biennially in the OHS or they may be referred to certain reputable centers that offer this service.

## PERIODIC SPECIFIC MEDICAL EXAMINATIONS

This type of examination involves a large segment of the medical surveillance of workers exposed to certain hazardous substances. Special attention is given those target organs or organ systems that may potentially exhibit the untoward effects of the absorption, ingestion, or inhalation of noxious substances. Further, the examiner seeks out possible effects from exposure to various forms of energy with which the worker is identified in his or her job.

The "specific" periodic examination is conducted on persons who may have occupational contact with asbestos, mercury, lead, a known carcinogen, or any other element or compound for which tissue change or excessive exposure has been recorded. Guidelines are provided by two sources: The standards promulgated by the U.S. Department of Labor and the criteria documents published by NIOSH of the U.S. Department of Health and Human Services.

As an example of the specificity called for in the periodic assay of a worker, the following procedures comprise, in part, both the interval history to be obtained and the periodic examination to be conducted on an employee exposed to vinyl chloride (11).

### Medical Surveillance

A program of medical surveillance shall be instituted for each employee exposed, without regard to the use of respirators, to vinyl chloride in excess of the action level.

1. At the time of initial assignment or upon institution of medical surveillance:
   a. A general physical examination shall be performed, with specific attention to detecting enlargement of the liver, spleen or kidneys, or dysfunction in these organs and for abnormalities in skin, connective tissues and the pulmonary system

b. A medical history shall be taken, including the following topics:
   (1) Alcohol intake
   (2) Past history of hepatitis
   (3) Work history and past exposure to potential hepatotoxic agents, including drugs and chemicals
   (4) Past history of blood transfusions
   (5) Past history of hospitalizations
c. A serum specimen shall be obtained and determinations made of the following:
   (1) Total bilirubin
   (2) Alkaline phosphatase
   (3) Serum glutamate oxalacetic transaminase (SGOT)
   (4) Serum glutamate pyruvic transaminase (SGPT)
   (5) Gamma glutamyl transpeptidase.

2. Examinations provided in accordance with this paragraph shall be performed at least
   a. Every 6 months for each employee who has been employed in vinyl chloride or polyvinyl chloride manufacturing for 10 years or longer
   b. Annually for all other employees.
3. Each employee exposed to an emergency shall be afforded appropriate medical surveillance.
4. A statement of each employee's suitability for continued exposure to vinyl chloride, including use of protective equipment and respirators, shall be obtained from the examining physician promptly after each examination. A copy of the physician's statement shall be provided each employee.
5. If any employee's health would be materially impaired by continuous exposure, each employee shall be withdrawn from possible contact with vinyl chloride.
6. Laboratory analyses for all biologic specimens included in medical examinations shall be performed in laboratories licensed under 42 CFR Part 74.

A less detailed guide for periodic appraisal is the criteria document for beryllium (12). It is not feasible to include all the advised examination procedures—physical, hematologic, biochemical, and the like—for every work substance potentially productive of unwanted biologic effects. Such consolidated bodies of knowledge have been compiled and are commercially available. Each work material will have its own unique effects when constant exposure exceeds the threshold limit value as determined by research and clinical observation. OHSs must have available for staff use, in writing, preferably in a manual, the following desiderata: (1) the type of examination (complete or partial, general, or specific); (2) the interval history items to be reviewed; (3) the periodicity; (4) the organ system or organs to be given special scrutiny; (5) the hematologic, urine, biochemical, fecal, radiographic, cytologic, or breath analytic procedures to be completed; (6) acceptable levels for each test result; (7) the interval between a test productive of an abnormal level and the repetition of the test; (8) the time of specimen collection (e.g., at the end of the workweek, before the beginning of the shift, after a weekend, after a shower); (9) the personnel to be notified in the event of persistently abnormal findings, such as industrial hygienist, worker, supervisor, safety director, department head, plant manager; and (10) other action to be taken (e.g., removal from job assignment, closure of operation, conduct of more sophisticated laboratory analyses, or examination of co-workers).

The question that arises in the event of abnormal findings of any type, physical or analytic, is how quickly the worker must be removed from contact with the toxicant. In the case of new pneumoconiotic findings, where there is a long period of latency between first exposure and clinical evidence of absorption or change, there need be no emergency removal from the work source, but clearly the work site must be evaluated and the workers protected. If, however, the worker is in contact with a noxious material that is producing evidence of intoxication for the first time and if a repeat test confirms the abnormal finding, the incumbent should be assigned to other work until the job is studied and the cause of overexposure is identified.

Rarely should action be taken on the basis of only a single test result. Many variables may give a false-positive finding, and reporting such a result without confirmation creates unwarranted anxiety. One recalls a serodiagnostic test for syphilis that was returned as strongly positive on an employee and the subsequent apprehension, anger, and distress resulting when the finding was reported before reversal was established through more sophisticated analytic methods. If the employee manifests evidence of one or more other disease processes that may influence or cause synergistic interaction with the work-generated clinical change, special study is indicated, preferably in consultation with the worker's private physician.

**Physical Fitness Examinations**

A physical fitness examination is usually requested by a department head because of observed changes in the worker's performance, excessive absence for illness, personality or behavioral change, repeated injury, or any altered work habit that may have a medical basis. As in the conduct of the preplacement examination, the physician determines if the incumbent is physically or emotionally fit to carry out the tasks called for in his or her job description. The medical conclusion is added to other evidence obtained by the department head, such as attendance records, production levels, or previous performance evaluations, and administrative action taken. The examiner or the medical director usually states only, in his or her opinion, the incumbent is fit or unfit to perform the expected duties. The examiner may, however, recommend illness-related action. Frequently the examiner meets informally with the department head before a report or a recommendation is submitted. The worker may request that his or her representative be present at all deliberations; a worker representative should not be present during the actual examining process, which is a physician-worker relationship.

### Mandatory Partial Examinations

Certain work exposures indicate periodic partial examinations only, for complete clinical reviews are unnecessary. Crane operators require visual acuity determinations, workers in noisy environments require audiometry, and certain workers in dyestuff manufacturing require cytologic examination of urine sediment. A single procedure, in the hands of a skilled examiner or specialist, provides greater protection than a complete medical examination performed by a dispirited practitioner in a desultory, uncaring manner merely to meet the obligations of an examination schedule.

## COUNSELING PROGRAM

An OHS must be prepared to assist management in the recognition of employees with work difficulties and in the method of referral to the medical arm of the company. Not only should the physicians and nurses be skilled in identifying behavioral problems, but they should also be able to offer affected employees reassurance and supportive counseling.

As determined by a needs assessment, mental health specialists can be added to the staff on a full-time or part-time basis to provide short-term assistance to troubled workers. Special skill may be needed to uncover a problem from its concealment or discoloration by supervisory prejudice, supposedly rational explanations, or protective shielding. In counseling, it is important that one know the work scene and production patterns and expectations, so that there is acceptance of the counselor by the employee in a situation that already is tenuous because of the nature of the difficulty, and the disinclination of most workers to concede deficits in themselves.

Mental health programs should not be limited exclusively to a one-to-one counselor-patient operation, but should include other activities, such as helping managers understand human problems, helping supervisors relate to workers, and holding group sessions in stress management (13). This form of outreach can stop many problems before they require medical or counseling attention, because it helps an enlightened managerial body interact more effectively with its staff.

While many professionals in OM believe that the counseling function should be an inherent program element in OH (14), most counseling efforts are carried out in industry through employee assistance programs (EAPs) that are usually staffed by professionally trained clinical psychologists or social workers (15). In some instances, when the emphasis is on alcohol or substance abuse, the counselors may be recovering or recovered alcoholics or drug abusers whose personal experience enhances their effectiveness as counselors. Personal problems in behavior, family dysfunction, disagreements with supervisors, or even troubles with budgets may be brought to the EAP for reevaluation. Complete confidentiality is maintained, and, if indicated, referral to appropriate community sources of continuing care may be made.

The EAP may be located on-site in the organization, or it may be a facility in the community supported by several companies or a free-standing mental health care agency accepting referrals from multiple sources.

## ADMINISTRATION

The OHS in business and industry is an organizational unit like any other department or division, and must assume responsibility for a great number of functions that are not clinical. The proper exercise of these functions permits not only smooth and efficient delivery of day-to-day services but also an effective response to emergent needs. No specific program for OH administrators has been developed, so that those persons who serve in this capacity have moved either from hospital administration or business management. Many OHSs are not of sufficient size to warrant such a position, so that the medical director assumes this managerial role as is done in many academic clinical departments. Administration of an OHS includes many activities, and all will be discussed briefly.

### Budget Development

A budget must be prepared annually to cover the business year cycled by the company, such as fiscal year, calendar year, or federal fiscal year. Certain categories are traditional, and although the headings may vary from organization to organization, the required expenditures can be subsumed under some commonly understood designations (Table 5).

Many companies, in anticipation of growth by virtue of new markets, new technology (e.g., the electronics industry), new products, expansion, merger or acquisition, or even downsizing, may request a 2-, 3-, or 5-year plan with a supportive budget. Difficult though it is to forecast needs many years in advance, particularly in light of the yet-to-be-determined relationship of OM to managed care, one's surmise, always optimistic, will probably

**TABLE 5.** *Categories of expenditure for budget development*

- I. Labor
  - A. Salaries
    - 1. Professional, consultant, paramedical, support staff
    - 2. Plan for merit increases or reclassification
  - B. Benefits
    - 1. Social Security or special retirement fund payments
    - 2. Unemployment and disability insurance taxes
    - 3. Group life, hospitalization, and medical care insurance
    - 4. Uniforms and laundry service
    - 5. Meals (if furnished)
    - 6. Moving expenses (if authorized)
- II. Materials
  - A. Capital equipment
  - B. Depreciation of equipment
    - 1. Maintenance (instrument calibration) service
    - 2. Repairs
  - C. Office supplies, expendable
  - D. Medical supplies, expendable
  - E. Industrial hygiene supplies, expendable
  - F. Printing—forms, health educational materials, etc.
  - G. Video, film, CD-Rom rental or purchase for staff development and health education program
  - H. Personal protective devices for staff members (field use)
- III. Overhead
  - A. Rent, electricity, heat, air conditioning, gas, water, ventilation
  - B. Telecommunications, postage, freight
  - C. Fire, theft, professional liability insurance
  - D. Building repair, maintenance, alterations
  - E. Custodial service
  - F. Data-processing time charge (only if dependent upon a mainframe computer
  - G. Diagnostic, therapeutic, industrial hygiene instrument maintenance
  - H. Staff vacancy advertising
  - I. Record storage
- IV. Medical care
  - A. Special extramural examinations
  - B. Special immunization interpretation service
  - C. Extramural radiographic interpretation service
  - D. Blood Bank
  - E. Patient transportation
  - F. Optical dispensing (departmental charge back)
- V. Contingency fund
  - A. Petty cash for emergency purchases
  - B. Meals for official visitors
  - C. Gifts, if appropriate
- VI. Staff development
  - A. Continuing professional education
    - 1. Travel and lodging (conferences)
    - 2. Course tuition or fee, conference registration
    - 3. Professional books and journal subscriptions
    - 4. Materials for professional presentations—artwork, slides, exhibits, posters, etc.
    - 5. Honoraria to invited speakers at staff meetings
  - B. Professional society memberships
  - C. Staff retreats
  - D. Overtime, when required
- VII. Research
  - A. Personnel
  - B. Supplies

make good sense as additional program elements will be expected. Future projections are rendered somewhat intangible by virtue of the conversion of the United States from a manufacturing to a service and information economy, but new legislation, new toxicity evaluations, and new public mandates will demand broader clinical and laboratory examinations.

### Physical Plant

An OHS receives considerable use, particularly in heavy industry where workers wear clothing and boots heavy with occupational material soil. The dirt, oil, grease, and dust from the clothing and exposed skin surfaces are transferred to the furniture, the equipment, and the walls. Frequent cleaning and repair are needed. Ideally, tiled walls, stainless steel work surfaces, and mottled, dark flooring materials allow the best wear.

### Disaster Planning

There is a strong medical component in every disaster plan, because severe injuries can be sustained following earthquakes, floods, fires, explosions, volcanic eruptions, or toxic chemical releases.

A plan involves provision of emergency medical care facilities at points away from the primary OHS, since that particular installation may be rendered useless. The medical director should develop the plan jointly with the security or safety director or the person directly responsible for disaster planning, to coordinate all efforts, to establish a list of available personnel, and to establish lines of authority. Reciprocal arrangements for medical facility use can be made with adjacent plants, unless the neighboring installation has great fears of industrial espionage. Those organizations having substances in use or on stream that are unique in their biologic effect, such as hydrofluoric acid (16), should have specific antidotal or treatment supplies available at multiple sites where they can be checked at established intervals.[5]

### Manuals

Every OHS should have a policy and procedure manual in which directives for all aspects of the program may be found. A loose-leaf compendium of this type includes not only the objectives and functions of the department but also a description of all responsible positions and sections, program elements, record forms,

[5]For additional information concerning medical preparedness see ref. 128.

**TABLE 6.** *Suggested outline for a manual of policies and procedures for an occupational health service*

| |
|---|
| 1. Introduction, including authority for OHS |
| 2. Objectives |
| 3. Program components |
| 4. Preplacement medical examinations |
| 5. Periodic medical examinations |
| 6. Specialized programs |
| 7. Emergency medical care |
| 8. Subsequent care of workers with acute or chronic disorders |
| 9. Counseling |
| 10. Radiography |
| 11. Health education |
| 12. Wellness program |
| 13. Medications and prescriptions |
| 14. Industrial hygiene |
| 15. Epidemiology/biostatistics |
| 16. Medical documentation |
| 17. Reports |
| 18. Appointment system |
| 19. Personnel management |
| 20. Staff development |
| 21. Supply management and control |
| 22. Budget preparation |
| 23. Training programs for plant personnel |
| 24. Field training of students |
| 25. Relationship with federal, state, and local health-care agencies |
| 26. Research |

formats for reports, and professional clinical procedures in some detail. A suggested outline appears in Table 6.

### Personnel Management

Although the human resources department is charged with the responsibility of recruitment, testing, employment, and subsequent actions regarding personnel, including promotion, demotion, disciplinary action, evaluation, reclassification, termination, and retirement (service or disability), each department participates in the action taken on its own workers. Specific requests for the carrying out of personnel functions are initiated by the OHS, and in cooperation with the department of human resources a change or move is completed.

In contradistinction to the customary mode of seeking of staff personnel by other company divisions, the OHS usually is familiar with potential or prospective OH professionals and can assist the human resources department in the recruitment process. Advertising in the appropriate journals is always helpful in the location of candidates to fill vacancies in professional positions.

### Staff Development

Professionals avoid stagnation by a constant update of knowledge and skills. Of particular importance in the industrial arena is the constant acquisition of new information by members of the OHS staff. The company itself, in order to remain competitive, must enlarge, adapt new manufacturing methods, diversify, discard products in low demand, and so forth. The medical area must behave comparably and, through a system of personal and group growth, remain current in the practice of their particular disciplines.

Staff meetings are mandatory for the exchange of information among section supervisors and should be held regularly. Such sessions should provide a permissive climate so that all members feel free to contribute to the updating and progress of the OHS.

Continuing education for both physicians and nurses has been mandated in many states, and staff members should be encouraged to attend conferences or seminars that relate to their roles in the department. Provision for reimbursement of attendant costs is noted in the preparation of the departmental budget. It is desirable that on the return of a staff member from a course or conference that a report be made at a staff meeting so that others may benefit from the learning opportunity.

### The Internet

In recent times, the professional societies representing members of the OH team have offered informational resources for their members, and others interested in the OH specialties, through web sites on the Internet or other on-line service providers. Considerable material is available for perusal or downloading including such areas as professional objectives, current and forthcoming society publications, notices of upcoming conferences, changes in work environmental standards, instructions to prospective authors concerning manuscript formats, news or press releases, responses to frequently asked questions, and membership applications.

Through CompuServe and its Special Internet Groups one can leave messages for colleagues in the form of a question, a news item, or merely the announcement of something of concern to fellow practitioners or investigators. Web sites of interest to OH professionals appear in Table 7.

The use of computer resources will aid the staff member in keeping apprised of developments within the various specialties even before certain material may be published in the associations' journals (17).[6]

[6]Considerable software is available in all aspects of OH. The most recent version of a landmark publication appeared early in 1996, which is not only a directory prepared for the American College of Occupational and Environmental Medicine, but a publication that offers comparison tables that "point computer users to the classes of software which might meet their needs." Included in the work is a discussion of information management, personal computer (PC)–based hardware and generic PC software, CD-ROM sources for OM physicians, and specific items for use in clinic management, ADA compliance, screening, health promotion and epidemiology, among others, plus a glossary that defines the main terms unique to computer usage. (See refs. 129, 130.)

**TABLE 7.** *Web sites on the Internet of interest to occupational health professionals*

| Organization | Web site |
|---|---|
| Al-ANON and ALATEEN | http://www.solar.rtd.utk.edu/ran-anon/ |
| Alcoholics Anonymous, information about resources/self | http://www.moscow.com/ |
| American College of Occupational and Environmental Medicine | http://www.acoem.org/ |
| American College of Preventive Medicine | http://www.acpem.org/acpm/ |
| American Conference of Governmental Industrial Hygienists | http://www.acgih.org/ |
| American Medical Association | http://www.ama-assn.org/ |
| American Public Health Association | http://www.apha.org/ |
| Environmental Protection Agency (Governmental Information Locator Service) | http://epa.gov/gils/ |
| Join Together (national resource center for communities fighting substance abuse) | http://www.jointogether.org/jointogether.html/ |
| Medical Resources on the Internet | http://www.vifp.monash.edu.au/medical/eval.html/ |
| Med Help International | http://medhlp.netusa.net/ |
| Mine Safety and Health Administration | http://www.msha.gov/ |
| MSDS | gopher://atlas.chem.utah.edu/msds/ |
| National Cancer Institute | http://www.nci.nih.gov/ |
| National Institutes of Health | http://www.nih.gov/ |
| National Library of Medicine | http://www.nlm.nih.gov/ |
| OSHA Technical Manual | http://www.osha-slc.gov/oshnews/index.html/ |
| OSHA News Releases | http://www.osha.gov/media/ |
| OSHA What's New | http://www.osha.gov/wutsnew.html/ |
| Physician's Guide to the Internet | http://www.webcom.com/pgi/ |

Note: For a complete list of 583 web sites pertinent to occupational and environmental medicine, see Leopold (133). The classification of web sites follows the 50 categories utilized in McCunney (134). E-mail addresses are included.

### Lecture Series

In some organizations outside lecturers are invited to address the staff on topics of contemporary OH concern or on subjects immediately pertinent to clinical problems presented by workers. Information related to new program elements of the OHS, or to newly initiated services of community agencies will augment the staff's body of knowledge. Speakers from adjacent or regional universities are ideal source personnel for such intramural training presentations.

## REPORTS

An OHS can provide superlative service, but if no one is informed of the size of the patient load or the scope of the program, it may be difficult to substantiate requests for increased funding or personnel. A combined statistical and narrative report should be prepared for the head of the next higher echelon at least on a monthly basis, and could include the data derived from, or descriptions of the topics enumerated in, Table 8.

It has been the practice of some seasoned occupational health physicians to include in a report a narrative description of a particularly interesting or unusual employee/patient visit, with all identifying data of the individual appropriately disguised or changed in order to retain the privileged aspect of the relationship. The purpose is twofold: to add a human touch to an otherwise arid listing of numbers, and to familiarize the managerial reader with some of the difficulties presented to an OHS for resolution. Further, some of the behavioral problems jointly facing supervisors and the OHS may reveal areas of mismanagement worthy of top-level knowledge.

Reports need not be jejune, for an OHS is concerned with the work and home lives of employees, and some relating of staff experiences in the carrying out of assigned functions can be most revealing of the morale factors present among the employee force.

### Medical Records

A chronologic record on each person who visits the medical unit is initiated with the first visit. The record should be a compilation of all the data acquired in the process of investigating or measuring the employee's health.

Many OH physicians, as do private practitioners, include in the employee's record some of the nonmedical information that can broaden the understanding of the individual as a person, beyond an inventory of health status determinations. Clippings from local newspapers or house organs can be included, as can description of awards received, family additions, hobby pursuits, and records of travel, among other news items.

Some of the standards promulgated by the Department of Labor under the OSH Act of 1970 call for record retention for prescribed periods of time. For example, the final standard, Occupational Exposure to Lead, requires that medical records be maintained for at least 40 years, or for

**TABLE 8.** *Suggested topics for inclusion in monthly and annual departmental reports*

| |
|---|
| Statistical report for period of _____ to _____, 199_ |
| Number of applicants examined |
| Number of applicants accepted for employment |
| Number of employees receiving care |
| Number of employee visits |
| Number of visits for occupational injury |
| Number of visits for nonoccupational injury |
| Number of visits for occupational illness |
| Number of visits for nonoccupational illness |
| Number of clinical laboratory procedures |
| Number of diagnostic radiographic procedures |
| Number of immunizing injections given |
| Number of medications dispensed |
| Number of physical therapy procedures |
| Number of employees referred to community health care resources |
| Number of consultant visits of employees requested of community specialists, by medical specialty |
| Number of visits per employee per ____ |
| Number of illness absences per employee per ____ |
| Number of health education sessions held |
| Personnel of the OHS by discipline, with positional changes indicated |
| Current facilities |
| Attendance at professional meetings |
| Papers presented by staff members |
| Publications by staff members |
| Illness absences by department |
| Illness absences by occupation (job title) |
| Illness absences by gender |
| Illness absences by marital status |
| Illness absences by ethnicity |
| Illness absences by health status classification |
| Illness absences by shift |
| Visits by diagnostic category |
| Visits by diagnostic category by department |
| Visits by diagnostic category by occupation (job title) |
| Visits by diagnostic category by gender |
| Visits by diagnostic category by marital status |
| Visits by diagnostic category by ethnicity |
| Visits by diagnostic category by health status classification |
| Visits by diagnostic category by shift |
| Cost per employee visit |
| Cost per employee per year |
| Conclusions |
| Recommendations |

the duration of employment plus 20 years, whichever is longer (18). Other considerations enter into the matter, for in the standard Occupational Exposure to Cotton Dust, again as an example, the following is specified (19), in essence:

**Record Keeping**

1. Medical surveillance
   a. The employer shall establish and maintain an accurate medical record for each employee subject to medical surveillance
   b. The record shall include
      (1) The name, social security number, and description of the duties of the employees
      (2) A copy of the medical examination results including the medical history, questionnaire response, results of all tests, and the physician's recommendation
      (3) A copy of the physician's written opinion
      (4) Any employee medical complaints related to exposure to cotton dust
      (5) The type of protective devices worn and length of time worn
      (6) A copy of this standard and its appendices, except that the employer may keep one copy of the standard and the appendices for all employees, provided that he or she references the standard and appendices in the medical surveillance record of each employee
   c. The employer shall maintain this record for at least 20 years.
2. Availability
   a. The employer shall make available upon request all records required to be maintained to the assistant secretary (of the Department of Labor) and the director (of the National Institute for Occupational Safety and Health) for examination and copying
   b. Employee exposure measurement records and employee medical records ... shall be provided upon request to employees, designated representatives and the assistant secretary.
3. Transfer of records
   a. Whenever the employer ceases to do business, the successor employer shall receive and retain all records required to be maintained
   b. Whenever the employer ceases to do business and there is no successor employer to receive and retain the records for the prescribed period, these records shall be transmitted to the director
   c. At the expiration of the retention period for the records required to be maintained, the employer shall notify the director at least 3 months prior to the disposal of such records and shall transmit those records to the director if the director requests them within that period.

Each criteria document developed by NIOSH for transmission to the Department of Labor carries recommendations regarding medical records that differ with the noxious agent under discussion. Even though few of the criteria documents have been converted to promulgated standards,[7] it is easier to develop records as exposure

[7]To date, the only standards issued in final form are those covering asbestos (29 CFR Part 1910-1001), coal tar pitch volatiles (§ 1002), lead (§ 1 or 5), coke oven emissions (§ 1029), blood-borne pathogens (§ 1030), cotton dust (§ 1042), and 22 carcinogens labeled as one of four classes: potential cancer hazard, cancer hazard, cancer-suspect agent, or may cause cancer. Periodically some of the standards are stayed by the court.

with a work material becomes known in an operation rather than attempting to retrofit the record to past data. Medical records can be admitted as evidence at workers' compensation hearings or in subsequent third-party suits, so it must be remembered that any notation may be subject to public review.

With the development and issue of the standard promulgated by the Department of Labor on access to medical records, it is now permitted that the worker and the government have access to employer-maintained medical and toxic exposure records. Following considerable comment and testimony on its development, the standard allows employees to examine and copy their own records and to designate which other persons may review them (20).

## COMPUTERIZED MEDICAL RECORDS

As one looks toward temporal change, one sees multiple alterations in the format of medical practice and possibly in the configuration of OM. As two reviewers expressed it, "It will only be a matter of time before computerized patient records, distance continuing medical education classes, telemedicine, virtual surgery, and myriad health education interactive programs transform the way medicine and public health are practiced and received" (21). While the computerization of patents' records is undergoing consideration, the issue was of sufficient currency as to warrant exploration by the Committee on Governmental Affairs of the U.S. Senate (22).

It was pointed out that most health care providers today maintain medical records in manual, paper-intensive systems from which it is difficult to retrieve information and that require huge amounts of physical storage space. There are barriers to automating medical records and developing a systems framework to support health care reform: the lack of standards, the cost of automation, the security and privacy issues arising from the use of such automated medical information, and the reluctance of health care professionals to use new technology. It was concluded that, in overall health care reform, strong federal leadership will be required to ensure that adequate steps are taken to design, develop, and implement a systems framework that supports a nationwide program (22).

The practice of OM is not nationwide in the same sense of overall health care that would affect the population of the United States. Multinational companies, however, do have labor forces in the hundreds of thousands, with a certain mobility of workers among different facilities.

In early 1995, a lengthy conference was held, the Eleventh International Symposium on the Creation of Electronic Health Record Systems and Global Conferences on Patient Cards (23). Innumerable papers were presented that reviewed many aspects of the concept of computerized patient records (CPRs). As pointed out by Burstein (24), in designing a CPR, one must mesh the two worlds of computers and medicine. The CPR has several distinct advantages over a paper record and the design of the system should capitalize on these strengths. There are limitations not present in the paper record, but these can be worked around in the design phase. An electronic system makes all data available for research, quality improvement, reports, financial review, etc.

Information in a patient's record is diverse, coursing from descriptive episodes in a medical history to numerical data in laboratory reports to qualitative character findings in certain test procedures. A coding scheme must be developed that allows transfer of the diversity of the data. Some systems have the ability to put in free text alongside the coded entry so that a comprehensive and accurate description need not be lost.

In the creation of an electronic record system, avenues for information collection and analysis can be integrated into the system so that access to database sources—National Library of Medicine, Centers for Disease Control and Prevention, etc. (see Staff Development, above)—is possible. As expressed by Burstein, "The electronic medical record provides a natural springboard into this new world of shared electronic information, and the design of the record should have the ability to incorporate these avenues as a basic part of its structure" (24).

But what is a CPR? Waegemann (25), the executive director of the Medical Records Institute has offered workable definitions. The CPR is achieved by using the traditional medical record components on paper and converting them into the computer format. Such change is accomplished by the scanning process, wherein paper records, complete with the required legal "attributes" (signature of person entering data and the data), are converted from the standard clinical record page to the digital format. Such conversion does not require the staff person to alter the usual method of entering notes into the record. As expressed by Waegemann, "Through a combination of document imagining, OCR (Optical Character Recognition) scanning and the scanning of image-based documents such as x-rays, EKGs, fetal strips, etc., a computerized medical record is created in look-up format (document images) and working format (OCR images and limited computer input)." The end result of this CPR system is that it retains the function of the customary paper record with the added advantages of electronic availability vs. physical distribution of paper records to users, computer storage vs. manual record assembly, filing, and retrieval, and service as an intermediate step in the creation of electronic medical records or the higher level electronic patient record systems. The CPR allows collection of all records, many of which may have been kept in separate departmental files, e.g., EEG, EKG, etc.

The system has seen limited use, for the CPR remains a "look-up" record.

The electronic medical record (EMR) is created on the computer, the care provider developing the system through appropriate software using the customary modalities of the keyboard, mouse, touch-screen, voice recognition device, sound recording device, or pen computing service (25). At times scanned paper documents may be added. The differences between the EMR system and the traditional paper record is seen in these features: (a) The structure is defined by computer processes rather than by chronologic document entries. (b) It can be active (rather than passive) by providing interactive aids in decision making through knowledge coupling, decision support, and other functions. (c) It can provide further functions such as patient education, automatic reporting to registries (cancer, reportable diseases), price and effectiveness comparisons, care plan development, claim generation with automatic coding, and patient management functions such as appointment scheduling and referrals. (d) It can provide compliance with documentation standards in security, authentication, data integrity, protection against unauthorized use, and auditability (25).

The electronic patient record system (also called the computer-based patient record) covers information from birth to death, including prenatal and postmortem data. The scope is wider than the medical record and includes information of treatment by all health-related disciplines such as dentistry, podiatry, physical therapy, and even the treatment offered in alternative medicine (acupuncture, chiropractic, and the like). Required is the linkage of records from care at multiple sources to form "a continuous chronology of a patient's health care experiences" (25). Standard coded formats are needed in drug nomenclature procedures performed, outcomes, etc., so that the data are utilizable in analytic or research endeavors.

The electronic health record—the first use of the word *health* in this connotation—collects comprehensive information concerning the individual's health, data often not gathered in medical records. Included would be behavioral characteristics concerning smoking, drinking, exercising, and eating, and wellness information obtained from parents, sports trainers, and other ancillary professionals, such as exercise physiologists or biofeedback therapists. Such a record is multidisciplinary and multienterprise.

Hurdles exist in the world of medical records that might, and do, affect the introduction of any electronic system into a health care source. Standards are created by multiple standards organizations (9), not one. Technical developments are still in progress concerning hardware in such areas as speech input, repository strategies, and interspersability. Some states have yet to legalize paperless medical record systems and to address the issues of confidentiality and security. Lastly, caregivers must be convinced that not using the computer will be disadvantageous (25).

The question remains of the adaptability of such systems to OH care. It is not possible to estimate current usage in various OSHs, but computers have certainly entered most care facilities and their use could be extended to allow development of one or another of the electronic formats. In light of the Occupational Safety and Health Administration (OSHA) mandates discussed earlier concerning the lengthy retention of records, computerization would certainly make obsolete the space- and personnel-demanding storage of paper records, which, in themselves, may not always guarantee legibility over decades.

Factors to be considered in the possible conversion of the traditional format are primarily user acceptance and enthusiasm, costs, size of work force covered by an OHS, and availability of technical assistance in the installation, training, and maintenance of electronic systems in remote industrial facilities as secondary factors. An aggressive, far-sighted management can mandate the change in systems, with or without the concurrence of the OH professionals involved.

In essence, it is believed that an electronic record, in one configuration or another, will be the standard in most OHSs as thinking modernizes to keep the parent company competitive in all areas. It has been concluded by one observer that "unless consensus is found, not only within professions but also between professions, records will remain fragmented, largely usable only by single individuals or groups and yielding information from aggregate analysis of very limited value" (26). With the current disarray of medical care, in general, computerization of records must be part of the solution to health care in the United States.

The issue of confidentiality of records has always been a primary concern in an OHS, and only rarely has the breaching of confidentiality been justified; if the public health is endangered, then some medical material may have to be relayed (27,28). It is believed that with the installation of safeguards, an electronic record system can preserve the confidential nature of information entered into the record, and allay fears of professionals who guard scrupulously this ethical principle. The issue was of sufficient merit that bills were introduced in Congress as it was felt that "computerized record keeping poses an undeniable threat to the traditional confidentiality of physicians' and hospitals' information systems" (29). To date, no further action has been taken with such privacy legislation.

Conferences concerning the electronic patient record continue to be held, primarily as arranged by the Medical Records Institute of Newton, Massachusetts. With its inception in 1981, the institute, patterned somewhat after an academic organization, has been a force in the movement toward an electronic health record. Its mission state-

**TABLE 9.** *Mission of the medical records institute*

1. Promote electronic health record systems and identify building blocks and strategies for their implementation
2. Participate in organizations concerned with the creation of electronic health records, and help to shape its overall vision
3. Act as a clearinghouse of information on national and international developments by publishing and distributing newsletters, books, and other materials related to health care information technology, as well as sponsoring national and international symposia and seminars
4. Conduct applied research and coordinate projects related to the creation of electronic patient record systems
5. Support, coordinate, and foster the process of creating standards which cover the creation of electronic patient records
6. Participate in, and contribute to creation of a national and global information infrastructure for health care
7. Support the acceleration of telemedicine and foster its links to electronic health record systems
8. Bridge efforts between the United States and other regions of the world in developing electronic patient record systems
9. Act as a voice of conscience on aspects of confidentiality, security and social impact

Reprinted with permission from Steve Dreskin, Medical Records Institute, Newton, Massachusetts.

ment summarizes the current efforts in the conversion of the time-honored paper record to the computer-based, electronic model (Table 9).

Records of personnel exposure to toxic materials have been created (30), and further adaptations to electronic record keeping are seen in Accusafe Pro, an injury and illness reporting system, and Training Tracker, a system that schedules, tracks, and records training activities and requirements [as mandated by OSHA, the Environmental Protection Agency (EPA), and the Department of Transportation (DOT)], which are available from the National Safety Council, Itasca, Illinois.

### Public Relations

The OHS needs to establish close working relationships with members of the medical community. Service is provided to persons who are the private patients of practitioners in the area. It is not completely understood that occupational medicine is preventive medicine, and the maintenance of continuing contact by frequent telephone inquiries with local physicians who are treating employees prevents misunderstandings. Since most practitioners have little knowledge of industry, it is helpful to invite community practitioners to visit the OHS and tour the more hazardous operating areas of the plant, so that they might see—and learn—first-hand the kinds of work demands made of their patients.

Such visits, coupled with lunch in the company's cafeteria, would allow employees to see their physicians at their place of work and to realize that some fusion of two bodies of knowledge—work and medicine—must result and be helpful in the rendering of medical care. The same kind of invitation can be extended to the executives of various community health agencies concerned with specific organ system disorders or discrete disease entities, e.g., cancer, heart, lung, multiple sclerosis, Alzheimer's disease, and arthritis, or those concerned with rehabilitation and job placement, such as Goodwill Industries. In the latter case, familiarization with prospective work sites may foster a larger move into industry of persons with disabilities.

### Transportation of Patients

Many problems can arise in connection with the transport of ill or injured employees, either to a source of care or to their homes. Some medical departments, particularly those units in large organizations divided into many buildings located over a wide area, maintain their own ambulances to bring injured workers to the central medical facility. These same vehicles may be used to take workers to community hospitals or clinics. If an ambulance is maintained, it should be completely equipped to allow delivery of emergency care in the field by trained personnel—physicians, nurses, physicians' assistants, or emergency medical technicians.

## HEALTH EDUCATION AND EMPLOYEE EDUCATION

The OSH Act of 1970 states that there shall be "programs for the education and training of employers and employees in the recognition, avoidance, and prevention of unsafe or unhealthful working conditions"(31). Through various educational institutions, labor unions, and official and voluntary health agencies, a considerable number of seminars, workshops, conferences, and congresses have been held to teach both professional persons and workers about the hazards of employment and the mechanisms of disease prevention.

It is the duty of the more articulate members of the OHS to conduct a program in health education. The effort may be targeted toward a change in health behavior, so that illness, particularly of an occupational origin, can be averted. Workers must know the nature of the toxicants to which they are exposed, the diseases that may result from undue contact, the procedures involved in medical surveillance, the meaning of various test results, and the measures to be taken to avoid the ill effects from the absorption, ingestion, or inhalation of toxic substances.

Despite the engagement of the company in legal defense, in the continued use of potentially hazardous materials, or the belief of inflexible executives that informing is dangerous, the medical staff must apprise workers of risks, hazards, and available protection (32,33).

The transmission of health information goes beyond the dissemination of knowledge relating to work-site hazards. All people are in need of material relating to their health status, particularly counsel in the area of preventive medicine. The government health agencies have been issuing innumerable publications over the years, but recently the Congress has been concerned with what is termed consumer health informatics (34,35). The increasing demand for health information has driven the development of informatics systems, such systems being the union of health care content with the speed and ease of technology (35). While many people obtain health information through the use of personal computers in their homes, other points of public access are found in libraries, clinics, hospitals, and physicians' waiting rooms. The systems have involved a range of technologies from telephones to interactive online systems.

Studies of the value of informatics systems have shown the systems' abilities to respond to consumers' information needs quickly and efficiently, and reduce the need for some unnecessary medical services, thus lowering health care costs (34). The information often is so customized that consumers may review the pros and cons of elective surgery or provide physicians with preoperative health information, potentially avoiding unnecessary preoperative tests.

It is anticipated that a forward-thinking OHS will investigate the value of these systems and install the particular modality that will meet the needs of the company's or plant's population. The time may come soon when merely having an employee/patient view a videotape of a certain disorder or its treatment choices will seem old-fashioned. Currently, six federal government departments are involved in consumer health informatics (35).

## SERVICE TO SMALL BUSINESS

About half of the private-sector members of the labor force work in firms employing fewer than 100 workers (36). Small establishments are covered by fewer regulations; those with ten employees or less need not comply with the OSH Act. Accordingly, this segment of workers has been singularly deprived of OHSs. To fill this need, a private clinic located in a large industrial area often develops a number of "accounts," meaning that a certain set of services is provided to a company on a fee-for-service basis or for a per-capita charge. Often these services are limited to the performance of examinations and the provision of emergency medical or surgical care. Little is included in the way of environmental health services, health education, counseling, or consultation on specific problems of the work group. Occasionally, a clinic of this type has its physicians spend a predetermined number of hours per day at a plant to examine new employees or consult with the occupational health nurse on certain clinical problems.

A group of companies may establish a clinic, contract for its operation, and function as sole users and codirectors of the facility. In other situations, a small plant may call upon its workers' compensation underwriter for consultation in safety, occupational medicine, occupational health nursing, or industrial hygiene.

Occupational medicine is appearing in the United States more and more as a new department in large general medical clinics and hospitals, and also in free-standing occupational medicine clinics. They provide quality care in the clinic or occupational medical service, but little professional help is provided at the work site. These clinic-based services usually have many different specialists available.

Small businesses or new businesses beginning operation would be helped regarding occupational safety and concerns by obtaining pertinent publications from OSHA (37,38).

## RELATED ADMINISTRATIVE FUNCTIONS

It is the function of the medical director or a designee to provide consultative assistance to department heads and top executives when interpersonal or motivational problems arise, and when they may have medical or illness-related causes for their appearance and persistence. Through either the application of sound epidemiologic analysis of data or the interviewing of individual workers who manifest counterproductive behavior styles, the problems and their causes can be identified, and with the help and new insights of managers the trends toward ineffectiveness—and lower profits—can be counteracted.

The OHS has a unique opportunity for doing health-related environmental research. It has a captive population with good baseline data. It has both a frequently updated set of medical records on each subject and access to industrial hygiene records, including individual exposure histories. Nearby university staffs are often available to provide help with biostatistics, toxicology, or epidemiology, as needed, if these disciplines are not represented in the OHS. Opportunities for short-term field experience can be offered to graduate students in a variety of health disciplines. With research and education in the on-site OHSs of industry, investigators and staff will realize professional growth, with resultant benefits to workers and industry.

The OHS should make every effort to cooperate with employee organizations. Such action not only improves morale and increases worker confidence in the OHS, but it also permits early resolution of many grievances related to medical action or lack of action—grievances that might otherwise result in formal complaints and become a source of friction between labor and management (39).

## MANAGEMENT MODELS

The organization and operation of most OHSs up to the recent past have followed the traditional departmental head-and-staff configuration, as indicated earlier. But changes have been initiated, and many of the services in this country have begun to be viewed not as profit centers comparable to other company departments but as business operations that can be costly. That a closer look is needed is given evidence by some of the postgraduate seminars held early in 1996 as part of the American Occupational Health Conference (40–42).

Total Quality Management (TQM), at times called Quality Circles (QC), Total Quality (TQ), or Total Quality Improvement (TQI), is a system whose objective is to succeed by continually improving a product or service. The history of management styling has been well traced from cottage industries (43), through the Industrial Revolution with its mass production (44), the concept of scientific management as initiated by Frederick Taylor (45,46), the use of motion study by the Gilbreths (47), the introduction of mental health principles in preventive management (48), up to quality control as conceived by Shewhart of Bell Telephone Laboratories (43). W. Edwards Deming went to Japan shortly after the conclusion of World War II to "teach statistical process control methods to Japanese workers and managers," methods that were based on the assumption that the system is the source of 85% of quality problems, not the workers (43). The application of his principles led to the success of Japanese industry in the decades following.

Quality is a management system issue and not one of technology. As reviewed by Roughton (49), quality efforts must be led by management, must become the fundamental responsibility of all employees, and must focus on problem prevention. A new paradigm, or belief system,[8] was created for quality, which means conformance to customer requirements and specifications, fitness for use, buyer satisfaction, and value at an affordable price. Inherent in TQM are communication, cross-departmental cooperation in problem resolution, constant retraining, management commitment, and statistical control.

With such typical industrially based precepts, is the concept applicable to the operation of an OHS? TQM has been adapted by the Joint Commission on Accreditation of Health Care Organizations, which bespeaks the expectations of this accrediting body of organizations involved in the provision of health services. An OHS, or any health facility, or even a university (51), can alter its management style as noted by several writers (49,52–57). Primarily, in a conversion to TQM, if the effort is made, in customer satisfaction, and in the case of an OHS, the employees who seek service or who are directed to the source of service through legislative surveillance mandates are the customers. While they do not come away with a purchased product, they will come away with feelings regarding the care given, and these feelings, if negative, can soon permeate a work force and the OHS will fail in its mission.

An excellent way of seeking information from the body of potential users of OH service offerings is through an occupational health advisory committee whose membership comprises representatives from the OHS; union officials; representatives of nonunionized employee associations; management personnel; members of the military if the organization is part of the defense structure; rotating representatives from various departments; and personnel from subcontractors if their work on company premises is of sufficient duration, if adherence to industrial hygiene principles govern their operation, and if the OHS is their source of emergency medical care. Through stimulated discussion at the meetings of the committee it can be readily learned if the OHS is being accepted for quality in the services provided, or is being avoided because of poor experience in past contacts.

The other element of special worth in the move to TQM has been touched on earlier. Staff meetings should not only allow but also encourage "group think," where the OHS personnel can express their ideas freely as to indicated changes that will produce quality in the staff/patient relationship. There must be a complete sense of freedom for all staff members to express their feelings regarding both policy and procedures. It is the staff that has the greatest number of diagnostic/therapeutic contacts with employees and it is they who can recognize if a certain procedure is devoid of all patient satisfaction.

While TQM has not entered the American health care industry in toto, it is Pierce's (58) contention that TQM is the future and that the concept must be incorporated into our culture.

[8]Paradigm, in this sense, as defined, is a philosophical and theoretical framework of a scientific school or discipline within which theories, laws, and generalizations and the experiments performed in support of them are formulated (50).

## CURRENT ISSUES

### Changing Work Force

While the structure and functions of an OHS may seem stable and fully subject to replication by any organization, certain societal, industrial, and geopolitical changes have had their effects on the mission of the in-plant service. Because of the new waves of immigration to the United States, the demographics of the work force have been altered. Refugees and persons seeking asylum have come to the United States for fear of persecution in their homelands in Southeast Asia, Cuba, and Central America. In addition, both legal and undocumented migrant laborers have crossed the southern border to swell the ranks of the service work force. In each of fiscal years 1992 and 1993, nearly a million immigrants to the United States were admitted (59).

Apart from these additions, there have been losses of jobs and reemployment elsewhere of some of the dischargees. According to the U.S. Department of Labor, over the period from January 1991 to December 1993, 4.5 million workers were displaced from jobs they held for 3 or more years (60). However, nearly seven in ten workers were reemployed when surveyed in February 1994. While this factor may or may not involve immigrants, it does imply radical changes in the work force.

Although many new arrivals establish small businesses in ethnic enclaves in the big cities, great numbers do obtain employment in large companies. Language poses a problem in communication and in a need for interpreters (61). Care must be given the selection of persons providing this function, for the translator may interject personal opinions or judgments or may even demonstrate a prejudice based on social class differences. Over 40 years ago, the eminent anthropologist Margaret Mead (62) wrote:

> It is possible to point out that in any program involving popular education in public health, the problem of language is a serious one—exact meanings must be explored, questions of adapting old words to new ideas, as opposed to coining new words, must be weighed, choice must be made among racial dialects, issues such as the use of a world-language or the elevation of a local language to a level at which the literature of the world may be expected to be translated into it—all must be taken into consideration.

There must be an awareness on the part of the health-care provider of the vast cultural differences between a certain segment of the immigrant population and our own citizenry. As an example of one in-coming group, Locke (63) has written of the Koreans: "The family-centered, traditional Korean immigrant finds the free-style, aggressive, individualistic way of life in the United States incompatible with that of the homeland.... Thus some have a tendency to isolate themselves from the dominant culture and stay within the Korean community."

Ideally, staff members should be bilingual, having skills in the second language most represented in the work force, as is seen in flight personnel engaged in intercontinental travel. Not only will communication be facilitated, but there can be an understanding of native beliefs in folk medicine still possessed by persons migrating to the United States (64–66).

A new modality has been devised to enable translation of languages foreign to American parlance. The multimedia medical language translator (MLT), currently used by the U.S. military, is distributed as a CD-ROM disk (compact disk read-only memory). The MLT is a computer-based system, run on a laptop computer, that "allows the physician to determine which language the patient is familiar with, to ask questions and give directions or explanations in that language (via the recorded voice of a native speaker), and to have the patient's responses translated to English" (67). The system makes possible the asking of questions common for physical examinations, the offering of basic explanations of diagnoses, the indicating of the therapy to be undertaken, and the responding to a patient's common questions such as, "Can I take a walk?"

Some 43 languages are available and for those literate in Russian, Chinese, or English, nearly 2,000 phrases are included. Examples of languages strange to most American practitioners are Azerbaijani, Farsi, Macedonian, Navajo, Rwandan, Urdu, and Yupik. The voices used in this "mouse-driven" system are those of women and men who are native speakers of the language, employing natural inflections, the most courteous phrasing, and essentially an unaccented form of speech. No robotic, synthesized voice sounds are used. The MLT has been a result of the work of Lee M. Morin of the U.S. Navy. It is anticipated that the system will be made available commercially.

Several disease entities may be discovered at the preplacement medical evaluation (68). Most disturbing has been the rise in tuberculosis rates, as noted earlier, a disease once considered conquered in the United States. The Department of Health and Human Services identifies immigrants and refugees from high-prevalence countries as one of the groups at risk for infection and disease (9,69,70). Chest radiography for asymptomatic populations has been discontinued except in certain situations involving exposure to fibrogenic dusts. With the recrudescence of tuberculosis, however, a return to this form of case finding is necessary if immigrants continue to enter the work force, particularly as employees in health care institutions.

Immigrants suffering posttraumatic stress disorder (71) while trying to preserve native belief systems in a foreign country provide challenges to occupational physicians that almost equal the early experiences of Hull House's Dr. Alice Hamilton with the emigrés of the 1890s (72).

## ADDICTIVE BEHAVIOR

Without question, chemical dependency and drug addiction are affecting every physician's practice including practitioners in industry. With the passage of the Drug-Free Workplace Act of 1988 (73), it was required that all grantees and contractors of federal agencies certify that they will provide drug-free workplaces. As nearly all educational institutions and many manufacturers receive government funds, the act has virtually universal applicability. A policy statement and a drug awareness program are required. Although not mandated, possible components of such a program may include employee education, employee assistance (either the establishment of or enhancement of an existing EAP), supervisory training, and drug detection. The federal government, in order to avoid erroneous accusation of illicit drug use by an employee, has relied on the placement of a physician between the laboratory conducting the drug testing and the employer. The physician who serves in this role, the medical review officer (MRO), must have knowledge of substance-abuse disorders and appropriate medical training to interpret and evaluate positive test results.

In industry the role of the MRO is assumed by the medical director or a designate, and in most instances a seasoned occupational physician will find the new functions parallel ongoing activities. Of prime importance to the public are entities subject to the requirements of the DOT. Six of its agencies have promulgated regulations on drug-testing programs that affect both the public and private sectors, including four million employees and 200,000 entities. While the MRO's treatment of negative test results is administrative, the positive-test report-verification process comprises these functions: reviewing positive report documents; notifying employees of positive test results; providing an opportunity for the employee to discuss the test results; reviewing medical records, history, and other biomedical factors; processing employees' requests for retesting; and authorizing testing of a "split sample" for drug metabolites (74).

As the effective date of the DOT regulations was January 2, 1990, some experience with MROs and drug testing at the work site has been logged. Educational programs have been held to train physicians as MROs (75), and drug testing has been introduced in different kinds of industrial activities. Interestingly, a program for the testing of house physicians beginning training has been initiated (76), civilian pilots have been tested (77), and although preemployment testing is a popular type of screening, other programs exist, including postaccident, reasonable suspicion, posttreatment, random, and voluntary testing (78).

While the issue still is debated as to its relationship to the workplace, employers have found that random drug testing is a deterrent to both frequent and occasional use of illicit drugs (79). It is the feeling, however, that the deterrent value of screening is uncertain, and that testing programs are not efficient mechanisms for linking drug users to assistance programs (80). The entire matter of such testing remains contentious and warrants much further study, particularly in light of efforts to legalize the sale of certain controlled drugs for either general or therapeutic use.

Alcohol testing has been mandated by the Omnibus Employee Testing Act of 1991, part of the 1992 DOT and Related Agencies Appropriations Act (81). In a further effort to decrease accidents and fatalities, breath alcohol testing of persons in "safety-sensitive" positions was required as part of the preemployment examination, postaccident, at random intervals, on return to duty and follow-up, and when there is reasonable suspicion. Employers with 50 or more workers were to have implemented these procedures by January 1, 1995, and companies with fewer than 50 in safety-sensitive positions were to have the testing in place one year later. The mandate applies to about seven million persons. If the test results are positive for alcohol misuse, the regulations allow the employer to remove immediately the worker from a safety-sensitive position. These generally mandated requirements are part of the increasing workload of an OHS created by progressive, preventive medicine legislation.

## WELLNESS PROGRAMS

Most OHS program elements in the past have been directed toward the prevention of work-related disease. In the past decade, motivated by a desire for containment of rising medical care costs, industry has moved away somewhat from health education as identified since the early years of this century—apart from compliance with right-to-know legislation—to efforts called work-site wellness programs or employee fitness programs. Although occupational medical practitioners have been conducting such activities for years, the new catch phrases have attracted managerial attention and support. In place of targeting solely plant interiors that have atmospheric contaminants, the movement is directed to identifying factors that place the employee's health at risk, most having their origin in an unhealthful lifestyle (82,83).

The programs have frequently combined two undertakings: the ascertainment of certain health deficits (e.g., hypertension, coronary artery disease, obesity) and the institution of measures aimed at correcting or reversing the course of these adverse clinical findings. A battery of examinations or tests is conducted, the employee is told the results, and is then encouraged to participate in program segments that will stay the disease process or forestall the future onset of serious illness (Table 10).

While a multitude of benefits has been proclaimed following the introduction of wellness programs—less

**TABLE 10.** *Elements of a wellness (fitness) promotion program*

| |
|---|
| Clinical measurements and screening |
| Blood glucose level |
| Blood pressure |
| Breast examination |
| Fecal occult blood |
| One-second forced expiratory volume |
| Oral examination (smokers) |
| Prostatic specific antigen (PSA), as indicated |
| Rectal examination |
| Serum cholesterol level, HDL cholesterol level, and triglycerides |
| Skin-fold thickness determination |
| Spine flexibility |
| Vital capacity |
| Weight determination |
| Promotional activities |
| Accident prevention (seat-belt use) |
| AIDS education |
| Blood pressure control or treatment |
| Cancer risk reduction |
| Cardiopulmonary resuscitation |
| Dental care improvement |
| Drug abuse education or referral |
| Exercise |
| Family involvement |
| Improved nutrition |
| Lowering cholesterol level |
| Mental health counseling |
| Self-examination |
| Skin protection |
| Smoking cessation |
| Stress management |
| Weight control |

absenteeism and turnover; lower blood pressure, heart rate, serum cholesterol, and triglyceride values; and fewer back problems, in addition to increased productivity and morale—definitive long-term results have not really met rigorous research design demands in their development or certain confounding variables have precluded solid conclusions (84). Further, the participants in such programs appear to be somewhat healthier and more concerned with fitness and health matters than nonparticipants (85). A sedentary lifestyle was estimated to cost every citizen $1,900 as a subsidy from the public (86). The primary focus of a wellness program could well be the initiation of regular exercise as a personal health ritual.

Much recent literature has reviewed the economic aspects of wellness programs in industry (87–91).

## CROSS-SPECIALTY MOVES

A change that may dilute the effect of an in-plant OHS is the increased interest in occupationally related disorders and in the work environment itself by primary care physicians and internists. The Institute of Medicine has been studying the rate of the former (92). The American College of Physicians has emphasized in a position paper that to the extent that they care for persons of working age, all physicians are engaged in the practice of occupational medicine (93). Studies by the Institute of Medicine are continuing relative to the shortage of physicians trained in occupational medicine and to the establishment of regional centers where physicians could have access to an occupational and environmental exposure and disease database (Frazier J, personal communication, 1990). Other observers have indicated the need for involvement of the practicing physician in health issues of their working patients and even those persons living in industrial communities (94–99).

The accelerated concern may either lead to a greater investment of time in the private practitioner's office so that more workers are seen extramurally and with greater insight, or a number of knowledgeable internists may provide in-plant consultation services. This move is positive, and the implication hints at divided responsibilities for worker care.

## REMAINING ISSUES

Many other potential influences on the configuration and program objectives of today's OHS warrant consideration. The practice of medicine today is seen as a quandary in motion. Solo physicians are forming or joining groups as a defense position against the inroads of managed care. Health insurance underwriters are merging and the large hospital chains are getting larger as they buy not only local hospitals but long-established health/hospital insurance organizations. There is fear on the part of health care providers that significant decisions in medical care will be replaced exclusively by cost considerations of the various modalities of diagnosis and treatment, the directives for these elements in medical practice coming exclusively from lay finance controllers. There is concern that the public sector in health care will gradually be placed in private hands and that the health of the public at large may suffer. Leaders in medicine have expressed great apprehension regarding the conversion to truly untested formulations of the delivery of care, as seen in such article titles as "Managed Care—A Work in Progress" (100), "Health of the Public—The Private-Sector Challenge" (101), and "Health Care Crisis From a Trauma Center Perspective" (102).[9] The effect on contemporary OHSs is not determinable at this time of transition.

The pertinent question at this point in the vortex is the position of OM as it will relate to the new format of medical care. Will the functions of an OH be transferred to the health maintenance organization (HMO) with which the employer has contracted care of the work force? Or will the

[9] An excellent post–World War II history of the reconfiguration of the medical care model is seen in Richmond and Fein (131).

OHS remain and mature further because of the lack of OM background seen in most HMOs? Those growing organizations, in some instances, have OM departments, but rarely, as noted previously, do the professionals of such a section visit a plant. Without visitation to the work site there cannot be the close and bilaterally highly rewarding physician/patient relationship that allows the surfacing of personal problems and their therapy, resulting in the return to productive, effective work. In an effort to understand the forthcoming relationship, if any, the American College of Occupational and Environmental Medicine is soliciting material that, it is hoped, will clarify the position of the OM specialty in the years ahead (103).

Other aspects of the move to managed care may affect the delivery of OH services. Academic institutions are merging their patient resources, and university hospitals are adding smaller community hospitals to their teaching bases (104). How will managed care affect residency training programs? There is no present answer, or, as expressed by one medical academician, "No process currently exists to monitor nationwide the effects of managed care on residency training, and one needs to be developed" (105). A large HMO wants its new physicians "to come to them with information systems skills, a knowledge of epidemiology and a variety of psychosocial skills" (104). How many medical education programs so train their students?

If the new system utilizes a capitated payment strategy (capitation) will health status determine the rates (106,107)? Will the OHS be asked to submit privileged information at the time of conversion so that individual rates can be determined, if health status is a factor? Also, if the primary care physician sees patients on a fixed-rate basis in the capitation model, is the OHS likely to provide more primary care—care, that is, for nonoccupational illnesses or injuries? As a greater number of visits of a patient under capitation does not increase the provider's income, will the caseload of the OHS grow now that the community physician's cry—the OHS is "taking my patients away"—will no longer hold? Answers may never be forthcoming (108).

Efforts have been made, however, to look at the relationship between managed care and workers' compensation. This aspect of managed care has been defined as "the active process of reducing work related injuries and assuring that when an injury does occur, the employee can find medical care and return to work quickly and safely" (109). A more basic meaning is expressed for managed care in this connotation as "an umbrella term that usually describes a mix of services, discounts, and aggressive oversight" (110). The head of a Massachusetts-based provider of workers' compensation services has suggested that the better-managed programs should comprise these elements (110):

- A network, carefully screened, of primary care providers and occupational medicine specialists, that may not necessarily be connected to the regular network providing health services to the company's employees.
- Case-management expertise including ongoing contact and personal attention.
- Return-to-work expertise including physical therapists, rehabilitation consultants and facilities, and knowledgeable counsel concerning temporary light-duty placement.
- Review of billing practices and the services provided.
- Reviews of loss data, case-management practices, and vendor relationships.

While workers' compensation management has been lax, and fraud has been prevalent, a tightening of supervisory functions over the system may allow managed care to limit the excessive therapy costs attendant currently on work injuries.

## INTERNATIONAL OCCUPATIONAL HEALTH SERVICE

As American companies establish facilities abroad, and as the work population bases comprise both expatriates from the United States and native workers, different considerations arise in the creation of the OHS by the multinational company. The questions of risk assessment and resource assessment are paramount, for the American employees overseas expect the same quality care as received at their home base. Certain country-related medical issues and cultural differences must be understood. Problems of patient transport arise in selecting referral sites away from the installation. A solution, as offered by Moore (111) is to provide a level of care comparable to the Western equivalent of a middle-level hospital in the employee's home country, i.e., the country in which the company is operating. The many issues of interactional OH are covered elsewhere (112).

## MULTIPLE NATIONAL SITES OF AN OCCUPATIONAL HEALTH SERVICE

Somewhat in parallel with the establishment of OHSs abroad by a multinational company is the development of medical programs within an organization at its numerous small manufacturing locations. As most of the preventive health care will be provided by local physicians, care must be exercised in the selection and retention of such practitioners. Hathaway (113) has described well the role of the corporate medical director and the need for good local office management, the continuing education of the community physicians who provide service, and the ongoing basic requirements of impartiality, objectivity, and fairness in situations where the worker may be the private patient of the local physician. Good communications are mandatory in the transmission of examination results to site management. Adverse recommendations—those perceived as adverse—will be accepted more readily by employees and organized bargaining units if they know that they have been treated fairly and honestly in the past by the site physician. Policies vary in the relationship of the corporate medical director to those outlying plants that have their own in-house staffs. Whether such an installation can be granted autonomy in operations or must remain in constant contact with the headquarter's medical arm will vary with the management skills[10] of the corporate office and the educational attainment of the distant plant personnel in OH. Wellness programs at diverse settings have been cited (89).

## OUTSOURCING OCCUPATIONAL HEALTH CARE

With the downsizing of industry, the merging of large companies, and the movement of manufacturing to foreign labor sites, some organizations have either minimized their in-house OH capability, or have contracted out for services from neighboring clinics. While the external professionals might be equally qualified as to medical or nursing specialty certification, they are not part of the in-house body of employees, and are viewed as outsiders. While the functions of an OH program such as preplacement examinations, medical surveillance, and care for injured employees can be obtained, there is missing the close relationship that develops between OHS staff members and workers. Such a relationship is needed, as indicated earlier, to allow employees the freedom and willingness to bring personal problems to the OHS for solution.

While job-generated injuries and their resulting fiscal cost result in the greater publicity and rationale for preventive-program improvement, most of the traumatized workers get well. The unattended psychosocial problems that coexist when OH services are contracted externally are the difficulties that will persist, impairing work relationships and lowering productivity. Most employees will not seek assistance for their emotional problems, particularly if they must go outside the plant premises for such professional aid. It is only the contact with workers at an on-site facility that will create a milieu where confidences can be shared, where physical problems psychogenic in origin can be recognized for their true etiology, and appropriate therapy can be initiated. It is this kind of biopsychosocial orientation in medicine that brings the greatest satisfaction to perceptive professionals in OH. External facilities cannot create this ongoing sense of shared concerns.

[10]That managerial skills are both needed and attainable in the world of science is given testimony by Badawy (132), a disciple of the eminent economist Peter Drucker.

## PRERETIREMENT COUNSELING

An activity rarely introduced as an OHS function is the counseling of personnel who are about to retire. The writer has had the experience of meeting with workers due for separation and preparing them for the health considerations of the future. Such counseling is not commonplace but is deeply appreciated by those persons about to separate from contacts of a lifetime.

The various anatomic and physiologic changes attendant upon aging are discussed and professional care for the early appearance of various disease states is encouraged. In light of possible changes in health insurance coverage, the preretirees are encouraged to have needed surgery performed now before possible postretirement insurance variance. Considerable emphasis is placed on lifestyle as it relates to smoking, alcohol and drug abuse, weight gain, and lack of exercise. Continuing immunization is encouraged and some of the traditional misconceptions about sex and age are decompressed. Hobbies, travel, interests, and the volunteering of service to community agencies are advocated. If an outplacement service is offered or desired, contact—with authorization—can be made with the new employer concerning accumulated health record information. Like all conferences, many attendees will come to the lectern with questions they did not wish to ask in front of co-workers.

## TELEMEDICINE

Although tried successfully several years ago at one of the nation's airports, it is only recently that telemedicine has seen renewed interest as a modality of extending medical care. Originally thought to be the savior of rural medicine, now its uses have advanced beyond its most popular application in radiology to dermatology, cardiology, oncology, and neurology (114). By definition, telemedicine includes both the diagnosis and treatment of distant patients and the use of distant resources to care for patients who are close at hand.

It is entirely conceivable that subdispensaries or aid stations widely peripheral to a headquarters OHS could employ this technology, saving much lost time in operations through the avoidance of patient transport. The factors productive of this medical system are the explosive growth and development of digital technologies, high-speed communications, and imaging protocols, along with cost reductions in computing equipment, increased use of the Internet, and changes in the economics and organization of health care (114). Systems of telemedicine can answer former U.S. Surgeon General Koop's hope that, "We must find ways to overcome the intellectual isolation that takes place as soon as young men and women graduate from their residence programs" (115).

## REHABILITATION AND TODAY'S TECHNOLOGY

Most observers believe that with the remarkable changes in technology and electronics, persons with disabilities should find placement in gainful employment, for jobs are becoming less labor-intensive. Despite rehabilitation efforts, a majority of disabled Americans, ages 16 to 24, are not working, a number that has remained unchanged since 1986, and despite the fact that a majority of nonemployed persons with disabilities in this age group want to work (116).

The factors causing changes in the nature of work are the global economy, new technology, and population shifts. The postindustrial world has formally defined labor forces, is highly organized, has developed infrastructures capable of responding to the populace's needs, is extremely energy-intensive, is technologically innovative, and is increasingly geared to the provision of services rather than the production of goods (116). Further, there is a growing demand for administrative and professional services, and occupations acquiring nonroutine, face-to-face interactions. The new labor groups are knowledge workers and service workers, where most in demand are people with qualitative knowledge-based skills and the ability constantly to learn and relearn. The capacity to adapt to change is the needed capability of a worker in this society.

The task facing rehabilitation counselors today, in light of the changes in the work world, is enormous. Routine manufacturing jobs are gone. Counselors must be aware of a particular client's economic needs and the job benefits. The restructuring of industry means little, if any, job security; therefore, clients must expect frequent job change and fierce competition when seeking new jobs. Multiple skills are needed. A rehabilitation client must know how to look for a job and how to cope with job loss and extended periods of unemployment. Advice will be needed on the seeking of a second job, most likely part-time and with limited benefits. Personal flexibility and adaptive skills are needed particularly in those individuals with disabilities.

These new views of today's work are needed by the OH professional because it is often he or she who assists in the placement effort and who can suggest the mode of reasonable accommodation. Prejudice against job applicants has not disappeared even though ADA's intent was to see full utilization of persons with impairments. What will be most difficult in this service society, where learning and relearning skills are mandatory, is the placement of those with prior learning difficulties, current learning disabilities, mental health problems, and family obligations, and those who are lacking educational resources in the community and job choice. The OHS can be of distinct aid in working with community rehabilitation counselors in familiarizing them with the vagaries and the chameleon characteristics of today's workplace, as individuals with disabilities are referred to industry.

## THE CONTEMPORARY SCENE

Many other potential influences on the in-plant facility require noting, in the areas of demands on the staff and the needs for additional skills. Medicine is being reshaped by increased organizational control, as noted in some detail above, which has led to conflict (117), and the threat of rationing of medical care will surely lead to heated discussion at all legislative levels (118). These changes may increase the workload of OHS staff.

The rise of the occupational health nurse (OHN) to positions of leadership in the delivery of in-plant care has been accelerated by both the economics as seen by employers and the paucity of trained occupational physicians (119). OHNs far outnumber other professionals serving in-plant care facilities.

Occupational physicians can be the target of lawsuits by the injured workers they treat, so they must minimize their personal liability for malpractice (120).

An issue somewhat beyond the control of the OHS but consistently vexing is certification for work, or absenteeism certification, as practiced by outside professionals (121,122). In most instances the individual certifying a return to work has little knowledge of the physical or emotional demands of the patient's job and thus renders judgments that are often based on biased descriptions offered by the recovering worker.

Of utmost importance to the physician who directs an OHS are management skills, and only recently has this element been added to curricula in occupational medicine (123,124). The medical director is a department head with the same organizational responsibilities as any other unit chief for planning, budget development, administration, personnel management, and the like. No longer can the physician rely on clinical capabilities alone. While they are used in the care of employees, they count little in the organization and operation of an in-plant service.

Other problems remain: the HIV-infection epidemic; the intrusion of legislators, rather than ergonomists, in attempted solution of difficulties with the ubiquitous video display terminal; the possible development and acceptance of a generic standard for exposure monitoring; hazardous waste management; and the preparation of business travelers for the hazards of assignment abroad, including terrorism.

To brighten the contemporary scene, however, new leadership in the U.S. Department of Labor in the mid-1990s strengthened the weakened Occupational Safety and Health Administration, resulting in increased citations for a broad variety of infractions of existing legislation, and with the assistance of concerned individuals and organizations, has been able to defeat destructive legislation proposed by uncaring members of Congress.

An OHS within a plant serves a mixed population of workers differing in origin, previous health care, job demands, age, gender, and perception of the work ethic. A sensitive professional staff can help managers accomplish the mission established by the organization, be it a service or product or a new truth in science. Such a goal can be accomplished only through dedication, responsibility, and commitment to quality preventive health care.

## REFERENCES


1. Occupational Safety and Health Act of 1970. Public Law 91-596, 91st Congress, S.2193, December 29, 1970, Sec. 6(b)(7).
2. Task Force Report: periodic (vs. annual health examination). *Can Med Assoc J* 1979;12:1193.
3. Couch MHA, ed. *Health assessment For adults.* North Ryde, Australia: CCH International, 1989;201.
4. Cox RAF, Edwards FC, McCallum RI, eds. *Fitness for work—the medical aspects,* 2nd ed. Oxford, England: Oxford University Press, 1995;9.
5. Energy Technology Committee of the American Occupational Medical Association. Guidelines for use of routine x-ray examinations in occupational medicine. *J Occup Med* 1979;21:500–502.
6. Andersson GBJ, Fine LJ, Silverstein PA. Musculoskeletal disorders. In: Levy BS, Wegman DH, eds. *Occupational health—recognizing and preventing work-related disease,* 3rd ed. Boston: Little, Brown, 1995;455–487.
7. Centers for Disease Control and Prevention. *Reported tuberculosis in the United States, 1995.* Atlanta: Centers for Disease Control and Prevention, 1996.
8. *Tuberculosis—costly and preventable cases continue in five cities.* Report #GAO/HEHS 95-11. Washington, DC: U.S.General Accounting Office, 1995.
9. Evens RG. Appropriateness of routine chest radiography. *JAMA* 1996; 275:326.
10. Felton JS, Voss H. Cardiopulmonary evaluation studies in an occupational health program. *J Occup Med* 1972;14:552–555.
11. Occupational safety and health standards for general industry. Vinyl Chloride 29 CFR 1910 §1910.1017(k), 1995.
12. National Institute for Occupational Safety and Health. *Criteria for a recommended standard—occupational exposure to beryllium.* DHEW (NIOSH) publication HSM 72-10268. Washington, DC: U.S. Department of Health, Education, and Welfare, 1972.
13. Felton JS, Swinger H. Mental health outreach of an occupational health service in a government setting. *Am J Public Health* 1973;63: 1058–1063.
14. Pilling K. EAPs—occupational health on the chEAP? *Occup Med (Oxf)* 1993;43:119–120.
15. Amarol TM. EAP utilization rates. *Employee Assistance* 1996;8:27–30.
16. Matsuno K. The treatment of hydrofluoric acid burns. *Occup Med (Oxf)* 1996;46:313–317.
17. Connor E. Online with physicians assessing the Internet. *JAMA* 1996; 276:1218.
18. Occupational Safety and Health Standards. *Lead.* 29 CFR 1910 §1910.1025, (n)(1)(iii) and (iv).
19. Occupational Safety and Health Standards. *Cotton dust.* 29 CFR 1910 §1910.1043, (k)(1–4).
20. Occupational Safety and Health Standards. *Access to employee exposure and medical records.* 29 CFR 1910 §1910.1020.
21. Langlieb AM, Soman S. A review of Harris LM, ed. *Health and the new media:* technologies transforming personal and *public health.* Rahway, NJ: Laurence Erlbaum Associates, 1995. *JAMA* 1996;275:1932.
22. Reilly FW. *Benefits and barriers to automated medical records.* Testimony before the Committee on Governmental Affairs, U.S. Senate. Report #GAO/Y-AIMD-94-117. Washington, DC: U.S. General Accounting Office, 1994.
23. Toward an electronic patient record '95. *Proceedings of Eleventh International Symposium on the Creation of Electronic Health Records Systems and Global Conference on Patient Cards,* March 14–19, 1995. Disney's Contemporary Resort, Orlando, Florida. Newton, MA: Medical Records Institute, 1995.
24. Burstein TL. Challenges in conforming a diverse patient record to a structured database—lessons in compromising. In: Toward an electronic patient record '95. *Proceedings of Eleventh International Symposium on the Creation of Electronic Health Records Systems and Global Conference on Patient Cards,* March 14–19, 1995. Disney's Contemporary Resort, Orlando, Florida. Newton, MA: Medical Records Institute, 1995;325–327.
25. Waegemann CP. The electronic medical record as the basis for integrated delivery systems. In: Toward an electronic patient record '95. *Proceedings of Eleventh International Symposium on the Creation of Electronic Health Records Systems and Global Conference on Patient Cards,* March 14–19, 1995. Disney's Contemporary Resort, Orlando, Florida. Newton, MA: Medical Records Institute, 1995; 53–61.
26. Williams JG. Capturing clinical data: the importance of the clinical interface. In: Toward an electronic patient record '95. *Proceedings of Eleventh International Symposium on the Creation of Electronic Health Records Systems and Global Conference on Patient Cards,* March 14–19, 1995. Disney's Contemporary Resort, Orlando, Florida. Newton, MA: Medical Records Institute, 1995;307–309.
27. Rischitelli DG. The confidentiality of medical information in the workplace. *J Occup Environ Med* 1995;37:583–596.
28. Smith JF. Occupational medical records. *AAOHN J* 1994;42:18–22.
29. Marwick C. Increasing use of computerized recordkeeping leads to legislative proposal for medical privacy. *JAMA* 1996;276:270,272.
30. Lyon M, Martin JB. Automating occupational protection records systems. Appl Occup Environ Hyg 1996;11:377.
31. Occupational Safety and Health Act of 1970. Public Law 91-596, 91st Congress, S.2193, December 29, 1970, Sec. 21(c)(1).
32. Tepper LB. The right to know; the duty to inform. *J Occup Med* 1980; 22:433.
33. Occupational Safety and Health Standards. *Hazard communication* 29 CFR 1910 §1910.1200; see also *Chemical hazard communication,* OSHA 3084, and *Hazard communication guidelines for compliance.* OSHA 3111. Washington, DC: U.S. Department of Labor, Occupational Safety and Health Administration, 1995.
34. *Consumer health informatics—emerging issues.* Report to the chairman, Subcommittee on Human Resources and Intergovernmental Relations, House Committee on Government Reform and Oversight. Report #GAO/AIMO-96-86. Washington, DC: U.S. General Accounting Office, July 26, 1996.
35. Taylor PT. *Consumer health informatics—emerging issues.* Testimony before the Subcommittee on Human Resources and Intergovernmental Relations, Committee on Government Reform and Oversight, PH. Report #GAO/T-AIMD-96-134. Washington, DC: U.S. General Accounting Office, July 26, 1996.
36. Wiatrowski WJ. Small businesses and their employees. *Monthly Labor Rev* 1994;117:29–35.
37. *OSHA handbook for small businesses,* revised. OSHA 3209. Washington, DC: U.S. Department of Labor, Occupational Safety and Health Administration, 1990.
38. *OSHA help for new businesses.* Fact Sheet No. OSHA 91-43. Washington, DC: U.S. Department of Labor, Occupational Safety and Health Administration, 1991.
39. Felton JS. How the occupational physician works with the unions. *Occup Med (Oxf)* 1997;47:117–119.
40. *The organization and operation of clinic-based occupational medical programs.* Postgraduate Seminar #8. American Occupational health Conference, San Antonio, TX, April 29, 1996.
41. *Update for clinic-based occupational medicine programs.* Postgraduate Seminar, #14. American Occupational Health Conference, San Antonio, TX, April 29, 1996.
42. *The strategic management of occupational health services.* Postgraduate Seminar #18. American Occupational Health Conference, San Antonio, TX, April 29, 1996.
43. Widtfeldt AK, Widtfeldt JR. Total quality management in American industry. *AAOHN J* 1992;40:311.
44. Toynbee A. *Lectures on the Industrial Revolution in England.* London, Rivingtons, 1884.
45. Taylor FW. *Scientific management.* New York: Harper & Row, 1947.
46. Kakar S. *Frederick Taylor:* a study in personality and innovation. Cambridge, MA: MIT Press, 1970.
47. Gilbreth FB. *Motion study.* New York: Van Nostrand, 1911.
48. Bloomfield M. Preventive management: the next step in industrial relations. In: Elkind HB, ed. *Preventive management:* mental hygiene in industry. New York, B.C. Forbes, 1931.
49. Roughton J. Integrating a total quality management system into safety and health programs. *Profess Safety* 1993(June);32.
50. *Merriam-Webster's collegiate dictionary,* 10th ed. Springfield, MA: Merriam Webster, 1993;842.
51. El-Ahraf A, Gray D, Maguib H. Partners for quality in a university setting: California State University-Dominguez Hills and Xerox Corpo-

ration. In: Hoffman AM, Julius D, eds. *Total quality management:* implications for higher education. Maryville, MO: Prescott, 1995; 164–195.
52. Rooney E. TQM/CQI in business and health care. *AAOHN J* 1992;40: 319.
53. Widtfeldt AK. Quality and quality improvement. *AAOHN J* 1992;40: 326.
54. Yarborough CM III. System for quality management. *J Occup Med* 1993;35:1096–1105.
55. Moser R Jr. Quality management in occupational and environmental health programs. *J Occup Med* 1993;35:1103–1105.
56. Weinstein MB. Improving safety programs through total quality. *Occup Hazards* 1996;58:42–46.
57. Pritham CH. Quality improvement process/outcomes research. *J Rehab Res Dev* 1996:33:vii–viii.
58. Pierce FD. *Total quality for safety and health professionals.* Rockville, MD: Government Institutes, 1995.
59. *World almanac and book of facts 1995.* Rahway, NJ: World Almanac (Funk & Wagnalls), 1994;385.
60. *Worker displacement during the early 1990s.* USDL 94-434. Washington, DC: U.S. Department of Labor, Bureau of Labor Statistics, News, September 14, 1994;1.
61. Putsch RW III. Cross-cultural communication—the special case of interpreters in health care. *JAMA* 1985;254:3344–3348.
62. Mead M. *Cultural patterns and technical change.* New York: Mentor, 1955;289.
63. Locke DC. *Increasing multicultural understanding.* Newbury Park, CA: Sage, 1992;115.
64. Anderson JN. Health and illness in Philippino immigrants. *West J Med* 1983;139:811–819.
65. Fitzpatrick-Nietschmann J. Pacific islanders—migration and health. *West J Med* 1983;139:848–853.
66. Lin T-Y. Psychiatry and Chinese culture. *West J Med* 1983;139: 862–867.
67. Gunby P. Computer-based medical translator system helps bridge language gap between physician, patient. *JAMA* 1995;274:1002–1004.
68. Hoang GN, Erickson RV. Guidelines for providing medical care to Southeast Asian refugees. *JAMA* 1982;248:710–714.
69. Goldsmith MF. Forgotten (almost) but not gone, tuberculosis suddenly looms large on domestic scene. *JAMA* 1990;264:1852–1886.
70. Strategic plan for the elimination of tuberculosis in the United States. *JAMA* 1989;261:2941–2942.
71. Paughan DM, White-Baughan J, Wong S. Posttraumatic stress disorder in Southeast Asian refugees. *West J Med* 1989;150:201.
72. Hamilton A. *Exploring the dangerous trades.* Boston: Little, Brown, 1943;70–72.
73. Public Law 100-690, Title V, Subtitle D; 41 U.S.C. 70, et seq.
74. Clark HW. The role of physicians as medical review officers in workplace drug testing programs. *West J Med* 1990;152:514–521.
75. Upfal MJ, Markell B. Training and proficiency in the medical review of job applicant drug screens. *J Occup Med* 1992;34:1189–1196.
76. Lewy RM. Pre-employment drug testing of house staff physicians at a large urban hospital. *Acad Med* 1991;66:618–619.
77. Lindseth PD, Lindseth G. Attitudes toward urinalysis drug testing within a civilian pilot training program. *Aviat Space Environ Med* 1995;66:837–840.
78. Morland J. Types of drug-testing programs in the workplace. *Bull Narc* 1993;45:85–113.
79. DuPont RL, Griffin DW, Siskin BR, Shiraki S, Katze E. Random drug tests at work: the probability of identifying frequent and infrequent users of illicit drugs. *J Addict Dis* 1995;14:1–17.
80. Hanson M. Overview on drug and alcohol testing in the workplace. *Bull Narc* 1993;45:3–44.
81. Levitt S. Department of Transportation 1995 Regulations for Alcohol Testing. *AAOHN J* 1996;44:139–140.
82. Cyster R, McEwen J. Alcohol problems at work: a new approach? *Public Health* 1988;102:373–379.
83. Schilling RF II, Gilchrist LD, Schinke SP. Smoking in the workplace: review of critical issues. *Public Health Rep* 1985;100:473–479.
84. Conrad KM, Blue CL. Physical fitness and employee absenteeism-measurement considerations for programs. *AAOHN J* 1995;43:577–587.
85. Conrad P. Who comes to worksite wellness programs? A preliminary review. *J Occup Med* 1987;29:317–320.
86. Keeler EB, Manning WG, Newhouse JP, Sloss EM, Wasserman J. The external costs of a sedentary lifestyle. *Am J Public Health* 1989;79: 995–981.
87. Anspaugh DJ, Hunter S, Mosley J. The economic impact of corporate wellness programs—past and future considerations. *AAOHN J* 1995; 43:203–210.
88. Helmer DC, Dunn LM, Eaton K, Macedonio C, Lubritz L. Implementing corporate wellness programs—a business approach to program planning. *AAOHN J* 1995;43:558–563.
89. Foran M, Campanelli LC. Health promotion communications system—a model for a dispersed population. *AAOHN J* 1995;43:564–569.
90. Saphire LS. Comprehensive health promotion—opportunities for demonstrating value added to the business. *AAOHN J* 1995;570–573.
91. Stokols D, Pellatier KR, Fielding JE. Integration of medical care and worksite health promotion. *JAMA* 1995;273:1136–1142.
92. Institute of Medicine, National Academy of Sciences. *Role of the primary care physician in occupational and environmental medicine.* Washington, DC: National Academy Press, 1988.
93. *Role of internist in occupational medicine.* Philadelphia: American College of Physicians; and Washington, DC: Department of Health and Public Policy; 1984:1.
94. Council on Long-Range Planning and Development of the American Medical Association. The future of general internal medicine. *JAMA* 1989:262:2119–2124.
95. Freund E, Seligman PJ, Chorba TL, Safford SK, Drachman JG, Hull HF. Mandatory reporting of occupational diseases by clinicians. *JAMA* 1989;262:3041–3044.
96. Fried RA. The family physician looks at occupational health information. *Am J Prev Med* 1987;3:110–115.
97. Glick JA. The occupational physician and the community physician: a team? *Del Med J* 1986;58:185–187.
98. Kottke TE. A strategy to define the role of the primary care physician in occupational and environmental medicine. *J Gen Intern Med* 1989; 4:320–324.
99. Rountree P, Fields MR, Coleman MA. Occupational medicine: a challenge for the primary care physician. *J Arkansas Med Soc* 1989;86: 243–246.
100. Ellwood PM Jr, Lunaberg GD. Managed care—a work in progress. *JAMA* 1996;276:1083–1086.
101. Showstack J, Lurie N, Leatherman S, Fisher E, Inui T. Health of the public—the private-sector challenge. *JAMA* 1996;276:1071–1074.
102. Tranquada RE. Health care crisis from a trauma center perspective. *JAMA* 1996;276:940–946.
103. *Request for proposal for a free-standing course in managed care's impact on occupational medicine.* Arlington Heights, IL: American College of Occupational and Environmental Medicine, 1996.
104. Wilson CB. Survival by merger—what will it take for academic medical centers to survive in the managed-care marketplace? *Stanford Med* 1996;13:31–32.
105. Mattix H. Managed care and residence training. *JAMA* 1996;276: 109–126.
106. Fowles JB, Weiner JP, Knutson D, Fowler E, Tucker AM, Ireland M. Taking health status into account when setting capitation rates. *JAMA* 1996;276:1316–1321.
107. Bodenheimer TS, Grumbach K. Capitation or decapitation—keeping your head in changing times. *JAMA* 1996;276:1025–1031.
108. Burgel BJ. Primary care at the worksite. *AAOHN J* 1996;44:238–242.
109. Shore M. cited in Daiker B. Managed care in workers' compensation—analysis of cost drivers and vendor selection. *AAOHN J* 1995; 43:422–427.
110. Workers' Comp Update. *Saf Health* 1995;152:26–27.
111. Moore CE. International occupational health care. *J Occup Med* 1994;36:419–427.
112. Fleming LE, Herzstein J, Bunn WB III, eds. *Issues in international occupational and environmental medicine.* Beverly Farms, MA: OEM Press, 1979, in press.
113. Hathaway JA. Medical programs for multiple domestic sites. *J Occup Med* 1994;36:428–433.
114. Phillips DF. Physicians put promise of telemedicine to the test: reports from rural practitioners, anesthesiologists. *JAMA* 1996;276: 267–268.
115. Koop CE. Cited in Skolnick AA. Experts explore emerging information technologies' effects on medicine. *JAMA* 1996;275:669–670.
116. Ryan CP. Work isn't what it used to be: implications, recommendations, and strategies for vocational rehabilitation. *J Rehabil* 1995;61:8–15.

117. Burchell RC, White RE, Smith HL, Piland NF. Physicians and the organizational evolution of medicine. *JAMA* 1988:260:826–831.
118. Drexler M. Medical-care rationing may be in America's future. *San Francisco Chronicle* 1990(August 2):A25.
119. Wachs JE, Parker-Conrad JE. Occupational health nursing in 1990 and the coming decade. *Appl Occup Environ Hyg* 1990;4:200–204.
120. Postal LP. Suing the doctor: lawsuits by injured workers against the occupational physician. *J Occup Med* 1989:31-891–896.
121. Holleman WL, Holleman MC. School and work release evaluation. *JAMA* 1988;260:3629–3634.
122. Mayhew HE. Nordlund DJ. Absenteeism certification: the physician's role. *J Fam Pract* 1988;6:651–655.
123. Cordes DH, Rea DF, Vuturo A, Rea J. Management roles for physicians: training residents for the reality. *J Occup Med* 1988;30:863–867.
124. Fallon LF Jr, Brandt-Rauf PW. An overview of management. *Occup Med* 1989:1–10.
125. Management schools make environment part of their business. *Chemecology* 1996;25:4–5.
126. Persival L, Quaker SB, Lamm SH, et al. A case study of dermatitis based on a collaborative approach between occupational physicians and industrial hygienists. *Am Ind Hyg Assoc J* 1995;56:184–188.
127. Canadian Task Force on the Periodic Health Examination. *Clinical preventive health care.* Ottawa: Canada Communication Group, 1994.
128. Beall T. When disaster strikes—ready or not? *California Physician* 1995;12:26–32.
129. Peterson KW, David LF, eds. *Directory of Occupational Health & Safety Software*, Version 9.0. ISBN 1-885190-03-4. Charlottesville, WA: Occupational Health Strategies, 1996.
130. Pisaniello D, Brooks B. The Internet and OHS. Part 1: overview and users prospective. *J Occup Health Safety Aust NZ* 1995;11: 467–470; Part 2. OHS-related Internet tools and resources. *J Occup Health Safety Aust NZ* 1995;11:601–606; Part 3. Networking the global OHS community. *J Occup Health Safety Aust NZ* 1996; 12:25–30.
131. Richmond JB, Fein R. The health care mess—a bit of history. *JAMA* 1995;273:69–71.
132. Badawy MK. *Developing managerial skills in engineers and scientists:* succeeding as a technical manager, 2nd ed. New York: Van Nostrand Reinhold, 1995.
133. Leopold RS. *The 1997 OEM Internet companion.* Beverly Farms, MA: OEM Press, 1997.
134. McCunney RJ, ed. *A practical approach to occupational and environmental medicine,* 2nd ed. Boston: Little, Brown, 1994.

*Environmental and Occupational Medicine, Third Edition*, edited by William N. Rom.
Lippincott–Raven Publishers, Philadelphia © 1998.

CHAPTER 135

# On the Ethical Practice of Environmental and Occupational Medicine

Sheldon Wilfred Samuels

## PURPOSE AND HISTORY

This chapter discusses the intertwined traditions in the social and intellectual history of medicine and philosophy that are critical to understanding ethical issues in occupational and environmental medical practice and research. Understanding these patterns of thought enables the reader to address moral issues. The objective is to reduce dependence on others and avoid a repetition of centuries of agonizing discovery. The physician's own discovery of how to judge what is moral and what is not, and the resulting confidence in recognizing the ethical choice and doing "the right thing," is of paramount importance. For this purpose, the references not only lend weight to the author's arguments, but more importantly should be read to be fully appreciated for their relevance.

This chapter also presents a time-tested rational framework—a model similar to traditional medical practice—within which the author's conclusions on what is ethical can be used to challenge and test the reader's own discoveries. The emotions explicit and implicit in the rhetoric with which these conclusions are expressed are drawn from his own discoveries. They are part of what the author believes is true, as well as an attempt to persuade. Rhetoric is part of the dialectic of discovery. It moves us to open the doors of our minds, and sets the pace at which we progress. But neither the framework nor the conclusions can escape the ultimate test, the test of fruitfulness.

Discovering for oneself the "right thing" is difficult. Acting upon this discovery is more difficult. It is often painful and unsuccessful, especially when action must be taken alone. While we should seek the support of others and seek consensus and professional solidarity, none of us can lean only upon these often hollow and sometimes rotted reeds.

It is easier to do the right thing now than it was in the past. All the negative aspects of the history of industrial medicine are unlikely to be repeated.

## UNDERSTANDING ETHICS: THE SCIENCE OF "OUGHT"

Some philosophers conclude that ethics, the discipline that should prescribe how we or our institutions ought to act, is based on the world as we might find it. In this case, ethics would be an empirical science.

Others believe that the *ought* is not necessarily derived from a description of what is, leaving a gap in the process of discovery that must be bridged either by operational assumptions, or requires rational dialectic. In this case, ethics would be a theoretical science.

In either case, how certain and objective are the findings? We begin to answer the question by rejecting the historically persistent myth that rules of clear thinking associated with scientific endeavors must be abandoned in dealing with issues of moral and social value. Nor can ethics exist separate from our niche-view: the total of our views on the scientific and moral nature and purpose, if any, of the human niche, as developed in our lives and in lives past. That total governs how we perceive ethical issues. Nor can it be understood apart from logics that

S. W. Samuels: Ramazzini Institute for Occupational and Environmental Health Research, Solomons Island, Maryland 20688.

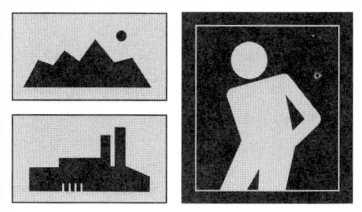

guide the construction and application of systems of ethics. Yet we are not required to answer all the questions philosophers have asked for the past 3,000 years prior to making a judgment. The totality of the historic experience provides a basis for our assumptions, the analysis of which may be productive.

In this discussion, the poet's observation is not necessarily less concrete or objective than an observation based on the measures of the scientist, for while quantification enables precision, precision is not the same as certainty or objectivity. It is the utopian poet-philosopher who has given us the key to the conceptual framework by which science approaches certainty and objectivity: the axiomatic method, or the use of those postulated schemes called "models."

The optimistic worlds of "as if," the systems of hypotheses, have never been restricted to poets. The same axiomatic method has been used in medical practice, from the time of the physicians of Cos to the theoretical biologists and the current practitioners of quantitative risk assessment. An early observer of the use of models in medical practice, Aristotle (1), stated, "The physician ... sets about his work ... by forming for himself a definite picture ... of health ... and this he holds forward as the reason and explanation of each subsequent step he takes."

Yet the system need not appear like an exercise of Euclid, or bear the straitjacket forms and special language of mathematics and symbolic logic. We can use simple, clear exposition to postulate empirical information, or postulate presumptions about the empirical. This takes two forms: observations that presume that we correctly perceive the world as it is, and presumptions that make no pretense of reality (but permit us to act as if fact is established).

Presumptions bridge gaps in knowledge, systematize our experience, and are retained only as long as they are valuable (heuristic). Most important of all, this basic construct of clear thinking permits us to act without solving in advance recurring issues that defy certainty and objectivity. The predicted or experienced consequences of the chosen action, not its presumptions, test its value (2).

Ethical models are not essentially different from the models of medical practice. Consequences we think are good (have moral value), true (have scientific value), and passionate (have aesthetic value) are separable as thoughts and distinctly understood. But when brought into being, they are integrated by the creative action itself, although in that process passion does not always yield pleasure, truth does not always flow from logic or consistency, and actions believed good are not always what we ought to do. Intuition and reason, even strict deduction and calculation, do not always result in certainty or objectivity.

Systems of ethical axioms, to be useful, must in the first steps in their construction presume ethical principles in which we have confidence, and touch a relevant portion of the empirical universe of *as is, to be more than a game.*

*What is an ethical principle? We begin to find the answer by looking to people and their institutions, where the identity, confidence, and relevance of our principles will be tested.*

## WHO IS JUDGED?

The literature purporting to describe or prescribe an ethical basis for the behavior of the physician and allied practitioners often confuses the individual and an organization or treats them the same. Corporations, unions, trade associations, and professional societies differ from each other and from the individual member (who, in fact, may participate in such social structures simultaneously). What generally is not understood is that the differences are reflected in the moral collectiveness of their actions, even in the possibility that an act can be judged morally as group or personal behavior.

For example, a body such as a corporation is per se only a form. Forms are not morally responsible. Such bodies become morally responsible in the unlikely event that every member freely, rationally, and equally determines actions taken in the name of the form. Only actual or potential decision makers are morally responsible. Moral judgments apply to the judgments of a society—its individuals—rather than its forms. Individuals, separately or collectively, act and make decisions. Institutions may crystallize, structurally incorporate, and impose these acts and decisions as part of a system of mores. However, mores are not generated in a structureless void.

If the mores are to be consistent with a system of morals, the enforcing institutions must often themselves be changed. This change has more than one source, but the constant dialectic between the individual and his/her institution is a very effective source of change. Failure to act to effect change may be an immoral omission when participation in decision making is possible.

There is a lesson in ancient philosophy lost in the modern quest for understanding what is and what is not ethical. In *The Republic,* Plato reminds us that there is an organic relationship between individual behavior and the character of the institution or social structure in which the behavior takes place: "And must not the tyrannical man be like the tyrannical state and the democratical man like the democratical state?" asked Socrates (3).

What Plato tells us is that the organic relationship means, that, in a sense, the reality of the social system is seen in the mirror of the individual, and vice versa. But is it what we ought to see? That is the question of ethics. Does the system of social mores determine right and wrong?

Relative ethics tells us that it does, and that as the system changes, whatever recrystallization of mores may result, so does what is morally acceptable change.

The application of this view to occupational and environmental medicine, to the question of who should live and who should die in our attempt to manage the risks of an industrial society, has its own language: cost-benefit analysis, socially acceptable risk, hazard pay, market regulation, risk perception modification, accident-prone workers. This language does not upset most of us. Most of us do not understand that its moral grammar is shared with totalitarianism, collectivism, and cannibalism. For some, this language expresses the politically correct ideas of leaders in occupational and environmental health policy. For others, it is a system rejected by its own consequences.

Whether we subscribe to this view or not, it is a matter of observation that moral judgments draw on ethical principles that guide the behavior and mold the value systems of different people. Every culture has shared moral forces, because it needs them. In every human society the morally good is not derived from solipsistic passion and impulse that would negate social control of behavior and negate the survival of society itself.

Are these principles mere ethnocentricities? Or is there another, more fundamental source of standards not relative to a given culture or set of cultures at a given time? Are there no absolute standards?

There is more than one possible culture and, therefore, more than one set of ethical axioms. Biologically, however, there is only one kind of man and woman: human. To determine which set of ethical axioms will best preserve human life does not require us to go beyond deciding which have been more successful in this regard. The preservation of life is, then, an absolute standard that transcends cultural change.

## THE ALTERNATIVE TO RELATIVISM

The alternative to ethical relativism, to seek some criterion outside of the cultural context from which to judge the individual's activity and the social system itself, is seen in nature. We may see either a positive and bullish response to the need to live or a negative and bearish response that may incompletely—and therefore incorrectly—characterize the state of nature (i.e., survival of the fittest). Whether what we see in nature is the pseudo-Darwinistic myth of the jungle, or another selection and interpretation of the same data (i.e., survival of the fit) that may also be incomplete, both hypotheses are scientifically (but not both morally) defensible.

Our initial moral refraction biases the selection of the hypothesis. The *ought* is not simply derived from the *is*. Rather, our interpretation of the *is* reflects a polarization in philosophic outlook that at any given time essentially determines the ought. The identification of presumably absolute, objective generic criteria, such as the needs for life, are easily obscured by the current moral condition of the observer. Nevertheless, a dialectic version of this method or dialectic methods dependent on reason alone may permit us to avoid the issue of cultural relativity.

If ethical questions must be answered in terms of currently prevailing mores, moral uncertainty generated by the shifting position of relativism will yield uncertain and shifting answers. Answers based on unchanging ethical values are more likely to be morally certain. But historic, unresolved conflicts between those who take an absolutist view and those who take a relativist view of ethical values (and within each camp) make it difficult—but not impossible—to construct an operative set of prescriptions or ethical axioms from which morally certain behavior can be derived.

Relativistic uncertainty is typified by the perception that preferences or ethical opinions are problems solved by politics or war. If an ethical axiom is not dictated or politically compromised, according to this view, there is no way of reaching a conclusion. The rational alternative to the politics or war pessimism suggested here extends the concept of axiom so that it is used in the science of how we ought to behave in the same way we use it in other sciences.

Does this system work? It has worked in the past. There has been a steady if gradual expansion of the codes (systems of axioms) protecting human life, beginning with the family, clan, and tribe, extended to the ethnic and racial group, which now includes the heterogeneous nation and family of nations. Laws (systems of axioms) against the killing of "barbarians," extended to genocide, now include the worker, the worker's community, and even other species. While these constantly revised axiomatic systems are most apparent to us in the West, the same kind of cultural change is occurring throughout the world. This is because these changes are seen by the great masses, more importantly, by the peer group leaders of the great masses, to bear fruit in the protection of life, or what Schweitzer (4) and Goethe before him called reverence for life.

The progress of human society, perhaps more latent in some parts of the world than in others, is measured by the advance of absolute standards. Although formulated with less precision (but no less certainty and objectivity) than in some other sciences, axioms derived from these standards need not be obscure. No intervening deity, felicific calculus, or existential intuition is needed. While moral judgments are made in a specific cultural context and vary from other moral judgments on similar issues in another context, the ethical axioms that guide these judgments must and can have in common an historically justified transcendent, a universal source or need to be met, the achievement of which determines whether or not the axiom is fruitful: life preservation.

## THE EVOLUTION OF A NEW DISCIPLINE

An institutional expression of the expanding circle within which we preserve life is the rise of medical ethics or bioethics as a specialty of medicine. It is not regulated like cardiology or internal medicine. Admission to its professional organizations, none of which (interestingly) have a professional code of ethics, has few restrictions. It is, however, a discipline-in-the-making as professional and public expectations for virtue in public affairs rise to ever-higher levels. In the United States, besides the traditional medical school professorships in medical ethics, academic centers have been established to serve a growing employment market for ethicists. In conjunction with departments of philosophy, specialists are being trained in the counseling arts, law, and social sciences essential to the administration of codes of ethics (which increasingly take the form of laws and regulations for the protection of patients, research subjects, and practitioners).

For many, the rise of this new professional has become still another excuse for ignoring the obligation of each practitioner to understand the moral or immoral or amoral content of his or her own decisions. Admittedly, the case can be made that for most choices the ethical choice is clear. Society could not function at any level in its hierarchy without the bulk of our acts being consistent with some form of ethical behavior, whether by reason, education, imitation, regulation, or altruistic instinct. Most choices we make are relatively simple or require little examination. The complex situations with which we are continually confronted, while fewer, almost never yield simple choices, even when the medical judgments and the ethical questions are clear. Increasingly, referrals are made to ethicists specializing in the problems of medicine in much the same way patients or problems are referred to a medical specialty. This is a hazardous practice.

An ethicist can provide dialectical skills to help us maintain objectivity in our perception of the choices, to loosen the bonds of our emotions. The ethicist is seldom qualified to make the "right" decision for us, but should be able to challenge our ideas and motives, ask questions, impart understandings, make critical distinctions, and impose internal coherence and external applicability on our perceptions as a system.

None of us can understand everything, making the most effective process of ethical choice, as Bernard Gert (5) notes, an interdisciplinary team effort. Rarely are the requisite arts and sciences coupled in one person. Even the best-known medical ethicist, Hippocrates, sought help from outside his profession.

Born in 460 B.C., Hippocrates was a physician (who integrated environmental perspectives in his work) and a philosopher (who sought to understand how medicine ought to be practiced) (6). The code of ethics ascribed to him, embodied in the Hippocratic Oath, included the admonition that "whatever, in connection with my professional practice, or not in connection with it, I see or hear, in the life of men, which *ought* not be spoken of abroad, I will not divulge, reckoning that all such should be kept secret" (7).

The word *ought* implies a moral judgment to be made by the physician, not for the physician by an ethicist, regarding the confidentiality of patient information divulged under the cloak of the patient-physician relationship. Then, as now, physicians continuously make moral judgments in the practice of medicine through action or inaction, with knowledge or ignorance, willingly or not. Responsibility cannot be delegated, except when the physician fails to function qua physician, because of the high moral content of choices made in the normal practice of medicine.

To help him make such judgments, Hippocrates sought the guidance of a popular school of ethicists, the Sophists. His contemporary, Socrates (8) (born 469 B.C.), is said (by Plato) to have admonished him, "You are going to commit your soul to the care of a man whom you call a Sophist. And yet I hardly think that you know what a Sophist is; and, if not, then you do not know … whether (that) to which you commit yourself be good or evil."

This guidance is as useful today as it was 25 centuries ago to Hippocrates. But the warning about sophists needs to be addressed not only to the practitioner as an individual who must make a choice, but also to the community that would judge that choice. Assignment of primary responsibility for review of the judgment made, then as now, resided in the community of physicians. "He who … judges rightly will judge of the physician as a physician," enjoined Socrates (9). A generation later, a student in the Academy of Plato, Aristotle (10), clarified the advice: "The physician ought to be called to account by physicians."

## THE LADDER OF SOCIAL JUSTICE

A hierarchy for assigning responsibility has evolved, in which we are obligated to accept a level of responsibility determined by where we each stand on the ladder of social justice. This ladder has structured a process remarkably resilient from the priestly cults of pre-Hippocratic medicine to contemporary Western medicine.

The ladder helps us to decide who ought to meet a different and often conflicting range of needs—from the provision of family health care to safe tools and the design of a workstation—by helping us allocate moral responsibility. On this ladder, those most able to act are rationally obligated to rise to the highest rung of responsibility so that they may act first in pursuit of a moral objective. They are obligated to act before others, because they are best or uniquely able to do so. This does not mean that only they should act. When those with special obligations fail to act, or need assistance, the obligation falls on the shoulders of those on the next rung (11).

Thus, the responsibility to make a judgment traditionally is shared. A 15th-century code forbade the "physician to make a grave or even a qualified prognosis about his patient's disease without consultation with a colleague" (12). Both the physician and the community of physicians must know, then, what is believed, the niche-view, of those to whom they "commit their souls" when seeking assistance from those further down on the ladder on how to determine what is good or evil.

The ladder doesn't tell us how to act, a direction found in what we mean by rational. By rational, we mean an action that logically follows another. We also mean, Bernard Gert (13) teaches us, actions taken to avoid pain, disability, death, and loss of pleasure. Reason clearly is never passive. It appears to be an agent of life itself.

An application of the ladder is found in the axioms of the Occupational Safety and Health Act of 1970. The act provides "that employers and employees have separate but dependent responsibilities and rights with respect to achieving safe and healthful working conditions." An employee has a duty to comply with rules uniquely "applicable to his own actions and conduct." The employer has duties based on a unique ability to enable compliance with rules applicable to an entire workplace. Government has a separate duty based on its unique abilities, e.g., to mandate rules if reason fails.

In distributing our obligations on the ladder, we seldom use force. We make a judgment and argue for that choice. The method of that argument poses ethical problems of its own. Germaine Grisez (14) emphasizes that "the immorality of sophistic arguments includes that of deception, but (also) the additional immorality of miseducation," a frequent pitfall of specialists pressing for a course of action among those who do not share their special knowledge.

The pitfall is greater when the physician ventures into the broader community, especially when the argument becomes part of an adversarial process within an organization, in administrative hearings, or in the courts.

## THE NATURE OF CODES

If the physician needs a framework for making an ethical choice—a guide, a *code*—some care is justified in understanding what a code is. Whether based on rational analysis, a moral sense, or an intuition accreted from experience, the codes have been designed to protect not only the patient, but also the professional.

The 15th century code that enjoined the physician to consult with a colleague protected the physician as it did the patient. By the 15th century, the hospital and medical school environments fostered communities of physicians in which they could seek protection. Codes of ethics became an expression of community responsibility, but less so to society-at-large than to the subcommunity that is the profession.

In cultures of the East, social and religious sanctions, and to a lesser extent, the legal systems enforced professional behaviors consistent with Buddhist belief in the eight-fold path to righteous living, the fifth fold of which was righteous livelihood, or with Confucian traditions of professional responsibility (15). In such settings, the physician responded directly to the community-at-large (16).

In cultures of the West, the intervening profession organized the response to the community with a code of ethics devised to guide behavior. While they may be consistent with ethical principles, the codes are not the same as a system of ethics.

Often ethical codes are promulgated private extensions of our legal system. Yet they ought not be confused with laws, despite the fact that in the case of physicians and some other licensed professionals the codes may be given legal status enforceable by restrictions of practice.

On the one hand, immoral acts that these codes may proscribe need not be forbidden by law; nor is an act that is made illegal by these codes necessarily immoral. On the other hand, the acts such codes sanction are not necessarily moral, and the acts they would ban may be morally justified.

If there is such a tenuous relationship between such codes and our systems of law and ethics, why are they important? The codes reflect a crystallization of mores, which themselves can be judged by moral dicta now and used in evolving legal requirements. More, because the codes can be changed, they can be a meaningful tool in molding future professional group behavior, voluntary or mandatory, to become ethically consistent (e.g., consistent with an idea of the good society or the protection of life).

Even when not legally enforceable, the codes have become both an important mode of individual or group self-regulation and self-defense, not on the ends of medical practice, which are seldom questioned, but the heatedly debated means. In this debate, the separatist thesis is persistent: a positive answer to the question formulated by Alan Gewirth (17), "Does the professional's end of providing valued services justify his using *any* means positively related to his expertise?" If the answer is no, and we seek moral limits to the means that may used to attain the valued end, what are they?

Schuman (18), defending separatism, berates nonoccupational physicians when they perform occupational services and support ethical practices, such as those governing the traditional physician-patient relationship. "The time has come," he contends, when they must be guided by "the rules of the game." While limits to the means are arguable, the separatist thesis is irrational and therefore morally wrong, counters Gewirth (17), if "the actions in question … violate anyone's moral rights (except) to prevent infringements of (equal or) more important rights."

The traditional patient-physician relationship is based on rights of the patient seldom less important than any rights or obligation of the physician. Thus, correctly, the thesis has been abandoned as a formal policy by the professional organizations of occupational physicians. In practice, especially in the social allocation of historically persistent unnecessary risks and of efforts to ameliorate their effects, the thesis still lives as an artifact of an historically persistent caste system (19). The caste system is accepted as a norm and defended by sophistical pleas that confuse mores with morals and ideals with utopia.

## CODES AS SOCIAL THERAPY

Nearly a century ago, Emile Durkheim (20) described a social disease or systemic disorder: anomie. A symptom of this disease is the endemic community crisis in which organic relationships (such as patient-physician relationships) are not protected. Regulating professional behavior can correct anomie by restoring organic social solidarity.

How do we construct a regulatory code that is effective or practical for this purpose? Does being "practical" eliminate codes based on ethical principles, allegedly because they would be utopian and divorced from the real world?

Utopian worlds have utopian ideals. We need ideals for the world in which we live. A moral principle that is not practical is not a moral principle. There are not two realities, only one. If the ideal and the practical are bifurcated, then there is no possibility of an ethical code of behavior, since it would not be universally or always applicable. It would have little value in the real world. Professional behavior could never be judged morally with any degree of certainty.

Codes of professional conduct, as artifacts of a culture, may not reflect mores consistent with ethical standards. Codes typically assume, often falsely, that compliance defines ethical behavior. Most codes are constructed eclectically from a sense of what is right and wrong in actual practice and determined by consensus in a professional society.

Are codes constructed and determined in this fashion sufficient to guide courses of action that ought to prevail, as distinct from actions that do prevail? Or is a clear sense of what is ethical an essential, but frequently missing, element in its design?

For example, do these codes ethically resolve the role of the physician (or other practitioner) if, as Thomas Szasz proposed, he is merely "an agent of the party that pays him and thus controls him," even if that means, for example, an employer-dependent "obligation to truth telling"? (21). Can such a role be consistent with an ethical code?

A recent survey of the codes promulgated by the American Professional Associations for Physicians, Nurses, and Hygienists, and the International Commission on Occupation Health (18) shows widespread rejection of the Szasz position. But while words such as *inform, integrity,* and *ethical* are used extensively in all of them, the International Commission code specifically details what the physician is to tell both the patient and the physician's employer. Truth-telling itself is not fully addressed in any of the codes.

There are clinical situations in which telling a partial truth to a patient or a patient's family may be justified in order to allow hope or buffer despair, or even to protect the quality of life. The failure to fully disclose information in the workplace often has less benign causes, reflecting the caste system that blankets both the worker and the physician (corporate, union, government, or academic). But it is also a failure to understand or address critical ethical, legal, and social realities. This is most obvious in relation to pledges of confidentiality and the doctrine of voluntary informed consent.

All the codes encourage unjustified partial truth because they fail to deal with conflicts in protecting the confidentiality of data or records with the need to obey the law. They fail to specifically mandate that workers and others be told clearly and directly difficult-to-digest truths: unauthorized access to most personal, family, and medical information is not the critical issue. Authorized access through court, insurance company, and employer demands for access may result in employment, insurance, and workers' compensation discrimination.

Repeating the phrase "voluntary informed consent" in codes of ethics does not close the gap with reality.

## THE SOPHISTRY OF ASSUMED AUTONOMY

At the base of any decision is the ability to make a rational choice or exercise rationally the freedom to will and to act. Harald Ofstad (23) states the ethical consequence of our failure to provide for more than physical ability or freedom to act, to protect the voluntariness or autonomy of action: "Moral guilt can be attributed only to a person who had it in his power to act in an ethically better way than he did.... He must have committed the wrong act, and he must have had the power to act otherwise and he must believe that he has this power (or conversely) ... he did not believe that he lacked this power.

Aristotle (24) would not let us forget the key social issue of effective power: "Those things, then, are thought involuntary which take place under compulsion or owing to ignorance." But compulsion and ignorance are part of everyone's life. Thus the worker, patient, or research subject who signs such forms cannot necessarily be held responsible for any adverse consequence of the approval. As Beasley and Graber (25) point out, "Autonomy is clearly a notion that allows of gradation."

When no effective effort is made to ensure that the signatory understands what is being signed, or that family, legal advisor, or in-plant peer group or union, economic, and employer pressures that create compulsions that result in involuntary signatures are controlled, autonomy does not effectively exist. Consequent action in which autonomy is assumed is immoral. The moral mistake shifts from the signer to the solicitor!

Sophistry takes place in not recognizing the obvious: rational acts, as we claimed before, are not only logical, they are also actions taken to avoid pain, disability, loss of pleasure, and death. Also, the seldom qualified pronouncements ex cathedra by the guardians of the doctrine of voluntary informed consent lead us to forget that all our thoughts, passions, and actions are products of multiple vectors, of which those that might enable unconstrained action are few. Yet it does not follow that we ought always to act as if what Gewirth (15) calls "the thesis of hard determinism" is always the case, i.e., all events, including even the agent's own choices, are caused by choices beyond the agent's control.

There is almost always some degree of autonomy, but the semilogical fallacies in its discussion allow blame to fall not on the patient-subject or physician-researcher, but on a fictitious third agent: luck or chance. It is deterministic, but not "hard" determinism, to believe that chance never exists, although it may be heuristically assumed in the face of ignorance of causation. It is ironic that being called a determinist in the forums of the ethicists is tantamount to having one's parentage questioned. Yet this is the position taken by Newton, Einstein (26), Planck (27), Bernard (28), Darwin (29), Freud, and others more ancient, who have shaped our understanding of causation. Determinism is justifiably abhorrent only within the (equally abhorrent) single cause–single effect etiologic paradigm (as in genetic determinism) (30).

It is clear, however, that our developing open society frees us of fetters once important, but less important now. This has enhanced the potential to be free, not freed us totally. Nevertheless, it is often heuristic to act as if autonomy exists when it has been protected.

The ethically responsive action when consent is sought is to mandate analysis of the context in which it is sought, and to devise and apply methods from this analysis that enhance both the voluntariness and informativeness of the effort. This means three safeguards must be in place:

1. Protection for those who might refuse consent (such as confidentiality of the solicitation itself, private or in-home solicitation) and use of agents other than those of the government, investigative agency, employer, or union.
2. Effective efforts to educate, not just the paragraph or two of jargon and promises that cannot be kept, which characterizes most efforts to inform the prospective subject.
3. Oversight of the process through a community or other relatively neutral structure not associated with the workplace, the physician, or the sponsoring institution.

These are also safeguards against conflicts of interest.

## BALANCING INTERESTS

Ethical behavior balances human emotions to achieve a state of equity between competing interests. The emotions we seek to mediate are often rooted in the domestic and social economies. Economics measures emotional behavior in a marketplace, but other sets of emotions are in play on another stage. There are social and ethical risks to the mediation of emotions inherent in conflicts of interest that occur when we participate in two or more groups, or represent two or more interests, that cannot share an identical set of perspectives. The conflict impairs judgment and constrains freedom of action.

Judgment is never fully objective, that is, absolute or isolatable. Judgment can never be value-free (lose social context) or detached from either the judge or the object. It is always relative to (a) the group with which we most identify (thus the secondary group is always the lesser served) and (b) the distance or detachment we are able to construct for the purposes of maximizing a "cold" gaze on the choice before us.

Conflicts of interest result in a loss of freedom to act by the group itself, since we are always bound to affect in some way or to some degree the decisions of a group in which we participate either as an observer or decision maker. There are no passive bystanders or observers in the dynamics of a group. In a kind of Heisenberg effect, we change the group just by watching and change it more when our response to what is observed is anticipated (correctly or incorrectly) even by acting as if we are just blotting papers.

The risk of dual involvement is ethical only if it is necessary to protect the well-being of the greater community or is culturally impacted and very difficult to eliminate, and another risk with a higher priority would clearly result by failure to take the risk of dual involvement.

Conflicting interests may consciously and ethically be structured or included, for example in a governing body, to ensure representation of these interests in policy making. Often, however, recusal is a remedy in cases when the conditions of ethical risk are not present.

Conflicts of interest and truncated autonomy are central not only to issues of confidentiality and other patient or research subject rights. They are important in the personal dilemmas of the physician in which the professional's freedom of will is the issue, not his moral conduct.

A study by the Conference Board (31) found that many corporate physicians are troubled by "insufficient management interest in employee health and health care programs and by insensitivity to ethical standards." These physicians specifically charged that management demanded breaches of confidentiality and classification of occupational disease as nonoccupational, and withheld from them information on work environment hazards.

When the patient is an institution, e.g., a government, corporation, or union, do all the rights of the patient extend to that institution? If the physician is to function as a physician, the answer may be no. Rights imply obligations. As we have claimed before, an institution may only be an empty form without moral responsibility and, therefore, no rights. Laws to the contrary notwithstanding, a degree in medicine does not automatically confer the rights of a physician. If a physician is unable to make ethical decisions, then he or she is not a physician and is unable to claim a patient–physician relationship with the institution.

## THE ETHICS OF GENETIC TESTING

An issue often discussed in environmental and occupational medicine is genetic testing, which will increasingly become a mainstay of medicine, beyond its original function in the diagnosis of genetically based disease. It has become integral to wellness programs and risk assessment for regulatory purposes. Information once gathered through family histories is being supplemented by genetic testing.

The Centers for Disease Control and Prevention (CDC) already is focusing its efforts through state health departments on preventing disease, disability, and death among workers and others with specific genotypes through medical, behavioral, and environmental interventions. The CDC has devised methods for targeting specific genetic risk factors (32).

The list of genetic differences with impacts associated with specific environments, but which may be neither the necessary nor sufficient cause of disease (such as G6PD deficiency), is rapidly growing. While the number of workers is small in percentile terms for each marker, the total number of workers being identified as susceptible to an environmentally evoked disorder or disease is large and growing larger. This compounds the problem of equitably distributing the burden of risk and control.

Fortunately, there is a long history of dealing with the pertinent issues in medical ethics. Unfortunately, these issues can be only partially resolved without legislation. Genetic testing—if regulated only by the existing informed consent, confidentiality, discrimination, and privacy laws and codes—poses the greatest threat to an open society that has ever emanated from a technology (15). It is clear that its abuse cannot be separated from the mercantilism that dominates wellness programs and the failure to legislate new approaches to insuring health care, workers' compensation, disability, and rehabilitation.

Absent legislation, the key protection in place is the traditional patient-physician relationship. This safeguard has grown from the life-preserving needs of the patient. Altering the relationship, characterized chiefly by confidentiality and patient advocacy, may put life itself at risk. The Hippocratic code and tradition, which extends this relationship to the community, is justified by the need to preserve the life of others as well as that of the patient. The right of the patient and the community to expect a protected patient-physician relationship is paralleled by an obligation not only to protect privacy but also to affirmatively provide information needed by the patient and the community.

Conflict with the right to privacy may arise in the right of society (including employers) to gain access to information useful in protecting societal needs, some of which are economic, legal, and public health needs. The conflict is recognized in an associated controversy: the rights to know health status, ambient and workplace exposures, the effects of exposures, and control measures. Clearly, the right of access by all parties to environmental data and records must be fully protected, since they may provide information essential to decisions that may reduce risk and thus preserve life.

The right of access is always qualified; while the records and data may have information important to the protection of other lives, the same information may be used inappropriately (e.g., ignoring scientific uncertainties in dose reconstruction, misinterpreting genotypic expression, and understating the role of environment in phenotypic expression) or for discrimination. The potential for abuse in job discrimination and social degradation warrants special regulatory measures to protect privacy while at the same time enabling research and high-risk management. Thus, a need to know must be decided (by a neutral body) on a case-by-case basis in which the motives, use, level of understanding, and capacity to do harm qualifies the right of access.

## ETHICS AND RESEARCH

With genetic testing increasingly common in research, there is renewed attention to the protection of research subjects. Fortunately, there is a well-defined body of guidelines and rules for researchers. Unfortunately, the guides and rules are not consistent with each other, let alone with ethical principles.

Prevailing government policy on ethical issues in their protection is based on the Belmont Report of the National Commission for the Protection of Human Subjects of Biomedical and Behavioral Research, published in 1979 (33). This report was intended to provide a practical ethical basis for the Common Rule for the protection of research subjects adopted by 16 federal agencies on June 11, 1991 (34).

The Belmont Report ably and clearly applies principles of ethics by three interrelated mechanisms: informed consent, risk/benefit assessment, and the selection of subjects for research. Of these three, the informed consent mechanism and its administration is most critical, since it shapes the response to the other two in regard to the key ethical principle of autonomy. The report restated this principle for use as an ethical standard: "To give weight to autonomous persons' considered opinions and choices [is to respect autonomy].... Voluntariness decides the validity of informed consent, requiring conditions free of coercion and undue influence.... Unjustifiable pressures usually occur when persons [are] in positions of authority ... especially where possible sanctions are involved."

The Common Rule requires protection for vulnerable populations. However, this protection does not include populations vulnerable because of coercive relationships in the workplace. While community representatives are required members of the institutional review boards charged with enforcing these protections, this generally has not resulted in membership for representatives of the worker or the worker's family or peer group, who would be knowledgeable about the the realities of "voluntary" consent. Thus the Common Rule fails the standard of the Belmont Report.

Government policy on tissue collection and storage for genetic research is guided by a supposedly "unofficial" document: The Consensus Statement on informed consent developed by the National Institutes for Health and the Centers for Disease Control and Prevention (35). The Belmont Report is at variance with this policy. The consensus statement fails to meet the Belmont standard, since it, too, fails to take into consideration coercive economic and social influences (e.g., consent as a condition of employment or insurance).

Neither the Common Rule nor the consensus statement prohibits the withholding of obvious truths that must be made known to the subject (e.g., confidentiality can never be guaranteed in the face of court-ordered discovery or public health needs).

Neither adequately addresses the need for specific protections in health care insurance and employment discrimination, or the need for controlling the environmental factors in phenotypic expression. Neither provides clear guidance in the workplace setting for the institutions on which the existing system of protections are constructed: the institutional review boards. These decentralized instruments of delegated governmental responsibility consistently ignore the conditions and agent under which and by whom a signature is solicited, reflecting more often the legal and financial needs of the institutions that appoint them than the needs of the research subject or patient.

Suppose the research subject is fully informed and all coercive influences are removed. Then a risk/benefit assessment is possible, since the necessary conditions have been met under which such an assessment can ethically take place. The outcome is positive. The subject wishes to participate.

In this hypothetical situation, the critical ethical question then is, "Who will be selected by the investigator for participation in the study and thus become a beneficiary of the program?"

The Belmont Report sets a fairness standard: "An injustice occurs when some benefit to which a person is entitled is denied without some good reason." The report notes that "Social justice requires that a distinction be drawn between classes of subjects that ought, and ought not, to participate in any particular kind of research, based on the ability of members of that class to bear burdens and on the appropriateness of placing further burdens on already burdened persons."

Age is often given as a positive or negative reason for differential treatment. Retired workers will have little or no risk from insurance and workers' compensation discrimination, and may clearly benefit, e.g., from specialized medical management that is part of the research protocol. Older workers in the employment market, if postresearch medical care is provided by the developing system, might share this scenario. However, there is a tendency to make arbitrary judgments of populations based on arbitrary age cutoffs that are not medically justified (36) and do not take into consideration adverse effects on individual ability and need (and therefore right) to work.

Distribution of the benefit, then, might fruitfully follow the formulation of the Belmont Report: "(1) to each person an equal share, (2) to each person according to individual need, (3) to each person according to individual effort, (4) to each person according to societal contribution, and (5) to each person according to merit."

Since the Common Rule and Consensus Statement do not provide an ethical basis for the conduct of research, the researcher is obligated to go beyond mere compliance with the law. Specific protocols that fit the ethical needs of the population being studied are necessary.

## THE ETHICS OF RISK ASSESSMENT

Like genetic testing, but with a much shorter history, risk assessment, especially quantitative methods, is another example of a technology being abused. Traditional methods of evaluating risk as the first step in its management have been transformed, often inappropriately, into increasingly precise quantitative risk assessment. In doing so, its practitioners typically ignore guidelines enabling ethical considerations found (ironically) in the Supreme Court decision that established it as a tool of public policy. A plurality in the Court (37) made clear that the requirement to determine significant risk need not be "a mathematical straitjacket," but can be "based on policy considerations…" risking error on the side of overprotection rather than underprotection."

This is hardly descriptive of the mythic value-free science or chimeric precision assumed by most of its proponents, who not only often obscure the scientific uncertainties and subjectivity assumed in its methods, but the values implicit in their methods (Table 1). The mainstream of assessors fall into a category Kristine Shrader-Frechette (38) calls "naive positivists," who "base their position on a number of doubtful presuppositions, such as the pure-science ideal and the fact-value dichotomy" or "complete neutrality and objectivity."

The doctrine of acceptable risk at the heart of most risk assessment-management schema assigns risk through the presumption of a class of so-called voluntary risks, in which the prevalent sophistry is to confuse historically persistent risks with autonomous acceptance, even though a rational, fully informed, and freely acting person

**TABLE 1.** *Value-impacted axioms in risk assessment*

| |
|---|
| Thresholds of toxic effects in populations (never found) |
| Levels of observed effects (depend on methods) |
| Statistical confidence factors (arbitrary by definition) |
| Exact risk extrapolations (seldom fit data) |
| Zero risk tolerances (exist only with zero exposure) |
| Margins of safety (always speculative) |
| Control feasibility (depends on values) |
| Measurement methods (choice of instruments) |
| Physiologic norms (abstractions from averages) |
| Biologic end points (valuing an effect) |
| Lifestyle and genetic homogeneity (never found) |

would not accept unnecessary risks assigned by caste categories associated more with the color of one's collar than feasible regulation. A risk differential is assigned by the assessor based on calculating from a narrow selection of risks associated with past work practice or historically prevalent exposure to a toxic substance in the workplace. The total burden of risk—including social, economic, cultural, and habitat risks—typically are ignored. The resultant selected burden of risk is then distributed by caste: different levels of risk for different sets of humans as marked by genome, age, socioeconomic status, geographic location, ethnicity, or occupation. Allocation of risk by caste assumes that there are humans whose needs and, thus, generic rights are different than others.

The concept of "acceptable risk," widely if not universally used in standard-setting, promotes unnecessary risks by arbitrarily assigning, for example, an "acceptable" risk ratio of one death per thousand in setting a permissible exposure level for workers, compared to one death for each million other members of the same community.

Other examples of irrational (immoral) risk allocation are the acceptance of risk differentials within a caste, as between adults and more vulnerable children (setting one standard for both when stronger protection is needed for children), between the work and community environments, between "guest" (or other less empowered workers) and indigenous workers, and risks (greater than we have set for ourselves) imposed by our market demands for products made in countries where workers are less protected.

Unnecessary risks are never morally acceptable. A risk is ethically "acceptable" only if it is necessary to protect life (or well-being) and freedom or is (a) culturally impacted and very difficult to eliminate or control in a short time, and (b) another biologically adverse hazard has a higher priority for control within a rational abatement scheme. The concept of socially acceptable risk disregards the necessity of a risk in favor of a crystallization of relative values drawn from discriminatory mores. The concept of necessary risk uses an absolute standard in which the right to life is given a priority over other rights within the realm of feasible protection.

Risk assessment techniques use a variety of dose-response models with different risk assessment characteristics based on assumptions, some of which are currently untestable. A "straight line" model, a choice common to the labor and environmental movements, yields estimates useful in making a case for control of low doses of toxic agents. While chosen for regulatory purposes, other configurations may be in better accord with some data. In the face of uncertainty, and the arbitrary nature of the choice, these models are justified if the obligation to conserve life is greater than other obligations.

Most assessors demand of statistical data a 95% confidence level to reduce the chance of false-positive findings. This mathematical artifice with no empirical justification has tremendous moral impact on regulation because of the increased chance of false negatives when it is used to judge studies of small samples for relatively rare diseases (a frequent case in occupational studies). Carl Cranor (39) correctly notes, "Use of the 95% rule in many circumstances may well protect commercial manufacturers and sellers of a substance better than potential victims."

More than other problems examined in this chapter, because of the formal axiomatic methods routinely used, risk assessment illustrates how sets of axioms, models of scientific explanation, or assessments of data must not be confused with invariable reality. The sophistry is found when the models are discussed as if they are the truth, rather than sets of assumptions about individuals, risks, and their control, based (at best) on limited information discardable when found unheuristic. The social and economic values implicit in the selection and use of these axioms guide the policy judgments of those who govern, manage,and control (Table 1). These values, not scientific data alone, determine environmental and biologic norms and standards in the community and workplace (40).

It is an obligation of the assessor to disclose the arbitrary nature of his assumptions, the reasons for their choice, and the implications for the assessment and subsequent management, rather than the cloaked imposition of personal values on the public under the guise of science. These values, judgments based on them, and the axioms selected must be judged by their reasonableness or success in avoiding the risk of pain, disability, and death.

## THE CRITICAL RIGHT-TO-KNOW

No matter how we choose to manage risk in our industrial society, the simple right to know is perhaps most critical. Without it, there can be no effective autonomy or direction in which even the most mythically free being could venture to cast aside bonds of a closed society, negative emotions, unfruitful mores or traditions that stand in the way of the physician and of the whole of the community of science to humanely meet the future.

This right and other rights discussed here are what Alan Gewirth (41) calls "specifications of the rights to freedom and well-being." Freedom and well-being are generic or human or fundamental rights because they are the necessary conditions by which we act as humans. Generic rights are generic human needs, and Gewirth's idea of well-being is an idea of life.

Life is not the only generic human need. Life preservation, therefore, is not the only absolute ethical standard of conduct. Freedom is the other need. Life and freedom are, in many circumstances, antinomies that, at best, exist in a balance of the moment. To preserve both life and freedom means that the quest for moral certainty in a changing society is an unending dialectic. No code of ethical behavior, nor any single judgment or ethical axiom, can be immune from change by interpretation or amendment. While ethical principles remain absolute, specific ethical axioms may change as we know more about their consequences. Thus not all specifications of the generic rights are equal. The right to know is paramount.

## REFERENCES


1. Aristotle. De Partibus Animalium. In: Smith, Ross, eds. *The works of Aristotle,* vol 5. Oxford: 1939; and In: Woodger JH. *The axiomatic method in biology.* Cambridge: 1937.
2. Woodger JH. *The axiomatic method in biology.* Cambridge: Cambridge University Press, 1937.
3. Socrates. In: Plato's *The Republic* (Jowett, trans.). New York: Modern Library.
4. Schweitzer A. *The philosophy of civilization.* New York: Prometheus, 1957.
5. Gert B. Morality, moral theory and applied and professional ethics. *Prof Ethics* 1992;1:5–24.
6. Hippocrates. On the air, water and places. In: *Ancient medicine.* New York: Regency, 1919.
7. Castiglioni A. *A history of medicine,* 2nd ed. New York: Knopf, 1958; 154–155.
8. Socrates. In: Protagoras. *Dialogues of Plato* (Jowett, trans.). New York: Random House, 1937;1:84.
9. Socrates. In Charmides. 171, 1:21, *ibid.*
10. Aristotle. In: McKeon, ed. *Politics, the basic works of Aristotle*. New York: Random House, 1941;1191.
11. Samuels SW. Ethics in the workplace: a framework for moral judgment. In: *ILO encyclopedia of occupational health and safety,* 4th rev. ed. Geneva: ILO, 1998;19.9–19.11.
12. Castiglioni A, Samuels SW. Ethics in the workplace: a framework for moral judgment. In: *ILO encyclopedia of occupational health and safety.*
13. Gert B. Defending irrationality and lists. *Ethics* 1993;103(2):329–336.
14. Grisez GG. The concept of appropriateness: ethical considerations in persuasive argument. *J Am Forensic Assoc* 1965;2(2):53.
15. Rosement H. Human rights: a bill of worries. In: de Barry WJ. *Confucianism and human rights.* New York: Columbia University Press, 1998;54–66.
16. McNeil WH. *Plagues and peoples.* Garden City, NY: Anchor/Doubleday, 1976.
17. Gewirth A. Professional ethics: the separatist thesis. *Ethics* 1986;96: 282.
18. Schuman BJ. Commentary on ethics. *JAMA* 1980;224:2417.
19. Samuels SW. A moral history of a caste of workers. *Environ Health Perspect* 1996;104(5):991–998.
20. Durkheim E. *The division of labor*. New York: Free Press, 1947.
21. Szasz T. The moral physician. *Center Magazine* 1975(Mar/Apr):9.
22. Brodkin CA, Frumkin H, et al. AOEC position paper on the organizational code for ethical conduct. *J Occup Environ Med* 1996;38(9): 869–881.
23. Ofstad H. Responsibility and freedom in contemporary philosophy in Scandinavia. In: Olson RE, Paul AM, eds. Baltimore: Johns Hopkins University Press, 1972;291.
24. Aristotle. *Nichomachean ethics.*
25. Beasley AD, Graber GC. The range of autonomy: informed consent in medicine. *Theor Med* 1984;5:31.
26. Einstein A. Reply to criticisms. In: Schilpp, ed. *Albert Einstein:* philosopher-scientist. La Salle, Canada: Open Court, 1949;666.
27. Planck M. *Where is science going?* 1987 edition. Woodbridge: Oxbow, 1933:145.
28. Bernard C. Lecons sur les phenomenes de la vie commune aux animaux et vegetaux. In: Greene HC, ed. *An introduction to the study of experimental medicine.* New York: Schuman, 1949:vii.
29. Darwin C. *Origin of the species.* New York: Modern Library 1948:101.
30. Samuels SW. Philosophic perspectives: community, communications and occupational disease causation. *Int J Health Services* 1998;28(1): 153–164.
31. Conference Board. *Industrial roles in health care.* New York: 1974.
32. Ottman R. Gene-environment interaction and public health. *Am J Hum Genet* 1995;56:821–823.
33. The Belmont Report Ethical Principles and Guidelines for the Protection of Human Subjects. *OPPR Rep* 1979(April 18):15-11–15-19.
34. The Common Rule Federal Policy for the Protection of Human Subjects. 10 CFR 745, June 18, 1991.
35. Clayton EW, et al. Consensus statement: informed consent for genetic research on stored tissue samples. *JAMA* 1995;274:1786–1792.
36. Cassel CK. The limits of setting limits. In: Homer P, Holstein M, eds. *A good old age.* New York: Simon and Schuster, 1990.
37. *IUD (Industrial Union Department) vs. API (American Petroleum Institute) (1980)*: 448 0.5 607 Supreme Court, Washington, DC.
38. Shrader-Frechette K. In: Mayo, Hollander, eds. *Reductionist approaches to risk in acceptable evidence.* Oxford: 1991;218–248
39. Cranor CF. Moral issues in risk assessment. *Ethics* 1990;101:123–143.
40. Samuels SW. Ethical and metaethical criteria for an emerging technology: risk assessment. *Occup Med* 1997;47:241–246.
41. Gewirth A. Human rights and the workplace. In: Samuels SW, ed. The environment of the workplace and human values. *Am J Ind Med* 1986;9(1):31–38.

*Environmental and Occupational Medicine, Third Edition,* edited by William N. Rom.
Published by Lippincott–Raven Publishers,
Philadelphia, 1998.

# CHAPTER 136

# New Frontiers in Environmental Health Research

Kenneth Olden and Janet Guthrie

Virtually all diseases have both a genetic and an environmental component. Thus, both environmental health research and human genome research are vitally important for fulfilling the public health mission of the United States. Unfortunately, one cannot say in every case which environmental factors are the most important contributors to ill health, nor can one say which individuals are either most susceptible or most resistant. As a consequence, public health protection is often based on broad and expensive programs of public education, immunization, and treatment where possible, or environmental controls and regulations. This leaves policy makers in the uncomfortable position, particularly in times of scarce resources, of having to decide whether to relax environmental controls and appear uncaring, or to continue to spend large amounts of money on programs whose impact on public health is uncertain.

This question of cost of intervention versus benefit of the program is most problematic in environmental health protection programs targeted at low levels of exposures. Scientists agree that high levels of exposure to environmental toxicants are detrimental to human health. However, except for the special circumstances of increased susceptibility, sharp disagreements exist among scientists concerning the effects of low levels of environmental pollutants on human health and disease incidence. Since most environmental pollutants now occur at relatively low levels in air, water, soil, and food, some argue that stringent environmental regulatory practices are not necessary to protect human health.

The limitations discussed above derive, in part, from a need to define better the genetic and environmental components of disease. Technological advances hold the promise of real progress in relieving the bottleneck depicted in Fig. 1. Many of today's devastating illnesses and disabilities will in the future be prevented or cured as we come to understand the molecular mechanisms by which toxicants act; as the many types of susceptibilities that affect disease development and progression, including gene-environment interactions, are defined; as current exposure assessment methods are improved and strengthened; as our understanding is expanded from predicting effects of single exposures to predicting effects of multiple exposures; and, finally, as this information is translated into prevention and treatment strategies.

Unfortunately, investment in environmental health research stagnated in the 1980s and early 1990s (specifically from 1983 to 1992). Most distressing, the decrease in constant dollars occurred at the very time when extraordinary advances were within our grasp, advances that could have revolutionized and enhanced the cost-effectiveness of the practice of medicine and environmental health risk assessment. While the resources for the conduct of environmental health research are beginning to grow again, the decade or more of underfunding has left a large chasm between scientific opportunities and the capacity of the National Institute of Environmental Health Sciences (NIEHS) to exploit the new science to

K. Olden: National Institute of Environmental Health Sciences and National Toxicology Program, National Institutes of Health, Research Triangle Park, North Carolina 27709-2233.

J. Guthrie: Office of Policy, Planning, and Evaluation, National Institute of Environmental Health Sciences, Research Triangle Park, North Carolina 27709-2233.

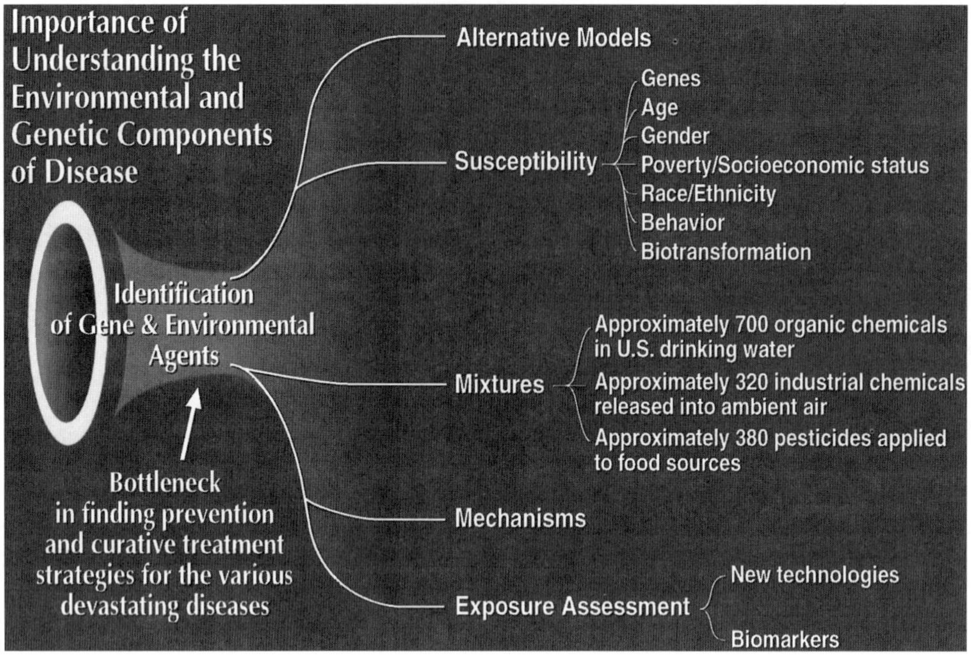


**FIG. 1.** The bottlenecks in advancing environmental health.

improve human health. We have entered the era of molecular toxicology in which scientific opportunities have converged with public health and regulatory needs. The remarkable advances in our understanding of human genetics provides an unprecedented opportunity to determine the causes of the various chronic and devastating diseases. Failure to pursue promising areas of investigation will result in loss of opportunity to reduce serious illness.

In considering research needs and opportunities, we have focused on areas of fundamental knowledge and practical issues relevant to understanding the role of the environment in the etiology of human illness. The areas of emphasis represent issues (shown in Table 1) where major information gaps exist, where reasonable research questions can be formulated, where technologies are available, and where understanding offers the potential to significantly improve public health and regulatory policy.

**TABLE 1.** *Environmental health research needs*

| |
|---|
| Gene-environment interaction |
| Susceptibility |
| New approaches to toxicologic testing |
| Mechanisms of toxicity |
| Prevention/intervention |
| Endocrine modulation |
| Mixtures |
| Poverty as a risk factor |
| Exposure assessment |
| Exposures and children |
| Clinical efforts |

## GENE–ENVIRONMENT INTERACTION

Efforts to control environmentally caused illness must be based on an understanding of the human–environment interaction at the molecular level. The complexities associated with interactions between humans and their environment can now be unraveled using the tools of modern biology and epidemiology.

Good health depends on the proper functioning of genes that control cellular growth, differentiation, and death. When critical genetic material is altered, the functions over which it exerts control can go awry, leading to birth defects, cancer, neurobehavioral abnormalities, and other diseases and dysfunctions. Human health also depends on a complex network of chemical signals between cells. The molecules that transmit signals are primary targets to toxic substances in the environment. Identification of the role of individual protein messengers and receptors in cellular determination, growth, differentiation, and responsiveness, and understanding the ability of environmental chemicals to interact with these critical proteins are important NIEHS research priorities.

Over the past 20 years, using the tools of recombinant DNA technology, researchers have identified a number of genes involved in the development of specific diseases such as cystic fibrosis and sickle cell anemia. However, these discoveries have been of the single gene variety (i.e., an alteration in just one gene causes a disease). Today we seek the causes and prevention of more common diseases, such as cancer, Alzheimer's, Parkinson's, osteoporosis, and asthma, that appear to arise from a complex interplay between several inherited genetic alterations and the environment rather than from a single gene. But before we can prevent or improve the treatment of such diseases, we need a better understanding of individual function of critical genes involved in the growth and development of humans and the ability of environmental agents to interact with and damage these genes. Analyzing these complexities and teasing apart the genetic and environmental components involved represents a daunting challenge and an important scientific opportunity. The tools and technology developed by molecular geneticists are being used by environmental health scientists to help in the discovery of genes modulated by the environment.

## SUSCEPTIBILITY

Research is urgently needed to determine the genetic, behavioral, and developmental basis for the wide variation in individual responsiveness to exposures to environmental toxicants. There are indications that differences in responsiveness can be related to age, gender, lifestyle, or genetic predispositions; yet this possibility is rarely taken into consideration by environmental regulatory agencies in human health risk assessment. The identification of disease predisposition genes, the determination of how these genes function normally, and how loss of function of these genes predisposes to disease are vitally important research issues. Their discovery will pave the way for development of novel strategies for prevention, early detection, and treatment; however, bigger challenges are presented by attempts to identify genetic predisposition resulting from inheritance of a complex of several genes. Also, identification of the nongenetic factors—environmental and dietary exposures, behavior, lifestyle, and infectious agents that influence whether the presence of altered susceptibility genes actually lead to disease—offers tremendous potential to improve human health.

The NIEHS proposes to greatly expand its molecular genetics research on susceptibility genes for environmentally induced diseases through the new Environmental Genome Project. This genome project, which makes use of technology developed by the human genome efforts, will acquire a population database on the sequence diversity for the environmental disease susceptibility genes.

Genetic approaches used in the past have identified many susceptibility genes for environmental diseases. An individual with a defect in such a gene has an elevated risk of becoming ill after an environmental exposure. The molecular mechanisms of susceptibility are not well understood; however, we are now able to categorize many of the susceptibility genes into five broad classes: genes controlling the distribution and metabolism of toxicants; genes for the DNA repair pathways; genes for the cell cycle control system, including apoptosis; genes for metabolism of nucleic acid precursors; and genes for signal transduction systems controlling expression of the genes in the other classes. The NIEHS Environmental Genome Project will be a broad, multicenter effort to obtain information about DNA sequence diversity for the U.S. population on all of the environmental disease susceptibility genes now recognized (greater than 200). The project will be expanded as additional susceptibility genes are discovered.

The availability of a population database on environmental disease gene diversity will allow us to conduct much more focused molecular epidemiology that can relate environmental exposures and disease to individual susceptibility genotype. Ultimately, information from such medical genetic epidemiology will allow us to greatly enhance public health through better prevention strategies for environmental diseases. The Environmental Genome Project will provide information for future research on molecular mechanisms of susceptibility gene products. The project will also foster development of new high-throughput technology for the application of genetics in medical epidemiology as a function of environmental exposure.

## NEW APPROACHES TO TOXICOLOGIC TESTING

There is considerable pressure on both government and industry to cut costs and increase the speed of toxicologic testing and evaluation. Thus, we need to continue our effort to develop new and better carcinogenicity and toxicity test systems. While we have greatly improved test methods, they are still too costly and too time-consuming for use in screening the thousands of natural and synthetic environmental chemicals requiring toxicity assessment. Opportunities now exist to develop alternative testing methods by incorporating knowledge of molecular and cellular mechanisms associated with the toxic or carcinogenic process.

Technical advances have always played a key role in improving our ability to prevent and treat disease and are equally important in the discovery process in environmental health research. Technical improvements in mouse genetics have now overcome an important impediment in biomedical research: the lack of animal models in which to study the development of human diseases. New methods in animal genetics allow the study of diseases in a way that was impossible just 30 years ago. These new techniques provide the remarkable ability to introduce mutations into the genetic material of mice that can be passed to their offspring. Investigators can now insert any mutation they choose into the mouse genome. They can also transfer genes from one animal species to another, and they can express or inactivate genes at a different time and in different than normal tissue. Using such approaches, researchers have developed a knockout mouse lacking the estrogen receptor (1,2), and are on the verge of developing transgenic mouse models containing the human breast cancer susceptibility genes BRCA1 and BRCA2 (3,4). These are likely to be the three most important animal models needed to determine the role of the environment in the development of breast and ovarian cancers.

For decades the identification of potential human carcinogens has relied on epidemiologic methods and the use of long-term rodent bioassays. Both methodologies present significant limitations, but the search for suitable alternative methods has only been partially successful. In the rodent bioassays, mice are fed large amounts of a single chemical; in contrast, human diets consist of small amounts of several natural and synthetic chemicals. These differences in exposures raise considerable uncertainties about whether the data derived from animal tests can be applied directly to humans. Moreover, the current rodent bioassay for assessing carcinogenicity is too costly ($2–6 million per chemical, depending on the route of exposure) and too time-consuming (taking up to 5 years to plan, interpret, and peer review).

However, recent revolutionary advances in the recognition of specific genes that play critical roles in the induction and development of cancer, together with the development of methods with which to manipulate the mammalian genome, have provided new approaches for distinguishing between carcinogens and noncarcinogens. Selected transgenic mouse lines have been identified that provide new approaches to identifying carcinogens. The NIEHS has focused on the p53 deficient and Tg·AC (zetoglobin promoted v-Ha-*ras*) lines and has evaluated their response to specific chemicals (5–7). The results to date suggest that the combination of the two models can be used in the identification of transpecies carcinogens. Other transgenic models may also be appropriate for evaluation at this time. For example, the *ras* H2 model developed in Japan is presently being evaluated by researchers at the Central Institute for Experimental Animals and the National Institute of Health Sciences of Japan (8). In the Netherlands, researchers at the National Institute of Public Health and Environmental Protection have developed an xpa repair-deficient/p53-deficient mouse for use in similar studies (9).

Preliminary data indicate that these transgenic animal models can reduce the time required for a cancer bioassay from 2 years to 6 months. While it is still uncertain as to what extent these models can be used in lieu of the 2-year rodent bioassay, the best guess is that they will greatly reduce our dependency on this assay, with considerable savings in both time and cost. Also, the new models may be more relevant to human risk assessment in terms of dosimetry, mechanism, and genetic background. While there are reasons for excitement concerning the potential impact that these genetically engineered models can have on environmental health research, it is important to emphasize that they represent only the first generation; better models will be developed.

For example, with advances in recombinant DNA technology, combinatorial chemistry, and structure-based prediction, it should be possible to develop high-throughput screening procedures to evaluate large numbers of chemicals for their effects on DNA or particular biologic processes. Using such an approach, it should be possible to screen thousands of chemicals per year.

Also, current databases can be used more effectively for predicting toxicity using mathematical modeling and structural biology approaches. Over a decade of National Institutes of Health (NIH)/NIEHS-supported research has culminated in the ability to present three-dimensional models that assess the similarity or homology between different toxicant metabolizing enzymes. These enzymes represent one of the most important ways in which biologic systems convert ingested harmful environmental substances into less toxic, easily excretable compounds. Understanding how similar, or different, these critical enzymes are across species is important in extrapolating the toxicology results in rodents to their relevance for the human condition. These structure-activity studies represent substantial progress toward rationalizing and predicting individual, strain, and species differences in toxicant metabolism. In turn, it may be possible to link such findings to individual differences in susceptibility to toxicants. In addition, knowledge of the structural basis of metabolizing enzyme specificity may lead to the rational design of inhibitors that modulate this metabolism.

## MECHANISMS OF TOXICITY

Environmental health research can also capitalize on recent developments in molecular and cell biology to develop a mechanistic understanding of the toxic action of environmental agents. We must find and elucidate important pathways using smart assays. Under this scheme the actual biologic events that lead to toxicity will be determined. Insights into molecular mechanisms involved in carcinogenesis or other disease processes are important in several ways: (a) they can provide a more rational basis for assessing human risk based on data obtained in animals; (b) knowledge of mechanisms can suggest new laboratory procedures for use in epidemiologic studies to more precisely identify the causes of human illnesses; (c) insights into the mechanism of disease initiation can increase understanding of the wide person-to-person variation in risk to disease; and (d) information on mechanisms of action of environmental agents can lead to development of molecular medicine strategies to prevent, detect, and treat various diseases.

## PREVENTION/INTERVENTION

Knowledge of mechanisms is also a prerequisite for prevention/intervention using molecular medicine approaches. The field of environmental toxicology has historically limited its prevention efforts to behavioral modification designed to reduce exposure. While this remains the most pragmatic approach, behavioral intervention is not possible in some cases because the causative agent cannot be readily controlled.

Although much progress is being made in the laboratory in defining the environmental basis of diseases and dysfunctions, this knowledge and technology is not being effectively translated into the practice of medicine. The recent creation of the clinical program within the NIEHS underscored the importance of translating discoveries made in the laboratory to benefit individuals and populations in terms of improved health status and reduced health care costs.

Current efforts by NIEHS-supported scientists are transforming today's opportunities into tantalizing possibilities for the future. These possibilities include developing techniques to pinpoint molecular events that, when blocked by specific probes, will prevent the progression of disease, working with regulatory agencies to use mechanistic data for classifying carcinogens and other toxicants without the use of traditional bioassays, and using computational graphics and molecular studies that may permit accurate predictions of which chemicals may damage specific parts of DNA or interact with specific receptors, thereby significantly advancing the field or predictive toxicology.

## ENDOCRINE MODULATION

Research is needed to develop methodologies for screening environmental pollutants and natural products for endocrine-disrupting effects and for assessing the health effects of these exposures. Although the possibility for human health effects of these hormonally active agents remains hypothetical, their pervasiveness and persistence in the environment make this an area of significant public health concern (10–13). These chemicals can potentially alter the balance of physiologic systems of complex organisms whose coordination is controlled by delicately balanced neuroendocrine mechanisms.

Animal studies have demonstrated that exposure of the fetus to endocrine-disrupting chemicals can profoundly disturb organ development. Field studies have shown an association between exposure to endocrine-disrupting chemicals in the environment and developmental anomalies in fish, birds, reptiles, and other wildlife species. These anomalies include feminization of male fish, birds, and mammals, decrease in reproductive potential, and underdeveloped genitalia. Human exposure to synthetic estrogen (e.g., diethylstilbestrol) during early development caused reproductive organ dysfunction, abnormal pregnancies, cancers of the reproductive tract, and decreased fertility in females.

Given the large numbers of hormonally active chemicals released into the environment over the past 50 years, more research is needed concerning the health consequences associated with chronic exposure to low doses of mixtures of endocrine-disrupting chemicals during the various stages of development. Exposure during the development of the embryo, fetus, and neonates is of particular concern because the consequences may be both more striking and more permanent.

The potential benefits of research in this area extend beyond women. The expanded study of environmental factors in diseases of women is expected to provide multiple benefits, not limited to the obvious goal of developing new prevention strategies to decrease disease prevalence and severity. A heightened understanding of the mechanisms through which environmental agents disrupt normal physiologic processes will undoubtedly lead to greater insights into the biologic phenomena and pathways themselves. Data on such phenomena could then be used in the design of new disease and prevention strategies. Progress in the area of reproductive and developmental toxicology translates into better health throughout later life for men and women equally.

## MIXTURES

Investigation of the mechanisms and health effects of mixtures is another area where lack of information is a serious problem. The data on exposure and toxicology of mixtures is inadequate for assessing health risk. The current toxicologic databases were developed using single chemicals in animal bioassays, whereas humans are exposed at a variety of levels to large numbers of chemicals either concurrently or sequentially via multiple pathways. Mixtures of chemicals are ubiquitous in ground and surface water, and in air, food, and soil. For example, 700 organic chemicals have been identified in the drinking water supply of the United States, 40 of which are possible carcinogens; 320 toxic industrial chemicals are released into ambient air, of which 60 are possible carcinogens; and approximately 380 pesticides are applied to food sources, 66 of which have been identified as actual or potential carcinogens. Furthermore, the problem of mixtures is not limited to chemical interactions since health outcome may also be influenced by physical or biologic agents. For example, risk of radon-induced lung cancer is increased in cigarette smokers, and people infected with hepatitis B virus are more susceptible to aflatoxin-induced liver cancer.

Thus, our inability to say whether agents act in an additive, synergistic, or antagonistic fashion creates real problems in health risk assessment. Depending on the assumptions made regarding the nature of the interaction between components, risk may be seriously over- or underestimated with dire economic or public health consequences, respectively.

## POVERTY AS A RISK FACTOR

The health needs of socioeconomically disadvantaged populations will require special attention if the United States is to improve public health and reduce health care costs. Health survey analyses have shown that major disparities exist between the health status of the overall population of the United States and that of its socioeconomically disadvantaged groups, especially African-Americans, Hispanic/Latinos, American Indians, and Pacific Islanders (14). The most striking health disparities involve shorter life expectancy and high cancer rates, birth defects, infant mortality, asthma, diabetes, kidney disease, and cardiovascular dysfunctions.

While behavioral and lifestyle factors and access to health care services are important contributors to the excess morbidity and mortality among socioeconomically disadvantaged populations, environmental and occupational exposures, over which such individuals have little control, are likely to play prominent roles (15). Economically and politically disenfranchised people are more likely to have toxic waste sites located near their homes, the poor are more likely to work at hazardous occupations, and low-income neighborhoods are more likely to be found near polluting industries (16). Consequently, people in the lower socioeconomic strata may also be more likely to experience long-term and higher levels of exposure to a wider variety of hazardous environmental agents than those in the middle or upper socioeconomic strata.

While the putative role of the environment in the overall health status of the poor has emerged as a legitimate public health issue, wider acceptance and reordering of national priorities are unlikely to occur unless research can better establish the link between disproportionate exposure to environmental carcinogens and toxicants and the disproportionate morbidity and mortality experienced by the poor. For economic reasons, environmental remediation efforts are rarely undertaken unless a link is presumed to exist between exposure to environmental toxicants and human illness or injury. To date, the preponderance of evidence comes from known occupational exposures of specific subpopulations (e.g., radon exposure of uranium miners, asbestos exposure of persons working in the building industry, and vinyl chloride exposure of plastics workers). However, if the problem is shown to be more general than workplace exposures and possibly compounded by both living and working in hazardous environments over many years, a more general environmental health protection policy may be required.

## EXPOSURE ASSESSMENT

A major challenge is to strengthen the links between fundamental science, toxicology, epidemiology, and risk assessment. To make environmental health research findings more applicable to human risk assessment, monitoring of human exposure to specific chemicals must be undertaken using improved and highly sensitive analytical procedures. Operationally, this could be achieved by expansion of the National Health and Nutrition Examination Survey (NHANES IV) for selected environmental contaminants. For example, monitoring the exposure of the U.S. population to the chemicals listed in the National Toxicology Program's Biennial Report on Carcinogens could be a top priority of such a national survey. One can now measure many of these chemicals in body tissues such as blood and urine. The survey should include information concerning the nature of the exposure, estimated number of persons exposed, and demographic information such as age, gender, socioeconomic status, race or ethnicity, and geographic region. Such real-world exposure assessment would be far more useful than estimation of exposure based on the Environmental Protection Agency (EPA) toxic release and production information. Estimation of exposure using this indirect approach is, at best, only a reflection of the potential for human exposure. Also, such an approach dose not take into account the biologically effective dose and individual differences in uptake and metabolism of various chemicals. Utilizing biomarker measurements in national surveys of the population would provide human exposure information far superior to what we have now.

## EXPOSURES AND CHILDREN

Research on the health effects of environmental exposures on children must become a higher priority. Currently, most of the health risk estimates for children are based on studies in adult humans and animals; these data are neither adequate nor appropriate for evaluating health risks to children. The risk of exposure to developing embryos, neonates, infants, young children, and adolescents all need to be evaluated. Children's risk may differ qualitatively and quantitatively from that of adults for a number of reasons, including differences in metabolism, pharmacokinetics, physiology factors, development, diet, and physical environment. Children are not miniature adults; they have their own unique environments, biology, and behaviors, which may increase their exposure or risk to environmental toxicants.

## CLINICAL EFFORTS

Clinical and epidemiologic studies are necessary components of environmental health research. Also, greater involvement of health care practitioners is important. The current group of health care providers are relatively unaware of the impact of environmental agents on the health of their patients, or of the means to prevent, diagnose, or treat environmentally caused diseases. The three primary goals of a clinical program should be the following:

1. To translate advances in understanding of environmental causes of diseases into prevention/intervention strategies;
2. To develop hospital-based case-control studies to examine associations between various exposure markers and clinical outcomes;
3. To train physicians in environmental and occupational medicine.

Translation of basic research into clinical studies of disease prevention, diagnosis, and treatment is crucial to the ultimate goals of research in environmental health and to affecting a discernible improvement in human health.

The clinical program in environmental health research is relatively new, although epidemiologic studies have been done for decades. For example, the NIEHS is sponsoring a large, multicenter, placebo-controlled randomized trial of succimer treatment for the prevention of lead-induced alterations in cognitive functions, neuromotor development, and behavior. The trial was started in 1994, and is scheduled to be completed in 1999. Also, NIEHS has developed intramural clinical research activities using the resources of two regional medical centers. Presently, there are two active protocols—one on sperm quality in men newly exposed to azidothymidine (AZT) and protease inhibitors, and the other on lung fibrosis in women who have had bone marrow transplants following chemotherapy for breast cancer. A third on asthma prevention is currently in the planing stages and is expected to get under way in the summer of 1997.

## SUMMARY

Environmental health policy decisions are only as good as the scientific foundation on which they are founded, that is, the data and models used in assessing the risk, and the assumptions made in the absence of facts. Extrapolations from animal models to assess possible human impacts leaves room for many uncertainties, and reasonable assumptions can turn out to be disastrously wrong. And risk assessment can be uncomfortably imprecise when mechanisms are poorly understood and epidemiologic data is sparse or absent. The guiding principal should be good science for good decisions.

## REFERENCES

1. Lubahn DB, Moyer JS, Golding TS, Couse JF, Korach KS, Smithies O. Alteration of reproductive function but not prenatal sexual development after insertional disruption of the mouse estrogen receptor gene. *Proc Natl Acad Sci USA* 1993;90:11162–11166.
2. Couse JF, Curtis SW, Washburn TF, et al. Analysis of transcription and estrogen insensitivity in the female mouse after targeted disruption of the estrogen receptor gene. *Mol Endocrinol* 1995;9:1441–1454.
3. Futreal PA, Liu Q, Shattuck-Eidens D, et al. BRCA1 mutations in primary breast and ovarian carcinomas. *Science* 1994;266:120–122.
4. Miki Y, Swensen J, Shattuck-Eidens D, et al. A strong candidate for the 17q-linked breast and ovarian cancer susceptibility gene BRCA1. *Science* 1994;266:66–71.
5. Spalding JW, Momma J, Elwell MR, Tennant RW. Chemically induced skin carcinogenesis in a transgenic mouse line (TG.AC) carrying a v-Ha-*ras* gene. *Carcinogenesis* 1993;14(7):1335–1341.
6. Tennant RW, Spalding J, French JE. Evaluation of transgenic mouse bioassays for identifying carcinogens and noncarcinogens. *Mutat Res* 1993;165:119–127.
7. Tennant RW, French JE, Spalding JW. Identifying chemical carcinogens and assessing potential risk in short-term bioassays using transgenic mouse models. *Environ Health Perspect* 1995;103(10):942–950.
8. Yamamoto S, Matsumori K, Kodama Y, et al. Rapid induction of more malignant tumors by various genotoxic carcinogens in transgenic mice harboring a human prototype c-Ha-ras gene than in control non-transgenic mice. *Carcinogenesis* 1996;17:2455–2464.
9. de Vries A, Canny T, Van Oostram M, et al. Increased susceptibility to ultraviolet-B and carcinogens of mice lacking the DNA excision repair gene XPA. *Nature* 1995;377:169–173.
10. McLachlan JA, ed. *Estrogens in the environment II:* influence on development. New York: Elsevier, 1985.
11. Newbold RR, McLachlan JA. Diethylstilbestrol associated defects in murine genital tract development. In: McLachlan JA, ed. *Estrogens in the environment.* New York: Elsevier Science, 1985;288–318.
12. Colburn T, Clement C, eds. *Chemically induced alterations in sexual and functional development:* the wildlife/human connection. Advances in Modern Environmental Toxicology, vol 21. Princeton, NJ: Princeton Scientific, 1992.
13. Newbold RR. Cellular and molecular effects of developmental exposure to diethylstilbestrol: implications for other environmental estrogens. *Environ Health Perspect* 1995;103(suppl 7):83–87.
14. Olden K, Poje GV. Environmental justice emerges as a national issue. *Health Environ Dig* 1996;9:77–79.
15. Sexton K, Olden K, Johnson B. Environmental Justice: the central role of research in establishing a credible scientific foundation for informed decision making. *Toxicol Ind Lett* 1993;9:685–727.
16. Bullard RD, Wright BH. The politics of pollution: implications for the black community. *Phylon* 1986;47:71–78.

# Subject Index

Page numbers in *italic* indicate figures. Page numbers followed by "t" indicate tables.

**I**

**P**

## Q

**T**

**X**



**Y**



**Z**